Saunders DICTIONARY & ENCYCLOPEDIA OF LABORATORY MEDICINE AND TECHNOLOGY

JAMES L. BENNINGTON, M.D.
Chairman, Department of Anatomic Pathology and Clinical Laboratories
Children's Hospital of San Francisco

Associate Editors

George Brecher, M.D. *Hematology*
Wie-Shing Lee, Ph.D. *Mycology, Parasitology, Virology*
Bruce Mackay, M.D., Ph.D. *Anatomy, Pathology*
Nathan J. Smith, M.D. *Medicine*
Earle H. Spaulding, Ph.D. *Bacteriology*
Norbert W. Tietz, Ph.D. *General and Clinical Chemistry*

W.B. SAUNDERS COMPANY
Philadelphia London Toronto Mexico City Rio de Janeiro Sydney Tokyo

W. B. Saunders Company: West Washington Square
Philadelphia, PA 19105

1 St. Anne's Road
Eastbourne, East Sussex BN21 3UN, England

1 Goldthorne Avenue
Toronto, Ontario M8Z 5T9, Canada

Apartado 26370—Cedro 512
Mexico 4, D.F., Mexico

Rua Coronel Cabrita, 8
Sao Cristovao Caixa Postal 21176
Rio de Janeiro, Brazil

9 Waltham Street
Artarmon, N.S.W. 2064, Australia

Ichibancho, Central Bldg., 22-1 Ichibancho
Chiyoda-Ku, Tokyo 102, Japan

Library of Congress Cataloging in Publication Data

Bennington, James L.
Saunders dictionary & encyclopedia of laboratory medicine and technology.

1. Diagnosis, Laboratory—Dictionaries. 2. Medical technology—Dictionaries. I. Brecher, G. (George) II. W. B. Saunders Company. III. Title. IV. Title: Saunders dictionary and encyclopedia of laboratory medicine and technology. V. Title: Dictionary & encyclopedia of laboratory medicine and technology. VI. Title: Dictionary and encyclopedia of laboratory medicine and technology. [DNLM: 1. Diagnosis, Laboratory—Dictionaries. QY 13 S257]
RB37.B453 1984 616.07′56′0321 83-4615

ISBN 0-7216-1714-X

The use of portions of the text of the 19th edition of the *United States Pharmacopeia* is by permission of the USP Convention. The Convention is not responsible for any inaccuracy of quotation or for any false or misleading implication that may arise from separation of excerpts from the original text or by obsolescence resulting from publication of a supplement or a revised edition of the *Pharmacopeia.*

Some of the words appearing in this dictionary are proprietary names (trademarks), even though no reference to this fact is made in the text. The appearance of any name without designation as a trademark is therefore not to be regarded as a representation by the editors or publisher that it is not a trademark or is not the subject of proprietary rights.

Saunders Dictionary & Encyclopedia of Laboratory Medicine and Technology ISBN 0-7216-1714-X

Last digit is the print number: 9 8 7 6 5 4 3 2 1

Preface

During the last several decades there has been an explosive growth in the field of laboratory medicine due to the combination of an insatiable demand by physicians for new and improved diagnostic procedures and an infinite capacity of modern technology to supply this demand through creation of increasingly sophisticated laboratory methods and instruments.

The advances in laboratory medicine that have made possible its rapid growth have also been responsible for revolutionary changes in the size, scope, and complexity of its vocabulary. Just a few years ago, the full lexicon of laboratory medicine occupied a relatively small portion of the standard medical dictionary. Today, the terminology of laboratory medicine is fully as great as that of nonlaboratory medicine and is of paramount importance for effective medical communication.

The *Dictionary and Encyclopedia of Laboratory Medicine and Technology* was created to provide in a single source comprehensive and authoritative definitions of the terms used in this field. By concentrating on this vocabulary, we have endeavored to produce a reference work that meets the exacting demands of specialists in the various disciplines of laboratory medicine and technology, as well as the needs of those outside the laboratory who use its services. This work was prepared to serve laboratorians, clinicians, nurses, allied health and public health personnel, basic scientists, and students preparing for careers in health care fields.

We have attempted to provide comprehensive coverage of currently used methods and techniques for laboratory analysis in the areas of clinical chemistry, biochemistry, toxicology, hematology, blood banking, bacteriology, virology, mycology, parasitology, immunology, cytology, histology, immunohistochemistry, electron microscopy, electrocardiography, electromyography, ultrasonography, radiology, nuclear medicine, and respiratory medicine. For each test, assay, or examination, the basic principles of the method or instrumentation, or both, used for analysis are discussed, along with the conditions that affect the accuracy and precision of detection and measurement, fundamentals of quality control, reference values, pathophysiologic alterations that produce abnormal values, and the clinical use of some applications of the procedures.

Terms related to other important aspects of laboratory medicine are also covered in detail, and include biostatistics, laboratory safety, normal gross and microscopic anatomy and physiology, diseases, syndromes, important toxic agents, frequently prescribed drugs, physiologic mechanisms, laboratory computers, electronics and instrumentation, quality control, taxonomy of microorganisms, dyes and stains, bacteriologic media, laboratory physics, biochemistry, oncology, and radiation therapy.

The terms included in the *Dictionary and Encyclopedia of Laboratory Medicine and Technology* were selected by medical editors from an exhaustive search of textbooks, glossaries, and journal publications in each area defined in the book. They also come from two other Saunders dictionaries, *Dorland's Illustrated Medical Dictionary* and the Miller and Keane *Encyclopedia and Dictionary of Medicine, Nursing, and Allied Health,* whose definitions formed the basis of many terms included in the present volume. The definitions were written by the dictionary staff, the medical editors, and leading authorities. Every definition was reviewed by two or more editors before approval for inclusion.

Completion of this dictionary required more than six years and represents a vast number of hours of research, writing, review, and mechanical preparation by the staff at Saunders and the medical editors. Suggestions, contributions, and corrections are welcomed for preparation of the second edition.

My special thanks go to all members of the dictionary staff at Saunders for their efforts; to Melonia Musser-Brauner, Marie Low, and Donna Kennedy for their organizational work on the project; and to two individuals in particular who helped make this work a reality: to John Hanley, President of the Saunders Company, for his confidence in this concept, and to Renee Munoz, Managing Editor, for her dedication to the dictionary, editorial skills, and unfailing patience and good humor.

JAMES L. BENNINGTON, M.D.

Contents

Notes on the Use of This Book

INTRODUCTION

SCOPE

The scope of this dictionary covers the medical fields of particular interest to laboratorians and others who need to be familiar with the technology of modern medical laboratories. Many anatomic terms and diseases and conditions have also been included for the convenience of those who would seek further explication of a specific anatomic site or pathologic condition referred to in a technical definition.

An encyclopedic approach was used to define certain terms considered basic to a particular field or whose complexity demanded more than a concise dictionary definition.

STYLE

We have tried to follow accepted conventions regarding such matters as abbreviation and nomenclature style for the specific fields defined in the dictionary, although readers will note that what is standard usage in one field may not be in another. For example, adoption of SI units (International Units), certain abbreviations (e.g., P_{CO_2}, $P_{A_{CO2}}$), and nomenclature such as nonproprietary names, chemical names, and trademarks are not consistently used by nor are familiar to all workers in all fields.

Terms are given in the singular form, with the plural spelling occasionally following the pronunciation. However, when a term is most commonly used in the plural form it is defined there; for example, the definition appears at *mitochondria* rather than on the singular form, *mitochondrion.* Also, when a term is referred to by its initials or acronym, the primary definition is found at the abbreviation; thus, *VDRL test* is at *VDRL,* not *Venereal Disease Research Laboratory.*

FORMAT

ALPHABETIZATION

The dictionary's alphabetic style is based on a strict letter sequence that disregards spaces or hyphens occurring between words, as, for example, in the following sequence: *analog, analog computer, analog data, analog multiplexer, analogous, analogous structures, analog signal, analog-to-digital converter, analogue, analogy.*

An exception is found with eponymic terms, when the apostrophe ('s) is disregarded in considering the alphabetic sequence; thus, *Fick's law* precedes *Fick principle.*

When the spelling of two words is identical, proper names (capitalized entries) precede the common noun (lower-cased entry), as when *Bacterium* precedes *bacterium.*

Arrangement of Terms

Following the lead of many biomedical dictionaries, terms are defined herein primarily where logic dictates; that is, most terms composed of a noun modified by a descriptive or eponymic designation are defined at the adjective or eponym. In those instances in which current usage dictates otherwise, or when placement is less clear, a cross-reference has been inserted to guide the reader; our primary aim was not uniformity but rather reader convenience and assistance. Thus, for example, the definition for *thymic tumors* appears at *thymic,* not *tumors,* and that for *Romanowsky's stain* is at *Romanowsky's,* not *stain.*

Form

Primary entries generally contain the following elements: name of term (in boldface type), pronunciation (in parentheses), plural form, etymology (in brackets), descriptive definition, and any synonyms, applicable trademarks, cross-references, and subentries.

[NA] identifies anatomic terms that are listed in the *Nomina Anatomica,* and [USP] identifies drugs listed in the *United States Pharmacopeia.* Coded numbers are given for enzymes (assigned by the Enzyme Commission) and for dyes (assigned by the *Colour Index*).

Compound Terms

Compound terms are usually listed separately rather than clustered under the first word; for example, there are separate entries for *linear attenuation coefficient, linear energy transfer,* and *linear equation.* When compound words are clustered under the first word, it is to facilitate access to related information; thus entries such as *heat of combustion, heat of reaction,* and *heat of solution* are subentries under the primary word *heat,* as is also the term *molar heat capacity.* Such arrangements allow the reader access to related terms that would otherwise be scattered alphabetically throughout the book.

Cross-References

The many cross-references in this dictionary are in part a consequence of the multiplicity of abbreviations, acronyms, trademarks of generic drugs and products, and synonyms that seem to particularly characterize laboratory medicine. At such entries the reader is directed to the primary term by the word "See."

The reader will also find cross-references to definitions of related information at the end of the primary term. These are indicated by use of the cross-referenced term in italics, as for example, at the end of *genetic code:* "See also *mutation, nucleic acid, protein synthesis,* and *wobble hypothesis.*" "Also called" information includes both italicized and nonitalicized terms: if the term is not italicized, it is included in the dictionary as a point of information but does not have a separate entry. Cross-references listed as part of "See under" indicate that the term is defined elsewhere, but only within the definition to which the reader is being directed: thus, at the term *erythrocuprein,* the reader is directed to "see under *copper storage protein,*" where *erythrocuprein* is defined.

Pronunciation

Indicated in parentheses after the name of the term, pronunciation employs the use of simple phonetic respelling. Diacritical markings to distinguish vowel sounds are used sparingly; occasionally an alternate pronunciation is also provided.

An unmarked vowel ending a syllable is long (gra′dĕ-ent).

An unmarked vowel in a syllable ending with a consonant is short (sek′shun).

A long vowel in a syllable that must end with a consonant is indicated by a macron (nōz′pēs).

A short vowel that constitutes or ends a syllable is marked with a breve (ep″ĭ-nef′rin).

The syllable *ah* is used for the sound of *a* in open, unaccented syllables (ah-fer′ĕ-sis).

The primary accent in a word is indicated by a single accent; the secondary accent is indicated by a double accent.

Abbreviations

An effort has been made to keep the use of abbreviations to a minimum. Ones that are found, primarily as part of the etymology, include:

Ar.	Arabic	L.	Latin
A.S.	Anglo Saxon	M.W.	molecular weight
dim.	diminutive	N.A.	Nomina Anatomica
cf.	compare (L. *confer*)	N.L.	New Latin
C.I.	Colour Index	O.E.	Old English
E.C.	Enzyme Commission	pl.	plural
e.g.	for example (L. *exempli gratia*)	Port.	Portuguese
Fr.	French	p.p.	past participle
Ger.	German	sing.	singular
Gr.	Greek	Sp.	Spanish
i.e.	that is (L. *id est*)	Swed.	Swedish
It.	Italian	USP	United States Pharmacopeia

DICTIONARY & ENCYCLOPEDIA OF LABORATORY MEDICINE AND TECHNOLOGY

James L. Bennington, M.D., *Editor*

Renee Munoz, *Managing Editor*

EDITORIAL ASSISTANT

Meredith A. Allen

EDITORIAL ASSISTANCE

Terry Russell
Terry Murray
Cynthia Fazzini
Douglas Anderson
Livia Berardi
Wendy Phillips

PROOFREADERS

Charlie Brown, *Supervisor*
Bob Young
Jim Leonard
Kate Mason
Dennis Dolan
Betty Gittens
Patricia Schilling
Douglas Anderson
Pearl Babb

PRODUCTION

Bob Butler, *Production Manager*

ILLUSTRATIONS

Ray Duglas
Linda Maugeri

DESIGN

Nina McDaid Ikeda
Bill Donnelly

COPY EDITOR

David Harvey

OFFICE ASSISTANCE

SAUNDERS

Donna Davis Ciccotelli
Janet Jurkowski
Mary L. Booth
Marcia Cohen
Richard Valenci
Jane Ligums
Annette Davis
Jay Valenci
Kathleen Collier
Melanie Cann
Jennifer Norris Peterson

EXTERNAL

Judy Fletcher
Secretary to Dr. Bennington
Nancy Pastrick
Karen Reeves
Secretaries to Dr. Tietz

INTERNATIONAL COMPUTAPRINT CORPORATION

John Macalino
Leslie Logan
The Commercial Division

Associate Editors

Assistant Editors

MICHAEL J. AMINOFF, M.D.

Professor of Neurology, University of California, San Francisco, School of Medicine; and Director of the Clinical Neurophysiology Laboratories, University of California Medical Center, San Francisco, California
Neurology

MARY C. BOWLING, M.T. (ASCP)*

Supervisory Biologist of the Laboratory of Pathology, National Cancer Institute, National Institutes of Health, Bethesda, Maryland
Histotechnology

BYRON W. BROWN, Jr., Ph.D.

Professor of Biostatistics, Stanford University; and Head of the Division of Biostatistics, Stanford University School of Medicine, Stanford, California
Statistics

H. JOACHIM BURHENNE, M.D.

Professor and Head of the Department of Radiology, University of British Columbia; and Director of Radiology, Vancouver General Hospital, Vancouver, British Columbia, Canada
Radiology

STEPHEN K. CARTER, M.D.

Vice President of Anti-Cancer Research, Pharmaceutical Research and Development Division, Bristol-Myers Company; and Adjunct Clinical Professor of Medicine, New York University Medical School, New York, New York
Oncology

ROBERT P. ERICKSON, M.D.

Professor of Human Genetics and of Pediatrics and Communicable Diseases, University of Michigan School of Medicine, Ann Arbor, Michigan
Genetics

HAROLD I. GRIFFEATH, M.D.

Corporate Medical Director, Castle & Cook, Inc.; and Associate Clinical Professor of Medicine, University of California, San Francisco, School of Medicine, San Francisco, California
Cardiology

DAVID P. HOLMAN, M.D.

Associate Clinical Professor of Medicine, University of California, San Francisco, School of Medicine; and Chief of Pulmonary Medicine and Director of the Pulmonary Laboratory, Children's Hospital of San Francisco, San Francisco, California
Pulmonary Function

THOMAS M. JACKSON, M.D.

Director of Clinical Laboratories, Children's Hospital of San Francisco, San Francisco, California
Blood Banking

EILEEN B. KING, M.D.

Clinical Professor of Pathology, University of California, San Francisco, School of Medicine; and Director of the Curriculum in Exfoliative Cytology, University of California Medical Center, San Francisco, California
Cytology

JEROLD M. LOWENSTEIN, M.D.

Chairman of the Department of Nuclear Medicine, Pacific Medical Center; and Clinical Professor of Medicine, University of California, San Francisco, School of Medicine, San Francisco, California
Nuclear Medicine

ROBERT G. MILLER, M.D.

Adjunct Associate Professor of Neurology, University of California, San Francisco, School of Medicine; and Chief of the Clinical Service of Neurology and Director of Neuromuscular Research, Children's Hospital of San Francisco, San Francisco, California
Neurology

NORMAN V. STEERE, C.S.P., P.E.

Laboratory Safety and Design Consultant, Norman V. Steere & Associates, Inc., Minneapolis, Minnesota
Laboratory Safety

DANIEL P. STITES, M.D.

Professor and Vice Chairman of the Laboratory Medicine Department, University of California, San Francisco, School of Medicine; and Director of the Clinical Immunology Laboratory, University of California Medical Center, San Francisco, California
Immunology

GEORGE E. WESTLAKE, M.D.

President, Georger Westlake Associates, Kentfield; and Chief of Pathology, Shriners Hospital for Crippled Children, San Francisco, California
Instrumentation

* Retired.

Consultants

N. V. BHAGAVAN, PH.D.

Professor and Chairman, Department of Biochemistry and Biophysics, University of Hawaii School of Medicine; and Consultant Biochemist, Kaiser Medical Center, Honolulu, Hawaii
Biochemistry

ROBERT V. BLANKE, PH.D.

Professor of Pathology, Virginia Commonwealth University School of Medicine; and Director of the Hospital Toxicology Laboratory, Medical College of Virginia, Richmond, Virginia
Toxicology

SATI C. CHATTORAJ, PH.D.

Associate Professor of Biochemistry; and Director of the Research Division of the Department of Obstetrics and Gynecology, Boston University School of Medicine, Boston, Massachusetts
Endocrinology

JOHN F. KACHMAR, PH.D.

Associate Professor of Biochemistry, Rush Medical School, and Department of Related Health Sciences, Rush Presbyterian–St. Luke's Medical Center; and Senior Attending Scientist, Biochemistry, and Consultant in Clinical Biochemistry, Laboratory Clinical Services, Presbyterian–St. Luke's Hospital, Chicago, Illinois
Clinical Chemistry

ALAN D. RINKER, M.S.

Supervisor of RIA/Immunochemistry Laboratory, Department of Pathology, University of Kentucky Medical Center, Lexington, Kentucky
General Support—Chemistry

JOSEPH W. WILSON, PH.D.

Associate Professor of Chemistry, University of Kentucky, Lexington, Kentucky
General Chemistry

DONALD S. YOUNG, M.B., PH.D.

Head of the Section of Clinical Chemistry, Mayo Clinic; and Professor of Laboratory Medicine, Mayo Medical School, Rochester, Minnesota
Clinical Chemistry

Contributors

ARTHUR E. BURGESS, Ph.D.
Associate Professor of Radiology, University of British Columbia, Vancouver, British Columbia, Canada

JEROME S. BURKE, M.D.
Pathologist, Department of Anatomic Pathology, City of Hope National Medical Center, Duarte, California

SIMEON T. CANTRIL, M.D.
Chief of Radiation Therapy Services, Children's Hospital of San Francisco; and Assistant Clinical Professor of Radiology, University of California, San Francisco, School of Medicine, San Francisco, California

WALTER S. CEGLOWSKI, Ph.D.
Professor of Microbiology, and Director of the Clinical Immunology Laboratory, Temple University School of Medicine, Philadelphia, Pennsylvania

ERNEST H. Y. CHU, Ph.D.
Professor of Human Genetics, University of Michigan School of Medicine, Ann Arbor, Michigan

RICHARD J. COHEN, M.D.
Chief of Hematology/Oncology, Children's Hospital of San Francisco; and Clinical Professor of Medicine, University of California, San Francisco, School of Medicine, San Francisco, California

THOMAS V. COLBY, M.D.
Assistant Professor of Pathology, Stanford University School of Medicine, Stanford, California

PETER L. COOPERBERG, M.D.
Associate Professor of Radiology, University of British Columbia; and Section Chief of Ultrasound, Vancouver General Hospital, Vancouver, British Columbia, Canada

KENNETH R. CUNDY, Ph.D.
Professor of Microbiology, and Director of the Clinical Microbiology Laboratories, Temple University School of Medicine, Philadelphia, Pennsylvania

FRANK A. DOLBEARE, Ph.D.
Biomedical Scientist, Lawrence Livermore National Laboratory, Livermore, California

CHARLES J. EPSTEIN, M.D.
Professor of Pediatrics and Biochemistry, and Director of the Division of Pediatric Genetics, University of California, San Francisco, School of Medicine, San Francisco, California

GARY FAGAN, B.S.
Research Associate in Immunology, Clinical Immunology Laboratory, University of California Medical Center, San Francisco, California

STEPHAN D. FIHN, M.D., M.P.H.
Assistant Professor of Medicine, University of Washington, Seattle, Washington

MICHAEL A. FRIEDMAN, M.D.
Associate Professor of Medicine, Cancer Research Institute, University of California Medical Center, San Francisco, California

MURIEL M. GLUCKSON, M.S.
Genetic Counselor and Research Associate in Pediatrics and Genetics, St. Vincent's Hospital & Medical Center, New York, New York

JACQUELINE S. HART, M.D.
Lieutenant Colonel, U.S. Army, Hematology/Oncology Service, Bellaire, Texas

MICHAEL R. HENDRICKSON, M.D.
Associate Professor of Pathology, Stanford University School of Medicine, Stanford, California

J. KENNETH HOOBER, Ph.D.
Professor of Biochemistry, Temple University School of Medicine, Philadelphia, Pennsylvania

EDWARD L. HOWES, M.D.
Chief of the Department of Anatomic Pathology, San Francisco General Hospital; and Professor of Pathology and Ophthalmology, University of California, San Francisco, School of Medicine, San Francisco, California

S. M. JACKSON, M.D.
Head of Radiation Oncology, Cancer Control Agency of British Columbia, Vancouver, British Columbia, Canada

PAUL JURKOWSKI, M.D.
Captain, U.S. Army, Fort Hood, Texas

RICHARD L. KEMPSON, M.D.
Professor of Pathology, Stanford University School of Medicine; and Co-Director of Surgical Pathology, Stanford University Medical Center, Stanford, California

MORTON KLEIN, Ph.D.
Professor of Microbiology, Temple University School of Medicine, Philadelphia, Pennsylvania

GERALD B. KOLSKI, M.D., PH.D.

Assistant Professor of Pediatrics, University of Pennsylvania School of Medicine; and Clinical Director of Allergy, Children's Hospital of Philadelphia, Philadelphia, Pennsylvania

MARIA M. KORETZ, PH.D.

Director of Statistics and Epidemiology for Cancer Control, Northern California Cancer Program, Palo Alto, California

MICHAEL KRUPP, B.S.E.E.

Engineer and Computer Consultant, Children's Hospital of San Francisco, San Francisco, California

F. R. MARGOLIN, M.D.

Chairman of the Department of Radiology, Children's Hospital of San Francisco; and Clinial Professor of Radiology, University of California, San Francisco, School of Medicine, San Francisco, California

BRIAN H. MAYALL, M.D.

Director of the Program for Analytical Cytology, Lawrence Livermore National Laboratory, Livermore; and Professor of Laboratory Medicine, University of California, San Francisco, School of Medicine, San Francisco, California

THEODORE MILLER, M.D.

Associate Professor of Pathology, University of California, San Francisco, School of Medicine, San Francisco, California

R. M. NAKAMURA, M.D.

Chairman of the Department of Pathology, Scripps Clinic and Research Foundation; and Adjunct Professor of Pathology, University of California, San Diego, La Jolla, California

J. ROBERT NEWLAND, D.D.S.

Associate Professor of Pathology, University of Texas Health Science Center at Houston, Dental Branch, Texas Medical Center, Houston, Texas

W. S. NICHOLS, M.D.

Department of Pathology, Scripps Clinic and Research Foundation; and Assistant Clinical Professor of Pathology, University of California, San Diego, La Jolla, California

NELSON G. ORDONEZ, M.D.

Associate Professor of Pathology, Associate Pathologist, and Director of Immunocytochemistry Laboratory, University, of Texas System Cancer Center, M.D. Anderson Hospital and Tumor Institute, Texas Medical Center, Houston, Texas

CHARLES PAVIA, PH.D.

Assistant Member and Staff Scientist, Trudeau Institute, Saranac Lake, New York

ALLAN PONT, M.D.

Chairman of the Department of Medicine, Children's Hospital of San Francisco; and Associate Clinical Professor of Medicine, University of California, San Francisco, School of Medicine, San Francisco, California

BRUCE RICHARDSON, M.D., PH.D.

Assistant Professor of Medicine, Section of Rheumatology, University of Michigan Medical School, Ann Arbor, Michigan

RICHARD W. SAGEBIEL, M.D.

Professor of Pathology and Dermatology, University of California, San Francisco, School of Medicine; and Co-Director of the Melanoma Clinic, University of California Medical Center, San Francisco, California

NANETTE SMITH, M.D.

Practitioner in Family Practice, Elk City, Idaho

PETER E. SMOUSE, PH.D.

Professor of Human Genetics, University of Michigan School of Medicine, Ann Arbor, Michigan

ALAN SOLINGER, M.D.

Assistant Professor of Medicine, University of Cincinnati College of Medicine, Cincinnati, Ohio

GREGORY A. STEPHENS, PH.D.

Assistant Professor, School of Life and Health Sciences, University of Delaware, Newark, Delaware

VIBEKE STRAND, M.D.

Assistant Clinical Professor, University of California, San Francisco; Practitioner in Internal Medicine and Rheumatology, San Francisco, California

CLIVE R. TAYLOR, M.D., D.PHIL.

Professor of Pathology, University of Southern California School of Medicine; and Chief of Immunopathology, University of Southern California Medical Center, Los Angeles, California

HARRIETTE D. VERA, PH.D.*

Manager of Quality Control, Bioquest Division, Becton, Dickinson & Co., Cockeysville, Maryland

SANDRA L. WATKINS, M.D.

Resident, Department of Pediatrics, University of Washington School of Medicine, Seattle, Washington

LEONARD J. ZUBRZYCKI, PH.D.

Professor of Microbiology, Temple University School of Medicine, Philadelphia, Pennsylvania

* Retired.

Writers

DAVID AHARONY, PH.D.
Clinical Chemistry

DEBORAH E. ALLEN, PH.D.
Pulmonary Function, Cardiology, Neurology

MICHÈLE DE GEORGE, B.S.
Genetics

PATRICIA DESOUSA, B.S.
Anatomy

MARY ANN DI GIROLAMO, B.S., M.T. (ASCP)
Hematology, Blood Banking

CHARLES J. GEYER, B.S.
General Support, Most Fields

TIMOTHY J. HAYES, PH.D.
Immunology, Virology, Mycology

EILEEN HINKS, PH.D.
Microbiology

PAUL JURKOWSKI, M.D.
Medicine

LORAN M. KILLAR, B.S.
Cytology

VIRGINIA MILLER, PH.D.
Neurology

LEONARD N. NORCIA, PH.D.
Biochemistry

KATHARINE PLAUT, M.S.
Bacteriology

WILLIAM R. RATE, PH.D.
Medicine, Oncology

JANET L. ROBINSON, A.B., M.T. (ASCP)
Parasitology, Medical Terminology

MARCA LEONISE SIPSKI, M.D.
Medicine

JONATHON SPEARS, PH.D.
Anatomy, Histotechnology, Blood Banking

BRIAN STANG, M.D.
Medicine

DONALD L. WARKENTIN, PH.D.
Clinical Chemistry

A

A symbol for *absorbance, activity* (radiation), *adenosine, admittance, alanine, alveolar gas, ampere, area, mass number.*

Å abbrev. See *angström.*

Ã abbrev. for cumulated activity. See under *dose estimate.*

$\mathbf{A^{1\%}_{1cm}}$ an obsolete expression; see *absorptivity.*

AI abbrev. See *a. I* under *angiotensin.*

AII abbrev. See *a. II* under *angiotensin.*

AIII abbrev. See *a. III* under *angiotensin.*

a symbol for *absorptivity,* acceleration, *activity* (chemical), *arterial blood,* atto-.

a- (a) [Gr. *a-* (before vowels, *an-*) without, not] a prefix word element to denote no, not, or without, e.g., apnea. See also *an-.*

α the Greek lower case letter alpha; symbol for: (1) optical rotation, (2) angular acceleration, (3) the heavy chain of IgA, (4) solubility coefficient.

α- a designator for: (1) an anomer of a carbohydrate, e.g., α-D-glucose; (2) one constituent of the plasma globulin fraction or other proteins migrating electrophoretically with this fraction, e.g., α-fetoprotein; (3) a substituent group of a steroid that projects below the plane of the ring, e.g., 3α-hydroxy-5α-androstan-17-one (androsterone).

AA abbrev. See *amino acid, arachidonic acid, atomic absorption.*

AAA abbrev. See *American Association of Anatomists.*

AAAS abbrev. See *American Association for the Advancement of Science.*

AAB abbrev. See *American Association of Bioanalysts.*

AABB abbrev. See *American Association of Blood Banks.*

AACC abbrev. See *American Association for Clinical Chemistry.*

AACIA abbrev. See *American Association for Clinical Immunology and Allergy.*

AAEE abbrev. See *American Association of Electromyography and Electrodiagnosis.*

AAI abbrev. See *American Association of Immunologists.*

AAM abbrev. See *American Academy of Microbiology.*

AAMI abbrev. See *Association for the Advancement of Medical Instrumentation.*

AAN abbrev. See *American Association of Neuropathologists.*

AAP abbrev. See *American Association of Pathologists.*

$\mathbf{(A\text{–}a)P_{CO_2}}$ abbrev. See *alveolar-arterial carbon dioxide difference.*

AAPA abbrev. See *American Association of Pathologist Assistants.*

AAV abbrev. for adeno-associated virus.

ab- (ab) [L. *ab* away from] a prefix word element to denote off, or away from, e.g., abnormal.

abacterial (a″bak-te′re-al) free from bacteria.

A band the dark-staining zone of a striated muscle sarcomere. It is formed by parallel myosin myofilaments, and by actin myofilaments that penetrate the A band to a depth that varies with the state of contraction of the myofibril. The central portion of the A band not occupied by actin myofilaments is the H zone, with the M line at its center. The A band is so named because it is anisotropic in polarized light. Its length does not alter when the myofibril contracts. See also *skeletal m.* under *muscle.*

abarognosis (a″bar-og-no′sis) [*a-* neg. + Gr. *baros* weight + *gnōsis* knowledge] loss of ability to perceive differences in weight or pressure.

abasia (a-ba′ze-ah) [*a-* neg. + Gr. *basis* step + *-ia*] an inability to walk.

abatement (ah-bāt′ment) a decrease in the severity of a pain or symptom.

ABB abbrev. See *American Board of Bioanalysis.*

Abbé test plate (ab′a) [Ernst Karl *Abbé,* German physicist, 1840–1905] a glass slide used to examine optical lenses and microscope objectives for their adequacy of correction of spherical or chromatic aberration, sharpness or definition, and flatness of field. The slide is ruled with several series of fine parallel lines and has a wedge-shaped coverglass for determination of optimal coverslip thickness.

ABC abbrev. See *American Blood Commission.*

abdomen (ab-do′men) [L., possibly from *abdere* to hide] the portion of the body that lies between the thorax and the pelvis. It contains the abdominal cavity, which is separated from the chest by the diaphragm, and is lined by the peritoneum. The cavity holds the stomach, large and small intestines, liver, spleen, pancreas, kidneys, appendix, gallbladder, urinary bladder, and other structures.

abdomin/o (ab-dom′ĭ-no) [L. *abdomen* the belly] a word element used in combining form to denote a relationship to the abdomen, e.g., abdominal.

abdominal (ab-dom′ĭ-nal) [L. *abdominalis*] pertaining to the abdomen.

abdominal regions 1. nine regions that are subdivisions of the surface of the abdomen (see the accompanying illustration).

2. nine regions into which the abdomen is divided by four of Addison's planes. The upper transverse plane is the transpyloric plane, the lower is the transtubercular plane, and the two vertical planes are the lateral sagittal planes. See also *Addison's planes.*

abdominal scan a procedure in nuclear medicine for examining the stomach and small intestine, which employs a scintillation camera or rectilinear scanner. The scan is used primarily for the detection and localization of Meckel's diverticulum. In the procedure, sodium pertechnetate Tc 99m is injected intravenously and is actively taken up by the gastric mucosa, including any ectopic gastric mucosa found in Meckel's diverticulum. The radionuclide also localizes some intestinal intussusceptions, obstructions, and duplications.

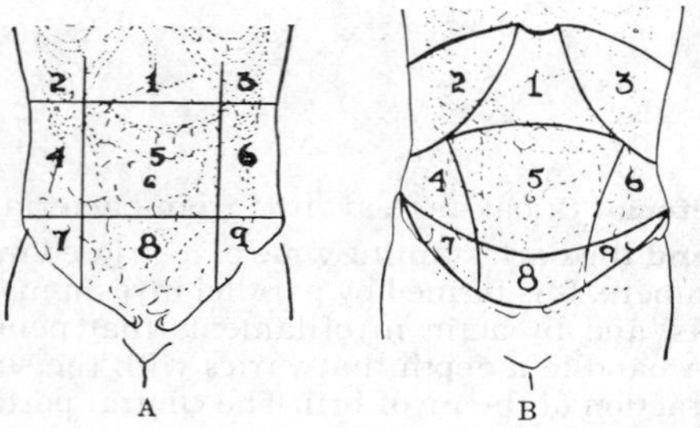

Abdominal regions. Regions of the abdomen bounded according to the standard (A) and a variant (B) system: 1 indicates the epigastric region; 2, right hypochondriac; 3, left hypochondriac; 4, right lateral (lumbar); 5, umbilical; 6, left lateral (lumbar); 7, right inguinal (iliac); 8, pubic (hypogastric; and 9, left inguinal (iliac). (From Dorland's Illustrated Medical Dictionary. 26th ed. Philadelphia, W. B. Saunders Co., 1981).

abdominal zones three zones into which the surface of the abdomen is divided by transverse planes: the epigastric zone, above the transpyloric plane; the hypogastric zone, below the transtubercular plane; and the umbilical (mesogastric) zone, which is in between the two.

abducent (ab-du′sent) [L. *abducens,* from *abducere* to draw away] abducting; drawing away from.

abducent nerve cranial nerve VI; a slender motor nerve that arises in the pons and runs forward in the lateral wall of the cavernous sinus into the orbit. It innervates the lateral rectus muscle. See also *cranial nerves.*

abduct (ab-dukt′) [L. *abducere* to draw away] to move a part away from the median plane (central axis) of the body or, in the case of the fingers and toes, away from the axial line of a limb.

abduction (ab-duk′shun) [L. *abductio*] the act of abducting or the state of being abducted.

abductor (ab-duk′tor) [L.] a muscle, such as the deltoid, that moves a bone away from another part (away from the median plane).

Abell method see under *cholesterol assays.*

aberrant (ab-er′ant) [L. *aberrans,* from *ab* from + *errare* to wander] wandering or deviating from the usual or normal course; an atypical element, group of elements, or characteristic.

aberrant rest see *choristoma.*

aberration (ab″er-a′shun) [L. *aberratio,* from *ab-* + *errare* to wander] 1. deviation from the usual course or condition.

2. in an optical system, any deviation from a perfect image; see *chromatic aberration* and *spherical aberration.*

3. see *chromosomal aberration.*

abetalipoproteinemia (a-ba″tah-lip″o-pro-tēn-e′-me-ah) [*a-* neg. + *beta* + *lipoprotein* + Gr. *haima* blood + *-ia*] a rare genetic disorder, transmitted as an autosomal recessive trait, that is characterized by an absolute deficiency of beta lipoproteins (LDLs), prebeta lipoproteins (VLDLs), and chylomicrons. It is thought to be due to deficient synthesis of apoprotein B. Onset occurs in the first year of life, with steatorrhea, growth failure, acanthocytosis, retinitis pigmentosa, hereditary ataxia, severe fat malabsorption, distal sensory loss, and visual disturbances.

Diagnosis is based on demonstration of very low serum cholesterol concentrations (<50 mg/100 ml) and virtually absent blood plasma triglycerides (<10 mg/100 ml). Electrophoresis and ultracentrifugation reveal no LDLs, VLDLs, or chylomicrons. There is no specific treatment, although massive doses of vitamins E or A may delay or retard the neurologic sequelae. There is significant disability with skeletal and muscular deformities and the prognosis is poor. Also called *Bassen-Kornzweig syndrome.*

ABG abbrev. for arterial blood gases.

ablate (ab-lāt′) [L. *ablatus* removed] to remove, especially by cutting; to destroy wholly.

ablatio (ab-la′she-o) [L.] detachment.

a. placentae, premature detachment of the placenta; see also *a. placentae* under *abruptio.*

ablation (ab-la′shun) [L. *ablatio*] the removal of a tissue by cutting, burning, or other means.

abnormal (ab-nor′mal) [*ab-* + L. *norma* rule] not normal; a deviation from the usual structure, position, condition, behavior, or rule.

ABO abbrev. for the three major blood systems. See under *blood groups* and *blood typing.*

Abopon (ah′bo-pon) trademark for a water-soluble (gum or crystalline solid) mounting medium used in histology in the form of a saturated solution in pH 7 phosphate buffer. This medium preserves crystal violet amyloid stains and acetic orcein stains.

abort (ah-bort′) [L. *abortus,* from *aboriri* to miscarry] 1. to halt the progress of a disease.

2. to halt the progress of a pregnancy. See also *abortion.*

abortion (ah-bor′shun) [L. *abortio*] the termination of pregnancy at any point in fetal development; more precisely, the termination of pregnancy before the twenty-first week of gestation. Termination after this time and before the twenty-ninth week is called premature labor. Before the twelfth week, abortion is usually performed by progressive dilation of the cervical opening and scraping or suctioning out of the uterine lining. After the sixteenth week and up to the twenty-first week, injections of saline, glucose, or prostaglandin solutions into the amniotic sac is the technique of choice.

complete a., an abortion in which the uterus is emptied completely of the fetus, placenta, and decidual lining. With spontaneous abortion this usually occurs only during the first 6 wk of pregnancy or after the fourteenth week.

habitual a., the spontaneous termination of three or more pregnancies in the same patient. It may be the result of organic or psychiatric disease.

incomplete a., an abortion in which fragments of placental tissue remain in the uterus. The retained tissue often becomes infected and is liable to hemorrhage, posing a severe danger to the patient.

Incomplete abortions are most likely to occur between the sixth and fourteenth weeks of pregnancy. Treatment is removal of the retained tissue and initiation of therapy for any infection or bleeding.

induced a., the deliberate termination of pregnancy by mechanical or chemical means.

missed a., a spontaneous abortion in which the

products of conception are retained within the uterus; the abortion is unknown to patient or physician at the time of occurrence. Diagnosis is made by noting a progressive decrease in uterine size, a lack of audible fetal heart sounds, and negative pregnancy tests.

A severe complication of missed abortion is the development of extensive intravascular coagulation and subsequent clotting defects owing to the release of thromboplastin by the dead fetus. This is most likely to occur if the fetus has been dead for several weeks late in the pregnancy.

septic a., a serious infection of the uterus, its surrounding tissues, and often the abdomen, which occurs after induced abortion (especially illegal abortion). The infection is characterized by extreme pelvic and lower abdominal tenderness, with peritonitis and paralysis of peristaltic motion in the bowel (ileus). Fever is often very high with rapid fluctuations. Bowel flora, including anaerobic streptococci, bacteroides, coli-aerogenes group or enterococci, and *Clostridium perfringens,* are common agents.

spontaneous a., an abortion that is not intentionally induced. It is due to disease in the mother or to pathology of the ovum, sperm, or fertilization and implantation processes. Spontaneous abortions may be the result of chromosomal abnormalities; especially common patterns found in aborted fetuses are autosomal trisomies. When chromosomal defects are not found, gross developmental abnormalities are often noted in the fetus. Maternal disease, including infection, endocrine abnormalities, and anatomic abnormalities, may also cause spontaneous abortions; trauma is not as common a cause as is widely held.

therapeutic a., an induced abortion. Common medical indications are severe maternal cardiac or renal disease, advanced tuberculosis, chronic hypertension with vascular pathology, and cancer in the organs of conception. Psychiatric disorder is also an indication for abortion in some instances. Imminent fetal disease may be included in some definitions of therapeutic abortion, as in those instances of maternal rubella infection in the first 20 wk of pregnancy, diagnosed lethal hereditary conditions, or exposure to teratogenic agents.

threatened a., a condition of impending expulsion of the products of conception. There is slight bleeding and/or brown vaginal discharge, often accompanied by cramping pelvic pain that signals a partial separation of the placenta from uterine tissue (and possible subsequent abortion). Threatened abortion is a clinical state that either may progress to actual abortion or may remit, the remainder of the pregnancy being uneventful.

tubal a., the extrusion of the fetus and placental tissues through the ostium of the uterine tube into the abdomen. This occurs in ectopic (tubal) pregnancies. Clinically, a tubal abortion is manifested by prolonged, intermittent, cramping abdominal pain with uterine (vaginal) bleeding. Blood also escapes into the peritoneal cavity, producing peritoneal irritation and rectal pressure. The severity of pain increases as separation progresses to the extrusion, with severe pain and rectal straining, and often with fainting while at stool.

Laboratory diagnosis is aided by findings of a slightly elevated white blood cell count with either gradual, progressive anemia or sudden falls in the hemoglobin or hematocrit. Radioimmunoassay for the β-subunit of human chorionic gonadotropin (hCG) is usually positive with tubal pregnancy, while standard measurements of urinary total hCG may not be.

abortive (ah-bor'tiv) [L. *abortivus*] 1. incompletely developed.

2. causing an abortion.

abortus (ah-bor'tus) [L.] a dead or nonviable fetus; one weighing less than 500 g at birth.

abortus fever see *brucellosis.*

ABO typing see *blood typing.*

abrasion (ah-bra'zhun) [L. *abrasio,* from *abradere* abrade] 1. the wearing away of material from a surface by friction.

2. an area of the body surface from which the epidermis or mucous membrane has been scraped away.

abreaction (ab"re-ak'shun) [*ab-* + *reaction*] the release of painful emotion through the recall of repressed memories. A basic technique employed in freudian psychotherapy, abreaction is especially valuable for individuals with independent personalities who cope well with stress.

abreuography (ab"roo-og'rah-fe) [Manoel de *Abreu,* Brazilian physician, 1892–1962] see *photofluorography.*

abruptio (ab-rup'she-o) [L., from *abrumpere* to break off] a tearing or separation of a tissue from its supports.

a. placentae, the premature separation (before delivery of the baby) of the placenta from the uterine wall. Separation before onset of labor occurs in about 0.2 percent of pregnancies and, if complete, results in fetal death unless delivery is immediate. Incomplete separation is not always incompatible with live delivery of the infant. Abruptio placentae may occur in association with maternal renal disease, chronic hypertension, and the syndrome of supine hypotension. Clinically, the process is manifested by abdominal pain and bleeding from the vagina. The uterus is tender and often firmly contracted. Maternal complications may include severe hemorrhage, shock, poor clotting secondary to low fibrinogen levels, disseminated intravascular coagulation, acute renal cortical or tubular necrosis, and death. Laboratory findings are limited to a modest increase in leukocytes (20,000 cells/cm^3) and a falling hematocrit.

ABS abbrev. See *alkylbenzene sulfonate.*

abscess (ab'ses) [L. *abscessus,* from *ab-* away + *cedere* to go] a circumscribed collection of necrotic cellular debris, inflammatory cells, and organisms surrounded by a zone of inflamed tissue. The contents of the abscess are semiliquid (pus). The cause is usually an irritant such as a staphylococcus that lacks spreading factors. An abscess contains large numbers of neutrophils, whose lysosomal enzymes digest the damaged tissue, converting it to a soft material that becomes more fluid with the influx of water. As the pressure rises within an abscess, it tends to expand by the route of least resistance, such as a fascial plane; this extension can be minimized surgically by incision and drainage. If the body's natural defense mechanisms can control the infection while it is still localized, the abscess may be converted to a cyst surrounded by a layer of dense fibrosis. An abscess heals by scarring.

amebic a. of liver, an abscess produced by *Enta-*

moeba histolytica, which represents a serious complication of amebiasis. The abscess contains a characteristic brown, pastelike exudate ("anchovy paste") instead of pus. The abscess may rupture into the peritoneal cavity, and secondary abscesses may develop in the lungs. Pain in the right hypochondrium is a common and striking symptom. Diagnostic procedures include a histologic identification of the parasite, an amebic indirect hemagglutination or gel diffusion (precipitin) test, and ultrasonic or radioisotopic scanning. See also *amebiasis.*

brain a., a focal, suppurative lesion of the brain, often occurring in the temporal lobe or the cerebellum. Brain abscesses usually are caused by direct spread of infection from an adjacent area such as the ear or paranasal sinus, and less commonly are metastatic (from a lung infection) or result from the direct implantation of septic material consequent to trauma. Common etiologic agents include anaerobic streptococci and *Staphylococcus aureus.* Other anaerobes (particularly *Bacteroides*) or Enterobacteriaceae are sometimes implicated.

Headache and symptoms of increased intracranial pressure are conspicuous clinical features, together with fever, seizures, and the subsequent development of localized neurologic symptoms. In other instances, patients present with focal signs and symptoms similar to those seen with other structural lesions, such as tumors.

Demonstration of the abscess is by various radiographic and isotopic techniques: CT and radionuclide scans are the most accurate and useful. CT scans in particular are helpful in visualizing the lesion and following its course during therapy. Lumbar puncture is potentially dangerous because of the increased intracranial pressure; the cerebrospinal fluid shows only a mild pleocytosis, an elevated protein concentration, and normal glucose, and these findings are not particularly helpful diagnostically.

Therapy includes the use of antimicrobial agents; excision of superficial, encapsulated lesions; and aspiration of the contents of those that are inaccessible. The mortality rate is about 40 percent, and many survivors are left with residual deficits.

Cf. *cerebral epidural a.* and *subdural e.* under *empyema.*

Brodie's a., a chronic, walled-off collection of necrotic debris and inflammatory cells that occurs most commonly as a punched out area in the metaphysis of the long bones caused by localized chronic osteomyelitis. These abscesses may be sterile or may act as a reservoir for the bacteria, leading to chronic osteomyelitis. They may remain in existence for years.

cerebral epidural a., an accumulation of granulomatous tissue and pus on the outer surface of the dura, separating it from the cranial bone. Epidural abscesses are usually secondary to a chronic sinus or ear infection that is often accompanied by osteomyelitis of adjacent bone. Common etiologic agents include streptococci and a variety of gram-negative organisms.

These abscesses are limited in size by the close adherence of the dura to bone; thus, there is rarely enough necrotic debris to produce increased intracranial pressure or focal neurologic signs. Typical symptoms include fever, pain, and local tenderness.

Diagnosis is often difficult, and an epidural abscess is usually discovered during surgery for a related condition such as subdural empyema. The CSF is generally sterile and contains few cells. Treatment is with antimicrobial agents, but attention must also be directed toward the underlying cause.

hepatic a., a localized collection of pus within the hepatic parenchyma, most commonly resulting from bacterial infection produced by enteric bacilli (particularly *Escherichia coli* and *Klebsiella* species) and pyogenic gram-positive cocci (particularly *Staphylococcus aureus*). Bacterial hepatic abscess is most often an extension of biliary tract infection, but may also be spread as the result of other infections (e.g., subphrenic abscess, appendicitis, septicemia). Typically, there is acute febrile illness with hepatomegaly and right upper quadrant tenderness; jaundice occurs in about 20 percent of cases and usually indicates infection of the biliary tract.

Laboratory diagnostic procedures include radionuclide scanning, which can detect about 80–90 percent of hepatic abscesses, but may miss those smaller than 2 cm in diameter. Ultrasonography may be particularly helpful in distinguishing an abscess from a solid tumor. About 40 percent of blood cultures are positive.

See also *amebic a. of liver.*

lung a., a localized, suppurative pulmonary infection that produces necrosis of the lung parenchyma. Characteristically, the abscess ruptures into a bronchus, forming a cavity with an air-fluid level as its contents are expectorated.

The primary factor predisposing to the formation of a lung abscess is aspiration of infected material, usually in an individual in an altered state of consciousness (brought about by general anesthesia, drug overdose, diabetic coma, cerebrovascular accident, seizure disorder, or other debilitating illnesses). Other processes underlying its formation are periodontal disease or gingivitis, bronchiectasis, secondary infection of a pulmonary embolus or infarct, bronchial obstruction (with bronchogenic carcinoma frequently the obstructing lesion), direct extension of subdiaphragmatic abscess or other intraabdominal infection into the lower lobes of the lungs, trauma, or infection of bullae or cysts. The location of the abscess, most commonly unifocal in nature, depends to a large extent on the underlying cause. The most common sites are the posterior segments of the right upper lobe and the superior segments of the right lower lobe.

During its development, the clinical manifestations of lung abscess resemble those of acute bronchopneumonia although they are not quite as insidious in onset. These include anorexia, malaise, septic fever, chills, prostration, frequent pleuritic pain, and periodic expectoration of a purulent, fetid sputum. Later complications include empyema (with or without secondary bronchopleural fistula), local spread of the infection, pericarditis, pyo- or tension pneumothorax, hemorrhage into the abscess, and metastatic abscesses, particularly to the brain.

Diagnosis is based primarily on consideration of the signs and symptoms (especially the purulent, foul-smelling sputum) in combination with chest radiographic findings of a cavity with an air-fluid level. Bronchoscopy, tomography, bacterial and cytologic examination of the sputum, and serial radiography may be of additional value in the differential diagnosis.

subphrenic a., a collection of pus beneath the diaphragm.

abscissa (ab-sis′ah) [L. *ab-* from + *scindere* to cut] the x-coordinate value of a point on a graph; the perpendicular distance from the point to the y-axis. Usually, the x-coordinate is used for the independent variable. Cf. *ordinate.*

absence (ab′sens) [L. *absens,* from *abesse* to be absent] the temporary impairment of consciousness.

absence attack a type of primary generalized epilepsy, of idiopathic origin, usually occurring in children aged 4–5 yr or in older adolescents. The attacks are typically abrupt in onset and consist of a transient loss or impairment of consciousness with minimal motor manifestations.

The electroencephalogram (EEG) during an attack is characterized by paroxysmal, bilaterally synchronous spike and wave activity at 3 Hz. This activity becomes generalized polyspike and polyspike wave discharges during nonrapid eye movement (REM) sleep, with fewer episodes of spikes occurring during REM sleep than during waking.

Absence attacks can be provoked by hyperventilation, alkalosis, ketogenic diet, and a low blood sugar concentration. The prognosis for seizure cessation is correlated with a negative history of tonic-clonic (grand mal) attacks, an intelligence quotient (IQ) above 90, and no family history of seizures.

Formerly called *petit mal attack.* See also *epilepsy.*

atypical a. a., a type of epileptic attack characterized clinically by very brief impairment of consciousness, and electroencephalographically by slow-wave and spike activity having a frequency of 2 Hz or less.

Absidia (ab-sid′e-ah) [L. *absis* arch] a genus of mucormycosis(zygomycosis)-causing fungi that are zygomycetes belonging to the family Mucoraceae, order Mucorales. Morphologically, *Absidia* are characterized by branching sporangiophores that arise between nodes (swollen areas) along a stolon and by rhizoids that arise directly from the nodes. This differs from *Mucor,* which has no rhizoids, and from *Rhizopus,* which has rhizoids in a different location. There is only one medically important species, *A. corymbifera.* See also *Mucor* and *Rhizopus.*

A. corymbifera, a species of fungi, belonging to the class Zygomycetes, that causes zygomycosis. Also called *A. ramosa* and *Mucor corymbifer.* See also *phycomycosis.*

absolute (ab′so-lūt) [L. *absolutus,* from *absolvere* to set loose] free from limitations; unlimited; uncombined.

absolute alcohol an extremely hygroscopic, transparent, colorless, volatile liquid with characteristic odor and burning taste, consisting of ethyl alcohol (ethanol) and containing no more than 0.005–0.01 percent by volume of water. Also called *anhydrous alcohol* and *dehydrated alcohol.*

absolute eosinophil count a quantitative measure of eosinophils in the peripheral blood. This test was used widely at one time to gauge the eosinopenic response to adrenocorticotropic hormone, but has largely been replaced by direct measurements of cortisol in the blood. It is still used, however, to determine the degree of eosinophilia, particularly in allergies. For this purpose, either an automated flow-through differential counter or a direct eosinophil count is performed. The flow-through differential counter counts 10,000 white blood cells (WBC) and hence gives a more accurate total count than can be obtained from computing the total eosinophils from a 100-cell differential and total WBC. To obtain an absolute eosinophil count using the direct count, all eosinophils in 1 mm^3 are counted, usually in a special hemocytometer chamber using a staining solution such as Randolph's stain, which both enhances staining of eosinophils using phloxine and lyses the red cells. An eosinophil count derived from a differential count is unimportant unless the percentage of eosinophils is quite high. See also *differential leukocyte count automation.*

absolute temperature (T) temperature measured on a scale having a zero point at absolute zero. See also *temperature.* Cf. *customary temperature.*

absolute temperature scale a temperature scale having a zero point at absolute zero, either the Kelvin temperature scale or the Rankine temperature scale.

absolute value the numerical magnitude of a number, denoted $|x|$. For $x \geq 0$, $|x| = x$; for $x \leq 0$, $|x| = -x$. For example, $|10| = 10$ and $|-10| = 10$.

absolute zero the temperature (0°K, −273.15°C, or −459.69°F) at which physical systems are in their lowest possible energy states (ground states). An object at absolute zero has no heat energy to be extracted; thus, its temperature cannot be lowered.

absorb (ab-sorb′) [L. *absorbere* to swallow or suck] to take up material or radiation by the process of absorption.

absorbance (A) (ab-sor′bans) 1. the term used to express the extent of light absorption when radiant energy is passed through a solution; usually applied in ultraviolet and visible spectrophotometry. $A = \log_{10}(I_0/I)$, where I_0 is the intensity of light transmitted through the pure solvent and I is the intensity of light transmitted through the solution, when both are contained in identical absorption cells. Formerly called *absorbency, extinction,* and *optical density.*

2. in radiology, a rarely used term that denotes a measure of the ability of a medium to absorb radiation, expressed as the logarithm of the quotient of the intensity of radiation entering the medium divided by the energy leaving it. It is the negative logarithm of transmittance.

absorbefacient (ab-sor″bĕ-fa′shent) [L. *absorbere* + *faciens,* from *facere* to make] 1. causing absorption.

2. an agent that promotes absorption.

absorbency (ab-sor′ben-se) see *absorbance.*

absorbency index the former term for absorptivity.

absorbent (ab-sor′bent) [L. *absorbens,* from *absorbere* to swallow] a material, usually with some degree of porous structure, that is able to: (1) take in and incorporate by chemical or molecular means or to remove or suck up by spongelike action; (2) absorb a liquid or gas from the medium in which it exists; or (3) absorb electromagnetic radiation of specific wavelengths.

absorber (ab-sor′ber) any matter used to absorb radiation for a particular purpose. An absorber may be used as a safety device to guard against unnecessary exposure to radiation, to determine the characteristics of a particular type of radiation, or to remove a specific component from a source of complex radiation. The penetrability of radiation may also be expressed in terms of the thickness of a specific absorber (e.g., aluminum) required to reduce the intensity by a specified percentage (e.g., half-value layer).

absorption (ab-sorp′shun) [L. *absorptio*] 1. in chemistry, a process in which a substance is taken up in bulk by a material (absorbent) and held in pores or interstices in the interior, as opposed to adsorption, a process in which a substance is bound at the surface of a material (adsorbent). Cf. *adsorption.*

2. in physics, a process in which the energy of a particle of radiation is completely dissipated within a material. The particle is not transmitted, reflected, or scattered. See also *interaction of radiation with matter.*

3. in photometry, the physical uptake of infrared, visible, or ultraviolet light by a chemical compound. The energy of each absorbed photon is transferred to the atom or molecule, thus placing it in an excited state. Absorption of infrared photons produces transitions between different rotational or vibrational states in the molecule. Visible or ultraviolet absorption produces electronic transitions in atoms. The wavelengths of light absorbed are characteristic of a particular compound. See also *absorbance* and *absorptivity.*

4. in immunology and serology, the use of reagents to remove or neutralize antibodies in sera or other fluids. The appropriate antigen reagent is added in the form of washed erythrocytes, enzyme-treated erythrocytes, formalinized erythrocytes, cell stromata, or soluble antigens, after which the resulting antigen-antibody complexes are removed. Absorption is used to remove antibodies from antisera when making specific reagent antisera, to confirm the specificity of an antibody, or to isolate a single antibody from a fluid.

5. in physiology, the passage of chemical substances into or across tissues, such as the passage of nutrients from the intestine through the intestinal mucosa into the portal circulation or lymphatic system; the passage of substances from the lumen of the renal tubule into the peritubular capillaries (tubular reabsorption); or the passage of materials through the skin.

Intestinal absorption is the process by which foods are absorbed into the blood stream. In the lumen of the stomach and intestines, digestive enzymes break down complex food substances into small molecules that can be absorbed. Carbohydrates are broken down into monosaccharides. Glucose and galactose are absorbed by carrier-mediated transport coupled with the diffusion of sodium ions along the concentration gradient; the latter is produced by a different active transport mechanism that pumps sodium ions from the mucosal cells into the intestinal lumen. Fructose is absorbed by facilitated diffusion, and other hexoses and pentoses are absorbed by passive diffusion. Proteins are broken down to amino acids, which are absorbed by three active transport mechanisms for L-amino acids: one for neutral amino acids, one for basic amino acids, and one for the imino acids proline and hydroxyproline. Nucleic acids are broken down to purine and pyrimidine bases (which are absorbed by active transport) and pentoses. Fats are broken down to monoacylglycerols, glycerol, cholesterol, and free fatty acids, all of which enter the mucosal cells by passive diffusion. Free fatty acids with less than 10–12 carbon atoms pass directly into the portal circulation. Other free fatty acids, monoacylglycerols, and most of the cholesterol are reesterified in the mucosal cells, forming triacylglycerols and cholesterol esters, which are then formed into chylomicrons and passed into the lymphatic circulation. Some electrolytes, minerals, and vitamins, such as chloride, iron, and vitamin B_{12}, are also absorbed by special active transport mechanisms.

absorption cavities spaces appearing in compact bone as a result of osteoclastic erosion.

absorption cell see *cuvet.*

absorption coefficient an obsolete term for *absorptivity.*

absorption constant an obsolete term for *absorptivity.*

absorption of erythrocyte antibodies a technique for the removal or neutralization of red cell antibodies from plasma or serum. By reacting the antibody with appropriate antigenic material (washed erythrocytes, enzyme-treated erythrocytes, formalinized erythrocytes, stromata, or soluble antigen), the antibody becomes attached, and is thus removed from the serum. The time, temperature, and number of absorptions required for antibody removal depend on the nature of the antibody being removed.

This technique is used to confirm antibody specificity, to remove cold- or warm-reacting autoagglutinins, to remove unwanted antibodies, to remove a single antibody from a serum with multiple antibodies, and to sensitize cells for elution studies.

absorption peak the wavelength of maximal electromagnetic absorption by a chemical substance; used to identify specific elements, radicals, or compounds.

absorption spectrum the spectrum resulting from electromagnetic energy at various wavelengths that has passed through an absorbing medium. The intensity at certain characteristic wavelengths (absorption lines) is reduced by absorption due to a specific atom, molecule, or ion.

absorptive (ab-sorp′tiv) capable of or pertaining to absorption.

absorptive cell a tall, columnar cell situated on the luminal surface of the villi in the small intestine. These cells have basally located oval nuclei. A striated border of microvilli serves to increase the surface area for absorption.

absorptive state the metabolic state of the body for a period of several hours after a meal, during which time glucose, amino acids, and fatty acids are being absorbed in the small intestine; the blood levels of glucose, insulin, lipids, and many nutrients are elevated; and glycogen and fat are being synthesized. Cf. *postabsorptive state.*

absorptivity (*a*) (ab″sorp-tiv′ĭ-te) a measure of the light energy absorbed by a solution, expressed in terms of absorbance per unit concentration and per unit light path length; $a = A/bc$, where A is absorbance, b is path length in centimeters, and c is the concentration. A variety of concentration units have been used. When c is expressed in grams per liter, a is called specific absorptivity. When c is expressed in moles per liter, a is replaced by ϵ, the molar absorptivity; and when c is grams per 100 ml, a is $E^{1\%}_{1cm}$, called absorbency index, which is now an obsolete term. Other terms such as absorption constant, absorption coefficient, and extinction coefficient are also obsolete. By Beer's law, absorptivity is independent of concentration and light path in the ideal situation, but varies with light wavelength used, with temperature, and with the chemical properties of the solution, such as pH and solute/solvent interaction. The measured absorptivity depends on the spectrophotometer used, especially in regard to half-band width and stray light in the instrument.

molar a. (ϵ), the absorbance value of a solution with a concentration of 1 mol/l, when measured in a cuvet with a 1-cm light path.

specific a. (*a*), the absorbance value of a solution with a concentration of 1 g/l when measured in a cuvet with a 1-cm light path.

abstinence (ab′stĭ-nens) [L. *abstinentia,* from *abstinere* to abstain] denial of the appetites; a refraining from use of or indulgence in food, alcohol, or coitus.

ABTS trademark for a colorless compound that is an oxygen acceptor used in some enzymatic glucose determinations. It is the diammonium salt of 2,2′-azino-di-(3-ethyl-benzthiazoline)-6-sulfonic acid.

ABVD abbrev. for Adriamycin, bleomycin, vinblastine, and dacarbazine, a major established cancer chemotherapy drug regimen. For more information, see the specific drug (listed under its generic name) and *Appendix A.*

Ac 1. symbol for the chemical element *actinium.* 2. abbrev. See *acetyl.*

ac abbrev. for *ante cibum* (before meals).

-ac (ak) a suffix word element used in combining form to denote pertaining to, e.g., cardiac.

ACA (eponym from Automatic Clinical Analyzer) trademark for a discrete clinical chemistry analyzer with prepackaged reagents; see under *clinical chemistry automation.*

acacia (ah-ka′she-ah) [L., Gr. *akakia*] [USP], the dried, water-soluble, gummy exudate from the tree *Acacia senegal.* A white or yellowish white powder or flakes, it is used as a suspending agent for pharmaceutical preparations and as an emulsifier. Also called *gum arabic.*

AcAcOH abbrev. for acetoacetic acid. See under *ketone bodies.*

Academy of Clinical Laboratory Physicians and Scientists (ACLPS) a professional organization of clinical laboratory scientists and teachers.

acanth/o (ah-kan′tho) [Gr. *akantha* a thorn or prickle] a word element used in combining form to denote thorny or spiny, e.g., acanthocyte.

acanthamebiasis (ah-kan″thah-me-bi′ah-sis) infection by amebas of the genus *Acanthamoeba.*

Acanthamoeba (ah-kan″thah-me′bah) [*acanth-* + *amoeba*] a genus of free-living amebas of the order Amoebida, which generally inhabit fresh water or moist soil. They have been found as human parasites; certain strains, such as *A. castellani,* are highly pathogenic and may cause a fatal meningoencephalitis. Infection is often acquired by swimming in freshwater lakes that harbor the species.

acanthella (ak″an-thel′ah) [N.L., dim. of Gr. *acantha* thorn] the simple, second-stage larva of the immature Acanthocephala, or thorny-headed worms.

acanthiomeatal line (ah-kan″the-o-me-a′tal) [Gr. *akanthion* little spine + L. *meatus* path] a line passing through the acanthion and the auricular point, i.e., between the bottom of the nose and the center of the opening of the ear (the external auditory meatus); used in radiographic positioning.

acanthion (ah-kan′the-on) [Gr. *akanthion* little spine] a point in the midsagittal plane at the base of the nose, the anterior nasal spine; used as an anatomic landmark.

Acanthobdella (ah-kan″tho-del′ah) [*acantho-* + Gr. *baella* leech] a genus of leeches, of the order Acanthobdellidea, class Hirudinea. These are the only leeches that have spines on the body surface.

Acanthocephala (ah-kan″tho-sef′ah-lah) [*acantho-* + Gr. *kephalē* head] a phylum of exclusively parasitic animals, the thorny- or spiny-headed worms. These worms have an anterior proboscis covered with thornlike retractable spines, used for attachment to the digestive tract of the host.

acanthocyte (ah-kan′tho-sit) [*acantho-* + Gr. *kytos* hollow vessel] an erythrocyte characterized by irregularly spiculated projections that vary in length and position, associated with abetalipoproteinemia, alcoholic liver disease, and postsplenectomy state, and occasionally with other conditions. Also called *acanthoid cell* and *spur cell.* See also *astrocyte.* Cf. *echinocyte.*

acanthocytosis (ah-kan″tho-si-to″sis) [*acantho-* + Gr. *kytos* hollow vessel + *-osis* condition] the presence of distorted red blood cells (acanthocytes) in a peripheral blood smear, found primarily in individuals with abetalipoproteinemia and occasionally in those with anemia secondary to cirrhosis. See also *abetalipoproteinemia.*

acanthoid cell (ah-kan′thoid) [*acantho-* + Gr. *eidos* form] see *acanthocyte.*

acantholysis (ak″an-thol′ĭ-sis) [*acantho-* + Gr. *lysis* a loosening] the loss of intercellular connections in the epidermis that is associated with formation of epidermal vesicles in pemphigus vulgaris, pemphigus foliaceus, and other skin disorders.

acanthor (ah-kan′thor) the first larval stage in the life cycle of the Acanthocephala, or thorny-headed worms.

acanthosis (ak″an-tho′sis) [*acantho-* + *-osis* condition] a hyperplastic thickening of the stratum spinosum layer of the skin.

a. nigricans, a hyperkeratotic lesion of the skin that is velvety, darkened, and wartlike. It is usually found in the axillae, groin, or neck. In adults these lesions are often an indicator of an internal malignancy, commonly an adenocarcinoma. Their course usually parallels growth or remission of the carcinoma. Similar lesions may also be congenital or develop in childhood or at puberty, in which case they do not indicate malignancy.

acapnia (a-kap′ne-ah) [*a-* neg. + Gr. *kapnos* smoke + *-ia*] a term that in the strictest sense denotes a lack of carbon dioxide in the blood; conventional usage, however, is as a synonym for hypocapnia (hypocarbia). See also *hypocapnia.*

acariasis (ak″ah-ri′ah-sis) [Gr. *akari* mite + *-iasis*] infestation with mites. See also *scabies.*

Acarus (ak′ah-rus) [L.; Gr. *akari* mite] a genus of small mites that cause itch, mange, and other skin diseases.

acaryote (a-kār′e-ōt) [*a-* neg. + Gr. *karyon* kernel] a nonnucleated cell.

acatalasia (a″kat-ah-la′ze-ah) [*a-* neg. + *catalase* + *-ia*] an inborn error of metabolism that results in the congenital absence of catalase. Acatalasia appears to arise from several different allelic mutations. Affected individuals fail to produce detectable bubbles of oxygen when hydrogen peroxide is applied to mucous membranes. The defect may be associated with recurrent infections of the oral cavity. It was originally associated with Orientals but has now been described in Caucasians. Also called acatalasemia.

accelerant (ak-sel′er-ant) [L. *accelerans* hastening] see *catalyst.*

accelerated idioventricular rhythm (AIVR) three or more consecutive QRS complexes of ventricular origin; the definition is usually limited to those with a rate of 50–100 beats/min. It occurs in 12–25 percent of patients after acute myocardial infarction, usually 2–3 da after the attack.

accelerator (ak-sel′er-a″tor) [L. *accelerare* hasten] 1. an agent or apparatus that is used to increase the rate at which an object proceeds or a substance acts, or at which some reaction occurs. It often refers specifically to a device that speeds up charged subatomic particles to extremely high rates. Such a procedure produces x-rays or nuclear reactions and may be used for irradiation, research, or the production of radionuclides. Betatrons, cyclotrons, and high-energy linear accelerators are examples of such devices. See also *cyclotron* and *linear accelerator.*

2. any nerve or muscle that hastens the performance of a function.

3. any of a group of chemicals used in the vulcanization of rubber; they frequently cause dermatitis in workers.

4. in histology, a chemical that speeds the polymerization of an epoxy resin embedding medium used in electron microscopy.

5. see *accentuator.*

accelerator globulin (AcG) see *Factor V.*

accelerin (ak-sel′er-in) the former coagulation Factor VI, once thought to be an activated form of Factor V but no longer considered as one of the coagulation factors.

accentuator (ak-sen′chu-a″tor) [L. *accentus* accent] any of a number of chemicals used to heighten the intensity, selectivity, or crispness of a stain, e.g., phenol, aniline, barbital, and chloral hydrate. Also called *accelerator.*

acceptor (ak-sep′tor) [L., from *accipere* to receive] 1. a substance that can accept electrons, protons, or molecules (simple or complex), forming new or modified chemical entities.

2. a substance that unites specifically with either hydrogen or oxygen in an oxidoreduction reaction and so allows the reaction to proceed toward completion.

access (ak′ses) [L. *accessus,* from *accedere* to arrive] 1. a means or path of approach.

2. in electronic data processing, memory access; the movement of data between the central processing unit (CPU) and a storage device.

accessory cells lymphoid cells, usually macrophages, that supplement the action of T and B lymphocytes and participate in the formation of antibodies and other aspects of the immune reaction, especially cell-mediated immunity.

accessory nerve cranial nerve XI; a motor nerve with two portions: a cranial root arising in the medulla, and a spinal root mainly arising in the cervical spinal cord. The spinal root ascends through the foramen magnum and meets the cranial root at the foramen lacerum; both leave the cranial cavity through the foramen, but the cranial root is distributed with the vagus nerve. In the neck, the spinal root is generally referred to as the accessory nerve; it innervates the sternomastoid and trapezius muscles. See also *cranial nerves.*

accessory spleen a common condition in which a person has extra splenic tissue, usually smaller than but functionally identical to the regular spleen. It becomes clinically relevant in the treatment of diseases such as hereditary spherocytosis or thrombocytopenic purpura in which complete removal of the spleen is the standard treatment.

access time in computer terms, the amount of time needed for a particular memory location to be reached and the data to appear after being requested.

AcCHS abbrev. See *acetylcholinesterase.*

accident (ak′sĭ-dent) an unplanned and sometimes injurious or damaging event that interrupts the normal progress of an activity. Causes may include human, energy, and environmental factors, and they may be simultaneous or time-sequenced events and contribute directly or indirectly to the accident.

accidental coincidence in coincidence detection of positron emissions, as in a positron camera or PET scanner, a count that is produced by the detection of two photons from unrelated events within the resolving time interval of the system and not by the simultaneous detection of the two 511-keV photons produced by the annihilation of a positron. Such counts contribute to the background noise.

acclimation (ak″lĭ-ma′shun) the adaptive changes that allow an organism to compensate functionally for a single environmental stressor (such as one produced in a controlled laboratory setting). The compensatory mechanisms begin to act within a period of several days to weeks following exposure to the stressor. Cf. *acclimatization.*

acclimatization (ah-kli″mah-tĭ-za′shun) the adaptive biochemical and physiologic processes and the behavioral, morphologic, and anatomic changes in an organism that result in an increased tolerance to repeated or continued exposure to complex environmental stressors such as seasonal changes. These compensatory mechanisms begin to act within several days to several weeks after initial exposure to the stressors. Cf. *acclimation.*

accommodation (ah-kom″o-da′shun) [L. *accommodare* to fit to] 1. the process by which the refractory power of the lens of the eye is altered during the viewing of objects at various distances. The refractory power of the lens changes as the shape of the lens alters with contraction or relaxation of the ciliary muscles. These changes, which are reflexly evoked in response to a blurred image on the retina, are mediated by parasympathetic fibers of the third cranial nerve. When evoked, the reflex occurs equally and simultaneously in both eyes. As focus is directed for near vision, accommodation is accompanied by convergence of the eyes and constriction of the pupils.

2. in neurophysiology, the phenomenon by which the rate of change of the membrane potential during stimulation alters the threshold voltage at which excitation eventually occurs. For example,

the more slowly a stimulus depolarizes the membrane, the greater the depolarization needed to initiate an action potential. This phenomenon is generally attributed to the outward potassium current overcompensating for the inward sodium current induced by subthreshold depolarization of the membrane. The net current flowing across the membrane is outward for sustained depolarizations; This tends to counteract the effect of an induced depolarization and raises the threshold for action potential development.

accumulator (ah-kūm′u-la″ter) the register in a computer that holds data being manipulated by arithmetic and logical operations. Large computers usually have several general-purpose registers that perform the functions of both the accumulator and the index registers.

accuracy (ak′ur-ah-se) [L. *accuratus,* from *accurare* to take care of] the closeness with which results agree with a known true value of the quantity being measured, or a value that is accepted as true. In the laboratory, true values are unknown and reference standards are used for comparison.

ACD abbrev. See *acid-citrate-dextrose.*

AC-DC, ac/dc capable of using either alternating or direct current as a power source.

A cell see *alpha cell.*

acellular (a-sel′u-lar) [*a-* neg. + *cellular*] not cellular in structure; without cells.

acentric (a-sen′trik) [Gr. *akentrikos* not centric, from *a-*negative + *kentron* center] a term referring to a chromosome or chromatid that has no centromere. Cf. *dicentric* and *monocentric.*

acephalous (a-sef′ah-lus) headless.

acephalus (a-sef′ah-lus), pl. *acephali* [*a-* neg. + Gr. *kephalē* head] a headless fetus.

acervulus (ah-ser′vu-lus), pl. *acervuli* [L., dim. of *acervus* a heap] 1. calcareous matter found in or near the pineal body, choroid plexus, and other parts of the brain. Also called *brain sand.*

2. an asexual fungal body composed of a stroma of vegetative hyphae and closely packed condiophores embedded within the tissue of an infected plant.

acetabul/o (as″ĕ-tab′u-lo) [L. *acetabulum* vinegar-cruet] a word element used in combining form to denote the hip socket, e.g., acetabulectomy.

acetabulum (as″ĕ-tab′u-lum) [L. "vinegar cruet," from *acetum* vinegar] the hip socket, the cup-shaped depression on the lateral side of the hip bone in which the head of the femur articulates.

acetal (as′ĕ-tal) 1. one of a class of compounds having the general formula $RCH(OR')_2$, usually formed by the reaction of an aldehyde with two molecules of an alcohol or with one molecule of a dihydric alcohol with the removal of one molecule of water. The reaction is reversible.

2. a colorless liquid, $CH_3CH(OC_2H_5)_2$, formed by the reaction of acetaldehyde with ethyl alcohol. Also called 1,1-diethoxyethane.

acetaldehydase (as″et-al-dĕ-hi′dās) an enzyme that reversibly catalyzes the conversion of acetic aldehyde to acetic acid. See also *aldehyde dehydrogenase* and *aldehyde oxidase.*

acetaldehyde (as″et-al′dĕ-hīd″) ethanal, a colorless, volatile, flammable liquid with a pungent odor, CH_3CHO, synthesized by the controlled oxidation of ethanol. In alcoholic fermentation, pyruvate is decarboxylated to acetaldehyde, which is reduced to alcohol. It is used as a chemical reagent and in the manufacture of acetic acid, perfumes, and flavors. Vapor or liquid may cause irritation of mucous membranes, lacrimation, photophobia, anosmia, conjunctivitis, corneal injury, rhinitis, headache, bronchitis, pneumonia, and unconsciousness.

In vivo acetaldehyde is produced from alcohol by the action of several enzymes in the liver, including alcohol dehydrogenase. The blood concentration of acetaldehyde remains low even in chronic alcoholics, although many of the symptoms of alcohol aversion therapy with disulfiram have been attributed to the accumulation of acetaldehyde.

Also called acetic aldehyde and ethyl aldehyde.

acetamide (ah-set′ah-mīd) a white crystalline substance, CH_3CONH_2, used in organic synthesis and as a general solvent when melted.

acetaminophen (as″et-ah-min′o-fen) [USP], an analgesic and antipyretic drug, *N*-acetyl-*p*-aminophenol, a metabolite of phenacetin, used in many over-the-counter pain relievers. It acts by inhibiting prostaglandin synthesis. Acetaminophen is largely excreted in the urine after conjugation to glucuronic or sulfuric acid; hydrolysis yields *p*-aminophenol. Some of the drug is hydroxylated and conjugated with glutathione, and excreted. When this pathway is overloaded, causing glutathione depletion, the hydroxylated metabolite may produce hepatic necrosis, although the latter may not appear until 2–6 da after ingestion. Phenobarbital and diphenhydramine increase the rate of this hydroxylation.

A dose of 10 g may be fatal. A serum concentration of 120–300 μg/ml 4 hr after ingestion is associated with a 50 percent chance of hepatic necrosis. In view of the serum half-life of 12 hr or more, hepatic coma is likely to develop if treatment is not initiated.

Trademarks, *Datril* and *Tylenol.*

acetaminophen assays 1. spot test for urine. The specimen is acidified and boiled; acetaminophen is hydrolyzed to *p*-aminophenol, which is coupled with *o*-cresol to produce indophenol blue. This test is an extremely sensitive indicator of acetaminophen or phenacetin.

2. gas chromatography. Acetaminophen and the internal standard *N*-butyryl-*p*-aminophenol are extracted from samples into ether, and the extract is evaporated to dryness. Both compounds are acetylated by heating the residue in acetic anhydride and pyridine and then chromatographed, using a cyclohexane dimethanol succinate column packing and a flame ionization detector. The sample concentration is proportional to the acetaminophen–internal standard peak height ratio. The sensitivity is 5 ng/ml.

3. liquid chromatography. An internal standard dissolved in acetonitrile is added directly to serum, causing protein precipitation. After centrifugation, a portion of the supernatant is injected onto a reverse-phase column, and detection accomplished at 254 nm. The sensitivity is 25 ng/ml.

acetanilid (as″ĕ-tan′ĭ-lid) [*acetic* + *aniline*] an analgesic antipyretic drug, *N*-phenylacetamide. It has now been replaced by two other aniline derivatives, acetaminophen and phenacetin, which are less likely to produce methemoglobinemia.

acetate (as′ĕ-tāt) the anion, salt, or ester form of acetic acid.

acetazolamide (ah-set″ah-zol′ah-mīd) [USP], a diuretic drug, $C_4H_6N_4O_3S_2$, and prototype of a class of sulfonamide drugs that inhibit the enzyme carbonic anhydrase in a noncompetitive manner. When given orally, it is rapidly absorbed from the gastrointestinal tract and is bound to plasma proteins. The drug inhibits H^+ formation in the renal tubule while increasing HCO_3^- secretion; this is probably why Na^+, as well as some K^+, secretion increases, while chloride secretion decreases. As a consequence of the above factors, the urine volume increases and becomes alkaline. As the plasma pH drops, metabolic acidosis occurs. Other effects include transient respiratory acidosis and depression of cerebrospinal fluid formation, both via the inhibition of local carbonic anhydrase.

As a carbonic anhydrase inhibitor acetazolamide reduces the formation of aqueous humor in the eye, causing a drop in intraocular pressure, which is a desired therapeutic effect in the treatment of glaucoma.

High doses (more than 1000 mg) in humans may cause drowsiness and paresthesia.

See also *diuretics* and *thiazide diuretics.* Trademark, *Diamox.*

Acetest (ah′sĕ-test) trademark. See under *ketone bodies tests.*

acetic acid (ah-se′tik) a colorless crystalline or liquid substance, CH_3COOH; a component of vinegar, used in the preparation of astringents. It is also used to decalcify hard tissue (bone) prior to staining. It is soluble in alcohol, ether, and water and has a pungent odor. Pure acetic acid is also called glacial acetic acid because its melting point (16.7°C) is close to room temperature, and it may solidify in a cold room. When sugar is fermented in air, acetic acid is produced by the oxidation of acetaldehyde; in the absence of air, fermentation yields ethanol, produced by the reduction of acetaldehyde. Also called *ethanoic acid* and *vinegar acid.*

acetic acid–alcohol-formalin a solution of acetic acid, alcohol, and formaldehyde used as a fixative for glycogen and cytoplasm. Also called Tellyesniczky's fixative.

acetic aldehyde see *acetaldehyde.*

acetic anhydride (ah-se′tik an-hi′drīd) a liquid, $(CH_3CO)_2O$, which forms acetic acid when added to hot water. It is a colorless, refractive, irritating, and corrosive liquid with a strong odor. It is used as an acetylating agent and also as a dehydrating reagent in organic synthesis.

acetic orcein (ah-se′tik or′se-in) orcein dissolved in acetic acid, used in making squash preparations of polytene chromosomes. It both fixes and stains chromosomes in smeared, suspended, or crushed cell forms. Specimens are immersed in the solution, placed in an alcohol vapor chamber until the coverslip is easily removed (impression smears may be immersed), counterstained, cleared, and mounted.

acetoacetic acid (AcAcOH) (as″e-to-ah-se′tik) 3-oxobutanoic acid, CH_3COCH_2COOH, one of the ketone bodies that occur in trace amounts in normal urine, and in elevated amounts in the urine of individuals with diabetes mellitus (especially in ketoacidosis) or starvation due to incomplete fatty acid oxidation. Also called acetylacetic acid, *diacetic acid,* and β-ketobutyric acid. See also *ketone bodies.*

acetoacetyl (ah-se″to-as′ĕ-til) the acyl radical of acetoacetic acid.

acetoacetyl-CoA the coenzyme A thioester of acetoacetic acid; an important compound of intermediary metabolism. It has a number of functions, e.g., in fatty acid synthesis in microorganisms, in fatty acid oxidation in the liver, in biogenesis of steroids and cholesterol, in ketone body formation in the liver, in ketone body catabolism in muscle and other appropriate tissues, and in the catabolism of some amino acids.

acetoacetyl-CoA reductase an enzyme of the oxidoreductase class (D-3-hydroxyacyl-CoA:$NADP^+$ oxidoreductase, EC 1.1.1.36) that catalyzes the reaction D-3-hydroxyacyl CoA + $NADP^+$ $\rightleftarrows$ 3-oxoacyl-CoA + NADPH. It is a part of the fatty acid synthetase complex.

Acetobacter (ah-se″to-bak′ter) [L. *acetum* vinegar + Gr. *baktērion* little rod] a genus of nonpathogenic gram-negative bacilli belonging to the group of acetic acid bacteria. These organisms are found on fruits and vegetables, and especially in souring juices and alcoholic beverages.

aceto-carmine a stain composed of carmine and acetic acid, formerly used in staining squash preparations of chromosomes; acetic orcein is now preferred.

acetohexamide (as″ĕ-to-heks′ah-mīd) [USP], one of the sulfonylureas, used as an oral hypoglycemic agent in the control of mild, maturity-onset diabetes mellitus. See also *sulfonylurea.* Trademark, Dymelor.

acetoin (ah-set′o-in) see *acetylmethylcarbinol.*

acetoin test see *Voges-Proskauer test.*

acetolysis (as″ĕ-tol′ĭ-sis) [L. *acetum* vinegar + Gr. *lysis* a loosing] a solvolysis reaction in which acetic acid as solvent reacts with a solute molecule, resulting in cleavage and acetylation of the solute molecule, for example $CH_3COOH + CH_3(CH_2)_3Br \rightarrow CH_3COO(CH_2)_3CH_3 + HBr$. See also *solvolysis.*

acetone (as′e-tōn) [acronym from *acet*ic + ke*tone*] 2-propanone, dimethylketone, $CH_3—CO—CH_3$; a colorless, highly flammable liquid with a characteristic taste and odor that is miscible with water. Acetone is an excellent laboratory and industrial solvent; however, because it can attack a variety of plastic materials used about the laboratory and home (such as eyeglass frames and nylon hosiery), it should be used with care. Serious poisoning is rare, but prolonged topical use causes erythema; extended inhalation can give rise to bronchial irritation and narcosis. In histology, it is used as a fixative, particularly in enzyme studies.

Acetone is one of the three "ketone bodies" formed by the nonenzymatic decarboxylation of acetoacetate. It is normally present in small amounts in urine but is found in greatly increased amounts in the urine of uncontrolled diabetics.

See also *ketone bodies.*

acetone bodies see *ketone bodies.*

acetonitrile (as″ĕ-to-ni′tril) a colorless, flammable liquid with an ethereal odor, ethanenitrile, CH_3CN, an important polar solvent; M.W. 41.05. It is metabolized to formate and thiocyanate and is toxic when ingested or inhaled.

acetophenazine maleate (as″ĕ-to-fen′ah-zēn) [USP], a piperazine-type phenothiazine major tranquilizer used in the management of psychotic disorders. See also *phenothiazine tranquilizers.* Trademark, *Tindal.*

acetrizoate (as'ĕ-tri-zo'āt) a radiopaque contrast medium used as acetrizoate sodium in cystography and hysterosalpingography. It is a water-soluble triiodobenzene derivative. Trademark, *Cystokon.*

acetyl- (AC) (as'ĕ-til, ah-sēt'il) [L. *acetum* vinegar + Gr. *hylē* matter] a prefix word element in organic chemistry to denote the acetyl group (CH_3CO—), e.g., acetylcholine.

***N*-acetylaspartic acid** (as"e-til-ah-spahr'tik) a derivative of L-aspartic acid that, along with the free acid and L-glutamine and γ-aminobutyrate, is present in large quantities in brain tissues.

acetylation (ah-sēt"ĭ-la'shun) the introduction of an acetyl group into a molecule.

acetylcholine (ACh) (as"ĕ-til-ko'lēn, ah-se"til-ko'lēn) acetylethanoltrimethylammonium hydroxide, the acetic acid ester of choline, which exists in solution as 2-(acetyloxy)-*N,N,N*-trimethylethaniminium cation, $CH_3COOCH_2CH_2N(CH_3)_3^+$; M.W. 146.23. Acetylcholine is normally present in many parts of the body and has important physiologic functions. It is one of several different mediators of chemical transmission of synaptic activity in the central nervous system. It is the mediator at all synapses between pre- and postganglionic autonomic fibers, at all postganglionic parasympathetic and some postganglionic sympathetic terminals, and at the neuromuscular junctions, where it is released by nerve impulses. Acetylcholine is inactivated by hydrolysis by acetylcholine esterase to choline and acetate. Compounds resistant to hydrolysis by choline esterase have been prepared and are used in medicine as parasympathomimetic agents.

The actions of acetylcholine are divided into muscarinic and nicotinic effects. The stimulatory effect of acetylcholine on smooth muscle and glands is referred to as muscarinic, as it is mimicked by muscarine; this effect is blocked by atropine. The effect of acetylcholine on autonomic ganglia is mimicked by nicotine and is thus referred to as nicotinic; it is not blocked by atropine. Atropine thus has important clinical uses based on its effects on secretions, smooth muscle, or the central nervous system.

See also *atropine.*

acetylcholinesterase (AcCHS, AChE) (as"e-til-ko"lin-es'ter-ās) one of the two species of enzymes of the hydrolase class (acetylcholine acetylhydrolase, EC 3.1.1.7) that hydrolyze the acetylcholinium cation (from acetylcholine chloride or bromide) to acetate + choline. The enzyme is found principally in nerve tissue (gray matter), erythrocytes, and skeletal muscle (motor end-plates). It is differentiated from the serum/plasma (liver) enzyme, acetylcholine acylhydrolase, EC 3.1.1.8 (see *cholinesterase*).

Substrate specificity is directed to the acetyl acyl, but some variety is allowed to the alkyl group: acetyl-β-methylcholine and 3,3'-dimethyl acetate serve as substrates. The enzyme is inhibited by many compounds, including physostigmine (eserine), prostigmine, its substrate acetylcholine, morphine, citrate, and fluoride, and by a number of organophosphate compounds such as tetraethyl pyrophosphate (TEPP) and di-isopropylphosphofluoridate (DFP). The enzyme functions to inactivate (hydrolyze) acetylcholine formed at neurohumoral junctions, causing depolarization of the muscle fiber, preventing unproductive firing of the neuron, and permitting further impulses to be transmitted.

There is little interest in the enzyme in clinical diagnosis, unlike the plasma (serum) enzyme (cholinesterase).

Also called *cholinesterase,* "true" or red cell cholinesterase, and Type I cholinesterase.

acetylcholinesterase assays see *cholinesterase* assays.

acetyl-CoA the active form of coenzyme A, composed of the acetyl group joined through a thiol ester linkage to coenzyme A. It is an important reactant in the citrate synthase reaction, the initial step in the tricarboxylic acid (Krebs) cycle. See also *tricarboxylic acid cycle.*

acetyl-CoA acyltransferase an enzyme of the transferase class (acyl-CoA:acetyl-CoA *C*-acyltransferase, EC 2.3.1.16) that catalyzes the reaction acyl-CoA + acetyl-CoA $\rightleftarrows$ CoA + 3-oxoacyl-CoA. The equilibrium constant favors the reverse reaction, which is important in the fatty acid oxidation pathway, leading to the cleavage of acetyl-SCoA from the acid and the formation of a CoA derivative of a fatty acid two carbons shorter. In the metabolism of leucine, the enzyme cleaves α-methylacetoacetyl-SCoA to acetyl-CoA and propionyl CoA. A genetic defect in the enzyme, transmitted as an autosomal recessive trait, causes β-ketothiolase deficiency, which leads to severe metabolic acidosis. Also called *β-ketothiolase.*

acetylene (ah-set'ĭ-lēn) 1. a colorless gas with an ethereal odor, ethyne, HC≡CH; M.W. 26.02. It burns with a hot, brilliant white flame, and is used as a fuel. An oxygen-acetylene flame, as used in some flame photometers and in oxyacetylene welding torches, produces a temperature of about 3000°C. Mixtures of 2.5–80 percent acetylene in air are explosive.

2. see *alkyne.*

acetylene dichloride 1,2-dichloroethene, a colorless, volatile liquid with an ethereal odor, *sym*-dichlorethylene, CHCl=CHCl; M.W. 96.95. Both the *cis-* and *trans-*isomers are used as industrial solvents. It is moderately toxic by ingestion, inhalation, or skin absorption; produces irritation and narcosis at high concentrations; and is highly flammable.

acetylene trichloride see *trichloroethylene.*

***N*-acetylgalactosamine** (as'e-til-gah-lak-tos'ah-mēn) a derivative of 2-deoxy-2-amino-D-galactose in which the acetyl group replaces one H on the amino group. It is a constituent of glycoproteins, proteoglycans, and glycosaminoglycans. See also *galactosamine.*

β-*N*-acetyl-D-galactosaminidase (as"e-til-gah-lak"tos-ah-min'ĭ-dās) the recommended name for the enzyme hexosaminidase; at present, however, it is not widely used. See also *hexosaminidase.*

***N*-acetylglucosamine** (as'ĕ-til-gloo-kos'ah-mēn) the *N*-acetyl derivative of glucosamine, a constituent of glycoproteins and proteoglycans, the structural unit of chitin. See also *glucose.*

***N*-acetylmannosamine** (as'ĕ-til-mah-nos'ah-mēn) the *N*-acetyl derivative of mannosamine, a constituent of glycoproteins. See also *mannosamine.*

acetylmethylcarbinol (as"ĕ-til-meth"il-kar'bĭ-nol) a keto-isomer of aldol, $CH_3 \cdot CHOH \cdot CO \cdot CH_3$, formed from glucose by certain bacteria and detected in broth culture by the Voges-Proskauer reaction. Also called *acetoin.*

***N*-acetylmuramic acid** (as″e-til-mu-ram″ik) 3-*O*-lactyl-*N*-acetylglucosamine, a peptidoglycan consisting of an acetylated six-carbon amino sugar (*N*-acetyl-D-glucosamine), linked to the three-carbon lactic acid. It is a major building block of the polysaccharide backbone of bacterial cell walls.

***N*-acetylneuraminate** (as″ĕ-til-nur-ah-min′āt) the *N*-acetyl derivative of neuraminic acid, a nine-carbon keto-sugar molecule that can exist in pyranose form; created biosynthetically from derivatives of pyruvate and mannosamine. It is an important constituent of glycoproteins and is one of a group of compounds referred to as sialic acids. See also *sialic acid.*

acetylsalicylic acid (ASA) (as″ĕ-til-sal″ĭ-sil′ik) [USP], aspirin; the most important and commonly used antipyretic analgesic drug. It relieves mild pain and lowers elevated body temperature. Aspirin is very rapidly absorbed and works to reduce inflammation and pain at its origin, not through a central nervous system control. In platelets it has been shown that aspirin specifically inhibits prostaglandin biosynthesis by tissue; this has been postulated to be the mode of action by which aspirin produces many of its effects (prolonged bleeding time, gastric irritation, and reduced inflammation, among others). In addition to the effects on prostaglandin synthesis, overdosage may produce dizziness, ringing of the ears, alteration of body temperature, gastrointestinal effects, hyperventilation, and other CNS effects. In severe poisoning, respiratory alkalosis occurs, which may convert to a metabolic acidosis, particularly in young children, with corresponding changes in serum electrolytes.

ASA is rapidly hydrolyzed to acetic and salicylic acids. The latter is then metabolized and excreted in the urine. The most common assay procedures are designed to detect the salicylic acid metabolite. Because of its wide use, ASA is commonly encountered in overdosage, especially in children.

AcG abbrev. for accelerator globulin. See *Factor V.*

ACh abbrev. See *acetylcholine.*

achalasia (ak″ah-la′ze-ah) [*a-* neg. + Gr. *chalasis* relaxation + *-ia*] see *cardiospasm.*

AChE abbrev. See *acetylcholinesterase.*

ache (āk) a constant, often dull pain frequently found with inflammation or other disease of deep structures.

Achilles tendon (ah-kil′ēz) [Gr. *Achilles,* a Greek hero whose mother held him by the heel to dip him in the Styx] see *Achilles t.* under *tendon.*

achiral (a-ki′ral) [*a-* neg. + Gr. *cheir* hand] pertaining to a molecule or environment that is symmetric (identical to its mirror image). In an achiral environment, a pair of enantiomers (which are each chiral) have identical physical and chemical properties.

achlorhydria (ah″klor-hi′dre-ah) [*a-* neg. + Gr. *chlōros* green + *hydōr* water + *-ia*] the absence of "free" hydrochloric acid in the gastric secretion in the basal condition and after maximal stimulation. Achlorhydria is not established until stimulation tests have been performed. "False" achlorhydria refers to those conditions in which hydrochloric acid has been secreted but has subsequently been neutralized by other components of the gastric residue. See also *anacidity* and *gastric function tests.* Cf. *hypochlorhydria.*

Acholeplasma (a-ko-lĕ-plas′mah) [*a-* neg. + Gr. *cholē* bile + *plasma* anything formed] a genus of mycoplasmas, class Mollicutes, family Acholeplasmataceae. The nonmotile spherical cells (minimum diameter, 125–220 nm) are filamentous, gram-negative, and bounded by a triple-layered membrane rather than a true cell wall. Colonies on a solid medium have a diameter of up to 3 mm and a "fried egg" appearance. Sterols are not required for growth. These organisms are resistant to penicillins. *A. laidlawii* is the best studied of the five recognized species. As a group, they are characterized as free-living saprophytes in soil and sewage, and as parasites with a wide host range among mammals and birds.

A. laidlawii, a species whose colonies are present in relatively short filaments, 2–5 μm long. Cells contain carotenoid pigments and are facultative anaerobes. The parasitic occurrence in the nasal cavities of cattle and swine, the sinuses of chicken, and oral cavities of humans challenges its role as a true saprophyte. It is present in sewage, manure, humus, and soil.

Acholeplasmataceae (a-ko″lĕ-plas″mah-ta′se-e) one of two families (with Mycoplasmataceae) in the order Mycoplasmatales, distinguished because the organisms do not require sterol for growth.

acholuria (ah-ko-lu′re-ah) [*a-* neg. + Gr. *cholē* bile + *ouron* urine + *-ia*] the absence of bile pigment (bilirubins) in the urine. The term is most often used to describe those diseases in which serum bilirubins are elevated but no bilirubin is excreted by the kidneys, e.g., acholuric jaundice of hemolytic disease.

acholuric (ah-ko-lu′rik) characterized by acholuria.

achondroplasia (ah-kon″dro-pla′ze-ah″) [*a-* neg. + Gr. *chondros* cartilage + *plassein* to form + *-ia*] a congenital skeletal disorder, transmitted as an autosomal dominant trait, that results from a disturbance of the endochondral ossification in the epiphyseal plates of the long bones. It occurs about once in 10,000 births; about 80 percent are new mutations. Abnormalities include short-limbed dwarfism, slightly enlarged head size, bulging forehead, and "scooped-out" nose bridge. Intelligence is normal and life expectancy about average.

achromasia (ak″ro-ma′se-ah) [*a-* neg. + Gr. *chrōma* color + *-ia*] 1. the lack of normal skin pigmentation. 2. the lack of staining of tissues or cells.

achromate (ah-kro′māt) a person who is totally color-blind.

achromatic (ak″ro-mat′ik) [*a-* neg. + Gr. *chrōmatikos* pertaining to color] 1. without color. 2. staining with difficulty, said of cells or tissues. 3. containing achromatin. 4. refracting light without breaking it into its component colors.

achromatic lens a lens designed to eliminate chromatic aberration and transmit light without separating it into its constituent colors. This can be achieved by combining a lens of low-dispersion glass with a thin lens of opposite curvature made from high-dispersion glass.

achromatic spindle the nonstaining part of the mitotic figure (the chromosomes stain deeply). See also *spindle.*

achromatophil (ak″ro-mat′o-fil) [*a-* neg. + Gr. *chrōma* color + *philein* to love] 1. having no affinity for stains.

2. an organism or tissue element that does not stain easily.

achromia (a-kro′me-ah) [*a-* neg. + Gr. *chrōma* color + *-ia*] absence of normal color; specifically, a condition of the erythrocytes in which their centers are paler than normal (central achromia). See also *hypochromia.*

Achromobacter (a-kro″mo-bak′ter) [*a-* neg. + Gr. *chrōma* color + *baktērion* little rod] the name for a genus of gram-negative bacteria of uncertain classification, but closely related to *Alcaligenes.*

achromocyte (a-kro′mo-sīt) [*a-* neg. + Gr. *chrōma* color + *kytos* hollow vessel] a red cell (usually a reticulocyte) with markedly diminished hemoglobin due to hemolysis during preparation of the smear.

achromophil (a-kro′mo-fil) [*a-* neg. + Gr. *chrōma* color + *philein* to love] see *achromatophil.*

Achucárro's stain (ach″oo-kah′rōz) [Nicolás *Achucárro,* Spanish histologist, 1881–1918] a tannin silver stain for impregnating connective tissue, particularly astrocytes. It stains protoplasmic astrocytes dark-gray to violet, neurofibrils black, connective tissue pale, and other structures reddish to violet. This stain is mainly of historical interest as the forerunner of Hortega's method for astrocytes.

achylia (a-ki′le-ah) [Gr. *achylos* juiceless, from *a-* neg. + *chylos* juice + *-ia*] the absence of hydrochloric acid and enzymes in the gastric secretions.

acid (as′id) [L. *acidus* sour] 1. sour to the taste; having properties opposite to those of an alkali.

2. a proton (H^+) donor (the common Brönsted-Lowry definition), e.g., acetic acid and hydrochloric acid; an electron pair donor (the most general, Lewis definition), e.g., BF_3. In aqueous solution, a strong protic acid dissociates completely to form an anion (the conjugate base of the acid) and the hydronium ion (H_3O^+). An aqueous solution of an acid has a pH below 7.0 and turns litmus paper from blue to red. Two important reactions of acids are: (1) the reaction with a base to form a salt, and (2) the reaction of an aqueous solution of an acid with an active metal to form hydrogen gas and a metallic salt. For more information, see the specific acid.

acid alcohol a solution of hydrochloric acid in ethyl alcohol, used in histology as a decolorizing agent, especially in techniques for demonstrating acid-fast microorganisms.

Acidaminococcus (as″id-ah-mēn″o-kok′kus) [*acid* + *amino* + Gr. *kokkos* seed, grain] a genus of the family Veillonellaceae; amino acids (especially glutamic acid) can serve as its sole energy source for growth. As in other members of the family, the cells are anaerobic and gram-negative. They are nonmotile and often present as oval- or kidney-shaped diplococci.

A. fermentans, the species that, although present in the intestinal tracts of humans and a wide variety of animals, is probably not pathogenic. It is the only species recognized in this genus at present.

acid anhydride 1. a compound having the general formula R—CO—O—CO—R′ and formed by the removal of one molecule of water from two carboxylic acid molecules or two carboxyl groups in the same molecule (to form a cyclic anhydride). Also called carboxylic anhydride. See also *functional groups.*

2. a compound formed by removal of water from two molecules of an inorganic oxo acid, e.g., pyrophosphoric acid. The high-energy bonds between phosphate groups in nucleoside di- and triphosphates are anhydride linkages.

3. an oxide of a nonmetal that reacts with water to form an acid, e.g., sulfur dioxide (SO_2), which forms sulfurous acid (H_2SO_3); sulfur trioxide (SO_3), which forms sulfuric acid (H_2SO_4); carbon dioxide (CO_2), which forms carbonic acid (H_2CO_3); and phosphorus pentoxide (P_2O_5), which forms phosphoric acid (H_3PO_4).

acid anhydride method a histochemical method used to demonstrate the presence of COOH groups in protein using paraffin sections and preferably Carnoy's fixative. The ketone is detected by use of an Ashbel-Seligman reagent, 2-hydroxy-3-naphthoic acid hydrazide (NAH).

acid-base balance the condition of homeostasis of the body with regard to the combined net rates of production and input of acid and base and excretion of acid and base from the body, by which pH and the content of acids and bases are maintained at normal physiologic levels. The acid-base status of an individual is indicated by the blood pH, P_{CO_2}, and various derived measurements. The normal range of pH in extracellular fluid is 7.35–7.45 (H^+ concentration, 36–44 nmol/l. An intricate system of buffers and controls maintains the pH in a healthy individual within this normal range. In a diseased state, however, the body's capacity to maintain a normal pH may be impaired, and significant and sometimes dangerous changes in pH may result. If the pH drops below 7.35, acidosis exists; if the pH rises above 7.45, alkalosis exists. It is important to note that acidosis or alkalosis does not occur spontaneously but is always the result of some other disease or insult to the individual.

The major buffer system in the extracellular fluid involves carbon dioxide, carbonic acid, and bicarbonate: as expressed by the formula $CO_2 + H_2O \rightleftarrows H_2CO_3 \rightleftarrows H^+ + HCO_3^-$. The lungs are involved in the excretion or retention of carbon dioxide (CO_2), whereas the kidneys are the predominant organ regulating the amount of bicarbonate (HCO_3^-) in the body. Therefore, diseases that affect the lungs or kidneys can cause changes in the acid-base balance or pH of body fluids, and result in acidosis or alkalosis.

Respiratory problems that result in decreased ventilation, such as chronic lung disease, severe asthma, or drug overdose, can cause retention of CO_2 during exhalation. As more CO_2 is retained, the pH of extracellular fluid falls and respiratory acidosis develops. In an acute condition, the P_{CO_2} is increased, the pH low, and the HCO_3^- concentration near normal. In time, however, the body attempts to bring the pH back to normal: the kidneys respond by reabsorbing HCO_3^-. Therefore, arterial blood gases eventually show lowered pH and increased P_{CO_2} and HCO_3^-. (Even though the pH is still decreased, it is closer to normal than initially.) This process of responding to acidosis or alkalosis by involving other organs to normalize the pH is known as compensation.

Respiratory alkalosis occurs when a person hyperventilates, exhaling too much CO_2 and causing the pH of extracellular fluids to rise. The usual cause of respiratory alkalosis is psychogenic (hyperventilation) and can be corrected acutely. However, in rare cases when the cause is a chronic problem of the central nervous system, the kidneys again become involved in compensation, and levels of serum HCO_3^- decrease. Arterial blood gases thus show increased pH and lowered P_{CO_2} and HCO_3^-.

Metabolic acidosis occurs following an insult to the body that causes an increased production of acids, a decreased excretion of acids, or a loss of base (HCO_3^-). The acids that accumulate in a diseased state may be organic acids, e.g., acetoacetic acid in diabetic ketoacidosis, lactic acid in hypoxia or shock, or amino acids in renal retention. Other acids may also be retained, such as Po_4 and So_4 in renal disease. A loss of base may also lead to metabolic acidosis, for example, in prolonged diarrhea. In acute metabolic acidosis, decreased pH, decreased P_{CO_2}, and decreased HCO_3^- concentrations are observed. The body again attempts to bring the pH closer to normal, or compensate, by increasing the respiratory rate. The person hyperventilates, causing more CO_2 to be exhaled, further lowering the P_{CO_2}. The respiratory system begins compensation almost immediately, much more rapidly than do the kidneys.

At times it is diagnostically important to know if the cause of metabolic acidosis is an accumulation of organic acids or a loss of HCO_3^-. This can be established by checking electrolytes and determining the anion gap. The anion gap is determined by using the formula $[Na^+] - [Cl^-] + HCO_3^-$. If this gap is greater than a range of 7–16 (mean, 12), the acidosis is caused by unmeasured anions, most often from organic acids.

Metabolic alkalosis is a less common problem. In severe vomiting, continuous nasogastric suction, or prolonged use of diuretics, the body loses too much Cl^-, and the kidneys respond by retaining HCO_3^-. As more HCO_3^- accumulates, the pH rises and metabolic alkalosis occurs. Compensation is through the lungs and therefore occurs quickly: the person breathes more slowly and exhales less CO_2, and the P_{CO_2} increases. Intracellular potassium deficiency is also a cause of metabolic alkalosis (see *hypokalemic a.* under *alkalosis*). In metabolic alkalosis, arterial P_{CO_2}, pH, and HCO_3^- are increased.

NANETTE SMITH, M.D.

acid-base diagram a graph that shows the interrelationship (as shown by the Henderson-Hasselbalch equation) between acid-base parameters (HCO_3^- concentration, pH, and P_{CO_2}), and allows calculation

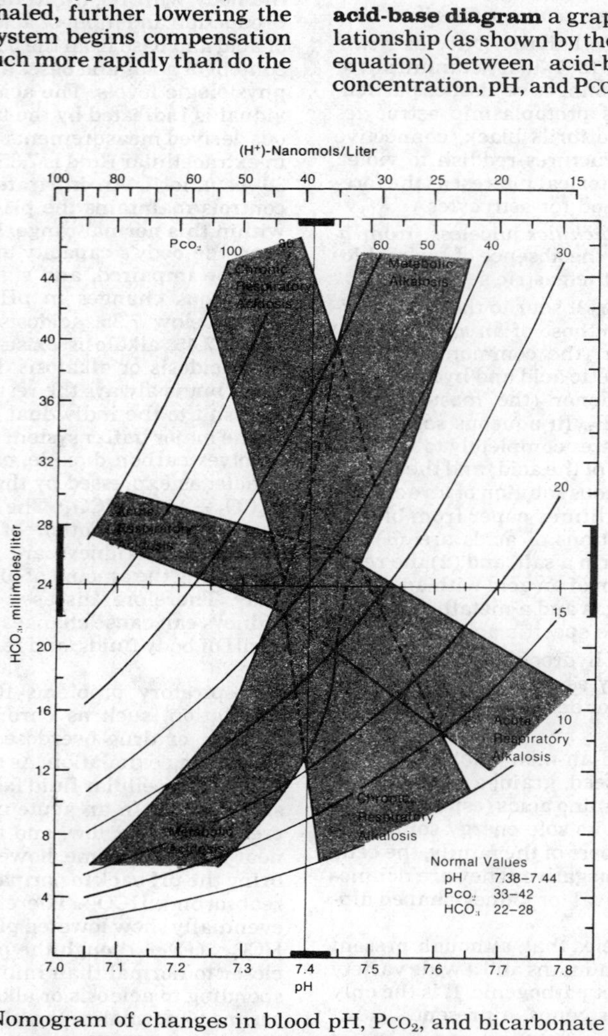

Acid-base diagram. Nomogram of changes in blood pH, P_{CO_2}, and bicarbonate concentration in various disease states. (From Chapman, W. H. et al.: The Urinary System: An Integrated Approach. Philadelphia, W. B. Saunders Co., 1973.)

of these if at least two are known. It displays all combinations of these variables and can be of great clinical use in defining the family of values (particularly the limits) that characterize a specific acid-base disorder such as respiratory acidosis. See the accompanying illustration. Cf. *Siggard-Anderson alignment nomogram.*

acid-base indicator one of a group of organic dyes that are weak acids (or weak bases) in aqueous solution, and which have different colors, depending on whether they are present as the free acid (or base) or as the conjugate ionic form. They are used to locate the end point of the neutralization reaction between an acid and a base. Indicators change their color over a narrow pH range centered about the pK_a of the indicator. The accompanying table lists typical indicators that are used over a variety of pH ranges.

acid - citrate - dextrose (ACD) anticoagulant-citrate-dextrose [USP], a citrate anticoagulant used for the collection and preservation of whole blood in the liquid state. ACD is no longer in common use in transfusion therapy because of the associated low levels of 2,3-diphosphoglycerate, which in turn result in increased hemoglobin-oxygen affinity and reduced delivery of oxygen to tissues. It has been replaced by citrate-phosphate-dextrose (CPD) or CPD-adenine for this use. ACD is currently used in apheresis procedures as a safe and rapidly reversible anticoagulant.

acid dye a dye that contains acidic functional groups, usually sulfonic acid groups, which combine with basic sites in cellular constituents, e.g., eosin.

acid elution test see differential staining under *fetal hemoglobin tests.*

acidemia (as″ĭ-de′me-ah) [*acid* + Gr. *haima* blood + *-ia*] an increased hydrogen ion concentration of the blood, which produces a pH below 7.35. Cf. *acidosis.*

acid-fast not readily decolorized by acid after staining; said of certain bacteria, particularly *Mycobacterium tuberculosis,* the tubercle bacillus, and *M. leprae,* the leprosy bacillus. These are resistant to simple staining methods, but do take certain dyes that bind tightly to the lipids of the cell and then are not removed by decolorization with acid. *M. tuberculosis* is also alcohol-fast. Some species of *Nocardia,* bacterial spores, hair cortex, keratohyalin, sperm, and some lipofuscins (particularly ceroid) exhibit acid-fastness.

Exposure to some substances such as pyridine or HCl-methanol reduces or eliminates acid-fastness, as does ultraviolet radiation (for mycobacteria). It has also been noted that the property of acid-fastness in bacterial strains is gradually lost when they are grown on inadequate artificial media.

acid-fast staining methods one of two general methods that use either carbolfuchsin or fluoro-

ACID BASE INDICATOR. SELECTED INDICATORS

Indicator	Color Change: *Acid Form*	Color Change: *Base Form*	pH Transition Range: *Acid Form Predominant at pH*	pH Transition Range: *Base Form Predominant at pH*
Picric acid	colorless	yellow	0.1	0.8
Paramethyl red	red	yellow	1.0	3.0
2,6-Dinitrophenol	colorless	yellow	2.0	4.0
Bromphenol blue	yellow	blue	3.0	4.6
Congo red	blue	red	3.0	5.0
Methyl orange	red	yellow	3.1	4.4
Ethyl orange	red	yellow	3.4	4.5
Alizarin red S	yellow	purple	3.7	5.0
Bromcresol green	yellow	blue	3.8	5.4
Methyl red	red	yellow	4.2	6.2
Propyl red	red	yellow	4.6	6.6
Methyl purple	purple	green	4.8	5.4
Chlorophenol red	yellow	red	4.8	6.4
Paranitrophenol	colorless	yellow	5.0	7.0
Bromcresol purple	yellow	purple	5.2	6.8
Bromthymol blue	yellow	blue	6.0	7.6
Brilliant yellow	yellow	orange	6.6	8.0
Neutral red	red	amber	6.7	8.0
Phenol red	yellow	red	6.7	8.4
Metanitrophenol	colorless	yellow	6.7	8.6
Phenolphthalein	colorless	pink	8.0	9.6
Thymolphthalein	colorless	blue	9.3	10.6
2,4,6-Trinitrotoluene	colorless	orange	12.0	14.0

From Fischer, R. B., and Peters, D. G.: Basic Theory and Practice of Quantitative Chemical Analysis. Philadelphia, W. B. Saunders Co., 1968, p. 285.

chrome dyes to identify acid-fast bacteria in sections or smears.

Carbolfuchsin is a solution of basic fuchsin and phenol in dilute alcohol. In the Ziehl-Neelsen method, smears or sections are stained in steaming carbolfuchsin for a few minutes or are stained at low temperatures for several hours. The Kinyoun method is a fast, cold carbolfuchsin stain for smears. Acid alcohol is used for decolorizing, and methylene blue is the usual counterstain. Acid-fast material appears red against a light blue background.

The auramine-rhodamine method uses these two fluorochromes in aqueous solution with phenol and glycerol. Acid alcohol or alcohol is used for decolorizing, and potassium permanganate is the counterstain. Under the fluorescence microscope, acid-fast material appears bright yellow or reddish-yellow against a dark background.

Acid-fast bacteria are more easily seen with the fluorochrome method; this permits the use of lower magnification. Although the sensitivity of detection with this method is higher than other staining methods, the specificity is not as good. Both methods stain some nonviable bacteria. The procedure is used in the identification of the tubercle bacillus and other mycobacteria.

acid formaldehyde hematin see *formalin pigment.*

α_1-acid glycoprotein see *orosomucoid.*

acid halide see *acyl halide.*

acid hematin see under *hematin.*

acid hydrolases a term used to refer to hydrolases that are optimally active at acid pH. Lysosomes contain several acid hydrolases.

acidic (ah-sid′ik) of or pertaining to an acid; acid-forming; containing acid.

acidic dye see *acid dye.*

acidified serum test a test for paroxysmal nocturnal hemoglobinuria (PNH). In this procedure, a patient's red cells are washed and incubated in acidified serum from the patient. PNH cells are abnormally sensitive to lysis by complement, which is activiated via the alternative pathway and bound to red cells in acidified serum. PNH is indicated by hemolysis, which is measured by the absorbance at 540 nm of the supernatant serum. Also called *Ham's test.* See also *sucrose hemolysis test.*

acidify (ah-sid′ĭ-fi) to render acid, as by addition of a strong acid.

acidimetry (as-ĭ-dim′ĕ-tre) [L. *acidus* acid + Gr. *metron* measure] the determination of the concentration of free acid in an acidic solution by titrating with a standard solution of base of known strength.

acid ionization constant (K_a) the equilibrium constant for the dissociation of an acid in water. The expression is $K_a = [H^+][A^-] / [HA]$, where the brackets denote concentration or activity, HA is an undissociated acid, and H^+ and A^- are its ions.

acidity (ah sid′ĭ-te) [L *aciditas*] the quality of being acid or sour.

acid number a measure of the amount of free acid in substances (such as waxes, fats, oils, resins, and plasticizers); the milligrams of potassium hydroxide required to neutralize 1 g of the substance dissolved in hot 95 percent ethanol using phenolphthalein as an indicator. Also called *acid value.*

acidophil (as′id-o-fil″) [L. *acidus* acid + Gr. *philein* to love] 1. acidophilic.

2. one of the acid-staining cells, especially of the anterior pituitary, which stain with eosin in routine preparations.

3. an organism that grows well in a highly acid medium.

acidophilic (as″id-o-fil′ik) 1. readily stained with acid dyes.

2. growing in highly acid media; said of microorganisms.

acidophilic body a rounded, densely eosinophilic refractile body usually located in an hepatic sinusoid and thought to represent a degenerating hepatocyte. It is characteristic of hepatic cell damage and is most commonly seen in viral hepatitis. Cf. *Councilman's bodies.*

acidophilic normoblast see orthochromatic normoblast under *normoblast.*

acid orcein (as′id or′se-in) a simple staining method for elastic fibers. Paraffin sections are stained in an alcohol solution containing orcein and concentrated hydrochloric acid. Elastic fibers stain dark brown to brownish-black. The various counterstains used include polychrome methylene blue (the Taenzer-Unna method), hematoxylin and eosin, azure A, toluidine blue, and van Gieson's picrofuchsin.

acidosis (as″ĭ-do′sis) [*acid* + *-osis* condition] a physiologic state or condition resulting from the accumulation of acid in, or the loss of base from, the body. See also *acid-base balance, metabolic acidosis, potassium acidosis,* and *respiratory acidosis.* Cf. *alkalosis.*

acidotic (as″ĭ-dot′ik) pertaining to or characterized by a condition of acidosis.

acid perfusion test see *Bernstein test.*

acid phosphatase (ACP) an enzyme of the hydrolase class (orthophosphoric-monoester phosphohydrolase, EC 3.1.3.2); one of a group of related phosphate transfer enzymes, each of which has optimal activity at a pH below 7.0. Individual enzymes are found in yeasts, milk, erythrocytes, platelets, bone marrow, liver, spleen, and pancreas, and especially in the prostate gland. Activity is also present in semen and urine. The optimal pH for activity is influenced by the enzyme source (tissue) and depends on the relative acidity of the substrate acted upon. The intracellular enzyme is located within organelles (lysosomes). Mammalian acid phosphatase is quite unstable, especially at temperatures above 37°C and pH levels above 7.0. Reducing the pH to below 6.0 (e.g., with citrate buffer) enhances stability. Serum ACP in healthy individuals derives from histiocytes and epithelioid tissue and from formed elements in blood.

Measurements of ACP activity in serum are important in detecting prostatic carcinoma that has metastasized. Moderate elevations occur in Paget's disease and hyperparathyroidism with skeletal involvement, and with invasion of the bones by a variety of malignant neoplasms, such as carcinoma of the breast. Increase in the nontartrate-inhibited (but cupric ion–inhibited) enzyme may be observed in Gaucher's disease, Niemann-Pick disease, various prepubertal conditions, and myelocytic leukemia.

cupric ion–inhibited a. p., an ACP isoenzyme form

that is markedly inhibited by cupric ions (Cu^{2+}) at a concentration of 1.0 mmol/l. This includes the ACP produced by red cells (which constitutes most of the ACP found in normal serum) but does not include prostatic ACP.

prostatic a. p. (PAP) the ACP form or isoenzyme produced by cells of the prostate gland. It shows maximal activity at pH 4.8–6.0 (depending on substrate) and is inhibited by tartrate ions. This property is used to demonstrate its presence. Radioimmunassay methods and isoelectric focusing techniques are now being developed in the hope of making the procedure more specific for the prostatic enzyme and to improve its sensitivity for detecting early nonmetastatic cancer of the prostate gland.

tartrate-inhibited a. p., ACP isoenzyme forms that are markedly inhibited by L-tartrate at a concentration of 20 mmol/l. This fraction is usually considered to include prostatic ACP, although tartrate-inhibited ACP is also present in platelets and some other tissues. It has also been found in the serum of females with breast cancer.

acid phosphatase assays 1. methods used to determine ACP activity in serum. These are based largely on the cleavage of phosphate esters and the measurements of the products formed (either the phosphate or, more commonly, the aromatic alcohol). In methods that are not specific for prostatic acid phosphatase (PAP), ACP activity may be determined in reaction mixtures with and without added tartrate. The difference between the two values gives a close estimate of the amount of the prostatic enzyme. Methods using thymolphthalein phosphate or α-naphthyl phosphate are claimed to be more specific for the prostatic enzyme.

In the Bessey-Lowry-Brock (BLB) method, ACP cleaves the substrate *p*-nitrophenylphosphate (PNPP) to liberate *p*-nitrophenol (PNP). NaOH is added to stop the reaction and convert PNP to its colored form, which is determined photometrically.

Reference ranges for total ACP are: for males, 2.5–11.7 U/l; and for females, 0.3–9.2. Reference ranges for tartrate-inhibited ACP are: for males, 0.2–3.5 U/l; and for females, 0–0.05. In the Gutman and Gutman method, ACP hydrolyzes phenylphosphate to phosphate ions and phenol, which is assayed. In the Babson method, ACP hydrolyzes α-naphthylphosphate to phosphate ions and naphthol, which is subsequently diazotized to a colored compound. In the Roy, Brower, and Hayden method, ACP hydrolyzes thymolphthalein monophosphate (TMP), and the liberated thymolphthalein is converted to its colored form by addition of alkaline carbonate. This method gives considerably lower values than other methods, but it is the most specific of the enzymatic methods for PAP.

2. radioimmunoassay. This procedure has been introduced recently to improve both sensitivity and specificity of the assay for the diagnosis of carcinoma of the prostate. Initial results indicate that RIA may be able to detect a greater number of cases of carcinoma of the prostate than enzymatic methods. Also, these methods measure the amount (as opposed to activity) of the enzyme. The reference ranges differ with the method employed but are most commonly considered to be less than 4.0 ng/ml.

acid phosphatase deficiency an inborn error of metabolism, transmitted as an autosomal recessive trait, caused by a deficiency of lysosomal ACP. The deficiency presents in the neonatal period and is rapidly fatal. It can be detected by prenatal analysis of amniotic fluid.

acid phosphatase staining demonstration of acid phosphatase in frozen or freeze-dried sections. In one method, sections are fixed and then incubated in a buffered solution of glycerophosphate and lead nitrate. As the enzyme decomposes the glycerophosphate, insoluble lead phosphate is formed, which is then converted to black lead sulfide. In a second method, frozen sections are incubated with naphthyl acid phosphate and diazonium salt. Free naphthol is liberated by the enzyme and an azo dye is formed.

acid seromucoid (as′id se″ro-mu′koid) see *orosomucoid.*

aciduria (as″ĭ-du′re-ah) [*acid* + Gr. *ouron* urine + *-ia*] the presence of acid in the urine, which may be produced by diets high in meat proteins (leading to the intake of elevated amounts of phosphates and sulfates) and certain fruits (e.g., cranberries). It can be induced intentionally by the administration of certain chemicals, e.g., acid phosphate, used for the treatment of urinary calculi that tend to form in an alkaline urine, ascorbic acid, and ammonium chloride. Maintenance of an acid urine is also part of the treatment of certain urinary tract infections.

Aciduria is a reflection of metabolic acid-base disturbances, e.g., metabolic acidosis, respiratory acidosis, and potassium depletion. The aciduria of potassium depletion eventually occurs despite a metabolic alkalosis, and is known as paradoxical aciduria. It is caused by an increased Na^+-H^+ exchange, as the depleted K^+ cannot adequately compete with the H^+ for the Na^+. The condition generally is not reversed until intracellular potassium levels have been restored.

Other circumstances in which an acid urine may be found include congenital aminoacidurias of various types (see also *aminoacidopathy*), cachexia, severe liver disease, ketoacidosis, and following administration of protein hydrolysates.

acid value see *acid number.*

acinar (as′ĭ-nar) [L. *acinarius*] pertaining to, affecting, or resembling an acinus. See also the illustration accompanying *contour.*

acinar cell carcinoma a malignant tumor of the acinar cells of the exocrine pancreas. This neoplasm is uncommon compared with the usual duct cell carcinoma of the pancreas; most reported cases have occurred in children, although adults may also be affected. The tumor may be difficult to identify by routine light microscopy, but ultrastructurally the cells contain large secretory granules. A rare instance has been reported of lipase-secreting acinar cell carcinoma that produces polyarthropathy.

acinar cells exocrine cells that form acini, as in the pancreas and salivary glands.

Acinetobacter (as″ĭ-net″o-bak′ter) [Gr. *akinestos* unable to move + *baktērion* little rod] a genus of bacteria of the family Neisseriaceae, consisting of strictly aerobic, gram-negative coccobacilli. Organisms of the genus are oxidase-negative, catalase-positive, and nonmotile, and do not reduce nitrate. They are widespread in nature, are part of the indigenous flora of humans and lower animals, and have been recovered from nearly every clinical source. They are opportunistic pathogens in that they are generally benign, although in compromised hosts they sometimes cause severe primary infections. The genus consists of a single species, *A. calcoaceticus,* which is divided into two biotypes. It contains organisms formerly classified as *Achromobacter, Herellea, Mima,* and *Moraxella.*

A. calcoaceticus anitratus, the strain consisting of those organisms that form acid from glucose oxidatively. These organisms are occasional opportunistic pathogens, causing infections especially in debilitated hospital patients. Formerly called *Acinetobacter anitratum, Bacterium anitratum,* and *Herellea vaginicola.*

A. calcoaceticus lwoffi, the strain consisting of organisms that do not form acid from glucose or lactose. They are part of the normal flora of the skin and genitals but are also considered to be occasional opportunistic pathogens of the skin, and have been associated with infections resulting from intravenous catheterizations. Formerly called *Acinetobacter lwoffi, Mima polymorpha,* and *Moraxella lwoffi.*

acinic (ah-sin'ik) pertaining to an acinus.

acinic cell tumor of the lung a bronchogenic carcinoma composed of cells that appear clear by light microscopy, stain with the PAS procedure following diastase digestion, and contain electron-dense granules. The serous cell of the peribronchial glands is believed to be the cell of origin.

acinic cell tumor of the salivary gland a salivary gland tumor composed of neoplastic serous cells; see also *salivary gland tumors.*

aciniform (ah-sin'ĭ-form) [L. *acinus* grape + *forma* form] having the shape of an acinus, or grape.

acinotubular (as"ĭ-no-tu'bu-lar) [L. *acinus* grape + *tubulus* little tube] composed of tubular acini or of tubules ending in acini.

acinous (as'ĭ-nus) [L. *acinosus*] 1. resembling a grape.

2. pertaining to or affecting an acinus or acini.

acinus (as'ĭ-nus), pl. *acini* [L. grape] a general term used in anatomic nomenclature to designate a small, saclike structure, particularly pertaining to the arrangement of secretory cells in exocrine glands. See also *alveolus.*

ACLA abbrev. See *American Clinical Laboratory Association.*

aclasis (ak'lah-sis) [*a-* neg. + Gr. *klasis* a breaking] pathologic continuity of structure.

diaphyseal a., see under *enchondroma.*

ACLPS abbrev. See *Academy of Clinical Laboratory Physicians and Scientists.*

acne (ak'ne) [possibly a corruption of Greek *akmē* a point or of *achnē* chaff] a papular or nodular skin disorder, with or without inflammation, that is most common in adolescence and early adult life. Acne is thought to be caused by the buildup of keratin and fatty acids in the sebaceous glands surrounding the hair follicles. If this buildup causes rupture of the follicle wall, an inflammatory reaction ensues, with formation of the typical red, pustular acne lesion. If the material remains within the follicle, the lesion is known as a comedo. Comedones, which are papular, are white when the skin surface is unbroken and black if open to the air. A bacterial agent, *Propionibacterium acnes,* is thought to be responsible for the increase in free fatty acids found in these lesions, whereas the activity of the sebaceous glands and production of keratin is primarily under hormonal (androgen-stimulated) control. In selected patients with resistant acne, antibiotics—most often tetracyclines—are used. Estrogen therapy is rarely indicated.

a. vulgaris, a chronic inflammatory disease of the pilosebaceous apparatus, the lesions occurring most frequently on the face, chest, and back. The inflamed glands may form small pink papules, which sometimes surround comedones so that they have black centers, or form pustules or cysts. The cause is unknown, but it has been suggested that many factors, including certain foods, stress, hereditary factors, hormones, drugs, and bacteria, especially *Corynebacterium acnes, Staphylococcus albus,* and *Pityrosporon ovale,* play an etiologic role. Also called common acne.

acneiform (ak-ne'ĭ-form") a term describing any skin disorder that resembles acne.

ACNM abbrev. See *American College of Nuclear Medicine.*

ACNP abbrev. See *American College of Nuclear Physicians.*

aconitase (ah-kon'ĭ-tās) see *aconitate hydratase.*

aconitate hydratase (ah-kon'ĭ-tāt hi'drah-tās) an important iron-containing (Fe^{2+}) enzyme of the lyase class (citrate [isocitrate] hydro-lyase, EC 4.2.1.3) that plays a part in the tricarboxylic acid (Krebs) cycle. It catalyzes the reactions citrate (or isocitrate) $\rightleftarrows$ *cis*-aconitate + H_2O. Also called *aconitase.*

aconitine (ah-kon'ĭ-tēn) 16-ethyl-1,16,19-trimethoxy-4-(methoxymethyl)aconitane-3,8,10,11,18-pentol 8-acetate 10-benzoate, the major alkaloid of the drug aconite, derived from the roots or leaves of *Aconitum napellus* (monkshood). It has a toxic effect on the nervous system, causing paresthesias. It was once given internally for fever and as an oral anesthetic.

acou/o (ah-koo'o) [Gr. *akouein* to hear] a word element used in combining form to denote hearing, e.g., acoumetry.

acoumeter (ah-koo'mĕ-ter) [*acou-* + Gr. *metron* measure] an instrument for measuring the accuracy or acuteness of the hearing.

acoustic (ah-koos'tik) [Gr. *akoustikos,* from *akouein* to hear] pertaining to sound or to the sense of hearing.

acoustic coupler a type of electronic device (modem) used to connect a peripheral device to a computer through a phoneline. The connection is made by dialing the telephone number of the computer and placing the telephone handset on the acoustic coupler.

acoustic impedance the product of the density of a substance and the speed in the substance. The intensity of a sound wave reflected from an acoustic interface is proportional to the intensity of the incident wave and to the difference between the acoustic impedances of the materials on either side of the interface.

acoustic interface a surface separating two substances having different acoustic impedances, and thus reflecting sound waves.

acoustic lens an element of some ultrasound probes that refracts the sound beam produced by the transducer crystal and focuses the beam.

acoustic neuroma a benign tumor of Schwann cells (neurilemma) arising from the auditory division of the eighth cranial nerve, usually in the cerebellopontine angle. Symptoms vary with the size and exact location, but the most common are tinnitus, deafness, vertigo, disturbances in balance, headache, and upper neck or facial pain or sensory disturbances.

acoustic radiation a tract of fibers that originates in the medial geniculate nucleus and passes below the lentiform nucleus to terminate in Heschl's gyrus of the temporal lobe.

acoustic shadow in an ultrasonogram, an area behind an attenuating object where the acoustic signal is reduced. Acoustic shadows must be distinguished from areas of low reflectivity.

ACP abbrev. See *acid phosphatase.*

acquired (ah-kwird′) [L. *acquirere* to obtain] incurred as a result of factors acting from or originating outside the organism; not inherited. For diseases or conditions beginning with this adjective, see the noun.

acquired immune deficiency syndrome (AIDS) a recently identified syndrome characterized by immunodeficiency associated with severe opportunistic infection and malignancy and affecting mostly young male homosexuals. Almost all the reported cases have occurred in North America, but some European cases have also been identified. Although the etiology is not understood, the possibility of a viral cause has been suggested. Not all those affected are homosexuals, but a high degree of sexual activity and high incidence of sexually transmitted diseases appear to be associated with the syndrome.

For some months prior to emergence of the infection or neoplasm, many patients have prodromal symptoms, including malaise, fever, gastrointestinal disturbances, and lymphoma. The most common opportunistic infection is pneumonia due to *Pneumocystis carinii*, but in some cases the organism has been a virus (cytomegalovirus or herpes simplex), fungus (*Candida, Cryptococcus, Aspergillus*), bacterium (*Mycobacterium*), or parasite (*Toxoplasma gondii, Giardia lamblia*). In spite of initial response to therapy, the infections tend to recur and the mortality from AIDS is over 50 percent. Patients with severe opportunistic infections exhibit skin test anergy, low T cells, reduced ratios of helper T to suppressor T cells, and reduced lymphocyte blastogenetic responses.

The neoplasm in most of the reported cases has been Kaposi's sarcoma, although some patients have had lymphoma or a carcinoma. Kaposi's sarcoma associated with AIDS has shown more of a tendency for lymph nodal and visceral involvement than usually occurs with this tumor; the mortality rate is exceedingly high.

See also *Kaposi's sarcoma.*

ACR abbrev. See *American College of Radiology.*

acr/o (ak′ro) [Gr. *akron* extremity; *akros* extreme] a word element used in combining form to denote a relationship to the extremities, top, or extreme point, e.g., acrodermatitis.

acrania (a-kra′ne-ah) [a- neg. + Gr. *kranion* skull + *-ia*] partial or complete absence of the cranium.

Acremonium (ak″rĕ-mo′ne-um) a genus of imperfect fungi, frequently isolated from human eumycotic mycetoma, now considered to be the proper name for *Cephalosporium.*

acridine (ak′ri-dēn) [L. *acer* sharp] a colorless crystalline solid, dibenzo[*b,e*]pyridine (10-azaanthracene); M.W. 179.21. It occurs in coal tar and is used in the manufacture of several dyes such as acriflavine and proflavine (which were formerly employed as antiseptics) and the acridine fluorescent dyes used in histology. Acridine has a noxious odor and is extremely irritating to the skin and mucous membranes.

a. hydrochloride, a red-brown salt of acriflavine, also used as an antiseptic and bacteriostatic agent.

acridine orange (AO) a basic fluorochrome dye, tetramethyl acridine; C.I. 46005. It binds nonspecifically to nucleic acids, proteins, polysaccharides, and glycosaminoglycans.

acridine orange method a histologic method in which fresh frozen sections or smears are fixed in Clarke-Carnoy acetic alcohol and stained with a dilute solution of acridine orange in buffered Ringer's solution. RNA shows red fluorescence, DNA green. In exfoliative cytology, this technique is used for staining tumor cells, which have abnormal nuclear DNA content. Because they are metabolically active, large amounts of cytoplasmic RNA are present. Metabolically active noncancerous cells are also stained.

acridine red 3B a basic fluorochrome dye belonging to the pyronin class; C.I. 45000.

acridine yellow a basic fluorochrome dye; C.I. 46025. It can be used to form Schiff-type reagents, which are used in the Feulgen reaction.

acriflavine (ak″rĭ-fla′vēn) [L. *acer* sharp + *flavus* yellow] an orange acridine dye used as a topical antiseptic and bacteriostatic agent, a basic fluorochrome dye; C.I. 46000. It is used in histology as a substitute for basic fuchsin in preparing Schiff-type reagents.

acroanesthesia (ak″ro-an″es-the′ze-ah) [*acro-* + *an-* neg. + Gr. *aisthēsis* sensation + *-ia*] anesthesia of the extremities.

acrocentric (ak″ro-sen′trik) [*acro-* + Gr. *kentron* center] see *subtelocentric.*

acrocephalosyndactyly (ak″ro-sef″ah-lo-sin-dak′tĭ-le) [*acrocephaly* + *syndactyly*] a group of inherited, congenital malformations, including premature closure of sagittal and coronal sutures, that are found in Apert's, Pfeiffer's, and Carpenter's syndromes. These conditions are characterized most often by acrocephaly, extensive syndactyly, hypertelorism, and hypoplasia of the maxilla. Also reported are malformations of the hard and soft palate, ankylosis of the joints, and polydactyly. Ocular complications include poor lid approximation, ophthalmoplegia, and optic atrophy. Treatment includes surgical correction of syndactyly and cleft palate. Prognosis must be guarded, as infant mortality is high.

acrocephaly (ak″ro-sef′ah-le) [*acro-* + Gr. *kephalē* head] the short, high skull that results from premature closure of the coronal suture. Also called *tower skull.* See also *acrocephalosyndactyly* and *craniostenosis.*

acrochordon (ak″ro-kor′don) [*acro-* + Gr. *chordē* string] a pedunculated skin tag that occurs principally on the neck, upper chest, and axillae in females of middle age or older.

acrocyanosis (ak″ro-si″ah-no′sis) [*acro-* + *cyanosis,* from Gr. *kyanos* blue *-osis* condition] an arteriolar, vasospastic disorder characterized by symmetric, uneven cyanosis of the hands and feet. It is both uncommon and benign. Symptoms include coldness and profuse sweating of the digits. The etiology is unknown. The cyanosis is intensified by cold temperatures and relieved by warmth. Those affected can lead normal lives, and usually no treatment is necessary.

acrodermatitis (ak″ro-der″mah-ti′tis) [*acro-* + Gr. *derma* skin + *-itis* inflammation] an inflammation of the skin of the hands and feet that may be associated with several disorders, including psoriasis and zinc deficiency. With zinc deficiency the disorder is more properly called acrodermatitis enteropathica, and the inflammation is accompanied by ulceration and hyperkeratosis of the skin and by gastrointestinal disturbance (diarrhea and weight loss), as well as disorders in white blood cell function.

acrodynia (ak″ro-din′e-ah) [*acr-* + Gr. *odynē* pain + *-ia* condition] a now uncommon disorder, primarily occurring in infants and young children, that is characterized by extreme irritability, insomnia, widespread erythema, hypertension, and loss of teeth. This condition is thought to occur as a result of chronic poisoning with mercury, which in the past has been associated with the use of mercury-containing teething powders, vermifuges, diaper rinses, and calomel. Fever, increases in white blood cell counts, and albuminuria are frequent. Laboratory diagnosis is confirmed by the demonstration of greater than 0.1 mg/da of mercury in the urine.

acrolein (ak-ro′le-in) [L. *acer* acrid + *oleum* oil] a volatile acrid liquid, $CH_2{=}CHCHO$, derived from the decomposition of glycerine. It is a simple, unsaturated aldehyde. Also called acrylaldehyde, acrylic aldehyde, allyl aldehyde, and propenal.

acromegaly (ak″ro-meg′ah-le) [*acro-* + Gr. *megas, megalos* great] a condition characterized by periosteal overgrowth, cortical thickening, coarsening of the facial features, excessive sweating, and hypertension, caused by the abnormally increased synthesis and secretion of growth hormone by the growth hormone–producing cells of the anterior pituitary. It most frequently occurs in adults and is due to the presence of a benign but functioning pituitary adenoma. The abnormal increase in growth hormone occurs after closure of the epiphyses, and results in excessive growth of the hands, feet, jaws, and internal organs.

Laboratory results include elevated concentrations of serum phosphorus (inorganic, >4.5 mg/100 ml) and urinary calcium. Glycosuria and hyperglycemia resistant to the administration of insulin are also seen. The basal metabolic rate (BMR) is usually elevated, whereas serum thyroxine concentrations are reduced. The most valuable laboratory test is direct radioimmunologic determination of increased concentrations of growth hormone in plasma (>10 ng/ml), which is not suppressed by the glucose tolerance test. X-rays and CT scans may reveal sella turcica enlargement, frontal sinus expansion, and thickening of the skull or long bones. Vertebral spur formation and dorsal kyphosis are also seen.

See also *gigantism.*

acromion (ah-kro′me-on) [*acro-* + Gr. *ōmos* shoulder] [NA], the lateral extension of the spine of the scapula, which projects over the shoulder joint and forms the highest point of the shoulder. Also called acromion process.

acropachy (ak′ro-pak″e) [*acro-* + Gr. *pachys* thick] a clinical sign characterized by clubbing of fingers and toes, caused by swelling of soft tissues and changes in the distal bone periosteum. Acropachy is often associated with hyperthyroidism and Graves' disease.

acropachyderma (ak″ro-pak″e-der′mah) [*acro-* + Gr. *pachys* thick + *derma* skin] a condition marked by thickening of the skin over the face, scalp, and extremities; clubbing of the extremities; and deformities of the long bones.

acroparesthesia (ak″ro-par″es-the′ze-ah) [*acro-* + *paresthesia*] an abnormal sensation in the distal parts of the limbs, such as tingling, numbness, or pins and needles.

acropetal (ah-krop′ĕ-tal) [*acro* + L. *petere* to seek] 1. rising toward the top.

2. produced successively in the direction of the top, the top member being the youngest.

acrophobia (ak″ro-fo′be-ah) [*acro-* + Gr. *phobos* fear + *-ia*] an obsessive, abnormal fear of heights. Although many healthy people fear heights to some extent, acrophobic individuals may be severely limited in their activity because of this fear.

acrosclerosis (ak″ro-sklĕ-ro′sis) [*acro-* + Gr. *sklērōsis* hardening] a combination of Raynaud's disease and scleroderma of the distal parts of the extremities, especially of the digits, and of the neck and face, particularly the nose.

acrosomal (ak′ro-so-mal) pertaining to the acrosome.

acrosomal granule a single large granule found in the Golgi apparatus of spermatocytes, formed by the fusion of several small granules whose appearance marks the first signs of spermatozoic differentiation.

acrosomal vesicle a large vacuole surrounding the acrosomal granule, which later adheres to the outer surface of the nuclear envelope.

acrosome (ak′ro-sōm) [*acro-* + Gr. *sōma* body] the caplike structure that invests the anterior part of the head of a spermatozoon. It contains enzymes that are important in fertilization.

acrosome reaction that series of observable, structural changes undergone by a sperm when in the vicinity of an ovum in the oviduct. Specifically, many openings appear in the sperm head membrane, through which the contents of the acrosome appear to be released. The functional changes of the sperm are called *capacitation.*

acrospiroma (ak″ro-spi-ro′mah) a tumor of eccrine sweat gland origin. It commonly occurs as a solitary, well-circumscribed dermal nodule, firm in consistency and measuring up to 2 cm, though a few are larger. Acrospiromas are usually benign. Also called clear cell hidradenoma, eccrine acrospiroma, and eccrine adenoma.

acrylamide (ah-kril′ah-mīd) a colorless, odorless, crystalline solid, propenamide, $CH_2{=}CH_2{-}CONH_2$; M.W. 71.08. It can be stored in the cold or dark but readily polymerizes at its melting point (84.5°C) or when irradiated with ultraviolet light. Acrylamide is highly toxic and irritating and can be absorbed through the skin, producing a polyneuropathy that affects both motor and sensory nerves. Symptoms include numbness, weakness, paresthesia, tremor, and loss of coordination. It is used in making several polymers; see *polyacrylamide.*

acrylamide gel electrophoresis electrophoresis carried out in acrylamide gel, often used for the study of individual proteins in serum, particularly genetic variants and enzymes. Preconcentration of samples with low protein content is unnecessary with this method.

Three gel layers are constructed, differing in composition and pore size: separation gel, spacer gel, and bottom separation gel. The actual ion separation is based on the charge and molecular size and takes place in the bottom gel layer. A recent variation on this technique, which involves the use of a continuous buffer system rather than the space and sample gel, has been used successfully.

See also *electrophoresis.*

acrylonitrile (ak″rĭ-lo-ni′tril) a colorless liquid, 2-propenenitrile, $H_2C{=}CHC{\equiv}N$; M.W. 53.06. Acrylonitrile is used in making acrylic plastics and synthetic fibers and as a grain fumigant. Flammable, explosive, and highly toxic, it behaves as cyanide when ingested or inhaled.

ACS abbrev. See *American Cancer Society, American Chemical Society, Association of Clinical Scientists.*

ACS grade a grade of purity of chemicals that meets the specifications of the Committee on Analytical Reagents of the American Chemical Society (ACS); see under *reagent grade.*

ACT abbrev. for activated clotting time.

ACTH abbrev. See *adrenocorticotropic hormone.*

ACTH-RF abbrev. for adrenocorticotropic hormone releasing-factor. See *corticotropin-releasing factor.*

Actidil (ak′tĭ-dil) trademark. See *triprolidine hydrochloride.*

Actifed (ak′tĭ-fed) trademark for a combination of pseudoephedrine hydrochloride and triprolidine hydrochloride.

actin/o (ak′tĭ-no) [Gr. *aktis, aktinos* a ray] a word element used in combining form to denote relationship to a ray or to some forms of radiant energy, e.g., actinogenesis.

actin (ak′tin) [L. *actus* motion + *-in*] a contractile protein present in muscle and other cells. Actin forms thin microfilaments 5 nm in diameter, each consisting of a double-stranded helix with a turn every 36 nm. It can be detected cytochemically by its reaction with heavy meromyosin. In striated muscle, parallel arrays of actin myofilaments interdigitate with myosin myofilaments to produce the characteristic banding pattern of the myofibril and provide the ultrastructural basis for the sliding filament mechanism of contraction. The actin filaments are supported at their midpoint by the Z band, and occupy the I band and extend between the myosin filaments into the A band for a distance that varies with the state of contraction of the myofibril. Actin myofilaments are numerous in smooth muscle cells and are present in small numbers in myofibroblasts. Actin filaments are present in most other cells in varying quantities: they form the terminal web and microvillus cores in absorptive epithelial cells, and produce the contraction ring that constricts the cytoplasm between dividing cells. See also *muscle.*

actinic (ak-tin′ik) pertaining to light that is energetic enough to produce a given chemical effect, e.g., initiate a photochemical reaction.

actinic keratosis see *actinic k.* under *keratosis.*

actinide (ak′tĭ-nīd) a group of chemical elements including actinium (atomic number 89) and the succeeding 5f transition elements (atomic numbers 90–103). Originally the term included only the elements after actinium. The term is used as both a noun and an adjective.

actinium (Ac) (ak-tin′e-um) a silvery-white radioactive metallic element; atomic number 89; most stable isotope Ac-227 (half-life, 21.6 yr.); a 6d transition element; oxidation state +3. It occurs in uranium ores.

Actinobacillus (ak″tĭ-no-bah-sil′lus) [*actino-* + L. *bacillus* small rod] a genus of fermentative, nonmotile, gram-negative bacilli that are part of the normal microflora of animals and also cause granulomatous lesions. These organisms are sometimes recovered from human infectious processes in mixed culture. There is no growth on MacConkey agar.

A. actinomycetemcomitans, a catalase-positive, indole- and oxidase-negative species that is frequently isolated from actinomycotic-like lesions of humans. Its pathogenic role is uncertain, however, as such cultures are usually mixed.

A. equuli, a bacterium that is part of the normal oral flora of horses. It has also been found to cause disease in horses and in pigs, and has been associated with cases of human infection. The cells are generally rod-shaped but vary with the medium.

A. lignieresii, a species that usually has rod-shaped cells, although this varies with the medium. This organism may cause granulomatous lesions in the throat and mouth of cattle (wooden tongue), and in the lungs and skin of sheep. There are reports of the species having been isolated from human lesions.

actinodermatitis (ak″tĭ-no-der″mah-ti′tis) [*actino-* + Gr. *derma* skin + *-itis*] dermatitis from exposure to x-rays.

Actinomadura (ak″tĭ-no-mad′ŭ-rah) [*actino-* + *madura,* from *madura foot,* a name for mycetoma] a genus of microorganisms of the family Nocardiaceae, formerly included in the *Nocardia* genus. These organisms are aerobic actinomycetes with a cosmopolitan distribution, which may cause mycetoma in humans.

A. madurae, a species that may cause an actinomycotic mycetoma, characterized by a raised border around the sinus openings in the infected site, often with bone and muscle involvement. The granules (microcolonies) are the largest seen in mycetoma. The colony morphology is dry, white, and wrinkled, with a flat periphery. Microscopically, long branched filaments with chains of arthrospores are found. This microorganism is gram-positive and not acid-fast. Formerly called *Nocardia madurae.*

A. pelletieri, a species that can cause actinomycotic mycetoma, a clinical syndrome of localized swollen and deformed lesions. *A. pelletieri* causes craterlike nodules in the draining sinuses, with a granulomatous inflammatory reaction. The granule (a microcolony of fungus in the lesion) is small and a garnet red color. The colony morphology is pink to red in color, dry, and granular. Microscopically, branched filaments are seen with a few arthrospores. *A. pelletieri* is not acid-fast and is gram-positive.

Actinomyces (ak″tĭ-no-mi′sez) [*actino-* + Gr.

mykēs fungus] one of five genera of bacteria belonging to the family Actinomycetaceae. These organisms are gram-positive, stain irregularly, are nonacid-fast and nonmotile, and do not form spores. They grow fine, straight, or wavy filaments that vary in length and degree of branching. They are facultative anaerobes, but increased CO_2 is required for optimal growth. Some species, and possibly all, are low-grade pathogens for human beings and lower animals. There are five major accepted species.

A. bovis, a facultatively anaerobic bacterium that causes "lumpy jaw," an actinomycosis of the jaw, tongue, and maxillary bone in cattle. Colonies of the organism called sulfur granules are seen on direct examination of the infected tissues, but in culture it is a short gram-positive rod and may show branching. *A. bovis* is catalase-negative and belongs to serologic group B. Unlike most *Actinomyces* species, *A. bovis* is not a soil saprophyte but rather a normal inhabitant of animal mucous membranes.

A. congolensis, see *D. congolensis* under *Dermatophilus.*

A. israelii, a microaerophilic to anaerobic bacterium that causes actinomycosis in humans and occasionally causes infections in cattle. On brain heart infusion blood agar plates, spiderlike colonies appear, which with age form a "molar tooth" gray colony. Microcolonies may be composed of branching filaments, serologic group D, types 1 and 2. Microscopically, long, gram-positive branching rods are seen. *A. israelii* is not acid-fast and is catalase-negative.

A. naeslundii, an inhabitant of the human oral cavity that may be responsible for some cases of human infection. Its microcolonies usually are spider-form with dense centers of tangled filaments and radiating filaments. It is catalase-negative; its serologic group is A, types 1 and 2. *A. naeslundii* is a normal resident of the human oral cavity and is occasionally incriminated in a disease process.

A. odontolyticus, a natural inhabitant of the human oral cavity, which has been found in caries. It closely resembles *A. naeslundii.*

A. viscosus, a bacterium found in the human oral cavity; it has not been proven pathogenic for humans, but produces periodontal disease in laboratory animals. Its microcolonies on brain heart infusion agar have dense centers with filaments around the edge (growth in 18-24 hr). Serologically, it belongs to group F, types 1 and 2.

actinomyces (ak″tĭ-no-mi′sez), pl. *actinomycetes* an organism of the genus *Actinomyces.*

Actinomycetaceae (ak″ti-no-mi″se-ta′se-e) a family of bacteria in the Actinomycetes. Such organisms are gram positive, resemble diphtheroids, and form branched, easily fragmented filaments in tissue. They are nonmotile and do not form spores. All five genera in this family (the anaerobic *Actinomyces, Arachnia,* and *Bifidobacterium,* and the aerobic facultative *Bacterionema* and *Rothia*) are important in human microbial ecology.

Actinomycetales (ak″tĭ-no-mi″se-ta′lēz) an order of bacteria composed of elongated cells that tend to form branching filaments, sometimes forming a mycelium, and, in some families, true spores. Two families do not form a mycelium: the gram-positive Actinomycetaceae and the acid- and alcohol-fast Mycobacteriaceae. The six producers of mycelium include one family, Nocardiaceae, that contains important human pathogens; the others are mostly soil saprophytes.

actinomycete (ak″tĭ-no-mi′sēt), pl. *actinomycetes* any member of the order Actinomycetales.

thermophilic a., one of the species of the genus *Thermoactinomyces* and any of the species within the *Microbispora* and *Micropolyspora* genera capable of good growth at 45°–60°C. One of the thermophilic actinomycetes, *Micropolyspora faeni,* is the primary agent of farmer's lung, an allergic pneumonitis acquired by inhalation of large numbers of the spores of this species, which thrives on overheated grain.

Actinomycetes (ak-tĭ″no-mi′sēts) a large collection of gram-positive species of bacteria, interrelated by chemically and serologically similar cell wall constituents. The coryneform bacilli are club shaped, whereas the members of the order Actinomycetales are filamentous and sometimes branching. The coryneform group contains the pathogenic *Corynebacterium diphtheriae* and the diphtheroids. Among the Actinomycetales, the *Actinomyces, Mycobacterium,* and *Nocardia* genera are of medical interest.

actinomycetoma (ak-tin″o-mi-sĕ-to′mah) [*actinomycete* + Gr. *-ōma* swelling] see under *mycetoma.*

actinomycin (ak″ti-no-mi′sin) [*Actinomyces* + *-in*] a large, complex family of antibiotics obtained from cultures of various species of *Streptomyces,* which are active against bacteria and fungi. Some, especially actinomycins C (cactinomycin) and D (dactinomycin), are used to inhibit the growth of malignant cells, and dactinomycin is also employed as an immunosuppressant. Actinomycin also is useful in the study of protein synthesis, as it alters the structure and function of DNA. See also *antibacterial agents.*

a. C, a highly toxic antibiotic produced by *Streptomyces chrysomallus,* formerly used as an antineoplastic. Also called *cactinomycin.*

a. D, an antibiotic extracted from *Streptomyces parvullus,* which is capable of blocking DNA-dependent RNA synthesis, and therefore is useful in cell physiology studies. It has been employed as a radiomimetic agent to treat hematologic malignancies, but its severe toxic effects prevent its use in the treatment of bacterial or viral infections. It has considerable antiviral, antibacterial, and antitumoral potency. Also called dactinomycin. Trademark, Cosmegen. For more information, see *Appendix A.*

actinomycosis (ak″tĭ-no-mi-ko′sis) [*actino* + Gr. *mykēs* fungus + *-osis* condition] a noncontagious, infectious disease in humans and animals, usually caused by *Actinomyces* species. Generally, it involves the head and neck regions; less often, the lung and intestinal tract. It is characterized by suppurating lesions of the lymph nodes draining the mouth, beginning as a painless, tumorlike mass or mycetoma (lumpy jaw). The drainage often contains dense microcolonies of the fungus, called sulfur granules. The most important species causing human actinomycosis is *A. israelii;* the species of lumpy jaw in cattle is *A. bovis.* Surgical drainage and chemotherapy are effective. Cf. *mycetoma.*

actinomycotic (ak″tĭ-no-mi-kot′ik) pertaining to or caused by actinomycosis.

actinomycotic mycetoma see under *mycetoma.*

actinophage (ak-tin′o-fāj) [*actino-* + Gr. *phagein*

to eat] a virus that infects and causes the lysis of actinomycetes.

Actinoplanaceae (ak″tĭ-no-plah-na′se-e) a family of bacteria of the order Actinomycetales, containing aerobic, gram-positive organisms that form filaments bearing spores in sporangia. The colonies are mycelial and white to colored.

Actinoplanes (ak″tĭ-no-pla′nēz) [*actino-* + Gr. *planēs* one who wanders] a genus of bacteria of the family Actinoplanaceae, of the actinomycetes. The organisms are chemoorganotrophic and aerobic. The majority of the species form brilliantly colored colonies on most agar media.

actinotherapy (ak″tĭ-no-ther′ah-pe) [*actino-* + Gr. *therapeia* treatment] treatment of disease by rays of light, especially ultraviolet rays.

action (ak′shun) [L. *actio*] any performance of function or movement either of a part or organ or the whole body.

action potential (ak′shun) [L. *actio,* from *agere* to do] an abrupt, transient reversal in the resting membrane potential of an excitable cell that is due to temporary changes in the membrane conductances (the product of the permeability and the ion concentration) of sodium and potassium ions. An action potential is actively propagated as a wave of excitation that passes along a nerve or muscle fiber in a regenerative, nondecremental manner. Any externally applied factor (chemical, mechanical, or electric stimuli) that causes a sudden increase in the membrane sodium permeability can trigger an action potential.

When the action potential is recorded from an intracellular electrode, two distinct phases—membrane depolarization and repolarization—are seen. These changes in membrane potential are correlated in time with the changes in membrane sodium and potassium conductances that occur. When the membrane potential of the excitable cell is reduced (i.e., the membrane polarity begins to reverse) to or beyond a critical threshold voltage, an increase of several thousand-fold in the sodium conductance occurs; in a positive feedback, regenerative cycle, the membrane becomes increasingly more permeable to sodium ions as the action potential progresses. At this upstroke of the action potentials, sodium ions diffuse into the cell at an increasingly rapid rate, causing the abrupt loss of the negative (with respect to the exterior) resting potential that is known as depolarization. The membrane potential changes from the resting potential of approximately –90 mV to +25–45 mV during depolarization.

Immediately afterward, the membrane once again becomes relatively impermeable to sodium ions (sodium inactivation), and potassium conductance in turn increases 30-fold. As a result, as inward sodium ion diffusion ceases and potassium ions leave the cell, the resting potential is restored (repolarization). Following repolarization, the membrane becomes hyperpolarized (for 50 msec to several seconds) because potassium ion permeability is temporarily still greater than normal.

In a muscle fiber or unmyelinated axon, the generation of an action potential in one region causes local current flow (movement of sodium and potassium ions in a circuit) between this active region and the adjacent inactive region of membrane. The membrane is depolarized to threshold, and the action potential is thus propagated without decrement to the adjacent regions of the membrane. In myelinated axons, local current flow occurs only at the uninsulated nodes, and the action potential leaps along the membrane from one node to the next (saltatory conduction).

The term action potential is also applied to the summated action potentials recorded extracellularly from a group of cells that are firing at nearly the same time (a compound action potential).

biphasic a. p., any action potential that has two phases.

cardiac a. p., changes in the transmembrane electric potential that occur with the depolarization and repolarization of an excitable cell of the heart. After an initial spike, during which the cell is depolarized from a resting membrane potential of –85 to –100 mV to approximately +20 mV, the potential remains on a plateau for several hundred milliseconds before repolarization occurs. The duration of the cardiac action potential is therefore 20–50 times longer than that of skeletal muscle or peripheral nerves.

compound muscle a. p., a group of muscle fiber action potentials that occur almost simultaneously within the pickup zone of an extracellular recording electrode, and thus appear as a summated, multipeaked action potential. In electromyography, compound action potentials are commonly produced by electrical stimulation of the motor nerve supplying the muscle fibers.

For more information on the types of compound action potential, see the specific names, e.g., *blink responses, F wave, H wave,* and *M wave.*

compound nerve a. p., a group of nerve fiber action potentials that occur almost synchronously, recorded from the trunk of a sensory, motor, or mixed nerve as a summated, multipeaked action potential. In electroneurography, it is commonly evoked by nerve stimulation. The number and size of the peaks of the resulting potential vary with the fiber types (the conduction velocities of the individual fibers), the number of fibers stimulated, and the distance between the stimulating and recording electrodes.

monophasic a. p., any action potential with only a single phase; it is represented in recordings of electric activity by one deflection either above or below the baseline.

muscle a. p., the self-propagated wave of depolarization that spreads without decrement along a muscle fiber membrane in both directions from the end-plate region. It is triggered when the end-plate potential reaches a critical threshold and initiates the processes within a muscle fiber that lead to its contraction. Although when strictly defined, the term muscle action potential refers to the reversal in potential recorded intracellularly from a single fiber, it is also used more loosely to refer to a compound muscle action potential.

polyphasic a. p., any action potential with a minimum of five distinct phases, or deflections, above or below the baseline.

serrated a. p., any action potential with a waveform characterized by several changes in direction relative to the baseline without actually crossing it.

activated charcoal see *activated c.* under *charcoal.*

activated complex an unstable, high-energy transition state in a chemical reaction, intermediate between the products and the reactants. Its energy is at the top of the energy barrier that separates the reactants and products of a reaction, or a particular step in a reaction. The reaction will proceed to products when at least this much energy (the activation energy) is supplied.

activated lymphocyte any lymphocyte that is in an active state; it has either been stimulated by an antigen or mitogen, or is producing antibody while taking part in a cell-mediated immune reaction. The process of activation involves a complex series of biochemical reactions that are initiated by changes produced in the cell membrane after antigen or mitogen interact with lymphocyte membrane receptors. See also *lymphocyte*.

activated partial thromboplastin time (aPTT) a coagulation test that has superseded the partial thromboplastin time test (PTT) in the clinical hematology laboratory. The term aPTT is interchangeable with PTT in daily usage. See under *partial thromboplastin time test*.

activation (ak″tĭ-va-shun) in electroencephalography, a procedure used to enhance or elicit normal or abnormal, especially paroxsymal, electric activity of the brain. Such techniques as hyperventilation, auditory and photic stimulation, natural sleep, sleep deprivation, and drug-induced sleep are used in the diagnosis of various brain disorders, including tumors and epilepsy. In the past, drugs used in activation procedures have included leptazol, bemegride, chlorpromazine, and imipramine. In some cases, clinical seizure may be induced by these techniques; however, this is justified only when surgical intervention is contemplated. Also called *provocation*. See also *auditory stimulation, hyperventilation, photic stimulation*, and *s. deprivation* under *sleep*.

photometrazol a., in electroencephalography, an activation technique used to induce myoclonic jerking or polyspike discharge. It consists of an intravenous injection of 50 mg of leptazol every 30 sec; each dose is followed by photic stimulation at about 15 flashes/sec for up to 10 sec, until bilateral myoclonic jerks are evoked, accompanied by polyspike discharges or spike and wave activity on the electroencephalographic record. See also *photometrazol threshold*.

activation analysis see *neutron activation analysis*.

activation energy see under *activated complex*.

activator (ak′tĭ-va″tor) 1. an effector molecule that increases the catalytic activity of an enzyme when it binds to an allosteric site.

2. a substance that stimulates the development of a particular structure in the embryo. Egg activation is the response of the egg to sperm penetration (and to various artificial stimuli) and the beginning of embryonic development. See also *fertilization*.

3. see *inducer*.

active (ak′tiv) characterized by action; not passive.

active transport a movement of solutes (ions or molecules) across cell membranes that is coupled to the input of energy. Generally, this type of transport refers to the movement of solute against an electrochemical gradient. Integral proteins that span the membrane are involved in these processes. The proteins contain binding sites on one side of the membrane for the substances to be transported, which then are released on the opposite side as a result of a conformational change in the proteins.

There are two types of active transport. In direct or primary active transport, the free energy required to move ions or molecules across a membrane against a concentration gradient is provided directly by the hydrolysis of ATP. An example is the Na^+, K^+-dependent ATPase, which establishes the sodium and potassium gradients and membrane potentials in nerve cells, muscle fibers, and other cells. This type of system is often referred to as a pump. In indirect or secondary active transport, the transport of one solute against its concentration gradient is coupled to that of another down its gradient. An example of indirect active transport is the absorption of glucose by the kidneys and intestinal mucosa, which is driven by and dependent on the simultaneous absorption of sodium. This type of system is referred to as indirect, as it employs the concentration gradient of sodium initially established by the hydrolysis of ATP during activity of Na^+, K^+-ATPase.

Transport in which two solutes move in the same direction is called symport or cotransport; antiport refers to movement of two solutes in opposite directions.

See also *facilitated diffusion*.

J. KENNETH HOOBER, PH.D.

activity (ak-tiv′ĭ-te) [L. *activus* active, from *agere* to do] 1. the state of being active or the extent of some function or action.

2. (symbol a), a thermodynamic quantity that denotes the effective concentration of a substance in a chemical system; it can be expressed as the product of the concentration of the substance and its activity coefficient (a measure of its deviation from ideality).

3. (symbol A), a measure of the strength of a radioactive source, defined as the number of atoms that disintegrate per unit time. It is given in units of curies, millicuries, or microcuries, as the number of recorded counts per unit time. Also called *radioactivity*.

4. a measurement of the catalytic activity of an enzyme preparation, expressed in micromoles per time unit. The common international enzyme unit (U) for expressing the activity of enzymes has the dimension of micromoles of substrate consumed per minute. A new unit used in the SI system, the katal (kat), is moles per second (kat $= 6 \times 10^7$ U).

5. see *optical activity*.

activity determination a potentiometric measurement performed on biologic fluids that compares the activity of an ion in an unknown solution with that in standard solutions. This is done by measuring the potentials produced by an ion-selective electrode against those produced by some reference electrode. An example is the pH determination using a pH meter—the measurement of hydrogen ion activity. The term is also applied to the measurement of the catalytic properties of enzymes.

activity ratio the ratio of the number of records in a computer file that are accessed or modified to the total number of records in the file.

cumulated a. ($\widetilde{A}$), see under *dose estimate*.

actomyosin (ak″to-mi′o-sin) a contractile protein formed by the interaction of actin and myosin found in large quantities in muscle cells and present as microfilaments in many cell types.

actuate (ak′choo-āt) [L. *actuare*, from *actus* an act] to put a mechanism into motion or action.

acu/o (ak'u-o) [L. *acus* needle] a word element used in combining form to denote sharpness, e.g., acupuncture.

acupuncture (ak"u-pungk'chūr) [*acu-* + L. *punctura* a prick] a form of therapy, originated by the Chinese, that involves piercing specific peripheral nerves with needles to relieve the discomfort associated with painful disorders, to induce surgical anesthesia, and for therapeutic purposes. Recent studies have shown that the procedure may mitigate pain through the release of enkephalin, a naturally occurring endorphin that has potent opiatelike effects. Acupuncture is still undergoing evaluation in the West and the extent of its usefulness in Western medicine is not yet clear.

acute (ah-kūt') [L. *acutus* sharp] 1. sharp.

2. having a short and relatively severe course, used to describe the progress of a disease. For diseases or conditions beginning with this adjective, see the noun. Cf. *chronic.*

acyclovir (a-si'klo-ver) a guanosine analog used in the treatment of herpes infections. It is an important, relatively safe antiviral agent and appears to be specific for virus-induced enzymes. A sensitive thymidine kinase appears to be central to the antiviral activity of this drug against herpes simplex and varicella-zoster viruses and to the selectivity of its action; the sensitivity of Epstein-Barr virus may be due to its highly sensitive DNA polymerase rather than to any thymidine kinase. See also *antiviral agent.*

acyesis (a"si-e'sis) [*a-* neg. + Gr. *kyēsis* pregnancy] 1. sterility of the female.

2. absence of pregnancy.

acyl (as'il) [*acid* + *-yl*] a radical formed by removing a hydroxyl group from an organic acid. RCO— is the general formula. The R group may be aliphatic, alicyclic, or aromatic. An example is acetyl, CH_3CO—. The term may be used alone as a general term or in combination to describe a specific class of compounds, as in acyl halide.

acylation (as"ĕ-la'shun) any process that involves the substitution of an acyl group into a molecule.

acylcarnitine (as'il-kar'nĭ-tēn) an *O*-ester of carnitine that mediates the transfer of fatty acyl groups from the cytoplasm to the mitochondrial matrix for oxidation purposes. Carnitine is L-3-hydroxy-4-trimethylammonium butyrate and is capable of coupling to a fatty acyl group in a high-energy linkage.

Fatty acids that enter the cell must be activated before they are metabolized. This activation process consists of a fatty acid reacting with coenzyme A (CoASH) to form acyl coenzyme A thioester (fatty acyl CoA). The mitochondrial membranes are impermeable to acyl CoA thioesters; however, this transport is accomplished by carnitine, which functions as a shuttle within the mitochondrial membranes. It accepts a fatty acyl group at the cytoplasmic side to form acylcarnitine and gives up the acyl group at the matrix side to CoASH to form fatty acyl CoASH and carnitine. In a similar fashion, carnitine is used in the transport of acetyl groups from the mitochondrial matrix to the cytoplasm, where the two carbon fragments can be used for either fatty acid or cholesterol synthesis.

acyl carrier protein see under *carrier protein.*

acyl coenzyme A a compound identical in structure to acetyl coenzyme A, except that it is made from long-chain fatty acids instead of the two-carbon acetic acid. It is also like acetyl CoA in being a high-energy thiol ester. It is the activated form of a fatty acid that can enter biosynthetic and biodegradative reactions.

acyl halide (as'il hal'īd) a compound formed by replacement of the —OH group of a carboxylic acid with a halogen atom. Also called *acid halide.*

acyloxy group (as"il-ok'se) the organic group (RCOO—) formed by the removal of a hydrogen from a carboxylic acid.

acyl peroxide (as'il per-ok'sīd) an organic compound containing two acyloxy (RCOO—) groups bonded together. See also *functional groups.*

***N*-acylsphingosine** (as"il-sfing'go-sēn) see *ceramide.*

acylsphingosine deacylase (a'sĭl-sfing'go-sēn de-a'sĭl-ās) an enzyme of the hydrolase class (*N*-acylsphingosine amidohydrolase, EC 3.5.1.23) that catalyzes the reaction *N*-acylsphingosine + $H_2O \rightleftarrows$ sphingosine + a fatty acid anion. A genetic deficiency of the enzyme, transmitted as an autosomal recessive trait, results in lipid accumulation in lysosomes, a condition known as Farber's disease. Also called *ceramidase.*

AD abbrev. for *alcohol dehydrogenase.*

ad- (ad) [L. *ad* to, toward] a prefix word element to denote toward, addition to, nearness, or intensification, e.g., adrenal.

ADA abbrev. See *adenosine deaminase.*

adactyly (a-dak'tĭ-le) [*a-* neg. + Gr. *daktylos* finger] congenital absence of the fingers or toes.

1-adamantanamine (ad"ah-man-tan'ah-mēn) see *amantadine.*

adamantinoma (ad"ah-man"-tĭ-no'mah) [*adamantine,* from Gr. *adamantinos* like a diamond + *ōma* swelling] see *ameloblastoma.*

adamantoblast (ad"ah-man'to-blast) [Gr. *adamas, diamond* + *blastos* germ] see *ameloblast* and *ameloblastoma.*

adaptation (ad"ap-ta'shun) [L. *adaptare* to fit] 1. the response of the eye to changing ambient light levels; see *dark a.* and *light a.*

2. the decline in the firing frequency of a neuron, particularly a receptor, under conditions of constant stimulation.

3. any evolutionary change in the behavioral, morphologic, anatomic, or physiologic characteristics of a species that improves its fitness. These changes are sometimes acquired through the process of natural selection over generations of exposure to an environmental stress (genetic adaptation). However, natural selection does not lead inevitably to adaptation.

4. the capacity for or process of adjusting to other organisms or to specific environmental conditions, particularly adverse ones. These adjustments are usually predetermined responses to the specific climatic stresses encountered (physiologic adaptation).

dark a., increase in sensitivity of the eye. The process occurs gradually, taking 5–10 min for the cones (color vision) to adapt, and 30–60 min for the rods (black and white vision). Also called scotopic adaptation.

light a., reduction in sensitivity of the eye in response to bright illumination. Also called photopic adaptation.

adapter (ah-dap'ter) 1. a device by which incompatible devices can be connected.

2. the device inserted in a centrifuge cup to allow a smaller sample holder to be used.

adaptive (a-dap'tiv) being capable of adaptation.

adaptive enzyme any enzyme formed as a response to the availability of a specific subtrate for the enzyme. Also called inducible enzyme.

adaptometer (ad"ap-tom'ĕ-ter) [*adaptation* + Gr. *metron* measure] an instrument for measuring the time required for retinal adaptation, i.e., for regeneration of rhodopsin. Adaptometers are used to detect night blindness, vitamin A deficiency, and retinitis pigmentosa.

ADC abbrev. See *analog-to-digital converter.*

ADCC abbrev. See *antibody-dependent cell-mediated cytotoxicity.*

addict (ad'ikt) [L. *addictus* given over, from *addicere* to sentence, award] a person who is dependent on a substance for psychologic or physiologic reasons. Such dependence includes the desire to avoid the unpleasant effects of withdrawal as well as the desire for the sensations caused by using the substance. When the physiology of addicts is altered by use of and/or withdrawal from the substance, they are said to be physically dependent. Dependence in the absence of physical dependence is known as psychologic dependence.

addiction (ah-dik'shun) the state of being given up to some habit. The term refers particularly to a drug dependence characterized by tolerance and physical dependence, and by detrimental effects on the individual and society. See also *drug d.* under *dependence.*

Addis count (ad'is) [Thomas *Addis,* San Francisco physician, 1881–1949] quantitative determination of the red blood cell count, white blood cell count, and casts in an aliquot of a 12-hr urine specimen. Designed to assess the degree of activity of chronic glomerulonephritis, this procedure is now seldom used as a diagnostic test; however, many physicians consider it helpful in following pediatric renal disease.

Addison's anemia (ad'ĭ-sonz) [Thomas *Addison,* English physician, 1793–1860] see *pernicious a.* under *anemia.*

Addison's disease [Thomas *Addison*] see *primary h.* under *hypoadrenocorticism.*

addisonian crisis (ad"ĭ-so'ne-an)[Thomas *Addison*] symptoms of fatigue, nausea and vomiting, weight loss, hypotension, and collapse, which accompany an acute attack of Addison's disease.

Addison's planes [Christopher *Addison,* English anatomist, 1869–1951] a group of imaginary planes used as anatomic landmarks of the thorax and abdomen. The vertical planes are the median (midsagittal) plane, the two spinous planes passing through the anterior superior iliac spines, and two lateral sagittal planes midway between the spinous planes and the median plane. Two transverse (horizontal) planes pass through the jugular notch of the sternum and the upper edge of the pubic symphysis. The transthoracic, transpyloric, and transtubercular planes (going from top to bottom) are spaced at equal intervals between them. See also *abdominal regions.*

Addison's point [Christopher *Addison*] the midpoint of the epigastric region.

addition reaction in organic chemistry, a reaction in which groups are attached to carbon atoms at a double or triple bond (or to a single bond in a strained ring), thus decreasing the degree of unsaturation of the substrate, e.g., $Br_2 + CH_2 = CH_2 \rightarrow CH_2BrCH_2Br$. See also *elimination reaction* and *substitution reaction.*

additive (ad'ĭ-tiv) [L. *additivus,* from *addere* to add] 1. characterized by addition.

2. a substance such as a flavoring agent, preservative, or vitamin, which is added to another substance to improve its flavor or appearance, to retard deterioration, to increase its nutritional value, and so forth.

address in computer terminology, the specific location of a particular piece of information, or the name or number that identifies a register, memory location, or storage device.

adduct (ah-dukt') [L. *adductus,* from *adducere* to draw toward] 1. to draw toward the median plane or (for the fingers and toes) toward the axis or axial line of a limb.

2. a chemical compound formed when two species are chemically added, or a complex compound formed by the unbonded association of two molecules.

adduction (ah-duk'shun) the act of adducting or the state of being adducted.

adductor (ah-duk'tor) [L.] a muscle, such as the pectoralis major, that moves a bone toward another part (toward the median plane).

Adelomycetes (ah-de"lo-mi-se'tēz) [Gr. *adēlos* invisible, obscure + *myketes* fungi] see *Deuteromycetes.*

aden/o (ad'ĕ-no) [Gr. *adēn, adenos* gland] a word element used in combining form to denote gland, e.g., adenocarcinoma.

adendritic (a"den-drit'ik) [*a-* neg. + Gr. *dendron* tree] lacking dendrites.

adenine (ad'e-nēn) [Gr. *adēn* gland] 6-aminopurine, $C_5H_5N_5$. One of the purine base constituents of both classes of nucleic acids (DNA and RNA). Adenine is present in adenosine, AMP, ADP, ATP, and cyclic AMP, and it pairs with thymine in DNA and uracil in RNA.

adenine arabinoside (ara-A) see *vidarabine.*

adenitis (ad"ĕ-ni'tis) [*aden-* + *-itis* inflammation] inflammation of a gland. The term is commonly used to refer to inflammation of a lymph node, more properly termed lymphadenitis.

adenoacanthoma (ad"ĕ-no-ak"an-tho'mah) endometrial adenocarcinoma, usually well differentiated, with benign squamous differentiation. The term adenoacanthoma has also been used to refer to mixed adenosquamous carcinoma; consequently, the term is a confusing one.

adenocarcinoma (ad"ĕ-no-kar"si-no'mah) [*adeno-* + *carcinoma,* from Gr. *karkinos* crab + *-oma* swelling] a malignant neoplasm originating from glandular epithelial cells or in which the neoplastic cells form glandular structures. It may be classified according to the predominant pattern of cell arrangement (such as papillary or alveolar) or by cell product (such as mucinous).

adenofibroma (ad″ĕ-no-fi-bro′mah) [*adeno-* + L. *fibra* thread + Gr. *ōma* swelling] a benign ovarian neoplasm composed of glandular elements in an abundant fibrous stroma.

adenohypophysis (ad″ĕ-no-hi-pof′ĭ-sis) [*adeno-* + *hypophysis*] the part of the pituitary gland, embryologically derived from the craniopharyngeal diverticulum (Rathke's pouch), that includes the anterior lobe. See also *hypophysis.*

adenoid/o (ad′ĕ-noid-o) [Gr. *adenoeidēs* glandlike, from *adēn, adenos* gland + *eidos* form] a word element used in combining form to denote adenoids, e.g., adenoiditis.

adenoid cystic carcinoma a malignant salivary tumor, most common in the parotid gland. The cells display a cribriform arrangement that becomes more solid with loss of differentiation. This tumor frequently infiltrates widely and surgical eradication may be difficult or impossible. Metastases initially involve regional nodes, but distant spread may ensue. Also called *cylindroma.* See also *salivary gland tumors.*

adenoma (ad″ĕ-no′mah) [*adeno-* + Gr. *-oma* swelling] a term used to denote a benign epithelial neoplasm that forms glandular structures, e.g., thyroid adenoma, or a benign epithelial neoplasm derived from a glandular epithelium but not producing a glandular pattern e.g., adrenocortical adenoma. See also *polyp, polyposis,* and the specific adenoma.

adenomatoid (ad″ĕ-no′mah-toid) [*adenoma* + Gr. *eidos* form] resembling adenoma.

adenomatoid tumor a rather uncommon benign neoplasm that arises from the serosal surface of the epididymis or uterine tube. It has a distinctive histologic appearance: tubular channels lined by cuboidal cells are set in a stroma of loose connective tissue. Ultrastructurally, the cells resemble mesothelial cells.

adenomatosis (ad″ĕ-no″mah-to′sis) [*adenoma-* + *-osis* condition] the formation of numerous adenomatous growths.

adenomatous (ad″ĕ-nom′ah-tus) a term used to describe those hyperplasias whose glands exhibit budding and branching. See also *adenomatous h.* under *hyperplasia.*

adenomyoma (ad″ĕ-no-mi-o′mah) [*adeno-* + Gr. *mys* muscle + *ōma* swelling] 1. a benign neoplasm composed of endometrial, glandular, and stromal elements and smooth muscle.

2. the occurrence of adenomyosis within a uterine leiomyoma.

adenomyosis (ad″ĕ-no-mi-o′sis) [*adeno-* + Gr. *mys* muscle + *-osis* condition] the presence of benign endometrial glands and stroma deep within the myometrium and not in continuity with the endometrium lining the uterine cavity.

adenopathy (ad″ĕ-nop′ah-the) [*adeno-* + Gr. *pathos* disease] a disease of a gland. Cf. *lymphadenopathy.*

adenosine (A) (ah-den′o-sēn) 6-amino-9-β-D-ribofuranosyl-9H-purine, a nucleoside composed of adenine and ribose; M.W. 267.24. Also called 9-β-D-ribofuranosyl-adenine. See also *adenine.*

adenosine arabinoside see *vidarabine.*

adenosine 3′, 5′-cyclic monophosphate see *cyclic adenosine monophosphate.*

adenosine deaminase (ADA) (ah-den′o-sēn de-ah′min-ās) an enzyme of the hydrolase class (adenosine aminohydrolase, EC 3.5.4.4) that catalyzes the reaction adenosine + $H_2O \rightleftharpoons$ inosine + NH_3. Some individuals with combined immunodeficiency syndrome are deficient in adenosine deaminase. See also *adenosine deaminase deficiency.*

adenosine deaminase assays determinations of the serum ADA activity performed by incubating serum with buffered adenosine (substrate) and measuring the ammonia formed with the Berthelot reaction.

adenosine deaminase deficiency a metabolic disorder, transmitted as an autosomal recessive trait, that is characterized by a relative or absolute deficiency of the enzyme adenosine deaminase. This enzyme catalyzes the deamination of adenosine to inosine and provides a revitalization pathway for purines. Deficiencies of this enzyme have been found in many individuals with severe combined immunodeficiency, an immunologic disorder with severe abnormalities of T-cell function and somewhat milder B-cell dysfunction. The mechanism of this association is unknown. Those affected with adenosine deaminase deficiency display abnormal Hassall's corpuscles and increased susceptibility to bacterial and viral infections. Bone lesions, including radiolucent bands in long bones and abnormalities of the spine, scapulas, and pelvis, are also seen.

adenosine diphosphate (ADP) (ah-den′o-sēn di-fos′fāt) a nucleotide, adenosine-5′-pyrophosphate, that occurs in all cells, where it is involved in energy metabolism and other processes. Its structure is represented as A — P ∾ P, where A is the adenosine nucleoside moiety, P is a phosphate group, ∾ represents a high-energy phosphate bond (an acid anhydride bond between phosphate groups), and — represents the ester linkage of the adenosine monophosphate (AMP) moiety. Hydrolysis of the high-energy bond, yielding AMP and inorganic phosphate, ADP + $H_2O \rightarrow$ AMP + P_i, releases 36,000 J/mol. The production of ADP by the hydrolysis of adenosine triphosphate (ATP) drives many biochemical processes. ADP is also produced in the regeneration of ATP from AMP, the first step of which is the reaction ATP + AMP $\rightleftharpoons$ 2 ADP, catalyzed by AMP kinase.

ADP is converted back to ATP primarily by the tricarboxylic acid (TCA) cycle and oxidative phosphorylation. ADP is an activator of the enzymes 6-phosphofructokinase and isocitrate dehydrogenase; thus, its concentration is one variable regulating glycolysis and the TCA cycle; it also induces platelet aggregation and causes clot retraction.

See also *adenosine triphosphate* and *platelet.*

adenosine monophosphate (AMP) (ah-den′o-sēn mon″o-fos′fāt) a nucleotide, adenosine-5′-phosphate, that occurs in all cells, where it is involved in energy metabolism and other processes. It is an effector involved in the regulation of the enzymes phosphofructokinase and glycogen phosphorylase, which in turn are involved in glucose metabolism. Also called *adenylic acid.* See also *adenosine diphosphate* and *adenosine triphosphate.*

adenosine 3′,5′-monophosphate see *cyclic adenosine monophosphate.*

adenosine triphosphatase (ATPase) (ah-den′o-sēn tri-fos′fah-tās) an enzyme of the hydrolase class (ATP phosphohydrolase, EC 3.6.1.3) that catalyzes the reaction ATP + $H_2O \rightleftarrows$ ADP + orthophosphate. The reaction releases energy that can be used for cell activities such as muscle contraction, maintenance of concentration gradients, transport of molecules across cell membranes, and regulation of calcium concentrations. Also called *adenylpyrophosphatase* and *myosin* (for the enzyme present in muscle).

adenosine triphosphate (ATP) (ah-den'o-sēn tri-fos'fāt) a nucleotide, adenosine-5'-triphosphate, that occurs in all cells, where it functions as the "common currency" of energy. Its structure is represented as A — P ∾ P ∾ P, where A is the adenosine nucleoside moiety, P is a phosphate group, ∾ represents a high-energy phosphate bond (an acid anhydride bond between phosphate groups), and — represents the ester linkage of the adenosine monophosphate (AMP) moiety. ATP is also represented as AMP ∾ P ∾ P. Hydrolysis of the terminal bond, yielding adenosine diphosphate (ADP) and inorganic phosphate (P_i), ATP + $H_2O \rightarrow$ ADP + P_i, releases 36,800 J/mol. Hydrolysis of the inner bond, yielding AMP and inorganic pyrophosphate (PP_i), ATP + $H_2O \rightarrow$ AMP + PP_i, releases 40,600 J/mol. Both of these reactions are used to drive biologic processes, which would be thermodynamically unfavorable if not coupled to the hydrolysis of ATP.

Thus, ATP provides the energy for molecular synthesis, for muscular contraction, and for the active transport of molecules and ions across cell membranes against concentration gradients. ATP also serves as a source of phosphate in phosphorylation reactions: ATP + X $\rightleftarrows$ ADP + X ∾ P, where X is a metabolite such as glucose, creatinine, or another nucleotide. Most of the ATP is produced from ADP by the tricarboxylic acid cycle and oxidative phosphorylation; some is produced by glycolysis.

adenosis (ad"ĕ-no'sis) [*aden-* + *-osis* condition] a nonneoplastic glandular hyperplasia, or the abnormal formation or location of glandular tissue.

a. of breast, one of the most common types of epithelial hyperplasia and hypertrophy of the breast, characterized by proliferation of small ducts and lobules in the breast; it is often seen in association with cystic disease of the breast. The ducts may end blindly (blunt duct adenosis), or the glands may be compressed and distorted by dense sheets of collagen (sclerosing adenosis). Adenosis is not associated with an increased risk of developing breast carcinoma. See also *cystic disease of breast.*

vaginal a., the occurrence of benign mucus-forming epithelium or glands within the mucosa of the vagina, commonly the middle third. The glands resemble those of the endocervix and may originate from mesonephric remnants. Symptoms, if present, are usually produced by excessive mucus secretion.

***S*-adenosyl-L-homocysteine** (SAH) (ah-den'o-sil ho"mo-sis'tēn) a product of transmethylation reactions utilizing *S*-adenosyl-L-methionine (SAM). See also *S-adenosyl-L-methionine.*

***S*-adenosyl-L-methionine** (SAM) (ah-den'o-sil mĕ-thi'o-nēn) an activated methyl donor compound formed from adenosine triphosphate (ATP) and methionine in which the *S* atom of methionine is bound to the ribose of adenosine. It is a high-energy compound serving as a methyl donor in transmethylation reactions. Products of transmethylation are the methylated acceptor and *S*-adenosyl-L-homocysteine (SAH).

adenovirus (ad"ĕ-no-vi'rus) [*adeno-* + *virus*] one of a group of double-stranded DNA viruses that may cause a latent infection of the tonsils and adenoids in children, as well as various respiratory infections in adults. Adenovirus was initially isolated from a tissue culture of adenoids in plasma. The virus particle is not enveloped and has an icosahedral capsid with 252 capsomeres. Projecting from the capsid are 12 fibers with terminal knobs. Adenovirus contains no lipid and is relatively resistant to heat and acid, which may explain its survival in the throat and respiratory and alimentary tracts (it can also be found in human feces). At present, 33 serotypes have been accepted; three candidate viruses, types 34, 35, and 36, are under consideration as additional serotypes. The adenovirus replicates its viral DNA and assembles the virion within the nucleus of the host cell. Adenovirus can transform host cells into a malignant state in vitro.

Adenovirus occurs most commonly in acute respiratory disease (ARD); types 3, 4, and 7 are most often responsible for epidemics of ARD in military recruits, and types 1, 2, 3, and 5 are most often encountered in pediatric patients. Clinical symptoms include pharyngitis, cough, headache, fever, and lymphadenopathy. In children, the adenovirus may spread to the lower respiratory tract. Adenovirus may also cause epidemic keratoconjunctivitis (type 8) and has been associated with various alimentary tract disorders, as well as acute hemorrhagic cystitis and meningoencephalitis; see also the accompanying table.

Pathologically, the virus multiplies in the local area of infection and has an incubation period of 5–7 da. Adenovirus infection usually results in high specific antibody titers; this acquired immunity is long-lasting. Adenovirus infections most often occur in the summer and winter seasons.

Human adenovirus is species-specific, spreading from human to human. However, this virus can also survive for a limited time in sewage, swimming pools, or similar environments. All adenoviruses account for less than 5 percent of the total human viral respiratory diseases.

Laboratory diagnosis of adenovirus infection is made by recovery of the virus from throat, feces, or conjunctiva. The virus may be cultured in human epithelial cell cultures, primary embryonic kidney cells, or HeLa cells. In these cell lines, the adenovirus causes the rounding, swelling, and aggregating of culture cells after 2–4 wk. The isolated virus may then be identified serologically by a complement-fixation test, and can be serologically typed by the hemagglutination inhibition test.

adenylate (ah-den-ĭ'lāt) the anion of adenylic acid, or a salt or ester of adenylic acid.

adenylate cyclase (ah"-den-ĭ'lāt si'klās) an enzyme of the lyase class (ATP pyrophosphate-lyase [cyclizing], EC 4.6.1.1.) that catalyzes the reaction ATP $\rightleftarrows$ cyclic AMP + pyrophosphate. The enzyme occurs in plasma cell membranes and is activated by hormones, e.g., epinephrine, vasopressin, glucagon, and corticotropin, with the resultant cyclic AMP serving as an important metabolic regulator. Also called *adenyl cyclase.* See also *cyclic adenosine monophosphate.*

adenylate kinase (ah-den-ĭ'lāt ki'nās) an enzyme of the transferase class, (ATP:AMP phosphotransferase, EC 2.7.4.3.) that catalyzes the reaction ATP + AMP = 2 ADP. It occurs predominantly in muscle

ADENOVIRUS. ILLNESSES MOST COMMONLY ASSOCIATED WITH ADENOVIRUS INFECTIONS

DISEASE	INDIVIDUALS MOST AT RISK	PRINCIPAL IMMUNOTYPE
Acute febrile pharyngitis	Infants, young children	1,2,3,5,6,7
Pharyngoconjunctival fever	School age children	3,7,14
Acute respiratory disease	Military recruits	3,4,7,14,21
Pneumonia	Infants, young children	1,2,3,7
Pneumonia	Military recruits	4,7
Epidemic keratoconjunctivitis	Any age group	8,11,19
Pertussis-like syndrome	Infants, young children	5
Acute hemorrhagic cystitis	Infants, young children	11

From Lennette, E. H., and Schmidt, N. J.: Diagnostic Procedure for Viral, Rickettsial and Chlamydial Infections. Washington, DC, American Public Health Association, 1979, p. 230.

and is of great importance in energy metabolism. Also called AMP kinase and *myokinase.* See also *adenosine diphosphate.*

adenyl cyclase (ad′ĕ-nil si′klās) see *adenylate cyclase.*

adenylic acid (ad″ĕ-nil′ik) see *adenosine monophosphate.*

adenylosuccinate (ad″ĕ-nil-o-suk′sĭ-nāt) a derivative of adenylic and succinic acids, which is an intermediate in the synthesis of AMP and is cleaved to form adenylic acid plus fumaric acid.

adenylpyrophosphatase (ad″ĕ-nil-pi″ro-fos′fah-tās) see *adenosine triphosphatase.*

adenylyl (ad′ĕ-nĭ-lil) a term for adenylic acid when it is being named as a substituent on some parent group or as an ester.

adenylylation (ad″ĕ-nĭ-lĭ-la′shun) the process of transferring a 5′-adenylyl group from adenosine triphosphate to form a phosphodiester linkage with another compound, such as a tyrosine in a protein molecule. The glutamine synthetase enzyme of *Escherichia coli* is regulated by adenylylation and deadenylylation.

ADH abbrev. See *alcohol dehydrogenase, antidiuretic hormone.*

adherence (ad-hēr′ens) [L. *adhaerens,* from *adhaerere* to stick to] 1. the act or quality of sticking to something.

2. the ability of certain bacteria with special surface macromolecules to cling to specific receptors on some animal and human cells, thus promoting the selective colonization of body surfaces by normal flora.

adhesion (ad-he′zhun) [L. *adhaesio,* from *adhaerere* to stick to] 1. the property of firm attachment.

2. the stable joining of parts to each other.

3. the union of two surfaces that are normally separate; also, any fibrous band or structure that connects them.

adiaspiromycosis (ad″ĭ-ah-spi″ro-mi-ko′sis) a rare pulmonary disease that involves the development of nonreplicating adiaspores from the inhaled aleuriospores of saprophytic soil fungi belonging to the genus *Emmonsia,* chiefly *E. parvum* and *E. crescens.* It may be mistaken for the tissue phase of *Coccidioides immitis.* This condition is commonly found in rodents and small animals, and is rarely reported in humans. Also called *adiasporosis* and haplomycosis.

adiasporosis (ad″ĭ-ah-spor-o′sis) see *adiaspiromycosis.*

Adie's pupil (a′dēz) [William John *Adie,* British neurologist, 1886–1935] a pupil that responds to accommodation and convergence in a very slow, delayed manner; when accommodation is relaxed, the pupil remains constricted for an excessive time, dilating very gradually. Initially there is usually the complaint of unequal pupils or visual blurring. Examination often reveals no other abnormality except for depressed or absent tendon reflexes in the legs. There is no specific treatment. Also called tonic pupil.

adip/o (ad′ĭ-po) [L. *adeps, adipis* fat] a word element used in combining form to denote fat, e.g., adiposis.

adiphenine hydrochloride (ah-di′fen-ēn) a synthetic parasympatholytic drug used as a smooth muscle relaxant. Adverse reactions are similar to those of atropine.

adipic (ah-dip′ik) pertaining to adipose.

adipocyte (ad′ĭ-po-sit″) [*adipo-* + Gr. *kytos* hollow vessel] a fat cell; a signet ring–shaped cell with a single, large lipid inclusion and displaced nucleus and cytoplasm.

adipokinesis (ad″ĭ-po-ki-ne′sis) [*adipo-* + Gr. *kinēsis* motion, from *kinein* to move] the mobilization of fat in the body, often with the release of free fatty acids into the blood.

adipolysis (ad″ĭ-pol′ĭ-sis) [*adipo-* + Gr. *lysis* dissolution] see *lipolysis.*

adipolytic (ad″ĭ-po-lit′ik) see *lipolytic.*

adiponecrosis (ad″ĭ-po-nĕ-kro′sis) [*adipo-* + Gr. *nekrōsis* death] inflammation and cell death in fatty tissue associated with pancreatic disease such as pancreatitis and ancinar carcinoma.

adipose (ad′ĭ-pōs) [N.L. *adiposus* fatty] composed of or pertaining to fat, as in adipose tissue.

adipose tissue fatty tissue, fat; a type of connective tissue made up of cells containing large amounts of cytoplasmic lipid supported by a delicate matrix of collagen fibrils. Fat cells are the principal site of energy storage in mammals. In routine histologic processing, lipid solvents remove the fat, leaving vacuolated cells.

brown a. t., a type of adipose tissue whose main function is heat production. Although plentiful in hibernating animals, in the human body it is confined to small deposits in the vicinity of the limb girdles that are gradually replaced with white adipose tissue as the individual ages. The cells of brown adipose tissue contain many mitochondria and are directly innervated by sympathetic adrenergic neurons. Brown adipose tissue is not influenced by starvation or overfeeding, but rapidly mobilizes lipid in response to cold.

adiposis (ad″ĭ-po′sis) [*adipo-* + *-osis* condition] a condition marked by deposits or degeneration of fatty tissue.

a. dolorosa, a poorly defined disorder of painful subcutaneous lipomas sometimes associated with evidence (such as motor weakness, decreased cutaneous sensation, and asthenia) of a peripheral neuropathy. There may be accompanying obesity. Siblings may be affected.

a. hepatica, fatty degeneration of the liver.

adipsia (a-dip′se-ah) [*a-* neg. + Gr. *dipsa* thirst + *-ia*] an absence of thirst; abnormal avoidance of drinking.

aditus (ad′ĭ-tus), pl. *aditus* [L.] [NA], a general term for the entrance or opening to an organ or structure.

adjacent (ad-ja′sent) next to, adjoining, lying near.

adjuvant (ad′ju-vant) [L. *adjuvans,* from *adiuvare* to aid] 1. assisting or aiding.

2. a substance that aids another, such as an auxiliary remedy. In immunology, the term refers to any substance that enhances the potency of an antigen and results in a superior immune response. There are two types: those that possess the ability to enhance both cellular and humoral response to a large number of antigens (general potentiation), and those that strengthen specific responses to only a few antigens (specific potentiation). Adjuvants work by several mechanisms, including prolongation of antigen release, improving immunogenicity by antigen denaturation, recruitment of other immunocompetent cells, and induction of inflammation.

ad lib abbrev. for *ad libitum* (as desired).

admittance (*A*) (ad-mit′ans) the reciprocal of impedance, the peak current divided by the peak voltage in an alternating current circuit. The unit of admittance is the reciprocal ohm (Ω^{-1}) or mho.

ADN-B assay see *anti-DNase B assay.*

adnexa (ad-nek′sah) [L. "connected parts," from *adnectere* to connect to] appendages; accessory organs or adjunct parts (such as the eyelids and the lacrimal glands in the eyes).

adnexal (ad-nek′sal) pertaining to adnexa.

adnexal neoplasms a group of neoplasms that develop from pilosebaceous structures and eccrine and apocrine ducts and glands in the dermis. They are classified according to their structure of origin, histologic appearance, and histochemical properties.

Adnexal neoplasms of the skin, which are often benign, include trichoepithelioma, pilomatrixoma, cylindroma, syringocystadenoma papilliferum, syringoma, eccrine spiradenoma, and nevus sebaceus.

For more information, see the specific neoplasm.

adoral (ad-o′ral) [*ad-* + L. *os, oris* mouth] 1. situated near the mouth.

2. directed toward the mouth.

ADP abbrev. See *adenosine diphosphate, automatic data processing.*

ADP/ATP ratio a measure of the phosphate potential. This ratio is of importance metabolically in the regulation of cellular metabolism to permit oxidative phosphorylation with the formation of ATP, or in the expenditure of ATP in the biosynthesis of storage fuels, namely, glycogen and triacylglycerols.

adren/o (ah-dre′no) [*ad-* + L. *ren* kidney] a word element used in combining form to denote a relationship to the adrenal glands, e.g., adrenomegaly.

adrenal/o (ah-dre′nal-o) [*ad-* + L. *renalis* pertaining to the kidneys] a word element used in combining form to denote a relationship to the adrenal glands, e.g., adrenalectomy.

adrenal (ah-dre′nal) pertaining to or originating from the adrenal gland.

adrenal cortex the outer portion of the adrenal gland, which produces the corticosteroid hormones; see also under *adrenal glands.*

adrenal cortical hyperplasia see *Cushing's syndrome.*

adrenal crisis see *primary h.* under *hypoadrenocorticism.*

adrenal function test see *adrenocorticotropic hormone stimulation test* and *dexamethasone suppression test.*

adrenal glands paired endocrine glands located atop the kidneys. They lie within the renal fascia, are roughly conical in shape, and receive a rich arterial supply. Each gland consists of a yellow cortex and a slender gray core, the medulla. In the adult the cortex consists of three concentric zones of cells. The outer layer is thin and sometimes incomplete; termed the zona glomerulosa, its cells form round clusters. In the middle zone, the zona fasciculata, the polyhedral cells form radial columns separated by fenestrated sinusoids. In the innermost zone, the zona reticularis, the cords of cells are irregularly arranged.

The cells of the adrenal cortex form steroid hormones and ultrastructurally possess cytoplasmic lipid, considerable quantities of smooth (agranular) endoplasmic reticulum, and, frequently, mitochondria with tubular cristae. Aldosterone is formed in the zona glomerulosa and is the most important mineralocorticoid hormone: it functions in the regulation of extracellular fluid volume and potassium metabolism. Release of aldosterone is regulated by the renin-angiotensin system and potassium. Two other types of corticosteroid hormone are formed in the inner zones of the cortex. Glucocorticoids, principally cortisol (hydrocortisone), regulate protein, carbohydrate, lipid, and nucleic acid metabolism. Androgens stimulate male secondary sex characteristics. Release of hormones from the zonae fasciculata and reticularis is effected by the adrenocorticotropic hormone (ACTH) of the anterior pituitary. The two most common disorders of the adrenal cortex are Addison's disease and Cushing's syndrome.

The adrenal cortex is embryologically of mesodermal origin, developing during the second month of embryonic life as a proliferation of cells on the dorsal wall of the coelomic cavity. It is then invaded by the medullary cells, which are of ectodermal derivation. The fetal adrenal cortex degenerates during the first two postnatal weeks, and residual cells proliferate to produce the characteristic zonation of the adult cortex.

Cells of the adrenal medulla are chromaffin cells and sympathetic ganglion cells. The former produce epinephrine (adrenaline) and norepinephrine (noradrenalin); their release is controlled by sympathetic nerves that synapse on the medullary cells. The hormones act similarly, aiding the body in coping with emergency situations by increasing cardiac output, elevating blood pressure, stimulating respiration, and accelerating glycogenolysis with a resulting increase in blood glucose and lactic acid.

Also called *suprarenal glands.* See also *adrenal tumors.*

adrenaline (ah-dren′ah-lēn) see *epinephrine.*

adrenal insufficiency see *hypoadrenocorticism.*

adrenal medulla the central part of the adrenal gland, which produces epinephrine and norepinephrine; see also under *adrenal glands.*

adrenal scan a procedure in nuclear medicine for imaging the adrenal glands, which utilizes a scintillation camera or a rectilinear scanner. The cholesterol analogs iodocholesterol I 131 and iodine-131-6β-iodomethyl-19-norcholesterol are concentrated by the normal adrenal cortex and by functioning adenomas, but not by carcinomas. The uptake of the imaging agent by normal tissue can be suppressed by administration of dexamethasone during the course of the study; tumor uptake is not suppressible.

Normal adrenal glands are bilaterally visualized 5–7 da after administration of the imaging agent. Hyperfunctioning glands are visualized earlier, and exhibit greater uptake. Unilateral visualization is due to the destruction of one adrenal gland or to an adenoma causing Cushing's syndrome; with cortisol-producing carcinomas neither gland can be visualized. Unequal visualization of the two glands is seen in unilateral pheochromocytoma or medullary hyperplasia, and in adenomas that produce aldosterone or androgens; visualization of these adenomas is improved by dexamethasone administration.

Posterior views are used and a high-energy collimator is necessary. Thyroid uptake of free ^{131}I is blocked by administration of iodine (Lugol's) solution or potassium perchlorate.

adrenal tumors neoplasms of the adrenal glands. Adenomas of the adrenal cortex are usually single, small encapsulated neoplasms. In primary aldosteronism (Conn's syndrome), the tumor is typically a small adenoma. In 10 percent of patients with Cushing's syndrome, the responsible lesion is an adrenal cortical adenoma, but more frequently the cortex shows hyperplasia: adenocarcinoma of the cortex is present in fewer than 20 percent of cases.

Most large tumors arising from the adrenal cortex are carcinomas—aggressive tumors with a high frequency of recurrence and a propensity for metastasis, particularly to liver, regional lymph nodes, and lungs. A minority are accompanied by clinical evidence of hypersecretion, such as Cushing's syndrome or virilism. Virilizing tumors in young children are usually malignant.

Embryologically and functionally, the adrenal medulla is part of the sympathetic nervous system. Approximately 50 percent of primary neuroblastomas develop within the gland; most of the others occur in the retroperitoneum or mediastinum. An occasional neuroblastoma is seen in an adult, but more than 80 percent of those affected are children under age 5 yr. The tumors are soft and hemorrhagic; most patients have metastases at the time of diagnosis, and more than two-thirds die within 3 yr. Histologically, the small round cells resemble lymphocytes, but they tend to form rosettes, and ultrastructurally have dendritic processes containing dense-core granules and microtubules. The amount of catecholamine formed by cells of a neuroblastoma may be detected by determination of the urinary concentrations of total catecholamines, homovanillic acid (HVA levels are generally more elevated than VMA in this tumor) and vanillylmandelic acid (VMA). Rarely, a neuroblastoma undergoes differentiation. If areas of differentiation are detected in sections of a neuroblastoma, the tumor is a ganglioneuroblastoma. The end stage of the differentiation process is the benign ganglioneuroma, which may be seen in older individuals.

Most pheochromocytomas arise within the adrenal gland. A minority of these tumors are malignant, but the histology of a particular tumor provides little indication of its potential behavior unless invasion of surrounding tissues or blood vessels can be demonstrated. The figure of 10 percent is often applied to this neoplasm, as roughly 10 percent are malignant, 10 percent are bilateral, and 10 percent are extraadrenal. It affects primarily adults. Other endocrine neoplasms may be present. The tumor cells are usually of moderate size, although pleomorphic forms are also common. The tumor displays the chromaffin reaction. Clinically, intermittent episodes of hypertension are characteristic, and the diagnosis can be confirmed by measurement of urinary catecholamines, metanephrines, and VMA.

For more information, see *ganglioneuroblastoma, ganglioneuroma, neuroblastoma,* and *pheochromocytoma.*

adrenergic (ad″ren-er′jik) [*adren-* + Gr. *ergon* work + *-ic*] 1. activated by, characteristic of, or secreting epinephrine or substances with similar activity; the term is also used to refer to those postganglionic sympathetic nerve fibers that liberate norepinephrine in response to a nerve impulse.

2. an agent that produces such an effect. Also called *sympathomimetic.* Cf. *cholinergic.*

adrenergic fibers postganglionic fibers of the sympathetic nervous system that release the neurotransmitter norepinephrine (noradrenalin) or, in some cases, dopamine, at their terminals. They innervate the heart, smooth muscle, and certain glands. Cf. *cholinergic fibers.*

adrenergic receptors postsynaptic membrane receptors in the central and sympathetic nervous systems that are stimulated by catecholamine neurotransmitters. In the sympathetic system, these are divided into two types: alpha (α) and beta (β) receptors; the β-receptors are further divided into β_1- and β_2-receptors.

Stimulation of the α-receptors produces vasoconstriction in the skin and viscera, causing a rise in blood pressure and also relaxing the gastrointestinal tract. Stimulation of β_1-receptors produces an increase in both the heart rate and the force of contractions. Stimulation of β_2-receptors produces vasodilation in skeletal and smooth muscles and also dilation of the bronchioles.

The various catecholamines have different effects: norepinephrine stimulates mainly α-receptors; isoproterenol, mainly the β-receptors; metaproterenol, mainly the β_2-receptors; and epinephrine, both α- and β-receptors.

Each type of receptor can be selectively blocked. Phentolamine and phenoxybenzamine are primarily α-blockers and cause peripheral vasodilation. Propranolol is a β-blocker, which produces a decrease in heart rate and output but can precipitate bronchospasm. Metoprolol, primarily a β_1-blocker, is less likely to produce bronchial constriction.

Also called *adrenoreceptor.*

adrenochrome (ad-re′no-krom″) [*adreno-* + Gr. *chrōma* color] an oxidation product of adrenaline, 1-methyl-3-hydroxy-5,6-indolinedione, and possibly an intermediate product in the chromaffin reaction.

adrenocortical (ad-re″no-kor′te-kal) [*adreno-* + *cortical,* from L. *cortex* bark] pertaining to or arising from the cortex of the adrenal gland.

adrenocortical insufficiency see *hypoadrenocorticism.*

adrenocorticotropic (ah-dre″no-kor″ti-ko-trop′ik) [*adreno-* + L. *cortex* bark + Gr. *tropos* a turn] having a stimulating effect on the adrenal cortex.

adrenocorticotropic hormone (ACTH) (ad-re″no-kor″te-ko-trop′ik) a single-chain polypeptide hormone produced by the anterior pituitary; M.W. 4507. It is the major regulator of adrenal cortical activity. It binds to receptors on the surface of the adrenal cortical cell, and through a cyclic AMP–mediated process stimulates the synthesis of corticosteroids from cholesterol. ACTH secretion is in turn controlled by corticotropin-releasing factor, which is secreted by the hypothalamus in response to low cortisol concentrations and stress. There is a circadian rhythm, which causes ACTH to be elevated in early morning and depressed in late afternoon and early evening. Increased concentrations are observed in Addison's disease, congenital adrenal hyperplasia, bilateral adrenalectomy, ectopic ACTH-secreting tumors, stress, electroshock therapy, hypoglycemia, and surgery. Decreased concentrations are seen in adrenal cancer and panhypopituitarism.

ACTH determinations are very useful in confirming the presence of an ectopic ACTH-producing tumor and in differentiating primary from secondary adrenal insufficiency, being elevated in the former and either normal or low in the latter. Reference ranges for ACTH are <90 pg/ml for samples drawn in the morning.

ACTH can also be demonstrated in tissue sections by use of immunoperoxidase techniques.

Also called *corticotropin.* See also *adrenocorticotropic hormone stimulation test, cortisol, dexamethasone suppression test,* and *metyrapone stimulation test.*

adrenocorticotropic hormone assays determination of the ACTH concentration in plasma by radioimmunoassay. Specimen collection must be properly timed because of the circadian variation in ACTH levels. To preserve ACTH from degradation by plasma proteases, the specimen must be maintained at 4°C and analyzed rapidly. The test is useful in differentiating primary from secondary adrenal insufficiency, in the differential diagnosis of Cushing's disease, and in the evaluation of tumors producing ectopic ACTH, such as oat cell carcinoma of the lung.

adrenocorticotropic hormone–releasing factor (ACTH-RF) see *corticotropin-releasing factor.*

adrenocorticotropic hormone stimulation test a functional test used mainly to distinguish between Addison's disease (primary adrenocortical insufficiency) and hypopituitarism. In a common procedure, a dose of 25 units of aqueous ACTH in normal saline is administered intravenously over 6–8 hr on 2–3 successive da. A normal response is a two- to fivefold increase in 17-hydroxycorticosteroids, a two- to threefold increase in 17-ketogenic steroids, and a twofold increase in 17-ketosteroid excretion in urine. Plasma cortisol levels should double within the first 30 min and should reach values of 36 to 60 μg/dl after 5 hr. In Addison's disease, there is little or no response to ACTH stimulation, whereas a gradual rise (staircase response) is observed in primary hypopituitarism after successive stimulations.

In the short stimulation test, administration of ACTH or 250 μg of cosyntropin (Cortrosyn, a synthetic polypeptide with ACTH-like activity) results in a normal increment of plasma cortisol of at least 7 μg/dl over the initial baseline of at least 5 μg/dl after 30 min. The response observed with this test is less consistent than that of the standard test.

These tests may also be of use in distinguishing Cushing's syndrome due to adrenocortical hyperplasia (a three- to fivefold increase in output of adrenal cortical hormones) from Cushing's syndrome due to adenocarcinoma (little or no response to stimulation).

If the test is performed in a case of suspected primary adrenal insufficiency, the patient is also given 2 mg/da of dexamethasone to prevent a fatal adrenal crisis.

See also *cortisol, cosyntropin, Cushing's syndrome* and *primary h.* under *hypoadrenocorticism* (Addison's disease).

adrenocorticotropic hormone suppression test see *dexamethasone suppression test.*

adrenodoxin (ah-dre″no-dok′sin) an iron-sulfide protein of the adrenal gland, which is involved in steroid hydroxylation reactions in cytochrome P_{450} systems. See also *iron-sulfide protein.*

adrenogenital (ad-re″no-jen′ĭ-tal) [*adreno* + L. *genitalis* pertaining to generation] pertaining to the adrenal gland and the reproductive organs.

adrenogenital syndromes a group of disorders characterized by the excess production and secretion of adrenal androgens, which results in virilization. The characteristics depend on the age at which the disease first becomes clinically apparent. In infants and children the syndrome may be due to benign or malignant adrenal neoplasms, but it most often occurs as a result of congenital adrenal hyperplasia. In adults, females are most frequently affected, displaying hirsutism, baldness, acne, deepening of the voice, amenorrhea, and increased masculinity.

Adrenogenital syndromes in adults may be due to acquired defects in adrenal hormone synthesis (especially glucocorticoids and mineralocorticoids), leading to increased adrenocorticotropic hormone (ACTH) secretion and adrenal hyperplasia with excess production and elaboration of adrenal androgens. Urinary 17-ketosteroid levels are increased, pregnanetriol excretion is elevated, and 17-hydroxycorticosteroid excretion is decreased. Plasma levels of testosterone and androstenedione are elevated. Diagnosis is accomplished via the suppression of 17-ketosteroid excretion by dexamethasone.

Virilizing neoplasms may also cause adult adrenogenital syndrome. Adrenal adenomas and adenocarcinomas may be implicated. In this situation, however, 17-ketosteroid excretion is unaffected by administration of dexamethasone. These neoplasms may be detected by renal tomography or adrenal venography. Treatment requires adrenalectomy and adrenal hormone replacement.

Also called adrenal virilism. See also *congenital adrenal h.* under *hyperplasia* and *virilism.*

adrenoreceptor (ah-dre″no-re-sep′tor) [*adreno-* + L. *receptor* receiver] see *adrenergic receptors.*

Adriamycin (a″dre-ah-mi′sin) trademark. See *doxorubicin.*

Adriamycin cardiomyopathy see *anthracycline cardiotoxicity.*

adsorb (ad-sorb′) [*ad-* + L. *sorbere* to suck up] to attract and retain other material on the surface.

adsorbate (ad-sor′bāt) a substance taken up on a surface by adsorption.

adsorbed plasma plasma from which the vitamin K–dependent factors have been removed; fibrinogen and Factors V, VIII, IX, and XI are left intact. It is used in the partial thromboplastin time substitution test or as a diluent of the plasma to be examined in the prothrombin test, to avoid decreasing the concentration of fibrinogen or Factor V. Commonly used adsorbents are barium sulfate and aluminum hydroxide.

adsorbent (ad-sor′bent) 1. pertaining to or characterized by adsorption.

2. an agent that attracts other materials or particles to its surface. In chromatography, an adsorbent is the supporting medium on which a mixture of solute molecules or particles is placed. The unknown substances are separated into component parts by their different rates of migration on or through the medium. Also called *sorbent.* See also *chromatography.*

gastrointestinal a., a substance, usually a powder, taken to adsorb gases, toxins, and bacteria in the stomach and intestines (e.g., activated charcoal and kaolin).

adsorption (ad-sorp′shun) the attachment of one substance to the surface of another; the concentration of a substance in a liquid or gas onto a surface in contact with the liquid or gas, resulting in a relatively high concentration of the substance at the surface. Cf. *absorption.*

chemical a., a process of adsorption in which the adsorbate is held to the surface by bonds of the strength of chemical bonds. The molecules of the adsorbate are usually dissociated or otherwise altered; e.g., hydrogen (H_2) is chemically adsorbed in the form of free atoms. The alteration of molecular structure by chemical adsorption is the mechanism of surface catalysis. Also called *chemisorption.* Cf. *physical a.*

physical a., a process of adsorption in which the adsorbate is held to the surface of the adsorbant by weak bonds (van der Waals forces) without alteration of the chemical structure of the adsorbate molecules. Also called *physisorption.* Cf. *chemical a.*

adsorption chromatography chromatography in which a chemical mixture is separated by passage through an adsorbent; the different compounds in the mixture have differing affinities for the adsorbent, thus allowing migration at different rates. Silica, alumina, and magnesium are most often used as the adsorbents, but diatomaceous earth, sucrose, and charcoal are also used. Column, thin-layer, and paper chromatography make use of this principle.

Substances such as sterols, carotenoids, lipids, and vitamins are often separated by this method. Tables are available to aid in the choice of appropriate solvents for use with a particular solute and sorbent.

See also *chromatography.*

adulteration (ah-dul″ter-a′shun) [L. *adulterare* to corrupt] the addition of an impure, cheap, or unnecessary ingredient to cheapen or falsify a preparation; the term is also used in a legal sense to refer to incorrect labeling, including dosage not in accordance with the label.

adult hemoglobin the normal hemoglobins found in adult blood. These include hemoglobin A (90–96 percent), hemoglobin A_2 (approximately 2.5–3.6 percent), hemoglobin F (less than 2.5 percent), hemoglobins A_{1a} (0.2 percent), hemoglobin A_{1b} (0.5 percent), and A_{1c} (4.0 percent). See also *hemoglobin.*

adult respiratory distress syndrome (ARDS) acute respiratory failure, usually occurring in an individual with no previously known lung disease, that is characterized by potentially lethal deficits in oxygenation of the arterial blood. Unlike respiratory failure secondary to acute or chronic airway obstruction, CO_2 retention is rarely, if ever, present, and then only as a terminal event.

Initiating causes of ARDS include inhaled substances (e.g., gastric acid in aspiration, phosgene gas) and blood-borne agents (e.g., bacterial endotoxins, fibrin microemboli). The pathophysiologic mechanism appears to be damage to the pulmonary capillaries, which results in increased permeability of the capillary endothelium. Extravasation of fluid and red cells into the interstitial lung tissue and alveoli ensues, accompanied by micro- and macroatelectasis. Clinical findings include prominent respiratory distress, severe arterial hypoxemia with hypocarbia, diffuse radiologic densities, and falling lung compliance. Mortality is high unless the underlying cause can be corrected.

adventitia (ad″ven-tish′e-ah) [N.L., from L. *adventicius* from without] outermost; denoting the layer of loose connective tissue that forms the outermost covering of an organ, particularly a blood vessel.

adventitious (ad″ven-tish′us) 1. accidental or acquired, as opposed to natural or hereditary.

2. not found in the normal or usual place, such as roots arising from the leaves of a plant.

Aedes (a-e′dēz) [Gr. *aēdēs* unpleasant] a genus of mosquitoes characterized by the short palpi and pointed abdomen of the female. These insects serve as intermediate hosts for *Wuchereria bancrofti,* which causes a type of filariasis. The species *A. aegypti* is the main vector of the togavirus infections dengue, yellow fever, and chikungunya fever.

AEM abbrev. See *analytical e. m.* under *electron microscope.*

aer/o (a′er-o) [Gr. *aēr, aeros* air or gas] a word element used in combining form to denote a relationship to air or gas, e.g., aerobic.

aerated (a′er-āt″ed) [L. *aeratus*] 1. filled with air; as an inflated lung.
2. charged with carbon dioxide (in reference to a liquid).
3. oxygenated (in reference to blood).

aeration (a″er-a′shun) 1. the exchange of carbon dioxide for oxygen in the blood that takes place in the lungs.
2. the charging of a liquid with air or gas.

Aerobacter (a″er-o-bak′ter) [*aero-* + Gr. *baktērion* little rod] a former name for *Enterobacter aerogenes.*

aerobe (a′er-ōb) [*aero-* + Gr. *bios* life] a microorganism that grows best, or only, in the presence of air. Most aerobes prefer the natural oxygen atmosphere but can grow satisfactorily when the oxygen tension is reduced considerably (facultative); others require the full amount and are known as strict aerobes. Cf. *anaerobe.*

aerobic (a-er-o′bik) 1. having molecular oxygen present in atmospheric concentration.
2. growing only in the presence of molecular oxygen by deriving energy from oxidation, using molecular oxygen as the final electron acceptor.

aerobic capacity the greatest oxygen uptake (sometimes expressed per unit of body weight) achieved during a period of maximal activity or work. Because it is a reflection of the ability of the cardiopulmonary system to deliver oxygen to the body tissues and of the ability of the working muscles to utilize the available oxygen, it can be used as an index of work capacity.

The aerobic capacity can be estimated using the following equation: max $\dot{V}O_2 = 1.29\ [(L/H - 60)\exp(-0.00884\ T)]^{1/2}$, where L is the load at submaximal work in kilopond meters per minute, H is the heart rate at the end of 5–6 min at L, and T is the age in years.

Also called maximal oxygen uptake.

aerobiosis (a″er-o-bi-o′sis) [*aero-* + Gr. *biosis* way of life] the process of living in an atmosphere of molecular oxygen.

Aerococcus (a′e-ro-kok″kus) [*aero-* + Gr. *kokkos* seed, grain] a genus of gram-positive cocci bacteria of the family Streptococcaceae. The organisms have a strong tendency for tetrad formation, are microaerophilic, and produce primarily lactic acid from glucose. They are usually α-hemolytic and susceptible to bacitracin. Like enterococci and staphylococci, they grow in 6.5 percent NaCl broth. They have been isolated from the blood of some individuals with endocarditis and from the urine of some individuals with urinary tract infections. The genus contains a single species, *A. viridans.*

aeroembolism (a″er-o-em′bo-lizm) [*aero-* + L. *embolismus,* from Gr. *embolimos* intercalated] the obstruction of a blood vessel by air or gas.

aerogenic (a″er-o-jen′ik) [*aero-* + Gr. *gennan* to produce] producing gas; said of bacteria that form free gaseous products.

Aeromonas (a″er-o-mo′nas) [*aero-* + Gr. *monas* unit] a genus of bacteria of the family Vibrionaceae, of which one species, *A. hydrophila,* may infect humans. It occurs as small, rod-shaped cells with polar flagella. The normal habitat is water; some species are pathogenic for fish and amphibians. *Aeromonas* organisms are gram-negative, facultative anaerobes, are catalase- and oxidase-positive, and ferment glucose.

A. hydrophila, a species that includes a number of subspecies, one of which (subspecies *hydrophila*) is pathogenic for frogs, causing "red leg disease." Fish and reptiles may also be infected. Human infections are not uncommon and occur in a number of forms: cellulitis and wound infection, a cholera-like disease, septicemia, and urinary tract infections.

A. salmonicida, the etiologic agent of furunculosis in salmonid fishes, but not recovered from human specimens. The organism is unable to grow at 37°C and is nonmotile.

aeropathy (a″er-op′ah-the) [*aero-* + Gr. *pathos* disease] a general term, rarely used, that refers to disease related to changes in the atmospheric pressure. See also *decompression sickness.*

aerophagia (a″er-o-fa′je-ah) [*aero-* + Gr. *phagein* to eat] the swallowing of air, which normally occurs in small amounts when an individual eats or drinks but may be excessive in those with various gastrointestinal or liver disorders. Depending on the postural position, the air will be either regurgitated (leading to eructation) or forced down the intestinal tract (leading to flatulence). See also *eructation.*

aerophil (a′er-o-fil″) [*aero-* + Gr. *philein* to love] an organism that requires air for growth.

aerophilic (a″er-o-fil′ik) requiring air for proper growth.

aerosol (a′er-o-sol″) [acronym from *aero-* + *solution*] 1. a gaseous suspension of extremely small particles of a liquid or solid.
2. airborne particles in the form of droplets or a fine mist. They are produced by coughing or sneezing, by microorganisms, and in the laboratory by use of a blender, centrifuge, or Bunsen burner. Airborne particles of relatively small diameter (approximately 5 μm or less) can penetrate to the lower respiratory tract.
3. a solution of a drug that can be atomized into a fine mist for inhalation therapy.
4. a material dispensed from its container as a mist, spray, or foam by a pressurized propellant.

aerosol generator a device that produces a fine (aerosol) spray.

aerosol therapy the local introduction, by inhalation into the respiratory airways, of therapeutic agents in the form of fine droplets or particles suspended in air. Aerosols can be produced manually, by squeezing a bulb, or by use of compressed oxygen or air. Those aerosols commonly employed in treatment of various respiratory disorders may contain bronchodilators such as isoproterenol, components of pulmonary surfactant, adrenocortical steroids, or mucolytic or proteolytic enzymes (such as crystalline trypsin, hyaluronidase, deoxyribonuclease, lysozyme, or streptokinase) or drugs (such as acetylcysteine).

An advantage of this form of therapy is that the droplet or particle size can be adjusted (by use of appropriate nebulizers and baffles) so that a high concentration of the therapeutic agent can be delivered to the specific portion of the respiratory tract requiring treatment. Only slight systemic absorption and few undesirable side-effects will occur. A serious disadvantage is that the aerosol does not reach completely obstructed portions of the lung, often the areas most in need of treatment.

aerotaxis (a″er-o-tak′sis) [*aero-* + Gr. *taxis* arrangement] a movement of an organism in response to the presence of molecular oxygen.

aerotolerant (a″er-o-tol′er-ant) able to survive or to grow slowly in an aerobic environment; said of certain anaerobic microorganisms.

aerotropism (a″er-ot′ro-pizm) [*aero-* + Gr. *tropos* a turning] the movement of an organism toward a supply of air.

AES abbrev. See *American Electroencephalographic Society.*

AFB abbrev. for acid-fast bacillus.

afebrile (a-feb′rĭl) [*a-* neg. + Fr. *febrile* feverish, from L. *febris* fever] without fever.

affective (ah-fek′tiv) [L. *affectare* to strive for, from *afficere* to do (something) to] pertaining to or arousing the emotions. In psychology, the term is used to contrast emotional states with those that have organic or cognitive causes.

afferent (af′er-ent) [*ad-* + L. *ferre* to carry] carrying toward the center, as an afferent nerve carries impulses into the central nervous system. Cf. *efferent.*

affinity (ah-fin′ĭ-te) [L. *affinitas* relationship, neighborhood] 1. inherent likeness or relationship.

2. the tendency of an element to combine with a second particular element rather than a third, even though conditions are equally favorable for combination; a special attraction for a specific element, organ, or structure.

3. in immunology, the binding strength of a single antibody combining site for a ligand; e.g., IgG has 2 affinity binding sites, whereas IgM has 10 affinity binding sites per antibody molecule. Cf. *avidity.*

4. in thermodynamics, a driving force; specifically, the negative of the reaction potential, which is generally known as the reaction free energy, ΔG.

5. in chromatography, the selective attraction of the adsorbent for specific types of compounds.

6. the energy released when a neutral atom in the gaseous state acquires an additional electron, becoming negatively charged. Also called electron affinity.

affinity chromatography any form of chromatography in which the components of the sample are separated on the basis of chemical affinity for a substance, such as a binding protein or an immunoglobulin, that is immobilized on an inert substrate and forms reversible, noncovalent bonds with molecules in the sample.

affinity constant the equilibrium constant for the binding of a drug to a drug receptor (the reciprocal of the dissociation constant).

affinity label see under *affinity labeling.*

affinity labeling a method of studying the active site of enzymes using a chemical inhibitor that has all the structural requirements of a good substrate. It can bind covalently to the enzyme active site with a parallel loss of enzyme activity. Subsequent structural studies are particularly useful in identifying residues present in the active site. The inhibitor itself is called an affinity label or Trojan Horse inhibitor. The same principle employing immunochemical techniques is also used to identify amino acid residues at the combining site on an antibody.

afibrinogenemia (a″fi-brin″o-jĕ-ne′me-ah) [*a-* neg. + *fibrinogen* + Gr. *haima* blood + *-ia*] the deficiency or absence of fibrinogen (Factor I) in the blood. It can be inherited as an autosomal recessive trait, affecting both sexes equally, or can result from an increased conversion of fibrinogen to fibrin due to pathologic conditions such as severe disseminated intravascular coagulation or an acquired decreased synthesis of fibrinogen. Individuals affected with this disorder bruise and bleed easily, often severely. Whole blood clotting time, prothrombin and thrombin time, and partial thromboplastin time are prolonged. Replacement therapy is with cryoprecipitate. See also *Factor I* and *hypofibrinogenemia.* Cf. *dysfibrinogenemia.*

aflatoxicosis (af″lah-tok″sĭ-ko-sis) poisoning by ingestion of the mycotoxin aflatoxin, primarily aflatoxin B_1 and G_1. In fish, birds, and domestic animals, the hepatotoxic effects of aflatoxin ingestion are well documented and range from acute hepatic necrosis to the development of hepatocellular carcinoma. In humans, chronic aflatoxin B_1 poisoning has been implicated in the high incidence of primary liver cancer in individuals in Africa and Asia. See also *aflatoxin.*

aflatoxin (af″lah-tok′sin) [acronym from *A*spergillus *fla*vus *toxin*] a highly toxic and carcinogenic factor produced by mold contamination of soil-contacted foodstuffs (e.g., peanuts). It is usually produced by *Aspergillus flavus* and *A. parasiticus* and has been identified as a highly unsaturated molecule with a coumarin nucleus.

Aflatoxin B_1 and G_1 are the parent compounds and are the most potent carcinogens; aflatoxin B_1 has also been shown to suppress DNA, RNA, and protein synthesis in rat liver cells. Other known compounds include the dihydro derivatives of aflatoxins B_1 and B_2, aflatoxin B_2 and G_2, and the hydroxylated derivatives of aflatoxin B_1, aflatoxins P_1, M_1, and Q_1.

AFP abbrev. See *alpha$_1$-fetoprotein.*

after-discharge the prolonged, repetitive firing of a neuronal pool that persists for a period ranging from milliseconds to minutes after a transient initial stimulus has ceased. In the case of motor neurons, the initial stimulus is usually a muscle contraction.

aftergilding (af″ter-gild′ing) the histologic application of gold salts to nerve tissue after fixation and hardening.

afterglow (af′ter-glo) the continuation of the fluorescence of an intensifying screen after x-ray excitation of the phosphors has ceased. The types of phosphor that cause afterglow are no longer used. Also called *screen lag.*

afterload (af″ter-lōd) the load against which a muscle contracts. The afterload on the heart is approximated by the arterial pressure. Increasing afterload decreases cardiac performance by reducing stroke volume. Cf. *preload.*

A/G abbrev. See *albumin/globulin ratio.*

Ag 1. symbol for the chemical element silver.

2. abbrev. See *antigen.*

agammaglobulinemia (a-gam″ah-glob″u-lĭ-ne′me-ah) [*a-* neg. + *gamma globulin* + Gr. *haima* blood + *-ia*] see *hypogammaglobulinemia.*

agar (ahg′ar) a complex acidic polysaccharide extracted from *Gelidium cartilagineum, Gracilaria confervoides,* and related red algae seaweeds. It has the property of melting at 80°–100°C and solidifying into a gel at 45°C. Agar is nontoxic for, and attacked by, very few bacteria; thus, it is used universally in a concentration of 1.5–2.0 percent as a gel in the preparation of solid culture media for the cultivation of microorganisms. In histology, agar is employed for orientation of small specimens prior to dehydration and infiltration with paraffin. Additional uses are as a bulk laxative, in making emulsions, and as a supporting medium for immunodiffusion tests and for immunoelectrophoresis. See also *culture media.*

birdseed a., a differential medium used for the identification of yeasts. It is prepared by adding an extract of seeds of *Guizottia abyssinica,* the Indian thistle plant (a common ingredient in birdseed), to an agar medium. The formation of brown colonies due to the production of phenol oxidase is presumptive evidence for the presence of *Cryptococcus neoformans.*

bismuth sulfite a., a culture medium used to isolate *Salmonella* species, especially *S. typhi,* from feces and other clinical material.

blood a., a medium containing blood (usually sheep blood), used for primary plating of specimens and subculturing of colonies. It supports the growth of most medically important bacteria and is especially useful for identifying bacterial hemolysis.

Bordet-Gengou a., a solid culture medium containing infusion from potato and enriched with blood and glycerol, used for the isolation of *Bordetella pertussis.*

brain-heart infusion a., a solid medium containing infusions of calf brain and beef heart, which is suitable for the cultivation of many kinds of pathogenic microorganisms, including bacteria, yeast, and molds.

brilliant green a., a highly selective primary isolation medium used for enteric pathogens such as *Salmonella* species.

chocolate a., a bacterial culture medium used as the primary plating medium for cultures of spinal fluids and eye fluids, for gonococcal cultures, and for other specimens that may contain fastidious organisms, e.g., *Hemophilus influenzae* or *Neisseria* species. It contains blood that has been heated or autoclaved, giving it a chocolate-brown color. Heating frees hematin and also destroys an enzyme that inactivates the nucleoside V factor required for the growth of certain bacterial species, notably *H. influenzae.*

Christensen's urea a., a medium of simple composition used for the detection of urease production, an important characteristic of the *Proteus* genus.

citrate a., an aerobic differential medium containing citrate and bromthymol blue, used to determine the ability of gram-negative bacilli, particularly the Enterobacteriaceae, to utilize citrate as the sole source of carbon.

cystine trypticase a., an aerobic differential medium used for the culture of fastidious pathogenic bacteria. The fermentation of glucose, lactose, maltose, and sucrose, which is used to identify species of *Neisseria,* may be determined by the individual addition of these sugars.

deep a., agar in an upright test tube, usually as a solid culture medium that contains 1.5–2 percent agar.

egg-yolk a., a medium containing trypticase and egg yolk, used for the isolation and identification of strains of *Clostridium.*

eosin-methylene blue (EMB) a., a differential medium used for the primary isolation of Enterobacteriaceae species.

Hektoen enteric a., a selective medium used for the primary isolation and identification of enteric pathogens, especially coliform organisms, *Salmonella,* and *Shigella.*

laked blood a., a solid culture medium containing blood that has been hemolyzed to release hemin.

lysine-iron a., an aerobic differential medium used to determine lysine decarboxylase and lysine deaminase of the Enterobacteriaceae, especially for the genera *Proteus* and *Providencia.*

MacConkey a., an agar culture medium containing peptone, lactose, bile salts, neutral red, and crystal violet, which is useful for the isolation of enteric bacilli from fecal cultures. Colonies of lactose-fermenting organisms appear red; nonfermenters are yellow or colorless.

Martin-Lester a., a modification of chocolate agar containing antibiotics, used for the transport and primary isolation of *Neisseria gonorrhoeae* and *N. meningitidis.*

Middlebrook 7H10 a., a complex medium used for the primary isolation of mycobacteria and for antimicrobial susceptibility testing. Middlebrook 7H11 agar is very similar: 0.1 percent casein hydrolipate is substituted for glucose. See also *mycobacteria.*

Mueller-Hinton a., a culture medium used for the primary isolation of *Neisseria gonorrheae* and *N. meningitidis;* it is also employed widely for antibiotic and sulfonamide susceptibility testing.

nutrient a., a nutrient broth gelled by the addition of agar. It has a simple composition: only beef extract and peptone.

phenylalanine a., a medium used to test for phenylalanine deaminase activity by bacteria, an important characteristic of *Proteus* and *Providencia* species.

phenylethyl alcohol blood a., a selective medium used for the primary isolation of anaerobic bacteria and gram-positive cocci, and for the separation of gram-positive cocci from a mixture containing gram-negative bacilli.

rabbit blood a., a medium containing rabbit blood, used to characterize hemolysis by *Hemophilus parahemolyticus.*

Sabouraud's dextrose a. (Emmon's modification), a medium containing antibiotics, used for the cultivation and identification of fungi.

sheep blood a., a medium containing sheep blood, used for the primary culture of clinical specimens and the characterization of hemolysis by group A *Streptococcus.*

Thayer-Martin a., a modification of chocolate blood agar containing antibiotics, used for the transport and primary culture of *Neisseria gonorrhoeae* and *N. meningitidis.*

triple sugar iron (TSI) a., a medium containing peptones (2 percent), glucose (0.1 percent), sucrose (1 percent), lactose (1 percent), ferrous ammonium sulfate (0.02 percent), sodium thiosulfate (0.02 percent), NaCl (0.5 percent), phenol red (0.0025 percent), and agar (1.3 percent), used for the preliminary screening of enteric bacilli. The medium is tubed as slants; the inoculum is both streaked on the surface and stabbed into the butt of the tube. Fermentation of the various sugars may be determined by examining growth and acid production on the surface (aerobic) and in the butt (anaerobic).

The sugar concentrations are critical: the amount of glucose is only one-tenth that of lactose and of sucrose. Consequently, organisms fermenting only glucose acidify the butt but do not produce enough acid to neutralize the alkaline end-products that accumulate in the aerobic slant portion. Production of hydrogen sulfide causes the formation of black ferrous sulfide along the stab line. Gas production (H_2 and CO_2) causes bubbles in the agar. TSIA reactions are very important in the identification of the Enterobacteriaceae.

xylose-lysine-deoxycholate (XLD) a., a highly selective medium for the direct inoculation of fecal specimens, used for isolating intestinal pathogens, especially *Shigella.*

agar cutter a device for cutting and preparing agar-coated plates for techniques such as radial immunodiffusion, electrophoresis, and immunoelectrophoresis.

agar diffusion method see *antibacterial agent susceptibility testing.*

agarose (ahg′ar-ōse) a sulfate-free fraction of agar, used in electrophoresis and as a special-purpose culture medium.

agarose gel electrophoresis a convenient method of electrophoresis of general applicability that uses a purified, essentially neutral fraction of agar called agarose as a medium, usually at concentrations of 0.5–1.0 g/100 ml. Specimens (1.0–3.0 μl) may be added into precut wells or as streaks of specimen dissolved in warm agar. Electrophoresis time may vary from 30 to 90 min. Agarose has a lower affinity for proteins than does paper and some other media and provides good clarity for scanning. The medium has been used for separation of serum proteins, hemoglobin variants, lipoprotein fractions, and lactate dehydrogenase isoenzymes. See also *electrophoresis.*

agar plate count an approximate determination of the number of bacteria present in a specimen or inoculum. The procedure is performed by spreading a measured specimen across a Petri dish containing an agar medium, and counting the number of colonies of bacteria that develop after a certain time. The more usual method of counting, however, is by pour plate. See also *pour p.* under *plate.*

AGE abbrev. See acrylamide gel and agarose gel electrophoresis under *electrophoresis.*

age-adjusted rate the prevalence rate of a disease or a death rate adjusted for the age structure of the population. The age-specific rate is determined for each age group and multiplied by the fraction of population in the age group, giving the incidence in the age group; these are summed to give the age-adjusted rate.

aged serum a reagent containing Factors VII, IX, X, XI, and XII. The serum is prepared by incubating normal serum for 24 hr at 37°C.

agenesis (a-jen′ĕ-sis) [*a-* neg. + Gr. *genesis* production] the failure of an organ or tissue to form during embryogenesis, owing to the absence of the anlagen of an organ. The term also refers to the primary absence of an organ, as opposed to the lack of that organ through maldevelopment, disease, or atrophy. Cf. *aplasia.*

agent (a′jent) [L. *agens,* from *agere* to do] a substance by which a reaction or process is accomplished.

Agent Orange see *chlorophenoxy herbicides.*

age-specific rate the incidence of disease or a death rate for persons of a specific age.

agglutination (ah-gloo″tĭ-na′shun) [L. *agglutinatio,* from *agglutinare* to glue to] 1. the action of an agglutinating substance.

2. the clumping of cells that are distributed diffusely in a fluid. It is caused by agglutinins, antibodies developed against that specific cell type, and is seen when a bacterial culture is treated with serum from an animal immunized against that particular organism or when a suspension of cells, particularly blood cells, is exposed to antisera. This phenomenon is commonly employed in blood banking as an indicator of antigen-antibody reaction between red cells and specific antiserum or donor plasma. See also *antiglobulin tests,* and *compatibility tests.*

agglutinin (ah-gloo′tĭ-nin) 1. an antibody that causes agglutination (clumping) of cells, particularly red blood cells.

2. any substance that causes agglutination, such as the lectins phytohemagglutinin and concanavalin A.

aggregation (ag″rĕ-ga′shun) 1. a massing or clumping of material, as in platelet aggregation.

2. a mass or clump of material.

aggregometer (ag″grĕ-gom′ĕ-ter) [L. *aggregare,* from *ad-* + *gregis* crowd + Gr. *metron* measure] an instrument used to measure platelet aggregation, generally by a photometer that registers changes in the optical density of a platelet suspension during aggregation. The platelet suspension is prepared from citrated blood by centrifugation, which removes red cells and concentrates the platelets. Aggregation is induced by addition of adenosine diphosphate (ADP), collagen, viper venom, and ristocetin or other agents. The pattern of reaction to different aggregating agents is used in distinguishing between different types of platelet dysfunction.

aging (āj′ing) 1. the gradual changes in the structure of any organism that occur with the passage of time, that do not result from disease or other gross accidents, and that eventually lead to the increased probability of death as the individual grows older. Cf. *senescence.*

2. the slow deterioration of chemical reagents or their containers, or of rubber, plastics, or biologic specimens; usually caused by air oxidation under the influence of heat, light, or trace impurities. All of these are sources of systematic variance in the performance of laboratory procedures.

agitation (aj-ĕ-ta′shun) [L. *agitatio* in motion, from *agitare* to drive to and fro] gentle shaking or stirring, usually by mechanical means.

Agkistrodon (ag-kis′tro-don) [Gr. *agkistron* fishhook + *odōn* tooth] a genus of venomous snakes, including *A. contortrix* (the copperhead) and *A. piscivorous* (the water moccasin) of North America. Their venom is not highly poisonous and causes few fatalities. The technically preferred name of this genus is *Ancistrodon.*

AGL abbrev. for acute granulocytic leukemia. See *acute myelogenous l.* under *leukemia.*

aglycone (a-gli′kōn) [*a-* neg. + Gr. *glykys* sweet + *ōn* being] the noncarbohydrate group of a glycoside molecule. This can be a phenolic compound, or a purine or pyrimidine base attached to sugar through a nitrogen atom, a phosphate group of a sugar phosphate, or some other type of group. Also called *genin.*

agnogenic (ag″no-jen′ik) [Gr. *agnōs* unknown, obscure + *genesis* origin] of unknown origin or etiology.

agnosia (ag-no′ze-ah) [Gr. *agnōsia* ignorance, from *a*- neg. + *gignōskein* to know] the inability to recognize sensory stimuli or their import despite preserved elementary perception. Agnosia may affect any of the senses (e.g., visual, auditory, tactile) and may also involve time and location. For example, individuals with auditory agnosia may be unable to recognize sounds although they are not deaf. The basis of agnosia is poorly understood; it is thought to be caused by organic disease affecting integrative pathways within the cerebral hemisphere.

agonadal (a-gon′ah-dal) [*a*- neg. + *gonad*] possessing no sex glands, or caused by the absence of sex glands.

agonal (ag′o-nal) [Gr. *agōnia* struggle, anguish, from *agōn* struggle, contest] pertaining to death or extreme suffering.

agonist (ag′o-nist) [Gr. *agōnistēs* combatant, from *agōn* contest] 1. a prime mover; a muscle opposed in action by another muscle, called the antagonist.

2. an effective drug, when considered in relation to its antagonist, that competes for the receptors and nullifies its effect. A partial agonist also competes for the receptors and has a weaker effect than the agonist, e.g., morphine (agonist), nalorphine (partial agonist), and naloxone (antagonist). Cf. *antagonist.*

agoraphobia (ag″o-rah-fo′be-ah) [Gr. *agora* market place + *phobos* fear + *-ia*] the obsessive, pathologic fear of being alone in large, open spaces.

agranular endoplasmic reticulum (ah″gran′u-lar en″do-plas′mik re-tik′u-lum) endoplasmic reticulum composed of membranes without attached ribosomes, plentiful in cells that form steroid hormones. See also *endoplasmic reticulum.*

agranulocytosis (a-gran″u-lo-si-to′sis) [*a*- neg. + *granulocyte,* from L. *granum* grain + Gr. *kytos* hollow vessel + *-osis* condition] a severe form of granulocytopenia (depression or lack of mature granulocytes in the peripheral blood) leading to overwhelming and, in the preantibiotic era, frequently fatal bacterial infections. It is frequently associated with the use of aminopyrinine compounds or phenothiazines. Onset is sudden and marked by sore throat, fever and chills, and prostration; unfavorable signs include confusion, jaundice, drowsiness, and a leukocyte count lower than 1.0×10^9 cells/l.

Treatment involves the use of antibiotics and sulfonamides and isolating the offending agent and discontinuing its use; the reappearance of myelocytes and metamyelocytes in the blood indicates a favorable prognosis. See also *granulocytopenia.*

agraphia (a-graf′e-ah) [*a*- neg. + Gr. *graphein* to write + *-ia*] the loss of ability to write properly or to communicate by writing, due to a lesion involving certain parts of the cerebral hemisphere, usually on the left (the dominant hemisphere for most individuals). Agraphia may be associated with other disorders of language or with abnormalities of spatial perception. A cerebrovascular accident, or stroke, is one common cause. To establish that the condition is agraphia when (as is frequently the case) there is paralysis of the right arm, it must be shown that the patient cannot write with the left hand.

A/G ratio see *albumin/globulin ratio.*

Agrobacterium (ag″ro-bak-te′re-um) [Gr. *agros* field + *baktērion* small rod] a genus of gram-negative, aerobic, rod-shaped bacteria of the family Rhizobiaceae. The organisms are positive for oxidase, nitrate, and MacConkey's medium; are motile; and oxidize glucose. Containing several species that are plant pathogens, the genus has one species, *A. radiobacter,* that has been isolated from clinical specimens. This species is not considered pathogenic but is easily confused with other bacteria of similar characteristics; it can be distinguished by its production of 3-ketolactose.

ague (a′gu) [Fr. *aigu* sharp] see *malaria.*

agyria (a-ji′re-ah) [*a*- neg. + Gr. *gyros* ring + *-ia*] see *lissencephaly.*

AHA abbrev. See *American Hospital Association.*

ahaptoglobinemia (a-hap″to-glo″bĭ-ne′me-ah) [*a*- neg. + *haptoglobin* + Gr. *haima* blood + *-ia*] the absence of haptoglobin in the blood serum, usually an indication of hemolytic disease. Haptoglobin is absent in most individuals when red cell destruction reaches twice the normal rate. Ahaptoglobinemia occurs congenitally in approximately 4 percent of the black population.

AHD abbrev. for autoimmune hemolytic disease. See *autoimmune hemolytic a.* under *anemia.*

AHF abbrev. for antihemophilic factor. See *Factor VIII.*

AHG abbrev. for antihemophilic globulin (see under *Factor VIII*), antihuman globulin.

A-H interval the time required for an impulse to be conducted through the atrioventricular (A-V) node of the heart, approximately equal to 50–150 msec in the normal adult. It is measured on the His bundle electrogram from the lower atrial deflection to that of the His bundle (H) spike. Determination of the A-H interval can be definitive in diagnosing A-V block.

βAIB abbrev. See *β-aminoisobutyric acid.*

AID abbrev. for acute infectious disease, artificial insemination donor, *autoimmune disease.*

AIDS abbrev. for *acquired immune deficiency syndrome.*

AIHA abbrev. See *autoimmune hemolytic a.* under *anemia.*

air (ār) [L. *aer*] the gaseous mixture that composes the earth's atmosphere.

air foil a curved or shaped piece of metal located across the bottom front of a laboratory hood. It is designed to provide a sweeping velocity along the floor of the hood, minimizing eddy currents that allow contaminants to escape from the hood.

air monitor a device that detects the presence of hazardous agents in the air. Air monitors are available for detecting explosive gases, noxious gases, chemicals, and radioactivity, and they may be set to sound a warning when unsafe levels are reached.

air quality standards ambient levels of air pollutants set by governmental agencies as targets for air pollution control. The standards take into account air quality effects on the health of the general population and of sensitive groups within the population, as well as effects on vegetation, structures, and materials. Pollutants for which standards have been set include sulfur dioxide, nitrogen dioxide, carbon monoxide, hydrogen sulfide, sulfuric acid, hydrogen fluoride, lead, suspensions of beryllium particulates, and total oxidants (ozone, peroxyacyl nitrates).

air spaces a general term for the alveoli, alveolar sacs, and alveolar ducts of the respiratory tracts.

airway conductance (GAW) the inverse (reciprocal) of airway resistance. It varies linearly with the lung volume during the respiratory cycle, increasing as the airways dilate and decreasing as they constrict. Cf. *airway resistance.*

specific a.c. (SGAW), the airway conductance per unit of lung volume, normally amounting to 0.22–0.24 sec^{-1} cm H_2O^{-1} in the adult nonsmoker.

airway resistance (RAW) the energy needed to overcome the frictional resistance to the flow of air through the respiratory airways. It is expressed as the pressure difference between the two ends of the airways (the atmospheric pressure of the mouth or nose minus the alveolar pressure) divided by the airflow. Volume-displacement whole body plethysmography is commonly used to determine alveolar pressure, whereas flow is simultaneously measured with a pneumotachograph; resistance can then be calculated as centimeters of water per liter per second (cm H_2O/l/sec). Airway resistance can also be partitioned into the contribution of airways of various diameters to the total resistance. The upper airways can contribute 50 percent of the total resistance, whereas 10–30 percent of the resistance can be provided by airways of a diameter less than 2 mm.

The physical factors (transmural pressure, compliance, dynamic changes during the respiratory cycle) and physiologic factors (nervous and chemical regulation of airway diameter) governing the dynamic compression or constriction of the airways and lungs normally affect the resistance; pulmonary obstructive disease can increase the resistance to the point at which breathing becomes difficult. Cf. *airway conductance.*

specific a. r. (SRAW), the airway resistance per unit of lung volume. The use of the body plethysmograph for measurement of airway resistance permits a simultaneous measurement of the total lung volume. Airway resistance can then be related to the degree of lung inflation at the time of the resistance measurement. Lung inflation increases airway diameter and lessens resistance to airflow. Specific airway resistance allows a more accurate comparison of the resistance to airflow in different individuals, and in the same individual over time.

airways (aw) the series of irregularly branching, heterogeneous passageways that compose the conducting system of the respiratory tract, beginning with the nares and mouth and extending to (and including) the respiratory bronchioles.

AIVR abbrev. See *accelerated idioventricular rhythm.*

Ajellomyces (ah″jĕ-lo-mi′sēz) a genus of fungi of which the species *A. dermatitidis* is the sexual stage or so-called perfect state of *Blastomyces dermatitidis,* the causative agent of North American blastomycosis. It can be obtained in culture by pairing two cultures that are heterothallic. Ascospores develop within asci, hence the classification of *B. dermatitidis* as an ascomycete. *Ajellomyces* is considered to be the same genus as *Emmonsiella.*

akathisia (ak″ah-the′ze-ah) [*a-* neg. + Gr. *kathisis* a sitting down + *-ia*] a restless, uncontrolled motor activity, most often seen as a side-effect of the phenothiazine group of drugs, that usually occurs soon after therapy with these agents has been initiated. See also *tardive d.* under *dyskinesia.*

Akeridae (ah-ker′ĭ-de) a family of snails serving as intermediate hosts for some helminths that infect humans, such as *Haminoea antillarum guadelupensis.*

akinesia (a-ki-ne′ze-ah) [*a-* neg. + Gr. *kinesis* motion + *-ia*] slowness in the initiation and execution of voluntary movements, as well as the tendency to stop such movements suddenly and unexpectedly. This disorder of motor control is a sign of extrapyramidal dysfunction, which is most frequently associated with parkinsonism.

akinesthesia (a-kin″es-the′zhe-ah) [*a-* neg. + Gr. *kinein* to move + *aisthesis* perception + *-ia*] absence of a sense of movement.

akinetic (a″kĭ-net′ik) pertaining to, characterized by, or causing akinesia.

akinetic apex a cardiac apex that has totally ceased to move during the pressure-volume changes of the cardiac cycle. It is a sign of ischemic dysfunction or damage to the left ventricular myocardium. Echocardiographic and angiographic techniques are used to reveal this lack of movement.

Al symbol for the chemical element *aluminum.*

-al a suffix word element in chemistry to name organic compounds in which the principal functional group is an aldehyde, e.g., propanal (CH_3CH_2CHO).

ALA abbrev. for *δ-aminolevulinic acid.*

Ala abbrev. See *alanine.*

ala (a′lah), pl. *alae* [L. "wing"] [NA], a general term for a winglike structure or process. For example, the ala nasi is the flaring expansion that forms the outer side of each nostril.

alanine (Ala or A) (al′ah-nēn) 2-aminopropanoic acid, $CH_3CH(NH_2)COOH$, a naturally occurring nonessential amino acid, present in many proteins; M.W. 89.09. Alanine is important in nitrogen export from muscle (glucose-alanine cycle) and in the transport of nitrogen from the intestinal tract to the liver. As a substrate for alanine transaminase, alanine functions in nitrogen transfer reactions. Its source is the proteins of the diet and synthesis from pyruvate. Also called *α-alanine* and *α-aminopropionic acid.* See also under *amino acids.*

α-**a.**, see *alanine.*

β-**a.**, 3-aminopropanoic acid, $H_2NCH_2CH_2COOH$, one of two *β*-amino acids of physiologic importance; M.W. 87.10. As a component of the vitamin pantothenic acid, it is a constituent of coenzyme A and is found in carnosine (*N-β*-alanyl-L-histidine) and in anserine (*N-β*-alanyl-3-methyl-L-histidine). The catabolism of cytosine and uracil may serve as a major source of *β*-alanine in the mammalian system.

alanine aminotransferase (ALT) (al′ah-nēn ahme″no-trans′fer-ās) an enzyme of the transferase class (alanine transaminase, L-alanine:2-oxoglutarate aminotransferase, EC 2.6.1.2). Of considerable interest in clinical medicine, the enzyme is one of two aminotransferases that catalyze the transfer of amino groups in the interconversion of amino acids and α-oxoacids. ALT catalyzes the reversible transamination reaction: L-alanine + α-ketoglutarate ⇄ pyruvate + L-glutamate. The equilibrium slightly favors the formation of alanine. It is normally found in plasma, bile, cerebrospinal fluid, and saliva; it is present in urine only if a kidney lesion is present.

The enzyme is present in relatively high concentrations in the liver and kidney; it is also found in skeletal muscle, heart, and pancreas. ALT is present in the serum of healthy persons at about 6–25 U/l, if measured at 30°C. Enzyme activity increases to 30–50 times normal in persons with viral or toxic hepatitis, and to values some 20 times normal in cases of infectious mononucleosis. In the early stages of liver disease it trails the aspartate aminotransferase (AST), but in later stages of the acute phase and during recovery, the De Ritis ratio (ALT/AST) is greater than 1.0. There are no, or only minor, elevations in myocardial infarction.

Also called *glutamate-pyruvate transaminase* (GPT) and *serum glutamate-pyruvate transaminase* (SGPT).

alanine aminotransferase assays 1. continuous monitoring spectrophotometric methods using coupled enzyme reactions. The activity of ALT in serum is determined at pH 7.8 and a temperature of either 30° or 37°C. The specimen is added to a buffered reaction mixture containing alanine, 2-oxoglutarate, lactate dehydrogenase, and NADH. The pyruvate produced by the ALT-catalyzed reaction is reduced to lactate by lactate dehydrogenase, with NADH serving as a reducing cofactor. The reaction is monitored by measuring the decrease in absorbance per minute (ΔA/min) of NADH at 340 nm as it is oxidized to NAD^+. The activity in International Units (U) is equal to the number of micromoles of NADH oxidized per minute. This method is now widely accepted in clinical laboratories.

2. two-point colorimetric methods in which the pyruvate produced is measured by the formation of a colored product. The specimen is added to a buffered reaction mixture containing 2-oxoglutarate, alanine, and 2,4-dinitrophenylhydrazine. The pyruvate formed reacts with 2,4-dinitrophenylhydrazine to form a yellow dinitrophenylhydrazone with an absorbance that can be measured at 505 nm. The substrate 2-oxoglutarate and other oxoacids in the reaction mixture also form hydrazones, causing reagent blanks with high absorbances. Because the absorbance of the reaction mixture is not a linear function of the pyruvate concentration, a standard curve must be used to determine the ALT activity. This method is rarely used today and is considered obsolete.

β-alanine-α-ketoglutarate transaminase (al″-ah-nēn ke″to-gloo′tah-rāt trans-am′ĭ-nās) see *aminobutyrate aminotransferase.*

alaninemia (al″ah-ne-ne′me-ah) [*alanine* + Gr. *haima* blood + *-ia*] the presence of excess alanine in the blood, which may have a number of causes, including a deficiency of several enzymes. See also *aminoacidopathy* and *hyper-β-alaninemia.*

β-alaninemia see *hyper-β-alaninemia.*

β-alanine-oxoglutarate aminotransferase (al″-ah-nēn ok″so-gloo′tah-rāt) see *aminobutyrate aminotransferase.*

β-alanine transaminase (al′ah-nēn trans-am′ĭ-nās) see *aminobutyrate aminotransferase.*

β-alaninuria (al″ah-ne-nu′re-ah) [*alanine* + Gr. *ouron* urine + *-ia*] a hereditary condition in which excesses of β-amino acids (β-alanine, β-aminoisobutyric acid, and taurine) occur in the urine and blood. See also *hyper-β-alaninemia.*

alanyl (al′ah-nil) the acyl radical derived from or relating to alanine.

alar (a′lar) [L. *alaris*] pertaining to an ala, or wing.

alar plate bilateral dorsal thickenings of the embryonic neural tube that develop into sensory areas of the brain stem and spinal cord.

alastrim (ah-las′trim) [Port., from *alastrar* to spread] a mild form of smallpox caused by a stable variant of the classic smallpox virus.

alb/o (al′bo) [L. *albus* white] a word element used in combining form to denote white, e.g., albinism.

alb abbrev. See *albumin.*

Albers-Schönberg disease (al′berz shern′berg) [Heinrich Ernst *Albers-Schönberg,* Hamburg radiologist, 1865–1921] see *osteopetrosis.*

Albert-Linder bone sectioning a method used to prepare sections of undecalcified bone tissue for histologic examination for alkaline phosphatase. Small pieces of bone are fixed in alcohol and infiltrated with tropical ester wax. Each section is coated with celloidin as it is cut and is then treated as an ordinary celloidin section.

albicans (al′bĭ-kans), pl. *albicantia* [L., from *albicare* to whiten] white.

albinism (al′bĭ-nizm) the congenital absence of normal pigment (apparent in the hair, skin, and eyes), caused by a defect of melanin precursors; it may be total or partial.

Albright's syndrome (awl′brīts) [Fuller *Albright,* Boston physician, 1900–1969] a syndrome characterized by polyostotic fibrous dysplasia, irregular zones of skin pigmentation, and endocrine dysfunction with precocious puberty, the last-named usually in females. See also *polyostotic fibrous d.* under *dysplasia* and *precocious p.* under *puberty.*

albumin/o (al-bu′min-o) a word element used in combining form to denote protein, e.g., albuminuria.

albumin (al-bu′min) a group of proteins found in nearly every animal and in many vegetable tissues; M.W. 40,000 (egg albumin) and 69,000 (human serum albumin). Albumin is characterized by its solubility in water and in dilute and moderately concentrated salt solutions and its coagulability by heat. It is the most abundant protein in human plasma, being present normally to an extent of 3.5–4.7 g/dl. It can be produced by a number of methods; the purest preparations are generally produced by alcohol fractionation. Albumin has been used to treat shock from trauma such as burns and hemorrhage. Its large molecules cannot cross capillary wall membranes, and thus it helps to maintain the colloidal osmotic pressure in the vascular compartment; this, in part, accounts for maintenance of a normal blood volume. It also binds ions such as calcium, magnesium, and toxic heavy-metal ions; transports large organic anions such as drugs, bilirubin, and poorly soluble hormones (e.g., cortisol); and serves as a protein and amino acid reserve. See also *hypoalbuminemia.*

aggregated a., a colloidal suspension of aggregated human serum albumin having a particle size range of about 10–60 μm; it is used in nuclear medicine for pulmonary perfusion imaging. Formerly, iodine-131–labeled aggregated albumin was the most commonly used imaging agent; this has now been replaced by technetium-99m–labeled aggregated albumin. When injected into a vein, about 90 percent of the particles become lodged in the first downstream capillary bed, the pulmonary capillaries and arterioles. The radionuclide distribution demonstrates areas of adequate perfusion. Also called *macroaggregated a.*

b s a. (BSA), purified albumin, prepared from bovine serum, and available as dry crystalline material or in the form of solutions of varied concentration. In clinical chemistry, dilutions of commercially prepared protein standard solution made with crystalline bovine serum albumin, sold in ampoules with protein content given in terms of milligrams of protein-nitrogen per milliliter of solution, are used for standardizing protein assays.

chromated Cr 51 serum a., a radiopharmaceutical used to measure gastrointestinal protein loss.

iodinated I 125 serum a. (human), [USP], a radiopharmaceutical used for plasma volume determinations. Also called ^{125}I-HSA, IHSA, RISA.

iodinated I 131 serum a. (human), [USP], a radiopharmaceutical used for plasma volume and cardiac output determinations. Also called ^{131}I-HSA, IHSA, and RISA.

macroaggregated a. (MAA), see *aggregated a.*

a. microspheres, sterile particles of human serum albumin, 10–35 μm in diameter, used in nuclear medicine for pulmonary perfusion imaging. The microspheres are labeled with technetium-99m. When injected into a vein, the microspheres become trapped in the first capillary bed the circulation passes through, that of the lungs. The radionuclide distribution shows areas of the lungs that are adequately perfused.

normal serum a. (human), [USP], a sterile, pyrogen-free albumin fraction used to treat shock or hypoproteinemia.

albumin assays 1. direct colorimetric measurement using dyes (e.g., bromocresol green or bromocresol purple) that bind tightly to albumin. These are the most commonly used assays because of their simplicity and ease of automation.

2. measurement by a colorimetric reaction employing the biuret reagent after globulins have been removed by salt precipitation; an obsolete procedure.

3. separation of the serum proteins by electrophoresis, followed by staining and densitometric determination of the albumin fraction.

4. immunochemical techniques using reagents with antibodies specific for albumin (e.g., nephelometry or radial immunodiffusion). This procedure and serum protein electrophoresis give the most accurate results.

albumin/globulin (A/G) ratio the ratio of albumin and globulin concentrations in serum, usually determined by protein electrophoresis. A low A/G ratio may occur in cirrhosis, hepatitis, and other liver diseases, reflecting a diminished capacity of the liver to synthesize albumin and also, but not invariably, an increase in the immune-globulin fraction. The measurement of the A/G ratio has largely been discontinued in favor of procedures that quantitate the individual protein components of body fluids, as such values are more useful clinically.

albuminocytologic dissociation (al-bu″mĭ-no-si″to-loj′ik) a marked increase of protein concentration in the cerebrospinal fluid without any corresponding increase in cell count. It occurs most frequently in the Guillain-Barré syndrome, but may also be present as a nonspecific finding in a variety of other neurologic disorders.

albuminoid (al-bu′mĭ-noid″) [*albumin* + Gr. *eidos* form] 1. resembling albumin.

2. a scleroprotein.

3. a group of fibrous proteins, which are insoluble in neutral solvents and dilute acids and bases. Included are the elastins (in tendons), keratins (in hair and feathers), and collagens (in cartilage). Such materials are generally present in structures that have a protective or supportive function.

albumin slide adhesive albumin preparations used to attach tissue sections to slides. One is Mayer's egg albumin, a 1:1 mixture of egg white and glycerin, which is smeared in a thin, even coat on slides before the sections are mounted.

albumin suspension test a blood grouping test in which red cell agglutination by blood group antibodies is determined in the presence of albumin.

albuminuria (al″bu-mĭ-nu′re-ah) [*albumin* + Gr. *ouron* urine + *-ia*] the presence in the urine of serum albumin. The term is sometimes used instead of proteinuria when there is a very high concentration of albumin in the plasma protein that has leaked through the glomeruli. This condition may follow immune complex nephritis.

Alcaligenes (al″kah-lij′ĕ-nēz) a genus of motile (peritrichous), gram-negative aerobic bacilli commonly found in water and soil. Within the hospital, strains of *Alcaligenes* are recovered from moist items such as respirator reservoirs and hemodialysis systems; they constitute a part of the normal human skin microflora, and occur in clinical specimens with or without the probability of clinical significance. *Alcaligenes* is a constituent of the collection of gram-negative bacteria referred to as "water bacteria." The genus is characterized as glucose-nonfermenting, oxidase-positive, and urease-negative.

A. faecalis, the species of *Alcaligenes* most often isolated from the hospital environment and from human sources, especially sputum and urine.

Alcian blue 8GX trademark for a blue, water-soluble basic phthalocyanin dye; C.I. 74240. It is used at varying pHs as a specific stain for mucopolysaccharides.

alcohol (al′ko-hol) [Arabic *al-koh'l* a sublimate] 1. any of a class of organic compounds containing the OH (hydroxyl) group attached to a saturated carbon that is not attached directly to another functional group (other compounds such as enols and phenols also contain an OH group but these are not classified as alcohols). An alcohol may be classified as primary, secondary, or tertiary, depending on the number of carbons attached to the carbon bearing the OH (see also *primary, secondary,* and *tertiary*). The term is extended to compounds that contain more than one OH group. They are distinguished as monohydric, dihydric, trihydric, or polyhydric alcohols, depending on the number of hydroxyl groups present. See also *ethanol* and *methanol.*

2. the common name for ethanol.

3. [USP], a preparation containing not less than 92.3 percent and not more than 93.8 percent of ethanol by weight, corresponding to not less than 94.9 percent and not more than 96.0 by volume, at 15.56°C, of C_2H_5OH; used as a topical anti-infective and solvent.

alcohol assays gas chromatography. The specimen is diluted 10-fold with diluent working solution (1-propanol and water), and 1-μl samples are injected into a gas chromatograph equipped with a polar column and flame ionization detector. Samples of standard alcohol solutions (methanol, ethanol and 2-propanol) diluted with the same working solution are then injected. The peak-area or peak-height ratios of the 1-propanol to the respective alcohol in the sample are compared with the ratios of the corresponding alcohol standard solutions. This method is sensitive to 100 mg/l of alcohol in blood. Larger volumes of dilute specimens can be used to determine lower concentrations. See also *ethanol assays.*

alcohol dehydrogenase (AD, ADH) (al'ko-hol de-hi'dro-jen-ās) an enzyme of the oxidoreductase class (alcohol:NAD oxidoreductase, EC 1.1.1.1), a widely distributed enzyme found in human liver, where it catalyzes the oxidation of primary and secondary alcohols to aldehydes in the presence of NAD^+. This enzyme catalyzes the conversion of methanol to formaldehyde, a hazardous compound responsible for the toxic effects of methanol. The measurement of the activity of this enzyme in body fluids has no common clinical usage, although it has been suggested as another parameter for hepatic disease. Its activity can be determined by following the increased absorbance of the NADH formed during the reaction. The enzyme is used as a reagent in the determination of ethanol. See also *ethanol.*

alcohol fixation a method of tissue fixation. Generally, alcohol fixation is not effective when used alone, but absolute alcohol may be used to preserve glycogen, tissue mast cells (in some species), and pigments, and to fix blood and tissue films and smears. Methyl alcohol is most often used for the latter purpose at concentrations of 80–100 percent. Ethyl alcohol (60–80 percent) may also preserve some proteins and enzymes in an undenatured state if kept at very low temperatures (–20° to –25°C). Alcohol is a slow tissue penetrator, but its rate can be increased when formalin is added. Some important alcohol fixatives are Carnoy's and Newcomer's.

alcoholic (al"ko-hol'ik) [L. *alcoholicus*] 1. a term used to describe any substance containing alcohol or those disorders related to alcohol use.

2. a term for a person who abuses alcohol. What constitutes abuse is difficult to define; many people consider an alcoholic to be one whose drinking interferes with social relationships, job, or health. Such impairment in the individual's life style is almost always accompanied by the inability to stop drinking.

alcoholic cardiomyopathy a clinical entity seen in alcoholic individuals that is characterized by cardiomegaly, arrhythmias, congestive heart failure, and thromboembolisms occurring in the absence of other known causes of heart disease. Without abstinence from alcohol, approximately 40 percent of patients die within 3 yr after the first appearance of symptoms. Those affected may have myoglobinuria and elevated serum concentrations of creatine kinase and aldolase. Electrocardiographic tracings are usually distinctive. See also *alcoholic m.* under *myopathy* and *alcoholic polyneuropathy* under *neuropathy.*

alcoholic cirrhosis a term used in the etiologic classification of cirrhosis to describe a form of cirrhosis that corresponds approximately to micronodular cirrhosis. See also *cirrhosis.*

alcoholic formalin a histologic fixative in which alcohol is substituted for distilled water as the diluent of formaldehyde solution; this cuts fixation time in half and results in greater hardening. The alcohol causes the loss of fats and lipids, improved preservation of glycogen, poorer preservation of iron-bearing pigments (e.g., heme), and sometimes lysis of erythrocytes and eosinophilic granules.

alcoholic hepatitis acute or chronic inflammation of the liver in response to ethanol-induced parenchymal necrosis. Histologic features of the acute form include zonal necrosis in the periphery of the hepatic acinus, infiltrates of polymorphonuclear neutrophils in and around areas of necrosis, steatosis, and alcoholic hyaline. The chronic form shows such additional histologic features as portal fibrosis with invasion of lobules and central hyaline sclerosis. See also *cirrhosis* and *hepatitis.*

alcoholic hyaline see under *Mallory bodies.*

alcoholism (al'ko-hol-izm) a disorder of alcohol abuse, with impairment of the affected individual's health, social interactions, or job. Alcoholism is perhaps the most serious illness in the United States, in terms of its associated morbidity and mortality, affecting as much as 10 percent of the population. It is a major contributor to accidental and intentionally caused deaths. Associated diseases include pancreatitis, hepatitis, cirrhosis, central nervous system disease, and (very probably) several forms of cancer, most notably esophageal carcinomas.

ALD abbrev. See *aldolase.*

Aldactone (al-dak'tōn) trademark. See *spironolactone.*

aldaric acid (al-dah'rik) a sugar acid formed by oxidation of both terminal carbon atoms of a monosaccharide to carboxyl groups. Aldaric acids have the general formula $COOH(CHOH)_nCOOH$.

aldehyde (al'dĕ-hīd) [*al*cohol + L. *de* away from + *hyd*rogen] any one of a large class of reactive compounds that are derived from the primary alcohols by oxidation or dehydrogenation and contain a carbonyl group with a hydrogen attached, —CHO. Acetaldehyde is one example. See also *functional group.*

aldehyde dehydrogenase (al'dĕ-hīd de-hi'dro-jen-ās) an enzyme of the oxidoreductase class (aldehyde:NAD^+ oxidoreductase, EC 1.2.1.3) that catalyzes the reaction aldehyde + NAD^+ + $H_2O \rightleftarrows$ acid + NADH. The enzyme is found in animal tissues and catalyzes the oxidation of various aldehydes, including the conversion of acetic aldehyde to acetic acid. Formerly called *acetaldehydase.*

aldehyde fixatives fixative solutions possessing one or more aldehyde groups that are of use in light and electron microscopy and in certain enzyme studies. They include glyoxal, glutaraldehyde, formaldehyde, paraformaldehyde, crotonaldehyde, hydroxyadipaldehyde, methacrolein, acetaldehyde, and succinaldehyde. The usefulness and application of each is dictated by such factors as the quality of cytologic fixation, rate of penetration, preservation of enzyme systems, reaction with embedding media, and reaction to electron bombardment. Aldehyde fixatives cross-link, like formalin, with active hydrogen, amino, and imino groups of proteins, as well as with the indoles, catecholamines, and hydroxyl groups of polyalcohols. See also *fixative.*

aldehyde fuchsin (al′de-hīd fook′sin) a histologic stain for elastin, pancreatic and hypophyseal beta cell granules, and the Australia antigen (hepatitis B antigen). Paraffin sections fixed in formalin or Bouin's fluid are oxidized in iodine, bleached in thiosulfate, stained in aldehyde-fuchsin solution (0.5 g of basic fuchsin, 100 ml of 70 percent alcohol, 1 ml of hydrochloric acid, and 1 ml of paraldehyde), and counterstained with hematoxylin and orange G, with Masson's trichrome, or with van Gieson's stain.

Elastic fibers, mast cell granules, gastric chief cells, pancreatic beta-cell granules, some of the hypophyseal beta-cell granules, mucins, and acid mucopolysaccharides are stained a violet-to-purple color. Alpha-cell granules in the pancreas or hypophysis are counterstained. The aldehyde-fuchsin solution keeps about 2 wk.

aldehyde oxidase (al′dĕ-hīd ok′sĭ-dās) an enzyme of the oxidoreductase class (aldehyde:oxygen oxidoreductase, EC 1.2.3.1) that catalyzes the reaction aldehyde + H_2O + O_2 ⇄ acid + superoxide. Physiologically, the enzyme is found in liver tissue and catalyzes the oxidation of acetic aldehyde. Formerly called *acetaldehydase.*

Alder-Reilly anomaly (al′der ri′le) [Albert von *Alder,* German physician, born 1888; William Anthony *Reilly,* U.S. pediatrician, born 1901] a genetic condition, transmitted as a dominant trait, that is characterized by the presence of abnormally large, azurophilic, metachromatically staining granules in granulocytes, lymphocytes and monocytes. See also *Alder-Reilly bodies* and *mucopolysaccharidosis.*

Alder-Reilly bodies [Albert von *Alder;* William Anthony *Reilly*] abnormally large azurophilic granules, composed of mucopolysaccharides, that occur in Alder-Reilly anomaly. The granules either are found in granulocytes, lymphocytes, and monocytes, or occur in only one type of leukocyte, usually the lymphocyte. They can be distinguished from normal azurophilic granules by metachromatic staining with toluidine blue.

Alder-Reilly bodies are also present in diseases of mucopolysaccharide metabolism (mucopolysaccharidoses) such as Hurler's disease, Hunter's syndrome, and Sanfilippo's syndrome. Morquio's disease (mucopolysaccharidosis IV) is distinguished by aggregates of the metachromatically staining granules. The granules are reported to be absent in Scheie's syndrome (mucopolysaccharidosis I S), a disorder closely related to Hurler's syndrome. Apparently they do not interfere with the function of leukocytes. Also called Alder bodies and Reilly bodies.

aldicarb (al′dĭ-karb) an extremely toxic carbamate insecticide, acaricide, and nematocide, 2-methyl-2-(methylthio)propanal *O*-[(methylamino)carbonyl] oxime, $CH_3SC(CH_3)_2CH{=}NOCONHCH_3$. It can be ingested or absorbed through the skin, and produces cholinesterase inhibition with symptoms that resemble poisoning by organophosphate compounds. Atropine (but not pralidoxime) is used to treat carbamate poisoning. Trademark, Temik.

aldimine (al′dim-ēn) an imine derived from an aldehyde; i.e., the carbon of the carbon-nitrogen double bond has a hydrogen attached. See also *imine* and *Schiff base.*

aldofuranose (al″do-fu′rah-nōs) an aldose having the furanose ring structure. See also *furanose.*

aldohexose (al″do-hek′sōs) any of a class of sugars that contain six carbon atoms and an aldehyde group on carbon–1, such as glucose or galactose.

aldolase (ALD) (al′do-lās) an enzyme of the lyase class (fructose bisphosphate aldolase, EC 4.1.2.13) that catalyzes the reaction D-fructose-1,6-bisphosphate ⇄ D-glyceraldehyde 3-phosphate + dihydroxyacetone phosphate. The reaction is reversible but favors formation of fructose-1,6-bisphosphate (fructose-1,6-diphosphate, FDP) from the two triose phosphates. This is one of the reactions in the Embden-Meyerhof pathway in which glucose is converted to pyruvate, which is then converted either to acetyl-CoA or lactate. Acetyl-CoA enters the citric acid cycle in the aerobic utilization of glucose as fuel. The conversion of glucose to lactate (glycolysis) is anaerobic and is important in skeletal muscles. The enzyme is present in all cells and in high concentration in skeletal muscle. Three forms of ALD are recognized: A, B, and C, differing in reactivity to FDP and fructose-1-phosphate (F-1-P) as substrates. A is found primarily in skeletal muscle and has only weak activity toward F-1-P; B occurs in the liver, kidneys, and leukocytes, and has considerably more activity toward F-1-P; C is found in the brain and is an embryonic form. A and C have tetrameric structures, and hybrid forms involving A and C are found in some tissues. The B enzyme is often referred to as the fructose-1-phosphate aldolase because of its greater reactivity toward F-1-P.

Serum ALD activity is elevated in a number of conditions associated with muscle wastage (Duchenne dystrophy, limb-girdle dystrophy), but is normal when the muscle pathology is neurogenic in origin (polio, multiple sclerosis). ALD serum levels rise remarkably in response to cortisone and adrenocorticotropic hormone therapy. The use of ALD measurements in muscle, heart, and liver diseases has decreased owing to the difficulties in determining the activity of the enzyme and because of its relatively low sensitivity compared with creatine kinase and liver enzymes, respectively.

The activity ratio of the A to B form has been used in the differential diagnosis and detection of cancer. The ratio is about 2.8 in healthy individuals, 1.3 for uncomplicated acute hepatitis, more than 18 for primary hepatoma, 12 for cancer without liver metastasis, and 7 when liver metastases are present.

aldolase assays methods for the determination of ALD activity, most commonly carried out on the enzyme in serum, although levels in tissues, especially in dystrophic muscle, are of clinical interest. In the outdated colorimetric procedure performed manually, the reaction is pushed to the right (fructose-1,6-biphosphate to triose phosphates) with the use of hydrazine as trapping agent. The triose phosphate hydrazones are hydrolyzed with NaOH, and the triose phosphates converted to brown-red 2,4-dinitrophenylhydrazones and measured at 540 nm. Two continuous monitoring methods are available. In one, the ALD reaction is coupled to the glyceraldehyde-3-phosphate dehydrogenase reaction, and the oxidation of the triose phosphates by NAD^+ is followed by measuring the NADH formed by its absorbance at 340 nm. In the other approach, the ALD is coupled to the glycerol-3-phosphate dehydrogenase reaction, and the reduction of triose phosphates is followed by measuring NADH consumption at 340 nm. In both systems triose phosphate isomerase is added to favor rapid interconversion of the two triose phosphates.

Aldomet (al′do-met) trademark. See *methyldopa.*

aldonic acid (al-don′ik) a sugar acid formed by oxidation of the aldehyde functional group of an aldose to a carboxyl group. Aldonic acids have the general formula $COOH(CHOH)_nCH_2OH$.

aldopentose (al″do-pen′tōs) any of a class of sugars that contain five carbon atoms and an aldehyde group, such as arabinose and ribose.

aldopyranose (al″do-pi′rah-nōs, al″do-peer′ah-nōs) an aldose having the pyranose ring structure. See also *pyranose.*

aldose (al′dōs) any monosaccharide having an aldehyde group (—CHO, see *functional group*) in the open-chain form. Aldoses usually exist in the cyclic hemiacetal form, the result of a reversible intramolecular reaction between the aldehyde group and a hydroxyl group in the same molecule. See also specific aldoses such as *galactose, glucose, mannose,* and *ribose.* Cf. *ketose.*

aldosterone (al″do-ster′ōn) one of the most powerful mineralocorticoids, 11β,21-dihydroxy-3,20-dioxopregn-4-en-18-al. It is the principal electrolyte-regulating steroid secreted by the adrenal cortex. Aldosterone reflects both electrolyte and water metabolic changes. It increases reabsorption of sodium and excretion of potassium in the kidney, and appears to increase the movement of sodium into and potassium out of body cells. It is primarily regulated by the renin-angiotensin system and possibly in a limited way by corticotropin. About 200 μg/da are secreted by the adrenals. Its secretion is inversely related to extracellular fluid (especially plasma) volume and to total body sodium. Lack of sodium in the diet may increase aldosterone concentration to five times above the reference range. Normal secretion varies with the time of day; it is lowest in the afternoon.

Reference values for plasma aldosterone (normal salt diet) are: for individuals recumbent for at least 2 hr, 1–7 ng/dl of plasma; and for those standing for at least 4 hr, 3–28. Such assays are useful in the diagnosis and treatment of patients with overproduction of this steroid hormone (aldosteronism).

aldosterone assays radioimmunoassay, using specific antisera. Like other steroids, aldosterone is not antigenic. It is made antigenic by conjugating with a protein (e.g., bovine serum albumin). To raise highly specific antisera, the protein should preferably be conjugated to C_6 of aldosterone. In the radioimmunoassay procedure, aldosterone is extracted from plasma, purified by chromatography (if the antibody is not specific), and incubated in the presence of radiolabeled aldosterone along with the antisera to aldosterone. Following separation of the antibody bound from the unbound aldosterone (by dextran-coated charcoal, Florisil, or double antibody techniques), final quantitation is made by comparing the percentage bound or unbound with a standard curve (run parallel with the sample) suitable for the range of estimation.

aldosteronism (al″do-ster′o-nizm″) overproduction of the steroid hormone aldosterone. It may be primary (due to adrenal adenoma, carcinoma, or bilateral cortical hyperplasia) or secondary (due to extraadrenal diseases such as congestive heart failure, nephrotic syndrome, or cirrhosis with ascites). Aldosteronism results in sodium retention, potassium loss, and, ultimately, hypertension.

aldotransferase (al″do-trans′fer-ās) see *transaldolase.*

aldotriose (al″do-tri′ōs) a monosaccharide with a free aldehyde functional group and three carbon atoms; D- and L-glyceraldehyde are the only examples.

aldrin (al′drin) a chlorinated cyclodiene insecticide that is rapidly metabolized to dieldrin. See also *chlorinated hydrocarbon pesticides.*

Aleppo boil (ah-lep′o) [*Aleppo,* Syria] cutaneous leishmaniasis, a type of ulcer or sore caused by *Leishmania tropica.* Also called Baghdad sore, Delhi sore, and oriental sore.

alert check a laboratory quality control check; see *limit check.*

alerting response a nonspecific response evoked by several types of stimuli. It consists of a widespread transient discharge on the electroencephalogram that reaches maximal amplitude at the vertex of the skull (V wave). During sleep, this response forms the vertex sharp transient of a K complex.

If the stimulus is novel to the patient, a sudden change in ongoing electroencephalographic activity (e.g., a decrease in alpha activity) may also be recorded. The alerting response is diminished if a given stimulus is reported several times. See also *evoked potential, K complex,* and *vertex sharp transient.*

aleukemia (a″lu-ke′me-ah) [*a-* neg. + Gr. *leukos* white + *haima* blood + *-ia*] 1. the absence or deficiency of leukocytes in the blood.

2. aleukemic leukemia; that is, leukemia without large numbers of circulating malignant cells.

aleuriospore (ah-lu′re-o-spōr) [Gr.; *aleuron* flour + *spora* seed] a terminal or lateral asexual fungal spore similar to a conidium except that it is not shed (not deciduous), being released only by the dissolving of its attachment to the mycelium. This type of conidial formation is recognized as the holothallic ontogeny. Spores produced by dermatophytes are either micro- or macroaleuriospores.

macroaleuriospore, see *macroconidium.*

alexia (ah-lek′se-ah) [*a-* neg. + Gr. *lexis* word + *-ia*] see *dyslexia.*

alexin (a-lek′sin) [Gr. *alexein* to ward off] a nonspecific, thermolabile substance, which is found in fresh serum and plasma and which combines with a specific sensitizer to produce cell lysis. See also *complement.*

alga (al′gah), pl. *algae* [L. "seaweed"] any individual organism of the algae.

algae (al′je) [L.] a group of simple plants commonly found in upper layers of bodies of water. Most are unicellular and contain chlorophyll. Algae perform nearly half of the world's total photosynthesis. In the laboratory, some species are used as a source of agar for culture media.

algesi/o (al-je′ze-o) [Gr. *algēsis* sense of pain] a word element used in combining form to denote pain or excessive sensitivity to pain, e.g., analgesia.

algesia (al-je′ze-ah) [Gr. *algēsis* a sense of pain + *-ia*] an increased sensitivity to pain or a perception of pain produced by stimuli that normally are not painful.

-algia (al′je-ah) [Gr. *algos* pain + *-ia* condition] a suffix word element to denote pain, e.g., arthralgia.

algin (al′jin) sodium alginate, a purified carbohydrate (sodium mannuronate) extracted from species of brown algae and used as a stabilizing colloid in numerous pharmaceuticals, cosmetics, and foods. See also *alginic acid.*

alginate (al′jĭ-nāt) a salt of alginic acid extracted from marine kelp. Calcium, sodium, and ammonium alginates have been used as foam, clot, or gauze for absorbable surgical dressings. Soluble alginates, such as sodium, potassium, and magnesium alginates, form a viscous sol that can be changed into a gel by a chemical reaction with compounds such as calcium sulfate; this property makes them useful as materials for taking dental impressions.

alginic acid (al″jin′ik) a polysaccharide polymer of mannuronic acid, polymannuronic acid, that is present in large quantities in the cell walls of algae. See also *algin.*

ALGOL (al′gol) [acronym from *algo*rithmic *o*riented *l*anguage] a high-level computer language, similar to FORTRAN, that is used primarily for scientific applications. The coding for its calculations resembles algebra.

algorithm (al′go-rith″um) [Muhammad ibn-Musa *al-Khwarizmi,* Arab mathematician, 780–850 A. D., author of a treatise on algebra] an explicit procedure for solving a mathematical problem; a series of well-defined operations, such as a computer program, that can be proved always to produce an answer, at least to a specific degree of approximation, in a finite number of steps. Cf. *heuristic method.*

algor mortis (al′gor) [L. "coldness of death"] the gradual decrease in body temperature after death, as it drops to that of its environment.

alicyclic (al″ĭ-sik′lik) being homocyclic (having only carbons in the ring) and not aromatic.

alicyclic hydrocarbon a hydrocarbon that has both cyclic structure and aliphatic properties; only carbon atoms are joined to form one or more nonaromatic rings. These hydrocarbons are classified as one of three types: cycloparaffins, cycloolefins, or cycloacetylenes.

aliesterase (al-ĕ-es′ter-ās) see *carboxylesterase.*

align (ah-līn′) [Fr. *aligner* to put in a straight line] 1. to place in a straight line; to aim along a particular line.

2. to adjust a tuned electronic circuit for maximal response.

alignment (ah-līn′ment) the act of arranging in a line, or the state of being arranged in a line.

alignment chart see *nomogram.*

alimentary (al″ĕ-men′tar-e) [L. *alimentarius,* from *alere* to feed] pertaining to food or nutritive material, or to the organs of digestion.

alimentary tract that part of the digestive tract formed by the esophagus, stomach, and small and large intestines. Also called alimentary canal. See also *gastrointestinal tract.*

alimentation (al″ĕ-men-ta′shun) the giving or receiving of nourishment.

aliphatic (al″ĕ-fat′ik) [Gr. *aleiphar, aleiphatos* oil] a term that can be applied to any nonaromatic organic compound, as in aliphatic hydrocarbon and aliphatic alcohol. The term was formerly used to refer to compounds containing no rings, being synonymous with acyclic. Many animal and vegetable fats (from which the term aliphatic is derived) have long-chain alkyl groups and are thus aliphatic compounds.

aliphatic acid one of the straight- or branched-chain carboxylic acids, e.g., acetic acid.

aliphatic alcohol one of the straight- or branched-chain alcohols, including ethanol, methanol, and butanol; they are widely used as industrial solvents.

aliphatic hydrocarbon a hydrocarbon that contains no aromatic rings. Aliphatic hydrocarbons are subdivided into alkanes, alkenes, and alkynes.

aliquot (al′ĕ-kwot) [L. "some, several"] 1. in mathematics, an exact divisor of a number.

2. in clinical chemistry and immunology, a measured portion of a sample, reference solution, etc., that has the same composition as the whole.

alizarin (ah-liz′ah-rin) [Arabic *ala sara* extract] a red mordant dye, 1,2-dihydroxyanthraquinone; C.I. 58000.

alizarin red S a mordant dye, the sulfonic acid derivative of alizarin; C.I. 58005. It forms red-orange lakes with calcium ions and is used in histology primarily for the demonstration of calcium deposits in tissues and for the vital staining of long bones. The injected dye is deposited at sites of calcification. Alizarin red S also forms scarlet lakes with aluminum and other metal ions.

alkalemia (al″kah-le′me-ah) [*alkali* + Gr. *haima* blood + *-ia*] a decreased hydrogen ion concentration of the blood, which produces a pH above 7.45. Cf. *alkalosis.*

alkali (al′kah-li) [Arabic *al qalīy* potash] any compound that in water has a pH of greater than 7.0. Strong alkalis in solution are corrosive to the skin and mucous membranes. See also *base.*

alkali denaturation test see under *fetal hemoglobin tests.*

alkali metals the metals of group IA in the periodic table: lithium, sodium, potassium, rubidium, cesium, and francium.

alkalimetry (al″kah-lim′ĕ-tre) [*alkali* + Gr. *metron* measure] the quantitative chemical analysis of the concentration of base or one particular free base in solution, as by titration with acid.

alkaline (al′kah-līn) basic; having a pH greater than 7.0 (when referring to an aqueous solution); having the properties or reactions of an alkali. See also *pH.*

alkaline phosphatase (ALP) an enzyme of the hydrolase class (orthophosphoric acid monoester phosphohydrolase, EC 3.1.3.1) that consists of relatively nonspecific enzyme species active only in an alkaline medium at about pH 9.5–10.5. Such enzymes are found in blood plasma or serum, liver, bone, kidney, mammary gland, placenta, spleen, lung, intestines, leukocytes, adrenal cortex, and seminiferous tubules, and in some malignant tissues. These enzymes catalyze the transfer of the phosphate group from one organic phosphate ester to an alcohol or water. When the phosphate acceptor is water, the reaction is essentially the hydrolysis of the ester to an alcohol and the HPO_4^{2-} group. Only monoesters of *o*-phosphoric acid can serve as substrates, although some pyrophosphates, such as

ALKALINE PHOSPHATASE. ALP INCREASES IN VARIOUS DISORDERS

DISORDER	ALP ACTIVITY
Osteitis deformans (Paget's disease of bone)	10–25 times normal
Extrahepatic obstruction	3–10 times normal
Viral hepatitis	2–3 times normal
Intrahepatic obstruction	2–2½ times normal
Bone cancer	Marked increase
Hodgkin's disease, congestive heart failure, ulcerative colitis, regional enteritis, intraabdominal bacterial infection	Moderate increase
Osteomalacia	Moderate increase
Osteoporosis	Normal
Fanconi's syndrome	Slight to moderate increase
Primary hyperparathyroidism	Slight to moderate increase

ATP, are also acted upon. Divalent cations, such as zinc, manganese, magnesium, or cobalt, must be present as activators. The exact function of the ALP enzymes in the organism is still not understood, but current evidence suggests that they are involved in the transport of metabolites across cell membranes, in the calcification process during bone formation, and in lipid transport.

Activity of some ALP preparations increases with time after freezing and thawing or after reconstitution of lyophilized preparations, probably as a result of disaggregation of phospholipid complexes formed with the enzyme.

The changes in ALP activity in serum are useful in the clinical diagnosis of many illnesses, especially hepatobiliary diseases and bone diseases with increased osteoblastic activity. Furthermore, ALP activity in leukocytes is increased in Down's syndrome, idiopathic myelofibrosis, and polycythemia vera. It is also increased in other diseases, as shown in the accompanying table. Activity is decreased in sickle cell disease and paroxysmal nocturnal hemoglobinuria. There are also transient elevations during the healing of fractures and the third trimester of pregnancy. Reference ranges for healthy, growing children are 1.5–2.5 times those of adults, owing to increases in bone isoenzyme.

See also *leukocyte alkaline phosphatase.*

alkaline phosphatase assays methods for determining the ALP activity in serum. Most current assays for ALP (two-point assays and the continuous monitoring assays) use the substrate *p*-nitrophenylphosphate (pNPP) as substrate, the activator $MgCl_2$, and 2 amino, 2 methyl-1-propanol (AMP) or diethanolamine (DEA) as buffer and phosphate acceptor. A reaction pH between 10.1 and 10.5 is used, depending on the reaction temperature and type of buffer. In continuous monitoring methods, the yellow color of the *p*-nitrophenol (pNP) formed by the reaction is measured at 402–410 nm. In the two-point methods, NaOH is added to stop the reaction and bring out the full color of pNP. The color is then read, and the enzyme activity is calculated using pure pNP as standard.

Thymolphthalein monophosphate and phenolphthalein monophosphate have also been used as substrates, and tris(hydroxymethyl)aminomethane has been used as buffer and phosphate acceptor. The measured activity expressed in International Units per liter (U/l) varies with the combination of substrate, buffer, pH, and reaction temperature (30° or 37°C) used.

alkaline phosphatase isoenzyme electrophoresis electrophoresis at an alkaline pH, usually on cellulose acetate or agarose, to separate the alkaline phosphatase (ALP) isoenzymes, followed by staining and qualitative assessment of the pattern. There are five distinct isoenzymes: those produced by liver, bone, intestine, kidneys, and placenta. The Regan isoenzyme is produced by various carcinomas. An additional "fast liver" band is often noted when there is significant hepatocellular jaundice. Human ALP isoenzymes are relatively stable at room temperatures but will denature rapidly at 56°C, with the exception of the placental and Regan enzymes, which are resistant to denaturation even at 65°C.

The primary purpose of the procedure is to determine whether the hepatic or osseous isoenzyme form is responsible for an elevation in total serum ALP. This is difficult because these isoenzymes have partially overlapping electrophoretic mobility and thus cannot easily be quantitated. The intestinal isoenzyme is run in parallel to the sample to provide a reference point.

The activity of other liver enzymes, such as γ-glutamyl transferase (GGT) or 5′-nucleotidase (5′NT), helps in interpretation of the ALP isoenzyme pattern, as these enzymes are not increased in bone disease.

alkaline phosphatase staining procedures for determining the presence of the enzyme alkaline phosphatase in cells. In the Gomori method, a monophosphate ester and calcium are reacted with the enzyme to form insoluble calcium phosphate. The calcium phosphate is then reacted with a lead or cobalt salt and ammonium sulfide to form an insoluble black precipitate. The Burstone azo-coupling method involves the reaction of a naphthol phosphate ester with the enzyme and the simultaneous coupling of the liberated naphthoic anilide with a diazonium salt (such as fast blue B) to produce an insoluble azo dye. This technique works best with freeze-dried tissue, and permits precise localization of alkaline phosphatase activity.

As with any enzymatic procedure, care must be taken to avoid inactivating the enzyme. Fixation should be in acetone, ethanol, or cold calcium-formalin, and frozen sectioning should be used to avoid denaturing the enzyme.

alkaline tide the rapid increase in blood pH and serum bicarbonate concentration and the decrease in the serum chloride concentration that accompanies the secretion of hydrochloric acid into the stomach during and after a meal.

alkalinuria (al″kah-lin-u′re-ah) [*alkaline* + Gr. *ouron* urine + *-ia*] an alkaline condition of the urine.

alkaloid (al′kah-loid″) [*alkali* + Gr. *eidos* form] one of a large group of organic basic substances found in plants. They are very bitter, many are pharmacologically active, some are deadly poisons, and others are medically useful. Most contain a heterocyclic ring, such as pyridine, quinoline, isoquinoline, pyrrole, purine, or tropine. They are given trivial names ending in -ine. Alkaloids used as drugs include atropine, caffeine, cocaine, codeine, ephedrine, morphine, nicotine, papaverine, pilocarpine, quinine, vinblastine, and vincristine. The term is also applied to synthetic substances (called artificial alkaloids) that have structures similar to plant alkaloids, such as procaine.

alkalosis (al″kah-lo′sis) [*alkali* + Gr. *-osis* condition] a physiologic state or condition resulting from the accumulation of base in, or the loss of acid from, the body. See also *acid-base balance, metabolic alkalosis,* and *respiratory alkalosis.* Cf. *acidosis.*

hypokalemic a., the metabolic alkalosis caused by a depletion of intracellular K^+. The decrease in K^+ results in an increase in the NA^+-H^+ exchange, and thus in increased H^+ excretion by the renal tubules and increased absorption of HCO_3^-, causing extracellular alkalosis. The urine pH in this condition is acid, despite the presence of a metabolic alkalosis. Serum K^+ concentrations may be low-normal until at least 20 percent of the intracellular K^+ is depleted, at which time values below normal are generally observed.

nonrespiratory a., see *metabolic alkalosis.*

alkane (al′kān) a saturated hydrocarbon. See also *cycloalkane* and *paraffin.* Cf. *alkene* and *alkyne.*

alkannin paper (al-kan′in) filter paper dipped in an alcoholic solution of alkannin. Alkalis turn the paper blue; acids turn it red.

alkapton bodies (al-kap′tōn) [*alkali* + Gr. *kaptein* to gulp] a class of substances found in some urines, which are easily oxidized to give the urine a brown-black color, especially if the pH is alkaline. The most common is homogentisic acid. See also *alkaptonuria* and *homogentisic acid.*

alkaptonuria (al″kap-to-nu′re-ah) [*alkaptone* + Gr. *ouron* urine + *-ia*] a recessively inherited condition resulting in the excretion in the urine of alkapton bodies (most commonly, homogentisic acid, HGA), which cause the urine to turn dark on standing, especially after the addition of alkali. The condition may occur without other symptoms or, in long-standing cases, may be associated with pigmentation of the ears (ochronosis) and arthritic symptoms. Alkaptonuria is caused by a deficiency of the enzyme HGA oxidase, leading to the abnormal metabolism of the amino acids phenylalanine and tyrosine. It was one of the first inborn errors of metabolism identified. See also *aminoacidopathy.*

alkaptonuria tests tests to detect the presence of homogentisic acid (HGA) based on its reducing properties. In the silver nitrate ($AgNO_3$) test, $AgNO_3$ solution is added to urine, followed by a few drops of dilute ammonia water (NH_4OH). The presence of HGA reduces silver, resulting in the formation of a brown-black or black precipitate of elemental Ag, even before the addition of ammonia. In Benedict's reagent test, HGA reduces Benedict's qualitative reagent to form a yellow cuprous oxide precipitate. In the ferric chloride ($FeCl_3$) test, the addition of $FeCl_3$ solution drop-wise to the urine causes the formation of a transient blue color. Melanogens in urine are differentiated from HGA, inasmuch as the $AgNO_3$ reduction proceeds very slowly and requires excess NH_3, Benedict's reagent is not reduced, and the $FeCl_3$ test results in the formation of a brown-black precipitate.

alkene (al′kēn) an aliphatic hydrocarbon containing one or more carbon-carbon double bonds. Also called *olefin.* See also *cycloalkene.* Cf. *alkane* and *alkyne.*

alkenyl (al-kēn′il) the name applied to a hydrocarbon substituent having a carbon-carbon double bond; e.g., the ethenyl group, $CH_2{=}CH$—, is an alkenyl group.

alkoxide ion (al-kok′sīd) the name of the class of anions having a negative oxygen with an alkyl group attached to it, RO^-. Sodium methoxide, $CH_3O^-Na^+$, is a specific example.

alkoxy (al″kok′se) the name applied to the class of substituents, RO—, in which R is an alkyl group. Acylic ethers are named as alkoxy hydrocarbons; e.g., $CH_3OCH_2CH_2CH_3$ is 1-methoxy-propane.

alk phos abbrev. See *alkaline phosphatase.*

alkyl (al′kil) the radical that results when an alkane loses one hydrogen atom.

alkylate (al′kĭ-lāt) to add an alkyl group to a compound.

alkylating agent (al′kĭ-lāt-ing) a substance or chemical that acts by transfer of an alkyl group, such as a methyl or ethyl, from one compound to an important group such as an amino, carboxyl, sulfhydryl, or phosphate compound whose function is thereby impaired. Many alkylating agents are used as chemotherapeutic agents in the treatment of cancer, and act to inhibit DNA synthesis by the insertion of an ethyl or methyl group into a nucleotide, thus preventing cell replication. Most are highly toxic. See also *chemotherapy.* Cf. *biologic alkylating agent.*

alkylation (al″kĭ-la′shun) the substitution or addition of an alkyl group into an organic compound.

alkylbenzene sulfonate (ABS) (al″kil-ben′zēn sul′fo-nāt) the generic term for the branched-chain alkylaryl sulfonate–type of synthetic detergent. Resistant to microbial decomposition, these substances are being replaced by the more biodegradable linear alkyl sulfonates (LAS).

alkyl group (al′kil, al′kel) an organic substituent group formed by the removal of a hydrogen from an alkane, e.g., the methyl group. Cf. *aryl group.*

alkyl peroxide a peroxide that contains two alkyl radicals, R_1—O—O—R_2. See also *functional group.*

alkyne (al′kīn) an aliphatic hydrocarbon with one or more triple bonds, e.g., ethyne. Cf. *alkane* and *alkene.*

ALL abbrev. See *acute lymphocytic l.* under *leukemia.*

all/o (al′o) [Gr. *allos* other] a word element used in combining form to denote reversal or a condition varying from the normal, or different, other, e.g., allosteric, allorhythmia.

allantoic acid (ah-lan′to-ik) an intermediate in the

degradation of allantoin to urea during the catabolism of purines in animals.

allantoin (ah-lan′to-in) a white crystallizable substance, 5-ureidohydantoin, $C_4H_6N_4O_3$, the diureide of glyoxylic acid. Allantoin is the urinary excretion end product of purine metabolism in most mammals and many lower animals, but not in primates, which excrete uric acid. It is produced from uric acid by the enzyme urate oxidase (uricase).

allantois (ah-lan′to-is) [N.L., from Gr. *allas, allantos* sausage + *eidos* form] an initially tubular ventral diverticulum of the hindgut of the embryos of reptiles, birds, and mammals. In humans, the allantois is vestigial, except that its blood vessels give rise to those of the umbilical cord. In the eggs of reptiles and birds, however, it expands to a large sac for storing urine and, after fusing with the chorion, provides for gas exchange.

allele (ah-lēl′) [Ger. *Allel,* from Gr. *allēlōn* of one another] one of two or more alternate forms of a gene at the same site in a chromosome, which determine alternate characteristics in inheritance. The demonstration that different, inherited forms of a trait are allelic defines a gene. In normal eukaryotic cells, chromosomes occur in homologous pairs so that two loci are present for each gene. If the same allele is present on both, the individual is homozygous; if different alleles are present, the individual is heterozygous.

multiple a., an alternate allele found in a population at a single locus. The classic example of multiple allelism is the series of alleles that determines the ABO blood group. Multiple allelism at a locus with a relatively high frequency of compound genotypes may be an important source of clinical heterogeneity for many genetic disorders. See also *polymorphism.*

allelic (ah-le′lik) pertaining to alleles.

allelic exclusion the expression of one phenotype to the exclusion of the other possibility in cells that have alternate alleles for one genetic locus. It is a rare occurrence, although well known for immunoglobulin genes.

Allen correction (al′len) In absorption spectrophotometry, a technique of making corrections for interfering substances. Absorbance is measured at the peak wavelength and at two other wavelengths equidistant from the peak. Values for the latter are averaged and then subtracted from the peak reading, thus yielding a corrected absorbance reading. Such a correction must be applied to both the sample and the standards, and the shape of the absorption curve and the interference must be known before its application. It should not be used if the background reading is not linear across the measured region.

allergen (al′er-jen) [*allergy* + Gr. *gennan* to produce] 1. a substance capable of producing allergy or hypersensitivity; an antigen that causes sensitization by IgE antibody. Allergens trigger the production of antibodies, which in turn sensitize mast cells. On reexposure the combination of allergen and IgE antibody may cause the release of chemicals that can produce various unpleasant symptoms, ranging from sneezing and rash to potentially fatal anaphylactic shock.

2. the purified protein(s) of some food, bacterium, or pollen, used to test whether a patient is hypersensitive to those substances.

allergic (ah-ler′jik) pertaining to allergy.

allergic purpura see *allergic p.* under *purpura.*

allergoid (al′er-goid) [*allergy* + Gr. *eidos* form] chemically modified allergens that produce IgG antibodies rather than the usual IgE antibody, and thus less serious allergic symptoms.

allergology (al″er-gol′o-je) [*allergy* + *-logy,* from Gr. *logos* reasoned speech] the branch of medicine devoted to the study of allergy: its etiology, diagnosis, and treatment.

allergy (al′er-je) [Ger. *Allergie,* from Gr. *allos* other + *ergon* action work] an abnormal and individual hypersensitivity to substances that ordinarily are harmless, acquired by exposure to a particular allergen.

Allescheria (al″es-ke′re-ah) a genus of pathogenic fungi of the order *Ascomycetes.* The medically relevant species *A. boydii* is now classified as a member of the genus *Petriellidium* (see under *Petriellidium*).

allescheriosis (al″es-ke″re-o′sis) see *petriellidiosis.*

alligator clip (al′ĭ-ga″tor) a spring clip with toothed jaws used to make temporary electric connections, such as with test leads.

alloalbuminemia (al″o-al-bu″mĭ-ne′me-ah) [*allo-* + *albumin* + Gr. *haima* blood + *-ia*] an asymptomatic genetic trait in which the serum albumin is a variant type with abnormal electrophoretic mobility. See also *bisalbuminemia.*

alloantibody (al″o-an′tĭ-bod″e) see *isoantibody.*

alloantigen (al″o-an′tĭ-jen) see *isoantigen.*

allobarbital (al″o-bar′bĭ-tal) an intermediate-acting barbiturate used in some sedative preparations. See also *barbiturate.*

Allodermanyssus (al″o-der″mah-nis′sus) [*allo-* + Gr. *derma* skin + *nyssein* to prick] a genus of blood-sucking mites.

A. sanguineus, an external parasite of mice and rats, and a vector of *Rickettsia akari,* the cause of rickettsialpox in humans.

allogeneic (al″o-jĕ-ne′ik) pertaining to the genotypes of two individuals from the same species who are not genetically identical and are antigenically distinct. Cf. *syngeneic* and *xenogeneic.*

allogeneic graft see *allogeneic g.* under *graft.*

allograft (al′o-graft) see *allogeneic g.* under *graft.*

alloimmune (al′o-ĭ-mūn′) see *isoimmune.*

alloimmunization (al″o-im″u-nĭ-za′shun) see *isoimmunization.*

allometric (al″o-met′rik) [*allo-* + Gr. *metron* measure] pertaining to a changing relationship between the size of different body parts as the organism grows.

allometry (al-lom′ĕ-tre) [*allo-* + Gr. *metron* measure] the relationship between the size and rate of growth of the parts of an organism or between a part and the whole organism, either for the same organism over time or for a series of related organisms. Also called *heterauxesis* and *heterogony.*

allophanamide (al″o-fan-am′id) see *biuret.*

alloploidy (al″o-ploi′de) [*allo-* + *ploidy,* from Gr. *-ploos* -fold (as in *diploos* twofold) + *eidos* form] the state of having any number of chromosome sets derived from different ancestral species.

allopolyploidy (al″o-pol′e-ploi″de) [*allo-* + Gr. *polys* much, many + *ploidy*] the state of having more than two sets of chromosomes derived from different ancestral species.

allopurinol (al″o-pu′rin-ol) [USP], an inhibitor of the enzyme xanthine oxidase, which catalyzes the conversion of hypoxanthine to xanthine and xanthine to uric acid, the last two steps in the catabolism of purines. Allopurinol is metabolized to an isomer of hypoxanthine, oxipurinol (alloxanthine), which also inhibits xanthine oxidase. It is used to treat gout and uric acid nephropathy due to either primary or secondary hyperuricemia (associated with blood dyscrasias, or with cancer chemotherapy). Trademark, Zyloprim.

allosteric (al″o-ster′ik) [*allo-* + Gr. *stereos* solid] referring to a phenomenon whereby the conformation (three-dimensional structure or folding pattern) of an enzyme (usually oligomeric) or other protein is altered by combination with a small molecule, referred to as an effector, which results in either increased or decreased activity by the enzyme. The binding of these effectors, which may be substrate or nonsubstrate molecules, is associated with the regulation of enzyme activity.

allosteric activation see under *allosteric effectors.*

allosteric effectors reagents that bind reversibly to an enzyme at specific sites other than their substrate-binding sites (active centers), hence the term allosteric sites. At constant enzyme and substrate concentrations, the binding of a negative effector reduces the reaction rate (allosteric inhibition), whereas the binding of a positive effector increases the rate (allosteric activation). If the effector is the substrate itself, the effect is said to be homotropic; if other than the substrate, it is said to be heterotropic.

allosteric inhibition see under *allosteric effectors.*

allosteric site see under *allosteric effectors.*

allostery (al″o-ste′re) the condition in which the binding of a compound to one subunit of a regulatory enzyme at other than the substrate binding site causes a change in conformation of the enzyme. This affects the affinity of the enzyme for substrate and increases (or decreases) the overall rate of reaction.

allothreonine (al″o-thre′o-nīn) a stereoisomer of the amino acid threonine. 2-Amino-3-hydroxybutanoic acid exists as four stereoisomers: D- and L-threonine and D- and L-allothreonine.

allotrope (al′o-trōp) an allotropic form.

allotropic (al″o-trop′ik) having the relation of allotropy.

allotropy (ah-lot′ro-pe) [Gr. *allotropia* variety, from *allo-* + *tropos* a turn] the existence of two or more forms of a substance in the same physical state (solid, liquid, or gas). This may be due to different crystal structures or to a different number of atoms in the molecule (e.g., oxygen, O_2, and ozone, O_3, or the various allotropes of liquid sulfur). The term polymorphism is often used when referring to different crystalline phases; allotropism is used when referring to elements.

allotype (al″o-tīp) any of the alternate traits determined by allelic genes, e.g., the ABO blood types.

alloxan (al′ok-san) a reddish, crystalline oxidation product of uric acid. It causes selective destruction of the beta cells of the pancreatic islets in laboratory animals, producing an animal model of diabetes mellitus. It can also be used as a histologic stain for demonstrating amino acids, substituting for ninhydrin in the ninhydrin-Schiff reaction.

alloxan-Schiff reaction a histochemical reaction used to demonstrate protein. Amino groups on protein undergo oxidative deamination to aldehyde by reaction with alloxan; the aldehyde groups then react with Schiff reagent. Proteins stain magenta. See also *ninhydrin-Schiff reaction.*

alloy (al′loi) [Fr. *aloyer* to mix metals] a mixture of two or more metals.

allyl- (al′il) [L. *allium* garlic + Gr. *hylē* matter] a prefix word element in organic chemistry to denote the 2-propenyl group ($CH_2{=}CHCH_2$—), e.g., allylamine.

allyl alcohol a colorless, flammable liquid with a pungent odor, 2-propen-1-ol, $CH_2{=}CH{-}CH_2OH$; M.W. 58.08. Allyl alcohol is used in industrial chemical synthesis. It is toxic when ingested or inhaled and is a strong eye and skin irritant, causing tearing, blurred vision, and corneal damage.

Alocinma (al″o-sin′mah) a genus of freshwater snails found in India and China that serves as the first intermediate host of the human liver fluke *Clonorchis sinensis;* it is sometimes treated as a subgenus of the genus *Bulima.*

alopecia (al″o-pe′she-ah) [Gr. *alōpekia* a disease in which the hair falls out] baldness; loss of hair. Baldness may be due to scarring (cicatricial) following trauma, radiation, antineoplastic chemotherapy, severe fungal or bacterial infections, or systemic diseases; this type is permanent. Nonscarring balding may be classified as alopecia universalis (generalized hair loss), alopecia totalis (total hair loss), or alopecia areata (patchy hair loss). The causes of this type of baldness include systemic diseases, drug reactions, and infections. Many forms of alopecia follow a genetic pattern and are of unknown causes.

ALP abbrev. See *alkaline phosphatase.*

alpha (A, α) (al′fah) the first letter of the *Greek alphabet;* used to denote plasma proteins in the alpha electrophoretic band, e.g., alpha-fetoprotein, and one of a group of related entities, e.g., alpha radiation.

alpha$_1$-acid glycoprotein see *orosomucoid.*

alpha-adrenergic receptor see under *adrenergic receptor.*

alpha$_2$-antiplasmin (an″tĭ-plas′min) a plasma protein that is the principal inhibitor of fibrinolysis; M.W. 67,000. It binds to plasmin, forming a 1:1 stoichiometric complex. Normal levels of alpha$_2$-antiplasmin are sufficient to inactivate half the plasmin that can be generated from circulating plasminogen. In pathologic states, such as disseminated intravascular coagulation, the capacity of alpha$_2$-antiplasmin may be exceeded. The excess plasmin is then bound by alpha$_2$-macroglobulin. See also *a. III* under *antithrombin, alpha$_1$-antitrypsin, alpha$_2$-macroglobulin,* and *C1 esterase inhibitor.*

alpha$_1$-antitrypsin a blood plasma protein synthesized in the liver, the major inhibitor of trypsin in serum; M.W. 40,000–50,000. It also acts on chymotrypsin, collagenase, elastase, and leukocyte-derived proteases, and in fact is the major inhibitor of enzymatic proteolysis. Alpha$_1$-antitrypsin has the capacity to act as a weak variant of antithrombin and binds to thrombin, plasmin, Factor XIa, and urokinase, but its physiologic role in coagulation is probably minor. It migrates with the alpha$_1$-globulin band in electrophoresis.

There are identifiable genetic variations of the protein, the normal phenotype being MM; deficiency appears to be tied to the autosomal recessive gene Z. Congenital deficiency is associated with increased incidence of panlobar emphysema in adults (especially females), hepatitis in neonates, and cirrhosis in children.

See also *a. III* under *antithrombin, alpha$_1$-antiplasmin, alpha$_2$-macroglobulin,* and *C1 esterase inhibitor.*

alpha$_1$-antitrypsin assays 1. trypsin inhibitory capability (TIC) assay, a functional assay of capacity for trypsin inhibition. The rate of hydrolysis of a substrate such as α-*N*-benzoyl-DL-arginine-*p*-nitroanilide is determined in a reaction mixture containing a trypsin preparation of known activity both with and without the addition of a serum specimen. The TIC is the difference in hydrolysis rates per unit volume of added serum expressed as micromoles per minute per milliliter (μmol/min/ml). About 80–90 percent of the TIC is due to alpha$_1$-antitrypsin. Reference ranges are: for the MM genotype, 2.1–3.8 U/ml; for the MZ phenotype, 1.05–2.1; and for the ZZ phenotype, 0.5–0.7.

2. routine serum protein electrophoresis. Protein staining in the alpha$_1$ band is due almost entirely to alpha$_1$-antitrypsin.

Patients with MM phenotype show a normal alpha$_1$ band, and those with the ZZ phenotype show no alpha$_1$ band, whereas those with an MZ phenotype show an alpha$_1$ band with half-normal stain intensity. Heterozygotes with an M allele and another variant allele show two light-staining bands, one with normal mobility and another moving faster or slower.

3. radial immunodiffusion or electroimmunodiffusion using an antiserum specific for alpha$_1$-antitrypsin.

alpha$_1$-antitrypsin deficiency a genetic defect resulting in a serum alpha$_1$-antitrypsin concentration that is only about 10 percent of normal, leading in most cases to severe pulmonary disease in adults or hepatic disease in infants and children.

Many alleles of this gene (called Pi for protease inhibitor) have been discovered by means of protein electrophoresis. The common allele is Pi^M, for which about 90 percent of the population is homozygous (genotype MM). The most common aberrant allele is Pi^Z; the ZZ genotype is linked with the deficiency. The MM phenotype exhibits an average serum alpha$_1$-antitrypsin concentration of about 210 mg/dl, as opposed to 120 for MZ heterozygotes, and 25 for ZZ homozygotes.

See also *alpha$_1$-antitrypsin assays.*

alpha band in electroencephalography, the frequency band of 8–13 Hz. Also called alpha frequency.

alpha$_1$ (α_1) band in electrophoretograms of serum, the first band with a mobility less than that of albumin. It is composed of at least three components; alpha$_1$-antitrypsin, alpha$_1$-lipoprotein, and orosomucoid (alpha$_1$-acid glycoprotein), which are present at concentrations of 2.5, 3.6, and 0.9 g/l, respectively, in human serum. Only alpha$_1$-antitrypsin stains with the usual protein stains; the lipid in alpha$_1$-lipoprotein and the carbohydrate moiety in orosomucoid do not bind dyes, giving rise to very weak staining reactions. See also *protein electrophoresis.*

alpha cell an acidophilic cell, i.e., a cell that stains best with acid dyes. Also called *A cell.*

a. c. of hypophysis, small, rounded, acidophilic cells of the anterior hypophysis, consisting of two populations of cells. The classic Romeis' alpha cells are predominantly found in clusters in the posterolateral parts of the lobe, and stain immunohistochemically for growth hormone (GH). The second population of acidophilic cells are interspersed between other cell types, and stain for prolactin.

a. c. of pancreas, a term applied to the acidophilic cells of the pancreatic islets. These cells are less numerous than the beta-islet cells. They contain spherical dense-core secretory granules, and secrete glucagon.

alpha (α) chain the heavy chain of IgA immunoglobulin; see also *immunoglobulin.*

alpha-chain disease a type of heavy-chain disease in which an incomplete IgA is synthesized that has partial H chains and no L chains. The paraprotein is usually found in the serum and urine. Clinical features include chronic diarrhea, steatorrhea, weight loss, hypocalcemia, and lymphadenopathy. Progressively immature plasma cells and lymphocytes are present in the small bowel, and constitute a lymphoma-like disease in the intestine. Diagnosis is by immunoelectrophoresis. See also *heavy-chain disease.*

alpha decay a mode of radioactive decay mediated by the strong nuclear force undergone by heavy elements (beyond lead in the periodic table). The general equation for the nuclear reaction is ${}^{A}_{Z}X \rightarrow {}^{A-4}_{Z-2}Y + {}^{4}_{2}\mathrm{He}$, where X is the parent radionuclide and Y is the daughter nuclide (decay product).

So that mass and charge are conserved, the sum of the mass numbers (superscripts) and atomic numbers (subscripts) on both sides of the equation must balance; the daughter nuclide has two less protons and two less neutrons than the parent.

For most nuclides there are several alpha decay modes. The alpha emission may leave the daughter nuclide in the ground state, or the daughter nuclide may be left in an excited state, in which case it will rapidly decay to the ground state, emitting one or more gamma rays. In either case, the difference between the mass of the parent nuclide and the mass of the reaction products (daughter nuclide and alpha particle) is equal to the kinetic energy of the alpha particle plus the recoil energy of the daughter nuclide plus the gamma-ray energies. Thus, a particular radioisotope emits alpha particles at a few discrete kinetic energies.

alpha-delta sleep pattern in electroencephalography, a pattern of electric activity, recorded from some individuals with insomnia; it consists of long periods of alpha-frequency activity occurring on a background of delta activity during non–rapid eye movement (NREM) sleep.

alpha$_1$-fetoglobulin (fe″to-glob′u-lin) see *alpha$_1$-fetoprotein.*

alpha$_1$-fetoprotein (AFP) an alpha$_1$-globulin present in appreciable amounts in the serum of the fetus, infant, and normal pregnant female. High concentrations (1000 ng/ml) are almost diagnostic of hepatocellular carcinoma in adults. Although they often do not reach the levels found in association with hepatocellular carcinoma, elevated concentrations of plasma AFP are found in association with a variety of malignant neoplasms and inflammatory and regenerative conditions. In fetuses with open spina bifida or anencephaly, AFP leaks into the amniotic fluid and maternal serum, and its measurement is of significant diagnostic value. Ataxia-telangiectasia and tyrosinosis have also been associated with elevated AFP concentrations. In children older than 1 yr and in normal adults, serum values are less than 30 ng/ml and are detectable by radioimmunoassay. Alpha$_1$-fetoprotein can be demonstrated in tissue sections by means of immunoperoxidase techniques. Also called *alpha$_1$-fetoglobulin.*

alpha$_1$-fetoprotein assays the determination of AFP in serum or amniotic fluid. One method is the Ouchterlony double diffusion method, in which a sample of the patient's serum is reacted with anti-AFP antibodies and the precipitin line is compared with that obtained with a standard reference sample. A newer approach is determination by radioimmunoassay. Reference ranges for this technique vary greatly, but are around 2–25 ng/ml. Enzyme-linked immunospecific assays (ELISA), in which an enzyme is utilized as a marker in place of a radioactive isotope, have also been used.

alpha$_1$-globulin a group of serum proteins that migrate with the alpha$_1$-electrophoretic band. Examples include alpha$_1$-antitrypsin, alpha$_1$-acid glycoprotein, and alpha$_1$-lipoprotein.

alpha granules platelet granules; oval, membrane-bound granules 0.15–0.4 μm in diameter that are found in the cytoplasm of platelets. They can be classed as lysosomes, peroxisomes, and undifferentiated granules containing fibrinogen and platelet factor 4. The platelet-dense body, a round, very electron-dense granule containing serotonin, catecholamine, nucleotides, and calcium ions, appears to be formed from undifferentiated alpha granules as a result of the uptake of serotonin from plasma.

alpha$_1$-inhibitor see *alpha$_1$-antitrypsin.*

α-level see *significance level.*

alpha$_2$-macroglobulin (α_2M) (mak″ro-glob′u-lin) a large, dimeric plasma protein; M.W. 820,000. It inhibits a wide variety of proteolytic enzymes, including trypsin, plasmin, thrombin, kallikrein, elastase, collagenase, and cathepsins, forming an irreversible complex that is rapidly cleared by the reticuloendothelial system. The bound enzyme retains a fraction of its proteolytic activity, especially against small substrates. α_2M provides one-fourth of the normal thrombin-inhibiting activity of plasma. Plasmin bound to α_2M may also play a role in normal fibrinolysis.

Reference ranges for alpha$_2$-macroglobulin in plasma are: for adult males, 0.15–0.35 g/dl; and for adult females, 0.17–0.42. Values for infants are 2.5 times those of the adult; they continue to rise until puberty, then fall to the adult level between the ages of 15 and 22 yr. Increased concentrations of α_2M are seen in nephrosis, liver disease, and diabetes.

See also *a. III* under *antithrombin, alpha$_1$-antitrypsin, alpha$_2$-antiplasmin,* and *C1 esterase inhibitor.*

alpha$_2$-macroglobulin inhibitor see under *antithrombin.*

alphameric (al″fah-mer′ik) see *alphanumeric.*

alpha motor neuron a motor nerve cell whose myelinated axon innervates extrafusal skeletal muscle fibers.

alphanumeric (al″fah-nu-mer′ik) referring to a set of characters that contain both letters and digits and, in some contexts, special characters (arithmetic operators and punctuation). Also called *alphameric.*

alpha particle the particle emitted from the nucleus in alpha decay, which is a helium-4 nucleus (^{4}He or α), composed of two protons and two neutrons. Most alpha particles are emitted with kinetic energies of 3–9 MeV and have a range of 3–9 cm in air or 25–45 μm in water or soft tissue. They produce dense ionization along a short, straight track, having 25 times the specific ionization produced by beta particles.

Because of the short range, alpha radiation from external radiation sources is not hazardous; however, alpha emitters, such as radium, radon, uranium, or plutonium, that enter the body by inhalation or ingestion, are extremely hazardous.

See also *interaction of radiation with matter.*

alpha-particle detector a radiation detector used to detect and count alpha particles. The device is usually a proportional counter with a 0.001-in. nylon or polyester film window. A discriminator circuit is used to separate the large pulses produced by alpha particles from the smaller beta-particle pulses. See also *proportional counter.*

alphaprodine hydrochloride (al″fah-pro′dēn) [USP], a synthetic narcotic analgesic, similar in effect to morphine and meperidine but having a short duration of action. It is used for obstetric analgesia and during minor surgery. As with other opiates it is addicting; overdoses produce respiratory depression, which can be reversed by administration of an antagonist such as levallorphan. Trademark, Nisentil.

alpha receptor see under *adrenergic receptor.*

alpha rhythm in electroencephalography, rhythmic electric activity having a frequency of 8–13 Hz, that is recorded from posterior regions of the head and is attenuated or abolished with visual attention; it is also temporarily attenuated by other stimuli, including mental concentration. It is best recorded in adults during relaxed wakefulness when the eyes are closed. In healthy adults, the mean frequency is 9–10 Hz. The characteristics of the rhythm appear to be genetically determined, and some normal subjects show no alpha rhythm (M; minus or minimum), whereas others show persistence (P) of the rhythm when the eyes are open.

The alpha rhythm begins to appear at age 24–36 mo. Recordings from depth electrodes suggest that there are multiple independent sources of this rhythm within the occipital lobes. The rhythm is usually asymmetric and asynchronous between the cerebral hemispheres, with the greater amplitude appearing in the nondominant hemisphere, and exact synchrony between the two hemispheres is rare.

Changes in the alpha rhythm are of diagnostic value only when previous electroencephalographic records of the patient are available for comparison. The mean frequency of the rhythm may slow with age, with administration of anticonvulsant drugs, with metabolic disorders, with impairment of consciousness, and with any type of cerebral disease (such as neoplasms, abscesses, and head injuries). In some comatose patients, rhythm of alpha frequency is widespread over the cerebral hemispheres and does not attenuate to sensory stimuli, unlike normal alpha rhythm; such alpha-pattern coma is particularly evident following brain stem or cardiopulmonary stroke, and usually indicates a poor prognosis for survival.

alpha$_1$-seromucoid (sēr″o-mu′koid) see *orosomucoid.*

alpha streptococcus any species of *Streptococcus* that produces alpha hemolysis; see under *Streptococcus.*

alpha thalassemia see under *thalassemia.*

alpha variant rhythm in electroencephalography, rhythmic activity that resembles alpha rhythm in its distribution over the head and responsiveness to stimuli, but differs from it in frequency. See also *alpha rhythm.*

fast a. v. r., an alpha variant rhythm having a frequency of 14–20 Hz.

slow a. v. r., an alpha variant rhythm having a frequency of 3.5–6 Hz.

alphavirus one of a group of small (60 nm), spherical togaviruses with a lipoprotein envelope and isocahedral core containing a single molecule of single-stranded RNA. Members are identified by immunologic cross-reactions, and many antigenic types have been determined.

Alphaviruses were formerly the group A arboviruses, or arthropod-borne viruses, so named because they are maintained by biologic transmission to vertebrate hosts through arthropod vectors. Many cause disease in humans, ranging from an influenza-type infection to encephalitis.

The alphavirus has proved valuable in the study of multiplication of RNA viruses because of its single RNA strand and the ease with which it is isolated.

See also *eastern equine e.* and *western equine e.* under *encephalitis.*

alphazurine 2G (al″fah-zur′ēn) see *patent blue V.*

Alport's syndrome [Arthur Cecil *Alport,* South African physician, 1880–1959] a hereditary disorder, transmitted as both autosomal dominant and X-linked traits, that is characterized by sensorineural deafness and hereditary nephritis. It may result from abnormal glycopeptide synthesis in renal basement membranes. Renal disease initially appears as recurrent hematuria and slowly progresses to renal insufficiency. There are occasional associated findings including cataracts, hyperprolinemia, and platelet abnormalities. Diagnosis is based on urinalysis, kidney biopsy, and hearing testing. Treatment is supportive, but corticosteroids are ineffective.

ALS abbrev. See *amyotrophic lateral s.* under *sclerosis* and *antilymphocyte serum.*

ALT abbrev. See *alanine aminotransferase.*

ALT/AST ratio the ratio of alanine aminotransferase (ALT) to aspartate aminotransferase (AST). Normally and in the case of myocardial infarction it is less than 1.0, but in viral hepatitis and necrotic liver diseases it may become greater. Also called *De Ritis ratio.*

Alternaria (awl″ter-na′re-ah) [L. *alternus* one after the other] a genus of dematiacious Fungi Imperfecti of the order Moniliales. This genus is characterized by muriform conidia in chain formation, a dark brown color, and germ tube formation. Each conidium has a pronounced dark spot at the attachment to the next conidium. *Alternaria* can cause cutaneous alternariosis in humans; it is also a common allergen in human bronchial asthma.

alternating (awl′ter-nāt″ing) occurring in regular succession; alternately direct and reversed.

alternating current (AC) an electric current that periodically reverses direction. The standard line current obtained from a wall socket is alternating current having a sinusoidal waveform and an effective voltage (root-mean-square voltage) of 115 V or 230 V. Alternating current is used because its voltage can be stepped up and down by transformers; it thus can be transmitted at high voltage to reduce power losses. X-ray machines and all electronic equipment require direct current for their internal components and have a circuit called the power supply, which converts alternating to direct current.

alternation of generations the occurrence in the life cycle of all plants, and some fungi and algae, of an alternating succession of haploid and diploid phases. The diploid stage or sporophyte produces haploid spores by meiosis. These divide and develop into male and female haploid organisms or gametophytes, which produce haploid gametes. Male and female gametes unite to form a diploid zygote, which divides and develops into a sporophyte. Also called *heterogony* and *metagenesis.*

alternative complement pathway (al-ter′nah-tiv) an amplification loop involving activation of the third component of complement C3 without the initial cascade of the C1, C2, or C4 components of complement. It also involves the serum proteins Factors B, D, and P (properdin).

The activation sequence involves the interaction of the C3 fragment C3b with Bb—the activated fragment of B produced by cleavage of B by the enzyme D, a serum protease. The interaction requires a favorable cell surface or macromolecule for stability and further activation. Substances that favor activation of the alternative pathway are aggregated IgA or IgE, polysaccharides, endotoxin, inulin, zymosan, cobra venom factor, and rabbit red blood cells.

The alternative complement pathway activation involves the interaction of C3b and Bb to form a C3 convertase, which can cleave C3 to form more C3b and C3a, an anaphylatoxin. The C3b thus formed can interact with the C3bBb complex to produce a C5 convertase. This can lead to activation of the late-acting components of the complement pathway C5 through C9. Properdin acts to stabilize the initial C3bBb complex and favors the formation of the C5 convertase by the addition of more C3b to the activated complex. The dissociation of the C3bBb complex with fluid-phase destruction of C3b and Bb is promoted by the inhibitor of the alternative pathway β-1-H, a serum glycoprotein. Nephritic factor C3NeF is an antibody to the C3bBb complex that is found in normal individuals, but is present in high concentrations in those with membranoproliferative glomerulonephritis. It promotes activation of the alternative pathway by protecting C3bBb complex from degradation by β-1-H and C3b inactivator.

The alternative complement pathway has a number of similarities to the classical pathway and on evolutionary terms is thought to have evolved first. Factor B and the complement component C2 have a number of common points in that both are heat-sensitive glycoproteins and both act as C3 convertases in cleavage and interaction with other complement components.

Assays of the alternative pathway take advantage of the fact that EGTA (ethyleneglycoltriacetic acid) binds Ca^{2+} more strongly than Mg^{2+} and prevents activation of the classical pathway (which requires Ca^{2+}) without affecting activation of the alternative pathway. Several methods have been utilized for studying the hemolytic activity of the alternative pathway; one method takes advantage of the fact that rabbit red blood cells act as a favorable surface for activation of the alternative pathway. In the presence of serum and MgEGTA, a measurement of rabbit red blood cell lysis will give a measure of hemolytic activity of the alternative pathway. Activation of the pathway can also be determined using radial immunodiffusion or laser nephelometry to measure levels of the components Factor B and properdin and the breakdown products of Factor B.

Hereditary dificiencies of the components of the alternative pathway have not been described, although an instance of low Factor B activity has been noted in a patient with C2 deficiency. A deficiency of C3bINA (C3b inactivator) has been described, and is associated with consumption of C3 and a clinical picture of recurrent infections similar to C3 deficiency.

Also called *properdin system.* See also *classical complement pathway, complement,* and the accompanying illustration.

GERALD B. KOLSKI, M.D., PH.D.

alternative hypothesis (H_1) a hypothesis about the parent population of a statistical sample that is inconsistent with the null hypothesis (H_0). The object of a statistical test is to produce evidence against the null hypothesis and in favor of accepting the alternative hypothesis. See also *hypothesis testing.*

ALU abbrev. See *arithmetic and logic unit.*

alum (al'um) [L. *alumen*] 1. [USP], an odorless, colorless, crystalline substance; it has local astringent and styptic properties and a sweetish taste, and is soluble in water but insoluble in alcohol. Alum may refer either to potassium alum, $AlK(SO_4)_2 \cdot 12H_2O$ or to ammonium alum, $AlNH_4(SO_4)_2 \cdot 12H_2O$, or $NaCrSO_4 \cdot 12H_2O$. Alums are frequently used as topical agents.

2. a generic term for a member of a class of double sulfates that crystallize as dodecahydrates and contain a trivalent metal ion such as Al, Fe, or Cr, and a monovalent ion such as Na, K, or NH_4.

alum carmine see *carmine.*

alumina (ah-loo'mĭ-nah) see *aluminum oxide.*

aluminosis (ah-loo"mĭ-no'sis) [*aluminum* + *-osis* condition] a form of pneumoconiosis that may appear in workers exposed to fine aluminum dust. The septal edema, appearance of inflammatory cells in

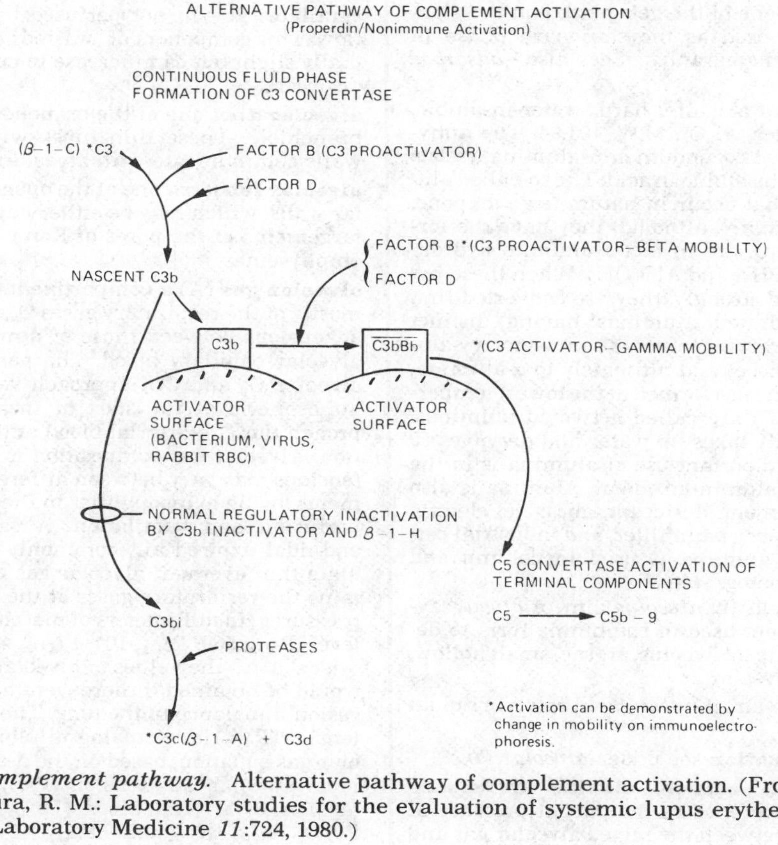

Alternative complement pathway. Alternative pathway of complement activation. (From Tucker, E. S., III, and Nakamura, R. M.: Laboratory studies for the evaluation of systemic lupus erythematosus and related disorders. Laboratory Medicine *11*:724, 1980.)

the alveolar walls, and obliterative endarteritis that initially develop lead to a diffuse interstitial fibrosis accompanied by pleural thickening. See also *pneumoconiosis.*

aluminum (Al) (ah-loo′mĭ-num) [L. *alumen* alum] a very light, whitish, lustrous, metallic element; atomic number 13; atomic weight 26.981; Group III of the periodic table; oxidation state +3. It is the most abundant of the metallic elements and is found in clays, feldspars, and micas. Aluminum is obtained commercially from bauxite. It is quite malleable and ductile, and is used as the pure metal or as alloys in the manufacture of a variety of industrial and consumer products. Aluminum hydroxide is used in medicine as a gastric antacid.

aluminum carbonate, basic an aluminum hydroxide–aluminum carbonate gel used as a gastric antacid.

aluminum hydroxide a white powder, $Al(OH)_3$, which forms a gel by absorbing water; M.W. 77.99. It is used chemically as an adsorbent and chromatographic medium, and medicinally as a gastric antacid. Also called *hydrated alumina.*

aluminum hydroxide gel the gel formed by aluminum hydroxide and water, used in the clinical laboratory as an adsorbent and chromatographic matrix. In tests of blood coagulation, the gel is mixed with plasma, incubated, and centrifuged; this results in a supernatant that is deficient in prothrombin and Factor VII but that does contain Factors V, VIII, XI, and XII. In immunology, it is used as an adjuvant of 2 percent $Al(OH)_3$, which adsorbs protein antigens and forms a precipitate. Aluminum hydroxide gel is one of the gels placed on the glass or plastic plate used as the stationary phase in thin-layer chromatography. See also *adsorbed plasma.*

aluminum oxide a white, hard, water-insoluble, crystalline powder, Al_2O_3; M.W. 101.94. The anhydrous oxide, called corundum or α-alumina, resists hydration and is insoluble in acid. The so-called alumina hydrates that occur in nature (e.g., diapone, gibbsite, and bauxite), although they have the formulas $Al_2O_3 \cdot xH_2O$, are in fact aluminum hydroxides such as $Al(OH)_3$ and $AlO(OH)$. When these hydrates are heated strongly, they are converted first to partially hydrated aluminas having distinct structures and varying amounts of water (γ-alumina is one of these) and ultimately to α-alumina. The group of aluminas formed at the lowest temperatures (200°–500°C) are called activated aluminas. γ-Alumina readily takes up water and dissolves in acid. The most important use of alumina is in the manufacture of aluminum metal. Alumina is also used as an adsorbent, desiccant, abrasive, electric insulator (ceramics), paint filler, and industrial catalyst. Activated alumina is used in column and thin-layer chromatography.

alveol/o (al-ve′o-lo) [L. *alveolus,* dim. of *alveus* cavity] a word element used in combining form to denote a relationship to alveolus, air sac, small hollow, or cavity, e.g., alveolar.

alveolar (al-ve′o-lar) [L. *alveolaris*] referring to an alveolus.

alveolar air equation see under *alveolar* P_{O_2}.

alveolar-arterial carbon dioxide difference (A-aP_{CO_2}) the difference in the partial pressure of carbon dioxide between the mixed alveolar gas and mixed arterial blood, normally equal to –0.4 mmHg in the young adult. The difference is influenced by factors, such as the presence of multiple pulmonary emboli, that lead to a high ventilation-perfusion ratio in a significant portion of the lungs, but it remains relatively unaffected by venous admixture or diffusion limitations.

alveolar bone a thin layer of bone, continuous with the maxilla and mandible, that surrounds the roots of the teeth to form sockets. The bone is penetrated by many foramina through which course the blood vessels, nerves, and lymphatics supplying the teeth.

alveolar cell a surface epithelial cell that lines the walls of pulmonary alveoli. Also called *pneumocyte* or *pneumonocyte.*

type I pneumocyte, one of the cells that form a very thin (about 200 nm) sheet of cytoplasm covering the alveolar basal lamina. The primary function of these cells is to provide an epithelial covering that is permeable to gases. Also called squamous alveolar epithelial cell.

type II pneumocyte, one of the large, roughly cuboidal epithelial cells that occur singly or in groups of two to four among the type I cells. These cells secrete a phospholipid substance, which acts as a surfactant (it lowers the surface tension at the air-fluid interface). The cells contain numerous large (up to 1 μm in diameter) multilamellar bodies. Also called *granular pneumocyte* and great or granular alveolar cell.

alveolar cell carcinoma see *bronchiolar carcinoma.*

alveolar dead space the volume of inspired air that ventilates alveoli not perfused by capillary blood flow. This component of "wasted ventilation" is normally slight but can increase in certain pulmonary disorders.

alveolar duct one of the branches of a respiratory bronchiole. These thin tubes with discontinuous walls communicate with alveolar sacs and alveoli.

alveolar fenestra one of the openings in the alveolar walls, which may be either new channels or enlargements of the pores of Kohn, that occurs with emphysema.

alveolar gas (A) a compartment of gas, consisting mostly of the respiratory gases O_2, CO_2, N_2, and H_2O at tensions between those of atmospheric air and alveolar capillary blood. The partial pressures of alveolar O_2 and CO_2 approach values close to the atmospheric at the start of inspiration, and approach those of arterial blood at the end of expiration. Alveolar gas composition is nonuniform; gas tensions may vary between different lung compartments owing to inequalities in the balance between perfusion and ventilation. A sample of resting end-tidal expired air, commonly used to approximate the "average" alveolar gas composition, contains the respiratory gases at the following partial pressures (in millimeters of mercury, mmHg) at sea level: $P_{A_{N_2}}$, 569; $P_{A_{O_2}}$, 104; $P_{A_{CO_2}}$, 40; and $P_{A_{H_2O}}$, 47.

ideal a. g., the values of alveolar gas tension that would be obtained if there were no ventilation-perfusion imbalance in the lung. The ideal alveolar O_2 tension ($P_{A_{O_2}}$) is calculated as follows from the alveolar gas equation, based on the assumption that the ideal alveolar CO_2 tension ($P_{A_{CO_2}}$) approaches its tension in arterial blood (Pa_{CO_2}): (ideal) $P_{A_{O_2}} = P_{I_{O_2}} - (Pa_{CO_2}/R) + 0.209\ Pa_{CO_2}[(1-R)/R]$, where $P_{I_{O_2}}$

is the O_2 tension of inspired air and R is the respiratory quotient.

alveolar line the vertical line that passes down the center of the face from the nasion to the alveolar point.

alveolar macrophage a phagocytic cell located in the alveoli of the lungs. It has the function of clearing the lungs of foreign material, such as microorganisms and dust. Large numbers of these cells are observed in heavy cigarette smokers or individuals who live or work in a dusty atmosphere. Also called *dust cell* and pulmonary macrophage.

alveolar P_{CO_2} (P_{ACO_2}) the partial pressure of carbon dioxide in alveolar gas. The mean alveolar P_{CO_2} is approximately equal to 40 mmHg (and to the arterial P_{CO_2}) in a healthy individual at rest at sea level. Also called alveolar CO_2 tension.

alveolar P_{O_2} (P_{AO_2}) the partial pressure of oxygen in alveolar gas. As it varies in different alveoli, during each breath, and from one breath to another, a mean value for alveolar P_{O_2} at sea level is commonly calculated. The equation used is: $P_{AO_2} = F_{IO_2}(713) - P_{ACO_2}\,[F_{IO_2} + 1 - F_{IO_2}/R_E]$; where F_{IO_2} is equal to the fraction of oxygen in the inspired air, P_{ACO_2} is equal to the mean alveolar P_{CO_2} (estimated as the arterial P_{CO_2}), and R_E is equal to the respiratory exchange ratio. Mean alveolar P_{O_2} is normally equal to 104 torr in an individual at rest. Also called alveolar O_2 tension.

alveolar point the most forward point of the upper jaw, the point of the alveolar process in the midsagittal plane. Also called *prosthion.*

alveolar pore see *alveolar p.* under *pore.*

alveolar soft part sarcoma an uncommon soft tissue tumor, so named because of a resemblance between the groups of tumor cells and alveoli. Some cells of these tumors contain cytoplasmic crystals that are PAS-positive and diastase-resistant and ultrastructurally are distinctive rhomboid structures with a fine periodicity. Most alveolar soft part sarcomas occur in females and involve the lower extremity, although other sites can also be affected. Growth is often slow, but metastases ultimately appear, sometimes many years after the primary tumor has been excised. Small, dense-core granules are present in some tumor cells; the possibility that this tumor represents a form of paraganglioma has been suggested, but neither normal paraganglial tissues nor paragangliomas occur in the limbs, and the histogenesis is still unknown.

alveolar ventilation ($\dot{V}_A$) the amount of air that enters the alveoli per minute, usually determined by subtraction of the total dead-space volume from the respiratory minute volume. An alveolar ventilation of 4 l/min is normally adequate to maintain the P_{AO_2} and P_{ACO_2} within physiologic limits when ventilation-perfusion ratios are nearly uniform throughout the lungs. The P_{ACO_2} varies inversely with alveolar ventilation; this value is usually considered indicative of the level of alveolar ventilation. Cf. *total ventilation.*

alveolitis (al″ve-o-li′tis) [*alveol-* + *-itis* inflammation] an inflammation of the respiratory alveoli, most commonly due to a hypersensitivity (immune reaction) to an inhaled antigen, e.g., hypersensitivity to moldy hay or vegetable matter in persons with farmer's lung. The resulting nodular inflammation of the alveoli is accompanied by a vascular inflammation and bronchiolitis. Immune complexes and cellular immunity contribute to pathogenesis. Clinically, the disorder is manifested acutely by shortness of breath, fever and chills, coughing, and nausea; a more chronic form results in severe respiratory compromise with progressive fibrosis of the lungs. Other antigens that may provoke an allergic alveolitis in sensitive individuals are the molds found in air conditioners and those on sugar cane, tree bark, and mushrooms.

Laboratory diagnosis is aided by findings of a leukocytosis with a shift to the left, elevated levels of serum immunoglobulins, and positive skin tests for sensitivity to specific antigens.

See also *hypersensitivity p.* under *pneumonitis.*

alveolus (al-ve′o-lus), pl. *alveoli* [L., dim. of *alveus* cavity] a general term used to designate a small saclike dilation. It is generally used alone to designate a pulmonary alveolus. See also *lung.*

dental a., in the maxilla and mandible, the cavity in the alveolar bone into which the roots of the teeth are inserted.

pulmonary a., a small, thin-walled pouch that protrudes from the walls of the respiratory bronchioles, alveolar ducts, and alveolar sacs; the site of gas exchange with the blood. There are approximately 300 million pulmonary alveoli divided between the two lungs, each with an average diameter of 250 μ, providing a surface area of 40–100 m². See also *alveolar cell.*

Alzheimer's disease (altz′hi-merz) [Alois *Alzheimer,* German neurologist, 1864–1915] an atrophic process that progressively involves the brain, with degeneration of nerve cells, leading to mental changes gradually evolving (over a period of 10 yr or more) from subtle intellectual impairment to dementia and death from intercurrent disease. Most of those affected are over age 40.

Two distinctive histologic changes are the presence of so-called senile plaques, which contain amyloid, and neurofibrillary tangles. In the early stages of the disease, the amount of alpha activity recorded on the electroencephalogram is reduced. As the disease progresses, irregular theta activity appears and delta waves of high amplitude may appear infrequently.

Also called *presenile dementia.*

Alzheimer's fibrillary degeneration [Alois *Alzheimer*] a type of degeneration of cortical nerve cells in which argyrophilic material condenses on and within the cell body in a basketwork configuration. It is seen in Alzheimer's disease and in the aging brain. Also called Alzheimer's basket cells.

Am symbol for the chemical element *americium.*

AMA abbrev. See *American Medical Association.*

amacrine (am′ah-krin) [*a-* neg. + Gr. *makros* long + *is, inos* fiber] having no long processes; said of some neurons.

amacrine cells small, multipolar nerve cells, common in the retina and olfactory bulb, that do not possess an axon.

Amanita (am″ah-ni′tah) [Gr. *amanitai* a kind of fungus] a genus of mushrooms of the family Agaricaceae with several highly poisonous species. Members of the genus produce two groups of sulfur-containing cyclic peptides, the phallotoxins and amatoxins. The phallotoxins act on the endoplasmic reticulum of liver cells, whereas the amatoxins act on the nucleus. *A. phalloides* (also called destroying angel, death cup) contains the peptide toxin phalloidin and amanitin. *A. muscaria* (fly agaric) produces the potent poison muscarine, as well as ibotenic acid, a psychotropic compound. See also *mycetismus.*

amanitin a very potent poison derived from various mushrooms of the genus *Amanita,* with three forms: α, β, and γ, each a heat-stable cyclopeptide. On ingestion, amanitin causes salivation, vomiting, cyanosis, and convulsions. An early effect is hepatic glycogen mobilization; carbohydrate, lipid, and protein metabolism enzymes are inhibited. Small amounts can be detected by thin-layer or paper chromatography. It should not be confused with "amanitine," an obsolete synonym for choline.

α-a., a toxic polypeptide, found in the poison mushroom *Amanita phalloides,* that is used experimentally to differentiate among the three RNA polymerases. It preferentially inhibits RNA polymerase II, which catalyzes messenger RNA transcription and, at higher concentrations, inhibits RNA polymerase III, which catalyzes the transcription of transfer RNA and 5S ribosomal RNA. RNA polymerase I, which catalyzes the transcription of 45S ribosomal RNA, is not affected.

amantadine (ah-man'tah-dēn) 1-adamantanamine, an antiviral agent that prevents the penetration and uptake of certain RNA membrane viruses. When used prophylactically, amantadine has been shown to be effective against influenza A. However, in view of the necessity for repeated administration, immunization is a preferred method of viral control. Useful derivatives of amantadine include methyl-1-adamantane methylamine hydrochloride (rimantadine) and *N*-methyl 1-adamantanespiro-3-pyrrolidine hydrochloride. See also *antiviral agent.*

amaurosis (am"aw-ro'sis) [L., from Gr. *amaurōsis* darkening] blindness, especially that resulting from a degenerative process of the spine, optic nerve, or brain.

ambenonium chloride (am"be-no'ne-um) [USP], a cholinesterase-inhibiting drug used to treat myasthenia gravis. For adverse reactions, see the similar drug *neostigmine.*

Amberlite (am"ber-līt) trademark for a variety of ion-exchange resins. They are synthetic polymers available in strong acid, weak acid, strong base, and weak base forms; each is available in different grades varying in terms of porosity and exchange capacity.

ambi- (am'be) [L.] a prefix word element to denote both, on both sides, about, e.g., ambidextrous.

ambient (am'be-ent) [L. *ambiens,* present participle of *ambire* to surround] surrounding; encompassing; prevailing.

ambient temperature the temperature of the surrounding environment.

ambly/o (am'ble-o) [Gr. *amblys* dull] a word element used in combining form to denote dull or dim, e.g., amblyopia.

Amblyomma (am"ble-om'ah) [*ambly-* + Gr. *omma* eye] a genus of ticks, of which the species *A. americanum* (the Lone Star tick) is a known vector of Rocky Mountain spotted fever. It is commonly found in the southern United States, especially Texas and Louisiana. See also the illustration under *tick.*

amblyopia (am"ble-o'pe-ah) [*ambly-* + Gr. *ōps* eye + *-ia* condition] a dimness or dullness of vision in the absence of an external lesion of the eye.

nutritional a., a reduction in visual acuity due to insufficient intake of an essential nutrient. The optic nerve is primarily affected, especially in the region of the papillomacular bundle. There is a slowly progressive blurring and dimming of vision, often with a central bilateral scotoma, which may advance to optic atrophy and irreversible blindness.

This disorder occurs primarily in chronically undernourished persons. A similar condition (tobacco-alcohol amblyopia) is found among chronic abusers of tobacco and alcohol. In both cases, the deficient nutrients may be difficult to identify; however, most of those affected respond to balanced diets that are especially rich in thiamine and riboflavin. In mild cases, proper nutrition may lead to dramatic reversal of the symptom, but severe cases may be irreversible.

Also called nutritional optic neuropathy.

amboceptor (am"bo-sep'tor) [*ambo-* + L. *capere* to take] literally, the substance with two receptors, Ehrlich's term for the bacteriolytic or hemolytic substance present in serum that combines with complement to effect cell lysis, i.e., antibody. The term is currently employed to refer to the antibody used in complement fixation to sensitize sheep erythrocytes.

Ambrosia (am-bro'zhe-ah) [L., from Gr. *ambrotus* immortal] a genus of annual weeds, of which *A. elatior* (common ragweed) and *A. trifida* (giant ragweed) are important species. The weed produces large amounts of wind-borne pollen and is a primary cause of hay fever.

ambulatory (am'bu-la-tor"e) [L. *ambulare* to walk] capable of walking or moving about.

AMEA abbrev. See *American Medical Electroencephalographic Association.*

ameba (ah-me'bah) [L. *amoeba,* from Gr. *amoibē* change] a minute protozoon of the subphylum Sarcodina. It is a single-celled, nucleated mass of protoplasm that changes shape by extending cytoplasmic processes called pseudopodia, which it uses to move about and absorb nourishment. Most amebas are free-living in soil or water, but the following are parasitic in the human mouth and intestine: *Entamoeba coli, E. hartmanni, E. histolytica, E. gingivalis, Dientamoeba fragilis, Endolimax nana,* and *Iodamoeba bütschlii.* The soil amebas *Acanthamoeba* and *Naegleria* are pathogenic for the upper respiratory tract and central nervous system of lower animals and humans, and are the etiologic agents of primary amebic meningoencephalitis.

amebiasis (am"e-bi'ah-sis) infection with amebas, most often due to *Entamoeba histolytica,* a tissue-invading ameba that is parasitic in the human intestine. It causes colitis in severe cases, characterized by the painful passage of bloody, mucoid stools, but more often is a mild or even asymptomatic condition.

Human infection results from the ingestion of food or water contaminated with infective cysts. The cysts pass through the stomach and lodge in the small intestines, where excystation occurs, resulting in free trophozoites. A sufficient number of amebas, suitable enteric bacteria (to provide low O_2 reduction potential), and other metabolic requirements are necessary for the trophozoites to multiply outside the tissues. Under proper conditions, the trophozoites then penetrate the mucous membrane of the cecum, appendix, ascending colon, sigmoid colon, and rectum, causing small abscesses and ulcers. If the amebas enter the radicles of the portal vein, they may be carried to the liver, and although most will be destroyed, those that survive may cause amebic hepatitis, and ultimately liver abscess. Other extraintestinal sites of *E. histolytica* infection are the lungs (most commonly a direct extension of hepatic infection), spleen, skin, and genitourinary tract, and areas such as the brain and pericardium, which are penetrated through blood-borne seeding.

Most cases of amebiasis are asymptomatic. Symptoms include ill-defined gastrointestinal complaints, diarrhea, constipation, fatigue, slight fever, and mild aches and pains. In severe cases, extreme pain and tenderness of the entire abdomen, weight loss, dehydration, and moderate-to-profuse diarrhea are present.

Laboratory diagnosis requires identifcation of the cysts or trophozoites in the stools; cysts are commonly found in formed stools, trophozoites in unformed stools. Both direct wet mounts and concentration methods should be used. Polyvinyl alcohol (PVA) fixative is the recommended method for the preservation of trophozoites; PVA-fixed specimens can be stained by iron-hematoxylin or trichrome stains. Several specimens should be examined before negative results are reported.

The distinguishing morphologic characteristics of *E. histolytica* cysts are one to four spherically shaped nuclei, a minute central karyosome, even peripheral chromatin, a chromatoid body with rounded ends, and glycogen masses. The trophozoites are characterized by a nucleus with a central karyosome, a single even layer of chromatin, and inclusions of red blood cells.

Also called *amebic dysentery* and *protozoal dysentery.*

amebic (ah-me′bik) pertaining to or of the nature of an ameba.

amebic dysentery see *amebiasis.*

amebic granuloma see *ameboma.*

ameboid (ah-me′boid) [*ameba* + Gr. *eidos* form] resembling an ameba in form or movement.

ameboid movement a type of single-cell locomotion resembling that of an ameba. It occurs by the extention and retraction of the cytoplasmic processes (pseudopodia) of the cell.

ameboma (am″e-bo′mah) a granulomatous, tumorlike mass produced by localized inflammation due to infection by amebas (*Entamoeba histolytica*). It often develops in the wall of the large intestine prior to the formation of an amebic ulcer. Also called *amebic granuloma.*

AMegL abbrev. See *acute megakaryoblastic l.* under *leukemia.*

amelia (ah-me′le-ah) [*a-* neg. + Gr. *melos* limb + *-ia*] the congenital malformation that results in the complete absence of one or more extremities. In the 1960s, this usually sporadic condition appeared in many children born to mothers who had taken the drug thalidomide, used particularly in West Germany and the British Commonwealth. Few cases have been observed since thalidomide was withdrawn from the market. Cf. *phocomelia.*

ameloblast (ah-mel′o-blast″) [Old Fr. *amel* enamel + Gr. *blastos* germ] a tall epithelial cell oriented toward the dental papilla, which elaborates the enamel matrix of the teeth. These cells constitute the innermost layer of the enamel organ.

ameloblastoma (ah-mel″o-blas-to′mah) an epithelial odontogenic tumor of the jaw, the histology of which is reminiscent of the enamel organ. Several histologic subtypes have been described, but all have epithelial nests and cords within a connective tissue stroma. The tumor tends to infiltrate adjacent tissues and may be difficult to eradicate; recurrence is common, but metastases are infrequent. Also called *adamantinoma.*

amenorrhea (ah-men″o-re′ah) [*a-* neg. + Gr. *mēn* month + *rhoia* flow] the absence of menstruation, defined as primary if no menstrual period has occurred by age 16 yr, or secondary if normal menstruation ceases as a result of disease, altered physiology, or pharmacologic agents.

Amenorrhea may be caused by structural abnormalities of the vagina (e.g., lack of a vaginal opening), uterus (e.g., hypoplasia or aplasia), or ovaries. Such abnormalities in turn may be congenital or may be the result of disease, trauma, or medical and surgical therapy. Alterations in hormonal function, either congenital or acquired (through infection, trauma, or neoplasia), may result in amenorrhea. Dysfunction of the hypothalamus, pituitary, or ovaries is often the cause of amenorrhea, but thyroid or adrenal neoplasias or dysfunction are occasionally the cause of the primary form. Amenorrhea arises normally during pregnancy, during breastfeeding, and after menopause. It may accompany marked losses of body weight in starvation or anorexia nervosa. Emotional stress may also be associated.

Laboratory studies often aid in diagnosis. Especially important are the determinations of hormone levels, including plasma triiodothyronine (T_3), thyroxine (T_4), thyroid-stimulating hormone (TSH), follicle-stimulating hormone (FSH), luteinizing hormone (LH), prolactin, free testosterone, and estradiol and also the measurement of urinary 17-ketosteroids (an indication of adrenal function).

American Academy of Microbiology (AAM) a professional organization of microbiologists.

American Association for Clinical Chemistry (AACC) a professional organization of clinical chemists.

American Association for Clinical Immunology and Allergy (AACIA) a professional organization of immunologists and allergists.

American Association for the Advancement of Science (AAAS) a professional organization of scientists.

American Association of Anatomists (AAA) a professional organization of anatomists.

American Association of Bioanalysts (AAB) a professional organization of bioanalysts.

American Association of Blood Banks (AABB) a professional organization for blood banks.

American Association of Electromyography and Electrodiagnosis (AAEE) a professional organization of electromyographers.

American Association of Immunologists (AAI) a professional organization of immunologists.

American Association of Neuropathologists (AAN) a professional organization of neuropathologists.

American Association of Pathologist Assistants (AAPA) a professional organization of pathologist assistants.

American Association of Pathologists (AAP) a professional organization of pathologists.

American Blood Commission (ABC) a professional health organization.

American Board of Bioanalysis (ABB) an agency that certifies the different levels of bioanalysts.

American Cancer Society (ACS) a professional health organization.

American Chemical Society (ACS) a professional organization of chemists.

American Clinical Laboratory Association (ACLA) a professional organization of clinical laboratory personnel.

American College of Nuclear Medicine (ACNM) a professional organization of nuclear physicians.

American College of Nuclear Physicians (ACNP) a professional organization of nuclear physicians.

American College of Radiology (ACR) a professional organization of radiologists.

American Electroencephalographic Society (AES) a professional organization for electroencephalography.

American Hospital Association (AHA) a professional organization for hospital personnel.

American Medical Association (AMA) a professional organization of physicians.

American Medical Electroencephalographic Association (AMEA) a professional organization of medical electroencephalographers,

American Medical Technologists (AMT) a professional organization of medical technologists.

American National Red Cross (ANRC) a professional health care society.

American Osteopathic Association (AOA) a professional organization of osteopaths.

American Public Health Association (APHA) a professional health care organization.

American Radium Society (ARS) a professional organization of radiologists.

American Registry of Radiologic Technologists (ARRT) a professional organization for the certification of radiologic technologists. Those individuals with specialty certification in Radiation Therapy Technology are designated Registered Technologist, RT T(ARRT); those with specialty certification in Nuclear Medicine Technology are designated Registered Technologist, RT N(ARRT); and those with specialty certification in Radiography are designated Registered Technologist, RT R(ARRT).

American Roentgen Ray Society (ARRS) a professional organization of radiologists.

American Society of Allied Health Professionals (ASAHP) a professional organization of allied health professionals.

American Society of Clinical Laboratory Technicians (ASCLT) a professional organization of clinical laboratory technicians.

American Society of Clinical Pathologists (ASCP) a professional organization of clinical pathologists.

American Society of Cytology (ASC) a professional organization of cytologists.

American Society of Hematology (ASH) a professional organization of hematologists.

American Society for Medical Technology (ASMT) a professional organization of medical technologists.

American Society for Microbiology (ASM) a professional organization of microbiologists.

American Society of Radiologic Technologists (ASRT) a professional society of radiologic technologists.

American Standard Code for Information Interchange (ASCII) see *ASCII.*

American Type Culture Collection (ATCC) a long-standing organization originally established as a central depository for reference cultures of bacteria and fungi under scientific society sponsorship. At present, it is a large institution containing several departments with highly specialized personnel and equipment for maintaining and distributing a wide variety of biologic materials, including authenticated reference strains of algae, bacteria, fungi, protozoa, bacteriophages, and animal and human viruses. Also available are tissue cell lines of hybridomas, human tumor cells, and other cell banks. Recent additions include bacterial and yeast recombinant DNA host strains and related plasmids.

americium (Am) (am″ĕ-ris′e-um) [from *America*] a synthetic radioactive element; atomic number 95; most stable isotope ^{243}Am (half-life, 8800 yr); a 5f transition element (actinide or rare earth); oxidation states +3 through +6.

Ames test see under *mutagenicity test.*

amethyst violet a safranian dye, used as a nuclear stain in some histochemical preparations; C.I. 50225.

ametropia (am″ĕ-tro′pe-ah) [Gr. *ametras* disproportionate + *ōps* eye + *-ia*] a condition of the eye in which parallel rays fail to come to a focus on the retina.

amidase (am′ĭ-dās) a subclass of enzymes of the hydrolase class (EC 3.5) that catalyze the hydrolysis of carbon-nitrogen bonds other than peptide bonds, e.g., those in amide, amidine, and nitrile compounds. Some of the clinically important amidases are *arginase, guanase, guanine deaminase, penicillinase,* and *urease.*

amide (am′id, am′id) [*ammonia* + *-ide*] an organic compound containing the —$CONH_2$, —CONHR, or —$CONR_2$ functional group. Amides are named with the suffix -amide, as in ethanamide, CH_3CONH_2, or -carboxamide, as in benzenecarboxamide. See also *sulfonamide.*

amidobenzene (am″ĕ-do-ben′zēn) see *aniline.*

amikacin (am″ĭ-ka′sin) a semisynthetic aminoglycoside antibiotic with a broad spectrum of activity against gram-negative bacilli. This agent is less active on a weight-to-weight basis than is gentamicin or tobramycin; however, this feature is counterbalanced by the higher blood levels achievable with amikacin. Organisms resistant to gentamicin and tobramycin are usually sensitive to amikacin. Clinical usage includes treatment of sepsis caused by gram-negative bacilli known or suspected to be resistant to gentamicin or tobramycin. See also *aminoglycoside* and *antibacterial agents.*

amine (ah-mēn′, am′in) an organic compound of nitrogen, derived from ammonia (NH_3) by replacement of one or more of the hydrogen atoms with alkyl or aryl groups. Primary, secondary, or tertiary amines are produced when one, two, or three hydrogen atoms, respectively, are replaced.

amine oxidase (flavin-containing) (ah-mēn′ ok′sĭ-dās) an enzyme of the oxidoreductase class (EC 1.4.3.4) that catalyzes the oxidation of primary, secondary, or tertiary amines to the corresponding aldehyde, ammonia, and hydrogen peroxide. Compounds oxidized include serotonin, norepinephrine, epinephrine, and dopamine. The enzyme is a copper-containing flavoprotein. Also called *monoamine oxidase* (MAO).

amino- (ah-me′no) a prefix word element in organic chemistry to denote an amino group (—NH_2) as a substituent when it is not the principal functional group in a polyfunctional compound, e.g., aminoacetic acid, the systematic name for glycine.

aminoacetic acid see *glycine.*

amino acid (ah-me′no) an organic compound containing both an amino group (NH_2) and a carboxyl group (COOH). Those occurring in proteins are α-amino acids, having the amino group located on the carbon atom adjacent to the carboxyl group. They are represented as $RCH(NH_2)COOH$, in which R represents the remainder of the molecule. β-amino acids and γ-amino acids also occur (e.g., β-alanine, γ-aminobutyric acid), but not as components of proteins. Amino acids exist in aqueous solution at physiologic pH largely as dipolar ions (zwitterions) having both positively and negatively charged groups. They are amphoteric, capable of reacting with both acids and bases, and may act as buffers over limited pH ranges. Except for glycine, the alpha carbon atom of α-amino acids is asymmetric so that both D- and L-stereoisomeric forms can exist. D-Amino acids occur in plants and microorganisms and are constituents of some antibiotics such as gramicidin, but in animal tissues practically all amino acids have the L-configuration. Amino acids are the principal constituents of protein molecules, where they are linked together by peptide bonds into long chains containing from 50 to many thousands of amino acids. Some 40 different amino acids have been isolated from various proteins—20 of these amino acids are specified by the genetic code and occur regularly in all proteins; the rest are produced by posttranslational enzymatic modification (see the accompanying table for lists and formulas). Those that cannot be synthesized in the animal organism at a rate adequate to meet normal growth requirements are termed essential amino acids and must be supplied in the diet. Those considered essential for vertebrates are: histidine, isoleucine, leucine, lysine, methionine, phenylalanine, threonine, tryptophan, and valine.

Congenital defects in amino acid metabolism are responsible for a variety of pathologic conditions, such as phenylketonuria, tyrosinosis, histidinemia, maple syrup urine disease, and cystinuria (see also *aminoacidopathies*). Some of these result in mental retardation, so that early detection and treatment is important. Routine testing of newborns for such genetic defects is often performed (see also *genetic screening*).

In blood plasma, amino acids account for the largest nonprotein nitrogen (NPN) fraction after urea. The amino acid concentration in plasma is relatively stable, with transient elevations occurring after high-protein meals. A slight elevation may be found in persons with diabetes mellitus or impaired renal function. Significantly elevated levels are seen only in severe liver disease, especially massive hepatic necrosis caused by toxic agents.

Normally, α-amino acid nitrogen (AAN) accounts for only 1–2 percent of total urinary nitrogen excretion, mostly in the form of peptides or conjugated forms (bound AAN). The urinary output of amino acids is of great clinical significance. Increased levels of specific amino acids may indicate the presence of inborn errors of amino acid metabolism. More commonly, aminoaciduria indicates some underlying generalized disease, such as liver failure, metal poisoning, acute tubular necrosis, severe wasting, or a congenital disease.

Individual amino acids may be determined by specific microbiologic or chemical tests. Chromatography is useful for the simultaneous determination of several amino acids in mixtures. In large-scale determinations, automatic amino acid analyzers separate amino acids by ion-exchange column chromatography, and then determine the individual concentrations by color reactions and spectrophotometric analysis.

For more information, see the specific amino acid, its assay method, or the metabolic disorder.

glucogenic a. a., a group of amino acids giving rise on catabolism to carbon skeletons that can enter pathways of glucose synthesis. Such glucose synthesis occurs during fasting or during times of low carbohydrate intake when fatty acids are the principal fuel.

ketogenic a. a., a group of amino acids giving rise on catabolism to carbon skeletons that can enter pathways of 3-oxobutyrate synthesis. Such ketone body formation occurs during fasting or during times of low carbohydrate intake when fatty acids are the principal fuel. The ketogenic amino acids include leucine, isoleucine, lysine, phenylalanine, tyrosine, and tryptophan. Of these, only leucine is purely ketogenic; and the rest are both ketogenic and glucogenic. See also *glucogenic a. a.*

modified a. a., a group of amino acids that are residues of amino acids in proteins (e.g., histones) that have another moiety covalently attached. Among those detected are mono-, di-, and tri-ε-*N*-methyllysines, ω-*N*-methylarginine, 3-methylhistidine, α-*N*-acetylserine, ε-*N*-acetyllysine, *O*-phosphoserine, *O*-phosphothreonine, *N*-phospholysine, and N^3-phosphohistidine.

amino acid–activating enzyme see under *aminoacyl-tRNA hydrolase.*

amino acid analyzer an analytic instrument that uses ion-exchange chromatography to separate, identify, and measure quantities of individual amino acids and related compounds present in biologic extracts, protein hydrolysates, or urine.

amino acid assays determinations of the total amounts of amino acids in urine, plasma, or hydrolyzed proteins. This is conventionally specified in terms of the α-amino acid nitrogen (AAN), using spectrophotometry of the colored product formed by reaction with 1,2-naphthoquinone-4-sulfonic acid or with 1-fluoro-2,4-dinitrobenzene (FDNB).

Proteins are removed from plasma or urine speci-

AMINO ACID. IMPORTANT EXAMPLES OF AMINO ACIDS

NAME	SYMBOL	FORMULA	COMMENTS	pK_1 (α-COOH)	pK_2	pK_3	pI
ALIPHATIC, UNCHARGED R-GROUPS							
Glycine	Gly	NH_2CH_2COOH	Simplest amino acid; optically inactive; used as buffer	2.34	9.60		5.97
Alanine	Ala	CH_3CHNH_2COOH	Substrate for alanine transaminase (GPT, ALT)	2.34	9.69		6.00
Serine	Ser	$HOCH_2CHNH_2COOH$	Involved in "active center" of many enzymes. Hydroxyl may be phosphorylated	2.21	9.15		5.68
Leucine	Leu	$CH_3CH(CH_3)CH_2CHNH_2COOH$	Branched chain R-group, which is hydrophobic; faulty metabolism in "maple syrup" disease; ketogenic; essential	2.36	9.60		5.98
Isoleucine	Ile	$CH_3CH_2CH(CH_3)CHNH_2COOH$	See leucine; partly ketogenic; essential	2.36	9.60		6.02
Valine	Val	$CH_3CH(CH_3)CHNH_2COOH$	See leucine; partly ketogenic; essential	2.32	9.62		5.96
Threonine	Thr	$CH_3CHOHCHNH_2COOH$	Essential	2.09	9.10		5.60
Cysteine	Cys	$HSCH_2CHNH_2COOH$	Functional sulfhydryl (-SH) group; free -SH necessary for activity of many enzymes	1.96	8.18 (thiol)	10.28 (α-NH_3^+)	5.07
Cystine	Cys–Cys	$S-CH_2CHNH_2COOH$ / $S-CH_2CHNH_2COOH$	Oxidized form of cysteine; insoluble at neutral pH; forms one type of kidney stone; may link two peptide chains, as in insulin	1.65 2.26	7.85 (α-NH_3^+) 9.85 (α-NH_3^+)		5.06
Methionine	Met	$CH_3-S-CH_2CH_2CHNH_2COOH$	Contains sulfur; methyl group transfer agent; essential	2.28	9.21		5.74
AROMATIC AND HETEROCYCLIC UNCHARGED R-GROUPS							
Phenylalanine	Phe	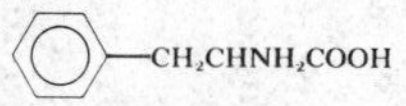	Metabolism deficient in phenylketonuria; essential	1.83	9.13		5.48
Tyrosine	Tyr	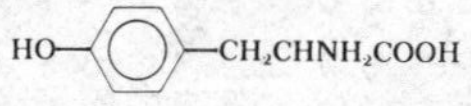	Usually nonessential; intermediate in synthesis of catecholamines, thyroxine; functional phenolic hydroxyl; reacts with Folin reagent in quantitative protein assay	2.20	9.11 (α-NH_3^+)	10.07 (phenolic OH)	5.66
Tryptophane	Trp	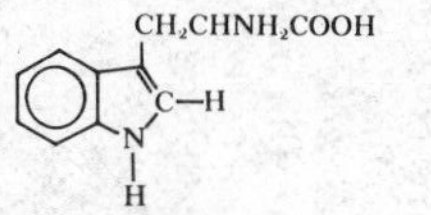	Essential; contains indole ring system; metabolites involved in carcinoid disease	2.83	9.39		5.89
DICARBOXYLIC, ACIDIC R-GROUPS							
Aspartic acid	Asp	$HOOC-CH_2CHNH_2COOH$	Substrate for aspartate transaminase (GOT)	1.88	3.65 (β-COOH)	9.60 (α-NH_3^+)	2.77
Glutamic acid	Glu	$HOOC-CH_2CH_2CHNH_2COOH$	Substrate for both GOT and GPT	2.19	4.25 (γ-COOH)	9.67 (α-NH_3^+)	3.22

BASIC AMINO ACIDS, BASIC R–GROUPS							
Lysine	Lys	$H_3NCH_2CH_2CH_2CH_2CHNH_2COOH$	Terminal NH_2 referred to as ξ (epsilon) NH_2; essential	2.18	8.95 (α-NH_3^+)	10.53 (ξ-NH_3^+)	9.74
Arginine	Arg	$H_2N{-}C({=}NH){-}NH{-}CH_2CH_2CH_2CHNH_2COOH$	Involved in urea synthesis; the basic group is guanidine	2.17	9.03 (α-NH_3^+)	12.48 (guanidinium)	10.76
Histidine	His	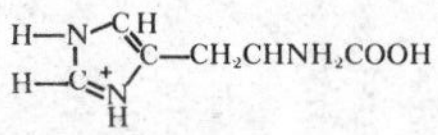	R-group represents imidazole; ring ⪰ NH ionizes at physiological pH; in hemoglobin it ionizes on oxygenation	1.82	6.00 (imidazolium)	9.17 (α-NH_3^+)	7.59
IMINO ACIDS (RING⪰NH REPLACES NH_2)							
Proline	Pro	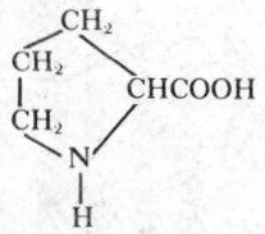	Important constituent of collagen and gelatin	1.99	10.60		6.30
Hydroxyproline	Hyp	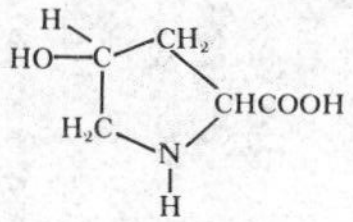	Present in collagen; urine output used as an index of bone matrix metabolism	1.92	9.73 (α-NH_3^+)		5.83
AMINO ACID AMIDES							
Glutamine	Gln	$H_2NC({=}O){-}CH_2CH_2CHNH_2COOH$	Storage form of ammonia in tissues	2.17	9.13		5.65
Asparagine	Asn	$H_2NC({=}O){-}CH_2CHNH_2COOH$		2.02	8.80		5.41
MISCELLANEOUS AMINO ACIDS							
Thyroxine	T_4	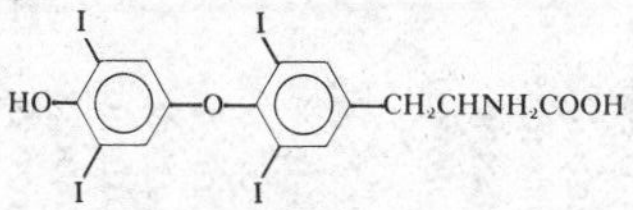	Thyroid hormone; contains 4 iodine atoms				
Triiodothyronine	T_3	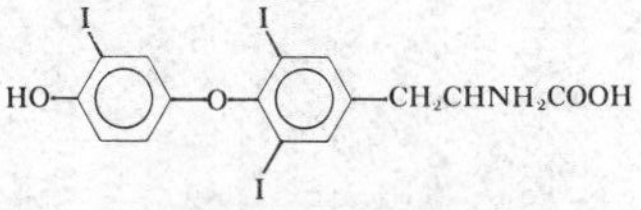	Thyroid hormone; more active than T_4; contains only 3 iodine atoms				
β-Alanine		$H_2N{-}CH_2CH_2COOH$	Constituent of pantothenic acid (a vitamin)	3.60	10.19 β-NH_3^+		6.90
Dihydroxyphenylalanine	DOPA	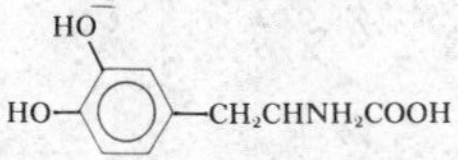	Intermediate in synthesis of catecholamines				
γ-Aminobutyric acid	GABA	$H_2NCH_2CH_2CH_2COOH$	Metabolite of Glu; regulates nerve impulses in brain	4.03	10.56 γ-NH_3^+		7.30
Ornithine		$H_2N(CH_2)_3CHNH_2COOH$	Intermediate in urea synthesis				
Phosphoserine		$H_2O_3P{-}O{-}CH_2CHNH_2COOH$	In casein and other phosphoproteins	1.94	8.65 α-NH_3^+	10.76 γ-NH_3^+	9.70
Pyrrolidone carboxylic acid	PCA	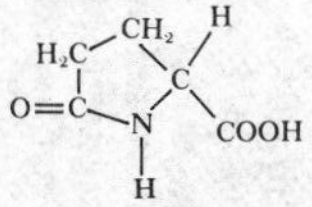	Cyclicized form of Glu; rare, used to terminate peptide chains, as at N-terminal end of L-chains in γ globulins	1.95		10.64 α-NH_3^+	6.30

All p*K* values measured at 25°C.
Modified from Tietz, N. W.: Fundamentals of Clinical Chemistry. 2nd ed. Philadelphia, W. B. Saunders Co., 1978, pp. 267-269.

mens by precipitation with tungstic acid and subsequent filtration. Ammonia is removed from urine by making it alkaline and boiling. For the naphthoquinone sulfonate method, urea must also be removed from urine specimens by ion-exchange column chromatography.

FDNB reacts with primary α-amino acids to form yellow *N*-2,4-dinitrophenyl (DNP) derivatives, which have absorption maxima near 356 nm. The imino acids proline and hydroxyproline form DNP-imino acids, which have maxima at 370 nm. The absorbance at 420 nm (similar for both) is used for quantitation. The molar absorptivity of the DNP derivatives of the commonly occurring amino acids ranges from 0.86 to 1.09 times that of glycine, with the exception of lysine (1.97) and ornithine (2.23). The naphthoquinone sulfonate reaction produces an orange-brown product, which is quantitated at 470 nm. Different amino acids produce differing color intensities per mole; thus, a mixture of glycine and glutamic acid is generally used as a standard.

The most precise method for assaying amino acids employs the gasometric ninhydrin (triketohydrindene hydrate) reaction. One mole of CO_2 is liberated per mole of amino acid (aspartic acid yields two moles). Either the liberated CO_2 is measured gasometrically, or the other products of the reaction, ammonia and hydrindentin, are reacted under acid conditions to form a blue product that is measured colorimetrically. Proline and hydroxyproline, however, do not react.

aminoacidemia (ah″me″-no-as″ĭ-de′me-ah) [*amino acid* + Gr. *haima* blood + *-ia*] an excess of amino acids in the blood. See also *aminoacidopathy.*

amino acid fractionation assays screening tests for specific amino acids, using various types of chromatography or high-voltage electrophoresis (HVE), that are primarily employed in detecting disorders of amino acid metabolism. Examples of chromatographic techniques include: paper or thin-layer chromatography (used for screening for metabolic disorders) and ion-exchange chromatography (most often used for quantitation of specific amino acids). Gas-liquid chromatography can also be employed but has not found widespread use.

The most commonly used screening test is one-dimensional or two-dimensional thin-layer chromatography, using cellulose or silica gel plates with ninhydrin as the staining reagent. For one-dimensional chromatography, the most popular developing solvent is a 12:3:5 mixture of *n*-butanol–acetic acid–water. For two-dimensional chromatography, the first solvent contains ammonia to increase the mobility of amino acids with basic side-chains; the second method contains acid to increase the mobility of amino acids with acidic side-chains.

aminoacidopathy (ah-me″no-as″ĭ-dop′ah-the) [*amino acid* + Gr. *pathos* suffering] any of a large number of inherited or acquired disorders of metabolism or transport of amino acids or their catabolites. Most can be divided into two large classes: inherited defects of amino acid catabolism and inherited defects of renal acid transport. The disorders in both classes are due to a genetic defect in a single enzyme or renal membrane transport protein. A few disorders are combinations of both types of defect. There are also several benign perinatal adaptive traits in which aminoaciduria occurs, owing either to high protein intake or other transient causes.

In the defects of amino acid catabolism, lack of activity of a specific enzyme causes a metabolic block. As a result, the substrate and (in some disorders) several metabolites accumulate in the blood; when the transepithelial transport mechanisms for the substances in the renal tubules become saturated, they are excreted in the urine. In most of these disorders, the accumulating substance is an amino acid whose concentration is increased in plasma and urine; in others, catabolites such as keto acids, ketones, and organic acids accumulate. In some cases, the substrate does not accumulate because there is no reabsorption in the kidneys; blood levels are low, but urine levels are increased.

These disorders are detected by screening tests (paper or thin-layer chromatography) for the presence of the amino acid in urine or by neonatal genetic screening (e.g., Guthrie bacterial inhibition assay in PKU). Positive identification is made by demonstration of elevated blood and/or urine levels of the accumulating substance, using chemical tests or column chromatography.

For some of the disorders, such as phenylketonuria (PKU), treatment consists of dietary restriction of the involved amino acid (in PKU, phenylalanine). This removes the substrate from the blocked metabolic pathway and prevents development of the associated pathology. For other disorders, no treatment is possible.

In the defects of amino acid transport, the active mechanism for renal tubular transport of a specific group of amino acids is defective. This causes a very high renal clearance of the amino acid and high urine levels (aminoaciduria) associated with normal blood levels.

For more information, see the accompanying tables and the specific disorders; see also *genetic screening.*

D-amino acid oxidase an enzyme of the oxidoreductase class (D-amino acid:oxygen oxidoreductase [deaminating], EC 1.4.3.3). It is found in the liver and kidneys and catalyzes the oxidative deamination of D-amino acids to α-keto acids and free ammonia. It has a tightly bound FAD group and uses molecular oxygen for the reaction. This enzyme presumably functions in degrading D-amino acids, which arise from bacterial peptide metabolism in the body. It is of minor importance in amino acid metabolism and has no known clinical application.

L-amino-acid oxidase an enzyme of the oxidoreductase class (L-amino acid:oxygen oxidoreductase [deaminating], EC 1.4.3.2). This enzyme is similar to D-amino acid oxidase in its distribution and function, but oxidizes L-amino acids rather than D-amino acids. It is found in large amounts in some snake venoms.

amino acid sequencer (se′kwen-ser) an automated apparatus used in determining the amino acid sequence of polypeptides. The *N*-terminal amino acid residue is removed and identified using the Edman degradation reaction. This step is automatically repeated 30–40 times, thus determining the sequence.

In a typical sequencer, the reagents are spread by centrifugal force over the wall of a rapidly spinning cup. Reagents are introduced at the bottom of the cup and removed by a scoop from a groove at the top. The peptide is dissolved in a suitable solvent (e.g., trifluoroacetic acid), spread over the wall of the cup, and dried. Then, phenylisothiocyanate (PITC) dissolved in heptane is spread and dried. A buffer of pH

9.0–9.5 (e.g., Quadrol, *N, N, N', N'*-tetrakis(2-hydroxypropenyl)ethylenediamine) is added, resulting in the formation of the phenylthiocarbamyl (PTC) derivative of the peptide within 15–30 min at 55°C. When the excess PITC and buffer are washed away, the PTC-peptide is cleaved by the addition of acid in a nonaqueous solvent (e.g., butyl chloride). This acidification produces the original peptide less its *N*-terminal residue and the anilinothiazolone derivative of the *N*-terminal amino acid, which is removed in the solvent and converted to the phenylthiohydantoin (PTH) derivative by the addition of water.

The PTH–amino acids are identified by chromatography, using a cation-exchange resin such as sulfonated styrene-divinylbenzene copolymer. The PTC–amino acids are sequentially eluted from the resin by using a series of buffers with increasing pH and identified by reaction with ninhydrin, which forms a colored compound with an absorption maximum at 570 nm for the primary amino acids and at 440 nm for the imino acids (proline and hydroxyproline).

Some systems use variations of this procedure. In solid-phase sequencers, the peptide is bonded (at the C-terminal end) to a resin. Some sequencers use gas chromatography or high-pressure liquid chromatography to separate the PTC–amino acids. Fluorescamine can be used instead of ninhydrin to identify the primary amino acids by fluorometry.

Also called amino acid sequenator.

aminoaciduria (ah-me″no-as-ĭ-du′re-ah) [*amino acid* + Gr. *ouron* urine + *-ia*] the presence of an excess of one or more amino acids in the urine, such as occurs in disorders of amino acid metabolism; see also *aminoacidopathy.*

neutral a., see *Hartnup disease.*

no-threshold a., an aminoacidopathy in which there is abnormal metabolism of an amino acid with no renal threshold. The amino acid is present in the urine but not in the blood, as in homocystinuria.

primary overflow a., an aminoacidopathy in which abnormal amino acid metabolism results in the accumulation of one or more amino acids in the blood at concentrations exceeding the renal excretion threshold, so that the amino acids are excreted in the urine, e.g., phenylketonuria.

renal transport a., an aminoaciduria caused by the defective renal tubular transport of one or more amino acids, e.g., cystinuria or Hartnup disease. The plasma concentrations of these amino acids are normal.

aminoacyl-histidine dipeptidase (ah-me″no-a′sil his′tĭ-din di-pep′tĭ-dās) an enzyme (a metalloprotein) of the hydrolase class (aminoacyl-L-histidine hydrolase, EC 3.4.13.3) that catalyzes the reaction carnosine (and other aminoacyl-L-histidine dipeptides) + H_2O ⇄ alanine (or other amino acid) + L-histidine. A genetic defect in the enzyme causes carnosinemia, with an accumulation of carnosine in the blood and possible mental retardation. Also called *carnosinase.*

aminoacyl-tRNA hydrolase a group of enzymes of the hydrolase class (aminoacyl-tRNA aminoacylhydrolase, EC 3.1.1.29) that catalyze the reaction amino acid + tRNA + ATP ⇄ aminoacyl-tRNA + AMP + PP_i. The enzymes are known as amino acid–activating enzymes, and each is highly specific for one amino acid and for its corresponding tRNA.

The transfer of an amino acid to its tRNA occurs in two separate steps on the enzyme catalytic site. In the first step, ATP reacts with the amino acid, with displacement of pyrophosphate, to form an enzyme-bound intermediate. In the second step, the activated amino is transferred to its tRNA with subsequent release of AMP and formation of an aminoacyl-tRNA.

aminoanthraquinone dyes a group of oil-soluble histologic dyes used as fat stains. They include the Sudan dyes violet R (C.I. 61100), blue GN (C.I. 61520), blue G (C.I. 61525), and green BB (C.I. 62545), as well as Oil blue N (C.I. 61555), carycinel red, and coccinel red.

aminobenzene (am″ĭ-no-ben′zēn) see *aniline.*

***p*-aminobenzoic acid** (PAB, PABA) vitamin B_x, $H_2NC_6H_4COOH$, widely distributed in nature as a B complex factor; M.W. 137.13. PABA is an essential metabolite for the synthesis of folic acid by plants and many microorganisms. Sulfonamides are antagonists of PABA because of their similar structures, and can be used as antibacterial agents because they block folic acid synthesis, which is essential for bacterial growth. However, this inhibition of bacterial growth by sulfonamides may be overcome by adding PABA to the growth medium. PABA also absorbs ultraviolet light and is used as a topical sunscreen.

aminobutyrate aminotransferase (ah-me″no-bu-ti′rāt ah-me″no-trans′fer-ās) an enzyme of the transferase class (4-aminobutyrate:2-oxoglutarate aminotransferase, EC 2.6.1.19) that catalyzes the reaction β-alanine (or 4-aminobutyrate) + 2-oxoglutarate ⇄ malonic semialdehyde (or succinate semialdehyde) + L-glutamate. A congenital deficiency of this enzyme causes hyper-β-alaninemia, characterized by the accumulation of β-alanine, β-aminoisobutyric acid, and γ-aminobutyric acid in the blood, resulting in mental retardation and somnolence. Excretion of β-aminoisobutyric acid and taurine is increased. Also called β-alanine:α-ketoglutarate aminotransferase and *β-alanine transaminase.*

γ-aminobutyric acid (GABA) 4-aminobutyric acid, $H_2NCH_2CH_2CH_2COOH$, a neurotransmitter present in the central nervous system. It is formed by decarboxylation of the α-carboxyl group of L-glutamate, which is catalyzed by the pyridoxal phosphate–dependent enzyme, glutamate dehydrogenase. GABA is involved in regulating neural activity in the brain, as an inhibitory neurotransmitter. It is also present in the kidneys, heart, and lungs.

γ-aminobutyric acid shunt a metabolic pathway occurring in nerve tissue that bypasses the 2-oxoglutarate dehydrogenase step of the tricarboxylic acid cycle. Glutamate, produced from 2-oxoglutarate by aspartate aminotransferase, is deaminated to produce GABA, which serves as a neurotransmitter. GABA is then catabolized first to succinic semialdehyde by aminobutyrate aminotransferase and then to succinate by aldehyde dehydrogenase. Roughly 10 percent of the 2-oxoglutarate goes into the GABA shunt.

ε-aminocaproic acid (EACA) a synthetic amino acid and analog of lysine, which inhibits the conversion of plasminogen to plasmin and the activation of plasminogen by urokinase in the urine. It is used to

Aminoacidopathy, Table 1. Metabolic Disorders of Amino Acids (Aminoacidopathies) and of Organic Acids

Conditions	Enzyme Defect	Elevated Metabolite*	Mode of Inheritance†
Alkaptonuria	Homogentisate 1,2-dioxygenase (homogentisic acid oxidase)	2,5-Dihydroxyphenylacetic acid (U) (homogentisic acid)	AR
Argininemia	Arginase	Arginine (B, SF)	AR
Arginosuccinic aciduria	Arginosuccinate lyase	Arginosuccinic acid (B, U)	AR
Branched chain ketoaciduria (maple syrup urine disease)			
Classic type	2-Oxoisovalerate dehydrogenase (branched chain keto acid decarboxylase)	Leucine, isoleucine, valine (S, U)	AR
Thiamine-responsive type	2-Oxoisovalerate dehydrogenase (branched chain keto acid decarboxylase)	Leucine, isoleucine, valine (B)	AR
Citrullinemia	Arginosuccinate synthetase	Citrulline (B, U), ammonia, methionine (B)	AR
Cystathioninuria	Cystathionine γ-lyase (cystathionase)	Cystathionine (B, U)	AR
Histidinemia	Histidine ammonia-lyase (histidase)	Histidine (B,U), imidazole derivatives (U)	AR
Homocystinuria			
I	Cystathionine β-synthase	Methionine, homocystine (B, U)	AR
II	5,10-Methylenetetrahydrofolate reductase ($FADH_2$)	Homocystine, cystathionine (B, U)	AR
III	Tetrahydropteroylglutamate methyltransferase (defect in coenzyme synthesis)	Homocystine, cystathionine (B, U), methylmalonic acid (U)	AR
Hydroxyprolinemia	4-Oxoproline reductase (hydroxyproline oxidase)	Hydroxyproline (S, U)	AR
Hyperammonemia			
I	Ornithine carbamoyltransferase (ornithine transcarbamylase)	Ammonia (B), glutamine (B, U)	X-Linked
II	Carbamoyl-phosphate synthetase (ammonia)	Ammonia (B)	AR
Hyperglycinemia (isolated)	Glycine synthase (glycine decarboxylase)	Glycine (B, U)	AR
Hyperlysinemia	Saccharopine dehydrogenase (lysine ketoglutarate reductase)	Lysine (B, U)	AR
Hyperornithinemia	Unknown	Ornithine, lysine, ammonia (B), homocitrulline (U)	AR

Hyperprolinemia			
I	Pyrroline-5-carboxylate reductase (proline oxidase)	Proline (S, U), hydroxyproline, glycine (U)	AR
II	1-Pyrroline-5-carboxylate dehydrogenase	Proline (S, U), hydroxyproline, glycine (U); pyrroline-5-COOH (U)	AR
Isovalericacidemia	Isovaleryl-CoA dehydrogenase	Isovaleric acid and isovalerylglycine (U)	AR
Lysine intolerance	Lysine dehydrogenase (lysine:NAD oxidoreductase)	Lysine, homoarginine (B, U)	AR
β-Methylcrotonylglycinuria	Methylcrotonyl-CoA carboxylase (holocarboxylase synthetase)	β-Methylcrotonylglycine and β-hydroxyisovalerate (U)	AR
α-Methyl-β-hydroxybutyricaciduria	Acetyl-CoA acetyltransferase (acetoacetyl-CoA thiolase)	α-Methyl-β-hydroxybutyric and α-methylacetoacetic acids (U)	AR
Methylmalonic acidemia			
(mut)	S-Methylmalonyl-CoA mutase	Methylmalonic acid (S, U), glycine (B, U)	AR
(cbl B)	Cob(I)alamin adenosyltransferase	Methylmalonic acid (S, U), glycine (B, U)	AR
5-Oxoprolinuria	Glutathione synthetase	5-Oxoproline (S, U)	AR
Phenylalaninemia ("lethal")	Dihydropteridine reductase	Phenylalanine (S) and bioperin (S)	AR
Phenylketonuria (three types)	Phenylalanine 4-monooxygenase (phenylalanine hydroxylase)	Phenylalanine (S)	AR
Propionic acidemia	Propionyl-CoA carboxylase	Propionic, β-hydroxypropionic, methylcitric acids (U), glycine (B, U)	AR
Sarcosinemia	Sarcosine dehydrogenase	Sarcosine (B, U)	AR
Sulfite oxidase deficiency	Sulfite oxidase	Sulfocysteine, sulfite, thiosulfate (U)	AR
Tryptophanuria	Tryptophan 2-3 dioxygenase‡ (tryptophan pyrrolase)	Tryptophan (B, U)	X-Linked
Tyrosinemia	4-Hydroxyphenylpyruvate dioxygenase	Tyrosine (B,U)	AR
Valinemia	Valine-3-methyl-2-oxovalerate aminotransferase (valine transaminase)	Valine (B, U)	AR

* B = blood; S = serum; SF = spinal fluid; and U = urine.
† AR = autosomal recessive.
‡ Enzyme defect not confirmed.

Aminoacidopathy, Table 2. Amino Acid Transport Disorders

Condition	Biochemical Defect	Elevated Metabolites (excreted)	Mode of Inheritance*
Blue diaper syndrome	Tryptophan malabsorption	Indoleacetamide, indolactic acid, indoleacetylglutamine, indican	AR
Cystinuria			
I	Dibasic amino acid nonabsorption	Cystine, lysine, ornithine, arginine	AR
II	Lysine malabsorption	Cystine, lysine (heterozygotes)	
III	Dibasic amino acid malabsorption	Cystine, lysine (heterozygotes)	
Hartnup disease	Neutral amino acid malabsorption	Neutral amino acids (alanine, threonine, serine, glutamine, histidine, isoleucine, leucine, valine, phenylalanine, tyrosine, tryptophan)	AR
Oasthouse urine disease	Methionine malabsorption	Methionine, α-hydroxybutyric acid	AR

*AR = autosomal recessive.

control increased fibrinolytic activity that results from primary fibrinolysis and is not associated with disseminated intravascular coagulation.

***p*-aminodimethylaniline** dimethyl-*p*-phenylenediamine, $(CH_3)_2NC_6H_4NH_2$, a reagent used in bacteriology in the indophenol (cytochrome) oxidase test to identify organisms and particularly to distinguish species of *Neisseria, Pseudomonas,* and *Vibrio.*

aminoglutaric acid see *glutamine.*

aminoglutethimide (ah-me″no-gloo-teth′ĭ-mīd) a drug formerly employed as an anticonvulsant, now used for the suppression of adrenal function. It blocks the conversion of cholesterol to Δ^5-pregnenolone, a step in the synthesis of adrenal steroid hormones and is used in the treatment of Cushing's syndrome. It is also used as a cancer chemotherapeutic drug; for more information, see *Appendix A.*

aminoglycosides (am″ĭ-no-gli-ko′sidz) a group of clinically useful bacterial antibiotics containing an inositol substituted with two amino or guanidino groups and with one or more sugars and amino sugars. The best known early member of the group is streptomycin; others include kanamycin, neomycin, tobramycin, gentamicin, and amikacin.

STRUCTURE. Aminoglycoside antibiotics, derived from either *Streptomyces* or *Micromonosporum* species, contain two or more amino sugars joined by glycosidic linkage to a central hexose. They are identified by variations in side-chains of the amino sugars attached to the central hexose.

MECHANISM OF ACTION. Aminoglycosides are bactericidal and inhibit protein synthesis by binding to the 30S subunit of bacterial ribosomes, which may result in detachment of messenger RNA from ribosomes or incorrect assembly of polypeptides by the misreading of transfer information.

RESISTANCE. Resistance to aminoglycosides can be mediated by aminoglycoside-modifying enzymes. Such enzymes are coded for by transferable plasmids, which have been found in *Staphylococcus aureus* and in many genera of gram-negative bacteria, including members of the family Enterobacteriaceae and *Pseudomonas* and *Hemophilus* species. The enzymes either acetylate, adenylate, or phosphorylate hydroxyl or amino groups at various positions on the aminoglycoside molecule, resulting in inactivation of the aminoglycoside. Cross-resistance may occur. Resistant organisms are usually isolated from patients in hospital areas where aminoglycoside usage is highest. Other mechanisms of resistance include loss of permeability to aminoglycosides or alterations in ribosomal binding sites.

CLINICAL USE. There are six aminoglycosides currently in clinical usage: streptomycin, neomycin, kanamycin, gentamicin, tobramycin, and amikacin. Their activity is primarily directed against, and they are used to treat serious infections with, aerobic gram-negative bacilli and *S. aureus.* Although poor activity is exhibited against certain streptococci, including enterococci, synergistic bactericidal activity may be obtained by combining an aminoglycoside with an inhibitor of cell wall synthesis. Tobramycin and gentamicin exhibit activity against *Klebsiella, Enterobacter,* and *Serratia* species. In vitro, tobramycin is more active than gentamicin against *Pseudomonas aeruginosa.* Amikacin has the broadest spectrum of activity against gram-negative bacilli, and resistance occurs infrequently. Streptomycin is active against *Mycobacterium tuberculosis.*

LABORATORY TESTING. In vitro susceptibility testing of amikacin is affected by inoculum size. The in vitro aminoglycoside susceptibility of *P. aeruginosa* is affected by high concentrations of cations, particularly magnesium and calcium, and this may result in an elevated minimal inhibitory concentration (MIC) because of aminoglycoside antagonism.

The in vitro activity of all aminoglycoside antibiotics is inhibited in an environment of low pH; a change from neutral pH to a pH range of 6–6.4 can result in an increase of MIC. Variable effects for different aminoglycosides are observed at alkaline pH. Increases in MIC are observed when sensitivity testing is performed in an atmosphere that is anaerobic or of lowered oxygen tension.

Peak serum aminoglycoside concentrations are achieved approximately 30 min after intramuscular injection and 15–30 min after the termination of intravenous infusion. All aminoglycosides have the ability to induce ototoxicity and nephrotoxicity. Aminoglycosides accumulate rapidly in patients with compromised renal function, increasing the risk of toxicity. Determination of serum aminoglycoside levels is essential in order to verify therapeutic expectations and detect possible toxic drug levels. Monitoring includes obtaining a trough serum level, collected immediately preceding an antibiotic dose, and a peak serum level, collected 15–30 min after the termination of the intravenous dose. Several methods are available for the determination of aminoglycoside serum levels, including bioassay, radioimmunoassay, and EMIT homogeneous enzyme immunoassay.

See also *antibacterial agents.*

***p*-aminohippurate** (PAH) (am″ĭ-no-hip′u-rāt) a synthetic substance used to estimate effective renal plasma flow (ERPF). When injected into a patient, PAH is both filtered by the glomeruli and secreted by the tubular cells. At low blood concentration (1 mg/dl), more than 90 percent of the plasma is cleared of PAH in one passage through the kidneys. From the plasma flow and the hematocrit, the total blood flow through the kidneys can be calculated. At high concentrations of PAH it is possible to measure the maximal rate of transport, which is a measure of effective tubular mass.

***p*-aminohippurate clearance test** a test used as a measure of renal blood flow and excretory capacity. It consists of the administration of a relatively high intravenous "priming dose" of PAH to achieve a conveniently measurable plasma concentration, followed by an infusion of a weak solution given slowly throughout the test to maintain this level. Three urine samples are taken at accurately timed intervals, a blood specimen being taken before the test and at the middle of each urine collection period. The three PAH clearance values are calculated, averaged, and reported in milliliters per minute (ml/min) and/or in milliliters per minute per square meter (ml/min/m²) of body surface area. Because performance of the test is technically difficult and requires the services of a physician, it is not performed routinely in clinical laboratory practice. Reference ranges for PAH clearance are 600–700 ml/min or 350–400 ml/min/m² of body surface. Because about 10 percent of the blood circulating through the kidneys does not come into contact with functional cells, the clearance value underestimates the actual plasma flow, which is usually about 750 ml/min.

β-aminoisobutyric acid (βAIB) a metabolite formed in the degradation of pyrimidines; most is excreted in the urine. There is a hereditary phenotypic variation, 5–10 percent of Caucasians and up to 95 percent of Mongolians being "high βAIB excretors." Transient high βAIB excretion may be produced by malignancies, burns, fasting, and other conditions with a high catabolic rate. Elevated concentrations are also seen in the aminoacidopathy, hyper-β-alaninemia.

δ-aminolevulinate (ALA) dehydratase see *porphobilinogen synthase* and *porphobilinogen dehydratase assays.*

δ-aminolevulinate synthase an enzyme of the transferase class (succinyl-CoA:glycine *C*-succinyltransferase, decarboxylating, EC 2.3.1.37) that catalyzes the reaction succinyl-CoA + glycine ⇄ δ-aminolevulinate + CoA + CO_2, the first step in the synthesis of porphyrins. This step requires pyridoxal phosphate; it is the committed step as well as the regulation step of the porphyrin synthesis pathway.

δ-aminolevulinic acid (ALA) a metabolic intermediate in the production of heme, synthesized from succinyl–coenzyme A and glycine in the presence of pyridoxal phosphate and ALA synthase. Two molecules of ALA form porphobilinogen. See also *porphyrin.*

δ-aminolevulinic acid assay the determination of the serum concentration of ALA, often used as a screening test to detect lead intoxication. The effect of interfering thiol compounds is eliminated by adding iodoacetamide to serum. After precipitation of protein, the supernatant solution is treated with acetate buffer, acetylacetone, and sodium hydroxide. A pyrrole condensation product is formed, and after addition of Ehrlich's reagent, the absorbance of the resulting color is read at 553 nm with a high-resolution spectrophotometer. The blank is prepared from the same serum without the addition of acetylacetone. In adult males, the reference value is 19 μg/dl (SD ± 4); children's values may be slightly lower.

6-aminopenicillanic acid (ah-me′no-pen″ĭ-sil-a′-nik) a nucleus of the penicillin molecule, produced in special culture media or by certain mutant cultures of *Penicillium notatum.* This inactive precursor can be modified chemically to produce a variety of penicillins with specific desired properties. They fall into two classes, penicillins resistant to penicillinase and those with a broader antibacterial spectrum.

aminopeptidase (cytosol) an enzyme of the hydrolase class (α-aminoacyl-peptide hydrolase [cytosol], EC 3.4.11.1) that catalyzes the reaction aminoacyl-peptide + H_2O ⇄ amino acid + peptide. It is a zinc-containing enzyme of broad specificity and hydrolyzes most L-peptides, splitting off an *N*-terminal residue with a free amino group. It does not act on lysyl and arginyl peptides. Aminopeptidase is commonly known as leucine aminopeptidase (LAP). See also *leucine aminopeptidase.*

aminophenol (ah-me″no-fe′nol) one of three isomers (*ortho-*, *meta-* or *para*-aminophenol) used in dyeing and in the manufacture of dyes and drugs; M.W. 109.12. All are white crystalline solids, which turn brown with age or exposure to light. They are moderately toxic, and may cause skin sensitization, dermatitis, and methemoglobinemia.

aminophylline (ah-me″no-fil′in) [USP], theophylline ethylenediamine, a bronchodilator used to treat bronchial asthma, chronic bronchitis, and emphysema. See also *theophylline.*

β-aminopropionitrile (ah-me″no-pro-pi″o-ni′tril) a toxic compound, $H_2N—CH_2—CH_2—CN$, present in the seeds of certain leguminous plants; when ingested, it produces lathyrism. See also *lathyrism.*

aminopterin sodium (am″ĭ-nop′ter-in) a cytotoxic drug, 4-aminofolic acid, an antimetabolite of folic acid formerly used in cancer chemotherapy, now replaced by methotrexate. For more information on methotrexate, see *Appendix A.*

aminopurine (ah-me″no-pu′rēn) a general term that describes a compound having a purine ring system with an amino group attached. Examples are adenine and guanine.

aminopyrine (ah-me″no-pi′rin) a pyrazolone derivative related to phenylbutazone. It was formerly used as an analgesic and antipyretic, and can cause habituation and agranulocytosis.

***p*-aminosalicylic acid** (PAS) a white, crystalline, heat-labile powder used as an antibacterial agent in the treatment of tuberculosis in combination with isoniazid. Like sulfonamides, it interferes with the enzymatic conversion of *p*-aminobenzoate (PABA) to folic acid. Except for tubercle bacilli, most of the mycobacteria population either are resistant or develop resistance to it. PAS is only bacteriostatic and is ineffectual against intramacrophage bacilli. See also *antibacterial agents.*

aminosuccinic acid (ah-me″no-suk′sĭ-nik) see *aspartic acid.*

aminotransferase (am″ĭ-no-trans′fer-ās) any of a group of enzymes that catalyze the transfer of amino groups in the interconversion of α-amino acids and α-oxoacids (α-keto acids). The α-amino group is reversibly transferred to the α-carbon atom of one of three α-keto acids (pyruvate, α-ketoglutarate, or oxaloacetate), yielding as products an amino acid (alanine, glutamate, or aspartate) and the α-keto analog of the original donor amino acid. Aspartate, glutamate, and alanine aminotransferases are important in laboratory medicine. Also called *transaminase.* For more information see the specific enzyme.

amitosis (am″ĭ-to′sis) [*a-* neg. + *mitos* thread + *-osis*] direct cell division by simple cleavage of the nucleus without the formation of a mitotic spindle. Cf. *mitosis.*

amitotic (am″ĭ-tot′ik) of the nature of amitosis; not occurring by mitosis.

amitriptyline (am″ĭ-trip′tĭ-lēn) a derivative of the tricyclic compound dibenzocycloheptadiene, which is used as an antidepressant. For toxicity, see *tricyclic antidepressant.* Trademark, *Elavil.*

amitriptyline and nortriptyline assays 1. a colorimetric procedure for the determination of amitriptyline and nortriptyline in biologic fluids. These drugs are extracted from alkalinized specimens with *n*-hexane, back-extracted into acidic aqueous solution, and oxidized to anthraquinone by refluxing. The anthraquinone is quantitated by spectrophotometry at 250 nm.

2. gas chromatography (GC) or high-pressure liquid chromatography (HPLC); these methods are

more sensitive and also separate these compounds from each other and from other tricyclic antidepressants.

amitrole a herbicide, 3-amino-1*H*-1,2,4,-triazole, with low acute toxicity. Experimentation using animals has shown that amitrole inhibits peroxidase activity in the liver and thyroid, and that continuous administration produces thyroid tumors.

AML abbrev. See *acute myelogenous l.* under *leukemia.*

AMM abbrev. for agnogenic myeloid metaplasia; see *myeloid metaplasia.*

ammeter (am′me-ter) [*ampere* + *meter*] an instrument for measuring electric current. See also *voltmeter.*

AMML abbrev. for acute monomyelocytic leukemia. See *monomyelocytic l.* under *leukemia.*

ammonemia (ah-mo″ne′me-ah) [*ammonia* + Gr. *haima* blood + *-ia*] the presence of greater than normal concentrations of ammonia or its compounds in the blood.

ammonia (ah-mo′ne-ah) [from Egyptian god *Ammon,* near whose temple in Egypt it was formerly obtained] a colorless gas, NH_3, with a penetrating pungent odor, soluble in water (28 percent at 30°C), alcohol, and ether; M.W. 17.03. In water solution, it forms ammonium hydroxide, NH_4OH, a weak base with a pK_a of 9.25. It is prepared commercially by the catalyzed reaction of nitrogen and hydrogen (the Haber process), and is used mainly for the manufacture of fertilizer and explosives.

In the human body, ammonia is produced primarily by the deamination of glutamine, glutamate, and adenosine monophosphate. It is also produced in the gut from nitrogenous compounds in food by enzymes and intestinal bacteria, and is absorbed by the intestinal mucosa and transported to the liver. Ammonia is highly toxic; normally, the conversion of ammonia to urea by the liver maintains an extremely low plasma ammonia concentration (about 35–85 μg/dl as ammonia nitrogen [NH_3-N] or 25–60 μmol/l as ammonia). In acidosis, ammonia is synthesized by the kidneys from amides and excreted in the urine as NH_4^+ to preserve sodium ions. The average urinary excretion of NH_4^+ in humans is 20–70 mg of ammonia nitrogen (1.5–5.0 mmol)/da.

Blood ammonia determinations are performed to help detect existing or impending hepatic coma, although this test is of limited value in these situations. Plasma ammonia levels are also increased in Reye's syndrome.

ammonia assays 1. titration methods. The specimen is alkalinized and ammonia is distilled into a standard solution of hydrochloric acid or boric acid; the excess acid is measured by back titration in the presence of an appropriate acid-base indicator.

2. microdiffusion using a Conway microdiffusion cell. The ammonia is collected in the center well in standard acid and measured by back titration, as in method 1, or colorimetrically, as per method 4.

3. column chromatography. Ammonia is isolated by capture on a strongly acidic cation exchange resin (such as Dowex 50W-X4 or 50-X12, Na form), followed by elution with sodium chloride and measurement of a blue color after formation of indophenol. In a similar approach, a sulfonated polystyrene cation exchanger, sodium form (Permutit), is used, followed by the addition of sodium phenoxide in the presence of hypochlorite and nitroprusside, which simultaneously elutes the ammonium ion from the column and reacts with ammonia to produce a stable blue color.

4. colorimetric methods. The specimen (or the ammonia isolated from the specimen as in method 1) is treated with Nessler or Berthelot reagent, and the color produced is measured spectrophotometrically. The latter reaction is more sensitive.

5. enzymatic method. Glutamate dehydrogenase (EC 1.4.1.3) catalyzes the reductive amination of oxoglutarate to L-glutamate in the presence of ammonia and NAD(P)H. Ammonia is quantitated by measuring the decrease in absorbance at 340 nm due to consumption of NAD(P)H.

6. selective ion electrode. See *glass e.* under *electrode.*

In measuring plasma ammonia, a key problem is the collection and preservation of the specimen so that the true level of NH_3 (or NH_4^+) is not altered by the ammonia produced by the enzymatic deamination of amides in the sample.

Specimens for ammonia analysis may be preserved for short periods by placing them immediately into ice water: freezing preserves the specimens for several days. Alternately, trichloroacetic or tungstic acid filtrates may be prepared to maintain the original ammonia concentration.

ammoniacal silver nitrate test a colorimetric test for melanogens in urine. A solution of $AgNO_3$ (3 g/100 ml) is added to a urine sample, followed by enough dilute ammonia solution (2 ml of concentrated NH_4OH/100 ml) to almost dissolve the AgCl precipitate. If melanogens are present, the solution slowly darkens owing to the reduction of the ammoniacal silver nitrate by melanogens and the concomitant oxidation of melanogens to a dark pigmented material. The test may serve to distinguish melanogens from homogentisic acid, which, if present, will cause darkening of the solution even before the ammonia is added.

ammoniacal silver solutions solutions formed by adding an alkali or a carbonate to a silver nitrate solution, which produces a precipitate of silver oxide or silver carbonate, to which strong ammonia water is added until the precipitate dissolves because of formation of the diamminesilver ion, $[Ag(NH_3)_2]^+$. These solutions should be prepared just before use, as age or exposure to light, formaldehyde, or alcohol causes the formation of silver nitride (Ag_3N), silver azide (AgN_3), or silver fulminate (CNOAg), compounds that are very sensitive explosives. Explosions may be detonated by the slight shock of pouring the solution down the drain. Adding an excess of chloride inactivates the solution by precipitating the silver.

ammonium (ah-mo′ne-um) 1. the NH_4^+ ion; it forms salts analogous to those of the alkaline metals.

2. the ion formed by protonating an amine, as in dimethylammonium chloride, $(CH_3)_2NH_2^+Cl^-$.

3. a cation in which the positive atom is a nitrogen with four alkyl or aryl groups attached, as in tetramethylammonium chloride, $(CH_3)_4N^+Cl^-$; also called quaternary ammonium compounds.

ammonium oxalate (ah-mo′ne-um ok′sah-lāt) odorless, colorless crystals or white granules, $(NH_4)_2C_2O_4$. Mixed with potassium oxalate, the compound is used as an anticoagulant in blood collection (see also *double oxalate*).

ammonium sulfate a salt, $(NH_4)_2SO_4$, formerly used widely to separate albumins from other proteins, and the major classes of globulins. Albumins are insoluble in highly concentrated or saturated salt solutions. Individual globulins will precipitate in $(NH_4)_2SO_4$ solutions that are 25–75 percent saturated.

ammoniuria (ah-mo″ne-u′re-ah) [*ammonia* + Gr. *ouron* urine + *-ia*] an excess of ammonia in the urine.

amnesia (am-ne′ze-ah) [Gr. *amnēsia* forgetfulness] the loss of memory; the inability to remember past experiences or to retain new ones. Amnesia may be retrograde when all experiences before a certain point (e.g., the trauma that caused the condition) are forgotten, and anterograde if experiences after that point in time cannot be recalled. Amnesia may have many causes, including trauma; infarction (stroke); subarachnoid hemorrhage; seizures; encephalitis and meningitis; cerebral neoplasms; metabolic, nutritional, or toxic disorders, including alcoholism; degenerative disorders; and hysteria.

transient global a., the temporary loss of ability to form long-term memory traces while the ability to perform previously learned tasks remains intact. Complete recovery occurs after a few hours, but amnesia for events that occurred during the episode persists. This disorder may be due to bilateral transient ischemia of the temporal lobes or hippocampus. During an attack, the electroencephalogram may be normal or may show focal slow activity originating from the temporal lobes.

amni/o (am′ne-o) [Gr. *amnion* amnion] a word element used in combining form to denote amnion (the sac in which the embryo develops), e.g., amniocentesis.

amniocentesis (am″nē-o-sen-te′sis) [*amnio-* + Gr. *kentēsis* packing] a diagnostic procedure used to obtain amniotic fluid for examination. It involves insertion of a long needle into the amniotic sac through the abdominal wall for withdrawal of the fluid. Ultrasound is used prior to amniocentesis to visualize the fetus and placenta and to ascertain the number of fetuses present. Amniocentesis is indicated for the antenatal diagnosis of chromosomal abnormalities or inborn errors of metabolism, and is usually performed in the fourteenth week of gestation for these purposes. It is also indicated in the assessment and management of Rh isoimmunization syndrome, to estimate fetal lung maturity and determine the risk of infant respiratory distress syndrome, and to remove excess amniotic fluid in polyhydramnios—it is then usually performed in the third trimester. See also *antenatal diagnosis, lecithin-sphingomyelin ratio,* and *Rh isoimmunization syndrome.*

amniography (am″ne-og′rah-fe) [*amnio-* + Gr. *graphein* to record] radiographic localization of the placenta using a water-soluble iodinated contrast medium injected into the amniotic fluid.

amnion (am′ne-on) [Gr. *amnion*] the innermost of the two fetal membranes. It lines the chorion and encloses the amniotic fluid in which the fetus is suspended.

amnionitis (am″ne-o-ni′tis) [*amnion* + *-itis* inflammation] inflammation of the amniotic membrane of the placenta.

amnioscope (am′ne-o-skōp″) an endoscope that, by passage through the abdominal wall into the amniotic cavity, permits direct visualization of the fetus and amniotic fluid.

amniotic (am″ne-ot′ik) pertaining to the amnion.

amniotic cavity the cavity enclosed within the amnion, in which the embryo develops.

amniotic fluid the fluid (500–1500 ml) that surrounds the fetus in the amniotic sac; it serves to cushion the fetus against injury from blows or sudden movement, as well as to maintain a constant body temperature.

The volume of amniotic fluid increases when the fetus is affected by severe hydrops fetalis, congenital obstruction of the esophagus or upper gastrointestinal tract, anencephaly, or defects of the central nervous system. The volume decreases in the conditions of fetal bilateral renal agenesis, obstruction of the urinary tract, or placental insufficiency, as fetal urine contributes significantly to the volume. Initially the fluid is clear and slightly alkaline; later it becomes cloudy. Excessive cloudiness or discoloration, however, may indicate fetal distress or disease.

In the early stages of gestation, the electrolyte composition of the fluid is similar to that of fetal plasma: hormones, minerals, proteins, enzymes, and lipids are present in varying proportions as gestation progresses. Later, concentrations of sodium and chloride gradually decrease, while urea, creatinine, and uric acid concentrations rise to two to three times those of maternal serum. The concentration of potassium is relatively stable, as are those of calcium, phosphorus, and glucose during the second and third trimesters. Total protein and albumin decrease to one-twentieth of normal serum near term; the concentration of amino acids is slightly lower or the same as that of maternal serum, the globulins may increase slightly, and fibrinogen is absent. The concentration of aspartate aminotransferase is found to double between the second and third trimesters, that of lactate dehydrogenase is usually lower than that in maternal serum, that of alkaline phosphatase increases with the length of the gestation period, and that of bilirubin generally decreases. Other substances present are oxyhemoglobin, nonheme iron, prostaglandins, and the lipids lecithin and sphingomyelin (whose ratio is a measure of fetal lung maturity, as is lecithin alone; see also *lecithin/sphingomyelin ratio*).

Highly elevated levels of lactate dehydrogenase (2–20 times) or the presence of methemalbumin are indicative of present or impending fetal death.

See also *amniocentesis.*

amniotic sac the fluid-filled sac enclosing the fetus.

amobarbital (am″o-bar′bĭ-tal) [USP], a moderately long-acting barbiturate used both as a sedative and to control convulsions. See also *barbiturate.*

A-mode echo see under *echocardiography.*

amodiaquine hydrochloride (am″o-di′ah-kwin) [USP], one of the 4-aminoquinoline group of antimalarial drugs; it kills schizonts infecting red blood cells and when used with the 8-aminoquinoline, primaquine, it is a drug of choice to kill the exoerythrocytic forms of the parasite. It is also used to treat amebiasis, particularly when the liver is infected.

Adverse effects include upset stomach and visual disturbances, whereas overdoses may cause shock and convulsions as well as heart and respiratory failure.

AMonoL abbrev. See *monocytic l.* under *leukemia.*

amorph (ah'morf) [*a-* neg. + Gr. *morphē* form] a mutant gene that has no effect on the phenotype; an inactive allele.

amorphic (a-mor'fik) amorphous.

amorphous (ah-mor'fus) [Gr. *amorphos*] having no definite form; shapeless; noncrystalline; without the lattice structure characteristic of the crystalline solid state.

amount of substance a physical quantity, the number of particles of a specified elementary entity (e.g., atoms of an element, molecules of a compound, or electrons) that are contained in a system. The International System (SI) unit of amount of substance is the mole (mol), which contains the same number of particles as the number of atoms in 1 g of pure carbon-12 (Avogadro's number, 6.02×10^{23}). See also *osmolality.*

amoxapine (ah-mok'sah-pēn) an antidepressant having effects similar to those of the tricyclic antidepressants such as amitriptyline. It is a dibenzoxazepine compound that is chemically related to the antipsychotic agent loxapine. Amoxapine has fewer anticholinergic side-effects than do tricyclic antidepressants, although it can produce extrapyramidal reactions like those produced by the antipsychotics.

amoxicillin (a-moks"ĭ-sil'in) a semisynthetic penicillin similar to ampicillin. It is more readily absorbed from the gastrointestinal tract and suitable for oral use. See also *antibacterial agents* and *penicillins.*

AMP abbrev. See *adenosine monophosphate.*

3',5'-AMP see *cyclic adenosine monophosphate.*

amp abbrev. See *ampere, ampule.*

amperage (am'per-ij) the electric current (measured in amperes) flowing in a circuit.

ampere (A) (am'pēr) [André M. *Ampère,* French physicist, 1775–1836] the International System (SI) unit of electric current, which carries a charge of 1 coulomb (C) through a conductor in 1 second.

ampere-second (A·s) a coulomb (C) of electric charge, the amount that flows in 1 second through a conductor and carries a current of 1 ampere. See also *milliampere-second.*

amperometry (am"pēr-om'ĕ-tre) an analytic technique used in clinical chemistry that involves measuring the current that flows through an electrochemical cell when a constant electric potential is applied to the electrodes. Amperometry using the Clark oxygen electrode may be employed to measure the Po_2 in blood. A modified Clark oxygen electrode in conjunction with an immobilized enzyme can also be used for the determination of other analytes such as glucose, uric acid, and ethanol. Amperometric end-point determination can also be performed in the coulometric titration of Cl^-.

amphetamine (am-fet'ah-min) dl-1-phenyl-2-aminopropane, a colorless, volatile liquid as the free base. Salts take the form of white, odorless, crystalline powders. The drug was first synthesized to replace ephedrine as an antiasthmatic. It was also used as a central nervous system stimulant, which increases blood pressure and reduces appetite. Present clinical use is limited to the treatment of narcolepsy and hyperactivity in children. Abuse leads to increasing tolerance and may result in a psychosis characterized by compulsive behavior, paranoia, hyperactivity, hallucinations, and violent actions. Abstinence results in severe depression, hallucinations, and suicidal tendencies. The action of amphetamine is probably due to an inhibition of uptake of norepinephrine, resulting in an increase of norepinephrine at synapses and increased stimulation. Cf. *dextroamphetamine* and *levamphetamine.*

a. adipate, a soluble salt used for oral administration.

a. sulfate, a soluble salt used for oral administration. Trademark, *Benzedrine.*

amphetamine assays methods for determining the concentration of amphetamines in biologic fluids. Amphetamine and related amines are extracted from urine by organic solvents such as ether or chloroform:isopropanol mixture at a pH above 9. A screening procedure uses thin-layer chromatography with ninhydrin-phenylacetaldehyde spray detection. Quantitative methods use gas-liquid chromatographic separation of these amines or their derivatives (Apiezon L column). Reagents for the detection of amphetamine by EMIT immunoassay or radioimmunoassay techniques are commercially available.

amphi- (am'fī) [Gr. *amphi* around, on both sides] a prefix word element to denote around or about, double, or on both sides, e.g., amphipathic.

amphiarthrosis (am"fe-ar-thro'sis) [*amphi-* + Gr. *arthrōsis* joint] a form of articulation that permits little motion, in which the apposed surfaces of bone are connected by fibrocartilage.

amphibolic (am"fe-bol'ik) [Gr. *amphibolos* doubtful] 1. uncertain.

2. having both an anabolic and catabolic function.

amphibolic pathway a group of metabolic reactions with a dual function, providing small metabolites for further catabolism to end products or for use as precursors in synthetic, anabolic reactions. The tricarboxylic cycle system is an example. See also *anabolism* and *catabolism.*

amphicyte (am'fe-sit) [*amphi-* + Gr. *kytos* hollow vessel] see *satellite cell.*

amphid one of the small sensory organs located in the cephalic or cervical region on the sides of roundworms (nematodes).

Amphimerus (am-fim'er-us) a genus of trematodes (flukes) that is parasitic for mammals. For example, the species *A. noverca* infests the biliary duct of dogs, foxes, and occasionally hogs and humans, and *A. pseudofelineus* infects cats and coyotes. The latter is identical to *Opisthorchis guayaquilensis* in humans.

amphipath (am'fe-path) a molecule showing amphipathic properties; a molecule having both a hydrophobic and a hydrophilic end. Soaps and many synthetic detergents have this property.

amphipathic (am"fe-path'ik) [*amphi-* + Gr. *pathos* feeling] of or relating to molecules containing regions or groups with both hydrophilic, polar properties and hydrophobic, nonpolar properties. Sodium oleate and phosphatidyl choline are two examples. Also called *amphiphilic.*

amphiphile (am"fe-fil') [*amphi-* + Gr. *philos* loving] an amphipathic molecule, i.e., a molecule that possesses both hydrophilic and hydrophobic moieties.

amphiphilic see *amphipathic.*

amphiprotic (am″fe-pro′tik) pertaining to substances capable of acting either as a proton donor when a base (a proton acceptor) is present or as a proton acceptor when an acid (a proton donor) is present. Also called *amphoteric.*

amphitrichous (am-fit′rĕ-kus) [*amphi-* + Gr. *thrix* hair] having polar flagella.

amphixenoses diseases that may occur in humans and other vertebrates.

ampho- (am′fo) [Gr. *amphō* both] a prefix word element to denote both, e.g., amphogenic.

ampholyte (am′fo-lit) [*ampho-* + *electrolyte*] a molecule or substance that can ionize to form either anions or cations, and therefore can be either basic or acidic, e.g., water.

amphophil cell (am′fo-fil) a cell that stains readily with acid or basic dyes.

amphophilic (am″fo-fil′ik) [*ampho-* + Gr. *philein* to love] having an affinity for both acid and basic dyes.

amphoteric (am″fo-ter′ik) [Gr. *amphoteros* pertaining to both] capable of acting either as an acid or as a base; combining with both acids and bases; containing both proton-donating and proton-accepting groups. See also *amphiprotic.*

amphoteric dye a dye in which the colored substance contains both anionic and cationic groups and forms salts with both acidic and basic tissue constituents.

amphotericin B (am″fo-ter′ĭ-sin) [USP], a polyene antibiotic derived from broth cultures of strains of *Streptomyces nodosus.* It occurs as an odorless powder that is yellow to orange in color. Amphotericin B is used parenterally in the treatment of systemic fungal infections and topically for superficial candidiasis. It is the drug of choice in the treatment of amebic meningoencephalitis and protothecosis, and is also an alternative in the treatment of American cutaneous leishmaniases. Kala azar (*Leishmania donovani*) and Oriental sore (*L. tropica*), also leishmaniases, do not respond to this drug.

ampicillin (amp″ĭ-sil′in) [USP], a semisynthetic penicillin that is more active than penicillin G against many gram-negative bacilli; it is less active against gram-positive organisms than is penicillin G. Ampicillin can be given orally. See also *antibacterial agents* and *penicillins.*

amplification (am″plĭ-fĭ-ka′shun) [L. *amplificatio*] 1. the process of making larger.

2. in electronics, the production of an output that has the same waveform as the input but a larger amplitude.

3. in gene cloning, the increase of plasmid DNA relative to bacterial DNA by blocking bacterial DNA replication, e.g., with chloramphenicol.

gene a., the increase in number (relative to the rest of the genome) of those genes needed for specialized functions in certain differentiated cells. Before amplification, these genes may be present in the genome either as one copy or in multiple copies. Amplification is a selective process, occurring only during a portion of the total life cycle and only in certain types of cells.

The best documented experiments demonstrating amplification involve *Xenopus* embryos and the amplification of the genes for 18S and 28S rRNA. Prior to amplification, these genes are present as 500 copies in the haploid genome. In the oocyte the genes are amplified 1000 times: at meiosis, there are 2 million copies of the genes. The amplified DNA is slowly lost during early cleavage. There appears to be a specific regulatory mechanism that increases these genes to accommodate the massive rRNA synthesis of oogenesis.

In insect larvae, a different type of amplification occurs in salivary glands and certain other tissues. Homologous chromosomes undergo multiple rounds of DNA replication during meiosis until each chromosome contains about 1000 parallel molecules. The giant chromosomes are called polytene chromosomes. There is no duplication of the highly repeated sequences but a duplication of the entire genome; this can be considered selective amplification of unique sequence DNA. See also *polytene chromosome.*

Gene amplification appears to be involved in the acquisition of resistance to the drug methotrexate in cultured cells. Cf. *repeated DNA sequences.*

amplification factor in electronic amplifiers, the ratio of output voltage to input voltage, which, for a linear amplifier, is constant regardless of signal size, up to the capacity of the amplifier. Also called *gain.*

amplifier (am′plĭ-fi″er) a device that increases the amplitude of a signal without altering the waveform, particularly an electronic circuit that produces an output having (ideally) the same waveform as the input. Either the voltage, current, or power amplitude can be amplified. The ratio of the output amplitude to the input amplitude is called the (voltage, current, or power) gain or amplification factor. When several amplifier circuits are connected in a cascade, each is usually called an amplifier stage, and the whole circuit is called an amplifier.

audio a., an amplifier with a bandpass of about 20 Hz–20 kHz.

buffer a., an amplifier (generally having a unit gain) used to isolate the input source from the load.

complementary symmetry a., a transistorized amplifier that uses two complementary transistors (one *npn* and one *pnp*) having identical characteristics. The same input is applied to both transistors, which are biased so that they cut off at zero input. Thus, one amplifies the positive half of the signal and the other the negative half.

Darlington a., a two-stage transistor amplifier configuration that consists of two directly connected common-collector stages (the emitter of the first transistor being connected to the base of the second one). This amplifier has a very high input impedance (greater than 1 MΩ) and a low output impedance. The two transistors are usually produced as a single component.

difference a., an amplifier whose output is proportional to the difference of the voltage applied to its two inputs (one inverting and one noninverting). It can be used to subtract analog signals or as a temperature-compensated direct current amplifier.

direct-coupled a., an amplifier that can amplify a direct current signal; it usually has a very wide bandwidth: 0 Hz–100 kHz.

electrometer a., a direct current amplifier with an extremely high input impedance (usually about 10^{16}

Ω) so that it draws a current of less than 10^{-12}A from the source. It is used to amplify the voltage output of signal sources (e.g., the pH glass electrode or the flame ionization or electron capture detectors of a gas chromatograph) that have high output impedance and would be overloaded by an amplifier drawing more current.

linear a., an amplifier that produces an output voltage directly propotional to the input voltage over its functional range.

lock-in a. (LIA), a complex electronic component used to separate signals from noise, which operates on the principle of phase-sensitive detection. The output is proportional to the amplitude of the input and also to the phase angle between the input signal and a reference signal. The input is usually the chopped output of a transducer; the reference signal is a square wave of the same frequency. All noise is filtered out of the input except that at the same frequency as the reference signal and in phase with it. An LIA can extract a clear noise-free signal from noise 50 dB above the signal level.

logarithmic a., an amplifier whose output is the logarithm of the input. This is accomplished using an operational amplifier and a nonlinear device such as a diode or transistor in the feedback loop. Multiplication (or division) of analog signals can be accomplished by conversion to logarithmic signals, summing (or differencing), and converting with an antilog amplifier, which also uses nonlinear feedback.

operational a. (op amp), a versatile amplifier used as a basic component of many types of electronic instruments. It has two inputs (one inverting and one noninverting) and one output, and is generally contained on a single integrated circuit. The ideal operational amplifier has infinite gain, input impedance, and bandwidth, and zero output impedance so that the operating characteristics of the circuit are entirely determined by the feedback loop between the output and the input.

The operational amplifier can be used to construct many different types of circuits depending on the type of feedback employed, such as an inverting or noninverting amplifier. The gain is determined by the ratio of the feedback resistor to the input resistor, a voltage follower (a unity gain buffer amplifier), a differential amplifier, a summing circuit, an integrator, or a differentiator.

Amplifiers of this type are commonly used in instrumentation that requires calibration based on a blank value and a single standard value. The zero value is adjusted using a bias voltage as input to a summing amplifier, and the slope of the output is adjusted by changing the gain of the amplifier. These adjustments are made by the operator, using controls labeled variously as zero or blank and gain or scale.

See also *analog computer* and *differentiator.*

power a., an amplifier or amplifier stage that has a high power gain but usually no voltage gain, which is used to supply sufficient power to the load and to match the impedance of the load.

push-pull a., an amplifier that uses two identical vacuum tubes or transistor amplifiers operating 180° out of phase. The input is split by a transformer with a grounded center tap in the secondary winding; the positive part of the input is amplified by one tube and the negative part by the other. The outputs are combined by another transformer. The circuit delivers four times the power of an amplifier that uses a single tube.

amplitude (am′plĕ-tūd) [L. amplitudo] 1. largeness or fullness; width or breadth of range or extent.

2. the maximal deviation of a time-varying quantity from its average or baseline value. In the electromyographic recording of an action potential, the difference in voltage between the baseline and peak voltage (the most negative peak in the case of compound muscle action potentials), or between the most positive and the most negative peak (peak-to-peak amplitude); usually measured in microvolts.

ampule (am′pūl) [Fr. *ampoule,* from L. *ampulla* bottle] a small, sealed glass container used to preserve a sterile, measured quantity of a compound or solution; it is often employed for injectable, parenteral solutions and drugs or prepackaged test reagents.

ampulla (am-pul′lah), pl. *ampullae* [L. "a bottle"] a general anatomic term for a dilation of a tubular structure such as a canal or duct.

membranaceous a., the dilated ends of the three semicircular ducts that open into the utricle of the membranous labyrinth of the inner ear. See also *semicircular ducts.*

osseous a., the recesses at the ends of the semicircular canals, in the petrous portion of the temporal bone, which house the correspondingly formed ampullae of the semicircular ducts.

a. of Vater, a small papilla on the posteromedial wall of the second part of the duodenum, on which the common bile duct and the main pancreatic duct open by a common orifice.

amputation (am″pu-ta′shun) [L. *amputare* to cut off, or to prune] the removal of a limb or other appendage or outgrowth of the body.

amputation neuroma see *amputation n.* under *neuroma.*

AMS abbrev. for *amylase.*

amsacrine (am′sah-krēn) a cancer chemotherapeutic drug. For more information, see *Appendix A.*

AMT abbrev. See *American Medical Technologists.*

amu see *atomic mass unit.*

amyctic (ah-mik′tik) [Gr. *amyktikos*] caustic or irritating.

amyelia (a″mi-e′le-ah) [*a-* neg. + Gr. *myelos* marrow + *-ia*] the congenital absence of the spinal cord.

amygdala (ah-mig′dah-lah) [Gr. *amygdalē* almond] the subcortical, almond-shaped complex of nuclei, anatomically one of the basal ganglia, that is located in the dorsomedial temporal pole of the cerebrum. As a functional part of the limbic system, the amygdala receives impulses from the hypothalamic and thalamic nuclei, brain stem reticular formation, olfactory bulb, cingulate gyrus, hippocampus, and limbic cortex; major outflow back to these same (and additional) areas is via the stria terminalis. Also called amygdaloid nucleus. See also *limbic system.*

amygdalase (ah-mig′dah-lās) see *β-D-glucosidase.*

amyl/o (am′ĭ-lo) [Gr. *amylon* starch] a word element used in combining form to denote starch, e.g., amylase.

amyl (am′il) [Gr. *amylon* starch] in trivial chemical names, a five-carbon substituent group, generally used with a symbol to identify the kind of branching in the substituent (e.g., *n*-amyl, *iso*-amyl).

a. nitrite, [USP], a flammable, clear, yellowish liquid with a fruity odor, used as a coronary vasodilator in the treatment of angina pectoris.

amylase (am'ĭ-lās) [*amyl-* + *-ase*] a generic name for the group of enzymes of the hydrolase class that catalyze the hydrolysis of poly-D-glucans, such as starch and glycogen, into smaller molecules. Both straight-chain and branched-chain polyglucans are hydrolyzed, the point of attack being the α-1,4-glycosidic links between the D-glucose residues. Maltose and residual glucose are the products of the hydrolysis of straight-chain polyglucans; with branched-chain starches, limit dextrins are also produced.

Two types of amylases are recognized. The α-amylases (AMS) or endo-amylases (1,4-glucan 4-glycanohydrolase, EC 3.2.1.1), which attack the glucoside bonds anywhere along the polyglucan chain, are found in animals and include the human salivary and pancreatic amylases. The β-amylases (EC 3.2.1.2), or exo-amylases, are found in plants and bacteria and can only split the terminal two glucose residues (maltose) from the reducing end of the polyglucan.

As a result of the action of amylase, products with considerably increased reducing capacity accumulate; the breakdown of the starch macromolecule results in the formation of smaller fragments, dextrins, with measurable decrease in the turbidity and viscosity of the starch solution, as well as loss of ability to form the characteristic blue-colored complex with molecular iodine (the dextrin-iodine color is purple or pink).

Human amylase, present in serum as well as pancreatic and salivary gland fluids, is a metalloenzyme with an absolute requirement for calcium ions. Optimal activity is obtained only in the presence of a variety of inorganic anions, the most effective being Cl^- at 0.01 mol/l. The pH optimum, using the traditional starch substrates, is 6.9–7.0. The human serum enzyme is filterable through the glomerulus and is found in urine. Some six or seven isoenzymes of human amylase are recognized; at least three forms originate from the pancreas and three from the salivary glands. The existence of macroamylases is well established. These are not filterable through the glomerulus, and appear to be complexes formed between the ordinary amylase molecule and immune globulins (IgG, IgA) or glycoproteins. Their presence in serum is not associated with any clinical symptoms, although serum amylase levels may be six to eight times normal.

Clinically, amylase assays are most useful in the detection of pancreatitis. Reference values for amylase in serum have a range of 60–180 Somogyi units or 65–290 U/l. In acute pancreatitis, values usually have a range of 550 to over 2000 Somogyi units, peaking at 24–30 hr and then dropping to normal within 2–3 da. Values above 1000 units are frequently associated with obstruction. At the same time, the urine amylase activity increases but the elevation persists longer (4–7 da). Normal urine amylase activity has a range of 1000 to 5000 or 6000 Somogyi units/da or 45–275 units/hr. Reference values for newer methods are expressed in International Units per liter (IU/l) and are consistently lower, depending on the method involved.

amylase assays 1. saccharogenic methods. The classic method for amylase activity measurements has been the saccharogenic method of Somogyi. In this procedure, starch, amylase, amylopectin, or glycogen is hydrolyzed by amylase with the production mainly of glucose and maltose but also of other reducing fragments of starch. The reaction rate is measured by determining the quantity of the reducing materials formed during a fixed incubation period. The units are expressed as milligrams of reducing substances measured as glucose per 100-ml specimen. The method is cumbersome and time-consuming, and is rarely used today.

2. dye-labeled starch methods. Amylose or amylopectin linked covalently by a triazine bridge to a red or blue dye serves as the substrate. The reaction rate is measured by determining colorimetrically the amount of dye released in a fixed time period. Results are reported in arbitrary dye units.

3. coupled enzyme methods. In the first example of such a procedure, α-glucosidase is added to convert maltose and maltotriose to glucose, which is then measured by either the glucose oxidase/peroxidase or hexokinase/glucose-6-phosphate dehydrogenase (G-6-PD) methods. The total glucose formed is a measure of amylase activity. Results may be reported in International Units. In a second such method, tetramaltose is used as a substrate that is hydrolyzed by amylase to two molecules of maltose. The maltose is then reacted with maltose phosphorylase to produce glucose-1-phosphate, which is then converted to glucose-6-phosphate (G-6-P) by phosphoglucomutase. The G-6-P is quantitated by the G-6-PD reaction. The activity measured with this method may also be reported in International Units. The latest enzyme-coupled amylase method employs *p*-nitrophenol glycosides of varying chain length, predominantly *p*-nitrophenol hexaglucosides and heptaglucosides. This substrate is hydrolyzed by amylase to shorter chain *p*-nitrophenol glycosides, which are then hydrolyzed by α-glucosidase to free *p*-nitrophenol; the latter can be measured photometrically.

4. miscellaneous methods. Older methods took advantage of the blue color that was produced between amylase and iodine. For example, in the amyloclastic method, the decrease in the quantity of starch was measured by a decrease in the blue starch-iodine color during a fixed incubation period, and in the chronometric method, the time required to completely hydrolyze a fixed quantity of starch was used as a measure of amylase activity. Both types of methods have been discontinued in the United States today.

amylasuria (am"ĭ-lās-u're-ah) [*amylase* + Gr. *ouron* urine + *-ia*] an excess of amylase in the urine, observed in pancreatitis.

Amylochrome trademark for a dye-labeled starch that is designed to serve as an amylase substrate for use in colorimetric assays of the enzyme activity. It consists of amylose bonded to Cibachron Blue F3GA. The dye is bonded to every second or third D-glucose residue at carbon 2. In the test procedure, a suspension of the water-insoluble substrate is incubated with the sample. The color of the water-soluble fragments, which are split off by action of the enzyme, can be measured photometrically after removal of the unreacted substrate by filtration or centrifugation.

amylo-1,6-glucosidase an enzyme (dextrin 6-α-D-glucosidase, EC 3.2.1.33) found in muscle and liver that hydrolyzes the 1,6-glycoside bonds in various polysaccharides such as starch and glycogen. This enzyme allows complete digestion of glucans after the reaction of α- or β-amylases. The enzyme has no clinical applications. Its genetic absence is found in Type III glycogen storage disease (Forbes' limit dextrinosis). Also commonly called *debranching enzyme.*

amyloid (am'i-loid) [*amylo-* + Gr. *eidos* form] 1. resembling starch; characterized by starchlike staining properties.

2. a substance produced by the action of sulfuric acid on cellulose, which gives a blue color when treated with iodine.

3. an abnormal extracellular protein complex deposited in a variety of tissues (e.g., kidney, spleen, liver, adrenal glands), especially in and about blood vessels, characterizing several disease states (amyloid disease). Amyloid is a hyalinlike material appearing grossly translucent and structureless, which stains with iodine and a variety of metachromatic dyes such as methyl violet, gentian violet, and methyl green. Tissue slices containing amyloid deposits stain mahogany-brown with iodine; the color changes to blue on acidification with 1 percent sulfuric acid. The affinity of amyloid substances for Congo Red is the basis of a (now obsolete) clinical test for amyloid disease (Congo Red test); intravenously injected dye is removed from plasma by amyloid-containing tissue. Amyloid is insoluble in water and acid, but soluble in strong alkali. Its chemical nature has not been established; in many cases, it appears to be composed of small fibrils, constituted of immunoglobulin fragments (aminoterminal variable portions of the kappa and lambda light chains) associated with sulfated glycoproteins. The source may be abnormally functioning plasma cells. However, amyloid deposits occur that are composed of other types of proteins.

amyloidosis (am"ĭ-loi-do'sis) the disease group characterized by the accumulation of amyloid, a homogeneous eosinophilic material, in various body tissues, divided (mainly for descriptive purposes) into the following categories: (1) primary, (2) secondary, (3) familial, (4) associated with multiple myeloma, and (5) associated with familial Mediterranean fever. Amyloidosis occurs most frequently in association with chronic infections such as syphilis or leprosy; in such cases, it is called secondary. When no other disease is present, it is called primary amyloidosis.

amyloid staining 1. Congo red method. Paraffin sections fixed in formalin or alcohol are stained with an alkaline alcoholic Congo red solution and differentiated in alkaline alcohol. Amyloid stains pink to red and exhibits a green birefringence (dichroism) using polarized light.

2. fluorescent stain. Paraffin sections are stained first in alum hematoxylin, which quenches nuclear fluorescence, and then in thioflavine T. They are then differentiated in acetic acid. Using a UG5 exciter filter and a colorless ultraviolet barrier filter in the fluorescence microscope, amyloid appears clear yellow on a blue background. No other tissue components stain yellow except mast cell granules.

3. electron microscopy. Amyloid appears as aggregates of randomly arranged filaments 7.5 nm in diameter having a 10-nm periodicity.

amylopectin (am"ĭ-lo-pek'tin) a D-glucosan polysaccharide found, along with amylose, in varying proportions in nearly all starches. It is a branched polymeric molecule that contains both α-1,4-links and α-1,6-glycosidic bonds, and which gives a red-to-violet color with iodine. Potato, wheat, and ordinary corn starch contain about 80 percent amylopectin and 20 percent amylose. It has also been called *α-amylose.*

amylopectinosis (am"i-lo-pek"tĭ-no'sis) see *brancher deficiency.*

amylorrhea (am"ĭ-lo-re'ah) [*amylo-* + Gr. *rhoia* flow] the presence of an abnormal amount of starch in the stool.

amylose (am'ĭ-lōs) a glucosan polysaccharide found, along with amylopectin, in varying proportions in almost all starches. Amylose is a linear polymer that gives a deep blue color with iodine. It contains α-1,4-linkages between glucose units and a terminal hemiacetal (free aldehyde) group. Wheat, potato, and normal corn starch contain about 20 percent amylose and 80 percent amylopectin. Also called *β-amylose.*

α-amylose see *amylopectin.*

β-amylose see *amylose.*

amyotonia (a"mi-o-to'ne-ah) [*a-* neg. + Gr. *mys* muscle + *tonos* tension + *-ia*] a term used to describe weakness and hypotonia in infants, more recently recognized as a symptom complex rather than a single diagnostic entity.

amyotrophic lateral sclerosis see *amyotrophic lateral s.* under *sclerosis.*

amyotrophy (ah"mi-ot'ro-fe) [*a-* neg. + Gr. *mys* muscle + *trophē* nourishment] a painful wasting, weakening, and atrophy of muscle tissue, most often affecting the deltoid muscle.

diabetic a., weakness and wasting of the thigh and pelvic girdle muscles, usually on the basis of a neurogenic lesion. It is sometimes accompanied by pain and sensory loss, and is associated with diabetes mellitus.

neuralgic a., a condition characterized by pain, weakness, and sensory loss in the shoulder, arm, and hand. The onset is usually acute; the etiology appears to be an inflammatory lesion in the brachial plexus. Electromyography and myelography may aid in diagnosis, especially to exclude a spinal cord or nerve root lesion. The prognosis for recovery is good. Also called brachial neuritis, brachial plexus neuropathy, and Parsonage-Turner syndrome.

an- (an) [Gr.; before consonants, *a-*] a prefix word element to denote no, not, or without, e.g., anesthesia.

See also *a-*.

an/o (a'no) [L. *anus* anus] a word element used in combining form to denote anus, e.g., anorectal.

ANA abbrev. See *antinuclear antibody.*

ana- (an'ah) [Gr. *ana* up, back, again] a prefix word element to denote up, again, backward, or excessive, e.g., anabolism.

anabolic (an"ah-bol'ik) [Gr. *anabolikos*] pertaining to anabolism.

anabolic steroids steroid hormones that act to enhance the buildup of tissue mass by increasing anabolic pathways. Androgens, particularly testosterone, are considered the most potent anabolic steroids.

anabolism (ah-nab'o-lizm") [Gr. *anabolē* something built up] any constructive process by which

ANAEROBE, TABLE 1. INCIDENCE OF VARIOUS ANAEROBES AS NORMAL FLORA IN HUMANS

		NONSPORE-FORMING BACILLI								COCCI	
		Gram-positive					*Gram-negative*			
	CLOSTRIDIUM	*Actinomyces*	*Bifidobacterium*	*Eubacterium*	*Lactobacillus*†	*Propionibacterium*	*Bacteroides*	*Fusobacterium*	*Gram-positive*	*Gram-negative*
Skin	0	0	0	±	0	2	0	0	1	0
Upper respiratory tract*	0	1	0	±	0	1	1	1	1	1
Mouth	±	1	1	1	1	±	2	2	2	2
Intestine	2	±	2	2	1	±	2	1	2	1
External genitalia	0	0	0	U	0	U	1	1	1	0
Urethra	±	0	0	U	±	0	1	1	±	U
Vagina	±	0	1	±	2	1	1	±	1	1

* Includes nasal passages, nasopharynx, oropharynx, and tonsils.
† Includes anaerobic, microaerophilic, and facultative strains.
U, Unknown; 0, not found or rare; ±, irregular; 1, usually present; 2, usually present in large numbers.
From Sutter, V. L., et al.: Wadsworth Anaerobic Bacteriology Manual. 3rd ed. St. Louis, C. V. Mosby Co., 1980, p. 5.

simple substances are converted by living cells into more complex compounds. Cf. *catabolism.*

anabolite (ah-nab′o-līt″) any product of anabolism or an intermediate in an anabolic process.

anacidity (an″ah-sid′ĭ-te) [*an-* neg. + *acidity*] the absence of hydrochloric acid in the gastric secretion, defined as the failure of the pH to fall below 7.0 (or 6.0) after stimulation with histamine, betazole, or pentagastrin. When pH 6.0 is used as the criterion, virtually every adult with pernicious anemia will exhibit anacidity. See also *achlorhydria* and *gastric function tests.*

anacrotism (ah-nak′rŏ-tizm) [*ana-* + Gr. *krotos* beat + *-ism*] a pulse anomaly evidenced by the presence of one or more notches on the ascending limb of the pulse tracing.

anaerobe (an-a′er-ōb) [*an-* neg. + Gr. *aēr* air + *bios* life] a microorganism that can multiply only in the absence of oxygen (O_2); most often, the term refers to anaerobic bacteria. Anaerobes play a major role in maintaining the biologic cycles of nature, and the number of species so involved is enormous. Comparatively few of them, however, are significant factors in human ecology, yet these species constitute a large part of the normal microbiota of mucous membranes and of skin (Table 1). Indeed, anaerobic bacteria are very numerous in the colon, where they constitute 99.9 percent of the microbial population. The mouth and vagina also harbor a constant anaerobic flora.

Generally, anaerobes growing on healthy mucous membrane surfaces act as harmless commensals and injure tissue only under conditions involving the reduction of host resistance or tissue integrity. Thus, anaerobes are classic opportunistic pathogens (Table 2). Systemic factors such as malignancy, immunologic deficiency states, immunosuppressive therapy, and some types of antibiotic therapy may favor sufficient multiplication of anaerobes to result in clinical infection. More often, the predisposing factor is trauma, surgical or accidental, which removes the natural barrier and allows access to deep tissues. Such an event introduces large numbers of these bacteria into previously sterile areas that provide the low O_2 tension and rich pabulum conducive to their rapid multiplication.

The origin of some anaerobic infections, however, is not from the host's own flora but is external. The etiologic agents in this instance are for the most part spore-forming species, the clostridia, whose habitat is soil, plants, and the marine environment. One such disease is botulism, a food poisoning due to ingestion of *Clostridium botulinum* toxin. Two important clostridial infections are gas gangrene and tetanus (lockjaw), which result from the entrance of spores in deep tissues at the time of traumatic injury. The first of these is often a fulminating myonecrosis and toxemia caused by a mixture of anaerobic species, predominantly *C. perfringens,* whereas tetanus is primarily a neurotoxic disease caused by *C. tetani.*

ANAEROBIOSIS. Anaerobic species vary widely in their susceptibility to the inhibitory and lethal effects of oxygen. Some are obligate anaerobes, meaning they are able to grow only at very low oxidation-reduction potentials, and brief exposure to oxygen may be lethal. Others are moderately anaerobic, as is *C. perfringens.* Some are called microaerophilic because the best growth occurs at a zone of moderately high O_2 tension, although full exposure to oxygen is inhibitory. Finally, there are aerotolerant species that produce colonies, although small, on the surface of aerobically incubated agar plates.

The toxicity of oxygen for anaerobes is due to the absence of the cytochromes needed for electron transport to O_2. Instead, they have flavoprotein enzymes that reduce O_2 to hydrogen peroxide and superoxide, but most strains do not produce the catalase, peroxidases, and superoxide dismutase needed to break down these toxic products. Consequently, oxygen is inhibitory or lethal.

CLINICAL SPECIMENS. Successful recovery of obligately anaerobic bacteria from clinical material requires special methods, some developed only in recent years. Specimens should be collected in "gassed-out" (O_2-free) tubes, inoculated to prere-

ANAEROBE, TABLE 2. INCIDENCE OF SPECIFIC ANAEROBES IN VARIOUS INFECTIONS (WADSWORTH MEDICAL CENTER EXPERIENCE 1973–1978)

SPECIMEN SOURCE OR TYPE OF INFECTION		B. FRAGILIS	B. THETAIOTAOMICRON	OTHER BILE-RESISTANT† BACTEROIDES	B. MELANINOGENICUS SS. MELANINOGENICUS	B. MELANINOGENICUS SS. INTERMEDIUS	B. MELANINOGENICUS, NO SUBSPECIES	B. ASACCHAROLYTICUS	BILE-SENSITIVE‡ SACCHAROLYTIC BACTEROIDES	B. UREOLYTICUS	OTHER BACTEROIDES SP. §
Blood	(58)	48	10	9	2	0	0	0	7	0	7
Central nervous system	(6)	0	0	0	0	17	0	0	0	0	17
Wound infections following head and neck surgery	(49)	0	0	0	45	53	14	4	82	4	49
Dental	(8)	0	0	0	13	13	0	0	25	0	13
Human bites	(18)	0	0	0	28	50	0	0	44	6	22
Animal bites	(16)	0	0	0	0	13	0	13	6	0	13
TTA and pleural fluid	(143)	4	1	3	20	31	4	3	47	9	36
Miscellaneous soft tissue infections above the waist	(41)	5	0	0	0	22	5	10	34	10	70
Intra-abdominal infections	(114)	54	32	33	8	12	4	9	17	5	29
Perirectal abscess	(15)	73	53	33	13	0	0	13	20	7	27
Decubitus ulcers	(16)	56	25	31	0	19	25	13	25	0	31
Foot ulcers	(70)	39	11	10	6	13	6	13	19	7	19
Miscellaneous soft tissue infections below the waist	(37)	24	8	10	3	11	0	5	14	3	14
Osteomyelitis	(32)	6	6	0	6	3	13	3	13	13	31

Note: Numbers in parentheses indicate number of specimens surveyed. Other numbers in this table represent numbers of isolates per 100 specimens containing anaerobes. TTA indicates transtracheal aspirates.
† *B. distasonis, B. vulgatus, B. ovatus, B. uniformis, B. splanchnicus, B. eggerthii.*
‡ *B. ruminicola* ss. *brevis, B. ruminicola* ss. *ruminicola, B. oralis, B. bivius, B. disiens.*
§ Includes nonspeciable *Bacteroides* sp. Includes nonspeciable *Fusobacterium* sp.
From Sutter, V. L., et al.: Wadsworth Anaerobic Bacteriology Manual. 3rd ed. St. Louis, C. V. Mosby Co., 1980, p. 8.

duced culture media and, of course, incubated anaerobically. A convenient anaerobic environment is provided by placing the culture tubes and plates in a jar in which is placed a packet that contains an H_2-CO_2 generator. Laboratories handling large numbers of anaerobic cultures employ a plastic glove box or chamber filled with an O_2-free gas mixture.

An infectious process is to be suspected clinically of being anaerobic in nature when it meets the following criteria: (1) the infected area is a mucous membrane or adjacent to it; (2) a foul odor is present; (3) there is traumatic injury or known immunologic deficiency; (4) immunosuppressive drugs are being used; (5) there has been previous administration of an aminoglycoside antibiotic; and (6) enterocolitis is present that could be due to oral antibiotic therapy.

The frequency with which various types of anaerobes are cultured from suspected anaerobic infections is quite uniform throughout the United States. Nonsporulating gram-negative bacilli predominate, about half belonging to the *Bacteroides fragilis* group. Members of the *B. melaninogenicus–B. asaccharolyticus* group are also frequent and important isolates.

Among the gram-positive nonsporulating species, two predominate: *Propionibacterium acnes* and *Eubacterium lentum. Clostridium* species are not often recovered from endogenous infections in sufficient numbers or in circumstances that suggest an etiologic role. However, the exogenous clostridial diseases mentioned earlier are notorious, despite their relatively uncommon occurrence, because of their severity and life-threatening nature. Thus, they continue to require continuous control measures and surveillance. In recent years, toxigenic strains of *C. difficile*, a normal bowel inhabitant, have been idenitifed as responsible for many cases of pseudomembranous colitis following administration of certain antibiotics.

Anaerobic cocci account for 25–30 percent of the anaerobes recovered from clinical specimens. They are primarily species of *Peptococcus or Peptostrep-*

tococcus, the former being about twice as frequent as the latter.

IDENTIFICATION. Most of the commonly encountered anaerobes in clinical specimens can be identified presumptively, and adequately for therapeutic guidance, by means of the following rapid and relatively simple methods: (1) observation of O_2 susceptibility (obligately anaerobic, moderately anaerobic, microaerophilic or aerotolerant); (2) microscopic appearance; (3) cultural characteristics; (4) a few biochemical tests; and (5) antibiotic susceptibility patterns. Frequently, the results of two or three of these methods, plus evaluation of species significance, are sufficient for the purpose of clinical management. Definitive species identification, however, can become quite involved; for this, analysis of metabolic products by gas-liquid chromatography is becoming increasingly helpful.

ANTIBIOTIC THERAPY. Many anaerobic infections respond adequately to penicillin G. However the *B. fragilis* group is largely resistant, and so are some strains of *C. perfringens*, *C. ramosum*, and *C. innocuum*, all of which are important pathogens. Clindamycin is very effective against many anaerobic species, although some strains of *C. perfringens* and *B. fragilis* are resistant. Chloramphenicol is broadly inhibitory for anaerobes in vitro but is not generally employed clinically because of the toxic side-reactions. Vancomycin is useful in the treatment of *C. difficile* enterocolitis.

Although many species have predictable susceptibility patterns, antibiotic susceptibility testing is an important adjunct of anaerobic clinical microbiology. The methods used for anaerobes are based on the standard procedures of aerobic testing but modified to fulfill their special nutritional and environmental requirements. The value of susceptibility results is reduced somewhat by the fact that most anaerobic infections are polymicrobial. Metronidazole, a synthetic amebacide and trichomonacide, is highly inhibitory for *Bacteroides* and *Fusobacterium*, and its clinical use appears to be increasing.

facultative a., an organism that can grow well under both aerobic and anaerobic conditions.

obligate a., an organism that cannot grow in the presence of molecular oxygen and that requires a low oxidation-reduction potential (E_h).

anaerobic (an″a-er-o′bik) 1. lacking molecular oxygen.

2. growing in the absence of molecular oxygen.

anaerobic bacteria culture bacteriologic culturing for anaerobes. Close attention to basic principles and methods is necessary for the successful recovery and identification of pathogenic anaerobes. This includes the sites and techniques for specimen collection, transportation of the specimens to the laboratory, primary culturing followed by secondary tests for recovery and identification, and interpretation of this information.

Specimens should be obtained for identification of anaerobic infection if any of the following indications are present: (1) wound or abscess pus, which may produce a foul or fetid odor; (2) an infection close to or within a mucous membrane; (3) necrotic tissue; (4) inflammation of a normally sterile area; and (5) human or animal bite. Owing to the presence of a normal flora of anaerobic bacteria, certain areas of the body are not appropriate for anaerobic specimen collection, e.g., the nose, throat, skin, feces, mucous membranes, vagina, urethra, and rectum.

When an anaerobic infection is suspected, a specimen should be obtained in a manner that avoids contamination with normal flora, molecular oxygen, and other high redox potential (E_h) contaminants; extremes in pH; dryness; and low temperatures. Recovery of aspirate or fluid by syringe is the optimal procedure. Abscess drainage or pus in a sealed syringe can be transported well to the laboratory. Tissue and blood are also good specimens for anaerobic bacteriology. The least desirable specimen is a swab.

Rapid transport of specimen from patient to laboratory for primary culturing is critical. For transportation, "gassed out" (prereduced) tubes, which are sterilized glass test tubes with a rubber stopper and a screw cap, are ideal. Some tubes contain a small amount of anaerobic brain heart infusion broth to protect anaerobic bacteria from harmful environmental effects.

In the anaerobic bacteriology laboratory, the objective is to grow all anaerobic bacteria that may be present in the specimen in contrast to the facultative or microaerophilic microorganisms that may also be present. First, a Gram stain of the specimen is prepared to observe the different morphologic types. This initial information will be compared with the culture results 48 hr later; however, the Gram reaction does not indicate whether a microorganism is anaerobic, facultatively aerobic, or microaerophilic. Primary culturing should include: (1) an enriched brain heart infusion broth; (2) two enriched brain heart infusion blood agar plates, one incubated aerobically and one incubated anaerobically; and (3) a laked blood agar plate. Anaerobic media should be stored anaerobically and inoculation performed anaerobically; an anaerobic chamber (glove box) is useful for these procedures. After 48 hr of incubation at 37°C in a jar or chamber, the cultures are examined for growth of anaerobic bacteria. Comparing the growth on aerobic and anaerobic plates will indicate whether a particular type of organism is anaerobic or facultative.

If an anaerobic bacterium is present, secondary culturing is used to identify the microorganism after its aerotolerance is checked by growing the bacterium both aerobically with 10 percent CO_2 and anaerobically. The tests used for identification include the utilization of certain sugars, growth on bile medium, casein digestion, catalase activity, lipase and lecithinase production on egg yolk agar, esculin hydrolysis, gelatin digestion, indole production, nitrate reduction, and starch hydrolysis. Gas-liquid chromatography may also be used to identify volatile fatty acids and alcohols produced during incubation in brain heart infusion–glucose broth.

See also *anaerobe* and *Gram stain*.

anaerobic chamber an apparatus with a controlled environment that supplies a suitable working area for the cultivation, transfer, and storage of anaerobic bacteria, anaerobic media, and associated equipment. This chamber may be a flexible plastic bag with a support frame, or a rigid cabinet. Gloves and sleeves sealed into the walls of the chamber allow external manipulation of the chamber's contents. Entrance and exit from the chamber is accomplished through use of a double door portal system in which the area between the doors may be atmospherically evacuated and subsequently filled with the desired anaerobic gases (similar to the control of water during entrance to and exit from a subaquatic submarine). Inside the anaerobic chamber there is usually a 37°C incubator for the growth of anaerobic cultures, an enclosed heated block for loop sterilization (an open flame cannot be used because of explosive gases that may be present), and various media and equipment necessary for working with anaerobic bacteria.

Anaerobiosis is maintained in a similar manner to the GasPak anaerobic jar system, in that palladium catalyzes the reaction $2H_2 + O_2 \rightarrow H_2O$. The anaerobic chamber is initially filled with 80 percent nitrogen, 10 percent hydrogen, and 10 percent carbon dioxide. The hydrogen aids in the removal of molecular oxygen, the carbon dioxide assists microbial growth, and the nitrogen provides the basis for an inert reduced anaerobic environment. Owing to the production of water by this reaction, silica gel desiccant is added and periodically regenerated with heat to control the humidity inside the chamber. Anaerobiosis is monitored with various redox dyes such as methylene blue (redox potential, +11 mV) and resazurin (redox potential, –42 mV). The anaerobic environment is circulated with fans to maintain homogeneity.

See also *anaerobic bacteria culture*. Cf. *anaerobic jar*.

anaerobic jar a tightly sealed environmental chamber that can maintain an anaerobic (oxygen-free) atmosphere, used for the incubation and storage of anaerobic bacterial cultures. The jar has a removable lid for the addition or removal of culture media, usually in the form of agar Petri dishes. There are two general procedures for generating an anaerobic atmosphere. One method involves removing oxygenated air from the jar through a vacuum and replacing the air with anaerobic gases; common types of jars used in this method include Brewer and Torbal jars. The other method utilizes a hydrogen-generating package combined with a catalyst to remove molecular oxygen; this is the GasPak jar system and is the most commonly used anaerobic jar.

The Brewer jar used in the first method utilizes plasticine to seal the lid to the jar. Oxygenated air is vacuumed out, anaerobic gases (80 percent N_2, 10 percent H_2, and 10 percent CO_2) are added, and a catalyst is heated electrically to remove any additional molecular oxygen. The Torbal jar is similar to the Brewer jar except that a rubber O ring is used to seal the lid to the jar and no heat is needed for the catalyst.

In the second method, the lid of the GasPak is sealed to the jar with a rubber O ring; a hydrogen-generating package inside the jar is activated with the addition of water. The package contains magnesium and zinc chloride pellets, which produce the following reaction: $Mg + ZnCl_2 + 2H_2O \xrightarrow{NaCl} MgCl_2 + Zn(OH)_2 + H_2\uparrow$. As hydrogen gas is generated, it combines with oxygen to form water. Catalyzing this reaction are palladium-coated alumina pellets attached to the bottom of the lid, which cause the following reaction: $2H_2 + O_2 \xrightarrow{palladium} H_2O$. While molecular oxygen is converted to water, the atmosphere becomes anaerobic. A methylene blue indicator strip is generally used to detect anaerobiosis. When methylene blue becomes colorless, there is a redox potential of less than 11 mV. Often an absorbent paper is added to the jar to remove some of the excess moisture.

See also *anaerobic bacteria culture*. Cf. *anaerobic chamber*.

anaerobiosis (an-a″er-o-bi-o′sis) [*an-* neg. + Gr. *aēr* air + *biōsis* way of life] 1. life in the absence of molecular oxygen.

2. the establishment of a strictly anaerobic environment, as for the cultivation of obligately anaerobic bacteria.

anaerogenic (an-a″er-o-jen′ik) [*an-* neg. + Gr. *aēr* air + *gennan* to produce] producing little or no gas. In bacteriology, the term is used to refer to an organism that does not produce gas from the breakdown of carbohydrate.

anal (a′nal) [L. *analis*] pertaining to the anus.

analbuminemia (an″al-bu″mĭ-ne′me-ah) [*an-* neg. + *albumin* + Gr. *haima* blood + *-ia*] a state or condition characterized by very low concentrations or the absence of albumin in the blood (plasma). It is seen only rarely and is associated with edema and increased concentrations of serum lipids, normally transported by albumin. The condition reflects an inborn impairment in the synthesis of this protein.

anal canal the short passage, less than 2 in. long, that connects the rectum with the exterior; its orifice is the anus. The anal canal is surrounded by thickened, circular smooth muscle and, outside this, by skeletal muscle, to form an efficient sphincter mechanism. The canal lies in front of the sacrum and coccyx, behind the bulb of the penis in the male and the lower vagina in the female. The lower half of the anal canal is lined by epidermis continuous with that of the surrounding skin. Longitudinal folds of mucosa in the upper half constitute the anal columns. A segment of transitional epithelium at the anorectal junction is probably of cloacal derivation, and a number of branching anal glands open through it. See also *gastrointestinal tract*.

anal columns vertical folds (numbering 6–10) in the mucous membrane of the anal canal, which contain terminal branches of the superior rectal vessels.

analeptic (an″ah-lep′tik) [Gr. *analēpsis* a repairing] originally, any drug that acted to restore most body functions depressed by disease or poisoning; the term is now employed for any of a group of central nervous system stimulants (e.g., pentylenetetrazol or picrotoxin) formerly used to antagonize respiratory or circulatory depression arising from an overdose of a depressant or general anesthetic. In large doses analeptics produce convulsions, and they are often used experimentally for this purpose.

anal fissure a superficial ulcerated laceration of the anal canal, which usually occurs in the posterior midline. It causes pain on defecation and spasm of the external anal sphincter. The condition may be associated with chronic diarrhea and nervous tightening of the anus. Symptoms include pain and passage of bright red blood during defecation.

Anoscopic examination reveals the ulcer. Initial treatment is with stool softeners. If there is no improvement within 30 da, surgery is indicated.

anal fistula a tract that usually leads from the anal canal to an opening of the skin near the anus. It is characterized by chronic purulent discharge and abscess formation, commonly caused by rupture or inadequate drainage of an abscess. A barium test and sigmoidoscopy are useful in detecting underlying disorders such as regional enteritis and ulcerative colitis. Treatment is surgical and requires excision of the tract.

analgesia (an″al-je′ze-ah) [*an-* neg. + Gr. *algēsis* sense of pain + *-ia*] the relief of pain or absence of sensibility to pain caused by neurologic disease, analgesic medications (e.g., aspirin, acetaminophen, opiate derivatives), or other methods (e.g., audioanalgesia, acupuncture, hypnosis). Analgesia is a major component of anesthesia.

analgesic (an″al-je′zik) 1. pertaining to analgesia.
2. an agent that alleviates pain without causing loss of consciousness, e.g., aspirin, acetanilide, and phenacetin. Excessive amounts (or lesser amounts in particularly sensitive people) may cause symptoms of nausea, vertigo, sweating, coma, and even death.

analgesic neuropathy see *analgesic n.* under *neuropathy.*

analog (an′ah-log) [Gr. *analogos* in proportion, from *ana-* + *logos* proportion] 1. something that corresponds in some respect to something else in function or appearance but not necessarily in origin. Examples are cortisol and dexamethasone, both of which affect the pituitary output of adrenocorticotropic hormone through the feedback loop, yet have different structures. Cf. *homologue.*
2. in biology, an analogous structure or organ; see *analogous structure.*
3. pertaining to electronic equipment in which the output is a continuous function (the transfer function) of the input and in which information is represented by continuously variable voltage (or current) levels. Cf. *digital.*

analog computer an electronic device containing circuits that perform mathematical operations (e.g., addition, negation, multiplication, division, differentiation, integration) on analog signals. The output is a specified mathematical function of the input. Cf. *digital computer.*

analog data data represented by the value of a continuous physical variable such as electric voltage, current, or resistance, or the optical density of a photographic film.

analog multiplexer a set of multiple channel switches used in computers for routing many analog or digital signals to a single input point.

analogous (ah-nal′o-gus) 1. corresponding or similar to in some respect.
2. in biology, relating to analogous structures or organs. Cf. *homologous.*

analogous structures structures that have the same function or appearance but are unrelated in evolutionary origin, e.g., the eyes of humans and of octopuses. Cf. *homologous structures.*

analog signal an electric quantity that may represent information such as AC or DC current, frequency or pulse duration, voltage, time position, or pulse amplitude.

analog-to-digital converter (ADC, A/D converter) an electronic device that converts an analog signal (input voltage) to digital data (a binary number) that can be processed by a digital computer. The most important characteristics of an A/D converter are the accuracy of and rate of conversion.
There are two types of inaccuracy in the conversion process: quantization and equipment error. Quantization error is the error inherent in representing the analog signal by discrete numbers and is reflected in the number of bits used for conversion. This type of error is about 10 percent for a 3-bit converter, 1 percent for a 7-bit converter, and 0.1 percent for a 10-bit converter. Equipment error is the error produced by circuit nonlinearities, variations in component values, or random noise.
In an integrator type A/D converter, the digital output is produced by counting the pulses produced by a clock circuit. At the start of the conversion period, the counter is reset and the input voltage is applied to the integrator circuit, where it charges a capacitor at a constant rate. When the counter overflows, a reference voltage is applied to the integrator, and it discharges the capacitor at the same rate until the charge reaches zero, when the clock is stopped.
The number of counts stored is equal to the ratio of the input voltage to the reference voltage times the full scale count (unless the input voltage was greater than the reference voltage; then, the counter overflows a second time and the overrange condition is turned on). This type of circuit, although slow, is quite accurate because variations in the components have the same effect in integrating the two voltages, and thus cancel out.
The successive approximation type A/D converter is faster but more complicated. The counter is connected to a digital-to-analog (D/A) converter, which produces a voltage that is compared with the input voltage. During the conversion process, the control logic circuit resets the counter and then determines the correct value of each bit in sequence starting with the overrange indicator bit, then the most significant bit, and so forth, down to the least significant bit. At each step the bit is set to 1 and, if the analog value of the count is less than the input voltage, the next bit is processed; otherwise, the bit is set to zero and the next bit is processed. The conversion time of this type of circuit is proportional to the number of bits rather than, as with the integrator type, to the full-scale count.
The parallel type A/D converter is the fastest type of converter, but it is also the most complex and least accurate. There is a separate comparator circuit and reference voltage (produced by a voltage divider circuit) for each voltage level that can be represented. Logic circuits determine the digital output from all the comparisons at once. The counting time is thus independent of the number of bits, but the circuit complexity is proportional to the full-scale count.

analogue (an′ah-log) see *analog.*

analogy (ah-nal′o-je) [Gr. *analogia* equality of proportion] 1. a correspondence between two otherwise dissimilar things. Cf. *homology.*
2. the inference (reasoning by analogy) that if two things correspond in one respect they also correspond in some other respect.

anal stricture a fibrotic narrowing of the anal canal, often associated with laxative abuse or previous surgery. A barium test may be useful in detecting underlying disease such as regional enteritis. Treatment is aimed at dilation of the stricture and the correction of any underlying disorder.

anal tumors neoplasms of the anal canal. Anal squamous carcinoma is relatively uncommon compared with rectal adenocarcinoma: the ratio of the two is roughly 1:9. Approximately 20 percent of anal tumors arise at the anorectal junction from cloacal remnants and are designated cloacogenic carcinomas; most resemble urothelial cancers, but a more aggressive variant histologically resembles cutaneous basal cell carcinoma. Inguinal lymph node metastases develop in 40 percent of squamous carcinomas of the anal canal; pelvic and mesenteric nodes are involved slightly less often.

analysis (ah-nal'ĭ-sis), pl. *analyses*[*ana-* + Gr. *lysis* dissolution] 1. separation into component parts or elements. Cf. *synthesis.*

2. determination of whether a chemical element, compound, or functional group is present in a substance, or the determination of its relative or absolute quantity.

qualitative a., determination of the presence or absence, in mixtures or solutions, of elements, specific compounds, or functional compound groups.

quantitative a., the accurate determination of the quantity of a chemical element, compound, or functional group present in a specimen.

semiquantitative a., the determination of the quantity of a chemical element, compound, or functional group that is present in a specimen, using a measurement of limited precision that is frequently rapid and simple. Examples are reagent strip tests carried out in urinalysis, the results of which are generally reported using a 4–6 level scale (negative, 1+, 2+, 3+, and 4+).

analysis of variance (ANOVA) a statistical procedure for comparing the means of several random variables, which are assumed to have normal distributions with the same variance σ^2.

In a completely randomized experiment (also called a one-way layout), there are k independent random samples having sample sizes n_i, means $\overline{X}_i$, and sum of squares SS_i($n_i - 1$ times the sample variance s_i^2) taken from parent populations with means μ_i and variances σ^2. The error sum of squares $SS_e = \Sigma_i SS_i$ is independent of the sample means and is an estimator of $(N-k)\sigma^2$, where N is the total of the sample sizes.

Under the null hypothesis that all the population means are the same (this is sometimes called the omnibus hypothesis), the sum of the mean squares $SS_H = \Sigma_i n_i (\overline{X}_i - \overline{X}_{tot})^2$ is independent of the grand mean $X_{tot} = \Sigma_i n_i \overline{X}_i / N$ and is an estimator of $(k-1)\sigma^2$. The statistic $F = (N-k)SS_H/(k-1)SS_e$ has the F distribution with $k-1$ degrees of freedom in the numerator and $N-k$ degrees of freedom in the denominator. The null hypothesis can be rejected at the α level of significance if F exceeds the upper α percentile $F_{\alpha,k-1,N-k}$. The sum of SS_e and SS_H is the total sum of squares SS_{tot}, which is the total squared deviation of data points from the grand mean calculated as $\Sigma X^2 - N\overline{X}_{tot}^2$. The name analysis of variance comes from the process of breaking down the total variation SS_{tot} into the two independent variations SS_e and SS_H.

A $k-1$ dimensional confidence ellipsoid for the means is given by the equation $\Sigma_i n_i(\overline{X}_i - \overline{X}_{tot} - \mu_i + \overline{\mu})^2 < (k-1)F_{\alpha,k-1,N-k}\,SS_e/(N-k) = c^2$, where $\overline{\mu} = \Sigma_i n_i \mu_i / N$. An equivalent but more convenient formulation is called Scheffé's test. A contrast is defined as a linear combination $\Sigma_i a_i \mu_i$ or $\Sigma_i a_i \overline{X}_i$, in which the coefficients a_i sum to zero. For values μ_i falling inside the confidence region, every contrast falls in the interval $(\Sigma_i a_i X_i - \Sigma_i a_i \mu_i)^2 < c^2\,\Sigma_i a_i^2/n_i$. This test permits after-the-fact examination of the data to discover significant contrasts among means. Each Scheffé interval, however, is much wider than that which would be used to test one particular contrast (or $k-1$ independent contrasts) chosen for examination before the data were collected. In testing for one particular contrast $t_{\alpha/2,N-k}$ would be used in place of $F_{\alpha,k-1,N-k}$ in computing c^2.

In the randomized blocks experiment (or two-way layout), each variable has a mean that is the sum of two independent effects usually called the treatment effect (which is the effect being examined) and the block effect (the average over the subject's control group or block, which has been made uniform with respect to some control variable, e.g., age, weight, or sex).

In this design, a sum of squares for blocks SS_B and a sum of squares for treatments SS_T (both calculated like SS_H in the one-way layout) are subtracted from SS_{tot} to give SS_e. If there are k treatments and n blocks, then SS_T has $k-1$ degrees of freedom, SS_B has $n-1$, and SS_e has $(k-1)(n-1)$. The null hypothesis that the treatment means are identical is rejected if $F = (n-1)SS_T/SS_e$ exceeds $F_{\alpha,k-1,(k-1)(n-1)}$; this percentile is also used in calculating confidence intervals for contrasts by the same procedure used with the one-way layout.

In the most general ANOVA experimental design, the population means can be any linear functions of the effects. The treatment or block effects are estimated using least-square linear regression, and an F statistic is formed from the sum of squares for the effects of interest and the error sum of squares. This includes linear regression as a special case.

analyte (an'ah-lit") in clinical chemistry, the system component being measured by an analysis, e.g., potassium in a serum potassium assay or total lipids in a serum lipids assay.

analytic (an"ah-lit'ik) [Gr. *analytikos*] 1. pertaining to separation into factors, components, or elements.

2. pertaining to or used in a chemical analysis.

analytical balance a balance capable of weighing substances with a high degree of accuracy and precision. The common analytical balances have a weighing range of up to 200 g and a reproducibility of ± 0.5 mg. Semimicrobalances have a weighing range of up to 100 g and a reproducibility between ± 0.1 and 0.01 mg, whereas microbalances have a range of 5–20 g and a reproducibility of up to 0.1 μg.

analytical reagent grade (AR) a degree of chemical purity that meets specifications established by the American Chemical Society. See also *reagent grade.*

analytic cytology see *cytometry.*

analyzer (an'ah-li"zer) 1. a device, such as a Nicol prism, attached to a polarizing apparatus that extinguishes the ray of light polarized by the polarizer.

2. a sensory receptor together with its central connections, by means of which sensitivity to stimulation is differentiated.

3. in clinical chemistry, an automated instrument that performs analytic procedures. See also *clinical chemistry automation.*

anamnesis (an"am-ne'sis) [Gr. *anamnēsis* a recalling] 1. recalling to memory, recollection.

2. the complete history of a patient, including data on previous illnesses and the patient's family and environment.

3. in immunology, the heightened immune re-

sponse that occurs on second exposure to an antigen. Also called *immunologic memory*.

anamnestic (an″am-nes′tik) [Gr. *anamnēstikos*] pertaining to anamnesis.

anamnestic response the rapid reappearance of antibody or cellular immunity in the blood following introduction of an antigen to which the individual had previously developed a primary immune response.

anamorph (an′ah-morf″) an organ of asexual or somatic reproduction, which can be specialized or generalized but is neither morphologically nor karyologically sexual. Cf. *teleomorph*.

anaphase (an′ah-fāz) [*ana-* + Gr. *phasis* phase] that stage in mitosis and the first and second meiotic divisions, following the metaphase, during which the centromere splits and the chromatids, which were lined up on the spindle, begin to move apart toward opposite poles of the spindle. See also *meiosis* and *mitosis*.

anaphase lag an abnormality in cell division in which a chromosome does not remain attached to the spindle fibers, and so cannot move to a daughter cell and is lost. This gives rise to a monosomic cell line. Cf. *nondisjunction*.

anaphoresis (an″ah-fo-re′sis) [*ana-* + Gr. *phorēsis* a being borne] the passage of charged particles toward the anode (positive pole) in electrophoresis.

anaphylactic (an″ah-fĭ-lak′tik) pertaining to anaphylaxis.

anaphylactic shock see *anaphylactic s.* under *shock*.

anaphylactoid shock (an″ah-fĭ-lak′toid) an abrupt, systemic reaction that resembles anaphylactic shock but is not usually initiated by an antigen-antibody reaction. The presence in serum of colloids such as peptone, agar, and kaolin has been observed to cause this type of shock.

anaphylatoxin (an″ah-fĭ″lah-tok′sin) a polypeptide cleaved from the C3a and C5a components of complement during complement fixation. It causes mast cells to degranulate and release pharmacologically active mediators such as histamine, which in turn greatly increase vascular permeability.

anaphylatoxin inactivator an alpha-globulin enzyme found in human serum; M.W. 300,000. It attacks and stops the biologic functions of the C3a and C5a fragments of the complement molecules C3 and C5 by removing the carboxyl terminal arginine from each molecule.

anaphylaxis (an″ah-fĭ-lak′sis) [*ana-* + Gr. *phylaxis* protection, from *phylax* guard] the systemic manifestation of an immediate hypersensitivity reaction to a foreign antigen. Characteristically, it involves the interaction of the foreign antigen with reaginic IgE antibody on the surface of a mast cell or basophil. The antigen-antibody reaction produces degranulation of the mast cell, with release of the mediators histamine, SRS-A (slow-reacting substance of anaphylaxis), ECF-A (eosinophilic chemotactic factor of anaphylaxis), and others. The mediator release leads to systemic reactions including generalized urticaria (hives), flushing, angioedema, upper airway edema, bronchospasm, circulatory collapse with shock and hypotension, gastrointestinal symptoms of bowel spasm and diarrhea, and uterine contractions. The major life-threatening problem usually is laryngeal edema and shock.

The most common causes of anaphylaxis include bee and wasp stings, drugs, heterologous serum, and hyposensitization. Immediate treatment usually involves maintenance of the airway and circulation, with concomitant administration of epinephrine by injection. Maintenance of blood volumes may require administration of intravenous colloid or saline.

A history of anaphylaxis to insect venom requires skin testing, which begins with prick testing with the offending venom. If prick testing is negative, dilute intradermal skin testing is warranted. If this test is negative, anaphylaxis is less likely, although still possible, with exposure to the venom of the insects tested. Similar skin testing can be done with penicillin G and with benzoylpenicilloyl-polylysine. Penicillin skin testing should not be performed unless desensitization with penicillin or therapy with penicillin is planned, as the skin testing procedure itself can be sensitizing or produce serious anaphylaxis.

See also *immediate hypersensitivity*.

GERALD B. KOLSKI, M.D., PH.D.

anaplasia (an″ah-pla′ze-ah) [*ana-* + Gr. *plassein* to form] the failure of parenchymal cells to differentiate and develop normal, mature, specialized, functional, and morphologic characteristics: a characteristic of many malignant tumors. Also called *undifferentiation*. Cf. *differentiation*.

anaplastic (an″ah-plas′tik) characterized by anaplasia.

anaplerotic (an″ah-plĕ-rot′ik) [Gr. *anaplērōsis* a filling up, from *plērēs* full] relating to a sequence of enzymatic actions in central metabolic cycles (e.g., the tricarboxylic acid cycle) by which intermediates are produced from catabolic products of a substrate needed for the growth of an organism. The mechanism thus serves to replenish an intermediate depleted during growth.

anasarca (an″ah-sar′kah) [N.L., from *ana-* + Gr. *sarx* flesh] a generalized edema.

anastalsis (an″ah-stal′sis) [Gr., from *ana-* + *stalsis* contraction] 1. an upward-moving wave of contraction without a preceding wave of inhibition, occurring in the alimentary canal in addition to the peristaltic wave.

2. styptic action.

anastigmat (an″ah-stig′mat) [*an-* + *a-* neg. + *stigmato* marks, spots] a lens system that is corrected for astigmatism.

anastomosis (ah-nas″to-mo′sis) [Gr. "opening, outlet"] 1. a communication or connection between two vessels.

2. an opening created by surgical, traumatic, or pathologic means between two normally distinct spaces or organs. See also *arteriovenous s.* under *shunt*.

anatomic (an″ah-tom′ik) pertaining to anatomy, or to the structure of the body.

anatomical snuff box a triangular depression on the dorsal aspect of the hand when the thumb is fully extended. It is bordered laterally by the tendons of extensor pollicis brevis and abductor pollicis longus, and medially by the tendon of extensor pollicis longus.

anatomic dead space a collective name for the extraalveolar structures of the respiratory tree (mouth, nose, pharynx, larynx, trachea, bronchi, and bronchioles), which with each breath are filled with a volume of air (approximately 150 ml) not involved in gaseous exchange. It is normally a constant component of, and is nearly equal in magnitude to, the physiologic dead space.

anatomist (ah-nat′o-mist) a specialist in anatomy.

anatomy (ah-nat′o-me) [Gr. anatomē, from *ana-* + *temnein* to cut] 1. the science of the structure of the animal body and the form and relations of its parts. Anatomy may be studied macroscopically (gross anatomy) and microscopically (histology).

2. dissection of an organized body.

3. the resolution of different structures into their molecular or atomic elements by means of optical instruments using different electromagnetic waves.

applied a., the study of those aspects of anatomy that are useful in the diagnosis and treatment of disease.

comparative a., the study of similarities and differences in the structure of animals or plants.

developmental a., the study of the embryologic formation and maturation of anatomic structures.

general a., the study of the structure and compositions of the body and its tissues.

gross a., the study of those anatomic structures that are distinguishable with the naked eye. Also called *macroscopic a.*

histologic a., see *microscopic a.*

macroscopic a., see *gross a.*

microscopic a., the microscopic study of body structures and tissues; histology.

morbid a., see *pathologic a.*

pathologic a., the anatomic study of abnormalities in the function, structure, or appearance of tissues. Also called *morbid a.*

physiologic a., the study of the structural basis for the function of cells, tissues, and organs.

radiologic a., the study of the anatomy of organs and tissues through their visualization on x-ray films.

Anatrichosoma an aphasmid, Capillaria-like nematode (worm), of which the species *A. cutaneum* (also called *Trichosoma cutaneum*) is parasitic in monkeys. It may rarely cause creeping eruption in humans.

anchorage dependence (ang′ker-ij) the requirement of some cultured cells for a rigid support to which they must attach in order to proliferate. See also cell culture.

anchorage independence the ability of cultured cells to divide and form colonies when suspended in a gel.

ancrod (an′krod) see under *thrombolytic agents.*

Ancylidae a family of mollusks, *Ferrissia tenuis* (limpets), which serve as intermediate hosts of *Schistosoma haematobium.* These mollusks are found in western India.

Ancylostoma (an″kĭ-los′to-mah) [Gr. *ankylos* crooked + *stoma* mouth] a genus of nematode parasites, of which the species *A. duodenale* is the common European or Old World hookworm. See also *hookworm.*

AND (& or $\wedge$) a logical relation whose result is *true* only if all arguments are *true;* otherwise, the result is *false.* Cf. *NAND.*

Andersen's disease (an′der-sonz) [Dorothy Hansine *Andersen,* New York pathologist, born 1901] see *brancher deficiency.*

"AND" gate an electronic circuit that calculates the logical "AND" function; its output is *true* if, and only if, all inputs are *true.*

andr/o (an′dro) [Gr. *anēr, andros* man] a word element used in combining form to denote man or male, e.g., androgen.

androblastoma (an″dro-blas-to′mah) a tumor of specialized gonadal stroma occurring in the ovaries or testes (when it occurs in the ovaries, it is called *arrhenoblastoma*). See also *gonadal-stromal tumors* and *Sertoli-Leydig cell tumors.*

androgen (an′dro-jen) [*andro-* + Gr. *gennan* to produce] a group of C-19 steroid hormones that exert profound influence on the male genital tract and are concerned with the development and maintenance of secondary male sex characteristics, such as beard growth, deepening of the voice at puberty, muscle and bone development, body strength, and sexual drive.

Testosterone is mainly secreted by the testes in males, and to a lesser extent by the adrenal glands in both sexes and by the ovaries in females. Females normally have a small percentage of male hormones in the same way that males produce female sex hormones, the estrogens. Dihydrotestosterone and androstanediol are predominantly formed by peripheral conversion of testosterone. In normal females, the functions of androgens, other than being estrogen precursors, are not well defined.

androgenesis (an″dro-jen′ĕ-sis) [*andro-* + Gr. *genesis* production] the situation in which the female pronucleus is present but makes no contribution. This is not a normal condition in any animal, although some species of salamanders and sea urchins attain full development as haploid individuals containing only the parental genome. In mammals, development of the fertilized egg with only male genetic information (by removal of a female pronucleus) can occur normally. See also *fertilization.* Cf. *gynogenesis.*

android (an′droid) [*andr-* + Gr. *eidos* shape] a term used to describe the typical male pelvis, which is angular, has a narrowing of the anteroposterior portion of the inlet, and has the greatest contraction at the outlet. Characteristically, the bones are thick. This pattern is also found in approximately 23 percent of females. Cf. *gynecoid.*

androstanediol (an″dro-stān′di-ol) a potent plasma androgen, 3α,17β-dihydroxy-5α-androstane, which is produced from testosterone and dihydrotestosterone in the liver and peripheral tissues.

androstenediol (an″dro-stēn′di-ol) a plasma androgen, 3β,17β-dihydroxyandrost-5-ene; it may be derived from plasma dehydroepiandrosterone or secreted by the adrenals, the ovaries, or both.

androstenedione (an″dro-stēn′di-ōn) 4-androstene-3,17-dione, a steroid that is an important prehormone for plasma testosterone. It is derived from the ovaries and adrenals.

androsterone (an-dros′ter-ōn) a weak androgen and primary metabolic product of testosterone, 3α-hydroxy-5α-androstan-17-one, which is excreted in the urine of both males and females. Its determination (along with that of total 17-ketosteroids) may be a measure of testicular function or may help to differentiate types of adrenogenital syndromes. Reference ranges for androsterone in urine (by gas chromatography) are: for males, 2.0–5.0 mg/da; and for females, 0.5–3.0. See also *17-ketosteroids* and *17-ketosteroid assays.*

-ane (ān) a suffix word element in organic chemistry used when the alkane itself is the parent compound, e.g., $ClCH_2CH_3$, chloroethane. Cf. *-ene* and *-yne.*

anechoic (an-ĕ-ko′ik) [*an-* neg. + *echoic*] not producing echoes; the term is applied to a chamber with nonreflecting walls used to measure sound or, in an ultrasonogram, is applied to regions that do not produce echoes.

anemia (ah-ne′me-ah) [Gr. *an-* neg. + *haima* blood + *-ia*] a reduction below normal in the quantity of hemoglobin or in the volume of packed red cells per 100 ml of blood. This occurs when the normal equilibrium between red cell loss (through senescence, bleeding, or destruction) and red cell production is disturbed. If the erythrocytes produced are microcytic (as in thalassemia), the number of red cells per cubic millimeter may be normal or elevated, yet the individual is considered anemic because of a lowered hemoglobin level. Sometimes a mild increase in erythrocyte destruction can be fully compensated for by increased production, and the number of erythrocytes and the quantity of hemoglobin per unit of blood are then normal. This condition is referred to as compensated hemolytic anemia.

aplastic a., pancytopenia resulting from hypoplasia or aplasia of the bone marrow, which is usually replaced by fat cells. The primary defect probably resides in the stem cells. Erythrocyte, granulocyte, and platelet levels may not be equally affected; a low platelet count, often the most remarkable feature, affects bleeding time, capillary fragility, or clot retraction tests, while other coagulation tests remain normal. The few erythrocytes produced are usually normal but can be macrocytic. The major types of aplastic anemia include acquired aplastic anemia, congenital aplastic anemia, and Fanconi's anemia.

ACQUIRED APLASTIC ANEMIA. This form may be caused by injury to bone marrow tissue from ionizing radiation, chemicals, drugs, or infections (viral hepatitis). Affected individuals may have an idiosyncratic sensitivity to these agents, the prognosis being most favorable when an offending agent can be identified and removed. No cause can be established in about 50 percent of cases. Some cases of acquired aplastic anemia develop into paroxysmal nocturnal hemoglobinuria (PNH) and leukemia.

CONGENITAL APLASTIC ANEMIA. Congenitally derived aplastic anemia may affect only the hematopoietic cell compartment or may be associated with other congenital abnormalities. Some cases arise without any familial history of the disease.

FANCONI'S ANEMIA. Transmitted as an autosomal recessive trait, Fanconi's anemia is a congenital form of pancytopenia with hyperpigmentation and malformations such as hypoplasia of the kidneys and spleen, as well as an absent or hypoplastic thumb and radius, small stature, hypogonadism, microcephaly, and mental retardation. Also called congenital pancytopenia, constitutional infantile panmyelopathy, Fanconi's pancytopenia, and pancytopenia-dysmelia syndrome. Pancytopenia without physical anomaly is often termed familial hypoplastic anemia.

The following anemias are often incorrectly grouped with aplastic anemia: (1) Diamond-Blackfan anemia, (2) myelophthisic anemia, (3) refractory anemia, and (4) aregenerative anemia.

aregenerative a., a term ambiguously applied to both refractory anemia and aplastic anemia in which the regeneration of erythrocytes is defective; its use should be discouraged. See also *aplastic a.* and *refractory a.*

autoimmune hemolytic a. (AIHA), an acquired hemolytic anemia due to the coating of the red cells by immunoglobulins and complement, predominantly C3. The immunoglobulins act as autoantibodies against the body's own red cells. This abnormality is thought to be caused by a change in the red cell membrane or in the immune system, and results in the loss of self-recognition. The cells may become spherocytic and are removed prematurely from the circulation by the spleen. The increased destruction of red cells may be partially or completely compensated for by increased erythropoiesis, with reticulocytosis and mild-to-moderate macrocytosis (compensated hemolytic anemia).

AIHA may be idiopathic or secondary to lymphocytic malignancies, other neoplastic disorders, autoimmune disorders (primarily lupus erythematosus), infections, or drugs. Antibodies may be of the warm or cold type, depending on their temperature optimum; the warm type (maximally active at 37°C) is more common. Cold autoantibodies are maximally active at 2°–4°C.

Also called *autoimmune hemolytic disease* (*AHD*). See also *autoimmune disease* and *paroxysmal cold hemoglobinuria.*

Biermer's a., see *pernicious a.*

blood loss a., anemia caused by acute or chronic blood loss. In acute blood loss, the hematocrit is initially normal or may even increase (hemoconcentration) until the plasma volume gradually expands. Normochromic normocytic anemia develops over the ensuing 20–72 hr as interstitial fluid enters the circulation and restores the original blood volume. In chronic blood loss, an iron deficiency usually develops unless the hemorrhage is internal rather than external. See also *iron deficiency a.*

a. of chronic disease, anemia that accompanies chronic infection and inflammatory or neoplastic diseases. It is usually normocytic and normochromic, although in some cases it may be slightly microcytic or hypochromic. This form may be associated with reduced serum iron and reduced iron-binding capacity, abundant iron in reticuloendothelial storage sites, and impaired marrow response ("relative marrow failure"). Unaffected by iron therapy, anemia of chronic disease disappears only with cure of the underlying disease. Also called by the following less desirable names: anemia of chronic disorders, hypoferremic anemia, hypoferremic anemia with reticuloendothelial siderosis, and therapeutic anemia.

a. of chronic renal failure, anemia that regularly accompanies renal insufficiency. It is usually normocytic and normochromic, and unlike anemia of chronic disease is not associated with hypoferremia.

congenital atransferrinemia, an extremely rare condition, transmitted as an autosomal recessive trait, in which an absence of transferrin in the plasma prevents delivery of iron to the bone marrow and thus impedes hemoglobin synthesis. Severe hypochromic microcytic anemia results, and death may occur in childhood from excessive iron deposition in tissues, particularly the myocardium, liver, and spleen. Transfusion of normal plasma or purified transferrin has shown promising results in producing reticulocytosis and a rise in hemoglobin. Also called congenital transferrin deficiency.

congenital dyserythropoietic a. (CDA), a group of rare, familial, refractory anemias characterized by ineffective erythropoiesis (erythroid marrow hyperplasia and normal or only slightly elevated absolute reticulocyte counts), red cell multinuclearity, and secondary siderosis. Three types are recognized, although others probably exist.

In CDA I, almost all nucleated red cells are abnormal, with both double nuclei or incompletely divided nuclear segments. Internuclear chromatin bridges are seen between pairs of normoblasts, and megaloblastic features are common.

In CDA II, there are late polychromatophilic or orthochromic erythroid cells with two to seven normal nuclei. The red cells are lysed by acidified normal sera owing to a naturally occurring IgM antibody. Note that only 30 percent of normal sera contain sufficient antibody to lyse CDA II cells effectively. Consequently, laboratories should ensure that sera tested for that ability is available, stored in small aliquots in the frozen state. The sucrose hemolysis is negative (see *paroxysmal nocturnal hemoglobinuria*). Also called *HEMPAS* (*hereditary erythroblastic multinuclearity with a positive acidified serum*).

In CDA III, there are giant erythroblasts up to 50 μm in diameter, which contain as many as 12 nuclei, with prominent basophilic stippling.

congenital hypoplastic a., see *Diamond-Blackfan a.* and *pure red cell aplasia* (under *anemia*).

Cooley's a., see *thalassemia*.

Diamond-Blackfan a., a progressive anemia of unknown etiology; encountered in the first year of life, it is not accompanied by leukopenia and thrombocytopenia, and is usually responsive to corticosteroids. Also called congenital pure red cell aplasia. See also *pure red cell aplasia* (under *anemia*).

Estren-Damashek a., an obsolete term for congenital aplastic anemia without developmental abnormalities.

factor deficiency a., an undesirable term for anemia caused by a deficiency of vital hematopoietic raw material, such as iron, vitamin B_{12}, or folic acid.

Fanconi's a., see under *aplastic a.*

folic acid (folate deficiency) a., a megaloblastic anemia due to a decreased intake of folic acid (in alcoholics), to inappropriate diet (in infants), to impaired absorption (in persons with sprue and celiac disease), to an increased requirement (in pregnant females), to metabolic inhibitors used in the chemotherapy of malignant disease (such as 6-mercaptopurine), and, rarely, to other causes. See also *megaloblastic a.*

hemolytic a., any of a large group of anemias produced by an increased rate of red cell destruction without sufficient compensation in bone marrow activity. The reticulocyte count is always elevated. Classification of hemolytic anemia is usually based on whether the anemia is congenital or acquired, as it may result from congenital, intrinsic (corpuscular) defects of the erythrocytes that predispose them to destruction, or from acquired, extrinsic (extracorpuscular) mechanisms. Classification of acquired hemolytic anemia is subdivided according to cause.

ACQUIRED HEMOLYTIC ANEMIA. This form involves the uncompensated premature destruction of erythrocytes due to extrinsic hemolytic factors such as antibodies (in transfusions and erythroblastosis fetalis), chemicals, infectious agents (malaria, clostridia, mechanical injury (from vascular prostheses, damaged blood vessels), physical agents (thermal injury, radiation), hypophosphatemia, or liver disease. Paroxysmal nocturnal hemoglobinuria, an acquired condition, is sometimes classified here, although it is probably due to a stem cell defect that results in abnormalities of red cells, white cells, and platelets.

CONGENITAL HEMOLYTIC ANEMIA. This form is characterized by a shortened life span of erythrocytes due to an inherited intrinsic defect of the cell, resulting in an abnormal cell membrane (e.g., hereditary spherocytosis or elliptocytosis), an enzyme abnormality, or abnormal hemoglobin.

hereditary spherocytosis (HS), a disease in which a hereditary defect of the red cell membrane results in a spherical shape and a shortened cell survival time owing to splenic entrapment. Splenectomy restores normal or near-normal red cell survival and cures the anemia, although the spherocytosis persists.

hypochromic a., anemia with a disproportionate reduction of red cell hemoglobin (mean corpuscular hemoglobin concentration, 31 or less) compared with red cell volume; anemia characterized by hypochromic erythrocytes. It is generally associated with microcytosis, although hypochromia without microcytosis can also occur in refractory anemia or hemopoietic dysplasia of older people. Slight microcytosis without hypochromia may also occur, particularly in anemia of chronic disease.

The classic hypochromic microcytic anemias are iron deficiency anemia and thalassemia. The degree of hypochromia is more marked in iron deficiency anemia than in thalassemia at the same level of microcytosis; this discrepancy has led to the development of a number of indices facilitating the differential diagnosis of iron deficiency anemia and thalassemia. The most commonly used is computed as MCV (in fluid) $\times$ PCV $\times$ 0.1. A value of less than 13 suggests thalassemia; 14 or above suggests iron deficiency anemia. However, because hypochromia is generally slight in thalassemia, and often minor even in iron deficiency anemia, microcytosis is a much better diagnostic index.

iatrogenic a., physician-connected anemia; i.e., anemia due to a physician's treatment. Cf. *nosocomial a.*

iron deficiency a., the most commonly encountered clinical anemia, characterized by low or absent iron stores, low serum iron concentration, low transferrin saturation (low total iron-binding capacity), elevated transferrin, low hemoglobin concentration or hematocrit, and hypochromic microcytic red blood cells. It is generally symptomatic of an underlying condition associated with chronic blood loss, as dietary deficiency of iron is rare, except in infants receiving an unsupplemented milk diet for long periods or similarly selective nutrition. Malabsorption of iron may occur after gastrointestinal surgery, particularly subtotal gastrectomy, and may also cause iron deficiency anemia. For differential diagnosis from thalassemia, see *hypochromic a.*

leukoerythroblastic a., an anemia accompanied by

a variable number of immature erythroid and myeloid cells in the circulation. A leukoerythroblastic blood picture is a nonspecific manifestation of a variety of insults to the bone marrow leading to the release of immature cells of both the red and white cell series; thus, "leukoerythroblastic anemia" is not a disease entity. Also called *leukoerythroblastosis.*

macrocytic a., anemia characterized by macronormoblastic erythropoiesis and the release of larger than normal erythrocytes into the circulation. Macrocytic anemia should be distinguished from megaloblastic anemia, which is also characterized by the presence of large red cells, but which has a marrow population of red cell precursors with abnormal nuclear maturation and excess cytoplasm. See also *megaloblastic a.*

Mediterranean a., see *thalassemia.*

megaloblastic a., anemia characterized by the presence of macrocytes in the circulation and megaloblasts in the bone marrow. Asynchrony of maturation in the erythroblasts, caused by impaired DNA synthesis, results in delicate chromatin, abundant cytoplasm that contains more hemoglobin than normal for the stage of nuclear development, and deformed red cells (anisocytosis and poikilocytosis). The neutrophils tend to be hypersegmented.

The condition is usually due to the deficient absorption of vitamin B_{12} or folate, which may be caused by inadequate dietary intake of folic acid, malabsorption of folic acid or vitamin B_{12}, or an increased requirement for folic acid (especially during pregnancy). It can also be due to a lack of intrinsic factor, a substance produced in the stomach that is necessary for the absorption of vitamin B_{12} (pernicious anemia). Administration of the deficient vitamin restores normal hemopoiesis, and may have to be given indefinitely in some cases (e.g., pernicious anemia); in the absence of intrinsic factor or malabsorption, it can be administered parenterally.

microangiopathic hemolytic a., a hemolytic process due to intravascular fragmentation of the red blood cells, which is caused by microcirculatory lesions or the insertion of prosthetic devices into the heart or major vessels. It is found in conditions such as disseminated intravascular coagulation, thrombotic thrombocytopenic purpura, malignant hypertension, other renal lesions, and uremic hemolytic syndrome of childhood. The common denominator appears to be deposition of the fibrin strands on injured endothelium, particularly on arterioles or surfaces of prostheses. When red cells are forced against the fibrin strands by sufficiently rapid blood flow, schiztocytes eventually result; they are indicative of, though not invariably present in, the disorders named. See also *schiztocyte.*

microcytic a., anemia characterized by a majority of smaller than normal red cells, which results in a greater decrease in the quantity of hemoglobin and volume of red cell mass than in the number of red cells. Simple microcytic anemia is seen in association with various chronic diseases.

In hypochromic microcytic anemia, most erythrocytes have both reduced size and reduced concentration of hemoglobin. Thus, the mean corpuscular volume (MCV), mean corpuscular hemoglobin (MCH), and mean corpuscular hemoglobin concentration (MCHC) are all lower than normal (less than 80, 31, and 30, respectively). Red cells on a blood smear show increased central pallor. The condition is primarily associated with iron deficiency and thalassemia.

microdrepanocytic a., see *thalassemia.*

myelophthisic a., anemia due to the replacement of hemopoietic marrow, usually by metastatic carcinoma, often associated with a leukoerythroblastic peripheral blood picture. The term occasionally refers to anemias with marrow infiltrations that develop by fungal, tuberculous, or other granulomatous processes associated with a leukoerythroblastosis.

normochromic a., a descriptive term for anemia in which the hemoglobin content of the red cells measured by the mean corpuscular hemoglobin concentration (MCHC) is in the normal range. The term usually refers to anemias that are also normocytic.

normocytic a., an anemia in which the individual erythrocytes are not altered in size, but in which the number of erythrocytes per cubic millimeter of blood is diminished.

nosocomial a., hospital-connected anemia; e.g., caused by the taking of blood from a patient for laboratory tests. Cf. *iatrogenic a.*

pernicious a. (PA), a megaloblastic anemia occurring at all ages, but commonly in later life; it is caused by vitamin B_{12} deficiency due to malabsorption secondary to the failure of the gastric mucosa to secrete intrinsic factor.

The underlying anatomic lesion is an atrophic gastritis with histamine-fast achlorhydria and the disappearance of parietal cells. A smooth tongue (atrophy of papillae) is common. Unless treated early, demyelinization of the dorsal and lateral columns of the spinal cord develops (see *subacute combined degeneration of the s. c.* under *spinal cord*). There is probably a genetic component that predisposes certain individuals to this condition.

Also called Addison's anemia, addisonian anemia, and Addison-Biermer or Biermer's anemia. See also *megaloblastic a.*

pure red cell aplasia, an anemia caused by the isolated depletion of erythroid tissue in three forms: (1) congenitial (see *Diamond-Blackfan a.*); (2) acquired, which is often associated with certain histologic forms of thymoma; or (3) transient cessation of red cell production (see *erythroblastopenia*). Also called *erythroid aplasia.*

refractory a., an anemia usually associated with the depression of granulocytes and platelets. The bone marrow has normal or increased cellularity but cannot produce a normal number of mature erythrocytes, granulocytes, and platelets, and is sometimes associated with ringed sideroblasts and a leukoerythroblastic peripheral blood picture. This contrasts with aplastic anemia, in which the marrow is hypocellular and is largely or completely replaced by fat cells.

A particular type is refractory anemia with excess myeloblasts (RAEM). It is closely related to hemopoietic dysplasia, and sometimes is also referred to as preleukemia or dysmyelopoietic syndrome.

refractory sideroblastic a., see *sideroblastic a.*

sideroachrestic a., see *sideroblastic a.*

sideroblastic a., a heterogeneous group of disorders characterized by ringed sideroblasts (normoblasts with aggregates of nonheme iron in the mitochondria) in the marrow.

The disease may be acquired or hereditary, with erythroid marrow hyperplasia associated with ineffective erythropoiesis, resulting in low reticulocyte counts. The anemia is hypochromic and microcytic in the inherited form, and commonly normocytic or macrocytic in the idiopathic form. Acquired sideroblastic anemia occurs in persons of both sexes above the age of 50. Leukemia is a known complication.

HEREDITARY SIDEROBLASTIC ANEMIA. This form includes a heterogenous group of sideroblastic anemias in which inheritance, in most but not all families, is sex-linked via the X chromosome. Also called congenital sideroachrestic anemia and hereditary iron-loading anemia.

ACQUIRED SIDEROBLASTIC ANEMIA. This form may be idiopathic or secondary to a variety of diseases. Normoblastic hyperplasia of the bone marrow, ringed sideroblasts, and mostly normochromic, macrocytic erythrocytes are characteristic. The mean corpuscular volume (MCV) is elevated, whereas the mean corpuscular hemoglobin concentration (MCHC) is normal or slightly reduced. A small population of hypochromic cells is usually present; stippling of red blood cells may be prominent. Idiopathic refractory sideroblastic anemia (IRSA) occurs in individuals of both sexes older than age 50. Leukemia sometimes develops in affected persons. Also called refractory anemia with sideroblastic bone marrow, refractory normoblastic anemia, *refractory sideroblastic anemia*, and *sideroachrestic anemia*. See also *erythroleukemia* under *leukemia*.

unstable hemoglobin disease, a congenital hemolytic anemia, due to autosomal inheritance of one of many kinds of unstable hemoglobin, which precipitates in vivo or in vitro as Heinz bodies. The anemia can be mild or severe and may be exacerbated by infections and oxidative drugs. Also called unstable hemoglobin hemolytic anemia and congenital (or idiopathic) Heinz-body hemolytic anemia. See also *hemoglobinopathy*.

anemic (ah-ne′mik) characterized by anemia.

anencephaly (an″en-sef′ah-le) [*an*-neg. + Gr. *enkephalos* brain] a congenital malformation of the nervous system characterized by the absence of the cranial vault, the complete or nearly complete absence of the forebrain, pituitary, and midbrain, the absence of the overlying skin and membranes, and rachischisis of the spine. Anencephaly and spina bifida cystica are considered to be a single entity. See also *neural tube defects* and *s. b. cystica* under *spina bifida*.

anergy (an′er-je) the diminished reactivity to a specific antigen that results in diminished immediate and/or delayed hypersensitivity to that antigen.

anesthesia (an″es-the′ze-ah) [*an*- neg. + Gr. *aisthēsis* sensation] the loss of feeling or sensation due either to a disease process or to drugs administered to permit painless surgery or to relieve severe pain.

The use of the electroencephalogram (EEG) to monitor the depth of anesthesia has been impeded by the lack of precise definition of anesthetic levels and by the differences in the EEG changes observed with different anesthetic agents.

anesthesiology (an″es-the″ze-ol′o-je) [*anesthesia* + *-logy*] the specialty of medicine that deals with the administration of anesthetic agents and the care of the patient receiving such agents.

anesthetic (an″es-thet′ik) 1. pertaining to, characterized by, or producing anesthesia.

2. a drug used to abolish pain. Such drugs may be divided into general anesthetics (including inhalational anesthetics and intravenous anesthetics) and local anesthetics.

aneucentric (an″u-sen′trik) a term denoting an aberration that produces a chromosome with two or more centromeres.

aneuploid (an′u-ploid) [*an*- + *euploid*] referring to a chromosome number (and, by extension, to nuclear DNA content) other than euploid or polyploid. It also includes instances of normal chromosome number with unbalanced chromosomal translocation.

aneuploidy (an″u-ploi′de) any deviation from an exact multiple of the haploid number of chromosomes, which can be seen in a karyotype. The most common clinically significant aneuploidy is one too many chromosomes (trisomy, as in Down's syndrome). Aneuploidy is a common finding in malignant neoplasms.

aneurysm/o (an-u-riz′mo) [Gr. *aneurysma* a widening] a word element used in combining form to denote an aneurysm, e.g., aneurysmotomy.

aneurysm (an′u-rizm) [Gr. *aneurysma* a widening] a localized abnormal dilation of any blood vessel. This lesion may be variously classified and described according to its location as arterial (including aortic) or venous. It may also be classified by its gross appearance e.g., a berry aneurysm, a small (usually <1–1.5 cm in diameter), spherical, often congenital aneurysm, found in the circle of Willis. Finally, aneurysms may be described as dissecting (more correctly, dissecting hematomas) when blood enters the wall of an artery and separates various layers of the vessel wall. Clinically, aneurysms are described according to their etiology. Known causes include arteriosclerosis, syphilis, infection, and cystic medionecrosis, all of which can cause a focal weakness which predisposes to dilation of the blood vessel wall. Since pressure within the lumen of a vessel increases with the cube of its diameter, the pressure at a site of dilation rises, promoting still further dilation and weakening of the wall of the vessel. The tension in the vessel wall is proportional to Pr/δ, where P is the intravascular pressure, r is the vessel radius, and δ is the wall thickness. As the aneurysm expands, r increases and δ decreases as the wall is stretched; eventually the tension exceeds the wall strength and the aneurysm bursts. Associated systolic hypertension is not an uncommon finding.

Laboratory tests reveal leukocytosis, elevated lactic dehydrogenase (LDH), and electrocardiographic changes. Radiographs reveal an abnormal contour with changes in wall thickness. Pleural or pericardial effusion may also be seen. CT scans and radionucleotide angiocardiography may also be valuable diagnostic procedures.

Complications of aneurysms include impaired blood flow, thrombosis, emboli, intravascular hematoma, and rupture, which can be followed by sudden death. Suspected aneurysms should be examined with x-rays, ultrasonography, CT scans, and aortography. Cardiac and renal function status should also be evaluated.

See also berry *aneurysm*.

aneurysmal (an″u-riz′mal) pertaining to or resembling an aneurysm.

aneurysmal bone cyst a benign lesion of bone, usually solitary, that is often located in the metaphyses of long bones. It is composed of distended, blood-filled spaces that may have an endothelial lining separated by connective tissue partitions containing osteoid, osteoclasts, and hemosiderin. The cause is unknown; many patients give a history of trauma, but the cyst occasionally forms a component of other bone lesions. Treatment is by surgical resection, curettage, or radiation therapy.

aneusomatic (an″u-so-mat′ik) a term applied to any organism having cells with different numbers of individual chromosomes; for instance, the germ line may maintain chromosomes lost in the somatic line (by diminution).

ANF abbrev. See *antinuclear factor.*

Anger camera [after its inventor, Hal O. *Anger*] an eponymic term for scintillation camera, named for its developer. See also *scintillation camera.*

angi/o (an′je-o) [Gr. *angeion* vessel] a word element used in combining form to denote a vessel, e.g., angionecrosis.

angiitis (an″je-i′tis), pl. *angiitides* inflammation of a vessel, more commonly called vasculitis; see *vasculitis.*

angina (an-ji′nah) [L. *angere* to strangle] 1. any disease marked by choking or suffocation, particularly diseases of the throat.

2. a term now used almost exclusively to denote *angina pectoris.*

Ludwig's a., see *Ludwig's angina.*

a. pectoris, a sensation of discomfort or tightness, most often felt retrosternally, that typically appears on exertion; it is usually relieved by rest and sublingual nitroglycerin. Cold, strong emotion, and heavy meals are additional factors that can precipitate or worsen an attack. Classic angina pectoris is caused by a discrepancy between oxygen demand and supply to the myocardium due to a fixed atherosclerotic lesion in one or more coronary arteries. The pain can be located in various areas of the chest and may radiate to the neck or jaws, or down the arms (usually the left arm). In each attack the pain is always in the same place, lasts for about the same time, and is of similar intensity. (Any variation in the pain constitutes unstable angina.) Pain that can be localized to a point at the heart apex is not angina. During an attack, the individual may be hypertensive with an increased heart rate. A fourth heart sound is commonly heard. Usually, there is no evidence of heart disease between attacks.

Resting electrocardiographic studies often show ST segment depression during attacks. Exercise ECG testing is considered positive for angina when a 1.0-mm downsloping or horizontal depression of the ST segment occurs for at least 0.08 sec in one or more leads; at least 75 percent of individuals with positive test results have significant disease. Thallium-201 and technetium pyrophosphate scans may reveal myocardial ischemia. A MUGA nuclear ventriculogram can also demonstrate ischemia or infarction of a heart wall. Coronary arteriography is often used with patients whose stress ECG suggests obstruction of a main coronary artery, in order to determine suitability for bypass surgery.

Treatment of angina pectoris should involve correction of the underlying risk factors. Causative activities and conditions (e.g., smoking, mental stress, obesity) should be decreased or terminated. Nitroglycerin tablets relieve acute attacks; long-acting nitrates also relieve pain. Propranolol, verapamil, and nifedipine are also used. None of these drugs, however, halts the progression of the atherosclerotic process. Coronary artery bypass surgery has been employed for treatment; the ideal candidate has severe angina pectoris with localized obstruction of an artery. Prognosis depends on the degree of obstruction of vessels, number of vessels involved, age of the patient, and ventricular function.

Prinzmetal's a., see *variant a.*

variant a., a sensation of discomfort and tightness similar to angina pectoris; however, unlike angina pectoris, it occurs at rest and is caused by coronary artery spasm with or without physical blockage of the coronary arteries. Spasm may be induced by cold, ergot-derived drugs, or mechanical irritation to the artery. Variant angina represents less than 10 percent of angina cases and is more apt to develop in females under age 50. During an attack, the individual may be hypotensive and faint. Ventricular arrhythmias may be present.

The stress ECG and resting ECG during attacks show elevation of the ST segment. Coronary arteriography can demonstrate spasm as the cause of angina; multiple views of the arteries should be obtained.

Treatment involves avoidance of cold exposure, and therapy with sublingual nitroglycerin or long-acting nitrates. Beta blockers may aggravate this form of angina. Alpha-adrenergic blockers or slow channel Ca^{2+}, e.g., verapamil or nifedipine, blockers can be tried if nitroglycerin is unsuccessful.

Also called *Prinzmetal's a.*

angiocardiography (an″je-o-kar″de-og′rah-fe) [*angio-* + Gr. *kardia* heart + *graphein* to write] a technique used to view the internal structure of the heart and great vessels by taking a series of radiographs after the radiodensity of the blood passing through these structures has been increased. It is used in the diagnosis of congenital and acquired defects in cardiac function and anatomy (particularly those of the cardiac valves) such as stenotic valves, valvular regurgitation and prolapse, patent ductus arteriosus, preductal coarctation of the aorta, atrial or atrioventricular septal defect, myocardial hypertrophy, and transposition of the great vessels.

In the procedure, a bolus of radiopaque contrast medium (usually a solution of the sodium and meglumine salts of organic iodine compounds) is rapidly injected via a catheter that has been introduced into a peripheral vessel and advanced to a site upstream from and as close as possible to the vessel or chamber under examination. Serial films at multiple views (view selection being dependent on the suspected nature of the cardiac defect) are usually required to adequately assess the function of the heart and pattern of blood flow through its chambers and the great vessels.

Potential complications of the technique include inadvertent mechanical trauma to the heart during catheterization and possible adverse hemodynamic, toxic, and allergenic effects of the contrast material.

forward a., see *venous a.*

radionuclide a., a procedure in nuclear medicine, that obtains successive images of the chest as a bolus of a blood-labeling agent (e.g., ^{99m}Tc-pertechnetate, ^{99m}Tc-serum albumin, ^{99}Tc–red blood cells, or ^{113m}In-transferrin) passes through the heart and major vessels and distributes throughout the blood pool.

Transit (also called flow or dynamic) studies use a scintillation camera that has computerized data analysis or videotape recording. Images are obtained either at end-systole and end-diastole or regular intervals throughout the pumping cycle. Irregularities in myocardial contraction can be detected.

A static scan may be performed with a rectilinear scanner or scintillation camera. Pericardial effusion can be seen as a separation of the heart blood pool from the lung and liver pools; a mediastinal tumor can be identified as vascular from its blood pool.

Also called *blood pool scan.* See also *cardiac output, cardiac shunt detection,* and *ejection fraction.*

retrograde a., the radiologic examination of the left ventricle of the heart to demonstrate mitral valve insufficiency or aortic stenosis. A radiopaque contrast medium is introduced directly into the left ventricle through a catheter, which is passed from a peripheral artery through the aorta and aortic valve and into the left ventricle. Also called left ventriculography and retrograde cardioangiography.

selective a., angiocardiography using a catheter passed under radioscopic control from a peripheral vein through the vena cava into the right atrium, right ventricle, or pulmonary artery.

venous a., angiocardiography in which the contrast medium is injected as a bolus into one of several peripheral veins. Exposures are made after the medium travels to the heart. Also called *forward a.*

angioedema (an″je-o-e-de′mah) see *angioneurotic e.* under *edema.*

angiogram (an′je-o-gram″) [*angio-* + Gr. *gramma* drawing] a radiograph of blood vessels that have been filled with a radiopaque contrast medium, or a scintillation photograph of the blood vessels.

radionuclide cerebral a., see under *brain scan.*

angiography (an″je-og′rah-fe) [*angio-* + Gr. *graphein* to write] 1. the radiographic examination of blood vessels after the introduction of a radiopaque contrast medium. See also *angiocardiography.*

2. the study of the vessels. See also *arteriography* and *venography.*

cerebral a., the radiographic examination of the blood vessels of the brain. One of the water-soluble iodinated contrast media is introduced by injection into a carotid or vertebral artery or by brachial or femoral catheterization. During the time it takes the medium to pass through the cerebral circulation, several films are made that show arterial circulation (arteriograms) or venous circulation (venograms).

peripheral a., the radiologic examination of the peripheral vascular structures. See also *arteriography, lymphography,* and *venography.*

visceral a., the radiologic examination of the viscera after the introduction of a contrast medium into the vessels supplying the organs of interest. See also *abdominal a.* under *aortography.*

angiokeratoma (an″je-o-ker″ah-to′mah) [*angio-* + Gr. *keras* horn + *-oma*] a disease of the skin characterized by telangiectasias or warty growths in groups, together with thickening of the epidermis.

diffuse a., a rare inherited disorder of glycosphingolipid metabolism, transmitted as an X-linked recessive trait, that is characterized by partial or total deficiency of a specific lysosomal hydrolytic enzyme—α-galactosidase—which leads to the systemic accumulation of trihexosyl ceramide. The anatomic and physiologic abnormalities of the disease are related to the progressive storage of this glycophospholipid in the lysosomal system of endothelial, pericytic, and smooth muscle cells of blood vessels throughout the body. Glycophospholipid is also stored in ganglion cells; in the perineural cells of the atuonomic nervous system; in the reticuloendothelial, myocardial, and connective tissue cells; and in the epithelial cells of the cornea, glomeruli, and renal tubules.

The disease is usually manifested during adolescence or young adult life by a characteristic, albeit protean, clinical syndrome of recurring "shooting" pains in the lower extremities, renal disease, and multiple punctate, papular, telangiectatic skin lesions (angiokeratomas) that tend to cluster on the lower trunk, thighs, and scrotum. The syndrome may be incompletely manifested. Skin lesions, in particular, are sometimes absent, and a variety of organic and psychiatric disorders should be considered before establishing the diagnosis. Renal failure, usually occurring in the third or fourth decade, is the major cause of death in hemizygous males. The initial manifestation of renal involvement is usually proteinuria, but progression to azotemia may occur before renal damage is suspected. Apart from the renal failure, coronary ischemic or cerebral vascular accidents represent the second most frequent cause of death in this group of patients.

Heterozygous females are usually asymptomatic. Opacities of the cornea due to dystrophy of the corneal epithelium, visible only by slit-lamp examination, are found in 80 percent of those affected. Some have slight skin changes and/or pain in the lower extremities. Heterozygous females may develop renal failure, but this is extremely rare.

By light microscopy, the affected cells are seen to be enlarged and contain abundant cytoplasm filled with numerous clear, small, uniform vacuoles, imparting a foamy appearance. In paraffin-embedded sections, the vacuoles do not stain with periodic acid–Schiff (PAS) or other histochemical stains; however, if the tissue is examined under polarized light before being processed through lipid-soluble solutions or stained with Sudan black or oil red O, the presence of lipid material can be demonstrated in the cells. The ultrastructural features are quite characteristic: round or ovoid vacuoles consisting of numerous single, membrane-bound, osmiophilic inclusions measuring 0.3–10 μm in diameter are present in all cell types, and have a concentric myelin-like structure of laminated membranes, and a regular arrangement of alternately light and dark leaflets with a periodicity of 4–5 nm ("zebra bodies"). At present, there is no effective treatment.

Also called *Fabry's disease* and hereditary dystopic lipidosis. See also *sphingolipidoses.*

NELSON ORDONEZ, M.D.

angiolipoma (an″je-o-lĭ-po′mah) [*angio-* + Gr. *lipos* fat + *-oma* tumor] a variant of lipoma in which numerous capillaries are admixed with the mature fat cells.

angioma (an″je-o′mah) a benign tumor formed by the proliferation of blood vessels (hemangiomas) or lymph vessels (lymphangiomas).

angiomatosis (an″je-o-mah-to′sis) [*angi-* + Gr. *-oma* tumor + *-osis* condition] the presence of multiple angiomas. See also *hereditary hemorrhagic t.*

under *telangiectasia, Sturge-Weber syndrome,* and *von Hippel–Lindau disease.*

angiomyolipoma (an″je-o-mi″o-lĭ-po′mah) see under *renal tumors.*

angioneurotic edema (an″je-o-nu-rot′ik) see *angioneurotic e.* under *edema.*

angiopathy (an″je-op′ah-the) [*angio-* + Gr. *pathos* diseases] a term used to describe any disease of blood vessels.

diabetic a., a condition, frequently seen in diabetics, that is characterized by occlusive alterations in the walls of the blood vessels. A hyaline material accumulates in the capillaries, resulting in a thickening of the basement membrane; paradoxically, the basement membrane is more permeable than normal. The lesions are most commonly in the vasculature of the skin, retinas, renal glomeruli, and nerves. Clinical complications include cutaneous ulcers and infections, blindness, renal failure, and peripheral neuropathy. Atherosclerotic lesions are the major pathologic changes seen in the larger vessels. Myocardial infarction may result. Treatment involves control of the diabetic condition in addition to that directed at the local lesions.

angiosarcoma (an″je-o-sar-ko′mah) [*angio-* + *sarcoma*] a malignant neoplasm of endothelial cells. It can occur in individuals of any age and may arise in any location, but is most common in the skin, liver, and bones. A broad range of differentiation is displayed, ranging from low-grade tumors with vessels whose endothelial cells show minimal cytologically malignant features to anaplastic solid tumors with no evidence of vessel formation. The diagnosis in the more anaplastic tumors may be difficult or impossible, but demonstration of Factor VIII–related antigen can be helpful. Angiosarcomas of the skin are seen in chronic lymphedematous extremities, notably the arm following a radical mastectomy on the same side as the mastectomy. Angiosarcomas of the liver have been related to exposure to the fumes of vinyl chloride, as well as to arsenic ingestion and use of Thorotrast as a contrast medium in radiology. These tumors are typically aggressive and have a poor prognosis. Also called hemangioendotheliosarcoma and *hemangiosarcoma.*

Angiostrongylus (an″je-o-stron′jĭ-lus) [*angio-* + Gr. *strongylos* round] a genus of roundworms of which the species *A. cantonensis* (lungworm), found in Australia and the Pacific Islands, is normally parasitic in the domestic rat. Human infection is thought to be caused by ingestion of infected prawns and crabs, which serve as paratenic transport hosts. The worms measure 17–25 mm long by 0.25–0.36 mm wide, and are delicate and filiformed. Their larvae migrate from the stomach to the central nervous system and cause an eosinophilic meningitis.

angiotensin (an″je-o-ten′sin) a class of polypeptide hormones derived from an angiotensinogen precursor (substrate) by action of the proteolytic enzyme renin, which is secreted by the juxtaglomerular (JG) cells of the nephrons. These hormones include angiotensin I (AI), angiotensin II (AII), and angiotensin III (AIII).

Renin is secreted in response to hypovolemia, a decrease in blood pressure, or an increased stimulation of the renal sympathetic nerves. It acts on angiotensinogen to release the decapeptide AI. Although AI has been shown under experimental conditions to exhibit a slight vasopressor activity, it has no established physiologic role other than to serve as a precursor to AII. It is cleaved to form the physiologically active octapeptide AII by a converting enzyme (a dipeptidyl carboxypeptidase) present in vascular endothelial cells, primarily in the lungs. An aminopeptidase (one of the angiotensinases) acts on AII to form the heptapeptide AIII, which also exhibits physiologic activity.

This class of hormones plays a major role in regulation of the extracellular fluid volume, blood pressure, and sodium balance of the body.

a. I (AI), a decapeptide, the physiologically inactive form of angiotensin. As blood circulates through the small vessels of the lungs (and elsewhere), a converting enzyme formed by the endothelial cells of the pulmonary vasculature splits off histadyl-leucine from angiotensin I to form angiotensin II.

a. II (AII), an octapeptide hormone formed by the action of converting enzyme on angiotensin I. It is the most powerful vasoconstrictor known. AII has a variety of roles: it acts on the adrenal cortex to increase the rate of aldosterone secretion, it exerts a negative feedback effect on the juxtaglomerular cells to decrease the rate of renin secretion, it acts on receptor areas in the diencephalon that in turn stimulate an increase in water intake and vasopressin secretion, and it modulates sympathetic function through its action on peripheral adrenergic neurons (thus facilitating catecholamine synthesis and release). Finally, AII acts on the area postrema (and other circumventricular organs of the brain) to cause an increase in blood pressure; the physiologic significance of this last action is as yet uncertain. AII is inactivated by the enzyme angiotensinase.

The normal plasma level of AII in a supine subject on a normal sodium diet is approximately 25 pg/ml.

a. III (AIII), a heptapeptide formed by the action of an aminopeptidase on angiotensin II (AII). It exerts approximately 40 percent of the vasoconstrictor activity of AII but has at least an equally potent effect on stimulation of aldosterone release.

angiotensin I–converting enzyme (kinase II) an enzyme (EC 3.4.15.1, recommended name dipeptidyl carboxypeptidase) found at the membrane of endothelial cells of pulmonary vessels. It catalyzes the conversion of angiotensin I to angiotensin II by cleavage of two terminal amino acids. See also *angiotensin.*

angiotensinogen (an″je-o-ten′sin-o-jen) a serum alpha$_2$-globulin secreted in the liver that, when acted on by renin, yields angiotensin I. See also *angiotensin.*

angle (ang′g′l) [L. *angulus*] 1. the geometric figure formed by two rays (half lines) extending from a point (the vertex) or by two half planes extending from a line.

2. the amount of rotation around the vertex that moves one ray to the other. Angles are measured in a dimensionless unit, the degree (symbol °), which is 1/360 of a full circle, or the radian (abbrev. rad), which is $1/2\pi$ of a full circle. Degrees can be further divided into minutes (symbol, ′), which are one-sixtieth of a degree, and seconds (symbol, ″), which are one-sixtieth of a minute; however, decimals are more commonly used, e.g., 25°30′45″= 25.5125°. See also *solid angle.*

3. in anatomy, the area or the point of junction of two intersecting borders or surfaces.

angle board a small inclined plane used in radiographic positioning of the head.

angle head a centrifuge head with holes that support the tubes at an angle to the plane of rotation.

angle of incidence in optics, the angle that the incident ray makes with the perpendicular to the reflecting or refracting surface at the point where the ray intersects the surface.

angle of reflection in optics, either of the two equal angles made by incident and reflected rays with the line perpendicular to the reflecting surface at the point of reflection.

angle of refraction in optics, the angle that a refracted ray makes with a line perpendicular to the refracting surface at the point of refraction.

angström (Å) (ang′strem) [Anders Jonas *Angström*, Swedish physicist, 1814–1874] an obsolete unit of length, 10^{-10} meter, commonly used in microscopy, optics, and spectroscopy. The preferred International System (SI) units are the nanometer (nm), equal to 10Å, and the picometer (pm), equal to 0.01Å. Also called Angström unit. See also *nanometer* and *picometer.*

anhidrosis (an″hi-dro′sis) [*an-* neg. + Gr. *hidrōs* sweat + *-osis*] an abnormal absence or deficiency of sweating.

anhydrase (an-hi′drās) see *dehydratase.*

anhydration (an″hi-dra′shun) the state of not being hydrated; loss of water. See also *dehydration.*

anhydride (an-hi′drīd) [*an-* neg. + Gr. *hydōr* water] a chemical compound formally derived from an acid or base by the removal of a molecule of water. There are acidic and basic anhydrides in organic chemistry. A metal oxide that reacts with water to form a metal hydroxide is called a basic oxide or basic anhydride, e.g., calcium oxide (CaO). A nonmetal oxide that reacts with water to form an acid is called acidic oxide or acidic anhydride; e.g., sulfur trioxide (SO_3) is the acidic anhydride of sulfuric acid (i.e., it reacts with water to form sulfuric acid). In organic chemistry, an acid anhydride can be formed by removing a molecule of water from two carboxyl groups; e.g., acetic anhydride [$(CH_3CO)_2O$] is the anhydride from acetic acid (CH_3COOH). See also *acid anhydride.*

anhydrous (an-hi′drus) deprived of or lacking water.

anhydrous alcohol see *absolute alcohol.*

Anichkov's myocyte (an-nich′kofs) [Nikolai Nikolaevich *Anichkov,* Russian pathologist, born 1885] a mesenchymal cell found in the Aschoff body in rheumatic fever, and in the heart in various forms of cardiac necrosis. The nucleus contains a central bar of chromatin with thread-like segmentations. Origin of the cell is controversial, but it may be an altered fibroblast or macrophage. Also called *Anitchkow's cell.* See also *Aschoff body.*

aniline (an′ĭ-līn) [Arabic *al-nil* indigo] a colorless, oily liquid, $C_6H_5NH_2$, from coal tar and from indigo, that is made commercially by reducing nitrobenzene. Freely soluble in alcohol, benzene, and ether, aniline is only slightly soluble in water. Combined with other substances, especially chlorine or chlorates, it forms aniline colors or dyes. Owing to its toxicity, it is a significant cause of serious industrial poisoning associated with bone marrow depression, as well as methemoglobinemia. Aniline is also an important substance for drugs. Also called *amidobenzene* and *aminobenzene.*

aniline blue a blue acid dye, a mixture of sulfonated triphenyl methanes; C.I. 42755. It is used in histology in stains for connective tissue and cytoplasmic granules. See also *Gomori's method for chromaffin, Heidenhain's azan stain,* and *Mallory's collagen stain.*

anilinism (an′ĭ-lin-izm) aniline poisoning, marked by methemoglobinemia, vertigo, muscular weakness, cyanosis, and digestive derangement. Anemia and jaundice may appear after the individual's recovery from the acute symptoms.

animal (an′i-mal) [L., from *anima* life, breath] 1. a living organism of the kingdom Animalia having sensation and the power of voluntary movement, and requiring oxygen and organic food for existence.

2. pertaining to such an organism.

animal cell culture see *cell culture.*

animalcule (an″i-mal′kūl) [N.L. *animalculum*] any minute or microscopic animal organism.

anion (an′i-on) [Gr. *anion* going up, from *ana* up + *ion* going] an ion that carries a negative charge; in an electric field, it is attracted by and travels to the anode (positive pole). Anions are indicated by a minus sign, as in Cl^-. See also *ion.* Cf. *cation.*

anion-exchange resin see under *ion-exchange resin.*

anion gap a quantity equal to the concentration of undetermined ions (cUA^-) in plasma. It is equal to the sum of the undetermined anions minus the sum of the undetermined cations: $cUA^- = (cPr^- + cOrg^- + ctPO_4^- + 2cSO_4^{2-}) - (cK^+ + 2cCa^{2+} + 2cMg^{2+})$, where c indicates the concentration expressed in milliequivalents per liter (mEq/l); Pr^- indicates proteinate; Org^- indicates various organic anions (such as lactate, β-hydroxybutyrate); and tPO_4^- indicates total inorganic phosphate. In the laboratory the cUA^- can simply be estimated by using the formula $cUA^- = cNa^+ - (cCl^- + cHCO_3^-)$.

The reference range for venous plasma (cUA^-) is 5-14 mmol/l.

Decreases may be caused by a low cPr^- or by an analytical error in determining cNa^+, cCl^-, or $cHCO_3^-$ (or $ctCO_2$). Increases may be due to elevations of $ctPO_4^-$ and cSO_4^{2-} in renal failure; to negatively charged amino acids in renal failure; and increases in lactate in shock, muscular exercise, or in the lactic acid syndrome; to hydroxybutyrate or acetoacetate in diabetic acidosis or starvation; to formate during methanol poisoning; and to cPr^- in states of dehydration.

Also called anion deficit.

anionic dye (an″i-on′ik) see *acid dye.*

anion interference in flame photometry, a low reading due to incomplete dissociation of the anion being measured from complexes formed with anions in the specimen. For example, calcium can be bound in calcium phosphate, which is nonvolatile and dissociates poorly in the flame.

anionotropy (an″e-on-ot′ro-pe) [*anion* + Gr. *tropos* a turning] the process by which an anionic group (e.g., Cl^-) moves from one part of a molecule to another. Cf. *prototropy.*

anisakiasis (an″is-ah-ki′ah-sis) gastrointestinal

disease due to infection with the nematode parasite *Anisakis;* intestinal lesions, abscess, and obstructions have been reported.

Anisakis (an′ĭ-sa′kis) a parasitic nematode that infests sea mammals and, in its larval stage, some fish. Ingestion of contaminated fish has led to human infection; *A. marina* is believed to be the species involved.

anise oil (an′is) [L. *anisum*] [NF], a volatile oil distilled from the dried, ripe fruit of *Pimpinella anisum* or of *Illicium verum,* used as a flavoring agent for drugs. This oil was formerly used as a carminative and expectorant.

aniso- (an-i′so) [Gr. *anisos,* from *an-* neg. + *isos* equal] a prefix word element to denote unequal or dissimilar, e.g., anisocytosis.

anisochromia (an″i-so-kro′me-ah) [*aniso-* + Gr. *chrōma* color] variations in the staining intensity of erythrocytes caused by unequal hemoglobin content.

anisocytosis (an-i″so-si-to′sis) [*aniso-* + Gr. *kytos* hollow vessel + *-osis* condition] a variation in the size of cells, particularly of erythrocytes, that is a common feature of a number of anemias and of cancer cells, which sometimes vary in size well beyond the physiologic limits seen in benign cells.

anisonucleolinosis (an-i″so-nu″kle-o-lin-o′sis) [*aniso-* + L. *nucleoli* small kernels + *-osis* condition] a variation in the size of nucleolini present in the nucleoli of a particular cell type.

anisonucleosis (an-ĭ″so-nu″kle-o′sis) [*aniso-* + *nucleus* kernel, pit + *ōsis* condition] variation in the size of the nuclei of a cell type, found especially in cancer cells.

anisotropic (an-i″so-trop′ik) [*aniso-* + Gr. *tropos* a turning] having unlike properties in different directions; e.g., a doubly refracting crystal has a different index of refraction in the direction of one of the crystal axes from that in the other two directions.

anisotropy (an″i-sot′ro-pe) the quality or condition of being anisotropic (varying in the value of some physical property with the direction in which the measurement is taken).

Anitchkow's cell see *Anichkov's myocyte.*

ankle (ang′k′l) the joint between the leg and the foot; the hinge joint formed between the tibia and fibula and the talus.

ankyl/o (ang′kĭ-lo) [Gr. *ankylos* bent or crooked] a word element used in combining form to denote crooked, bent, or stiff, e.g., ankylosis.

ankyloglossia (ang″kĭ-lo-glos′e-ah) [*ankylo-* + Gr. *glossa* tongue + *-ia*] a congenital malformation that results in an inability to elevate the tip of the tongue because of shortening of the lingual frenum. In North America, this condition affects 1 in 300 children. Treatment is not required in the milder forms, but if the defect interferes with function, the frenum may be clipped. Also called *tongue-tie.*

ankylosing (ang″kĭ-lo′zing) pertaining to ankylosis.

ankylosing spondylitis see *ankylosing s.* under *spondylitis.*

ankylosis (ang″kĭ-lo′sis) [Gr. *ankylōsis,* from *ankyloun* to bend] immobility and consolidation of a joint due to injury, disease, or a surgical procedure; the union of two or more bones that are normally separate.

anlage (ahn′lah-geh, an′lāj), pl. *anlagen* [Ger. "a laying on"] the earliest observable grouping of blast cells from which an organ or tissue develops. Also called *primordium.*

anneal (ah-nel′) [O.E. *anǣlan,* from *an* on + *ǣlan* to kindle] to expose a material or reaction to controlled heating for a specific time, and then to cooling at a predetermined rate. Annealing is used to soften and strengthen certain metals in order to make them less brittle and more easily fabricated or bent. In molecular genetics, the process is used to form hybrid nucleic acid molecules; see *hybridization.*

Annelida (ah-nel′ĭ-dah) [N.L., from *anellus* little ring] a phylum of invertebrates of the sub-kingdom Metazoa, the segmented worms, which have bilateral symmetry and a chitinous body covering. One class, *Hirudinea,* the leeches, is of medical interest as they are parasitic for a number of organisms, including humans.

annellophore (an-nel′o-fōr) [L. *anellus* little ring + Gr. *phoros* bearing] a conidiophore that produces a series of conidia (annellospores), each of which proliferates through the end of the previous spore. The successive ringlike scars give the tip of the conidiophore an annellated appearance. Cf. *phialide* and *sterigma.*

annular (an′u-lar) [L. *annularis,* from *anulus* ring] pertaining to or shaped like an annulus.

annulate lamellae (an′u-lāt lam-el′le) [L. *annulatis*] an occasional cytoplasmic component made up of stacks of membranes exhibiting small pores at regular intervals along their length, believed to represent reduplication of the nuclear envelope.

annulus (an′u-lus), pl. *annuli* [L. "a ring," dim. of *annus* a year, orginally a circuit] 1. a ring; a plane geometric figure bounded by two concentric circles.

2. in cytology, the ring-shaped nuclear pores of plant and animal cells.

3. the ringlike structure at the junction of the middle piece and principal piece of the tail of a mature spermatozoon.

anodal (an-o′dal) pertaining to the anode.

anodal block in nerve conduction studies, a localized conduction block caused by inadvertent placement of the anodal stimulating electrode between the recording electrodes and the cathode. The axolemma becomes hyperpolarized, and the action potential cannot be propagated beyond this point on the nerve. See also *conduction block.*

anode (an′ōd) [Gr. *ana* up + *hodos* way] 1. in an electrochemical cell, the electrode at which the oxidation half-reaction occurs, i.e., the positive electrode in an electrolytic cell and the negative electrode in a voltaic cell.

2. the positive electrode of devices such as electron tubes, x-ray tubes, and electrophoretic cells. In an x-ray tube, vacuum tube, or gas discharge tube, the anode collects the electrons emitted from the cathode. In an x-ray tube, the electrons, which are accelerated to a high speed by the high voltage between the anode and cathode, collide with a small area of the anode, the target (usually made of tungsten), and produce the x-rays. The rest of the anode is a large copper bar, which carries away the large amount of heat produced by stopping the electrons (99 percent of their energy). The x-ray beam is emitted in a direction perpendicular to the electron

stream. The face of the anode is tilted 10°–20° from the beam direction so that the large area of the anode (the electronic focal spot) that the electrons strike produces a narrow beam. The focal spot area as it appears from the beam direction is called the optical focal spot.

3. one of the terminals of a junction diode, silicon-controlled rectifier, or silicon-controlled switch.

rotating a., an x-ray tube anode composed of a tungsten disk about 7.5 cm in diameter attached to a spindle, which is spun at 3000–10,000 rpm. The edge of the disk has a beveled target face. Because the target area moves along the edge of the disk, more heat can be dissipated, and larger kilovoltage and milliamperage can be used than with the stationary anode.

stationary a., an x-ray tube anode composed of a large copper bar with a 2 mm–thick tungsten target set in the beveled end.

anode voltage the voltage between the anode and cathode of a vacuum tube.

anodic stripping voltammetry a variation of polarography in which one of the electrodes is a graphite rod coated with mercury. When negative potential is applied to it, the trace metal ions of the sample are reduced and plate the electrode. The time taken varies with the concentration but is usually 1–30 min. After this a polarogram is recorded with a nonpolarizable cathode and the plated electrode acting as the anode. Oxidation strips the metals off the anode in an order based on each metal's individual redox potential. The current flow is a function of the amount of metal present. This method therefore allows for both qualitative and quantitative measurement of trace metals, and permits very dilute samples to be used owing to the plating step, which further concentrates the sample.

anomalous (ah-nom′ah-lus) [Gr. *anōmalos*] irregular, marked by deviation from the natural order. The term is applied particularly to congenital and hereditary defects.

anomalous innervation a distribution or supply of nerves to a muscle that is aberrant or that deviates from the common pattern. Anomalous innervation is a potential source of confusion in interpretation of findings from nerve conduction studies, and should be suspected when the evoked potentials actually recorded differ from those expected.

anomaly (ah-nom′ah-le) a marked deviation of shape, position, or structure from the normal standard, especially as a result of congenital or hereditary defects. See also *deformation* and *malformation.*

anomer (an′o-mer) [Gr. *ana* up + *meros* part] one of a pair of carbohydrate stereoisomers, e.g., α-D-glucofuranose and β-D-glucofuranose, that differ only in the configuration at the hemiacetal or hemiketal carbon (anomeric carbon) (see the accompanying illustration). Anomers therefore are also epimers and diastereomers. They are designated as α- if the hydroxyl groups on the anomeric carbon and the reference carbon are on the same side in the Fischer projection; otherwise, as β-. See also *Fischer projection.*

anomeric (an″o-mer′ik) pertaining to an anomer.

Anopheles (ah-nof′ĕ-lēz) [Gr. *anōphelēs* hurtful] a genus of mosquitoes characterized by especially long, slender palpi; they are vectors in the transmission of malaria and encephalitis.

anophthalmia (an″of-thal′me-ah) [*an-* neg. + Gr. *ophthalmos* eye + *-ia*] a congenital malformation that results in complete absence of the eye because of the failure of the optic vesicle to form. Anophthalmia is usually associated with other serious craniofacial abnormalities.

Anoplocephalidae (an″o-plo-sĕ-fal′ĭ-de) a family of medium-sized or large tapeworms of the order Cyclophyllidea, subclass Cestoda, that are commonly parasitic in various herbivorous animals and man. Species of medical importance are *Bertiella studeri* and *B. mucronata.*

Anoplura (an″o-plu′rah) [Gr. *anoplos* unarmed + *oura* tail] an order of insects, the sucking lice, characterized by the absence of wings, a compressed body, and mouth parts adapted for piercing and sucking. The species *Pediculus humanus corporis* (body louse), *P. capitis* (head louse), and *Phthirus pubis* (pubic or "crab" louse) frequently infest humans. The body louse in particular is an important carrier of disease; it may transfer trench fever (*Rickettsia quintana*) and epidemic typhus (louse-borne typhus; *Rickettsia* prowazekii) to humans through its bite or feces, or by being crushed on the skin.

anorexia (an′o-rek″se-ah) [Gr. "want of appetite"] the lack or loss of appetite for food. Anorexia may be of psychologic origin, as in anorexia nervosa, or it may occur as a side-effect of some chemotherapeutic treatments for cancer, in renal failure, in ketosis, in hypopituitarism, or during treatment with sympathomimetic amines to suppress appetite in obesity.

anorexia nervosa a condition of unknown cause that is characterized by distorted body image and

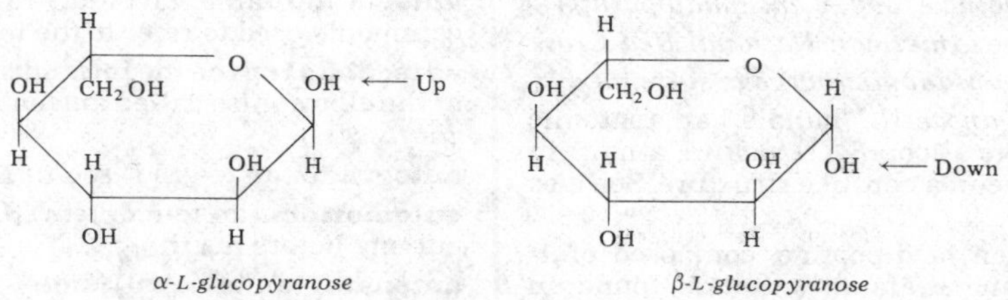

Anomer. α-L-Glucopyranose and β-L-glucopyranose. (From Banks, J. E. Naming Organic Compounds. 2nd ed. Philadelphia, W. B. Saunders Co., 1976.)

extreme refusal to eat, sometimes to the point of death; it occurs most often in females aged 15–30 yr. Those affected experience hunger yet refuse to eat; the hiding of uneaten food and self-induced vomiting are common practices. The individual appears emaciated, develops secondary amenorrhea, and may show laboratory evidence of mineral and vitamin deficiencies, iron deficiency anemia, decreased 17-ketosteroids, and decreased gonadotropin concentration. Initial treatment involves hospital admission to correct the nutritional deficiencies. Long-term psychotherapy is often necessary; relapse is common.

anorexic (an″o-rek′sik) 1. pertaining to anorexia; having no appetite.

2. a drug that suppresses the appetite, prescribed in the treatment of obesity. Amphetamines and some other similar compounds (such as diethylpropion, fenfluramine, and mazindol) affect dopaminergic and serotoninergic neurotransmission and suppress the appetite over a period of a few weeks. It should be noted that there is a risk of abuse with these drugs, and they have no ability to maintain a permanent weight loss. Also called anorectic and anorexigenic.

anoscope (a′no-skōp) [*anus* + Gr. *skopein* to examine] a speculum or endoscope used in direct visual examination of the anal canal.

anosmia (an-oz′me-ah) [*an-* neg. + Gr. *osmē* smell + *-ia*] the absence of the sense of smell.

ANOVA (acronym from *an*alysis *o*f *va*riance) see *analysis of variance.*

anovular (an-ov′ular) [*an-* neg. + L. *ovulum,* dim. of *ovum* egg] not accompanied by the discharge of an ovum.

anovulation (an″ov-u-la′shun) failure to ovulate, resulting in an anovulatory menstrual cycle in which the endometrium shows proliferative changes without an ensuing secretory pattern. The ovarian follicles degenerate instead of being extruded, and the resulting abrupt fall in estrogen levels may disturb the normal rhythm of menstrual flow.

anoxemia (an″ok-se′me-ah) [*an-* neg. + *oxygen* + Gr. *haima* blood + *-ia*] see *hypoxemia.*

anoxia (ah-nok′se-ah) [*an-* neg. + *oxygen* + *-ia*] the absence of oxygen in inspired air, arterial blood, or tissues. The term is sometimes used incorrectly to indicate a condition in which oxygen supply is less than that required for life, in contrast to hypoxia, in which the oxygen supply is lowered but still compatible with life. See also *hypoxia.*

anoxic (ah-nok′sik) pertaining to or characterized by anoxia.

anoxic encephalopathy (ah-nok′sik en-sef″ah-lop′ah-the) see *anoxic e.* under *encephalopathy.*

ANRC abbrev. See *American National Red Cross.*

ANS abbrev. See *autonomic nervous system.*

ansa (an′sah), pl. *ansae* [L. "handle"] an anatomic term used to denote a looplike structure; a hairpin turn or sharp curve in a cordlike structure. See also *loop.*

anserine (an-sēr′ēn) a dipeptide, composed of 1-methylhistidine and α-alanine, that is found in muscle. Its function is not yet understood.

ANSI abbrev. See *American National Standards Institute.*

ant/i (an′ti) [Gr. *anti* against] a word element used in combining form to denote counteracting, effective against, or opposing, e.g., antacid, antiamebic.

Antabuse (an′tah-būs) trademark. See *disulfiram.*

antacid (ant-as′id) [*ant-* + L. *acidus* sour] an agent that partially neutralizes or removes acid from the gastric lumen. Antacids are weak bases divided into two classes, systemic and nonsystemic. The systemic compounds produce metabolic alkalosis. A common agent of this kind is sodium bicarbonate, which titrates part of the acid and thus causes the increase in pH; the sodium is then absorbed. The nonsystemic antacids are those that remove hydrogen ions from the gastric contents; the cation remains insoluble. Calcium carbonate, magnesium, and aluminum salts are commonly used nonsystemic antacids. Antacids increase the gastric pH; above 4.5, pepsin activity is inhibited. The major clinical usage is in the treatment of peptic ulcer and hyperchlorhydria.

antagonism (an-tag′o-nizm) [Gr. *antagōnisma* struggle] opposing action between similar things, as between muscles, medicines, or organisms.

microbial a., the inhibition of one microorganism by another. It can be due to a metabolic competitive action, the effect of by-products such as low pH or E_h, or the production of an antibiotic. Cf. *antibiosis.*

antagonist (an-tag′o-nist) [Gr. *antagōnistēs* an opponent] 1. a muscle that acts in opposition to the action of another muscle, its agonist.

2. a substance that tends to nullify the action of another, particularly a drug that nullifies the action of another drug (an agonist) by competitive binding on the same receptors; e.g., naloxone is an antagonist of morphine. Cf. *agonist.*

antazoline (an-ta-zo′lēn) an antihistamine that has been used as antazoline chloride or antazoline phosphate in the treatment of allergy. It causes drowsiness, dry mouth and throat, and lassitude.

ant bite a bite from ants of the order Hymenoptera, which sting or spray venom into the wound caused by their bite. Stinging ants found in the temperate zones do not produce especially damaging lesions. However, the bite of the fire ant (*Solenopsis saevissima richeteri*), which is found in the southeastern United States, produces intense burning and itching, and the bite of species of the large black ants (*Paraponera clavata*), found in the tropics, produces a lesion with agonizing pain that lasts for several hours. Characteristic alkylated piperidine components of the venom may cause severe immediate and delayed anaphylactic reactions.

ante- (an′te) [L. *ante* before] a prefix word element to denote before or forward in time or place, e.g., antefebrile.

antecubital (an″te-ku′bĭ-tal) in front of the elbow; commonly used to refer to the fossa in this location.

antecubital space the intermuscular space in front of the elbow. Also called antecubital fossa and *cubital fossa.*

antegrade (an′te-grād) see *anterograde.*

antemortem (an″te-mor′tem) [L.] performed or occurring before death.

antenatal (an″te-na′tal) [ante- + L. *natus* born] occurring or formed before birth; during pregnancy.

antenatal diagnosis the diagnosis of genetic defects before birth, using amniocentesis and diagnostic ultrasonography. Ultrasonography is used to locate the fetus and placenta for facilitation of the amniocentesis procedure, to diagnose multiple pregnancies, and to estimate gestational age from fetal biparietal diameter and amniotic fluid volume.

Amniocentesis can be used in a variety of diagnostic procedures. The specimen obtained contains cells from the amnion and fetal skin, as well as the gastrointestinal, respiratory, and urinary tracts. These cells are cultured for karyotyping in order to detect chromosomal aberrations or to determine the fetal sex in cases in which the mother is a carrier of a severe X-linked disorder and there is a 50 percent chance that a male child will be affected.

Chemical analysis can detect certain inborn errors of metabolism; for example, Tay-Sachs disease can be determined from a decreased concentration of hexosaminidase A observed in cultured fetal fibroblasts, and neural tube defects can be identified by an increased concentration of alpha-fetoprotein (AFP) in the amniotic fluid (ultrasonography can demonstrate anencephaly and some other open neural tube defects).

There are many indications for amniocentesis in the diagnosis of potential chromosomal abnormalities, including a maternal age of greater than 35 yr (when there is a significantly increased risk of Down's syndrome), a previous child with a chromosomal abnormality, one parent who is a balanced translocation carrier, and a mother who is a habitual aborter. It is also indicated when the mother is a carrier of a severe X-linked disorder, or when both parents are carriers of an autosomal inborn error of metabolism detectable by amniotic fluid analysis.

Amniocentesis is also performed to assess and evaluate Rh isoimmunization and fetal lung maturity (see also *Rh isoimmunization syndrome* and *lecithin-sphingomyelin ratio*).

Also called *prenatal diagnosis.*

antepartum (an″te-par′tum) [L.] performed or occurring before parturition.

anter/o, anteri/o (an′ter-o, an-ter′ĭ-o) [L. *anterior* before] a word element used in combining form to denote front or before, e.g., anterior.

anterior (an-ter′e-or) [L. "before," neut. of *anterius*] situated in front of or in the forward part of an organ. The term may also refer to the ventral surface of the body.

anterior axillary line the vertical line that passes through the anterior axillary fold.

anterior chamber of the eye that portion of the anterior segment of the eyeball in front of the iris and the pupil. Filled with aqueous humor, it is bounded anteriorly by the cornea and part of the sclera, and posteriorly by the iris, part of the ciliary body, and the portion of the lens present in the pupil.

anterior horn cell a large, multipolar motor neuron found in the anterior (ventral) horns of the spinal cord gray matter. These cells are arranged in columnar groupings that extend longitudinally through particular segments of the cord. The axon of an anterior horn cell emerges from the anterior horn of the cord as an α- or γ-efferent axon.

anterior oblique see *left anterior oblique* or *right anterior oblique.*

anterior perforated substance an important landmark on the ventral surface of the brain that is caudal to the divergence of the medial and lateral olfactory striae at the base of the olfactory trigone. Medially, the substance is bordered by the diagonal band of Broca. Numerous small arteries that arise from the anterior and middle cerebral arteries pierce this substance at the surface of the brain to supply deeper structures. See also *posterior perforated substance.*

anterior superior iliac spine [NA], a blunt projection formed by the anterior end of the iliac crest.

anterograde (an′ter-o-grād″) [*antero-* + L. *gredi* to go] moving or extending forward, such as with the blood flow. Also called *antegrade.* Cf. *retrograde.*

anterolateral (an″ter-o-lat′er-al) pertaining to an oblique radiographic projection in which the central ray passes through a part (e.g., a knee) from the anterior medial surface to the posterior lateral surface.

anteromedial (an″ter-o-me′de-al) pertaining to an oblique radiographic projection in which the central ray passes through a part (e.g., a knee) from the anterior lateral surface to the posterior medial surface.

anteroposterior (AP) (an″ter-o-pos-te′re-or) in radiology, pertaining to a projection made by passing the x-ray beam from front to back through the subject. Cf. *posteroanterior.*

Anthela (an′thĕ-lah) a genus of caterpillars, found in Australia, whose hairs may cause keratoconjunctivitis.

anthelix (ant′he-liks) [*ant-* + Gr. *helix* coil] [NA], a semicircular prominence of the external ear, parallel and anterior to the helix on the lateral aspect of the pinna.

anthelmintic (ant″hel-min′tik) [*ant-* + Gr. *helmins* worm] destructive to worms; an agent that destroys worms.

anthelmycin (an-thel-mi′sin) an antibiotic substance produced by *Streptomyces longissimus,* which is destructive to worms.

anthocyanidin (an″tho-si-an′ĭ-din) a glucoside of cellobiose prepared from dried fruit and flower products, which is used in histology as a nuclear stain. These dried products, which are extracted from the same plants as the anthocyanins, are added to slightly acidic water for use. Cf. *anthocyanin.*

anthocyanin (an″tho-si′ah-nin) [Gr. *anthos* flower + *kyanos* blue] any of a group of fruit and flower pigments, usually glucosides of glucose, that are used in histology as nuclear stains. Chief among these are myrtillus from the juice of the European whortleberry (*Vaccinum myrtilus*) and sambucin from the juice of the black elderberry (*Sambucus niger*). Cf. *anthocyanidin.*

Anthomyia (an″tho-mi′yah) a genus of small black houseflies. Two species of medical importance were formerly assigned to this genus; see under *Fannia.*

anthrac/o (an′thrah-ko) [Gr. *anthrax* coal] a word element used in combining form to denote coal dust, e.g., anthracosis.

anthracene (an′thrah-sēn) 1. a colorless, crystalline hydrocarbon, $C_6H_4(CH)_2C_6H_4$, which is derived from coal tar and used in the manufacture of anthracene dyes. Large anthracene crystals have also been used in scintillation detectors to detect beta radiation.

2. a ptomaine obtained from cultures of *Bacillus anthracis.*

anthracene blue a mordant dye that may be used as an aluminum lake in place of alum hematoxylin in histologic stainings; it may also be used instead of carmine in Best's carmine procedure for glycogen.

anthracometer (an″thrah-kom′ĕ-ter) [*anthraco-* + Gr. *metron* measure] an instrument for measuring carbon dioxide in the air.

anthracosilicosis (an″thrah-ko-sil″ĭ-ko′sis) [*anthraco-* + *silicon* + *-osis*] an occupational lung disease caused by inhalation of coal dust (anthracosis) and fine particles of silica (silicosis). It is sometimes encountered in anthracite coal miners. See also *anthracosis* and *silicosis.*

anthracosis (an-thrah-kō′sĭs) [*anthraco-* + *-osis*] a form of pneumoconiosis caused by accumulation of carbon dust in the lungs. The carbon dust drains into the alveolar macrophages and lymphatic channels, blackening them. Present in most urban dwellers, carbon dust does not impair respiration or predispose to infection.

When coal dust, a form of carbon dust, accumulates in large amounts in the lungs of coal workers, it may result in a form of anthracosis called *coal worker's pneumoconiosis* (CWP). This condition is characterized by focal emphysema and pulmonary fibrosis, the result of long-term exposure to coal dust; diffuse nodular pulmonary deposition of the coal dust results in the formation of "coal macules" along the respiratory bronchioles.

Diagnosis is based on a patient history of more than 15 yr in the mining industry and an x-ray pattern of widely spaced small nodules. CWP may progress to a disabling chronic obstructive pulmonary disease, with progressive fibrosis, massive distortion of lung structure, and functional impairment.

Also called *black lung disease.*

anthracotic (an″thrah-kot′ik) pertaining to or affected with anthracosis.

anthracotic pigment a black pigment composed of inhaled particulate material, predominantly carbon, that accumulates in the lungs and regional lymph nodes of urban dwellers. Grossly, the involved tissues appear black, but there is usually no significant inflammatory response to the pigment. See also *anthracosis.*

anthracycline cardiotoxicity damage to the myocardium caused by administration of an anthracycline drug, notably doxorubicin (Adriamycin). The cardiotoxic effects are dose-related and may lead to heart failure and death. Attempts to limit the toxicity by restricting the cumulative dose (to 550 mg/m^2) lead to underutilization of the drug in individuals who could tolerate considerably higher doses, and fail to protect those who develop cardiotoxicity at a lower dose. Noninvasive methods have shown limited reliability in monitoring the cardiac function of patients receiving anthracyclines; endomyocardial biopsy via the transvenous route with grading by electron microscopy is currently the most effective procedure for detecting and quantitating myocardial muscle fiber alterations and determining the level at which administration of the drug should be discontinued. Myocardial damage can be significantly reduced by lowering the peak plasma levels through continuous intravenous infusion of Adriamycin over a 1- to 4-da period. Also called Adriamycin cardiomyopathy and anthracycline cardiomyopathy.

anthrapurpurin a mordant dye; C.I. 58255. Although used principally as a histologic reagent for calcium, it is also employed as a nuclear stain. Anthrapurpurin forms scarlet lakes with aluminum and calcium.

anthrax (an′thraks) [Gr. *anthrax* coal, carbuncle] a disease caused by *Bacillus anthracis,* primarily in domestic animals. Human infection, rare in the United States, sometimes occurs in workers who come into contact with contaminated animal wool or hides. Wool-sorter's disease is a pulmonary infection acquired by inhalation of, or from contact with, spores on wool. Cutaneous infection, highlighted clinically by the presence of a "malignant pustule," results from the contact of broken skin with contaminated hides.

anthropo- (an′thro-po) [Gr. *anthrōpos* man] a word element used in combining form to denote relationship to man or to a human being, e.g., anthropoid.

anthropoid (an′thro-poid) [*anthropo-* + Gr. *eidos* shape] a term used to describe the apelike pelvis, which has an oval pelvic inlet with a long anteroposterior dimension and a narrow transverse diameter. This pattern is found in approximately 28 percent of all females.

anthropomorphism (an″thro-po-mor′fizm) [*anthropo-* + Gr. *morphē* form] the attribution of human characteristics to nonhuman objects.

anthroponoses diseases that now occur only in humans, but which originally began as diseases in other species.

anthropozoonosis (an″thro-po-zo″o-no′sis) a disease of either humans or animals that may be transmitted from one species to another, e.g., an infection, such as anthrax, rabies, or brucellosis, that may be passed to humans from other vertebrates.

antiallotype (an″te-al′o-tīp) in immunology, the antibodies formed in response to allotype antigens, either as blood cells, blood proteins, or other tissues. These antibodies are found predominantly in infants, occasionally in healthy adults, and more frequently in persons who have received multiple blood transfusions. Severe reactions have occurred to blood transfusions containing antibodies to allotypes of IgA.

antianxiety (an″te-ang-zi′ĕ-te) dispelling anxiety; anxiolytic.

antianxiety drug a sedative-hypnotic drug prescribed for the treatment of anxiety; those most commonly prescribed are the benzodiazepines, diazepam (Valium), and chlordiazepoxide (Librium). Phenobarbital and meprobamate have also been used for anxiety, but both can produce tolerance and physical dependence; phenothiazine major tranquilizers and tricyclic antidepressants are also given. Also called *anxiolytic* and *minor tranquilizer.*

antiarrhythmic agent (an″tĭ-ah-rith′mik) a drug, such as lidocaine, procainamide, quinidine, propranolol, and disopyramide, used in the treatment of cardiac arrhythmias.

antibacterial (an″tĭ-bak-te′re-al) 1. destroying or suppressing the growth of bacteria.

2. an agent that destroys or suppresses the growth of bacteria.

antibacterial agents chemicals that destroy or inhibit the growth of bacteria in concentrations not significantly injurious to the host; consequently, they can be used as chemotherapeutic agents to prevent and treat bacterial infections. Most of the clinically useful antibacterial drugs are produced by microorganisms; these are the antibiotics. Some antibiotics or their core structures can be modified chemically to add or augment one or more desirable property. These are known as semisynthetic antibiotics, and many of them have lower toxicity, greater resistance to destruction by stomach acidity, better absorption from the gut, or a broader spectrum of susceptible species than the parent molecule. Some of the useful antibacterial agents, however, do not come from microorganisms but have been synthesized entirely in the chemical laboratory, e.g., sulfonamides.

MECHANISMS OF ACTION. Antibacterial agents act either by interfering with a normal function of the cell or by damaging its structural integrity. Vulnerable functions and sites include folic acid, cell wall, protein, and nucleic acid synthesis; cell membrane integrity; and some phases of carbohydrate metabolism.

FOLIC ACID SYNTHESIS. Folic acid is an essential cofactor for both human and bacterial cells, which must have it to synthesize purines and, ultimately, DNA. Whereas humans can absorb preformed folic acid from the diet, most bacteria lack this capacity and thus must synthesize the cofactor themselves. Sulfonamides are structurally related to *p*-aminobenzoic acid (PABA), which is a precursor of folic acid. The resemblance is so close that sulfonamides compete with PABA as a substrate for the enzyme tetrahydropteroic acid synthetase, which catalyzes a necessary step in building folic acid. An interesting and important advance in chemotherapy occurred when it was discovered that another synthetic antibacterial, trimethoprim, inhibits in similar manner another step in folic acid synthesis, catalyzed by dihydrofolate reductase. Double sequential blockage by these folic acid antagonists results in a synergistic action and affects a broad spectrum of microorganisms (see *sulfonamide* and *trimethoprim*).

CELL WALL SYNTHESIS. A number of commonly used antibiotics inhibit one of the steps in the biosynthesis of peptidoglycan, the structure that makes bacterial cell walls rigid. The synthesis of this complex molecule involves several steps: synthesis of precursors, attachment of those precursors to a membrane lipid carrier, lining up polymers outside the cell membrane, and cross-linking polymers to form a three-dimensional network.

The penicillin and cephalosporin groups of antibiotics block the cross-linking steps, which results in growth inhibition rather than cell death. The exact mechanism by which penicillins and cephalosporins kill growing cells is not completely understood, but lysis of bacterial cells by penicillin is known to be dependent on the presence of one or more autolytic enzymes. When the activity of lytic enzymes is blocked, penicillin is only bacteriostatic.

Other antibiotics affect cell wall synthesis by a variety of mechanisms. Cycloserine is a structural analog of D-alanine, a component of the peptidoglycan tetrapeptide, and blocks two consecutive steps involving D-alanine. Fosfomycin, a structural analog of phosphoenolpyruvate, inhibits the first stage of peptidoglycan synthesis by interfering with the synthesis of cell wall precursors. Although it has no clinical use, fosfomycin is a valuable research tool. Vancomycin blocks elongation of the peptidoglycan backbone, whereas bacitracin prevents conversion of an inactive form of the lipid carrier to the active form.

All the antibiotics named above inhibit cell wall synthesis by interfering in some way with building up the structure of the essential component, peptidoglycan. However, there is a synthetic compound, isoniazid, that has quite a different mechanism of affecting cell wall synthesis. It inhibits the synthesis of mycolic acids, which are part of the outer layer of the peptidoglycan cell wall of mycobacteria and certain other related bacteria, and has a lethal effect. The specificity and the consequences of this mechanism explain why isoniazid is an effective chemotherapeutic agent for tuberculosis—but only for TB and a few other diseases caused by mycolic acid–containing species.

Polymyxins are antibiotics that act like cationic detergents by damaging cell membranes so that there is leakage of cytoplasmic constituents. They also bind to the lipopolysaccharide of gram-negative organisms; this property may explain why gram-negative organisms are more susceptible than gram-positive organisms.

PROTEIN SYNTHESIS. This action takes place on ribosomes involving translation, through transfer RNA, of a messenger RNA (mRNA) sequence into a corresponding polypeptide sequence. The ribosomes of bacterial cells have a sedimentation constant of 70S, and consist of two subunits with sedimentation constants of 50S and 30S (in contrast to the 80S, with 60S and 40S subunits, of eukaryotic ribosomes). In general, the antibiotic susceptibility of ribosomes of eukaryotic mitochondria resembles that of bacteria.

A number of antibiotics inhibit protein synthesis by binding to specific sites on the ribosomes. Tetracycline, for example, binds to the 30S subunits and blocks the attachment of aminoacyl transfer RNA to the acceptor site on the messenger RNA–ribosome complex. Chloramphenicol and clindamycin, however, bind to the 50S subunit and block peptide transfer to the growing polypeptide. Erythromycin acts in a third manner by binding to free ribosomes; this allows initiation of protein synthesis but not elongation of polypeptide chains. Finally, there are the various aminoglycosides which, although they do not bind to identical sites, characteristically cause misreading of the messenger RNA code.

NUCLEIC ACID SYNTHESIS. Nalidixic acid, a synthetic compound used for the treatment of urinary tract infections, inactivates an enzyme involved in DNA replication. This mechanism differs from that of the rifamycin antibiotics (including the semisynthetic derivative rifampin). These prevent initiation of the transcription of DNA into RNA by inhibiting bacterial RNA polymerase. It is important to note that the rifamycins do not inhibit eukaryotic RNA polymerase, because this selective action is lacking in certain other agents that also interfere with DNA replication or transcription, such as actinomycin or mitomycin. Because these antibiotics inhibit nucleic acid synthesis in both eukaryotic cells and bacterial cells, they cannot be used as antibacterial agents.

An entirely different mode of action is exhibited

Antibacterial Agents. Classification of Antibacterial Agents by Mode of Action

Mechanism of Action	Agent
Inhibition of folic acid synthesis	Dapsone Sulfonamides Trimethoprim
Damage to cell wall	Bacitracin Cephalosporins Cephamycins Cycloserine Penicillins Vancomycin
Damage to cell membrane	Polymixins
Inhibition of protein synthesis	Aminoglycosides Chloramphenicol Clindamycin Erythromycin Spectinomycin Tetracycline
Inhibition of nucleic acid synthesis	Nalidixic acid Rifampin
Other	
Inhibition of mycolic acid synthesis	Isoniazid
Interference with carbohydrate metabolism	Nitrofurantoin

by the synthetic urinary tract agent, nitrofurantoin. This drug interferes with early stages of bacterial carbohydrate metabolism by inhibiting coenzyme A.

In the accompanying table, the most important antibacterial agents are arranged according to their mode of action. For descriptions of the agents, see the specific entries.

Development of Resistance. Resistance to antibiotic agents may arise in two ways: (1) by genetic transfer of extrachromosomal DNA, called plasmids or episomes, which carry the genes for new enzymes; and (2) by a mutation that alters a cell constituent in a manner that favors the selection of resistant organisms. The former mechanism of resistance may result in multiple drug resistance owing to the existence of multiple genes on the extrachromosomal element.

Plasmids. Genetic elements controlling resistance are called resistance or R factors. These consist of two components, the R determinant for drug resistance and the resistance transfer factor (RTF), which is responsible for transfer of the R determinant. Bacterial conjugation is required for transfer of R factors and is mediated by specific pili determined by genes on the plasmid. The role of R factors in resistance to antibiotics has clinical significance in that transfer of drug resistance can occur within the human intestinal tract by a variety of organisms. The growth of organisms carrying R factors is favored when exposure to antibiotics occurs. Several drug-resistance determinants can be transferred on R factors, including resistance to the aminoglycosides, sulfonamides, chloramphenicol, tetracyclines, and ampicillin.

Enzymatic inactivation of aminoglycosides, chloramphenicol, and penicillins is mediated by transferable plasmids. Enzymes that destroy penicillins or cephalosporins, called beta-lactamases, hydrolyze the beta-lactam ring of penicillin or cephalosporin molecules, rendering them inactive. Beta-lactamases have different affinities for the different types of penicillins or cephalosporins. In gram-negative bacteria, resistance to penicillin can be mediated by either chromosomal genes (mutation) or extrachromosomal genes (plasmid). The important mechanism of resistance in clinical isolates, however, is that of R factor–mediated beta-lactamase production.

Aminoglycosides may be enzymatically modified so that they can no longer interact with their target. Inactivation occurs by acetylation of amino groups, or phosphorylation or adenylation of hydroxyl groups. Chloramphenicol resistance occurs as a result of the presence of a plasmid coding for an inactivating enzyme, chloramphenicol acetyltransferase.

Mutations to resistance occur with a frequency of 1 in 10^5–10^{10} cell divisions, depending on the bacterial species and the antibacterial agent. Resistance results from alterations in the metabolism or structure of the cell, the degree of resistance varying with the nature of the change and the species. Mechanisms of mutational resistance include decreased permeability to the drug, modification of the bacterial receptor site for the drug, and increased synthesis of an essential metabolite whose structure is sufficiently related to that of the drug to compete with it for a specific receptor site.

Decreased permeability is an important mechanism in resistance to sulfonamides or tetracyclines. Modification of the drug receptor site may lead to resistance to penicillins, cephalosporins, streptomycin, erythromycin, rifampin, sulfonamides, and trimethoprim. An increase in the concentration of *p*-aminobenzoic acid results in resistance to sulfonamides.

Synergism and Antagonism. Synergism is observed when the combined effect of two antibacterial agents is greater than the sum of their independent activities. For example, the combination of a penicillin with an aminoglycoside is synergistic in vitro against a variety of organisms. The exact mechanism of synergy between penicillin and aminoglycosides in unclear, although it may involve enhanced penetration of the aminoglycoside into a bacterium whose cell wall has been damaged by penicillin. An example of the use of penicillin-aminoglycoside combinations is in the treatment of enterococcal endocarditis.

Sulfonamides and trimethoprim, as stated above, are synergistic because they inhibit sequential steps in the bacterial folic acid synthetic pathway. This combination has several clinical uses, such as in the treatment of urinary tract infections for which high concentrations and combined actions are needed to achieve good clinical results.

Antagonism is observed when the combined effect of two antibacterial agents is less than the sum of their independent effects. Antagonism has been observed in vitro with combinations of penicillin and tetracycline or penicillin and chloramphenicol. However, there are only a few well-documented clinical reports of in vivo antagonism in the medical literature.

The effectiveness of antibacterial combinations may be evaluated in the laboratory by testing multiple "checkerboard" combinations of drugs, using a broth dilution method.

See also *bacteria, aminoglycosides, cephalosporins, macrolides, nitrofurans, penicillin, polyene antibiotics, polymyxins, sulfonamide, tetracyclines*, and the individual antibiotics and antibacterial agents.

antibacterial agent susceptibility testing the use of methods such as agar and broth dilution tests, disk diffusion tests, and automated procedures to evaluate the in vitro susceptibility of an isolated pathogen to a variety of antibacterial agents. Because of their simplicity and adaptability, disk diffusion tests are commonly used in the routine laboratory.

Dilution Tests. In agar or broth dilution tests, serial dilutions of an antibacterial agent are prepared in agar or broth, respectively, and are inoculated with a suspension of a known concentration of a microorganism. Following incubation, the lowest concentration at which there is no visible growth is determined. This concentration is referred to as the minimum (or minimal) inhibitory concentration (MIC). The agar dilution test can conveniently test a number of strains simultaneously and can easily detect bacterial contamination.

A minimal bactericidal (or lethal) concentration (MBC or MLC) can be determined from broth dilution tests by subculturing to antibiotic-free agar from tubes showing no visible growth after overnight incubation. The lowest concentration of a drug that kills more than 99.9 percent of the initial inoculum is defined as the MBC (or MLC).

There are some problems with broth dilution tests. They are unsuitable for the testing of sulfonamides and trimethoprim because susceptible organisms go through several generations before inhibition, leading to obscuring of the end point. When the preferable agar dilution test is performed, a medium free of antagonists of sulfonamide and trimethoprim activity, such as thymidine, thymidine phosphorylase, *p*-aminobenzoic acid, or lysed horse blood, should be used.

Broth dilution tests with aminoglycosides against *Pseudomonas aeruginosa* may yield low MIC values because of low concentrations of magnesium and calcium ions in broth media, including Mueller-Hinton broth. The media may be supplemented to physiologic levels with filter-sterilized calcium and magnesium salts.

Dilution studies of *Staphylococcus aureus* with beta-lactamase–resistant antibiotics (such as methicillin, oxacillin, or nafcillin) should be incubated at 35°C to detect resistant strains.

Combinations of two drugs (synergistic studies) may be tested by preparing tubes of broth containing selected combinations of the two drugs. After overnight incubation, tubes with no visible growth are subcultured to antibiotic-free media to determine the MBC (or MLC) of the different combinations.

Generally, a microorganism is considered to be susceptible if the MIC is at least two to four times less than the average peak blood concentration of an antibacterial agent. Uncomplicated urinary tract infections respond to urine levels of antibiotics rather than to blood levels.

Microtitration techniques for determining MICs have been developed and are miniaturized versions of the broth dilution procedure performed in test tubes. Such techniques conveniently test a number of antibiotics against a single organism. Automated methods for preparation of microtitration plates containing antibiotics are available. Prepared plates can also be obtained commercially.

Disk Diffusion Test. In the disk diffusion test of Bauer, Kirby, Sherris, and Turck, agar plates are inoculated with a standardized suspension of a microorganism. Antibiotic-containing disks are applied to the agar surface. Following overnight incubation, the diameters of the zones of inhibition or clearing surrounding the disks are measured. Zone diameters are interpreted as sensitive (susceptible), indeterminate (or intermediate), or resistant. Different zone standards have been established for each drug, based on a linear relationship between MIC and zone diameter and on the averge peak serum level of the antibiotic.

The different disks used for the disk diffusion test should represent a member of each of the different groups of antibiotics in clinical use. Staphylococci must be tested with both a penicillinase-labile penicillin (e.g., benzylpenicillin) and a penicillinase-resistant penicillin (e.g., nafcillin or oxacillin). Test strains of gram-negative bacilli should include *Pseudomonas* species and selected Enterobacteriaceae. Cephalothin should be included as a representative of the cephalosporin group of antibiotics. Because of their extended spectrum of activity, cefamandole and cefoxitin disks should be used against selected isolates resistant to the remaining cephalosporins.

Cross-resistance between aminoglycosides occurs but has frequent exceptions; therefore, separate testing of aminoglycosides, such as gentamicin and

ANTIBACTERIAL AGENT SUSCEPTIBILITY TESTING

Gram-positive Organisms		Gram-negative Bacilli	
Staphylococcus	*Enterococcus*	*Enterobacteriaceae*	*Pseudomonas*
Cephalothin	Ampicillin	Ampicillin	Carbenicillin
Chloramphenicol	Cephalothin	Cefamandole	Chloramphenicol
Clindamycin	Chloramphenicol	Cefoxitin	Gentamicin
Erythromycin	Erythromycin	Cephalothin	Tetracycline
Gentamicin	Penicillin G	Chloramphenicol	Sulfonamides
Methicillin	Tetracycline	Gentamicin	Tobramycin
Penicillin G		Nalidixic acid*	
Tetracycline		Nitrofurantoin*	
Vancomycin		Sulfonamides*	
		Tetracycline	
		Tobramycin	
		Trimethoprim	
		Sulfamethoxazole	

* Used in the treatment of urinary tract infections.

tobramycin, may be indicated for selected isolates. Aminoglycoside alternatives (such as amikacin), to which resistance is infrequent, may be held in reserve for selected isolates. Tetracycline is the representative of the tetracycline group of antibiotics. Lincomycin and clindamycin can be used interchangeably. A suggested battery of antibacterial agents that can be used for routine susceptibility testing of clinical isolates is shown in the accompanying table.

Adherence to procedures established in 1979 by the National Committee for Clinical Laboratory Standards (NCCLS), and to strict quality control using recommended strains of *Pseudomonas aeruginosa, S. aureus,* and *Escherichia coli,* is essential.

There are limitations to the disk diffusion procedure. The technique has been standardized only for microorganisms that grow rapidly on the standard medium (Mueller-Hinton broth). Fastidious, slow-growing organisms cannot be tested with the standardized disk diffusion test because the results are not applicable. Standardized NCCLS modifications of the disk diffusion test do exist and are available for testing *Hemophilus influenzae, Neisseria gonorrhoeae,* and *Streptococcus pneumoniae.*

Disk diffusion test results may not be applicable to body fluids other than serum, e.g., spinal fluid or urine. Broth or agar dilution techniques should be employed to obtain precise, quantitative information. The disk diffusion test does not measure bactericidal activity; such information may be important in neutropenic or in otherwise immune-compromised individuals, or in those with endocarditis. In these situations, the broth dilution test may be performed; this yields both MIC and MBC (or MLC) values.

AUTOMATED TESTS. Automated systems for susceptibility testing are capable of yielding either MIC results or interpretive results (such as susceptible, intermediate, or resistant), or both. Automated systems utilize either light scattering or optical density measurements of growth in the presence of antimicrobial agents. Several systems have been extensively evaluated in collaborative studies: Autovac, MS-2, and Auto Microbic. Automated methods for preparation of microtitration plates for broth dilution tests are also available.

TESTING OF ANAEROBES. Susceptibility testing of anaerobes is indicated for isolates from individuals with endocarditis, brain abscesses, or infections requiring prolonged therapy (e.g., osteomyelitis), or in infections that are persistent or recurrent despite appropriate antimicrobial therapy. Agar dilution methods are currently recommended as a reference method. Broth dilution methods are available, as are broth disk methods for laboratories that cannot perform agar or broth dilution.

Antibiotics that should be tested against anaerobes are carbenicillin, cefoxitin, chloramphenicol, clindamycin, and penicillin. Aminoglycosides are generally inactive against anaerobes.

SPECIAL PROCEDURES. Some special procedures may be of use during therapy. These include: (1) measurement of bactericidal activity of an antibiotic (MBC or MLC); (2) determination of the effect of drug combinations (synergistic studies); (3) measurement of therapeutic levels of antibiotics; (4) measurement of the bactericidal activity of patient serum against the isolated pathogen (serum bactericidal level of Schlichter test); and (5) determination of beta-lactamase production by a clinical isolate.

Combinations of antibacterial agents are often used to treat enterococcal endocarditis or serious gram-negative infections. The activity of drugs in combination is determined by testing multiple combinations of drugs in broth. A combination is synergistic when the effect observed is greater than the sum of the effects observed with the two drugs independently. A combination is additive (indifferent) when the combined effect equals the sum of the effects produced by the drugs independently, or is equal only to that of the most active drug in the combination. Antagonistic combinations are combinations that are less effective than the most active drug alone.

ASSAYS. A number of methods, such as biologic, immunologic, enzymatic, and chromatographic assays, are available for the assay of antibacterial agents in biologic fluids. Biologic assays can be performed with minimal equipment and at low cost, but require 2–4 hr to perform. Rapid results can be provided by immunologic and enzymatic assays. Peak and trough samples are required, and aminoglycoside levels must be monitored, as discussed previously.

The Schlichter test is often used to measure serum bactericidal levels in patients being treated with one or more antibiotics. Dilutions of the serum are tested against the individual's own infecting organism. Bactericidal activity in serum is measured by subculturing the contents of the clear tubes to antibiotic-free medium. Samples are obtained just before an antibiotic dose (trough) and when the peak level is expected (usually 15–30 min after an intravenous infusion and about 1 hr after an intramuscular injection). Generally, peak bactericidal dilutions of 1:3 or more are desirable in bacterial endocarditis.

Several tests are available for determining beta-lactamase production in *S. aureus, H. influenzae,* and *N. gonorrhoeae.* The acidometric method is based on an increased acidity observed when the beta-lactam ring is hydrolyzed to yield a carboxyl group. In the rapid iodometric method, a starch-iodine mixture is decolorized as a result of the ability of the penicilloic acid to reduce iodine. A third method involves the production of a colored substance from a chromogenic cephalosporin substrate.

antibiosis (an″tĭ-bi-o′sis) [*anti-* + Gr. *bios* life] a type of microbial antagonism resulting from the production of an antibiotic by one member of a mixed microbial population. It is a natural dynamic process in distinction to the addition of a cell-free antibiotic substance to susceptible microorganisms. Cf. *microbial a.* under *antagonism.*

antibiotic (an″ti-bi-ot′ik) [*anti-* + Gr. *bios* life] 1. destructive of life.

2. a chemical substance produced by living microorganisms, which has the capacity, in dilute solutions, to inhibit the growth of or to kill other microorganisms. Antibiotics such as penicillin, which are sufficiently nontoxic to the host, are used as chemotherapeutic agents in the treatment of infectious diseases in humans, animals, and plants. Antibiotic substances usually do not destroy viruses, and are also added to specimens to be examined for viruses in order to suppress bacterial growth.

Some antibiotics are capable of chemical modification with improvement in antibacterial or pharmacologic properties, e.g., semisynthetic penicillins.

The clinically useful antibiotics can be classified into groups according to the mechanism of action: (1) folic acid synthesis inhibitors (sulfonamides and trimethoprim); (2) cell wall synthesis inhibitors (penicillins, cephalosporins, cephamycins, vancomycin, and bacitracin); (3) cell membrane inhibitors (polymyxins); (4) protein synthesis inhibitors (aminocyclitols, which include aminoglycosides and spectinomycin, tetracyclines, erythromycin, clindamycin, and chloramphenicol); and (5) nucleic acid inhibitors (nalidixic acid, rifampin).

For more information, see *antibacterial agents* and the individual antibiotics.

antibiotic antitumor drugs see *actinomycin D, dactinomycin,* and *mithramycin.*

antibody (an″tĭ-bod″e) a glycopeptide found in the serum, which may be either native or foreign to the host. It is capable of binding specifically to a wide array of natural and synthetic antigens, including proteins, carbohydrates, nucleic acids, lipids, or other chemicals. Antibodies consist of four polypeptide chains: two heavy or H chains (M.W. 50,000–70,000), and two light or L chains (M.W. 25,000). These are joined by disulfide bonds to form a four-chain basic structure. Each chain is subdivided by intrachain disulfide links that fold the chains into domains. The amino terminal domain of H and L chains is responsible for antigen binding and structurally shows a high degree of variability, giving rise to its name of the variable, or V, domain. The other domains show considerable homology of sequence between molecules and have been called constant, or C, domains. The constant regions are responsible for determining the immunoglobulin class or light-chain type, as well as the biologic function of the molecule. For example, complement fixation takes place on the second constant domain. The subscripts H and L are added to denote heavy- and light-chain domains; on the H chain, the C domains are numbered starting from the amino terminal.

At the junction of the C_H1 and C_H2 domains lies a distinct sequence of amino acids that forms a flexible region called the hinge region. Papain, a proteolytic enzyme, cleaves the H chain at this site to produce the Fab and Fc fragments.

The unique structure of the antibody molecule produces two antigen-binding sites per molecule, giving the antibody the ability to cross-link and agglutinate antigens. The individual antigen specificity seen in antibodies is due to variation in the amino acid sequence in certain regions of the V domain. There are three of these "hypervariable" regions in the V_L domain and four in the V_H domain. Amino acid substitutions within these hypervariable regions determine the antigen specificity and are detectable as "idiotypes," or unique antigenic determinants on the molecule. The origin of the diversity of these variables sequences is debatable, but there is evidence that at least some of the sequences are coded by V region genes, which are located on the same chromosome as the C region genes. The two groups are separated by a long stretch of DNA, and synthesis of an antibody molecule requires splicing the genes together. Other theories accounting for the variability propose that mutations occur during ontogeny, giving rise to the almost limitless diversity observed.

The amino acid sequences of the variable region determine not only antigenic specificity but also the binding affinity. The affinity is a measure of the strength of the binding between antibodies (Ab) and antigens (Ag): $Ab + Ag \rightleftarrows AbAg$. The association constant, or affinity (K), is $K = \frac{AbAg}{(Ab)(Ag)}$. The affinity of antibodies for antigens is heterogeneous and is dependent on factors such as temperature, pH, and the ionic strength of the solvent.

The exquisite specificity and the high affinity of Ag-Ab interactions, coupled with the unique ability of antibodies to cross-link antigens, are utilized in many routine laboratory tests, such as immunodiffusion, blood typing, and hemagglutination assays. These tests rely on the ability of the antibody to identify substances specifically and to cause a visible reaction such as precipitation in gels, or agglutination as in blood typing.

Antibodies are produced by a subpopulation of

lymphocytes known as B cells, which arise in the bone marrow and then migrate to other locations in the host such as the spleen, lymph nodes, or Peyer's patches of the gut. The first antibodies are of the IgM class, followed by IgG and IgA. The B lymphocytes exist in these organs in a resting state until the appropriate antigen comes into contact with the cells. Then, in a process that often involves other lymphocytes known as T cells, as well as macrophages, the B cell is induced to proliferate and mature to an antibody-secreting plasma cell.

On first contact with an antigen, this process takes a minimum of 3–4 da and results in production of an IgM antibody. As this primary response continues, two phenomena are observed. With time, the affinity of the antisera for the antigen increases, and the IgM produced may switch to IgG. Each B cell makes antibodies of only one specificity but may change the H-chain class while retaining the same specificity. On secondary challenge with the same antigen, a different response is observed. Production of antibody is seen much sooner, in response to a lower dose of antigen, and more antibody is produced over a longer period. The antibody made in this secondary response is usually IgG.

See also *immunoglobulin.*

BRUCE RICHARDSON, M.D., PH.D.

antibody-dependent cell-mediated cytotoxicity (ADCC) an important type of cell-mediated immunity (CMI) in which antibodies or antigen-antibody complexes bind macrophages to target cells promoting cell-mediated cytotoxicity. In addition to macrophages, immature and mature neutrophils, immature monocytes, eosinophils, and null or K cells can also bind to target cells coated with antibody, and exert cytotoxic effects. T cells are not directly involved in this process; their only involvement is the role of helper T cells in producing antibody. Cytolysis occurs primarily by direct cell contact, or, with mature macrophages and neutrophils, by phagocytosis.

In ADCC involving macrophages, neutrophils, and K cells, IgG antibodies (all subclasses) bind the killer cell to the target cell; opsonic binding (to the target cells first) is 10,000 times as effective as cytophilic binding (to the killer cells first). In ADCC involving basophils and eosinophils, homocytophilic antibodies bind first to the Fc receptors of the killer cells. ADCC can also be mediated by preformed immune complexes, as in ADCC of schistosomes by macrophages mediated by IgE complexes.

See also *cell-mediated immunity.*

antibody detection in testing blood-group antibodies, the identification of erythrocyte antibodies that are responsible for incompatibility in antibody screening and crossmatching. Several different temperatures and suspending mediums are used. Common techniques include the antiglobulin test, enzyme technique, high-protein (albumin) technique, low-ionic-strength medium test (LISS), and saline technique. Antibody screening routinely includes the following steps: a saline incubation at room temperature, a saline or albumin incubation at 37°C, the antiglobulin test performed on the incubated (37°C) saline and albumin samples, and, if required, the enzyme technique. The red blood cells used for antibody detection are from group O donors and contain as many common antigens as possible, including Rh, MNs, Lewis, Duffy, Kell, Kidd, Lutheran, and P.

ANTIGLOBULIN TEST. For details of this procedure, see *antiglobulin tests.*

ENZYME TECHNIQUE. This is a one- or two-stage technique that enhances antibody-antigen reactions. It is useful in detecting weak blood-group antibodies, such as Rh, Kidd, Lewis, and P, which are sometimes missed with routine methods. Enzymes may damage other blood-group determinants, such as MNs and Duffy, and therefore fail to detect them, as well as enhance cold autoagglutinins. In the one-stage procedure, used for screening, identification, and crossmatching, the enzyme is mixed directly with the cells and serum and incubated at 37°C, the cells washed, and the solution tested with antiglobulin serum. The two-stage technique, a more sensitive but time-consuming procedure for the detection and identification of antibodies, involves pretreating the red cells with the enzyme, reacting these cells with the test serum, and incubating, washing, and testing with antiglobulin serum as in the one-stage technique. The commonly used enzymes include bromelain, trypsin, papain, ficin, and multienzyme preparations. See also *a. of erythrocyte antibodies* under *absorption, antibody identification, elution,* and *titration technique.*

HIGH-PROTEIN TECHNIQUE. This is a test that uses bovine albumin to enhance the agglutination of warm-reacting antibodies (IgG and complement-binding IgM). Bovine albumin is added to a tube containing a mixture of serum and a 2–5 percent suspension of erythrocytes. The mixture is incubated at 37°C, centrifuged, and read for agglutination. As albumin can also enhance rouleaux formation, microscopic examination of the sample is required. Albumin can also suppress hemolysis.

LOW-IONIC-STRENGTH MEDIUM TEST (LISS). This method employs a low-ionic-strength reaction mixture composed of normal saline, phosphate buffer, and glycine instead of normal saline as the final suspending medium for the detection of red cell antibodies. The use of LISS shortens the time of incubation to 10 min and increases the uptake of certain antibodies.

SALINE TECHNIQUE. This is a technique that utilizes normal saline as a suspending medium. After erythrocytes are washed, a 2–5 percent suspension of erythrocytes in saline is added to serum and incubated at the desired temperature (4°, 15°, 18°, or 37°C). The mixture is then centrifuged and read for agglutination or hemolysis.

antibody excess zone that area during a precipitin reaction where antibody is present that is not bound to antigen. Free antibody is detectable in the supernatant.

antibody identification the definitive identification of red cell antibodies that are responsible for incompatibility in antibody screening and crossmatching. The results and techniques of antibody detection are essential for proper antibody identification. The techniques include the antiglobulin tests, enzyme technique, high-protein (albumin) technique, incubation in low-ionic-strength medium test (LISS), and the saline technique (for more information, see under *antibody detection*). In addition, the results obtained from a panel of red blood cells are required. The red cells in the panels are group O red cells containing multiple antigenic determinants so that the panel gives a distinctive reaction pattern for each antigen.

anti-*Chlamydia* antibody tests assays for antibodies against *Chlamydia* species. The most commonly used test is complement fixation, which measures antibodies to 2-keto-3-deoxyoctanoic acid, an antigen common to both species of the genus (*C. psittaci* and *C. trachomatis*). It is especially useful in the diagnosis of lymphogranuloma venereum and psittacosis (systemic infection); it is of little use in the diagnosis of trachoma (superficial infection). Titers of 1:8 or 1:16 are considered significant, although a higher titer (1:64 or greater) is much more conclusive. A fourfold rise in titer from acute to convalescent serum is most supportive of diagnosis, but in the case of lymphogranuloma venereum the patients do not present in time to obtain these two samples. Among sexually active individuals, 5–10 percent of males and 15–20 percent of females have significant titers. Titers as high as 1:64 are rare in the normal population but do occur in sexually active females. The complement-fixation test is more applicable in diagnosing psittacosis, as acute and convalescent sera usually can be obtained. Background titers vary in different populations; 10–20 percent of veterinarians may have significant titers.

The microimmunofluorescence test is useful in the diagnosis of ocular or genital infection. The test uses the patient's serum and chlamydial organisms grown in yolk sac fixed to a slide. It has the advantage of giving a positive reaction with IgG and IgA as well as IgM. Testing acute and convalescent sera for a fourfold rise in titer is best for confirming diagnosis. As with the complement-fixation test, the physician must judge whether the microimmunofluorescence titer is significant in instances in which only one serum sample is available.

anticholinergic (an″tĭ-ko″lin-er′jik) blocking the transmission of postganglionic cholinergic nerve impulses, as in an anticholinergic agent such as a beta blocker. Also called antimuscarinic and atropinic.

anticholinesterase (an″tĭ-ko-lin-es′ter-ās) [*anti-* + *cholinesterase*] a substance that inhibits one of the cholinesterases; see *cholinesterase inhibitor.*

anticoagulant (an″tĭ-ko-ag′u-lant) a substance that inhibits coagulation of the blood. Those used to prevent clotting of blood specimens for laboratory analysis include EDTA, citrate, oxalate, and fluoride, which make calcium unavailable to the clotting process, and heparin, which inactivates thrombin and several other clotting factors. Anticoagulant preservatives used for storing blood products include ACD (acid citrate dextrose), CPD (citrate phosphate dextrose), CPD-adenine, and heparin. The anticoagulants administered therapeutically to prevent thromboembolic disease are heparin, which must be given parenterally, and the oral anticoagulants (warfarin, dicumarol, and congeners), which inhibit the hepatic synthesis of vitamin K–dependent clotting factors.

anticoagulant–citrate dextrose [USP], an anticoagulant used for the storage of whole blood; see *acid-citrate-dextrose.*

anticoagulant – citrate - phosphate - dextrose [USP], an anticoagulant used for the preservation of whole blood; see *citrate-phosphate-dextrose.*

anticodon (an″tĭ-ko-don) a triplet of nucleotides on transfer RNA molecules, which binds to the complementary codon on messenger RNA during the translation process on ribosomes. The amino acid carried by the tRNA is then inserted into the growing polypeptide chain. Thus, the sequence of codons specifies the sequence of amino acids. Some anticodons can bind to several codons; see also *wobble hypothesis.* Cf. *codon.*

anticonvulsant (an″tĭ-kon-vul′sant) any of a group of drugs used for the control of epileptic seizures. Most act by attenuating the propagation of nerve impulses; they either modify the transport of sodium, potassium, and calcium ions across cell membranes or they modify the release and uptake of neurotransmitters at synapses.

For tonic-clonic (grand mal), focal, and psychomotor seizures, the most commonly used drugs are phenytoin, phenobarbital, primidone, and carbamazepine; for absence (petit mal) seizures, ethosuximide and valproate. Clonazepam and valproate are used for minor motor seizures.

anti-D antibody against the D (or Rh_O) antigen; see also *Rh_O (D) immune globulin.*

antidiuretic (an″tĭ-di″u-ret′ik) 1. suppressing the rate of urine formation.

2. an agent that suppresses urine formation.

antidiuretic hormone (ADH) a cyclic polypeptide, consisting of eight amino acids, that is formed in the hypothalamus and is stored in the posterior lobe of the pituitary and released as necessary. ADH raises the blood pressure by stimulating smooth muscle in the walls of small blood vessels to contract. It also conserves body water by promoting reabsorption of water in the distal convoluted tubules of the kidney, thus resulting in more concentrated urine. Also called *vasopressin.*

anti-DNA antibody assays tests for the presence of antibodies to native, double-stranded DNA, which is particularly important in the diagnosis of systemic lupus erythematosus (SLE). The most sensitive test for the detection and quantitation of anti-DNA antibodies is radioimmunoassay, although tanned cell hemagglutination, ELISA, and immunofluorescence are also employed. Anti-DNA antibody levels correlate well with the activity of the disease. Antibody titers decrease with remission and rise with exacerbation. See also *systemic l. erythematosus* under *lupus.*

anti-DNase B (ADN-B) assay a neutralization test for anti-DNase B antibodies, utilizing the enzyme streptococcal DNase B as the antigen, in sera from patients who have had an infection with group A beta-hemolytic streptococci.

A constant amount of the enzyme is added to different dilutions of the patient's serum and incubated. DNA is then added and the mixture reincubated. If anti-DNase B antibodies are present, the DNase B is neutralized and is no longer able to depolymerize the DNA. The presence of polymerized DNA can be detected by adding alcohol, which causes polymerized DNA to clot; methyl green dye retains its color when combined with polymerized DNA but fades when combined with unpolymerized DNA.

Although not as widely used, the ADN-B test is better than the antistreptolysin (ASO) test for detecting a streptococcal infection, because it is positive in more cases of streptococcal sequelae (especially chorea) and is not subject to the conditions that cause false-positive results in the ASO tests.

The ADN-B titer is particularly useful in the diagnosis of sequelae because it reaches a peak later than the ASO titer yet remains elevated for a longer period. An elevated level of DNase in the patient's serum can cause a false-negative result because anti-DNase B antibody is specific for streptococcal DNase; however, this condition is rare in patients with streptococcal infection.

A rise in titer by two dilution increments between acute and convalescent sera is considered significant. If an acute serum is not available, the titer can be compared with the upper limit of normal value, as in the case of ASO antibody.

See also *antistreptolysin O tests*.

antidote (an′tĭ-dōt) [L. *antidotum*, from Gr. *anti-* + *didonai* to give] a remedy given to counteract the effects of a poison or toxin.

antidromic (an″tĭ-drom′ik) [Gr. *antidromein* to run in a contrary direction] conducting impulses in a direction opposite to the normal.

antidromic conduction the propagation of an action potential or of the stimulus used to generate an action potential in a direction opposite to normal, e.g., in peripheral sensory nerve fibers, from the spinal cord to the receptor. Antidromic impulses do not pass the first synapse, as synapses permit only orthodromic conduction. Cf. *orthodromic conduction*.

antifactor Xa See *a. III* under *antithrombin*.

antifol (an″tĭ-fōl) an agent or compound that interferes with the synthesis of folate coenzymes, thus acting as a folate antagonist; an antimetabolite. Most antifols are structural analogs of folic acid, such as the most widely used, methotrexate. See also *methotrexate*.

antifungal agent (an″tĭ-fung′gal) a substance that is destructive to fungi, suppresses the growth or reproduction of fungi, or is effective against fungal infections. Agents employed in fungal disease chemotherapy include antibiotics of the polyene group (amphotericin B, candicidin, and nystatin), the imidazoles (clotrimazole, miconazole, and ketoconazole), griseofulvin, and the synthetic compounds fluorocytosin and tolnaftate. Also called *fungicide*. For more information, see the specific agent.

antigen (an′tĭ-jen) [*antibody* + Gr. *gennan* to produce] a protein, glycoprotein, complex polysaccharide, or nucleic acid that is recognized as foreign and thereby elicits an immunologic response from a host. Antigens may be divided into T cell–independent and T cell–dependent antigens. The latter cannot stimulate antibody formation without help of the T cell, whereas T cell–independent antigens do not require participation of the T cell for antibody formation. T cell–independent antigens tend to have repetitive sequences in their antigenic determinants. Examples include pneumococcal polysaccharide and dextran. Complex antigens tend to be T cell–dependent.

Immunogenicity. An antigen's ability to stimulate an antibody or cellular immune response is termed its immunogenicity. The complexity, size, charge, solubility, digestibility, dose, and route of administration of an antigen all affect its immunogenicity. Complex antigens tend to be more immunogenic; they have more antigenic determinants and tend to elicit an augmented, arrayed antibody response. The larger the size, the more immunogenic the antigen is, especially with regard to proteins. However, this is probably secondary to the increased number of antigenic determinants. Low-molecular-weight proteins (M.W. <1000) are usually nonimmunogenic unless they act as haptens. Substances that cannot be digested usually are not immunogenic, which is probably secondary to the inability of the macrophage to process the antigen. The dose of antigen is very important in determining the response of the host. Very small doses of antigen, as well as very large doses of antigen, may produce tolerance (termed low-dose and high-dose tolerance, respectively).

Antigen may produce a different immunologic response, depending on the route of administration or the mode of presentation. Intravenous or oral administration of antigen might produce tolerance, whereas subcutaneous administration might cause antibody production. If the antigen is administered with an adjuvant, it will probably be more immunogenic than without an adjuvant.

In addition to exogenous antigens, there are also antigens endogenous to an individual. These may take the form of particular proteins inherent to a particular organ, such as the heart, or particular hormones or receptors. These autoantigens are the basis for the various autoimmune diseases.

Individuals also have a unique genetic constitution with unique antigens that affect the immune response and transplantation reactions.

Immune Response to an Antigen. The antigen is processed by the monocyte-macrophage. The processed antigen can then induce a specific response in the lymphocyte population. In the T-cell population, a specific receptor or recognition unit is induced, and the cell proliferates and/or releases soluble factors. B cells respond to the processed antigen directly or through T lymphocyte–derived factors, and differentiate to plasma cells, which produce specific antibody. The initial antibody that is produced to a first antigen exposure is usually of the IgM subclass; an array of antibodies with different binding affinities is usually produced. After the initial IgM response, IgG and IgA follow.

The antibody produced is specific for a particular site on the antigen called the antigenic determinant, which binds to the variable region of the immunoglobin molecule. The affinity is determined by the strength of the interactions between the antigenic determinant and the amino acid configuration in the variable region. Some low-molecular-weight molecules (haptens) can act as antigenic determinants if they are bound to a larger macromolecule called a carrier. The lymphocyte response usually involves a specific B-lymphocyte antibody production response to the hapten and a T-lymphocyte response specific for the carrier protein.

Laboratory Methods for Antigen Detection. Most antigen detection methods require a specific interaction with specific antibody. Even though the interaction of the antibody with the antigen is the primary event in a number of these methods, a secondary event is needed for detection and quantitation.

1. Immunoprecipitation—Antigen detection is commonly performed qualitatively using double-diffusion precipitin reactions, such as in the Ouchterlony method in which precipitin bands form when antigen-antibody complexes precipitate. To measure new antigen synthesis, radiolabeled amino acids can be added to the in vitro or in vivo system, and the presence of radiolabeled antigen can be de-

termined using autoradiography of the immune precipitates.

2. Counterimmunoelectrophoresis (CIE)—This method has been used to detect small levels of antigen, such as organisms like *Hemophilus influenzae* in cerebrospinal fluid. It takes advantage of immunoprecipitation and electrophoresis.

3. ELISA—Various methods utilize enzyme-linked immunoassays to detect antigen. Antibodies linked to enzymes are used to detect antigens. After interaction of the antigen with antibody, the enzyme linked to antibody is used to generate a colorimetric reaction.

4. Complement fixation—In this procedure, a known antiserum, which has the ability to fix complement, is reacted with antigen. It is then added to sheep red blood cells that have been sensitized with antibody. The amount of antigen present determines how much complement is used up (fixed), and the decrease in complement available for lysis of the sheep RBCs is a function of the antigen present initially.

5. RAST inhibition—To test for the presence of allergen in an extract, a RAST inhibition assay is performed. Known allergen is fixed to a solid support or disk, after which a known IgE against the allergen is added, which binds to the allergen. A radiolabeled anti-IgE is then introduced, which binds to the IgE. The amount of radioactivity bound to the disk is the control. If an unknown allergen is reacted with the IgE before binding with the disk, the amount of IgE bound in the fluid phase can be washed away. When the radiolabeled anti-IgE is added, the amount bound will be decreased by the amount of fluid phase allergen in the unknown.

See also *autoimmune disease, immune response,* and *immunogenicity.* Cf. *immunogen.*

GERALD B. KOLSKI, M.D., PH.D.

antigen-binding site (region) that portion of the antibody molecule that binds the antigen.

antigenic (an-tĭ-jen′ik) having the properties of an antigen.

antigenic competition that which occurs between two closely related antigens when given at the same time, causing the immune response to either one to be suppressed.

antigenic deletion the loss or masking of antigenic determinants in daughter cells of cells whose parent tissue normally carries them. It may result from neoplastic or other mutational change in the parent tissue, or it may be due to the loss or repression of genetic material from the cell.

antigenic determinant the structural part of an antigen that determines the specificity of an antigen-antibody reaction. These are chemically active surface groupings of amino acids in globular proteins and sugar side-chains in polysaccharides. The most critical part is called the immunodominant point. Also called antigenic determinant group and epitope.

antigenic modulation the shifting of antigenic sites on a cell's surface, caused by the presence of bound antibody.

antigenic shift the major changes or mutations of viral surface chemistry that occur every so often and cause vaccines and immunizations against viruses to lose their protective value. Such changes often precede influenza pandemics. Also called antigenic drift.

antigen presentation a probable function of macrophages, whereby a small amount of the processed antigen bound to the surface of the macrophage is presented in a concentrated form to the lymphocytes or other immunocompetent cells.

antigen processing a probable activity of macrophages, in which they partially degrade the particulate antigens prior to presentation to other lymphoid cells.

antigen recognition the process of antigenic determinants binding to specific receptors on a lymphocyte plasma membrane. The cellular receptors are probably antibody or antibodylike in nature.

antigen-specific helper factor a factor that augments the antibody response of B cells against a specific antigen; M.W. 50,000–70,000. These factors are produced by the helper T-cell population; many require macrophages for their effect and have antigen combining sites. Their target cell is either the macrophage or the B cell. Many serologically cross react with immunoglobulin or cell-surface alloantigens. These factors induce IgM and IgG responses of B cells in vivo and in vitro.

antigen-specific suppressor factor a factor, probably a protein, that suppresses humoral or cell-mediated immune responses to a specific antigen; M.W. 40,000–60,000. The target cells—or at least those that have been identified—are T cells. These factors appear to have an antigen-binding site. Their genes are located in the major histocompatibility complex.

antiglobulin (an″tĭ-glob′u-lin) an antibody directed against a serum globulin, usually referring to one directed against another antibody (gamma globulin). See also *antiglobulin tests.*

antiglobulin tests direct and indirect assays to detect antierythrocyte antibodies or other red cell-coating serum proteins that do not form the necessary lattice to agglutinate the cells; used most frequently to detect anti-Rh antibodies in red cell typing and to diagnose hemolytic disease of the newborn and autoimmune hemolytic anemia. The tests involve the use of Coombs reagents, which may be antiimmunoglobulins, or nongamma Coombs reagents, which are directed against complement components; the latter type is useful in cases of autoimmune hemolytic anemia, in which only complement components bind to the red cell. Also called *Coombs' test.*

DIRECT ANTIGLOBULIN TEST. This antiglobulin test detects the in vivo sensitization of red blood cells. The cells to be tested should be thoroughly washed with saline, mixed with antiglobulin serum, and centrifuged immediately. Agglutination indicates a positive reaction. Negative reactions should be allowed to sit at room temperature for a few minutes and then be recentrifuged to detect C3d and IgA antibodies. As with all antiglobulin tests, the adequacy of the test sera should be checked with a suspension of known sensitized red blood cells. The direct antiglobulin test is utilized to aid in the diagnosis of hemolytic disease of the newborn and autoimmune hemolytic anemia, and to investigate possible transfusion reactions. Also called direct Coombs' test.

INDIRECT ANTIGLOBULIN TEST. This test utilizes antiglobulin serum to detect the in vitro sensitization of red blood cells by serum. The test is performed as an integral part of the crossmatch and used to detect and identify unexpected erythrocyte antigens. Test serum is incubated with red blood cells at 37°C. The medium usually contains albumin or a low ionic salt solution to lower its dielectric constant. After incubation, the cells are washed thoroughly with saline, mixed with antiglobulin serum, and centrifuged. Agglutination indicates the presence of incomplete sensitizing antibodies in the serum. Negative reactions should be confirmed with known sensitized check cells. Also called indirect Coombs' test.

antihemophilic factor (AHF) (an″tĭ-he″mo-fil′ik) see *Factor VIII.*

antihemophilic factor B see *Factor IX.*

antihemophilic factor C see *Factor XI.*

antihemophilic globulin (AHG) see *Factor VIII.*

antiheparin factor see *platelet factor 4.*

antihistamine (an″tĭ-his′tah-men) any substance, usually a substituted ethylamine, that is a structural analog of histamine and counteracts the action of excess histamine in body tissues; a histamine antagonist. Chlorpheniramine maleate, promethazine, and tripelennamine hydrochloride are examples. Drowsiness and dizziness, skin rash, dryness of mouth, and digestive disorders may be side-effects. Muscular twitching, medullary and cord convulsions, coma, and respiratory failure may result from excessive doses. Gas chromatography or thin-layer chromatography may be used to detect antihistamines after extraction of an alkalinized specimen with organic solvents. There does not appear, however, to be any clinical indication for routine measurements.

antihyaluronidase (AH) (an″tĭ-hi-ah-lu-ron′ĭ-dās) an antibody directed against hyaluronidase.

antihyaluronidase assays a test for the antibody antihyaluronidase in the serum of individuals who have had a group A streptococcal infection. It is an enzyme neutralization test that utilizes streptococcal hyaluronidase as the antigen.

In this procedure, a constant amount of streptococcal hyaluronidase is added to twofold serial dilutions of the patient's serum. After incubation, a constant amount of potassium hyaluronate is added and allowed to incubate, and a fixed amount of 2N acetic acid is added as an indicator.

Any antihyaluronidase antibodies present in the patient's serum will neutralize the streptococcal hyaluronidase, thus preventing it from breaking down the potassium hyaluronate. Also, the potassium hyaluronate will clot in the presence of the acetic acid. The titer is the reciprocal of the highest dilution of the patient's serum with a definite clot: a fourfold rise in titer between acute and convalescent sera is indicative of infection. In the absence of acute or convalescent serum, however, a titer of 512 suggests infection, 256 is equivocal, and 128 is negative.

The AH assays may be used with the antistreptolysin O (ASO) test, and is especially useful in cases of acute glomerulonephritis caused by a pyodermic strain of streptococci because these strains produce low levels of ASO antibody. The test is not subject to the factors that can cause false-positive results in the ASO test. The major disadvantage of the AH test is that it is not as reproducible as the ASO or anti-DNAse B (ADN-B) tests. See also *anti-DNAse B assay* and *antistreptolysin O test.*

antihypercholesterolemic (an″tĭ-hi″per-ko-les′ter-ol-e″mik) 1. effective against hypercholesterolemia.

2. an agent that prevents or relieves hypercholesterolemia.

antihypertensive (an″tĭ-hi″per-ten′siv) 1. effective against hypertension.

2. an agent that reduces high blood pressure.

antiinfective capable of killing infectious agents or preventing them from spreading and producing infections. Cf. *infective.*

antiinflammatory (an″te-in-flam′ah-to″re) 1. counteracting or suppressing inflammation.

2. an agent that reduces inflammation. Such substances are generally divided into two classes, steroid antiinflammatory drugs (e.g., cortisone) and nonsteroidal antiinflammatory drugs (e.g., aspirin).

anti-Lewisite see *dimercaprol.*

antilymphocyte serum (ALS) serum containing antibodies, which are directed against lymphocyte antigens and which generally cause suppression of the immune response. It is used to suppress resistance to tissue grafts (heterografts, xenografts, secondary allograft rejection), although certain T lymphocytes are resistant to it.

antimatter (an″tĭ-mat′er) matter composed of the antiparticles of ordinary matter, e.g., positrons and antiprotons.

antimetabolite (an″tĭ-mĕ-tab′o-līt) a substance whose structure closely resembles that of another substance necessary for normal growth or physiologic functioning, and which interferes with the utilization of the essential metabolite, e.g., sulfanilamide ($H_2NC_6H_4SO_2NH_2$), antagonizes the utilization of *p*-aminobenzoic acid ($H_2NC_6H_4COOH$) as a result of its similar chemical structure. Methotrexate is an antimetabolite of folic acid.

antimicrobial (an″tĭ-mi-kro′be-al) referring to killing microorganisms or the suppression of their multiplication or growth. See also *antibacterial.*

antimicrosomal antibodies (an″ti-mi″kro-so′mal) see *thyroid microsomal antibodies.*

antimitochondrial antibody one of the antibodies (IgG, IgA, or IgM) directed against a lipoprotein of the inner mitochondrial membrane. These antibodies are present in sera from 90 percent of those with primary biliary cirrhosis but are usually not found in any other type of chronic obstructive jaundice. Occasionally, sera from an individual with chronic aggressive hepatitis are positive.

antimitochondrial antibody assays the test to detect antibody to mitochondria. It involves indirect immunofluorescence using the patient's serum and unfixed cryostat sections of rat kidney as the substrate. The antibody is also detectible by complement fixation. See also *complement fixation* and *indirect immunofluorescence.*

antimode (an′tĭ-mōd) in statistics, the minimum lying between two modes of a bimodal probability density.

antimony (Sb) (an′tĭ-mo″ne) [L. *antimonium; stibium*] a silvery-white, semiconducting metallic element; atomic number 51; atomic weight 121.75; Group V of the periodic table; oxidation states −3, +3, +5. It is used as an *n*-type dopant in silicon semiconductors; compounds with Group III elements, e.g., gallium antimonide, are also semiconductors.

Trivalent and pentavalent antimony are highly toxic; like arsenic, they bind to sulfhydryl groups of proteins and inactivate enzymes. Symptoms of antimony poisoning include dermatitis, gastrointestinal irritation, hypothermia, and irregular respiration. Trivalent antimony salts are used medicinally in the treatment of schistosomiasis.

a. hydride, see *stibine.*

a. trichloride, a compound, $SbCl_3$, that yields a blue color when combined with vitamin A, used in some histologic preparations.

antimony assays 1. the Reinsch test. In this test, antimony salts are reduced to metallic antimony by metallic copper. Concentrated hydrochloric acid and a copper foil strip or wire spiral are added to a sample, which is then heated for several hours. Metallic antimony, bismuth, arsenic, selenium, tellurium, and some sulfides are deposited on the copper; all but bismuth and antimony dissolve in potassium cyanide solution.

2. a semiquantitative method. This process follows the first method, with conversion of the antimony into stibine (SbH_3) by reaction with hydrochloric acid, stannous chloride, and sodium iodide. The stibine gas is then bubbled through a solution of silver diethyldithiocarbamate to produce a red color that can be measured at 510 nm.

3. atomic absorption spectroscopy. The antimony in a processed specimen is converted to stibine (SbH_3), which is then swept into a nitrogen-entrained hydrogen diffusion flame of an atomic absorption spectrophotometer fitted with an appropriate lamp.

antimony stains histologic techniques used to demonstrate the presence of antimony in tissue. Antimony reacts with 9-methyl-2,3,7-trihydroxy-6-fluorone (pH 4.0) to form a red precipitate. This chemical also reacts with cerium, germanium, and iron, however, and is more often used for the Turchini reaction to distinguish DNA (blue) from RNA (rose).

antimorph (an′ti-morf) a mutant allele that acts to create a phenotype that is antagonistic or opposite to that of the normal allele.

antimorphic (an″tĭ-mor′fik) in genetics, antagonizing or inhibiting normal activity; acting in a manner opposite to that of the normal allele; of or pertaining to an antimorph.

antimutagen (an″tĭ-mu′tah-jen) any substance that antagonizes the mutagenic effects of another substance.

antineoplastic (an″tĭ-ne″o-plas′tik) 1. inhibiting or preventing the development of neoplasms; checking the maturation and spread of malignant cells.

2. an agent that has such properties.

antineutrino (an″tĭ-nu-tre′no) a particle with little or no mass, no charge, and a spin of 1/2. It shares with an electron the energy emitted in negative beta decay and also serves to conserve momentum. It is the antiparticle of the neutrino. Other antineutrinos are associated with muon production and possibly with tau meson production.

antinuclear antibody (ANA) (an″tĭ-nu′kle-ar) an autoantibody that reacts with the nuclear components, usually in nucleoproteins. It is found in several rheumatic conditions, especially systemic lupus erythematosus, rheumatoid arthritis, Sjögren's syndrome, and polymyositis, as well as occasionally in hepatic disease, pulmonary disease, lymphoma, chronic leukemia, chronic ulcerative colitis, infectious mononucleosis, autoimmune hemolytic anemia, and some drug reactions. ANA is usually detected by indirect immunofluorescence. Formerly called *antinuclear factor.*

antinuclear antibody assay immunofluorescence testing to demonstrate ANA in serum. In the procedure, 2- to 4-μm liver sections from young rats are prepared, placed on slides, and air dried. Test serum diluted with saline is added to the surface, after which the slide is incubated in a humidifying dish at room temperature. During this time the slide is washed twice in NaCl using gentle agitation, and the exposed part of the slide is wiped dry. The appropriate fluorescein-conjugated antiglobulin is added, left to stand briefly, and then washed again. When the slide is dry, a fluorescence microscope is used to look for bound fluorescent dye. If positive (with 64-fold dilution), titration may be performed to find the highest dilution at which the result is still positive. The morphologic characteristics may also be reported as homogeneous, speckled, diffuse, nucleolar, or (most frequently) mixed.

antinuclear factor (ANF) see *antinuclear antibody.*

antioxidant (an″tĭ-ok′sĭ-dant) a substance that retards or inhibits the oxidation of another substance to which it is added.

antiparallel (an″tĭ-par′ah-lel) in genetics, pertaining to the fact that the two strands of DNA in a chromosome run in opposite directions. Progressing in one direction along the chromosome, one strand reads from the 3′ to the 5′ end (3′ → 5′), and the other from the 5′ to the 3′ end (5′ → 3′).

antiparietal cell antibody assays tests for antibodies directed against intracytoplasmic canalicular antigens of gastric parietal cells or against intrinsic factor, found primarily in individuals with pernicious anemia. The most common tests are indirect immunofluorescence or complement fixation; the latter is less sensitive. In the indirect immunofluorescence test, various dilutions of the patient's serum are reacted with unfixed sections of gastric fundal mucosa (usually rat) as the substrate. Fluorescein-labeled antihuman immunoglobulin is then added. Because the cytoplasm of the parietal cells stains in a way that can be confused with antibodies occurring against mitochondria, a test on kidney cells should be performed as a control.

Parietal cell antibodies are found in more than 90 percent of individuals with pernicious anemia. They are also found in a number of other conditions, e.g., chronic thyroiditis, Sjögren's sicca syndrome, atrophic gastritis, and gastric ulcer, and in the normal population. The incidence increases with age and is more common in females than in males.

See also *pernicious a.* under *anemia.*

antiparticle (an″tĭ-par′ti-k'l) one of two particles differing only in having opposite electric charges and magnetic moments. When antiparticles collide, their mass is totally converted to radiation and sometimes lighter particle-antiparticle pairs. For example, the collision of an electron and a positron produces two gamma rays, each having the energy equal to the electron mass, 511 keV.

antipernicious anemia factor the former name for vitamin B_{12}. See *cyanocobalamin* and *vitamin B_{12}.*

antiphylaxis see *anaphylaxis*.

antiplasmin (an″tĭ-plaz′min) see *alpha₂-antiplasmin*.

antiplatelet antibodies (an″tĭ-plāt′let) platelet autoantibodies or isoantibodies. Platelet autoantibodies, which are generally IgG immunoglobulins, are the cause of idiopathic thrombocytopenic purpura (ITP). Even though their presence in virtually all cases of ITP is considered to be established, these autoantibodies are difficult to demonstrate. At present, one of the most sensitive tests for their detection is a quantitative antiglobulin consumption test. Platelet isoantibodies form after multiple transfusions. They are of particular importance in causing shortened platelet survival in patients with aplastic anemia and leukemia who require multiple transfusions of platelets.

Sensitization to a platelet antigen (Pl^{A1}), when present in donor blood but absent from recipient blood, leads to platelet destruction. In such instances, the donor's Pl^{A1} antigen is apparently transferred to the recipient's own platelets, which are then destroyed by the recipient's anti-Pl^{A1} antibodies. Isoantibodies are best demonstrated with a complement-fixation test.

antiport (an″tĭ-port) a transport protein that simultaneously moves two substances in opposite directions. See also *active transport*. Cf. *symport* and *uniport*.

antipsychotic drug (an″tĭ-si-kot′ik) a drug used for the management of manifestations of psychotic disorders, particularly for the treatment of schizophrenia. There are several chemical classes of antipsychotic drugs (phenothiazines, thioxanthines, dibenzapines, butyrophenones, and indolones), which vary widely in potency and side-effects but produce similar effects in equivalent doses: amelioration of the symptoms of schizophrenia by affecting disturbed thought processes and reducing tension, excitement, anxiety, and (in some cases) paranoia, delusions, and hallucinations.

These effects are probably all produced by the same mechanism, the blockade of dopaminergic receptors in the central nervous system, which reduces dopaminergic neurotransmission. This mechanism also produces the motor side-effects (extrapyramidal side-effects) experienced by 5–60 percent of patients, depending on the drug taken. These side-effects include dystonia (muscular contractions in the face, neck, and back) and parkinsonian-like symptoms (both of which sometimes respond to antiparkinsonian drugs), akathisia (motor restlessness), withdrawal dyskinesia, and tardive dyskinesia (involuntary movements such as tongue twitching and chewing), which occurs in about 20 percent of patients treated for long periods with antipsychotic medications. About 60 percent of cases of tardive dyskinesia are irreversible; in the rest, there is some remission when the drug is no longer given. Many of these drugs also have strong anticholinergic side-effects (dry mouth, blurred vision, constipation), and some also have α-adrenergic blocking activity. Also called *major tranquilizer* and *neuroleptic*.

antipyrine (an″te-pi′rēn) [*anti-* + Gr. *pyr* fire] [USP], a pyrazolone derivative related to phenylbutazone. It has been used as an analgesic and antipyretic; it is now used in analgesic ear drops.

anti-Rh titer the amount of anti-Rh antibody present in serum. It is usually determined by serial dilutions using the direct antiglobulin test; see under *antiglobulin tests*.

antisense (an′tĭ-sens) in molecular genetics, the DNA strand with the same sequence as the mRNA to which it was transcribed. Cf. *sense strand*.

antisepsis (an″tĭ-sep′sis) [*anti-* + Gr. *sēpsis* putrefaction] any procedure that reduces to a significant degree the microbial flora of skin or mucous membranes. Its purpose is to reduce the person-to-person transmission of infectious disease by eliminating or reducing the number of any pathogenic microorganisms present. Antiseptics differ from disinfectants, which also kill microorganisms but which are employed on inanimate objects, not people. Because antiseptics must not irritate the skin or mucous membranes, they are weaker than disinfectants and show only low-level activity. Yet, to qualify as an antiseptic, the cidal action must be rapid and strong enough to produce substantial reduction in the microbial population.

RECOMMENDED ANTISEPTICS. Only four chemicals are recommended as antiseptics in the 1981 guidelines of the U.S. Center for Disease Control: (1) aqueous 3 percent hexachlorphene; (2) aqueous iodophors; (3) aqueous 4 percent chlorhexidine; and (4) ethyl or isopropyl 70–90 percent alcohol.

Hexachlorophene is not recommended for use in nurseries except during outbreaks of *Staphylococcus* because it may be absorbed through the skin of newborn infants. As it is water-insoluble, repeated applications of hexachlorophene are needed to accumulate even inhibitory concentrations in the fatty acids of skin. The antibacterial spectrum is distinctly gram-positive; indeed, continued usage sometimes results in replacement of the normal gram-positive flora by gram-negative flora. It is a 6-chlorinated biphenyl compound.

Iodophors have a broader spectrum and act rapidly, but tend to cause skin dryness. The staining associated with iodine is moderate and temporary. Iodophors are complexes of elemental iodine with large organic molecules that release free iodine slowly.

Chlorhexidine is a *bis*-diguanide with rapid gram-positive activity and better killing of gram-negatives than hexachlorophene. This compound, like the other two chemicals, is marketed in combination with detergents in order to provide good cleaning action, a very important part of infection control.

Alcohol, unlike the other three, is not used for handwashing, but is the most rapidly cidal and has the broadest spectrum. Therefore, wiping the hands with an alcohol sponge, or rubbing them with an alcoholic lotion or foam, is a very important means of reducing the spread of infection by hospital and other patient-care personnel.

HANDWASHING PROCEDURES. Ordinary plain handwashing removes the transient microbial flora almost completely. The transient flora of the hands are microorganisms picked up during daily activities; the numbers and types vary greatly. Most significant is the fact that the pathogens responsible for hospital-acquired infections are part of this type of flora. There is also a permanent or resident flora, but it is entirely different. On the hands, it consists largely of just two types, the aerobic *Staphylococcus epidermidis* and anaerobic *Propionibacterium* species that are sequestered in the hair follicles and sebaceous glands. As the acetone-soluble substances these flora produce are inhibitory for a number of pathogens, the skin's resident flora are in fact part of the skin's defense mechanism, and attempts to dislodge them with strenuous surgical scrubbing are contraindicated.

Plain handwashing, however, is not adequate for infection control in high-risk areas of the hospital, such as surgery, intensive care units, and nurseries. Antiseptic procedures not only are indicated, but may be the most important single procedure in the prevention of hospital-acquired infections.

Surgical scrub procedures can be carried out satisfactorily with sponge application of any one of the recommended antiseptic-detergents. A plain soap scrub followed by an alcohol dip was widely used at one time, and produces the greatest and most rapid reduction in skin flora, although it is not so long-lasting as the antiseptic-detergent scrubs employed today. The drying effect of alcohol on skin can be largely overcome by incorporating an emollient such as cetyl alcohol.

The best antiseptic for skin preps is alcohol containing a solution of 0.5–1.0 percent iodine. The cidal effect is rapid, broad-spectrum, and lasting.

Cf. *disinfection* and *sterilization*.

antiseptic (an″tĭ-sep′tik) 1. preventing decay or putrefaction.

2. a substance that inhibits the growth and development of microorganisms without necessarily destroying them. Cf. *disinfectant*.

antiserum (an″tĭ-se′rum) a serum that contains antibody or antibodies against a particular antigen. It may be obtained from an animal that has been immunized either by injection of antigen into the body or by infection with microorganisms containing the antigen, or, rarely, by passively administered antibody from another immune subject.

anti–smooth muscle antibody antibody (usually IgG, occasionally IgM) directed against a component of hepatic cells that cross reacts with smooth muscle. Anti–smooth muscle antibodies are present in sera from 40–70 percent of persons affected with active chronic hepatitis, 50 percent of those with primary biliary cirrhosis, and 28 percent of those with cryptogenic cirrhosis. They are also found in persons with acute viral hepatitis, infectious mononucleosis, asthma, yellow fever, and some malignant tumors. Less than 2 percent of the normal population has these antibodies.

anti–smooth muscle antibody assay a test to detect antibody against smooth muscle. It involves indirect immunofluorescence using the patient's serum and unfixed cryostat sections of a substrate such as rat stomach. Various dilutions of the patient's serum are tested to determine the antibody titer. In active chronic hepatitis, titers have a range of 80–320, and are lower (less than 80) in other conditions involving anti–smooth muscle antibodies. See also *anti–smooth muscle antibody* and *indirect immunofluorescence*.

antistatic spray a product that inhibits the buildup of static electricity between a microtome knife and a tissue specimen embedded in paraffin.

antistreptolysin O tests 1. a neutralization test used to detect ASO antibody in serum; the most widely used serologic test for the detection of streptococcal infections and poststreptococcal disease. The original ASO test procedure was developed by Todd, whose name is still used to express the levels of antibody titer measured by the test (Todd Units). Traditionally, titers above 166 Todd Units are considered elevated, although higher values are used by many clinical investigators, depending on the historical prevalence of group A streptococcal infections.

The assay is based on the ability of ASO antibody to block the lysis of erythrocytes by streptolysin O. The test is performed by adding a constant amount of reduced streptolysin O to various dilutions of the test serum. After incubation, during which time the antigen and antibody combine, a constant amount of erythrocytes is added. If ASO is present in the serum, the streptolysin O will be neutralized and the erythrocytes will not lyse. The end point is the highest dilution of serum showing no hemolysis. Sometimes an end point of 50 percent hemolysis is used, although this is not widely accepted.

A number of substances other than ASO neutralize the hemolytic capability of streptolysin O, producing false-positive results. These substances include serum beta-lipoprotein produced in liver disease and growth products from the growth of bacteria such as *Bacillus cereus* and *Pseudomonas* species in serum specimens. Also, the oxidation of reduced streptolysin O eliminates its ability to lyse erythrocytes.

High ASO titers may indicate recent infection or persistence of antibody from a previous infection. Eighty percent of rheumatic fever patients have a significant rise in titer within 2 mo of an attack. ASO titers are common among the normal population; thus, only high titers (250 Todd Units in adults, 333 Units in children) are considered evidence of recent infection.

2. a particle agglutination test, which is used less frequently than the neutralization test. This involves coating particles (e.g., latex, treated erythrocytes, or certain bacteria) and mixing them with diluted test serum on a slide; if ASO is present, the particles agglutinate. Erythrocytes may be utilized as particles because the streptolysin O is in the oxidized state and thus is nonhemolytic. The advantage of the agglutination test is that lipoproteins, oxidized streptolysin O, or bacterial growth products do not give false-positive results.

The streptozyme test is a particle agglutination test in which erythrocytes are coated with a crude mixture of streptococcal antigens. It is good for screening but has limited value as a quantitative test. ASO titers are elevated in 80 percent of acute cases of rheumatic fever. Because 20 percent of the cases do not show a rise in ASO titer, other tests should also be performed. The rise in titer does not reach its peak until 3–5 wk after infection, with the titer returning to preinfection levels 6 mo to 1 yr later. A rise in titer of two dilution increments between acute and convalescent sera is considered significant. If acute serum is not available, comparison with an upper limit of normal value can be used to determine significance. The upper limit of normal is a titer not exceeded by 85 percent of the normal population with no apparent streptococcal disease. As this varies widely with age group, season of year, and geographic location, each laboratory must establish an upper limit of normal for a given population.

antithrombin (an″tĭ-throm′bin) [*anti-* + *thrombin*] a general term for substances that possess the ability to inactivate thrombin. Antithrombin III and heparin are recognized antithrombins. Antithrombins I, II, IV, V, and VI are no longer considered to be separate entities, and now fall under antithrombin III. See also *heparin.*

a. III (AT III), an alpha$_2$-globulin synthesized in the liver, which is widely distributed throughout the body fluids. It is a naturally occurring inhibitor of the clotting process and is the principal physiologic mechanism for inactivating thrombin and other serine proteases—Factors IXa, Xa, XIa, and XIIa—as well as acting as the cofactor of heparin (heparin cofactor).

AT III reacts stoichiometrically with the activated coagulation factors: one molecule of AT III inactivates one molecule of activated factor, forming a covalent and physiologically irreversible complex. It also inactivates trypsin, chymotrypsin, and plasmin.

Normal levels of antithrombin III are 80–100 percent. Decreased levels are seen in disseminated intravascular coagulation, liver disease, and congenital disorders; there is some tendency toward thrombosis when AT III levels are 60–80 percent of normal. Increased levels are seen in individuals with hemorrhagic disorders or in those receiving anticoagulants.

Also called *antifactor XA* and *Factor Xa inhibitor.* See also *alpha$_2$-antiplasmin, alpha$_1$-antitrypsin, alpha$_2$-macroglobulin,* and *C1 esterase inhibitor.*

antitoxin (an″tĭ-tok′sin) [*anti-* + Gr. *toxicon* poison] an antibody that neutralizes the soluble toxic protein products of a microorganism (usually bacteria), zootoxin (spider or bee venom), or phytotoxin (e.g., ricin of the castor bean).

antitoxoplasma antibody tests tests for antibody to *Toxoplasma gondii* in serum. One of the most reliable is the Sabin-Feldman dye test, but its dependence on the use of live organisms limits its feasibility in the routine serology laboratory. Indirect hemagglutination, complement fixation, and immunofluorescence are commonly used. Indirect hemagglutination titers greater than 256 and indirect immunofluorescence titers greater than 64 may be clinically significant. IgM antibody is indicative of an acute infection. See also *Sabin-Feldman dye test.*

antitragus (an″tĭ-tra′gus) [*anti-* + *tragus*] [NA], a small tubercule of the external ear opposite the tragus and continuous with the anthelix on the lateral aspect of the pinna.

α_1-antitrypsin see *alpha$_1$-antitrypsin.*

antitubular basement membrane antibodies antibodies that may cause direct tubulointerstitial damage in the kidneys when they fix to tubular basement membranes. Deposits of immunoglobulin and complement may be found in the interstitium during biopsy examination.

antitumor enzymes a new class of enzymes having application in both tumor and immunosuppressive therapy. One example is L-asparaginase, which, while possessing only limited clinical value, has produced remissions in acute lymphoblastic leukemia. It acts by depleting L-asparagine, an important amino acid, and results in the destruction of those tissues possessing lowered amounts of asparagine synthetase. The use of these enzymes as chemotherapeutic agents ideally evokes selective destruction of the tumor cells.

antivenin (an″tĭ-ven′in) [*anti-* + L. *venenum* poison] an antiserum against the venom of a poisonous animal or an extract of immunoglobulins from such a serum. Antivenin is usually produced by hyperimmunization of horses with the specific venom, and is used as a passive immunizing agent to treat poisoning from animal venom. There are several antivenins available: antivenin (Crotalidae) polyvalent [USP] for the treatment of snakebite by pit vipers, antivenin (*Micrurus fulvius*) [USP] for coral snakebite, and antivenin (*Latrodectus mactans*) [USP] for the black widow spiderbite.

antiviral agent (an″tĭ-vi′ral) any chemotherapeutic drug that either prevents multiplication of or is lethal to a virus. Ideally, an antiviral agent should be nontoxic to humans, long-lasting, and soluble, and should have a broad spectrum of antiviral activity. Two major problems in the development of antiviral therapy are that viruses use many host cell enzymes, so that many inhibitors of viral multiplication are toxic for the host cell, and that viral multiplication is almost over before the symptoms of the disease are present. Antiviral agents may be classified in three categories: inhibitors of early steps in viral infection, inhibitors of nucleic acid synthesis, and miscellaneous inhibitors.

Amantadine is an inhibitor of early steps in viral infection in that it prevents fusion of the virion envelope with the cell membrane and the subsequent uncoating of viral nucleic acid. Amantadine is effective against influenza A if administered prophylactically or within 1 da of the onset of symptoms, and is also useful in treatment of Parkinson's disease. The drug does have side-effects on the central nervous system.

Inhibition of nucleic acid polymerization is the most effective mechanism for the inhibition of viral replication because viruses require either new or modified polymerases. One type of nucleic acid synthesis inhibitor is the nucleoside analog. Vidarabine (ara-A) is an analog of deoxyadenosine. In the host cell, Ara-A is modified to a triphosphate ester, which then inhibits both DNA and RNA polymerases. Ara-A has been shown to be useful in the topical treatment of herpes keratitis. Parenteral vidarabine is also indicated in the treatment of patients with proved herpes simplex encephalitis, infants with culture-proved disseminated or central nervous system herpes simplex, and other herpes infections in immunocompromised patients. Nausea is a side-effect of systemic administration. Idoxuridine (IUDR) is an analog of thymidine and is therefore an inhibitor of nucleic acid synthesis. This antiviral agent is useful in the treatment of herpes keratitis; however, IUDR is toxic and immunosuppresive and systemic use should be discouraged.

Ribavirin blocks the formation of guanylic acid; it is useful in the treatment of herpes keratitis, as well as in the systemic treatment of hepatitis A and influenza A and B. It can cause reversible anemia and is teratogenic, which precludes extended systemic administration.

Another type of nucleic acid synthesis inhibitor includes drugs that inhibit DNA polymerase. Phosphonoacetic acid inhibits DNA polymerase of herpes virus and, less effectively, adenovirus. The benzimidazole derivatives inhibit multiplication of picornaviruses by altering control of the viral RNA synthesis. These drugs are not effective in vivo, and their use results in drug-resistant and drug-dependent viral mutants.

Methisazone blocks translation of late mRNA in poxvirus-infected cells. It is effective both prophylactically and therapeutically in the treatment of poxvirus. An occasional side-effect of the drug is vomiting. One of the more promising antiherpes compounds is acyclovir, which was formerly referred to as acycloguanosine. Its limited toxicity and the lack of metabolic degradation on systemic administration enhance its prospects as an antiviral agent. It has been approved for topical use in genital herpes infections and may be approved soon for parenteral use.

Interferon, an antiviral host protein produced in response to a virus infection, is probably the most effective early defense available against viral infections. Three different types of interferon have been identified (see *interferon*). There are certain antiviral agents that act by inducing host interferon production. They are double-stranded RNA polynucleotides known as poly (I)·poly (C). Polynucleotide is most useful prophylactically, intranasally, or topically. Systemic administration of polynucleotides is complicated by their side-effects on hematopoiesis and liver function. Interferon production is high following a single dose; however, the host is refractory to a second dose, with a temporary lack of interferon production.

Anton test (an'ton) in bacteriology, the instillation of a culture into the conjunctival sac of a rabbit to identify *Listeria monocytogenes.* This test was formerly used to determine the pathogenicity of clinical isolates; it currently is not often employed.

antr/o (an'tro) [L. *antrum;* Gr. *antron* cave] a word element used in combining form to denote relationship to an antrum or sinus, e.g., antronasal.

antrum (an'trum), pl. *antrums, antra* [L.; Gr. *antron* cave] a cavity or chamber; used as a general anatomic term to refer to a cavity within a bone, e.g., tympanic antrum.

mastoid a., see *tympanic a.*

pyloric a., the expanded portion of the pyloric part of the stomach between the angular incisure and the pyloric canal.

tympanic a., an air sinus in the petrosal portion of the temporal bone that communicates with the tympanic cavity and the mastoid cells. Also called *mastoid a.*

ANTU abbrev. See *α-naphthylthiourea.*

anuclear (ā-nu'cle-ar) having no nucleus; said of a cell, such as a red blood cell. Also called *anucleated,* and *enucleated.*

anucleated (a-nu'cle-āt"ed) see *anuclear.*

anuresis (an"u-re'sis) 1. retention of urine in the bladder.

2. see *anuria.*

anuria (ah-nu're-ah) [*an-* neg. + Gr. *ouron* urine + *-ia*] no output of urine from the body. Also called *anuresis.*

anus (a'nus), pl. *anus* [L.; said to have originated from an Anglo-Saxon word meaning "to sit"] the distal orifice of the digestive tract.

anxiolytic (ang"zi-o-lit'ik) 1. dispelling anxiety.

2. see *antianxiety drug.*

AO abbrev. See *acridine orange.*

AOA abbrev. See *American Osteopathic Association.*

aort/o (a-or'to) [N.L. *aorta,* from Gr. *aortē* something hung, suspended] a word element used in combining form to denote the aorta, e.g., aortitis.

aorta (a-or'tah) [N.L.] the main systemic arterial trunk. It arises from the left ventricle, ascends to the level of the second right costal cartilage as the ascending aorta, then curves to the left and backward to the lower border of the fourth thoracic vertebra as the aortic arch. From there it descends anterior to the vertebral column and behind the diaphragm as the thoracic and abdominal descending aorta. It ends at the level of the fourth lumbar vertebra by bifurcating to form the common iliac arteries.

aortic (a-or'tik) of or pertaining to the aorta.

aortic aneurysm see under *aneurysm.*

aortic arch syndrome progressive thrombotic encroachment on the origins of the major branches of the aortic arch. Pulses are weak or absent in the head, neck, or arms, and there may be ischemia in these areas.

aortic bodies a pair of small chemoreceptor organs located on each side of the thoracic aorta, composed of richly innervated epithelial cells that contain secretory-type granules. They respond to changes in the blood gases and pH, and initiate reflex adjustments in respiratory and cardiac function. Also called *glomera aortica.*

aortic dissection the separation of the tunica intima from the adventitia of the aorta, with the associated destruction of the tunica media. The dissection is a result of a tear in the tunica intima, which permits blood (under significant arterial pressure) to enter the vessel wall.

Several classifications of aortic dissection have been proposed, all based on the observation that most dissections (more than 95 percent) arise from one of two locations: the ascending aorta or the descending thoracic aorta. Three types are commonly recognized under the DeBakey system: Type I, in which the dissection extends beyond the ascending aorta and aortic arch; Type II, which does not extend beyond the ascending aorta; and Type III, which begins in the descending thoracic aorta and extends distally and (rarely) proximally to the arch.

Deterioration of the aortic tunica media is considered the primary pathologic lesion. It is found in young individuals with hereditary medial degeneration such as Marfan's syndrome), but the peak incidence is in the sixth or seventh decade, occurring with a 2:1 ratio of males to females. It is almost invariably associated with significant hypertension. The most common presenting symptom is a "severe tearing" pain located in the anterior thorax.

Diagnosis is made principally by chest x-ray, computed tomography, and aortic angiography. Medical therapy is employed initially to reduce the systolic blood pressure and thereby reduce the major force contributing to further aortic dissection. Subsequently, surgical therapy may be indicated, especially in proximal dissection.

Also called dissecting aneurysm and dissecting hematoma.

aortic regurgitation the reflux of blood (from aorta to left ventricle) across an incompetent aortic valve during diastole, and the hemodynamic consequences of this retrograde flow. Aortic regurgitation may accompany congenital cardiac defects. It may also be acquired as the result of a variety of primary diseases that affect the valve leaflets or wall of the aortic root, the most prevalent of which is rheumatic fever.

The overall hemodynamic consequence of chronic aortic regurgitation is a volume overload (and to a lesser degree, a pressure overload) on the left ventricular myocardium. It thus is associated with dilation and hypertrophy of the left ventricle that is often of greater severity than that encountered in any other form of valvular heart disease.

Individuals experiencing chronic aortic regurgitation often remain asymptomatic despite the presence of severe ventricular enlargement and retrograde flow. Once ventricular decompensation or coronary insufficiency ensue, however, exertional dyspnea, orthopnea, paroxysmal nocturnal dyspnea, nocturnal angina, thoracic pain, or palpitations frequently become manifest. At this stage, those affected are at the risk of sudden death.

The characteristic auscultatory finding in chronic aortic regurgitation is a high-pitched decrescendo diastolic murmur that begins with the second heart sound. A systolic ejection murmur and Austin Flint diastolic murmur are also commonly heard when the regurgitant flow is severe. Other clinical findings when the regurgitation is chronic and severe include water-hammer (Corrigan's), bisferiens, and Quincke's pulses; Traube's and Duroziez's signs; elevated systolic arterial and decreased aortic diastolic pressures. By echocardiography there is often markedly increased left ventricular end diastolic volume and (if "increased velocity" is meant) left ventricular ejection velocity; an exaggerated motion of the interventricular septum and posterior left ventricular wall; and a fluttering of the mitral valve during diastole. The ST segment and T-wave changes characteristic of a left ventricular volume overload are common electrocardiographic findings.

In most cases, medical management fails to ameliorate the inevitable downhill course of the disease, and surgical intervention (replacement of the defective valve with an artificial one) becomes necessary.

Also called aortic insufficiency.

aortic stenosis obstruction to outflow of blood from the left ventricle by narrowing of the aortic valve. It may be congenital or may be secondary to rheumatic endocarditis. Symptoms do not appear until the valve orifice is reduced to about one-third of normal; while this is developing, the left ventricle compensates by hypertrophy. Most individuals with this condition do not experience significant dyspnea on exertion or angina until they are over 40 yr. If surgical replacement of the valve is undertaken, it should be performed before the onset of left ventricular failure. See also *subaortic stenosis.*

aortic valve the valve composed of three semilunar cusps or segments (posterior, right, and left) that guards the aortic orifice of the left ventricle of the heart and prevents backflow into the ventricle.

aortitis (a″or-ti′tis) [*aort-* + *-itis*] an inflammation of the aorta, which may be caused by septicemia, syphilitic aortitis, or tuberculosis. Aortitis can lead to a weakening of the aortic wall and to changes that may result in a reduction of the blood supply to the innominate, left common carotid, and left subclavian arteries. The clinical manifestations of aortitis include syncope, fainting related to the turning of the head, temporary blindness, loss of memory, and atrophy of facial skeletal muscles. Diagnosis is based on clinical symptoms, aortic arch angiography, and analysis of peripheral blood.

aortography (a″or-tog′rah-fe) [*aorto-* + Gr. *graphein* to write] the radiologic examination of the thoracic or abdominal aorta after introduction of a contrast medium. This procedure may be used to aid in diagnosing aortic aneurysm, atherosclerosis, aortic occlusion or narrowing, and aortic valve deformity or insufficiency. See also *arteriography.*

abdominal a., aortography of the abdominal aorta and its branch vessels. Also called lumbar aortography.

catheter a., a type of aortography in which the contrast medium is introduced at the desired point through a catheter placed into the aorta.

selective visceral a., a type of catheter aortography in which the catheter is moved into several branches of the aorta, such as the renal, celiac, and superior mesenteric arteries, and an arteriogram of each branch is made in turn.

thoracic a., arteriography of the thoracic aorta and its branch vessels.

translumbar a., a type of abdominal aortography in which the contrast medium is injected through a long needle passed percutaneously directly into the aorta.

AP abbrev. See *anteroposterior.*

apallic syndrome (a-pal′ik) see *persistent vegetative state.*

Apathy's gum syrup medium (ap′ah-thēz) a water-soluble mounting medium used in histology consisting of acacia, cane sugar, and distilled water shaken together at 55°–60°C. Thimerosal (Merthiolate) or thymol is added as a preservative; while warm, the solution is placed in a vacuum chamber for a few minutes to remove air bubbles. Potassium acetate or sodium chloride may also be added to prevent bleeding of crystal violet stains used for amyloid. The index of refraction may vary from 1.417 to 1.52, depending on the type of sugar used and on additional ingredients.

apatite (ap′ah-tīt) a calcium phosphate–containing mineral. Hydroxyapatite is the major constituent of bone and tooth enamel. See also *hydroxyapatite.*

APB abbrev. for atrial premature beat. See *premature atrial contraction.*

APC abbrev. for aspirin, phenacetin, and caffeine (an antipyretic and analgesic drug compound); atrial premature contraction (see *premature atrial contraction*).

APD abbrev. for atrial premature depolarization. See *premature atrial contraction.*

aperture (ap′er-chūr) [L. *apertura,* from *aperire* to open] 1. an opening, or orifice.

2. the diameter of a microscope objective lens or the (adjustable) diameter of the iris diaphragm of a camera lens. See also *f number* and *numerical aperture.*

apex (a′peks), pl. *apexes, apices* [L.] 1. a general anatomic term used to denote the top of a body, organ, or part, or the pointed end of a conical structure.

2. the point of greatest activity or of greatest response to stimulation, as when a muscle is electrically stimulated.

apex beat the palpable outward movement of the anterior chest wall produced by the beating heart. Normally it is in a location superior and medial to the point of intersection of the fifth intercostal space and the midclavicular line. It is usually produced by transmission to the chest wall of the counterclockwise rotation of the heart during isometric left ventricular contraction. The portion of the left ventricle that produces the apex beat is medial to the actual apex of the heart.

In the normally functioning heart, the apex beat often coincides with the point of maximal impulse (PMI). The character, extent, and amplitude of the beat can vary with particular cardiac disorders. Also called apical thrust and cardiac impulse.

apexcardiogram (a″peks-kar′de-o-gram) [*apex* + Gr. *kardia* heart + *gramma* drawing] the graphic record of precordial movements over the region of the left ventricular apex. The time course and shape of the characteristic peaks and nadirs of the apexcardiogram are determined primarily by the timing and the amplitude of changes in left intraventricular pressure during the cardiac cycle. The time course and shape generally fall into three broad patterns: normal, hyperdynamic, or sustained.

The hyperdynamic pattern can be seen in conditions in which stroke volume is elevated. This occurs after exercise in normal subjects and also in mitral regurgitation. It has a systolic wave of normal configuration, but increased amplitude and a higher than normal diastolic, rapid filling (F) wave; the F wave may also have a sharp peak. The sustained pattern, which can be seen in conditions with left ventricular hypertrophy, has a prominent presystolic (a) wave, followed by a dome-shaped systolic wave.

apexcardiography (a″peks-kar″de-og′rah-fe) [*apex* + Gr. *kardia* + *graphein* to write] a noninvasive technique used to record the pulsations of the precordium in the region of the left ventricular apex. With the patient in partial left lateral recumbency, a transducer tambour or funnel is placed over the apex. This transducer senses the movement of the soft body tissue enclosed in the intercostal space. The characteristic, reproducible recording obtained, the apexcardiogram, is used in conjunction with other noninvasive diagnostic techniques to assess the status of left ventricular function. Apexcardiography can be utilized to record precordial movements at locations other than over the apex. See also *apexcardiogram.*

Apgar score (ap′gar) [Virginia *Apgar,* American anesthesiologist, 1909–1974] a method for determining an infant's condition at birth by scoring the heart rate, respiratory effort, muscle tone, reflex irritability, and color. The infant is rated on a scale of 0–2 on each of the five items, the highest possible cumulative score being 10. Each of the factors is rated 60 sec after birth and again 5 min later.

The Apgar score is useful as a predictive measure of neonatal difficulties. It is estimated that of the infants with scores of 2 or less at birth, 78 percent do not survive the neonatal period; of those with scores of 8 or greater, only about 1 percent die in the first 28 da of life.

APHA abbrev. See *American Public Health Association.*

aphagia (ah-fa′je-ah) [*a-* neg. + Gr. *phagein* to eat + *-ia*] impaired swallowing.

aphakia (ah-fa′ke-ah) [*a-* neg + Gr. *phakos* lentil + *-ia*] a congenital malformation of the eye in which there is an absence of the lens due to failure of the lens placode to form. The abnormality is probably caused by failure of lens induction or from degeneration of the lens vesicle during the fetal period.

aphasia (ah-fa′ze-ah) [*a-*neg. + Gr. *phasis* speech + *-ia*] a difficulty or impairment in the formulation or comprehension of speech. There are several clinical varieties of aphasia. In expressive or motor aphasia (of Broca), there is a primary disturbance of speech production. In receptive aphasia (also called Wernicke's aphasia), there is impaired comprehension of words and an impairment of language-dependent behavior. Global or total aphasia is characterized by loss of most or all language functions. Several dissociative speech syndromes have also been described and are due to disconnection (by a lesion) of the different parts of the brain involved in speech production or comprehension. Lesions of the central nervous system located in regions responsible for speech production or comprehension will lead to aphasia. Also called *dysphasia.*

Broca's a., an inability to speak and write, with relatively intact ability to comprehend spoken and written language. A result of disease involving the posterior part of the inferior frontal gyrus (Broca's area), this disorder is often associated with right hemiparesis or hemiplegia, and occurs most commonly in strokes that involve the middle cerebral artery. Cf. *Wernicke's a.*

Wernicke's a., an inability to understand spoken or written communication, although the ability to speak and write remains relatively normal. There may be verbal and grammatical errors in speech, however, and the utterance of incorrect or nonexistent words. The disorder is a result of a disturbance in function of a portion of the temporal lobe in the posterior one-third of the left superior temporal gyrus, known as Wernicke's area. Cf. *Broca's a.*

aphasmid (a-faz′mid) [Gr. *a-* neg. + *phasmid*] a nematode belonging to the class Aphasmidia, which lacks phasmids (olfactory receptors). Cf. *phasmid.*

aphonia (a-fo′ne-ah) [*a-*neg. + Gr. *phōnē* voice] loss of the ability to speak, caused by a loss of voice intensity. Rarely, this condition may be due to paralysis of the respiratory muscles, as in poliomyelitis or polyneuritis; it is more commonly caused by paralysis of the vocal cords. Incomplete impairment of phonation is referred to as dysphonia. Cf. *dysphonia.*

aphtha (af′thah), pl. *aphthae* [L.; Gr.] a small ulcer; the term especially refers to the whitish spots in the mouth found in aphthous stomatitis. Also called *canker sore.*

aphthous (af′thus) pertaining to or characterized by aphthae.

aphthous fever a disease that can be transmitted from animals, primarily cloven-hoofed animals and especially cattle, to humans. The etiologic agent is the foot-and-mouth virus. Humans are very rarely affected; the infection may be asymptomatic or there may be fever and vesiculations of the palms, soles, and oropharyngeal mucosa. The course of the disease is usually self-limited. Also called foot-and-mouth disease.

aphthous stomatitis a common disorder of the oral cavity characterized by one or more small whitish lesions, surrounded with a red border, which ulcerate before healing. The lesions are painful and may last 1 wk or more. The origin is unknown, but suggested causes include hormonal imbalance, immunologic disorder, heredity, microbes, allergies, local traumatic injury, and emotional stress. The herpes simplex virus was formerly thought to be a cause but this is now considered unlikely. Also called *aphtha* and *canker sore.*

aphthovirus (af″tho-vi′rus) a picornavirus that causes aphthous fever (foot-and-mouth disease) in cloven-footed animals, especially cattle. See also *aphthous fever* and *picornavirus.*

apiamine (a″pe-ah′mēn) a 16-residue polypeptide that is the toxin of bee venom. The toxin is believed to function as a negative effector in synapses, similar to strychnine. Also called *bee venom toxin.*

apical (ap′ĭ-kal) pertaining to or located at the apex.

apical abscess see *periapical abscess.*

apical canaliculi see *apical c.'s* under *canaliculus.*

apical lordotic view see *lordotic view.*

Apis [L. *apis* bee] a genus of bees, family Apidae, of which the species *A. mellifera* is the common honeybee. The stinging apparatus of this insect injects a painful venom, which may produce anaphylactic shock in allergic individuals.

aplanatic (ap″lah-nat′ik) [*a-* neg. + Gr. *planatikos* wandering] correcting or not affected by spherical aberration.

aplanatic lens a lens corrected for spherical aberration, which produces a flat visual field of focus.

aplasia (ah-pla′ze-ah) [*a-* neg. + Gr. *plassein* to form] the failure of an organ or tissue to develop, such as a congenital malformation caused by the failure of the anlagen of an organ to differentiate to form the organ. Cf. *hypoplasia.*

congenital thymic a., see *DiGeorge's syndrome.*

aplastic (ah-plas′tik) [*a-*neg. + Gr. *plassein* to form] pertaining to or characterized by aplasia; having no tendency to develop into new tissue.

aplastic anemia see *aplastic a.* under *anemia.*

aplastic crisis a sudden, transient disappearance of erythroblasts from the bone marrow, which develops in certain hemolytic states and infections.

apnea (ap-ne′ah) [*a-* neg + Gr. *pnoia* breathing] a cessation of breathing in the end-expiratory position. Apnea can occur after an overdose of depressants, periodically during sleep, following an episode of cerebral thrombosis or embolism, or as the result of various neurologic disorders associated with the medulla or pons (particularly neurons of the reticular activating system). In normal individuals the activity of the respiratory centers is also temporarily arrested during the act of swallowing (deglutition apnea).

posthyperventilation a., the cessation in pulmonary ventilation caused by a lowering of arterial Pco_2 through hyperventilation. It occurs only in anesthetized individuals or in individuals with damage to the pons.

sleep a., the periodic cessation of respiration during sleep in adults and newborns (most commonly in premature infants). In healthy sleeping adults, periods of apnea up to 150 sec in length can occur. These apneic episodes can lead to sudden awakening, impaired respiratory gas exchange, or changes in the cardiovascular system; they may be the result of upper airway obstruction (at the pharyngeal level) or impaired central respiratory control during sleep.

apneic (ap-ne′ik) pertaining to or characterized by apnea.

apneusis (ap-nu′sis) [*a-* neg. + Gr. *pneusis* breathing] arrest of breathing in the end-inspiratory position. In the absence of overriding input from the vagi and pneumotaxic center of the pons, the unrestrained activity of neurons in the apneustic center causes a breathing characterized by sustained inspiratory spasms occasionally interrupted by a brief expiratory gasp.

apneustic (ap-nu′stik) pertaining to or characterized by apneusis.

apo- (ap′o) [Gr. *apo* from] 1. a prefix word element to denote separation from.

2. a prefix word element in biochemistry to denote the polypeptide (protein) portion of a complex molecule, e.g., apoenzyme and apoferritin.

3. a prefix word element in genetics to denote the protein (aporepressor), which, together with a corepressor, may cause genetic repression.

apochromatic (ap″o-kro-mat′ik) [*apo-* + Gr. *chrōma* color] free from chromatic and spherical aberration. See also *apochromatic o.* under *objective.*

apocodeine (ap″o-ko′dēn) a derivative of apomorphine used as an emetic.

apocrine (ap′o-krin) [Gr. *apokrinesthai* to be secreted] denoting that type of exocrine glandular secretion in which the apical cytoplasm, as well as accumulated secretory products, is delivered from the cell. Cf. *holocrine* and *merocrine.*

apocrine carcinoma a carcinoma of the apocrine gland cells, seen particularly in the axillary and perianal regions.

apocrine metaplasia the metaplastic alteration of mammary epithelium to an apocrine sweat gland–type epithelium.

apocrine sweat glands branched tubular glands found mainly in the axilla, areola of the breast, and anogenital region. The tubules of the gland are lined by eosinophilic cells that form a type of sweat rich in protein. The secretion becomes odoriferous when acted on by skin bacteria.

apoenzyme (ap″o-en′zīm) the protein moiety of an enzyme without the cofactor necessary for catalysis. The cofactor can be a metal ion, an organic molecule, or a combination of both.

apoferritin (ap″o-fer′ĭ-tin) a colorless protein constituted of 24 identical units, which is found in the mucosal cells of the small intestine; M.W. 445,000. It functions to facilitate absorption of Fe(II) from the gut into the mucosal cells, where the iron, oxidized to the ferric form, Fe(III), binds with the apoferritin to form ferritin, the mucosal storage form of iron. Ferritin is an iron-storage protein that contains a shell of protein subunits surrounding a core of ferric hydroxyapatite $[Fe_9O_9(OH)(H_2PO_4)]$. Iron is then released and passed in the reduced form through the cell wall into the plasma, where it binds to apotransferrin to form transferrin. *Cf. transferrin.*

apolipoprotein (ah″po-lip″o-pro′tēn) [*apo-* + Gr. *lipos* fat + *protein*] any of a group of proteins that, when associated with lipids such as triglycerides, phospholipids, cholesterol, and cholesterol esters, form the various lipoproteins found in plasma and tissue; M.W. 6500–250,000. Some of these proteins function as cofactors, inhibitors, and activators for certain enzymes and are involved in the structural stability of the lipoproteins. They also transport cholesterol, phospholipids, and triglycerides between tissues, and possess specific binding sites that are recognized by the peripheral tissues involved in their metabolism.

Until recently, most of the characterization of the various lipoproteins involved cholesterol and triglyceride determinations and lipoprotein electrophoresis. However, the isolation of several of the apolipoproteins has made it possible to develop specific assays for individual apoproteins. Preliminary results indicate that such measurement of specific apolipoproteins may correlate clinically better than the tests mentioned above.

APOLIPOPROTEIN A-1. The main component of high-density lipoprotein (HDL), chylomicrons, and intestinal very-low density lipoprotein (VLDL), it has as one of its functions the activation of the enzyme lecithin–cholesterol acyltransferase (LCAT); M.W. 28,000. It contains a C-terminal glutamine.

APOLIPOPROTEIN A-2. A component of HDL, its function is unknown; M.W. 17,000. It is composed of two identical monomers joined by a disulfide bridge, and contains a C-terminal glutamine.

APOLIPOPROTEIN B. The major component of low-density lipoprotein (LDL), it is present also in chylomicrons and VLDL; M.W. 250,000. It appears to have a specific receptor in the peripheral tissues.

APOLIPOPROTEIN C-1. A component of chylomicrons, VLDL, and HDL, it activates lipase and lecithin–cholesterol acyltransferase; M.W. 6630. It is characterized by a C-terminal serine.

APOLIPOPROTEIN C-2. A component of chylomicrons, VLDL, and HDL, it activates extrahepatic lipoprotein lipase; M.W. 8837. It contains a C-terminal glutamic acid.

APOLIPOPROTEIN C-3. A component of chylomicrons, VLDL, and HDL, its possible function is the inhibition of lipoprotein lipase activity; M.W. 8764. It contains a C-terminal alanine. Several polymorphic forms differing in sialic acid content are known.

APOLIPOPROTEIN D. A component of HDL_3, it may function as an activator of lecithin–cholesterol acyltransferase; M.W. approximately 20,000. Also referred to as the thin-line peptide.

APOLIPOPROTEIN E. A component of chylomicrons, chylomicron remnants, VLDL, and HDL, it may be involved in cholesterol transport; M.W. 32,000–39,000. It is arginine-rich and is present in excess quantity in the β-VLDL fraction in type III hyperlipoproteinemia.

See also *chylomicron* and *lipoprotein.*

apomorphine hydrochloride (ap″o-mor′fin) [*apo-* + *morphine*] [USP], a morphine derivative used as a centrally acting emetic. It directly affects the vomiting center of the medulla oblongata.

aponeur/o (ap-o-nu′ro) [Gr. *aponeurōsis,* from *neuron* tendon, sinew] a word element used in combining form to denote aponeurosis (a type of tendon), e.g., aponeurositis.

aponeurosis (ap″o-nu-ro′sis), pl. *aponeuroses* [Gr.] [NA], a flat, white sheet of dense, fibrous connective tissue, generally associated with the attachment of muscles to their insertions.

palmar a., a fan-shaped sheet of fibrous connective tissue in the palm, radiating to the bases of the fingers from the distal end of the flexor retinaculum.

plantar a., a sheet of dense fibrous connective tissue extending forward from an attachment on the medial calcaneal tuberosity to insert mainly into the deep transverse ligament.

apophyseal (ap″o-fiz′e-al) pertaining to an apophysis.

apophysis (ah-pof′ĭ-sis), pl. *apophyses* [Gr. "an offshoot"] 1. an outgrowth or swelling, especially of bone such as a process, tubercle, or tuberosity.

2. in mycology, a swollen fungal filament.

apoprotein (ap″o-pro′tēn) the protein component or polypeptide chain of a protein-containing complex, freed of or separate from all ligands or prosthetic groups, such as a lipoprotein or transferrin. Cf. *apoenzyme.*

apoptosis (ap″o-to′sis) [Gr. "dropping off," as of leaves from trees] a naturally occurring, nonpathologic form of cell death distinct from necrosis, characterized by condensation of the nucleus and cytoplasm, extensive blebbing, and breaking up of the cell into a number of membrane-bound fragments (apoptotic bodies), which are then either phagocytosed by neighboring cells or shed into a lumen. Cf. *necrosis.*

aposiderin (ah″po-sid′er-in) [*apo-* + Gr. *sidēros* iron + *-in*] a granular, iron-negative pigment formed by the removal of iron from hemosiderin. It is produced by the action of very acid fixatives, and resists extraction even by strong acids and alkalis. Aposiderin can be distinguished from lipofuscin as it gives a negative Schmorl reaction.

apothecium (ap″o-the′se-um) [N.L., from Gk. *apothēkē* storehouse] a fungal ascocarp that is open and cup-shaped and contains the spores on its exposed surface.

apparatus (ap″ah-ra′tus), pl. *apparatus, apparatuses* [L., from *ad-* to + *parare* to make ready] 1. an arrangement of a number of parts that together perform some special function.

2. in anatomy, a number of structures or organs that act together in serving some particular function.

apparent power the product of the effective (rms) voltage and the effective (rms) current in an alternating current circuit, usually stated in units of volt-amperes (VA) or kilovolt-amperes (kVA). In a purely resistive load, the apparent power dissipation (in kilovolt-amperes) is equal to the average power dissipation (in watts). In a partially inductive or capacitative load, the voltage and current are out of phase, and the average power is less than the apparent power.

append/o, appendic/o (ah-pen′do, ah-pen′dĭ-ko) [L. *appendix,* from *appendere* to hang upon] a word element used in combining form to denote the appendix, e.g., appendicitis.

appendage (ah-pen′dij) an appendix, an adjunct or subordinate part attached to a larger part.

appendicitis (ah-pen″dĭ-si′tis) [*appendic-* + *-itis* inflammation] an inflammation of the vermiform appendix characterized by pain in the right lower abdominal quadrant, anorexia, malaise, slight fever, and constipation or diarrhea. Appendicitis usually occurs between ages 15 and 30 yr; it is one of the most common causes of emergency acute abdominal operations. Most often, the inflammation is initiated by obstruction of the lumen by a fecalith, followed by infection, edema, and ischemia. *Escherichia coli* and other normal bowel flora are the usual pathogens.

Laboratory studies may show leukocytosis (10,000–20,000 μl) with a shift to left, pyuria, and microscopic hematuria. If the appendix ruptures, complications may include peritonitis, abscess formation, and septicemia. Treatment consists of surgical removal of the appendix.

appendix (ah-pen′diks), pl. *appendices, appendixes* [L., from *appendere* to hang upon] 1. an appendage.

2. the vermiform appendix, a small diverticulum attached to the base of the cecum where the teniae coli come together. The appendix in adults is generally 5–12 cm long and 5–8 mm thick, and is suspended by a small mesentery through which vessels pass. It may be retrocecal or retroileal, or can overlap the brim of the pelvis.

In lower animals the appendix is relatively long and well developed, but in humans it is largely rudimentary, significant only for its rich content of lymphoid tissue (as part of the gut-associated lymphoid tissue) and its vulnerability to occlusion by fecal contents and consequent inflammation. An acutely inflamed appendix is a surgical emergency.

a. epididymis, a small, stalked appendage on the head of the epididymis, usually considered to be a remnant of the mesonephros.

epiploic a's., small appendages of peritoneum, arranged along the teniae of the colon, which are filled with adipose tissue.

a. testis, a small, oval, sessile body on the upper end of the testis or head of the epididymis; a remnant of the upper end of the paranephric duct. It is homologous with the fimbriated end of the uterine tube of the female.

apposition (ap″o-zish′un) [L. *appositio*] the placement or position of adjacent structures or parts so that they can be in contact; the deposition of successive layers on those already present, as in cell walls.

appositional growth growth by addition of material near the surface or end of a substance, the characteristic growth pattern of rigid materials such as bone. Cf. *interstitial growth.*

apraxia (a-prak′se-ah) [Gr. "inaction," from *a-* neg. + *praxis* action] an impairment of the ability to execute a movement upon command that can be performed spontaneously. It is usually produced by a lesion in the frontal or parietal lobes of the brain.

Apresoline (ah-pres′o-lēn) trademark. See *hydralazine hydrochloride.*

aprobarbital (ap″ro-bar′bĭ-tal) an intermediate-acting barbiturate used as a sedative. See also *barbiturate.*

AProL abbrev. See *promyelocytic l.* under *leukemia.*

apronalide (ah-pro′nah-lid) a sedative no longer in use that may induce thrombocytopenic purpura. Its effects have been studied extensively.

aprotic (a-pro′tik) a term used to denote a substance that does not possess dissociable protons.

aprotic solvent a solvent that has no proton for hydrogen bonding, e.g., acetone ($CH_3 \cdot CO \cdot CH_3$), hydrocarbons, and dimethyl sulfoxide ($((CH_3)_2SO)$). Cf. *protic solvent.*

aPTT abbrev. for activated partial thromboplastin time. See *partial thromboplastin time test.*

Apt test a test used to differentiate neonatal blood from maternal blood. One volume of specimen (vomitus or stool in which the blood is red) is mixed with water and centrifuged, and the clear supernatant mixed with sodium hydroxide. The color change is observed after 2 min. Maternal blood containing hemoglobin A changes from pink to yellow-brown, whereas neonatal blood containing hemoglobin F remains pink.

APUD (acronym from *a*mine *p*recursor *u*ptake and *d*ecarboxylation system) a diffuse system of cells, scattered throughout the body, that synthesizes structurally related peptides (usually biogenic amines) which function as hormones or neurotransmitters. The system includes the chromaffin system, hypothalamus, hypophysis, thyroid, parathyroids, lungs, gastrointestinal tract, and pancreas.

Examples of substances produced include epinephrine, norepinephrine, dopamine, serotonin, enkephalin, somatostatin, neurotensin, and substance P. The actions of the substances produced by these cells may affect contiguous cells, nearby groups of cells, or distant cells. It is thought that the APUD system may act as a link between the nervous and endocrine systems, providing further enhancement of the homeostatic control mechanisms.

See also *diffuse neuroendocrine system.*

aq abbrev. See *aqua.*

aqua (aq) (ak′wah), pl. *aquae* [L.] water.

aqua regia a solution made up of three parts concentrated hydrochloric acid and one part concentrated nitric acid.

aque/o (ak′we-o) [L. *aqua* water] a word element used in combining form to denote water, e.g., aqueous.

aqueduct (ak′wĕ-duct″) [L. *aquaeductus,* from *aqua* water + *ductus* leading] a passage or channel.

cerebral a., the narrow channel in the midbrain connecting the third and fourth ventricles and containing cerebrospinal fluid. Also called aqueduct of Silvius.

a. of cochlea, a canal in the temporal bone between the scala tympani and the subarachnoid space.

vestibular a., a canal in the temporal bone between the vestibule of the internal ear and the posterior cranial fossa. It gives passage to the endolymphatic duct.

aqueous (a′kwe-us) [L. *aqua* water] 1. watery; prepared with water.

2. the aqueous humor of the eye.

aqueous humor the colorless, transparent fluid that occupies the anterior chamber of the eye. Produced by the ciliary body (processes), this fluid enters from the posterior chamber and leaves via the trabecular network and Schlemm's canal. It maintains the proper ocular pressure and nourishes the cornea (which is nonvascular). Blockage of drainage elevates the intraocular pressure and is the cause of glaucoma. The pH is 7.4, the protein concentration is low (50 mg/dl), the ionic Ca^{2+} concentration is 1.7 mmol/l, but Na^+, K^+, Cl^-, and CO_2 are present at concentrations close to those in plasma.

Aqueous humor provides a convenient specimen in postmortem toxicologic analysis for specific substances, but the results must be interpreted cautiously.

aqueous mounting media a group of semipermanent mounts used in histology, including the simple syrups, gum arabics, glycerol gelatins, and lactophenol acid media. Their refractive indices are usually rather low (around 1.42).

aqueous solution a solution containing water as solvent.

aquocobalamin (ak″wo-ko-bal′ah-min) vitamin B_{12b}, an analog of cyanocobalamin, in which the cyanide ion is replaced with a water molecule. See also *vitamin B_{12}*.

AR abbrev. for analytical reagent grade; see *reagent grade.*

Ar symbol for the chemical element *argon.*

-ar (er) [L. *-aris*] a suffix word element to denote a relationship of pertaining to, e.g., glandular.

ara-A abbrev. for adenine arabinoside. See *vidarabine.*

arabinose (ah-rab′ĭ-nōs) a reducing aldopentose, obtained from vegetable gums by acid hydrolysis. It is present in large quantities in free or combined form in plums, prunes, and cherries. Alimentary pentosuria can result from ingestion of these fruits, as evidenced by the presence of arabinose and other reducing sugars in urine.

ara-C abbrev. for cytosine arabinoside. See *cytarabine.*

arachidonate (ar″ah-kid′on-ate) any salt, ester, or anion form of arachidonic acid.

arachidonic acid (AA) (ah-rak″ĭ-don′ik) all-*cis*-5,8,11,14-eicosatetraenoic, a naturally occurring, polyunsaturated fatty acid in animal tissues. It is an important precursor of prostaglandins and is quite abundant in animal phospholipids. See also *prostaglandin.*

Arachnia (ah-rak′ni-a) [Gr. *arachnion* a cobweb] a genus of bacteria of the family Actinomycetaceae, of the actinomycetes. The organisms are gram-positive, anaerobic or microaerophilic, nonsporulating rods, forming thin branching filaments but no mycelium; catalase is not produced. They are normal inhabitants of mammalian and human mucous membranes and skin, and are one of the causative agents of actinomycosis in humans and animals. The genus contains a single species, *A. propionica.*

arachnid (ah-rak′nid) any member of the class Arachnida.

Arachnida (ah-rak′nĭ-dah) [Gr. *arachnē* spider] a class of the Arthropoda, which includes the spiders, ticks, mites, and scorpions. Some members produce venoms that can be transmitted to humans by bites or stings; others serve as hosts or intermediate hosts to microorganisms that are human parasites.

arachnidism (ah-rak′nĭ-dizm) the condition produced by the bite of a venomous spider, such as the black widow spider (*Latrodectus mactans*) or the brown recluse spider (*Loxosceles reclusa*). It may be either a systemic reaction or a necrotic local lesion. Systemic arachnidism initially involves little swelling or redness at the site of the bite, but it is followed by dizziness, weakness, tremors, nausea, severe headache, cold perspiration, feeble pulse, constipation, and other symptoms. *L. mactans* antivenin is available for cases of severe envenomization. In necrotic arachnidism, the bitten area becomes swollen and ischemic with deep necrosis and a granulomatous center. Fever, restlessness, jaundice, and convulsions may occur. Healing is slow, with scar tissue formation at the site of the bite and occasional disfigurement. A less serious dose of venom may cause only a rash. Complete immunity is developed upon recovery from both types. Also called *arachnoidism.*

arachnodactyly (ah-rak″no-dak′tĭ-le) [*arachno-* + Gr. *daktylos* finger] a condition characterized by abnormal length of fingers (spider fingers) and toes; it is seen in individuals with Marfan's syndrome and homocystinuria.

arachnoid (ah-rak′noid) [Gr. *arachnoeidēs* like a cobweb] see *arachnoid mater.*

arachnoid granulation a projection of the arachnoid membrane into the superior sagittal sinus; cerebrospinal fluid passes into the blood stream via perforations of the membrane.

arachnoidism (ah-rak′noi-dizm″) see *arachnidism.*

arachnoiditis (ah-rak″noid-i′tis) [*arachnoid* + *-itis*] an inflammation of the arachnoid membrane.

arachnoid mater the middle of the three meningeal membranes covering the brain and spinal cord. It is separated internally from the pia mater by the CSF-filled subarachnoid space and externally from the dura mater by the subdural space.

The arachnoid mater bridges the sulci of the cerebral hemispheres, forming a connective tissue support for the blood vessels that cross the subarachnoid space to reach the pia mater. The basement membranes and tight junctions between cells of the arachnoid act as a barrier for diffusion of some materials between the subdural and subarachnoid spaces. Fingerlike projections of the arachnoid (arachnoid granulations or villi) protrude into the superior sagittal, transverse, and other venous sinuses within the cranial vault. These projections represent a modification of the diffusion barrier, and provide the CSF with a return access to the general circulation.

arachnoid villi minute diverticuli of the subarachnoid space that penetrate the dura mater and fuse with the endothelial cells lining the intradural venous sinuses. See also *arachnoid granulation.*

Araldite (ah-ral′dīt) trademark for an epoxy resin used for tissue embedding. It is very thick and polymerizes with minimal shrinkage; its hardness may be controlled by the amount of dibutyl pthalate added.

Aran-Duchenne disease (ar-ahn′ doo-shen′) [François Amilcar *Aran,* French physician, 1817–1861; Guillaume Benjamin Amand *Duchenne,* French neurologist, 1801–1875] a disorder of adults that is characterized by progressive spinal muscular atrophy and degeneration of the anterior horn cells at different levels of the spinal cord. There is wasting and weakness of the muscles of the limbs and trunk, and fasciculations of affected muscles are commonly seen. The cause is unknown, the disorder is progressive, and there is no treatment. Although the outcome is often fatal, cases with a more benign course and long survival period after diagnosis are sometimes encountered. Also called motor neuron disease and progressive spinal muscular atrophy.

Araneae (ah-rān′e-e) [L. *aranea* spider] an order of the Arachnida, composed of the spiders and divided into the suborders Labidognatha and Orthognatha. The cephalothorax, which bears four pairs of walking legs, is separated from the unsegmented abdomen, and the first pair of appendages form two poison fangs. All spiders produce venom, but most are incapable of harming humans; those that do may cause either systemic or necrotic arachnidism. Large tarantulas (family Aricularidae) are an example of the former, the black widow spider, *Lactrodectus mactans,* an example of the latter.

arbitrary (ar′bĭ-trar″e) chosen for convenience, by whim, or at random. An arbitrary unit or classification may suit the immediate purpose but have little to do with relevant theory or convention.

arborescence (ar″bo-res′ens) [L. *arborescens*] a highly branched or ramified structure that is shaped like a tree.

arborescent (ar″bo-res′ent) exhibiting arborescence, branching like a tree; a form of some bacterial or fungal growth in a deep agar test tube culture. The term is also used to describe the appearance of the edge of some bacterial colonies on solid media.

arborization (ar″bor-ĭ-za′shun) [L. *arbor* tree] a branching formation or arrangement resembling a tree or shrub. Examples include the branching termination of certain nerve cell processes, one form of termination of a nerve fiber when in contact with a muscle fiber, or the treelike appearance of capillary vessels in inflamed conditions.

arbovirus (ar″bo-vi′rus) [from *ar*thropod-*bor*ne + *virus*] a virus that multiplies in both arthropods and vertebrates, and is transmitted from the former to the latter by their bites. Arboviruses are also referred to as the arthropod-borne viruses and the arbovirus group. This ecologic group, however, contains more than 350 different viruses of diverse antigenic composition and virion structure. It is generally agreed that there are arboviruses in the families Togaviridae, Bunyaviridae (all members), Reoviridae, and Rhabdoviridae. Some virologists also include members of the Arenaviridae family.

The most clinically significant arbovirus family is the Togaviridae, which contains most of the members of the former antigenic groups A and B arboviruses. Group A is now the genus *Alphavirus,* group B the genus *Flavivirus.* Togaviruses have an icosahedral core, a single-stranded RNA molecule, and a glycoprotein envelope. They are endemic in tropical climates and may become epidemic during the summer in temperate climates.

Bunyaviridae members are single-stranded RNA viruses that are larger than togaviruses, have helical symmetry, are enveloped, and contain their own transcriptase in the virion. Among the many human diseases caused by Bunyaviridae viruses are sandfly fever, California encephalitis, and Rift Valley fever.

Orbivirus is the only virus of the family Reoviridae that infects humans. It is a spherical particle with an icosahedral symmetry, has a double-stranded segmented RNA, does not have a true envelope, and contains transcriptase in the virion. *Orbivirus* causes Colorado tick fever.

The Rhabdoviridae are a group of bullet-shaped viruses that contain single-stranded RNA. The rabies virus belongs to this group and may be transmitted by both wild and domestic animals.

Human infections with arboviruses vary in severity; some may be subclinical or may produce a harmless undifferentiated fever. When arbovirus infections progress to a more serious state, four types of clinical disease may appear: (1) Fever and arthraglia, with or without a rash, is the most common and is often referred to as dengue fever. This is characterized by a sudden onset of fever, chills, headache, conjunctivitis, lymphadenitis, and back and joint pain. The fever may be intermittent. (2) Another type of arbovirus infection is hemorrhagic fever, in which the individual bleeds from all orifices. This is accompanied by thrombocytopenia and hypotensive shock; it is often lethal. (3) Hemorrhagic fever with hepatitis is known as yellow fever. Usually, the gastrointestinal tract is hemorrhagic; black vomit is sometimes seen. Both blood pressure and pulse rate drop and the affected individual is jaundiced. (4) Encephalitis is the fourth type of arbovirus disease in which the virus first becomes systemic through viremia. The patient has symptoms similar to hemorrhagic fever, with the addition of neck rigidity and mental confusion.

Arbovirus results in type-specific immunity that is long-lasting, which could explain why these infections are endemic only in the tropics, where there are a great many different serotypes of this virus. The viruses multiply in the reticuloendothelial system. Arbovirus diseases may be controlled through reduction of exposure to the vector, reduction of the vector, and immunization. An attenuated strain of yellow fever virus has been shown to be very effective, with minimal side-effects. Protection is long-lasting and boosters are suggested every 10 yr.

Laboratory diagnosis of arboviruses may be made by isolation of the virus or by serologic methods. For isolation of the virus, specimens should be collected from blood, cerebrospinal fluid, or infected organs within 4 da of illness. The baby mouse is the laboratory host of choice. It should be inoculated intracerebrally and observed for 21 da for illness or death.

Serologically, the unidentified virus should be screened against polyvalent sera to determine the viral group. Further serologic identification may then be continued with type-specific sera within a viral group. The complement-fixation test, fluorescent antibody test, and hemagglutination inhibition tests may be applied to identify viral antigens. Neutralization of virus with specific antiserum in a mouse lethality assay, using acute and convalescent sera, is diagnostic for the disease in question.

arceau rhythm see *mu rhythm.*

arch (arch) [L. *arcus* bow] a structure with a curved or bowlike outline.

zygomatic a., the arch formed by the fused articulation of the zygomatic portion of the temporal bone and the temporal portion of the zygomatic bone.

-arche (ar′ke) [Gr. *archē* origin, beginning] a suffix word element to denote first, beginning, or original, e.g., menarche.

archil (ar′kil) roccellin; a violet dye derived from the lichen *Roccella tinctoria,* which is used as an indicator dye for litmus paper. The dye turns blue with bases and red with acids.

Arctiidae a family of tiger moths, order Lepidoptera, which possess poison hairs that may cause urticating dermatitis in humans.

arcuate (ar′ku-āt) [L. *arcuatus* bow-shaped, from *arcus* bow] shaped like an arch or arc; arranged in arches.

ARDS see *adult respiratory distress syndrome.*

area (A) (a′re-ah), pl. *areae, areas* [L. "piece of level ground"] 1. a limited space on a surface, usually measured in square units.

2. a region; for example, a motor area of the brain.

aregenerative (ah″re-jen′er-a″tiv) characterized by absence of regeneration.

Arenaviridae (ah″re-nah-vi′rĭ-de) a family of spherical viruses that contain a single strand of RNA and ribosomes.

arenavirus (ah″re-nah-vi′rus) [L. *arena* sand + *virus*] any of the members of the family Arenaviridae. These enveloped viruses have cellular ribosomes resembling grains of sand, which they pick up during budding from the host cell. The nucleic acid of arenaviruses is single-stranded, segmented RNA. There are four arenaviruses that cause human disease; Junin virus, Argentinian hemorrhagic fever; Machupo virus, Bolivian hemorrhagic fever; Lassa virus, Lassa fever; and lymphocytic choriomeningitis virus, lymphocytic choriomeningitis.

arene (ăr′ēn) the generic term for an aromatic hydrocarbon, e.g., benzene, naphthalene.

areola (ah-re′o-lah), pl. *areolae* [L., dim. of *area* space] 1. any minute space in a tissue. See *areolar connective tissue.*
2. a circular zone of a different color that surrounds a central point, such as the darkened area around the nipple of the mammary gland.

areolar (ah-re′o-lar) 1. pertaining to or containing minute spaces or areas.
2. pertaining to the areola.

areolar connective tissue loose connective tissue characterized by a relatively high ratio of cells to collagen.

ARF abbrev. See *acute r. f.* under *renal failure, acute r. f.* under *respiratory failure.*

Arg abbrev. See *arginine.*

Argas (ar′gas) a genus of ticks with a thin or flattened body and no dorsal shield.

Argasidae (ar-gas′ĭ-de) a family of soft-bodied ticks of the superfamily Ixodoidea, distinguished from the hard-bodied ticks (Ixodidae) by the absence of the scutum. The genera are *Antricola, Argas, Ornithodoros,* and *Otobius.*

argentaffin (ar-jen′tah-fin) [L. *argentum* silver + *affinis* having affinity for] pertaining to tissues that stain readily with silver. Argentaffin-positive cells have the ability to reduce silver salts in the dark without requiring the addition of a reducing agent. See also *argentaffin cell.* Cf. *argyrophil.*

argentaffin cell a polypeptide-forming endocrine cell that can be demonstrated with the argentaffin reaction. The term is often used to refer to serotonin-producing cells of the gastrointestinal tract or bronchi, but other enterochromaffin cells are also argentaffin-positive. See also *APUD.*

argentaffinoma (ar″jen-taf″ĭ-no′mah) see *carcinoid tumor.*

argentaffin reaction a staining procedure employing the reduction of ammoniacal silver solutions to metallic silver, used to demonstrate polypeptide-synthesizing endocrine cells (APUD cells). The reaction is of low specificity. A greater number of these cells can be demonstrated by pretreatment with a reducer (the argyrophil reaction).

Argentinian hemorrhagic fever an acute, sometimes fatal disease caused by the arenavirus Junin virus and probably transmitted by contact with the urine of infected rodents. Its symptoms include chills, fever, severe muscle pain, leukopenia, diffuse hemorrhages, shock, oliguria, and neurologic abnormalities.

argentum (ar-jen′tum) [L.] see *silver.*

arginase (ar″jĭ-nās) an enzyme of the hydrolase class (L-arginine amidinohydrolase, EC 3.5.3.1) that catalyzes the reaction L-arginine + $H_2O \rightleftarrows$ L-ornithine + urea. It also attacks α-*N*-substituted L-arginine and canavanine. Arginase is found in the mammalian liver. The enzyme is part of the Krebs-Henseleit urea cycle.

arginine (Arg or R) (ar′jĭ-nēn) a naturally occurring basic α-amino acid, 2-amino-5-guanidinopentanoic acid, $NH_2C(=NH)NH(CH_2)_3CH(NH_2)COOH$ M.W. 174.20. Arginine is essential in the rat diet but is not essential for humans; it is present in many proteins. It supplies the amidine group for the synthesis of creatine and is involved in urea synthesis (urea cycle). Arginine can be converted to ornithine, glutamate, proline, and hydroxyproline. Its sources are the proteins of the diet, synthesis from glutamate, and synthesis in the urea cycle from ornithine. Also called *guanidino-aminovaleric acid.* See also under *amino acids.*

argininemia (ar-jĭn-in-ē′mē-ah) [*arginine* + Gr. *haima* blood + *-ia*] an inborn error of metabolism, transmitted as an autosomal recessive trait, in which the concentration of arginase is low in tissues and that of arginine elevated in the blood and cerebrospinal fluid. It is characterized by spastic paraplegia, epileptic seizures, hyperammonemia (an inconsistent finding), and severe mental retardation. See also *aminoacidopathy.*

argininosuccinate (ar″jĭ-nĭ-no-suk′sĭ-nāt) an intermediate formed during the condensation of aspartate and citrulline in the argininosuccinate synthetase reaction of the urea cycle. Normally, no traces of argininosuccinate are found in the blood, urine, or cerebrospinal fluid. However, in the occurrence of argininosuccinic aciduria, a block or deficiency of the enzyme that converts argininosuccinate to arginine, argininosuccinate lyase, the blood concentration may rise to 4 mg/100 ml, with a urinary excretion of 2.5–9.0 g/da.

argininosuccinate lyase an enzyme of the lyase class (L-argininosuccinate arginine-lyase, EC 4.3.2.1) that is an integral part of the urea cycle. It catalyzes the cleavage of argininosuccinate to arginine and fumarate, and is found in the liver, kidney, brain, red blood cells, and plasma. The enzyme activity in plasma is increased markedly in parenchymal liver disease (up to 100-fold). A genetic deficiency results in argininosuccinate accumulation in the blood and its excretion in the urine; it is associated with hyperaminoacidemia and hyperammonemia, and leads to mental retardation or, in severe cases, to death. Also called argininosuccinase. See also *argininosuccinic aciduria.*

argininosuccinate lyase assays determination of enzyme activity in plasma performed by the Takahara method. The specimen is incubated for 1 hr at 37°C at neutral pH with argininosuccinate as substrate. After protein precipitation, the supernatant is reacted with 2,4-dichloronaphthol, and the red-colored complex is measured spectrophotometrically at 515 nm. The reference range is 0–4 units (a unit being μmoles of arginine per 100 ml of specimen per hour).

argininosuccinate synthetase an enzyme of the

ligase class (L-citrulline:L-aspartate ligase [AMP-forming], EC 6.3.4.5). It is an integral part of the Krebs-Henseleit urea cycle that catalyzes the reaction ATP + L-citrulline + L-aspartate ⇄ AMP + pyrophosphate + L-argininosuccinate. A genetic deficiency of this enzyme results in citrullinemia with citrulline and ammonia accumulation in the blood.

argininosuccinate synthetase deficiency a disorder of citrulline metabolism, transmitted as an autosomal recessive trait, that is due to a relative or absolute deficiency of argininosuccinate synthetase. Those affected with this very rare disease have hyperammonemia and increased concentrations of citrulline in the blood, urine, and cerebrospinal fluid. Mental retardation, central nervous system dysfunctions, protein intolerance, vomiting, convulsions, coma, and death in the neonatal period are common. Screening for carriers and prenatal detection of affected fetuses are considered possible. Also called *citrullinemia.* See also *aminoacidopathy.*

argininosuccinic acidemia the accumulation of high levels of argininosuccinic acid in the blood, usually due to the aminoacidopathy argininosuccinic aciduria.

argininosuccinic aciduria a disorder of argininosuccinic acid metabolism, transmitted as an autosomal recessive trait, that is due to the relative or absolute deficiency of the enzyme argininosuccinate lyase (argininosuccinase). This results in accumulations of argininosuccinic acid in the urine and blood, and intermittent hyperammonemia, especially after the ingestion of protein meals. Those affected have a variety of clinical syndromes, including: (early onset) seizures, lethargy, pulmonary dysfunction, and early death; (late onset) mental and physical retardation, hepatomegaly, protein intolerance, and ataxia; and (subacute) mental retardation, central nervous system dysfunction, and trichorrhexis nodosa. Urine screening may be more efficient than blood screening. Detection of carriers and prenatal screening are considered feasible. Low-protein diets may offer variable relief. See also *aminoacidopathy.*

arginyl (ar′jĭ-nil) the acyl radical derived from or relating to arginine.

argon (Ar) (ar′gon) [Gr. *argos* inert] an inert, gaseous element, atomic number 18; atomic weight 39.948; Group O of the periodic table (the noble gases); oxidation state 0 (no compounds). It is used as an inert atmosphere in gasflow proportional counters, in Geiger-Müller counters, in some positron cameras, and as carrier gas in gas chromatography.

AR grade abbrev. for analytical reagent grade. See under *reagent grade.*

argument (ar′gu-ment) [L. *argumentum* evidence] 1. an independent variable of a mathematical function.

2. a variable or constant available to a computer subroutine. The subroutine returns information to the calling program by changing the values of some of the arguments. In most languages, a subroutine cannot change the values of constant arguments.

Argyll Robertson pupil (ar-gīl′ rob′ert-son) [Douglas Moray Cooper Lamb *Argyll Robertson,* Scottish physician, 1837–1909] a pupil that is miotic and responds to accomodative effort, but not to light. It is encountered in syphilitic meningitis and other forms of late syphilis.

argyremia (ar″jĭ-re′me-ah) [Gr. *argyros* silver + *haima* blood + *-ia*] the presence of silver or silver salts in the blood.

argyria (ar-jir′e-ah) [Gr. *argyros* silver] poisoning by prolonged use of, or contact with, silver and silver salts absorbed from the lungs or gastrointestinal tract. If absorption is local, grayish patches may form on the skin and conjunctiva; if general, there is widespread pigmentation and sometimes the presence of a metallic luster. The hue may range from gray to one suggesting marked cyanosis. Also called *argyrosis.*

argyrophil (ar-ji′ro-fil) [Gr. *argyros* silver + *philein* to love] capable of binding silver salts, which may then be reduced by light or by a reducing agent to give a black deposit of silver; said of cells and tissues. Cf. *argentaffin.*

argyrosis (ar″jĭ-ro′sis) [Gr. *argyros* silver + *-osis* condition] see *argyria.*

Arias-Stella cells [Javier *Arias-Stella,* Peruvian pathologist, born 1920] dysplastic cells found in aneuploid hypersecretory endometrial glands, e.g., in the presence of ectopic pregnancy and trophoblastic disease. Their occurrence in early pregnancy is called the Arias-Stella phenomenon or reaction.

Arias syndrome (ar′e-as) [Irwin Monroe *Arias,* U.S. physician, born 1926] see *C.-N. s., type 2,* under Crigler-Najjar syndrome.

ariboflavinosis (a-ri″bo-fla″vĭ-no′sis) deficiency of riboflavin (vitamin B_2). Clinical signs are poorly defined, but when severe they include lesions of the lip (angular stomatitis), tongue, skin (scaling seborrheic dermatitis), and eyes, along with corneal or other eye changes. Ariboflavinosis occurs most often in association with other vitamin B complex deficiencies.

arithmetic (ah-rith′mah-tik; ah-rith-met′ik) [Gr. arithmētikē, from *arithmos* number] 1. the mathematics of real numbers in addition, subtraction, multiplication, division, and exponentiation.

2. pertaining to the process of arithmetic.

arithmetic and logic unit (ALU) the circuitry in the central processing unit of a digital computer that performs arithmetic operations, logical operations, and comparisons on binary-coded data. See also *digital computer.*

arithmetic mean the arithmetic average; the sum of a group of items divided by the number of items i.e., $\Sigma_i x_i / n$, where $x_1, x_2, \ldots, x_n$ are the items and n is the number of items. See also *mean.* Cf. *geometric mean.*

arithmetic operation in computer programming, one of the fundamental arithmetic operations: addition, subtraction, multiplication, division, and exponentiation. See also *operation.*

Arizona a genus of bacteria of the tribe Salmonelleae, family Enterobacteriaceae. The organisms are malonate-positive, and many ferment lactose rapidly. Found originally in reptiles, they also occur in fowl and other domestic animals, and have been isolated from dried egg powder and other food sources. Infection with the single species of the genus, *A. hinshawii,* can produce gastroenteritis, enteric fevers, bacteremia, and local infections resembling salmonellosis. Formerly called *Salmonella arizonae.* See also *Enterobacteriaceae.*

Arlex gelatin an aqueous histochemical mounting medium. It is formed by heating Arlex D-sorbitol syrup and gelatin in a boiling water bath and then adding potassium acetate and merthiolate. It has a pH of 6.0+; preparations set quickly but remain sticky for some time.

arm (arm) [L. *armus* shoulder] 1. the upper extremity from shoulder to elbow, as distinguished from the forearm; the term is popularly used to refer to the extremity from shoulder to hand.

2. an armlike part, e.g., the portion of the chromatid extending from the centromere of a mitotic chromosome in either direction.

Armanni-Ebstein cells [Luciano *Armanni,* Italian pathologist, 1839-1903; Wilhelm *Ebstein,* German internist, 1836-1912] cells of the straight part of the proximal convoluted tubule of the kidney containing an accumulation of glycogen, seen occasionally in diabetes.

armed macrophage a type of phagocytic cell able to destroy other cells, owing either to the presence of cytophilic antibodies (IgG or IgM) or to arming factors from T cells. If injected with tumor cells at the same site, such cells may produce a strong degree of rejection.

Armigeres (ar-mij′er-ēz) a genus of mosquitos that may transmit human diseases.

A. obturbans, a species that has been found to carry the dengue virus in Japan.

Armillifer (ar-mil′ĭ-fer) a genus of endoparasites, family Porocephalidae, order Porocephalida.

A. armillatus, a species, found in Africa, whose adult members are found in the lungs and trachea of the python (*Python sebae* and *P. regius*) and whose larvae occur in the internal organs of monkeys and lions and occasionally of humans. Called the "tongue worms," this small group of bloodsucking arthropods has separate sexes and generally lives in the respiratory tract. Also called *Porocephalus armillatus* and *Porocephalus constrictus.*

A. moniliformis, a species, found in China, the Philippines, and other Asian islands, that is parasitic to humans.

Arneth count (ar-nāt′) [Joseph *Arneth,* German physician, 1873–1955] an expression of the ratio of the number of lobes or segments (from one to five) of the nucleus of a polymorphonuclear leukocyte (PMN). On the average, 5 percent of PMNs have one lobe, 35 percent have two, 41 percent have three, 17 percent have four, and 2 percent have five. The least mature PMNs have the fewest number of lobes because they pass through a band, nonsegmented stage as they develop from myelocytes.

Because an Arneth count is reported starting with the percentage of PMNs with the fewest lobes, a "shift to the left" indicates an increase in more immature forms, most commonly observed in the leukocytosis of bacterial infections. A "shift to the right" is equivalent to a hypersegmentation of PMNs, and accompanies vitamin B_{12} or folic acid deficiencies associated with megaloblastic anemias, although it occurs in other conditions.

The complete Arneth formula now is seldom determined and is an obsolete laboratory measurement, no longer included in many standard textbooks of hematology. The hypersegmentation of PMNs, however, remains a useful diagnostic sign of folic acid or vitamin B_{12} deficiency, and an increased band count (above 5 percent) may be an indicator of bacterial infection.

Arnold-Chiari malformation [Julius *Arnold,* German pathologist, 1835–1915; Hans *Chiari,* German pathologist, 1851–1916] a congenital anomaly in which the posterior cerebellum and medulla oblongata (which is lengthened and flattened) are caudally displaced and extend through the foramen magnum into the spinal canal. It may be accompanied by internal hydrocephalus, aqueductal stenosis, meningomyelocele, and flattening of the base of the skull (platybasia). Patients may present with symptoms and signs of syringomyelia, increased intracranial pressure, pyramidal or cerebellar deficits, lower cranial nerve abnormalities, or some combination of these features. Treatment is surgical.

aromatic (ar″o-mat′ik) [L. *aromaticus,* from Gr. *arōmatikos*] 1. having an aroma.

2. in chemistry, denoting a compound characterized by the presence of one or more benzene rings or other rings having aromatic character. Aromatic character, which is not limited to benzene, is associated with the delocalization of π electrons in a planar cyclic molecule; for example, pyrrole, thiophene, pyridine, and purine are considered to be aromatic compounds. See also *aromatic ring.*

aromatic acid any of a group of organic acids containing a carboxyl group (—COOH) and a benzene or other aromatic ring, e.g., benzoic acid.

aromatic amine an organic compound that contains a free or substituted amino group attached to an aromatic ring. The systematic generic names for this class of compounds are arylamine (in the IUPAC system) and arenamine (in the *Chemical Abstracts* system).

aromatic compound any compound that contains an aromatic ring, e.g., pyrrole, pyrimidine. See also *aromatic ring.*

aromatic hydrocarbon an organic compound containing an aromatic ring; because of resonance stabilization, these compounds are less reactive than unsaturated aliphatic hydrocarbons. The simplest are benzene, naphthalene, anthracene, phenanthrene, and their derivatives.

aromaticity (ar″o-ma-tis′ĭ-te) the quality that renders aromatic rings especially stable, owing to resonance stabilization or delocalization of π electrons. See also *aromatic.*

aromatic ring the resonance-stabilized ring characteristic of aromatic organic compounds. Most aromatic rings are planar six-membered rings (e.g., benzene or pyridine) or planar five-membered rings containing a hetero atom with an unshared electron pair (e.g., furan or pyrrole). Although aromatic rings are unsaturated, they do not undergo the addition reactions characteristic of alkenes; instead, aromatic compounds are characterized by substitution reactions. Many organic compounds, such as naphthalene and purine, contain several aromatic rings fused together.

array 1. a collection of data items of the same type. An array can be one-dimensional to n-dimensional. A one-dimensional array consists of a column of data items and is known as a vector; a two-dimensional array consists of rows and columns of data items and is known as a matrix. See also *matrix* and *vector.*

2. in electrophysiology, the placement or arrangement of electrodes.

arrector (ah-rek'tor), pl. *arrectores* [L.] raising, or that which raises.

arrector pili (ah-rek'tor pi'li), pl. *arrectores pilorum*[L. "raiser of hair"] a small band of smooth muscle attached to the connective tissue sheath that surrounds a hair follicle. Contraction of these muscles can cause the hair to rise vertically and produce the appearance called goose flesh (cutis anserina).

arrhenoblastoma (ah-re"no-blas-to'mah) [*arrheno-* + Gr. *blastos* germ + *-oma*] a tumor of specialized gonadal stroma arising in the ovaries. Also called *androblastoma.* See also *gonadal-stromal tumors* and *Sertoli-Leydig cell tumors.*

arrhythmia (ah-rith'me-ah) [*a-* neg. + Gr. *rhythmos* rhythm] an abnormality of the rate or rhythm of heartbeats. Abnormalities of rhythm include those caused by an abnormally located pacemaker, abnormal conducting pathways, or a dysfunctional sinus pacemaker, as well as abnormalities of conduction of electric impulses through the atrioventricular node and the bundle of His and its branches. Also called *dysrhythmia.*

ARRS abbrev. See *American Roentgen Ray Society.*

ARRT abbrev. See *American Registry of Radiologic Technologists.*

ARS abbrev. See *American Radium Society.*

arsanilic acid *p*-aminobenzene arsonic acid, a compound used as a food additive for domestic animals; its derivatives are used to treat amebiasis; see *carbarsone.*

arsenate (ar'sĕ-nāt) a salt of arsenic acid, H_3AsO_4; usually a salt with AsO_4^{3-} as the anion.

arsenic (As) (ar'sĕ-nik) [Gr. *arsenikon* yellow orpiment (arsenic trisulfide)] a silvery-gray, crystalline, semiconducting element; atomic number 33; atomic weight 74.9216; Group V of the periodic table; oxidation states –3, +3, +5. It is used in metallic alloys, in semiconductor devices, and in various toxic compounds as a pesticide. Most arsenic compounds are toxic; the arsenic(III) ion is more so than arsenic(V). Arsenic binds to sulfhydryl groups and thus denatures and inactivates proteins, including enzymes. It is rapidly cleared from the blood. Symptoms of acute arsenic poisoning include edema, gastrointestinal irritation, muscle spasms, and coma; chronic poisoning causes fatigue and damage to skin and nerves.

Arsenic occurs naturally in the environment and in food. Individuals generally have less than 50 μg/l of arsenic in their urine, although arsenic workers may have 200 μg/l. Acute poisoning causes levels of up to 1.0 mg/l or more.

arsenic assays 1. a screening test in which concentrated hydrochloric acid and pure copper foil or wire spiral are added to a urine sample, and the solution is heated to simmering for 1–2 hr. The copper is then rinsed with distilled water and examined for color changes. Gray or black deposits on the surface of the copper may mean the presence of arsenic, selenium, some sulfur compounds, antimony, bismuth, or tellurium. Mercury produces a light gray or silvery film that becomes shiny when rubbed. If no change in the copper is noted, the presence of arsenic, antimony, mercury, and selenium in quantities of 25 μg/l, 1 mg/l, 500 μg/l, and 500 μg/l or more, respectively, is ruled out. Also called *Reinsch test.*

2. a quantitative test in which the sample is digested in strong acid. Arsine (AsH_3) is liberated (in a closed system) by the addition of hydrochloric acid, stannous chloride, and sodium iodide. It is then reacted with a color reagent such as diethyldithiocarbamate, and the concentration is measured spectrophotometrically.

3. flameless atomic absorption spectrophotometry of an acid-digested sample.

4. neutron activation analysis for the determination of minute quantities of arsenic in hair and nail samples.

arsenic stain a histologic procedure to demonstrate the presence of metallic salts of arsenic in tissue. Following fixation in a formalin solution containing copper sulfate, the tissue is washed vigorously in water and embedded in paraffin. Sections exhibit green granules of Scheele's green, the cupric salt of arsenic. Granules are soluble in acid or ammonium hydroxide. Granular Paris green or green cupric acetoarsenite with the same solubility may be obtained by using cupric acetate instead of copper sulfate. A light safranin may be used as a counterstain.

arsine (ar'sin) arsenic trihydride or hydrogen arsenide, AsH_3, a very poisonous gas. Upon inhalation of as little as 0.5 ppm, it may cause hemolysis, jaundice, gastroenteritis, and nephritis. Those involved in the smelting of certain metals or those exposed to arsenic-containing chemicals risk the development of severe hemolytic anemia if arsenic-containing compounds are subjected to reducing conditions.

arsphenamine (ars-fen'ah-min) an arsenical; the first arsenical specific for the treatment of syphilis, yaws, and *Spirillum* infections, it was later replaced—first by arsenoxide, then by penicillin.

ART abbrev. for *absolute retention time*(see under *retention time*), automated reagin test.

arteri/o (ar-te're-o) [L. *arteria,* from Gr. *artēria*] a word element used in combining form to denote artery, e.g., arteriosclerosis.

arterial (ar-te're-al) pertaining to an artery or to the arteries.

arterial (a) blood blood present in or taken from an artery: blood that has been oxygenated during passage through the lung, at which time CO_2 is partially removed by diffusion into the alveoli. As arterial blood passes through the capillaries in the tissues, it gives off O_2 and picks up CO_2 and other metabolites, becoming venous blood. This is recycled through the lung, where it is again converted to arterial blood. As a result of these processes, the $ctCO_2$ of arterial blood is about 2 mmol/l lower and the O_2 content 2 mmol/l higher than in venous blood. The pH of human venous blood is about 0.03 pH less than in arterial blood, owing to the accumulation of acidic metabolites. Heparinized arterial blood is the preferred specimen for blood gas (Po_2; Pco_2) and pH determinations.

arterial cone see *c. arteriosus* under *conus.*

arterialized blood blood from a limb that has been warmed before sampling; the forearm, hand, and fingers may be placed in a 45°C water bath for several minutes, or a towel dipped in 45°C water may be wrapped around the forearm. Blood drawn in such a manner is similar to arterial blood in terms of its

P_{O_2}, $ctCO_2$, and pH. It is used when arterial blood is not available.

arterial P_{CO_2} (Pa_{CO_2}) the partial pressure of carbon dioxide in arterial blood, approximately equal to 40 mmHg in the healthy subject at rest at sea level. Also called arterial CO_2 tension. See also *blood gas analysis.*

arterial P_{O_2} (Pa_{O_2}) the partial pressure of oxygen in arterial blood, approximately equal to 90 mmHg in the healthy individual at rest at sea level. Also called arterial O_2 tension. See also *blood gas analysis.*

arterial pressure the force exerted by the blood against the walls of the arteries, by convention expressed as millimeters of mercury (mmHg) above atmospheric pressure. Because the pumping action of the heart is pulsatile, ejection of blood into the arteries is intermittent and causes a pressure pulse. The aortic arterial pressure thus fluctuates between a peak systolic pressure level of about 120 mmHg, reached at maximal left ventricular stroke output, and a minimal diastolic pressure of about 80 mmHg at late ventricular diastole. The pulse pressure is equal to the difference between these two pressure levels. The mean arterial pressure is the average pressure level during the cardiac cycle, measured by integration of the area under a tracing of the pressure pulse, or calculated as the diastolic pressure + (pulse pressure/3).

Pulse pressure is slightly augmented in the large- to medium-sized peripheral arteries owing to summation of a pressure wave that has been reflected from the smaller arteries with the oncoming wave. Mean pressure progressively decreases in the smaller arteries, and the pulse pressure becomes progressively more damped.

See also the accompanying illustration.

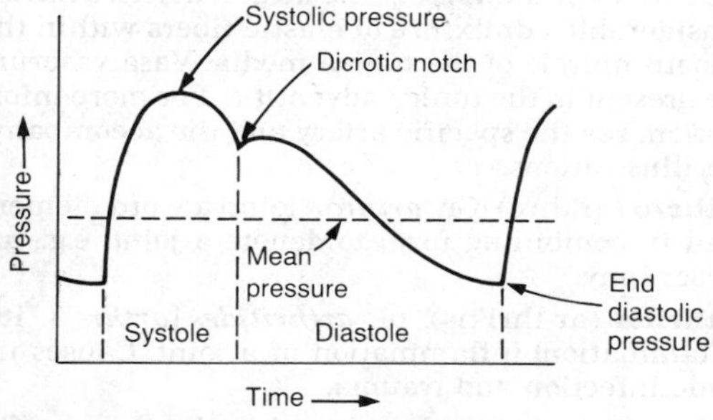

Arterial pressure. Diagram illustrating a portion of the aortic arterial pulse wave. (Modified from Ruch, T. C., and Patton, H. D.: Physiology and Biophysics, Vol. II. 20th ed. Philadelphia, W. B. Saunders Co., 1974.)

arteriogram (ar-te′re-o-gram″) [*arterio-* + Gr. *gramma* a writing] a radiogram produced by arteriography.

arteriography (ar″te-re-og′rah-fe) [*arterio-* + Gr. *graphein* to write] the radiologic examination of arteries and their branches after introduction of a contrast medium into the blood stream. This procedure is frequently used as a diagnostic aid for vascular abnormalities such as malformation, occlusion, tumor, or atherosclerosis. It may be designated by the specific artery into which the medium is directed, as illustrated in the following subentries.

coronary a., a procedure used to visualize the coronary arteries by the introduction of a contrast medium. The sequential or motion picture films that can be made may be used to detect atherosclerosis, occlusion, and malformations of the coronary arteries.

peripheral a., arteriography of the extremities after injection of a contrast medium into the subclavian or femoral artery.

selective a., the introduction of contrast material, usually by catheter, into the opening of a vessel that arises from the aorta for the purpose of radiologic examination.

selective visceral a., see *selective visceral a.* under *aortography.*

transfemoral a., a type of catheter abdominal aortography in which the catheter is introduced by way of the femoral artery.

arteriol/o (ar-te-re-ōl′o) [N.L. *arteriola,* dim. of *arteria*] a word element used in combining form to denote a small artery or arteriole, e.g., arteriolosclerosis.

arteriole (ar-te′re-ōl) [N.L. *arteriola,* dim. of L. *arteria* artery] the smallest branch of an artery, just proximal to a capillary.

afferent a., a branch of the interlobular artery that supplies a renal glomerulus.

efferent a., an arteriole formed by the confluence of the renal glomerular capillaries. It divides into the capillaries of the vasa recta, which invests the renal tubule.

arteriolosclerosis (ar-te″re-o″lo-sklĕ-ro′sis) [*arteriolo-* + Gr. *sklēros* hard + *-osis* condition] see under *arteriosclerosis.*

arterionephrosclerosis (ar-te″re-o-nef″ro-skle-ro′sis) see *nephrosclerosis.*

arteriopathy (ar-te″re-op′ah-the) [*arterio-* + Gr. *pathos* disease] any disease of an artery.

hypertensive a., the widespread involvement of the smaller arteries and arterioles, associated with hypertension and characterized primarily by hypertrophy of the tunica media.

arteriosclerosis (ar-te″re-o-sklĕ-ro′sis) [*arterio-* + Gr. *sklēros* hard + *-osis* condition] a generic term used to describe pathologic changes in arteries characterized by the hardening and thickening of the arteries and their loss of normal elasticity. There are three main forms, arteriolosclerosis, atherosclerosis, and Mönckeberg's medial calcific sclerosis.

arteriolosclerosis, a term encompassing two forms of arteriolar disease that are usually related to elevations of blood pressure, hyaline and hyperplastic arteriolosclerosis.

Hyaline arteriolosclerosis is most common in elderly individuals having moderate elevation of systolic blood pressure (benign hypertension); it is also encountered in normotensive as well as hypertensive diabetic individuals. The disease is characterized by irregular thickening of the basement membrane and intimal and medial collagenization of arteriolar walls. The resulting narrowing of the arteriolar lumens causes reduced blood supply to the affected tissues. Also called presenile arteriosclerosis and senile arteriosclerosis.

Hyperplastic arteriolosclerosis is related to severe elevations of blood pressure (malignant hypertension). This form is characterized by the proliferation of myofibroblasts to form concentric, laminated (onion skin) thickenings of arteriole walls with progressive narrowing of lumens. The basement membranes of the arterioles are thickened and reduplicated, and frequently, necrosis and deposition of fibrinoid are seen in the walls. Vessels showing predilection for this form of arteriolar disease include those of the kidney, lung, and gallbladder, and the peripancreatic, periadrenal, and intestinal arterioles. Also called hypertensive arteriosclerosis.

atherosclerosis, the most common form of arteriosclerosis, occurring with highest frequency in affluent societies. It is a slowly progressive vascular disease characterized by the focal formation of atheromata in the intima of muscular arteries, primarily those of large and medium size. The atheroma is composed of a core of cholesterol and cholesterol esters and a covering of fibrous plaque; its growth causes a reduction in blood flow and a weakening of affected arteries. The atheroma may become calcified and ulcerated, undergo internal hemorrhage, and form a nidus for overlying thrombosis. Atherosclerosis is the major cause, along with superimposed thrombosis, of coronary heart disease, cerebrovascular accidents, and gangrene of the lower extremities (arteriosclerosis obliterans). Its incidence increases with age.

Mönckeberg's medial calcific sclerosis, a form of arteriosclerosis of unknown etiology, characterized by ringlike calcifications within the media of muscular arteries that are small to medium in size. The vessels most severely affected are the femoral, tibial, radial, and ulnar arteries. The lesions do not compromise vascular lumens and are of relatively little clinical significance. Also called medial calcinosis.

arteriosclerotic (ar-te″re-o-sklĕ-rot′ik) pertaining to or characterized by arteriosclerosis.

arteriosclerotic heart disease see *atherosclerotic heart disease.*

arteriovenous (AV) (ar-te″re-o-ve′nus) both arterial and venous; referring to or affecting both an artery and a vein.

arteriovenous malformations of the central nervous system abnormal connection between an artery or arteries and the venous system, which may occur anywhere in the central nervous system and its surrounding meninges. Intracranial bleeding is the first manifestation of about half of those with such malformations, and may lead to focal neurologic deficits or occasionally to death. In other individuals, headaches, progressive sensory or motor impairment, or seizures may signal the presence of the lesion, which is visualized by CT scan and arteriography. Definitive treatment is surgical when feasible.

The Sturge-Weber syndrome consists of associated cutaneous (facial) and intracranial meningeal hemangiomas. Those affected may be neurologically asymptomatic, or may have seizures, focal deficits, and intellectual decline.

For more information, see *Sturge-Weber syndrome.*

arteritis (ar″tĕ-ri′tis), pl. *arteritides* [*arteri-* + *-itis*] inflammation of the arteries, usually accompanied by acute or chronic inflammatory cell infiltration around the vessel walls. It may often result in arterial wall destruction with hemorrhage into the surrounding tissues, as well as partial or full occlusion of the artery with resultant ischemic damage to the tissues supplied by that artery and its branches. Arteritis is a component of many connective tissue disorders (e.g., systemic lupus erythematosus, rheumatoid arthritis), rheumatic fever, allergic reactions, and some infectious diseases. The pathogenesis is believed to stem from the deposition of antigen-antibody complexes in the walls of the vessels involved.

temporal a., a chronic, generalized inflammatory disease of unknown etiology that principally involves the temporal, occipital, and other cranial arteries of the external carotid system. Most cases occur in persons over the age of 60. Manifestations include headache, scalp tenderness, myalgia, fever, malaise, anorexia, weight loss, and a thickened, tender temporal artery.

Laboratory findings include an elevated erythrocyte sedimentation rate (ESR), leukocytosis, and mild anemia. Temporal artery biopsy usually shows inflammatory cells, including giant cells, throughout the wall. Treatment involves administration of corticosteroids. Serious but infrequent complications include blindness, stroke, and coronary occlusion.

artery (ar′ter-e) [L. *arteria;* Gr. *artēria,* from *aēr* air + *tērein* to keep, because the arteries were supposed by the ancients to contain air, or from Gr. *aeirein* to lift or attach] a vessel that carries blood away from the heart to various parts of the body. The wall of an artery typically consists of an outer coat (tunica adventitia), a middle coat (tunica media), and an inner coat (tunica intima). A wavy internal elastic lamina separates the tunicae intima and media. In larger arteries, a less prominent external elastic lamina can also be identified. The thickness of the various layers, particularly the tunica media, varies with the caliber of the vessel. The largest arteries have a considerable admixture of elastic fibers within the smooth muscle of the tunica media. Vasa vasorum are present in the tunica adventitia. For more information, see the specific artery and the accompanying illustrations.

arthr/o (ar′thro) [Gr. *arthron* joint] a word element used in combining form to denote a joint, e.g., arthrography.

arthritis (ar-thri′tis), pl. *arthritides* [*arthr-* + itis inflammation] inflammation of a joint. Causes include infection and trauma.

arthrocentesis (ar″thro-sen-te′sis) [*arthro-* + Gr. *kentēsis* a pricking] surgical puncture of a joint cavity in order to aspirate synovial fluid for examination.

arthrochondritis (ar″thro-kon-dri′tis) inflammation of the cartilage of a joint.

Arthroderma (ar″thro-der′mah) [*arthro-* + Gr. *derma* skin] a genus of fungi that belongs to the family Gymnoascaceae, order Eurotiales. It is the perfect stage of the *Trichophyton* and *Chrysosporium* genera. The hyphae around the gymnothecia are dichotomously branched; individual cells have a dumbbell-like appearance. *Arthroderma* are similar to *Nannizzia.* See also *Trichophyton.*

arthrodia (ar-thro′de-ah) [Gr., from *arthrōdēs* well articulated] a type of synovial joint that allows only a gliding motion, e.g., a shoulder joint.

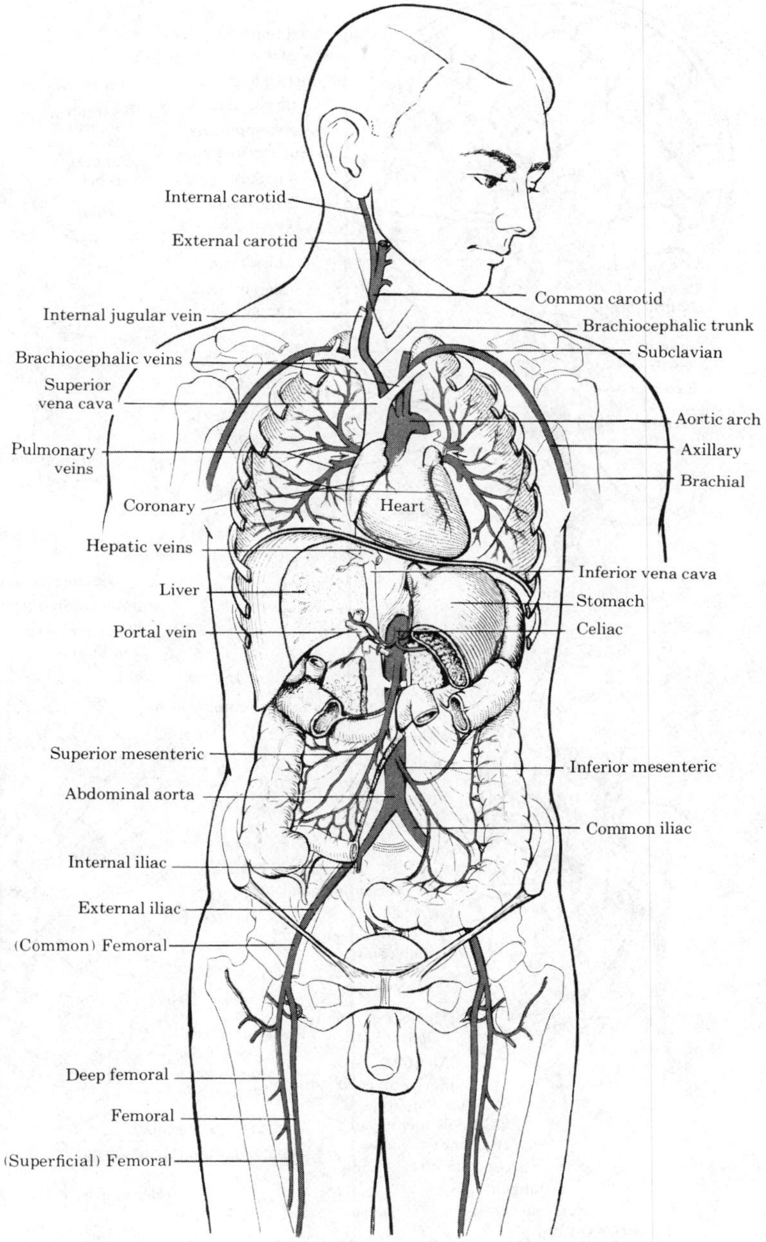

Artery, Figure 1. Principal arteries of the body and pulmonary veins. (From Dorland's Illustrated Medical Dictionary. 26th ed. Philadelphia, W. B. Saunders Co., 1981.)

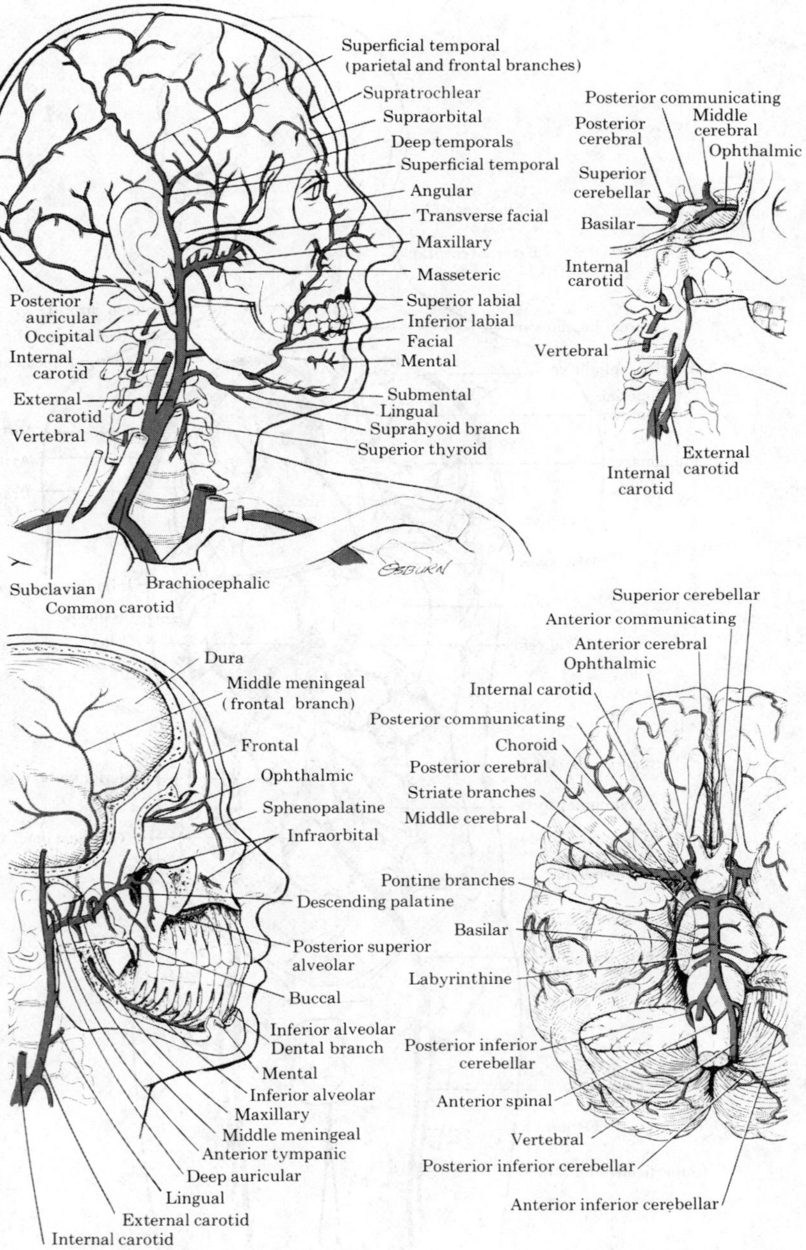

Artery, Figure 2. Arteries of the head, neck, and base of the brain. (From Dorland's Illustrated Medical Dictionary. 26th ed. Philadelphia, W. B. Saunders Co., 1981.)

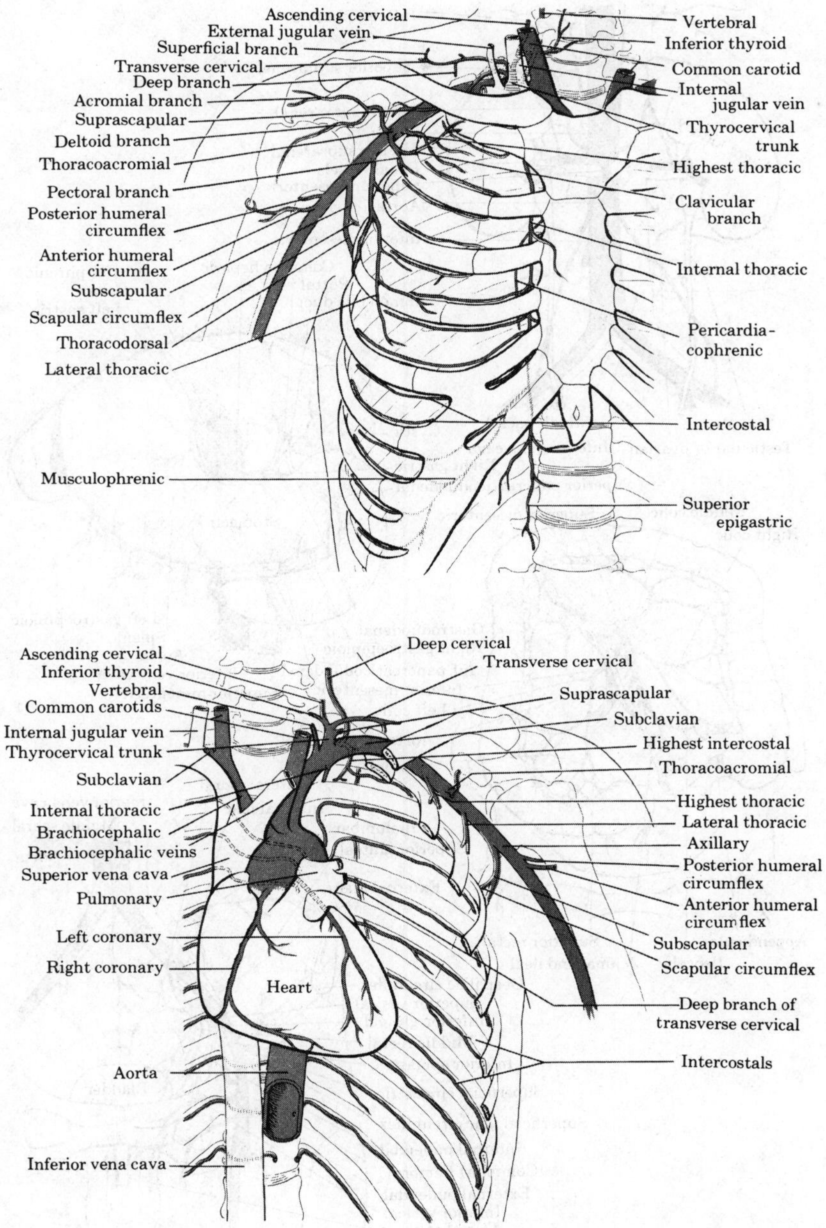

Artery, Figure 3. Arteries of the thorax and axilla. (From Dorland's Illustrated Medical Dictionary. 26th ed. Philadelphia, W. B. Saunders Co., 1981.)

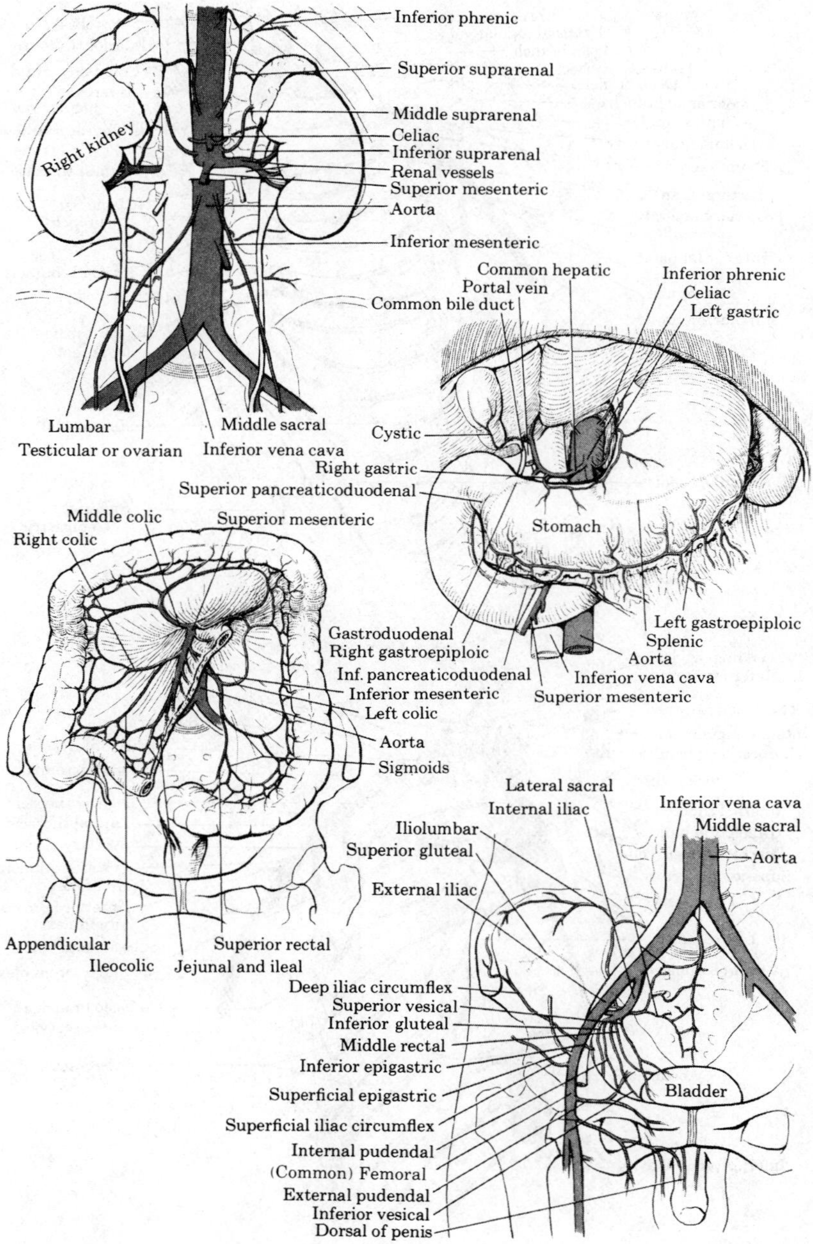

Artery, Figure 4. Arteries of the abdomen and pelvis. (From Dorland's Illustrated Medical Dictionary. 26th ed. Philadelphia, W. B. Saunders Co., 1981.)

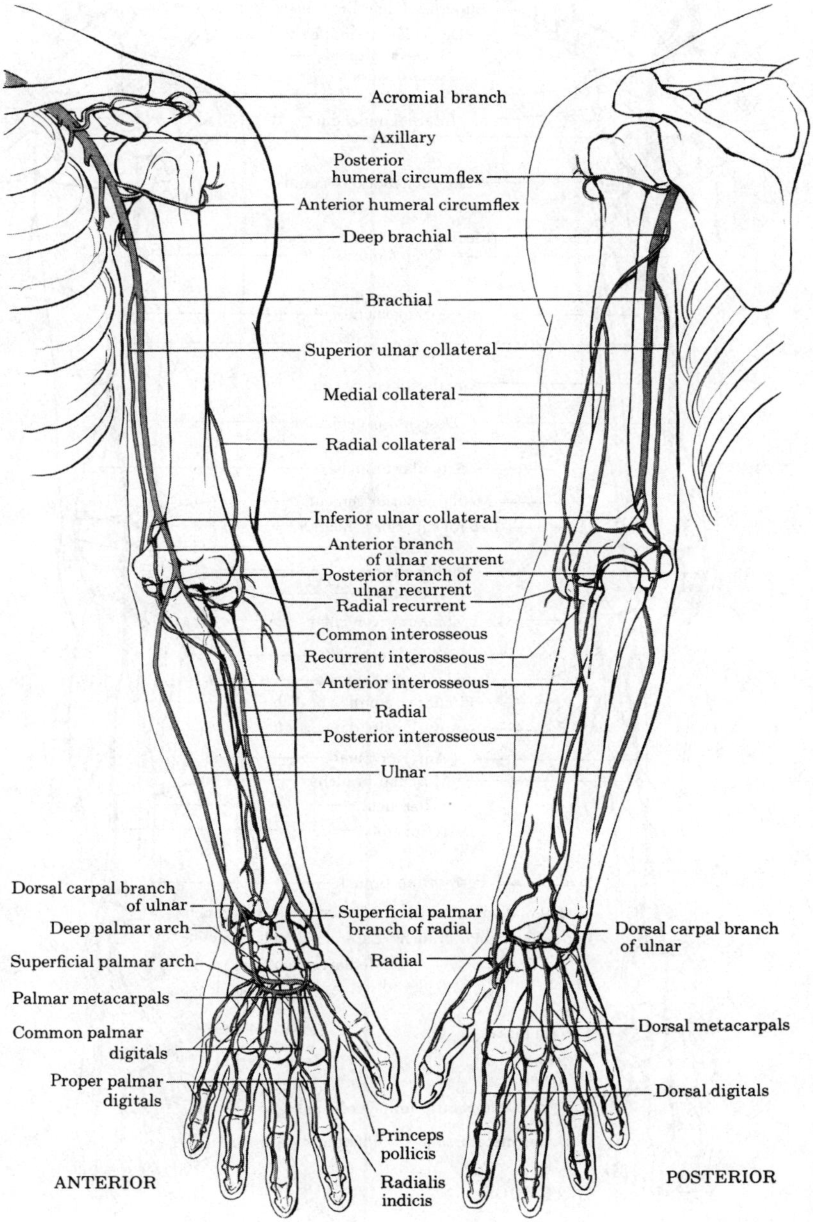

Artery, Figure 5. Arteries of the upper extremity. (From Dorland's Illustrated Medical Dictionary. 26th ed. Philadelphia, W. B. Saunders Co., 1981.)

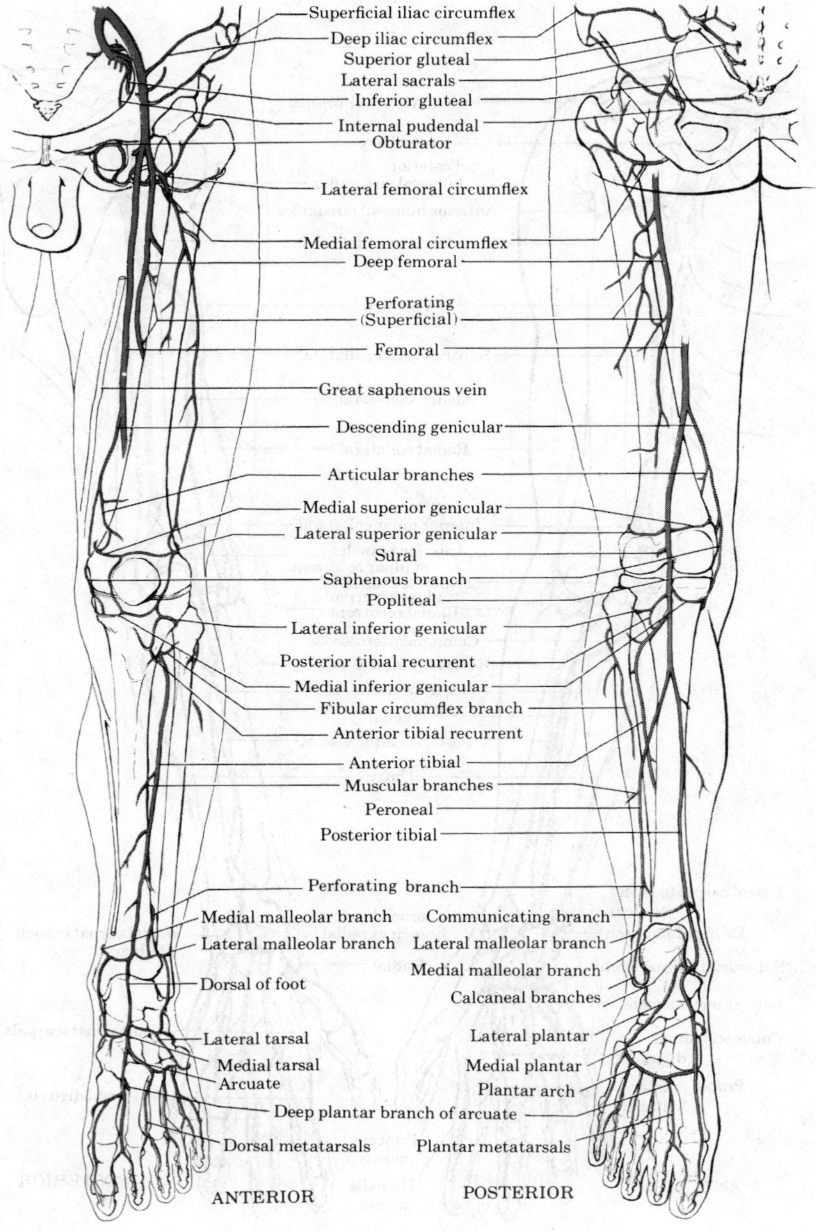

Artery, Figure 6. Arteries of the lower extremity. (From Dorland's Illustrated Dictionary. 26th ed. Philadelphia, W. B. Saunders Co., 1981.)

arthrodial (ar-thro′de-al) pertaining to an arthrodia.

arthroendoscopy (ar″thro-en-dos′ko-pe) see *arthroscopy.*

arthrogram (ar′thro-gram) [*arthro-* + Gr. *gramma* drawing] a radiograph of a joint made after the injection of a contrast medium.

arthrography (ar-throg′rah-fe) [*arthro-* + Gr. *graphein* to write] the radiographic examination of a joint after contrast injection. Also called *arthroendoscopy.*

air a., arthrography that uses air as the contrast medium. Also called *pneumoarthrography.*

double-contrast a., arthrography after injection of both a water-soluble iodinated contrast medium, such as diatrizoate, and air into the capsular space. The opaque contrast agent drains into the lower part of the joint, leaving only a thin coating on the portion of the joint that is uppermost in the view.

opaque a., arthrography after injection of a water-soluble iodinated contrast medium.

arthropathy (ar-throp′ah-the) [*arthro-* + Gr. *pathos* disease] a general term used to describe any joint disease.

neurogenic a., a destructive disease of joints due to impaired proprioception, pain, and temperature perception, which inhibits normal protective joint reflexes. There are a variety of causes, including tabes dorsalis (of syphilis), diabetic neuropathy, syringomyelia, neoplasms of and injury to the spinal cord, and congenital insensitivity to pain. Following the loss of the protective reflexes, there is increased trauma and stress on joint movement, which leads to cartilage degeneration, subchondral bone fractures, and osteophyte proliferation. Treatment is directed at the underlying process and at the restoration of joint stability. Also called *Charcot's joint.*

osteopulmonary a., the clubbing of fingers and toes and enlargement of ends of the long bones that occurs in cardiac or pulmonary disease. Also called hypertrophic pulmonary osteoarthropathy.

Arthropoda (ar-throp′o-dah) [*arthro-* + Gr. *pous* foot] a phylum of the animal kingdom composed of bilaterally symmetric organisms that have a hard, jointed exoskeleton and paired, jointed legs. It includes, among others, the classes Chilopoda, Arachnida, Crustacea, and Insecta. There are at least 740,000 species which have been divided into 12 classes. Many of the species are very important as parasites or carriers of organisms such as protozoa, worms, bacteria, viruses, Rickettsiae, and spirochetes that can cause diseases in humans (see the accompanying table). They may be mechanical but are usually biologic vectors (true hosts). Arthropods may themselves invade tissue, release toxins, or produce harmful allergic reactions.

arthroscopy (ar-thros′ko-pe) [*arthro-* + Gr. *skopein* to examine] the examination of the interior of a joint with an arthroscope.

arthrospore (ar′thro-spōr) [*arthro-* + Gr. *sporos* seed] an asexual spore formed by hyphal fragmentation leading to a chain of spores (conidia). There are two kinds of thallic-arthric development, which involves conversion of preexisting hyphal elements into deciduous conidia: (1) holoarthric development, in which all wall layers of the fertile hypha are involved in the formation of the conidial wall, e.g., *Geotrichum candidum;* and (2) enteroarthric development, in which the conidia differentiate within the outer wall layer of the fertile hypha, while certain segments of the preexisting hypha are not converted into conidia but instead degenerate. Such degeneration aids in the eventual release of the endogenous conidia, e.g., *Coccidioides immitis.*

arthrosynovitis (ar″thro-sin″o-vi′tis) [*arthro-* + *synovitis*] inflammation of the synovial membrane of a joint.

Arthus reaction (ar-toos′) [Nicolas-Maurice *Arthus,* French physiologist, 1862–1945] the development of an inflammatory lesion and necrosis marked by edema and hemorrhage at the site of an injection of a soluble antigen to which the individual is already sensitized. Antigen-antibody complexes form in the presence of complement, anaphylatoxins are released, neutrophils aggregate and release cytolytic lysosomal enzymes, and the vessel walls become abnormally permeable. Fibrin, platelets, and neutrophils plug the vessels. An Arthus-type reaction is any hypersensitivity state in which the antibody-antigen complexes begin the lesion. Also called Arthus phenomenon.

articul/o (ar-tik′u-lo) [L. *articulus* joint] a word element used in combining form to denote a joint, e.g., articulation.

articular (ar-tik′u-lar) [L. *articularis,* from *articulus* joint] pertaining to a joint.

articular capsule the saclike envelope that encloses the cavity of a synovial joint. It attaches to the periosteum of the bones and is composed of dense, fibrous tissue lined by the synovial membrane. The capsule may thicken to form ligaments holding the joint together. Also called joint capsule and synovial capsule.

articulate (ar-tik′u-lāt) [L. *articulatus* jointed] 1. divided into or united by joints.

2. enunciated into words and sentences; use of clear, expressive language.

articulated (ar-tik′u-lāt″ed) connected by movable joints; consisting of separate segments joined so as to be movable on each other.

articulation (ar-tik″u-la′shun) [L. *articulatio*] 1. the place of union or junction between two discrete objects, particularly between two or more bones of the skeleton. Also called *joint.*

2. the percentage of nonsense syllables that can be correctly repeated by the listener in an auditory test.

artifact (ar′tĭ-fakt) [L. *ars* art + *factum* made] 1. in histology or microscopy, any structure or feature that has been introduced by processing a tissue. Cf. *fixation artifact.*

2. in radiology, a substance or structure not naturally present in living tissue, but forming an authentic image that appears in a radiograph. Causes include motion of the subject during radiologic examination, contamination of the subject's clothing or skin, or foreign objects such as prostheses or medals.

3. in electroneurography, electromyography, and electroencephalography, any unwanted potential difference generated by a source other than the tissue under examination. When recorded on the oscilloscope screen or paper tracing, it is referred to as noise. In nerve conduction studies, the potential difference produced between the two recording electrodes (as a result of flow of part of the stimulating

ARTHROPODA. SOME IMPORTANT DISEASES TRANSMITTED BY ARTHROPODS

ARTHROPOD GROUP	DISEASE	VECTOR OR INTERMEDIATE HOST	VERTEBRATE RESERVOIR OF DISEASE*	DISEASE DISTRIBUTION
Crustacea				
Copepods	Diphyllobothriasis	*Cyclops* spp.	Dog, bear	Scandinavia, northern United States, Finland, Russia
	Dracunculosis	*Cyclops* spp.	Carnivores probably	Africa, India, Middle East
Crabs, crayfish	Paragonimiasis	Fresh-water crabs, crayfish	Carnivores?	Asia, Africa, Philippines, Pacific Islands, South America
Arachnida				
Mites	Scrub typhus (Tsutsugamushi disease)	*Trombicula* spp.	Rodents	Far East, Southwest Pacific, Philippines
	Rickettsialpox	*Allodermanyssus*	Mice	United States
Ticks	Tularemia	*Dermacentor* spp.	Rabbits	North America, Europe, Japan
	Rocky Mountain spotted fever	*Dermacentor* spp. and other Ixodid ticks	None	Canada, United States, Central and South America
	Q-fever	*Dermacentor, Boophilus*	Cattle, sheep, goats, bandicoot	Probably world-wide
	Colorado tick fever	*Dermacentor*	Wild rodents, porcupine	Western United States
	Tick-borne viral encephalitis	*Ixodes*	Various mammals and birds	Northern Europe and Asia
	Relapsing fever	*Ornithodoros*	Monkeys, squirrels, rats	Africa, Asia, America, Europe
	Babesiosis	Ixodid ticks	Rodents	Eastern and Western United States
Insecta				
Lice	Epidemic typhus	*Pediculus humanus*	None	Europe, Asia, Africa, Central America, United States
	Trench fever	*Pediculus humanus*	None	Central Europe
	Louse-borne relapsing fever	*Pediculus humanus*	None	Europe, Asia, Africa
Fleas	Plague	*Xenopsylla cheopis*, other rodent fleas	Rodents	World-wide
	Murine typhus	*Xenopsylla cheopis*	Rats and other rodents	Tropics and subtropics
	Dipylidiasis	Cat and dog fleas	Cats, dogs	World-wide
Bugs	Chagas' disease (South American trypanosomiasis)	*Triatoma, Panstrongylus*	Carnivores, rodents, armadillo	South America, Central America, North America
Beetles	Hymenolepiasis	Flour beetle†	Mice, rats	World-wide

Flies, gnats	African sleeping sickness	*Glossina* spp. (tsetse flies)	Herbivores?	Africa
	Onchocerciasis	*Simulium* spp. (black flies)	None	Africa, Mexico, Central and South America
	Tularemia	*Chrysops* (deer flies)	Rabbits	North America, Europe, Japan
	Loiasis	*Chrysops* spp.	Monkeys	Tropical Africa
	Leishmaniasis (all kinds)	*Phlebotomus* spp. (Sandfly)	Dogs and cats in various areas	Asia, Mediterranean, East Africa, southern Mexico, Central and South America
	Bartonellosis (Verruga peruana)	*Phlebotomus* spp. (Sandfly)	?	Peru, Colombia, Ecuador, (1700-10,000 feet)
Mosquitoes	Malaria	*Anopheles* spp.	None	World-wide
	Yellow fever	*Aedes aegypti*†	Monkeys	Africa, Central and South America
	Dengue fever	*Aedes* spp.	?	Tropics and subtropics
	Western equine encephalomyelitis	*Culex* spp.	Birds, horses	United States, southern Canada, Argentina
	Venezuelan equine encephalomyelitis	" "	Rodents, horses	Southern United States, Central and South America
	St. Louis encephalomyelitis	*Culex* spp.	Birds, horses	United States
	Eastern equine encephalomyelitis	*Aedes* and *Mansonia* spp.	Birds, horses	United States, Canada, West Indies, Central America
	Japanese B encephalomyelitis	*Culex* spp.	Birds, domestic animals	Far East
	Filariasis, bancroftian	*Culex, Aedes, Anopheles*	?	Tropical Africa, South Pacific, Australia, Asia
	Filariasis, Malayan	*Anopheles, Mansonia*	Monkeys? Cats?	India, Malaysia

* Other than humans.
† Important but not only vector.
From Markell, E., and Voge, M.: Medical Parasitology. 5th ed., Philadelphia, W. B. Saunders Co., 1981, pp. 276–278.

current in their vicinity) is recorded as the stimulus artifact. A small stimulus artifact is retained as a useful indication of when the stimulus was applied. An artifact may also be caused by volume conduction of a stimulating current to the surrounding tissues (electric or shock artifact), by movement of the recording electrodes (movement artifact), by the power line, or by distortion or malfunction of the instrumentation used in examination.

artificial (ar'ti-fish"al) [L. *ars* art + *facere* to make] made by human intervention; not natural or pathologic.

artificial kidney a popular name for an extracorporeal hemodialyzer employed to remove substances usually excreted in the urine from the blood.

artificial language a restricted, rigorously defined language for communication with computers, as opposed to the natural languages of humans.

artificial respiration the maintenance or restoration of respiration by manual, mouth-to-mouth, or mechanical means after spontaneous breathing has become inadequate (hypoventilation) or has stopped completely (apnea). Before any of the methods of artificial ventilation can be effectively employed, an open airway must be established by backward tilting of the victim's head; forward displacement of the jaw; endotracheal intubation; tracheotomy; or removal of a source of airway obstruction by clearing the mouth and oropharynx in any of several ways (including finger probe or forceps; back,

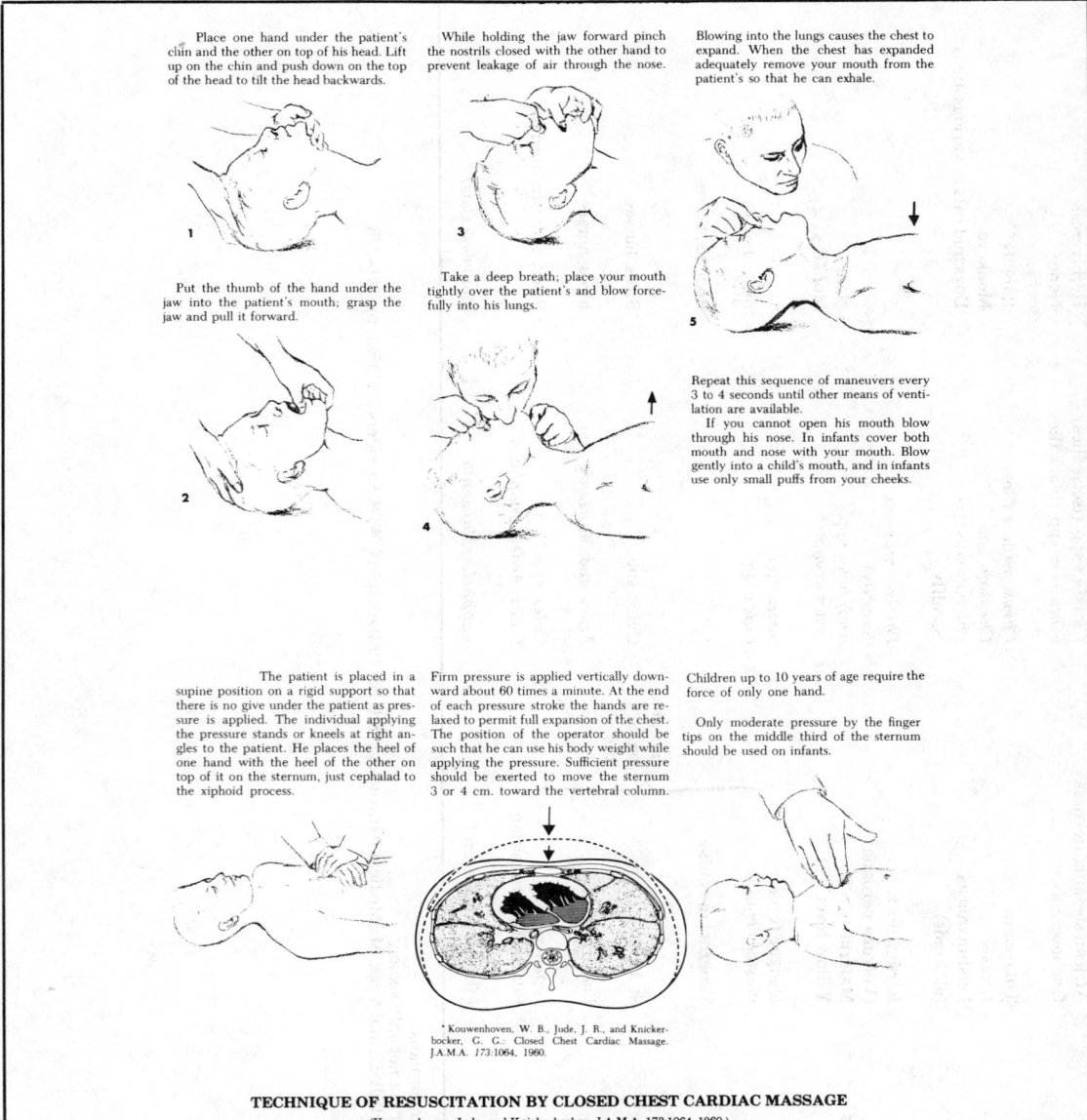

Place one hand under the patient's chin and the other on top of his head. Lift up on the chin and push down on the top of the head to tilt the head backwards.

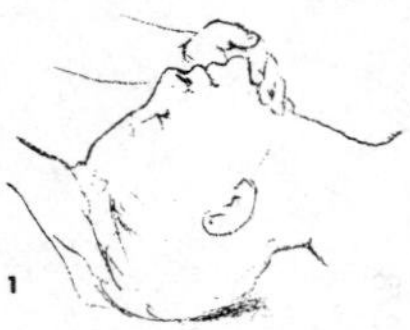

Put the thumb of the hand under the jaw into the patient's mouth; grasp the jaw and pull it forward.

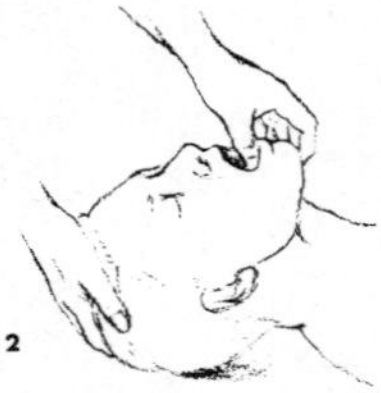

While holding the jaw forward pinch the nostrils closed with the other hand to prevent leakage of air through the nose.

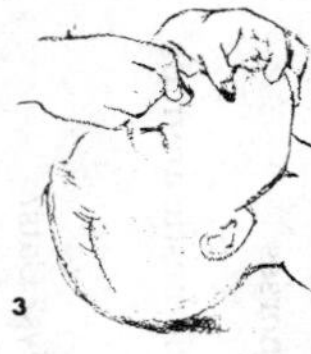

Take a deep breath; place your mouth tightly over the patient's and blow forcefully into his lungs.

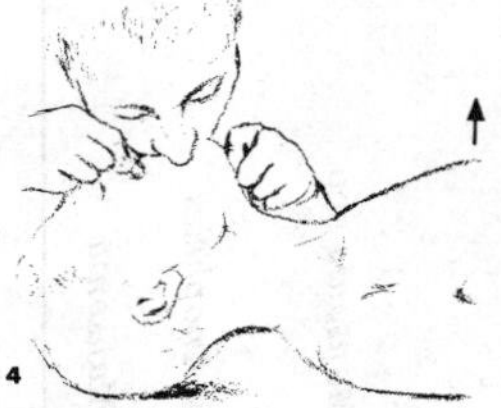

Blowing into the lungs causes the chest to expand. When the chest has expanded adequately remove your mouth from the patient's so that he can exhale.

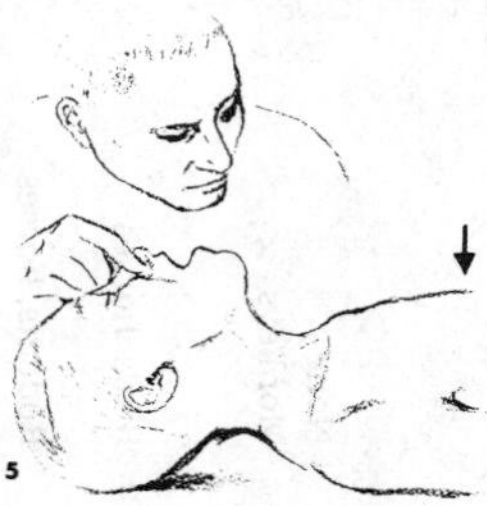

Repeat this sequence of maneuvers every 3 to 4 seconds until other means of ventilation are available.

If you cannot open his mouth blow through his nose. In infants cover both mouth and nose with your mouth. Blow gently into a child's mouth, and in infants use only small puffs from your cheeks.

The patient is placed in a supine position on a rigid support so that there is no give under the patient as pressure is applied. The individual applying the pressure stands or kneels at right angles to the patient. He places the heel of one hand with the heel of the other on top of it on the sternum, just cephalad to the xiphoid process.

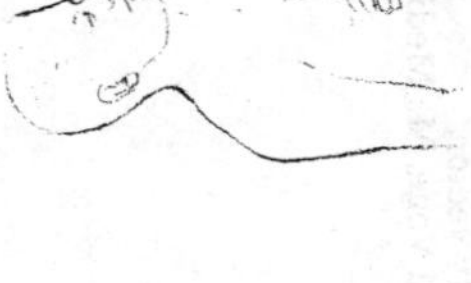

Firm pressure is applied vertically downward about 60 times a minute. At the end of each pressure stroke the hands are relaxed to permit full expansion of the chest. The position of the operator should be such that he can use his body weight while applying the pressure. Sufficient pressure should be exerted to move the sternum 3 or 4 cm. toward the vertebral column.

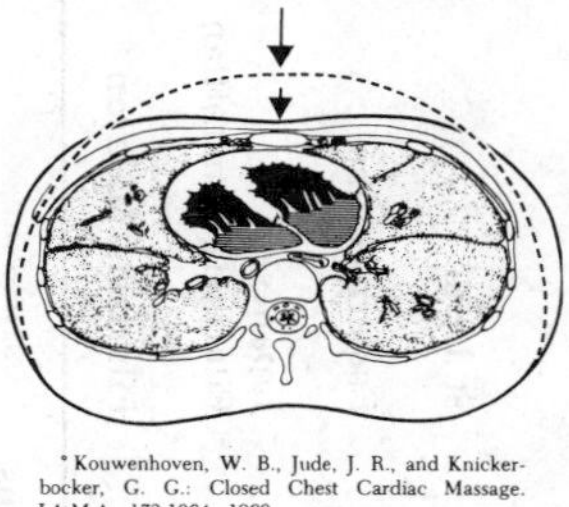

* Kouwenhoven, W. B., Jude, J. R., and Knickerbocker, G. G.: Closed Chest Cardiac Massage. J.A.M.A. *173*:1064, 1960.

Children up to 10 years of age require the force of only one hand.

Only moderate pressure by the finger tips on the middle third of the sternum should be used on infants.

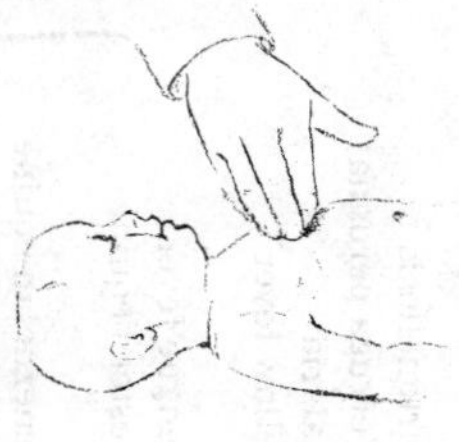

TECHNIQUE OF RESUSCITATION BY CLOSED CHEST CARDIAC MASSAGE

(Kouwenhoven, Jude, and Knickerbocker, J.A.M.A. 173:1064, 1960.)

Artificial respiration. (From Dorland's Illustrated Medical Dictionary. 26th ed. Philadelphia, W. B. Saunders Co., 1981.)

chest, or abdominal thrust; tracheotomy; or cricothyrotomy).

The manual and mouth-to-mouth (also mouth-to-nose or mouth-to-stoma) methods can be initiated immediately and require little or no special apparatus. Of the various manual methods, the Silvester and arm-lift back-pressure (Holger-Nielsen) methods provide the most adequate ventilation. These methods include a phase in which an additional inflating force (an active expansion or pulling of the thorax into the range of the inspiratory capacity) is produced.

In all manual methods, the air is pushed out of the lungs by the rhythmic, manual compression of the rib cage, with the victim placed in a variation of the prone or supine position. The compression is repeated every 3–5 sec. Elastic recoil of the lungs and thorax restores them to their normal resting positions. Most manual methods fail to produce an adequate tidal volume in unconscious, apneic individuals, especially those with mechanical breathing problems.

The mouth-to-mouth method is preferred for use as an immediate, temporary means of artificial respiration. Obstruction of the airways can be more readily detected; the operator can sense in his own airways the compliance and resistance of the victim's lungs (safe inflation pressures are therefore used); and the degree of inflation of the thorax can be seen by the practitioner, as shown in the accompanying illustration.

Mechanical respiration is accomplished by use of hand-inflated devices (anesthesia bags or bellows) or by use of automatic cycling machines (respirators) that create positive or negative pressures to inflate the lungs forcibly.

Also called *resuscitation.* See also *respirator* and *ventilator.*

Artyfechinostomum (ar″te-fek″ĭ-nos′to-mum) see *Paryphostomum.*

-ary (er′e) [L. *-arius*] a suffix word element to denote pertaining to, e.g., submaxillary.

aryepiglottic (ar″e-ep″i-glot′ik) [Gr. *arytaina* ladle + *epiglottis*] pertaining to the arytenoid cartilage and to the epiglottis.

aryepiglottic fold the first of three pairs of lateral folds of the mucosa at the laryngeal entrance. It stretches between the arytenoid cartilage and the epiglottis.

aryl- (ar′il) [from *ar*omatic + *-yl*] a prefix word element to denote aromatic groups, e.g., arylesterase.

arylaminopeptidase (ar″il-ah-me″no-pep′tĭ-dās) see under *leucine aminopeptidase.*

arylesterase (ar″il-es′ter-ās) an enzyme of the hydrolase class (aryl-ester hydrolase, EC 3.1.1.2), which catalyzes reactions such as: phenyl acetate + $H_2O \rightleftharpoons$ phenol + acetate. It occurs in normal serum and acts on many phenolic esters.

aryl-ester hydrolase see *arylesterase.*

aryl group (Ar-) (ar′il) an organic substituent group formed by the removal of a hydrogen from a carbon in a ring of an aromatic compound, e.g., the phenol group. Cf. *alkyl group.*

arylsulfatase (ar′il-sul″fah-tās) a group of enzymes (aryl-sulfate sulfohydrolase EC 3.1.6.1) that hydrolyze sulfate esters of aromatic hydroxy compounds to SO_4^{2-} and the free phenol. In mammals arylsulfatases are found in the liver, pancreas, kidneys, and immature monocytes. Several species of mollusks and *Aerobacter* serve as commercial sources of the enzyme. Partially purified preparations are used in analytic endocrinology to hydrolyze sulfates of various steroids prior to analysis. Three isoenzyme types are recognized: types A and B are present in cell lysosomes; type C is found in the microsomes. Normally, only types A and B are found in the urine. Isoenzymes A and B hydrolyze *p*-nitrocatechol sulfate but do not hydrolyze *p*-nitrophenyl sulfate nor *p*-acetylphenyl sulfate; isoenzyme C attacks the last two substrates more rapidly than it attacks the first. Urinary levels of A and B are increased in many malignant diseases.

Deficiency of lysosomal arylsulfatase activity is associated with two genetic diseases. In metachromatic leukodystrophy (a neurodegenerative sulfatide lipidosis), cerebrosulfatide accumulation has been attributed to a deficiency of arylsulfatase A activity. This enzyme splits sulfate from β-D-galactosyl-3-sulfate-β-D-glucosyl ceramide. The latter cerebroside sulfate is not a true arylsulfate; thus, it is possible that two different (but similar and related) enzymes are involved. In mucopolysaccharidosis type VI (Maroteaux-Lamy syndrome), greatly reduced levels of isoenzyme B are found in many tissues and cultured fibroblasts. Again, a different enzyme may be involved and the relation between it and true arylsulfatase B is not known at present.

The activity of the arylsulfatases may be determined in urine, white cells, tissues, and cultured skin fibroblasts. Increases in arylsulfatase in serum and urine have been reported to be associated with bladder tumors and myeloid leukemia.

Also called *phenol sulfatase.*

arylsulfatase test a method used to differentiate various species of mycobacteria, mainly the rapid growers. *Mycobacterium fortuitum* and *M. chelonei* give a strong positive reaction, whereas other Group IV rapid-growing mycobacteria are weakly positive or negative.

arytenoid (ar″ĕ-te′noid) [Gr. *arytainoeides,* from *arytaina* ladle + *eidos* form] shaped like a jug or pitcher.

arytenoid cartilage one of the paired cartilages, pyramidal in shape, that form part of the skeletal framework of the larynx. Located at the posterior aspect of the larynx, it articulates at its posterior and lateral surfaces with the cricoid and corniculate cartilages.

arytenoiditis (ar-it″ĕ-noi-di′tis) inflammation of the arytenoid muscle or cartilage.

AS abbrev. for aortic stenosis, *auris sinistra* (left ear).

As symbol for the chemical element *arsenic.*

ASA abbrev. See *acetylsalicylic acid.*

ASAHP abbrev. See *American Society of Allied Health Professionals.*

asbestos (as-bes′tos) [Gr. "unquenchable"] a fibrous, incombustible group of impure magnesium silicate minerals, which appear white, gray, green or brown in color. Types include chrysotile and fine amphibole asbestos such as crocidolite and amosite. Inhalation of the fibers (particularly by those who handle the material) causes pulmonary fibrosis: the fibers are deposited in the terminal bronchioles, where they are phagocytized. Extended exposure (usually 10-20 yr but sometimes a shorter period) may result in hypertrophic conjuctivitis, diffuse pulmonary fibrosis, pleural thickening with and without calcification, and mesothelioma. The incidence of bronchogenic carcinoma is greatly increased when asbestos exposure is combined with smoking.

asbestos body a deposit of protein, calcium, and iron salts that forms around an inhaled fiber of asbestos, forming a beaded rod with club-shaped ends. Because this coating is primarily ferritin, these asbestos bodies have been called ferruginous bodies. There is evidence that the coating process goes on inside lung macrophages, and that the change from an asbestos fiber to an asbestos body reduces the fibrogenicity of the particle.

asbestosis (as″bĕs-to′sis) [*asbestos* + *-osis* condition] a diffuse, fibrous pneumoconiosis caused by prolonged exposure to asbestos. It is one of several asbestos-related diseases.

Asbestosis is a fibrosing process that gradually (after a long latency period) takes the form of a diffuse, but nonuniform, interstitial and alveolar fibrosis that tends to be most prevalent in the basal portions of the lower lobes of the lungs. Because inflammatory tissue becomes interposed between the alveolar walls and pulmonary capillaries, gaseous exchange is impaired. This impairment is evident clinically as a decreased CO diffusing capacity. Other signs include a decreased vital capacity, basal rales, dyspnea, and productive cough. The disease process continues after asbestos exposure has ceased. A large percentage of patients with mesothelioma have had clinically significant exposure to asbestos. There is no effective therapy.

See also *mesothelioma* and *pneumoconiosis.*

ASC abbrev. See *American Society of Cytology.*

ascariasis (as″kah-ri′ah-sis) [*ascaris* + *-iasis*] infection with the giant roundworms of the species *Ascaris lumbricoides.* Light infections usually cause minor damage, although reinfection may produce hypersensitivity to *Ascaris* antigen, accompanied by high IgE levels. It is most common in children in rural subtropical areas, and in both children and adults in tropical areas. An early phase of pulmonary involvement occurs owing to larval migration to the lungs. In the prolonged intestinal/abdominal phase caused by the adult worms, there is poor digestion, diarrhea, bowel inflammation, or blockage of the bile ducts. Reexposure and subsequent reinfection is a serious problem.

Diagnosis is made by identification of eggs from the stools, or from clinical manifestations. Treatment with piperazine citrate, pyrantel, or mebendazole causes evacuation of adult worms.

Ascaridoidea (as″kah-rĭ-doi′de-ah) [*Askaris* + Gr. *eidos* form] a superfamily of phasmid nematodes, many of which are parasitic for humans. Ascaridoidea is characterized by worms that have three-lipped mouths, lack a buccal capsule, and reproduce sexually. It includes the genera *Ascaridia, Ascaris, Toxocara, Toxascaris,* and *Lagochilascaris.*

Ascaris (as′kah-ris) [L.; Gr. *askaris*] a genus of large, intestinal, nematode parasites of the superfamily Ascaridoidea. These worms have three-lipped mouths with no buccal capsule, and reproduce sexually. Severe infections may cause obstructions in the body, or may penetrate the liver, lungs, and intestinal walls. See also *ascariasis* and *Ascaridoidea.*

A. alata, see *T. canis* under *Toxocara.*

A. canis, see *T. canis* under *Toxocara.*

A. lumbricoides, the largest and most common species of *Ascaris,* known as the eelworm or roundworm, and particularly found in moist, warm, or temperate regions. These worms require no intermediate host and their eggs remain viable for months. Infection is usually through the mouth from polluted soil, food, or drink.

A. mystax, see *T. cati* under *Toxocara.*

A. suum, the swine *Ascaris.* Human infection is very rare. Also called *A. suilla,* and *A. suis.*

***Ascaris* pneumonitis** bronchopneumonia with cough, wheezing, fever, eosinophilia, and migratory infiltrates that occurs during the passage of *Ascaris lumbricoides* larvae through the lungs. See also *Löffler's syndrome.*

ascending (ah-send′ing) [L. *ascendere* to climb] having an upward course.

ascending chromatography paper chromatography in which the solvent front moves upward; see also *paper chromatography.*

ascertainment (as″-er-tān′ment) in genetic studies, the method by which persons are selected for inclusion in the study. When, as is usual, families come to the attention of the investigator because of the genetic defect of some member (the proband), the families at risk but with no affected children are not included in the study; this procedure is known as the bias of ascertainment. The simplest method of correcting for this bias is to omit the proband from the calculations by determining the incidence of the defect in the siblings of each proband. For the exact probabilities corresponding to the different methods, see *single a.* and *truncate a.*

complete a., any method by which every individual suffering from a specific disease (usually genetic) is identified in a given population at a given time.

incomplete a., see *multiple a., single a.,* and *truncate a.*

multiple a., any method in which some families are ascertained more than once through different affected children.

single a., any method by which there is a very low probability that any family will be ascertained more than once; the probability of ascertainment of a given family is proportional to the number of affected children. For an autosomal recessive trait, the sampling distribution is binomial.

truncate a., any method by which every affected child in the population (or a random sample of them) is selected for inclusion in the study. For an autosomal recessive trait, the frequency of affected children in each family size will have a truncated binomial distribution (no families with zero affected children are ascertained).

Aschoff body (ash′of) [Karl Albert Ludwig *Aschoff,* German pathologist, 1866–1942] a microscopic, lemon-shaped focus of chronic inflammation seen particularly in the heart, and less often around joints in rheumatic fever. Aschoff bodies consist of a central zone of necrosis surrounded by lymphocytes, plasma cells, and large, often multinucleated cells that are probably of histiocytic origin. They heal by fibrosis. Also called Aschoff's nodule. See also *Anichkov's myocyte.*

ASCII (as′ke) [acronym from *A*merican *S*tandard *C*ode for *I*nformation *I*nterchange] a standard character code used by many computer systems for the transmission of information over data links and to and from peripheral devices. The full ASCII code (also called extended ASCII and USASCII) includes upper case and lower case alphabetic characters, and numeric, special, and control characters. A parity check bit is usually added; in this case each character takes up a full byte. The high-order three bits are in the column heading above the character, and the low-order four bits are in the row heading; e.g., the ASCII code for A is 1000001 (binary) or 41 (hexadecimal). The decimal equivalent is 16 times the column number plus the row number; e.g., A is $16 \times 4 + 1 = 65$. There is also a six-bit ASCII code that has no lower case letters. See also *Extended Binary Coded Decimal Interchange Code.*

ascites (ah-si'tēz) [L.; Gr. *askitēs,* from *askos* bag] the excessive accumulation of free fluid ($\approx$5-10 l) within the peritoneal cavity. There is abdominal distention, loss of tone of abdominal muscles, severe protein loss, and electrolyte imbalance. Most frequently, ascites is the result of subacute or chronic disease processes involving the liver and/or the portal circulation (e.g., portal hypertension due to cirrhosis). Other causes include congestive heart failure, nephrotic syndrome, decreased hepatic synthesis of serum albumin, constrictive pericarditis, carcinomas, or tuberculosis. The production of ascitic fluid is an incompletely understood process; it is thought to involve hypoalbuminemia with decreased plasma oncotic pressure or high portal venous pressure. This, according to Starling's hypothesis, causes a flux of fluid from the blood vessels to the extravascular spaces. Other contributory factors are thought to include lymphatic obstruction, renal sodium retention, and increased aldosterone secretion.

Ascitic fluid is a watery fluid containing protein (mostly albumin) in the range of 1–2 g/100 ml. Other solutes, including glucose and electrolytes, occur in concentrations essentially equivalent to those found in plasma. The fluid is usually clear and straw-colored. Cloudy fluid suggests infection; blood-tinged fluid may be associated with malignancy or tuberculosis. Protein concentrations of 3–4 g/100 ml suggest liver or systemic disease; higher concentrations suggest malignancy or infection.

Ultrasonography may confirm the clinical impression of ascites, and may help estimate the volume and indicate the best location for paracentesis. The recovered fluid is assessed for its protein content and the presence of blood cells, and is examined cytologically; it is also stained and cultured for bacteria and examined for the presence of amylase. Removal of the fluid is usually an ineffective therapeutic procedure because rapid reaccumulation occurs, leading to accentuated protein loss.

ascitic (ah-sit'ik) pertaining to ascites.

ascitic fluid an accumulation of fluid in the abdominal cavity; see also *ascites.*

ASCLT abbrev. See *American Society of Clinical Laboratory Technicians.*

ascocarp (as'ko-karp) a structure, found in many ascomycete fungi, which supports the ascus, the sac containing the sexual spores.

ascomycetes (as"ko-mi-se'tēz) [Gr. *askos* bag + *mykes* fungus] a group of perfect fungi belonging to the division Eumycota. These fungi are distinguished by the formation of the sexual spore, the ascospore, in a sac or ascus during reproduction. In most members the asci are borne by an ascocarp. Organisms commonly called yeasts and mildews, and cheese, jelly, and fruit molds are included. Several organisms of this class are also pathogenic for humans, and cause disorders including blastomycosis, candidiasis, aspergillosis, and dermatophytosis.

Ascomycotina (as"ko-mi"ko-te'nah) ascomycete fungi, a subdivision of the Eumycota. These fungi are characterized by the production of sexual spores (ascospores) contained in a sac (ascus) that is often supported by an organ called an ascocarp.

ascorbate (ah-skor'bāt) an anionic form or salt or ester of ascorbic acid.

ascorbic acid vitamin C, a carbohydrate derivative, which can be synthesized from glucose. Although not a carboxylic acid, it has an enediol group, making it a good reducing agent; it behaves as a weak acid ($pK'_{a_1} = 4.30$). The naturally occurring vitamin is the L- isomer, L-ascorbic acid. Its exact metabolic/physiologic role is as yet unknown, but a complete absence of vitamin C intake leads to failure of connective tissue cells to form their collagenous matrices, resulting in the disease scurvy. Ascorbic acid is known to be required for the hydroxylation of some metabolites and some adrenal steroid hormone intermediates. It is synthesized by all mammals (except guinea pigs and primates) from D-glucuronic acid. In humans, ascorbic acid is slowly metabolized by conversion to oxalate.

The U.S. recommended daily allowance for adults is 45 mg/da, except during pregnancy (60 mg) or lactation (80 mg). Massive doses have been advocated for the treatment of the common cold, but its usefulness for this purpose has not been established or adequately supported by available data.

ascorbic acid assays determination of ascorbic acid in biologic specimens using either a redox titration or a colorimetric method. The titration using a redox indicator, such as 2,6-dichlorophenol-iodophenol in acid solution, is rapid and convenient, but end points may be difficult to detect owing to rapid fading of the color. In the colorimetric method, ascorbic acid is oxidized to dehydroascorbic acid, which is then converted to a 2,4-dinitrophenolhydrazone, which develops a red color and can be measured spectrophotometrically in acid solution. This procedure does not, however, differentiate between biologically active vitamin C and any inactive diketogulonic acid. The latter is a relatively minor component in normal blood specimens, but may be present in urine and natural products such as juices. For the assessment of blood levels, plasma (heparin, oxalate, EDTA) or serum specimens are preferred, although whole blood may be used. Buffy coat (leukocyte) levels are a sensitive and convenient indicator of tissue levels. Ascorbic acid assays should be performed immediately after collection of the specimen, although the vitamin C content remains stable in whole blood for 3 hr when refrigerated, or for 2 wk in protein-free filtrates prepared with either 6 g/100 ml of metaphosphoric acid or 10 g/100 ml of trichloroacetic acid and stored at –20°C.

Reference ranges for plasma specimens are 0.6–2.0 mg/100 dl, the lower values being found in older persons with subclinical deficiency. Low plasma concentrations do not necessarily indicate low tissue levels of vitamin C, leukocytes being the better specimen for this purpose.

ascospore (as′ko-spōr) a sexual spore formed within a special sac, or ascus, as in ascomycetous fungi. See also *spore.*

ASCP abbrev. See *American Society of Clinical Pathologists.*

ascus (as′kus), pl. *asci* [Gr. *askos* a bag] a special, spore-bearing sac filled with ascospores in members of the ascomycete fungi.

ASD abbrev. See *atrial septal defect.*

-ase (ās) [from diast*ase*] a suffix word element to denote an enzyme, e.g., lipase.

asepsis (a-sep′sis) [*a-* neg. + Gr. *sēpsis* decay] 1. the complete absence of microbial contamination or infection.

2. the exclusion of microorganisms.

aseptic (a-sep′tik) free from infection or septic material; sterile.

asexual (a-seks′u-al) [*a-* neg. + L. *sexualis,* from *sexus* sex] 1. without sex, not sexual.

2. in reference to spores, those produced vegetatively without the union of nuclei in a sexual process.

ASH abbrev. See *American Society of Hematology.*

Ashby differential agglutination method the earliest satisfactory technique for measuring red cell survival, no longer in common use. Individuals are given transfusions of immunologically compatible but distinct red cells (such as O cells to an A or B recipient, or M cells to an MN recipient). Samples are taken at appropriate intervals. Enumeration of the free red cells after agglutination of the recipient's cells with suitable antisera provides a direct measurement of the decline of donor cells over time.

asialoglycoprotein (ah″si-a″lo-gli″ko-pro′te-in) a class of serum glycoproteins with the terminal sialic acid residues removed, exposing a terminal galactose that permits binding by liver cells. Normal human serum contains 1–5 μg/ml of asialoglycoproteins, but serum from patients with hepatic cirrhosis or hepatitis may have two to three times this amount. These facts support the view that hepatic binding of asialoglycoproteins is a normal physiologic process that furthers the degradation of plasma glycoproteins.

asiderosis (ah″sid-er-o′sis) [*a-* neg. + Gr. *sidēros* iron + *-osis* condition] a deficiency of the iron reserves of the body.

Askanazy cell (as″kan-āz′e) [Max *Askanazy,* German pathologist, 1865–1940] see *Hürthle cell.*

ASM abbrev. See *American Society for Microbiology.*

ASMT abbrev. See *American Society for Medical Technology.*

Asn abbrev. See *asparagine.*

ASO abbrev. See *antistreptolysin O tests.*

Asp abbrev. See *aspartic acid.*

asparagic acid (as-par′ah-jik) see *aspartic acid.*

asparaginase (as-par′ah-gĭ-nās″) an enzyme of the hydrolase class (L-asparagine amidohydrolase, EC 3.5.1.1) that catalyzes the reaction L-asparagine + H_2O ⇄ L-aspartate + NH_3. It is used as a cancer chemotherapeutic drug; trademark, Elspar. For more information, see *Appendix A.*

asparagine (Asn or N) (as-par′ah-jēn) [Gr. *asparagos* asparagus] α-aminosuccinamic acid, a monoamide of aspartic acid, $H_2NCOCH_2CH(NH_2)$-COOH, a naturally occurring nonessential amino acid; M.W.132.12. It occurs as an amino acid residue in many proteins. Asparagine is found in asparagus and in many kinds of seeds. Some glycoproteins have asparagine-linked polysaccharides; in proteins, it destabilizes α-helical and β-structures. Asparagine is active as a diuretic and is used in the culture media of certain bacteria. Its source is the proteins of the diet and biosynthesis from aspartate and glutamine by the enzyme asparaginase synthetase. See also under *amino acids.*

asparaginic acid (as-par′ah-jin-ik) see *aspartic acid.*

asparaginyl (as-par′ah-jin″il) the acyl radical derived from or relating to asparagine.

aspartate (as-par′tāt) a salt or the anionic form of aspartic acid.

aspartate aminotransferase (AST) an enzyme of the transaminase class (L-aspartate:2-oxoglutarate aminotransferase, EC 2.6.1.1) that catalyzes the reaction L-aspartate + α-oxoglutarate ⇄ oxaloacetate + L-glutamate. The enzyme in serum is also known as serum glutamate–oxaloacetate transaminase (SGOT, GOT).

AST is found in both cell cytoplasm and mitochondria. Mild tissue damage causes a rise in cytoplasmic AST activity in the serum; severe trauma also raises mitochondrial AST activity in the serum. Present in normal plasma, bile, cerebrospinal fluid, and saliva, AST is found in urine only if a kidney lesion is present. The enzyme is present in high concentrations in the heart, liver, skeletal muscle, kidneys, and pancreas, and its activity in plasma increases for 6–8 hr following a myocardial infarction (peaking at 24–36 hr). Other conditions that may cause increases in plasma AST activity are given in the accompanying table, with elevations above the upper limit of normal. AST changes in CSF are fairly nonspecific, but its activities do increase in cerebrovascular damage.

Also called *aspartate transaminase.*

aspartate aminotransferase assays 1. continuous monitoring spectrophotometric methods using coupled enzyme reactions. The activity of AST in serum is determined at pH 7.8 and a temperature of either 30° or 37°C. The specimen is added to a reaction mixture containing aspartate, 2-oxoglutarate, malate dehydrogenase, and NADH. The oxaloacetate produced by the AST-catalyzed reaction is reduced to malate by malate dehydrogenase, with NADH serving as a reducing cofactor. The reaction is monitored by measuring the decrease in absorbance per minute (ΔA/min) of NADH at 340 nm as it is oxidized to NAD^+. The activity in International Units (U) is equal to the number of micromoles of NADH oxidized per minute. This method is now widely accepted in clinical laboratories.

2. two-point colorimetric methods in which the oxaloacetate produced is measured by the formation of a colored product. The specimen is added to a buffered reaction mixture containing 2-oxoglutarate, aspartate, and 2,4-dinitrophenylhydrazine. The oxaloacetate formed reacts with the 2,4-dinitrophenylhydrazine to form a yellow dinitrophenylhydrazone with an absorbance that can be measured at 505 nm. The substrate 2-oxoglutarate and other oxoacids in the reaction mixture also form hydrazones, so that the reagent blanks have a high absorbance. Because the absorbance of the reaction mix-

ASPARTATE AMINOTRANSFERASE. CONDITIONS CAUSING ELEVATION IN AST ACTIVITY

CONDITION	INCREASED CONCENTRATION
Viral hepatitis, toxic hepatitis, and other necrotic liver diseases	3–50 or even 100×
Infectious mononucleosis	Up to 20×
Intrahepatic cholestasis	Up to 20×
Muscular dystrophy	Up to 8×
Dermatomyositis	Up to 8×
Primary liver carcinoma	5–10×
Metastatic liver carcinoma	5–10×
Acute pancreatitis	2–5×
Crushed muscle injuries	2–5×
Gangrene	2–5×
Hemolytic disease	2–5×
Pulmonary emboli	2–3×
After alcohol intake	Slight increase
Delirium tremens	Slight increase
Medication (opiates, salicylates, ampicillin)	Slight increase

ture is not a linear function of the oxaloacetate concentration, a standard curve is used to determine the AST activity. In another procedure, oxaloacetate is coupled to a diazonium salt, e.g., Azoene fast violet B, to form a red product. The absorbance of reagent blanks is minimal; however, there is still a deviation from linearity because of product inhibition of AST by oxaloacetate. Both methods are rarely used today and are considered obsolete.

aspartate kinase an enzyme of the transferase class (ATP:L-aspartate 4-phosphotransferase, EC 2.7.2.4) that catalyzes the reaction ATP + L-aspartate ⇄ ADP + 4-phospho-L-aspartate, the first step in the metabolism of aspartic acid. Also called *aspartokinase*.

aspartate transaminase see *aspartate aminotransferase*.

aspartic acid (Asp, D) (as-par′tik) 2-aminobutanedioic acid, $HOOCCH(NH_2)CH_2COOH$, a naturally occurring, nonessential, dibasic amino acid; M.W. 133.10. It occurs widely in proteins and serves as a nitrogen donor for urea and adenine synthesis; β-alanine and the pyrimidine ring are formed from it. *N*-Acetylaspartate may serve as a neurotransmitter in the brain. Aspartic acid functions in a shuttle (malate-aspartate shuttle) of electrons between cytosol and mitochondria. It is used in culture media and as a sweetener. Its source is the proteins of the diet and biosynthesis from oxaloacetate.

The biosynthesis of aspartic acid involves the important transamination reaction glutamic acid + oxaloacetic acid ⇄ α-ketoglutaric acid + aspartic acid; its breakdown involves the reverse of this reaction. The enzyme that catalyzes the transamination reaction is aspartate aminotransferase, AST, and its clinical determination involves the use of aspartic acid as a substrate.

Also called *aminosuccinic acid* and *asparaginic acid*. See also *amino acids*.

aspartokinase (as-par″to-ki′nās) see *aspartate kinase*.

aspartyl (as-par′til) the acyl radical derived from or relating to aspartic acid.

β-aspartylacetylglucosaminidase (as-par″til-as″-ĕ-til-gloo″kōs-am′ĭ-nĭ-dās″) an enzyme of the hydrolase class (EC 3.2.2.11) that catalyzes the reaction 1-β-aspartyl-2-acetamido-1,2-dideoxy-D-glucosylamine + H_2O ⇄ 2-acetamido-2-deoxy-D-glucose + L-asparagine. The enzyme is present in seminal fluid and lysosomes. A genetic deficiency of the enzyme, transmitted as an autosomal recessive trait, is the cause of aspartylglucosaminuria. See also *mucolipidoses*.

aspartylglucosaminuria (as-par″til-gloo-kos-am″-ĭ-nu′re-ah) [*aspartylglucosamine* + Gr. *ouron* urine + *-ia*] a hereditary disease, transmitted as an autosomal recessive trait, that is caused by a deficiency of the enzyme β-aspartylacetylglucosaminidase. It is one of the mucolipidoses. The disorder is found primarily in individuals in Finland and is characterized by severe mental retardation, coarse features, diarrhea, and frequent infections.

aspect (as′pekt) [L. *aspectus*, from *aspicere* to look forward] 1. that part of a surface facing in any designated direction.

2. the look or appearance.

aspergilloma (as″per-jil-o′mah) [*Aspergillus* + Gr. -ōma swelling] a condition caused by colonizing organisms of the genus *Aspergillus*, in which a fungus ball or balls form in ectatic bronchi, commonly in the upper lobes of the lungs. The symptoms produced are similar to those of allergic aspergillosis, but crises of severe hemoptysis may occur periodically. Aspergilloma frequently arises as a complication of preexisting cavitary pulmonary disease. Radiographically, the fungus ball is characterized by a uniform, nondense, round or oval shape, with a radiolucent crest (Monod's sign) over the upper portion.

aspergillosis (as″per-jil-o′sis) [*Aspergillus* + *-osis* condition] any disease of humans and animals that is caused by species of the genus *Aspergillus*. Of the very many species recognized, only seven or eight are pathogenic for humans, and of these, *A. fumigatus* is the most important, being responsible for about 90 percent of infections. Other noteworthy species include *A. flavus, A. niger, A. nidulans, A. terreus*, and *A. clavatus*.

These saprophytic molds are widespread in soil, particularly in decaying vegetation such as compost. Many species are thermotolerant and consequently are selectively adaptable to the high body temperature of birds. Generally, human contact occurs by inhalation of airborne spores.

Aspergilli show a wide range of disease manifestations in humans; most organs can be involved in infections. In immunologically competent persons; however, clinical manifestations are predominantly allergic in nature, and true infection is absent. Most often, multiplication of the mold in tissues occurs only in the presence of a predisposing debilitating disease such as leukemia (about 5 percent of leukemics develop aspergillosis). Other predisposing conditions in which aspergilli act as opportunists are immunosuppressive therapy and pulmonary tuberculosis.

Clinical Disease. Aspergillus may act on the lungs in three ways: as allergens, as saprophytes, or invasively. Acting as allergens, the spores may cause asthma and bronchitis in sensitized individuals, a condition called allergic aspergillosis. These spores rarely germinate in the bronchial passages. Symptoms include intermittent fever, cough, chills, aches, pain, and sputum eosinophilia.

In atopic sensitized individuals, the inhaled spores settle in the medium-sized bronchi, where reactions to inhalation of the antigen may be manifested in two ways: (1) An acute asthmatic reaction may occur in the bronchi, sometimes accompanied by rhinitis and a transient eosinophilia. This reaction is mediated by reaginic antibody (IgE). Up to 40 percent of such individuals give an immediate wheal-and-flare reaction to the antigen in an intradermal test. Precipitins are rarely found; if found, they are usually weak.

(2) The other way in which reactions may be manifested involves more prolonged antigenic exposure, which results in a more severe asthmatic reaction accompanied by pulmonary eosinophilia. This is caused by the development of Type I (immediate) hypersensitivity followed by the appearance of Type III (Arthus-type) reactions in the bronchi. Circulating antibody combines locally with antigen and forms complexes. Because there is an antigen (spore) excess in the bronchi, these complexes result in extensive tissue damage in the peribronchial area. Polymorphonuclear cells and lymphocytes infiltrate the damaged tissue. Sputum plugs are expectorated, and the *Aspergillus* fungus can be isolated from these plugs. Skin testing shows two reactions in this situation: an immediate wheal-and-flare reaction and a delayed Arthus-type reaction. Precipitins are present in approximately 90 percent of those affected.

As saprophytes, the spores may occur in lung cavities or in dead areas of lung tissue where they can grow to form a fungal ball or aspergilloma. This chronic form of the disease may be accompanied by hemoptysis and cough. A fungus gains entry to a necrotic area of the lung, such as an old tuberculous cavity or an infarct, where it grows in the form of a ball of mycelia. The upper lobes of the lung are most often invaded. Radiographs usually show a mobile mass separated from the cavity by a crescent of air. Sputum cultures are generally negative. Precipitating antibodies are usually found. Skin tests are negative unless the person is hypersensitive to *Aspergillus*. In the United States, the most common species of *Aspergillus* that causes aspergilloma is *A. niger*; in England and Europe, it is *A. fumigatus*.

Invasive or systemic aspergillosis occurs in immunologically compromised hosts when fungal elements invade the living lung tissue and reach one or several other organs. Symptoms of pulmonary aspergillosis resemble pneumonia, with fever, cough, leukocytosis, and respiratory distress. Invasive aspergillosis is secondary to other diseases, such as leukemias and lymphomas. Often, three factors are found to contribute to invasive aspergillosis: a decreased host resistance, a constant local port of entry of the fungus, and disruption of the normal microbial flora as a result of antimicrobial therapy.

Other variations of aspergillosis include aural, commonly caused by *A. niger*; cutaneous, especially involving the nails; cardiac, often a complication of heart surgery; and central nervous system infection.

Laboratory Diagnosis. Direct examination of sputum may demonstrate long, branching septate hyphae or numerous tangled masses of hyphae, as well as the typical conidiophores topped by an expanded, spore-bearing vesicle. In most cases of aspergilloma, direct examination of sputum is negative. Biopsy material may be digested with potassium hydroxide, thus making branched mycelia visible, but use of a sterile saline–antibacterial antibiotic allows subsequent culturing of the same specimen.

Because *Aspergillus* is airborne and ubiquitous, repeated positive cultures are desirable in order to be confident of an etiologic role. The organism will grow at 37°C on common mycologic laboratory media; however, it is sensitive to cycloheximide. Species identification of *Aspergillus* is made microscopically. The conidiophore is short, green to brown in color, and gradually enlarges to form a flask-shaped vesicle. Sterigmata are produced on the vesicle, which turn upward and parallel the conidiophore. The long, unbranched chains of the conidia may be green.

Serologically, skin reactions and immunodiffusion are useful identification tools, especially if the culture is negative. There are different serologic reactions, depending on the type of aspergillosis present. All atopic individuals are skin test–positive. Precipitin formation by immunodiffusion is useful in those patients with pulmonary eosinophilia, severe allergic aspergillosis, and aspergillomas. When aspergillomas are surgically removed, the precipitin bands disappear. For invasive aspergillosis, the patient usually has a defective immune system, and thus the demonstration of antibodies is poor. To increase the sensitivity of immunodiffusion tests for aspergillosis, a battery of antigens from several species of *Aspergillus* should be used and the serum should be concentrated. The recent and promising ELISA procedure (enzyme-linked immunoabsorbent assay) is being used to detect both IgE and IgG antibodies in patients' sera.

Aspergillus (as″per-jil′us) [L. *aspergere* to scatter] a genus of monomorphic molds, containing many species of saprophytes, which is very widely distributed in nature. Species known to reproduce sexually (by ascospores) are placed in the class Ascomycetes. Other species for which a sexual phase has not been demonstrated are considered "fungi imperfecti" or Deuteromycetes. Most of the seven species capable of causing human aspergillosis are imperfect, but some, e.g., *A. nidulans*, produce ascospores.

The distribution of *Aspergillus* spores is ubiquitous; they are especially abundant in warm, damp, decaying vegetation. The elevated temperatures of compost favor strains able to grow at the high body temperature of birds, contributing to the frequency of aspergilli as etiologic agents in birds.

Aspergillus is always filamentous in form. Microscopically, these molds are characterized by the occurrence of a single conidiophore arising from a septate hypha. This aerial conidiophore terminates in a swollen vesicle that bears single or double protuberances, called sterigmata or phialides, from each of which extends a single and sometimes long chain of small, round conidia, as in a chain of beads, as shown in the accompanying illustration.

Primary contact of humans with *Aspergillus* is by inhalation. Therefore, when a disease state results, the organ first and most often involved is the lung. About 90 percent of the cases of human *Aspergillus* are due to one species, *A. fumigatus.*

See also *aspergillosis.* For more information, see the accompanying table.

A. clavatus, a species found in soil and manure, which is associated with malt worker's lung, an allergic alveolitis that results from exposure to spores from germinating malting barley. Its cultures produce the antibacterial substance patulin.

A. flavus, a species or group of closely related molds best known for the production in foodstuffs of potent mycotoxins called aflatoxins. There is good evidence for believing that aflatoxin B_1 is carcinogenic (producing hepatocarcinomas). Sensitization to the antigens of this species can cause allergic bronchopulmonary aspergillosis as well as primary and opportunistic infections of the nasal sinuses and lungs. See also *aflatoxin.*

A. fumigatus, a species of thermotolerant mold found in soils and manure, which is responsible for 90 percent of infections in humans, including the most severe cases of aspergillosis. The organism has been found in the nose, ears, lungs, and other organs; it may also be one of the species producing the allergic syndromes known as malt worker's disease. Its cultures produce the antibiotics fumagillin and helvolic acid; growth can occur at temperatures of up to 50°C. See also the accompanying illustration.

A. nidulans, a species of *Aspergillus* that causes localized lesions, usually on the hands and feet, and is found especially in the tropics. This species is an uncommon cause of pulmonary aspergillosis. See also *mycetoma.*

A. niger, a species that may cause some cases of pulmonary aspergillosis, and which is frequently the etiologic agent of otomycosis (fungal infection of the ear) in humans. Its colonies are white, floccose, and fast-growing. The mycelium is first yellow and then black, with the profuse production of black conidia.

A. terreus, a thermotolerant mold and an etiologic agent of allergic aspergillosis, which has also been implicated in some cases of aspergillosis of the lungs and (rarely) primary cerebral aspergillosis in humans. On Czapek-Dox agar, it produces fast-growing, floccose-to-velvety colonies that are cinnamon-buff to wood brown in color.

aspergillus antibody tests assays for antibodies to aspergillus organisms in individuals with pulmonary conditions caused by aspergillus infection. The most common test is immunodiffusion, although countercurrent electrophoresis is also used, especially for screening. Precipitins (antiaspergillus antibodies) are found in more than 90 percent of fungus ball cases and in 70 percent of cases of allergic bronchopulmonary aspergillosis.

In the immunodiffusion test, only those sera that

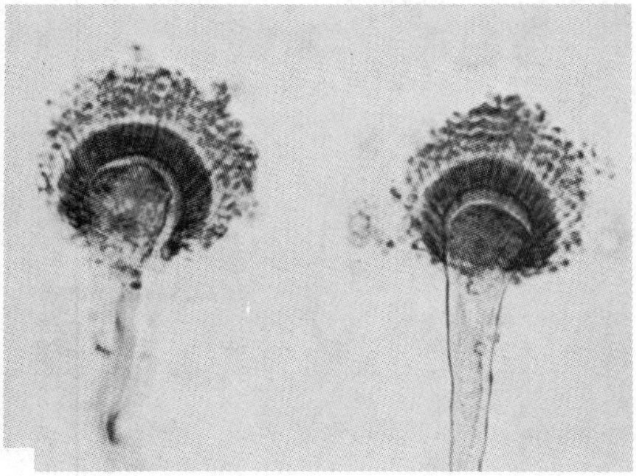

Aspergillus fumigatus. Conidiophores from Sabouraud's glucose agar, ×825. (From Conant, N. F.: Manual of Clinical Mycology. Philadelphia, W. B. Saunders Co., 1971.)

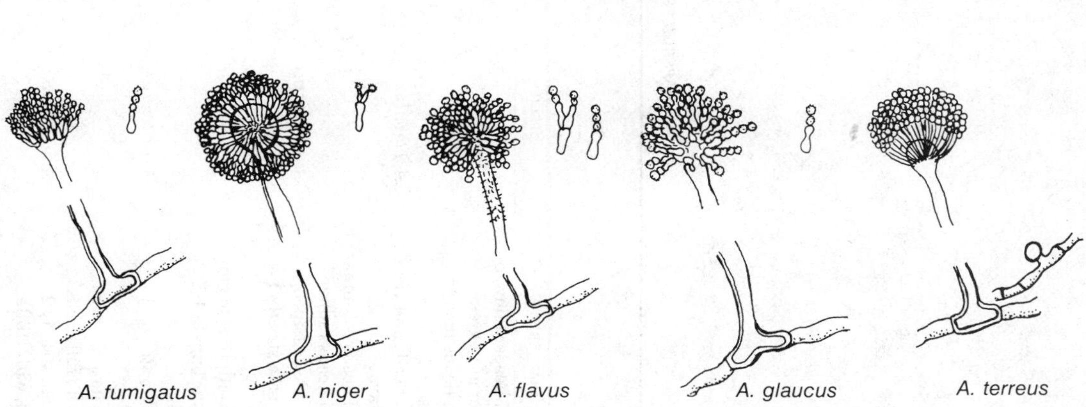

Aspergillus. Identification of the most common species of *Aspergillus.* (From Larone, D. H.: Medically Important Fungi: A Guide to Identification. Hagerstown, MD, Harper & Row, 1976.)

ASPERGILLUS. CHARACTERISTICS OF *ASPERGILLUS* SPECIES GROWN ON CZAPEK-DOX MEDIUM*

CHARACTERISTIC	SPECIES	COLONY COLOR: *Surface*	COLONY COLOR: *Reverse (none to:)*	MAX. CONIDIOPHORE LENGTH	MAX. VESICLE DIAM. (μm)	NO. OF ROWS OF STERIGMATA	CONIDIA (μm)	ASCOSPORE COLOR
Conidial heads yellow, or blue- or gray-green								
Conidial heads in other shades								
Conidial heads and vesicles clavate	*A. clavatus*	Pale blue- or gray-green	Brown	2–3 mm 10 mm+	50 180	1	3.5–4.5 × 2.4–3.0	–
Conidial heads columnar								
Conidial heads radiate								
Vesicles flask shaped, sterigmata strictly 1 rowed	*A. fumigatus*	Dark blue-green	Brown	300 μm	30	1	2.5–3.5	–
Vesicles elliptical to globose, sterigmata 1–2 rowed								
Sterigmata strictly 1 rowed	*A. restrictus*	Green to dark olive	Dark green	150 μm	12	1	4.5–5.5 × 3.0–3.5	–
Sterigmata 1–2 rowed without Hülle cells								
Sterigmata strictly 2 rowed, with Hülle cells	*A. nidulans*	Dark cress green	Purplish red	130 μm	10	2	3.0–3.5	Red

Cleistothecia present	*A. glaucus* group							
Cleistothecia absent								
Ascospores rough	*A. amstelodami*	Olive green†	Yellow	350 μm	25	1	4.5–5.0 × 3.5–4.0	Colorless
Ascospores smooth, ridges absent	*A. repens*	Dull green†	Maroon	1 mm	40	1	5.0–6.0	Colorless
Ascospores smooth, ridges thin, flexuous	*A. chevalieri*	Gray-green†	Maroon	850 μm	35	1	4.5–5.5	Colorless
Sterigmata 1–2 rowed	*A. flavus*	Yellow to dark green	Red-Brown	2 mm	65	1–2	3.5–4.5	–
Sterigmata 2 rowed	*A. versicolor*	Yellow to blue-green	Wine red	500 μm	16	2	2.0–3.0	–
Conidial heads brown to black	*A. niger*	Brown to black	Yellow	6 mm	100	2	5.5–8.0	
Conidial heads pale cinnamon to orange-brown	*A. terreus*	Cinnamon brown	Brown	250 μm	16	2	1.8–2.4	–
Conidial heads white to cream							–	
Conidial heads radiate	*A. candidus*	White to cream	Pale pink or yellow	1 mm	40+	2	2.5–3.5	–
Conidial heads columnar	*A. carneus*	White to vinaceous	Brown	1 mm	9	2	2.4–2.8	–

* *A. glaucus* series and *A. restrictus* grown on 20% sucrose.
† To yellow or orange according to density of cleistothecia.
Modified from Austwick, P., and Longbottom, J. L.: Medically Important *Aspergillus* Species. *In* Lennette, E. H., et al. (eds.). Manual of Clinical Microbiology. Washington, DC, American Society for Microbiology, 1980, p. 625.

form lines of identity with known positive serum from a confirmed aspergillosis case should be considered positive. Occasionally, bands of nonidentity are associated with aspergillosis, especially when C-reactive protein is present in the serum. These should disappear after addition of sodium citrate; if they do not, further study is warranted. Sera from patients with fungus balls and allergic bronchopulmonary aspergillosis generally do not have to be concentrated to give a positive immunodiffusion test result, whereas sera from cases of suspected invasive aspergillosis often do (three to four times) to detect precipitins.

aspermia (a-sper′me-ah) [*a-* neg. + Gr. *sperma* seed + *-ia*] the failure of formation or of the emission of semen. Cf. *azoospermia*.

aspheric (a-sfer′ik) [*a-* neg. + Gr. *sphaira* sphere] not spherical; said of a lens with a surface that is not spherical.

asphyxia (as-fik′se-ah) [Gr. "a stopping of the pulse"] the occurrence of apnea and death secondary to severe arterial hypoxemia and tissue hypoxia as a result of the absence of oxygen in the inspired air, or the blockage or cessation of the respiratory air exchange. See also *adult respiratory distress syndrome* and *Raynaud's disease*.

asphyxial (as-fik′se-al) pertaining to asphyxia.

asphyxiant (as-fik′se-ant) a substance that can deprive tissues of oxygen without affecting the mechanics of respiration.

chemical a., a gas that interferes with the utilization of oxygen by the body. For example, carbon monoxide combines readily with hemoglobin, thus reducing the amount available for oxygen transport and consequently the concentration of oxygen in the blood. Another example is cyanide, which combines with ferric iron in enzymes and the cytochrome system and interferes with cellular respiration.

simple a., a physiologically inert gas whose presence in sufficient quantity (20–30 volumes percent) prevents tissues from receiving adequate oxygen. Examples are carbon dioxide, helium, hydrogen, nitrogen, nitrous oxide, and aliphatic hydrocarbons.

asphyxiation (as-fik″se-a′shun) the occurrence of apnea and death secondary to severe arterial hypoxemia and tissue hypoxia caused by the absence of oxygen in the inspired air or the blockage or cessation of respiratory air exchange.

aspidium oleoresin (as-pid′e-um o″le-o-rez′in) a dark-green, thick liquid, extracted from the rhizomes of *Dryopteris filix-mas* (male fern), which was formerly used as a vermifuge or anthelmintic in the treatment of tapeworm infection. After administration, the worms are evacuated. It is toxic and in large doses may cause vomiting, weakness, convulsions, coma, blindness, jaundice, and kidney damage.

aspirate (as′pĭ-rāt) [L. *aspirare* to breathe upon] 1. to treat by aspiration; to remove by suction.

2. the substance or material obtained by aspiration. See also *aspiration b.* under *biopsy*.

aspiration (as″pĭ-ra′shun) [L. *aspiratio*, from *aspirare*] 1. the act of inhaling.

2. the removal of fluids or gases from a cavity by the application of suction. It may refer to treatment given to a patient or to the drawing up of a sample into a pipet.

tracheal a., a clinical procedure performed to suck out tracheal secretions. This procedure is often initiated to remove tracheal secretions, to prevent postoperative atelectasis, or to obtain bronchopulmonary secretions for microbiologic examination and culture, especially if the patient is affected with a lung disease that does not produce expectoration. Tracheal aspiration through intubation is accomplished by passing a nasal catheter past the larynx and into the trachea. Tracheal aspiration by percutaneous catheterization involves passing a large-bore, thin-walled needle through the cricothyroid membrane or a high intercartilaginous space. This direct approach may be preferred in debilitated patients and yields culture specimens that are free of oral microbial flora. Uncommon complications of this technique may be subcutaneous or mediastinal emphysema, cardiac arrhythmia, or tracheal bleeding.

aspiration cytology see *needle aspiration cytology*.

aspirator (as′pĭ-ra″tor) an apparatus used to remove fluids or gases from a cavity by suction.

aspirin (as′pĭ-rin) see *acetylsalicylic acid*.

asplenia (a-sple′ne-ah) the absence of a spleen; see under *hyposplenism*.

asporogenic (as″po-ro-jen′ik) [*a-* neg. + *sporogenic*] nonspore-forming; not produced from spores.

asporous (a-spo′rus) [*a-* neg. + Gr. *sporos* seed] without spores, especially the highly resistant endospores of bacteria.

ASRT abbrev. See *American Society of Radiologic Technologists*.

assassin bug one of a species of cone-nosed bugs, family Triatomidae, that has been implicated as a carrier of Chagas' disease through its bites.

assay (as-sa′) the measurement of the quantity of a chemical constituent, or of the activity of an enzyme, or of the pharmacologic or biologic potency of a drug in a biologic specimen.

biologic a., see *bioassay*.

immune a., see *immunoassay*.

assembler (ah-sem′bler) a computer program that produces a machine-language program (the object program) from an assembly-language program (the source program).

assembly language (ah-sem′ble) a computer programming language in which each machine language instruction in the object program is directly specified by the programmer. Operation codes and addresses are specified by using symbolic labels, which are translated into numerical form by the assembler.

assignment statement in computer programming, a statement that evaluates an expression and assigns the computed value to a variable, thus changing its value. In some languages (e.g., FORTRAN), the assignment statement is written: *variable* = *expression*, e.g., X = Y + 2. Other forms are X := Y + 2; (PASCAL) and LET X = Y + 2 (BASIC).

assimilation (ah-sim″ĭ-la′shun) [L. *assimilatio*, from *ad* to + *similare* to make like] the process of changing digested food into living tissue; anabolism.

association (ah-so″se-a′shun) [L. *associatio*, from *ad* to + *socius* a fellow] 1. the coordination of the functions of similar parts.

2. a group of people organized for a common activity or interest.

3. see *correlation.*

association constant a mathematical expression of the ratio of bound antibody sites to unbound sites, yielding a measure of the affinity of binding between an antigen and an antibody.

association fibers nerve fibers that interconnect portions of the cerebral cortex within a hemisphere. Short association fibers interconnect neighboring gyri; long fibers interconnect more widely separated gyri and are arranged into bundles or fasciculi.

Association for the Advancement of Medical Instrumentation (AAMI) a professional organization for medical instrumentation.

Association of Clinical Scientists (ACS) a professional organization of clinical scientists.

assortative mating nonrandom mating; the selection of a mate with a preference for a particular genotype. Cf. *random mating.*

negative a. m., the tendency for persons with dissimilar genotypes to mate more frequently than by chance alone.

positive a. m., the tendency for persons with similar genotypes to mate more frequently than by chance alone. Members of subpopulations (e.g., those determined by ethnic groups, religions, intelligence) are more likely to mate within their own subgroup than outside it.

assortment (ah-sort′ment) the random distribution and combination of the chromosomes in the gametes at anaphase I of meiosis. Each chromosome in each gamete may be of paternal or maternal origin, or both (if a cross-over occurred).

independent a., the random distribution to the gametes of genes that are located on different chromosomes (i.e., not linked). The statement that this occurs is Mendel's second law.

AST see *aspartate aminotransferase.*

astasia (as-ta′ze-ah) [*a-* neg. + Gr. *stasis* stand] motor incoordination with an inability to stand.

astatine (At) (as′tah-tēn) [Gr. *astatos* unstable] a radioactive element; atomic number 85; most stable isotope, ^{210}At (half-life, 8.3 hr); Group VII of the periodic table (the halogens); oxidation states −1, +1, +5.

asteatosis (as″te-ah-to′sis) [*a-* neg. + Gr. *stear* tallow + *-osis*] any disease in which persistent, dry scaling of the skin suggests scant or absent sebum.

aster (as′ter) [L., from *Gr. astēr* star] a set of short microtubules that radiate from each centriole during mitosis and meiosis. See also *spindle.*

asterixis (as″ter-ik′sis) [*a-* neg. + Gr. *stērixis* a fixed position] a clinical sign that consists of a coarse, flapping tremor best elicited when the individual is asked to extend the arms, dorsiflex the hands, and spread the fingers. It is most frequently seen in hepatic encephalopathy but may also occur in other metabolic encephalopathies.

asteroid (as′ter-oid) [Gr. *astēr* star + *eidos* form] star-shaped; resembling the aster.

asteroid body a stellate inclusion occasionally seen in the large multinucleated cells of granulomas in sarcoidosis, berylliosis, and other granulomatous disorders.

asthenia (as-the′ne-ah) [Gr. *asthenēs* without strength + *-ia*] lack or loss of strength and energy; weakness. It is found as a presenting symptom of many medical disorders.

-asthenia (as-the′ne-ah) a suffix word element to denote lack of strength, e.g., neurasthenia.

asthma (az′mah) [Gr. "panting"] a reversible respiratory disorder characterized by the presence of airflow limitation within the airways of the lungs, secondary to bronchial smooth muscle contraction (bronchoconstriction), mucosal edema, and excessive airway secretions. These three factors reduce the patency of the airways and increase both the resistance to airflow and the respiratory muscle energy expenditure for a given level of ventilation. Asthma occurs in response to a wide variety of inciting agents, most of which belong to the categories of: (1) inhaled allergens; (2) infectious agents; (3) physical irritants, such as dusts and chemical vapors, and even cold air; and (4) emotions. Often, several inciting agents work together to produce an asthmatic episode in an individual who would have been relatively asymptomatic had only one of the agents been operating alone. Emotions provide an example of this additive effect, contributing to the airway constriction in an allergic person who is at the same time exposed to inhaled allergens and is emotionally distraught. Emotions alone seldom, if ever, cause significant asthma.

Asthmatic individuals possess significantly increased airway reactivity as compared with normal persons. This hyperreactivity results in constriction of the airways in response to concentrations of inhaled, active substances that are lower than those needed to evoke the same response in normal individuals. The state of hyperreactivity can be tested and demonstrated by having an asthmatic individual inhale small, controlled quantities of either histamine or methacholine while the response is carefully monitored with forced expiratory efforts into a spirometer. A fall in the forced expiratory volume in 1 sec (FEV-1) of more than 20 percent occurs at concentrations much lower than those necessary to achieve the same results in normal persons.

Hyperreactive airways respond with bronchoconstriction to provocation through two distinct and experimentally demonstrable pathways. Histamine, released from mast cells within the airway mucosa following an antigen-antibody (IgE) reaction on the mast cell surface, stimulates smooth muscle contraction either directly or through a vagal reflex arc that starts with rapidly adapting sensory receptors (often called irritant receptors) located just beneath the mucosal surface. This vagal reflex arc can also be initiated by nonimmune mechanisms that act on the sensory receptors, such as dusts and chemicals, and can be blocked with local anesthetics and parasympatholytic drugs.

Asthmatic episodes occur in a wide spectrum of severity, from mild episodes that are barely perceptible to the patient to very severe episodes that culminate in respiratory failure and death. A typical episode is associated with respiratory distress, a wheezing sound during breathing, coughing, hyperventilation in the early phases (despite the airway obstruction and increased work of breathing), and increased mucus production. Physiologically, resistance to airflow is elevated, flow rates on spirometry are reduced, and vital capacity is often reduced. The lungs become overinflated because of the impaired emptying, the distribution of ventilation throughout the lungs is quite uneven, and respiratory gas exchange deteriorates. In the late stages of an acute, severe episode, hypoxemia occurs early, followed considerably later by carbon dioxide retention, the latter reflecting severe airway obstruction and fatigue.

The term asthma has been used for years to designate *any* disorder associated with wheezing and airway obstruction. Efforts are being made by some physicians to limit the term to episodic, truly reversible bronchoconstriction and to avoid using the term when the obstruction is relatively fixed and accompanies emphysema and/or chronic bronchitis. (Bronchospasm accompanying the latter is often referred to as asthmatic bronchitis.) The three disorders—bronchial asthma, chronic bronchitis with bronchospasm, and obstructive emphysema—are included together in the commonly used term chronic obstructive pulmonary disease (COPD).

Status asthmaticus refers to a particularly severe episode of asthma, usually requiring hospitalization, that does not respond adequately to ordinary therapeutic measures. It has been clinically defined, in ways that some authorities consider imprecise, as a failure to achieve improvement in wheezing and substantial reduction in airway obstruction after two therapeutic doses of subcutaneous epinephrine.

See also *bronchospasm, chronic obstructive pulmonary disease, emphysema,* and *forced expiratory volume.*

asthma crystals see *Charcot-Leyden crystals.*

asthmatic (az-mat′ik) [L. *asthmaticus*] pertaining to asthma.

asthmatic bronchitis see under *asthma.*

astigmatism (ah-stig′ma-tizm) [*a-* neg. + Gr. *stigma* spot] an aberration of an optical system, such as the lens of the eye or the electronic lens of a cathode ray tube, that distorts the circular symmmetry of a pattern because of the inequality of refraction in different planes (e.g., vertical and horizontal).

astigmometer (as″tig-mom′ĕ-ter) [*astigmatism* + Gr. *metron* measure] an apparatus used in measuring astigmatism of the eye.

astomatous (as-tom′ah-tus) [*a-* neg. + Gr. *stoma* mouth] having no mouth, as in certain ciliates.

astr/o (as′tro) [Gr. *astron* star] a word element used in combining form to denote resemblance to a star; e.g., astrocyte.

Astra Blue 4R a triarylmethane dye, similar to Alcian Blue 8GX, that is specific for acid mucopolysaccharides.

Astracyanine B a dark blue triaminoditolylphenylmethane basic dye used for staining acid mucopolysaccharides; C.I. 42705.

astringent (ah-strin′jent) [L. *astringens,* from *ad-* to + *stringere* to bind] 1. causing contraction of the tissues and the arrest of bleeding or secretion.

2. an agent, especially one for topical application, having such effects.

astroblastoma (as″tro-blas-to′mah) [*astro-* + Gr. *blastos* germ + *ōma* swelling] a rare tumor of mature astrocytes that generally occurs in the cerebrum of young persons. Some consider it a form of gemistocytic astrocytoma. It may dedifferentiate into a glioblastoma.

astrocyte (as′tro-sīt) [*astro-* + Gr. *kytos* hollow vessel] one of the supporting cells of the central nervous system (glial cells). An astrocyte has a number of cytoplasmic processes that branch and ramify to envelop neurons and attach to the walls of blood vessels or the membranes enclosing the brain and spinal cord (pia mater, ependyma). Although two forms of astrocytes are traditionally recognized, they are variants of a single cell type. Fibrous astrocytes are principally present in the white matter and have long, thin cytoplasmic processes. Protoplasmic astrocytes are mainly found in gray matter and have short branching processes. In routine histologic preparations, only the nuclei of astrocytes are readily seen by light microscopy. Many special stains have been developed to demonstrate astrocytic cells by impregnation with metals such as silver and gold. Astrocytes participate in the process of repair following injury to the central nervous system. Collectively, these cells are called *astroglia.*

astrocyte staining histologic methods for the demonstration of astrocytes. Cajal's gold-sublimate method and Mallory's phosphotungstic acid–hematoxylin are the most commonly used methods; several silver impregnation methods using ammoniacal silver solutions can also be used. See also *Cajal's gold-sublimate method* and *phosphotungstic acid–hematoxylin.*

astrocytoma (as″tro-si-to′mah) [*astro-* + Gr. *kytos* hollow vessel + *ōma* swelling] a brain or cord tumor (glioma) composed of astrocytes. The degree of differentiation is commonly expressed in four grades, I through IV; tumors of grades III and IV are often termed glioblastoma multiforme. In adults, astrocytomas are usually located in the cerebrum, whereas cerebellar astrocytomas occur in children. The astrocytoma is the most common primary tumor of the central nervous system. See also *brain tumors* and *g. multiforme* under *glioblastoma.*

gemistocytic a., an astrocytoma in which the cells are plump with hyalinized, eosinophilic cytoplasm and short, blunt processes. The cells are closely packed and may form perivascular rosettes. Although found in the cerebrum of adults in pure form, gemistocytic astrocytomas are more commonly a component of a fibrillary tumor. This type of astrocytoma is well differentiated but may in time become a glioblastoma.

pilocytic a., an astrocytoma composed of elongated cells that form a uniform intersecting pattern in the adult type, but are irregularly grouped in the juvenile form (also called polar spongioblastoma); this tumor occurs in the vicinity of the third ventricle. The pattern does not have any particular prognostic significance.

astroglia (as-trog′le-ah) [*astro-* + *neuroglia,* from Gr. *neuron* nerve + *glia* glue] glial tissue made up of astrocytes.

asym- a prefix word element in organic chemistry to denote one of two constitutional isomers that is asymmetric, e.g., *asym*-dichloroethane (1,1-dichloroethane, CH_3CHCl_2). Also called *unsym-.* Cf. *sym-.*

asymmetric (a″sim-met′rik) pertaining to asymmetry.

asymmetric carbon atom a carbon atom with four different substituents. In general, a structure with n asymmetric carbon atoms (chiral centers) has 2^{n-1} pairs of enantiomers. In special cases, however, some of the configurations are meso compounds (molecules that are achiral, although they have asymmetric atoms) that replace a pair of enantiomers. Any atom that is the source of the optical activity of a chiral molecule can be called an asymmetric atom. Examples are the nitrogen of an ammonium compound with four different groups attached, or the phosphorus of an optically stable phosphine with three different groups attached. Cf. *chiral center* and *pseudoasymmetric carbon atom.*

asymmetry (a-sim′ĕ-tre) [Gr. *asymmetria* disproportion, from *a*-neg. + *symmetria* symmetry] 1. lack or absence of symmetry. An asymmetric object has neither a symmetry plane nor a symmetry axis. Asymmetric molecules have nonidentical mirror images called enantiomers. Cf. *dissymmetry.*

2. a dissimilarity in paired organs on opposite sides of the body.

3. in electroencephalography, cerebral electric activity of unequal amplitude, frequency, configuration, or distribution over homologous regions of the two sides of the scalp.

asymptote (as′im-tōt″) [Gr. *asymptōtos,* from *a*-neg. + *sympiptein* to fall together] a straight line that is approached arbitrarily closely in the limit by a given curve as the curve approaches infinity.

asynapsis (ah-sĭ-nap′sis) [*a*- neg. + Gr. *synapsis* conjunction] the failure of homologous chromosomes to pair during meiosis.

asynchronism (a-sin′kro-nizm) see *asynchrony.*

asynchronous (a-sin′kro-nus) [*a*- neg. + L. *synchronus,* from Gr. *synchronos,* from *syn* together with + *chronos* time] not occurring at the same time; of an electric circuit, not controlled by regular timing signals, operating at a speed determined by the characteristics of the circuit.

asynchronous data transmission a method of coordinating the data transmission between a computer and a peripheral device. The bits of each character are regularly spaced between special start and stop signals used to synchronize the receiving device. This method is used for aperiodic character transmission to and from remote terminals. Also called start/stop synchronization. Cf. *synchronous data transmission.*

asynchrony (a-sin′kro-ne) 1. the occurrence at different times of events normally occurring together; a disturbance of coordination.

2. in electroencephalography, the nonsimultaneous occurrence of cerebral electric activity recorded from different areas of the scalp on the same or opposite sides of the head, or from corresponding regions of both sides of the scalp.

3. in hematology, a difference in rate of maturation of the nucleus and cytoplasm of a bone marrow cell, resulting in an atypical form of the cell.

asystole (a-sis′to-le) [*a*- neg + Gr. *systolē* contraction] the absence of cardiac contraction; cardiac standstill or arrest.

At symbol for the chemical element *astatine.*

AT III abbrev. see a. III under *antithrombin.*

ATA abbrev. See *atmosphere absolute.*

Atabrine (at′ah-brīn) trademark. See *quinacrine hydrochloride.*

ataractic (at″ah-rak′tik) [Gr. *ataraktos*] 1. pertaining to or producing ataraxia (calmness, serenity). Also called ataraxic.

2. see *tranquilizer.*

Atarax (at′ah-raks) trademark. See *hydroxyzine.*

ataxia (ah-tak′se-ah) [Gr. *ataxia* failure of order] a general term for disturbances in the coordination of voluntary movements, characterized by errors in their rate, range, strength, and direction. The coordination of motor activity may be impaired by lesions in the cerebellum or cerebellar peduncles, or by weakness or sensory disturbances.

cerebellar a., an ataxia that results from dysfunction of the cerebellum, such as by tumor, abscess, vascular lesion, drug intoxication, or hereditary degenerative disease. Depending on the region of the cerebellum involved, there may be ataxia of gait or incoordination of the limbs on one or both sides. Other signs of cerebellar dysfunction may include dysarthria, disturbances of eye movements, and muscular hypotonia.

Friedreich's a., a type of hereditary ataxia characterized by the progressive degeneration of the spinal cord, cerebellum, and peripheral nerves; in some cases there is also fibrosis of the myocardium. Symptoms usually appear in late childhood as staggering gait and difficulty in standing. Clumsiness, intention tremor, slurred speech, and skeletal deformities (pes cavus, kyphoscoliosis) may occur. Tendon reflexes are absent, but the plantar reflexes are extensor. Numerous abortive or incomplete forms of the disorder exist. There is no medical treatment that influences its course. See also *spinocerebellar degeneration.*

a. telangiectasia, a genetic disorder, transmitted as an autosomal recessive trait, that is characterized by cerebellar ataxia, oculocutaneous telangiectasia, and immunologic defects. This disease is thought to result from defective DNA repair mechanisms, with increased susceptibility to chromosome breakage on exposure to radiation. It is considered that this accounts for the high incidence of malignancies, especially leukemia and lymphomas, in affected individuals. There may also be a generalized defect of cellular differentiation, which results in gonadal dysgenesis, early development of senile lesions, and expression of oncofetal antigens.

Persons affected display truncal incoordination in infancy, which progresses to severe disability. Vascular lesions develop on the bulbar conjunctiva, ears, and nose. There is a marked T-cell dysfunction with impaired cell-mediated immunity and thymic hypoplasia. B-cell function is also decreased with deficiences of serum IgA and IgE, resulting in recurrent sinopulmonary infection. Diagnosis is based on the clinical picture, immunologic findings, and demonstration of oncofetal proteins. Treatment is supportive and the prognosis is poor, with death frequently occurring in the third decade from pulmonary infections or malignancy.

ATCC abbrev. See *American Type Culture Collection.*

-ate (āt) [L. *-atus* ending of the past participle of first conjugation verbs] 1. a suffix word element to denote the object of a process, e.g., hemolysate, homogenate; possession of a structure, e.g., dentate, corticate; being shaped like, e.g., lanceolate; or a process involving some object, e.g., aerate, pollinate. This suffix also occurs in words formed from Latin participles, e.g., coagulate.

2. a suffix word element in inorganic chemistry to denote a complex anion. In common names, *-ate* indicates the anion of an oxo acid in which the central atom has the higher of the two common oxidation states, e.g., sulfate, the common name for tet-

raoxosulfate (SO_4^{2-}). Cf. *-ide* and *-ite.* See also *coordination compound.*

3. a suffix word element used in naming salts, esters, or anions, of organic and inorganic acids ending in -ic, e.g., acetic acid, sodium acetate (salt), methyl acetate (ester); phosphoric acid, phosphate (anion), glucose-6-phosphate (ester).

4. a suffix word element used in naming salts of alcohols, phenols, and thiols, e.g., sodium phenolate.

atel/o (at′ĕ-lo) [Gr. *atelēs* incomplete] a word element used in combining form to denote incomplete or imperfect, e.g., atelomyelia.

atelectasis (at″e-lek′tah-sis) [*atel-* + Gr. *ektasis* expansion] the failure of lungs to expand adequately at birth (congenital atelectasis) or the collapse of a lung or portions of the lungs that were previously inflated (acquired atelectasis).

Atelectasis in the newborn (atelectasis neonatorum) may be primary or congenital, and consists of incomplete expansion of the lungs at birth. It may also develop after adequate inflation has occurred (secondary atelectasis), commonly in association with respiratory distress syndrome or as a consequence of the excessive pulmonary secretions that may accompany respiratory infections.

The most common causes of acquired atelectasis are complete obstruction of segments of the airways beyond the tracheal bifurcation (obstructive atelectasis), or extrinsic compression of the lungs due to the elevation in intrapleural pressure that accompanies partial or complete filling of the pleural cavity with air (pneumothorax), blood (hemothorax), tissue fluids (hydrothorax, neoplastic effusion), a tumor, or an abnormally elevated diaphragm (compressive atelectasis). It can also occur during anesthesia, following extracorporeal perfusion of the lungs in open heart surgery, or postoperatively.

Atelectasis reduces ventilatory functions to varying degrees, depending on the extent of the collapse. If the affected volume is slight (and the rest of the lung is normal), the total lung, functional residual, and vital capacities are reduced, but the ventilatory capacity drops only slightly. In acute atelectasis the patient may show symptoms of tachypnea, severe dyspnea, and hypoxemia. Massive atelectasis commonly produces an immediate hyperventilation of the contralateral (unaffected) lung and a drop in arterial P_{O_2} and P_{CO_2}.

Reexpansion of the collapsed lung parenchyma is nearly always possible; however, if reinflation is not accomplished after collapse of a large volume of the lungs (massive collapse), death usually follows.

The presence of atelectasis can be confirmed radiographically, and bronchoscopy can be used to establish its specific etiology.

a. neonatorum, the collapse of lung parenchyma in newborns; it is present at birth (primary or congenital) or occurs subsequent to initial (often inadequate) expansions of the lungs (secondary). The respiratory failure that leads to the primary type may be the result of such adverse intrauterine conditions as kinking of the umbilical cord, hypoxia, retroplacental hemorrhage, or premature separation of the placenta. Adequate respiration is never established, and the infants die. The secondary type is related to the respiratory distress syndrome or is caused when some primary disease such as respiratory infection or aspiration leads to obstruction of the airway.

obstructive a., the collapse of localized segments of lung parenchyma, a lobe, or an entire lung that is caused by complete obstruction of portions of the bronchi or bronchioles. The obstruction may be caused by excessive secretions (caused by bronchiectasis, bronchial asthma, or chronic bronchitis, or occurring in comatose patients), by a solid object such as a bronchial neoplasm or aspirated foreign body, or by inflammation. Because the air trapped distal to the obstruction is rapidly absorbed by the pulmonary capillary blood, a negative pressure develops in the alveoli, causing them to collapse. If the parenchymal tissue is not pliant enough to collapse, the negative pressure leads to filling of the alveoli with edematous fluid.

Hyperventilation of adjoining areas, an increased resistance to blood flow in the collapsed segments, and a hypoxia-induced vasoconstriction that leads to shunting of the blood flow toward adequately aerated areas all contribute to the maintenance of ventilatory capacity despite the presence of atelectasis.

AT/GC ratio the value determined by the amount of adenine + thymine divided by the amount of guanine + cytosine in a given deoxyribonucleic acid. Also called *base ratio.* See also *nucleic acid.*

ather/o (ath′er-o) [Gr. *athērē* gruel, porridge] a word element used in combining form to denote a yellowish plaque, fatty substance, or paste, e.g., atheroma.

atheroma (ath″er-o′mah) [*ather-* + Gr. *ōma* swelling] a mass of degenerated fatty or lipid material found with necrosis of a fibrous plaque in the arterial wall in atherosclerosis. It undergoes a number of changes as the disease progresses: calcification, internal hemorrhaging, ulceration, and, occasionally, superimposed thrombosis. See also *atherosclerosis* under *arteriosclerosis.*

atherosclerosis (ath″er-o″skle-ro′sis) [*athero-* + Gr. *sklēros* hard + *-osis* condition] see under *arteriosclerosis.*

atherosclerotic heart disease the most common form of heart disease, characterized by the localized deposition of fibrous and lipid tissue in the large- and medium-sized blood vessels supplying the heart. Males are affected more often than females; the peak incidence is between 50 and 60 yr (for males), and 60 and 70 yr (for females). Coronary angiography is the most accurate means of diagnosis. In certain cases, surgery can be performed to bypass the lesions. The condition can lead to angina pectoris, myocardial infarction, and sudden death. Also called *arteriosclerotic heart disease* and *coronary heart disease.*

athetosis (ath″ĕ-to′sis) [Gr. *athetos* not fixed + *-osis*] repetitive involuntary, slow, sinuous, writhing movements.

athlete's foot see *tinea pedis.*

Ativan trademark. See *lorazepam.*

atlas (at′las) [Gr., from the giant *Atlas,* who, in Greek mythology, bears the world on his shoulders] 1. [NA], the first cervical vertebra. It is essentially a ring of bone, devoid of body or spine but with paired transverse processes each of which encloses a transverse foramen. Large superior facets articulate with the occipital condyles.

2. a collection of illustrations on one subject, such as anatomy.

atm abbrev. See *atmosphere.*

atm/o (at′mo) [Gr. *atmos* steam or vapor] a word element used in combining form to denote relationship to steam or vapor, e.g., atmosphere.

atmosphere (at'mos-fēr) [Gr. *atmos* steam + *sphaira* sphere] 1. the gaseous envelope that surrounds the earth. The specific composition is as follows:

COMPOSITION OF THE ATMOSPHERE (%)

Nitrogen	78.09
Oxygen	20.95
Argon	0.93
Carbon dioxide	0.03
Neon	1.8×10^{-3}
Helium	5.24×10^{-4}
Krypton	1.0×10^{-4}
Hydrogen	5.0×10^{-5}
Xenon	8.0×10^{-6}
Ozone	1.0×10^{-6}
Radon	6.0×10^{-18}

2. (abbrev. atm), the average atmospheric pressure at sea level, 101.325 kilopascals (kPa), 760 millimeters of mercury (mmHg), 1033 centimeters of water (cm H_2O), or 14.7 pounds per square inch (psi).

atmosphere absolute (ATA) the pressure exerted by the atmosphere at sea level; also called atmosphere.

atmospheric monitoring the measurement of concentrations of potentially toxic materials in the breathing zones of employees or students. It is recommended to evaluate the effectiveness of ventilation systems and techniques if quantities of toxic or irritating materials are being used, or if workers are experiencing physiologic effects that may be caused or increased by exposure to chemicals. See also *permissible exposure limits* and *threshold limit values.*

atocia (ah-to'se-ah) [*a*- neg. + Gr. *tokos* birth] sterility in the female.

atom (at'om) [Gr. *atomos* indivisible, from *a*- neg. + *tomos* cut, piece] the smallest particle of a chemical element, composed of a nucleus and electrons. The nucleus is made up of protons and neutrons bound together by the "strong force" and is very small (about 1 fm). In a neutral atom there is one electron for every proton. In the ground state the electrons fill the lowest energy quantum states. An atom ranges in size from 30 to 300 pm.

The lower energy electrons are always localized near the nucleus, but the outer or valence electrons may be in quantum states that surround two atoms (a covalent bond) or many atoms (in a crystal). These bonding electrons hold the molecule or crystal together. See also *bond* and *element.*

atomic (ah-tom'ik) pertaining to an atom.

atomic absorption (AA) spectrophotometer an instrument for performing atomic absorption spectrophotometry. It consists of a light source, sample atomizer, monochromator, and detector.

The light source is usually a hollow cathode lamp, a neon or argon glow-discharge tube with a cathode that is lined with the metal being assayed. Gas ions striking the cathode cause metal atoms to sputter off and be ionized by other collisions, emitting light. For easily vaporized metals such as sodium or mercury, vapor discharge lamps may be used.

The sample atomizer is a total consumption burner, a premix burner, or a furnace. The total consumption burner produces a hotter flame, but large variations in droplet size produce a noisy signal owing to light scattering. The premix (or laminar flow) burner has a more uniform droplet size and a long flame that produces a longer optical path length and thus greater analytic sensitivity. The graphite furnace permits measurements with the highest sensitivity, but matrix interference is more severe than with flame methods, and sample throughput is lower because the furnace must cool down between measurements.

The monochromator is a grating or prism device with a narrow bandpass, usually adjustable down to 0.2 nm. The detector is usually a photomultiplier tube.

A single-beam instrument has only one optical path and is subject to several types of measurement error. To correct these, two types of double-beam instrument are used. In one, the beam emitted by the lamp is chopped, with one beam going through the flame and the other around it. The beams are recombined and pass through the monochromator to the detector, as in a conventional double-beam spectrophotometer. This compensates for instabilities in the light source and flame. In the other type of instrument, two light sources are used. Both pass through the flame but via separate monochromators. One beam is on an absorption line of the analyte. The other is used to determine the absorbance of the flame at a different wavelength; this compensates for various matrix interferences and is especially important in photometers that use a furnace for sample atomization.

atomic absorption spectrophotometry an analytic method used for high-sensitivity measurements (detection limits on the order of 1 ng/l) of metals such as calcium, iron, lithium, copper, zinc, arsenic, lead, and beryllium. In the process, a sample is vaporized and the concentration of a metal is determined from the absorption of light at one of the strong emission lines of the element.

There are three types of interference found in atomic absorption methods: chemical, matrix, and ionization. Chemical interference is due to the presence of compounds or complexes formed between the analyte and the anions in the sample that are not dissociated in the flame. This problem is usually overcome by adding some other metal with a greater affinity for the interfering anion. Matrix interference is due to the effects of solvents on background absorption or droplet size, or it is due to refractory salts in the sample that absorb much of the flame energy in their decomposition. Ionization interference results when atoms of the analyte are excited to energy levels above the ground state, and emit radiation at the wavelength used for measurement. This is usually overcome by lowering the temperature of the flame.

atomic mass see *atomic weight.*

atomic mass unit (amu) a unit of mass equal to one twelfth of the mass of an atom of the carbon isotope ^{12}C. The absolute value of 1 amu $= 1.66041 \times 10^{-27}$ kg. The absolute masses of atoms are expressed as multiples of the amu. For potassium, the amu multiplied by the atomic weight of potassium (39.102) equals 1.66041×10^{-27} kg $\times$ 39.102 $= 6.9925 \times 10^{-26}$ kg (the absolute mass of one potassium atom). The atomic weight of an element and the average mass per atom expressed in atomic mass units have the same value. Also called *dalton.*

atomic number (Z) the whole number representing the number of units of positive charge (number of protons) in the nucleus of an atom.

atomic spectrum the distribution of spectral lines (either absorption or emission) in the x-ray region caused by intraatomic transitions of orbital electrons between quantized energy levels. Each chemical element has a characteristic atomic spectrum that can be used to quantitate it in compounds and mixtures.

atomic weight (A.W., at wt.) the mass of an atom of a specific isotope of a chemical element relative to the mass of the carbon isotope ^{12}C, which is assigned an atomic weight of exactly 12. The atomic weight of a chemical element is the sum of the atomic weights of the isotopes multiplied by their natural abundances; thus, it is the relative average mass of the atoms in the naturally occurring mixture of isotopes. The term is imprecise—a better term is relative atomic mass—but its use is firmly established and generally accepted. Also called *atomic mass.* See also *molecular weight.*

atomization (at″om-ĭ-za′shun) the act or process of breaking up a liquid into a spray of drops.

atomizer (at′om-iz″er) an instrument for breaking up a liquid into a spray of fine droplets. In the flame photometer, a high-velocity gas is passed over the upper end of a capillary tube whose lower end is in the sample. The sample is drawn through the capillary tube and emerges as a fine mist. This enters the flame, and the emission or absorption of light by atoms in the sample is measured.

atony (at′o-ne) [L. *atonia,* from *a-* neg. + Gr. *tonos* tension] the absence of normal tone or normal resistance to passive elongation or stretching. The term is usually applied to the bladder or the GI tract, e.g., gastric atony in diabetic neuropathy with gastroparesis.

atopen (at′o-pen) an allergen that causes an atopic allergy.

atopic (a-top′ik) [*a-* neg. + Gr. *topos* place] 1. ectopic; out of place.
2. referring to an atopen or to atopy; allergic.

atopic allergen any allergen that causes a state of atopy; an atopen. Common ones include plant pollens, fungal spores, animal hair, dust, and insect debris.

atopic keratoconjunctivitis inflammation of the cornea and conjunctiva in which the skin of the eyelids is dry and appears scaly, and the conjunctiva is pale and slightly swollen. Scarring may result. Serum IgE is usually present in the subepithelial mast cells, and many eosinophils are found.

atopy (at′o-pe) [Gr. *atopia* strangeness] a predisposition to the development of IgE-mediated hypersensitivity reactions to common antigens: atopic individuals are more prone to develop diseases such as atopic dermatitis, allergic rhinitis, urticaria, and asthma. The characteristic triad of diseases seen in atopic patients (atopic dermatitis, allergic rhinitis, and asthma) may all occur in the same patient, although there are often only one or two. A predisposition to atopy is thought to be inherited because the incidence of atopy is higher in families with a history of the condition. Atopic persons tend to have higher than normal concentrations of total serum IgE, eosinophilia in the peripheral blood, and evidence of IgE sensitization to antigens, as demonstrated by skin tests or bronchial provocation testing.

The etiology for this predisposition is not well established. Individuals with atopic diseases may have some autonomic nervous dysfunction, as manifested by hyperresponsiveness to cholinergic and α-adrenergic stimuli and hyporesponsiveness to β-adrenergic stimuli. This theory is consistent with the increased reactivity in atopic individuals (especially asthmatics) to methacholine on bronchial challenge, and to the decreased β-adrenergic response seen in the white blood cells of atopic patients, but it does not explain the increased propensity for formation of IgE antibodies and development of immediate hypersensitivity reactions.

Also called atopic allergy. See also *immediate hypersensitivity.*

GERALD B. KOLSKI, M.D., PH.D.

ATP abbrev. See *adenosine triphosphate.*

ATPase abbrev. See *adenosine triphosphatase.*

Atrax (a′traks) a genus of tarantula-like spiders (funnel-web spiders) of Australia, family Dipluridae. The venom of several species, including *A. robustus* and *A. formidabilis* (tree funnel-web spider), is harmful to humans. Several individuals bitten by *A. robustus* have died from the bite.

atresia (ah-tre′ze-ah) [*a-* neg. + Gr. *trēsis* a hole + *-ia*] a congenital absence or closure of a normal body orifice or tubular structure; the term is also applied to the retrogression of ovarian follicles, e.g., corpora atretica.

a. ani., see *i. anus* under *imperforate.*

biliary a., an obliteration or hypoplasia of the bile ducts due to arrested fetal development. The condition results in persistent jaundice and liver damage (biliary stasis and cirrhosis) with associated splenomegaly as the portal hypertension progresses.

esophageal a., a lack of continuity of the esophagus due to failure in development. There is commonly an associated tracheoesophageal fistula. Clinical features include hypersalivation, gagging, vomiting during feeding, cyanosis, and dyspnea.

follicular a., the degeneration and resorption of an ovarian follicle.

intestinal a., a congenital occlusion of the intestine. It can occur at any level, and symptoms vary with the obstructed site.

mitral a., congenital absence of the left atrioventricular orifice.

pulmonary a., a congenital narrowing of the orifice between the pulmonary artery and right ventricle, commonly associated with tetralogy of Fallot, transposition of the great vessels, or other cardiovascular anomalies. It is characterized by cardiac hypertrophy, decreased pulmonary vascularity, and right ventricular atrophy.

tricuspid a., the congenital absence of the passage that normally lies between the right atrium and right ventricle (tricuspid orifice) of the heart, accompanied by hypoplasia of the right ventricle. There may also be transposition of the pulmonary artery and aorta, narrowing of the pulmonary artery (pulmonary stenosis), and communication between the right and left ventricles (ventricular septal defect).

Circulation is maintained through an atrial septal defect so that blood flows from the right to the left atrium to the left ventricle to the aorta. Blood reaches the lungs through a patent ductus arteriosus or through the ventricular septal defect from the left to the right ventricle to the pulmonary artery.

Diagnosis of the condition is suggested by the presence of left axis deviation on the electrocardiogram, accompanied by right atrial enlargement, left ventricular hypertrophy, and cyanosis, and can be confirmed by cardiac catheterization. Surgical correction is possible in those having normal pulmonary artery anatomy and adequate left ventricular function.

atret/o (ah-tre′to) [Gr. *atrētos* not perforated, from *a-* neg. + *trētos* perforated] a word element used in combining form to denote imperforate or closed, or the absence of a normal opening, e.g., atretic.

atretic (ah-tret′ik) without an opening; pertaining to atresia.

atretic follicle a degenerated ovarian follicle following ovulation.

atri/o (a′tre-o) [L. *atrium* hall] a word element used in combining form to denote atrium, e.g., atrioventricular.

atrial (a′tre-al) pertaining to an atrium.

atrial appendage see *auricle*.

atrial arrhythmia any variation in the rate or pattern of the normal sinus rhythm of the heartbeat resulting from disordered impulse formation within the atria. Atrial arrhythmias can be initiated subsequent to reentry of the cardiac impulse, or to an alteration of the normal automaticity of the sinoatrial node or of potential pacemaker sites outside the node (ectopic sites) in atrial tissue.

The presence of an atrial arrhythmia, its type, the mechanisms responsible for triggering or aggravating it, and the severity of the disturbances in function likely to be a consequence of the arrhythmia can be established through use of diagnostic techniques such as recording of the jugular venous or arterial pulse, carotid sinus massage, phonocardiography, and electrocardiography.

For more information on specific arrhythmias, see the individual entries (e.g., *atrial f.* under *fibrillation, atrial f.* under *flutter*, and *atrial p. d.* under *premature depolarization*.

atrial fibrillation see *atrial f.* under *fibrillation*.

atrial flutter see *atrial f.* under *flutter*.

atrial premature beat (APB) see *premature atrial contraction*.

atrial premature contraction (APC) see *premature atrial contraction*.

atrial premature depolarization (APD) see *premature atrial contraction*.

atrial septal defect (ASD) a common congenital anomaly characterized by an abnormal opening in the septum between the right and left atria. It may occur in one of three locations: the endocardial cushion near the atrioventricular valves (ostium primum); the fossa ovalis (ostium secundum, the most common form); or near the entry of the superior vena cava (sinus venosus). The openings create a left-to-right shunt, causing an increased volume load in the right side of the heart. Clinical manifestations include systolic and diastolic murmurs and fixed splitting of second heart sounds. Complications, which usually appear later in life, are exertional dyspnea, atrial arrhythmias, pulmonary hypertension, cardiac failure, and right-to-left shunting that leads to cyanosis. Diagnosis is made on the basis of clinical findings, electrocardiography, echocardiography of septal motions, cardiac catheterization, and radiographs. Surgical correction is the recommended treatment.

atrichous (ah-trik′us) [Gr. *atrichos* hairless, from *a-* neg. + *thrix* hair] 1. having no hair.
2. having no flagella; said of bacteria.

atrioventricular (A-V, AV) (a″tre-o-ven-trik′u-lar) [*atrio-* + L. *ventriculus* stomach, ventricle] pertaining to an atrium and ventricle of the heart.

atrioventricular (A-V) block an impairment in the conduction of excitatory impulses from the atria to the ventricles, usually occurring in the junctional tissues of the A-V node or the bundle of His, and consisting of three degrees of block.

first-degree A-V b., the mild impairment of conduction from atria to ventricles marked by abnormal slowing of the wave of depolarizaton passing through the conduction pathways. First-degree A-V block presents as a prolonged P-R interval in the electrocardiogram. A clinical sign is a soft first heart sound. It is often present for years and produces no symptoms; it also occasionally occurs after acute inferior myocardial infarction, although the block itself seldom requires therapy.

second-degree A-V b., a form of block in which some but not all atrial beats are followed by a ventricular beat. Second-degree block may result in a slowing of the ventricular rate and is observed in two types. Type I A-V block occurs within the A-V node. The P-R interval increases with each beat until a P wave is not conducted to the ventricles, resulting in a long R-R interval. This type of block often accompanies a transient condition such as acute rheumatic fever or acute inferior myocardial infarction. It can progress to a complete block but usually requires no therapy, although a temporary pacemaker is indicated in rare cases. Type II A-V block is a relatively rare and much more serious condition, involving a lesion below the A-V node associated with His bundle or bundle branch disease. This type of block does not present with a gradually lengthening P-R interval; rather, there is abrupt failure to conduct one or more complexes. Affected individuals usually have symptoms associated with bradyarrhythmias, and there is often progression to complete block.

third-degree A-V b., complete blockage of A-V conduction with separate pacemakers for the atria and the ventricles. There usually is dramatic slowing of the ventricular rate, as the ventricles are paced by a low idioventricular pacemaker. The electrocardiogram shows regular R-R intervals and QRS complexes that are widened to about 0.12 sec (unless the ventricular pacemaker is in the His region, resulting in a narrow QRS). The block itself generally occurs distal to the A-V node and has a poor prognosis without pacemaker therapy. Also called *complete heart block* and *third-degree heart block*.

atrioventricular bundle part of the conducting system of the heart. The A-V bundle (bundle of His) begins in the atrioventricular node, runs to the upper end of the muscular part of the interventricular septum, and divides into right and left (bundle) branches, which form a network of fine (Purkinje) fibers within the ventricles beneath the endocardium.

left b. branch, a fascicle of Purkinje fibers that

gives off many fine branches to the papillary muscles of the left ventricle as it courses along the left margin of the interventricular septum. See also *heart.*

right b. branch, a discrete, narrow fascicle of Purkinje fibers that runs along the interventricular septum to the right ventricular apex. Its many fine branches invest the papillary muscles of the right ventricle.

atrioventricular node see *atrioventricular n.* under *node.*

atrioventricular valve a heart valve between the atrium and ventricle; see under *heart.*

atrium (a′tre-um) [L. "hall"] an external hall or entrance chamber, used anatomically to indicate a chamber that allows access to another structure or organ. When used alone, the term usually indicates an atrial chamber of the heart.

Atromid-S (at′ro-mid) trademark. See *clofibrate.*

Atropa (at′ro-pah) a genus of solanaceous plants of which the species *A. belladonna,* commonly called "nightshade," is the source of various alkaloids. These are primarily atropine, which is used to block the parasympathetic nerves, and scopolamine, which is also a parasympathetic blocking agent that may in addition produce stimulation of the central nervous system.

atrophic (ah-trof′ik) pertaining to atrophy.

atrophy (at′ro-fe) [Gr. *atrophia* lack of nourishment] 1. a wasting away; a decrease in the size of a cell, tissue, organ, or part. It may result from factors such as a loss of or reduction in endocrine stimulation of sex organs or endocrine glands, inadequate nutrition, diminished blood supply, or decreased workload and loss of innervation of muscle. Cf. *hypoplasia* and *hypertrophy.*

2. to undergo atrophy or to cause atrophy.

atropine (at′ro-pin) [USP], a white crystalline alkaloid found in *Atropa belladonna* and other plants of the nightshade family. It blocks the cholinergic receptors in smooth muscles and thus relieves smooth muscle spasms. Also, because it reduces secretions, it is administered as a preanesthetic to reduce salivary and bronchial secretions. Small doses are a central nervous system stimulant; overdoses may cause confusion, hallucinations, CNS depression, and death due to paralysis. Atropine is given as an antidote to cholinesterase-inhibiting poisons, organophosphate insecticides, and chemical warfare nerve gases.

attachment (ah-tach′ment) 1. the state of being fixed or attached.

2. the means or device by which something is fixed or stabilized.

3. in virology, the process of bonding between a virus and the plasma membrane of a cell. Viral receptor sites must be present on the cell in order for this to take place.

attachment plaque the region of a desmosome where tonofilaments attach to the cell membrane.

attenuated (ah-ten″u-āt′ed) [L. *attenuare* to weaken, from *ad-* + *tenuare* from *tenuis* weak, thin] 1. weakened or decreased virulence; the term is usually applied in microbiology to pathogenic microorganisms that have been modified by repeated culturing under relatively unfavorable conditions until the virulence level is significantly reduced. Attenuated microorganisms were, and still are, used for immunization against infectious diseases, e.g., Pasteur's anthrax and rabies vaccines, and the BCG vaccine against tuberculosis.

2. in histology, a cell with thinned out cytoplasm, e.g., type I pneumocyte, perineural cell.

attenuation (ah-ten″u-a′shun) [L. *attenuare* to thin, from *ad-* to + *tenuis* thin] 1. the act of thinning or weakening.

2. the reduction of the pathogenicity of an organism for a particular host, such as by the adaptation of the organism to another host or to a culture medium, a process used in the preparation of live vaccines.

3. the reduction in the intensity of a beam of radiation by absorption or scattering processes.

4. in electroencephalography, a decrease in amplitude (desynchronization) of the electric activity recorded from the brain. This may be a transient decrease resulting from stimulation of the brain or may reflect a pathologic condition. The term is also used for a reduction in the sensitivity of an EEG channel.

attenuation coefficient see *linear attenuation coefficient* and *mass attenuation coefficient.*

attenuator (ah-ten′u-a-tor) in electronics, a device that reduces the size of a signal.

atto- (a) (at′to) [Danish *atten* eighteen] a prefix attached to International System (SI) units to make a unit that is one-quintillionth of the basic unit (10^{-18} unit).

attribute (at′trĭ-būt) in statistics, an often nonquantifiable characteristic of some members of a population, which is recorded as present or absent in individual data.

at. wt. abbrev. See *atomic weight.*

atypia (a-tip′e-ah) [N.L., from *a-* neg. + Gr. *typos* type or model] a general term used to describe the deviation from the normal or typical type. See also *cellular atypia* and *dysplasia.*

atypical (a-tip′ĭ-kal) 1. irregular; not conforming to type.

2. in microbiology, referring to strains of unusual type.

3. in cytology, a general term indicating a cell that is not normal. The cause of the atypia may be reactive, hyperplastic, inflammatory, dysplastic, or neoplastic change.

atypical hyperplasia see *atypical h.* under *hyperplasia.*

atypical mycobacterium a term frequently used to designate strains isolated from clinical specimens and elsewhere that differ from *Mycobacterium tuberculosis* and *M. bovis.* Because these strains are not in reality atypical, but rather are characteristic of several definitive species, use of the term should be avoided.

atypical repetitive spike-and-slow waves see *three-Hertz spike and slow waves.*

Au [L. *aurum*] symbol for the chemical element *gold.*

Au Ag abbrev. See *Australia antigen.*

Auchmeromyia (awk″mer-o-mi′yah) [Gr. *auchmeros* without rain, dirty + *myia* fly] a genus of flies of the family Calliphoridae.

A. luteola, a species, found in tropical Africa, that has a bloodsucking larval stage specifically parasitic for humans. These insects have five pairs of posterior processes and characteristic posterior spiracles, and can tolerate wide variations in climate. See also *Congo floor m.* under *maggot.*

audi/o (aw′de-o) [L. *audire* to hear] a word element used in combining form to denote hearing, e.g., auditory.

audiogram (au′de-o-gram″) [*audio-* + Gr. *gramma* to write] a graph that charts the sound intensity of the threshold of audibility (in decibels) versus frequency in the range of 125–8000 Hz.

audiology (aw″de-ol′o-je) [*audio-* + Gr. *logos* reason, speech] the study of hearing disorders, including the measurement of hearing function and the rehabilitation of those with impaired hearing.

audiometer (aw″de-om′ĕ-ter) [*audio-* + Gr. *metron* measure] an instrument used by an audiologist in testing human ear function. It produces precisely defined sounds conveyed to the ear by earphones or by bone conduction. Pure tones are generated that cover the frequency range of 125–8000 Hz in octave or half-octave steps at sound pressure levels covering the range of 0–110 dB re 2×10^{-4} dyne/cm^2 in 5-dB steps. This includes frequencies critical for understanding speech and loudnesses from the minimal audible pressure for healthy young ears to levels loud enough to produce discomfort.

Most audiometers also generate white noise, which can be added to the signal tone in 5-dB increments to test the ability to hear a tone against the noise background. Some audiometers also have a speech circuit that enables the audiologist to produce speech with a calibrated sound level for intelligibility testing.

audiometry (aw″de-om′e-tre) the measurement of hearing; see also *audiometer.*

auditory (aw′dĭ-to″re) [L. *auditorius*] pertaining to the sense of hearing.

auditory evoked potential see *brain stem auditory e. p.* under *evoked potential.*

auditory nerve the eighth cranial nerve, a sensory nerve consisting of two portions: the vestibular nerve concerned with equilibrium and the cochlear nerve, the nerve of hearing.

auditory ossicles a chain of three small, movable bones—individually called the malleus, incus, and stapes—of the middle ear; these bones transmit the vibrations of the tympanic membrane to the perilymph of the inner ear (cochlea).

auditory stimulation an activation technique used to induce changes in the electroencephalogram by music, rhythmic nonmusical sounds (clicks), random taps, or pure tones. In normal children and adults, a burst of one or two high-voltage slow waves (K complex) may be elicted by auditory stimulation during sleep, while vertex waves may be elicited during the awake state. In individuals with some types of epilepsy, sudden auditory stimulation produces abnormal EEG activity and/or myoclonic attacks.

auditory tube the channel between the tympanic cavity and the nasopharynx that permits equalization of air pressure on opposite sides of the tympanic membrane. Also called *eustachian tube* and *pharyngotympanic tube.*

auditory vesicle see *otic vesicle.*

audit trail 1. the stepwise trace from a line of data in a report back to the documentation of those actions or transactions that caused that line of data to be generated.

2. in accounting, the trace from a line in a financial statement back to specific general ledger accounts, then back to books of original entry (such as cash receipts), then back to the source documents of the transaction (such as customer receipt form).

Auerbach's plexus (ow′er-bahks) [Leopold *Auerbach,* German anatomist, 1828–1897] see *myenteric p.* under *plexus.*

Auer rod (ow′er) [John *Auer,* American physician, 1875–1948] a rod-, lozenge-, or needle-shaped inclusion found within the cytoplasm of myeloid and occasionally monocytic leukemic cells that stains like the azurophilic cytoplasmic granules from which they originate by fusion. Auer rods give a positive reaction with peroxidase, PAS, and acid phosphatase, and on electron microscopy have a characteristic periodicity. They occur in 5 percent of acute myelogenous leukemias and in monomyelocytic leukemias, but their presence in pure monocytic leukemia has been questioned. These inclusions may also occur in refractory anemia with excess myeloblasts, a type of hemopoietic dysplasia (preleukemia). Auer rods have never been seen in lymphocytic leukemia or in the blood of healthy individuals.

Auger effect (oh-zhay) [Pierre Victor *Auger,* French physicist, born 1899] one of the two processes by which an atom left in an excited state by electron-capture nuclear decay can return to the ground state. A photon is emitted as an electron drops from an outer orbital to the orbital vacated by the electron capture. In the Auger effect, this photon is totally absorbed by another electron in the same atom, which gains enough energy to be ejected from the atom. The electron (Auger electron) has a kinetic energy equal to the energy of the photon minus the binding energy of the electron. In the alternate process, the photon, termed a fluorescent x-ray, is emitted.

Auger electron [Pierre Victor *Auger*] the orbital electron that is ejected from an atom by interaction with fluorescent x-ray photons emitted from the same atom, a process referred to as an internal photoelectric effect. See also *Auger effect.*

aura (aw′rah) [L. "breath"] a subjective sensation or motor phenomenon that marks the onset of an epileptic attack. The sensation may involve hallucinations or perceptual illusion. The aura is part of the seizure and by its nature indicates the part of the brain from which the seizure is initiated. See also *epilepsy.*

aural (aw′ral) 1. [L. *auris* ear] pertaining to or perceived by the ear.

2. [*aura*] pertaining to an aura.

auramine (aw′rah-mēn) a yellow fluorochrome dye, commonly used in Schiff reagents; C.I. 41000.

auramine-rhodamine stain see under *acid-fast staining methods.*

aurantiasis (aw″ran-ti′ah-sis) [N.L. *aurantium* orange + *-iasis*] a yellowness of skin caused by intake of large amounts of food containing carotenes.

Aureobasidium (aw-re″o-bah-sid′ĭ-um) [L. *aureus* golden + Gr. *basidion,* dim, of *basis* step, base] a genus of imperfect fungi of the family Dematiaceae, order Moniliales, that is usually considered a soil contaminant. Morphologically, the fungus forms a yeastlike colony, which turns from creamy white to pink to dark brown. The conidia are ovoid and are produced directly from mycelium on short denticles.

Aureomycin (aw″re-o-mi′sin) trademark. See *tetracycline.*

auricle (aw′rĕ-k′l) [L. *auricula* a little ear] 1. the external part of the ear; the pinna or flap of the ear.

2. the ear-shaped prolongation of an atrium of the heart. Also called *atrial appendage.*

auricular (aw-rik′u-lar) [L. *auricularis*] pertaining to the ear or to the auricle of an atrium of the heart.

auricular line a vertical line (parallel to the midcoronal plane) passing through the auricular point.

auricular point the center of the opening of the ear (the external auditory meatus); used as an anatomic landmark.

auricular region the region on the side of the head that surrounds the ear.

aurin tricarboxylic acid (aw′rin) see *chrome violet CG.*

auriscope (aw″rĭ-skōp) [L. *auris* ear + Gr. *skopein* to examine] an otoscope, an instrument used for examining the ear.

aurothioglucose (aw″ro-thi″o-gloo′kōs) [USP], a gold-containing drug used to treat rheumatoid arthritis. Adverse reactions are due to gold toxicity. Also called *gold thioglucose.* See also *gold* and *gold assays.*

auscultation (aws″kul-ta′shun) [L. *auscultare* to listen to] the act of listening (usually with a stethoscope) to sounds produced by the body, a procedure performed to ascertain the presence of any abnormal function or structure of the internal organs. Sounds heard with auscultation include those produced by the heart, lungs, and gastrointestinal tract, and those produced by pathologic structures (including bruits heard over narrowed or tortuous vessels and arteriovenous malformations, and the rubs heard over inflamed or enlarged organs such as the pleura, liver, or spleen).

auscultatory (aw-skul′tah-to″re) [L. *auscultare* to listen to] pertaining to auscultation.

Australia antigen (Au Ag) the former name for hepatitis B surface antigen, the envelope of the hepatitis B virus found in the serum of infected patients. The antigen was named Australia by its discoverers because it was first identified in the blood of an Australian aborigine. See also *hepatitis antigen.*

Australorbis (aws″trah-lor′bis) a genus of snails. See *Biomphalaria.*

A. glabratus, see *B. glabrata* under *Biomphalaria.*

autism (aw′tizm) [Gr. *autos* self + *-ism*] extreme self-absorption and egocentricity with failure to form interpersonal relationships. Thought, the major content of which is subjective, is regulated by affective needs or desires rather than by reality.

infantile a., a condition appearing in children and characterized by failure to develop any form of social communication. It is a poorly understood disorder of unknown cause, although an organic basis is suspected, and in a few cases atrophic lesions have been found on the left side in the medial temporal lobe. Diagnosis is usually made by the time the child is aged 4–5 yr. Affected children are preoccupied with inanimate objects, shun interpersonal contact, and may be self-aggressive; many are retarded. The autistic qualities are generally carried into adult life, and improvement is rare; there is no treatment. Also called autistic childhood psychosis.

autistic (aw-tis′tik) pertaining to or exhibiting autism.

auto- (aw′to) [Gr. *autos* self] a prefix word element to denote self, e.g., autogenous.

autoadsorption (aw″to-ad-sorp′shun) a technique used to remove cold-reacting autoantibodies from a patient's serum so that compatibility testing for alloantibodies may be performed. To increase their sensitivity the patient's red blood cells (either untreated or treated with enzymes) are incubated in the cold with his or her own serum. Cold-reacting autoantibodies adsorb onto the red cells and are removed from the serum.

autoagglutination (aw″to-ah-gloo″tĭ-na′shun) 1. the clumping or aggregation of an individual's cells by autoantibodies in his or her own serum, as in autohemagglutination. Autoagglutination occurring at low temperatures is called cold agglutination.

2. the clumping of a particulate antigen after suspension in a solution of electrolyte. This property is an important source of error in bacterial agglutination tests.

autoagglutinin (aw″to-ah-gloo′tĭ-nin) an autoantibody that produces autoagglutination.

autoallergy (aw″to-al′er-je) a specific immunity to the body's own antigens; see *autoimmunity.*

AutoAnalyzer (aw″to-an′a-līz-er) trademark for a continuous-flow clinical chemistry analyzer; see under *clinical chemistry automation.*

autoantibody (aw″to-an′tĭ-bod″e) antibody that reacts with an individual's own endogenous antigenic determinants.

warm a., that antibody directed against an individual's own red blood cells which is optimally reactive at 37°C. There are two types of warm autoantibodies: (1) a rare and harmless type, which is nonspecific and produces a positive direct antiglobulin test but does not reduce red cell life span in vivo; and (2) a type that causes autoimmune hemolytic anemia, which, when a specificity can be shown, is most often an anti-Rh antibody. This also produces a positive direct antiglobulin test; it can be identified with some difficulty by eluting the anti-Rh antibody and reacting with known cells.

autoantigen (aw″to-an′tĭ-jen) a self-antigen that stimulates the production of autoantibody in the organism in which it occurs, often resulting in an autoimmune disease.

autocatalysis (aw″to-kah-tal′ĭ-sis) [*auto-* + Gr. *katalysis* dissolution] a catalytic reaction enhanced by a product of that same reaction. An example is the conversion of a proenzyme (zymogen) to the active enzyme by the action of the enzyme on the proenzyme, e.g., the cleavage of trypsinogen by trypsin, forming more trypsin.

autochthonous (aw-tok′tho-nus) [Gr. *autochthōn* sprung from the land itself, from *auto-* + *chthōn,* land] 1. found in the place of formation; not taken to a new site, as in a disease contracted locally.

2. indigenous, as in the common microflora of the body.

autochthonous graft see *autologous g.* under *graft.*

autoclave (aw′to-klāv) [*auto-* + L. *clavis* key] 1. an apparatus for the decontamination of infectious wastes or the sterilization of media, reagents, or equipment by steam under pressure. It is fitted with a gauge that automatically regulates the pressure and thus the degree of heat to which the contents are subjected. Autoclaving is the most effective method of destroying all types of microorganisms. The amount of time articles are left in the apparatus and the degree of temperature may be regulated, depending on the material and the degree of sterility necessary. See also *sterilization*.

2. to sterilize material in an autoclave.

autocorrelation function a mathematical property of statistical sequences useful in characterizing the ability of coded aperture collimators to produce adequate tomographic images from a stationary imaging device such as a scintillation camera; it describes the degree to which different points in the same image are correlated. See also *coded aperture imaging*.

autofluorescence (aw″to-floo″o-res′ens) fluorescence in cells produced by substances that are normally present in them.

autofluoroscope (aw″to-floo′o-ro-skōp″) a scintillation camera that produces a picture composed of a 14-by-21 array of squares. The brightness of each square is proportional to the number of counts detected in that area of the image by a separate crystal and photomultiplier tube. See also *scintillation camera*.

autogeneic (aw″to-jen-e′ik) see *autogenous*.

autogeneic graft see *autologous g.* under *graft*.

autogenous (aw-toj′ĕ-nus) [*auto-* + Gr. *genesis* origin] self-generated; originating in the body. In transplantation immunology, the term refers to tissue transferred or transplanted within one individual. Also called *autogeneic*. See also *autogeneic g.* under *graft*.

autogenous vaccine any vaccine made from the patient's own disease-producing microorganisms, as opposed to stock vaccines made from standard cultures. It is made by culturing the organisms collected from the diseased individual, which are then killed and inoculated back into that same individual.

autograft (aw″to-graft) see *autologous g.* under *graft*.

autohemagglutination (aw″to-hēm″ah-gloo″tĭ-na′-shun) the agglutination or clumping of red blood cells in autologous plasma or serum.

autohemagglutinin (aw″to-hēm-ah-gloo′tĭ-nin) [*auto-* + Gr. *haima* blood + L. *agglutināre* to glue to + *-in*] a hemagglutinin that causes the clumping or agglutination of autologous erythrocytes.

autohemolysin (aw″to-he-mol′ĭ-sin) [*auto-* + Gr. *haima* blood + *lysis* destruction] a type of antibody or related factor with the ability to lyse autologous erythrocytes.

autohemolysis (aw″to-he-mol′ĭ-sis) hemolysis of red blood cells observed during incubation in their own plasma.

autohemolysis test a test used in the diagnosis of hereditary spherocytic anemia (hereditary spherocytosis, HS). Defibrinated or heparinized blood is incubated for 24 and 48 hr with and without added glucose. Normally, autohemolysis is less than 3.5 percent after 48 hr without glucose, and less than 0.6 percent with glucose. Autohemolysis is increased in HS in the absence of added glucose, and is markedly reduced in the presence of added glucose.

The test was also used previously in the diagnosis of nonspherocytic congenital hemolytic anemias to distinguish between type 1 (moderate autohemolysis corrected by glucose) and type 2 (marked autohemolysis not corrected by glucose). The availability of specific enzymatic assays for nonspherocytic hemolytic anemias has made the autohemolysis test obsolete for this purpose.

autohemotherapy (aw″to-he″mo-ther′ah-pe) [*auto-* + Gr. *haima* blood + *therapeia* treatment] treatment by reinjection of the individual's own blood.

autoimmune (aw″to-im-mūn′) directed against the body's own tissue.

autoimmune disease a disease in which the host produces an immune response against self antigens. With the advent of more sensitive tests, an increasing number of diseases and disease entities have been found to be characterized by autoantibodies. Autoimmune diseases are listed in the accompanying table.

The reason for the formation of autoantibodies is still largely speculative; four theories exist. (1) Formation appears secondary to tissue destruction and release of autoantigens that had previously been sequestered. This is true of antimyocardial antibody following a myocardial infarction and has been proposed as the reason for antithyroglobulin antibodies in Hashimoto's thyroiditis. It is often difficult to decide whether the tissue destruction elicits autoantibody formation or the autoantibodies promote tissue destruction. Most studies indicate some evidence of T-suppressor cell dysfunction in affected patients, but their role in pathogenesis is unclear. (2) Normal cells are transformed by viruses; the cell then presents the autoantigen and a virally transformed neoantigen that the host recognizes as foreign. The antidouble-stranded DNA in systemic lupus erythematosus (SLE) was once thought to be secondary to a "C"-type virus infection with the double-stranded DNA containing viral and host genome. (3) Transformation of autoantigens is known to occur secondary to administration of drugs such as α-methyldopa. The Rhesus (Rh) antigen is altered by α-methyldopa, and this leads to an autoimmune hemolytic anemia. (4) Cross-reacting antigens are also thought to occur in infections with certain beta-hemolytic streptococci. Cross-reaction between streptococcal antigens and the myocardium is though to be the basis for rheumatic myocarditis.

The autoimmune disease for which the most information is available is SLE. Autoantibodies in SLE are directed against nuclear antigens (i.e., antinuclear antibody (ANA) and anti–double-stranded DNA antibodies). The LE cell first used as a diagnostic test for SLE is thought to be a cell that phagocytizes the antibody-bound nucleus of another cell (see also *lupus erythematosus cell*). The clinical manifestations include systemic vasculitis with high titers of the autoantibodies ANA and anti-DNA. Immune complexes between DNA and antibody formed in SLE activate complement and lead to multiorgan tissue destruction. Central nervous system and renal involvement are the most serious manifestations. The renal disease is also characterized by inflammatory cellular infiltration of glomeruli triggered by immune complex deposition.

AUTOIMMUNE DISEASE. ANTIBODIES IN ORGAN-SPECIFIC AUTOIMMUNE DISEASES

DISEASES	ANTIGEN INVOLVED	METHODS FOR DETECTION OF ANTIBODY
Organ-Specific, Endocrine		
Autoimmune thyroiditis, primary myxedema, thyrotoxicosis	Thyroglobulin	Immunofluorescence test (IFT) (indirect)–methanol-fixed human thyroid
		Passive hemagglutination
		Latex agglutination
	Cytoplasmic microsome	IFT (indirect)–unfixed human hyperplastic thyroid tissue
		Passive hemagglutination
		Complement fixation
Thyrotoxicosis	Thyroid cell surface antigen	Bioassay–mouse thyroid stimulation in vivo
		Radioimmunoassay with inhibition of *TSH-tissue receptor
Addison's disease	Adrenal cell cytoplasm	IFT (indirect)–unfixed human adrenal cortex
Parathyroid	Parathyroid cytoplasmic antigen	IFT (indirect)–human parathyroid gland
Early onset diabetes	Islet cell	IFT on human or guinea pig pancreas
Alimentary Tract Diseases		
Atrophic gastritis	Parietal cell microsomes	IFT (indirect)–human or mouse gastric mucosa substrate
Pernicious anemia	Intrinsic factor	Radioactive vitamin B_{12} binding assay
Sjögren's syndrome	Salivary duct cells	IFT (indirect)–unfixed human salivary gland
Ulcerative colitis	Colon, lipopolysaccharide	IFT (indirect)–human or rat colon
Celiac disease	Reticulin	IFT (indirect)–rat kidney and liver
Crohn's disease	Reticulin	IFT (indirect) –rat kidney and liver
Liver Diseases		
Chronic aggressive hepatitis	Smooth muscle (actin)	IFT (indirect)–rat gastric mucosa, human cervical tissue
	Liver/kidney microsomal	IFT (indirect)–rat kidney and liver
Primary biliary cirrhosis	Mitochondrial	IFT (indirect)–rat kidney, unfixed
Neuromuscular Diseases		
Myasthenia gravis	Skeletal or heart muscle	IFT (indirect)–rat skeletal muscle and calf thymus
	Acetylcholine receptor	Radioimmunoassay
Demyelinating diseases (i.e., multiple sclerosis)	Myelin	IFT (indirect)–mammalian spinal cord
Dermatologic Diseases		
Pemphigus vulgaris	Prickle cell desmosomes	IFT (direct and indirect)–human skin peroxidase-labeled antibody
Bullous pemphigoid	Epithelial basement membrane	IFT (direct and indirect)–human skin peroxidase-labeled antibody
Cicatricial pemphigoid	Epithelial basement membrane	IFT (direct) on biopsy of mucous membrane–indirect on human skin
Dermatitis herpetiformis	Reticulin	IFT (indirect)–rat kidney and liver
Others		
Autoimmune hemolytic anemia	Red cell	Coombs' antiglobulin test (direct and indirect)
Goodpasture's syndrome	Glomerular and lung basement membrane	IFT (direct)–biopsy of patient's kidney
		IFT (indirect)–patient's serum on human kidney substrate
		Radioimmunoassay on serum

Modified from Nakamura, R. M., Chisari, F. V., and Edgington, T. S.: Laboratory tests for diagnosis of autoimmune diseases. *In* Stefannini, M. (ed.): Progress in Clinical Pathology. New York, Grune & Stratton, Inc., 1975.

The animal most useful as a model for SLE is the New Zealand black (NZB) mouse. These mice appear to have a premature failure of the thymic function that predisposes them to an autoimmune disease similar to SLE. A deficiency of T-suppressor cells occurs early, and for this reason T-suppressor function in SLE has been extensively studied.

Rheumatoid arthritis is an autoimmune disease that primarily involves the synovial lining of joints. The etiologic agent of rheumatoid arthritis is unknown; however, an IgM rheumatoid factor (RF) is found in affected areas and in serum. RF reacts with IgG, and probably as a result of this autoimmune phenomenon the joints are damaged. The combination of RF, IgG, and complement causes an inflammatory response in joints and other tissues.

Ankylosing spondylitis is a type of rheumatic disease, similar to rheumatoid arthritis, which affects the sacroiliac and spinal joints. This particular autoimmune disease has an association with the HLA antigen HLA-B27. Other systemic autoimmune diseases include Sjögren's syndrome, necrotizing angiitis, polymyositis, and progressive systemic sclerosis.

Some autoimmune diseases, such as autoimmune hemolytic anemia, affect specific organs. In this disease, the red blood cells are coated by autoantibodies. When complement is also present, the antibody–red blood cell complex is rapidly taken up by macrophages in the spleen—a process that explains anemia. Other organ-specific autoimmune diseases affect the thyroid gland (acute thyroiditis, Hashimoto's thyroiditis, or Graves' disease), pancreas, adrenals, parathyroids, central nervous system, or myoneural function (myasthenia gravis).

Laboratory Diagnosis. Many autoimmune diseases are characterized by the formation of immune complexes. There are a variety of nonspecific tests for the detection of soluble immune complexes in biologic fluids, which make use of the increased molecular weight and decreased solubility of the immune complex; they include cryoprecipitation, polyethylene glycol (PEG) precipation, and ultracentrifugation.

Specific tests make use of the ability of immune complexes to fix and bind complement and to react with antiglobulins or cell-surface receptors. Among these are assays utilizing C1q or rheumatoid factor (RF) as a specific reagent and those using complement receptors on Fc receptors on specific cells.

Two assays that are routinely performed involve the use of C1q, which binds to immune complexes containing IgG_1, IgG_2, IgG_3, or IgM and also to polyanionic substances including DNA and certain bacterial endotoxins. In the C1q precipitin assay, immune complexes are detected by a precipitin reaction in a gel diffusion test. In the more widely used ^{125}I-C1q binding assay, serum is incubated with EDTA, which dissociates C1 into its subcomponents C1q, C1r, and C1s, and then is mixed with ^{125}I-labeled C1q. Free C1q is then separated from that bound to immune complexes by PEG precipitation, and the radioactivity in the bound fraction is quantitated. This test is very sensitive and does not give false positive results with DNA or bacterial endotoxin, which are soluble in PEG.

There are several tests using either monoclonal or polyclonal RF (antibodies that react with the Fc portion of IgG molecules) as a specific reagent for immune complexes. These include solid-phase radioimmunoassay, latex agglutination, gel diffusion, and quantitative immunoprecipitation.

Raji cells are human lymphoblastoid cells from a patient with Burkitt's lymphoma that have been grown in cell culture; they express receptors for C1q, C3b, C3d, and the Fc portion of IgG. The binding of immune complexes that have also bound complement by these cells is the basis of immunofluorescence assay or radioimmunoassay for immune complexes. This binding is primarily at complement receptors. An assay method that depends on Fc receptors is the platelet aggregation test, which is based on the ability of soluble immune complexes to cause platelet aggregation.

Diagnosis of organ-specific autoimmune diseases is aided by serologic tests for the presence of antibodies to tissue-specific antigens. Antibodies against thyroid epithelium, thyroglobulin, and CA-2 (the "second colloid antigen") are seen in thyroid autoimmune diseases. Antiparietal cell antibodies are seen in atrophic gastritis. Antismooth muscle, and antimitochondrial antibodies are seen in some forms of chronic liver disease. Antiglomerular basement membrane (anti-GBM) antibodies occur in Goodpasture's syndrome, a glomerulonephritis. Antitubule BM antibodies also occur in Goodpasture's syndrome as well as in renal transplant patients. Among the most important autoantibodies are ANA in SLE and antiacetylcholine receptor (AChR) antibodies in myasthenia gravis.

Laboratory diagnosis of SLE involves two procedures: demonstration of the LE cell and detection of ANA (some laboratories no longer perform the LE cell test). There are several specificities of ANA, and certain antibodies are specific for certain diseases.

The preferred method of detection of ANA is by the fluorescent method. In this procedure, an appropriate section (e.g., rodent liver or kidney) is fixed and mounted on slides that are then treated with the test serum. After washing, fluorescein-conjugated antihuman gamma globulin is added and the slides examined with a fluorescence microscope. The serum dilution at which staining occurred and the pattern of fluorescence are important for detection. There are several other methods for detecting antibodies to DNA and nucleoprotein, including radioimmunoassay (RIA) and hemagglutination tests. The RIA involves radiolabeling DNA and then using the radiolabeled DNA and the patient's heat-inactivated serum in an incubation to produce antigen-antibody complexes. Subsequently these immune complexes are detected either by precipitation with $(NH_4)SO_4$ or by filtration of the complexes through cellulose ester filters. The counts present in the precipitates give a measure of the antibody present. The hemagglutination assay involves adsorption of DNA and soluble nucleoprotein onto formalinized human erythrocytes. The treated cells are then used to test for the presence of a hemagglutinating antibody to DNA. Neither RIA nor hemagglutinating assay is widely used in clinical laboratory, however.

Serologic diagnosis of rheumatoid arthritis involves methods that detect aggregated IgM antibodies to IgG. All of the methods involve a particulate indicator system containing a large quantity of IgG molecules to which the RF binds. On binding of the RF, the indicator system agglutinates or flocculates. The particles used include latex, erythrocytes, charcoal, and bentonite.

Myasthenia gravis is a disease in which antibodies have been detected to the receptor for acetylcholine, a neurotransmitter. It appears to be directly involved in the decreased responsiveness of the muscle with the development of muscular weakness. A sensitive radioimmunoassay has been developed utilizing the binding of α-bungarotoxin, a low–molecular weight toxin to acetylcholine receptors (AChR). The ^{125}I-α-bungarotoxin binds to the AChR. After incubation with the unknown serum, an antibody against human gamma globulin is added. If there is an antibody against the AChR, it will be precipitated along with the ^{125}I-α-bungarotoxin and AChR. The radioactivity of the precipitate will be a measure of the level of antibody against AChR. As long as the antibody is not against the site of the receptor that binds α-bungarotoxin, the method should be fairly reliable. At present, interference with bungarotoxin has not been a problem.

GERALD B. KOLSKI, M.D., PH.D.

autoimmunity (aw″to-im-mu′nĭ-te) a state in which an immune response is generated against components of the individual's own body. This failure to distinguish between what is actually foreign and what is self can lead to the production of either antibodies or cell-mediated immunity directed against various host cells, tissues, or organs. Accordingly, this antiself immune response may have a harmful effect, resulting in the destruction of host components and the production of disease by concomitant loss of normal physiologic function.

This inability to maintain self-recognition without immune reactions against oneself is probably related to a breakdown in several normal control mechanisms. One such evasion can occur when usually inaccessible or sequestered antigens (e.g., sperm, lens antigens of the eye) become exposed to the immune system after some protective cellular or tissue barrier has been broken. These formerly hidden antigens are now in intimate contact with cells of the immune system, and consequently initiate an immune reaction.

Another possibility for circumvention of self-tolerance is for a tissue antigen to be altered by a chemical agent, drug, or infectious microorganism (e.g., virus), producing a form that the body's immunocompetent cells perceive as foreign. This occurs in experimental autoimmune thyroiditis, in which anti-thyroglobulin antibodies and inflammatory lesions are produced in rabbit thyroid glands after injection with chemically modified (using Freund's adjuvant) homologous thyroglobulin.

Normally, nonimmunogenic drugs may act as haptens after binding to host protein. Such complexes may be capable of eliciting an immune reaction that damages cells coated with the drug; this occurs in penicillin allergy. Similarly, in certain tissue culture systems, virally infected cells are able to bring about changes on cell membranes with the appearance of new cell surface antigens that may act as transplantation antigens.

Autoimmunity may arise as a result of immune responses to antigens that cross react with antigens of various normal tissue components. Human colon possesses an antigen similar to a polysaccharide antigen present on *Escherichia coli.* It is possible that the inflammatory disease of the large bowel, known as colitis, in which anticolon antibodies are found, is mediated by an immune reaction against the cross-reacting bacterial antigen. In a similar fashion many patients with rheumatic fever, a disease regularly preceded by repeated infections with group A beta-hemolytic streptococci, have circulating antimyocardial antibody that cross reacts with a streptococcal cell membrane.

The development of self-tolerance occurs during the fetal and neonatal period when tissue antigens present themselves to the immune system and are recognized as self. As an individual's defense system matures, the induction of an immune reaction against these antigens usually does not occur, whereas antigens that were not manifested during early life and that gain entry into the body are treated as foreign. However, the immune system is a highly complex and intricate network involving interaction among various populations and subpopulations of lymphocytes as well as other leukocytes. Effector mechanisms, such as antibody production and the vast array of T cell–induced mediators of cellular immunity, are controlled both by components of the immune system and by certain host-derived hormonal factors. Any breakdown in these "built-in" regulatory systems that is due to improper recognition of monitoring signals could markedly affect the outcome of an immune response and result in the classic features of autoimmune phenomena, namely, loss of tolerance and immunologic self-injury.

Autoimmunity can be either a temporary and reversible state or one that is chronic, debilitating, and even life-threatening. In clinical medicine there is intense study of a wide spectrum of illnesses ("autoimmune diseases"), such as systemic lupus erythematosus and rheumatoid arthritis, in which antihost tissue reactions closely associated with these disorders are believed to play a major role in the underlying pathogenetic mechanisms. It now appears that attempts at preventing autoimmune phenomena may depend heavily on artificial manipulation of the immune system rather than on the currently employed drug treatments that are sometimes ineffective and deleterious to the patient.

CHARLES PAVIA, PH.D.

autoinfection (aw″to-in-fek′shun) an infection due to an agent already present in the body, often the transferral of an agent from one area of the body to another.

autoinoculation (aw″to-ĭ-nok″u-la′shun) inoculation with antigens, usually microorganisms, from one's own body.

autologous (aw-tol′o-gus) [*auto-* + Gr. *logos* relation] related to or derived from self; referring to products or components of the same individual, such as grafts or antigens. See also *autogenous.*

autologous graft see *autologous g.* under *graft.*

autologous transfusion the transfusion of one's own blood or blood components, thereby eliminating risks (e.g., hepatitis and alloimmunization) associated with homologous blood transfusion.

predeposit a. t., blood that is obtained from a patient and stored for later reinfusion.

autolysis (aw-tol′ĭ-sis) [*auto-* + Gr. *lysis* dissolution] the spontaneous disintegration of tissues or of cells by the action of their own enzymes, such as occurs after death and in some pathologic conditions. Cf. *cytolysis.*

autolysosome (aw″to-li′so-sōm) see *autophagic vacuole.*

automate (aw′to-māt) [Gr. *automatos* self-acting, spontaneous] to replace manual procedures by those using instrumental process control.

automated activated partial thromboplastin a partial thromboplastin time reagent prepared from rabbit brain tissue and micronized silica (as particulate activator) formulated for use in automated and semiautomated coagulation systems.

automated slide staining the use of any of a variety of commercially available machines used to stain histologic, cytologic, or hematologic slides automatically. This is accomplished either by moving slides through various chemical and stain solutions or by applying these solutions seqentially to stationary slides.

automatic (aw″to-mat′ik) 1. spontaneous, involuntary.

2. self-moving; self-regulating.

automatic data processing (ADP) a general term applied to all uses of computers.

automation (aw″to-ma′shun) 1. the automatic control of a process or piece of equipment. In the clinical laboratory, fully automated instrumentation refers to equipment that performs an entire procedure, including sample pickup, mixing of reagents, incubation, and the acquisition and recording of data, without human intervention. See also *blood cell count automation, clinical chemistry automation, cytometry, differential leukocyte count automation, microbiology automation,* and *radioimmunoassay automation.*

2. the installation of automated equipment.

automatism (aw-tom′ah-tizm) repetitive motor activity performed without full awareness or control, often as part of a seizure in individuals with psychomotor epilepsy.

Automeris a genus of moths of which the species *A. io,* which is found in the United States, causes a dermatitis reaction by means of the irritant hairs on its larva.

automutagen (aw″to-mu′tah-gen) any chemical substance, formed as a metabolic product by an organism, which is capable of inducing mutations.

autonomic (aw″to-nom′ik) [Gr. *autonomos,* from *auto-* + *nomas* law] self-controlling; not subject to voluntary control.

autonomic nervous system (ANS) the part of the nervous system that regulates the activity of the viscera. The peripheral efferent portion of the ANS is composed of pre- and postganglionic neurons. The preganglionic neurons have their cell bodies in the brain or spinal cord; their axons terminate on nerve cell bodies (ganglia) within either the thoracic or the abdominal cavity, or in close proximity to or in the visceral organ; these myelinated fibers have a diameter of 1–3 μ (B fibers). The postganglionic fibers originate in the ganglia and terminate directly on either cardiac muscle, smooth muscle, or glandular tissue; these unmyelinated fibers have a diameter of less than 1 μ (C fibers).

There are two divisions of the ANS, the sympathetic and parasympathetic nervous systems. The preganglionic fibers of the sympathetic system arise from cells within the first thoracic to second or third lumbar segments of the spinal cord, whereas those of the parasympathetic system emerge from the brain in cranial nerves III, VII, IX, and X (oculomotor, facial, glossopharyngeal, and vagal nerves, respectively) and the second, third, and fourth sacral spinal nerves.

The neurotransmitter of preganglionic fibers is acetylcholine. The neurotransmitters of the postganglionic fibers vary; acetylcholine is released from the parasympathetic fibers, and acetylcholine, norepinephrine, or epinephrine from the sympathetic fibers. Recent evidence suggests that dopamine, 5-hydroxytryptamine, and adenine nucleotides may also be released by some autonomic fibers.

The ANS is relatively independent of conscious thought (hence the name autonomic, i.e., self-governing), although activity from higher brain structures (such as the cerebral cortex) can modulate ANS activity. The ANS functions in the reflex activity that maintains a stable internal environment of the body; this activity is controlled by regulatory centers within the hypothalamus and medulla oblongata. The ANS maintains a basal level of activity (autonomic tone) that can be either increased or decreased by central structures.

Most visceral organs are innervated by both divisions of the ANS. However, the adrenal medulla, spleen, pilomotor muscles, sweat glands, and blood vessels of the viscera, skin, and skeletal muscle are innervated only by the sympathetic division. Generally, where dual innervation exists, the parasympathetic and sympathetic systems act antagonistically: activity of the parasympathetic system promotes vegetative function, and activity of the sympathetic system favors those functions necessary for vigorous muscle activity.

See also *parasympathetic nervous system* and *sympathetic nervous system.*

autophagic (aw-to-fa′jik) pertaining to autophagy.

autophagic vacuole a digestive vacuole formed in the cytoplasm when primary lysosomes fuse with a membrane-bound sac of worn-out organelle material. Also called *autolysosome, autophagosome,* and *cytolysosome.*

autophagosome (aw″to-fag′o-sōm) see *autophagic vacuole.*

autophagy (aw-tof′ah-je) [*auto-* + Gr. *phagein* to eat] the process by which cells dispose of worn-out organelles. The material is enclosed within a membrane, and primary lysosomes fuse with it to form an autophagic vacuole in which digestion occurs. See also *lysosome.*

autoplast (aw′to-plast) [*auto-* + Gr. *plastos* formed] see *autologous g.* under *graft.*

autoploidy (aw″to-ploi′de) the state of having two or more chromosome sets as the result of multiplying the haploid set.

autoprothrombin I (aw″to-pro-throm′bin) see *Factor VII.*

autoprothrombin II see *Factor IX.*

autoprothrombin IIA a competitive inhibitor of Factor Xa, formed by the action of thrombin on a vitamin K–dependent plasma protein. It is unlike known coagulation factors, and is a precursor of a serine esterase.

autoprothrombin III see *Factor X.*

autopsy (aw′top-se) [Gr. *autopsia* seeing for oneself, from *auto-* + *opsis* sight] the examination of a body after death. The autopsy provides extensive information about human illnesses and the morphologic changes they produce in tissues and organs. The modern autopsy brings to bear on the study of disease a wide range of morphologic and laboratory techniques to: (1) determine the cause of the death; (2) evalute incompletely known disorders or discover new diseases; (3) serve as an educational function through demonstration of tissue alterations (gross, microscopic, microbiologic, biochemical) as they relate to pathogenesis and to the natural or therapeutically altered cause of disease; and (4) collect data for statistical analyses of disease incidence. When the cause of death is not known or if the death occurred under suspicious circumstances, a coroner or medical examiner can order an autopsy to be performed. Without such an order, an autopsy cannot be performed without the permission of the deceased's next of kin. Also called *necropsy* and *postmortem examination.*

autoradiograph (aw″to-ra′de-o-graf) a photograph made by autoradiography.

autoradiography (aw″to-ra″de-og′rah-fe) the imaging of an object using alpha or beta particles emitted by the object itself to expose a photographic film or emulsion. The object most frequently used is tissue labeled with a radioactive compound that is incorporated into the cell. Microscopic sections of the labeled tissue are mounted on a glass slide and placed in direct contact with the photographic emulsion. After appropriate exposure and development of the photographic emulsion, the tissue is stained to demonstrate its histologic features. Reduced silver grains in the photographic emulsion resulting from exposure to charged particles emitted by radioactive decay are revealed as black grains. When the specimen is examined with a microscope, the tissue sections can be viewed together with the overlying emulsion to determine in which cells the radioactive tracer compound is localized.

Autoradiography can be performed at the macro level, using large pieces of tissue to demonstrate the localization of a radioactive compound in various tissues or organs. It can also be performed at the subcellular level, using specimens prepared for and examined by electron microscopy.

An example of a radioactively labeled compound used frequently in autoradiography is tritium-labeled thymidine, a compound incorporated into the nucleus only during DNA synthesis. It is used in cell kinetic studies to determine the number of cells synthesizing DNA, the number of cells in the growth fraction and length of the cell cycle, and the various cell cycle components. A number of other radioactively labeled tracers are used with the technique of autoradiography. Examples of their uses include the study of RNA and protein synthesis, and the metabolism of carbohydrates, lipids, hormones, minerals, and drugs.

Also called *radioautography.*

contact a., an autoradiographic technique in which one microscope slide that is carrying the radioisotope-labeled tissue and another that is covered with photographic emulsion are clamped together.

dip-coating a., a method in which the microscope slide and tissue are dipped into and coated with a liquid photographic emulsion. Also called liquid emulsion coating autoradiography.

film stripping a., a method in which a sheet or strip of photographic film is applied to the microscope slide and the radioisotope-labeled tissue.

thick-layer a., a dip-coating method that uses a thick photographic emulsion to record the tracks of alpha particles when working with radioisotopes that are weak alpha-emitters, such as thorium or radium.

two-emulsion a., a method for distinguishing between low-energy beta particles from one radioisotope and high-energy beta particles from a second radioisotope in the autoradiographs of tissues containing two radioisotopes, usually ^{3}H and ^{14}C. Two layers of photographic emulsion or two different emulsions are used. Beta particles emitted by the two different sources can be distinguished because the lower energy particles cannot penetrate to the outer or second layer of the emulsion.

autoradiolysis (aw″to-ra″de-ol′ĭ-sis) [*auto-* + L. *radius* ray + Gr. *lysis* destruction] the chemical decomposition of a substance, such as a radiopharmaceutical, due to the action of ionizing radiation emitted by the substance. The dissociation may be directly produced by the emitted particles or indirectly by free radicals produced by them.

autoregulation (au″to-reg″u-la′shun) [*auto-* + L. *regulare* to regulate, from *regula* pattern] the intrinsic ability of a tissue to adapt to changes in the conditions that influence its function without intervention of external control mechanisms. An example is the capacity of many vascular beds (renal, mesenteric, cerebral, liver, myocardial, skeletal muscle) to maintain their blood flow independent of changes in perfusion pressure. A relatively constant blood flow is maintained by changes in vascular resistance. These changes may represent a response of the blood vessels to a local buildup of metabolites (metabolic theory) or an intrinsic reaction of vascular smooth muscle to stretch (myogenic theory).

The heart also exhibits autoregulation. A balance between right and left ventricular outputs is maintained and cardiac function is matched to the body's vascular capacity and total blood volume as a result of heterometric autoregulation. Homeometric autoregulation of the myocardium allows the circulation to adjust to demands such as heavy exercise without significant changes in the size of the heart or in central venous pressure.

autosome (aw′to-sōm) [*auto-* + Gr. *soma* body] any chromosome that is not a sex chromosome. The 46 chromosomes in normal humans are composed of 22 homologous pairs of autosomes and 2 sex chromosomes. See also *karyotype.*

autotomography (aw″to-to-mog′rah-fe) [*auto-* + Gr. *tomos* a slice + *graphein* to write or draw] a technique used in pneumoencephalography. During the exposure, the patient nods his head from side to side while the forehead remains resting on the film holder. The midline structures (the fourth ventricle, cerebral aqueduct, and basal cisternae) are clearly imaged while the lateral ventricles are blurred out.

autotransformer (aw″to-trans-for′mer) a transformer that has only one winding, which is tapped somewhere along its length. The whole winding acts as the primary, and the part between the tap and one end acts as the secondary (or vice versa). As with other transformers, the ratio of the input and output voltages is equal to the ratio of the number of turns in the primary and secondary coils.

variable a., an autotransformer that has multiple

taps selected by a switch or a continuously movable tap, so that the output voltage can be varied.

autotroph (aw'to-trōf) [*auto-* + Gr. *trophē* nourishment] an autotrophic organism; one that is self-nourishing. The term denotes microorganisms that do not require organic carbon and nitrogen as a source of energy but are able to form carbohydrates and protein from CO_2 and inorganic salts. Also called *lithotroph*. See also *chemoautotroph* and *photoautotroph*. Cf. *heterotroph*.

autotrophic (aw"to-trof'ik) pertaining to autotrophs.

aux/o (awk'so) [Gr. *auxein* to increase] a word element used in combining form to denote growth or increase, e.g., auxotroph.

auxanography (awks"an-og'rah-fe) [Gr. *auxanein* to increase + *graphein* to write] the procedure that involves selecting the best medium for the growth of a microbe. Disks or drops of various substrates are placed on a culture plate; the largest microbial colonies develop on the spot that contains the best medium. Auxanography is also useful in the carbohydrate assimilation testing of yeasts.

auxesis (awk-se'sis) [Gr. *auxēsis* growth] an increase in the size of an organism; the term is specifically used to denote growth caused by an increase in individual cell volume without any increase in cell numbers.

auxochrome (awk'so-krōm) [*auxo-* + Gr. *chrōma* color] a chemical group that, if introduced into a chromogen, converts the latter into a dye; examples include —COOH, —OH, and $—NH_2$.

auxocyte (awk'so-sīt) [*auxo-* + Gr. *kytos* hollow vessel] a cell, such as a primary oocyte or spermatocyte, just before its nucleus enters meiotic prophase.

auxotroph (awk'so-trōf) [*auxo-* + Gr. *trophē* nourishment] a microorganism that, through mutation, has lost an essential enzyme or component and thus can grow only if the culture medium contains the missing growth factor. With the discovery of auxotrophy in 1940, biochemical mutants became an important microbiologic tool in the study of biosynthesis.

auxotrophic (awk"so-trof'ik) 1. requiring a growth factor that is not required by the parental or prototype strain; said of mutant microorganisms.
2. requiring specific organic growth factors in addition to the carbon source present in a minimal medium.

AV abbrev. See *arteriovenous, atrioventricular.*

A-V block see *atrioventricular block.*

Aventyl (ah-ven'til) trademark. See *nortriptyline.*

average (av'er-ij) the arithmetic mean of a set of numbers. See also *arithmetic mean* and *mean.*

average gradient a measure of film latitude; the average slope of the H and D curve (density versus log relative exposure) between two specified density values, usually the net density values (total density with the base and fog densities subtracted) of 0.25 and 2.0.

average life the average time of existence in a specific form of an elementary particle, nucleus, or atom. The term is also used specifically to refer to the average of the individual lives of all the atoms in a radioactive compound: average life is the reciprocal of the decay constant, or 1.443 times the radioactive half-life. Also called *lifetime* and *mean life.*

average potential reference in electroencephalography, a reference point obtained by joining all leads from the active scalp electrodes through equal high-resistance resistors to a single point. This is then used as a common reference. The reference point has a potential that is the average of the individual potentials of the various active scalp electrodes. Each EEG amplifier is connected to an active electrode (via input terminal 1) and to the average reference point (via input terminal 2) to record the EEG. Also called *Goldman-Offner reference.*

avian (a've-an) [L. *avis* bird] of or pertaining to birds.

avidin (av'ĭ-din) a glycoprotein in egg white that combines with biotin to block its absorption into the body, thus producing a biotin deficiency; M.W. 68,000. It is a tetramer; each subunit contains a specific binding site for biotin.

avidity (ah-vid'ĭ-te) [L. *avidus* greedy, eager] the binding strength of an antibody for an antigen. The term refers to the sum of the binding affinities of all the individual combining sites on the antibody. See also *affinity.*

avidity testing a procedure in which cells and serum are combined on a slide to determine the speed and intensity with which an antigen and its antibody react. Macroscopically apparent agglutination is the end point.

avirulence (a-vir'u-lens) [*a-* neg. + L. *virulentus* poisonous] lack of virulence; lack of competence of an infectious agent to produce pathologic effects.

avirulent (a-vir'u-lent) not virulent, as in a pathogenic organism that lacks the ability to produce pathologic effects.

avitaminosis (a-vi"tah-mĭ-no'sis) [*a-* neg. + *vitamin* + *-osis* condition] vitamin deficiency; see under *hypovitaminosis.*

A-V node see *atrioventricular n.* under *node.*

Avogadro's number (av-o-gad'rōz) [Amadeo *Avogadro,* Italian physicist, 1776–1856] the number of particles in 1 mole of a substance, 6.02246×10^{23}.

avulsion (ah-vul'shun) [L. *avulsio,* from *a* away from + *vellere* to pull] the tearing away of a structure or part.

A.W. abbrev. See *atomic weight.*

aw abbrev. See *airways.*

A wave the deflection in the bundle of His electrocardiogram that is the result of depolarization of the atria.

a wave see under *jugular venous pulse.*

***a* wave** see under *electroretinogram.*

axenic (a-zen'ik) [*a-* neg. + Gr. *xenos* a foreigner or stranger] not contaminated by or associated with any foreign organism. The term is used to refer to pure cultures of microorganisms such as the cultivation of *Entamoeba histolytica* without a symbiont.

axial (ak'se-al) 1. of or pertaining to the axis of a structure; in radiology, a view or projection directed from the base to the vertex or vice versa.
2. in chemistry, pertaining to a substituent group of a cyclohexane ring compound that lies farther from the plane of the ring than does the other (equatorial) substituent on the same carbon atom. See also *conformation.*

axill/o (ak'sĭ-lo) [L. *axilla* armpit] a word element

used in combining form to denote armpit, e.g., axillary.

axilla (ak-sil'ah), pl. *axillae* [L.] [NA], the armpit; the anatomic space bounded medially by the upper lateral chest wall, and laterally by the inner aspect of the upper arm. The anterior fold is formed by the lower border of the pectoralis major muscle and the posterior fold by the latissimus dorsi and teres major muscles. The space contains fat and several groups of lymph nodes, and is traversed by the axillary artery and vein and by the cords and branches of the brachial plexus.

axillary (ak'sĭ-lar"e) pertaining to the axilla.

axillary artery the continuation of the subclavian artery. It begins at the outer border of the first rib and ends at the lower border of the teres major muscle by becoming the brachial artery.

axillary line see *midaxillary line.*

axillary projection an anteroposterior projection of the axillary portion of the breast and of the axillary lymph nodes, used in routine mammography.

axillary region the armpit (axilla) and the region of the chest bordering on it.

axiolateral (ak"se-o-lat'er-al) pertaining to a radiographic projection in which the central ray is between the axial and lateral projections. It is used particularly for views of the cranium or mandible.

axis (ak'sis), pl. *axes* [L. "axle"] 1. [NA], the second cervical vertebra. The odontoid process projects upward from its body to articulate with the anterior arch of the atlas.

2. a line about which a revolving body turns or about which a structure would turn if it did revolve; a line around which specified parts of the body are arranged.

axis cylinder see *axon.*

axis of rotation an imaginary straight line around which a rotating body turns; the points on the axis remain stationary.

axolemma (ak"so-lem'ah) [Gr. *axōn* axis + *eilēma* sheath] the surface or plasma membrane of an axon.

axon (ak'son) [Gr. *axōn* axle, axis] the main process of a nerve cell, along which impulses (action potentials) are conducted away from the cell body. Axons vary in diameter and length; at their distal end, usually some distance from the cell body, they branch to form synapses with other nerve cells or their processes, or with specialized effector cells. Axons are sheathed by an insulating cover provided by the plasma membrane and cytoplasm of Schwann cells in the peripheral nervous system, and oligodendrocytes in the central nervous system. Around unmyelinated axons the layer is thin; around myelinated axons there is a multilayered wrapping called the myelin sheath. Also called *axis cylinder.* See also *nerve, Schwann cell,* and *synapse.*

axonal (ak'so-nal) pertaining to an axon.

axonal degeneration see *wallerian degeneration.*

axoneme (ak'so-nēm) [Gr. *axōn* axle + *nēma* thread] 1. the core structure of cilia and flagella, composed of microtubules that are arranged longitudinally in a precise arrangement with a constant number. Two single microtubules are positioned centrally and nine doublets of microtubules are radially arranged. This pinwheel appearance is often referred to as a 9 + 2 configuration.

2. an elongated cilium that forms the core of the tail of a spermatozoon.

3. the axial thread of a chromosome.

axon hillock the conical expansion of an axon at its point of attachment to the body of the nerve cell.

axonotmesis (ak"son-ot-me'sis) [Gr. *axōn* axis + *tmēsis* a cutting apart] an injury to a nerve fiber of sufficient severity to cause complete degeneration of the segment distal to the damaged area. Muscle action potentials cannot be evoked by stimulation at any point along the axon. This condition may be the result of prolonged entrapment or compression of the nerve.

axon staining methods see *Bodian's method* and *Holzer's method.*

axoplasm (ak'so-plasm) [Gr. *axōn* axis + *plasma* anything formed or molded] the cytoplasm of an axon.

Ayerza's disease (ah-yer'thaz) [Abel *Ayerza,* Buenos Aires physician, 1861–1918] a form of polycythemia vera marked by chronic cyanosis, chronic dyspnea, chronic bronchitis, hepatosplenomegaly, and hyperplasia of bone marrow; it is associated with sclerosis of the pulmonary artery. See also *p. vera* under *polycythemia.*

Ayoub-Shklar method see under *keratin staining.*

aza- (a'zah) a prefix word element in organic chemistry to denote the replacement of a methylene group (—CH_2—) in a carbon chain by an imino group (—NH—), e.g., $CH_3CH_2CH_2NHCH_2CH_3$ is 3-azahexane (ethyl *n*-propyl amine).

azacyclonol hydrochloride (a"zah-si'klo-nōl) an isomer of pipradol used as a tranquilizer in the treatment of confusional states and hallucinations.

5-azacytidine (ah"zah-si'tĭ-dēn) a cancer chemotherapeutic drug. For more information, see *Appendix A.*

8-azaguanine (az"ah-gwan'īn) a triazolo analog of guanine; it is an antimetabolite of purine and thus blocks nucleic acid synthesis. It is used as an antineoplastic compound. Also called guanazolo.

azan stain [acronym from *Az*okarmin B and *An*ilinblau W] see *Heidenhain's azan stain.*

azaserine (a"zah-ser'ēn) L-serine diazoacetate (ester), an antibiotic compound, $C_4H_7N_3O_4$, produced by a species of *Streptomyces.* It is used to suppress immune response in cases of autoimmune disease and in the treatment of acute leukemia.

azathioprine (a"zah-thi'o-prēn) a nitroimidazole derivative of mercaptopurine. Because it is used to kill cells during the active phase of DNA synthesis, it is a "phase-specific drug." It interferes with purine synthesis and is used as an immunosuppressive drug in patients with autoimmune diseases and those undergoing transplant rejection.

azeotrope (a"ze-o-trōp) [*a*- neg. + Gr *zein* to boil + *tropēa* turn, or turning] a mixture of two liquid components that boil at a constant temperature without change in the composition of the vapor or liquid phases. For example, a mixture containing 4.5 percent water (b.p., 100.0°C) and 95.5 percent ethyl alcohol (b.p., 78.4°C) boils at 78.1°C at atmospheric pressure. Also called azeotropic solution.

azeotropic (a"ze-o-trop'ik) pertaining to or characterized by azeotropy.

azeotropic solution see *azeotrope.*

azeotropy (a″ze-ot′ro-pe) a property indicated by the absence of any change in the composition of a liquid mixture when it is boiled under a given pressure.

azide (az′id) 1. a compound that contains the group $—N_3$, as in ethyl azide, $CH_3CH_2—N_3$. Like cyanide, it inhibits cytochrome oxidase. It can produce lesions in the white matter and other parts of the brain.

2. the azide ion, N_3^- or $-N{=}N^+{=}N^-$.

3. a salt of hydrazoic acid, HN_3, containing the azide ion.

azinphosmethyl (az″in-fos-meth′il) a highly toxic organothiophosphate insecticide, phosphorodithiotic acid *O,O*-dimethyl *S*-[(4-oxo-1,2,3-benzotriazin-3(4H)-yl)methyl] ester. Also called guthion. See also *organophosphate compounds.*

azo- (a′zo) [Fr. *azote* nitrogen, from Gr. *azoōs* lifeless] a prefix word element in organic chemistry to denote the presence of the azo group —N=N—, in a molecule, e.g., azomethane, $CH_3—N{=}N—CH_3$.

azobenzene (az″o-ben′zēn) an orange-red crystalline product of the reduction of nitrobenzene, soluble in alcohol and ether but only slightly so in water. It is the parent substance of azo dyes and some pH indicators.

azobilirubin (az″o-bil″ĭ-ru′bin) the product formed when bilirubin is treated with diazotized sulfanilic acid. Two similar, but not identical, azobilirubins are formed for each bilirubin molecule, both containing two pyrrole groups of the heme molecule. Azobilirubins are indicator pigments with a red-violet color at pH below 6.0 and a blue color above pH 7.5. Both pigments are used for assaying bilirubin in serum and other biologic fluids, as the intensity of the color is directly proportional to the concentration of bilirubin in the specimen.

azo coupling reaction the chemical reaction of a diazonium salt with an aromatic compound to produce an azo dye: $\phi—N^+{\equiv}N + Cl^- + \phi' \rightarrow \phi—N{=}N—\phi' + HCl$, where ϕ denotes an aromatic ring. This reaction is widely used in histochemistry for localization of enzymes (where ϕ' is a naphthol or phenol liberated from an ester by the enzyme), for localization of proteins (where ϕ' is the phenol group of tyrosine, the imidazole group of histidine, or the indole group of tryptophan), and for localization of other phenolic and heterocyclic substances such as chromaffin, neurotransmitters, and hormones. The reaction can be blocked by acetylation using a 1:1 mixture of acetic anhydride and absolute alcohol.

azo dye a group of synthetic dyes that have —N=N— as their chromophoric group, produced from amino compounds by the processes of diazotization and coupling. By varying the chemical composition, it is possible to produce acid, basic, direct, or mordant dyes. This general group is subdivided into monazo, diazo, triazo, and tetrazo, according to the number of —N=N— groups in the molecule.

azolitmin paper (az″o-lit′min) filter paper saturated with a solution of azolitmin, the purified coloring matter from litmus; acids turn the color of the paper from purple to bright red (pH 4.8), alkalis turn it blue (pH 8.0).

azoospermia (a-zo″o-sper′me-ah) [*a-* neg. + Gr. *zōos* living + *sperma* seed + *-ia*] the absence of spermatozoa in the semen, or the failure of formation of spermatozoa. Cf. *aspermia.*

azoprotein (az″o-pro′te-in) 1. protein linked to any substance by an azo bond, —N=N—.

2. in immunochemistry, a protein coupled through a diazo bond to a hapten, which then becomes immunogenic.

azot/o (az′o-to) [Fr. *azote* nitrogen, from Gr. *azoōs* lifeless] a word element used in combining form to denote urea or nitrogen, e.g., azoturia.

azote (az′ōt) [Fr.] the name (used only in French) for nitrogen; proposed by Lavoisier because a nitrogen atmosphere does not support life; the source of the prefixes azo- and azoto-.

azotemia (az″o-te′me-ah) [Fr. *azote* nitrogen + Gr. *haima* blood + *-ia*] a condition involving an elevated serum concentration of nonprotein nitrogenous (NPN) compounds, primarily urea (45 percent of NPN), but also amino acids, uric acid, creatinine, creatine, and ammonia. It is produced by the diminished filtration of these compounds by the kidney in prerenal, renal, and postrenal azotemia. See also *uremia* (symptomatic azotemia).

postrenal a., azotemia resulting from urinary tract obstruction.

prerenal a., azotemia produced by inadequate perfusion of the kidneys. It is due to dehydration, shock, diminished blood volume (hypovolemia), or congestive heart failure, which causes a reduction in the glomerular filtration rate (GFR).

renal a., azotemia produced by renal disease, such as acute glomerulonephritis, or acute renal failure, which results in reduced glomerular function. Significant azotemia does not occur until the GFR has been reduced by more than 50 percent.

Azotobacter (ah-zo′to-bak″ter) [*azoto-* + Gr. *baktērion* little rod] a genus of aerobic bacteria that are gram-negative, free-living, and nitrogen-fixing; they occur in soil and water, and on leaf surfaces. Members of this genus, together with some blue-green algae, are the principal agents of aerobic nitrogen fixation (fertilization) of soil and water.

azotorrhea (az″o-to-re′ah) [Fr. *azote* nitrogen + Gr. *rhoia* flow] excessive loss of nitrogen in the feces.

azoturia (az″o-tu′re-ah) [Fr. *azote* nitrogen + Gr. *ouron* urine + *-ia*] an excess amount of urea or other nitrogen compounds in the urine.

azure (azh′ūr) [O. Fr. *azur*] any of three metachromatic basic thiazin dyes: azure A (C.I. 52005), azure B (C.I. 52010), and azure C (C.I. 52002). They are used as nuclear stains and as metachromatic stains for acid mucopolysaccharides. The orthochromatic colors are blue for azure B and blue-violet for azure A and azure C. The metachromatic colors are purple-red for azure A, violet for azure B, and red for azure C.

azure-eosin stains routine histologic stains, which may be substituted for hematoxylin and eosin (H and E) methods. The nuclear stain is a basic thiazin dye, such as azure A or methylene blue, and the plasma stain is an acid xanthine dye, such as eosin Y or phloxine B. The Romanowsky stains (Giemsa stain, Wright stain) used for blood cells are also azure-eosin stains. These techniques demonstrate bacteria (particularly rickettsiae) in tissues better than do H and E stains.

azuresin (azh″u-rez′in) a complex of the dye azure A bound to a carboxylic cation exchange resin. Trademark, *Diagnex Blue.* See under *tubeless gastric analysis test.*

azurophilic (azh″u-ro-fil′ik) [O. Fr. *azur* + Gr. *philein* to love] staining well with blue aniline dyes.

azurophilic granule a cellular element that stains purple-blue with Wright-Giemsa stain and is seen in granulocytes, monocytes, and immature erythrocytes. The granules in promyelocytes and monocytes are primary lysosomes containing the lysosomal enzymes acid phosphatase, myeloperoxidase, indoxylesterase, and β-glucuronidase. They are positive for the histochemical stain myeloperoxidase and negative for alkaline phosphatase. The granules are smaller in monocytes than in granulocytes and do not all contain peroxidase.

In the erythroid series, the granules appear by light microscopy as purple dust visible only after hemolysis. The inclusions are either enlarged lysosomes or remnants of karyorrhexis, and occur either in severe anemia or as artifacts. In lymphocytes, azurophilic inclusions are, at least in part, lysosomes. In granulocytes, they are also called *primary granules.* See also *granules of developing neutrophils.*

azygography (az″ĭ-gog′rah-fe) [Gr. *azygos* unpaired + *graphein* to record] radiography of the azygous venous system.

azygos lobe a small accessory lobe of the right lung, formed from the right upper lobe when its medial part becomes separated from the remainder of the lobe by a fissure containing the terminal portion of the azygos vein. The azygos lobe varies in size, and it may include the apex. It is supplied by a branch or branches from the apical bronchus.

azygos vein a vein that drains blood from the right posterior intercostal veins and lumbar region, and ends in the superior vena cava just above the pericardium. Its position is somewhat variable.

azygous (az′ĭ-gus) [Gr. "unpaired," from *a-* neg. + *zygon* yoke] having no fellow; unpaired.

azymia (ah-zim′e-ah) [Gr. *azymos* unleavened + *-ia*] a physiologic condition in which an enzyme that is normally present is absent.

B

B symbol for *bel, blood, boron, magnetic induction.*

B-5 a histologic fixative solution utilizing mercuric chloride and formaldehyde buffered with sodium acetate. Good preservation of cellular detail is achieved without overhardening of tissue. Tissue should be stored in 70 percent alcohol.

b symbol for barn, *base.*

β the Greek lower case letter *beta.*

β- a designator for: (1) an anomer of a carbohydrate, e.g., *β*-D-glucose; (2) a constituent of the beta plasma protein fraction, e.g., *β*-lipoprotein; (3) a substituent group of a steroid that projects above the plane of the ring, e.g., cholest-5-en-3*β*-ol (cholesterol); (4) in aliphatic compounds, the carbon separated from a carboxyl by one other carbon.

Ba symbol for the chemical element *barium.*

Babès-Ernst granules (bah′bāz ernst′) [Victor *Babès,* Romanian bacteriologist, 1854–1926; Paul *Ernst,* German pathologist, 1859–1937] see *metachromatic granule.*

Babesia (bah-be′ze-ah) [Victor *Babès*] a genus of protozoa belonging to the Haemosporidia. It rarely infects humans but often causes malaria-like disease in horses, sheep, and cattle, e.g., Texas cattle fever.

babesiosis (bah-be″ze-o′sis) [*Babesia* + *-osis* condition] an infection with a protozoan of the genus *Babesia,* which has long been known as a parasite of domestic and wild animals, causing such economically important diseases as Texas cattle fever and malignant jaundice in dogs. Human infection results when the organism (most commonly *B. microti*) is transferred from a rodent by hard tick vectors (usually of the genus *Ixodes*). Those affected experience malaria-like fever, chills, myalgia, hemolytic anemia, and splenomegaly.

Diagnosis is based on demonstration of intraerythrocytic parasites in Giemsa-stained peripheral blood smears. The unique basket shapes and tetrads present, which are due to parasite budding, may help in the identification. Recovery is the rule, although carrier states may be prolonged. Chloroquine phosphate or pentamidine is used in treatment.

Also called babesiasis.

Babinski sign (bah-bin′ske) [Joseph François Felix *Babinski,* physician in Paris, 1857–1932] a sign elicited by a tactile stimulus applied to the lateral aspect of the sole, consisting of dorsiflexion of the great toe while the other toes are spread outward. This contrasts with the planter flexion (bending downward) of the toes seen in normal adults in response to this stimulus. The sign is considered to be indicative of an upper motor neuron or pyramidal tract lesion when found in patients older than 18 mo, but is a normal finding in infants.

bacampicillin (bah-kamp″ĭ-sil′in) a semisynthetic carbonate ester of ampicillin that is completely hydrolyzed to ampicillin in the blood and tissues. It is used like ampicillin.

Bachman test (bahk′man) [George William *Bachman,* U.S. parasitologist, born 1890] an intradermal skin test used to diagnose trichinosis. In the procedure, powdered antigen from trichina larvae in a dilution of 1:5000–10,000 is injected. After 15–20 min the site is checked: when positive, there is a small, white swelling surrounded by a flat, irregular zone of wheal-and-flare reaction. (This denotes past or present infection, regardless of the intensity of the reaction.)

Many false-positive reactions have been reported. Although the test can be helpful, definitive diagnosis depends on demonstration of the larvae in muscle biopsy tissue.

See also *trichinosis.*

Bacillaceae (bas″il-la′se-e) a family of bacteria containing endospore-forming rods (one genus is spherical). Two of the recognized genera are important in human ecology—the aerobic–facultatively anaerobic *Bacillus* and the anaerobic *Clostridium.* Most species in both genera are soil saprophytes or insect pathogens, although a few can cause disease in animals and humans by infection or production of exotoxins. See also *Bacillus* and *Clostridium.*

bacillary (bas′ĭ-la″re) referring to bacilli or to rod-like forms.

bacillary dysentery see *shigellosis.*

bacille Calmette-Guérin (BCG) (bah-sēl′ kal-met′ ga-ran′) [Albert *Calmette,* French bacteriologist, 1863–1933; Camille *Guérin,* French bacteriologist, 1872–1961] a strain of *Mycobacterium bovis* that became attenuated through hundreds of subcultures on an unfavorable bile-glycerine medium. The strain, commonly referred to as BCG, is sufficiently avirulent to be used as a living culture for the immunization of humans against tuberculosis. See also *BCG vaccine.*

Bacillus (bah-sil′us) [L. "little rod"] a genus of bacteria of the family Bacillaceae. Its many species consist of aerobic–facultatively anaerobic, spore-forming, rod-shaped cells, the great majority of which are gram-positive and motile. One species, *B. anthracis,* is highly pathogenic for humans and animals; another, *B. cereus,* causes food poisoning. The remainder are primarily soil saprophytes, but a number of them are infrequent causes of human infections. Many organisms historically called *Bacillus* are now classified in other genera.

B. anthracis, a species that is the etiologic agent of anthrax in humans and lower animals, consisting of large, gram-positive, nonmotile, spore-forming rods. Typical cells are square-ended and form chains of two or three bacilli. Virulence is associated with: (1) an unusual capsule composed of D-glutamic acid, which is antiphagocytic and probably responsible for the rough, Medusa-head colonies on solid media; and (2) potent exotoxin composed of three proteins or lipoproteins, each with its own toxic action. See also *exotoxins.*

B. brevis, a species that is the source of the polypeptide antibiotic gramicidin.

B. cereus, a usually saprophytic species that is widespread in soil but is also responsible for outbreaks of food-borne illness. These occur after extensive bacterial multiplication and secretion of an enterotoxin in foods, especially fried rice and dairy products. *B. cereus* must be distinguished in the laboratory from *B. anthracis,* which it resembles closely. *B. cereus* produces penicillinase; thus, unlike *B. anthracis,* it is resistant to penicillin and the cephalosporins.

B. polymyxa, a species that is a saprophytic soil and water microorganism, producing the polymyxins, a group of cyclic polypeptide antibiotics. It is also involved in the retting of flax.

B. pyocyaneus, see *P. aeruginosa* under *Pseudomonas.*

B. stearothermophilus, a thermophilic species that produces very resistant spores. Its optimal growth temperature is about 55°C. The organism is widely used to test for quality control of autoclave sterilization.

B. subtilis, an aerobic, spore-forming species that is rarely pathogenic to humans. It produces the antibiotic bacitracin. Spores are widespread in nature and frequently contaminate laboratory media, food, and hospital liquids.

B. typhi, an obsolete name for *Salmonella typhi;* see *S. typhi* under *Salmonella.*

bacillus (bah-sil′us), pl. *bacilli* [L. "little rod"] any rod-shaped bacterium.

anthrax b., see *B. anthracis* under *Bacillus.*

Bang's b., an obsolete name for *Brucella abortus;* see *B. abortus* under *Brucella.*

Battey bacilli, formerly unclassified mycobacteria now known as *Mycobacterium intracellulare.* They are of Runyon Group III nonphotochromogens that may produce a pulmonary or tubercular-like disease in humans. See also *M. intracellulare* under *Mycobacterium.*

Bordet-Gengou b., an obsolete name for *Bordetella pertussis;* see *B. pertussis* under *Bordetella.*

coliform b., a general term without precise meaning, first used by Escherich in 1886 to include those gram-negative bacilli that closely resemble *Escherichia coli,* particularly in the fermentation of lactose with gas. At present it generally refers to certain groups of enteric bacilli in the intestinal tract of humans and/or lower animals; usually included are: *Citrobacter, E. coli, Edwardsiella, Enterobacter, Klebsiella,* and *Serratia.*

colon b., see *E. coli* under *Escherichia.*

Döderlein's b., an obsolete and ill-defined term for aciduric, gram-positive rods commonly found in the vagina, which may be composed of mixtures of *Lactobacillus acidophilus, L. casei, L. cellobiosus, L. fermentum,* or even *Leuconostoc mesenteroides.*

Ducrey's b., an obsolete name for *Hemophilus ducreyi;* see *H. ducreyi* under *Hemophilus.*

dysentery bacilli, a vernacular term for the gram-negative, nonmotile, enteric bacilli of the genus *Shigella.* These organisms are the cause of bacillary dysentery.

enteric b., a vernacular term for a bacterium belonging to the family Enterobacteriaceae. Also called enterics and enterobacteria.

Friedländer's b., see *K. pneumoniae* under *Klebsiella.*

fusiform b., a bacillus that is tapered at both ends.

Gärtner's b., an obsolete name for Salmonella *enteritidis;* see *S. enteritidis* under *Salmonella.*

glanders b., see *P. mallei* under *Pseudomonas.*

Hansen's b., an obsolete name for the leprosy bacillus; see *M. leprae* under *Mycobacterium.*

Hofmann's b., an obsolete name (along with *Corynebacterium hofmannii* for *C. pseudodiphtheriticum;* see *C. pseudodiphtheriticum* under *Corynebacterium.*

Klebs-Löffler b., an obsolete name for *Corynebacterium diphtheriae;* see *C. diphtheriae* under *Corynebacterium.*

Koch-Weeks b., an obsolete name for *Hemophilus aegyptius;* see *H. aegyptius* under *Hemophilus.*

Morax-Axenfeld b., see *M. lacunata* under *Moraxella.*

paracolon b., an obsolete term for any member of a loose collection of enteric bacilli having in common the biochemical characteristic of delayed fermentation of lactose. *Paracolobactrum,* once the genus name for this group, is no longer in use; instead, the constituent species have been assigned to recognized genera and species according to their aggregate biochemical reactions.

Shiga b., see *S. dysenteriae* under *Shigella.*

tetanus b., see *C. tetani* under *Clostridium.*

tubercle b., see *M. tuberculosis* under *Mycobacterium.*

bacitracin (bas″ĭ-tra′sin) [acronym from *Bacillus* + *Tracy,* the name of a patient from whom a culture producing this antibiotic was isolated] a cyclic polypeptide antibiotic derived from *Bacillus licheniformis.* In vitro, it is bactericidal for many gram-positive species and for *Neisseria* species. It affects cell wall synthesis by inhibiting an early step involving a membrane-bound phospholipid intermediate. Because of its nephrotoxicity, bacitracin is used only as a topical antibiotic. See also *antibacterial agents.*

bacitracin disk test an antibiotic susceptibility test used for classification of beta-hemolytic streptococci. Disks containing a measured amount (0.04 units) of bacitracin are placed on a blood agar plate inoculated with beta-hemolytic streptococci. Any zone of inhibition regardless of size is positive for group A beta-hemolytic streptococci.

back (bak) the posterior part of the trunk from the neck to the pelvis. Also called dorsum.

backbone (bak′bōn) 1. the vertebral column.

2. in a polymer, the core of the molecule from which side-chains project.

backcross (bak′kros) the mating of an F_1 (offspring) heterozygote to one of the homozygous P_1 (parental) individuals. A double backcross, mating an F_1 individual heterozygous at two loci and the P_1 double homozygote, is also performed because it is very informative in the analysis of certain gene linkages. In addition, backcrosses may involve individuals of the P_1 genotype rather than the P_1 individual itself. Cf. *testcross.*

backflow (bak′flo) see *regurgitation.*

background (bak′grownd) effects that obscure a phenomenon under investigation, and from which the phenomenon must be differentiated in order to be measured.

background activity 1. in radionuclide imaging, the activity in tissue areas surrounding a region of interest.

2. in the measurement of radioactivity, those counts caused by instrument noise, power line surges, cosmic radiation, and other sources of extraneous radiation. Also called *background radiation.*

3. in electroencephalography, the general setting of electric activity from which more specific normal

or abnormal patterns of activity can be distinguished.

background count the count rate obtained by a radiation detection device while the sample to be measured is absent, although all other conditions are the same. The background count is subtracted from the measured sample count in order to remove the influence of extraneous radiation and provide a true measure of the radioactivity of the sample.

background erase a control present in some rectilinear scanners that deletes counts recorded below a preselected background count rate. Background erase may improve image resolution but involves the loss of a certain amount of data. Excessive erasure may seriously distort images. See also *rectilinear scanner.*

background interference in spectrophotometry, interference with the absorbance reading of the sample owing to the absorbance of the background (cuvet and reagents), which varies with wavelength. It can sometimes be eliminated or corrected for by using a reagent blank or measurements at several wavelengths. See also *Allen correction* and *blank.*

background radiation see *background activity.*

backlash (bak′lash) the difference between the actual value of a quantity, usually the wavelength setting of a spectrophotometer, when the dial controlling this quantity is turned to a given position by a clockwise rotation and when it is turned to the same position by a counterclockwise rotation.

back pressure the pressure exerted by the damming back of blood in a heart chamber or its tributary vessels when the forward flow of blood has been obstructed. For example, the back pressure caused by mitral stenosis or a failing left ventricular myocardium can result in congestion in the pulmonary circulation.

backscatter (bak′skat-er) radiation deflected by scattering processes at angles greater than 90 degrees to the original direction of the beam of radiation.

backscatter peak a peak in the gamma-ray spectrum, recorded with a scintillation detector, that is produced by incident photons that undergo Compton scattering before detection. The minimum energy of a backscatter event is the difference between the photopeak energy and the Compton edge.

baclofen (bak′lo-fen) β-(aminomethyl)-*p*-chlorohydrocinnamic acid, an analog of the neurotransmitter γ-aminobutyric acid (GABA) used as a muscle relaxant for the management of spinal spasticity caused by multiple sclerosis or spinal cord injury. It acts by inhibiting both monosynaptic and polysynaptic reflexes at the spinal level. Adverse reactions include nausea, drowsiness, dizziness, weakness, confusion, and hypotension. Trademark, Lioresal.

Bactec system (bak′tek) an automated device that detects bacterial growth by measuring the amount of radioactive $^{14}CO_2$ given off by bacteria growing in a ^{14}C-labeled culture medium, such as ^{14}C-glucose. This system detects bacterial growth faster than routine procedures (usually within 6 hr) and can use smaller samples. See also *microbiology automation.*

bacteremia (bak″ter-e′me-ah) [Gr. *bakterion* little rod + *haima* blood + *-ia*] the presence of bacteria in the blood stream. It may be a transient event associated with trauma such as a dental procedure. Persistent or recurrent bacteremia indicates that the microorganisms have been released from a site of local infection. See also septicemia.

bacteri/o (bak-te′re-o) [Gr. *baktérion* little rod] a word element used in combining form to denote bacteria, e.g., bacteriuria.

bacterial (bak-te′re-al) pertaining to or caused by bacteria.

bacterial adherence originally, the tendency of bacteria to cling to a surface; in recent years, however, the term refers more particularly to the tendency to cling to the mucous membranes of the intestinal wall, oral cavity, or urinary bladder. Many bacteria have on their surfaces macromolecules with an affinity for specific receptors on certain tissue cells, e.g., *Escherichia coli* for intestinal epithelium. Pili and other structures are involved. Selective adherence is recognized as playing a major role in the colonization of microorganisms on tissue surfaces and in the establishment of the normal microflora of the body.

bacterial agar method see under *cell block preparation.*

bacterial capsule an envelope of tightly associated gel-like material that surrounds a bacterial cell. It is composed of simple polysaccharides containing repeating sequences of two or three sugars and often uronic acids. The presence of a capsule is associated with increased virulence of pathogenic bacteria, as it often protects the bacteria from phagocytosis.

The capsules can be demonstrated by negative staining with India ink, and are seen as a clear zone between the medium and the more refractile cell body. Different antigenic strains in a bacterial species often have immunologically distinct capsules. Common microorganisms that produce large capsules include *Cryptococcus, Pneumococcus,* and *Klebsiella.*

bacterial culturing see *clinical bacteriologic specimens* and *culture media.*

bacterial endaortitis see *bacterial endarteritis.*

bacterial endarteritis infection of an artery by bacteria, resulting in a buildup of vegetations of the endothelial lining, often with formation of aneurysms. It may result from the metastasis of bacterial endocarditis.

bacterial genetics see *bacterial g.* under *genetics.*

bacterial opsonin an antibody that, by interaction with bacteria, renders the bacteria more susceptible to phagocytosis by leukocytes. Also called *bacteria-opsonin* and *bacteriotropin.*

bacterial pathogenicity the ability of a microorganism to produce disease in humans, animals, or plants. Bacterial infections may be clinically apparent, with signs and symptoms; more often they are subclinical infections with no clinical manifestations. In either instance, the host usually makes a specific humoral and/or cellular immunologic response.

Pathogenicity of a microorganism has little meaning except in relation to a particular host. The meningococcus, for example, is a primary pathogen for humans but is incapable of even colonizing the tissues of lower animals; thus, it is highly virulent for humans but nonpathogenic for lower animals. Conversely, many animal pathogens lack pathogenicity for humans, although some may colonize tissue surfaces for a time as inconsequential parasites.

Bacteria vary greatly in their pathogenic potential. Some species are characterized as primary pathogens because a very small number of cells can initiate a disease process in susceptible individuals. Others are moderately pathogenic in that larger numbers of bacteria, as well as a certain portal of entry, are required for infection to occur. Still others have such low-grade potential that infection occurs only if certain host factors favor multiplication of the bacteria. The term virulence is used to express this quantitative aspect of pathogenicity.

Host factors greatly influence the ability of a given bacterial species to produce disease. Age is one such factor: species that behave as low-grade pathogens in the adult may be highly virulent in the newborn. Another example is opportunistic infections due to low-grade pathogens or even commensals in hospitalized patients whose resistance is low or whose specific immune mechanisms are suppressed.

Immunologic reactivity on the part of the host, e.g., hypersensitivity reaction, may also contribute to the pathogenic process and heighten the apparent virulence of a parasitic microorganism. The role of hypersensitivity is most pronounced in chronic infections such as tuberculosis. Some pathogens induce the host to make other types of humoral or cell-mediated responses that become part of the disease pattern. Examples include postinfectious sequelae with the formation of immune complexes, as in acute glomerulonephritis, and the occurrence of cross-reactivity between host tissue and certain microbial antigens associated with antibody production, as in rheumatic fever.

HOST-PARASITE RELATIONSHIPS. Pathogenicity may also be viewed as the result of a host-parasite relationship that is detrimental to the host. In the absence of disease there is a delicately balanced equilibrium between the bacterial parasite and the host, a good example being the normal microbial flora of the human body, which persists without tissue invasion under normal circumstances. These organisms are successful parasites, because they obtain all their needs from, and do not destroy, the host. Highly virulent organisms, however, may produce fatal disease, ending the relationship. Less virulent strains may cause temporary illness and be eliminated from the tissues by the body's defenses, or survive for a long time without harming carrier hosts (if transmitted to another human host, however, their full pathogenic potential may become evident).

MECHANISMS OF PATHOGENICITY. A wide spectrum of pathogenic mechanisms exists among bacteria. Two important pathogenic factors are toxigenicity and invasiveness. Toxigenicity reflects the ability to produce toxins. Toxins are divided into two main types. Toxic products that are secreted into the growth medium or tissues are called exotoxins. Endotoxins are those that are integral parts of the bacterial cell surface and produce their principal effects when the microbes lyse or break down. Invasiveness refers to the capacity of an organism to enter the host tissues and multiply and spread throughout them. Some bacterial diseases are produced by a combination of the toxigenic and invasive properties of the same organism (see Tables 1 and 2).

ATTACHMENT AND ADHERENCE. Attachment of bacteria to the surface of host tissue cells is an important step in the initiation of many infections. This may involve specific interaction between complementary receptor sites on the surface of the parasite and host cell membrane. Less specific mechanisms may involve pili (fimbriae) or the presence of sticky exopolymers at the microbial cell surface that promote the adherence of microbes to epithelial cells or certain tissue surfaces (e.g., tooth enamel). The first step in the pathogenesis of disease is achieved once an organism adheres to a cell surface and is able to persist and multiply.

Some diseases follow the pattern of adherence, growth, and localized exotoxin production. This is the case with diphtheria and cholera: the causative

BACTERIAL PATHOGENICITY, TABLE 1. EXOTOXINS THAT DETERMINE THE PATHOGENICITY OF SOME HUMAN BACTERIAL PARASITES

DISEASE	SOURCE OF EXOTOXIN	ACTIVITY
Diphtheria	*Corynebacterium diphtheriae*	Inhibits protein synthesis (ADP ribosylating)
Botulism	*Clostridium botulinum*	Anticholinergic
Tetanus	*Clostridium tetani*	Anticholinergic; blocks inhibitory synapses (?)
Gas gangrene	*Clostridium perfringens*	Cytolytic (necrotizing, hemolytic)
Staphylococcal food poisoning	*Staphylococcus aureus*	Stimulates brain or peripheral nerves to produce vomiting (?)
Scarlet fever	Streptococci, group A	Cytotoxic to blood vessels
Whooping cough	*Bordetella pertussis*	Necrotizing to bronchial epithelium; produces lymphocytosis
Cholera and *E. coli*, traveler's diarrhea	*Vibrio cholerae*, *Escherichia coli*	Alters water and electrolyte balance in intestine, accumulation of cAMP (ADP ribosylating)

BACTERIAL PATHOGENICITY, TABLE 2. INVASIVE FACTORS THAT INFLUENCE THE PATHOGENICITY OF SOME HUMAN BACTERIAL PARASITES

INVASIVE FACTOR	SOURCE	ACTIVITY
Capsules	*Streptococcus pneumoniae, Hemophilus influenzae, Klebsiella pneumoniae, Bacillus anthracis, Staphylococcus aureus, Pasteurella pestis*	Antiphagocytic
M protein at cell surface	Streptococci, group A	Antiphagocytic
Extracellular enzymes*		
Hyaluronidase	Streptococci, group A	Lysis of tissue group substance
Coagulase	*Staphylococcus aureus*	Clots fibrin
Kinase	Staphylococci, streptococci	Lysis of fibrin
Collagenase and lecithinase	*Clostridium perfringens*	Lysis of collagen, connective tissue (necrotic), and erythrocytes

* The extent of the role played by individual extracellular enzymes in the pathogenesis of human infections is uncertain.

organisms do not invade the deeper tissues. Exotoxin can act locally and also be absorbed into the circulation and/or spread along nerve pathways to body sites remote from the original focus of infection. Other organisms produce powerful exotoxins or proteolytic enzymes that help them to further invade and destroy deeper tissue when introduced into a wound or otherwise compromised sites of infection. One such example is clostridial myonecrosis (gas gangrene).

Another frequent pathogenic pattern is that of adherence to the mucosal cells lining the respiratory, gastrointestinal, and genitourinary tracts, with subsequent penetration of the cells. Intracellular growth of the organisms results in destruction of the epithelial cells, e.g., gonorrhea, shigellosis, and salmonellosis.

ANTIPHAGOCYTIC MECHANISMS. Following infection exhibiting any one of these patterns of pathogenesis, most organisms are eliminated locally by phagocytic cells and/or by the macrophages in such locations as the alveolar spaces of the lungs, sinusoidal spaces of the liver, and regional lymph nodes. If not halted at the lymph node level, they reach the circulation and are carried to other organs with or without persistent bacteremia.

Some organisms can produce invasive disease, primarily because of the nature of their capsule or some other surface component that is antiphagocytic. It may enable the bacterium to resist the engulfment stage of the phagocytic process, e.g., *Streptococcus pneumoniae* (pneumococcus), or it may enable some engulfed pathogens to resist destruction by phagocytic cells; thus, they not only survive but also multiply. An example is *Mycobacterium tuberculosis.*

ENDOTOXINS. Cell wall structural components contributing to pathogenicity are the lipopolysaccharide complex (LPS or endotoxin) common to almost all gram-negative bacteria and peptidoglycans from gram-positive bacteria such as streptococci and staphylococci. These materials share such biologic activities as pyrogenicity, localized Shwartzman reactivity, and complement activation. LPS has additional effects on the circulatory system and other tissues; its action is better understood than that of the peptidoglycans. The toxic moiety of LPS seems to be primarily associated with the lipid A portion of the molecule and does not vary in degree of activity from one organism to another.

EXOTOXINS. Exotoxins and other extracellular products may play a significant role in pathogenicity. These toxins are proteins and, in general, are produced by gram-positive bacteria. Some gram-negative organisms, however, produce powerful exotoxins such as exotoxin A from certain strains of *Pseudomonas aeruginosa,* the enterotoxins of some of the enteric pathogens including *Vibrio cholerae* and enterotoxic *Escherichia coli,* and the neurotoxin of *Shigella dysenteriae.* Exotoxins are found within and without the bacterial cell and may be secreted without breakdown of the bacterial cell, although cell lysis of cultures often increases exotoxic activity. Exotoxins are much more potent than endotoxins, and they are highly specific in their site of action. Typical exotoxins block or otherwise abnormally affect biosynthetic or neurologic transmission pathways (see Table 1). This may produce profound pathophysiologic effects. Examples of such gram-positive exotoxins are the tetanus and botulinum toxins, as well as enterotoxins from *Staphylococcus aureus* and *Clostridium perfringens.* Additional related extracellular products elaborated by many gram-positive bacteria are proteolytic and saccharolytic enzymes. These may contribute to the invasive qualities of the organisms by destruction of tissues and by increasing their penetrability. Such enzymes are frequently included with the exotoxins that are nonenzymatic in nature, or thought not to be enzymatic.

KENNETH R. CUNDY, PH. D.

bacterial susceptibility testing see *antibacterial agent susceptibility testing.*

bacterial virus see *bacteriophage.*

bactericidal (bak-tēr″i-si′dal) [*bacteri-* + L. *caedere* to kill] having the capacity to kill bacteria. Cf. *bacteriostatic.*

bactericide (bak-tēr′ĭ-sīd) an agent that kills bacteria.

bacterid (bak′ter-id) a sterile skin eruption caused by bacterial infection elsewhere in the body, generally an allergic response to a bacterial antigen. Examples are erythematous rashes and urticaria associated with group A streptococcal infections.

pustular b., an originally sterile cutaneous vesicular lesion that has become infected by a pyrogen; it most often occurs on the palm or sole.

bacteriemia (bak-tēr″e-e′me-ah) [*bacteri-* + Gr. *haima* blood + *-ia*] see *bacteremia.*

bacterin (bak′ter-in) a vaccine consisting of a suspension of killed bacteria. Such vaccines generally are used as a preventive measure to stimulate the production of antibodies by active immunization, but sometimes are also employed in the treatment of persistent low-grade infection.

bacterioagglutinin (bak-te″re-o-ah-gloo′tĭ-nin) an agglutinin that causes bacteria suspended in an electrolyte to clump. Also called bacterial agglutinin.

bacteriocin (bak-te′re-o-sin) any of a group of proteins released by certain bacteria that kill other strains of the same species or different species, (e.g., the colicins of *Escherichia coli*). Bacteriocins attach to specific receptors on susceptible cells and induce a specific metabolic block, such as the cessation of nucleic acid or protein synthesis, or of oxidative phosphorylation.

bacteriocinogen (bak-te″re-osin′o-jen) a plasmid responsible for the formation of bacteriocins produced by specific strains of bacteria, which can inhibit the growth of a limited number of other strains. Bacteriocinogens have been isolated from *Escherichia, Proteus,* and *Bacillus* organisms. The larger of these plasmids are conjugative; smaller bacteriocinogens are not. Normally, the formation of bacteriocinogenic bacteria is repressed, but ultraviolet radiation can induce the release of the bacteriocin much as it can induce temperate phage to become infectious. See also *bacteriocin* and *colicinogen.*

bacterioclasis (bak-te″re-ok′lah-sis) [*bacterio-* + Gr. *klasis* breaking] see *bacteriolysis.*

bacteriogenic (bak-te″re-o-jen′ik) [*bacterio-* + Gr. *gennan* to produce] 1. caused by bacteria.
2. of bacterial origin.

bacterioid (bak-te′re-oid) see *bacteroid.*

bacteriologic (bak-te″re-o-loj′ik) pertaining to bacteriology.

bacteriologic specimens see *clinical bacteriologic specimens.*

bacteriologist (bak-te″re-ol′o-jist) an individual involved primarily in studying and working with bacteria.

bacteriology (bak-te″re-ol′o-je) [*bacterio-* + *-logy*] the science and study of bacteria. Cf. *microbiology.*

automated b., see *microbiology automation.*

clinical diagnostic b., the science and practice of collecting specimens from persons or the environment, examining them for bacteria or evidence of bacterial infection, and evaluating the results.

medical b., the branch of bacteriology that deals chiefly with the microorganisms causing disease in humans.

public health b., the branch of bacteriology that deals chiefly with the spread and prevention of bacterial diseases in the environment and among populations, including animal and arthropod reservoirs.

sanitary b., the branch of public health bacteriology that deals with safe water supplies, sanitation in public eating establishments, and sewage disposal.

systematic b., the branch of bacteriology that studies the nomenclature and classification of bacteria.

bacteriolysin (bak-te″re-ol′ĭ-sin) a substance capable of lysing bacteria. It may be an antibody acting in the presence of complement, a bacteriophage, or a chemical compound.

bacteriolysis (bak-te″re-ol′ĭ-sis) [*bacterio-* + Gr. *lysis* dissolution] the lysis of a bacterial cell.

bacteriolytic (bak-te″re-o-lit′ik) having the capacity to act as a bacteriolysin.

bacterio-opsonin (bak-te″re-o-op′so-nin) [*bacterio-* + Gr. *opsōnein* to buy victuals] see *bacterial opsonin.*

bacteriopexy (bak-te″re-o-pek′se) [*bacterio-* + Gr. *pēxis* fixation] the immobilization of bacteria by histiocytes or other phagocytes. Also called bacteriopexia.

bacteriophage (bak-te′re-o-faj″) [*bacterio-* + Gr. *phagein* to eat] any virus that infects a bacterium. As with plant and animal viruses, there are many types of bacteriophages, with structures ranging from simple to complex; both DNA and RNA bacteriophages occur. They are usually species-specfic. Most groups of bacteria have bacteriophages.

Bacteriophages are obligate intracellular parasites. The virus particle (virion) binds to a specific site on the bacterial cell surface; the phage nucleic acid is injected into the host cell where it is replicated by host (and in some cases, viral enzymes also) and translated to form new viral proteins. The nucleic acid and viral proteins then self-assemble into new virions, and the host cell is lysed, releasing new infectious virus particles. Some viruses, called temperate phages, can also have their nucleic acid incorporated into the host chromosome. In this process (lysogeny), the viral DNA may replicate with the host cell DNA for many cycles until virions are produced and lysis occurs.

See also *bacteriophage g.* under *genetics.*

bacteriophage genetics see *bacteriophage g.* under *genetics.*

bacteriopsonic (bak-te″re-op-son′ik) capable of increasing the susceptibility of bacteria to phagocytosis.

bacteriostasis (bak-te″re-os′tah-sis) [*bacterio-* + Gr. *stasis* stoppage] the inhibition of bacterial growth produced by physical, chemical, or biologic agents.

bacteriostat (bak-te′re-o-stat″) 1. an agent that inhibits the growth of bacteria; the preferred usage is *bacteriostatic agent.*
2. see *chemostat.*

bacteriostatic (bak-te″re-o-stat′ik) 1. inhibiting the growth or multiplication of bacteria.
2. an agent that inhibits the growth or multiplication of bacteria. Cf. *bactericidal.*

bacteriostatic agent an inhibitor of the multiplication of bacteria.

bacteriotherapy (bak-te″re-o-ther′ah-pe) [*bacterio-* + *therapy*] the treatment of disease by the introduction of bacteria or their products into the body.

bacteriotoxic (bak-te″re-o-tok′sik) toxic to bacteria.

bacteriotropic (bak-te″re-o-trop′ik) [*bacterio-* + Gr. *tropos* a turning] having the capacity of a bacteriotropin, i.e., making bacteria more susceptible to phagocytosis. See also *bacterial opsonin.*

bacteriotropin (bak-te″re-ot′ro-pin) see *bacterial opsonin.*

Bacterium (bak-te′re-um) [L., from Gr. *baktērion* little rod] a name formerly given a genus composed of nonspore-forming, rod-shaped bacteria that are not necessarily closely related; these organisms are now placed in other genera.

bacterium any of a group of prokaryotic organisms that differ from cyanobacteria (the other division of prokaryotic organisms) in their pigment systems and lack of aerobic photosynthesis. Bacteria differ from eukaryotes in many ways. They divide by binary fission and not mitosis. Their genetic material is a single loop of naked, double-stranded DNA, whereas in eukaryotes DNA is associated with basic proteins in chromosomes and enclosed in a nuclear envelope. Bacterial ribosomes are smaller (70S) than eukaryotic cytoplasmic ribosomes (80S), and they differ in their sensitivity to antibiotics. Finally, bacteria lack all internal membrane-bound organelles, such as the Golgi apparatus, lysosomes, the endoplasmic reticulum, the nuclear membrane, mitochondria, and chloroplasts. Bacteria are divided into many groups on the basis of differences in structure, staining properties, morphology, ability to sporulate, and mechanism of energy metabolism, as well as atmospheric and other growth requirements.

STRUCTURE AND MORPHOLOGY. Bacteria typically possess a cell envelope that includes the cell or plasma membrane and a cell wall with associated proteins and polysaccharides. The cell membrane is a trilaminar structure composed of protein and lipid; it is an osmotic barrier, and functions in both active and passive transport of nutrients. Various enzymatic activities have been found to be associated with membrane proteins. The cell wall is composed of a network of polysaccharide chains called peptidoglycans, unique to bacterial cells. It is responsible for maintaining cell shape; all bacteria with the exception of *Mycoplasma* and *Halobacterium* have a rigid cell wall. In hypertonic media (e.g., 20 percent sucrose), either hydrolysis of peptidoglycan by lysozyme or prevention of cell wall synthesis with penicillin converts bacteria into osmotically sensitive spheres. Under such conditions, gram-positive organisms become protoplasts and gram-negative organisms become spheroplasts.

A variety of lipids, polysaccharides, and proteins may be found in the cell envelope of different bacteria. Significant differences in peptidoglycan content, cell wall mass, and other envelope components may be observed between gram-positive and gram-negative organisms. The cell envelopes of gram-positive organisms may contain teichoic or teichuronic acids covalently linked to cell wall peptidoglycan, and lipoteichoic acids that are membrane-bound. Gram-negative bacteris, on the other hand, possess a thinner cell-wall peptidoglycan layer, as well as an outer membrane that overlies the peptidolglycan layer and consists of lipopolysaccharide and phospholipids. The lipopolysaccharide layer is also called endotoxin because of its toxicity and firm binding to the cells. It consists of lipid A, responsible for toxicity, and polysaccharide O antigen, responsible for antigenic specificity of different bacterial strains.

Polysaccharide or polypeptide capsules or slime layers are formed by some bacteria. Capsules of pathogenic bacteria play a role in their pathogenicity by allowing the bacteria to evade phagocytic cells in vivo.

The cytoplasm present with the cell membrane of bacteria contains nuclear DNA that is not enclosed by a nuclear membrane. Mesosomes, invaginations of the plasma membrane, can be observed in many bacteria and may be involved in cell division, secretion, or electron transport.

The cytoplasm also contains ribosomes composed of RNA and protein. Bacterial ribosomes have a sedimentation constant of 70S. The 70S monomer can be dissociated into 50S and 30S subunits. Cytoplasmic inclusion bodies, representing accumulations of food reserves, may be present. Specialized structures, called chromatophores, are present in photosynthetic bacteria.

Flagella, pili, or both may be present on the surface of bacteria. Flagella are long, thin, helical protein filaments that are responsible for motility. They may be distributed over the entire surface (peritrichous), be present in either one pole (monotrichous) or two poles (amphitrichous), or be present as a tuft of several polar flagella (lophotrichous). Pili are hairlike helical filaments, of which there are two types: common pili, which may play a role in the adherence of bacteria to surfaces, and sex pili, which function in bacterial conjugation, allowing the transfer of genetic material between bacteria. Pili may also play a role in the twitching or gliding motion exhibited by certain nonflagellated bacteria.

Bacteria have a size of 0.2–10 μm, varying with the species. Most bacteria of medical importance are approximately 1 μm (for comparison, an erythrocyte measures about 8 μm). As the average resolution of the light microscope is about 0.3 μm, most bacteria can be visualized by means of light microscopy. Some bacteria, such as spirochetes, can be visualized by special silver staining techniques.

The shapes of bacteria vary, appearing as spheres (cocci), rods (bacilli), spirals (spirochetes), or commas (vibrios). Depending on the type of cell division observed, cocci can be observed as chains, tetrads, or clusters. Rods may appear morphologically different: e.g., short rods, or rods with rounded, tapered, or square ends. Because *Mycoplasma* lack a rigid cell wall, they are extremely pleomorphic.

Bacteria that form spores are limited to a few genera, including species of *Bacillus, Clostridium,* and *Sporosarcina.* Spores are generally formed under conditions of inadequate nutrition. They tend to be resistant to heat, drying, freezing, toxic chemicals (e.g., some antiseptics and disinfectants), and radiation. By means of the light microscope, spores can be seen as an unstained area within the parent bacterial cells. Structurally, spores consist of an inner spore wall and a thick cortex, both containing peptidoglycan, and an outermost coat, containing a keratinlike substance. Spores will germinate under certain conditions, such as activation by heat or when present in a favorable environment.

METABOLISM—MAJOR ENERGY PATHWAYS. Bacteria can be divided into two large groups based on their carbon source requirement: autotrophic (lithotrophic) bacteria and heterotrophic (organotrophic) bacteria. Autotrophs require only water, inorganic salts, and carbon dioxide for growth; e.g., they can utilize carbon dioxide as a sole carbon source, and synthesize essential organic metabolites from it. Heterotrophs, which include all known human pathogens, require organic molecules, such as glucose, as a carbon source. Autotrophs and heterotrophs are either photosynthetic or chemosynthetic, depending on whether they obtain energy from light or oxidation-reduction reactions, respectively.

In heterotrophs, carbohydrates are metabolized by several different systems: (1) glycolysis (Embden-Meyerhof-Parnas pathway); (2) the phosphogluconate pathway (hexosemonophosphate shunt); and (3) the Entner-Doudoroff pathway. Glycolysis is the major metabolic pathway used by bacteria to catabolize glucose.

Heterotrophs extract energy by either fermentation or respiration. Fermentation, a type of metabolism in which organic compounds serve as both electron donors and electron acceptors, occurs in the absence of oxygen and is a less efficient mechanism. Products of fermentation vary with the bacterial species. Such products, e.g., alcohol or various types of organic acids, are useful in industry (e.g., ethanol production from glucose) and for the identification of bacteria in the clinical laboratory (e.g., lactic acid or propionic acid producing bacteria, mixed acid fermentation, butanediol fermentation).

There are two types of respiration in heterotrophs: aerobic and anaerobic. Aerobic respiration differs from fermentation in that oxygen, rather than an organic molecule, is the ultimate electron acceptor. Obligate aerobes and facultative anaerobes carry out aerobic respiration. In anaerobic respiration, oxidized inorganic compounds are used as the terminal electron acceptor. Obligate anaerobes utilize sulfates or carbonates for this purpose, whereas certain facultative anaerobes can use nitrates.

Growth Requirements. Bacteria require carbon and nitrogen sources and inorganic ions for growth. In addition, some bacteria require growth factors, such as amino acids, vitamins, purines, pyrimidines, and coenzymes.

Bacteria differ in their requirement for oxygen. Obligate aerobes need oxygen for growth, whereas obligate anaerobes grow only in the absence of oxygen. Facultative anaerobes can grow under both aerobic and anaerobic conditions. Microaerophilic organisms require conditions of lowered oxygen tension.

Bacteria grow optimally within a specified range of temperatures. Most bacteria are mesophiles: i.e., they grow optimally at temperatures near 37°C. Psychrophiles prefer very low temperatures (30°C and below); thermophiles prefer higher temperatures (50°C and above).

Stages of Bacterial Growth. Bacterial growth can be divided into lag, exponential, and stationary phases. The lag phase can be observed when stationary phase cells are transferred to fresh media. This phase is characterized by an increase in cell size that precedes cell division. The length of the lag phase is dependent on the organism and the medium. Cells divide at a constant rate in the phase of exponential or logarithmic growth. The doubling time of bacterial cells varies with the organism and the medium used. The stationary phase is reached when inhibitory products accumulate or when nutrients are no longer available to the cell.

Growth can be defined by bacterial cell mass or cell number. Methods for determining cell mass include dry weight or nitrogen content measurement and turbidometric techniques. Bacterial cell numbers are determined by direct count of cells (using a bacterial counting chamber or an electronic particle counter, such as a Coulter counter) or viable count of colony-forming units, measured by making dilutions of a culture and counting colonies growing on solid media.

Bacteria that are important in clinical medicine are classified in the accompanying table. For more information, see the specific genera.

acid-fast b., a bacterium that resists decolorization by acids after staining by dyes such as carbol fuchsin or auramine (a fluorochrome), especially mycobacteria and *Nocardia.*

aerobic b., a type of bacterium that requires oxygen for growth, such as the tubercle bacillus, *Mycobacterium tuberculosis,* and some spore-forming bacilli.

anaerobic b., a type of bacterium that can grow only in the absence of molecular oxygen, such as *Clostridium* and *Bacteroides.* See also *anaerobe.*

autotrophic b., a microorganism that can fulfill all its nutritional requirements by the utilization of CO_2 and inorganic salts.

beaded b., a bacterium that has deeply staining granules along the rod.

bifid b., a branching, rod-shaped organism, especially *Bifidobacterium.*

chemoautotrophic b., a bacterium that uses reduced inorganic compounds as substrates for respiratory metabolism, especially H_2, NH_3, NO_2^-, Fe^{++}, and reduced sulfur compounds (H_2S, S, $S_2O_3^{2-}$), and CO_2 as its principal carbon source. Substrate oxidation yields adenosine triphosphate (ATP) through oxidative phosphorylation.

chemoheterotrophic b., a heterotrophic microorganism that requires organic compounds as energy sources. The mechanisms of energy production are similar to those of higher animals.

chromogenic b., a microorganism that produces pigmented colonies on solid culture media.

denitrifying b., a microorganism that is able to reduce nitrates to nitrites, ammonia, or nitrogen gas.

facultative b., a term generally referring to a facultative anaerobe, i.e., a type of bacterium that can grow either in the absence or presence of atmospheric oxygen, changing its metabolism according to the environment.

gram-negative b., a type of bacterium that loses its violet stain when treated with organic solvent and therefore shows the counterstain in the Gram stain procedure. See also *Gram stain.*

gram-positive b., a type of bacterium that retains the initial violet color in the Gram stain procedure. See also *Gram stain.*

heterotrophic b., a microorganism that obtains its carbon and energy for growth from organic compounds.

higher bacteria, an informal term most often applied to filamentous bacteria that seem to be intermediate between bacteria and fungi.

hydrogen b., a facultative chemoautotroph that can use H_2 as an energy source with end products such as H_2O, H_2S, and CH_4. Hydrogen bacteria are sometimes assigned to a special genus, *Hydrogenomonas,* but in many strains the autotrophic character is facultative. These are phenotypically identical with certain chemoheterotrophic genera such as *Pseudomonas.*

CLASSIFICATION	ORGANISM
Kingdom:	Prokaryotae
Division:	The Bacteria
The Spirochetes	
Family:	Spirochaetaceae
Genera:	*Treponema*
	Borrelia
	Leptospira
Spiral and Curved Bacteria	
Family:	Spirillaceae
Genera:	*Spirillum*
	Campylobacter
Gram-negative Aerobic Rods and Cocci	
Family:	Pseudomonadaceae
Genus:	*Pseudomonas*
Family:	Rhizobiaceae
Genus:	*Agrobacterium*
Uncertain affiliation:	*Alcaligenes*
	Acetobacter
	Brucella
	Bordetella
	Francisella
	Legionella
Gram-negative Facultatively Anerobic Rods	
Family:	Enterobacteriaceae
Genera:	*Escherichia*
	Edwardsiella
	Citrobacter
	Salmonella
	Shigella
	Klebsiella
	Enterobacter
	Hafnia
	Serratia
	Proteus
	Yersinia
	Arizona
	Providencia
Family:	Vibrionaceae
Genera:	*Vibrio*
	Aeromonas
	Plesiomonas
Uncertain affiliation:	*Chromobacterium*
	Flavobacterium
	Hemophilus
	Pasteurella
	Actinobacillus
	Cardiobacterium
	Streptobacillus
	Calymmatobacterium
	Capnocytophaga
	Kingella
	Eikenella
	Achromobacter
Gram-negative Anerobic Bacilli	
Family:	Bacteroidaceae
Genera:	*Bacteroides*
	Fusobacterium
	Leptotrichia
Gram-negative Cocci and Coccobacilli	
Family:	Neisseriaceae
Genera:	*Neisseria*
	Branhamella
	Moraxella
	Acinetobacter

BACTERIUM. (*Continued*)

CLASSIFICATION	ORGANISM
Gram-negative Anerobic Cocci	
Family:	Veillonellaceae
Genus:	*Veillonella*
Gram-positive Cocci	
Family:	Micrococcaceae
Genera:	*Micrococcus*
	Staphylococcus
Family:	Streptococcaceae
Genus:	*Streptococcus*
Family:	Peptococcaceae
Genera:	*Peptococcus*
	Peptostreptococcus
Endospore-forming Rods and Cocci	
Family:	Bacillaceae
Genera:	*Bacillus*
	Clostridium
Gram-positive Asporogenous Rods	
Family:	Lactobacillaceae
Genus:	*Lactobacillus*
Uncertain affiliation:	*Listeria*
	Erysipelothrix
Actinomycetes and Related Organisms	
Family:	Coryneform group
Genus:	*Corynebacterium*
Family:	Propionibacteriaceae
Genera:	*Propionibacterium*
	Eubacterium
Family:	Actinomycetaceae
Genera:	*Actinomyces*
	Arachnia
	Bifidobacterium
Family:	Mycobacteriaceae
Genus:	*Mycobacterium*
Family:	Actinoplanaceae
Genus:	*Actinoplanes*
Family:	Dermatophilaceae
Genus:	*Dermatophilus*
Family:	Nocardiaceae
Genera:	*Nocardia*
	Nocardiopsis
	Actinomadura
Family:	Streptomycetaceae
Genus:	*Streptomyces*
The Rickettsias	
Family:	Rickettsiaceae
Genera:	*Rickettsia*
	Rochalimaea
	Coxiella
Family:	Bartonellaceae
Genus:	*Bartonella*
Family:	Chlamydiaceae
Genus:	*Chlamydia*
The Mycoplasmas	
(Class: Mollicutes)	
Family:	Mycoplasmataceae
Genera:	*Mycoplasma*
	Ureaplasma
Family:	Acholeplasmataceae
Genus:	*Acholeplasma*

lysogenic b., a bacterial cell that harbors in its genome the genetic material (prophage) of a temperate bacteriophage and thus reproduces the bacteriophage in cell division. If the prophage matures and replicates, it lyses its host cell and is free to infect other cells.

mesophilic b., a bacterium that grows best in a midrange (30°–45°C), including temperatures found in the human body.

nitrifying b., a bacterium that uses reduced inorganic nitrogen compounds present in the soil as energy sources, converting NH_3 to NO_2^- (*Nitrosomonas, Nitrosospira, Nitrosococcus*) or NO_2^- to NO_3^- (*Nitrobacter, Nitrococcus,* or *Nitrospina*).

organotropic b., a bacterium that is highly selective of the type of tissues it infects. For example, pneumococcus is especially invasive of the lower respiratory tract, causing pneumonia.

psychrophilic b., a bacterium that grows best at 15°–18°C. Facultative psychrophiles can grow also in the mesophile range and, although slowly, at temperatures near or below 0°C.

pyogenic b., a microorganism that, when it infects an organism, produces suppuration.

rough b., a variant form of a bacterium characterized by dry, wrinkled colonies on solid media and/or the formation of granular clumps in liquid media.

smooth b., a bacterium characterized by smooth, glossy colonies on solid media.

sulfur b., an obligate or facultative chemoautotroph that utilizes elemental sulfur, hydrogen sulfide, or partially reduced oxides as energy, such as *Thiobacillus.*

thermophilic b., a bacterium that grows best at a temperature above 40°C, with an optimal range of 50°–70°C.

toxigenic b., a bacterium that produces a toxin; the term usually refers to soluble exotoxin production.

water b., a term applied to gram-negative bacteria capable of fast growth in all types of water, that can produce a pyrogenic reaction or infection in humans. Water bacteria have attracted attention in recent years when there have been cases of heavy contamination of hemodialysis fluid or flood-caused disease in immunologically compromised patients in hospitals. Members of the *Pseudomonas, Achromobacter, Flavobacterium, Aeromonas, Acinetobacter,* and *Serratia* genera are the most common of the water bacteria.

bacteriuria (bak-te″re-u′re-ah) [*bacteri-* + Gr. *ouron* urine + *-ia*] the presence of bacteria in the urine.

bacteroid (bak′tĕ-roid) 1. resembling a bacterium.
2. a structure or organism resembling a bacterium.
3. sometimes used to denote a member of the genus *Bacteroides.*

Bacteroidaceae (bak″tĕ-roi-da′se-e) [Gr. *baktērion* rod + Gr. *eidos* form] a family of gram-negative, anaerobic bacteria. It includes the genera *Bacteroides, Fusobacterium,* and *Leptotrichia,* the first two of which contain human pathogens.

Bacteroides (bak-tĕ-roi′dēz) [Gr. *baktērion* rod + Gr. *eidos* form] a genus of bacteria of the family Bacteroidaceae. These organisms consist of gram-negative, obligately anaerobic, nonspore-forming rods that are nonmotile or motile with peritrichous flagella. They metabolize carbohydrates or peptone, producing succinic, lactic, acetic, formic, and propionic acid, but not butyric acid, as major products. *Bacteroides* are normal inhabitants of the human oral, respiratory, intestinal, and urogenital cavities. Indeed, *Bacteroides* species predominate numerically in the colons of many humans and animals. Some species are potential pathogens, causing a variety of life-threatening infections including bacteremias and abscesses in all regions of the body. More than 20 species have been described. Identification is based on morphology, biochemical characteristics, fluorescence, and susceptibility to antibacterial agents.

B. corrodens, a species that produces colonies on agar media that lie in surface depressions. It is probably a normal inhabitant of the mucous membranes of humans and animals.

B. fragilis, a species that consists of a group of closely related gram-negative, nonsporulating, strictly anaerobic bacilli containing five species, four of which had previously been regarded as subspecies of *B. fragilis: B. vulgatus, B. distasonis, B. ovatus,* and *B. thetaiotamicron.* Collectively, they are the most commonly encountered anaerobic bacteria in clinical specimens. It is the numerically dominant species (group) in the normal colon microflora of persons on a protein diet, but is also present normally in the throat and vaginal tract.

B. fragilis itself is the most important anaerobic species causing human infection, followed by *B. thetaiotamicron.* It is most frequently implicated in intraabdominal infections, but is also encountered in many other sites on and in the body. *B. fragilis* is more resistant to antibiotics than any other anaerobe, but is usually sensitive to clindamycin, chloramphenicol, and metronidazole.

B. funduliformis, see *F. necrophorum* under *Fusobacterium.*

B. melaninogenicus, a species having the distinctive property of producing colonies that are brown to black in color on laked blood agar. It consists of three subspecies, *melaninogenicus, intermedius,* and *asaccharolyticus.* This species is part of the normal flora of the mucous membranes and is an important pathogen in oral, pulmonary, and soft tissue infections, as well as brain abscesses. It is susceptible to penicillin. Both vitamin K and hemin are required for growth by most strains; hemin is also a prerequisite for the development of the characteristic brown pigment (hematin).

bacteroides (bak″tĕ-roi′dēz) a member of the genus *Bacteroides.*

bacteruria (bak″te-ru′re-ah) see *bacteriuria.*

Bactrim (bak′trim) trademark for a combination of *sulfamethoxazole* and *trimethoprim.*

BAEP abbrev. for brain stem auditory evoked potential. See *brain stem auditory e. p.* under *evoked potential.*

bagassosis (bag″ah-so′sis) [Fr. *bagasse* + *-osis*] a respiratory disorder caused by inhaling the dust of bagasse, the waste product left after the sugar has been removed from sugar cane. It is one of the pneumoconioses. See also *pneumoconiosis.*

bag-box circuit a spirometer circuit used in pulmonary function tests that consists of a Neoprene balloon suspended within a sealed tank connected to a spirometer. The individual either inspires from a mixture of gases in the balloon or, if expired gas samples are to be collected, inhales from the tank and exhales into the balloon. Tidal volume can be recorded with the spirometer even when gases are inhaled or exhaled from the balloon, because the box surrounding the balloon is connected to the spirometer. Bag-box circuits are used in pulmonary function tests in which a mixture of inspired gases with a composition radically different from that of atmospheric air is used, or in which the gases used are soluble in the water jacket of the more conventional spirometer. This spirometer circuit can be used in both single-breath and steady-state breathing experiments.

Baker's acid hematein test (ba'kerz) [John Randal *Baker,* English zoologist, born 1900] a histologic procedure for demonstrating phosphoglycerides that is generally used for, but probably is not specific for, phospholipids. It yields dark blue to blue-black phospholipids, blue-black to pale blue galactolipids (from the brain), and brown or dark to pale blue mucin.

Baker's cyst [William Morrant *Baker,* British surgeon, 1839–1896] a cystic swelling in the popliteal space produced by herniation of the synovial membrane of the knee joint. Any condition that gives rise to increased intraarticular pressure, such as degenerative joint disease, can predispose to its development. Untreated, this cyst may grow in size to 10 cm or larger, and can insinuate into the soft tissues and muscles of the upper calf. It has a fibrous wall, usually lined by synovium, and contains mucoid fluid. Treatment is simple excision.

Baker's formol calcium [John Randal *Baker*] a histologic fixative used to preserve lipids, especially phospholipids. Tissue specimens can be stored in the same fluid.

Baker's pyridine extraction test [J. R. *Baker*] a histologic method to remove phospholipids. Extracted and nonextracted tissues are stained with Baker's acid hematein or Sudan black B to verify the presence of phospholipids.

Baker's Sudan black method [J. R. *Baker*] a staining procedure used to demonstrate the presence of Golgi bodies in cells. In the procedure, formalin-fixed tissue is chromated in potassium dichromate. After being infiltrated with gelatin and embedded, blocks are hardened in formalin and cut on a freezing microtome. Sections are stained in Sudan black B, washed briefly in alcohol, and counterstained with alum carmine. Solid Golgi bodies and neutral fats appear dark blue; chromatin, red to pink; cytoplasm, pale gray-blue; and Golgi vacuoles, colorless.

BAL abbrev. for British anti-Lewisite. See *dimercaprol.*

Balamuth buffer solution (bal'a-mūth) a solution used in Balamuth medium consisting of K_2HPO_4 and distilled water.

Balamuth culture medium a monophasic culture medium used to grow *Entamoeba histolytica* or other intestinal amebae. It consists of dehydrated egg yolk, distilled water, and saline, which are heated until coagulation occurs and then filtered. After autoclaving and chilling, the medium is filtered again through a Buchner funnel, and Balamuth buffer solution is added. Liver extract may or may not be added. The medium is then placed in tubes and reautoclaved, after which it may be inoculated with fresh stool, obtained via enema, proctoscopic aspirate, or saline-cleaned specimen. Incubation is at 37°C. Unused media should be refrigerated and may be kept for about 1 mo.

balan/o (bal'ah-no) [Gr. *balanos* an acorn] a word element used in combining form to denote the glans penis or glans clitoridis, e.g., balanoposthitis.

balance (bal'ans) [L. *bilanx*] 1. an instrument for weighing.

2. the harmonious adjustment or performance of functions. In physiology, for example, the term refers to a condition in which the input and output rates of some component are equal for a given period of time.

negative b., in physiology, the condition resulting when the output of a particular component is greater than the input; thus, the overall rate of gain is negative. Cf. *positive b.*

positive b., in physiology, the condition resulting when the input of a particular component is greater than the output; thus, the overall rate of gain is positive. Cf. *negative b.*

balance account a detailed description of all intake plus production (input) and all excretion plus metabolic conversion (output) of a component or components over a given period of time.

balanitis (bal″ah-ni'tis) [*balano-* + *-itis*] a general term for an inflammation of the glans penis, most often due to infection by *Trichomonas vaginalis,* herpes simplex virus, or *Chlamydia trachomatis* (TRIC agents).

balanoposthitis (bal″ah-no-pos-thi'tis) [*balano-* + Gr. *posthē* prepuce + *-itis*] a general term for an inflammation of the glans penis and prepuce in an uncircumcised male. The condition is characterized by soreness, irritation, and discharge, and may be due to a number of infectious agents such as *Neisseria gonorrhoeae, Candida albicans,* and herpes simplex virus, or it may be due to contact dermatitis, psoriasis, or an allergic drug reaction. Diabetes mellitus is a predisposing cause for *Candida* infection. Complications include phimosis.

Laboratory analysis should include testing for sexually transmitted diseases, cultures of the discharge, and urinary glucose testing to detect diabetes. Treatment is directed at the underlying disorder.

Cf. *balanitis* and *sexually transmitted diseases.*

balantidiasis (bal″an-tĭ-di'ah-sis) [Gr. *balantidion* little bag + *-iasis*] an infection with the ciliated intestinal protozoan *Balantidium coli.* It results from ingestion of cysts that have come from stools of the carriers, which include rats, swine, and humans. The organism invades the mucosa and submucosa of the terminal ileum and colon, producing abscesses and ulcerations. Persons affected may be asymptomatic or have alternating episodes of constipation and diarrhea. Occasionally, severe dysentery may result, with bloody stools and colic; rarely, there is fatal intestinal perforation.

Diagnosis is based on identification of trophozoites or cysts in stools; repeated attempts may be required for identification. Tetracycline or diiodohydroxyquin is the treatment of choice.

See also *B. coli* under *Balantidium.*

Balantidium (bal″an-tid'e-um) [Gr. *balantidion* little bag] a genus of ciliated protozoa of the class Ciliata, which are parasitic in the digestive tract of invertebrates and vertebrates.

B. coli, a species that is the largest protozoon parasite of humans; in its trophozoite form, it is 50–200 μ long by 40–70 μ wide. A round, deeply staining micronucleus lies in the inner curvature of the narrow, bean-shaped macronucleus. Trophozoites feed on the bacteria and mucus of the lumen or the cells of the intestinal wall of the large intestine, and ulcers form as they burrow into tissue and establish colonies. Individual trophozoites encyst as fecal material undergoes dehydration. Infection usually occurs through the exposure of an individual to contaminated feces. Diagnosis is made by demonstrating the presence of the parasite in the feces. Also called *Holophyra coli* and *Paramecium coli.*

Balbiani chromosome (bal-be-ah′ne) [Edouard Gérard *Balbiani,* French embryologist, 1823–1899] see *polytene chromosome.*

Balbiani ring [Edouard Gérard *Balbiani*] a puffed section of a polytene chromosome, considered the site of RNA transcription. Because the chromonemata may be spun laterally in a series of loops, it gives the appearance of a portion of a lampbrush chromosome.

baldness (bawld′nes) see *alopecia.*

ball (bawl) a more or less spherical mass.

ballismus (bah-liz′mus) [Gr. *ballismos* a jumping about, dancing] violent flinging movements of the limbs, often affecting only one side of the body (hemiballismus).

ballistocardiogram (BCG) (bah-lis″to-kar′de-o-gram″) the record obtained by ballistocardiography.

ballistocardiography (bah-lis″to-kar″de-og′rah-fe) a noninvasive technique used to measure the recoil movements of the body that result from the motion of the blood within it. This movement varies according to the cardiac output and myocardial performance, as it is determined primarily by the acceleration given to the blood upon ejection from the left ventricle.

Because of the technical difficulties inherent in the accurate measurement of such a complex variable, ballistocardiography is not an extensively used diagnostic technique and is being supplanted by newer diagnostic methods.

ballooning degeneration (bah-lo͞on′ing) a form of cell degeneration in which influx of fluid causes swelling and vacuolation of the cytoplasm.

balsam (bawl′sam) [L. *balsamum;* Gr. *balsamon;* Hebrew *basam* spice] a resinous, fragrant, gummy mixture that contains oils, resins, terpenes, and usually cinnamic and benzoic acids. See also *Canada balsam* and *Peruvian balsam.*

Bancroft's filarial worm (ban′krofts) [Joseph *Bancroft,* English physician in Australia, 1836–1894] see *W. bancroft* under *Wuchereria.*

Bancroft's filariasis [Joseph *Bancroft*] infection with the filarial worm *Wuchereria bancrofti,* the adults of which reside in the lymphatic system, producing recurrent lymphangitis with fibrosis and obstruction. In extensive obstruction, chronic edema may result, progressing to elephantiasis.

Human infection is transmitted by bloodsucking mosquitoes of the genera *Anopheles, Culex, Mansonia,* and *Aedes.* Infective larvae are introduced into humans during blood meals of the mosquito; they develop into mature adults in the lymphatics (especially those of the abdominal cavity), causing inflammatory reactions and progressive obstruction of the lymphatic channels by scar tissue. The mature females liberate sheathed microfilariae that migrate through the lymph and circulatory system; these enter the mosquitoes as they feed and mature into infective larvae.

Laboratory diagnosis requires identification of microfilariae from blood films. *Wuchereria* infections are characterized by sheathed microfilariae (measuring 244–296 μm), with graceful sweeping curves and a tail tapering to a delicate point (terminal nuclei are absent). There are two biologically different forms: night-biting *Culex pipiens fatigans* and various species of *Anopheles* are the main vectors of the nocturnal periodic form of the microfilariae, and day-biting *Aedes polynesiensis* transmits the subperiodic form of the microfilariae in various Pacific islands.

See also *elephantiasis.* Cf. *Malayan filariaris.*

band [band] 1. a strip that binds or constricts a part.

2. a range of definitely limited electromagnetc frequencies.

3. transverse zones across an elongated structure, produced by a symmetric arrangement of the component molecules, as in myofibrils and collagen fibrils. See also *collagen* and *myofibril.*

band cell a slightly immature, "young" neutrophil characterized by a nucleus that is not segmented but forms a continuous band. Normally, less than 5 percent of neutrophils in the peripheral blood are "bands." Increased numbers (a shift to the left) indicate increased granulocytopoiesis, usually due to bacterial infections or inflammatory disease (see *Arneth count*). Lesser degrees of notching of the band nucleus, indicating the beginning of segmentation, make classification of bands somewhat subjective, with some laboratories reporting "nonfilament" counts (up to 16 percent in normals) instead, because the absence of filaments between lobes of the polymorphonuclear leukocyte is more easily determined. Also called *band form* and *band neutrophil.*

band form see *band cell.*

band neutrophil see *band cell.*

bandpass (band′pas) the range of frequencies passed by a filter or of wavelengths of light used by a spectrophotometer or colorimeter; specifically, the range in which the intensity (transmittance) is at least one-half the peak value. Also called *bandwidth* and *half bandwith.*

bandpass filter a filter that transmits a certain portion of the spectrum of energies. All other parts of the spectrum are blocked, or at least attenuated.

band spectrum an absorption or emission spectrum that contains groups of spectral lines too closely spaced to be resolved by the spectrophotometer being used. Each unresolved group of lines is thus seen as a band or peak.

All substances except rarefied gases of atoms or simple molecules exhibit band spectra because of interactions between molecules or between parts of the same molecule, which split the energy levels for each electronic orbital or rotational or vibrational mode into many closely spaced levels.

bandwidth (band′width) see *bandpass.*

Banti's disease (ban′tēz) [Guido *Banti,* Italian pathologist, 1852–1925] a term formerly used for a syndrome characterized by congestive splenomegaly, leukopenia, and anemia.

BAO abbrev. See *basal acid output.*

bar (bahr) a unit of pressure defined as 1 million

dynes per square centimeter, which is equal to 100 kilopascals (kPa).

baragnosis (bar″ag-no′sis) [Gr. *baros* weight + *a-* neg. + *gnōsis* knowledge] loss or impairment of the ability to perceive differences in weight or pressure.

barber's itch (bahr′berz) see *tinea barbae.*

barbital (bar′bĭ-tal) a barbiturate used in some sedative preparations. Barbital is commonly employed in clinical chemistry and histology as a buffer for the pH range of 7–9; the maximal buffer capacity is at pH 8.

barbiturate (bar-bit′u-rāt, bar″bĭ-tūr′āt) any one of the drugs derived from barbituric acid or thiobarbituric acid. All produce central nervous system depression by interfering with oxygen consumption in the brain and other tissues. Increasing dosages produce first sedation, then sleep, and then anesthesia; overdoses may produce respiratory and renal failure, shock, coma, and death. Alcohol and other depressants potentiate these effects. All are habit-forming and most are subject to federal narcotics control.

Barbiturates are classed by their clearance time as long-, intermediate-, short-, or ultrashort-acting. The last group is used as basal and general anesthetics, e.g., thiopental. Many of the intermediate- and short-acting barbiturates are used alone or in combination with other drugs as sedatives or sleeping pills.

Phenobarbital, mephobarbital, or metharbital is used to control epileptic seizures; phenobarbital (and mephobarbital, which is metabolized to phenobarbital) for generalized tonic-clonic and cortical focal seizures, especially in children; and metharbital for infantile myoclonic spasms. Several barbiturates are used to control convulsions due to poisoning or drug overdose.

Barbiturates can induce changes in the electroencephalogram (EEG). Such changes are characterized by spindles in the beta (>13/Hz) frequency and usually have a range of 18–24 Hz. In normal individuals, this activity is symmetric and located frontocentrally. Accompanying the increase in beta activity, there may be changes in electric activity associated with sleep. With barbiturate overdose, the EEG may be characterized by a suppression-burst pattern or electrocerebral silence, depending on the dose taken. Asymmetry in barbiturate-induced beta activity may indicate localized cerebral disease or damage.

barbiturate assays 1. ultraviolet spectrophotometry. Barbiturates are extracted as weak acids from blood, serum, urine, or gastric contents at pH 6.5 into methylene chloride and then extracted back into alkaline aqueous solution. Barbiturates have a characteristic absorption spectrum. The non-ionized form in acid solution has almost no absorption between 230 and 270 nm; the first ionized form at pH 9.8–10.5 has an absorption maximum at 240 nm; and the second ionized form at pH 13–14 has an absorption maximum at 252–255 nm and a minimum at 234–237 nm. *N*-Methylbarbiturates, e.g., mephobarbital, have no second ionized form. The barbiturate concentration is determined from the differences in the absorbance at 260 nm of the first and second ionized forms.

2. immunoassay, EMIT homogeneous enzyme immunoassay, or radioimmunoassay for barbiturates in urine. These are used for suspected drug abuse or drug overdose monitoring. EMIT is also used for monitoring serum phenobarbital therapeutic drug levels.

3. gas chromatography. Barbiturates are extracted as above and *N*-methylated with trimethylanilinium hydroxide (TMAH). The different barbiturates are quantitated relative to an internal standard (e.g., aprobarbital) by gas chromatography, using a nonpolar silicone stationary phase and a flame ionization detector. The sensitivity of this procedure is about 0.1 mg/dl.

4. colorimetric test. Barbiturates complex with mercury(II), and the complex can be extracted into chloroform. Diphenylthiocarbazone is added, and turns from green to orange if these drugs are present at concentrations greater than approximately 1 mg/dl.

barium (Ba) (ba′re-um) [L., from Gr. *baros* weight] a pale yellowish or silvery-white metallic element; atomic number 56; atomic weight 137.34; Group II of the periodic table (the alkaline earths); oxidation state +2. Soluble salts are poisonous, causing gastrointestinal distress, muscular paralysis, decreased pulse rate, and cardiac arrhythmias; insoluble salts, such as barium sulfate, are not toxic.

b. sulfate, [USP], a white powder, $BaSO_4$, odorless and tasteless; used in the radiographic examination of the digestive tract. It is administered orally or by enema.

barium test see under *gastrointestinal series.*

barn (barn) [from "big as a barn"] a unit of area, 10^{-24} cm^2, used to measure absorption or scattering cross sections in nuclear physics. It is approximately the thermal neutron capture cross section of a copper nucleus.

Barnett-Bourne acetic alcohol–silver nitrate (bahr-net′boorn) a histologic fixative used in demonstrating vitamin C, bile pigment in liver tissue, or hemorrhagic infarcts.

barometer (bah-rom′ĕ-ter) [Gr. *baros* weight + *metron* measure] an instrument that measures atmospheric pressure. A mercury barometer indicates the pressure by the height of a column of mercury, the weight of the column per unit cross-sectional area being equal to the atmospheric pressure. An aneroid barometer indicates the pressure by the expansion or contraction of an aneroid capsule, a thin-walled, disk-shaped, partially evacuated box.

barometric pressure (bar″o-met′rik) the pressure exerted by the atmosphere on a surface.

baroreceptor (bar″o-re-sep′tor) a group of fine sensory nerve endings, usually found in the wall of a vessel. When stimulated by stretching, baroreceptors convey information on changes in pressure within the vessel.

baroreflex (bar″o-re′fleks) see *baroreceptor r.* under *reflex.*

barosinusitis (bar″o-si″nū-si′tis) a symptom complex due to differences in environmental atmospheric pressure and the air pressure in the paranasal sinuses.

Barr body (bahr) [Murray Llewellyn *Barr,* Canadian anatomist, born 1908] a small mass of intensely staining chromatin seen in the nucleus of the female cell during interphase. Variably shaped, it is adjacent to the inner surface of the nuclear membrane. The number of Barr bodies is always one less than the number of X chromosomes: one in the normal female and XXY (Klinefelter's syndrome) male; zero in the normal male or XO (Turner's syndrome) female; and two in the XXX (superfemale) female. The X chromosomes do not replicate simultaneously, and the X chromosome that forms the Barr body replicates late.

Barr body test [Murray Llewellyn *Barr*] a procedure to determine the presence or absence of Barr bodies in cells for assessment of the number of X chromosomes in the karyotype (the number of Barr bodies is one less than the number of X chromosomes). This test has been largely supplanted by the performance of karyotyping, as structurally abnormal X chromosomes (causing abnormalities of sexual differentiation) give nearly normal Barr bodies.

barreling distortion (bar′el-ing) a distortion of scintillation camera images resembling the distortion produced by a point source when the source is placed too close (less than 1m) to the detector in transmission phantom imaging of bar patterns; the images of the bars are curved like barrel staves.

Barrett's epithelium (bar′ets) [N. R. *Barrett,* English surgeon, born 1903] a type of heterotopic columnar epithelium that replaces the normal squamous epithelium of the esophagus. It is associated with peptic ulceration, inflammation, and stricture and an increased risk of development of esophageal adenocarcinoma. Radiography, esophagoscopy, and biopsy are useful in establishing the diagnosis and should be used in conjunction with cytologic examination to monitor the patient for the possible development of cancer.

Barrett's esophagus the occurrence of gastrointestinal-type columnar epithelium (Barrett's epithelium) within the esophagus.

barrier-layer cell see under *photocell.*

Barrnett-Seligman dihydroxydinaphthyl disulfide (DDD) method (bar-net′ se′lig-man) a histologic procedure for demonstrating sulfhydryl and disulfide groups. The sites of reaction stain according to the intensity of the reaction from weak (pink) to medium (red or blue-red) to strong (blue).

Barrnett-Seligman indoxyl esterase method a histologic method for demonstrating nonspecific esterase, lipase, and cholinesterase by producing indigo on hydrolysis in the presence of air.

Barroso-Moguel and Costero silver method (bar-o′so mo-gel′ kos-ter′o) a histologic procedure used on tissue from carotid body tumors to demonstrate argentaffin cells, which turn black. All other structures are pale purple. It is not thought to be specific enough for regular use.

Bart's hemoglobin (Hb Barts) (bahrts) an abnormal hemoglobin, composed of four gamma chains, that results from a reduction of alpha-chain synthesis with an increased production of beta chains. The hemoglobin has a very high oxygen affinity, which prevents effective oxygen delivery. Most normal newborn infants have levels of less than 0.5 percent of Bart's hemoglobin. In the heterozygous state, hematologic changes are extremely mild, whereas the homozygous state (the absence of alpha chains) is incompatible with life beyond the fetal stage (hydrops fetalis). See also *hemoglobin* and *thalassemia.*

bartholin/o (bar′to-lin-o) a word element used in combining form to denote Bartholin's glands, e.g., bartholinitis.

Bartholin's cyst (bar′to-linz) [Caspar Thomèson *Bartholin,* Jr., Danish anatomist, 1655–1738] a small, round mass found in the labium minus, caused by blockage of the excretory ducts of Bartholin's glands. It is a common condition that can occur at any age and is quite painful. The cyst is filled with a mucinous secretion, unless complicated by a secondary infection, in which event the cyst becomes filled with pus.

Bartholin's glands [Capsar Thomèson *Bartholin,* Jr.] paired glands found in the lateral walls of the vestibule. They open on the inner surface of the labia minora on either side of the vaginal opening, and secrete a lubricating mucus.

bartholinitis (bar″to-lin-i′tis) [*Bartholin* + *-itis*] inflammation of the Bartholin glands.

Bartonella (bar″to-nel′ah) [A. L. *Barton,* Peruvian physician, 1871–1950] a genus of bacteria in the family *Bartonellaceae.* The genus contains a single species, *B. bacilliformis.*

B. bacilliformis, the only species in the *Bartonella* genus. This small aerobic coccobacillus is found in and on human erythrocytes and in the cytoplasm of fixed tissue cells. It is also found in the tissues of sandflies of the genus *Phlebotomus* but does not occur in nonhuman vertebrates. *B. bacilliformis* is stained weakly by aniline dyes (but is gram-negative); it is well visualized by the Giemsa stain. Unlike malarial parasites, it shows a rigid cell and is motile by means of polar flagella. *B. bacilliformis* can be grown in cell-free media. A human pathogen, it is the cause of bartonellosis.

Bartonellaceae (bar″to-nel-a′se-e) [A.L. *Barton*] a family of polymorphic, gram-negative bacteria of the Rickettsiales that is parasitic in or on the erythrocytes of humans and other vertebrates. It includes two genera, *Bartonella* and *Grahamella.*

bartonellosis (bahr″to-nel-o′sis) an infection by *Bartonella bacilliformis.* It has two distinctly different clinical manifestations, which occur as sequential stages of one infection. These are Oroya fever, a severe febrile hemolytic anemia, and verruga peruana, a benign skin eruption of hemangioma-like nodules. The geographic distribution of bartonellosis is restricted primarily to Colombia, Peru, and Ecuador. Sandflies are the vector. Penicillin, streptomycin, and chloramphenicol are antibiotics effective in the treatment of bartonellosis. Also called *Carrión's disease, Oroya fever,* and *verruga peruana.*

Bartter's syndrome (bahrt′erz) [Frederic C. *Bartter,* U.S. physiologist, born 1914] a syndrome of secondary hyperaldosteronism occurring most frequently in children and adolescents. It is due to increased production of renin, with juxtaglomerular cell hyperplasia and hypokalemia. Edema and hypertension are absent, and a tendency to hyponatremia due to salt wastage may be present.

bas/o (ba′so) a word element used in combining form to denote a base or foundation, e.g., basophil.

basal (ba′sal) referring to or located near a base. The term is sometimes used specifically to refer to the minimal level at which the essential life activities of an organism can be continued. In histology it refers to the lowest layer of cells in an epithelium.

basal acid output (BAO) the rate of acid secretion (millimoles of titratable acidity per hour) by the stomach in the basal condition (with the individual at rest, fasting, and calm). See also *gastric function tests.*

basal body a modified centriole that serves as the base of a cilium or flagellum. It differs from a centriole in being closed by a basal plate at the end from which the cilium grows. Also called *basal granule, blepharoplast,* and *kinetosome.*

basal cell a cell located at the base of stratified squamous or pseudostratified epithelium, resting on the basal lamina.

basal cell carcinoma a skin neoplasm, common on sun-exposed areas, that arises from the epidermis of hair-bearing skin. Histologically, the cells are similar to those of the basal layer of the epidermis. They form compact nests of hyperchromatic cells, and may display a tubular or cystic architecture or contain foci of squamous differentiation. The neoplasm is common in individuals with xeroderma pigmentosum, and in those with the nevoid basal cell carcinoma syndrome. Basal cell carcinomas rarely metastasize but can infiltrate aggressively; depending on their location, they may recur and may be difficult to eradicate. Also called basal cell epithelioma.

basal cell nevus syndrome a condition, transmitted as an autosomal dominant trait, that is characterized by the occurrence in childhood of multiple basal cell carcinomas associated with abnormalities of bone (including jaw cysts), eyes, nervous system (medulloblastoma), and reproductive system. Also called nevoid basal cell carcinoma syndrome.

basal feet dense bundles of microfilaments that are arranged perpendicular to the basal body of a cilium. Their particular orientation imposes a structural asymmetry on the basal body that may be related to the direction of the ciliary beat.

basal ganglia the large masses of gray matter buried in the central white matter core of the cerebral hemisphere. The components are the amygdaloid complex, the claustrum, and the corpus striatum, which include the caudate and lentiform nuclei. Also called the *basal nuclei.*

basal granule see *basal body.*

basal lamina an electron-dense filamentous sheet on which epithelial cells rest. Although commonly thought of as synonymous with the basement membrane, it is more precisely a component of that membrane. The basal lamina is 50–100 nm thick and contains glycoproteins similar to those of collagen, as well as some glycosaminoglycans. It appears to be formed by the epithelial cells, and an intact basal lamina is necessary to preserve the architecture of the epithelium during regeneration. Basal laminae of epithelial and endothelial cells in the pulmonary alveolus and renal glomerulus fuse to form a combined diffusion barrier. A basal lamina may also be seen around muscle cells and Schwann cells.

2. that part of the gray matter in the neural tube of embryos that later develops into the motor neurons.

basal metabolic rate (BMR) the rate of energy utilization (in kilocalories per hour, kcal/hr) in a subject under basal conditions: absolute rest (relaxed but awake, recumbent, minimal psychic or physical stimulation), and in the postabsorptive state.

basal metabolic rate test a test measuring the oxygen consumption by a patient over a period of 2–6 min under basal conditions, i.e., postabsorptive state, recumbent, awake, and relaxed. This test was formerly much used to diagnose possible abnormalities in thyroid function, values obtained being raised in hyperthyroid and depressed in hypothyroid states. Because of technical difficulties in doing the test and because many extraneous factors affect the results obtained, its use as a thyroid function test has been replaced by other tests.

basal metabolism (BM) that process of energy exchange in a human or an animal measured by heat loss during a postabsorptive period when the individual is in the resting state. It reflects the energy requirements of those cellular and tissue processes associated with vital activities of the resting organism, e.g., the metabolic activity of the brain, muscle, kidneys, liver, and other cells, plus the heat released as a result of the mechanical work represented by the contraction of the muscles involved in respiration, circulation, and peristalsis.

The basal metabolism is not the minimal degree of metabolism necessary for mere maintenance of life, since during the sleep state the metabolic rate may be lower than that in the basal state.

See also *basal metabolic rate.*

basal nuclei see *basal ganglia.*

basal plate 1. parachordal cartilage, embryologic precursor of part of the base of the occipital bone.

2. the ventral portion of the embryonal neural tube that forms the motor nuclei of the brain stem and spinal cord.

basal projection a radiologic projection of the base of the skull in which the central ray is perpendicular to the infraorbitomeatal line. Also called full basal projection. See also *Schüller position.* Cf. *subbasal projection.*

base (bās) [L., Gr. *basis*] 1. the lowest part or foundation of anything; see also *basis.*

2. the main ingredient of a preparation.

3. in chemistry, a species that yields hydroxide ions when dissolved in water, e.g., NaOH (Arrhenius definition); a species that can combine with a proton, e.g., NH_3 (Bronsted definition); and a species (molecule or ion) that can donate a pair of electrons to form a bond with an acid, e.g., $CaO + SO_3 \rightarrow CaSO_4$ (Lewis definition).

4. one of the terminals of a junction transistor or unijunction transistor.

5. the insulator at the bottom of a vacuum tube that supports the electrodes, pins, and envelope.

6. the insulator that supports the circuit of a printed circuit board.

7. the radix of a number system. See under *number system.*

8. (symbol b), a unit of length of single-stranded nucleic acid molecules defined as one nucleotide residue. Cf. *base pair.*

purine and pyrimidine b.'s, nitrogenous heterocyclic compounds occurring naturally as constituents of nucleic acids and purine and pyrimidine nucleotides and nucleosides. The structures of major bases are shown in the accompanying illustration; some two dozen modified bases, known to occur in various transfer RNAs, are not shown. For metabolic products of the bases, see under *purine* and *pyrimidine.*

Basedow's disease (bas'e-dōz) [Carl Adolph von *Basedow,* German physician, 1799–1854] see *Graves' disease.*

base excess (BE) the amount of strong acid or base (measured in millimoles) that is necessary to titrate

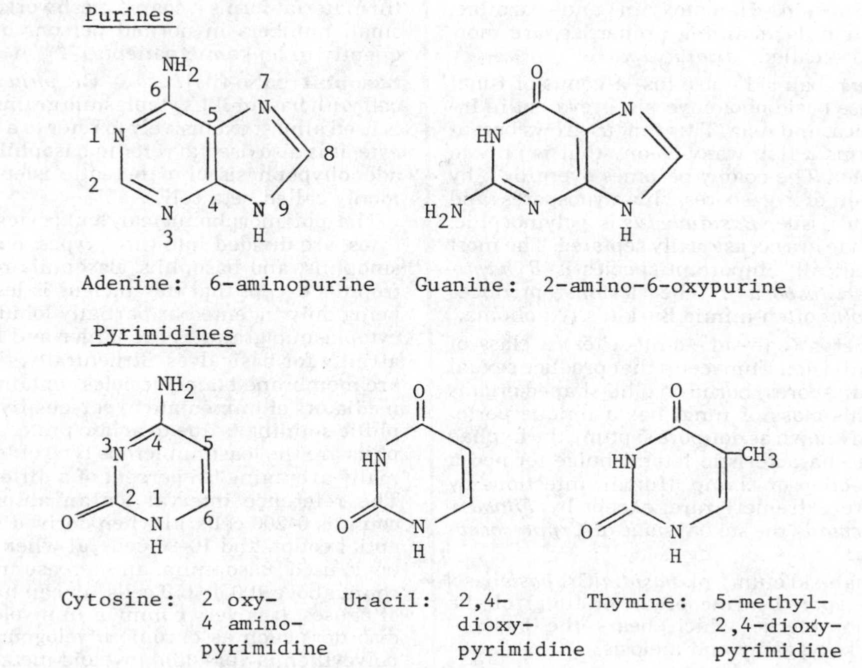

Purine and pyrimidine bases. Chemical structures for adenine, guanine, cytosine, uracil, and thymine. (From Bhagavan, N. V.: Biochemistry. 2nd ed. Philadelphia, J. B. Lippincott Co., 1978.)

a 1-l sample of whole arterial blood to a pH of 7.4 and thus to restore its normal acid-base balance. The sample is fully saturated with O_2 and held at 37°C and a P_{CO_2} of 40 mmHg (by equilibration) throughout the titration. The base excess, negative in acidosis and positive in alkalosis, can be read from the Siggaard-Andersen alignment nomogram as the point of intersection of the base excess line and the line connecting the measured pH and P_{CO_2} values, taking the hemoglobin concentration into account. The reference range for normal adults is +3 to –3 mmol/l.

base ionization constant (K_b) the equilibrium constant for the protonation of a base in water. The expression is $K_b = [BH^+][OH^-]/[B]$, where brackets denote concentration or activity, BH^+ is the protonated base, and B is the free base.

baseline (bās′līn) 1. a known value or quantity in comparison with which an unknown is measured or assessed, such as a baseline urine sample. In continuous-flow types of automated analysis, the term refers to the absorbance of the reagent solutions when all contaminants have been removed that absorb light at the measured wavelength.

2. the horizontal axis of a graph.

3. a DC voltage level that is treated as the zero level of an electric signal.

4. with reference to an electric signal of biologic origin, the voltage that is recorded when the system is in the resting state.

baseline steady state in an AutoAnalyzer, the transmittance reading produced during normal operation with no standards, controls, or unknowns being aspirated, and any reaction product from previous samples having been washed out.

basement membrane the thin, continuous layer at the base of epithelia that can be demonstrated by light microscopy with periodic acid–Schiff or silver impregnation methods. See also *basal lamina.*

base pair (bp) a unit of length of double-stranded nucleic acid molecules defined as one nucleotide residue in each strand.

base pairing the term used in molecular biology to describe the pairing of nitrogenous bases in the polynucleotide chains by hydrogen bonds in a specific manner. The pairing occurs between a purine base of one strand and a pyrimidine base of another strand in DNA, RNA, and DNA/RNA hybrid molecules. In DNA the complementary base pairs are adenine with thymine and guanine with cytosine. In RNA, the pairs are adenine with uracil and guanine with cytosine. See also *nucleic acid.*

base ratio see *AT/GC ratio.*

BASIC (ba′sik) a high-level but easy-to-learn computer language that has immediate syntax correction when a program line is entered. Enhanced and extended versions are available that allow efficient programming for many scientific and business applications. BASIC is offered as both a compiled and an interpreted language.

basic (ba′sik) 1. pertaining to or having the properties of a base.

2. capable of neutralizing acids.

basic anhydride a metal oxide that reacts with water to form a hydroxide, e.g., calcium oxide (CaO).

basic dye a dye in which the colored substance is cationic and forms salts with anionic tissue constituents, e.g., nucleic acids and acid mucopolysaccharides. Examples are methylene blue, toluidine blue, and basic fuchsin. Hematoxylin and carmine, which have similar staining properties, are mordant dyes. Also called *cationic dye.*

Basidiobolus (bah-sid″ĭ-ob′o-lus) a genus of fungi that can cause basidiobolomycosis, prevalent in Indonesia, Africa, and Asia. This fungus grows best at 30°C and forms a flat, waxy colony that is gray to yellow in color. The colony becomes overgrown by the production of zygospores, chlamydospores, and sporangia. In tissue, *Basidiobolus* is polymorphic, and the hyphae are occasionally septated. The most common medically important species is *B. haptosporus* (*meristosporus*). The lesions produces by *Basidiobolus* often mimic Burkitt's lymphoma.

Basidiomycetes (bah-sid″e-o-mi-se′tēz) a class of fungi of the division Eumycetes that produce sexual spores (basidiospores) borne on club-shaped organs (basidia). This class of fungi has a unique perforated septum known as dolipore septum; the hyphae often bear a characteristic lateral bulge termed a clamp connection or clamp. Human infections by this class are extremely rare, except by *Filobasidiella neoformans,* the sexual stage of *Cryptococcus neoformans.*

basidium (bah-sid′e-um), pl. *basidia* [Gr. *basis* base] the clublike spore-bearing organ of fungi of the class Basidiomycetes, which bears the basidiospores after karyogamy and meiosis.

basilar (bas′ĭ-lar) [L. *basilaris,* from *basis* base] pertaining to a base or basal part.

basilar artery the artery formed by the junction of the two vertebral arteries at the lower border of the pons. It divides at the upper border of the pons into the two posterior cerebral arteries.

basilar membrane the thin sheet of fibrous connective tissue that forms a partition along the length of the cochlear duct of the inner ear. It stretches from the tip of the osseous spiral lamina to the spiral ligament, and separates the scala media from the scala tympani. The organ of Corti rests on it.

basilic vein (bah-sil′ik) [L. *basilicus,* from Gr. *basilikos* royal] the vein that begins on the back of the hand and runs up the medial side of the forearm and upper arm to the lower border of teres major, from where it continues as the axillary vein.

basipetal (ba-sip′ĕ-tal) [L., from Gr. *basis* + L. *petere* to seek] descending toward the base; developing in the direction of the base, so that the lower part is the youngest, as a spore.

basis (ba′sis), pl. *bases* [L.; Gr.] 1. the lower, basic, or fundamental part of an object.

2. [NA], in anatomy, a general term used to designate the base of a structure or organ, or the part opposite to or distinguished from the apex.

basket (bas′ket) 1. a large axon terminal that covers a considerable area of the surface of the postsynaptic cell. Also called *calyx.*

2. a band of material with some resemblance to amyloid that is deposited on or within cortical neurons in presenile dementia. Also called neurofibrillary degeneration.

basket cell 1. a cell of the cerebellar cortex whose axons give off sprays of fine branches that enclose adjacent Purkinje cells in basketlike fashion.

2. see *myoepithelial cell.*

3. the nucleus of a ruptured or degenerated leukocyte as seen in a blood smear, in which the chromatin material forms a coarse meshwork. It is found in small numbers in normal persons and more frequently in leukemic patients.

basophil (ba′so-fil) [*baso-* + Gr. *philein* to love] any cell with basophilic cytoplasmic granules. The term is used almost exclusively to refer to a type of leukocyte; it is also used to refer to basophilic cells of the adenohypophysis or pancreatic islets (more commonly called beta cells).

The polymorphonuclear leukocytes, or granulocytes, are divided into three types: neutrophils, eosinophils, and basophils. Basophils resemble neutrophils except that the nucleus is less segmented, being only indented or partially lobulated, and the cytoplasmic granules are larger and have a strong affinity for basic dyes. Structurally, these granules are membrane-bound vesicles containing chemical mediators of immediate hypersensitivity. The basophilic staining is due to acidic proteoglycans. Basophils are the least numerous type of leukocyte, normally averaging 0.5 percent of a differential count. The reference interval for an absolute basophil count is 0–200 cells/μl when derived from a differential count, and 10–80 cells/μl when flow cytometry is used. Basophilia, an increase in the absolute count above 100 or 150 cells/μl, can have a number of causes. It is very common in myeloproliferative disorders such as chronic myelogenous leukemia, polycythemia vera, and myeloid metaplasia; it may also occur with many other disorders, including ulcerative colitis and varicella, and following the administration of drugs such as estrogens and antithyroid medications.

Basophils and mast cells (found in tissue) are two distinct cell types that have a similar physiologic role: they are involved in immediate hypersensitivity responses. Both have cell surface receptors for IgE. When bound IgE molecules are cross-linked by reaction with specific antigens, chemical mediators of immediate hypersensitivity are released, leading to clinical manifestations such as anaphylaxis, bronchial asthma, and urticaria.

Basophils and mast cells also respond to the activated complement components C3a and C5a, to basic lysosomal proteins released by neutrophils, and to at least one lymphokine and to several kinins; each probably acts by means of a specific cell surface receptor. Many mediators are released by basophils, including biogenic amines (histamine), acidic tetrapeptides (eosinophil chemotactic factors of anaphylaxis, ECF-A), prostaglandins and other products of arachidonic acid metabolism (slow-reacting substance of anaphylaxis, SRS-A; prostaglandin D_2, PGD_2; hydroxyheptadecatrienoic acid, HHT; and hydroxyeicosatetraenoic acid, HETE), a lipid (platelet-activating factor, PAF), and an acidic proteoglycan (heparin). Histamine, SRS-A, and PGD_2 induce smooth muscle contraction; histamine and SRS-A also increase vascular permeability. ECF-A, HETE, and HHT are all chemotactic for eosinophils. PAF causes platelet aggregation and the release of effector substances from platelets. Heparin is an anticoagulant. Histamine, heparin, and ECF-A are preformed substances stored in the granules for release. The others are synthesized when the basophil is stimulated during immediate hypersensitivity responses.

See also *eosinophil* and *neutrophil.*

basophil chemotactic factor (BCF) a lymphocyte-derived factor that is an attractant for basophils. It appears to be distinct from eosinophil chemotactic factors (ECF) and polymorphonuclear neutrophil chemotactic factor (NCF).

basophilia (ba″so-fil′e-ah) 1. having an affinity for basic dyes.

2. the reaction of immature erythrocytes to basic dyes. The degree of basophilia depends on the relative quantities of residual ribonucleic acid and hemoglobin in the cell cytoplasm. Reticulocytes normally exhibit no appreciable basophilia because residual RNA is minimal. Young reticulocytes released in accelerated (stimulated) erythropoiesis have varying degrees of basophilia recognizable in routine Giemsa-stained smears, the degree of basophilia reflecting the amount of residual RNA or "youthfulness" of the reticulocyte.

3. an increased number (above 50/mm^3) of basophils in the peripheral blood (basophil leukocytosis). This may occur in hypothyroidism, certain hypersensitivity reactions, and some myeloproliferative disorders and chronic infections.

basophilic (ba″so-fil′ik) staining readily with basic dyes.

basophilic erythroblast see basophilic normoblast under *normoblast.*

basophilic granular degeneration see *basophilic stippling.*

basophilic granule the characteristic granule of basophilic leukocytes. These granules stain blue-black and metachromatically with basic dyes (owing to the presence of mucopolysaccharides); brick red with toluidine blue, methyl violet, or methylene blue; and yellow with neutral red, safranine, or methylene azure. The granules are primary lysosomes that contain dehydrogenase, diaphorase, peroxidase, and other lysosomal enzymes.

In electron microscopy, they appear as dense, membrane-bound vesicles. Inclusions may appear as granules, lamellae, or crystalloids. In mast cells, the fine particles are arranged in parallel rows forming lamellae that curl back on themselves, sometimes in the shape of cylinders. Both mast cells and basophilic granules contain large amounts of histamine and heparin. The granules are readily soluble in water. After exposure to water or laser irradiation, crystals that differ from Charcot-Leyden crystals appear in basophils but not in mast cells.

basophilic leukocyte see *basophil.*

basophilic metamyelocyte an immature basophil in the metamyelocyte stage of development, containing dark purple granules that are more numerous than in the basophilic myelocyte.

basophilic myelocyte an immature basophil at the myelocytic stage of development.

basophilic normoblast see under *normoblast.*

basophilic stippling the presence of minute basophilic granules in reticulocytes. These granules vary widely in size and number, and are clumps of ribosomes that aggregate during the drying of reticulocytes in preparation of blood smears. Increased stippling is seen in lead poisoning, thalassemia, and other severe anemias, even in rapidly dried smears, presumably owing to the aggregation of RNA prior to preparation of the smear. Also called *basophilic granular degeneration.*

Bassen-Kornzweig syndrome (bas′en korn′zwīg) [Frank A. *Bassen,* U.S. physician, born 1903; Abraham L. *Kornzweig,* U.S. physician, born 1900] see *abetalipoproteinemia.*

batch processing (bach) in automatic data processing, a method of processing in which a group of programs and all of the required input data are submitted together and run on the computer without interaction with the user. Cf. *interactive processing.*

bath (bath) 1. the application of water or other medium to the body for cleansing or therapeutic purposes; see also *water bath.*

2. a piece of laboratory equipment or apparatus in which a body or object may be immersed.

bathochromic shift (bath′o-kro″mik) a shift in the absorption peak of a chromophore to a longer wavelength.

bathophenanthroline (bath″o-fen-an′thro-lēn) a histologic reagent utilized for the high molar absorptivity of its complex with iron, specifically Fe^{2+} ions. Iron stains red with this reagent.

Batten's disease (bat′enz) [Frederic Eustace *Batten,* English ophthalmologist, 1865–1918] see *juvenile amaurotic familial i.* under *idiocy.*

battery (bat′er-e) 1. any set, series, or grouping of similar things, such as a battery of tests.

2. a set of electrochemical cells, connected in series, that is used as a source of direct-current electric power; also a single cell used as a power source. A battery acts as a constant-voltage source in series with a resistance (the internal resistance); thus, the voltage drops as the current drain increases.

alkaline b., a battery similar to the carbon-zinc battery but having a higher capacity, longer shelf life, and lower internal resistance. The electrodes are zinc and manganese dioxide; the electrolyte is potassium hydroxide.

carbon-zinc b., the familiar flashlight battery. The electrodes are zinc and carbon; each cell develops 1.5 V.

mercury b., a battery with electrodes made from zinc amalgam and mercuric oxide–zinc. This type of battery is suitable for use as a voltage reference, because each cell produces exactly 1.35 V, and the voltage remains almost constant throughout the life of the battery.

nickel-cadmium b., a rechargeable battery with electrodes made from nickel hydroxide and cadmium when charged, and nickel and cadmium oxide when discharged. Each cell produces 1.3 V.

Battey bacillus (bat′e) [*Battey,* a tuberculosis hospital in Rome, Georgia] see *M. intracellulare* under *Mycobacterium.*

baud (bawd) [J. M. E. *Baudot,* French inventor, 1845–1903] a unit of data transmission defined as the number of code elements transmitted per second. For Morse code, it is the number of dots, dashes, and spaces per second; for binary signals, a baud equals 1 bit/sec.

Bauer reaction (bou′er) a variant of the periodic acid–Schiff reaction that uses chromic acid instead of periodic acid as the oxidizer. It was one of the first glycol-aldehyde oxidative reactions to be utilized in histochemistry and is the reaction used in the Gridley fungus stain.

Baumé's (hydrometer) scale (Bé) (bo-māz′) [Antoine *Baumé,* French chemist, 1728–1804] a scale for expressing the specific gravity of fluids. At 60°F, with fluids heavier than water, specific gravity =

145 ÷ 145 − n and for those lighter than water, specific gravity = 140 ÷ 130 + n (n = Baumé scale reading).

Baumgartner method (baum′gahrt-ner) see under *platelet adhesiveness test.*

Bayes's theorem a consequence of the definition of conditional probability: $P(B|A) = P(A|B)\,P(B)/P(A)$, where $P(A)$ and $P(B)$ are the conditional probabilities of two events, A and B, and $P(A|B)$ and $P(B|A)$ are the conditional probabilities of A given that B has occurred and of B given A.

In medicine, Bayes's theorem is used to determine the predictive value of a positive test result, $P(B|A)$, where B is the event "the person has disease," and A is the event "the person's test is positive." $P(B)$, the a priori probability that the person has disease, is the prevalence rate of the disease in the population to which the test is administered. $P(A)$, the probability of a positive test result, is given by the formula: $P(A) = P(A|B)P(B) + P(A|\text{not } B)\,P(\text{not } B)$, where $P(A|B)$ is the diagnostic sensitivity of the test, the probability of a correct test result for persons known to have disease; $P(\text{not } A|\text{not } B)$ is the diagnostic specificity of the test, the probability of a correct test result for persons known not to have disease; $P(\text{not } B) = 1 - P(B)$, and $P(A|\text{not } B) = 1 - P(\text{not } A|\text{not } B)$.

The predictive value of the test is the number that is useful to the clinician, whereas the diagnostic specifity and sensitivity are the numbers determined in clinical trials of the test. Moreover, the predictive value varies with the prevalence rate, which depends on the patient population seen by a particular clinic, and on the criteria for selecting patients for the test, e.g., whether the test is primarily for diagnosis or for screening. See also *sensitivity* and *susceptibility.*

BB abbrev. for the isoenzyme of creatine kinase that contains two B subunits. See under *creatine kinase isoenzymes.*

BCD abbrev. See *binary coded decimal.*

BCE abbrev. for basal cell epithelioma.

B cell see *B l.* under *lymphocyte.*

BCF abbrev. See *basophil chemotactic factor.*

BCG abbrev. See *bacille Calmette-Guérin, ballistocardiogram, bromocresol green.*

BCG vaccine a live but dried and attenuated preparation of bacille Calmette-Guérin, used widely throughout the world for active immunization against human tuberculosis. The vaccine is safe when properly prepared and administered; the immunity that follows is relative rather than solid. Intracutaneous or multiple puncture administration results in a local superficial ulceration lasting a few weeks; the individual becomes tuberculin-positive.

BE abbrev. for bacterial endocarditis (see under *endocarditis*), *barium enema* (see under *enema*), *base excess.*

Be symbol for the chemical element *beryllium.*

beaker (bēk′er) a common item of laboratory glassware, having the shape of a cylindrical cup, usually with a lip for pouring.

beam (bēm) a nearly unidirectional emission of electromagnetic or acoustic radiation or of particles. The production of an x-ray beam involves two processes: beam restriction (delimitation) and filtering. Beam restrictors (collimators, cones, or diaphragms) are lead or iron devices with adjustable apertures that limit the area of the beam. Filters are thin aluminum plates that absorb the softer (lower-energy) photons, increasing the penetrability of the beam and improving the radiographic contrast.

beam alignment adjustment of the electron beam of the cathode ray tube.

beam splitting the division of a light beam into two separate beams by placement of a stationary or rotating half-silvered mirror or prism in the optical path. In a double-beam spectrophotometer, this is used to direct one beam through the sample and one beam through the blank.

beat (bēt) a throb or pulsation, as of the heart or an artery. See also *pulse.*

Beauvaria (bo-var′e-ah) a genus of imperfect fungi, family Moniliaceae, order Moniliales. Common soil fungi, these organisms are often pathogenic for insects, especially beetles. The species *B. bassiana* was the first microorganism shown to be specifically responsible for a disease process, in 1835, producing muscardine in silkworms.

beauvariosis (bo-var″e-o′sis) a disease caused by organisms of the genus *Beauvaria,* which may attack the lungs.

Beaver direct smear method an egg-counting method used to estimate the worm burden from fecal specimens. This procedure is used primarily for the evaluation of hookworm, *Ascaris,* and *Trichuris* infections. The method is rapid and requires no correction for stool consistency, but it does call for a calibrated, photoelectric light meter.

In the procedure, a fecal sample is mixed with water or saline and stirred until a 1-mg preparation (determined by previous calibration) is obtained. The preparation is counted (in terms of eggs per milligrams of feces) and reported as a light or heavy infection, depending on the patient's age and condition, the bulk of the stool specimen, and the duration of the infection.

Becker's muscular dystrophy (bek′erz) an inherited condition, transmitted as an X-linked recessive trait, that is a somewhat more benign condition than Duchenne's muscular dystrophy; in comparison with the latter, the onset of symptoms occurs later in life, it pursues a milder course, and it tends to be more variable. The serum creatine concentration is also less elevated. Persons affected may continue to have walking mobility beyond late adolescence, and often live to the sixth decade. See also *muscular d.* under *dystrophy.*

Beck's triad (beks) [Claude Schaeffer *Beck,* Cleveland surgeon, born 1894] high venous pressure, low arterial pressure, and quiet heart action, characteristic of cardiac compression.

Beckwith-Wiedemann syndrome (bek′with vēd′ĕ-man) [John Bruce *Beckwith,* U.S. pathologist, born 1933; Hans Rudolf *Wiedemann,* German pediatrician, born 1915] a syndrome characterized by macroglossia, omphalocele, adrenal cytomegaly, gigantism, and hyperplastic visceromegaly. Nephroblastoma has been associated with this syndrome in several infants.

becquerel (Bq) (bek-rel′) [Antoine Henri *Becquerel,* French physicist, 1852–1908] the proposed new International System (SI) unit of radioactivity, the quantity of a radionuclide that undergoes one decay per second (1 s^{-1}). One curie (Ci) equals 3.7×10^{10} Bq; 1 μCi equals 37 kBq.

bedbug (bed′bug) see *Cimex.*

Bedsonia (bed-so′ne-ah) a generic name formerly used for several species now placed in the genus *Chlamydia;* see *Chlamydia.*

beef tapeworm see *T. saginata* under *Taenia.*

Beer's law (bērz) [August *Beer,* German physicist, 1825–1863] stated as: the absorbance of monochromatic light by a solution is proportional to the absorptivity, the light-path length, and the concentration. The absorptivity depends on the wavelength of the light, the solute, and the solvent, but not on the concentration.

The variation of absorbance with concentration was discovered by Beer; the variation with path length, by Bouguer and Lambert. The law is often called by any combination of the three names.

See also *absorptivity* and *spectrophotometric assays.*

bee sting injection with the venom of bees of the order Hymenoptera: either bee (bumblebee, honeybee) or vespid (yellow jacket, hornet, wasp). The venom of these insects contains peptides and nonenzymatic proteins such as kinins and mellitin, mediators of inflammation such as histamine and serotonin, and enzymes. Phospholipase A is the main toxin in bee venom, whereas in vespid venom it is the incompletely characterized protein antigen 5.

Local pain and inflammation are the usual reaction; however, in hyperimmune individuals, anaphylaxis can result from just one sting. The treatment of choice for anaphylactic shock is subcutaneous epinephrine. Skin tests can be performed to detect sensitization using the intradermal injection of diluted species-specific venom; IGE antibody detection using the radioallergosorbent test (RAST) can be performed, but is less sensitive.

bee venom toxin see *apiamine.*

Behçet's syndrome (ba′sets) [Hulusi *Behçet,* Turkish dermatologist, 1889–1948] a chronic, recurring disease of unknown etiology, characterized by severe inflammation of the eyes, optic atrophy, and aphthous lesions of the mouth and genitals. These are often accompanied by a diffuse vasculitis, arthritis, and varied central nervous system involvement. Corticosteroids are moderately effective in treatment.

behenic acid (be-hen′ik) a fatty acid, *n*-docosanoic acid. It is present in oil of black mustard and other plant-seed oils.

BEI abbrev. for serum butanol–extractable iodine. See under *thyroxine assays.*

bejel (bej′el) [Arabic *bajal*] a name used in the Near East for chronic, nonvenereal, treponemal infection of childhood. It is characterized by early mucocutaneous lesions, a latent period, and late complications including soft gummy tumors (gummas) of bone and skin.

bel (B) (bel) [Alexander Graham *Bell,* U.S. inventor, 1847–1922] a unit of relative power intensity used for acoustic or electric power. It is equal to the base 10 logarithm of the ratio of the measured power to some reference power level. A change of 1 B is a 10-fold power increase. The decibel (0.1 B) is more commonly used.

Belascaris (bĕ-las′kah-ris) an obsolete name for the genus *Toxocara.*

belladonna (bel″ah-don′ah) [It. "fair lady"] an anticholinergic and antispasmodic drug extracted from the deadly nightshade *Atropa belladonna.* It contains the pure substances atropine, hyoscyamine, and scopolamine.

Bell-Magendie law (bel ma-zhen′de) [Sir Charles *Bell,* Scottish physiologist in London, 1774–1842; François *Magendie,* French physiologist, 1783–1855] stated as: the fibers running in the ventral roots of the spinal cord are motor and those in the dorsal roots are sensory.

bemegride (bem′ĕ-grīd) a central nervous system stimulant formerly used in the treatment of barbiturate poisoning. Overdosage can cause convulsions. Trademark, Megimide.

benactyzine hydrochloride (ben-ak′tĭ-zēn) a mild anticholinergic drug used in combination with meprobamate as an antidepressant. Adverse reactions to benactyzine include dizziness and anticholinergic effects, e.g., blurred vision, dry mouth. See also *meprobamate.*

Benadryl (ben′ah-dril) trademark. See *diphenhydramine hydrochloride.*

Bence Jones protein (bens jōnz) [Henry *Bence Jones,* English physician, 1814–1873] an abnormal protein often found in the urine of patients with multiple myeloma and Waldenström's macroglobulinemia. Such proteins are characterized by their unusual solubility properties: when heated, they will precipitate (coagulate) in the temperature range of 40°–60°C and then redissolve on further heating to 80°–100°C. They are known to be monomers or dimers of immunoglobulin light (L) chains, with molecular weights of 25,000 or 50,000, and can be either kappa (κ) or lambda (λ) chains. In any one individual they are identical; i.e., they are the products of a single clone of plasma cells. In 60–70 percent of patients, Bence Jones protein is accompanied by elevations of plasma immunoglobulin levels. In 20 percent of cases, only Bence Jones proteins are found.

Bence Jones protein tests 1. serum protein electrophoresis. Bence Jones protein or other paraproteins appear as a narrow (monoclonal) band (M component) with an electrophoretic mobility somewhere between the alpha$_2$- and gamma globulins. Bence Jones protein can be identified as κ or λ light chains by immunochemical methods.

2. Bradshaw's test, a simple screening procedure. Acidified diluted urine is layered over concentrated HCl; a distinct ring at the interface suggests the presence of Bence Jones protein.

3. the thermal method or heat test, another screening procedure. Bence Jones protein precipitates at pH 4.9 at a temperature of 40°–60°C and redissolves when heated to 80°–100°C.

Bence Jones proteinuria the presence of Bence Jones protein in the urine.

Benditt hypothesis (ben′dit) a hypothesis that the collagen-producing smooth muscle cells forming the stroma of the atherosclerotic plaque are abnormal and represent a benign smooth muscle tumor. The basis for this hypothesis is the finding that in many atherosclerotic plaques the proliferating smooth muscle cells are apparently monoclonal in origin.

bendroflumethiazide (ben″dro-floo″mĕ-thi′ah-zīd) [USP], see under *thiazide diuretics.*

bends (bendz) see *decompression sickness.*

bene- (ben′e) [L. *bene* well] a prefix word element to denote good, e.g., benign.

Benedict's solution (ben′ĕ-dikts) [Stanley Rossiter *Benedict,* U.S. physiologic chemist, 1884–1936] a term referring to two reagents (a quantitative and a qualitative) devised for use in the examination of urine specimens for the presence of reducing sugars and/or substances. Both solutions contain cupric sulfate dissolved in a solution of sodium sulfate and sodium citrate, although the concentration of the salts differs in the two reagents. When the clear, dark blue qualitative reagent is heated with the test specimen, the sugar or other reducing material reduces the Cu^{2+} ion, and a yellow-to-red precipitate (hydrated cuprous oxide) is formed. The quantitative reagent also contains some potassium thiocyanate (KCNS) and a trace of ferrocyanide. The solution is titrated into the urine specimen until no more cupric ion is reduced.

Bengston's method (beng′stonz) a modification of Macchiavello's rickettsiae stain; rickettsiae stain red and other bacteria stain blue.

benign (be-nīn′) [L. *benignus* kind] favorable, mild, kindly; in oncology, the opposite of malignant. Benign neoplasms are usually well circumscribed, are often encapsulated, and by definition do not invade locally and do not metastasize. Rarely, benign tumors cause death through infection or inanition associated with neglect, hemorrhage (e.g., massive retroperitoneal hemorrhage from a renal angiomyolipoma), disseminated intravascular coagulation seen in some vascular neoplasms, and expansion at a critical anatomic site, which causes interference with essential body functions (e.g., intracranial meningioma, intracardiac myxoma).

In a number of tumor systems, benign neoplasms may undergo malignant change. The frequency with which this occurs is not known, but some carcinomas are known to arise from a preexisting benign tumor (e.g., a colon carcinoma arising from a villous adenoma). Cf. *malignant.*

benign intracranial hypertension (BIH) a condition, most often found in children or young women, that is characterized by elevated intracranial pressure with headache, nausea, vomiting, papilledema, occasional sixth nerve palsy, and the absence of other neurologic signs. A number of etiologic factors have been identified, including intracranial venous sinus thrombosis; ingestion of large amounts of vitamin A; administration of steroids, tetracycline, or nalidixic acid; chronic emphysema; and various metabolic and hematologic disorders. More commonly, however, BIH occurs idiopathically in otherwise healthy subjects or in overweight females with a history of menstrual dysfunction.

In the idiopathic disorder, the cerebrospinal fluid is of normal composition but is under increased pressure; arteriograms demonstrate patency of the venous sinuses and veins, and CT scans show small or normal-sized ventricles. The underlying causes must be treated if known. In most cases, treatment with drugs to reduce CSF formation is helpful, but it may be necessary to use steroids, repeated lumbar punctures, or various shunting procedures to lower the intracranial pressure and so prevent permanent visual damage.

Also called *pseudotumor cerebri.*

Bennett's sulfhydryl method (ben′ets) a histologic staining procedure to demonstrate sulfhydryl sites (red), which uses mercury orange as the primary reagent.

Bennhold's Congo red method (ben′holdz) [H. *Bennhold,* German physician, born 1893] a histologic staining procedure to demonstrate amyloid as red to pink; nuclei, blue; elastic tissue, light red. It has been modified by Puchtler.

Bensley's aniline-acid fuchsin-methyl green method (benz′lēz) [Robert Russell *Bensley,* Canadian-born U.S. anatomist, 1867–1956] a histologic staining procedure for the demonstration of cytoplasmic granules and organelles. Nuclei stain green; mitochondria are crimson; zymogen granules are red. This method may also be used to demonstrate pancreatic islet cells. Alpha granules stain a deep red; beta granules are green. The method is occasionally employed for other glands, such as the hypophysis and thyroid.

Bensley's osmic dichromate fluid [R. R. *Bensley*] a histologic fixative containing acetic acid, osmium tetroxide, and potassium dichromate, used in staining procedures to demonstrate cytoplasmic granules and organelles.

Bensley's safranin acid violet [R. R. *Bensley*] a method that employs neutral stains to differentiate pancreatic islet cells.

bentonite (ben′ton-īt) [from Fort *Benton,* Montana] [USP], a type of siliceous earth, a native hydrated aluminum silicate that swells to 12 times its volume when water is added. It is used as a bulk laxative, as a base for skin preparations, and to detect antibodies. See also *bentonite flocculation test.*

bentonite flocculation test a test for detecting the presence of serum antibody based on the ability of bentonite to adsorb protein, carbohydrate, and nucleic acids. The adsorbed antigens may remain stable for 3–6 mo; negative and positive control sera are added to a slide, with simple flocculation the criterion for antibody presence. This test may be used for trichinella, DNA, and rheumatoid factor antibodies.

benzalkonium chloride (ben″zal-ko′ne-um) a mixture of alkylbenzyldimethylammonium chlorides with the general formula $[C_6H_5CH_2N(CH_3)_2R]Cl$. A white or yellowish-white powder or gel, soluble in water, it has an aromatic odor and a bitter taste. It is used as a topical antiseptic and as a fungicide.

Benzedrine (ben′zĕ-drēn) trademark. See *a. sulfate* under *amphetamine.*

benzene (ben′zēn) a colorless, volatile, liquid aromatic hydrocarbon, C_6H_6, obtained mainly from the cracking and reforming of petroleum and used mainly in the production of rubber and plastics such as polystyrene and nylon. It has a characteristic odor and burns with a yellow, sooty flame. Benzene is a common solvent used in the manufacture of many organic compounds. Inhalation of fumes in laboratory operations (even in low concentrations) is hazardous and may cause fatal poisoning or leukemia and other blood disorders. Changes in peripheral blood cell counts and in bone marrow are frequently apparent. Bacterial infection, especially bronchopneumonia, may follow benzene poisoning, with fatal results. Because it is readily absorbed by inhalation or through the skin and because it is a recognized carcinogen, it must be used with extreme caution. In histology, benzene has been used as a clearing agent to replace alcohol in tissues following dehydration; because of its toxicity, it is no longer in general use. Formerly called benzol. See also *aromatic hydrocarbon.*

benzene assays 1. a semiquantitative color test. Benzene, toluene, and xylene are extracted from acidified blood samples into carbon tetrachloride and reacted with Marquis' reagent. A red color indicates the presence of one of these three solvents. The color is compared with standards having concentrations in the range of 0–30 μg/ml.

2. gas chromatography using a flame ionization detector. See also *head space analysis.*

benzene hexachloride (BHC) the trivial name for *1,2,3,4,5,6-hexachlorocyclohexane.*

benzidine (ben′zĭ-dēn) *p*-Diaminodiphenyl, NH_2-$C_6H_4C_6H_4NH_2$, a colorless, grayish-yellow, or white crystalline powder. It is used in the manufacture of dyes (especially Congo red), and has been employed in tests for occult blood, in microscopic staining, and as a reagent. Its use is now limited because it is classified as a carcinogen.

benzidine method for myoglobin peroxidase a histologic procedure for demonstrating myoglobin peroxidase in striated and smooth muscles. Dark blue microcrystalline masses are shown at I-band level.

benzoate (ben′zo-āt) a salt or ester of benzoic acid.

benzocaine (ben′zo-kān) [USP], a water-insoluble local anesthetic, ethyl *p*-aminobenzoate, used in cough drops, ointments, and suppositories as a surface anesthetic for skin and mucous membranes.

benzodiazepine (ben″zo-di-az′ĕ-pēn) any of a number of psychoactive compounds that are derivatives of 5-phenyl-2H-1,4-benzodiazepine. Benzodiazepine drugs are classified as minor tranquilizers and are the type of drug most frequently prescribed for the treatment of anxiety. Some are also used to treat muscle spasms, convulsions, and alcohol withdrawal syndrome, and to calm patients undergoing minor surgery.

The most common side-effects are drowsiness, confusion, and loss of coordination. In combination with other central nervous system depressants such as alcohol and barbiturates, the effects of benzodiazepines are additive. Benzodiazepine overdoses are often taken, alone or with alcohol, either accidentally or intentionally; the symptoms produced include stupor, coma, and respiratory depression.

See also *chlordiazepoxide, clonazepam, clorazepate, diazepam, flurazepam hydrochloride,* and *oxazepam.*

benzodiazepine assays 1. thin-layer chromatography. Benzodiazepines are extracted from alkalinized blood or urine samples into relatively polar solvents such as ether or chlorobutane. They may be separated into strong bases (flurazepam), weak bases (diazepam), and neutrals (clonazepam) by reextraction into mild or strong acid. A polar developing solvent and iodoplatinate spray reagent are used.

2. gas chromatography, using a nonpolar column and a flame ionization detector or an electron capture detector, which improves the sensitivity of the assay.

3. high-pressure liquid chromatography (HPLC), using a reverse-phase column, buffered acetonitrile as the mobile phase, and an ultraviolet detector set at 240 nm. It is important to measure the parent drug together with active metabolites.

4. EMIT homogeneous enzyme immunoassays for benzodiazepines in serum specimens or benzodiazepine metabolites in urine specimens.

benzoflavine (ben″zo-fla′vēn) a histologic stain; C.I. 46065. It is a fluorescent basic primary amine dye, which may be used as a Schiff reagent in the Feulgen reaction.

benzoic acid (ben-zo′ik) benzenecarboxylic acid, C_6H_5COOH, a white, crystalline substance; a weak acid with limited solubility; M.W. 122.12. It is mildly irritating to skin, mucous membranes, and eyes. It occurs naturally in benzoin resin and is used as a food preservative (as sodium benzoate), as a dye mordant, in tobacco curing, and as an antifungal agent. Ingested benzoic acid is excreted as hippuric acid. Benzoic acid may produce gastrointestinal intolerance or allergic reaction; its concentration in foods is limited by law to 0.1 percent. Highly purified benzoic acid is used as an acid-base standard and as a colorimetric standard.

benzoin (ben′zō-in, ben′zoin) 1. [USP], a balsamic resin with an aromatic odor obtained from trees of the genus *Styrax;* used in a tincture as a topical protectant. Also called benzoin resin.

2. 2-hydroxy-1,2-diphenylethanone, used in organic synthesis.

benzol (ben′zol) an obsolete term for *benzene.*

benzonatate (ben-zo′nah-tāt) [USP], a nonnarcotic, antitussive drug related to the local anesthetic tetracaine. It reduces the cough reflex by anesthetizing the stretch receptors of the pharynx, trachea, lungs, and pleura. Adverse reactions include drowsiness, dizziness, nausea, and nasal congestion. Overdosage may cause convulsions and respiratory depression.

benzo[a]pyrene (ben″zo-pi′rēn) a yellow crystalline solid, a polycyclic aromatic hydrocarbon containing five fused benzene rings; M.W. 252.30. It occurs in coal tar, cigarette smoke, and air pollution, and is a potent procarcinogen that undergoes metabolic activation to an aryl epoxide, the direct-acting carcinogen.

benzo sky blue method a histologic staining procedure (after Kerenyi-Taylor) for demonstrating beta-cell granules of the anterior pituitary. Formalin-fixed sections are initially stained with benzo sky blue color, followed by hematoxylin-eosin staining. Beta-cell granules appear a bluish purple; alpha cell granules, red; and chromophobe cytoplasm, pink.

benzoyl- (ben′zo-il) a prefix word element in organic chemistry to denote the acyl group formed from benzoic acid, the benzenecarbonyl group (C_6H_5CO—), e.g., benzoyl chloride (C_6H_5COCl).

benzoylaminoacetic acid (ben″zo-il-ah-me″no-ah-se′tik) see *hippuric acid.*

benzoylation (ben″zo-il-a′shun) the treatment of tissue sections with benzoyl chloride and pyridine, which makes hydroxyl and amine groups and aldehydes nonreactive. It thus blocks the periodic acid–Schiff reaction.

benzoylecgonine (ben″zo-il-ek′go-nēn) one of the two principal metabolites of cocaine (ecgonine methyl ester benzoate) formed by enzymatic hydrolysis in the liver (the other is ecgonine). Because only about 10–20 percent of a dose of cocaine is excreted unchanged, drug abuse screening tests for the use of cocaine determine primarily excreted benzoylecgonine, using radioimmunoassay, EMIT homogeneous enzyme immunoassay, thin-layer chromatography, or gas-liquid chromatography.

benzoylglycine (ben″zo-il-gli′sin) see *hippuric acid.*

benzoyl oil red O see *oil red O.*

benzoyl peroxide [USP], a white, granular, crystalline solid, $(C_6H_5CO)_2O_2$, soluble in organic solvents and used to induce skin peeling in the treatment of acne vulgaris.

benzphetamine hydrochloride (benz-fet′ah-mēn) a derivative of amphetamine that has a similar central nervous system stimulating effect and potential for abuse. See also *amphetamine* and *amphetamine assays.*

3,4-benzpyrene (benz-pi′rēn) a colorless, oil-soluble dye sometimes used in histology to demonstrate lipids. It is highly fluorescent in ultraviolet light, giving a blue color. It is a carcinogenic, polycyclic hydrocarbon.

benzthiazide (benz-thi′ah-zīd) [USP], see under *thiazide diuretics.*

benztropine mesylate (benz′tro-pēn) [USP], an anticholinergic and antihistaminic drug used in the palliative treatment of Parkinson's disease and of parkinsonian adverse reactions to antipsychotic drugs. Adverse effects include dryness of the mouth, blurring of vision, nausea, vomiting, nervousness, and constipation; confusion, disorientation, and hallucinations may also develop, especially in older persons. The drug may increase the likelihood of heat stroke. Trademark, Cogentin.

benzyl- (ben′zil) a prefix word element in organic chemistry to denote the phenylmethyl group (C_6H_5-CH_2-), e.g., benzylamine.

benzyl alcohol [NF], a clear, colorless, oily liquid, $C_6H_5 \cdot CH_2OH$, occurring in balsam of Peru, tolic balsam, and storax. It is used as a bacteriostatic in solutions for injection and is also applied topically as a local anesthetic. Also called *phenylcarbinol* and phenylmethanol.

benzylamine (ben″zil-ah′mēn) an amber liquid, benzenemethenamine, $C_6H_5CH_2NH_2$, used in the manufacture of dyes, plastics, and drugs; M.W. 107.15. It is a strong irritant of the skin and mucous membranes.

benzylpenicillin (ben″zil-pen-ĭ-sil′in) see *p. G.* under *penicillin.*

bephenium hydroxynaphthoate (bĕ-fen′e-um) [USP], an anthelmintic agent used to treat the *Ancylostoma duodenale* hookworm and, less successfully, *Necator americanus.* Vomiting and nausea are possible side-effects.

Bereitschaftspotential (ber-it′shafts-po-ten′shal) [Ger.] see *readiness potential.*

bergamot oil (ber′gah-mot) a volatile oil, brownish-yellow to green in color and obtained from the rind of fresh fruit of *Citrus bergamia,* that is used as a perfuming agent. Bergamot oil does not extract aniline dyes and is compatible with celloidin preparations. It clears from 95 percent alcohol.

Berg's chelate removal method (bergz) a histochemical staining method used to demonstrate inorganic triphosphatases. It can stain phosphatases that act on substrates that are not soluble in Gomori-type solutions. Modifications of this technique may be used to demonstrate alkaline polyphosphatase and neutral triphosphatase.

Berger's disease (bār-zhāz′) [J. *Berger,* French physician, 20th century] a disease that is characterized histologically by mesangial proliferative glomerulonephritis. Although it can occur in individuals of any age, it most commonly affects children and young adults. There are diffuse mesangial immune complex deposits containing IgA commonly associated with IgG and C3. The etiology is unknown. The clinical presentation is usually of repeated episodes of macroscopic hematuria, often associated with nonspecific upper respiratory infections. In between the hematuric episodes there usually is persistent proteinuria and microscopic hematuria, although the urinary sediment may return to normal. The prevailing belief that Berger's disease is benign has not been supported by long-term studies; a significant number of patients, especially adults, develop chronic renal failure. In approximately half of those receiving renal transplants, the disease recurs in the donor kidney.

Also called *IgA nephropathy.* See also *glomerulopathy.*

Bergey's classification (ber′gēz) [David Hendricks *Bergey,* U.S. bacteriologist, 1860–1937] a system of classification of bacteria based on *Bergey's Manual of Determinative Bacteriology.* Classification in the eighth edition (1974) consists of 19 parts, divided according to gram reaction, metabolism, and morphology, with each part further subdivided into families, genera, and species.

beriberi (ber″e-ber′e) [Singhalese "I cannot," signifying that the person is too ill to do anything] a disease caused by a thiamine (vitamin B_1) deficiency, common where polished (white) rice and extensively milled grains have been dietary staples (China, Philippines, India, Southeast Asia). It is rarely seen in the United States, where diets are greatly varied and wheat flour is thiamine-enriched. There are three forms of beriberi: an acute form with heart failure; a less acute, wet form with prominent peripheral edema; and a dry form with peripheral neuritis, paralysis, and atrophy of the muscles.

Laboratory findings include absent urinary thiamine in acute cases, decreased erythrocyte transketolase activity, and increases in pyruvic acid. Diagnosis is based on clinical evidence and demonstration of thiamine insufficiency.

berkelium (Bk) (berk′le-um, ber-ke′le-um) [from *Berkeley,* California] a cyclotron-produced metallic radioactive element; atomic number 97; most stable isotope, Bk-247 (half-life, 1.4×10^3 yr); a 5f transition actinide element; oxidation states +3 (the most common), +4.

Bernstein test (bern′stēn) [L. M. *Bernstein,* U.S. physician, born 1923] a diagnostic procedure performed to confirm gastric reflux as the cause of substernal pain. The esophagus is perfused with either a normal saline solution or a weak hydrochloric acid solution; if identical substernal pain is felt, the result is considered positive. Also called *acid perfusion test.*

Bernthsen's methylene violet (bernt′senz) [Heinrich August *Bernthsen,* German biochemist, 1855–1931] a weakly basic dye derived from methylene blue and used in the polychrome methylene blue stains, especially MacNeal's tetrachrome stain.

berry aneurysm (ber′e) a saccular dilation of an intracranial artery that characteristically forms at vessel bifurcations located near the circle of Willis, and is presumed to be due to a developmental anomaly of the vessel wall. The most common site is at the junction of the internal carotid and posterior communicating arteries. The rupture of a berry aneurysm, which may be precipitated by hypertension, is an important cause of intracranial hemorrhage. Clinically, this rupture is manifested by severe headache and/or loss of consciousness, and death can occur. See also *aneurysm.*

berry cell see *echinocyte.*

Berthelot reaction (ber′tĕ-lo) [Pierre Eugène Marcellin *Berthelot,* French chemist, 1827–1907] the reaction of ammonia with Berthelot's reagent (an alkaline solution of phenol and hypochlorite) to form a stable, deep blue product, phenol-indophenol, used in colorimetric methods for measuring ammonia and urea.

Bertiella (ber″te-el′lah) a genus of tapeworms of the family Anoplocephalidae.

B. mucronata, a species of tapeworm similar in form to *B. studeri,* but with a different arrangement of genitals, and eggs that are shaped differently. This species is indigenous to warm climates of Latin America. Human infections have been recorded resulting from contact with imported monkeys.

B. studeri, a species that measures 275–300 mm in length and as much as 10 mm in width, found mostly in children. The eggs are irregular ovoids, with a bicornuate protrusion on an inner shell and delicate middle envelope. Infections can be acquired from the accidental ingestion of certain mites containing the cysticercoid larval stage of the worm. Diagnosis may be made from identification of the eggs in the host feces.

berylliosis (ber-il″le-o′sis) beryllium poisoning, usually involving the lungs and less often the skin, subcutaneous tissue, lymph nodes, liver, and other structures. Beryllium fumes, its oxide and salts, and finely divided dust all may cause a tissue reaction when inhaled or implanted in the skin. Individual sensitivity to the element is an important factor. Of the two types, acute and chronic, the chronic form, called beryllium granulomatosis, is marked by focal granulomas in the alveolar septa and spaces. In the less common acute form, granulomatous reaction is not present. Because the disease is histologically similar to tuberculosis and sarcoidosis, history of exposure and the clinical signs are useful indicators. See also *pneumoconiosis.*

beryllium (Be) (ber-il′le-um) [Gr. *bēryllos* beryl] a gray metallic element; atomic number 4; atomic weight 9.01218; Group II of the periodic table (the alkaline earths); oxidation state +2. It is highly toxic; inhalation of beryllium dust produces pneumonitis and granulomatous lung disease (berylliosis); contact can also cause dermatitis, skin ulcerations, and conjunctivitis.

beryllium granulomatosis the chronic form of berylliosis; see under *berylliosis.*

Besnier-Boeck disease (bez′ne-a bek) [Ernest *Besnier,* French dermatologist, 1831–1909; Caesar P. M. *Boeck,* Norwegian dermatologist and syphilologist, 1845–1917] see *sarcoidosis.*

Bessey-Lowry-Brock unit (BLB unit) (bes′e lou′re brok) [Otto Arthur *Bessey,* U.S. biochemist, born 1904; Oliver Howe *Lowry,* U.S. pharmacologist and biochemist, born 1910; M. J. *Brock*] a unit of measurement of enzyme activity for acid or alkaline phosphatase defined as the quantity of activity, in 1 l of serum, which hydrolyzes 1 mmol of substrate (*p*-nitrophenylphosphate) in 60 min at 37°C.

Best's carmine stain (bests) [Franz *Best,* German pathologist, 1878–1920] a highly selective stain for glycogen, which stains a color that is pink to red. Mucin, fibrin, and mast cell granules stain also, but only faintly.

Stock solution is prepared by dissolving carmine, potassium carbonate, and potassium chloride in boiling distilled water; after cooling, strong ammonia water is added. When the solution has ripened at room temperature for 24 hr, it is refrigerated, and it remains stable for 1–2 mo.

Staining solution is two parts of stock solution, three parts of strong ammonia water, and three parts of methyl alcohol; it is stable only for 1 da. Sections are rinsed in methyl alcohol after staining.

See also *glycogen staining.*

Best's disease a congenital disease of the eye, transmitted as an autosomal dominant trait and characterized by macular degeneration leading to visual impairment. Ophthalmoscopic indications include a vitelline lesion that may be present at birth, progressing to the formation of yellow masses in the macular area and deep, irregular pigmentation. Also called vitelline macular dystrophy.

beta (B, β) (ba′tah) the second letter of the *Greek alphabet;* used to denote plasma proteins in the beta electrophoretic band, e.g., beta-lipoprotein, and one of a group of related entities, e.g., beta radiation.

beta activity in electroencephalography, any pattern of electric activity having a frequency greater than 13 Hz. It can often be recorded during wakefulness from the frontocentral regions of the head, when it is usually less than 30 μU in amplitude and can sometimes be attenuated by tactile stimuli or contralateral movement. Beta rhythms having other patterns of distribution or responsiveness are also well described. Beta activity occurs independently of the alpha rhythm and is often inversely related to the amount of alpha activity.

Beta activity with a characteristic frequency of 18–24 Hz can be induced by drugs such as barbiturates and benzodiazepine compounds. The integrated amount of beta activity (15–30 Hz) induced by the intravenous administration of amobarbital has been used as a measure of sedation threshold in the diagnosis of types of psychosis (see *sedation threshold*). Focal spontaneous beta activity or asymmetric drug-induced beta activity may suggest cerebral damage or disease. Generalized fast activity of 25–32 Hz occurring in high amplitude bursts has been held to characterize the electroencephalogram from those affected with Lowe's syndrome (oculocerebrorenal syndrome).

Also called beta rhythm.

beta-adrenergic antagonist see *beta-adrenergic blocking agent.*

beta-adrenergic blocking agent any drug that blocks the action of epinephrine and like compounds at the β-adrenergic receptors on cells of effector organs. There are two types of receptors, β_1-receptors in the myocardium and β_2-receptors in bronchial and vascular smooth muscle. The principal effects of β-adrenergic stimulation are increased heart rate and contractility, vasodilation of the arterioles that supply the skeletal muscles, and relaxation of bronchial muscles. β-Adrenergic blocking agents have opposite effects.

Beta-blockers are used to treat angina pectoris, hypertension, and cardiac arrhythmias, and to reduce the long-term risk of mortality and reinfarction after the acute phase of a myocardial infarction has passed. Beta-blockers are also prescribed for glaucoma and for prophylaxis of migraine.

The most widely used β-blocker is propranolol; it is nonselective, affecting both types of β-receptors, and can produce bronchospasm in persons with asthma or chronic obstructive pulmonary disease. Other nonselective β-blockers are nadolol and timolol. Cardioselective β-blockers (atenolol and metoprolol) preferentially block β_1-receptors and are less likely to produce bronchospasm.

Also called *beta-adrenergic antagonist* and *beta-blocker.*

beta-adrenergic receptor see under *adrenergic receptor.*

beta band in electroencephalography, activity with a frequency greater than 13 Hz.

beta basophil see *b. c. of hypophysis* under *beta cells.*

beta-blocker see *beta-adrenergic blocking agent.*

beta cells basophilic cells that stain most readily with basic dyes.

b. c. of hypophysis, large, granular basophilic cells of the anterior hypophysis. As with the acidophilic cells, there are two cell populations. The beta cells are ovoid and PAS-positive, and immunohistochemically stain for adrenocorticotropin (ACTH) and lipotropin (LPH), the precursor for melanocyte-stimulating hormone (MSH). The $beta_2$ cells are angular with small subplasmalemmal granules and are situated in the anterocentral parts of the lobe. They stain positively for thyroid-stimulating hormone (TSH).

b. c. of pancreas, the granular basophilic cells of the pancreatic islets. Making up about 75 percent of the cells in an islet, these cells contain crystalloid secretory granules, and secrete insulin.

beta decay a mode of radioactive decay, mediated by the weak force, in which beta particles are emitted. For nuclides with a high proportion of neutrons to protons, the emitted particle is an electron, and the general equation for the reaction is ${}^{A}_{Z}X \rightarrow {}_{Z+1}^{A}Y + e^- + \bar{\nu}$, where X is the parent radionuclide, Y is the daughter nuclide (decay product), e^- is an electron, and $\bar{\nu}$ an antineutrino.

So that mass and charge are conserved, the mass numbers (superscripts) and atomic numbers (subscripts) on both sides of the equation must balance. The particle reaction occurring in the nucleus is the conversion of a neutron to a proton: $n^o \rightarrow p^+ + e^- + \bar{\nu}$. The daughter nuclide has one less neutron and one more proton than the parent. For pure beta emitters, the decay process leaves the daughter nuclide in the ground state, and the emitted beta particles have a continuous spectrum of energies ranging from zero to E_{max}, the difference between the mass of the parent nuclide and the combined mass of the daughter nuclide and the electron. When the beta particle energy is below E_{max}, the rest of the decay energy is carried away by the antineutrino.

For some nuclides there are decay modes in which the beta emission can place the daughter nuclide in an excited state. In the transition to the ground state, gamma rays or internal conversion electrons are emitted. The internal conversion electrons produce sharp peaks in the beta energy spectrum.

For nuclides with a high proportion of protons to neutrons, the emitted particles are a positron (e^+) and a neutrino (ν). The nuclear equation is ${}^{A}_{Z}X \rightarrow {}_{Z-1}^{A}Y + e^+ + \nu$, and the particle equation is $p^+ \rightarrow n^o + e^+ + \nu$. Because the proton is lighter than the neutron, this process can occur only if the parent nuclide is heavier than the daughter by at least two electron masses; otherwise, a proton-rich nuclide must decay by electron capture.

Betadine (ba′tah-dīn) trademark. See *povidone-iodine.*

beta emitter a radioactive nuclide that undergoes beta decay by emitting a beta particle.

$beta_{1A}$-globulin see *C3b.*

beta hemolysis see *beta h.* under *hemolysis.*

betaine (be′tah-ēn) *N,N,N*-trimethylamino glycine, glycine betaine. Other trimethylamino acids are also known as betaines. The compound can supply methyl groups biologically and is thus a lipotropic agent.

beta-lipoprotein see *low-density l.* under *lipoprotein.*

beta-lysin a relatively heat-stable yet highly reactive cationic protein that lyses most gram-positive bacteria but does not destroy streptococci or gram-negative bacteria. It is released from platelets during coagulation and concentrates in the serum. The primary site of action is the cell membrane. Increased amounts of beta-lysin appear during the acute phase of an infection.

betamethasone (ba″tah-meth′ah-sōn) a synthetic anti-inflammatory corticosteroid (9α-fluoro-16β-methylprednisolone), a potent glucocorticoid with no mineralocorticoid activity. See also *corticosteroid.*

$beta_2$-microglobulin (β2m) a molecule present on the surface of cells, noncovalently linked to HLA A, B, and C antigens; M.W. 11,800. Structurally, it is homologous to a constant region (CH_3) of IgG.

This molecule has been remarkably preserved throughout ontogeny, suggesting that it serves an integral function in membrane surface receptors. In murine lymphoid cells, β_2-microglobulin is intimately associated with H2 D and K antigens but not Ig; in human cell lines it is associated with HLA A, B, and C antigens but is distinct from DR, DRW, and Ig antigens, and Fc and C3b receptors. Incubation of lymphoid cells with interferon enhances levels of surface membrane–associated β2m, as well as HLA antigens without a change in DR reactivity or the expression of new antigens. β_2-Microglobulin is synthesized and released into the supernatant of cell culture lines. Mitogen stimulation by phytohemagglutination, concanavalin A, and (less so) pokeweed mitogen increases production of β2m, suggesting that it is predominantly associated with T-cell proliferation. Stimulation with staphylococcal protein A, B cell mitogen does not increase β2m synthesis.

Similarly, antibody to β2m inhibits the mixed lymphocyte reaction (MLR), T-cell proliferation in response to antigens such as purified protein derivative (PPD), and cell-mediated lymphocytotoxicity (CML). β_2-Microglobulin may serve as part of the poorly characterized "T-cell receptor." Its concentration is readily measured by radioimmunoassay, and samples may be preserved at –20° and –80°C with acceptable stability. Clinically, elevated levels of β2m have been described in the sera of patients with rheumatoid arthritis and Sjögren's syndrome, in synovial fluid of patients with rheumatoid arthritis, and in salivary fluid of patients with Sjögren's syndrome, which suggests local production by infiltrating lymphoid cells. β_2-Microglobulin has been reported to be elevated in the sera of patients with Crohn's disease and active liver disease, reflecting ongoing inflammation. It is associated with a variety of carcinomas and lymphoid malignancies and may serve as a marker of tumor antigen. Elevated serum levels of β2m were initially described as indicative of renal tubular damage, and continue to be useful in monitoring renal function in acute nephrotoxicity and after transplantation. Diminished tubular function leads to increased urinary β2m; reduced glomerular filtration rate causes elevated serum β2m.

VIBEKE STRAND, M.D.

beta particle a particle emitted from the nucleus in beta decay, consisting of either a positron or an electron. The particles interact with nuclei (producing bremsstrahlung) and with orbital electrons (producing ionization and excitation). Positrons lose most of their kinetic energy by these interactions and then combine with electrons, producing two 511-keV gamma rays.

Beta particle energies range up to about 3 MeV and have a range of up to 10 m in air or 1 mm in water or soft tissue. The scattering by nuclei gives the beta particle a winding track unlike the straight track of an alpha particle.

Radioisotopes that are both beta and gamma emitters are shielded with an inner layer of plastic and an outer layer of lead. The plastic stops the beta particles with the emission of minimal bremsstrahlung.

Also called *beta ray.* See also *interaction of radiation with matter.*

beta radiation the emission of beta rays.

beta ray see *beta particle.*

beta receptor see under *adrenergic receptor.*

beta streptococcus any species of *Streptococcus* that produces beta hemolysis. See also *Streptococcus.*

beta thalassemia see under *thalassemia.*

beta-thromboglobulin a protein contained in the alpha granules of platelets (together with platelet factor 4 and platelet-derived growth factor).

betatron (ba′tah-tron) a circular magnetic induction electron accelerator; used for supervoltage (megavoltage) radiation therapy. The electron beam is used to produce x-rays in the energy range of 1–100 MeV.

betazole hydrochloride (ba′tah-zōl) [USP], an analog of histamine, 3-(β-aminoethyl)pyrazole, that is used as a diagnostic aid in gastric function tests. Like histamine, it stimulates gastric acid secretion, but its other histamine-like effects (dilation of capillaries, stimulation of smooth muscle contractions) are less prominent. Side-effects include flushing, headache, and hives. Trademark, *Histalog.*

Bethesda unit (bĕ-thez′dah) [from *Bethesda,* Maryland] a measure of inhibitor activity. One unit of inhibitor is the amount that will inactivate 50 percent or 0.5 unit of a coagulation factor during the incubation period. See also *inhibitor assay.*

Betke stain (bet′ke) see under *fetal hemoglobin tests.*

Betke-Kleihauer test (bet′ke kli′hou-er) see under *fetal hemoglobin tests.*

Betz cell area (betz) the motor area of the cerebral cortex.

Betz cells [Vladimir Aleksandrovich *Betz,* Russian anatomist, 1834–1894] large, pyramidal ganglion cells forming one of the layers of the motor area of the gray matter of the brain.

BeV abbrev. for billion electron volts; see *giga electron volt.*

bevatron (bev′ah-tron) a machine that accelerates protons.

bezoar (be′zōr) [Persian] a coagulation or concretion that forms within the stomach; it is composed of food and mucus, vegetable matter (phytobezoar), or hair (trichobezoar). These masses often form following partial gastrectomy, especially if the vagus innervation has been removed. Improper mastication and the cellulose from citrus fruits have also been implicated. Trichobezoars are most commonly encountered in young children under emotional stress who ingest pulled-out hair. Affected individuals complain of nausea, vomiting, loss of appetite, and a feeling of fullness. Abdominal pain, with ulceration and bleeding, may also occur. Vigorous gastric lavage or surgery may be required to remove the masses.

BFP abbrev. See *biologic false-positive.*

BFU-E abbrev. for burst-forming units–erythrocyte, a hematopoietic stem cell that gives rise to the erythrocyte. See also under *stem cell.*

BG abbrev. for blood glucose, bone graft.

BHBA abbrev. for β-hydroxybutyric acid. See under *ketone bodies.*

BHC abbrev. for benzene hexachloride; see 1,2,3,4,5,6-*hexachlorocyclohexane.*

BHI abbrev. See brain-heart infusion *a.* under *agar.*

Bi symbol for the chemical element *bismuth.*

bi- (bi) [L. *bi* two] a prefix word element to denote two or twice, e.g., bifid.

bi/o (bi′o) [Gr. *bios* life] a word element used in combining form to denote life, e.g., bioenergetics.

Bial's reagent (be′alz) [Manfred *Bial,* German physician, 1870–1908] a solution of orcinol, hydrochloric acid, and ferric chloride, used to detect the presence of pentose in urine. Formulations in use vary; e.g., one is composed of 1.5 g of orcinol, 500 g of fuming HCl, and 20–30 drops of 10 g/dl of $FeCl_3$, and another of 1.0 g of orcinol, 500 ml of concentrated HCl, and 1.5 ml of 1 g/dl of $FeCl_3$. See also *pentose assays.*

bias (bi′as) 1. a source of systematic variance (error) in laboratory procedures that can affect test results. It may involve consideration of such factors as: (1) personal bias, due to unconscious personal characteristics, such as one person consistently reading a meniscus mark lower than another; (2) laboratory bias, usually due to differences in standards, reagents, methods, environmental factors, or instrumentation, which cause one laboratory's results to be consistently higher or lower than those of another; (3) interindividual bias, due to differences in parameters between races, sexes, ages, health, and related factors; and (4) intraindividual bias, or variations in data for any one individual over a period of time. Bias may also refer to the observed average difference between two laboratory methods.

2. a voltage established between the emitter and the base of a transistor, or the cathode and the grid of a vacuum tube, for the purpose of controlling the device's operating conditions. The bias voltage is generally constant.

3. in statistics, the difference between the mean of the sampling distribution of a point estimate and the value of the parameter. See also *unbiased e.* under *estimate.*

bibulous (bib′u-lus) [L. *bibulus,* from *bibere* to drink] 1. absorbent or spongy.

2. having the property of absorbing moisture. Cf. *hygroscopic.*

bicameral (bi-kam′er-al) [*bi-* + L. *camera* chamber] having two chambers.

bicarbonate (bi-kar′bo-nāt) the HCO_3^- anion or any salt that contains this anion. Bicarbonate ions constitute the second largest fraction of anions in the plasma. The bicarbonate content of blood (plasma), which is defined to include carbonate (CO_3^{2-}) and carbamino compounds ($RCNHCOO^-$), may be determined by titration with acid, though it is more easily calculated from pH and Pco_2 values, or from pH and total CO_2 values, using the Henderson-Hasselbalch equation. The bicarbonate content can be approximated from the value of the total CO_2 minus 1.2 mmol (the average concentration of carbonic acid).

Bicarbonates facilitate the transport of CO_2 from the tissues to the lung and are part of the blood buffer system. A primary bicarbonate deficit is called metabolic acidosis and may be caused by excess production of organic acids (e.g., in diabetes), decreased excretion of acid (e.g., in renal failure), administration of acid salts, or loss of bicarbonate (e.g., in diarrhea). A primary carbonate excess is termed metabolic alkalosis and is caused by a loss of H^+ (due to vomiting, diuretics, or gastric lavage), administration of alkaline salts, or the presence of potassium deficit (e.g., due to insufficient potassium intake, loss of gastrointestinal secretions, extensive burns). Reference values for plasma bicarbonate are 23–28 mmol/l for males and 21–27 mmol/l for females.

Bicarbonates are also secreted by the pancreas and liver into the duodenum under stimulation by secretin; they serve to neutralize the acid chyme emptied from the stomach into the duodenum.

bicarbonate buffer system a mixture of bicarbonate and carbonic acid, which buffers noncarbonic acid or base in blood. The effect of the addition of a strong acid to the system is minimized by the HCO_3^- reacting with the added H^+ to form H_2CO_3, a weakly dissociated acid; if base (OH^- or HPO_4^{2-}) is added, it is removed by reacting with the H_2CO_3 to form $H_2O + HCO_3^-$ or $H_2PO_4^- + HCO_3^-$, respectively. The net result is a change in the ratio of HCO_3^-/H_2CO_3 and a relatively small change in pH. The buffer capacity of this system in the human organism is quite high, because it is an "open system"; i.e., a large quantity of H_2CO_3 is available from metabolic reactions, and the lungs can either retain or remove large quantities of formed carbonic acid, depending on the need.

Bicarbonate can also be excreted or retained by the kidney, in accordance with need. The ability to retain or eliminate carbonic acid (by the lungs) and bicarbonate (by the kidneys) increases the buffer value 20 times over that of a regular bicarbonate buffer of equal concentration.

biceps (bi′seps) [*bi-* + L. *caput* head] a muscle with two heads; either of two muscles (in the arm and the thigh) that flex the forearm and the lower leg.

biconcave (bi-kon′kāv) [*bi-* + L. *concavus* hollow] having two concave surfaces on opposite sides of a structure; an example is the red blood cell.

biconvex (bi-kon′veks) having two convex surfaces, as the opposite sides of a structure.

bicuspid (bi-kus′pid) [*bi-* + L. *cuspis* point] 1. having two cusps or points.

2. a bicuspid valve.

3. a premolar tooth.

bicuspid aortic valve a common congenital anomaly, occurring in about 2 percent of the population, that is characterized by two aortic valve cusps instead of the normal three. The condition is associated with other cardiac defects, most frequently coarctation of the aorta. Possible life-threatening complications include infective endocarditis and calcification leading to stenosis. A midsystolic murmur may be heard upon auscultation, and aids in clinical detection. The condition is usually asymptomatic, however, and is found incidentally at autopsy.

bicuspid valve see *bicuspid aortic valve* and *mitral v.* under *valve.*

bicycle ergometer (bi′sik′l er-gom′ĕ-ter) a bicycle used in exercise stress testing to measure the work capacity of the subject. Although the rate of pedaling is controlled by the subject, the work can be adjusted by increasing the resistance to pedaling. This method of stress testing offers the following advantages: the electrocardiogram is less distorted, precordial measurements and expired air collections can be readily made, and intravenous catheters can be maintained in place during testing. See also *stress testing.*

bid abbrev. for *bis in die* (twice a day).

Biebrich scarlet (be′brik) [from *Biebrich,* Germany] a histologic stain, useful for demonstrating sex chromatin, basic protein, and connective tissues, which may also be used in Shorr stains; C.I. 26905.

Biebrich scarlet–picroaniline blue a histologic staining procedure used to stain mucus light blue; erythrocytes, orange-scarlet; muscle, pink; and connective tissue, renal glomerular stroma, basement membranes, and reticulum blue. When iron hematoxylin is used, nuclei stain gray to black.

Bielschowsky-Jansky syndrome (be″el-shou′ske yan′ske) [Max *Bielschowsky,* German neuropathologist, 1869–1940; *Jan Jansky,* Czech psychiatrist, 1873–1921] the late infantile form of familial amaurotic idiocy, thought to be transmitted as a recessive trait, that is characterized by cerebromacular degeneration, lipid storage in the brain, and demyelination. It occurs most frequently in children aged 3–4 yr, with progressive mental deterioration, visual impairment leading to blindness, seizures, and myoclonic jerking. Weakness, spasticity, and cerebellar ataxia are also seen. There is no known cure. Also called *Bielschowsky syndrome,* Dollinger-Bielschowsky syndrome, and late infantile amaurotic familial idiocy. See also *amaurotic familial i.* under *idiocy.*

Bielschowsky's method (be″el-shou′skēz) [Max *Bielschowsky*] a diamine silver impregnation technique for differentiating reticular fibers. Formalin-fixed sections are sensitized with silver nitrate before impregnation with diamine silver in diffuse white light. The diamine silver is developed with formalin, toned with acidic gold chloride, and treated with sodium thiosulfate to remove any unreduced silver. The reticular fibers appear as threads brown to black in color, whereas associated collagen fibers appear lavender to gray.

Bielschowsky syndrome see *Bielschowsky-Jansky syndrome.*

Biermer's anemia (bēr′merz) [Anton *Biermer,* German physician, 1827–1892] see *pernicious a.* under *anemia.*

bifascicular block (bi″fah-sik′u-lar) [*bi-* + L. *fasciculus* diminutive of *fascis* bundle] an imprecise term for the obstruction of two of the three main conduction pathways in the ventricles, e.g., a right bundle branch block with a left anterior hemiblock. This condition implies a lesion that has left a single pathway for atrioventricular conduction.

bifid (bi′fid) [L.] 1. cleft into two parts or branches. 2. a bacterial rod with one or both ends forked; see *Bifidobacterium.*

Bifidobacterium (bi″fid-o-bak-te′re-um) a genus of the family Actinomycetaceae in which bifurcated V- and Y-shaped forms are common. These organisms are gram-positive, stain irregularly, are anaerobic, and ferment glucose to acetic and L(+)-lactic acid. They are found in the feces of humans (particularly infants), lower animals, and insects, and are nonpathogenic, except for the newly added species *B. eriksonii.*

B. bifidum, an obligate anaerobe, possibly bacteriophagic, that is found in the alimentary tract and feces of infants and adults.

B. eriksonii, an infrequent isolate from subcutaneous and pulmonary abscesses in humans. More often, it is recovered from human feces.

B. infantis, a species composed of small, thin, coccoid cells, sometimes with central granules, which are the predominant bifidobacteria in the feces of breast-fed infants. The combination of increased acidity and overgrowth by *B. infantis* in the intestine appears to result in diminished enteric colonization by *Escherichia coli* and perhaps other invasive bacteria.

bifid tongue a congenital malformation in which the anterior part of the tongue is divided by a longitudinal fissure.

bifurcation (bi″fur-ka′shun) [L. *bifurcatio,* from *bi-* + *furca* fork] 1. division into two branches.

2. the point at which a single structure divides into two branches, particularly as in the aorta or trachea.

bigeminy (bi-jem′ĭ-ne) [L. *bigeminum* twin] the condition of occurring in pairs; the term is used particularly with reference to the heart rhythm, consisting of heartbeats in a succession of pairs.

ventricular b., a pattern of arrhythmia that consists of coupled ventricular beats, in which alternate QRS complexes commonly are ventricular premature depolarizations.

BIH abbrev. See *benign intracranial h.* under *hypertension.*

bil/i (bil′ĭ) [L. *bilis* bile] a word element used in combining form to denote bile, e.g., biliary.

bilateral (bi-lat′er-al) [*bi-* + L. *latus* side] having two sides, or pertaining to both the right and left sides.

bilateral symmetry see *bilateral s.* under *symmetry.*

bile (bīl) [L. *bilis*] a liquid produced by the liver, clear greenish–yellow to golden brown in color, that is important in digestion, and particularly in fat emulsification. Its formation depends on active secretion by liver cells into the bile canaliculi; it is then concentrated and stored in the gallbladder until needed. The major components of bile are conjugated bile salts, cholesterol, phospholipid, bilirubin diglucuronide, and electrolytes. It is alkaline because of its bicarbonate content. Also called *gall.*

bile acids products of cholesterol metabolism in the liver, containing one, two, or three OH groups at positions 3, 7, or 12, and a carboxyl group at the end of the side-chain. Conjugated to glycine or taurine, they form bile salts. Examples include cholic acid (3,7,12-hydroxy), lithocholic acid (3-hydroxy), deoxycholic acid (3,12-hydroxy acid), and chenodeoxycholic acid (3,7-hydroxy acid). They are water-soluble, have a bitter taste, and aid in the absorption of fat from the intestine.

Increased concentrations of bile acids are found in the serum of individuals with hepatitis and obstructive jaundice. These are caused by a deficiency in the conjugation of bile acids with glycine and taurine, and by the inability of the liver to remove bile acids from the enterohepatic circulation.

Bile acid determinations are presently thought to be the most sensitive measure of liver function.

See also *bile salts.*

bile acids assays methods for the determination of bile acids in biologic specimens. Partition chromatography, gas chromatography alone, or coupled with mass spectroscopy, and radioimmunoassay have been used for quantitative assay of bile acids in serum. The Pettenkofer reaction has been used to detect increased concentrations of bile acids in urine; a red-purple color is produced when cholic acid reacts with fructose or furfural in the presence of sulfuric acid.

bile canaliculi see *bile canaliculi* under *canaliculus.*

bile duct a channel that carries bile.

common b. d., a channel formed by the union of the common hepatic and cystic ducts, which enters the duodenum with the main pancreatic duct at the ampulla of Vater.

hepatic b. d., the main canal through which bile leaves the liver. The right and left hepatic ducts fuse in the porta hepatis to form the common hepatic duct.

interlobular b. d., a system of channels forming a network in the portal tracts, through which bile passes to the porta hepatis. These channels eventually fuse to become the hepatic ducts.

bile duct carcinoma a carcinoma arising from cells of the biliary passages. It may be intra- or extrahepatic. The better differentiated tumors show duct formation, but more solid forms are difficult to distinguish from liver cell carcinomas, and mixed patterns occur. It may also be hard to differentiate between a primary intrahepatic bile duct carcinoma and metastatic disease. As with liver cell carcinoma, bile duct carcinoma can arise in a cirrhotic liver.

Also called *cholangiocarcinoma.*

bile ductules short, thin canals situated at the periphery of the classic hepatic lobule, into which the bile canaliculi empty. Their walls are formed of hepatocytes on one side and ductule cells on the other; the latter become more cuboidal as the ductule approaches the portal canal. These ductules penetrate the limiting plate to empty into the interlobular bile ducts. Also called *canals of Hering, cholangioles,* and terminal ductules.

bile infarct a focus of liver cell necrosis due to the accumulation of intracytoplasmic bile secondary to biliary duct obstruction. The distribution is usually periportal.

bile lake an accumulation of bile as a result of leakage from a duct in the hepatic parenchyma. It is caused by obstruction of the larger biliary ducts.

bile pigment demonstration in tissue see under *bilirubin demonstration in tissue.*

bile pigments any of the colored materials present in the bile, including bilirubin, biliverdin, D-urobilins, D-urobilinogens, L-stercocobilin, L-stercobilinogen, bilifuscin, biliprasin, choleprasin, bilihumin, bilicyanin, mesobiliviolin, mesobilirubin, and some coproporphyrinogen. All are metabolic breakdown products of porphyrins originating from the reticuloendothelial system (liver, bone marrow) and are reduced or oxidized by passage through the gastrointestinal system into a variety of pigmented and colorless products. Approximately 0.5–2.1 mg of bile pigment is excreted in the urine and as much as 250 mg in the feces of a normal adult each day. See also *stercobilin* and *urobilin.*

bile salts glycine or taurine conjugates of bile acids (e.g., glycocholate or taurocholate) formed in the liver and secreted in bile. Their function is to emulsify dietary fat and increase the action of lipases. After secretion into the intestinal tract, most bile salts are reabsorbed by the small intestine, enter the enterohepatic circulation, and return to the liver for secretion. See also *bile acids.*

bile solubility test a test for the differentiation of pneumococci from other streptococci. A sample of a broth culture is incubated at pH 7.4–7.6 with sodium deoxycholate. A decrease in turbidity (positive test) indicates lysing of the cells. Pneumococci are positive, whereas other viridans streptococci are negative.

Bilharzia (bil-har′ze-ah) [Theodor Maximilian *Bilharz,* German physician, 1825-1862] a genus of flukes more commonly called *Schistosoma;* see *Schistosoma.*

bilharziasis (bil″har-zi′ah-sis) see *schistosomiasis.*

biliary (bil′e-a-re) pertaining to the bile ducts or to the gallbladder.

biliary cirrhosis cirrhosis associated with intra- or extrahepatic obstruction of the large bile ducts (primary biliary cirrhosis), or with a chronic, nonsuppurative, destructive cholangitis (secondary biliary cirrhosis).

primary b. c., a progressive hepatic disease of unknown etiology, occurring mainly in middle-aged females. It is characterized by chronic nonsuppurative cholangitis, with eventual progression to cirrhosis, portal hypertension, and, frequently, esophageal varices. The onset is insidious, usually beginning with pruritis and followed by obstructive jaundice with elevation of serum alkaline phosphatase levels; late in the course of the disease there is hypercholesterolemia associated with xanthomas of the skin (xanthomatous biliary cirrhosis). Serum IgM and IgG are elevated and the mitochondrial antibody test is positive in the great majority of those affected. Rheumatoid arthritis, autoimmune thyroiditis, and Sjögren's syndrome may be associated. Also called chronic nonsuppurative cholangitis and xanthomatous biliary cirrhosis. See also *cirrhosis.*

secondary b. c., a true cirrhosis, with hyperplastic, hepatic parenchymal nodules separated by a fibrous meshwork. It occurs late in the course of prolonged bile duct obstruction due to such conditions as impacted stone, fibrous stricture, or tumor.

biliary obstruction any obstruction of the bile ducts, accompanied by decreased passage of bile to the duodenum and elevated concentrations of serum bilibrubin.

bilirubin/o (bil″ĭ-roo′bin-o) a word element used in combining form to denote bilirubin (bile pigment), e.g., hyperbilirubinemia.

bilirubin (bil″ĭ-roo′bin) [*bili-* + L. *ruber* red] an orange-red-brown pigment, insoluble in water but soluble in chloroform, hexane, benzene, and other organic solvents. Solutions in chloroform give an absorption maximum at 453 nm, with a molar absorptivity of 60,700 $\pm$ 800. It is the main pigment in bile, is found in many gallbladder stones, and is present in serum. Bilirubin is the product of the breakdown of hemoglobin and other heme-containing proteins and is formed in the reticuloendothelial (RE) cells of the spleen. The decomposition of 1 g of hemoglobin provides the heme from which 35 mg of bilirubin is formed. After heme-iron is removed as Fe^{3+}, the protoporphyrin-IX ring is oxidatively severed at the methyne (=CH—) bridge between the two pyrroles that carry the vinyl groups, forming a linear tetrapyrrole structure in which the pyrroles are linked by (=CH—) bridges. The bilirubin precursor thus formed is a green pigment, called biliverdin. The middle methyne bridge is then reduced by NADPH to ($—CH_2—$) to form bilirubin IXα.

Because of the two methyne bridges, several geometric isomers are possible. The common form of bilirubin is referred to as 4Z,15Z bilirubin IXα, with the H on the bridges transformed to the pyrrole nitrogens. This form permits hydrogen bonding between the carboxyethyls on rings II and III and the pyrrole nitrogen atoms, leading to an apolar structure highly insoluble in water. It can be transformed by irradiation with blue light to the 4E,15Z and 4Z,15E isomers, which cannot form such internal hydrogen bond compounds and thus are more soluble.

After formation in the RE cells, bilirubin is transported to the liver in the form of a bilirubin-albumin complex. It is actively transported into the parenchymal liver cells, where most is reacted with D-glucuronate (and perhaps with other carbohydrates) to form water-soluble mono- and diglucuronides (conjugates). Conjugation occurs on the carboxyethyl groups, which prevents inner hydrogen bonding and thus increases water solubility. The water-soluble conjugates are actively transported from the parenchymal cells into the bile canaliculi for excretion via the bile into the gastrointestinal tract. There the bilirubin is reduced by intestinal microorganisms to various urobilins and urobilinogens. Some of these are reabsorbed into the enterohepatic circulation and excreted by the kidneys. Urobilin is partially responsible for the brown color of stool.

The reference range for bilirubin in serum in nonjaundiced patients is 0.2–1.0 mg/dl, with 0.0–0.2 mg in the conjugated form. Normally, none is seen in urine (under 0.02 mg/dl). Elevations of serum bilirubin are reflected in clinical jaundice, which can be caused by hemolytic disorders (such as acquired hemolytic anemia), reticulocytosis, parenchymal liver disease, obstruction of the bile excretory pathways, or by a deficiency of the enzyme UDP-glucuronate:bilirubin-glucuronosyltransferase (UDP-glucuronyl transferase).

conjugated b., bilirubin diglucuronide that has been conjugated in the liver and is soluble in water. In the analytical procedure, it couples with diazotized sulfanilic acid, in aqueous solution without the presence of an organic solvent or a coupling agent; hence, also called direct bilirubin.

unconjugated b., the lipid-soluble form of bilirubin that circulates in loose association with the plasma proteins en route to the liver from its site of formation in the reticuloendothelial cells. It will not react with diazotized sulfanilic acid without the presence of an organic solvent or a coupling agent; hence, also called indirect bilirubin.

bilirubin assays 1. spectrophotometric determination as azobilirubin, a colored product formed on diazotization of bilirubin with Ehrlich's diazo reagent. Azobilirubin is reddish-violet in color at moderately acid or neutral pH conditions and has an absorption maximum at 540 nm. Azobilirubin is blue in strongly acid or alkaline solution.

Several methods have been devised to measure both the conjugated (direct) and total bilirubin. In the Malloy-Evelyn method, the conjugated bilirubin is measured 1 min after the addition of Ehrlich's diazo reagent, whereas measurement of total bilirubin requires the addition of methanol as accelerator and a reaction time of 15 min. In the Jendrassik-Grof method, the caffeine-benzoate serves as an accelerator instead of methanol. The blue azobilirubin is measured at 600 nm. This method is now preferred because of its greater sensitivity and greater reproducibility.

2. a direct spectrophotometric method used for micro- or ultramicroanalysis. In the serum of newborn infants, which does not contain interfering lipochromes, the bilirubin concentration is approximately proportional to the difference between the absorbances at 455 (bilirubin) and 575 nm, which corrects for the absorbance due to any hemoglobin present. More accurate corrections may be made using the measured absorptivities of hemoglobin and bilirubin at these wavelengths.

A bilirubinometer is a differential spectrophotometer specially designed for this assay. It takes readings at wavelengths of 454 and 540 nm (or 461 and 561 nm), where the absorptivity of oxyhemoglobin is equal to that of bilirubin.

3. screening tests for bilirubin in urine. There are several qualitative reagent strip tests and a reagent tablet test (Icotest) that can be made semiquantitative by using serial dilutions; they use the azobilirubin reaction employing a variety of diazo reagents. Large amounts of phenothiazines give a false positive reaction. The drugs phenazopyridine, ethoxazene, and salicylate and high levels of urobilin or indican give a masking red color.

A different test is based on the oxidation of bilirubin to green biliverdin by Fouchet's ferric chloride–trichloroacetic acid reagent. Urobilin, urobilinogen, indican, and salicylates may give masking colors.

bilirubin demonstration in tissues histologic procedures to demonstrate bilirubin, hematoidin, and bile pigments in tissue sections. The Gmelin reaction results from treating tissue sections with 50 percent nitric acid in ethanol, which produces a series of color changes observable under the microscope, ranging from green to blue to violet and ending with yellowish-brown. The test may give false-negative results; all negative results should be repeated.

The Hall method utilizes the reaction of Fouchet's reagent with bilirubin, which is oxidized to biliverdin. Hydrated sections are stained with Fouchet's reagent, counterstained with van Gieson's solution, and mounted. Pigment deposits (biliverdin) appear olive to emerald green in color; collagen, red; and muscle, yellow.

bilirubinemia (bil″ĭ-roo-bĭ-ne′me-ah) [*bilirubin* + Gr. *haima* blood + *-ia*] the presence of excess bilirubin in the blood.

bilirubin encephalopathy see *kernicterus.*

bilirubinuria (bil″ĭ-roo-bĭ-nu′re-ah) [*bilirubin* + Gr. *ouron* urine + *-ia*] the presence of direct bilirubin in the urine; large amounts give it a dark color. Bilirubinuria is seen in forms of liver disease that cause serum elevation of bilirubin, and may precede the appearance of jaundice.

biliverdin (bil″ĭ-ver′din) [*bili-* + L. *viridis* green] a green pigment, the first bile pigment formed in the breakdown of heme, containing all interpyrrole bridges in the methyne (—CH=) form. It is reduced to bilirubin, a yellow pigment containing the middle bridge in the methylene (—CH_2—) form, by the enzyme biliverdin reductase. The enzyme is present in large excess, so that biliverdin is not demonstrable even in severe hemolysis. However, very rare cases of biliverdin pigmentation have been reported in patients with biliary carcinoma and subacute hepatic necrosis. The biliverdin green is a much more intense color than is the bilirubin yellow. Also called *dehydrobilirubin.*

billion electron volts (BeV) see *giga electron volt.*

Bilopaque (bil′o-pāk) trademark. See under *tyropanoate.*

bimodal (bi-mo′dal) of a probability density, having two modes; of any graph having two maxima (peaks). See also *mode.*

bimolecular (bi″mo-lek′u-lar) relating to, formed from, or involving two molecular species.

binary (bi′na-re) [L. *binarius* of two] 1. made up of two elements or two equal parts.

2. pertaining to the base 2 number system, or the number 2. See also *number system.*

binary acid an acid that contains only two elements, e.g., HCl.

binary addition the addition of binary numbers. Like decimal numbers, they are added digit by digit, and 0 + 0 = 0, and 0 + 1 = 1. But in binary arithmetic, 1 + 1 = 10; that is, a zero with a 1 carried over to the next column.

binary code a code that uses two code elements represented symbolically by 0 and 1 and electrically by the absence or presence of a pulse.

binary coded decimal (BCD) pertaining to the representation of decimal numbers in which each decimal digit is represented by four binary digits (bits). Two methods of weighting the bits are used, 8421 and 4421. By adding the weights of the four positions, any decimal number from 0 through 9 can be obtained; e.g., 0110 represents 6. The decimal digits 0–9 correspond to the hexadecimal digits 0–9. Some computers have instructions that perform arithmetic operations on BCD data. Most calculators and digital instruments use BCD arithmetic.

binary coded decimal addition normal decimal addition carried out by logic circuitry on decimal numbers in binary coded form.

binary digit 0 or 1, the only two digits in the binary number system.

binary fission the cleaving of a cell by transverse division into two cells of approximately equal size.

binary variate a random variable having only two possible values. See also *binomial distribution.*

binding energy (bīnd′ing) the energy required to remove a particle from a system; in particular, the energy required to separate the particles of an atomic nucleus, which is equal to the mass defect (the sum of the masses of the constituent protons and neutrons minus the mass of the nucleus) converted to energy using the equation $E = mc^2$.

binocular (bi-nok′u-lar) [L. *bini* two + *oculus* eye] 1. pertaining to both eyes.
2. having two eyepieces, as in a microscope.

binomial (bi-no′me-al) [*bi-* + L. *nomen* name] composed of two names or terms.

binomial coefficient the number of different combinations of k elements that can be formed from a set of n elements; written $\binom{n}{k}$ or $_nC_k$; determined by the formula $\binom{n}{k} = n!/k!(n-k)!$ where $n!$ is n factorial, $n \times (n-1) \times \ldots \times 2 \times 1$, and $0! = 1$.

binomial distribution the probability distribution of the number X of successes in n independent identical trials, when each trial has only two possible outcomes (traditionally called success and failure). The probability of X successes is $P(X = x) = \binom{n}{x} P^x(1-p)^{n-x}$, where p is the probability of success for each trial and $\binom{n}{x}$ is a binomial coefficient.

The mean of the binomial distribution (the average number of successes in n trials) is np; the standard deviation is $\sigma = \sqrt{np(1-p)}$.

Exact values of the cumulative binomial distribution are tabulated for small sample sizes; for large sample sizes, the normal approximation is used. The left tail probability $P(X \leq x)$ is approximated by the area under the standard normal curve to the left of $(x + \frac{1}{2} - np)/\sigma$. The right tail probability $P(X \geq x)$ is approximated by the area under the standard normal curve to the right of $(x - \frac{1}{2} - np)/\sigma$. A rule of thumb is that np and $n(1-p)$ should both be at least 5 when this approximation is used.

binomial nomenclature the current system of scientific classification of organisms, in which each receives two names, one for its genus, the second for its species.

binuclear (bi-nu′kle-ar) [*bi-* + L. *nucleus* nut] having two nuclei, the result of an abnormal mitosis.

binucleate (bi-nu′kle-āt) see *binuclear.*

bioaccumulation (bi″o-ah-kūm″u-la′shun) the process by which some environmental contaminant becomes concentrated in exposed organisms. Chemicals showing high bioaccumulation ratios are either lipophilic and accumulate in fatty tissues, or are substances that resist all types of degradation.

bioassay (bi″o-as′a) the determination of the quantity of a chemical, drug, vitamin, or other physiologically active or toxic material by its effect on a living organism, on a physiologic activity of an animal, or on an isolated organ preparation from an animal compared with the effect of known quantities of standard preparations of the compound under investigation. In special applications, plants or microorganisms may serve as test agents. Also called *biological assay.*

bioavailability (bi″o-ah-vāl″ah-bil′ĭ-te) the percentage of and rate at which a physiologically active compound (such as drugs, vitamins, or hormones) is available for action on a target tissue.

biochemical (bi″o-kem′ĕ-kal) pertaining to biochemistry.

biochemical energetics the study of the energy transformations involved in those biochemical reactions that synthesize cellular constituents from food molecules, provide energy to drive cellular processes and maintain body temperature, and generally maintain organisms in a steady-state condition.

A reaction proceeding toward equilibrium can do work or supply energy, and the further the concentrations of the reactants and products are removed from equilibrium, the greater is the amount of energy obtained from each mole of reactant. The energy liberated or consumed by a reaction occurring at a constant temperature and pressure (as in all biochemical systems) is given by the Gibbs free-energy change (ΔG) for the reaction. Exergonic reactions, those that liberate free energy (ΔG is negative), can proceed spontaneously. Endergonic reactions, those that take up free energy (ΔG is positive), cannot proceed spontaneously; for such a reaction to occur, it must be coupled to an exergonic reaction with a larger free-energy change so that the overall ΔG is negative. The overall free-energy change for a series of reactions is equal to the sum of the free-energy changes of the individual reactions. Examples of exergonic processes are oxidation of carbohydrates, fats, and proteins, and fermentation. Examples of endergonic processes are movement, maintenance of concentration gradients across membranes, synthesis of cellular constituents, and storage of fats and carbohydrates.

The free-energy change is defined by the equation $\Delta G = -RT \ln (K_{eq}/Q)$, where R is the gas constant (8.314 J/mol·K), T is the absolute temperature, Q is the reaction product (the product of the concentrations of the products divided by the product of the concentrations of the reactants) at the prevailing (physiologic) conditions, and K_{eq} is the equilibrium constant (the reaction product at equilibrium). Using the standard free-energy change: $\Delta G° = -RT \ln K_{eq}$, the free-energy change is given by $\Delta G = \Delta G° + RT \ln Q$. For oxidation-reduction reactions, $\Delta G°$ can also be determined from the difference $\Delta E°$ in the standard electrode potentials of the two half reactions using the equation $-\Delta G° = nF\Delta E°$, where n is the number of electrons transferred and *F* is the Faraday constant (96,500 C).

biochemistry (bi″o-kem′is-tre) the science that utilizes chemical, physical, or biologic techniques to study the chemical nature and behavior of living matter.

biodegradability (bi″o-de-grād″ah-bil′ĭ-te) the susceptibility of a chemical compound, such as a detergent or pesticide, to decomposition by the action of microorganisms or other natural environmental processes.

biodegradable (bi″o-de-grād′ah-b′l) susceptible of degradation by biologic processes, such as bacterial or other enzymatic action.

bioenergetics (bi″o-en″er-jet′iks) the area of biochemistry that deals with the study of the energy transformations in living organisms.

bioequivalence (bi″o-e-kwiv′ah-lens) the equivalent biologic effect of two or more drugs.

biohazard (bi′o-haz″ard) biologic hazards that are related to infectious agents found in clinical microbiology laboratories. Exposure to pathogenic microorganisms can occur by the mechanisms listed in the accompanying table.

biohazard sign a sign bearing the biohazard symbol. Such signs should be posted on the doors of laboratories performing work with infectious agents that require special conditions for containment. Labels with the biohazard symbol are required for the interstate shipping of microorganisms. See also *biohazard symbol.*

biohazard symbol an international symbol warning of infectious or potentially infectious hazards. See also the accompanying illustration.

biologic (bi-o-loj′ik) pertaining to biology.

biological alkylating agent (bi″o-loj′ĭ-kal) a substance that can add or substitute an alkyl radical under the conditions present in a living organism (pH, hydration, temperature, ionic concentration). Some alkylating agents of this type are the ethylene imines, nitrogen mustards, and sulfonic acid esters, which act to suppress specific mechanisms of immunity. Cf. *alkylating agent.*

biological assay see *bioassay.*

Biological Matrix Reference Materials see under *reference materials.*

biologicals (bi″o-loj′ĭ-kalz) medicinal preparations made from living organisms or their products and used in the diagnosis, prevention, or treatment of disease. These include killed or attenuated microorganisms (vaccines) or their products (toxoids, microbial antigens), antibodies (antitoxins, immune globulins, antivenoms), extracts of plants or foods (allergens), or some antimicrobial agents (antibiotics).

biological safety cabinet a device for the containment of infectious aerosols generated by many microbiologic procedures. Three classes of cabinets are available: class I and class II cabinets are partial containment cabinets; class III cabinets provide maximal containment. The cabinets used in the routine clinical microbiology laboratory are usually class II cabinets. See also *biosafety.*

Biological Stain Commission a nonprofit organization that tests stains and supplies information about them. It issues certificates to stains and dyes

BIOHAZARD. OCCURRENCE AND PREVENTION OF EXPOSURE TO PATHOLOGIC MICROORGANISMS IN THE CLINICAL LABORATORY*

ROUTES OF INFECTION	EXAMPLES	METHODS FOR PREVENTION
Airborne	Aerosols created by spills or breakage of containers, removal of culture tube caps, centrifuges, blenders; grinding of tissues	Biologic safety cabinet; safety centrifuge cups
Ingestion	Mouth pipeting; failure to wash hands; eating, drinking, or smoking in the laboratory	Mechanical pipeting devices; hand-washing facilities; separate areas for eating, drinking, and smoking
Direct inoculation	Accidents involving needles and syringes or broken glassware; scratches or bites of laboratory animals	Proper disposal of needles and broken glassware; care in animal contacts
Skin contact	Contact with cuts or scratches on skin; contact with conjunctiva	Disinfection of laboratory benches; covering cuts or scratches with gloves or bandages; emergency eye wash; laboratory coats
Insect vectors	Contact with insects; laboratory studies involving vectors or infected animals	Insect and rodent control; fly screens; animal rooms

* Information regarding containment levels for infectious agents in clinical microbiology laboratories may be found in *Classification of Etiologic Agents on the Basis of Hazard,* obtainable from the Centers for Disease Control, Office of Biosafety, Public Health Service, U.S. Department of Human Services, Atlanta, Georgia.

Biohazard symbol. An international symbol warning of infectious or potentially infectious hazards.

that designate them as reliable for use for the purposes tested.

biologic false-positive (BFP) a positive result on a serologic test for syphilis (STS), such as the VDRL or rapid plasma reagin (RPR) tests, when syphilis is not present. BFPs occur in 10–50 percent of tested individuals in various populations; the VDRL test usually is weakly reactive, the reactive titer being less than 1:8.

Acute BFP is associated with infectious disease such as bacterial and mycoplasmal pneumonias, subacute bacterial endocarditis, varicella, infectious mononucleosis, and scarlet fever. Chronic BFP is associated with immune complex diseases such as systemic lupus erythematosus, and with leprosy. It also occurs in pregnancy.

biology (bi-ol′o-je) [*bio-* + *-logy*] the study of life and living organisms.

population b., the study of the relationships among organisms in populations. It includes taxonomy, population genetics, ethnology, and ecology.

bioluminescence (bi″o-loo″mĭ-nes′ens) the emission of light as a consequence of the cellular oxidation of some substrate (luciferins) in the presence of an enzyme (luciferases). It is present in bacteria, fungi, protozoa, and species belonging to 40 different orders of animals.

biomass (bi′o-mas) the sum total of living organisms of a particular region, system, or culture medium; in bacteriology, the term refers to the dry weight or volume of microorganisms in a culture.

biomechanics (bi″o-mĕ-kan′iks) the application of mechanics (the physics of forces and motion) to living organisms, such as is involved in the analysis of the stresses and forces involved in locomotion.

biomedical engineering the engineering discipline that deals with the development of biomedical technology, particularly prosthetic devices to replace body parts or assist in performing body functions.

biometry (bi-om′ĕ-tre) [*bio-* + Gr. *metron* measure] the mathematical and statistical analysis of biologic data.

Biomphalaria (bi-om″fah-la′re-ah) a genus of orblike shelled snails of the family Planorbidae, some species of which are the chief molluscan intermediate hosts of the parasitic worm *Schistosoma mansoni,* that cause schistosomiasis in humans. Also called *Australorbis.*

B. glabrata, the host species for *S. mansoni* in parts of the Western hemisphere. Also called *Australorbis glabrata.*

bionics (bi-on′iks) an applied science that uses biologic knowledge to improve the performance of electric or mechanical devices such as computers, sensors, robots, etc.

biophysics (bi″o-fiz′iks) the physics of living organisms, particularly the study of their structure and motion.

biopsy (bi′op-se) [*bio-* + Gr. *opsis* vision] the surgical removal and examination, usually microscopic, of tissues, cells, or fluid from the living body. This procedure is performed to establish or confirm a diagnosis.

aspiration b., a biopsy that involves the use of a biopsy needle to remove a sample of tissue. Small-bore needles are generally used for obtaining a cell suspension, which is best examined as a cytologic preparation. Large-bore needles are most often employed to obtain a well-formed core of tissue that can be processed as any other small tissue biopsy. See also *biopsy n.* under *needle.*

cone b., a conical-shaped incisional biopsy of the cervix, which includes a circular portion of the ectocervix around the os in continuity with the endocervical canal and subjacent stroma. See also the accompanying illustration.

excisional b., a diagnostic procedure in which the entire lesion, along with a cuff or rim of normal tissue, is removed with a scalpel. This biopsy is used to obtain preliminary information for planning the nature and extent of subsequent therapy; in some

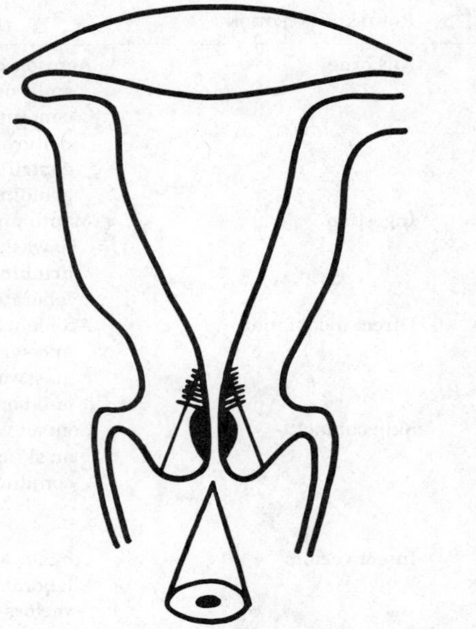

Cone biopsy. Illustration showing cone biopsy for endocervical disease. (From DiSaia, P. J., and Creasman, W. T.: Clinical Gynecologic Oncology. St. Louis, C. V. Mosby Co., 1981.)

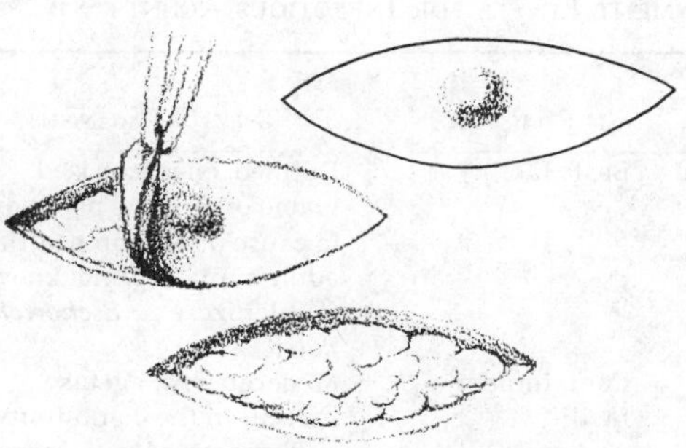

Excisional biopsy. Illustration showing excisional biopsy. (From Nealon, T. F., Jr.: Fundamental Skills in Surgery. 2nd ed. Philadelphia, W. B. Saunders Co., 1971.)

situations, it may be the definitive therapy. See also the accompanying illustration.

fine-needle b., see *needle aspiration cytology.*

incisional b., a preliminary diagnostic procedure used to obtain information for planning the nature and extent of subsequent therapy. Performed with a punch or scalpel, this biopsy involves the removal of a sample of tissue from a lesion. Usually, the specimen is taken at the margin of the lesion so that it includes adjacent normal tissue. In some situations, however, the specimen is taken at the base or center of the lesion; e.g., in the case of a cutaneous tumor suspected of being a verrucous carcinoma, when it is essential to search for evidence of invasion. See also the accompanying illustration.

punch b., any method used to obtain a small, cylindric specimen of tissue (e.g., skin) for examination; it employs a special instrument designed to cut such specimens.

thin-needle b., see *needle aspiration cytology.*

biopterin (bi-op′ter-in) a naturally occurring pteridine, 2-amino-4-hydroxy-6-(1,2-dihydroxypropyl) pteridine.

biosafety (bi″o-sāf′te) the safe handling of microorganisms that are known to cause or have the potential to cause disease in humans. The Centers for Disease Control and the National Institutes of Health, of the U.S. Department of Health and Human Services, have made recommendations applicable to microorganisms and to clinical materials known to contain, or which may contain, agents infectious for humans. Specific microorganisms are assigned to one of four biosafety levels on the basis of the potential hazard of the agent and of the laboratory function or activity (see the accompanying table).

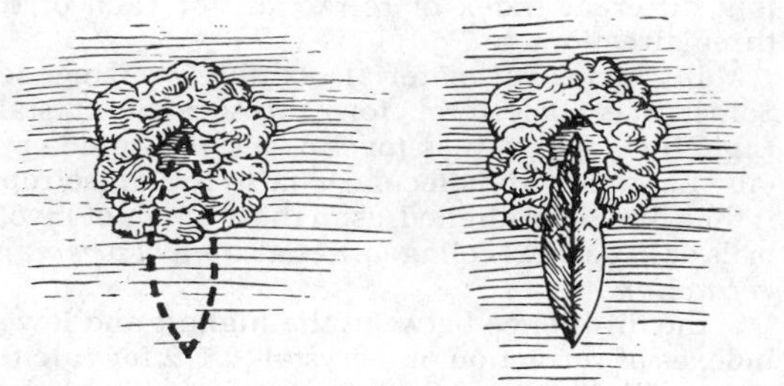

Incisional biopsy. Illustration showing biopsy technique for incisional biopsy. The specimen should contain both normal and abnormal tissue. (From Nealon, T. F., Jr.: Management of the Patient with Cancer. Philadelphia, W. B. Saunders Co., 1965.)

biosynthesis (bi″o-sin′thĕ-sis) the processes of chemical synthesis that occur in living organisms.

biotin (bi′o-tin) a colorless, crystalline, water-soluble compound, hexahydro-2-oxo-1H-thieno[3,4-d]-imidazole-4-pentanoic acid. It is widely distributed in nature, in both animals and plants; food sources are liver, yeast, molasses, and milk. Mainly, it occurs in a combined form, bound to proteins. Biotin deficiency can be produced by a diet containing large amounts of raw egg white. Avidin, a protein in egg white, binds biotin very strongly to form a compound that is not absorbed by the body. The biochemical function of biotin is to serve as a coenzyme in carbon dioxide fixation or carboxylation reactions; it is involved, for example, in the carboxylation of pyruvic acid to form oxaloacetic acid. Also called *vitamin* B_7; formerly called *coenzyme R* and *vitamin H.*

biotin assays a microbiologic assay with *Lactobacillus plantarum,* performed in the same manner as a niacin assay after the sample has been enzymatically treated or acid-hydrolyzed to release all bound biotin. See also *niacin assays.*

biotransformation (bi″o-trans″for-ma′shun) the sequence of chemical reactions undergone by a compound (e.g., a drug or environmental contaminant) in a biologic system. The process is usually due to enzymatic metabolic reactions occurring primarily in the liver but also in extrahepatic tissues. Hydrolysis, oxidation, reduction, or conjugation may be involved in these reactions.

biotype (bi′o-tip) 1. a group of individuals possessing the same genotype.

2. any one of a number of strains of a species of microorganisms having physiologic characteristics that can be differentiated. Clinically, it is possible to define biotypes as biochemical fingerprints by which many of the known bacterial species can be further subgrouped for epidemiologic study.

biparietal (bi″pah-ri′e-tal) pertaining to the two parietal eminences or bones.

biparietal hump see *vertex sharp transient.*

biperiden (bi-per′ĭ-den) [USP], a synthetic anticholinergic drug that is used to reduce the akinesia, rigidity, and tremor of parkinsonism and to reduce the extrapyramidal side-effects of antipsychotic drugs, such as reserpine or phenothiazines. Adverse reactions include blurred vision, dry mouth, and gastric irritation. Symptoms of overdosage are similar to those of atropine poisoning. Trademark, Akineton.

b. hydrochloride, the salt used for oral administration.

b. lactate, the salt used for intramuscular or intravenous administration.

biphasic (bi-fāz′ik) 1. having both gametophyte (haploid) and sporophyte (diploid) generations. See also *alternation of generations.*

2. pertaining to a culture system for the isolation

BIOSAFETY. SUMMARY OF RECOMMENDED CONTAINMENT LEVELS FOR INFECTIOUS AGENTS

BIOSAFETY LEVEL	PRACTICES AND TECHNIQUES	SAFETY EQUIPMENT	FACILITIES	TYPES OF ORGANISMS
1	Standard microbiologic practices	None; primary containment provided by adherence to standard laboratory practices during open bench operations	Basic facility	Defined, characterized, viable organisms not known to cause disease in healthy adult humans or not known to colonize, e.g., *Escherichia coli* K12
2	Level 1 practices plus: protective gloves and coats when conducting procedures with infectious agents; decontamination of all infectious waste; biohazard signs; limited access	Partial containment equipment (i.e., Class I or II biological safety cabinets) used to isolate mechanical and manipulative procedures that produce readily detectable aerosols	Containment facility	Moderate-risk agents present in the community and associated with human disease of varying severity, e.g., *E. coli, Staphylococcus aureus, Pseudomonas aeruginosa*
3	Level 2 practices plus: special laboratory clothing; controlled access	Partial containment equipment used to isolate all procedures that may produce aerosols	High containment facility	Indigenous or exotic agents that may cause serious and potentially lethal infections, e.g., *Mycobacterium, tuberculosis, Brucella* species
4	Level 3 practices plus: entrance through change room where street clothing removed and laboratory clothing donned; shower on exit; all wastes decontaminated on exit from facility	Total containment equipment (i.e., Class III biological safety cabinets) used to isolate all procedures and operations involving infectious materials	Maximum containment facility	Dangerous and exotic agents that pose a high risk of life-threatening disease, e.g., Lassa fever virus

Information courtesy of Centers for Disease Control, Public Health Service, Atlanta, Georgia.

of pathogenic microorganisms derived from blood on both solid and liquid media.

biphenyl (bi-fen′il, bi-fe′nil) phenylbenzene, $(C_6H_5)_2$, a colorless crystalline compound, used as a heat transfer agent and in the synthesis of the halogenated biphenyls and some dyes. Also called *diphenyl.*

bipolar (bi-po′lar) 1. having two poles; having processes at both poles. See also *bipolar cell.*

2. pertaining to both poles; also to bacterial staining confined to the poles (ends) of the organism.

bipolar cell a neuron with two processes emerging symmetrically from opposite sides of the cell body. The axon may be short (bipolar cells of the retina) or long (bipolar ganglion cells of the inner ear). In cells of the dorsal root ganglia and cranial nerve sensory ganglia, the two processes fuse to form a pseudounipolar neuron.

bipolar neuron see *bipolar cell.*

bipyridyl (bi-pĕr″ĭ-dil) a term sometimes used to denote a class of herbicides in which two pyridine rings are joined to form several isomers. Examples are paraquat and diquat, in which the *N* atoms are quaternized and substituted with alkyl groups.

birefringence (bi″re-frin′jens) [*bi-* + L. *refringere* to break up] 1. double refraction, a property of certain anisotropic media, such as the uniaxial crystal calcite, in which light polarized in one direction (the optic axis) travels at a different velocity from light polarized in the other directions. In effect, the crystal has two different indexes of refraction. A beam of light entering the crystal perpendicularly to the optic axis is split into two beams: one, the extraordinary ray, is polarized in the direction of the optic axis (in calcite, its index of refraction (*n*) is 1.486); the other, the ordinary ray, is polarized perpendicularly to the optic axis (in calcite, *n* is 1.658). In calcite, the ordinary ray is refracted more than the extraordinary ray. In biaxial crystals there is a different index of refraction for each of the three directions.

Many biological materials exhibit birefringence. Some, like cholesterol, form anisotropic crystals. Lipid bilayers, such as myelin, act like liquid crystals. Large macromolecular chains are anisotropic if the chains are aligned, as in the A bands of myofibrils or in corneal collagen. See also *nicol prism* and *refraction.*

2. the difference between the highest and lowest indexes of refraction of a crystal (0.172 for calcite).

crystalline b., birefringence that occurs in systems in which the bonds between molecules or ions have a regular asymmetric arrangement; it is independent of the refractive index of the medium.

flow b., birefringence exhibited by substances in solution and flowing; e.g., it is seen in solutions of long, thin molecules, such as nucleoproteins, when molecules are lined up in the path of least resistance to current flow.

form b., birefringence produced by regular orientation of submicroscopic asymmetric particles in a substance or object, differing in refractive index from the surrounding medium; it is the most common form that occurs in organisms. Such birefringence disappears when the object is dipped into a medium with the same refractive index.

strain b., double refraction observed occasionally in isotropic structures when they are subjected to tension or pressure.

birefringent (bi″re-frin′jent) [*bi-* + L. *refringere* to break up] having the property of birefringence; being doubly refractive in plane-polarized light.

birthmark (berth′mark) a congenital blemish or spot on the skin, usually visible at birth or shortly after. Birthmarks are most commonly a superficial vascular anomaly and usually regress with time. See also *nevus.*

vascular b., see *hemangioma* and *nevus.*

bis- (bis) a prefix word element to denote two or twice, e.g., bisalbuminemia.

bisacodyl (bis″ah-ko′dil) [USP], a contact laxative that stimulates the mucosa of the colon, thus inducing reflex peristalsis.

bisacodyl tannex a complex of bisacodyl and tannic acid used in single- or double-contrast radiography of the large bowel. It is administered in both the preparatory cleansing enema and the barium (positive contrast) enema to increase peristalsis and to obtain better coating. This preparation is not given to children under 10 yr of age or to patients with ulcerative colitis. Trademark, Clysodrast.

bisalbuminemia (bis″al-bu″mĭ-ne′me-ah) a polymorphism of serum albumin indicated by a double albumin peak in the serum protein electrophoretic pattern. The variant albumins differ from normal albumin (albumin A) either in electric charge or in forming dimers. This condition is transmitted as an autosomal dominant trait, and does not present significant clinical abnormalities.

Bisalbuminemia strictly refers only to the heterozygous state in which both normal and abnormal albumin are present. Alloalbuminemia refers to the homozygous state, and paralbuminemia refers to both. An acquired temporary bisalbuminemia may occur with diabetes mellitus, nephrotic syndrome, hyperamylasemia, or penicillin therapy.

bis(2-chloroethyl)sulfide (bis″klo″ro-eth″il-sul′fide) a highly toxic chemical war gas, which causes severe skin and eye burns and blisters. Also called *mustard gas* and Yperite.

bisection (bi-sek′shun) [*bi-* + L. *sectio* a cut] a division into two parts by cutting. Also called *hemisection.*

bishydroxycoumarin (bis″hi-drok″se-koo′mahrin) the former name for *dicumarol.*

Bismarck brown (biz′mark) [Prince Otto Edward Leopold von *Bismarck*-Schoenhausen, German statesman, 1815–1898] any of a group of basic azo dyes that do not diffuse in aqueous mounting media and are largely permanent. These dyes are used in histology for staining nuclei in the contrast staining of fats; they may also be used for the metachromatic staining of mucin and cartilage matrix (brownish yellow). Two major members are Bismarck brown R (C.I. 21010) and Y (C.I. 21000).

bismuth (Bi) (biz′muth) [L. *bismuthum,* from Ger. *wismuth,* from *weisse Masse* white mass] a brittle crystalline metal with a reddish tinge; atomic number 83; atomic weight 208.980; Group V of the periodic table; oxidation states +3, +5. It is soluble in nitric and hydrochloric acids and is obtained as a by-product from tin, lead, and copper ores. Various bismuth compounds have been used in medicines, particularly for distress of the gastrointestinal tract; however, as their therapeutic efficacy is doubtful, former medical uses are of historical interest only. Because bismuth is not easily absorbed, toxicity is not severe, but toxicity from chronic exposure occurs with symptoms of weakness, decreased appetite, fever, rheumatic-like pain, and foul breath. Miners may be affected by a radioactive isotope, ^{214}Bi.

bismuth aluminate a fine powder, $Bi_2(Al_2O_4)_3$, used as a gastric antacid; M.W. 771.88.

bismuth assays 1. the Reinsch test, in which bismuth salts are reduced to metallic bismuth by metallic copper. Concentrated hydrochloric acid and a copper foil strip or wire spiral are added to a sample, then heated for several hours. Metallic bismuth, arsenic, antimony, selenium, tellurium, and some sulfides are deposited on the copper; all but bismuth and antimony dissolve in potassium cyanide solution.

2. a semiquantitative method that follows the first method with the color reaction for bismuth. The deposit is dissolved in nitric acid, and an orange product is formed by reaction with quinine sulfate and potassium iodide. The color intensity is compared with standard solutions processed in the same way.

bisphosphatidylglycerol (bis-fos″fah-ti-dil-glis′er-ol) an ester of two phosphatidic acids with an additional molecule of glycerol. Also called *cardiolipin* and *diphosphatidylglycerol.*

2,3-bisphosphoglycerate (DPG; 2,3-DPG) (bis-fos″fo-glis′er-āt) a diphosphate ester of glyceric acid. It is a product of glucose metabolism and binds strongly to deoxygenated hemoglobin (deoxyhemoglobin). A high concentration of 2,3-bisphosphoglycerate decreases the oxygen affinity of hemoglobin. Also called *2,3-diphosphoglycerate.*

bisphosphoglycerate phosphatase an enzyme of the hydrolase class (EC 3.1.3.13) that catalyzes the reaction 2,3-bisphospho-D-glycerate + $H_2O \rightleftarrows$ 3-phospho-D-glycerate + orthophosphate. The reaction is important in the regulation of the oxygen affinity of hemoglobin. Also called *diphosphoglycerate phosphatase.*

bisphosphoglyceromutase (bis-fos″fo-glis″er-o-mu′tās) an enzyme of the transferase class (3-phospho-D-glyceroyl-phosphate: 3-phospho-D-glycerate phosphotransferase, EC 2.7.5.4) that catalyzes the reaction 3-phospho-D-glyceroyl-phosphate + 3-phospho-D-glycerate ⇄ 3-phospho-D-glycerate + 2,3-bisphospho-D-glycerate. The reaction is a shunt mechanism in the Embden-Meyerhof pathway of glycolysis in erythrocytes. A genetic deficiency of the enzyme, transmitted as an autosomal recessive trait, causes a hemolytic anemia. Also called *2,3-diphosphoglycerate mutase.*

bis-trimethylsilylacetamide (BSA) (bis-tri-meth″il-sil″il-ah-sēt′ah-mid) a silylation reagent used in gas chromatography, $CH_3CON[Si(CH_3)_3]_2$.

Repeated use fouls flame ionization detectors. See also *silylation.*

bis-trimethylsilyltrifluoroacetamide (BSTFA) (bis-tri-meth″il-sil″il-tri-floo″or-o-ah-sēt′ah-mid) a volatile silylation reagent, $CF_3CON[Si(CH_3)_3]_2$. It is miscible with most solvents used in gas chromatography, so no additional solvent is necessary for derivatization. See also *silylation.*

bisulfate (bi-sul′fāt) 1. pertaining to the HSO_4^- ion.
2. a compound containing this ion. Also called hydrogen or acid sulfate, e.g., $NaHSO_4$, sodium bisulfate, sodium hydrogen sulfate, or sodium acid sulfate.

bisulfite (bi-sul′fīt) 1. pertaining to the HSO_3^- ion.
2. a compound containing this ion. Also called acid or hydrogen sulfite, e.g., $NaHSO_3$, sodium bisulfite, sodium hydrogen sulfite, or sodium acid sulfite.

bit (bit) 1. a binary digit, 0 or 1, used in the base 2 number system.
2. a unit of information equivalent to knowing which of two equally probable possibilities has occurred.
3. a switch in a computer memory or logic circuit that has two states (off and on), representing the bits 0 and 1. The bits of computer memories are commonly grouped into bytes and words. See also *information* and *number system.*

bite-wing film (bīt′wing) a dental x-ray film, held inside the mouth by having the patient bite on a fin attached to the center of the film. It is used for interproximal projections showing the crowns and necks of the teeth. See also *dental radiography.*

bithionol (bĭ-thi′o-nol) 2,2-thiobis(4,6-dichlorophenol), a grayish-white, odorless powder. It is soluble in acetone, alcohol, and ether, and is used as a local antiseptic; when applied to the skin, it may induce photoallergic contact dermatitis. Bithionol is also used orally in treatment of infections of *Fasciola hepatica* (a liver fluke) and *Paragonimus westermani* (a lung fluke). Given orally for a period of 10–30 da, egg counts of stools and sputum become negative after a few days of treatment. Side-effects include diarrhea, nausea, vomiting, abdominal pain, and (occasionally) urticarial rash. Trademarks, Actamer and Lorothidol.

Bithynia (bi-thin′e-ah) the former name for a genus of snails now considered part of the genus *Bulima.*

biting house fly see *Stomoxys.*

Bitot's spots (be′tōz) [Pierre A. *Bitot,* Bordeaux physician, 1822–1888] whitish or foamy-gray superficial spots on the conjunctiva of the eyes, formed of keratinized epithelium and associated with, but not specific for, vitamin A deficiency.

biuret (bi′u-ret) [L. *bis* twice + *urea*] a derivative of urea, $H_2NCONHCONH_2$ formed by heating urea to 180°C. It is soluble in ethanol, partially soluble in water (2 g/100 g of water at 25°C). Aqueous solutions react (chelate) with Cu(II) ions and NaOH to form a reddish-violet complex, which absorbs light in the ranges of 305–310 and 540–550 nm. Also called *allophanamide, carbamylurea,* and *dicarbamylamine.*

biuret reaction a chemical reaction that occurs in an alkaline medium between cupric ions and any compound containing at least two —NHCO—, —$NHCH_2$—, —NHC(NH)—, —NHCS—, or similar groups joined together directly or through a single carbon or nitrogen atom. An example is the reaction with biuret ($NH_2CONHCO_2NH_2$), which gave the reaction its name. The copper in the reagent is thought to chelate to two pairs of such —NHCX— centers to form a colored complex absorbing at 540–545 nm and also at 300–310 nm.
The reaction is widely employed in colorimetric tests for fibrinogen, albumin, and total protein in plasma or serum. Tripeptides and higher polypeptides react, but amino acids and dipeptides do not. The purplish color obtained varies somewhat with the type of protein.

bivalent (bi-va′lent) 1. in chemistry, having a valence of 2. Also called *divalent.*
2. in genetics, the structure that is formed during the first meiotic prophase by the synapsis of two homologous chromosomes.

Bk symbol for the chemical element *berkelium.*

blackbody (blak′bod-e) an idealized object that is a perfect absorber and emitter of electromagnetic radiation. All incident radiation is absorbed, and the emission spectrum is completely determined by the temperature of the blackbody.

blackbody radiation the radiation emitted by a blackbody, which is described by the Planck radiation law: $E = 2\pi h\nu^3/c^2(e^{h\nu/kT} - 1)$, where ν is the frequency, T is the absolute temperature, h is Planck's constant, c is the velocity of light, k is Boltzmann's constant, and E is the radiated power per unit frequency interval per unit area. The total energy at all frequencies is given by the Stefan-Boltzmann law: $E = \sigma T^4$, where σ is the Stefan-Boltzmann constant, 5.6699×10^{-8} W/m²·K⁴.
Blackbody radiation is in thermal equilibrium with the emitting blackbody. Sunlight is primarily blackbody radiation at a temperature of about 5700 K. The redder emission of an incandescent lamp has a temperature of about 3000 K. Below 2000 K, most of the radiation is emitted as infrared and radio waves.

black box a term originally applied to electronic components and now used for any physical system that can be described in terms of an input, an output, and a function (the transfer function) connecting the output and the input. A "black box approach" is an investigation of the systems named above by measurement of the output (response) for various values of the input (stimuli) to determine the transfer function without any investigation of the actual internal mechanisms that connect the input and output.

black death see *plague.*

black lead see *input terminal 1.*

black light electromagnetic radiation that is invisible to the human eye, such as ultraviolet light or infrared light.

black lung disease see under *anthracosis.*

black periodic acid method a histologic staining procedure that may be used to demonstrate smooth and striated muscle stroma, mucosal basement membranes, reticulum, starch, glycogen, and mucins, as well as other substances. Cytoplasm turns grayish pink or red; nuclei, deeper red; and glycogen and starch granules, mucins, fungi cell walls, and muscle stroma, black.

black sickness see *kala-azar.*

blackwater fever the syndrome of intravascular hemolysis, hemoglobinuria, and acute renal failure, which can occur in acute falciparum malaria, especially in individuals in whom a previous infection was treated with quinine. The cause has not been definitely established, but it probably involves sensitization to malarial antigens or to quinine; deposition of immune complexes leads to acute tubular necrosis.

Persons affected are treated with chloroquine, or primaquine and sulfonamides for chloroquine-resistant infection; quinine is not used. Hemodialysis may be required for treatment of acute renal failure.

Also called West African fever.

black widow spider see *Lactrodectus.*

bladder (blad′er) [A.S. *blaedre*] 1. a hollow musculomembranous sac, especially one serving as a receptacle for secretion, as the gallbladder or urinary bladder; the term is often used alone to designate the urinary bladder.

2. anything resembling such a sac.

3. a blister or cyst filled with air or serous fluid.

urinary b., a muscular, epithelium-lined sac in the pelvis that receives urine from the kidneys through the ureters and retains it until, by contraction of the smooth muscle in its wall, the urine is voided through the urethra. When the bladder is empty, it is roughly a three-sided pyramid with the apex located inferiorly. It has a superior surface, a pair of inferolateral surfaces, and a posterior surface or base. Each surface is roughly triangular, but as the bladder fills it becomes more spherical and the margins of the sides are no longer evident. The distended bladder comes into relation with the pelvic side-walls and the fascia transversalis above the pubis. Peritoneum clothes the superior surface and a small part of the base before being reflected onto the rectum in the male and uterus in the female. In the male, the base is largely covered by the seminal vesicles. The lowest part of the bladder, surrounding the urethral orifice, is termed the bladder neck; in the male it rests on the prostate, and in the female, on the fascia covering the sphincter urethrae.

The interior of the bladder can be visualized radiologically by a cystogram, and can be inspected through a cystoscope and the ureters catheterized for retrograde pyelography. The bladder surface is wrinkled when it is empty, with the exception of the trigone, a triangular area on the posterior surface with the ureteral orifices at its upper angles and the internal orifice of the urethra at its lower angle. The uvula is a bulge located, in the male, immediately above the urethral orifice, produced by the median lobe of the prostate.

The bladder is lined by transitional epithelium supported by a submucosal layer of connective tissue that is generally termed the lamina propria. The muscularis of the bladder is thick, and in some areas two poorly defined smooth muscle layers can be discerned.

bladder tumors neoplasms of the bladder, of which 97 percent are epithelial. The incidence of papillomas (low-grade, probably benign, papillary tumors composed of transitional cells) varies, depending on the criteria of the pathologist making the diagnosis. Most tumors are transitional cell carcinomas. Infrequent adenocarcinomas and squamous carcinoma occur; they can also be admixed with a transitional cell carcinoma. Some mucinous adenocarcinomas arising in the superior part of the bladder are of urachal derivation. In children, the most common tumor is a rhabdomyosarcoma, typically displaying a botryoid appearance; these are aggressive neoplasms that indicate a poor prognosis for the patient. Bladder sarcomas in adults are usually leiomyosarcomas. Occasionally a pheochromocytoma arises within the bladder wall.

Most transitional cell carcinomas are papillary. Histologic assessment includes assigning a histologic grade to the tumor (usually on a scale of 1 to 4) and determining whether invasion is present and, if so, whether there is lymphatic or muscular extension. Aggressive tumors infiltrate into perivesical soft tissue and spread to regional nodes or more distant sites. Metastases occur in more than 30 percent of cases overall; the rate exceeds 50 percent for tumors that are deeply invasive.

blanch (blanch) to become pale.

blank (blangk) [Fr. *blanc* white] 1. in spectrophotometric analyses (e.g., in clinical chemistry), a cuvet prepared containing a solution identical in composition and content to that in the sample cuvet except for absence of the analyte being measured. The solution in the blank cuvet will have been treated identically (heating, mixing) to the solution in the sample cuvet. The cuvets containing the sample and/or standards are read in the spectrophotometer against the blank cuvet set at 100 percent transmittance. Such a blank is commonly referred to as a "reagent blank." A sample blank contains the specimen (e.g., serum or urine) in a diluent but no color reagent, in an attempt to correct for pigment and/or turbidity in the sample.

2. to turn off the beam of a cathode ray tube (CRT) by applying a large negative voltage to the accelerating electrode.

3. in automatic data processing, a code character that represents a space in a character string.

blast/o (blas′to) [Gr. *blastos* germ] a word element used in combining form to denote a bud or budding, an embryonic stage, or a formative element, cell, or layer, e.g., blastocyst or blast cell.

blast (blast) [Gr. *blastos* germ] an early stage in cellular development before appearance of the definitive characteristics of the mature cell.

blast cell a term used to designate a multipotential cell, particularly a primitive myeloid or lymphoid precursor cell.

blast cell leukemia see *stem cell l.* under *leukemia.*

blast crisis the acute phase of chronic myelogenous leukemia. The patient's condition suddenly worsens; the white cell count becomes extremely elevated with a high percentage of blast forms in both the blood and bone marrow. Death usually follows. Also called *blastic transformation.* See also *chronic myelogenous l.* under *leukemia.*

blastema (blas-te′mah) [Gr. *blastēma* shoot] 1. the primitive tissue from which cells are formed.

2. a group of cells capable of giving rise to a part or the whole of an organ either through normal development or through regeneration.

blastic (blas′tik) pertaining to the blast stage in cellular development.

blastic transformation see *blast crisis.*

blastocyst (blas′to-sist) [*blasto-* + Gr. *kystis* bladder] the stage of embryonic development entered by the mammalian embryo near the time of implantation into the wall of the uterus, consisting of a hollow ball of cells with a small cluster of cells adhering to the inner surface, as shown in the accompanying illustration.

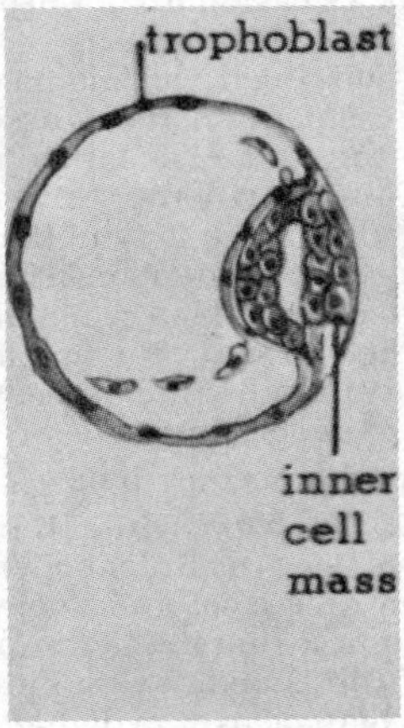

Blastocyst. One stage in the formation of the blastocyst and its embedding in the uterine wall. (From Ham, A. W.: Histology. 7th ed. Philadelphia, J. B. Lippincott Co., 1974.)

blastocyte (blas′to-sīt) an undifferentiated cell of the blastula or morula stage of the embryo.

blastoma (blas-to′mah) [*blast-* + *-oma* tumor] a neoplasm composed of primitive cells responsible for the development of a given organ (blastema).

blastomere (blas′to-mēr) [*blasto-* + Gr. *meros* a part] one of the cells produced by cleavage of a fertilized ovum. Also called *cleavage cell.*

Blastomyces (blas″to-mi′sēz) [*blasto-* + Gr. *mykēs* fungus] a genus of thermal dimorphic imperfect fungi, of the Ascomycetes class, that is one of the true pathogenic fungi. It grows in mycelial form at room temperature and as a yeastlike form at body temperature.

B. brasiliensis, see *P. brasiliensis* under *Paracoccidioides.*

B. dermatitidis, a species that is the causative agent in blastomycosis. It has large multinucleate cells, 8–10 μm in diameter, and occurs in the tissues as a unicellular budding yeast, usually separated from the parent cell by a large septum. On a culture medium at 25°C, *B. dermatitidis* appears in its mycelial form, with varied coloring: white, tan, or dark brown. Its ascomycetous state is *Ajellomyces dermatitidis.* See also *North American b.* under *blastomycosis.*

blastomycin (blas″to-mi′sin) a sterile broth filtrate of a culture of *Blastomyces dermatitidis,* used for skin testing in the diagnosis of blastomycosis. Because of cross reactions with other fungal antigens, the test is not considered conclusive.

blastomycosis (blas″to-mi-ko′sis) [*blasto-* + Gr. *mykēs* fungus] a general term used in some parts of the world for any infection caused by budding yeasts in tissue; the term is often used alone to refer to North American blastomycosis.

European b., a disease of the lungs, bone, and central nervous system caused by the fungus *Cryptococcus neoformans;* see *cryptococcosis.*

North American b., a chronic granulomatous and suppurative fungal disease caused by the dimorphic fungus *Blastomyces dermatitidis.* This disease usually begins with a pulmonary infection, which may spread to skin and bone. Although the infection is called North American blastomycosis, it is found worldwide.

Epidemiology. North American blastomycosis is most often found in 20- to 40-yr-old males, usually living in rural settings. Most cases are found in the southeastern and north central United States. Although the disease also occurs in dogs, there is no evidence of spread from canines to humans, or from one person to another. This illness does not usually occur in epidemics, unlike histoplasmosis and coccidioidomycosis.

Pathogenic Mechanisms. North American blastomycosis is initiated by the inhalation of spores, probably from soil, and may disseminate by invading the blood vessels and lymphatics. In this state, the fungus is in the yeast phase and usually ends up in skin, bone, and any mucous membrane.

Clinical Diagnosis. The disease most often begins with an insidious onset of low-grade fever, cough, nonpleuritic chest pain, anorexia, malaise, and weight loss. Erythema nodosum lesions may occur, as well as papular lesions, which can break down, ulcerate, drain, and spread out. Pus and yeast cells are found at the periphery of such lesions, while the central area of the lesion represents healing.

Examination of the sputum or biopsy material from the advancing margin of skin ulcers may reveal typical budding yeast organisms. This disease must be differentiated from other chronic and suppurative pulmonary diseases such as tuberculosis and sarcoid and pulmonary neoplasms, as well as other fungal diseases.

Laboratory Diagnosis. The diagnosis of blastomycosis depends on histopathologic direct examination and culture. Initially, the aspirated material from the periphery of the skin lesions is examined microscopically in 6 percent potassium hydroxide solution. The yeast is a thick-walled spherical cell with broad-based budding. Stained *B. dermatitidis* are multinucleate, whereas *Histoplasma capsulatum* and *Cryptococcus neoformans* are uninucleate. In pulmonary blastomycosis, a first morning sputum is optimal for detection of the presence of yeast cells. Specimens are cultured on blood agar without cyclohexamide at 37°C and Sabouraud's agar at 25°C. Growth of *B. dermatitidis* is slow and may range from a few days to a month. The colony morphology is usually flat, glabrous, and white-tan in color, with concentric rings. There is no reliable skin test. Problematically, serology is nonspecific owing to a high cross-reactivity with antigenic components of the organisms causing histoplasmosis and coccidioidomycosis. Two tests, complement-fixation (CF) and immunodiffusion (ID), have been used in the serodiagnosis of blastomycosis. The CF test is less specific than the ID test; however, in documented cases the CF test may provide prognostic value. There is a good fluorescent antibody test specific for the yeast phase of *B. dermatitidis.*

Treatment. Treatment of blastomycosis involves amphotericin B, to which the fungus is highly susceptible. In spinal fluid, the disease is treated with direct injections of both amphotericin B and hydrocortisone. Other therapies include the less toxic hydroxystilbamidine.

South American b., a skin disease caused by the

imperfect fungus *Paracoccidioides brasilensis;* see *paracoccidioidomycosis.*

blastospore (blas'to-spōr) a spore formed by budding in yeast and yeastlike cells.

blastula (blas'tu-lah) [L.] an early embryonic stage following cleavage of the fertilized ovum. It consists of one cell layer (the blastoderm), which surrounds a fluid-filled cavity (the blastocele).

blastulation (blas"tu-la'shun) the development of the morula into the blastula by formation of the cleavage cavity (blastocele). See also *embryonic development.*

Blatta (blat'ah) a genus of insects, order Blattaria—the cockroaches. Cockroaches often serve as intermediate hosts of certain helminths. *B. orientalis,* the black beetle, is a common European species.

Blattidae (blat'ĭ-de) a family of cockroaches. Cockroaches have a cosmopolitan distribution and are primarily found in unsanitary environments; they feed on excrement and sputum, and may transmit disease by depositing feces or regurgitating on human food. They sometimes serve as intermediate hosts of the tapeworm *Hymenolepis diminuta.*

bleach (blēch) an agent that whitens a material by chemically oxidizing or reducing colored substances to colorless forms. Most bleaches are toxic and strong oxidizing agents, such as hydrogen peroxide and sodium hypochlorite (chlorine bleach). Some bleaches function by reducing dyes or pigments to colorless leuko forms.

bleaching (blēch'ing) the act or process of removing stains or color by chemical means.

bleb (blĕb) a large, flaccid vesicle, usually at least 1 cm in diameter. Blebs are generally filled with fluid such as serum or blood, although they may contain air when located on the surface of the lung.

bleeding (blēd'ing) 1. the act of losing blood; the escape of blood from an injured vessel.

2. in histology, the diffusion of dye into the medium; often a problem with aqueous mounting media.

blennorrhea (blen"o-re'ah) [Gr. *blennos* mucus + *rhoia* flow] a free discharge from a mucous membrane surface, especially a gonorrheal discharge from the urethra, vagina, or conjunctiva caused by infection.

b. adultorum, gonorrheal ophthalmia; acute and severe purulent ophthalmia due to gonorrheal infection.

b. neonatorum, see *o. neonatorum* under *ophthalmia.*

bleomycin sulfate (ble"o-mi'sin) an antineoplastic drug that is a mixture of glycopeptide antibiotics isolated from *Streptomyces verticillus,* which inhibits DNA synthesis and, to a lesser extent, RNA and protein synthesis. It is often used in combination with other chemotherapeutic agents such as vincristine, doxorubicin, and cisplatin. Trademark, Blenoxane. For more information, see *Appendix A.*

blephar/o (blef'ah-ro) [Gr. *blepharon* eyelid] a word element used in combining form to denote an eyelid or eyelash, e.g., blepharoptosis.

blepharitis (blef"ah-ri'tis) [*blephar-* + *-itis*] an inflammation of the eyelids.

ulcerative b., blepharitis marked by small ulcerated areas along the eyelid margin, multiple suppurative lesions, and loss of lashes.

blepharoplast (blef'ah-ro-plast") [*blepharo-* + Gr. *plassein* to form] see *basal body.*

blepharoptosis (blef"ar-op-to'sis) [*blepharo-* + Gr. *ptōsis* a fall] drooping of an upper eyelid; ptosis.

blind (blīnd) lacking the sense of sight. For practical or legal purposes, the term has been used to refer to a condition in which visual acuity for distant vision is 20/200 or less in the better eye with best correction, or in which the widest diameter of visual field subtends an angle of less than 20°. For social purposes, the term may be used to refer to a condition in which vision is insufficient to permit individuals to support themselves in an occupation, making them dependent on others or on various devices.

blind spot in the retina, the exit site of the optic nerve, so called because there are no receptors at this point.

blink responses the evoked compound muscle action potentials elicited from the two orbicularis oculi muscles by percutaneous electric or mechanical stimulation of the supraorbital nerve (a branch of the trigeminal nerve).

An early ipsilateral response (the R_1 wave) occurs with a latency of 9–11 msec, and a late bilateral response (the R_2 wave), associated with a visible twitch of the muscles, is recorded with a latency of 28–32 msec. Both responses are transmitted through the polysynaptic components of the blink reflex, a reflex arc integrated in the brain stem, with an afferent pathway through the main sensory fibers of the trigeminal nerve and an efferent pathway via the motor fibers of the facial nerve. Elicitation of the blink responses can be used clinically to identify a conduction abnormality in either of these two arms of the reflex.

blister (blis'ter) [L. *vesicula*] a localized collection of fluid in the epidermis, which separates and elevates the horny upper layers from the underlying parts; a vesicle.

fever b., a lesion on the skin or mucous membrane due to infection with herpes simplex virus. Fever blisters often accompany fever and most commonly appear about the lips or nose.

block (blok) 1. an obstruction or stoppage.

2. a term used to express an obstruction of the passage of muscular or nervous impulses.

3. regional anesthesia.

4. in automatic data processing, a group of consecutive memory locations, or records in a file that are input or output as a single unit.

5. see *atrioventricular block.*

blockade (blok-ād') in histochemistry, a chemical reaction that alters a particular reactive group so that it will not be stained. For example, amino and hydroxy groups can be protected by forming benzoic acid or acetic acid esters (benzoylation or acetylation); this blocks the PAS reaction.

block diagram a diagram in which the major subunits of a system are represented as rectangles containing the subunit names, and interactions between the subunits (signal, information, activity, or energy flows) are represented by connecting lines. Arrowheads on the connecting lines indicate the direction of flow. See also *flow chart.*

blocking (blok'ing) 1. in electroencephalography, the temporary obliteration (desynchronization) of electric activity recorded from the brain in response to the physiologic stimulation of the individual or to the electric stimulation of the brain.

2. the temporary unresponsiveness of an amplifier resulting from input overload.

3. see under *embedding.*

blocking antibody an antibody that can compete with another antibody from a different class or group for the same antigenic determinant. The competitive inhibition of blocking antibodies is due to similarities in antibody specificity. Blocking antibodies are also capable of blocking cell-mediated reactions on sensitized lymphocytes, thus permitting the growth of tumor cells. Blocking antibodies of IgG class interfere with IgE-mediated allergic reactions and are thought to be the primary mechanism of desensitization to allergens.

blood (B) (blud) [L. *sanguis, cruor;* Gr. *haima*] the fluid that circulates through the heart, arteries, capillaries, and veins. Blood is the chief means of transport within the body, carrying oxygen from the lungs to the body tissues and carbon dioxide from the tissues to the lungs. It also carries absorbed nutrients from the digestive system to the tissues, carries waste products from the tissues to the kidneys and bowel for excretion, and carries fluid to and from the tissues, thus maintaining proper fluid balance throughout the body. The average pH of human blood is about 7.40.

In response to trauma or infection, blood cells and antibodies carried in the blood are brought to a point of infection, or blood-clotting substances are carried to a break in a blood vessel. The blood also carries hormones from the endocrine glands to the target organs, and it assists in the regulation of body temperature by carrying excess heat from the interior of the body to the surface layers of the skin, where the heat is dissipated to the surrounding air.

Blood is composed of two main parts: (1) plasma, the fluid portion, which consists primarily of water in which are dissolved proteins and many inorganic and organic substances carried by the blood to and from the tissues; and (2) blood cells, the particles suspended in the plasma, making up about 45 percent of total blood volume and including erythrocytes (red blood cells), leukocytes (white blood cells), and thrombocytes (platelets). The red and white blood cells are also known as corpuscles.

See also *erythrocyte, leukocyte, plasma,* and *platelet.*

citrated b., blood treated with sodium citrate which prevents its coagulation.

cord b., the blood contained in the vessels of the umbilical cord at the time of birth.

occult b., see *occult blood.*

peripheral b., blood obtained from parts of the body that are some distance from the heart. Examples are blood drawn from the earlobe, fingertip, heel pad, or antecubital vein.

blood-air barrier the physical barrier to the diffusion of gas from alveoli to the erythrocytes, consisting of the surfactant that lines the alveoli, the alveolocapillary membrane, the plasma in the capillary, and the membrane and intracellular fluid of the erythrocyte. This pathway does not normally form a significant barrier to gaseous diffusion, except in conditions under which it is lengthened or altered (alveolocapillary block) because of factors such as the growth of fibrous tissue, presence of extraalveolar cells, dilation of the capillaries, presence of intraalveolar and interstitial edema fluid, or change in shape of the erythrocytes.

blood bank a facility for the collection, processing, storage, and distribution of blood, blood components, and blood products. Most blood banks provide a comprehensive transfusion service that includes crossmatching and testing of blood components, as well as consultation concerning their use.

blood bank technology specialist a medical technologist with training in blood banking. Educational preparation involves completion of an approved 1-yr program; graduates are certified by the American Society of Clinical Pathologists, and are designated MT (ASCP) SBB.

blood-brain barrier the functional barrier, separating the blood from the parenchyma of the central nervous system, which prevents the entry of large molecules into the central nervous system. It appears to result from tight junctions between the endothelial cells of the nonfenestrated capillaries and between choroidal ependymal cells.

blood buffering capacity the maximal quantity of hydrogen ions that combines with the solutes normally present in a liter of blood, with a range of 45–53 mEq/l in the healthy adult. It can be estimated as the total number of bicarbonate and phosphate ions, negative charges on the plasma proteins and on hemoglobin, and other minor blood buffers.

blood cell any cellular element of the blood including erythrocytes, leukocytes, and (in some contexts) platelets.

blood cell count a count of the number of red blood cells (RBC) and white blood cells (WBC) per unit volume in a sample of venous blood. A complete blood count (CBC) also includes measurement of the hematocrit, hemoglobin, and erythrocyte indices (MCV, MCH, and MCHC). These counts are usually performed by automated instruments (see *blood cell count automation*); in most laboratories, manual methods are no longer used for routine work. The manual methods involve use of a counting chamber (hemacytometer), which is a glass slide with platforms holding up the ruled cover glass and forming a chamber exactly 0.1 mm deep. The blood sample is diluted 1 in 200 for the red cell count and 1 in 20 for the white cell count, using either a Thoma pipet or a test tube and disposable pipets. For the white cell count the diluting fluid contains acetic acid to lyse red cells. The fluid is placed in the counting chamber so that it completely fills the chamber, and the cells are allowed to settle.

Red cells are counted in five small squares 0.2 mm on a slide (a total volume of 0.02 μl). Because the dilution is 1 in 200, this is equivalent to 10^{-4} μl of blood, so the count is multiplied by 10,000 to give the number of cells per microliter. White cells are counted in four large squares 1.0 mm on a side (a total volume of 0.4 μl), equivalent to 0.02 μl of blood, so the count is multiplied by 50 to give the number of cells per microliter.

Blood cell counts are among the most commonly performed laboratory tests. They are of great utility in the diagnosis of primary blood diseases, as well as in a variety of infections and acute and chronic diseases in which the blood counts are affected secondarily.

See also *differential leukocyte count,* the accompanying table, and *Appendix C.*

blood cell count automation the counting of each

BLOOD CELL COUNT

COMPONENT	REFERENCE RANGES
Red cell count	3.8–5.8 million/mm³
White cell count	4,500–11,000/mm³
Platelet count	150,000–450,000 mm³
Hemoglobin	13.5–18.0 g/dl (males); 12.0–16.0 (females)
Hematocrit	39.8–52.0 ml/100 ml of blood (males); 34.9–46.9 (females)
Red cell indices	
Mean corpuscular hemoglobin	26.4–34.0 pg
Mean corpuscular hemoglobin concentration	31.5–35.8%
Mean corpuscular volume	80.5–100.0 μm³

of the formed elements of the blood—red blood cells (RBC), white blood cells (WBC), and platelets—by electronic instruments. The cells are detected by one of two general methods: the voltage pulse method (Coulter method) or the electro-optical method. Various instruments are available. The basic models perform red cell counts and white cell counts, whereas the more advanced models routinely measure four parameters: red blood cell count, white blood cell count, blood hemoglobin concentration, and mean corpuscular volume (MCV). From these parameters three other red cell indices are calculated: hematocrit (HCT = MCV × total RBC), mean corpuscular hemoglobin (MCH = Hb/RBC), and mean corpuscular hemoglobin concentration (MCHC = Hb/Hct). Other models also make platelet counts simultaneously.

VOLTAGE PULSE COUNTER. In these instruments, a blood sample is diluted in an isotonic, EDTA-anticoagulated solution and is drawn through a narrow aperture. An electric current flowing between two platinum electrodes located on either side of the aperture passes through the solution (a conductor), not through the blood cells suspended in it. Each time a cell passes through the aperture, a voltage pulse (current decrease) occurs and is recorded. The magnitude of the pulse is proportional to the portion of the aperture occluded by the cell, i.e., the volume of saline replaced by the nonconducting cell as it passes through the aperture, as well as the cross-sectional area of the cell, which is influenced by shape and deformability.

When two or more cells pass through the aperture simultaneously, a single large pulse is produced; small pulses are produced by subcellular particles. A discriminator circuit rejects pulses that are excessively large or small, accepting only those with pulse heights falling between two preset voltage levels. The cell suspension is drawn through the aperture by a column of mercury, which is pulled up a glass tube by a vacuum pump. As the mercury rises between two contacts, a precisely determined volume flows through the aperture and a cell count is recorded.

The red cell count is performed on a dilution of whole blood containing both red cells and white cells. Because there are usually 500 red cells per white cell, the error produced by counting white cells with red cells is negligible. However, when the white cell count is above 5×10^{10} l, a significant error is introduced, which must be corrected. In the more advanced models, the MCV is determined by a circuit that averages the pulse heights of all the counts; this is proportional to the cell volume. The size distribution of the cells is also determined from the distribution of the signal pulses produced in counting the cells. A more sophisticated model also determines the red cell distribution width (RDW).

During calibration, the instrument may be adjusted using the hemoglobin concentration or hematocrit; the hemoglobin value determined by cyanmethemoglobin standards is thought to be a better reference method than the microhematocrit. (Macrohematocrits are too variable for calibration purposes.) It has been shown that means of the MCV, MCH, and MCHC are so constant in normal, and even in many patient, populations (because most anemias are normocytic and normochromic) that the average of 20 determinations does not differ more than 1 percent from established standard values, and thus can be used for calibration checks. A reference hemoglobin determination is needed to guard against dilution errors that would remain undetected.

The white cell count is determined by counting a blood sample diluted in an isotonic solution to which saponin has been added; this lyses the red cells but not the white cells. The hemoglobin concentration is determined in a hemoglobinometer. Whole blood is diluted and lysed with saponin. The diluted sample is pumped through the hemoglobinometer, where a modified Drabkin's reagent is added. The hemoglobin is converted to cyanmethemoglobin by the reagent, and the hemoglobin concentration is then determined by standard photometric methods. More advanced instruments can determine the WBC and Hb from the same sample dilution.

ELECTROOPTICAL COUNTERS. These instruments detect cells optically while a diluted sample is drawn through an illuminated flow cell; some instruments use a laser beam for illumination. The light scattered by the individual cells is detected and recorded.

Some of the instruments determine the MCV from the pulse height (similar to the voltage pulse counters) and compute the hematocrit (packed cell volume, PCV) as the MCV × RBC. Others accumulate the pulses over a fixed period of time and thus determine a value proportional to the PCV, computing the MCV as the PCV/RBC.

A manual method for determining hematocrit involves filling a capillary tube with whole blood; the proportion of the length of the packed red cell column to the length of the whole blood (red cell plus plasma) column is determined visually or electro-optically.

PLATELET COUNTING. Platelet counts are determined by any of these automated systems using either whole blood or platelet-rich plasma. The more sophisticated instruments have the capacity to determine a platelet count, platelet hematocrit (PCT), mean platelet volume (MPV), and platelet distribution width PDW). The size measurements of platelets determined from samples diluted from EDTA-anticoagulated blood are probably unreliable because of swelling of platelets. (It should be noted that most of these parameters have not yet been approved by the U.S. Food and Drug Administration.) Additionally, these instruments are capable of detecting white cell sizes and distribution.

SOURCES OF ERROR. The major sources of error in blood cell counting are dilution, sampling, and calibration. In all three categories, automated methods are superior to manual methods. The large dilutions required are performed by accurate automated dilutors. The sampling error obeys Poisson statistics; the coefficient of variation (CV) is $(100/\sqrt{n})$ percent, where n is the cell count. Thus, a manual method counting 500 cells has an inherent CV of approximately 4.5 percent. The overall CV of manual methods in routine work is in the range of 10–15 percent. Automated counters can reliably perform measurements with a CV in the range of 1–3 percent.

Error may also be introduced by the presence of cold agglutinins. The agglutination of a portion of red cells by cold agglutinins gives erroneously high MCV and also low red cell counts. The spurious macrocytosis is proportionally greater than the reduction in the erythrocyte counts, so that an unusually high MCHC often pinpoints the error, which can then be corrected by prewarming the blood sample. Erroneous hemoglobin values may be caused by the failure of red cells to lyse in the reagents.

See also *cytometry.*

blood-cerebral barrier see *blood-brain barrier.*

blood clot blood that has lost its fluidity because of coagulation, i.e., the conversion of fibrinogen to fibrin. The contracted meshwork of fibrin retains the red cells, white cells, and platelets from which the serum has been expressed. See also *blood coagulation, thrombosis,* and *thrombus.*

blood component any of those elements in whole blood that may be extracted or separated for specific therapeutic use, including whole blood, packed red blood cells, leukocyte-poor red blood cells, frozen red blood cells, washed red blood cells, platelet concentrate, granulocyte concentrate, cryoprecipitate, and plasma. Other components, which are available commercially, are prepared from large pools of plasma. These derivatives include normal serum albumin, plasma protein fraction, Factor VIII, prothrombin complex, and $Rh_0(D)$ immune globulin. The use of individual components allows the treatment of specific conditions or the continuation of therapy while avoiding transfusion reaction to other unnecessary components. For more information, see the specific component.

blood culture the microbiologic examination of blood, performed to determine the presence or absence of microorganisms when sepsis is suspected. Blood is one of the most clinically useful specimens received by the microbiology laboratory.

Blood is normally sterile, and the presence of any microorganisms in it represents contamination; transient bacteremia, e.g., as produced by dental work; or an active infection. Two types of infectious processes can be characterized: bacteremia, which may develop secondary to several infectious diseases such as pneumonia, wounds, meningitis, peritonitis, and nephritis; and septicemia, the persistence of microorganisms in blood, which is a more serious condition indicating some type of intravascular infection such as endocarditis. In a particular stage of some infectious diseases, microorganisms spread to other organs and tissues through the blood.

To obtain a proper blood culture specimen, several concepts should be considered. First, there may be several factors in the serum that prevent the growth of bacteria in culture. Such factors include antibiotics administered from an external source or from endogenous inhibitory cells and cellular products normally present in the serum. For this reason, a blood specimen is diluted at least 1:10 in a growth medium. Second, the timing and the number of blood specimen collection are important in obtaining optimal results. The greatest number of bacteria in an infection are found shortly before an expected temperature rise. When bacteria enter the circulation, there is a lag of 1–2 hr before the body temperature changes. Third, contamination of the specimen with extraneous bacteria should be avoided by ensuring skin antisepsis before venipuncture, using an aseptic technique while blood is being drawn, and immediate transfer of the blood into the transporting medium. Usually, 5 ml of blood is added to 45 ml of broth; however, less may be used in the case of very young children. Finally, each blood specimen is collected in duplicate to allow both aerobic and anaerobic cultures.

The blood cultures should be incubated for at least 7 da at 37°C and examined daily for growth. Growth in the blood culture bottle may be indicated by turbidity and gas bubbles (gram-negative bacilli), cotton ball–like turbidity on top of the erythrocyte sedimentation layer (streptococci), a pellicle on the surface of the medium (*Bacillus,* fungi), hemolysis (certain streptococci, *Clostridium*), or subtle changes in the medium (*Hemophilus*).

On both the first and seventh days of incubation, all blood cultures should be subcultured onto blood agar for anaerobic incubation and onto chocolate agar for CO_2 incubation. This allows for growth and identification of certain microorganisms that do not cause visible changes in the initial culture medium. In cases of suspected low-grade endocarditis, blood cultures should be incubated for at least 14 da. Any culture that grows from a blood specimen should be identified and examined for antimicrobial susceptibility.

Some common microorganisms that can be isolated from bacteremic patients include *Streptococcus pneumoniae, Staphylococcus aureus, Pseudomonas aeruginosa,* any members of the Enterobacteriaceae, *Hemophilus influenza, Neisseria meningitidis, Bacteroides* species, and *Clostridium* species.

See also *bacteremia, septicemia,* and *septic shock.*

blood film see *blood smear.*

blood fluke see *Schistosoma.*

blood gas analysis analysis of blood specimens to determine their content (concentration) of gaseous carbon dioxide (CO_2) and oxygen (O_2), usually expressed in terms of partial pressure (or tension). The measurement of pH is frequently included. The parameters measured are as follows: pH, which is the measure of free hydrogen ion concentration $[H^+]$ (or, more accurately, H^+ activity) expressed as the negative logarithm of $[H^+]$; Po_2, which is measured as partial pressure of O_2 in the specimen, expressed in millimeters of mercury (mmHg); and Pco_2, which is measured as partial pressure of CO_2 in the specimen, expressed in millimeters of mercury. In addition, two other useful parameters may be calculated if whole blood is used as a specimen: So_2, which is fractional saturation of hemoglobin with oxygen—it is calculated by use of a nomogram from the measured Po_2, corrected to pH 7.4, temperature 37°C, and base excess zero (it may also be determined spectrophotometrically); and Po_2 (0.5) or P_{50}, which is the partial pressure of oxygen at half-saturation of hemoglobin—it is calculated from the measured value of Po_2 and the calculated value of So_2 by the equation

$$\log Po_2\ (0.5) = \log Po_2 - \left(\frac{1}{2.7}\right)\left(\log \frac{So_2}{1-So_2}\right).$$

This parameter is a measure of the affinity between O_2 and the patient's hemoglobin.

In the past, each of the three first-mentioned parameters was individually determined with special instruments. Currently, technology has made available a number of instruments that can measure these parameters simultaneously on a single small specimen with good precision and accuracy (see *Clark oxygen e.* under *electrode, glass e.* under *electrode,* and *Pco_2 e.* under *electrode*).

The manner in which specimens of blood are obtained for blood gas analysis is important to the accuracy of the test results. Arterial blood samples are the specimens of choice. They may be taken from an indwelling arterial catheter or may be obtained by an arterial puncture. Peripheral venous blood is not recommended as a specimen because it does not present a true picture of pH and blood gas state.

During the process of drawing blood for gas analyses, care is taken to avoid exposure of the blood to the atmosphere (anaerobic collection). The amount of blood drawn may vary from 0.1 to 0.5 ml, depending on the type of blood gas instrument used in the laboratory. The sample is usually collected in a heparinized vacuum tube or plastic syringe, as unclotted blood is required for analysis. Care must be exercised that the amount of heparin used is not excessive, because it can lower pH values.

It is important that the type of blood specimen be identified correctly, as Po_2 and Pco_2 values and reference ranges for venous and arterial blood differ considerably.

Po_2 and So_2 are both related to oxygen transport in the blood. Po_2 represents the sum of the oxygen dissolved in the blood (usually small amount) plus the oxygen in combination with hemoglobin (oxyhemoglobin), the form in which most of the oxygen is carried in the blood. Adequate oxygen transport, therefore, depends on a normal amount of hemoglobin and a normally functioning hemoglobin. Both Po_2 and So_2 must be evaluated to determine the adequacy of oxygen delivery to the tissues.

It is important to remember that although the normal Po_2 for a middle-aged person is 83–108 mmHg (11.0–14.0 kPa), some patients with chronic obstructive pulmonary disease can tolerate Po_2 values as low as 70 mmHg without signs of hypoxia.

The measurement of pH and Pco_2 is required to aid in the assessment of a patient's acid-base status (especially the establishment of respiratory status), to establish whether acidosis or alkalosis exists, and if so to establish its severity and degree of compensation.

It is most useful in the investigation of acid-base dyscrasias of mixed pathology. Pco_2 will tend to fall to compensate for a metabolic acidosis and increase to compensate for a metabolic alkalosis.

Pulmonary acidosis is characterized by a rise of Pco_2 from its normal value of 36–45 mmHg (4.85–6.1 kPa) to values of about 60–80 mmHg (hypercapnia). Narcosis develops at levels around 100 mmHg. Causes of pulmonary acidosis include pneumonia and emphysema.

The Po_2 is an indicator of the availability of oxygen for oxygenation of tissue. When the Po_2 falls to about 60 mmHg, hypoxemia and cyanosis develop; these become severe at 40 mmHg, with death possible at levels of 20 mmHg. Causes of low Po_2 are: pneumonia, emphysema, cardiac (left ventricular) failure, asthmatic bronchospasm, and low O_2 content in inspired air. See also *acid-base balance, Henderson-Hasselbalch equation, pH,* and *p. p. of oxygen* under *partial pressure.*

blood gases a term used to refer to the respiratory gases oxygen and carbon dioxide in arterial blood. Both gases are measured with appropriate electrodes, along with the pH of the sample. From the pH and Pco_2, using the Henderson-Hasselbalch equation, the blood bicarbonate content is derived. The three values together allow an assessment of the acid-base status of the patient. The oxygen tension (Po_2) reflects the lungs' ability to oxygenate arterial blood. Arterial blood-gas analysis in respiratory failure, for example, demonstrates hypoxemia and one of the acid-base abnormalities known as respiratory acidosis, which is characterized by elevated carbon dioxide tension ($>$ 42 torr) and reduced pH ($<$7.35).

blood groups red cell phenotypes grouped by their antigenic structural characteristics, which are under the control of various allelic genes. The cell membrane properties that provide the specific antigenicity of the blood groups are called agglutinogens, as they agglutinate or clump in the presence of their specific antibody.

ABO BLOOD GROUP. This group was first described by Landsteiner in 1900. It involves two antigens, A and B, which are coded by allelic genes located on the short arm of chromosome 9. There is also an allele (O) that does not code for either antigen. Thus, there are four possible phenotype groups: type O (genotype OO), in which neither antigen appears; type A (genotypes AA and AO), in which antigen A is expressed; type B (genotypes BB and BO), in which antigen B is expressed; and type AB (genotype AB), in which both antigens are expressed. All individuals produce antibodies against the A or B antigens that are lacking on their own red cells. Thus, type O individuals have both anti-A and anti-B antibodies in the serum; type A have anti-B; type B have anti-A; and type AB have neither.

The antigenic substances on the red cell membrane are glycosphingolipids. The proteins coded by the A and B genes are glycosyltransferases that attach specific sugars, *N*-acetyl-D-galactosamine for the A antigen and D-galactose for the B antigen, to the glycolipid molecule. The substrate for both of these glycosyltransferases is called the H substance; it is a glycosphingolipid produced by the addition of an L-fucose residue to a precursor molecule. This reaction is catalyzed by a fucosyltransferase controlled by the H gene, which is not linked with the A and B genes. Type O individuals express the H substance on their red cells. For this reason, the ABO group is sometimes referred to as the ABH group.

The H gene has an inactive allele h. The rare hh individuals do not produce the H substance and thus cannot produce the A or B antigen; they appear to be type O, regardless of their ABO genotype—a condition termed the "Bombay phenotype" (type O_h).

Many individuals also secrete soluble counterparts of the A, B, and H antigens in their body fluids and secretions. These are glycoproteins produced by the same enzymes that produce A, B, and H cellular antigens acting on a glycoprotein whose production is controlled by the secretor locus. Homozygous (se/se) individuals lack the capacity to secrete the ABH antigens.

LEWIS BLOOD GROUP. This group consists of two antigenic species, Le^a and Le^b, which are closely related to the ABO system. The Lewis genes control the addition of an additional fucose residue to the H substance. Lewis antigens have resulted in occasional hemolytic reactions but do not present the transfusion problems associated with the ABO system.

MNS BLOOD GROUP. One of the first groups discovered after the ABO system, this consists of at least three alleles that produce complex agglutinogens. Terminal *N*-acetylneuraminic acid residues are an important determinant in the MNS system in which carbohydrates provide the antigenic specificity as in the ABO system. The MNS system is rarely of clinical importance, except in those infrequent cases in which isoimmune antibodies have been elicited, as in transfusion or hemolytic disease of the newborn.

P BLOOD GROUP. This is a highly antigenic group thought to consist of three alleles, P_1, P, and P^k. The system can stimulate the production of hemolytic isoimmune antibodies and, like the ABO system, it bases its specificity on cell surface glycolipid antigens.

RH BLOOD GROUP. This is the most important blood group involved in transfusions after the ABO system. Its various antigenic components are highly immunogenic and capable of eliciting a hemolytic transfusion reaction; indeed, the Rh blood group is the most frequent cause of hemolytic disease of the newborn. It consists of at least three pairs of closely linked genes among which, some authorities believe, there is crossing over.

The system is further complicated by notational controversy between the Wiener system of notation (rh-hr) and the Fisher-Race system (CDE), which indicates the genetic constituents of the blood type. Another system, a numerical one, has been proposed by Rosenfeld. In it, antigens are numbered in the order of discovery. Typically, 85 percent of all Caucasians are Rh positive (i.e., Rh_0 or D-positive), although strong racial differences in distribution prevail for all the antigens of the Rh system. Antibodies against the Rh system rarely occur naturally. In the case of Rh_0(D), the antigen appears to be a protein constituent of the cell membrane, and not a surface feature like that of the ABO system.

OTHER BLOOD GROUPS. Among the other blood groups that may be encountered in blood banking, most are of little clinical significance unless they elicit the production of isoimmune antibodies. Four examples may be cited, the first of which is the Lutheran blood group system. This system has two alleles, Lu^a and Lu^b (anti-Lu^b is the predominant antibody). Another system is the Kell (K) system, which is frequently implicated in hemolytic disease of the newborn. K antibodies are not usually detected except by indirect antiglobulin screening test. The allelic k is called Cellano after the individual who was first found to display the antibody. The antigen is almost ubiquitous (99.8 percent), thus causing severe problems when blood is needed for those who have anti-K. Racial differences are marked for some Kell antigens, e.g., the Sutter (Js^a) antigen, which is found in 20 percent of blacks, and in less than 0.1 percent of Caucasians. The Duffy (Fy) system is another lesser group and consists of four alleles: Fy^a, Fy^b, Fy, and Fy^x. The Fy antigen is found in as many as 90 percent of blacks and in 3 percent of Caucasians.

The final example is the Kidd system (JK), first observed in a case of hemolytic disease of the newborn, which is present as two alleles, JK^a, and JK^b. Anti-JK^a and anti-JK^b are notorious for implication in severe, particularly delayed, hemolytic transfusion reactions.

Numerous other blood groups have been described, although the numbers of individuals exhibiting the antigen often are extremely limited. These groups provide powerful tools for the study of genetics and anthropology but have little clinical significance.

blood group substances glycoproteins found in saliva or other body fluids that have the same specificity as the red cell antigens expressed by the individual. Genes that determine blood group specificities do not direct the synthesis of the antigens themselves, but rather direct the synthesis of glycosyltransferases, which transfer specific monosaccharides from uridine diphosphate or guanosine diphosphate to precursor substances. These precursors are oligosaccharides bound to glycolipids on the red cell membrane and glycoproteins in body fluids.

This chemical relationship applies to the ABO, H, and Le systems, with a similar relationship found in the P system. In the MNS system, and probably the RH system, two panterminal amino acids forming the backbone of the peptides in the precursor substances appear to be involved in the determination of the blood group specificities.

In the RH system (as well as in most other systems), substances with the same antigenic specificities as the red cells are not present in body fluids, so that the source of extractable antigenic material is limited to the red cell itself.

blood island one of the areas in the mesenchyme of the yolk sac where erythropoiesis first occurs. See also *yolk sac*.

blood lancet a small, pointed instrument used to puncture a child's fingertip or heel to obtain a blood sample. It is commercially available in disposable sterile packets.

blood loss anemia see *blood loss a.* under *anemia.*

blood poisoning see *septicemia.*

blood pool scan see *radionuclide a.* under *angiocardiography.*

blood pressure the force exerted against the wall of a vessel by the blood, conventionally expressed as millimeters of mercury (mmHg) or centimeters of H_2O (cm H_2O) above atmospheric pressure. The blood pressure in the systemic vasculature system depends on the force of contraction of the ventricles, the degree of vessel compliance and vascular resistance, and the volume and viscosity of the blood. Also, the hydrostatic pressure exerted by the weight of the column of blood above it increases the pressure in a vessel, particularly a vein, located below the heart. Thus, the position of the heart (tricuspid valve) by convention is used as the zero reference level for blood pressure measurement.

The term blood pressure usually refers to arterial pressure and is conventionally recorded as two values: systolic pressure, which is the arterial pressure measured during systole (the ejection phase of the cardiac cycle), and diastolic pressure, which is the arterial pressure measured during diastole (the filling phase of the cardiac cycle). Reference ranges are under constant review, although it is generally considered that, in adults, a value of 140/90 or greater (systolic/diastolic) represents hypertension.

See also *arterial pressure, capillary pressure,* and *venous pressure.*

blood smear a thin film of blood that is spread on a slide, dried quickly, and fixed. Also called *blood film.*

blood typing the determination of ABO and Rh antigens and antibodies, routinely performed on all blood donor and recipient blood specimens.

Testing for A and B red cell antigens is generally done on a slide. For this procedure, a 10 percent suspension of cells in saline or whole blood is mixed with commercial antiserums, using a separate, clean stick for each antiserum-cell mixture, and is observed for agglutination. Testing for serum anti-A and anti-B antigens is generally done in tubes. For this procedure, serum is mixed with red cells of known ABO type, either commercial cells or freshly prepared 2–5 percent suspensions of washed cells in saline. The tubes are mixed by shaking and then incubated and centrifuged. The supernatant is observed for signs of hemolysis, and the cells are examined for agglutination. The results are interpreted according to the accompanying table.

Of the Rh antigens, only $Rh_0(D)$ is routinely tested; a slide or rapid tube test is generally used for this procedure. An immunologically inert, high-protein medium resembling the anti-$Rh_0(D)$ serum is used as a control. In the slide tests, a suspension of cells in serum or plasma is mixed with anti-D serum or the control; each combination is mixed with a separate, clean stick and observed for agglutination. In the tube tests, the cell suspension and antiserum or control are mixed and centrifuged, and the cell button is resuspended in saline and observed for agglutination. A positive result for either type of test consists of agglutination with the antiserum and none with the control. Some specimens react with the antiserum to a variable degree, but are not agglutinated and therefore cannot be categorized as either Rh-positive or Rh-negative. These are subjected to a direct antiglobulin test (direct Coomb's test) in order to demonstrate D antigen; if the AGT is positive, the subject is termed Rh-variant or D^u.

blood urea clearance see *urea clearance.*

blood urea nitrogen (BUN) see *urea nitrogen.*

blood vessel a channel for carrying blood; an artery, vein, or capillary.

blood volume measurements two procedures in nuclear medicine that determine the volume of both the plasma and red blood cells of an individual. The plasma is labeled with ^{131}I or ^{99m}Tc human serum albumin, and the patient's red cells are labeled with ^{51}Cr sodium chromate (the chromium(VI) ion binds to hemoglobin).

A known volume of labeled plasma or red cells is injected, and 15 min (longer for patients with splenomegaly) is allowed for the complete mixing of the labeled material in the circulation, at which time a sample is withdrawn and its radioactivity is measured. The counts per minute (cpm) of the injected plasma or red cells, divided by the counts per minute per milliliter of plasma or red cells in the 15-min sample, gives the total volume of plasma or red cells.

If both the plasma volume and the red cell volume are measured, the total blood volume is their sum and the mean circulatory hematocrit is the red cell volume divided by the total volume. The mean circulatory hematocrit is about nine-tenths of the venous hematocrit, although this proportion can vary widely. If only one measurement is performed, approximate values for the other can be estimated from the hematocrit.

Reference ranges vary widely according to age, sex, and body build, but repeat measurements are reproducible to within 5 percent unless there are changes in the individual's clinical status. These

Blood Typing. ABO Blood Typing

Blood Group	Reaction of Cells with Antiserum*		Reactions of Serum with Cells		
	Anti-A	*Anti-B*	*A cells*	*B cells*	*O cells*
O	−	−	+	+	−
A	+	−	−	+	−
B	−	+	+	−	−
AB	+	+	−	−	−

* + indicates agglutination; − indicates no agglutination.

measurements are used to evaluate blood or fluid losses from trauma, burns, or surgery, and to detect abnormalities such as polycythemia.

bloom (bloom) a surface texture on a colony of microorganisms, which appears velvety or powdery owing to aerial projections of hyphae.

Bloom's syndrome (bloomz) [David *Bloom,* U.S. dermatologist, born 1892] a hereditary condition, transmitted as an autosomal recessive trait, that is characterized by dwarfism, photosensitivity, and butterfly telangiectatic erythema of the face, with many defects of skin pigmentation, keratinization, dentition, and development. There is a markedly increased frequency of chromosomal breakage and malignancy.

Blount's disease (bluntz) [Walter Putnam *Blount,* U.S. orthopedist, born 1900] an aseptic necrosis of the medial condyle of the tibia, which sometimes causes lateral bowing of the legs.

blowback (blo'bak) ignition of the fuel-oxidant mixture in the premix chamber of a burner, usually caused by too lean a mixture.

blowfly (blo'fli) an insect of the family Calliphoridae. These flies are large and are often metallic green, copper, or blue in color. The maggots of this insect cause myiasis in domestic animals and humans.

blue (bloo) [Fr. *bleu*] a spectral color that corresponds to the perceived hue of monochromatic light having a wavelength between 455 and 492 nm (i.e., between violet and green).

blue diaper syndrome a rare disorder in infants, probably transmitted as an autosomal recessive trait, that involves the intestinal absorption of tryptophan and the resulting excretion of tryptophan breakdown products (primarily indoles) in the feces and urine. These indoles may be further degraded by hydrolytic enzymes to form a blue pigment, indigotin. Affected infants may show disorders of growth, increased levels of calcium in the blood and kidneys, widespread renal abnormalities, and recurrent infections. Carriers of this trait may exhibit a slight increase in urinary indoles. No pellagra-like symptoms are seen. Also called *tryptophan malabsorption syndrome.* See also *aminoacidopathy.*

blue dome cyst of breast see under *cystic disease of breast.*

blueing (bloo'ing) the treatment of tissue stained with alum hematoxylin with an alkaline solution to turn the stain blue. A solution of lithium carbonate, bicarbonate, ammonium hydroxide, Scott's tap water, potassium, or sodium acetate is used if plain tap water is not sufficiently alkaline.

blue nevus a melanocytic cutaneous hamartoma; see *blue n.* under *nevus.*

cellular b. n., see *cellular blue n.* under *nevus.*

malignant b. n., see *malignant blue n.* under *nevus.*

blue rubber bleb disease a syndrome of systemic manifestations associated with gastrointestinal bleeding. There are cutaneous hemangiomas (primarily of the trunk and arms), and lesions of the liver, spleen, lung, adrenals, and central nervous system.

blunt duct adenosis see *a. of breast* under *adenosis.*

blunt end an end of a double-stranded DNA molecule where both strands end at the same point (there is no single-stranded tail).

blurring (blur'ing) 1. any indistinctness of a radiographic image, such as that produced by the motion of body parts during the exposure, or by magnification of the image. See also *unsharpness.*

2. in body-section radiography, the smearing out of the image of every object that lies out of the focal plane. See also *tomography.*

BM abbrev. for *basal metabolism,* bowel movement, buccomesial.

β2m see *beta$_2$ microglobulin.*

B-mode see under *echocardiography* and *ultrasonography.*

BMR abbrev. See *basal metabolic rate.*

BNDD see *Bureau of Narcotics and Dangerous Drugs.*

boat (bōt) the least stable conformation of cyclohexane and other six-membered rings. See under *conformation.*

Bodansky unit (bo-dan'ske) [Aaron *Bodansky,* U.S. biochemist, 1887–1961] a measure of alkaline phosphatase activity defined as the quantity of catalytic activity in 100 ml of specimen that can split off 1 mg of phosphate-phosphorus from β-glycerophosphate in barbital buffer at pH 8.6 in 60 min at 37°C. The Bodansky unit has also been used to express the activity of acid phosphatase, which is measured at pH 5.0.

Bodian's method (bo'de-anz) [D. *Bodian,* U.S. neuroanatomist, born 1910] a histologic staining method for nerve fibers and argyrophilic substances. Formalin-fixed paraffin sections are incubated at 37°C for 48 hr in a 1 percent aqueous Protargol solution containing 5 g of clean copper shot per 100 ml of solution. The sections are then rinsed, reduced in hydroquinone–sodium sulfite solution, toned with gold chloride, developed with sodium thiosulfate, and fixed in oxalic acid. Nerve fibers and nuclei stain black against a blue background.

body (bod'e) 1. the trunk, or animal frame, with its organs.

2. a cadaver or corpse.

3. the largest and most important part of any organ. See also *corpus* and *soma.*

4. any mass or collection of material.

body cavity a visceral space within the body. Specifically the thoracic cavity or abdominopelvic cavity.

body fluids the fluids present in the various anatomic compartments of the body. They differ in the type and quantity of solutes dissolved in the solvent water and in the ease with which their water exchanges or equilibrates with water in other compartments.

FLUID VOLUMES. In the adult human, the total water mass is about 57 percent of the total body mass, which is equivalent to about 43 kg of water in a 75-kg adult. In newborns, water may amount to about 75 percent of the total weight, whereas in obese persons the water content may be less than 45 percent of the total mass because of the increased fat content in the tissues. The various water compartments, such as the vascular (blood), plasma, intracellular, interstitial, secretory (transcellular), cerebrospinal, osseous (bone), and joint, are separated from each other by membranes and structures of varied permeability. Although the compartments vary in size (volume) and composition of fluid, there is always some interchange of solvent and solute between the compartments.

The measurement of body fluid volumes is based on the application of the dilution principle. The volume of any compartment can be measured by introducing into the compartment a known quantity of a substance that cannot leave the compartment readily, and permitting adequate time for complete mixture throughout the compartment. The extent of dilution of the indicator or tag substance is a measure of the total fluid volume in the respective compartment.

TOTAL BODY WATER. Urea, antipyrene, deuterium oxide (^2H_2O = D_2O), and tritium oxide (^3H_2O = T_2O) are materials that can serve as tags, because they can diffuse into and become dispersed in all the water in all compartments. A known quantity of tag is administered intravenously and, after allowing time for dispersion throughout the entire body, a specimen of blood (plasma) is obtained and analyzed for concentration of the tag. T_2O can be conveniently assayed in a scintillation counter and is thus the tagging material of choice. D_2O can be assayed by measurement of density or by infrared spectrophotometry; urea and antipyrene are analyzed chemically. The volume of all body fluid compartments in a 70-kg male is about 66 l, of which about 44 l is water; 14 l is fat, with the remainder being other solids.

TOTAL BLOOD (INTRAVASCULAR) VOLUME. A sample of red cells from a subject is incubated in vitro with radioactive ferrous, chromium, or phosphate ions as tagging agents. The cells are washed free of unbound tagging material and reintroduced into the subject; after allowing time for mixing, a blood specimen is obtained and the concentration of radioactive tag measured. The value for the blood volume is obtained by multiplying the measured volume by the factor 1.1 (a necessary correction factor). If the hematocrit is known, plasma volume may be calculated from the blood volume value. Blood volume is about 5200 ml for a 75-kg individual.

PLASMA VOLUME. The tag materials may be radioactive iodinated serum albumin (RISA) or one of several vital dyes that bind to plasma proteins, such as Evans blue. These are administered intravenously and remain confined within the blood vessel walls. After about 20 min for admixture with all the blood, a specimen is obtained and the plasma volume calculated on the basis of the dilution of the tag. Again, if the hematocrit is known, total blood volume may be calculated. Plasma volume for a 70-kg individual is about 3000 ml.

EXTRACELLULAR WATER. For this measurement the tag must diffuse throughout all the noncellular water inside and outside the capillaries, but not across cell membranes. Suitable tag materials are ^{24}Na, chloride, bromide, thiocyanate, inulin, or sucrose. Not all membranes separating the many extracellular spaces are equally permeable to all the tag materials; thus, the ^{24}Na space and the CNS^- space may not be identical. Extracellular volume for a 70-kg person may vary from 8 to 22 l.

INTERSTITIAL FLUID VOLUME. This parameter cannot be measured directly; it must be calculated by subtracting plasma volume from the total extracellular fluid volume (ECFV). The value varies by what is included in the ECFV. For a 70-kg person, the interstitial fluid volume (ISFV) amounts to some 12–14 l and includes the cerebrospinal fluid volume (CSFV) of about 150 ml, joint fluids, secretory fluids (gastric, pancreatic), and the fluid bathing the cells.

INTRACELLULAR FLUID. This is also calculated by difference: total body water minus extracellular volume.

COMPOSITION OF BODY FLUIDS. Many inorganic and organic chemical species are present in all body fluids but in varying concentrations. The sodium ion is primarily an extracellular cation, whereas potassium and magnesium are primarily intracellular cations. The interstitial fluids are very low in protein, whereas plasma and intracellular fluids are relatively rich in protein. Cellular phosphate is present mainly in the form of organic ester-phosphate, whereas in interstitial fluids and plasma the phosphate is predominantly in the inorganic form. See also the accompanying table.

body-section radiography a term for any method of focal-plane radiography. See also *tomography.*

body surface area (BSA) the surface area of the human body, which is related to weight and height. It may be determined by consulting a nomogram (see *nomogram*) or by the formula: $\log A = (0.425 \log W) + (0.725 \log H) - 2.144$, where A is body surface area in square meters, W is patient weight in kilograms, and H is patient height in centimeters. Renal clearance rates are approximately proportional to patient body surface area but must be corrected for deviations from the average adult body surface area of 1.73 m^2.

body wall the limiting structure surrounding a visceral space, such as the abdominal wall.

Boeck's disease (beks) [Caesar P. M. *Boeck,* Norwegian dermatologist and syphilologist, 1845–1913] see *sarcoidosis.*

Boeck-Drbohlav-Locke egg-serum medium (bek der'bo-lahv lok) a buffered culture medium to which eggs, serum, and rice powder are added, which is used for the cultivation of amebae.

Boettcher cells (bet'sher) [Arthur *Boettcher,* German anatomist, 1831–1889] small cells that lie on the basilar membrane of the cochlear duct and provide mechanical support for the sensory cells of the organ of Corti.

Bogaert's disease (bo'gertz) see *cerebrotendinous xanthomatosis.*

Bohr effect (bor) [Christian *Bohr,* Danish physiologist, 1855–1911] the displacement of the oxygen-hemoglobin dissociation curve to the right or left by a change in blood pH. A decrease in pH, caused by an increase in blood CO_2 tension or acidity, decreases the affinity of the hemoglobin for oxygen; this is evidenced by a shift in the curve to the right. A decrease in the pH of blood perfusing metabolically active tissues would thus promote the unloading of oxygen at these sites.

Bohr equation [Christian *Bohr*] the mathematical formula that allows for the calculation of the physiologic dead space (V_D) for any gas, and therefore for an estimation of the volume of the conducting airways and those alveoli with impaired perfusion that contribute to dead space. If it is assumed that arterial P_{CO_2} (Pa_{CO_2}) is equal to alveolar P_{CO_2}, the equation for CO_2 can be expressed as: $V_{D_{CO_2}} = V_T \cdot [Pa_{CO_2} - P_{E_{CO_2}}]/Pa_{CO_2}$, where $P_{E_{CO_2}}$ is equal to the CO_2 tension in a sample of the total volume of alveolar gas collected during a single expiration.

BODY FLUIDS. AVERAGE CONCENTRATIONS IN HUMAN EXTRACELLULAR FLUID

	PLASMA (mEq/l)	PLASMA (mEq/kg H_2O*)	INTERSTITIAL FLUID (mEq/kg H_2O**)
Ions			
Na^+	141	150	144
K^+	4 to 5	4 to 5	4 to 5
Ca^{++}	5	5	3
Mg^{++}	2	2	1.5
H^+	4×10^{-5}	4×10^{-5}	4×10^{-5}
Total cation	152	161	153
Cl^-	103	110	114
HCO_3^-	26	27	28
$HPO_4^=$ and $H_2PO_4^-$	2	2	2
$SO_4^=$	1	1	1
Proteinate	16	17	4
Organic acids	4	4	4
Total anion	152	161	153
Water			
Volume per measured unit	940 ml/l	1000 ml/kg H_2O	1000 ml/kg H_2O
Concentration (as osmolality)		289 mOsm/kg H_2O	288 mOsm/kg H_2O
Potential difference (calculated)		(−) ⟵	1 mv ⟶ (+)

* Values in previous column divided by 0.94 to correct for nonwater volume of plasma.
** Calculated from previous column, assuming a Donnan factor of 0.96 for univalent ions and 0.92 for divalent ions, and recognizing that for Ca^{++} and Mg^{++} greater proportions are protein-bound in plasma than in interstitial fluid.
Modified from Brenner, B., and Rector, F.: The Kidney. 2nd ed. Philadelphia, W. B. Saunders Co., 1981, p. 95.

For any gas (G), the equation is expressed as: $V_{DG} = (F_{EG} - F_{AG}) \times V_T / (F_{IG} - F_{AG})$, where F_{EG}, F_{AG}, and F_{IG} are the fractional concentrations of that gas in the expired, alveolar, and inspired gas, respectively.

Bohr magneton (μ_B) [Niels Henrik David *Bohr,* Danish physicist, 1885–1962] a unit of magnetic moment defined as $eh/4\pi mc$ (where h is Planck's constant, c is the velocity of light, m is the electron mass, and e is the electron charge), which is equal to 9.274×10^{-24} J/T.

boil (boil) 1. see *furuncle.*

2. to convert a liquid into vapor by means of heat.

boiling point (b. p.) the temperature at which the vapor pressure of a liquid equals the atmospheric pressure, and bubbles form in the liquid.

bol/o (bol′o) a word element used in combining form to denote to throw or cast off, e.g., anabolism.

Boletus (bo-le′tus) [L.; Gr. bolītēs] a genus of basidiomycetous Hymenomycetes mushrooms; some of the species are edible, some poisonous.

Boling burner (bo′ling) a three-slot burner for an atomic absorption photometer that can efficiently atomize a solution.

Boltzmann constant (k) (boltz′mahn) [Ludwig Eduard *Boltzmann,* Austrian physicist, 1844–1906] the gas law constant divided by Avogadro's number: 1.38066×10^{-23} J/K. It is the average energy per unit temperature of a single degree of freedom, e.g., the x, y, or z component of the velocity or rotational or vibrational mode of a molecule.

bolus (bo′lus) [L., from Gr. *bolos* lump] 1. a rounded mass of food or a pharmaceutical preparation ready to be swallowed, or such a mass passing through the gastrointestinal tract.

2. a concentrated mass of pharmaceutical preparation given intravenously.

3. in radiation therapy, a mass of tissue-equivalent material placed around irregular or curved areas of the body between the source of radiation and the skin to obtain an even distribution of dosage in the tissue. Materials used include rice, beeswax, Vaseline gauze, and bags of water.

bombardment (bom-bard′ment) exposure of a body or substance to ionizing radiation.

Bombay blood group (bom-ba′) [from *Bombay,* India] a rare blood group determined by the Hh locus, which is also involved in the expression of the ABO blood group. The phenotype is characterized by the lack of H antigen—the precursor of A and B blood group antigens. The very rare homozygotes (O_hO_h) cannot express A or B, even though the genes may be present.

Bombidae (bom′bĭ-de) a family of bees, including the bumblebee, *Bombus californicus.* The sting is toxic, producing local pain and swelling. In hypersensitive people, allergic reactions can occur as a result of the sting; see *bee sting.*

bond (bond) 1. the strong attractive force that links two atoms of a chemical compound. These bonds are classified generally as either covalent or ionic. A pair of dots or a line between atoms is used to represent a single covalent bond, e.g., H—O—H or H:O:H. Also called chemical bond.

2. a weaker force linking atoms of the same or different molecules, e.g., a hydrogen bond.

coordinate covalent b., a covalent bond in which both electrons of the shared pair are contributed by the same atom, the donor atom. (The other atom is the acceptor atom.) The bond is sometimes indicated by an arrow pointing from the donor atom to the acceptor atom, for example, $H_3N \rightarrow BF_3$. See also *Lewis acid.*

covalent b., a bond in which the electrons are shared (not transferred) between two atoms, e.g., the C—H bonds in methane, CH_4. If two electrons are shared, it is called a single covalent bond; four shared electrons are designated a double covalent bond; and six shared electrons form a triple covalent bond. Covalent bonds may also be classified as polar or nonpolar, depending on whether the electrons are unevenly (with the charge distribution nearer to one atom of the bond) or evenly shared. Also called *electron pair b.*

electron pair b., see *covalent b.*

high-energy b., a chemical bond that on hydrolysis releases considerable amounts of free energy. Examples of high-energy bonds are the two pyrophosphate anhydride bonds in ATP and the thioester bond in acetyl CoA.

hydrogen b., a weak bond, primarily electrostatic, between a hydrogen atom and a highly electronegative atom (such as oxygen or nitrogen) in another molecule or a different part of the same molecule. Hydrogen bonding can have important effects on the physical properties, such as the melting and boiling points, of a compound (e.g., the high boiling point of water is caused by hydrogen bonding). Hydrogen bonding influences the structure and reactivity of many large molecules of importance in biochemistry; e.g., some substrates are bound, in part, to enzymes by hydrogen bonds, and the helical structure of DNA is maintained by hydrogen bonds between the base pairs, adenine and thymine and guanine and cytosine.

ionic b., the type of bond that occurs when an electron is transferred completely from one atom to another to form two ions. The strong attraction that occurs between two oppositely charged ions is called an ionic bond; e.g., the bonds between sodium ions and chloride ions in NaCl are ionic bonds.

metallic b., the type of bond found in a metallic crystal. In a metal, the valence electrons are not bound to specific atoms and flow freely as a "sea of electrons" around a lattice of positively charged atomic cores (nuclei and inner-shell electrons). The attraction between the delocalized valence electrons and the positive atomic cores is referred to as the metallic bond.

peptide b., an amide linkage, —CONH—, formed when the amino group of one amino acid is joined with the carboxyl group of another amino acid with the elimination of water to form a peptide. See also *peptide.*

pi (π) b., the bonding molecular orbital formed by the interaction of two atomic orbitals that do not lie along the internuclear axis but at some angle (usually perpendicular) to it. The typical π bond is formed by the overlap of two parallel p orbitals, but π bonds can also result from the overlap of d orbitals and p orbitals (as in the P=O bond). According to molecular orbital theory, the carbon-carbon double bond in an alkene, for example, can be considered to be a combination of a π bond and a σ bond. Likewise, the carbon-carbon triple bond in an alkyne is the combination of two mutually perpendicular π bonds and a σ bond.

sigma (σ) b., the bonding molecular orbital formed by the overlap of two atomic orbitals along the internuclear axis. According to molecular orbital theory, the carbon-carbon single bond, in an alkane for example, is a σ bond. One of the bonds of a single, double, or triple bond is a σ bond; any others are π bonds.

bond energy the amount of energy needed to break a particular chemical bond to yield two atoms or free radicals (not two ions).

bonding a method of controlling the static electricity developed during transfer of solvents, in which ignitable vapors may be produced. An important safety measure, bonding can be provided by metallic contact during filling operations, by a bond wire between metal dispensing and receiving containers, or by other conductive paths having an electric resistance not greater than 10^6 ohms. The procedure is required by regulatory standards except when the container involved is made of glass or other nonconducting material, or when it is filled through a closed system.

bone (bōn) [L. *os;* Gr. *osteon*] the hard, rigid form of connective tissue that constitutes most of the skeleton of vertebrates. Bones maintain the external form of the human body and, with the joints, provide a framework of levers on which muscles and tendons insert and act to produce movements. Some skull and thoracic bones protect internal organs. Many of the spaces in the interior of bones are filled with bone marrow.

There are 206 bones in the human body, and they vary greatly in size and shape. Long bones have a shaft and two ends: the long bones in the fingers are small compared with those of the thighs (femur). Other bones are described according to their shape—short, flat, or irregular. Small bones that develop in tendon are sesamoid bones. The shaft, or diaphysis, of a long bone is a hollow cylinder with a central cavity, the medullary canal. Cavities in bones make them lighter without significantly diminishing their strength, and the sinuses in some skull bones contribute to the resonance of the voice. Bones are covered over most of their surface by a fibrous membrane, the periosteum, and within synovial joints by a layer of articular cartilage.

The dry, inert appearance of the bones of a skeleton is misleading. Living bone is a dynamic vascular tissue that bleeds when it is cut and dies when it is severely injured. It is biochemically active and contains most of the body's calcium and phosphorus. Calcium metabolism is controlled by thyroid and parathyroid hormones, and when calcium is extracted from bones they may become porous (osteoporosis).

Bone develops in the embryo from mesenchyme. A few of the skull bones form by direct ossification of mesenchyme (mesenchymal bones), but usually a cartilage model is formed first and is then progressively ossified (osteochondral bones). The areas where bony tissue is being formed are centers of ossification; there are several in the larger bones. The primary center in a long bone is in the shaft. Secondary or epiphyseal centers appear later in the ends of the long bones, and are separated from the diaphyseal center by a zone of epiphyseal cartilage that disappears only when growth in length is complete. An increase in the girth of a long bone occurs by the deposition of new bone under the periosteum, with progressive remodeling by resorption from the wall of the medullary cavity. Bone-forming cells are osteoblasts; multinucleated cells that resorb bone are osteoclasts.

The outer layer of a bone is dense and solid (compact or cortical bone), but in the interior many fine plates of bone form a spongelike structure (cancellous bone), and bone marrow is present in the interstices. Microscopically, bone is composed of flattened lamellae arranged concentrically around a central canal to form a cylindric haversian system. Irregular interstitial lamellae fill in the spaces between haversian systems, and concentric lamellae are present at the outer and inner surfaces of the bone. Osteocytes reside in small lacunae within the haversian systems and communicate with one another by cytoplasmic processes in fine canaliculi; the osteocytes are osteoblasts that became entombed within the haversian systems during their formation. They depend for their nutritive requirements on material that passes along the canaliculi from blood vessels in the central canals of the haversian systems. In response to hormonal stimulation, the osteocytes break down the matrix in the walls of the lacunae, freeing the mineral component of the bone.

For more information, see the specific bone (the major bones are defined and listed alphabetically) and *bone tumors.*

bone cell see *osteoblast, osteoclast,* and *osteocyte.*

bone conduction the conduction of sound to the inner ear through the cranial bones rather than through the external auditory meatus and middle ear.

bone marrow the soft pulpy material that fills the medullary cavity of bones. It is found in the ends of long bones and is also interspersed between the trabeculae of flat bones.

Red marrow is found in all areas of the skeleton throughout gestation. After birth, however, the red marrow in the long bones is gradually replaced with fat and, in the adult, the latter predominates; the red marrow then persists only in the vertebrae, ribs, sternum, pelvis, clavicles, scapulae, cranial bones, and proximal epiphyses of the humeri and femora.

Interspersed among the reticular framework of the red marrow are hematopoietic tissue, mature blood cells, and small nodules of lymphoid tissue. Blood is supplied to the red marrow of a bone via the nutrient artery of that bone, and leaves via its accompanying vein. The artery branches out to terminate in thin-walled, cell-lined sinusoids called vascular sinuses. Within the meshwork of reticulin fibers of the marrow there are hematopoietic cells between the sinuses. Each group of cells probably belongs to a single clone. Groups of cells of the erythroid series lie close to the adventitial surface of the vascular sinuses, with the more mature cells at the periphery of the clusters. Each erythrocytic cluster surrounds a macrophage. Megakaryoblasts also lie adjacent to the walls of the sinuses.

Differentiation in the granulocytic series occurs deep within the hematopoietic cords. Once these cells have developed to the metamyelocyte stage, they migrate toward the sinuses and cross the wall to enter the circulation.

Groups of cells of the lymphocytic series and monohistiocytic series concentrate around the arterial vessels that penetrate the hematopoietic cords.

There appear to be two types of stem cells: one that gives rise to undifferentiated lymphocytes and a second that gives rise to red blood cells, platelets, monocytes, and granulocytes.

The reticular cells, which invest the vascular sinuses and the endothelial cells of the sinuses, move apart to create openings, permitting egress of cells into the circulation. Evidence exists that the withdrawal of the reticular cells is in part influenced by erythropoietin.

See also *erythrocytic series, granulocytic series, lymphocytic series,* and *monohistiocytic series.*

bone marrow aspiration a procedure for obtaining a specimen of marrow cells for histologic examination. The iliac crest and sternum are the common locations. Under local anesthesia, a needle is introduced into the marrow cavity and a syringe is attached; approximately 2 cc of marrow is forcibly aspirated and transferred to a tube containing heparin or EDTA to prevent clotting. Small particles of marrow (marrow granules) can be separated and smeared between glass slides; smears of the more fluid portion of the aspirate are also prepared. These preparations, generally treated with Wright stain, allow assessment of the cells present in the marrow and their relative proportions. See also the accompanying table.

bone marrow biopsy a procedure for obtaining a specimen of bone marrow for histologic examination. It allows determination of the cellularity of the marrow, as well as the relative proportions of the component cells and the presence of granulomas or tumor deposits. In this procedure, a core of bone is obtained (usually at the posterior superior portion of the ilium) with a cutting needle and is fixed in formalin and decalcified for preparation of paraffin-embedded sections. If electron microscopy of the marrow cells is desired, the contents of the marrow spaces should be removed under a dissecting microscope and fixed in glutaraldehyde. See also *bone marrow differential* and *myeloid/erythroid ratio.*

bone marrow depression a reduction in the hematopoietic cells of the bone marrow that leads to the depletion of the mature cell lines in the circulating blood. It is often the result of neoplastic growth or the use of therapeutic drugs. Aplastic cases can occur if the stem cell compartment is suppressed and the offending agent cannot be removed. Also called *myeloid depression.*

bone marrow differential count examination and enumeration of the various hematopoietic cells seen on a bone marrow film. The nucleated cells commonly found in normal bone marrow include granulocytes, granulocyte precursors, erythroid precursors, lymphocytes, lymphocyte precursors, monocytes, megakaryocytes, and reticulum cells. Between 300 and 500 cells must be examined to determine the differential count, which, in conjunction with a bone marrow biopsy and myeloid/erythroid ratio, provides an accurate evaluation of the state of the bone marrow. Abnormal results are obtained in patients with anemia, leukemia, and other blood disorders.

bone marrow scan a procedure in nuclear medicine. It is similar in technique to a bone scan but uses an agent that localizes in the bone marrow, most commonly technetium-99m sulfur colloid, which is taken into cells of the reticuloendothelial system by phagocytosis. Bone marrow scans are used in the differential diagnosis of various myeloproliferative diseases and hemolylic anemias, and to identify areas with reduced bone marrow function due to metastatic malignancy, infarction, radiation therapy, or chemotherapy.

bone scan a scintillation camera scan or rectilinear scan of the skeleton, which produces minified ante-

BONE MARROW ASPIRATION. DIFFERENTIAL CELL COUNTS OF BONE MARROW IN PERCENT OF TOTAL NUCLEATED CELLS

	BIRTH	1 MONTH	>4 MONTHS		ADULT	
	Mean SD	*Mean SD*	*Mean*	*Range*	*Mean*	*Range*
Normoblasts, total	14.5 ± 7.2	8.0 ± 5.0	23.1		25.6	(18.4-33.8)
Pronormoblasts	0.02 ± 0.06	0.10 ± 0.14	0.5	(0-1.5)		(0.2-1.3)
Basophilic	0.24 ± 0.24	0.34 ± 0.33	1.7	(0.2-4.8)		(0.5-2.4)
Polychromatophilic	13.1 ± 6.8	6.9 ± 4.4	18.2	(4.8-34.0)		(17.9-29.2)
Orthochromatic	0.69 ± 0.73	0.54 ± 1.88	2.7	(0-7.8)		(0.4-4.6)
Neutrophils, total	60.4 ± 8.7	32.4 ± 7.7	57.1		53.6	(49.2-65.0)
Myeloblasts	0.31 ± 0.31	0.62 ± 0.50	1.2	(0-3.2)		(0.2-1.5)
Promyelocytes	0.79 ± 0.91	0.76 ± 0.65	1.4	(0-4.0)		(2.1-4.1)
Myelocytes	3.9 ± 2.9	2.5 ± 1.5	18.3	(8.5-29.7)		(8.2-15.7)
Metamyelocytes	19.4 ± 4.8	11.3 ± 3.6	23.3	(14.0-34.2)		(9.6-24.6)
Bands	28.4 ± 7.6	14.1 ± 4.6				(9.5-15.3)
Segmented	7.4 ± 4.6	3.6 ± 3.0	12.9	(4.5-29.0)		(6.0-12.0)
Eosinophils	2.7 ± 1.3	2.6 ± 1.4	3.6	(1.0-9.0)	3.1	(1.2-5.3)
Basophils	0.12 ± 0.20	0.07 ± 0.16	0.06	(0-0.8)	0.1	(0-0.2)
Lymphocytes, total	15.6	49.0	16.0	(4.8-35.8)	16.2	(11.1-23.2)
Transitional	1.2 ± 1.1	2.0 ± 0.9				
Small (mature)	14.4 ± 5.5	47.0 ± 9.2				
Plasma cells	0.00 ± 0.02	0.02 ± 0.06	0.4	(0.2-0.6)	1.3	(0.4-3.9)
Monocytes	0.88 ± 0.85	1.01 ± 0.89			0.3	(0-0.8)
Megakaryocytes	0.06 ± 0.15	0.05 ± 0.09			0.1	(0-0.4)
Reticulum cells					0.3	(0-0.9)
M:E Ratio	4.4	4.4	2.9	(1.2-5.2)	2.3	(1.5-2.3)

Modified from Mauer, A. M.: Pediatric Hematology. New York, McGraw-Hill Book Company, 1969; and Wintrobe, M. M., et al.: Clinical Hematology. 7th ed. Philadelphia, Lea & Febiger, 1974.

rior and posterior whole body images and other localization films. The bone agents of choice are the technetium-labeled phosphates ^{99m}Tc-pyrophosphate and ^{99m}Tc-diphosphonate, which are chemically absorbed by the hydroxyapatite crystals of the bones of the body.

Sites of new bone growth or repair (as seen with fractures, primary or metastatic osteoblastic tumors, and Paget's disease) appear as hot lesions on the scan, whereas sites of complete bone destruction by osteolytic tumors appear as cold lesions. Conditions of osteomyelitis, arthritis, and osteolytic tumors can increase tracer accumulation. Because Tc-labeled phosphates are excreted in the urine and are retained in the kidneys and bladder, these structures may also appear on the scan.

Bone scans are most frequently used for the detection, localization, and staging of metastatic bone tumors, and for planning of therapy. Scans also indicate osteomyelitis and certain fractures, such as stress fractures, more readily than do conventional x-rays.

bone sclerosis see *bone s.* under *sclerosis.*

bone tumors neoplasms of bone. The most common benign bone tumors are those forming cartilage; the most frequent primary malignant tumor of bone, other than hemopoietic disorders of the bone marrow cells, is osteosarcoma. The differential diagnosis of a bone tumor must include consideration of reactive and inflammatory processes, as well as metastatic neoplasms. A classification that is a modification of the World Health Organization's categorization of bone tumors is shown in the accompanying table.

Biopsy of a bone lesion is mandatory before treatment is begun. A needle biopsy is sometimes suitable, but it is often necessary to obtain an open biopsy for the adequate assessment of a lesion. The tissue should be selected carefully, if possible including a soft area to allow a rapid histologic assessment. The pathologist must make use of all the available clinical and radiologic information in reaching a tissue diagnosis.

Osteomas are benign masses of periosteal bone that occur most frequently in the skull, especially within the sinuses. They may be multiple but rarely cause symptoms. An osteoid osteoma can involve any bone but is more common in the diaphysis of the femur or tibia. This lesion has a small central nidus of closely packed osteoid trabeculae surrounded by dense sclerotic bone. It is often painful, and may recur if excision is not complete. There are similarities between osteoid osteoma and the benign solitary osteoblastoma of bone, but the latter (which has been called a giant osteoid osteoma) is larger and shows a predilection for the bones of the vertebral column. It is highly vascular and consists of broad trabeculae of osteoid and bone; it must not be confused with osteosarcoma.

Osteosarcoma makes up approximately 15 percent of all bone tumors. It is characterized by the presence of malignant osteoid, bone, and, in some instances, cartilage formation. It is particularly a tumor of childhood and adolescence, and accounts for more than 50 percent of deaths from bone cancer in this age group. A small number have been reported as arising in previously irradiated areas, and in bone affected by Paget's disease. Trauma has not been proved to be an etiologic factor. Approximately 60 percent of osteosarcomas arise in the metaphyseal region of a long bone, particularly adjacent to the knee or shoulder. Spread occurs through the blood stream. Generally 5-yr survival figures are less than 20 percent. Occasionally a well-differentiated osteosarcoma occurs in an older patient within the cortex of a long bone (parosteal). Such tumors indicate a much better prognosis for the patient, with more than 80 percent surviving at least 5 yr.

Chondroma or enchondroma is a benign tumor of cartilage cells that occurs in the medullary cavity of bones, particularly those of the hand or foot. It rarely recurs after curettage or excision. In Ollier's disease and Maffucci's syndrome, chondromas are multiple, and in the latter syndrome they are liable to become sarcomatous. Approximately 20 percent of malignant bone tumors are chondrosarcomas; pelvic bones are a common site. Most patients are adults; males are more often affected than females. Histologic grading of a chondrosarcoma can be useful in assessing the prognosis. The primary tumor usually exhibits a slow, expansile growth, and distant spread occurs late and through the blood stream. Figures for 10-yr survivals indicate that from one-third to two-thirds of patients will be alive at that time. In mesenchymal chondrosarcomas, malignant cartilage is present admixed with clusters of small, round to spindle-shaped mesenchymal cells. Mesenchymal tumors such as rhabdomyosarcoma are occasionally identified within a chondrosarcoma; the tumor is then described as being dedifferentiated. Malignant cartilage- and bone-forming tumors may arise within soft tissues (extraskeletal).

Osteoclast-like multinucleated giant cells occur in many benign and nonneoplastic bone lesions and can be a component of malignant bone tumors, but they are particularly numerous in the so-called osteoclastoma or giant cell tumor. In reaching the diagnosis, clinical and radiologic features must be taken into consideration, since a giant cell reparative granuloma or hyperparathyroidism can present a similar histologic appearance. Most patients with a giant cell tumor of bone are young adults; it is rare in children. Giant cell tumor of bone arises in the epiphysis and spreads through the metaphyseal region, being seen most frequently in the lower femur and upper tibia. Areas of stroma simulating a fibrosarcoma are an ominous prognostic sign. At least 15 percent of giant cell tumors exhibit malignant behavior.

Ewing's sarcoma is a small cell tumor arising in bones of adolescents and young adults, often of the extremities. The radiologic findings may strongly suggest the diagnosis but alone are not sufficient to make the diagnosis and biopsy must be performed. The pathologist must distinguish the tumor from other small cell neoplasms occurring in young patients. In the proper clinical context, the diffuse sheets of closely packed small round cells with frequent areas of necrosis are highly suggestive. Electron microscopy may be helpful in excluding other possibilities from the differential diagnosis. Glycogen stains should be clearly positive. Ewing's tumor is aggressive, and 5-yr survival figures are around 20 percent but are rising with improved combination forms of therapy. Metastases appear to have a preference for bones as well as for the lungs. Ewing's tumor of bone must be distinguished from lymphoma, (primary bone lymphomas are usually seen in older patients and are often large cell lymphomas). Myeloma also occurs in older adults and tends to involve bones of the skull, pelvis, ribs, and vertebral column (see *multiple myeloma*).

Tumors of the connective tissue elements of bone are not particularly common, and they appear similar microscopically to the same tumor types arising in soft tissues. The most common are benign and malignant tumors of fibroblasts and of endothelial cells.

bony ankylosis (bōn'e) the union of two or more bones that are normally separate.

Boolean algebra (bool'e-an) [George *Boole,* British mathematician, 1815–1864] an algebraic system used in symbolic logic. The logical operations in a digital computer are based on the Boolean system at both the hardware and software levels. See also *logical operation.*

Boolean function [George *Boole*] a mathematical function that has one of two values, true or false. See also *logical operation.*

booster (boo'ster) 1. an amplifier inserted into a cable or transmission line to boost weak signals.

2. a second immunization, given after an appropriate time interval, that continues the protection of a previously immunized person from certain disease agents. There is a rapid, dramatic increase in serum antibody on reimmunization in comparison with the initial primary response to the first inoculation. See also *anamnestic response* and *booster d.* under *dose.*

bootstrap loader (bōōt'strap) a method for loading a computer's main control program (operating system) into memory, perhaps after a power failure. The bootstrap loader is a small program that may be in read-only memory (ROM) or may be manually entered; it loads the operating system into memory from peripheral storage and starts execution.

borate (bo'rāt) 1. one of a number of compounds in which each boron atom is bonded to three or four oxygen atoms. Anhydrous borates can be made by fusing boric acid and metal oxides. These compounds have a variety of structures including some cyclic and some polymeric chains. They are similar structurally to the silicates. Examples are $K_3B_3O_6$, $Na_2B_4O_7$, and CaB_2O_4.

2. an ester of boric acid. See also *borax* and *boron assays.*

borax (bo'raks) [L., from Arabic *būaq,* Persian *būrah*] sodium borate; the term refers both to the naturally occurring hydrated form, $Na_2B_4O_7 \cdot 10H_2O$, and to the anhydrous sodium borate used in commerce. Borax occurs as hard, odorless crystals that effloresce in dry air; it is soluble in water but insoluble in most organic solvents. It has a variety of uses in industry, and is a common ingredient in cleaning solutions. Chronic exposure may lead to borism; 5–10 g is acutely toxic. See also *boric acid* and *boron.*

Borchgrevink method (bōrch'grĕ-vink) see under *platelet adhesiveness test.*

border (bōr'der) a boundary line, edge, or surface.

borderline lesion see *atypical hyperplasia.*

Bordetella (bōr″dĕ-tel'ah) [J. J. B. V. *Bordet*] a genus of minute, gram-negative aerobic coccobacilli. The three recognized species are mammalian parasites and pathogens of the respiratory tract of humans and/or lower animals. The most important species is *B. pertussis,* the cause of whooping cough in humans; the others are *B. parapertussis,* a closely re-

Bone Tumors. Modified World Health Organization Classification of Tumors of Bone

I. Bone-forming tumors
- A. Benign
  1. Osteoma
  2. Osteoid osteoma and osteoblastoma (benign osteoblastoma)
- B. Indeterminate
  1. Aggressive osteoblastoma
- C. Malignant
  1. Osteosarcoma (osteogenic sarcoma)
  2. Juxtacortical osteosarcoma (parosteal osteosarcoma)
  3. Periosteal osteosarcoma

II. Cartilage-forming tumors
- A. Benign
  1. Chondroma (enchondroma)
  2. Osteochondroma (osteocartilaginous exostosis)
  3. Periosteal chondroma
  4. Chondroblastoma (benign chondroblastoma, epiphyseal chondroblastoma)
  5. Chondromyxoid fibroma
- B. Malignant
  1. Chondrosarcoma
  2. Mesenchymal chondrosarcoma
  3. Dedifferentiated chondrosarcoma

III. Giant cell tumor (osteoclastoma)

IV. Marrow tumors
1. Ewing's sarcoma
2. Malignant lymphoma
3. Myeloma

V. Vascular tumors
- A. Benign
  1. Hemangioma
  2. Lymphangioma
  3. Glomus tumor (glomangioma)
- B. Intermediate or indeterminate
  1. Hemangioendothelioma
  2. Hemangiopericytoma
- C. Malignant
  1. Angiosarcoma

VI. Other connective tissue tumors
- A. Benign
  1. Desmoplastic fibroma
  2. Lipoma
- B. Malignant
  1. Fibrosarcoma
  2. Malignant fibrous histiocytoma
  3. Liposarcoma
  4. Malignant mesenchymoma
  5. Undifferentiated sarcoma

VII. Other tumors
1. Chordoma
2. "Adamantinoma" of long bones
3. Neurilemoma (schwannoma, neurinoma)
4. Neurofibroma

VIII. Unclassified tumors

IX. Tumor-like lesions
1. Solitary bone cyst (simple or unicameral bone cyst)
2. Aneurysmal bone cyst
3. Juxta-articular bone cyst (intra-osseous ganglion)
4. Metaphyseal fibrous defect (non-ossifying fibroma)
5. Eosinophilic granuloma
6. Fibrous dysplasia and ossifying fibroma
7. "Myositis ossificans"
8. "Brown tumor" of hyperparathyroidism

Reproduced with permission from Spjut, H. J.: Histologic Classification of Primary Tumors of Bone. In M. D. Anderson Hospital and Tumor Institute, Houston: *Management of Primary Bone and Soft Tissue Tumors.*

lated organism, and *B. bronchiseptica,* which is primarily an animal parasite and pathogen.

B. bronchiseptica, a species similar to *B. pertussis* except that it is motile and grows more rapidly. It causes bronchopneumonia in rodents and dogs, and is occasionally found in human respiratory and wound infections.

B. parapertussis, a species resembling *B. pertussis* that is also a cause of whooping cough. It is distinguished from *B. pertussis* by the readiness with which it grows on simple culture media.

B. pertussis, a species that is the cause of whooping cough in humans. Isolates from clinical specimens can be grown only on special culture media, such as Bordet-Gengou agar. Virulent strains possess a capsule of unknown nature and produce a soluble dermonecrotic exotoxin, as well as a lymphocyte-promoting factor. This organism is found only in humans and has a remarkable affinity for ciliated bronchial epithelial cells. See also *exotoxins* and *whooping cough.*

Bordet-Gengou agar (bōr-da′ zhahn-goo′) [Jules Jean Baptiste Vincent *Bordet,* Belgian bacteriologist, 1870–1961; Octave *Gengou,* French bacteriologist, 1875–1957] see *Bordet-Gengou a.* under *agar.*

Bordet-Gengou phenomenon [J. J. B. V. *Bordet;* O. *Gengou*] complement fixation, which was first used to detect antibodies against *Bordetella pertussis;* see *complement-fixation test.*

boric acid (bo′rik) a colorless or white, odorless, crystalline solid, H_3BO_3, that is stable in air and soluble in boiling water, alcohol, and glycerine. Weak water solutions are used as a mild antiseptic and eyewash. Epigastric pain, vomiting, weak pulse, unconsciousness, cyanosis, and paroxysms of strangling precede death in lethal ingested doses, which can range from 8 to 30 g.

borism (bor′izm) poisoning by a boron compound. See also *borax, boric acid,* and *boron.*

Bornholm disease (bōrn′hōm) [from the Danish island *Bornholm*] see *epidemic p.* under *pleurodynia.*

boro- (bo′ro) [L. *borium* boron] a prefix in chemistry to denote compounds in which boron is present as a substituent, e.g., borosilicate.

boron (B) (bo′ron) [L. *borium*] a nonmetallic element occurring as a crystal or a powder; atomic number 5; atomic weight 10.811; Group III of the periodic table; oxidation state +3. Some boron compounds are toxic; the boron hydrides (boranes), boric acid, and borates can cause damage to the lungs, kidneys, and central nervous system.

boron assays quantitative methods for the determination of boron and borate salts utilizing colorimetric procedures. Boron-free glassware must be used. A simple urine screening test, which makes use of commercially available paper treated with turmeric yellow, may be used to test for elevated boron levels (3–10 mg/l). The turmeric yellow on the paper combines with borates to form a characteristic brownish-red color, changing to blue after exposure to ammonia fumes. The normal concentration for borate in urine is less than 2 mg of borate/l. Toxic effects do not appear until a level of about 10 mg/l is reached.

boron trifluoride-methanol a solution of boron trifluoride in methanol (BF_3-MeOH), used as an esterifying agent in histology. It prevents the basic dye staining of nucleic acids, fatty acids, protein carboxyls, and polysaccharide carboxyls. It is corrosive to the skin, has a pungent, corrosive odor, and decomposes in water. This solution is also used to prepare fatty acid methyl esters for gas-liquid chromatography.

borosilicate glass (bo″ro-sil′ĭ-kāt) a type of heat-resistant glass with low alkali content and a boric oxide content of about 5 percent. It has a high tensile strength, a low thermal coefficient of expansion, and a softening point of about 600°C; the continuous-use temperature is about 480°C. It is commonly used for laboratory glassware. Trademarks, Kimax and Pyrex.

Borrelia (bŏ-rel′e-ah) [from Amédée *Borrel,* French bacteriologist in Strasbourg, 1867–1936] a genus of bacteria in the family Spirochaetaceae. These spirochetes have a central axial filament surrounded by a cytoplasmic membrane, contractile protoplasm with 15–20 parallel fibers, and a delicate, foamy, elastic envelope. Contractions of fibers make the cell rotate. The helical cells are up to 1 μm wide by 25 μm long (usually 0.2–0.5 by 3–20 μm). They are gram-negative and strict anaerobes. Generally parasitic or living on mucous membranes, they are the cause of relapsing fever in humans and other animals. Species designations are based on their respective arthropod vectors (ticks and lice). They are sometimes transmitted by rodents. See also *spirochete.*

B. duttonii, the species that causes endemic relapsing fever in humans in Africa. Its vector is the arthropod *Ornithodoros moubata,* which transmits the microorganism in the saliva from human to human.

B. hermsii, the species that causes endemic relapsing fever in humans in the western United States and Canada. Its vector is the tick *Ornithodoros hermsii,* which is transported mainly by rodents.

B. hispanica, the species that causes endemic relapsing fever in humans in North Africa and the Mediterranean area. Its vector is the large tick *Ornithodoros erraticus erraticus,* which lives in animal burrows and stables and transmits the organism as the tick is feeding.

B. parkeri, the species that causes endemic relapsing fever in humans in the western United States. Burrowing rodents, such as ground squirrels, carry the tick vector *Ornithodoros parkeri,* which transmits the organism in its bite.

B. persica, the species that is the etiologic cause of endemic relapsing fever in humans in the Middle East and Central Asia. Its vector is the tick *Ornithodoros tholozani.*

B. recurrentis, the species that cause epidemic relapsing fever in humans, a disease found worldwide. Its vector is the human body louse, *Pediculus humanus,* which transmits the organism when the louse's infested coelomic fluid is rubbed onto the skin (such as during scratching). The organsim is highly invasive; large numbers appear in the blood and urine during febrile episodes. An endotoxin is probably responsible for the necrotic and hemorrhagic lesions that are produced. A remarkable feature of *B. recurrentis* is its capacity to produce a series of antigenically distinct mutants, which develop rapidly to cause a succession of clinical relapses.

B. turicatae, the species that causes endemic relapsing fever in humans in Mexico and the United

States. Rodents carry the tick vector *Ornithodoros turicata,* which transmits the organism in its bite.

B. venezuelensis, a species that causes endemic relapsing fever in humans in South and Central America. Its vector is the tick *Ornithodoros rudis.*

boss (bos) a rounded eminence, as on the surface of a bone or tumor.

bothridium (both-rid′ē-um) one of the four slitlike suckers symmetrically placed around the anterior end of the scolex of tetraphyllidean tapeworms. Also called phyllidea.

bothrium (both′re-um) [Gr. *bothrion* pit] a grooved sucker. Ventral and dorsal bothria attach the scolex to the mucosa. They are characteristic of the fish tapeworm, *Diphyllobothrium latum.*

***Bothrops atrox* serine proteinase** see *reptilase.*

botryoid (bot′re-oid) [Gr. *botrys* bunch of grapes + *eidos* form] shaped like a bunch of grapes.

botryoid rhabdomyosarcoma a descriptive term applied to a rhabdomyosarcoma arising in a submucosal location, particularly the genitourinary tract. Submucosal proliferation of neoplastic cells with associated inflammation and edema results in the development of a polypoid gelatinous tumor with a fancied resemblance to a small bunch of grapes. In sections, the tumor cells are concentrated in a layer (cambium layer) subjacent to the epithelium. Also called *botryoid sarcoma* and *sarcoma botryoides.* See also *rhabdomyosarcoma.*

botryoid sarcoma see *botryoid rhabdomyosarcoma.*

botryomycosis (bot″re-o-mi-ko′sis) [Gr. *botrys* bunch of grapes + *mykēs* fungus + *-osis*] a chronic disease of the skin characterized by lesions containing pus and sulfur granules, so called because it was mistakenly believed to be due to a fungus called "botryomycetes." The usual cause is *Staphylococcus aureus.* The lesions may spread to internal organs.

bottleneck (bot″l-nek) any point at which movement, progress, or a chemical reaction is slowed because of a restriction or deficiency.

botulin (bot′u-lin) [L. *botulus* sausage] see *botulinum toxin.*

botulinum toxin (bot″u-li′num) a potent exotoxin produced by germinating spores and growing vegetative cells of *Clostridium botulinum.* The thermolabile neurotoxin (inactivated in 10 min at 100°C) is not inactivated by gastric acid or proteolytic enzymes of the stomach and upper gastrointestinal tract, but is absorbed from the GI tract into the blood stream where it travels to neuromuscular junctions and peripheral autonomic synapses. Botulinum toxin binds to the presynaptic terminals, thus blocking the release of acetylcholine by the nerve endings. This results in a decrease of skeletal muscle function, which may progress to paralysis, respiratory failure, and cardiac arrest.

There are seven immunologically distinct forms of botulinum toxin (A–G). In the United States, type A neurotoxin causes 62 percent of all cases of botulism; type B, 28 percent; and type E, 10 percent. Types A and B are associated with uncooked meats or improperly canned vegetables, whereas type E is associated with seafood. Type A botulinum toxin is a protein (M.W. 900,000) consisting of a neurotoxin (M.W. 150,000), a hemagglutinin, and a nontoxic portion.

See also *exotoxins.*

botulism (bot′u-lizm) a neuroparalytic disease caused by the anaerobic, gram-positive, spore-forming bacterium *Clostridium botulinum* and its toxins. There are three types of botulism disease: classical food-borne, wound, and infant botulism.

Clinical Disease. Food-borne botulism, the most common form of the disease, is an intoxication (not an infectious disease) following ingestion of preformed toxin with food that may not appear or taste spoiled. In the United States, the principal source is improperly canned or preserved foods, especially home-canned vegetables; of the seven forms of toxin, A and B are most often responsible.

Clinical symptoms begin 18–36 hr after ingestion when absorbed toxin reaches susceptible cholinergic nerve endings. The botulinum toxin inhibits skeletal muscle function, which initially affects the small muscles of the eyes, larynx, and pharynx, leading to speech and swallowing difficulties, blurring of vision, and pupillary dilation. Patients may feel weak and dizzy and often complain of dryness of the mouth, nausea, and vomiting, but fever is usually absent. As the botulism advances, there is a weakness in the extremities, and impairment of respiration, and cardiac arrest may occur. Death from respiratory failure can occur 1–7 da after onset of the symptoms. The fatality rate of botulism is around 21 percent.

Wound botulism is a rare infection caused by *Clostridium botulinum* growing in skin lesions. The spores do not readily germinate in the wound, requiring proper anaerobic conditions and time for germination (4–14 da).

Infant botulism is actually a type of food-borne infection and intoxication. Infants in the first weeks of life are susceptible because the microbial flora of their gastrointestinal tract is sparse and unstable. Clinical symptoms include weakness, constipation, cranial nerve abnormalities, and a sudden cessation of breathing.

Laboratory Diagnosis. In food-borne botulism, the organism can be recovered in anaerobic cultures from the food when available or from the patient's feces. Because nontoxigenic strains exist, it is necessary to demonstrate toxin production. Injection of about 0.4 ml of food extract, fecal extract, and serum intraperitioneally into mice usually results in flaccid paralysis in 24 hr and death in 3 da. Fecal extract in suspected infant botulism is both cultured and tested for toxigenicity. In wound botulism, swabs from the wound, as well as serum and feces, are processed in the same manner.

Prevention and Treatment. Botulism may be prevented by cooking food sufficiently to inactivate the toxin. The disease is treated with antitoxin, but this only inactivates the unbound toxin. Respiratory assistance may be necessary.

See also *exotoxins.*

Bouchard's nodes (boo-sharz′) [Charles Jacques *Bouchard,* French physician 1837–1915] cartilaginous and bony enlargements of the proximal interphalangeal joints of the fingers, seen in degenerative joint disease. Such nodules in the terminal interphalangeal joints are called *Heberden's nodes.*

Bouguer's law (boo-gāz) [Pierre *Bouguer,* French mathematician, 1698–1758] see *Beer's law.*

Bouin's fluid (bwanz′) [Paul *Bouin,* French anatomist, 1870–1962] a general-purpose fixative and fixative of choice for testicular tissue, composed of a mixture of saturated picric acid, formaldehyde, and glacial acetic acid. Most stains can be used on tissue fixed in Bouin's fluid but this fixative is particularly suitable for trichrome connective tissue stains. It penetrates tissues slowly and must be removed before staining. Bouin's fluid does not harden tissue to the extent that formalin does and does not produce formalin hematin pigment, but it does tend to lyse blood cells. Tissues should not be allowed to remain in the solution longer than 24 hr and should be stored in 70 percent alcohol. See also *fixative.*

Bouin's picroformol–acetic fixative [P. *Bouin*] a histologic fixative composed of saturated picric acid, formalin, and glacial acetic acid.

Bourneville's disease (boor-ne-vēz′) [Désiré-Magloire *Bourneville,* French neurologist, 1840–1909] see *tuberous s.* under *sclerosis.*

bouton (boo-taw′) [Fr.] button; a knoblike swelling or enlargement, such as those found on nerve fibers.

b. en passant, a synapse formed by a bulblike expansion along the course of an axon. Also called bouton de passage.

terminal b., see *b.'s terminaux.*

b.'s terminaux, synaptic swellings at the termination of axons.

boutonneuse fever (boo-ton-uhz′) [Fr. pimply] an acute febrile disease caused by the *Rickettsia conorii* organism, which is found in humans in the Mediterranean area, India, and South and East Africa. The vector is a tick (*Rhipicephalus sanguineus*). Symptoms of a primary skin lesion (eschar or tache noire), lymph node inflammation, and rash are followed by chills and fever. Tetracycline drugs are used to treat the fever, as for Rocky Mountain spotted fever.

bovine (bo′vīn) [L. *bos, bovis* ox, bullock, cow] referring to, characteristic of, or derived from cattle or oxen.

bovine serum albumin (BSA) 1. purified albumin, prepared from bovine serum, and available as dry crystalline material or in the form of solutions of varied concentration.

2. in clinical chemistry, a commercially prepared protein standard solution made with crystalline BSA, sold in ampules with protein content given in terms of milligrams of protein nitrogen per milliliter of solution.

bowel (bow′el) [Fr. *boyau,* from L. *botellus* sausage] see *intestine.*

Bowen's disease (bo′enz) [John Templeton *Bowen,* U.S. dermatologist, 1857–1941] a term in common usage as an equivalent for intraepithelial squamous carcinoma of the epidermis of the body; see *intraepidermal s. c. c.* under *squamous cell carcinoma.*

Bowie's stain (bo′ēz) see under *juxtaglomerular granules staining.*

Bowman's capsule (bō′manz) [Sir William *Bowman,* English physician, 1816–1892] the thin-walled, proximal expansion of a renal tubule, which surrounds a tuft of capillaries to form the renal glomerulus. See also *kidney.*

Bowman's glands [Sir William *Bowman*] see *olfactory glands.*

Bowman's membrane [W. *Bowman*] a thin layer of the cornea, about 30 μm thick, that is composed of a feltwork of collagen fibrils. It is found between the anterior layer of epithelium and Descemet's membrane.

Boyden chamber (boi′den) an apparatus used to detect and quantify leukocyte chemotaxis. It consists of two chambers separated by a millipore filter. The cells are placed in the upper chamber, and an agent to provide the chemotactic stimulus is placed in the lower. After incubation, the filter is stained, cleared, and examined microscopically for migrating cells. The response is determined as the number of leukocytes that have moved through the filter or a specified distance into the filter. Migration of various types of granulocytes, including neutrophils and eosinophils, as well as monocyte-macrophage chemotaxis, can be analyzed with this apparatus.

Boyle's law (boilz) [Robert *Boyle,* British physicist, 1627–1691] stated as: the volume of a given mass of a perfect gas held at a constant temperature varies inversely with the pressure under which it is measured; if the volume (V) is decreased, the pressure (P) increases by the same proportion, so that the product PV is a constant if the temperature stays constant.

BP abbrev. See *blood pressure.*

bp abbrev. See *base pair.*

b. p. abbrev. See *boiling point.*

BPH abbrev. for *benign prostatic hyperplasia.*

BPL abbrev. See *β-propiolactone.*

Bq abbrev. See *becquerel.*

Br symbol for the chemical element *bromine.*

brachi/o (bra′ke-o) [L. *brachium,* from Gr. *brachiōn* arm] a word element used in combining form to denote arm, e.g., brachial.

brachial (bra′ke-al) [L. *brachialis,* from *brachium* arm] pertaining to the arm.

brachial artery the continuation of the axillary artery. It begins at the lower border of the teres major muscle, runs down the arm, and ends below the elbow joint by dividing into the radial and ulnar arteries.

brachial neuritis a disorder of uncertain cause that is characterized by pain, weakness, and sensory and reflex changes in the arms, shoulders, or neck, due to dysfunction of the brachial plexus. Brachial neuritis may occur after a viral illness or inoculations, or without specific antecedents. It is usually self-limiting, with near-complete or complete recovery after several weeks or months. There is no specific treatment. Also called *neuralgic amyotrophy.*

brachiocephalic (brak″e-o-sĕ-fal′ik) [*brachio-* + Gr. *kephalē* head] pertaining to the arm and head.

brachiocephalic artery the largest branch of the aortic arch. It ascends to the level of the right sternoclavicular joint, where it divides into the right common carotid and right subclavian arteries. Also called the innominate artery.

brachiocephalic vein one of the paired large trunks in the base of the neck and upper thorax, each formed by junction of the internal jugular and subclavian veins of that side. Also called the innominate vein.

brachy- (brak′e) [Gr. *brachys* short] a prefix word element to denote short, e.g., brachycephaly.

brachycephalic (brak″e-sĕ-fal′ik) [*brachy-* + Gr. *kephalē* head] having a short, wide head, with a cephalic index of 81.0–85.4.

brachytherapy (brak″e-ther′ah-pe) [*brachy-* + Gr.

therapeia treatment] radiation therapy that uses an implanted radioisotope radiation source. See also *radiation therapy.*

Bradshaw's test (brad′shawz) [Thomas Robert *Bradshaw,* English physician, 1857–1927] a test for Bence Jones protein in urine; see *Bence Jones protein tests.*

brady- (brad′e) [Gr. *bradys* slow] a prefix word element to denote slow, e.g., bradycardia.

bradyarrhythmia (brad″e-ah-rith′me-ah) [*brady-* + *a-* neg. + Gr. *rhythmos* rhythm] a general term denoting a slowing of the heart rate to fewer than 60 beats/min. It is commonly the result of conditions such as sinus bradycardia, second-degree atrioventricular block, or complete A-V block.

bradycardia (brad″e-kar′de-ah) [*brady-* + Gr. *kardia* heart] a slow heart rate; usually applied to adult humans when the heart rate is less than 60 beats/min. Cf. *tachycardia.*

junctional b., see *nodal b.*

nodal b., a slow heart rate with the stimulus arising in or near the atrioventricular node. Also called *junctional b.*

sinus b., a slow heart rate with the impulse originating in the sinoatrial node.

bradycardia-tachycardia syndrome a form of sick sinus syndrome characterized by interruption of sinus bradycardia or other bradyarrhythmia, with recurrent episodes of one or several forms of supraventricular tachyarrhythmia. After cessation of the tachyarrhythmia, a long pause may precede the resumption of the normal sinus rhythm or another escape rhythm. The syndrome is associated with an increased incidence of cerebral or other systemic thromboemboli. It may also occur as a complication of acute myocardial infarction. A pacemaker may be indicated.

bradykinin (brad″e-ki′nin) [*brady-* + Gr. *kinein* to move] a naturally occurring nonapeptide that is split from a serum alpha$_2$-globulin precursor by the enzyme kallikrein. Bradykinin is the final product of the kinin system. Among its effects are slow, sustained contraction of smooth muscles, increased vascular permeability, increased mucous gland secretions, and pain. It contributes to hay fever, angiodema, and asthma symptoms.

Bragg curve (brag) [Sir William Henry *Bragg,* British physicist, 1862–1942; and his son, Sir William Lawrence *Bragg,* British physicist, 1890–1971] a plot of the specific ionization produced by a beam of alpha particles or other heavy charged particles, a function of the residual kinetic energy of the beam. The specific ionization gradually increases as the beam loses energy and then rises in a sharp peak (the Bragg peak) just as all the energy is lost. Thus, most of the beam energy is deposited near the depth at which the beam is stopped.

Bragg reflection [Sir W. H. *Bragg; Sir W. L. Bragg*] the specular reflection of x-rays by parallel planes of atoms in a crystal lattice. The rays reflected from successive planes constructively interfere (reinforce each other) when the angle θ between the incident (or reflected) ray and the crystal planes, the distance d between the crystal planes, and the wavelength λ of the x-rays are related by Bragg's law: $n\lambda = 2d \sin \theta$, where n is any integer. Any such angle θ is called a Bragg angle. See also *x-ray crystallography.*

brain (brān) [Anglo-Saxon *braegen*] the part of the central nervous system that is contained within the cranial cavity. It is continuous with the spinal cord through the foramen magnum in the base of the skull. The functions of the body are controlled or influenced by cells of the brain through processes of neurons that leave the brain through the cranial nerves or pass to the spinal cord, where they influence the activity of cells, giving rise to the spinal nerves. Constant monitoring of activities of various parts of the body is necessary so that the brain can coordinate motor activity; it receives this information through sensory neurons that enter the spinal cord through the dorsal roots of the spinal nerves, or that reach the brain directly in cranial nerves.

The brain of an adult weighs about 1400 g and almost fills the cranial cavity. Its blood supply comes from the paired internal carotid and vertebral arteries that communicate over the base of the brain in the arterial circle of Willis, and then ramify on the surface and give off numerous branches that penetrate to the interior.

There are five interconnected divisions of the brain. The largest is the cerebrum, which has right and left halves—the cerebral hemispheres—partially separated by a longitudinal fissure. At the base of the fissure, a broad sheet of connecting fibers, the corpus callosum, extends between the two hemispheres. The cerebellum lies beneath the posterior part of the cerebrum, and also has right and left hemispheres that are united by a median portion called the vermis. The three other parts of the brain form a stem to which the cerebrum and cerebellum are attached. From above, they are the midbrain, the pons, and the medulla oblongata, which is continuous with the spinal cord.

The areas of the brain that are filled with nerve cell bodies have a gray color, whereas those made up of nerve cell processes appear white. In the cerebrum and cerebellum, much of the gray matter is on the surface, forming the cortex, whereas in the brain stem the surface is white matter and most of the nerve cells are grouped in its interior. There are many deep grooves, or sulci, on the surface of the cerebrum, so that the cortex forms an undulating layer whose area is some five times greater than the cerebral surface. The ridges between sulci are called gyri. The surface of the cerebellum has a distinctive foliated appearance from the presence of many deep, parallel fissures that increase the area of its cortex.

Each cerebral hemisphere is subdivided into four lobes. The anterior part is the frontal lobe, and the posterior part the occipital lobe; the parietal lobe lies between the two, with the temporal lobe below it. The frontal, occipital, and temporal lobes have pointed tips or poles. A deep, oblique sulcus located roughly midway between the frontal and occipital poles is the central sulcus. The gyrus immediately in front of it is the precentral gyrus, which contains the cells that control individual movements on the opposite side of the body. It is often called the motor area of the cerebral cortex. Sensory information is processed in the sensory area, located in the postcentral gyrus immediately behind the central sulcus. In the motor and sensory areas the body is more or less represented upside down, the area for the head being in the lower part of the gyrus, with the upper limb, trunk, and lower limb above it. Other areas of the cortex known to be concerned with par-

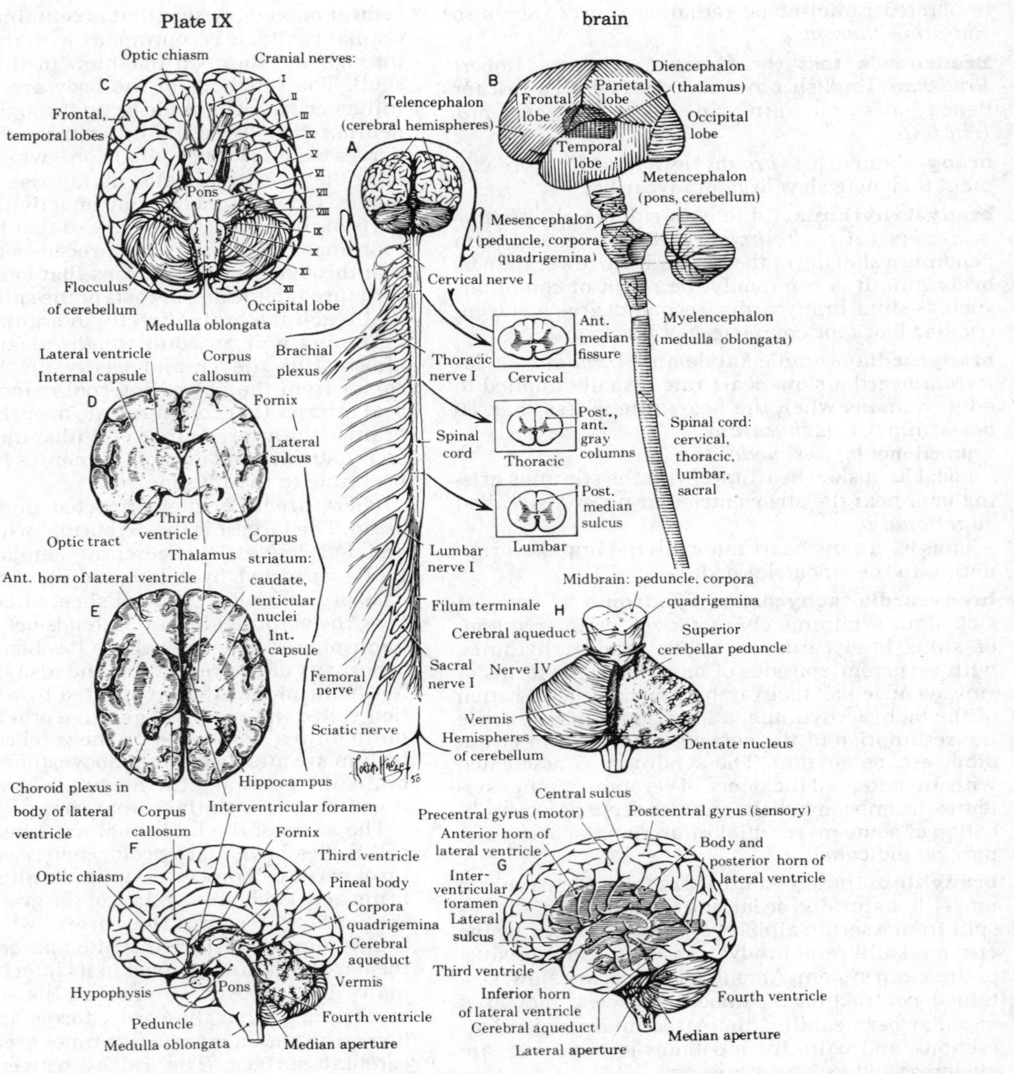

Brain. Various aspects and sections of brain and spinal cord. (From Dorland's Illustrated Medical Dictionary. 26th ed. Philadelphia, W. B. Saunders Co., 1981.)

ticular functions include the occipital lobe (vision) and the upper part of the temporal lobe (hearing). The physiology and anatomic correlates of higher intellectual functions, such as memory, learning, and language, are still poorly defined. The cerebellum is primarily concerned with coordinating the body's movements.

Large collections of gray matter in the interior of the cerebral hemispheres constitute the basal nuclei. In lower animals lacking a motor cortex, the basal ganglia are well developed, and in humans their function is probably the regulation of movement. The thalamus is a large, ovoid mass of gray matter located above the midbrain; it receives sensory impulses from the opposite half of the body and transmits most of them to the sensory cortex.

A system of cavities (ventricles) and communicating channels within the brain and spinal cord is lined by a layer of specialized ependymal cells that are remnants of the embryonal neuroepithelium. In the ventricles it is modified to form the choroid plexuses, whose cells take up fluid from the blood capillaries and secrete it into the ventricles as cerebrospinal fluid (CSF).

The brain and spinal cord are enclosed in three concentric connective tissue membranes, the meninges. The outermost is the dura mater: it is adherent to the inner surface of the bones that form the cranial cavity, and projects into clefts in the brain as supporting partitions, the largest of which is the falx cerebri in the longitudinal fissure. The middle membrane is the arachnoid; it bridges across the sulci, whereas the innermost membrane, the pia, closely invests the brain surface. At many points, the arachnoid and pia separate to enclose a subarachnoid space that is filled with CSF. The major functions of the CSF include the provision of physical support or buoyancy for the brain, the distribution of biologically active substances intracerebrally, and the control of the brain's chemical environment. It also has an excretory function for the brain. There are free communications between the CSF and intercellular spaces within the brain; the so-called "blood-brain barrier," which protects the brain from certain harmful substances in the blood stream, depends for its integrity on tight junctions between the endothelial cells of brain capillaries.

See also the accompanying illustration.

brain death syndrome the state in which brain function, including autonomic control, is totally and permanantly abolished. Criteria for establishing the loss of brain function are reviewed and revised as new technologies develop. The American Neurological Association (ANA) guidelines state that brain death may be declared if, after appropriate measures to remedy hypothermia and/or circulatory collapse, the patient remains comatose, is unable to breathe spontaneously, and is without cephalic reflexes (e.g., pupillary, corneal, audioocular, and oculocephalic reflexes). The electroencephalogram must be isoelectric for at least 30 min when recorded after the clinical signs have persisted for 6 hr or longer. Persistence of clinical signs should be verified after an additional interval of at least 6 hr; an interval of 48 hr or longer is required in cases involving drug effects. These criteria may not apply to children under the age of 5 yr.

In instances of ambiguity, evidence for the absence of cerebral blood flow or the absence of cerebral metabolism should be sought. Cerebral blood flow can be studied by various angiographic or isotopic techniques; cerebral metabolism is evaluated by measuring the cerebral metabolic rate of oxygen, or the arteriovenous difference in oxygen concentration across the brain, or by other similar approaches.

Also called *irreversible coma.* See also *electrocerebral inactivity, evoked potential,* and *Harvard criteria of irreversible coma.*

brain sand see *corpora arenacea.*

brain scan a procedure in nuclear medicine for examining the brain that utilizes a scintillation camera or rectilinear scanner. Ionic radiopharmaceuticals, which cannot cross the blood-brain barrier, localize in areas of tissue damage or destruction, such as occurs in brain tumors, cerebrovascular accidents (CVA), abscesses, contusions, or hematomas. These injured areas appear as hot lesions with a tumor-to-brain uptake ratio of 10:1 to 20:1. Sodium pertechnetate Tc-99m is the most commonly used agent, but technetium Tc 99m pentetate sodium (^{99m}Tc-DTPA), ^{113m}In-DTPA, ^{169}Yb-DTPA, and ^{99m}Tc-glucoheptonate are also used.

A radionuclide cerebral angiogram is usually performed prior to the static scans. Normal anterior views (with the camera head tipped 15°–20° forward) are taken with the scintillation camera at intervals of 2–3 sec for at least 30 sec after the intravenous injection of a bolus of ^{99m}Tc-pertechnetate. An asymmetric pattern of activity may indicate an area of ischemia on the side that has decreased activity.

Static scans are made 1–3 hr after injection. Normal anterior, lateral, and posterior views (with the head tipped 15°–45° forward) are routinely made. A vertex view, which aids in detecting parasagittal lesions, is also commonly obtained. Delayed views made 2–6 hr after injection may help to detect low-grade astrocytomas, metastatic lesions, CVAs, early infarcts, abscesses, and subdural hematomas. (Richly vascular tumors, such as high-grade astrocytomas and meningiomas, show better on the angiogram or on early views.)

Slight malpositioning, such as a 10° rotation of the head, can produce abnormal scans. Potassium perchlorate is given before the procedure to block pertechnetate uptake by the choroid plexus, and atropine may be administered to block uptake by the salivary glands and nasal mucosa when the vertex view is used.

brain stem the stemlike portion of the brain that connects the cerebral hemispheres with the spinal cord. It is composed of the pons, medulla oblongata, and mesencephalon; some also consider the diencephalon to be one of the components. For more information, see the specific components and *brain.*

brain stem auditory evoked potential (BAEP) see *brain stem auditory e. p.* under *evoked potential.*

brain waves the fluctuations of electric potential in the brain, as recorded by electroencephalography. See also *electroencephalography.*

braking radiation (bra′king) see *bremsstrahlung.*

branch (branch) 1. a division or offshoot from a main stem, especially of blood vessels, nerves, or lymphatics; also called *ramus.*

2. a point in a computer program at which a decision is made and the flow of control can be passed to a statement other than the next in sequence.

3. See *branching decay.*

branched chain a chain of atoms, usually carbon, having one or more side-chains attached.

branched-chain aminoaciduria see *maple syrup urine disease.*

branched-chain α-ketoacid decarboxylase see *2-oxoisovalerate dehydrogenase.*

branched-chain α-ketoacid dehydrogenase see *2-oxoisovalerate dehydrogenase.*

branched-chain ketoaciduria see *maple syrup urine disease.*

brancher deficiency (branch′er) a hereditary disorder, transmitted as an autosomal recessive trait, that is characterized by the abnormal metabolism, deposition, and structure of glycogen. There is a deficiency of 1,4-α-glucan branching enzyme, resulting in the generalized deposition of amylopectin, an abnormal form of glycogen. The symptoms result from the inadequacy of liver glycogen stores. Cirrhosis, portal hypertension, hepatosplenomegaly, liver failure, and amylopectin deposition in the kidneys, heart, muscles, and nervous system often lead to death before puberty. Demonstration of enzyme deficiency prenatally in amniotic cells or postnatally in cultured skin fibroblasts or muscle biopsies is diagnostic. Also called *amylopectinosis* and glycogenosis type IV. See also *glycogenoses.*

brancher enzyme see *1,4-α-glucan branching enzyme.*

branchial (brang′ke-al) [Gr. *branchia* gills] pertaining to the gills of a fish or the homologous parts of other organisms.

branchial cyst see *branchial c.* under *cyst.*

branchial region in lower animals, a term used to

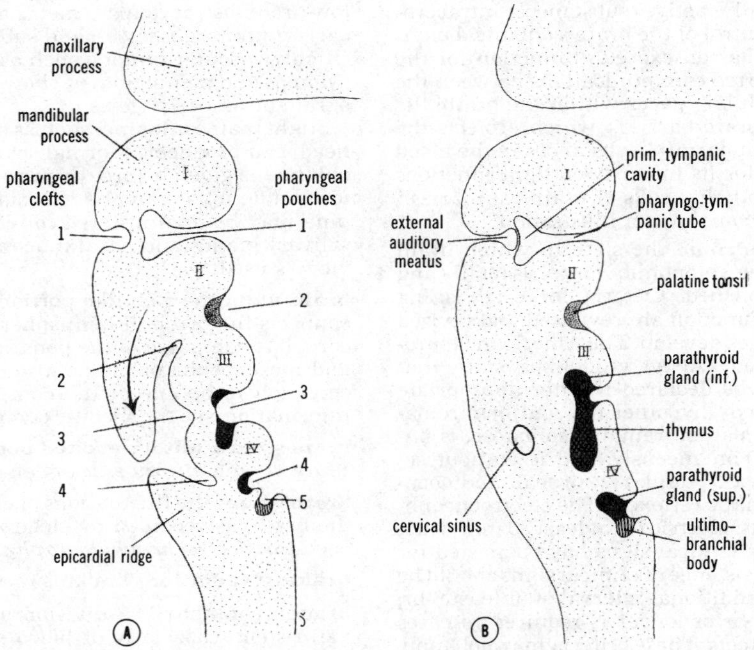

Branchial region, Figure 1. *A,* Schematic representation of the development of the pharyngeal clefts and pouches. Note how the second arch grows over the third and fourth arches, thereby burying the second, third, and fourth pharyngeal clefts. *B,* The remnants of the second, third, and fourth pharyngeal clefts from the cervical sinus. Note also the differentiation of the epithelium in the wall of the entodermal pharyngeal pouches (modified after Starck). From Langman, J.: Medical Embryology. 4th ed. Baltimore, Williams & Wilkins Co., 1981.)

refer to the region of the gill clefts; in human embryology it refers to the primitive pharynx, which undergoes a significant sequence of alterations between the third and eighth weeks.

In the developing embryo, the primitive pharynx is part of the cephalic (headward) end of the developing alimentary canal; it is separated from the oral cavity by the buccopharyngeal membrane, which ruptures at the end of the third week. The wall of the pharynx thickens through proliferation of its mesodermal cells, and a series of four clefts appears in the outer aspect of each lateral wall. At the same time, five pouches develop on each inner wall (Fig. 1). The clefts and pouches grow toward one another but do not meet, remaining separated by a bar of mesoderm (pharyneal arch) within which an artery, a nerve, muscles, and a strip of cartilage develop. Some of the cartilage persists to form mature bone or cartilage. The muscles derived from a particular arch may attach to adjacent structures, but retain their nerve supply from the nerve of that arch. Cells proliferate in the branchial pouches to form the primordia of endocrine glands, which migrate to their permanent locations.

The first pharyngeal arch gives rise to the incus, malleus, mandible, and muscles of mastication; its nerve is the mandibular division of the trigeminal. The stapes, styloid process, upper part of the hyoid bone, and related muscles develop from the second arch, and the muscles are innervated by the facial nerve. The remainder of the hyoid is derived from the third arch, together with the stylopharyngeus muscle, which is supplied by the glossopharyngeal nerve. From the fourth and fifth arches come the laryngeal cartilages and the cricothyroid and pharyngeal constrictor muscles, which are innervated by the superior laryngeal branch of the vagus nerve. The tissue of the second pharyngeal arch grows over the third and fourth arches to enclose the cervical sinus, a cavity that is usually obliterated but occasionally persists as a lateral cervical (branchial) cyst. (See Fig. 2.)

The first pharyngeal pouch develops into the pharyngotympanic tube, and the first cleft forms the external auditory canal; the two remain separated by the tympanic membrane. The second pouch disappears, but the palatine tonsil forms at its site. Cells from the third pouch form the primordia of the thymus and inferior parathyroid glands, and parathyroid tissue is occasionally drawn down into the mediastinum as the thymus descends. The superior parathyroids come from the fourth pouches, and the fifth gives rise to the C cells of the thyroid.

While these events are taking place, the tongue develops from proliferations of mesoderm of the arches and anterior wall of the pharynx, and the thyroid gland appears as a group of cells close to the base of the tongue that burrow down through the neck, temporarily retaining a connection with the pharynx through the thyroglossal duct.

branching decay (branch′ing) radioactive decay in which a nuclide may decay in more than one mode. Each mode has a characteristic decay constant.

branching enzyme see *1,4-a-glucan branching enzyme.*

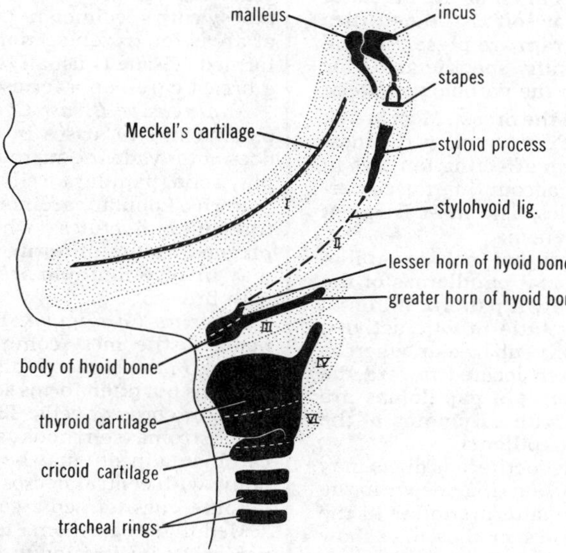

Branchial region, Figure 2. A drawing showing the definitive structures formed by the cartilaginous components of the various pharyngeal arches (modified after Giroud). (From Langman, J.: Medical Embryology. 4th ed. Baltimore, Williams & Wilkins Co., 1981.)

branching fraction the fraction of substance decaying in a particular mode.

branching ratio the ratio of two branching fractions.

Branhamella (bran″hah-mel′ah) [Sara Elizabeth *Branham,* U.S. bacteriologist, born 1888] a genus of bacteria of the family Neisseriaceae. These organisms are generally nonpathogenic and are common commensals on the mucous membrane, especially the nasopharynx. *Branhamella* consists of a single species, *B. catarrhalis.*

B. catarrhalis, a nonpathogenic species found in secretions of the normal pharynx and frequently confused with meningococci or gonococci. Unlike them, it does not ferment glucose. Microscopically, it is also gram-negative and forms pairs of cocci whose adjacent sides are flattened. Although generally considered nonpathogenic, the species can occasionally cause otitis media and respiratory disease in children and adults. Formerly called *Neisseria catarrhalis.*

Brasil's fixative (brah-zilz′) a solution of formalin, picric acid, ethanol, and trichloroacetic acid. It is used as a fixative for surgical pathology specimens and is often preferred to other picroformol fixatives, such as Bouin's fluid, because of its alcoholic base. See also *fixatives.*

brazilin (braz′ĭ-lin, brah-zil′in) an acid-base indicator, extracted from Brazil wood, that is used as a biologic stain, which turns yellow in acid solutions and carmine red in alkali; C.I. 75280.

BrdU abbrev. See *5-bromodeoxyuridine.*

breadboard a prototype of an electronic circuit in which the components are connected in the most convenient manner, usually with temporary connections.

breakbone fever (brāk′bōn) see *dengue.*

break-even point the level of activity of an operation at which total revenue equals total cost.

breast (brest) 1. the anterior aspect of the chest. 2. one of the mammary glands, which embryologically is a modified sweat gland. The breast remains rudimentary in the male but enlarges in the female to form an elaborate structure with 15–20 lobes, each passing their secretion into a duct that converges on the nipple. The histology of the breast varies with its functional activity. It is most highly developed in the childbearing years, especially during and following pregnancy. Secreting alveolar cells are evident only when milk is being formed. A complex interplay of ovarian and pituitary hormones influences the development and functional activity of the normal breast.

The breast lies within the superficial fascia of the anterior thorax and extends into the axilla (axillary tail). It is separated from the pectoral muscles by deep fascia. Fibrous septa intervene between the lobes of the breast and attach to the overlying skin. The secretions of the lobes drain into lactiferous ducts that traverse the nipple. The nipple is surrounded by a circle of colored skin, the areola, under which there are apocrine and sebaceous glands. Active alveolar cells are columnar with a few apical microvilli and contain many lipid droplets; duct cells are cuboidal. Myoepithelial cells are present between the alveolar and small duct cells and their basal lamina to aid in the expression of secretion into the larger ducts.

The lymphatics of the breast begin as capillaries in the lobules and continue as interlobular connective tissue that drains into a network in the skin around the nipple, and then into the pectoral, axillary, and parasternal lymph node groups.

See also *breast tumors.*

breast specimen radiography the radiographic examination of a biopsy specimen of the breast to confirm that calcifications or soft tissue densities demonstrated in a mammogram are present in the biopsy specimen, and to identify specific areas for microscopic examination by the pathologist.

breast tumors neoplasms of the breast. Most breast tumors are epithelial. Breast carcinoma is the most common malignant neoplasm affecting females in the United States, currently accounting for 26 percent of all cancers in females. The most frequent benign tumor is the fibroadenoma.

benign epithelial b. t., tumors that include papillomas and adenomas. Intraductal papillomas of the breast display an orderly growth pattern, minimal cellular pleomorphism, and little mitotic activity. Solitary papillomas are usually subareolar, whereas multiple papillomas are often located toward the periphery of the breast. Multiple papillomas are more frequently associated with carcinoma of the breast than with a solitary papilloma.

Adenomas occurring in the lactiferous ducts may be papillary or solid. Those occurring deeper in the breast may have a tubular pattern similar to the ductules of the inactive lobules, or they may show secretory (lactating) changes.

Fibroadenoma is the most common benign breast tumor. It is usually seen in younger females, in whom it forms a sharply delimited nodule that is generally less than 4 cm when excised. Sections show branching ducts within a fibrous stroma. Malignant transformation is exceedingly rare. The term giant fibroadenoma was formerly used for cystosarcoma phyllodes.

Cystosarcoma phyllodes, an uncommon connective tissue tumor of the breast, occurs in an older age group of females than does fibroadenoma, and is usually benign, although some grow to giant proportions. The cut surface displays a nodular appearance and is sharply demarcated from the adjacent normal or compressed breast tissue. The ductal elements present within the tumor are benign, and the prominent histologic feature is the cellularity of the stroma. Usually it is fibrous, but it can have a liposarcomatous or other mesenchymal appearance. The tumor may recur, particularly if it has been enucleated under the impression that it was a fibroadenoma. Frankly sarcomatous histologic features are an indication that metastasis may develop, but this is unusual.

malignant b. t., tumors that include breast carcinomas and the relatively rare sarcomas. Breast carcinomas may arise from duct cells or from the terminal secretory units of the breast lobules. More than 70 percent are infiltrating duct cell carcinomas. Studies of whole organ sections of breasts have shown that the carcinomas are often multicentric. Breast carcinoma is more common in females living in affluent societies, and is more likely to occur in individuals who are single, nulliparous, and/or those with a family history of breast cancer.

A number of histologic types have been defined, and their identification has some bearing on the prognosis, as has histologic grading. Frequently a breast carcinoma contains a combination of histologic patterns. It may then be classified according to the predominant pattern, but if more than one component is extensive, multiple diagnoses are indicated.

Breast carcinoma is frequently diagnosed from a frozen section or a needle biopsy. When a mammogram fails to provide a firm diagnosis, excisional biopsy with specimen radiography prior to selection of areas for frozen section evaluation is often performed. Tissue is usually routinely submitted from a breast carcinoma for estrogen receptor studies.

Noninvasive Breast Carcinoma. Intraductal carcinoma in situ arises in the mammary ducts and does not invade the surrounding stroma. It may display solid, papillary, cribriform, or comedo growth patterns. Lobular carcinoma in situ involves the intralobular ductules, which in sections appear plugged by the uniform, round cells. The process may involve multiple areas of the breast or affect both breasts.

Invasive Carcinoma. Invasive duct cell carcinoma is the most common malignant neoplasm arising in the breast. It displays a variety of growth patterns but often forms solid nests, glandlike structures, or cords of cells. There may be extensive fibrous stroma (scirrhous carcinoma). Areas of ductal carcinoma in situ may be present. A duct cell carcinoma with central necrosis within the nests of cells is sometimes termed a comedo carcinoma.

Medullary carcinoma makes up approximately 5 percent of infiltrating breast carcinomas. Those affected are usually younger than 50 yr. The cells have more cytoplasm than in a typical intraductal carcinoma, and they form diffuse aggregates that are often associated with a prominent infiltrate of small lymphocytes. This type of breast cancer is believed to have a more favorable prognosis than invasive duct cell carcinoma despite its frequent poor differentiation and numerous mitoses.

Mucinous carcinoma of the breast is characterized by large quantities of extracellular mucin, and in microscopic sections, nests of cells appear to float within a mucinous sea. This tumor has been called colloid carcinoma. In pure form, a mucinous carcinoma is considered to possess a better prognosis than invasive duct cell carcinoma.

Tubular carcinoma of the breast is made up of cells forming well-defined tubules within a fibrous stroma. The ductlike structures are haphazardly distributed, and there may be foci of dysplasia or intraductal carcinoma, features important in differentiating the tumor from sclerosing adenosis. Tubular carcinomas are considered to have a relatively good prognosis.

Inflammatory carcinoma is a variant of invasive duct cell carcinoma, and represents approximately 1 percent of all breast carcinomas. It is characterized by redness and warmth without pain of the affected breast, and histologically by the presence of tumor emboli in the dermal lymphatics. Recently the histologic definition has been expanded to include the presence of tumor emboli in lymphatics of the breast parenchyma as well as the skin. Inasmuch as the histologic recognition of dermal lymphatic tumor emboli appears to be more significant than the clinical skin changes as an indicator of prognosis, a number of authors have proposed that the term inflammatory carcinoma be abandoned in favor of the term dermal lymphatic carcinomatosis of the breast. Historically, the disease has been characterized by rapid growth and wide dissemination, leading to early death; with newer therapeutic regimes, however, there are reports of increased survival.

Invasive lobular carcinoma arises within the terminal secretory units, which include the terminal ducts, lobules, and acini of the breast parenchyma, and the tumor cells are similar to those of lobular carcinoma in situ. Almost 10 percent of breast carcinomas are invasive lobular carcinomas; such tumors are often bilateral. The cells tend to form slender columns (Indian-file arrangement) within the fibrous connective tissue stroma. Mitotic figures are frequently sparse. Sections of a lymph node containing metastatic lobular carcinoma can be misinterpreted as diffuse large cell lymphoma because of the uniformity of the cells and the absence of any architectural pattern.

Paget's disease of the breast is an epidermotropic form of breast cancer that involves the skin of the nipple, and an underlying carcinoma composed of similar cells usually can be demonstrated.

The behavior of carcinoma of the female breast is related to a number of factors including the size of the primary tumor, its location within the breast, and the presence and extent of axillary lymph node involvement. Radiotherapy, chemotherapy, and hormonal treatments may be employed when the tumor is more advanced.

Carcinoma of the male breast is not common in North America, where it makes up approximately 1 percent of all breast cancers. Gynecomastia does not appear to be a precancerous condition. Cancer of the male breast tends to be located close to the nipple and is more aggressive in behavior than is carcinoma of the female breast. The prognosis is influenced by the size of the tumor and the occurrence of axillary lymph node metastasis: 10 percent of the patients in whom the latter are found survive for at least 10 yr.

See also *estrogen receptor.*

breath (breth) [M. E. *breeth, breth*] the air taken in and expelled by the expansion and contraction of the thorax and the vertical movement of the diaphragm.

breath holding a voluntarily or reflexively produced apnea, usually with the glottis closed. Voluntary breath holding, when prolonged maximally, is involuntarily terminated at the breaking point, determined by the levels of arterial Po_2 and Pco_2. In human adults, this breaking point (in professional divers) occurs 1–2.5 min after the onset of breath holding. The duration of voluntary apnea can be increased by preliminary hyperventilation, particularly with the use of oxygen.

Involuntary breath holding is a reflex action that occurs during swallowing, periodically in crying infants, and in some diving mammals at the onset of a dive.

breathing (brēth′ing) 1. the inspiration and expiration of air into and out of the lungs. See also *respiration.*

2. evaporation of a liquid through a permeable substance such as polyethylene.

breathing frequency (*f*) the number of respiratory cycles (an inspiration followed by an expiration) that occur per unit of time. Also called *respiratory rate.*

breathing zone the space in which atmospheric monitoring samples are likely to be most representative of the inhalation exposure of a person. Samples should be taken as near as possible to the nose of the individual whose exposure is being evaluated.

Brecher-Cronkite method (brech′er krong′kit) a method for enumerating blood platelets; see under *platelet count.*

Brecher's new methylene blue technique (brech′erz) [George *Brecher,* U.S. hematologist, born 1913] a hematologic staining method for the demonstration of reticulocytes in blood. The reticulum stains a deep blue; erythrocytes are light greenish blue.

breeder reactor (brēd′er) a nuclear reactor that produces more atoms of fissionable plutonium (which can be used as fuel) than the uranium consumed in the process.

bregma (breg′mah) [L., from Gr. "front part of the head"] a point at the top of the skull where the sagittal and coronal sutures meet; it is used as an anatomic landmark.

bremsstrahlung (brem′strah-lung) [Ger. "braking radiation"] penetrating electromagnetic radiation produced by the rapid deceleration of a rapidly moving charged particle (such as an electron or beta particle) in the electric field of another charged particle (usually a nucleus). The spectral distribution of bremsstrahlung is continuous. The effect of bremsstrahlung in stopping beta particles in tissue is minor because of the low atomic number of most atoms in tissue. Most x-ray beams have a large bremsstrahlung component.

Brenner tumor (bren′er) [Fritz *Brenner,* German pathologist, born 1877] a tumor of the ovary that is usually small, unilateral, and benign. It is composed of solid or cystic nests of epithelial cells resembling transitional cells separated by a fibrous stroma. The histogenesis is uncertain, but an origin from the serosal surface (mesothelium) of the ovary is postulated. See also under *ovarian tumors.*

Brethine (breth′ēn) trademark. See *terbutaline sulfate.*

brevicollis (brev″ĭ-kol′is) [L. *brevis* short + *collum* neck] see *Klippel-Feil syndrome.*

bridge (brij) 1. a protoplasmic structure that unites or connects separate cells, or adjacent elements within a cell.

2. see *pons.*

conjugation b., in bacterial genetics, the F pilus, the tip of which attaches to become the connection between male (F+) and female (F–) cells. Because F pili are hollow, the conjugation bridge offers a possible, but not proved, mechanism for the transfer of genetic material from one bacterium to another. See also *conjugation.*

bridging necrosis see under *hepatitis.*

bright contrast in phase contrast microscopy, when two sets of rays (one passing through the objective, the other through an annular phase plate) are added and the object appears brighter than the surroundings. Also called negative contrast.

Brill's disease (brilz) [Nathan Edwin *Brill,* U.S. physician, 1860–1925] see *recrudescent t.* under *typhus.*

brilliant cresyl blue a basic dye of the oxazine group; C.I. 51010. It has a strong affinity for nucleic acids and is used primarily for staining blood to demonstrate platelets and reticulocytes.

brilliant crocein (kro′se-in) an acid dye used as a histologic stain; C.I. 27290.

brilliant green a basic dye, one of the triphenylmethane dyes used mainly as a component of bacteriologic media; C.I. 42040. It has a bacteriostatic effect on *Escherichia coli.*

brilliant purpurin R an acid dye used as a histologic stain; C.I. 23510. It is employed principally for plasma and collagen stains.

Brill-Symmers disease (bril sim′erz) [N. E. *Brill;* Douglas *Symmers,* U.S. physician, 1879–1952] see *nodular l.* under *lymphoma.*

Brill-Zinsser disease (bril zin′ser) [N. E. *Brill;* Hans *Zinsser,* U.S. bacteriologist, 1878–1940] see *recrudescent t.* under *typhus.*

British thermal unit (BTU) any of several units of heat defined as the amount of heat necessary to raise 1 lb of water 1°F (which varies with the initial temperature of the water); all are approximately equal to 1055 J.

broad fish tapeworm see *D. latum* under *Diphyllobothrium.*

broad-spectrum effective against a wide range of microorganisms; referring to antimicrobial drugs.

Broders' index (bro′derz) [Albert Compton *Broders,* U.S. pathologist, 1885–1964] a classification of the degree of malignancy of tumors based on histologic features. Four grades are identified. Grade I is the most differentiated and grade IV the least differentiated. In general, the poorer the degree of differentiation, the greater the biologic aggressiveness of the neoplasm and the poorer the patient's prognosis.

Brodie's abscess (bro′dēz) [Sir Benjamin Collins *Brodie,* English surgeon, 1783–1862] see *Brodie's a.* under *abscess.*

broken cell preparation a preparation of the surviving components of broken cells used for in vitro metabolic studies. Disruption of the plasma membrane of cells in order to release cellular constituents can be accomplished by suspending a cell suspension or tissue fragments in a suitable isotonic medium. The suspension is subjected to ultrasonic vibration or fragmentation with a mechanical blender or mortar and pestle. Such preparations may contain nuclei, mitochondria, microsomes, other cellular organelles, plasma membrane fragments, and constituents of the cytosol. Specific fractions can be obtained by gradient ultracentrifugation. Also called homogenates.

brom/o (bro′mo) [Gr. *brōmos* stench] 1. a prefix word element to denote the presence of bromine.

2. a prefix word element, specifically in organic chemistry, to denote bromine as a substituent, e.g., bromomethane (CH_3BR).

bromate (bro′māt) the BrO_3^- ion or a salt of bromic acid. Moderately toxic, bromates are strong oxidizing agents and thus can be a fire hazard. Accidental ingestion may cause nausea, diarrhea, abdominal pain, renal injury, and marked methemoglobinemia.

bromelain (bro′mĕ-lān) an enzyme of the hydrolase class (EC 3.4.22.4). It is a thiol proteinase, which preferentially cleaves peptide bonds containing lysine, alanine, tyrosine, or glycine. Bromelain is prepared from the pineapple plant and is used in conjunction with ficin in the treatment of inflammation and edema of soft tissues.

bromide (bro′mīd) any binary compound of bromine that contains the bromide ion (Br^-); a salt of hydrobromic acid (HBr). Bromides were once widely used as antiepileptics, sedatives, and hypnotics, but have been abandoned because of their low therapeutic index. An overdose may cause serious mental disturbance, as bromides displace chlorides from body fluids and produce central nervous system depression. Serum concentrations above 100 mg/dl are toxic. Alcoholics are more susceptible than most individuals.

bromide assays the gold chloride test. Protein is removed from serum samples by precipitation with trichloroacetic acid and by filtration. Gold trichloride is added. It reacts with bromide to form gold tribromide ($AuBr_3$), which is yellow at bromide concentrations of about 25 mg/dl and red-brown at levels above 50 mg/dl. The sample bromide concentration is proportional to the absorbance at 440 nm and can be determined by photometry.

bromination (bro″mĭ-na′shun) the introduction of bromine into a compound. In histochemistry bromination is used to block the reactivity of many substances, notably tyrosine groups, glycogen, aldehyde, and ethylenes.

bromine (Br) (bro′mēn) [L. *bromium, brominium, bromum,* from Gr. *brōmos* stench] a reddish-brown, nonmetallic, volatile liquid element; atomic number 35; atomic weight 79.909; Group VII of the periodic table (the halogens); oxidation state −1, +1, +5, +7. Bromine gives off suffocating vapors, is highly toxic, and is a severe skin irritant. It is soluble in most common organic solvents.

Bromide (Br^-) replaces chloride (Cl^-) in body tissues, which produces sedation and depression of the central nervous system. Chronic poisoning (brominism) can produce skin rashes, ataxia, and delirium. Although organic and inorganic bromides have been used as sedatives and anticonvulsants, they have a low therapeutic index. Methyl bromide, a fumigant, can produce the symptoms of brominism, as well as pulmonary edema and convulsions.

brominism (bro′min-izm) poisoning by excessive use of bromine or its compounds. This condition occurs when the bromine concentration in the body fluids is high enough to have a toxic and depressant action on the central nervous system. The toxic level varies with each individual, and is also somewhat dependent on chloride intake because the bromide ions and the chloride ions are equally absorbed and distributed throughout the same fluid compartments. This means that a person with a limited salt intake accumulates bromine more quickly, so severe poisoning could occur after ingestion of an amount of bromine that would be relatively harmless for a person with a normal or high salt intake. In the past many cases of brominism resulted from the indiscriminate use of patent medicines containing bromide. Another frequent cause is methyl bromide, a pesticide. The symptoms of bromine poisoning include acne, coldness of arms and legs, fetid breath, sleeplessness, impotence, headache, irritability, emotional instability, malaise, and mental aberrations such as hallucinations, amnesia, and disorientation.

Treatment consists of immediate curtailment of bromine ingestion and elimination of the substance from the body using diuretics; administration of chloride if not contraindicated by cardiac or renal disease; and in severe, acute poisoning, dialysis.

bromism (bro′mizm) see *brominism.*

bromocresol green (BCG) (bro″mo-kre′sol) a pH indicator, tetrabromo-*m*-cresolsulfonphthalein, with a pH range of 3.8 (yellow) to 4.6–4.7 (green) to 5.5 (blue). Like many other indicators, BCG binds to protein anions and is used as an indicator in dye-binding methods for determining serum albumin.

bromocresol purple a pH indicator, dibromorthocresol sulfonphthalein, with a pH range of 5.2 (yellow) to 6.8 (purple).

5-bromodeoxyuridine (BrdU) (bro′mo-de-ok-se-u′rĭ-dēn) a structural analog of thymidine with a bromine atom replacing the methyl group that occupies position 5 in the pyrimidine ring of thymidine. The presence of BrdU in a cell culture medium selectively inhibits the expression of differentiated properties of some types of cells. In addition, there are certain genes that become expressed in the presence of BrdU.

The incorporation of BrdU in DNA causes the mispairing of bases, thus increasing the probability of mutation. BrdU in DNA shifts its maximal absorption of light from 260 nm in the ultraviolet spectrum to longer wavelengths near the violet end of the visible light spectrum. The DNA is then susceptible to radiation damage from ordinary fluorescent light. This property can be used to select for auxotrophic mutants.

See also *cell culture.*

bromoderma (bro″mo-der′mah) [*bromo-* + Gr. *derma* skin] a skin eruption caused by bromides that occurs only after their chronic use for many months.

bromodiphenhydramine hydrochloride (bro″-mo-di″fen-hi′drah-mēn) [USP], a drug with antihistaminic and anticholinergic activity that is used in cough and cold preparations. Side-effects include drowsiness, dizziness, and dryness of the mouth, nose, and throat.

bromomethane (bro″mo-meth′ān) see *methyl bromide.*

bromophenol blue (bro″mo-fe′nol) a pH indicator, tetrabromophenolsulfonphthalein, with a pH range of 3.0 (yellow) to 4.6 (blue).

bromothymol blue (bro″mo-thi′mol) a pH indicator, dibromothymolsulfonphthalein, with a pH range of 6.0 (yellow) to 7.6 (blue).

brompheniramine maleate (brom″fen-ir′ah-mēn) [USP], an antihistamine, the bromine analog of chlorpheniramine. Trademark, Dimetane.

Bromsulphalein (BSP) (brom-sul′fah-lin) trademark. See *sulfobromophthalein sodium.*

bronch/o, bronchi/o (brong′ko, brong′ke-o) [Gr. *bronchos* windpipe] a word element used in combining form to denote a bronchial passage, e.g., bronchitis.

bronchial (brong′ke-al) [L. *bronchialis*] pertaining to one or more bronchi.

bronchial adenoma a term formerly used for bronchial carcinoid.

bronchial carcinoid a term applied to a tumor that arises within the respiratory passages from cells of the diffuse endocrine system, with histology usually similar to that of carcinoid tumors in other locations. Some peripheral lung tumors, however, are composed of spindle-shaped cells, and distinction from a poorly differentiated adenocarcinoma or intermediate variant of small cell undifferentiated (oat cell) carcinoma may be difficult by light microscopy alone. Ultrastructurally, the cells of a bronchial carcinoid contain dense-core granules; the degree of variation in granule caliber among these tumors, coupled with the range of secretory products that can be demonstrated within the tumor cells using immunocytochemical procedures, suggests that some heterogeneity exists among these neoplasms.

Perhaps 5 percent of those with a bronchial carcinoid have clinical manifestations of excess serotonin production (carcinoid syndrome). Most bronchial carcinoids are of a low grade of malignancy, and the majority are small at the time of diagnosis. Extrathoracic metastases are uncommon. The term atypical carcinoid has been applied to carcinoid tumors with more anaplastic features; such tumors appear to be more aggressive. Small clusters of cells similar to those of a carcinoid tumor are referred to as tumorlets.

A bronchial carcinoid should not be equated with small cell undifferentiated (oat cell) carcinoma, as the two differ in their histology, biologic behavior, and response to therapy. Any relationship that may exist between the two neoplasms has not yet been clearly defined.

See also *carcinoid tumor* and *lung tumors.*

bronchial tree the main bronchi and their branches down to the terminal bronchioles.

bronchiectasis (brong″ke-ek′tah-sis) [*bronchi-* + Gr. *ektasis* dilatation] the abnormal, permanent dilation of the bronchi. When caused by bronchial obstruction from factors such as tumor, mucus impaction, or inhalation of foreign bodies, the condition may be reversible if the obstruction is removed. Persons affected by chronic bronchitis, emphysema, and asthma are often found to have localized bronchiectasis, whereas those suffering from cystic fibrosis characteristically have widespread and severe bronchiectasis. Dilation of the airways may produce long, tubelike enlargements (cylindroid bronchiectasis), irregular pockets (saccular bronchiectasis), or fusiform shapes (fusiform bronchiectasis) at the termination of the bronchi.

bronchiol/o (brong-ki′o-lo) [L. *bronchiolus*] a word element used in combining form to denote bronchiole or small bronchus, e.g., bronchiolitis.

bronchiolar (brong′ke-o″lar) pertaining to bronchioles.

bronchiolar carcinoma a type of adenocarcinoma of the lung in which the tumor cells typically spread along the existing connective tissue framework of alveoli, forming glandular and papillary structures. The neoplastic cells are tall and columnar, and they show ultrastructural features of cells of the distal respiratory passages, including the nonciliated bronchiolar (Clara) cell. Also called *alveolar cell carcinoma* and bronchiolo-alveolar cell carcinoma.

bronchiolar cell any of the tall, rounded, nonciliated cells interspersed among the ciliated cells that line the distal bronchioles. These cells protrude into the lumen to the tips of the cilia, contributing to the scalloped appearance of the bronchioles in cross section and form a protein component of surfactant. Also called *Clara cell.*

bronchiole (brong′ke-ōl) [L. *bronchiolus*] one of the finer subdivisions of the respiratory tree (1 mm or less in diameter). It can be distinguished from a bronchus by the absence of cartilage, glands, and continuous smooth muscle, and by the presence of simple columnar epithelium.

respiratory b., a subdivision of a terminal bronchiole that possesses alveolar outpouchings. It gives rise to alveolar ducts, 2–11 in number.

terminal b., the smallest bronchiole, concerned solely with gas conduction.

bronchiolitis (brong″ke-o-li′tis) [*bronchiol-* + *-itis*] an inflammation of the bronchioles, usually due to viral infection. Bronchiolitis most often occurs in young children, with occasional epidemics seen among those younger than 18 mo. The common etiologic agents include respiratory syncytial virus, parainfluenza virus, influenza virus, adenovirus, and *Mycoplasma pneumoniae.* The infectious agent initially causes an upper respiratory tract infection that results in epithelial necrosis, edema, exudate production, and, eventually, obstruction. There is a rapid onset of respiratory distress, tachycardia, hacking cough, cyanosis, wheezing, and, in some cases, fever.

Diagnosis is made by a combination of clinical symptoms, an increased white blood cell count with a high percentage of lymphocytes, and analysis of serum electrolytes and blood gases. Bronchiolitis must be distinguished from asthma. Mortality is less than 1 percent. Recovery usually occurs within 5 da.

bronchiolitis fibrosa obliterans a complication of bronchitis that occurs when the airways are blocked by purulent secretions, with an ingrowth of vascular connective tissue from the wall of terminal bronchi obliterating the airway.

bronchitis (brong-ki′tis) [*bronch-* + *-itis*] inflammation of the tracheobronchial tree.

acute b., an acute inflammation of the respiratory mucosa, primarily centered in the lower trachea and major bronchi. Predisposing factors to an attack are bacterial or viral infections (frequently a common cold), inhalation of irritants, and possibly exposure to cold. These factors may render the respiratory mucosa more susceptible to secondary bacterial infections; the bacterial agents commonly involved are *Staphylococcus aureus, Hemophilus influenzae,* pneumococci, or streptococci. Recurrent bronchitic attacks frequently are a complication of diseases that impair the clearance function of the bronchial epithelium and may indicate the presence of a focus of infection (e.g., hypertrophied tonsils, chronic sinusitis).

The respiratory mucosa affected by acute bronchitis is hyperemic, thickened, and edematous, and its surface becomes covered by a stringy mucus. As the attack worsens, an inflammatory infiltrate begins to accumulate, along with a mucopurulent exudate containing large numbers of leukocytes and bacterial aggregates.

The initial symptoms of an uncomplicated acute bronchitic attack include malaise, sore throat, low-grade fever, chills, and muscle and back pain. There is initially dry cough, which usually becomes progressively more productive. When a bacterial infection is superimposed, the sputum becomes increasingly mucopurulent. If airway obstruction is also present (due to retained secretions and bronchial wall edema), dyspnea may also be noted. The pulmonary signs in acute, uncomplicated bronchitis are generally limited to scattered rales of a varying quality or wheezing. Diagnosis is usually made on the basis of these signs and symptoms, chest radiographs or blood gas analysis are indicated only if the symptoms are intense and persistent, or if an underlying pulmonary disorder is present.

asthmatic b., see under *asthma.*

chronic b., a pathologic condition characterized by a chronic hypersecretion of mucus in the bronchial tree in association with a recurrent productive cough not attributable to a specific disease. Chronic bronchitis refers both to a clinical circumstance in which the symptoms are relatively mild and more readily susceptible to therapeutic management, and to a syndrome of irreversible airway obstruction that, if sufficiently severe, can lead to hypoxemia, hypercapnia, cor pulmonale (right ventricular hypertrophy), and respiratory failure. Chronic bronchitis and pulmonary emphysema (the other major chronic obstructive pulmonary disease) commonly coexist, perhaps in a relationship of mutual predisposition. The most prominent morphologic features associated with chronic bronchitis are the presence of an excess of mucus in the tracheobronchial tree and a marked hypertrophy of the bronchial goblet cells and mucous glands. (Because of this mucous gland hypertrophy, the Reid index in this condition generally exceeds 0.36.)

The major cause of chronic bronchitis is cigarette smoking. The effect of smoking appears to be exacerbated by residence in an urban area; by exposure to cold, moist climatic conditions; or by occupational exposure to mineral organic dusts, chemicals, or noxious gases. In addition, recent evidence suggests that various clinical circumstances (age, obesity, mitral stenosis, left venticular failure, ascites, prolonged recumbency) aggravate any tendency toward a diminished patency of the small airways caused by a prexisting chronic bronchitis.

The patient diagnosed as a chronic bronchitic typically is a male, age 45–65, cigarette smoker, and frequently from a lower economic level. The symptoms that characteristically lead the patient to seek medical advice are a shortness of breath (dypsnea), particularly on exertion, associated with an expiratory wheeze, a productive cough, frequently with hemoptysis, and an increase volume of sputum expectorated that reaches a peak in the early morning.

A definitive diagnosis of chronic bronchitis is based on: (1) elimination of other pathologic conditions possibly contributory to these patient complaints or clinical features, accompanied primarily by (2) a quantitative measurement of the extent of airway obstructions (the FEV_1 is commonly used as measure of the obstruction to expiratory air flow), and (3) an identification of any accompanying imbalance in the ventilation-perfusion ratio (commonly demonstrated by single breath nitrogen exhalation tests). Plain x-ray films of the chest seldom contribute to a definitive diagnosis but may reveal a slight degree of hyperinflation of the lungs, or increased pulmonary marking; these patterns are not characteristic and cannot be attributed to chronic bronchitis alone. Those abnormalities found on bronchographic examination may be considered more characteristic: an abrupt, truncated termination of (obliterated) bronchioles, a slight bronchial dilation on inspiration and collapse on expiration, and an enlargement of the bronchial mucous glands to such an extent that they admit the radiopaque medium.

The FEV_1 in chronic bronchitis commonly is slightly or moderately reduced and exhibits a progressive diminution that is clinically detectable on a yearly basis. The expiratory reserve volume may be reduced, whereas the residual volume is frequently increased. Dynamic compliance may drop markedly as breathing frequency is increased, and recoil pressure and resistance may be elevated. This pattern of clinical features is consistent with a picture of obstruction of the terminal airway units and a concomitant nonuniformity of the $\dot{V}/\dot{Q}$ ratio in these peripheral airways. When the obstruction and $\dot{V}/\dot{Q}$ derangement are severe, the bronchitis may be complicated by a chronic hypoxemia and hypercapnia, and often progresses to chronic cor pulmonale. Other complications of chronic bronchitis that may make it a lethal condition are a superimposed and recurrent bronchopulmonary infection (commonly bronchopneumonia) or the development of emphysema. These complicating conditions can lead to bronchiolitis, bronchiolar and bronchial obliteration, abscess formation, bronchiolectasis, and eventual respiratory and right ventricular failure.

See also *chronic obstructive pulmonary disease.*

bronchocandidiasis (brong″ko-kan″dĭ-di′ah-sis) candidiasis of the respiratory tree, occurring in a mild afebrile form manifested as chronic bronchitis, and in a usually fatal form resembling tuberculosis.

bronchoconstrictor (brong″ko-kon-strik′tor) a stimulus such as a chemical (e.g., acetylcholine, histamine, nicotine, serotonin) or an irritant (cigarette smoke, dust, sulfur dioxide) that directly or reflexly acts to reduce the caliber of the bronchial tree. Bronchoconstrictor drugs are administered clinically to test the reactivity of the airways.

bronchodilator (brong″ko-di-la′tor) a chemical (e.g., epinephrine, isoproterenol) or other agent that acts to widen the diameter of the bronchial lumen. Bronchodilators are administered clinically to test the sensitivity of the airways in diagnosing conditions such as asthma or bronchitis. They are also used to relieve the bronchospasm that occurs in these and other disease conditions that decrease the resistance of the bronchial airways.

bronchoesophagoscopy (brong″ko-ĕ-sof″ah-gos′ko-pe) endoscopic examination of the bronchi and esophagus.

bronchography (brong-kog′rah-fe) [*broncho-* + Gr. *graphein* to write] radiologic examination of the bronchial tree after instillation of a contrast medium, such as propyliodone in oil suspension or iodized oil. It is used in the investigation of chronic pneumonia and bronchitis; bronchial obstruction; pulmonary tumors, cysts, and cavities; hemoptysis; and bronchocutaneous fistulae.

The contrast medium can be introduced by supraglottic or infraglottic instillation, transglottic intratracheal intubation, and percutaneous cricothyroid or percutaneous transtracheal catheterization. During introduction of the medium, the patient is rotated into various positions so that the medium will evenly coat the bronchial passages; they may be done under fluoroscopic control. The patient is premedicated with a sedative, an anticholinergic or adrenergic to reduce bronchial secretions, and a local anesthetic to inhibit the cough reflex.

Cope method, a method of percutaneous transtracheal bronchography. A cannula threaded on a metal needle is inserted through the front of the neck and passed down the trachea, and the needle is withdrawn.

In nonselective bronchography, the contrast medium is instilled at this point. In selective bronchography, the cannula is replaced, using the Seldinger technique, with a catheter that is passed into a particular bronchial segment for aspiration of secretion samples, followed by instillation of the contrast medium.

bronchopathy (brong-kop′ah-the) [*broncho-* + Gr. *pathos* disease] a general term for disease of the bronchi.

bronchopneumonia (brong″ko-nu-mo′ne-ah) [*broncho-* + Gr. *pneumonia* lung disease] an infection of the lungs, usually originating in the bronchioles and characterized by patchy consolidation of lobular tissue. It is caused by bacteria and other microorganisms, especially *Mycoplasma pneumoniae.* Suppurative exudate fills the bronchi, bronchioles, and alveolar spaces. The severity of the disease depends on the virulence of the etiologic agent and the susceptibility of the host, which is greatest in the young and elderly. The distinction between lobar and bronchopneumonia is unclear and of little clinical significance; it is more important to determine the type of pathogen responsible so that appropriate chemotherapy can be selected.

bronchopneumopathy (brong″ko-nu-mop′ah-the) [*broncho-* + Gr. *pneumon* lung + *pathos* disease] any disease involving the bronchi and lungs.

bronchopulmonary (brong″ko-pul′mo-ner″e) [*broncho-* + L. *pulmo, pulmonis* lung] pertaining to the bronchi and lungs.

bronchopulmonary lavage see *bronchopulmonary l.* under *lavage.*

bronchopulmonary segment one of the subdivisions of the lobes of the lungs, partially separated by connective tissue septa. See also *lung.*

bronchoscopy (brong-kos′ko-pe) [*broncho-* + Gr. *skopein* to examine] clinical examination of the lumen of the tracheobronchial tree with a lighted optical instrument, the bronchoscope. This procedure may be used to examine bronchial obstructions suspected from clinical findings, unresolved pneumonia, unexplained hemoptysis, suspected carcinoma, foreign bodies, abscesses, and aspiration pneumonia.

Originally, this procedure employed a rigid, hollow metal tube with an illumination system at the distal end. Rigid-tube bronchoscopy is now preferred only for the retrieval of large biopsy samples and in the management of tracheal stenosis. More recently, fiberoptic bronchoscopes with flexible bidirectional light systems have been used.

Either instrument may be equipped with suction catheters, bronchial brushes, and various types of biopsy and forceps attachments, which facilitate the recovery of washings for bacterial or fungal culture and cytologic examination. Visible lesions may be biopsied directly. Brush biopsies may be recovered from specific lung segments. These biopsies can reveal up to 50 percent of lung neoplasms and may confirm a diagnosis of bronchogenic carcinoma or tuberculosis.

See also *endoscopy.*

fiberoptic b., a clinical technique used to examine the bronchi through the use of a portable, flexible tube containing specialized glass fibers capable of delivering illumination to the interior of the bronchi and returning a magnified image. This instrument may be modified to obtain specimens for microbiologic, cytologic, and pathologic evaluation. It is employed for the same purpose as the rigid bronchoscope, but because of its flexibility and smaller diameter, it is more easily manipulated into upper lobe bronchi and can reach to the subsegmental bronchi level.

Although it is a relatively simple procedure, fiberoptic bronchoscopy still carries attendant risks such as hypoxemia, cardiac stress, hemorrhage, bacteremia, fever, and pneumonia, and thus its use should be evaluated against potential risks. In certain conditions, percutaneous fine-needle aspiration may be more appropriate.

bronchospasm (brong′ko-spazm) a spasmodic contraction of the bronchial smooth muscle that commonly occurs in asthmatics. Bronchospasm may be provoked by inhalation of potential irritants such as allergens, gases, particles, or fumes, or may be the result of bronchial infection (acute viral bronchitis), psychologic stress, mechanical irritation of the airways, or severe exercise. As a consequence of the spasm, the diameter of the airways is reduced, resulting in reduced flow rates during both inspiratory and expiratory efforts, provided the chest wall and diaphragm are performing normally. The bronchospasm that accompanies chronic bronchitis is often referred to as asthmatic bronchitis. See also *asthma.*

bronchospirometry (brong″ko-spi-rom′ĕ-tre) [*broncho-* + L. *spirate* to breath + *metrum* measure] a technique used to evaluate the function of the individual lungs through insertion of a catheter into one (usually the left) main bronchus. Both lungs can also be studied through use of a double-lumen catheter (such as Carlen's catheter). Conventional spirometric techniques, or techniques for measuring the ventilatory rate and gas exchange, may then be employed. See also *spirometry.*

bronchostenosis (brong″ko-stĕ-no′sis) [*broncho-* + Gr. *stenōsis* a narrowing] a stricture or cicatricial diminution of the caliber of a bronchus.

bronchus (brong′kus) [L.; Gr. *bronchos* windpipe] one of the system of tubular air passages that connect the functional portions of the lungs with the upper respiratory tract. The two main bronchi are formed by the bifurcation of the trachea: each extends downward and to the side to enter the hilum of its lung. Because of the asymmetry of the heart, the left bronchus has to travel farther to reach the hilum, and as a result is longer, thinner, and more horizontal than the right main bronchus.

Within the hilum, each main bronchus divides to form secondary bronchi, one for each lobe. Within a lobe, the secondary bronchus continues to undergo dichotomous division; after about 10 subdivisions, the bronchi are roughly 1 mm in diameter and become bronchioles.

The larger bronchi are lined by respiratory (pseudostratified ciliated columnar) epithelium, supported by a loose submucosal connective tissue that contains mucus-forming glands; their walls contain rings of cartilage and layers of smooth muscle.

See also the accompanying illustration.

Brönsted-Lowry acid (bron′sted lou′re) [Johannes Nicolaus *Brönsted,* Danish chemist, 1879–1947; Thomas Martin *Lowry,* English chemist, 1874–1936] a substance that can donate a proton (H^+) to another molecular species. The molecular species accepting

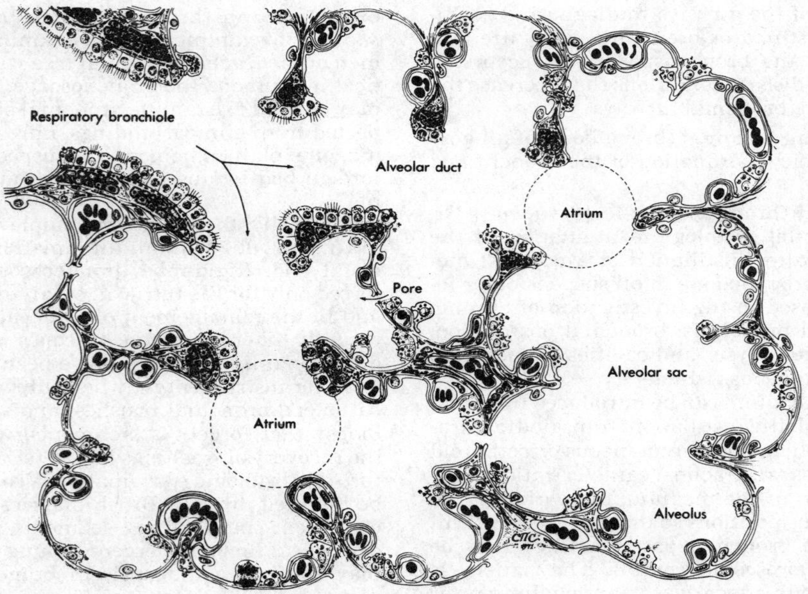

Bronchus. Drawing of the respiratory subdivisions in the lung, showing a respiratory bronchiole, alveolar ducts, and subdivisions. Smooth muscle (dark cells) ends in the alveolar ducts. The atria (circled) are spaces bounded by the termination of the alveolar duct on one end and the openings of the alveolar sacs on the other. In addition, major features of the alveolar walls are presented. (From Weiss, L., and Greep, R.: Histology. 4th ed. New York, McGraw-Hill Book Co., 1977.)

the proton is referred to as a Brönsted-Lowry base. For example, in the reaction $NH_3 + H_2O \rightarrow NH_4^+ + OH^-$, H_2O is the acid and NH_3 is the base; in the reverse reaction, NH_4^+ is the acid and OH^- is the base. See also *acid* and *base.*

Brönsted-Lowry base see under *Brönsted-Lowry acid.*

broth (broth) a liquid culture medium for the cultivation of microorganisms. See also *culture media.*

chopped meat b., a medium used for the cultivation of anaerobic bacteria, especially species of *Clostridium.*

GN (gram-negative) b., an enrichment medium for the primary culture of fecal specimens. It contains sodium deoxycholate and citrate, which retard the growth of some Enterobacteriaceae such as *Escherichia coli* but not that of *Salmonella* and some *Shigella* strains.

Mueller-Hinton b. (MHB), a medium containing beef infusion, used especially to determine the antibiotic sensitivity of bacteria.

nutrient b., a basal medium consisting of beef extract and peptone for the culture of microorganisms.

sodium chloride (6.5 percent) b., a broth medium for the selective identification of enterococci within group D streptococci. Staphylococci and gram-negative bacilli can also grow in this high concentration of NaCl. See also *Streptococcus.*

thioglycollate-135C b., a thioglycollate medium that contains no indicator or yeast extract and is used as a general utility medium for the growth of both aerobic and anaerobic bacteria.

Todd-Hewitt b., a medium that contains beef heart infusion, used for the growth of streptococci and especially for grouping beta-hemolytic streptococci.

trypticase soy with agar b., a medium that contains a small amount of agar, used for the primary culture of fastidious bacteria, including anaerobes.

brow-down position a radiographic position used in pneumonencephalography. The patient is prone, with the forehead and nose resting on the table. Posteroanterior, half-axial posteroanterior (25°–30° cranial angulation of the central ray), and lateral projections are routinely used.

brown atrophy the occurrence in tissues (e.g., in the liver, heart, and spleen) of atrophy and intracellular accumulation of lipofuscin. See also *lipofuscin.*

Brown-Brenn technique (broun bren) a staining method for demonstrating the presence of bacteria in tissue specimens. Sections are stained in basic crystal violet, followed by Gram's iodine. After partial drying, the sections are decolorized with ether-acetone and counterstained with basic fuchsin. The sections are finally differentiated with dilute picric acid in acetone. Gram-positive bacteria appear black; gram-negative bacteria, red; and nuclei and mast cell granules, red on a yellow background.

brown fat see *brown a. t.* under *adipose tissue.*

brownian motion (brou′ne-an) [Robert *Brown,* British botanist, 1773–1858] the random, dancing, zig-zag movements of minute, microscopic particles suspended in a liquid. This motion is due to collisions of the particles with the individual random-moving molecules of the solvent.

brown recluse spider see *L. reclusa* under *Loxosceles.*

Brown-Séquard's syndrome (broun· sa-karz′) [Charles Edouard *Brown-Séquard,* French physiologist 1817–1894] paralysis and loss of vibratory and joint sensation on one side of the body and of pain and temperature sensation on the other, due to a lesion involving one side of the spinal cord.

brown tumor see *osteitis fibrosa cystica.*

brow-up position a radiographic position used in pneumoencephalography. The patient is supine with the orbitomeatal line vertical. Projections used are half-axial anteroposterior (25°–30° caudad or 10° cranial angulation of the central ray), direct anteroposterior, and lateral.

Brucella (broo-sel′ah) [Sir David *Bruce,* English physician, 1855–1931] a genus of nonmotile, nonspore-forming, gram-negative coccobacilli or short rods. They are aerobic and require biotin, niacin, thiamine, and sometimes serum for growth. Brucella organisms are common parasites of cattle, swine, goats, and sheep, tending to localize in placental tissue and mammary glands, and are capable of causing acute or chronic illness. They have a marked ability to multiply within phagocytic cells. Infection spreads to humans through contact with tissue or consumption of unpasteurized milk or cheese. Species identification is difficult. Isolates that produce nonhemolytic colonies on blood agar, and which are oxidase-positive, glucose- and lactose-negative, and agglutinated by *Brucella* antiserum, may be considered a species of *Brucella.* See also *brucellosis.*

B. abortus, the species that is the most common cause of brucellosis (undulant fever) in humans in the United States. It is the causative agent of infectious abortion of cattle, which constitutes the animal reservoir of infection. The species was formerly called *Bang's bacillus* because it was first isolated from cattle in Denmark by Bang in 1897.

B. canis, a species that is pathogenic for dogs and transmissible to humans, in whom it can produce brucellosis.

B. melitensis, a species that is the causative agent of brucellosis (undulant fever) that occurs primarily in goats and sheep. It was first identified in 1904 when it was isolated from the milk and urine of healthy goats.

B. suis, a species, found primarily in swine, that is capable of producing severe disease in humans.

brucella (broo-sel′ah) an individual organism of the genus *Brucella.*

brucella agglutination test an assay for the detection of antibodies to *Brucella* species, used for a presumptive diagnosis of brucellosis. It is an agglutination test that utilizes dilutions of the patient's serum and an antigen prepared from the organism. Titers of 1:160 or higher usually are indicative of acute infection. If the test is negative and brucellosis is still suspected, a test for blocking antibodies should be performed.

The blocking antibody test involves the ability of the patient's serum to block agglutination of the *Brucella* antigen by known, positive serum. The agglutination test can only back up the diagnosis of brucellosis; isolation of the organisms is necessary for confirmation. High titers can occur in healthy individuals repeatedly exposed to *Brucella,* such as slaughterhouse workers. Cross reaction may occur with *Vibrio cholerae, Francisella tularensis,* and *Yersinia enterocolitica.*

brucellin (broo-sel′in) a preparation of soluble antigens from cultures of *Brucella.* Individuals with brucellosis develop hypersensitivity of the delayed type. Development of an edematous area in 6–12 hr is a positive reaction, indicating past exposure.

brucellosis (broo″sel-o′sis) an infection of humans caused by species of *Brucella.* The invariable source is contact with animals or their products. In the United States, it is largely an occupational disease; from 1965 to 1977, 70 percent of cases occurred in workers in the meat-processing and livestock industries. Recently, *B. canis* infections, presumably from contact with infected dogs, have been recognized.

Incubation periods are long—several weeks in duration, with insidious onset of malaise, fever, chills, sweats, fatigue, and headache. The fever is characteristically intermittent (undulant fever). Bacteremia is detected in about 20 percent of cases. Secondary manifestations are protean in nature. Chronic infection is common.

The organisms are not easily cultivated, so that laboratory diagnosis is often based on serologic findings. *Brucella* species are susceptible to the tetracyclines.

Also called *abortus fever, Malta fever, Mediterranean fever,* and *undulant fever.*

Bruch's membrane (brooks) [Karl Wilhelm Ludwig *Bruch,* German anatomist, 1819–1884] a thin layer of loose collagen and elastin fibrils in the choroid of the eye. Its inner surface is the basal lamina of the pigment epithelium, and its outer surface interdigitates with the choriocapillaris.

brucine (broo′sēn) [from *Brucea,* a genus of shrubs named for James *Bruce,* Scottish explorer, 1730–1794] a poisonous alkaloid similar to strychnine, formerly used as a cardiac stimulant.

Brudzinski's sign (bro͞od-zin′skēz) [Jósef *Brudzinski,* Polish physician, 1874–1917] in patients with meningitis, a term that refers either to flexion of both knees and hips in response to forward flexion of the patient's neck, or to the passive flexion of the hip on one side when the knee on the other is extended while that hip is flexed.

Brugia (bro͞og′e-ah, broo′je-ah) [S. L. *Brug,* Dutch parasitologist, 1879–1946] a genus of filarial nematodes, family Onchocercidae, that includes many parasites infecting both humans and domestic animals. Adult worms coil in pairs in the lymphatic glands, tissues, and body cavities; the sheathed "larvae" (microfilariae) used for identification are found in the blood. Adult *Brugia* nematodes are distinguished from *Wuchereria* nematodes by their size (*Brugia* males are smaller: the males are 25 mm by 100 μ; the females, 60 mm by 190 μ) and because they have fewer anal and postanal papillae than do the *Wuchereria.*

B. malayi, the only species of *Brugia* that is parasitic in humans; it causes Malayan filariaris and elephantiasis, usually of the limbs. The organism is transmitted by species of *Mansonia* and *Anopheles* mosquitoes in China, India, Malaysia, and Indonesia, and by *Aedes togoi* in Japan.

The life cycles of *B. malayi* and *Wuchereria bancrofti* are very similar, except that the principal mosquito vectors of *B. malayi* are species of the genus *Mansonia.* The adult forms are delicate white worms, usually found coiled and paired in the dilated lymphatics. The males measure 13–23 mm long; the females, 43–55 mm. The microfilariae are sheathed, averaging 177–230 μm long and 5–6 μm wide. The body nuclei extend almost to the end of the tail, a characteristic that distinguishes *B. malayi* from *W. bancrofti* microfilariae. *B. malayi* microfilariae also possess two terminal nuclei, in addition to those in the tail, which differentiate it from other microfilariae.

Also called Malayan filarial worm.

bruit (broo-e′, bro͞ot) [Fr.] an abnormal sound or murmur heard in auscultation of the cardiovascular system. It is commonly due to obstruction or turbulence in the blood flow.

placental b., a soft, blowing auscultatory sound produced by blood flow in the placenta. Also called placental souffle.

Brunner's glands (brun′erz) [Johann Conrad *Brunner,* Swiss anatomist, 1653–1727] tubuloalveolar glands located in the submucosa of the duodenum. These mucus-producing glands empty into the intestinal crypts, and serve to lubricate and coat the duodenal lining and to reduce the acidity of the gastric contents as they enter the duodenum.

brush border a specialization of the free surface of certain epithelial cells consisting of tiny cylindric processes (microvilli) that greatly increase the surface area; they are noted especially on the cells of the proximal convoluted tubule of the kidney and on the intestinal absorptive epithelium. Also called *striated border.* See also *microvillus.*

brushes in electroencephalography, a pattern of electric activity recorded during sleep from the brain of premature infants with a conceptional age of 32–35 wk. This pattern is characterized by rhythmic activity at 8–20 Hz superimposed on slow-wave activity at 0.8–1.5 Hz. Brushes occur in rolandic and occipital brain areas and disappear in the first few postterm weeks of life. Also called spindlelike fast rhythms.

brush specimens cytologic specimens obtained from the bronchial tree, gastrointestinal tract, or genitourinary tract. The procedure involves guiding a small brush to the lesion using a radiopaque catheter under radioscopic control or a fiberoptic endoscope under visual control.

Bruton's disease (broo′tonz) [Ogden Carr *Bruton,* U.S. pediatrician, born 1908] see *x-linked h.* under *hypogammaglobulinemia.*

BSA abbrev. See *bis-trimethylsilylacetamide, body surface area, bovine serum albumin.*

BSAP [acronym from *b*rief, *s*mall, *a*bundant *p*otentials] a recruitment pattern that consists of overly abundant motor unit potentials with a small amplitude and a short duration. In electromyography, the use of this descriptive term is discouraged; it should be replaced by a more quantitative statement of the specific amplitude, duration, number of phases, and recruitment frequency of the action potentials.

B-5 sodium acetate–sublimate formalin a histologic fixative consisting of formalin, mercuric chloride, and sodium acetate. Fixation is usually complete within 2–24 hr, but the tissue does not become overhard until after several days. Specimens should be stored in a 70 percent alcohol solution.

BSP abbrev. for *Bromsulphalein;* see *sulfobromophthalein sodium.*

BSP excretion test see under *dye excretion tests.*

BSTFA abbrev. See *bis-trimethylsilyltrifluoroacetamide.*

BT abbrev. for bladder tumor, bleeding time, brain tumor.

BTPS conditions of a gas a volume of gas that is at body temperature (usually taken as 37°C) and ambient pressure, and that is saturated with water vapor (usually considered to be at a partial pressure of 47 torr). The gas in the lungs exists under these conditions.

BTU abbrev. See *British thermal unit.*

bubo (bu′bo) [L., from Gr. *boubōn* groin] a tender, enlarged, and inflamed lymph node, especially in the axilla or groin. It may be caused by a variety of infections including plague, syphilis, gonorrhea, lymphogranuloma venereum, and tuberculosis.

bubonic (bu-bon′ik) characterized by or pertaining to buboes.

bubonic plague see *bubonic p.* under *plague.*

bucc/o (buk′o) [L. *bucca* cheek] a word element used in combining form to denote the cheek, e.g., buccal.

buccal (buk′al) pertaining to or directed toward the cheek.

buccal cavity that part of the oral cavity between the teeth and gingiva medially and the cheek laterally.

buccal glands small, mixed salivary glands in the submucosa of the cheek.

buccal region the region of the cheek overlying the buccinator muscle.

buccopharyngeal membrane in the developing embryo, the membrane produced by the fusing of the ectoderm and endoderm at the cephalic end of the primitive gut tube; it covers the opening into the foregut, which later develops into the mouth.

Bucky grid (buk′e) [Gustav P. *Bucky,* German radiologist in America, 1880–1963] see *Bucky-Potter g.* under *grid.*

buclizine hydrochloride (bu′klĭ-zēn) an antihistamine and central nervous system depressant that is used to suppress nausea and vomiting. Adverse reactions include drowsiness, dryness of the mouth, headache, and nervousness.

Budd-Chiari syndrome (bud ke-ar′e) [George *Budd,* London physician, 1808–1882; Hans *Chiari,* Austrian pathologist, 1851–1916] a rare condition that results from obstruction of the major hepatic veins. Initially there is vague right upper quadrant pain, which progresses within weeks or months to ascites, hepatomegaly, and, ultimately, hepatic failure. The condition is often caused by spontaneous thrombosis of the hepatic veins (as in association with polycythemia) or obstruction of the venous system by a neoplasm. A number of cases have been reported in females taking oral contraceptives.

Laboratory studies show markedly elevated aspartate aminotransferase and slightly elevated serum bilirubin. Hepatic scintiscanning shows isotope concentration in the caudate lobe of the liver. Hepatic venography and liver biopsy are also useful to determine the extent of the obstruction and evaluate the possibility of surgical treatment.

budding (bud′ing) 1. a form of cell division in which the parent cell divides unequally, putting out a budlike process that becomes the daughter cell, e.g., the process of multiplication in one-celled fungi or in spores.

2. in some simple metazoans, an asexual reproductive process in which a small part of the parent's body separates to become a new individual.

3. the process by which certain viruses acquire an outer membrane (the viral envelope or coat). The virus codes for certain proteins that are treated like membrane proteins of the host cell and inserted in the plasma membrane. When these coat proteins bind to the nucleoprotein core of the virus to form the virion, a portion of the host-cell membrane is pinched off to form the viral coat.

4. the process by which a new blood vessel arises from a preexisting vessel.

Buerger's disease (berg′erz) [Leo *Buerger,* U.S. physician, 1879–1943] see *thromboangiitis obliterans.*

buffer (buf′er) 1. a chemical system that prevents or minimizes changes in the concentration of some chemical moiety.

2. a system constituted of a solution of a weak acid (proton donor) or weak base (proton acceptor) and one of its salts. Buffers resist changes in the hydrogen ion concentration of the solution by reacting with added acid or base. Those of interest in clinical chemistry are phosphate, acetate, bicarbonate/carbonate, citrate, glycine, acid phthalate, diethylbarbiturate (Veronal), tris (hydroxymethyl) aminomethane (Tris), diethanolamine (DEA), and 2-amino-2-methyl-1-propanol (AMP).

The effective range of a buffer equals the $pK_a \pm$ 1.0 pH unit. The buffer capacity is greatest when the pH equals the pK_a.

The buffer capacity is expressed by the buffer value, which is equal to the amount of acid or base (expressed in millimoles) required to cause a change in pH of one unit. Buffers used in electrophoretic procedures are frequently described in terms of ionic strength, which equals one-half of the sum of the numbers obtained by multiplying the concentration (in moles per liter) of each ion by the square of its ionic charge.

Buffers are important in electrophoretic procedures, in the pH regulation of many chemical tests and procedures (e.g., enzyme activity measurements), and as physiologic buffers in maintaining the pH of body fluids and cellular contents. Buffers accurate to 0.005 pH units are used as primary standards in the standardization of pH meters.

If exposed to air, the pH of a buffer above pH 7.0 gradually decreases due to absorption of CO_2. See also *Henderson-Hasselbalch equation.*

4. in a computer, a storage area that is used to hold input or output data while waiting for an I/O device to finish an operation.

buffer base the total concentration of buffer anions (plasma and red blood cell bicarbonate and phosphate, hemoglobin, plasma proteins) in whole blood, normally equal to 45–50 mEq/l. Because the whole blood buffer base is altered only when the fixed acid concentration of the blood changes, it is used clinically as an index of the degree of metabolic disturbance in the body's acid-base balance. See also *base excess.*

buffer capacity (β) a measure of the capacity of a buffer to resist a pH change when acid or base is added; it is the number of equivalents of strong base (acid) required to cause a unit change in pH in 1 l of a buffer solution. Also called *buffer value* and Van Slyke buffer value.

buffer system the total of all conjugate acid-base pairs that help regulate the pH of any chemical system, and in particular that of the extracellular and intracellular fluids of the body. In order of decreasing capacity, the most important buffer systems of the body are: (1) bicarbonate/carbonic acid in plasma, having a buffer value (β) of about 56.6 mmol/l; (2) hemoglobin in erythrocyte fluid (the imidazole group of histidine residues are proton acceptors), with a β of about 53 mmol/l; (3) plasma protein, with a β of about 7.7 mmol/l; (4) plasma phosphate, $H_2PO_4^-/HPO_4^{2-}$ (with a β of 0.4 mmol/l); and (5) 2,3-diphosphoglycerate in erythrocyte fluid, with a β of about 10 mmol/l. See also *base excess* and *buffer base*.

buffer value see *buffer capacity*.

buffy coat (buf'e) the thin layer of white blood cells formed between the plasma and red cell layers following centrifugation of anticoagulated whole blood.

buffy coat smear a smear made from the buffy coat obtained by centrifugation of anticoagulated, fresh whole blood. It is used in the diagnosis of lupus erythematosus (LE) to identify LE cells; for the identification of abnormal blood cells that occur in very small numbers; and for the detection of protozoans (e.g., *Leishmania donovani*) or fungi (e.g., *Histoplasma capsulatum*) in peripheral blood.

bug (bug) 1. in computer terminology, a program error or a problem in an operation.
2. an insect of the order Hemiptera.

bulb (bulb) [L. *bulbus*, from Gr. *bolbos*] a rounded mass or enlargement.

end b., a spherical expansion of the peripheral termination of a sensory nerve, particularly the tactile corpuscle known as the end bulb of Krause.

olfactory b., the elliptic anterior end of the olfactory nerve, which lies on the cribriform plate of the ethmoid and receives olfactory nerves from the nasal epithelium.

b. of penis, the enlarged posterior continuation of the corpus spongiosum. It lies under and is adherent to the perineal membrane, and is covered by the bulbospongiosus muscle. Also called bulb of urethra.

b. of vestibule, a body consisting of paired, elongated aggregates of erectile tissue in the female. These masses lie under and are adherent to the perineal membrane and lower part of the vagina, and are connected by a commissure of similar tissue.

bulbar (bul'bar) 1. pertaining to a bulb.
2. pertaining to or involving the medulla oblongata.

bulbar palsy see *bulbar p.* under *palsy*.

bulbourethral (bul"bo-u-re'thral) pertaining to the bulb of the penis.

bulbourethral glands small paired glands whose ducts enter the proximal urethra. Also called *Cowper's glands*.

bulbus (bul'bus), pl. *bulbi* [L.] a rounded mass, or enlargement.

bulbus cordis in the developing embryo, the cephalic portion of the primitive heart loop that forms the major part of the right ventricle, together with the outflow tracts of both ventricles and the proximal pulmonary artery and aorta.

bulimia (bu-lim'e-ah) [L., from Gr. *bous* ox + *limos* hunger] insatiable hunger; an eating disorder that occurs most often in adolescent or young adult females, in which there is a pattern of eating binges interspersed with periods of normal eating or rigid dieting. The binges may be accompanied by induced vomiting and followed by periods of depression and self-criticism.

Bulimus (bu-li'mus) a genus of small freshwater snails that contains first intermediate hosts for the human liver flukes in the genera *Clonorchis* and *Opisthorchis*. The genera *Alocinma, Bulinus,* and *Parafossarulus* are sometimes classified as subgenera of *Bulimus*.

Bulinus (bu-li'nus) a genus of freshwater snails, found in North Africa and Asia Minor, that contains several species serving as intermediate hosts for the human blood fluke *Schistosoma hematobium*.

bulla (bul'ah), pl. *bullae* [L.] a large blister or cutaneous vesicle.

Bullis fever (bul'is) [after Camp *Bullis*, Texas, where soldiers suffered attacks of the disease in 1942] a febrile disease characterized by neutropenia and persistent lymphadenitis that is spread by the bite of *Amblyomma americanum*, the Lone Star tick; the causative organism is *Rickettsia rickettsii* or a closely related species. See also *Rickettsiaceae*.

BUN abbrev. for blood urea nitrogen. See *urea nitrogen*.

bundle bone (bun'd'l) a type of bone in the alveolar processes of the maxilla and mandible, so called because the fibers of the periodontal membrane continue into it.

bundle branch block failure of the right, left, or major divisions of the left bundle to conduct a wave of depolarization along its pathway to activate the ventricular muscles. A true block can be demonstrated on an electrocardiogram when: (1) a P wave precedes the QRS complexes with an interval of at least 0.12 sec to indicate conduction above the division of the bundle branches; (2) the QRS wave is longer than 0.11 sec; and (3) the Q wave is absent with a wide R wave in leads I, V_5 and V_6 for a left branch block, and the R wave is tall and late in V_1 for a right branch block.

left b. b. b., an obstruction of the wave of depolarization in the left bundle branch, which alters the characteristics of activation of the left ventricle. The sequence of activation is affected from its onset: the QRS complex is greatly prolonged, with the R wave often absent in right precordial leads and the Q wave absent in leads X, I, V_5, and V_6. Left bundle branch block is almost always an abnormal condition, and is often associated with calcific aortic valve disease or with disease or infarction involving the left ventricle.

right b. b. b., interruption of transmission in the right bundle branch, which affects both the time and manner of activation in the right ventricle. Excitation of this chamber occurs through its anterior and inferior attachments to the interventricular septum, resulting in late asynchronous activation. Graphically, this produces an increased duration of the QRS complex, distortion and delay of the R wave in lead V_1 and broadening of the S wave in I, V_5 and V_6, and slowing of the late rightward loop on vectorcardiogram. Repolarization of the ventricle is often affected, indicated by a distortion of the T wave. Right bundle branch block may be asymptomatic and is often associated with hypertrophy of the right ventricle.

bundle of His see *atrioventricular bundle.*

Büngner's bands (bing′nerz) [Otto von *Büngner,* German neurologist, 1858–1905] dense, round cords of proliferating Schwann cells that remain following degeneration of a peripheral axon. If regeneration occurs, the cells envelop the sprouting axons. If regeneration does not take place, the bands are replaced by connective tissue.

Bunsen burner (bun′sen) [Robert Wilhelm Eberhard von *Bunsen,* German chemist, 1811–1899] a gas burner often used in laboratories, in which the gas is mixed with air before ignition to give complete oxidation.

Bunsen coefficient [R. W. E. von *Bunsen*] the number of milliliters of gas (STP) dissolved in a milliliter of liquid at atmospheric (760 mmHg) pressure and at a specified temperature. Also called *solubility coefficient.*

Bunyaviridae (bun″yah-vēr′ĭ-de) [from *Bunyawera,* Africa] a large, antigenically related group of viruses that are carried by arthropods. They are large (90–100 nm), enveloped, spherical viruses containing single-stranded RNA, which develop in the cytoplasm and mature by budding through cytoplasmic membrane systems such as the Golgi apparatus. Most are carried by mosquitoes but some are tickborne. Members of this family produce a number of diseases of humans and domestic animals, including Rift Valley fever and California encephalitis.

bunyavirus (bun′ya-vi″rus) a member of the Bunyaviridae.

buoyant density (boi′ent) the density at which a macromolecule reaches an equilibrium during high-speed centrifugation when suspended in a medium containing a density gradient. Cesium chloride and sucrose have been used to establish flotation media with such a density gradient.

bupivacaine hydrochloride (bu-piv′ah-kān) [USP], a local anesthetic similar to mepivacaine and lidocaine but having a longer duration of action (4–10 hr). It is used to induce several types of conduction anesthesia: peripheral nerve, sympathetic, caudal, and epidural blocks. Trademark, Marcaine.

Bureau of Narcotics and Dangerous Drugs (BNDD) formerly, a division of the U.S. Department of Justice that regulated and controlled the distribution of narcotics and drugs on the Controlled Drug List. This responsibility now rests with the Drug Enforcement Agency (DEA) in the Justice Department.

Bureau of Radiologic Health a division of the U.S. Department of Health and Human Services concerned with the regulation of radiation from consumer products, and the radiation produced in therapeutics, industrial research, and electronic products. Other related aspects of radiologic health are now under the auspices of the Environmental Protection Agency.

buret (bu-ret′) [Fr.] a common item of laboratory volumetric glassware. It consists of a glass tube marked off in graduated intervals and with a glass or Teflon stopcock at the bottom. Burets are used to measure an amount of liquid, as in titration. Capacities range from 1 ml to several hundred, with intervals of 0.05–0.1 ml. Burets holding 10 ml or less are called *microburets.*

burette (bu-ret′) see *buret.*

Burkitt's lymphoma a form of malignant lymphoma, falling within the category of undifferentiated lymphomas and composed of a proliferation of small, noncleaved cells. Most are B-cell neoplasms. It is endemic in areas of equatorial Africa where most of the patients are children with jaw lesions. It occurs sporadically in other parts of the world, including the United States, where abdominal involvement is the commonest presentation. An association with the Epstein-Barr virus has been demonstrated. Many cases respond to chemotherapy. See also *Epstein-Barr virus* and *malignant l.* under *lymphoma.*

burn (bern) tissue injury caused by heat, electricity, or corrosive chemicals. Burns have been traditionally classified into three categories: (1) first degree, when the damage is limited to the outer layer of the epidermis; (2) second degree, when the damage extends through the epidermis to the dermis but rapid regeneration of the epithelium is possible; and (3) third degree, when both the epidermis and dermis are destroyed, and the wound is considered an open one from which fluid and plasma proteins may be lost. In a newer terminology, burns are categorized as partial thickness (encompassing first- and second-degree burns) or full thickness (third-degree burns).

The affected area shows cell damage caused by increased cellular metabolism, the inactivation of temperature-dependent enzymes, and vascular injury. The area becomes reddened as the capillaries dilate, and increased capillary permeability and the formation of serous or protein-rich exudates follow, and may blister on the skin surface. Tissue necrosis may ensue. Severe insults may cause outright necrosis and coagulation of the vessels, and show little evidence of exudation.

In persons with major burns covering more than 25 percent of the body surface, systemic reactions are more significant than local tissue injury. The most important of these is the potential for the development of shock due to the loss of fluid, protein, and red cells from the intravascular compartment because of exudate from the burn surface. Balanced electrolyte solutions and albumin are administered as necessary to correct fluid volume deficit. The most frequent cause of death in seriously burned individuals is burn sepsis. In the past, staphylococci and streptococci were the infectious agents most frequently isolated. Recently, gram-negative organisms, such as *Pseudomonas aeruginosa* and *Proteus* species, *Providencia stuartii,* and *Enterobacter cloacae,* have been involved in epidemics of burn sepsis.

burner (ber′ner) a device for burning or vaporizing something, or the part of a lamp, stove, or furnace from which the flame issues. See also names of specific burners, e.g., *Bunsen burner.*

burn-in the operation of an electronic component or device before it is placed in service, in order to allow its operating characteristics to stabilize and any defects to be discovered.

burr cell (bur) see *echinocyte.*

burs/o (ber′so) [L., from Gr. "a wine skin"] a word element used in combining form to denote a bursa, e.g., bursitis.

bursa (ber′sah) [L., from Gr. "a wine skin"] a sac or saclike cavity filled with fluid, situated in tissues where friction would otherwise develop, such as over a joint or bony prominence.

b. of Fabricius, an appendix-like outgrowth of the avian cloaca (hindgut) that has been found to be the site of production or preconditioning of B lymphocytes in birds; the central lymphoid organ for the avian B-cell immune system. As yet, no equivalent structure has been found in humans. Removal of the bursa by hormonal or microsurgical techniques prior to hatching renders the bird profoundly hypogammaglobulinemic in later life.

omental b., see *lesser sac of p.* under *peritoneum.*

"bursa-equivalent" tissue a hypothetical site of extramedullary differentiation of B lymphocytes in mammals equivalent to the bursa of Fabricius in birds; as yet no such structure has been identified and its existence is questionable. See also *B l.* under *lymphocyte.*

bursitis (ber-si′tis) [*burs-* + *itis*] inflammation of a bursa. It is most commonly seen in the subdeltoid, trochanteric, olecranon, and prepatellar bursae. There is inflammation, pain, and a restriction of motion in the affected area. Bursitis may become chronic, leading to calcification and fibrosis.

Diagnosis is based on clinical examination, radiography and examination of fluid aspirated from the affected area.

burst (berst) in electroencephalography, any pattern of electric activity, of abrupt onset and termination, that differs from background activity in amplitude, frequency, and/or configuration. Cf. *paroxysm.*

burst-suppression see *suppression-burst activity.*

busulfan (bu-sul′fan) [USP], tetramethylene dimethanesulfonate, a white crystalline powder, which is slightly soluble in water and alcohol. It is used as a cancer chemotherapeutic drug; trademark, Myleran. For more information, see *Appendix A.*

busulfan lung a reactive process in the lungs that occurs as a complication of prolonged busulfan treatment. It begins with hyperplasia of type II of alveolar epithelial cells and leads to interstitial and alveolar fibrosis. The most prominent clinical features are dyspnea, particularly on exertion, and a diffuse mottling on the chest x-ray. A reduction in vital and total lung capacities may also be present. Steroid therapy may partially relieve the symptoms.

butabarbital (bu″tah-bar′bĭ-tal) [USP], an intermediate-acting barbiturate used in sedative preparations. See also *barbiturate.*

butalbital (bu-tal′bĭ-tal) [USP], a barbiturate used in sedative preparations. See also *barbiturate.*

butane (bu′tān) *n*-butane; a straight-chain 4-carbon alkane, C_4H_{10}. It is a colorless, flammable, stable gas derived from petroleum, and it has a characteristic odor. It is often used as fuel for laboratory burners.

butanoic acid (bu″tah-no′ik) see *butyric acid.*

butanol (bu′tah-nol) see *butyl alcohol.*

butanol-extractable iodine (BEI) an obsolete procedure originally used for the quantitation of thyroid hormones in serum and involving butanol extraction to remove most of the nonthyroidal iodine. The procedure has been replaced by more specific and sensitive tests; see *thyroxine assays.*

butanone (bu′tah-nōn) see *methyl ethyl ketone.*

butaperazine (bu″tah-per′ah-zēn) a piperazine-type phenothiazine major tranquilizer used in the management of psychotic disorders. See also *phenothiazine tranquilizers.*

butorphanol tartrate (bu-tōr′fah-nōl) a synthetic narcotic agonist-antagonist used to treat severe pain. The analgesic effect is similar to that of morphine; it also causes respiratory depression. Adverse reactions include sedation, nausea, headache, vertigo, and the production of withdrawal effects when it is given to narcotic addicts. Overdose effects can be reversed by naloxone.

butt (but) the bottom and thickest part of an agar or gelatin slope for the culture of bacteria. A stab inoculation of this portion produces a microaerophilic or anaerobic culture medium.

buttock (but′ok) one of the two gluteal prominences on the posterior aspect of the lower trunk.

butyl- (bu′til) 1. a prefix word element in organic chemistry to denote the C_4H_9 group. Used in this way, the term can mean the *n*-butyl, the *iso*-butyl, the *sec*-butyl, or the *tert*-butyl group.

2. in current IUPAC usage, a prefix word element in organic chemistry to denote the $CH_3CH_2CH_2$-CH_2— group (referred to as the *n*-butyl group in earlier usage).

***iso*-butyl** a prefix word element in organic chemistry to denote the 2-methylpropyl group, —CH_2CH-$(CH_3)_2$, e.g., *iso*-butyl alcohol.

***sec*-butyl-** a prefix word element in organic chemistry to denote the 1-methylpropyl group, —CH-$(CH_3)CH_2CH_3$, e.g., *sec*-butylamine, *sec*-butyl alcohol.

***t*-butyl-** see *tert-butyl-.*

***tert*-butyl-** a prefix word element in organic chemistry to denote the 1,1-dimethylethyl group, —C-$(CH_3)_3$, e.g., *tert*-butylamine *tert*-butyl alcohol. Also called *t-butyl-.*

butyl alcohol any of four isomers: *n*-butyl alcohol (1-butanol, $CH_3(CH_2)_3OH$), *sec*-butyl alcohol (2-butanol, $CH_3CH_2CH(OH)CH_3$), *iso*-butyl alcohol (2-methyl-1-propanol), or *tert*-butyl alcohol (2-methyl-2-propanol, $(CH_3)_3COH$); M.W. 74.12. All are flammable liquids (*tert*-butyl alcohol melts at 25.6°C) used as industrial solvents and in the preparation of chemical intermediates. Their vapors may be irritating to the eyes, skin, and respiratory tract.

butyl methacrylate $H_2CC(CH_3)COO_4H_9$, a colorless liquid; polymers of this compound are used for tissue embedding.

butyric acid (bu-tir′ik) a saturated, weakly ionized, 4-carbon, monocarboxylic fatty acid, *n*-butyric acid, $CH_3CH_2CH_2COOH$; an oily liquid with a rancid odor. It is found in butter (especially when rancid); in sweat, feces, and urine; and in trace amounts in the blood and tissues. Also called *butanoic acid.*

butyrophenone tranquilizers (bu″tĭ-ro-fe′nōn) a group of major tranquilizers that are derivatives of butyrophenone (1-phenyl-1-butanone). See also *droperidol* and *haloperidol.*

***b* wave** see under *electroretinogram.*

bypass (bi′pas) an auxiliary flow; a shunt.

bypass capacitor a capacitor connected in parallel with a circuit element. It provides a low-impedance path around the element for high-frequency signals or noise.

byssinosis (bis″ĭ-no′sis) [Gr. *byssos* flax + *-osis*] an occupational asthmatic condition caused by the inhalation of organic dusts such as cotton, flax, or hemp dust, with bronchoconstriction secondary to pharmacologically active, histamine-releasing substances. There is a tightness of the chest, shortness of breath, wheezing, and coughing. It may be diagnosed by immunologic tests (e.g., skin tests) using the suspect antigen, and by examination of the sputum for the inhaled dust; in polarized light, the crystals are brightly shining, rectangular, and prism-shaped. Characteristically, symptoms often are not apparent until after the individual has left work, or they worsen on the first day back at work following a weekend or holiday. Also called cotton dust asthma, cotton mill fever, and Monday fever. See also *pneumoconiosis.*

byte (bīt) a group of eight binary bits (of information). Word and byte are sometimes used interchangeably: in a computer that processes 16 bits of information as its fundamental unit, a word would be composed of 2 bytes. The byte is a useful designation for indicating memory or storage capacity, as an eight-bit byte can represent either a decimal digit or an alphanumeric character in the ASCII code.

C

C symbol for *capacitance, carbon, Celsius* (*centigrade*) *temperature scale, complement, compliance, coulomb, cysteine, cytidine, heat capacity* (see under *heat*).

C-1, C-2 abbrev. for first, second cervical vertebrae.

C1, C2–C9 the nine discrete protein components or precursor molecules of the complement system; see under *complement.*

C1 esterase inhibitor an inhibitor of the complement system that blocks $C1_S$ (a subunit of the first protein to react in the complement system), and blocks the precursor form of kallikrein, the action of plasmin, and the activation of Hageman factor. Individuals who lack the C1 esterase inhibitor suffer from angioedema of the larynx. See also *alpha*$_2$*-antiplasmin, alpha*$_1$*-antitrypsin, alpha*$_2$*-macroglobulin,* and *a. III* under *antithrombin.* Cf. *complement pathway.*

C1q radioassay a method for detecting serum immune complexes involving the interaction of C1q, a protein of the complement system, and aggregated IgG. There are two types: (1) the C1q-binding test, in which the sample to be assayed is incubated with soluble radiolabeled C1q (the C1q that is bound to immune complexes is precipitated with polyethylene glycol and the precipitate is measured for radioactivity); and (2) the C1q deviation test, in which the remaining free C1q (unbound) is attached to sensitized red blood cells and the radioactivity of the red blood cells is measured.

C3b a product that results when complement component C3 breaks down upon storage. It can cause falsely elevated values of C3 in radial immunodiffusion tests because it reacts with antiserum to C3, but it diffuses more rapidly than C3 because of its lower molecular weight. Formerly called *beta*$_{1A}$*-globulin.*

c 1. symbol for *centi-,* molar concentration, *specific heat capacity* (see under *heat*), the velocity of light. 2. abbrev. for *cum* (with).

CA symbol for *cancer, cathode.*

Ca symbol for the chemical element *calcium.*

Cabot ring (kab'ot) [Richard Clarke *Cabot,* Boston physician, 1868–1939] a threadlike filament in the shape of a single or double ring, which is present in red blood cells in individuals with severe anemia. It represents a remnant of the mitotic spindle, and stains bright red or purple with Wright stain.

cacao oil (kah-ka'o) see *theobroma oil.*

cachectic anergy the transient, lessened reactivity to allergens that occurs as a result of debilitation in a sensitized individual. Also called absolute anergy and negative anergy.

cache memory (kash) a small, high-speed memory used for the temporary storage of data in a digital computer. It differs from a scratch-pad memory in that it has a larger capacity.

cachexia (kah-kek'se-ah) [Gr. *kachexia* bad condition of the body] a symptom complex consisting of progressive weakness, loss of appetite, anemia, and malnutrition, which can accompany any chronic disorder that causes a negative nutritional balance.

cacodylic acid (kak"o-dil'ik) a weak acid, hydroxydimethyl arsine oxide, $(CH_3)_2AsOOH$; M.W. 137.99. Cacodylic acid is highly toxic and is used as a herbicide. It has a pK_a of 6.2; cacodylic acid/cacodylate solution is used as a buffer in the pH range 5.0–7.4, particularly as a pH 7.4 buffer for glutaraldehyde fixation for electron microscopy.

cactinomycin (kak"tin-o-mi'sin) see *a. C* under *actinomycin.*

CAD abbrev. for coronary artery disease.

cadaver (kah-dav'er) [L., from *cadere,* to fall, to perish] a dead body; the term is generally used to refer to a human body preserved for anatomic study.

cadaverine (kah-dav'er-in) [L. *cadaver* corpse] $NH_3^+(CH_2)_5(NH_3)^+$, a polyamine formed by decarboxylation of lysine during the bacterial fermentation of protein. It has an unpleasant odor. See also *polyamine.*

cadmium (Cd) (kad'me-um) [Gr. *kadmeia* calamine a zinc ore in which cadmium is found] a silvery-white, soft metallic element; atomic number 48; atomic weight 112.40; a 4d transition element; oxidation state +2. The metal is obtained from zinc ores and is used in the manufacture of alloys, in storage batteries, and in electroplating. Industrial exposure to dust or fumes, or ingestion of cadmium-contaminated water or food stored in cadmium-plated containers, may result in severe poisoning. Acute manifestations include irritation of the respiratory tract, vertigo, headache, dyspnea, intestinal symptoms, and sometimes fatal pulmonary edema. Chronic exposure produces renal and hepatic disorders, pulmonary fibrosis, emphysema, anemia, skeletal deformities such as softening of the bones, and yellowing of the teeth.

cadmium assays colorimetric, spectrometric, or electrochemical methods for determination of cadmium in biologic specimens after digestion, using oxidizing acids and heat. Most commonly, atomic absorption spectrophotometry or anodic stripping voltammetry are used. Flameless atomic absorption spectrophotometry (graphite furnace) presently appears the best procedure for quantitative measurement of cadmium in blood or urine.

cadmium telluride detector a cadmium telluride semiconductor gamma-ray radiation detector. See under *solid-state radiation detector.*

CAE abbrev. for cellulose acetate electrophoresis; see under *electrophoresis.*

café au lait spot (kah'fa o la) a pigmented macule of a distinctive light-brown color, seen on the skin of individuals with neurofibromatosis and Albright's syndrome.

caffeine (kah-fēn') [Ger. *Kaffein,* from *Kaffee* coffee] 1,3,7-Trimethylxanthine; an odorless, bitter, white powder soluble in water, alcohol, and chloroform. Caffeine is extracted from coffee beans, tea leaves, and kola nuts, and is used as a central nervous system stimulant. It is also a purine analog that is mutagenically active in microbial systems and can inhibit the activity of the enzyme DNA polymerase. Mild cerebral symptoms such as insomnia, anxiety, headache, tremor, and nausea are sometimes produced; the ingestion of an excessive dose may cause focal or generalized convulsions. Also called methyltheobromine and thein.

caffeine assays assays for caffeine in biologic materials. Caffeine may be tested for in an acid ether extract from a variety of specimens by microscopic or colorimetric tests. In biological material, it is commonly measured by ultraviolet spectrophotometry, gas chromatography, or high performance liquid chromatography after extraction with organic solvents. Due to its widespread occurrence in food and beverages, it frequently interferes in many drug assays, particularly in the assay for the asthmatic drug, theophylline, which is chemically similar to caffeine.

CAH abbrev. for chronic active hepatitis. See under *hepatitis.*

CAHEA abbrev. See *Committee on Allied Health Education and Accreditation.*

caisson disease (ka'son) [from the pressurized watertight compartment used in underwater construction] see *decompression sickness.*

Cajal's formol ammonium bromide solution (ka-halz') [Santiago Ramón y *Cajal,* Spanish histologist, 1852–1934] a fixative solution containing ammonium bromide and formalin, used to fix nervous tissue for the demonstration of astrocytes by gold sublimate or silver impregnation methods.

Cajal's gold-sublimate method a classic histologic technique for astrocytes. Following fixation of nervous tissue in formalin ammonium bromide, 15–30-μm frozen sections are cut. These are placed in freshly prepared gold sublimate solution (a 1:1 mixture of 1 percent gold chloride and 5 percent mercuric chloride). Proper impregnation is determined microscopically; astrocytes are dark purple against a light background. The sections are then rinsed and fixed in sodium thiosulfate solution. Astrocytes stain black, nerve cells are pale red, nerve fibers are unstained, and the background is light brown.

Cajal's uranium silver method a histologic staining procedure used to demonstrate the Golgi complex in tissues. Tissue is fixed in a solution of formalin and uranyl nitrate, washed in distilled water, and impregnated with silver nitrate. Silver is reduced in a hydroquinone, formalin, and sodium sulfite solution, and the sections are washed and embedded. In mounted sections, the Golgi complex appears black. This is an experimental technique recommended for use on tissue from young animals.

Cal abbrev. for the obsolete unit *Calorie,* replaced by the *kilocalorie* (kcal).

cal abbrev. See *calorie.*

calamine (kal'ah-mīn) [USP], a pink, odorless, powdered form of zinc oxide, containing 0.5 percent ferric oxide, used in a lotion or paste as a topical protectant and astringent.

calcane/o (kal-ka'ne-o) a word element used in combining form to denote the calcaneus (heel bone), e.g., calcaneitis.

calcaneus (kal-ka'ne-us) [L., from *calx* heel] the largest of the tarsal bones that forms the prominence of the heel. It has three articular facets for the talus, which lies above it, and an anterior facet for the cuboid. The surface that supports the talus is expanded by a projecting shelf, the sustentaculum tali.

calcemia (kal-se'me-ah) [*calcium* + Gr. *haima* blood + *-ia*] excessive calcium in the blood; see *hypercalcemia.*

calci/o (kal'se-o) a word element used in combining form to denote calcium, e.g., calcification.

calcicosis (kal"sĭ-ko'sis) [L. *calx* lime + *-osis* condition] a pneumoconiosis due to the inhalation of marble dust.

calciferol (kal-sif'er-ol) see *vitamin D.*

calcific (kal-sif'ik) forming or depositing calcium salts. See also *calcific d.* under *density.*

calcific aortic stenosis a narrowing of the orifice of the aortic valve by the deposition of calcium in previously damaged valve leaflets.

calcification (kal"sĭ-fĭ-ka'shun) [*calci-* + L. *facere* to make] the deposition of calcium salts, mostly calcium phosphates, as needle-shaped hydroxyapatite crystals in body tissues. This occurs normally in growing bones and teeth, and may be seen in aging cartilage. In teeth, the crystals are larger hexagonal plates, and ameloblasts aid in their deposition.

dystrophic c., the accumulation of calcium salts in diseased tissues, as in chronic tuberculosis, damaged heart valves, or atherosclerotic plaques.

metastatic c., the pathologic calcification of normal tissue, e.g., alveoli, renal tubules, arterial walls, and other tissues, as may occur in hyperparathyroidism, certain tumors, leukemia, or Addison's disease.

calcific concretions round, dark-staining aggregations observed in the cytologic examination of the sputum of individuals having chronic pulmonary diseases, such as tuberculosis. Similar concretions develop in prostatic glandular hyperplasia and may be observed in urine sediments.

calcinosis (kal"sĭ-no'sis) the abnormal deposition of calcium salts as nodules in muscles, tendons, and beneath the skin. The condition may be due to hypercalcemia or result for a local disturbance following infection, or it may be secondary to scleroderma or dermatomyositis. The deposits stain a deep blue with hematoxylin and eosin, and black with von Kossa's stain.

calcipenia (kal"sĭ-pe'ne-ah) [*calci-* + Gr. *penia* poverty, need] a deficiency of calcium in the body; see *hypocalcemia.*

calcite (kal'sīt) a mineral, the hexagonal-rhombohedral crystal form of calcium carbonate, $CaCO_3$. It is a uniaxial crystal with doubly refracting properties. Also called Iceland spar. See also *birefringence* and *Nicol prism.*

calcitonin (kal"sĭ-to'nin) a polypeptide hormone consisting of a single chain of 32 amino acids, produced by the parafollicular (C) cells of the thyroid gland. Calcitonin lowers the concentrations of calcium and phosphate in plasma, inhibits bone resorption, and is an antagonist to parathyroid hormone; it also produces histologic changes in the osteoclast including the disappearance of the ruffled border, membrane changes, and the separation of the osteoclast from the bone surface. Formerly called thyrocalcitonin. See also *thyroid tumors.*

calcium (Ca) (kal'se-um) [L. *calx* lime] a silvery-white, moderately soft metal; atomic number 20; atomic weight 40.08; Group II of the periodic table (the alkaline earths); oxidation state +2. Calcium is found in all body tissues. About 99 percent of body calcium occurs in the bones and teeth, in which calcium salts, primarily hydroxyapatite, are an essential component supplying structural strength. The calcium ion (Ca^{2+}) is found in the extracellular fluid (ECF) at a concentration of approximately 2.5 mmol/l (5 mEq/l). It is required for all reactions in blood coagulation except contact initiation, and is referred to as coagulation Factor IV. Ca^{2+} is excluded from the interior of all cells (concentrations of 10–100 nmol/l) by an ATP-driven active transport mechanism, which pumps in Mg^{2+}. Ca^{2+} plays an important role in muscle contraction: it is pumped from the sarcoplasm into the lumen of the sarcoplasmic reticulum (SR), where it is bound by the protein calsequestrin. Release of acetylcholine at the myoneural junction causes the propagation of an action potential along the sarcolemma and T tubules, followed by release of Ca^{2+} from the SR into the sarcoplasm. Binding of Ca^{2+} causes a conformational change in troponin, which is the immediate trigger of muscle contraction. Calcium also acts as an intracellular second messenger for hormones, a function mediated by the protein calmodulin.

The ECF Ca^{2+} concentration is controlled by a negative feedback mechanism involving parathyroid hormone (PTH), calcitonin, and vitamin D. PTH increases the rate of reabsorption of Ca^{2+} from the tubular fluid in the kidneys and of resorption of Ca^{2+} from bone. PTH also causes an increase in the conversion of 25-OH-D_3 to 1,25-OH-D_3 (the most active form of vitamin D) in the kidneys, which acts to increase the absorption of Ca^{2+} in the intestine. Calcitonin is a physiologic antagonist of PTH that causes a decrease in the resorption of Ca^{2+} from bone, primarily by decreasing osteoclast activity and preventing osteoclast formation.

In serum, calcium may be present either as nondiffusible protein-bound calcium or as diffusible calcium. The diffusible form may be either complexed or ionized (the physiologically active form). Most of the nondiffusible form is bound to protein, but binding activity changes with some disease states and pH changes.

Tentative reference ranges are: for serum total calcium, 2.12–2.60 mmol/l (8.5–10.4 mg/dl); and for serum-ionized Ca^{2+}, 1.15–1.42 mmol/l (4.5–5.7 mg/dl). The degree of ionization is dependent on serum pH. The urine calcium output on average calcium intake is 2.0–7.5 mmol/da (80–300 mg/da).

calcium-45 (^{45}Ca, Ca-45) a reactor-produced radionuclide that decays by beta emission with a half-life of 163 da. It has been used as a tracer of calcium metabolism.

calcium acetate formalin formaldehyde-based histologic fixation fluid that contains calcium acetate; it improves the preservation of phospholipids and provides a buffering effect.

calcium assays determination of the calcium concentration in specimens of serum, urine, stool, or bone. Blood specimens must be serum or heparinized plasma; blood collected with EDTA or oxalate is unsuitable for analysis (see the two methods described below). A screening test for calcium in urine is the Sulkowitch test, in which oxalate buffered with acetate (Sulkowitch reagent) is added to the specimen. The degree of the turbidity is a semiquantitative measure of the amount of calcium present in the sample. Quantitative determination of calcium in urine may be performed by atomic absorption spectrophotometry (AAS) or one of the colorimetric methods described under *total c. a.* Stool specimens are ashed in a muffle furnace, the residue is dissolved in acid, and the calcium concentration is measured by AAS. Bone specimens may be assayed by x-ray fluorescence spectroscopy.

ionized c. a., methods for determining the concentration (or activity) of calcium not complexed to plasma proteins or other complexing agents. The most commonly used methods use ion-selective electrodes. Alternately, the calcium concentration in a serum ultrafiltrate or gel (molecular sieve) eluate may be determined by one of the methods for determining total calcium, which is a measure of the ultrafiltrable calcium.

total c. a., 1. titration methods. Calcium is precipitated with oxalate and determined by redox titration with permanganate (MnO_4^{2-}) or cesium (II). Alternately, complexometric titration with EDTA may be performed, using a fluorescent end-point indicator such as calcein, murexide, Cal-Red, or Eriochrome Black T. These methods are now obsolete.

2. colorimetric methods. A colored product is formed by using a dye, such as *o*-cresolphthalein complexone, calcein plasmo-corinth B, or glyoxal-bis-(2-hydroxyanil)-GBHA, and quantitated by colorimetry. These methods are used by most automated analyzers. Alternately, calcium may be precipitated with chloranilic acid and the precipitate centrifuged and washed. The purple chloranilic acid is released by adding EDTA and the color is measured spectrophotometrically.

3. atomic absorption spectrophotometry (AAS). Lanthanum or strontium chloride is added to the diluted specimen to bind interfering phosphate ions. Absorption at 422.7 nm is a measure of calcium concentration. The assay may be performed with or without previous protein precipitation. The method is highly accurate and is the recommended reference procedure.

calcium carbonate a colorless crystalline powder, $CaCO_3$; M.W. 100.09. It is used medicinally as a gastric antacid and as a dietary calcium supplement.

calcium deposit demonstration histologic methods for the localization of insoluble calcium salts (calcium phosphate, calcium carbonate, hydroxyapatite) in tissue sections. The two general methods are the reaction of the calcium with a dye (e.g., alizarin red S) to form a dye lake, and the reaction of the carbonate or phosphate with a heavy metal which results in an insoluble precipitate.

Alizarin red S staining at pH 4.2 produces a doubly refracting orange-red calcium lake. In von Kossa's method, sections are reacted with silver nitrate in bright light (preferably sunlight), resulting in silver carbonate or silver phosphate. Treatment with sodium thiosulfate reduces any unbound silver. Sections are counterstained with nuclear fast red and mounted. Calcium deposits appear black on a pink-to-red background.

calcium disodium edetate a chelating agent used in the treatment of lead poisoning; the calcium disodium salt of ethylenediaminetetraacetic acid (EDTA). Excessive doses may cause kidney damage.

calcium gluconate a calcium salt of gluconic acid, $Ca[HOCH_2(CHOH)_4COO]_2$, occurring as odorless, tasteless, white crystalline granules or powder. It is used in tablet form or by intravenous injection as a source of supplemental or therapeutic calcium.

calcium orotate the most assimilable form of calcium, used as a nutritional supplement; it is able to penetrate cells better than other forms of calcium.

calcium oxalate a salt, CaC_2O_4, that may be present as crystals in urine or may be the major component of renal calculi. The usual crystalline form is small, colorless, and octahedrous. Calcium oxalate is soluble in dilute hydrochloric acid.

calcium oxalate tests tests for the identification of calcium oxalate, e.g., in calculi. The calculus is pulverized, and calcium oxalate identified by any one of several chemical tests.

1. Dissolve a portion of the stone in HCl, 0.6 mol/l, add 0.5 ml of saturated sodium acetate, and adjust the pH to approximately 5.0 with acetic acid, 1.7 mol/l; a white precipitate indicates presence of calcium oxalate.

2. The powdered calculi is heated to convert oxalate to carbonate, and HCl, 0.6 mol/l, is added. Effervescence on heating indicates presence of oxalate. This test is valid only in the absence of carbonate.

3. A portion of the powdered stone is dissolved in HCl, 0.6 mol/l, and magnesium dioxide is added, which oxidizes the oxalate to CO_2. Effervescence indicates the presence of oxalate.

calcium red see *nuclear fast red.*

calciuria (kal″se-u′re-ah) [*calci-* + Gr. *ouron* urine + *-ia*] the presence of calcium in the urine.

calculus (kal″ku-lus) [L. "pebble"] an abnormal concretion of chemical deposits within hollow organs or passages of the body, especially in the renal and biliary systems. The composition of calculi can be analyzed by x-ray diffraction, infrared spectrophotometry, and chemical analysis. Also called *stone,* as in kidney stones or gallstones. See also *cholelithiasis* and *urolithiasis,* and *renal calculi* and *gallstones.*

articular c., a calculus deposit occurring in a joint, formed from sodium urate or calcium urate. Also called *joint c.*

biliary c., a gallstone (see *cholelithiasis*).

calcium oxalate c., a hard, rough calculus composed of calcium oxalate; calcium phosphate may be mixed in the same stone. Calcium stones are the most common type of urinary calculi, accounting for 75–85 percent of all kidney stones.

calcium phosphate c., a hard stone composed of calcium phosphate, usually hydroxyapatite, $Ca_5(PO_4)_3OH$, or bushite, $CaHPO_4$. See also *calcium oxalate c.*

cholesterol c., a calculus composed of cholesterol. It is the most common type of biliary calculus, making up about 80 percent of all gallstones. Although some cholesterol stones are almost pure cholesterol, most also have some admixture of calcium salts, bile acids, bile pigments, fatty acids, proteins, or phospholipids.

cystine c., a soft urinary calculus composed of cystine, occurring infrequently (about 1 percent of all kidney stones) in some individuals with cystinuria. See also *cystinuria.*

joint c., see *articular c.*

lacrimal c., a calculus formed in a lacrimal gland or duct.

pigment c., a gallstone composed primarily of bile pigments (calcium bilirubinate, complex bilirubin polymers, and other organic and inorganic solids); this type makes up about 20 percent of all gallstones. Formation of these stones is associated with an increase in unconjugated bilirubin in the bile due either to increased excretion or to the action of bacterial β-glucuronidase occurring in bacterial infection secondary to invasion of liver flukes.

renal c., a calculus lying within the caliceal system or pelvis of the kidney, which is too large to pass into the ureter. The most frequent type of calculus is the calcium oxalate calculus (pure or in combination with phosphate). The next most frequent are the calcium phosphate and magnesium ammonium phosphate (struvite) calculi. Approximately 5 percent of renal calculi are uric acid and urate calculi, 1 percent are cystine calculi, and a small number are xanthine calculi. Calculi do not usually become large enough to obstruct the renal pelvis. Also called *nephrolithiasis.*

salivary c., a calculus formed in a salivary gland duct.

struvite c., a urinary calculus composed of struvite (magnesium ammonium phosphate, $MgNH_4PO_4$), which makes up about 10–15 percent of all kidney stones. Struvite stones are formed from urinary tract infections by bacteria, usually *Proteus* species, that produce urease, and they are found primarily in females. See also *urinary c.*

uric acid c., a calculus formed from uric acid. It is hard and is yellow or reddish-yellow in color and makes up 5–8 percent of all kidney stones. Uric acid stones occur in conditions in which there is excessive excretion of uric acid, e.g., gout, Lesch-Nyhan syndrome, and those who have myelo- or lymphoproliferative disorders who are being treated by chemotherapy. Also called urate calculus.

urinary c., a calculus found in any part of the urinary tract. Urinary calculi are most often composed of calcium oxalate and calcium phosphate (together making up about two-thirds of all those analyzed), followed in frequency by mixtures of calcium phosphate and magnesium ammonium phosphate, uric acid and urates, and cystine and xanthine. Such stones are more common in males than females and most often occur after the second decade of life.

Often, the cause for renal calculus formation is unclear. Approximately 25 percent of calcium-containing calculi occur in individuals with normal concentrations of serum and urine calcium. In slightly more than 40 percent of those affected, urine calcium is elevated in the presence of normal serum calcium, with no known explanation for the formation of the calculi. Those who also have high serum calcium usually have an unidentified cause of hypercalcemia, including hyperparathyroidism, malignancy, sarcoidosis, Paget's disease, excess intake of vitamin D or of calcium and antacids, and prolonged bed rest.

Uric acid stones are formed in the presence of high urinary levels of uric acid, especially in urine of low pH. This may occur in individuals afflicted with gout or prolonged diarrhea, or in those who have myeloproliferative or lymphocytic malignancies that have been treated with chemotherapy.

Magnesium ammonium phosphate (struvite) stones usually are formed in the alkaline urine of individuals infected with urea-splitting organisms, most commonly *Proteus* species. These organisms split urea in urine to produce an alkaline urine.

Other factors involved in the formation of urinary calculi include geographic residence (in the United

States, they are found most frequently in the Southeast); diets high in oxalate, calcium, lactose, and purines; use of antacids, vitamin D, and carbonic anhydrase inhibitors; urinary obstruction; and dehydration.

vesical c., a calculus in the urinary bladder or gallbladder.

Caldwell-Moloy classification (kald′wel mo-loi′) [William Edgar *Caldwell,* U.S. obstetrician, 1880–1943; Howard Carman *Moloy,* U.S. obstetrician, 1903–1953] the classification of female pelves as gynecoid, android, anthropoid, and platypelloid.

Caldwell-Moloy method see under *pelvimetry.*

Caldwell projection (kald′wel) [Eugene Wilson *Caldwell,* U.S. radiologist, 1870–1918] a projection used in radiology of the frontal and anterior ethmoidal sinuses. In the original method, the patient's forehead and nose rest on the film, and the central ray is directed through the glabella with a caudal angulation of 23° to the glabellomeatal line. In the modified method, the orbitomeatal line is perpendicular to the film, and the central ray is directed 15° caudad through the nasion.

calefacient (kal″e-fa′shent) [L. *calidus* warm + *facere* to make] causing a sensation of warmth; an agent that so acts.

calibrate (kal′ĭ-brāt) 1. to adjust a system or process so that it performs within specified tolerance limits.

2. to determine correction factors to be applied to readout or to the indication of a measuring device or instrument or to the results of an analytical method.

calibration (kal″ĭ-bra′shun) the process of testing and adjusting a measuring device so that it can be used to make measurements that are accurate to within a specified tolerance. As such devices or instruments are used to measure reference standards of known values, either they are adjusted to read out the correct values, or correction factors are derived for conversion of the measured values.

calibration curve a function relating some conveniently measured physical parameter to the precisely known concentration of some analyte. Ideally, the function is a straight line, but often it is not. The coordinate axes are usually arithmetic, but may be logarithmic, or even more complex, e.g., the logit function. In spectrophotometry, the measured parameter is light absorbance (or logarithm of percent transmittance). Also called *standard curve.*

calibration materials see *reference materials.*

California encephalitis virus a bunyavirus causing California encephalitis; see also *arbovirus.*

californium (Cf) (kal″ĭ-fōr′ne-um) [from the University of *California,* where it was first produced] a synthetic, radioactive element, atomic number 98; most stable isotope ^{251}Cf (half-life, 800 yr); a 5f transition element (actinide); oxidation state +3.

calix (ka′liks), pl. *calices, calyces* [L.] see *calyx.*

call (kawl) in computer programming, to execute a subroutine.

Call-Exner body (kawl ek′sner) [F. von *Call,* Austrian physician, 1844–1917; Sigmund *Exner,* Austrian physiologist, 1846–1926] a small accumulation of eosinophilic material surrounded by a ring of granulosa cells, seen in maturing ovarian follicles and in granulosa cell tumors.

calling sequence the sequence of instructions in an assembly-language program used to transfer control to a subroutine, and to provide it with its required arguments and a return address.

Calliphora (kah-lif′o-rah) [Gr. *kallos* beauty + *phoros* bearing] a genus of flies, the blow flies or bluebottle flies, which have been implicated as the cause of facultative nasopharyngeal or intestinal myiasis in humans. See also the accompanying illustration.

Calliphoridae (kal″ĭ-fōr′ĭ-de) a family of Diptera commonly called blowflies or bluebottle flies. The adults are medium to large in size, and metallic green, blue, or copper in color, with plumose antennae. They feed on carrion, excrement, and garbage, and may transmit dysentery by contaminating food. Larvae of the same species can cause myiasis.

Callitroga (kal″ĭ-tro′gah) see *Cochliomyia.*

callosity (kah-los′ĭ-te) [L. *callositas,* from *callositatis* thick-skinned] see *callus.*

callus (kal′us) [L.] 1. localized hyperplasia of the horny layer of the epidermis due to pressure or friction; also called callosity.

2. the formation of cartilage and bone within granulation tissue at a fracture site during the process of repair. An unorganized network of woven bone is formed about the ends of a broken bone; it is absorbed as repair is completed (provisional callus), and is ultimately replaced by true bone (definitive callus).

calmodulin a protein, with four binding sites for Ca^{2+}, that mediates the action of Ca^{2+} as an intracellular second messenger in all eukaryotic cells; M.W. 16,700. Binding of calcium to calmodulin causes a conformational change, converting it to an active form that can bind to various effector enzymes, converting them in turn to an active conformation. One example is the Ca-dependent ATPase, which pumps Ca^{2+} out of cells and is turned on by activated calmodulin.

calomel (kal′o-mel) [L. *calomelas,* from Gr. *kalos* fair + *melas* black] *mercurous chloride.* See also *calomel e.* under *electrode.*

calor (ka′lor) [L.] heat; one of the classic signs of inflammation.

Calorie (Cal) (kal′o-re) [Fr., from L. *calor* heat] an obsolete unit of heat, 1000 calories (cal), used to measure the energy produced by the metabolism of food; the calorie counted by dieters. Because of confusion between the terms Calorie and calorie, the unit kilocalorie (kcal) should be used instead. Also called kilogram calorie and large calorie.

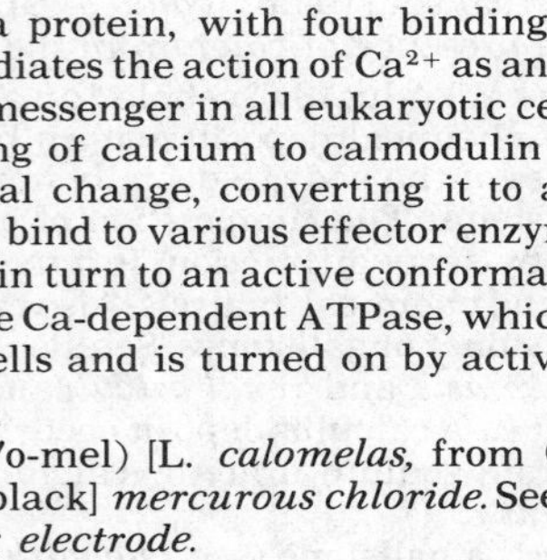

Calliphora. The species *C. vomitoria.* (From Dorland's Illustrated Medical Dictionary. 26th ed. Philadelphia, W. B. Saunders Co., 1981.)

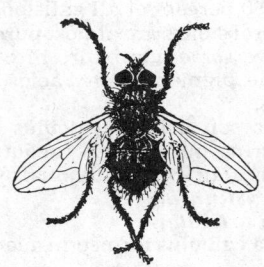

calorie (cal) 1. a derived unit of heat, 4.184 joules (J).

2. formerly, any of several units of heat, all approximately equal to 4.18 J; defined as the quantity of heat required to raise 1 g of water 1° Celsius, which varies with the initial temperature. Also called gram calorie, small calorie, and standard calorie.

calorimeter (kal″o-rim′ĕ-ter) [L. *calor* heat + Gr. *metron* measure] an instrument used for measuring the amount of heat absorbed or released by a process such as a chemical reaction. In physiology, the term refers to an apparatus for measuring the amount of heat produced by an individual.

calsequestrin (kal″sĕ-kwes′trin) [*calcium* + *sequester* + *-in* a chemical suffix] a calcium-binding protein on the inner surface of the sarcoplasmic reticulum of muscle cells. It facilitates storage of Ca^{2+} within the sarcoplasmic reticulum.

Calvé-Perthes disease (kal-va′ per′tez) [Jacques *Calvé,* French orthopedist, 1875–1954; Georg Clemens *Perthes,* German surgeon, 1869–1927] osteochondrosis of the epiphysis at the head of the femur.

Calymmatobacterium (kah-lim″ah-to-bak-te′re-um) [Gr. *kalymma* a hood or veil + *baktērion* little rod] a genus of bacteria consisting of a single species, *C. granulomatis,* which causes granuloma inguinale, a sexually transmitted disease.

C. granulomatis, the pathogenic, gram-negative, encapsulated species responsible for granuloma inguinale, an ulcerative spreading lesion of the skin of the genitals, groin, and anus. When seen in Wright-stained smears of lesions, of the bacteria are typically massed within large mononuclear cells where they become the Donovan bodies. When first isolated, *C. granulomatis* cannot grow on artificial media. It is antigenically related to *Klebsiella pneumoniae,* and extracts are used to prepare skin test antigen. See also *g. inguinale* under *granuloma* and *sexually transmitted diseases.*

calyx (ka′liks), pl. *calyces* [Gr. *kalyx* cup of a flower] a cup-shaped organ or cavity.

major c., an extension of the renal pelvis into which minor calyces empty. There are three to five major calyces in the human kidney.

minor c., a funnel-shaped membranous sac that forms a cap over the tip of a renal medullary pyramid, and channels urine into a major calyx.

camera (kam′er-ah) [L. "chamber"] 1. a box, chamber, or compartment.

2. any enclosed space or ventricle.

3. a device for making photographs; by extension, any stationary detector imaging device, e.g., a scintillation camera.

camera lucida an optical instrument that uses a system of mirrors or prisms to project an image of an object on a surface where a tracing is made.

cAMP abbrev. See *cyclic adenosine monophosphate.*

Camp-Gianturco method (kamp jan-tur′ko) in radiography, a method used to obtain a parietoorbital projection of the optic canal. With the patient prone, the head is turned so that one eye socket is next to the film. The head is placed either horizontally or inclined 15° caudally, using an angle block. A metal device called a Camp-Gianturco optic canal localizer is placed against the head for alignment so that the central ray passes vertically through the optic canal.

camphor (kam′for) [L. *camphora;* Gr. *kamphora*] a colorless, crystalline ketone that sublimes readily; M.W. 152.23. It has a penetrating characteristic odor and pungent taste, is derived from the tree *Cinnamomum camphora,* and is used topically as a rubefacient and antipruritic. Severe poisoning may occur from ingestion of solid camphor, spirit of camphor, or camphorated oil. Nausea, vomiting, diarrhea, convulsions, and renal failure may occur depending on the severity of the poisoning.

camphor assays ultraviolet spectrophotometry or gas chromatography following separation of camphor from biologic specimens by extraction or steam distillation.

CAMP test (kamp) a test for the presumptive identification of group B beta-hemolytic streptococci. A culture of streptococcus is streaked on a sheep or bovine blood-agar plate near a streak of beta-lysin–producing *Staphylococcus aureus.* Group B streptococci produce a substance (CAMP factor) that enlarges the zone of lysis formed by the staphylococcal beta-hemolysin. A CAMP disk test is also available.

Campylobacter (kam″pĭ-lo-bak′ter) [Gr. *kampylos* curved + *bactērion* little rod] a genus of bacteria of the family Spirillaceae; it consists of gram-negative, thin, curved rods (0.2–0.8 μm wide by 0.5–5.0 μm long) or (occasionally) long, spiral rods or S-shaped or gull-winged forms. The organisms are motile, with a single polar flagellum at one or both ends. They are microaerophilic or anaerobic and oxidase-positive. The genus includes pathogenic species that cause human systemic disease, abortion, and enteritis, as well as abortion in cattle. Nonpathogenic species occur in both humans and cattle.

C. fetus, the microaerophilic type species, occurring as three subspecies, two of which are pathogenic in humans. Formerly called *Vibrio fetus.*

C. fetus intestinalis, the subspecies that is the most common human pathogen in this genus. It causes septicemic infections and enteritis, especially in elderly, debilitated, and immunosuppressed individuals. The organism is usually isolated from blood culture incubated under microaerophilic conditions. It is oxidase- and catalase-positive, grows at 25°C, and requires an anaerobic or 10 percent CO_2 atmosphere.

C. fetus jejuni, a subspecies that is one of the common causes of bacterial gastroenteritis in otherwise healthy children, but less often in adults. The organism can be isolated readily from stool and rectal specimens on blood agar plates containing several antibiotics. Colonies are seen as flat and gray or raised and mucoid. Growth is microaerophilic, requiring 10 percent CO_2. The organisms are oxidase- and catalase-positive, and do not grow at 25°C. Erythromycin is the drug of choice for treatment.

C. sputorum, a nonpathogenic subspecies found as a normal inhabitant of the human oral cavity. The organisms are oxidase-positive and catalase-negative.

Canada balsam (kan′ah-dah) a turpentine procured from the liquid rosin of the balsam fir, *Abies balsamea.* It may be used as a mounting medium for tissues stained with hematoxylin-eosin stains, but is not suitable for use with basic aniline dyes, Prussian blue, or acid fuchsin.

Canada balsam may be prepared by heating with water; it solidifies to a clear and hard (but brittle) rosin. It is soluble in a number of solutions such as chloroform and xylene, and takes several months to dry to a sufficient degree of hardness. Its refractive index in solution is 1.523.

Canada-Cronkhite syndrome (kan′ah-dah krong′-kīt) [Wilma-Jeanne *Canada,* U.S. radiologist; Leonard W. *Cronkhite,* Jr., U.S. internist, born 1919] familial polyposis of the gastrointestinal tract, which is associated with alopecia, nail dystrophy, and hyperpigmentation of the skin. See also *familial p.* under *polyposis.*

canal (kah-nal′) [L. *canalis* channel] a relatively narrow tubular passage or channel. For more information, see the specific canal.

canaliculitis (kan″ah-lik″u-li′tis) [L. *canaliculus,* from *canalis* channel + *-itis* inflammation] inflammation of the lacrimal ducts, with tearing and inflammation of the conjunctiva. It is most often caused by *Actinomyces israelii,* fusobacteria, *Candida albicans,* or *Aspergillus* species.

canaliculus (kan″ah-lik′u-lus), pl. *canaliculi* [L. dim. of *canalis*] 1. an extremely narrow tubular passage or channel.
2. [NA], in anatomy, a general term used to denote various small channels, especially bile canaliculi.

apical canaliculi, tubular invaginations of the apical cell membrane of cells of the proximal convoluted tubule of the kidney, through which protein molecules are absorbed.

bile canaliculi, the smallest channels of the biliary system, situated between adjacent hepatocytes. Microvillar specializations of the hepatocyte plasma membrane protrude into the lumen, and tight junctions unite the membranes of the adjacent hepatocytes so that bile can empty only into the intralobular or terminal ductules.

canals of Hering see *bile ductules.*

cancellous (kan′sĕ-lus) [L. "a lattice"] of reticular, spongy, or latticelike structure; generally used to refer to bony tissue.

cancellous bone see *spongy bone.*

cancer (CA) (kan′ser) [L. "crab"] a term that by common usage has come to encompass all forms of malignant neoplasms. See also *neoplasm.*

cancer management therapy see the specific type of therapy (i.e., *chemotherapy, hormonal therapy, immunotherapy, radiation therapy*).

cancer promoter see *tumor p.* under *promoter.*

cancer staging see *tumor staging.*

candela (cd) (kan-del′ah) [L. *candēla* candle] the International System (SI) unit of luminous intensity, defined as 1/60 of the luminous intensity of a source of blackbody radiation at the temperature of the freezing point of platinum.

candicidin B (kan″dĭ-si′din) a polyene antibiotic produced by strains of *Streptomyces griseus.* It is not absorbed systemically and produces few toxic effects; it is useful only in the treatment of vaginitis due to *Candida.*

Candida (kan′dĭ-dah) [L. *candidus* glowing white] a genus of candidiasis-causing fungi that may exist in yeast and mycelial forms. Presently, *Candida* is classified within the family Cryptococcaceae, Fungi Imperfecti; however, some members of this genus reproduce sexually. It is commonly part of the normal flora of the alimentary tract and mucocutaneous regions, but can also cause a variety of infections, especially in patients whose immune defenses have been compromised.

Candida grows on glucose peptone agar and should be incubated at both 24° and 37°C because yeasts can vary in their temperature requirements. The culture morphology reveals cream-colored colonies, usually without mycelia. Microscopically, the *Candida* yeast cell is a single budding microorganism without a capsule. For production of mycelia, *Candida* should be grown on cornmeal agar with Tween 80 (polysorbate 80); the inoculum should be either cut into the agar or covered with a sterile coverslip.

C. albicans and *C. stellatoidea,* two common human pathogens, can be differentiated by a sucrose assimilation test and by sensitivity to cycloheximide.

C. albicans, the species that is the most common etiologic agent of candidiasis. The colony morphology on Sabouraud's dextrose agar at 25°C after 3 da is creamy-colored and smooth in appearance. Microscopically, short, ovoid yeast cells, pseudohyphae, and internodal blastospores are seen. It also produces chlamydospores on cornmeal agar and germ tubes in serum.

C. guilliermondi, a species that has been isolated from certain systemic candidiases, e.g., endocarditis in patients undergoing cardiovascular surgery. The colony morphology on Sabouraud's dextrose agar at 25°C after 3 da is thin, flat, and cream to pink in color. Microscopically, short, ovoid yeast cells are seen. A pseudomycelium may be present. Ascospore-forming strains of *C. guilliermondi* have been assigned to the genus *Pichia.*

C. krusei, a species of *Candida* whose colony morphology is flat, dull, dry, and green to yellow in color. Microscopically, the yeast cells are cylindric and ovoid in shape. Mycelia appear branched in a treelike manner.

C. parapsilosis, a species that occasionally causes paronychias, endocarditis, or otitis externa. The colony morphology is soft, smooth, and white. Microscopically, yeast cells are ovoid, and a thin pseudomycelium may be present in addition to blastospores.

C. pseudotropicalis, a species of *Candida* characterized by soft, smooth, white colonies on agar. Microscopic examination shows elongated yeast cells lying parallel to one another.

C. stellatoidea, a species associated with vaginitis. The colony morphology is small, smooth, and white to cream in color. Microscopically, yeast cells may be ovoid or elongated. A branched pseudomycelium and blastospores, as well as chlamydospores, may be present.

C. tropicalis, a species of *Candida* that is associated with vaginitis or bronchopulmonary and systemic candidiasis. The colony morphology is white and smooth. Microscopically, globoid or ovoid yeast cells are seen, as well as an abundant pseudomycelium and blastospores.

candidal (kan′dĭ-dal) pertaining to or caused by *Candida.*

candida precipitin test an immunodiffusion test to detect antibodies against the fungus *Candida.* If the reaction of the patient's serum and whole-cell antigens is positive, from one to seven precipitin lines may form. Systemic candidiasis should be suspected when a series of serum samples converts from negative to positive or shows an increase in the number of precipitins. Positive reactions may also reflect colonization by *Candida* species.

candidemia (kan″dĭ-de′me-ah) the presence of *Candida* species in the blood, usually as a complication of indwelling intravascular lines, burns, or surgery. See also *candidiasis.*

candidiasis (kan″dĭ-di′ah-sis) any fungal infection involving the genus *Candida.* The clinical manifestations range from acute to chronic and may be localized or systemic. The *Candida* organism most likely to produce candidiasis in various regions of the body is influenced by antibiotic therapy, diet, pregnancy, endocrine disorders, defective cell-mediated immunity, and pH. Although candidiasis involves a wide spectrum of clinical diseases, it is convenient to divide them into oral, vaginal, pulmonary, alimentary, cutaneous, and systemic forms.

CLINICAL DISEASE. Oral candidiasis (thrush) is the overgrowth of *Candida albicans* in the mouth. This form often affects newborns and adults as a result of low local pH or antibiotic or immunosuppressive therapy. A pseudomembrane that is gray to white in color covers the tongue and other oral surfaces, and contains fungi in the mycelial and yeast growth phases. Removal of the pseudomembrane leaves a red, oozing base. In addition, a chronic mucocutaneous candidiasis with persistent or recurrent candidal infections of the mucous membranes, skin, and nails is found in persons who have some underlying endocrinopathies.

Vaginal candidiasis is often associated with diabetes, pregnancy, and broad-spectrum antibiotic therapy. A white, curdlike discharge, inflammation, and pruritus are present, and a pseudomembrane forms on the vaginal mucosa. A high proportion of healthy females can harbor *C. albicans* in their vaginal tracts and develop vaginitis. *C. albicans* are classified as sexually transmitted diseases.

Pulmonary candidiasis is characterized by a chronic bronchitis with cough, rales, and peribronchial thickening. It is infrequent, but when pulmonary candidiasis occurs as a primary infection, those infected have a cough, low-grade fever, night sweats, weight loss, and mucoid sputum. Lung lesions resemble miliary tuberculosis and may involve one or both lobes. Pulmonary candidiasis is often secondary to septicemia and is usually fatal.

Alimentary candidiasis may result from extended oral candidiasis, a genetic defect, or various types of chemotherapy. The mucous membrane of the esophagus may be destroyed, resulting in an irregular and ragged esophageal outline on radiography. Enteric disease has been associated with the presence of *Candida;* however, demonstration of invasion of the intestinal mucosa with this yeast is considered a prerequisite for the diagnosis of intestinal candidiasis. Perianal involvement with *Candida* is a common complication of diaper rash in infants.

Cutaneous candidiasis is most often seen at the axillae and groin, in folds under the breasts, and between the fingers and toes. The lesions give the appearance of scalded skin with an erythematous base and scalloped border. Cutaneous candidiasis is often associated with either metabolic disorders or moist, warm, constricted environments.

Systemic candidiasis is secondary to a primary debilitating disease and may involve the urinary tract, heart valves (as in endocarditis), central nervous system (as in meningitis), or blood (as in septicemia). This form of candidiasis has a poor prognosis.

LABORATORY DIAGNOSIS. Candidiasis is diagnosed by clinical observation and laboratory identification. Superficial infections of the skin and mucous membranes caused by *Candida* species are best diagnosed by a combination of culture and microscopy. The isolation of a pathogenic species from normally sterile tissue is significant; however, the microscopic demonstration of yeasts and hyphae in tissue is conclusive evidence of disease.

Candida grows on most laboratory media at room temperature. *C. albicans,* the yeast most commonly involved in disease in humans, produces a germ tube after incubation in serum at 37°C for 2 hr. On cornmeal agar, *C. albicans* produces chlamydospores. Other biochemical tests involving carbohydrate fermentation and assimilation for the differentiation of the various *Candida* species are also available.

The serologic diagnosis of candidiasis is evolving as a tool for laboratory diagnosis, as well as for determination of the progress of the disease. The principal cell wall antigens of *C. albicans,* called glucomannans, are sometimes found in healthy individuals but are indicative of an immunologically sensitive state. High titers of antibodies to intracellular antigens of *Candida* are indicative of systemic disease. Antibodies may be demonstrated by precipitin tests in agar.

Also called *candidosis.*

candidid (kan′dĭ-did) see *moniliid.*

candidosis (kan″dĭ-do′sis) see *candidiasis.*

canker (kang′ker) an ulceration, especially of the lip or oral mucosa. See also *aphthous stomatitis* and *stomatitis.*

canker sore see *aphtha.*

cannabinoid (kah-nab′ĭ-noid) Δ^9-tetrahydrocannabinol, the psychoactive compound in marijuana and related compounds. An EMIT homogeneous enzyme immunoassay for cannabinoids in urine is a simple test for marijuana use. Other methods utilize gas chromatography–mass spectroscopy or gas-liquid chromatography after extensive separation and concentration procedures.

Cannabis (kan′ah-bis) [Gr. *kannabis* hemp] a genus of flowering plants; the species *C. sativa* produces a fiber, hemp, which is used to make canvas and rope. The resin produced by flowering tops (hashish) or the dried leaves are smoked or ingested for euphoric and psychedelic effects, which are produced by the active ingredient Δ^9-tetrahydrocannabinol (Δ^9-THC) and its isomers. Increased heart rate, dry mouth and throat, conjunctival vascular congestion, hunger, and occasionally dizziness and nausea accompany euphoria and heightened concentration on the present environment. Acute toxicity may result in paranoia, disorientation, perceptual alterations, and short-term memory loss. Also called *marijuana.*

See also *cannabinoid assays.*

cannabism (kan″ah-bizm) cannabis intoxication. Acute marijuana toxicity is marked by nausea, hallucinations, anxiety, disorientation, paranoid ideation, and short-term memory loss.

cannon wave (kan′on) an exaggerated (giant) wave in the jugular venous pulse. It occurs in conditions such as premature ventricular contraction or complete heart block, whenever right atrial systole is coincident with a closed tricuspid valve.

cannula (kan′u-lah) [L. dim. of *canna* "reed"] a tube for insertion into a duct or cavity; during insertion its lumen is usually occupied by a trocar.

cannulation (kan″u-la′shun) the introduction of a tube into a body duct, cavity, or tubelike organ.

venous c., the introduction of a catheter into a major vein to administer blood products or fluids, to measure central venous pressure, or to administer hyperalimentation nutrients. This procedure is most frequently performed when it is impossible to use a large vein percutaneously (such as in obese or very young patients or those in shock), or when large amounts of fluid must be administered rapidly. The most common sites of venous cannulation are the subclavian, internal and external jugular, and saphenous veins. The procedure involves surgical insertion of the catheter, which is sutured in place. Intravenous infusion is started immediately. Side-effects of the presence of an indwelling venous cannula include septicemia and other nosocomial infections and phlebitis. Local pain, edema, erythema, and fevers of unknown origin are all indications for removing the cannula.

cantharidin (kan-thar′ĭ-din) the anhydride of cantharidic acid, the active component of blistering toxins produced by certain beetles such as *Cantharis vesicatoria.* Contact with human skin causes slowly forming blisters. Taken internally, it causes nausea, diarrhea, and cramps. Cantharidin was formerly used as a vesicant.

canthomeatal line (kan″tho-me-a′tal) see *orbitomeatal line.*

canthus (kan′thus), pl. *canthi* [L., from Gr. *kanthos*] either of the corners of the eye, where the upper and lower eyelids meet; used as an anatomic landmark.

inner c., the canthus nearer to the nose. Also called nasal canthus.

outer c., the canthus nearer to the temple. Also called temporal canthus.

CAP abbrev. See *College of American Pathologists.*

cap (kap) 1. any anatomic structure shaped like a cap, or one that covers the anterior end of another structure.

2. the structure that terminates the 5′ end of many cytoplasmic mRNA molecules in eukaryotic cells. There is a triphosphate bridge between the 5′ positions of a 7-methylguanosine (m^7G) residue and the first nucleotide transcribed from the nuclear DNA. Also, the first nucleotide (and in some cases the second) is methylated at the 2′ position. The cap terminates the mRNA with free 3′-hydroxy groups at each end so that the mRNA is not attacked by the 5′-exonucleases.

capacitance (kah-pas′ĭ-tans) 1. the capability to store an electric charge.

2. (abbrev. C), the ratio of the stored charge (Q) to the voltage across a capacitor (V); that is, $C = Q/V$. The unit of capacitance is the farad (F), 1 coulomb per volt (1 C/V).

capacitation (kah-pas″ĭ-ta′shun) the functional change undergone by a sperm when in the female reproductive tract; it involves the release of enzymes and an increase in respiratory metabolism. The corresponding structural changes are called the acrosome reaction.

capacitor (kah-pas′ĭ-tor) an electric component having a fixed or variable value of capacitance. In essence, it consists of two parallel plates that are electric conductors separated by an electrical insulator, the dielectric.

A charge (Q) on the plates ($+Q$ on one, $-Q$ on the other) produces an electric field between the plates and a proportional polarization in the dielectric. The more the dielectric can be polarized, the greater the dielectric constant (ϵ) and the more charge stored for a given voltage. The charge is proportional to the product of voltage (V) and capacitance (C). If A is the plate area and d is the plate separation, $C = \epsilon A/d$.

The instantaneous current (i) flowing through a capacitor is the product of the time rate of change of the voltage (V) and the capacitance. Therefore, a capacitor does not conduct direct current, but it does pass alternating current.

Large capacitors, such as the filter capacitors of power supplies, can store enough charge to deliver a serious electric shock for hours after the equipment has been turned off. Such a charge should be safely discharged before the equipment is worked on.

Formerly called *condenser.* See also *reactance.*

ceramic c., a capacitor that has a ceramic dielectric.

disk c., a small, thin, low-capacitance capacitor that has leads attached at the edge.

electrolytic c., a capacitor in which a metal plate and an electrolyte solution or paste are the conducting plates, and a thin layer of oxide on the surface of the plate is the dielectric.

junction c., a capacitor consisting of a reverse-biased *pn* junction. See also *varactor d.* under *diode.*

Mylar c., a capacitor that has a Mylar film dielectric sandwiched between rolled metal foil plates.

paper c., a capacitor that has an oiled paper dielectric sandwiched between metal foil plates. This sandwich is rolled up and enclosed in an insulating covering.

variable c., a capacitor consisting of two metal plates separated by air, the distance between which can be adjusted. Also called trimming capacitor.

capacity (kah-pas′ĭ-te) [L. *capacitas,* from *capere* to take] 1. the power to hold, retain, contain, or absorb.

2. the potential volume available for storage or containment. For more information, see the specific capacity.

3. the mental ability to accomplish tasks, or to understand.

4. the maximal quantity that can be determined by a measuring device.

Capillaria (kap″ĭ-la′re-ah) a genus of nematode worms, family Capillaridae, order Trichinellida, that parasitizes a wide variety of animals, usually without intermediate hosts. The uniformly cylindric body is very thin.

C. hepatica, the most common species of *Capillaria* that parasitizes mammals, especially rats. After passage through an intermediate host (dog or cat), it may infect humans, producing a syndrome clinically indistinguishable from visceral larva migrans. The females are 20 mm long by 0.1 mm wide; the males are half as long. *C. hepatica* eggs are 51–67.5 μm long by 30–35 μm wide and are pitted;

infection usually occurs when the eggs are ingested. Larvae migrate to the connective tissue of the liver where they mature, and can then produce eosinophilia, hepatomegaly, and pneumonitis.

C. philippinensis, a species that may infest the human intestine; it is found in individuals in the Philippines. It causes a disease resembling a malabsorption syndrome, with intractable diarrhea and emaciation. The female (2.5–4.3 mm long) produces bioperculated eggs or eggs without shells; first-stage larvae may develop in utero. The males (2.3–3.17 mm long) have a tail with ventrolateral expansions and two pairs of papillae.

capillarity (kap″ĭ-lăr′ĭ-te) the action by which the surface of a liquid is elevated or depressed, depending on the relative attraction of the molecules of the liquid for each other and for those of the solid, and being especially observable in capillary tubes. The extent of elevation or depression is proportional to the surface tension of the liquid. All liquids that wet (adhere to) the containing surface (e.g., glass capillary tube) will rise. If the liquid does not adhere to the surface (i.e., does not wet it), a depression of the liquid surface occurs, as observed with mercury and glass.

capillary (kap′ĭ-lăr″e) [L. *capillaris* hairlike] 1. pertaining to or resembling a hair.

2. any of the minute blood vessels that form networks connecting arterioles with venules, permitting the exchange of various substances, fluids, gases, and solutes between the blood and tissues. The wall is one endothelial cell thick and semipermeable. See also *lymphatic.*

capillary fragility the escape of red cells through the capillary walls. The number of petechiae (punctate hemorrhages) formed under the negative pressure produced by application of a suction cup or positive pressure from occluding venous outflow is indicative of the degree of fragility. Increased capillary fragility occurs because of a decreased number or abnormal function of platelets (thrombocytopenic purpura) or because of vasculitis (vascular purpura).

capillary fragility test a test used to measure vascular integrity, which consists of two forms, negative- and positive-pressure methods. In the negative-pressure method, a suction cup is applied to the skin; capillary resistance is the least negative pressure required for 1 min to elicit one or more petechiae. In the positive-pressure method, the venous blood flow is occluded by use of a tourniquet (see *tourniquet test*). This test is of doubtful diagnostic value, as a significant number of healthy individuals exhibit capillary fragility, whereas some patients with thrombocytopenia do not.

Caplan's syndrome (kap′lanz) [Anthony *Caplan,* English physician, 20th century] the association between seropositive rheumatoid arthritis and progressive pulmonary fibrosis, especially the type seen in coal worker's pneumoconiosis, silicosis, and asbestosis.

capneic (kap′ne-ik) [Gr. *kapnos* smoke] referring to incubation of bacterial cultures under increased carbon dioxide tension, e.g., in a candle-extinguishing jar.

-capnia (kap′ne-ah) [Gr. *kapnos* smoke] a suffix word element to denote carbon dioxide, e.g., hypercapnia.

Capnocytophaga (kap″no-si-tof′ah-gah) [Gr. *kapnos* smoke + *kytos* hollow vessel + *phagein* to eat] a genus of bacteria consisting of gram-negative, facultatively anaerobic rods that occur in normal and diseased sites in the human oral cavity. The organisms are thin, fusiform rods that require CO_2 for growth; growth is slow and the colonies are quite small. Gliding motility can be observed by darkfield microscopy. These organisms ferment glucose, sucrose, and maltose but not xylose or mannitol. Reactions to catalase and oxidase are negative. The organism has been associated with systemic disease in debilitated individuals. There are three species in the genus: *C. gingivalis, C. ochracea,* and *C. sputigena.*

capnohepatography (kap″no-hep″ah-tog′rah-fe) [Gr. *kapnos* smoke + *hēpar, hēpatos* liver + *graphein* to record] radiography of the liver after intravenous injection of carbon dioxide gas.

capping (kap′ing) 1. providing with a protective or obstructive covering.

2. in immunology, the accumulation of cell surface antigens at one pole of a cell, often as a result of cross-linking by specific antibody to these antigens. It frequently takes place on lymphocytes but also occurs with aggregated proteins in protozoa and other cells.

capreomycin (kap″re-o-mi′sin) a polypeptide antibiotic used in the treatment of tuberculosis. It is given by intramuscular injection and is generally used only in treatment-resistant diseases, usually in combination with ethambutol or isoniazid.

capric acid (kap′rik) a rancid-smelling fatty acid, $CH_3(CH_2)_8COOH$, from butter. Also called *decanoic acid.*

caproic acid (kah-pro′ik) a fatty acid, $CH_3(CH_2)_4$-$COOH$, that occurs in milk fat and some plant oils, used in the manufacture of artificial flavors. Also called *hexanoic acid.*

caprylic acid (kah-pril′ik) a fatty acid, $CH_3(CH_2)_6$-$COOH$, from goat and cow milk fat and some seed oils, used in the manufacture of perfumes. Also called *octanoic acid.*

capsid (kap′sid) [L. *capsa* a box] the protein coat that surrounds the nucleic acid (DNA or RNA) core of viruses. The capsid and core together form the nucleocapsid. Capsids have either helical or icosahedral symmetry. In either case they are made up of a large number of small protein units (protomers), which are associated in structural units (capsomers). Helical capsids generally have only a single type of protomer; icosahedral capsids may have several. Helical capsids form a cylinder made of protomers arranged in a spiral around the axis. In icosahedral capsids, the protomers make up an icosahedron, the regular geometric solid with 20 identical equilateral triangles for faces. See also *capsomer* and *icosahedral symmetry.*

capsomer (kap′so-mer) [L. *capsa* a box + Gr. *meros* part] one of the morphologic units of a viral capsid, each composed of a group of identical protein subunits (protomers) held together by noncovalent bonds. In icosahedral viruses, the capsomers at the vertices have five neighbors and are called pentons or pentamers; those on the faces have six neighbors and are called hexons or hexamers. Pentons consist of five protamers; the hexons, three or six. Each icosahedral capsid has 12 pentons and a multiple of

10 hexons, making a total of 10 $T = 2$ capsomers, where T is the triangulation humber. The possible values of T are given by $T = h^2 + hk + k^2$, where h and k are integers; the first few values being 1, 3, 4, 7, ...

capsular space the space between the visceral and parietal layers of the glomerular capsule. It is continuous with the lumen of the renal tubule. Also called *Bowman's space.*

capsule (kap′sūl) [L. *capsula* a little box] 1. a soluble container enclosing an orally administered dose of medicine.

2. in anatomy, a general term for a fatty, fibrous, or membranous structure enclosing an organ or part, such as the kidney or a synovial joint; see also *articular capsule.*

3. see *bacterial capsule.*

4. a layer of fibrous tissue that surrounds some benign tumors.

capsule cell see *satellite cell.*

capsulitis (kap″su-li′tis) [*capsula* + *-itis*] inflammation of a capsule.

adhesive c., an adhesive inflammation between the joint capsule and the peripheral articular cartilage of the shoulder, with obliteration of the subdeltoid bursa; it is characterized by increasing pain, stiffness, and limitation of motion.

capture cross section (kap′cher) that section of an atomic nucleus where the capture of an incident particle is probable, measured in barns.

caput (kap′ut) [L. "head"] 1. the head, comprising the cranium and face.

2. a general term applied to the chief extremity of an organ or part.

Carazzi's hematoxylin (kah-rat′sēz) a weak alum hematoxylin solution occasionally used in histology.

carb/o (kar′bo) [L. "coal," "charcoal"] a word element used in combining form to denote a single carbon atom in a functional group, e.g., carboxylic acid (—COOH), carboxamide ($—CONH_2$), carbonitrile (—C≡N), or carbaldehyde (—CHO).

carbachol (kar′bah-kol) carbamylcholine chloride or choline chloride carbamate, used only as an ophthalmic solution and applied topically to the conjunctiva to constrict the pupil.

carbamate (kar′bah-māt) an ester or salt of carbamic acid (aminomethanoic acid) having the general formula H_2NCOOR (for a salt R would equal a metal ion); the alkyl carbamates are also called urethans. One class of carbamates is used as insecticides and herbicides. These show reversible inhibition of cholinesterases and varying degrees of toxicity; they may cause tearing of the eyes, salivation, convulsions, and death upon ingestion or dermal contact. Atropine is used as an antidote.

carbamazepine (kar″bah-maz′e-pēn) [USP], an iminostilbene that is chemically related to the tricyclic antidepressants. It is used as an anticonvulsant for controlling temporal lobe or generalized tonic-clonic seizures; it is also used to treat trigeminal and glossopharyngeal neuralgias. Frequent adverse reactions include drowsiness, dizziness, nausea, vomiting, and ataxia. Infrequent severe reactions can occur, including drug allergy, bone marrow depression, and cardiac, renal, or hepatic damage. Before treatment, a complete blood count (including platelet and reticulocyte counts) should be obtained, as well as baseline serum iron concentration, liver function tests, urinalysis, and eye examination; these tests are repeated periodically during therapy.

carbamazepine assay determination of carbamazepine serum concentration, usually for therapeutic drug monitoring. Methods used include high-pressure liquid chromatography (HPLC), gas chromatography, and EMIT homogeneous enzyme immunoassay.

carbamide (kar′bah-mīd) carbamic acid amide, a formal but infrequently used name for urea.

carbamino–carbon dioxide (kar-bah-me′no) the carbon dioxide that is reacted with undissociated aliphatic amino groups to form carbamino compounds: $R \cdot NH_2 + CO_2 \rightleftarrows R \cdot NH \cdot COO^- + H^+$. A fraction of the CO_2 in plasma, approximately 0.2 mmol/l, is thus bound to the plasma proteins. The contribution of this form of bound CO_2 to the transport of CO_2 in blood is slight when compared with that due to other forms of CO_2 transport. In the erythrocyte, approximately 1.5 mmol/l of CO_2 is carried as carbamino-CO_2, mostly as carbaminohemoglobin.

carbaminohemoglobin (kar-bah-me′no-he″moglo″bin) the product of the reaction of amino groups of hemoglobin with carbon dioxide, forming $—NH—COO^-$ groups. It makes a modest contribution to CO_2 transport in the blood.

carbamoyl (kar′bah-moil) the radical NH_2—CO—. Also called *carbamyl.*

carbamoyl phosphate an important precursor molecule, $H_2N \cdot CO \cdot PO_3^{2-}$, used in the biosynthesis of urea and the pyrimidine bases.

carbamoyl-phosphate synthetase (ammonia) an enzyme of the ligase class (carbon dioxide:ammonia ligase, EC 6.3.4.16), which catalyzes the reaction $2\ ATP + NH_3 + CO_2 + H_2O \rightleftarrows 2\ ADP + PO_4 + H_2N–CO–OPO_3H_2$. Occurring principally in the mitochondria of the liver, the reaction is the first step in a series of reactions of the urea cycle, and thus is important in the removal of ammonia from the blood. Also called carbamoyl-phosphate synthase and CPS I. (This enzyme should be distinguished from carbamoyl-phosphate synthetase (glutamine-hydrolyzing), EC 6.3.5.5; also called CPS II.) Cf. *urea cycle.*

carbamoyl-phosphate synthetase I deficiency a disorder of glycine and glutamine metabolism, transmitted as an autosomal recessive trait, that is due to a relative or absolute deficiency of the enzyme carbamoyl-phosphate synthetase I, which is the first enzyme in the urea synthesis sequence of steps. Serum urea nitrogen may be very low in these cases. Affected individuals have severe hyperammonemia and a rapidly fatal course after birth. Clinically, there is protein intolerance, vomiting, lethargy, mental retardation, central nervous system dysfunction, ataxia, and coma. Many features of the disease are similar to those of nonketotic hyperglycinemia or several organic acidurias. Also called *hyperammonemia II.* See also *aminoacidopathy.*

carbamylurea (kar″bah-mil-u-re′a) see *biuret.*

carbanion (karb-an′i-on) an ion having a negatively charged carbon atom with an unshared pair of electrons, e.g., ethyl anion ($CH_3CH_2^-$). Salts of such anions have names ending in -ide, e.g., lithium ethanide.

carbarsone (kar′bar-sōn) [USP], *N*-carbamoylarsanilic acid, an arsenical that has been used as an antiamebic in the treatment of amebic dysentery.

carbaryl (kar′bah-ril) 1-naphthyl-*N*-methylcarbamate, an insecticide with relatively low acute toxicity. As this substance inhibits cholinesterase activity, exposure to it can be monitored by measuring the degree of inhibition of this enzyme.

carbaryl assays detection of carbaryl in blood by measurement of cholinesterase activity, which correlates inversely with carbaryl concentration. The insecticide can also be detected by extraction, followed by Florisil column purification, deprivatization, and gas chromatography using a relatively polar column and an electron capture detector.

carbenicillin (kar-ben″ĭ-sil′in) a disodium α-carboxyl benzyl penicillin that inhibits cell wall synthesis in susceptible bacteria. This is a semisynthetic, broad-spectrum, penicillinase-susceptible antibiotic that should be used only when absolutely necessary, and given intravenously. It is effective in treatment of *Pseudomonas* infections, which are known for their resistance to antibiotics. Excessive use of the drug may select for even more resistant strains of *Pseudomonas* species. In addition, a superinfection with another microorganism may result. Carbenicillin is also effective against *Proteus, Enterobacter, Serratia,* and some anaerobic bacteria. Adverse reactions include transient rashes, increased serum transaminase levels, and possible neurotoxicity. See also *antibacterial agents* and *penicillins.*

c. indanyl sodium, an α-carboxy ester of carbenicillin useful for the oral treatment of urinary tract infections, especially those due to *Pseudomonas aeruginosa.* It can also be combined with an aminoglycoside in treating acute leukemia patients who have unexplained fever and severe gram-negative infections.

carbinol (kar′bĭ-nol) 1. an older name for methanol.

2. a term used in the naming of alcohols as substituted methanols; e.g., by this method, $(CH_3CH_2)_3$-COH is triethylcarbinol and $C_6H_5CH_2OH$ is phenylcarbinol.

carbinoxamine maleate (kar″bin-ok′sah-mēn) [USP], an antihistamine used in cough and cold preparations. Drowsiness is one side-effect. Trademark, Clistin.

Carbitol (kar′bĭ-tol) trademark for a series of solvents of mono- and dialkyl ethers of diethylene glycol having the general formula, $ROCH_2CH_2OCH_2$-CH_2OR' and including diethylene glycol monoethyl ether (Carbitol), diethylene glycol monomethyl ether (methyl Carbitol), diethylene glycol monobutyl ether (butyl Carbitol), and diethylene glycol diethyl ether (diethyl Carbitol).

carbohydrate (kar″bo-hi′drāt) a term applied to the saccharides, which are polyhydroxy aldehydes or ketones; so called because they are composed of carbon, hydrogen, and oxygen, and in most saccharides the latter two occur in the proportions found in water; i.e., the generic formula is $(CH_2O)_n$. In physiologic conditions they are mostly in the cyclic hemiacetal form. They are classified into mono-, di-, tri-, poly-, homopoly-, and heteropolysaccharides. Carbohydrates in food are an important and immediate source of energy for the body; 1 g of carbohydrate yields four calories. They are present, at least in small quantities, in most foods, but the chief sources are sugars and starches. The simple sugars (monosaccharides) include glucose, fructose, and galactose, which is produced by the digestion or hydrolysis of lactose. The double sugars (disaccharides) include sucrose, maltose, and lactose. All ripe fruits and many vegetables contain some natural sugars. The starches are present in such foods as rice, wheat, and potatoes.

Carbohydrates may be stored in the body as glycogen for future use. If they are eaten in excessive amounts, however, the body changes them into fats, and stores them in that form.

For more information, see the specific carbohydrate.

carbohydrate identification tests 1. qualitative methods for the identification of sugars. These include the fermentation test, the glucose oxidase (Clinistix) and galactose oxidase tests, Seliwanoff's test for fructose, and Bial's test for pentoses. See also *fermentation test, fructose assays, galactose assays, glucose assays,* and *pentose assays.*

2. separation and identification using paper or thin-layer chromatography, with pyridine-*n*-butanol or pyridine-ethyl acetate as the developing solvent and dinitrosalicylic acid as the spray agent. Reference samples are run in parallel so that the migration of the specimen spots can be compared with the migration of a standard.

carbolfuchsin–methylene blue staining method (kar″bol-fook′sin) see under *acid-fast staining methods* and *Ziehl-Neelsen stain.*

carbolic acid (kar-bol′ik) an obsolete name for phenol; see *phenol.*

carbolism (kar′bol-izm) phenol poisoning; see under *phenol.*

carbolxylene (kar″bol-zi′lēn) a mixture of carbolic acid (phenol) and xylene, in the ratio of 1:3, used for clearing microscopic sections.

carbomycin (kar″bo-mi′sin) one of the macrolide group of antibiotics produced by *Streptomyces halstedii.* It is inhibitory for gram-positive bacteria. See also *antibacterial agents* and *macrolides.*

carbon (C) (kar′bon) [L. *carbo* coal, charcoal] a nonmetallic element; atomic number 6; atomic weight 12.0111, group IV of the periodic table; common oxidation state +4; other states +2 (in carbenes, e.g., carbon monoxide), –2, and –4 (in carbides). Carbon has two crystalline allotropes, diamond and graphite. The amorphous forms of carbon, such as charcoal and carbon black, are actually microcrystalline forms of graphite.

Its common inorganic forms are oxides of carbon, carbon disulfide, carbon tetrachloride, and carbonate salts. In both inorganic and organic compounds, carbon usually forms four covalent bonds. The bond angles at a carbon atom are approximately equal. If there are four single bonds, each bonded atom is at one vertex of a regular tetrahedron with the carbon atom at the center, and the bond angles are 109.5°. If there are one double and two single bonds, the structure is an equilateral triangle, and the bond angles are 120°. If there are two double bonds or one single and one triple bond, the structure is linear and the bond angle is 180°.

Because of the strength of the carbon-carbon single bond (about 83 kcal/mol), carbon can form the long stable chains that are the skeletons of organic compounds.

carbon-11 (^{11}C, C 11) a cyclotron-produced radionuclide. It decays by positron beta decay with a half-life of 20.3 min, producing 511-keV (annihilation radiation) gamma rays. Because of the short half-life, it has been used only in facilities equipped with a cyclotron.

carbon-12 (^{12}C, C 12) a stable isotope of carbon with a natural abundance of 98.89 percent. It is used to define the atomic mass unit, which is exactly one-twelfth the mass of a carbon-12 nucleus.

carbon-13 (^{13}C, C 13) a stable isotope of carbon with a natural abundance of 1.11 percent.

carbon-14 (^{14}C, C 14) a radionuclide that decays by beta decay with a half-life of 5770 yr. It occurs naturally, being formed by cosmic ray bombardment of nitrogen. Carbon 14 is used as a tracer for in vitro procedures such as radioimmunoassay, and for procedures that include autoradiography.

carbonate 1. the CO_3^{2-} anion. In water it is in equilibrium with bicarbonate ion (HCO_3^-), the pK'_a for the acid/base pair, (HCO_3^-/CO_3^{2-}), being 10.34. With the exception of those of the alkali metals, all carbonate salts are insoluble. Many occur as important minerals (e.g., Iceland spar, which is $CaCO_3$).

2. an organic ester containing this group.

carbonate dehydratase an enzyme of the lyase class (carbonate hydro-lyase, EC 4.2.1.1) that catalyzes the reaction $CO_2 + H_2O \rightleftarrows H_2CO_3$. It is a zinc-containing protein that occurs mainly in red blood cells and renal parenchymal cells. It is important in facilitating the transfer of CO_2 from tissues to blood and from blood to alveolar air, and in maintaining rapid equilibrium between $CO_2 \rightleftarrows H_2CO_3 \rightleftarrows HCO_3^-$ in the kidney. Also called *carbonic anhydrase.*

carbon bisulfide see *carbon disulfide.*

carbon dioxide a colorless, odorless, noncombustible gas, CO_2, present in air at 0.027–0.036 percent by volume; M.W. 44.01. It is produced by the combustion of fossil fuels and any type of organic materials, by the processes of respiration and fermentation, and by the action of heat or acid on carbonates; CO_2 itself does not support combustion. The gas is used commercially in carbonated beverages, in fire extinguishers, as a refrigerant and freezing agent (dry ice), as an aerosol propellant, and as an inert (nonoxidizing) atmosphere.

Carbon dioxide is nontoxic but is an asphyxiant, producing narcosis at concentrations of 3 percent and loss of consciousness within several minutes at concentrations of 7–10 percent. The loss of consciousness is primarily due to oxygen deprivation and is preceded by dizziness, headache, confusion, and dyspnea. An excess of CO_2 in the blood (hypercapnia) stimulates the respiratory center, causing hyperventilation in order to increase the exhalation of CO_2.

In vertebrates, the CO_2 produced by cellular respiration diffuses to the capillaries and is transported by the blood to the lungs for removal. A small fraction is carried in the plasma as dissolved CO_2, carbonic acid ($HHCO_3$), bicarbonate (HCO_3^-), or carbamino compounds ($RNHCOO^-$). The larger fraction is carried in erythrocytes as carbamino-CO_2 bound to deoxgenated hemoglobin.

See also *p. p. of carbon dioxide* under *partial pressure.*

c. d. with oxygen, [USP], a mixture of 5 percent (by volume) carbon dioxide with 95 percent oxygen, used to stimulate respiration during recovery from anesthesia and in cases of asphyxia or carbon monoxide poisoning.

solid c. d., a white crystalline solid that sublimes at atmospheric pressure at –78.48°C, passing into the gas phase without passing through the liquid phase. Skin contact can produce serious frostbite, burns, and blistering. Solid CO_2 is used as a refrigerant; solid carbon dioxide [USP], also called carbon dioxide snow, is used in the treatment of certain skin lesions. Also called *dry ice.*

carbon dioxide combining power a measurement of the total CO_2 that can be bound as HCO_3^- at a P_{CO_2} of 40 mmHg at 25°C by serum, plasma, or whole blood.

carbon dioxide combining power measurements the measurement of the carbon dioxide in serum or plasma equilibrated with a gas mixture with a P_{CO_2} of 40 mmHg and then analyzed for total CO_2 (see *carbon dioxide concentration assays*). Because this measurement includes dissolved CO_2, the value must be corrected by subtracting the concentration of dissolved CO_2 (cdCO_2), which is dependent on temperature. The test has largely been replaced by more accurate procedures that measure the concentration of total CO_2 ($ct$$CO_2$). The value for the combining power may even be misleading in respiratory disorders, as the specimen has been modified by equilibration to a normal P_{CO_2} of 40 mmHg (as opposed to the true P_{CO_2} of the patient being tested).

carbon dioxide concentration ($ct$$CO_2$) the combined concentrations of bicarbonate (HCO_3^-), carbamino CO_2, carbonic acid ($HHCO_3$), and dissolved CO_2 in plasma or erythrocytes, usually expressed in millimoles per liter (mmol/l). The $ct$$CO_2$ value is not always very useful by itself, as a high $ct$$CO_2$ may indicate compensated respiratory acidosis (retention of CO_2) or metabolic alkalosis (increased HCO_3^-), whereas a low $ct$$CO_2$ is present in compensated respiratory alkalosis (decrease of CO_2 from hyperventilation) or metabolic acidosis (decrease in CO_2 due to compensatory hyperventilation). Measurement of both pH and P_{CO_2} is required to delineate the underlying cause.

Reference values for $ct$$CO_2$ in various components of blood are: for venous plasma (serum), 23–29 mmol/l; for capillary plasma (serum), 21–28; for venous (whole) blood, 22–26; and for arterial (whole) blood, 19–24.

Also called total CO_2. Formerly called CO_2 content.

carbon dioxide concentration assays 1. Natelson microgasometer method. The specimen is treated with lactic acid to release CO_2 and other gases, the pressure (P_1) of which is measured manometrically. The gas mixture is then exposed to sodium hydroxide, which absorbs CO_2, and the pressure (P_2) is measured. The total concentration ($ct$$CO_2$) is proportional to the P_1–P_2 difference corrected for the ambient temperature by application of a conversion factor. This technique is a microversion of the classic Van Slyke technique.

2. AutoAnalyzer I method. Sulfuric acid releases CO_2 and HCO_3^- and carbamino ($RCNHCOO^-$) ions. A fixed aliquot of this gas passes into an alkaline buffer solution containing phenolphthalein, resulting in a decreased intensity of the red color. The method has several disadvantages, although it has been widely used.

3. AutoAnalyzer II method. This procedure is similar to the AutoAnalyzer I method except that it employs a more stable reagent consisting of TRIS-buffer [tris(hydroxymethol)aminomethane], with cresol red as indicator. The color change is directly proportional to the CO_2 concentration.

4. electrochemical method. CO_2 in a serum specimen is released by sulfuric acid. The rate of release of CO_2, which is proportional to the $ctCO_2$, is monitored by a P_{CO_2} electrode.

carbon dioxide dissociation curve the graphic representation of the relationship between the CO_2 content of whole blood (expressed in milliliters per 100 ml of blood) and the P_{CO_2} to which the blood is exposed. The relationship is nearly linear throughout the physiologic range. The curve is shifted toward the X axis (decreased CO_2 content at the same P_{CO_2}), with increases in the saturation of hemoglobin with O_2 (the Haldane effect).

carbon dioxide fixation the reduction of carbon dioxide (CO_2) to the oxidation level of a carbohydrate. Carbon dioxide fixation allows a capable organism, including algae, green plants, and autotropic bacteria, to obtain all its carbon source from CO_2. This process, which occurs in total darkness, requires energy from the high-energy phosphate bond of adenosine-5′-triphosphate and reducing power from nicotinamide adenine dinucleotide phosphate. The first main step is the reduction of CO_2 to two molecules of 3-phosphoglyceric acid (a 3C intermediate), using ribulose diphosphate, a C5 intermediate, as a substrate and ribulose diphosphate carboxylase as a catalyst. The molecules of 3-phosphoglyceric acid may be further reduced through the Calvin cycle, which includes additional pentose metabolism and the production of glyceraldehyde-3-phosphate. Glyceraldehyde-3-phosphate is an active intermediate of glycolysis.

carbon dioxide output ($\dot{V}_{CO_2}$) the quantity of CO_2 eliminated from the entire body by expiration, usually expressed as a rate in millimeters per minute. CO_2 output is calculated on the basis of measurements of the volume and composition of mixed expired air, using the following equation: $\dot{V}_{CO_2} = \dot{V}_E \times [F_{E_{CO_2}} (1 - F_{I_{CO_2}}) - F_{I_{CO_2}} (1 - F_{E_{CO_2}})]/(1 - F_{I_{O_2}} - F_{I_{CO_2}})$, where $\dot{V}_E$ is the flow rate of the expired air, $F_{E_{CO_2}}$ and $F_{E_{O_2}}$ are the fractional content of CO_2 and O_2 in the expired air, and $F_{I_{CO_2}}$ and $F_{I_{O_2}}$ are the fractional content of CO_2 and O_2 in any inspired air. Cf. *carbon dioxide production.*

carbon dioxide production the quantity of CO_2 produced at the cellular level by metabolic processes. Cf. *carbon dioxide output.*

carbon dioxide response curve the graphic representation of the respiratory response to the inhalation of a constant or an increasing concentration of carbon dioxide, commonly plotted as alveolar ventilation (in liters per minute, l/min, or liters per square meter per minute, $l/m^2/min$) vs. alveolar P_{CO_2} (torr) or percent CO_2. The curves are determined to establish whether certain drugs (depressants such as meperidine or morphine), procedures, or changes in the state of the body (such as changes in arterial P_{O_2}, blood pressure, arterial blood pH, body temperature, or state of arousal) have altered the sensitivity of the respiratory mechanism to carbon dioxide.

carbon dioxide tension see *p. p. of carbon dioxide* under *partial pressure.*

carbon disulfide a colorless, flammable liquid, CS_2, insoluble in water; used in the manufacture of rayon and rubber, and as a fumigant to preserve stored foodstuffs from rodents. It is an acute fire and explosion hazard. Acute exposure produces burning, irritation, blistering, and numbness. Severe neurologic disorders develop with chronic exposure to fumes, resulting in neuritis, pain, parkinsonian palsy, gastric disturbances, and psychosis. Exposure can occur by absorption through the skin as well as by other routes. Carbon disulfide is used in histology as a clearing agent (solvent) but only infrequently because of its odor and toxic fumes. Also called *carbon bisulfide.*

carbon disulfide assays 1. colorimetric methods. Carbon disulfide (CS_2) is separated from biologic specimens using steam distillation followed by identification using a variety of colorimetric tests, such as the lead acetate test in which CS_2 is indicated by a black precipitate formed when lead acetate and potassium hydroxide are added to the distillate and boiled.

2. gas chromatography; see *head space analysis.*

carbon gelatin mass a suspension of fine carbon particles in a gelatin solution for injection into the vascular system of an organ in order to study its circulatory system. The carbon particles do not pass through the capillaries, so afferent and efferent vessels may be injected and studied. After injection, the organ is cooled and fixed in formalin. It may then be used as a gross specimen or sectioned for histologic study.

carbonic acid (kar-bon′ik) a weak, dibasic acid, H_2CO_3, formed by the reaction of CO_2 with water: $CO_2 + H_2O \rightleftarrows H_2CO_3$. As an unstable compound it is found only in equilibrium with CO_2 and H_2O and cannot be isolated in the pure state. The acid is also in equilibrium with the bicarbonate ion ($H_2CO_3 \rightleftarrows HCO_3^- + H^+$), which in turn is in equilibrium with the carbonate ion ($HCO_3 \rightleftarrows H^+ + CO_3^{2-}$). Organic carbonates are esters of this acid; inorganic carbonates (e.g., Na_2CO_3) and inorganic bicarbonates (e.g., $NaHCO_3$) are its salts.

The dissociation constants for carbonic acid in aqueous solution are $pK_1 = 6.37$ and $pK_2 = 10.25$. The pK_1 for carbonic acid in serum is 6.10 (average), due to the relatively high ionic strength.

In blood gas chemistry, the term dissolved CO_2-($cdCO_2$) includes, by definition, the physically dissolved (gaseous) CO_2 and the undissociated carbonic acid.

carbonic anhydrase see *carbonate dehydratase.*

carbonic anhydrase inhibitor one of a group of chemicals, commonly sulfonamide drugs such as acetazolamide and the thiazides, that noncompetitively inhibit the activity of blood carbonic anhydrase (carbonate dehydratase). When used therapeutically as diuretics, they can cause metabolic acidosis, depression of aqueous humor and cerebrospinal fluid formation, and a transient respiratory acidosis, in addition to their effects on renal tubular secretion of hydrogen ions. See also *acetazolamide, carbonate dehydratase,* and *thiazide diuretics.*

carbonium ion (kar-bo′ne-um) an ion having a positively charged (and usually trivalent) carbon atom. The preferred term describing this class of ions is carbocations, and they are named as carbenium ions. For example, $CH_3CH_2^+$ is the ethyl cation by itself; in combination with an anion like perchlorate, it is ethylcarbenium perchlorate.

carbon monoxide a colorless, odorless, tasteless gas, CO, produced by incomplete oxidation of hydrocarbons and organic materials under conditions of limited oxygen supply; M.W. 28.01. It is a component of coal gas and water gas, and of exhaust and flue gases. CO is highly flammable, burning with a blue flame. It can be prepared conveniently in the laboratory by dropping concentrated H_2SO_4 onto a solution of formic acid. CO is highly poisonous because it has a stronger affinity for hemoglobin than O_2; the carboxyhemoglobin thus formed renders the Hb unavailable for O_2 transport. It is a product of Hb degradation; 0.45 mmol (10 ml) being produced per 24 hr. See also *carboxyhemoglobin.*

fractional uptake of c. m., the uptake of CO from a standardized sample of inspired gas, which is used as an index of the diffusing capacity of the lung for CO. It is computed from the following equation: fractional CO uptake = $(F_{I_{CO}} - F_{E_{CO}})/F_{I_{CO}}$, where $F_{I_{CO}}$ and $F_{E_{CO}}$ are the concentrations of CO in the inspired and expired air samples, respectively. Deviation from the normal range of 0.35–0.58 (depending on age and sex) can be used as an indication of change in the surface area for diffusion.

carbon monoxide assays the level of carbon monoxide in a specimen, primarily of whole blood, analyzed by microdiffusion or spectrophotometry. The microdiffusion method involves release of carbon monoxide from hemoglobin with dilute sulfuric acid or lactic acid–ferricyanide solution. The amount of carbon monoxide, if any, is then estimated by the silvery-black film on the palladium chloride that is contained in the diffusion chamber. For spectrophotometry, a hemolysate of blood is treated with sodium hydrosulfite; methemoglobin and oxyhemoglobin are reduced, but carboxyhemoglobin is unaffected. The carboxyhemoglobin then has absorption bands substantially different from deoxygenated hemoglobin and can be analyzed with a narrow bandpass spectrophotometer, using a standard calibration curve.

carbon tetrachloride a colorless, dense liquid, CCl_4. It is slightly soluble in water and is used as a degreasing or cleaning agent, as a solvent, and as a fire extinguisher fluid. In histology, it can be used as a solvent for paraffin. It is toxic when ingested, inhaled, or absorbed through the skin. Chronic poisoning can occur from repeated exposure to small quantities, leading to liver or kidney damage.

carbon tetrachloride assays methods for detecting halogenated hydrocarbons; carbon tetrachloride, chloroform, and related compounds give similar reactions in many tests. Carbon tetrachloride may be detected by various colorimetric methods (see under *chloroform*) and especially by gas chromatography that employs the head space technique (see also *head space analysis*).

carbonyl (kar′bo-nil, kar′bo-nēl) [*carbon* + Gr. *hylē* matter] 1. the organic functional group C=O, occurring in aldehydes, ketones, and carboxylic acids and their derivatives.

2. a term describing a metal complex in which at least one ligand is carbon monoxide (a metal carbonyl), e.g., nickel carbonyl, $Ni(CO)_4$.

carbonylhemoglobin see *carboxyhemoglobin.*

carbophenothion (kar″bo-fen″o-thi′on) an organophosphate compound, phosphorodithioic acid *S*-[[(4-chlorophenyl)thio]methyl] *O,O*-diethyl ester, used as an insecticide and miticide. It is a highly toxic cholinesterase inhibitor. Trademark, Trithion.

Carborundum (kar″bo-run′dum) trademark for abrasives and refractory materials made of silicon carbide or fused alumina.

Carbowax (kar′bo-waks) trademark for polyethylene glycol (PEG) and methoxypolyethylene glycol, which are used as water-soluble solvents, lubricants, reverse osmosis agents, and fluids for heating baths. The approximate polymer molecular weight is specified by an accompanying number, e.g., Carbowax 4000.

In gas chromatography, Carbowax is used as a polar stationary phase, being especially useful in separating hydrocarbons, alcohols, amines, and solvents.

In histology, Carbowax is used as an embedding medium; it is especially suitable for preserving lipids, neutral fats, and the acid-fastness of leprosy and tuberculosis bacteria (*Mycobacterium leprae* and *M. tuberculosis*). Because it is water-soluble, no dehydration or clearing is necessary.

Tissue blocks and sections must be protected from water. The sections are floated out on a 4:5:1 diethylene glycol–water–formalin medium or on a solution of 0.02 percent gelatin, 0.02 percent potassium dichromate.

See also *polyethylene glycol.*

carboxy- (kar-bok′se) a prefix word element in organic chemistry to denote the —COOH group when it must be treated as a substituent in polyfunctional compounds. It is incorrectly used in the word carboxyhemoglobin, a complex between hemoglobin and carbon monoxide, which is better called carbon monoxide hemoglobin or carbonylhemoglobin.

carboxyhemoglobin (Hb CO) (kar-bok″se-he″mo-glo′bin) a compound of hemoglobin and carbon monoxide, joined by a covalent bond analogous to that between hemoglobin and O_2. Because carbon monoxide has about 210 times the affinity for hemoglobin that oxygen has, the formation of carboxyhemoglobin makes hemoglobin unavailable for transport of oxygen; hypoxia or anoxia may result. Carbon monoxide is normally generated in the catabolism of heme, but the amount of carboxyhemoglobin formed is negligible. Its spectral absorbance maxima are 568–572 and 537–540 nm. Inhalation of increased amounts of CO in the air results in anoxia, with symptoms varying from headache (about 20 percent of total Hb in the form of Hb CO) to coma and convulsions (about 40–50 percent) and death (about 79–80 percent). The skin takes on a cherry-red color from the Hb CO. The anoxia is readily reversible by oxygen treatment, but the associated effects of the poisoning—hemorrhage, edema, necrosis—may persist. Also called *carbonylhemoglobin.* See also *carbon monoxide.*

carboxyhemoglobinemia (kar-bok″se-he″mo-glo″-bin-e′me-ah) the presence of carboxyhemoglobin in the blood.

carboxyl (kar-bok′sil) the monovalent group, —COOH, occurring in those organic acids termed carboxylic acids.

carboxylase (kar-bok′sil-ās) one of several enzymes of the carboxy-lyase subclass (EC 4.1.1) that catalyzes the removal of carbon dioxide from the carboxylate group of α-keto acid and other carboxylic acids, e.g., pyruvate, aspartate.

carboxylate ion (kar-bok′sil-āt) a carboxylic acid anion.

carboxylesterase (kar-bok″sil-es′ter-ās) an enzyme of the hydrolase class (carboxylic-ester hydrolase, EC 3.1.1.1) that catalyzes the reaction carboxylic ester + $H_2O \rightleftharpoons$ alcohol + carboxylic acid anion. The enzyme acts on glycerol esters of short-chain fatty acids, esters of monohydric alcohols, and esters of dibasic acids. Also called *aliesterase*.

carboxylic acid (kar″bok-sil′ik) the class of organic acids composed of one or more carboxyl groups attached to an aliphatic carbon chain. Fatty acids (e.g., butyric acid), amino acids (e.g., valine), and hydroxy acids (e.g., lactic acid) are examples of monocarboxylic acids. Tartaric, oxalic, and glutamic acids have two carboxyl groups; citric acid is a tricarboxylic acid.

The carboxylic acids are moderately weak, with pK values with a range of about 2.0–5.0. If several electrophilic groups are attached to the carbon adjacent to the carboxyl, the acid strength may be considerably increased (e.g., trichloroacetic acid).

carboxyl terminal see *C-terminal*.

carboxymethylcellulose (kar-bok″se-meth″il-sel′u-lōs) an ion-exchange resin used to separate proteins by chromatography. See also ion-exchange chromatography under *chromatography*.

carboxypeptidase (kar-bok″se-pep′tĭ-dās) a group of enzymes of the hydrolase class (metallo-carboxypeptidases, EC 3.4.17) that hydrolyze the peptide bond closest to the carboxyl end of a polypeptide chain, liberating a free amino acid and a smaller peptide chain. The enzymes are formed in the pancreas and contain zinc or cobalt.

carbromal (kar-bro′mal) a sedative used in sleeping pills. It acts by releasing bromide, which displaces chloride and interferes with the transmission of nerve impulses. Chronic use can cause brominism, which is characterized by delirium, delusions, drowsiness, dermatitis, speech defects, and unsteady gait.

carbuncle (kar′bung-k′l) [L. *carbunculus* little coal] a large, indurated, deeply situated infection commonly occurring in dense fibrous tissue such as in the superficial neck or back. It is usually due to infection with coagulase-positive *Staphylococcus aureus*. A carbuncle often results from coalescence of several furuncles (boils), and it tends to develop multiple drainage sites. It is more common in debilitated individuals and diabetics. Carbuncles may produce fever, leukocytosis, and bacteremia. Treatment is drainage and antibiotic therapy. See also *furuncle*.

carcin/o (kar′sin-o) [Gr. *karkinos* a crab] a word element used in combining form to denote cancer, e.g., carcinogenic.

carcinoembryonic antigen (CEA) (kar″sĭ-no-em″bre-on′ik) a glycoprotein secreted as part of the glycocalyx of gastrointestinal cells of the 2- to 6-mo-old human fetus; M.W. 200,000. CEA is an oncofetal antigen that reappears in certain neoplasms as one manifestation of the neoplastic transformation. It was originally described as a specific antigen for adenocarcinoma of the colon, but now is known to be present in small amounts in the secretions of the adult colonic mucosa and pancreaticobiliary system; many tumors, primarily those derived from gastrointestinal and pulmonary tissue of ectodermal origin, produce CEA. Moderately elevated serum concentrations of the antigen also occur in nonneoplastic conditions, such as alcoholic cirrhosis, inflammatory bowel syndrome, and in association with cigarette smoking. Thus, CEA is not a diagnostic test for cancer; it is used primarily as a measure of the response of a cancer to therapy. A persistent elevation of CEA after surgical resection of a tumor suggests residual tumor or metastasis. A rising CEA level following therapy is indicative of a recurrence and may precede by months the clinical signs of a relapse.

CEA is measured by radioimmunoassay. The reference range for CEA in plasma is $1.34 \pm 0.16\ \mu g/l$. It can also be demonstrated immunochemically by the immunoperoxidase method.

carcinogen (kar-sin′o-jen) [*carcino-* + Gr. *gennan* to produce] an agent or process that significantly increases the incidence of malignant neoplasms in a population. Carcinogens fall into three classes: chemicals (polycyclic aromatic hydrocarbons, aflatoxin B_1, nitrosamines, and certain aromatic amines and azo dyes), viruses, and ionizing radiation (x-rays and ultraviolet light). Some 80–90 percent of all human neoplasms are considered to be caused by environmental exposure to chemical carcinogens. A variety of screening assays have been developed to detect chemical carcinogens, including the salmonella-mediated mutagenesis assay (Ames assay), the sister chromatid exchange assay, and the micronucleus test, as well as traditional laboratory animal toxicity tests.

Many carcinogens are inert compounds that must be metabolically activated to exert their biologic effects. Activation occurs by microsomal mixed-function oxidases, an enzyme complex found in highest concentration in the liver that predominantly functions in drug detoxification. Activated carcinogens are highly reactive substances that are capable of interacting with cellular macromolecules (primarily), as well as nucleic acids and proteins, and that produce neoplastic transformation. Most carcinogens are mutagens.

There are federal standards for handling some of the known and suspected carcinogens, and the principles adopted by the Occupational Safety and Health Administration (OSHA) could be useful for setting up and operating laboratories in which any highly toxic or pathogenic material is to be handled. The standards call for establishment of a "regulated area" as the contaminable work area and for controlling the movement of personnel, equipment, and air into and out of the regulated area; they specify washing of the hands, forearms, face, and neck on each exit from the regulated area and before engaging in other activities, and for showers after the last exit of the day. There are also specifications relating to clean and dirty change areas, protective clothing, signs, training, emergency procedures, and medical surveillance (OSHA Standards 1910.1003–1910.1017).

See also *mutagen* and *mutagenicity test*.

carcinogenesis (kar″sĭ-no-jen′ĕ-sis) [Gr. *karkinos* cancer + *genesis* production] the production of neoplasms.

carcinogenic (kar″sĭ-no-jen′ik) [*carcino-* + Gr. *gennan* to produce] capable of causing cancer.

carcinoid syndrome a complex, variable constellation of signs and symptoms produced by biologically active substances (e.g., serotonin, bradykinin, histamine, prostaglandins) released in large quantities by carcinoid tumors that have metastasized, usually with extensive hepatic involvement.

Clinical features include (1) flushing of the face and neck with a feeling of warmth or intense heat; (2) gastrointestinal symptoms caused by mechanical obstruction due to metastasis of the tumor; (3) cardiac lesions in about 50 percent of all cases, including plaquelike fibrotic proliferation on the endocardium of the valvular cusps and cardiac chambers, especially on the pulmonary and tricuspid valves; and (4) asthmalike attacks of bronchoconstriction in about 33 percent of the cases. The physiologic basis of the flushing and cardiac lesions is not definitely known; the flushing may be due to bradykinin or prostaglandins; serotonin or bradykinin may be involved in the genesis of the cardiac lesions.

The chemical abnormality of diagnostic significance is the marked elevation of urinary excretion of the serotonin metabolite 5-hydroxyindoleacetic acid (5-HIAA). Normally, 2–8 mg/da of 5-HIAA is excreted, but in carcinoid syndrome as much as 1000 mg/da may be excreted–the excretion is generally above 50 mg/da, which is the sensitivity of the qualitative screening test.

carcinoid tumor a term that, when used precisely, denotes a neoplasm of serotonin-forming argentaffin (Kulchitsky's) cells. However, the term is frequently also used loosely for any endocrine tumor of the gastrointestinal tract or lungs without documentation of the hormone(s) produced. The carcinoid tumor is found most frequently in the gastrointestinal tract and lungs and also occurs infrequently in other locations (e.g., the ovary).

Histologically, carcinoid tumors are characterized by round cells with eosinophilic cytoplasm, and by small, round nuclei arranged in sheets or ribbons, or in a cribriform pattern, frequently in association with a densely sclerotic stroma. Some particularly aggressive carcinoid tumors histologically resemble poorly differentiated adenocarcinomas. Tumors histologically identical to the typical carcinoid and which do not produce serotonin but do produce hormonal polypeptides or biologically active amines are designated as APUD tumors or neuroendocrine tumors, and are frequently further classified by cell type (e.g., islet cell tumor) or by secretory product (e.g., insulinoma).

With electron microscopy, dense-core granules 200–400 nm in diameter can be seen in varying numbers in the cytoplasm of carcinoid tumor cells. Such granules are generally pleomorphic in carcinoids of the small bowel. An uncommon variant is the goblet cell carcinoid seen in the appendix, in which tumor cells contain both mucin and dense-core neurosecretory granules. Although many carcinoid tumors do not metastasize, all should be regarded as at least potentially malignant.

Also called *argentaffinoma.*

carcinoma (kar″sĭ-no′mah), pl. *carcinomas* [Gr. *karkinōma* from *karkinos* crab, cancer] a malignant neoplasm of epithelial cells. Carcinomas are designated according to the cell of origin (e.g., squamous carcinoma, renal cell carcinoma), and may be further subclassified as adenocarcinomas if they are of gland cell origin (e.g., adenocarcinoma of colon). Some tumors are named descriptively (e.g., adenoid cystic carcinoma, spindle squamous carcinoma). Mixed forms occur (e.g., mucoepidermoid carcinoma, adenosquamous carcinoma). A tumor in which an apparent admixture of epithelial and mesenchymal elements is present may be termed a carcinosarcoma, but spindle cell transformation of a carcinoma must be excluded before this diagnosis can be considered valid. The term carcinoma in situ indicates an epithelial malignancy that has not yet become invasive.

Carcinomas spread by local infiltration; they form distant metastases by vascular embolization, predominantly through lymphatic channels, although blood vessel invasion can also lead to dissemination.

Some indication of the potential behavior of a carcinoma may be obtained by an assessment of the histologic features, notably the degree of differentiation of the component cells and the amount of mitotic activity. The result can be expressed as a histologic grade. For example, the Broders system allocates tumors to one of four grades, ranging from grade 1, in which the cells appear relatively normal and there is scanty mitotic activity, to grade IV, in which the tumor is poorly differentiated and may be anticipated to behave aggressively.

Clinical assessment of the extent of a carcinoma may be expressed by a tumor staging system such as the general TNM system, or by one devised for a particular tumor type, such as the Dukes staging system for adenocarcinomas of the colon.

For more information, see the specific carcinoma, *tumor grading,* and *tumor staging.*

carcinoma in situ a morphologically recognizable preinvasive stage of certain malignant epithelial neoplasms (carcinomas). Because the term carcinoma denotes invasion, the concept of carcinoma in situ is considered to be a contradiction in terms. Preinvasive carcinoma may be observed in a number of sites, most frequently the uterine cervix, external genitalia, skin, lungs, and breast, and prostate. This lesion is believed to be a stage in the continuum from dysplasia to invasive carcinoma. In sites where it can be detected by cytologic screening, e.g., the cervix, treatment while the tumor is still in the preinvasive stage has substantially reduced the incidence of invasive carcinoma. See also *cervical intraepithelial neoplasia* and *dysplasia.*

carcinomatosis (kar″sĭ-no-mah-to′sis) the condition of widespread dissemination of cancer throughout the body. Also called *carcinosis.* See also *metastasis.*

carcinomatous (kar″sĭ-nom′ah-tus) pertaining to carcinoma or cancer.

carcinosarcoma (kar″sĭ-no-sar-ko′mah) a neoplasm with malignant epithelial and mesenchymal components. The diagnosis can be considered valid only if an epithelial tumor with reactive stroma can be excluded. Carcinosarcomas most frequently arise in the respiratory tract or bladder. They are highly aggressive neoplasms.

embryonal c., an obsolete term for nephroblastoma; see *nephroblastoma.*

carcinosis (kar″sĭ-no′sis) see *carcinomatosis.*

cardi/o (kar′de-o) [Gr. *kardia* heart] a word element used in combining form to denote the heart or cardiac orifice, e.g., carditis.

cardia (kar′de-ah) [Gr. *kardia* heart] 1. an obsolete term for the heart or heart region.

2. the part of the stomach that adjoins the esophageal orifice.

cardiac (kar′de-ak) [L. *cardiacus,* from Gr. *kardiakos*] 1. pertaining to the heart.
2. a cordial or restorative medicine.
3. pertaining to the portion of the stomach adjacent to the esophagus.

cardiac arrest the sudden cessation of mechanical heart function usually associated with ventricular standstill or ventricular fibrillation. A third mechanism is electromechanical dissociation in which there is electrical activity of the ventricles (QRS complexes) but no associated mechanical heart function. All three types are accompanied by loss of arterial blood pressure, loss of tissue perfusion, and brain death unless cardiac function is promptly restored. It may occur in any type of heart disease, but most commonly is observed in association with coronary heart disease, particularly acute myocardial infarction. Intoxication with digitalis, quinidine, and other cardioactive drugs is also a cause.

cardiac catheterization the passage of a catheter via a vein or artery into the chambers of the heart. This procedure may be used to measure the cardiac output and pressures and the oxygen content of blood in the heart chambers, or to introduce radiopaque contrast media for cardioangiographic studies of the structural components of the heart. It is helpful in establishing a definite diagnosis to determine if surgery is necessary and to plan the optimal surgical approach.

cardiac cycle the electrical and mechanical events that occur in the interval between the beginning of one heart contraction and the beginning of the next. Each contraction (the mechanical events) is initiated by an action potential that spontaneously arises in the sinoatrial node, spreads throughout the atrial myocardium, and passes through the atrioventricular node and down the A-V bundle of His and its branches to excite the ventricles (the electric events).

The mechanical events of each cardiac cycle can be divided into those that occur during a period of contraction (systole) and those that are part of the period of relaxation (diastole) that follows. During the initial third of diastole, the aortic and pulmonary (semilunar) valves are closed, and the pressure in the atria exceeds that in the relaxed ventricles. During this period, venous blood pours into the atria and then through the open A-V valves to rapidly fill the ventricles. During the middle third of diastole, a period known as diastasis, the inflow reaches a near standstill. In the final third of diastole, the atria contract, causing an additional forceful inflow that serves to "prime" the already almost full ventricles before they contract.

When systole (ventricular contraction) begins, intraventricular pressure rises rapidly. When pressure within the ventricles exceeds intraatrial pressure, the A-V valves are forced to close (producing the first heart sound). As the semilunar valves are also closed (because pressure in the aorta and pulmonary artery still exceeds that in the ventricles), the ventricles are essentially sealed chambers at this point. This time during which the ventricles are contracting but no blood is emptying from them (or when tension is generated but no shortening of the myocardial fibers occurs) is known as the period of isometric or isovolumic ventricular contraction. When pressure in the ventricles reaches a level that exceeds that in the aorta and pulmonary artery (normally at a left ventricular pressure greater than 80 mmHg and a right ventricular pressure greater than 8 mmHg), the semilunar valves are forced open, and ventricular volume decreases as blood is rapidly ejected into the aorta and pulmonary artery. During the last quarter of systole, the ventricular musculature is still contracted, but little outflow occurs.

At the onset of ventricular relaxation (diastole), intraventricular pressure begins to decline rapidly to a level less than that in the arteries, and the semilunar valves snap closed (the second heart sound). As the ventricular myocardium continues to relax (a period of isometric relaxation), pressure within the ventricles declines to a diastolic minimum that is less than the pressure in the atria, the A-V valves open, and a new cycle begins.

At an average heart rate of 75 beats/min, all the events of one cardiac cycle occur within 0.8 sec.

cardiac dilation enlargement of the heart by stretching of one or more of its chambers; see *cardiomegaly.*

cardiac enlargement see *cardiomegaly.*

cardiac glycoside any one of a group of glycosides occurring in certain plants, such as *Digitalis purpurea* (the foxglove), *Strophanthus,* and *Urginea,* which have an inotropic effect on the heart. See also *digitalis glycosides.*

cardiac index the cardiac output per square meter of body surface. Under basal conditions, it is equal to 2.5–4.2 $l/min/m^2$.

cardiac massage the rhythmic compression of the heart, either directly or through the closed chest; it is performed to maintain an effective circulation in cardiac asystole or ventricular fibrillation.

When external massage is to be used, the patient is placed in a supine position, and the heel of one hand is placed on the sternum in a position just above the xiphoid process; the heel of the other hand is placed over the first. Downward thrusts of pressure are rhythmically applied, at a rate of 60–80 thrusts/min in an adult, with a force sufficient to depress the sternum 4–5 cm. If the thorax is already open, the ventricles can be squeezed manually to deliver blood into the aorta (open chest massage).

cardiac muscle see *cardiac m.* under *muscle.*

cardiac output (CO) the volume of blood delivered from the left ventricle into the aorta per unit of time, generally expressed in liters per minute (l/min). It is equal to the product of the stroke volume and the heart rate. Because it increases in direct proportion to body surface area, the normal resting value of cardiac output varies from approximately 4.5–6.0 l/min in the average adult. The Fick oxygen and indicator-dilution methods are the techniques most commonly used to measure this quantity.

cardiac output measurements the methods used to measure the volume of blood pumped by the heart each minute. Two of the most generally accepted techniques used in cardiac catheterization laboratories are based on the Fick principle: the Fick oxygen method and the indicator-dilution method. A third method utilizes radionuclide scanning.

FICK OXYGEN METHOD. In this procedure, the cardiac output (CO), measured in liters per minute, is equal to the O_2 consumption, measured in milliliters per minute, divided by arteriovenous O_2 difference across the lungs, measured in milliliters per liter of blood. The O_2 consumption is estimated by measuring the amount of O_2 extracted by the lungs per unit of time. The arteriovenous O_2 difference is the difference in oxygen saturation of the mixed venous and arterial blood. Arterial blood can be sampled from any convenient artery. Mixed venous blood is best sampled from the pulmonary artery. The O_2 saturation of the sampled blood is measured by standard laboratory techniques.

INDICATOR-DILUTION METHOD. A small bolus of indicator (usually a dye such as indocyanine green) is injected into the pulmonary artery or a large vein. A peripheral artery is sampled to record the concentration of the dye during its first pass (and subsequent recirculation). This information is used to chart a time-concentration curve of the dye in the artery. CO (in milliliters per minute) can then be calculated through use of the following equation: $CO = (i \times 60)/(\bar{c} \times t)$, where i is the amount of dye injected (in milligrams), $\bar{c}$ is the mean concentration of the dye in each milliliter of blood during its first pass, and t is the duration (in seconds) of the first-pass curve. Through planimetry, $\bar{c} \times t$ can be determined as the area under the first-pass curve. Computer methods are also available for performing all necessary calculations. Another more commonly used indicator-dilution technique, thermodilution, utilizes cold saline as an indicator. The saline is continually infused via a catheter, and the temperature of the blood-injectate mixture downstream from the injection site is monitored via a thermistor that is affixed to the outside of the catheter. The cardiac output is a function of the flow rate of the injected saline, multiplied by the quantity $[(T_B - T_I)/(T_B - T_M) - 1]$, where T_B, T_I, and T_M are the body, injectate, and blood-injectate mixture temperatures, respectively. Use of the thermodilution technique is particularly appropriate when repeated cardiac output measurements must be performed.

RADIONUCLIDE METHOD. In nuclear medicine, in vivo cardiac output can be measured as follows: a bolus of radioactive tracer (generally ^{99m}Tc human serum albumin) is injected into a vein, passes through the heart, and equilibrates throughout the blood within 10 min. Activity over the heart is counted throughout the first passage of the bolus and is then counted at equilibrium using a scintillation probe or a scintillation camera that has computerized data analysis. The cardiac output is the equilibrium activity multiplied by the total blood volume divided by the integrated activity measured during the first pass of the bolus.

Cardiac output can also be calculated from measurements made by quantitative left ventricular angiography; see also *blood volume measurements* and *Fick principle.*

cardiac shunt detection a nuclear medicine procedure involving radionuclide angiocardiography. Shunts can be detected with the serial scinitillation photographs or the time-activity curves produced by a gamma camera that has computerized data analysis.

A right-to-left shunt is indicated when activity from an intravenously injected bolus reaches the aorta as it reaches the lungs.

A left-to-right shunt is indicated when the lung activity persists owing to recirculation through the shunt after activity appears in the aorta. The C_2/C_1 ratio (the activity at twice the peak time divided by the peak activity) provides a qualitative measure; a ratio greater than 35 percent indicates a shunt. An improvement on this is the QP/QS ratio (the ratio of pulmonary to systemic circulation), which is calculated by the computer from the areas under the lung recirculation peak to the area under the initial peak.

cardiac silhouette an image of the heart on a radiograph. See also *cardiomegaly.*

cardiac tamponade a pathologic compression or constriction of the heart caused by an accumulation of fluid within the relatively noncompliant pericardial sac. If uncorrected, pericardial tamponade can initially lead to impairment in filling of the right ventricle, resulting in a compromised stroke volume and cardiac output, and then to a drop in systemic arterial pressure. Coronary artery filling pressure and coronary blood flow decrease, leading to myocardial ischemia and a further decline in myocardial function.

Pericardial tamponade occurs in acute and chronic forms, depending on the underlying cause of the fluid accumulation. The acute form may result from hemopericardium (owing to such factors as pericardial tumors, chest wall trauma, acute myocardial infarction, and aortic aneurysm) or from an acute pericarditis of diverse etiologies. Parasitic and tuberculous infections, and various noninfectious conditions such as myxedema, uremia, neoplasia, and irradiation, can lead to the chronic form.

The constellation of physical manifestations most characteristic of tamponade are decreased arterial and pulse pressure, elevation of the systemic venous pressure (often visible as a noticeable distention of the cervical veins and a steep x and/or y descent on the jugular venous pulse), paradoxical pulse (a drop in systolic arterial pressure greater than 10 mmHg during inspiration), and a decrease in the intensity of heart sounds upon auscultation.

In general, radiographic and electrocardiographic features of pericardial tamponade are neither specific nor diagnostic. Electrical alternans (a change in the amplitude of the QRS complex occurring with every other beat) may be seen. More valuable diagnostic procedures include echocardiography and right heart catheterization. The nature of clinical management depends on the etiology of the tamponade and the physical status of the patient. In those acutely affected, pericardiocentesis and hemodynamic support may be essential before other time-consuming diagnostic and therapeutic measures can be carried out.

cardioangiography (kar″de-o-an″je-og′rah-fe) [*cardio-* + Gr. *angeion* vessel + *graphein* to record] see *angiocardiography.*

Cardiobacterium (kar″de-o-bak-te′re-um) [*cardio-* + Gr. *baktērion* small rod] a genus of bacteria consisting of faculatively anaerobic rods that are gram-negative, possibly with some stain retention. The organisms are part of the normal flora of the nose and throat and are a causative agent of endocarditis. They are pleomorphic, frequently occur in rosette clusters, and are oxidase-positive, catalase-negative, and nonmotile. Acid is produced from glucose, mannitol, sucrose, and maltose, but not from xylose or lactose. The genus contains a single species, *C. hominis.*

cardiocentesis (kar″de-o-sen-te′sis) [*cardio-* + Gr.

kentēsis puncture] surgical puncture of a chamber of the heart.

Cardiografin (kar″de-o-graf′in) trademark. See under *diatrizoate.*

cardiogram (kar′de-o-gram″) [*cardio-* + Gr. *gramma* a writing] a tracing of a cardiac event produced by cardiography. See also *electrocardiogram.*

cardiography (kar″de-og′rah-fe) [*cardio-* + Gr. *graphein* to record] the graphic recording of a physical or functional aspect of the heart; see *echocardiography, electrocardiography, phonocardiography,* and *vectorcardiography.*

cardiolipin (kar″de-o-lip′in) [*cardio-* + Gr. *lipos* fat] 1,3-bisphosphatidylglycerol, a substance extracted from beef hearts and an important lipid component of mammalian tissue membranes. It is used as an antigen in serologic flocculation and precipitation tests for syphilis. Why infection with the treponeme of syphilis produces antibody (Wassermann) to a normal constituent of host tissue is not understood, but it appears to be an autoimmune response. Also called *Wassermann antigen.* See also *Wassermann reaction.*

cardiology (kar″de-ol′o-je) [*cardio-* + *-logy*] the study of the heart and its functions.

cardiomegaly (kar″de-o-meg′ah-le) [*cardio-* + Gr. *megas* large] enlargement of the heart or portions of it, an indication of the presence of cardiovascular disease and dysfunction. Cardiomegaly frequently occurs secondary to (and may be the first obvious manifestation of) cardiovascular disorders such as pulmonary hypertension, coronary heart disease, valvular disease, left ventricular failure, arteriovenous fistulas, and cardiomyopathy. Its presence can be detected clinically by electrocardiography, echocardiography, and radiologic (calculation of the relative cardiac volume) and angiographic examination. Also called *cardiac dilation* and *cardiac enlargement.* See also *relative cardiac volume.*

cardiomyopathy (kar″de-o-mi-op′ah-the) [*cardio-* + Gr. *mys* muscle + *pathos* disease] an array of diseases principally involving the myocardium. Primary cardiomyopathies are those in which the underlying pathologic process (if known) directly affects the myocardium, rather than any other structures. Secondary cardiomyopathies are those in which other cardiovascular abnormalities or pathologic processes (e.g., hypertension or sarcoidosis) lead to the myocardial abnormalities.

Cardiomyopathies can be classified as functional or etiologic. The functional impairments can be divided into three categories: hypertrophic, restrictive, and congestive. Etiologies of cardiomyopathies include infiltrative, metabolic (nutritional, due to electrolyte imbalance or altered metabolism or endocrine), fibroplastic, hematologic, toxic, inflammatory, genetic, and idiopathic processes.

Individual cardiomyopathies frequently provide a distinct hemodynamic and clinical picture that allows for positive diagnosis by techniques such as cardiac catheterization, radionuclide scanning studies, electrocardiography, echocardiography and phonocardiography, and the chest x-ray.

For more information, see the specific cardiomyopathy, e.g., *alcoholic cardiomyopathy, amyloidosis, anthracycline cardiotoxicity, idiopathic hypertrophic s. s.* under *subaortic stenosis, Löffler's endocarditis,* and *sarcoidosis.*

Adriamycin c., see *anthracycline cardiotoxicity.*

cardioplegia (kar″de-o-ple′je-ah) [*cardio-* + Gr. *plēgē* stroke + *ia*] interruption of myocardial contraction, as by use of chemical compounds or cold in cardiac surgery.

cardiopulmonary (kar″de-o-pul′mo-ner-e) [*cardio-* + L. *pulmo, pulmonis* lung] pertaining to the heart and lungs.

cardiopulmonary resuscitation (CPR) see *artificial respiration.*

cardiospasm (kar′de-o-spazm″) a neuromotor disorder that affects the lower two-thirds of the esophagus. It is characterized by failure of the esophagogastric sphincter to function with swallowing and, in extreme cases, by obstructive regurgitation. As a result of the uncoordinated and ineffective neuromuscular activity, the vestibule (lowermost portion) of the esophagus may remain contracted despite an oncoming peristaltic wave. The esophagus may become progressively elongated, flaccid, dilated, and sometimes tortuous (megaesophagus). The genesis of cardiospasm may involve a functional or anatomic abnormality in the parasympathetic innervation of Auerbach's plexus. Also called *achalasia.*

cardiotachometer (kar″de-o-tah-kom′ĕ-ter) [*cardio-* + Gr. *tachos* speed + *metron* measure] an instrument for continuously portraying or recording the heart rate.

cardiotocography (kar″de-o-to-kog′rah-fe) [*cardio-* + Gr. *tokos* childbirth + *graphein* to record] the monitoring of the fetal heart rate and uterine contractions, as during delivery.

cardiotoxic (kar″de-o-tok′sik) [*cardio-* + Gr. *toxicon* poison] having a poisonous or deleterious effect on the heart.

cardiovascular (kar″de-o-vas′ku-lar) [*cardio-* + L. *vasculum* vessel] pertaining to the heart and blood vessels.

cardiovascular system the heart and blood vessels considered together; see *circulatory system.*

cardioversion (kar″de-o-ver′zhun) [*cardio-* + L. *vertere* to turn] a treatment for certain arrhythmias by the delivery of a brief electric shock to the heart through two paddle electrodes placed on the chest wall or the exposed heart. It can be used as an elective procedure to convert paroxysmal supraventricular tachycardia, ventricular tachycardia, atrial flutter, or atrial fibrillation to a normal sinus rhythm. Cardioversion differs from the emergency procedure using electric discharge to convert ventricular fibrillation (*defibrillation*) in that the shock with cardioversion is programmed to avoid the vulnerable period of the cardiac cycle. This is usually accomplished by having the QRS of the electrocardiogram trigger the discharge.

cardioverter (kar″de-o-ver′ter) a machine that delivers a direct-current shock to restore normal sinus rhythm in atrial fibrillation and other arrhythmias.

cardiovirus (kar″de-o-vi′rus) a picornavirus that causes a rare cephalomyocarditis in humans. See also *picornavirus.*

carditis (kar-di′tis) [*cardio* + *itis*] an inflammation of the heart. See also *endocarditis* and *myocarditis.*

card punch a computer output device that punches data output by the program into punched cards.

card reader a computer input device that reads punched cards, which are stacked in a hopper and fed past a row of 12 photocells that sense the punches in each column of the card. A card reader that can also punch cards (after they are read) is called a card read punch. See also *mark sense reader.*

Carey's Ranvier technique (ka′rēz) a variant of Ranvier's gold chloride method for staining motor end-plates and peripheral nerve endings. Thin slices of muscle are incubated for a short time in fresh lemon juice before being transferred into a gold chloride solution. After toning in gold chloride, the tissue is reduced in formic acid. Nerve fibers and endings appear black on a background that ranges from red to purple.

caries (ka′re-ēz, kār′ēz) [L. "rottenness"] the decay of the calcified tissues of the teeth. The major etiologic factor in dental caries is dental plaque, which consists of acidogenic bacteria in a glucan matrix that adheres to the surface of the teeth. In the presence of carbohydrates, acidogenic bacteria produce acid that demineralizes the enamel and dentin of the teeth.

carina (kah-ri′nah, kah-re′nah), pl. *carinae* [L. "keel"] a ridgelike structure.

c. of trachea, a prominent, hook-shaped process of the lowest tracheal cartilage, which forms a prominent ridge between the two bronchi.

carinate (kar′ĭ-nāt) [L. *carina* a keel] keel-shaped (ridged); having a keel-shaped process.

cariogenesis (kār″e-o-jen′e-sis) the development of caries.

carisoprodol (kar-i″so-pro′dol) the *N*-isopropyl derivative of meprobamate, used as an analgesic and skeletal muscle relaxant. High concentrations result in central nervous system depression and, with increasing amounts, drowsiness, double vision, and increased heart rate.

carmalum (kar-mal′um) see *carmine.*

carmine (kar′min) a red stain; C.I. 75470. It is the dye lake formed by the mordant dye carminic acid complexed with an aluminum salt. Carmine was formerly employed as a nuclear stain, but is now primarily used in Best's carmine stain for glycogen and the mucicarmine stain for mucin. Also called *alum carmine* and *carmalum.*

chrome alum c., a dark blue nuclear stain that contains carmine with chrome alum as a mordant. Eosin or van Gieson's picrofuchsin is used as a counterstain.

lithium c., a solution containing carmine and thymol dissolved in saturated lithium carbonate solution. It is used in the Gram-Weigert stain.

carmine gelatin mass an injectable gelatin mass used in histology to make casts of the vasculature of an organ or tissue. It is composed of a neutral mixture of carmine, ammonia, and gelatin.

carminic acid (kar-min′ik) a natural red mordant dye; C.I. 75470. It is extracted from cochineal, dried insects of the species *Coccus cacti.* See also *carmine.*

carmustine (kar-mus′tēn) a cancer chemotherapeutic drug. For more information, see *Appendix A.*

carnitine (kar′ni-tin) L-3-hydroxy-4-(trimethylammonium) butyrate, a compound that serves as an acyl carrier, transporting acyl groups across the inner mitochondrial membrane and equilibrating acyl CoA on both sides of the membrane. See also *acylcarnitine.*

carnosinase (kar′no-sĭ-nās) see *aminoacyl-histidine dipeptidase.*

carnosine (kar′no-sin) a dipeptide, β-alanylhistidine, composed of β-alanine and histidine and found in the skeletal muscle of vertebrates.

carnosinemia (kar″no-sĭ-ne″me ah) [*carnosine* + Gr. *haima* blood + *-ia*] an inherited condition, transmitted as an autosomal recessive trait, that is characterized by the presence of excessive amounts of carnosine in the blood and urine. Caused by a genetic deficiency of the enzyme carnosinase (aminoacyl-histidine dipeptidase), carnosinemia results in progressive neurologic damage, severe mental retardation, and myoclonic seizures.

carnosinuria (kar″no-sĭ-nu′re-ah) [*carnosine* + Gr. *ouron* urine + *-ia*] an aminoaciduria characterized by excess of carnosine in the urine; it occurs in carnosinemia or may be dietary in origin, especially in young children.

Carnoy's fixative (kar′noiz) an alcohol–acetic acid or alcohol–chloroform–acetic acid fixative; see under *fixative.*

carotene (kar′o-tēn) [L. *carota* carrot] one of four isomeric pigments (α-, β-, γ-, and δ-carotene), having colors from violet to red-yellow to yellow, found in many fruits and vegetables such as carrots, sweet potatoes, and leafy vegetables. They are fat-soluble, unsaturated aliphatic hydrocarbons that are converted to vitamin A in animals by an enzyme in the intestinal wall and the liver. β-Carotene is the major precursor (provitamin) of vitamin A in humans. The reference range for β-carotene in serum depends on the method used but is about 60–200 μg/100 ml.

carotene assays see *vitamin A and carotene assays.*

carotenemia (kar″o-te-ne′me-ah) [*carotene* + Gr. *haima* blood + *-ia*] the presence of carotene in the blood, sometimes occurring in sufficient amounts to cause yellowing of the skin.

carotenoid (kah-rot′ĕ-noid) any of a group of pigments, yellow to deep red in color, that chemically consist of tetraterpene (polyisoprene) hydrocarbons. Carotenoids are synthesized in plants (giving color to the tomato and carrot, for example) and in some animals; they concentrate in animal fat when eaten (where they are called lipochromes). Examples are β-carotene, lycopene, and xanthophyll.

carotid (kah-rot′id) [Gr. *karōtis,* from *karos* deep sleep] relating to the carotid artery, the principal artery of the neck.

carotid artery, common one of the principal arteries of the head and neck. The right artery begins at the bifurcation of the brachiocephalic artery; the left arises from the aortic arch. Each ascends in the neck to divide at the level of the upper border of the thyroid cartilage into external and internal carotid arteries. The carotid sinus is a dilation of the vessel at the site of its bifurcation, and may be confined to the proximal internal carotid artery. The carotid body lies behind the point of division of the common carotid artery.

carotid artery, external an artery that arises from the common carotid at the level of the upper border of the thyroid cartilage. It passes upward and forward, then backward, and in the parotid gland divides into the superficial temporal and maxillary arteries.

carotid artery, internal an artery that begins at the bifurcation of the common carotid artery, ascends to the base of the skull, and passes through the carotid canal in the temporal bone to enter the cavernous sinus. It supplies the greater part of the cerebrum and the eye, together with adjacent tissues.

carotid body a small neurovascular structure that lies in the bifurcation of each common carotid artery. It contains innervated epithelial cells that are sensitive to the oxygen and carbon dioxide tensions and pH of the blood: decreased O_2 tension, or an increased CO_2 tension and decreased pH, generate an increased frequency of nerve impulses to the brain, resulting in appropriate respiratory and cardiovascular compensatory responses. The epithelial cells of the carotid body are chemoreceptors, containing numerous small, dense granules that represent stored catecholamines and 5-hydroxytryptamine. Also called *glomus caroticum.*

carotid sinus a dilation of the internal carotid artery above its site of origin at the carotid bifurcation. Pressure-sensitive afferent nerve terminals (baroreceptors), which arborize in its wall, initiate reflex adjustments in cardiovascular function that buffer transient changes in blood pressure.

carotid sinus syndrome the occurrence of faintness or loss of consciousness (carotid sinus syncope) brought about by an accentuated reflex response (a bradycardia and peripheral vasodilation) to carotid sinus stimulation. Enlargement of the lymph nodes in the neck, a tight collar, or any factor that causes pressure to be exerted within or on the carotid sinus can evoke the episodes. This exaggerated response may be due to an increase in the sensitivity of the carotid sinus baroreflex caused by aging, arteriosclerosis, or drugs such as digitalis. See also *carotid sinus r.* under *reflex.*

carp/o (kar′po) [L., from Gr. *karpos*] a word element used in combining form to denote the carpus (wrist), e.g., carpal.

carpal tunnel syndrome (kar′pal) a peripheral entrapment neuropathy that occurs when the median nerve is compressed as it passes through the carpal tunnel at the wrist. Any factor that reduces the diameter of the tunnel or increases the size of its contents can lead to the syndrome. The principal symptoms—pain, paresthesia, and muscle weakness—tend to increase in severity at night. Surgical decompression may be required for relief of the symptoms.

carpus (kar′pus) [L., from Gr. *karpos*] [NA], the eight small bones of the wrist that are interposed between the distal ends of the radius and ulna proximally and the metacarpal bones distally. From lateral to medial, the proximal row of carpal bones is made up of the scaphoid, lunate, triquetral, and pisiform; the distal row contains the trapezium, trapezoid, capitate, and hamate.

carrier (kar′e-er) 1. an instrument or apparatus for transporting something.

2. an individual who harbors the specific organism of a disease without noticeable symptoms and thus acts as a transmitter of the infection; the condition of such a person is known as carrier state.

3. referring to an electron carrier, a substance in a cell that can accept one or two electrons and so be reduced and then be reoxidized.

4. in genetics, one who carries a recessive gene, either autosomal or sex-linked, together with its normal allele, i.e., one who is heterozygous for a recessive gene. As female carriers of X-linked disorders are mosaics of affected and normal cells, special carrier tests are sometimes available, e.g., for muscular dystrophy and hemophilia. See also *Lyon hypothesis.*

5. in nuclear medicine, a substance to which a radioisotope label can be attached and by which it is carried in the body (e.g., albumin and red blood cells are used to carry ^{99m}Tc).

6. also in nuclear medicine, an unwanted isotope that will compete with the useful isotope, when labeling a compound; ^{99}Tc is a carrier of ^{99m}Tc. Pure isotope is said to be carrier-free.

7. a molecule to which a substance may be reversibly attached for transport, as across an intracellular membrane.

8. in immunology, a substance (usually a protein) that can join with a hapten, thereby enabling the hapten to stimulate an immune response.

carrier-free in nuclear medicine, a term used to describe the pure form of a radioisotope of an element that is essentially undiluted by its stable isotopes.

carrier gas in gas chromatography, an inert gas such as nitrogen or helium that carries the sample molecules through the column.

carrier-mediated transport see *active transport* and *facilitated diffusion.*

carrier protein a protein that serves to transport a specific molecule or group of molecules in blood, in body fluids, or in cytoplasm. Specific carrier proteins are known for fatty acids in blood (albumin), fatty acids in cytoplasm (fatty acid binding protein), retinol in blood (retinol binding protein), some anions in blood, anions in cells (ligandin), hormones in blood, haptens in blood, and other substances. Two important carrier proteins are acyl carrier protein, a part of the fatty acid synthetase enzyme complex, which serves to hold the lengthening acyl chain during synthesis; and sterol carrier proteins, several carriers that hold intermediates from squalene to cholesterol during the biosynthesis of cholesterol.

Carrión's disease (kar-e-onz′) [Daniel A. *Carrión,* a student in Peru who inoculated himself and died of the disease, 1850–1885] see *bartonellosis.*

cartilage (kar″tĭ-lij) [L. *cartilago*] a specialized fibrous connective tissue that serves as temporary or permanent skeletal tissue. Cartilage forms a temporary fetal skeleton, and functions both as a model and growth mechanism for bone development. The solid but resilient consistency of cartilage is a function of the secretion by its constituent cells (chondrocytes) of complex protein-polysaccharides, forming a gel that accumulates in its matrix, which also includes collagen and elastic fibrils. Types of cartilage include *elastic cartilage, fibrocartilage,* and *hyaline cartilage;* see also *epiphyseal plate.*

cartilage bone any bone that develops within cartilage; in contrast to membrane bone, ossification takes place within a cartilage model. Also called endochondral bone.

caruncle (kar′ung-k′l) [L. *caruncula,* dim. of *caro* flesh] a small fleshy eminence.

hymenal c.'s, small elevations of mucous membrane around the vaginal opening, remnants of the ruptured hymen.

urethral c., a tender, congested nodule of the tissue

adjacent to the female external urethral meatus, where it may be a focus of granulomatous inflammation or a sclerosing hemangioma; seen particularly in older persons.

casanthranol (kah-san′thrah-nōl) a purified extract of cascara sagrada, an irritant cathartic used in laxatives. It contains anthranol glycosides, which are absorbed in the small intestine and hydrolyzed to anthraquinones. These compounds are then excreted into the large intestine, where they increase peristalsis by irritation of the mucosa.

cascade (kas-kād′) any system composed of a group of subsystems acting sequentially in which there is amplification of the signal, information, or effect at each stage. In electronics, the term is applied to multistage amplifiers. In biochemistry, it is applied to pathways in which there is a sequence of enzymes, each of which converts the next one in the sequence to an active form; examples are blood coagulation and the complement system. Because each enzyme molecule can rapidly act on thousands of molecules of substrate, there is a very large gain at each stage. Thus, activation of only a few molecules of the first component of the system can result in formation of macroscopic amounts (on the order of 10^{20} molecules) if there are enough steps in the cascade.

cascara sagrada (kas-kar′ah sah-grah′dah) [Sp. "sacred bark"] [USP], the dried bark of *Rhamnus purshiana,* an irritant cathartic used in laxatives. See also *casanthranol.*

caseation (ka″se-a′shun) [L. *caseus* cheese] the precipitation of the phosphoprotein casein, seen in mycobacterial infection. See also *tuberculosis.*

case-control study see under *retrospective study.*

case history the collected data concerning an individual and his or her family and environment. It usually includes the person's medical history and any other information that may be useful for analytic and diagnostic or instructional purposes.

casein (ka′sēn, ka′se-in) [L. *caseus* cheese] a phosphoprotein that is the principal protein of milk. Casein is used in the diet to enrich the protein content. When treated with acid or certain enzymes, the protein is broken down to small peptides or free amino acids, forming a casein hydrolysate that is used in the preparation of media for bacterial cultures.

casein agar a culture medium made of skim milk. It is principally used to identify *Nocardia asteroides, N. brasiliensis,* and *Streptomyces,* and to differentiate between some agents of mycotic mycetoma.

casein hydrolysate a common source of amino acids for making relatively rich culture media for microorganisms. Acid hydrolysates are usually deficient in tryptophan and glutamine; enzymatic hydrolysates contain all the amino acids.

caseous (ka′se-us) [L. *caseus* cheese] resembling cheese or curd; cheesy.

caseous necrosis see *caseous n.* under *necrosis.*

Casoni's skin test (kah-so′nēz) [Tomaso *Casoni,* Italian physician, 1880–1933] a test for past or present echinococcosis (hydatid disease). Hydatid cyst fluid is injected intradermally; the immediate or delayed production of a wheal-and-flare reaction is a positive response.

cassette (kah-set′) [Fr. "a little box"] 1. a light-proof device for holding x-ray film during exposure, the tube side being a radiolucent material and the back a hinged lead plate. Film is placed between them, sandwiched between two intensifying screens.

2. a light-proof container for holding photographic film.

cast (kast) 1. a rigid casing used for immobilizing a body part.

2. a structure formed by deposition of material in a body cavity so that the deposit takes the form of that cavity. Casts may remain in the site or be dislodged and expelled from the site of formation. Bronchial casts are composed of fibrin that is deposited in bronchioles and expelled in the sputum. Urinary casts, composed of material deposited in renal tubules and washed out in the urine, are associated with various kidney diseases. Casts are further classified by materials trapped in their matrices; for specific types, see under *urinary cast.*

Castellanella (kas″tel-ah-nel′ah) [Sir Aldo *Castellani,* Italian-born physician, 1879–1971] a former name for the genus *Trypanosoma.* See *Trypanosoma.*

Castellania (kas-tel-a′ne-ah) [Sir Aldo *Castellani*] an obsolete name for the genus *Candida;* see *Candida.*

casting (kast′ing) see under *embedding.*

castor bean (kas′tor) the common name for *Ricinus communis,* a plant grown for ornamental purposes and for its oil (castor oil, ricinus oil). A powerful allergen called pomace is formed during extraction of the castor oil. The seeds of the bean are highly toxic; ingestion may produce vomiting, collapse, convulsions, bleeding from the lungs and mucous membranes, and possibly death. Inhalation of the dust irritates the respiratory tract, and contact causes dermatitis and urticaria.

castor oil [USP], a fixed oil obtained from the seed of *Ricinus communis,* used internally as a cathartic and externally as an emollient in seborrheic dermatitis and other skin diseases.

castrate (kas′trāt) to deprive an individual of the gonads, rendering that individual incapable of reproduction.

castration (kas-tra′shun) excision of the gonads, or their destruction by agents such as radiation or infection.

female c., removal of the ovaries, or bilateral oophorectomy.

male c., removal of the testes, or bilateral orchiectomy.

castration cells enlarged and vacuolated anterior pituitary gonadotropes in gonadal insufficiency or castration.

CAT acronym from computerized axial tomography, the former name for *computed tomography.*

cata- (kat′ah) [Gr. *kata* down] a prefix word element to denote down, lower, under, against, or along with, e.g., catabolism.

catabolic (kat″ah-bol′ik) pertaining to catabolism; destructive. Cf. *anabolic.*

catabolism (kah-tab′o-lizm) [Gr. *katabolē* a throwing down] any destructive process by which complex substances are converted by living cells into simpler compounds with the liberation of energy.

catabolite (kah-tab′o-lit) any product of catabolism or of a destructive metabolic process.

catabolite activator protein (kah-tab′o-līt ak′tĭ-va″tor) a protein required for initiation of transcription in RNA synthesis. It binds cAMP and then complexes with the promoter of the operon as a prerequisite to action of RNA polymerase.

catacrotism (kah-tak′ro-tizm) [*cata-* + Gr. *krotos* beat] a pulse anomaly in which a small additional wave or notch appears in the descending limb of the pulse tracing.

catalase (kat′ah-lās) an enzyme of the oxidoreductase class (hydrogen-peroxide:hydrogen-peroxide oxidoreductase, EC 1.11.1.6.) that catalyzes the reaction $2H_2O_2 \rightleftarrows O_2 + 2H_2O$. It is widely distributed, with high activity in the liver, kidneys, and erythrocytes. Its catalytic action is one of the fastest of any known enzyme; presumably it functions to protect the cell constituents from hydrogen peroxide formed by various oxidation reactions. Catalase is found in almost all cells, except for certain bacteria such as most obligate anaerobes and the lactic acid bacteria. Its determination has diagnostic applications in cases of oral gangrene resulting from a genetic deficiency of the enzyme, transmitted as an autosomal recessive trait. In microbiology, production of this enzyme is used to differentiate between the genera of *Streptococcus* and *Staphylococcus.*

catalase test a test for the production of catalase by bacteria. A slant culture (incubated at 35°C for 18–24 hr) is treated with 3 percent hydrogen peroxide. The presence of gas bubbles indicates a positive reaction. Micrococci, staphylococci, most species of *Bacillus,* and anaerobic diphtheroids are catalase-positive; streptococci, pneumococci, and most *Actinomyces* are catalase-negative.

catalepsy (kat′ah-lep″se) [Gr. *katalēsis*] a condition of diminished responsiveness usually characterized by a trancelike state and muscle rigidity; an individual remains passive in any position. Catalepsy may occur in organic and psychologic disorders and under hypnosis.

catalysis (kah-tal′ĭ-sis) [Gr. *katalysis* dissolution] the increase in the velocity of a chemical reaction or process that is produced by the presence of a substance not itself consumed or permanently altered in the process.

catalyst (kat′ah-list) any substance that brings about catalysis; i.e., it can increase the rate at which a chemical reaction will proceed without affecting the equilibrium state for the reaction. The catalyst is neither consumed nor altered during the reaction. Inorganic catalysts are used extensively in industrial processes and in laboratory determinations. A protein catalyst of biologic origin is called an enzyme. See also *enzyme.*

negative c., a term used incorrectly to describe a decrease in the velocity of a chemical reaction, produced by a substance that is not itself consumed. "True" negative catalysts do not exist, because these compounds are either changed in the course of the reaction, or force the reaction to take its normal, uncatalyzed pathway. Inhibitors are sometimes incorrectly called negative catalysts. See also *inhibitors.*

catalytic (kat″ah-lit′ik) [Gr. *katalyein* to dissolve] causing catalysis.

catalyze (kat′ah-līz) to cause or produce catalysis.

catalyzer (kat′ah-līz″er) see *catalyst.*

catamnesis (kat″am-ne′sis) [*cata-* + Gr. *mnēsis* remembering] the follow-up history of a patient after discharge from treatment or a hospital.

cataphasia (kat″ah-fa′ze-ah) [*cata-* + Gr. *phasis* speech] a speech disorder marked by constant repetition of a word or phrase.

cataphoresis (kat″ah-fo-re′sis) [*cata* + Gr. *phorēsis* bearing] the passage of charged particles toward the negative pole (cathode) in electrophoresis.

cataphoretic (kat″ah-fo-ret′ik) of, or referring to, cataphoresis.

cataplectic (kat″ah-plek′tik) 1. pertaining to or characterized by cataplexy.
2. having a sudden, overwhelming onset.

cataplexy (kat′ah-plek″se) [Gr. *kataplēxis* amazement] a condition in which there are abrupt attacks of muscular weakness and hypotonia triggered by an emotional stimulus such as mirth, anger, fear, or surprise. It is often associated with narcolepsy. Also called cataplexis.

Catapres (kat′ah-pres) trademark. See *clonidine hydrochloride.*

cataract (kat′ah-rakt) [L. *cataracta,* from Gr. *katarrhēgnynai* to break down] an opacity of the lens of the eye or its capsule. Most cataracts are due to the natural aging process of the body, but they may also be caused by injury to the eye, exposure to intense heat or radiation, intrauterine infection of the fetus, side-effects of certain drugs, or inherited factors. The only effective treatment available at present is surgical removal.

catatonia (kat″ah-to′ne-ah) [*cata-* + Gr. *tonos* tension + *-ia*] a condition marked by: (1) excessive and sometimes violent motor activity and excitement, or (2) generalized inhibition of motor activity with stupor and marked muscle rigidity or flexibility. It may be a major diagnostic cue to catatonic schizophrenia or severe anxiety neurosis.

cat-bite fever an infectious disease of humans caused by *Pasteurella multocida;* it is transmitted by the bite of a cat and marked by the formation of an abscess at the site of inoculation. It should not be confused with cat-scratch disease.

cat's cry syndrome see *cri du chat syndrome.*

catechol (kat′e-kol) *o*-dihydroxybenzene, a compound that gives the catecholamines their name. The name catechol is shortened from pyrocatechol; the term originally referred to a larger compound catechin from which pyrocatechol is derived by heating.

catecholamine (kat″ĕ-kol-am′in) one of the dihydroxyphenylalkylamines, a group of compounds (dopamine, norepinephrine, and epinephrine) serving as hormones and neurotransmitters, that are found in the adrenal medulla, neurons, and brain; they are synthesized in a chain of reactions starting with L-tyrosine. This precursor is hydroxylated to 3,4-dihydroxyphenylalanine (dopa), which is then decarboxylated to dopamine. Norepinephrine acts as a neurotransmitter in other regions of the central nervous system and in sympathetic postganglionic neurons. The adrenal medulla has almost the exclusive capacity to convert norepinephrine to epinephrine, which is the true medullary hormone, and has important effects on metabolism, as well as on the cardiovascular system.

The metabolism of catecholamines occurs via two major processes, catechol-O-methylation and *N*-deamination. These result in a mixture of products such as metanephrine, normetanephrine, and vanillylmandelic acid (VMA) from epinephrine and norepinephrine, and homovanillic acid (HVA) from dopamine. The plasma concentration of catecholamines and their urinary metabolites indicate the functional status of the adrenal medulla and may also indicate the overall peripheral sympathetic activity.

The plasma concentration of catecholamines reflects the balance between synthesis, release, uptake, catabolism, and excretion at the time of sampling. The urinary concentration of the catecholamines and their metabolites is an indication of the overall long-term activity of the sympathetic system. Assay methods are available for catecholamines proper (total or individual catecholamines) in plasma and in urine. Methods for catecholamine metabolites such as vanillylmandelic acid (VMA), homovanillic acid (HVA), and metanephrines are primarily applied to urine specimens.

Reference ranges for catecholamines in urine, using the trihydroxy indole (fluorometric) method are: for norepinephrine, 30 ± 13 (1 SD) μg/da, and for epinephrine, 5.6 ± 3.1. Free catecholamines in urine, using high-pressure liquid chromatography with electrochemical detection, are: for norepinephrine, 14–80 μg/da; for epinephrine, 0.5–20; and for dopamine, 65–400. Reference ranges for catecholamines in plasma, using a radioenzymatic assay, are: for epinephrine, less than 88 pg/ml; for norepinephrine, 104–548; and for dopamine, less than 136. Values are lower in the supine position. Increased values of norepinephrine are found in individuals with certain neural tumors. Values for total urinary metanephrines are: 0.3–0.9 mg/da; and for urinary VMA 1.8–7.1 mg/d or 1.5–7.0 μg/mg of creatinine.

See also *dopamine, epinephrine, metanephrine,* and *norepinephrine.*

catecholamine assays 1. radioenzymatic assay of unconjugated catecholamines in plasma, spinal fluid, or urine. The enzyme catechol-O-methyltransferase catalyzes the transfer of a radiolabeled methyl group from ^{3}H-methyl-*S*-adenosyl-L-methionine to norepinephrine, epinephrine, and dopamine. Thin-layer chromatography is subsequently utilized to isolate the resulting methylated derivatives, normetanephrine, metanephrine, and 3-methoxytyramine. Some procedures separately oxidize the two metanephrines to vanillin before counting. Methoxytyramine is not oxidized by periodate and is counted directly after chromatography.

2. radioimmunoassay of total catecholamines in plasma or urine utilizing an antibody that completely crossreacts with metanephrine. Following hydrolysis of the conjugates, two procedures are used to quantitate the free amines. One procedure measures metanephrines following enzymatic conversion of epinephrine to metanephrine, whereas the other first converts norepinephrine to epinephrine to yield a total measurement of both amines. Subtraction then gives a measure of norepinephrine.

3. liquid chromatography with electrochemical detection. Unconjugated catecholamines are specifically extracted and purified from biological fluids by several methods including alumina adsorption, cation exchange chromatography, boric acid–gel adsorption, or ion-pair partition chromatography. The purified amines are resolved using reverse phase high-pressure liquid chromatography and quantitated by amperometric detection.

categorical data (kat″ĕ-gor′ĭ-kal) data composed of observations described only as belonging to one of several categories. See also *scale.*

catharsis (kah-thar′sis) [Gr. *katharsis* a cleaning] 1. a cleansing or purgation.

2. the bringing into consciousness and the emotional reliving of a forgotten (repressed) painful experience as means of releasing anxiety and tension.

catheter (kath′ĕ-ter) [Gr. *kathetēr*] a flexible tube introduced into a blood vessel or the lumen of a hollow organ for the purpose of introducing or removing fluids, or performing certain measurements. The term is often used to refer to a urinary catheter, introduced into the bladder via the urethra.

catheterization (kath″ĕ-ter-ĭ-za′shun) the employment or passage of a catheter.

cathexis (kah-thek′sis) [Gr. *kathexis*] the amount of mental or emotional energy spent on an object, idea, or function.

cathode (kath′ōd) [Gr. *kata* down + *hodos* way] 1. in an electrochemical cell, the electrode at which the reduction half-reaction occurs, i.e., the negative electrode of an electrolytic cell and the positive electrode of a voltaic cell. Cf. *anode.*

2. the negative electrode of devices such as electron tubes, x-ray tubes and electrophoretic cells.

3. the electrode through which a current leaves a nerve or other substance.

4. a terminal of a junction diode, silicon-controlled rectifier, or silicon-controlled switch.

cathode ray electrons produced from the cathode of an x-ray, gas, or vacuum tube and moving at high speed in straight lines unless deflected by a magnetic or electric field.

cathode-ray tube (CRT) a vacuum tube used in oscilloscopes, computer terminals, and television sets to produce images. A beam of electrons emitted from the cathode and accelerated and focused by anode elements is directed by an electric or magnetic field to a position on a phosphor-coated screen that glows when hit by the beam.

cathodoluminescence (kath″o-do-loo″mĭ-nes′ens) the emission of light by a material when it is bombarded by high-energy electrons. Examples are the image on a television set or on the fluorescent screen of a transmission electron microscope. In the scanning electron microscope, cathodoluminescence can be used to image uncoated specimens, provided the detector is sufficiently sensitive; however, the image is of low resolution and intensity, and fades rapidly because of beam damage and contamination of the surface of the specimen.

cation (kat′i-on) [Gr. *kata* down + *iōn* going] a positively charged ion; a chemical moiety with a deficiency of one or more electrons. Under the influence of an applied electric field, cations migrate to the negative electrode (cathode). Symbols for cations indicate the numerical values of the charge of the ion, e.g., NH_4^+ (ammonium) or Fe^{3+} (ferric ion). Cf. *anion.*

cation-exchange resin see under *ion-exchange resin.*

cationic dye (kat″i-on′ik) see *basic dye.*

cation interference in flame photometry, erroneous readings due to the presence of cations in the specimen other than the one being measured. These occur because of the direct transfer of energy between excited atoms without the emission of radiation.

cat liver fluke see *O. felineus* under *Opisthorchis.*

cat-scratch disease an acute infectious disease of unknown etiology, usually transmitted by close contact with cats. Young children are most commonly affected, and experience tender regional lymphadenopathy and sterile suppuration. Encephalitis is a rare complication. Laboratory tests often reveal an elevated erythrocyte sedimentation rate and leukocytosis. Eosinophilia may be present. Intradermal skin testing with an antigen preparation from suppurative lymph nodes gives a tuberculin-like reaction. Biopsy of an individual node can confirm the diagnosis. Most cases are benign and self-limited, but lymphadenopathy may persist for several months in the absence of any other symptoms.

caud/o (kaw′do) [L. *cauda* tail] a word element used in combining form to denote a tail or the lower part of the body, e.g., caudal.

cauda (kaw′dah), pl. *caudae* [L.] [NA], a tail or tail-like appendage, or a structure resembling such an appendage.

c. equina, [NA], the loose bundle of spinal nerve roots that descend from the lower spinal cord and lie in the vertebral canal below the cord, surrounding the filum terminale.

c. nuclei caudati, [NA], an arcuate, subcortical mass of gray matter, located within each cerebral hemisphere along the floor of the anterior and central part of the lateral ventricle. Functionally and anatomically one of the basal ganglia, the structure is commonly grouped with the putamen as the striate body. As part of a system for voluntary motor control, it receives and sends projections to a neuronal circuit that originates in the motor cortex, and passes through the basal ganglia and the ventroanterior nucleus of the thalamus, and back to the cortex. Also called *caudate nucleus.*

caudad (kaw′dad) [*caud-* + *-ad*] toward the tail; in human anatomy, toward the feet. Cf. *cephalad* and *craniad.*

caudal (kaw′dal) [L. *cauda* tail] 1. pertaining to a tail.

2. denoting a position more toward the tail; in human anatomy, the same as inferior.

caudate (kaw′dāt) [L. *caudatus*] having a tail.

caudate nucleus see *c. nuclei caudati* under *cauda.*

caumesthesia (kaw″mes-the′ze-ah) [Gr. *kauma* burn + *aisthēsis* perception] a sensation of burning heat even though the body temperature is not elevated.

caus/o (kaw′so) [Gr. *kausos* heat] a word element used in combining form to denote burn, e.g., causalgia.

causalgia (kaw-zal′je-ah) [*caus-* + *-algia*] a persistent, severe burning pain of the skin that may follow traumatic injury to a peripheral nerve.

causative (kawz′ah-tiv) effective or responsible as a cause or agent, e.g. a positive agent in infectious disease.

cause (kawz) [L. *causa*] that which brings about a condition or produces an effect.

caustic (kaws′tik) [L. *causticus,* from Gr. *kaustikos*] 1. burning or corrosive; usually strongly alkaline; destructive to living tissues.

2. chemically similar to sodium hydroxide, as in caustic soda and caustic potash.

3. an escharotic or corrosive agent. Also called *cauterant.*

cauter/o (kaw′ter-o) [L. *cauterium* cautery, from Gr. *kautērion*] a word element used in combining form to denote heat or burn, e.g., cautery.

cauterant (kaw′ter-ant) 1. any caustic material or application.

2. caustic.

cauterization (kaw″ter-ĭ-za′shun) the destruction of tissue by means of heat, electricity, or chemical agents. See also *electrosurgery.*

cautery (kaw′ter-e) [L. *cauterium,* from Gr. *kautērion*] 1. cauterization.

2. an instrument or agent used in cauterization.

caveolae (ka-ve-o′le), sing. *caveola* [L.] small vesicular pits roughly 50 nm in diameter, formed by invagination of the cell membrane in the process of uptake of extracellular material. Also called pinocytotic vesicles.

cavernous sinus one of a pair of intracranial venous channels, approximately 2 cm long by 1 cm wide, which are located on either side of the body of the sphenoid. It is so named because of its spongy composition, which probably reflects a plexiform architecture during development. The cavernous sinus is traversed by the internal carotid artery with its accompanying sympathetic nerves, and is indented by the oculomotor, trochlear, ophthalmic, and maxillary divisions of the trigeminal, and by the abducent nerves.

Blood enters the sinus from the ophthalmic veins, the central vein of the retina, and the cerebral veins, and it drains into the superior and inferior petrosal sinuses and through emissary veins. The cavernous sinuses are connected in front and behind the sella turcica by communicating veins.

Because of its location, the cavernous sinus is vulnerable to the spread of infection from the ear, paranasal sinuses, upper nasal cavity, and face. Cavernous sinus thrombosis is a serious condition that can lead to meningitis or to secondary effects from obstruction of the ophthalmic and retinal veins, or from involvement of the cranial nerves that are intimately related to the sinus wall.

cavitation (kav″ĭ-ta′shun) [L. *cavitas* hollow space] the formation of air- or fluid-filled spaces within the lungs, involving the destruction of lung parenchyma, usually as a sequela of granulomatous disease (tuberculosis or histoplasmosis) or neoplasia.

The central portions of tumors or dense granulomatous disease lose their sustaining blood supply, become necrotic, and are coughed out, to be replaced by air if there are nearby bronchial communications.

cavity (kav′ĭ-te) [L. *cavitas* hollow space] 1. a hollow space or a potential space within the body or an organ.

2. a destructive lesion of the calcified tissues of a tooth; see *dental caries.*

3. see *cavity resonator.*

cavity resonator an enclosed space with metallic walls in which electromagnetic radiation is produced, which has a resonant frequency that is determined by the geometry of the cavity. See also *waveguide.*

cavography (ka-vog'rah-fe) radiographic visualization of the inferior or superior vena cava by injection of a radiopaque medium.

Cb symbol for the chemical element *columbium.*

CB agar abbrev. for chocolate blood agar. See *chocolate a.* under *agar.*

C banding centromeric or constitutive heterochromatin banding; see under *chromosome banding.*

CBC abbrev. See *complete blood count.*

CBG abbrev. for corticosteroid-binding globulin. See *transcortin.*

C cell a pale-staining cell found at the periphery of follicles of the thyroid gland. It makes up fewer than 1 percent of the parenchymal cells of the thyroid. Usually it lies within the follicle, resting on the basal lamina and rarely reaching the lumen. Ultrastructurally, C cells contain numerous dense-core granules roughly 200 nm in caliber. Similar cells form the ultimobranchial body in avian species; in humans, they migrate from the distal pharynx in the early embryo and enter the developing thyroid. The C cell forms calcitonin and is the proliferating cell in medullary carcinoma of the thyroid. Also called *parafollicular cell.*

CCU abbrev. for coronary care unit.

CCV abbrev. See *conductivity cell volume.*

CD abbrev. See *carbonate dehydratase, circular dichroism.*

CD_{50} abbrev. See *median curative d.* under *dose.*

Cd symbol for the chemical element *cadmium.*

cd abbrev. See *candela.*

CDA abbrev. See *congenital dyserythropoietic a.* under *anemia.*

CDC abbrev. See *Center for Disease Control.*

cDNA abbrev. See *complementary DNA.*

CDP abbrev. See *cytidine diphosphate.*

CDP-choline cytidine diphosphate choline, an intermediate in the biosynthesis of phosphatidylcholine and sphingomyelin.

CDP-diglyceride cytidine diphosphate diglyceride, an intermediate in the biosynthesis of phosphatidylglycerols, phosphatidylinositides, and phosphatidylcholines.

CDP-ethanolamine cytidine diphosphate ethanolamine, an intermediate in the biosynthesis of phosphatidylethanolamine.

Cdyn abbrev. See *dynamic c.* under *compliance.*

Ce symbol for the chemical element *cerium.*

CEA abbrev. See *carcinoembryonic antigen.*

cec/o (se'ko) [L. *caecus* blind] a word element used in combining form to denote the cecum (the first part of the large intestine), e.g., cecotomy.

cecal (se'kal) [L. *caecalis*] 1. ending in a blind passage.
2. pertaining to the cecum.
3. pertaining to the blind spot in the field of vision.

cecum (se'kum) [L. *caecus* blind, from *intestinum caecum* blind gut] the pouchlike proximal end of the large intestine, approximately 5 cm long by 7.5 cm wide; it is considered to be the portion of the proximal colon below the level of the ileocecal valve. The cecum is in continuity with the ascending colon: the two merge imperceptibly. The appendix attaches to the base of the cecum where the taenia coli come together. The cecum is located in the right iliac fossa on the psoas muscle, just above the lateral part of the inguinal ligament. Part of the greater omentum may intervene between it and the anterior abdominal wall. The cecum is entirely covered by peritoneum but has no mesentery.

cedar oil (se'dar) a volatile oil from cedar wood, used as a clearing agent in microscopic techniques; the thicker fraction is used as the immersion medium with oil-immersion objectives. It may also be boiled and concentrated for use as a histologic mounting medium.

cefaclor (sef'ah-klōr) a cephalosporin antibiotic active against gram-positive cocci (except enterococci) and gram-negative bacilli, especially *Hemophilus influenzae;* it is more active than cephalexin. Cefaclor can be administered orally. See also *antibacterial agents* and *cephalosporin.*

cefamandole (sef"ah-man'dōl) a second-generation cephalosporin antibiotic with an extended antibacterial spectrum of activity. It is less active against the common gram-positive cocci than cephalothin, but it has an enhanced spectrum against gram-negative bacilli. Organisms inhibited include *Hemophilus influenzae, Enterobacter* species, *Escherichia coli,* and *Klebsiella* species. See also *antibacterial agents* and *cephalosporin.*

cefoperazone (sef"o-per'ah-zōn) a new wide-spectrum parenteral cephalosporin that combines many of the properties of cefamandole and piperacillin; it has as wide an in vitro antibacterial spectrum as either agent, and greater activity than either. Cefoperazone is active against *Hemophilus, Neisseria,* most of Enterobacteriaceae, and the majority of *Pseudomonas aeruginosa* strains. It is less active than cephalothin or cefamandole against *Staphylococcus aureus* and beta-hemolytic streptococci, and less active than piperacillin against enterococci. This agent can be used effectively in the treatment of infections due to enterobacteria, susceptible *P. aeruginosa,* and perhaps *Hemophilus* and *Neisseria.* Urinary excretion is low so that high blood levels occur. See also *antibacterial agents* and *cephalosporins.*

cefotaxime (sef"o-tak'sēm) a semisynthetic cephalosporin antibiotic that has a wider spectrum of antibacterial activity than do previously available cephalosporins. It is parenterally administered. Cefotaxime is highly resistant to degradation by beta-lactamases, and therefore is more active against many strains of enteric gram-negative bacilli, including some multiple drug-resistant strains responsible for hospital-acquired infections. For such infections, this drug may be as effective as some of the aminoglycosides, and less toxic.

cefoxitin (sĕ-foks'ĭ-tin) an antibacterial agent derived from cephamycin. The methoxy group on the beta-lactam ring confers greater resistance to the beta-lactamase of certain gram-negative bacilli. Cefoxitin is more active than cephalothin against certain gram-negative organisms, but is less active against *Enterobacter* species and *Hemophilus influenzae.* Active against *Proteus vulgaris* and *Bacteroides fragilis* in vitro, cefoxitin is less active than cefamandole and other cephalosporins against gram-positive bacteria. See also *antibacterial agents* and *cephamycin.*

-cele (sēl) [Gr. *kēlē* hernia] a suffix word element to denote a hernial swelling or protrusion, e.g., meningocele.

celestin blue B (sĕ-les'tin) a mordant dye used as a histologic stain to demonstrate eosinophil leukocyte granules and to form iron lakes for selective nuclear staining; C.I. 51050.

celi/o (se'le-o) [Gr. *koilia* belly] a word element used in combining form to denote the abdomen, e.g., celiac.

celiac (se'le-ak) [Gr. *koilia* belly] pertaining to the abdomen.

celiac artery a short, wide branch of the abdominal aorta that arises just below the aortic opening of the diaphragm. Less than 2 cm long, it divides into the left gastric, hepatic, and splenic arteries. The celiac artery is embryologically the artery of the foregut, and through its branches it supplies the lower esophagus, stomach, proximal duodenum, liver, gallbladder, pancreas, and spleen.

celiac disease see *celiac s.* under *sprue.*

celiac sprue see *celiac s.* under *sprue.*

celiocentesis (se"le-o-sen-te'sis) [*celio-* + Gr. *kentēsis* puncture] puncture into the abdominal cavity.

celioparacentesis (se"le-o-par"ah-sen-te'sis) [*celio-* + Gr. *para* beyond + *kentēsis* puncture] paracentesis of the abdominal cavity.

celiopathy (se"le-op'ah-the) [*celio-* + Gr. *pathos* disease] a general term for disease of the abdomen.

celioscopy (se"le-os'ko-pe) [*celio-* + Gr. *skopein* to examine] examination of a body cavity, especially the abdominal cavity, through a celioscope.

cell (sel) [L. *cella* compartment] the structural unit of living organisms. A cell is a complex collection of molecules with many different activities that are integrated to form a functional unit. In multicellular organisms, most cells have become specialized to perform specific functions; this usually entails some structural modification, hence the wide variety of sizes and shapes of cells in the human body.

There are two basic classes of cell. They are distinguished on the basis of complexity of structure. The more simple do not possess a nucleus and are termed prokaryotes (*pro-* before + *karyon* nucleus): they include bacteria and cyanobacteria. In contrast, the chromatin material in eukaryotes (*eu-* true) is separated from the rest of the cell by the nuclear envelope (composed of two membranes). The higher degree of organization in eukaryotic cells is also evident in segregation of components of

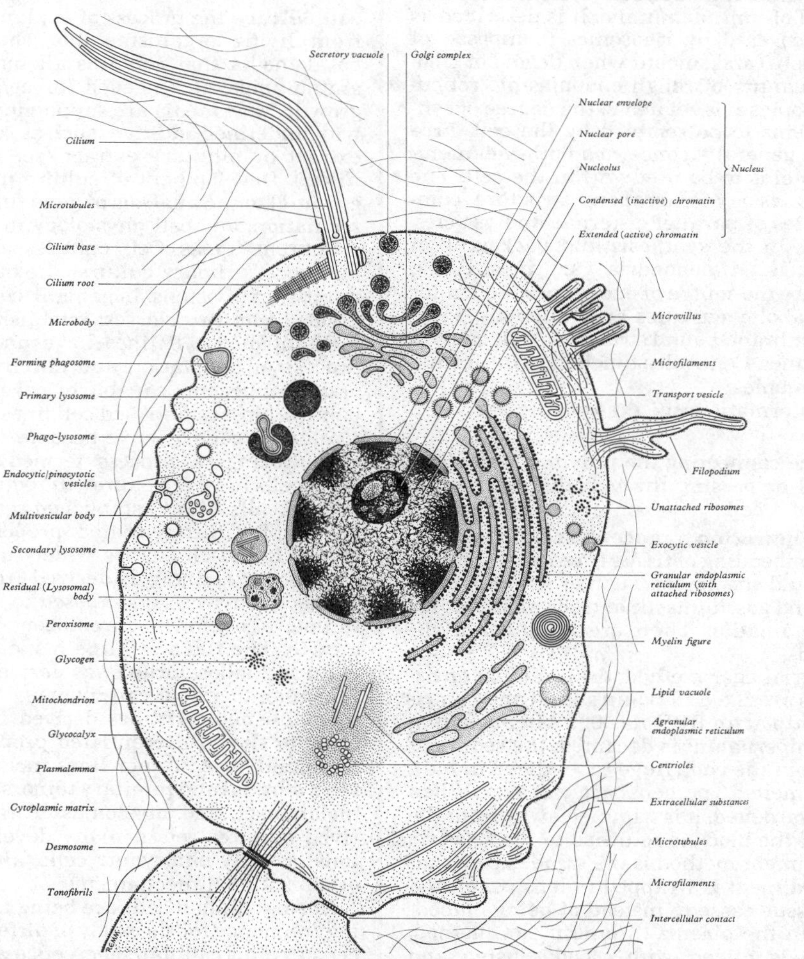

Cell. A composite diagram showing the principal structures found within tissue cells. Only a proportion of the features illustrated are present in any specific cell type. (From Williams, P. L., and Warwick, R.: Gray's Anatomy. 36th ed. Philadelphia, W. B. Saunders Co., 1980.)

the cytoplasm by a system of membranes to form the various organelles. They include mitochondria, endoplasmic reticulum, chloroplasts, Golgi complex, lysosomes, and centrioles, as shown in the accompanying illustration. Cells with specialized activities may contain unique cytoplasmic structures, as in the myofilaments of muscle cells. Most of the information required to direct the activities of a cell is contained in the chromosomes, coded in the sequences of nucleotides of the DNA molecules, and conveyed by RNA molecules to the cytoplasm. Within the nucleus, the nucleoli are involved in the synthesis of ribosomes. In eukaryotic cells, DNA also is present in mitochondria and chloroplasts.

The cytoplasm is the part of a cell that surrounds the nucleus and is enclosed by the plasma membrane. It consists of a continuous aqueous solution (cytosol) and the organelles and inclusions suspended in it, and is the site of most of the chemical activities of the cell, including cellular metabolism and synthesis.

Specialized cellular differentiation related to specific function is manifested in cytoplasmic structure. By conventional light microscopy, the cytoplasm appears relatively homogeneous, but electron microscopy reveals its complex organization.

The endoplasmic reticulum is a system of tubular canals formed of unit membrane. It is described as rough when covered by ribosomes (composed of RNA and protein) and smooth when devoid of ribosomes. The quantity of rough endoplasmic reticulum in the cytoplasm is related to the degree of synthesis of proteins to be secreted by the cell. Free ribosomes are generally concerned with the manufacture of proteins to be used within the cell. The Golgi complex is a membranous structure composed of a series of parallel cisternae and vesicles. It participates in the synthesis and packaging of various products. Mitochondria vary in size and number and are the source of energy production for the cell's metabolic activities and functions. Lysosomes are membrane-bound structures that contain digestive enzymes. Centrioles function in the formation of microtubules.

For more information, see the specific parts of a cell.

cell axis a line connecting the proximal and distal sides of a cell or passing through the centrosome and nucleus of a cell.

cell block preparation a processing technique for the paraffin embedding of tissue fragments and sediment from fluid specimens, such as sputum, effusions, urine, and gastrointestinal tract washings for histologic examination. There are a number of different methods.

In the bacterial agar method, the sediment or tissue fragments are fixed in Bouin's fluid and centrifuged for 10 min at an RCF of 600 *g*. After standing for 2 hr, the supernatant is decanted; the sediment is removed from the centrifuge tube, sliced in half, and placed in melted 3 percent bacterial agar. When the agar has hardened, it is trimmed away from the cell block and the block is returned to the fixative. The fixed sediment method is the same except that the packed sediment is wrapped in lens paper and placed in a tissue cassette instead of being embedded in agar. In the plasma-thrombin clot method, the sediment is mixed with blood plasma and thrombin. Following clot formation, it is wrapped in lens paper and placed in a cassette. Another method involves the preparation of a collodion bag for lining the tube in which the fluid is centrifuged. After decanting the supernate, the bag is tied just above the sediment and the sample is placed directly in the tissue cassette.

After processing by any of these methods, the block is dehydrated, cleared, embedded in paraffin, sectioned, and stained by means of routine histologic techniques.

cell body the part of a neuron around the nucleus as distinguished from its axon and dendrites. Also called *perikaryon*.

cell coat see *glycocalyx*.

cell count determination of the number of cells in a given volume of fluid. Cells can be counted directly in specially designed devices (see *counting chamber*) or by an automated cell counter. See also *cytometry*.

total c. c., in bacteriology, the total number of cells, living or dead, in a fixed sample.

viable c. c., in bacteriology, the number of living cells in a fixed sample. This may be determined by inoculating a medium and counting the colonies produced (see *counting plate*), or by staining a bacterial suspension with a vital stain and counting the cells directly (see *counting chamber*).

cell culture the process of explanting animal cells from living organisms into chemically defined basal media that contains all major ions, sugars, amino acids, etc., needed for cellular survival or growth. Most media are supplemented and fortified with undefined additives such as serum and embryo extract or pituitary extract (see also *culture medium*). Development of culture methods has been essential to the analysis of gene function, metabolic regulation, and cell physiology in animal cells.

CULTURE TYPES. Cell cultures are rather unstable—most primary cultures die out after a limited number of divisions. In general, cell cultures can be divided into two classes: established and primary.

Established cell lines have undergone a major process of adaptation and chromosomal changes, and have become capable of permanent growth in culture. Most established cell lines are derived from malignant cells or have become malignant during subculturing (a process termed transformation). Such cells have fewer growth requirements than do normal cells. Many established cells in culture cannot display differentiated properties. Two lines, mouse L and HeLa, are widely used for research. The mouse L line was derived from subcutaneous connective tissue and exposed to 20-methylcholanthrene, a chemical carcinogen, to acquire rapid growth. The HeLa cell line, a standard line in most culturing laboratories, was derived from a human malignant cervical carcinoma.

Established cell lines derived from tumors continue to show differentiated properties in culture. Frequently used tumor lines include those derived from adrenal and pituitary tumors, neuroblastomas, melanomas, and myelomas. Teratocarcinoma derived cultures retain many developmental potentials of early embryonic cells, although they lack organizational mechanisms.

Normal diploid cells are being used with increasing frequency for the study of differentiation. These cells exhibit cellular senescence after a number of divisions characteristic for each cell type and species. Normal cells used in culture include those derived from cartilage, heart muscle, liver, mammary gland, and thyroid, all of which exhibit their own characteristic differentiated properties.

In primary cultures, the cells are mainly of three types: fibroblast-like (thin and elongated), epithelial-like (polygonal in sheets), or epithelioid (roundish and individually membraned). Fibroblastic cells usually form only monolayers because of contact inhibition; in contrast, cells of neoplastic cell origin are able to form masses and crowd the culture.

CULTURING TECHNIQUES. Tissue fragments are first dispersed into single cells, usually with the aid of trypsin. The trypsin is removed and, using a capillary tube, the cell suspension is placed into a flat-bottomed dish or flat-sided bottle containing appropriate medium. After a lag period, cells attach to the bottom and divide, giving rise to the primary culture (anchorage dependence). Cultures can be maintained by serial passes into fresh media (secondary cultures). Cells may be freed for subculturing from the glass by trypsin or the chelating agent ethylenediaminetetraacetic acid (EDTA). Oncogenic viruses, radiation, and chemical treatment can produce mutation of cultured cells (see *Ames test*). The cells may also transform spontaneously during serial transfer. Transformed cells have many properties absent in untransformed cells, including increased saturation density, decreased serum requirement, decreased anchorage dependence, increased efficiency of clone formation, formation of chromosomal abnormalities, and absence of aging.

DIFFERENTIATION OF CELLS IN CULTURES. Culture conditions are defined as permissive if they allow differentiation or as nonpermissive if they do not. Experiments demonstrate that the expression of differentiated properties by cultured cells is under environmental control.

It appears that cells committed to a specific differentiation pathway can return to that capacity when transferred to nonpermissive media for many generations. When put back into permissive conditions, they revert to their original differentiation pattern. Thus, there is a distinction between the commitment to a particular pathway of differentiation (epigenotype) and the actual expression of differentiated properties (epiphenotype). Therefore, commitment in cells occurs long before overt expression, and changes in epiphenotype can be caused by changes in growth conditions.

The drug 5-bromodeoxyuridine (BrdU) inhibits certain differentiated properties in cultured cells and induces the expression of others. Incorporation of BrdU into either strand of DNA is sufficient to block differentiation. One theory postulates the mode of action of BrdU to be modification of the interaction between DNA and regulatory proteins. Most of the effects of BrdU on cell culture differentiation are reversible.

CELL CULTURE AGING. Unless cells in culture overcome some barrier to immortality, which is revealed by the ability to grow in very sparse cultures with high cloning efficiency, they become senescent and die. Cellular senescence is absent in transformed cells. Senescence depends on the number of cellular divisions rather than on a length of time; it is attributed to the accumulation of unrepaired damage to cell constituents.

Another factor determining senescence is terminal differention. When a cell differentiates to its final state, it may stop DNA synthesis and cell division (e.g., erythrocytes and skeletal muscle cells) and become senescent. Possibly transformation may prevent aging by preventing terminal differentiation.

MAPPING IN CULTURED CELLS. Genetic mapping of mutations in cell cultures is simpler than classic breeding approaches and offers a means by which to examine genetic organization. Germinal mutations and somatic mutations induced by mutagens are recognizable in culture.

The location of genetic markers can be studied in cultures by using cellular hybridization techniques. Hybrid cells can express many parental genes in isolation.

As viruses cannot replicate apart from living cells, animal cell cultures are used for laboratory studies on viral multiplication. The choice of species, tissue and type of culture depends on the virus and the experimental objectives.

See also *cloning, hybrid c.* under *cell,* and *somatic cell g.* under *genetics.*

cell cycle a succession of changes that occurs in DNA content as a newly divided daughter cell progresses through a series of cell cycle stages until the cell again undergoes mitosis. The phases of the cell cycle, proposed to explain the synthesis of DNA during the interphase period, are G_1 (a presynthetic gap), followed by S (a DNA synthetic period), then G_2 (a postsynthetic gap), and M (a brief mitotic period). During M phase, the nuclear membrane begins to disappear, chromatin condenses into chromosomes (prophase), the chromosomes align in parallel in the equatorial plane of the spindle (metaphase), the chromosomes separate into pairs and move to opposite poles (anaphase), and the final process of cytokinesis takes place, in which the cell body divides into two, the nuclear membrane appears, the chromosomes become more diffuse, and the nucleolus reappears (see also *mitosis*). Cells that leave the mitotic cycle become quiescent (G_0); they may remain in that state until stimulated to return to cycling, or they may remain in G_0 as functionally differentiated cells (such as epithelial cells, fibroblasts, leukocytes, and myocytes).

The duration of the cell cycle varies from 8 hr in rapidly proliferating embryonic cells to more than 100 hr in some slow-growing tumors. Variation in the length of the cell cycle is due to variation in the length of G_1, which ranges from zero in embryonic cells to more than 100 hr in slowly proliferating tissue. The S phase is generally 6–8 hr; G_2, 2–6 hr; and mitosis, approximately 1 hr.

Although this description of the cell cycle applies to eukaryotic cells (i.e., those cells with a true nucleus, seen in molds and higher organisms), prokaryotic cells (e.g., bacteria) also have a replication cycle. It includes a brief period of initiation of DNA synthesis followed by DNA synthesis and cell division; the entire cycle can be accomplished in as little as 20 min for *Escherichia coli.*

CHEMICAL AND MORPHOLOGIC CHANGES DURING THE CELL CYCLE. Proteins (including many enzymes and membrane and cytoplasmic proteins) are synthesized at a fairly uniform rate through most of the cell cycle, except during M phase. The enzymes and proteins necessary for initiating and carrying out DNA synthesis are synthesized late in G_1 and early in S. Proteins and other macromolecules required in mitotic operation are synthesized in G_2 or prophase of M.

Regarding nucleic acids, RNA is synthesized actively through G_1, S, and G_2 phases, but this activity almost ceases during M phase. The deoxynucleotides required for DNA synthesis are produced in late G_1 and on into S phase. Nuclear DNA is synthesized only during S phase, whereas mitochondrial DNA (which represents a very small fraction of total cellular DNA) is synthesized throughout the cell cycle. The amount of DNA at the end of S is equal to twice the amount of DNA of the G_1 cell.

Membrane components such as proteins, lipoproteins, and glycoproteins are synthesized at a uniform rate except during mitosis. Both membrane area and cell volume generally show a uniform increase during the cell cycle.

METHODS OF STUDYING CELL CYCLE PHASE DURATION. Several methods have been devised to analyze cell cycle length and phase duration. The study of cell cycle time and phase duration (called cell kinetics) contributes to an understanding of the timing of biochemical events in the cell cycle, the effect of various drugs (especially antitumor drugs) on proliferating cells, and the optimization of cancer chemotherapy.

1. Percent labeled mitoses (PLM): Cells are labeled for a short period, e.g., 30 min, with a radiolabeled DNA precursor (usually thymidine). At intervals during the cell cycle, the number of mitotic cells labeled is noted by autoradiography and compared with the total number of mitotic cells observed. PLM can be used to calculate phase duration and cell cycle time.

2. Mitotic index (MI): The number of mitotic cells is counted and compared with the total number of cells in the sample. A high MI indicates rapid cell proliferation (i.e., a short cell cycle time) and that a large fraction of the population is cycling.

3. Labeling index (LI): Cycling cells are labeled with radiolabeled DNA precursor for a period of time (usually less than 1 hr). The cells are immediately fixed for autoradiographic analysis. The fraction of cells labeled is considered to represent those in S phase.

4. Flow cytometry (FCM): Flow cytometers can be used to determine DNA content in single cells. Cells are stained with a fluorescent DNA-specific stain (e.g., chromomycin A3, Hoechst 33258, propidium iodide). The stained cells are then analyzed for fluorescence as they flow rapidly (5×10^4 cells/min) in single file through an exciting light from a bright source (laser or mercury arc lamp). Fluorescent signals (proportional to DNA content) from hundreds of thousands of cells are amplified and accumulated in a few minutes, and are used to generate a histogram. G_1 and G_2 + M cells form discrete populations in the histogram, in which G_2 + M has twice the DNA content of the G_1 population; S phase forms a broad distribution between G_1 and G_2. FCM can generally distinguish cells in G_1 from cells in G_0 (noncycling cells) by special staining techniques.

5. Radioactivity per cell in S (RCSi): Cells are given a pulse label of thymidine. Labeled thymidine is then washed from the cells, and unlabeled thymidine is added. Cells are collected periodically during a time exceeding cell cycle length and are analyzed and sorted electronically with a cell sorter (a special flow cytometer that permits individual cells with a given fluorescence value to be separated from all the rest). G_1, S, and G_2 + M cells are sorted and counted in a scintillation counter for radioactivity. The cohort of labeled cells moves out of S phase, through G_2 and mitosis, into G_1, and eventually back into S phase. Duration of cell cycle phases can be determined from this sequence of measurements.

6. Double-label techniques: Cells may be labeled at two discrete periods during the cell cycle with different types of radiolabel (e.g., ^{14}C and ^{3}H-thymidine). Tissue (or cells) is removed at intervals beginning shortly after the second labeling. Duration of S phase and cell cycle time can be determined.

7. Cell cycle inhibitors: Some chemical agents prevent further cycling of cells by blocking the cells in a specific phase. Alternately, the deprivation of certain nutrients (e.g., certain amino acids) will arrest cells in G_0. Many protein synthesis inhibitors block cells in G_1 or G_2 (e.g., 5-azacytidine, cycloheximide, puromycin). Others, which interfere with DNA synthesis, block the cells in S phase (e.g., doxorubicin (Adriamycin) 5-fluorouracil, hydroxyurea). Still other agents (colchicine, cytochalasin B, vincristine) interfere with the mitotic process and thus prevent cell division. Information on the blocking reaction to various agents has been used in the design of antitumor drugs.

8. Temperature-sensitive mutants: Some mutant cell lines are blocked at specific points in the cell cycle when they are grown at a certain temperature (the nonpermissive temperature); these cells return to normal cycling when the cells are returned to the permissive temperature. Blocking cells for a period of time allows them to pile up in a given phase. When the block is removed, the cells may cycle through the phases in synchronization, i.e., all cells enter the same phase at the same time. The rate of progression of cells from the blocked phase may be followed by the methods described above.

Also called *replication cycle.*

FRANK A. DOLBEARE, M.D.

cell-cycle inhibitor a chemical agent capable of preventing further cycling by blocking specific phases of the cell cycle. See also *cell cycle* and *chemotherapy.*

cell cycle time the time required to complete one cell cycle; see under *cell cycle.*

cell death the irreversible cessation of the ordered molecular processes within the cell.

cell differentiation the process by which specialized cell types develop from pluripotent embryonic cells.

cell division the process by which almost all multicellular organisms increase their number of cells for growth and replacement. For more information, see *cell cycle, meiosis,* and *mitosis.*

cell envelope in bacteriology, a term used to include the cell membrane plus the cell wall. In eukaryotic cells, the term refers to a double membrane around an organelle (e.g., nuclear envelope, chloroplast envelope).

cell-free system a preparation obtained from a broken cell preparation by differential centrifugation. The centrifugation separates unbroken cells, diverse cellular organelles, and subcellular particles. The structures of these particles can be assessed by light, phase contrast, and electron microscopy, and by histochemical and cytochemical methods, as well as by their metabolic contributions to cellular processes.

cell fusion see *cellular h.* under *hybridization.*

cell junction regions of the cell membranes between apposed cells specialized to provide for cohesion between these cells or for intercellular communication. Although these junctions are most numerous between epithelial cells, they are present in most other tissues, including muscle and nerve. See also *desmosome, nexus, zonula adherens,* and *zonula occludens.*

cell kinetics see under *cell cycle.*

cell line a population of animal cells that develops on repeated secondary cultivation for an indefinite time. A cell line arises from a cell strain when some cells become altered; their morphology changes, they grow faster, and they are able to start a culture from only a few cells. The development of cell culture methods was essential for progress in animal virology.

established c. l., a group of cultured cells that have undergone a major process of adaptation to become capable of indefinite growth. These cells do not have the property of contact inhibition and do not undergo senescence. Most established cell lines are of neoplastic cell origin or acquire such properties during adaptation. They also have unstable karyotypes. Two widely used lines are the HeLa and mouse L cell lines. Also called permanent cell line. See also *cell culture.*

cell-mediated immunity (CMI) that aspect of the host defense system in which immunity is mediated primarily by lymphocytes, although cells such as macrophages, neutrophils, eosinophils, and other less well defined cell types known as killer (K) cells and natural killer (NK) cells may also play a role. The population of lymphoid cells chiefly responsible for CMI is referred to as thymus-derived lymphocytes or T cells. Pre–T cells originate in the bone marrow and migrate to the thymus, where they undergo differentiation and become immunocompetent.

A cell-mediated immune response is initiated by introduction of antigen into the host. Usually after initial processing of antigen by macrophages, T cells become antigen-sensitive in peripheral lymphoid tissue, such as the periarteriolar areas of the spleen or the thymus-dependent deep cortical areas of the lymph nodes that drain the site of foreign antigen deposition. On subsequent exposure to antigen, the previously sensitized T cells are transformed into lymphoblasts, which do not secrete appreciable amounts of immunoglobulin and do not contain antibody in the cytoplasm. During this period of blast transformation the T cells enlarge; proliferate; undergo DNA, RNA, and protein synthesis; and eventually divide.

These sensitized T cells are specific for a given antigen and eventually give rise to a population of cells that express various biologic activities. They include the production of helper or suppressor (regulator) T cells for T-T and T-B cell interaction, and the induction of cytotoxic cells capable of destroying target cells possessing the corresponding relevant antigen. This effector process occurs either directly or indirectly through the elaboration of cell products known as lymphokines. Cytotoxic lymphocytes can also be generated in vitro during a mixed lymphocyte culture or in vivo during the rejection of an allograft, tumor cell, or virally transformed or chemically modified target cell. In addition, in certain cytoxicity systems, especially those involving histocompatibility (transplantation) antigens or viral antigens, the recognition and destruction of target cells by sensitized T cells is genetically restricted. The formation of an array of biologically active lymphokines by antigen-sensitized T cells is believed to be an in vitro correlate of cellular immunity. These diverse mediators include chemotactic factors for macrophages, neutrophils, and eosinophils; mitogenic and/or growth factors for other lymphocytes; a factor that both activates and inhibits the migration of macrophages; and the antiviral agent interferon.

Some of the antigen-stimulated T cells become memory cells, which express an antigen rechallenge with greatly enhanced responses. As a result of the swift recall, increased numbers of cells participate in CMI reactions to expedite the disposal of the undesirable antigenic material, such as an infecting microogranism.

Human T cells have the unique property of forming spontaneous rosettes with uncoated sheep red blood cells, and the T-lymphocyte membrane shares an antigenic determinant with the brain previously designated (in the mouse) as theta (θ) but now referred to as Thy 1. In addition, T cells can be nonspecifically activated in vitro following attachment of mitogens, such as the plant lectins concanavalin A and phytohemagglutinin, to their cell surface.

Besides T lymphocytes there are other leukocytes that may participate in cellular immunity. Macrophages perform an accessory function in the expression of effector mechanisms initiated by T cells. As previously noted, macrophages become activated in response to the release of lymphokines by sensitized T cells, such as macrophage activating factor and migration inhibition factor, which mobilize and then inhibit further movement of these cells. Activated macrophages express different properties and metabolic characteristics than do normal macrophages. These activated phagocytes prevent the multiplication of certain intracellular organisms, have increased antimicrobial activity, regulate lymphocyte responses, and are inhibitory or cytotoxic in various tumor models.

In addition, K cells are important in some CMI reactions. These cells are morphologically indistinguishable from small lymphocytes but lack surface immunoglobulin. They possess cytotoxic activity for easily detectable target cells coated with specific antibody. In the antibody-dependent cell-mediated cytotoxicity reaction (ADCC), antibody molecules link the target and effector (K) cell receptors.

Another recently described effector mechanism of CMI is the NK cell. It functions primarily in the nonspecific direct killing of virally transformed cells, allografts, and tumors. These cells may be important in protection against the spontaneous development of neoplastic diseases in humans.

Our early knowledge of CMI stems from the late 19th-century work of Robert Koch, who first described the classic delayed hypersensitivity reaction. In attempting to develop a vaccine for tuberculosis, he observed that repeated inoculations of a culture filtrate of *Mycobacterium tuberculosis* or of dead mycobacterial organisms into the skin of tuberculous guinea pigs elicited 24–48 hr later a local, raised, erythematous lesion, which sometimes became necrotic.

It has subsequently been shown that the lesion of delayed hypersensitivity arises from a massive influx mostly of macrophages as a result of a specific response of sensitized lymphocytes following intradermal injection of antigen. It has also been demonstrated that this reactivity, unlike humoral or antibody-mediated immunity, could be passively transferred to normal individuals with living lymphoid cells from sensitized hosts, but not with serum. Modern immunologists tend to use CMI synonymously with delayed hypersensitivity.

CMI plays a vital role in host defense against various infectious agents, such as bacteria, viruses, fungi, and parasites; it probably provides protection against tumor development; and it is responsible for a phase of transplant rejection. Drastic alteration or suppression of immunocompetent cells (e.g., by drugs, congenital defects, malnutrition, certain infections, and malignancies) can considerably modify normal CMI reactivity and may thus be either beneficial or harmful to the host.

See also *immunity.*

CHARLES PAVIA, PH.D.

cell membrane the structure that surrounds a cell and provides the boundary or barrier between the cytoplasm and the cell's environment. The membrane consists of a double layer of amphipathic lipid molecules (a lipid bilayer), in which the molecules in each layer are oriented with their nonpolar, hydrophobic hydrocarbon fatty acid portions toward the interior and their polar, hydrophilic ends exposed on the surfaces. Embedded into this bilayer are proteins that have nonpolar regions on their surfaces and thus dissolve into one membrane. Because they span the membrane, some proteins are exposed on both surfaces. These proteins are important for transport processes. Proteins that cannot be dissociated without destruction of the membrane are called integral proteins. Those that are only loosely associated are called peripheral proteins. The lipid bilayer is fluid at growth temperatures, thereby permitting the proteins to diffuse freely within the plane of the membrane. The remarkable stability of the membrane is provided by the attractive forces between surrounding water molecules, which prevents the escape of membrane components.

The membrane, 6–9 nm thick, appears in electron micrographs of fixed and stained preparations as a dark-light-dark image called the unit membrane.

Also called *cytoplasmic membrane* and *plasma membrane.*

J. KENNETH HOOBER, PH.D.

cellobiase (sel″o-bi′ās) see *β-D-glucosidase.*

cellobiose (sel″o-bi′ōs) a disaccharide, β-D-glucopyranosyl-(1→4)-β-D-glucopyranose, obtained by the partial hydrolysis of cellulose. It is the repeating unit of cellulose, a linear homopolymer of glucose.

celloidin (sĕ-loi′din) a nitrocellulose histologic embedding medium. Because the embedding process is slow and requires comparatively thick sections (10–15 μm), it is used only rarely, primarily for teeth and bones (which may crumble when paraffin is used) and for eyes (paraffin may cause detachment of the retina).

cellophane (sel′o-fān) a transparent film of regenerated cellulose. It is used as a dialysis membrane, as wrapping material, and for bandages and compresses.

cellophane tape method see *Scotch tape method.*

Cellosolve a tradename for mono- and dialkyl ethers of ethylene glycol and their derivatives, widely used as industrial solvents. The terms Cellosolves and Cellosolve refer to this family of compounds: Cellosolve alone refers to 2-ethoxyethanol, and, when combined with a modifier, e.g., methyl Cellosolve, to other members of the family. Examples are ethylene glycol monoethyl ether (2-ethoxyethanol, Cellosolve, Cellosolve solvent), ethylene glycol monobutyl ether (butyl Cellosolve), and ethylene glycol monomethyl ether (methyl Cellosolve). Inhalation of methyl Cellosolve produces neurologic symptoms and macrocytic anemia. The ether linkage is thought to be stable in vivo. Nevertheless, CNS depression, kidney damage, and acidosis may occur.

cell proliferation the replication of cells. See also *cell cycle.* Cf. *growth.*

cell sap see *cytosol.*

cell separation methods cytologic methods for separating cancer cells from fluids, such as blood, that also contain many other cells. Red blood cells are removed by hemolysis using acetic acid, saponin, or streptolysin O, or by sedimentation using fibrinogen, dextran, phytohemagglutinin, or hemolymph heteroagglutinin to speed up the process.

Filtering techniques make use of differences in filter pore size to separate cells of larger or smaller diameter than a given pore diameter.

Flotation techniques (differential centrifugation) are used alone or in combination with hemolysis or sedimentation to isolate cancer cells using their low specific gravity. Phagocytes, such as neutrophils, can be removed with a magnet after the specimen is incubated with a colloidal suspension of carbonyl iron.

See also *flotation techniques.*

cell strain a population of animal cells that develops from a primary culture by reseeding serially; the number of transfers is usually limited. The characteristics of the parent cell are retained in culture. See also *cell culture.*

cell surface receptor a binding or reaction site on the surface of the cell membrane for lectins, proteins, or other substances. These sites may undergo changes in conformation or reactivity during the course of the cell cycle.

cell theory the hypothesis that all living beings —animals, plants, or protozoa—are composed of cells and cell products, and that growth and reproduction occur as a result of cell division.

cellular (sel′u-lar) pertaining to cells or composed of cells.

cellular atypia the cytologic manifestation of certain abnormal forms of cellular activity. Associated terms include atypical hyperplasia, atypical metaplasia, anaplasia, basal cell hyperactivity, dysplasia, hyperplasia, metaplasia, prosoplasia, reserve cell hyperplasia, subcolumnar cell hyperplasia, transitional zone, and subcylindric cell hyperplasia. As the term cellular atypia is used to denote structural changes ranging from nonneoplastic to malignant neoplastic, its use causes much confusion and misunderstanding.

cellular immunity see *cell-mediated immunity.*

cellular inclusions 1. cell components that are not organized units of living substance (cell organelles), but instead are lifeless collections of cell products or metabolites such as stored fat, pigments, or secretory droplets.

2. in virology, accumulations of virions or viral components in the nucleus and/or cytoplasm of cells; often, they are referred to as inclusion bodies.

cellular swelling one of the first signs of cell injury. When sodium builds up in the cell and the plasma membrane increases in permeability, the cell increases in size from influx of fluid.

cellulase (sel′u-lās) an extracellular enzyme of the hydrolase class [1,4-(1,3;1,4)-β-D-glucan 4-glucanohydrolase, EC 3.2.1.4] that catalyzes the cleavage of 1,4-β-glucosidic linkages in cellulose and other β-D-glucans. It is secreted by some bacteria and is a useful tool in bacterial identification.

cellulitis (sel″u-li′tis) an inflammation that is not localized. It is usually acute, and is caused by an irritant that liberates factors favoring spread. For example, hemolytic streptococci produce hyaluronidase, which breaks down hyaluronic acid in the connective tissue ground substance, promoting further spread of the infection. See also *inflammation.* Cf. *abscess.*

cellulose (sel′u-lōs) a carbohydrate, $(C_6H_{10}O_5)_n$, a polymer of glucose (joined by β-1,4-glucoside linkages) forming the skeleton of most plant structures and of plant cells.

cellulose acetate a thermoplastic resin of cellulose partially esterified by acetic acid, formed by treating cellulose with acetic anhydride. It is used in nontoxic films and coatings or is spun into fibers. Cellulose acetate film is a widely used electrophoretic medium.

cellulose caprate a pale yellow, resinous mounting medium widely used for the preparation of slides in histology. It is a neutral ester with a refractive index of 1.486 in solution.

cell wall a rigid structure outside of and protecting the cell membrane, present in all plant cells and in many bacteria and other types of cells. It is composed chiefly of cellulose in plants, and of peptidoglycan in bacteria. See also under *bacterium.*

celosomia (se″lo-so′me-ah) [Gr. *kēlē* hernia + *sōma* body + *-ia*] a congenital fissure or absence of the sternum, with hernial protrusion of the viscera.

Celsius temperature scale (C) (sel′se-us) [Anders *Celsius,* Swedish astronomer, 1701–1744] the customary scale of temperature on which water freezes at 0°C and boils at 100°C. Also called *centigrade temperature scale.* See also *temperature.*

cement line a name applied to lines that are visible in microscopic examination of bone in cross section and which mark the boundaries of the haversian systems. Such lines are layers of bone matrix with little collagen and no canaliculi.

cement substance a hypothetical substance once believed to hold apposed cell membranes together.

cementum (se-men′tum) [L.] [NA], a dense connective tissue that covers the dentine layer at the root of a tooth and assists in tooth support. Its calcified intracellular matrix is arranged in a system of flattened lamellae and associated lacunae and canaliculi, superficially resembling that of compact bone.

cenobium (se-no′be-um) [Gr. *koinobios* living in communion with others] several cells of a unicellular organism that remain together after division, forming a clump.

censored observation (sen′sōrd) in statistics, an observation whose value is bounded in some sense but not completely determined in a study or experiment. For example, the relapse-free survival time for a patient who is disease-free at the end of the study is known to be at least as long as the disease-free period during which the patient has been observed, but the additional time before relapse is not known; this value is called right-censored. An example of left-censoring is the case of a 12-yr-old female who reports that she menstruates; with regard to her menarche, it is known from her report only that onset occurred at an age younger than 12.

Centers for Disease Control (CDC) a major agency of the United States Public Health Service, concerned with the research and control of communicable, vector-borne, and other related diseases and of work-related diseases. It was established in 1946 as the Communicable Disease Center, an outgrowth of a center for malaria control set up in Atlanta, Georgia, during World War II; in 1970 the name was changed to the present one. Through the years the CDC's responsibilities have expanded to include epidemiology, surveillance, detection, laboratory science, ecologic investigations, training, and disease control methods for an increasing variety of health problems. Among its major tasks today are the licensing of qualified clinical laboratories for interstate commerce, the maintenance of laboratories as reference centers for microorganisms and infectious diseases, and the operation of extensive research programs in the detection and control of disease.

-centesis (sen-te′sis) [Gr. *kentēsis*] a suffix word element to denote a surgical puncture to remove fluid, e.g., amniocentesis.

centi- (sen′tĭ) [L. *centum* hundred] 1. a combining form meaning 100, as in centipede.

2. (abbrev. c), a prefix attached to units of measurement to make a unit that is one-hundredth of the basic unit.

centigrade temperature scale (sent′ĭ-grād) [*centi-* + L. *gradus* step] see *Celsius temperature scale.*

centigram (cg) (sen′tĭ-gram) [Fr. *centigramme*] a unit of mass equal to one-hundredth of a gram (10^{-2} g, 10^{-5} kg).

centiliter (cl) (sen′tĭ-le″ter) [Fr. *centilitre*] a unit of volume equal to one-hundredth of a liter (10^{-2} l).

centimeter (cm) (sen′tĭ-me″ter) [Fr. *centimètre*] a unit of length equal to one-hundredth of a meter (10^{-2} m), about 0.3937 in.

centimeter-gram-second (cgs) system a coherent system of measuring units in which the centimeter, gram, and second are the base units. Derived units of the cgs system are products and quotients of the base units, e.g., the dyne ($1\ g \cdot cm/sec^2$) and the erg ($1\ g \cdot cm^2/sec^2$). Although cgs units are still commonly used in the scientific literature, especially in theoretical work, International System (SI) units are now preferred for reporting data. See also *International System.*

centimorgan (cMo) (sen′tĭ-mōr′gan) [Thomas Hunt

Morgan, American zoologist, 1866–1945] the unit of measure of crossover frequency; 1 percent = 1 centimorgan. Also called *map unit.* See also *crossover frequency.*

centipede (sen′tĭ-pēd) see *Chilopoda.*

centipoise (cP) (sen′tĭ-poiz) a unit of dynamic viscosity equal to one-hundredth of a poise (0.01 P).

centistoke (cSt) (sen′tĭ-stōk) a unit of kinematic visocity equal to one-hundredth of a stoke (0.01 St).

central (sen′tral) pertaining to a center; located at the midpoint.

central canal a small canal running the length of the spinal cord; within the medulla oblongata, it opens into the fourth ventricle. The canal is filled with cerebrospinal fluid and is lined with ependymal cells.

central limit theorem stated as: the sampling distribution of the mean of a random sample from an arbitrary probability distribution with mean μ and variance σ^2 approaches the normal distribution as the sample size increases. The limiting normal distribution has mean μ and variance σ^2/n, where n is the sample size. The mean of a sequence of (not necessarily identically distributed) random variables also has a limiting normal distribution, as long as the individual variances are approximately the size of the average variance. In this case the limiting normal distribution has a mean and variance equal to the averages of the means and variances of the variable in the sequence.

This theorem justifies the use of the normal distribution as the approximate distribution of the mean of a large sample. It also explains why a variable that is the average of many small independent effects has an approximately normal distribution.

central nervous system (CNS) that portion of the nervous system consisting of the brain and spinal cord. See also *brain* and *spinal cord.*

central nervous system tumors neoplasms of the central nervous system, which make up approximately 9 percent of all primary tumors. Approximately 85 percent of CNS tumors arise in the brain, and the remainder arise in the spinal cord. Many intracranial tumors are metastatic carcinomas, but the exact incidence of these is difficult to determine. Most intracranial tumors in adults arise above the tentorium, whereas in children 70 percent are infratentorial. CNS tumors may lead to a focal neurologic deficit (due to compression, distortion, or infiltration), to increased intracranial pressure, to a general impairment of cerebral function, or to seizures. Gliomas rarely metastasize, but spread through the cerebrospinal fluid sometimes occurs.

Tumors of the intrinsic cells of the CNS are collectively designated as gliomas. The most common form of glioma is the astrocytoma which is graded histologically on a scale of 1–4. Glioblastoma multiforme is a synonym for tumors of grades 3–4. Some 45–55 percent of primary intracranial neoplasms are glioblastomas, and 20 percent are low-grade astrocytomas. In children, gliomas mainly involve the cerebellum and brain stem. Astrocytomas of the spinal cord are more common in the upper half of the cord. Subtypes of astrocytomas include gemistocytic tumors in which the cells are large and angulated with eosinophilic cytoplasm, and pilocytic tumors, in which the cells are elongated; these appearances may be seen within an otherwise typical astrocytoma. Glioblastomas display a varied histologic picture but are usually cellular with pleomorphic undifferentiated cells and frequent mitotic figures. Capillaries within the tumor may contain unusually plump endothelial cells. Glioblastomas are aggressive tumors, most patients surviving for less than 2 yr from the time of diagnosis. In contrast, more than half of patients with differentiated astrocytomas survive longer than 2 yr with adequate (surgical) treatment.

Oligodendrogliomas are much less common than astrocytomas, making up roughly 5 percent of intracranial tumors. They are composed of uniform round cells with clear cytoplasm. Astrocytic cells can be identified in 50 percent of oligodendrogliomas. Usually the tumor grows slowly, although a few are aggressive. Metastasis can occur through the CSF, but distant spread is rare. Treatment is surgical. Fifty percent of the tumors recur. The mean postoperative survival time is about 5 yr.

The most common tumor of the spinal cord is the ependymoma. It represents more than 60 percent of tumors in this location, but makes up only 6 percent of intracranial gliomas. It can occur at any age, but most persons with ependymomas of the cord are adults. Ependymomas arise from the walls of the ventricles and grow into the ventricle or adjacent brain, although frequently the tumor does not appear to be connected with the ventricular system. Histologically, the cells form rosettes. With the electron microscope, cilia projecting into small acinar spaces and perivascular rings of cell processes rich in intermediate filaments can be seen.

Medulloblastomas arise in the cerebellar vermis and roof of the fourth ventricle of children, in whom they make up more than 40 percent of intracranial gliomas, and in the cerebellum or cerebrum of adults. Sections of the tumor show sheets of hyperchromatic cells, round to carrot-shaped, occasionally forming rosettes. In at least half of persons affected the cells spread through the CSF, and infrequent distant metastases may involve bones or lymph nodes. The tumors are radiosensitive; surgery combined with radiotherapy can prolong life for more than 5 yr in many cases.

Other primary tumors of the CNS are uncommon. Those of particular interest are the choroid plexus papilloma (which arises in the lateral ventricles), the cerebral neuroblastoma, and the medulloepithelioma; all occur primarily in children.

Meningiomas are tumors of arachnoid cells. Most meningiomas occur in adults, particularly females; they may arise at any site within the meninges, most often the parasagittal region. Meningiomas account for roughly 15 percent of all intracranial tumors and roughly 25 percent of tumors arising within the spinal canal. Typically, a meningioma is a well-circumscribed lesion that grows slowly and appears histologically benign. Psammoma bodies are often present within the tumor. Approximately 10 percent of meningiomas recur, but authentic malignant examples are rare. Other soft tissue neoplasms may arise in, or secondarily involve, the meninges.

Neurofibromas are encapsulated tumors derived from Schwann cells and occur most frequently in relation to the acoustic nerve. Multiple neurofibromas are found in persons with neurofibromatosis (von Recklinghausen's disease).

central processing unit (CPU) the portion of a

computer holding the circuits that interpret and carry out the instructions to the computer.

central ray that part of the primary x-ray beam directed from the x-ray tube to the center of the film or object being radiographed.

central tendency in statistics, a number that describes the center of a distribution of measurements. Central tendency is usually measured by the arithmetic mean, the median, or the geometric mean of the measurements.

central vein the vein that forms the axis of the classic lobule in the liver. This smallest subdivision of the hepatic veins is the hub from which the rays of sinusoids radiate to the portal area of the lobule.

centric fusion (sen′trik) see *robertsonian translocation.*

centrifugal (sen-trif′u-gal) [L. *centrum* center + *fugere* to flee] moving away from a center, as in centrifugal force. Cf. *centripetal.*

centrifugal analyzer an automated chemical analyzer that uses centrifugal force to transfer and mix liquids, and monitors the resulting reactions in a centrifuge. A photometer detects the reaction progress. A separate module is required for dispensing samples and reagents. See also *clinical chemistry automation.*

centrifugal flotation a method of separating helminth parasites and eggs from feces, in which the material is suspended in a medium heavier than the parasites so that they float when centrifuged. Zinc sulfate is commonly used as the floating medium (sp. gr. 1.180).

centrifugal force a force defined as the product of the mass of an object and its radial acceleration. It is equal and opposite to the centripetal force. For an object undergoing circular motion, the centrifugal force is $mr\omega^2$, where m is the mass, r is the radius, and ω is the angular velocity. See also *relative centrifugal force.*

centrifugation (sen″tri-fu-ga′shun) the process of separating components of a mixture on the basis of differences in densities of the different components using a centrifuge. See also *density gradient centrifugation.*

centrifuge (sen′tri-fūj) [L. *centrum* center + *fugere* to flee] a laboratory device that applies a relatively high centrifugal force (up to 25,000 *g*) to a specimen, causing its separation into different fractions according to their specific gravities. See also *ultracentrifuge.*

centrilobular (sen″trĭ-lob′u-lar) referring to the region around the central vein in a hepatic lobule.

centriole (sen′tre-ōl) an organelle composed of microtubules found near the nucleus in eukaryotic cells. It is a cylinder 150 nm in diameter and 300–500 nm long, which in cross section appears as a pinwheel of nine blades, each composed of three microtubules extending the length of the centriole.

During cell division, the centriole replicates, and the two centrioles move to opposite poles of the cell. Spindle fibers form between the chromosomes and the centrioles, and the chromosomes move to the poles of the cell along these fibers. Centrioles also replicate and move toward the cell surface to form the basal bodies of cilia.

centripetal (sen-trip′e-tal) [L. *centrum* center + *petere* to seek] moving toward a center. Cf. *centrifugal.*

centripetal force (sen-trip′ĕ-tal) the radial component of the force acting on an object.

centroacinar cells (sen″tro-as′ĭ-nar) the terminal duct cells of the pancreas that are incorporated into acini.

centromere (sen′tro-mēr) the constricted portion of the chromosome, usually chromomeric, at which the chromatids are joined and by which the chromosome is attached to the spindle during cell division. According to its location, a centromere is said to be metacentric (central), submetacentric (off center), or acrocentric (near one end). Also called *kinetochore* and *primary constriction.* See also *chromosome.*

centromere interference the inhibition by the centromere of nearby crossovers.

centromeric bands (C bands) (sen″tro-mer′ik) bands produced by several chromosome-staining techniques. They are used for human karyotyping, especially when chromosomal rearrangements at or near centromeres are suspected. Normal variants of centromeric bands are common. Also called constitutive heterochromatin bands. See also *chromosome banding.*

centrosome (sen′tro-sōm) a specialized area of condensed cytoplasm that contains the centrioles. Also called *centrosphere.*

centrosphere (sen′tro-sfēr) see *centrosome.*

Centruroides (sen″troo-roi′dēz) a genus of scorpions native to Mexico and the southwestern United States, whose venom is a dangerous neurotoxin.

cenurosis (sen″u-ro′sis) infection by a cenurus, the larva of the tapeworm genus *Multiceps.*

cenurus (sen-u′rus) the larva of the tapeworm genus *Multiceps,* which is sometimes parasitic in humans.

cephal/o (sef′ah-lo) [Gr. *kephalē* head] a word element used in combining form to denote head, e.g., cephalometry.

cephalad (sef′ah-lad) [*cephal-* + *-ad* toward] toward the head. Also called *craniad.* Cf. *caudad.*

cephalexin (sef″ah-lek′sin) an acid-stable derivative of cephalosporin. The use of cephalexin may be indicated for the treatment of pneumococcal or streptococcal infections in individuals with penicillin hypersensitivity, and for certain urinary tract infections due to susceptible strains of *Escherichia coli* and *Proteus* species. This antibiotic may be given orally, intramuscularly, or intravenously, but oral administration in most appropriate. Trademark, *Keflex.* See also *antibacterial agents* and *cephalosporins.*

cephalgia (sef″al′je-ah) [*cephal-* + Gr. *algos* pain + *-ia*] see *headache.*

cephalhematoma (sef″al-he″mah-to′mah) [*cephal-* + Gr. *haima, haimatos* blood + *-oma*] a blood-filled swelling or hematoma beneath the pericranium in the skull, seen most frequently in newborn infants.

cephalic (sĕ-fal′ik) [L. *cephalicus,* from Gr. *kephalikos*] pertaining to the head or to the head end of an organism.

cephalic index 100 times the maximal breadth of the skull divided by its maximal length.

cephalic vein the vein that runs up the radial border of the forearm and anterolateral aspect of the upper arm over the deltoid to join the axillary vein just below the clavicle.

cephalin (sef'ah-lin) [Gr. *kephalē* head] 1. a crude extract of brain tissue with a high content of phospholipids (phosphoglycerides) precipitable by ethyl alcohol, primarily phosphatidyl ethanolamine and some related compounds. It is used as a clotting agent in laboratory coagulation studies.

2. the trivial name for *phosphatidyl ethanolamine, phosphatidyl inositol,* or *phosphatidyl serine.*

cephalin-cholesterol flocculation test a diagnostic test of liver function in which serum specimens from individuals with various types of intrinsic hepatic disease react with a cephalin-cholesterol suspension to produce a flocculent precipitate, which is graded from 0 to 4+. Positive test results occur when the gamma-globulin levels are increased along with a concomitant decrease in albumin concentrations. The test is obsolete and rarely used.

cephaloglycin (sef"ah-lo-gli'sin) one of the cephalosporin group of antibiotics, useful against some gram-negative bacilli and staphylococci. Cephaloglycin is not absorbed well after oral administration. It has a limited use in the treatment of certain urinary tract infections. See also *antibacterial agents* and *cephalosporins.*

cephalometer (sef"ah-lom'ĕ-ter) [*cephalo-* + Gr. *metron* measure] an instrument for measuring the head; an orienting device to position the head for radiographic examination and measurement.

cephalometry (sef"ah-lom'ĕ-tre) measurement of the dimensions of the head.

fetal c., measurement of the cephalic diameter of the unborn fetus.

roentgen c., see *roentgen p.* under *pelvimetry.*

ultrasonic c., fetal cephalometry by B-mode ultrasound scanning, used to determine the age and weight of a fetus by measurement of the biparietal diameter.

cephalopathy (sef"ah-lop'ah-the) [*cephalo-* + Gr. *pathos* disease] a general term for disease of the head.

cephalopelvimetry (sef"ah-lo-pel-vim'ĕ-tre) see *roentgen p.* under *pelvimetry.*

cephaloridine (sef"ah-lŏr'ĭ-dēn) one of the cephalosporin group of antibiotics useful in treating individuals with penicillin hypersensitivity. Cephaloridine is effective against pneumococcal and streptococcal infections, as well as viridans endocarditis. It may also be used to treat gonorrhea and syphilis, but not meningococcal meningitis. This antibiotic should be administered intramuscularly. The most common adverse effect is nephrotoxicity (tubular necrosis). See also *antibacterial agents* and *cephalosporins.*

cephalosporins (sef"ah-lo-spŏr'inz) a group of antibiotics derived from the mold *Cephalosporium* (*Acremonium*). Cephalosporins consist of a beta-lactam ring and a dihydrothiazine ring. The cephalosporin nucleus, 7-aminocephalosporanic acid, can be modified with different side-chains to produce cephalosporins with different pharmacologic and antibacterial properties. They are commonly grouped in "generations." First-generation cephalosporins, all having a similar antibiotic spectrum, include cephalothin, cefazolin, cephapirin, cephalexin, cephradine, and cefaclor. Second-generation cephalosporins, such as cefamandole and cefoxitin, have a broader spectrum with more activity against certain gram-negative bacteria. Third-generation cephalosporins, such as cefoperazone, cefotaxime, and moxalactam, have an even wider spectrum with activity against most enteric gram-negative bacilli and a high resistance to inactivation by beta-lactamases.

MECHANISM OF ACTION AND RESISTANCE. Like the penicillins, cephalosporins inhibit cell wall synthesis, but the mechanism of killing is not well defined. Resistance to antibiotic inhibition or killing may be due to the presence of beta-lactamases (cephalosporinases), permeability barriers, alterations in target sites, or a defect in autolytic enzymes.

CLINICAL USE. Cephalosporins are indicated for individuals allergic to penicillin. They are useful for treatment of pneumococci, staphylococci, and *Klebsiella* species. Cefaclor is more active against gram-negative bacilli and is especially useful against *Hemophilus influenzae, Escherichia coli,* and *Proteus mirabilis.* Cefamandole has a broad spectrum of activity against gram-negative bacilli including *H. influenzae, Enterobacter* species, *E. coli,* and *Klebsiella* species. Because of cefamandole's broader spectrum of activity, it should be included along with an older cephalosporin, such as cephalothin, when testing clinical isolates in the laboratory.

CEPHAMYCINS. The cephamycins are similar to the cephalosporins in structure and also inhibit cell wall synthesis, but they are derived from *Streptomyces* species. Cefoxitin, derived from cephamycin, is more active than cephalothin against certain gram-negative organisms but is less active against *Enterobacter* species and *H. influenzae.* It is also active against indole-positive *Proteus* species and *Bacteroides fragilis* in vitro. It is less active than cefamandole and the older cephalosporins against gram-positive bacteria.

See also *antibacterial agents.*

Cephalosporium (sef"ah-lo-spo're-um) the former name for the genus *Acremonium.*

cephalostat (sef'ah-lo-stat") a head-positioning device that ensures reproducibility of the relations among an x-ray beam, a patient's head, and an x-ray film.

cephalothin (sef'ah-lo-thin) a broad-spectrum semisynthetic cephalosporin antibiotic. Cephalothin is resistant to penicillinase and useful in individuals who are allergic to penicillin. It is effective against some of the gram-negative bacilli, e.g., *Arizona, Klebsiella pneumoniae, Proteus mirabilis,* staphylococci, pneumococci, and streptococci. Cephalothin may cause pain at the site of intramuscular injection; however, nephrotoxicity is rare. See also *antibacterial agents* and *cephalosporins.*

cephamycins (sef"ah-mi'sinz) a group of antibiotics structurally related to the cephalosporins. They are produced by certain streptomycetes. See also *antibacterial agents, cefoxitin,* and *cephalosporins.*

cephapirin (sef"ah-pi'rin) an antibacterial agent similar in activity and pharmacokinetics to cephalothin. See also *antibacterial agents* and *cephalosporins.*

cephradine (sef'rah-dēn) an antibacterial agent similar in structure and activity to cephalexin. Like the latter, cephradine can be administered orally and parenterally. See also *antibacterial agents* and *cephalosporins.*

cera (se'rah) [L.] see *wax.*

ceramidase (ser-am'ĭ-dās) see *acylsphingosine deacylase.*

ceramide (ser'ah-mīd) an *N*-acyl derivative of sphingosine (4-sphingenine), occurring as an intermediate in the biosynthesis or degradation of sphingolipids. In natural products, the acyl group is derived from a long-chain fatty acid with 18–24 carbon atoms.

ceramide hexoside see *cerebroside.*

ceramide lactoside a glycolipid, ceramide-linked 1': β-1 to the glucosyl residue of lactose. This material accumulates in tissues as a result of the genetic deficiency of the lysosomal enzyme lactosyl-β-D-galactoside galactohydrolase. The disease is known as ceramide lactoside lipidosis or lactosylceramidosis. Also called *cytolipin H* and *lactosyl ceramide.* See also *ceramide lactoside lipidosis* and *sphingolipidoses.*

ceramide lactoside lipidosis a disorder of sphingolipid metabolism, suspected to have a familial transmission pattern characterized by a relative or absolute deficiency of the enzyme lactosyl-β-D-galactoside galactohydrolase; it results in the accumulation of ceramide lactoside. Individuals with this disorder experience progressive brain damage, spleen and liver enlargement, and a variety of blood disorders. Also called lactosylceramidosis. See also *sphingolipidoses.*

ceramide trihexosidase an enzyme of the hydrolase class, an α-D-galactosidase, that catalyzes the reaction ceramide-glucose-galactose-galactose + H_2O ⇄ galactose + ceramide-glucose-galactose. A deficiency of the enzyme, transmitted as an X-linked trait, leads to the accumulation of ceramide trihexoside in plasma and tissues, a condition known as diffuse angiokeratoma (Fabry's disease).

Ceratophyllus (ser"ah-tof'ĭ-lus) [Gr. *keras* horn + *phyllon* leaf] a genus of fleas in the family Ceratophyllidae; the species *C. gallinae* and *C. nigu* are primarily parasites of hens but also infest dogs, cats, and humans. They do not attach to the skin except while feeding.

Ceratopogonidae (ser"ah-to-po-gon'ĭ-de) a family of insects commonly known as biting midges, no-see-ums, punkies, and black gnats. They are smaller than mosquitoes, though similar in form. Most are plant parasites, feeding on fruit juices, but some attack humans. Their bite can produce swelling and open, exuding lesions. The blood-sucking *Culicoides* is the most important genus, with species that are significant pests in North America and England; some are also the vector of filarial nematode worms. Antennae are hairy in both sexes, but only the female has sucking mouthparts. Other pest genera are *Ceratopogon, Forcipomyia,* and *Leptoconops.*

cercaria (ser-kār'e-ah), pl. *cercariae* [Gr. *kerkos* tail] the free-living larva of trematode parasites that is liberated from the host mollusk (snail or clam). In some trematode species, cercaria can directly penetrate the skin of the vertebrate host; in others, they encyst on aquatic vegetation and are ingested by either vertebrate or arthropod hosts.

cercarial dermatitis (ser-ka're-al) infestation of skin by cercariae, the larvae of schistosome flukes, which are parasites of fish, birds, and mammals. Humans may become affected while swimming in infested waters. The dermatitis may vary from transient urticaria to macules to a papular rash, which subsides in a few days. Individuals living in endemic areas are usually immune, as they carry a constant low-grade schistosomal infection; travelers to the region are more commonly affected. See also *schistosomiasis.*

Cercospora (ser-kos'por-ah) a genus of fungus of which the species *C. apii* is a common plant pathogen; it may be the etiologic agent of cercosporamycosis in humans.

cercosporamycosis (ser"ko-spōr"ah-mi-ko'sis) a fungal infection in humans. It occurs in individuals in Indonesia and is characterized by extensive subcutaneous lesions containing a brown mycelium.

cerebell/o (ser"ĕ-bel'o) a word element used in combining form to denote the cerebellum, e.g., cerebellopontine.

cerebellomedullary cistern (ser"e-bel"o-med'u-lar"e) the enlarged subarachnoid space between the cerebellum and medulla oblongata, continuous below with the spinal subarachnoid space. Cerebrospinal fluid enters this space from the fourth ventricle. It can be tapped by means of a needle inserted through the posterior atlantooccipital membrane (cisternal puncture).

cerebellum (ser"ĕ-bel'um) [L. dim. of *cerebrum* brain] [NA], the largest part of the hindbrain, located in the posterior cranial fossa behind the pons and medulla oblongata. It consists of three lobes, a single median lobe and paired lateral lobes, which are connected with the brain stem by three pairs of peduncles. The cerebellum functions in the coordination of movement. See also *brain.*

cerebr/o (ser'ĕ-bro) a word element used in combining form to denote the cerebrum (brain), e.g., cerebral.

cerebral (ser'ĕ-bral, sĕ-re'bral) pertaining to the cerebrum.

cerebral artery thrombosis a term to denote the occlusion of a cerebral artery by a local thrombotic process. Cerebral artery thrombosis results in ischemic necrosis of cerebral tissue supplied by that vessel; the extent and distribution of the necrosis depends on the artery involved and the amount of collateral circulation available. See also *cerebrovascular accident.*

cerebral cortex the thin layer of gray matter that covers the surface of the cerebral hemispheres. It has many folds (gyri) that serve to increase its surface area. The cortex is made up of six distinct cell layers and has various functional areas, such as motor, sensory, and association areas. The cortex is involved with higher mental functions, general movement, sensory perception, behavioral reactions, association, and integration.

cerebral edema see *cerebral e.* under *edema.*

cerebral herniation a term used to describe the shift or herniation of brain tissue from one part of the cranial cavity to another, caused by increased intracranial pressure. Herniation of a temporal lobe through the opening formed by the right and left edges of the tentorium may occur as a result of increased intracranial pressure above the tentorium, and can be accompanied by herniation of the brain stem through the foramen magnum. Clinical signs include unilateral third cranial nerve palsy (dilation and abduction of one eye with ptosis of the ipsilateral lid), hemiplegia, stupor, and coma. Death eventually results from respiratory arrest, as the brain stem centers controlling respiration are compromised. Also called temporal lobe or uncal herniation.

cerebral palsy (CP) see *cerebral p. syndromes* under *palsy.*

cerebritis (ser″ĕ-bri′tis) [*cerebr-* + *-itis* inflammation] inflammation of the cerebrum.

cerebrocuprein (ser″ĕ-bro-ku′pre-in) see *copper storage protein* and *superoxide dismutase.*

cerebronic acid (ser″ĕ-bron′ik) a 24-carbon, 2-hydroxy saturated fatty acid that occurs as a constituent of brain cerebrosides.

cerebrosclerosis (ser″ĕ-bro-skle-ro′sis) pathologic firmness of the substance of the cerebrum.

cerebroside (ser′ĕ-bro-sīd″) a derivative of sphingosine in which the amino group is linked to an acyl group, and the alcohol group is connected by a glycosidic linkage to a hexose, either D-glucose or D-galactose. Accumulation of some cerebroside or cerebroside derivatives in tissues such as the cerebrum, liver, spleen, and lymph nodes is seen in sphingolipidoses such as Gaucher's and Tay-Sachs diseases. Also called *ceramide hexoside* and *glycosyl ceramide.*

cerebroside β-galactosidase see *galactosylceramidase.*

cerebroside β-glucosidase see *glucosylceramidase.*

cerebroside lipidosis see *Gaucher's disease.*

cerebroside sulfatide one of the subclass of cerebrosides containing sulfate esterified to the hexose moiety, usually on the C-3 of galactose. Found largely in medullated nerve fibers, these esters may accumulate in the white matter of the brain in metachromatic leukodystrophy. Also called *sulfatide.*

cerebrospinal (ser″ĕ-bro-spi′nal) pertaining to the brain and spinal cord.

cerebrospinal fluid (CSF) a clear, colorless fluid that fills spaces within and around the central nervous system. It occupies the lateral ventricles, third ventricle, aqueduct, fourth ventricle, and the slender canal of the spinal cord, and bathes the exterior of the brain and cord, occupying discrepancies in contour between their surfaces and the surrounding bony confines. The internal and external circulations communicate through three small foramina in the wall of the fourth ventricle; if these become obstructed, hydrocephalus results. Where the surface of the brain is angular, the subarachnoid space containing the CSF enlarges to form a cistern.

The CSF is formed from plasma by an ultrafiltration process that takes place in the choroid plexuses of the ventricles. About 500 ml is formed in a day, and as the total volume in the CNS is approximately 150 ml, there must be a rapid turnover. Some fluid also reaches the CSF from the cells of the brain by a transependymal route, but the mechanisms involved are unclear. Absorption of the CSF occurs through the arachnoid villi into the venous sinuses. A rise in venous pressure is rapidly followed by a rise in CSF pressure.

Specimens for study can be obtained by lumbar puncture, or, when necessary, by cisternal puncture.

cerebrospinal fluid assays important diagnostic procedures for many pathologic conditions of the central nervous system, such as meningitis, neurosyphilis, encephalitis, and brain tumor. These diseases can alter the composition of the CSF, including its appearance, volume, pressure, and protein, glucose, and electrolyte concentrations. Chemical tests are performed on clear fluid specimens. If turbidity is present, the sample first must be centrifuged and the precipitate removed. The reference ranges for CSF constituents in the healthy adult are listed in Table 1.

The clinical assays used to determine CSF constituents are largely those used for plasma; however, because of the low protein concentration of CSF (except in the presence of a few diseases), direct measurement in many cases may be made without having to precipitate the protein. For some constituents, concentration of the specimen may be required to obtain adequate precision. Table 2 lists some methods and basic principles.

cerebrospinal fluid culture the microbiologic analysis of cerebrospinal fluid as an aid to the diagnosis of meningitis. Because flora are not normally found in the CSF, recovery of any microorganisms is a significant finding. CSF should be inoculated only on enriched media and incubated both aerobically and at increased levels of CO_2 for at least 2 da. Meningitis represents a medical emergency, so CSF cultures should be undertaken as soon as possible in suspected cases. Although meningitis can be caused by a variety of microorganisms, the more common pathogens are *Hemophilus influenzae, Neisseria meningitidis, Streptococcus pneumoniae,* and the yeast *Cryptococcus neoformans.* See also *Gram stain.*

cerebrospinal fluid electrophoresis electrophoresis of CSF proteins, performed in a manner similar to serum protein electrophoresis, with the inclusion of a concentration step prior to the application of the sample. Owing to the low concentration of protein in spinal fluid, the degree of concentration required is usually 50- to 100-fold. The primary purpose of the test is to detect increases in the gamma-globulin fraction of the protein, specifically IgG, and any discrete banding in the gamma-globulin region (oligoclonal banding) that may be present.

Oligoclonal banding can best be seen when agarose is used but it can also be demonstrated by use of cellulose acetate. Visualization of banding is facilitated by staining the gel with stains such as amido black or Coomassie blue. For greater sensitivity, research-oriented techniques such as isoelectric focusing or polyacrylamide gel electrophoresis can be used, although they are less practical for a clinical laboratory.

See also *oligoclonal banding* and *protein electrophoresis.*

cerebrospinal fluid pressure pressure in the CSF system, which ranges between 70 and 200 mm of H_2O in normal individuals lying in a horizontal position. CSF pressure is affected by various pathologic conditions (brain tumor, hemorrhage, infec-

CEREBROSPINAL FLUID ASSAYS, TABLE 1. REFERENCE VALUES FOR LUMBAR CSF

	VALUE
Appearance	Clear, colorless
Volume	90–150 ml
Specific gravity	1.006–1.008
Cells	0–10 mononuclear cells or lymphocytes/mm^3
Glucose	40–70 mg/dl
Total protein	15–45 mg/dl (by biuret or turbidimetric methods), 8–32 mg/dl (by column methods)
Albumin	10–30 mg/dl
Gamma globulins	About 8% of total protein, with IgG 0.8–6.4 mg/dl
Total osmolality	280–290 mOsm/kg
Sodium	140–154 mmol/l
Potassium	2.0–3.5 mmol/l
Calcium	1.2–1.3 mmol/l
Magnesium	1.1–1.3 mmol/l
Chloride	118–132 mmol/l
Fluid pressure	130 mm H_2O
pH	7.3–7.4
P_{CO_2}	40–50 mmHg
P_{O_2}	40–44 mmHg
Creatinine	0.5–1.2 mg/dl
Urea	6–16 mg/dl
Glutamine	6–16 mg/dl
Lactate	10–18 mg/dl

Note: The clinical assays used to determine CSF constituents are largely those used for plasma; only when different methods are used are they listed here.

tion, hydrocephalus) in which either the rate of secretion (by the choroid plexus) or absorption (through the arachnoid villi) of the CSF is altered.

cerebrotendinous (ser″ĕ-bro-ten′dĭ-nus) pertaining to the cerebrum and tendons.

cerebrotendinous xanthomatosis a rare hereditary disorder, transmitted as an autosomal recessive trait, that is characterized by abnormal cholesterol metabolism and bile acid formation. Cholestanol (5α-cholestan-3β-ol) is found in greatly increased concentrations in the nervous system and blood. There is progressive ataxia, mental degeneration, cataracts, and multiple xanthomas, especially on

CEREBROSPINAL FLUID ASSAYS, TABLE 2. CLINICAL TESTS FOR CSF CONSTITUENTS

CONSTITUENT	COMMENT
Pressure	CSF allowed to rise in sterile manometer tube while lumbar puncture performed, before specimen removed for analysis
Volume	Volume measured by using radioactive tracers such as ^{99m}Tc-inulin or DTPA inserted through lumbar puncture needle
Appearance	Specimen examined against light: should appear clear and colorless
Cells	In clear specimen, leukocyte count performed in hemocytometer; turbid specimen examined under microscope for presence of other cell types; under suspicion of bacterial disease, CSF should be cultured and smear examined
Glucose	Glucose analyzed without delay after obtaining specimen: should be measured enzymatically as for plasma
Total protein	1. Turbidimetric methods, which measure turbidity when proteins are precipitated with reagents such as trichloroacetic or sulfosalicylic acids 2. Biuret method, based on formation of pink complex between peptide bonds and cuprous ions 3. Lowry method, based on formation of blue complex of phosphomolybdic acid, catalyzed by cuprous ion and tyrosine, tryptophan, and cysteine residues of the proteins 4. Column methods (Sephadex), which separate proteins from other CSF constituents and thus allow their quantitation by absorbance measurements at 220 nm
Specific proteins	Major fractions analyzed by electrophoresis; specific proteins quantitated immunochemically
Glutamine	Determination based on glutamyl transferase reaction, catalyzed by glutamine synthetase, in which glutamine reacts with hydroxylamine and product gives colored complex with Fe^{3+} salts

Note: Other constituents are measured by procedures regularly applied to plasma or serum samples.

tendons. Genital infantilism, lip and tongue paralysis, and premature atherosclerosis are also seen. Although progressive, this disease may not become clinically evident until after age 30 yr. The specific defect in cerebrotendinous xanthomatosis is unknown and no therapy has proved effective. Also called *Bogaert's disease, van Bogaert's disease,* and van Bogaert-Scherer-Epstein disease.

cerebrovascular accident (CVA) the development of an acute neurologic deficit due to a disturbance in the blood supply to the brain. CVAs are classified as thrombotic, embolic, or hemorrhagic. A thrombus or embolus in one of the cerebral arteries may cause an infarction of brain tissue supplied by that vessel. Alternately, rupture of a vessel will lead to focal damage as the blood clot destroys and compresses surrounding areas of the brain. Prognosis and treatment vary with the type of CVA.

An understanding of the anatomy of the brain and its circulation is important in studying CVA, because the type of neurologic deficit usually indicates the area of the brain in which vascular injury has occurred. The major arteries supplying the brain are the internal carotids, whose branches supply much of the cerebral hemispheres, and the vertebral and basilar arteries, which supply the brain stem and cerebellum. There is an extensive collateral circulation throughout the brain, and often the effects of damage to a vessel are not as severe as might be anticipated because uninvolved collateral vessels can provide some circulation to the ischemic tissue.

Atherosclerosis affecting the blood vessels of the brain causes the development of plaques and thrombi within these vessels. If a thrombus completely occludes an artery and no collateral blood flow is present, the area distal to the occlusion will infarct, resulting in a CVA. The onset of such a thrombotic event is usually sudden, but the symptoms may progress over the next several hours or days if the occlusion becomes more extensive. Many cerebral thromboses are preceded by transient ischemic attacks (TIA). A TIA occurs when there is partial occlusion of a vessel, resulting in temporary ischemia to an area of the brain. The person will show symptoms of a focal neurologic loss, as in a stroke, but the symptoms will usually only last minutes or hours and will always clear within 24 hr. TIAs can recur, however, because the thrombus persists in the artery; approximately one-third of those experiencing TIAs will have a stroke at a later time. Treatments of TIA may involve surgical removal of the thrombus if it is accessible; alternatively, administration of an anticoagulant or aspirin may prevent further TIAs or the development of a major stroke.

Embolic strokes occur when an embolus breaks loose into the circulation and lodges in one of the vessels of the brain, causing its occlusion. Embolic CVAs are seen frequently in persons with chronic atrial fibrillation, prosthetic heart valves, or a mural thrombus (a clot along the wall of the heart) following a myocardial infarction. Emboli may also originate from atheromatous plaques, particularly from the major vessels in the neck, which may be suggested by the presence of an audible bruit over the carotid vessels in the neck. Embolic strokes occur suddenly but are often preceded by TIAs. Those patients with the cardiac or vascular diseases mentioned above may be given prophylactic anticoagulants to prevent the occurrence of an embolic CVA.

Hemorrhagic strokes carry the worst prognosis. Hemorrhage usually occurs because of hypertension, an underlying bleeding disorder, or rupture of an aneurysm (a weakness in the vessel wall). Onset of symptoms is rapid and usually accompanied by a severe headache. If bleeding is extensive, the neurologic deficit will increase rapidly, and coma or death may ensue.

The hallmark of a CVA is the sudden loss of neurologic function. The type and the severity of deficit are related to the location and extent of infarction, or hemorrhage. The classic sign is hemiparesis (weakness of one side of the body), which usually occurs on the side of the body opposite to the intracranial damage. The clinical presentation is highly variable, however, and at times may be complex. Damage in the anterior portion of the brain most often results in hemiparesis, sensory deficits, aphasia, and changes in personality and behavior. Compromise within the posterior portion of the brain and brain stem often leads to visual disturbance, dizziness, vertigo, dysarthria, and motor and sensory deficits involving the limbs on both sides. Unfortunately, these distinctions are not always entirely accurate, and the anatomic localization of an infarct can be difficult. Extensive damage in any part of the brain may cause coma and death.

Laboratory tests useful in evaluation of a CVA include computerized tomography (CT) and examination of the cerebrospinal fluid. The CT scan will show hemorrhagic areas of the brain acutely and will reveal infarcted areas after several days. A lumbar puncture to check for blood in the CSF can also be helpful diagnostically, but should not be performed if there is a significant increase in intracranial pressure. Arteriography may be used to demonstrate pathologic alterations of the cerebral vessels; this is usually performed if surgery is contemplated. Radionuclide brain scans can be used to look for bleeding or infarction if a CT scan is not available.

The mortality from CVAs averages about 20 percent but rises with age. Of those who survive, almost two-thirds have major disability. Recovery of function is usually unpredictable but most commonly begins in the first weeks following the attack.

Also called *stroke.*

STEPHAN D. FIHN, M.D., M.P.H.
NANETTE SMITH, M.D.

cerebrum (ser′ĕ-brum, sĕ-re′brum) [L.] [NA], the largest part of the human brain. It is composed of two hemispheres united by the corpus callosum. See also *brain.*

Cerithidia (ser″ĭ-thid′e-ah) a genus of freshwater snails, of which the species *C. cingulata* serves as an intermediate host for the fluke *Heterophyes heterophyes* in Japan. Also called *Tymphonotonus microptera.*

cerium (Ce) (se′re-um) [L., from the asteroid *Ceres*] a metallic element, atomic number 58; atomic weight 140.12; a 4f transition element (lanthanide or rare earth); common oxidation states +3, +4. It is used industrially in ignition devices and as a catalyst and reducing agent.

cerium oxalate see *cerous oxalate.*

ceroid (se′roid) an insoluble complex of oxidized polyunsaturated lipids, which accumulates in the lysosomes of macrophages in the gastrointestinal tract in some malabsorption states and in the liver following liver-cell injury. It has also been described in animals deficient in vitamin E. Ceroid is a pale, acid-fast pigment that gives a yellow-green fluorescence, and it can be stained with oil red O.

cerous oxalate (se′rus) a mixture of oxalates of cerium, neodymium, praseodymium, lanthanum, and other elements; formerly used as an antiemetic. Also called *cerium oxalate.*

Certified Reference Materials see under *reference materials.*

certified stains those stains that have been tested for specific purposes by the Biological Stain Commission and are then designated as generally reliable for those purposes. See also *Biological Stain Commission.*

certified standards although not officially recognized, a term used for reference substances available for laboratory use that are certified by a recognized and accepted organization as to their suitability for clinical use. Examples are standards for bilirubin and cyanomethemoglobin, certified by the College of American Pathologists. Depending on the purity of these materials and the organization issuing the certificate, these compounds may be categorized as *primary reference material* or *secondary reference material;* see under *reference materials.*

cerulein (se-roo′le-in) a decapeptide amide isolated from the skin of frogs; it is a peptide analog of cholecystokinin and gastrin. In mammals it is a powerful stimulant of gallbladder contraction.

ceruloplasmin (sĕ-roo″lo-plaz′min) a deep blue–colored, copper-containing glycoprotein, with eight atoms of copper per molecule (four as Cu^{+}), that has properties of an enzyme of the oxidoreductase class (iron(II):oxygen reductase, EC 1.16.3.1), catalyzing the reaction $4Fe^{2+} + 4H^{+} + O_2 = 4Fe^{3+} + 2H_2O$. It also catalyzes the oxidation of polyphenols, polyalcohols, and polyamines. It occurs in the alpha$_2$-globulin electrophoretic fraction in plasma, and is the primary vehicle for copper transport and maintenance of the optimal levels of Cu^{2+} in the tissues.

One of the "acute-phase reaction" proteins, ceruloplasmin in plasma increases in concentration in such conditions as physiologic stress, infectious disease, pregnancy, and intake of oral contraceptives. Of most clinical interest is the considerably lowered value found in hepatolenticular degeneration (Wilson's disease), a congenital disease associated with defective copper metabolism.

The EC recommended name for this enzyme is *ferroxidase.*

ceruloplasmin assays 1. immunochemical methods using radial immunodiffusion (RID), electroimmunodiffusion, or nephelometry.

2. colorimetric methods that measure the blue hue of the protein at 605 nm.

3. enzymatic methods that measure the rate of oxidation of ferrous iron (Fe^{2+}) to ferric iron (Fe^{3+}) by ceruloplasmin and the binding of Fe^{3+} to apotransferrin to form the pinkish-red transferrin, which absorbs at 460 nm.

4. enzymatic methods that measure the rate of oxidation of *p*-phenylene diamine by ceruloplasmin. The O_2 consumed can be measured with a Warburg apparatus, or the oxidation product can be quantitated colorimetrically at 530 nm.

cerumen (sĕ-roo′men) [L., from *cera* wax] the brownish, waxlike secretion produced by ceruminous glands within the external meatus of the ear; also called earwax.

cerumin/o (sĕ-roo′mĭ-no) a word element used in combining form to denote cerumen, e.g., ceruminosis.

ceruminous (sĕ-roo′mĭ-nus) of or pertaining to the cerumen.

ceruminous gland a gland in the skin of the external auditory canal that secretes earwax. Largely limited to the cartilaginous areas of the canal and meatus, the glands are modified apocrine sweat glands.

cervic/o (ser′vĭ-ko) [L. *cervix* neck] a word element used in combining form to denote the neck, often the neck of the uterus (cervix), e.g., cervicitis.

cervical (ser′vĭ-kal) [L. *cervicalis,* from *cervix* neck] pertaining to the neck or to the uterine cervix.

cervical canal a fusiform passageway, flattened at each end and broader in the middle, that connects the vaginal cavity with the uterine cavity.

cervical culture the microbiologic analysis of a cervical specimen as a laboratory procedure to aid in the control, diagnosis, and subsequent treatment of infectious diseases of the genital tract. The female genital tract has a normal flora consisting of staphylococci, micrococci, and gram-positive rods; occasionally there are lactobacilli, diphtheroids, *Bacteroides* species, and anaerobic gram-positive cocci.

A cervical culture is plated onto differential and selective media to decrease the growth of normal flora, and onto enriched media to encourage the growth of certain pathogens that survive well in vivo but have special growth requirements in vitro. Pathogens that can be isolated from such cultures include coliform bacilli, enterococci, group B streptococci in the pregnant female, *Clostridium* species, *Mycobacterium* species, and any of the microorganisms involved in sexually transmitted diseases, such as *Neisseria gonorrhoeae, Hemophilus vaginalis, Candida albicans,* and *Treponema pallidum* (a spirochete visualized only microscopically and not recovered culturally). The endocervix may be the site of an anaerobic infection and should also be cultured.

See also *Gram stain* and *normal flora.*

cervical intraepithelial neoplasia (CIN) a spectrum of intraepithelial changes in the cervix, which ranges from what has traditionally been defined as mild dysplasia to carcinoma in situ. According to this concept, Grade I CIN corresponds to mild dysplasia, Grade II to moderate dysplasia, and Grade III to severe dysplasia and carcinoma in situ. See also *carcinoma in situ* and *dysplasia* and the accompanying illustration.

cervical rib an extra rib derived from the costal element of the seventh cervical vertebra. Depending on its length, it may extend into the posterior triangle of the neck and end blindly, or it may connect with the first rib or sternum. The subclavian vessels pass above it and are prone to compression from contraction of the scalenus anterior.

cervical rib syndrome a disorder characterized by cervical rib compression of the brachial plexus or the subclavian artery. This disorder may give rise to

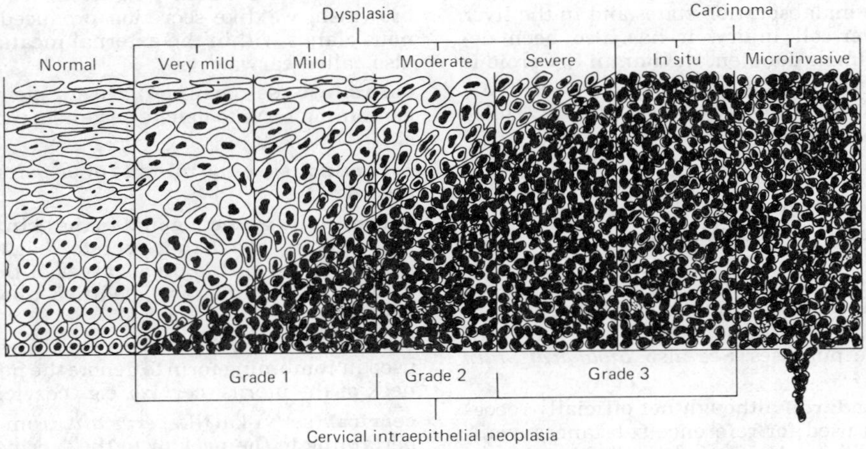

Cervical intraepithelial neoplasia. (From Blaustein, A.: Pathology of the Female Genital Tract. New York, Springer-Verlag, 1977.)

vascular, motor, or sensory disturbances in the extremities.

cervical scraper an instrument used to obtain specimens for cytologic study from the uterine cervix. Commercially prepared plastic and wooden scrapers are available, or a tongue depressor cut to fit the contour of the cervix may be used. The scraper should be rotated 360° to obtain the specimen.

cervical somatosensory evoked potential see *spinal somatosensory e. p.* under *evoked potential.*

cervicitis (ser″vĭ-si′tis) an acute or chronic inflammation of the cervix that occurs in at least three-fourths of all females at some time in their lives. Symptoms include urinary frequency and urgency, vaginal discharge, low back pain, dysmenorrhea, and pain with intercourse. Common causative organisms include *Candida albicans, Neisseria gonorrhoeae, Chlamydia trachomatis,* and herpes simplex virus; sexually transmitted infections and trauma to the cervix may also be implicated. Chronic cervicitis can lead to infertility, abortion, and intrapartum infection.

Laboratory studies include cervical culture to identify the specific organism, along with a cervical smear to rule out cervical cancer.

See also *sexually transmitted diseases.*

cervix (ser′viks), pl. *cervices* [L.] [NA], a term denoting the neck of the body (the portion connecting the head and trunk), or the neck of any organ or structure. See also *uterus.*

cesium (Cs) (se′ze-um) [L. *caesium,* from *caesius* sky blue] a soft, silvery-white metallic element; atomic number 55; atomic weight 132.905; Group I of the periodic table (the alkali metals); oxidation state +1. Cesium melts at slightly above room temperature (28.4°C). It is used in photocells and as a hydrogenation catalyst. Its physiologic localization is like that of potassium.

cesium-137 (^{137}Cs, Cs 137) a reactor-produced radionuclide with a half-life of 30.0 yr. It has two beta-decay modes: the major mode (93.5 percent) has a maximal beta-particle energy of 510 keV; the other has an energy of 1180 keV. The decay is accompanied by the emission of 662 keV gamma rays, which have a half-value layer of 0.5 in. of lead.

Cesium-137 is used as a brachytherapy radiation source in the form of removable interstitial implants or sources for intercavitary application. Because of the moderately long half-life, dose adjustments are necessary only once a year; because cesium-137 has a lower gamma-ray energy than radium, it requires less shielding.

Cestoda (ses-to′da) a subclass of the class Cestoidea. It is composed of the true tapeworms, which have a scolex and proglottids, and includes all of the cestodes that parasitize humans and other animals.

cestode (ses′tōd) any tapeworm or platyhelminth of the class Cestoidea, especially those of the subclass Cestoda. These worms are the true segmented tapeworms, having a scolex and a series of hermaphroditic body segments. The adult tapeworm anchors to the wall of the small intestine by the scolex, and absorbs the host's digested food through its skin. Infection occurs when larvae are ingested along with intermediate host tissue such as inadequately cooked beef, pork, or fish. The two orders containing human parasites are Pseudophyllidea and Cyclophyllidea.

cestodiasis (ses″to-di′ah-sis) an infection with cestodes (tapeworms). Currently, only six cestode parasites are known to affect humans with any frequency: *Taenia saginata, T. solium, Diphyllobothrium latum, Hymenolepsis nana, H. diminuta,* and *Dipylidium caninum.* Ordinarily, the presence of adult cestodes in the human intestine does not result in symptoms. Heavy infections may cause anemia, weight loss, and abdominal pain. Rarely, larval tapeworms may lodge in the muscles, connective tissue, or brain, where they calcify and produce a variety of symptoms including pain, seizures, and neurologic disorders.

Diagnosis is accomplished by microscopic examination of shed segments. Radiologic studies and serologic tests may be helpful. For more information, see the specific parasite.

cetyl (se′til) the saturated alkyl group containing 16 carbons, $CH_3(CH_2)_{15}$—.

cetyltrimethylammonium bromide (se″til-tri-meth″il-ah-mo′ne-um) hexadecyltrimethylammonium bromide, a cationic surfactant compound.

CF abbrev. for complement fixation.

Cf symbol for the chemical element *californium.*

CFU abbrev. See *colony-forming units.*

CFU_{EOS} abbrev. for colony-forming units–eosinophil, a hematopoietic stem cell that gives rise to the eosinophil. See also under *stem cell.*

CFU_{MEG} abbrev. for colony-forming units–megakaryocyte, a hematopoietic stem cell that gives rise to the platelet. See also under *stem cell.*

CFU_{NM} abbrev. for colony-forming units–neutrophil-monocyte, a hematopoietic stem cell that gives rise to the neutrophil and monocyte. See also under *stem cell.*

CFU-E abbrev. for colony-forming units–erythrocyte, a hematopoietic stem cell that gives rise to the erythrocyte. See also under *stem cell.*

CG abbrev. See *chorionic gonadotropin.*

cg abbrev. See *centigram.*

CGD abbrev. See *chronic granulomatous disease.*

CGL abbrev. for chronic granulocytic leukemia. See *chronic myelogenous l.* under *leukemia.*

cGMP abbrev. See *cyclic guanosine monophosphate.*

cgs system abbrev. See *centimeter-gram-second system.*

Chaddock's sign (chad′oks) [Charles Gilbert *Chaddock,* U.S. neurologist, 1861–1936] dorsiflexion of the big toe (extensor plantar response) produced by stroking the foot on its lateral aspect under the malleolus. It is positive in lesions of the pyramidal tract.

Chaetomium (ke-to′me-um) a genus of ascomycetous fungus. The species *C. globosum* is frequently isolated from skin scrapings; it may contaminate cultures of dermatophytes.

chafe (chāf) to irritate the skin, usually a constant frictional rubbing; the rubbing sloughs off epithelial cells more quickly than they are produced.

Chagas' disease (chag′as) [Carlos *Chagas,* physician in Brazil, 1879–1934] see *American t.* under *trypanosomiasis.*

chagoma (chah-go′mah) an inflamed nodule appearing within a few days at the site of insect inoculation of the parasite in Chagas' disease. Lymph vessels draining the site may become blocked with scar tissue and produce edema in the area.

chain (chān) a collection of objects linked together in linear fashion or end-to-end; used in chemistry to refer to a linear assembly of atoms or moieties that are connected by covalent bonds. When applied to a reaction, it indicates a series of successive stages initiated by a primary reaction.

chaining (chān′ing) in automatic data processing, the storage of data in a linked list. Each item of the list contains the address of the next item on the list so that the list can be followed even though the items are not stored in sequence.

chain reaction a chemical or nuclear reaction, which, once initiated, continues or multiplies because one or more of the reaction products propagates the reaction.

chair (chār) the most stable conformation of cyclohexane and many other six-membered rings; see under *conformation.*

chalasia (kah-la′ze-ah) [Gr. *chalasis* relaxation] relaxation of an orifice, e.g., the cardiac sphincter.

chalazion (kah-la′ze-on) [Gr. "small lump"] a persistent granulomatous inflammation of a meibomian gland, which results from occlusion of its duct. It forms a firm swelling on the upper or lower lid. Initially, it may be indistinguishable from a sty; however, with progression it can compress the cornea and distort the vision. Most resolve spontaneously within several months.

chalcogen (kal′ko-jen) [Gr. *chalkos* copper; from copper ores, such as chalcocite, Cu_2S] the generic term for an element in Group VI of the periodic table, i.e., oxygen, sulfur, selenium, tellurium, or polonium.

chalcogenide (kal′ko-jĕ-nīd″) the generic term for an oxide, sulfide, selenide, telluride, or polonide.

chalicosis (kal″ĭ-ko′sis) [Gr. *chalix* gravel] pneumoconiosis due to the inhalation of particles of stone.

challenge (chal′enj) to administer a substance to a patient in order to observe whether there is a normal physiologic response. Examples include administration of (1) an antigen to evoke an immunologic response in a previously sensitized individual, (2) a hormone to evoke the normal response, and (3) a chemical compound to see if it is normally metabolized by the body.

chalone (ka′lōn, kal′ōn) [Gr. *chalan* to relax] a large number of diverse substances present in biologic fluids and tissues. Like hormones, they affect the rates of cellular reactions; however, unlike true hormones, chalones are not produced by specific glands. True chalones are polypeptides that inhibit cellular proliferation and are target organ–specific; e.g., skin chalones inhibit the proliferation of skin cells yet are not species-specific.

chamaecephaly (kam″e-sef′ah-le) [Gr. *chamai* low + *kephalē* head] the condition of having a low, flat head, i.e., having a cephalic index of 70 or less.

Chamberland filter (shahm-ber-lah′) [Charles Edouard *Chamberland,* French bacteriologist, 1851–1908] see *Chamberland f.* under *filter.*

chancre (shang′ker) [Fr. for "canker," a destructive sore, from L. *cancer* crab] 1. the primary sore of syphilis; a painless, hardened, eroded papule that occurs at the entry site of the infection, usually 2–3 wk after exposure.

2. a papular lesion that occurs at the site of entry of infection in skin tuberculosis or sporotrichosis.

chancroid (shang′kroid) an acute localized venereal disease caused by *Hemophilus ducreyi.* After transmission through sexual contact, *H. ducreyi* has an incubation period of 3–5 da. Initially, there is a vesiculopustular lesion, which advances and breaks to form a dirty, grayish-white ulcer with an overhanging edge. This lesion is painful and bleeds easily. There may also be lymphadenopathy, fever, chills, and malaise. Although it is unusual in the United States, chancroid is endemic in most of the rest of the world. The male-to-female ratio of the disease is 10 to 1. Diagnosis is made by culturing *H. ducreyi.* Also called *soft chancre.*

Chang's aniline-acid fuchsin method (changz) a histologic technique for the demonstration of mitochondria. It is a variation on Altmann's method for use on frozen dried tissue. Mitochondria stain bright red; collagen, red or purplish; erythrocytes, dark red; cytoplasm, light pink; and nuclei, slightly green.

channel (chan′el) [L. *canalis* a water pipe] 1. a duct, cut, or groove through which a fluid flows.

2. in information theory, any pathway over which information can be transmitted.

3. in a digital computer, a circuit that moves data between subunits.

character (kar′ak-ter) 1. a quality or attribute indicative of the nature of an object or an organism; in genetics, the expression of a gene or group of genes as seen in phenotype.

2. in computer programming, a letter, digit, special symbol (e.g., +, $), or blank that can be used by a computer program. The totality of characters recognized by the program is called the character set and is usually defined by the computer language. In the ASCII code, a character is represented in memory by a seven- or eight-bit code. See also *ASCII* and *binary coded decimal.*

acquired c., a noninheritable modification produced in an animal as a result of its own activities or of environmental influences.

dominant c., a mendelian character that is expressed when it is present in a single copy. See also *mendelian c.*

mendelian c., in genetics, a separate and distinct trait that is inherited in accordance with Mendel's laws, i.e., a trait primarily controlled by one gene. See also *dominant c., mendelian i.* under *inheritance, Mendel's laws, recessive c.,* and *sex-linked c.*

monogenic c., see *mendelian c.*

primary sex c., those characters of the male and female directly concerned in reproduction.

recessive c., a mendelian character that is not expressed phenotypically in the presence of its dominant allele, i.e., it is expressed only when homozygous. See also *mendelian c.*

secondary sex c., those characters specific to the male or female but not directly concerned with reproductive function, e.g., facial hirsutism in the male.

sex-conditioned c., an autosomal trait whose full expression is conditioned by the sex of the individual, e.g., male pattern baldness.

sex-limited c., an autosomally transmitted character that is expressed in only one sex.

sex-linked c., a trait controlled by a gene located on a sex chromosome; in humans, it is on the X or Y chromosome. Sex linkage has become synonymous with X linkage. See also *X-linked c.* Cf. *Y-linked c.*

X-linked c., a trait controlled by a gene located on the X chromosome. In males, who have only one X chromosome, the trait is always expressed whether it is dominant or recessive. See also *X-linked dominant i.* and *X-linked recessive i.* under *inheritance.*

Y-linked c., a trait controlled by a gene located on the Y chromosome, which is therefore exhibited only by males and is transmitted from a father to all his sons. Other than genes determining maleness, no clinically significant Y-linked characters have been identified in humans. Cf. *sex-linked c.*

character density in automatic data processing, the number of characters stored per unit length or per unit area.

characteristic (kar″ak-ter-is′tik) 1. see *character.*

2. typical of an individual or other entity.

3. an inherent property or operational parameter of a device.

characteristic curve see *H and D curve.*

characteristic fluorescent ray an x-ray photon emitted from the patient or surrounding objects by the same process as are characteristic rays.

characteristic ray an x-ray photon emitted from the target of an x-ray tube by an electron transition to the K level from a higher level. It has one of a few definite wavelengths that are characteristic of each element in the target.

charcoal (char′kōl) carbon derived by charring wood or other organic materials, such as bone.

activated c., [USP], a highly adsorbent amorphous form of carbon prepared by the destructive distillation of organic matter, followed by heating to 800°–900°C with steam or carbon dioxide. This produces a material with a honeycomb, porous internal structure possessing a surface area of approximately 900 m^2/g. It is used as a filter medium and to purify gases and liquids.

In medicine, activated charcoal is used as an agent to minimize gastrointestinal absorption after ingestions of many poisons. The usual dose is a slurry of 5–6 teaspoons in a glass of water given after gastric lavage or emesis (when indicated).

Charcot-Böttcher crystalloids (shar-ko′bet′cher) [Jean Martin *Charcot;* Arthur *Böttcher,* German anatomist, 1831–1889] slender filamentous structures, 10–25 μm long, unique to the Sertoli cells of the testes in the human. Their origin and function are unknown.

Charcot's joint (shar-kōz′) [Jean Martin *Charcot,* French neurologist, 1825–1893] see *neurogenic a.* under *arthropathy.*

Charcot-Marie-Tooth disease (shar-ko′ mah-re′ to͞oth) [J. M. *Charcot;* Pierre *Marie,* French physician, 1853–1940; Howard Henry *Tooth,* English physician, 1856–1925] the term for the dominant form of peroneal muscular atrophy; see *peroneal muscular atrophy.*

Charcot-Leyden crystals (shar-ko′ li′den) [Jean Martin *Charcot;* Ernst Victor von *Leyden,* German physician, 1832–1910] crystalline structures found in tissues containing large numbers of eosinophils; their composition is similar to that of eosinophilic granules. They are commonly found in the lung tissues of individuals with bronchial asthma, helminthiasis, and other conditions with hypereosinophilia or intestinal amebiasis. They can also be produced in vitro from eosinophils. Also called *asthma crystals.*

charge (charj) a basic property of elementary particles that determines the strength of their interaction with the electromagnetic field. Charge may be positive or negative, but each particle has an integral number of charge quanta (the proton has +1, the electron −1, and the neutron 0). The International System (SI) unit of charge is the coulomb (C). The charge quantum is 1.602×10^{-19}C. The charge of an object is the difference between the number of positive and negative quanta of its particles.

charged particle an elementary particle that carries an electric charge, e.g., a proton or an electron.

charge-transfer complex a complex formed between two molecules or between two parts of one molecule in which one acts as an electron donor, partially transferring electronic charge to the other, which acts as the electron acceptor. See also *π-complex.*

Charles' law (sharlz) [Jacques Alexandre César *Charles,* French physicist, 1746–1823] stated as: the volume of a given mass of a perfect gas is directly proportional to its absolute temperature when the pressure is held constant. Also called *Gay-Lussac's law.*

chart (chart) a record of data in graphic or tabular form.

chart recorder (chart) an electromechanical device that draws a graph of an electric signal on a strip of chart paper. A pen moves back and forth in response to the signal while the chart paper is driven at a constant speed by an electric motor.

The simplest type of pen movement is the galvanometer type used in most electrocardiographs. It works like a large voltmeter, with the pen at the point of the meter needle. Most laboratory recorders have a more complicated movement that uses a servomotor connected to a potentiometer to drive the pen. A reference voltage is stepped down by the potentiometer and compared with the input signal. The error voltage is applied to the servomotor, which moves the pen and potentiometer until the system reaches the null point (zero error voltage).

Two important performance characteristics of chart recorders are the pen response (the time taken by the pen in crossing the chart after the input jumps from zero to full-scale) and the step-response time (the time taken by the pen to reach an equilibrium after a jump in the input signal).

Also called *strip-chart recorder.*

Chassard-Lapiné position (shas-ard′ lap-e-na′) a radiographic position used to obtain superoinferior projections of the opacified urinary bladder or colon or of the pelvic outlet. The patient sits on the film, abducts the thighs, and bends forward as far as possible. The central ray projects vertically through the symphysis pubis.

chassis (chas′e, shas′e) a metal frame (usually grounded) on which the components of an electronic device are mounted.

chaulmoogra oil (chaul-moo′grah) a fixed oil expressed from the ripe seeds of *Taraktogenos kurzii, Hydnocarpus wightiana,* and *H. anthelmintica;* formerly used in the treatment of leprosy.

CHD abbrev. for coronary heart disease.

check bit (chek) a binary check digit.

check digit a redundant digit in a computer word or code group used to check the accuracy of the other digits of the word or group. See also *parity bit.*

Chédiak-Higashi syndrome (sha′de-ak hĭ-gash′e) [Moisés *Chédiak,* French physician, 20th century; Ototaka *Higashi,* Japanese physician, 20th century] a multisystem disorder, transmitted as an autosomal recessive trait, that is characterized by recurrent infections, hepatosplenomegaly, partial albinism, central nervous system abnormalities, and a high incidence of lymphoreticular malignancies. Both intracellular killing of organisms and neutrophil chemotaxis are abnormal.

The most obvious laboratory findings are giant cytoplasmic granular inclusions in the leukocytes and platelets on peripheral blood smears. There is no treatment other than antibiotic therapy for infections. Most affected individuals die during childhood from infection or neurologic deterioration, although a few survive to the third decade.

cheek (chēk) a fleshy protuberance, especially the fleshy portion of the sides of the face.

cheese washer's disease a type of hypersensitivity pneumonitis caused by the spores of *Penicillium casei,* developed by cheese workers. Also called cheese worker's disease.

cheil/o (ki′lo) [Gr. *cheilos* lip] a word element used in combining form to denote lip, edge, or brim, e.g., cheilitis.

cheilitis (ki-li′tis) [*cheil-* + *-itis*] inflammation of the lips.

cheilosis (ki-lo′sis) [*cheil-* + *-osis*] fissuring and dry scaling of the vermilion surface of the lips and angles of the mouth. It may be due to riboflavin deficiency and it is also caused by malfitting dentures.

chelate (ke′lāt) [Gr. *chēlē* claw] the complex (coordination compound) formed between a central metal ion and an organic ligand with more than one binding site (donor atom). The result is one or more rings that include the metal. Originally used as an adjective, as in chelate ring, the term is now used as a noun and as a verb meaning to form a chelate ring. The ligand that binds the metal may be called a chelating agent. Ethylenediaminetetraacetic acid (EDTA) is a common chelating agent, and, as the calcium disodium salt, is used in the treatment of lead poisoning. Other chelating agents are employed in the titrimetric determination of metals and to remove metallic ions from solutions and soils. Some naturally occurring chelates are chlorophyll (Mg), vitamin B_{12} (Co), and hemoglobin (Fe); the metallic part of the chelate is given in parentheses.

chelating agent (ke′lāt-ing) an organic compound (e.g., EDTA) that can bind metal ions by forming two or more coordinate bonds with cations. See also *chelate.*

chelation (ke-la′shun) the formation or presence of bonds from two or more atoms within the same ligand to a single central atom. An example is EDTA, which can bind one or two Ca^{2+} with a high binding affinity.

chem/o (ke′mo) [Gr. *chēmeia* chemistry] a word element used in combining form to denote chemistry, a chemical, or a drug, e.g., chemotherapy.

chemical (kem′ĭ-kal) 1. of, or pertaining to, chemistry.

2. a substance made up of chemical elements and characterized by a definite molecular composition.

incompatible c.'s, two or more chemicals that are likely to react vigorously or violently with each other; the term is generally used in reference to the storage of chemicals and to recommendations for segregation in order to avoid reactions in case of spill or fire. For example, there should be separate storage for combustible materials not compatible with strong oxidizers, particularly if the combustible and the oxidizer are liquids and are stored in large glass bottles, which are susceptible to breakage. If the combustible is acetic acid and the oxidizer is sulfuric acid, they should be stored in separate areas or cupboards, if possible, or at least in bottle carriers or containers designed for breakage protection and spill limitation.

National Fire Protection Association regulations (NFPA 49-1975 and NFPA 491M) contain information on identification of hazardous chemicals and on storage recommendations for segregating incompatible chemicals.

chemical bond see *bond.*

chemical interference the interference of one chemical entity (e.g., drug) in the analysis of another chemical entity or physiologic function. Various types of chemical interference are recognized:

1. a direct interference of a chemical compound with the chemical reaction used to qualitatively or quantitatively analyze a specific analyte (e.g., ascorbic acid in the glucose oxidase-peroxidase reaction).
2. in atomic absorption spectrophotometry, the interference caused by the formation of highly refractory compounds that do not dissociate in the flame.
3. the effect of a chemical compound on the quantitative composition of the body or a body fluid in regard to a specific analyte (e.g., administration of epinephrine will cause a change in the blood glucose level).

chemically clean relatively free of actual or potential organic and/or inorganic constituents that may alter the result of a chemical analysis, generally applied to laboratory ware used in analytical work.

chemical shift the shift in the NMR frequency of a nucleus in a compound due to diamagnetic shielding by the electrons in the compound.

chemical waste used or discarded chemicals. Standards for the handling, storage, and transportation of chemical waste in laboratories are subject to the same provisions as standards for the chemicals themselves. Quantities of flammable and combustible liquid wastes being held for disposal must be included in the total inventory subject to storage limits, according to National Fire Protection Association regulations (NFPA 56C-1980 and NFPA 45-1981). See also *hazardous waste.*

chemiluminescence (kem″ĭ-loo″mĭ-nes′ens) the emission of light by molecules in excited states produced by a chemical reaction, as in fireflies.

chemiluminescence assays see *nonradioisotopic i.* under *immunoassays.*

chemiosmotic hypothesis (kem″e-oz-mot′ik) a theory explaining the coupling of electron transport to ATP synthesis in oxidative phosphorylation. Each of the three transfers of an electron pair along the electron transport chain (accompanied by reductions of ubiquinone, cytochrome c, and molecular oxygen) produces a transfer of two to four protons across the mitochondrial inner membrane from the matrix to the intermembrane space. Energy for ATP synthesis is provided by the flow of protons back across the membrane.

The original chemiosmotic hypothesis supposed that this proton gradient is directly created by the electron transfer as protons are released on the outer side of the membrane while the reduced coenzymes NADH, $FMNH_2$, and QH_2 (ubiquinol) are reoxidized. An alternate theory, the conformational hypothesis, supposes that the protons are released by membrane proteins on the outer side upon oxidation, and then undergo a conformational change, accepting protons on the matrix side. This is similar to the Bohr effect in hemoglobin.

See also *oxidative phosphorylation.*

chemisorption (kem″e-sorp′shun) see *chemical a.* under *adsorption.*

chemistry (kem′is-tre) [Gr. *chēmeia*] the study of the chemical elements and their compounds, especially the physical properties of the compounds and their reactions. Branches of the science include biological chemistry, clinical chemistry, and geochemistry.

analytical c., the branch of chemistry that deals with the qualitative and quantitative chemical analysis of unknown specimens; it includes instrumental analysis.

clinical c., see *clinical chemistry.*

inorganic c., the branch of chemistry that deals with all chemical elements and their compounds, except hydrocarbons and their derivatives. Generally included are also carbides and other relatively simple carbon compounds such as carbon-oxygen and carbon-sulfur compounds in the form of oxides of carbon, metallic carbonates, and carbon disulfide, as well as some carbon-nitrogen compounds such as hydrogen cyanide and metallic cyanides.

organic c., the branch of chemistry that deals with hydrocarbons (compounds containing hydrogen and carbon) and their derivatives. A large portion of these compounds occur in living organisms.

physical c., the branch of chemistry that applies physical laws and physical methods to the study of chemistry, e.g., the study of reaction kinetics, thermodynamics, or electrochemistry.

chemoattractant (ke″mo-ah-trak′tant) see *chemotactic factor.*

chemoautotroph (ke″mo-au′to-trōf) an autotroph that can obtain energy by oxidation of inorganic chemicals. A few bacteria are chemoautotrophs. Also called *chemolithotroph.* See also *autotroph* and *photoautotroph.*

chemoautotrophic (ke″mo-au″to-trōf′ik) pertaining to chemoautotrophs.

chemodectoma (ke″mo-dek-to′mah) [*chemo-* + Gr. *dektos* to be received or accepted + *-oma*] any chromaffin negative tumor of the chemoreceptor system, primarily the carotid body, aortic pulmonary bodies, or glomus jugulare. See also *carotid body tumor* and *paraganglioma.*

chemoheterotroph (ke″mo-het′er-o-trōf″) see *heterotroph.*

chemokinesis (ke″mo-kin′ĕ-sis) the reaction by which cells increase their rate of locomotion or turning in response to chemical substances. Cf. *chemotaxis.*

chemolithotroph (ke″mo-lith′o-trōf) see *chemoautotroph.*

chemoorganotroph (ke″mo-or′gah-no-trōf″) see *heterotroph.*

chemoreceptor (ke″mo-re-sep′tor) a receptor, sense organ, or sensory nerve ending that reacts to chemical stimuli; some such stimuli participate in gustation and olfaction, others respond to changes in pH, P_{CO_2}, and P_{O_2}, as well as osmolality of blood and other body fluids.

central c., one of the chemosensitive neurons that lie just beneath the ventral surface of the medulla near the bilateral points of exit of the ninth and tenth cranial nerves. They are sensitive to changes in the carbon dioxide and hydrogen ion concentrations in the cerebrospinal fluid that bathes them. When these concentrations increase, the receptors act to excite the medullary inspiratory centers to cause a compensatory increase in the rate and depth of respiration.

peripheral c.'s, the aortic and carotid bodies.

chemostat (ke′mo-stat) an apparatus that maintains a carefully controlled environment, used to keep bacterial populations in a steady state of continuous cell division for many generations. See also *continuous flow c.* under *culture.*

chemosterilant (ke″mo-ster′ĭ-lant) a chemical compound or a process, such as gamma radiation, that causes sterility; used to control insects and other pests.

chemosynthesis (ke″mo-sin′the-sis) [*chemo-* + Gr. *synthesis* a putting together] the synthesis of carbohydrate from carbon dioxide and water by utilizing energy derived from chemical reactions rather than from absorbed light. It is characteristic of certain bacteria and fungi. Cf. *photosynthesis.*

chemotactic (ke″mo-tak′tik) of or pertaining to chemotaxis.

chemotactic factor a chemical substance that induces chemotaxis. Also called *chemoattractant* and *chemotactin.* See under *chemotaxis.*

chemotactin (ke″mo-tak′tin) see *chemotactic factor.*

chemotaxis (ke″mo-tak′sis) [*chemo-* + Gr. *taxis* arrangement] the directed motion of cells in response to a chemical concentration gradient. The term is sometimes more narrowly defined as the reaction by which cells orient themselves along a gradient, as opposed to chemokinesis, the reaction by which cells increase their rate of locomotion or turning in response to chemical substances.

All types of leukocytes exhibit chemotaxis; these cells crawl along surfaces with an ameboid movement toward the greater concentration of several possible chemicals, extending a ruffled pseudopod, called a lamellapodium, in response to products formed in immunologic reactions. They sense a chemical gradient by comparing the concentration at different points on their surfaces, using specific receptors.

Many chemotactic agents have been discovered. Among the natural agents are the activated complement component C5a, which is chemotactic for all leukocytes except lymphocytes; fibrinopeptides and fibrin degradation products, chemotactic for neutrophils and monocytes; kallikrein, chemotactic primarily for neutrophils; and various bacterial products, some lipid, and some protein, chemotactic for all leukocytes except lymphocytes. In addition there are chemotactic lymphokines released by T lymphocytes (see *lymphokine*) and ECF-A released by basophils and mast cells.

Several important diseases involve abnormalities of leukocyte chemotaxis. Chédiak-Higashi syndrome is the primary example of a genetic disorder in which there is an intrinsic cellular defect that hinders leukocyte locomotion as well as lysosomal degranulation and bacterial killing. Genetic deficiency of complement component C3 or C5 causes an absence of chemotaxis in response to complement activation. Defects of T lymphocytes or basophils that prevent them from making or releasing chemotactic factors also can reduce chemotaxis. Two serum inhibitors of chemotaxis, chemotactic-factor inactivator (CFI) and cell-directed inhibitor (CDI), have been described. Elevated serum concentration of these inhibitors, seen in individuals with various infections and malignancies, leads to deficient chemotaxis.

Cf. *chemokinesis.*

chemotaxis assays 1. Boyden chamber assays. In these tests a chemical gradient is established across a Millipore filter, and the response of leukocytes is measured by the number of cells crossing the filter (or moving a set distance into it). See also *Boyden chamber.*

2. agarose migration assay. The cells and chemoattractant are placed in two reservoirs in an agarose plate. The amount of movement of the cells toward the reservoir containing the attractant is a measure of chemotaxis.

chemotherapy (ke″mo-ther′ah-pe) [chemo- + Gr. *therapeia* treatment] the treatment of disease by chemical agents, i.e., drug treatment as opposed to other treatment modalities.

The term is often used to refer to the use of drugs in the treatment of cancer to achieve the selective killing of tumor cells. Such chemotherapy is based on the principles of the "cell-kill hypothesis" derived from experimental studies of tumors: (1) the survival of an animal with a transplantable tumor is inversely related to either the number of tumor cells inoculated or the number remaining after treatment; (2) a single tumor cell is capable of multiplying and eventually killing the host; (3) for most drugs, a clear relationship exists between the drug dose and killing of tumor cells; and (4) a given drug dose kills a constant fraction, not number, of tumor cells, regardless of the cell numbers present at the time of therapy. Thus, the maximal opportunity for achieving cure exists during the early stage of the disease. It is more difficult to eradicate disseminated than localized cancer, and much easier to control small tumors than larger ones.

The first-order kinetics of neoplastic cell kill are valid only when all tumor cells are similarly exposed and both the growth fraction and the ratio of drug-sensitive to permanently drug-resistant cancer cells are the same. Because large tumors have nonuniform blood supplies with mixtures of hypoxic and oxic cells and many chemotherapeutic agents kill only oxygenated cells, and because pharmacologic sanctuaries exist for many drugs, this concept can be applied only in a general sense in most therapeutic situations.

In humans, the side-effects of chemotherapy on normal tissue are also based on the cell-kill hypothesis. For clinically detectable neoplasms, reduction in tumor size can be used as an approximation of cell kill. For leukemias, the basic parameter is reduction in percentage of leukemic cells. For solid tumors, objective response is a percentage reduction of measurable lesions. In an attempt to represent cell kill, volume reduction is approximated because most clinical lesions can be measured only in two dimensions.

A complete response implies no apparent tumor, but the threshold for measurement varies with the technique. For humans, the calculated tumor burden resulting in the death of the host is approximately 10^{12} tumor cells. A tumor 1 cm in diameter contains approximately 10^9 cells. Thus, in a tumor containing 10^{11}–10^{12} cells, a two- to three-log cell kill may result in objective regression, but 10^9 cells still remain. Because such a hypothetical 1-cm tumor nodule may not be detected clinically, other measures of cell kill must be used. In animals, duration of response correlates with cell kill. In both human leukemias and solid tumors, duration of response and/or host survival represent the best clinical correlates of cell kill.

CELL KINETICS. Renewing cells that are synthesizing DNA go through a series of phases known as the cell cycle. At the completion of mitosis (M) the cell spends a variable length of time in a "resting" phase (G_1), during which the synthesis of DNA for cell replication is suspended while synthesis of RNA and protein continues. In late G_1 (the G_1-S conversion), an unknown signal initiates a burst of RNA synthesis, and shortly thereafter the period of DNA synthesis (S phase) begins, after which the cell is committed to undergo division or remain polyploid. Next, the cell ceases DNA synthesis during the G_2 phase before entry into mitosis, although RNA and protein synthesis continue. In mitosis, the rates of protein and RNA synthesis diminish abruptly while the genetic material is segregated into daughter cells. In addition to actively dividing cells, there is also a population of nondividing cells, which are said to be in the G_0-phase. If such cells have not undergone terminal differentiation, they may reenter the cell cycle and proliferate. Cells in G_0 are, for the most part, refractory to cancer chemotherapeutic agents.

Tumor growth is dependent on the proliferating pool (growth fraction) of cells in the tumor. The rate of growth and the doubling time of small tumors depend largely, but not entirely, on the percentage of cells in the mitotic cycle. Particularly in larger tumors, rate of growth is also contingent on the number of tumor cells spontaneously dying or becoming differentiated. Tumor cells may be proliferating more or less rapidly than sensitive normal cell populations, and they may have more or less cells in the drug-sensitive phases of the cell cycle. However, this does not explain all successes and failures of drug therapy.

PHARMACOKINETICS. Another reason for success or failure of chemotherapy may be related to the pharmacologic disposition of drugs in patients. A drug cannot influence the tumor in a favorable way unless it reaches the tumor site and remains there in tumoricidal concentration for a sufficiently long period to kill the tumor cells. In general, the purpose of pharmacokinetic studies is to tell the physician how to obtain an effective concentration (C) of drug at the target site for sufficient time (T) to bring about the desired effect. This is referred to as the optimal $C \times T$ and, in most cases, can be approximated for treatment of human tumors from experimental studies on the delivery of the drug to the organs or tissues of interest.

The effectiveness of an antitumor agent is directly related to its $C \times T$, which is markedly affected by drug dosage and schedule of administration; the tumor cells and, to some degree, the critical normal tissues present variable targets. Knowledge of cell kinetics of normal tissue (which should remain relatively constant) and of tumor populations can help to determine the most effective means of obtaining an optimal $C \times T$, which is defined as the $C \times T$ that kills the maximal number of tumor cells with minimal lethality in cells of normal tissue.

RESISTANCE. Resistance to cancer chemotherapy may be either natural (innate) or acquired. Natural resistance means that the tumor is resistant from the outset of treatment. Acquired resistance occurs after therapy has begun as a result of epigenetic or genetic phenomena. Treatment selectively destroys the sensitive population, with subsequent overgrowth of the resistant population. In advanced tumors, in which the neoplastic cell burden is high, heterogeneity of sensitivity is likely. Spontaneous mutants have been shown to arise in response to various antimetabolites in mammalian cells. Other factors that contribute to natural drug resistance include a low-growth fraction and long generation time of the tumor, and the failure of drugs to enter pharmacologic sanctuaries.

Clinical resistance involves host as well as tumor factors. The toxicity to normal tissues, such as bone marrow, limits the drug doses that can be administered. Many drugs are highly active in vitro at concentrations that could never be used in humans because of normal tissue dose restrictions.

Some of the factors, at a cellular level, that may explain why certain tumor cells are resistant and others sensitive to chemotherapy include: (1) variability in membrane transport of drug into the cell; (2) extent of phosphorylation of purine and pyrimidine analogs; (3) extent of catabolism, e.g., deamination, decarboxylation, phosphorolysis, hydrolysis, reduction, oxidation, or esterification of drug to inactive forms; (4) altered affinity of target enzymes for inhibiting drugs; (5) different pathways of precursor utilization for DNA synthesis by tumor cells; (6) extent of repair of drug-induced damage; (7) drug induction of enzymatic activity in tumor or normal tissue; (8) distribution of drug receptors in cell surfaces, cytoplasm, or nucleus; (9) immune inactivation of antigenic drugs; and (10) fraction of cell population in drug-sensitive phases of the mitotic cycle. In any given case of acquired resistance, more than one of these factors may be involved.

For the large majority of anticancer drugs, administered singly or in combination, bone marrow suppression represents the most important dose-limiting factor. Therefore, as a minimal requirement, complete blood counts should be determined immediately before each course when intermittent chemotherapy is applied. Because single-agent as well as multi-agent chemotherapy is most effective when administered in full dosage, it is advisable when possible to prolong the interval between courses rather than reduce the dosage.

Severe marrow suppression may require adequate supportive measures, but sophisticated techniques are available in only a limited number of centers. Repeated platelet transfusions are usually considered necessary in case of petechiae or bleeding tendency, or when the platelet level is below 25,000/mm^3. In patients with severe granulocytopenia (less than 1000/mm^3), gram-negative septicemia often occurs and specific antibiotics such as gentamicin plus carbenicillin are indicated, especially when the body temperature rises above 38°C. In this situation, repeated granulocyte transfusions have proved very helpful in the control of infection in more than 80 percent of patients.

In susceptible tumors, a rapid destruction of bulky tumor masses can produce, through an increased purine and pyrimidine breakdown, uric acid nephropathy. To prevent this serious complication, adequate fluid intake, alkalinization of urine, and oral administration of allopurinol (300–350 mg/da) are indicated during the first period of induction chemotherapy.

DRUG ADMINISTRATION. The route of administration is an important variable in the delivery of the required dose of chemotherapy. Many factors relate to the logistics and mechanics of drug delivery. An oral drug formulation cannot be given to a patient who is vomiting, unconscious, or dysphagic. Prolonged daily drug administration precludes intravenous administration for ambulatory patients. Hospitalization is required for a continuous infusion of drug, unless a portable infusion pump is used. Prolonged intravenous administration becomes technically difficult because of inaccessible veins.

The intrathecal route has been used with methotrexate and cytosine arabinoside. Leukemia that has spread to the central nervous system has been controlled by the direct delivery of effective drugs that are relatively unable to cross the blood-brain barrier.

Direct intracavitary drug instillation is effective in controlling malignant neoplastic effusions. It is unclear whether the mechanism of action is by the induction of a nonspecific inflammatory response resulting in fibrous adhesion of the parietal and visceral surfaces, or by a direct cytotoxic effect.

The intraarterial route has been used for delivery of a high drug concentration to areas of bulk disease. Fluorinated pyrimidines have been administered via the hepatic artery for treatment of metastatic colorectal carcinoma to the liver. Intraarterial infusion of phenylalanine mustard has been used for extremity melanomas, and intraarterial doxorubicin (Adriamycin) for extremity sarcomas. The therapeutic advantage of this route of administration has not been proven.

DRUG DOSAGE. The optimal drug dosage is a critical variable in the management of cancer patients. The treatment objective is to provide the maximal therapeutic benefit and the minimal amount of morbidity. Because anticancer drugs are only relatively selective for neoplastic cells as compared with nonneoplastic cells, most of the agents have a narrow therapeutic index.

The cancer chemotherapist must choose drug dose(s) within a narrow range because of the dose-response relationship and the low therapeutic index for most antitumor drugs. The determination of the most appropriate dose is a complex clinical judgment that should be based on the therapeutic goal, the patient's anticipated tolerance to chemotherapy, and the characteristics of the drugs to be used.

The therapeutic goal may be expressed as a risk-benefit ratio; the morbidity of the treatment must be balanced with its potential benefits. In a patient with advanced cancer who will die shortly if untreated, the highly aggressive use of drugs is warranted if a significant survival potential exists. If survival without treatment can be expected to be long, greater caution must be exercised with drugs. In adjuvant trials where drugs are given to some patients who are already cured of their tumor, there must be cognizance of both acute toxic dangers and long-term side-effects.

MECHANISM OF ACTION. Cytotoxic drugs, like ionizing radiation, do not kill tumor cells directly, but impair cell division and thereby cell proliferation. A number of fundamental molecular processes must continue to take place for cells to proliferate. The genetic material, DNA, must be replicated without error once every cycle. This requires an adequate supply of purine and pyrimidine nucleotides as building blocks, the enzyme DNA polymerase, and an intact DNA template to direct the synthesis of complementary RNA, a process catalyzed by RNA polymerase. RNA is then translated into proteins through a complex polymerization reaction that takes place on the ribosomes in the cell cytoplasm. The sequence of nucleotides of the messenger RNA determines the sequence whereby amino acids, attached to their specific transfer RNA, are positioned in the growing protein. After the cells have replicated their DNA, thereby having a double complement of genetic material, they undergo mitosis. The various chemotherapeutic agents interfere with one or other of these essential cellular processes.

Alkylating agents act by the transfer of alkyl groups to biologically important cell constituents such as amino, carboxyl, sulfhydryl, or phosphate groups whose function is then impaired. Antimetabolites interfere with the synthesis of building blocks for nucleic acid. The plant alkaloids produce mitotic arrest by binding to a cytoplasmic precursor of the spindle, and many of the antibiotics bind selectively to DNA, forming complexes that block the formation of DNA-dependent RNA. The nitrosoureas exhibit alkylating agent activity. The enzyme L-asparaginase has the unique property of depleting asparagine in tumor cells. The precise mode of action of the hormones is unknown.

DRUGS IN CURRENT USE. A total of 39 drugs, including hormonal agents, are now commercially available in the United States (See *Appendix A*), along with their major indications and toxicity patterns. Also listed are 13 agents that are still investigational but have demonstrated evidence of meaningful anticancer activity. There are a large number of other investigational drugs currently under study, but they have not as yet clearly demonstrated anticancer activity.

chemotroph (ke′mo-trōf) a microorganism that derives energy from chemical reactions.

chemotropism (ke-mot′ro-pizm) [*chemo-* + Gr. *tropos* a turning] the tendency of an organism to move toward or away from an increased chemical concentration.

chenodeoxycholate (ke″no-de-ok″se-ko′lāt) any salt, ester, or dissociated form of chenodeoxycholic acid.

chenodeoxycholic acid (ke″no-de-ok″se-ko′lik) a $3\alpha,7\alpha$-dihydroxy-5β-cholanic acid, produced in the liver from cholesterol; it occurs as the third most abundant acid in human bile.

chenopodium oil (ke″no-po′de-um) a volatile oil obtained by steam distillation of fresh overground parts of the flowering and fruiting plants of *Chenopodium ambrosiodes,* L. (Chenopodiaceae). It contains 65 percent of ascaridole, an active anthelmintic principle, and is used as an anthelmintic.

Chen's test a test for demonstrating the presence of sympathomimetic amines. One percent of drug in 1 percent acetic acid is treated with one drop of 1 percent $CuSO_4$ and one drop of 2 molar NaOH. Ephedrine and metanephrine give a purple color, adrenaline and isoprenaline a green to green-brown color.

Cherry-Crandall procedure (cher′e cran′dal) see under *lipase assays.*

cherry-red spot the choroid appearing as a red circular area surrounded by abnormal gray-white retina as viewed through the fovea centralis. It is seen in Tay-Sachs disease and other storage diseases. In Tay-Sachs, it is due to stored sphingolipid. Also called Tay's spot.

cherubism (cher′ŭ-bizm) a hereditary condition, thought to be transmitted as an autosomal dominant trait, that appears in children aged 3–5 yr as a progressive bilateral swelling of the angle of the mandible, which imparts a cherubic look to the face. The maxilla or entire jaw may also be involved, and submandibular lymphadenopathy is common. On histologic examination, the condition is identical to central giant cell reparative granuloma. Also called familial fibrodysplasia of the jaw.

chest (chest) see *thorax.*

chest tube a tube inserted into the thoracic cavity for the purpose of removing air or fluid. It is attached to a closed drainage system so that normal intrapleural pressure is maintained.

Cheyne-Stokes respiration (chān stōks) [John *Cheyne,* Scottish physician, 1777–1836; William *Stokes,* Irish physician, 1804–1878] an abnormal pattern of breathing characterized by a rhythmic recurrence (every 45 sec to 3 min) of a series of inspiratory-expiratory cycles having a gradually waxing and then waning tidal volume. The series is regularly interrupted by periods of apnea. This pattern of periodic breathing is most often associated with metabolic encephalopathy, bilateral cerebral hemisphere damage, or circulatory disorders (congestive heart failure), which result in an increased feedback sensitivity of the central nervous system respiratory control mechanism or in an increased lag time between the transport of blood from the lungs to the medullary and arterial chemoreceptors.

CHF abbrev. See *congestive heart failure.*

chi (X, χ) (ki) the twenty-second letter of the *Greek alphabet.*

χ the Greek lower case letter *chi.*

χ^2 a statistic used to measure goodness of fit. See also *chi-squared test.*

χ_e symbol for *electric susceptibility.*

χ_m symbol for *magnetic susceptibility.*

Chiari-Frommel syndrome (ke-ar′e from′el) [Johann Baptist *Chiari,* German obstetrician, 1817–1854; Richard *Frommel,* German gynecologist, 1854–1912] a syndrome that occurs most often in first-time mothers and is characterized by amenorrhea, persistent lactation, uterine hypoplasia, and an atrophic endometrium. It is due to a disturbance in secretion of prolactin. Laboratory studies reveal increased levels of luteinizing and luteotropic hormones. Cf. *Forbes-Albright syndrome.*

Chiari's net (ke-ar′ēz) [Hans *Chiari,* Austrian pathologist, 1851–1916] a network of fine fibers occasionally found on the wall of the right atrium. It represents remnants of the right valve of the sinus venosus and the septum spurium.

chiasm (ki′azm) [Gr. *chiasma*] in anatomy, an X-shaped crossing of two structures such as nerves, tendons, or muscles. Also called *chiasma.* See also *optic chiasm.*

chiasma (ki-as′mah), pl. *chiasmata* [Gr. "an X-shape," from the letter chi] 1. an X-shaped crossing; also called *chiasm.*

2. in genetics, an X-shaped junction where nonsister chromatids are in contact during the prophase of meiosis. Chiasmata are thought to be the visible signs of recombination (crossing over). They appear during the diplotene stage and move toward the ends of the chromatids (a process called terminalization); the homologous chromosomes then separate.

chickenpox (chik′en-poks) a highly contagious viral disease caused by the varicella-zoster virus. The portal of entry is the respiratory tract in which the virus can multiply, progress to viremia, and then disseminate to the skin and internal organs. A fever appears after an incubation period of 2–3 wk, followed by the appearance of a maculopapular eruption on the skin of the face and trunk that becomes vesicular. Chickenpox is relatively benign in children, but may be complicated with pneumonitis and encephalitis in adults. Once infected, the patient develops life-long immunity from external reinfection. The virus has a remarkable capability of latency, however, persisting in the dorsal root or cranial nerve ganglia; upon subsequent activation, it causes the disease herpes zoster. Also called *varicella.* See also *herpesvirus.*

chief cell (chēf) 1. one of the types of cuboidal epithelial cells that line the gastric glands; pepsinogen and intrinsic factor are its secretory products. Also called *peptic cell* and *zymogenic cell.*

2. see *pinealocyte.*

3. see *principal cell.*

Chievitz's organ (che′wits-ez) [Johan Henrik *Chievitz,* Danish anatomist, 1850-1901] an embryonic epithelial outgrowth behind the parotid gland. It may merge into the gland or disappear entirely. Also called organ of Chievitz.

Chiffelle and Putt method (chif-el′ put) a histologic procedure utilizing Sudan IV or Sudan Black B in propylene glycol for the demonstration of lipids. Cytoplasm does not stain; neutral fats, myelin, mitochondria, and lipids stain either reddish-orange (with Sudan IV) or greenish-black (with Sudan Black B).

chigger (chig′er) the six-legged red larva of mites of the family Trombiculidae. These larvae attach to the skin of humans and other vertebrates when feeding, and produce severe dermatitis and allergic reactions. Some species are vectors of the rickettsiae of scrub typhus. Also called *harvest mite* and *red mite.* See also *E. alfreddugèsi* under *Eutrombicula.*

chikungunya (chik″un-gun′yah) [Bantu "that which bends up"] an arboviral disease characterized by a sudden onset of fever, chills, headache, conjunctivitis, back pain, and (especially) joint pain. A maculopapular rash may or may not appear. The virus that causes this disease belongs to the genus *Alphavirus;* the transmitting vector is the mosquito.

chilblain (chil′blān) a mild form of cold injury that usually occurs on the fingers, toes, or nose. The lesions are red and itchy, and form a blister. Warmth usually exacerbates the condition.

childbed fever (chīld′bed) a postpartum infection of the uterus, usually transmitted to patients by contamination from the hands or clothing of an attendant during delivery. It is most often a bacterial infection caused by *Streptococcus pyogenes.*

This disease had an important role in the history of infectious disease control. Its indirect transmission was not recognized until the 1840s when physicians were implicated in the prevalence of childbed fever in hospitals because they moved from patient to patient with unwashed hands. Also called puerperal sepsis.

Chilomastix (ki″lo-mas′tiks) a genus of trophozoite protozoa, with three flagella projecting from the rounded anterior region and a fourth within the cytostome. They encyst in pear- or lemon-shaped forms. They are found in the intestines of vertebrates but are nonpathogenic.

Chilopoda (ki-lop′o-dah) [Gr. *cheilos* lip + *pous* foot] a class of centipedes within the phylum Arthropoda. Members have one pair of legs and one pair of spiracles on each segment of the body posterior to the head, and gonads on the last segment. The first pair of legs is modified to form claws equipped with a venom gland and duct. Bites are not fatal, but the venom and other secreted fluid is histolytic and may cause painful swelling and papules.

chimera (ki-me′rah) [Gr. *chimaira* a mythologic fire-spouting monster with a lion's head, goat's body, and serpent's tail] an organism that consists of two or more cell lineages descended from different zygotes. Cf. *mixoploid.*

blood group c., the result of exchange of blood cells across the placenta between dizygotic twins or between mother and fetus; the chimera has two different blood cell lines and thus two different blood groups. This condition occurs rarely in humans.

dispermic c., a chimera that results from fertilization of an ovum by two spermatozoa that combine with the ovum nucleus and the second polar body, or with the two daughter nuclei of an abnormal division of the ovum nucleus.

heterologous c., a chimera in which the cell lines come from organisms of different species.

homologous c., a chimera in which the cell lines come from conspecific organisms.

isologous c., a chimera in which the cell lines have the same genotype, as from identical twins.

radiation c., an organism with immunologic characteristics of host and donor after a bone marrow graft from an antigenically different donor, the host having first been subjected to irradiation to inhibit an immune response to the donor cells.

chimerism (ki-mĕr′izm) the quality of being a chimera; in genetics, the presence in an individual of cells of different genetic origin, as of blood cells derived from a dizygotic twin.

chin (chin) the anterior prominence of the lower jaw.

Chinese restaurant syndrome see under *monosodium glutamate.*

chip (chip) 1. a small piece, usually a fragment broken off a larger object.

2. the silicon substrate of a single integrated circuit.

bone c.'s, small pieces of cancellous bone used to fill bony defects.

chir/o (ki′ro) [Gr. *cheir* hand] a word element used in combining form to denote the hand, e.g., chiromegaly.

chiral (ki′ral) in chemistry, pertaining to a molecule that cannot be superimposed on its mirror image. The mirror images (enantiomers) are distinguished by their chirality or handedness.

chiral center 1. the center of dissymmetry or handedness in a molecule. It often is an atom with four different substituents, but it can be another type of atom or even a point in space between atoms.

2. an asymmetric carbon atom (one with four different substituents) or another asymmetric atom, such as the nitrogen of a quaternary amine or the sulfur of an optically stable sulfoxide.

chirality (ki-ral′ĭ-te) [Gr. *cheir* hand] in chemistry, the handedness of a chiral molecule as specified by its optical rotation or absolute configuration.

chi-squared (χ^2) distribution (ki skwārd) a theoretical frequency distribution that plays a central role in statistical theory and applications. It can be characterized as the probability distribution of the sum of the squares of a number (n) of independent normally distributed variables having mean zero and standard deviation one. The parameter n is called the number of degrees of freedom. The mean of the χ^2 distribution is n and the standard deviation is $\sqrt{2n}$. The distributions for two or more degrees of freedom have a single mode at $n/2 - 1$ (the density becomes infinite at $\chi^2 = 0$ for one degree of freedom). See also *normal distribution.*

chi-squared (χ^2) test a statistical hypothesis test that employs the theoretical chi-squared distribution. In particular, the term is often used for a test applied to categorical (nominal scale) data where $\chi^2 = \Sigma_i (O_i - E_i)/E_i$, with O_i the number of sample individuals in category i and E_i the number expected according to the null hypothesis. The sampling distribution of the χ^2 statistic is approximately the χ^2 distribution with $n - m$ degrees of freedom, where n is the number of categories and m is the number of sample statistics used in estimating the expected number of individuals in each category. The null hypothesis is rejected at the significance level if the χ^2 statistic exceeds the upper α percentile point of the χ^2 distribution.

The χ^2-tests of independence and homogeneity are applied to data classified on two nominal scales. The data are arranged in an $r \times k$ contingency table.

The null hypothesis of independence is that the two scales measure independent random variables; therefore, the expected number of individuals in each cell is the product of the totals for that cell's row and column divided by the sample size. The number of degrees of freedom is $rk - r - (k - 1) = (r - 1)(k - 1)$ because there are rk categories, and r row totals and $k - 1$ column totals are used in determining the expected frequencies. (One column total is redundant because both the row and the column totals add up to the sample size.) The hypothesis of homogeneity is that the K samples, from K populations, all have the same distribution with regard to the row variable; the test is identical to that for independence.

The χ^2-test of goodness of fit is applied to determine whether the data are consistent with some theoretical probability distribution that predicts the expected relative frequency (p_i) in each category. The expected frequencies are $E_i = Np_i$, where N is the sample size. If the null hypothesis completely specifies the theoretical distribution, the number of degrees of freedom is one less than the number of categories (because the sample size is used in determining expected frequencies). If the null hypothesis specifies only a family of distributions with one or more unspecified parameters (e.g., binomial or Poisson), one degree of freedom (in addition to the one for the sample size) is subtracted for each parameter that must be estimated from the data in order to compute the expected relative frequencies.

The significance level of the χ^2-test is only an approximation of the true probability of a type I error. The approximation is good for large samples. A traditional guideline is that the sample size must be large enough so that every expected frequency is at least five.

When the test statistic has only one degree of freedom, as with a 2 × 2 contingency table, Yates' correction for continuity is used. The formula for χ^2 is modified to $\chi^2 = \Sigma_i(|O_i - E_i| - 1/2)^2/E_i$.

See also *contingency table* and *Fisher's exact test.*

chitin (kī'tĭn) [Gr. *chitōn* tunic] a white, insoluble, horny polysaccharide, the principal organic constituent of the exoskeleton of some insects and crustacea; it is also found in certain fungi. On hydrolysis it yields a linear homopolymer of β-(1→4)-2-acetamido-2-deoxy-D-glucose (an *N*-acetyl-D-glucosamine).

Chlamydia (klah-mid'e-ah) [Gr. *chlamys* cloak] a genus representing a widespread group of nonmotile, gram-negative, obligately intracellular bacteria. Because chlamydiae are quite small and replicate only within susceptible cells, they were previously considered to be viruses. Some of the characteristics that distinguish chlamydiae from other pathogens are listed in Table 1. Chlamydiae may be viewed as gram-negative bacteria that lack important pathways for the production of energy, and as a consequence are restricted to growth in an intracellular environment where the host cell provides the necessary adenosine triphosphate.

Chlamydiae have a unique developmental cycle that distinguishes them from all other microorganisms. This replicative cycle gives rise to the characteristic inclusion observed in the cytoplasm of the host cell. The elementary body represents the infectious particle that is taken up by the host cell. The small body within the phagosome undergoes reorganization into a reticulate body (initial body). Within this membrane-bound vacuole, the reticulate bodies grow by means of binary fission. Eventually the vacuole becomes filled with elementary bodies, resulting in the typical inclusion. The subsequent release of elementary bodies and the lysis of the host cell permit infection of surrounding cells.

The genus *Chlamydia* contains two species: *C. trachomatis* and *C. psittaci.* Criteria for distinguishing between them are summarized in Table 2. *C. trachomatis* is capable of inducing trachoma, inclusion conjunctivitis, lymphogranuloma venereum (LGV), and a significant proportion of genital infections.

Chlamydial infection of the neonate, in addition to causing inclusion conjunctivitis, may also lead to pneumonia some weeks after birth, presumably through the drainage of infectious organisms via the nasolacrimal ducts. Adults with inclusion conjunctivitis may manifest symptoms of upper respiratory infection, although pneumonia does not develop.

LABORATORY DIAGNOSIS. Direct examination smears prepared from tissues or scrapings may be examined with Macchiavello or Giemsa stain. The typical inclusions can be observed in *C. trachomatis* infections of the conjunctiva, urethra, and cervix. Chlamydiae have distinctive staining properties in that the elementary bodies stain purple with Giemsa stain and red with Macchiavello stain, in contrast to the blue host cell cytoplasm. The reticulate bodies stain blue with Giemsa stain.

Immunofluorescence using broadly reactive antisera is thought to be a more sensitive method than direct examination of stained preparations. Inclusions appear as well-defined, yellow-green, fluorescent masses within the cytoplasm of epithelial cells; they are observed with greater frequency in acute, severe infections than in chronic ones.

Chlamydia grow well in the yolk sac of embryonated eggs. However, few medical laboratories have the capacity for routine isolation of chlamydia by this means. The most frequently employed means of isolation, particularly of *C. trachomatis,* is inoculation into cell cultures. Usually, cell cultures (the McCoy cell line has been found most useful) are treated with either x-ray or selected drugs to arrest cell division. Centrifugation is used to bring chlamydia in

Chlamydia, TABLE 1. COMPARISON OF CHLAMYDIAE WITH OTHER PATHOGENIC AGENTS

	CHLAMYDIAE	BACTERIA	RICKETTSIAE	MYCOPLASMAS	VIRUSES
Growth outside host cell	0	+	0*	+	0
Independent protein synthesis	+	+	+	+	0
Generation of metabolic energy	0	+	+	+	0
Rigid cell envelope	Variable	+	+	0	Variable
Antibiotic susceptibility	+	+	+	+	0
Mode of reproduction	Fission	Fission	Fission	Fission	Host cell synthesis of subunits; then assembly of virion
Nucleic acids	DNA & RNA	DNA & RNA	DNA & RNA	DNA & RNA	DNA OR RNA, not both

* Except *Rochalimaea quintana.*
From Davis, B. D., et al.: Microbiology. 3rd ed. New York, Harper & Row, 1980, p. 777.

Chlamydia, TABLE 2. DIVISION OF CHLAMYDIAE INTO SPECIES

PROPERTY	*C. trachomatis*	*C. psittaci*
Susceptibility to sulfonamides	Sensitive	Resistant
Type of inclusion produced	More compact	More diffuse
Presence of glycogen in inclusion	Yes	No
% G + C	~44%	~41%
Principal hosts	Humans	Birds and mammals
Diseases induced	Trachoma Inclusion conjunctivitis Lymphogranuloma venereum Urethritis Mouse pneumonitis	Ornithosis, psittacosis Many clinical and subclinical diseases of mammals and birds

Adapted from Gordon, F. B., and Quan, A. L.: Occurrence of glycogen in inclusions of the psittacosis-lymphogranuloma-venereum-trachoma agents. J. Infect. Dis. *115*:186, 1965, by permission of The University of Chicago Press.

the inoculum into intimate contact with the cells. Beginning at 3 da and continuing to 10 da, the cell cultures are observed for the production of inclusions, which are visualized by conventional or immunofluorescent staining.

Strains of *C. psittaci* of avian origin can be grown in cell culture, mice, or embryonated eggs. Because a significant number of laboratory-acquired infections have been documented, the isolation of this agent should be attempted only in laboratories having the requisite containment facilities and technical expertise.

Serologic tests are available. The chlamydiae possess group-, species-, and type-specific antigens that are believed to be cell wall–associated. *C. trachomatis* occurs as 15 immunotypes, which have been designated A, B, Ba, C through K, and L1, L2, and L3. Type-specific antigens can best be identified by the immunofluorescence technique.

Chlamydial infection induces a variety of antibodies. In humans the most likely and widely utilized procedure for detecting them is the complement-fixation test, using the group antigen. Acute- and convalescent-phase sera should be collected and tested at the same time to confirm a rise in titer. This procedure is useful for diagnosing psittacosis, LGV, and genital chlamydial infections. For trachoma, the more sensitive immunofluorescent assay technique is preferred.

See also *anti-chlamydia antibody tests, inclusion c.* under *conjunctivitis, lymphogranuloma venereum,* and *trachoma.*

WALTER S. CEGLOWSKI, PH.D.

C. psittaci, a species endemic in a wide variety of birds and important economically because it can cause the death of large flocks of poultry. The disease, first called psittacosis because of its identification with the parrot family, is now given the more general name of ornithosis. Human infection occurs from contact with infected birds, and can cause severe and fatal pneumonia. The organism is resistant to sulfonamides but is susceptible to tetracycline. See also *ornithosis.*

C. trachomatis, a species responsible for a variety of diseases of the mucous membranes of the ocular and urogenital areas. The most widely seen disease is trachoma, the greatest single cause of blindness worldwide. Others are conjunctivitis, urethritis, and lymphogranuloma venereum. Transmission occurs from direct contact during birth or infant care, or from venereal contact. The organism is susceptible to sulfonamides and broad-spectrum antibiotics such as tetracyclines, chloramphenicol, and rifamycin. See also *lymphogranuloma venereum* and *trachoma.*

chlamydia, pl. *chlamydiae.* any member of the genus *Chlamydia.*

Chlamydiaceae (klah-mid″e-a′se-e) a family within the rickettsias, that consists of small, gram-negative bacteria with a unique, obligately intracellular developmental cycle. These organisms are parasites of birds and mammals (including humans) in which they may cause various diseases, and are occasionally found in arthropods. The family contains a single genus, *Chlamydia.*

chlamydiosis (klah-mid″e-o′sis) a general term for an infection caused by *Chlamydia.*

chlamydospore (klam′ĭ-do-spōr′) [Gr. *chlamys* cloak + Gr. *sporos* seed] a large, round, thick-walled asexual spore formed within a fungal hypha or from terminal hyphal cells. It is not shed. See also *spore* and the accompanying illustration. Cf. *conidium.*

chloasma (klo-az′mah) [Gr. *chloazein* to be green] see *melasma.*

chlor/o (klor′o) [Gr. *chlōros* green] 1. a prefix word element to denote green, e.g., chlorophyll, or the presence of chlorine.

2. a prefix word element in organic chemistry to denote compounds in which chlorine is present as a substituent, e.g., chloromethane (CH_3Cl).

chloracne (klōr-ak′ne) an acnelike condition of the skin marked by keratin-containing cysts; caused by exposure to chlorinated compounds such as biphenyls, naphthalenes, and some herbicides, which affect the sebaceous glands.

chloral (klo″ral) trichloroacetaldehyde, CCl_3CHO, a colorless, oily liquid with a pungent odor; M.W. 147.40. It is formed by chlorination of ethyl alcohol or acetaldehyde, and reacts readily with water to form chloral hydrate, $CCl_3CH(OH)_2$.

chloral hydrate [USP], $CCl_3CH(OH)_2$, a transparent, crystalline substance with an aromatic, penetrating odor and a bitter taste, formed by the action of water on chloral. In medicine, it is used as a sedative. With overdose, it causes respiratory failure, circulatory collapse, or yellow atrophy of the liver. Chloral hydrate is also used in histology as a preservative in Mayer's alum hematoxylin and occasionally as a fixative. It decomposes to chloroform in the presence of strong alkalis. Trademark, Noctec.

chloral hydrate assays the Fujiwara pyridine-alkali screening test. A specimen of urine is reacted with pyridine and sodium hydroxide at 100°C; a red color in the pyridine layer indicates chloral hydrate or similar compounds, e.g., chloroform, trichloroethylene.

Chloral hydrate is rapidly metabolized to trichloroethanol. This active metabolite can be extracted into diethylether from serum, blood, or urine. Pyridine and sodium hydroxide are added to the extract, and a colored reaction product is formed after heating. The absorbance at 368 nm is used for quantification.

chlorambucil (klo-ram′bu-sil) an alkylating agent [USP] of the nitrogen mustard group that is used as a cancer chemotherapeutic drug. Trademark, Leukeran. For more information, see *Appendix A*.

chloramine-T (klo′rah-mēn) *N*-chloro-*p*-toluenesulfonamide sodium salt, an antibacterial substance used as a topical antiseptic. It is also used to facilitate iodination of hormones and fibrinogen by radioactive iodine in competitive-binding assays.

chloramphenicol (klo″ram-fen′ĭ-kol) an antibiotic, a derivative of dichloroacetic acid, that is produced by a species of *Streptomyces*. Chloramphenicol is a bacteriostatic agent with an antibacterial spectrum similar to those of the tetracyclines. It inhibits protein synthesis by binding to the 50S subunit of the bacterial ribosome, thus preventing attachment of the amino acid–containing end of the aminoacyl-transfer RNA to its binding region. As a consequence, peptide bond formation is prevented. Organisms can become resistant to chloramphenicol by producing the enzyme acetyltransferase, which acetylates the antibiotic to an inactive diacetyl derivative. Such resistance is mediated by transferable plasmids.

Chloramphenicol is a broad-spectrum antibiotic readily absorbed from the intestine, and is active against many genera of aerobic and anaerobic bacteria, spirochetes, rickettsiae, chlamydiae, and mycoplasmas. Clinical indications include brain abscesses, meningitis with ampicillin-resistant *Hemophilus influenzae* or aerobic gram-negative bacilli, typhoid fever, or infections with *Bacteroides fragilis* or a rickettsia. The antibiotic is toxic because of inhibition of mammalian mitochondrial protein synthesis. Because it is especially damaging to bone marrow and can cause either reversible bone marrow depression or, if continued, fatal aplastic anemia, it is not used when an alternate form of therapy is available.

See also *antibacterial agents*.

chloranil (klo′rah-nil, klōr-an′il) 2,3,5,6 tetrachloro-1,4-benzoquinone, crystallized as yellow leaflets from acetic acid. It is soluble in alcohol, ether, and benzene, but is insoluble in cold alcohol and water. Chloranil is used as a fungicide, in electrodes for pH measurements, and as a dehydrogenating reagent in organic synthesis. Also called *tetrachloroquinone*.

chloranil assays methods for determination of chloranil in biologic specimens. After extraction with hexane or acetone, this substance can be detected by colorimetric tests or thin-layer chromatography and quantitated by spectrophotometry or gas-liquid chromatography.

chloranilate method (klōr-an′ĭ-lāt) a histologic staining procedure for the demonstration of calcium. Small yellow-brown crystals are formed that produce a brilliant birefringence when viewed in polarized light.

chlorate (klo′rāt) any salt of chloric acid ($HClO_3$) or a compound containing the chlorate ion (ClO_3^-). Chlorates are explosively unstable substances. The sodium and potassium salts are the most common forms. Both are strong oxidizing agents and the latter is also used therapeutically in mouthwashes, throat lozenges, and dentifrices. In chlorate poisoning, intravascular hemolysis may result in emboli, nephritis, and dyspnea. Methemoglobinemia is commonly seen.

chlorate assays a colorimetric test for chlorate in biologic materials. Chlorate and other toxic anions are separated by dialysis or filtration following ammonium sulfate deproteinization. Free chlorate in the presence of concentrated hydrochloric acid liberates iodine from sodium iodide (I^- is oxidized to iodine, I_2). Iodine then reacts with starch to form a deep blue color.

chlorazepate (klo-raz′e-pāt) a benzodiazepine minor tranquilizer, available as monopotassium and dipotassium salts. See also *benzodiazepine*.

chlorazol black E (klōr′ah-zōl) an acid dye, used mainly in plant histology and for staining protozoa; C.I. 30235.

chlorazol black E stain a simple procedure for

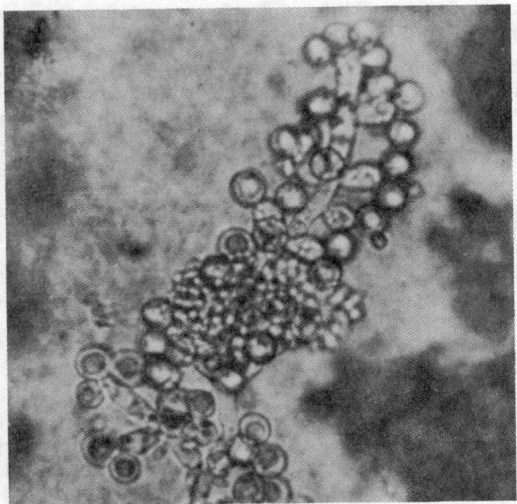

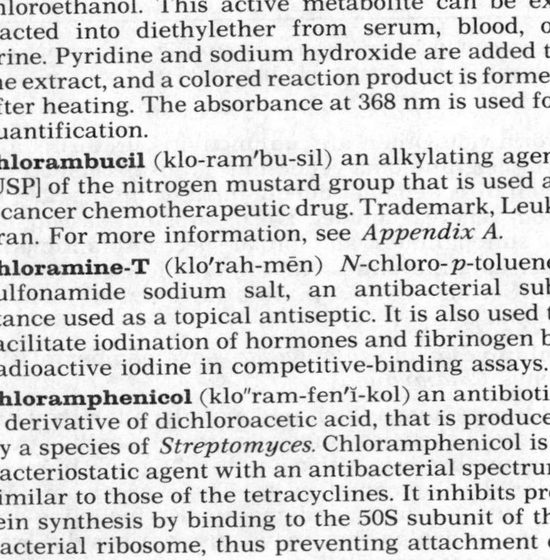

Chlamydospores. Live colony of *Candida albicans,* which has produced a thick-walled chlamydospore and small blastospores on cornmeal agar. (From Freeman, B. A.: Burrow's Textbook of Microbiology. 21st ed. Philadelphia, W. B. Saunders Co., 1979.)

fixing and staining protozoan parasites in fresh fecal samples and tissues. This method is considered as good as Heidenhain's hematoxylin and trichrome stains and takes less time. The stain is prepared by grinding chlorazol black E and a basic solution. When a smooth paste is obtained, and the solution has settled for 4–6 wk, a black cherry–colored liquid is formed. Permanent stained films are prepared by making a fecal smear, then staining with this stain. The protozoa in fresh fecal specimens stain green to gray-green; in old stools, organisms are gray to black. Nuclei, chromatoid bodies, karyosomes, and cell membranes stain dark green to black. Also called *Kohn's one-step staining technic.*

chlorbenside (klor′ben-sīd) a miticide, 1-chloro-4-[[(4-chlorophenyl)-methyl]thio] benzene. Its human toxicity is similar to that of the chlorinated hydrocarbon pesticides (e.g., DDT); it is also a skin irritant. Trademarks, Chlorparacide, Chlorsulphacide, and Mitox.

chlorcyclizine hydrochloride (klōr-si′klĭ-zēn) [USP], a long-acting antihistamine used in antiallergy preparations. Drowsiness is one side-effect.

chlordane (klōr′dān) a chlorinated hydrocarbon pesticide used to disinfect bodies, bedding, and other areas from lice, cockroaches, fleas, and stinging ants. Contact with skin causes moderate irritation, and chlordane is poisonous when ingested, with effects similar to those of DDT.

chlordiazepoxide (klōr″di-az″ĕ-pok′sīd) [USP], one of the benzodiazepine minor tranquilizers; frequently prescribed for treatment of anxiety. It is the drug of choice for the alleviation of alcohol withdrawal symptoms and for management of delirium tremens. The maximal blood concentration from therapeutic dosages is about 1.0 μg/ml. For toxicity, see *benzodiazepine.* Trademark for chlordiazepoxide hydrochloride, *Librium.*

chlordiazepoxide assays 1. spectrometry. Chlordiazepoxide is extracted from neutralized or alkalinized blood or urine into an organic solvent, and then reextracted into strong acid. The concentration is determined from the difference in absorbance at the peak (245 nm) and the minimum (290 nm) for both the sample and a reference solution. Other benzodiazepines and their metabolites interfere.

2. gas chromatography; a nonpolar or intermediate-polarity stationary phase and an electron capture detector are used. The ratio of the peak areas of chlordiazepoxide and of the internal standard (e.g., flurazepam) in the sample and reference solution, extracted as in method 1, are used to determine the concentration. Other benzodiazepines may interfere. Concentrations as low as 0.3 μg/ml can be detected.

See also *benzodiazepine assays.*

chloride (Cl) (klo′rīd) a salt of hydrochloric acid; the Cl^- anion. In mammals it is the major extracellular anion. Its presence in the body is important in the regulation of water distribution, anion and cation balance, and osmotic pressure.

Reference values for serum or plasma are 98–106 mmol/l, being slightly less just after meals. The concentration in red cell fluid is 49–54 mmol/l. Spinal fluid values are 118–132 mmol/l. Urinary excretion varies considerably, being usually 110–250 mmol/da. For the concentration of chloride in sweat, see *sweat tests.* An approximate check on the accuracy of chloride values in serum can be obtained by determining the difference between the value for sodium and the combined concentrations of chloride and carbon dioxide when all values are expressed in millimoles per liter (see also *anion gap*).

Low concentrations of chloride are found in the serum of patients with chronic pyelonephritis and Addison's disease, especially during addisonian crises. Low serum chloride concentrations may also occur with metabolic acidosis associated with increased production or diminished excretion of acids, as observed in lactic acidosis, renal failure, or diabetic acidosis. Prolonged vomiting may also cause loss of chloride ions and a reduction of its serum concentration.

Increased serum chloride concentrations may be observed with dehydration and in conditions causing decreased renal blood flow, e.g., congestive cardiac failure. Excess treatment with, or absorption of, chloride may also increase the serum concentration.

chloride methods 1. coulometric-amperometric titration. This is probably the most useful procedure, as it can be used over the whole range of physiologic values and is capable of great accuracy. An acid solution (HNO_3 with CH_3COOH) is added to the specimen to provide a solution of high conductivity, to make the solution less polar, to provide a sharper end point, and to equalize the reaction rate over the whole electrode surface. The silver ions produced by the current combine with the chloride ions to form insoluble AgCl. The surge of conductivity that occurs when all the Cl^- has combined with Ag^+, owing to the production of excess free Ag^+, trips a relay that stops an automatic timer and the production of Ag^+. Since the current (and thus the production of Ag^+) is constant, the time needed to reach the titration end point is a measure of chloride concentration. The instruments designed for such measurements are called chloridometers. Other halides are also measured by this technique.

2. mercurimetric titration method. The methods presently used are essentially modifications of the procedure originally described by Schales and Schales. A serum specimen is treated with sodium tungstate to produce a protein-free solution. This is then titrated with mercuric nitrate, with diphenylcarbazone as an indicator. The chloride ions react with the free mercuric ions to form undissociated mercuric chloride, and any excess mercuric ions combine with diphenylcarbazone, producing a blue-violet color. The chloride concentration is calculated from the titration data, which are related to values obtained with a standard solution. The method may be used for urine and cerebrospinal fluid as well as for serum. Bromide ions also react with mercuric nitrates, and thus are also measured.

3. colorimetric technique using mercuric thiocyanate. This procedure is widely used with the AutoAnalyzer. The principle depends on the combination of Cl^- with Hg^{2+} from mercuric thiocyanate to form $HgCl_2$ with the release of free SCN^-. This, in turn, combines with Fe^{3+} in the ferric nitrate reagent to form $Fe(SCN)_3$, a reddish-colored complex with an absorption peak at 480 nm. The procedure as commonly used is limited in range and linearity and is most useful for serum specimens between 80 and 120 mmol/l.

4. colorimetric technique using ferric perchlorate. This procedure has also been adapted to the Auto-

Analyzer and has greater linearity. A colored complex is formed by ferric perchlorate and chloride ions, with an absorbance maximum at about 340 nm. This technique has the advantage that it avoids the use of toxic Hg ions.

chloride shift a movement of chloride ions from blood plasma into red cells, which balances a movement of bicarbonate out of the red cells and thus reestablishes electrical neutrality. The bicarbonate is produced by the enzyme carbonic anhydrase from the carbon dioxide produced by cellular metabolism. Because of the chloride shift, the chloride concentration is about 1 mmol/l lower in venous plasma (1 percent) than in arterial plasma. See also *isohydric shift.*

chloridometer (klo″rĭ-dom′ĕ-ter) [*chloride* + Gr. *metron* measure] an instrument devised for measuring the content of chloride ions in solution, particularly in serum or urine, by titration with electrically generated silver ions. Several different types of chloridometers are commercially available. See also *chloride methods.*

chlorinated (klo′rĭ-nāt″ed) charged with chlorine. Chlorinated water contains dissolved chlorine in several oxidation states. In chlorinated hydrocarbons, the chlorine is part of the molecule, having replaced hydrogen atoms.

chlorinated hydrocarbon pesticide one of a group of pesticides that are toxic by ingestion or absorption through the skin. These pesticides act as central nervous system stimulants and nerve poisons, causing dizziness, headaches, and (in high doses) loss of coordination, tremor, and convulsions. The chlorinated cyclodienes can cause convulsions without warning symptoms. Although acute poisoning resulting in death is rare in humans, these substances are of concern, as many are persistent in the environment, are stored in body fat, and may have carcinogenic potential. Also called *organo-chloro pesticides.*

chlorinated hydrocarbon pesticide assays gas or thin-layer chromatography. These pesticides can be extracted from blood or ground-up tissue into hexane; after clean-up procedures, they are detected by GLC using a nonpolar stationary phase and an electron capture detector. They can also be detected by TLC, using hexane or carbon tetrachloride as the solvent and phenoxyethanol as the spray reagent.

chlorine (Cl) (klo′rin, klo′rēn) [L. *chlorum* or *chlorinum,* from Gr. *chlōros* green] a yellowish-green, gaseous, nonmetallic element with a suffocating odor; atomic number 17; atomic weight 35.45; Group VII of the periodic table (the halogens); oxidation state –1. Chlorine is a highly irritating gas that can cause fatal pulmonary edema. It is used for the chlorination of drinking water, as a bleach, and as a disinfectant. See also *chloride.*

chlormerodrin (klōr-mer′o-drin) an organomercury compound formerly used as a diuretic.

chlormerodrin Hg 197 [USP], an imaging agent formerly used for kidney scans and brain scans. It is protein-bound in the blood and is localized in the liver and spleen, although most goes to the kidneys where it is excreted. It has been largely replaced by technetium 99m that contains pharmaceuticals with better properties for brain and kidney scanning.

chlorobenzilate (klo″ro-ben′zil-āt) a miticide, 4-chloro-α-(4-chlorophenyl)-α-hydroxybenzeneacetic acid ethyl ester, similar in toxicity to chlorbenside.

chlorofluorocarbon (klo″ro-floo″or-o-kar′bon) see *fluorocarbon.*

chloroform (klo′ro-form) [L. *chloroformum,* from *chlorine* + *formyl*] [NF], a clear, colorless, volatile liquid, $CHCl_3$; a halogenated hydrocarbon with a strong, characteristic, ethereal smell and a sweetish burning taste. It is used as a solvent and a cleaning agent; it was formerly employed as an anesthetic. It has some bacteriostatic action but is not a reliable disinfectant. Effects of chloroform poisoning, which may be fatal, include necrosis and fat accumulation in the liver, kidney damage, asphyxia, and cardiac failure. Also called *trichloromethane.*

chloroform assays tests for chloroform in brain, liver, body fat, or blood. Tissue suspected of containing chloroform is homogenized and steam-distilled. The distillate may be tested by a variety of colorimetric procedures including the Fujiwara test and the resorcinol test. Chloral hydrate, carbon tetrachloride, and certain other compounds give similar results and must be ruled out by specific tests. Alternately, a homogenized specimen can be subjected to microdiffusion in a Conway cell. The diffusate is then tested by colorimetric methods. A more specific method is gas chromatography, utilizing the head space technique.

In the Fujiwara test, chloroform and other volatile chlorinated hydrocarbons in distillate from tissue cause pyridine to develop a pink to dark-red color in the presence of NaOH solution, the intensity indicating the amount of chloroform present. Owing to the sensitivity of the test, a blank determination must always be performed and compared with the test sample. In the resorcinol test, resorcinol and sodium hydroxide are added to a distillate of homogenized tissue. A color that is yellowish-pink to red on warming indicates chloroform or other chlorinated hydrocarbons. The solution exhibits a greenish fluorescence when diluted.

chloroform-methanol a mixture of chloroform and methanol used for the fixation of tissues and the concurrent extraction of lipids from the tissue. These two procedures are generally performed at 60°C in a 1:2 chloroform-methanol solution.

chloroguanide hydrochloride (klo″ro-gwan′īd) an antimalarial drug taken as a suppressive by persons entering malarial areas. It kills the parasite in the asexual-erythrocytic state and inhibits the development of the sexual cycle in the mosquito, especially in the case of malaria caused by *Plasmodium falciparum.* Side-effects include nausea, vomiting, diarrhea, anemia, anorexia, and malaise. This agent has a tendency to cause resistant strains of parasites to develop. Also known as proguanil. Trademark, Paludrine.

chlorohydrocarbon (klor″o-hi″dro-kar′bon) any chlorine-substituted hydrocarbon, e.g., chloroform or carbon tetrachloride. Many are commonly used laboratory solvents. Excessive acute or chronic exposure to these compounds can cause damage to the kidneys and liver.

chlorohydrocarbon assays (klo″ro-hi″dro-kar′-bon) see *halogenated hydrocarbon assays.*

chloroma (klo-ro′mah) [*chloro-* + *-oma*] granulocytic leukemia, usually the acute form, occurring as discrete masses in organs or tissues. It is so named because the presence of myeloperoxidase, a green pigment with high peroxidase activity, gives the tumor a distinctive greenish hue. The color is not always evident; when present, it tends to fade after the tumor has been exposed to air for an hour or two; it can be restored by the application of hydrogen peroxide or sodium metabisulfite.

Chloromycetin (klo″ro-mi-se′tin) trademark. See *chloramphenicol.*

chlorophenol red (klo″ro-fe′nol) a pH indicator, dichlorosulfonphthalein, with a pH range of 5.2 (yellow)–6.8 (red).

chlorophenoxy herbicides (klo″ro-fen-ok′se) a group of compounds that act as plant growth hormones. In animals, toxic symptoms include tenseness, muscular weakness and twitching, and irritation of the skin, eyes, and mucous membranes. In massive doses, ataxia, convulsions, coma, and death due to ventricular fibrillation occur. These compounds can also produce contact dermatitis and chloracne, and some contain a highly teratogenic impurity, dioxin (TCDD). In the military, these substances have been used under the name Agent Orange. See also *dioxin* and the chlorophenoxy compounds *2,4-D, 2,4,5-T,* and *silvex.*

chlorophyll (klo′ro-fil) [*chloro-* + Gr. *phyllon* leaf] the green substance of plants by which photosynthesis is accomplished; it is usually localized in intracellular organelles called chloroplasts. There are many types: *chlorophyll a* is bluish green in color and is the major pigment in plants that release oxygen in photosynthesis; chlorophyll b is yellowish green in color; chlorophyll c occurs in many marine algae; and chlorophyll d occurs in red algae.

chloropicrin (klo″ro-pik′rin) trichloronitromethane, CCl_3NO_2, a colorless or yellowish nonflammable liquid with a strong odor. It is used as a soil fumigant and as an agent for disinfecting cereals and grains. Human mucous membranes, especially the eyes, are very sensitive to it, and deep inhalation may be fatal. Chloropicrin has been used as a war gas, producing vomiting and pulmonary edema. It has also been used occasionally in solution with alcohol as a blocking agent for sulfhydryl groups in histologic preparations.

Chloropidae (klo-rop′i-de) a family of very small flies in the order Diptera. These flies are usually less than 3 mm long and have short antennae and rudimentary basal lobes on their wings. Two genera, *Hippelates* and *Siphunculina,* are attracted to the eyes of humans and animals and may transmit conjunctivitis.

chloroplast (klo′ro-plast) [*chloro-* + Gr. *plastos* formed] any one of the chlorophyll-containing organized cell bodies in higher plants. Photosynthesis occurs in these organelles.

chloropsia (klo-rop′se-ah) [*chloro-* + Gr. *opsis* vision + *-ia*] a defect of vision in which objects appear to have a greenish tinge.

chloroquine (klo′ro-kwin) [USP], one of the 4-aminoquinoline group of antimalarial drugs; it kills the schizonts infecting the red blood cells, and is a drug of choice when used with the 8-aminoquinoline primaquine that kills the exoerythrocytic forms of the parasite. It is also used to treat amebiasis, particularly when the liver is infected. Adverse effects include upset stomach and visual disturbances; overdoses may cause shock, convulsions, and heart and respiratory failure.

chlorothiazide (klo″ro-thi′ah-zīd) a thiazide diuretic used to treat edema or hypertension. See also *thiazide diuretics.* Trademark, *Diuril.*

Chlorothion (klo″ro-thi′on) trademark for a moderately toxic organothiophosphate insecticide, *O,O*-dimethyl *O*-(3-chloro-4-nitrophenyl)thionophosphate. See also *organophosphate compounds.*

chlorous acid reagent (klo′rus) a combination of $NaClO_2$, water, and acetic acid; sometimes used in histology to block aldehydes in the periodic acid, ninhydrin, Schiff, and Feulgen reactions.

chlorphenesin carbamate (klor-fen′ĕ-sin) a centrally acting muscle relaxant.

chlorpheniramine maleate (klōr″fen-ir′ah-mēn) [USP], an antihistamine having anticholinergic and sedative side-effects. It is used for the treatment of allergic reactions and as an ingredient in many cough and cold preparations. Common side-effects are sedation, excitation (in children), and dizziness and hypotension (in the elderly). It should not be taken by persons having glaucoma, bronchial asthma, or an enlarged prostate. Overdoses may cause hallucinations, convulsions, or death, especially in children. Trademarks, *Chlor-Trimeton* and *Teldrin.*

chlorphentermine hydrochloride (klōr-fen′ter-mēn) a sympathomimetic amine similar to the amphetamines used as diet pills (anorexic). Overdosage may cause confusion, restlessness, hallucinations, panic states, gastrointestinal distress, circulatory collapse, convulsions, and coma. Trademark, Pre-sate.

chlorpromazine (klōr-pro′mah-zēn) [USP], an alkyl-type phenothiazine major tranquilizer; used in the management of psychotic disorders and other psychiatric conditions, to control nausea and vomiting, and to cure intractable hiccups. It is used as the free base in suppositories and as chlorpromazine hydrochloride [USP] orally or parenterally. See also *phenothiazine tranquilizers.* Trademark *Thorazine.*

chlorpromazine assays 1. the urine ferric chloride screening test; see *phenothiazine tranquilizers assays.*

2. ultraviolet spectrophotometry. Chlorpromazine is extracted from an alkalinized blood specimen into acid. The concentration is determined from the absorbance at 225 nm.

3. gas chromatography. The drug and its metabolites plus 2,4-dichlorpromazine as internal standard are extracted from alkalinized plasma by organic solvents. After clean-up by differential extraction, the drugs are injected onto a moderately polar column with an electron capture detector. Sensitivity is 0.01 ng/ml.

chlorpropamide (klōr-pro′pah-mīd) [USP], one of the sulfonylureas, used as an oral hypoglycemic agent in the control of mild noninsulin-dependent diabetes mellitus. Trademark, *Diabinese.* See also *sulfonylurea.*

chlorprothixene (klōr″pro-thik′zēn) [USP], one of the thioxanthene major tranquilizers used in the management of psychotic disorders. See also *phenothiazine tranquilizers.* Trademark, *Taractan.*

chlortetracycline (klōr″tet-rah-si′klēn) a tetracycline antibiotic produced by *Streptomyces aureo-*

faciens. It is the drug of choice in the treatment of a number of bacterial, rickettsial, chlamydial, and mycoplasmal diseases. Trademark, *Aureomycin.* See also *antibacterial agents* and *tetracyclines.*

chlorthalidone (klōr-thal′ĭ-dōn) [USP], a thiazide-like diuretic; see under *thiazide diuretics.* Trademark, *Hygroton.*

Chlor-Trimeton (klōr-tri′mĕ-ton) trademark. See *chlorpheniramine maleate.*

chlorzoxazone (klōr-zok′sah-zōn) a skeletal muscle relaxant used for the relief of muscle spasm. It inhibits reflex arcs at the spinal cord and brain stem levels. Trademark, Paraflex.

choana (ko′a-nah), pl. *choanae* [L., from Gr. *choanē* funnel] 1. any funnel-shaped cavity. 2. [pl.] [NA], the posterior nasal apertures; the paired openings between the nasal cavity and the nasopharynx.

chocolate agar (chok′o-lat) see *chocolate a.* under *agar.*

chocolate cyst a cyst containing dark, chocolate-brown, thick fluid, representing inspissated, thickened old blood. In the ovary, such cysts are usually due to endometriosis.

choke (chōk) see *inductor.*

chol/e, chol/o (ko′le, ko′lo) [Gr. *cholē* bile] a word element used in combining form to denote relationship to the bile, e.g., cholangiogram.

cholagogue (ko′lah-gog) [*chol-* + Gr. *agōgos* leading] an agent that stimulates the flow of bile into the duodenum, especially one that does so by stimulating the gallbladder to contract. See also *cholecystokinin-pancreozymin, fatty meal,* and *sincalide.* Cf. *choleretic* and *cholecystagogue.*

cholangiocarcinoma (ko-lan″je-o-kar′sĭ-no′mah) see *bile duct carcinoma.*

cholangiogram (ko-lan′je-o-gram″) a radiograph of the bile ducts after contrast medium injection.

cholangiography (ko-lan″je-og′rah-fe) [chol- + Gr. *angeion* vessel + *graphein* to write] the radiologic examination of the biliary tract, in particular of the bile ducts, after the introduction of a radiopaque contrast medium. See also *cholecystography* and *cholegraphy.*

delayed operative c., operative cholangiography performed after cholecystectomy. Also called operative T-tube cholangiography and postcholedochotomy cholangiography.

direct c., cholangiography in which the contrast medium is instilled directly into the biliary system. See *operative c., percutaneous transhepatic c.,* and *postoperative c.*

intravenous c., see *intravenous c.* under *cholecystography.*

operative c., cholangiography performed as a routine part of biliary tract surgery, either before or after exploration of the biliary tract. The surgeon injects a water-soluble iodinated contrast medium, e.g., diatrizoate, directly into the common bile duct through a needle, a cystic duct catheter, or (after cholecystectomy) a T tube. This examination demonstrates both the extrahepatic and the major intrahepatic ducts. it also reveals the presence of stones that were not palpable or other duct obstructions, and indicates the condition of the sphincter of Oddi. Also called immediate cholangiography. See also *choledochography.*

percutaneous transhepatic c., cholangiography in which a water-soluble iodinated contrast medium, e.g., diatrizoate, is injected directly into the hepatic bile duct by way of a needle inserted through the abdominal wall and liver. It is used in jaundiced patients when the ducts are dilated and when oral or intravenous cholangiography would be ineffective. Also called transabdominal cholangiography and transhepatic cholangiography.

postoperative c., cholangiography in which a water-soluble iodinated contrast medium, e.g., diatrizoate, is introduced through an indwelling T tube that drains the common bile duct. The day before the examination, the T tube is clamped to avoid air bubbles in the ducts. Patient preparation and positioning are as described for cholecystography. Also called T-tube cholangiography.

cholangiole (ko-lan′je-ōl) [*chol-* + Gr. *angeion* vessel + *-ole* dim. suffix] see *bile ductules.*

cholangiotomogram (ko-lan″je-o-to′mo-gram) a body-section radiograph (tomogram) of the bile ducts.

cholangitis (ko″lan-ji′tis) [*chol-* + Gr. *angeion* vessel + *-itis*] inflammation of the bile ducts, characterized by right upper abdominal pain, jaundice, and fever with chills (collectively known as Charcot's triad). Most frequently the condition is precipitated by choledocholithiasis (gallstone in the common bile duct) or by biliary surgery. Bacterial infection may occur and most commonly involves *Escherichia coli* from lymphatic, blood, or intestinal regurgitation routes. Persons affected appear to be very ill and may pass dark, bile-stained urine.

Laboratory findings include a mild-to-moderate degree of leukocytosis, often with a left shift, and a rise principally in conjugated serum bilirubin (2–4 mg/100 ml). Serum alkaline phosphatase, leucine aminopeptidase, and 5′-nucleotidase levels are elevated, indicating extrahepatic obstruction. Serum amylase may be increased if there is pancreatic involvement, but serum aspartate aminotransferase (SGOT) generally remains below 200 units. A cholecystogram or intravenous cholangiogram may be helpful in diagnosis. Blood cultures should be performed to monitor septicemic complications.

sclerosing c., a rare bile duct disease of unknown etiology in which there is benign, noninfectious, chronic, inflammatory narrowing of the ducts. In approximately one-third of persons affected, the condition occurs in association with other diseases, primarily ulcerative colitis, but also Crohn's disease (regional enteritis), retroperitoneal fibrosis, and Riedel's thyroiditis.

suppurative c., a severe bacterial cholangitis in which there is complete bile duct obstruction. Septicemia, shock, and mental confusion or delirium are common. Also called obstructive cholangitis.

cholate (ko′lāt) a salt, ester, or ionic form of cholic acid; see also *cholic acid* and *glycocholate.*

Cholebrine (ko′le-brin) trademark. See *iocetamic acid.*

cholecalciferol (ko″le-kal-sif′er-ol) 9,10-secocholesta-5,7,10(19)-trien-3β-ol, a substance synthesized by the irradiation of its provitamin, 7-dehydrocholesterol. In the body, ultraviolet light acts with an enzyme in the skin to convert 7-dehydrocholesterol to cholecalciferol. In the liver, cholecalciferol is converted to 25-hydroxycholecalciferol, which in turn is converted in the kidney into the physiologically most active metabolite 1,25-dihydroxycholecalciferol. Because the latter is transported in the blood stream to act at a distance from its site of production, it is considered by many authorities as a hormone. The hormone acts on intestine and bone to increase the plasma calcium and phosphate concentration. Its formation in the kidney is regulated by a negative feedback loop involving these two ions and parathyroid hormone. As the active hormone is formed in the kidney, hypocalcemia may develop in cases of chronic renal failure (acquired or hereditary). The vitamins D_2 and D_3 and their 25-hydroxylated forms show some intrinsic activity in intestine and bone. 25,26-Dihydroxy- and 24,25-dihydroxycholecalciferols are generally considered to be inactive metabolites. Main sources of cholecalciferol include fish liver oils, eggs, milk, and butter. The recommended daily allowance (RDA) is 400 USP units. Also called vitamin D_3; see under *vitamin D*.

cholecyst (ko′le-sist) [*chole-* + Gr. *kystis* bladder] the gallbladder.

cholecystagogue (ko″le-sis′tah-gog) [*cholecyst* + Gr. *agōgos* leading] an agent that stimulates the gallbladder to contract and empty bile into the duodenum. Cf. *cholagogue*.

cholecystangiography (ko″le-sis-tan″je-og′rah-fe) see *cholecystocholangiography*.

cholecystectasia (ko″le-sis″tek-ta′ze-ah) [*cholecyst* + Gr. *ektasis* distention] distention of the gallbladder.

cholecystitis (ko″le-sis-ti′tis) [*cholecyst* + *-itis*] an acute or chronic inflammation of the gallbladder.

Acute cholecystitis is most frequently associated with obstruction of the outflow of the gallbladder due to a blockage of the cystic duct by a gallstone. Bacterial infection develops secondary to the obstruction. Persons affected experience pain in the right upper quadrant, often associated with nausea and vomiting. Potential complications include empyema, gangrene, gallbladder perforation, and formation of internal biliary fistulas. White blood cell counts and serum bilirubin, serum transaminase, and alkaline phosphatase levels may all be elevated. Diagnosis is usually accomplished by intravenous cholangiography, or infrequently by radiographic demonstration of a radiopaque gallstone.

Chronic cholecystitis is frequently associated with gallstones. Usually it does not result from repeated acute attacks but develops insidiously. Symptoms (including variable right upper quadrant pain, biliary colic, flatulence, and nausea) may be present or may intensify after meals, especially those rich in fatty foods. Laboratory tests are nonspecific. Diagnosis may be supported by nonvisualization of the gallbladder on oral cholecystography.

cholecystocholangiography (ko″le-sis″to-ko-lan″je-og′rah-fe) injection of a radiopaque medium for radiographic examination of the gallbladder and bile ducts. Also called *cholecystangiography*. See also *cholangiography* and *cholecystography*.

cholecystogram (ko″le-sis′to-gram) a radiograph of the gallbladder.

cholecystography (ko″le-sis-tog′rah-fe) [*cholecyst* + Gr. *graphein* to write] radiologic examination of the biliary tract, in particular of the gallbladder, after intravenous or oral administration of a radiopaque contrast medium. It demonstrates the ability of the liver to clear the contrast medium from the blood and excrete it in the bile; the ability of the gallbladder to fill, concentrate bile, and empty; and the presence of bile duct obstructions, such as gallstones, strictures, tumors, or other anomalies of the ducts.

The day before the examination, a high-fat–containing meal is eaten to empty the gallbladder. The intestinal tract is cleared of gas and fecal material by administration of cleansing enemas and, if necessary, cathartics.

A scout (plain) film of the abdomen may be obtained to determine whether the intestinal tract is clear and to locate radiopaque stones. After administration of the contrast medium and its concentration in the gallbladder (see below), films demonstrating the gallbladder are made using the left anterior oblique (prone) position and the right lateral decubitus or erect positions to observe mobility or stratification of filling defects.

After these cholecystograms have been made, a fatty meal or synthetic cholagogue (e.g., sincalide) may be administered to determine the emptying rate of the gallbladder and to obtain radiographs that demonstrate the extrahepatic bile ducts (cholangiograms). These films are obtained 5–20 min after the fatty meal.

Also called *cholegraphy*.

intravenous c., cholecystography in which the contrast medium is administered intravenously by injection or by drip infusion. The medium is carried by way of the hepatic artery to the liver, where it is rapidly excreted. Except when liver function is impaired, the bile ducts can be visualized after about 30 min, and the gallbladder after 2–3 hr. This examination is used when it is necessary to distinguish gallbladder disease from distal bile duct obstruction, when the patient has been cholecystectomized, or in the diagnosis of cystic duct obstruction. Iodipamide meglumine (Cholografin) is the currently used contrast medium. Also called *intravenous cholangiography*. See also *urography*.

oral c., cholecystography in which the contrast medium is administered by mouth; it is ingested after a low-fat evening meal, and the patient should not eat, smoke, or chew gum until after the cholecystography procedure 10–15 hr later. The contrast medium is absorbed by the duodenum and carried by the portal vein to the liver, where it is conjugated with glucuronic acid and excreted. It is then concentrated and stored by the gallbladder.

Lack of visualization of the gallbladder may be due to lack of intestinal absorption, vomiting or diarrhea, inadequate liver function, biliary duct obstruction, or failure of the patient to follow instructions. A repetition of the study is usually indicated.

Iopanoic acid (Telepaque), iocetamic acid (Cholebrine), ipodate sodium, and ipodate calcium (Oragrafin) are contrast media used in oral cholegraphy. The usual dose is 3 g of any of these. Double doses are no longer recommended.

Also called *Graham-Cole test*.

cholecystokinin-pancreozymin (CCK-PZ) (ko″lē-sis″tō-kin′in) [*cholecyst* + Gr. *kinein* to move] a hormone secreted by the mucosa of the upper intestine, which stimulates contraction of the gallbladder and secretion of pancreatic enzymes. Formerly it was thought that this action was due to two different hormones, cholecystokinin and pancreozymin.

choledoch/o (kol′ĕ-dok-o) a word element used in

combining form to denote the common bile duct, e.g., choledochography.

choledochogram (ko-led′ŏ-ko-gram) a radiograph of the common bile duct made by choledochography.

choledochography (ko-led″o-kog′rah-fe) [*choledochus* + Gr. *graphein* to write] radiographic examination of the common bile duct; a specialized procedure in operative cholangiography in which the x-ray film in a sterile enclosure is placed directly under the common bile duct to obtain better definition.

choledocholithiasis (ko-led″ŏ-ko-lĭ-thi′ah-sis) [*choledochus* + Gr. *lithos* stone + *-iasis*] the presence of a calculus in the common bile duct. The crystalline stone is usually nonopaque and may appear as a negative shadow in a duct filled with radiopaque medium. See also *cholelithiasis.*

choledochus (ko-led′o-kus) [*chole-* + Gr. *dochos* receptacle] the common bile duct.

cholegraphy (ko-leg′rah-fe) [*chole-* + Gr. *graphein* to write] a general term for radiologic examinations of the biliary tract following administration of a radiopaque contrast medium, which may be given orally, intravenously, by percutaneous transhepatic puncture, by direct injection during surgery, or through an indwelling T tube left for postoperative drainage. See also *cholangiography, cholecystangiography, cholecystocholangiography, cholecystography,* and *choledochography.*

cholelithiasis (ko″le-lĭ-thi′ah-sis) [*chole-* + Gr. *lithos* stone + *-iasis*] the presence of gallstones (calculi) in the gallbladder or bile duct, formed from the constituents of bile, usually bilirubin or cholesterol. Often a result of abnormalities of the bile (especially an excess of cholesterol), stones may also be caused by inflammation due to chemical irritation, bacterial infection, or stasis from obstruction of the outflow tract.

cholemia (ko-le′me-ah) [*chole-* + Gr. *haima* blood + *-ia*] bile or bile pigment in the blood.

choleperitoneum (ko″le-per″ĭ-to-ne′um) [*chole-* + *peritoneum*] see *bile p.* under *peritonitis.*

cholera (kol′er-ah) [Gr. from *cholē* bile] an acute infectious enteritis, which is endemic in India and Southeast Asia and periodically spreads to other parts of the world in pandemics. The causative organism, *Vibrio cholerae,* produces an extremely potent enterotoxin (choleragen) that acts on the epithelial cells of the small bowel to cause massive loss of intestinal fluid and electrolytes (the loss of fluid from the gut may reach 10–15 l/da). Infection occurs from feces-contaminated water and food, producing severe nausea, vomiting, diarrhea, and abdominal cramps. "Rice-water" stools occur, containing mucus, epithelial cells, and many (10^6 or more per milliliter) cholera vibrios, and these stools are diagnostic of the disease. Shock and death may occur if cholera is untreated.

Treatment with intravenous fluids supplemented with electrolytes is almost always effective if started promptly. Tetracycline therapy reduces fluid loss and also eliminates the organism from the feces in many cases. Mild forms of the disease often go unrecognized. It is now known that gastric acidity is an important defense mechanism against cholera, so that disease production is probably the consequence of the heavy contamination of food or drink, or of achlorhydria in the host.

pancreatic c., see *Verner-Morrison syndrome.*

choleragen (kol′er-ah-jen) an extremely potent enterotoxin produced by pathogenic strains of *Vibrio cholerae,* including some non-01 strains. It is a protein molecule that acts on the epithelial cells of the small bowel by stimulating adenylate cyclase activity, causing hypersecretion of chloride and bicarbonate and massive accumulation of fluid and diarrhea. See also *exotoxins* and *V. cholerae* under *Vibrio.*

choleretic (ko″ler-et′ik) 1. pertaining to the secretion of bile by the liver.

2. an agent that increases the flow of bile by stimulating its secretion by the liver. Cf. *cholagogue.*

cholescintigram (ko″le-sin′tĭ-gram) a radionuclide scan of the gallbladder.

cholestasis (ko″le-sta′sis) [*chole-* + Gr. *stasis* stoppage] morphologically, the presence of excess bile pigment within hepatocytes and Kupffer cells and of bile thrombi in canaliculi. The distribution is usually centrilobular when it is indicative of acute disease including large duct biliary obstruction; various forms of acute hepatitis; drug-induced jaundice; and miscellaneous disorders, e.g., jaundice due to anabolic or contraceptive steroids, cholestatic jaundice of pregnancy, and idiopathic types. When cholestasis is periportal, it is usually due to long-standing large biliary duct obstruction or late-stage primary biliary cirrhosis.

cholesteatoma (ko″le-ste″ah-to′mah) a cystlike mass occurring most often in the middle ear cavity; it is lined with keratinizing stratified squamous epithelium and filled with cholesterol-containing desquamated debris. Cholesteatomas are usually the result of chronic otitis media and are frequently associated with perforations of the tympanic membrane.

Otoscopic examination reveals white debris in the middle ear. Erosion of surrounding bone, a complication of cholesteatoma, may also be visualized by otoscopic examination or may be demonstrated radiographically.

cholesterol (ko-les′ter-ol) [*chole-* + Gr. *stereos* solid] cholest-5-en-3-β-ol, the principal steroid in higher animals, synthesized by all cells from acetyl CoA; M.W. 386.64. It is found in all body tissues, especially in animal fats and oils. Its concentration in the serum (plasma) of healthy young persons is on the order of 140–225 mg/dl, although the reference range in the United States is generally given as 140–250 mg/dl. About three-fourths of the serum cholesterol is esterified with unsaturated long-chain fatty acids; the remainder is present in the free cholesterol form. The cholesterol concentration in serum increases to values as high as 450 mg/dl with age and as the aftermath of poor nutritional habits.

Serum cholesterol is associated with the high-density (HDL) and low-density (LDL) lipoprotein fractions in a ratio of 1:3. High-serum total cholesterol and low HDL cholesterol concentrations are considered high-risk factors for arteriosclerosis. A low-serum cholesterol level may be caused by an inherited deficiency of LDL or HDL, or by impaired liver function. Cholesterol is a component of one type of gallstone.

cholesterol assays 1. the Abell method, one of the

most accurate and precise methods for assaying cholesterol in plasma. The cholesterol esters in the specimen are saponified with alcoholic KOH to form free cholesterol. The free cholesterol is then extracted into petroleum ether, the solvent is evaporated under nitrogen, and the residue is treated with Liebermann-Burchard reagent (acetic anhydride, concentrated sulfuric acid, and acetic acid) after cooling the test tube to 25°C. The amount of cholesterol is determined by measuring the green color at 620 nm. See also *Liebermann-Burchard reaction.*

2. Zak-Zlatkis-Boyle method. In this procedure, samples are extracted with acetone-alcohol, and the dried residue containing the total cholesterol is dissolved in acetic acid and treated with an $FeCl_3$-H_2SO_4 color reagent to give a red-violet color that can be measured at 550 nm.

3. automated methods. These are generally colorimetric methods for total cholesterol that do not use a saponification step. In one method, interfering substances are removed from an isopropanol extract of serum by zeolite, and the total cholesterol is determined by reaction with ferric chloride–sulfuric acid reagent. Other methods use the enzymatic method listed below. See also *Liebermann-Burchard reaction.*

4. enzymatic methods. These are relatively specific and accurate for the determination of total cholesterol but are inferior to the Abell method. Cholesterol esters are hydrolyzed by an esterase, and the free cholesterol is oxidized by molecular oxygen to cholest-4-ene-3-one and hydrogen peroxide in the presence of the bacterial enzyme cholesterol oxidase. The peroxide is then determined by a peroxidase reaction that converts 4-aminopyrene and phenol to a quinoneimine dye, which is quantitated photometrically. Cholesterol esters can also be determined using hydrolysis by cholesteryl ester hydrolase prior to the oxidase reaction. Some other plasma sterols are also oxidized by cholesterol oxidase.

cholesterolemia (ko-les″ter-ol-e′me-ah) [*cholesterol* + Gr. *haima* blood + *-ia*] an elevated concentration of cholesterol in the blood. Hypercholesterolemia may be seen in atherosclerotic vascular disease, diabetes, cholestasis, and the hyperlipemia characteristic of nephrotic syndrome. Moderately increased levels can occur as a result of excessive dietary intake. See also *hyperlipoproteinemia.*

cholesterol ester storage disease an extremely rare familial disorder characterized by the abnormal metabolism of cholesterol esters. The primary metabolic defect is thought to be a relative deficiency of acid lipase (complete deficiency causes Wolman's disease). Hepatomegaly secondary to very high concentrations of cholesterol esters is seen; however, patients may be otherwise asymptomatic. Diagnosis is based on liver biopsy, and carrier detection and prenatal diagnosis are considered feasible. There is no available treatment. See also *Wolman's disease.*

cholesterolosis (ko-les″ter-ol-o′sis) deposition of abnormal amounts of cholesterol in the tissues. In the gallbladder, the folds of the mucosa become streaked with yellow, cholesterol crystals, simulating the appearance of a ripe strawberry ("strawberry gallbladder"). The condition is common, occurring to some degree in at least 15 percent of cholecystectomy specimens, and it may precede or accompany the formation of a cholesterol gallstone.

cholesterol staining methods 1. the Schultz method for cholesterol, a modification of the Liebermann-Burchard reaction for steroids. Formalin-fixed frozen sections are treated with iron alum solution for several days, oxidizing cholesterol to oxycholesterol. Sections are then treated with a drop of a 1:1 acetic acid–sulfuric acid mixture and examined immediately under a microscope. Cholesterol turns a characteristic blue-green color. This method is specific (only carotene gives the same color) but insensitive (cholesterol must occur in 5–25 percent concentration to show even a faint color). The color lasts 30–60 min.

2. the Lewis-Lobban modification of the Schultz method. A 0.5 percent solution of iron alum in 80 percent sulfuric acid is used instead of the acetic acid–sulfuric acid mixture employed in the Schultz method. Androgens turn blue-green to brown-green with absorption peaks at 655 and 605 nm, which can be determined with a microspectroscope. Pregnenolone, pregnanedione, methyltestosterone, and estradiol turn strong-to-moderate colors in the range of purple to pink. Cholesterol turns a weak red. See also *digitonin method.*

cholesteroluria (ko-les″ter-ol-u′re-ah) [*cholesterol* + Gr. *ouron* urine + *-ia*] the presence of cholesterol in the urine.

cholestyramine resin (ko-les′tir-ah-mēn) [USP], a basic anion-exchange resin used in the treatment of hypercholesterolemia and of partial biliary obstruction. It acts by binding bile acids in the intestines, preventing their absorption and causing their fecal excretion. This reduces serum bile acid levels and causes an increase in the metabolism of cholesterol to bile acids. Adverse reactions include constipation and interference with fat digestion and absorption. Prolonged interference with fat absorption can cause a deficiency of vitamins A, D, K, and E. Trademark, Questran.

cholic acid (ko′lik) a bile acid, $3\alpha,7\alpha,12\alpha$-trihydroxy-5β-cholan-24-oic acid. It is quantitatively the most important of the several bile acids. It is synthesized in the liver from cholesterol, stored there bound to coenzyme A, and converted to glycine and taurine conjugates (bile salts) just prior to secretion into bile.

choline (ko′lēn) 1. the (2-hydroxyethyl)trimethylammonium ion, $(CH_3)_3N^+CH_2CH_2OH$. It has several biochemical roles: it is a component of several important membrane lipids, including phosphatidylcholine (PC) and sphingomyelin; it is a component of the neurotransmitter acetylcholine; and it serves as a methyl group donor. (The methyl groups can be transferred, in several steps, to *S*-adenosylmethionine or to 5,10-methylene-tetrahydrofolate for use in the synthesis of other compounds.) Choline is also known as a lipotropic agent because it has been shown to promote the transport of excess fat from the liver under certain conditions in laboratory animals, apparently by supplying choline necessary for lipid synthesis. Choline has been included in the B vitamin complex; combined deficiency of choline and all other methyl group donors causes cirrhosis of the liver in some animals, such as the guinea pig, which have a low capacity for choline synthesis. However, no human deficiency syndrome has been described, and, unlike compounds normally considered as vitamins, choline does not serve as a cofactor in enzymatic reactions.

Choline has been administered as a therapeutic agent in order to increase acetylcholine synthesis in certain neurologic disorders, including tardive dyskinesia, Huntington's chorea, Tourette's disease, Friedrich's ataxia, and Alzheimer's disease. The effectiveness of choline for these conditions is yet to be established.

2. choline base; (2-hydroxyethyl)trimethylammonium hydroxide; M.W. 121.18.

cholinergic (ko″lin-er′jik) pertaining to the neurotransmitter acetylcholine. The term is particularly used to describe nerve fibers that release acetylcholine at their terminals, physiologic effects produced by stimulation of these nerve fibers, acetylcholine receptors on the postsynaptic membrane, and drugs that imitate the effects of acetylcholine. Cf. *adrenergic.*

cholinergic fibers the neurons of the autonomic nervous system that release the neurotransmitter acetylcholine at their terminals. All preganglionic neurons of both the parasympathetic and sympathetic divisions of the autonomic nervous system are cholinergic, as are all postganglionic neurons of the parasympathetic nervous system. Most postganglionic sympathetic neurons are adrenergic; only those that innervate the sweat glands (with the exception of those in the hands and feet) and portions of the systemic vasculature (the sympathetic cholinergic vasodilators, principally to the skeletal muscles) are cholinergic. See also *cholinergic receptors.* Cf. *adrenergic fibers.*

cholinergic receptors postsynaptic membrane receptors in the central and autonomic nervous systems that are stimulated by the neurotransmitter acetylcholine. Two types of cholinergic receptors exist in the autonomic system: muscarinic receptors, which are stimulated by the poison muscarine, and nicotinic receptors, which are stimulated by nicotine.

Muscarinic receptors are those stimulated by postganglionic fibers of the parasympathetic nervous system or by the cholinergic fibers of the sympathetic nervous system. These receptors are activated by the drug pilocarpine, which can produce sweating and vasodilation (sympathomimetic effects) and salivary and bronchial secretion, constriction of the pupil of the eye, slowing of heart rate, and stimulation of smooth muscles (parasympathomimetic effects). Muscarinic receptors are blocked by the drug atropine, which also has central effects, and also by atropine substitutes such as propantheline, which do not.

Nicotinic receptors are those stimulated by all autonomic preganglionic fibers, by the splanchnic fibers that innervate the adrenal medulla and stimulate release of the hormones epinephrine and norepinephrine, and by the motor nerves innervating striated muscle. There are three types of drugs that block nicotinic receptors: (1) ganglion blockers, e.g., trimethaphan, which occupy receptor sites in the autonomic ganglia, and prevent the transmission of nerve impulses, producing a potent hypotensive effect; (2) competitive neuromuscular blockers, e.g., tubocurarine, which occupy receptor sites on the motor end-plate of skeletal muscle, producing paralysis; and (3) depolarizing neuromuscular blockers, e.g., succinylcholine, which stimulate the motor end-plate receptors in very small doses. Larger doses produce depolarization of the postsynaptic membrane (an effect produced experimentally by acetylcholine), also causing paralysis.

See also *cholinesterase inhibitors.*

cholinesterase (CHS) (ko″lin-es′ter-ās) 1. an enzyme of the hydrolase class (acylcholine acylhydrolase, EC 3.1.1.8) that catalyzes the reaction acetyl (or other acyl) choline + $H_2O \rightleftharpoons$ choline + acetate (or other carboxylic acid anion).

The enzyme shows moderate substrate specificity, and hydrolyzes butyryl esters more rapidly than propionyl or acetyl esters; benzoylcholine and thiocholine esters can also serve as substrates. Enzyme activity is inhibited by alkaloids such as eserine (physostigmine), prostigmine, and morphine; by a variety of organophosphate compounds such as diisopropylfluorophosphate (DFP), Parathion, Sarin, and tri-*o*-cresyl phosphate; and by chemicals such as citrate, fluoride, and borate (but not by acetylcholine as is the case for true cholinesterase).

Isoenzyme studies suggest the presence of more than seven forms, all with similar mobility but with varying molecular masses, which appear to be forms with a differing degree of aggregation of a basic unit. Of more interest are the genetic variants, controlled by different alleles, possessing weaker enzyme activity, but with increased resistance to inhibition by dibucaine or fluoride.

The enzyme is of considerable interest in clinical diagnosis, not only in the detection of possible succinylcholine sensitivity, but also in monitoring persons in contact with organophosphate insecticides. The measurement of cholinesterase activity may be important in patients with liver disease, as the enzyme is synthesized by this organ. Also called CHS, PCE, *pseudocholinesterase,* and serum or plasma cholinesterase. See also *cholinesterase assays* and *pseudocholinesterase deficiency.*

2. formerly a general term for any enzyme that hydrolyzes choline esters to release free choline. This included two enzyme entities now known as cholinesterase (EC 3.1.1.8) and *acetylcholinesterase* (EC 3.1.1.7).

cholinesterase assays determination of the activity of pseudocholinesterase (CHS or PCE) in blood plasma or of acetylcholinesterase (AcCHS) in erythrocytes or hemolyzed blood. This assay is a sensitive indicator of exposure to organophosphate or carbamate insecticides. Although a 20 percent drop in activity (to 80 percent of the preexposure value) indicates significant exposure, the first symptoms appear with only a 40 percent drop, and serious neuromuscular effects do not appear until there is a 80 percent drop in activity. The assay is also used to identify individuals who are sensitive to the anesthetic succinylcholine because of low plasma cholinesterase activity. This low activity may be caused by parenchymatous liver disease or by an inactive or weakly active enzyme due to a genetic defect (pseudocholinesterase deficiency). The two abnormal forms of the enzyme can be identified by determining the dibucaine number (DN) and fluoride number (FN). These measure the percentage inhibition of the enzyme of dibucaine or fluoride and identify the abnormal genotypes $E_1^aE_1^a$, and $E_1^fE_1^f$.

The activity of the enzyme depends on the substrate, temperature, and pH used for the assay. A temperature of 25° or 37°C and pH in the range of 7.4–8.1 are used. The amount of substrate hydrolyzed can be determined by the amount of acid liberated from the optimum substrates acetylcholine (for

AcCHS) or butyrylcholine (for CHS or PCE). The acid can be determined by the pH change produced as measured by a pH meter or (for reagent strip tests) by an indicator such as phenol red, or it can be determined by titration with a base while maintaining a constant pH (pH-stat).

Nonphysiologic, synthetic substrates are also used. The hydrolysis of benzoylcholine to benzoic acid and choline produces a linear change in the ultraviolet absorbance at 240 nm. The formation of thiocholine by hydrolysis of acetylthiocholine and butyrylthiocholine can be measured by its reaction with 5,5′-dithiobis(2-nitrobenzoic acid) (DTNB) (Ellman reaction). Thiocholine displaces 5-mercapto-2-nitrobenzoic acid (5-MNBA) from DTNB. The 5-MNBA concentration is determined by its absorbance at 410 nm.

See also *organophosphate compounds* and *pseudocholinesterase deficiency.*

cholinesterase inhibitors a group of compounds that inhibit the activity of one or both of the cholinesterase enzymes—acetylcholinesterase (in nerves and erythrocytes) and pseudocholinesterase (in blood plasma). Those that are reversible (competitive) inhibitors, such as the drugs neostigmine, pyridostigmine, and echothiophate, compete with acetylcholine for the same binding site on the enzyme. The resulting accumulation of acetylcholine at neural synapses produces both nicotinic and muscarinic cholinergic effects. These drugs are used to treat glaucoma (by reducing intraocular pressure) and myasthenia gravis, and to reverse the effects of cholinergic receptor blocking agents such as tubocurarine. Carbamate insecticides are also reversible inhibitors. The organophosphorus insecticides, such as tri-*ortho*-cresyl phosphate, diisopropylfluorophosphate and others, behave as irreversible inhibitors; a phosphonium ion is formed that binds to the enzyme to form a stable, undissociating intermediate, incapable of binding acetylcholine. They are thus more toxic. Some affect the plasma enzyme only, and some affect both the plasma and the red cell enzyme. Also called *anticholinesterase.* See also *organophosphate compounds.*

Cholografin (ko″lo-gra′fin) trademark. See under *iodipamide.*

choluria (ko-lu′re-ah) [*chol-* + Gr. *ouron* urine + *-ia*] the presence of bile in the urine; discoloration of the urine with bile pigments.

chondr/o (kon′dro) [Gr. *chondros* cartilage] a word element used in combining form to denote cartilage, e.g., chondroblastoma.

chondralgia (kon-dral′je-ah) [*chondr-* + Gr. *algos* pain + *-ia*] pain in a cartilage. Also called chondrodynia.

chondritis (kon-dri′tis) [*chondr-* + *-itis*] inflammation of a cartilage.

chondroblast (kon′dro-blast) [*chondro* + Gr. *blastos* germ] a cell that forms cartilage.

chondroblastoma (kon″dro-blas-to′mah) [Gr. *chondros* cartilage + *blastos* germ + *-oma*] a benign, cartilaginous tumor, most commonly occurring at the epiphyses of the femur, tibia, or humerus of adolescent males. In a radiograph, this tumor appears as an area of radiolucency with mottled calcification, and is sometimes confused with giant cell tumors. See also *bone tumors.*

chondrocalcinosis (kon″dro-kal″si-no′sis) [*chondro-* + *calx* lime + *-osis*] a joint disease characterized by recurrent and transient attacks of acute arthritis and the presence of calcium-containing salts in articular cartilage. These salts include calcium pyrophosphate, calcium hydroxyapatite, and calcium orthophosphate. When calcium pyrophosphate dihydrate salts are found in joint fluid and there is acute or chronic synovitis, the term pseudogout is used. The cause of the deposition of the calcium salts is not clear, but the condition is known to be associated with diabetes mellitus, hyperparathyroidism, hemochromatosis, and Wilson's disease. A familial pattern has been described. Incidence increases with age.

Large or small calcium crystals may be found within leukocytes or floating free within synovial fluid. There is radiographic evidence of the presence of the calcium-containing salts in the cartilaginous structures of one or more joints. Radiographs may also reveal linear calcification in articular cartilage. The diseased cartilage is most probably the source of the crystals, which show weakly positive birefringence, as opposed to the sodium urate crystals of gout, which are negatively birefringent.

chondrocyte (kon′dro-sit) [*chondro-* + Gr. *kytos* hollow vessel] a cell of mature cartilage.

chondrodermatitis (kon″dro-der″mah-ti′tis) an inflammatory process involving cartilage and skin, often occurring as a painful nodule on the helix of the ear.

chondrodysplasia (kon″dro-dis-pla′ze-ah) [*chondro-* + Gr. *dys* abnormal + *plassein* to form + *-ia*] see *enchondroma.*

chondrodystrophy (kon″dro-dis′tro-fe) a disorder of cartilage formation.

chondroitin sulfate (kon-dro′ĭ-tin) a glycosaminoglycan (mucopolysaccharide) composed of a chain of alternating residues of *N*-acetyl-D-glucosamine (GalNAc) and D-glucuronic acid (GlcUA) in which the GalNAc residues are sulfate esters. There are two types: chondroitin sulfate A (or chondroitin 4-sulfate), in which the sulfate group is esterified to the C-4 hydroxyl group of GalNAc, and chondroitin sulfate C (or chondroitin-6-sulfate), in which it is esterified at C-6. Condroitin sulfate B was applied to a compound, now called dermatan sulfate, which is the same as chondroitin-6-sulfate except that the GlcUA residue is epimerized at C-5 to form L-iduronic acid. The general formula for both of the chondroitin sulfates is $[(1\rightarrow 3)\text{-}\beta\text{-GalNAc-}(1\rightarrow 4)\text{-}\beta\text{-GlcUA}]_n$.

Chondroitin sulfates are the predominant glycosaminoglycans in cartilage, bone, and blood vessels; they also occur in the skin, cornea, and other connective tissues.

chondroitin sulfate staining see *mucopolysaccharide staining.*

chondroma (kon-dro′mah) see *enchondroma.*

chondromatous exostosis (kon-drom′ah-tus) see *osteochondroma.*

chondromyxoid (kon″dro-mik′soid) [*chondro-* + Gr. *myxo-* mucus + *eidos* form] composed of cartilaginous and myxoid connective tissue.

chondromyxoid fibroma a benign bone tumor that usually occurs within the long bones of young adults. It is solid and cellular, and contains cartilaginous areas and giant cells within a myxoid stroma.

Care must be taken not to mistake it for chondrosarcoma.

chondroporosis (kon″dro-po-ro′sis) [*chondro-* + Gr. *poros* a passage] the formation of sinuses or spaces in cartilage.

chondrosarcoma (kon″dro-sar-ko′mah) [*chondro-* + Gr. *sarx, sarcos* flesh + *-oma*] a malignant neoplasm derived from cartilage cells or their precursors, typically occurring in the pelvic girdle, thoracic cage, and proximal femur and humerus of adults (predominantly males). Two forms are distinguished: the peripheral, which grows out from the bone, and the central, which arises from the medullary cavity. See also *bone tumors.*

CHOP abbrev. for cyclophosphamide, hydroxydaunorubicin (Adriamycin), Oncovin, and prednisone, a major established cancer chemotherapy drug regimen. For more information, see the specific drug (listed under its generic name) and *Appendix A.*

chopped meat medium see *chopped meat b.* under *broth.*

chopper (chop′er) a device that intermittently interrupts a signal, producing a square wave, so that the signal can be amplified by an AC-coupled amplifier. This may either be an electronic circuit that chops the output of a detector, or a mechanical device, as in some colorimeters, where there is a fan whose blades interrupt the light beam.

chord/o (kor′do) [Gr. *chordē* cord] a word element used in combining form to denote relationship to a cord, e.g., chorditis.

chorda (kor′dah) [L.; Gr. *chordē*] any cord or sinew.

c. tendineae cordis, [NA], fibrous, white, connective tissue cords that arise from the papillary muscles of the ventricles and insert onto the atrioventricular valve leaflets. They keep the valve centered and prevent eversion of the cusps during systole.

c. tympani, [NA], a branch of the facial nerve carrying taste fibers for the anterior two-thirds of the tongue; it also carries preganglionic parasympathetic secretory fibers to the submandibular ganglion, which relays them to the submandibular and sublingual glands. The nerve arises as the facial nerve descends behind the middle ear, and proceeds through a bony canal to enter the tympanic cavity opposite the upper part of the tympanic membrane. It then reenters the temporal bone and descends along the spine of the sphenoid to pass deep to the lateral pterygoid before joining the lingual nerve.

chordoma (kor-do′mah) a neoplasm that arises from persisting notochord cells. Roughly half occur in the sacrococcygeal region and a third occur in the region of the body of the sphenoid. A sacral tumor tends to form a large presacral soft tissue mass, whereas cranial tumors are more likely to infiltrate the sphenoid, ethmoid, and occipital bones, and often involve cranial nerves. The tumors are gelatinous with hemorrhagic areas. Sections show a variable histologic appearance, but typically nests and ribbons of cells lie within a myxoid stroma. Large vacuolated "physaliferous" cells can usually be found. There is a strong likelihood of recurrence following resection of a chordoma, often years after surgery, and as many as half of the individuals affected develop metastases.

chorea (ko-re′ah) [L., from Gr. *choreia* dance] purposeless, unpredictable, rapid, highly complex, jerky movements that appear well coordinated but actually are performed involuntarily. Chorea occurs as a dominant symptom in a number of disease states such as Huntington's chorea and Sydenham's chorea.

Huntington's c., a hereditary, progressive disease, transmitted as an autosomal dominant trait, that is characterized by choreic movements and mental deterioration. The brain appears atrophied, and neuronal degeneration is seen in the caudate and other deep nuclei. Deficiency of glutamic acid decarboxylase and the inhibitory transmitter α-aminobutyric acid (GABA) in the basal ganglia have been reported. Huntington's chorea usually appears in middle life, with development of irregular, jerky, choreic movements of the limbs, neck, and face, which may interfere with speech and gait. Dementia may develop before, with, or after the onset of the motor disorder, and progressively becomes more profound.

Diagnosis is made primarily on the basis of clinical findings and family history. Computed tomography of the brain may be helpful in detecting caudate nuclear atrophy. The electroencephalogram is also informative. It is characterized by low-voltage activity: alpha rhythm may be absent and the background activity may be in the range of beta activity. Visual evoked potentials to flash stimuli show abnormal amplitudes with normal spike latencies. Abnormalities in the electroencephalogram are of no value in predicting the development of the disease in the offspring of those affected.

No treatment is available to halt the progression of the disease, and death often occurs about 15 yr after the onset of symptoms. Because 50 percent of the children of those affected are at risk of developing the disease themselves, genetic counseling is important.

Sydenham's c., a disorder of the central nervous system that primarily affects young people and is often associated with rheumatic fever. It is of finite duration and is characterized by rapid, involuntary, nonrepetitive, jerky movements without neurologic dysfunction. The speech and walking gait may be impaired, and mild muscle weakness and emotional lability are common. This disorder is considered to be an inflammatory complication of group A streptococcal infections. Laboratory findings may reveal a lingering streptococcal infection but are otherwise normal. Usually this disorder spontaneously terminates within 3 mo. Also called chorea minor, rheumatic chorea, and St. Vitus' dance.

choreoathetosis (ko″re-o-ath″ĕ-to′sis) abnormal movements having some of the features of both chorea and athetosis.

chori/o (ko′re-o) a word element used in combining form to denote the chorion (the extraembryonic membrane), e.g., choriocarcinoma.

chorioadenoma destruens (ko″re-o-ad″ĕ-no′mah des-troo′enz) a form of hydatidiform mole in which molar chorionic villi penetrate into the myometrium and/or parametrium. Rarely, they metastasize. The most common site of metastasis is the lungs. Also called *invasive mole.*

chorioamnionitis (ko″re-o-am″ne-o-ni′tis) an inflammation of fetal membranes most commonly due to bacterial infection.

choriocarcinoma (ko″re-o-kar″sĭ-no″mah) a malignant neoplasm of trophoblastic epithelium showing

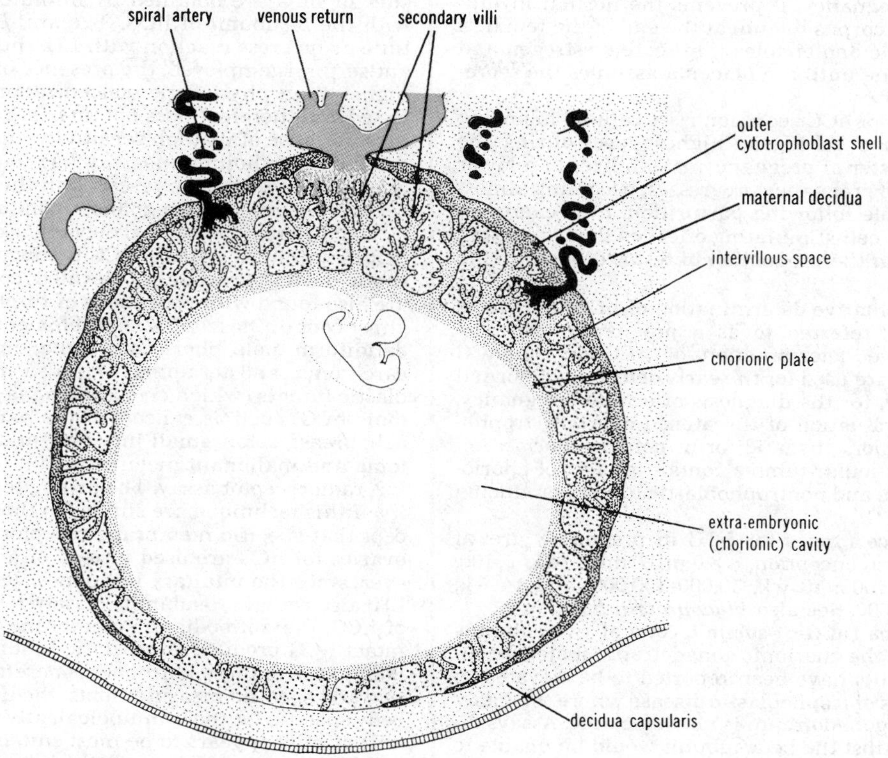

Chorion. Schematic representation of the human embryo at the beginning of the second month of development. At the embryonic pole the villi are numerous and well formed; at the abembryonic pole they are few in number and poorly developed (modified after von Ortmann). (From Langman, J.: Medical Embryology. 4th ed. Baltimore, Williams & Wilkins, 1981.)

differentiation toward both cyto- and syncytiotrophoblastic cells. Such tumors may be gestational (arising from products of conception) or nongestational (arising from germ cells of the gonads or extragonadal sites in individuals of either sex).

Human chorionic gonadotrophin (hCG), which is produced by normal syncytiotrophoblast, is also produced by the neoplastic syncytiotrophoblastic cells of a choriocarcinoma. This provides a biochemical marker that can be used as a diagnostic aid and for followup of patients during and after treatment.

The great majority of choriocarcinomas are gestational in origin. Of these, 50 percent are associated with a hydatidiform mole, 25 percent with an abortion, 22 percent with a normal pregnancy, and a small number with ectopic pregnancies. The remainder are of nongestational origin. Untreated, this tumor is generally aggressive and metastasizes widely, most frequently to the lungs, liver, kidneys, and brain.

chorioepithelioma (ko″re-o-ep″ĭ-the″le-o′mah) see *choriocarcinoma.*

choriomeningitis (ko″re-o-men″in-ji′tis) cerebral meningitis with lymphocytic infiltration of the choroid plexus. See also *lymphocytic choriomeningitis.*

chorion (ko′re-on) [Gr.] in the developing embryo, the outermost extraembryonic membrane. See also the accompanying illustration.

c. frondosum, the persisting villi on the chorionic sac of the developing fetus that, together with the decidua basalis, form the placenta; see *placenta.*

c. laeve, the smooth (nonvillous) portion of the chorion that surrounds the developing embryo.

chorionic (ko″re-on″ik) pertaining to the chorion.

chorionic carcinoma see *choriocarcinoma.*

chorionic cavity see *extraembryonic c.* under *coelom.*

chorionic gonadotropin (CG, hCG) human chorionic gonadotropin, a polypeptide hormone normally produced by synctiotrophoblastic epithelial cells of the human placenta, a sialoglycoprotein, M.W. 56,000 (protein core); carbohydrate content 40 percent, sialic acid content 9 percent. Like thyroid-stimulating hormone (TSH), follicle-stimulating hormone (FSH), and luteinizing hormone (LH), hCG consists of two nonidentical subunits, denoted alpha and beta, along with a protein core and carbohydrate side-chain. The alpha subunit is essentially identical to the alpha subunits of the pituitary FSH, LH, and TSH. The beta subunits of these hormones differ in amino acid sequence and are responsible for target organ specificity and immunologic properties. For this reason, the use of antisera against the beta subunit for the RIA of hCG overcomes the problems of cross reaction with other structurally similar glycoprotein hormones.

hCG is similar in function to luteinizing hormone. During pregnancy, it prevents the normal involution of the corpus luteum at the end of the female's sexual cycle and enables it to secrete estrogen and progesterone until the placenta assumes the secretory activity.

The rate of hCG secretion rises rapidly following conception, reaching its highest level during the first trimester of pregnancy; it stabilizes at a lower level as the pregnancy progresses, becoming almost undetectable following parturition. hCG exerts an interstitial cell-stimulating effect on the fetal testes, resulting in the production of testosterone in male fetuses.

The qualitative determination of hCG in urine is commonly referred to as a pregnancy test. The quantitative determination of hCG or the hCG β-subunit are used for the early detection of normal pregnancy, for the diagnosis of ectopic pregnancy, and for evaluation of threatened abortion, trophoblastic tumors (hydatidiform mole or choriocarcinoma), testicular tumors containing foci of choriocarcinoma, and nontrophoblastic tumors producing ectopic hCG.

Reference ranges for hCG in pregnancy are: at 7–10 da postconception, $>$ 3.0 mIU/ml; 30 da, $>$ 100; 40 da, $>$ 2000; 10 wk, 50,000–100,000; and 14 wk, 10,000–20,000. See also *glycoprotein hormones.*

c. g.-alpha (hCG-α) subunit, one of two subunits present in the chorionic gonadotropin molecule; alpha subunits have been reported to be elevated in some cases of trophoblastic disease where the intact chorionic gonadotropin is not detectable. Assays directed against the beta subunit would be unable to detect some of these conditions.

c. g.-beta (hCG-β) subunit, one of two subunits present in the chorionic gonadotropin molecule. All specific hormonal and specific immunologic properties of hCG derive from the unique beta chain. The alpha chain is identical to the alpha chains in thyroid-stimulating hormone (TSH), follicle-stimulating hormone (FSH), and luteinizing hormone (LH). As a result, quantitative procedures for hCG-β (as opposed to procedures for total hCG) do not show cross reaction with TSH, FSH, or LH.

chorionic gonadotropin assays 1. immunologic tests and radioimmunoassay, used primarily for detection of pregnancy. The immunologic method is based on hemagglutination (or latex agglutination) inhibition and is available as a tube test or slide test. In the tube test, the hCG-containing specimen competes with hCG-coated red blood cells for binding with anti-hCG antibodies. A positive agglutination means that no detectable hCG is present in the specimen (i.e., absence of pregnancy). The slide test is based on the same principle but uses hCG-coated latex particles.

Commercially available immunologic tests that utilize latex particles, or erythrocytes coated with hCG and an antibody against hCG, are capable of measuring hCG levels as early as 1 or 2 da after the first missed menstrual period. However, sensitivity of those methodologies generally cannot be increased beyond 0.5 IU/ml, as greater sensitivity results in immunologic cross reactions with pituitary gonadotropins. The anti-hCG sera generally used for the radioimmunoassay of hCG show a cross reaction with various glycoprotein hormones, especially LH, so that it is sometimes difficult to assess which hormone is being measured in the sample. Antibodies directed against the specific antigenic sites of hCG are obtained by immunizing rabbits with the β-subunit of hCG. The anti-β-hCG shows little or no cross reaction with LH; thus, when this antiserum is employed, the presence of LH even in higher than physiologic concentrations is not detected and therefore does not interfere in β-hCG assays. Because of its high sensitivity and specificity, the β-hCG radioimmunoassay has found wide application in diagnostic research in the field of placental function and pregnancy monitoring.

In addition to the normal elevations of serum and urine concentrations of β-hCG produced by the placenta during pregnancy, elevated concentrations are also found with neoplasms of trophoblastic origin or containing trophoblastic elements such as hydatidiform mole, choriocarcinoma, embryonal cell carcinoma, and teratoma, and also in nontrophoblastic tumors (which on occasion may produce ectopic hCG) such as cancers of the pancreas, stomach, breast, colon, small intestine, and nephroblastoma and malignant melanoma.

2. radioreceptor assay. The principle and sensitivity of this technique are similar to those of RIA except that specific membrane receptors from ovine ovaries for hCG are used instead of antisera. However, since the pituitary hormones, TSH, FSH, and LH, also contain α-subunits closely related to those of hCG, the antibodies or membrane receptors for intact hCG produce nonspecific binding and cross reaction with these hormones. Therefore, for sensitive and specific measurements, the use of an antibody specific for the immunologically potent β-subunit of hCG appears to be most suitable.

3. bioassay tests. This method is based on the injection of urine into test animals. If hCG is present in the urine, it produces corpora lutea and corpora hemorrhagica in the ovaries of mice and rabbits, hyperemia in the ovaries of rats, and secretion of sperm and ova in toads and frogs. Although this procedure is very sensitive to the presence of hCG, it is costly, time-consuming, and not very reproducible; it has largely been abandoned in favor of the faster and more reliable immunologic methods.

chorionic somatomammotropin (CS, hCS) a peptide hormone secreted by the placenta; see *placental lactogen, human.*

chorionic villi numerous branching projections from the external surface of the chorion, each covered by trophoblast and containing a fibrovascular core. The chorionic villi provide for exchange between the maternal and fetal circulations. Also called *placental villi.*

choristoma (ko″ris-to′mah) [Gr. *chōristos* separated + *-oma*] a mass of tissue in which the cellular elements are histologically normal but present in abnormal proportions and are located in a part of the body where these tissues are not normally found. Also called *aberrant rest.* Cf. *hamartoma.*

choroid (ko′roid) [*chorion* + Gr. *eidos* form] the thin, dark brown, pigmented vascular coat of the eye; the portion of the uvea from the ora serrata to the optic nerve. It provides nutritional and vascular support for the eyeball.

choroideremia (ko-roi″der-e′me-ah) [*choroid* + Gr. *erēmia* destitution] a hereditary primary choroidal degeneration, transmitted as an x-linked trait. In males it eventually leads to blindess as degeneration of the retinal pigment epithelium progresses to complete atrophy. In females it is nonprogressive and vision is usually normal.

choroiditis (ko″roi-di′tis) [*choroid + itis*] 1. inflammation of the choroid as an accompaniment of meningitis. The choroid plexus becomes congested and infiltrated with inflammatory cells, and eventually may become covered with exudate.

2. a form of posterior uveitis characterized by inflammation of the choroid, which frequently extends to involve the retina (chorioretinitis). Granulomatous infections (especially toxoplasmosis and histoplasmosis) and intraocular parasites may be implicated, but frequently the cause is unknown. Persons affected experience blurred vision, metamorphopsia (distortion of object shape and size), and photophobia. Diagnosis may be accomplished by ophthalmoscopic examination. Skin tests, radiographs, blood counts, and stool examination may be required to demonstrate the infectious nature of the disease.

choroid plexus a series of vascular folds of the pia mater projecting into the lateral, third, and fourth ventricles of the brain; they are important in the production of cerebrospinal fluid. These folds are composed of blood vessels, capillaries, nerve fibers, pia mater, and the ependymal cell lining of the ventricles. The blood supply is derived from branches of the internal carotid arteries and posterior cerebral arteries. The capillaries drain into venous plexuses, which join to form the choroidal vein. The pia mater does not form a complete sheet between the ependymal cells and the capillary endothelium. However, the tight junctions between the ependymal cells are an important component of the blood-brain barrier.

chr abbrev. for chronic.

Christeller reaction (kris′tel-er) a reaction used to demonstrate gold in tissue sections using stannous chloride.

Christensen's urea agar (kris′ten-senz) see *Christensen's urea a.* under *agar.*

Christmas disease (kris′mas) [Stephen *Christmas,* 20th century, an English boy in whom the disease was first studied in detail] see *h. B* under *hemophilia.*

Christmas factor see *Factor IX.*

chrom/o-, chromato- (kro′mo, kro-mat′o) [Gr. *chrōma, chrōmatos* color] a word element used in combining form to denote relationship to color, e.g., chromatography.

chromaffin (kro′maf-in, kro-maf′in) [*chromium* + L. *affinis* having an affinity for] pertaining to cells or tissues that undergo the chromaffin reaction by virtue of their content of epinephrine or norepinephrine. They include cells of the adrenal medulla, tumors (pheochromocytomas) derived from the adrenal medulla and the paraganglia, and small clusters of cells near the sympathetic ganglia. Enterochromaffin cells also undergo the chromaffin reaction; however, this is because of the presence of serotonin, not of epinephrine or norepinephrine.

chromaffin body see *paraganglion.*

chromaffin cells cells that stain yellowish-brown with chromium salts. They synthesize and release catecholamines and are found primarily in the adrenal medulla and paraganglia.

chromaffin reaction the formation of a yellow-brown coloration in the cytoplasm of certain cells by chromic acid or dichromate fixation. This chromaffin reaction is based on the oxidation of epinephrine and norepinephrine, which are neurotransmitters and hormones, to form a pigment similar to melanin. The pigment is found in chromaffin granules, which are the secretory vacuoles containing the neurotransmitter.

chromate (kro′māt) the CrO_4^{2-} ion or a salt containing this ion. Chromate esters, the product of the reaction of $HCrO_4^-$ with alcohols, are known. Chromates are corrosive oxidizing agents and can cause dermatitis and ulceration of exposed tissues.

chromate method a histologic procedure for the demonstration of lead, in which lead salts are converted to yellow chromate crystals.

chromatic (kro-mat′ik) 1. pertaining to color; stainable with dyes.

2. pertaining to chromatin.

chromatic aberration a defect of an optical system in which different colors are focused at different points. It may be partially corrected by using multiple lenses that compensate for each other. Microscope objective lenses corrected in this manner are called achromatic lenses.

chromatid (kro′mah-tid) one of the two filaments joined at the centromere that make up a chromosome, as visualized during metaphase. They separate into daughter filaments during anaphase, going to opposite poles of the dividing cell.

chromatid interference deviation from the expected ratio of the proportion of double crossovers involving 2, 3, or 4 chromatids of a tetrad. A 1:2:1 ratio would be expected by chance if the crossovers did not interact.

chromatin (kro′mah-tin) the material of which chromosomes are composed, a complex of DNA and histones. Chromatin is found in the cell nucleus and is the carrier of the genes. The uncoiled, less readily stained chromatin is called extended chromatin or euchromatin; the tightly coiled, more readily stained chromatin is condensed chromatin or heterochromatin. See also *Barr body, euchromatin,* and *heterochromatin.*

sex c., the Barr body, the inactivated X-chromosome, which remains in the form of heterochromatin in the cells of normal females.

chromatinic body (kro″mah-tin′ik) the nuclear material of a prokaryotic cell that consists of aggregates of deoxyribonucleic acid. It is found in bacterial cells.

chromatin-negative a term used to refer to an individual with cell nuclei that lack typical Barr bodies, usually signifying a genetic male but also found in Turner's (XO) and other sex chromosomal abnormalities.

chromatin-positive a term used to refer to an individual whose cell nuclei contain typical Barr bodies in more than 20 percent of nuclei in buccal smears, usually signifying a genetic female but also occurring in a variety of sex chromosomal abnormalities.

chromation (kro-ma′shun) the use of dichromate fixatives. See also *chromaffin.*

chromatogram (kro-mat′o-gram) originally, the pattern of bands produced by the separation of substances by column chromatography. The procedure was so named by the Russian botanist Mikhail Tswett, who was the first to use the technique to separate plant pigments, producing colored bands. By extension, the term also refers to the record produced by any form of chromatography, such as the stained filter paper or plate produced by paper or thin-layer chromatography, the output of the chart recorder in gas chromatography, or high-pressure liquid chromatography.

chromatograph (kro-mat′o-graf) 1. the apparatus used in chromatography.

2. to use chromatography for the separation of substances.

chromatography (kro″mah-tog′rah-fe) [*chromato-* + Gr. *graphein* to write] any of a diverse group of techniques used to separate mixtures of chemical compounds into individual components based on differences in their relative affinities for two different media: one is the mobile phase (e.g., a moving fluid [solvent] or a moving gas) and the other, the stationary phase or sorbent (e.g., a porous solid, gel, or liquid bound to a porous inert solid support).

TECHNIQUES. In column chromatography, the stationary phase is packed in a glass or plastic tube; the sample, dissolved in a solvent, is added at the top. As the solvent moves through the packing, the sample components that have greater solubility in the solvent or less affinity for the sorbent travel faster and farther down the column. This results in separation of the components into bands along the column. The different isolated components are then washed out of the column (eluted) in successive aliquots of the same or different solvents.

There are two methods of column chromatography in which there is a continuous flow of the mobile phase through the column; both methods have been automated. The sample is injected at one end, and the components, separated by their passage through the column, are quantitated by a detector at the other end.

In gas chromatography (GC) the mobile phase is an inert gas, usually helium or nitrogen; in liquid chromatography (LC) the mobile phase is a liquid (water or organic solvent). A special form of liquid chromatography is high-pressure (or high-performance) liquid chromatography (HPLC) in which the mobile phase is pumped through the column at high pressures (about 1000 psi). The stationary phase in this technique is either a liquid bound to a solid or a liquid through which the mobile phase percolates.

In thin-layer chromatography (TLC), the stationary phase is a thin layer of adsorbent gel coated on a glass or plastic plate. The sample is applied in a small spot at the base of the plate, and the plate is made to stand on edge in a solvent. As the solvent rises in the gel by capillary action, the sample components move at different rates and are separated into different spots. The plate is removed from the solvent, dried, and stained to visualize the components.

A similar technique is paper chromatography, in which the thin-layer plate is replaced by a specially prepared sheet of filter paper.

Both techniques can be performed in one or two directions. In the latter approach, after one solvent development step, the TLC plate (or paper) is rotated 90° and developed again; different solvents may be used for each direction of separation, thus improving the quality of separation.

METHODS OF SEPARATION. Generally, molecular species can be separated by virtue of three properties: solubility, charge, and size. In adsorption chromatography, the stationary phase is an adsorbent, such as silica gel, alumina, magnesium silicate, diatomaceous earth, porous polymers, sucrose, cellulose, or charcoal; the mobile phase is a solvent or a mixture of solvents. Sample components are separated by differences in solubility and in strength of binding to the adsorbent. This method is used primarily for non-ionic compounds such as lipids and carbohydrates.

In ion-exchange chromatography, the stationary phase is an ion-exchange resin and the mobile phase is a buffer solution. An anion-exchange resin has many covalently bound positively charged groups (R_3N^+—) and binds anions; a cation-exchange resin with negative groups (COO^-, SO^-_3) binds cations. The pH of the buffer solution determines the ionization of the sample components, and thus their degree of binding with the resin. This method is used to separate ions and ionic compounds such as amino acids and to remove interfering ionic substances from specimens before analysis.

In gel-filtration chromatography, the stationary phase is a gel with an accurately controlled pore size. As the sample moves through the gel with the mobile phase, smaller molecules frequently become trapped for a time in the pores while larger molecules pass unimpeded. The sample components are thus separated by differences in molecular size and shape. Commonly used stationary phases are cross-linked dextrans (Sephadex), agarose (Sepharose), or polyacrylamide gels. This method is also called exclusion, gel-permeation, molecular-exclusion, molecular-sieve, or size-exclusion chromatography.

In partition chromatography (also called liquid-liquid chromatography), the stationary and mobile phases are immiscible liquids, and the sample components are separated on the basis of their partition coefficients (the ratio of the solubilities in the two phases).

For more information on the specific types of chromatography, see *gas chromatography, high-pressure liquid chromatography,* and *thin-layer chromatography.*

chromatolysis (kro″mah-tol′i-sis) [*chromato-* + Gr. *lysis* dissolution] disintegration of the Nissl substance of a nerve cell resulting from transection of its axon. See also *Wallerian degeneration.*

chromatophil (kro-mat′o-fil) any cell or tissue constituent having a high affinity for a stain.

chromatophilic granules see *Nissl bodies.*

chrome (krōm) [Fr., from Gr. *chrōma* color] 1. the element chromium.

2. a chromium alloy plating, such as chrome steel or chrome-molybdenum steel.

3. any of several brilliantly colored inorganic pigments containing chromium.

chrome alum hematoxylin-phloxine method a histologic method for the differential staining of the alpha and beta cells of the pancreas and hypophysis. Paraffin sections of tissue fixed in Bouin's fluid are dehydrated, refixed in Bouin's fluid for 12–24 hr, oxidized in permanganate, decolorized in bisulfite, stained with chrome alum hematoxylin, and counterstained with a 0.5 percent solution of phloxine B, followed by immersion in 5 percent phosphotungstic acid. Pancreatic and hypophyseal alpha cells are stained red; beta cells, blue.

chrome violet CG a histologic stain that turns aluminum salts dark red; C.I. 43810. Also called *aurin tricarboxylic acid.*

chromic (kro′mik) [Gr. *chrōma* color] pertaining to chromium, or to compounds containing the trivalent form of chromium.

chromic acid the common name for chromium trioxide or chromic anhydride, CrO_3, a dark purple crystalline solid. It is a corrosive oxidizer that is irritating to skin and mucous membranes. True chromic acid, H_2CrO_4, exists only in solution. In histology, chromic acid is used as an oxidizing agent; see also *Bauer reaction* and *Gridley stain.*

chromic phosphate P 32 colloid a radiopharmaceutical used for the palliative treatment of malignant neoplastic pleural or peritoneal effusions in patients who do not respond to radiation therapy or chemotherapy. The chromic phosphate is an insoluble precipitate that is instilled directly into a body cavity, where the emitted beta radiation is thought to kill free-floating malignant cells or those that have seeded the serous membrane.

chromium (Cr) (kro′me-um) [L., from Gr. *chrōma* color] a steel-gray, lustrous, hard metallic element; atomic number 24; atomic weight 51.996; a 3d transition element; common oxidation states +2, +3, and +6.

Chromium is an essential trace element; the adult human body contains about 6 mg, distributed through all tissues. Evidence suggests that Cr^{3+} is involved in the effect of insulin on glucose transport. In industry it is used in stainless steel alloys, in chrome plating, and in chrome pigments. Chromates, chromic acid, and other chromium (VI) compounds constitute industrial hazards; they are skin and lung irritants that cause ulceration of the skin and mucous membranes and are carcinogenic.

chromium-51 (^{51}Cr, Cr 51) a gamma-emitting radioactive isotope of chromium with a half-life of 27.8 da. The hexavalent form (sodium chromate Cr 51) attaches in vitro to the globin portion of the hemoglobin molecule, and thus is very useful in tagging red blood cells for studies of red cell life span, blood volume, bone and renal blood flow, and gastrointestinal blood loss. The trivalent chromic ion can also label platelets and leukocytes for cell survival and thrombus studies.

chromium assays a quantitative test for chromium in the plasma or urine. The specimen is ashed by treatment with HNO_3 and H_2O_2 and oxidized with saturated bromine water mixed with NaOH. Phenol water is added to remove excess Br_2, and 1,5-diphenylcarbonhydrazide reagent is then added to form a red chelate complex with an absorbance at 543 nm. Atomic absorption spectrophotometry (AAS) with graphite furnace, using a wavelength of 357.9 nm, is currently the preferred method.

Chromobacterium (kro″mo-bak-te′re-um) [*chromo-* + *baktērion* little rod] a genus of bacteria that consists of gram-negative, facultatively anaerobic rods. These organisms are motile with polar and lateral flagella. They normally occur in soil and water, but also are potential pathogens and can cause local and systemic infections and abscesses, predominantly in tropical climates. Most strains produce a violet pigment, causing colonies to appear black on blood agar. Carbohydrates are fermented, and reaction to catalase is positive and to oxidase negative. The type species is *C. violaceum.*

chromoblastomycosis (kro″mo-blas″to-mi-ko′sis) a chronic granulomatous infection of skin and subcutaneous tissue caused by dematiacious fungi belonging to the genera *Phialophora, Cladosporium,* and related species. This subcutaneous mycosis is probably initiated by a dermal injury and is common in the Americas, Africa, Southeast Asia, Australia, the Soviet Union, and Japan. The five organisms that most commonly cause chromoblastomycosis are *Phialophora verrucosa, Fonsecaea pedrosoi, F. compactum, Wangiella dermatidis,* and *Cladosporium carrionii.* All have been isolated from wood and soil.

Clinical Diagnosis. The cutaneous lesions develop first as small papules or nodules that become ulcerated. Growth is very slow and occurs by peripheral extension, while the center of the lesions heal with scar formation. The lesions may remain flat or may become raised above the surface on a small stalk. Older lesions may be verrucous, papillomatous, or crusted, and can be confused with older forms of tuberculosis, sarcoidosis, leishmaniasis, syphilis, or blastomycosis. Continued extension produces the characteristic lobulated masses known as "cauliflower" lesions.

Although the disease is painless, a secondary painful infection may develop, which usually causes the patient to seek treatment. Satellite lesions may develop as a result of scratching, and the fungus probably spreads through the lymphatic or blood system.

In tissue, these fungi are seen as clusters of brown, thick-walled cells known as sclerotic cells ("corps fumagoides"). These cells are often septate and are found within giant cells or extracellularly among polymorphonuclear leukocytes. Histologically, chromoblastomycosis appears granulomatous, with nodules containing giant cells and surrounded by a zone of inflammatory cells. In advanced stages of the disease, the epidermis becomes thickened due to epithelial hyperplasia and the influx of inflammatory cells.

Laboratory Diagnosis. Direct examination of pus or scales from the surface of the lesion digested in 10 percent potassium hydroxide frequently reveals the fungus. Sclerotic cells are characteristic of chromoblastomycosis. The fungus may be grown on Sabouraud's glucose agar, with and without cycloheximide. It is possible to distinguish the pathogenic species from saprophytes by their ability to grow at 37°C, by their inability to assimilate lactose, and by their inability to liquefy gelatin. The demonstration of precipitating antibodies in the sera of infected patients may aid in establishing the diagnosis; however, the cross-reactivity of antigens makes species identification a problem.

chromogen (kro′mo-jen) 1. one of a group of chemical species that can form a particular colored material or can be identified by such a reaction with an appropriate reagent; e.g., 17,21-dihydroxy-20-oxosteroids such as cortisone and cortisol are referred to as Porter-Silber chromogens because they form a yellow color on reaction with phenylhydrazine and sulfuric acid. Cf. *chromophore.*

2. a microorganism having the ability to produce color or pigment. In clinical bacteriology, the term is often used to describe strains of the *Mycobacte-*

rium genus that produce a carotenoid pigment resulting in colonies yellow to red in color on the appropriate solid media.

chromogenesis (kro″mo-jen′ĕ-sis) [*chromo-* + Gr. *genesis* production] the formation of pigments or colors by chemical reaction or by the action of living organisms such as bacteria.

chromogenic (kro″mo-jen′ik) capable of producing color or pigment.

chromomere (kro′mo-mēr) [*chromo-* + Gr. *meros* part] any one of the beadlike granules occurring in series along the chromonema of a chromosome. It is most easily seen when the chromosome is partially uncoiled during the leptotene or zygotene stages of meiosis. These granules give polytene chromosomes their banded appearance.

chromomycosis (kro″mo-mi-ko′sis) see *chromoblastomycosis.*

chromonema (kro″mo-ne′mah), pl. *chromonemata* [*chromo-* + Gr. *nēma* thread] the thin, threadlike form of an uncoiled chromosome seen in interphase, early prophase, and late telophase, as opposed to the tightly coiled metaphase chromosome.

chromophil (kro′mo-fil) [*chromo-* + Gr. *philein* to love] an easily stainable cell.

chromophobe (kro′mo-fōb) [*chromo-* + Gr. *phobein* to be frightened by + *-ia*] any cell, structure, or tissue that does not stain readily. The term is applied especially to those cells of the anterior pituitary that contain few secretory granules, either because they are in an inactive phase of their secretory cycle, or because their secretion is being released rapidly.

chromophobe adenoma a pituitary adenoma composed of cells with pale-staining cytoplasm. The cells may nevertheless contain secretory granules demonstrable by electron microscopy, and many chromophobe adenomas are functioning neoplasms. See also *chromophobe.*

chromophore (kro′mo-fōr) 1. the part of a molecule that is responsible for the absorption of visible light and causes a compound to appear colored. One group of chromophores consists of conjugated double and triple bonds. (Usually 10 or more are necessary for absorption of visible light.) Other chromophores contain hetero atoms (usually nitrogen, oxygen, or sulfur) and absorb at longer wavelengths than analogous structures containing only carbon atoms. A replacement of side-groups that does not affect the structure of the chromophore usually produces only a slight shift of the absorption band.

2. one or more functional groups that, when placed in a structure (a chromogen) containing several aromatic rings, form a system of conjugated double bonds that absorb visible light. For example, in azo dyes (such as orange G), the chromophore is the azo group and the chromogen is azobenzene; in thiazine dyes (such as methylene blue), the chromophores are —N= and —S^+=, and the chromogen is the phenothiazine nucleus.

chromoprotein (kro″mo-pro′te-in) a colored, conjugated protein containing an organic prosthetic group that is linked to a metal ion. Examples are the red hemoglobin of the higher animals, the blue hemocyanin of many lower animals, and the red and blue pigments of seaweeds. Chromoproteins have respiratory functions and are closely related to the green chlorophyll of the higher plants.

chromosomal aberration (kro″mo-so′mal) an irregularity in the number or composition of chromosomes that may alter an embryo's course of development, usually through loss, duplication, exchange, or rearrangement of genetic material. Changes that take place in only one chromosome are called intrachromosomal or homosomal. Those involving two or more are interchromosomal or heterosomal.

chromosomal RNA (cRNA) small RNA molecules found in eukaryotic chromatin of the nucleus and presumed to have structural roles. The amount of cRNA found in each cell is highly variable.

chromosome (kro′mo-sōm) [*chromo-* + Gr. *sōma* body; from its intense staining capacity] a separate, deeply staining, threadlike structure found in the nucleus of all plant and animal cells. Higher organisms are termed eukaryotes (truly nucleated) in contrast to bacteria and viruses, which are prokaryotes (organisms without a nucleus). The eukaryotic chromosome is a complicated structure composed of deoxyribonucleic acid (DNA), several different types of proteins, and some ribonucleic acid (RNA). A prokaryotic chromosome consists of naked DNA or, in some viruses, naked RNA. DNA (or RNA) is the molecule containing coded information that directs the growth and development of a living organism and is transmitted from parents to offspring.

The chromosomes of higher organisms are most frequently studied when the cell is ready to divide into two cells. Before somatic cell division (mitosis) begins, replication of DNA occurs and the chromosomes are duplicated. As cell division proceeds, the chromosome threads become compactly coiled and condensed, making them visible under a microscope after appropriate staining. Each duplicate chromosome forms into a pair of rods (sister chromatids) joined at the centromere (sometimes called the kinetochore, spindle attachment, or primary constriction), which is essential for the normal movement of the chromosome. The genetic constitution of a chromatid is a double helix of DNA. The sister chromatid pairs separate, with one of each going into one of two daughter cells. Each receive a complete set of chromosomes exactly like those of the original unduplicated cell.

Each species (kind of organism) has a characteristic number of chromosomes in every body cell. Human beings typically have 46 chromosomes (23 pairs), of which 44 are autosomes (nonsex chromosomes) and 2 sex chromosomes (two X chromosomes in the female and an X and a Y chromosome in the male). In humans and other mammals the Y chromosome is male-determining. In the gonads of both sexes, by the process of meiosis (reduction division), the somatic cell (body cell) chromosome number making up two basic sets (diploid) is reduced to half (haploid) in the gametes. In humans, for example, the egg cell has 22 autosomes and 1 X chromosome; the sperm has 22 autosomes plus either 1 X or 1 Y chromosome. The diploid chromosome number of 46 is restored after fertilization, and the sex chromosome constitution is either XX or XY.

Chromosome numbers vary greatly between and within groups of organisms. Chromosome size also varies in different organisms, ranging from a fraction of a micrometer to more than 30 μm in length. Human chromosomes range in size from somewhat larger than 5 μm to less than 1 μm, the range varying between cells.

A typical chromosome in mitosis is identified morphologically both by its total length and by the position of the centromere, which determines the relative lengths of its arms. In human chromosomes the short arm is designated p and the long arm q. A chromosome in which the centromere is more or less in the middle is called metacentric; a chromosome in which the centromere is at the very end is telocentric; and chromosomes intermediate between these two may be called submetacentric or subtelocentric. In an acrocentric chromosome the centromere is located very near the end.

Besides the centromere (primary constriction), a chromosome may contain a secondary constriction, which appears as a narrowing or an unstained gap in the chromosome. Usually, a secondary constriction represents the nucleolus organizer region where the ribosomal RNA genes are located; in other instances it may contain heterochromatin with highly repetitive short sequences of DNA.

With the banding techniques now available, each individual human chromosome can be identified. The locations of hundreds of genes have now been mapped to specific regions of human chromosomes. Variations in both chromosome number and structure, observed in plants and animals (including humans), can lead to abnormalities in that particular individual; for example, Down's syndrome is the result of trisomy 21.

See also *chromosome banding* and *karyotype*.

ERNEST H. Y. CHU, PH.D.

homologous c.'s, 1. chromosomes that are structurally identical and have the same sequence of genes (although possibly different alleles) along their lengths.

2. a pair of chromosomes that join to form a bivalent during meiosis, even though they match along only part of their lengths, e.g., in humans, the X and Y chromosomes. Also called *heteromorphic chromosomes.*

Philadelphia c. (Ph^1), an acquired abnormal chromosome that arises from translocation from chromosome 22, usually to chromosome 9. It is seen in 85 percent of adult patients with chronic myelogenous leukemia and is present in myeloblasts, erythroblasts, and megakaryoblasts, all of which arise from the same stem cell. The chromosome is absent from lymphocytes and usually persists in the cells of patients in remission.

ring c., an aberrant chromosome that has pieces deleted from both ends, with the ends of the remaining piece joined to form a ring.

sex c., a chromosome responsible for sex determination. In mammals there are two types: the X (female) chromosome and the Y (male) chromosome, which are not homologous. Each cell of a normal individual has two sex chromosomes: XX individuals are female; XY are male. The Y chromosome is male-determining (with rare exceptions), even in the presence of multiple X chromosomes.

somatic c., any chromosome that is not a sex chromosome. Also called *autosome.*

chromosome banding the use of various physical and cytochemical treatments of cytologically fixed chromosome preparations with differential staining or fluorescence techniques; the chromosomes take on an alternate light- and dark-banded appearance. The banded chromosome permits definitive identification and delineation of all the chromosomes and chromosomal segments of humans and many other organisms. With appropriate techniques, more than 2000 bands can be demonstrated in the early mitotic chromosomes of the human complement, but the total number of observable bands decreases as the chromosomes continue to condense as they approach full metaphase. In most chromosome structural rearrangements, the positions of chromosome breaks and exchanges can be identified. The banding patterns also allow certain inferences to be made concerning the chemical composition, physical state, and functional significance of different regions of eukaryotic chromosomes. The most commonly used techniques for longitudinal differentiation of eukaryotic chromosomes are Q, G, R, and C banding.

Q BANDS. When human chromosomes are stained with quinacrine HCl (Atabrine) or quinacrine mustard and studied with a fluorescence microscope, they show bands of different degrees of brightness. The brightness of the Q bands is positively correlated with the adenine-thymine (AT):guanine-cytosine (GC) ratio for that particular region; the AT-rich regions fluoresce brightly, whereas the GC-rich regions quench the fluorescence.

G BANDS. When chromosome preparations are pretreated with a salt solution at 60°C or with proteolytic enzymes (usually trypsin or pronase) and stained with a Giemsa solution, G bands appear. Still other agents, including urea and strong bases, can produce banding patterns that can be visualized by the Giemsa stain. These results indicate that solubilization of some chromosomal proteins may be involved in producing the bands. However, DNA is also attacked by some of the Giemsa banding procedures. The actual mechanisms involved in the various methods are still unknown. Most of the G bands coincide with bands visualized by the quinacrine fluorescence method; the brightly fluorescent Q bands are now darkly stained, whereas the Q dark regions are now lightly stained.

R BANDS. The letter R refers to reverse banding, which involves pretreatment of chromosome preparations with hot (85°–90°C) alkali and subsequent staining with Giemsa. The banding pattern is the reverse of G banding: bands that are dark with R banding are light with G banding, and vice versa.

C BANDS. Constitutive heterochromatin is found in the chromosomes of practically all higher organisms, both plants and animals. It is the common form of heterochromatin that is composed of highly repetitive sequences of DNA and is present in the proximity of centromeres and telomeres, in the nucleolus organizer regions, in secondary constrictions, and in other regions such as the distal end of the long arm of the human Y chromosome. It is so designated to distinguish it from facultative heterochromatin, which is euchromatin that has been heterochromatinized, e.g., the genetically inactive X chromosome of the mammals (see *Barr body* and *Lyon hypothesis*).

Constitutive heterochromatin is naturally differentiated by darker staining areas during interphase and prophase of cell division. In metaphase, it usually appears as lightly stained or unstained regions of the chromosomes, with special methods needed to make constitutive heterochromatin visible in metaphase chromosome preparations. These methods for C banding usually involve treatment of chromosomes with acid, alkali, or elevated temperature before Giemsa staining. It is presumed that the cellular DNA is denatured by these treatments. An overnight incubation at 60°C in saline-citrate solution presumably renatures the DNA. Therefore, it is reasoned that the highly repetitive DNA sequences such as constitutive heterochromatin renature under these conditions, whereas low repetitive DNA and unique DNA sequences do not, resulting in differential staining reaction.

There is a considerable variation in the size of C bands in human chromosomes, which does not seem to affect the phenotype of the individual.

See also *karyotype.*

ERNEST H. Y. CHU, PH.D.

chromosome complement the normal set of chromosomes found in all somatic (diploid) cells of normal individuals of a given species. In humans, it consists of 46 chromosomes: 22 homologous pairs of autosomes and 2 sex chromosomes (two X chromosomes in females and one X and one Y chromosome in males). See also *karyotype.*

chromosome map a diagram that describes the sequence and distance of genetic traits on a chromosome. See also *linkage map.*

chromosome nomenclature the terminology established by the Denver (1960), Chicago (1966), and Paris (1971) Nomenclature Conferences for the description of karyotypes. At the time of the Denver Conference, the autosomes could not be unambiguously identified and were classified into seven groups identified by the letters A–G. The autosomes are now numbered 1–22 in order of decreasing size and are identified on the basis of the Paris Conference banding pattern ideogram.

A chromosome complement is indicated by giving the total number of chromosomes and the sex chromosome constitution; e.g., 46,XX (female) and 46,XY (male) are the normal chromosome complements. A + or – placed in front of an autosome number indicates the addition or loss of a whole chromosome; e.g., 47,XX, +21 indicates trisomy 21, as in Down's syndrome. A + or – sign placed after a structure indicates that it is larger or smaller than normal; e.g., 5p– indicates deletion of part of the short arm, as in cri du chat syndrome.

In general, an abnormality may be indicated by the symbol for the abnormality followed by the affected chromosome or chromosomes in parentheses, followed by the bands where the chromosome breakage occurred in a second parenthesis; e.g., t(2;6)(q34;p12) describes a translocation between chromosomes 2 and 6, with the breaks at band 4 of region 3 of the long arm of chromosome 2 and at band 2 of region 1 of the short arm of chromosome 6.

See also the accompanying table of chromosome nomenclature symbols.

chromotrope 2R a red acid dye used in some histologic procedures as a plasma and connective tissue stain; C.I. 16570.

chromotropic acid (CTA) 4,5-dihydroxy-2,7-naphthalenedisulfonic acid; M.W. 356.33. CTA is used as a reagent in several laboratory procedures such as methanol and triglyceride assays.

chromoxane cyanin R (kro-mok′sān) a mordant blue dye; C.I. 43820.

chromoxane pure blue B a mordant blue dye; C.I. 43830.

chromoxane pure blue BLD an acid mordant dye

CHROMOSOME NOMENCLATURE. NOMENCLATURE SYMBOLS RESULTING FROM THE CHICAGO (1966) AND PARIS (1972) CONFERENCES

SYMBOL	MEANING
Chicago Conference Recommendations	
A-G	Chromosome groups (Denver Conference)
1-22	Autosome numbers (Denver Conference)
X, Y	Sex chromosomes
diagonal (/)	Separates cell lines in mosaics
plus sign (+) or minus sign (–)	When placed immediately before the autosome number or group or letter designation, indicates the particular chromosome is extra or missing. When placed immediately after the arm or structural designation, indicates that the particular arm or structure is larger or smaller than normal.
question mark (?)	Questionable identification of chromosome or chromosome structure.
ace	acentric
cen	centromere
dic	dicentric
end	endoreduplication
h	secondary constriction or negative staining region
i	isochromosome
inv	inversion
inv (p+q–) or inv (p–q+)	pericentric inversion
mar	marker chromosome
mat	maternal origin
p	short arm of chromosome
pat	paternal origin
q	long arm of chromosome
r	ring chromosome
s	satellite
t	translocation
tri	tricentric
repeated symbols	duplication of chromosome structure
Paris (1972) Conference Additions	
del	deletion
der	derivative chromosome
dup	duplication
ins	insertion
inv ins	inverted insertion
rcp	reciprocal translocation
rec	recombinant chromosome
rob	Robertsonian translocation
ter	terminal or end
p ter	end of short arm
q ter	end of long arm
:	break (no reunion)
::	break and join
-	from—to

Modified from Raphael, S. S.: Lynch's Medical Laboratory Technology. 3rd ed. Philadelphia, W. B. Saunders Co., 1976, p. 1370.

used in histologic staining procedures, especially for beryllium; C.I. 43825.

chron/o (kron′o) [Gr. *chronos* time] a word element used in combining form to denote time, e.g., chronology.

chronaxy (kro′nak-se) [*chron-* + Gr. *axios* fit] the minimal duration of current flow at double the rheobase voltage necessary to stimulate a threshold muscle contraction. Chronaxy values are characteristic for different tissues and thus can be used to compare tissue excitabilities. In clinical electroneurography and electromyography (EMG), the measurement of chronaxy is used to establish the state of innervation of a muscle (the presence of denervation or reinnervation) or to confirm EMG findings.

chronic (kron′ik) [L. *chronicus,* from Gr. *chronos* time] persisting over a long period of time. For most diseases or conditions beginning with this adjective, see the noun. Cf. *acute.*

chronic granulomatous disease (CGD) a genetic disorder usually transmitted as an X-linked inherited trait (an autosomal recessive form also occurs). It is characterized by severe and repeated infections of the skin, lymph nodes, liver, lungs, and bones with catalase-positive organisms (such as staphylococci, *Klebsiella, Aerobacter, Escherichia coli, Pseudomonas, Aspergillus, Proteus, Serratia, Salmonella,* and *Candida*). Most parameters of host defense, such as lymphocyte function and delayed hypersensitivity, are normal. However, circulating phagocytes (i.e., polymorphonuclear leukocytes) and macrophages fail to generate hydrogen peroxide, which, together with halide ions and peroxidase, is necessary to destroy phagocytized bacteria. Catalase-negative microorganisms are killed normally; viruses are also handled normally. Failure to kill the catalase-positive organisms leads to chronic infections with granuloma and abscess formation.

Laboratory tests for this disorder include demonstration of catalase-positive microorganism survival after phagocytosis, normal killing of catalase-negative bacteria, and no increase in O_2 consumption, glucose oxidation, or halide fixation following phagocytosis. Further, nitroblue tetrazolium (NBT) is not reduced (colorless to deep blue) by the polymorphonuclear leukocytes and macrophages of affected individuals. The abnormal leukocyte function can also be detected by a sensitive chemiluminescence assay.

chronic obstructive pulmonary disease (COPD) a term applied to a group of overlapping disorders of lung function that share an element of irreversible expiratory airflow obstruction. The three entities most commonly included are emphysema, chronic bronchitis, and chronic asthma in adults.

Emphysema is a pathologic term that refers to the destruction of alveolar spaces, usually accompanied by the loss of the natural elastic recoil of the lung and weakening of the walls of bronchiolar airways. Chronic bronchitis is a clinical term that refers to the daily production of sputum for a continuous period of 3 mo during two successive years. Pathologically, this is manifested by hypertrophy of mucous glands in the bronchial wall and chronic bronchial inflammation. Emphysema and chronic bronchitis frequently coexist in varying degrees and are often considered together, as their individual clinical features are difficult to separate. On occasion, symptoms are episodic and somewhat reversible, suggesting an asthmatic component. However, pulmonary function may never return to normal, and this chronicity may make differentiation from COPD impossible.

Obstruction to airflow results from several factors. The caliber of larger airways may be diminished by mucous gland hypertrophy and the increased production of bronchial secretions. The removal of these secretions is hampered by impairment of normal clearance mechanisms such as ciliary activity and cough. The obstruction in smaller airways, caused by damage and fibrosis, is made worse by increases in intrathoracic pressure that occur during exhalation. The smaller airways are more susceptible to compression and collapse because of weakening of the intrinsic rigidity of their walls and loss of the normal elastic recoil of the lung, including elastic fibers that support the patency of these airways. If an asthmatic component is present, there may be smooth muscle hypertrophy in these airways during exacerbations, with further reduction of the internal diameter owing to spasm. In emphysema, loss of elastic recoil is a major cause of obstruction in all airways.

The single most important cause of COPD is smoking, which impairs the lungs' natural defenses against infection. There is clearly a differential susceptibility to COPD among smokers, but almost all chronic smokers demonstrate some impairment of pulmonary function. Other causes, which frequently coexist with tobacco exposure, include exposure to fumes and dust in the workplace. Relatively rare genetic conditions, such as alpha$_1$-antitrypsin deficiency and cystic fibrosis, are also associated with COPD.

The predominant symptom of COPD is dyspnea. Initially this may be experienced only with exertion, but with progression of the disease it becomes present at rest. Affected individuals are more prone to respiratory infections, including bronchitis and pneumonia. Episodic worsening of breathlessness and cough may also occur in the absence of overt infection.

The physical findings depend on the severity of the condition. The individual may demonstrate labored breathing, often with halting speech. There may be weight loss or cyanosis. The chest tends to be overexpanded, and breath sounds frequently are diminished. Rales and rhonchi may be present.

Diagnosis is based on the clinical presentation and results of spirometry, which show reduction in expiratory flow rates and volumes with normal or slightly increased total lung capacity and residual volume. The main complications of COPD are respiratory failure, overwhelming infections, and right-sided heart failure. When symptoms are present chronically at rest, the prognosis is usually poor.

STEPHAN D. FIHN, M.D., M.P.H.

chronotropic (kron″o-trop′ik) [*chrono-* + Gr. *tropikos* turning] affecting the time or rate, such as a drug that increases the heart rate.

chronotropism (kro-not′ro-pizm) having an effect on a periodic movement such as the heart rate.

CHR reaction [Ger. *Cercarienhullenreaktion*] a precipitin reaction that occurs when living cercariae of *Schistosoma mansoni* are placed in serum from an infected host. A translucent irregular envelope around each immobilized organism is seen under a light microscope.

Chrysomyia (kris″o-mi′yah) [Gr. *chrysos-* gold + *myia* fly] a genus of screwworm flies of the family Calliphoridae that occurs geographically in Africa, Australia, and parts of Asia. The species *C. bezziana,* widely distributed in Asia and Africa, may cause severe and disfiguring myiasis in humans. The adult fly is bluish-green with dark thoracic stripes and often carries pathogenic microorganisms on its external parts or in its digestive tract. When it lays its eggs on an open cut or mucous membrane of a mammal, the larvae can burrow into the wound, causing myiasis. Lesions produced in the sinuses as a result of bone erosion are particularly severe.

Chrysops (kris′ops) [Gr. *chrysos* gold + *ōps* eye] a genus of bloodsucking flies of the family Tabanidae; these flies have prominent eyes, a broad head, and large wings, each with a black band. Two species (mango flies) serve as intermediate host of the microfilaria *Loa loa,* and a third (the deerfly) transmits tularemia.

Chrysosporium (kris″o-spōr′ĭ-um) a genus of imperfect keratinophilic soil fungi related to the dermatophytes. Some species have been isolated in individuals with dermatophytosis.

chrysotile (kris′o-til) a fibrous, hydrated magnesium silicate, the most widely used form of asbestos. See also *asbestos.*

CHS abbrev. See *cholinesterase.*

Chvostek's sign (h-vos′teks) [Franz *Chvostek,* Austrian surgeon, 1835–1884] a spasm of the facial muscles seen in tetany, which is caused by tapping the muscles or the branches of the facial nerve. It may result from hypocalcemia or hypomagnesemia. Also called Chvostek-Weiss sign.

chyl/o (ki′lo) [L. *chylus* juice] a word element used in combining form to denote relationship to chyle, e.g., chylomicron.

chyle (kīl) [L. *chylus* juice] the milky fluid taken up by the lacteals (lymphatic ducts) from the intestine. Chyle consists of lymph and droplets of triglycerides (chylomicrons) in a stable emulsion. It passes into the vascular system via the thoracic duct, becoming mixed with the blood.

chylomicron (ki″lo-mi′kron) [*chylo-* + Gr. *mikros* small] a stable droplet of aggregated lipids and proteins, 0.1 to 0.5 μm in diameter. They consist mainly of triglycerides (80–95 percent) formed from food lipids, cholesterol (2–5 percent), phospholipids (3–6 percent), and protein (1–2 percent). They originate in the intestinal lymphatic vessels (lacteals) and are found in blood during and after meals, giving serum a milky appearance. Chylomicrons carry long-chain fats (triglycerides) and cholesterol from the intestine to adipose cells for storage and to working cells for catabolism. Observance of the presence or absence of chylomicrons in fasting serum is of assistance in the phenotyping of various hyperlipoproteinemias. A large increase in the number of chylomicrons in serum characterizes type I familial hyperlipoproteinemia caused by low or absent lipoprotein lipase activity. A lesser increase is found in types III and V hyperlipoproteinemia.

chylomicronemia (ki″lo-mi″kron-e′me-ah) [*chylo-* + Gr. *mikros* small + *haima* blood + *-ia*] an excess of chylomicrons in the blood.

chyloperitoneum (ki″lo-per″ĭ-to-ne′um) [*chylo-* + Gr. *peritonaion,* from *per* around + *teinein* to stretch] the presence of effused chyle in the peritoneal cavity.

chylopleura (ki″lo-ploo′rah) [*chylo-* + Gr. *pleura* rib, side] see *chylothorax.*

chylopneumothorax (ki″lo-nu″mo-tho′raks) [*chylo-* + Gr. *pneumōn* lung + *thōrax* chest] the presence of chyle and air in the pleural cavity.

chylothorax (ki″lo-tho′raks) [*chylo-* + Gr. *thōrax* chest] accumulation of lymph in the thoracic cavity as a result of damage to the thoracic duct.

chyluria (ki-lu′re-ah) [*chylo-* + Gr. *ouron* urine + *-ia*] the presence of chyle in the urine, giving it a milky appearance. Chyluria is produced by an obstruction of lymph flow and the rupture of lymphatic vessels into the renal tubules. Also called *galacturia.* Cf. *lipiduria.*

chyme (kīm) [Gr. *chymos* juice] the semifluid, homogeneous, creamy material that is produced in the stomach by the gastric digestion of food.

chymosin (ki′mo-sin) a proteolytic, milk-curdling enzyme of the hydrolase class (EC 3.4.23.4) that converts soluble casein K to paracasein, which forms a curd with calcium. It is found in the fourth stomach of the calf and other ruminants. Formerly called *rennin.*

chymotrypsin (ki″mo-trip′sin) an enzyme of the hydrolase class (EC 3.4.21.1) that catalyzes the cleavage of polypeptides to smaller peptide units. It is secreted by the pancreas in the form of chymotrypsinogen and is activated by the action of trypsin in the small intestine. It attacks preferentially peptide bonds located next to tyrosine, tryptophan, phenylalanine, or leucine residues. Decreased chymotrypsin activity in the stool may indicate pancreatic duct obstruction or cystic fibrosis.

C.I. abbrev. See *Colour Index.*

Ci abbrev. See *curie.*

Ciaccio's fluid (chah′chōz) [Carmelo *Ciaccio,* Palermo pathologist, 1877–1956] a histologic fixative whose composition varies somewhat, depending on its use. It usually contains potassium dichromate solution, formalin, small amounts of formic acid or acetic acid, and (possibly) mercuric chloride.

Ciaccio's method [Carmelo *Ciaccio*] a technique for demonstrating saturated and unsaturated phospholipids, or mixtures of cholesterol and cholesterol esters with oleic acid, in which fresh tissue is treated with formaldehyde and chromate prior to paraffin embedding. The lipid substances are rendered resistant to extraction and can be stained with Sudan dyes.

Ciaccio-positive lipids [Carmelo *Ciaccio*] lipids that stain with Ciaccio's method, i.e., those that remain after prolonged chromating and paraffin embedding and retain the capacity to stain with oil-soluble dyes.

Cib abbrev. for L. *cibus* (food).

cib/o (si′bo) [L. *cibus* food] a word element used in combining form to denote meals, e.g., cibophobia.

cicatrix (sik-a′triks, sik′ah-triks), pl. *cicatrices* [L.] a scar, the new fibrous tissue formed in the healing of a wound.

CICU abbrev. for cardiac intensive care unit, coronary intensive care unit.

Cicuta (sik′u-tah) a genus of umbelliferous plants, including the water hemlocks. The roots and stems of these plants contain cicutoxin, a resinous toxin that can cause death within minutes after ingestion.

cicutoxin (sik″u-tok′sin) a very poisonous, resinous, polyunsaturated alcohol produced in the roots and stems of the water hemlock (*Cicuta maculata* and *C. virosa*).

CID abbrev. See *cytomegalic inclusion disease.*

-cidal (si′dal) a suffix word element to denote killing capacity, e.g., bactericidal.

CIE abbrev. See *counterimmunoelectrophoresis.*

CIEP abbrev. See *counterimmunoelectrophoresis.*

CIF abbrev. for cloning inhibitory factor. See under *proliferation inhibitory factor.*

ciguatoxin (se″gwah-tok′sin) [sp. (orig. Taino) *cigua* a poisonous snail + L. *toxicum* poison, from Gr. *toxicos* of or for the bow] an ichthyosarcotoxin found in some marine fishes that consume plant material containing the toxin or a precursor. The toxin is an inhibitor of cholinesterase and consumption of toxic fish produces numbness, spasms, convulsions, paralysis, and, infrequently, death. Also called ciguatera toxin.

Ci-hr abbrev. See *curie-hour.*

ciliary (sil′e-er″e) [L. *ciliaris,* from *cilium* eyelash] pertaining to cilia or the eyelashes and to certain structures of the eye.

ciliary body the thickened region of the uvea connecting the iris and the ora serrata, concerned with suspension of the lens and accommodation. It encompasses the ciliary muscle, the ciliary processes, and the ciliary ring.

ciliary muscle a ring of smooth muscle that lies deep to the anterior part of the sclera of the eye, made up of radial and circular fibers. The radial fibers arise from the corneoscleral junction and pectinate ligament, and radiate posteriorly and inward to the ciliary processes and choroid. The ring of circular fibers lies internal to the radial fibers at the periphery of the iris. The ciliary muscle allows the lens to become more convex as the eye accommodates for near vision.

Ciliata (sil″e-a′tah) a class of protozoa characterized by the presence of cilia throughout their life cycle. The cells usually have a macronucleus and one or more micronuclei. The only species of medical importance is *Balantidium coli.*

ciliocytophthoria (CCP) (sil″e-o-si″tof-tho′re-ah) the nonspecific destruction of the ciliated bronchial cells of the respiratory tract. The distal ciliated portion of the cell pinches off, resulting in the formation of anucleated ciliated tufts and nucleated cytoplasmic pieces. This occurs in inflammatory conditions of the lungs, particularly viral infections, as well as in bacterial infections; it may also arise in the female genital tract where the source of the ciliated cells may be the cervix, endometrium, or fallopian tube.

cilium (sil′e-um), pl. *cilia* [L.] a motile, hairlike projection on the free surface of many animal cells. It is larger than a microvillus and has a more complex internal structure. Most cilia are approximately 0.2 μm in diameter and 5–10 μm long. The so-called stereocilia on cells of the epididymis and inner ear do not contain microtubules and are unusually long microvilli. A cilium has an internal structure (axoneme) consisting of nine peripheral microtubule doublets and two central microtubules. The peripheral microtubules terminate at the base of the cilium in the basal body, which is similar in structure to a centriole. Cilia are well developed on the surface of many of the epithelial cells of the respiratory tract and uterine tube, and they beat in waves (metachronal rhythm). Cilia are also characteristic of the ciliate class of Protozoa, where they serve as an organ of locomotion.

cimetidine (si-met′ĭ-dēn) a drug used in the treatment of peptic ulcer. It acts by blocking the stimulation of histamine H_2-receptors of the parietal cells. Trademark *Tagamet.*

Cimex (si′meks) [L. "bug"] a genus of insects in the family Cimicidae, commonly known as bedbugs. They lack true wings and have an ovate, flattened body and four-jointed antennae. Although two species are known to invade human dwellings, it has not been proved that bedbugs disseminate disease, with the doubtful exception of relapsing fever. Their bite, during which they ingest blood, may produce edema and inflammation in sensitive victims.

CIN abbrev. See *cervical intraepithelial neoplasia.*

cinchonidine sulfate (sin-ko′nĭ-dēn) the salt of an alkaloid similar to quinine. It is extracted from cinchona bark and has been used to treat malaria. Cinchonidine is a stereoisomer of cinchonine.

cinchonine sulfate (sin′ko-nin) the salt of an alkaloid similar to quinine. It is extracted from cinchona bark and has been used to treat malaria. It is a stereoisomer of cinchonidine.

cinchophen (sin′ko-fen) a synthetic quinoline 2-phenylcinchoninic acid, chemically related to quinine; formerly used as an analgesic.

cine/o (sin′e-o) [Gr. *kinēsis* movement] a word element used in combining form to denote movement, e.g., cineradiography.

cineangiocardiography (sin″e-an″je-o-kar″de-og′rah-fe) [*cine-* + Gr. *angeion* vessel + *kardia* heart + *graphein* to record] the visualization of injected medium flowing through the heart by means of cineangiography.

cineangiography (sin″e-an″je-og′rah-fe) [*cine-* + Gr. *angeion* vessel + *graphein* to record] the photographic recording of fluoroscopic images of the blood vessels by motion picture techniques.

cinebronchography (sin″ĕ-brong-kog′rah-fe) [*cine-* + Gr. *bronchos* windpipe + *graphein* to record] the making of a motion picture record of successive radiographic images during bronchography. This technique can be used to study functional changes in bronchial caliber. See also *bronchography.*

cinefluorography (sin″ĕ-floo″or-og′rah-fe) [*cine-* + N.L. *fluor* a mineral + Gr. *graphein* to record] see *cineradiography.*

cinemicrography (sin″ĕ-mi-krog′rah-fe) [*cine-* + Gr. *mikros* small + *graphein* to record] the making of motion pictures of a small object through the lens system of a microscope.

cinephlebography (sin″ĕ-flĕ-bog′rah-fe) [*cine-* + Gr. *phlebos* vein + *graphein* to record] cineradiography of the veins after administration of a contrast medium, which, with the technique of ascending functional cinephlebography, is introduced into a vein in a foot. Its progress is then observed as it courses through the tibial, popliteal, and iliac veins.

cineradiography (sin″ĕ-ra″de-og′rah-fe) [*cine-* + L. *radius* ray + Gr. *graphein* to record] the making of a motion picture record of successive radiographic images, employing an image amplifier and a specifically mounted camera. It is used to study functional movement in angiocardiography, coronary arteriography, and for esophageal and urinary tract examination.

cinerins (sin′ĕ-rinz) see under *pyrethrins.*

cingulate gyrus (sin′gu-lāt) [L. *cingulum* girdle] a long, curved bundle of fibers occupying the medial surface of each cerebral hemisphere superior to the corpus callosum. It is thought to be a sensorimotor association area of the limbic system.

cingulum (sin′gu-lum), pl. *cingula* [L. "girdle"] a long, curved bundle of association fibers within the gyrus cinguli of a cerebral hemisphere. Fibers entering and leaving it confer a spiked appearance, which may be seen when it is dissected.

C.I. number abbrev. See under *Colour Index.*

circadian (ser″kah-de′an) [L. *circa* about + *dies* day] referring to a period of 24 hr.

circadian rhythm the rhythmic repetition of certain activities or processes in living organisms at about the same time each day.

circinate (ser′sĭ-nāt) [L. *circinatus,* from *circinare* to make round] circular, shaped like a ring.

circle (ser′k′l) [L. *circulus*] a round figure, structure, or part.

circle of confusion the blurred image of a point source produced by an optical system, used as a measure of image sharpness or definition.

circle of Willis [Thomas *Willis,* English anatomist and physician, 1621–1675] a polygonal anastomosis between the two internal carotid and the two vertebral arteries that interconnects with the anterior and posterior cerebral arteries and the anterior and posterior communicating arteries; it provides the arterial blood supply to the brain.

circuit (ser′kit) [L. *circuitus,* from *circumire* to go around] 1. a path or interconnecting array of paths for electric current, or wiring and components that make up a functional unit.

2. in electric circuit theory, a closed path. The algebraic sum of the voltage drops around a circuit must be zero. See also *Kirchoff's laws.*

open c., a circuit in which the path has been broken, such as by an open switch or by a defective component, so that no current can flow.

short c., an unintentional, low-resistance connection between two points of a circuit. A short circuit between the output terminals of a power source will overload it and cause a fuse to blow or a circuit breaker to trip.

circuit breaker a resettable electromagnetic device used to protect an electric circuit against current overloads. Like a fuse, it opens the circuit (trips) when the current rating is exceeded.

circuitry (ser′kĭ-tre) the collection of electric circuits in a device.

circulating anticoagulants (ser′ku-lāt″ing) see *coagulation factor inhibitors.*

circulation (ser″ku-la′shun) [L. *circulatio*] movement in a regular or circuitous course that returns to the point of origin, such as the movement of blood through the heart and blood vessels.

circulation time the time it takes for blood to flow between two designated points in the circulatory system. The arm-to-tongue circulation time is measured clinically by injection of a bile salt preparation (Decholin) into the antecubital vein; the end point occurs at the first sensation of a bitter taste. Circulation time decreases with increasing blood velocity but varies directly with the circulating blood volume; thus, it tends to be increased above the normal value of 9–16 sec when cardiac output is reduced or when systemic or pulmonary venous congestion is present.

circulatory (ser′ku-lah-to″re) pertaining to the circulation.

circulatory overload hypervolemia subsequent to overtransfusion or overinfusion of intravenous fluids. A rapid increase in blood volume may result in congestive heart failure with coughing, dyspnea, and cyanosis, and may cause a rapid rise in systolic blood pressure.

circulatory system the heart, blood vessels, and lymph vessels considered as a whole. Blood is pumped from the right side of the heart through the pulmonary arteries to the lungs, where it is oxygenated and returned through the pulmonary veins to the left side of the heart. From there the blood is pumped through the systemic arteries to the tissue capillary beds, where it releases oxygen to and takes up carbon dioxide from the tissues, and also provides them with nutrients and removes wastes. The blood returns to the right side of the heart through the systemic veins. Some of the fluid leaves the cardiovascular system in the capillary beds and is returned via the lymphatic system.

circumflex (ser′kum-fleks) [L. *circumflexus* bent about] curved like a bow.

circumscribed (ser′kum-skrībd) [L. *circum* around + *scribere* to write] bounded or limited; confined within a certain space.

circumvallate (ser″kum-val′āt) [L. *circum* around + *vallare* to wall] surrounded by a trench; the term is used to refer to one type of papilla found on the tongue.

cirrhosis (sir-ro′sis) [Gr. *kirrhos* orange yellow + *-osis*] a disease affecting the entire liver in which the normal hepatic architecture is permanently destroyed, frequently to the extent that preexisting portal tracts and central veins cannot be identified. Morphologically, cirrhosis is characterized by expanding parenchymal nodules separated by encircling bands of fibrous tissue. The parenchymal nodules are usually yellowish-tan, hence the name. The term cirrhosis is reserved for livers affected by both nodular regeneration of hepatocytes and fibrosis. The major clinical effects of cirrhosis include portal vein hypertension and disturbances of hepatocyte function. Cirrhosis may be active or inactive, depending on the degree of ongoing liver cell injury and necrosis, as judged by clinical, laboratory, and histologic parameters.

Cirrhosis is an end stage for a number of different destructive processes affecting the liver. The established causes of cirrhosis are listed in the table below. Unproved causes include autoimmune disease, certain toxins, parasitic disease, and malnutrition. Chronic recurring injury to the liver appears to be a necessary precondition for cirrhosis to develop. The key factor predisposing to cirrhosis appears to be the destruction of hepatic architecture and loss of the normal relationships between portal tracts, hepatocytes, and central veins. Chronic recurring and ongoing injury, e.g., chronic alcoholism, can usually be demonstrated in well-documented cases.

ESTABLISHED CAUSES OF CIRRHOSIS

- Alcoholism
- Biliary disease
  - Primary biliary cirrhosis
  - Secondary biliary cirrhosis
- Drugs and toxins
- Intestinal bypass
- Metabolic disease
  - Aketolipoproteinemia
  - α_1-Antitrypsin deficiency
  - Cystic fibrosis
  - Glycogen storage disease (types III and IV)
  - Hemochromatosis
  - Hereditary fructose intolerance
  - Wilson's disease
- Venous outflow obstruction
  - Budd-Chiari syndrome
  - Venoocclusive disease
- Viral hepatitis
- Other
  - Hereditary hemorrhagic telangiectasia
  - Idiopathic
  - Sarcoidosis

Cirrhosis cannot be classified according to its etiology because there are many cases with no identifiable cause, and therefore a simple morphologic system of classification is generally used. In macronodular cirrhosis, the nodules are generally larger than 0.3 cm in diameter, whereas in micronodular cirrhosis they are usually smaller than 0.3 cm; mixed macro- and micronodular forms of cirrhosis occur. Alcoholic cirrhosis is generally associated with a micronodular pattern, whereas cirrhosis caused by chronic hepatitis B infection is usually macronodular. There are many exceptions, however, and for any case the cause of the cirrhosis cannot be identified solely on the basis of the nodule size. Some individuals with cirrhosis are asymptomatic and die of unrelated causes; most have an inactive cirrhosis with little or no ongoing hepatic necrosis. When the etiology of the cirrhosis is unknown and no overt evidence of liver disease preceded its development, the term cryptogenic cirrhosis has been applied. Some etiologies are associated with specific hepatocellular changes, such as intracellular globules found in alpha$_1$-antitrypsin deficiency and the aldehyde-fuchsin positive ground-glass hepatocytes in chronic hepatitis B infections. In many individuals, a combination of clinical history, specific biochemical markers, and morphology is needed before an etiology for the cirrhosis can be confidently assigned.

The clinical effects of cirrhosis can be divided into the categories of functional disturbances of the hepatocytes and hemodynamic alterations. In the latter, progressive scarring and regenerative nodules combine to compress and occlude portal and hepatic veins, and arteriovenous communications develop between the hepatic arterial system and both the portal and hepatic veins. As a consequence of these alterations in the hepatic vasculature, some of the portal venous blood bypasses the hepatic cells, elevating the portal vein pressure and resulting in portal hypertension. This leads to dilation of the collateral vessels between the portal vein and the systemic venous system. The most significant site at which this occurs is between the short gastric and esophageal veins. The resulting markedly dilated esophageal veins (esophageal varices) are prone to rupture and may result in massive, often fatal, gastrointestinal hemorrhage; rupture of esophageal varices is a significant cause of death in cirrhotic individuals.

Abnormal hepatic cell function is mainly caused by marginally adequate perfusion of blood secondary to the above-described vascular alterations, although in some instances the ongoing insult that initially caused the cirrhosis also contributes to the abnormal function. Hepatic failure may occur if the residual liver cells can no longer maintain adequate function. Decreased hepatic cell function is also associated with decreases in certain serum proteins, notably albumin and clotting factors; the decreased serum albumin contributes to the ascites commonly seen in cirrhotics, and decreased clotting factors can result in hemorrhagic states, which may complicate bleeding esophageal varices.

A constellation of altered central nervous system functions, termed hepatic encephalopathy (see under *encephalopathy*), is often observed in persons in the late stages of cirrhosis. It is associated with increased serum ammonia, which is probably due both to shunting of amines from the intestine past the liver and to the decreased ability of the cells to metabolize it.

The presence of cirrhosis per se is a major risk factor in the development of hepatocellular carcinoma. The association occurs regardless of the etiology of the cirrhosis, although persons with macronodular cirrhosis are thought to be at slightly greater risk than those with micronodular cirrhosis.

For more information, see the specific cirrhosis.

THOMAS V. COLBY, M.D.

cirrus (sir'rus), p. *cirri* [L. "curl"] a slender, usually flexible, appendage, such as one of the stiff, spikelike organs of locomotion of ciliate protozoa. The term refers to fused protozoa cilia from several rows or to the muscular retractile copulatory organ or certain trematodes.

cis- (sis) [L. "on the same side"] a prefix word element in organic chemistry to denote a chemical compound in which the two substituent groups referred to are on the same side of a line passing through a double bond or of a plane passing through a ring, e.g., *cis*-2-butene. See also *isomerism.* Cf. *trans-*.

cis configuration the location of two alleles on the same chromosome of a homologous pair. Cf. *trans configuration.*

cisplatin (sis'plah-tin) a cancer chemotherapeutic drug; trademark, Platino. For more information, see *Appendix A.*

cistern (sis'tern) [L. *cisterna* reservoir] a closed space serving as a reservoir for lymph or other body fluid, especially one of the enlarged subarachnoid spaces containing cerebrospinal fluid. The term is also used to refer to the flattened sacs enclosed by the endoplasmic reticulum of cells.

great c., see *cerebellomedullary cistern.*

cisterna (sis-ter'nah) [L.] see *cistern.*

cisternal puncture (sis-ter'nal) the insertion of a hollow needle into the cisterna magna of the subarachnoid space to withdraw cerebrospinal fluid or to inject a radiographic contrast medium, as in pneumoencephalography or myelography. Cf. *lumbar puncture.*

cisternography (sis″ter-nog′rah-fe) an imaging study of the spaces (cisterns) of the brain that are filled with cerebrospinal fluid. The CSF is labeled with a radionuclide or with an x-ray contrast medium. Cf. *cerebral p.* under *pneumography.*

radionuclide c., cisternography that uses a radiopharmaceutical injected into the CSF by lumbar puncture. Sagittal and lateral views are taken at 4, 24, and 48 hr. This procedure is useful in the evaluation of hydrocephalus and the detection of CSF leaks. The preferred radiopharmaceutical is ^{111}In-DTPA (In 111 pentetate), which has a half-life long enough to accommodate the 48-hr study. Alternatives are ^{99m}Tc-DTPA (which has a short half-life) and ^{169}Yb-DTPA (which subjects the patient to a high radiation dose). In the past, ^{131}I-HSA (human serum albumin) was frequently used for this procedure.

cis-trans test [L. *cis* on this side + *trans* on the other side] a genetic complementation test used to determine whether two mutations are both on the same functional unit. If two mutations are in different coding sequences, normal function is observed when they are combined, as one wild-type copy of the information is present. If both mutations are in the same coding unit, however, normal function is impeded as long as the two mutations remain in separate cistrons (trans). If the wild-type sequences cross over into one cistron (cis), normal function results.

cistron (sis′tron) [L. *cis* + *trans* + *-on* particle, quantum] the smallest unit of genetic material that must be intact to function as a transmitter of genetic information, i.e., to determine the sequence of amino acids of one polypeptide chain. The cistron is defined by the cis-trans test. The gene as traditionally conceived is identical to the cistron. Cf. *muton* and *recon.*

citrate (sit′rāt) any salt or anionic form of citric acid; it occurs naturally in large quantities in citrus fruits.

citrate agar gel electrophoresis a method used to separate hemoglobin F (Hb F) from Hb A, Hb S from Hb D and Hb G, and Hb C from Hb E and Hb O. Electrophoresis of a hemolysate is performed at pH 6.25 on citrate agar gel. This is in contrast to paper and ordinary agar gel electrophoresis, which are performed at pH 8.6 where these combinations coincide: Hb F and Hb A; Hb S, Hb D, and Hb G; and Hb C, Hb E and Hb O.

citrate-phosphate-dextrose (CPD) anticoagulant-citrate-phosphate-dextrose [USP], the most commonly used citrate anticoagulant for the collection and preservation of whole blood in the liquid state. A modified acid citrate dextrose (ACD) solution, 1 l of CPD contains 3.27 g of citric acid, 26.3 g of sodium citrate, 25.5 g of glucose, and 2.22 g of $NaH_2PO_4 \cdot H_2O$.

For blood transfusion, 450 ml of whole blood is collected into a sterile plastic bag containing 63 ml of CPD solution; the red cells can be stored for up to 21 da. CPD maintains a higher pH and level of 2,3-DPG throughout the storage period than does ACD. Adenine (CPDA-1) can be added to a modified CPD solution to improve the maintenance of ATP levels in blood and prolong the storage life of erythrocytes from 21 da to 35 da.

citrate-phosphate-dextrose-adenine (CPDA-1) a recently approved anticoagulant preservative consisting of the most commonly used anticoagulant, citrate-phosphate-dextrose (CPD) with adenine added. Whole blood stored in this preservative has an extended shelf-life, up to 35 da, because the adenine allows the red blood cells to synthesize adenosine triphosphate (ATP) during storage. See also *citrate-phosphate-dextrose.*

citrate test in microbiology, the ability of an organism to grow on a medium, using citrate as its sole carbon source. In a positive reaction, the metabolic products formed from citrate cause a rise in pH of the medium, which turns the bromthymol blue indicator from green to blue. It is used for differentiation of organisms of the *Enterobacter* group. See also *IMViC tests.*

citric acid (sit′rik) 2-hydroxy-1,2,3-propanetricarboxylic acid, $CH_2(COOH)C(OH)(COOH)CH_2COOH$, a tribasic crystalline acid from citrus fruits and other plant and animal sources, or produced by the fermentation of sugars; M.W. 192.12. In animals, it is a component of the citric acid cycle that produces ATP by oxidative phosphorylation. Citric acid is used as an acidulant in beverages, confectionery, and effervescent powders and tablets; as a flavoring agent; and to adjust the pH of foods. Its potassium salt (potassium citrate) is used in potassium deficiencies and as a systemic alkalizer, sudorific, diuretic, and expectorant. Its use as an anticoagulant for clinical laboratory test specimens has been discontinued because of the large water shifts that it produces. Citrate is used in various buffers in the clinical laboratory.

Citrate has been measured by a variety of techniques in both plasma and urine because of its role in intermediary carbohydrate metabolism, but more often to assess toxicity from infusion of a large quantity of citrated blood.

citric acid assays 1. methods based on the reaction of citric acid with an oxidizing agent (permanganate, manganese dioxide, or vanadic acid) and bromine to produce pentabromoacetone, which, after isolation, can be determined by titration of bromine by various colorimetric methods (such as reaction with iodine, forming a yellow iodine complex), or radiometrically, using bromine-82.

2. enzymatic methods. Citric acid is oxidized by citrate dehydrogenase using methylene blue as hydrogen acceptor. Decolorization of the dye is measured and serves as an index of citric acid concentration. Another enzymatic method uses citrate lyase, resulting in the formation of acetate and oxalacetate. The latter is reduced by NADH in the presence of malate dehydrogenase. The decrease in absorbance due to the oxidation of NADH is a measure of citrate concentration.

citric acid cycle see *tricarboxylic acid cycle.*

Citrobacter (sit″ro-bak′ter) [L. *citrus* lemon + Gr. *baktērion* little rod] a genus of gram-negative, facultatively anaerobic, rod-shaped bacteria of the family Enterobacteriaceae. The organisms are motile and can use citrate as a sole carbon source. They ferment lactose, produce gas and H_2S on triple sugar iron agar, and produce β-galactosidase, but they lack lysine decarboxylase. The organisms may occur harmlessly in normal feces but have also been associated with diarrhea and secondary infections in debilitated individuals. Occasionally, severe primary septic infections occur. See also *Enterobacteriaceae.*

C. diversus, a species that ferments adonitol and is inhibited by potassium cyanide.

C. freundii, a species that does not ferment adonitol and is not inhibited by potassium cyanide.

citrovorum factor (sit-ro′vo-rum) see *folinic acid.*

citrulline (sit-rul′lēn) 2-amino-5-ureidopentanoic acid, $H_2NCONH(CH_2)_3CH(NH_2)COOH$, an amino acid first isolated from watermelon juice. It is an intermediate in the synthesis of arginine and urea in the liver, but ordinarily does not occur naturally in proteins.

citrullinemia (sit-rul″ĭ-ne′me-ah) [*citrulline* + Gr. *haima* blood + *-ia*] the presence of large amounts of citrulline in the blood, usually accompanied by citrulline in the cerebrospinal fluid and urine. It is most commonly due to a deficiency of the enzyme argininosuccinate synthetase. See also *aminoacidopathy* and *argininosuccinate synthetase deficiency.*

citrullinuria (sit-rul″ĭ-nu′re-ah) [*citrulline* + Gr. *ouron* urine + *-ia*] the presence of large amounts of citrulline in the urine, usually accompanied by citrulline in the blood and cerebrospinal fluid. It is most commonly due to a deficiency of the enzyme argininosuccinate synthetase. See also *aminoacidopathy* and *argininosuccinate synthetase deficiency.*

Civatte body (siv-at′) [Achille *Civatte,* French dermatologist, 1877–1956] see *colloid body.*

CK abbrev. See *creatine kinase.*

CK_1, CK_2, CK_3 abbrev. for the isoenzymes of creatine kinase. See under *creatine kinase.*

Cl symbol for the chemical element *chlorine.*

cl abbrev. See *centiliter.*

CLA abbrev. for certified laboratory assistant.

Cladosporium (klad″o-spo′re-um) a genus of imperfect fungi of which the species *C. carrionii* is an agent of chromomycosis and *C. bantianum* (*C. trichoides*) is the most common cause of phaeohyphomycosis of the brain.

Cladothrix (klad′o-thriks) [Gr. *klados* branch + *thrix* hair] the former name for a genus of sheathed bacteria now classified as *Sphaerotilus.*

Clara cell (klah′rah) [M. *Clara,* Austrian histologist, 20th century] one of the nonciliated epithelial cells that protrude into the lumen of the terminal and preterminal bronchioles. It secretes the protein component (hypophase) of pulmonary surfactant. See also *bronchiolar carcinoma.*

Clara's hematoxylin (klah′rahz) [M. *Clara*] a dilute hematoxylin stain used in a number of histologic procedures. It may be used to demonstrate keratin and keratohyalin, as well as enterochromaffin cells and eosinophils. This stain is susceptible to blockade reactions and also reacts with iron.

clarificant (klar-if′ĭ-kant) an agent that clears liquids of turbidity by removing or aiding in the removal of suspended matter. Also called clarifying agent.

clarify (klar′ĭ-fi) [L. *clarificare* to render clear] to clear of turbidity or of suspended matter.

Clarke's fluid (klarks) a fixative solution of methanol and glacial acetic acid. Also called Carnoy A.

Clarke-Hadfield syndrome (klark had′fēld) [Cecil *Clarke,* English physician, 20th century; Geoffrey *Hadfield,* English pathologist, born 1889] congenital pancreatic infantilism characterized by hepatomegaly, bulky stools, and extensive atrophy of the pancreas; it occurs in undersized and underweight children.

Clark oxygen electrode [Leland C. *Clark,* Jr., U.S. biochemist, born 1918] see *Clark oxygen e.* under *electrode.*

Clark rule [Cecil Henry Douglas *Clark,* English chemist, 20th century] a rule under which a drug dose for a child is obtained by multiplying the adult dose by the child's weight in pounds and dividing the result by 150.

Clark test a gynecologic procedure performed in the diagnostic evaluation of postmenopausal vaginal bleeding. A sound is passed into the uterus, and if an endometrial or cervical neoplasm is present, bleeding from the vagina will occur.

clasmatosis (klaz″mah-to′sis) [Gr. *klasma* a piece broken off + *-osis* condition] the breaking off of parts of a cell.

class (klas) 1. a term used in the taxonomic classification of organisms; it is a subdivision of phylum and is in turn divided into orders.

2. in statistics, a group of data, all of which have one particular value or a set of values falling between certain limits (the class limits).

classical complement pathway a biochemical pathway that involves activation of the serum complement components C1, C4, C2, C3, and C5 through C9, in that order. The initiation of activation involves the binding of C1q, the hexavalent portion of C1 that is rich in carbohydrate, glycine, and hydroxylysine, to the Fc portion of an immunoglobulin. The immunoglobulins involved must be bound to antigen and must have a site to fix complement. The complement-fixing antibodies are IgM, IgG1, and IgG3 (IgG2 weakly binds complement).

The accompanying illustration shows the initial sequence of activation in which C1q on binding to an antibody activates the C1r portion of C1, causing C1r to cleave C1s and generate an esterase. This esterase then cleaves C4 into two fragments, C4a and C4b. C4b binds to the activated cell surface and promotes immune adherence. C2 is also cleaved by C1s into two fragments, C2a and C2b. In the presence of Mg^{2+}, C2a is absorbed onto C4b and forms the C3 convertase C4b2a. C4b2a cleaves C3 into C3a (a fluid-phase anaphylatoxin) and C3b (the large-molecular-weight fragment that binds to C4b2a to form the C5 convertase C4b2a3b). The C3b generated on C3 cleavage by C4b2a is important in opsonization, and may be involved as an opsonin on a cell surface even if it does not interact further with the C4b2a complex. It also may be important as a source of C3b for utilization in alternative pathway activation. The C5 convertase C4b2a3b cleaves C5 into C5a and C5b. C5a is an anaphylatoxin with very strong chemoattractant activity for polymorphonuclear leukocytes. C5b is rapidly inactivated if it does not interact with C6. The bimolecular complex of C5b and C6 interacts with C7 to form a trimolecular complex capable of binding to a cell surface. With the addition of C8 and C9, the membrane attack complex is completed. The actual membrane attack complex consists of a dimer of C5b-C9. With the completed complex, lysis occurs.

There are a number of regulatory proteins in-

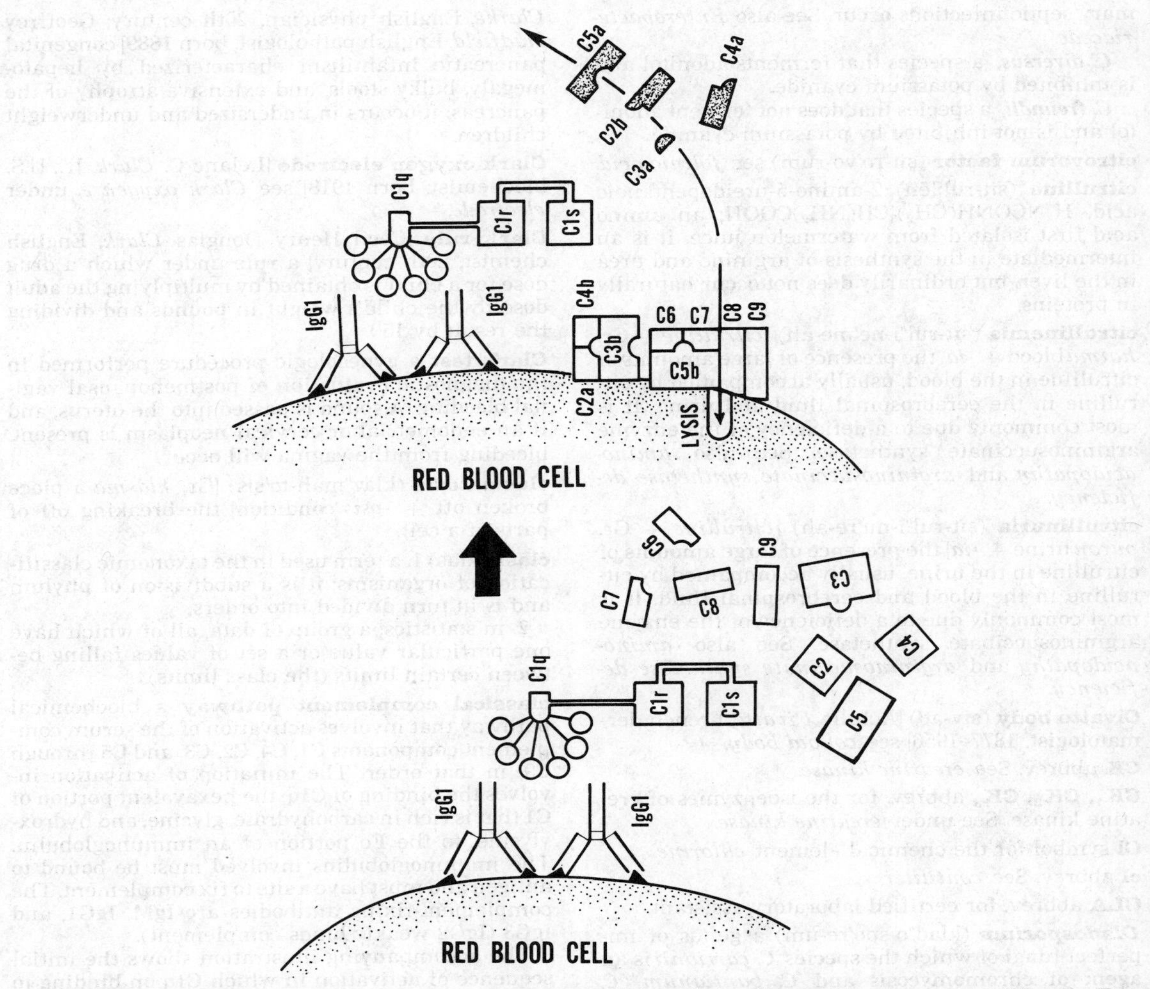

Classical complement pathway. Schematic representation of the classical complement pathway. Two molecules of IgG, termed a "doublet," combine with homologous antigenic determinants on a red blood cell surface and activate the first complement component by interacting with C1q. This is followed by C1r and C1s activation. The reaction sequence of the classical complement pathway is C1,4,2,3,5,6,7,8,9. This biochemical pathway leads to the formation of a "hole" in the cell membrane, leading to cell swelling and lysis. Although C9 is not essential for lysis, it accelerates the lytic reaction. This in contrast to the alternative, or properdin, pathway, which provides a mechanism to mediate the bactericidal and opsonic effects of complement without requiring specific antibody. Both pathways follow a similar course from the C3 step forward. (From Dorland's Illustrated Medical Dictionary. 26th ed. Philadelphia, W. B. Saunders Co., 1981.)

volved at various points in the sequence. C1q inhibitor inhibits binding of C1q to the Fc fragment of immunoglobulin. C1 inhibitor inhibits the activated C1r or C1s esterases. Its absence is associated with increased production of C2 kinin, a fragment cleaved from activated C2 by plasmin. C2 kinin is trypsin-labile but builds up in individuals with C1 inhibitor deficiency or hereditary angioneurotic edema (HANE). The next inhibitor of consequence is C3b inactivator, an endopeptidase that cleaves C3b into C3d and C3ca, a precursor of C3e. C3e mobilizes polymorphonuclear leukocytes from the bone marrow. A fluid-phase regulator of the anaphylatoxins C5a and C3a is carboxypeptidase B, a zinc-containing enzyme that cleaves arginine residues from the C terminus of these compounds. There are three inhibitors of the membrane attack complex (MAC) C5b-C9: antithrombin III, MAC inhibitor, and lipoprotein. It is believed that these inhibitor substances resemble the surfaces of membranes and that they inhibit binding to a cell surface.

Deficiencies of the classical components have been described and can be grouped. Deficiencies of C2 and C4 have been associated with an increase in lupus-like syndromes. C3, C3bINA, and C5 deficiencies have been associated with recurrent infection by bacteria. Opsonization is a problem with C3 and C3bINA deficiency, and activation of complement with generation of chemoattractants is a problem with C5 deficiency. C6 through C8 deficiencies have been associated with recurrent *Neisseria* infections, both gonococcal and meningitides. It is not entirely clear why *Neisseria* species seem to cause so much trouble for these patients, but the association would indicate that bacterial lysis and inactivation is not complete without the late-acting components.

Assays for the classical complement components are hemolytic (activity) assays or immunochemical assays. Hemolytic assays involve the activation of sheep red blood cells (RBC) with antisheep RBC antibody followed by the addition of excess amounts of the complement components other than the one to be detected. The component to be assayed is added at the appropriate time in the activation sequence. Standards and unknowns are added and the amount of lysis used as a measure of the component activity. Radial immunodiffusion using antibodies against the appropriate component to be studied can also be used to measure many of the individual components.

See also *alternative complement pathway* and *complement.*

GERALD B. KOLSKI, M.D., PH.D.

classification (klas″ĭ-fĭ-ka′shun) the systematic division of entities into related groups having similar characteristics. The branch of biology concerned with the classification of all living organisms is called taxonomy. The system of classification is a hierarchic one, originated by Linnaeus in 1758, which has six levels of classification: phylum, class, order, family, genus, and species. At each level, one or more of these taxonomic groups (taxa) are collected to form a single taxon at the level above.

The lowest level is the species, which is generally the finest division that is feasible. In higher organisms, a species constitutes a single interbreeding population. In bacteria, a species is often a group of distinct biotypes or subspecies; each of these is composed of strains with very similar phenotypic traits. All the members of a species, however, possess one or more stable and fundamental characteristics not present in other closely related species.

The discoveries of microbial genetics have had a major impact on the taxonomy of microorganisms, particularly of bacteria. Comparisons of the base composition of their DNA revealed wide variation in the amounts of guanine and cytosine (G + C) present (the G + C composition, or ratio, ranges from 30 to 70 moles percent). When a species with phenotypic properties very similar to those of the others in that genus is found to have a very dissimilar G + C composition, the species is removed from the genus. This happened to the former *Lactobacillus bifidus,* which was taken out of the lactic acid bacteria group and renamed *Propionibacterium bifidus.*

No organism is named by its species alone; every species must be assigned to a genus, and an organism is designated by giving both its generic and species names. This practice is termed the binomial system of nomenclature. These names are Latin or latinized forms of other words and are always italicized with the generic name capitalized, e.g., *Escherichia coli.* When the context makes clear which genus is being referred to, the initial of the generic name is used, e.g., *E. coli.*

Classification is intended to reflect the phylogeny of organisms. Each taxon should be a monophyletic grouping. Organisms are assigned to different taxa when new findings clearly show the lines of evolutionary descent. The species name is not changed when a species is assigned to a new genus.

In some taxa, additional levels of classification are used. The level tribe may be inserted between genus and family. The prefix sub- denotes a level immediately below, e.g., suborder below order; super- denotes a level immediately above, e.g., superorder. See the accompanying table for suffixes used to indicate the levels of taxa.

Organisms were originally divided into two kingdoms: plants (Plantae) and animals (Animalia). As the study of microorganisms progressed, protozoa were placed in the animal kingdom, whereas fungi and bacteria were classified as plants. Because of the myriad of inconsistencies that appeared, Haeckel proposed in 1866 a third kingdom, Protista, although this was not adopted for many years. The protists, which include algae as well as fungi, protozoa, and bacteria, have in common the characteristic of a simpler organization than that of higher organisms. They are essentially unicellular, for multicellular protists show very little differentiation. A recent proposal would divide living organisms into a total of five kingdoms, adding prokary-

CLASSIFICATION. SUFFIXES USED IN BIOLOGIC NOMENCLATURE

TAXON	ANIMALIA	PLANTAE	FUNGI
Phylum (Division)	-a	-phyta	
Subphylum (Subdivision)	-a	-phytina	-mycotina
Class	-ea	-phyceae	-mycetes
Subclass	-ia	-phycidae	-mycetidae
Superorder	-eda		
Order	-ida	-ales	-ales
Suborder	-ina	-ineae	-ineae
Superfamily	-edae		
Family	-idae	-aceae	-aceae
Subfamily	-inae	-oideae	-oideae
Tribe	-ini	-eae	-eae
Subtribe		-ineae	-ineae

Note: No standard suffixes are used for genera and species.

otes (Prokaryotae or Monera), fungi (Fungi), and single-celled eukaryotes (Protista) to the metazoa (plants and animals).

-clast (klast) [Gr. *klastes* breaker] a suffix word element to denote a break, or the process of breaking down, e.g., osteoclast.

clathrate (klath′rāt) [L. *clathrare* to furnish with a lattice] in chemistry, an inclusion compound in which molecules of one type are trapped in cavities within the crystal lattice of another substance or in cavities within macromolecules. Also called clathrate compound and inclusion complex.

claudication (klaw″dĭ-ka′shun) [L. *claudicatio*] lameness or limping.

intermittent c., the presence of pain, weakness, or cramping in a muscle mass when stressed by exercise, and the absence of these symptoms when the muscles are at rest. It most commonly occurs in the calf muscles. Intermittent claudication may be neurogenic in etiology, but much more commonly is caused by inadequate blood supply due to occlusive artery disease. If the condition is advanced, treatment must be surgical. See also *a. obliterans* under *arteriosclerosis* and *t. obliterans* under *thromboangiitis.*

claustrum (klaws′trum), pl. *claustra* [L. "a barrier"] a thin sheet of gray matter interposed between the insula and the putamen, and separated from them by fibers of the external capsule. It is continuous rostrally with the anterior perforated substance and the amygdala.

clavate (kla′vāt) [L. *clavatus* club] pertaining to the clava, the tuberculum nuclei gracilis; club shaped.

Claviceps (klav′ĭ-seps) [L. *clava* club + *caput* head] a genus of parasitic ascomycetous fungi that infest the seeds of various plants. *C. purpurea* produces a number of toxic ergot alkaloids and is the etiologic agent of ergotism, which may occur as acute or chronic poisoning. These toxins are used in the extraction of pharmacologic agents.

clavicle (klav′ĭ-k′l) [L. *clavicula* bolt, fastener, dim. of *clavis* key] an elongated bone that lies horizontally in the root of the neck; it articulates medially with the sternum and first costal cartilage (sternoclavicular joint) and laterally with the acromion of the scapula (acromioclavicular joint).

clavicul/o (klah-vik′u-lo) [L. *clavicula* bolt] a word element used in combining form to denote the clavicle (the collarbone), e.g., clavicular.

clavicular (klah-vik′u-lar) pertaining to the clavicle.

clavicular region the region of the front of the chest that overlies a clavicle.

clean-catch collection method a procedure for obtaining a urine specimen for bacterial culture having minimal contamination with bacteria from the external genitalia or the rectum. For males, the glans is exposed, cleaned with antiseptic, and dried. The urine stream is started and a midstream specimen is caught in a sterile screw-cap container without stopping the stream until after the container is removed. For females, the labia minora are held apart using sterile gloves. The area in and around the urinary meatus is cleansed with sterile soapy water and rinsed. Then the urine stream is started and a midstream specimen caught. Neither the urine stream nor the specimen container should touch the perineum.

cleaning solution any solution used for cleaning laboratory glassware; it usually refers to a solution of sodium dichromate in concentrated sulfuric acid, used to clean glassware from grease, lipids, and other organic matter by oxidation. At times heating is necessary for effective cleaning.

clear (klēr) 1. to free from anything that obscures or darkens.

2. transparent; without discoloration or turbidity.

3. in histology, to remove alcohol from a specimen; see also *clearing.*

clearance 1. the act of clearing; specifically, the volume of blood per unit time cleared of a substance.

2. the space between two structures.

clear cell a cell whose cytoplasm appears empty. The term is sometimes used to refer to secretory cells in sweat glands that have sparse ribosomes and abundant glycogen; however, any cell that contains much glycogen or lipid can have this appearance in histologic sections.

clear cell carcinoma a descriptive term for a tumor composed of cells whose cytoplasm appears clear in routine hematoxylin and eosin-stained paraffin sections. The appearance can result from the presence of abundant glycogen or lipid within the cells, as in many renal cell adenocarcinomas, or it may be produced by degenerative changes with influx of fluid that distends the cytoplasm. The term is sometimes used as a synonym for certain adnexal and salivary tumors, and for the so-called "mesonephric" carcinoma of the ovary. See also *ovarian tumors.*

clear cell sarcoma a soft tissue neoplasm initially held to be histogenetically related to tendons and aponeuroses, but now believed to be a tumor of melanocytes that have become sequestered in the soft tissues during embryonic migration from neural crest to skin. The tumor arises in the distal extremities; more than 70 percent recur or metastasize. Fewer than half the tumors have demonstrable melanin by light microscopy, but premelanosomes generally can be found with electron microscopy. Most of those affected are young adults.

clearing in histology, the process of removing alcohol (dealcoholization) or other dehydrating agents from tissue specimens. This procedure is performed prior to embedding or mounting; the clearing agent is miscible in the embedding or mounting medium. Clearing agents used before mounting have a high refractive index so that the tissue becomes transparent when immersed.

Xylene is commonly used before mounting; toluene, methyl salicylate, and terpineol are alternatives. Xylene, toluene, chloroform and dioxane are the most widely used agents for clearing before embedding.

For electron microscopy, propylene oxide is generally used for clearing; it is miscible with the epoxy resins used for plastic embedding.

clearing factor lipase see *lipoprotein lipase.*

cleavage (klēv′ij) the quality of splitting along a definite plane or planes.

c. lines of skin, a series of imaginary lines on the surface of the body, the direction of which is determined by the orientation of the parallel bundles of collagen fibers in the reticular dermis. The lines are roughly horizontal in the neck and trunk and longitudinal in the limbs. A surgical incision made in the direction of a cleavage line will heal with minimal scarring. Also called Langer's lines.

c. of ovum, the process by which the unicellular ovum, through a series of mitotic divisions, is transformed into a multicellular mass of blastomeres; each has a nuclear cytoplasmic ratio comparable to that of a general somatic cell.

cleavage cell see *blastomere.*

cleft (kleft) a fissure or elongated opening, especially one occurring in the embryo or derived from a failure of parts to fuse during embryonic development. See also *branchial region.*

cleft lip a common congenital defect of the head and neck, which may occur alone or in association with cleft palate. It may or may not be associated with other anatomic defects, but has no connection with mental retardation. This condition is thought to arise as a developmental defect of the first branchial arch and usually causes no disability, although it may be cosmetically distressing. Also called *harelip.*

cleft palate the most common developmental abnormality of the head and neck, occurring in 1 of every 650–750 live births. It often occurs with cleft lip; cleft lip with or without cleft palate is etiologically distinct from isolated cleft palate. The extent of the defect may vary from involvement of only the soft palate to a complete cleft in both the hard and soft palates as well as the lip. This defect may occur by itself or in combination with a number of genetic syndromes, including trisomy 13 or Apert's syndrome.

cleft tongue a rare congenital malformation of the tongue that results from incomplete fusion of the lateral lingual swellings.

cleistothecium (klīs″to-the′se-um) [*Gr. kleisis* closure + *thēkē* case] a fruiting body (ascocarp) produced by some ascomycetes in which there is no pore for the escape of the ascospores: they are released when the carp walls disintegrate.

Cleland's reagent (kle′landz) [Wallace W. *Cleland*] see under *dithiothreitol.*

CLH abbrev. for chronic lobular hepatitis. See under *hepatitis.*

click (klik) a brief, sharp sound, especially any of the short clicking heart sounds during systole. It is indicative of various heart conditions.

ejection c., a high-frequency clicking sound that occurs early in systole at the time of maximal opening of the semilunar valves. Ejection clicks can be auscultated and recorded in pathologic conditions in which the semilunar valves are deformed (as in congenital, rheumatic aortic, or pulmonic stenosis) or the roots of the great vessels are dilated (as in systemic or pulmonary hypertension). Also called ejection sound.

midsystolic c., a high-frequency clicking sound or sounds in systole characteristically heard and recorded in mitral valve prolapse (click murmur syndrome). The click occurs coincident with maximal prolapse when the valve motion is abruptly checked.

clidinium bromide (klĭ-din′e-um) a quaternary ammonium compound with anticholinergic and antispasmodic activity, used in adjunctive therapy for peptic ulcer and in combination with the antianxiety agent chlordiazepoxide (Librium). It has the typical anticholinergic adverse reactions of dry mouth, blurred vision, and drowsiness.

clindamycin (klin″dah-mi′sin) a macrolide antibiotic related to lincomycin; see *lincomycin.*

cline (klīn) [Gr. *klinein* to slope] in population genetics and ecology, a gradual change in a phenotype character and/or gene frequency over the geographic range of a population.

clinic (klin′ik) [Gr. *klinikē* medical practice at the bedside] 1. an institution situated in a hospital that treats patients on an outpatient basis in a medical specialty; a group practice of physicians in one area of medicine.

2. a meeting held to analyze actual cases or concrete problems in a particular discipline.

clinical (klin′ĭ-k′l) pertaining to a clinic or to the bedside; pertaining to or founded on the actual observation and treatment of patients, as distinguished from research studies or pathologic or laboratory findings.

clinical bacteriologic specimens biologic materials by which medical microbiology laboratories provide clinicians with information needed for the proper management of infections in their patients. Several steps are involved, and each must be carried out correctly to achieve the intended result—determination of the presence or absence of pathogens.

The first step is selection and collection of the specimen; this is the responsibility of the clinical team, as is also partly true of the next step, which is transport of the specimen to the laboratory. When received, speed is of the essence; some specimens are, or should be, examined directly by microscopy and the findings reported to the clinician at once.

The major step in the laboratory, also to be performed promptly, is inoculation of the primary culture. In recent years there has been great emphasis on, and much progress in, the development of rapid culture methods that allow earlier inoculation of isolates to secondary and special identification media. Each culture is examined at least once each day for a period of time appropriate for the type of specimen. An additional advantage of rapid methodology is the early initiation of antibiotic profile testing, an essential part of proper handling of most clinical bacteriologic specimens.

The final steps are bacteriologic evaluation of the results of the foregoing work, prompt reporting of them to the clinician, and filing them along with others from the same source so that they remain readily available for future reference and retrieval. Sometimes it is also advisable to keep for several days or a few weeks certain isolates of particular interest for further study.

COLLECTION. All microbiology laboratories should provide hospital personnel with detailed instructions for collection and transport of specimens. Criteria for acceptability of specimens should be included. Specimens that are not acceptable for culture are saliva, 24-hr pooled sputum or urine, feces for acid-fast bacilli, and Foley catheter tips; specimens obtained from sites that contain contaminating normal flora are not acceptable for anaerobic culture. However, such specimens should not be discarded without prior consultation with the physician or nursing supervisor. It is best if a member of the clinical staff consults with the microbiology laboratory staff before attempting to collect a specimen for isolation of an unusual bacterial pathogen.

Specimens should be collected with minimal chance of contamination. For those obtained by needle aspiration, skin contamination can be minimized by application of 0.5 percent tincture of iodine followed by 70 percent alcohol; tender areas may be cleansed instead with sterile saline. Tissues, aspirates, or body fluids rather than swabs should be submitted for bacteriologic examination whenever possible. For specimens that must be collected with swabs, calcium alginate or polyester swabs should be used, as cotton may be inhibitory. One of the buffered, nonproliferating transport media available commercially should be employed for the transport of swabs to prevent drying. Oxygen-free transport media are available for transport of fluids or material on swabs for anaerobic culture.

Appropriate types of specimens from various anatomic sites are listed in Table 1, and detailed information on specimen collection is found in Appendix B.

DIRECT EXAMINATION. Gram-stained smears are used to aid in the selection of appropriate culture media, to screen for acceptability, and to give the physician immediate information about the absence or presence of bacteria and their morphology. Direct smears also serve as a quality control measure because the same morphotypes observed in the preculture smear should be recovered later in culture. Smears should also be examined for the number and type of cells (e.g., white blood cells, squamous epithelial cells) present. Special stains are useful for certain bacteria: Giemsa (e.g., *Borrelia, Chlamydia*); Giménez (e.g., *Rickettsia*); Dieterle (e.g., *Legionella*); and modified acid-fast stains (e.g., *Legionella, Nocardia*).

Other microscopic procedures include darkfield microscopy (useful for spirochetes), methylene blue preparations (useful for stools), and direct fluorescent antibody techniques (useful for a number of bacteria including *Legionella, Bordetella*).

Serologic procedures, such as counterimmunoelectrophoresis or latex agglutination, may be used to detect bacterial antigens in cerebrospinal fluid, serum, or urine.

INOCULATION. Many satisfactory media are available commercially for the primary culturing of clinical specimens (see *culture media*). They have been developed in ever-growing numbers in order to encompass the broad nutritional requirements of various bacterial pathogens and to facilitate the growth of particular types. The basic isolation medium is blood agar; its rich composition supports growth of a majority of pathogenic species, and it is the most widely used of the nutrient types of media. A second category is the differential media; these may have some selective action for one or more groups of bacteria, but the principal purpose is to differentiate pathogenic varieties from related nonpathogenic ones; one example is MacConkey agar. Selective media, the third type, may or may not have differenti-

CLINICAL BACTERIOLOGIC SPECIMENS, TABLE 1. SPECIMEN-COLLECTING SITES

ANATOMIC SITE	SPECIMEN
Body fluids*	Peripheral blood; joint, pericardial, peritoneal, pleural fluids
Central nervous system	Brain biopsy,* cerebrospinal fluid (CSF), shunt fluid*
Ear	External ear swabs, internal ear (swabs or fluid)*
Eye	Conjunctival or corneal scrapings, swabs of conjunctival scrapings, surgical specimens*
Gastrointestinal tract	Duodenal contents, feces, rectal swabs, gastric aspirates
Genital tract	
Female	Amniotic fluid; products of conception; cervical, vaginal, urethral secretions; intrauterine devices (IUD); inguinal lymph node aspirates; cul de sac (culdocentesis)*; endometrial aspirates*; vaginal cuff aspirates*; Bartholin gland aspirates*; specimens for darkfield examination
Male	Inguinal lymph node aspirates, penile lesions, prostatic fluid, urethral discharge, specimens for darkfield examination
Respiratory tract	
Upper tract	Nasopharyngeal swabs or aspirates, swabs of anterior nares, throat swabs, swabs of epiglottis, sinus aspirates,* dental abscesses*
Lower tract	Expectorated or induced sputum, tracheal aspirates, bronchoscopy brushes or washings,† lung aspirates or biopsies,* transtracheal aspirates*
Urinary tract	Voided urine, catheterized urine, collection from catheter, cystoscopy specimens,* suprapubic aspirates*
Wounds	Superficial wounds (burns, rashes), swabs of decubitus ulcers, aspirates of pus from abscesses or deep wounds,* sinus tract aspirates*

* Appropriate for isolation of anaerobic bacteria.
† Double-lumen catheters available; anaerobic cultures appropriate if these catheters are used.

ating properties, but they are formulated to favor one or more genera or species and/or suppress the growth of others. Suppression is accomplished by the incorporation into a standard formulation of a chemical such as phenylethyl alcohol or an antibiotic with the desired selective inhibitory action. Finally, some primary culture media are mainly enrichments, in that substances (such as serum, vitamin K, cysteine, or larger amounts of iron) are added to satisfy specific nutritional needs of a particular species. Table 2 is a summary of useful information about the primary plating media in common use at present.

Safety precautions must be followed with all specimens, and certain types of specimens should be handled in a biological safety cabinet. Swab specimens may be transferred to one section of a culture plate; liquid specimens may be similarly transferred with a sterile pipet. For viscous specimens, such as sputum, a loop or swab is used. Platinum or stainless steel bacteriologic loops are also used to spread the inoculum so as to produce isolated colonies. (See also *biohazard* and *biological safety cabinet*).

INCUBATION. Plates are incubated inverted to prevent water condensation. Generally, specimens are incubated aerobically at 35°C with a humidity of about 70 percent. Certain bacteria grow optimally or exclusively at temperatures other than 35°C (e.g., *Campylobacter jejuni,* 42°C; *Yersinia enterocolitica,* room temperature). Certain bacteria may require or be stimulated by CO_2 (usually 5–10 percent). CO_2 incubators, candle jars, or CO_2-generating systems are available commercially. Anaerobic atmospheres are required for anaerobic bacteria (see *anaerobes*).

EXAMINATION OF CULTURES. The microbiology laboratory should report the presence of significant isolates as rapidly as possible. Preliminary identification of microorganisms includes characterization of the colony morphology and growth on selective media. Colonies should be examined with an illuminated magnifying lens.

Rapid methods for identification are available and include tests such as the coagulase test for staphylococci and serotyping of presumptive colonies of *Salmonella* and *Shigella* species in a stool specimen.

Miniaturized versions of conventional media are available for the identification of Enterobacteriaceae, nonglucose-fermenting gram-negative bacilli, *Neisseria* species, and anaerobes. A number of automated systems are also available for the identification of Enterobacteriaceae (such as Vitek Automicrobic System and Abbott MS-2).

All clinical microbiology laboratories should prepare, use routinely, and revise frequently a manual of procedures for identifying those microorganisms encountered most often in the clinical specimens it receives. Appendix B contains practical information about some important, but relatively uncommon, pathogenic species.

See also *microbiology automation* and *microbiology identification systems.*

clinical chemistry the application of aspects of chemical science to the study of chemical processes in humans and animals, both in health and disease. It encompasses the study of the physical-chemical laws governing the biochemical reactions in which the multitude of inorganic and organic chemical moieties participate. It also involves analytical chemistry as applied to the measurement of the concentrations of metabolites and other body constituents in health and disease. Such studies make an increasing contribution to the understanding and diagnosis of disease processes. Clinical chemistry also includes the development of analytical methods, the design of automated apparatus, and the establishment of statistical and quality assurance procedures.

clinical chemistry automation the performance of clinical chemical analyses or tests with the use of mechanical and/or electronic instruments. Partial automation refers to the use of automatic pipetting devices or diluters and such devices as flow-through cuvets, with manual performance of the other steps of the procedure. In fully automated equipment, all steps are performed automatically, including sampling of specimens and reagents, mixing, selection of wavelength or filter, photometric readings, and any pertinent calculations. Automated equipment may consist of separate modules, each performing one or a limited number of operations, or it may be of a nonmodular form, with all subunits combined in one integrated instrument. Versatility may vary. Some are designed to perform only one specific type of test procedure, such as radioimmunoassay or enzyme assays. Some enzyme analyzers can carry out only end-point measurements, others only reaction-type measurements, and others can perform both types of analytical procedures.

The fully automated, general-purpose instruments presently available are based on two essentially different principles. These are continuous flow analyzers and discrete sample analyzers. The centrifugal analyzers, the DuPont *aca,* the Hitachi 705, and the Eastman Kodak Ektachem are each unique examples of the latter, as each sample is analyzed separately in its own discrete cuvet, test tube, or slide.

CONTINUOUS FLOW ANALYZERS. In these instruments, the chemical reactions take place in a continuously flowing stream of fluid. Specimen aliquots are drawn up from sample cups in a sample carousel at preset intervals and are introduced into a stream with diluent (sample or donor stream). Protein is separated from the analyte by dialysis through a semipermeable membrane against a reagent stream that accepts the analyte (recipient stream).

The movement of fluid is maintained by a peristaltic pump, the rollers of which move over a bank of flexible, plastic tubes through which the reagents, specimens, and diluents are dispensed. Tubes of varying diameter permit delivery of required reagent volumes. Mixing is provided by flow-through helical glass coils. Air bubbles segment the flowing stream to separate samples and to minimize carryover between samples. The reaction time is controlled by the length of the transmission tubing and delay coils, which may be immersed in a heating bath for some reactions. The reaction mixture then enters the flow-through cuvet in the double-beam photometer. Interference filters provide wavelength selection. The results are presented on a recorder or in the form of a printout, depending on the complexity of the instrument. All operations are performed by separate modules (sampler, peristaltic pump, dialyzer, colorimeter, recorder). With

Medium	Incubation Atm[a]	Incubation Type[b]	Inhibitor/Indicator	Purpose
Blood agar (BA) (5% defibrinated sheep blood in a nutrient agar base)	CO_2 or ANO_2	N		Growth of most medically significant bacteria; determination of hemolysis depends on source of erythrocytes; will not support growth of *Haemophilus, N. gonorrhoeae, C. granulomatis,* mycobacteria, *Leptospira, Mycoplasma, Borrelia, Treponema, Rickettsia, Chlamydia, B. pertussis, F. tularensis,* or *L. pneumophila*
Enteric agars				Selective agars for *Enterobacteriaceae;* support growth of some other gram-negative rods (i.e., *Pseudomonas, Acinetobacter*); inhibitory for most gram-positive bacteria; differentiate lactose (and sucrose in EMB)-fermenting and nonfermenting gram-negative bacilli
MacConkey agar	O_2	D	Bile salts, crystal violet/lactose-neutral red	Formula available without crystal violet supports growth of staphylococci and enterococci.
Deoxycholate agar	O_2	D	Desoxycholate/lactose-neutral red	
Eosin-methylene blue agar	O_2	D	Eosin Y-methylene blue, lactose, sucrose	
Selective agars for streptococci and staphylococci				
Phenylethyl alcohol	CO_2	S	Phenylethyl alcohol (2.5 mg/ml)	Isolation of streptococci and staphylococci; inhibition of most gram-negative bacteria
BA (Columbia base) + colistin, nalidixic acid	CO_2	S	Colistin (15 μg/ml), nalidixic acid (15 μg/ml)	Supports all gram-positives and inhibits most gram-negatives: staphylococci may appear later than streptococci (P. Ellner, personal communication).
Mannitol salt	O_2	S, D	NaCl/mannitol-phenol red	Isolation of staphylococci, most other bacteria inhibited
Selective agars for enteric pathogens				For isolation of *Salmonella* and in some cases *Shigella.* At least 2 types should be used, preferably one of moderate selectivity (M) and one of high selectivity (H). In some studies, HE and XLD appear to be the most useful.
Bismuth sulfite agar	O_2	S, D	Brilliant green, bismuth sulfite/ferrous sulfite	Isolation of *S. typhi* and other *Salmonella.* Inhibits most other *Enterobacteriaceae,* including *Shigella*
Brilliant green agar	O_2	S, D	Brilliant green/lactose, sucrose-phenol red	Isolation of *Salmonella;* inhibits most other *Enterobacteriaceae* including *Shigella*
Hektoen enteric agar	O_2	S, D	Bile salts, sodium deoxycholate (DC)/ferric ammonium citrate (FAC); sodium thiosulfate (STS); lactose, sucrose salicin bromthymol blue, Andrade indicator	Isolation of most *Enterobacteriaceae* including *Shigella* and some other gram-negative bacilli; differentiation of lactose/sucrose fermenters and nonfermenters and HS producers and nonproducers

Medium	Incubation Atm[a]	Type[b]	Inhibitor/Indicator	Purpose
Desoxycholate citrate agar	O_2	S, D	DC, sodium citrate (SC)/ferric citrate (FC) lactose, neutral red	Isolation of *Salmonella* and some *Shigella*
Salmonella-Shigella agar	O_2	S, D	Bile salts, brilliant green/FC, SC, STS, lactose, neutral red	Isolation of *Salmonella,* some *Shigella,* and some other gram-negative bacilli, differentiation of lactose fermenters
Xylose lysine desoxycholate agar	O_2	S, D	DC/STS, FAC, L-lysine, xylose, lactose, sucrose, phenol red	Similar to HE
Enteric enrichment broth				
GN broth	O_2	E	DC, citrate	Enrichment for *Salmonella* and *Shigella*
Selenite F broth	O_2	E	Selenium salts	Enrichment for *Salmonella*
Tetrathionate broth	O_2	E	Bile salts, tetrathionate	Enrichment for *Salmonella;* some *Shigella* may also grow.
Chocolate blood agar (choc)	CO_2	N	A 10-unit bacitracin disk or 5 units of bacitracin per ml for isolation of *Haemophilus* from mixed cultures; for other organisms, no antibiotic	Growth of all bacteria that grow on blood agar as well as *Haemophilus* and *N. gonorrhoeae;* should prepare with 1% Iso Vitale X
Selective agars for pathogenic neisseriae				
Thayer-Martin agar (modified)	CO_2	S	Vancomycin (3.0 μg/ml), colistin (7.5 μg/ml), nystatin (12.5 units/ml), trimethoprim (5 μg/ml)	Isolation of *N. meningitidis, N. gonorrhoeae,* and *N. lactamica;* most other bacteria will not grow (except some *C. fetus* subsp. *jejuni* and *Kingella denitrificans*).
Transgrow	CO_2	S	As above, except dextrose increased to 0.15%; agar increased to 2%	For transport as well as isolation of *N. gonorrhoeae, N. meningitidis,* and *N. lactamica*
Anaerobic agars				
Anaerobic BA	ANO_2	N		Growth of all anaerobic bacteria; should contain yeast extract, vitamin K_1, and hemin.
Anaerobic kanamycin-vancomycin laked BA	ANO_2	S	Kanamycin (100 μg/ml), vancomycin (7.5 μg/ml)	Isolation of *Bacteroides*
Enrichment broth				For enrichment of low numbers of bacteria and for isolation of fastidious bacteria
Prereduced brain-heart infusion broth	O_2	E		
Thioglycolate (without indicator)	O_2	E		Supplement with 10% animal serum, 10% Fildes enrichment, or 5 mg of hemin per ml.
Chopped meat-glucose	O_2	E		Supplement with 0.5 μg of menadione per ml

[a] O_2, Air, aerobic incubation; CO_2, incubation with 3 to 10% CO_2; ANO_2, incubation under anaerobic conditions.
[b] Types of media: nutrient (N), differential (D), selective (S), and enrichment (E).
Modified from Isenberg, H.D., et al.: Collection and Processing of Bacteriologic Specimens (Cumitech 9). Washington, DC, American Society for Microbiology, 1979, pp. 15-16. Also see Cumitech 9 for a simplified guide to the presumptive identification of the species commonly present in clinical specimens.

standard instrumentation, only end-point procedures can be carried out, and the continuous flow principle limits to some degree the types of procedures that can be developed. The simpler instruments can do only one or two procedures at one time; advanced models (e.g., SMA 6/60, SMA 12/60) can do 6 (12) tests per hour on each of 60 specimens. The SMAC (a computer-linked instrument) can do 20 of a possible 40 tests developed for the instrument per specimen at a rate of about 180 specimens per hour.

DISCRETE SAMPLE ANALYZERS. In essence, these instruments automate (or mechanize) a manual procedure, step by step, without significant changes in the original manual method. Each test is performed in a separate test tube or cuvet, which is transported on a conveyer or in a carousel past the various stations, where specimens, diluents, and reagents are dispensed. Time is allowed for mixing, incubation, and color development, after which the absorbance of the reaction mixture is measured by a built-in filter photometer or spectrophotometer. Instruments vary in complexity. Some perform only one test at a time, others as many as 30 different tests simultaneously. In some analyzers, the tubes serve also as cuvets, in which case a mechanism is provided to wash and dry the tubes. The more sophisticated computer-assisted or computer-controlled instruments permit performance of individual tests or test combinations as may be desired.

CENTRIFUGAL ANALYZERS. In these instruments, specimens and reagents are dispensed in appropriate volumes into separate radially aligned wells cut into uniquely designed centrifugal rotors. The number of specimens processed varies with the rotor size (15–36). As the rotor is spun, the reactants are forced outward by the centrifugal force into a transparent reaction chamber, which also serves as a cuvet. This causes mixing of the specimens with the reagents, and thus initiation of the reaction. The rotor spins over a fixed light beam, which passes through the cuvet. A photometer measures the light transmission through the cuvet, which is referenced against a blank. Measurements are made for each cuvet once for each revolution of the rotor, and several consecutive readings are averaged.

In the case of end-point reactions, a built-in computer compares absorbance (A) readings and converts the ΔA values to concentration values, which are printed out. In reaction rate measurements, the average A change per second throughout the linear range is calculated and converted to final results. Only one specific method can be carried out at a time, but changeover time to a new procedure is minimal, as the next rotors can be loaded with specimens and reagents while specimens in the first rotor are being analyzed.

EASTMAN KODAK EKTACHEM. This analytical system employs a singular technology in which all reagents are contained in dry form in several layers of a small slide. A 10-μl drop of serum is dispensed onto the porous top layer, which then spreads evenly to a uniform thickness. Proteins and lipids are retained in the top spreading layer, while the other solutes dissolved in the serum water percolate to lower layers that contain the buffered reagents. After color development, the slide is scanned by a reflectance spectrophotometer, and the readings are converted to the appropriate test result with the aid of a microprocessor. Most methods currently available are colorimetric, but the use of ion-specific electrodes makes the determination of cations such as Na^+ or K^+ possible. Fluorometric and immunoassay methods are under development.

DUPONT ACA (AUTOMATIC CLINICAL ANALYZER). In this type of discrete analyzer, a transparent reagent pack, which contains all required reagents in individual compartments, is obtained from the manufacturer for each individual test. The packet also serves as reaction vessel and as a cuvet.

The instrument is loaded with packets in the order in which the tests are to be performed, with those for any one specimen grouped together. The specimen and diluent are automatically dispensed into the appropriate reaction packet for each test ordered, the seals of the reagent compartment in the packets are broken by applying pressure against the compartments, and the packet content is mixed by vibrating action. During the fixed reaction time incubation, the individual packets move along a chain in a temperature-controlled environment, and the packet is then mechanically compressed to form a 1.0-cm pathlength cuvet. The absorbance of the reaction mixture in the cuvet is measured at two wavelengths (to correct for turbidity and interference by other chromogens) by a filter photometer. A computer-readable code on the packet identifies the test to be performed, and programs the instrument to add the appropriate volume of diluent and to select the correct filter for the photometric measurement. The final result is presented in the form of a printed report. Some packets contain microchromatographic columns to remove proteins or other interfering substances.

COMPUTER CONTROL. Many fully automated instruments are controlled by a built-in microprocessor or computer and can also be interfaced with a laboratory-based computer or a hospital information system. Depending on the type of microprocessor or computer, its role may include such tasks as start-up calibration of the instrument, performance of diagnostic and trouble-shooting procedures, automatic sample identification by use of machine-readable labels, calculation of test results, and performance of calculations for special test procedures such as clearances. Some computers are capable of monitoring rate curves of enzyme reactions and calculating the enzyme activity on the basis of the linear portion of the reaction rate curve. Some instruments are provided with microprocessors that allow insertion of stat samples in the middle of a routine run or the performance of selected test procedures on a multitest instrument. More sophisticated computer systems allow reporting of test results together with a reference range stratified by the age and the sex of the patient, printout of cumulative summary reports, display and storage of patient and quality control data, flagging of abnormal test results, and performance of a variety of management functions.

JOHN F. KACHMAR, PH.D.

clinical chemistry quality control efforts to assure that the analytical quality of test results provided by the clinical chemistry laboratory meets quality control (QC) standards and is appropriate for their medical application and interpretation. These efforts include a broad spectrum of plans, policies, and procedures, including the monitoring of performance parameters. QC can be divided into internal and external programs, involving practically every activity of the clinical laboratory from sample acquisition, processing, and analysis to reporting of laboratory test results. Programs should be designed to prevent and detect preanalytical errors related to activities such as patient identification and patient preparation, as well as specimen collection, processing, and storage. Furthermore, they should detect analytical errors through proper selection and use of standard and control materials, use of a suitable analytical protocol, verification of reference ranges, and selection and maintenance of appropriate instrumentation, as well as the hiring and training of competent personnel.

The most visible aspect of a QC program is the introduction of control specimens into each analytical run and the plotting of the results on control charts (most commonly, Levy-Jennings charts). Control material should have a matrix similar to that of the test specimens, and should have previously established values for analytes in the normal and abnormal range that correspond to values observed in patient specimens. The observed results are best displayed on QC charts, on which they are plotted versus the time (or the day) that the control value was obtained. Rejection criteria should be set so that there is minimal probability for false rejection of an analytical run that is in control, and also to ensure that the probability for error detection —either systematic or random error—is very high. Control charts indicating a wide scatter of results with values outside the performance limits on either side of the mean can reveal excessive random errors, whereas systematic errors can be detected by the observance of consecutive results found on one side of the mean. Such shifts and trends require corrective action. Their cause could be deterioration of reagents, use of inappropriate standards, a change in control material, a technical problem in the procedure, or instrument failure such as drifts.

Other internal QC procedures include clinical correlation of all test results obtained on one patient; use of calculation, such as anion gap, osmolal gap, and use of the Henderson-Hasselbalch equation for correlation of pH, Pco_2, and total CO_2; delta checks, i.e., the calculation of the difference in laboratory values compared with previous values obtained on the same patient; and limit checks, i.e., confirmation that test results are within physiologic range and are compatible with life.

The analytical quality of test results should also be monitored by external quality assurance programs, several of which are sponsored by professional societies, the Centers for Disease Control, state agencies, and various manufacturers (see under *quality control*).

clinical laboratory a laboratory in which procedures in clinical chemistry, hematology, histology, serology, cytology, microbiology, immunology, and so forth are performed.

Clinical laboratories should meet one of two regulations established by the National Fire Protection Association, depending on their location and activities: (1) NFPA 56C-1980, which is referenced in both CAP (College of American Pathologists) and JCAH (Joint Commission on Accreditation of Hospitals) accreditation standards, applies to laboratory rooms or spaces in which flammable, combustible, or oxidizing materials are to be used in health care occupancies or in buildings occupied at any time by four or more patients who are anesthetized, immobilized, or otherwise incapable of self-preservation in case of fire. The regulation is not intended to apply to those areas in which oxygen is administered; to blood donor rooms in which flammable, combustible, or otherwise hazardous materials normally used in laboratory procedures are not present; to clinical service areas not using hazardous materials; or to isolated frozen-section laboratories in which flammable liquids are not used. Laboratories in separate or detached buildings separated by construction resistive to a 2-hr fire do not need to comply with this regulation. (2) NFPA 45-1981 applies to all other laboratory rooms or spaces for testing, analysis, research, instruction, or similar activities that involve the use of chemical materials.

c. l. maximum area, the maximum area permitted for clinical laboratories in hospitals. No such maximum area is recommended by NFPA regulation 56C-1980; NFPA 45-1981, however, has maximum area standards for laboratories that range up to 20,000 ft^2, depending on fire resistance of separations from other areas.

Clinical Laboratory Management Association (CLMA) a professional organization of clinical laboratory managers.

Clinical Laboratory Scientist see under *medical technologist.*

clinical microbiology quality control a program established to ensure a consistently high quality of laboratory results in the clinical microbiology laboratory. The Joint Commission on Accreditation of Hospitals (JCAH), the Centers for Disease Control (CDC) of the U.S. Public Health Service, the College of American Pathologists (CAP), and state health departments have developed guidelines and standards for QC that should be consulted when setting up a program for the clinical laboratory.

A satisfactory QC program includes periodic reviews of methods being used for the collection, transport, and processing of specimens; surveillance of equipment, reagents, stains, biologicals, culture media, and susceptibility testing materials; and frequent evaluation of personnel performance.

SPECIMENS. Quality assurance begins with the proper handling of specimens; it is the responsibility of the microbiologist to provide a manual containing criteria for their proper collection and transport. Especially important is the preparation of body sites to eliminate contamination with normal flora; information regarding proper containers and transport media must also be included. Adherence to these criteria should be monitored by close liaison with the nursing and medical staff. Request slips for specimen collection should be completed accurately and in full, and should include both the time of collection and the person responsible for it. The laboratory should establish criteria for acceptance of specimens, and rejection of those specimens that were collected or transported improperly or labeled inadequately.

Instruction for the proper handling of specimens in the laboratory should be established and maintained by means of an operating manual. If specimens are to be forwarded to a referral laboratory, it is necessary to follow that laboratory's criteria for collection techniques and transport material. Priorities should be established for the preferential processing of certain types of specimens when a large number arrive at the same time.

Specimens should be examined microscopically and Gram-stained prior to culture to avoid the work-up of specimens badly contaminated with normal flora: a complete identification of organisms from contaminated specimens yields results that may be misleading and are of no clinical value. Gram stains are also useful as a mechanism of QC in that subsequent culture results can be correlated with organisms seen in preculture smears.

SURVEILLANCE OF EQUIPMENT. All equipment used in the clinical microbiology laboratory should be monitored regularly and good records kept. A preventive maintenance program is essential. Temperature-controlled equipment, CO_2 incubators, and anaerobic jars or chambers must be monitored daily. Autoclaves should be tested with spore strips in accordance with national standards, and heat-sensitive tape should be used with each load. Biological safety cabinets should undergo efficiency monitoring at least semiannually. A good quality control program also requires the periodic calibration and maintenance checks of centrifuges and the frequent cleaning and inspection of microscopes. A usage record for each fluorescent microscope should be kept. Automated and semiautomated instruments should be included in the preventive maintenance schedule.

REAGENTS, STAINS, BIOLOGICALS, AND IDENTIFICATION SYSTEMS. Current regulations require that reactivity of reagents, stains, and biologicals be checked by means of appropriate controls each day of use. The CDC and state departments of health can provide information regarding the use of appropriate controls. Each new lot of materials should be monitored before being placed into use. Expiration dates must be strictly adhered to. Commercial packaged identification systems (e.g., API, Minitek) must be monitored with appropriate controls. Each new batch must be tested for proper reactions. Automated identification systems (e.g., MS-2, AMS) should be monitored according to the manufacturer's instructions. All data must be recorded and all discrepancies investigated.

CULTURED MEDIA. Whether they are prepared by the user or supplied commercially, every different batch of culture media is subject to QC surveillance. They should be stored properly to prevent dehydration and contamination. Each batch must be checked with appropriate test organisms. The monitoring of media requires the maintenance of stock cultures, which can be obtained from the state department of health or the American Type Culture Collection (ATCC). The keeping of records of the lot numbers of commercially prepared media is necessary for communication with the manufacturer when there are relevant QC problems.

SUSCEPTIBILITY TESTING. The disk diffusion test should be performed in a standardized manner according to criteria recommended by the National Committee for Clinical Laboratory Standards (NCCLS). Both the disks and the media used for disk diffusion testing should be checked using QC organisms recommended by the NCCLS. Appropriate QC procedures for automated susceptibility testing (e.g., Autobac, AMS, MS-2) must be performed according to the manufacturer's instructions. Broth dilution tests, either prepared by the user or supplied by a manufacturer as frozen or dried trays, must be monitored using organisms appropriate for these tests.

PERSONNEL. Personnel must have access to laboratory procedure manuals that have been reviewed and updated periodically by the supervisor. An important phase of quality assurance is the monitoring of the performance of laboratory personnel. The supervisor should review all outgoing laboratory results, as well as QC records. A satisfactory proficiency testing program allows the technologists to become familiar with organisms encountered only occasionally in the clinical laboratory. Frequent workshops, seminars, and other continuing education programs are also valuable aspects of a good QC program.

clinical spectrum the range of symptoms exhibited by individuals with a specific disease. Persons being reported on may vary from those who are asymptomatic or mildly symptomatic and have not seen a doctor, to those hospital patients who may be seriously involved with life-threatening disease. It should be noted that data about one part of the spectrum cannot necessarily be extrapolated to the rest of the spectrum.

clinical toxicology a medical practice oriented toward the clinical management of diseases associated with exogenous toxic substances. It concerns the prevention, epidemiology, diagnosis, and treatment of the immediate, continuing, and delayed effects of acute or chronic exposure to such substances.

clinical trials experiments performed on human beings for the comparative evaluation of the efficacy of two or more therapies. It is only in the last 30 yr that the current types of clinical trials have come into common use, although studies with some of these characteristics have been performed for the last several centuries, an example being the demonstration of effectiveness of citrus fruit in the management of scurvy by James Lind in 1747.

PRINCIPLES OF DESIGN. The central considerations in designing a clinical trial are the same as the requirements for performing a good experiment: absence of bias, determination and maximization of precision, definition of the range of validity, and simplicity of design.

Bias is the statistical term for systematic error; if it is present, no conclusion can be drawn about the source of the observed difference. For example, if in testing treatments A and B, all males are assigned to A and all females to B, it cannot be determined whether the superiority of response in one group is due to the treatment or to the sex of the patient. The sources of bias are legion and may be obvious or quite subtle. To help prevent bias, a technique of patient allocation, called randomization, is employed. Randomization is a systematic procedure for allocating patients to two or more treatments by chance so that each possible set of assignments has equal probability of occurring. However, because each possible grouping has the same probability of occurring, there is a chance of allocating in a "biased" manner; e.g., there is a small but finite probability of assigning all males to one group and all females to another. The larger the number of patients involved, the smaller the likelihood of the above event happening. For small samples, it is frequently advisable to "block," i.e., assign randomly within a subset that is expected to react similarly: e.g., separately randomize males to treatment A or B, and females to treatment A and B.

Precision is the second consideration in designing a good experiment. It is a function of the inherent variability of the components of the trial, such as variation among human beings and reliability of measuring instruments; of the number of units observed; and of the design of the experiment. It is important to be able to measure random errors utilizing the standard error, because the magnitude of the random errors sets an upper limit on the detectable difference in response to treatment; the more precise the measurement, i.e., the smaller the standard error, the smaller the difference that can be statistically verified. A general method of improving precision, though not always the best, is to increase sample size. A greater sample size is thus required to detect a small therapeutic improvement than is required to detect a large one.

It is important to determine the range of validity, i.e., the population of interest for applying the findings of the trial. For example, if a clinical trial is performed on patients with acute nonlymphocytic leukemia (ANLL) at university hospitals, the findings may not be applicable to the general population with ANLL. As ANLL is not uncommon, it is frequently treated in community hospitals, with university hospitals receiving only the more complicated cases; the latter patients are not representative of ANLL patients at large, and findings of studies performed on them cannot be generalized to the former patients. The population of interest should be determined before initiation of the study, and only patients who are part of that population should be eligible for entry into the study.

Finally, the trial should be as simple as possible in design while still meeting the above criteria. A complex study may be difficult to administer properly, resulting in weak adherence to specified procedures and poor overall data quality.

APPLICATIONS. A variety of randomization schemes exist. For a large study, unrestricted (simple) randomization is appropriate. For two treatments under study, simple randomization is the conceptual equivalent of a coin toss; in practice, a random number table is used. A possible scheme might be:

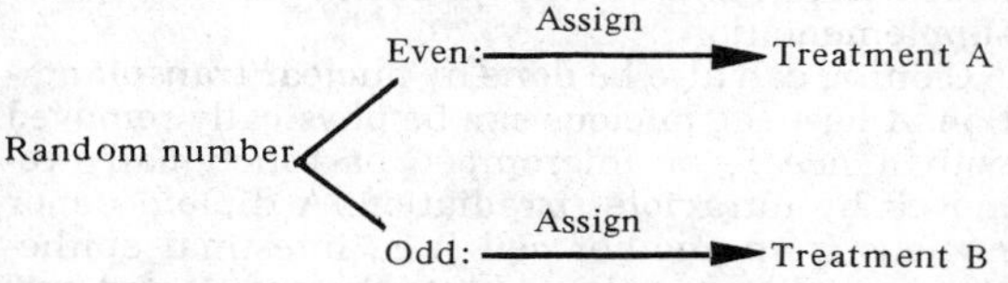

Although this scheme is appealingly simple, it may result in an unbalanced assignment, although the probability for the latter is small with large samples.

To avoid the problem of unbalanced assignments, particularly with small studies, restricted randomization may be performed. The simplest method is using permutation sets of the treatments to randomize consecutive groups of patients. For example, with two treatments, all the possible orderings (i.e., permutation sets) are A,B and B,A and random numbers are picked to select a permutation set:

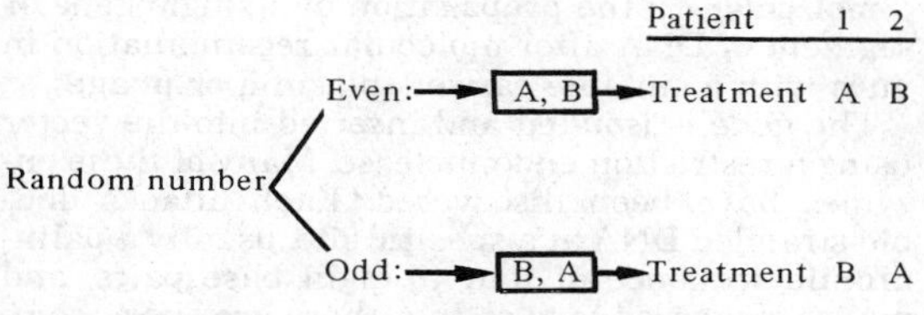

This simple scheme results in balanced assignments but is predictable; thus, biases may creep in. To avoid predictability, larger permutation sets or permutation sets of variable size can be employed, with selections of size of set and particular set by random number.

A technique used to prevent observer bias is masking (blinding). It implies that certain individuals involved in the randomized study do not know what specific treatment a particular individual is receiving. It is imperative to mask when the measurement of response is subjective to any degree. Blinding of a study can be at several levels: single blind—the patient does not know to which treatment he or she has been assigned; double blind—neither the patient nor the person administering therapy knows to which treatment group the patient belongs; triple blind—neither the patient nor the treatment administrator nor the response evaluator knows to which treatment group the patient belongs.

Masking is not always realistic. For example, a randomized surgical study cannot be double blind because the surgeons must know which procedures they are performing. Indeed, even single-masked conditions cannot always be maintained, in that patients frequently know which treatment they have received from the side-effects experienced.

The number of participants enrolled in a study, i.e., the sample size, depends on the size of the response difference of interest to the clinician, the number of research questions asked, and the level of decision error that is tolerable. In general, the smaller the difference and the error level and the greater the number of questions, the greater must be the sample size. The required sample size determines study duration through the accrual rate. Thus, the differences sought and the number of questions asked must be such as to make the study worthwhile, i.e., clinically significant, but not so demanding as to make it unfeasible by being unrealistically long.

Matching is another technique that may be used when there is much variation of response among participants and when factors are known that influence outcome. Individuals who are as similar as possible with respect to these factors may be selected and randomly assigned treatment. Identical twins are frequently a good match. A person can act as his or her own match if the treatments have no carry-over effect. This is a precision-enhancing technique.

MARIA M. KORETZ, PH.D.

clinician (klin-ish′an) a physician who works in a clinic or employs clinical methods.

Clinilab (klin′ĭ-lab) trademark for an automated instrument that performs routine urinalysis. Urine is automatically aspirated and delivered to the test modules. The specific gravity is measured by determining the time that it takes a drop of urine to fall through an immiscible liquid, the drop being detected by photocells. Six other parameters—pH, protein, glucose, ketone bodies, bilirubin, and occult blood—are measured by standard reagent strip tests. The color change of the reagent strip is detected by photocells that measure the change in reflectance. A 2-ml sample is required. The results are printed on data tags and affixed onto the specimen tube.

Clinistix (klin′ĭ-stiks) see under *glucose assays*.

Clinitest (klin′ĭ-test) see under *glucose assays* and *reducing substances in urine.*

Clinoril (klin′o-ril) trademark. See *sulindac.*

clinoscope (kli′no-skōp) [Gr. *klinein* to recline + *skopein* to examine] an instrument for measuring the paralysis of the ocular muscles, as shown by torsion of the eyeballs.

Clitocybe (kli-tos′ĭ-be) a genus of poisonous club fungi. *C. gigantea* is the source of clitocybine; *C. nebularis,* the source of nebularine. Ingestion of *C. illudens,* the orange jack-o-lantern mushroom, causes mycetismus gastrointestinalis, but is not usually fatal unless large quantities are eaten.

clitoris (klit′o-ris, kli′to-ris) [Gr. *kleitoris*] a small, elongated, erectile body located at the anterior part of the vulva in the female. Embryologically, it corresponds to the dorsal part of the penis.

CLL abbrev. See *chronic lymphocytic l.* under *leukemia.*

CLMA abbrev. See *Clinical Laboratory Management Association.*

cloaca (klo-a′kah), pl. *cloacae* [L. "drain"] 1. in zoology, a common passage for fecal, urinary, and reproductive discharge.

2. in mammalian embryology, the terminal end of the hindgut before division into rectum, bladder, and genital primordia.

cloacal membrane (klo-a′kal) in the embryo, a membrane that separates the cloaca from the exterior. It is formed from a fusion of ectoderm and entoderm; with development of the perineum, it is separated into the urogenital and anal membranes, which subsequently rupture.

cloacogenic (klo″ah-ko-jen′ik) [L. *cloaca* drain + Gr. *gennan* to produce] originating from the cloaca or from persisting cloacal remnants.

cloacogenic carcinoma a carcinoma arising in the anal glands, which are embryologic remnants of the cloacal epithelium. Some cloacogenic carcinomas resemble transitional cell carcinomas; others are histologically similar to cutaneous basal cell carcinomas but behave aggressively. Metastases are initially to inguinal or pelvic lymph nodes.

clock (klok) 1. a device that measures time.

2. an electronic circuit that produces a regular series of timing pulses (clock pulses), which are used to synchronize the actions of independent circuits.

clofibrate (klo-fi′brāt) [USP], an antilipidemic drug used in the treatment of hyperlipidemia, particularly hypertriglyceridemia. It primarily reduces levels of very-low-density lipoproteins (VLDL) but also reduces low-density lipoprotein (LDL) and cholesterol levels. Side-effects include the potentiation of anticoagulant drugs, and an increase in the incidence of gallstones and possibly of liver tumors. Trademark, *Atromid-S.*

clomipramine hydrochloride (klo-mip′rah-mēn) an antidepressant; see under *tricyclic antidepressant.*

clonal (klo′nal) pertaining to a clone.

clonazepam (klo-naz′ĕ-pam) [USP], a benzodiazepine drug used for the control of minor motor and myoclonic seizures and also for petit mal seizures not responsive to ethosuximide. See also *benzodiazepine.*

clone (klōn) [Gr. *klōn* young shoot or twig] 1. the genetically identical progeny produced by asexual reproduction of a single organism, cell, or gene; e.g., plant cuttings, a cell culture descended from a single cell, or genes reproduced by recombinant DNA technology.

2. to establish or produce such a line of progeny.

clonic (klon′ik) [Gr. *klonos* turmoil] pertaining to or characterized by clonus. The term is often used to describe the jerking movements that follow the tonic phase of a major motor seizure.

clonidine hydrochloride (klo′nĭ-dēn) an imidazoline derivative used in the treatment of hypertension. It acts by stimulating the alpha-adrenergic receptors in the central nervous system, which produces a reduction in sympathetic activity and a decrease in heart rate and blood pressure. Common adverse reactions are dryness of mouth, sedation, and drowsiness. Trademark, *Catapres.*

cloning (klo′ning) the generation of a genetically homologous population (of cells or DNA sequences) from a single progenitor.

cellular c., the derivation of a cell line from a single cell. Clones can be obtained from most cell lines by transferring cells to a new culture at very high dilution. The cells that survive divide mitotically to form colonies. The efficiency of the mitotic divisions can be increased with the addition of similar cells that are incapable of multiplication because of previous treatment by irradiation or mitomycin, but are still metabolically active. The irradiated cells provide growth factors that enable the unirradiated cells to survive and multiply. The efficiency can also be increased by introducing individual cells into very small volumes of media, such as in a capillary tube, which allows cell products to accumulate in concentration.

Media used in cloning techniques are those used for cell cultures. The media contain all major ions, sugars, amino acids, vitamins, and so forth, that are needed for cell survival and multiplication with added serum and/or embryo extract for undefined supplementation.

Cloning can also be done by nuclear transplantation. A host egg nucleus can be physically removed with a needle or micropipet, or functionally removed by ultraviolet irradiation. A diploid donor nucleus from another cell (e.g., intestinal epithelium) can be transplanted into the enucleated egg; the egg begins parthenogenetic development. A small percentage of the nuclei support some development from enucleated eggs. The frequency of successful transplants increases when serial transfer procedures are done. In serial transfers, the egg that receives the donor nucleus is allowed to cleave and form a blastula, which is then dissociated and used as a source of nuclei for the next transplantation. Blastulas may represent a better source of nuclei than adult cells because blastula nuclei are more capable of the rapid DNA synthesis needed for early embryonic development.

molecular c., the propagation of a single gene or segment of DNA after molecular recombination in vitro with a suitable carrier (plasmid or phage).

The gene is isolated and inserted into the vector using a restriction endonuclease. Many of these enzymes have been discovered. Each attacks double-stranded DNA at a specific site, usually a palindromic sequence of four to eight base pairs, and makes staggered cuts so that there are short, complementary sequences of single-stranded DNA on the cut pieces making so-called sticky ends. The endonuclease makes cuts in a mixture of DNA containing both the vector and the potential genes. When the ends have reannealed and the nicks have been closed with a DNA ligase, some of the genes will have been inserted into the vector DNA. The recombinant DNA can then be cloned in a bacterial culture.

Two kinds of vectors may be used to clone foreign DNA: plasmids and viruses. With a bacterial virus (phage) carrier, the recombinant DNA is used to infect the bacteria and produce a plaque. The phage recovered from the plaque is a clone. The cloned fragment of DNA can be extracted from the phage by cutting the inserted sequence out with a restriction endonuclease. DNA from animal tumor virus can transduce spliced DNA into cultured animal cells, allowing eukaryotic gene expression in a cell culture.

After propagation, cloned segments can be identified, primarily by hybridization with a radioactive cDNA or RNA probe; occasionally an auxotrophic mutant can be used. Homology between probe and clone can be seen by autoradiography after a Southern blot electrophoretic procedure.

Advances in molecular cloning include the insertion and expression of eukaryotic genes into prokaryotes and animal viruses and the insertion and expression of prokaryotic DNA into eukaryotic cultured cells. Both procedures give insight into genetic regulation and cellular differentiation.

Also called *recombinant DNA.* See also *cell culture* and *cellular h.* under *hybridization.*

cloning inhibitory factor (CIF) see under *proliferation inhibitory factor.*

clonorchiasis (klo″nor-ki′ah-sis) see *opisthorchosis.*

Clonorchis (klon-or′kis) [Gr. *klōn* branch + *orchis* testicle] the former name for a genus of flukes that included the common liver fluke, *C. sinensis;* see *Opisthorchis.*

C. sinensis, see under *Opisthorchis.*

clonus (klo′nus) [Gr. *klonos* turmoil] alternative involuntary muscular contraction and relaxation in rapid succession. Clonus is usually elicited by a sudden muscle stretch in an individual with spasticity, especially at the ankle.

Cloquet's node [Jules Germain *Cloquet,* French surgeon, 1790–1883] the highest of the deep inguinal lymph nodes. Also called Cloquet's gland.

clorazepate (klo-raz′ĕ-pāt) a benzodiazepine minor tranquilizer, available as the salts clorazepate monopotassium and clorazepate dipotassium. See also *benzodiazepine.*

closed fracture a simple fracture, a break of bone with no open skin wound.

closing volume the level of lung inflation at which airway closure occurs in the lower (dependent) lobes of the lungs while the airways to the upper lobes are still open. In the normal young adult, this occurs at about 10–12 percent of vital capacity (beginning from residual volume) as intrapleural pressure begins to exceed intraluminal pressure.

Measurement of closing volume is made by deliberately creating a different gas composition (usually nitrogen or a radioactive inert gas such as xenon-133) in the dependent and upper portions of the lungs. The lung volume (in liters or milliliters above residual volume) at which a change in concentration of the gas in the expired air occurs is equal to the closing volume. This technique is useful in the detection of obstructive airway disease; closing volume is abnormally high under these conditions.

clostridiopeptidase A (klos-trid″e-o-pep′tĭ-dās) see *collagenase.*

Clostridium (klo-strid′e-um), pl. *clostridia* [N.L., from Gr. *klōstēr* spindle] a large genus of anaerobic and aerotolerant, gram-positive, spore-forming bacilli. Microscopically, these organisms often appear swollen with central, subterminal, or terminal spores. The hundred or more *Clostridium* species are widely distributed in soil and water and on vegetation; some of them are part of the normal microbiota of the intestinal tracts of humans and lower animals. Their sensitivity to oxygen varies widely. *C. tetani* requires strictly anaerobic conditions; *C. perfringens* is much less fastidious; and *C. tertium* produces colonies, although small, on aerobic plates. As a genus, *Clostridium* lacks catalase, peroxidase, and superoxide dismutase, but does possess flavoprotein enzymes that reduce oxygen to hydrogen peroxide and superoxide, which are toxic compounds. Thus, oxygen is inhibitory or lethal for these organisms. Most species produce abundant gas, some are highly saccharolytic, and others are predominantly proteolytic.

The pathogenicity of clostridia is due to the effects of numerous enzymes, some of which are very destructive, or, in the case of a few species, to powerful exotoxins. The species *C. botulinum* (botulism) and *C. tetani* (tetanus) are solely responsible for these two diseases. Gas gangrene (clostridial myonecrosis) is generally a mixed infection by histotoxic species, characterized by extensive and rapid enzymatic destruction of tissue locally combined with systemic toxicity. Considerable attention is presently being directed to the recently recognized pseudomembranous colitis caused principally by toxigenic strains of *C. difficile* and associated with the oral administration of certain antibiotics. The clostridia of botulism, tetanus, and gas gangrene are exogenous, but most of clostridial infections are endogenous. The species involved are part of the normal flora and act as opportunists when lines of defense are violated or the host's immunologic system is weakened by neoplastic disease, diabetes mellitus, or immunosuppressive drugs.

About 10 percent of the anaerobes isolated from human clinical specimens are clostridia. Approximately 80 percent are represented by five species: *C. perfringens,* accounting for 45–50 percent; *C. ramosum,* 15–20 percent; and *C. difficile, C. clostridiiforme,* and *C. innocuum,* 4–6 percent each.

The presence of *C. perfringens* in a clinical specimen can be suspected by direct microscopic examination, and presumptively identified within 24 hr by double-zone hemolysis on blood agar. Fluorescent antibody reagent is commercially available for *C. novyi, C. septicum,* and *C. sordellii,* which are also etiologic agents of gas gangrene. Toxin production can be determined 24 hr after injection of a chopped meat broth culture or, for *C. perfringens,* by Nagler's reaction test.

Generally, however, species identification is based on biochemical reactions with increasing use in recent years of gas-liquid chromatography.

See also *anaerobes, exotoxins, Nagler's reaction,* and the accompanying table.

CLOSTRIDIUM. DIFFERENTIAL CHARACTERISTICS OF COMMONLY ENCOUNTERED CLOSTRIDIA[a]

Species[b]	Spores	Egg Yolk Agar		Growth on Aerobic Blood Agar	Gelatin Hydrolysis	Milk Digestion	Indole Production	Carbohydrate Fermentation						Principal Fermentation Products
		LEC	*LIP*					*Glucose*	*Maltose*	*Lactose*	*Sucrose*	*Salicin*	*Mannitol*	
C. bifermentans	OS	+	–	–	+	+	+	+	+	–	–	V	–	A, (p), (ib), (b), (iv), (v), (ic)
C. botulinum[c]														
Group I	OS	–	+	–	+	+	–	+	+	–	–	V	–	A, P, IB, B, IV, (v), (ic)
Group II	OS	–	+	–	+	–	–	+	+	–	–	V	–	A, P, B
Group III	OS	V	+	–	+	–	–	+	V	–	–	–	–	A, B
C. butyricum	OS	–	–	–	–	–	–	+	+	+	+	+	–	A, (p), B
C. cadaveris	OT	–	–	–	V	–	+	+	–	–	–	–	–	A, (p), (ib), B, (iv)
C. chauvoei	OS	–	–	–	+/-	–	–	+	+	+	+	–	–	A, B
C. clostridiiforme	OS	–	–	–	–	–	–/+	+	+	V	+	V	–	A
C. difficile	OS	–	–	–	V	–	–	+	–	–	–	V	+	A, p, IB, B, IV, V, IC
C. histolyticum	OS	–	–	V	+	+	–	–	–	–	–	–	–	A
C. innocuum	OT	–	–	–	–	–	–	+	–	–	V	+	+	A, B
C. limosum	OS	+	–	–	+	+	–	–	–	–	–	–	–	A
C. novyi A	OS	+	+	–	+	–	–	+	V	–	–	–	–	A, P, B, (v)
C. novyi B	OS	+	–	–	+	+	–	+	+	–	–	–	–	A, P, B, (v)
C. paraputrificum	OT	–	–	–	–	–	–	+	+	+	+	+	–	A, (p), B
C. perfringens	OS	+	–	–	+	+	–	+	+	+	+	V	–	A, (p),
C. ramosum	R/OT	–	–	–	–	–	–	+	+	+	+	+	V	A
C. septicum	OS	–	–	–	+	–	–	+	+	+	–	+	–	A, B
C. sordellii	OS	+/-	–	–	+	+	+	+	+	–	–	–	–	A, (p), (ib), (b), (iv), (ic)
C. sphenoides	RS/T	–	–	–	–/+	–	+/-	+	+	V	+/-	+	+	A
C. sporogenes	OS	–	+	–	+	+	–	+	+	–	–	V	–	A, (p), (ib), B, IV, (ic)
C. subterminale	OS	–	–	–	+	+	–	–	–	–	–	–	–	A, (p) IB, B, IV
C. tertium	OT	–	–	+	–	–	–	+	+	+	+	+	+	A, B
C. tetani	RT	–	–	–	+	–	V	–	–	–	–	–	–	A, p, B

[a] Key: +, positive reaction; –, negative reaction; V, variable reaction; /, either/or; O, oval; R, round; S, subterminal; T, terminal; LEC, lecithinase production; LIP, lipase production. Fermentation products: A, acetic; B, butyric; F, formic; IB, isobutyric; IC, isocaproic; IV, isovaleric; P, propionic; V, valeric; ( ) = May or may not be present; capital letters = major peaks, lower case = minor peaks.

[b] Other characteristics: toxin neutralization test is required for identification of *C. botulinum* Groups I, II, III, and for *C. novyi A* and *B. C. chauvoei* is pathogenic for herbivores. *C. innocuum, C. perfringens,* and *C. ramosum* are nonmotile. *C. bifermentans* is urease negative; *C. sordellii* is urease positive; *C. clostridiiforme* and *C. sphenoides* are usually gram negative; and *C. ramosum* is frequently gram negative. *C. perfringens* has a double zone of hemolysis. Spores are seldom observed in *C. clostridiiforme, C. perfringens,* and *C. ramosum.*

[c] Group I contains proteolytic strains (A, B, F, G); group II, types C and D; group III, nonproteolytic strains (B, E, F).

Modified from Lennette, E. H., et al.: Manual of Clinical Microbiology. 3rd ed. Washington, DC, American Society for Microbiology, 1980, p. 423.

C. botulinum, a species consisting of large, motile, gram-positive rods; it is widely distributed in soil and on vegetation, often as very resistant spores. These organisms are grouped into seven types, A–G, based on the production of antigenically distinct neurotoxins. The vegetative forms from germinated spores of types A, B, E, and F cause botulism in humans. See also *botulinum toxin, botulism,* and *exotoxins.*

C. clostridiiforme, one of the species commonly isolated from clinical specimens. It was formerly called *Bacteroides clostridiiforme* and was later classified in the genus *Clostridium* when endospore production was found. Because *Bacteroides* species are gram-negative, whereas the clostridia are generally gram-positive, it is apparent that this species is only weakly gram-positive, a trait shared by several other clostridial species.

C. difficile, a species, relatively inert in biochemical identification tests, that has come into prominence since the introduction of lincomycin and clindamycin, as use of these antibiotics (as well as a number of others) can produce a pseudomembranous colitis. *C. difficile* is part of the normal colon flora but ordinarily is held in check by other more susceptible microbial species. These are suppressed by the administered antibiotic, thus allowing *C. difficile* to grow in large numbers and produce a protein exotoxin in sufficient amounts to cause disease. Laboratory identification of the species is based on biochemical tests and gas-liquid chromatography.

C. histolyticum, a pathogenic species sometimes recovered from cases of gas gangrene associated with other clostridial species. Some strains have the ability to grow aerobically on agar. *C. histolyticum* fails to ferment carbohydrates, and produces potent proteolytic enzymes that cause severe lysis of tissues.

C. innocuum, one of the species commonly isolated from cases of gas gangrene and other anaerobic infections. It is not toxigenic and its etiologic significance is unclear. The spores are oval and terminal; identification is based on biochemical tests and gas-liquid chromatography.

C. novyi, one of the species commonly associated with gas gangrene. Type A produces lipase.

C. perfringens, a species that is a highly gram-positive, aerotolerant, nonmotile bacillus. *C. perfringens* is grouped into five serotypes, A–E, according to the range of exotoxins produced. It can be differentiated from other clostridial species by lactose fermentation, tests for motility, nitrate reduction, and Nagler's reaction test for lecithinase activity.

Types A, C, and D are pathogenic for humans: type A causes gas gangrene, necrotizing colitis, and food poisoning; type C causes enteritis necroticans. The opportunities for human contact with this species are abundant, as it is ubiquitous in soil and marine environments; 80 percent of environmental isolates are type A. Many clinical isolates come from sites where there is no indication of infection; *C. perfringens* apparently can persist in the body but must be present in large quantities to produce disease.

Twelve exotoxins have been described for this species; alpha toxin (lecithinase) is common to all types of *C. perfringens* but is produced in the greatest amount by type A. It is capable of breaking down not only lecithin but also cephalin and sphingomyelin, and consequently affects many organs. Other toxins include the lethal and necrotizing beta (types B, C), epsilon (types B, D); the hemolytic delta (types B, C) and theta (mainly type C) and the destructive enzymes mu (hyaluronidase), nu (deoxyribonuclease), lambda (proteinase; types B, E), and kappa (collagenase; types A, C, E). Types A and C also release an enterotoxin during sporulation in the large intestine that causes the food poisoning associated with this species.

C. perfringens is best known as the species most frequently involved in two types of clostridial wound infections, cellulitis and gas gangrene or myonecrosis. The strains responsible for cellulitis are of low virulence; the infection remains localized without systemic manifestations and only soft tissues are infected. Gas gangrene is a much more severe, invasive, and muscle-destructive disease with life-threatening systemic toxemia. Both of these are mixed infections, but *C. perfringens* usually plays the dominant role.

This species is often recovered from fecal (approximately 10 percent) and vaginal (5 percent) specimens in the absence of disease. These endogenous sources account for the frequency with which *C. perfringens* gains entrance to wounds below the diaphragm and causes uterine infections associated with septic abortions. Because *C. perfringens* is an invasive organism, bacteremia is a common complication of uterine infections and gas gangrene. Bowel organisms are probably the source of the bacteremia that often occurs in persons with lowered resistance and weakened immunity.

C. perfringens is second only to *Staphylococcus* as a cause of food poisoning. In the case of the *Clostridium,* large numbers of organisms must be ingested for there to be sufficient bacterial multiplication in the large intestine to produce disease. A cholera-like enteritis results.

Tentative laboratory identification of *C. perfringens* is easily made because of the formation of a characteristic double zone of hemolysis surrounding its colonies on blood agar. The inner zone around moist colonies is clear; the outer ring is a distinct discolored and incompletely hemolytic area. The cells are plump and surrounded by a definite capsule; spores are absent. Species confirmation is based on a biochemical test pattern, a positive Nagler reaction (opacity around colonies on egg yolk agar), and the absence of motility.

Formerly called *C. welchii.* See also *gas gangrene* and *Nagler's reaction.*

C. ramosum, one of the species frequently isolated from clinical specimens. It is highly fermentative, is nontoxigenic, and shows terminal spores in stained smears. Gas-liquid chromatographic analysis of fermentative products is useful in identification, for it shows acetic acid as the only principal organic acid. Gelatin is not hydrolyzed and milk is not digested. Isolates are frequently gram-negative, and spores are seldom seen.

C. septicum, a toxigenic species present in about 20 percent of gas gangrene specimens. It resembles *C. perfringens* but is lecithinase-negative. *C. septicum* septicemia is associated with the presence of malignancy.

C. tetani, a species found in the soil and in the feces of various animals. It produces a potent neurotoxin (tetanospasmin) when spores of the organism germinate after entering a wound, causing tetanus.

C. tetani is a strict anaerobe; thus, spores introduced into a wound will not germinate unless the oxidation-reduction potential is low, as in deep penetrating wounds such as nail punctures. Its spores are terminal and round at the end of a long, thin bacillus ("drumstick" spore). This species is inert with respect to the biochemical tests used for identification of clostridia.

Although there are several serologic types of *C. tetani,* they all share a single neurotoxin, which is extremely toxic for humans and most lower animals. It acts by combining with ganglioside-containing membranes of the central nervous system, producing sustained muscular spasms, probably by blocking the normal postsynaptic inhibitor.

See also *tetanospasmin* and *tetanus.*

***Clostridium histolyticum* collagenase** see under *collagenase.*

clot (klot) 1. a semisolidified mass, as of blood or lymph. See also *coagulation.*

2. to form such a mass.

clothing fire safety procedures procedures to follow in cases of clothing fires, in which laboratory personnel should be thoroughly indoctrinated. The single most important instruction is to immediately drop to the floor and roll. Rolling on the floor or other horizontal surface smothers the fire, keeps flames out of the eyes and face, and reduces the inhalation of smoke and heat. Fire blankets and safety showers are of secondary importance. National Fire Protection Association regulations contain additional information on this subject (NFPA 45-1981 and NFPA 56C-1980).

clot lysis the breakdown (liquefaction) of a blood clot, primarily by fibrinolysis. This occurs normally about 72 hr after coagulation. Earlier clot lysis is abnormal and is indicative of the presence of fibrinolysis. See also *euglobulin lysis test.*

clot retraction a stage in normal clot formation, normally occurring within 1 hr of initial coagulation. As the pseudopods of platelets adhering to fibrin strands shorten, the coagulum reduces and expresses serum. At a normal hematocrit, the clot reduces to almost half its size, retraction being almost complete within 4 hr and fully complete within 24 hr. If the platelet count is very low or if the individual has thrombasthenia, retraction is reduced or absent. Erythrocytosis, fibrinolysis, or abnormal fibrinogens also interfere with normal clot retraction. See also *syneresis.*

clotrimazole (klo-trim′ah-zōl) [USP], an antifungal agent used in the treatment of dermatophyte and *Candida* infections of the skin. Administered in cream and ointment form, clotrimazole is also available as a suppository for vaginal candidiasis. It has not been approved for systemic use.

clotting time (klot′ing) see *partial thromboplastin time test* and *prothrombin time test.*

cloudy swelling (kloud′e) an early stage of toxic degenerative changes, especially in the protein constituents of organs in infectious diseases. The tissues appear swollen, parboiled, and opaque but revert to normal when the cause is removed. Such an appearance is characterized by slight swelling of the cell and granularity and cloudiness of the cytoplasm.

clove oil (klōv) [L. *clavus* a nail or spike] [USP], a volatile oil distilled with steam from cloves, the dried flower buds of *Eugenia caryophyllus.* It is used as a topical dental analgesic and flavoring agent, and also as a germicide and counterirritant. In histology, clove oil is used as a clearing agent and as a differentiator in the Bowie stain for juxtaglomerular granules.

cloxacillin sodium (kloks″ah-sil′in) [USP], a semisynthetic, penicillinase-resistant penicillin. It is much less potent than penicillin G but is useful against penicillin-resistant staphylococci and other gram-positive cocci. Cloxacillin is well absorbed orally and has an achievable serum level of about 8 mg/ml orally and 14 mg/ml intramuscularly. Adverse reactions include gastrointestinal upset and hypersensitivity. See also *antibacterial agents* and *penicillins.*

CLS abbrev. for Clinical Laboratory Scientist. See under *medical technologist.*

clubbing (klub′ing) an enlargement of the terminal phalanges of the digits caused by edema, proliferative changes, and increased vascularity. Clubbing of the digits may be seen in conditions such as bronchogenic carcinoma, lung sepsis, bronchiectasis, congenital heart disease, subacute bacterial endocarditis, regional enteritis, ulcerative colitis, liver abscesses, biliary cirrhosis, and certain neoplasms.

clubfoot (klub′foot) see *talipes.*

clump (klump) an aggregation as of bacteria caused by the action of agglutinins (agglutination).

clumping (klump′ing) the aggregation of particles, such as bacteria, into irregular masses.

clysis (kli′sis) [Gr. *klysis*] the administration of fluid by infusion to replace lost body fluid, supply nutriment, or raise blood pressure.

-clysis (kli′sis) [Gr. *klysis*] a suffix word element to denote irrigation or washing, e.g., enteroclysis.

clyster (klis′ter) [Gr. *klystēr* a syringe] an enema.

CM abbrev. for *cras mane* (tomorrow morning).

Cm symbol for the chemical element *curium.*

cm abbrev. See *centimeter.*

cmc abbrev. See *critical micelle concentration.*

CM-cellulose abbrev. See *carboxymethylcellulose.*

CMF abbrev. for cyclophosphamide, methotrexate, and fluorouracil, a major established cancer chemotherapy drug regimen. For more information, see the specific drug (listed under its generic name) and *Appendix A.*

CMFVP abbrev. for cyclophosphamide, methotrexate, fluorouracil, vincristine, and prednisone, a major established cancer chemotherapy drug regimen. For more information, see the specific drug (listed under its generic name) and *Appendix A.*

CMI abbrev. See *cell-mediated immunity.*

CML abbrev. See *chronic myelogenous l.* under *leukemia.*

cMo abbrev. See *centimorgan.*

CMOS abbrev. See *complementary metal oxide semiconductor logic.*

CMP abbrev. for cytidine monophosphate. See *cytidine-5′-phosphate.*

CMP-*N*-acetyl-D-neuraminate cytidine monophosphate-*N*-acetyl-D-neuraminate, an activated donor molecule functioning in the transfer of sialyl groups (*N*-acetylneuraminate) to receptor molecules.

CMRR abbrev. See *common mode rejection ratio.*

CMV abbrev. See *cytomegalovirus.*

Cnephia (ne′fe-ah) a genus of black flies in the family Simuliidae, with a short, stout body and a highly arched thorax. Several species feed on the blood of domestic animals and humans.

CNMT abbrev. for certified nuclear medicine technologist. See under *nuclear medicine technologist.*

CNS abbrev. See *central nervous system.*

CNV abbrev. See *contingent negative variation.*

CO abbrev. See *cardiac output.*

Co symbol for the chemical element *cobalt.*

Co I abbrev. for coenzyme I. See *nicotinamide adenine dinucleotide.*

Co II abbrev. for coenzyme II. See *nicotinamide adenine dinucleotide phosphate.*

CoA abbrev. See *coenzyme A.*

coacervate (ko-as′er-vāt) [L. *coacervatus* heaped up] the viscous liquid phase that separates from a colloid in the phenomenon of coacervation.

coacervation (ko-as″er-va′shun) the separation of a mixture of two liquids, one or both of which are colloids, into two phases, one of which (the coacervate) contains the colloidal particles, the other being an aqueous solution.

coagulant (ko-ag′u-lant) [L. *coagulans*] promoting, accelerating, or causing the coagulation of blood; also, an agent with this activity.

coagulase (ko-ag′u-lās) a bacterial enzyme that causes citrated (or oxalated) plasma to coagulate. Staphylococci appear to be the only bacteria producing this enzyme, and a positive coagulase test is generally considered the best evidence that a strain is pathogenic for humans. The tube test demonstrates "free" coagulase, whereas a coagulase slide test demonstrates "bound" coagulase or clumping factor.

coagulase test a test for the production of coagulase by bacteria. Rabbit plasma is mixed with a culture of staphylococci. Clumping in a slide test indicates the presence of bound coagulase (clumping factor); clotting in a tube test indicates extracellular coagulase. Most strains of *Staphylococcus aureus* are coagulase-positive; *S. epidermidis* and *Micrococcus* are coagulase-negative.

coagulate (ko-ag′u-lāt) [L. *coagulare*] to cause to clot, or to become clotted.

coagulation (ko-ag″u-la′shun) [L. *coagulatio*] the sequential process by which the multiple coagulation factors of the blood and the platelets interact, ultimately resulting in the formation of an insoluble blood clot, which aids in the stoppage of blood flow. The blood clot consists of a mesh of fine threads of fibrin in which are embedded erythrocytes, leukocytes, and small amounts of serum.

Coagulation may be divided into three stages: stage 1, the formation of activated Factor X (Xa) via the intrinsic and extrinsic pathway; stage 2, the formation of thrombin from prothrombin by Factor Xa in the presence of Factor V and Ca^{++}; and stage 3, the formation of fibrin from fibrinogen, stabilized by Factor XIIIa. In vivo, the mechanism is triggered by the platelets via the intrinsic pathway; however, in vitro coagulation can proceed without platelets via either pathway.

Blood clotting involves 12 factors whose absence, diminution, or excess may lead to abnormalities of the clotting mechanism, and which are designated by Roman numerals I–V and VII–XIII; VI is no longer considered to have a clotting function.

See also *coagulation pathways* and under *Factor*. Cf. *anticoagulant*.

coagulation factor one of 12 substances in the plasma essential to the clotting process, and hence to maintenance of normal hemostasis. The factors are designated by Roman numerals I–V and VII–XIII, to which the notation "a" is added to indicate the activated state. For more information on all 12 factors, see the table accompanying *Factor I*.

coagulation factor assays see *factor assays*.

coagulation factor inhibitors antibodies in the plasma that are capable of neutralizing coagulation factors and producing severe bleeding. Inhibitors have been reported to Factors V, VIII, IX, XI, and XIII; inhibitors to Factor VIII are most common. Factor IX inhibitors occur in 5–10 percent of individuals with Factor IX deficiency after a previous transfusion; the inhibitors to Factors V, XI, and XIII usually occur in those without the corresponding factor deficiency. Also called *circulating anticoagulants*. See also *Factor VIII inhibitor* and *lupus anticoagulant*.

coagulation pathways a series of enzymatic interactions leading to the formation of thrombin and the subsequent cleavage of the soluble plasma protein, fibrinogen, to form the insoluble fibrin clot. The initiation of the sequence can occur by two mechanisms, designated as the extrinsic and intrinsic pathways. Although these pathways are studied as two distinct entities, they probably interact in vivo from the beginning of the clotting process.

The extrinsic pathway involves a series of enzymatic reactions that are initiated by the release into the circulation of tissue factor (Factor III), a lipoprotein present in blood vessels and other tissues. Tissue factor forms a complex with Factor VII, which then activates Factor X to Xa, the lower case letter a indicating the activated form. Factor Xa, bound to a phospholipid surface (platelets) through the action of Factor V, activates Factor II (prothrombin) to form thrombin, with the thrombin cleaving fibrinogen to form fibrin. The intrinsic pathway involves a series of enzymatic reactions initiated by the activation of Factor XII by a negatively charged surface, presumably subendothelial collagen fibers, in the presence of kallikrein and high-molecular-weight kininogen. Factor XIIa and high-molecular-weight kininogen then activate Factor XI to XIa, which, in the presence of Ca^{++}, activates Factor IX to IXa. Factor IXa activates Factor X in the presence of a phospholipid surface, platelets, Ca^{++}, and Factor VIII. Factor Xa, bound to the platelets' surface by Factor V, then activates Factor II to form thrombin, with the thrombin cleaving fibrinogen to form fibrin. Once Factor X is activated, both the intrinsic and extrinsic pathways share a common pathway.

See also the accompanying illustration.

coagulation time test see *partial thromboplastin time test* and *prothrombin time test*.

coagulative (ko-ag′u-la″tiv) associated with or promoting the process of coagulation; of the nature of coagulation.

coagulative necrosis cell death in which there is retention of the basic cell shape but loss of the nucleus. The cell becomes a dense, homogeneous, acidophilic mass.

coagulum (ko-ag′u-lum), pl. *coagula* [L.] a clot or curd.

coal a black, solid, combustible, inhomogeneous material composed mostly of high–molecular-weight organic macromolecules that have aromatic rings connected with aliphatic cross-links. Much of the oxygen and nitrogen and some of the sulfur present in coal are included in the organic network as ether linkages, phenolic groups, pyridine rings, etc. Coal also contains smaller amounts of small molecules (M.W. < 1000) and inorganic compounds. It is mined as an important fuel and for other raw materials, such as coal tar, derivatives of which are used in industry and medicine. Exposure of workers to coal dust often leads to pulmonary fibrosis, with chronic bronchitis and emphysema (pneumoconiosis or anthrosilicosis—"black lung").

coal tar 1. a dark brown–black viscous liquid produced by the destructive distillation of coal. It has an odor of moth balls and a sharp, burning taste. Coal tar is a mixture of aromatic compounds (benzene, toluene, naphthalene, anthracene, and their phenol and arylamine derivatives); pyridine and other nitrogenous heterocyclic compounds; and complex compounds such as the coal tar dyes (e.g., pararosaniline). It is used as raw material for the manufacture of plastics, drugs, and other organic chemicals.

2. [USP], a 1–5 percent solution applied topically to treat eczema, psoriasis, and dermatosis.

coal worker's pneumoconiosis (CWP) see under *anthracosis*.

coarctate (ko-ark′tāt) [L. *coarctare* to straighten or tighten] 1. to press close together; contract.

2. pressed close together; restrained.

coarctation (ko″ark-ta′shun) [L. *coarctatio*, from *cum* together + *arctare* to make tight] a condition in which a structure is narrowed, thus restricting passage through its lumen; a constriction.

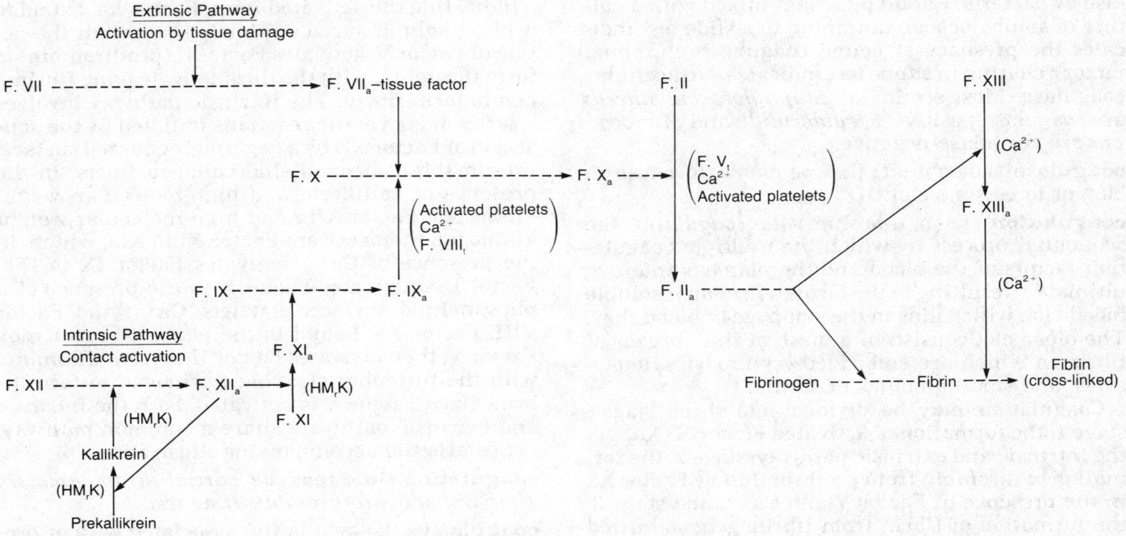

Coagulation pathways. F. V_t indicates thrombin-activated Factor V; F. VIII_t indicates thrombin-activated Factor VIII; HM_rR indicates high-molecular-weight kininogen; and parentheses indicate cofactor(s) for activation. (Courtesy of Marc A. Shuman, M.D.)

coarctation of the aorta a congenital area of constriction in the aorta, usually located distal to the insertion of the ductus arteriosus and origin of the subclavian artery. It occurs most frequently in males and is associated with Turner's syndrome and other cardiac abnormalities, most commonly a bicuspid aortic valve.

Classic signs include a midsystolic murmur, hypertension in the upper extremities, and hypotension in the lower extremities. Collateral circulation increases to help shunt blood to the lower body. Life-threatening hazards include left ventricular failure, endarteritis, cerebral aneurysm rupture, and rupture of the aorta. Diagnosis is made using clinical signs, electrocardiography, radiography, and angiography.

postductal c. of the a., a form of coarctation characterized by constriction distal to the insertion of the ductus arteriosus. Symptoms are manifested later in life, as fetal circulation is altered and collateral circulation forms in utero.

preductal c. of the a., a form of coarctation characterized by constriction proximal to the insertion of the ductus arteriosus. Symptoms develop early in life because fetal circulation is not substantially altered and collateral channels do not form until after birth.

coarsening (kōrs′en-ing) having a pattern that is abnormally coarse, as in describing the radiographic appearance of the gastric rugae or the texture of the skin.

coat (kōt) [L. *cotta* a tunic] a membrane or other structure covering or lining a part or organ; see also *buffy coat* and *tunica.*

Coats' disease (kōts) [George *Coats,* London ophthalmologist, 1876–1915] chronic progressive retinopathy, usually affecting male children, in which the fundus reveals an exudative retinal detachment associated with telangiectatic blood vessels and multiple hemorrhages. It may lead to total retinal detachment, iritis, glaucoma, and cataract.

cobalamin (ko-bal′ah-min) a name used for vitamin B_{12}, but more properly referring to that portion of vitamin B_{12} which contains the corrin ring, the 5,6-dimethylbenzimidazole residue, and cobalt, but not the cyanide or analogous ligands.

cobalt (Co) (ko′bawlt) [L. *cobaltum*] a silvery-gray, hard, ductile, ferromagnetic metallic element; atomic number 27; atomic weight 58.93; a 3d transition element; oxidation states +1 through +5 (+2 and +3 are most common). It is used in many high-temperature and magnetic alloys. Cobalt(III) is the central constituent of vitamin B_{12}. There is one natural isotope, ^{59}Co, and eight artificial isotopes, of which ^{60}Co is most important. The daily requirement is 0.2 μg; the daily intake, 4–8 μg. Inhalation of cobalt dust in industrial settings may produce asthma and pulmonary symptoms. The average level of cobalt in serum is 0.12–0.20 μg/dl. Most of the ingested cobalt is excreted; excessive amounts, however, may accumulate to cause polycythemia, goiter, cardiomyopathy, and nerve damage.

cobalt-57 (^{57}Co, Co 57) a cyclotron-produced radionuclide with a half-life of 270 da. It decays by electron capture, emitting gamma rays, most of which are the 122-keV and 136-keV emissions used for counting. See also *cyanocobalamin Co 57.*

cobalt-60 (^{60}Co, Co 60) a reactor-produced radionuclide with a half-life of 5.2 yr. It undergoes beta decay with the emission of 1.173-MeV gamma rays. Cobalt-60 is used as a gamma-ray source in megavoltage radiation therapy.

cobalt assays quantitative colorimetric assay. Following digestion with an oxidizing acid or ashing of the sample to remove interfering substances, the digest is made alkaline with ammonium hydroxide, and a specific violet-to-pink color is obtained by adding a solution of the *p*-nitrophenylhydrazone of diacetylmonoxime. Alternately, after removal of iron, copper, and nickel interferences, blue-colored cobalt thiocyanate can be formed and the concentration determined by measuring the absorbance at 625 nm.

cobaltinitrite method (ko″bawl-tĭ-ni′trāt) a histologic staining procedure that uses a cobaltinitrite reagent (cobaltous nitrite, sodium nitrite, and acetic acid) to demonstrate potassium as birefringent, chrome-yellow potassium cobaltinitrite crystals.

cobaltous chloride a salt, $CoCl_2$, formerly used to treat certain anemias; it produces polycythemia by stimulating erythropoietin production. Presumably cobaltous chloride inhibits enzymes involved in oxidative metabolism, thereby causing tissue hypoxia, which results in increased secretion of erythropoietin.

COBOL [acronym from *co*mmon *b*usiness *o*riented *l*anguage] a computer programming language designed for business applications in which the program has the appearance of plain English. Although it is less efficient and more difficult to use than newer programming languages, most business programs are still written in COBOL.

cobra (ko′brah) a term applied to several poisonous snakes of the genus *Naja,* family Elapidae, that are capable of expanding their neck regions to form a hood, and that have immovable hollow fangs. Native to Africa and Asia, cobras produce a venom having both neurotoxic and hemotoxic properties; it is a potent anticoagulant and causes hyperglycemia, coronary vessel dilation, and cardiac arrest. Antivenins are available through poison control centers or zoo administrators.

cocaine (ko′kān) [*coca* + *-ine*] [USP], an alkaloid, methylbenzoylecgonine, obtained from leaves of the coca tree, *Erythroxylon coca,* and other *Erythroxylon* species. Cocaine blocks nerve conduction in a manner similar to that of other local anesthetics; however, it also blocks the reuptake of norepinephrine at nerve terminals, producing sympathomimetic effects including increased cardiac rate, dilated pupils, and constricted blood vessels. Its vasoconstrictive property makes it useful as a topical anesthetic for surgery on the mucous membranes. Cocaine is also a central nervous system stimulant that produces euphoric excitement; abuse and dependence constitute a major drug problem. Hydrolysis of the drug in the gastrointestinal tract makes oral administration of therapeutic doses ineffective; it is, however, readily absorbed through the mucous membranes.

c. hydrochloride, [USP], the salt form of cocaine.

cocaine assays determination of cocaine in biologic specimens. After extraction from ammoniacal solution, cocaine can be quantitated by colorimetry, spectrophotometry, thin-layer chromatography, or gas-liquid chromatography. For urine assays, both heterogeneous and homogeneous immunoassay procedures are available. The latter are primarily directed toward benzoylecgonine, a major metabolite.

cocaine metabolite assay see under *benzoylecgonine.*

cocarboxylase (ko″kahr-bok′sĭ-lās) see *phosphorylated t.* under *thiamine.*

cocarcinogen (ko″kar-sin′o-jen, ko-kar′sin-o-gen″) [*co-* with, together + *carcinogen,* from Gr. *karkinos* crab + *gennan* to produce] an agent that is not in itself carcinogenic but increases the effect of a carcinogen, perhaps by rendering tissue more susceptible to the primary carcinogen, or by encouraging the multiplication of transformed cells. Many substances that were considered cocarcinogens are now considered to be promoters. See also *tumor p.* under *promoter.*

cocc/i, cocc/o [Gr. *kokkos* grain, seed] a word element used in combining form to denote relationship to coccoid bacteria, e.g., streptococci.

coccal (kok′al) resembling or pertaining to cocci.

Coccidia (kok-sid′e-ah) [pl. of N.L. *coccidium,* from *coccus* grain, seed] a subclass of sporozoa exhibiting alternation of generations with sexual and asexual stages of the life cycle. It contains the order Eucoccidia, which contains the suborders Eimeriina (including the parasitic species of the genera *Eimeria, Isospora,* and *Toxoplasma*) and Haemosporina (including *Plasmodium, Haemoproteus,* and *Hepatocystis*).

coccidioidal granuloma (kok-sid″e-oi′dal) see *coccidioidomycosis.*

Coccidioides (kok-sid″e-oi′dez) [N.L. *coccidium* + *-oides,* from Gr. *eidos* form] a genus of pathogenic imperfect fungi that grows as a mycelium with arthrospores in soil and as a spherule with endospores in tissue. The most important of its species is *C. immitis,* the etiologic agent of coccidioidomycosis.

coccidioidomycosis (kok-sid″e-oi″do-mi-ko′sis) [*Coccidioides* + Gr. *mykēs* fungus + *-osis* condition] a systemic mycosis, occurring in primary and secondary forms, that is caused by the organism *Coccidioides immitis;* it usually results in a flu-like illness. About 100,000 individuals are affected annually; 80-95 percent of those in areas where coccidiomycosis is endemic are skin-test positive. Many cases are asymptomatic.

EPIDEMIOLOGY. *C. immitis* is a soil saprophyte found in semiarid regions of the southwestern United States as well as Mexico and Central and South America. The fungus grows 3-4 in. below the surface of the soil, and following rainfall comes closer to the surface. On drying, arthrospores disseminate, and susceptible persons acquire the disease from inhaled spores or the infection of open skin lesions. Transmission in humans from a draining sinus has also been demonstrated.

PATHOGENIC MECHANISMS. The incubation period is 1–4 wk. Infection within the lungs may be pneumonic, involve hilar nodes, or both. Usually, the infection is self-limiting, although it becomes disseminated to bone, subcutaneous tissues, and the meninges in 5 percent of those affected.

Clinically, coccidioidomycosis is a variable flu-like illness, producing fever, cough, bone and joint pain, weight loss, chest pains, and sore throat. Some patients may develop erythema nodosum and erythema multiforme. These cutaneous manifestations are prognostic signs that the disease has probably become disseminated. The pulmonary manifestations usually disappear rapidly (95 percent of the time). Chronic pulmonary disease may be associated with significant exertional dyspnea, hemoptysis, or pleural effusion.

LABORATORY DIAGNOSIS. *C. immitis* grows within 4 da on enriched Sabouraud's medium at room temperature. Intraperitoneal injection of mice with the organism results in the appearance of spherules in pulmonary and splenic areas within 2 wk. Sputum and biopsy material may also show spherules, with endospores. Recently, special media have been developed to replace mice for the conversion of the growth pattern of the organism from mycelia to spherules. Microscopically, mycelia with boxcar-like arthrospores are characteristic of *C. immitis.*

There are several serologic tests available: the tube precipitin (TP), complement-fixation (CF), latex agglutination (LA), and immunodiffusion (ID) tests. The TP test is positive in more than 90 percent of the primary symptomatic cases. The CF test becomes positive later than the TP test, and it is most effective in determining disseminated disease. The ID test gives results that usually correlate with those observed with the CF test. The LA is a highly sensitive rapid test, but is not as specific as the TP test.

Also called desert rheumatisim, *San Joaquin Valley fever,* and *valley fever.*

coccidiosis (kok″sid″e-o′sis) [N.L. *coccidium* + *-osis* condition] an acute or chronic diarrhea of humans or animals, caused by several genera of sporozoa of the subclass Coccidia.

coccidium (kok-sid′e-um), pl. *coccidia* [N.L., from *coccus* grain] any organism of the order Coccidia.

coccobacillus (kok″o-bah-sil′us) [*cocco-* + L. *bacillus* small rod] an unusually short form of bacillus that is intermediate between the coccus and bacillus in shape.

coccoid (kok′oid) [*cocc-* + Gr. *eidos* form] resembling a coccus; globular.

coccus (kok′us), pl. *cocci* [L., from Gr. *kokkos* grain, seed] a bacterial cell with a spherical shape.

coccyg/o (kok′sĭ-go) [Gr. *kokkyx* cuckoo, whose bill the coccyx is said to resemble] a word element used in combining form to denote the coccyx (the tailbone), e.g., coccygeal.

coccyx (kok-siks), pl. *coccyges* [Gr. *kokkyx,* a cuckoo, the coccyx] the small bone at the lower end of the vertebral column formed by the fusion of four rudimentary vertebrae.

cochlea (kok′le-ah) [L. "snail shell"] 1. anything of spiral form.

2. [NA], a conical structure, resembling a snail's shell, that constitutes the anterior part of the labyrinth of the inner ear. It consists of a system of fluid-filled membranous tubes coiled within a bony canal that spirals around a central pillar. Within the cochlea is the sensory organ of hearing. See also *ear.*

cochlear duct (kok′le-ar) see *s. media* under *scala.*

Cochliomyia (kok″lĭ-o-mi′yah) a genus of flies (family Calliphoridae) whose larvae (maggots) develop in decaying flesh or in living tissue.

C. hominivorax, a species, the primary screwworm, that is found from the southern United States to northern Chile. It is an obligate myiasis-producing fly for which humans are the favored host. Infection with this worm may produce aural, ophthalmic, genitourinary, nasopharyngeal, or integumentary myiasis.

cockroach (kok′rōch) [Sp. *cucaracha*] see *Blattidae.*

cocoa butter see *theobroma oil.*

cocurrent (ko-kur′ent) pertaining to two streams flowing in the same direction, such as the sample streams on the two sides of the dialyzing membrane of an AutoAnalyzer.

code (kōd) [L. *codex* something written] 1. a set of rules governing conduct.

2. a system of representing information, which consists of a group of symbols and a set of rules for interpreting the meaning of sequences of the symbols. Examples are the various binary codes used by computers (the instruction set, binary integers, floating-point numbers, character codes) and the genetic code used by living organisms (the sequence of purine and pyrimidine bases along DNA molecules). See also *genetic code.*

coded aperture imaging a method of gamma-ray imaging used to produce tomographic images of the distribution of a radioisotope in the body. In the procedure, a coded aperture plate having a pattern of holes (several patterns are used) is inserted between the source and detector. Only the rays that pass through the holes contribute to the image; the rest are absorbed by the coded aperture plate. This coded image is reconstructed by projecting it through the coded aperture plate onto a screen. This reverses the imaging process, reconstructing a tomographic image in which the radioisotopic distribution of a single body plane is in sharp focus on the screen and the images of other planes are out of focus.

The same geometric relationship holds between the focal plane in the body, the coded aperture, and the detector in the original setup, and the screen, aperture, and film in the projection setup.

codeine (ko′dēn) [L. *codeina*] a colorless or white crystalline alkaloid, morphine-3-methyl ether, derived from the opium poppy but primarily prepared by methylation of morphine. Codeine is a metabolite of morphine and produces the morphinelike effects of analgesia, euphoria, and respiratory depression; it is also used to relieve coughing. Although its addiction potential is less than that of morphine or heroin, codeine is frequently abused. Also called *methylmorphine.*

codeine assays determination of codeine in biologic specimens. After extraction from alkaline solution, codeine can be detected by a variety of colorimetric procedures and quantitated by colorimetry, spectrophotometry, and thin-layer or gas-liquid chromatography. Both heterogeneous and homogeneous immunoassay procedures are available. As codeine is a metabolite of morphine, specificity of the assay procedure may be of prime importance.

coding (kōd′ing) 1. in statistics, the conversion of data to a more manageable form by the addition, subtraction, multiplication, or division of a constant to all members of the list of data.

2. in computer programming, a translation of logic and text of a program into computer-readable language.

3. in genetics, the relationship between the sequences of nucleotides in nucleic acids and amino acids in proteins.

coding triplet see *codon.*

Codman's triangle (kod′manz) [Ernest Amory *Codman,* Boston surgeon, 1869–1940] a triangular area visible radiographically, caused by the space left by the elevation and calcification of the periosteum at the border of a subperiosteal tumor.

codocyte (ko′do-sīt) see *target cell.*

codominance (ko-dom′ĭ-nans) the full expression of both alleles in a gene pair in the heterozygote, without either being influenced by the other; e.g., a person with the blood group AB shows I^A and I^B genes codominantly.

codon (ko′don) a series of three adjacent nucleotides in one polynucleotide chain of a DNA or RNA molecule, which directs the insertion of a specific amino acid in the growing polypeptide chain during protein synthesis. Also called *coding triplet* and *triplet.* See also *translation.*

coefficient (ko″ĕ-fish′ent) 1. a factor that serves as a multiplier in an algebraic equation.

2. a multiplier in a chemical equation; the number placed before a chemical formula that indicates how many molecules of that compound enter into the reaction.

coefficient of inbreeding see *inbreeding coefficient.*

coefficient of variation (CV) the standard deviation expressed as a percentage of the mean: $CV = (\sigma/\mu) \times 100$ percent, where μ is the mean and σ the standard deviation. The coefficient of variation is commonly used as a measure of precision for laboratory procedures. It is most useful when variation is proportional to the magnitude of the measured quantity and/or a dimensionless measure is needed for comparison on differing scales. Also called *relative standard deviation.*

Coelenterata (se-len″ter-a′tah) [Gr. *koilos* hollow + *enteron* intestine] a phylum of aquatic invertebrates that includes the hydras, jellyfish, sea anemones, and corals. Some species (*Physalia,* the Portuguese man-of-war) are equipped with nematocysts, stinging cells that inject a toxin capable of producing a burning pain, shock reaction, muscle cramps, paralysis, convulsions, and death.

coelom (se′lom) [Gr. *koilōma*] a cavity within the embryo, particularly the intraembryonic coelom or body cavity.

extraembryonic c., a cavity (chorionic cavity) that forms in the extraembryonic mesoderm and becomes filled with fluid. It is lined by the chorion and surrounds the embryo, yolk sac, connecting stalk, and amniotic cavity. It is obliterated when the amniotic cavity expands and the amnion fuses with the chorion.

intraembryonic c.'s, paired cavities that form on each side of the early embryo within the lateral mesoderm. They are initially in open connection with the extraembryonic coelom, but lose this connection and fuse to form a continuous body cavity with folding of the embryo. The pericardial, pleural, and peritoneal cavities develop from the intraembryonic coelom. Also called *coelomic cavity.*

coelomic cavity (se-lom′ik) see *intraembryonic c.* under *coelom.*

coenurus (se-nu′rus) [Gr. *koinos* common + *oura* tail] the generic name for the larvae of the tapeworm genus *Multiceps,* of the family Taeniidae, which are occasionally parasitic in humans and cause coenurosis.

coenzyme (ko-en′zim) an organic nonprotein molecule, frequently a phosphorylated derivative of a water-soluble vitamin, that is necessary for the activity of an enzyme. The coenzyme binds with the associated protein (apoenzyme) to form the active enzyme (holoenzyme). Important coenzymes are nicotinamide adenine dinucleotide (NAD, formerly coenzyme I or DPN), nicotinamide adenine dinucleotide phosphate (NADP, formerly coenzyme II or TPN), coenzyme A (phosphopantetheine), pyridoxal phosphate, thiamin pyrophosphate, and flavine adenine dinucleotide (FAD).

coenzyme I (Co I) see *nicotinamide adenine dinucleotide.*

coenzyme II (Co II) see *nicotinamide adenine dinucleotide phosphate.*

coenzyme A (CoA) a coenzyme composed of 4-phosphopantothenic acid, β-mercaptoethylamine, and adenosine-3′,5′-biphosphate. It serves as an acyl group transfer coenzyme, with the acyl group linked to the —SH group. Acetyl CoA, the activated form of acetate, is a key participant in the citrate synthase reaction, which is the initial step in the tricarboxylic acid (Krebs) cycle. See also *tricarboxylic acid cycle.*

coenzyme Q see *ubiquinone.*

coenzyme R the former name for vitamin B_7; see *biotin.*

coeur en sabot (ker on să-bo′) [Fr. "boot-shaped heart"] a heart appearing on a radiograph to have an increased transverse diameter and an elevated and rounded apex, vaguely resembling a wooden shoe. It is characteristic of the tetralogy of Fallot.

cofactor (ko′fak-tor) an element or principle (e.g., a coenzyme) with which another material (e.g., an enzyme) must unite or associate in order to function.

cognition (kog-nish′un) [L. *cognitio,* from *cognoscere* to know] the mental process by which individuals become aware of objects of thought and experience. Cognition is a broad term that includes all aspects of comprehension, judgment, memory, and reasoning.

coherent (ko-hēr′ent) 1. sticking together.

2. orderly and comprehensible.

3. in physics, pertaining to two waves that have the same wavelength and a definite (nonrandom) phase relationship so that interference effects can be produced by superimposing them. A laser produces coherent light; different parts of the beam are in phase. Other light sources are incoherent.

4. pertaining to a system of units, such as the International System (SI), in which the derived units are formed as a product or quotient of base units, as opposed to a noncoherent system in which conversion factors are necessary for the expression of the derived units in terms of the base units. One noncoherent unit, the liter, has been adopted for use in the International System. The coherent unit of volume is the cubic meter (m^3) because the meter is the base unit of length.

cohesion (ko-he′zhun) [L. *cohaesio,* from *con-* + *haerere* to stick] the forces of attraction that hold an object together or cause particles to clump or stick together.

cohesive termini (ko-he′siv) the short, single-stranded complementary ends of double-stranded DNA fragments that are cleaved by certain restriction endonucleases. The fragments can reanneal, joining end to end. Also called cohesive ends. See also *restriction endonuclease.*

cohort (ko′hort) [one of 10 units of a Roman legion, consisting of 300–600 soldiers] in statistics, a group of individuals who share a common characteristic, such as date of birth. In prospective studies, cohorts of subjects are followed over a period of years. The natural course of the process under study, e.g., a disease, is followed in individuals. This method avoids one type of misleading inference that can occur in cross-sectional studies in which the data obtained refer to the condition of the subjects at a single time and different stages of the disease or other process as seen in different individuals.

cohort labeling a method of labeling red cells of a single age for quantitative measurement of life span. In the procedure, when ^{59}Fe, ^{75}Se-selenomethionine, or ^{14}C-glycine is administered to a subject, it is rapidly incorporated into hemoglobin, thus labeling a cohort of newly formed red cells of approximately the same age. The erythrocyte life span is then recorded by plotting the radioactivity of the red cells until the last labeled cells disappear at 135–150 da. Normally, almost all the labeled cells live about 110 da, after which their number rapidly declines, with approximately half disappearing by 120 da. Cohort methods are more time-consuming than the more widely used random labeling methods (see *red cell survival test*); however, they are better able to distinguish a shortened red cell life span from low-intensity random red cell destruction.

cohort study see under *prospective study.*

coil (koil) 1. a helix.

2. a number of turns of wire around an air or iron core. Also called *choke* and *inductor.*

coincidence (ko-ĭn′si-dens) a group of two or more events occurring at the same time, which may or may not have a causal relationship.

coincidence correction (ko-in′sĭ-dens) a procedure by which the actual count accumulated by a radiation detection device can be adjusted to correct for coincidence losses. If r_t and r_o are the true counting rate and the observed counting rates and τ is the resolving time of the device, then $r_t = r_o/(1 - r_o\tau)$. The resolving time can be determined by calibrating with a source of known activity. Coincidence correction is also required for some particle counters, e.g., blood cell counters, that allow more than one particle through the counting orifice at one time.

coincidence error the loss of data by a detector as a result of its inability to respond to two events within a certain period of time—the resolving time for that instrument.

coincidence sum peak a peak in a gamma-ray spectrum caused by the simultaneous detection of two incident photons produced by the decay of one atom. This process is important only in the gamma well counter, which surrounds the source and can intercept both photons. Iodine-125, for example, produces a sum peak at 56 keV, which contains about half as many counts as the 28-keV photopeak, which corresponds to the single photon energy. Either two windows, or one that includes both peaks, should be used.

coin lesion a round, sharply delineated pulmonary radiodensity scan on a chest radiograph.

coinlike (koin′lik) shaped like a coin, i.e., a cylinder with a diameter several times the thickness. See also the illustration accompanying *contour.*

coitus (koi′tus) [L., from *coire* to go together] the act of sexual union; copulation.

col/o (ko′lo) [Gr. *kolon* colon] a word element used in combining form to denote the large intestine or colon, e.g., colonoscopy.

Colcemid (kol′sĕ-mid) trademark for a deacetylated *N*-methyl derivative of colchicine, used as a mitotic poison, especially in preparing karyotypes.

Colcher-Sussman method (kōl′cher sus′man) see under *pelvimetry.*

colchicine (kol′chi-sēn) [from *Colchis,* a city in Asia Minor] [USP], an alkaloid isolated from *Colchicum autumnale* (the autumn crocus or meadow saffron). It blocks microtubule formation by binding to tubulin monomers, preventing their polymerization. Colchicine and its derivatives are used in the laboratory for cytologic studies to arrest cell division in midmetaphase by disrupting the mitotic spindle fibers. Clinically, it is used to provide relief from acute attacks of gout and in conjunction with uricosuric agents (probenicid or sulfinpyrazone) and xanthine oxidase inhibitors (allopurinol) prophylactically to prevent acute attacks.

cold 1. a relatively low temperature as compared with a normal one; the lack of heat. A total absence of heat is absolute zero, at which all molecular action ceases.

2. a lay term for an acute and highly contagious virus infection of the upper respiratory tract; see also *rhinitis.*

cold agglutinin an agglutinin that reacts best below 37°C, often most strongly at temperatures of 0°–4°C; it is progressively weaker at higher temperatures. Also called *cold-reacting antibody.*

cold agglutinin syndrome a condition in which there is a high titer of cold agglutinins (1/1000–1/100,000). The antigens involved are the I, i, and Pr red cell antigens: polysaccharide antigens related to the ABO and Lewis blood groups. The cold agglutinins cause intravascular agglutination when the blood is cooled in peripheral parts of the body exposed to cold; they also cause mild hemolytic anemia as a result of complement fixation. On exposure to cold, the hands, feet, ears, and nose may turn a darker color and become painful; with rewarming the symptoms are reversed.

This syndrome occurs in two distinct clinical settings. In the first, chronic cold agglutinin disease of the elderly, there is a gradual onset and chronic course. The agglutinins usually contain monoclonal κ light chains. This condition may also be due to the presence of lymphoma in some individuals. In the second setting, postinfectious cold agglutinin syndrome, the syndrome follows infection with *Mycoplasma pneumoniae* or infectious mononucleosis. The course is self-limited, with manifestations disappearing in 2–3 mo (the agglutinins are not monoclonal and may be IgM, IgA, or IgG).

In addition to the high titer of cold agglutinins, those affected are also found to have large amounts of C3d, which results in a positive direct antiglobulin test.

Also called cold hemagglutinin disease.

cold agglutinin test a test to detect antibodies that cause the agglutination of erythrocytes at temperatures below 37°C. The test is performed by incubating human group O erythrocytes with dilutions of the patient's serum at 4°C. Cold agglutinins are found in patients with infectious mononucleosis, *Mycoplasma pneumoniae* infection, chronic parasitic infections, or lymphomas.

cold-knife conization see *conization.*

cold lesion in gamma-ray photography or scanning, a lesion that takes up less radionuclide than does the surrounding tissue, causing it to appear darker in the picture. Cf. *hot lesion.*

cold-reacting antibody see *cold agglutinin.*

cold room a refrigerated area large enough for laboratory personnel to enter.

cold sore a lesion caused by the herpes simplex virus, usually seen on the border of the lips or nostrils.

Cole's hematoxylin (kōlz) a hematoxylin stain variant that is prepared from a solution of hematoxylin, warm distilled water, 1 percent iodine in 95 percent ethanol, and saturated aqueous ammonium alum.

Coleman's Schiff reagent (kōl′manz) a variation of the traditional Schiff reagent that is 0.5 percent basic fuchsin, rather than 1 percent, and contains less acid. This reagent is generally used to stain fungi in Gridley's stain.

Coleoptera (kol″e-op′ter-ah) [Gr. *koleos* sheath + *pteron* wing] the order of insects that includes beetles. Their bodies have a leathery integument and two pairs of wings, the front pair being nonfunctional for flight but serving as horny coverings for the hind pair. Some species act as hosts for pathogenic helminths, such as *Gongylonema pulchrum, Macracanthorhynchus hirudinaceus,* and *Hymenolepis diminuta.* The volatile substance cantharidin, concentrated in the genitalia of some beetles, produces irritation or blisters on contact with human skin.

colestipol hydrochloride (ko-les′tĭ-pōl) a basic anion-exchange resin used in the treatment of hypercholesterolemia. It acts by binding and causing the excretion of bile acids; this increases the synthesis of bile acids from cholesterol and reduces serum cholesterol. Trademark, Colestid.

colic (kol′ik) [Gr. *kōlikos*] 1. pertaining to the colon. 2. acute spasmodic abdominal pain, such as intermittent visceral pain with fluctuations corresponding to smooth muscle peristalsis.

renal c., intermittent and acute pain usually resulting from the presence of one or more calculi in the kidney or ureter. The pain begins in the kidney region and radiates forward and downward to envelop the abdomen, genitalia, and legs. Other symptoms include nausea, vomiting, diaphoresis, and a frequent urge to urinate.

colicin (kol′ĭ-sin) [*coli* (from *Escherichia coli*) + *-cin* (adapted from L. *caedere* to kill)] a term for a bacteriocin produced by any strain of *Escherichia coli.* Owing to inaccurate historical nomenclature, however, colicin E_3 is actually produced by *Shigella sonnei* and is active against *E. coli.* Colicins are the prototype bacteriocin and are the best studied. They have been useful in investigating the physiology of many bacteria, as well as in typing various strains according to colicin susceptibility.

Colicin E_1 and colicin K kill specific bacteria by uncoupling electron transport from active transport of amino acids, disrupting the cell membrane, and eventually inhibiting macromolecular synthesis. Colicin E_2 is an endonuclease that degrades DNA in susceptible bacteria. Colicin E_3 inhibits protein synthesis by binding and cleaving ribosomal 16S RNA. Colicin E_4 affects energy metabolism through proteolytic activity.

See also *bacteriocin.*

colicinogen one of the bacterial plasmids called bacteriocinogens that regulate the production of bacteriocin in bacteria. Colicinogen is the term used for such plasmids when they are detected in strains of *Escherichia coli.* They may also be conjugative, i.e., act as sex factors. See also *bacteriocinogen.*

coliform (ko′li-form) [*Escherichia coli* + *-form*] a general term referring to various enteric gram-negative bacilli. See also *coliform b.* under *bacillus* and *E. coli* under *Escherichia.*

colinearity (ko-lin″e-ar′ĭ-te) in genetics, the property that describes the linear relationship between the units of triplet sequence of nucleotides in DNA (or in RNA transcribed from it) and the corresponding sequence of amino acids in the polypeptide chain. However, some stretches of DNA molecules may not code for any peptide, and the final assembly of messenger RNA and DNA in higher organisms may require a considerable amount of processing, namely, deletion and splicing of selected segments.

colipase (ko-li′pās) a noncatalytic protein of pancreatic juice that functions to prevent the denaturation of pancreatic lipase on the interface of triglycerides and water and to promote its action; M.W. 10,000.

coliphage (kol′ĭ-fāj) any of the bacteriophages that infect *Escherichia coli.* This group of viruses has been widely used in studies of virus replication and viral genetics.

colistimethate sodium (ko-lis″ti-meth′āt) [USP], the penta(methanesulfonate) derivative of colistin, the form for parenteral use. See also *colistin sulfate.*

colistin sulfate (ko-lis′tin) [USP], an antibiotic of the polymyxin group. It has a cyclopolypeptide structure containing α-γ-diaminobutyrate and is produced by a strain of *Bacillus polymyxa.* It is effective against many of the enteric bacilli and similar gram-negative bacteria, but its use is limited by its toxic nature. Also called colimycin or polymyxin E. See also *antibacterial agents* and *polymyxin.*

colitis (ko-li′tis) [*col-* + *-itis*] a nonspecific term used to refer to inflammation of the colon. It should be reserved for inflammatory diseases (e.g., ulcerative colitis, ischemic colitis) and should not be used for functional disorders (e.g., spastic colon), more properly described as *irritable bowel syndrome.*

amebic c., see *amebiasis.*

granulomatous c., see *regional i.* under *ileitis.*

ischemic c., a disorder, primarily found in individuals older than 50 yr, that is due to impaired arterial blood flow to the intestines. Intestinal involvement may be focal or widespread, and is characterized by mucosal and submucosal ulceration and hemorrhage. A variety of conditions may precipitate ischemic colitis, including aortic surgery, atherosclerosis, vasculitis, and coagulation disorders.

mucous c., see *irritable bowel syndrome.*

pseudomembranous c., an acute disease of the intestinal tract characterized by mucosal necrosis and replacement by a membranelike exudate. It has been associated with a variety of conditions, including gastrectomy, vascular collapse with bowel anoxia, and staphylococcal overgrowth following preoperative bowel "sterilization" with wide-spectrum antibiotics (clostridial infections have also been implicated). Increasing numbers of cases have also been linked to therapy with the drugs lincomycin and clindamycin. Those affected experience a rapid onset of abdominal pain, nausea, and profuse bloody diarrhea, with fever, dehydration, and abdominal tenderness.

Laboratory tests reveal leukocytosis, thrombocytopenia, and renal abnormalities. X-rays may reveal the presence of gas. Diagnosis is confirmed by proctoscopic demonstration of yellow-white plaques, edematous walls, and membranes composed of fibrin, mucus, and cellular elements. The mortality associated with this disease is high.

radiation c., damage to the large intestine that occurs following radiation therapy. Mucosal thickness decreases with progressive epithelial sloughing, leading to crypt abscesses and ulceration. In severe instances, there is vascular degeneration and ischemia, and perforation can occur.

Most often there is diarrhea and intestinal bleeding, and a variety of malabsorption disorders may occur. Diagnosis is based on patient history, clinical picture, sigmoidoscopy, barium studies, and angiography. Prognosis is based on the extent of damage, the course of underlying malignancy, and the patient's age.

spastic c., see *irritable bowel syndrome.*

ulcerative c., a recurrent, acute inflammatory process that involves part or all of the large intestine. It may extend to the rectum, and infrequently crosses the ileocecal valve into the terminal ileum. Usually the process is confined to the mucosa.

The prevalence of ulcerative colitis in the United States is fewer than 100 individuals per 100,000 population. There is a peak incidence between the ages of 15 and 30 yr, and a smaller increase around age 60. The condition is slightly more common in females than in males, and may present or become aggravated during pregnancy. The incidence is lower in blacks and higher in Jewish persons. There is no convincing evidence of a relationship between ulcerative colitis and socioeconomic status. The cause is not known, but it has been suggested that ulcerative colitis might be the final common pathway of a variety of pathologic processes involving the colon. Infectious agents have not been proven to be associated with the disorder. A familial occurrence has been demonstrated, indicating that genetic factors may be involved.

Diarrhea, often with the passage of blood and mucus in the stools, is the common presenting symptom, and the patient may complain of pain during defecation. Vomiting, weight loss, and fever are also seen. The diagnosis is made by barium enema, sigmoidoscopy, and biopsy; the histologic features vary with the stage of the disease. The process begins with regressive changes in the epithelium of the mucosal crypts, accompanied by a migration of neutrophils from the lamina propria into the intestinal lumen. Foci of necrosis develop within mucosal glands (crypt abscesses) and extend and coalesce to produce a distinctive hyperemic, shaggy, ulcerated mucosa. Subsequently, a chronic inflammatory response is superimposed, but fibrosis is not conspicuous. It is unusual for the process to involve the deeper layers of the wall of the colon.

The clinical course is quite variable, but typically is one of progression with exacerbations and remissions. The course is more severe when the disease first appears in young individuals and when the early symptoms are severe. The more extensive the involvement, the poorer the prognosis; the outlook is better when only the sigmoid and rectum are affected. Lesions may develop in other tissues. In the liver, fatty change occurs in roughly half those affected, and a few develop cirrhosis. One person in four has skin lesions, usually erythema nodosum, and less commonly, pyoderma gangrenosum. Some 10 percent of those affected have an associated arthritis, and rarely systemic amyloidosis. Longstanding ulcerative colitis is recognized to be a precancerous lesion, and 6 percent of those affected develop adenocarcinoma of the colon, usually after having the disease for at least 10 yr; the 5-yr survival rate for those with carcinoma is roughly 20 percent.

Ulcerative colitis must be differentiated from Crohn's disease (regional enteritis), which primarily involves the small intestine but may also occur in the colon (regional colitis). The two conditions are often grouped together under the generic term inflammatory bowel disease, and it has even been suggested that they may represent different responses to a common etiology, although the evidence favors their not being related. A comparison of the features of the two disorders is shown in the accompanying table.

Cf. *Crohn's disease.*

colitose (kol'ĭ-tōs) 3,6-dideoxy-L-galactose, an unusual sugar found in the O-specific chains in the lipopolysaccharides of certain serotypes of *Salmonella* and *Escherichia coli.*

collagen (kol'ah-jen) [Gr. *kolla* glue + *gennan* to produce] a protein present in the connective tissue throughout the body in the form of slender fibrils of high tensile strength and distinctive periodicity. It is formed by fibroblasts, as are the other basic elements of connective tissue, elastin and the proteoglycans of the ground substance. Other mesenchymal cells can also form collagen.

Collagen fibrils aggregate to form bundles and sheets that vary in density and in their relative proportions of elastin and ground substance, depending on the functional requirement of the tissue. Thus, collagen is densely packed in tendons but is sparse in the vitreous humor of the eye and the stroma of myxoid tumors. Thin sheets of collagen (reticulin) form a supporting network for the cells of the bone marrow, lymph nodes, thymus, and spleen; collagen is also present in the basal lamina of epithelia.

Collagen fibrils are formed in the extracellular space from tropocollagen filaments that are synthesized within fibroblasts from glycine, hydroxyproline, and other amino acids. Because collagen is the only human protein that contains appreciable amounts of hydroxyproline, its quantity within a tissue may be measured indirectly by the amount of hydroxyproline the latter contains.

At least four types of collagen, differing slightly in amino acid composition, are found in the human body. A tropocollagen filament is approximately 300 nm long and is formed by the wrapping of three helical chains of amino acids. Overlapping of the tropocollagen filaments produces the 67-nm periodicity of the collagen fibril. Under certain conditions, collagen can dissociate and recombine with the filaments in register to form segment-long-spacing (SLS) collagen. Collagenases formed by fibroblasts and other cells including neutrophils and macrophages can cleave tropocollagen molecules

ULCERATIVE COLITIS. REGIONAL AND ULCERATIVE COLITIS COMPARED

	REGIONAL ENTERITIS	ULCERATIVE COLITIS
Natural History		
Occurrence in animals	pigs, dogs	none
Occurrence in humans	worldwide	worldwide
Incidence (U.K. & N. Amer. gen. white)	0.8–1.8 cases per 100,000	4.6–6.5 cases per 100,000
(non-white)	? less in Am. negro	? less in non-white
(Jews)	9× higher than general white	2–4× higher than general white
Prevalence	9 cases/100,000	80 cases/100,000
Male to female ratio	1:1	1:1.3–1.5
Familial occurrence	1–2% of cases	1–2% of cases
Age at onset	15–55 equal rate	peaks 20–40 and 65
Annual death rate (U.K. & N. Amer. white)	0.08–0.11 deaths per 100,000	0.05–0.9 deaths per 100,000
Etiology	unknown	unknown
Macroscopic Features		
Distribution of lesions	1. stomach to anus 2. principally terminal ileum and cecum 3. discontinuous lesions	1. ileum to anus 2. principally rectosigmoid 3. continuous lesions
Length of diseased organ	unchanged	decreased
Diameter of diseased organ	decreased	unchanged
Thickness of bowel wall	markedly increased	unchanged
Ulceration	yes	yes
Vascular congestion	yes	yes
Muscular hypertrophy	usually	sometimes
Serosal changes	yes	no
Ileocecal valve	constricted	loose, patulous
Mesentery	short, thick, indurated	unchanged
Adhesions	frequent	rare
Fistulas	common	uncommmon
Carcinomatous change	rare	frequent (2–5% of cases)
Microscopic Features		
Inflammation distribution	all layers	mucosa and submucosa
Ulcers	deep clefts	shallow
Mucin production	normal or increased	normal or decreased
Mast cell infiltrate	minimal	increased
Lymphocytosis	extreme	extreme
Histiocytic proliferation	extensive	none
Collagen production	extensive	scanty if any
Crypt abscesses	rare	common
Pseudopolyps	absent	common
Lymphangitis	early obliterative	none
Lymph node hyperplasia	moderate	moderate
Lymph node granulomas	present	absent
Extraintestinal Lesions		
Liver granulomata	present	absent
Sclerosing cholangitis	rare	frequent
Erythema nodosum	occasional	occasional
Arthritis (nonspecific)	3–10% of cases	25% of cases
Spondylitis	2% of cases	2% of cases
Amyloidosis	rare	rare

From Mottet, N. K.: Histopathologic Spectrum of Regional Enteritis and Ulcerative Colitis. Philadelphia, W.B. Saunders Co., 1971, p. 237.

during processes of resorption for remodeling or repair of connective tissue.

collagenase (kol-laj′e-nās) a proteinase with a specificity for collagen. Vertebrate collagenase (EC 3.4.24.7) refers to a group of Zn^{2+}-containing enzymes occurring ubiquitously in animals. All preferentially cleave a single bond in native collagen at a site between a glycine residue and a leucine or isoleucine residue, leaving a large N-terminal fragment (75 percent) and a small C-terminal fragment (25 percent). Most are secreted in an inactive form that requires activation by proteolytic enzymes. They are involved in collagen resorption during tissue repair and are secreted by fibroblasts, neutrophils, and other cells.

Clostridium histolyticum collagenase (EC 3.4.24.3; also called clostridiopeptidase A) cleaves helical regions of native collagen into small fragments, preferentially attacking the —Gly bond in the sequence Z—Pro—X—Gly—Pro—X. This enzyme breaks down the collagen framework of muscles, facilitating the spread of the organism to deeper tissues in gas gangrene. Many bacteria produce similar collagenases.

collagen diseases a group of diseases or conditions that are clinically distinct and etiologically unrelated, but that have as a common feature a widespread inflammatory damage to connective tissue. Collagen diseases do not include the genetic disorders in which the collagen molecule can be abnormal, e.g., osteogenesis imperfecta, Ehlers-Danlos syndrome. A frequently associated occurrence in collagen diseases is the deposition of a fibrinoid substance (an amorphous, eosinophilic substance composed primarily of fibrin) along the connective tissue fibers.

Each condition classified as a collagen disease has a nonspecific pattern of renal, cardiovascular, gastrointestinal, pulmonary, musculoskeletal, and cutaneous involvement that establishes its specific clinical designation.

For more information, see the entries on individual collagen diseases, such as *dermatomyositis, systemic l. erythematosus* under *lupus, polymyositis, rheumatic fever, rheumatoid arthritis,* and *scleroderma.*

collagenous fibers (kol-laj′ĕ-nus) thick (1–10 μm) fibers composed of bundles of cross-linked collagen fibrils, which are found in all types of connective tissue. They provide the tensile strength of tissues such as tendons and ligaments, and form the matrix on which calcium phosphate is deposited in bone. See also *collagen.* Cf. *reticular fibers.*

collagen staining methods specific histologic stains for collagen, which has an affinity for acid aniline dyes, such as acid fuchsin or aniline blue, under strongly acidic conditions. In some methods, picric acid serves as both the acidifier and as a plasma stain; see *van Gieson's stain.*

In other methods, the stain is preceded by mordanting in phosphotungstic or phosphomolybdic acid; see *Gomori's trichrome stain, Heidenhain's azan stain, Mallory's collagen, Masson's trichrome method,* and *Movat's pentachrome method.*

collapse (ko-laps′) [L. *collapsus*] 1. to break down or flatten.

2. a state of extreme prostration.

collateral (kŏ-lat′er-al) [*con-* + L. *latus* side] 1. secondary or accessory; not direct or immediate.

2. a small side-branch, as of a blood vessel or nerve.

collateral ventilation the entrance of gas into alveoli with obstructed airways through collateral channels (presumably the alveolar pores or Lambert's canals) from adjacent ventilated alveoli. As this gas is alveolar (low in oxygen and high in carbon dioxide) and not fresh air, little change results in the O_2 saturation of the blood flowing past these alveoli.

collector (kŏ-lek′tor) one of the terminals of a junction transistor.

College of American Pathologists (CAP) a professional organization of pathologists.

colliculus (kol-lik′u-lus), pl. *colliculi* [L.] a small elevation or mound.

inferior c., the caudal pair of the four eminences that constitute the corpora quadrigemina on the tectum of the mesencephalon. These structures are involved with relaying auditory information and the localization of sound; they receive tonotopically organized input from the lateral lemniscus and project ipsilaterally via the inferior brachium to the medial geniculate body. The paired inferior colliculi are connected by a substantial commissure; they project to the brain stem and spinal cord via fibers to the superior colliculus.

superior c., The rostral pair of the four eminences that make up the corpora quadrigemina on the tectum of the mesencephalon. Long thought to be associated primarily with visual reflexes, those structures appear to integrate vision with a broad array of body activities.

2,4,6-collidine (kol′ĭ-dēn) the trivial name for 2,4,6-trimethylpyridine, used as a buffer in histology. Also called *s*-collidine.

colligative (kol′ĭ-ga″tive) [L. *colligare* to bind together] a term used to refer to properties of solutions that depend only on the number of free particles present, either ions or undissociated molecules. Four colligative properties of solutions are recognized: osmotic pressure, vapor pressure depression, boiling point elevation, and freezing point depression. They are all interrelated and the value of any one can be used to determine the values of the others. Measurements are usually expressed in osmoles per liter (osmol/l) or osmoles per kilogram. See also *osmometer.*

collimate (kol′ĭ-māt) [L. *collimare,* misspelling of *collineare* to direct along a straight line] 1. to make parallel.

2. to adjust the line of sight of an optical instrument.

3. to use a collimator.

collimator (kol″ĭ-ma′tor) 1. a device that produces a beam of parallel rays of light or other radiation.

2. a device that produces a beam of limited cross section. In radiography, a collimator is an adjustable beam delimiter attached to the x-ray tube housing at the port. Two pairs of movable iron or lead shutters form a rectangular aperture through which the primary beam passes. All new diagnostic x-ray machines are required by federal regulations to have an automatic collimator, which limits the beam to the exact site of the film.

3. in nuclear medicine, a device placed in front of the detector of a scintillation camera or rectilinear scanner to absorb gamma rays traveling in inappro-

priate directions. The collimator is analogous to a camera lens in that it forms the image, but it does not focus the rays by bending them as a lens does. The collimator consists of one or more holes surrounded by walls (usually referred to as septa) of lead or another dense metal.

In multihole collimators (also called multichannel collimators), the holes are usually arranged in a uniform array with hexagonal spacing.

The rectilinear scanner is used with a multichannel focused collimator, in which all the holes are tapered, the conical sides pointing toward a common apex called the focus. In the focal plane, the fields of view of all the holes overlap so that only gamma rays emitted from a small circle centered at the focus reach the detector. The radius of this circle, called the geometric radius of view, provides one measure of the spatial resolution of the collimator. As the detector is scanned over an organ, only emissions from a point in the focal plane are recorded while the detector axis is within the geometric radius of view of the point. Above or below the focal plane, the fields of view overlap only partially or not at all. This produces a tomographic effect: emissions from a point outside the focal zone are recorded at widely dispersed points on the scan so that the image is blurred.

When magnification or minification is not required, the scintillation camera is used with a parallel-hole multichannel collimator. Each point of the detector sees only points in the narrow cone visible through one collimator hole. The spatial resolution of the collimator is best in the plane of the collimator face where the radius of view is restricted to the size of a hole.

The image is magnified by a converging collimator in which the cylindric holes are aimed at a point behind the object and minified by a diverging collimator in which the holes are aimed away from a point behind the detector. Both collimators produce some distortion of the image because more distant parts of the object are more magnified (minified), as are parts nearer the perimeter of the image.

The pinhole collimator has a single small aperture located some distance from the detector. It produces an inverted image that has a magnification factor equal to the ratio of the aperture-detector distance to the aperture-object distance. This collimator magnifies nearby objects and minifies those farther away; thus, when used for magnification, the distortion is opposite that of a coverging collimator.

Because the intrinsic resolution of the camera is related to the size of the image, magnification improves the overall system resolution, whereas minification reduces it. The radius of spatial resolution of the pinhole collimator is proportional to the magnification and the aperture size. The resolution of the converging and diverging collimators is proportional to the product of the magnification and the detector-object distance.

The sensitivity of a collimator is measured by its geometric efficiency, the detector response to a uniform plane source, which is proportional to the area of the collimator holes. It is independent of distance in air and falls off exponentially in a scattering medium.

The septal penetration fraction is the ratio of the gamma rays that pass through the septa to those passing through the holes. The septa must be thick enough so that the penetration fraction, which increases with gamma-ray energy, is kept below 5–10 percent.

Spatial resolution, sensitivity, and septal penetration are conflicting parameters. The resolution improves with hole number and collimator thickness, whereas sensitivity improves with hole area and collimator thinness. Therefore, different collimators are used for different applications. High resolution is used to detect small lesions, high sensitivity to detect large ones.

collision (ko-lĭ′zhun) in studies of peripheral nerve conduction velocity, a conduction block caused by the propagation of two action potentials toward one another from opposite portions of the nerve. When the two potentials meet, their refractory periods prevent propagation in either direction from the point of interaction.

collodion (kol-lo′de-on) [L. *collodium,* from Gr. *kollōdēs* glutinous] [USP], a clear or slightly opalescent, highly flammable, syrupy liquid compounded of pyroxylin (chiefly nitrocellulose), ether, and alcohol, which dries to a transparent, tenacious film; used as a topical protectant and as a bag for processing fluids to prepare cell blocks for histologic examination.

colloid (kol′oid) [Gr. *kollōdēs* glutinous] 1. a suspension of particles so small (1 nm–1 μm) that they do not settle out by gravity.

2. any material, such as a foam, with one finely divided phase dispersed in another. Also called colloidal dispersion, emulsion, or suspension.

3. the iodinated glycoprotein (thyroglobulin) stored within the thyroid follicles. It is formed and degraded by the surrounding follicular cells.

colloidal (kol-loi′dal) pertaining to a colloid or to the dispersed phase of a colloid.

colloidal gold a stable gold colloid formerly used to identify and quantitate cerebrospinal fluid proteins. Abnormal precipitation of the gold is produced in CSF from individuals with abnormal CSF protein in composition, caused by diseases such as syphilis, multiple sclerosis, poliomyelitis, and encephalitis.

colloidal iron stain a histologic staining method for acid mucopolysaccharides and acidic epithelial mucins, which are stained deep blue. Paraffin sections are immersed in Müller's colloidal iron solution and then in acidic potassium ferrocyanide. Acidic polysaccharides bind the colloidal iron, which is then demonstrated by the Prussian blue reaction. Müller's colloidal iron stock solution is prepared by adding 4.4 ml of 29 percent ferric chloride solution to 250 ml of boiling water; boiling is continued until the dark red ferric oxide colloid is formed. Before use, 20 ml of stock solution is combined with 15 ml of water and 5 ml of glacial acetic acid.

colloidal osmotic pressure see under *osmotic pressure.*

colloid body a homogeneous, eosinophilic, hyalinized body, round to oval in shape, that averages about 10 μm in diameter. These structures represent degenerated epidermal basal cells and are seen in the lower epidermis and papillary dermis in lichen planus, discoid lupus erythematosus, and, on occasion, in other skin diseases with damage to basal cells. Colloid bodies contain glycoprotein (PAS-positive, diastase-resistant) and immunoglobulins, complement, and fibrin. Also called *Civatte body* and *hyaline body*.

colloid-osmotic lysis see *osmotic hemolysis*.

coloboma (kol″o-bo′mah), pl. *colobomas, colobomata* [L, from Gr. *kolobōma*] the congenital absence or defect of any portion of the eye. Typical colobomas arise from failure of closure of the fetal optic fissure. Uninherited atypical colobomas involve areas of the eye that do not originate from the embryonic cleft.

colon (ko′lon) [Gr. *kolon*] the major portion of the large intestine, between the cecum and rectum; see *large intestine*. See also *colon tumors*.

colonization (kol″ŏ-nĭ-za′shun) the establishment and growth of an exogenous microorganism in or on a host; immune or clinical manifestations may or may not follow colonization.

colonoscope (ko-lon′o-skōp) an elongated, flexible fiberoptic endoscope that permits visual examination of the entire colon.

colonoscopy (ko″lon-os′ko-pe) [*colon* + Gr. *skopein* to examine] a diagnostic procedure, performed transabdominally during laparotomy, or transanally, to visualize the entire length of the colon from anus to cecum by means of a flexible fiberoptic endoscope. Transanal colonoscopy, with instruments 105–185 cm in length, may be used to visualize the entire colon in approximately 80 percent of individuals, producing a complication rate (bleeding and perforation) of less than 1 percent.

Some of the uses of fiberoptic colonoscopy include polyp removal, confirmation of lesions unresolved radiographically, examination for sources of bleeding, periodic evaluation of the colon following removal of a typical polyp or a partial colonic resection for cancer, and examination of the colon in patients with chronic inflammatory bowel disease.

colon tumors neoplasms of the colon; most are epithelial.

Benign epithelial neoplasms of the colon are usually polypoid and are generally referred to as adenomatous polyps. Adenomatous polyps occur at any level of the colon and are often pedunculated. A spectrum of histologic patterns is seen in these tumors, ranging from the tubular adenoma through the tubulovillous adenoma to the villous adenoma (see under *adenoma* and *polyp*).

The incidence of adenocarcinoma of the colon is considerably higher in Europe and North America than it is in economically underdeveloped countries such as areas of Africa and South America. Dietary factors have been implicated in its genesis. Most adenocarcinomas of the colon arise in preexisting adenomatous polyps). The incidence of adenocarcinoma of the colon in persons with familial polyposis is extremely high: virtually all those affected eventually develop malignant transformation of one or more adenomatous polyps (see *polyposis*). The better differentiated adenocarcinomas form well-defined glands, but with loss of differentiation there is a transition to more solid forms, and spindle cell transformation can occur. Clinical staging of colonic adenocarcinoma is generally based on the method of Dukes (stage A tumors are confined to the wall of the colon, stage B tumors have infiltrated transmurally to reach pericolic fat, and stage C tumors also involve lymph nodes). Both the histologic grade and the stage of the tumor influence the patient's prognosis: 5-yr survival rates are above 90 percent for well-differentiated tumors having only superficial invasion of the submucosa, in contrast to less than a 30 percent survival rate for individuals with stage C tumors. The location of the adenocarcinoma also influences prognosis. Tumors of the distal colon are more aggressive and likely to give rise to lymph node metastasis than those of the proximal colon.

Endocrine neoplasms arising in the colon are generally designated as carcinoid tumors, although immunocytochemical studies show that not all form serotonin. The Grimelius stain is usually positive, but argentaffin and argyrophil procedures may be negative. Coexistence of a carcinoid tumor and an adenocarcinoma of the colon is a rare occurrence. Large cell lymphoma may be primary within the colon, although lymphomas are less common in this location than in more proximal segments of the gastrointestinal tract.

Smooth muscle tumors are the most frequent mesenchymal neoplasms arising in the colon, but they are nevertheless uncommon tumors in this location. Leiomyomas are the most common mesenchymal tumor of the colon but are rare except in the rectum. Leiomyosarcomas can occur at any level of the large intestine.

See also *polyp*.

colony (kol′o-ne) [L. *colonia*, from *colere* to dwell] a mass of individual cells of bacteria or yeasts on the surface of a solid nutrient medium, arising from a single organism or small number of organisms, and visible to the naked eye or by low-power microscopy. Characteristics of the colony, although influenced by the nature of the culture medium and conditions of incubation, are relatively constant for the organism and constitute one of the most important initial steps in identifying microbial species. Colonies are classified according to surface texture (rough, R; smooth, S; mucoid, M), size, shape, elevation from the surface of the medium, pigmentation, and description of borders.

mucoid (M) c., a large, dome-shaped, and shiny colony of bacteria or yeasts, which may be drawn out in viscous strings by a needle. The mucoid nature of this type of colony is due to the capsular polysaccharides produced by the bacteria. Also called M-type.

raised c., a bacterial colony with a thick center that diminishes uniformly to the edge.

rough (R) c., a colony that shows a wrinkled, dry surface; also called R-type.

smooth (S) c., a colony that shows a moist, glistening, rounded, regular surface. It is the form normally shown by microorganisms. Also called S-type.

colony-forming unit (CFU) 1. any of several hematopoietic stem cells that have been identified by their ability to give rise to monoclonal colonies in the spleen when transplanted into isogeneic, lethally irradiated mice. Included in this class are the pluripotent myeloid stem cell (CFU-S) and the precursors of neutrophils and monocytes (CFU_{NM}), eosinophils (CFU_{EOS}), erythrocytes (CFU_{E}), and megakaryocytes (CFU_{MEG}). See also *stem cell*.

2. in microbiology, a term used to estimate the number of bacteria or yeasts by counting the colonies on a solid medium. One bacterium is considered equal to one colony, but use of the term CFU recognizes the likelihood that some colonies have developed from two or more organisms that were

attached or were close to each other when inoculated.

colony-stimulating activity (CSA) see *colony-stimulating factor.*

colony-stimulating factor (CSF) any of several substances produced by blood monocytes, tissue macrophages, and stimulated lymphocytes, required for differentiation of the CFU_{NM} cells into granulocyte and monocyte cell colonies in vitro. Release of the factor from macrophages may be stimulated by endotoxin from gram-negative bacteria. CFU is demonstrable in blood and urine and appears to play a physiologic role in the in vivo regulation of granulocytopoiesis. Also called *colony-stimulating activity.*

color (kul′or) [L.] 1. a property of visible light that subsists in the wavelengths of its components.

2. a property of an object, the color of the light it transmits or reflects when illuminated with white light.

3. a perception, the response of the visual system to colored light. See also *color vision* and *spectrum.*

complementary c.'s, a pair of colors, e.g., blue and orange or red and green, that produce an achromatic hue when mixed.

primary c.'s, 1. the three colors—red, yellow, and blue—that can be mixed to produce any hue.

2. the three colors—red, green, and blue—that correspond to the maximal sensitivity of the three types of color receptor in the eye.

spectral c., a perceived hue that can be produced by monochromatic light and also by combinations of wavelengths that produce the same ratios of stimulation of the visual pigments.

Colorado tick fever a benign arthropod-vector disease caused by the RNA virus *Orbivirus.* It is characterized by headache, ocular pain, backache, muscle and joint pain, nausea, and leukopenia. The disease is transmitted by the wood tick *Dermacentor andersoni* and occurs in the Rocky Mountain states. Laboratory identification of *Orbivirus* infection involves the serologic detection of virus antigens by immunofluorescence of a peripheral blood smear. There are approximately 2000 cases annually.

color blindness defective color vision due to the partial or total lack of function of one or more types of color receptors (cones). The vision is trichromatic if there is at least partial function in all three types, dichromatic if in only two, and monochromatic if only one type functions. Color blindness is also classified as protanopia (no red vision), deuteranopia (no green), tritanopia (no yellow), protanomaly (weak red vision), deuteranomaly (weak green), and tritanomaly (weak yellow).

The two most common types are protanopia and deuteranopia, which are jointly referred to as red-green color blindness. The incidence of protanopia is 2 percent in males and 0.04 percent in females; that of deuteranopia is 6 percent in males and 0.36 percent in females. Both types are X-linked mendelian traits; their loci are closely linked to the loci for hemophilia A and glucose-6-phosphate dehydrogenase deficiency.

Several other color blindness traits occur very rarely: monochromatic blue color blindness and tritanomaly (both X-linked), total color blindness (an autosomal recessive trait in which all cones are missing), and tritanopia (an autosomal dominant trait). Color blindness can also be due to nongenetic conditions.

Also called *parachromatopsia.*

colorectitis (ko″lo-rek-ti′tis) [*colo-* + L. *rectum* straight + *-itis* inflammation] inflammation of the colon and rectum; coloproctitis.

colorimeter (kul″or-im′ĕ-ter) [*color* + Gr. *metron* measure] an optical instrument that measures absorbance of light by a sample or transmittance of light through a sample; the term is generally applied to instruments having a relatively wide bandwidth. A filter or other device limits the light falling on the sample to the range of frequencies in which the absorbance is measured. Many automated chemistry devices use colorimeters for measurement. Also called *filter photometer.* Cf. *spectrophotometer.*

colorimetric (kul″or-ĭ-met′rik) pertaining to the determination of the concentration of a sample solution by measuring its absorbance of a particular color (wavelength band) of light.

colorimetry (kul″or-im′ĕ-tre) the analysis or measurement of color by means of a colorimeter. See *colorimeter.*

color index an obsolete measurement: the ratio of hemoglobin concentration per red cell to the normal hemoglobin concentration. See *mean corpuscular hemoglobin concentration.*

color index number (C.I. number) see under *Colour Index.*

color vision the perception of colored light by the visual system. There are three types of color receptors (cones) in the retina, which differ in the color to which their visual pigment (iodopsin) is most sensitive. The absorption peaks of the three different iodopsins are in the blue-violet, green, and yellow-red regions of the spectrum. White light stimulates the three types of cones equally.

The perception of hue or color corresponds to the ratios of stimulation of the three types of cone. The primary colors (red, green, and blue) correspond to the maximal sensitivity of a single type of cone. The other 150 discernible hues correspond to mixtures of the primary colors and include the nonspectral colors between red and blue, e.g., purple. Saturation is the amount of white light mixed with a pure hue, and brightness is the intensity of the light.

The secondary retinal elements mix the signals from the cones. Certain horizontal cells (red-green cells and blue-yellow cells) are depolarized by one color and hyperpolarized by its complement so that a mixture of the two is sensed as white. Other neurons of the visual system called opponent cells (found in the ganglion cell layer, the lateral geniculate nucleus, and the striate cortex) respond to the difference between color received by the center of a field and that received by its surrounding receptors.

colostrum (kŏ-los′trum) [L.] the thin, yellowy, milky fluid secreted by the mammary gland a few days before or after parturition. It contains up to 20 percent protein, including immunoglobulins, representing the antibodies found in maternal blood. Colostrum contains more minerals and less fat and carbohydrate than does milk. It also contains many colostrum corpuscles, and usually coagulates on boiling owing to a large amount of lactalbumin.

Colour Index (C.I.) a publication of the (British) Society of Dyers and Colourists and the American

Association of Textile Chemists and Colorists that lists almost 8000 dyes and dye intermediates. It gives the chemical composition and physical and chemical properties of each dye and a list of its synonyms. Each dye that is a pure chemical substance is assigned a unique number, its Colour Index number (also called color index number, C.I. number) by which it may be specified; e.g., eosin Y, C.I. 45380. Dyes that are chemical mixtures have no C.I. number.

colp/o (kol′po) [Gr. *kolpos* womb, vagina] a word element used in combining form to denote the vagina, e.g., colposcope.

colpectasia (kol″pek-ta′ze-ah) [*colp-* + Gr. *ektasis* distention + *-ia*] distention or dilation of the vagina.

colpocytology (kol″po-si-tol′o-je) the quantitative and differential study of cells exfoliated from the epithelium of the vagina.

colpomicroscope (kol″po-mi′kro-skōp) [*colpo-* + Gr. *mikros* small + *skopein* to examine] an instrument similar to a colposcope but having higher magnification.

colposcope (kol′po-skōp) [*colpo-* + Gr. *skopein* to examine] a stereoscopic endoscope with a magnification of 4X–2OX, used to examine the uterine cervix. The focal distance is such that the instrument is far enough from the vaginal introitus to permit ease in examination and the carrying out of procedures such as biopsy of colposcopically defined abnormalities.

colposcopy (kol-pos′ko-pe) endoscopic examination of the uterine cervix for abnormal vascular patterns or epithelial configurations indicative of neoplasia. Biopsies may be obtained directly from the abnormal epithelium under visual control.

A weak acetic acid solution is applied to the cervix to dissolve mucus, and Schiller's iodine stain is applied to differentiate nonstaining (nonglycogenated) tissue. The transformation zone and adjacent areas of the portio are examined for signs of dysplasia or intraepithelial neoplasia.

columbium (Cb) (ko-lum′be-um) a former name for the chemical element *niobium.*

columella (kol″u-mel′lah), pl. *columellae* [L.] in molds, a supportive structure that extends into the sporangium, forming the central axis of the spore case, and around which the spores are arranged.

column (kol′um) [L. *columna*] an anatomic part in the form of a pillarlike structure.

columnar epithelium (kō-lum′nar) an epithelium composed of tall, cylindrical cells. It is usually a simple epithelium: stratified columnar surfaces are seen in some of the larger salivary ducts but are uncommon. Simple columnar epithelium lines the gastrointestinal tract, where many of the cells possess numerous apical microvilli and are united by junctional complexes at their luminal margins.

coma (ko′mah) [L., from Gr. *kōma*] a state in which an individual appears to be asleep but cannot respond adequately to externally applied stimuli or to inner needs. The degree of responsiveness and the state of the corneal, pupillary, pharyngeal, tendon, plantar, and brain stem reflexes vary with the degree of coma.

Coma is a symptomatic expression of a disease. It can result from extremes in body temperature; metabolic disorders (e.g., diabetes, drug overdose, hepatic dysfunction, uremia); cerebral infection; epilepsy; and neoplastic, vascular, or traumatic disorders of the brain. The presence of coma implies dysfunction of the brain stem or both cerebral hemispheres.

A complete neurologic examination is important in assessing the extent of central nervous system impairment. The electroencephalogram is also useful in monitoring the patient: it may help to exclude a seizure disorder or structural cerebral lesion as the cause of the coma, it can provide a guide to the depth of coma, and—when recorded appropriately—it can indicate the degree of irreversible brain damage that has occurred.

Treatment of the comatose patient depends on the cause of the coma, but immediate management is directed at the evaluation and maintenance of vital functions. Care of such patients should include regular monitoring of all vital signs and the maintenance of respiration and an adequate circulation. In some cases the patient may require artificial respiration. Fluid and electrolyte balance must be maintained, at least initially, by intravenous administration. Loss of bladder control requires an indwelling catheter. The patient should be turned at least every 2 hr; this reduces pressure on the skin, prevents formation of decubitus ulcers, and helps to preserve respiratory function. Orthopedic deformities can be minimized by maintaining good alignment of body parts, and daily physical therapy helps to maintain mobility of the joints. Further management depends on the cause of the coma. With the advent of sophisticated artificial life support systems, the comatose patient can be maintained for extended periods of time.

See also *brain death syndrome, consciousness disorder,* and *electrocerebral inactivity.*

alcoholic c., stupor or coma accompanying severe alcoholic intoxication.

diabetic c., see *diabetic coma.*

hepatic c., coma accompanying cerebral damage resulting from degeneration of liver cells, most commonly that associated with cirrhosis of the liver.

irreversible c., see *brain death syndrome.*

coma dépassé (ko′mah da″pah-sa′) [Fr.] literally, a state beyond coma; see *brain death syndrome* and *electrocerebral inactivity.*

comatose (ko′mah-tōs) pertaining to or being in a coma.

coma vigil see *apallic syndrome.*

combination (kom″bĭ-na′shun) the number of ways in which *r* objects can be selected (without regard to ordering) from a set of *n* objects. See also *binomial coefficient.*

combined immunodeficiency (kom-bind) see under *immunodeficiency.*

comb rhythm (kōm) see *mu rhythm.*

combustible (kom-bus′ti-b′l) capable of burning. Cf. *flammable, noncombustible,* and *nonflammable.*

combustible gas an inexact term that refers to any flammable gas. See also *flammable gas.*

combustible gas detector an instrument for detecting and measuring concentrations of flammable gases or vapors. Also called combustible gas analyzer, explosion meter, and flammable vapor detector.

combustible liquid an organic liquid having a flash point at or above 37.8°C (100°F). Combustible liquids having flash points below 93.4°C (200°F) have storage limits set by National Fire Protection Association (NFPA) and Occupational Safety and Health Administration (OSHA) standards for laboratories. Such regulated combustible liquids include Class II and IIIA combustible liquids: Class II liquids have flash points at or above 37.8°C (100°F) and below 60°C (140°F), and Class IIIA liquids have flash points at or above 60°C (140°F) and below 93.4°C (200°F). (Class IIIB liquids have flash points at or above 93.4°C (200°F).)

combustible vapor vapor emitted by combustible or flammable liquids but not in sufficient concentration for flame to propagate through the vapor-air mixture. See also *flammable limits.*

combustion (kom-bust'yun) the process of burning in which heat is released in glowing or flaming form. Glowing combustion is usually a condensed-phase reaction, and flame is usually a gas-phase reaction. Glowing combustion cannot be extinguished by dry chemicals or halogenated extinguishing agents, which act by suppressing the chain reactions produced by flames. If combustion is confined so that an appreciable pressure rise occurs, the process is called an explosion. It is called detonation if the combustion wave propagates at supersonic speed.

comedo (kom'ĕ-do), pl. *comedones* a noninflammatory papule, most frequently associated with acne vulgaris, that is characterized as a hyperkeratotic thickening of the epithelium of the duct of a sebaceous gland with the retention of sebum. Comedones frequently progress to inflammatory papules and pustules. The initial stimulus to comedo formation is unknown, but *Propionibacterium acnes* or *Staphylococcus epidermidis* may play a role. See also *a. vulgaris* under *acne.*

comet cell (kom'et) in cytology, an epithelial cell, usually of urothelial origin, that is characterized by a dark, homogeneous, degenerating nucleus and a cytoplasmic elongation or tail. It is often present in the urine in cystitis and can be mistaken for a cell of transitional cell carcinoma in situ. It also resembles cells infected with human polyomavirus and may in fact be a manifestation of this viral infection. Also called decoy cell.

command (kŏ-mand') in computer programming, a machine-language instruction or high-level language statement.

commensal (kŏ-men'sal) [L. *com-* together + *mensa* table] denoting two organisms living together without harm to either, with one or both deriving benefit from the arrangement.

commensalism (kŏ-men'sal-izm") a relationship between organisms living together by which neither is harmful to the other and one derives some benefit such as protection or nourishment. Cf. *parasitism.*

comment (kom'ent) a part of a computer program, ignored by the computer but printed in program listing, that explains the program to the reader.

comminuted (kom'ĭ-nūt"ed) [L. *comminutus,* from *com-* together + *minuere* to diminish] broken or crushed into small pieces, as a comminuted fracture.

comminuted fracture a fracture in which the bone is splintered or crushed.

commissure (kom'ĭ-shūr) [L. *commissura* a joining together] a site of union of corresponding parts. The term is also used in a general sense to designate such a junction of corresponding anatomic structures, frequently, but not always, across the midplane of the body.

Committee on Allied Health Education and Accreditation (CAHEA) an organization that establishes standards for allied health education and accredits allied health programs.

common (kom'un) 1. pertaining equally to two or more; joint.
2. occurring most frequently; ordinary.

common bile duct see *common b. d.* under *bile duct.*

common carotid artery see *common c. a.* under *carotid artery.*

common logarithm a logarithm to the base 10. Also called briggsian logarithm.

common mode rejection ratio (CMRR) the ability of a differential amplifier to reject artifact or interference potentials common to both inputs (common mode signals) while amplifying potential differences between the two inputs (differential signals).

common mode signal two signals that appear equally at both input terminals of a differential amplifier. Interference or artifact potentials frequently occur as common mode signals.

common reference see *average reference m.* and *referential m.* under *montage.*

common storage an area of computer memory that can be used by more than one program, such as that defined by the COMMON statement in FORTRAN.

communicable (kŏ-mu'nĭ-kah-b'l) capable of being transmitted from one person to another.

commutator (kom'u-ta"tor) a device consisting of conducting brushes that contact a rotating shaft. It is used in electric motors and generators, where it has the dual function of transferring power to the rotating armature windings and reversing the polarity of the current during the cycle.

compact (kom-pakt') dense; having a dense structure.

compact bone the hard outer layer, cortex, or dense portion of mature bone. Compact bone appears as a solid, continuous mass in which spaces can be seen only with magnification. Cf. *spongy bone.*

comparison film (kom-par'ĭ-son) a radiograph of a normal part taken for comparison with a radiograph of the matching part on the other side, which is suspected of being abnormal; the term also refers to a previously taken radiograph that is being compared with a later film of the same part.

comparison operation in high-level computer languages, an operation in which two numeric or character string variables are compared, giving a result that is a logical variable. For example, $X < Y$ is true if, and only if, the value of X is less than the value of Y. (For character strings the "less than" symbol means "preceding in alphabetical order [in the collating sequence]".) See also *operation.*

compartment (com-part'ment) a small enclosure within a larger space.

compartmental analysis (kom"part-men'tal) a mathematical technique for describing the flow of a radioisotope-labeled tracer in the body, which is used for tracer dilution and blood flow measurements. The tracer is assumed to have a uniform concentration throughout one or more compartments. It flows out of the compartment at a rate proportional to its concentration, and goes into another compartment or is excreted. A compartment need not correspond with an anatomic organ or space. When the tracer is eliminated at two different rates by two different mechanisms, it can be treated as being in two different compartments.

The measured volume of the compartment, the amount of tracer administered divided by its concentration after dilution, is called a space. The total amount of a substance, the space multiplied by the concentration, is called the pool. A plot is made of the logarithm of the activity of the tracer in all compartments as a function of time. For a single compartment, the rate constant is the slope of the plot. For two or three compartments, a straight line is fitted to the last part of the curve; its slope is one rate constant. The line is subtracted from the original plot and the process is repeated. This process, called the peeling technique, is shown in the accompanying illustration.

Computer programs are available to treat larger systems, but the problem is mathematically ill-conditioned (small data errors make large differences in the determined rates) unless the rates are very different.

compatibility tests various procedures employed to determine the compatibility of a specific donor's blood with a recipient's serum. The procedures include testing the recipient's blood for ABO and Rh blood groups and screening the recipient's serum for the presence of red blood cell antibodies. After the recipient's blood group has been determined and screened for unexpected antibodies, donor blood of the same ABO and Rh groups or compatible with that of the recipient is selected for crossmatch.

Crossmatching is performed with the recipient's serum and a suspension of washed donor cells. After the serum and cells are mixed, they are centrifuged and examined for hemolysis and agglutination. Albumin or a low-ionic-strength salt solution is added to the crossmatch tubes at this point, altering the dielectric constant of the medium and enhancing antigen-antibody reactions. The tubes are incubated at 37°C to detect the presence of any clinically significant antibodies in the recipient's serum against the donor blood. Following an incubation period, the crossmatch tubes are again centrifuged and examined for hemolysis or agglutination; if neither is observed, the cells are subjected to an antiglobulin test to detect any antibodies that might be coating the cells without causing agglutination. Following a thorough washing with saline, antiglobulin serum is added to the cells and the tubes are again centrifuged and examined for agglutination. If there is none, the activity of the antiglobulin serum is checked by adding sensitized red cells and recentrifugation. Agglutination or hemolysis at any point, except with the sensitized check cells, indicates an incompatibility.

in vivo c. t., a technique performed to predict the in vivo survivability of red cells that are incompatible in an in vitro crossmatch. This procedure is resorted to only if the patient's antibodies cannot be determined and a transfusion is urgently needed. Cells of the least compatible unit are tagged with ^{51}Cr, and their short-term survival after transfusion is measured by counting the residual radioactivity in the circulating red cells. If these cells survive, other units are then transfused. See also *red cell survival test.*

compatible (kom-pat′i-b′l) capable of harmonious coexistence; not inconsistent with; the term is used to denote substances that do not react chemically when mixed.

Compazine (kom′pah-zēn) trademark. See *prochlorperazine.*

compensation (kom″pen-sa′shun) [L. *compensatio,* from *com-* together + *pensare* to weigh] 1. the counterbalancing of any defect of structure or function.

2. in cardiology, the maintenance of an adequate blood flow.

competence (kom′pĕ-tens) 1. the ability of an organ or part to perform its assigned functions adequately.

2. in embryology, the ability of a part of an embryo to react to inductive stimuli by differentiation in a given direction.

competition (kom″pĕ-tish′un) 1. the phenomenon of two structurally similar molecules attempting to bind to the same site on a third molecule, usually an enzyme. Such a binding is mutually exclusive. See also *competitive inhibition.*

2. the interaction that results when organisms share the same limited environmental resources.

competitive inhibition (kom-pet′ĭ-tiv) in enzyme kinetics, inhibition in which the substrate and inhibitor compete for the same catalytic site on the enzyme owing to structural resemblance. The overall inhibition is dependent on the concentration of the inhibitor, the ratio of inhibitor to substrate, and

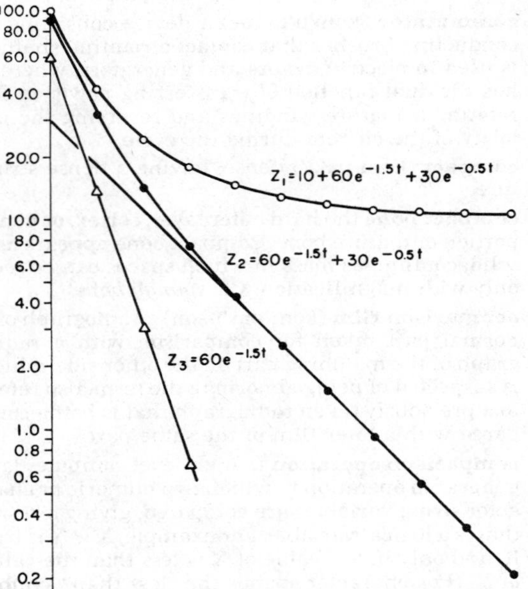

Compartmental analysis. Illustration of the "peeling technique" for estimating decay constants. (From Wagner, H. N.: Principles of Nuclear Medicine. Philadelphia, W. B. Saunders Co., 1968.)

the affinity of the inhibitor for the enzyme. Many drugs are competitive inhibitors of enzymes.

competitive protein-binding (CPB) assays radioassays; the term is usually restricted to those employing a binding protein that is not an antibody. Examples of plasma proteins used include corticosteroid-binding globulin (CBG) for the assay of cortisol and progesterone; sex hormone–binding globulin (SHBG) for the assay of estradiol, testosterone, and dihydrotestosterone; and thyroxine-binding globulin (TBG) for the assay of thyroxine. Target tissue containing specific receptors for different hormones may be used for the same purpose, e.g., uterus (for estrogens), prostate and seminal vesicles (for dihydrotestosterone), thymus (for glucocorticoids), and kidney and toad bladder (for mineralocorticoids). See also *immunoassay* and *radioimmunoassay.*

compile (kom-pīl′) to produce a machine-language program (the object program) from a high-level language program (the source program).

compiler (kom-pi′ler) a computer program that translates a computer program written in a high-level language, such as FORTRAN, BASIC, or PL/I, into a machine-language program. Cf. *interpreter.*

compile time pertaining to events that occur during compilation of a computer program, e.g., setting initial values for variables or allocating static storage. Cf. *execution time.*

complement (C) (kom′plĕ-ment) [L. *complementum,* from *complere* to fill] a complex system of at least 11 proteins and glycoproteins that is the chief humoral mediator of antigen-antibody reactions. Complement was originally defined as the serum factor or factors that cause the lysis of antibody-coated bacteria. This function is now known to be accomplished by nine proteins, the complement components C1–C9, which are activated in a cascade (the classical complement pathway); the result is the formation of a hole in the cell membrane that allows the influx of water and causes the cell to burst. Certain activated complement components are also involved in other biologic functions: enhancement of phagocytosis (opsonization), viral neutralization, mediation of anaphylaxis, leukocyte chemotaxis, increased vascular permeability, and modulation of the immune response. All these effects combine to produce a coordinated inflammatory response against bacterial infection.

THE CLASSICAL PATHWAY. This pathway is activated with the binding of C1 to antibody-coated surfaces. C1 binds to a specific site on the Fc portion of the heavy chain of IgG or IgM; for binding to IgG to occur, there must be two IgG molecules bound side by side. C1 binding results in development of enzymatic activity, and the activated protein is termed C1 esterase, which cleaves C2 and C4. The fragments C2a and C4b bind together on the cell membrane surface; the complex $C\overline{42}$ that is formed has enzymatic activity and cleaves C3, producing a fragment C3b that combines with $C\overline{42}$ to form C423, which acts as a C5 convertase. Cleavage of C5 results in the sequential binding of C5b, C6, C7, C8, and C9 at another site on the surface of the cell membrane. They form a structure with a hydrophilic center that allows the passage of water and ions through the membrane. At each enzymatic step in the pathway, the number of molecules involved is amplified because each enzyme molecule can cleave many substrate molecules; hence, the term "cascade" is applied to the process. This pathway and the one described below are shown in the accompanying illustration.

THE ALTERNATIVE PATHWAY. The complement system can also be activated via another pathway, which bypasses the early components C1, C2, and C4; it involves three serum glycoproteins called properdin factors B, D, and P. The exact initiating events are unknown, but material such as bacterial cell walls and lipopolysaccharide endotoxin can interact with B, D, and C3 to produce small amounts of C3b. Once C3b is generated, it combines with B and D in the presence of Mg^{2+} to form a C3b-dependent C3 convertase (C3bBb), which, like C423 in the classical pathway, cleaves C3 to form more C3b. C3b then combines with C3bBb and P to produce a C5 convertase that activates the late-acting components.

The formation of C36 that results in the formation of C3bBb and more C3b constitutes a positive feedback loop that greatly amplifies the production of C3b. This feedback loop can also operate to amplify the classical pathway.

BIOLOGIC FUNCTIONS. The other functions of the complement system are mediated by fragments of complement released during activation of the sequence. A fragment of C2, called C2 kinin, has kininlike activity and increases vascular permeability. C3a, released by the cleavage of C3, is an anaphylatoxin that causes the release of mediators of immediate hypersensitivity from basophils and mast cells. C5a is a major chemotactic factor for neutrophils and macrophages; it also has anaphylatoxic activity. C4b binds to viruses, preventing attachment to host cells.

C3b and a smaller fragment C3d split off from C3b by C3b inactivator have specific membrane receptors on a variety of cells. The C3b receptors on macrophages and neutrophils cause the phagocytosis of coated cells. Those on B lymphocytes trigger antibody synthesis. C3b receptors also occur on erythrocytes, eosinophils, and basophils; the physiologic function of these receptors is unclear, but the erythrocyte receptors are involved in immune adherence. A distinct C3d receptor occurs on B lymphocytes, monocytes, and immature neutrophils.

INHIBITORS OF COMPLEMENT. There are several serum proteins that inhibit a particular point in the complement cascade. C1 esterase inhibitor binds stoichiometrically to C1 esterase and eliminates its enzymatic activity. C3b inactivator cleaves C3b. It acts in concert with B1H, which inactivates the convertases of the alternative pathway, to regulate the alternative pathway. Other less well-characterized inhibitors include C6 inactivator, anaphylatoxin inactivator, C4-binding protein, and C1q-binding protein.

See also *alternative complement pathway, classical complement pathway,* and the accompanying table.

complement assays 1. the whole complement titer or CH_{50} assay, the usual screening assay for complement. Erythrocytes are coated with antibody in the absence of complement, dilutions of the serum to be tested are then added to the standardized suspension in the presence of divalent cations, and the percentage of lysis is scored. The values are expressed by (CH_{50}), hemolytic complement units per milli-

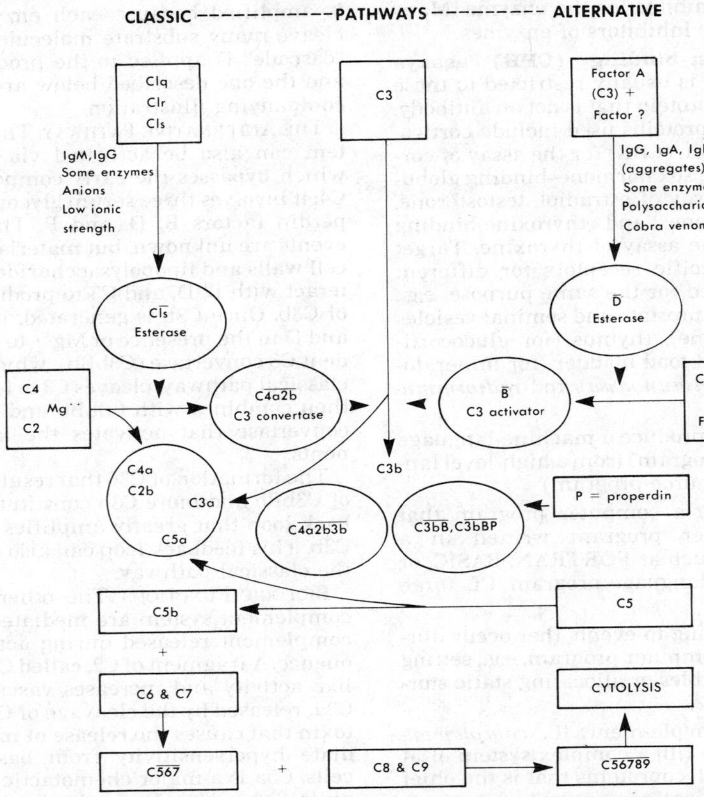

Complement. Comparison of the classical and alternative pathways of activation of complement. Proenzymes are in the squares, activated enzymes are in the ovals, activated components in liquid phase are in the circle, and the remaining components are in rectangles. C3 and C3b play double roles in the activation process and serve as amplifiers. Properdin (P) serves as a stabilizer for C3bB and thus enhances the reaction. (From Henry, J. B.: Clinical Diagnosis and Management. 16th ed. Philadelphia, W. B. Saunders Co., 1979.)

liter, which is the dilution of serum required to lyse 50 percent of the erythrocytes in the assay.

2. immunoassays, usually radial immunodiffusion tests, for complement components or complement inhibitors. Reagent plates for C3, C4, C5, properdin factor B, and C1 inhibitor are commercially available. Antibody to the specific component of complement to be quantitated is prepared and suspended into agar, and known standards of complement and the unknown test serums are placed into appropriate wells in the agar. These antigens diffuse from the wells into the agar; a visible precipitin line forms where antigen and antibody react at an optimal antigen-antibody ratio.

3. functional tests for individual components of complement. This method is similar to the hemolytic assay used in the CH_{50} assay. Pure preparations of the individual complement components are added sequentially until lysis of the antibody-coated erythrocytes occurs. The component that produces lysis is the one missing from the patient's serum.

complementary (kom″plĕ-men′tă-re) supplying a lack or making something complete; accessory.

complementary bases a pair of bases, one purine and one pyrimidine, that are connected to each other by hydrogen bonds in complementary nucleic acid strands. The pairs are adenine-thymine and guanine-cytosine in DNA, and adenine-uracil and guanine-cytosine in RNA. See also *nucleic acid.*

complementary DNA (cDNA) single-stranded DNA that is synthesized from an RNA template by the enzyme reverse transcriptase. Complementary DNA may be radioactively labeled and hybridized with cellular DNA, and the kinetics of hybridization may be used to measure the number of copies of specific genes in various types of cells. Such cDNA probes are also useful in DNA recombination and cloning techniques.

complementary genes two independent pairs of nonallelic genes, neither of which produces its effect without the appropriate alleles of the other being present. Also called complementary factors.

complementary metal oxide semiconductor (CMOS) logic a type of logic circuitry that uses both *p*-channel and *n*-channel metal oxide semiconductor field effect transistors (MOSFETs) in a complementary arrangement in each logic circuit so that only one power supply voltage is necessary. CMOS logic has a lower power consumption (but also a slower switching speed) than emitter-coupled logic (ECL) or transistor-transistor logic (TTL). Because of its low-power consumption, CMOS logic is often used in portable battery-powered computing devices, and allows such features as "constant memo-

Complement. Congenital Abnormalities of Complement

Defect	Associated Disease
C1q	Combined immunodeficiency disease
C1s	Systemic lupus erythematosus (SLE)
C1r	SLE-like
C2	Some normal Some with glomerulonephritis Some with SLE-like diseases
C4	SLE-like
C3	Recurrent pyogenic infections
C5	SLE-like disease
C5 dysfunction	Syndrome in infants with diarrhea, dermatitis, infections
C6	Gonococcemia
C7	Raynaud's phenomenon
C8	Gonococcemia
C1s inhibitor deficiency	Hereditary angioneurotic edema
C3b inactivator deficiency	Recurrent infections (also known as Type 1 C3 hypercatabolism)
C3 hypercatabolism, Type 2	Partial lipodystrophy, glomerulonephritis

From Bellanti, J. A.: Immunology II. Philadelphia, W. B. Saunders Co., 1978, p. 148.

ry" by supplying a power to the memory circuits even with the power switch off.

complement-fixation test a very sensitive serologic test, performed as a two-stage procedure, that is used to measure a wide variety of antigens and antibodies. In the first stage, the test antigen (or antibody) is mixed with the patient's heated (complement-inactivated) serum. If the specific antibody for the test antigen (or antigen for test antibody) is present, an antigen-antibody complex forms. A known amount of complement is then added. If antigen-antibody complexes are present, the complement pathway will be activated and complement consumed (fixed). In the second stage, antibody-coated sheep red cells are added. If an Ag-Ab complex was formed and complement consumed, there is no lysis, indicating a positive test result (CFT+); a negative test result, expressed as CFT–, indicates that hemolysis has occurred.

complement inactivation the destruction of activity of complement, usually produced in the laboratory by heating serum to 56°C for 30 min.

complement lysis sensitivity test the most accurate and sensitive test for paroxysmal nocturnal hemoglobinuria; red cells are lysed by a smaller concentration of isoimmune antibodies than are normal cells in the presence of complement. See also *sucrose lysis test.*

complete antibody (kom-plēt′) a term for the Rh antibody that is capable of directly agglutinating Rh-positive erythrocytes in physiologic saline, which indicates that the antibody is multivalent, i.e., possesses two or more reactive groups. The definition may be extended to include a number of other globulins with similar agglutinating, but not necessarily type-specific, features. Also called saline active antibody.

complete blood count (CBC) a measure of the hematologic parameters of the blood, consisting of hemoglobin, hematocrit, red cell indices (MCV, MCH, MCHC), red cell count, white cell count, differential leukocyte count, and sometimes a platelet count. See also *blood cell count* and *differential leukocyte count.*

complete heart block see *third-degree A-V b.* under *atrioventricular (A-V) block.*

complete penetrance the appearance of the effect of a dominant gene or of homozygous recessive genes in all individuals heterozygous for the dominant gene or homozygous for the recessive gene.

complex (kom′pleks) [L. *complexus* woven together, entwined] 1. complicated; not simple.

2. the sum or combination of various things, like or unlike, as a complex of symptoms.

3. in electrocardiography, that portion of an ECG tracing that represents the systole of an atrium or ventricle.

4. in electroencephalography, any sequence of waves that can be distinguished from background activity and that has a characteristic or consistent form.

5. in psychology, a term used for a group of associated, partially or wholly repressed ideas that can evoke emotional forces that influence an individual's behavior, usually operating outside of awareness.

6. in biochemistry, a reversible association of chemical compounds held together by weak chemical bonds, such as an enzyme-substrate complex (an association of an enzyme and one or more substrates that is the reacting moiety in an enzyme-catalyzed reaction), an antigen-antibody complex, or a hapten-antibody complex. The term can also refer to the association of a number of enzymes, activators, and coenzymes to effect a complex biochemical reaction, as in the pyruvate dehydrogenase complex, a system of three enzymes and five coenzymes that transforms pyruvate to acetyl CoA in the first step of the tricarboxylic acid cycle.

7. in inorganic chemistry, any compound consisting of a central atom surrounded by a set of ligand atoms. In the classical use of the term, a complex is an ion or molecule in which a metal atom or ion is

joined by coordinate covalent bonds to several nonmetallic ions or molecules called ligands, coordinating groups, or complexing agents. The metal, which is usually a transition metal, is called the central metal or the coordinated metal ion or atom. It acts as Lewis acid, accepting an unshared electron pair from an atom in each ligand. The number of these bonds formed by the central metal is called the coordination number; it is usually 4 or 6.

Six-coordinate complexes (the most common) have octahedral geometry; the six ligands are located along three orthogonal (perpendicular) axes, the metal at the center of the octahedron. Four-coordinate complexes have square planar geometry (with ligands at the corners of a square) or tetrahedral geometry (at the vertices of a tetrahedron).

Many enzyme prosthetic groups contain a six-coordinate complex in which the central metal ion forms four bonds to a planar ring (such as a porphyrin or corrin ring) and two vertical bonds to other groups of the protein or the prosthetic group.

Stereoisomerism, a consequence of the spatial arrangement of the ligands about the metal, is possible for some complexes. Individual stereoisomers may be chiral or achiral; a pair of stereoisomers may be enantiomers or diastereomers. When, because of the nature of the ligands, a complex exists in only two diastereomeric forms, they are called *cis*-(when the two like ligands are on adjacent vertices of the complex) and *trans*- (when they are on opposite vertices).

Some ligand molecules can form more than one bond (from different atoms) to the central metal. Such a complex is called a chelate (although some authorities use the term chelate only as an adjective referring to the ligand, as in chelate ring, chelate complex, and chelate effect).

See also *coordination compound.*

π-c., an adduct formed between two molecules or two parts of one molecule in which the bond between them involves electron-pair donation from a π-orbital in the donor to a σ-orbital in the acceptor, or from a σ- to a π-orbital, or from a π- to a π-orbital. See also *charge-transfer complex.*

complex number a number of the form $z = a + bi$, where a and b are real numbers, called the real part, Re(z), and the imaginary part, Im(z), respectively; and i is a symbol usually thought of as the square root of –1. The complex numbers obey ordinary rules of arithmetic with the additional rule that $i^2 = -1$. Every algebraic equation (polynomial) has a solution in the set of complex numbers.

For some purposes, complex numbers are represented in polar form: $z = re^{i\theta}$, where r and θ are real numbers called the modulus or absolute value, $r = |z|$, and the argument, $\theta = \arg z$. They are defined by the equations $a = r\cos\theta$ and $b = r\sin\theta$.

compliance (C) (kom-pli′ans) distensibility, or the ease with which a structure or substance is deformed when subjected to a pressure or force. The compliance of a hollow viscus (such as an air- or fluid-filled organ) is the unit change in volume (ΔV) produced by the application of a unit pressure difference (ΔP) across its wall ($\Delta V/\Delta P$).

When measured under static conditions (static compliance), the compliance of the lungs is equivalent to the change in lung volume (or volume of air that enters the lungs) resulting from the unit pressure change exerted on the lungs by contraction of the respiratory muscles (and reflected by the resulting change in intrapleural or airway pressure) at specific degrees of lung inflation. Static compliance (measured with the respiratory muscles relaxed) is normally determined by calculating the slope of the linear approximation to the pulmonary pressure-volume curve at any point (usually in the tidal volume range) and is expressed in units of liters per centimeter of water (l/cm H_2O). Because the pressure-volume curve is curvilinear, compliance decreases with increasing lung volumes. The absolute value for static compliance in the steepest portion of the pressure-volume curve is about 0.2 l/cm H_2O in the healthy lung; this value is dependent on lung size and therefore is less in newborns or in individuals with one lung.

Disorders such as interstitial pulmonary fibrosis and pulmonary edema effect a decrease in specific lung compliance, larger transpulmonary pressures being required to inflate the lungs to tidal volume. Specific compliance is increased in emphysema and in asthma during a bronchospasm.

See also *pressure-volume curve.* Cf. *elastance.*

dynamic c. (Cdyn), the pulmonary compliance measured during breathing. It is equal to the ratio between the tidal volume and the difference in intrapleural pressure between the two extremes of tidal volume (end-expiration and end-inspiration) when there is zero gas flow. The intrapleural pressures are recorded at these two points as the subject performs a series of inspiratory-expiratory cycles of gradually increasing depth. The slope of the line that connects the two points (the curve of the volume versus the intrapleural pressure changes) is considered to represent the dynamic compliance. More accurately (especially at higher breathing frequencies), it is a measure of the pressure difference needed to overcome tissue and airway resistance and produce a unit change in airflow.

In individuals with healthy lungs, the pressure required to overcome resistance, at lower respiratory rates, is low relative to that required to overcome the elastic recoil (because airflow is slow). More pressure is required to produce a given change in flow at higher breathing frequencies. The pressure-volume curve measured at increasingly faster respiratory rates thus becomes a loop, with a narrow portion at the lower flows and increasingly wider portion as flow increases. In healthy lungs, the slope of the line joining the pressures at end-expiration and end-inspiration (the dynamic compliance) is essentially equal to the static compliance at frequencies below 60–90 cycles/min. However, in persons with pulmonary disorders that result in an increased tissue or airway resistance, such as emphysema or chronic bronchitis, the dynamic compliance is less than the compliance measured under static conditions.

Also called frequency-dependent compliance.

specific c., the static lung or chest wall compliance per unit lung volume (usually functional residual capacity, vital capacity, or total lung capacity). Calculation of this standardized value of static compliance allows for comparison of individuals of different sizes.

static c. (Cst), the pulmonary compliance measured under static conditions when breathing is suspended and gas flow in the airways is zero. When measured under these conditions, the force or pressure acting to distend the lungs is solely a reflection of that needed to overcome the elastic recoil of lung and chest wall tissue; static compliance is thus a measure of elastic recoil.

Pulmonary static compliance in unanesthetized humans can be measured by determining the relative difference in intrapleural pressure (the pressure within an intraesophageal balloon) measured at end-expiration and that measured with the respiratory muscles relaxed following inspiration of a known volume of gas. The airway closes following inspiration by holding the breath. These measurements are repeated using increasingly larger (or smaller) lung volumes.

In both methods for determining compliance, the volume history of the lungs prior to measurement must be specified (compliance at a given volume is decreased following deflation and increased after an inflation). The static compliance is taken as the slope ($\Delta V/\Delta P$) of the pressure-volume curve, usually in the tidal volume range.

complication (kom″plĭ-ka′shun) [L. *complicatio,* from *cum* together + *plicare* to fold] a pathologic process occurring in the course of a disease that is not an essential part of the disease process.

component (kom-po′nent) 1. a constituent element or part of a larger system.

2. in clinical chemistry, a constituent that is being measured. Measurements are specified in terms of the system (e.g., serum), the component (e.g., glucose), and the kind of quantity (e.g., substance concentration).

3. any of the distinct chemical substances forming a mixture or solution.

4. any electric or electronic device, such as a resistor, transistor, capacitor, or integrated circuit, that has well-defined operating characteristics and can be connected to other components to make an electronic circuit.

5. the projection of a vector in a given direction; see under *vector.*

compos mentis (kom′pos men′tis) [L.] sound of mind; sane.

compound (kom′pownd) [L. *componere* to place together] 1. made up of diverse elements; a substance made up of two or more materials.

2. in chemistry, identical molecules considered collectively.

3. (kom-pownd′), to make up from component parts or substances.

compound B see *corticosterone.*

compound E see *cortisone.*

compound F see *cortisol.*

compound fracture bone breakage that produces puncture of the skin by bony fragments. Also called open fracture.

compound S see *11-deoxycortisol.*

compound X a term referring to metacentric, attached X chromosomes or multiple X chromosomes, which are inherited together and determine sex in some nonmammalian species.

compressed gas storage storage of gas under high pressure. Compressed gas cylinders can be extremely hazardous if exposed to fire, or if a fall or other impact ruptures the cylinder, valve, or regulator. National Fire Protection Association standards require the cylinders to be in racks or secured in position. Quantities of flammable gases stored for use within laboratories are limited by regulations (NFPA 56C-1980 and NFPA 45-1981). Multiple-cylinder systems and storage of flammable and oxidizing gases are generally required to be located outside the laboratory or in a separate room with specified fire resistance and ventilation.

compressed spectral assay (CSA) in electroencephalography, a quantitative method of expressing the amount of activity in each frequency band of a selected segment of the electroencephalogram (EEG). The electric activity recorded from pairs of scalp electrodes is analyzed into frequency components using Fourier transform methods, and plotted as intensity (proportional to the square of the voltage) on the ordinate and frequency (measured in hertz) on the abscissa of a graph.

This method of frequency spectral analysis is useful in the the primary analysis of the EEG. Because CSA lacks sensitivity to transient events, however, and because it does not account for subject variability caused by differing states of arousal, the technique is significantly less accurate than visual inspection of polygraph tracings in differentiating between normal and abnormal activity.

compression (kom-presh′un) [L. *compressio,* from *comprimere* to squeeze together] 1. the act of pressing together; an action exerted on a body by an external force that tends to diminish its volume and increase its density.

2. in embryology, the shortening or omission of certain stages during development.

3. in radiography, pressure applied to a part during radiographic examination in order to move aside obscuring structures or to contain contrast medium in the tissue or organ of interest, e.g., ureteric compression applied during excretory urography to keep the contrast medium from flowing out of the kidneys and down to the bladder.

compression fracture a fracture due to traumatic compression of bone.

compromised (kom′pro-mizd) lacking adequate resistance to infection, or lacking the ability to mount an adequate immune response.

Compton edge (komp′ton) [Arthur Holly *Compton,* U.S. physicist, 1892–1962; winner of the Nobel prize in physics for 1927] the maximal energy of a Compton scattered electron, which occurs when the photon is scattered through an angle of 180°. In a gamma-ray spectrum produced with a scintillation detector, there is a broad peak covering the energies below the Compton edge. This is due to photons with the primary photopeak energy that are scattered out of the crystal so that only part of their energy is detected. If E is the photopeak energy in keV, then the Compton edge, T_{max} (in keV), is given by the formula $T_{max} = E^2/(255 + E)$.

Compton effect [Arthur Holly *Compton*] the change in the wavelength of x- or gamma-radiation due to the interaction of an incident photon with an orbital electron of an atom, which produces a recoil electron and a scattered photon of reduced energy. This type of interaction is quite probable between gamma rays of intermediate energies (between 0.5 and 1.0 MeV) and absorbers of medium-to-low atomic numbers.

Compton photon [Arthur Holly *Compton*] a photon that has undergone Compton scattering.

computed tomography (CT) (kom-pu′ted) a radiologic imaging device that utilizes computer processing to generate an image (CT scan) of the tissue density in a transverse plane of the patient's body.

Since the introduction of CT in 1972, its use has grown rapidly: common clinical uses include the diagnosis of tumors, infarction, cysts, and other space-occupying lesions. Examination of abdominal organs, such as the prostate, adrenal gland, pancreas, and retroperitoneal tissues, has also become possible with the new high-speed scanners. Because the procedure is noninvasive and has better contrast resolution, it has clear advantages over some radiographic contrast studies. The better spatial resolution of CT as compared with scintillation imaging has led to its use in place of some radionuclide studies.

IMAGING PROCESS. The CT scan is a two-dimensional image that corresponds to a tissue slice of finite thickness (about 10 mm). The scan is divided into a square matrix of pixels (picture elements); the corresponding regions in the tissue slice are called voxels (volume elements). Newer equipment uses a 512 × 512 pixel matrix. For a 20 cm–wide head scan, the pixel area is 0.4 × 0.4 mm.

During a scan, the x-ray tube or detectors are moved around the patient, so that the x-ray attenuations along many lines in the tissue slice can be determined and stored in the computer. Each attenuation value is the sum of the attenuation values for the voxels lying in a straight line across the scan.

A computer program called the reconstruction algorithm solves the mathematical problem of determining which voxel values have the observed sums. One type of algorithm, the algebraic reconstruction technique (ART), solves the equations algebraically. Other methods use Fourier transforms to achieve equivalent results. When the attenuation value (μ) has been determined for each voxel, it is converted to a CT number (also called Hounsfield unit) using the formula: CT number = $k(\mu - \mu_w)/\mu_w$, where μ_w is the attenuation value of water and k is a calibration constant chosen so that dense bone has a CT number of +1000 and air a CT number of −1000. Water has a CT number of 0.

CT SCANNER. The scanner consists of three major components: gantry, computer, and operating console. The gantry assembly contains the patient support, a high-capacity rotating anode x-ray tube, and a detector array.

CT technology has grown rapidly, with advances in both complexity of equipment and efficiency of computer programs. First-generation scanners have a single detector and operate in a rotate and translate mode. In the translation, the tube and detector move in synchronization past the patient, stopping at equal intervals to record a sequence of attenuation values on parallel lines across the scan (a view). The line between the tube and detector is rotated in 1° steps through 180° so that 180 views are acquired, a process that takes 3–5 min.

Newer scanners use a fan beam, which spreads out from the tube to an array of detectors so that many attenuation values can be recorded simultaneously, as shown in the accompanying illustration. Because the scan lines of a view are not determined in sequence and are not equally spaced, more sophisticated reconstruction programs are required. In second-generation scanners, the beam is not as wide as the reconstruction diameter, so that both rotations and translations are still necessary but scan time is reduced to about 20 sec. Third-generation scanners have a wider detector array so that no translation is required, whereas fourth-generation scanners have a stationary circular array of 1000 detectors so that only the tube moves.

With first-generation scanners, only cerebral scans could be performed. The latest scanners perform rapidly enough to stop the motion of the abdominal visera and other organs, and thus have many more applications than first-generation scanners.

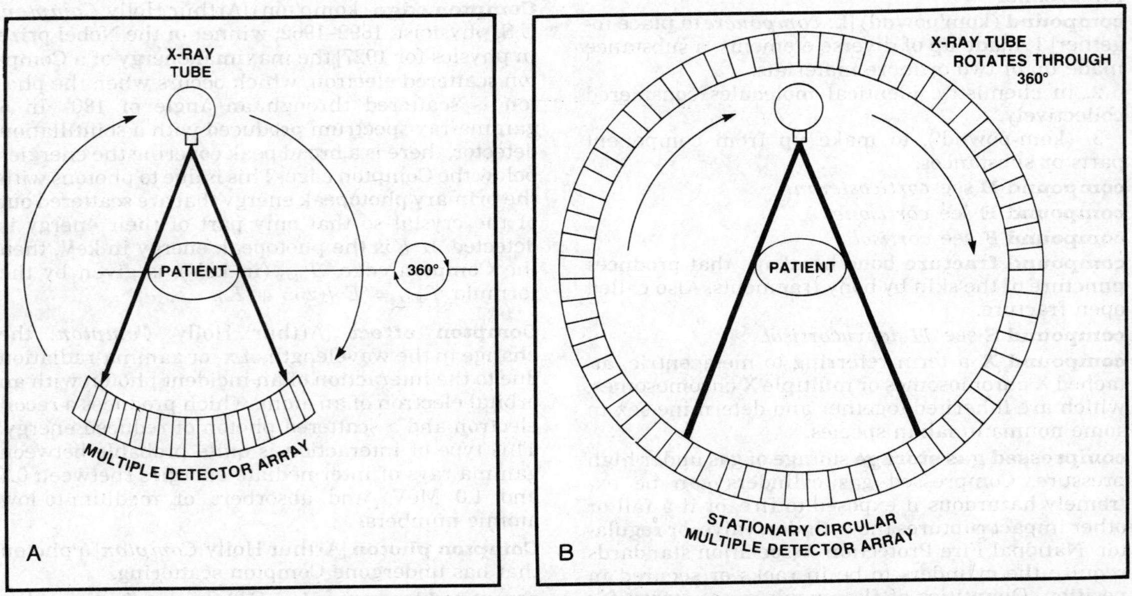

Computed tomography. *A,* Continuously rotating pulsed fan-beam scanning typical of third-generation CT scanners; *B,* scanning scheme of fourth-generation scanners. (From Seeram, Euclid: Computed Tomography Technology. Philadelphia, W. B. Saunders Co., 1982.)

There are two types of detectors, scintillation crystals and gas-filled detectors. The various types of crystals include sodium iodide (NaI), cesium iodide (CsI), and bismuth germanate ($Bi_4Ge_3O_{12}$, BGO). A gas-filled detector array consists of a stack of conducting plates separated by high-pressure xenon gas, and functions as a bank of ionization chambers.

There are two collimators in the scanner. The prepatient collimator limits the beam to plane of the tissue slice. Collimators placed in front of the detectors function like a Bucky grid to absorb scattered x-rays.

The operating console has controls for setting the kilovoltage, milliamperage, scan time, and slice thickness. There are also remote terminals that enable the physician to retrieve images from the computer memory and to manipulate them to obtain more information. Brightness, contrast, and magnification can be adjusted; regions of interest (ROI) can be defined; and a histogram of the CT numbers of the pixels in the ROI can be generated, and the mean and standard deviation of the CT numbers computed. Another feature enables the computer to subtract one image from another. The range of CT numbers in an image can be displayed on the video screen using either a gray scale or a false color scale in which the different colors represent different densities.

RESOLUTION. The resolution of low-contrast structures in CT is limited by statistical noise that is a consequence of the finite number of photons contributing to the calculation of each CT number. The noise has a Poisson distribution so that the noise-relative standard deviation is inversely proportional to the square root of the number of photons detected. To reduce the pixel size to one-half the width (one-fourth the area), it would be necessary to quadruple the radiation dose to the patient to maintain the same noise level or to tolerate twice the noise at the same dose level.

Formerly called *computerized axial tomography* (*CAT*) and *computerized transaxial tomography* (*CTAT*).

computer (kom-pu′ter) an electronic device that performs specified mathematical operations on the input. See also *analog computer* and *digital computer.*

general-purpose c., a digital computer that can be programmed to perform a wide variety of tasks.

special-purpose c., a computer designed to perform a particular task.

computer graphics the area of computer science involved with pictorial communication; the computers using cathode ray tube (CRT) display terminals or plotters for output, and light pens, joy sticks, or graph tablets for input. With interactive computer graphics systems, the graphics programs can convert roughly sketched lines and curves to mathematically exact shapes, and can produce rotated views and other pictorial processing.

computerized axial tomography (CAT) (com-pu′ter-izd) a former name for *computed tomography.*

computerized transaxial tomography (CTAT) a former name for *computed tomography.*

con- (kon) [L., from *cum* with] a prefix word element to denote together or with, e.g., concentrate.

Con A abbrev. See *concanavalin A.*

conc abbrev. See *concentrated.*

concanavalin A (Con A) (kon″kah-nav′ah-lin) a glycoprotein found in jack beans, *Canavalia ensiformis,* which is used in immunology as a mitogen to stimulate lymphocytes. It is also a lectin or hemagglutinin for certain animal erythrocytes. Con A binds specifically to polysaccharides with α-D-glucopyranosyl or α-D-mannopyranosyl residues. It has been used to stimulate T cells, and under appropriate conditions can activate suppressor T cells. It can also stimulate the release of histamine from mast cells or basophils.

concatenation (kon-kat″ĕ-na′shun) [*con-* + L. *catenare* to link, from *catena* chain] 1. a sequence of closely connected events or objects.

2. (symbol | |), in computer programming, the joining of two bit or character strings end-to-end to make one string. For example, if A and B are two three-character strings with the values "OUT" and "PUT," the result of the operation A| |B is the six-character string "OUTPUT."

Concato's disease (kon-kah′tōz) [Luigi Maria *Concato,* Italian physician, 1825–1882] progressive malignant polyserositis with large effusions into the pericardium, pleura, and peritoneum.

concave (con′kāv) [L. *concavus* hollow] pertaining to a line or surface that curves toward the viewer, such as the surface of a sphere as viewed from the inside. Cf. *convex.*

concentrate (kon′sen-trāt) [con- + L. *centrum* center] 1. to bring to a common center, to gather together at one point; to focus.

2. to increase the concentration of a solution as by the evaporation of a solvent; to condense.

3. a solution prepared by increasing its concentration.

concentrated (conc) (kon′sen-tra″ted) 1. pertaining to a solution that contains a relatively large amount of solute.

2. referring to arbitrary or conventional concentrations of certain common acids and bases. The concentrations commercially used are those compatible with convenience of manufacture or storage and are often close to saturation (e.g., 96 percent sulfuric acid or 28 percent ammonia water). See also the accompanying table.

concentration (kon″sen-tra′shun) [L. *concentratio*] the amount (which may be expressed as mass, volume, number of moles, number of equivalents, etc.) of a solute to the mass or volume of solvent or solution. See the specific types of concentration: *mass concentration, molality, molarity, mole fraction,* and *normality.* See also *pH.*

concentration procedures the process of separating protozoan cysts or helminth eggs in stool specimens. A variety of methods are used, in which the parasites are separated either by settling out of an aqueous suspension as a result of gravity or centrifugation, or by flotation to the top of a suspension in a liquid of high specific gravity. Usually, formalin-fixed specimens are employed.

conception (kon-sep′shun) [L. *conceptio*] the onset of pregnancy, marked by implantation of the blastocyst; the formation of a viable zygote.

conceptional age (kon-sep′shun-al) the age of an infant calculated in weeks from the first day of the mother's last menstrual period until birth (the estimated gestational age) plus the number of weeks since birth (legal age).

concha (kong′kah), pl. *conchae* [L., from Gr. *kon-*

CONCENTRATED. STRENGTHS OF CONCENTRATED SOLUTIONS OF ACIDS AND BASES

ACID OR BASE	SPECIFIC GRAVITY	% BY WEIGHT	WEIGHT (g/l)	APPROXIMATE MOLARITY
Hydrochloric acid (HCl)	1.19	37	440	12.1
Sulfuric acid (H_2SO_4)	1.84	96	1730	18
Nitric acid (HNO_3)	1.42	70	990	15.7
Acetic acid (CH_3COOH)	1.06	99.5	1060	17.4
Ammonium hydroxide (NH_4OH)	0.880	29	250	15–17
Sodium hydroxide (saturated solution) (NaOH)	1.50–1.53	about 50	600–700	15–18
Potassium hydroxide* (saturated solution) (KOH)	1.55	about 50	800	14

* Saturated solutions made from the usual CP potassium hydroxide will vary in strength, chiefly because of the variable amount of carbonate that such solutions contain.

Modified from Tietz, N.W.: Fundamentals of Clinical Chemistry. 2nd ed. Philadelphia, W.B. Saunders Co., 1976, p. 39.

chē] a shell; used in anatomic nomenclature to designate a structure or part that resembles a shell in shape, particularly the nasal conchae or turbinate bones.

concordance (kon-kōr′dans) in genetics, the occurrence of a given trait in both members of a twin pair. Cf. *discordance.*

concretion (kon-kre′shun) [L. *concretio,* from *con-* + *crescere* to grow] 1. a calculus or inorganic mass.

2. the abnormal union of adjacent parts.

concussion (kon-kush′un) [L. *concussio*] 1. a violent jar or shock.

2. a transient and immediate loss of consciousness due to a head injury.

condensation (kon″den-sa′shun) [L. *condensatio,* from *con-* + *densare* to make thick] 1. the process of becoming more compact.

2. the process of passing from a gaseous to a liquid or solid state.

condenser (kon-den′ser) [L. *condensare* to make thick] 1. an apparatus for condensing gases or vapors.

2. in optics, a system of lenses or mirrors that gathers the maximum amount of light from the source and directs it through the specimen to the microscope objective.

3. see *capacitor.*

Abbe c., a compound lens used to direct light through the objective of a compound microscope.

darkfield c., the condenser of a darkfield microscope.

conditional jump (kon-dish′un-al) in a digital computer, a machine-language instruction that either specifies the address of the next instruction or permits the normal execution of instructions in sequence, depending on whether a specified condition is satisfied.

In some computers the conditions tested are whether the contents of the accumulator are less than, equal to, or greater than zero, or are even or odd, and whether the last operation produced an overflow. In other computers there is a comparison register set by special comparison operations and by arithmetic overflows.

Also called branch on condition or conditional branch. Cf. *unconditional jump.*

conditional probability the probability of an event *B* given that another event *A* has occurred, denoted $P(B|A)$. For example, if *B* is the event "a person has disease," and *A* is the event "a person has a positive test result," then $P(A|B)$ (which is called the diagnostic sensitivity of the test) is the probability that the test can correctly identify a person who is known to have the disease, whereas $P(B|A)$ is the probability that a person who has a positive test also has the disease (which is the predictive value of a positive test result). See also *Bayes's theorem* and *probability.*

conductance (G) (kon-duk′tans) 1. the ability of a circuit to conduct electricity, the reciprocal of resistance. The unit of electric conductance is the mho.

2. the ability of an object to conduct heat. Thermal conductance is the temperature difference divided by the heat flow.

conduction (kon-duk′shun) [L. *conductio*] the transfer of energy or information via a material medium.

conduction defect a general term for any disorder of the conducting system of the heart.

conduction electron an electron that contributes to the electric conductivity of a metal or an intrinsic semiconductor. In metals, conduction electrons behave approximately like free electrons, moving freely through the crystal in response to an applied electric field.

conduction time see *latency.*

conduction velocity the speed (distance per unit of time) of transmission of an action potential along the fiber of a muscle or nerve, generally expressed as meters per second (m/sec). The speed of conduction increases with increasing axon diameter. Myelinated somatic afferent and efferent axons (A fibers) in some mammals conduct with a maximal velocity of up to 125 m/sec, myelinated efferent preganglionic autonomic B fibers at velocities of 3–15 m/sec, and unmyelinated postganglionic sympathetic C fibers at 0.3–2.0 m/sec.

conductivity (kon″duk-tiv′ĭ-te) 1. the capacity of a material to conduct a flow of electricity or heat; the conductance per unit area of material.

2. the ability of protoplasm to transmit an electric impulse throughout the cell from the point of stimulus.

water c., a measure of purity of water, since the purity of water is inversely related to its conductivity and directly related to its resistance. It is generally expressed in mhos. High-purity water for trace metal work should have a conductivity of $< 10^{-7}\ \Omega^{-1}$ (or greater than 10 MΩ resistance).

conductivity cell volume (CCV) a relationship between the electric conductivity of whole blood and the packed red cell volume (PVC). This concept was devised as an attempt to measure the PCV directly from the change of conductivity of a saline solution by introducing a fixed volume of blood. The method did not prove to be satisfactory and has been abandoned.

conductometry (kon″duk-tom′ĕ-tre) measurement of the conductivity of a solution using alternating current (100–3000 Hz) to avoid electrode polarization. At a fixed voltage, the conductivity is proportional to the current. Conductometry is used to determine the end points of many types of titrations and to detect the presence of electrolytes in water.

conductor (kon-duk′tor) a material medium, such as an electric wire, that conducts energy.

condyle (kon′dīl) [L. *condylus,* from Gr. *kondylos* knuckle] a rounded projection of bone.

condyloma (kon″dĭ-lo′mah), pl. *condylomata* [Gr. *kondylōma* knuckle or knob] a general term used to describe proliferative hyperkeratotic exophytic lesions of stratified squamous epithelium, seen particularly on the penis, mucosa of the female genitalia, and skin of the perianal region. Lesions begin as small, elevated, soft nodules, which grow and coalesce, eventually producing cauliflower-like excrescences.

c. accuminatum, a form of verruca; a papillary, cauliflower-like growth that occurs on the glans or prepuce of the penis, on the mucosal surfaces of the female genitalia, and around and within the anus. Such growths usually are sexually transmitted. Viral particles consistent with the papovavirus group have been identified by electron microscopy in these lesions.

giant c. of Buschke-Lowenstein, a low-grade, verrucous, squamous carcinoma that resembles a giant condyloma. Such lesions typically arise on the vulva, glans or foreskin of the penis, and perineum. Also called verrucous carcinoma.

c. latum, a form of the secondary stage of syphilis, affecting the moist skin or mucosa about the genitals and anus; the lesions are papular or plaquelike. Also called flat condyloma.

cone (kōn) [L. *conus,* from Gr. *kōnos*] 1. a funnel-shaped structure, made from light metal with a radiopaque lining and attached over the x-ray tube aperture to center the radiation beam and control scattering, determine source-to-film distance, and improve detail visibility. It may be equipped with adjustable diaphragms. Collimators have largely replaced cones on modern equipment.

2. a solid figure or body with a circular base tapering to a point.

3. one of the retinal photorceptors. See under *photoreceptor.*

4. see *conus.*

cone biopsy see *conization.*

cone-nosed bug see *Triatoma.*

confabulation (kon-fab″u-la′shun) the recitation of imaginary events and experiences to fill gaps in memory.

confidence interval (kon′fĭ-dens) a type of statistical interval estimate for an unknown parameter μ. The end points of the interval are called upper and lower confidence limits. The confidence limits are determined so that, whatever the true value of μ may be, the probability is $1 - \alpha$ that the limits will contain (encompass, straddle) μ. The percentage $100(1 - \alpha)$ is called the confidence coefficient; α is called the confidence level.

It is often said that the confidence interval calculated from a particular random sample has a $100(1 - \alpha)$ percent probability of containing μ; however, this is a loose description that is not technically correct: μ is a definite (although unknown) parameter of the population and either is or is not contained in any specific interval. However, if a large number of random samples are taken, $100(1 - \alpha)$ percent of the various confidence intervals calculated from the series or random samples will contain μ, and 100α percent will not.

For examples, see under *analysis of variance, linear regression, rank sum test, signed rank test,* and *t distribution.*

confidence level the probability that a confidence interval (i.e., the interval estimate) will contain the true value of the statistical parameter estimated.

configuration (kon-fig″u-ra′shun) 1. the actual components of a piece of equipment or operational unit as opposed to other available options, e.g., the input/output devices and operating system programs used in a computer system.

2. in organic chemistry, the relative order in which the atoms of a molecule are arranged in space in a particular stereoisomer. One can refer to the configuration of a molecule as a whole or to the configuration of an individual chiral center in a molecule. Enantiomers have opposite (mirror image) configurations; diastereomers have different but not opposite configurations. Absolute configuration refers to the configuration of a molecule or chiral center relative to some observable standard, like a left-handed helix. The R and S nomenclature symbols specify absolute configuration. Relative configuration refers to the relationship between the configuration of a particular molecule and a reference compound.

conformation (kon″for-ma′shun) the particular shape of an entity. In chemistry, any of the various shapes that a molecule can assume by rotating about its single bonds (without breaking bonds or rotating about double or triple bonds) and by stretching and bending bonds. The many different conformations possible for most molecules have different energies as a consequence of different degrees of angle strain, steric hindrance, electronic repulsion, etc. The energy difference between the different possible conformations is generally less than the available thermal energy (15–20 kcal/mol at room temperature), and the molecules are constantly shifting between conformations. Thus an equilibrium mixture of all the conformers results, with the more stable conformers being favored. The term conformers (here synonymous with conformational isomers and rotamers) usually refers only to those structures or isomers that can be interconverted by rotation about a single bond.

The conformations produced by rotations about one single bond are typified by those of ethane. (The accompanying illustration shows a Newman projection along the C—C bond axis, in which the hydrogens bonded to the carbon atom in front are shown with bonds drawn to the center of the circle, and those bonded to the carbon in back, with lines to the circumference.) Owing to repulsion between bonding electrons, the eclipsed conformation is 3 kcal/mol less stable than the staggered conformation. This energy barrier to free rotation is increased when a larger group is substituted for a hydrogen atom. Any rotational conformation intermediate between eclipsed and staggered is called a skewed conformer.

If a methyl group is substituted on both carbons (giving *n*-butane), several distinct staggered conformers are possible. The *anti* conformer, in which the methyl groups are 180° apart (Newman projection), is 0.8 kcal/mol more stable than the *gauche* conformer, in which the methyl groups are 60° apart.

The conformational forms of cyclohexane and its derivatives and of other six-membered ring compounds, such as those present in the pyranose forms of sugars, are very important. Only three such conformers are free of angle-bending strain (all bond angles = 109.5°). These are the chair, the boat, and the twist-boat (or twist), which are shown in the accompanying illustration. The chair is the more common form, being about 6 kcal/mol more stable than the other two.

In the chair conformation of cyclohexane, substituents or hydrogen atoms may occupy either axial or equatorial positions. At each carbon atom two substituent positions may occur (the hydrogen atoms in cyclohexane). The positions closest to the "plane" of the ring are called equatorial positions; the others (perpendicular to that "plane") are the axial positions. In substituted cyclohexane (e.g., methylcyclohexane), the conformer with the substituent in the equatorial position tends to be more stable by about 1.7 kcal/mol.

conformer (kon-for′mer) a specific conformation of a molecule, e.g., the chair conformation of cyclohexane. See under *conformation.*

confusion (kon-fu′zhun) a mental state characterized by disturbed orientation to time, place, and person. Affected individuals may interpret sensory stimuli abnormally, have hallucinations and a shortened attention span, be drowsy, and show agitated behavior; disordered states of consciousness may also occur. Causes include both physiologic and psychologic disorders. See also *consciousness disorder.*

congener (kon′jĕ-ner) [*con-* + L. *genus* race] something closely related to another thing, as a chemical compound closely related to another in composition and exerting similar or antagonistic effects.

congenital (kon-jen′ĭ-tal) [L. *congenitus* born together] existing at, and usually before, birth; the term is often used to refer to conditions present at birth regardless of the reason why they are present. For diseases or conditions beginning with this adjective, see the noun.

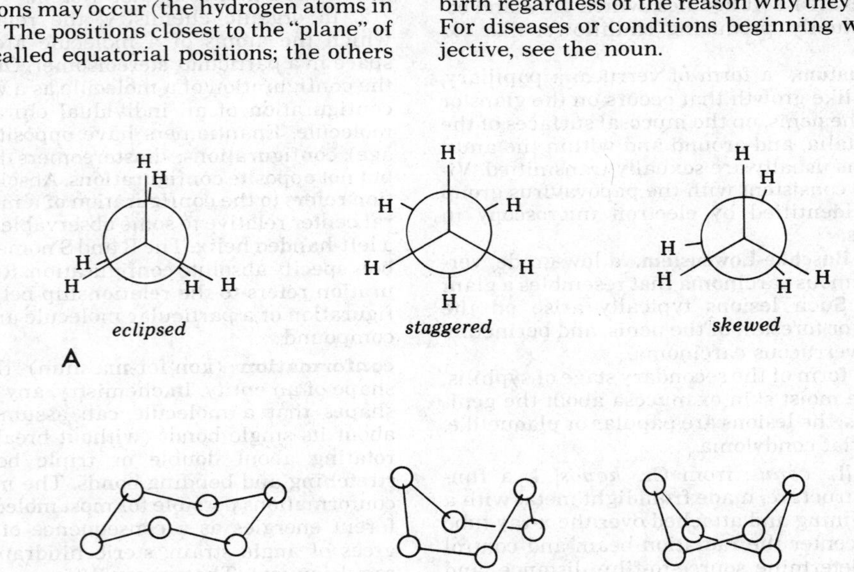

Conformation. *A,* Conformers of ethane. *B,* Conformers of cyclohexane. (From Banks, J. E.: Naming Organic Compounds. 2nd ed. Philadelphia, W. B. Saunders Co., 1976.)

congestion (kon-jes′chun) [L. *congestio,* from *congerere* to heap together] the abnormal accumulation of fluid in an organ or part: usually blood, congestion is also occasionally caused by the accumulation of bile or mucus.

congestive heart failure (CHF) a state in which there is circulatory congestion secondary to heart failure. When the volume of blood delivered into the systemic circulation is chronically reduced, and when one or both ventricles fail to expel the normal fraction of blood delivered to it, a complex sequence of adjustments occurs that ultimately results in an abnormal accumulation of fluid. Thus initially there may be heart failure without congestion, but if the process continues, congestive heart failure will ensue rapidly or gradually.

Although the term congestive heart failure usually denotes failure of both ventricles, typically it is dysfunction of the left side that results in failure of the right side. Venous congestion usually involves both the pulmonary and systemic beds, but congestion may be limited to either.

SIGNS AND SYMPTOMS. An individual frequently seeks medical attention because of breathlessness, which worsens with activity demanding an increased cardiac output. This symptom results from elevated pulmonary venous and capillary pressures that force fluid into the interstitium of the lung, thus increasing the work of breathing. When the left ventricular end-diastolic pressure is severely elevated, the fluid transudes into the alveolar spaces, causing pulmonary edema. Orthopnea (dyspnea when supine) and paroxysmal nocturnal dyspnea (nighttime episodes of pulmonary edema) are other symptoms of pulmonary venous congestion. Cough and wheezing are common and may be mistaken for symptoms of primary pulmonary problems. Right-sided heart failure elevates systemic venous pressure; its principal symptoms are peripheral edema and abdominal discomfort from hepatic enlargement.

Physical examination demonstrates a variety of additional signs and symptoms. A lowered cardiac output may cause the person to appear pale and clammy, and tachycardia and tachypnea may be found. The presence of alveolar fluid may be detected as rales on lung examination. Systemic venous hypertension is demonstrated by elevated jugular venous pressure, liver engorgement, and peripheral edema. The heart is frequently enlarged. Auscultation usually reveals a third heart sound, which is an indication of reduced left ventricular compliance. A fourth heart sound may also be present. The chest radiograph usually confirms cardiac enlargement and shows venous redistribution or frank pulmonary edema. The electrocardiogram is usually abnormal, as it is affected by a major underlying disorder.

TREATMENT. Treatment of CHF is aimed at correcting the basic physiologic derangements. The patient is allowed to sit upright and may be given oxygen to improve pulmonary gas exchange. Diuretics are given to reduce venous hypertension and cardiac filling, and thus myocardial work. Sometimes a drug that improves myocardial contractility, such as digoxin, is given. Sodium restriction is usually indicated. When the acute symptoms are abated, a thorough search for the etiology of heart failure is undertaken. Although the prognosis depends on the underlying cause, the outlook is serious; less than 50 percent of those individuals affected with congestive heart failure are alive 5 yr after onset of the condition.

STEPHAN D. FIHN, M.D., M.P.H.

Congo Corinth (kon′go) an acid azo dye; C.I. 22145. It is used in histology to demonstrate amyloid.

Congo floor maggot see *A. luteola* under *Auchmeromyia* and *Congo floor m.* under *maggot.*

Congo red an acid disazo dye; C.I. 22120. It is used in histology as a stain for amyloid and was formerly used in clinical chemistry in a test for amyloidosis.

Congo red test an obsolete test for demonstrating the possible presence of amyloidosis. It is based on the rate of removal of the dye from the peripheral circulation by amyloid deposits in tissues. Pure parenteral-grade Congo red dye is injected intravenously (4.5 mg/kg of body weight, up to 100 mg), and blood specimens are taken at 3–4 min and at 60 min. Acetone is added to the specimens to remove serum proteins, and the dye is measured photometrically in the clear supernatant. The concentration in the 3–4-min specimen is assumed to equal 100 percent dye retained; reference values for the 60-min specimens are 60–70 percent retention. Retention of only 20–25 percent is highly indicative, and 35–40 percent is suggestive of amyloid deposits. Proteinuria may invalidate the test.

coni/o (ko′ni-o) [Gr. *konis* dust] a word element used in combining form to denote dust, e.g., pneumoconiosis.

conical (kon′ĭ-kal) [Gr. *kōnikos*] having the shape of a cone. A conical object has a circular outline when viewed along its axis, and a triangular outline in projections perpendicular to the long axis. See also the illustration accompanying *contour.*

conidial (ko-nid′e-al) pertaining to or of the nature of conidia; bearing conidia.

Conidiobolus (ko-nid″e-ob′o-lus) [Gr. *konidion* a particle of dust + *bolos* lump] a genus of fungi similar to *Entomophthora,* characterized by globose, multinucleated conidia. Zygospore formation has not yet been demonstrated in *C. coronatus.* The conidia are forcibly discharged from the tips of conidiophores. Two species are recognized to cause entomophthoromycosis: *C. coronatus* and *C. incongruus.*

conidiospore (ko-nid′e-o-spōr″) [Gr. *konidion* a particle of dust + *sporos* seed] a conidium, an asexual spore; see *conidium.*

conidium (ko-nid′e-um), pl. *conidia* [N.L., from Gr. *konis* dust] an asexual spore of fungi borne on hyphal (filamentous) branches either at the tip or laterally. These spores occur singly or in clusters, and vary considerably in size, shape, and color. Examples of conidia include the blastospore, arthrospore, aleuriospore, and phialospore; and macro- or microconidia (most often used in reference to the dermatophyte characteristics). The terms conidium and aleuriospore are sometimes used interchangeably. See also *macroconidium.*

coniine (co′ne-ēn) a very toxic alkaloid, 2-propylpiperidine, obtained from poison hemlock (*Conium maculatum*) and fool's parsley (*Ethusa cynapium*). It affects motor nerve endings, resulting in general paralysis and eventual respiratory paralysis and asphyxia.

coniofibrosis (ko″ne-o-fi-bro′sis) [*conio-* + L. *fibra* fiber + *-osis* condition] pneumoconiosis with growth of connective tissue in the lungs.

coniosis (ko″ne-o′sis) [*conio-* + *-osis* condition] a diseased state due to inhalation of dust, e.g. pneumoconiosis.

Coniosporium (ko″ne-o-spōr′e-um) [N.L., from *conio-* + Gr. *sporos* seed] a genus of saprophytic fungi. The species *C. corticale* (*Cryptostroma corticale*) grows on the bark of certain trees such as the maple, and may cause coniosporosis, an allergic lung disease.

coniosporosis (ko″ne-o-spo-ro′sis) [*Coniosporium* + *-osis* condition] a pneumonitis characterized by asthmatic symptoms, fever, night sweats, and acute pneumonitis. It is caused by the inhalation of *Cryptostroma corticale* spores, which commonly grow on the bark of maple trees. Small, cream-colored granulomas are formed in the lung by the spores, which remain dormant. The condition is seen primarily in workers who strip logs of bark. Also called *cryptostromosis.*

Conium (ko-ni′um) [L., from Gr. *koneion*] a genus of umbelliferous plants. The species *C. maculatum,* poison hemlock, produces the alkaloid coniine, a potent toxin that causes death from paralysis and asphyxia.

conization (kon″ĭ-za′shun) the technique or process of taking a biopsy of the uterine cervix in which a cone of tissue is excised from the base surrounding the cervical os, with the apex in the endocervical canal (see the illustration accompanying *cone biopsy*). The cone is cut out with a cold knife, as electrocautery distorts the tissue and makes it unsatisfactory for histologic diagnosis.

Diagnostic conization is employed when cervical smears indicate the presence of cervical intraepithelial neoplasia and the extent or invasiveness of the carcinoma cannot be determined by colposcopy and punch biopsy.

conjugate (kon′ju-gāt) [L. *conjugatus* yoked together] 1. paired or equally coupled; working in unison, as in conjugate eye movements.

2. a diameter of the pelvic inlet; generally used alone to denote the true internal conjugate diameter as distinct from the external or diagonal conjugates.

c. acid-base pairs, in an acid-base reaction, the proton donor (acid) and the base formed from it by proton removal, or the proton acceptor (base) and the acid formed from it by proton transfer; e.g., in the reaction CH_3COOH (acetic acid) + OH^- (hydroxide ion) ⇄ CH_3COO^- (acetate) + H_2O, acetic acid and acetate are a conjugate acid-base pair, as are hydroxide and water. Acetate can be called the conjugate base of acetic acid, or acetic acid can be called the conjugate acid of acetate.

conjugate acid the chemical species formed by the addition of a proton to its conjugate base; e.g., the ammonium ion (NH_4^+) is the conjugate acid of the base ammonia (NH_3).

$$NH_3 + H^+ \rightleftharpoons NH_4^+$$

Base (a proton acceptor)	Proton	Conjugate acid (a proton donor)

conjugate base the chemical species formed by removal (dissociation, ionization) of a proton from another species (its conjugate acid).

conjugated protein the class of complex proteins characterized by the presence of one or more nonprotein molecules (prosthetic groups) linked to the polypeptide chains of the protein by forces other than those operating in simple salt formation. This class includes the nucleoproteins, chromoproteins (e.g., hemoglobin), glycoproteins, phosphoproteins, lipoproteins, and metalloproteins.

conjugate redox pair see *redox couple.*

conjugation (kon″ju-ga′shun) 1. the act of joining together.

2. in bacterial genetics, a form of sexual reproduction by direct cell contact in which a donor bacterium contributes some or all of its DNA (in the form of a replicated set) to a recipient, which then incorporates the new genetic information into its own chromosome by recombination, and passes the recombined set on to its progeny by replication. See also *bacterial g.* under *genetics.*

3. in chemistry, the joining together of two compounds to produce another compound, such as the combination of a toxic product with some substance in the body to form a detoxified product, which is then eliminated (e.g., as sulfate or glucuronide ester).

4. the condition resulting from the presence of two or more unsaturated groups connected by a single bond. The double bonds in 1,3-pentadiene are conjugated, for example; those in 1,2-pentadiene and 1,4-pentadiene are not. Acrolein, $CH_2{=}CH{-}CH{=}O$, also has conjugated double bonds.

conjunctiv/o (kon″junk-ti′vo) [L. *conjunctivus* serving to connect] a word element used in combining form to denote the conjunctiva, e.g., conjunctivitis.

conjunctiva (kon″junk-tī′vah), pl. *conjunctivae* [L.] the delicate membrane that lines the eyelids and covers the exposed surface of the sclera.

conjunctivitis (kon-junk″tĭ-vi′tis) [*conjunctiva* + *-itis* inflammation] an acute or chronic inflammation of the conjunctiva of the eye. It may be caused by a number of organisms, including staphylococci, chlamydiae, rickettsiae and other bacteria, viruses, and parasites, as well as by trauma and allergy. This disorder is characterized by injection and redness of the conjunctiva, clear-to-purulent discharge, swelling of the eyelid, lymph node involvement, and itching. Dust or air pollution may aggravate the condition. Diagnosis is based on culture and staining of the discharge, especially with Gram or Wright stains.

adult gonococcal c., an uncommon form of conjunctivitis that is frequently severe and purulent. Adults acquire this infection through self-inoculation from a genital gonorrheal infection or through exposure to a gonorrheal contact. The infection is similar to that seen in infants (ophthalmia neonatorum). It tends to be unilateral, with serous discharge and swelling of the eyelids; bulbar infection may develop within several days. Corneal ulceration, abscess formation, and blindness are potential complications. Treatment requires parenteral antimicrobial therapy. See also *sexually transmitted diseases.*

allergic c., a chronic, recurrent bilateral inflammation of the conjunctiva associated with exposure to environmental antigens, e.g., hay fever. It is characterized by tearing, itching, redness, photophobia, and a stringy discharge with many eosinophils. The symptoms often occur in the spring when trees and grasses are pollinating; they abate after the summer. Also called vernal conjunctivitis.

granular c., see *trachoma.*

inclusion c., an acute inflammation of the conjunctiva, usually due to an infection with serotypes of *Chlamydia trachomatis* characteristic of genital infection. In infants, this disease (also called inclusion blennorrhea or TRIC ophthalmia neonatorum) occurs 5–14 da after birth and leads to redness, mucopurulent discharge, swelling of the eyelid, and chemosis. Pupillary hypertrophy and keratitis, usually without corneal scarring, are also seen. Babies with this disease may have associated infections of the upper respiratory tract, as well as pneumonia and genital infections. In adults, inclusion conjunctivitis occurs in sexually active individuals through self-inoculation with genital secretions. It is characterized by redness, irritation, and discharge. Mild keratitis and lymphadenitis may occur, but permanent damage is rare. Some cases become chronic or result in scarring of the conjunctiva and formation of a corneal pannus that lead to an acute trachoma.

Diagnosis is based on clinical findings and demonstration of epithelial-cell inclusion bodies in conjunctival scrapings. Also called *swimming pool c.* See also *Chlamydia* and *sexually transmitted diseases.*

c. neonatorum, see *o. neonatorum* under *ophthalmia.*

swimming pool c., see *inclusion c.*

connective tissue (kŏ-nek′tiv) the tissue that binds together and provides support for the organs and other structures of the body. It is derived from mesoderm and consists primarily of bundles of collagen fibrils with a matrix of proteoglycans (ground substance) and varying numbers of elastin fibrils. In loose connective tissue there is an admixture of fat, whereas dense connective tissue is principally collagenous. The fibrils and ground substance are formed by fibroblasts. Connective tissue also contains blood and lymph vessels, and various transient cells including macrophages and mast cells.

connective tissue nevus see *connective tissue n.* under *nevus.*

connector (kŏ-nek′tor) 1. a device that makes a detachable electric and mechanical connection between electric cables.

2. a device used to join, fasten together, or establish communication between two objects.

Conn's syndrome (konz) [Jerome W. *Conn,* U.S. internist, born 1907] see *primary h.* under *hyperaldosteronism.*

Conray (kon′ra) trademark. See under *iothalamate.*

consanguineous (kon″san-gwin′e-us) sharing a common ancestor(s).

consanguineous mating mating occurring between relatives; this type of assortative mating disturbs the Hardy-Weinberg equilibrium of genotype frequencies by increasing the proportion of homozygotes at the expense of the heterozygotes. Only first- and second-cousin mating involves enough common genes to carry a sufficiently increased risk of producing offspring homozygous for a deleterious recessive trait. Consanguinity can expose recessive genes to selection and eventual loss, permanently altering gene frequencies in the population. See also *consanguinity* and *inbreeding coefficient.*

consanguinity (kon″sang-gwin′ĭ-te) [L. *consanguinitas*] kinship by descent from a common ancestor. Consanguinity is measured by the coefficient of inbreeding (F), which is the probability that an individual is homozygous for alleles derived from the same ancestral source. The coefficient of inbreeding for first-cousin matings is 1/16.

Consanguineous matings have an increased risk of producing offspring homozygous for a deleterious recessive trait. For instance, congenital deafness is found in high frequencies in consanguineous communities.

consciousness (kon′shus-nes) the state of being conscious; responsiveness of the mind to impressions made by the senses, so that there is external awareness.

consciousness disorder any deviation from the normal state of awareness and responsiveness to one's self and the environment; terms such as confusion, stupor, delirium, and coma have been used to describe these abnormal situations. There is no universal agreement on the definition of any of these terms; in fact, each term generally has a different meaning when used by medical personnel, psychiatric workers, or the lay public. Thus, although these terms have some clinical usefulness, it is best to describe specifically what the individual can and cannot do rather than apply an ill-defined label to his or her condition.

Confusion is described as a condition in which the attention span is shortened and external stimuli are misinterpreted. A confused individual is often drowsy, bewildered, and mildly disoriented. In a severe case, the person may be markedly disoriented and quite out of touch with his or her environment. It is important to distinguish confusion from dysphasia or language disorders. In the latter cases, the person exhibits inappropriate speech but other behavior and responses are normal.

In delirium, the individual is confused, agitated, fearful, and irritable. Illusions and hallucinations are common and often difficult to control. Delirium may occur in persons withdrawing from alcohol; it also occurs in those with drug overdoses, certain medical illnesses, central nervous system infections and injuries, metabolic disorders, and toxic disorders.

Stupor is a state of markedly decreased alertness, characterized by unresponsiveness from which the person can be aroused only by repeated, vigorous stimulation. It is often seen as a prelude to coma and sometimes noted in psychiatric disorders.

One of the most frequently seen consciousness disorders is coma. In coma, a person is unconscious (i.e., not responsive either to external stimuli or to internal sensations or needs) and cannot be aroused. Coma is not a disease in itself: it is a symptom of some other underlying medical or neurological disorder. The causes may be metabolic, such as hypoglycemia, hypoxia, electrolyte abnormalities, drug overdoses, or hepatic or uremic encephalopathy. Structural abnormalities in the CNS can also cause coma if they involve both cerebral hemispheres or the brain stem. Examples of structural problems are lesions such as subdural or epidural hematomas, neoplasms, abscesses, or intracerebral hematomas. The extent of structural injury to the brain stem can be assessed in comatose patients by evaluation of certain neurologic signs. Reactions such as pupillary responses, motor activity to painful stimuli, eye movements, and respiratory status will vary, depending on the area of the brain or brain stem that has been damaged.

Initial treatment of a comatose person includes maintaining an adequate airway and circulation. If there has been trauma to the head and neck, the cervical spine must be protected until further evaluation is carried out. Historical information obtained from persons accompanying the patient is helpful in defining the causes of coma. Laboratory evaluation of the comatose patient includes checking levels of serum glucose, calcium, electrolytes, and arterial blood gases. Determination of BUN and a complete blood count also are usually performed. Depending on the history and suspected diagnosis, a toxicology screen may be performed on serum, urine, or gastric contents, and a CT scan of the brain or skull and cervical spine radiographs may be obtained.

The cause of coma is not always immediately obvious. However, if neurosurgical intervention is needed, prompt diagnosis and initiation of therapy are essential. A detailed physical examination, together with laboratory information, are often helpful in this regard. In all cases, glucose must be given intravenously as soon as possible (but after a blood sample has been obtained for glucose determination) in case hypoglycemia is the underlying cause; delay may lead to permanent damage.

NANETTE SMITH, M.D.

consensual (kon′sen′shu-al) [L. *consensus* agreement] excited by reflex stimulation. The term is used with special reference to the reflex pupillary response of one eye when a stimulus is applied to the other.

consensual light reflex see *light r.* under *reflex.*

console (kon′sōl) the part of a computer used by the operator to supervise and control its operations. It can be used to correct errors, to change storage content, and to communicate with the central processing unit.

consolidation (kon-sol″ĭ-da′shun) [L. *consolidatio*] the process of becoming solidified or more dense, as occurs in the lungs in pneumonia.

consolidation therapy continued treatment of acute leukemia after induction of complete remission to prolong the remission.

conspecific (kon″spĕ-sif′ik) 1. of or referring to the same species.

2. considered to be a member of the same species.

constant (kon′stant) [L. *constans* standing together] 1. unchanging.

2. a value that is not subject to change; in a mathematical equation, it refers to a quantity that has a fixed value, whereas in a computer program it refers to a numeric, logical, or character datum that can be used but not changed by the program.

constant (C) region the carboxyl-terminal region of an immunoglobulin chain. It is the same in all immunoglobulins of a particular subclass; the variable region at the amino-terminal end of each chain is the same for all immunoglobulins produced by a given cell or clone of cells but is different for chains produced by different cells, and it confers antigenic specificity. The constant region of a light chain is denoted C_L; that of a heavy chain, C_H. The C_H region is further divided into three homology units (C_H1, C_H2, and C_H3) for α, β, and γ heavy chains, and four units (C_H1 to C_H4) for ϵ and μ heavy chains.

constitution (kon″stĭ-tu′shun) [L. *constitutio,* from *constituere* to fix] 1. the make-up or functional habit of the body.

2. the order in which the atoms of a molecule are joined together.

constitutional (kon″stĭ-tu′shun-al) affecting the whole constitution of the body; not local.

constitutive enzyme an enzyme that is synthesized by a cell regardless of the presence of substrate.

constitutive heterochromatin method see C banding under *chromosome banding.*

constriction (kon-strik′shun) [*con-* + L. *stringere* to draw] a constricted part or place; a stricture.

constructable (kon-struk′tah-b′l) pertaining to a solution of a mathematical problem that can be obtained by a known procedure. Cf. *algorithm* and *constructive proof.*

constructive proof (kon-struk′tiv) in mathematics, a proof that supplies an explicit procedure for solving a problem (even a procedure requiring an infinite number of steps). Cf. *algorithm* and *existence proof.*

consumption (kon-sump′shun) [L. *consumptio* a wasting] 1. the act of consuming, or the process of being consumed.

2. a wasting away of the body; once applied especially to pulmonary tuberculosis.

consumption coagulopathy see *disseminated intravascular coagulation.*

contact (kon-takt) [L. *contactus* a touching together] 1. the mutual touching of two bodies.

2. the completion of an electric circuit.

3. a person who has been sufficiently near an infected person to have been exposed to the transfer of infectious material.

contact catalysis catalysis produced by adsorbing the reactants onto a surface, e.g., catalysis by colloidal platinum. Also called heterogeneous catalysis.

contact inhibition the cessation of movement or cell division that occurs when cells come into contact with one another. Neoplastic transformation is accompanied by a decreased sensitivity to contact inhibition.

contact sensitivity a type of delayed hypersensitivity reaction in which an individual is sensitized by skin contact with a chemical and then develops a skin reaction when subsequently exposed to the same chemical. An example of one chemical that causes this reaction is dinitrochlorobenzene (DNCB), which is sometimes used to test for a delayed hypersensitivity response in an individual who shows anergy to skin tests.

contagion (kon-ta′jun) [L. *contagio* contact, infection] 1. the spread of disease from one person to another.

2. a contagious disease.

contagious (kon-ta′jus) capable of being transmitted from one person to another.

container size limitations regulatory standards for sizes of glass containers and containers of flammable liquids in laboratories.

Glass containers for chemicals may be hazardous if the containers are large or easily broken, or if the chemicals are corrosive, irritating, toxic, or flammable. Gallon-sized glass bottles are particularly susceptible to breakage; the use of safety cans or breakage protection for such bottles should be considered if spills would present severe hazards. Gallon-sized glass bottles are prohibited for the storage of flammable liquids having flash-point temperatures below 22.8°C (73°F) by NFPA (National Fire Protection Association) and OSHA (Occupational Safety and Health Administration) standards, unless the required liquid purity (such as analytical reagent grade or higher) would be affected by storage in metal containers, or if the liquid would cause excessive corrosion of the metal container. One pint is the maximal allowable size of glass containers for Class IA flammable liquids, such as ethyl ether, and 1 qt is the maximal allowable size for Class IB flammable liquids, such as acetone and alcohol, unless there is a need for larger containers and glass is needed for purity.

Containers of flammable liquids in laboratories are limited to a maximal size of 18.9 l (5 gal). The maximal size of container permitted in instructional laboratories is 3.8 l (1 gal).

containment (kon-tān′ment) a term used to describe methods for managing infectious agents in the laboratory environment where such agents are being handled or maintained. The purpose of these procedures is to reduce the exposure of laboratory workers, visitors, and the outside environment to potentially hazardous agents. Containment involves a combination of good microbiologic techniques and appropriate safety equipment and facility design. See also *biohazard* and *biological safety cabinet.*

contaminant (kon-tam′ĭ-nant) [L. *contaminare* to bring into contact] something that causes contamination.

contamination (kon-tam″ĭ-na′shun) [L. *contaminatio,* from *con-* + *tangere* to touch] 1. the presence of any extraneous material that makes a substance or preparation impure. Assays with high sensitivity but low specificity are most affected by contaminants.

2. the soiling or pollution by inferior material, as by the introduction of organisms into a wound, or sewage into a stream.

3. the deposition of radioactive material where it may be dangerous to humans or other living species, or may interfere with clinical radiation measurements.

continence (kon′tĭ-nens) [L. *continentia,* from *continere* to refrain] the ability to exercise voluntary control over natural impulses, such as the urge to defecate or urinate.

contingency table (kon-tin′jen-se) a table used to display statistical data classified according to two nominal scales (qualitative characteristics), each consisting of a number of mutually exclusive categories.

An $r \times k$ contingency table contains r rows, which correspond to the r categories of one scale, and k columns, which correspond to the k categories of the other. Each item is the observed number of individuals that are members of both the row and the column categories. Each row or column total gives the number of individuals in the associated category.

Statistical analysis of the contingency table often involves procedures based on the chi-squared distribution. See also *chi-squared test.*

contingent negative variation (CNV) (kon-tin′jent) in electroencephalography, a small negative potential recorded from the frontocentral area of the brain, which may be demonstrated in subjects performing a task requiring attention and expectancy. For example, the task may consist of two stimuli, one a warning stimulus and the second a stimulus to which the subject must make a response. The CNV occurs between the first stimulus and the response. Occurrence of the CNV is not related to the modality or intensity of the stimulus, but its amplitude does show a positive correlation to the degree of attention displayed by the subject. The fact that it is poorly developed in young children may be related to their degree of distraction and fatigue during testing.

The CNV is usually recorded from the vertex of the scalp with a reference electrode placed on the mastoid bone. When using this derivation, care must be taken to eliminate the recording potentials produced by vertical eye movements.

Because of the ease with which the CNV can be diminished and/or reestablished, it has been used as a clinical tool in the evaluation of individuals with psychiatric disorders.

The wave is slow to develop in those with anxiety, its amplitude is generally of lower voltage in hysterical than in obsessional patients, and its duration is longer in psychotic patients than in normal subjects. Such findings, however, have no diagnostic relevance.

Also called expectancy wave.

continuous (kon-tin′u-us) [L. *continuus*] 1. unbroken, uninterrupted, or unceasing.

2. in mathematics, pertaining to a continuous function. See also *continuous function.*

3. in statistics, pertaining to a random variable that can assume any value in a continuum. Cf. *discrete.*

continuous flow culture see *continuous flow c.* under *culture.*

continuous function a mathematical function with no jumps; i.e., $f(x) - f(y)$ approaches zero as x approaches y, where $f(x)$ is the value of the function at the point x.

continuous positive airway pressure (CPAP) see *continuous p. p. b.* under *positive pressure breathing.*

continuous spectrum an absorption or emission spectrum distributed over a wide range of frequencies, which does not have well-defined bands or lines. It is typified by the blackbody radiation emitted by an incandescent object.

continuous x-ray spectrum the part of an x-ray beam that consists of a continuous range of wavelengths. It is the bremsstrahlung emitted by cathode electrons striking the target of an x-ray tube.

contour (kon′toor) [Fr.] the outline or shape of a part. Terms used in describing the contours of parts and structures are shown in the accompanying illustration.

contra- (kon′trah) [L. *contra* against] a prefix word element to denote against or opposite, e.g., contralateral.

contractile (con-trak′tĭl) [*con-* + L. *trahere* to draw] having the ability to contract.

contractile ring constriction produced by microfilament action that appears during anaphase

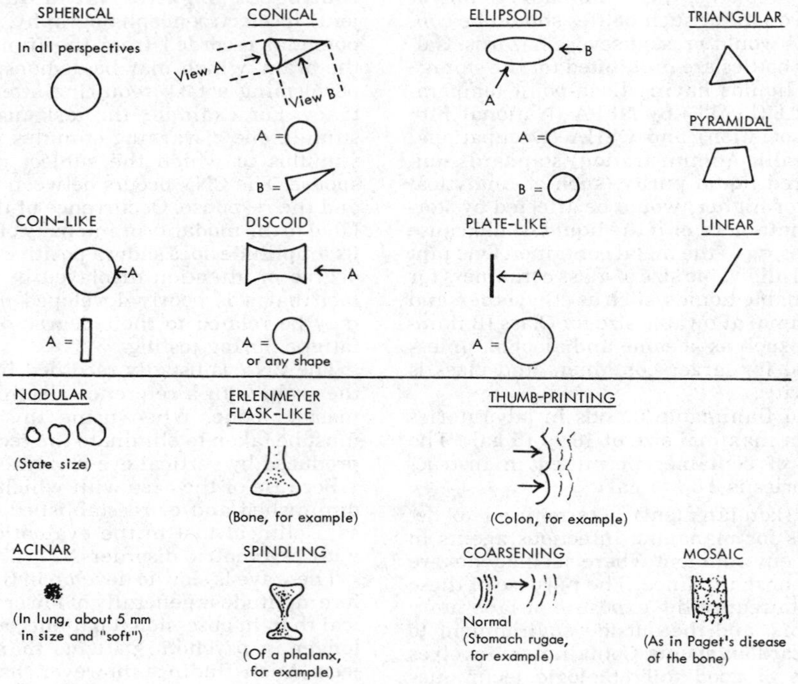

Contour. Illustrations of terms often used in description of contour or architecture. (From Meschan, I.: Synopsis of Analysis of Roentgen Signs in General Radiology. Philadelphia, W. B. Saunders Co., 1976.)

and telophase of cell division and causes the cleavage into two cells. See also *mitosis.*

contractility (kon″trak-til′ĭ-te) the capacity to shorten in response to a stimulus.

contraction (kon-trak′shun) [L. *contractus* drawn together] 1. a reversible shortening or development of tension in a muscle that is normally accompanied by muscle action potentials. In striated muscle fibers, contraction is the result of the orderly interdigitation of cross-bridges of the contractile proteins actin and myosin.

2. a single beat of the atrium or ventricle of a heart.

contracture (kon-trak′chur) [L. *contractura*] 1. a prolonged, involuntary state of muscle contraction that is electrically silent. Relaxation does not occur, owing to an inhibition of the active transport of calcium ions back into the cisterns of the sarcoplasmic reticulum. Contracture can develop following muscle exercise in patients with phosphorylase deficiency (McArdle's disease). It is also a common artifact in muscle biopsies.

2. a joint deformity produced by fixed muscle shortening with fibrosis.

Dupuytren's c., thickening and shortening of the palmar fascia, which results in flexion deformity of one or more fingers. Also called palmar fibromatosis.

ischemic c., a contraction deformity of a muscle due to impaired circulation from pressure, injury, or cold.

Volkmann's c., a contraction deformity of the fingers and sometimes the wrist, with loss of power, that develops rapidly after a severe ischemic injury, usually in the region of the elbow joint.

contraindication (kon″trah-in″dĭ-ka′shun) any condition that renders a particular line of treatment improper or undesirable.

contralateral (kon″trah-lat′er-al) [*contra-* + L. *latus* side] situated on or affecting the opposite side. Cf. *ipsilateral.*

contrast (kon′trast) the degree to which light and dark areas of an image differ in brightness or in optical density. In radiology, it is the difference in optical density in a radiograph that results from a difference in radiolucency or penetrability of the subject. Extreme contrast, resulting in an image in blacks and whites, is called high or short-scale contrast. Low contrast, resulting in an image in shades of gray, is called long-scale contrast. Contrast that is too high can wash out faint but significant shadows.

The properties of both the x-ray beam and the film control contrast. Increasing the kilovoltage reduces the contrast; reducing the exposure (milliampere-seconds) secondarily reduces the contrast by reducing the density. The contrast due to film sensitivity is the gradient by which density increases with log exposure (shown by the H and D curve of the film). A film with low contrast has wide latitude.

contrast media substances introduced into or around a body part so that the part can be radiographically visualized. A radiopaque medium has an x-ray absorptivity significantly greater than body tissues, a radiolucent medium significantly less. Radiopaque media are compounds containing barium or iodine, that because of their high atomic numbers (56 and 53) have approximately 400 times the absorptivity of the atoms of soft tissue. In contrast, radiolucent media are gases: air, oxygen, helium, carbon dioxide, nitrous oxide, and nitrogen, that because of their low density have approximately 1/750 times the absorptivity of soft tissue.

Barium sulfate is an insoluble salt used in colloidal suspension for examination of the gastrointestinal tract. It coats the mucosa or fills the lumen, and it is not absorbed by the intestines nor does it interfere with physiologic function.

WATER-SOLUBLE IODINATED MEDIA. These contrast media are organic compounds with a high iodine content. Most contain a benzene ring substituted with iodine at the 2, 4, and 6 positions and organic radicals at the 1, 3, and 5 positions; an example is diatrizoate, 3,5-bis(acetylamino)-2,4,6-triiodobenzoate. Diatrizoate and iothalamate are excreted primarily by the kidneys; they are administered intravenously in angiography or intravenous urography. They are also introduced into body cavities by catheterization in cystography or hysterosalpingography, and injected into tissues or cavities in transhepatic cholangiography, splenoportography, and arthrography.

Some water-soluble iodinated media are selectively excreted by the liver. Iopanoic acid, iocetamic acid, trypanoate, and ipodate are absorbed by the intestines, transported to the liver, and excreted in the bile. These are used in oral cholecystography; iodipamide is used in intravenous cholangiography.

FAT-SOLUBLE CONTRAST MEDIA. Oily or fat-soluble contrast media include propyliodone (Dionosil), used in bronchography; ethiodized oil (Ethiodol), used in lymphangiography; and iophendylate (Pantopaque), used in myelography.

RADIOLUCENT MEDIA. These media are utilized in pneumoencephalography and ventriculography; for double-contrast procedures, as in arthrography; and for dual contrast procedures, as in retroperitoneal gas insufflation in urography.

contrast media reaction any of the side-effects to the iodine-containing intravascular injections of contrast media in x-ray examinations of tissues, organs, and organ systems. These occur in a small but significant number of individuals. The cause and mechanisms of contrast reactions remain unexplained, despite extensive investigation. True allergic responses have not been demonstrated, and many reactions must be considered to be of an idiosyncratic or chemotoxic nature related to the hypertonicity of the solution, and probably involving the release of histamine.

Routinely, after intravenous injection of contrast agents, individuals experience mild flushing, nausea, a metallic taste, and some warmth or tingling sensations. These reactions are thought to be mild, and they occur with sufficient frequency (50 percent) to be anticipated; no therapy is required.

More severe reactions necessitating immediate treatment occur in approximately 2 percent of individuals; life-threatening reactions arise with a frequency of approximately 0.1 percent. Deaths as a direct result of contrast injections do occur, but fortunately are rare. Current estimates place the mortality rate at 1 in 50,000 examinations.

Severe reactions are of two major types. One type consists of generalized anaphylactoid reactions, characterized by airway spasm, hives, hypotension, laryngeal edema, vasodilation, and tachycardia. The patient is usually conscious; treatment involves immediate establishment of an airway and ventilation followed by epinephrine, corticosteroid, and antihistamine injections. The second type is the cardiovascular reaction, which may include cardiopulmonary arrest, profound bradycardia, apnea, loss of consciousness, and shock. Treatment involves immediate establishment and maintenance of an airway, ventilation, and restoration of cardiac output utilizing standard cardiopulmonary resuscitation techniques. The vagus reaction is characterized by hypotension and bradycardia; this responds to intravenous atropine in moderately large doses.

Proper preparation for and prompt recognition of contrast media reactions can prevent death or serious permanent disability in all but rare instances.

FREDERICK R. MARGOLIN, M.D.

contrecoup (kon-trĕ-koo′) [Fr. "counterblow"] see *contracoup c.* under *contusion.*

control (kon-trōl′) [Fr. *controle* a register] 1. a limitation or restraint.

2. the elimination or restriction of the spread of infectious agents or pests.

3. a standard of comparison. In scientific experiments, a control consists of a procedure or study group identical to that of the experiment except for the absence of the one factor being studied. See also *control group.*

4. in clinical chemistry, a sample with known values used to determine the accuracy of a method. See also *reference materials.*

control group in statistics, a group of individuals similar to the study group in every important respect except for exposure to a particular risk factor or treatment.

controlled substance (kon-trōld) a term for a substance subject to federal regulation of its manufacture, sale, or distribution because of the potential for, or proved evidence of, abuse; because of its potential for psychic or physiologic dependence; because it constitutes a public health risk; because of the scientific evidence of its pharmacologic effect; or because of its role as a precursor of other controlled substances.

control materials see under *reference materials.*

control panel a panel that holds the meters and other readout devices for indicating the status of an electronic system, and the switches and dials for controlling its operation.

control system an automatic system in which the output is forced to follow a preset program or is maintained at a desired value despite external perturbing forces.

contusion (kon-tu′zhun) [L. *contusio,* from *contundere* to bruise] a bruise; a superficial injury without a break in the skin.

contrecoup c., injury resulting from a blow on another site, such as a cerebral injury caused by a blow to the opposite side of the head.

conus (ko′nus), pl. *coni* [L., from Gr. *kōnos*] 1. a cone.

2. [NA], a general term used to denote a structure that resembles a cone.

c. arteriosus, [NA], the anterosuperior portion of the right ventricle of the heart, which is delimited from the rest of the ventricle by the supraventricular crest. It joins the pulmonary trunk, thus forming the outflow tract for blood in the right ventricle. Also called *arterial cone* and *infundibulum of heart.*

c. medullaris, [NA], see *c. terminalis.*

c. terminalis, the cone-shaped lower end of the spinal cord at the level of the upper lumbar vertebrae. Also called *c. medullaris.*

convalescence (kon″vah-les′ens) [L. *convalescere* to become strong] the stage of recovery from an illness, operation, or injury.

convection (kon-vek′shun) [L. *convectio,* from *convehere* to convey] a flow of heat carried by the bulk movement of fluid (a convection current), which exchanges material between warmer and cooler regions.

convergence (kon-ver′jens) 1. the quality of approaching or aiming toward the same point.

2. in physiology, the coordinated movement of the two eyes toward fixation on the same near point.

3. in biology, the evolution of similar structures or similar life strategies in unrelated species because of adaptation to similar ecologic habitats.

4. in mathematics, the property of having a limit. An infinite sequence converges to a limit if, for any specified error (no matter how small) beyond some point in the sequence, all the terms differ from the limit by less than the specified error.

5. in a multibeam cathode ray tube, the condition in which the electron beams intersect at a specified point.

conversational mode (kon″ver-sa′shun-al) a mode of data transmission between a computer program and a user at a remote terminal in which the program and user interact in a question-and-answer or request-and-response manner.

conversion (kon-ver′zhun) [*con-* + L. *versio* turning] 1. in automatic data processing, the process of translating from one data code to another or from one storage medium to another, e.g., from binary to decimal or from punched cards to magnetic tape.

2. the change in the numerical value of a measurement corresponding to a change in the units of measurement.

3. see *internal conversion.*

conversion coefficient the ratio of the probabilities of emission of conversion electrons and gamma rays in an isomeric transition.

conversion electron an electron emitted by a radionuclide in an internal conversion decay process.

conversion ratio see under *protein-bound iodine 131 test.*

convex (kon′veks) [L. *convexus*] pertaining to a line or surface that curves away from the viewer, such as the surface of a sphere as viewed from the outside. Cf. *concave.*

convoluted (kon′vo-lut-ed) [L. *convolutus*] rolled together or coiled.

convoluted tubule the contorted portion of the renal tubule that precedes the loop of Henle (the proximal convoluted tubule) or the portion that follows the loop of Henle (the distal convoluted tubule). See also *kidney.*

convolution (kon″vo-lu′shun) [L. *convolutus* rolled together] a tortuous irregularity or elevation caused by a structure being infolded upon itself, as the convolutions of the gray matter on the surface of the brain.

convulsant (kon-vul′sant) an agent that produces convulsions by acting on the central nervous system (the cerebrum, brain stem, cerebellum, or spinal cord), either directly or indirectly through asphyxia or chemical change.

convulsion (con-vul′shun) [L. *convulsio,* from *convellere* to pull violently] 1. a violent, involuntary contraction or series of contractions of the voluntary muscles.

2. tonic-clonic attack; see under *seizure.*

Conway cell (kon′wa) [E. J. *Conway,* Irish biochemist, born 1894] see under *microdiffusion analysis.*

coolant (koo′lant) a cooling agent, usually a liquid or gas, used to transfer heat away from a system.

Cooley's anemia (koo′lēz) [Thomas Benton *Cooley,* U.S. pediatrician, 1871–1945] see under *thalassemia.*

Coombs' test (kōōmz) [R. R. A. *Coombs,* British immunologist, born 1921] see *antiglobulin tests.*

coordinate (ko-or′dĭ-nat) one of a set of numbers that specifies the location of a point. Two coordinates locate a point in a plane; three, a point in space.

cartesian c.'s, coordinates that are the distances of a point from two orthogonal (perpendicular) axes in a plane or from three orthogonal planes in space. The intersection of the axes (or planes) is called the origin.

The two-dimensional coordinates are usually given the symbols x and y and the names abscissa (the horizontal distance in graphs) and ordinate (vertical distance), respectively. The three-dimensional coordinates are symbolized x, y, and z.

polar c.'s, plane coordinates that give a point's distance from the origin (r) and the angle (θ) between its radius vector and some fixed direction. The transformation from cartesian to polar coordinates is given by the equations $x = r\cos\theta$ and $y = r\sin\theta$.

spherical polar c.'s, space coordinates that give a point's distance from the origin (r), longitude (ϕ), and colatitude (θ). The transformation to cartesian coordinates is given by the equations $x = r\cos\phi \sin\theta$, $y = r\sin\phi \sin\theta$, and $z = r\cos\theta$.

coordination (ko-or″dĭ-na′shun) [L. *coordinatio,* from *co-* with + *ordinare* to arrange in order] the harmonious functioning of muscles and muscle groups in performing complex movements.

coordination compound 1. a species in which a central atom is surrounded by a set of ligand atoms. In this very general definition, coordination compound and complex are synonymous terms.

2. a neutral, ionic compound formed between a complex ion and other ions. As with other ionic compounds, the cation is named first. In the name of the complex ion, anionic ligands are named first and always have the suffix -o; neutral ligands are next; then cationic ligands; and finally the central metal atom (with the suffix -ate if the whole complex is an anion). The number of each kind of ligand present is designated with the prefixes *di-, tri-, tetra-,* etc. For complicated ligands, the prefixes *bis-, tris-, tetrakis-* are used; bridging ligands have the prefix *μ-*.

The oxidation number of the central metal ion in Roman numerals or the complex ion charge in Arabic numerals is given in parentheses after the name. Water and ammonia as neutral ligands are given the special names aquo and ammine. Some examples are chlorotriaquoplatinum(III) bromide, $[Pt(H_2O)_3Cl]Br$, and hexachloroplatinate (2-) ion, [Pt-

$Cl_6]^{2-}$. In the formula, the complex is enclosed in brackets and the central metal comes first.

coordination number the number of ligand atoms bonded to the central metal ion of a complex.

CO_2 output see *carbon dioxide output.*

COPD abbrev. See *chronic obstructive pulmonary disease.*

Cope method (kōp) see under *bronchography.*

Copepoda (ko-pep′ŏ-dah) [Gr. *kōpē* oar + *pous* foot] a subclass of crustaceans including some parasites of fishes and amphibians. Some species (*Diaptomus* and *Cyclops*) are intermediate hosts of the broad fish tapeworm *Diphyllobothrium latum* and the nematode *Dracunculus medinensis.* Humans are infected by the last-named two after eating raw or poorly cooked infected fish.

Coplin jar (kop′lin) [W. M. L. *Coplin,* U.S. physician, 1864–1928] a wide-mouthed container made of glass or other material that is used in histology laboratories for the storage or staining of tissue sections. The jars are usually slotted for 5–15 slides.

copolymer (ko-pol′ĭ-mer) a polymer formed by the combination of two chemically different monomers.

copper (Cu) (kop′er) [M.E. *coper,* from L. *cuprum,* from Gr. *Kypros* Cyprus] a reddish, malleable, ductile, metallic element, atomic number 29; atomic weight 63.54; a 3d transition element; oxidation states +1, +2, +3 (rare). It is a good conductor of heat and electricity. Copper is an essential trace element, occurring in several redox enzymes including cytochrome aa_3, lysyl oxidase, ferroxidase (ceruloplasmin), and dopamine hydroxylase. Its absence tends to impair the production of red cells, mitochondrial function, and erythrocyte survival time, and it leads to a decrease in the catalytic action of copper-containing enzymes.

Copper is present in the body in a number of forms: bound to albumin, plasma alpha$_2$-globulin, ceruloplasmin (the copper transport protein), or in the so-called copper storage proteins—erythrocuprein, cerebrocuprein, are increased. hepatocuprein, now known to be superoxide dismutases.

The most useful medical application of copper determination is in the diagnosis of Wilson's disease (hepatolenticular degeneration). In this condition, total serum copper is decreased, while urinary and tissue copper content are increased.

Copper salts can be poisonous, causing nausea, vomiting, headache, diarrhea, abdominal pain, liver injury and jaundice, and hemolytic shock, if untreated.

Reference ranges for copper in serum are: for birth to 6 mo, up to 70 μg/dl; 6 yr, 90–190; 12 yr, 80–160; adult males, 70–140; and adult females, 80–155. Values in blacks are 8–12 percent higher than in whites, and may exceed 200 μg/dl during pregnancy or in females on oral contraceptives.

copper assays 1. atomic absorption spectrophotometry. Copper in serum may be measured directly after dilution of the specimen or with the addition of a suitable organic solution to minimize viscosity problems. Copper has also been complexed with pyrrolidine dithiocarbamate and extracted into an organic solvent, which allows concentration of copper if initially present at a low concentration. The resonance line of 324.7 nm is most often used because of the low interference from other elements and low noise level at this wavelength.

2. quantitative spectrophotometric method. Tissues are digested with acid, and other specimens are rendered protein-free with dilute acid. Oxalyldihydrazide, cuprizone (biscyclohexanoneoxalyl-dihydrazone), diethyldithiocarbamate, or 1,5-diphenylcarbohydrazide in a suitable solvent is reacted with the copper-containing solution, and the absorbance of the mixture is recorded spectrophotometrically.

copper deposit demonstration histologic methods for the localization of copper deposits in tissues, as occurs in Wilson's disease. In Mallory's hematoxylin method, sections are stained in a fresh, unoxidized hematoxylin solution without mordant. Nuclei stain bluish-gray and copper stains a clear blue. In Uzman's rubeanic acid method, paraffin or cryostat sections are stained in a solution of rubeanic acid (dithiooxamide, $H_2NCSCSNH_2$), which forms a chelate with copper and other ions. Copper stains dark greenish-black. Linquist's method stains copper red-brown with rhodanine (*p*-dimethylaminobenzylidine rhodanine).

copperhead (kop′er-hed) a poisonous snake, *Agkistrodon contortrix,* of the pit viper family; see also *snakebite.*

copper storage protein one of a group of cellular proteins for copper storage in the body: erythrocuprein in erythrocytes, cerebrocuprein in brain, and hepatocuprein in the liver. All three proteins are colorless and contain two atoms of copper per molecule; M.W. 33,600.

The precise role of these proteins is not yet clear. They act as superoxide dismutases and may function as storage proteins, but this is not established. Ceruloplasmin may be the circulating storage protein for copper.

copper sulfate a compound, $CuSO_4$. The anhydrous salt is grayish-white, but it is hygroscopic and readily absorbs water to form the blue pentahydrate, $CuSO_4 \cdot 5H_2O$. Soluble in water, its astringent and caustic action led to its former use as an emetic, an astringent, an antihelmintic, and, when mixed with lime, a fungicide. When retained in sufficient quantities, copper sulfate may produce shock, jaundice, and kidney damage. Also called cupric sulfate.

coprecipitin (ko″pre-sip′ĭ-tin) a normally unbound antigen that precipitates with an antigen-antibody complex.

copremesis (kop-rem′ĕ-sis) [Gr. *kopros* dung + *emesis* vomiting] the vomiting of fecal matter.

Coprinus (kop′rĭ-nus) a genus of the class Basidiomycetes, rarely isolated from endocarditis and meningoencephalitis infections. It is commonly called the inky cap mushroom.

coproantibody (kop″ro-an′tĭ-bod″ē) antibodies (chiefly IgA) found in the lumen of the gastrointestinal tract and associated with immunity to intestinal infection.

CO_2 production see *carbon dioxide production.*

coprolith (kop′ro-lith) [Gr. *kopros* dung + *lithos* a stone] a hard fecal concretion in the intestine.

coprophil (kop′ro-fil) [Gr. *kopros* dung + *phileín* to love] a microorganism that lives in fecal matter; said especially of intestinal bacteria.

coproporphyria (kop″ro-por-fīr′e-ah) any porphyria in which coproporphyrin levels are elevated. There are two types: an extremely rare, largely asymptomatic erythropoietic coproporphyria and a hepatic porphyria that is transmitted as an autosomal dominant trait. See *hereditary coproporphyria* under *porphyria.*

coproporphyrin (kop"ro-por'fir-in) [Gr. *kopros* dung + *porphyra* purple] a tetra-carboxylated porphyrin with four isomers, only two of which occur naturally. The isomer of type III is a by-product of heme synthesis. Small amounts are normally excreted in the feces. High levels are excreted in the feces and urine in coproporphyria. The amount of coproporphyrin in urine is a parameter in assessing lead poisoning, which may be indicated by amounts greater than 200 μg/da in adults or 2 μg/kg/da in children.

coproporphyrin assay see under *porphyrin assays.*

coproporphyrinogen (kop"ro-por"fi-rin'o-jen) one of several colorless porphyrin precursors, formed by the enzymatic decarboxylation of the acetic acid side-chains of uroporphyrinogen, that readily give rise to coproporphyrin by oxidation. Coproporphyrinogen I differs from coproporphyrinogen III in a manner analogous to the structure of their respective precursors, uroporphyrinogens I and III. Coproporphyrinogen III is also the immediate precursor of protoporphyrin IX in the biosynthesis of heme. Increased concentrations are observed in several porphyrias.

coproporphyrinogen oxidase an enzyme of the oxidoreductase class (EC 1.3.3.3) that catalyzes the reaction coproporphyrinogen III $+O_2 \rightleftarrows$ protoporphyrinogen IX + 2 CO_2. A genetic deficiency of this enzyme, transmitted as an autosomal dominant trait, results in hereditary coproporphyria characterized by the massive excretion of coproporphyrin III.

coproporphyrinuria (kop"ro-por"fir-in-u're-ah) [*coproporphyrin* + Gr. *ouron* urine + *-ia*] the presence of coproporphyrin in the urine.

coprostanol (ko-pros'tah-nol) a steroid alcohol, 5β-cholestan-3β-ol; M.W. 388.65. It is formed by the reduction of cholesterol by intestinal bacteria and is excreted in the feces. In the laboratory, it is used as an internal standard in the gas chromatographic analysis of some steroids. Also called *coprosterol.*

coprostasis (ko-pros'tah-sis) [Gr. *kopros* dung + *stasis* stoppage] fecal impaction.

coprosterol (ko-pros'tĕ-rol) see *coprostanol.*

coprozoic (kop"ro-zo'ik) living in fecal material. When free-living protozoan cysts are ingested, the wall of the cyst may be resistant to the digestive processes of the host, and so may encyst in the feces when the material leaves the host.

copy error a mutation that occurs as a result of mispairing during DNA replication.

cor (kōr) [L.] see *heart.*

coracoid (kor'ah-koid) [Gr. *korakoeidēs* crowlike] 1. like a crow's beak. See also *coronoid.*

2. phylogenetically, a bone of the pectoral girdle; in mammals it refers to the coracoid process, a hooked process of bone arising from the neck of the scapula.

coral snake (kor'al) a highly poisonous snake, *Micrurus fulvius,* that produces a potent neurotoxin; see also *snakebite.*

Corbin technique (kor'bin) a method of obtaining wide-angle frontal projections of the chest. The patient is erect and the central ray is directed anteroposteriorly. Two grid-front cassettes are held vertically in a frame so that they form a 45° angle with the central ray, and abut in the midsagittal plane. Because the object-film distance is increased with the closeness of the object to the midsagittal plane, the magnification is also increased, providing a panoramic view of these structures.

cord (kord) [L. *chorda;* from Gr. *chordē* string] 1. any long, rounded, flexible structure.

2. in anatomy, a columnlike arrangement of cells seen in certain tissues and in some neoplasms.

3. in bacteriology, mycobacteria compacted in curved, serpentine strands. Cord-forming strains of tubercule bacilli are more virulent than non-cord-forming types.

cord blood a specimen of blood obtained from the umbilical cord at the time of birth. In cases of suspected hemolytic disease of the newborn, the blood is tested for ABO group, Rh type, and sensitized red blood cells by the direct antiglobulin test.

cord factor trehalose-6, 6'-dimycolic acid, a mycoside produced by *Mycobacterium tuberculosis* that is toxic, stimulates the formation of granulomas, and inhibits the migration of polymorphonuclear leukocytes. The production of cord factor causes cultures of the bacilli to aggregate in serpentine cords.

cords of Billroth (bil'rōt) [Christian Albert Theodor *Billroth,* surgeon in Vienna, 1829–1894] see *splenic cords.*

Cordylobia (kor"di-lo'be-ah) a genus of tumbu flies; the species *C. anthropophaga,* native to tropical Africa, is a myiasis-producing fly for which humans are an obligate host. Infection results in multiple furuncles, each with a single maggot; removal of the maggots is curative.

core/o, cor/o (kor'e-o, kor'o) [Gr. *korē* pupil] a word element used in combining form to denote the pupil of the eye, e.g., corediastasis, coroscopy.

core (kor) [L. *cor* heart] 1. the central part of anything.

2. the central mass of necrotic matter in a furuncle (boil).

3. the part of a nuclear reactor inside the shielding and containment vessel where the nuclear reaction occurs.

air c., pertaining to an inductor or transformer (usually those for use at radio frequencies) in which the coils are wound around a tube of nonmagnetic material.

magnetic c., 1. a bar of magnetic material around which the coils of an inductor or transformer are wound. It increases the magnetic induction in the core and thus increases the inductance of the inductor or the coupling between the transformer windings.

2. a small ferrite ring used in magnetic core computer memories.

core antigen see *h. B core a.* under *hepatitis antigen.*

corectasis (kor-ek'tah-sis) [*core-* + Gr. *ektasis* a dilation] a pathologic dilation of the pupil of the eye.

core memory see *magnetic core memory.*

coremium (ko-re'me-um) a bundle of aerial hyphae projecting from the surface of a fungus culture, usually bearing spores.

corepressor (ko"re-pres'or) an effector molecule

that modifies a regulatory protein (activation), allowing it to bind to an operator to inactivate transcription. See also *negative control r.* and *positive control r.* under *repression.*

Cori's disease (ko′rēz) [Carl Ferdinand *Cori,* U.S. biochemist, born 1896; Gerty Theresa *Cori,* U.S. biochemist, 1896–1957] see *Forbes' disease* and *glycogenoses.*

coriphosphine O (kor″ĭ-fos′fēn) a basic primary amine dye, which is yellow and fluorescent in ultraviolet light; C.I. 46020. It may be used in histology to form Schiff reagents.

corium (ko′re-um) [L. "hide"] see *dermis.*

corn (korn) [L. *cornu* horn] a horny thickening of the skin, found on the feet at sites of localized pressure or friction. It forms a conelike mass pointing deeper into the skin, usually producing pain and irritation. Histologically, the basal layer is intact, the corium is mildly infiltrated by lymphocytes, and the epithelial surface is markedly hyperkeratotic.

corne/o (kor′ne-o) [L. *corneus* horny] a word element used in combining form to denote the cornea, e.g., corneitis.

cornea (kor′ne-ah) [L. *corneus* horny] [NA], the transparent structure that is the most anterior part of the fibrous coat of the eyeball. It provides most of the refraction of light rays entering the eye.

cornification (kor′nĭ-fĭ-ka′shun) [L. *cornu* horn + *facere* to make] conversion into keratin; hyperkeratosis.

cornmeal agar (korn′mēl) a deficient culture medium composed of water, cornmeal, and agar, used extensively for promoting sporulation. Chlamydospore formation by yeasts such as *Candida* is increased by incorporation of polysorbate 80 (Tween 80). Dextrose or glucose may be added for stimulating pigment production of *Trichophyton rubrum.*

corn oil a refined fixed oil (triglycerides) obtained from the embryo of *Zea mays;* used, [USP] grade, as a solvent and vehicle for various medicinal agents and as a vehicle for injections. It is an important food oil promoted as a source of polyunsaturated fatty acids in special diets, and may have approximately 54 percent of linoleic in its constituent fatty acids.

coron/o (kor′ŏ-no) [L. *corona* crown] a word element used in combining form to denote the heart, e.g., coronary.

corona (ko-ro′nah), pl. *coronas* or *coronae* [L. from Gr. *korōnē* crown] a crown; used in anatomic nomenclature to designate a crownlike eminence or encircling structure.

c. of glans penis, the rounded, proximal, projecting border of the glans penis that overhangs a grooved constriction, the neck of the penis.

c. radiata, 1. [NA], an expanding array of nerve fibers radiating from the internal capsule to every part of the cerebral cortex.

2. a layer of elongated follicle cells that surround the zona pellucida of an ovum.

coronal plane (ko-ro′nal) a vertical plane passing through the body from side to side (parallel to the midcoronal plane). Also called *frontal plane.*

coronary (kor′ŏ-nar″e) [L. *corona,* from Gr. *korōnē* crown] encircling in the manner of a crown; a term applied to such structures as vessels, nerves, and ligaments. It usually refers to the arteries that supply the heart muscle and, by extension, to a pathologic involvement of these arteries.

coronary artery, left the larger of the two arteries that arise from the ascending aorta to supply oxygenated blood to the myocardium. Emerging from the left aortic sinus, the artery passes between the pulmonary trunk and left atrial appendage. Once at the atrioventricular sulcus, it turns left and divides into the left descending artery, the circumflex artery, and occasionally the left marginal artery. The left descending artery appears as a continuation of the left coronary artery, proceeding down the interventricular sulcus to the apex and sending fine branches into the septum. From this artery arises the left diagonal branch, which supplies the anterior region of the left ventricle. The circumflex artery branches from the left coronary artery and proceeds in the left atrioventricular sulcus, supplying branches to the atrium and ventricle. The left marginal artery arises from the circumflex or perpendicular to its exit of the left coronary artery. It ramifies over much of the left ventricle, usually reaching the apex.

coronary artery, right the artery that supplies oxygenated blood to the myocardium of the right atrium, the right ventricle, and a portion of the atrioventricular septum. Emerging from the anterior aortic sinus, the artery proceeds anteriorly and to the right between the right atrial appendage and the pulmonary trunk. It then descends in the atrioventricular sulcus to the right margin of the heart. Branches ramify over the right heart to supply the atrium, conus, ventricle, and right side of the interventricular septum.

coronary heart disease see *atherosclerotic heart disease.*

coronary sinus the principal vein draining the myocardium. It opens into the right atrium between the tricuspid valve and the entrance of the inferior vena cava, and its orifice has a small, semilunar valve cusp.

coronary thrombosis thrombosis of a coronary artery. It generally occurs on a preexisting atherosclerotic plaque; a soft plaque with a core of cholesterol and cholesterol esters particularly has a tendency to ulcerate and promote thrombus formation. The thrombotic process further narrows the lumen and is liable to occlude the artery, and consequently interferes with oxygen delivery to the myocardium. Clinical effects depend on the location of the thrombosis, the suddenness with which it develops, and whether sufficient collateral flow exists. Coronary thrombosis is implicated in more than half the episodes of acute ischemic heart disease.

coronavirus (ko-ro″nah-vi′rus) a single-stranded RNA virus that is the second most frequent cause of the common cold. The term coronavirus refers to the petal-shaped peplomers, which resemble the appearance of the solar corona, that are contained in the viral envelope. The virion is spherical, whereas the nucleocapsid has a helical symmetry. The virion contains its own transcriptase. There are three human serotypes.

Clinically, coronavirus infections present a coldlike illness with sore throat, cough, malaise, chills, and low fever. Usually only the upper respiratory tract is infected. Coronavirus infections occur most often in the winter seasons.

The incubation period for coronaviruses is 2–5 da.

The acquired immunity is not strong, and reinfection may therefore be frequent, even though there are only a few serotypes.

Laboratory diagnosis is based primarily on serologic techniques such as hemagglutination inhibition and complement-fixation assays. When multiplying, the coronavirus buds internally into cytoplasmic vesicles, so that the outer plasma membrane of the host cell lacks viral antigens. The virions themselves may be present on the host cell surface, and thus react with antibody. Isolation and culturing of coronavirus are difficult and tedious.

coroner (kor′o-ner) [Fr. *corouner,* a local officer of the crown] an officer, either a physician specializing in forensic medicine or a trained lay investigator, who investigates violent, sudden, or unexplained deaths.

coronoid (kor′o-noid) [Gr. *korōnē* crow + *eidos* form] shaped like a crow's beak, e.g., hooked or curved, such as a coronoid process of the mandible or ulna.

coroscopy (ko-ros′ko-pe) [*coro-* + Gr. *skopein* to examine] see *retinoscopy.*

corps ronds (kor rawn) [Fr. "round bodies"] round, double-contoured dyskeratotic cells seen in the spinous cell layer of the epidermis in keratosis follicularis. See also *k. follicularis* under *keratosis.*

cor pulmonale (kor pul″mo-na′le) [N.L. "pulmonary heart"] right heart hypertrophy and subsequent right ventricular failure that is secondary to pulmonary hypertension. The pulmonary hypertension can be a consequence of a variety of conditions such as severe kyphoscoliosis, emphysema, and hypoxic vasoconstriction and/or thickening of the muscular layer of the pulmonary arteries and arterioles (particularly that occurring at high altitudes). The increased pulmonary vascular resistance increases the workload of the right heart, leading to hypertrophy and failure.

corpus (kor′pus), pl. *corpora* [L. "body"] a distinct mass (body) of material. The term is used in anatomic nomenclature to refer to the entire organism and is also applied to the main portion of an anatomic part, structure, or organ.

c. albicans, [NA], a white hyaline scar of the ovary formed from the involution of the corpus luteum. It develops either immediately following ovulation, if a pregnancy does not ensue, or after delivery, if a pregnancy does ensue.

corpora amylacea, small eosinophilic bodies found in prostatic glands and ducts. They form by the concentric layering of desquamated epithelial cells around inspissated prostatic secretion, and increase in number with age. If the flow of prostate secretion is sluggish, infection can develop and predispose to calcification of the corpora.

corpora arenacea, calcareous concretions deposited as concentric layers around extracellular debris in the pineal gland. Also called *brain sand.*

c. callosum, [NA], a commissure of transverse fibers deep in the longitudinal fissure that connects the cerebral hemispheres. It consists of white matter and roofs the lateral ventricles.

c. cavernosum clitoridis, [NA], paired masses of erectile tissue that fuse to form the body of the clitoris.

c. cavernosum penis, [NA], paired, elongated masses of erectile tissue that, with the crus, form the substance of the penis.

c. luteum, [NA], a yellow glandular mass in the ovary formed by an ovarian follicle that has matured and discharged its ovum. If the ovum is impregnated, the corpus luteum increases in size and persists for several months (corpus luteum of pregnancy); if impregnation does not occur, it degenerates, shrinks, and becomes scarred (corpora albicans). The cells of the corpus luteum secrete estrogens and progestins.

corpora quadrigemina, four rounded eminences on the posterior surface of the midbrain, consisting of the superior and inferior colliculi.

c. striatum, [NA], the striate body: one of the components of the basal ganglia; it consists of a subcortical mass of gray and white matter in front of and lateral to the thalamus in each cerebral hemisphere. The gray substance forms two principal masses, the caudate nucleus and the lentiform nucleus. The striate appearance of the area is produced by connecting bands of gray substance passing from one nucleus to the other through the white fibers of the internal capsule.

c. uteri, [NA], that part of the uterus above the cervix. See also *uterus.*

corpuscle (kōr′pus′l) [L. *corpusculum,* from *corpus* body] 1. in anatomy, a small mass or body.
2. a blood cell; see under *blood.*

corrected reticulocyte count see *reticulocyte production index.*

correction (kŏ-rek′shun) an adjustment made to a device or measured value in order to produce a more accurate result.

correlation (kor″ĕ-la′shun) most generally, the degree to which one variable can be predicted from another; the term is often used more specifically in statistics to refer to the degree of linearity in the relationship of two random variables (X and Y), as measured by the correlation coefficient ρ, which is the covariance of X and Y divided by the product of their standard deviations. For a random sample of n X,Y pairs, the sample correlation coefficient $r = \Sigma_i(X_i - \overline{X})(Y_i - \overline{Y})/(n-1)s_X s_Y$, where X and Y are the sample means, and s_X and s_Y are the sample standard deviations.

The possible values of ρ or r range from −1 to +1. When $r = \pm 1$, all the data points can be plotted on a straight line. When $\rho = \pm 1$, the parent population has this straight-line relationship.

The slope b of the linear regression of Y on X is equal to rs_X/s_Y (rs_y/s_X, for the regression of X on Y). The correlation coefficient measures how much of the variation of Y is explained by the regression equation. The variance $b^2 s_X^2 = r^2 s_Y^2$ of $b(X - \overline{X})$, the deviation from the mean $\overline{Y}$ of the values of Y predicted by the regression equation, explains the fraction r^2 (also called the coefficient of determination) of s_Y^2.

If the variables are positively correlated ($r > 0$), the regression equation has a positive slope, and Y increases with X. If the variables are negatively correlated, Y decreases as X increases.

The null hypothesis that X and Y are normally distributed and independent (and therefore uncorrelated, $\rho = 0$) can be tested with the statistic $(n-2)r^2/(1-r^2)$, the ratio of the explained variance of Y to the unexplained variance of Y, which under the null hypothesis has the F distribution with 1 degree of freedom in the numerator and $n-2$ degrees of freedom in the denominator. This is equivalent to the *t* test of the hypothesis that the slope of the regression line is zero.

If *X* and *Y* have the bivariate normal distribution with correlation coefficient ρ, approximate confidence intervals for *r* can be determined from the statistic *z*, which is approximately normally distributed with a mean of $\zeta + \rho/2(n - 1)$ and a variance of $1/(n - 3)$, where $r = \tanh z$ and $\rho = \tanh \zeta$.

If two variables are uncorrelated, no regression line provides a better least-squares fit than any other. Independent variables are always uncorrelated, but uncorrelated variables are not necessarily independent (unless they are also assumed to have a bivariate normal distribution).

Also called *association*. See also *linear regression* and *rank correlation coefficient*.

correlation coefficient a statistical measure of the degree to which two random variables (x and y) vary together. The most commonly used measure is the Pearson product moment correlation, the ratio of the covariance of x and y to the square root of the product of the variance of x and the variance of y. Other measures sometimes used are Spearman's and Kendall's coefficients. For each measure, the value may range between −1 (perfect negative correlation) to +1 (perfect positive correlation). A value of zero denotes no correlation.

corresponding ray (kor″ĕ-spon′ding) an x-ray emitted with the transition of an electron between the energy levels of an atom. The x-ray photon energy is the difference of the two energy levels, which is determined by the atomic number of the atom. The highest energy corresponding rays, those in which the transition is to the lowest (K) level, are called *characteristic rays*.

Corrigan's pulse (kor′e-ganz) [Sir Dominic John *Corrigan*, physician in Dublin, 1802–1880] see *water-hammer p.* under *pulse*.

corrin ring (kor′in) a large tetrapyrrole ring that chelates a cobalt atom and forms part of the cobalamin (vitamin B_{12}) molecule.

corrosion (kŏ-ro′zhun) [L. *corrosio*] 1. the process of dissolving or eroding a material, especially a metal or hard tissue, usually by chemical action.

2. a substance, e.g., rust, formed by such a process.

corrosion cast a technique whereby a substance is injected into the vascular system of an organ or tissue after it hardens and the tissue is then digested away, leaving the form of the vascular system. Many different substances, including rubber, neoprene latex, metals, and methacrylate plastics are used for casting.

corrosive (ko-ro′siv) [L. *con-* + *rodere* to gnaw] 1. having the power to corrode or wear away by chemical action.

2. any substance that damages or destroys living tissue, including some strong mineral acids and fixed alkalis. Common examples include bromine, iodine crystals, hydrochloric acid, and potassium hydroxide. To identify a corrosive that has been swallowed, the gastric contents can be evaluated for pH and for an excess of ions typical of strong acids and alkalis (Na^+, K^+, Cl^-, SO_4^{2-}, PO_4^{3-}).

corrosivity (kŏ″ro-siv′ĭ-te) a characteristic of chemical waste exhibited if a representative sample of the waste has either of the following properties: (1) it is aqueous and has a pH less than or equal to 2, or greater than or equal to 12.5; or (2) it is a liquid and corrodes steel at a rate greater than 6.35 mm/yr under specified test methods. If corrosivity is evident, the waste is classified as hazardous and is regulated by EPA/RCRA (Environmental Protection Agency/Resource Conservation and Recovery Act) standards.

cortex (kor′teks), pl. *cortices* [L. "bark, rind"] 1. an external layer, as the bark of a tree or the rind of a fruit.

2. [NA], the outer layer of an organ or other body structure, as distinguished from the internal substance.

cortic/o (kor′tĭ-ko) [L. *cortex* bark] a word element used in combining form to denote a cortex, e.g., corticosteroid.

cortical (kor′tĭ-kal) [L. *corticalis*] pertaining to a cortex or bark.

cortical bone the compact dense bone that is external to the inner cancellous bone.

cortical DC potential in electroencephalography, a steady or DC potential measured from the cortical surface with respect to an electrically indifferent area. In a healthy adult human, the cortical surface is 5–20 mV positive to the indifferent area. The amplitude of the potential is decreased by anoxia, anesthesia, and cerebral damage, and falls to zero at death.

The potential is thought to result from the potential difference between the apical dendrites and soma of the cortical pyramidal cells, but the cortical glial cells may also contribute.

corticifugal (kor″tĭ-sif′u-gal) [*cortic-* + L. *fugere* to flee] proceeding, conducting, or moving away from the cortex.

corticipetal (kor″tĭ-sip′ĕ-tal) [*cortic-* + L. *petere* to seek] proceeding, conducting, or moving toward the cortex.

corticobulbar (kor′tĭ-ko-bul′bar) pertaining to or connecting the cerebral cortex and the medulla oblongata and/or brain stem.

corticobulbar tract (kor″tĭ-ko-bul′bar) [*cortico-* + L. *bulbus* onion] one of the fascicles of nerve fibers from various areas of the sensorimotor cortex that project onto the motor nuclei of the cranial nerves in the mesencephalon, pons, and medulla oblongata. After leaving the cortex, the fibers pass through the genu of the internal capsule and crura cerebri before entering the pons and medulla oblongata. Most of the projections of these fibers are to contralateral nuclei. Also called corticonuclear tract.

corticoid (kor′tĭ-koid) [*cortico-* + Gr. *eidos* form] 1. any of the steroids produced by the adrenal cortex; see *corticosteroid*.

2. having an activity similar to that of corticosteroids.

corticospinal (kor″tĭ-ko-spi′nal) pertaining to or connecting the cortex of the brain and the spinal cord.

corticospinal tract (kor″tĭ-ko-spi′nal) [*cortico-* + L. *spina* spine, thorn] one of the bundles of nerve fibers that descend uninterrupted from the sensorimotor cortex to the anterior and lateral funiculi of the spinal cord. These fibers pass from the cerebral cortex through the posterior limb of the internal capsule, the crura cerebri, and the pons before decussating in the medulla oblongata as the pyramids and entering the spinal cord.

corticosteroid (kor″tĭ-ko-ste′roid) any of the steroid hormones produced by the adrenal cortex except for the sex hormones; principally, aldosterone, cortisol, and corticosterone, or synthetic analogs having similar activities, such as betamethasone, dexamethasone, methylprednisolone, prednisolone, prednisone, and triamcinolone. Both the corticosteroids and the steroid sex hormones are produced via biosynthetic pathways that begin with cholesterol. Corticosteroids are divided into two types: glucocorticoids, which affect carbohydrate metabolism, and mineralocorticoids, which affect electrolyte balance.

The glucocorticoids, chiefly cortisol but also cortisone, corticosterone, and 11-dehydrocorticosterone, are released in response to adrenocorticotropic hormone (ACTH) produced by the pituitary. The secretion of ACTH is controlled by three factors: negative feedback (ACTH secretion is suppressed by high plasma cortisol levels), a circadian rhythm (ACTH secretion increases during the normal sleep period and falls during the waking hours), and stress (severe stress, such as trauma, the release of pyrogens, hypoglycemia, or anxiety, causes the release of ACTH).

The glucocorticoids have many effects including inhibition of protein synthesis and acceleration of protein catabolism, stimulation of gluconeogenesis, increase in the synthesis and redistribution of fat, inhibition of allergic and inflammatory reactions, and suppression of immune response. Specific antiinflammatory effects include (1) the inhibition of leukocyte migration and degranulation; and (2) decreases in the number of circulating lymphocytes, in the size of the lymph nodes, thymus, and spleen, and in the production of antibodies. There is also an inhibition of the formation of granulation tissue.

Glucocorticoids are administered in conjunction with mineralocorticoids for endocrine disorders that result in adrenal insufficiency. They are also employed as antiinflammatory agents in a wide variety of conditions, including rheumatoid arthritis, collagen diseases, allergic diseases, bronchial asthma, eye inflammations, skin diseases, ulcerative colitis and regional enteritis, and edematous states. Prednisone in particular is used for the treatment of acute lymphocytic leukemia, Hodgkin's disease, and other lymphomas in a regimen that combines prednisone with an alkylating agent and a vinca alkaloid. Several corticosteroids are used for the palliative treatment of certain cancers of the breast, prostate, and ovary by adrenocortical suppression.

Abrupt withdrawal from corticosteroids can result in acute adrenal insufficiency. Prolonged corticosteroid therapy can cause many adverse reactions, including hypokalemic alkalosis and edema, hyperglycemia, increased susceptibility to infection, increased incidence of peptic ulcers in patients with rheumatoid arthritis, muscle weakness, steroid myopathy, osteoporosis and vertical compression fractures, the development of posterior subcapsular cataracts and glaucoma, and behavior disturbances ranging from euphoria, insomnia, and mood changes to severe depression or psychotic episodes. Short courses of corticosteroid therapy, however, rarely produce adverse reactions.

The mineralocorticoids, chiefly aldosterone but also 11-deoxycorticosterone (DOC) and 18-hydroxy-DOC, are released in response to angiotensin II, increased plasma potassium concentration, or decreased serum sodium concentration. Angiotensin I is produced from the plasma protein angiotensinogen by renin, which is released by the juxtaglomerular apparatus in the kidneys; it is then converted to angiotensin II by converting enzymes found primarily in the lungs. Aldosterone promotes the retention of sodium and water and the excretion of potassium. Angiotensin II and increased fluid volume and blood pressure all suppress renin release, acting as negative feedback loops to control aldosterone levels.

See also *adrenal glands* and *renin-angiotensin-aldosterone system.*

corticosteroid-binding globulin (CBG) see *transcortin.*

corticosterone (kor″tĭ-kos′ter-on) 11β,21-dihydroxy-pregn-4-ene-3,20-dione ($C_{21}H_{34}O_4$); a steroid hormone from the adrenal cortex with slight glucocorticoid and mineralocorticoid activities. Also called *compound B.* See also *corticosteroid* and *cortisol.*

corticotrope (kōr′tĭ-ko-trōp) [*cortico-* + Gr. *tropos* turn] a cell type in the adenohypophysis that produces adrenocorticotropic hormone (ACTH). In the classical nomenclature it is a basophil (β_1 cell of Romeis). The precursor molecule of melanocyte-stimulating hormone (β-lipotropin) has also been identified in corticotropes.

corticotropin (kor″tĭ-ko-tro′pin) see *adrenocorticotropic hormone.*

corticotropin-releasing factor (CRF) a releasing factor (polypeptide) that is liberated at nerve endings close to the median eminence of the hypothalamus in response to decreased cortisol blood levels or stressful stimulation. It is carried in the blood to the anterior lobe of the pituitary, where it causes the release of adrenocorticotropic hormone (ACTH) into the general circulation. Also called *adrenocorticotropic hormone–releasing factor.*

cortisol (kor′tĭ-sol) 11β,17,21-trihydroxypregn-4-ene-3,20-dione, the major glucocorticoid controlling the metabolism of carbohydrates; M.W. 362.47. It is synthesized in the zona fasciculata and zona reticularis of the adrenal cortex, and is the only naturally occurring steroid that exerts a negative feedback effect on the release of adrenocorticotropic hormone (ACTH) from the pituitary. When the level of cortisol drops beyond a certain point, it triggers the release of ACTH into the circulation and stimulates the adrenal cortex to produce steroids. When the level of cortisol increases to a certain point, the ACTH secretion diminishes.

11-Desoxycortisol is the immediate precursor of cortisol, which in turn is converted to cortisone. About 90 percent of cortisol is transported in the plasma bound to transcortin and albumin. The biologically active cortisol is the free form, and the protein binding serves to protect the cortisol from metabolism and excretion. Cortisol is metabolized in the liver to tetrahydrocortisol, cortol, and 11β-etiocholanolone. The secretion of cortisol is subject to a circadian rhythm, reaching a maximum early in the morning and minimum in the early evening. Cortisol is used pharmacologically as an antiinflammatory agent.

Cortisol determination is the single most useful means of diagnosing Cushing's syndrome due to either adrenal hyperplasia or adrenal tumors. Increased values are seen in Cushing's syndrome, adrenal carcinoma, pregnancy, obesity, and in females taking oral contraceptives. Decreased values are observed in primary adrenal insufficiency (Addison's disease) and secondary adrenal insufficiency (Sheehan's syndrome).

Reference values for cortisol in serum or plasma for radioimmunoassay are: for adults, 6–23 μg/dl in the early morning and 4–15 in the late afternoon. Somewhat higher values are observed for the fluorometric or competitive protein-binding techniques.

Also called compound F and *hydrocortisone.* See also *adrenocorticotropic hormone, adrenocorticotropic hormone stimulation test, dexamethasone suppression test,* and *metyrapone stimulation test.*

urinary free c., the unconjugated, nonprotein-bound cortisol that is directly eliminated by glomerular ultrafiltration in the kidneys. Because 90 percent of serum cortisol is bound to transcortin and 10 percent is free, and because most of the transcortin binding sites are saturated, small increases in cortisol can more easily be detected in the urine as free cortisol. Most important, urinary free cortisol represents the nonprotein-bound fraction that is biologically active.

This is a better and more sensitive diagnostic test for Cushing's disease than is the measurement of serum cortisol concentration. It is of greatest value in diagnosing a hyperfunctioning adrenal gland. Urinary free cortisol is also elevated during pregnancy; decreased values can be observed in patients with renal disease. Reference ranges for urinary free cortisol are 20–90 μg/da.

cortisol assays 1. radioimmunoassay (RIA) using an antibody specific for cortisol and an ^{125}I-cortisol tracer (tritium and selenium-75 labels have also been employed). Cortisol is assayed directly in the plasma or serum. Urinary-free cortisol can be assayed after methylene chloride extraction to remove the water-soluble cortisol conjugates. There is some cross-reactivity in the cortisol RIA with 11-deoxycortisol, desoxycorticosterone, and dexamethasone.

2. enzyme immunoassay. Cortisol is covalently linked to an enzyme, and the complex is allowed to compete with endogenous cortisol for sites on a cortisol-specific antibody. The enzymatic reaction is monitored at a wavelength suitable for the product generated. Typical enzymes employed are glucose-6-phosphate dehydrogenase, horseradish peroxidase, and alkaline phosphatase. The enzyme immunoassay can be either homogeneous (no separation required) or heterogeneous (separation step included). Appropriate standards are included to generate a standard curve, and the values for the sample are obtained by comparison with the standard curve.

3. fluoroimmunoassay. This is very similar to radioimmunoassay except that the antibody is tagged with a fluorescent label; the bound and free antigen are separated and then measured with a suitable fluorometer.

4. competitive protein binding (CBP) assay using transcortin, the binder that also recognizes corticosterone and 11-deoxycortisol, as well as cortisol. This assay is not used frequently because it requires an extraction and chromatographic separation, unlike RIA.

5. fluorometric assay that involves extraction by methylene chloride and the development of a fluorescence after the addition of ethanol-sulfuric acid. This method is no longer used because it is subject to various forms of interference and requires pretreatment of the sample.

6. assays for cortisol metabolites as well as intact cortisol. See *17-hydroxycorticosteroid assays* and *Porter-Silber assays.*

cortisone (kor′ti-sōn) 17,21-dihydroxy-pregn-4-ene-3,11,20-trione ($C_{21}H_{28}O_5$); a glucocorticoid with significant mineralocorticoid activity from the adrenal cortex. It is largely inactive in humans until converted to cortisol. Quantitatively, cortisone is not an important corticosteroid. The acetate derivative is used for its antiinflammatory properties in various conditions. Also called *compound E.* See also *corticosteroid.*

cortol (kor′tol) see under *hexahydrocortisol.*

cortolone (kor′to-lōn) a metabolite of cortisol, 3α,17α,20α,21-tetrahydroxypregnan-11-one, which is found in urine; M.W. 366.48. It is one of the so-called 17-ketogenic steroids.

Cortrosyn (kor′tro-sin) trademark. See *cosyntropin.*

Corynebacterium (ko-ri″ne-bak-te′re-um) [Gr. *korynē* club + *baktērion* little rod] a genus of microorganisms of the family Corynebacteriaceae, order Eubacteriales, made up of gram-positive, nonsporulating, nonmotile rods that are often club-shaped. The rods may be arranged in irregular groups resembling Chinese letters or pickets on a fence (palisade arrangement). Irregular staining with granules is commonly seen. These organisms are generally aerobic but may be facultatively anaerobic, and are catalase-positive.

Eight species are parasitic for humans or animals. Two are clearly pathogenic for humans, producing potent exotoxins: *C. diphtheriae* and *C. pseudotuberculosis.* Another species, *C. renale,* is an animal pathogen.

C. diphtheriae, the species that causes diphtheria in humans. The diphtheria bacillus is a straight or slightly curved rod that is frequently club-shaped when grown on artificial media. It does not stain uniformly because of the presence of metachromatic granules, and therefore has a beaded appearance. *C. diphtheriae* is identified by microscopic morphology, colony characteristics, and the production of a narrow band of hemolysis on blood agar. Also characteristic are the production of acid from glucose and maltose but not sucrose and the formation of exotoxin (although nontoxigenic strains occur). *C. diphtheriae* should be cultured on enriched blood infusion agar or chocolate agar. For a selective and differential medium, potassium tellurite can be added. In the presence of potassium tellurite, *C. diphtheriae* colonies appear gray or black.

Three distinct cultural types can be recognized in the clinical laboratory: *gravis, intermedius,* and *mitis.* It was thought at one time that these types correlated with the clinical severity of the cases most frequently yielding them, but this relationship is now considered invalid. Differentiation is based on morphologic and cultural characteristics, plus fermentation of starch by the *gravis* type.

Primary infection by *C. diphtheriae* in humans occurs in the upper respiratory tract when the organism is inhaled, colonizes, and produces exotoxin. Toxin production is dependent on the bacterium being infected with lysogenic bacteriophage that contains the necessary genetic information for its production. Diphtheria toxin inhibits protein synthesis by transferring an ADP-ribosyl group from NAD to an elongation factor (EF-2) that is responsible for advancing the ribosome along the mRNA molecule; it prevents polypeptide chain elongation. The toxin may become disseminated, and the resultant inflammatory response causes necrotic lesions and the characteristic diphtheritic pseudomembranes. In highly susceptible animals, a lethal dose is 0.1 μg/kg of body weight.

Treatment of diphtheria includes immediate antitoxin therapy combined with a primary skin test for anaphylaxis. Widespread active immunization for many years has reduced the reservoir for *C. diphtheriae* to occasional foci. In those areas where immunization was carried out thoroughly, the disease has been almost eliminated.

See also *exotoxins.*

C. hofmannii, an invalid species name for *C. pseudodiphtheriticum.*

C. minutissimum, a species that causes erythrasma, a superficial skin disease the scales of which fluoresce under Wood's light. The organism is difficult to grow in the laboratory, requiring tissue culture medium and fetal bovine serum for the production of fluorescence. The relationship of this species to the lipophilic corynebacteria is not certain; it probably relates to *C. xerosis.*

C. pseudodiphtheriticum, a nontoxigenic, nonfermentative species found in the nasopharynx of humans. It is not pathogenic.

C. pseudotuberculosis, a toxigenic species found in and pathogenic for a variety of lower animals. It causes ulcerative lymphangitis, abscesses, and chronic purulent infections in sheep, goats, and horses, and occasionally in humans.

C. renale, a species that causes cystitis and pyelonephritis in cattle.

C. tenuis, a species that is an etiologic agent of trichomycosis axillaris. Although the affiliation of this species is uncertain, it more likely belongs to the genera *Nocardia.*

coryneform group (ko-ri′nĕ-form) a group of bacteria containing four genera: *Corynebacterium, Arthrobacter, Cellulomonas,* and *Kurthia.* They are nonspore-forming, gram-positive, irregular rods. The *Corynebacterium* genus includes *C. diphtheriae,* the cause of diphtheria in humans, as well as plant pathogens and nonpathogenic organisms.

coryza (kŏ-ri′zah) [L., from Gr. *koryza* nasal mucus] an acute catarrhal condition of the nasal mucous membrane, with a profuse discharge from the nostrils.

coryzavirus (kŏ-ri′zah-vi″rus) [Gr. *koryza* nasal mucus + *virus*] see *rhinovirus.*

cos abbrev. See *cosine.*

cosine (cos) (ko′sin) a trigonometric function, the sine of the complementary angle, $\cos\theta = \sin(\theta - 90°)$ or $\cos\chi = \sin(\chi - \pi/2)$, where θ is in degrees and χ is in radians. See also *sine w.* under *wave.*

cosmic rays (koz′mik) [Gr. *kosmos* the universe] high-energy particles, primarily protons, electrons, and nuclei, that approach the earth from all directions. These primary cosmic rays are deflected toward the poles by the earth's magnetic field. Some collide with atoms in the atmosphere, producing secondary cosmic rays, primarily pions, electrons, and muons. Cosmic rays make up about half the natural background radiation (the other half coming from radioisotopes in soils and rocks). Exposure increases with increasing altitude and latitude, but the average annual whole-body dose is about 44 mrem/yr.

cost/o (kos′to) [L. *costa* rib] a word element used in combining form to denote the ribs, e.g., costochondral.

costal (kos′tal) [L. *costalis*] pertaining to a rib or ribs.

costal cartilage a band of hyaline cartilage situated on the ventral extremity of a rib. It serves to attach the true ribs to the sternum and the upper false ribs to the superior ribs.

costal element the outer part of the arch of a developing vertebra. In the thoracic region, each costal element develops into a rib. At other levels of the vertebral column in mammals, it remains rudimentary as a portion of the transverse process.

costovertebral angle (CVA) (kos″to-ver′tĕ-bral) the angle formed between the last rib and the vertebral column.

cosyntropin (ko″sin-tro′pin) a synthetic polypeptide whose physiologic actions are much like those of natural corticotropin. It is often used in the short adrenocorticotropic hormone (ACTH) stimulation test to screen for secondary hypoadrenalism. Trademark, *Cortrosyn.*

cotinine (ko′tĭ-nēn) an active metabolite of nicotine, which is eliminated by urinary excretion.

Cotlove titrator (kot′luv) an instrument used in the coulometric determination of chloride. See also *chloride methods.*

cotransport (ko-trans′port) see under *active transport.*

cotton (kot′n) [Arabic *qutn*] the fibers surrounding the seed of *Gossypium* species, used as an absorbant and woven into materials. Cottonseed contains the toxin gossypol. Dust inhaled by workers exposed to cotton fibers may cause byssinosis. See also *byssinosis.*

cotton-wool appearance a description of the radiographic image of sclerosis of bone interspersed with rarefied regions, characteristic of osteitis deformans (Paget's disease of bone).

cotton-wool spot white or gray soft-edged opacities in the retina composed of cytoid bodies; seen in hypertensive retinopathy, lupus erythematosus, and numerous other conditions.

cot value (kot) a measure of DNA sequence complexity and, indirectly, of genome size. The DNA is sheared into small fragments and is denatured and allowed to renature. The rate of renaturation depends on the effective concentrations of each of the distinct DNA sequences. This in turn depends on total DNA concentration, DNA sequence diversity, and DNA sequence repetitiveness. The progress of the renaturation is monitored by hypochromicity (ultraviolet light absorbance at 260 nm), nuclease digestion (using a single-stranded specific nuclease), or hydroxyapatite chromatography (double-stranded DNA will bind and single-stranded DNA will not bind under certain conditions). The DNA concentration is expressed in terms of moles of nucleotides per liter. The product of the initial concentration (C_0) and the time taken for half the DNA to renature ($t_{\frac{1}{2}}$) is the reciprocal of the renaturation rate constant and is termed the cot value.

A similar term, the rot value, is used for DNA:RNA hybridization experiments in which cDNA is hybridized with an excess of RNA; it is the product of the reaction time and the initial RNA concentration.

cotyledon of placenta (kot″ĭ-le′don) [Gr. *kotylēdōn,* a cup-shaped depression] one of the numerous (15–30) lobes separated by fissures on the maternal surface of the human placenta.

cough (kof) 1. a sudden and violent expiratory effort that explosively expels alveolar gas out through the glottis at velocities of 75–100 mph, usually to clear the airways of foreign matter. It is the culmination of a coordinated sequence of events mediated by the medulla and initiated by irritation of the respiratory passages. See also *cough r.* under *reflex.*

2. to produce such an expulsion of air.

dry c., cough without expectoration.

productive c., cough attended by expectoration of material from the bronchi.

cough plate a plate of culture medium exposed to droplet inoculation from an individual's cough. After incubation, the plate is examined for bacterial colonies, especially *Bordetella,* in suspected cases of whooping cough. The method has been replaced by use of a flexible wire swab passed through the nose.

coulomb (C) (koo′lom) [Charles Augustin de *Coulomb,* French physicist, 1736–1806] the International System (SI) unit of electric charge defined as 1 ampere-second (1A·s), which is equal to 6.24146×10^{18} times the elementary charge (the magnitude of the charge on the electron or proton). Cf. *electrostatic unit* and *faraday.*

Coulomb's law [Charles Augustin de *Coulomb*] stated as: that which gives the force between two electric point charges. The force is proportional to the product of the magnitudes of the charges and is inversely proportional to the square of the distance between the charges. For charges with the same sign, the force is repulsive; with opposite signs, it is attractive.

coulometer (koo-lom′ĕ-ter) an electrochemical cell used in coulometry.

coulometric titration (koo″lŏ-met′rik) a titration in which the titrant is generated by electric current and its amount determined by coulometry. For example, chloride can be assayed in a cell in which silver ions are generated by the current; they are consumed by forming a precipitate with chloride. The end point is determined by the potentiometric or amperometric detection of free silver ions at a second pair of electrodes.

coulometry (koo-lom′ĕ-trē) an instrumental method for determining the amount of a substance (e.g., a metal, metal ion, or anion) by measuring the quantity of electricity (in coulombs) needed to cause a quantitative electrochemical reaction. The equation that gives the relationship between the number of moles, *N,* of the substance and the quantity of electricity in coulombs (ampere-seconds), *Q,* is: $N = Q/96{,}487\ n$ (n is the number of electrons per molecule or ion involved in the reduction).

In direct coulometric methods, the material to be determined is oxidized or reduced directly at one of the electrodes. For example, in the determination of the concentration of Cu(II) in solution, it is reduced to metallic copper at the electrode by passing current through the solution. In indirect coulometric methods or coulometric "titrations," the ion to be determined reacts with a "titrant" being generated at an electrode. For example, Fe(II) can be determined by its reaction with Ce(IV), which is being continuously generated in solution from an excess of Ce(III), which is being oxidized at the electrode. The end point is detected by using a visual indicator or by electrochemical means.

See also *chloride assays.*

Coulter Counter (kōlt′er) [W. H. *Coulter,* U.S. engineer, 20th century] trademark for voltage pulse counters; see *blood cell count automation.*

Coumadin (koo′mah-din) trademark. See *w. sodium* under *warfarin.*

coumarin (koo′mah-rin) any of a group of derivatives of 4′-hydroxycoumarin, used as anticoagulant drugs for the prevention and treatment of venous thrombosis and pulmonary embolism. After oral administration, such drugs are absorbed from the gut and carried, bound to albumin, to the liver where they affect the synthesis of vitamin K–dependent coagulation factors (prothrombin and Factors VII, IX, and X). The prothrombin time is the best indication of drug efficacy. Vitamin K may serve as an antidote in case of hemorrhage resulting from coumarin administration. The most commonly used derivatives are warfarin (trademark, Coumadin) and dicumerol.

Councilman's body (kown′sil-manz) [William Thomas *Councilman,* U.S. pathologist, 1854–1933] a rounded, densely eosinophilic refractile body usually located in an hepatic sinusoid and thought to represent a degenerating hepatocyte. It is characteristic of hepatic cell damage and is most commonly seen in viral hepatitis. Also called *acidophilic body.*

Councilmania (kown″sil-ma′ne-ah) [Williams Thomas *Councilman,* U.S. pathologist, 1854–1933] the former name of the genus *Entamoeba.*

count (kownt) [L. *computare* to reckon] 1. a measurement that consists of enumerating a number of objects, e.g., a red blood cell count.

2. in radiation measurement, a single response of the radiation counter to a particle of ionizing radiation (the detected radioactivity is measured in counts per time unit).

count density the number of radiation particles detected by an instrument in a unit area of an image. For a scintillation camera, $CD = (R \times T)/A,$ and for a rectilinear scanner, $CD = R/(S \times LS)$, where CD is count density, R is count rate, T is image time, A is image area, S is scan speed, and LS is line spacing.

counter (kown′ter) 1. an instrument or apparatus by which a numerical value is computed for discrete events.

2. in electronics, a device or circuit that counts and records the number of pulses in a period of time. Also called *scaler.*

binary c., an electronic counter that uses a series of binary stages (flip-flops) to record the number of input pulses, and thus has binary number readout.

cell c., a device that automatically counts the number of cells or specific types of cells in a specimen. Also called *cytometer.* See also *blood cell count automation, cytometry,* and *differential leukocyte count automation.*

decade c., an electronic counter that uses circuits (decades) that can count nine inputs, reset to zero on the tenth, and produce an output (carry) to the next stage. It thus has decimal readout, which is usually coded as binary coded decimal (BCD) for the read-out device.

frequency c., an electronic counter that can count pulses and also determine frequencies by counting the pulses in a preset time interval.

radiation c., a device that records the rate of entry or the number of alpha, beta, or gamma particles entering its detector. See also *gamma well counter, Geiger-Müller counter, liquid scintillation counter, proportional counter,* and *scintillation counter.*

ring c., a synchronously controlled electronic counter circuit composed of flip-flops, which are arranged in a loop and connected so that only one can be on at a given time. With each clock pulse, the flip-flop that is on is turned off and the next one is turned on so that the on state moves around the loop. Also called *shift c.*

ripple c., an electronic counting circuit composed of an array of flip-flops in which clock pulses are applied only to the first flip-flop of the array. As each flip-flop changes state, its output is the input for the next flip-flop in the array. Because of the time required for the input to propagate along the array, a ripple counter is slower than a synchronous counter; its circuitry, however, is less complex. Cf. *synchronous c.*

shift c., see *ring c.*

synchronous c., an electronic counting circuit composed of an array of flip-flops to which clock pulses (input) are applied simultaneously so that all of the flip-flops change state in unison. Cf. *ripple c.*

countercurrent (kown″ter-kur′ent) one of two streams flowing in opposite directions.

countercurrent extraction a liquid–liquid separation process in which the two liquids flow in opposite directions, with solutes being exchanged between the two immiscible liquids.

countercurrent immunoelectrophoresis (CIE) see *counterimmunoelectrophoresis.*

counterimmunoelectrophoresis (CIEP or CIE) (kown″ter-im″u-no-e-lek″tro-fo-re′sis) a combination of immunodiffusion and electrophoresis that provides for the rapid (less than 2 hr) identification of antigens in blood, e.g., hepatitis B antigen and endotoxins and polysaccharides from bacteria. The sample and a specific antibody are placed in wells at opposite ends of an agarose plate and subjected to electrophoresis. The antigen will migrate toward the anode, the antibody moves in the opposite direction as a result of electroosmosis, and a line of precipitin is formed where they meet.

counterpulsation (kown″ter-pul-sa′shun) a technique for assisting the circulation and decreasing the work of the heart by synchronizing the force of an external pumping device with cardiac systole and diastole.

counterstain (kown′ter-stān) a second stain that provides a contrasting effect to another stain. For example, in the routine H and E stain for tissue sections, hematoxylin stains the nuclei blue, and eosin (the counterstain) stains the cytoplasm pink. In this example, the stains have different affinities, the hematoxylin being basophilic and the eosin acidophilic. In other cases, the counterstain colors tissues or microorganisms from which a first stain has been removed. An example is the Gram stain, in which bacteria are stained in crystal violet, placed in iodine solution (a mordant), then decolorized in acid alcohol and stained with safranine O. Gram-positive bacteria retain the crystal violet, but gram-negative bacteria do not and are counterstained by the safranine O.

count information density the count density of a rectilinear scanner. See also *count density.*

counting cadence (kownt′ing) in some models of the Coulter counter, the regular noise produced by the decade counters. Irregular cadence indicates improper function.

counting chamber a device for determining the number of microorganisms or cells in a given volume of medium or fluid. A glass block with a depression marked in grids is fitted with a special coverslip. A sample of cell suspension is introduced and the cells in each square counted under a microscope. Because the volume in each square is predetermined by the distance between glass block and coverslip, the number of cells per unit volume can be calculated.

counting plate in bacteriology, a plate that is ruled off in square centimeters. When placed on the plate, the number of colonies in representative square centimeters of a Petri dish culture are counted. The number of colonies per plate is calculated by multiplying the average count per square centimeter by 62.5 (the area of a standard Petri dish being 62.5 cm^2).

count rate the number of radiation particles detected by an instrument in a unit time period.

count rate meter see *rate meter.*

coup (koo) [Fr.] a stroke.

c. de sabre, a linear, circumscribed lesion of scleroderma on the forehead or scalp, so called because of its resemblance to the scar of a saber wound.

c. de soleil, see *sunstroke.*

coupling (kup′ling) 1. a pairing or joining.

2. an interaction that transfers energy or information from one system to another.

3. in genetics, the occurrence on the same chromosome in a double heterozygote of the two mutant alleles of interest, the normal alleles being on the homologous chromosome. The genes are said to be linked in coupling.

4. in electronics, the transfer of a signal between two circuits. The capacitor or transformer that passes the AC but not the DC signal between amplifier stages is called a coupling capacitor or transformer. An amplifier that has resistors coupling the stages and thus can amplify DC signals is called a direct-coupled amplifier.

5. the joining of two molecular species to form a chemical compound. The term is particularly used for radical coupling reactions, which join two free radicals; for oxidative coupling reactions, which join free radicals, such as phenoxy radicals produced by an oxidizing agent; and for azo coupling reactions, which join an arene and a diazonium salt to form an azo dye.

6. the interaction of proton spins with the spins of other nuclei in the molecule. This spin coupling splits the peaks of the NMR spectrum into multiplets.

7. the joining of two chemical reactions, the product of the first being a reactant in the second. A

biochemical pathway may be a series of coupled enzymatic reactions.

coupling capacitor a capacitor used to pass an alternating current signal without passing direct current. In effect, it passes the signal between two points with different DC levels (e.g., the output of an amplifier stage and the input of the next stage).

covalent (ko-va′lent) pertaining to chemical bonds formed by shared electron pairs. See *covalent b.* under *bond.*

covariance (ko-va′re-ans) the mean (expectation) of the products of the deviation from the mean of the coordinate values (X and Y) of a two-dimensional random variable. The covariance of a sample of n X, Y pairs is $\Sigma_i (X_i - \overline{X})(Y_i - \overline{Y})$, where $\overline{X} = \Sigma_i X_i/n$ and $\overline{Y} = \Sigma_i Y_i/n$.

coverglass (kuv′er-glas) a thin, transparent plate used to cover a tissue section mounted on a slide for microscopic examination. Also called *coverslip.*

coverslip (kuv′er-slip) see *coverglass.*

cow see *generator.*

Cowdry type A inclusion body (kow′dre) [Edmund Vincent *Cowdry,* U.S. pathologist, 1888–1975] an area of nucleic acid and protein in the nucleus of cells involved in viral synthesis, which is morphologically changed in a cell infected with herpes simplex virus to form a discrete intranuclear inclusion.

Cowper's glands (kow′perz) [William *Cowper,* English surgeon, 1666-1709] see *bulbourethral glands.*

cowpox (kow′poks) a self-limiting disease acquired by humans from cows and caused by poxviruses; the etiologic agent is *Poxvirus bovis.* It is characterized by pustular skin lesions commonly localized to the hands. Cowpox occurs in cows as ulcers around the udder and is spread by the process of milking. The virus enters the skin and eventually forms a vesicle. Regional lymphadenitis occurs, and fever may or may not be present. The English physician Jenner first demonstrated vaccination in 1798 when he showed that inoculation with material from cowpox lesions led to immunity against smallpox.

Laboratory diagnosis is made by injecting vesicular exudate into the chorioallantoic membrane of a chick embryo. Lesions form on the membrane if the virus is present. Most cases of cowpox cure spontaneously.

coxa (kok′sah) [L.] [NA], the part of the body lateral to and including the hip joint. The term is used loosely to denote the hip joint.

c. valga, a deformity of the hip joint in which the angle between the axis of the head and neck of the femur and the axis of the shaft is greater than normal (normal being 135°) and the neck appears thickened.

c. vara, a deformity of the hip joint in which the angle formed by the axis of the head and neck of the femur and the axis of its shaft is less than normal (normal being 135°) and the neck appears shortened.

coxal (kok′sal) referring to the hip joint.

coxalgia (kok-sal′je-ah) [L. *coxa* hip + Gr. *algos* pain + *-ia*] see *coxodynia.*

coxal region the region of the back and side that overlies the hip bone.

Coxiella (kok″se-el′ah) [Herald Rea *Cox,* U.S. bacteriologist, born 1907] a genus of bacteria-like cells of the family of Rickettsiaceae. They are short rods growing preferentially in the host cell, and are more resistant to drying and elevated temperatures than are other rickettsiae. *Coxiella* grows well in the yolk sac of chick embryos. The genus consists of a single species, *C. burnetii,* which causes a pneumonia-like disease called Q fever in humans. See also *Rickettsiaceae.*

C. burnetii, gram-negative rods, 0.4–1.0 μm, that are the cause of Q fever in humans. *C. burnetii* is antigenically distinct from the true rickettsiae. The organisms are unusually stable outside host cells and contaminate dust, especially around cattle sheds. The discovery of a sporogenic cycle in these organisms may explain this remarkable stability. Humans acquire the infection by inhaling contaminated particles, which invade cells in the blood vessels, spleen, and liver.

Fever, headache, shivering, malaise, and interstitial pneumonitis with upper respiratory tract involvement are common manifestations of the disease. Tetracyclines and chloramphenicol are used in treatment.

See also *Q fever.*

coxitis (kok-si′tis) [L. *coxa* hip + *-itis* inflammation] inflammation of the hip joint.

coxodynia (kok″so-din′e-ah) [L. *coxa* hip + Gr. *odynē* pain] 1. hip-joint disease.

2. pain in the hip. Also called *coxalgia.*

coxsackievirus (kok-sak′e-vi″rus) [*Coxsackie,* New York, the source of the original isolates in 1948] a virus that belongs to the Picornavirus family; a subdivision of the enteroviruses—small, single-stranded RNA viruses. Coxsackievirus has physical and chemical characteristics similar to those of the poliovirus but contains a greater portion of guanine in RNA. There are two subgroups, both infectious for humans, group A and group B.

Coxsackievirus A has at least 23 immunotypes. Because it is a type of enterovirus, it can survive the low pH of the stomach and grows well at 37°C. The most characteristic result of infection is widespread lesions and a flaccid paralysis. It has also been known to cause herpangina, hand-foot-and-mouth disease, meningitis, macular rash, vesicular pharyngitis, upper respiratory tract infection, the common cold, and occasionally Guillain-Barré syndrome. There are six immunotypes of coxsackievirus B. Viruses of this group can cause epidemic pleurodynia (Bornholm disease) and lesions of the heart (coxsackie B myopericarditis), pancreas, and central nervous system, sometimes resulting in spastic paralysis or Guillain-Barré syndrome. All the viruses included in group B grow readily in monkey kidney cells, whereas group A must grow in a special cell line, but both grow well in newborn mice. Both are resistant to acids, proteolytic enzymes, and bile. In primary cultures of monkey kidney, cytopathic effects result in rounded refractile cells that lyse and fail away from glass. Hemagglutination inhibition tests are also used for identification. See also *picornavirus.*

Cox vaccine (koks) [H. R. *Cox*] a vaccine for prevention of epidemic typhus. It is prepared by treating a yolk sac culture of *Rickettsia prowazekii* with formalin. It was highly effective in large-scale immunization of civilian and military populations during World War II. See also typhus under *vaccination.*

CP abbrev. for cerebral palsy (see under *palsy*), chemically pure.

cP abbrev. See *centipoise.*

CPAP abbrev. for continuous positive airway pressure. See *continuous p. p. b.* under *positive pressure breathing.*

CPD abbrev. See *citrate-phosphate-dextrose.*

CPDA-1 abbrev. See *citrate-phosphate-dextrose-adenine.*

CPD-adenine see *citrate-phosphate-dextrose-adenine.*

CPE abbrev. See *cytopathic effect.*

C peptide a 31–amino acid residue that is formed from proinsulin in the beta cells of the pancreas. Proinsulin is enzymatically degraded to C peptide and insulin, which are subsequently secreted into the circulation in equal amounts. C peptide is biologically not active. Measurement of C-peptide levels by radioimmunoassay allows assessment of pancreatic beta-cell secretory function, especially in cases in which insulin antibodies that are present interfere with insulin determinations.

CPH abbrev. for chronic persistent hepatitis. See under *hepatitis.*

CPK abbrev. for creatine phosphokinase. See *creatine kinase.*

cpm abbrev. for counts per minute, the scale calibration for many radiation survey meters.

CPPB abbrev. See *continuous p. p. b.* under *positive pressure breathing.*

CPR abbrev. for cardiopulmonary resuscitation. See under *artificial respiration.*

cps abbrev. See *cycle per second.*

CPU abbrev. See *central processing unit.*

CR abbrev. See *creatinine.*

Cr symbol for the chemical element *chromium.*

Crabtree effect (krab′tre) [H. G. *Crabtree,* English biochemist, 20th century] the inhibition of oxidative phosphorylation by high concentrations of glucose, found in isolated systems such as ascites tumor cells. The probable mechanism for this effect is the more effective competition by the glycolysis pathway for inorganic phosphate and NADH.

Craigie's tube method (kra′gēz) a method for separating motile from nonmotile bacteria. A tube of semisolid agar medium is prepared, and a length of glass tubing with a slanted bottom is inserted so that the top protrudes above the medium. A stab inoculation is made inside the glass tubing. After incubation, motile organisms can be isolated from the medium outside the tubing while nonmotile types remain inside. This method is also used for isolating phase variations of *Salmonella.*

cramp (kramp) a painful, involuntary muscle contraction, associated with the rapid firing of large number of motor units.

cramp discharge bursts of electric activity associated with muscle cramps. These discharges consist of spontaneous, repetitive high-frequency firing of motor units, similar to that seen in the maximal voluntary contraction of a muscle.

crani/o (kra′ne-o) [L. *cranium,* from Gr. *kranion* skull] a word element used in combining form to denote the skull, e.g., craniostenosis.

craniad (kra′ne-ad) [*crani-* + *ad* toward] toward the head. Also called *cephalad.* Cf. *caudad.*

cranial (kra′ne-al) [L. *cranialis*] pertaining to the cranium or the head end of the body.

cranial cavity the space within the skull that contains the brain. It is enclosed by the bones of the cranium.

cranial nerves 12 pairs of nerves that emerge from the brain and pass through openings in the floor of the cranial cavity to be distributed mainly to structures of the head and neck. One exception, the vagus nerve, extends to the thorax and abdomen. Some cranial nerves are motor, others sensory, and four carry both motor and sensory nerve fibers. For more information, see the specific cranial nerve.

craniocaudal projection (cra″ne-o-kaw′dal) [*cranio-* + L. *cauda* tail] a projection used in mammography. The patient sits erect with the breast supported by the film holder and the breast and nipple extended in profile. The central ray projects vertically. Also called craniocaudad projection.

craniometry (kra″ne-om′ĕ-tre) [*cranio-* + Gr. *metrein* measure] measurement of the dimensions of the skull and facial bones.

craniopharyngioma (kra″ne-o-fah-rin″je-o′mah) [*cranio-* + Gr. *pharyngos* pharynx + *-ema* swelling] a benign tumor of the pituitary region that histologically resembles the odontogenic adamantinoma and is consequently believed to arise from misplaced cells of the embryonal oral cavity carried upward by the craniopharyngeal diverticulum (Rathke's pouch). It constitutes 3 percent of all intracranial tumors; most patients are children or young adults. The tumor arises above the sella, and may grow large enough to fill the third ventricle and obstruct the flow of cerebrospinal fluid. The epithelial cells of the tumor form cords of columnar cells that enclose small microcystic spaces and are surrounded by a stroma of stellate cells. Areas of squamous cells and foci of calcification are common. The tumor is difficult to remove surgically because of its location and attachment to surrounding structures. Some success has been reported with combined surgery and radiotherapy.

craniosclerosis (kra″ne-o-sklĕ-ro′sis) [*cranio-* + Gr. *sklēros* hard] abnormal calcification and thickening of the cranial bones.

cranioscopy (kra″ne-os′ko-pe) [*cranio-* + Gr. *skopein* to examine] diagnostic examination of the head.

craniostenosis (kra″ne-o-stĕ-no′sis) [*cranio-* + Gr. *stenosis* narrowing] a deformation of the skull resulting from the premature closure of sutures and subsequent cessation of cranial growth. Radiographs show that the sutures are obliterated, the skull outline is abnormal, and a ridge is evident along the suture line. Involvement of the coronal and lambdoid sutures is termed oxycephaly; involvement of the sagittal sutures, scaphocephaly; fusion of the coronal suture, brachycephaly; and fusion of all sutures, microcrania.

craniosynostosis (kra″ne-o-sin″os-to′sis) premature ossification of the cranium, which results in obliteration of the sutures and in gross deformity of the skull or restricted growth of the brain.

craniotabes (kra″ne-o-ta′bēz) [*cranio-* + L. *tabes* a wasting] a reduction in mineralization of the skull, with abnormal softness of the bone, usually affecting the occipital and parietal bones along the lambdoid sutures. Craniotabes is seen most commonly in vitamin D deficiency in infants.

craniotomy (kra″ne-ot′o-me) [*cranio-* + Gr. *tomē* a cut] 1. any operation on the cranium.

2. puncture of the skull and removal of its contents to decrease the size of the head of a dead fetus and facilitate delivery.

cranium (kra′ne-um), pl. *crania* [L., from Gr. *kranion* the upper part of the head] the skeleton of the head, generally considered to be all the bones of the head except the mandible. It may also be construed, however, to mean only the eight bones forming the cranial cavity.

cras/o (kra′zo) [Gr. *krasis* a mixture, combination] a word element used in combining form to denote a mixture, e.g., dyscrasia.

crateriform (kra-ter′ĭ-form) [L. *crater* bowl + *forma* shape] depressed or hollowed like a bowl.

C-reactive protein (CRP) an acute-phase protein, named for its ability to bind the C polysaccharide in the cell wall of *Streptococcus pneumoniae,* that migrates with the gamma-globulin fraction in serum protein electrophoresis. It has also been shown to activate the classical complement pathway, to bind to T lymphocytes, and to inhibit clot retraction and platelet aggregration. CRP shows significant homology with IgG but is antigenically distinct.

Serum concentrations are elevated approximately up to one thousand-fold as a nonspecific response to inflammation. CRP has use as a more sensitive indicator than the erythrocyte sedimentation rate (ESR) for evaluating both the response to therapy and the severity of inflammation in common rheumatic diseases such as rheumatoid arthritis and systemic lupus erythematosus. The reference range is 10–37 μg/ml.

C-reactive protein assays 1. serologic methods to demonstrate reactivity to *Streptococcus pneumoniae* C-polysaccharide; gel diffusion techniques are the most widely used. Such methods lack the sensitivity to detect CRP in normal sera.

2. immunologic methods such as radioimmunoassay or fluoroimmunoassay; these highly sensitive methods are required for detection of the small amounts present in normal sera.

creatine (kre′ah-tēn, kre′ah-tin) [Gr. *kreas* flesh] a compound, *N*-methylguanidinoacetic acid, that provides a means of storing high-energy phosphate in vertebrate muscle and nerve tissue. Creatine kinase catalyzes the equilibration of high-energy phosphate charges stored in adenosine triphosphate (ATP) and phosphocreatine. The reaction ADP + phosphocreatine ⇄ ATP + creatine has a $\Delta G°$ of –3.0 kcal/mol and therefore tends to go to the right, keeping the ATP level high until the store of phosphocreatine is almost depleted. Thus, phosphocreatine provides a large store of energy for short periods of intense muscular activity.

creatine assays 1. measurement using a creatinine assay before and after treatment of the specimens with heat at an acid pH. The difference between the preformed creatinine and the total creatinine in the specimen is a measure of the creatine concentration. See also *creatinine assays.*

2. a coupled enzyme assay involving creatine kinase, pyruvate kinase, and lactate dehydrogenase. The change in the absorbance at 340 nm reflects the amount of NADH oxidized in the lactate dehydrogenase reaction and is a measure of the creatine in the specimen.

creatine kinase (CK) an enzyme of the phosphotransferase subclass (EC 2.7.3.2) that catalyzes the reaction creatine + ATP = phosphocreatine + ADP. The enzyme is activated by Mg^{2+} and Mn^{2+}, and by sulfhydryl agents. The reaction serves to transfer the energy stored in ATP to phosphocreatine, which is stored in muscle tissue. The equilibrium favors the reverse reaction with a pH optimum of 6.9–7.4. Increased CK activity in serum is associated with skeletal muscle disease (muscular dystrophy and poliomyelitis), and also with myocardial and cerebral infarction. A clinical diagnosis of any of these disorders is frequently confirmed by CK isoenzyme determination. Also called *creatine phosphokinase.*

creatine kinase assays methods for determining CK activity in serum. There are several methods using the reverse reaction: ADP + creatine phosphate → ATP + creatine. The creatine formed in the reaction is measured colorimetrically after addition of diacetyl and α-naphthol, or fluorometrically after addition of ninhydrin. In methods using the forward reaction, the acid-labile creatine phosphate, which is formed in the reaction, is hydrolyzed, and the inorganic phosphate is measured. Two continuous monitoring assays have been devised. In one, the ADP formed from ATP + Cr is reacted with phospho-enol pyruvate in the presence of pyruvic kinase to form pyruvate, which is measured with NADH and lactate dehydrogenase; in the other, the ATP formed from Cr-P + ADP is used to phosphorylate glucose to Gluc-6-PO_4, which is assayed by oxidation to 6-phosphogluconic acid by NADP in the presence of Gluc-6-PO_4-DH. The increase in $A_{340\ nm}$ due to the formation of NADPH is a measure of enzyme activity.

creatine kinase isoenzymes the isoenzymes of creatine kinase (CK). CK is a dimer with M (muscle) and/or B (brain) subunits; it exists in three isoenzyme forms: CK-MM (CK_3), CK-MB (CK_2), and CK-BB (CK_1). CK-MM is the predominant form found in the serum and accounts for approximately 95 percent of the total enzyme activity. It is found primarily in skeletal muscle. CK-MB is found in the cardiac muscle, tongue, diaphragm, and in small amounts in skeletal muscle (3–5 percent). CK-BB is present in the brain, smooth muscle, thyroid, lungs, and prostate.

The CK isoenzymes are assayed by electrophoresis to assess damage to the myocardium, which is indicated by increased amounts of CK-MB in serum. After a myocardial infarction, CK-MM and CK-MB enter the circulatory system as a result of damage to the cardiac muscle cells. Increased levels of these isoenzymes can be detected in the serum 4–6 hr after the infarct, with maximal concentrations usually occurring by 18–24 hr, and a return to normal within 36–72 hr.

Increased CK-MB is also seen after cardiac surgery and in infarct extensions, myocardial ischemia, Duchenne's muscular dystrophy, pericarditis, hypothyroidism and in long-distance runners.

Increases in the CK-MM isoenzyme are predominantly seen in Duchenne's muscular dystrophy, rhabdomyolysis, polymyositis, myocardial infarcts, myocardial ischemia, brain injury, chronic renal failure, severe shock, and biliary atresia. CK-BB is seen in the serum following renal failure, brain injury, and bowel infarcts and in the presence of certain malignancies.

Reference ranges for the CK isoenzymes in serum are 95–97 percent for CK-MM and 3–5 percent for CK-MB; CK-BB is not detected with most routine techniques.

See also *lactate dehydrogenase isoenzymes.*

creatine kinase isoenzymes electrophoresis electrophoresis at alkaline pH (8.6), usually on agarose or cellulose acetate, performed to separate the creatine kinase (CK) isoenzymes. The bands are visualized by coupling the CK reaction with the hexokinase and glucose-6-phosphate dehydrogenase reaction (G-6-PD) to form NADPH, which can be seen under ultraviolet light or measured fluorometrically. Alternately, the NADPH found can be used to reduce tetrazolium to a formazan dye, which can be measured photometrically.

creatine phosphate (kre′ah-tēn fos′fāt) see *phosphocreatine.*

creatine phosphokinase (CPK) (kre′ah-tēn fos″-fo-ki′nās) see *creatine kinase.*

creatinine (CR) (kre-at′ĭ-nēn, kre-at′ĭ-nin) a basic substance, $NH \cdot C(:NH) \cdot N(CH_3) \cdot CH_2$, creatine anhydride. Creatinine is formed by the spontaneous breakdown (in vivo) of phosphocreatine and is excreted in urine. It is removed from plasma by glomerular filtration, and to a minor degree by tubular secretion; a small amount is reabsorbed by the renal tubules. Therefore, creatinine clearance is approximately equal to, and is used for the determination of, the glomerular filtration rate (GFR).

creatinine assays 1. methods based on the Jaffe reaction in which creatinine reacts with alkaline picrate to produce an orange-red product, which is quantitated photometrically at 515–525 nm. A variety of noncreatinine chromogens are present in serum; they may be removed by adsorbing creatinine from an acidified, deproteinized specimen onto Lloyd's reagent, an aluminum silicate, and eluting it with alkaline solution.

2. a coupled enzymatic method in which creatinine is hydrolyzed to creatine by an amido hydrolase. The creatine formed is then phosphorylated by ATP in the presence of creatine kinase to form ADP, which reacts with phosphopyruvate to form pyruvate. Pyruvate is measured at 340 nm by the oxidation of NADH in the presence of LDH.

3. an enzymatic method in which creatinine is hydrolyzed by creatininase to form NH_3. This can be assayed by the Berthelot reaction or with glutamate dehydrogenase.

4. a kinetic method measuring the rate of formation of the Jaffe color with a sensitive spectrophotometer. With appropriate timing of the measurement, the reaction can be fairly specific for creatinine.

creatinine clearance (C_{cr}) a practical procedure for evaluating the glomerular filtration rate (GFR) of the kidneys. It measures the rate at which endogenous creatinine is cleared from the blood. The creatinine concentrations of a precisely timed (e.g., 4-hr, 24-hr) urine specimen (U) and of a plasma specimen (P) drawn during the urine collection period are measured. The clearance value, corrected to standard body surface area, is given by the formula: $C_{cr} = (U \times V) \times (1.73)/(P \times A)$, where V is the urine flow rate in milliliters per minute, A is the body surface area in square meters, and 1.73 is the standard surface area.

Reference values for creatinine clearance (when methods are used to measure creatinine concentrations that are based on the standard Jaffe reaction) are: for males, 85–125 ml/min of standard surface area; and for females, 75–115. When more specific creatinine procedures are used, the reference intervals increase to 97–137 ml/min for males and 88–128 ml/min for females.

The endogenous creatinine clearance test is a reasonably good estimate of the GFR, except in severe renal disease or in the presence of exogenous creatinine.

creatinine coefficient a number expressed as milligrams of creatinine excreted in urine in a 24-hr period per kilogram of body weight. The index reflects the fact that the rate of creatinine excretion is a function of body muscle mass. Reference values are: for males, 22–30; for females, 15–22; and for infants and children, 5–20.

creatinuria (kre-at″ĭ-nu′re-ah) [*creatine* + Gr. *ouron* urine + *-ia*] an increased concentration of creatine in the urine.

creeping eruption see under *larva migrans.*

creeping substitution of bone the formation of new bone by osteoblasts on the surfaces of necrotic bony trabeculae. This process occurs after the revascularization of bone disrupted by fracture, as at the head of the femur after fracture of the neck of the bone has disrupted the blood supply to its head. Bone grafts using bone fragments taken from elsewhere in the body take advantage of the process of creeping substitution to repair bony defects.

C region see *constant region.*

crenate (kre′nāt) [L. *crenatus* notched] scalloped or notched.

crenated cell (kre′nāt-ed) [L. *crenatus*] see *echinocyte.*

crenation (kre-na′shun) the formation of 10–30 abnormal spicules on the surface of an erythrocyte, caused by the accumulation of fatty acids or lysophosphatidylcholine on the erythrocyte surface that is due to altered erythrocyte metabolism or plasma composition. The crenated red cells are referred to as echinocytes. It is a common misconception that crenation is due to shrinkage of the cells in hypertonic solutions.

crenulate (kren′u-lāt) wavy or scalloped; crenate.

crepitation (krep″ĭ-ta′shun) [L. *crepitare* to crackle] a dry, crackling sound or sensation, such as that produced by approximating the ends of a fractured bone.

crepitus (krep′ĭ-tus) [L.] 1. discharge of flatus from the bowels.

2. crepitation.

3. a crepitant rale.

crescent (kres′ent) [L. *crescens*] 1. shaped like a new moon.

2. a crescent-shaped structure.

crescent cell a large, pale erythrocyte that becomes crescent-shaped as a result of peripheral blood film preparation. Also called *selenocyte.*

crescentic glomerulopathy (krĕ-sen′tik) see under *glomerulopathy.*

cresol (kre′sol) 1. one of the three isomeric methylphenols ($CH_3C_6H_4OH$): 2-methylphenol (*o*-cresol, a solid), 3-methylphenol (*m*-cresol, a liquid), or 4-methylphenol (*p*-cresol, a solid). The pure chemicals are white or colorless but darken rapidly on exposure to air and light. Cresols are highly toxic by ingestion or skin absorption. The effects of poisoning are similar to those produced by other phenols; see under *phenol*.

2. a colorless, yellowish to brownish-yellow, or pinkish liquid, which is a mixture of the three isomers with the meta form predominant and is used as a disinfectant. It contains not more than 5 percent phenol and is obtained from coal tar.

cresol assays see *phenol assays*.

cresol red a pH indicator, *o*-cresolsulfonphthalein, with a pH range of 7.2 (yellow)–8.8 (red).

crest (krest) [L. *crista* ridge] a projection or projecting structure or ridge, especially one surmounting a bone or its border.

iliac c., the expanded upper border of the ilium that provides for attachment of the anterolateral abdominal muscles and muscles of the lower extremity and of the lower back. The crest is often used as the source of bone marrow for clinical examination.

pubic c., the thick, rough anterior border of the body of the pubic bone.

cresyl blue (kres′il) see *brilliant cresyl blue*.

cresyl fast violet a basic oxazine dye used in histology for Nissl staining. Also called cresyl echt violet and Cresylechtviolett.

cresyl violet acetate a dye similar to cresyl fast violet.

cretinism (kre′tin-izm) a syndrome of irreversible mental retardation that results from a lack of thyroid hormone during the first year or two of life. The incidence is approximately 1 in 4000 births: 65 percent of infants with congenital hypothyroidism have hypoplasia or agenesis of the thyroid gland, 25 percent have an ectopic thyroid, and 10 percent have a defect in the pathway for thyroid hormone synthesis. Clinical manifestations include physical and mental retardation, deafness, dystrophy of bones and soft tissues, and lowered basal metabolism. Cretinism can be corrected and controlled by the prompt administration of thyroid hormone, provided irreparable damage to the central nervous system has not already occurred. Screening of newborns for hypothyroidism is now widely practiced. See also under *goiter*.

Creutzfeldt-Jakob disease (kroits′felt yak′ob) [Hans Gerhard *Creutzfeldt*, German psychiatrist, 1885–1964; Alfons Maria *Jakob*, German psychiatrist, 1884–1931] a type of subacute, spongiform viral encephalopathy characterized by progressive dementia, ataxia, and myoclonic jerks. The disease usually commences in late middle age and has a fatal outcome, generally within 1 yr of onset. There is no effective treatment.

Results of cerebrospinal fluid analysis are normal, but this disease is transmissible. The electroencephalogram may show a characteristic pattern of periodic sharp waves, which is helpful in supporting the clinical diagnosis.

See also *slow viruses*.

CRF abbrev. See *chronic r. f.* under *renal failure*, *chronic r. f.* under *respiratory failure*, *corticotropin releasing factor*.

cribriform (krib′rĭ-form) [L. *cribrum* sieve + *forma* form] perforated with small apertures, like a sieve.

cribriform plate a horizontal layer of perforated bone that forms the roof of each half of the nasal cavity. It is a part of the ethmoid bone. The plate has many small foramina for passage of the olfactory nerves.

cri du chat syndrome (kre du shah) [Fr. "cat's cry"] a hereditary condition caused by deletion of the short arm of chromosome 5 (5p–) and characterized by severe mental retardation, microcephaly, epicanthic folds, ocular hypertelorism, and round facies. It is named for the characteristic mewing, catlike cry produced by the afflicted infants.

Crigler-Najjar syndrome a severe form of congenital nonhemolytic jaundice caused by a complete deficiency of bilirubin UDP-glucuronyl transferase. The disease is rare, usually familial, and in such cases is transmitted as an autosomal recessive trait. Kernicterus develops in most of those affected, although it may not occur until after the neonatal period. Most affected individuals die in infancy or early childhood as a result of neurologic complications.

C.-N. s., type II, a mild form of congenital nonhemolytic jaundice caused by a partial deficiency of bilirubin UDP-glucuronyl transferase, which some investigators believe to be a variant of Crigler-Najjar syndrome. The disease is rare and is usually familial; when familial, it appears to be transmitted as an autosomal dominant trait with a variable penetrance. Kernicterus is uncommon, and most individuals with this syndrome survive to adulthood without neurologic signs or intellectual impairment. Also called *Arias syndrome*.

crin/o (krin′o) [Gr. *krinein* to separate] a word element used in combining form to denote secretion, e.g., crinogenic.

-crine (krin) [Gr. *krinein* to separate] a suffix word element to denote secretion, e.g., endocrine.

crinophagy (krin-of′ah-je) [*crino-* + Gr. *phagein* to eat] the process by which secretory granules in the prolactin-forming cells of the adenohypophysis are disposed of after the end of lactation. They fuse with lysosomes to form autophagic vacuoles within which they are broken down enzymatically.

Crippa's lead tetraacetate method (krip′az) a histologic staining procedure used to demonstrate mucins and mucoids. Aldehyde deposits formed by lead tetraacetate oxidation are stained red-purple by a Schiff reagent.

crisis (kri′sis), pl. *crises* [L., from Gr. *krisis* turning point, decision] 1. the turning point of a disease for better or worse; especially a sudden change for the better in the course of an acute disease.

2. a sudden paroxysmal intensification of symptoms in the course of a disease.

Addisonian c., an acute, life-threatening episode occurring in Addison's disease, which is characterized by glucocorticoid deficiency, extracellular fluid depletion, and hyperkalemia. Immediate correction of the electrolyte imbalance and administration of hydrocortisone are necessary.

blast c., see *blast crisis*.

celiac c., an attack of severe watery diarrhea and vomiting producing dehydration and acidosis, sometimes occurring in the infantile form of celiac disease.

thyroid c., see *thyroid crisis*.

crista (kris′tah), pl. *cristae* [L. "ridge"] 1. a projection or ridge, especially of a bone; also called crest and ridge.

2. one of the elaborate infoldings of the mitochondrial inner membrane.

c. ampullaris, the transverse ridge in the ampullae of the semicircular canals, which is covered by the sensory epithelium of the vestibular apparatus of the inner ear.

c. galli, a triangular crest projecting upward from the superior surface of the cribriform plate of the ethmoid bone, to which the falx cerebri attaches.

-crit (krit) [Gr. *krinein* to separate] a suffix word element to denote separation, e.g., hematocrit.

critical (krit'ĭ-k'l) 1. in a state of crisis; in danger of death.

2. in sufficient quantity to constitute a turning point.

critical angle the smallest angle of incidence at which total internal reflection occurs, expressed as $\sin^{-1}(n'/n)$, where n is the refractive index of the medium in which the light travels, and n' is the index of refraction of the medium on the other side of the reflecting interface. See also *refraction* and *total internal r.* under *reflection.*

critical illumination see under *illumination.*

critical mass the minimal mass of fissionable material needed for a self-sustaining fission chain reaction.

critical micelle concentration (cmc) a narrow concentration range of a solution of an amphiphilic compound above which stable colloidal aggregates (micelles) are formed and below which there are only free monomers.

critical path analysis a technique for determining the critical path through a network. See also *network.*

critical region see under *hypothesis testing.*

critical temperature the temperature above which a substance has no liquid phase. It is either a gas or a solid, depending on the pressure.

CRM abbrev. for *Certified Reference Materials, cross-reacting material.*

cRNA abbrev. See *chromosomal RNA.*

crocidolite (kro-sid'o-lit") a sodium ferrosoferric silicate having a blue color. A form of asbestos used industrially, crocidolite has been found to cause asbestosis and cancer. See also *asbestos* and *asbestosis.*

Crohn's disease (krōnz) [Burrill Bernard *Crohn,* New York physician, born 1884] an inflammatory disease of unknown etiology, originally described as limited to the terminal ileum, but subsequently recognized as frequently involving other portions of the intestinal tract also, and occasionally producing secondary involvement of lymph nodes, liver, skin, and joints. The disease is basically an acute or chronic inflammatory process that involves the full thickness of the bowel wall, and is usually associated with mucosal ulcers and crypt abscesses. Later in the course of the disease, noncaseating granulomatous inflammation develops. Involved areas may be separated by segments of normal bowel (skip areas). Obstruction and fistula formation are common complications. At times this disease may be confused with other forms of enteritis. Also called *regional enteritis.* Cf. *ulcerative colitis.*

cromolyn sodium (kro'mŏ-lin) a drug given as a powder for inhalation in the prophylactic treatment of bronchial asthma. It has no effect in an acute crisis. The probable mechanism of action is stabilization of mast cell membranes, thereby preventing the release of mediators of immediate hypersensitivity (histamine, SRS-A, etc.).

Crooke's hyalin change a cytologic change in the ACTH-producing cells of the anterior pituitary that reflects a negative feedback effect of excess glucocorticoids. It occurs in Cushing's disease or following administration of glucocorticoids. The homogeneous appearance of the cytoplasm of the Crooke's cells by light microscopy is produced by an accumulation of intermediate filaments. Also called Crooke's hyalin.

cross a mating between organisms that have different genes determining particular traits of inheritance.

cross activation the activation of genes from an undifferentiated cell resulting from its hybridization with a differentiated cell. See also *hybrid c.* under *cell.*

cross-assembler an assembler that, like a cross-compiler, produces a machine-language program to be run on a different computer.

cross-compiler a computer program running on a large computer that translates a high-level language program into the machine language of a minicomputer, which does not have the memory capacity required by the compiler.

cross-fire treatment radiation therapy in which two or more x-ray beams are directed at a tumor through separate portals of entry.

crossmatching see under *compatibility tests.*

crossover the exchange of material between homologous chromosomes during the first meiotic division, resulting in new combinations of genes. Also called crossing over. See also *bacterial g.* under *genetics.*

crossover frequency the frequency of crossovers between two genes, used as a measure of physical separation of the genes on the chromosome. It is expressed in percentage units or centimorgans (cMo); 1 cMo is equal to a crossover frequency of 1 percent; the total length of human chromosomes is about 3000 cMo. Genes on a chromosome may be so far apart as to appear unlinked (the recombination frequency is 50 percent), but linkage of each with intermediate genes may establish their co-linkage. Also called *map distance.*

cross product see *vector product.*

cross-reacting antigen an antigen that reacts with an antibody that did not specifically stimulate its formation.

cross-reacting material (CRM) an enzymatically inactive protein produced by a mutant gene that reacts antigenically with antibody against the unaltered protein. Thus, its serologic properties are like those of the enzyme produced by the normal allele. The specific activity of an enzyme can be examined by comparing catalytic activity with the total amount of CRM precipitated by antibody to the enzyme. This assay depends on the assumption that most single-substitution mutations, which inactivate an enzyme, do not change its antigenic properties.

cross reaction the reaction of an antibody with a heterologous antigen that did not specifically stimulate its formation. It may be weaker than a reaction with the inducing antigen. Such cross reactions provide some information about the composition of antigenic determinants, as structural similarities between specific antigens are necessary for a cross reaction to occur.

cross-reactivity the degree to which an antibody participates in cross reactions with antigens other than the one used to produce the antibody. This is a property of nearly all naturally derived antibodies.

cross-sectional survey a clinical survey in which the incidence of two diseases or a disease and a risk factor are determined at the same time. Unlike prospective or retrospective studies, it can show only association, not a causal relationship.

cross wall see *septum.*

Crotalidae (kro-tal′ĭ-de) the family of pit vipers, which includes the genera *Agkistrodon* (copperhead and water moccasin), *Bothops* (fer-de-lance), *Crotalus* (rattlesnake), and *Lachesis* (bushmaster). These snakes are characterized by a depression between the nostril and the eye and by long, retractable hollow fangs attached to a venom gland which can inject lethal venom into a bite. See also *snakebite.*

crotalin (kro′tah-lin) the venom of rattlesnakes and some other snakes. It produces a bradykinin-like action on blood vessels, which causes a fall in blood pressure and damage to capillary epithelium, and results in fluid and blood cell loss. Lymph nodes become dilated and filled with erythrocytes and phagocytic cells.

croton oil (kro′ton) [L., from Gr. *krotōn* tick] a thick, brownish-yellow, fixed oil obtained from the seeds of *Croton tiglium,* of the plant family Euphorbiaceae. It contains glycerides of stearic, palmitic, myristic, lauric, oleic, and tiglic acids, and croton resin. Croton oil acts as a drastic purgative and counterirritant, producing pustules and skin tumors with cutaneous application. It is unfit for human use but is employed as a standard irritant in pharmacologic research. Also called *tiglium oil.*

crot value (krot) the initiation concentration of RNA multiplied by time in the hybridization of cDNA to RNA. Cf. *cot value.*

croup (kroop) a general term for a group of infectious conditions characterized by a barking cough that is often accompanied by inspiratory respiratory sounds (stridor), expiratory rhonchi and wheeze, laryngeal obstruction, respiratory distress, and retraction of the accessory muscles of respiration. The most common form of the condition is acute laryngotracheobronchitis. Croup may also be associated with diphtheria, epiglottitis, foreign bodies, allergy, and laryngitis.

In acute laryngotracheobronchitis, there is viral inflammation of both the upper and lower respiratory tracts, most frequently associated with a parainfluenza infection, especially type 1. The disease primarily affects children aged 3 mo to 3 yr and tends to be seasonal.

Diagnosis is based on the characteristic clinical picture. Anteroposterior neck x-rays often show subepiglottic swelling and narrowing. Arterial blood gases may reveal hypoxia with or without hypercapnia. Diminished breath sounds and atelectasis may also be seen. In the absence of complications, the condition usually abates within several days.

Crouzon's syndrome (kroo-zawz′) [Octave *Crouzon,* French neurologist, 1874–1938] a craniofacial synostosis, transmitted as an autosomal dominant trait, in which both the sagittal and coronal sutures are closed at birth. The most common characteristics include hypertelorism, hypoplasia of the maxilla, low-set ears, and a parrot-beaked nose. Mental development is usually normal.

Treatment involves surgical correction that includes orthodontic treatment of malocclusion, widening of the coronal sutures, and (occasionally) bilateral frontal craniectomy. The outlook depends on the severity of cranial closure; prognosis is generally good.

crowded cell index see under *squamous cell index.*

crowding effect a phenomenon of tapeworm parasitism in which the size of the worms (notably *Dibothriocephalus latus*) is inversely proportional to the number present in the intestine.

CRP abbrev. See *C-reactive protein.*

CRT abbrev. See *cathode ray tube, corrected r. t.* under *retention time.*

CRT terminal a computer terminal that utilizes a cathode ray tube to display data from the computer. A keyboard, or possibly a light pen, may be incorporated to input data to the computer.

cruciate (kroo′she-āt) [L. *crux* cross] shaped like a cross.

crucible (kroo′sĭ-b′l) [N.L. *crucibulum* earthen pot] a vessel for melting refractory substances.

cruor (kroo′or), pl. *cruores* [L.] a blood clot.

crush syndrome (krush) the edema, oliguria, myoglobinuria, and other symptoms of renal tubular failure that follow crushing of a large muscle mass.

Crustacea (krus-ta′she-ah) [L. *crusta* shell] a large class of aquatic, water-breathing arthropods including the lobsters, crabs, shrimps, wood lice, water fleas, and barnacles.

cry/o (kri′o) [Gr. *kryos* cold] a word element used in combining form to denote cold, e.g., cryostat.

cryalgesia (kri″al-je′ze-ah) [*cry-* + Gr. *algēsis* pain + *-ia*] pain on application of cold.

cryoablation (kri″o-ah-bla′shun) [*cryo-* + L. *ablatio* removal] surgical resection or removal of a tissue through the application of extreme cold. This technique is increasingly being applied to patients with premature ventricular excitation, especially when it is due to Wolff-Parkinson-White syndrome. Following extensive electrophysiologic mapping, the anomalous excitation pathway is interrupted to prevent both delta waves and the subsequent arrhythmias.

cryobank (kri′o-bank″) a facility for freezing and preserving semen at low temperatures (usually –196.5°C) for future use.

cryobiology (kri″o-bi-ol′o-je) [*cryo-* + Gr. *bios* life + *-logy*] the science dealing with the effect of low temperatures on biologic systems.

cryocautery (kri″o-kaw′ter-e) [*cryo-* + Gr. *kautērion* branding iron] cold cautery.

cryocrit (kri′o-krit) [*cryo-* + Gr. *krinein* to separate] the relative amount of cryoglobulins in serum estimated by centrifuging the serum at 4°C in a hematocrit tube. See also *cryoglobulin.*

cryofibrinogen (kri″o-fi-brin′o-jen) a soluble complex of fibrinogen and protein fragments that precipitate in cold (4°C) or in heparinized plasma. They redissolve at around 37°C.

cryofibrinogenemia (kri″o-fi-brin″o-jen-e′me-ah) [*cryo-* + *fibrinogen* + Gr. *haima* blood + *-ia*] a hematologic condition in which precipitates of fibrinogen and plasma globulins form at cold temperatures. Vascular damage may result, manifested as purpura on the extremities and the face. Thromboembolic phenomena and a hemorrhagic diathesis may also be induced.

cryogenic (kri″o-jen′ik) [*cryo-* + Gr. *gennan* to produce] pertaining to or causing the production of low temperatures.

cryoglobulin (kri″o-glob′u-lin) [*cryo-* + L. *globulus* little ball] an abnormal serum protein that precipitates in the cold at less than 37°C and redissolves when warmed to 37°C. There are three types: type I consists of a single, monoclonal immunoglobulin; type II of a monoclonal immunoglobulin with antibody activity against a polyclonal immunoglobulin; and type III of mixed polyclonal immunoglobulins.

Cryoglobulins are detected by storing serum at 4°C and looking for the formation of a white precipitate or gel after a variable period of time. They usually precipitate within 24–72 hr, but the serum should be observed for at least 1 wk so that late-forming cryoglobulins may be detected. The reversibility of precipitate formation should be confirmed by warming the serum.

Cryoglobulins are indicative of a number of diseases. Types I and II are usually present in patients with monoclonal paraproteinemias, such as lymphoma or multiple myeloma, and occur in amounts greater than 5 mg/ml. Sometimes they are found as benign paraproteins in patients lacking any evidence of lymphoid malignancy. Type III indicates circulating immune complexes, is associated with rheumatoid disease and chronic infections, and is usually present in concentrations of less than 1 mg/ml. All types of cryoglobulins may be responsible for symptoms that occur as a result of changes in the cryoglobulin due to exposure to cold. These symptoms include Raynaud's phenomenon, vascular purpura, bleeding tendencies, cold-induced urticaria, and distal arterial thrombosis with gangrene. Types II and III may be associated with serum sickness–like syndrome characterized by polyarthritis, vasculitis, glomerulonephritis, or neurologic symptoms.

Cryoglobulins may cause errors in many serologic tests by removing certain substances with them when they precipitate. Complement fixation and coprecipitation of immunoglobulins are examples. Redissolving the precipitate does not restore the activity, especially of complement.

For more information, see the accompanying table.

cryoglobulinemia (kri″o-glob″u-lin-e′me-ah) [*cryoglobulin* + Gr. *haima* blood + *-ia*] the presence of cryoglobulin in the blood.

Cryokwik (kri′o-kwik) trademark for a fluorinated hydrocarbon used for quick freezing of specimens to be sectioned in a cryostat.

cryopathic hemolytic syndrome (kri″o-path′ik) an autoimmune disorder characterized by enhanced autoantibody activity at body temperatures below about 31°C. See also *cold agglutinin disease* and *paroxysmal cold hemoglobinuria*.

CRYOGLOBULIN. CLASSIFICATION OF TYPES OF CRYOGLOBULINS AND ASSOCIATED DISEASES

TYPE OF CRYOGLOBULIN	IMMUNOCHEMICAL COMPOSITION	ASSOCIATED DISEASES
Type I		
Monoclonal cryoglobulin	IgM	Myeloma
	IgG	Waldenström's macroglobulinemia
	IgA	
	Bence Jones protein	Chronic lymphocytic leukemia
Type II		
Mixed cryoglobulin	IgM-IgG	Rheumatoid arthritis
	IgG-IgG	Sjögren's syndrome
	IgA-IgG	Mixed essential cryoglobulinemia
Type III		
Mixed polyclonal cryoglobulin	IgM-IgG	Systemic lupus erythematosus
	IgM-IgG-IgA	Rheumatoid arthritis, Sjögren's syndrome
		Infectious mononucleosis
		Cytomegalovirus infections
		Acute viral hepatitis
		Chronic active hepatitis
		Primary biliary cirrhosis
		Poststreptococcal glomerulonephritis
		Infective endocarditis
		Leprosy
		Kala-azar
		Tropical splenomegaly syndrome

From Fudenberg, H. H., et al.: Basic & Clinical Immunology. 3rd ed. Los Altos, CA, Lange Medical Publications, 1980, p. 362.

cryophile (kri′o-fil) [*cryo-* + Gr. *philein* love] a microorganism that grows best at low temperatures.

cryoprecipitate (kri″o-pre-sip′ĭ-tāt) a fraction of plasma extracted by freezing and slow thawing, which contains high concentrations of Factor VIII, von Willebrand factor, and fibrinogen. It is used in treating hemophilia A and sometimes in preparing patients with von Willebrand's disease for surgery.

cryopreservation (kri″o-prez″er-va′shun) the use of freezing as a method of preservation.

cryoprobe (kri′o-prōb) an instrument for applying extreme cold to tissue.

cryoprotectant (kri″o-pro-tek′tant) an agent, such as glycerol or dimethylsulfoxide, used to protect organisms, blood cells, or cell cultures from damage while in the frozen state.

cryoprotein (kri″o-pro′tēn) any blood protein that precipitates on cooling, such as cryoimmunoglobulin or cryofibrinogen.

cryoscope (kri′o-skōp) [*cryo-* + Gr. *skopein* to examine] a freezing-point depression osmometer. See *osmometer*.

cryostat (kri′o-stat) [*cryo-* + Gr. *histanai* to halt] 1. a device by which temperature can be maintained at a very low level.

2. in pathology and histology, a chamber containing a microtome for sectioning frozen tissue under

controlled conditions. See also *cold m.* under *microtome.*

cryosurgery (kri″o-sur′jer-e) the application of extreme cold to tissues for their fusion, destruction, or removal. This procedure is used frequently in the treatment of retinal detachment, when a supercooled probe is applied to the sclera to fuse it to the retina. Cryosurgery has replaced diathermy as the preferred form of therapy. Other applications include removal of premalignant or disfiguring cutaneous and mucous membrane lesions, cataract removal, central nervous system surgery, and cardiac manipulation in conduction disorders. See also *cryoablation.*

cryotherapy (kri″o-ther′ah-pe) [*cryo-* + Gr. *therapeia* treatment] the therapeutic use of cold.

crypt/o (krip′to) [Gr. *kryptos* hidden] a word element used in combining form to denote hidden or concealed, e.g., cryptorchidism.

crypt (kript) [L. *crypta,* from Gr. *kryptos* hidden] a blind pit or tube on a free surface.

anal c., one of several small depressions of the lining of the anal canal, into which the duct of an anal gland opens.

c.'s of Lieberkühn one of the simple tubular invaginations in the mucosal lining of the intestine.

c.'s of Luschka, see *Luschka's ducts.*

tonsillar c.'s, deep, narrow indentations along the medial surface of the palatine tonsils. They are lined by stratified squamous epithelium and penetrate almost the entire depth of the tonsil.

cryptic (krip′tik) [Gr. *kryptikos* hidden] concealed, hidden, larval.

cryptic enzyme in bacteriology, an enzyme that can attack added substrate in a cell lysate but not in intact cells, owing to selective action of a permeability barrier.

cryptitis (krip-ti′tis) inflammation of the mucous membrane of the anal crypts.

Cryptococcaceae (krip″to-kok-ka′se-e) a family of imperfect fungi, class Deuteromycetes, the members of which remain yeastlike throughout most of their life cycle. A number of its genera, such as *Candida, Cryptococcus, Torulopsis,* and *Pityrosporum,* are medically important because of their pathogenicity for humans. However, some genera were removed from this family after the discovery of their sexual stages.

cryptococcal meningitis (krip″to-kok′al) infection of the meninges by organisms of the genus *Cryptococcus;* see *cryptococcosis.*

cryptococcosis (krip″to-kok-o′sis) [*Cryptococcus* + *-osis* inflammation] a subacute or chronic fungal disease caused by the pathogenic, yeastlike fungus *Cryptococcus neoformans.* Cryptococcosis may occur in pulmonary, systemic, or meningitic forms and usually affects debilitated patients. The etiologic agent, *C. neoformans,* is unique for its production of a large mucinous capsule in both tissue and culture; it may be present in very large numbers in pigeon droppings, since it has a predilection for the abundant creatine as a source of nitrogen. Also called *European blastomycosis* and *torulosis.*

Clinical Disease. There are five clinical variations of cryptococcosis—pulmonary, central nervous system, cutaneous, osseous, and disseminated. The portal of entry of the organism is usually the lungs; thus, it begins as a pulmonary disease. Pulmonary cryptococcosis is often asymptomatic; however, cough, low-grade fever, and pleuritic pain may be present. At this stage of infection, the yeast can be recovered from sputum and urine. The pulmonary lesions do not calcify upon healing, and it is probable that most lesions heal without forming "cryptococcoma" and without leaving other residual evidence of past cryptococcosis.

Cryptococcosis of the CNS is the most frequently recognized form of the disease. The lack of phagocytic cells in the spinal fluid, as well as the availability of nitrogen and other nutritional factors, seems to favor the development of chronic meningitis. Symptoms include headache, fever, and neck tenderness. Localized granulomas of the brain may also be present and cause severe symptoms such as epileptic seizures. CNS cryptococcosis may persist for months or even years.

Cutaneous cryptococcosis is characterized by papular or acneiform pustules of the skin. This form is seen more often in Europe than in the United States. It is thought to be a symptom of disseminated disease and not the result of a primary infection. Osseous cryptococcosis is relatively rare and is usually associated with other diseases of the bone. The yeasts cause multiple, disseminated, destructive lesions in bone, which result in swelling and pain. Joints are not usually infected.

In disseminated cryptococcosis, any organ of the body may be involved by granulomatous lesions, but especially the heart, testes, prostate, and eyes. When cryptococcosis spreads to the gastrointestinal tract, the disease mimics tuberculosis.

Diagnosis. On direct examination, *C. neoformans* can be recognized by its large characteristic capsule visible in India ink preparations. A cell wall, vacuoles, and budding forms, as well as a capsule, should be visible, enabling differentiation from white blood cells; see the accompanying illustration. With the Gridley fungal stain or the PAS stain, the diagnosis of cryptococcosis on histologic examination can usually be made, but further identification should be confirmed by use of a mucicarmine stain. *C. neoformans* grows well on Sabouraud's dextrose agar at 37°C, and produces urease. In addition, *C. neoformans* is unique among *Cryptococcus* species, and indeed among yeasts generally, in producing brown colonies on "birdseed agar," which is Littman oxgall agar containing an extract of seeds from the plant *Guizotia abyssinia* (common in birdseed mixtures). The brown-to-black color is due to the formation of melanin pigment in the cell wall, a reaction catalyzed by phenol oxidase.

Serologically, a latex agglutination test is used to detect cryptococcal antigen. Hyperimmune rabbit antiserum coated onto a suspension of latex beads is mixed with dilutions of serum or spinal fluid. A 1:8 antigen dilution with agglutination is indicative of infection. False-negative reactions are possible with the latex agglutination test. With pulmonary cryptococcosis, antigens are not usually present in spinal fluid or serum. In disseminated cryptococcosis, cryptococcal antigen is found in serum and urine. With meningitic cryptococcosis, antigen is present in the cerebrospinal fluid. There is also an immunofluorescent technique for the identification of *C. neoformans* in which antigen is fixed to a slide and the patient's serum or spinal fluid is added. This is followed by addition of fluorescein-labeled rabbit antihuman globulin. Fluorescence indicates the presence of antigen.

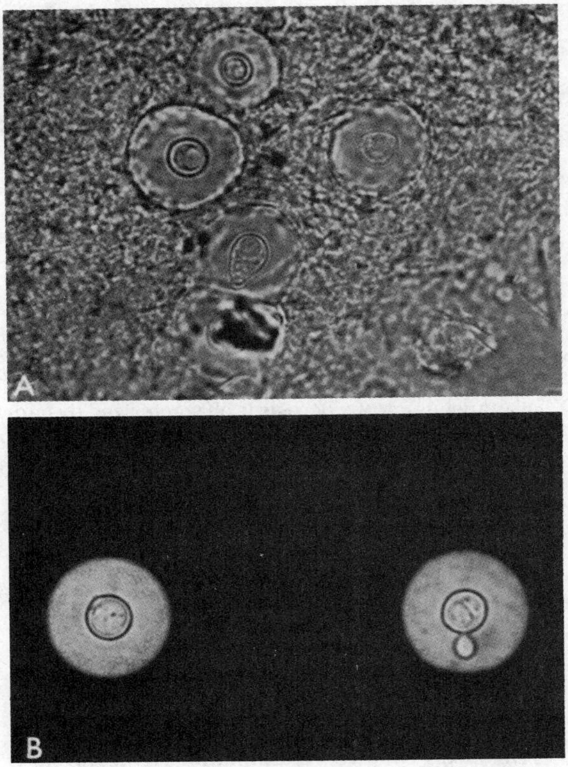

Cryptococcosis. The *Cryptococcus neoformans* organism: *A,* Pus containing the round, thick-walled, budding fungus surrounded by a capsule; ×850. *B,* India ink preparation of spinal fluid showing the budding fungus surrounded by a capsule; ×820. (From Conant, N. F., et al.: Manual of Clinical Mycology. 3rd ed. Philadelphia, W. B. Saunders Co., 1971.)

There are four serotypes of *C. neoformans,* designated A, B, C, and D. The serotype most commonly isolated from individuals in the United States is B. The serotypes most frequently found in soil are A and D. These can be distinguished by their ability to produce malic acid dehydrogenase. With the use of creatinine dextrose agar with blue dye, serotypes B and C produce ammonia and malic acid dehydrogenase, changing the indicator dye.

Cryptococcus (krip″to-kok′us) [*crypto-* + Gr. *kokkos* berry] a genus of round, yeastlike fungi of the family Cryptococcaceae, 3.5–7.0 μm in diameter, that are characterized by the production of a large capsule (1–30 μm) and the lack of a pseudomycelium. There are 8 species of *Cryptococcus: C. albidus albidus, C. albidus diffluens, C. gastricus, C. laurentii, C. luteolus, C. neoformans, C. terreus,* and *C. uniguttalatus.*

C. neoformans, a species that causes cryptococcosis in humans. It is identified by the formation of brown or black colonies on bird seed agar, or media containing dihydroxyphenylalanine or related substrates. The color reaction has been shown to be catalyzed by a phenol oxidase and result in melanin formation. Other important tests include assimilation of inositol, hydrolysis of urea, growth at 37°C, capsule formation, and no assimilation of malic acid for serotypes B and C. The perfect state of the serotypes A and D of *C. neoformans* is *Filobasidiella neoformans,* and the perfect state of serotypes B and C is *F. bacillispora.* See also *cryptococcosis.*

cryptomenorrhea (krip″to-men″o-re′ah) [*crypto-* + Gr. *mens* month + *rhein* to flow] the occurrence of menstrual symptoms without external bleeding, as in females with an imperforate hymen.

cryptophthalmos (krip″tof-thal′mos) [*crypto-* + Gr. *ophthalmos* eye] a rare congenital malformation that results from the failure of the eyelids to develop: the forehead skin continues over the eyes. The eyes are defective and smaller than normal.

cryptorchidism (krip-tor′kĭ-dizm) [*crypto-* + Gr. *orchis* testis + *-ism*] a congenital anomaly occurring in males that results in the incomplete descent of one or both testes. The undescended testis may be located in the abdominal cavity or anywhere along the path of descent of the testes. About 4 percent of full-term infants have a cryptorchid testis; usually, the testis has completely descended into the scrotum by age 1 yr. If it remains in the abdominal cavity, however, surgical correction should be performed, as delay beyond age 5 yr may inhibit subsequent spermatogenesis. An increased incidence of testicular neoplasms has been reported in males with uncorrected cryptorchid testes.

Cryptostroma (krip″to-stro′mah) [*crypto-* + Gr. *strōma* bed] a genus of fungi, one member of which, *C. corticale,* has been implicated in coniosporosis; see *coniosporosis.*

cryptostromosis (krip″to-stro-mo′sis) [*Cryptostroma* + *-osis* condition] see *coniosporosis.*

cryptoxanthin (krip″to-zan′thin) [*crypto-* + Gr. *xanthos* yellow] hydroxy-β-carotene, β-caroten-3-ol, a yellow carotenoid pigment that can be converted into vitamin A in the body; M.W. 552.85. It contains only one β-ionone ring and thus forms only one molecule of retinol after oxidative scission.

cryptozoite (krip″to-zo′īt) [*crypto-* + Gr. *zōon* animal] the first form of malarial plasmodia in the asexual exoerythrocytic cycle, initiated by the sporozoite in hepatic cells of the vertebrate host. The mature cryptozoic schizont divides and releases cryptozoic merozoites that may reinvade hepatic cells and reproduce to form a second generation of cryptozoites. See also *malaria.*

crystal (kris′tal) [Gr. *krystallos* ice] a solid in which the atoms or molecules are arranged in a regular repeating pattern. The repeating units, called unit cells, are identical parallelopipeds stacked in a space-filling array; the vertices of the unit cells are referred to as the crystal lattice or space lattice. The lattice points are occupied by identical ions, atoms, or molecules. In body-centered crystal structures there is another ion, atom, or molecule at the center of each unit cell (which may be different from the ones at the lattice points). In face-centered structures there is an atom or molecule at the center of each face of the unit cell.

All true solids are crystalline. Amorphous solids, such as glasses, resins, and polymers, are actually high-viscosity fluids that undergo very slow plastic flow.

For more information, see the specific crystal.

crystal cell a red blood cell that contains tetragonal crystals formed by aggregation of hemoglobins. The anomaly is found in up to 10 percent of circulating cells in splenectomized individuals with homozygous hemoglobin C disease.

crystal deposition disease a term used to embrace those diseases characterized by an inflammatory reaction to tissue deposits of crystals produced endogenously in primary or secondary metabolic abnormalities. They include gout and other metabolic disorders in which there is an accumulation of monosodium urate, as well as pseudogout and chondrocalcinosis, in which there is accumulation of calcium pyrophosphate dihydrate.

crystalline (kris′tah-lin) composed of crystals; having the structure of a crystal; resembling a crystal in shape, form, or clearness.

crystallization (kris″tah-lĭ-za′shun) the formation of crystals; conversion to a crystalline form.

crystallography (kris″tah-log′rah-fe) [*crystal* + Gr. *graphein* to write] 1. the branch of physics that deals with crystal structure.

2. the determination of the structure of a crystal; see *x-ray crystallography.*

crystalloid (kris′tah-loid) [*crystal* + Gr. *eidos* shape, form] 1. resembling a crystal.

2. a noncolloidal substance; a substance that, in solution, passes readily through animal membranes, lowers the freezing point of the solvent containing it, and is generally capable of being crystallized.

crystalluria (kris″tah-lu′re-ah) [*crystal* + Gr. *ouron* urine + *-ia*] the excretion of crystals in the urine.

crystal of Lubarsch (loo′barsh) [Otto *Lubarsch,* German pathologist, 1860–1933] an inclusion of closely packed dense filaments arranged in parallel arrays in the cytoplasm of a spermatogonium.

crystals in urine sediment crystals observed in the microscopic examination of urine sediment. Most crystals formed in a specimen at room temperature redissolve at 37°C. Of those remaining undissolved, only a few types are clinically significant.

Acid urine normally contains some crystals of urates, uric acid, and calcium oxalate. Alkaline urine normally contains some crystals of phosphates, ammonium biurate, and calcium carbonate. Numerous uric acid crystals suggest gout, but are also observed during cancer chemotherapy with agents that increase nucleoprotein turnover. Numerous oxalate crystals may indicate severe chronic renal disease or the presence of kidney stones. Cystine crystals suggest possible metabolic defects such as cystinosis or cystinuria. Tyrosine or leucine crystals are observed in acute liver failure. The crystals of some drugs may be noted with high-dosage therapy or with overdosage, and include the less soluble sulfonamides, ampicillin, mercaptopurine, and primidone. Diatrizoate crystals are commonly observed after urography.

crystals of Reinke cytoplasmic crystals found in the cytoplasm of the interstitial (Leydig) cells of the testes and ovarian hilus cells. They have variable shapes, are 2–3 μm thick and up to 20 μm in length, and are composed of macromolecules approximately 5 nm in diameter. The crystals are isotropic in polarized light.

crystal violet a basic dye, *N*-hexamethylpararosaniline; C.I. 42555. See also *triphenylmethane dyes.* Cf. *gentian violet* and *methyl violet.*

CS abbrev. See *chorionic somatomammotropin.*

Cs symbol for the chemical element *cesium.*

C&S abbrev. for culture and sensitivity.

CSA abbrev. See *colony-stimulating activity, compressed spectral assay.*

CSF abbrev. See *cerebrospinal fluid, colony-stimulating factor.*

Cst abbrev. See *static c.* under *compliance.*

cSt abbrev. See *centistoke.*

CT abbrev. See *computed tomography.*

CTA abbrev. See *chromotropic acid.*

CTAT abbrev. for computerized transaxial tomography, a former name for computed tomography.

***ct*CO_2** abbrev. for concentration of total carbon dioxide. See *carbon dioxide concentration.*

Ctenocephalides (te″no-sĕ-fal′ĭ-dēz) [N.L., from Gr. *kteis, ktenos* comb + *kephalē* head] a genus of fleas in the arthropod family Pulicidae, which commonly feed on carnivores (most importantly on cats, dogs, and humans), causing dermal irritation. The species *C. canis* and *C. felis,* the dog and cat fleas, respectively, may serve as intermediate hosts for the dog tapeworms *Dipylidium caninum* and *Dipetalonema reconditum* and for other tapeworms transmitted to mammalian hosts when the flea is ingested. *C. canis* may also be a mechanical vector of the yellow fever virus. See also the illustration under *flea.*

C-terminal see *carboxyl t.* under *terminal.*

CT number the unit of attenuation used for CT scans. Water has the CT number zero; air, −1000; and compact bone, +1000. Some systems use these values divided by two. Also called *Hounsfield unit.*

CTP abbrev. See *cytidine triphosphate.*

CTT abbrev. for computed transaxial tomography, a former name for *computed tomography.*

CTX abbrev. for *Cytoxan.* See *cyclophosphamide.*

Cu [L. *cuprum*] symbol for the chemical element *copper.*

cubic (ku′bik) 1. shaped like a cube.

2. designating the volume of a cube having edges of a stated unit of length; e.g., a cubic meter (m^3) is the volume of a cube with 1-m edges.

cubital (ku′bĭ-tal) pertaining to the elbow or the forearm.

cubital fossa see *antecubital space.*

cubital vein a vein of the cubital region.

median c. v., a communication between the cephalic and basilic veins that angles across the front of the elbow. It is frequently accessible for venipuncture.

cuboid (ku′boid) [Gr. *kyboeidēs*] 1. resembling a cube.

2. the cuboid bone.

cuboidal (ku-boi′dal) resembling a cube.

cuffing (kuf′ing) the formation of a cufflike surrounding border, as of leukocytes about a blood vessel, observed in certain infections.

culd/o (kul′do) [Fr. *cul-de-sac*] a word element used in combining form to denote a cul-de-sac (a blind pouch or cecum, or a cavity closed at one end), e.g., culdoscopy.

cul-de-sac (kul′dĕ-sahk) [Fr. "bottom of the sack"] 1. a blind pouch; a saclike cavity or tube open at only one end.

2. the rectouterine pouch (also called pouch of Douglas).

culdocentesis (kul″do-sen-te′sis) [*culdo-* + Gr. *kentēsis* puncture] a procedure involving aspiration of fluid from the rectouterine pouch by puncture of the vaginal wall. The value of this procedure for early detection of ovarian carcinoma is questionable.

culdoscope (kul′do-skōp) [*culdo-* + Gr. *skopein* to examine] an endoscope used in culdoscopy.

culdoscopy (kul-dos′ko-pe) direct visual examination of the female viscera through an endoscope introduced into the pelvic cavity through the posterior vaginal fornix.

Culex (ku′leks) [L. "gnat"] a genus of mosquitos in the family Culicidae characterized by a humpbacked, usually brown, body. Females have short palpi and a blunt-tipped abdomen; they deposit their eggs in masses on the surface of water. Some species are vectors of *Wuchereria bancrofti*, a filarial nematode parasite. Other members transmit viral encephalitis, including the Japanese, western and eastern equine, and St. Louis varieties.

Culicidae (ku-lis′ĭ-de) a family of mosquitos characterized by long wings with scales along the wing veins and posterior margin and an elongated, forward-thrusting probiscus, and having both aquatic larval and pupal forms. Subfamilies of medical importance include Anophelinae (containing the genus *Anopheles*) and Culicinae (containing the genera *Culex* and *Aedes*), which are vectors of filariasis and viral disease. Human malaria, however, is transmitted only by the genus *Anopheles.*

Culicoides (ku-lĭ-koi′dēz) a genus of biting flies of the family Ceratopogonidae. *C. austeni* and *C. grahami* are intermediate hosts of the parasitic roundworm *Dipetalonema perstans*; *C. fucens* and possibly other species are intermediate hosts of *Mansonella ozzardi.*

Cullen's sign (kul′enz) [Thomas Stephen *Cullen*, Baltimore surgeon, 1868–1953] a bluish discoloration around the umbilicus sometimes occurring with intraperitoneal hemorrhage, especially following rupture of the uterine tube in ectopic pregnancy. A similar discoloration can be seen in acute hemorrhagic pancreatitis.

cultivation (kul″tĭ-va′shun) [L. *cultivatio*] the propagation of living organisms, especially of cells in artificial media.

culture (kul′tūr) [L. *cultura*] 1. a growth of isolated microorganisms or of living tissue cells in a special laboratory medium capable of supporting growth.

2. the propagation of microorganisms or other living cells.

3. to induce the propagation of microorganisms or living tissue cells in media conducive to their growth. See also *clinical bacteriologic specimens* and *culture media.*

attenuated c., a culture of pathogenic microorganisms of weakened virulence. See also *attenuation.*

bacterial c., a culture of bacterial cells.

cell c., see *cell culture.*

chorioallantoic c., a culture grown on the chorioallantois of the developing chick.

continuous flow c., the cultivation of bacteria in a continuous flow of fresh medium to maintain bacterial growth in an actively multiplying or logarithmic phase. The instrument in which a continuous flow culture is grown is called a chemostat. By precisely controlling the flow of fresh medium and by stirring, the cell density remains constant. As the mass of cells is constant, culture growth is linear rather than exponential.

direct c., see *primary c.*

hanging-block c., a culture grown on a block of agar medium fastened to a coverglass, which is then inverted over a hollowed-out slide.

hanging-drop c., a culture in which cells are inoculated into a drop of fluid attached to a coverglass, which is then inverted over a hollowed-out slide. This technique is sometimes used for examining fungi in the natural state.

mixed c., a culture that contains more than one species or strain of organism.

needle c., see *stab c.*

plate c., a culture grown on a solid medium, usually agar or gelatin, in a Petri dish.

primary c., a culture made directly from a natural source, such as a clinical specimen, for microbiologic examination. Also called *direct c.*

pure c., a culture of a single species, without any contaminants.

radioisotopic c., the use of a liquid culture medium containing isotopically labeled carbohydrate, e.g., ^{14}C-glucose, to detect the growth of microorganisms. Metabolism of this or similar substrates releases $^{14}CO_2$, which can be measured by an automated system such as Bactec. This method has been applied widely in clinical microbiology for culturing blood specimens.

The major theoretical advantage is that it offers earlier detection of growth than do conventional methods. This procedure does not identify the organism that has grown; subsequent identification is made in the usual manner.

secondary c., a culture derived or subcultured from growth in a primary culture.

shake c., a culture made by inoculating melted (45°C) agar medium in a tube. Incubation of the resolidified culture allows the development of separated colonies. This method is applicable to obligate anaerobes.

slant c., a culture made on a slanting surface of a solidified medium in a tube, the latter being tilted to provide a greater surface area for growth. Also called *slope c.*

slope c., see *slant c.*

stab c., a culture in which a tube of solid medium is inoculated by means of a needle thrust into it. Also called *needle c.*

stock c., a culture of a microorganism kept as a reference strain by storage at a low temperature. Subcultures are made from it as needed.

streak c., a culture in which the surface of a solid medium is inoculated by drawing across it, in a zigzag fashion, a wire inoculating loop carrying the inoculum.

synchronized c.'s, multiple cultures in the same phase of the cell growth cycle. Methods used to obtain a synchronized culture include: delaying the initiation of DNA synthesis, depriving an auxotroph of a required nutrient, alternating the culture for short periods at 37° and 25°C, and/or mechanically separating the cells according to size by filtration.

tissue c., see *tissue culture.*

type c., a culture of any species of microorganism, usually maintained in a central collection of type or standard cultures.

culture media the fluid, solid, or semisolid formulations devised for the cultivation of microorganisms and tissue cells. Microbial culturing may be performed for many purposes other than the isolation and identification of organisms; it is used, for example, in sterility testing, food and water analyses, environmental control, production of biologicals (such as antibiotics and vaccines), vitamin and drug assays, and the detection of antimicrobial action in sera, chemicals, and other substances. There are many different media formulations available to the clinical laboratory, which can be divided into three types: (1) general-purpose formulations, which have a rich composition, such as trypticase soy, and are used for growing many varieties of pathogens (the standard blood agar used for primary isolation contains such a base, plus blood to provide further enrichment and also to detect hemolysis); (2) differential-selective media, which are each designed to promote the growth of one or a few pathogenic species and at the same time retard development of unwanted varieties, e.g., bismuth sulfite agar for *Salmonella;* and (3) special-purpose media, which often contain one test substrate for determining the production of one enzyme system, e.g., urea medium for the urease test.

Microorganisms require sources of nitrogen, carbon, oxygen, and many other elements. Autotrophs can utilize free nitrogen or inorganic compounds such as ammonia or nitrate; thus, satisfactory media for them are chemically simple. Conversely, heterotrophic organisms, which include the human pathogens, need more complex nitrogen sources. Some obtain nitrogen from protein, whereas others need a more available, intermediate form of digested protein, such as peptones.

Oxygen is supplied by air at the surface of media for cells that can utilize free oxygen. For organisms that must grow without free oxygen, media are kept in an atmosphere of O_2-free hydrogen, nitrogen, or other gases. These anaerobic organisms obtain oxygen from the constituents of the media. Carbon is supplied by incorporated carbohydrates or nitrogenous material that contains carbohydrates, or even from carbon dioxide, depending on the nature of the cells.

NATURE AND COMPOSITION. Historically, culture media were made with natural ingredients e.g., milk, eggs, meat, and potatoes, or infusions thereof. Most modern formulations, however, contain more defined nitrogenous components, such as the peptones described in the *U.S. Pharmacopeia,* and relatively pure salts and carbohydrates. The trend is toward the use of better defined and even entirely synthetic media.

Peptones are water-soluble protein hydrolysates derived from proteinaceous materials by hydrolysis or digestion with acid, alkali, or enzymes. Acids and alkalis tend to destroy the vitamin content, as well as some amino acids, and to increase the salt content, whereas enzymatic methods preserve the vitamin and amino acid content. For example, pure casein contains no carbohydrate and has a high tryptophan content, so a tryptic casein peptone can be used in media for fermentation and indole testing. A gelatin enzymatic digest should not contain fermentable carbohydrate or tryptophan because gelatin contains neither component. By contrast, peptones made from milk or meat should contain carbohydrates. The *U.S. Pharmacopeia* requires that media made with defined peptones be used in sterility testing and for determining the microbial attributes of pharmaceutical articles from raw materials to finished forms. Most microbiologic yeast extracts are really peptones; after growth of the yeast has occurred, the cells are digested by their own autolytic enzymes.

Infusions and extracts of meat and other tissues are undefined, water-soluble materials derived without added enzymes, usually after heat coagulation. The methods used and the time involved are often such as to permit uncontrolled enzymatic action by microbial contaminants. Consequently, these products are likely to vary from lot to lot in composition and nutritional quality.

Solidifying agents for culture media include gelatin and agar. Gelatin is now rarely used because of its low melting temperature. Most microbiologic grade agar is derived from red seaweeds, the *Rhodophyceae;* it must melt at 80°C and gel at no higher than 30°. Agarose is a polysaccharide dissociation product from agar and is incorporated into media for immunodiffusion tests; certain polyacrylic gels have also been used as solidifying agents.

Colorimetric indicators may be incorporated to show pH and E_h (redox potential) changes in media produced by microbial growth. The pH indicators in common use today are phenol red, bromcresol purple, and neutral red; these have replaced the more crude litmus and Andrade indicator. Phenol red probably has the most sensitive range for most pathogens. Methylene blue and resazurin are commonly used E_h indicators.

Selective agents are put in media to promote growth of some organisms while inhibiting growth of others in order to detect specific pathogens in a mixed flora and to aid identification. Dyes were probably employed first for this purpose, e.g., brilliant green inhibits gram-positive organisms and permits gram-negative organisms to grow. Sodium chloride in high concentrations inhibits most bacteria but is well tolerated by staphylococci. Some other salts in common use include sodium azide, citrates, and selenites. Crude bile salts, or purified bile salts such as sodium deoxycholate, are also good selective substances. Acid or alkali may be added to facilitate selective isolation; a pH of 8.0 is helpful for isolation of *Vibrio cholerae,* and a pH of 5.6 for isolating some fungi.

Antimicrobial agents are added to culture media for the selective isolation of microbial species or to inhibit bacterial contaminants in tissue cultures. Penicillin and streptomycin are effective, but solutions must be prepared aseptically and they deteriorate rapidly. Relatively stable agents such as chloramphenicol, nalidixic acid, sulfonamides, and neomycin are more practical because they can be added before sterilization.

Reducing agents such as cysteine and sodium thioglycolate are often incorporated to promote anaerobiosis, and the addition of a small amount (0.5–1.0 g) of agar per liter of liquid medium limits convection currents.

Enrichment media, with or without selective

agents, are designed to promote growth of pathogens when very few may be present. A good general enrichment medium for many kinds of organisms is thioglycolate medium without indicator. Enrichment media should not be confused with transport media, which "hold" the microbial flora of a specimen but do not encourage growth.

Maintenance media are those that support a satisfactory amount of growth and also provide long viability. Prolonged viability is aided by omission of carbohydrate or by adding calcium carbonate to neutralize acid as it is formed.

Assay media for determining the vitamin or amino acid content of serum or other materials generally consist of a water solution of many salts, vitamins, and amino acids, with omission of at least one necessary vitamin or amino acid. Great care must be taken in preparation because of chemical contamination from air, containers, and so forth.

Tissue and organ culture media are even more complex. Many contain mixtures of salts, vitamins, and amino acids, plus serum or plasma and antibiotics.

Protozoa and other small animals can be grown on media similar to those for bacteria. Some organisms of clinical importance include *Entamoeba histolytica, Trypanosoma cruzi, Trichomonas,* flukes, and even some stages of malaria parasites.

SELECTION. Appropriate choice of media depends on the number and kinds of specimens to be handled and the facilities available for preparation, testing, and storage. Some guidelines for selection of media from the hundreds available are as follows:

1. If the laboratory has limited facilities and personnel, use prepared commercial media.
2. Select defined media, rather than those with unidentified components.
3. Choose media with broad growth potential. The laboratory using the most kinds of media may not be the best.
4. Before adopting a new medium, compare it first with the one in use as a control.
5. When a selective medium is used for primary isolation, also include a nonselective one. When two selective media are employed, select ones with different levels of inhibition, e.g., the highly selective brilliant green agar with the less inhibitory XLD agar.

PREPARATION AND QUALITY CONTROL. Media can be made from the separate ingredients or from the dehydrated commercial powders that are mixtures of dry ingredients to which water, blood, and other ingredients are added. The water employed should be tested frequently, both chemically and bacteriologically, to determine if it is of suitable "USP Purified" quality. For preparing media from dry bases, the manufacturer's directions should be followed exactly.

Sterilization is accomplished usually by autoclaving and occasionally by filtration. Most media are sterilized at 121°C for 15 min, but more heat-sensitive ones should be autoclaved at 116°–118°C. Excessive heating is to be avoided, because it causes discoloration, fall of pH, and other damage. The final pH should be ± 0.2 of the desired figure when meter-tested at room temperature. Filtration of ingredient solutions and media may be with Seitz, membrane, or other filters. Filters and collection equipment must, of course, be sterile and handled aseptically.

Many media commonly used in clinically laboratories contain blood or other nonfilterable, heat-sensitive materials. These should be obtained aseptically from normal animals on antibiotic-free diets. Defibrinated sheep and rabbit blood are probably the most useful. Horse blood is popular, but group D streptococci may be mistaken for group A cocci when grown on horse blood plates. Human bank blood is convenient but contains citrate, glucose, and sometimes inhibitory drugs and antibodies.

Each lot of media in plates, tubes, or other containers should be tested for sterility and performance while the bulk of the lot is stored in the refrigerator in sealed containers. Representative samples should be incubated at 25°–32°C and examined after 48 hr. Performance tests are carried out at the same time. Each clinical laboratory should maintain a set of stock cultures that are stable and typical. For general-purpose media, qualitative tests are made with several different organisms suspended in broth. After incubation, colonies should be well separated, and their distribution should be similar to that on the control media.

Selective media can be tested both with cultures that grow well and with cultures that should be partially or completely inhibited. It is advisable to include also a nonselective medium as a second control. Biochemical test media for identification purposes are both positive and negative controls.

Additional quality control measures that affect culture media include checking of incubator temperatures, autoclaves, and biologic controls, pH meters and buffers, balances, and other equipment. Stored ingredients and dry bases should be checked regularly and discarded if outdated or visibly deteriorated, deterioration generally being due to access of moisture or to heat exposure. Most such materials can be stored satisfactorily at temperatures up to 30°C for months.

HARRIETTE D. VERA, PH.D.

nonpermissive c. m., media conditions that do not support the expression of differentiated properties by cultured cells. Cf. *permissive c. m.*

permissive c. m., media conditions that support the expression of differentiated properties by cultured cells. Such media usually contain a poorly defined additive, such as serum or embryo extract. Cf. *nonpermissive c. m.*

cumulative distribution (ku'mu-la"tiv) see *distribution function.*

cumulus (ku'mu-lus) [L.] a little mound.

cumulus oophorous (ku'mu-lus o-of'or-us) [L.] a mound of follicular cells that surrounds an ovum and is attached to one pole of the ovarian follicle.

cuneate (ku'ne-āt) [L. *cuneus* wedge] shaped like a wedge.

cuneiform (ku-ne'ĭ-form) [L. *cuneus* wedge + *forma* form] shaped like a wedge. One of the three tarsal bones is so named.

Cunninghamella (kun"ing-hah-mel'ah) a genus of fungi that can cause zygomycosis. This fungus has been isolated from disseminated infections as well as pulmonary infections in individuals with other debilitating diseases (e.g., leukemia or lymphoma). Morphologically, *Cunninghamella* forms a light gray colony that consists of vesicles and conidia borne on the surface of inflated conidiophores. The most common medically important species is *C. bertholletiae,* and not *C. elegans* as previously believed.

cupric (koo′prik) denoting copper in the +2 oxidation state or the Cu^{2+} cation.

cuprous (koo′prus) denoting copper in the +1 oxidation state or the Cu^{+} cation.

curare (ku-rah′re) [Carib *kurari*] one of a variety of highly toxic extracts from several botanical sources, including *Strychnos* and *Chondrodendron tomentosum*; composed of about 40 alkaloids, the most important of which is *d*-tubocurarine. Its effect of paralyzing skeletal musculature and producing apnea and cardiovascular collapse when absorbed through denuded skin or injected made it a widely used arrow poison among South American Indians. Tubocurarine is used as a muscle relaxant as an adjunct to anesthesia.

curariform (ku-rar′ĭ-form) having the skeletal muscle-relaxing action of curare; producing nondepolarizing neuromuscular block. See also *metocurine iodide, pancuronium bromide,* and *tubocurarine chloride.*

curarization (ku″rar-ĭ-za′shun) the administration of curare (usually tubocurarine) to induce muscle relaxation by its blocking activity at the myoneural junction.

cure (kūr) [L. *cura* care, from *curare* to take care of] 1. the course of treatment of any disease.
2. the successful treatment of a disease or wound.
3. a system of treating diseases.
4. a medicine effective in treating a disease.

curet (ku-ret′) [Fr. *curette* scraper] 1. an instrument for removing material from the uterine cavity.
2. to remove a growth or other material from a cavity or other surface with a spoon-shaped instrument.

curettage (ku″rĕ-tahzh′) [Fr.] the removal of a diseased surface with a curet or similar instrument.

endometrial c., the removal of endometrial tissue by scraping the surface of the uterine cavity, a procedure usually employed for the purpose of obtaining material for pathologic examination. It provides a more generous specimen than can be obtained by aspiration or jet washing.

curette (ku-ret′) [Fr.] see *curet.*

curie (Ci) (ku′re) [Marie Sklodowska *Curie,* Polish chemist in Paris, 1867–1934, the discoverer of radium, and Pierre *Curie,* French chemist, 1859–1906] a unit of radioactivity defined as that quantity of a radionuclide that undergoes 3.7×10^{10} disintegrations/sec (originally the radioactivity of 1 g of radium).

curie-hour (Ci-hr) [Marie and Pierre *Curie*] a unit of cumulated activity equal to the presence of 1 curie of radioactivity for 1 hr, i.e., 1.332×10^{14} disintegrations.

curium (Cm) (ku′re-um) [Marie and Pierre *Curie*] a silvery-white, metallic radioactive element; atomic number 96; most stable isotope, Cu-247 (half-life, 1.6×10^{7} million yr); a 5f transition element (actinide element); oxidization states +3 (the most common), +4.

Curling's ulcer (kur′lingz) [Thomas Blizard *Curling,* English physician, 1811–1888] an acute stress ulcer of the fundus and body of the stomach, first described in patients with extensive burn injuries.

current (kur′ent) [L. *currens* running] 1. any flow or rate of flow.
2. in physics, the rate of flow of a conserved quantity, the amount per unit time that flows across a surface or out of a region.
3. electric current, the electric charge per unit time flowing past a point in an electric circuit. The International System (SI) unit of current is the ampere (A), a flow of 1 coulomb of charge per second. See also *Ohm's law.*

current gain the ratio of the output current to the input current of an amplifier or amplifier stage.

current regulator an electronic circuit or other component that maintains a constant output current from a power source despite variations in the load.

Curschmann's spiral (koorsh′manz) [Heinrich *Curschmann,* physician in Leipzig, 1846–1910] coiled, basophilic plugs of mucus, sometimes found in the bronchi and sputum in individuals with bronchial asthma.

cursor (kur′ser) a mark on a display screen that indicates a position. The cursor is moved around on the display under control of the operator to mark points or regions of the display for computer processing.

curvature (kur′vah-tūr) [L. *curvatura*] deviation from a rectilinear direction.

greater c. of stomach, the longer of the two margins of the stomach, formed where the anterior and posterior surfaces meet. It extends from the esophageal opening to the pyloric sphincter and forms the upper left and lower borders of the stomach. The gastroepiploic vessels course along its length.

lesser c. of stomach, the shorter of the two margins of the stomach, formed where the anterior and posterior surfaces meet. It extends from the esophageal opening to the pyloric sphincter and forms the upper right border of the stomach. The left and right gastric arteries and their accompanying veins course along its length.

spinal c., deviation of the vertebral column from its normal direction or position; see *kyphosis, lordosis,* and *scoliosis.*

curve (kurv) [L. *curvum*] a smooth, continuous deviation from a straight line or plane surface. For more information, see the specific curve.

curve fitting the process of choosing a function or graph that describes some experimental data. Often a straight line is fitted by the least-square method. The fitted curve will describe the actual process, eliminating the experimental error, if the assumed function type (e.g., line, parabola, exponential) is the correct one. When used to calibrate a procedure, a series of specimens of known value are used to determine the response of the analytical process. If the resulting curve has an irregular function, the value of unknown specimens may be calculated graphically rather than by a mathematical function. See also *calibration curve.*

Curvularia (kur″vu-la′re-ah) a genus of soil saprophytes that are dark and typically curved, with conidia. They are brown pigmented in culture and appear in a mycelial form in tissue. This fungus is rarely a cause of human disease; however, rare cases of keratitis, mycetomas, endocarditis, allergies, and lung infections have been reported.

Cushing's disease (koosh′ingz) [Harvey Williams

Cushing, U.S. neurosurgeon, 1869–1939] Cushing's syndrome caused by the overproduction of adrenocorticotropic hormone (ACTH) by the pituitary, which results in increased concentrations of cortisol and other corticosteroids in plasma. Cushing's disease results most commonly from a pituitary basophil or chromophobe adenoma. See also *Cushing's syndrome.*

cushingoid (koosh′ing-oid) [Harvey W. *Cushing*] resembling Cushing's syndrome; said of signs and symptoms.

Cushing's syndrome [Harvey W. *Cushing*] abnormal overproduction of the major adrenal cortex glucocorticoid (cortisol) or related corticosteroids, resulting in a constellation of clinical signs and symptoms. There are several primary, well-established causes of excess production of adrenocorticosteroids, e.g., adrenocortical neoplasms (carcinomas or adenomas), which secrete cortisol autonomously (ACTH-independent); nonpituitary neoplasms, which secrete ACTH (ectopic ACTH production); and pituitary-hypothalamic dysfunction, which leads to the excess pituitary secretion of ACTH (Cushing's disease). Regardless of the cause, excess cortisol production leads to a variety of symptoms, including a "moon face," truncal obesity with "buffalo hump," muscle wasting and weakness, thin skin with striae, hypertension, glucose intolerance with glycosuria, osteoporosis, and emotional disorders. Linear bone growth may cease in affected children, and females may experience menstrual irregularities.

Laboratory tests reveal increases in plasma cortisol above the normal morning concentrations of 10–25 μg/100 ml, and a loss of diurnal decline in plasma cortisol concentrations. This results in an above-average 24-hr cortisol concentration. Elevations are also observed in the normal 24-hr concentrations of 17-hydroxycorticosteroids to levels above 10 mg/24 hr, and in 24-hr concentrations of free urinary cortisol to levels above 100 μg/24 hr. Eosinophil counts are reduced ($<50/\mu l$ of blood) and lymphocytes are under 20 percent. X-rays reveal osteoporosis and often kidney stones. Intravenous urograms, retroperitoneal pneumograms, polytomography, adrenal angiography, or ^{131}I-19-iodocholesterol scanning may help demonstrate an adrenal neoplasm or hyperplasia. Electrocardiographic tests often reveal evidence of hypertension, hypokalemia, and short P-R intervals. A variety of special tests may help to pinpoint the exact cause of Cushing's syndrome, e.g., radioimmunoassay of plasma concentrations of ACTH and cortisol, dexamethasone suppression tests, ACTH stimulation tests, and metyrapone stimulation tests.

Also called *adrenal cortical hyperplasia* and *hypercortisolism.* See also *hyperadrenalism, hyperadrenocorticism,* and *hypercorticism.*

-cusis (ku′sis) [Gr. *akousis* hearing] a suffix word element to denote hearing, e.g., presbycusis.

cuspid (kus′pid) [L. *cuspis* point] 1. having a single cusp or point.

2. a canine tooth.

customary temperature (*t*) **scale** a temperature scale having a zero point other than absolute zero, i.e., Celsius or Fahrenheit temperature. See also *temperature.* Cf. *absolute temperature.*

cutane/o (ku-ta′ne-o) [L. *cutis* skin] a word element used in combining form to denote the skin, e.g., subcutaneous.

cutaneous (ku-ta′ne-us) [L. *cutis* skin] pertaining to the skin.

cutdown (kut′down) the creation of a small incised opening, especially in a vein (venous cutdown), to facilitate venipuncture and permit the passage of an indwelling needle or cannula for withdrawal of blood or administration of fluids.

cuticle (ku′tĭ-k′l) [L. *cuticula,* from *cutis* skin] 1. the eponychium of the nail.

2. the acellular outer covering of some insects, composed of chitin.

3. the thin layer of keratinized anucleate cells on the outer surface of a hair shaft.

Cutie Pie a hand-held radiation survey meter used to detect or measure moderately high-level radiation fields that exceed the capacity of a Geiger counter survey meter. The detector is an ionization chamber with a direct-reading dial that can be calibrated to read in roentgens per minute.

cutis (ku′tis) [L. "skin"] [NA], the skin, the outer protective covering of the body, including the epidermis and the dermis.

cutoff frequency the low- and high-frequency levels at which the gain of an amplifier falls to 70.7 percent of its original value. The frequency response of an amplifier is the range between these low and high cutoff frequencies.

cuvet (ku-vet′) [Fr., from *cuve* vat, tub] the absorption cell used to hold a specimen during photometric and nephelometric determinations. For routine colorimetry a round glass test tube is commonly used; for precise spectrophotometric determinations, square or rectangular cuvets with parallel optically flat surfaces are used. The latter generally have a 1.0-cm path length and hold 0.1–3.0 ml of fluid. Glass cuvets are employed for measurements in the visible spectrum. Quartz cuvets are necessary for measurements at wavelengths below 340 nm. Disposable plastic cuvets are also used for some applications.

cuvette (ku-vet′) [Fr.] see *cuvet.*

CV abbrev. See *coefficient of variation.*

CVA abbrev. See *cerebrovascular accident, costovertebral angle.*

CVP abbrev. for cyclophosphamide, vincristine, and prednisone, a major established cancer chemotherapy drug regimen. For more information, see the specific drug (listed under its generic name) and *Appendix A.*

CVS abbrev. for cardiovascular system.

c wave see under *jugular venous pulse.*

***c* wave** see under *electroretinogram.*

CWP abbrev. for coal worker's pneumoconiosis. See under *anthracosis.*

cyan/o (si′an-o) [Gr. *kyanos* blue] 1. a prefix word element to denote generally the color blue, e.g., cyanosis.

2. in organic chemistry, a prefix word element to denote the —C≡N group when it must be treated as a substituent in a polyfunctional compound, e.g., cyanoacetic acid ($N{\equiv}CCH_2COOH$).

cyanide (si′ah-nid) 1. an alkyl cyanide, R—C≡N, or nitrile.

2. a salt of hydrogen cyanide, HCN (hydrocyanic

acid), e.g., sodium cyanide (NaCN) and potassium cyanide (KCN). When these salts react with acid, the highly poisonous hydrogen cyanide gas is generated.

3. the cyanide ion N≡C:⁻, which is highly toxic, the minimal lethal dose being 1.0 mg/kg. A blood level of 0.1 mg/dl may be lethal (normally, no detectable cyanide is present). Cyanide toxicity is due to inactivation of the cytochrome oxidase system, which blocks cellular respiration and produces asphyxia. Labored respiration, mental confusion developing into coma, and convulsions precede death. There may be permanent damage from tissue hypoxia in persons who survive. The blood and skin has a bright cherry-red color, which is due to cyanmethemoglobin. Sodium nitrite, which oxidizes hemoglobin to methemoglobin, has been used as an antidote. Methemoglobin strongly binds cyanide, producing cyanmethemoglobin, which removes cyanide from the tissues. Sodium thiosulfate is also given to provide sulfur for the rhodanase system of the liver; the liver converts the cyanide to thiocyanate, a relatively nontoxic metabolite, which is excreted in the urine. The cyanide group in organic compounds is not toxic unless it is released by metabolism; this occurs with the alkyl cyanides, but not with aromatic cyanide compounds. Cyanides and HCN are readily absorbed through the intestinal tract, lungs, and skin.

Cyanide-liberating glycosides, e.g., amygdalin, are contained in some seeds, especially those of the genus *Prunus.* Cyanide has a characteristic "peach pit" or "bitter almond" odor that may be detected in vomitus, or in body tissues at autopsy. It is reported that 20–40 percent of the population is congenitally insensitive to the odor.

cyanide-ascorbate test a test used to screen for anemia caused by glucose-6-phosphate dehydrogenase deficiency. It measures peroxidative degradation of hemoglobin. The test may also be positive in normal newborn infants, possibly because of a temporary deficiency of glutathione peroxidase.

cyanide assays 1. Prussian blue test. A specimen acidified with tartaric acid is steam-distilled into a small quantity of dilute NaOH solution, which will trap any CN^- present. The alkaline distillate is then treated with 1 percent $FeSO_4$ and $FeCl_3$ solutions. After being warmed carefully, the solution is acidified with dilute HCl. A precipitate of Prussian blue or a blue color of varying intensity (ferric ferrocyanide) will form if cyanide is present.

2. quantitative estimation with pyridine-barbituric acid. Cyanide is separated from blood, urine, or homogenized tissue by H_2SO_4 and trapped by dilute alkali (NaOH) through microdiffusion. Monobasic sodium phosphate and Chloramine-T solution are added to the absorbing solution to form cyanogen chloride with cyanide. Pyridine-barbituric acid produces a red color with cyanogen chloride by forming *N*-cyanopyridinium chloride, which is cleaved to form an anil of glutaconic aldehyde, which couples with barbituric acid. The color is read at 580 nm.

cyanmethemoglobin (HiCN) (si″an-met-he′mo-glo″bin) the stable complex formed by methemoglobin and cyanide. It is characterized by a Soret band at 416–419 nm and a secondary absorption peak at 541 nm. The standard method for assaying hemoglobin in whole blood uses potassium ferricyanide to oxidize all hemoglobin forms to methemoglobin, which is then converted to cyanmethemoglobin by adding potassium cyanide and measured spectrophotometrically at 540 nm. See also *hemoglobin assays.*

cyanoacrylate (si″ah-no-ah-kril′āt) a type of polymer formed by the polymerization of cyanoacrylic acid, $H_2C{=}C(CN)COOH$, when exposed to moisture. The polymer is formed as a tenacious film, with useful applications in the preparation of medical adhesives.

Cyanobacteria (si″ah-no-bak-tēr′e-ah) a division of prokaryotic organisms that have true aerobic photosynthesis like the green plants. Many are obligate phototrophs that cannot utilize organic compounds as energy and carbon sources. Although they are ecologically important in that they produce much of the atmospheric oxygen, they have no known medical importance, as none are animal or human pathogens. Also called *blue-green bacteria.* Formerly called *blue-green algae.*

cyanocobalamin (si″ah-no-ko-bal′ah-min) [USP], the form of cobalamin in which one of the ligands of the central cobalt atom is a cyanide group (N≡C⁻). Cyanocobalamin (commonly referred to as vitamin B_{12}) can be administered parenterally in pernicious anemia or following gastrectomy; in B_{12} malabsorption which may be due to sprue, gluten enteropathy, fish tapeworm infestation, blind loop syndrome, or ileal resection; and in hereditary transcobalamin II deficiency. It is also administered as part of the Schilling test for gastrointestinal absorption of vitamin B_{12}. See also *vitamin B_{12}.*

cyanocobalamin Co 57 [USP], a radiopharmaceutical used in the Schilling test of vitamin B_{12} absorption. It is identical to normal vitamin B_{12} except that the nonradioactive cobalt atom is replaced by cobalt-57.

cyanogen (si-an′o-jen) [*cyano-* + Gr. *gennan* to produce] ethane dinitrile, N≡C—C≡N; a flammable, highly toxic, colorless gas with a pungent odor. Its toxic effects are similar to those of hydrogen cyanide.

cyanol FF (si′ah-nol) a sulfonated triphenylmethane dye; C.I. 43535 used in histology for demonstrating hemoglobin. It produces a leuko dye after reduction with zinc and acid.

cyanopia (si″ah-no′pe-ah) [*cyano-* + Gr. *opsis* vision + *-ia*] a defect of vision in which objects appear tinged with blue. Also called cyanopsia.

cyanosis (si″ah-no′sis) [Gr. *kyanos* blue] a bluish coloration of the skin, mucous membranes, and nail beds caused by excessive concentration of deoxyhemoglobin in the blood. It can accompany polycythemia, methemoglobinemia, impaired pulmonary or cardiac function, and any condition that results in arterial hypoxia.

cybernetics (si″ber-net′iks) [Gr. *kybernētēs* helmsman] the science of the processes of communication and control in the animal, the machine, and organizations. In biology, the term refers to the processes of self-regulating control mechanisms.

cybrid (si′brid) a cytoplasmic hybrid; the viable cell resulting from the fusion of the enucleated cytoplasm of one cell with another complete cell. See also *cellular h.* under *hybridization.*

cyclamate (si′klah-māt) a salt of cyclamic acid, *N*-cyclohexylsulfamic acid, used as a nonnutritive sweetener. Owing to carcinogenicity demonstrated in animal testing, cyclamate has been banned in the United States.

cyclazocine (si-klaz′o-sēn) a benzomorphine derivative with analgesic and narcotic antagonist properties, which has been used to treat opiate addiction.

cycle (si′k′l) [Gr. *kyklos* circle] 1. a complete sequence of operations of a piece of equipment.

2. a metabolic pathway in which the reactions form a closed chain.

3. one period of a periodic waveform.

4. in electroencephalography, a complete sequence of potential changes making up an individual component of a sequence of several regularly repeated waveforms or complexes.

cycle per second (cps) an obsolete unit of frequency, now replaced by the *hertz* (Hz).

cyclic (sik′lik, sīk′lik) forming a closed curve or ring; in chemistry, the term is used to denote a compound with a ring of atoms joined by bonds.

cyclic adenosine monophosphate (cyclic AMP, cAMP, 3′,5′-AMP) a cyclic nucleotide, adenosine 3′,5′-cyclic monophosphate, which mediates the action of many hormones on their target organs. These hormones bind to their own specific plasma membrane receptor and subsequently activate a general membrane-bound enzyme, adenylate cyclase (EC 4.6.1.1.), which catalyzes the hydrolytic cyclization of ATP to cAMP. cAMP serves as the amplification step in these hormonal-mediated processes. Epinephrine, glucagon, ACTH, TSH, GH, LH, and a number of prostaglandins are all known to increase intracellular cAMP. The most reliable and common method to assay cAMP is by radioimmunoassay. Although cAMP measurement is not widely used in clinical laboratory work, its measurement in urine does have some applications.

cyclic AMP see *cyclic adenosine monophosphate.*

cyclic GMP see *cyclic guanosine monophosphate.*

cyclic guanosine monophosphate (cGMP, cyclic GMP, 3′:5′-GMP) a cyclic nucleotide that, like cyclic AMP, serves as an intracellular "second messenger," mediating the action of hormones; cyclic AMP and cyclic GMP have opposing functions in many cells. Also called *guanosine 3′:5′-cyclic phosphate.*

cyclic neutropenia a rare disorder, sometimes transmitted as a familial autosomal dominant trait, in which the number of circulating neutrophilic granulocytes diminishes, sometimes to zero, about every 21 da. It is due to a periodic failure of granulocytopoiesis in the marrow. The crises are sometimes characterized by fever, malaise, and oral or skin infections, but remit in 3–4 da.

cyclic nucleotides cyclic adenosine monophosphate (cAMP) and cyclic guanosine monophosphate (cGMP), cyclic 3′,5′-phosphates that function as second messengers. When hormones or neurotransmitters bind to specific receptors on target cells, this activates a membrane-bound enzyme, adenylate cyclase or guanylate cyclase, that produces cAMP or cGMP. These in turn inhibit or accelerate certain intracellular processes. The cAMP and cGMP concentrations often vary inversely with the same stimulus.

cyclitis (si-kli′tis) [Gr. *kyklos* ciliary body + *-itis*] a form of anterior uveitis characterized by inflammation of the ciliary body, which frequently extends to involve the iris (iridocyclitis). Many causes have been suggested, including viruses, granulomatous infections, trauma, and systemic diseases. Persons affected experience pain, photophobia, blurred vision, and lacrimation. Ciliary injection, turbid aqueous humor, and a dull swollen iris may be seen.

cyclitol (sik′lĭ-tol) a class of naturally occurring cycloalkanes that contains one hydroxyl group on each of three or more ring atoms. Its most important form is *myo*-inositol.

cyclization (si″klĭ-za′shun) a reaction that creates a ring in a molecule by the internal (or intramolecular) reaction between two functional groups on the same molecule.

cyclizine (si′klĭ-zēn) [USP], a drug with anticholinergic and antihistaminic effects, used as the free base, as cyclizine hydrochloride [USP], or as cyclizine lactate [USP] as an antiemetic. Adverse reactions include hives, restlessness, drowsiness, and dryness of the mouth, nose, and throat. Cyclizine increases the sedative effect of alcohol and other CNS depressants.

cyclo- (si′klo) [Gr. *kyklos* circle] a prefix word element used generally to denote roundness or repetition or to refer to the eye or the ciliary body of the eye, and specifically in organic chemistry to denote a ring compound, e.g. cyclohexane. Compounds containing multiple rings use the (Latin) multiplying prefixes bi-, ter-, quater-, etc., e.g., bicyclo[2.3.1]octane.

cycloalkane (si″klo-al′kān) a saturated hydrocarbon having a ring structure, e.g., cyclopropane, cyclohexane, Decalin (decahydronaphthalene).

cycloalkene (si″klo-al′kēn) an unsaturated, nonaromatic hydrocarbon having a ring structure, e.g., cyclopropene, cyclohexene, cyclohexadiene.

cyclobenzaprine hydrochloride (si″klo-ben′zah-prēn) a skeletal muscle relaxant related to the tricyclic antidepressants, used for short-term relief of muscle spasm. It reduces tonic somatic motor activity at the brain stem level. Adverse reactions include drowsiness, dryness of the mouth, and dizziness. This drug may interact with monoamine oxidase inhibitors (MAOI) and with alcohol, barbiturates, and other central nervous system depressants. Trademark, Flexeril.

cyclocryotherapy (si″klo-kri″o-ther′ah-pe) freezing of the ciliary body; used in the treatment of glaucoma.

cyclodiene hydrocarbon pesticides (si″klo-di′ēn) a group of pesticides that contain one or two norbornane rings, produced by Diels-Alder addition to hexachlorocyclopentadiene. Examples are aldrin, dieldrin, chlordane, and heptachlor. Symptoms of poisoning are generally similar to those produced by DDT, including headache, nausea, and tremors; however, convulsions can occur without warning symptoms. See also *chlorinated hydrocarbon pesticide assays.*

cyclodimerization (si″klo-di″mer-ĭ-za′shun) the reaction between two identical or similar monomers to form a cyclic structure (dimer). The dimerization of isoprene is an example.

cyclogeny (si-kloj′ĕ-ne) [*cyclo-* + Gr. *gennan* to produce] the developmental cycle of a microorganism.

cyclogram (si′klo-gram) [*cyclo-* + Gr. *gramma* mark] a tracing of the visual field made with a cycloscope.

cyclohexane (si″klo-heks′ān) a colorless, flammable liquid, C_6H_{12}; M.W. 84.16. It is the simplest strain-free alicyclic hydrocarbon (cycloalkane). High vapor concentrations are narcotic and irritating to the skin. See also *conformation.*

cycloheximide (si″klo-heks′ĭ-mīd) an antibiotic produced by *Streptomyces griseus* that inhibits protein synthesis in animal cells, many yeasts, some amebas, and some species of fungi. Cycloheximide blocks peptide bond formation in protein synthesis by preventing the transfer of activated amino acids from transfer RNA to the growing polypeptide chain. This antibiotic binds to the large ribosomal subunits of eukaryotic 80S ribosome and not prokaryotic 70S ribosomes, which explains its spectrum of activity and toxicity to humans. Although it is toxic, cycloheximide is useful as an agricultural fungicide and in selective media for fungi culture.

See also *antibacterial agents.*

cyclohexylamine (si″klo-hek-sil′ah-mēn) a colorless, flammable liquid with an unpleasant odor, cyclohexanamine; M.W. 99.17. It is a strong base and is used in organic syntheses. Cyclohexylamine is a skin sensitizer and irritant; high vapor concentrations are narcotic.

cyclomethycaine sulfate (si″klo-meth′i-kān) [USP], a local anesthetic applied topically to mucous membranes before examination, catheterization, or intubation. Adverse reactions include a stinging or burning sensation at the site of injection and allergic reactions. Trademark, Surfacaine.

cyclonite (si′klo-nīt) a white crystalline solid, *sym*-trimethylenetrinitramine, hexahydro-1,3,5-trinitro-1,3,5-triazine, a high explosive also used as a rat poison; M.W. 222.26. It is highly toxic when inhaled and produces convulsions in cases of severe poisoning.

cyclopentamine hydrochloride (si″klo-pen′tah-mēn) [USP], a sympathomimetic amine similar to ephedrine, used in nasal preparations. Adverse reactions include insomnia, nervousness, and increased blood pressure and heart rate. Trademark, Clopane.

cyclopentane (si″klo-pen′tān) a hydrocarbon, C_5H_{10}, in which all five carbon atoms are in a single ring.

cyclopentanoperhydrophenanthrene (si″klo-pen″tah-no-per-hi″dro-fen-an′thrēn) 1,2-cyclopentanoperhydrophenanthrene ($C_{17}H_{28}$), a tetracyclic sterane skeleton, consisting of a perhydro-phenanthrene ring; i.e., three saturated six-membered carbocyclic rings fused angularly, which are further fused to another saturated five-membered ring, the cyclopentane ring. The prefix "perhydro" means that all the necessary hydrogen atoms have been added to the phenanthrene ring system to make a saturated compound. The skeleton is common to sterols, bile acid, sex steroid hormones, corticosteroids, cardiac glycosides, sapogenins, and certain alkaloids.

cyclophosphamide (si″klo-fos′fah-mīd) [USP], an alkylating agent, 2-[bis(2-chloroethyl)amino]tetrahydro-2H-1,3,2-oxazaphosphorine-2-oxide. Cyclophosphamide is a white crystalline powder soluble in alcohol and water, which is used as a cancer chemotherapeutic drug. When metabolized, its nitrogen mustard component disrupts DNA activity by combining with guanine. It also suppresses the body's immune response. Trademark, *Cytoxan* (CTX). For more information, see *Appendix A.*

Cyclophyllidea (si″klo-fil-lid′e-ah) an order of cestode tapeworms that includes most of the tapeworms parasitic in humans. They are slender, long worms that have a few to many segments and a larval stage that develops in an intermediate host. There are no circulatory, respiratory, or skeletal organs, and no alimentary system. The scolex has four large, depressed suckers, a central apical rostellum (sometimes with hooks), and lateral genital pores. Families with species parasitic in humans are Anoplocephalidae, Davaineidae, Linstowiidae, Mesocestoididae, Dilepididae, Hymenolepididae, and Taeniidae. Also known as Taenioidea.

cyclopia (si-klo′pe-ah) [*cyclo-* + Gr. *opos* eye + *-ia*] a rare congenital malformation that results in partial or complete fusion of the eyes into one orbit. The condition may be accompanied by a proboscis above the eye, as well as other craniocerebral and craniofacial abnormalities. There is no treatment; the associated anomalies cause early death. Also called *synophthalmia.*

cyclopropane (si″klo-pro′pān) a colorless, flammable, and explosive gas, C_3H_6, with characteristic odor and pungent taste; the carbons of the molecule are linked in a three-membered ring. It is used as a general anesthetic.

Cyclops (si′klops) a genus of tiny crustaceans, order Eucopepoda, having a median eye, noncompound eyes, and rudimentary fifth legs. They are intermediate hosts for larvae of the human parasites *Dracunculus medinensis, Diphyllobothrium latum,* and *Gnathostoma spinigerum.* Humans are infected if they swallow water containing the crustacean, or eat uncooked fish that have ingested such water.

cycloscope (si′klo-skōp) [*cyclo-* + Gr. *skopein* to examine] a form of perimeter for mapping the visual fields.

cycloserine (si″klo-ser′ēn) [USP], an antibiotic produced by a strain of *Streptomyces garyphalus.* D-Cycloserine is similar in structure to D-alanine. It is a competitive inhibitor of alanine racemase and D-alanyl-D-alanine synthetase, sequential enzymes of peptidoglycan synthesis, and has a higher affinity than D-alanine for these enzymes.

Resistance may be due to lack of transport for D-cycloserine into the cell or to elevated levels of alanine racemase and D-alanyl-D-alanine synthetase. D-Cycloserine is used for the treatment of tuberculosis resistant to commonly used drugs.

See also *antibacterial agents.*

cyclothiazide (si″klo-thi′ah-zīd) [USP], see under *thiazide diuretics.*

cyclotron (si″klo-tron) an apparatus for accelerating charged particles such as deuterons, alpha particles, ^{3}He ions, or protons to extremely high energies. The particles are accelerated by a constant frequency-alternating electric field that is synchronized with their movement. They are then deflected in a spiral path by a constant magnetic field normal to their path. Cyclotrons are used to produce short-lived radionuclides for medical use.

-cyesis (si-e′sis) [Gr. *kyēsis* pregnancy] a suffix word element to denote pregnancy, e.g., pseudocyesis.

cylinder (sil′in-der) [Gr. *kylindros* a roller] a solid body shaped like a column, especially a cylindrical cast or cylindrical lens.

cylindric (sĭ-lin′drik) pertaining to or shaped like a cylinder.

cylindroid (sil′in-droid) [Gr. *kylindroeidēs* cylindric] 1. shaped like a cylinder.

2. a urinary cast of various origins, which tapers to a slender tail that is often twisted or curled upon itself.

cylindroma (sil″in-dro′mah) [Gr. *kylindros* cylinder + *-ōma* swelling] 1. a tumor of eccrine or apocrine gland origin that forms one or several nodules, usually on the scalp. Multiple nodules are seen in the dominantly inherited form, and the gross appearance of the lesions has led to the description of turban tumor. Sections show groups of hyperchromatic cells with basophilic cytoplasm separated by bands of connective tissue. The tumor is usually benign.

2. see *adenoid cystic carcinoma.*

cylindruria (sil″in-droo′re-ah) [Gr. *kylindros* cylinder + *ouron* urine + *-ia*] the presence of an increased number of casts in the urine.

cyproheptadine hydrochloride (si″pro-hep′tah-dēn) [USP], a serotonin and histamine antagonist with anticholinergic effects, used to alleviate symptoms of allergic rhinitis, vasomotor rhinitis, hives, and other allergic reactions. Adverse reactions include drowsiness, dizziness, gastrointestinal intolerance, and dryness of the mouth, nose, and throat. Because of its anticholinergic effects, this agent should be used with caution in individuals with asthma or increased intraocular pressure. Trademark, Periactin.

cyrtometer (sir-tom′ĕ-ter) [Gr. *kyrtos* bent + *metron* measure] a device for measuring the curved surfaces of the body.

Cys abbrev. See *cysteine.*

cyst/o (sis′to) [Gr. *kystis* sac, bladder] a word element used in combining form to denote the urinary bladder or a cyst, sac, or sac of fluid, e.g., cystic.

cyst (sist) [Gr. *kystis* sac, bladder] 1. any closed cavity or sac, normal or abnormal. Many are lined by epithelium, although cysts in some locations are lined by connective tissue or bone. Most cysts contain a liquid or semisolid material.

2. a stage in the life cycle of certain parasites during which they are enclosed within a protective sac, e.g., hydatid cyst.

branchial c., a cyst of the neck that arises through persistence of the embryonic cervical sinus (see *branchial region*), which may not become clinically apparent until adult life. It is usually lined by a squamous epithelium and contains keratin debris and cholesterol crystals. It forms a swelling at the anterior border of the sternomastoid muscle, usually just below the angle of the jaw. Also called branchial cleft cyst and branchiogenic cyst.

bronchial c., a spherical cyst arising in the respiratory system of children or young adults as a result of a developmental aberration of the primitive foregut. It is an accessory bronchial bud, with a wall lined by bronchial-type cells (epithelium, glands, muscle, cartilage). Large cysts may cause coughing, dyspnea, and pain. Also called bronchogenic cyst.

chocolate c., a cyst containing syrupy, dark brown contents, which results from the collection of inspissated blood following local hemorrhage. The term is used to describe blood-filled cysts of the ovary in ovarian endometriosis.

corpus luteum c., an ovarian cyst that forms because of delayed organization of the central cavity of the corpus luteum, and which in turn results in lack of regression of luteal cells. Continued progesterone production by the luteal cells causes delayed menstruation and abnormal uterine bleeding.

dentigerous c., a cyst of the jaw surrounding the crown of a tooth. It is caused by degenerative changes in enamel epithelium of unerupted teeth, and most often occurs in young adults. Cysts are unilocular and lined by stratified squamous epithelium.

dermoid c., a benign cystic ovarian teratoma.

gas c., see *p. cystoides intestinalis* under *pneumatosis.*

germinal inclusion c., a small cystic inclusion within ovarian stroma, lined by cuboidal cells. These cysts are commonly multiple and are thought to arise as a result of invaginations of the surface of the ovary that become pinched off to form cysts lined by mesothelium. The mesothelium subsequently undergoes metaplasia to a serous or mucinous epithelium and may represent precursors of serous and mucinous cystomas.

hydatid c., see *hydatid.*

c. of the jaw, a developmental cyst derived from ectodermal remnants. It may be classified as odontogenic (including periodontal, dentigerous, gingival) or nonodontogenic.

keratinous c., a cyst composed of layers of epithelial cells and epithelial debris; it is most often found on the scalp, neck, or back. It may be of pilar or epidermal origin. On physical examination, the cyst appears firm, elevated, and movable.

nabothian c., a mucus-filled cyst of the mucosa of the uterine cervix formed by stenosis of an endocervical gland, resulting in the intraluminal accumulation of mucus produced by the lining epithelial cells.

parathyroid c., a relatively common, usually small, and slow-growing cyst of the parathyroid glands. Rarely, one becomes sufficiently large to cause pressure symptoms, such as hoarseness from compression of the recurrent laryngeal nerve, or dysphagia.

pericardial c., an asymptomatic cyst of the pericardium, filled with clear fluid, that develops in the cardiophrenic angle. Also called celomic cyst and mesothelial cyst.

renal c., a cyst of the renal parenchyma that may arise anywhere along the nephron or in the collecting system. Renal cysts may be single or multiple and are of diverse pathogenesis including hereditary, developmental, and acquired origins. A proposed clinicopathologic classification of renal cysts is shown in the accompanying table.

tension c., a cyst that contains fluid under pressure. In the breast, tension cysts arise as a component of fibrocystic disease due to the secretion of fluid into cystically dilated lobules at a rate faster than the epithelium that lines the cyst can reabsorb the fluid. Such cysts may rupture, leaking their contents into adjacent stroma and producing inflammation and fibrosis.

theca-lutein c., an ovarian cyst in which theca interna cells line the cystic cavity. It usually occurs in association with hydatidiform mole. Large amounts of human chorionic gonadotropin (hCG)

RENAL CYST

CLASSIFICATION OF RENAL CYSTS

I. Renal dysplasia
- A. Multicystic dyplasia
  - 1. Unilateral multicystic kidney
  - 2. Bilateral multicystic dysplasia
- B. Focal and segmental cystic dysplasia
- C. Cystic dysplasia associated with lower urinary tract obstruction
- D. Familial cystic dysplasia

II. Polycystic disease
- A. Infantile polycystic disease
  - 1. Polycystic disease of early infancy
  - 2. Polycystic disease of childhood
  - 3. Congenital hepatic fibrosis
- B. Adult polycystic disease

III. Renal cysts in hereditary syndromes
- A. Meckel's syndrome
- B. Zellweger's cerebrohepatorenal syndrome
- C. Jeune's asphyxiating thoracic dystrophy
- D. Tuberous sclerosis complex and Lindau's disease
- E. Cortical cysts in syndromes of multiple malformations

IV. Renal cortical cysts
- A. Diffuse glomerular cystic disease
- B. Perpheral cortical microcysts
- C. Juxtamedullary cortical microcysts
- D. Simple cysts, solitary and multiple

V. Renal medullary cystic disorders
- A. Medullary sponge kidney
- B. Medullary cystic disease complex
  - 1. Familial juvenile nephronophthisis
  - 2. Medullary cystic disease
  - 3. Renal-retinal dysplasia

VI. Miscellaneous parenchymal renal cysts
- A. Inflammation and necrosis
  - 1. Medullary necrosis
  - 2. Lithiasis
  - 3. Tuberculosis
  - 4. Echinococcosis
- B. Neoplasia
  - 1. Cystic degeneration of carcinoma
  - 2. Multilocular cystadenoma (benign cystic nephroma)
  - 3. Dermoid cyst
- C. Endometriosis
- D. Traumatic intrarenal hematoma

VII. Extraparenchymal renal cysts
- A. Pyelogenic cyst (pelvic diverticulum)
- B. Parapelvic cyst (lymphangiectasia)
- C. Perinephric cyst

Modified from Bernstein, J.: An orientation to renal cysts. *In* Gardner, K. D., Jr. (ed.). Cystic Diseases of the Kidney. New York, John Wiley & Sons, 1976.

are responsible for its development. By radioimmunoassay, the serum concentration of the beta subunit of hCG is usually elevated. Spontaneous regression follows removal of the mole. See also *hydatidiform mole.*

thyroglossal c., a cystic remnant of a portion of the thyroglossal duct. It occurs in or close to the anterior midline of the neck, at any point on the path of migration of the thyroid gland from the base of the tongue to the front of the trachea. Roughly 50 percent are close to the hyoid bone. The cyst may connect to the surface through a thyroglossal fistula that is occasionally congenital but more commonly results from rupture of the cyst. Aberrant thyroid tissue can be present in such a cyst; thyroid carcinomas rarely occur in this location.

cystadenocarcinoma (sist-ad″ĕ-no-kar″sĭ-no′mah) [*cyst-* + Gr. *adēn* gland + *carcinoma*] a cystic adenocarcinoma, commonly of the ovary or pancreas, in which the cystic spaces are lined by a malignant neoplastic epithelium. The type of epithelium may be serous, mucinous, or mixed. See also *ovarian tumors.*

mucinous c., see mucinous tumors under *ovarian tumors.*

cystadenoma (sist″ad-ĕ-no′mah) [*cyst-* + Gr. *adēn* gland + *-ōma* swelling] an adenoma with extensive formation of cystic structures. Such tumors are seen in the ovary and occasionally in the pancreas. The cystic cavities are commonly filled with mucin or serous fluid. The lining epithelium may be serous or mucinous, and is usually smooth but may form papillary projections.

c. lymphomatosum, a benign tumor of the parotid or, rarely, the submandibular glands. It is composed of cylindrical oncocytic epithelial cells frequently arranged in papillary projections accompanied by a lymphoid stroma. Also called adenolymphoma and *Warthin's tumor.*

mucinous c., see mucinous tumors under *ovarian tumors.*

oncocytic papillary c., an uncommon benign tumor of the larynx, composed of mitochondria-rich cells.

serous c., see under *ovarian tumors.*

cystalgia (sis-tal′je-ah) [*cyst-* + Gr. *algos* pain + *-ia*] pain in the bladder.

cystathionase (sis″tah-thi′o-nās) see *cystathionine-γ-lyase.*

cystathionine (sis″tah-thi′o-nēn) an asymmetric thioether of homocysteine and serine, $COOH \cdot CH(NH_2) \cdot CH_2 \cdot CH_2 \cdot S \cdot CH_2 \cdot CH(NH_2) \cdot COOH$, which occurs as an intermediate in cysteine synthesis. An inherited defect of cystathionine-γ-lyase, a pyridoxal-phosphate enzyme that cleaves cystathionine to cysteine and homoserine, leads to the excretion of large amounts of cystathionine in the urine (cystathioninuria). No characteristic clinical manifestation has been noted in this abnormality. Cystathioninuria can also occur with disorders associated with remethylation of homocysteine, B_6-deficiency, liver disease, and tumors of the neural crest.

cystathionine-γ-lyase an enzyme of the lyase class (L-cystathionine cysteine-lyase [deaminating], EC 4.4.1.1) that catalyzes the reaction L-cystathionine + $H_2O \rightleftharpoons$ L-cysteine + NH_3 + 2-oxobutyrate. It is a pyridoxal-phosphate protein. A genetic deficiency of the enzyme causes cystathionuria. Some patients with this disorder have demonstrated physical or mental abnormalities, but no consistent clinical pattern is evident. Also called *cystathionase.* See also *cystathioninuria.*

cystathionine-β-synthase an enzyme of the lyase class (L-serine hydro-lyase [adding homocysteine], EC 4.2.1.22) that catalyzes the reaction L-serine + L-homocysteine ⇌ cystathionine + H_2O. It requires pyridoxal-phosphate as a coenzyme. A hereditary absence or deficient activity of the enzyme (due to vitamin B_6 deficiency) causes homocystinuria, as well as the excretion of the oxidized form of homocysteine and elevated plasma concentrations of methionine and homocysteine.

cystathioninuria (sis″tah-thi′o-nēn-ur′e-ah) [*cystathionine* + Gr. *ouron* urine] the excretion in the urine of cystathionine, an α-amino acid involved in the synthesis of cysteine. Normally, individuals have no detectable amounts of cystathionine in the urine. The condition occurs in the inherited disorders of cobalamin and folate deficiency (with homocysteinuria); it can also be secondary to pyridoxine deficiency, hepatic disease, neural crest tumors, and administration of thyroxine. Patients have also been described who excrete large amounts of cystathionine in the urine but have none of the above-mentioned disorders; it is believed that a defect in γ-cystathioninase activity, transmitted as an autosomal recessive trait, is responsible for these cases. Those affected with the latter form have sometimes shown a variety of signs and symptoms including retardation, endocrinopathies, convulsions, anemia, thrombocytopenia, nephrogenic diabetes insipidus, and immunoglycinuria; no consistent clinical pattern has emerged, and most individuals with the disorder show no adverse effects.

cysteamine (sis-te′ah-mēn) see *β-mercaptoethylamine.*

cystectasia (sis″tek-ta′ze-ah) [*cyst-* + Gr. *ektasis* dilation] dilation of the bladder.

cystectomy (sis-tek′to-me) [*cyst-* + Gr. *ektomē* excision] 1. excision of a cyst.

2. excision or resection of the bladder, usually with transplantation of the ureters into an isolated segment of the ileum.

cysteic acid methods (sis′te-ik) any of a number of methods for the histologic demonstration of cystine, based on the principle that, when combined with peracetic or performic acid, cystine turns to cysteic acid.

cysteine (Cys or C) (sis′te-ēn) 2-amino-3-mercaptopropanoic acid, $HSCH_2CH(NH_2)COOH$, a nonessential amino acid and constituent of most proteins; M.W. 121.16. It is easily oxidized to the disulfide form, cystine. The presence of a free thiol group in the cysteine residue is essential for the activity of many enzymes, and the disulfide bonds between cysteine residues on nearby sections of peptide chains give stability to protein structure. The pK'_a for the thiol group in cysteine is 10.80. It is present as a constituent of glutathione, which serves redox functions and also the transport of amino acids across cellular membranes by the γ-glutamyl transfer cycle. Its sources are the proteins of the diet and synthesis from serine and homocysteine. Cysteine is often present in urine but is not clinically significant, whereas the presence of cystine may lead to renal calculi. Also called *thiolaminopropionic acid.* See also under *amino acids.*

cysteinyl (sis′tēn-il) the acyl radical derived from or relating to cysteine.

cystic (sis′tik) [Gr. *kystis* sac, bladder] 1. pertaining to the urinary bladder or the gallbladder.

2. pertaining to or containing a cyst or cysts.

cystic disease of breast an involutional disease of the mammary parenchyma, characterized by dilation of lobules and the presence of lobular cysts (tension cyst of breast), usually lined by metaplastic apocrine epithelium. Cysts contain fluid that is yellow to brown in color; when viewed through an unruptured cyst wall, the fluid gives the cyst a blue appearance (blue dome cyst of breast). When cyst contents leak into the stroma, they produce inflammation and fibrosis. Duct ectasia and hyperplasia of the lobules and ducts frequently accompany this condition. Nipple inversion and discharge are not features, and calcifications are rarely detected mammographically. Rarely or formerly called Bloodgood's disease, chronic mastitis, fibroadenosis, *fibrocystic disease of breast,* fibrous mastopathy, mazoplasia, and Schimmelbusch's disease. See also *apocrine metaplasia* and *tension cyst of breast.* Cf. *duct ectasia of breast.*

cystic disease of lung a condition characterized by the formation of abnormally large (greater than 1 cm in diameter) airspaces in the lungs. Cystic degeneration of the lung parenchyma may be the result of a developmental anomaly, or may be acquired secondary to some other degenerative pathologic process.

There are two forms of cystic lesion of the lung: bronchogenic and alveolar. Bronchogenic cysts are relatively rare and are thought to be of congenital origin, presumably produced by the enforced expansion of poorly formed bronchi (when subjected to thrusts of inspiratory pressure) or by the isolation of nests of epithelial cells during embryogenesis (congenital bronchogenic cystic disease of the lung). These bronchogenic cysts are lined by bronchial epithelial cells, possess thin walls, are often filled with mucus, and may be found in the mediastinum or lung parenchyma, frequently adjacent to bronchi or bronchioles.

Alveolar cysts presumably arise as the result of the progressive rupture of alveolar walls that either are congenitally malformed or have deteriorated in the course of some disease process. Their walls are fragile, thin, and ill-defined. They are somewhat centrally located, often in multiple sites primarily in the upper lobes; they may be large enough to occupy an entire lobe (vanishing lung syndrome).

Bronchogenic and alveolar cysts are often asymptomatic, discovered incidentally on radiologic examination. When present, the symptoms referable to a cyst reflect its size and the condition of the rest of the affected lung. Both types of cyst have the potential to impair ventilatory function, rupture and cause pneumothorax or collapse, or provide primary loci for the development of infection.

cystic duct the small duct that connects the neck of the gallbladder with the common bile duct. The folds of its mucosal lining have a spiral arrangement (spiral valve of Heister).

cysticercoid (sis″tĭ-ser′koid) [*Cysticercus* + Gr. *eidos* form] pertaining to the larval form of tapeworms. The often encysted larvae have a small anterior bladder into which the head is invaginated and frequently a solid, elongated caudal portion.

cysticercosis (sis″tĭ-ser-ko′sis) [*Cysticercus* + *-osis* condition] infection with the encysted larvae of tapeworms, particularly of *Taenia solium.* Larvae are introduced into the body through ingestion of fecally contaminated food or by orogenital contamination, or they may be swallowed after regurgitation of larvae produced by a resident adult worm. The larvae migrate from the small intestine to almost any organ in the body, but most frequently to subcutaneous tissue, eyes, and brain. Surrounded by a fibrous capsule, the larvae evoke inflammatory reactions, sometimes resulting in fibrosis and necrosis of the capsule and larval caseation or calcification. Infestation of the brain may produce serious effects, including jacksonian epilepsy, disordered behavior, dysequilibrium, meningoencephalitis, and visual dysfunction. Larvae are not encapsulated in the eyes, but produce iritis, retinitis, palpebral conjunctivitis, and visual discomfort.

Cysticercus (sis″tĭ-ser′kus) [*cyst-* + Gr. *kerkos tail*] the genus name formerly applied to the larvae of tapeworms and used clinically to indicate this developmental stage.

C. bovis, the larva of *Taenia saginata,* the beef tapeworm.

C. cellulosae, the larva of *Taenia solium,* the pork tapeworm, which causes cysticercosis. The ovoid body is whitish in color and 6–18 mm in length, with an invaginated scolex. Also called pork measles or bladderworm.

cysticercus, pl. *cysticerci* a bladderworm, the larva of a tapeworm in which a head with one or more scolices develops by invagination into the bladder. Encysting may occur in this stage.

cystic fibrosis a systemic disease, transmitted as an autosomal recessive trait, that is characterized as a disorder of the exocrine glands and most prominently affects the pancreas, lungs, and sweat glands. The cause is unknown; it has been reported to occur in as many as 1 in every 1500 Caucasian births. All exocrine glands are affected, and there is secretion of high-protein viscous material, which obstructs the exocrine ducts.

The disease most frequently appears in infancy and is marked by disturbances of the gastrointestinal and pulmonary systems. Infants may have meconium ileus owing to obstruction of the small intestine by viscid secretions. There is pancreatic insufficiency, resulting in steatorrhea, azotorrhea, and foul stools. Biliary cirrhosis, cholelithiasis, and rectal prolapse may occur.

Pulmonary abnormalities account for the major morbidity and mortality associated with cystic fibrosis. There is diffuse obstruction of the lungs with tenacious, viscous secretions. This results in atelectasis, emphysema, and pulmonary infections, primarily involving *Staphylococcus aureus* and *Pseudomonas aeruginosa.* Sinusitis, chronic bronchitis, recurrent pneumonias, pulmonary abscesses, bronchiectasis, and cor pulmonale are also potential complications. Other manifestations include cyanosis, male sterility and decreased female fertility, and excessive sweat gland secretions of sodium and chloride, which leads to sodium depletion and heat intolerance.

The most important diagnostic test is the standard quantitative sweat test (see *sweat test*). Following pilocarpine iontophoresis, affected infants show elevated sodium and chloride excretion to >60 mEq/l (normal, 20–30 mEq/l). This test may be performed on persons of any age. A secondary test may be used to determine sodium and potassium concentrations in fingernail and toenail clippings; those affected have a threefold elevation of sodium and a twofold elevation of potassium. Pancreatic tests reveal decreased secretion of amylase, lipase, and proteolytic enzymes. Malabsorption states are also seen.

Adults who possess the cystic fibrosis trait have a 25 percent chance of passing on the disease to an offspring. Screening tests to detect carriers by measuring cellular sodium absorption in response to ouabain are currently being evaluated.

Effective treatment of pulmonary complications has permitted the survival of affected infants to reproductive age.

Also called *fibrocystic disease of the pancreas* and *mucoviscidosis.*

cystic fibrosis tests 1. see *sweat test.*

2. agar plate test, a semiquantitative test used to screen patients (usually infants) for cystic fibrosis. It tests for the presence of abnormal (elevated) levels of chloride in sweat. The patient's fingers and palm are pressed against the surface of an agar plate prepared to contain silver ions. If the Cl^- level is high enough, sufficient Cl^- will diffuse into the agar to react with the Ag^+ and form a fine precipitate of silver chloride, seen as a white handprint pattern against the agar background. The test is not very reliable and should be used only if the standard sweat chloride test is not available.

cystic hyperplasia see *cystic h.* under *hyperplasia.*

cystic hyperplasia of breast cystic disease of the breast associated with epithelial hyperplasia. See also *cystic disease of breast.*

cystic hyperplasia of endometrium see *endometrial h.* under *hyperplasia.*

cystic mastopathy see *cystic disease of breast.*

cystine (sis′tēn) [*cyst-* + *-ine*] 3,3′-dithiobis-(2-aminopropanoic acid), $[\text{—SCH}_2\text{CH(NH}_2\text{) COOH]}_2$, a naturally occurring, nonessential alpha amino acid contained in most proteins; M.W. 240.31. It can be formed by the oxidation of two molecules of cysteine and can readily be reduced again to cysteine. Along with methionine, it is the major sulfur-containing compound of proteins and occurs in high concentrations in the keratin of hair. Cystine disulfide bonds between cysteine residues on nonadjacent peptide chains help to give proteins their tertiary structure.

As cystine is relatively insoluble at the pH range characteristic of urine, it is frequently found in urine in crystalline form, but it is present in high amounts only in persons affected with cystinuria (a hereditary defect in tubular amino acid absorption). Cystinuric patients may also develop cystine kidney stones. Cystine is sometimes added to culture media to promote the growth of facultative organisms. The reference range for cystine excretion is 1–2 mg/kg/da.

cystinemia (sis″tĭ-ne′me-ah) [*cystine* + Gr. *haima* blood + *-ia*] an increase in the concentration of cystine in the blood. This condition may occur nonspecifically, or may be due to disorders of amino acid metabolism and transport. See also *aminoacidopathy.*

cystinosis (sis″ti-no′sis) [*cystine* + *-osis* condition] any of three genetic disorders in the metabolism of cystine, transmitted as autosomal recessive traits, that result in the deposition of cystine in body tissues. The urinary output may be normal or only slightly increased. Cystine accumulates in lysosomes; the molecular defect responsible for this is not known. The condition occurs in an early-onset or infantile nephropathic form, a late-onset juvenile or adolescent nephropathic form, and a benign or adult nephropathic form. The latter two forms are extremely rare.

cystinuria (sis″tĭ-nu′re-ah) [*cystine* + Gr. *ouron* urine + *-ia*] the most common group of disorders of amino acid transport, transmitted as autosomal recessive traits, that are due to the deficient transport of dibasic amino acids, cystine, lysine, ornithine, and arginine. Cystinuria occurs in 1 in every 10,000–15,000 births. This defect is expressed at two primary sites: in the intestine there is deficient absorption, and in the kidneys there is deficient reabsorption, the latter resulting in aminoaciduria. Because cystine is the least soluble of these amino acids, it tends to precipitate in the urinary tract, leading to the formation of renal, ureteral, and bladder calculi.

The peak time for expression of this disorder is between ages 10 and 30 yr. Three homozygous variants have been described: type I, characterized by total lack of intestinal dibasic amino acid transport; type II, characterized by lack of lysine transport but with some cystine transport in the intestine; and type III, characterized by some capacity for intestinal transport of all of the dibasic amino acids. Urinary tract stones are the primary threat in this disorder, with hematuria, flank pain, renal colic, infection, and renal destruction as complications.

Cystinuria should be suspected in patients with radiopaque urinary tract stones, which are less dense than calcium stones. The nitroprusside test should be performed on urine samples, The test is also positive in acetonuria and homocystinuria. The type of individual amino acids can be determined by electrophoresis or chromatography. If the concentration of cystine in the urine exceeds 250 mg/l, cystine crystals may form. Treatment is aimed at reducing cystine concentration in the kidney tubules by increasing urine volume through massive fluid intake (5–7 l/da.). To increase the solubility of cystine, the pH of the urine is raised by administering agents such as sodium bicarbonate and acetazolamide. Administration of D-penicillamine, which binds and solubilizes cystine, may be useful; however, because of systemic toxicity, it is recommended only in high-risk cases or in patients who do not respond satisfactorily to other means of therapy.

See also *aminoacidopathy.*

cystinuria tests 1. the nitroprusside test. Cystine is reduced by sodium cyanide to cysteine, which reacts with sodium nitroprusside (sodium nitroferrocyanide, $Na_2FeNO(CN)_5$) to form a magenta-colored product. Homocystine reacts identically, but ketone bodies also give a positive test. The safer reagent sodium borohydride can be substituted for sodium cyanide; this also eliminates interference from ketones. Homocystine also gives a positive reaction with silver nitroprusside, whereas cystine does not.

2. the lead acetate test. The urine specimen is boiled with alkali (40 percent w/v), which liberates sulfide from compounds containing mercapto groups. The sulfide reacts with lead acetate to form a black precipitate of lead sulfide. Proteinuria may give false-positive results.

3. paper or thin-layer chromatography for the separation of amino acids.

cystitis (sis-ti′tis) [*cyst-* + *-itis* inflammation] an acute or chronic infection of the urinary bladder, which occurs more often in females than in males. Acute cystitis is characterized by frequency and urgency of urination accompanied by burning and pain. Symptoms are usually milder in chronic cases. The infection is usually bacterial and is a result of ascending infection or, less commonly, hematogenous spread.

Laboratory studies show significant bacteriuria (in excess of 10^5/ml of urine), pyuria, and sometimes hematuria. Voided midstream urine collection, catheterization, and suprapubic needle aspiration may be helpful in obtaining uncontaminated bladder urine specimens for culture. In chronic cystitis, cystoscopy may be useful in detecting predisposing factors.

c. cystica, a benign proliferative disorder of the epithelium of the urinary bladder, in which groups of transitional epithelial cells in the superficial lamina propria surround a small cavity. These aggregates probably derive from von Brunn's nests.

c. follicularis, a chronic inflammation of the bladder wall characterized by the formation of lymphoid follicles within the lamina propria.

c. glandularis, a lesion of the bladder characterized by the presence of cystic nests of mucus-forming columnar epithelium within the lamina propria. It is often associated with cystitis cystica.

cystocele (sis′to-sēl) [*cysto-* + Gr. *kēlē* hernia] herniation of the urinary bladder into the vagina.

cystogram (sis′to-gram) [*cysto-* + Gr. *gramma* mark] the radiograph obtained by cystography.

voiding c., a radiograph of the urinary tract made while the patient is urinating.

cystography (sis-tog′rah-fe) [*cysto-* + Gr. *graphein* to write] a general term for radiologic examination of the lower urinary tract (the lower ends of the ureters, the bladder, and the urethra) after introduction of a contrast medium. See also *cystoureterography, cystourethrography, prostatography,* and *urography.*

radionuclide c., a procedure in nuclear medicine used primarily in pediatrics to detect vesicoureteral reflux. ^{99m}Tc-DTPA is introduced into the bladder in one of two ways: the direct method, by instillation through a catheter, or the indirect method, by intravenous injection and filtration by the kidneys. A series of scintillation scans is made; any reflux of urine into the ureters can be seen. A residual urine volume measurement is also performed.

retrograde c., cystography in which the contrast medium is introduced by way of a urethral catheter. A radiopaque, water-soluble, iodinated contrast medium, e.g., 10–30 percent diatrizoate meglumine (Hypaque-cysto, Cystografin) or 17 or 43 percent iothalamate meglumine (cysto-Conray), is commonly used; air can be used for negative-contrast studies (pneumocystography) or double-contrast studies.

After catheterization and drainage of residual urine, the bladder is filled with a radiopaque medium by either the contrast injection method or the contrast infusion method, in which the pressure and flow rate are controlled in order to make possible reliable comparisons with subsequent studies. Frontal, lateral, and oblique views demonstrate diverticula, filling defects (tumors, calculi), or vesicoureteral reflux. Voiding or postvoiding studies are then made to observe vesicoureteral reflux during voiding and the residual urine volume. In triple-voiding cystography, films are made after three voiding attempts; this permits better evacuation of an atonic bladder.

Cystokon (sis′to-kon) trademark. See *acetrizoate.*

cystolith (sis′to-lith) [*cysto-* + Gr. *lithos* stone] a bladder calculus.

cystometer (sis-tom′ĕ-ter) [*cysto-* Gr. *metron* measure] an instrument for studying the neuromuscular mechanism of the bladder by means of measurements of pressure and capacity.

cystometrography (sis″to-mĕ-trog′rah-fe) [*cysto-* + Gr. *metron* measure + *graphein* to record] the graphic recording of intravesical volumes and pressures.

cystopyelitis (sis″to-pi″ĕ-li′tis) [*cysto-* + Gr. *pyelos* trough + *-itis* inflammation] inflammation of the bladder and renal pelvis.

cystosarcoma phyllodes (sis″to-sar-ko′mah filo′dēz) [*cysto-* + Gr. *sarkos* flesh + *-oma* swelling] a distinctive fibroepithelial neoplasm of the breast without counterpart in other organs of the body. It occurs rarely in childhood and adolescence, is almost invariably unilateral, and frequently grows to massive proportions if untreated. The term cystosarcoma phyllodes is a poor one, as both benign and malignant variants of the lesion occur, but it is well established in the medical literature.

Histologically, cystosarcoma phyllodes resembles a fibroadenoma but differs in that the connective tissue stromal component is more cellular, pleomorphic, and, frequently, more mitotically active. The distinction between benign and malignant forms is best made by assessment of the stromal component. Those tumors that have well-defined, "pushing" borders, that have a stroma with low mitotic activity and little cellular atypia, and that show no glandular obliteration by stromal overgrowth are most likely benign. The epithelial component rarely shows carcinomatous change.

Approximately 20 percent of the tumors are malignant; recurrence of a histologically benign tumor is rare. For malignant tumors, the recurrence rate is 30 percent and the metastatic rate approximately 25 percent. When metastases occur, they may be in any site in the body, but are infrequent in regional lymph nodes.

Also called giant fibroadenoma.

cystoscope (sis′to-skōp) [*cysto-* + Gr. *skopein* to examine] an endoscope designed for passage through the urethra into the bladder to permit visual inspection of its interior.

cystoscopy (sis-tos′ko-pe) direct visual examination of the urinary tract and bladder with a cystoscope.

cystoureteritis (sis″to-u-re″ter-i′tis) [*cysto-* + Gr. *ourētēr* ureter + *-itis* inflammation] inflammation involving the urinary bladder and ureter.

cystoureterogram (sis″to-u-re′ter-o-gram″) [*cysto-* + Gr. *ourētēr* ureter + *gramma* mark] a radiograph of the bladder and ureter.

cystoureterography (sis″to-u-re″ter-og′rah-fe) radiologic examination of the bladder and ureters after the introduction of a radiopaque contrast medium.

cystourethrography (sis″to-u-re-throg′rah-fe) [*cysto-* + Gr. *ourēthra* urethra + *graphein* to record] radiographic examination of the bladder and urethra after the introduction of a radiopaque contrast medium using a syringe inserted into the urethral orifice. This is usually preceded by a cystoscopic examination and drainage of the bladder by catheter. It is useful in diagnosing urethral strictures, dilations, obstructions, diverticula, and, in females, urinary stress incontinence. Voiding studies (often using cineradiography) are usually made.

female c., cystourethrography of the female urethra and bladder, either by the contrast injection method (see above) or by the metallic bead chain method (chain cystourethrography), which is used to investigate stress continence. The chain is passed through the urethra into the bladder, and the bladder is drained and partly filled with a radiopaque contrast medium. Frontal and lateral rest and stress (with the patient performing the Valsalva maneuver) demonstrate the anatomic changes produced by the stress.

cystourethroscope (sis″to-u-re′thro-skōp) [*cysto-* + Gr. *ourēthra* urethra + *skopein* to examine] an instrument for examining the posterior urethra and bladder.

cystyl (sis′til) the divalent acyl radical derived from or relating to cystine.

cyt/o (si′to) [Gr. *kytos* hollow vessel; anything that contains or covers] a word element used in combining form to denote a cell, e.g., cytotrophoblast.

cytarabine (si-tăr′ah-bēn) [USP], cytosine arabinoside (ara-C), a synthetic pyrimidine antimetabolite used as an antiviral drug (see *antiviral agent*) and as a cancer chemotherapeutic drug (see *Appendix A*).

-cyte (sīt) [Gr. *kytos* hollow vessel] a suffix word element to denote a cell, e.g., leukocyte.

cytidine (C) (si′ti-dēn) a nucleoside, cytosine riboside, that is a constituent of RNA and cytidine nucleotides.

cytidine diphosphate (CDP) a nucleoside diphosphate compound that has both a product and a precursor relationship with cytidine triphosphate (CTP). It is thus functionally related to CTP.

cytidine monophosphate see *cytidine-5′-phosphate.*

cytidine-5′-phosphate (CMP) a mononucleotide formed from cytosine, ribose, and phosphoric acid. As a derivative, cytidine monophosphate *N*-acetylneuraminate (an ester of CMP with a sugar), it can act as a sialyl carrier and donor. Also called *cytidylic acid* and *cytidine monophosphate.* See also under *nucleotide.*

cytidine triphosphate (CTP) an energy-rich nucleoside triphosphate analogous to adenosine triphosphate. It is an important regulator molecule of many enzymatic reactions. CTP can form a number of intermediates important for biosynthesis, especially of complex lipids.

cytidylic acid (si″tĭ-dil′ik) see *cytidine-5′-phosphate.*

cytidylyl (si″tĭ-dil′il) a name for cytidylic acid when it is being named as a substituent on some parent group or as an ester.

cytoanalyzer (si″to-an″ah-li′zer) an electronic optical apparatus for the detection of malignant cells in smears. See also *cytometry.*

cytocentrifuge (si″to-sen′trĭ-fūj) a centrifuge used in cytology to concentrate cells from fluid specimens. A microscope slide is covered with a filter paper card having a 6-mm hole; this is covered with a plate having a matching hole and a tube leading to a sample chamber. When the centrifuge is spun, the sample is forced toward the slide. Cells sediment on the slide while fluid is absorbed by the filter paper. The slides are then removed and air-dried for Wright staining or wet-fixed with 95 percent ethanol for Papanicolaou staining. When samples have been prefixed with Saccomanno fixative, they can be air-dried after cytocentrifugation and subsequently stained by the Papanicolaou method.

cytochalasin (si″to-kah-la′sin) one of a number of complex biomolecules that contain both aromatic and aliphatic rings in their molecules and are used in cytologic research. The general effects of cytochalasin on cells are interference with cytoplasmic cleavage (cytokinesis), inhibition of cell movement, and cell enucleation (extrusion of the nucleus from a cell). The specific processes that cytochalasins inhibit include clot retraction (platelets), phagocytosis, platelet aggregation, cardiac muscle contraction, thyroid secretion, and growth hormone release.

cytochemistry (si″to-kem′is-tre) the branch of biochemistry that deals with the identification, localization, and study of the different chemical compounds and their activities within the cell. It includes the study of chromosomes, genes, cellular enzymes, and the complicated reactions of cell growth and reproduction. The term is used particularly to refer to studies that localize a biochemical process in a particular cell structure.

cytochrome (si′to-krōm) [*cyto-* + Gr. *chrōma* color] an electron transfer hemoprotein having a mode of action in which the transfer of a single electron is effected by a reversible valence change of the central iron atom of the heme prosthetic group between the +2 and +3 oxidation states. The heme group can be any tetrapyrrolic chelate of iron, not necessarily the protoheme-containing protoporphyrin IX that is found in hemoglobin.

Cytochromes are classified into four major groups; *a,* in which the heme prosthetic group contains a formyl side-chain; *b,* in which the heme prosthetic group does not contain a formyl side-chain and is not covalently bound to the protein; *c,* in which the heme prosthetic group is covalently bound to the protein; and *d,* in which the heme group has fewer conjugated double bonds than porphyrin, e.g., dihydroporphyrin. Well-established cytochromes are numbered with consecutive subscripts within groups, beginning with no subscript, e.g., cytochrome *c,* cytochrome c_1, and cytochrome c_2. New cytochromes are named according to the absorption maximum (in nanometers) of the α band of the iron(II) form in pyridine, e.g., cytochrome *c*-555. One important cytochrome of the *b* group is usually referred to by the trivial name "cytochrome P_{450}," which refers to the Soret peak of the reduced CO compound.

In eukaryotes, cytochromes are involved in two important functions. Those located in the inner mitochondrial membrane are involved in the electron transfer chain of oxidative phosphorylation. Electrons are transferred from ubiquinone to a complex involving cytochrome *b,* cytochrome c_1, and several iron-sulfur proteins; then to cytochrome *c;* next to a complex referred to as cytochrome *c* oxidase or cytochrome aa_3 (because it contains two cytochromes, *a* and a_3); and finally to molecular oxygen. These electron transfers are coupled to the synthesis of adenosine triphosphate (ATP); each pair of electrons transferred results in the production of three molecules of ATP. The other function involves cytochrome b_5 and cytochrome P_{450}, which are located in the endoplasmic reticulum. These cytochromes are involved in hydroxylation reactions carried out by mixed-function oxidases, enzymes that simultaneously oxidize two substrates. Molecular oxygen is activated by the transfer of an electron from NADH or NADPH via cytochrome b_5 or cytochrome P_{450}; it then attacks the second substrate. Such mixed-function oxidases are found in the liver, adrenal gland, and renal brush border. They are involved in the oxidation of a wide variety of compounds: they can introduce a hydroxy group at the terminal methyl group of an alkane or fatty acid, or at an *O*- or *N*-methyl group of many drugs, or at a ring carbon atom of many steroids and aromatic compounds. Such enzymes are important in the synthesis of steroid hormones and in the detoxification of many drugs and toxic substances.

Bacteria contain a wide variety of cytochromes involved in oxidative phosphorylation. Cytochromes related to eukaryotic cytochrome *c* are widely distributed, but many other cytochromes not found in eukaryotes occur in various species of bacteria.

cytochrome b_5 reductase an enzyme of the oxidoreductase class (NADH:ferricytochrome b_5 oxidoreductase, EC 1.6.2.2) that catalyzes the reaction NADH + H^+ + 2 ferricytochrome b_5 ⇄ NAD^+ + 2 ferrocytochrome b_5. It also catalyzes the reaction NADH + H^+ + 2 methemoglobin ⇄ NAD^+ + 2 hemoglobin. The ferricytochrome reaction is important in the electron transport system of the endoplasmic reticulum for the desaturation of fatty acids. The methemoglobin reaction reduces the amount of methemoglobin in erythrocytes. A hereditary deficiency of the enzyme, known as methemoglobinemia, can cause toxic accumulation of methemoglobin in red blood cells in infants or in adults treated with certain drugs or chemicals. Also called *methemoglobin reductase* and *NADH methemoglobin reductase.*

cytochrome b_5 reductase assays 1. quantitative method for assaying the enzyme present in erythrocytes. The enzyme present in a lysate of cells catalyzes the reduction of the blue dye 2,6-dichlorophenolindophenol by NADH. The decrease in color is measured at 600 nm.

2. quantitative method based on the reduction of methemoglobin (ferrihemoglobin). Ferricyanide is added to a specimen of lysed red cells, resulting in the oxidation of hemoglobin to methemoglobin, which then forms a complex with the ferrocyanide, a product of the reaction. The blue-violet–colored methemoglobin-ferrocyanide complex is easily re-

duced by Fe^{2+}-cytochrome-b_5 to form hemoglobin and Fe^{3+}-cytochrome-b_5. The latter is then reduced by NADH in the reaction catalyzed by the reductase; the Fe^{2+}-cytochrome-b_5 thus formed reduces additional methemoglobin. The reaction can be followed by measuring photometrically at 580 nm the amount of hemoglobin complex remaining.

3. screening procedure using the reduction of 2,6-dichlorophenolindophenol by NADH catalyzed by the enzyme in an erythrocyte lysate. The mixture is spotted on filter paper and the paper is examined for fluorescence (due to NADH), using a long-range ultraviolet lamp over a period of time. If enzyme activity is present, the degree of fluorescence decreases and should disappear after a specific time (compared with that of a controlled specimen). If fluorescence persists after a specified time, this is presumptive evidence for the absence or deficiency of the enzyme. Sodium nitrate is added to the reaction mixture to convert all hemoglobin to hemiglobin, thus preventing reduction of the dye by the hemoglobin.

cytochrome *c* oxidase an enzyme of the oxidoreductase class (ferrocytochrome *c*:oxygen oxidoreductase, EC 1.9.3.1) that transfers electrons from cytochrome *c* to oxygen in the reaction 4 ferrocytochrome $c + O_2 \rightleftarrows$ 4 ferricytochrome $c + 2\ H_2O$. It is a hemoprotein of the cytochrome *a* type and contains copper. Also called *cytochrome oxidase.*

cytochrome oxidase see *cytochrome c oxidase.*

cytoclasis (si-tok′lah-sis) [*cyto-* + Gr. *klasis* a breaking] the destruction of cells.

cytoclastic (si″to-klas′tik) pertaining to, characterized by, or causing the destruction of cells.

cytodiagnosis (si″to-di″ag-no′sis) diagnosis based on examination of cells.

cytogenetic map (si″to-jĕ-net′ik) a diagram that shows the locations of genes on chromosomes by giving their position relative to morphologically distinguishable features such as centromeres, bands, or satellites.

cytogenetics (si″to-jĕ-net′iks) the study of the structure and abnormalities of chromosomes and their effect on the genotype and phenotype of the individual. Chromosome abnormalities are clinically important because of their involvement in birth defects, mental retardation, and spontaneous abortion.

population c., the study of the various cytogenetic (chromosomal) abnormalities, their phenotypic consequences, and the frequency of such abnormalities in the population.

cytokine (si′to-kīn) [*cyto-* + Gr. *kinein* to move] a substance produced by one cell that affects the function of another cell or some chemical reaction. See also *lymphokines.*

cytokinesis (si″to-ki-ne′sis) [*cyto-* + Gr. *kinēsis* motion] the changes that take place in the cytoplasm during mitosis, meiosis, and fertilization; cytoplasmic division. See also *karyokinesis.*

cytolipin H (si′to-lip″in) see *ceramide lactoside.*

cytology (si-tol′o-je) [*cyto-* + *-logy*] the study of cells: their origin, structure, function, and pathology. A number of important laboratory disciplines, including cytogenetics, cytochemistry, quantitative cytology, and clinical or diagnostic cytology, have grown from this science. Clinical cytology is also referred to as cytopathology and is regarded as a division of anatomic pathology.

Cytopathology includes the analysis of cells that are spontaneously exfoliated; mechanically dislodged by irrigation, brushing, or scraping; or forcibly removed by needle aspiration. Cytologic methods have been extensively applied to the detection and diagnosis of cancer. The value of cytology is best recognized for its use in screening females for cervical cancer; it has played a significant role in the reduction of the incidence of and deaths from this form of cancer. Less well known is the fact that cytology provides valuable insights into the interpretation of nonneoplastic disease processes of many organ systems. Knowledge of cellular patterns of disease continues to increase, resulting in an ever-widening field of application for this diagnostic method.

See also *cytometry.*

cytolysis (si-tol′ĭ-sis) [*cyto-* + Gr. *lysis* dissolution] the destruction or dissolution of cells. Usually this connotes a response to external injury, such as that caused by certain chemical or microbial products. Cf. *autolysis.*

cytolysosome (si″to-li′so-sōm) see *autophagic vacuole.*

cytomegalic inclusion disease (CID) disease caused by cytomegalovirus (CMV), so-called because of the characteristic large intranuclear and small intracytoplasmic inclusions that are found in enlarged epithelial and mesenchymal host cells.

The classic form of CID is a congenital disease acquired in utero from the mother. Most infected infants are asymptomatic. Symptomatic newborn infants have hepatosplenomegaly, jaundice, purpura, microcephaly, cerebral calcifications, and chorioretinitis. There may be severe central nervous system sequelae resulting in blindness, deafness, quadriplegia, or mental retardation. Infection also can be transmitted from mother to infant perinatally in passage through the birth canal or from ingestion of the virus present in the mother's milk.

The disease is acquired by children or adults via respiratory droplet transmission or in blood or tissue donation; it can also be a sexually transmitted disease. Acquired CMV infection may be asymptomatic or may be a respiratory infection with pneumonia, cough, petechial rash, splenomegaly, and hepatomegaly. The condition may be life-threatening in physically debilitated or immunocompromised individuals.

cytomegalovirus (CMV) (si″to-meg″ah-lo-vi′rus) [*cyto-* + Gr. *megalos* large + *virus*] a group of double-stranded DNA viruses that belong to the Herpetoviridae family. Cytomegalovirus can cause three types of primary infections: a clinical syndrome in young adults similar to infectious mononucleosis, a subclinical infection with latency in various parts of the body, and a venereal disease resulting in a cervical carrier state. In the venereal disease state a fetus may become infected in utero or during delivery, a condition known as cytomegalic inclusion disease of the newborn. This disease may be fatal, or more frequently is asymptomatic until later in life but results in decreased intelligence. In children or adults with congenital or acquired defects of cellular immunity, CMV infections are frequent and occasionally severe; included are patients with cancer, particularly leukemia and lymphoma, and recipients of organ transplants and multiple blood transfusions. Recipients in these cases who undergo primary and not reactivated infections are more likely to develop symptoms. These include fever, leukopenia, thrombocytopenia, pneumonitis, hepatitis, chorioretinitis, and encephalitis. Death may occur as a result of a variety of complications.

Pathologically, the cytomegalic cell is enlarged and the nucleus distended by an acidophilic inclusion, which is separated from the nuclear membrane by a halo. Infected children secrete the virus into the saliva and urine. Congenital infection does not result in immunologic tolerance, and the newborn has a high titer of IgM and IgG; however, this immune response is not sufficient to prevent the disease.

Laboratory diagnosis of cytomegalovirus is made by isolation of the virus in culture. Specimens of urine, saliva, and milk should be examined. Human fetal fibroblasts should be used for virus isolation. Cytomegalic cells will appear within 4–6 wk. Centrifuged saliva or urine may be examined with Giemsa staining to identify exfoliated cytomegalic cells. Serologically, IgM to cytomegalovirus may be detected by indirect immunofluorescence.

See also *cytomegalic inclusion disease* and *herpesvirus.*

cytometer (si-tom′ĕ-ter) [*cyto-* + Gr. *metron* measure] a device used to count cells visually, such as a hemacytometer, or an automatic cell counter, such as a flow cytometer. See also *blood cell count, cytometry,* and *differential leukocyte count.*

cytometry (si-tom′ĕ-tre) the characterization and measurement of cells and cellular constituents for medical and biologic purposes. Modern cytometric systems rapidly and accurately measure large numbers of cells, thus enabling statistical precision in cell counting, analysis of the distribution of biologic properties among different types of cells, and detection of rarely occurring cells. Such capabilities have led to many clinical and research applications.

Cytometric systems measure one or more properties of individual cells. Typical properties are based on the amount, color, and spatial distribution of dyes used to stain the cells, but they may also include electrical impedance (as in erythrocyte and leukocyte counting) or light scattering, absorbance, and fluorescence of unstained cells.

Staining with colored or fluorescent dyes enhances the visibility of cells and subcellular components such as chromosomes. Although common stains may be used, special procedures in which the dye reacts specifically and quantitatively with particular molecules within the cell are more powerful. Examples include the Feulgen reaction for nuclear DNA, immunologic procedures for particular antigenic proteins, and cytoenzymatic methods for assaying the cellular activities of specific enzymes.

Cytometric systems may be based on flow or image principles. Either type of cytometer quickly generates large amounts of data. Computer processing assists in display and statistical analysis of the data.

In flow cytometers, cells are dispersed in fluid suspension and flow one at a time through a narrow beam of light, typically from a laser. Each cell generates optical signals that are measured and analyzed. The signals can be scattered light, which relates to the mass of the cell, and fluorescence, which relates to the amounts and molecular environments of the dyes used to stain the cell. Tens of thousands of cells are measured in a minute, yielding precise quantitative information about the cell population and enabling rare cells to be detected.

Flow cytometers also may sort cells by means of a droplet generation approach. If measurements associated with a particular cell satisfy some predetermined criteria, the droplet containing that cell is electronically deflected into a separate container. The sorted objects can be cultured, analyzed biochemically, or examined on a microscope slide.

In image cytometry, either cells are spread on microscope slides or histologic tissue sections are prepared; the cells are then imaged and analyzed. An automatic system scans a microscope image in a process resembling television. Dividing the image into a large number of small picture elements, it converts the average light intensity in each element into a digital value; the array of values is a digital image that is stored and analyzed by computer. The first task is to locate individual cells in the image and to separate them from adjacent cells. The cell image is then subdivided into nucleus and cytoplasm, which may be analyzed separately.

Image cytometers measure many different properties for each cell. Geometric properties, such as area, perimeter, and shape, are simple to calculate. The sum of the optical densities of all the picture elements of the cell estimates the amount of stain in the cell; when combined with an appropriate stain, it is a powerful measure of cellular molecular composition. Other properties, however, such as statistical estimates of texture, may be difficult to interpret.

Image cytometry can mimic human perception but with greater precision and objectivity; it also can measure cellular attributes, such as the statistical distribution of color, that do not have a counterpart in human perception. Measurement is slower than in flow cytometers, but more information about the spatial distribution and structural relationship of cellular components may be obtained from each cell. Also, the results are easier to relate to human experience.

The most common medical application of analytic cytology is in the hematology laboratory for automation of erythrocyte, leukocyte, differential leukocyte, and platelet counts. Other medical uses include determining ploidy, proliferative activity, and therapeutic response of tumors; classifying and grading leukemias and monitoring their chemotherapy; automatically prescreening and diagnosing exfoliative cytology specimens; detecting and sorting fetal blood cells in the maternal circulation; analyzing chromosomes and mapping genes; evaluating immunologic responses to transplants and to disease; determining bone marrow activity; and detecting metastatic cells in the circulation.

Also called *analytic cytology.*

BRIAN H. MAYALL, M.D.

cytopathic (si″to-path′ik) [*cyto-* + Gr. *pathos* disease] characterized by pathologic changes in cells.

cytopathic effect (CPE) a term applied to those morphologic changes that occur when a virus replicates in cell culture that are distinctive enough to aid in identification of the virus. Also called cytopathogenic effect.

cytopathogenesis (si″to-path″o-jen′ĕ-sis) the origin of pathologic changes in cells.

cytopathology (si″to-pah-thol′o-je) [*cyto-* + Gr. *pathos* disease + *-logy*] see under *cytology.*

cytopenia (si″to-pe′ne-ah) [*cyto-* + Gr. *penia* poverty] a reduction in the cellular elements of the blood. See also *pancytopenia.*

cytophilic (si″to-fil′ik) [*cyto-* + Gr. *philein* to love] having an affinity for cells, as in cytophilic antibodies.

cytophotometer (si″to-fo-tom′ĕ-ter) [*cyto-* + Gr. *photos* light + *metron* measure] a photometer for measuring localization of organic compounds within cells by measuring the light intensity transmitted through selected stained areas of cytoplasm.

cytophotometry (si″to-fo-tom′e-tre) the quantitative study of the localization of organic compounds within cells by means of microspectrophotometry. An example is the study of changes in a cell's DNA content throughout its life cycle, using the strong ultraviolet absorbance of DNA for quantitation.

cytoplasm (si′to-plasm) [*cyto-* + Gr. *plasma* something formed, from *plassein* to form] the protoplasm of a cell exclusive of that of the nucleus; see under *cell.* Cf. *nucleoplasm.*

cytoplasmic (si″to-plaz′mik) referring to or contained in the cytoplasm.

cytoplasmic membrane see *cell membrane.*

cytoplast (si′to-plast) [*cyto-* + Gr. *plastos* formed] an anucleate cytoplasm. See also *cellular h.* under *hybridization.*

cytosine (si-to-sēn) a nitrogenous pyrimidine base, oxyaminopyrimidine, that is a constituent of DNA and RNA and occurs in some cytidylyl compounds, e.g., CMP, CDP, and CTP. Its complementary purine base is guanosine.

cytosine arabinoside (ara-C) see *cytarabine.*

-cytosis (si-to′sis) [*cyto-* + *-osis* condition] a suffix word element to denote the condition of cells, e.g., leukocytosis.

cytoskeleton (si″to-skel′ĕ-ton) the internal framework of a cell, composed of microtubules and tonofilaments. The number and proportions of these components vary in different cells: tonofilament bundles are prominent in squamous epithelial cells, whereas microtubules are an important component of the axons of nerve cells where, in addtion to providing support, they facilitate axon transport.

cytosol (si′to-sol) the soluble phase of the cytoplasm as obtained by differential centrifugation of a broken cell preparation. Cellular organelles, fragments of plasma membrane, and nonmembranous insoluble components are excluded. Also called *cell sap.*

cytosome (si′to-sōm) [*cyto-* + Gr. *sōma* body] see *multilamellar body.*

cytostatic (si″to-stat′ik) [*cyto-* + Gr. *statikos* bringing to a standstill] 1. suppressing the growth and multiplication of cells.
2. an agent that suppresses cell growth and multiplication.

cytostome (si′to-stōm) [*cyto-* + Gr. *stoma* mouth] the opening in the membrane of certain ciliate protozoa, functioning in the intake of food particles.

cytotechnologist (si″to-tek-nol′o-jist) an allied health professional who specializes in cytologic procedures including the processing and staining of exfoliated cell specimens obtained from the female reproductive tract, oral cavity, or other body cavities. The specimens are examined for evidence of minute abnormalities that may indicate malignant disease, and for signs of inflammation, infection, and changes in hormonal status. Education preparation involves completion of an approved associate degree program. Cytotechnologists certified by the National Certification Agency for Medical Laboratory Personnel are designated CLSP(NCA), Clinical Laboratory Specialist (in cytogenetics); those certified by the Board of Registry of the American Society of Clinical Pathologists are designated CT(ASCP), Cytotechnologist.

cytotoxic (si″to-tok′sik) having a deleterious effect on cells.

cytotoxin (si″to-tok′sin) [*cyto-* + L. *toxicum* poison] a substance that has a specific destructive effect on cells, such as a nephrotoxin. Antibodies may also act as cytotoxins, e.g., in tissue transplantation immune reactions.

cytotrophoblast (si″to-trof′o-blast) [*cyto-* + Gr. *trophē* nutrition + *blastos* germ] in the developing embryo, a single sheet of cuboidal cells that forms the inner layer of the trophoblast. Also called *Langhans' layer.* Cf. *syncytiotrophoblast.*

cytotropic (si″to-trop′ik) [*cyto-* + Gr. *tropos* a turning] attracting cells; possessing an affinity for cells, particularly referring to antibodies that attach to the cell surface.

cytotropic antibody any of a class of antibodies that can bind to a limited number of mediator cells, such as basophils and mast cells, through the Fc segments. These antibodies appear to be mainly of the IgE class and have the ability to induce the release of a variety of vasoconstrictive amines important in immediate hypersensitivity reactions. They may be detected by radioimmunoassay, by assays of their effect on isolated target tissues, or by assays of the release of vasoactive amines from sensitized mediator cells.

cytotropism (si-tot′ro-pizm) 1. cell movement in response to external stimulation.
2. the tendency of viruses, bacteria, drugs, etc., to exert their effect on certain cells of the body.

Cytoxan (CTX) trademark. See *cyclophosphamide.*

Czapek-Dox agar (chah′pek doks) [Friedrich Johann Franz *Czapek,* Czeck botanist, 1868–1921; Arthur Wayland Dox, U.S. chemist, born 1882] one of the standard agar preparations used in medical mycology for the identification of certain fungi. It is a "deficient" medium often used for *Aspergillus* or *Penicillium.*

D

D symbol for *aspartic acid, debye, deuterium, diopter,* electric displacement.

$\bar{D}$ abbrev. See *mean d.* under *dose.*

D- a chemical prefix, written as a small capital D, that specifies the configuration of a stereoisomer by comparing its structure with D-glyceraldehyde (the standard). If there are more than two chiral (asymmetric) carbon atoms (i.e., more than two stereoisomers), the configuration for carbohydrates is determined by the asymmetric carbon most distant from the carbonyl functional group, and the symbol D_g is used; the configuration for amino acids is determined by the asymmetric carbon closest to the carbonyl group, and the symbol D_s is used. The mirror-image stereoisomers (enantiomorphs) are called L-. A more systematic way of specifying configuration known as the *R,S* system is coming into current usage; see under *isomerism.*

D_g- see under D-.

D_L abbrev. See *diffusing capacity of the lungs.*

D_M abbrev. See *membrane component of diffusion.*

D_s- see under D-.

(A-a)D_{N_2} the difference in the nitrogen tensions between mixed alveolar air and mixed arterial blood, equal to –4.0 mmHg in the normal young adult. The difference can be used as a specific indication of the presence of a significant lung volume possessing a low ventilation-perfusion ratio, as it is relatively unaffected by venous admixture or diffusion impairment.

(A-a)D_{O_2} the difference in the partial pressure of oxygen in mixed alveolar gas and mixed arterial blood, normally equal to 5–10 mmHg in the young adult. An increase in this quantity indicates an impairment in gas exchange within the lungs of a nonspecific etiology.

2,4-D one of the chlorophenoxy herbicides, (2,4-dichlorophenoxy)acetic acid; M.W. 221.04. It is used as a defoliant and weed killer. See also *chlorophenoxy herbicides.*

d symbol for atomic orbital with angular momentum quantum number 2, *day, deci-, deoxyribose,* dextro rotatory, relative to rotation of a beam of polarized light (now replaced by (+)), diameter.

***d*-** [abbrev. for *dextro-,* right] a chemical prefix that specifies a stereoisomer by the direction the polarization plane of light is rotated by a solution of the substance.

Δ the Greek capital letter *delta,* used in mathematics to indicate a difference; e.g., ΔE is the change in energy between two states.

δ the Greek lower case letter *delta;* symbol for the heavy chain of IgD.

DAC abbrev. See *digital-to-analog converter.*

dacarbazine (dah-kar′bah-zēn) a cancer chemotherapeutic drug. For more information, see *Appendix A.*

D/A converter abbrev. See *digital-to-analog converter.*

dacrocyte (dak′re-o-sīt″) [*dacro-* + Gr. *kytos* hollow vessel] see *teardrop cell.*

dacry/o (dak′re-o) [Gr. *dakryon* tear] a word element used in combining form to denote a tear, e.g., dacryops.

dacryoaden/o (dak″re-o-ad′ĕ-no) [*dacryo-* + Gr. *adēn* gland] a word element used in combining form to denote the lacrimal gland, e.g., dacryoadenitis.

dacryoadenitis (dak″re-o-ad″ĕ-ni′tis) [*dacryo-* + Gr. *adēn* gland + *-itis* inflammation] inflammation of a lacrimal gland.

dacryoblennorrhea (dak″re-o-blen″o-re′ah) [*dacryo-* + Gr. *blennos* mucus + *rhein* to flow] mucous discharge from the lacrimal apparatus.

dacryocyst/o (dak″re-o-sis′to) [*dacryo-* + Gr. *kystis* sac] a word element used in combining form to denote the lacrimal sac (tear sac), e.g., dacryocystitis.

dacryocystitis (dak″re-o-sis-ti′tis) [*dacryo-* + Gr. *kystis* sac + *-itis* inflammation] inflammation of the lacrimal sac, often secondary to nasal obstruction.

dacryocystography (dak″re-o-sis-tog′rah-fe) the radiographic or scintigraphic examination of the nasolacrimal drainage system to find the location of an obstruction.

In the radiographic examination, an oily radiopaque contrast medium (e.g., iophendylate [Pantopaque] or ethiodized oil [Ethiodol]) is injected into a lacrimal canal, and films are taken in the Caldwell, Waters, and lateral positions, showing the passage of the medium down the nasolacrimal duct.

In the scintigraphic examination, a drop of sodium pertechnetate Tc 99m solution is placed in the eye, and a series of scintigrams are made using a high-resolution micropinhole (1-mm aperture) collimator. Normally, the lacrimal sac and canal and the nasolacrimal sac and duct fill within 40 sec and are cleared within 5 min.

dactinomycin (dak″tĭ-no-mi′sin) see *actinomycin D.*

dactyl/o (dak′til-o) [Gr. *daktylos* a finger] a word element used in combining form to denote fingers or toes, e.g., dactylomegaly.

Dakin's solution (da′kinz) [Henry Drysdale *Dakin,* U.S. chemist, 1880–1952] an aqueous solution, containing sodium hypochlorite and sodium bicarbonate, that is used as a local antibacterial agent and to irrigate wounds.

dalapon (dal′ah-pon) 2,2-dichloropropanoic acid, a moderately toxic herbicide that is strongly irritating to the eyes and skin.

Dalmane (dal′mān) trademark. See *flurazepam hydrochloride.*

dalton (dawl′ton) [John *Dalton,* English chemist and physicist, 1766–1844] see *atomic mass unit.*

Dalton's law [John *Dalton*] stated as: the total pressure exerted by a mixture of nonreacting gases is equal to the sum of the partial pressures of the constituent gases.

dam abbrev. See *decameter.*

dAMP abbrev. See *deoxyadenosine-5′-phosphate.*

damping (dam′ping) a physical force, electric feedback, or other process that reduces (damps out) periodic oscillations of a physical system, such as a meter movement. If, in response to a sudden change in input, the meter overshoots the true value and then oscillates around it with exponentially decaying amplitude, it is said to be underdamped. If the damping force is increased beyond a certain point, the meter will no longer overshoot but will exponentially approach the true value with a time constant that increases with the damping force. The optimal condition is critical damping, the point between overdamping and underdamping at which the meter makes the fastest possible approach to the true value without overshoot.

D and C dilation (of cervix) and curettage (of uterus).

dandy fever (dan′de) see *dengue.*

Dandy-Walker syndrome (dan′de wal′ker) [Walter Edward *Dandy,* U.S. surgeon, 1886–1946; Arthur Earl *Walker,* U.S. surgeon, born 1907] the association of hydrocephalus, a posterior fossa cyst, and hypoplasia of the cerebellar vermis. In many cases the foramen of Magendie is not patent, and in some the foramina of Luschka are also obstructed, but this is not a constant finding. Shunting procedures may be helpful in treatment.

Dane's method see under *keratin staining.*

Dane particle (dān) [D. S. *Dane,* English physician, 20th century] a synonym for the hepatitis B virus, the causative agent of serum hepatitis. The Dane particle contains double-stranded DNA in its core, as well as DNA polymerase. See also *hepatitis.*

dansyl chloride (dan′sil) the acid chloride of 5-(dimethylamino)-1-naphthalenesulfonic acid. It is used in the sequencing and synthesis of polypeptide chains by reacting it with the *N*-terminal group of the chain so that it is blocked from reacting (in a synthesis) or so that the *N*-terminal residue can be identified (after hydrolysis). In histology, it is used as a fluorescent label; it reacts with acidic and basic side-groups of proteins and provides a stable fluorochrome-protein conjugate. See also *immunofluorescence techniques.*

danthron (dan′thron) dihydroxyanthraquinone, an irritant cathartic used as a laxative. It is absorbed in the small intestine and excreted in the large intestine, where it increases peristalsis by irritation of the mucosa.

dantrolene sodium (dan′tro-lēn) a skeletal muscle relaxant used for the management of spasticity due to cerebral palsy, stroke, multiple sclerosis, or spinal cord injury. It blocks muscle contraction by interfering with the release of calcium ions. Common adverse reactions include drowsiness, dizziness, weakness, and diarrhea. Because danrolene can produce serious liver damage and toxic hepatitis, liver function tests should be performed regularly during therapy, together with determination of serum concentrations of bilirubin and the liver enzymes alanine aminotransferase (ALT, SGPT), aspartate aminotransferase (AST, SGOT), and alkaline phosphatase. Trademark, Dantrium.

dapsone (dap′sōn) diaminodiphenyl sulfone, a synthetic drug used in the treatment of leprosy. Dapsone has bacteriostatic activity against *Mycobacterium leprae,* the etiologic agent of leprosy, and interferes with folic acid synthesis by the same mechanism as that of sulfonamides. Mild hemolytic anemia is observed in patients receiving high doses of dapsone. Resistance may occur years after the initiation of therapy. See also *antibacterial agents* and *sulfones.*

Darier's disease (dar-e-āz′) [Ferdinand Jean *Darier,* French dermatologist, 1856–1938] see *k. follicularis* under *keratosis.*

dark current the current produced by applying voltage to a darkened photodetector, i.e., one carefully shielded from all light sources. Most instruments have a method of compensating for this signal so that the readout device registers zero at zero light input. An important parameter for a detector is the change in dark current with ambient temperature change—the less the better.

darkfield microscope see *darkfield m.* under *microscope.*

darkground microscope see *darkfield m.* under *microscope.*

dark reactions the part of photosynthesis that occurs in the dark, the stage in which glucose and other reduced metabolites are produced from CO_2. Dark reactions follow the light reactions, the conversion of light energy to chemical energy in NADPH and ATP.

dark reactivation a type of DNA repair of the damage produced by ultraviolet light or alkylating agents. It involves excision of bases from the damaged strand and resynthesis of the strand, using the complementary strand as a template. See also under *DNA repair.* Cf. *photoreactivation.*

d'Arsonval meter (dar-son-val′) [Jacques Arsene *d'Arsonval,* French physicist, 1851–1940] the type of meter movement used in most electric meters. The pointer is attached to a movable coil, which is suspended between the poles of a horseshoe magnet and connected to a spring. A small current through the coil produces a magnetic field, and the pointer rotates until the torque produced by the spring cancels out the torque produced by the magnetic fields.

dartos (dar′tos) [Gr. "flayed"] a thin layer of nonstriated muscle fibers situated in the superficial fascia of the scrotum and continuous with the superficial fascia of the peritoneum. The dartos contributes to the septum of the scrotum, connecting with the raphe to create two cavities for the testes.

data (da′tah) [L., plural of *datum*] any information, particularly numerical, used for statistical inferences or processed by a computer; any collection of facts on which discussions or inferences are based.

data acquisition system a data processing system in which a central computer gathers and processes data from many remote terminals or automated testing devices.

database (da′tah-bās) a collection of computer files containing the operational data of an organization. The database system includes not only the stored information but also the data sublanguage (DSL), a group of subroutines used to retrieve, update, insert, and delete information; and the database administrator, the person responsible for the integrity of the data and programs.

data display the visual presentation of computer data on a display screen, such as a cathode ray tube (CRT) screen.

data processing operations performed on data,

usually referring to those done by a digital computer.

data reduction the process of transforming a large amount of raw data into a smaller amount of useful data.

Datril (da'tril) trademark. See *acetaminophen.*

daughter (daw'ter) 1. an atom or nucleus resulting from radioactive decay or fission.

2. a cell or cell nucleus resulting from cell division.

daunomycin (daw-no-mi'sin) see *daunorubicin.*

daunorubicin (daw"-no-roo'bi-sin) an anthracycline antibiotic produced in fermentation broths of *Streptomyces peucetius;* M.W. 527.51. The structure consists of a tetracyclic aglycone (daunomycinone) in glycoside linkage with an amino hexose sugar (daunosamin). It binds to DNA and has antineoplastic properties. Also called *daunomycin* and *rubidomycin.* See also *anthracycline cardiotoxicity* and *Appendix A.*

Davainea (da-va'ne-ah) [Casimir Joseph *Davaine,* French physician, 1812–1882] a former name for a genus of tapeworms of the family Davaineidae, now called *Raillietina.*

Davaineidae (da"va-ne'ĭ-de) a family of small tapeworms that are parasitic in humans and birds. The most important genus is *Raillietina.*

Davenport graph (dav'en-port) a graph of plasma bicarbonate concentration (expressed in milliequivalents per liter of plasma) versus plasma pH. Lines of equal P_{CO_2} are calculated from the Henderson-Hasselbalch equation for P_{CO_2} equal to 10, 15, 20, 30, 40, 60, 80, 120, and 160 torr. A buffer curve for normal plasma is also constructed. Comparison of this curve with one constructed from analysis of a patient's blood is used to determine the nature and degree of any deviation in acid-base balance.

Davidsohn differential test (da'vid-sōn) [Israel *Davidsohn,* U.S. pathologist, born 1895] see under *infectious mononucleosis.*

day (d, da) a unit of time equal to 24 hours.

dB abbrev. See *decibel.*

DC abbrev. See *direct current.*

dCMP abbrev. See *deoxycytidine-5'-phosphate.*

DDA a metabolite of DDT that is excreted in the urine and bile in free and conjugated form, and can be detected by gas chromatography.

DDE abbrev. for dichlorodiphenyldichloroethylene, the most common metabolite of DDT in humans. It accumulates in fatty tissue and is detected by thin-layer or gas chromatography.

DDT dichlorodiphenyltrichloroethane, a polychlorinated nondegradable contact insecticide; M.W. 354.50. It was previously used extensively for control of body lice and rat fleas in typhus epidemics, and in control of mosquitoes in malaria epidemics. Its unusual stability results in long-remaining residues in water, soil, and foodstuffs; it is toxic to vertebrates, resulting in damage to the liver and central nervous system, and death. It accumulates in fatty tissues and may do so in large quantities, as the stored DDT is nonreactive. It is thus passed in concentrated amounts through the food chain. Because of its long-lasting toxicity, all production and use in the United States was banned in 1971, except for use by the U.S. Public Health Service in an epidemic situation, or by a physician's prescription for control of body lice. See also *chlorinated hydrocarbon pesticides.*

DDT assays 1. gas chromatography; the method of choice. Serum is extracted with hexane, and the concentrated extract is subjected to gas chromatography using an electron capture detector. Tissues, particularly fat, require Florisil column clean-up of the extract prior to gas chromatography.

2. spot tests of chloroform extracts of suspect stomach contents. The application of alcoholic potassium hydroxide produces colors ranging from rose to bright blue to green to yellow if DDT or its metabolites are present. The subsequent addition of acetone results in a series of colors ranging from bright blue to bright purple to gray to yellow if DDT is present.

DDVP see *dichlorovos.*

de- (de) [L. from, down, off, away] a prefix word element to denote (1) reversal or a reverse process, e.g., decode; (2) removal, e.g., decarboxylation; (3) down or lowering, e.g., decline, decubitus; or (4) away or away from, e.g., deficiency.

deactivation (de"ak-tĭ-va'shun) the process of making or becoming inactive, as removal or loss of radioactivity from previously radioactive material.

deacylase (de-as'il-ās) a hydrolase that catalyzes the removal of an acyl group from a molecule.

deacylate (de-as'il-āt) to remove an acyl group from a molecule.

dead time the time interval after an event has been recorded by a device during which the device cannot respond to another event. In the operation of a Geiger-Müller counter, dead time is the time that elapses after a count before the tube can produce any pulse (as distinguished from the resolving time, the time required before it can produce a pulse large enough to be counted). See also *recovery time* and *resolving time.*

DEAE-cellulose abbrev. See *diethylaminoethylcellulose.*

deafferentation (de-af"er-en-ta'shun) the elimination or interruption of afferent nerve impulses, as by destruction of the afferent pathway.

dealcoholization (de-al"ko-hol-ĭ-za'shun) the removal of alcohol from an object, particularly from tissue specimens during histologic preparation. See also *clearing.*

deallergization (de-al"er-ji-za'shun) the desensitization of an allergic individual to any particular allergen.

deaminase (de-am'ĭ-nās) a sub-subclass of enzymes in the hydrolase class (EC 3.5.4) that catalyze the hydrolysis of carbon-nitrogen bonds in cyclic amidines, e.g., guanine deaminase. The name sometimes is also used more generally for any enzyme that catalyzes the removal of an amino group from an organic compound. Of the clinically important deaminases, only adenosine deaminase is measured in some clinical laboratories.

deaquation (de"ah-kwa'shun) [*de-* + L. *aqua* water] dehydration; the removal of water from anything.

death (deth) the irreversible cessation of normal life processes. The exact moment of biologic death is difficult to define; for legal purposes, it is usually defined as the abatement of detectable brain activity along with the cessation of other body functions. See also *brain death syndrome.*

crib d., see *sudden infant death syndrome.*

fetal d., the death of a fetus in utero.

death fever see *kala-azar* and *L. donovani* under *Leishmania.*

debranching enzyme (de-branch′ing) see *amylo-1,6-glucosidase.*

débridement (da-brēd′maw) [Fr.] the surgical removal of dead tissue and any foreign matter, often performed when anaerobic bacteria (e.g., *Clostridium perfringens*) initiate an infection. This procedure increases the concentration of oxygen in the wound, thereby inhibiting growth of anaerobes and killing them.

debris (dĕ-bre′) [Fr.] accumulated functionless fragments of worn-out material, such as degenerating cells and tissue in an area of acute inflammation.

debubbling (de-bub′ling) a process of removing air bubbles from a continuous-flow system. In an AutoAnalyzer the debubbler removes bubbles from the sample stream before it enters the cuvet in the colorimeter. The debubbler unit consists of an inverted glass "T," which is placed near the inlet of the cuvet. This allows air bubbles to rise and to flow into the "waste" stream, along with some portion of the reagent, while the remaining bubble-free volume is pumped into the cuvet and analyzed. Bubbles must be removed because their presence in the reaction stream gives rise to an irregular electric signal and thus a "noisy" record.

debug (de-bug′) to find and correct the errors in a computer program or electronic circuit.

debye (D) (dĕ-bi′) [Peter Joseph Wilhelm *Debye,* Dutch physicist, 1884–1966] a unit of electric dipole moment equal to 10^{-18} statcoulomb-centimeter (StatC·cm) or 3.3356×10^{-30} coulomb-meter (C·m).

deca- (dek′ah) [Gr. *deka* ten] 1. a combining form meaning 10.

2. (abbrev. da), a prefix attached to units of measurement to make a unit that is equal to 10 of the basic units.

decalcification (de-kal″sĭ-fĭ-ka′shun) 1. the process of loss of calcium from a bone or tooth.

2. in histology, the removal of calcium from a tissue by treating the material with a decalcifying agent. The calcium is freed from its salts and can then be washed out of the tissue. Common decalcifying agents include formic acid, nitric acid, trichloracetic acid, and EDTA. The tissue is immersed in a solution of the decalcifying agent until the process is completed, usually one to several days; the decalcification can be monitored by testing the flexibility of the tissue, by x-raying it, or by testing the solution for the presence of calcium with ammonium oxalate.

decameter (dam) (dek′ah-me″ter) a unit of length equal to 10 meters (10 m).

decamethonium bromide (dek″ah-mĕ-tho′ne-um) a quaternary ammonium compound used as a skeletal muscle relaxant and adjunct to surgical anesthesia. Like succinylcholine, it acts by depolarizing the motor end-plate.

decanoic acid (dek″ah-no′ik) see *capric acid.*

decantation (de″kan-ta′shun) [*de-* + L. *canthus* rim of a vessel] the pouring of a clear supernatant liquid from a container, leaving the sediment or precipitate.

decarboxylase (de″kar-bok′sĭ-lās) carboxy-lyase (EC 4.1.1), a general term for a large number of enzymes of the lyase class, which catalyze the removal of a carboxyl group (—COOH) from an organic compound to liberate carbon dioxide (CO_2); e.g., the reaction aspartate → alanine + CO_2 is catalyzed by the enzyme aspartate decarboxylase. In the clinical microbiology laboratory, lysine and ornithine decarboxylase reactions are used to differentiate among members of Enterobacteriaceae and other closely related gram-negative bacilli. In a positive test, the decarboxylase converts the substrate to a product that raises the pH of the medium; the color of the indicator (bromcresol purple) is changed from yellow to violet or purple.

De Castro's fluid (de kas′trōz) a solution of chloral hydrate, distilled water, ethanol, and nitric acid, used as a decalcifying agent.

decay (de-ka′) [*de-* + L. *cadere* to fall] the change of one nuclide into another nuclide or two nuclides, which may also be radioactive. See also the specific types of decay (e.g., *alpha decay, beta decay, radioactive decay*), *electron capture, fission,* and *isomeric transition.*

decay coefficient see *decay constant.*

decay constant (λ) the probability per unit time that a radionuclide will decay. Each radioactive species has a characteristic decay constant. During a time period (T), the fraction $e^{\lambda T}$ decays. Also called *decay coefficient, decay rate, disintegration constant,* and *radioactive constant.*

decay mode one of several types of decay that a particular radionuclide can undergo.

decay product a nuclide, which may be stable or radioactive, that results from the radioactive decay of a radionuclide. It is formed either directly or as the result of successive transformations in a radioactive series.

decay rate see *decay constant.*

decay scheme a chart of a parent radionuclide that shows its half-life, each decay mode, each daughter nuclide, and the type, energy, and abundance of each emitted radiation. The chart may be extended by treating radioactive daughters in the same way.

deceration (de″sĕ-ra′shun) [*de-* + L. *cera* wax] see *deparaffinization.*

decerebrate (de-ser′ĕ-brāt) 1. to eliminate cerebral function by transecting the brain stem or by ligating the common carotid arteries and the basilar artery.

2. an animal so prepared.

3. a person with brain damage that results in neurologic signs similar to those of a decerebrate animal.

deci- (d) (des′i) [L. *decem* ten] a prefix attached to units of measurement to make a unit that is one-tenth of the basic unit.

decibel (dB) (des′ĭ-bel) one-tenth of a bel, a unit of relative power intensity used for electric or acoustic power. It is equal to 10 times the base 10 logarithm of the ratio of power to some reference power; i.e., the decibel level is given by the formula $10 \log_{10}(P / P_0)$, where P is the power and P_0 is the reference power.

For acoustic measurements, the reference power is that of a wave having a sound pressure level (the root-mean-square pressure) of 2×10^{-4} dyn/cm^2. For electric power, the reference level is usually specified, e.g., decibels above 1 kilowatt (dBk), decibels above 1 watt (dBW), or decibels above 1 milliwatt (dBm).

decidua (de-sid′u-ah) [L., from *deciduus* falling off] the uterine mucosa after it undergoes distinctive epithelioid transformation of the endometrial stromal cells during pregnancy. The process of decidualization begins soon after conception and is completed by the end of the first month of gestation.

basal d., the decidual lining of the pregnant uterus deep to the developing embryo. It forms a compact layer adherent to the chorion frondosum and constitutes the maternal portion of the developing placenta.

capsular d., the decidual layer that covers the developing embryonic sac other than the area deep to the embryo. It covers the chorion laeve and, with expansion of the amniotic cavity, fuses with the parietal decidua.

parietal d., the decidua that lines the pregnant uterus other than in the area occupied by the developing embryo. Cf. *pseudodecidua.*

decidual (de-sid′u-al) pertaining to the decidua.

decidual cells swollen epithelioid endometrial stromal cells that develop during pregnancy. Similar transformation of endometrial stromal cells may be induced by exogenous estrogen and progesterone administration.

decidual membrane a term applied to a membrane of decidualized secretory endometrium. It is produced by separation of the superficial layer of decidua, including the compact and a portion of the spongy zones, from the underlying basal layer of decidua. The saclike membrane formed conforms to the contour of the uterine cavity. When disintegration does not occur during delivery, it may be expelled as a "decidual cast."

deciduous teeth (de-sid′u-us) [L. *deciduus,* from *decidere* to fall off] the temporary or "milk" teeth of mammals; in humans, there are 20 deciduous teeth, 4 incisors, 2 canines, and 4 molars in each jaw, which are shed and replaced with permanent teeth.

decigram (dg) (des′ĭ-gram) a unit of mass equal to one-tenth of a gram (10^{-1} g).

decile (des′īl) in statistics, one of the values that divides a sample or population of measurements into 10 equal parts; e.g., for a set of white blood counts, 30 percent will score below the third decile. See also *percentile* and *quantile.*

deciliter (dl) (des′ĭ-le″ter) a unit of volume equal to one-tenth of a liter or 100 milliliters.

decimal (dec′ĭ-mal) 1. pertaining to the base 10 number system or to the number 10.

2. a number, particularly a fractional one, represented in decimal form.

decimal reduction time (D) a term used in heat sterilization to denote the time required for a 10-fold reduction of viability of cells. It is useful in calculating the time required to sterilize bacterial suspensions. Also called *D value.*

decimeter (dm) (des′ĭ-me″ter) a unit of length equal to one-tenth of a meter (10^{-1} m).

decision table in computer programming, a table that specifies every contingency that can occur at a particular point in the program and the correct action to be taken.

decode (de-kōd′) to translate coded data into a more understandable form.

decoder (de-ko′der) 1. a device that converts coded data into a more useful form.

2. a circuit in the control unit of a digital computer that interprets the operation code of an instruction.

decolorize (de-kul′or-īz) 1. the removal of dye from tissue sections. Cf. *differentiation.*

2. the removal of color; bleaching.

decompensation (de″kom-pen-sa′shun) [*de-* + L. *compensare* to compensate] the failure of an organ or organ system to maintain homeostasis and dynamic equilibrium. Types of decompensation include cardiac (failure to maintain adequate circulation), renal (failure to maintain filtration and purification mechanisms), and pulmonary (failure to maintain adequate oxygenation).

decomposition potential (de″kom-po-zish′un) the voltage across an electrochemical cell at which current flows owing to electrolysis of water. See also *polarography.*

decompression (de″kom-presh′un) 1. return to normal environmental pressure after exposure to greatly increased pressure, as occurs in divers and underwater workers.

2. a manipulative or surgical procedure performed to decrease the pressure within or exerted on an organ or structure (e.g., colonic or cerebral decompression).

decompression sickness a disorder resulting from a rapid decrease in surrounding pressure (e.g., ascent from under water or to high altitude) that leads to the formation of gas bubbles (primarily nitrogen) in the tissues and blood vessels. As a person moves to an area of lower pressure, the respiratory blood gases come out of solution as minute bubbles. Oxygen and carbon dioxide are rapidly reabsorbed, but nitrogen, which has low solubility, accumulates in tissues, including joints, muscles, tendons, and ligaments. Clinically, there is a gradual (0.5–6 hr) onset of symptoms: pain in the major joints (commonly known as the "bends") is the most common. The skin may itch. In severe cases, there is neurologic impairment (including weakness, paralysis, hypesthesia, confusion, visual defects, and coma) and pulmonary involvement (with dyspnea, cough, and cyanosis, due to massive bubble embolism into the pulmonary arteries). Long-term sequelae of decompression sickness include aseptic bone necrosis and permanent neurologic deficits.

Treatment includes recompression to an atmospheric pressure greater than that of exposure and a slow return to normal ambient pressure. Divers can prevent decompression sickness by observing established limits for the depth and length of their dives, and controlling their rate of ascent.

Also called *bends* (when there is muscle and joint involvement) and *caisson disease.*

decontamination (de″kon-tam″ĭ-na′shun) a process whereby equipment, laboratory surfaces, or materials containing infectious or potentially infectious agents or radioactive materials are rendered harmless. Decontamination may include the use of incinerators, autoclaves, or disinfectants.

decortication (de″kor-tĭ-ka′shun) [L. *decorticare* to remove bark] the surgical removal of the outer layer from an organ or structure to free it from rigid encasement.

decoy cell (de′koi) an exfoliated superficial cell of the transitional epithelium of the urinary bladder that, through degenerative changes, has enlarged and become hyperchromatic. In cytologic preparations its appearance may give a mistaken impression of malignancy.

decrement (dek′rĕ-ment) [L. *decrementum*] subtraction or decrease; the amount by which a quantity is decreased.

decrementing response (dek″rĕ-ment′ing) utilizing supramaximal stimuli to a motor nerve, the decrease in amplitude of successive evoked compound muscle action potentials (M waves). During repetitive, low-frequency stimulation (usually 2 or 3 Hz), a decrement in amplitude greater than 10 percent of the first evoked potential indicates an abnormality in neuromuscular transmission. Cf. *incrementing response.*

decubitus (de-ku′bĭ-tus), pl. *decubiti* [L. "a lying down"] 1. a position assumed in lying down. In radiography, the term is applied only to horizontal ray projections. Cf. *recumbent.*

2. decubitus ulcer; see under *ulcer.*

dorsal d., lying on the back. Also called *supine.*

left lateral d., lying on the left side.

right lateral d., lying on the right side.

ventral d., lying face down. Also called *prone.*

decussate (de-kus′āt) [L. *decussare* to cross in the form of an X] 1. to cross or intersect in the form of the letter X.

2. pertaining to a decussation, an X-shaped crossing.

decussation (de″kus-sa′shun) [L. *decussatio* crossing over] the crossing of similar parts or structures in the form of an X.

decussation of the pyramids the crossing over of approximately three-quarters of the corticospinal fibers in the medulla oblongata; this generally occurs in the lower part of the anterior median fissure and is complete by the medullary-spinal junction.

deefferented states (de-ef′er-ent″ed) see *ventral pontine syndrome.*

DEEG abbrev. See *depth electroencephalogram* and *depth electrography.*

deep sleep see *s. stages* under *sleep.*

deerfly (dēr′fli) a common name for *Chrysops discalis,* which is known to transmit tularemia to humans. See also *Chrysops* and *tularemia.*

defecation (def″ĕ-ka′shun) [L. *defaecare* to cleanse of dregs] the expulsion of fecal matter from the rectum, brought about by reflex contraction of the rectum and relaxation of the internal (involuntary) and external (voluntary) anal sphincters.

defecography (def″ĕ-kog′rah-fe) radiologic examination, using cineradiography and spot films, of the rectum and anal canal during defecation following administration of a barium enema. It is used to evaluate fecal incontinence and abnormalities of colonic emptying.

defect (de′fekt) an imperfection, failure, or absence.

acquired d., an imperfection that arises secondarily after birth.

atrial septal d., see *atrial septal defect.*

congenital d., birth defect; a structural or chemical imperfection present at birth.

neural tube d., see *neural tube defect.*

septal d., see *septal defect.*

ventricular septal d., see *ventricular septal defect.*

defective virus a virus that is genetically defective and thus does not produce infectious progeny. These viruses may be helped to produce infectious progeny by coinfection with a helper virus, which is usually, but not necessarily, a related virus.

deferoxamine mesylate (dĕ″fer-oks′ah-mēn) [USP], an iron-chelating agent isolated from *Streptomyces pilosus.* It forms a stable complex with iron that is readily soluble in water, and is excreted primarily in the urine but also in the feces.

Deferoxamine is used to remove iron in the treatment of acute iron intoxication and chronic iron overload due to transfusion-dependent anemias, such as thalassemia major and aplastic anemia, and in the treatment of iron overload in patients with hemachromatosis who do not tolerate phlebotomy, the treatment of choice. It is also used to evaluate iron overload; a standard amount of deferoxamine removes larger amounts of iron when stores are high, and lesser amounts when they are low.

Also called *desferrioxamine.*

defibrillation (de′fib″rĭ-la′shun) the termination of ventricular fibrillation by delivery of an electrical shock (of up to 400 J of energy) directly to the heart, or transthoracically through use of paddle electrodes. Cf. *cardioversion.*

defibrillator (de-fib′rĭ-la″tor) a capacitor-discharge type of condenser that, when discharged, delivers a direct-current shock to the heart.

defibrination (de-fi″brĭ-na′shun) the removal of fibrin from the blood. Fibrin is removed from fresh whole blood samples by gently swirling the blood in a flask with glass beads. The red cells remain intact in the plasma, which is unchanged except for the removal of the fibrin. Defibrinated blood is used in the autohemolysin, Ham, and sucrose hemolysis tests, although heparinized blood can be substituted with identical results.

defibrination syndrome see *disseminated intravascular coagulation.*

deficiency (de-fish′en-se) 1. a lack or deficit.

2. in genetics, a deletion in a chromosome, sometimes occurring because of a translocation or inversion.

3. in immunology, referring to a functional defect in or lack of some element of host defense.

4. a dietary lack relating to the amount or quality of protein, essential amino acids or fatty acids, vitamins, or minerals.

5. reduced or absent enzyme activity due either to gene deletion or to the production of a defective enzyme.

deficit (def′ĭ-sit) a lack or deficiency. See also *pulse deficit.*

definition (def″ĭ-nish′un) the quality of sharpness of outline in an image, photograph, or radiograph.

deflection (de-flek′shun) 1. the bending of the electron beam in a cathode ray tube (CRT) by electrostatic or electromagnetic fields.

2. the movement of the pointer of a meter in response to an input.

deflection signal either of the signals that control the position of the dot on the face of a cathode ray tube. The horizontal dimension is controlled by the

X deflection signal, the vertical by the Y-deflection signal.

defoliant (de-fol′e-ant) a herbicide that kills plants by removing the leaves.

deformation (de″for-ma′shun) an abnormality of shape in a normally differentiated structure usually effected by extrinsic forces, e.g., an abnormal skull shape from prolonged in utero positional abnormalities.

deformity (de-for′mĭ-te) a congenital anomaly that consists of abnormal shaping of an initially correctly formed structure. It is usually due to an extrinsic process, e.g., the peculiar facies of Potter's syndrome, which results from a lack of amniotic fluid with consequent prolonged molding of the head by the uterus.

De Galantha's method for urates (de gal-an′thaz) a procedure for determining the presence of uric and urate crystals in tissue. Tissue must be fixed in alcohol to prevent the crystals from dissolving. Sections are placed in a 20 percent silver nitrate solution in bright sunlight until the urates appear reddish-brown. They are then reduced in a hot solution containing gelatin, hydroquinone, and silver nitrate until the urates are black; rinsed in hot water to remove the developer; and dehydrated.

degenerate code [L. *degenerare* to depart from] a code in which more than one code element stands for the same message element. The genetic code is degenerate; most of the amino acids are coded for by several different codons; e.g., UAU and UAC code for tyrosine.

degenerating myelin demonstration histologic methods for demonstrating the myelin degeneration that occurs when a nerve cell or its axon is damaged. In this process the complex lipids of the myelin sheath are broken down into neutral fats or fatty acids and removed by phagocytosis.

In the intermediate stage of degeneration (1–8 wk after the injury), the neutral fats are stained bright red with oil red O, whereas normal myelin stains pale orange-yellow. In the Marchi method, formalin-fixed tissue is oxidized in potassium dichromate solution and then stained in osmic acid. Degenerating myelin is not fully oxidized because of the oleic acid content, and stains black, whereas normal myelin is unstained.

Under a polarizing microscope, normal myelin is birefringent in formalin-fixed frozen sections, but degenerating myelin is isotropic.

degeneration (de-jen″er-a′shun) [L. *degeneratio*] deterioration; a change in quality from a more desirable to a less desirable state, particularly in reference to performing a biologic role. Some forms of cellular degeneration are characterized by the infiltration or accumulation of compounds such as amyloid or fat.

amyloid d., see *amyloidosis.*

axonal d., the reaction of a nerve cell to injury to its axon: it is characterized by central chromatolysis and eccentric displacement of the nucleus.

ballooning d., a form of hepatic cell degeneration in which the cell is swollen and the cytoplasm exhibits a granular appearance.

cloudy swelling d., see *cloudy swelling.*

Crooke's hyaline d., see *Crooke's hyaline change.*

fatty d., see *fatty change.*

feathery d., focal degeneration of isolated hepatic cells associated with cholestasis. Degenerating cells are swollen and contain scant cytoplasm arranged in thin strands.

fibrinous d., necrosis with the deposition of fibrin within a tissue.

hepatolenticular d., see *Wilson's disease.*

hyaline d., a regressive cellular change in which the cytoplasm takes on a homogeneous, glassy, eosinophilic appearance. The term is also used loosely to describe the histologic appearance of affected tissues. Also called hyalinosis and vitreous degeneration.

subacute combined d. of spinal cord, degeneration of the posterior and lateral columns of the spinal cord, caused by vitamin B_{12} deficiency. It is a progressive disease associated with pernicious anemia. Symptoms may include paresthesias, ataxia, unsteadiness of gait, and emotional disorders.

wallerian d., see *wallerian* degeneration.

degenerative index a quantitative evaluation of changes in the white blood cells such as toxic granulation, cytoplasmic vacuoles, pyknotic nuclear areas, and diffuse cytoplasmic basophilia.

deglutition (deg″loo-tish′un) [L. *deglutitio,* from *deglutire* to swallow] the act of swallowing.

deglycerolization (de-glis″er-ol-ĭ-za′shun) a technique used in blood banking to remove the glycerol cryoprotective medium in which frozen red blood cells are suspended. Thawed red blood cells are equilibrated with a hypertonic saline solution to remove intracellular glycerol, and then washed in progressively lowered concentrations of sodium chloride.

degradation (deg″-rah-da′shun) the breakdown of a chemical compound, e.g., a protein or other polymer, into component compounds.

degranulation (de-gran″u-la′shun) the release of granules from a cell or of the enzymatic contents from lysosomes.

degree (de-gre′) 1. an academic title awarded by a college or university.

2. a unit of measure of temperature—the centigrade or Celsius degree (°C), the Fahrenheit degree (°F), or the Kelvin degree (K). The Kelvin degree is now called the kelvin (K) and is used like other units of measurement.

3. a unit of measure of arcs and angles, 1/360 of a full circle.

degrees of freedom (df) a statistical parameter. See under *chi-square distribution, F distribution,* and *t distribution.*

dehiscence (de-his′ens) [L. *dehiscere* to gape] a splitting open; a split or gap in a structure, e.g., in a surgical incision.

dehydratase (de-hi′drah-tās″) one of the group of enzymes referred to as hydro-lyases (EC 4.2.1) that catalyze the removal of water from compounds containing a hydroxyl, leaving double bonds. Examples include carbonic anhydrase, enolase, fumarase, and serine dehydratase. Also called *anhydrase,* hydrase, and *hydratase.*

dehydrate (de-hi′drāt) to remove water from a substance.

dehydrated alcohol (de-hi′drāt-ed) see *absolute alcohol.*

dehydration (de″hi-dra′shun) [*de-* + Gr. *hydōr* water] 1. the removal of water from a substance.

2. the loss of body water in excess of intake. This may occur by decreased intake or increased loss, as

caused by sweating, diarrhea, or polyuria (as in uncontrolled diabetes). The acute effect is a decrease in plasma volume, which limits circulatory transport functions. Also called *anhydration, deaquation,* and hypohydration.

3. in histology, the process of removing water from tissue specimens after they have been fixed and washed so that they can be embedded in paraffin or another medium. Most dehydrating agents are immiscible in paraffin and must be cleared before embedding. Ethyl or isopropyl alcohol is routinely used. Acetone is also widely used and acts more quickly than alcohol.

Specimens are placed in successive baths, starting with about 75 percent ethanol (50 percent for delicate tissues) and finishing with several changes of absolute ethanol. Each bath is 10 times the volume of the specimen; five or six steps each requiring 1 hr are followed.

Ethylene glycol monoethyl ether (Cellosolve) may be used for dehydration and to store tissue. Dioxane and tetrahydrofuran are miscible in both water and paraffin and do not need to be cleared. Both are somewhat toxic, however, and are not used routinely.

dehydro- (de-hi′dro) a prefix word element in organic chemistry to denote a compound formed by (conceptual) subtraction of hydrogen from the reference compound. Although the number of hydrogen atoms removed and the sites from which they are removed should be specified (as in 7,8-didehydro-), they usually are not (as in dehydroascorbic acid and dehydrocholic acid). Often, the term refers to the removal of hydrogen from two adjacent atoms, leaving a double bond, e.g., 7-dehydrocholesterol.

dehydroascorbic acid (de-hi″dro-as-kor′bik) the oxidized form of ascorbic acid, produced when ascorbic acid is oxidized by air, especially in the presence of certain enzymes, metal ions, and heat. It is biologically active (antiscorbutic) because it can be reduced to ascorbic acid in the body. See also *ascorbic acid assays.*

dehydrobilirubin (de-hi″dro-bil″ĭ-roo′bin) see *biliverdin.*

dehydrocholic acid (de-hi″dro-ko′lik) [USP], a synthetic bile acid used as a physiologic laxative.

dehydrogenase (de-hi′dro-jen-ās) a large group of enzymes that catalyze oxidation-reduction reactions involving the transfer of hydrogen from a compound to a coenzyme or vice versa (e.g., NAD/NADH, NADP/NADPH). A specific dehydrogenase is named according to the compound acted on, e.g., isocitrate dehydrogenase and succinate dehydrogenase.

dehydrogenate (de-hi′dro-jen-āt) to remove hydrogen.

dehydrogenation (de-hi″dro-jen-a′shun) the removal of hydrogen from a substrate by its reaction with a hydrogen acceptor; formally, this reaction is an oxidation.

deionization (de-i″on-ĭ-za′shun) the removal of ions from solutions, especially by use of ion-exchange resins.

Dejerine-Sottas disease (deh″zher-ēn′ sot′tahz) [Joseph Jules *Dejerine,* French neurologist, 1849–1917; Jules *Sottas,* French neurologist, 1866–1943] a progressive distal neuropathy, transmitted as an autosomal recessive trait, that has its onset in childhood and manifests itself by weakness, distal muscle atrophy, loss of tendon reflexes, and distal loss of sensation. See also *peripheral n.* under *neuropathy.*

Delaney clause (de-la′ne) a section of the Food Additive Amendment of 1958 that provides that food additives that have been shown to cause cancer in any animal must be banned from interstate commerce.

delay the time required for a signal to pass through an electric circuit or between two points in space.

delay circuit an electric circuit that passes a signal pulse with a specified time delay. Delay circuits can be designed with either analog or digital components.

delayed hypersensitivity (DH) the cell-mediated response of a host to an antigen to which it has previously been exposed. There is a delayed response peaking at 24–48 hr after the intradermal injection of antigen, which is manifested by erythema and induration. The degree of induration at 48 hr is a measure of the delayed hypersensitivity response to that antigen. DH is not dependent on humoral antibody. The response requires specific recognition of the antigen by specific T lymphocytes, which are stimulated to produce lymphokines. Migration-inhibition factor (MIF) and other lymphokines attract mononuclear cells (monocytes and macrophages) to the area. This accounts for the histologic finding of mononuclear cell infiltration at the site of antigen injection.

For a delayed hypersensitivity response to give a positive reaction, a three-step process must occur: (1) a T lymphocyte specific for the antigen must recognize the antigen, (2) it must respond with lymphokine production, and (3) macrophages must respond to the lymphokine production and migrate to the site of inoculation. A negative delayed hypersensitivity reaction to an antigen can have several meanings: that the antigen was not recognized by the host because of either no prior exposure or inadequate sensitization, that the T lymphocyte recognized the antigen but did not produce lymphokines, or that the macrophage did not respond to the lymphokine production or did not respond in a normal manner.

The primary method of assessing DH reactions is the skin test. Antigens of a bacterium, fungus, or virus are injected intradermally, or chemically reactive compounds are applied to the skin. An inflammatory reaction 24–48 hr later indicates delayed hypersensitivity. Inability to respond to a battery of common antigens (anergy) can be further investigated by in vitro tests of the three steps of the DH process: lymphocyte transformation with blastogenesis, production and release of lymphokines by lymphocytes, and response of monocytes to lymphokines. In the first test, tritiated thymidine incorporation is measured in isolated lymphocytes after exposure to a specific antigen; the increase in radioactive counts per minute over control cultures without antigen is a measure of activation. In the second, supernatants from an antigen-lymphocyte culture can be utilized in assays for MIF and other lymphokines to determine if lymphocytes produce lymphokines to that antigen. In the third, monocytes are isolated from individuals to see whether they respond to the lymphokines produced. If any of the in vitro experiments are abnormal, but the individual still has a strong DH skin test, the skin test is always taken as a measure of appropriate cell-mediated immunity, as it combines all elements of the immune response.

Contact dermatitis is a common clinical example of delayed hypersensitivity reaction. Often, the offending chemical is a low-molecular-weight molecule that acts as a hapten, such as the test agent dinitrochlorobenzene (DNCB). The molecule binds to some protein in the skin, and the hapten-protein conjugate is antigenic. Sensitization can be transferred by lymphoid cells but not by serum. Contact dermatitis from poison ivy or oak is also a DH phenomenon.

A dialyzable material obtained from sensitized lymphocytes called transfer factor can transfer DH to another host. Whether this factor transfers antigenic specificity is controversial. The disease in which transfer factor has been used the most is chronic mucocutaneous candidiasis, although beneficial results are sporadic and not conclusive.

See also *antigen, lymphocyte,* and *transfer factor.* Cf. *immediate hypersensitivity.*

GERALD B. KOLSKI, M.D., PH.D.

delay line an electronic circuit having an output identical to the input except for being delayed by a fixed time interval. A transmission line can be used as a delay line, the delay being the time it takes a signal to propagate along the cable.

deletion (de-le′shun) 1. a chromosomal aberration in which part of a chromosome is lost, as in cri du chat syndrome, in which there is a deletion of part of the short arm of chromosome 5 (5p-)

2. see *antigenic deletion.*

deletion theory an early theory proposed by cancer researchers, which states that as neoplasms grow, they generally advance to more malignant and anaplastic forms, both in their histologic features and in their metabolic activity. Specifically, it was held that as neoplasms become more malignant, they revert to more primitive energy-producing systems (glycolysis) and exhibit less variation in their enzyme patterns. It was suggested that both phenomena occurred as the result of deletions of complex cellular organelles in dividing cells, with daughter cells reverting to less complex, less well differentiated states. Although this theory may be applicable to certain aspects of carcinogenesis, the alteration of DNA is now thought to be the most important basic initiating factor in carcinogenesis.

deliquescence (del″ĭ-kwes′ens) [L. *deliquescere* to grow moist] the property of certain solids to absorb sufficient moisture from the air to become liquid (forming an aqueous solution).

deliquescent (del″ĭ-kwes′ent) exhibiting deliquescence.

delirium (de-lir′e-um), pl. *deliria* [*de-* + L. *lira* furrow or track] a syndrome of acute onset characterized by disorientation, inability to reason with clarity and speed, inattentiveness, vivid hallucinations, restlessness, tremulousness, and increased autonomic nervous system activity that may lead to dilated pupils, conjunctival injection, rapid pulse, elevated temperature, sweating, and low urine output. Depending on the cause, the symptoms show a high degree of variability within and among individuals, and may persist for a period of from a few hours to 5 da. The mildest form, quiet delirium or hypokinetic delirium, in which motor or autonomic overactivity is lacking, often accompanies febrile disease. The more florid form is usually seen during withdrawal from chronic intoxication by a depressant agent such as alcohol. The most severe form, delirium tremens, has a mortality rate of 15 percent.

The electroencephalogram (EEG) obtained from delirious individuals may appear to show no abnormality, but in fact there is usually significant slowing of the basic rhythm. The dominant alpha rhythm of the waking state may be replaced by activity in the theta or delta ranges. This generalized slowing of the EEG subsides with the other symptoms. Focal activity indicating lesions within the central nervous system may also be present.

A destructive lesion in the brain is only one of many causes of delirium. The condition may complicate any medical or surgical illness, a variety of metabolic or toxic disorders, drug intoxication and withdrawal states, posttraumatic disorders, and sensory deprivation.

The care of the delirious individual should include protection against injury while the primary medical disease is controlled. Drugs that might be causing the disorder should be withdrawn unless the delirium is thought to represent a withdrawal effect in itself. Sedation may be necessary. Efforts should also be made to reduce fear and hallucinations by placing the patient in a familiar, lighted room and reducing sensory isolation. Vital signs must be monitored frequently, especially during the acute stage. Most delirious patients recover following appropriate care.

Delphian node (del′fe-an) [*Delphi,* a town of ancient Greece, seat of an oracle of Apollo] a lymph node encased in the fascia anterior to the thyroid isthmus, so called because it is exposed first at surgery and, if diseased, is indicative of disease in the thyroid gland.

delta (Δ, δ) (del′tah) the fourth letter of the *Greek alphabet.*

delta activity in electroencephalography, activity of a frequency less than 4 Hz. This is a normal finding during wakefulness and sleep in infants and during sleep in older individuals, but is an abnormal finding in awake adults. Also called delta rhythm.

intermittent rhythmic d. a., paroxysmal delta activity of relatively constant frequency that occurs synchronously over both cerebral hemispheres. It is best recorded over the occipital cortex in children and over the frontal cortex in adults. This activity is enhanced during drowsiness or by hyperventilation, and can be attenuated by attention. It probably relates to dysfunction of midline subcortical centers of the brain that influence activity of the cerebral cortex.

polymorphic d. a., continuous irregular delta activity that varies in amplitude and duration; it persists during sleep and shows no change with the physiologic state of the individual. This activity occurs with metabolic disorders, migraine, subcortical white matter encephalopathies, destructive cerebral lesions involving subcortical white matter, thalamic tumors, and acute or extensive lesions of the upper brain stem; it may also occur after a seizure. Its origin may relate to metabolic factors or to deafferentation of the cerebral cortex.

delta band in electroencephalography, a frequency band of less than 4 Hz.

delta check in clinical chemistry, a quality control check, performed manually or by a laboratory computer, that identifies unusually large differences between two consecutive test results for the same patient. Also called *previous value check.*

delta ray a charged particle scattered from matter by the passage of an alpha particle or other ionizing radiation. Cf. *secondary ray.*

demarcation (de″mar-ka′shun) [L. *demarcare* to limit] 1. a boundary, such as the edge or margin of an organ, tissue, or lesion.

2. a separation.

line of d., a discrete line separating two structures.

Dematiaceae (de-mat″ĭ-a′se-e) a family of the order Moniliales, soil-inhabiting fungi, that have brown to black conidia or hyphae. Some are the agents of the skin infection chromoblastomycosis. Five species are commonly isolated from individuals with the disease: *Fonsecaea pedrosoi, F. compactum, Wangiella dermatitidis, Phialophora verrucosa,* and *Cladosporium carrionii.* All exhibit a pigment dark brown to black in color and slow culture growth. Colonies of *F. pedrosoi, F. compactum, Cl. carrionii,* and *P. verrucosa* have a moldy look and show many dry aerial hyphae; *W. dermatitidis* is characterized by soft, moist colonies that exhibit a yeastlike phase. No antigenic patterns have been found by immunologic testing that differentiate these species but each strain does show variations in color, growth rate, and colony characteristics. See also *chromoblastomycosis.*

dematiacious (de-mat″e-a′shus) pertaining to fungi of the family Dematiaceae; dark toned, usually greenish-gray to black.

demeclocycline (dem″ĕ-klo-si′klēn) a broad-spectrum tetracycline antibiotic produced by *Streptomyces aureofaciens.* See also *antibacterial agents* and *tetracyclines.*

dementia (de-men′she-ah) [de- + L. *mens* mind] a form of organic brain disease characterized by progressive, and frequently irreversible, loss of cognitive function and failing memory. The specific clinical manifestations, rate of evolution, and duration are variable. Causes of this condition include Alzheimer's disease, Pick's disease, cerebral arteriosclerosis, Creutzfeldt-Jakob disease, Huntington's chorea, head injury, hydrocephalus, neoplasia, neurosyphilis, subdural hematoma, metabolic disorders, and certain nutritional deficiencies.

Diagnosis is primarily on clinical grounds. Radiography of the skull, lumbar puncture, computerized tomography, electroencephalography, and hematologic and biochemical screening tests may be helpful in determining the cause or extent of cerebral involvement. These procedures are important, because dementia may be secondary to a treatable condition (e.g., myxedema, vitamin B_{12} deficiency, pellagra, and normal-pressure hydrocephalus).

See also *organic brain syndrome.*

Demerol (dem′er-ol) trademark. See *meperidine hydrochloride.*

demethylchlortetracycline (de-meth″il-klōr″tet-rah-si′klēn) see *demeclocycline.*

demeton (dem′ĕ-ton) a highly toxic organothiophosphate insecticide, a mixture of phosphorothioic acid *O,O*-diethyl *O*-[2-ethylthio)ethyl] ester (demeton-O) and *O,O*-diethyl *S*-[2-(ethylthio)ethyl] phosphorothioate (demeton-S). See also *organophosphate compounds.*

demilune (dem′ĭ-lo͞on) [Fr. *demi* half + L. *luna* moon] 1. a half moon or crescent.

2. crescentic; crescent-shaped.

3. a group of serous cells at the periphery of an acinus of a mixed salivary gland.

demineralization (de-min″er-al-ĭ-za′shun) a decrease in mineral ions or organic salts in tissue, especially bone tissue.

Demodex (dem′o-deks) [Gr. *dēmos* fat + *dēx* worm] a genus of mites, the most common species of which is *D. folliculorum,* parasitic in humans and domestic animals. The mites burrow into the hair follicles or sebaceous glands of the face. Also called follicular mites.

demyelinate (de-mi′ĕ-lin-āt) to destroy or remove the myelin sheath of a nerve.

demyelinating diseases (de-mi′ĕ-lin-āt″ing) a group of neurologic disorders characterized by the destruction and loss of the myelin sheath of the nerve fibers. Multiple and diffuse sclerosis are two of the most common forms.

demyelination (de-mi″ĕ-lĭ-na′shun) the loss, attenuation, or dysfunction of the myelin sheath of an axon without accompanying destruction of the axis cylinder. Demyelination can occur focally near the nodes of Ranvier (paranodal demyelination) or more randomly and extensively over entire segments between nodes (segmental demyelination). It may occur in the central nervous system (e.g., encephalomyelitis, multiple sclerosis, progressive multifocal leukoencephalopathy) or in the peripheral nervous system (e.g., Guillain-Barré syndrome, metachromatic leukodystrophy, or nerve compression). Demyelination results in marked slowing of nerve conduction, complete failure of conduction (conduction block) in affected axons, or both. See also *degenerating myelin demonstration.* Cf. *wallerian degeneration.*

denaturation (de-na″chur-a′shun) 1. the partial or total alteration of the structure of a protein by the action of certain physical procedures (heating, agitation) or chemical agents. Denaturation is the result of the disruption of tertiary bonds, which causes the opening of the folded structure and the loss of characteristic physiologic, enzymatic, or physicochemical properties; it can be either reversible or irreversible.

2. the adulteration of ethanol by the addition of methyl alcohol or other toxic materials to render it unfit for consumption.

dendrite (den′drit) [Gr. *dendron* tree] a fine, branching extension of a neuron that generally serves as a postsynaptic element. It always conducts impulses toward the cell body.

dendritic (den-drit′ik) 1. branched like a tree.

2. pertaining to or possessing dendrites.

dengue (deng′e; Sp. *dānga*) [Sp.] an infectious febrile disease caused by a group B arbovirus (genus *Flavivirus*); it is usually transmitted by the *Aedes aegypti* mosquito. Dengue is endemic to the tropics and subtropics, especially the Caribbean, Central America, South America, and Southeast Asia. After an incubation period of 5-8 da, there is a sudden onset of chills, headache, high fever, prostration, joint and muscle pain, leukopenia, lymphadenopathy, and rash. The fever usually persists for 3-6 da; it may subside after 2-3 da and be followed by a second rapid increase in temperature, giving a saddleback appearance to the fever curve. The disease is self-limiting and is only rarely fatal. In addition to this classic form of the disease, an atypical mild form occurs. A severe, life-threatening hemorrhagic and/or shock syndrome can also occur.

The diagnosis can be confused with typhus, Colorado tick fever, or yellow fever; it is confirmed by viral isolation early in the disease or by later serologic tests. Treatment is symptomatic.

Also called *breakbone fever* and *dandy fever*.

hemorrhagic d., an acute, severe, infectious hemorrhagic fever caused by dengue viruses. There is some evidence that it may arise from an immunologic reaction in cases of a second infection with another serotype of the virus. This form of dengue is usually seen in urban epidemics; today, outbreaks are seen in Asian countries.

The World Health Organization has classified hemorrhagic dengue into four clinical grades: grade I exhibits the classic symptoms of dengue (nausea and vomiting, thrombocytopenia, hemoconcentration, and a positive tourniquet test); in grade II, there is spontaneous bleeding (often in the GI tract); in grade III, there is progression to circulatory failure (hypotension of $\leq$ 20 mmHg) and manifestations of restlessness and agitation; and in grade IV, there is profound shock, often with unmeasurable pulse and blood pressure. Groups III and IV, sometimes called dengue shock syndrome, are life-threatening.

Dennis' technique (den'is) a method for preparing a potent purified antigen from the fluid of hydatid cysts of the liver and lungs of cattle and sheep; used in an immunologic intradermal test for hydatid disease.

dens (denz), pl. *dentes* [L.] a tooth or toothlike structure. See also *odontoid p.* under *process.*

dense body (dens) an ultrastructural term without precise connotation, used to designate a discrete electron-dense inclusion, which may be of uncertain nature, within a cell.

dense deposit disease (DDD) a renal disorder in which zones of homogeneous electron-dense material are deposited centrally within the glomerular basement membranes and, to a lesser degree, in the mesangial matrix. Serum C3 is depleted, and the glomerular deposits stain weakly for C3 using immunofluorescence methods. An abnormal circulating *IgG* (C3 nephritic factor) can usually be demonstrated; it is probably an autoantibody acting against a component of the alternate complement system. In about 10 percent of patients, an association with partial lipodystrophy has been recognized. Patients with this disease are usually between the ages of 5 and 25 yr, and with few exceptions it progresses to renal failure. Also called mesangiocapillary glomerulonephritis, type II. See also *glomerulopathy.*

densimeter (den-sim'ĕ-ter) a device that measures the density or specific gravity of a fluid or solid. Also called *densitometer.*

densitometer (den″sĭ-tom'ĕ-ter) 1. an instrument that measures the absorbance of light. Some types are used to measure the photographic density of areas of developed x-ray plates or of film badges and thus the radiation recorded, and others to measure the density of staining of paper electrophoresis strips.

2. see *densimeter.*

densitometry (den″sĭ-tom'ĕ-tre) 1. measurement of the density, or of variations in the density, of an object.

2. measurement of the absorbance (optical density) of an object such as photographic film or a paper electrophoresis strip.

density (den'sĭ-te) [L. *densitas*] 1. (symbol ρ), mass per unit volume.

2. the amount of any unit per unit volume, area, or length, such as energy or information density.

3. (symbol *D*), the degree of blackening of photographic film, the logarithm of the opacity, i.e., the logarithm of the intensity (I_0) of the light incident on the film divided by the intensity of the light transmitted (I): $D = \log (I_0/I)$.

base d., the optical density of the film base, measured with the emulsion removed.

calcific d., the radiographic density of bones and tissues that contain calcium salts. This density is also called moderately radiopaque.

decreased d., a darker shadow on a radiograph produced by a less dense or a thinner substance. Also called *hyperlucency* and increased radiolucency.

increased d., a lighter shadow on a radiograph produced by a denser or thicker substance. Also called radiopacity.

intermediate d., a range of radiographic densities intermediate between moderately radiolucent (fatty tissue) and moderately radiopaque (bone). The densities of water, blood, muscle, connective tissue, cartilage, epithelium, and uric acid stones are included in this category.

radiographic d., the photographic density of a radiograph or the relative density of a part as seen in a radiograph.

water d., the radiographic density of water. See also *intermediate d.*

density function in statistics, a mathematical function that describes the distribution or frequency of occurrence of measurements on a scale for a specific population. The most familiar example is the gaussian or normal bell-shaped curve. The area under the curve over a given interval represents the probability that a randomly selected individual will have a measurement in that interval. The sample histogram approximates the theoretical density function. Also called *frequency distribution* and frequency function.

density gradient centrifugation a method of separating mixtures of substances in an ultracentrifuge, utilizing a density gradient established from the top to the bottom of the centrifuge tube. The tube is filled by means of a device that continuously decreases the concentration of a solute (usually cesium chloride or sucrose) as the tube is filled. The sample mixture (e.g., a cell homogenate) is placed on top of the solution and the tube is spun. Each component of the mixture sinks until it reaches the level at which its density matches that of the solution, a process sometimes referred to as equilibrium density gradient centrifugation. Zone density gradient centrifugation refers to the fractionation of cell homogenates into fractions (zones) of different density, such as mitochondria and microsomes.

dent/i (den'tĭ) [L. *dens, dentis* tooth] a word element used in combining form to denote teeth, e.g., dentigerous.

dental (den′tal) [L. *dentalis*] pertaining to a tooth or teeth.

dental caries see *caries.*

dental radiography radiographic examination of the teeth. Extraoral projections (the film is placed outside the mouth) and axial and semiaxial intraoral projections (with the film held in the occlusal plane) are used to demonstrate impacted teeth, trauma, and malocclusion. Two other intraoral methods are used: periapical projections to demonstrate lesions of the roots, and interproximal projections to demonstrate cavities in the crown and neck.

For a periapical projection, a small film packet is placed without being bent against the inside of three or four teeth and the adjacent gingiva. The central ray is directed perpendicular to the mesiodistal plane of the center tooth and to the line that bisects the angle formed by the film and the axis of the tooth. Seven films are commonly required for each arch.

Interproximal projections show the crowns and necks of both the upper and lower teeth. The slightly bent film is held behind the teeth by the bite-wing attached to the center of the film. The central ray is directed to the center of the film perpendicular to the horizontal axis of the film and angled ρ–10° caudad. Five or seven films are usually required.

dentate (den′tāt) [L. *dentatus* toothed] having teeth or saw-toothed projections on the margins.

dentate nucleus see *dentate n.* under *nucleus.*

denticle (den′tĭk′l) [L. *denticulus* a little tooth] 1. a small, toothlike process.

2. a relatively large body of calcified substance in the pulp chamber of a tooth.

denticulated (den-tik′u-lăt″ed) having minute teeth.

dentigerous (den-tij′er-us) [*denti-* + L. *gerere* to carry] relating to teeth or dental material.

dentigerous cyst a follicular cyst of the mouth or jaw that occurs because of the accumulation of fluid between the crown of a tooth and the reduced enamel epithelium. Ameloblastomatous transformation can result.

dentin (den′tin) [L. *dens* tooth] the chief substance or tissue of the teeth; it surrounds the tooth pulp and is covered by enamel on the crown and by cementum on the roots of the tooth. Dentin is similar to but harder and denser than bone, and consists of a solid organic substratum infiltrated with calcium salts. It is permeated by numerous branching spiral canaliculi or tubules that contain processes of the connective tissue cells (odontoblasts) lining the pulp cavity.

dentistry (den′tis-tre) the science and art of preventing, diagnosing, and treating diseases, injuries, and malformations of the teeth and associated structures of the oral cavity. Also called *odontology.*

dentition (den-tish′un) [L. *dentitio,* from *dentire* to teethe] the teeth in the dental arch; the term is ordinarily used to designate the natural teeth in their normal position.

Denver classification (den′ver) an obsolete classification of the human autosomes into seven groups: A (chromosomes 1–3), B (4 and 5), C (6–12 and X), D (13–15), E (16–18), F (19 and 20), and G (21 and 22). See also *chromosome nomenclature.*

deoxy- (de-ok′se) a prefix word element in organic chemistry to denote a compound formed by the (conceptual) removal of an oxygen atom (often a hydroxyl or keto group) from the reference compound, e.g., deoxyribose, deoxycortisone, deoxybenzoin. Formerly called *desoxy-.*

deoxyadenosine monophosphate (dAMP) (de-ok″se-ah-den′o-sēn) see *deoxyadenosine-5′-phosphate.*

deoxyadenosine-5′-phosphate (dAMP) a mononucleotide formed from adenine, deoxyribose, and phosphoric acid. Also called *deoxyadenosine monophosphate* and *deoxyadenylic acid.* See also under *nucleotide.*

deoxyadenylic acid (de-ok″se-ad″ĕ-nil′ik) see *deoxyadenosine-5′-phosphate.*

deoxycholate (de-ok″se-ko′lāt) any salt, ester, or dissociated form of deoxycholic acid.

deoxycholic acid (de-ok″se-ko′lik) 3α,12α-dihydroxy-5β-cholanoic acid, a bile acid formed by bacterial action in the gut on cholic acid. Deoxycholic acid forms molecular coordination compounds (so-called choleic acids) with many substances, and complexes with fatty acids have been studied extensively. See also *bile acid.*

11-deoxycorticosterone (de-ok″se-kor″tĭ-kos′ter-ōn) see *11-desoxycorticosterone.*

11-deoxycortisol (compound S) (de-ok″se-kor′tĭ-sol) a glucocorticoid that is formed in the zona fasciculata of the adrenal cortex. It possesses some mineralocorticoid activity and is an important intermediate in the synthesis of cortisol. It is formed by the enzymatic action of 21-hydroxylase on 17α-hydroxyprogesterone and is acted on by 11-β-hydroxylase to produce cortisol. The second most common enzymatic defect in the adrenogenital syndrome is the absence or deficiency of 11-β-hydroxylase, which leads to increased levels of 11-deoxycortisol.

Increased values are noted in adrenocortical carcinomas and following metyrapone administration. The response of 11-deoxycortisol and its urinary metabolite tetrahydro-S to metyrapone is helpful in assessing the pituitary-adrenal reserve, in differentiating adrenal hyperplasia from adrenal tumors, and in evaluating panhypopituitarism. Decreased levels are seen in Addison's disease and hypofunction of the anterior pituitary. Reference ranges for 11-deoxycortisol in plasma are: for baseline, 0.05-0.25 μg/dl; and for postmetyrapone, more than 7.0.

See also *metyrapone test* and *tetrahydro-11-deoxycortisol.*

deoxycytidine monophosphate (dCMP) (de-ok″se-si′tĭ-dēn) see *deoxycytidine-5′-phosphate.*

deoxycytidine-5′-phosphate (dCMP) a mononucleotide formed from cytosine, 2-deoxyribose, and phosphoric acid. It can be converted to and formed from deoxyuridine-5′-phosphate in the body. Also called *deoxycytidine monophosphate* and *deoxycytidylic acid.* See also under *nucleotide.*

deoxycytidylic acid (de-ok″se-si″tĭ-dil′ik) see *deoxycytidine-5′-phosphate.*

6-deoxy-L-galactose (de-ok″se-gah-lak′tōs) see *L-fucose.*

deoxyguanosine monophosphate (dGMP) (de-ok″se-gwan′o-sēn mon″o-fos′fāt) see *deoxyguanosine-5′-phosphate.*

deoxyguanosine-5′-phosphate (dGMP) a mononucleotide formed from guanine, deoxyribose, and phosphoric acid. Also called *deoxyguanosine monophosphate* and *deoxyguanylic acid.* See also under *nucleotide.*

deoxyguanylic acid (de-ok″se-gwan-il′ik) see *deoxyguanosine-5′-phosphate.*

deoxyhemoglobin (de-ok″se-he′mo-glo″bin) hemoglobin uncombined with oxygen. Also called reduced hemoglobin.

6-deoxy-β-L-mannose (de-ok″se-man′ōs) see *β-L-rhamnose.*

deoxyribonuclease (DNase, DNAase) (de-ok″se-ri″bo-nu′kle-ās) one of a group of enzymes, endodeoxyribonucleases (EC 3.1.21 and 3.1.22), found in bacterial, yeast, and mammalian tissues, that catalyze the degradation of deoxyribonucleic acid (DNA). The enzymes are important in the repair of defective DNA, acting by catalyzing the hydrolytic cleavage of a continuous polynucleotide chain near a site of distortion. The formed gap can then be filled in by a DNA polymerase. See also *endodeoxyribonuclease* and *endonuclease.*

d. I, an enzyme of the hydrolase class (EC 3.1.21.1) that catalyzes the hydrolytic cleavage of a strand of deoxyribonucleic acid on the 3′ side of certain phosphodiester linkages to yield 5′-phosphodinucleotide and 5′-phosphooligonucleotide end products. The enzyme functions in the repair of damaged DNA by exposing a faulty fragment for replacement. Formerly called streptococcal deoxyribonuclease.

d. II, an enzyme of the hydrolase class (EC 3.1.22.1) that catalyzes the hydrolytic cleavage of a strand of deoxyribonucleic acid on the 5′ side of certain phosphodiester linkages to yield 3′-phosphomononucleotide and 3′-phosphooligonucleotide end products. The enzyme is important in the repair of damaged DNA, acting by attacking the center of a faulty strand of DNA to expose the damaged fragment for replacement.

deoxyribonuclease digestion a method for the demonstration of DNA in tissues. Deoxyribonucleic acid can be located in the cell by comparing two slides of material stained with Giemsa stain, one of which has been previously treated with deoxyribonuclease. DNA will have been digested on the treated slide, and the areas that are stained blue in the control slide will be colorless.

deoxyribonuclease (DNase) test a test for the presence of deoxyribonuclease in bacteria. In the procedure, a medium containing deoxyribonucleic acid and toluidine blue is inoculated from a young agar slant. After incubation, a red zone around the inoculum indicates the presence of deoxyribonuclease.

deoxyribonucleic acid (DNA) (de-ok″se-ri″bo-nūk′la-ik) the molecule that is the repository of genetic information in all organisms with the exception of the relatively small number of viruses in which ribonucleic acid is used. The information coded in DNA determines the entire structure, physiology, and biochemistry of a living cell. The primary structure of DNA is a linear sequence of nucleotides joined by covalent bonds. This sequence specifies the primary structure of all RNA molecules (nucleotide sequence) and peptides (amino acid sequence) synthesized by the cell, and enzymes coded by DNA control the biochemical processes by which all the other cellular constituents are made. For the structure of DNA, see Figure 1.

The information in DNA is duplicated during the cell cycle, with one copy passed on to each of the daughter cells in mitosis. The molecular basis of this process depends on the two complementary linear strands joined by hydrogen bonds. The information content of either strand is completely determined by the other strand. During DNA replication, the two strands are separated and new complementary strands are synthesized using the old strands as templates. DNA replication has an extremely high copying fidelity; the entire DNA content of the cell is normally copied without error. Mistakes during the copying process (which occur in approximately 1 in 1000 cell divisions) or unrepaired damage to a cell's DNA result in mutations, changes in the genetic information. Most mutations are deleterious, but some are beneficial and are preserved in the process of evolution, leading to new traits and ultimately the production of new species.

STRUCTURE. DNA is a nucleotide polymer, each nucleotide being composed of a nitrogenous base, the five-carbon sugar deoxyribose, and a phosphate group. The combination of a sugar with a nitrogenous base without a phosphate group is known as a nucleoside. The nitrogenous base is linked to deoxyribose by an *N-β*-glycosidic linkage. There are two classes of nitrogenous bases, purines and pyrimidines. In the case of purines the linkage is between C-1 of the deoxyribose and N-9 of the purine; in pyrimidines the linkage is between C-1 of the sugar residue and N-1 of the pyrimidine. The purines are adenine (A) and guanine (G), and the pyrimidines are cytosine (C) and thymine (T). Some of these purines may be further altered, and it is believed that a particular pattern of modification (e.g., methylation) of selected bases may be a characteristic feature of a DNA molecule.

The monomeric units of nucleotides are linked by phosphodiester bonds between the third and fifth carbons of deoxyribose, with phosphate forming the diester bonds between the adjacent nucleotides. In DNA, two polynucleotide strands coil around each other to form a right-handed double helix. The deoxyribosyl residues, joined by phosphodiester bonds, give rise to spirals of the helix, while the bases project perpendicularly into the center of the double-stranded helix. The two polynucleotide strands of the double helix are held together primarily by hydrogen bonding between specific bases of the opposing strands. The structure is further stabilized by a hydrophobic stacking interaction between these base pairs. Both interactions, namely the hydrogen bonding between bases and the hydrophobic interaction due to base stacking, contribute to the stabilization of the double helix in a synergistic manner. The hydrogen bonds occur between specific complementary base pairs: A and T, G and C. Therefore, the two strands of DNA are complementary to each other; this means that once the sequence of one strand is specified, the sequence of the other strand is also specified as a result of base-pairing rules. (See Figure 2.)

The elegant structure of DNA was elucidated by Watson and Crick, who made use of several key facts discovered by other workers. These include the x-ray diffraction patterns obtained by Wilkins and

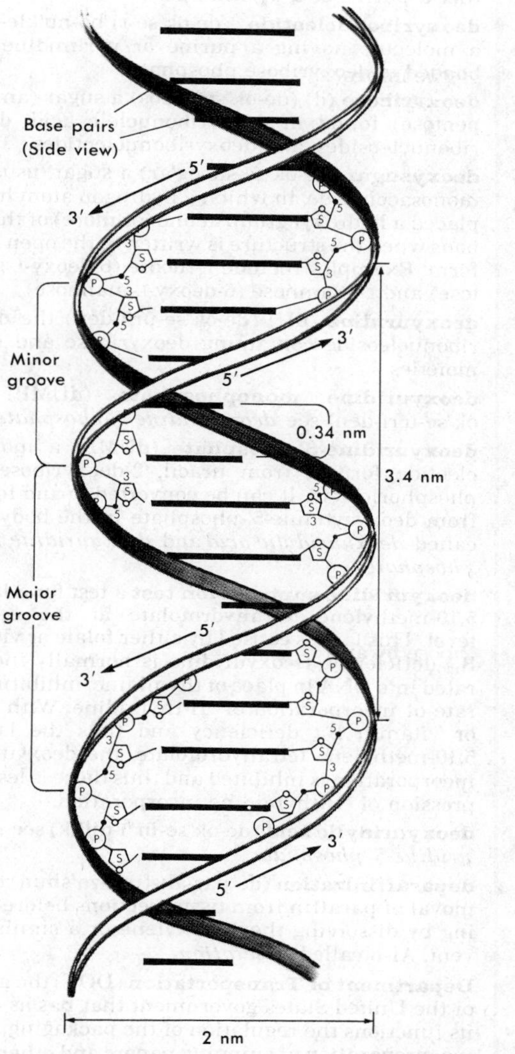

Deoxyribonucleic acid, Figure 1. The DNA double helix: the phosphate-ribose backbones are indicated as ribbons; the base pairs are flat structures stacked one on top of another, perpendicular to the long axis of DNA, and are therefore represented as horizontal lines in this side view. Note that the two strands are antiparallel and that the molecule has a minor and a major groove. The double helix gives one complete turn every 10 base pairs (3.4 nm). P indicates phosphate group, and S indicates sugar. (From DeRobertis, E. D., and DeRobertis, E. M., Jr.: Cell and Molecular Biology. 7th ed. Philadelphia, W. B. Saunders Co., 1980.)

Franklin, who used DNA from different sources and discovered a common repetitive pattern suggestive of a helical three-dimensional structure, and also Chargaff's observation ("Chargaff's rule") that DNA from different organisms showed the molar ratios of A to T and G to C to be close to one. The double helical model for DNA of Watson and Crick has now been confirmed as the correct structure by a variety of evidence. Rarely, DNA takes a different structure, Z structure.

Other features of the DNA structure are: (1) the distance between each base pair is 3.4 Å; (2) A-T base pairs are held together by two hydrogen bonds, whereas G-C base pairs are maintained by three; (3) the helical sugar-phosphate backbones make one revolution every 10 base pairs, resulting in a 36° rotation between adjacent base pairs; (4) the pitch of the helix is 34 Å; and (5) the two strands of DNA are antiparallel (meaning the 3′-5′ phosphodiester linkages run in opposite directions in the two strands). The DNA molecule also shows striking difference between the hydrophobic core of stacked bases and the hydrophilic exterior consisting of charged sugar-phosphate groups.

CHROMOSOME STRUCTURE. The DNA molecule exists in several different forms, namely, linear double-stranded, circular double-stranded, and, in some bacteriophages (ϕX174, for example), single-stranded circular forms. The double-stranded circular DNA is present in bacteria, chloroplasts, and mitochondria.

The DNA in higher organisms is associated with large amounts of protein (about four or five times the weight of DNA). Most of these proteins, known as histones, are basic proteins, rich in the basic amino acids arginine and lysine. These proteins are held in the grooves of the DNA helix by ionic bonds between the positively charged arginine and lysine residues of histones and the negatively charged phosphate groups of DNA. They form beadlike structures with DNA, which are termed nucleosomes. The exact function of these proteins, other than structural, is not known. In bacteria the DNA is complexed with much less protein and with protein having a very different amino acid composition from that of eukaryotic DNA-associated proteins.

The molecular weights of DNA from different sources vary considerably. For example, the DNA from the bacterium *Escherichia coli* has a molecular weight of about 3×10^9, whereas in the animal cell the molecular weight is between 10^{11} and 10^{12}.

FUNCTION. As DNA serves as the genetic material, it must be capable of four functions: (1) replication, (2) transcription, (3) recombination, and (4) mutation.

Replication. This process is required in order that the progeny and the parent cell will have identical properties. As noted earlier, the two strands of DNA are complementary to each other. In the replication process, each of the two parental strands are separated by unwinding, and each serves as a template for the synthesis of two new strands by complex enzymes termed DNA polymerases, according to the base-pairing rules of Watson and Crick. Thus, this process yields two identical daughter DNA molecules, each having one newly synthesized and one parental strand. This mode of duplication is known as semiconservative replication.

Transcription. This is a process by which the encoded information specified by the sequence of nucleotides in the DNA is copied in the form of ribonucleic acid (RNA). This RNA includes ribosomal, transfer, and messenger RNA (rRNA, tRNA, and mRNA); mRNA migrates to ribosomes and directs the order of incorporation of amino acids into polypeptide chains (translation). Thus, the amino acid sequence of proteins is specified by the sequence of nucleotides in DNA. Recent studies have shown that DNA (genes) of many higher organisms and animal viruses contain stretches of polynucleotides that are not translated into proteins. They are, however, transcribed into a high-molecular-weight RNA known as precursor messenger RNA. The interruptions not involved in directing the order of incorporation of amino acid residues into proteins are termed intervening sequences or introns, and the nucleotide sequences selected from precursor mRNA for directing protein synthesis are known as exons. The intervening sequences from precursor mRNA are removed by an enzymatic step called processing, and the remaining pieces are rejoined to yield mature mRNA. In eukaryotic cells it is the mature mRNA that migrates from the nucleus to the cytoplasm. Therefore, the RNA found in the nucleus is much larger than its cytoplasmic counterparts. The bacterial gene products are not fragmented in this manner.

Recombination and Mutation. These two processes acting on DNA are sources of genetic variability and are responsible for production of variability within species that, when subjected to natural selection, leads to the evolution of better adapted organisms. In recombination via sexual reproduction, the genes from both parents are exchanged and incorporated into the genes of the progeny, giving rise to variability in the assortment of parental genes. The term mutation implies alterations in the genetic material leading to changes in base sequences, which may involve alterations of bases or additions or deletions of bases. Mutations can occur as a result of high-energy radiation (e.g., x-rays, ultraviolet rays, gamma rays), chemicals, or errors in DNA replication. Mutations may cause a beneficial, harmless, or deleterious change, or no change, in the final expression of the gene.

A new and rapidly developing area of DNA research is the field of recombinant DNA, which makes possible the transfer of genetic information from one species to another. One method of producing recombinant DNA is by splicing selected pieces of DNA from one organism onto extrachromosomal pieces of DNA, namely, plasmid DNA of a bacterium. The plasmids are parasites (or symbiotes) and are able to reproduce by utilizing the bacterium's (host) replicative machinery. The recombinant DNA (DNA chimera) is then inserted into cells of the species from which the extrachromosomal DNA was originally derived. In the host, the recombinant DNA undergoes propagation, permitting the production of many identical copies of foreign DNA (known as cloning). In addition, the gene products (e.g., proteins) of the foreign DNA can be isolated. As the generation time of bacteria is short, large amounts of the desired gene product can be synthesized. The synthesis of human insulin and human growth hormone has been achieved by using recombinant techniques, which suggests the possibility of employing this type of technology in the diagnosis and therapy of human ailments.

See also *ribonucleic acid.*

N. V. BHAGAVAN, PH.D.

deoxyribonucleic acid staining see *Feulgen reaction* and *methyl green–pyronine stain.*

deoxyribonucleoside (de-ok″se-ri″bo-nu′kle-o-sīd) the glycosidic combination of deoxyribose with either a purine or a pyrimidine.

deoxyribonucleotide (de-ok″se-ri″bo-nu′kle-o-tīd) a molecule having a purine or pyrimidine base bonded to deoxyribose phosphate.

deoxyribose (d) (de-ok″se-ri′bōs) a sugar (an aldopentose) found in deoxyribonucleic acid, deoxyribonucleosides, and deoxyribonucleotides.

deoxysugar (de-ok″se-shoog′ar) a sugar, usually a monosaccharide, in which a hydrogen atom has replaced a hydroxyl group at one (or more) of the carbons when the structure is written in the open chain form. Examples include L-fucose (6-deoxy-L-galactose) and L-rhamnose (6-deoxy-L-mannose).

deoxyuridine (dU) (de-ok″se-ūr′i-dēn) the deoxyribonucleoside containing deoxyribose and uracil moieties.

deoxyuridine monophosphate (dUMP) (de-ok″se-u′rĭ-dēn) see *deoxyuridine-5′-phosphate.*

deoxyuridine-5′-phosphate (dUMP) a mononucleotide formed from uracil, 2-deoxyribose, and phosphoric acid. It can be converted to and formed from deoxycytidine-5′-phosphate in the body. Also called *deoxyuridylic acid* and *deoxyuridine monophosphate.*

deoxyuridine suppression test a test for a lack of 5,10-methylene tetrahydrofolate at the cellular level. This lack is caused by either folate or vitamin B_{12} deficiency. Deoxyuridine is normally incorporated into DNA in place of thymidine, inhibiting the rate of incorporation of ^{3}H-thymidine. With folate or vitamin B_{12} deficiency and thus the lack of 5,10-methylene tetrahydrofolate, the deoxyuridine incorporation is inhibited and thus there is less suppression of ^{3}H-thymidine incorporation.

deoxyuridylic acid (de-ok″se-ūr″ĭ-dil′ik) see *deoxyuridine-5′-phosphate.*

deparaffinization (de″par-ah-fin″ĭ-za′shun) the removal of paraffin from tissue sections before staining by dissolving them in xylene or a similar solvent. Also called *deceration.*

Department of Transportation (DOT) the agency of the United States government that has as one of its functions the regulation of the packaging, labeling, preparation of shipping papers and other documentations and shipping of hazardous materials, including waste chemicals. DOT regulations also include requirements for the training of personnel with responsibility for dealing with hazardous materials.

dependence (de-pen′dens) [L. *dependeo* to hang from] the state of having need or reliance on a person, object, or substance, so that loss or removal results in serious adverse effects.

drug d., the state of chronic intoxication with a drug taken for its psychic effects. The term encompasses both psychologic dependence, which refers to a compulsion to take the drug despite the risk of adverse consequences, and physical dependence, which implies that a specific syndrome of physical symptoms will follow abrupt withdrawal of the drug. The terms drug dependence and drug abuse are now preferred to the more controversial terms addiction and habituation.

dependent variable (de-pen′dent) 1. in mathematics, the variable specified by a function, i.e., y in $y = f(x)$.

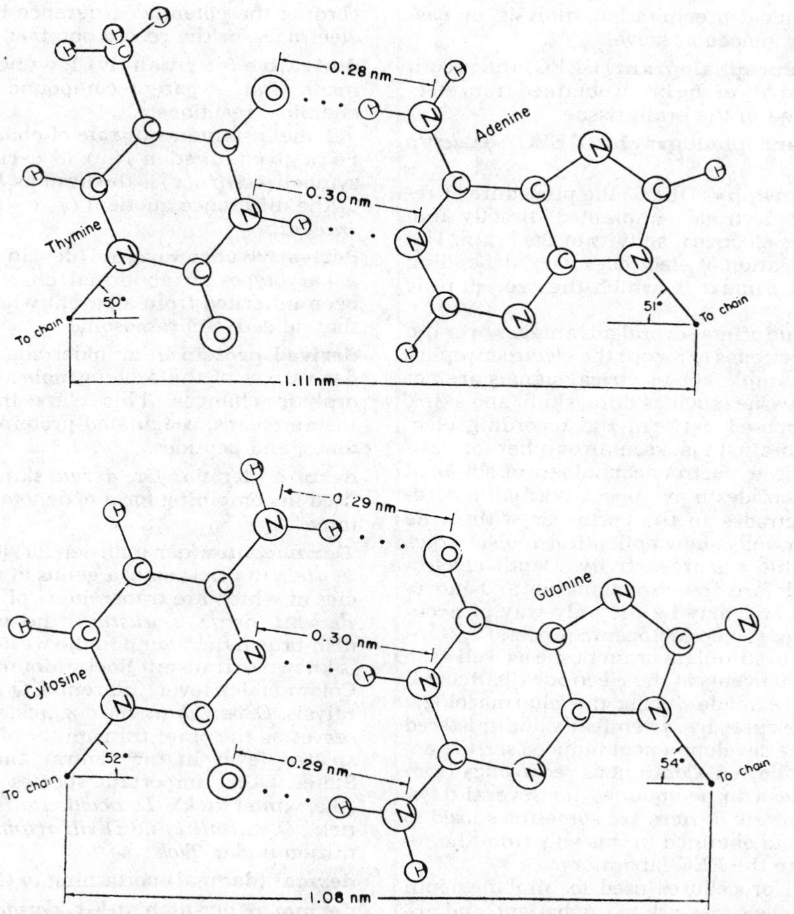

Deoxyribonucleic acid, Figure 2. The two base pairs in DNA. The complementary bases are thymine and adenine (T-A) and cytosine and guanine (C-G). Observe that between T and A there are two, and between C and G three, hydrogen bonds. (From Pauling, L., and Corey, R. B.: Specific hydrogen-bond formation between pyramidines and purines in deoxyribonucleic acids. Archives of Biochemistry and Biophysics *65*:164, 1956.)

2. in statistics, a stochastic variable whose distribution function depends on another variable. See also *independent variable* and *linear regression.*

depigmentation (de″pig-men-ta′shun) the loss of pigment (melanin) from the skin, as in albinism, partial albinism or vitiligo; also used as a synonym of *hypopigmentation.*

depletion (de-ple′shun) [L. *deplere* to empty] removal of a specific substance from the body or from some physical system.

depletion layer the region on both sides of a *p-n* junction in a semiconductor that is depleted of charge carriers. See also *diode.*

depolarization (de-po″lar-ĭ-za′shun) any decrease in the transmembrane potential of an excitable cell in which the interior of the cell becomes more positive than when under normal resting conditions. Cf. *hyperpolarization.*

deposit (de-poz′it) [*de-* down + L. *ponere* to place] 1. a sediment.

2. a pathologic accumulation of inorganic material in a tissue.

depressant (de-pres′ant) 1. diminishing any function or activity.

2. an agent that retards any function, especially a drug that slows a function of the body or calms and quiets nervous excitement; a sedative. Among the best known depressants are barbiturates. See also *tranquilizer.*

depression (de-presh′un) [*depressio; de-* down + L. *premere* to press] 1. a hollow or depressed area; downward or inward displacement.

2. a lowering of functional activity.

3. major depression; a clinical syndrome characterized by dysphoria, a loss of interest or pleasure in one's normal activities. Symptoms include appetite disturbance (usually loss of appetite, but also greatly increased appetite), sleep disturbance, withdrawal from friends and family, inability to concentrate, feelings of worthlessness or inadequacy, and suicidal ideation.

4. see *bone marrow depression.*

deproteinization (de-pro″tēn-ĭ-za′shun) the removal of protein from a solution as in the preparation of a protein-free filtrate of serum, by such means as chemical precipitation, dialysis, or passage through a molecular sieve.

depth electroencephalogram (DEEG) the record of electrical activity of the brain obtained from electrodes implanted in the brain tissue.

depth electroencephalography (DEEG) see *depth electrography.*

depth electrography (DEEG) the procedure of recording, from electrodes implanted directly into brain tissue, the electrical activity of the brain. The number and location of electrodes vary, depending on the clinical context in which the procedure is undertaken.

This technique offers several advantages over the use of scalp electrodes to record the electroencephalogram. For example, the electrical signals are not attenuated by tissue (such as dura, skull, and skin), which is interposed between the recording electrodes and the brain. In jacksonian or other forms of focal epilepsy, the electroencephalogram obtained from scalp electrodes may appear normal; recordings from electrodes in the cortex or within the brain, however, may show epileptiform discharges or electrographic seizure activity. Depth electrographic records are free from muscle and movement artifacts and may be the only way of accurately localizing the epileptogenic process.

It is possible to stimulate brain tissue as well as to record electrical events at the electrode tip. Recordings can also be made during the pharmacologic activation of seizures by systemically administered drugs. Thus, the development of induced seizure activity can be followed. Continuous recordings from depth electrodes can be obtained for several days, and radiotelemetric devices are sometimes used to transmit the data obtained in this way from the recording room to the EEG laboratory.

The surgical procedures used to implant depth electrodes involve some risk to the patient, and are recommended in the localization of an epileptic focus only in situations in which surgical therapy is possible and medical treatment has failed.

Also called *depth electroencephalography.* See also *s. surgery* under *stereotaxic.*

depth of field the range of distances from the camera or detector of a tomograph or rectilinear scanner, or from the lens of a camera or microscope, within which objects are sharply imaged; objects that are nearer or farther are blurred. Also called *depth of focus.*

depth of focus see *depth of field.*

de Quervain's thyroiditis (dĕ-kār-vanz′) [Fritz de *Quervain,* Swiss surgeon, 1868–1940] see *subacute t.* under *thyroiditis.*

der abbrev. See *derivative chromosome.*

derepression (de″re-presh′un) an increase in the synthesis of the product of a regulated gene by interference with the action of the repressor. Derepression can be produced by mutation of the repressor gene or of the operator gene or by an inducer that binds to the repressor, releasing it from the operator. See also *genetic regulation.*

De Ritis ratio see *ALT/AST ratio.*

derivation (der″ĭ-va′shun) [L. *derivatio,* from *derivare* to draw off] 1. the origin or source of a substance.

2. a lead in electrocardiography.

3. in electroencephalography, the process of recording the potential difference between a pair of electrodes, or the record obtained thereby.

derivative (de-riv′ah-tiv) 1. a chemical compound made from a parent compound by one or more chemical reactions.

2. the instantaneous rate of change of a function. For a given function $f(x)$, its derivative $f'(x)$ (also symbolized df/dx) is the limit as h approaches zero of the difference quotient $(f(x + h) - f(x))/h$. Cf. *integral.*

derivative chromosome (der) in the description of a karyotype, an abnormal chromosome that has been inherited from a parent who was a carrier of that defective chromosome.

derived protein in an older classification system, derivatives of the protein molecule formed by hydrolytic changes. This class includes proteans, metaproteans, coagulated proteins, proteoses, peptones, and peptides.

derm/o (der′mo) [Gr. *derma* skin] a word element used in combining form to denote skin, e.g., dermatome.

Dermacentor (der″mah-sen′tor) [Gr. *derma* skin + *kentein* to prick, stab] a genus of ticks, several species of which are transmitters of pathogens. *D. andersoni* (or *D. venustus*), the wood tick, a reddish-brown tick found in the western United States, is known to transmit Rocky Mountain spotted fever, Colorado tick fever, tularemia, Q fever, and tick paralysis. *D. variabilis,* the dog tick, a dark brown tick, serves as the chief transmitter of Rocky Mountain spotted fever in the central and eastern United States. Other important species are *D. albipictus* (the winter tick), *D. occidentalis* (the West Coast tick), *D. nuttallii,* and *D. silvarum.* See also the illustration under *Tick.*

dermal (der′mal) pertaining to the skin.

dermat/o (der-mah′to) [Gr. *derma, dermatos* skin] a word element used in combining form to denote skin, e.g., dermatosis.

dermatan sulfate (der′mah-tan) a glycosaminoglycan (mucopolysaccharide) found primarily in the skin but also in the lungs, tendons, and heart valves. It consists of alternating residues of L-iduronic acid and *N*-acetyl-D-galactosamine-4-sulfate. Glucuronic acid may replace some iduronic acid residues. Formerly called chrondroitin B sulfate.

dermatitis (der″mah-ti′tis) [*dermat-* + *-itis* inflammation] a general term used to describe superficial inflammation of the skin. The many symptoms include redness, edema, vesicles, crusting, scaling, and itching. There are numerous causes, including metabolic disturbances, nutritional inadequacies, allergic responses to various chemicals, physical processes and psychogenic factors.

actinic d., dermatitis that results from exposure to actinic radiation, such as that from the sun, ultraviolet waves, or x- or gamma radiation. Also called senile dermatitis and solar dermatitis.

allergic d., any inflammation of the skin due to allergy; see also *atopic d.*

atopic d., a chronic, superficial, pruritic inflammation of the skin in adults or children with a personal or family history of allergic manifestations. This disorder causes severe itching of the affected areas and may lead to dry, leathery, and lichenified patches of skin, especially on the flexor areas of the knees and elbows. The cause is unknown, but patients may react to numerous inhalants and foods on scratch and intradermal tests. Eosinophilia and increased serum concentrations of IgE may be present. Diagnosis often relies on a detailed personal history of environmental contacts with potential offending agents. Viral infections with herpes simplex or vaccinia are serious complications. Also called allergic dermatitis; allergic, atopic, or flexural eczema; infantile eczema in infants; and, in Great Britain, Besnier's prurigo.

contact d., an acute or chronic inflammation of the skin caused by direct contact with certain chemicals or other irritants. The lesions are usually well circumscribed and may be initially characterized by erythema and edema, progressing to become weeping, oozing, or crusty patches. Secondary bacterial infection of involved areas is common.

Contact dermatitis is considered to be an immunologically mediated type-IV delayed hypersensitivity reaction, which may require days to develop after exposure. Many agents can provoke the condition in sensitized individuals, including metal compounds, dyes, cosmetics, antibiotics, antihistamines, anesthetics, and other chemical compounds. Irritants, such as plant products (e.g., poison ivy), detergents, soaps, and solvents, may damage normal skin and exacerbate an existing dermatitis.

Skin patch tests can help identify the allergic agent but may be of limited value. Most lesions of this condition are self-limiting, and prevention is based on avoiding exposure to the offending agent. In severe cases, corticosteroid therapy may be required.

exfoliative d., an inflammatory condition of the skin characterized by extensive erythema, scaling, and frequently oozing of fluid from the affected surface. This form constitutes a severe manifestation of several types of dermatitis, including those due to contact with drugs or allergic reaction to drugs. It may be seen in individuals with vascular stasis, and can also occur in leukemia or lymphoma, including Sézary's syndrome. In some instances the cause is not known. See also *exfoliatin*.

d. herpetiformis, a skin disorder characterized by recurrent groups of erythematous lesions that are papular, vesicular, eczematous, or bullous. They are often symmetric; may affect the limbs, back, and scalp; and are often accompanied by itching and burning sensations. The cause is unknown, but the lesions may be associated with specific HLA antigen genotypes. Dermatitis herpetiformis may also affect the mucosa of the intestines, producing villous atrophy and causing a malabsorption syndrome.

d. medicamentosa, an acute or chronic inflammatory skin reaction to a drug. Almost any drug may lead to almost any type of dermatitis in susceptible individuals. The condition usually has an abrupt onset of erythematous lesions. Systemic symptoms (such as fever, headache) may also appear. Blood tests may reveal decreased white blood cell counts and anemia; patch tests are rarely definitive. Blood dyscrasias, symptoms of anaphylaxis, and hepatic, renal, and nervous disorders may be accompanying manifestations of toxicity.

photo contact d., an inflammation of the skin caused by exposure to sunlight after sensitization by some agent (e.g., a halogenated salicylamide or hexachlorophene) that is capable of acting as a hapten, which can cause persisting and recurrent reactions. See also *phototoxic contact d.*

phototoxic contact d., an inflammation of the skin caused by exposure to sunlight after contact with a phototoxic substance, such as coal tar, certain perfumes, cutting oils, and plants containing psoralens. See also *photo contact d.*

radiation d., an acute or chronic inflammation of the skin following exposure to ionizing radiation, most frequently following cancer radiation therapy. The acute form occurs approximately 3 wk after therapy and is characterized by erythema, blistering, and sloughing of skin, which progresses to scarring, fibrosis, and dermal atrophy. Hyper- or hypopigmentation may be seen.

seborrheic d., an inflammation of the superficial skin affecting the scalp and skin folds, most particularly those about the head and neck. This disorder may cause a diffuse scaling of a dry or greasy scalp (dandruff), with itching and formation of papules. Genetic and climatic factors may be involved. Selenium and sulfur shampoos (or, in severe cases, corticosteroids) may be indicated in the treatment.

stasis d., a chronic inflammation of the legs, primarily in older people, that is due to insufficient venous return of blood. Red, edematous, itching lesions often become infected and ulcerated. Lesions may become worse following injury, possibly owing to a reaction with heat-labile, complement-dependent 7S gamma globulin that is specific for epidermal cells.

Dermatobia (der"mah-to'be-ah) [*dermato-* + Gr. *bios* life] a genus of botflies, the most common species of which is *D. hominis* (the human botfly of South America). A large, stout fly (15–18 mm long), *D. hominis* is an obligate myiasis-producing fly for which humans are a favored host. Its eggs, deposited on mosquitoes and bloodsucking flies, are distributed to humans; when the eggs hatch the larvae burrow into the skin, causing painful lesions. Also called *warble fly*. See also the accompanying illustration.

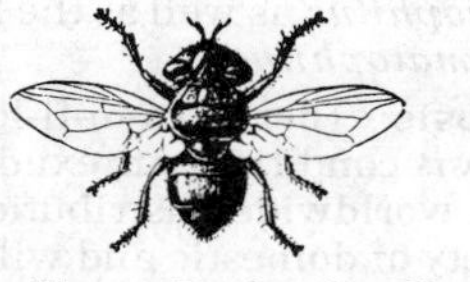

Dermatobia. (From Dorland's Illustrated Medical Dictionary. 26th ed. Philadelphia, W. B. Saunders Co., 1981.)

dermatofibroma (der"mah-to-fi-bro'mah) [*dermato-* + L. *fibra* fiber + Gr. *-ōma* swelling] a benign tumor of fibroblasts arising in the dermis. Also called subepidermal nodular fibrosis.

dermatofibrosarcoma protuberans (der"mah-to-fi"bro-sar-ko'mah) [*dermato-* + L. *fibra* fiber + Gr. *sarkos* flesh + *-oma* swelling] a slow-growing dermal tumor that begins as a plaque but, with growth, forms protuberant nodules. It can occur at any location but is most common on the trunk and proximal extremities. Typically, the histologic appearance is that of atypical spindle-shaped fibroblasts arranged in a storiform pattern. There is a strong tendency for local recurrence.

dermatoglyphics (der"mah-to-glif'iks) [*dermato-*

+ Gr. *glyphein* to carve] 1. the patterns of skin ridges on the fingers, palms, toes, and soles, used clinically in the study of congenital defects, such as in the diagnosis of Down's syndrome.

2. the study of skin ridge patterns.

dermatologic (der″mah-to-loj′ik) pertaining to dermatology; of or affecting the skin.

dermatology (der″mah-tol′o-je) the medical specialty concerned with the diagnosis and treatment of diseases of the skin.

dermatome (der′mah-tōm) [*derma-* + Gr. *tomē* a cutting, from *temnein* to cut] 1. an instrument for cutting thin slices of skin for skin grafts.

2. one of the overlapping areas of skin, each of which is supplied with afferent nerve fibers by a single spinal nerve.

3. in the developing embryo, the lateral portion of a mesodermal somite that produces the fibrous layer of the integument, the dens. Also called cutis plate.

dermatomycosis (der″mah-to-mi-ko′sis) [*dermato-* + Gr. *mykes* fungus + *-osis* condition] a general term for any fungal infection of the skin. Dermatomycosis may be caused by infection with a dermatophyte, by a cutaneous infection with species of *Candida,* or by a secondary spread of a systemic mycosis to the epidermis.

dermatomyositis (der″mah-to-mi″o-si′tis) [*dermato-* + Gr. *mys* muscle + *-itis*] a disease of unknown cause characterized by a maculopapular or eczemalike skin rash occurring concurrently with a symmetric weakening and atrophy of the muscles of the shoulders, hips, neck, and trunk. Although most cases are idiopathic, some are associated with malignant neoplasms or connective tissue disease. Involvement of the esophagus may produce dysphagia and symptoms typical of systemic sclerosis; Raynaud's disease is often found in persons with polymyositis. See also *polymyositis.*

Dermatophilaceae (der″mah-to-fil-a′se-e) a family of bacteria of the order Actinomycetales, one of the actinomycetes. The family contains the pathogenic genus *Dermatophilus,* as well as the less pathogenic genus *Geodermatophilus.*

dermatophilosis (der″mah-to-fi-lo′sis) [*Dermatophilus* + *-osis* condition] an exudative, pustular dermatitis of worldwide distribution that occurs among a variety of domestic and wild animals, and is caused by the actinomycete *Dermatophilus congolensis.* Acquired by animal contact, the uncommon human infection involves only the epidermis and develops as pustules, furuncles, and desquamative eczema. The lesions heal spontaneously or may be treated with sulfonamides or other specific antibiotics. Also called *strawberry foot rot* (in sheep) or *streptotrichosis* (in cattle).

Dermatophilus (der″mah-tof′ĭ-lus) [*dermato-* + Gr. *philein* to love] a genus of bacteria of the family Dermatophilaceae, of the order Actinomycetales. The organisms are aerobic, gram-positive, and non-acid-fast, forming a mycelium containing filaments that segment transversely and longitudinally to produce coccoid cells in packets, which become motile spores. The organisms produce catalase and are virulent for laboratory animals.

D. congolensis, the only species in the genus *Dermatophilus,* and the agent of dermatophilosis. It is unique among bacteria in that it forms filaments that segment in three planes, resulting in packets of coccoid cells that become motile spores. *D. congolensis* is a parasite of skin and does not invade vascular tissue. Human infections occur as pustules, furuncles, or desquamating eczema of exposed skin; they are acquired by contact with infected animals. This microorganism is nonacid-fast, urease- and oxidase-positive, and breaks down gelatin and casein. On agar, colonies initially appear white; with age they turn from yellow to orange. Formerly called *Actinomycetes congolensis* and *Streptothrix bovis.*

dermatophyte (der′mah-to-fīt) [*dermato-* + Gr. *phyton* plant] a filamentous fungus that is keratinophilic and often causes infections involving the epidermal tissue of humans and animals. It can penetrate and parasitize the skin, hair, and nails. There are three genera of dermatophytes, *Microsporum, Trichophyton,* and *Epidermophyton. Microsporum* infects only hair and skin; *Trichophyton* can infect hair, skin, and nails; and *Epidermophyton* can infect only skin and nails. Any single species can cause several different types of cutaneous infections.

The dermatophytes are a closely related and relatively homogeneous group of organisms with respect to appearance, physiology, taxonomy, antigenicity, growth requirements, and infectivity. They produce keratinase, which breaks down keratin. Most dermatophytes can be isolated from soil; however, through evolution a host specificity has developed. Dermatophytes are conveniently divided into three groups according to environmental predilection: anthropophilic (human) dermatophytes, which include *M. audouinii, T. rubrum, T. tonsurans, T. schoenleinii, T. mentagrophytes, T. violaceum,* and *E. floccosum;* zoophilic (animal) dermatophytes, which include *M. canis* and *T. verrucosum;* and geophilic (soil) dermatophytes, which include *M. fulvum* and *M. gypseum.* These groupings are important when considering sources of infection.

Human transmission of dermatophytes is usually indirect through such items as combs, brushes, and hats. Direct transmission from animals or soil to humans occurs frequently in some situations.

CLINICAL DISEASE. the pathologic changes caused by all dermatophyte infections have a common sequence. The infection in the horny layer of skin starts an incubation period when fungal hyphae grow in the stratum corneum. This may continue for several months. The infection then spreads centrifugally, resulting in a characteristic ringworm formation. An equilibrium is eventually reached when growth and death of the dermatophyte equalizes. A host-parasite relationship develops with the fungus, in which the immune system has no advantage. Depending on host conditions and the species of fungus involved, a prolonged refractory period may ensue.

Dermatophytes are temperature-sensitive in that body temperature (37°C) inhibits their growth. Another reason why they do not invade subcutaneous and deeper tissues is the presence of natural inhibitory substances found in blood and other body fluids. Reinfection is common and previous infection does not result in immunity.

Dermatophytoses are sometimes designated clinically by location on the body as: tinea capitis (ringworm of the scalp), tinea corporis (smooth skin), tinea cruris (groin), tinea unguium (nails), tinea pedis (feet), tinea barbae (beard), or tinea manuum (hand).

Laboratory Diagnosis. As dermatophytes are antigenically similar, there is no serologic assay for species identification. Direct examination of skin scrapings, hairs, or nail clippings and cultivation of the fungus on culture media are necessary for diagnosis of dermatophytosis. Specimens are cleared by heating in 10 percent KOH on a slide. They should reveal fungal hyphae and/or spores (conidia). Their locations in or on the hair aid identification. Examination of the culture growth is generally needed for genus and species identification. Some dermatophyte lesions fluoresce when the skin or scalp is examined under ultraviolet light (Wood's lamp), a useful diagnostic tool.

Dermatophyte. The Common Dermatophytes

			Species	Human Disease	Geographical Distribution
Invading the Hair and Hair Follicles	Small Spore Varieties	Ectothrix type	*Microsporum audouini* *	Prepuberal ringworm of the scalp; suppuration rare	Commonest in Europe, producing about 90 per cent of infections; in U.S. 50 per cent
			Microsporum canis *	Prepuberal ringworm of scalp and glabrous skin; suppuration not infrequent; kerion occasional; from pets	Uncommon in Europe; responsible for about half the infections in U.S.
			Microsporum gypseum	Ringworm of the scalp and glabrous skin; suppuration and kerion common; from soil	Relatively rare in U.S.; common in South America
			Microsporum fulvum	Ringworm similar to that of *M. gypseum*	Same as above
	Large Spore Varieties	Endothrix type	*Trichophyton tonsurans*	Black-dot ringworm of scalp and smooth skin; sycosis; onychomycosis; suppuration common; the hair follicles are atrophied	Common in Europe, Russia, Poland, Italy, Near East, but uncommon in U.S. until recently
			Trichophyton violaceum	Black-dot endothrix in both scalp and smooth skin; onychomycosis; suppuraton is the rule and kerion frequent	Common in Europe and Far East; rare in U.S.
		Ectothrix type	*Trichophyton mentagrophytes*	Commonest cause of intertriginous dermatophytosis of the foot ("athlete's foot"); ringworm of smooth skin; suppurative folliculitis in scalp and beard	Ubiquitous
			Trichophyton verrucosum	Ringworm of scalp and smooth skin; suppurative folliculitis in scalp and beard; from cattle	Ubiquitous
	No Spores in Hair		*Trichophyton schoenleinii*	Favus in both scalp and smooth skin; scutulum and kerion	Europe, Far East, Near East, Greenland, South Africa; rare in U.S.
Not Invading the Hair and Hair Follicles			*Epidermophyton floccosum*	Cause of classic eczema marginatum of crural region; causes minority of cases of intertriginous dermatophytosis of foot; not known to infect hair and hair follicles	Ubiquitous, but more common in tropics
			Trichophyton rubrum	Psoriasis-like lesions of smooth skin; tinea unguium and rare invasion of scalp hair; endothrix and ectothrix spores described; mild suppurative folliculitis in beard	Common in Far East, tropics, Europe, U.S.

* Infected hairs fluoresce under Wood's lamp.
Modified from Freeman, B.A.: Burrows' Textbook of Microbiology. 21st ed. Philadelphia, W.B. Saunders Co., 1979, p. 741.

Dermatophyte colonies appear on Sabouraud's medium in 1–2 wk. To reduce bacterial growth, the medium can be supplemented with antibiotics such as chloramphenicol and cyclohexamide.

For more information, see the accompanying table.

dermatophytid (der"mah-tof'ĭ-tid) [*dermato-* + Gr. *phyton* plant + *-id,* from *eidos* form] a secondary skin vesicle containing clear fluid that appears symmetrically on the hands as an allergic reaction to a fungal infection. Dermatophytid and bacterid reactions are generally called "id" reactions. See also *id reaction.*

dermatophytosis (der"mah-to-fi-to'sis) [*dermato-* + Gr. *phyton* plant + *-osis* condition] a specific term for a fungal infection of keratinized tissue (hair, nails, stratum corneum of skin) caused by species of *Microsporum, Trichophyton,* or *Epidermophyton.* The severity of dermatophytosis is dependent on the immune status of the host and the specific strain of fungus involved. See also *dermatophyte.*

dermatosis (der"mah-to'sis), pl. *dermatoses* [*dermat-* + *-osis* condition] a general term used to denote any skin disease.

dermis (der'mis) [L.] [NA], the corium; the thick, vascular connective tissue layer of the skin deep to the epidermis. See also *stain.*

dermoid cyst see under *ovarian tumors.*

DES abbrev. See *diethylstilbestrol.*

desalt (de-sawlt') to remove salt from a substance. Clinical specimens are sometimes desalted electrolytically before analysis, as, for example, urine in the determination of amino acids by thin-media chromatography or electrophoresis.

desaturation (de-sach"u-ra'shun) the introduction of a double bond into an organic compound, e.g., a saturated fatty acid.

Descemet's membrane (des-ĕ-māz') [Jean *Descemet,* French anatomist, 1732–1810] a thin, hyaline, acellular membrane between the stroma and endothelial layer of the cornea; the elastic properties of this layer act to distribute tension evenly over the cornea.

desensitization (de-sen"sĭ-tĭ-za'shun) a condition in which an organism does not react immunologically to a specific antigen; also, the process by which this condition is brought about.

desensitize (de-sen'sĭ-tiz) 1. to deprive of sensation; paralysis of a sensory nerve by section or blocking. 2. to remove antibody from sensitized cells or blood for the purpose of preventing allergy or anaphylaxis.

desferrioxamine (des-fer"e-oks'ah-mēn) see *deferoxamine mesylate.*

desiccant (des'ĭ-kant) [L. *desiccare* to dry up] an agent that promotes dryness, such as anhydrous calcium chloride, magnesium perchlorate, or silica gel. Desiccants are used to remove moisture from gaseous, liquid, or solid substances.

desiccate (des'ĭ-kāt) to render thoroughly dry.

desiccation (des"ĭ-ka'shun) the removal of water from a substance.

desiccator (des'ĭ-ka"tor) a vessel in which apparatus or substances are enclosed with a desiccant to be dried.

desipramine (des-ip'rah-mēn) a tricyclic antidepressant used as desipramine hydrochloride [USP] to treat major depression. In the body it is a metabolite of imipramine. See also *tricyclic antidepressant.* Trademarks, *Norpramin* and *Pertofrane.*

desipramine assays see *imipramine and desipramine assays.*

-desis (de'sis) [Gr. "binding"] a suffix word element to denote binding or fusion, e.g., arthrodesis.

deslanoside (des-lan'o-sīd) [USP], a digitalis glycoside, deacetyllanatoside C, which occurs as a white crystalline powder and is prepared by the alkaline hydrolysis of lanatoside C. Deslanoside is most often administered intravenously and is commonly used in the digitalization of patients suffering from heart failure and requiring rapid parenteral digitalis effect. Trademark, Cedilanid-D. See also *digitalis glycosides.*

desm/o (des'mo) [Gr. *desmos* band, ligament] a word element used in combining form to denote band, bond, or ligament, e.g., desmopathy, desmoplasia.

desmoid tumor an aggressive form of musculoaponeurotic fibromatosis, so named because of its tendon-like consistency. The lesion is best known for its occurrence in the anterior abdominal wall of females of childbearing age, but extraabdominal desmoids occur, and common locations for the latter are the neck, chest wall, and extremities. Desmoid tumors infiltrate aggressively but do not metastasize, and malignant transformation is rare. The lesions are not encapsulated, and, as the periphery is indistinct, pathologic evaluation of the surgical margins at the time of excision is advisable. It can be difficult, however, to distinguish the lesion from reactive fibrous tissue in frozen sections. The proliferating cells are fibroblasts and myofibroblasts, and they may form parallel bundles or be loosely arranged. Mitotic figures can usually be found, and the distinction of a cellular desmoid tumor from a low-grade fibrosarcoma can be difficult and sometimes is not possible. Because low-grade fibrosarcomas rarely metastasize, the location and size of a desmoid tumor determine the form of treatment.

17,20 desmolase (des'mo-lās) an enzyme catalyzing the conversion of 17αOH-pregnenolone to dehydroepiandrosterone in the biosynthetic pathway for testosterone. Defects of this enzyme cause male pseudohermaphrodism.

20,22 desmolase a complex of enzymes that catalyze the conversion of cholesterol to pregnenolone. The reaction involves cleavage of the side-chain in three successive oxidation reactions. Cytochrome P_{450} is a component of the system and NADPH is a secondary electron donor. This complex is involved in the biosynthetic pathway for testosterone. Enzymatic defects in this complex cause male pseudohermaphrodism.

20,22-desmolase deficiency a rare metabolic disorder due to a deficiency of 20,22-desmolase, resulting in a block in the synthesis of steroids from cholesterol. The disorder is characterized by adrenal insufficiency, hyperplasia, and lipid infiltration. Cortisol, aldosterone, sex hormones, and urinary steroids are not produced. Affected males are incompletely masculinized; both sexes develop salt wasting and usually die during infancy. This defect may be detected in utero and is thought to be genetically transmitted. Also called lipoid adrenal hyperplasia.

desmoplasia (des"mo-pla'ze-ah) [*desmo-* + Gr. *plasis* molding + *-ia*] the formation of fibrous tissue, a term applied particularly to the production of a fibrous stroma by a tumor, as in scirrhous breast carcinoma. The process is accompanied by fibroblastic activity and collagen production, and is at least partially the result of the creation of new fibrous tissue in response to the presence of the tumor.

desmosine (des′mo-sēn) a compound containing a pyridine ring with four lysine-related substituents attached. It is formed by the condensation of three molecules of allysine (the aldehyde derivative of lysine) and one molecule of lysine. Desmosyl residues (desmosine attached to protein by peptide linkages at its amino and carboxyl groups) serve as cross-linking agents in the structural protein elastin. See also *elastin.*

desmosome (des′mo-sōm) [*desmo-* + Gr. *sōma* body] a cell junction adapted for cell cohesion. The adjacent membranes are separated by a gap of about 20 nm within which there is material of low electron density bisected by an intermediate disk; the material presumably consists of cement substances such as sialic acid. On the inner aspect of each cell membrane, a dense plaque provides a site for the insertion of tonofilaments of the cytoskeleton. Desmosomes are particularly numerous and well developed in the stratified squamous epithelium of the epidermis. Also called *macula adherens.*

hemidesmosome, a structure corresponding to one-half of a desmosome and found in an epithelial cell, where it abuts on a basal lamina.

desmosterol (des-mos′ter-ol) cholesta-5,24-dien-3β-ol or 24-dehydrocholesterol, the immediate precursor of cholesterol.

desolvation (de″sol-va′shun) removal of a solvent.

desoxy- (des-ok′se) see *deoxy-.*

11-desoxycorticosterone (DOC) (des-ok″se-kor″-tĭ-kos′ter-ōn) 21-hydroxypregn-4-ene-3,20-dione, a corticosteroid with mineralocorticoid activity that is synthesized in the zona fasciculata of the adrenal cortex; M.W. 330.45. It is an important intermediate in the biosynthesis of aldosterone and corticosterone, and is not usually present to a great extent in the blood.

DOC is considerably less potent than aldosterone and helps to regulate salt and water metabolism, causing sodium retention and potassium loss. It can cause expansion of extracellular volume, increased blood pressure, and increased resorption of Na^+, Cl^-, and HCO_3^- in the distal tubule of the kidneys, in the gastrointestinal mucosa, and in the sweat and salivary glands. DOC concentration is increased in Cushing's syndrome, adrenal carcinoma, ACTH-like secreting tumors, and Cushing's disease. Decreased values are noted in adrenal insufficiency (Addison's disease) and panhypopituitarism (Sheehan's syndrome). The reference range for DOC in serum is 40–180 pg/ml, the mean evening level being 50 percent of the morning level.

It is administered as desoxycorticosterone acetate [USP] or desoxycorticosterone pivalate [USP] for replacement therapy in Addison's disease or salt-losing adrenogenital syndrome.

Also called 11-deoxycorticosterone. See also *mineralocorticoid.*

desquamation (des″kwah-ma′shun) [*de-* + L. *squama* scale] the shedding of layers, often used to describe the sheetlike loss of skin.

desquamative (des-kwam′ah-tiv) characterized by desquamation.

desquamative interstitial pneumonitis (DIP) see *desquamative interstitial p.* under *pneumonitis.*

desynapsis (de″sin-ap′sis) [*de-* + Gr. *synapsis* contact] the early separation of homologous chromosomes that have synapsed to form a bivalent, usually owing to lack of chiasmata.

desynchronization (de-sin″kron-i-za′shun) [*de-* + Gr. *synchronos* concurrent] loss of synchronization. See also *attenuation* and *blocking.*

desynchronized sleep (de-sin′kron-īzd″) see under *sleep* and *s. stages.*

detachment (de-tach′ment) [Fr. *détacher* to unfasten; to separate] the condition of being unfastened, disconnected, or separated. See also *retinal detachment.*

detail (de-tāl′, de′tāl) the degree to which small structures are visible in a radiograph.

detector (de-tek′tor) a device that senses the presence of something or measures the amount present; examples include the image detector of a scintillation camera, the light detector of a spectrophotometer, any device that detects radiation, and the various devices on gas or high-pressure liquid chromatographs that detect the presence of chemical compounds. See also specific types of detectors.

detector transfer function (DTF) see *modulation transfer function.*

detergent (de-ter′jent) [L. *detergere* to cleanse] an agent that has a cleansing action; e.g., soaps and synthetic detergents can both be considered as detergents. The term is most frequently applied to synthetic detergents, synthetic organic compounds with surface-active properties. Those most widely used are the linear alkyl sulfonates, which are anionic and biodegradable. Some of the cationic (alkaline) detergents are also very effective as antiviral and antibacterial agents, being widely used for skin antisepsis and for sanitizing food utensils.

determinant (de-ter′mĭ-nant) [L. *determinare* to bound or limit] 1. a factor responsible for the essential nature of an entity or event.

2. in mathematics, a function defined for square matrices that is used in solving linear equations. It has the following properties: (1) interchanging any two rows (or columns) of the matrix changes the sign of the determinant, (2) multiplying each element of a row by a constant multiplies the determinant by that constant, and (3) adding one row to another row (element by element) leaves the determinant unchanged.

determination (de-ter″mĭ-na′shun) in the developing embryo, the commitment of a part of the embryo to a single pathway of histogenesis, from which it does not normally diverge.

deterministic (de-ter″mĭ-nis′tik) pertaining to a process described by a law that completely specifies the effects in terms of a number of causes. Cf. *probabilistic.*

detoxication (de-tok″sĭ-ka′shun) see *detoxification.*

detoxification (de-tok″sĭ-fĭ-ka′shun) [*de-* + L. *toxicum* poison] reduction of the toxic properties of any toxic substance.

metabolic d., reduction of the toxic properties of a substance by chemical reactions carried out in the body, most commonly in the liver or kidneys.

detritus (de-tri′tus) [L., from *deterere* to rub away] particulate matter produced by or remaining after the wearing away or disintegration of a substance or tissue. Detritus can be organic or nonorganic, depending on the nature of the original material.

deutan (doo′tan) a person who has deuteranomaly or deuteranopia.

deuteranomaly (doo″ter-ah-nom′ah-le) defective color vision of the trichromatic type in which green vision is anomalous (weak).

deuteranopia (doo″ter-ah-no′pe-ah) [Gr. *deuteros* second + *an*-neg. + *ōpē* sight + *-ia*] defective color vision of the dichromatic type in which green cones are lacking. The full spectral range is perceived and the luminosity of colors is normal but some colors cannot be distinguished. See also *color blindness.*

deuterium (^2H or D) (doo-te′re-um) [Gr. *deuteros* second] the stable, mass two isotope of hydrogen. It may be used to make labeled compounds, which are detectable by mass spectroscopy. Also called heavy hydrogen.

Deuteromycetes (doo″ter-o-mi-se′tēz) [Gr. *deuteros* second + *mykēs* fungus] a class of fungi with only asexual spores that arise from spore-bearing hyphae without nuclear fusion. Most pathogenic fungi are Deuteromycetes. Also called *Adelomycetes* and *Fungi Imperfecti.*

deuteron (D) (doo′ter-on) [Gr. *deuteros* second + *-on* particle] the nucleus of a deuterium atom, which contains one proton and one neutron.

deuterosome (doo′ter-o-sōm″) [Gr. *deuteros* second + *sōma* body] see *procentriole organizer.*

develop (de″vel′op) 1. to undergo development.

2. to process exposed photographic film to bring out the latent image.

developer (de-vel′o-per) a solution of chemicals used in developing photographic film.

development (de-vel′op-ment) 1. the process of growth and differentiation.

2. the separation of a sample mixture in a chromatographic procedure. See also *chromatography.*

3. see *film processing.*

developmental genetics (de-vel″op-men′tal) the study of the genetic control of growth and development. Also called *phenogenetics.*

developmental jaw cyst a cyst that results from faulty jaw formation. In the embryo the jaws develop from the fusion of facial processes, which consist of a connective tissue core covered with a layer of epithelium. As these facial processes fuse, the epithelial covering degenerates and the adjacent connective tissue components unite. If the process of epithelial degeneration is incomplete, nests of epithelial cells remain in the connective tissue at the site of fusion and can give rise to developmental jaw cysts (also called fissural cysts).

The globulomaxillary cyst develops in the bones of the anterior maxilla between the lateral incisor and cuspid teeth at the site of fusion of the medial nasal process and the lateral palatal process (Fig. 1). It displays an inverted pear-shaped appearance when viewed on x-ray and can cause divergence of the adjacent teeth as it enlarges. Globulomaxillary cysts are lined by stratified squamous and ciliated columnar epithelia.

The median anterior maxillary cyst arises in the bones of the maxilla between the central incisor teeth at the site of the incisive canal (Fig. 2). It forms from remnants of the nasopalatine duct, an embryonic structure that joins the oral and nasal cavities. It is also called nasopalatine duct cyst.

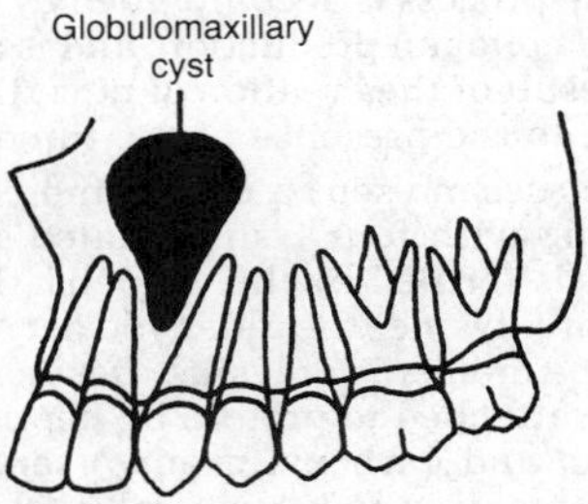

Developmental jaw cyst, Figure 1. Location of globulomaxillary cyst. (Courtesy of J. Robert Newland, D.D.S.)

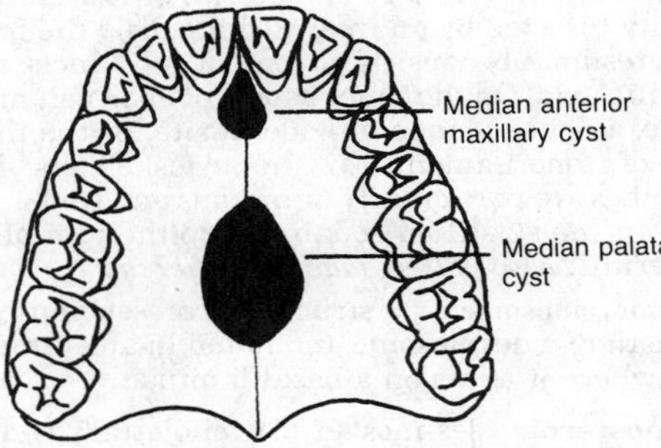

Developmental jaw cyst, Figure 2. Location of median anterior maxillary and median palatal cysts. (Courtesy of J. Robert Newland, D.D.S.)

The median palatal cyst is situated in the bones of the palate along the line of fusion of the lateral palatal processes of the maxilla. If this cyst enlarges, it produces a swelling in the roof of the mouth.

The median mandibular cyst develops at the site of fusion of the mandibular arches and is found between the roots of the central incisor teeth. Enlargement can displace the roots of these teeth.

J. ROBERT NEWLAND, D.D.S.

developmental synchronism the normal maturation of a cell or an organism in which the component parts differentiate simultaneously in a parallel fashion.

deviation (de″ve-a′shun) [L. *deviare* to turn aside] the distance between a statistical sample datum and some central point such as the sample mean. See also *mean deviation* and *standard deviation.*

device (dĕ-vis′) 1. a machine, instrument, or contrivance that performs a specific function.

2. in electronics, a discrete component, such as a resistor, transistor, or integrated circuit.

3. in automatic data processing, a subunit of a computer system, such as an input/output device.

dew (doo) moisture that condenses from the air.

Dewar flask (dyoo′er) [Sir James *Dewar,* Scottish physicist, 1842–1923] a vessel used to contain cryogenic liquids, such as liquid nitrogen or liquid helium. It has double walls, silvered on the interior, that form a chamber that is evacuated (to minimize heat transfer by radiation).

dew point the temperature at which dew forms.

dexamethasone (dek″sah-meth′ah-sōn) [USP], a synthetic glucocorticoid, a potent analog of cortisol. It is used as an antiinflammatory steroid with little salt-retaining action and also as a cancer chemotherapeutic drug. Trademark, Decadron. For more information, see *Appendix A.*

dexamethasone suppression test a suppression test used to differentiate between adrenocortical hyperplasia and adrenocortical carcinoma. One standard version of the test procedure involves administration of dexamethasone, a potent cortisol analog: 0.5 mg × 6/48 hr, which normally reduces the concentration of 17-hydroxycorticosteroids excreted in the urine to less than 4 mg/da, and total 17-ketogenic steroids to less than 7 mg/da. Free cortisol excretion decreases to less than 50 percent of the baseline. In patients with adrenocortical hyperplasia, a 2-mg dose reduces the elevated baseline levels of 17-keto-, 17-ketogenic-, and 17-hydroxycorticosteroids to less than 50 percent of the baseline, whereas the concentration of free cortisol is suppressed to more than 70 percent of the baseline. With an adrenal neoplasm or with ectopic adrenocorticotropic hormone-producing tumors, 17-keto-, 17-hydroxy-, and 17-ketogenic steroid execretion is maintained at a high level even after administration of an 8-mg dose. Also called *adrenocorticotropic hormone suppression test.*

dexbrompheniramine maleate (deks″brōm-fenir′ah-mēn) [USP], an antihistamine used in allergy medications.

dexchlorpheniramine maleate (deks″klōr-fenir′ah-mēn) [USP], the dextrorotatory optical isomer of chlorpheniramine maleate, an antihistamine used in allergy medications.

Dexedrine (dek′sĕ-drēn) trademark. See *dextroamphetamine.*

dextr/o [L. *dexter* right] a word used in combining form to denote right or to the right, e.g., dextrocerebral. Cf. *lev/o.*

dextran (deks′tran) a high-molecular-weight polymer of D-glucose; it has an open three-dimensional network structure that can be freely penetrated by water and that forms a highly viscous, sticky, slimy, gelatinous solution. Dextran is synthesized by enzymes (glycosyl transferases) on the cell surface of certain lactic acid bacteria. The polysaccharide backbone has α-(1→6) glycosidic linkages, and the backbones are connected in different species by α-(1→2), -(1→3), or -(1→4) glycosidic cross-links.

Commercial preparations (Sephadex, Bio-Gel) in bead form are widely used as molecular sieve chromatographic media. The degree of cross-linking determines the pore size.

Uniform-molecular-weight preparations of dextran from *Leuconostoc mesenteroides,* dextran 40 (M.W. 40,000), dextran 70, (M.W. 70,000), and dextran 75 (M.W. 75,000), are used as plasma volume expanders. Because dextran solution contains no clotting factors, excessive use may cause hemorrhagic diathesis.

Dextrans produced from sucrose by *Streptococcus mutans* contribute to the formation of dental plaque. The dextran traps the lactic acid and other acids produced by bacteria, which are the direct cause of dental caries.

dextrin (deks′trin) [L. *dexter* right] a mixture of hydrolysis products from the partial hydrolysis of starch by the enzyme amylase or hydrochloric acid, consisting of glucose, maltose, and dextrin proper (higher-molecular-weight carbohydrates containing glucose in α(1→4) and α(1→6) linkages). Dextrin is soluble in three parts of boiling water, less soluble in cold water, and insoluble in alcohol and ether. Dextrins are only mildly reducing, as only terminal glucose residues can react. Dextrins give a reddish-brown color with iodine. See also *α-dextrin, ϕ-dextrin,* and *erythrodextrin.*

α-dextrin a product of the partial hydrolysis of starch by amylases. Dextrins may contain five to nine or more glucose residues in α(1 → 4) linkages if generated from amylose and in both α(1 → 4) and α(1 → 6) linkages if generated from amylopectin or glycogen. Depending on the number of glucose residues, they may stain purple, red, pink, or remain colorless with iodine. Like glucose, dextrins are reducing compounds and are dextrorotatory. See also *erythrodextrin.*

ϕ-dextrin a phosphorylase limit dextrin, an end product of phosphorylase action on glycogen if phosphorylase is the only enzyme present that can act on glycogen. Phosphorolysis of 1,4 bonds proceeds along the glucose chain from the nonreducing end until a glucose residue of at least four units from a 1,6 branch point is reached, at which point the reaction stops. The limit dextrin residue containing these glucose stubs is referred to as ϕ-dextrin. In tissues, an oligosaccharide transferase shifts the glucose stubs to another side-chain, allowing additional phosphorolysis. The single branch-point residue remaining is split by a 1,6-glucosidase. See also *limit dextrin.*

α-dextrinase (deks′trin-ās) an enzyme in the intestinal mucosa, dextrin-6-α-D-glucanohydrolase (EC 3.2.1.10), that can hydrolyze 1,6 bonds as well as 1,4 bonds in branched polysaccharides, releasing glucose from α-dextrins. Also called limit dextrinase.

dextro- (deks′tro) a prefix word element used in chemistry to denote a dextrorotatory compound, e.g., dextroamphetamine. Cf. *levo-.*

dextroamphetamine (deks″tro-am-fet′ah-mēn) the optical isomer of amphetamine that has a greater central nervous system stimulating effect and a higher potential for abuse than amphetamine. It is used as dextroamphetamine phosphate [USP] or dextroamphetamine sulfate [USP] (Dexadrine) in the treatment of hyperactivity and minimal brain dysfunction in children and in treatment of narcolepsy. See also *amphetamine* and *amphetamine assays.* Cf. *levamphetamine.*

dextrocardia (deks″tro-kar′de-ah) [*dextro-* + Gr. *kardia* heart] location of the heart in the right hemithorax, with the apex pointing to the right. It occurs with or without transposition of abdominal viscera.

dextromethorphan hydrobromide (deks″tro-meth-or′fan) [USP], a synthetic derivative of morphine used as a cough suppressant, acting centrally to elevate the cough threshold. It has little analgesic effect and low toxicity, and is generally used in combination with other agents in preparations designed to relieve symptoms of common respiratory disease.

dextrorotatory (deks″tro-ro′tah-to″re) [*dextro-* + L. *rotare* to turn] pertaining to an optically active compound with a positive optical rotation, i.e., rotation to the right or clockwise as the observer looks toward the beam of polarized light. See also *optical activity.*

dextrose (deks′trōs) [USP], an outmoded chemical name for D-glucose, now also primarily used as the nonproprietary drug name for solutions of glucose given by intravenous administration.

dextrosuria (deks″tro-su′re-ah) [*dextrose* + Gr. *ouron* urine + *-ia*] the presence of higher than normal concentrations of dextrose (D-glucose) in the urine. Also called *glucosuria.*

dextrothyroxine sodium (deks″tro-thi-rok′sēn) [USP], D-thyroxine, the dextrorotatory stereoisomer of the hormone L-thyroxine, used for the treatment of hyperlipoproteinemia. It increases the catabolism and excretion of cholesterol by the liver. Side-effects are increased metabolism, an increased incidence of myocardial ischemia and other heart irregularities, and the potentiation of anticoagulant drugs.

df abbrev. See *degrees of freedom.*

DFOM abbrev. See *deferoxamine.*

DF^{32}P abbrev. See *diisopropyl phosphofluoridate.*

dg abbrev. See *decigram.*

dGMP abbrev. See *deoxyguanosine-5′-phosphate.*

DH abbrev. See *delayed hypersensitivity.*

dhobie itch (do′be) [Hindu "laundryman"] contact dermatitis due to laundry marking dye (bhilawanol oil) used by Indian washermen (dhobies).

DHR abbrev. for delayed hypersensitivity reaction.

DI abbrev. See *d. insipidus* under *diabetes.*

di- (di) [Gr. *dis* twice, double] a prefix word element to denote twice, e.g., dicarboxylic acid.

dia- (di′ah) [Gr. *dia* through] a prefix word element to denote through, between, apart, across, or completely, e.g., diaphragm.

diabetes (di″ah-be′tēz) [Gr. *diabētēs* a syphon, from *bainein* to go] a general term referring to disorders characterized by the copious production and excessive excretion of urine.

bronze d., see *hemochromatosis.*

d. insipidus (DI), an unusual type of diabetes characterized by the production of large quantities of urine that has low specific gravity but is normal in all other characteristics. It is caused by either a deficient neurohypophyseal production of vasopressin (ADH) or the abnormal response of the renal tubules to the action of vasopressin.

Diabetes insipidus due to the deficient production of vasopressin may be classified as primary or secondary. The primary defect, due to genetic factors, may be transmitted as a dominant trait or may occur spontaneously. The secondary form results from a functional destruction of the hypothalamus due to trauma, neoplasms, systemic infections, histiocytosis, or granulomatous disease. DI due to renal tubules that are unresponsive to the action of vasopressin is called nephrogenic DI. It is usually transmitted as an X-linked recessive trait or is associated with hyperuricemia. Several drugs, such as demeclocycline, may also induce this condition.

Individuals with DI exhibit increased, prolonged thirst and massive urinary output (4–20 l/da). Restriction of fluids leads to dehydration, fatigue, hypothermia, and shock; following fluid restriction, the urine is not concentrated. Polyuria associated with urine of a specific gravity of less than 1.006 is suggestive of this condition. There is hyperosmolarity of the plasma ($<$285–290 mOsm/kg). In the primary and secondary forms of this disorder, vasopressin falls below a level of 1–3 μU/ml in the plasma and 11–30 μU/hr in the urine. Those so affected exhibit rises in urine osmolarity following administration of 5 units of vasopressin. Failure to respond to vasopressin therapy indicates the presence of nephrogenic DI. Development of a radioimmune assay for arginine vasopressin may help to differentiate the true form of DI from similar clinical disorders (such as psychogenic polydipsia).

After diagnosis of this disease has been established, the possibility of brain lesions should be investigated by means of brain scans, CT scans, visual field tests, and encephalograms. Primary lung and breast neoplasms and bone lesions of xanthomatosis should also be sought. Pyelonephritis and hydronephrosis also are commonly observed in nephrogenic DI.

d. mellitus (DM), a chronic syndrome of impaired carbohydrate, protein, and fat metabolism secondary to insufficient secretion of insulin or to target tissue insulin resistance. It encompasses a heterogeneous group of disorders that vary in etiology, clinical manifestations, and patterns of inheritance. The classical symptoms of DM are polyuria, polydipsia, ketonuria, and rapid weight loss. Diagnosis is based either on the classical pattern of symptoms accompanied by hyperglycemia or on laboratory findings indicating a pattern of hyperglycemia or glucose intolerance. The acute metabolic derangements of DM can be controlled by appropriate therapy. However, diabetics are susceptible to a group of serious complications appearing later in life, including atherosclerosis, microangiopathy, retinopathy, nephropathy, and neuropathy, which produce considerable morbidity and premature mortality.

CLASSIFICATION. DM is classified into two major types. Type I, insulin-dependent (IDDM), is characterized by an abrupt onset of symptoms, insulinopenia, dependence on exogenous insulin to sustain life, and a tendency to develop ketoacidosis. The peak age of onset is 12 yr, but onset can occur at any age. IDDM was formerly called juvenile-onset diabetes (JOD). Type II, noninsulin-dependent (NIDDM), is characterized by a gradual onset with minimal or no symptoms of metabolic disturbance. Individuals with NIDDM do not develop significant ketosis. The peak age of onset is between ages 50 and 60 yr, but can occur in any age group and the diagnosis may be delayed for many years. NIDDM was formerly called adult-onset diabetes and maturity-onset diabetes. NIDDM is further divided into two subtypes, obese and nonobese NIDDM. Obesity is thought to be important in the etiology of the glucose intolerance of the former such type.

Gestational diabetes mellitus is defined as glucose intolerance with onset during pregnancy, and is thought to be due to metabolic and hormonal changes that occur during pregnancy. It is associated with an increased risk of perinatal complications and also with an increased tendency to develop glucose intolerance in the absence of pregnancy for 5–10 yr after the pregnancy.

Glucose intolerance can also occur secondary to many other diseases and conditions including pancreatic disease, endocrine disorders, hyperglycemia produced by chemical agents, genetic disorders, and malnutrition.

ETIOLOGY AND PATHOLOGY. Approximately 2–4 percent of the population of the United States has diagnosed DM; about 10 percent of diabetics have IDDM. IDDM is due to lack of insulin production by the beta cells of the pancreatic islets. It is thought that in most cases there is a genetic predisposition to beta-cell injury, which is possibly caused by viral infection or autoimmune reactions. Islet cell antibodies are detectable in about 75 percent of IDDM individuals at diagnosis. About one-third of patients have a period of remission lasting a few weeks or months, followed by a relapse that does not remit.

In NIDDM, the basal level of insulin may be low, normal, or elevated. Insulin release in response to a glucose load is generally delayed or reduced, but occasionally a brisk insulin response is present. The defect resulting in glucose intolerance is a resistance to insulin; this may be due to a decreased number of insulin receptors on target cells, a decreased affinity of the receptors for insulin, or to a postreceptor defect. NIDDM is strongly associated with obesity; about 80 percent of NIDDM patients are at least 25 percent over their ideal weight. The genetics of all types of DM are unclear.

CLINICAL MANIFESTATIONS. In undiagnosed or inadequately controlled IDDM, the lack of insulin causes hyperglycemia, protein wasting, and production of ketone bodies (acetoacetate, β-hydroxybutyrate, and acetone). The hyperglycemia causes glycosuria and osmotic diuresis, which in turn results in hyperosmolarity and dehydration. The final result is diabetic ketoacidosis, hyperosmolar coma, or a combination of both (see *diabetic coma*). Accompanying symptoms are the "three polys": polyuria, polydipsia, and polyphagia, plus weight loss, lassitude, paresthesias, leg cramps, and recurrent blurred vision due to altered osmolarity in the lens. If untreated, individuals may progress to nausea, vomiting, stupor, coma, and death.

The acute symptoms of NIDDM are usually mild, and diagnosis is occasionally based solely on laboratory findings. Individuals with NIDDM do not develop ketoacidosis, although in some cases they can develop hyperglycemic hyperosmolar nonketotic coma.

There are many long-term complications, which typically take 10–15 years to develop. Many pathologic changes occur in the basement membranes, small vessels, arteries, pancreas, kidneys, retinas, and peripheral nerves. Basement membrane thickening (BMT) occurs in the capillaries, renal tubules, Bowman's capsule, and peripheral nerves; this is thought to be due to the increased incorporation of carbohydrate in basement membrane glycoproteins, and results in an abnormal permeability to plasma proteins. BMT is the primary cause of diabetic microangiopathy.

Atherosclerosis is much more common in diabetics than in nondiabetics. Diabetics are five times more likely to have significant coronary atherosclerosis or to have a myocardial infarction. Pancreatic changes vary; in IDDM there is usually a reduction in the size and number of the islets, beta cell degranulation, and, in time, hyalin replacement of islets. Microangiopathy and BMT cause severe kidney damage; about 40 percent of insulin-dependent diabetics die from acute renal failure that is due to glomerular sclerosis, pyelonephritis, arteriolosclerosis, glycogen accumulation, or fatty change. Diabetic retinopathy is a leading cause of blindness; it begins as a nonproliferative retinopathy characterized by microaneurysms of the retinal capillaries, and may progress to proliferative retinopathy characterized by neovascularization and fibrosis. Symmetric peripheral neuropathy of sensory and motor nerves in the lower extremities is common; it is due to degeneration of the myelin, which may also occur in the central nervous system. Skin lesions such as diabetic xanthomas are also common.

LABORATORY TESTS. The diagnosis of DM is based on the finding of an elevated fasting glucose concentration (FBG), and/or an increased 2-hr postprandial value of an abnormal oral glucose tolerance test (OGTT). Formerly, the terms chemical and borderline were used to refer to individuals with abnormal values within these parameters but with no diabetic symptoms; these appellations have now been replaced by the term impaired glucose tolerance.

Current criteria for diagnosis of DM in children or nonpregnant adults are an elevated fasting blood glucose concentration on more than one occasion (plasma glucose >140 mg/dl) or an abnormal oral glucose tolerance test on more than one occasion. The plasma glucose may be 15 percent lower than the serum glucose concentration. The oral glucose load in the OGTT has been standardized at 75 g for adults and 1.75 g/kg of ideal body weight (maximum, 75 g) for children. The glucose values 2 hr after an oral glucose load may be increased with age over 50 yr; thus, the GTC must be interpreted with this in mind. Generally, a plasma glucose concentration of >200 mg/dl is diagnostic of DM. In normal individuals, 1-hr values of >200 mg/dl are consistent with a diagnosis of DM, but may be seen in other, nondiabetic conditions. A laboratory test used in monitoring control of hyperglycemia is the hemoglobin A_{1c} level, which gives an approximation of the average blood glucose level for the month preceding the test (see also *Hb* A_{1a}, *Hb* A_{1b}, *Hb* A_{1c} under *hemoglobin*).

Insulin and C peptide, which are secreted into the circulation on a 1:1 molar ratio, are both measurable by radioimmunoassay. The insulin radioimmunoassay can be useful in differentiating insulinopenic from insulinoplethoric forms of DM. The assay is also useful in differentiating the various causes of hypoglycemia. Patients who have received exogenous insulin develop antiinsulin antibodies but do not develop antibodies to C peptide. Thus the insulin radioimmunoassay cannot be used to measure insulin levels in patients who have previously received insulin therapeutically; however, C peptide radioimmunoassay can be used in its place as an indicator of insulin secretion.

diabetic (di″ah-bet′ik) 1. referring to or characterized by diabetes.

2. a patient manifesting the clinical symptoms of diabetes.

diabetic angiopathy see *diabetic a.* under *angiopathy.*

diabetic coma a state of unresponsiveness due to abnormal metabolic processes associated with diabetes mellitus. There are three recognized types of diabetic coma: hypoglycemic coma, due to the excessive administration of insulin or oral hypoglycemic agents (insulin reaction); hyperglycemic coma, due to a severe deficiency of insulin (the coma resulting from ketoacidosis); and hyperglycemic coma, due to a mild insulin deficiency (resulting from dehydration and prerenal azotemia and referred to as hyperosmolar diabetic coma). Differentiation among the various states is based on physical diagnosis and laboratory tests, including plasma determinations of glucose, bicarbonate, pH, and acetone, as well as urinary determination of glucose and acetone.

hyperosmolar d. c., a form of diabetic coma characterized by severe hyperglycemia in the absence of ketosis. It occurs most frequently in individuals with mild or undiagnosed diabetes mellitus. Ineffective insulin action decreases glucose utilization, increases glucagon levels and hepatic glucose output, and leads to a massive glycosuria and water loss. Hyperosmolarity and severe dehydration ensue.

Those affected with this condition experience a slowly developing polydipsia and polyuria. If fluid intake is reduced as a consequence of burns, systemic disease, or drug therapy, the condition is accelerated. Fluid loss leads to renal insufficiency and hyperosmolarity, mental confusion, and can lead to coma.

Laboratory findings include marked hyperglycemia, with a range of 800–2400 mg/100 ml. Dehydration may cause serum sodium levels to exceed 140 mEq/l. This may lead to serum osmolarity readings of 330–440 mOsm/kg. Prerenal azotemia is common, leading to blood urea nitrogen (BUN) levels of 90 mg/100 ml. Ketosis and acidosis are uncommon. Isotonic saline and potassium replacement therapy is recommended in the clinical management of this disorder.

Also called nonketonic hyperglycemic coma.

diabetic glomerulosclerosis see under *glomerulopathy.*

Diabinese (di-ab′ĭ-nēz) trademark. See *chlorpropamide.*

diacetic acid (di″ah-se′tik) see *acetoacetic acid.*

diacylglycerol (di-as″il-glis′er-ol) see *diglyceride.*

Diagnex Blue (di′ag-neks) trademark. See *azuresin.*

diagnosis (di″ag-no′sis) [*dia-* + Gr. *gnōsis* knowledge] 1. the determination of the nature of a case of disease.

2. the detection of errors or faults in computer programs or electronic circuitry.

clinical d., diagnosis based on the signs, symptoms, and laboratory findings obtained from examination of a patient by medical personnel.

cytologic d., diagnosis of disease by the microscopic examination of exfoliated cells.

differential d., the consideration of which of two or more diseases or conditions is affecting a patient. The process involves systematic comparison and decision analysis based on clinical, laboratory, and radiologic findings.

laboratory d., diagnosis based on the findings of laboratory examinations or measurements.

pathologic d., diagnosis made by a pathologist from the gross, microscopic, or electron microscopic, histo- or immunochemical, and cytologic examination of cells, tissues, or organs.

physical d., determination of disease by methods including visual inspection, palpation, percussion, and auscultation.

provocative d., the induction of a condition for the purpose of diagnosis, as the induction of a seizure to establish a diagnosis of epilepsy.

diagram (di′ah-gram) a simplified graphic representation of an object, system, or process.

diakinesis (di″ah-ki-ne′sis) [*dia-* + Gr. *kinēsis* motion] the last stage of the first meiotic prophase during which the chiasmata move to the ends of the bivalents and the nucleolus and nuclear membrane dissolve. See also *meiosis.*

dial unit (du) arbitrary units on the energy window setting of a rectilinear scanner.

dialysate (di-al′ĭ-sāt) the part of a mixture that passes through the semipermeable membrane in dialysis.

dialysis (di-al′ĭ-sis) [*dia-* + Gr. *lysis* dissolution] the process of separating some components of a solution having smaller molecular size from others of larger molecular size by the ability of the former to pass through a semipermeable membrane. The size of the molecules retained or allowed to pass through the membrane and their speed of passage are determined by the pore size of the membrane. This principle is employed in the clinical laboratory to separate crystalloids from interfering proteins and cells. See also *clinical chemistry automation* and *hemodialysis.*

dialyzer (di′ah-līz″er) 1. any type of apparatus that permits the separation of small-sized molecules from large-sized molecules by use of a semipermeable membrane (dialysis).

2. an apparatus that permits removal of some undesirable components from blood without loss of protein or formed elements. See also *hemodialyzer.*

3. a component of the AutoAnalyzer that permits the movement of small molecular components of blood (serum) to migrate from the sample stream into the reagent stream (dialysis) while directing proteins and formed elements to waste. See also *clinical chemistry automation.*

diamagnetic (di″ah-mag-net′ik) pertaining to materials in which the molecules or atoms have no intrinsic magnetic moment. An external magnetic field induces a weak opposing magnetization. Diamagnetic susceptibilities are typically about -10^{-5}. Such materials are repelled by a magnet.

diameter (di-am′ĕ-ter) the length of a straight line passing through the center of a circle and connecting opposite points on its circumference; the distance between two specified opposite points on the periphery of a structure such as the cranium or pelvis.

diamide (di-am′īd, di′ah-mid) 1. a compound that contains two amido groups.

2. hydrazine.

diamine (di′ah-mēn) a compound that contains two amino groups.

diaminodiphenyl sulfone (di-am″ĭ-no-di-fen′il) see *dapsone.*

Diamond-Blackfan anemia (di′ah-mond blak′fan) [Louis Klein *Diamond,* U.S. physician, born 1902; Kenneth D. *Blackfan,* U.S. physician, 1883–1941] see *Diamond-Blackfan a.* under *anemia.*

Diamox (di′ah-moks) trademark. See *acetazolamide.*

Diamyl (di-am′il) trademark for amylopectin coupled to Reactone Red 2B, a red dye. It is used as a substrate for determination of amylase activity.

diapedesis (di″ah-pĕ-de′sis) [*dia-* + Gr. *pēdan* to leap] the passage of blood cellular elements, both red cells and leukocytes, from the lumen of a blood vessel to extravascular tissue spaces without damage to the vessel itself. For leukocytes, the process involves active locomotion.

Diaphane solution (di′ah-fān) a coating fixative used for cytologic smears, consisting of a 3:2 mixture of 95 percent ethanol and Diaphane, a semisynthetic gum.

diaphor/o (di′ah-fo-ro) [Gr. *diaphorein* to carry through] a word element used in combining form to denote sweat, e.g., diaphoresis.

diaphoresis (di″ah-fo-re′sis) [Gr. *diphorēsis*] sweating, excessive sweating.

diaphragm (di′ah-fram) [Gr. *diaphragma* a partition-wall, barrier] 1. any separating membrane or structure.

2. the musculomembranous partition that separates the abdominal and thoracic cavities, and is involved with the process of respiration.

3. an adjustable opening that controls the size or shape of an x-ray beam.

eventration of the d., a congenital malformation that results from a defect in or insufficiency of the musculature of the diaphragm, which gives rise to a thin aponeurotic structure that may balloon into the thoracic cavity. There is upward displacement of the abdominal contents into an outpouching of the diaphragm.

field d., an iris diaphragm, placed below a microscope stage, that restricts light to the field of view.

iris d., a mechanical device that provides an aperture having a variable diameter that controls the amount of light entering a camera or that serves as a field diaphragm in a microscope.

Potter-Bucky d., see *Potter-Bucky g.* under *grid.*

diaphragma sellae (di″ah-frag′mah sel′e) [NA], the small, horizontal, circular fold of dura mater covering the sella turcica; it completely covers the pituitary except for a small aperture for the infundibular stalk.

diaphragmatic paralysis (di″ah-fram-at′ik) paralysis of the diaphragm. This condition may occur unilaterally or bilaterally. Unilateral diaphragmatic paralysis results from injury to the phrenic nerve that may result from trauma, inflammation, or neoplasm. This disorder is usually asymptomatic, although the individual may complain of dyspnea. Diagnosis may be confirmed by demonstration of an elevated hemidiaphragm on chest x-ray.

Bilateral diaphragmatic paralysis is far rarer and more serious. It may be due to upper cervical injuries, motor neuron disease, poliomyelitis, polyneuritis, or neoplasms. Individuals suffer severe breathing difficulties and often experience respiratory failure. Diagnosis may be established by measuring transdiaphragmatic pressure at the esophagus and stomach.

Also called phrenic nerve paralysis.

diaphysis (di-af′ĭ-sis), pl. *diaphyses* [Gr. "the point of separation between stalk and branch"] 1. [NA], the portion of a long bone between its ends; it consists of a tube of compact bone enclosing the medullary cavity.

2. that portion of a long bone formed from a primary ossification center.

diapophysis (di-ah-pof′ĭ-sis) [*dia-* + Gr. *apophysis* outgrowth] the true transverse process of a vertebra. See also *costal element.*

diapositive (di″ah-poz′ĭ-tiv) a positive image made from a regular (negative) x-ray film.

Diaptomus (di-ap′to-mus) a genus of copepod crustaceans, which serves as the first intermediate host of the larvae of the tapeworm *Diphyllobothrium latum.* They are very small and are an important food source for fish, through which the parasites are passed to humans. The most common, medically important species is *D. vulgaris.*

diarrhea (di″ah-re′ah) [*dia-* + Gr. *rhein* to flow] an increase in the volume, fluidity, and frequency of bowel movements beyond that which is normal for an individual. Diarrhea can be caused by many disorders, including various bacterial, parasitic, and viral infections; lactose deficiency; regional enteritis; ulcerative colitis; and food poisoning. Epidemics of contagious diarrhea are usually due to bacterial and viral infections. Acute, severe diarrhea may lead to electrolyte depletion, fluid loss with dehydration, and metabolic acidosis. Chronic diarrhea may result in malnutrition.

Stool examination should be performed to note the presence of blood, fat, and pus, and the degree of liquidity; microscopic examination should be performed to look for parasites. A decrease in stool pH (normally greater than 6.0) may be due to bacterial fermentation. Any electrolyte, acid-base, or dehydration disturbances must be carefully monitored.

diarthrosis (di″ar-thro′sis), pl. *diarthroses* [Gr. *diarthrōsis* a movable articulation] see *synovial j.* under *joint.*

diastasis (di-as′tah-sis) [Gr.] 1. the middle third of ventricular diastole, during which time the flow of blood from the atria into the already distended ventricles has nearly reached a standstill.

2. a separation of parts that are normally joined, especially bones that are normally attached to each other without existence of a true joint (the pubic symphysis) or the rectus abdominis muscles during pregnancy.

diastereoisomer (di″ah-ster″e-o-i′so-mer) see *diastereomer.*

diastereoisomerism (di″ah-ster″e-o-i-som′er-izm) the relationship between diastereomers.

diastereomer (di″ah-ster′e-o″-mer) one of a group of compounds that are stereoisomers (i.e., the atoms of which are bonded in the same sequence) but not enantiomers (mirror images); e.g., glucose and galactose or *cis*-2-butene and *trans*-2-butene. Diastereomers differ in their chemical and physical properties. Also called *diastereoisomer.* See also *isomerism.*

diastole (di-as′to-le) [Gr. *diastolē* a drawing asunder, expansion] the relaxation or period of relaxation of the atria or ventricles, during which time they are filling and expanding with the volume of blood to be ejected during systole (contraction). The duration of diastole, approximately equal to 0.5–0.6 sec, can be measured clinically as the time interval between occurrence of the second heart sound (closure of the aortic and pulmonic valves) and the first heart sound (closure of the A-V valves). Cf. *systole.*

diastolic (di″ah-stol′ik) of or pertaining to diastole.

diastolic murmur see under *murmur.*

diastolic pressure see under *arterial pressure.*

diathermy (di′ah-ther″me) [*dia-* + Gr. *thermē* heat] a form of therapy that uses high-frequency electric current produced in three forms: short wave, ultrasound, and microwave. It may be used to produce gentle heat, often in deep tissues. The production of intense heat can also be employed to remove warts surgically and to cauterize blood vessels.

diathesis (di-ath′ĕ-sis) [Gr. "arrangement, disposition"] a constitution or condition of the body that makes a tissue or tissues react in special ways to certain stimuli, thereby tending to make an individual more than usually susceptible to certain disorders.

hemorrhagic d., a predisposition to abnormal hemostasis.

diatom (di′a-tom) a unicellular microscopic alga, belonging to the family Diatomaceae, whose cell wall is made of silica. The skeletal siliceous remains of many species are mined for uses such as filtering and abrasive agents in the laboratory.

diatomaceous earth (di″ah-to-ma′shus) a soft, solid material that is composed of skeletons of diatoms deposited in the earth in earlier geologic times. White, gray, or pale buff in color, it is insoluble in water, acids, and dilute alkali. Containing about 88 percent silica, diatomaceous earth is used as an adsorbant in chromatography, for clarification of filtrates, as a filler in paper, as a heat insulator, and as a fire- and acid-resistant packing agent. Also called Cellite, *kieselguhr*, and Super-Cel.

diatrizoate (di″ah-tri-zo′āt) a radiopaque contrast medium used in urography, angiography, arthrography, and gastrointestinal studies. It is a water-soluble triiodobenzene derivative. A widely used medium, diatrizoate is available in many preparations of the meglumine or sodium salts, or mixtures of the two. Trademarks include Cardiografin, Cystografin, Gastrografin, Hypaque, Renovist, Renografin, and Sinografin (diatrizoate and iodipamide).

diauxic (di-awk′sik) pertaining to or characterized by diauxie; implying two periods of growth separated by a lag period.

diauxie (di-awk′se) [*di-* + Gr. *auxein* to increase in size] a phenomenon of bacterial growth in which an organism that is given a mixture of carbon sources grows exclusively on one until that compound is exhausted. After a lag period during which induced enzymes are formed, growth is resumed on a second carbon compound.

diaxon (di-ak′son) a nerve cell that has two axons.

diazepam (di-az′ĕ-pam) [USP], one of the benzodiazepine minor tranquilizers. A frequently prescribed antianxiety medication, diazepam is also used for treatment of status epilepticus and muscle spasm, for alleviation of alcohol withdrawal symptoms, and for calming patients undergoing minor surgery.

Diazepam and two active metabolites, desmethyldiazepam and oxazepam, have blood concentrations of 0.1–2.0 μg/ml following therapeutic dosages; they are bound to plasma proteins. Oxazepam glucuronide is excreted in the urine. For toxicity, see *benzodiazepine*.

Trademark, *Valium*.

diazepam assays 1. spectrophotometry. Diazepam is extracted from neutralized or alkalinized blood or urine into chloroform and then reextracted into strong acid. The concentration is determined from the difference in absorbance at the peak (near 240 nm) and at the minimum (near 265 nm) for both the sample and a reference solution. Other benzodiazepines and their metabolites interfere.

2. gas chromatography. A nonpolar or intermediate polarity silicone column and a flame ionization or electron capture detector are employed. The peak heights of diazepam in the sample and reference solution, extracted as in method 1, are used to determine the concentration. Many benzodiazepines and other basic drugs interfere; it may be necessary to use two columns for positive identification.

See also *benzodiazepine assays*.

diazinon (di-az′ĭ-non) *O,O*-diethyl-*O*-[6-methyl-2-(1-methylethyl)-4-pyrimidinyl] phosphorothioate, an organophosphate insecticide that is an acetylcholinesterase inhibitor and is highly toxic to humans.

diazo- (di-az′o) a prefix word element in organic chemistry to denote the diazo group ($=N^+=N^-$), e.g., diazomethane.

diazomethane (di-az″o-meth′ān) an extremely poisonous, carcinogenic, explosive, yellow gas, used as a methylation reagent in organic chemistry; M.W. 42.04. It is a resonance hybrid of the two structures: $CH_2=N^+=N^- \rightleftarrows CH_2^-{-}N^+\equiv N$.

diazomethane generator a laboratory device assembled from a series of tubes that is used to generate diazomethane gas. It is commonly employed as a methylation reagent for fatty acid analysis by gas-liquid chromatography.

diazonium salt (di″ah-zo′ne-um) a salt that contains a diazonium ion ($\phi{-}N^+\equiv N$) prepared from an arylamine by diazotization. There are many commercial diazonium salts used as azo coupling reagents, which are usually in a stabilized form (a stable diazotate) produced by reaction with alkali (forming the free base) or with zinc chloride (forming a diazo double salt).

diazo staining method a specific histochemical method for enterochromaffin cell granules. Formalin-fixed paraffin sections are stained with the stable diazonium salt of a dye, such as fast red B (C.I. 37125) or fast red GG (C.I. 37035). Both these salts stain enterochromaffin granules fiery orange-red, while staining argentaffin granules in carcinoid tumors brownish-red. See also *azo coupling reaction*.

diazotize (di-az′o-tīz) to prepare a diazonium salt from an arylamine ($\phi{-}NH_2$) by reaction with nitrous acid and excess mineral acid: $\phi{-}NH_2 + HNO_2 + HCl \rightarrow \phi{-}N^+\equiv N + Cl^- + 2H_2O$, where ϕ represents any aryl group.

dibasic acid (di-bā′sik) [*di-* + Gr. *basis* base] an acid that contains two replaceable hydrogen atoms, e.g., H_2SO_4.

dibenz[*a,h*]anthracene (di″benz-an′thrah-sēn) a polycyclic aromatic hydrocarbon containing five fused benzene rings, $C_{22}H_{14}$; M.W. 278.33. It occurs in coal tar, cigarette smoke, and air pollution, and is a potent procarcinogen that undergoes metabolic activation to an aryl epoxide, the direct-acting carcinogen.

dibenzepin hydrochloride (di-benz′ĕ-pin) a benzodiazepine used as an antidepressant.

Dibenzyline (di-ben′zĭ-lēn) trademark. See *phenoxybenzamine hydrochloride*.

diborane (di′bōr-ān) a highly toxic, flammable gas, B_2H_6, used as a reducing agent in the synthesis of other boron compounds and as a polymerization catalyst. Toxic effects include nausea and convulsions.

dibothriocephaliasis (di-both″re-o-sef″ah-li′ah-sis) see *diphyllobothriasis.*

Dibothriocephalus (di-both″re-o-sef′ah-lus) [*di-* + Gr. *bothrion* pit + *kephalē* head] see *Diphyllobothrium.*

1,2-dibromethane (di″bro-meth′ān) see *ethylene dibromide.*

dibucaine hydrochloride (di′bu-kān) [USP], a water-soluble amide-type, local anesthetic. It is one of the most potent, most toxic, and longest lasting of this group. It is infrequently used topically in ointments and sprays and by injection. Trademark, Nupercaine.

dibucaine number (DN) a parameter used to differentiate variant forms of plasma pseudocholinesterase. The dibucaine number represents the percentage inhibition of enzyme activity for a given substrate (butyryl choline, proprionyl thiocholine) in the presence of a standard concentration (8×10^{-6} mol/l) of dibucaine, under standard assay conditions. The normal form of enzyme shows 70–86 percent inhibition, whereas intermediate and atypical, weakly active variants show 48–60 percent, and under 30 percent, respectively.

DIC abbrev. See *disseminated intravascular coagulation.*

dicarbamylamine (di-kar′bah-mil-ah″mēn) see *biuret.*

dicarboxylic acid (di-kar″bok-sil′ik) an organic compound having two carboxyl groups (COOH).

dicentric (dic) (di-sen′trik) pertaining to, developing from, or having two centers. In genetics, this refers to a chromosome or chromatid with two centromeres. Cf. *acentric* and *monocentric.*

dichlobenil (di-klo′ben-il) a toxic herbicide, 2,6-dichlorobenzonitrile.

***p*-dichlorobenzene** (di-klo″ro-ben′zēn) a white, volatile (subliming) crystalline substance with a penetrating odor, 1,4-dichlorobenzene; M.W. 147.01. It is nonflammable, nontarnishing, and nonbleaching; it is used domestically to repel moths and kill fly larva, and agriculturally to fumigate soil. The vapors are irritating to the eyes, skin, and mucous membranes. Chronic exposure to high concentrations may produce liver damage.

dichlorodiethyl sulfide (di-klo″ro-di-eth′il) see *bis (2-chloroethyl) sulfide.*

1,1-dichloroethane (di-klo″ro-eth′ān) an oily, combustible liquid with the odor and taste of chloroform, CH_3CHCl_2, used as an industrial solvent and synthesis intermediate; M.W. 98.97. It is irritating to the eyes and mucous membranes. It acts as an anesthetic in high concentrations and can produce fatal liver and kidney damage. Also called ethylidene dichloride.

1,2-dichloroethane an oily, highly flammable liquid, CH_2ClCH_2Cl. Its use and toxicity are similar to those of 1,1-dichloroethane. Also called ethylene chloride and *ethylene dichloride.*

***sym*-dichloroethylene** (di-klo″ro-eth′il-ēn) see *acetylene dichloride.*

dichloromethane (di-klo″ro-meth′ān) see *m. chloride* under *methylene.*

(2,4-dichlorophenoxy)acetic acid (di-klo″ro-fen-ok″se-ah-se′tik) see *2,4-D.*

dichloropropene-dichloropropene mixture (di-klo″ro-pro′pēn) a highly toxic pesticide, a mixture of 1,3-dichloropropene and 1,2-dichloropropene, used as a soil fumigant for control of nematodes. It is highly irritating to the eyes, skin, and respiratory tract, and can produce fatal poisoning by ingestion, inhalation, or absorption through the skin.

dichlorvos (DDVP) (di-klor′vos) the generic name for 2,2-dichlorovinyldimethylphosphate, a toxic organophosphate insecticide and fumigant.

dichotomous (di-kot′o-mus) pertaining to dichotomy.

dichotomous variable a variable with only two possible categories. In statistics, it is often called a Bernoulli or binary variable.

dichotomy (di-kot′o-me) [Gr. *dicha* in two + *tomē* a cutting] a division or classification into two parts; in logic and statistics, a division of a class or population into two mutually exclusive groups. (Each member belongs to one and only one of the groups.)

dichroism (di′kro-izm) [*di-* + Gr. *chroa* color] the property of a material that allows it to reflect light of one color while transmitting light of other colors. This property is made use of in the diagnosis of amyloid in tissue sections using the Congo Red stain and viewing the sections under polarization.

circular d. (CD), a difference spectrum for a compound resulting from a plot of the wavelength of the light used versus the difference in intensities of absorption (molecular extinction coefficient) resulting from the use of left and right circularly polarized light. The circular dichroism in the neighborhood of optically active absorption bands can be related to the absolute configuration and the conformation of asymmetric molecules. See also *optical rotary dispersion.*

Dick test (dik) [George Frederick *Dick* (1881–1967) and Gladys Rowena Henry *Dick* (1881–1963), U.S. physicians] a test formerly used to determine the susceptibility of an individual to scarlet fever. In the procedure, purified erythrogenic toxin from group A streptococci is injected intradermally. Susceptibility (a positive response) is indicated by inflammation at the injection site after 24 hr, whereas in immune individuals, antitoxin produced from previous infection neutralizes the toxin, resulting in a negative response. The Dick test is no longer performed because the toxin is unavailable.

dicloxacillin (di-kloks″ah-sil′in) an antibacterial agent used against penicillin-resistant staphylococci. The drug can be administered orally. See also *antibacterial agents* and *penicillins.*

dicofol (di′ko-fol) a moderately toxic miticide, an analog of DDT, 1,1-bis(*p*-chlorophenyl)-2,2,2-trichloroethanol. See also *chlorinated hydrocarbon pesticides.*

Dicrocoelium (dik″ro-se′le-um) [Gr. *dikroos* forked + *koilia* bowel] a genus of flukes of which the most common species is *D. dendriticum.* This species is lancet-shaped and flat, measures 5–15 mm long, and is chiefly parasitic in sheep although it occasionally infects humans. Land snails and certain ants are intermediate hosts. Also called *lancet fluke.*

dicrotic notch (di-krot′ik) [Gr. *dikrotos* double beating] the small, sharp incisura or downward deflection that occurs in the descending portion of the arterial pressure contour just after the maximum systolic pressure has been reached. It is the result of the closing of the aortic valve following the ejection period.

dictyosome (dik′te-o-sōm) [Gr. *diktyon* net + *sōma* body] see *Golgi complex*.

dictyotene (dik′te-o-tēn) [Gr. *diktyon* net] the prolonged diplotene stage in oogenesis. The first meiotic division of human primary oocytes begins in utero, with some entering prophase as early as the third month of fetal life. Division is suspended in diplotene until the time of ovulation, when the first meiotic division is completed and is followed immediately by the second meiotic division.

dicumarol (di-koo′mah-rol) [USP], one of the coumarin group of oral anticoagulants, which acts by inhibiting the hepatic synthesis of vitamin K–dependent coagulation factors (Factors II, VII, IX, and X). Dicumarol is used in the prevention and treatment of thromboembolic disease. It is a natural product formed in spoiled silage, which causes hemorrhagic sweet clover disease in cattle. Formerly called *bishydroxycoumarin*.

dicyclomine hydrochloride (di-si′klo-mēn) [USP], a synthetic parasympatholytic drug used as an antispasmodic in the treatment of irritable bowel syndrome or acute enterocolitis. Adverse reactions are similar to those for other anticholinergics, e.g., dryness of the mouth, blurred vision, urinary retention, drowsiness, tachycardia, and increased blood pressure. Trademark, Bentyl.

Diego antigen (di-eg′o) the antigen responsible for the designation of the Diego blood group system. The antigen Di^a, inherited as a dominant character, is peculiar to people of monogolian extraction (excluding Eskimos). The absence of Di^a is now thought to imply the presence of antigen Di^b. Antibodies against Di^a or Di^b have caused hemolytic disease in newborn infants.

dieldrin (HEOD) (di-el′drin) the generic name for chlorinated cyclodiene hydrocarbon pesticide, 3,4,5,6,9,9-hexachloro-1a,2,2a,3,6,6a,7,7a-octahydro-2,7:3,6-dimethanonaphth[2,3-b]oxirene. The term refers both to the pure compound and to the commercially available product, which contains not less than 85 per cent of this compound and 15 per cent of active, related compounds. It is highly toxic if ingested, inhaled, or absorbed through the skin and is possibly carcinogenic. Serum levels may be measured by gas chromatography. See also *chlorinated hydrocarbon pesticides*.

dielectric (di″ĕ-lek′trik) an electric insulator, particularly one that can be polarized by an applied electric field. Permanent or induced molecular dipoles align with the field, producing a polarization (the net dipole moment per unit volume) proportional to the applied field strength for most materials. The proportionality constant is called the electric susceptibility (χ). In International System (SI) units, the dielectric constant (ϵ) is $1 + \chi$; in the electrostatic centimeter-gram-second system, it is $1 + 4\pi\chi$.

dielectric constant (ϵ) for an isotropic electric insulator, the ratio of the capacitance having that insulator as a dielectric to the same capacitor with vacuum as a dielectric.

dielectric strength the maximal electric potential gradient (usually expressed in volts per millimeter or volts per centimeter) that a dielectric material can withstand without breaking down (arcing over).

diencephalon (di″en-sef′ah-lon) [*dia-* + Gr. *enkephalos* brain] [NA], a midline region in the brain corresponding to the third ventricle and the structures surrounding it, including the thalamus, hypothalamus, metathalamus, and epithalamus. Its limits rostrally are a line from the foramen of Monro to the optic chiasm and caudally a line from the posterior commissure to the posterior border of the mamillary bodies.

diene (di′ēn) a hydrocarbon with two carbon-carbon double bonds.

-diene a suffix word element to denote a hydrocarbon with two carbon-carbon double bonds.

Dientamoeba (di-ent″ah-me′bah) a genus of flagellates that parasitizes the human intestines; formerly considered a unique intestinal ameba because it lacks a cyst stage and is binucleated. The species *D. fragilis,* which has a range of 5–20 μm in diameter, can cause diarrhea and gastrointestinal discomfort. Diagnosis requires identification of binucleate forms on iron hematoxylin–stained fecal films.

diet (di′et) [Gr. *diaita* way of living] the customary amount and kind of food and drink taken by a person from day to day, particularly one planned to meet specific nutritional requirements of the individual.

Dieterle's method (de′ter-lēz) a histologic technique originally used to demonstrate spirochetes but modified by the U.S. Public Health Service's Center for Disease Control for staining species of the *Legionella* organism. Slides are sensitized in uranyl nitrate, treated with gum mastic, incubated in silver nitrate, and developed in a solution of hydroquinone, sodium sulfite, acetone, formaldehyde, pyridine, and gum mastic. Bacilli stain black on a yellow-tan background. Although the technique stains *Legionella* species, it is not specific for them.

dietetics (di″ĕ-tet′iks) the science of nutrition as it pertains to the analysis and prescription of diets.

diethylamine (di-eth″il-ah′mēn) a colorless liquid with the odor of ammonia, *N*-ethylethanamine, $(C_2H_5)_2NH$; M.W. 73.14. It is highly flammable and strongly irritating to the skin and mucous membranes.

diethylaminoethylcellulose (DEAE) (di-eth″il-ah-mēn″o-eth″il-sel′u-lōs) an ion-exchange resin used to separate proteins by chromatography.

diethyldithiocarbamate (di-eth″il-di-thi″o-kar′-bah-māt) a salt of diethyldithiocarbamic acid (diethylcarbamodithioic acid, $(C_2H_5)_2NCS_2H$), a chelating agent used in the colorimetric assay of copper, arsenic, and other metals; M.W. 171.27.

diethylenetriaminepentaacetic acid (di-eth″il-ēn-tri″ah-mēn-pen″tah-ah-se′tik) see *DTPA*.

diethyl ether (di-eth′il) see *ether*.

diethylpropion hydrochloride (di-eth″il-pro′pe-on) a stimulant used as an anorexic that is similar to the amphetamines both in structure and in the risk of dependence and personality changes with prolonged use. Trademarks, Anorex, Regenon, Tenuate. See also *amphetamine assays*.

diethylstilbestrol (DES) (di-eth″il-stil-bes′trol) a synthetic estrogen, 3,4-bis(*p*-hydroxyphenyl)-3-hexene, that has therapeutic usefulness in the treatment of breast and prostate cancer. It has been linked to the occurrence of vaginal clear cell adenocarcinomas in the daughters of females given this compound during pregnancy. For more information, see *Appendix A*.

diethyl sulfate sulfuric acid diethyl ester, $(C_2H_5O)_2SO_2$, a highly toxic industrial chemical used in syntheses as an alkylating agent. It causes blistering of the skin and pulmonary edema and is possibly carcinogenic.

diethyltryptamine (DET) (di-eth″il-trip′tah-mēn) a hallucinogenic drug, the synthetic ethyl homologue of dimethyltryptamine (DMT). DET is less potent but longer-acting than DMT.

diff abbrev. for differential count.

differential (dif″er-en′shal) [L. *differre* to carry apart] 1. pertaining to or showing a difference or differences.

2. of or pertaining to differentiation.

3. in mathematics, for any function $f(x)$, the differential of f at x_0 is the linear function that is tangent to f at x_0. Conventionally, the differential (df) is expressed as a function of the variable (dx): $df = f'(x_0)$, where $f'(x_0)$ is the derivative of f at x_0. The value of $f'(x_0)$ is defined as the limit of $(f(x_0) - f(x_0)/(x - x_0)$ as x approaches x_0.

differential leukocyte count the relative numbers of different types of white cells in a representative blood sample, usually a stained peripheral blood smear. Normally occurring cells are polymorphonuclear (PMN) neutrophils, lymphocytes, monocytes, basophils, and eosinophils. Other types present in bone marrow occur in the peripheral blood under pathologic conditions, i.e., immature forms of granulocytes, lymphocytes, and monocytes.

Differential leukocyte counts results are customarily reported as percentages of the different cell types. However, the reporting of absolute numbers is preferable; they are calculated by multiplying the percentage value for each cell type by the total white count. In some automated differential counters the absolute numbers of the different cell types are determined directly.

The differential leukocyte cell count is performed routinely as part of the complete blood count (CBC). In normal human blood there are more neutrophils than lymphocytes; the reverse occurs in certain diseases, e.g., infectious mononucleosis. A "shift to the left" is seen when the granulocyte count is increased and there is an increased number of cells with less segmented nuclei, i.e., more immature cells. A decrease in the number of neutrophils is referred to as neutropenia and an increase as granulocytosis; a decrease in the number of lymphocytes is referred to as lymphocytopenia and an increase as lymphocytosis. Reference values are shown in the accompanying table.

Differential Leukocyte Count

Cell Type	Range	Percent
Total WBC	4500–11,000	
PMN		
neutrophils	4100–6500	36–66
Band		
neutrophils	100–2100	<5 or 0–5
Eosinophils	0–700	1–3
Basophils	0–150	0–1
Lymphocytes	1500–4000	24–44
Monocytes	200–950	2–8

differential leukocyte count automation the classification of white blood cells by automated equipment and the counting of the relative numbers of each type of cell. There are two basic types of differential counters: computer pattern recognition systems and continuous-flow systems.

Computer Pattern Recognition Systems. As in manual methods, the computer systems count 100–500 leukocytes in a Romanowsky-stained blood smear. The slide is moved on a motorized microscope stage, and color television images of each cell are processed by the computer program to determine the cell size, nuclear size, nuclear shape (number of lobes), nuclear density, cytoplasmic color and texture, and length of cell perimeter. These measurements are then compared with established criteria, for cell recognition, and the cell is classified as a neutrophil (further classified as a band or segmented neutrophil is some systems), eosinophil, basophil, monocyte, or lymphocyte. Cells that cannot be classified by the computer are left to be identified by the operator and are entered manually into the count at the keyboard.

These systems can reliably classify leukocytes using the standard classification, and take 1–2 min per slide. Programs that evaluate red cell morphology and estimate platelet numbers are being introduced. The sampling error ranges from 20 percent for segmented neutrophils to over 100 percent for the less frequent cell types.

Continuous-Flow Systems. These systems classify leukocytes by size and staining properties. In one continuous process, a blood sample is aspirated, a hemolyzing solution is added to lyse red cells, the white cells are fixed, the sample stream is divided into several channels where the cells are stained by specific histochemical methods, and the light scattering and absorption of the cells is used to classify them.

In the peroxidase channel, neutrophils, eosinophils, and monocytes are stained with 4-chloro-1-naphthol and hydrogen peroxide (the peroxide is broken down by peroxidase to water and oxygen, which oxidizes the naphthol to a colored quinone). Eosinophils are identified by their staining, which is more intense (higher absorption but less scattering) than that of mature neurophils. A special class of neutrophils (designated as "high peroxidase cells") are identified by their having both greater absorption and greater scattering. Monocytes stain only lightly and are differentiated by both absorption and scatter. Lymphocytes remain unstained and are identified as small lymphocytes and "large unstained cells."

In the nonspecific esterase channel, monocytes are stained with α-naphthyl butyrate and diazotized basic fuchsin (the esterase hydrolyzes the naphthyl ester; the naphthyl group is azo-coupled to the fuchsin). Large, intensely stained cells are identified as monocytes.

In a third channel, basophils are stained with the basic dye Alcian blue. Modifications using only two channels or even one channel have been introduced.

Routinely, 10,000 cells are counted in each channel, although for patients with very low white cell counts, as few as 1000 cells can still be counted. The value of the increased precision of routine counts provided by this technique is debatable (because the issue is seldom of medical significance), the ability to distinguish the return of normal, or persistence of abnormal, cells during leukopenia following chemotherapy in leukemia is often very valuable, and represents an advantage of the continuous flow system over the pattern recognition system in which at best 500 cells, and usually only 100 cells, are counted routinely.

Both the computer pattern recognition and the continuous-flow systems have only limited capabilities for recognizing or subclassifying abnormal cells. One advantage that some of the pattern recognition systems offer is the recording by the computer memory of the location of cells unidentifiable by the instrument, permitting later inspection for interpretation by a technologist or physician. The special categories of HPX and LUC of the continuous flow system correspond in part to immature cells. Thus, these categories, as well as a column marked "remainder" (a measure of the discrepancy, if any, between the sum of registration in the different channels and the total count), cannot be directly translated to the known categories of cells; however, they serve as a useful warning of the existence of, or high likelihood of, some cytologic abnormality.

differential medium see *differential m.* under *medium.*

differential segments (of sex chromosomes) the segments of the X and Y chromosomes that do not contain homologous sequences and therefore do not synapse or cross over during meiosis. Cf. *pairing segments.*

differentiation (dif″er-en″shē-a′shun) 1. the distinguishing of one thing or disease from another.

2. in embryology, the generally irreversible process by which immature cells and tissues mature and become specialized to carry out specific functions. During this process, differences between various cell types become evident histologically and biochemically.

3. in pathology, a term used in reference to neoplasms to indicate the extent to which the histologic specialization of a neoplasm corresponds to that of its nonneoplastic counterpart. For example, some carcinomas of the breast show a morphologic resemblance to breast ducts, others to breast lobules, and still others to both. The term also refers to the degree to which architectural and cytologic features of the tissue of origin are retained in a neoplasm. When there is total loss of such features, the tumor is referred to as undifferentiated or anaplastic. Cf. *anaplasia.*

4. an increase in morphologic or chemical heterogeneity.

5. the process of selective removal of dye from some cell structures while others are still strongly stained. In some staining techniques, the selective production of certain colors is achieved by altering the pH of the dye.

6. in mathematics, the process of obtaining the derivative of a function.

differentiator (dif″er-en′she-a″tor) an electronic circuit that produces an output waveform that is approximately the derivative of the input waveform. A triangular input produces a square wave output, and a square wave input produces a positive spike corresponding to the leading edge of the square wave and a negative spike corresponding to the trailing edge.

The accompanying illustration shows an integrator (left) and a differentiator (right), which use operational amplifiers (op amps, marked OA). The input impedance of the op amp is virtually infinite, so it draws no appreciable current, and the currents through the resistor and capacitor (i_i and i_f) are equal. Because the op amp has near-infinite gain, the input voltage is esentially zero. For the differentiator, $i_i = C \cdot dv_{in}/dt$ and $i_f = -v_{out}/R$; thus, the output is the negative of the time derivative of the input multiplied by the time constant (RC). For the integrator, $i_i = v_{in}/R$ and $i_f = -C \cdot dv_{out}/dt$; thus, the input is proportional to the derivative of the output, or the output is the integral of the input times $-1/RC$.

diffraction (dĭ-frak′shun) [L. *dis-* apart + *frangere* to break] the bending or breaking up into its component parts of a ray of light.

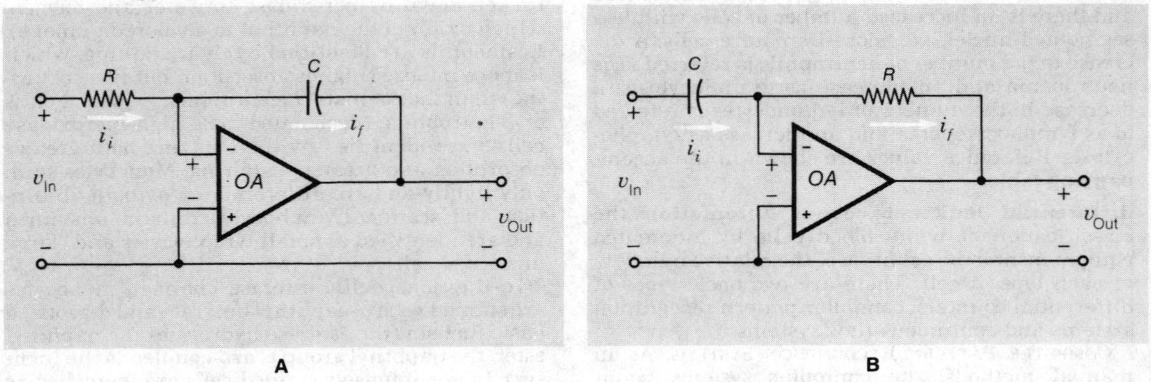

Differentiator. Operational amplifier circuits: *A,* integrator; and *B,* differentiator. (From Diefenderfer, A. J.: Principles of Electronic Instrumentation. 2nd ed. Philadelphia, W. B. Saunders Co., 1979.)

diffraction grating see *grating.*

diffusate (dĭ-fu'zāt) a product of diffusion; the material that passes through a membrane in dialysis, or that passes through a barrier in gaseous diffusion.

diffuse [L. *dis-* apart + *fundere* to pour] 1. (dĭ-fūs'), not definitely limited or localized; widely distributed.

2. (dĭ-fūz'), to pass through or to spread widely through a solution or a tissue or structure.

diffuse esophageal spasm a common disorder of the esophagus in which the normal peristaltic contractions are replaced by diffuse nonpropulsive contractions. A number of processes may be responsible, including neuromuscular disorders, mucosal irritation, and aging. Symptoms include chest pain (which may mimic angina pectoris) and dysphagia. Barium tests and esophageal manometry are useful in establishing the diagnosis.

diffuse illumination uniform lighting falling on an object from all directions.

diffuse interstitial fibrosis see *pulmonary f.* under *fibrosis.*

diffuse lymphatic tissue a term for the lymphoid cells dispersed within the mucosa and submucosa of the intestines. Also called gut-associated lymphoid tissue.

diffuse neuroendocrine system hormone-producing cells distributed singly or in small groups throughout many tissues of the body in addition to the cells concentrated within the major endocrine organs. Most of these cells, collectively termed the diffuse neuroendocrine system, form polypeptides and have been designated APUD cells because of their common properties of biogenic amine precursor uptake and decarboxylation (see the accompanying table). The hormones produced by cells of the system function in the control or modulation of neu-

DIFFUSE NEUROENDOCRINE SYSTEM. APUD CELLS OF THE DIFFUSE NEUROENDOCRINE SYSTEM

I. APUD cells of neural crest origin

Location	*Type*	*Main secretion*	
		Peptide	*Amine*
Thyroid	Parafollicular (C)	Calcitonin	5-HT, Da
Ultimobranchial body	C	Calcitonin	5-HT, Da
Carotid body	Type I Glomus	–	Da, NA
Sympathetic ganglia	SIF	–	NA
Adrenal medulla	Chromaffin	–	Ad
Adrenal medulla	Chromaffin	–	NA
Skin	Melanoblast	–	Promelanin
Urogenital tract	EC	–	5-HT
Urogenital tract	E	–	–

II. APUD cells of placodal or specialized ectodermal origin

Location	*Type*	*Main secretion*	
		Peptide	*Amine*
Hypothalamus	N pv	Oxytocin, CRF	–
	N so	Vasopressin	–
	N sch	–	–
	N dm/vm	TRF	–
	N arc	LHRF	Da
	N ant/post	SRF, CRF	–
	N periv	Somatostatin	–
Pineal gland	P	LHRF	5-HT, MT
Parathyroid	Chief	PTH	-
Pituitary	Somatotroph	Somatotropin	Da
	Mammotroph	Prolactin	Da
	Gonadotroph	Follitropin	Da
	Gonadotroph	Lutropin	Da
	Corticotroph	Corticotropin	–
	M	Melanotropin	T
	Thyrotroph	Thyrotropin	Da
Placenta	Endocrine	Gonadotropin	–
	Endocrine	Somatomammotropin	
	Endocrine	Corticotropin	–

III. APUD cells of disputed origin (possibly endodermal)

Location	*Type*	*Main secretion*	
		Peptide	*Amine*
Pancreas	A	Glucagon	5-HT
	B	Insulin	5-HT
	D	Somatostatin	Da
	D_1	VIP-like	Da
	P	Bombesin-like	–
	PP	Pancreatic polypeptide	Da
Stomach	A	Glucagon	–
	D	Somatostatin	–
	ECL	–	H?
	EC_1	Substance P	5-HT
	G	Gastrin, Enkephalin	–
	X	–	–
Intestine	D	Somatostatin	–
	D_1(H)	VIP	–
	EC_1	Substance P	5-HT
	EC_2	Motilin	5-HT
	EC_n	–	5-HT
	I	Cholecystokinin	–
	K	GIP	–
	L	Enteroglucagon	–
	N	Neurotensin	–
	S	Secretin	–
Lung	Kulchitsky (P_a)	–	–

Abbreviations: Ad, adrenalin; CRF, corticotropin-releasing factor; Da, dopamine; GIP, gastric inhibitory peptide; H, Histamine; 5-HT, 5-hydroxytryptamine; LHRF, Luteotropin-releasing factor (luteinizing hormone–releasing factor); MT, melatonin; NA, noradrenalin; N ant/post, Anterior and posterior nuclear "zones" of hypothalamus; Narc, nucleus arcuatus (nucleus infundibularis); N dm/vm, nucleus dorsomedialis/ventromedialis; N periv, nuclei periventriculares; N pv, nucleus paraventricularis; N sch, nucleus suprachiasmaticus; N so, nucleus supraopticus; PTH, parathyroid hormone; SIF, small intensely fluorescent; SRF, somatotropin releasing factor; T, tryptamine; TRF, thyrotropin releasing factor; VIP, vasoactive intestinal peptide; and –, unidentified.

Modified from Williams, P. L., and Warwick, R.: Gray's Anatomy. 36th ed. Philadelphia, W. B. Saunders, 1980, p. 1455.

rons of the peripheral nervous system, and the alternate term paraneuron has been suggested. The actions of this system are considerably slower and more prolonged than those of the autonomic nervous system.

diffuse septal cirrhosis a term that has been used in the anatomic classification of cirrhosis to describe a form of cirrhosis that corresponds approximately to micronodular cirrhosis.

diffusible (dĭ-fūz-′ĭ-b′l) capable of diffusing or of being diffused; susceptible of becoming widely spread.

diffusing capacity of the lungs (DL) the volume of gas (usually O_2 or CO) transferred across the pulmonary tissue-blood barrier each minute ($\dot{V}$) for each mean pressure gradient of 1 mmHg between the alveolar gas and capillary blood (P_{ACO}–P_{CCO}). The diffusing capacity of any gas (X) is represented by the equation: $D_{LX} = V_X/(P_{AX} - P_{CX})$.

The resistance to diffusion of gas between the alveolar air and the erythrocyte can be expressed as the summed resistances exerted by the individual components of the total diffusion capacity. This relationship is expressed mathematically as: $1/D_{LCO} = (1/D_M) + (1/\Theta V_C)$, where D_M is the membrane component of diffusion, the kinetic constant Θ represents the rate of combination of the gas with hemoglobin in the red blood cells for each 1 mmHg gradient of pressure, V_C is the pulmonary capillary blood volume, and the gas in this instance is CO. Any factor that contributes to a thickening of the alveolocapillary membrane (alveolocapillary block), a decrease in the surface area for gas exchange, or an abnormal ventilation-perfusion ratio would offer more resistance, and thus decrease the diffusing capacity.

d. c. of the l. for carbon monoxide (D_{LCO}), the measurement of diffusing capacity based on the rate of transfer of CO to the red blood cell. Although CO is not a physiologic gas, it is used in this procedure because it has a distribution in the lungs similar to that of O_2, but has an affinity for hemoglobin (Hb) 210 times that of O_2. Thus, the general formula for calculating the capacity need only consider milliliters of CO transferred per minute and the mean alveolar P_{CO}; because of the high Hb affinity, the mean pulmonary capillary P_{CO} is so small that it can be neglected.

Normally amounting to about 25 ml of CO/min/torr in the young adult, D_{LCO} increases with exercise and can vary with body size, body position, alveolar P_{O_2}, and the amount of Hb per unit volume of blood in the pulmonary capillaries.

Common methods used to test the pulmonary exchange of CO include the single-breath method and various methods based on a steady-state CO uptake; each method varies with respect to the method of determination of alveolar P_{CO} (P_{ACO}).

d. c. of the l. for oxygen (D_{LO_2}), the uptake of O_2 by the lungs per unit time for each 1 mmHg of driving pressure. Its direct measurement is complex and impractical because the P_{O_2} gradient along the capillaries, which changes nonlinearly and continuously, must be considered. It is commonly obtained indirectly by multiplication of the diffusion capacity for CO by a factor of 1.23 (derived from Henry's and Graham's laws).

single-breath d. c. of the l. ($D_{LCO}SB$), a method for measuring the rate of transfer of CO across the pulmonary tissue-blood barrier. One full inspiration of a mixture of CO (at a concentration of 0.3 percent) and helium in air is utilized. After a period of breath holding (usually about 10 sec), which allows for some CO to enter the red blood cells, a sample of the expired air is taken. Mean alveolar CO can be calculated from the concentration of CO in the initial and expired alveolar gas if the volume of the alveolar gas is also determined using the nonabsorbed tracer gas helium (the inspired alveolar CO concentration is calculated from the difference in helium concentrations in the inspired and expired air samples).

In a single subject, $D_{LCO}SB$ can vary with the lung volume during the breath-holding period and therefore is often expressed as the volume-corrected Krogh constant (D_{LCO} divided by lung volume). The uncorrected D_{LCO} measured by the single-breath technique varies from 20 to 41 ml of CO/min/torr in the normal young adult, depending on sex and body size.

steady state d. c. of the l. ($D_{LCO}SS$), a test of the rate of CO uptake during continuous rebreathing. Alveolar CO, the value needed for the denominator of the general equation for diffusing capacity, is variously computed on the basis of several assumed or measured quantities: measured arterial P_{CO_2} ($D_{LCO}SS_1$), a sample of end-tidal gas ($D_{LCO}SS_2$), an assumed value for the physiologic dead space ($D_{LCO}SS_3$), or an estimate of the mixed venous CO_2 ($D_{LCO}SS_4$).

For example, in the Filley method ($D_{LCO}SS_1$), simultaneous measurements of the inspired (F_{ICO}) and expired (F_{ECO}) concentrations, expired CO_2 concentration (F_{ECO_2}), arterial P_{CO_2} (Pa_{CO_2}), and minute volume are made. Mean alveolar CO (P_{ACO}) can then be calculated as follows: $P_{ACO} = P_B - 47\ [(F_{ECO} - rF_{ICO})/(1 - r)]$, where $r = (Pa_{CO_2} - F_{ECO_2})/Pa_{CO_2}$, and P_B is the barometric pressure.

diffusion (dĭ-fu′zhun) 1. the process of becoming widely spread.

2. in physics and chemistry, the movement of molecules in solution from a region of high concentration to one of low concentration. Diffusion is a thermodynamic process; the system spontaneously proceeds toward a state of maximal entropy in which each solute is evenly distributed throughout the volume of the solution.

Diffusion is governed by the equation $\partial c/\partial t = -D \cdot \partial c/\partial x$, where $\partial c/\partial t$ is the time rate of change of the concentration, $\partial c/\partial x$ is the concentration gradient, and D is the diffusion coefficient (diffusivity) for the substance. For diffusion across a membrane, the equation is $M = -D(C_1 - C_2)$, where M is the flow rate through the membrane, C_1 and C_2 are the concentrations on both sides of the membrane, and D is the diffusion coefficient.

facilitated d., see *facilitated diffusion.*

diffusion coefficient the amount of a substance diffusing across a unit area in a unit concentraton gradient. Also called *diffusivity.*

diffusion current the current in an electrochemical cell carried by ions diffusing toward the electrode where they are reduced. It is proportional to the concentration of the substance in solution and can be used to identify as well as quantify the substance. See also *polarography.*

diffusion method see *microdiffusion analysis.*

diffusion potential the potential across a membrane in an electrochemical cell that is caused by different rates of diffusion of anions and cations across the membrane. It is caused by the chemical properties of the ions and the membrane. A thermal diffusion potential is caused by a temperature difference across the membrane. Both types should be reduced as much as possible in measuring electrodes. Also called *liquid-liquid junction potential.*

diffusivity (dĭ″fu-siv′ĭ-te) see *diffusion coefficient.*

digastric (di-gas′trik) [*di-* + Gr. *gastēr* belly] having two bellies; pertaining to the digastric muscle.

digenetic (di″jĕ-net′ik) [*di-* + Gr. *genesis* generation] having two stages of multiplication during the life cycle: an asexual, larval stage, with the mollusk being the usual host, and a mature, sexual stage, with vertebrates as the final host. The classic example is the trematode (fluke).

DiGeorge's syndrome (de-jōrj′ez) [Angelo Mario *DiGeorge,* U.S. endocrinologist, born 1821] a condition caused by abnormal development of the third and fourth pharyngeal pouches, which give rise to the thymus and parathyroid glands. This disorder results in impaired cellular (T lymphocyte) immunity and hypocalcemia. It is one of the few immunodeficiency disorders with symptoms apparent at birth. The complete syndrome includes the following characteristics: (1) abnormal facies (e.g., hypertelorism, antimongoloid eye slant, shortened lip philtrum, and low-set, often notched ears), (2) hypoparathyroidism, (3) congenital heart disease (atrial and ventricular septal defects), (4) transposition of the great vessels, and (5) cellular immunodeficiency. The most frequent presenting sign is hypocalcemia, occurring within 24 hr of neonatal life and not responding to standard treatment. Infants surviving the immediate neonatal period are prone to recurrent or chronic infections with a variety of viruses, bacteria, fungi, or protozoa, which may result in pneumonia, chronic mucosal infections with *Candida,* or diarrhea.

T-cell immunity should be evaluated in newborns suspected of having DiGeorge's syndrome. The lymphocyte count is usually low ($<1200/\mu l$) but may be normal or elevated. T-cell rosettes are diminished, and peripheral blood lymphocytes may fail to respond to mitogens or allogenic cells. Hypoparathyroidism may be diagnosed by demonstrating low serum calcium with elevated serum phosphorus and absence of parathyroid hormone.

The treatment of T-cell deficiency associated with DiGeorge's syndrome is a fetal thymic transplant. Because those with DiGeorge's syndrome may develop graft-versus-host disease, fetal thymus glands older than 14 wk of gestation should not be used, and any blood products should be irradiated before administration. The hypocalcemia may be controlled with orally administered calcium with vitamin D or parathyroid hormone. If present, congenital heart disease may require immediate surgical correction. The prognosis for individuals with this syndrome depends on the severity of the congenital heart disease (if present) and the cellular immunodeficiency.

digestion (di-jes′chun) [L. *digestio,* from *dis-* apart + *gerere* to carry] 1. the process or act of converting food into chemical substances that can be absorbed and assimilated.

2. the subjection of tissues to prolonged heat and moisture so as to disintegrate and soften them.

digestion vacuole a cytoplasmic vacuole within which phagocytosed material is digested by lysosomal enzymes. See also *lysosome.*

digit (dij′it) [L. *digitus*] 1. a finger or toe.

2. one of the set of characters that represents nonnegative integers less than the base of a number system, e.g., in the decimal system, 0–9; in the binary system, 0 and 1.

digital (dij′ĭ-tal) 1. pertaining to or performed with a finger.

2. pertaining to numbers.

3. with reference to an electronic circuit or to data or signals, having only a finite number of values rather than a continuous range. Cf. *analog.*

digital cassette recorder the least expensive form of bulk storage used in microcomputer systems. It is a slightly modified audio cassette tape recorder that records and can be used to read back digital data under computer control. Its low rate of data transfer and long access time make floppy disks preferable, if the cost differential is justified.

digital computer an automated electronic calculating machine. Its physical components, called hardware, include an arithmetic-logic unit (ALU), controlling circuitry, a memory, and various peripheral machines. The nonphysical component, the software, consists of the principal programs that control the computer and its peripherals, and includes the language processors that implement user-written programs in languages such as FORTRAN.

The ALU is the computer's computer: it performs mathematical and logical operations such as addition and comparison. The controlling circuitry determines which operation will be done and how; its decision may be based on the results of previous operations. The memory can store both computational data and instructions that specify the computer's sequence of operations. The ALU, the controlling circuitry, and the memory are part of one machine called the central processing unit (CPU), and the details of the construction of the CPU are called the architecture.

The peripheral machines are used either for extending the capabilities of the computer or for communicating with the outside world. Disk drives, tape drives, and add-on memory augment the computer's data-storage space; specialized devices such as array processors or fast numerical processors can speed up certain operations. Data input to and output from the computer (I/O) are handled by video terminals, by printers, and possibly by specialized machines that may control an analytical system or an industrial process.

Digitalis (dij″ĭ-tal′is) [L., from *digitus* finger, for the fingerlike leaves of its flower] a genus of herbs. It includes the species *D. purpurea,* the purple foxglove, whose leaves furnish digitalis, and *D. lanata,* a Balkan species that yields digoxin and lanatoside.

digitalis (dij″ĭ-tal′is) 1. [USP], the dried leaf of *Digitalis purpurea,* used as a cardiotonic. The primary active principle is digitoxin.

2. a general term used to refer to any of the digitalis glycosides.

3. a general term for a finger-like structure.

digitalis glycosides a group of cardiotonic drugs extracted from leaves of the foxglove plant (*Digitalis*), of which the most commonly used is digoxin (Lanoxin). Together with similar compounds, such as the drug ouabain extracted from *Strophanthus gratus* seeds, they are called cardiac glycosides. Digitalis glycosides consist of a chain of three or four sugar residues (one residue in ouabain) bonded to an aglycone, which in turn consists of a steroid nucleus and an unsaturated lactone ring at C-17.

The primary effect of digitalis is to increase the force and velocity of myocardial contraction. This effect is produced by inhibition of the active transport of sodium and potassium ions across cell membranes and modulation of Ca^{2+}. It also acts indirectly on vagal activity to increase the refractory period of the atrioventricular node, the Purkinje fibers, and the sinoatrial node. A low serum potassium level potentiates some of the toxic effects of digitalis, although corrective potassium replacement alleviates some of these effects; high levels of potassium intensify atrioventricular block and may cause cardiac arrest.

Digitalis has a low therapeutic index: the effective dose is about 50 percent of the toxic dose and 25 percent of the lethal dose in some sensitive adults. The most common symptoms of overdosage are anorexia, nausea, vomiting (particularly in adults), visual disturbances, and cardiac arrhythmias including sinus bradycardia, sinus arrest, premature atrial and ventricular beats, ventricular tachycardia, paroxysmal atrial tachycardia, and atrioventricular dissociation and block.

Serum concentrations of cardiac glycosides are determined by radioimmunoassay, using antisera specific for the aglycone portion of the molecule. Because of cross-reactivity of the antisera, it must be known which glycoside the patient is taking. This assay may be helpful in evaluating any sign of toxicity or lack of therapeutic response, and in monitoring patients who are prone to digitalis toxicity or who have impaired renal function. Serum samples are obtained at least 6–8 hr after the last dose so that the postabsorptive concentration is determined.

The usual therapeutic range is 0.5–2.0 ng/ml for digoxin and 9–25 ng/ml for digitoxin, although the toxic and nontoxic ranges overlap. Some adults experience no toxicity at a digoxin concentration of 2.0–4.0 ng/ml, but others have toxic symptoms at concentrations of 1.5–2.0 ng/ml.

For more information, see also the particular drugs *deslanoside, digitalis, digitoxin, digoxin, gitalin,* and *lanatoside C.*

digitalization (dij″ĭ-tal-ĭ-za′shun) the process of establishing a safe and effective serum concentration of a digitalis glycoside in a patient.

digital radiography radiographic methods that use digital image processing. X-ray images are detected by a fluoroscopic screen, converted to digital form, and stored in a computer. Using this procedure, it is possible to make subtraction images without film processing: the computer cancels out obscuring shadows from the images that show opacified structures by subtracting the images made before injection of the contrast medium.

digital readout a device for displaying digital information, usually employing light-emitting diodes (LEDs), liquid crystal devices, or flowing filament (NIXIE) tubes.

digital subtraction angiography (DSA) a type of digital radiography used for examining the blood vessels. Computer processing produces a motion picture of contrast-injected vessels, with obscuring shadows subtracted from the images.

digital-to-analog converter (DAC, D/A converter) an electronic device that converts a digital (binary or binary coded decimal BCD) to an analog signal (output voltage) proportional to the number. The bits of the number are summed by a resistor network that adds in each bit with the correct weight; e.g., for a binary number, the *m*th bit gets weight 2^m.

digital voltmeter (DVM) a digital electronic device that measures AC and DC voltage; most DVMs also measure resistance and AC and DC current. The measured voltage is compared with an internal reference voltage, converted to digital form by an analog-to-digital converter, and then displayed with a digital readout. Outputs are often available so that the digital form can be fed directly to a computer in binary coded decimal (BCD) format.

digitize (dij′ĭ-tīz) to convert an analog measurement into a digital measurement, as with an analog-to-digital converter.

digitizer (dij′ĭ-tiz″er) a device that converts analog data into numerical data.

digitonin (dig″ĭ-to′nin) a saponin from *Digitalis purpurea,* which occurs as a white crystalline powder. It is used as a reagent to precipitate free cholesterol.

digitonin method a histologic method for determining the presence of cholesterol in tissue. Nonesterified cholesterol and some other 3-hydroxy steroids form a birefringent crystalline precipitate with digitonin. Formalin-fixed frozen sections are incubated in a dilute alcoholic solution of digitonin. Alternate paired sections are counterstained with oil red O or Sudan IV. When viewed with polarized light, nonesterified cholesterol is seen as doubly refractile needles or rosettes. In the counterstained sections, cholesterol esters and other lipids are stained but are not birefringent.

digitoxin (dij″ĭ-tok′sin) [USP], a digitalis glycoside that occurs as a white crystalline powder and is obtained from the plant *Digitalis purpurea* and other species of *Digitalis.* It consists of the aglycone digitoxigenin and three digitoxose sugar residues.

Digitoxin is used in the treatment of congestive heart failure, atrial fibrillation, atrial flutter, and paroxysmal atrial tachycardia. When administered orally, it is 90–100 percent absorbed and produces its peak effect in 4–12 hr.

Digitoxin is the most slowly excreted of the cardiac glycosides, having a half-life of 7–8 da. Unlike the other glycosides, it is primarily metabolized to inactive forms by the liver; however, one of the metabolites is digoxin. A small fraction of the unmetabolized drug is excreted in the bile (from which it is returned to the liver by enterohepatic circulation) and in the urine. Because it can be detoxified by the liver, its use is preferred for patients with renal insufficiency.

Trademark, Crystodigin. See also *digitalis glycosides.*

digitoxose (dij″ĭ-tok′sōs) 2,6-dideoxy-ribo-hexose, a sugar that occurs in digoxin, digitoxin, lanatoside C, and deslanoside; M.W. 148.16.

diglyceride (di-glis′er-īd) a lipid containing two fatty acids esterified to glycerol. Both 1,2- and 1,3-diacylglycerols are encountered. Diglycerides are metabolic intermediates in the formation and degradation of triglycerides and phospholipids. They can be found only in minute quantities. Also called *diacylglycerol.*

digoxin (dĭ-jok′sin) [USP], a digitalis glycoside that occurs as a white crystalline powder and is obtained from the plant *Digitalis lanata.* It consists of the aglycone digoxigenin and three digitoxose sugar residues. Digoxin is used in the treatment of congestive heart failure, atrial fibrillation, atrial flutter, paroxysmal atrial tachycardia, and cardiogenic shock.

When administered orally, digoxin is 50–85 percent absorbed and produces its peak effect in 1.5–5 hr; when administered intravenously, the peak effect is produced in 1–2 hr. Digoxin is excreted unchanged by the kidneys, the excretion being proportional to the glomerular filtration rate. In individuals with normal renal function, the half-life is about 36 hr. There is also some gastrointestinal excretion. Because digoxin is well absorbed and rapidly cleared, it is the most commonly used cardiac glycoside.

Trademark, *Lanoxin.* See also *digitalis glycosides.*

Di Guglielmo syndrome (de gōōl-yel′mo) [Giovanni *di Guglielmo,* Italian physician, 1886–1961] see *erythroleukemia* under *leukemia.*

dihydric alcohol (di-hi′drik) an alcohol containing two hydroxy groups, e.g., ethylene glycol. Also called *diol* and *glycol.*

dihydrobiopterin (di-hi″dro-bi-op′ter-in) an oxidized pterin cofactor produced from tetrahydrobiopterin during the conversion of phenylalanine to tyrosine by phenylalanine hydroxylase and converted back to tetrahydrobiopterin by the enzyme dihydropteridine reductase (which uses NAD as a cofactor).

dihydrocodeinone (di-hi″dro-ko′de-ĭ-nōn) see *hydrocodone.*

dihydroergotamine mesylate (di-hi″dro-er-got′-ah-mēn) [USP], a hydrogenated ergot alkaloid administered parenterally to treat migraine attacks. It stimulates the cranial arteries to constrict, and produces alpha-adrenergic blockade. Adverse reactions include nausea, vomiting, irregular heart rate, and numbness, tingling, and muscle pain in the extremities. Trademark, D.H.E. 45.

dihydrofolate (di-hi″dro-fo′lāt) the anionic form of dihydrofolic acid.

dihydrofolate reductase see *tetrahydrofolate dehydrogenase.*

dihydrofolic acid (di-hi″dro-fo′lik) a reduced form of folic acid formed in tissues, a reduced pteridine linked to *p*-aminobenzoic acid linked to glutamic acid. See also *folic acid.*

dihydrofolliculin (di-hi″dro-fol-lik′u-lin) see *17β-estradiol.*

dihydromorphinone hydrochloride (di-hi″dro-mor′fĭ-nōn) see *hydromorphone hydrochloride.*

dihydropteridine reductase (di-hi″dro-ter′ĭ-din) an enzyme of the oxidoreductase class (NADPH:-6,7-dihydropteridine oxidoreductase, EC 1.6.99.7) that catalyzes the reaction NADPH + 6,7-dihydropteridine ⇄ $NADP^+$ + 5,6,7,8-tetrahydropteridine. This enzyme is one of three enzymes involved in the hydroxylation of phenylalanine to tyrosine. A deficiency of this enzyme causes a variant form of phenylketonuria not treatable with low phenylalanine diet.

dihydropteridine reductase deficiency a disorder of phenylalanine metabolism, possibly familial, in which there is a relative or absolute deficiency of the enzyme dihydropteridine reductase. This results in a disease that resembles phenylketonuria but is not improved by dietary phenylalanine restriction. Central nervous system deterioration with retardation, spasms, and chorea appear early in life and progress to death within several years, despite early detection. Diagnosis is achieved by enzyme assay in cultured skin fibroblasts. See also *aminoacidopathy.*

dihydrosphingosine (di-hi″dro-sfing′go-sēn) the saturated analog of the monounsaturated compound sphingosine, present in some sphingolipids. It does not exist in free form. Also called *sphinganine.*

dihydrotestosterone (DHT) (di-hi″dro-tes-tos′ter-ōn) 17β-hydroxy-5α-androstan-3-one, a potent androgen, largely formed by the reduction of testosterone by the enzyme 5α-reductase in the prostate, seminal vesicles, and skin; M.W. 290.43. A smaller amount (less than 10 percent of the total DHT) is directly synthesized in the testes.

Dihydrotestosterone is more potent than testosterone and is active not only in the target tissue where it is formed, but also in other organs when transported by the blood. It is conjugated in the liver as the glucuronide and is largely transported bound to a testosterone-binding globulin, known as sex hormone–binding globulin (SHBG), which has a higher affinity for DHT than for testosterone. Testosterone is probably not just a prehormone for DHT, as not all target tissues possess the enzyme 5α-reductase (e.g., muscle).

Reference ranges for DHT in serum are: for adult males, 23–75 ng/dl; for adult females, 5–30; and for prepubertal children, < 10.

Also called 5α-dihydrotestosterone. See also *androgen.*

dihydroubiquinone (di-hi″dro-u-bik′wĭ-nōn) see *ubiquinol.*

dihydrouridine (di-hi″dro-u′rĭ-dēn) a pyrimidine nucleoside, a derivative of uridine, found in transfer RNA.

dihydroxyacetone phosphate (di″hi-drok″se-as′-ĕ-tōn) an intermediate in glycolysis. See also *triose phosphate.*

dihydroxycholecalciferol (di″hi-drok″se-ko″le-kal- sif′ĕ-rol) a group of active hydroxylated derivatives of cholecalciferol (vitamin D_3) numbered according to the carbon atom(s) on which a hydroxyl group is substituted. The most active of these is 1,25-dihydroxycholecalciferol. It is formed in the kidneys and is the true active form of vitamin D. The kidney also forms the 24,25-dihydroxy derivative, which has no vitamin D activity, but which is formed at the expense of the 1,25 compound. See also *cholecalciferol.*

3,4-dihydroxymandelic acid (DHMA) (di″hi-drok″se-man-del′ik) a common metabolite of epinephrine and norepinephrine, formed by oxidative deamination. DHMA is further metabolized by *O*-methylation at position 3 to vanillylmandelic acid, which is then excreted in the urine.

2,5-dihydroxyphenylacetic acid (di″hi-drok″se-fen″il-ah-se′tik) see *homogentisic acid.*

diiodothyronine (T_2) (di″i-o″do-thi′ro-nēn) a term used to describe a group of compounds that are metabolites of peripheral (extrathyroidal) triiodothyronine (T_3) and reverse T_3 (rT_3) monodeiodinations; M.W. 525.10. The following diiodothyronines have been found in thyroid tissue and circulating in the blood: 3,3′-L-diiodothyronine (3,3′ T_2), 3,5-L-diiodothyronine (3,5T_2), and 3′,5′-L-diiodothyronine (3′,5′ T_2). In contrast to T_3 and thyroxine (T_4), they appear to be calorigenically inactive. Diiodothyronines are found in the blood in a free form, bound to proteins, and as glucuronate and sulfate conjugates.

diiodotyrosine (DIT) (di″i-o″do-ti′ro-sen) 3,5-diiodo-4-hydroxy-β-phenylalanine, a precursor of triiodothyronine (T_3) and thyroxine (T_4); M.W. 433.92. DIT accounts for 25–42 percent of the total iodine in the thyroid gland, yet possesses no biologic activity. It is formed by a sequential iodination at positions 3 and 5 of the tyrosine residue on the thyroglobulin molecule in the thyroid follicular cell. Two molecules of DIT are coupled on the thyroglobulin molecule to form T_4, which remains bound to thyroglobulin until cleaved by a thyroglobulin protease, releasing free T_4. Similarly, one molecule each of monoiodotyrosine and DIT are coupled to form T_3. DIT is eventually deiodinated, and the iodide is recycled back into the iodide pool. Although DIT is found in small amounts in the serum, it is not normally measured. See also *monoiodotyrosine, thyroxine,* and *triiodothyronine.*

diisopropyl phosphofluoridate (di-i″so-pro′pil fos″fo-floor′ĭ-dāt) an ester of phosphofluoridic acid, $[(CH_3)_2CHO]_2POF$, extremely toxic in very low concentrations; M.W. 184.147. It acts by inhibition of acetylcholinesterase activity and causes mental confusion, constriction of the larynx, and marked contraction of the pupils. Derivatives have been prepared as war gases.

Radiolabeled diisopropyl phosphofluoridate ($DF^{32}P$) binds to red blood cells and some white blood cells. It is used in measurement of red cell mass and life span by the random labeling method. As ^{32}P is a pure beta emitter, it is more difficult to detect than ^{51}Cr labeling, and in vivo determinations cannot be done. $DF^{32}P$ does not elute from tagged red blood cells, which makes the results relatively easy to interpret. $DF^{32}P$ is also used for some leukocyte kinetics studies. Although it permits the most accurate method for red cell life span measurement, $DF^{32}P$ is not widely available and is rarely used for this purpose.

Also called diisopropylfluorophosphate (DFP) and isofluorphate. See also *red cell survival test.*

dikaryon (di-ka′re-on) [*di-* + Gr. *karyon* kernel] a growth stage in the mycelium of fungi, especially the Basidiomycetes, in which each cell has two haploid nuclei.

diktyoma (dik″te-o′mah) [Gr. *diktyon* net + *-oma*] a rare tumor of the ciliary body, so named because of its netlike histologic structure. It arises from embryonic retinal elements and is closely related to retinoblastoma. Diktyomas usually appear at birth or in the first few years of life, are single, unilateral, and grow slowly but infiltrate aggressively; metastases are unusual.

dil abbrev. See *dilute.*

Dilantin (di-lan′tin) trademark. See *phenytoin.*

dilatation (dil-ah-ta′shun) see *dilation.*

dilation (di-la′shun) [L. *dilatare* to spread out, enlarge] the condition in which a body opening or tubular organ is stretched or expanded beyond its normal boundaries or dimensions. Dilation of body tissues may occur in disease states, such as inflammation, tumor invasion, or the retention of products that are normally secreted. It can also be induced for therapeutic reasons, e.g., dilation of the endocervical canal, esophagus, or anus. See also *distention.*

Dilaudid (di-law′did) trademark. See *hydromorphone hydrochloride.*

diluent (dil′u-ent) [L. *diluere* to wash] 1. an inert substance added to a solution or a mixture of components to decrease the concentration of active substances or substances of interest.

2. diluting.

dilute (dĭ-lo͞ot′) [L. *diluere* to wash away] 1. to reduce the concentration of a solution.

2. pertaining to a solution that contains a relatively small amount of solute.

3. (abbrev. dil), specifying conventional concentrations of certain common acids and bases (e.g., 6 mol/l or 3 mol/l). Cf. *concentrated.*

dilution (dĭ-loo′shun) 1. the process of diluting, i.e., reducing the concentraton of the solute by adding additional solvent.

2. a diluted solution. For example, a 1/10 dilution is 1/10 of the concentration of the original solution, prepared by adding nine volumes of solvent to one volume of the original solution. Cf. *concentration.*

doubling d., a serial dilution in which the dilutions are 1/2, 1/4, 1/8, and so on.

log d., a serial dilution in which the dilutions are 1/10, 1/100, 1/1000, and so on; i.e., they vary by a factor of 10.

serial d., 1. the process of making dilutions of a solute in two or more steps, e.g., a 1/100 dilution made by first making a 1/10 dilution, which is again further diluted 1/10.

2. a series of diluted solutions of a solute in which the degree of dilution increases by a constant factor, e.g., 1/10, 1/20, 1/40, and so on, the factor in this case being 1/2.

dilution coefficient a number that expresses the relationship between the effectiveness and concentration of a disinfectant for a given organism. It is expressed by the equation $tc^n = k$, where t is the time required for killing of all organisms, c is the concentration of disinfectant, n is the dilution coefficient, and k is a constant. A disinfectant with a high dilution coefficient, e.g., phenol, is less effective at a low concentration than one with a low coefficient.

dilution test 1. a test used for determination of renal function. A large fluid load is administered, after which the volume and specific gravity of the urine excreted are followed for a specific period.

2. a test for bacterial sensitivity to antibacterial agents. See under *antibacterial agent susceptibility testing.*

dimefox (BFPO) (di′mĕ-foks) the generic name for bis(dimethylamido)phosphoryl fluoride, a highly toxic pesticide used on ornamental plants. It is a cholinesterase inhibitor.

dimenhydrinate (di″men-hi′drĭ-nāt) [USP], generic name for the salt of diphenhydramine and 8-chloro-theophylline; used for motion sickness. Trademark, *Dramamine.* See under *diphenhydramine* for toxicity.

dimension (dĭ-men′shun) a numerical expression, in appropriate units, of a linear measurement of an object, such as an organ or body part, or the units of a measurement. Dimension is also used in computer programming languages to indicate the number of rows and columns to be assigned for a data matrix.

dimer (di′mer) 1. a substance formed by the reaction of two identical molecules. The molecules may be joined by covalent bonds (e.g., maltose) or by weak interactions.

2. an oligomer formed by the reaction of two monomers.

3. the combined form of two monomeric units of immunoglobulin. The class of immunoglobulin most often found in the dimeric form is IgA.

4. a viral capsomer composed of two polypeptide units.

thymine d., two adjacent thymine molecules on a DNA chain that are linked by covalent bonds. Such dimers are frequently produced by ultraviolet light irradiation and prevent replication. A number of enzymes are involved in dimer removal and replacement by normal nucleotides. Defects in these repair mechanisms may lead to diseases such as xeroderma pigmentosum.

dimercaprol (di″mer-kap′rol) 2,3-dimercapto-1-propanol, an agent used in the treatment of acute arsenic or mercury poisoning; M.W. 124.21. It acts by forming a soluble, chelated compound with the metallic ion, which is then excreted in the urine. It was originally developed as an antidote for the arsenical war gas Lewisite. Also called British *anti-Lewisite* (BAL) and *dimercaptopropanol.*

dimercaptopropanol (di″mer-kap″to-pro′pan-ol) see *dimercaprol.*

dimerization (di″mer-ĭ-za′shun) the formation of dimeric molecules from their constituent monomers.

dimethicone (di-meth′ĭ-kōn) a poly(dimethylsiloxane) silicone polymer that can vary in physical properties from a viscous fluid to an elastic silicone rubber, depending on the molecular weight. It is used as an ointment base and topical protectant, and as a fluid soft tissue prosthesis or elastic surgical prosthesis. Trademark, *Silastic.*

dimethindene maleate (di″meth-in′dēn) [USP], an antihistamine with some anticholinergic activity, used in the treatment of allergic reactions. Common adverse reactions, include drowsiness; dizziness; dryness of the mouth, nose, and throat; and thickening of bronchial secretions. Trademark, Forhistal.

dimethoate (di-meth′o-āt) phosphorodithioic acid *O,O*-dimethyl *S*-[2-(methylamino)-2-oxoethyl] ester, an organophosphate insecticide, which is a highly toxic cholinesterase inhibitor. See also *organophosphate compounds.*

2,5-dimethoxy-4-methylamphetamine (DOM) (di″mĕ-thok″se-meth″il-am-fet′ah-mēn) a hallucinogenic drug known to users as STP. Its physiologic effects are similar to those of amphetamine. DOM abuse can cause acute panic reaction. It is a DEA (Drug Enforcement Agency) controlled substance.

***N,N*-dimethylacetamide** (DMAC) (di-meth″il-ah-se′tah-mīd) a colorless liquid, $CH_3CON(CH_3)_2$, which is miscible with water and most organic solvents; M.W. 87.12. It is used as an industrial solvent for plastics and resins. DMAC is a strong irritant to the skin, eyes, and mucous membranes. See also *N-methylformamide and N-methylacetamide assays.*

dimethylallyl diphosphate (di-meth″il-al′il) the initial acceptor molecule in the synthesis of all polyprenyl compounds. Also called *Δ^2-isopentenyl diphosphate.*

dimethylaminoazobenzene (di-meth″il-am″ĭ-no-az″o-ben′zēn) *N,N*-dimethyl-4-(phenylazo) benzenamine; a highly carcinogenic compound, a dye (butter yellow) that has been banned by the FDA from all foods.

7,12-dimethylbenz[*a*]anthracene (DMBA) (di-meth″il-benz-an′thrah-sēn) a synthetic polycyclic aromatic hydrocarbon, one of the most potent of this type of carcinogens, frequently used in experimental studies of carcinogenesis. It is a procarcinogen that requires metabolic activation to an aryl epoxide, the direct-acting carcinogen.

dimethyl ether (di-meth″il) $CH_3 \cdot O \cdot CH_3$, methyl ether, a colorless, highly flammable gas, used as a refrigerant and spray propellant.

***N,N*-dimethylformamide** (DMF) (di-meth″il-for′-mah-mīd) $HCON(CH_3)_2$, a colorless, flammable liquid, M.W. 73.09. It is miscible with water and most organic solvents and has been called a universal organic solvent. DMF is widely used in industry, particularly in the manufacture of synthetic fibers. The vapors can be absorbed through the skin or lungs and are highly irritating to the skin, eyes, and mucous membranes. In experiments with animals, DMF has produced liver damage. See also *N-methylformamide and N-methylacetamide assays.*

dimethylguanosine (di-meth″il-gwan′o-sēn) a purine nucleoside derivative of guanosine found in transfer RNA.

dimethyl ketone see *acetone.*

dimethylnitrosamine (DMN) (di-meth″il-ni-trōs′-ah-mēn) *N*-methyl-*N*-nitrosomethanamine, a liquid used as a rocket fuel and solvent. It is carcinogenic, is frequently used in experimental studies of carcinogenesis, and causes hepatic damage.

5,5-dimethyl-2,4-oxazolidinedione (DMO) (di-meth″il-ok″sah-zol″ĭ-dēn-di′ōn) a weak acid, $pK'_a = 6.13$, used in the measurement of intracellular pH because its concentration is easily quantitated. It is not metabolized in the body and does not bind to plasma proteins or cytoplasmic proteins. The free acid passively diffuses across cell membranes; the ionized form cannot cross the cell membranes. Thus the ratio of the intracellular and extracellular concentrations reflects the ratio of the intracellular and extracellular pH.

dimethyl sulfate (di-meth′il sul′fāt) sulfuric acid dimethyl ester, $(CH_3O)_2SO_2$, a highly toxic industrial chemical used in syntheses as an alkylating agent. It causes blistering and pulmonary edema and is possibly carcinogenic.

dimethyl sulfoxide (DMSO) (di-meth′il sul-fok′sīd) a highly polar, colorless, almost odorless, hygroscopic liquid, $(CH_3)_2SO$, that dissolves most organic substances and readily penetrates living cells. DMSO is absorbed rapidly from the skin or mucosa; in high concentrations it may relieve pain and swelling of acute inflammation and soft tissue injuries. However, its safety and effectiveness have not yet been established. It gives a garliclike odor to the breath and skin and can produce visual disturbances, headache, gastrointestinal intolerance, dermatitis, burning on urination, and severe hypersensitivity reactions. With prolonged use in animals, it has caused ocular lens opacities, and has also been shown to be teratogenic. The only approved indication is the instillation of a 50 percent solution into the bladder for interstitial cystitis. Self-medication with impure DMSO preparations can be dangerous.

***N,N*-dimethyltryptamine** (DMT) (di-meth″il-trip′tah-mēn) a hallucinogenic alkaloid that occurs in the bark resin of *Virola theidora,* a South American tree of the nutmeg family.

diminazene aceturate (di-min′ah-zēn) an antiprotozoal drug used for the treatment of *Trypanosoma gambiense* and *Babesia microti* infections. It is similar to pentamidine and superior to tryparsamide and suramin. Trademark, Berenil.

dimorphic (di-mor′fik) [*di-* + Gr. *morphē* form] occurring in two distinct forms.

dimorphic pathogenic fungi (di-mor′fik) pathogenic fungi that can grow in two different morphologic states—a yeast phase or a filamentous phase. Temperature and the tissue environment determine which stage of the organism will exist. Examples include *Blastomyces dermatitidis, Coccidioides immitis, Histoplasma capsulatum, Paracoccidioides brasilensis,* and *Sporothrix schenckii.*

dimorphism (di-mor′fizm) [*di-* + Gr. *morphē* form] 1. the property of having or existing in two or more forms.

2. the ability of a fungus to change from a filamentous stage to a yeast stage, or vice versa.

dinitrobenzene (di-ni″tro-ben′zēn) an industrial chemical, available as *o-*, *p-*, and *m-*isomers, all used in organic synthesis. The *meta* form is used as a reagent in the Zimmermann reaction for measuring 17-ketosteroids. All forms are highly toxic, producing methemoglobinemia and, with chronic exposure, liver damage.

dinitrochlorobenzene (DNCB) (di-ni″tro-klōr″o-ben′zēn) 1-chloro-2,4-dinitrobenzene, a compound derived by chlorination of nitrobenzene. When applied to the skin, it results in contact sensitivity, a type of delayed hypersensitivity reaction. DNCB is used in a confirmatory test for delayed hypersensitivity reactions.

dinitrogen tetroxide (di-ni′tro-jen) a colorless gas (b. p., 21.15°C), N_2O_4; M.W. 92.02. It exists in equilibrium with nitrogen dioxide, NO_2, a highly toxic red-brown gas.

dinitroorthocresol (DNOC) (di-ni″tro-or″tho-kre′-sol) a highly toxic pesticide. It is a cumulative poison that acts by uncoupling oxidative phosphorylation, producing fever, tachypnea, and tachycardia. DNOC can be assayed spectrophotometrically using the difference in its absorbance at 430 nm in neutral and acidic solutions.

dinitrophenol (DNP) (di-ni″tro-fe′nol) any one of the six isomeric compounds, $C_6H_3(OH)(NO_2)_2$, originally synthesized for use as dye intermediates. The 2,4 isomer is important in biochemistry because it is an agent that acts to uncouple oxidative phosphorylation, and thus increases the metabolic rate. Although it was formerly suggested for the treatment of myxedema and obesity, it is no longer used because it causes bone marrow suppression, agranulocytosis, cataracts, and calcification. Acute poisoning results in an increased metabolic rate and may be fatal. 2,4-Dinitrophenol is used as a chemical reagent, as an acid-base indicator, as a haptenic immunogen in immunology, and as an agent for weed control.

dinitrophenylhydrazine test (di-ni″tro-fen″il-hi′-drah-zēn) a test used to detect the presence of keto acids (oxo acids) in urine. 2,4-Dinitrophenylhydrazine is added dropwise to a clear urine specimen. The formation of a yellow or white precipitate within 10 min indicates the presence of a ketone or keto acid. If the possibility of ketonuria is eliminated by a preliminary screening test, a positive result indicates maple syrup urine disease (branched-chain ketoacids), phenylketonuria (phenylpyruvic acid), histidinemia (imidazolepyruvic acid), or methionine malabsorption syndrome (α-ketobutyric acid and other α-keto acids). See also *aminoacidopathy.*

dinucleotide (di-nu′kle-o-tīd) one of the cleavage products into which a polynucleotide or a nucleic acid may be split; a dinucleotide itself may be split into two mononucleotides. Some dinucleotides that occur as such in biological systems are synthesized de novo and have special functions. These dinucleotides contain moieties not found in nucleic acids; they include the redoxcoenzymes NAD, NADP, and FAD.

Dioctophyma (di-ok″to-fi′mah) a genus of nematode worms that are parasitic in mammals.

D. renale, a large nematode that is parasitic chiefly in dogs and rarely in humans. Males of the species have a range of 14–20 cm in length; females, 20–100 cm. Infection is thought to be caused by ingestion of contaminated fish. The adult worm lives in the kidney and causes severe renal and nervous disorders. Laboratory diagnosis requires microscopic identification of eggs found in urine sediment. Also called *Eustrongylus gigas.*

diode (di′ōd) 1. a vacuum tube with two electrodes, used as a rectifier.

2. a two-terminal semiconductor device, the *p-n* junction diode, which is used as a rectifier. It consists of a silicon or germanium crystal, half of which is doped with an *n*-type impurity (donor) and the other half with a *p*-type impurity (acceptor). The donor region is connected to a terminal called the cathode, the acceptor region to the anode. The extra valence electrons of donor atoms migrate across the *p-n* junction to fill the holes at acceptor atoms until the additional energy gained by having four valence electrons at each atom is offset by the energy of the electric field produced. The region on either side of the junction that is emptied of current carriers (electrons on the *n*-side, holes on the *p*-side) is called the depletion layer, and the voltage built up across the junction (approximately 0.7 V is silicon, 0.4 V is germanium) is called the junction potential.

When a reverse bias (positive cathode, negative anode) is applied, more electrons are attracted across the junction and the depletion layer is enlarged. Very little current can be conducted across the depletion layer because of the scarcity of current carriers. There are only a very few minority current carriers (holes on the *n*-side, electrons on the *p*-side).

A forward bias reduces the size of the depletion layer and eliminates it altogether when the junction potential is exceeded. The diode then conducts a current that is approximately proportional to the voltage. Thus, the diode can serve as a rectifier conducting current only when forward-biased.

The reverse bias cannot be increased indefinitely; at some point (the breakdown voltage), free electrons are accelerated strongly enough so that they can knock loose more valence electrons and produce a very large current (the avalanche effect). Because, in practice, the current is limited by the external circuit, the voltage cannot be increased above the breakdown level.

varactor d., a semiconductor diode used as a variable capacitor. It is operated with reverse bias so that the barrier layer acts as the dielectric of a capacitor. As the reverse bias increases, the width of the barrier layer increases, thus lowering the capacitance.

Zener d., a semiconductor diode that functions as a voltage regulator. It is connected across a direct-current voltage source in series with a current-limiting resistor. The diode is reverse-biased and operates at its breakdown voltage whenever the source voltage is above this level. It thus serves as a fixed voltage, which is independent of the source voltage.

diol (di′ol) a dihydric alcohol; also called *glycol.*

-diol a suffix word element in organic chemistry to denote the presence of two —OH groups, e.g., pregnanediol.

***gem*-diol** an alcohol having two hydroxyl groups on the same carbon atom.

Dionosil (di-on′o-sil) trademark. See under *propyliodone.*

diopter (D) (di-op′ter) [Gr. *dioptra* optical instrument for measuring angles] a unit equal to one reciprocal meter, which is used to express the refractive power of lenses as the reciprocal of the focal length in meters.

dioxane (di-ok′sān) 1,4-diethylene dioxide, a colorless, flammable liquid with an etherlike odor; M.W. 88.10. It is used as an industrial solvent, and in histology sometimes as a dehydrating agent; because it is miscible in all proportions with both water and wax, no clearing is necessary. Dioxane is highly toxic both by inhalation and by absorption through the skin. Acute effects include nausea, headache, and eye irritation. Chronic exposure may injure the kidneys and liver.

1,4-dioxane see *dioxane.*

dioxathion (di-ok″sah-thi′on) a highly toxic organothiophosphate insecticide and miticide, phosphorodithioic acid *S,S*-1,4-dioxane-2,3-diyl *O,O,O′,O′*-tetraethyl ester. See also *organophosphate compounds.*

dioxin (di-ok′sin) a highly toxic chlorinated aromatic hydrocarbon 2,3,7,8-tetrachlorodibenzo-*p*-dioxin (TCDD), that occurs as a contaminant in chlorophenoxy herbicides, particularly 2,4,5-T. Dioxin is about 500,000 times as toxic as 2,4,5-T and is highly teratogenic. It is approximately 400 times as toxic to a fetus as to its mother. It probably is also responsible for the chloracne that has been produced by heavy industrial exposure to 2,4,5-T. Dioxin has an environmental half-life of about 1 yr in the soil.

dioxygenase (di-ok′se-jen-ās) a group of enzymes (EC 1.13.11) that incorporate both atoms of O_2 into substances being oxidized. Most members of this subclass require either iron or copper ions for activity.

DIP abbrev. for *desquamative interstitial pneumonitis* (see under *pneumonitis*), *dual in-line package.*

dipalmitoylphosphatidylcholine (di-pal″mĭ-to-il-fos″fah-ti″dil-ko′lēn) a phospholipid that contains two palmitic acid chains. It is one of the lecithins necessary for lung function. See also *lecithin.*

Dipetalonema (di-pet″ah-lo-ne′mah) a genus of filarial nematode worms, several species of which are parasitic in humans.

D. perstans, a creamy-white, elongated filarial worm that is found in the tropical regions of the world and infects humans. The fly *Culicoides* serves as the intermediate host. Diagnosis requires identification of microfilariae in peripheral blood on Giemsa-stained blood films. Also called *Acanthoceilonema perstans.*

D. streptocercum, a nonpathogenic filarial worm found in Africa, whose microfilaria parasitizes the subcutaneous tissues of humans. The microfilariae are identified by staining the peripheral blood or cutaneous tissue juices with Giemsa stain. Also called *Acanthocheilonema streptocerca, Agamofilaria streptocerca,* and *Microfilaria streptocerca.*

dipetalonemiasis (di-pet″ah-lo-ne-mi′ah-sis) infected with nematodes of the genus *Dipetalonema.*

diphenadione (di-fen″ah-di′ōn) [USP], an indanedione derivative used as an oral anticoagulant. It is of limited use because of its very long half-life of 2–3 wk.

diphenhydramine hydrochloride (di″fen-hi′drah-mēn) [USP], an antihistamine (H_1-receptor blocker) with pronounced muscarinic anticholinergic side-effects. It is used in drugs prescribed for allergic reactions, motion sickness, and Parkinson's disease, and is also found in some over-the-counter sedative-hypnotics. Common adverse reactions include sedation, dizziness, gastrointestinal intolerance, and thickening of the bronchial secretions. Overdose reactions may vary from sedation to stimulation; children are particularly susceptible to overdoses and most frequently react with stimulation. Adverse reactions are aggravated by alcohol, sedatives, or tranquilizers. Diphenhydramine is assayed in biologic materials by injecting an extract from alkalinized blood or urine into a gas chromatograph with a flame ionization or nitrogen detector. Trademark, *Benadryl.*

diphenidol (di-fen′ĭ-dol) a drug used to alleviate symptoms of vertigo and nausea. Hallucinations and confusion are possible side-effects.

diphenoxylate hydrochloride (di″fen-ok′sĭ-lāt) a narcotic drug used, usually in combination with atropine, as an antiperistaltic. Overdosage causes symptoms similar to those caused by meperidine (of which it is a derivative) or by morphine.

diphenyl (di-fen′il, di-fe′nil) a toxic, colorless, crystalline compound, $(C_6H_5)_2$, two phenyl groups linked together by a single bond. Because of its fungistatic action against the *Penicillium* fungus, it is used to impregnate citrus fruit wrappers to prevent fruit decay, and in industry for organic synthesis. Diphenyl is metabolized to 4-hydroxydiphenyl, and as such is excreted either free or as a sulfate or glucuronide conjugate. Also called *biphenyl.*

diphenylhydantoin (di-fen″il-hi-dan′to-in) see *phenytoin.*

diphenylpyraline hydrochloride (di-fen″il-pi′rah-lēn) [USP], an antihistamine. Overdosage may cause central nervous system depression or stimulation, and possibly convulsions or stupor.

diphosphatidylglycerol (di-fos′fah-ti-dil-glĭ″ser-ol) see *bisphosphatidylglycerol.*

2,3-diphosphoglycerate (di-fos″fo-glis′er-āt) see *2,3-bisphosphoglycerate.*

2,3-diphosphoglycerate mutase (2,3-DPGM) see *bisphosphoglyceromutase.*

diphosphoglycerate phosphatase see *bisphosphoglycerate phosphatase.*

diphosphoinositide (di-fos″fo-in-o′sĭ-tīd) see under *phosphatidyl inositide.*

diphosphonate (di-fos′fo-nāt) one of several compounds used as chelating agents for ^{99m}Tc. ^{99m}Tc-diphosphonates are among the principal agents used clinically for bone scanning. These compounds contain two phosphonate (—P(O)$(OH)_2$) groups linked by P—C—P bonds. They are not broken down by phosphatase enzymes, which attack the P—O—P linkage of polyphosphates. See also *technetium Tc 99m diphosphonate.*

diphosphopyridine nucleotide (DPN) (di-fos″fo-pēr′ĭ-dēn) an obsolete name for nicotinamide-adenine dinucleotide (NAD).

diphtheria (dif-thēr′e-ah) [Gr. *diphthera* leather + *-ia*] an acute infectious disease caused by toxigenic strains of *Corynebacterium diphtheriae.* Infection is usually localized in the upper respiratory tract, although there is also a cutaneous form primarily found in individuals living in the tropics. Infections of the eyes, middle ear, or genitalia are rare and usually secondary. Systemic effects, primarily myocarditis and peripheral neuritis, are caused by the powerful exotoxin produced by the diphtheria bacilli. Fatalities may result from heart failure (secondary to myocarditis), shock, respiratory paralysis, or hypoxia.

Etiology. *C. diphtheriae* is a gram-positive bacillus that has been classified into three types: gravis, intermedius, and mitis, based on its colony appearance on tellurite medium and the ability to ferment starch and produce hemolysis on blood agar. Although the gravis and intermedius strains generally produce more toxic infections, toxigenic strains of the three types can produce diphtheria of serious epidemic proportions. The toxins of all three types are antigenically identical.

The diphtheria toxin is a protein produced by bacilli infected with a lysogenic bacteriophage. Avirulent strains of *C. diphtheriae* can become toxigenic by infection with the phage. The toxin is a proenzyme; proteolytic cleavage of the toxin produces two fragments, A and B. Fragment A is an enzyme that catalyzes the transfer of an ADP-ribosyl group from NAD to EF-2, an elongation factor involved in the translocation of the aminoacyl-tRNA and mRNA between sites on the eukaryotic ribosome. This inactivates EF-2 and stops protein synthesis. The other fragment (B) mediates entry of fragment A into the cell. A single molecule of the toxin can kill a cell.

Epidemiology. Diphtheria has a worldwide distribution. Epidemics occur primarily in urban environments, with the highest incidence and mortality found among the lower socioeconomic classes because of overcrowding and lack of immunization. Humans constitute the only significant reservoir of the diphtheria bacillus. The major mode of transmission of the infection from person to person is by droplets; nasopharyngeal secretions, fomites, dust, and milk have proved to be minor modes. During an epidemic, 15–20 percent of those infected are asymptomatic carriers. A carrier state may also exist for several days before and many weeks after clinical recovery.

Clinical Manifestations. Most serious infections begin as tonsilar (faucial) diphtheria. The infection usually begins on one tonsil and may spread to the other tonsil, uvula, soft palate, and pharyngeal wall. The diphtheria toxin causes necrosis of adjacent tissue, forming an exudate that contains fibrin, leukocytes, erythrocytes, necrotic epithelial cells, and diphtheria bacilli. As it congeals, the exudate forms a tough membrane (sometimes called the pseudomembrane) firmly attached to the underlying tissue, which will cause bleeding if forcibly removed. The membrane has a shiny white center and grayish-green periphery. Accompanying signs and symptoms at onset are low-grade fever, sore throat, general malaise, nausea and vomiting, and headache. The cervical lymph nodes are usually moderately tender.

In anterior nasal diphtheria, there is a mucopurulent discharge that irritates the skin around the nostrils and upper lips, sometimes producing crusting. There is a creamy-yellowish membrane in the nose. This form rarely has systemic complications, but it is an important source of infection in epidemics.

When faucial-laryngeal diphtheria spreads downward to the trachea and bronchi, dyspnea, stridor, and cyanosis are produced. The membrane may form casts in the main bronchi, causing death from hypoxia if the membrane cannot be removed by bronchoscopy.

Myocardial complications are due to toxic myocarditis produced by the diphtheria toxin. Acute circulatory failure occurs in about 9 percent of those with faucial or laryngeal diphtheria; acute electrocardiographic changes occur in about 25 percent. At the onset of myocarditis, there is a weak pulse and muffled heart sounds. ECG abnormalities include T-wave flattening and conduction disturbances including atrioventricular block, left bundle branch block, premature beats, and atrial fibrillation. Serum aspartate aminotransferase (AST, SGOT) levels correlate well with the severity of the myocarditis. The most common forms of nervous system involvement are cranial or peripheral nerve paralysis and peripheral neuritis.

Laboratory Identification. Direct examination of material from an exudate should be done with methylene-blue–stained smears to demonstrate metachromatic granules, which are suggestive but not diagnostic for diphtheria. Some of the specimen is cultured on Löffler's medium, blood agar, and cystine tellurite agar in a CO_2-rich environment. The agar gel diffusion (Elek) plate test or the guinea pig virulence test is used to identify toxigenic strains; this is the definitive basis for the laboratory diagnosis of diphtheria.

See also *C. diphtheriae* under *Corynebacterium, exotoxins,* and *vaccination.*

diphtheria bacillus see *C. diphtheriae* under *Corynebacterium.*

diphtheroid bacilli (dif′ther-oid) microorganisms

that closely resemble morphologically, and are commonly confused with, the diphtheria bacillus; they are usually members of the *Corynebacterium* genus (e.g., *C. hofmannii* or *C. pseudodiphtheriticum* and *C. xerosis*). They are nonpathogenic and do not form soluble toxins.

diphyllobothriasis (di-fil″o-both-ri′ah-sis) infected with tapeworms of the genus *Diphyllobothrium.* Formerly called *dibothriocephaliosis.*

Diphyllobothrium (di-fil″o-both′re-um) [*di-* + Gr. *phyllon* leaf + *bothrion* pit] a genus of large tapeworms in the family Diphyllobothriidae.

D. latum, a large tapeworm (10mm long), that is parasitic in humans and other fish-eating mammals. Human infection is caused by ingestion of uncooked fresh-water fish contaminated with larvae that have developed to maturity in the small intestine. Most infections produce no symptoms; however, some infected individuals develop a megaloblastic anemia resembling pernicious anemia due to competition by the tapeworm for the vitamin B_{12}. Laboratory diagnosis requires identification of the characteristic operculate egg (70 μ long by 50 μ wide) in the feces. Also called broad fish tapeworm and *Taenia latum.*

dipicolinic acid (di-pik″o-li′nik) pyridine-2,6-dicarboxylic acid, an intermediate in the bacterial synthesis of lysine and a calcium chelating agent. It is an important constituent (15 percent) of bacterial spores and is thought to be concerned with the transport of calcium, which has a high concentration in spores.

dipl/o (dip′lo) [Gr. *diploos* double] a word element used in combining form to denote double, twin, twofold, or twice, e.g., diploidy.

diplegia (di-ple′je-ah) [*di-* + Gr. *plēgē* stroke] paralysis of similar parts on both sides of the body.

diplochromosome (dip″lo-kro′mo-sōm) a chromosome that has four chromatids instead of two owing to a failure to separate into two daughter chromosomes in the anaphase state of meiosis. See also *nondisjunction.*

diplococcus (dip″lo-kok′us), pl. *diplococci* [*diplo-* + Gr. *kokkos* berry] a spherical bacterium occurring predominantly in pairs. The organisms may also assume a lancet or coffee bean shape.

diploë (dip′lo-e) [Gr. *diploē* fold] [NA], the spongy, cancellous bone found between the inner and outer plates of the bones of the cranium.

diploic vein (dĭ-plo′ik) one of the veins occupying the channels in the diploë of the cranial bones. These veins lack valves and communicate with the meningeal veins and the dural sinuses. They do not develop until the second year of life.

diploid (dip′loid) [*diplo-* + Gr. *eidos* form] 1. having two sets of chromosomes. Each chromosome (except the sex chromosome) has a homologue in the other set. By extension, the DNA content characteristic of diploid cells is referred to as diploid. All cells (except the gametes) of normal higher animals are diploid.

2. an organism or cell having two sets of chromosomes.

diploid number (2n) the number of chromosomes in the diploid set; there are 46 in humans; see also *karyotype.*

diploidy (dip′loi-de) the state of having two full sets of homologous chromosomes.

diplonema (dip″lo-ne′mah) [*diplo-* + Gr. *nēma* thread] 1. see diplotene.

2. a pair of chromosomes specially paired (synapsed) together in the diplotene stage of meiosis I. Also called *bivalent* or *tetrad.* See also *meiosis.*

diplont (dip′lont) [*diplo-* + Gr. *ōn* being] an individual having two sets of chromosomes (diploid).

diplopia (dĭ-plo′pe-ah) [*diplo-* + Gr. *ōpē* sight + *-ia*] double vision or the perception of two images of a single object.

Diplopoda (di-plop′o-dah) [*diplo-* + Gr. *pous* foot] a class of arthropods that comprises the millipedes. They possess segmental glands that secrete a cyanogenic compound capable of causing burning dermatitis. Some species of the genera *Julus* and *Fontaria* are the intermediate host of the tapeworm *Hymenolepis diminuta,* and other species of the genera *Julus* and *Polydesmus* have been found in the digestive and urinary tracts of humans.

diplosome (dip′lo-sōm) [*diplo-* + Gr. *sōma* body] a pair of centrioles before their separation.

diplotene (dip′lo-tēn) the stage of the first prophase of meiosis in which the sister chromosomes of the tetrads begin to separate. Also called *diplonema.* See also *meiosis.*

dipolar structure (di-po′lar) a compound in which there is separation of positive and negative charges, as in a zwitterion.

dipole (di′pōl) two separated electric charges or magnetic poles having equal magnitudes but opposite polarity, or referring to the electric or magnetic field produced by such a system.

Ionic or polar covalent bonds produce electric dipoles in molecules. These polar molecules are then able to bond electrostatically to both positive and negative ions or charged groups. Hydrogen bonds are an example of this type of bonding between dipoles. Dipoles can also be induced in molecules by the electric field of another dipole; the resulting weak attraction of the two dipoles produces the London (or van der Waals) force.

The intrinsic magnetic dipole moment of nuclei or of electrons is the property utilized in nuclear magnetic resonance (NMR) or electron spin resonance (ESR) spectroscopy.

See also *polar.*

dipole moment (μ) the product of the magnitude and the separation of charges in an electric dipole or of poles of a magnetic dipole. In chemistry, the debye (D) is commonly used to measure electric dipole strength, e.g., for water, $\mu = 1.85$ D. See also *magnetic moment.*

dips/o (dip′so) [Gr. *dipsa* thirst] a word element used in combining form to denote thirst, e.g., polydipsia.

Diptera (dip′ter-ah) [Gr. *dipteros* two-winged] an order of insects that includes flies, gnats, and mosquitoes having a single pair of wings.

dipterous (dip′ter-us) 1. possessing two wings.

2. pertaining to insects of the order Diptera.

Dipylidium (dip″ĭ-lid′e-um) [Gr. *dipylos* having two entrances] a genus of tapeworms.

D. canium, a species of tapeworm of worldwide distribution, commonly found in dogs and cats and occasionally in humans. Infection is caused by ingestion of contaminated fleas. The larvae (cysticercoids) develop in the small intestine. Children are usually infected through close association with infected pets. Diagnosis requires identification of eggs or proglottids in the feces. Also called *Taenia canina.*

dipyridamole (di″pĭ-rid′ah-mōl) a coronary vasodilator, chemically unrelated to nitrates, that is used in the treatment of chronic angina pectoris. Adverse reactions include headache, dizziness, nausea, and syncope. Trademark, *Persantine.*

diquat (di′kwat) 1,1′-ethylene,2,2′-dipyridylium dibromide, a quaternary ammonium compound generally used as a herbicide and defoliant. Toxic effects include inflammation and bleeding of the nasal mucosa and eye damage. Unlike paraquat, progressive pulmonary fibrosis does not occur.

diquat assays colorimetric methods for diquat in urine specimens. When sodium dithionite is added to the specimen, diquat is indicated by an apple-green color. For quantitative measurements, diquat is separated from the sample by column chromatography and reduced with sodium dithionite; the diquat concentration is measured by the absorbance at 379 nm.

direct access (di-rekt′) pertaining to a computer storage device, such as a disk or drum, that has approximately the same access time for every stored item, or pertaining to a file resident on such a device from which records can be requested at random. Cf. *sequential access.*

direct current (DC, dc, or d.c.) electric current that flows in only one direction, rather than alternately in both directions. Electronic instruments operate on direct current produced by a power supply or batteries.

pulsating d. c., an electric current that flows in only one direction but with varying voltage, such as is produced by rectification of alternating current.

direct light reflex see *light r.* under *reflex.*

direct memory access (DMA) a form of data transfer from a bulk storage device, such as a disk or magnetic tape drive, to the main memory of a minicomputer. The computer sends the input/output request to the device, which starts the operation, such as reading a disk sector. The data is transferred to memory without program control by a process called cycle stealing; as each word is read, one instruction cycle is used to transfer it to memory. The program running at the time is unaffected.

directory (di-rek′to-re) in computer programming, a file that contains the names and addresses of the files and programs in a library or database.

direct transport see under *active transport.*

Dirofilaria (di″ro-fĭ-la′re-ah) a genus of filarial nematode worms, many species of which are parasitic in humans.

D. conjunctivae, a filiarial worm that occasionally infects the eyes or subcutaneous tissues of humans and other mammals. It is probably the same species as *D. repens* and *D. tenuis.*

D. immitis, a creamy-white, slender filarial worm that parasitizes the heart, lungs, and subcutaneous tissues in dogs and cats, and occasionally humans. The females measure 25–30 cm long; the males, 12–18 cm. Infections are transmitted by mosquitoes. Also called dog heartworm and *Filaria sanguinis.*

dirofilariasis (di″ro-fil″ah-ri′ah-sis) infected with nematodes of the genus *Dirofilaria.*

dis- (dis) [L. *dis* apart], a prefix word element to denote reversal or separation, e.g., dislocation.

disaccharidase (di-sak′ah-rĭ-dās″) glycosidases, EC 3.2.1, a common name for any enzyme that hydrolyzes a *O*-glycosyl disaccharide to the constituent monosaccharides. Deficiency of one or more of these enzymes in the intestinal mucosa produces a variety of clinical symptoms. See also *disaccharidase deficiency, α-D-glucosidase* (maltase), *lactase, oligo-1,6-glucosidase* (isomaltase), and *sucrase.*

disaccharidase deficiency the absence or diminished activity of one or more of the disaccharidase enzymes located in the intestinal mucosa. This deficient activity gives rise to intolerance toward one or more of the disaccharides when ingested orally, resulting in such symptoms as cramps, diarrhea, nutritional insufficiency, electrolyte imbalance, and acidosis. The condition can be primary, due to an inborn deficiency of one or more enzymes (lactase, sucrase and isomaltase), a loss of activity with age (lactose intolerance), or a generalized deficiency; or it may be secondary to other diseases such as celiac sprue, or enteric inflammatory disease. All human infants are normally born with active intestinal lactase, but in a high percentage of blacks, Orientals, American Indians, and Semites, the enzyme activity decreases in early childhood, with a consequent development of lactose intolerance.

disaccharide (di-sak′ah-rīd) any of a class of sugars that yields two monosaccharides on hydrolysis. The most common disaccharides are maltose (glucose + glucose), lactose (glucose + galactose), and sucrose (glucose + fructose).

disaccharide tolerance test a procedure used to test whether a defect in the absorption of the disaccharides sucrose, isomaltose, or lactose is present and, when present, if it is due to a deficiency or an absence of the appropriate intestinal mucosal disaccharidase. A disaccharide dose of 2 g/kg of body weight or 50 g/m² of body surface is administered to the patient. If the disaccharide is hydrolyzed and the monosaccharides absorbed, a normal or near-normal type of glucose tolerance curve is obtained. If a deficiency is present, a flat curve is obtained, with the glucose rise less than 20 mg/dl.

disc/o (dis′ko) [L. *discus;* Gr. *diskos*] a word element used in combining form to denote relationship to a disk, or disk-shaped, e.g., discoid.

disc (disk) [L. *discus*] see *disk.*

disc electrophoresis (disk) see under *electrophoresis.*

discharge (dis-charj′) 1. a material that is emitted, e.g., a secretion or excretion.

2. the firing of a neuron or neurons.

3. removal of stored electrical energy from a battery or capacitor.

4. an electric current flow that produces a glow, arc, or corona.

discharge frequency the number of action potentials that repeat within a certain period of time, usually reported in impulses per second (hertz). When the potentials occur as a grouped discharge, the repetition rate of the entire group and of the individual potentials is usually specified.

disclosing solution (dis-klōz′ing) a solution that contains the dye erythrosin, which is used by dentists and dental personnel to demonstrate dental plaque. Disclosing solution stains the transparent plaque and thus facilitates its removal by making it visible. Dentists often prescribe disclosing solution for home use so that patients may remove plaque more efficiently and prevent dental caries. See also *caries* and *dental plaque.*

discocyte (dis'ko-sīt) [*disco-* + Gr. *kytos* hollow vessel] the normal disc form of an erythrocyte. Also called biconcave disc.

discography (dis-kog'rah-fe) [*disco-* + Gr. *graphein* to record] see *diskography.*

discoid (dis'koid) [*disco-* + Gr. *eidos* form] 1. shaped like a disk, cylindric.
2. shaped like an intervertebral disk; spool-shaped. See also the illustration accompanying *contour.*

discordance (dis-kor'dans) in genetics, the occurrence of a given trait in only one member of a twin pair. Cf. *concordance.*

discordant (dis-kor'dant) pertaining to the exhibition of a trait by only one of a pair of twins.

discrete (dis-krēt') [L. *discretus,* from *discernere* to separate] 1. made up of separated parts.
2. having a separate and distinct identity.
3. in mathematics, pertaining to a variable or a set, all of whose values are separated by more than some definite minimal separation.
4. in statistics, pertaining to a random variable that can assume only a finite or countable set of distinct values. Cf. *continuum.*

discriminator (dis-krim"ĭ-na'tor) an electronic circuit in which the output signal depends on the difference between the frequencies or voltages of an input signal and a reference signal.

disease (dĭ-zēz) [Fr. *des* from + *aise* ease] a well-defined disorder of the structure or functions of a living organism having a predictable course. Increasingly, the tendency is to use the term disease only for conditions that have or appear to have a single pathogenic mechanism, as distinguished from the term syndrome, which connotes only a recognizable pattern or constellation of signs and symptoms.

dish (dish) a shallow vessel of glass or other material for laboratory work. See also *Petri dish.*

disinfect (dis"in-fekt') [*dis-* + L. *inficere* to corrupt] to free from pathogenic organisms or to render them inert. The term is correctly applied to the treatment of inanimate objects or surfaces with heat or chemicals to reduce the risk of transmitting infection.

disinfectant (dis"in-fek'tant) a physical or chemical agent used to disinfect. To be useful, a disinfectant must kill microorganisms rapidly, preferably at a low concentration. Disinfectants are used in the control of infection in hospitals, other health care facilities, public health areas, and the food industry.

Most disinfectants act by dissolving lipids from the cell membrane or by denaturing protein. Phenol has been the standard disinfectant, and disinfectant potency has in the past often been expressed as the phenol coefficient. This standard, however, is valid only for phenolic compounds. See also *phenol coefficient.*

disinfection (dis"in-fek'shun) any practical procedure that significantly reduces the microbial contamination in the inanimate environment, e.g., air, water, instruments, and equipment. Disinfection can be carried out with a physical agent (usually heat) or a chemical disinfectant. Disinfection is distinct from antisepsis, which is similar in purpose but limited in application to the skin and mucous membranes; it also should not be confused with sterilization. Although a disinfection procedure can actually sterilize a solution or an object, it does not necessarily do so. Whether this happens depends on the presence or absence of resistant forms of microorganisms, strength of the disinfectant, degree of heating, length of exposure time, and amount of organic soil protecting microbes entrapped in it. The difference between sterilization and disinfection, then, is that disinfection procedures do not guarantee sterility as the end result.

SUSCEPTIBILITY TO DISINFECTION. Most vegetative bacterial and fungal cells, as well as the majority of pathogenic viruses, fall within the same general range of susceptibility to chemical disinfection. However, tubercle bacilli, chlamydospores of fungi, and the picornaviruses are significantly more resistant and require high-level disinfection. Disinfectants cannot be tested experimentally against hepatitis viruses because their host range is limited to humans and chimpanzees. For this reason and because of the serious nature of hepatitis in humans, surgical instruments and medical items used for known or suspected hepatitis patients should be sterilized. Bacterial endospores are by far the most resistant of all microbial forms. Spores of *Clostridium tetani,* the tetanus bacillus, can survive commonly used disinfection procedures for many hours or even days of constant exposure. Only a very few chemical disinfectants can destroy spores within a useful time period, and these strong disinfectants are in effect chemical sterilants.

Heat is a rapid, thorough, and simple method of disinfection, and fungi, bacteria, and most viruses are killed by boiling water within a few minutes. Common applications of heat disinfection are immersion of instruments in boiling water for 5 min and pasteurization of milk (62°C for 30 min). Tubercle bacilli are no more resistant to heat than other vegetative forms of bacteria and fungi. Bacterial spores, however, are extremely resistant and can survive boiling water for 2 hr or longer; therefore, boiling cannot be used when the complete absence of microorganisms is required.

PROCEDURES. Most disinfection is carried out with chemicals. Examples include chlorination of water, and numerous procedures used in hospital, clinic, and office practice for handling reusable instruments and equipment. Instruments and other items that will penetrate body tissues are considered "critical" (carrying a high risk of infection) and must be sterilized. This generally means autoclaving (see under *sterilization*). Some such items, however, are thermolabile and must be sterilized chemically. Certain instruments, such as laparoscopes, are considered "semicritical" and subjected to high-level disinfection. Instruments and equipment that contact surface mucous membranes and skin but do not penetrate them are also semicritical items. Noncritical items are equipment and instrument components that do not make direct contact with the body; for these, low-level disinfection suffices. Recommended disinfection procedures are listed below.

All chemical formulations listed are liquid except the gas ethylene oxide. The pasteurization procedure is carried out at a higher temperature than that used for the pasteurization of milk. With the exception of alcohol, all these chemicals are available as commercial products. Three of the four disinfectants in the low-level category become high-level agents when the concentration is increased from threefold to tenfold, and the exposure time lengthened from 10 min to 30 min. Alcohol rapidly kills tubercle bacilli because the high-lipid cell wall that is quite impermeable to aqueous germicides is no effective barrier against alcohol penetration. Iodophors are complexes of elemental iodine with a large organic molecule that slowly release free iodine.

RECOMMENDED DISINFECTION PROCEDURES*

High-level disinfection category (30 min)
Ethylene oxide (manufacturer's directions)
Glutaraldehyde, 2% aqueous
Formaldehyde, 8% — alcohol, 70%
Stabilized hydrogen peroxide, 6%, aqueous
Sodium hypochlorite, 1000 ppm, aqueous
Phenolic compounds, 3%, aqueous
Iodophors, 500 ppm, aqueous
Alcohol, ethyl or isopropyl, 70–90%
Pasteurization at 75°C
Low-level disinfection category (10 min)
Sodium hypochlorite, 100 ppm, aqueous
Phenolic compounds, 1%, aqueous
Iodophors, 100 ppm, aqueous
Quaternary ammonium compound-detergents, aqueous (manufacturer's directions)

*Source: United States Centers for Disease Control, "1981 Guidelines for Hospital Environmental Control" (Atlanta, GA: CDC, 1981).

MECHANISM OF DISINFECTION. Disinfectants kill microorganisms through several different mechanisms. Heat and strong disinfectants coagulate protein or otherwise denature it irreversibly. Glutaraldehyde and ethylene oxide are examples of strong (high-level) disinfectants that are alkylating agents acting primarily on nucleic acids. Some less strong chemicals are surface-active agents that disrupt cell membranes, e.g., phenolics and quaternary ammonium compounds. Others are oxidizing agents, or they combine with essential enzymes, proteins of cell membranes, and the like, so that growth cannot be demonstrated (the criterion of microbial death) after contact.

Cf. *antisepsis* and *sterilization.*

disintegration (dis″in-tĕ-gra′shun) [*dis-* + L. *integer* entire] 1. the process of breaking up or decomposing.

2. radioactive decay; see *decay.*

disintegration constant see *decay constant.*

disjunction (dis-junk′shun) the act or state of being disjoined; in genetics, the separation and moving apart of sister chromosomes in the first meiotic anaphase. Cf. *nondisjunction.*

disk (disk) [L. *discus,* from Gr. *diskos*] 1. a circular or rounded flat plate. For more information, see also the specific disk.

2. a direct-access mass storage device for digital computers in which information is stored magnetically in concentric tracks in the magnetic coating on a rotating disk. The read-write heads are moved mechanically to select the track. There are two types: hard disks, which have a capacity of up to hundreds of megabytes and are generally used with larger computers, and inexpensive floppy disks, which have a capacity of about 1 megabyte and are used with microcomputers.

disk diffusion test see under *antibacterial agent susceptibility testing.*

diskocyte (dis′ko-sit) [*disco-* + Gr. *kytos* hollow vessel] see *discocyte.*

diskogram (dis′ko-gram) [*disco-* + Gr. *gramma* mark] a radiograph of an intervertebral disk.

diskography (dis-kog′rah-fe) [*disco-* + Gr. *graphein* to record] the radiologic examination of an intervertebral disk after injection of a water-soluble iodinated contrast medium such as diatrizoate. It is used to demonstrate lesions of the disk such as a rupture of the nucleus pulposus. Also called *nucleography.*

cervical d., radiography of a cervical disk. The patient is supine, with the head elevated to reduce the spinal curvature; anteroposterior (10° cranial angulation) and lateral views are made.

lumbar d., radiography of a lumbar disk. With the patient in the lateral position and verified in a lateral view, the contrast medium is injected. Frontal views (direct and 10°–20° cranial angulation) are then made with the patient supine and the thighs flexed so that the back is flat against the table. Finally, weight-bearing flexion and extension lateral views are made with the patient erect.

dislocation (dis″lo-ka′shun) [*dis-* + L. *locare* to place] the displacement of any part, especially a bone.

congenital d., dislocation that exists from or before birth.

fracture d., a dislocation complicated by an adjacent fracture.

pathologic d., a dislocation that results from paralysis, synovitis, infection, or other disease.

disomic (di-so′mik) pertaining to disomy.

disomy (di′so-me) [*di-* + Gr. *soma* body] the normal condition of having two homologues of a given chromosome as opposed to one (monosomy) or three (trisomy). In the somatic cell chromosome complement of normal humans, all the autosomes are disomic, as is the X chromosome in females.

disorder (dis-or′der) a derangement or abnormality of function; a morbid physical or mental state.

disorganization (dis-or″gah-ni-za′shun) 1. the process of destruction of any organic tissue; any profound change in the tissue of an organ or structure that causes the loss of most or all of its proper characters.

2. in electroencephalography, an alteration in the frequency, form, distribution, and/or extent of the electric activity of the brain as recorded in an individual when related to activity recorded previously or to activity recorded from homologous regions on the opposite side of the head.

disorientation (dis-o″re-en-ta′shun) the loss of proper bearings so that the individual may not know where or who he or she is. The grasp of time, place, person, or situation may be affected, either singly or in combination. Disorientation is a conspicuous feature of confusional states.

spatial d., a condition in which an individual is unable to determine accurately spatial attitude in relation to the earth's surface. Spatial disorientation that is the result of extremely poor visibility (e.g., heavy snow, fog) may particularly affect automobile drivers and air crew members; it may also occur when the vision is otherwise restricted, resulting in vestibular illusions.

dispermy (di'sper-me) the penetration of one ovum by two sperm, which may result in triploidy. Cf. *monospermy.*

disperse (dis-pers') [*dis-* + L. *spargere* to scatter] to scatter or spread. The term is used especially when a finely divided substance is distributed more or less evenly in another, as the particles of a colloid, or when a collection of similar phenomena is separated into distinct components, as the different colors constituting white light.

disperse phase the suspended particles of a colloid.

dispersion (dis-per'zhun) [L. *dispersio*] 1. the property of being scattered or spread out.

2. the degree of scatter in statistical data. Any measure such as the range or standard deviation that describes this scatter may be said to measure dispersion.

3. the spreading of a spectrum produced by a prism or grating. Angular dispersion is the change in angle per unit wavelength of the dispersed beam; linear dispersion is the linear change per unit wavelength at the detector or slit.

colloidal d., a colloid.

molecular d., a solution, i.e., the distribution of the individual solute molecules among the molecules of the solvent.

displacement (dis-plās'ment) 1. removal from the normal position or place; ectopia.

2. a chemical reaction in which a constituent atom or group of atoms is displaced (set free) from a compound by another atom or group of atoms.

3. the distance that an object is moved.

display (dis-plā') the portion of any electronic device that shows the readout, such as a cathode ray tube, digital voltmeter, or strip chart recorder of a measuring instrument.

disposable (dis-pōs'ah-b'l) designed to be discarded after use.

disproportion (dis"pro-por'shun) a lack of the proper relationship between two elements or factors.

dissect (dĭ-sekt', di-sekt') [L. *dissecare* to cut up] to cut apart or separate; applied especially to the exposure of structures of a cadaver for anatomic study.

dissection (dĭ-sek'shun) [L. *dissectio*] the act or process of cutting apart. This term is often applied to cadavers being cut open to display anatomic features. Dissection can be blunt (separation of tissues along existing cleavage planes) or sharp (separation of tissues with a scalpel or scissors).

disseminated (dis-sem'ĭ-nat"ed) [*dis-* + L. *seminare* to sow] scattered; distributed away from a source, usually over a considerable area.

disseminated intravascular coagulation (DIC) a disturbance in the hemostatic balance, activated by a procoagulant stimulus, that produces the release of tissue factor into the circulation, or conditions that lead to endothelial cell injury and/or Factor XII activation. Both platelets and coagulation factors are consumed, fibrin is deposited in small vessels in many organs, and the fibrinolytic system is activated with the subsequent accumulation of fibrin (fibrinogen) degradation products in the circulation, which also inhibit clot formation.

DIC may accompany septicemia with gram-negative or occasionally gram-positive infection, premature placental separation, shock, and malignancies. It is associated with abnormal bleeding, anemia with red cell fragmentation (formation of schistocytes), thrombocytopenia, prolonged prothrombin and activated partial thromboplastin times, hypofibrinogenemia, and increased fibrin (fibrinogen) degradation products.

As DIC is a secondary disorder, treatment and subsequent removal of the primary diseases are essential for its control. If serious bleeding and thrombosis are present, or if the underlying disease cannot be managed effectively, anticoagulation with heparin and replacement of clotting factors with fresh frozen plasma, cryoprecipitate and platelet transfusions are utilized. If secondary fibrinolysis occurs, treatment with ϵ-aminocaproic acid (EACA) is indicated.

Also called *consumption coagulopathy* and *defibrination syndrome.*

disseminated sclerosis see *disseminated s.* under *sclerosis.*

dissemination (dis-sem'ĭ-na'shun) [*dis-* + L. *seminare* to sow] 1. the act of scattering or distributing over a considerable area, i.e., from a localized site to various organs or other parts of the body.

2. in microbiology, the scattering or shedding of microorganisms from an individual into the environment, as by a carrier.

Disse's space (dis'ez) [Joseph *Disse,* German anatomist, 1852–1912] the slender space that separates a hepatic sinusoid from the parenchymal cells of the liver. Also called space of Disse.

dissociation (dis-so"se-a'shun) [*dis-* + L. *sociatio* union] 1. the act of separating or state of being separated.

2. the separation of a molecule into two or more molecules, atoms, or ions produced by thermal or electromagnetic energy or by solvation. See also *photodissociation.*

dissociation constant (K_d) the equilibrium constant, expressed in terms of concentrations, for the dissociation of a molecule or an ion into parts. The dissociation constant for an acid is denoted K_a. The formula is: $K_a = [H^+][A^-]/[HA]$. The dissociation constant for a base is denoted K_b. The formula is $K_b = [OH^-][B^+]/[BOH]$. Also called *ionization constant.*

dissolution (dis"so-lu'shun) [L. *dissolutio,* from *dissolvere* to dissolve] the rate at which disintegration, measured in terms of the release of an active material (drug) into a test solution, occurs in vitro under standard conditions, e.g., as defined by USP.

dissolve (diz-zolv') to pass or to cause to pass into solution. A solvent dissolves a solute; a solute dissolves in a solvent.

dissymmetry (dis-sim'ĕ-tre) having no mirror symmetry. A dissymmetric object has no symmetry plane, but may have a symmetry axis. Dissymetric molecules have nonidentical mirror images called enantiomers. Cf. *asymmetry.*

dist/o (dis'to) [L. *distans* distant] a word element used in combining form to denote far, e.g., distal.

distal (dis'tal) farther from some reference point; in referring to a chromosome, farther from the centromere.

distal latency see *distal l.* under *latency.*

distention (dis-ten′shun) the state of being dilated or enlarged; the act of distending. See also *dilation.*

distill (dis-til′) [L. *destillare,* from *de* down + *stillare* to drip] to separate liquids by the process of distillation, e.g., by virtue of differences in boiling points.

distillate (dis′til-lāt) a liquid produced by distillation.

distillation (dis-til-la′shun) a process in which a mixture of liquids or solutes and liquids are heated; the more volatile components are vaporized, collected, and then condensed into one or more fractions. The distillate is thus separated from the less volatile components or solids present in the mixture.

destructive d., a process of thermal decomposition performed in the absence of oxygen in which the volatile components are separated from a combustible solid, e.g., coal tar from coal. Also called pyrolysis.

fractional d., a process in which several distillation fractions are collected. Each fraction consists of liquids or azeotropic mixtures that have boiling points lying within a narrow range of temperatures. The temperature of the condensing vapor is continuously monitored, and each time the temperature rises appreciably (indicating that a compound with a higher boiling point is condensing), the collection of a new fraction is begun.

molecular d., distillation performed in high vacuum (a pressure of about 10^{-6} atm) in which the distillate is condensed on a cooled plate near the surface of the liquid being vaporized (so named because in this process a molecule has a high probability of passing from the liquid phase to the condensation plate without colliding with another molecule). This process is used in the purification of substances that have high boiling points or that are sensitive to thermal decomposition, such as vitamins, steroids and other hormones, triglycerides, and other complex organic compounds.

vacuum d., a distillation performed at reduced pressure, which lowers the boiling point of the distillates and consequently reduces the possibility of thermal decomposition.

distilled oil see *volatile oil.*

Distoma (dis′to-mah) [*di-* + Gr. *stoma* mouth] a genus name formerly used for many species of trematode worms that have been classified into different genera and even superfamilies. The anglicized form of this term is now used to describe a morphologic type common to many trematodes. The species *D. pulmonum, D. ringeri,* and *D. westermani* are now termed *Paragonimus westermani.* See also *distome.*

distome (dis′tōm) a characteristic morphologic type of adult digenetic trematodes (flukes). The body has two suckers: an oral sucker and a ventral sucker or acetabulum. This term is used in a descriptive, not taxonomic, sense. Many species of this suborder are parasitic in humans, e.g., *Fasciola hepatica.*

distomiasis (dis″to-mi′ah-sis) a parasitic infection caused by several species of flukes that have a predilection for the intestines, liver, or lungs.

distortion (dis-tor′shun) [*dis-* + L. *torsio* a twisting] 1. any change in the shape of a radiographic image from the true shape of the structure; some causes include misalignment of the beam, structure, or film. See also *spatial distortion.*

2. in electronics, an undesired, nonrandom change in a waveform during amplification or transmission. Cf. *noise.*

distribution (dis″trĭ-bu′shun) [L. *distributio*] 1. the arrangement of objects or events in space or time.

2. branching to supply various tissues, as of an artery or nerve.

3. the area supplied by an artery or nerve.

4. the geographic range of an organism or disease.

5. in probability and statistics, a function or table that specifies the probability of occurrence for each value or range of values of a random variable; see also *probability distribution.*

reference d., in clinical chemistry, a probability distribution that represents the observable values in a reference class. The distribution is derived from the observed values of a sample group. Examples include those data collected for establishing the precision of a method or the normal range for a given population.

sample d., a function that specifies the cumulative number or proportion of sample measurements less than a given value for each possible value on the measurement scale.

distribution coefficient see *partition coefficient.*

distribution function a function that describes a probability distribution by giving the probability that the random variable will be less than the value of the argument; the integrated or cumulative form of the density function. Also called *cumulative distribution,* cumulative distribution function, and cumulative frequency distribution. See also *probability distribution.*

disulfide (di-sul′fīd) an organic compound containing the —S—S— group. See also *functional group.*

disulfide bond the chemical bond —S—S—, that connects two atoms of sulfur. Interchain and intrachain disulfide bonds, formed by the oxidation of two cysteine residues, are essential for the three-dimensional tertiary structure of proteins.

disulfiram (di-sul′fĭ-ram) [USP], bis(diethylthiocarbamyl)disulfide, a drug used to deter alcohol consumption; M.W. 296.54. It inhibits aldehyde dehydrogenase, thus causing the accumulation of acetaldehyde, a metabolite of ethanol, when alcohol is ingested. This produces nausea, vomiting, headache, weakness, and, in severe reactions, heart irregularities or failure. Toxic reactions also occur when disulfiram is taken in combination with phenytoin, metronidazole, or isoniazid. Trademark, *Antabuse.*

disulfiram assays ultraviolet spectrophotometry. Disulfiram is extracted into ethylene dichloride from a blood sample to which copper sulfate and pH 7.4 buffer have been added. The drug concentration is proportional to the difference in the absorbances at 270 and 320 nm.

disulfoton (di-sul′fo-ton) the generic name for *O,O*-diethyl *S*-[2-(ethylthio)ethyl]phosphorodithioate, a highly toxic, cholinesterase-inhibiting organophosphate pesticide. Trademarks, Di-Syston and Dithiosystox.

DIT abbrev. See *diiodotyrosine.*

dithionite (di-thi′o-nīt) the $S_2O_4^{2-}$ ion, a strong reducing agent. The commercial form is the salt sodium dithionite ($Na_2S_2O_4$). Also called hydrosulfite.

dithiothreitol (di-thi″o-thre′ĭ-tol) 1,4-dithiol-2,3-dihydroxybutane, used in protein and enzyme work to keep —SH groups in the reduced state. Some investigators also claim that it acts to stereoselectively reduce disulfide bridges. Dithiothreitol is optically active, and both the racemic and (−) forms are available. It is also referred to as optically active Cleland's reagent. The term Cleland's reagent used without qualification refers to *meso*-dithioerythritol, which is optically inactive.

In immunohematology, dithiothreitol is used to dissociate 19S IgM molecules into 7S subunits. Agglutinating IgM antibodies are inactivated, whereas IgG antibodies are not affected.

diuresis (di″u-re′sis), pl. *diureses* [Gr. *diourein* to urinate, to pass in urine] the increased excretion of urine, which may be produced by the excessive drinking of water or by the administration of diuretic agents. It may be due to hormonal imbalances, renal dysfunctions, or drug intoxication.

diuretic (di″u-ret′ik) [Gr. *diourētikos* promoting urine] an agent that increases the rate of formation of urine in the body; some common examples of substances having diuretic action are coffee, tea, ethanol, and water. Drugs that have a diuretic effect can be grouped into classes by their mechanisms of action.

Osmotic Diuretics. Substances such as mannitol are freely filtered in the glomerulus and are reabsorbed in the renal tubules only to a limited extent. Thus, osmotic diuretics increase the amount of osmotically active solute in the urine and consequently the urine volume. These compounds also increase the osmolality of plasma and therefore increase the diffusion of water from intraocular and cerebrospinal fluids. Osmotic diuretics are used for reducing the pressure and volume of these fluids.

Mercurial Diuretics. These are organometallic compounds, now rarely used, that inhibit the tubular resorption of sodium and chloride.

Carbonic Anhydrase Inhibitors. Acetazolamide and its congeners, compounds that are noncompetitive inhibitors of carbonic anhydrase, make up this class. Their action causes increased excretion of bicarbonate, sodium, and water in the proximal tubules.

Thiazides. This class of structurally related heterocyclic sulfonamides, typified by chlorothiazide, increases the renal excretion of sodium and its accompanying anion, chloride, by inhibiting the reabsorption of sodium in the distal tubules, thus increasing the excretion of water. Thiazides also increase the excretion of potassium, which can cause hypokalemia and thus require dietary potassium supplementation. These drugs are used to treat edema due to congestive heart failure, and chronic hepatic or renal disease; they are also used alone or in combination with other drugs to treat hypertension.

High-Ceiling (Loop) Diuretics. These chemically unrelated compounds, including ethacrynic acid and furosemide, increase the excretion of sodium and chloride primarily by inhibiting the resorption of chloride by active transport, which occurs in the ascending limb of the loop of Henle; electrolyte resorption is also inhibited in the proximal tubule. The excretion of potassium, magnesium, and calcium is also increased. High-ceiling diuretics produce a much higher level of diuresis than do other diuretics, and their effect is not altered by acid-base imbalances or hypoalbuminemia. As with the thiazides, they are used to treat edema and hypertension.

Aldosterone Antagonists. Spironolactone, a competitive antagonist of aldosterone at receptor sites in the distal tubules, is the only drug in this class. It causes an increase in the excretion of sodium and chloride and the conservation of potassium. It is used primarily to treat refractory edema and also for hyperaldosteronism.

Potassium-Sparing Diuretics. This class includes triamterene and amiloride, a group of drugs that block the aldosterone-independent exchange of sodium for potassium and hydrogen ions in the distal tubule. They increase sodium and chloride excretion with only a negligible increase in potassium excretion. These drugs are generally used in combination with a thiazide diuretic in individuals in whom there is concern about potassium depletion.

Diuril (di′u-ril) trademark for chlorothiazide; see under *thiazide diuretics*.

diurnal (di-er′nal) [L. *diurnus* daily] 1. pertaining to a daily occurrence, such as the variation of body temperature over a 24-hr cycle.

2. occurring during daylight hours rather than at night.

diuron (di′u-ron) a preemergence phenylurea herbicide, 3-(3,4-dichlorophenyl)-1,1-dimethylurea. It is irritating to the skin and respiratory tract. If metabolized to dichloroaniline, it can produce methemoglobinemia.

divalent (di-va′lent) see *bivalent*.

divergence (di-ver′jens) a spreading or bending apart; in ophthalmology, the term refers to simultaneous abduction of both eyes.

diverticulitis (di″ver-tik-u-li′tis) inflammation of a diverticulum, especially used to refer to inflammation of colonic diverticulum. The process in the colon usually begins within a single diverticulum when its narrow neck is obstructed by food residues. Inflammation develops within the obstructed diverticulum, and readily extends through the mucosa and thin covering of subserosal areolar tissue to the peritoneal surface. Peritonitis and bleeding may ensue, or the condition can become chronic, leading to fibrosis, distortion, and narrowing of the bowel wall, and the formation of adhesions.

The diagnosis can be confirmed by barium enema. In some patients, distinction from carcinoma is difficult by radiologic examination.

diverticulosis (di″ver-tik″u-lo′sis) a condition characterized by the presence of multiple diverticula of the bowel, particularly in the descending and sigmoid colon.

diverticulum (di″ver-tik′u-lum), pl. *diverticula* [L. *divertere* to turn aside] a general term used to describe the hernial protrusion of a pouch or sac of mucosal epithelium through a defect in the muscular coat of a hollow organ. Such protrusions may be congenital or acquired, and most commonly occur in the intestines, esophagus, and bladder.

colonic d., a herniation or saclike protrusion of the mucosa of the colon through the muscularis. These protrusions are seen most frequently in the sigmoid colon; the incidence increases with age (affecting 20–50 percent of individuals above age 50). The cause of this disorder is unknown, but is suspected to be related to the low-fiber, low-bulk diet of Western culture. Major complications are acute and chronic inflammation (diverticulitis) and hemorrhage. See also *diverticulitis* and *diverticulosis.*

epiphrenic d., a herniation of the esophageal mucosa that occurs most frequently just above the diaphragm. It is usually associated with motility disturbances and may occur in conjunction with achalasia and diffuse esophageal spasm. Dysphagia, intermittent vomiting, and pain are frequent symptoms. Complications include esophagitis and ulcerative bleeding. Diagnosis is based on endoscopic, radiographic, and fluoroscopic examination.

intestinal d., a herniation or outpouching of the mucosa and submucosa between mesenteric leaves, especially at the site of entry of a blood vessel. True (congenital) diverticula are rare (excluding Meckel's); false (acquired) are more common (more than 1 percent in radiographic studies). This lesion may occur in multiple sites, is most frequent near the ligament of Treitz, and is often associated with diverticula of the colon. It may be visualized on barium x-rays. Bleeding and inflammation are the primary complications.

Meckel's d., a diverticulum of the ileum, which results from the failure of the omphalomesenteric (vitellointestinal) duct to close and degenerate. The most common congenital anomaly of the gastrointestinal tract, it occurs in 1–2 percent of the population and may produce a pouch as long as 12 cm, which often contains heterotopic tissue, such as gastric mucosa. It is found in the terminal ileum, some 3 ft from the ileocecal valve. The diverticulum is symptomatic in approximately 4 percent of cases. Bleeding, pain, inflammation, and perforation are the most frequent complications. Acute inflammation may stimulate appendicitis. Laboratory diagnostic methods include radiographic studies with contrast media, and sodium pertechnetate Tc 99m nuclear scans to demonstrate hydrochloric acid–producing parietal cells in ectopic gastric mucosa.

pharyngoesophageal d., a herniation or outpouching of the esophageal mucosa and submucosa through the cricopharyngeal muscles. It is the most common type of esophageal diverticulum, and occurs three times more frequently in males than in females. This condition is thought to result from increased intrapharyngeal pressure produced by incoordination of muscular propulsion and relaxation during swallowing. Dysphagia, regurgitation of undigested food and nocturnal fits of coughing are the most common symptoms. Aspiration pneumonitis, fistula formation, and infection are the most frequent complications. Diagnosis is based on barium-swallow radiographic and fluoroscopic examination. Esophagoscopy is not usually required. Also called *Zenker's diverticulum.*

pulsion d., a herniation or saclike projection of mucosa and submucosa that protrudes through a defect or weakness in the musculature of a hollow or tubelike organ, e.g., pharyngoesophageal diverticulum. Cf. *traction d.*

traction d., a pouch in the mucosa of the midthoracic esophagus produced by external traction. Initiated by adhesions of inflamed lymph nodes to the esophagus in the region of the tracheal bifurcation, the diverticulum is formed when fibrosis and constriction develop, pulling the esophageal wall anteriorly and creating a sac. This lesion occurs most frequently after age 40 and is usually asymptomatic. Dysphagia, abscess, or fistula formation may occur. Diagnosis is based on radiologic and fluoroscopic examination. Cf. *pulsion d.*

division (dĭ-vizh'un) [L. *divisio*] 1. the act of separating into parts.

2. the state of being divided. The term is applied to certain major branches of the peripheral nervous system, i.e., the craniosacral and thoracolumbar divisions of the autonomic nervous system and the anterior and posterior divisions of trunks of the brachial plexus.

cell d., the fission of a cell; see *amitosis, meiosis,* and *mitosis.*

equational d., the second meiotic division; see under *meiosis.*

maturation d., see *meiosis.*

reduction d., the first meiotic division; see under *meiosis.*

Dixon's test (dik'sonz) [Wilfrid Joseph *Dixon,* U.S. statistician, born 1915] a test for determining whether a value may be considered an outlier and be excluded from the calculations for the mean and standard deviation of a set of values.

dizygotic (DZ) (dī"zi-got'ik) pertaining to or derived from two separate zygotes, as dizygotic (fraternal twins). Cf. *monozygotic.*

DL- a prefix in organic chemistry to denote racemic mixture, i.e., an equimolar mixture of D- and L-stereoisomers. See also *optical isomer.*

DL_{CO} abbrev. See *d.c. of the l. for carbon monoxide* under *diffusing capacity of the lungs.*

DL_{CO}SB abbrev. See *single breath d.c. of the l.* under *diffusing capacity of the lungs.*

DL_{CO}SS abbrev. See *steady state d.c. of the l.* under *diffusing capacity of the lungs.*

DL_{O_2} abbrev. See *d.c. of the l. for oxygen* under *diffusing capacity of the lungs.*

dl abbrev. See *deciliter.*

***dl*-** a prefix in organic chemistry to denote a racemic material, i.e., one which does not rotate polarized light, because it is an equimolar mixture of *d*- and *l*- forms (now often indicated by (±).

DLE abbrev. See *discoid l. erythematosus* under *lupus.*

D-L hemolysin see *Donath-Landsteiner antibody.*

D line a bright yellow doublet in the emission spectrum of sodium at 589.593 and 588.996 nm. It is commonly used for the measurement of the index of refraction or optical rotation. The measurement is symbolized n_D or α_D.

DLL abbrev. for dihomo-gammalinoleic acid. See *prostaglandin.*

DM abbrev. See *d. mellitus* under *diabetes.*

dm abbrev. See *decimeter.*

DMA abbrev. See *direct memory access.*

DMAC abbrev. See *N,N-dimethylacetamide.*

DMBA abbrev. See *7,12-dimethylbenz[a]anthracene.*

DMC di(*p*-chlorophenyl)methylcarbinol, a moderately toxic chlorinated hydrocarbon insecticide having toxicity similar to that of DDT. See also *chlorinated hydrocarbon pesticides.*

DMF abbrev. See *N,N-dimethylformamide.*

DMO abbrev. See *5,5-dimethyl-2,4-oxazolidinedione.*

DMSO abbrev. See *dimethyl sulfoxide.*

DMT abbrev. See *N,N-dimethyltryptamine.*

DN abbrev. See *dibucaine number.*

DNA abbrev. See *deoxyribonucleic acid.*

DNAase see *deoxyribonuclease.*

DNA complexity the total number of nucleotide pairs necessary to make one complete copy of all the base sequences within a genome or DNA preparation with no repetitions.

DNA ligase see *polydeoxyribonucleotide synthetase (ATP).*

DNA nucleotidylexotransferase (nu″kle-o-tīd′il-eks″o-trans′fer-ās) an enzyme of the transferase class (E.C. 2.7.7.31) that catalyzes the reaction n deoxynucleoside triphosphate + (deoxynucleotide)$_m$ ⇄ n pyrophosphate + (deoxynucleotide)$_{m+n}$. The enzyme is a polymerase that catalyzes the synthesis of larger nucleotide molecules and is used to characterize tumor cells. DNA nucleotidylexotransferase is present in the tumor cells of nearly all patients with T- and null-cell acute lymphoblastic leukemia and lymphomas. Cells of some patients with pre–B-cell lymphoblastic leukemia, acute undifferentiated leukemia, and chronic myelogenous leukemia in blast crisis may also be positive. Also called *terminal addition enzyme, terminal deoxynucleotidyl transferase,* and *terminal deoxyribonucleotidyl transferase.*

DNA nucleotidyltransferase an enzyme of the transferase class (deoxynucleosidetriphosphate: DNA deoxynucleotidyltransferase, EC 2.7.7.7), one of a group of enzymes important in the replicative synthesis and repair of DNA. It catalyzes the condensation of deoxyribonucleoside triphosphates to form a polynucleotide chain with the concomitant release of inorganic pyrophosphate, using a strand of existing DNA as a template. DNA nucleotidyltransferase requires a hydrogen-bonded complementary sequence as a primer. Also called *DNA polymerase.*

DNA polymerase see *DNA nucleotidyltransferase.*

DNA reassociation see *DNA renaturation.*

DNA renaturation the process by which complementary single strands of DNA reform into a double helix.

Renaturation is achieved by random collision of single-stranded fragments that contain complementary sequences. The rate of renaturation depends on the effective concentrations of the reacting species, which are dependent on the total concentration of DNA, its complexity, and the amount of DNA repeated sequences.

Measurement of the renaturation can be achieved by a number of methods. DNA can be fragmented into pieces of 400–500 nucleotides, heated (denatured) into separate strands, and then cooled, allowing complementary sequences to renature. The degree of repetition of the DNA can be found by measuring the cot value.

One method of monitoring DNA renaturation is by ultraviolet absorption. Single-stranded DNA absorbs ultraviolet light more strongly than double-stranded DNA, which absorbs less owing to base pairing (hypochromicity). Therefore, as renaturation proceeds, the amount of absorbed ultraviolet light decreases. Another method is by column chromatography. Using a hydroxyapatite column, renaturation mixtures can be monitored during the reaction. At low salt concentrations, double-stranded DNA sticks to the column while single-stranded DNA passes through. The bound DNA can be eluted with high salt concentrations.

Also called DNA-DNA hybridization and *DNA reassociation.* See also *cot value.*

DNA repair the repair of damages, i.e., structural change, in the DNA molecule. There are four main types of structural DNA alterations: (1) dimerization of two adjacent pyrimidine residues caused by ultraviolet light; (2) chemical alteration of bases by deaminating or monofunctional alkylating agents; (3) cross-links between strands caused by UV light and bifunctional alkylating agents; and (4) breaks of one or both strands, mostly by ionizing radiation.

Repair of the DNA molecule can be effected through several mechanisms. In direct repair, a return to the original structure results. This process can only reverse the pyrimidine dimerization. One direct repair mechanism, photoreactivation, involves irradiation of the cell with long UV or short visible light; this activates enzymes that cleave the dimers and restores the original pyrimidine configuration. In excision repair, which is a more general repair mechanism, the segment of the DNA strand with the alteration is excised. The gap is filled using the complementary strand as the template; the free ends are closed by ligase (also called *dark reactivation*). If during DNA replication the replication apparatus encounters an alteration site where there is an unrecognizable base, a gap is left; then a third mechanism, reconstructive postreplication repair, is used to eliminate the gap. The gaps of new DNA strands are filled by synthesis that does not copy a template, thus producing many mutations. Damages leading to this type of error-prone repair include those caused by UV light, carcinogens, and mutagens (also called *SOS repair system*).

The significance of DNA repair in humans is dramatized by defects of repair mechanisms in individuals with such diseases as xeroderma pigmentosum, ataxia telangiectasia, Fanconi's anemia, and Bloom's disease. Persons affected by these diseases frequently develop cancer and neurologic disorders that are probably the result of somatic mutations during error-prone repair.

DNAse see *deoxyribonuclease.*

DNA synthesis the replication of double-stranded DNA, producing new, complementary daughter strands from each existing parental strand. The old DNA serves as a template—a process known as semiconservative replication. Eukaryotic DNA molecules are too large to be replicated at only one site, so each molecule of DNA has several initiation sites (replicons) where replication begins.

The duplex uses unwinding proteins to separate the strands for replication. Unwinding requires a nick (hydrolysis of one phosphodiester bond by a swivel enzyme) in one strand to relieve the torque in the long DNA molecule. When the DNA is unwound, two identical replicating forks are created. Replication is bidirectional, with one strand growing in a $5' \rightarrow 3'$ direction and the other in a $3' \rightarrow 5'$ direction (it is synthesized as fragments, called Okazaki segments, in the $5' \rightarrow 3'$ direction, which are then joined). It can proceed simultaneously at each replicon.

DNA polymerase enzymes probably require the synthesis of short, complementary RNA primer sequences; the DNA is synthesized as an extension of

RNA by DNA polymerase III. The RNA primer is then degraded and replaced with DNA sequences by DNA polymerase I, and DNA ligase joins the 3′ and 5′ ends of the synthesized fragments.

After replication, some bases are modified; methylation of cytosine residues is common. In prokaryotes methylated bases serve in part as a device for identifying the DNA of the organism. In eukaryotes base modification may be involved in regulation and control mechanisms.

See also *deoxyribonucleic acid.*

DNCB abbrev. See *dinitrochlorobenzene.*

DNOC abbrev. See *dinitroorthocresol.*

DO abbrev. for diamine oxidase, Doctor of Osteopathy.

DOA abbrev. for dead on arrival.

DOC see *11-desoxycorticosterone.*

document (dok′u-ment) 1. to prepare documentation for a computer program.

2. a machine-readable form or record such as those read by a document reader or optical character recognition (OCR) reader.

documentation (dok″u-men-ta′shun) 1. papers such as manuals, flow charts, and program listings that explain the purpose, use, and maintenance of computer programs or systems.

2. procedure manuals, quality control records, and maintenance sheets that document and verify the correct performance of test procedures.

dog flea see under *Ctenocephalides.*

dog fly see *Stomoxys.*

dog hookworm see under *hookworm* and *larva migrans.*

dog louse a broad, short species of dog-biting lice, *Trichodectes canis,* belonging to the order Mallophaga.

dolichol (dol′ĭ-kol) one of a group of polyprenols (C_{80}–C_{100}) containing 16–20 isoprene units; the final isoprene unit is saturated and terminates in a hydroxyl group. Dolichol phosphate serves as a sugar carrier molecule for the formation of polysaccharide side-chains on glycoproteins in higher organisms.

dolichol phosphate dolichol esterified by its terminal hydroxyl group to phosphoric acid.

dolipore (dol′ĭ-pōr) an expanded liplike structure around the sides of the opening in the septum in hyphae, which prevents nuclear migration. This is characteristic of the Basidiomycetes.

doll's eye movements see *oculocephalic r.* under *reflex.*

DOM abbrev. See *dimethoxymethylamphetamine.*

domain (do-mān′) 1. a region of an immunoglobulin molecule consisting of 110 amino acids and 1 intrachain disulfide bond. All light chains have two domains, a constant (C_L) and a variable (V_L) region. The heavy chain of IgA or IgG contains four domains, a variable (V_H) region and a constant region with three domains (C_H1, C_H2, and C_H3). The heavy chain of IgM or IgE contains five domains, a variable (V_H) region and a constant region with four domains (C_H1, C_H2, C_H3, and C_H4). See also *immunoglobulin.*

2. the space occupied by a proteoglycan molecule of connective tissue ground substance.

dominant (dom′ĭ-nant) 1. exerting a controlling influence.

2. in genetics, pertaining to a trait that is expressed in both homozygous and heterozygous individuals, i.e., when either or both homologous alleles of a gene code(s) for the trait. The term is also applied to the allele or gene for a dominant trait. See also *autosomal dominant i.* and *X-linked dominant i.* under *inheritance,* and *codominance.* Cf. *recessive.*

dominant complementarity the necessity that the dominant alleles from more than one gene be present for the expression of some trait.

Donath-Landsteiner antibody (do′nat land′stiner) [Julius *Donath,* German immunologist, 1870–1950; Karl Landsteiner, Austrian physician in New York, 1868–1943] an antibody of the IgG type (with P specificity) characteristic of paroxysmal cold hemoglobinuria. The antibody is adsorbed to the red cell in the cold (less than 18°C) in the presence of complement, and lyses the red cell when the temperature is raised to 37°C. Also called D-L antibody or *D-L hemolysin.* See also *paroxysmal cold hemoglobinuria.*

Donnan potential (don′an) [Frederick George *Donnan,* English physical chemist, 1870–1956] see *membrane potential.*

Donohue's syndrome (don′o-hūz) a rare familial condition, transmitted as an autosomal recessive trait, that is characterized by mental retardation, severe failure to thrive, leprechaun facies, and endocrine disturbances such as sexual precocity and breast and clitoral enlargement. It is prevalent in, and possibly confined to, females. Those affected are hypoglycemic and demonstrate decreased urine concentrations of gonadotropin and elevated urine concentrations of 17-ketosteroid. Also called leprechaunism.

donor (do′nor) [Old French *doneur,* from *L. donator* giver] 1. one that gives; an individual who supplies blood or other tissue to be used in another body.

2. in chemistry, a substance or compound that contributes part of itself to another acceptor compound, e.g., hydrogen donor, electron donor.

3. in bacterial genetics, a cell that contributes genetic information to another recipient cell.

Donovan bodies (don′o-van) [Charles *Donovan,* Irish physician in India, 1863–1951] see under *C. granulomatis* and *Calymmatobacterium* and *g. inguinale* under *granuloma.*

dopa (do′pah) an amino acid, 3-(3,4-dihydroxyphenyl)alanine; M.W. 197.19. It occurs naturally in seedlings, pods, and the beans of broad and velvet beans. Dopa is produced by the hydroxylation of tyrosine by the enzyme tyrosine hydroxylase in the nerves and adrenal medulla, and is an intermediate in the synthesis of dopamine, norepinephrine, and epinephrine. The L form (levodopa) is used to treat Parkinson's disease.

dopamine (do′pah-mēn) 4-(2-aminoethyl)-1,2-benzenediol, one of the catecholamines; M.W. 153.18. Dopamine is found primarily in the brain, sympathetic ganglia, and retina, and also in the liver, lungs, and intestines. It is produced by the decarboxylation of dopa, and acts as a neurotransmitter in certain parts of the brain. A decrease in its production in the substantia nigra of the brain leads to Parkinson's disease, which is treated with L-dopa, as dopamine itself cannot cross the blood-brain barrier. Dopamine also inhibits the release of the prolactin-inhibitory factor from the hypothalamus. A small dose of dopamine selectively dilates the renal and splanchnic arteries, whereas larger doses increase the cardiac output and heart rate; above a certain dose, its vasoconstrictor and hypertensive effects are indistinguishable from those of norepinephrine. Dopamine is used to treat shock, including shock of cardiac origin. It is metabolized by the combined action of catechol *O*-methyl transferase (COMT) and monoamine oxidase (MAO) to homovanillic acid, which is excreted in urine. Dopamine is assayed directly or through its urinary metabolite. See also *catecholamine.*

dopamine β-hydroxylase see *dopamine β-monooxygenase.*

dopamine β-monooxygenase an enzyme of the oxidoreductase class (3,4-dihydroxyphenylethylamine, ascorbate:oxygen oxidoreductase [β-hydroxylating], EC 1.14.17.1) that catalyzes the synthesis of norepinephrine by the reaction 3,4-dihydroxyphenylethylamine (dopamine) + ascorbate + $O_2 \rightleftharpoons$ norepinephrine + dehydroascorbate + H_2O. Also called *dopamine β-hydroxylase.*

dopaquinone (do″pah-kwĭ-nōn′) an oxidation product of dihydroxyphenylalanine (dopa); it is converted by subsequent reactions to melanin. See also *melanin.*

dopa reaction a histochemical reaction for the enzyme tyrosinase (dopa oxidase), which catalyzes the oxidation of tyrosine and dopa to dopaquinone, which in turn polymerizes to form melanin. Frozen tissue slices are incubated for 24 hr at 20°–25°C in the presence of L-dopa at pH 7. Large confluent globules of melanin are formed around the melanin granules of melanocytes. The slices are then postfixed in calcium acetate–formalin and processed by paraffin section technique.

Doppler effect (dop′ler) [Christian Johann *Doppler,* Austrian physicist and mathematician, 1803–1853] a change in the observed frequency of a wave, e.g., light, sound, or radio, caused by the motion of the source relative to the detector. The amount of the change (compared with a stationary source) is called the Doppler shift and increases with increasing velocity.

Doriden (dor′ĭ-den) trademark. See *glutethimide.*

dormancy (dor′man-se) [L. *dormire* to sleep] 1. the state of being dormant.

2. in bacteriology, the property exhibited by some bacteria, and especially by bacterial spores, of remaining viable for long periods with minimal physical and chemical change, often in reaction to an unfavorable environment for growth.

dormant (dor′mant) [L. *dormire* to sleep] sleeping, inactive, quiescent.

Dorner stain (dōr′ner) a stain for the ascospore of perfect fungi and yeasts. Carbolfuchsin is heated with the fungus on a slide, cooled, and decolorized with acid alcohol. If ascospores are present, they retain the carbolfuchsin dye. Nigrosin is applied as a final step for the visualization of nonascospore material. With this procedure, the ascospores are red.

dors/o (dōr′so) [L. *dorsum* back] a word element used in combining form to denote the back or posterior portion of the body, e.g., dorsal.

dorsal (dōr′sal) [L. *dorsalis,* from *dorsum* back] 1. pertaining to the back.

2. denoting a position more toward the back; the same as posterior in human anatomy. Cf. *ventral.*

3. pertaining to the superior surface of the foot. (cf. *plantar*) or the back of the hand (cf. *palmar*).

dorsiflex (dōr′sĭ-fleks) to bend the foot or hand in a backward direction, i.e., away from the sole or palm.

dorsiflexion (dōr″sĭ-flek′shun) bending of the dorsal aspect of the hand or foot.

dorsoplantar (dor″so-plan′tar) pertaining to a radiographic projection of the foot, in which the central ray passes from the dorsal surface to the plantar surface or from the calf to the sole; the latter is also called *suroplantar.*

dorsum (dōr′sum), pl. *dorsa* [L.] the back, the dorsal surface of the body. The dorsum of the foot or hand is the surface opposite the sole or palm, respectively. The dorsum of the tongue is its upper surface.

dorsum sellae (dor′sum sel′e) [L.] [NA], a square plate on the sphenoid that forms the posterior wall of the sella turcica.

dosage (do′sij) determination of the quantity and frequency of doses.

dosage compensation the mechanism by which one X chromosome in each female cell is inactivated; it remains condensed during interphase so that no transcription can occur. The inactivation occurs in the embryo, and all clonal descendants have the same homologue (either maternal or paternal) inactivated. Also called *Lyon hypothesis.* See also *X chromosome.*

dose (dōs) [Gr. *dosis* gift, portion] a quantity to be administered at one time, such as a specified amount of medicine.

absorbed d., the amount of energy per unit mass absorbed by the body from ionizing radiation, expressed in rads.

air d. (E), the intensity of an x-ray or gamma-ray beam in air, expressed in roentgens. Also called exposure dose.

booster d., an amount of immunogen (vaccine, toxoid, or other antigen preparation), usually smaller than the initial dose, given to heighten and sustain the immune response to the immunogen. See also *anamnestic response* and *booster.*

depth d. (E_d), the intensity of radiation at a specified depth below the skin, expressed in roentgens or as a percentage of the intensity measured at the surface.

divided d., a fraction of the total drug prescribed, to be given at intervals, usually during a 24-hr period.

effective d. (ED), the dose of a drug that produces the intended therapeutic effect.

epilating d., the radiation dose that is large enough to produce a temporary or permanent loss of hair.

erythema d., the amount of radiation that will cause skin reddening, about 1000 roentgens.

exit d., the amount of radiation in an x-ray beam that has passed through the body, expressed in roentgens.

genetically significant d. (GSD), the average gonadal dose of mutagenic radiation received by any potential parent.

integral d., the total energy absorbed by the whole

body or by a region of the body, expressed in gram-rads (100 ergs).

lethal d. (LD), see *median lethal d.* and *minimum lethal d.*

loading d., a dose of a drug that immediately produces the desired steady-state concentration of a drug, which is then maintained with lower doses. Loading doses are used with drugs having a long half-life for which it would take several days to reach a steady state with a regimen of equal doses.

maximal permissible d. (MPD), the maximal permissible exposure to direct external radiation, calculated at 5 rem × (age at last birthday – 18).

mean d. ($\bar{D}$), the mean or average radiation dose (in rads) that is absorbed by an organ or by the whole body from the administration of a radiopharmaceutical. The mean dose can be calculated and used in dose estimates even when the organ or body is not being uniformly irradiated. See also *dose estimate.*

mean d. per unit cumulated activity (S), see under *dose estimate.*

median effective d. (ED_{50}), the amount necessary to produce an effect in half the test subjects.

median infectious d. (ID_{50}), the amount of pathogenic microorganisms that produces demonstrable infection in 50 percent of the test subjects.

median lethal d. (LD_{50}), the dose of an agent required to kill half a population administered that dose or exposed at that dose level.

minimal lethal d. (MLD), the smallest amount of a toxic substance that can cause the death of a laboratory animal.

radiation absorbed d., see *rad.*

radiation d., direct exposure to ionizing radiation, which is measured in rads or rems. The maximal allowable doses for workers in facilities licensed by the Nuclear Regulatory Commission (NRC) is 1.25 rem per calendar quarter (3.0 rem per quarter when documented on NRC Form 4); this amount should not exceed 5 rem × (age at last birthday – 18) in a worker's lifetime. The limits for exposure to the general public, or nonoccupationally exposed workers, are 0.5 rem/yr (as specified in Title 10 of the Code of Federal Regulations).

sensitizing d., a dose of a sensitizing antigen that makes an animal susceptible to anaphylactic shock or another hypersensitivity reaction on exposure to another dose of the same antigen.

skin d. (E_0), the amount of radiation, including backscatter from the patient, at the skin surface, expressed in roentgens or rads.

threshold d., the minimal dose of ionizing radiation that will produce a detectable effect.

threshold erythema d. (TED), the skin dose that will cause skin reddening in 80 percent of individuals exposed.

tissue tolerance d. (TTD), a dose of theraputic radiation considered to have an acceptably low rate of lethal complications or normal tissue necrosis.

tumor lethal d. (TLD), a dose of therapeutic radiation intended to completely destroy a tumor, expressed in rads.

dose account the accumulated lifetime occupational radiation exposure.

dose calibrator a device that measures radiation, generally an ionization chamber or scintillation counter, used to measure the radioactivity of a radiopharmaceutical agent before it is administered to a patient.

dose estimate an approximation of the radiation absorbed by a particular organ (the target organ) or by the whole body from an administered quantity of radionuclide-labeled agent; given in rads or in rads per microcurie of administered activity. This dose is the sum, for all the organs in which the agent localizes (source organs), of the product of the cumulated activity ($\tilde{A}$) and the mean dose per unit cumulated activity (S).

The cumulated activity is the total number of radioactive disintegrations (in microcurie-hours) that occur in a source organ. This is calculated from the fraction of the administered activity that localizes in the source organ and from the effective half-life of the agent in that organ.

The mean dose per unit cumulated activity is the radiation dose absorbed by the target organ (in rads) from disintegrations in the source organ (in μCi-hr). This depends on the number and energy of particles emitted by the nuclide, on the relative location of the source and target organs, and on the fraction per unit mass of the incident particles absorbed by the target organ. Values of S for each combination of nuclide, source, and target have been tabulated.

See also *Medical Internal Radiation Dose.*

dose rate 1. dose per unit time.

2. the number of ion pairs per unit time measured by an ionization chamber.

dosimeter (do-sim'ĕ-ter) [Gr. *dosis* portion + *metron* measure] a portable device that detects and measures the total exposure to radiation of the person wearing it. Persons subject to occupational radiation exposure wear film badges, thermoluminescent dosimeters, or ultraviolet fluorescent dosimeters, all of which require processing to be read, or pocket dosimeters, which do not.

pencil d., see *pocket d.*

pocket d., a pen-sized ionization chamber with an electrometer. The dosimeter is read by looking through an eyepiece at a scale and pointer that display the dose accumulated since the dosimeter was reset. Also called *pencil d.*

thermoluminescent d. (TLD), a crystal or glasslike substance that stores the energy of ionizing radiation and releases it as light when heated. Also called *thermoluminescent detector.*

ultraviolet fluorescent d., a substance that absorbs the energy of ionizing radiation as permanent molecular rearrangements. When exposed to ultraviolet light, it fluoresces, showing the accumulated dose.

dosimetry (do-sim'ĕ-tre) [Gr. *dosis* portion + *metrein* to measure] 1. the determination of the radiation exposure from a source of ionizing radiation, as with a dosimeter.

2. the calculation of a dose estimate.

DOT abbrev. See *Department of Transportation.*

dot product see *scalar product.*

dot scan the printed record produced by a rectilinear scanner.

double-beam photometer a colorimeter or spectrophotometer in which the light beam leaving the monochromator is split, with one beam passing through the specimen and the other through a blank. There are two types of design: one in which the two beams are chopped and alternately fall on the same photocell or photomultiplier tube, and another in which each beam is measured by a separate detector. Both designs eliminate variations in lamp intensity as a source of error; the first design also eliminates error due to differences in detector sensitivity.

double-blind (dub″l-blīnd) pertaining to an experiment in which neither subjects nor persons administering treatment know which subjects are in the treatment group and which are the controls. See also *clinical trials.*

double-contrast study a radiographic procedure in which both a radiopaque contrast medium and a radiolucent gas are introduced into a hollow organ or the capsule of a joint to highlight it. Cf. *dual-contrast study.*

double diffusion test see *Ouchterlony test.*

double discharge the occurrence of two action potentials of similar form and amplitude with a short interspike interval (approximately 2–20 msec). Also called doublet.

double helix the three-dimensional structure of double-stranded DNA. See also *deoxyribonucleic acid.*

double oxalate a mixture of ammonium oxalate and potassium oxalate (6:4), used to prevent coagulation of blood samples by removal of calcium ions from the blood. It has now been generally replaced by EDTA for cell counts and morphologic examination of the formed elements of the blood. Also called balanced oxalate.

double-pole double-throw (dpdt) switch a six-terminal electric switch that simultaneously connects two lines and makes a connection in both switch positions; i.e., a pair of input terminals is connected to either of two pairs of output terminals.

double-pole single-throw (dpst) switch a four-terminal electric switch that connects or opens two lines simultaneously.

double-precision variable a number that requires two computer words of storage.

doubling time see *generation time.*

Dowex (dow′eks) trademark for synthetic styrene-divinylbenzene copolymer ion-exchange resins.

Downey cell (dow′ne) [H. *Downey,* U.S. hematologist, 1877–1959] an abnormal lymphocyte seen in infectious mononucleosis; it is a large cell with a round, undifferentiated nucleus and occasionally nucleoli and basophilic cytoplasm.

Down's syndrome (downz) [John Langdon Haydon *Down,* English physician, 1828–1896] a group of physical, mental, and functional abnormalities that result from the presence of three (rather than the normal number of two) chromosomes designated as chromosome 21, the smallest of the human chromosomes. The physical abnormalities that give rise to the distinctive facial appearance associated with this condition include upslanting of the eye slits (palpebral fissures) with skin folds (epicanthic folds) at the inner sides, flatness of the bridge of the nose, and a tendency for protrusion of the tongue, especially in the very young. Minor abnormalities of the ears, hands, and feet may also be present, and overall stature is generally reduced. Of greater concern is the severe congenital heart disease that affects about 40 percent of affected children but which may be surgically correctable. Obstruction of the intestinal tract also occurs.

There are two important abnormalities of the nervous system. One is a diminution of muscular tone (hypotonia), which may produce a sense of floppiness or looseness; the other, the single most serious feature of Down's syndrome, is mental retardation, which is generally moderate but may vary from mild to severe. The rate of acquisition of skills and capabilities is often normal during the first few months of life but then decreases, so that the development of more advanced physical and intellectual skills (such as the abilities to construct sentences, walk up and down stairs alone, and dress oneself) may be delayed by a year or more. Persons with Down's syndrome have learned complex intellectual tasks such as reading, writing, and arithmetic calculations, but this does not occur in all instances. It is not possible during their first years of life to predict the ultimate level of intellectual and social accomplishment that those with this syndrome will achieve.

Individuals with Down's syndrome are more susceptible to infections. They also have an increased, although still low, likelihood of developing childhood leukemia. Despite these predispositions, those affected generally enjoy good health. If they survive the first year of life, their average life expectancy is now 55–60 yr.

At present, it is not known whether the mental retardation is the result of permanent changes in the structure of the brain or of a potentially reversible chemical imbalance. More generally, the manner by which the presence of an extra chromosome 21 (referred to as trisomy 21) produces any of the physical, neurologic, and functional abnormalities associated with Down's syndrome is not known, although only a small part of the chromosome actually seems to be involved.

The syndrome occurs in 1 in every 600–1000 newborn infants, and the probability of having an affected child rises with increasing parental age, particularly with maternal age. Thus, although about 1 in 1000 children born to women aged 25–30 yr have Down's syndrome, the proportion increases to 1 in 350 for 35-yr-old mothers and 1 in 100 for those aged 40. Because of this still unexplained risk associated with older mothers, prenatal diagnosis has been used to determine whether pregnant women, usually 35 yr or older, have chromosomally abnormal fetuses. Developed in the late 1960s, the prenatal diagnosis of Down's syndrome is based on the detection of an extra chromosome 21 in fetal cells grown from amniotic fluid taken about 15–16 wk after conception. With this information, the parents can decide whether to continue or terminate the pregnancy.

Down's syndrome usually is the result of a new genetic accident in which there is a failure of the two chromosomes 21 to separate from one another during formation of the egg or sperm. This abnormality in chromosome separation, the cause of which is unknown, is termed "nondisjunction" and results in the presence of three rather than two chromosomes 21 in the embryo after conception. Although most cases of Down's syndrome arise in this way, part of chromosome 21 is occasionally attached to one or the other chromosomes in the set to form a translocation chromosome. In these instances, it is sometimes possible for an otherwise unaffected parent to have a child with the syndrome and for several members of a family to be similarly affected. As with older mothers, prenatal diagnosis is available to families that carry such translocation chromosomes.

The attitude of society toward Down's syndrome has changed markedly in recent years. Nevertheless, much still remains to be accomplished in learning why trisomy 21 occurs, how it gives rise to the syndrome with its associated abnormalities, and what can be done to optimize the physical and mental development of affected individuals.

Also called *trisomy 21 syndrome.*

CHARLES J. EPSTEIN, M.D.

downtime a part of the scheduled operating time during which a computer or other device is inoperative owing to equipment or program malfunction; it is one of the critical parameters used in configuring a data processing system. Cf. *uptime.*

doxepin (dok′se-pin) a tricyclic compound used to treat major depression. See also *tricyclic antidepressant.* Trademark, *Sinequan.*

doxepin assays 1. ultraviolet spectrophotometry. Doxepin is oxidized to doxepin ketone, which is extracted into hexane and quantitated by its absorbance at 266 nm.

2. gas chromatography using a flame ionization detector and a column with a moderately polar silicone stationary phase. Doxepin and the internal standard (codeine) are extracted from alkalinized samples and subjected to chromatography. The sample doxepin concentration is proportional to the doxepin-codeine peak height ratio.

See also *amitriptyline and nortriptyline assays.*

doxorubicin (dok″so-roo′bĭ-sin) an anthracycline antibiotic produced by the fungus *Streptomyces peucetius caesius,* which is used as a cancer chemotherapy drug. The mechanism of action is not precisely known but seems to involve intercalation of doxorubicin between the base pairs of the DNA double helix. This may block DNA replication or transcription, or it may cause chain scission and the production of toxic free radicals. The maximal cytotoxic effect occurs in the S phase of the cell cycle, but some cytotoxic effects are also exerted in other phases. The most serious side-effect of doxorubicin therapy is a chronic, cumulative dose-related cardiomyopathy that leads to congestive heart failure; it does not respond to digitalis and is fatal in about 50 percent of those in whom it develops. Trademark, *Adriamycin.* See also *anthracycline cardiotoxicity* and *Appendix A.*

doxycycline (dok″se-si′klēn) a broad-spectrum antibiotic derived from oxytetracycline. Advantages of its use include a long half-life and less of an effect on normal bowel flora than other tetracyclines. See also *antibacterial agents* and *tetracyclines.*

doxylamine succinate (dok-sil′ah-mēn) [USP], an antihistamine used in the treatment of nausea and vomiting during pregnancy and as a sedative in preparations for nighttime relief of symptoms of the common cold. Adverse reactions include drowsiness, vertigo, epigastric distress, diarrhea, and nervousness. Trademark, *Bendectin.*

dpdt switch abbrev. See *double-pole double-throw switch.*

DPG; 2,3-DPG abbrev. for 2,3-diphosphoglycerate. See *2,3-bisphosphoglycerate.*

2,3-DPGM abbrev. for *2,3-diphosphoglycerate mutase.* See *bisphosphoglyceromutase.*

DPN abbrev. for the oxidized form of the redox coenzyme diphosphopyridine nucleotide, now called *nicotinamide adenine dinucleotide* (NAD).

DPNH abbrev. for the reduced form of the redox coenzyme diphosphopyridine nucleotide, now called reduced *nicotinamide adenine dinucleotide* (NADH).

dpst switch abbrev. See *double-pole single-throw switch.*

Drabkin's reagent (drab′kinz) a solution used in the cyanmethemoglobin method of measuring hemoglobin. It consists of sodium bicarbonate, potassium cyanide, and potassium ferricyanide in distilled water; because of the potassium cyanide, care must be exercised in the use and disposal of this solution.

dracontiasis (drak″on-ti′ah-sis) [Gr. *drakontion* little dragon] see *dracunculiasis.*

dracunculiasis (drah-kung″ku-li′ah-sis) an infection caused by tissue-invading nematodes of *Dracunculus medinensis,* the guinea worm, in the skin and subcutaneous tissue. The disease is endemic in tropical Africa and parts of India, and is common in Iran, Arabia, and Afghanistan.

Human infection is caused by drinking water contaminated with infected copepods (intermediate hosts) or by ingesting the infective crustacean. Following an incubation period of 8–12 mo, the fertilized females migrate to the lower extremities, where a lesion appears. When the infected person comes into contact with water, the lesion or blister ruptures and the larvae are liberated.

Many of the symptoms begin in the incubation period, when there may be erythema, generalized urticaria, severe pruritus, giddiness, dyspnea, and, occasionally, vomiting and diarrhea. As the worm reaches the skin, intense itching or burning sensations occur.

Laboratory diagnosis cannot be made until cutaneous lesions are present and the worms are below the skin surface. The larvae may be found in washings of the lesions (in which the gravid females discharge their young) or in synovial fluid. Serologic tests include complement-fixation and indirect immunofluorescence tests. Radiography may detect calcified worms.

Also called *dracunculosis, dracontiasis, dragon worm infection, guinea worm infection, medina infection,* and *serpent infection.*

dracunculosis (drah-kung″ku-lo′sis) see *dracunculiasis.*

Dracunculus (drah-kung′ku-lus) [L. "little dragon"] a genus of nematode worms.

D. medinensis, an elongate, cylindrical, threadlike worm, found in Africa and India, that is parasitic in humans. Infection is caused by drinking water containing contaminated copepods (minute crustaceans). The larval form of *D. medinensis* occurs in the crustacean *Cyclops,* which is found in stagnant surface water, e.g., the water in cisterns and step-down wells. When the water is drunk, the ingested *Cyclops* organisms are digested by gastric secretions, liberating larvae that then penetrate the intestinal mucosa, where the worms mature. It is the gravid female worm that migrates to the subcutaneous tissue, usually the legs and feet, a journey that takes about 8 mo. The female then emerges through the skin and deposits its larvae when the skin comes into contact with water. As warm water is necessary for the larva's development in the crustacean, dracunculiasis occurs in tropical areas. Also called dragon worm, guinea worm, serpent worm, and *Vena medinensis.* See also *dracunculiasis.*

Dragendorff's solution (drag′en-dorfs) [Georg Johann Noël *Dragendorff,* German physician, 1836–1898] see *iodobismuthate.*

dragon worm (drag′on) see *D. medinensis* under *Dracunculus.*

dragon worm infection see *dracunculiasis.*

drain (drān) 1. any device for removing fluid as it collects in a wound or cavity.
2. one of the terminals of a field effect transistor.

Dramamine (dram′ah-mēn) trademark. See *dimenhydrinate.*

Drechslera (drek′sler-ah) a genus of dematiacious fungi that can cause phaecohyphomycosis in humans and animals. One species, *D. hawaiiensis,* has been isolated from a patient with well-differentiated lymphocytic lymphoma who died of meningoencephalitis.

drench hose a device with a hand-operated valve on the end of a hose attached to the laboratory water supply system. Bench- or wall-mounted, it can be regulated to provide a controlled flow of water for emergency flushing of chemicals from the eyes or body.

drepanocyte (drep′ah-no-sīt) [Gr. *drepanē* sickle + *kytos* hollow vessel] see *sickled cell.*

drepanocytemia (drep″ah-no-si-te′me-ah) [*drepanocyte* + Gr. *haima* blood + *-ia*] see *sickle cell anemia.*

drepanocytic (drep″ah-no-sit′ik) pertaining to drepanocytes; having sickle-shaped red cells.

drepanocytosis (drep″ah-no-si-to′sis) [*drepanocyte* + *-osis* condition] an occurrence of drepanocytes in the blood.

drift a gradual shift from the original calibration setting of a measuring device. See also *antigenic drift* and *genetic drift.*

driving response see *photic driving.*

drom/o (drom′o) [Gr. *dromos* a course] a word element used in combining form to denote running or conduction, e.g., dromograph, syndrome.

dromostanolone propionate (dro″mo-stan′o-lōn) a cancer chemotherapeutic drug. Trademark, Drolban. For more information, see *Appendix A.*

droperidol (dro-per′ĭ-dol) one of the butyrophenone major tranquilizers; used as a preanesthetic and, in combination with fentanyl (a narcotic analgesic), as a neuroleptanalgesic (an agent that produces stupor and total analgesia). Adverse effects include hypotension, tachycardia, and extrapyramidal effects. Trademark, *Inapsine.*

droplet (drop′let) a diminutive drop, such as the particles of moisture expelled from the mouth in coughing, sneezing, or speaking, which may carry infection to others through the air.

d. nuclei, small particles of respiratory secretions that are expelled into the air by coughing. While they are suspended in air, evaporation reduces them to small, dry particles that can then remain airborne for long periods. This is one possible mechanism for the transmission of microbial diseases from one human to another.

Drosophila (dro-sof′ĭ-lah) [Gr. *drosos* dew + *philein* to love] a genus of flies; the fruitflies. The species *D. melanogaster,* a small fly often seen near decaying fruit, has been used extensively in experimental genetics.

drowsiness (drow′zĭ-nes) see *s. stages* under *sleep.*

drug (drug) 1. any chemical compound with therapeutic or medicinal qualities.
2. a narcotic.
3. to give or take a drug.

drug dependence see *drug d.* under *dependence.*

drug desensitization a drug tolerance that appears in response to rapidly repeated doses. Also called *tachyphylaxis.*

drug-induced thrombocytopenia a reduction in the amount of platelets in the circulating blood caused by the administration of drugs. Known mechanisms include the suppression of the hematopoietic stem cell compartment in the marrow and the formation of drug-induced antibodies.

Generalized marrow suppression is a predictable side-effect of many drugs used for cancer chemotherapy and immunosuppression owing to the drugs' cytotoxic effects (see *cancer chemotherapy*). When the marrow precursor cells are destroyed, severe thrombocytopenia develops quite rapidly, as there is no platelet storage reservoir and the maximal platelet life span is 10 da. Examples of such agents include the nitrogen mustards and other alkylating agents (e.g., busulfan, melphalan, cyclophosphamide), antimetabolites (e.g., purine and pyrimidine analogs such as 6-mercaptopurine, thioguanine, cytosine arabinoside), antimitotics (e.g., vinca alkaloids), certain antibiotics (e.g., daunorubicin, doxorubicin [Adriamycin], and some miscellaneous substances such as estrogens. Other drugs (e.g., chloramphenicol) cause marrow suppression by a poorly understood mechanism. A few (e.g., chlorothiazide) selectively suppress the megakaryocyte.

The formation of drug-induced antibodies occurs in only a small percentage of individuals exposed to a particular drug. This idiosyncratic hypersensitivity is presumably caused by some metabolite of the drug. The antibody has been of the IgG type in almost all documented cases. One model of this phenomenon, termed the "innocent-bystander hypothesis," postulates the attachment of the drug to a plasma protein or some carrier molecule, which then combines with an antibody directed against this complex. The resulting drug-antibody complex becomes attached to the platelet, which is then destroyed by the reticuloendothelial system. Drugs documented as causing some type of platelet antibody formation include quinine, quinidine, and digitoxin; many others that cause thrombocytopenia probably do so by some kind of immune reaction, but are incompletely documented.

drug interference in laboratory medicine, particularly in clinical chemistry, an alteration in the result obtained in a laboratory test owing to the effect of some drug (or one or more metabolites of the drug) being administered to the patient. A change may occur in the actual (true) value of the parameter being measured owing to some physiologic effect of the drug; alternately, the drug may cause an incorrect value for the measured quantity because of some interference in the analytic procedure. Also called pharmacologic interference.

drug-resistant resistant to the action of drugs; said of microorganisms.

drug screening assays methods used to identify the drugs present in specimens of blood, urine, or gastric contents from individuals suspected of drug abuse or from patients in coma with suspected drug overdose. Screening tests for drugs of abuse commonly utilize methods such as thin-layer chromatography (TLC), gas chromatography (GC), or a battery of enzyme immunoassays (EMIT assays). The number of drugs included in screening tests may vary from laboratory to laboratory but should include ethanol, and commonly abused drugs as well as widely used drugs, available with or without prescription. Screening procedures must have sufficient sensitivity to avoid false-negative results. Positive results are presumptive only, and frequently must be confirmed by more complex procedures that utilize GC, high-pressure liquid chromatography (HPLC), or gas chromatography–mass spectrometry (GC-MS) to identify and quantitate the drugs and their important metabolites.

In chromatographic assays the specimen preparation may include solvent extraction to separate three fractions containing acids (e.g., barbiturates), bases (e.g., opiates and amphetamines), and neutral or weak acids and bases from the biologic matrix. The enzyme immunoassays require no preparation of the specimen, but are directed toward specific drugs and thus have limited utility in screening procedures, except for confirmation.

drumstick (drum′stik) a dense, well-defined round mass about 1.5 μ in diameter, which is attached by a thin filament of nuclear membrane to the nucleus of a percentage of polymorphonuclear leukocytes (eosinophils or neutrophils) of females. It contains the Barr body and is present in normal females and in some individuals with sex chromosomal abnormalities such as Kleinfelter's syndrome (XXY). Drumsticks normally appear one to a cell and are best visualized on a thin blood smear of fresh capillary blood stained by the routine Wright method.

drumstick spore classically, the rounded terminal spore of *Clostridium tetani,* although a number of *Clostridium* species share this characteristic. Under the microscope, the small round body at one end of the long thin bacillus resembles a drumstick.

dry ice see *solid c. d.* under *carbon dioxide.*

drying agent see *desiccant.*

DSA abbrev. See *digital subtraction angiography.*

dsDNA abbrev. for double-stranded DNA. See under *deoxyribonucleic acid.*

dTDP abbrev. See *t. diphosphate* under *thymidine.*

DTF abbrev. for detector transfer function. See *modulation transfer function.*

DTH abbrev. for delayed-type hypersensitivity reaction. See *delayed hypersensitivity.*

dTMP abbrev. See *thymidine-5′-phosphate.*

DTPA a chelating agent. DTPA is a pentabasic acid that binds metal ions and is used in nuclear medicine to carry radionuclides, e.g., ^{99m}Tc, ^{111}In, ^{113m}In, and ^{169}Yb in body fluids (blood, cerebrospinal fluid, urine) for cisternography, brain imaging, and renal scanning. Chemical name, *diethylenetriaminepentaacetic acid.* Generic drug name, *pentetate.*

dTTP abbrev. See *thymidine triphosphate.*

dU abbrev. See *deoxyuridine.*

du abbrev. See *dial unit.*

dual-contrast study a radiographic procedure in which a radiopaque contrast medium is introduced into a cavity or passage in an organ, and a radiolucent gas is introduced into the body cavity surrounding the organ. The effect is to highlight both the surface and the luminal contours of the cavity. Cf. *double-contrast study.*

dual-in-line package (DIP) the most common package for integrated circuits. A standard DIP is a rectangular epoxy plastic brick about 0.3 in. wide and 0.8 in. long, with 14 or 16 electrical pins in two parallel rows along opposite sides. Standing on its pins, the package is about 0.4 in. high and slightly resembles a centipede.

Duane-Hunt relation (doo-ān′ hunt) the shortest wavelength emitted from an x-ray tube, shown by the formula $\lambda = 1240/V$, where λ is the wavelength in nanometers and V is the peak tube voltage in volts.

Dubin-Johnson syndrome see *type II h.* under *hyperbilirubinemia.*

Duchenne's disease (du-shenz′) [Guillaume Benjamin Amand *Duchenne,* French neurologist, 1806–1875] pseudohypertrophic muscular dystrophy. See *muscular d.* under *dystrophy.*

Ducrey bacillus (doo-kra′) [Augosto *Ducrey,* Italian dermatologist, 1860–1940] see *H. ducreyi* under *Hemophilus.*

duct/o (duk′to) [L. *ductus,* from *ducere* to draw or lead] a word element used in combining form to denote a passage, e.g., ductus.

duct (dukt) [L. *ductus,* from *ducere* to draw or lead] a passage with well-defined walls, especially a tube for the passage of excretions or secretions; see also *ductus.*

aberrant d., any duct that is not normally present or that takes an unusual course or direction.

alveolar d.'s, the small passages that connect the respiratory bronchioles with the alveolar sacs.

d. of Arantius, see *ductus venosus.*

bile d., see *bile duct.*

cochlear d., a spirally arranged membranous tube in the bony canal of the cochlea.

d. of Cuvier, one of two short venous trunks in the fetus that open into the sinus venosus; the right becomes the superior vena cava. Also called the common cardinal vein.

cystic d., the passage that connects the neck of the gall bladder and the common bile duct.

ejaculatory d., a canal formed by the union of the ductus deferens and the duct of the seminal vesicle, which enters the prostatic urethra.

endolymphatic d., a tubular prolongation of the saccule of the inner ear, which communicates with the endolymphatic sac. See also *ear.*

d. of Gartner, a small rudimentary duct in the broad ligament of the uterus parallel to the uterine tube. A remnant of the mesonephros, it is perpendicular to the transverse ducts of the epoophoron (10–15 in number), which open into it.

hepatic d., one of the canals that receive bile from the lobes of the liver and unite to form the common hepatic duct, which joins the cystic duct to form the common bile duct.

intercalated d., a slender initial portion of a duct system interposed between the acinus of a gland and its secretory duct.

interlobular bile d.'s, small biliary channels in the portal canals of the liver. They form a tortuous network that empties into the extrahepatic bile ducts at the porta hepatis.

lacrimal d., a narrow channel in each eyelid that begins at the punctum and leads to the lacrimal sac. Also called *lacrimal canaliculus.*

lactiferous d.'s, channels that convey milk secreted by the lobes of the breast to and through the nipples. Also called mammary ducts.

Luschka's d.'s, see *Luschka's ducts.*

lymphatic d.'s, channels for conducting lymph.

mesonephric d., an embryonic duct initiated in association with rudiments of the pronephric kidney. It is taken over as excretory duct by the mesonephros and develops into various ducts of the reproductive system in the male and into vestigial structures in the female. Also called *wolffian d.*

müllerian d., paired embryonic ducts formed from involution of the peritoneal epithelium. The ducts extend to the urogenital sinus and are the precursors of the uterine corpus, cervix, and fallopian tubes. Also called *paramesonephric d.*

nasolacrimal d., a duct that extends from the inner angle of the eye to the nasal cavity.

omphalomesenteric d., in the developing embryo, the narrow tube that connects the umbilical vesicle (yolk sac) with the midgut. Also called *vitelline duct* and vitellointestinal duct. See also *omphalomesenteric duct anomalies.*

pancreatic d., the main excretory duct of the pancreas, which usually unites with the common bile duct before entering the duodenum at the major duodenal papilla. See also *pancreas.*

paramesonephric d., see *müllerian d.*

parotid d., the duct that drains the parotid gland; it empties through a papilla on the oral surface of the cheek opposite the second superior molar. Also called *Stensen's d.*

prostatic d.'s, ducts from the prostate gland that open on either side into or near the prostatic sinuses on the posterior wall of the urethra.

salivary d.'s, the ducts that convey the saliva.

d. of Santorini, the accessory pancreatic duct that drains much of the head of the pancreas. It opens into the duodenum independently from the main pancreatic duct, approximately 2 cm above the ampulla of Vater. Also called accessory pancreatic duct.

semicircular d.'s, the long ducts of the membranous labyrinth of the ear.

Stensen's d., see *parotid d.*

sudoriferous d., the duct that leads from the secretory portion of a sweat gland to the surface of the skin. Also called sweat duct.

thoracic d., the common trunk of the lymph vessels, other than those of the right upper body. It ascends from the cisterna chyli and empties into the juncture of the left subclavian and left internal jugular veins.

thyroglossal d., in the embryo, the duct that forms as the developing thyroid migrates downward in the neck. Its upper end communicates with the primitive pharynx at the foramen cecum, where thyroid tissue rarely persists as a lingual thyroid. The duct usually shrivels to become a fibrous cord, but part of it may persist and subsequently become distended to form a thyroglossal cyst. See also *thyroglossal c.* under *cyst.*

vitelline d., see *omphalomesenteric d.*

Wharton's d., the duct that drains the submandibular gland and opens at the sublingual caruncle. Also called submandibular duct.

wolffian d., see *mesonephric d.*

duct ectasia of breast an inflammatory disorder that involves extralobular mammary ducts associated with periductal fibrosis and ductal dilation. Discharge from the nipple occurs in 15–20 percent of persons affected, and nipple inversion is common. Also called *periductal mastitis.*

ductus (duk'tus), pl. *ductus*[L.] [NA], a duct. See also *duct.*

d. arteriosus, a vessel in the embryo that connects the pulmonary trunk at its bifurcation with the arch of the aorta usually just below the left subclavian artery. It is derived from the persistent dorsal portion of the left sixth aortic arch, and serves to shunt blood that would otherwise have to pass through the developing lungs. At birth or shortly thereafter, the ductus becomes twisted; normally, it occludes and shrivels to a fibrous cord. Infrequently, it remains patent and may be symptomatic; see also *patent ductus arteriosus.*

d. deferens, [NA], the thick-walled continuation of the duct of the epididymis, which carries spermatozoa from the testis to the junction with the duct of the seminal vesicle. Also called *vas deferens.*

d. venosus, in the embryo, a vessel that connects the left umbilical vein with the inferior vena cava, enabling blood to bypass the developing venous system in the liver. After birth, the ductus venosus is obliterated and forms the ligamentum venosum. The left umbilical vein is also obliterated and forms the ligamentum teres of the liver. Also called *duct of Arantius.*

Duffy blood group system (duf'e) see under *blood groups.*

Dukes' classification (dūks) [Cuthbert Esquire *Dukes,* English pathologist, born 1890] a system of staging colorectal tumors, based on pathologic evaluation of the depth of invasion of the carcinoma and the presence or absence of metastases. It includes four stages: A, tumors confined to the mucosa and submucosa; B, tumors invading through the muscularis without lymph node involvement; C, tumors invading through the muscularis with regional lymph node metastases; and D, tumor metastasis to distant sites in liver, bones, or other parts of the body.

dullness (dul'nes) a clinical sign demonstrating diminished resonance on percussion; also, a peculiar percussion sound lacking the normal resonance.

Gerhard's d., a physiologic state of nonresponsiveness occurring after prolonged exposure to intellectual cohorts.

shifting d., dullness on abdominal percussion, the level of which shifts as the patient is rolled from side to side; it is indicative of free fluid in the abdominal cavity.

tympanitic d., resonance that is of a dull and diminished quality.

dumdum fever see *kala-azar* and *L. donovani* under *Leishmania.*

dummy in data processing, pertaining to an artificial address, instruction, or record. The value of a dummy item is not used; it only reserves a space or performs some similar function.

dummy variable a variable defined by the compiler that is used to supply the value of a constant to a subroutine. This prevents the alteration of the constant by the subroutine.

dUMP abbrev. See *deoxyuridine-5′-phosphate.*

dump (dump) a copy of the contents of part of a computer memory, usually in binary or octal form.

duoden/o (du″od′ĕ-no) [L. *duodeni* twelve] a word element used in combining form to denote the duodenum, e.g., duodenoscopy.

duodenal (du″o-de′nal, du-od′ĕ-nal) of, pertaining to, or situated in the duodenum.

duodenal contents examination the physical, microscopic, and/or chemical examination of duodenal contents aspirated through a double-lumen gastroduodenal tube positioned under radioscopic control. The specimen is obtained while the patient is in the fasting state.

The residual content is a gray, transparent or translucent, viscid fluid, which may be stained with bile or slight amounts of blood from the intubation. Food particles may indicate the presence of intestinal obstruction or a duodenal diverticulum. Sediment or large numbers of polymorphonuclear leukocytes and exfoliated epithelial cells usually indicate an inflammatory process in the duodenum, pancreas, or biliary tract.

The pancreatic enzymes trypsin, amylase, and lipase are rarely assayed; activities of all three are decreased in pancreatic deficiency.

See also *secretin test.*

duodenography (du″o-de-nog′rah-fe) [*duodeno-* + Gr. *graphein* to examine] radiographic examination of the duodenum.

hypotonic d., a procedure employed in the radiologic diagnosis of duodenal pathology, such as that due to carcinoma of the pancreas. An anticholinergic drug causes the duodenal loop to become hypotonic. When barium and air are introduced into the duodenum, there is maximal distention and enhanced visualization.

duodenoscopy (du″o-de-nos′ko-pe) [*duodeno-* + Gr. *skopein* to examine] an endoscopic procedure for observation of the duodenum. It can be used for cannulation of the ampulla of Vater and for retrograde injection of the pancreatic ducts to detect ductal carcinomas. Specimens for cytologic examination can also be obtained by this technique.

duodenum (du″o-de′num, du-od′ĕ-num) [M.L. *duodenum digitorum* of 12 fingerbreadths] [NA], the proximal 25 cm of the small intestine. It is retroperitoneal and, with the exception of its first 2.5 cm, lies on the posterior wall of the abdomen. It is shaped like a letter C, with the head of the pancreas enclosed within its concavity. For descriptive purposes, the duodenum is considered to have four parts. The first part (2.5 cm) is continuous with the stomach at the pyloric sphincter. It curves backward, to the right, and upward over the portal vein and inferior vena cava, then flexes sharply in its second part (7.5 cm). The second part descends in front of the renal vessels and medial margin of the right kidney. The common bile duct and pancreatic duct enter the second part at about its midportion; the accessory pancreatic duct enters slightly higher. The third part of the duodenum (10 cm) runs transversely to the left in front of the vena cava and aorta, and the fourth part ascends for about 2.5 cm along the left side of the aorta to become the duodenojejunal flexure, where suspension of the small bowel by a mesentery begins. The terminal part of the duodenum and the duodenojejunal flexure are held in position by the suspensory muscle of the duodenum, frequently called the ligament of Treitz. It includes a slip of skeletal muscle from the diaphragm and a fibromuscular band containing smooth muscle cells that blends with the retroperitoneal connective tissue near the origin of the celiac artery. It is possible that the muscle may exert some tension on the flexure, conferring a valvular effect.

As with the rest of the small intestine, the duodenum has mucosal villi and crypts. Its epithelial cells include mucus-forming goblet cells, absorptive cells, enterochromaffin cells, and, at the base of the crypts, Paneth cells. Brunner's glands are submucosal glands that form an alkaline secretion. They may extend over the pylorus into the distal gastric antrum but are not normally found in the jejunum or ileum.

duplication (doo″plĭ-ka′shun) a chromosomal aberration, the repetition of part of a chromosome. It may occur following an unequal crossover; in that case, one of the daughter cells (gametes) will have a deletion and the other a duplication. The latter is usually less harmful and the cell thus more likely to survive.

duplication deficiency a chromosomal aberration usually due to unequal crossing over. It may be considered a reciprocal translocation in which one chromosome has one gene sequence missing and another chromosome has the sequence duplicated. With segregation at mitosis or meiosis, daughter cells with absent or duplicated segments occur, with potentially harmful consequences.

duplicity theory (doo-plis′ĭ-te) the description of the light-sensing capacity of the retina as being composed of two divisions: the scotopic system, which functions at low levels of illumination, and the photopic system, which functions at high levels. Retinal rods and cones are the receptors for the scotopic and photopic systems, respectively. The degree of activation of the two systems depends on the properties of the stimulus and the levels of visual adaptation. Frequently, a stimulus can simultaneously stimulate both systems to some degree. See also *photoreceptor.*

Dupuytren's contracture (doo-pwe-trahnz′) [Baron Guillaume *Dupuytren,* French surgeon, 1777–1835] fibromatosis involving the fascia of the palm. It may coexist with plantar fibromatosis. In the hand, the process commonly involves the middle, ring, and little fingers; the index finger and thumb are infrequently involved. Most of those affected are over age 40 yr when the original symptoms appear as small fascial nodules composed of actively synthesizing myofibroblasts and loose, wavy bundles of collagen. Areas of myxoid stroma are common. The process may extend through the dermis, but the underlying tendons and muscles are not involved. With progression, the myofibroblasts organize into bundles and collagen accumulates, while the vascularity diminishes.

The process is found three times more frequently in males than in females, and is bilateral in 10 percent of those affected. Over the years, progressive contracture develops, and surgical correction is required in about one-third of cases. There is a tendency for recurrence following surgery, and physical therapy, particularly regular extension exercises, is important.

dur/o (du′ro) [L. *dura* hard] a word element used in combining form to denote the dura mater, e.g., dural.

dura mater (du′rah ma′ter) [L. "hard mother"] the outermost and strongest of the meninges that cover the brain and spinal cord. The dura covering the brain lines the interior of the skull and is intimately adherent to the inner surface of the cranial bones. In some areas, a meningeal layer of the dura can be identified; it provides sheaths for the cranial nerves as they leave the cranial cavity, encloses the venous sinuses, and is reduplicated inward as septa that support the brain (falx cerebri, tentorium cerebelli, falx cerebelli, diaphragma sellae).

At the foramen magnum the meningeal layer continues down the spinal canal, forming the spinal dura mater. It is separated from the periosteum lining the vertebral canal by the extradural space. Also known as the epidural space, the extradural space contains a small amount of fat, loose connective tissue, and a plexus of veins. Below the second sacral vertebra, the dura clothes the filum terminale. It also provides sheaths for the spinal nerves as they exit through the intervertebral foramina.

duration (du-ra′shun) 1. the time interval during which a stimulating electric current or voltage is applied to a sensory receptor, nerve muscle, or discrete area of the brain or spinal cord.

2. the time period, usually measured in milliseconds, until the waveform of an individual action potential or a complex of waveforms is terminated. The duration of an individual potential by convention (except in the case of the M wave) is measured from the initial deflection above or below the baseline to the final return of the waveform to the baseline.

3. the time interval from the start to the finish of a recurring sequence of waveform complexes, or stimuli.

Durham tube (dur′um) [Herbert Edward *Durham*, English bacteriologist, 1866–1945] a carbohydrate fermentation tube used to determine gas production by a bacterial culture. A small glass test tube is inverted in another tube containing a liquid medium. After inoculation and incubation, the gas produced by the growing culture is trapped and visible inside the inverted tube.

dust (dust) solid particles small enough to be capable of temporary suspension in the air and large enough to eventually settle out (approximately 10–50 μm in diameter). Numerous types of industrial dusts constitute a toxic hazard, e.g., metals, minerals (silica, asbestos, coal), organic materials (cotton), and toxic chemicals (pesticides). Many dust particles can serve as immunogens (allergens). See also *suspended p.'s* under *particulate.*

dust cell see *alveolar macrophage.*

D value see *decimal reduction time.*

DVM abbrev. See *digital voltmeter.*

DVT abbrev. for deep venous thrombosis. See under *thrombophlebitis.*

dwarfism (dwarf′izm) generalized retardation of growth, associated with many disorders including rickets, Hurler's syndrome, intestinal malabsorption, hypothyroidism, renal disease, congenital cardiac malformation, sexual precocity, chondrodystrophy, and pituitary growth hormone deficiency. Affected individuals typically have abnormally short extremities and may manifest any of the following: bone deformities, proteinuria, cyanosis, heart murmurs, or mental and physical deficiencies.

pituitary d., abnormally retarded growth and delayed sexual development in children that is the result of a deficiency in the production or secretion of growth hormone. Mental development is normal. There may also be reduced concentrations of other pituitary hormones (e.g., adrenocorticotropic hormone, gonadotropins, or thyrotropin. This condition is most frequently due to a craniopharyngioma but may also occur idiopathically. Affected infants are of normal size at birth but fail to grow normally. Hypoglycemia, thyroid and adrenocortical insufficiency, and deficient sexual maturation are common. Children may have wrinkled skin, appearing to age abnormally fast.

Laboratory findings include severely reduced concentrations of plasma growth hormone (by immunochemical methods), reduced serum or urinary gonadotropins (by radioimmunoassay), decreased serum protein-bound iodine, and a subnormal response of plasma corticosteroids to intravenous adrenocorticotropin. Skull x-rays, CT scans, and polytomography may be helpful in the diagnosis of pituitary neoplasms and craniopharyngiomas.

See also *hypopituitarism.*

dwarf tapeworm see *H. nana* under *Hymenolepis.*

***d* wave** see under *electroretinogram.*

Dy symbol for the chemical element *dysprosium.*

dyad (di′ad) a double chromosome resulting from the halving of a tetrad in the first meiotic division.

dye (di) a colored organic compound used in histology, hematology, and microbiology to selectively stain certain tissue or cell components so that they can be seen under the microscope. All dyes are composed of complex large molecules that contain many conjugated double bonds and thus absorb visible light; most are synthetic compounds produced from coal tar.

Many dyes bind to tissue or cell components by forming ionic bonds. Acid (anionic) dyes bind to cationic side groups of proteins; basic (cationic) dyes bind to anionic groups of proteins and nucleic acids. Components that specifically bind acid dyes are called acidophilic (or eosinophilic or oxyphilic); those that bind basic dyes are called basophilic.

Mordant dyes, such as hematoxylin, bind to tissues or cell components by forming a complex (called a lake) with a metal ion, such as iron or aluminum (the mordant). The dye lake binds to basophilic tissue constituents.

Fat-soluble dyes are neutral compounds that are much more soluble in neutral lipids than in water; components that bind these dyes are called sudanophilic.

Fluorescent dyes (fluorochromes) are acidic, basic, or fat-soluble dyes used in ultraviolet microscopy.

Metachromatic dyes are basic dyes that stain basophilic structures their own color but stain connective tissue a redder color, which is due to polymerization of the dye on acid mucopolysaccharides.

The nomenclature of dyes is confusing because a dye may be known by many synonymous trivial names (some quite dissimilar) and because quite different dyes can have similar names. Furthermore, some dyes are not pure compounds but mixtures of homologous compounds. Dyes that are pure compounds are unambiguously identified by their color index number.

Some dyes are used clinically as antiseptic and antibacterial agents; others are used as reagents in laboratory tests.

See also *chromophore, Color Index, staining,* and the individual dyes.

dye content the percentage of pure dye contained in a commercial preparation of a stain or dye.

dye excretion tests tests used in the evaluation of liver function that measure the ability of the hepatic parenchymal cells to remove a foreign dye from the blood and excrete it into the bile. Two dyes used in these tests are rose bengal (now used only as the radioactive tracers ^{125}I–rose bengal and ^{131}I–rose bengal) and indocyanine green (ICG, Cardio-Green). Sulfobromophthalein (Bromosulphthalein, BSP) has recently been discontinued. Use of these tests is rare. Their applications have mainly been in the differential diagnosis of hemolytic and hepatic jaundice, with normal tests being observed in hemolytic diseases. In liver disease, these tests are useful only in the absence of jaundice. The dose for the ICG excretion test is 0.5 mg/kg of body weight.

dyn abbrev. See *dyne.*

dynamic (di-nam′ik) [Gr. *dynamikos* powerful] 1. pertaining to force, energy, or power, or to the motion of a physical system in response to an applied force.

2. in motion; changing state.

dyne (dyn) (dīn) the centimeter-gram-second (cgs) unit of force equal to 1 gram-centimeter per second squared ($g \cdot cm/s^2$) or 10^{-5} newton (N).

dynein (di′ne-in) a large protein making up the arms on the A tubules in the axoneme of cilia and flagella. A Ca^{++} or Mg^{++} adenosine triphosphatase, it is important to the movement of cilia and flagella.

dyphylline (di-fil′in) a theophylline derivative used as a bronchodilator to treat bronchial asthma, chronic bronchitis, and emphysema. See also *theophylline.*

Dyrenium (di-ren′ĭ-um) trademark. See *triamterene.*

dys- (dis) [Gr.] a prefix word element to denote difficult, painful, abnormal, or bad, e.g., dyspnea.

dysarthria (dis-ar′thre-ah) [*dys-* + Gr. *arthroun* to utter distinctly + *-ia*] impaired articulation of speech, due to muscular weakness or incoordination. Often, speech is slurred and difficult to understand. This condition must be distinguished from dysphasia, a primary disturbance of language comprehension or expression that usually results from a lesion in the cerebral cortex.

dysaudia (dis-aw′de-ah) [*dys-* + L. *audire* to hear + *-ia*] impairment of the sense of hearing, which may be due to infection, cysts, tumors, wax impaction, allergy, trauma, or degenerative disorders.

dysautonomia (dis″aw-to-no′me-ah) [*dys-* + Gr. *autonomia* freedom to use its own laws] a general term used to describe a disturbance of autonomic function.

familial d., a genetic disease, transmitted as an autosomal recessive trait and occurring soon after birth, that is limited almost exclusively to Ashkenazi Jews and is characterized by dysfunction of autonomic processes. These include abnormal sweating, defective temperature control, decreased vasomotor control, skin blotchiness, dysphagia, recurrent vomiting, impaired growth, corneal ulceration and alacrima. Hyporeflexia and impaired pain and temperature appreciation are neuropathic features.

Diagnosis is based on the history, family background, clinical signs, and a lack of skin flares on exposure to histamine. Nerve conduction velocities may be slowed and a variety of nerve disorders are seen. Mortality is high and is often due to recurrent pulmonary infections. Treatment is symptomatic.

Also called familial autonomic dysfunction, familial dysautonomia, and *Riley-Day syndrome.*

dysbarism (dis′bar-izm) [*dys-* + Gr. *baros* weight + *-ism*] a general term applied to any disease, condition, or clinical syndrome that results from sudden exposure of the body to a change (usually pronounced) in ambient pressure. See also *decompression sickness.*

dysbasia (dis-ba′ze-ah) [*dys-* + Gr. *basis* step + *-ia*] difficulty or impairment in walking, especially when caused by a neurologic lesion.

dyschezia (dis-ke′ze-ah) [*dys-* + Gr. *chezein* to defecate + *-ia*] difficulty or pain upon defecation. There are a large number of possible causes, including inflammation, abscesses, ulcers, hemorrhoids, proctitis, and neoplasms.

dyschondroplasia (dis″kon-dro-pla′ze-ah) [*dys-* + Gr. *chondros* cartilage + *plassein* to form + *-ia*] see under *enchondroma.*

dyscrasia (dis-kra′ze-ah) [Gr. *dyskrasis* bad mixture + *-ia*] a term historically used to denote a disordered mixture of the humors, but now broadly applied in modern medicine to denote a disorder of a body system. The term is frequently used in hematology to refer to congenital disorders of a particular cell line, e.g., plasma cell and leukocyte dyscrasias.

dysdiadochokinesia (dis″di-ad″ŏ-ko-ki-ne′se-ah) [*dys-* + Gr. *diadochos* successive + *kinēsis* motion + *-ia*] the impaired ability to perform fine, rapid, alternating movements.

dysentery (dis′en-ter″e) [L. *dysenteria,* from *dys-* + Gr. *enteron* intestine] a general term used to refer to severe inflammation of the intestine (especially the colon). It is associated with vigorous outpouring of stools containing blood and mucus, abdominal pain, colic, and tenesmus.

amebic d., see *amebiasis.*

bacillary d., a disease characterized by the sudden onset of abdominal cramps, fever, and diarrhea. Severe infection commonly produces acute dysentery and intestinal ulceration. The lesions generally are confined to the terminal ileum and colon; systemic infection is rare, even in infants and children.

Transmission is by the oral-fecal route. The disease occurs as epidemics among populations subjected to malnutrition, poor sanitation, and overcrowding. It is caused by four species of *Shigella;* in recent years, most cases in the United States have been due to *S. sonnei. S. dysenteriae* is usually associated with a clinically severe form of the disease.

See also *shigellosis.*

epidemic d., a form of dysentery that becomes epidemic; it can be dangerous and even fatal in infants, children or the elderly.

Flexner's d., see *bacillary d.*

giardial d., see *giardiasis.*

protozoal d., see *amebiasis.*

Sonne d., a mild form of dysentery, caused by the *Shigella sonnei* bacillus.

sporadic d., dysentery that has a scattered pattern with no apparent connection.

viral d., a virus-caused dysentery that often occurs in epidemics; it is marked by acute, watery bouts of diarrhea.

dyserythropoiesis (dis″ĕ-rith″ro-poi-e′sis) [*dys-* + Gr. *erythros* red + Gr. *poiēsis* making] the production of abnormal red cells; the term is used only in describing congenital dyserythropoietic anemia.

dyserythropoietic congenital anemia (dis″ĕ-rith″ro-poi-et′ik) [*dys-* + Gr. *erythros* red + *poiein* to make] see *congenital dyserythropoietic a.* under *anemia.*

dysfibrinogenemia (dis″fi-brin″o-jĕ-ne′me-ah) [*dys-* + *fibrinogen* + Gr. *haima* blood + *-ia*] a qualitative abnormality in the fibrinogen molecule, usually transmitted as an autosomal dominant trait, by which coagulation is often inhibited (i.e., the prothrombin, thrombin, and reptilase times are prolonged). About 40 inherited qualitatively abnormal fibrinogens have been described, but the molecular defect has been elucidated in only one (fibrinogen Detroit). Functional abnormalities include abnormal aggregation of the fibrin monomers, which usually is asymptomatic. Less commonly, there is abnormal fibrinopeptide release, and rarely there is abnormal fibrin cross-linking. The latter two abnormalities are usually symptomatic, and produce bleeding, rarely thrombosis, or both.

dysfunction (dis-funk′shun) impaired or abnormal function.

dysfunctional bleeding (dis-funk′shun-al) a disordered rhythm of menstrual flow that results from hormonal imbalance.

dysgammaglobulinemia (dis-gam″mah-glob″u-lĭ-ne′me-ah) [*dys-* + *gammaglobulin* + Gr. *haima blood* + *-ia*] a selective deficiency in one or more classes of immunoglobulin. It usually results in an immunologic deficiency and an increased susceptibility to infectious disease. Dysgammaglobulinemia may occur with either abnormal synthesis or abnormal function of immunoglobulins.

dysgenesis (dis-jen′ĕ-sis) [*dys-* + Gr. *genesis* production] an abnormality due to defects that occur during the development of the embryo.

dysgerminoma (dis″jer-mĭ-no′mah) [*dys-* + L. *germen* germ + Gr. *-oma* swelling] a tumor of the ovary that appears histogenetically and histologically to be the counterpart of the seminoma in the male. Both are believed to be derived from primordial germ cells. Most individuals with dysgerminoma are young, the majority under age 30 yr; some are children. The tumors are solid and usually unilateral. A good prognosis is indicated for small dysgerminomas confined to the ovary. Once the ovarian capsule has been penetrated, however, spread to the peritoneum, regional lymph nodes, and distant sites is likely. Dysgerminomas are radiosensitive, so the prognosis is relatively good for patients with metastases.

The tumor cells appear similar to those of the testicular seminoma, forming diffuse sheets devoid of architectural patterns. The plentiful cytoplasm contains sparse organelles but abundant glycogen. Rarely, dysgerminomas contain multinucleated cells of the trophoblastic type that form chorionic gonadotropin, but most do not have any endocrine activity.

See also *ovarian tumors.*

dysglobulinemia (dis-glob″u-lĭ-ne′me-ah) [*dys-* + *globulin* + Gr. *haima* blood + *-ia*] any disorder of the blood globulins.

dysgonic (dis-gon′ik) [*dys-* + Gr. *gonē* seed] seeding poorly; said of bacterial cultures, especially species of *Mycobacterium* that grow sparsely on culture media. Cf. *eugonic.*

dyshidrosis (dis-hid-ro′sis) [*dys-* + Gr. *hidrōsis* a sweating] 1. difficulty in perspiring, which may be caused by a blockage of the opening of the eccrine sweat glands.

2. a disease of the hands and feet marked by the eruption of deep-seated, grainy vesicles that work their way to the skin surface and become larger. They appear often in summer, are recurrent, and often itch intensely. Also called pompholyx.

dyskaryosis (dis″kar-e-o′sis) [*dys-* + Gr. *karyon* nucleus + *-osis*] in cytology, abnormal changes in the nucleus of a cell with a well-differentiated cytoplasm. These changes may range from slight nuclear enlargement, with multinucleation and hyperchromasia (early or slight dyskaryosis), to bizarre nuclear shape and size (markedly enlarged) with significant hyperchromasia and variable chromatin patterns that may be coarse, granular, or filamentous (late or severe dyskaryosis). Such changes may have a number of causes including chemicals, cell division, and malignant transformation. The term dyskaryosis is often used to describe changes in cervical epithelial cells seen on a vaginal smear and may reflect pregnancy, premalignancy, malignancy, or a normal state.

dyskeratosis (dis″ker-ah-to′sis) [*dys-* + Gr. *keras* horn + *-osis* condition] the faulty and premature formation of keratin by epidermal cells. In acantholytic dyskeratosis, corps ronds are formed. In neoplastic dyskeratosis, or individual cell keratinization, masses of keratin accumulate in the cytoplasm, ultimately compressing the nucleus, which degenerates, leaving a homogeneous eosinophilic body. See also *k. follicularis* under *keratosis.*

dyskeratosis congenita a rare, sex-linked recessive disorder of the skin that affects males. It is characterized by areas of hyperpigmentation, hyperkeratosis of mucous membranes, hyperkeratosis of the palms and soles (often with nail loss), and atrophy of skin surfaces.

dyskinesia (dis″ki-ne′ze-ah) [Gr. *dyskinēsia* difficulty of movement] 1. disorder of movement.

2. abnormal involuntary movements.

tardive d., abnormal, repetitive movements, most frequently involving the lower part of the face, provoked by long-term use of antipsychotic drugs. Phenothiazine tranquilizers are commonly implicated; it is thought that the chronic blocking of dopaminergic receptors may result in their supersensitization. The disorder may first develop some years after the causative drug was taken by an individual, hence the designation tardive. In other persons, it first becomes manifest as the drug is withdrawn. There is no satisfactory treatment, and when the condition develops in adults, it is likely to be permanent.

dyslexia (dis-lek′se-170 ah) [*dys-* + Gr. *lexis* word

+ *-ia*] impairment of the ability to read, owing to difficulty in the visual recognition of words. The dyslexic person may be of normal intelligence with normal abilities in other areas, but often has problems organizing and understanding groups of letters and words. This condition may not have an obvious cause, or it may be due to a lesion in certain parts of the brain. Also called *alexia.*

dysmenorrhea (dis″men-o-re′ah) [*dys-* + Gr. *mēn* month + *rhein* to flow + *-ia*] abnormal or painful menstruation, which may first occur shortly after menarche or may appear later in life. Primary dysmenorrhea is generally of unknown etiology; however, dysmenorrhea appearing later in life usually has an identifiable cause such as salpingitis or endometriosis. Cramplike abdominal pain, nausea, urinary frequency, and irritability may all be present.

dysmorphism (dis-mor′fizm) [*dys-* + Gr. *morphē* form + *-ism*] a morphologic developmental abnormality, especially external, seen in individuals with syndromes of genetic or environmental origin. Dysmorphism can arise from single-gene disorders, chromosome disorders, disorders having multifactorial inheritance, and environmental teratogens.

dysmyelopoietic syndrome [*dys-* + Gr. *myelos* marrow + *poiein* to form] see *refractory a.* under *anemia.*

dysostosis (dis″os-to′sis) [*dys-* + Gr. *osteon* bone + *-osis* condition] abnormal fetal formation of bone, especially in the early transition from cartilage to bone. In many cases there is a congenital defect in the ossification process. Commonly affected areas include the cleidocranial, craniofacial, and mandibulofacial regions, and the metaphyseal areas. These abnormalities present a characteristic appearance on x-ray examination, bone form and density being affected.

dyspareunia (dis″pah-roo′ne-ah) [Gr. *dyspareunos* badly mated + *-ia*] the condition of painful or difficult sexual intercourse in women. The causes may be disease-related, mechanical, or psychological.

dyspepsia (dis-pep′se-ah) [*dys-* + Gr. *peptein* to digest + *-ia*] symptoms due to impairment of the process of digestion, generally associated with the intake of food. The symptoms are often vague, with complaints of gas, heartburn, pressure, and loss of appetite. The condition may be due to poor eating habits, irritating diet, allergy, drugs, or poisons. Defects in the digestive organs themselves, such as ulcers, inflammations, and tumors, can cause dyspepsia. Psychogenic factors including stress, nervousness, and exhaustion also are possible causes. See also *indigestion.*

dysphagia (dis-fa′je-ah) [*dys-* + Gr. *phagein* to eat + *-ia*] difficulty in swallowing, a general symptom of esophageal transport problems. The condition may be of motor or obstructive origin and may or may not be accompanied by pain. Radiographic examination and fiberoptic esophagoscopy can aid in detecting esophageal webs and in assessing cardiospasm. Monitoring esophageal pH provides evidence of gastroesophageal reflux. Esophageal manometry is used to diagnose achalasia, progressive systemic sclerosis, lower esophageal sphincter hypertension and hypotension, and diffuse esophageal spasm.

sideropenic d., see *Plummer-Vinson syndrome.*

dysphasia (dis-fa′ze-ah) [*dys-* + Gr. *phasis* speech + *-ia*] see *aphasia.*

dysphonia (dis-fo′ne-ah) [*dys-* + Gr. *phonē* voice + *-ia*] impaired vocal intensity or clarity, often with hoarseness or a breathy quality, that is due to laryngeal dysfunction (e.g., inflammation, infection, weakness, tumor, or edema). Dysphonia may be temporary after voice overuse or outbursts of hysteria. Laryngoscopic examination can often differentiate among the possible causes of the condition. Cf. *aphonia.*

dysphoria (dis-fo′re-ah) [Gr. "agitation"] restlessness, uneasiness. Cf. *euphoria.*

dysplasia (dis-pla′ze-ah) [*dys-* + Gr. *plassein* to form + *ia*] 1. an abnormal growth pattern or deranged development.

2. in histopathology, an epithelium in which there are cells with cytologic features of malignancy but insufficient changes to warrant the diagnosis of carcinoma in situ. The term is frequently used in connection with the uterine cervix to denote an epithelium in which there are cells with atypical cytologic features (dyskaryosis) but also some degree of maturation at the surface of the epithelium. Traditionally, cervical dysplasia is further categorized as mild, moderate, or severe, on the basis of the level in the epithelium to which cytologically atypical cells extend and their degree of atypia. There is no uniform agreement on the categorization of the degree of severity of dysplasia occurring in the cervix or other epithelia. See also *cervical intraepithelial neoplasia* and *dyskaryosis.* Cf. *carcinoma in situ.*

3. a congenital anomaly due to abnormal development of tissue structures. Such a dysplasia can be metabolic or nonmetabolic, be benign or premalignant, affect one or several organs, originate in one or several germ layers, and be hereditary, environmental, or multifactorial.

fibrous d., see *fibrous dysplasia.*

polyostotic fibrous d., a disorder of bone, of unknown cause, that is characterized by reddish-gray, gritty lesions, especially in the craniofacial bones and ribs. Fibromata are embedded in coarse fibrous bone, often associated with wide osteoid seams. Radiographs reveal radiolucent areas with a "ground-glass appearance"; the facial bones may show increased radiodensity. The course of this disease is highly variable. When associated with areas of pigmentation, endocrine dysfunction, and precocious puberty in females, the condition is referred to as Albright's syndrome. See also *Albright's syndrome.*

dyspnea (disp′ne-ah) [Gr. *dyspnoia* difficulty of breathing] shortness of breath or difficulty in breathing associated with a subjective awareness of discomfort with each respiratory effort. Dyspnea is often associated with abnormalities that cause a disproportion between the muscular effort required to breathe and the level of ventilation achieved, or with an increased discharge in lung irritation receptors subserved by vagal afferents.

cardiac d., distressful breathing (or subjective sensation of breathlessness) caused by, and often one of the earliest manifestations of, heart diseases such as left heart failure, mitral stenosis, aortic regurgitation, and angina.

exertional d., dyspnea produced by physical effort such as exercise. In persons who have conditions associated with cardiac or pulmonary disease, it often becomes extreme after only mild exertion.

paroxysmal nocturnal d., often-frightening episodes of acute respiratory distress with sensations of breathlessness and suffocation that suddenly appear at night. They are caused by prolonged assumption of the supine position and may waken individuals from sleep, causing them anxiously to seek relief. The bouts occur in those with left heart failure, owing to an aggravation of the pulmonary vascular congestion and the edema that accompany this condition.

dyspneic (disp-ne′ik) pertaining to or characterized by dyspnea.

dyspoiesis (dis″poi-e′sis) [*dys-* + Gr. *poiesis* making] impaired or abnormal formation and production. The term often refers to the pathologic development of blood cells in diseases such as anemias and leukemias.

dysprosium (Dy) (dis-pro′se-um) [Gr. *dysprositos* difficult to approach] a silvery metallic element; atomic number 66; atomic weight 162.50; a 4f transition element (lanthanide or rare earth); oxidation state +3. See also *rare earth elements.*

dysproteinemia (dis-pro″te-in-e′me-ah) [*dys-* + *protein* + Gr. *haima* blood + *-ia*] the presence of abnormal proteins in the blood, e.g. dysprothrombinemia.

dysprothrombinemia (dis″pro-throm″bĭ-ne′me-ah) [*dys-* + *prothrombin* + Gr. *haima* blood + *-ia*] a hereditary abnormality of the prothrombin (coagulation Factor II) molecule, transmitted as an autosomal recessive trait, that occurs in two forms: prothrombin Barcelona, and another variant in which only some molecules are abnormal and not convertible to thrombin. Both cause relatively mild hemorrhagic symptoms and a moderately prolonged prothombin time. Normal amounts of prothrombin are found on immunoassay.

dysrhythmia (dis-rith′me-ah) [*dys-* + Gr. *rhythmos* + *-ia*] disordered rhythm.

dyssynergia (dis″sin-er′je-ah) [*dys-* + Gr. *synergia* cooperation] impaired coordination affecting limb movements, speech, or walking; usually the result of cerebellar dysfunction.

dystaxia (dis-tak′se-ah) [*dys-* + Gr. *taxis* arrangement + *-ia*] see *ataxia.*

dystocia (dis-to′se-ah) [*dys-* + Gr. *tokos* birth + *-ia*] cessation of the progress of labor due to mechanical factors. The causes may be weakness of the expulsive action of the uterus, an abnormality in size or position of the fetus, or obstruction in the birth canal because of its size or shape or from the presence of an obstructing lesion such as a tumor.

dystrophy (dis′tro-fe) [Gr. *dystrophia,* from *dys-* abnormal + Gr. *trephein* to nourish] any disorder in which there is muscular wasting and hypotrophy. For more information, see the specific dystrophy.

dysuria (dis-u′re-ah) [*dys-* + Gr. *ouron* urine + *-ia*] a general term used to describe abnormalities in urination, including pain, burning, frequency, urgency, dripping, and pyuria. The underlying causes include such conditions as cystitis, urethritis, prostatitis, prostatic hypertrophy, neurogenic bladder, and psychosomatic illness.

Common procedures used to determine the etiology of dysuria include microscopic examination of the urine and urine culture. If a diagnosis cannot be established, more complex tests may be used, including excretory urography, voiding cystourethrography, cystoscopy, urethroscopy, and urodynamic studies.

DZ abbrev. See *dizygotic.*

E

E symbol for air dose (see under *dose*), *elastance, electric field vector, electromotive force* (voltage), *exa-, glutamic acid,* internal energy, mathematical expectation, redox potential.

***E*-** [Ger. *entgegen* opposite] a stereodescriptor used to indicate the configuration at a double bond, e.g., (*E*)-2-butene (*trans*-2-butene); see also *isomerism.*

E° symbol for standard potential. See under *Nernst equation.*

E_0 symbol. See *skin d.* under *dose.*

E_1 abbrev. See *estrone.*

E_2 abbrev. See *17β-estradiol.*

E_3 abbrev. See *estriol.*

E_4 abbrev. See *estetrol.*

E_d abbrev. See *depth d.* under *dose.*

E_h abbrev. See *redox potential.*

$E_{1cm}^{1\%}$ an obsolete abbrev. for extinction coefficient, equivalent to $A_{1cm}^{1\%}$. See under *absorptivity.*

e symbol for the base of natural logarithms: approximately 2.7182818285, *electron, elementary charge.*

e^- symbol for a negative electron.

e^+ symbol for *positron.*

ε the Greek lower case letter *epsilon;* symbol for: (1) the heavy chain of IgE, (2) permittivity (ϵ_0, the permittivity of vacuum), (3) molar absorptivity.

η the Greek lower case letter *eta;* symbol for viscosity.

EACA abbrev. for *ε-aminocaproic acid.*

Eadie-Hofstee equation (e′de hof′ste) see under *Lineweaver-Burk equation.*

e antigen see under *hepatitis.*

ear (ēr) [L. *auris;* Gr. *ous*] the organ of hearing. For descriptive purposes it is conveniently subdivided into external, middle, and inner portions. The auditory apparatus is anatomically contiguous with the peripheral vestibular apparatus that provides the brain with information concerning the position or state of motion of the head.

The external ear includes the auricle or pinna and the external auditory meatus. The auricle is covered by skin and its shape is maintained by a sheet of elastic cartilage. The curved rim of the auricle (the helix) leads inferiorly to the soft tip (lobule). The opening of the external auditory meatus is partially overlapped from in front by a posterior projection, the tragus. Sound waves are deflected by the auricle and transmitted via the external auditory meatus to the tympanic membrane at the inner end of the meatus.

The tympanic membrane is the lateral wall of the tympanic cavity or middle ear, an irregular space located within the temporal bone and filled with air that reaches it through the internal auditory canal (pharyngotympanic or eustachian tube). The auditory ossicles (malleus, incus, stapes) are three small bones that articulate to form a chain that transmits vibration of the tympanic membrane across the middle ear to the internal ear. The medial wall of the middle ear is the lateral wall of the internal ear and contains two openings, the oval window (fenestra ovalis, fenestra vestibuli) and below it the round window (fenestra rotunda, fenestra cochleae). In the posterior wall of the middle ear there is an irregular opening that leads into an air sinus in the petrous portion of the temporal bone called the mastoid antrum, with its adjacent mastoid air cells.

The internal ear lies within the petrous part of the temporal bone. It consists of a series of cavities, the bony labyrinth, which contain a system of communicating membranous sacs and ducts that constitute the membranous labyrinth. The component parts of the bony labyrinth are the vestibule, semicircular canals, and cochlea. They are filled with a fluid, perilymph, within which the membranous labyrinth is suspended.

The vestibule is the central part of the bony labyrinth; its lateral wall is perforated by the oval window, which is occupied by the footplate of the stapes. In the medial wall of the vestibule there is a small opening for the aqueduct of the vestibule, which contains a slender extension of the membranous labyrinth, the endolymphatic duct. The communication with the cochlea is in the anterior wall of the vestibule, and the openings of the semicircular canals are in its posterior part.

The three semicircular canals (anterior, posterior, lateral) lie behind the vestibule. They are approximately perpendicular to each other. The cochlea resembles a snail shell. It has a cone-shaped central pillar, the modiolus, surrounded by a spiral canal that is partially subdivided by a shelf of bone projecting from the modiolus. This bony ridge is the osseous spiral lamina and partially divides the spiral canal into upper (scala vestibuli) and lower (scala tympani) chambers.

The membranous labyrinth lies within the perilymph and is in turn filled with endolymph. Its contours are roughly similar to those of its bony confines. Two small sacs within the vestibule (the utricle and saccule) communicate with one another, and with the semicircular canals and cochlear duct, respectively. The semicircular ducts lie within the corresponding canals; each has an expanded end or ampulla where the thickened wall projects to form a crest. The epithelium of the crest contains strategically positioned sensory cells, termed hair cells because of the long microvilli on their apical surfaces. Afferent fibers of the vestibular portion of the eighth cranial nerve conduct information on the movements of the head from the hair cells to the vestibular cortex.

The spiral canal of the cochlea makes fewer than three turns around the modiolus, tapering as it ascends. From the tip of the projecting bony spiral lamina the basilar membrane extends to its outer wall, completing the separation of the scala vestibuli above and the scala tympani below. Above the basilar membrane, a slender vestibular membrane extends across the scala vestibuli, and the tunnel between the vestibular and basilar membranes is the duct of the cochlea.

The spiral organ (of Corti) is made up of a group of epithelial cells resting on the upper surface of the basilar membrane. They include the hair cells, and supporting cells that have various eponyms. Long apical microvilli on the hair cells are deformed by slight movements of the endolymph within the cochlear duct. The base of each hair cell synapses with afferent and efferent nerve terminations.

Sound waves channeled through the external auditory meatus cause the tympanic membrane to vibrate, the vibrations being transmitted and amplified by the chain of auditory ossicles. The footplate of the stapes is positioned in the oval window; its movements produce pressure waves within the perilymph that are transmitted to the basilar membrane, and through it to the hair cells and auditory nerve fibers.

Eaton agent (e′ton) [Monroe Davis *Eaton,* U.S. bacteriologist, born 1904] see *M. pneumoniae* under *Mycoplasma.*

Eaton-Lambert syndrome (e′ton lam′bert) [Lealdes McKendree *Eaton,* U.S. physician, 1905–1958; Edward Howard *Lambert,* U.S. physiologist, born 1915] a disorder of neuromuscular transmission that has been associated in many cases with a variety of cancers, particularly oat cell carcinoma. It is characterized clinically by muscle weakness and depression of muscle stretch reflexes in the legs. The disorder is due to impaired release of acetylcholine at nerve terminals.

Diagnosis is made by means of electrodiagnostic studies, which typically show reduction of the muscle action potential amplitude in response to a single stimulus to the nerve, and marked augmentation (200–900 percent) after a brief period (30 sec) of muscle exercise.

EBCDIC (eb′se-dik) [acronym from *e*xtended *b*inary *c*oded *d*ecimal *i*nterchange *c*ode] an eight-bit character code used primarily with IBM computers. See also *American Standard Code for Information Interchange.*

Ebner's gland (eb′nerz) [Anton Gilbert Viktor *Ebner* von Rofenstein, Viennese histologist, 1842–1925] a serous secreting gland of the posterior tongue associated with the circumvallate papillae.

Ebola virus (eb′o-lah) [from a river in Zaire] an RNA virus with a lipoprotein envelope, the etiologic agent of Ebola virus disease. Structurally, it is similar to the Marburg virus but without antigenic similarities. An infection with Ebola virus is immunogenic, although it is not known how long these antibodies last. See also *Ebola virus disease.*

Ebola virus disease a hemorrhagic fever similar to Marburg virus disease. After an incubation peroid of 4–16 da (average, 7 da), there is fever, gastrointestinal symptoms, and limb pain, followed by diarrhea, pharyngitis, and a dry cough. The mortality rate is high, death often occurring between da 4 and da 10. Initial diagnosis is made according to the clinical symptoms and results of serology tests. Rapid diagnosis is important. The virus should also be isolated in Vero cells and guinea pigs, and identified using immunofluorescence.

Ebstein's anomaly (eb′stīnz) [Wilhelm *Ebstein,* German physician, 1836–1912] a rare congenital condition characterized by the downward displacement of a malformed tricuspid valve. This results in a larger right atrium and a smaller right ventricle. Tricuspid valve regurgitation, a patent foramen ovale, or other atrial septal defects are also usually present. These anatomic changes may cause decreased right ventricular output, right-to-left shunt, arrhythmia, split heart sounds, and both systolic and diastolic murmurs. Symptoms are variable early in life, but the degree of cyanosis increases with age. Most of those affected live to their third decade, but mortality increases dramatically thereafter. Diagnosis is made by a combination of clinical signs, echocardiography, electrocardiography, and angiocardiography.

eburnation (e″bur-na′shun) [L. *ebur* ivory] see *bone s.* under *sclerosis.*

EBV abbrev. See *Epstein-Barr virus.*

EC abbrev. for *Enzyme Commission.*

ec- (ek) [Gr. *ek* out] a prefix word element to denote out or outside, e.g., ecchymosis.

ecchymosis (ek″ĭ-mo′sis), pl. *ecchymoses* [*ec-* + Gr. *chymos* juice + *-osis* condition] a hemorrhage into the skin greater than 3 cm in diameter. Cf. *petechia.*

ECCLS abbrev. See *European Committee for Clinical Laboratory Standards.*

eccrine gland (ek′rin) [*ec-* + *-crine,* from Gr. *krinein* to separate] one of the numerous ordinary sweat glands found in the skin anywhere on the body. See also *sweat glands.*

eccrine tumor a tumor that arises from the duct or secretory cells of the eccrine sweat glands of the dermis. Both adenomas and carcinomas occur. See also *adnexal neoplasms.*

EC detector abbrev. for electron capture detector; see under *gas chromatography.*

ECF abbrev. See *extracellular fluid.*

ECF-A abbrev. See *eosinophil chemotactic factor of anaphylaxis.*

ECG abbrev. See *electrocardiogram.*

ecgonine (ek′go-nin) a hydrolysis product and metabolite of cocaine. It contains both tertiary amino and carboxylic acid groups.

ech/o (ek′o) [Gr. *ēchō* a returned sound] a word element used in combining form to denote echoes, e.g., echocardiography.

Echidnophaga (ek″id-nof′ah-gah) [N.L., from Gr. *echidna* viper + *phagos* glutton] a genus of fleas of which the species *E. gallinacea,* the sticktight flea, is found throughout tropical and subtropical regions of the world; it has also been found in warm regions of the United States. These fleas attack humans, dogs, cats, rats, and poultry; they are thought to be reservoirs of *Yersinia pestis.*

echino- (e-ki′no) [Gr. *echinos* a prickly husk; hedgehog] a word element used in combining form to denote spiny, e.g., echinocyte.

echinococcosis (e-ki″no-kok-o′sis) [*echino-* + Gr. *kokkos* berry + *-osis* condition] an infection by tapeworms of the genus *Echinococcus.*

Echinococcus (e-ki″no-kok′us) [*echino-* + Gr. *kokkos* berry] a genus of tapeworms.

E. granulosus, a small tapeworm (2–8 mm long) that is chiefly parasitic in dogs and other carnivores. Infection in humans is caused by ingestion of the eggs, which develop into larvae and eventually into hydatid cysts, predominantly in the liver but also in other organs. Diagnostic tests include complement-fixation, flocculation, hemagglutination, and intracutaneous Casoni tests.

echinocyte (e-ki′no-sīt) [*echino-* + Gr. *kytos* hollow vessel] a spiculated red cell having 10–30 small projections evenly distributed over the cell surface. It occurs as an artifact in the preparation of blood smears, owing to changes in pH. It is occasionally found as a true in vivo alteration of erythrocytes in patients with renal failure and in those on heparin during cardiac bypass surgery. To determine whether the presence of echinocytes is an artifact, a fresh drop of blood placed between plastic coverslips is examined. Any echinocytes present with this technique are presumed to have been formed in vivo. Also called *berry cell, burr cell,* and *crenated cell.*

echinocytosis (e-ki″no-si-to′sis) [*echino-* + Gr. *kytos* hollow vessel + *-osis* condition] an irregularity in the form of an erythrocyte, which gives the cell a spiny appearance. See also *crenation* and *echinocyte.*

Echinostoma (ek″ĭ-nos′to-mah) [*echino-* + Gr. *stoma* mouth] a genus of parasitic flukes. *E. ilocanum* and E. *revolutum* are the most common species found in humans.

echinostomiasis (ē-kin″o-sto-mi′ah-sis) [*echino-* + Gr. *stoma* mouth + *-iasis*] an infection by various species of flukes of the genus *Echinostoma,* caused by the consumption of raw or improperly cooked freshwater snails and clams with encysted metocercariae. It rarely produces symptoms but may result in diarrhea.

echocardiogram (ek″o-kar′de-o-gram″) [*echo-* + Gr. *kardia* heart + *gramma* mark] the recording produced by echocardiography, commonly a film, paper copy, or videotape of the moving echoes that are displayed on an oscilloscope screen. The distance from the transducer to the portions of the heart examined is displayed along the ordinate (with the transducer and chest wall by convention at the top of the tracing), and time is displayed on the abscissa. The brightness of the recorded signal is related to the intensity of the reflected ultrasonic energy. See also the accompanying illustration.

echocardiograph (ek″o-kar′de-o-graph″) [*echo-* + Gr. *kardia* heart + *graphein* to record] an instrument used to record the echocardiogram.

echocardiography (ek″o-kar″de-og′rah-fe) a noninvasive technique for acoustic imaging of the heart. It is a highly useful diagnostic tool in the evaluation of ventricular function or of disorders such as idiopathic hypertrophic subaortic stenosis, atrial tumors, valvular stenosis or regurgitation, and congenital heart disease.

With the patient in a recumbent position, a transducer with a piezoelectric element is applied to the chest wall, usually near the left sternal border. The transducer emits short (1 μsec) pulses of ultrasonic (1–7 mHz) waves at a rate of 1000/sec. The ultrasonic beam, when directed toward the portion of the heart under examination, penetrates the chest wall and is reflected back from any interface between tissues with different acoustic impedances. The transducer also intermittently (for 999 μsec of every msec) acts as a receiver, detecting the reflected waves.

The echoes can then be displayed on an oscilloscope in the following ways. In the A (amplitude) mode, the distance of the interface from the transducer is displayed on the horizontal axis, and the strength of the reflected signal is displayed as spikes on the vertical axis. If the spikes of the A mode are reduced to an array of dots, with a brightness related to the echo intensity, the B (brightness) mode is recorded. Movement of the dots in either direction indicates movement (in a plane parallel to the beam) of the structures under study. A time factor is introduced by sweeping the B-mode echo across the oscilloscope screen (the M or motion mode). An M-mode scan can thus provide a record of the dimensions, thickness, and pattern of motion during each cardiac cycle of various structures in the heart.

The resolution of echocardiography depends on the sonic frequency of the test beam: the higher the frequency, the shorter the wavelength and the greater the resolution of the system. A drawback of ultrasound imaging is the relatively poor penetrating ability of high-frequency short-wavelength sound, as the depth in the chest that the beam can penetrate is greatly lessened. Thus in children, who have thinner, less dense chest walls than adults, a higher frequency sound wave is used to penetrate sufficiently while permitting greater resolution.

Frequencies of 1–7 MHz are commonly employed, with frequencies of 2–3 MHz typical of the values

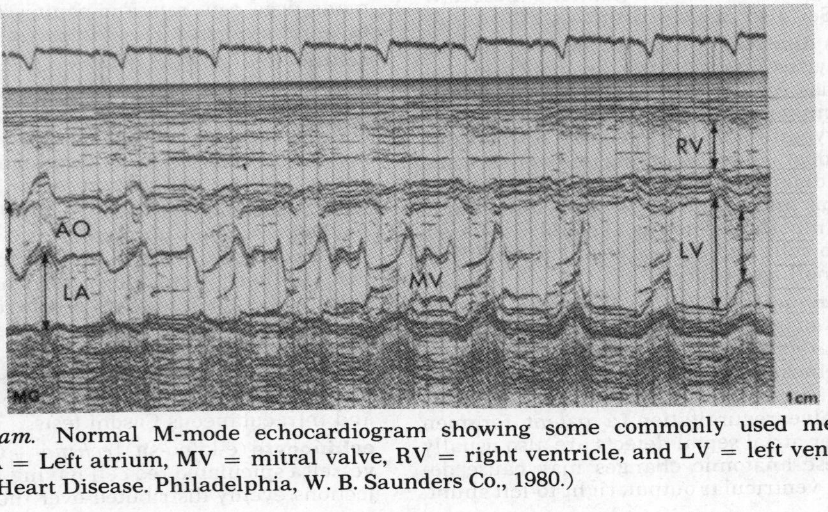

Echocardiogram. Normal M-mode echocardiogram showing some commonly used measurements; AO = aorta, LA = Left atrium, MV = mitral valve, RV = right ventricle, and LV = left ventricle. (From Braunwald, E.: Heart Disease. Philadelphia, W. B. Saunders Co., 1980.)

used in examining adults and 3–5 MHz in children. Most commercially available echocardiographs utilize a beam of 2.25 MHz in adults; this provides a resolution of 1–2 mm between points, yet still reserves sufficient penetrating power to provide adequate images. The higher frequencies employed in children resolve to less than 1 mm point to point.

contrast e., a technique in which the minute bubbles produced by the intravascular injection of a substance (the patient's blood, indocyanine green, 5 percent dextrose, or saline) are detected by echocardiographic techniques. It is used to determine whether right-to-left cardiac shunts are at the level of the atria or ventricles.

cross-sectional e., an echocardiographic examination produced by directing the rapidly moving ultrasonic beam across various axes of the heart. It allows for evaluation of the shape, spatial orientation, and lateral movement (in a plane perpendicular to the beam) of the heart. Long-axis studies are carried out by directing the beam along a plane parallel to the heart's greatest longitudinal axis. Views across the various planes perpendicular to the long axis (short-axis studies) can also be made. A variety of other cross-sectional views can be used to examine structures such as the pulmonary artery, arch of the aorta and base of the heart, papillary muscles, or right ventricular outflow tract.

One disadvantage of this technique is that the sampling rate is drastically reduced by the recording technique, which is usually restricted to 60 frames/sec; high-speed cinematography is being considered as a substitute method to eliminate this limitation. Also called real-time echocardiography.

Doppler e., an echocardiographic technique that utilizes the property of ultrasound waves in which the frequency of the reflected wave or echo is changed in proportion to the velocity of the moving object. Traditionally used with a continuous wave of ultrasound directed at blood flowing through the arteries and veins, Doppler techniques have permitted the evaluation of arterial obstructions, venous thrombosis, and blood flow patterns in central arteries. A recent advance has coupled Doppler technology with pulsed wave echocardiography; with this procedure, valvular regurgitation, stenosis, and intracardiac shunts can be detected.

echoencephalography (ek″o-en-sef″ah-log′rah-fe) [*echo-* + Gr. *enkephalos* brain + *graphein* to record] a method of A-mode ultrasonography in which pulses of ultrasound are transmitted through the head and are reflected from three structures: the skull boundaries on each side and the midline structures. A shift in the position of the midline echo may indicate the presence of a mass lesion such as a brain tumor or a subdural hematoma.

echogenic (ek″o-jen′ik) [*echo-* + Gr. *gennan* to produce] in ultrasonography, referring to areas of a sonogram that reflect ultrasound (produce echoes) and appear dark.

echogram (ek′o-gram) [*echo-* + Gr. *gramma* mark] see *sonogram.*

echography (ĕ-kog′rah-fe) [*echo-* + Gr. *graphein* to record] see *ultrasonography.*

echolucent (ek″o-loo′sent) [*echo-* + L. *lucere* to shine] see *sonolucent.*

echoophthalmography (ek″o-of-thal-mog′rah-fe) [*echo-* + Gr. *ophthalmos* eye + *graphein* to record] the use of ultrasonography in the examination of the eye and orbit.

echophonocardiography (ek″o-fo″no-kar″de-og′rah-fe) [*echo-* + Gr. *phōnē* sound + *kardia* heart + *graphein* to record] the combined use of echocardiography (cardiac ultrasound) and phonocardiography (recording of heart sounds and murmurs), usually in conjunction with a carotid pulse tracing and an electrocardiogram. This procedure is used in the evaluation of many heart disorders. See also *echocardiography* and *phonocardiography.*

echovirus (ek″o-vi′rus) [acronym from *e*nteric *c*ytopathic *h*uman *o*rphan + *virus*] an enterovirus that belongs to the picornavirus family, having 30 immunotypes. It consists of an outer capsid and a single strand of RNA without a lipid envelope.

The enteroviruses are termed echoviruses if they are found in the GI tract, produce cytopathic changes in cell cultures, and do not induce detectable pathologic lesions in suckling mice. Many echoviruses, however, are indistinguishable from other enteroviruses; therefore, those enteroviruses numbered 1–67 are still classified according to the tripart scheme, i.e., coxsackieviruses, polioviruses, and echoviruses. Agents 68–71 (to date) are now simply called enteroviruses, and all subdivisions have been dropped.

Echoviruses may be implicated in myocarditis, pericarditis, and upper respiratory tract and central nervous system infections. Echoviruses 1–9, 11–27, and 29–33 have been isolated in patients with viral meningitis, and types 2 and 11 in those with paralytic poliomyelitis.

ECI abbrev. See *electrocerebral inactivity.*

ECL abbrev. See *emitter-coupled logic.*

eclampsia (ĕ-klamp′se-ah) [Gr. *eklampein* to shine forth] a disorder that develops in the mother during the last trimester of pregnancy or immediately postpartum; it is characterized by the development of convulsions or coma in association with preeclampsia (hypertension, edema, and proteinuria). Laboratory tests show increased urea nitrogen, hemoconcentration, decreased serum protein, and reduced CO_2 content and combining power in the blood; urinalysis usually reveals proteinuria of 3+ to 4+. Cf. *preeclampsia.* See also *toxemia.*

eclipsed (e-klipst′) 1. pertaining to the least stable conformation of ethane (or one of its derivatives) in which the hydrogen atoms seem to overlap when viewed along the axis of the carbon-carbon bond.

2. referring to the bonds connecting two such overlapping hydrogen atoms (or substituent groups) to a carbon atom. See under *conformation.*

eclipse period (e-klips′) the period of time during the multiplication of a virus between the initial infection of the virus and the first appearance of new virions intracellularly.

ECM abbrev. for erythema chronicum migrans. See under *Lyme disease.*

ECoG abbrev. See *electrocorticogram* and *electrocorticography.*

E. coli see *E. coli* under *Escherichia.*

ecologic niche (e″ko-loj′ik) an organism's place in its environment. The niche may be considered physically as the actual habitat occupied by a population; more often, however, it is considered abstractly as a place along the spectrum of some ecologic variable, e.g., resource utilization.

ecology (e-kol′o-je) [Gr. *oikos* house + *-logy*] the branch of biology dealing with the interactions between organisms and their environment, and how the organisms' life strategies adapt them to their ecologic niches.

economic life the interval of time during which a piece of equipment has economic utility. Cf. *technologic life.*

Eco RI a restriction endonuclease from *Escherichia coli* that hydrolyzes double-stranded DNA between the GA site of the sequence GAATTC and the AG site of the palindromic complement. See also *restriction endonuclease.*

Eco RII a restriction endonuclease from *Escherichia coli* that hydrolyzes double-stranded DNA between the first GC site of the sequence GCCTGG and the second CG site of the palindromic complement. See also *restriction endonuclease.*

ecosystem (e′ko-sis″tem) a physical environment and the organisms that live there, considered as an interrelated unit.

ectasia (ek-ta′ze-ah) [Gr.] the expansion, dilation, or distention of a structure or organ.

-ectasia, -ectasis (ek-ta′ze-ah, ek′tah-sis) [Gr. *ektasis* stretching out + *-ia*] a suffix word element to denote stretching or dilation, e.g., sclerectasia.

ecto- (ek′to) [Gr. *ektos* outside] a prefix word element to denote out or outside, e.g., ectoderm.

ectoderm (ek′to-derm) [*ecto-* + Gr. *derma* skin] in the developing embryo, the outermost of the three primary germ layers; it remains chiefly as a sheet exposed on one surface throughout embryonic and fetal development. From it are differentiated the teeth, tongue, palate, salivary glands, hypophysis, anal canal, skin, mammary glands, nervous system, nose, eyes, and ears.

-ectomize (ek′to-mīz) [Gr. *ektomē* excision + *-izein* to render] a suffix word element to denote destruction or deprivation by excision, e.g., thyroidectomize.

-ectomy (ek′to-me) [Gr. *ektomē* excision] a suffix word element to denote removal, excision, or resection, e.g., laryngectomy.

ectoparasite (ek″to-par′ah-sīt) [*ecto-* + Gr. *parasitos* parasite] a parasite that is attached or embedded to the outside body of the host. Cf. *endoparasite.*

ectopia (ek-to′pe-ah) [Gr. *ektopos* displaced + *-ia*] the displacement or improper positioning, usually congenital, of a body organ or structure.

ectopic (ek-top′ik) 1. pertaining to or characterized by ectopia.

2. located in an abnormal position. Cf. *entopic.*

ectopic pregnancy a condition in which the fertilized ovum implants at a site other than the endometrium; its occurrence is about 1 in 200 gestations and is frequently associated with prior chronic pelvic inflammatory disease. Fallopian tubal pregnancies are by far the most common form of this condition, whereas ovarian or intraabdominal implantation is infrequent. The embryo commonly dies in the early weeks of pregnancy and the placental villi degenerate. Rupture of the tube is a frequent and serious complication; the resultant severe bleeding constitutes a medical emergency that requires prompt surgical intervention.

Laboratory studies of patients with ruptured tubal pregnancy may reveal anemia, an increased serum bilirubin, slight leukocytosis, and reticulocytosis. Posteroanterior radiographs and ultrasonography may reveal a pelvic mass. Pregnancy testing, culdoscopy, laparoscopy, and the obtaining of nonclotting blood on colpocentesis may also be useful in diagnosis. Concentrations of β-hCG are significantly lower than those observed at the same gestational age in a normal pregnancy.

See also *pregnancy tests.*

ectoplasm (ek′to-plazm) [*ecto-* + Gr. *plasma* a thing formed] a thin, shell-like layer of cytoplasm near the cell membrane, believed to have a gel-like consistency and sometimes containing filaments. Cf. *endoplasm.*

ectothrix (ek′to-thriks) [*ekto-* + Gr. *thrix* hair] a fungal invasion with vegetative hyphae growing inside the hair shaft and a sheath of arthrospores on the outside of the hair. Cf. *endothrix.*

ectothrix infection a fungal infection in which arthrospores form a sheath around a hair shaft under the cuticle of the hair. Fungi that cause ectothrix infections include *Microsporum audouinii, M. canis,* and *M. ferrugineum.* These fungal infections are Wood's lamp–positive.

ectozoon (ek″to-zo′on), pl. *ectozoa* [*ecto-* + Gr. *zōon* animal] an external parasite.

ectropion (ek-tro′pe-on) [Gr. *ektropion,* from *ek* out + *tropē* turning] the turning outward (eversion) of an edge or margin, applied particularly to the eyelid where the process can expose the palpebral conjunctiva. When applied to the cervix uteri, the term also refers to the eversion of endocervical columnar mucosa onto the ectocervix.

eczema (ek′ze-mah) [Gr. *ekzein* to boil out] a superficial inflammation of the skin, characterized by variable degrees of redness, itching, vesicles, and discharge, often with crusting and thickening as it progresses. The most common type is atopic eczematous dermatitis, caused by a sensitizing antigen in the diet or environment. See also *atopic d.* under *dermatitis.*

ED_{50} abbrev. See *median effective d.* under *dose.*

eddy current (ed′e) a circular current produced in a conductor by a changing magnetic field.

eddy-current loss power dissipated in forming eddy currents in the magnetic core of a transformer or inductor.

Edecrin (ĕ-dek′rin) trademark. See *ethacrynic acid.*

edema (ĕ-de′mah) [Gr. *oidēma* swelling] excessive accumulation of fluid in the tissue spaces. The principal disturbances that may induce edema include an elevated venous capillary pressure (as in the edema of heart failure), hypoproteinemia with reduced plasma oncotic pressure (as in the nephrotic syndrome), increased capillary permeability to fluids and proteins (as in the inflammatory response to tissue injury), failure of the lymphatics to remove fluid and protein adequately from the interstitial space (as in filariasis or other parasitic infections), and increased mucopolysaccharide content in the interstitial space (as in endocrine disorders such as myxedema).

angioneurotic e., acute, painless swelling of the subcutaneous tissue or submucosa of the face, hands, feet, genitalia, or viscera secondary to localized edema. It may be hereditary or a transient, sporadic condition caused by food or drug allergy.

Death may result if the edema develops in a critical area, e.g., the larynx.

Hereditary angioneurotic edema (HANE) is marked by a relative or absolute lack of C1 esterase inhibitor (C1 INH), which leads to increased vascular permeability, possibly through the mediation of the rest of the complement pathway. This deficiency can be detected by immunodiffusion techniques for C1 INH. Severe abdominal pain and vomiting are common in the familial condition and can help to distinguish it from the transient form. HANE is transmitted as an autosomal dominant trait and is thus manifest in heterozygotes. Usually, levels of C2 and C4 are reduced, even in the attack-free period. Some patients exhibit the presence of an abnormal C1 INH molecule that lacks activity. The disease has been successfully treated with EACA (ϵ-aminocaproic acid) and attenuated testosterone derivatives. Recently, an acquired form in association with lymphomas has been described.

Also called *angioedema.*

cerebral e., abnormal accumulation of fluid and associated volumetric enlargement of the tissue of the cerebrum. This may primarily involve the extravascular intercellular compartment of the brain (interstitial edema), or the cellular elements so that there is a reduction in the extracellular fluid space (cytotoxic edema).

A variable amount of cerebral edema can complicate (and sometimes threaten life in) conditions such as bacterial meningitis, intracranial tumor, serious head injury, and cerebral infarction, and may increase the neurologic deficit that occurs. On pathologic examination, the edematous cerebrum appears swollen, pale, and moist, with flattened gyri and narrowed sulci.

dependent e., a type of incompletely characterized edema that commonly affects the lower limbs, but may involve other body parts that are in a lowered or dependent position. It is often relieved by elevation of the affected part.

pulmonary e., a pathologic state in which there is an excessive, diffuse accumulation of fluid in the pulmonary interstitium and alveolar airspaces. Pulmonary edema is primarily precipitated by factors that cause an imbalance in the Starling equilibrium in the lung (the balance between the forces that favor filtration of fluid from the pulmonary capillary blood to the tissues and those that promote absorption of fluid into the capillary blood from the tissues and return of fluid to the circulation via the lymphatics). Among these factors are an increase in pulmonary capillary hydrostatic pressure (the cardiogenic forms of pulmonary edema, or those secondary to conditions such as mitral stenosis and left ventricular failure) and a decrease in plasma oncotic pressure (hypoalbuminemia secondary to hepatic and renal disease or dermatologic or nutritional disorders). The Starling equilibrium can also be upset by any factor that directly injures the alveolocapillary membrane, thus increasing its permeability. These factors include bacterial and viral infections, pulmonary embolism, shock lung, inhalation of noxious gases, immunologic disorders, or the presence of endogenous vasoactive agents. Less frequently, disorders that lead to less effective pumping by the pulmonary lymphatics can result in an abnormal accumulation of extravascular fluid. Diverse factors such as high altitude, eclampsia, anesthesia, cardioversion, cardiopulmonary bypass surgery, central nervous system disorders, and narcotic overdose can also lead to pulmonary edema through mechanisms that are as yet poorly understood.

The clinical manifestations of pulmonary edema may begin with a cough, wheezing, dyspnea, and a feeling of oppression in the chest. A rapid, shallow pattern of breathing becomes apparent, presumably a reflex response to stimulation of the pulmonary interstitial J receptors. In a severe, acute attack of pulmonary edema, the individual gasps for breath, becomes pale, sweaty, and cyanotic, and may expectorate a frothy, blood-tinged sputum. Diffusing capacity and gas exchange are impaired, leading to a progressively severe hypoxemia. Rhonchi and moist, bubbly, and fine crepitant rales become most markedly audible in the dependent portions of the lungs, and extend upward as the attack of edema worsens. Cardiac auscultation often reveals a third heart sound, and frequently an accentuation of the pulmonic component of the second sound. Pulmonary capillary wedge pressure may be elevated to values above 25–30 mmHg. Radiologic features commonly present include prominent and congested vessels, thickening of the interlobular septa (Kerley B lines), or confluent, patchy densities that may have the appearance of wings extending out from the mediastinum ("bat wing" perihilar shadows).

edetate (ed′ĕ-tāt) the nonproprietary drug name for the chelating agent ethylenediaminetetraacetate, the salt of edetic acid. See also *EDTA.*

calcium disodium e., a chelating agent used in the treatment of lead poisoning; the calcium disodium salt of ethylenediaminetetraacetic acid (EDTA). Excessive doses may cause renal tubular necrosis.

edetic acid (e-det′ik) the nonproprietary drug name for ethylenediaminetetraacetic acid; see *EDTA.*

edge packing a type of distortion in scintillation photographs. An image of a regular pattern of dots would have the dots packed together near the edges of the image.

Edinger-Westphal nucleus (ed′ing-ger vest′fahl) [Ludwig *Edinger,* German neurologist, 1855–1918; Carl Friedrich Otto *Westphal,* German neurologist, 1833–1890] see *Edinger-Westphal n.* under *nucleus.*

Edman reaction (ed′man) a procedure that results in the stepwise removal of amino acids from the amino terminus of a peptide, used in the sequencing of a purified peptide or protein. The treatment of a peptide or protein with phenylisothiocyanate (Edman's reagent) produces a coupling with the free alpha amino group of the *N*-terminal amino acid, giving the phenylthiocarbamyl (PTC) derivative of the peptide or protein. This is then cleaved to a peptide or protein with one less residue, and the thiazolinone of the *N*-terminal amino acid. This rearranges to the phenylthiohydantoin (PTH) derivative, which is extracted from the reaction mixture, converted to a volatile derivative, and identified by gas chromatography.

edrophonium chloride (ed″ro-fo′ne-um) [USP], a cholinesterase-inhibiting drug used in the differential diagnosis of myasthenia gravis, in the differentiation of myasthenic crisis from cholinergic crisis, and also as an antidote to curariform muscle relaxants such as tubocurarine, metocurine, and pancuronium. The duration of the effect is about 10 min. Adverse reactions are the cholinergic effects of excessive cholinesterase inhibition. Trademark, *Tensilon.*

EDTA a chelating agent, ethylenediaminetetraacetic acid (nonproprietary drug name, edetic acid), $(HOOCCH_2)_2NCH_2CH_2N(CH_2COOH)_2$, which chelates many divalent and trivalent metals; M.W. 292.24. The disodium and dipotassium salts are commonly used as anticoagulants for blood specimens and whole blood in clinical chemistry and hematology. EDTA acts by binding calcium ions necessary for the clotting process. Calcium disodium salt is used in the diagnosis and therapy of lead poisoning; it acts by binding lead (and, to a lesser extent, zinc and other ions), thus increasing their excretion in the urine.

Edwardsiella (ed-ward′se-el″ah) [Philip R. *Edwards,* U.S. bacteriologist, born 1901] a genus of *Salmonella*-like bacteria of the Enterobacteriaceae family, consisting of small gram-negative rods, motile with peritrichous flagella; H_2S-positive. They ferment only glucose and maltose. The species *E. tarda,* occasionally found in the human intestinal tract, can cause acute gastroenteritis and serious septic infections. See also *Enterobacteriaceae.*

Edwards-Patau syndrome (ed′wardz pah-tow′) [John Hilton *Edwards,* English geneticist, born 1928; Klaus *Patau,* U.S. cytogeneticist, 20th century] see *trisomy 18 syndrome.*

EDX abbrev. See *electrodiagnosis.*

EEE abbrev. See *eastern equine e.* under *encephalitis.*

EEG abbrev. See *electroencephalogram.*

effect (e-fekt′) 1. the result of a cause, agent, or action.

2. to produce a result.

effective current a measure of alternating current equal to the amount of direct current that would produce the same power in a resistive load: 0.707 of the peak current. Also called root-mean-square current.

effective half-life (T_{eff}) the time for half of an amount of a radioisotope to either decay or be excreted; its reciprocal is the sum of the reciprocals of the physical half-life (T_p) and of the biologic half-life (T_b), i.e., $1/T_{eff} = 1/T_p + 1/T_b$.

effective renal plasma flow (ERPF) a measure of the flow of blood through the kidney. The reference procedure is the clearance of *p*-aminohippuric acid (PAH). It may also be measured using ^{131}I orthoiodohippuric acid (OIH).

effective voltage a measure of the voltage of alternating current equal to the direct current voltage that would produce the same power in a resistive load: 0.707 of the peak voltage. Also called root-mean-square voltage.

effector (ĕ-fek′tor) 1. a muscle or gland that reacts to nerve impulses, producing an effect (contraction or secretion).

2. a cell that mediates an effect of the immune system; see *effector cells.*

3. a molecule that binds to an enzyme.

effector cells (ĕ-fek′tor) a general term used to describe lymphocytes that are the direct mediators of the immune response. The term includes antibody-secreting B cells, as well as lymphokine-producing and killer or cytotoxic T cells and null cells and monocytes. Effector cells are distinguished from regulatory cells such as helper T and suppressor T cells, which interact with effector cells to modulate their response.

efferent (ef′er-ent) [L. *effere* to carry away] conducting or conveying away from the center. The term is often used to describe the blood vessels flowing away from an organ, the lymphatics leaving a lymph node, or neurons leaving the central nervous system. Cf. *afferent.*

efficiency (e-fish′en-se) the relative ability to accomplish a task. In gas chromatography, efficiency is measured by the narrowness of peaks. See also *theoretical plate.*

efflorescence (ef″lo-res′ens) [L. *efflorescere* to bloom] the loss of water of hydration from a crystal to the air because the vapor pressure of the water is higher in the crystal than in the air.

effuse [L. *effusus,* from *ex* out + *fundere* to pour] 1. (ĕ-fūs′), spread out, profuse; said of bacterial growth that is thin, veil-like, and unusually widely spread.

2. (ĕ-fūz′), to pour out and spread widely.

effusion (ĕ-fu′zhun) [L. *effusio* a pouring out] 1. the escape of fluids into body spaces or cavities.

2. the fluid material (e.g., pericardial, peritoneal, pleural) that escapes into body spaces or cavities. See also the accompanying tables.

effusion cytology the study of cells in effusions using routine techniques of exfoliative cytology. The cells may be concentrated by sedimentation or centrifugation. If many red blood cells contaminate the specimen, they can be partially removed by hemolysis: this is particularly desirable if electron microscopy is to be used in addition to preparing conventional Papanicolaou-stained smears. By light microscopy, it is usually possible to distinguish between inflammatory and neoplastic processes; in the case of malignant neoplasms, the cell type of a tumor can frequently be identified.

egg (eg) the female gamete; see also *ovum.*

egg counts quantitative techniques for estimating the parasite burden in an individual. They are a useful diagnostic tool, making it possible to determine whether the infection is incidental, moderate, or heavy. Techniques have been developed for hookworm, *Ascaris,* and *Trichuris* that consist of counting the eggs found in the stool. See also *Beaver's direct egg-count technique* and *Stoll's dilution egg-count technique.*

egobronchophony (e″go-bron-kof′o-ne) [Gr. *aix, aigos* goat + *bronchos* windpipe + *phōnē* voice] a diagnostic sign occurring most frequently in lung tissue compression by pleural effusion, which can be detected by auscultation of the chest wall and lungs. It is characterized by increased vocal resonance and a high-pitched bleating quality of the transmitted voice. Also called *egophony.*

egophony (e-gof′o-ne) [Gr. *aigos* goat + *phōnē* voice] see *egobronchophony.*

egress (e′gres) [L. *egressus,* from *egredi* to go out] a continuous and unobstructed way of exit travel from any point in a building or structure to a public way. A means of egress consists of three separate and distinct parts: the way of exit access (such as a corridor), the exit (such as an enclosed stairwell), and the way of exit discharge (such as the passageway from the bottom of the stairwell to the street). Adequate means of egress from laboratories are important so that occupants can escape promptly in case of fire or other emergency.

EFFUSION, TABLE 1. CHYLOUS AND PSEUDOCHYLOUS EFFUSIONS

	CHYLOUS EFFUSION	PSEUDOCHYLOUS EFFUSION
Appearance	Milky: may form creamy top layer on standing	Milky to greenish—or "gold paint" appearance
Odor	Odorless	Variable from odorless to foul
pH	Alkaline	Variable
Extraction with ether after acidification with dilute HCl	Clearing and decrease in volume	Does not clear or decrease in volume
Microscopic examination	Lymphocytes plus fine fat droplets	Mixed cellular reaction with cholesterol crystals
Triglycerides	2x-8x serum triglycerides	Lower than serum triglycerides
Cholesterol	Lower than serum cholesterol	May be higher than serum cholesterol
Lipoprotein electrophoresis	Increased chylomicron band in relation to plasma	Chylomicrons scanty or absent
Effect of diet with no long-chain fatty acids	Decreased accumulation of lipid in effusion	No significant change in effusion
Ingestion of lipophilic dye	Dye appears in effusion	Dye does not appear in effusion
Culture	Always sterile	Usually sterile (check for tuberculosis or fungus)
Etiology	Damage or obstruction to thoracic duct	Chronic effusion of any cause (e.g., cyst fluid, rheumatoid disease, tuberculosis, myxedema)

From Henry, J. B.: Clinical Diagnosis and Management. 16th ed. Philadelphia, W. B. Saunders Co., 1979, p. 667.

Ehrlich's diazo reagent (ār′liks) [Paul *Ehrlich,* German bacteriologist, 1854–1915; co-winner of the Nobel Prize for his work in immunity] a sodium *p*-diazobenzenesulfonate solution, formed by mixing sodium nitrite, sulfanilic acid, and hydrochloric acid just before use. It is used primarily in the determination of bilirubin, which is measured spectrophotometrically as azobilirubin. See also *bilirubin assays.*

Ehrlich unit (EU) [Paul *Ehrlich*] a unit of urobilinogen quantity defined or equivalent to 1 mg of urobilinogen, as assayed by Ehrlich's method using *p*-dimethylaminobenzaldehyde as color reagent.

EI abbrev. See *eosinophilic i.* under *squamous cell index.*

EIA abbrev. for Electronics Industries Association, enzyme immunoassay (see *nonradioisotopic i.* under *immunoassays*).

EIA interface an interface between a computer and a specific system for transmitting digital information by wire. The interface specification (e.g., EIA RS-232-C or EIA RS-366) describes the cable connectors and the electrical signals, so that two machines with the same interface can be connected together with the standard cable.

Eikenella (i″ken-el′ah) a genus of bacteria that consists of gram-negative, facultatively anaerobic rods that do not ferment glucose. The organisms do not grow on MacConkey agar, are oxidase- and nitrate-positive, and are nonmotile. The colonies are tiny, and about one-half of isolates show the characteristic ability to "pit" or corrode the agar surface. The organism is part of the normal flora of mucous membrane surfaces but also occurs in human infections of the gums and soft tissues. The genus contains a single species, *E. corrodens.*

einsteinium (Es) (īn-sti′ne-um) [Albert *Einstein,* German-born theoretical physicist, 1879–1955; winner of the Nobel Prize for explanation of the photoelectric effect and the invention of special and general theories of relativity] a synthetic, metallic radioactive element; atomic number 99; most stable isotope ^{254}Es (half-life, 276 da); a 5f transition element (actinide element); oxidation states +2, +3.

Einthoven's law (īn′to-venz) [Willem *Einthoven,* Dutch physiologist, 1860–1927; winner of the Nobel Prize for his discovery of the mechanism of the electrocardiogram] stated as: the algebraic sum of the potential differences recorded in leads I and III of the electrocardiogram is equal to the electric potential in lead II at any instant in time.

Einthoven's triangle [Willem *Einthoven*] a diagram devised by Einthoven in which the axes of the standard limb leads of the electrocardiogram (leads I, II, and III) form an equilateral triangle, with the heart at its center and apices at the right shoulder, left shoulder, and left hip.

ejection (e-jek′shun) [L. *e* out + *jacere* to cast] 1. the act of ejecting or the state of being ejected. 2. something ejected.

ejection fraction the fraction of the blood that a heart chamber contains when filled, which is pumped out during contraction. The most significant ejection fractions are those of the ventricles, particularly the left ventricle. The passage through the heart of an intravenously injected bolus of a radiopharmaceutical such as ^{99m}Tc human serum albumin is recorded via a scintillation camera that has computerized data analysis. The activity of a region of interest that covers the left ventricle is

EFFUSION, TABLE 2. CAUSES OF PLEURAL, PERICARDIAL, AND PERITONEAL EFFUSIONS

PLEURAL

Transudates
- Congestive heart failure
- Hepatic cirrhosis
- Hypoproteinemia (e.g., nephrotic syndrome)

Exudates
- Neoplasms
  - bronchogenic carcinoma
  - metastatic carcinoma
  - lymphoma
  - mesothelioma (increased hyaluronate content of effusion fluid)
- Infections
  - tuberculosis (high percentage of lymphocytes with under 1% mesothelial cells)
  - bacterial pneumonia
  - viral or mycoplasmal pneumonia
- Trauma (may be associated with hemorrhagic effusion)
- Pulmonary infarct (may be associated with hemorrhagic effusion)
- Rheumatoid disease (low pleural fluid glucose in most cases)
- Systemic lupus erythematosus (LE cells occasionally present)
- Pancreatitis (elevated amylase activity in effusion fluid)
- Ruptured esophagus (elevated amylase activity and low pH in effusion fluid)

Chylous effusion
- Damage or obstruction to thoracic duct, e.g., trauma, lymphoma, carcinoma, tuberculosis

PERICARDIAL

Exudates
- Infections
  - bacterial pericarditis
  - tuberculosis
  - fungal pericarditis
  - viral or mycoplasmal pericarditis
- Neoplasms
  - metastic carcinoma or lymphoma

PERICARDIAL (continued)

Exudates (continued)
- Trauma (may be associated with hemorrhagic effusion)
- Myocardial infarct
- Hemorrhagic effusion
  - secondary to anticoagulant therapy
  - leakage of aortic aneurysm
- Metabolic (uremia, myxedema)
- Rheumatoid disease
- Systemic lupus erythematosus

PERITONEAL

Transudates
- Congestive heart failure
- Hepatic cirrhosis
- Hypoproteinemia (e.g., nephrotic syndrome)

Exudates
- Neoplasms
  - hepatoma
  - metastatic carcinoma
  - lymphoma
  - mesothelioma
- Infections
  - tuberculosis
  - primary bacterial peritonitis (may be superimposed on transudate)
  - secondary bacterial peritonitis (e.g., appendicitis, intestinal infarct)
- Trauma
- Pancreatitis
- Bile peritonitis (secondary to ruptured gallbladder or gallbladder or needle perforation of bile duct)

Chylous effusion
- Damage or obstruction to thoracic duct, e.g., trauma, lymphoma, carcinoma, tuberculosis, parasitic infestation

From Henry, J. B.: Clinical Diagnosis and Management. 16th ed. Philadelphia, W. B. Saunders Co., 1979, p. 668.

measured at the end of diastole and at the end of systole, either by triggering the camera exposures with an electrocardiogram or by computer analysis. The ejection fraction is the difference in activity divided by the end-diastolic activity.

ejection sounds high-pitched clicking sounds heard very shortly after the first heart sound, attributed to the forceful opening of a diseased pulmonic or aortic valve (valvular ejection sound); also heard in conditions with a dilated pulmonary artery or aorta (vascular ejection sound). Also called ejection click.

ejection time see left ventricular ejection time under *systolic time intervals.*

EKG abbrev. See *electrocardiogram.*

Ektachem (ek′tah-kem) trademark for a clinical chemistry analyzer that uses thin-film technology; see under *clinical chemistry automation.*

EL abbrev. See *erythroleukemia* under *leukemia.*

elaidic acid (el″a-id′ik) an unsaturated fatty acid, *trans*-9-octadecenoic acid, isomeric with oleic acid. The two isomers equilibrate under acidic conditions.

elastance (*E*) (e-las′tans) the tendency of a structure (e.g., lung, urinary bladder) to recoil or return to its original nonstretched position when a distending or compressing pressure or force has been removed. It is the reciprocal of compliance and is commonly expressed as a unit volume change per unit change in pressure. See also *elastic recoil of the lungs.*

elastase (e-las′tās) an endopeptidase of the hydrolase class (EC 3.4.21.11) that catalyzes the hydrolysis of elastin and polypeptides at peptide bonds containing uncharged nonaromatic side-chains, such as in leucine and serine. It is secreted as a proelastase by the pancreas and activated by trypsin, and is important in the digestion of proteins in the small intestine. The enzyme also degrades the mucopeptides of certain bacterial cell walls.

elastic (e-las′tik) [L. *elasticus,* from Gr. *elastos* ductile, beaten] 1. pertaining to a material that, when stretched, compressed, or distorted, returns to its original shape when released.

2. pertaining to the limits to which a material can be distorted and still resume its original shape.

elastica (e-las′tĭ-ka) [L.] a general term for the elastic tissue found in blood vessels, particularly the internal and external elastic laminae.

elastic fibers yellowish fibers, about 0.2–1.0 μm in diameter, found in connective tissue. They are composed of elastin, which is synthesized by fibroblasts. Elastic fibers give flexibility and resilience to tissues such as the walls of blood vessels, bronchial tree, and pulmonary alveoli; the yellow (flaval) ligaments of the vertebral column; the auricular cartilage of the external ear; and the dermis of the skin.

Viewed with a polarizing microscope, elastic fibers are seen to have a weak birefringence, which becomes stronger as they stretch. Under ultraviolet light, they have a yellowish autofluorescence. They frequently give a weak reaction with stains for amyloid. When elastic fibers degenerate with age, calcium salts or acid mucopolysaccharides may replace some of their material.

elastic fiber stains a group of empirical procedures that probably involve hydrogen bonding of the dye to elastin, although the exact mechanism is unknown. Acid solutions of basic dyes (fuchsin, hematoxylin, orcein) are most commonly used, but alkaline solutions of acid dyes also selectively bind to elastic fibers. Elastase, a pancreatic enzyme that digests elastin, may be used for specific identification. For more information, see the specific methods, e.g., *acid orcein, aldehyde fuchsin, resorcin fuchsin,* and *Verhoeff's stain.*

elasticity (e″las-tis′ĭ-te) the quality or condition of being elastic, i.e., of returning to the original shape after being deformed.

elastic lamellae fenestrated elastic sheets 2–3 μm thick in the tunica media of elastic (conducting) arteries. They are separated by collagenous fibers, smooth muscle cells, and fibroblasts.

external e. l., a thin elastic layer found between the tunica media and the tunica adventitia of the larger arteries.

internal e. l., a fenestrated elastic layer found between the tunica intima and tunica media of arteries, arterioles, and the larger veins.

elastic recoil of the lungs the tendency of the lungs to collapse and retract away from the chest wall, or the recoil pressure that develops as the result of lung inflation. The tendency of the elastic fibers in lung tissue to shorten to their original position after being stretched by lung inflation (potential energy being stored in the fibers during inspiration), and the tendency of the alveoli to collapse because of the surface tension of the fluid that lines them, both contribute to the development of recoil pressure.

At any lung volume, elastic recoil pressure is equal to the change in transpulmonary pressure (the difference between intrapleural and alveolar pressure) necessary to produce a given change in lung volume. It is determined from a plot of the static pressure-volume relationship of the lungs. At functional residual capacity (with the respiratory muscles relaxed), lung recoil pressure is balanced by an equal and opposite tendency of the chest wall to expand, and the total pressure in the airways and mouth is equal to zero. Pleural pressure is a negative 3–5 cm of H_2O at functional residual capacity (FRC), reflecting the normal recoil properties of the lungs.

Loss of elastic recoil properties of the lungs occurs in individuals who are emphysematous or asthmatic (with bronchospasm), and with advancing age.

Also called elastance of the lungs. Cf. *compliance.*

elastin (e-las′tin) [*elastic* + *-in*] a fibrous protein, the essential constituent of elastic fibers that give certain tissues the ability to stretch and return to their original shape without tearing or deforming. Elastic fibers occur in arterial walls and the vocal cords; in the pleura, tracheobronchial tree, and alveolar septa in the lungs; and also in certain ligaments and cartilages. As in collagen, approximately one-third of the residues in elastin are composed of glycine; there is also a high proportion of alanine, proline, and valine. Elastin differs from collagen, however, in that: (1) glycine does not occur in a tripeptide repeating unit, (2) it contains little hydroxyproline, and (3) it does not have a triple-helix structure.

The elastin molecule is formed by cross-linking of small globular subunits. The cross-links are of two types, both involving lysine residues. In one type, one lysine residue and three allysine (the ε-aldehyde of lysine) residues are condensed to form a desmosine or isodesmosine heterocyclic ring. The conversion of the ε-amino group of lysine to an ε-aldehyde group is catalyzed by the copper-containing enzyme lysyl oxidase. Copper deficiency in growing animals can produce deposition of defective elastin, which may lead to the rupture of major blood vessels. The other type of cross-link is formed by the condensation of a lysine residue with a hydroxylysine residue.

elastofibroma (e-las″to-fi-bro′mah) [*elastin* + L. *fibra* fiber + Gr. *ōma* swelling] a tumor consisting of both elastin and fibrous elements.

e. dorsi, an uncommon lesion located in most instances deep to the angle of the scapula, composed of fibrous tissue with many fragmented elastic fibers. It is suspected to be a peculiar response to prolonged irritation.

Elavil (el′ah-vil) trademark. See *amitriptyline.*

elbow (el′bo) [M.E. *elbowe*] 1. the bend of the arm. Also called cubitus.

2. any angular bend.

elbow joint the synovial hinge joint between the arm and forearm where the humerus articulates with the head of the radius and trochlear notch of the ulna.

electr/o [Gr. *ēlektron* amber (static electricity was found to be produced by rubbing cloth on amber)] a word element used in combining form to denote relationship to electricity, e.g., electrophoresis.

electric (e-lek′trik) of the nature of electricity.

electrical (e-lek′trĭ-kal) pertaining to electricity.

electrical alternans a change in the amplitudes of the QRS complex that occurs with alternate (or less commonly, with every two or three) heartbeats. This electrocardiographic feature, seen in pathologic conditions such as cardiac tamponade, pericardial effusion, pneumothorax, severe dysfunction of the cardiac muscle, and paroxysmal supraventricular tachycardia, is thought to be the result of a cyclic cardiac motion within the pericardium.

electrical artifact see under *artifact.*

electric field vector (E) the force per unit charge exerted on a stationary charge at a given point by the electromagnetic field; measured in volts per meter (V/m). Together, the electric field vector and the magnetic field vector describe the electromagnetic field. Also called electric field intensity, electric field strength, and electric vector.

electricity (e″lek-tris′ĭ-te) 1. the physical phenomenon that involves electric charges and the electromagnetic forces that act on them.
2. alternating current or direct current electric power.

electric potential the potential energy per unit charge of an electrostatic field; measured in units of volts (V). Also called *voltage* and, in electrochemistry, *electromotive force.*

electric potential difference the difference between the electric potentials of two points. Also called *voltage.*

electric susceptibility (χ or χ_e) the ratio of the polarization of a dielectric to the applied electric field. See also *dielectric.*

electrocardiogram (ECG, EKG) (e-lek″tro-kar′de-o-gram″) [*electro-* + Gr. *kardia* heart + *gramma* mark] a recording of the electrical activity of the heart. See also *electrocardiography.*

electrocardiograph (e-lek″tro-kar′de-o-graf″) [*electro-* + Gr. *kardia* heart + *graphein* to record] an instrument for recording electric potentials at the body surface that have been generated by the heart. See also *electrocardiography.*

electrocardiography (e-lek″tro-kar″de-og′rah-fe) the technique of measuring changes in the electrical activity of the heart using electrodes placed on the surface of the body. The recording of the depolarization and repolarization waves that pass over the heart muscle and its conducting system in each cardiac cycle is affected by the morphology of the heart and its chambers, the shape of the thorax, the conductivity of the body tissues through which the potential is recorded, and the electrical influence of neighboring cells on the potential. Electrode placement is shown in the accompanying illustration.

The electrocardiogram (ECG) presents a characteristic pattern of wave forms, which are referred to as the P wave, QRS complex, T wave, and U wave. The P wave corresponds to a wave of depolarization crossing the atria; the QRS complex, to the depolarization of the ventricles; and the T wave, to the repolarization of the ventricles. Sometimes the T wave is followed by the relatively low-amplitude, slow U wave, which is thought to originate from the repolarization of the papillary muscles.

P WAVE. The P wave originates at the sinoatrial (SA) node and moves primarily inferiorly and to the left, with a smaller component moving anteriorly to depolarize the right atrium; the duration of this wave is approximately 100 ms, with an amplitude of 0.2 mV in lead II. Following the P wave is a quiescent period of about 80 ms during which most of the cells of the atrioventricular (A-V) node become depolarized. No potential is recorded owing to the small number of cells involved, and thus a very small electric potential results.

QRS COMPLEX. The Q, R, and S waves, or the QRS complex, represent the wave of depolarization invading the ventricles and their septum. Initially, the wave of excitation courses from the left ventricular endocardium toward the center of the septum in its middle and apical portions. It then proceeds from right to left and from the endocardium to the epicardium in the apical walls of the ventricles. Activity terminates in the thin right ventricular wall while continuing to invade the central regions of the left ventricular wall, finally terminating in the basal septum and basilar regions of the left ventricular wall. These changes in the direction of the wave of depolarization result in the complex QRS waveform that mirrors their progression through the ventricles. The QRS complex usually lasts about 80 ms with an amplitude of about 1 mV in lead II.

T WAVE. The T wave represents the wave of repolarization across the ventricles as the cells return to their resting state. In most recording configurations the T wave has the same polarity as the QRS complex, indicating that repolarization follows a course opposite that of depolarization.

The earliest ECGs were recorded with bipolar leads using a triangular pattern of electrode placement. Named for its designer, the Einthoven triangle represents the axes of the bipolar limb leads I, II, and III, which measure potentials between the right arm and left arm, right arm and left leg, and left

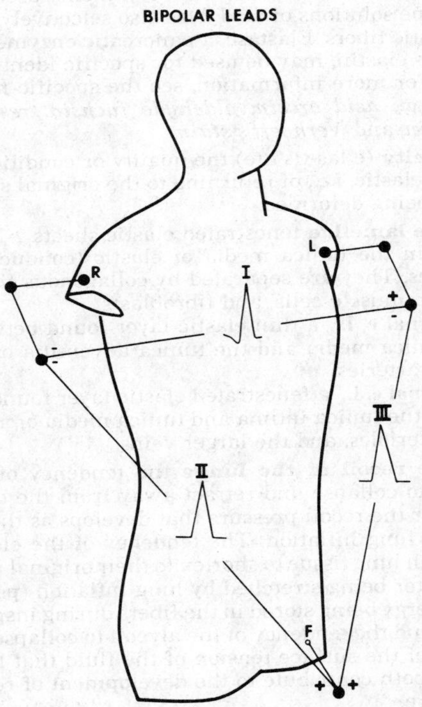

Electrocardiography. Electrode placements commonly used in electrocardiography and vectorcardiography are the bipolar limb leads I, II, and III, which are derived from the placement of electrodes on the right upper extremity (R), left upper extremity (L), and left lower extremity (F). (Modified from Braunwald, E.: Heart Disease. Philadelphia, W. B. Saunders Co., 1980.)

arm and left leg, respectively. The right leg is connected as the ground. A "central terminal" for the reference electrode was proposed by Wilson. In this arrangement, the three limb leads are interconnected and approximate a "zero terminal" for reference with exploring unipolar electrodes. This allows a determination of local unipolar voltage. Wilson's central terminal is used for recording unipolar limb leads and precordial unipolar leads V_1–V_6. An improvement on Wilson's central terminal was introduced by Goldberger in an effort to increase the amplitude of recorded potentials. The scheme utilized the interconnection of two limb leads as a reference electrode, with the exploring electrode on the third limb. This configuration augments the amplitude of the recorded potentials by about 50 percent, hence their designation as augmented leads — aV_r, aV_l, and aV_f for the right arm, left arm, and left leg (foot), respectively. Goldberger's leads are generally wired into most electrocardiographic recorders available commercially. Six precordial or chest leads (V_1–V_6) are routinely used in electrocardiography. These unipolar exploring electrodes are placed on the chest at defined positions extending from the right parasternal border at the fourth intercostal space (V_1) to the left midaxillary line.

A standard 12-lead ECG includes three bipolar limb leads (I, II, III), three augmented unipolar limb leads (aV_r, aV_l, aV_f) and six precordial leads (V_1–V_6). Certain conventions of recording are followed to facilitate easy analysis of the ECG. The amplifier should be calibrated so that a 1-mV potential results in a 1-cm deflection, and the recording paper movement should be 25 mm/sec.

ECG analysis requires substantial practical experience and familiarity with the various pathologic changes that may alter the electric potentials produced by the heart. Certain basic features of the recording should be noted to make such an analysis. Initially, the heart rate should be determined; the atrial and ventricular rates should be noted to help ascertain the rhythm and whether normal A-V conduction is present. The relationship of the P wave and QRS complex should be examined to determine whether they are constant or variable. Particular attention should be directed to the P-R interval, which may indicate abnormality in the conduction system. The shape, duration, and amplitude of the QRS complex is noted, which may be altered during premature systoles, in ventricular conduction defects, by ventricular hypertrophy, and following myocardial infarction. The Q-T interval is measured; it can be altered by disease, drugs, and imbalance of electrolytes. Changes in the S-T segments and T waves can indicate changes associated with myocardial infarction. Determination of the electrical axis of the heart can aid in the diagnosis of conduction defects, hypertrophy of the heart chambers, abnormal heart position, and myocardial changes following infarction. Many ECG abnormalities are nonspecific, and care must be taken to avoid overreading; as with most laboratory tests, clinical correlation is of major importance.

See also *cardiac cycle* and *vectorcardiography.*

ambulatory e., a method in which prolonged electrocardiographic recordings are made on a portable tape recorder while the patient engages in normal daily activities and keeps a diary of activities and accompanying symptoms. It is especially useful in the diagnosis and management of intermittent cardiac arrhythmias, to detect and relate the arrhythmias to daily activities and to drug treatment. Also called *Holter ECG recording.*

electrocautery (e-lek″tro-kaw′ter-e) [*electro-* + Gr. *kautērion* branding iron] an apparatus for cauterizing tissue that utilizes a resistance wire heated red- or white-hot by an electric current.

electrocerebral inactivity (ECI) (e-lek″tro-ser′ĕ-bral, e-lek″tro-sĕ-re′bral) [*electro-* + L. *cerebrum* brain] the lack of identifiable spontaneous or induced electrical activity from the cerebral cortex as recorded from a series of electrodes placed on the scalp. The temporary loss of cerebral activity often accompanies overdoses of such central nervous system depressants as barbiturates and benzodiazepines. It may also occur with hypothermia (body temperature below 32°C) and/or cardiovascular shock with a low cerebral perfusion pressure. Permanent loss of cerebral electrical activity, as recorded from the scalp, is one of the recommended criteria for establishing brain death.

The American Electroencephalographic Society has established guidelines for recording the electroencephalogram in cases of suspected brain death. The use of at least eight scalp electrodes and two ear lobe reference electrodes with impedances of 100–10,000 Ω is required. Recordings are made between electrodes that are at least 10 cm apart. Instrumental sensitivities of at least 2 μV/mm should be used for most of the recording, and a time constant of 0.3–0.4 sec used for part of the time. Intense noxious, auditory, and photic stimuli should be employed in an attempt to evoke electric potentials from the brain. The recording must be continued for at least 30 min and should be repeated after an interval of 6 hr or longer if there is doubt about ECI. When evaluating patients in intensive care units, care must be taken to identify, monitor, and eliminate artifacts originating from electrical equipment (respirators, dialysis units, cardiac pacemakers) and from the patient (electrocardiogram, muscular movements). In all cases, the integrity of the entire recording system must be tested. Telephone transmission of the electroencephalogram should not be used for determining whether there is ECI.

The significance of ECI in infants and children under age 5 is not clearly established.

Also called cerebral silence and electrocerebral silence (ECS). See also *brain death syndrome* and *evoked potential.*

electrochemical cell an apparatus having two electrodes placed in an electrolyte solution, possibly separated by an ion-selective membrane or a salt bridge. Electrochemical cells are used in pH, blood gas, and some glucose analyzers, and in chloride titrators. They can also be used to measure the amount of a chemical species present in the electrolyte solution by allowing the electrode reaction to proceed to completion and measuring the total charge transferred in the process (referred to as coulometry).

The voltage between the electrodes is determined by the oxidation-reduction reaction occurring at each electrode, the potential across the membrane or salt bridge, and the current flow through the cell. When the current flow is produced by the electrochemical reactions and is available as useful electric power, the cell is termed a galvanic cell. When sufficient voltage is applied by an external source to reverse the current flow and the electrode reactions, the cell is termed an electrolytic cell.

Because the electrode voltage is proportional to the concentration (more precisely the activity) of ions involved in the electrode reactions, an electrochemical cell can be used to measure the concentration of a specific ionic species or of other chemical compounds by means of coupled reactions. In such measurements, the electrode voltage is measured potentiometrically by determining the applied voltage that exactly balances the cell voltage producing a null current.

electrochemistry (e-lek″tro-kem′is-tre) the branch of physical chemistry and instrumental analysis that deals with relations involving electricity and chemical changes.

electrocorticogram (ECoG) (e-lek″tro-kor′tĭ-ko-gram″) [*electro-* + *cortico-*, from L. *cortex* + Gr. *gramma* mark] the record obtained from electrocorticography.

electrocorticography (ECoG) (e-lek″tro-kor″tĭ-kog′rah-fe) [*electro-* + *cortico-* + Gr. *graphein* to record] the technique of recording electrical activity from the cerebral cortex in humans or in animals. The electrodes are applied directly on or into the cortical tissue through openings cut into the skull. In contrast to recordings made from the scalp, the electrical activity recorded from the cortex in this way is not distorted by movement artifacts or attenuated by tissue, such as skull or skin, interposed between the electrode and the surface of the brain. Accurate placement of the electrodes can be attained because the cortical surface is visualized, although exposure of the cortical surface can itself cause changes in the normal electrical activity.

The main clinical application of this technique is in the localization of epileptiform discharges in patients in whom surgical treatment is possible. It is also used to check the persistence of potentially epileptogenic tissue after the main focus has been removed.

electrode (e-lek′trōd) [Gr. *ēlektron* amber + *hodas* way] an electric conductor through which electricity is applied to an object or through which an electric current enters or leaves a medium. In electrocardiography, electroencephalography, and electromyography, electrodes are metal plates or needles used to measure the electrical activity of living tissue.

In a vacuum tube, the electrodes are the conductors that control the flow of electrons through the tube. A diode has two electrodes: the cathode, which emits electrons, and the anode, which collects them. A triode, tetrode, or pentode has one, two, or three grids that control the electron flow by electrostatic attraction or repulsion.

In an electrochemical cell, the electrodes (or half-cells) at which the half-reactions occur are conductors in contact with the electrolyte solution. The anode is the electrode that accepts electrons from a chemical species (i.e., an oxidation occurs), and the cathode is the electrode that donates electrons to a chemical species (i.e., a reduction occurs). In an electrolytic cell the anode is positive with respect to the cathode, whereas in a galvanic cell, the anode is negative relative to the cathode. The voltage produced by the half-reaction at an electrode is called the electrode potential and is given by the Nernst equation.

active e., see under *exploring e.*

basal e., in electroencephalography, any electrode placed near the base of the skull. These are used to record electrical activity from areas of the brain that are inaccessible to electrodes placed on the scalp. See also *nasoethmoidal e., nasopharyngeal e.,* and *sphenoidal e.*

bipolar needle e., a recording electrode that consists of two wires (usually platinum), both insulated except at the tip and positioned side by side within the shaft of a metal needle. Although neither wire can technically be called the active or reference electrode (the tips are symmetric and equal in area), variations in voltage between them are measured. The outer surface of the shaft may be used as the ground electrode.

calomel e., a reference electrode used in electrochemistry that consists of a pool of mercury covered by a layer of calomel (Hg_2Cl_2). This is immersed in a potassium chloride solution of known concentration (which is often a saturated solution, although concentrations of 0.1, 1.0, 3.5, and 4.0 mol/l are also commonly used).

Clark oxygen e., an electrode used to determine the Po_2 in a sample of gas or liquid, most commonly a sample of blood. The electrode works on the polarographic principle: a constant voltage (−0.6 to −0.7 V) from an external source is applied to polarize the silver/silver chloride anode and the glass-encased platinum wire cathode, which are both in contact with a film of buffered KCl solution. A plastic (usually polypropylene), O_2-permeable membrane separates the blood sample from the two half-cells. When O_2 from the sample diffuses through the membrane, it is reduced at the cathode. The change in potential varies directly with the rate at which the O_2 is reduced, which in turn is directly proportional to the Po_2 of the sample.

common reference e., in clinical electroencephalography, a single reference electrode that is connected to input terminal two of several or all of the amplifiers in use.

concentric needle e., an electrode used in electroneuromyography to record the potential difference between a stainless steel hypodermic needle (reference electrode) and the uninsulated tip of a nichrome, silver, or platinum wire (active electrode) inserted into the hollow center of the needle. The tip is flush with the bevel of the needle. A separate surface electrode is used to ground the subject. Also called coaxial needle electrode.

contact lens e., an electrode made of a wire embedded in a glass or pliable lens, which is placed on a film of tears or an electrolyte solution covering the cornea and is used to record the electroretinogram.

cortical e., in electroencephalography, an electrode that is placed directly on or into the cerebral cortex of the brain. See also *electrocorticography.*

depth e., in electroencephalography, any electrode that is placed within the substance of the brain.

disk e., a disk-shaped (usually metal) surface electrode that is applied to the appropriate skin surface (in electroencephalography, the scalp; in electromyography, the skin overlying a superficial muscle) with collodion, paste, wax, or adhesive tape. A dome-shaped concavity in the center of some disk electrodes is used to contain electrically conductive electrolyte paste.

dropping mercury e., a type of indicator electrode

used in polarography. In this type, the anode is a pool of mercury at the bottom of the polarographic cell, and the cathode is a capillary tube filled with mercury, which slowly drips out so that the electrode surface is constantly renewed. See also *polarography.*

epidural e., an electrode placed on the dura mater that covers the cerebrum, used in recording the electrical activity from the brain.

exploring e., in electrodiagnosis, the electrode positioned nearest to the source of the recorded bioelectrical activity. Use of the terms active electrode or stigmatic electrode as synonyms for exploring electrode is discouraged in electroencephalography. In clinical electromyography, however, it is more often referred to as an active electrode.

e. of first kind, in electrochemistry, a metal electrode that is in contact with ions of the same metal in solution, the metal being oxidized or the ions reduced.

glass e., an indicator electrode used to selectively measure the activity (which is approximately equal to the concentration) of a specific ion in a solution, such as blood. Glass electrodes that are selective for hydrogen, alkali (group I) metals, or thallium are available.

The electrode has a thin (less than 0.1 mm) glass membrane, which can selectively bind or release one species of ion, and thus acts as if it were permeable to only that ion. The membrane encloses a reference solution of the ion and a reference (usually an Ag/AgCl) electrode. Some electrodes have the reference electrode plated on one side of the membrane and need no reference solution. When the membrane is immersed in the test solution, the specific ion diffuses through the membrane until the activity gradient balances the membrane potential, which is then proportional to the logarithm of the ion activity (pH, if the ion is H^+).

If the membrane is slightly permeable to another ion, a fraction (the selectivity ratio) of the activity of this ion will be added into the measured activity of the specific ion, producing a measurement error. Some of the Ph (H^+-selective) electrodes used in pH meters are available with a selectivity ratio of 10^{-15} against Na^+, allowing measurement of pH 13 to within 2 percent. Na^+-selective electrodes with a selectivity ratio of 0.001 against K^+ and K^+-selective electrodes with a selectivity ratio of 0.05 against Na^+ are available for measuring the serum concentration of these ions. An NH_4^+-selective electrode can be used to measure blood urea nitrogen (BUN) after the urea is hydrolyzed to NH_4^+ by urease.

hydrogen e., a reference electrode used in electrochemistry that consists of a platinum or gold electrode coated with porous platinum. The platinum adsorbs hydrogen and catalyzes the reversible half-reaction: $H^+ + e^- \rightleftharpoons \frac{1}{2} H_2$. Although the hydrogen electrode is used in the reference method for pH measurement, the pH glass electrode is used for routine measurements.

indicator e., in potentiometry, an electrochemical cell used to measure the concentration of a particular chemical species in the electrolyte solution; the electrode poential is directly proportional to the logarithm of the activity of that species. Cf. *reference e.*

indifferent e., see *reference e.*

inert e., in electrochemistry, a metal (usually gold or platinum) electrode that is not chemically involved in the half-reaction but serves only as a passive donor or acceptor of electrons.

intracerebral e., an electrode placed into the brain tissue that is used either to record the electrical activity from the brain or to stimulate the brain. Also called *depth e.*

ion-selective e. (ISE), a device used as an indicator electrode to measure the activity of an individual ion in a solution. It operates on the same principle as a glass electrode, but the glass membrane is replaced by some other type of barrier that is selectively permeable to the specific ion. In one type, the solid-state electrode, the ion-selective barrier is a crystal that contains the ion, whereas in the ion-exchange electrode the barrier is a liquid immiscible in water; ions are carried across the liquid layer by a carrier substance with a specific affinity for the ion. Solid-state electrodes are available to measure F^-, Cl^-, Br^-, I^-, S^{2-}, and Cu^{2+}.

The chloride-specific electrode is used to measure chloride in sweat; the fluoride electrode is used to measure fluoride in saliva. Ion-exchange electrodes are available to measure Ca^{2+} using dioctyl phosphate as the carrier, and to measure K^+ using the antibiotic valinomycin as the carrier. This K^+ electrode has a selectivity constant of 2×10^{-4} for Na^+.

monopolar needle e., a solid stainless steel wire, approximately 0.4 mm in diameter, coated with insulating material except at the tip. In monopolar needle electrode recording, the potential difference between the active electrode area at the tip (inserted in such tissue as a muscle) and a reference electrode (a surface electrode or uninsulated monopolar needle electrode inserted in subcutaneous tissue) is measured. A separate ground electrode is also used.

multilead e., an electrode that can be used to measure the territory of a motor unit. It is composed of a metal cannula into which are inserted a number of insulated wires (typically, 14). The uninsulated tips (recording surfaces) are positioned at apertures along the length of the cannula, flush with its outer surface.

nasoethmoidal e., a flexible electrode inserted between the nasal septum and the conchae to rest on the ethmoid bone. It is used in electroencephalography to record the electrical activity originating from the inferior portion of the frontal lobe.

nasopharyngeal e., an electrode inserted into the nose until its tip is in contact with the nasopharyngeal mucosa near the base of the sphenoid bone. It is used to record the electrical activity originating from the hypothalamus, upper brain stem, hippocampal gyrus, and anteromedial temporal lobe. A disadvantage in the use of these electrodes is that they give rise to artifacts on the electroencephalographic tracing. They are of greatest value in the investigation of patients with suspected temporal lobe seizures.

needle e., a recording or stimulating electrode with an outer shaft usually made of tempered stainless steel beveled into the shape of a needle, which can systematically explore the activity of individual motor or nerve units. When inserted into tissue, it allows for a much smaller pickup area for recording (usually less than 1.0 mm^2) than does a surface electrode.

pad e., a metal electrode covered with gauze, which is placed on the scalp, secured by pressure from a cap or headband, and used to record the electrical activity from the brain.

Pco_2 e., a pH electrode that is used to determine the Pco_2 of a sample of gas or liquid, most commonly a sample of blood. The electrode measures the pH of a film of bicarbonate solution that equilibrates with the Pco_2 of the sample. The solution is separated from the sample by a CO_2-permeable membrane (usually composed of Teflon or Silastic). After diffusing across the membrane, the CO_2 reacts with H_2O to form carbonic acid, decreasing the pH of the solution and creating a potential difference at the electrode. This potential difference changes linearly with the log Pco_2 of the sample. Also called *Severinghaus e.*

pH e., see under *glass e.*

Po_2 e., see under *Clark oxygen e.*

quinhydrone e., an indicator electrode used for pH measurement that consists of an inert electrode immersed in a saturated solution of quinhydrone (a 1:1 mixture of quinone and hydroquinone). The reaction quinone + $2H^+ + 2e^- \rightleftharpoons$ hydroquinone occurs at the electrode, and the electrode potential is proportional to the pH.

recording e., a conducting device used to monitor electric potential changes from a given tissue. The size, shape, and location of the electrode vary according to the intended function of the electrode. Of the two electrodes used to record electrical activity, the active or exploring electrode is closest to the source of the activity; the other is called the reference electrode. By convention, a negative potential difference at the exploring electrode relative to the reference one is seen as a positive deflection on the cathode ray screen.

reference e., 1. an electrode presumed to be at a constant potential, with which the changes in potential of another electrode can be compared. Of the two electrodes used in electrodiagnosis, the reference electrode is the more remote from the source of recorded activity, reducing the possibility that it will pick up activity identical to that recorded by the exploring electrode. Also called *indifferent e.*

2. in potentiometry, the electrode having a known electrode potential, e.g., a *calomel e., hydrogen e.,* or *silver/silver chloride e.* Cf. *indicator e.*

scalp e., an electrode placed on the surface of, or inserted into, the scalp. This is the most common type of electrode used for recording the electrical activity of the brain.

e. of second kind, in electrochemistry, a metal electrode coated with a layer of an insoluble salt of the same metal, e.g., a silver/silver chloride electrode.

Severinghaus e., see *Pco_2 e.*

silver/silver chloride e. (Ag/AgCl e.), a reference electrode used in electrochemistry that consists of a silver wire coated with silver chloride. This is immersed in a saturated silver chloride solution that also contains a known concentration of potassium chloride.

single-fiber needle e., a needle electrode with a minute recording surface, 25 μm in diameter, that allows the recording of action potentials from single, uninjured muscle fibers.

sphenoidal e., an electrode consisting of a needle or flexible wire insulated except at the tip and inserted perpendicular to the soft tissue on the surface of the sphenoid bone near the region of the foramen ovale. It is used to assess electrical activity originating from the anteroinferior portion of the temporal lobe, a region of the brain that may be the site of epileptogenic activity not detectable by electrodes placed on the scalp.

standard hydrogen e., a reference electrode. An inert metal such as platinum, which is covered with finely divided platinum, adsorbs hydrogen; reversible dissociation of hydrogen to hydrogen ions and electrons occurs on the surface, and the arrangement functions as a hydrogen electrode: $H_2 \rightleftharpoons 2H^+ + 2(e)$. The potential of this electrode is taken as zero volts when the solution containing the hydrogen ions is at unit activity and in equilibrium with hydrogen gas at unit fugacity (1 atm).

sternospinal reference e., a noncephalic reference in electroencephalography, formed by interconnecting two electrodes, one of which is placed over the right sternoclavicular junction and the other over the spinous process of the seventh cervical vertebra. The voltage between them is balanced by a potentiometer to reduce the artifacts on the electroencephalogram that arise from the electrical activity generated by the heart. Also called *Stephenson-Gibbs reference.*

stigmatic e., see under *exploring e.*

stimulating e., a conducting device through which an electric current is applied to a certain tissue to study its function. Two electrodes are used to stimulate; by convention in electroneuromyography, if the two stimulating electrodes are less than 5 cm apart and of somewhat equal size, they are referred to as bipolar. The cathode is smaller than the anode in monopolar stimulating electrodes, and the two are placed more than 5 cm apart. In nerve conduction studies, the cathode is used to depolarize the nerve under examination.

subcutaneous e., a conducting device that is inserted in tissue beneath the skin surface and used to stimulate or record electrical activity, e.g., a needle or depth electrode.

subdural e., an electrode placed under the dura mater covering the brain or spinal cord.

surface e., a conducting device that is affixed to the surface of the skin and used to stimulate or record electrical activity in the tissue beneath it. Contact resistance of the electrode with the skin is reduced through application of a conductive electrolyte paste or saline-soaked fabric between the two apposing surfaces. Skin impedance may also be reduced by abrasion of the skin at the application site. These electrodes can be constructed from various types of metal or fabric and have the configuration of a disk, rectangular plate, strip, ring, or prong, among others. They can be paired to localize the recording or stimulating area, used as reference electrodes in conjunction with monopolar needle electrodes, or used as ground electrodes. Thus, the size, shape, and separation of the various types of surface electrode are generally specified. Cf. *depth e.* and *needle e.*

tympanic e., an electrode inserted through the external auditory canal and placed on the tympanic membrane. It is used to record the electrical activity from the inferior or medial portion of the temporal lobe. In individuals with epileptic foci in these regions, localized spikes may be recorded from tympanic electrodes, especially at the onset of sleep.

electrode potential the voltage produced by an electrochemical half-cell compared with that produced by a hydrogen (H_2/H^+) half-cell at standard conditions (defined as 0.0 V); i.e., the voltage of the cell made up of the given electrode and the standard hydrogen electrode. The electrode potential depends on the temperature and the concentrations of the reactants. Also called *reduction potential.* See also *Nernst equation, redox potential,* and *standard electrode potential.*

electrode response time the time taken for an electrode to reach an equilibrium with the test solution, e.g., several seconds for a pH glass electrode.

electrode sensitivity in a pH meter, the change in the meter reading (in millivolts) per pH unit change in the test solution.

electrodiagnosis (EDX) (e-lek″tro-di″ag-no′sis) a general term applied to any clinical examination for abnormal function in peripheral nerves or muscles. Such examinations utilize techniques based on the recording of the response of these tissues to electrical stimulation, or on the recording of the spontaneous, insertional, and voluntary electrical activity of muscles.

electroencephalogram (EEG) (e-lek″tro-en-sef′ah-lo-gram″) [*electro-* + Gr. *enkephalos* brain + *gramma* mark] the record obtained in electroencephalography.

low-voltage e., the electroencephalographic record sometimes obtained from an awake normal individual that is characterized by low-voltage activity (< 20 μV) of mixed frequencies. The finding is of no diagnostic significance.

electroencephalograph (e-lek″tro-en-sef′ah-lo-graf″) [*electro-* + Gr. *enkephalos* brain + *graphein* to record] the instrument used to record the electroencephalogram. Usually it consists of a series of amplifiers and pen recorders. The Committee on Apparatus of the International Federation of Societies for Electroencephalography and Clinical Neurophysiology recommends specifications for the recorders used in clinical practice.

electroencephalographic activity (e-lek″tro-en-sef″ah-lo-graf′ik) any wave or sequence of waves that makes up the electroencephalogram.

electroencephalographic technologist an allied health professional trained to obtain interpretable electroencephalographic (EEG) recordings. This entails responsibility for the preparation of patients, the conduction of various EEG examinations, and the collection of information needed to interpret the tests. Educational preparation involves completion of a 2-yr approved program; graduates are certified by the American Board of Registration of Electroencephalograph Technologists and are designated R EEG T, Registered Electroencephalographic Technologist. Also called EEG technologist.

electroencephalography (e-lek″tro-en-sef″ah-log′rah-fe) the recording of the electric currents continuously developed in the brain, by means of electrodes applied to the scalp or surface of the brain or placed within the substance of the brain. These electric currents represent the summated excitatory and inhibitory postsynaptic potentials that occur over the dendrites and soma of cortical pyramidal cells. Changes in the membrane potentials of these cells, which are oriented perpendicularly to the cortical surface, result from continuous synaptic input from the thalamus, brain stem structures, and other cortical regions. The potentials thus establish a series of dipoles, the current of which overlaps in time and space. Electroencephalographic (EEG) potentials are present throughout life, varying with different states of consciousness in both health and disease.

Electroencephalography is a noninvasive technique that is medically useful in the diagnosis and treatment of epilepsy, the localization of tumors and other structural lesions of the brain, the investigation of individuals with neurologic disorders, the monitoring of those with metabolic disorders, the evaluation of comatose patients, the study of sleep and its disorders, and the assessment of patients with suspected brain death. It is of little use in the study of mental disorders that do not involve brain damage.

For clinical diagnosis in human subjects, electrodes are applied to the scalp with a conductive paste in a predetermined pattern (the most widely used being the International 10–20 system). The potential differences between various pairs of electrodes are amplified by high-gain differential amplifiers, and the output is recorded continuously by a paper-writing oscillograph or cathode ray oscilloscope. Standard recording parameters are amplifier calibration, 100 μV/cm of pen deflection; time constant, 0.3 sec; and recorder speed, 30 mm/sec. Records are obtained over a 30-min period with the patient relaxed but awake; note is made of eye openings and closings, and recording is continued during sleep or following an activation procedure (hyperventilation, photic stimulation, or drug injection), as this may alter the EEG patterns in diagnostically helpful ways. Care is taken to eliminate artifacts from the electrical activity of muscle and/or the heart. Records are usually analyzed visually, but computers are employed in some cases to permit more detailed analysis.

EEG patterns can be classified on the basis of dominant waveform frequency. The alpha frequency (8–13 Hz) is symmetric about the baseline, is recorded over the back of the head, and is the dominant frequency of the quiet, awake adult human. The beta frequency (> 13 Hz) typifies the record of the alert adult human and laboratory animal. The theta frequency (4–7 Hz), symmetric about the baseline, appears frequently over the frontal and temporal lobes, is a common pattern in juvenile humans, and occurs during rapid eye movement (REM) sleep in adult humans and laboratory animals. The delta frequency (< 4 Hz) characterizes slow-wave sleep in both adult and juvenile humans and in laboratory animals.

The dominant EEG pattern is unique to an individual, and varies with age and stage of arousal, but it otherwise tends to be stable in the absence of injury or disease. The EEG tends to slow, with theta and delta frequency dominating the record of awake patients with a variety of diffuse neurologic and metabolic disorders, decreased blood glucose or oxygen (O_2) saturation, or increased blood carbon dioxide (CO_2) levels.

For more information on particular EEG waveforms associated with disease states, see the specific pathology. See also *activation procedures, brain death syndrome, coma, electrocerebral inactivity, epilepsy, International 10–20 system, montage, sleep, spike,* and *wave.*

electroendosmosis (e-lek″tro-en″doz-mo′sis) see *electroosmosis.*

electroimmunodiffusion (e-lek″tro-im″u-no-dĭ-fu′zhun) see *counterimmunoelectrophoresis.*

electrolysis (e″lek-trol′ĭ-sis) [*electro-* + Gr. *lysis* release] 1. the dissociation of a chemical compound driven by an applied electric current.

2. destruction by means of electricity, as of hair.

electrolyte (e-lek′tro-līt) [*electro-* + Gr. *lytos* soluble] a substance that dissociates into ions when molten or in solution and thus becomes capable of conducting electricity; an ionic solute. In clinical chemistry, the term is used to refer to the major ions commonly measured in the extracellular fluid: sodium (Na^+), potassium (K^+), chloride (Cl^-), and bicarbonate (HCO_3^-).

electrolyte balance and homeostasis a complex interplay of physiologic mechanisms in which the body maintains the concentrations of inorganic ions in the body fluid compartments at preset levels. The major cations are sodium (Na^+), potassium (K^+), calcium (Ca^{2+}), and magnesium (Mg^{2+}); the major anions are chloride (Cl^-), bicarbonate (HCO_3^-), and phosphate (PO_4). For the nerves, muscle fibers, and other cells to function properly, intracellular and extracellular concentrations of the various ions must be tightly controlled. There are large variations between the intracellular and extracellular concentrations of certain electrolytes. The ratio of intracellular to extracellular K is 40:1, whereas that for Na is 1:30. Cl is mainly extracellular. Extracellular Ca and, to a lesser extent, PO_4 concentrations are controlled by parathyroid hormone (PTH), vitamin D, and calcitonin. Magnesium homeostasis is mostly a renal function. In clinical usage, the term electrolytes usually refers to Na, K, Cl, and HCO_3^-.

The normal resting electrical potential of the cell membrane of nerve and muscle fibers is maintained by a sodium-potassium pump, which actively transports Na out of cells and K into cells. The propagation of action potentials, which initiates nerve and muscle function, is associated with Na entering and K exiting the cell. Major alterations of electrolyte concentrations will disturb normal function of these tissues.

The concentration of electrolytes in the body fluid compartments is related to both the fluid volume of the compartments and the total solute content. Disturbances of electrolyte balance, such as severe diarrhea causing water and Na loss, bring homeostatic mechanisms into play that adjust both body water and electrolyte content so as to return electrolyte concentrations to normal. Generally, extracellular concentrations are preserved at normal levels, even when intracellular levels change.

Sodium concentration is a major determinant of plasma osmolality. The body adjusts osmolality by altering renal water conservation and loss. The hypothalamic peptide hormone vasopressin (also called antidiuretic hormone, ADH) inhibits renal water loss in situations of increased plasma osmolality. With the return of water to the circulation, osmolality is lowered and serum sodium concentration falls toward normal. ADH secretion is inhibited by decreased plasma osmolality, and the ensuing water loss from the circulation raises osmolality and sodium levels to normal. The adrenal steroid hormone aldosterone is extremely important in adjusting Na and K balance. A deficiency of serum sodium or deficient perfusion causes secretion by the renal juxtaglomerular apparatus of the enzyme renin, which cleaves a circulating plasma factor, producing angiotensin, which causes secretion of aldosterone. Aldosterone inhibits renal sodium loss but increases potassium loss. The ability of the kidneys to respond to circulating factors, as well as to intrinsic renal control mechanisms, is essential for electrolyte homeostasis.

Hyponatremia refers to low levels of serum Na. Mild hyponatremia is present when Na levels are less than 135 mEq/l and severe hyponatremia when Na concentration is less than 125 mEq/l. Hyponatremia can exist when there is an excess of plasma water and/or a deficiency of plasma Na content. Hyponatremia due to excess plasma water can be due to an inappropriate secretion of ADH, congestive heart failure, or hepatic disease. Causes of deficient extracellular Na content include gastrointestinal losses (diarrhea), renal losses (renal disease or use of diuretics), or a lack of aldosterone (hypoadrenalism). Transient hyponatremia can be induced by the use of intravenous hypotonic (low osmolality) fluids that overload the body's homeostatic mechanisms. The presence of severe hyperglycemia or hyperlipidemia may produce an artifactually low measured value of serum Na when the osmolality of the extracellular water is normal. This is known as pseudohyponatremia, and is due to an increase in either the nonwater volume (hyperlipemia) or the nonsodium solute (hyperproteinemia) of the serum.

Symptoms of hyponatremia can range from mild to severe, with confusion, seizures, coma, or death. The symptoms depend on the rapidity at which hyponatremia develops and on how low the Na level falls.

Hypernatremia exists when Na concentration is greater than 148 mEq/l. It is usually due to deficient extracellular water in the presence of normal or even decreased extracellular Na content. Thus, dehydration is the most common etiology. Normally, the body avoids hypernatremia from dehydration by increasing ADH secretion. This results in concentrated urine (high urine osmolality) and renal water conservation. The condition in which an individual is unable to produce ADH is called diabetes insipidus. Nephrogenic diabetes insipidus results when ADH is produced but does not function due to renal abnormalities; both conditions are rare. Most commonly, hypernatremia is caused by water and, occasionally, Na losses from the gastrointestinal tract, which overwhelm the water and Na conservation mechanisms. The symptoms of hypernatremia are similar to those of hyponatremia and result from the shrinkage of nerve tissue.

Hypokalemia refers to a decreased serum K concentration to levels below 3.5 mEq/l. Although 98 percent of total body K is intracellular, the extracellular K concentration generally reflects total body stores, and normal extracellular levels are essential for normal nerve and muscle function. Hypokalemia occurs when gastrointestinal and/or urinary K losses exceed K intake. Diarrhea, emesis, and renal disease are the usual etiologic factors. Use of diuretics causing renal potassium loss is the most common clinical cause. Occasionally, hypokalemia occurs as part of the body's response to avoid dehydration. In states of dehydration and decreased renal perfusion, aldosterone is secreted in large quantities. This results in Na and HCO_3^- preservation, but also in K diuresis and hypokalemia (hypokalemic alkalosis). The symptoms of hypokalemia are progressive muscle weakness and cardiac arrhythmias. Hypokalemia is particularly dangerous in patients taking digitalis compounds. The electrocardiogram in individuals with hypokalemia may show a prolonged QT interval and abnormal T waves or U waves.

Hyperkalemia occurs when serum K concentration exceeds 5.5 mEq/l. Generally, the kidneys maintain a K concentration of less than 5.5 mEq/l by increasing K excretion when the serum levels are excessive. Intrinsic renal disease may prevent renal potassium excretion, resulting in hyperkalemia. Another cause of hyperkalemia is a lack of aldosterone (hypoadrenalism). Hyperkalemia can also occur when the high levels of intracellular K are rapidly released into the circulation. Thus, trauma resulting in breakdown of muscle and other tissues, or severe hemolysis can induce hyperkalemia. Hyperkalemia is also encountered in the presence of acidosis. The body's cells buffer the extracellular acidosis by allowing hydrogen ions to enter cells. Electrical neutrality is preserved by allowing K ions to enter the circulation. Thus hyperkalemia results. A condition known as pseudohyperkalemia can occur in patients with very high platelet counts. When blood is drawn and the clot is forming, the platelets break down, releasing large amounts of K into the serum. When pseudohyperkalemia is suspected, blood that is drawn should not be allowed to clot. The plasma K concentration is then a true reflection of the concentration of extracellular K. Hyperkalemia results in neuromuscular dysfunction and serious cardiac arrhythmias or death. The ECG shows tall peaked T waves and a short QT interval.

NANETTE SMITH, M.D.
ALLAN PONT, M.D.

electrolytic cell (e-lek″tro-lit′ik) an electrochemical cell in which a voltage exceeding the cell electromotive force is applied from an external source. Current flows and the electrode half-reactions proceed in the opposite direction from the spontaneous direction. This can be used for electrolytic analysis in which a metal is plated on an electrode and, when the electrolysis is complete, weighed or analyzed.

electrolytic stripping the removal of a layer of plated metal or metal oxide tarnish by electrolysis.

electromagnet (e-lek″tro-mag′net) a temporary magnet made by passing an electric current through a coil of wire that is wrapped around an inner core.

electromagnetic radiation the propagation of the electromagnetic field, which moves in space at the velocity of light ($c = 3 \times 10^8$ m/s). Electromagnetic radiation includes radio waves; infrared, visible, and ultraviolet light; and x-rays and gamma rays. Its properties are determined by the frequency (ν), wavelength ($\lambda = c/\nu$), and polarization. An electromagnetic wave consists of quanta called photons, which may be considered to be particles. Every photon has an energy proportional to the frequency ($E = h\nu$, where h is Planck's constant).

electromagnetic unit (emu) the electromagnetic centimeter-gram-second (cgs) electric charge, which is equal to 10 coulombs (C). Also called abcoulomb.

electrometer (e″lek″trom′ĕ-ter) [*electro-* + Gr. *metron* measure] a voltmeter that has very high resistance and thus draws no appreciable current. See also *electrometer a.* under *amplifier.*

electromotance (e-lek″tro-mo′tans) see *electromotive force.*

electromotive force (EMF, emf, E) (e-lek″tro-mo′tiv) the total voltage (potential difference) across an electrochemical cell. Also called *electromotance.*

electromyogram (e-lek″tro-mi′o-gram) [*electro-* + Gr. *mys* muscle + *gramma* mark] the record obtained by electromyography.

electromyograph (e-lek″tro-mi′o-graf) [*electro-* + Gr. *mys* muscle + *graphein* to record] the instrument used in electromyography to record and study the intrinsic electric activity of skeletal muscle. It consists of a recording electrode that is usually inserted directly into the muscle and consists of an amplifier that boosts the signal level so the bioelectric potentials obtained can be recorded satisfactorily, and a cathode ray oscilloscope that displays the waveforms for visual analysis and recording. A loudspeaker system is attached so the potentials can be monitored acoustically.

electromyography (EMG) (e-lek″tro-mi-og′rah-fe) [*electro-* + Gr. *mys* muscle + *graphein* to record] an electrodiagnostic technique used primarily for the extracellular in situ recording of the electrical activity of skeletal muscle fibers at rest and during voluntary contraction, as well as during stimulation. The electromyographic examination can be a valuable guide in detecting injuries or diseases that affect the muscles, peripheral nerves, lower motor neurons in the spinal cord, and transmission of action potentials at the neuromuscular junction; it also aids in ascertaining the specific level of the neuraxis at which an underlying pathologic process is taking place. It may be used as a guide to prognosis or in following the progression of a disease process. It is important to recognize, however, that no electromyographic potential alone can be regarded as being pathognomonic of a particular disease or level of involvement. The information obtained through EMG must be considered in combination with the entire complement of relevant clinical and laboratory data when making a diagnosis.

BASIC COMPONENTS OF THE ELECTROMYOGRAPH SYSTEM. Recording electrodes form the essential link in any EMG system (see the accompanying illustration). They function as electric conductors that convert the flow of current (due to movement of ions) in the extracellular fluid surrounding nerve and muscle cells to the movement of electrons (and thus changing electric currents) in the wires connecting the other functional components of the EMG system. When it is necessary to systematically explore the activity arising from discrete areas of a muscle (as small as the individual fiber or motor unit), a needle electrode that can be inserted close to the source of the activity is used. Concentric needle electrodes (each consisting of a wire insulated except at the tip and inserted into the lumen of a stainless steel hypodermic needle) and monopolar needle electrodes (consisting of a stainless steel needle covered with insulation except at the tip) are most commonly used. Surface electrodes (affixed to the skin above the tissue to be studied) are used as reference or ground electrodes (in conjunction with needle electrodes). Surface electrodes are also utilized in the recording of evoked compound muscle action potentials in studies of either motor nerve conduction velocity or neuromuscular transmission. Sensory nerve conduction studies may be performed with either needle or surface electrodes.

Because the changes in electric potential recorded

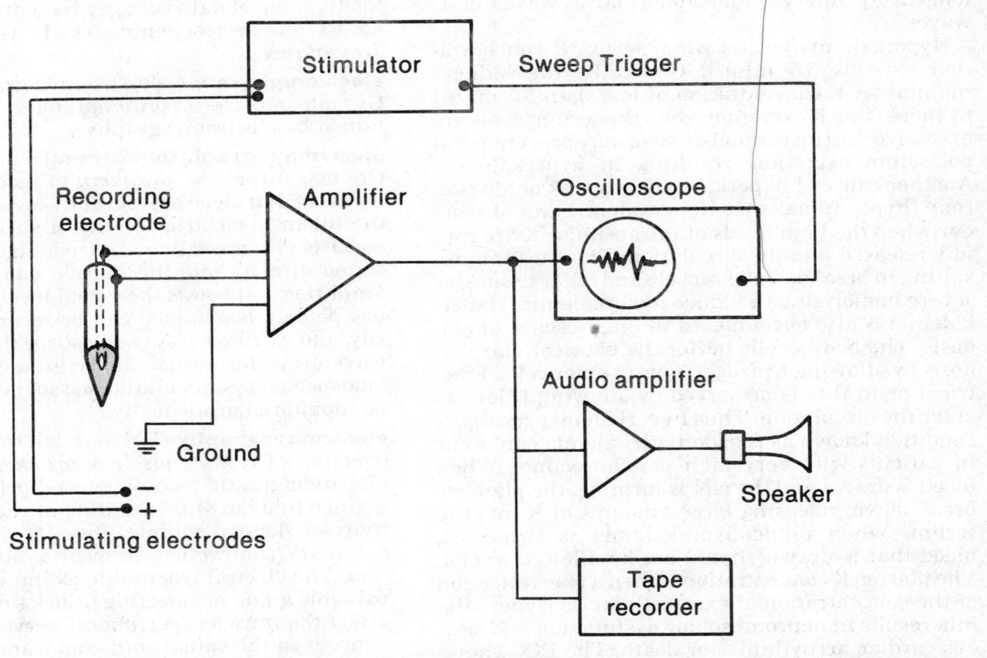

Electromyography. The components of an electromyograph system. (From Aminoff, M. J.: Electromyography in Clinical Practice. Menlo Park, CA, Addison-Wesley Publishing Co., 1978.)

from a muscle or nerve are small in amplitude (usually less than 5.0 mV), the signal must be magnified before it can be adequately displayed. This is accomplished by feeding the connections from the electrodes to the two input terminals of a differential amplifier: when calibrated, this amplifier is capable of magnifying the input signal by a selected and known amount, usually up to a million times the original input signal. The third input terminal of the amplifier is used to establish the patient's ground connection. The differential amplifier helps to eliminate powerline artifacts and other interference signals; it does this by amplifying any difference in potential between the two electrode inputs while simultaneously rejecting those signals, such as interference signals, that are common to both inputs when they are referenced to the ground terminal. In addition, the amplifier used in EMG must be capable of maintaining a uniform gain (the ratio between the output and input voltages) over the frequency range of the input; an amplifier with low- and high-frequency cutoff points of 2 and 10 kHz, respectively, is required.

The output from the amplifier is delivered to a cathode ray oscilloscope so that voltage changes can be visualized and recorded. The amplifier output is simultaneously fed to an audio monitoring system (an amplifier and loudspeaker) to enable the electromyographer to hear the electrical activity, because certain types of abnormal activity can be readily identified by their characteristic sound over the loudspeaker.

Some form of recording (usually a strip recorder, Polaroid camera, or motor-driven camera) is used to make a permanent graphic record of the electrical events displayed on the cathode ray screen. The recorded electrical activity can also be stored by means of a magnetic tape recorder (connected to the amplifier output), allowing for visualization, graphic recording, and detailed analysis at a later date.

Nerve stimulation is necessary to determine nerve conduction velocities. Surface electrodes are generally used to deliver the stimulus, but needle electrodes may also be employed. The stimulator is capable of passing a brief, square-wave pulse of current of controlled frequency (from 1 impulse/sec to the tetanizing frequency), voltage, and duration (0.05–1 msec) between the two stimulus electrodes. The stimulator output is made to trigger the sweep of the oscilloscope and thus appears as a readily identifiable, fixed "stimulus artifact" on the oscilloscope screen.

EXAMINATION PROCEDURE. The clinical findings on neurologic examination are commonly used to establish which muscles will be examined by electromyography. Those muscles are then systematically explored by inserting a needle electrode into multiple recording sites. After insertion, the electrode is allowed to remain in place for a brief period in several sites so that any spontaneous muscle activity may be recorded. The electrical activity is then recorded while the muscle is voluntarily and minimally contracted with the electrode left in position. Recordings of voluntary activity are also made at each stage of a gradual increase in the force of contraction until maximal voluntary effort is achieved. The electromyographer is thus able to look for any abnormalities in the pattern of electrical activity recorded during and immediately after electrode insertion, when the electrode is at rest within the muscle (spontaneous activity), and during voluntary muscle contraction of graded effort.

Healthy skeletal muscle typically exhibits a brief

burst of electrical activity when its fibers are stimulated by needle insertion or movement. A pattern of high-frequency repetitive discharges (bizarre high-frequency potentials) of constant amplitude can be seen on electrode insertion in conditions such as forms of muscular dystrophy, hyperkalemic periodic paralysis, chronic partial denervation, and polymyositis. In conditions in which myotonia is a feature, this discharge pattern appears to be composed of potentials resembling positive sharp waves and fibrillation potentials; it has an amplitude and frequency that waxes and wanes, giving rise to a characteristic decrescendo whine ("dive-bomber" sound) on the loudspeaker.

After insertional activity has ceased in healthy muscle at rest, no spontaneous activity (other than the end-plate noise that results when the electrode has been inadvertently placed in the end-plate region) can typically be recorded. In certain neuropathic disorders, spontaneous activity in the form of fasciculation and fibrillation potentials and positive sharp waves is a common finding. The bi- or triphasic fibrillation potentials have an amplitude of 20–300 μV, are usually up to 5 msec in duration, and fire at a rate of 2–20 per second. The fibrillation potential represents the spontaneous discharge of a single denervated muscle fiber. The sound over the loudspeaker, a high-pitched train of clicks, is characteristic. Although fibrillation potentials are infrequently recorded from normal muscle, they are common in neuropathies and may also be seen in progressive muscular dystrophy, polymyositis, and certain metabolic muscle disorders. Fasciculation potentials have similar dimensions to motor unit potentials (see below), occur singly or in repetition, and are heard as an abrupt, dull thud over the loudspeaker. Although characteristically found in anterior horn cell disease (such as that due to amyotrophic lateral sclerosis, syringomelia, or Werdnig-Hoffmann disease), fasciculation potentials are also seen in motor radiculopathies or neuropathies, and even occasionally in healthy muscles. Spontaneously occurring positive sharp waves have the same significance as fibrillations and are recorded in the same conditions. These potentials have an amplitude similar to that of fibrillation potentials, and discharge at a rate of 5–10 per second. Their duration may be as long as 100 msec. A repetitive firing of motor unit potentials, sometimes occurring in double, triple, or multiple discharge patterns, can also occur spontaneously in disorders such as tetany and myokymia.

Motor unit potentials are recorded during voluntary contraction of normal skeletal muscle. These compound action potentials represent the summed activity of the individual muscle fibers (usually about 10–15) within recording range of the needle electrode. They are typically bi- or triphasic in configuration, are 6–15 msec in duration, and have an amplitude of 200 μV to 3 mV. When the force of the voluntary contraction is increased, the firing rate of these potentials becomes progressively more regular and rapid as more motor units are recruited. When maximal voluntary effort is achieved, the so-called interference pattern of electrical activity results, a pattern in which the individual potentials can no longer be distinguished.

Changes in the size, shape, and number of these motor unit (voluntary) potentials can aid in the diagnosis of neuropathy and myopathy. For example, in myopathic disorders, motor unit potentials are reduced in amplitude and duration as muscle fibers are lost from the motor unit. The interference pattern is decreased in amplitude, but density of the recorded electrical activity is not reduced. In partially denervated muscle, the density of the interference pattern may become so reduced that individual motor units can again be recognized. With reinnervation, motor units become enlarged in amplitude and duration.

When certain abnormalities are present, the findings of this basic electromyographic examination may be supplemented by additional testing. For example, when myasthenia gravis or other defects of neuromuscular transmission are suspected, repetitive nerve stimulation may be utilized to demonstrate impaired neuromuscular transmission. Single-fiber electromyography, a sensitive and quantitative technique for the recording of action potentials of individual muscle fibers, can also be employed to investigate the state of functional integrity of the myoneural junction. Similarly, when some form of neuropathic disorder such as nerve entrapment, mononeuritis, or polyneuropathy is present, the results of nerve conduction studies (including the size and shape of evoked compound muscle action potentials) might also prove informative.

Additional information about these diagnostic techniques and their usefulness may be found under *nerve conduction studies.*

single-fiber e. (SFEMG), a technique used to assess the degree of functional integrity of neuromuscular transmission. A needle electrode is inserted to record the muscle action potentials from only one muscle fiber or from two or more individual fibers that are part of the same motor unit. This technique can also be used to measure the temporal variability between the potentials of two muscle fibers (the jitter) or to calculate the estimated fiber density of a motor unit.

electron (e) (e-lek′tron) [Gr. *ēlektron* amber] an elementary particle that has a negative unit charge, mass of 551 keV, and spin 1/2. The electrons of atoms are responsible for all their chemical properties. High-energy electrons emitted by nuclear decay are called beta particles. See also *beta decay.*

electron beam a narrow beam of electrons that is focused and deflected by electric or magnetic fields, as in a cathode ray rube (CRT) or electron microscope.

electron capture a type of radioactive decay in which a nuclide captures one of its inner shell electrons and a proton is converted to a neutron. In the process, the mass number of the nuclide is unchanged and the atomic number is decreased by one. A neutrino is always emitted. A gamma ray, characteristic x-ray, or Auger electron may also be emitted, depending on the specific nuclide.

electron capture (EC) detector a detector for a gas chromatograph. The current flowing through the ionized carrier gas is reduced by any compounds in the sample that bind (capture) electrons, e.g., halogenated compounds. See also under *gas chromatography.*

electron-dense opaque to the electron beam of an electron miscroscope, and therefore appearing dark on an electron micrograph.

electronegative (e-lek″tro-neg′ah-tiv) 1. having high electronegativity.

2. having a negative electric charge.

electronegativity (e′lek″tro-neg″ah-tiv′ĭ-te) in chemistry, the degree to which a chemical element can attract electrons.

electronic (e″lek-tron′ik) 1. pertaining to or carrying electrons. 2. pertaining to electrical circuitry that contains active components, such as transistors or integrated circuits.

electronic focal spot the area on the anode of an x-ray tube that is bombarded with electrons and produces x-rays.

electronics (e″lek-tron′iks) the branch of physics that deals with the behavior of electrons; the science and technology involved in the design and manufacture of electronic devices.

electronic voltmeter (EVM) a voltmeter in which the voltage being measured is amplified so that very little current is drawn from the circuit being tested. A typical EVM has an input resistance of 10 MΩ on DC ranges and 1 MΩ on AC ranges. Most also measure resistance but not current. An example is the vacuum tube voltmeter (VTVM).

electron lens the electric or magnetic fields used to focus an electron beam.

electron micrograph a photograph of an object made using an electron microscope.

electron microprobe an analytical instrument in which a beam of electrons scans the surface of a specimen, and collected electrons provide information on its composition. It differs from an analytical electron microscope in that the beam is considerably wider in diameter (several micrometers), providing a more homogeneous analysis; it must be targeted using light microscopic optics, and electron-micrographic images cannot be obtained.

electron microscope a microscope that uses electrons instead of light for illumination, thereby allowing much greater magnification and resolution than is possible with the light microscope. The electron microscope is correspondingly larger and more complex, and specimen preparation is more exacting. In the transmission electron microscope (TEM), the beam of electrons passes through the specimen, which is usually an extremely thin slice of tissue. The scanning electron microscope (SEM) provides an image of the surface of a specimen. The capabilities of the TEM and SEM can be combined in a single instrument (STEM). With the analytical electron microscope (AEM), the elemental composition of a specimen can be determined. See also the accompanying illustration.

analytical e. m. (AEM), an electron microscope in which a fine probe of electrons scans the surface of the specimen and emitted radiations are collected by detectors. A broad range of qualitative and quantitative determinations of the composition of the specimen can be recorded. At present, the AEM has limited practical application in service pathology.

scanning e. m. (SEM), an electron microscope that uses a beam of electrons to provide a three-dimensional image of the surface of a specimen. The SEM provides a depth of focus some 500 times greater than the light microscope and can give a resolution of better than 5 nm. In medicine the SEM has yielded interesting information on hematologic disorders and about surfaces such as those of the small intestine and the serous cavities; however, its contributions to patient care at present are limited in comparison with those of the TEM.

The electron beam is produced in the same way as in the TEM, using a tungsten filament, but alternatives with certain advantages are a lanthanum hexaboride electrode or a field emission system. The specimen is located at the foot of the column, and the electron beam scans a small area of the surface in a coordinated raster of fine lines. The surface of the specimen is positioned at an angle to the axis of the electron beam. The beam penetrates the surface for several micrometers, and the electrons collide with atoms of the specimen to give rise to several types of radiation, the most important of which are secondary and backscattered electrons. These electrons strike a detector that emits light, which is converted to an electron current and amplified by a photomultiplier to produce an image on a cathode ray tube. It can be examined by the operator sitting in front of the screen and can be photographically recorded (usually from a second screen, using Polaroid film).

In preparing biologic specimens for SEM, fixation of the surface is of paramount importance. Glutaraldehyde is widely used. The specimen is dehydrated in graded alcohols, and then the fluid is removed by freeze drying or more commonly by critical point drying. The dried specimen is mounted on a support stub, and its surface coated with a thin film of a heavy metal, such as gold, deposited using a vacuum evaporator or sputtering unit. The specimen is then ready for study.

transmission e. m. (TEM), an electron microscope in which the beam of electrons passes through the specimen to provide a magnified image of the area under study on a fluorescent screen. In clinical medicine the TEM has been particularly useful in evaluating renal biopsies and identifying and classifying many types of tumors, and, to a lesser degree, in studying entities such as infectious diseases.

The electrons are produced by passing an electric current through a pointed tungsten filament located at the top of a cylindric column. From 20 to 100 kV are used in most instruments, although larger and more powerful electron microscopes up to 2 MeV are available for the study of thicker sections. The electrons are formed into a slender beam that passes down the column, traversing the specimen, which is positioned at its midlevel, and impinging on the fluorescent screen located at its base. As the electrons pass through the specimen, some are deflected by denser areas, such as membranes. Electromagnetic lenses surround the column and alter the shape of the beam. Some of the lenses have at their center a small aperture (a disk with a central hole) that serves to screen off scattered electrons. The condenser lens or lenses located above the specimen control the illumination, the objective lens at the level of the specimen focuses the image, and the intermediate and projector lenses below the specimen magnify the image.

Much of the bulk of an electron microscope is taken up by the electrical controls, vacuum pumps (rotary and oil diffusion), and chilled water circulation for cooling. Photography is carried out by elevating the fluorescent screen, with the room darkened, to expose a photographic plate or film located beneath the screen. In some instruments, a 35-mm camera can be interposed higher in the column.

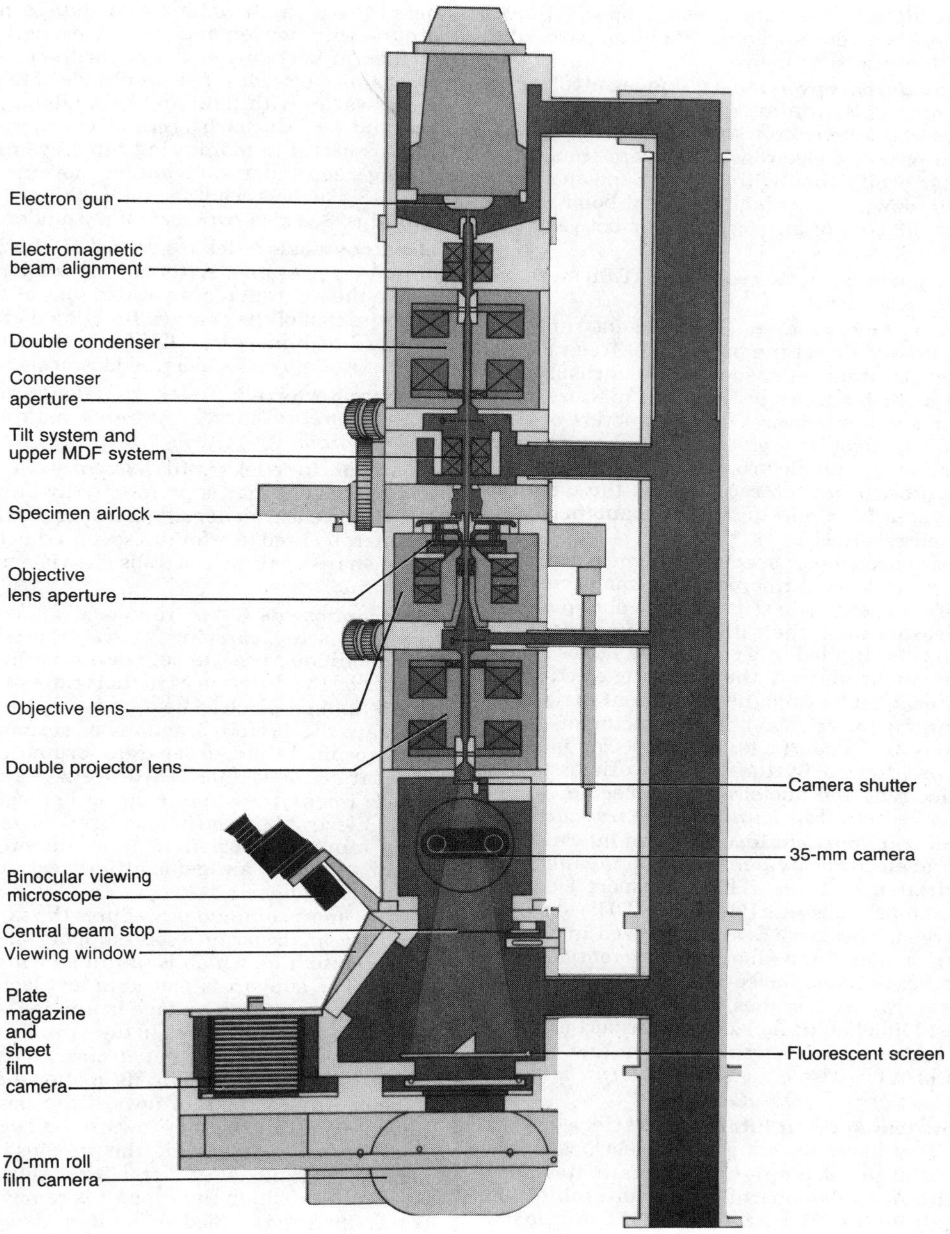

Electron microscope. Schematic drawing of electron microscope column. (Courtesy of Carl Zeiss, Inc.)

The image in the transmission electron microscope is black and white, and living material cannot be examined.

Preparation of specimens for examination with the TEM must be performed carefully, as any distortion introduced into the structure will be readily detectable. The initial and critical step is fixation. Most biologic specimens are fixed in a buffered solution of glutaraldehyde (e.g., 2 percent), and are then postfixed in 1 percent osmium tetroxide. Because the fixatives penetrate the tissues slowly, a specimen should not be larger than 1 mm in size or thickness. The fixed specimen is dehydrated in graded alcohols and is then embedded in an epoxy resin.

Once the resin has polymerized, sections approximately 1 mμ thick can be cut with glass knives, prepared by careful breaking of strips of glass, and stained with methylene blue or toluidine blue for examination with the light microscope. Thinner sections (of the order of 70 nm) are usually cut with diamond knives and mounted on small copper grids. To enhance image contrast, the sections are stained with solutions of heavy metals, usually lead (citrate or hydroxide) and uranium (acetate). Special procedures have been developed for handling particular types of biologic specimens.

electron microscopy 1. the techniques involved in the use of the electron microscope.
2. the use of an electron microscope.

electron pair two electrons in the same atomic or molecular orbital, one with spin up and the other with spin down. A covalent chemical bond results from the sharing of an electron pair between two atoms.

electron paramagnetic resonance (EPR) see *electron spin resonance.*

electron spin resonance (ESR) an instrumental method used to detect the presence of free radicals or other paramagnetic species, to measure the amount of such species present in a mixture, or to determine certain features of the structure of such species. The sample is placed in a magnetic field and irradiated with electromagnetic radiation. Energy absorbed from the radiation as the unpaired electron goes from one spin state to another is detected and recorded.

The esr spectrum is specified by measuring the absorption of a fixed microwave frequency over a range of magnetic field strengths. To obtain a standard measurement, the ratio of frequency to field strength is multiplied by a conversion factor to give the magnetic moment of the absorbing electrons as a g factor, which is magnetic moment divided by the Bohr magnetron (μ_B). The g factor of a free electron is 2.00. The g factor of an electron in a free radical is affected by the magnetic fields of the other electrons and nuclei in the molecule.

Also called *electron paramagnetic resonance.*

electron transport chain a system of intermediate carriers of electrons located in and on the inner mitochondrial membrane. They transport electrons from a reduced substrate (NADH, $FADH_2$) to molecular oxygen. The carriers are organized in a chain in order of their individual redox potentials; they include flavin mononucleotide (FMN), ubiquinone (CoQ), several cytochromes, and several iron-sulfur proteins. Mitochondrial electron transport is tightly coupled to oxidative phosphorylation and the formation of ATP. Also called *respiratory chain.* See also *oxidative phosphorylation.*

electron transport inhibitors a variety of compounds that block the transfer of electrons at specific sites of the electron transfer chain. Rotenone, piericidin A, and amobarbital (Amytal) inhibit the transfer from NADH to flavoprotein FP_1. Antimycin A_1 inhibits the transfer from cytochrome b to cytochrome c_1. Cyanide, hydrogen sulfide, and carbon monoxide inhibit the transfer from cytochrome c to cytochromes a and a_3. See also *oxidative phosphorylation inhibitors* and *oxidative phosphorylation uncouplers.*

electron volt (eV) a very small unit of energy defined as the kinetic energy acquired by an electron in moving through an electric potential difference of 1 volt (1.602192×10^{-19} J). It is a convenient unit for measurements of the mass and kinetic energy of elementary particles or for measurements of the ionization energy of atoms and molecules.

electrooculogram (EOG) (e-lek″tro-ok′u-lo-gram″) [*electro-* + L. *oculus* eye + Gr. *gramma* mark] the record of the changes in steady, resting electric potential of the eye obtained from electrodes placed near the two canthi of the eye. A change in potential occurs with movements of the eyeball owing to change in positions of the eye with respect to the recording electrodes. The amplitude of these fluctuations varies with light and dark adaptation of the eye and is reduced by retinal degeneration. The EOG is useful in monitoring rapid eye movements during sleep and in studying eye movements during activities such as reading and tracking of a moving stimulus. See also *corneoretinal p.* under *potential.*

electroosmosis (e-lek″tro-oz-mo′sis) the movement of liquid across an electrophoretic support medium due to the migration of hydrated ions of the charge opposite that of the charged functional group in the support medium (e.g., $—CH_2COO^-$ in cellulose acetate). Also known as electroendosmosis.

electropherogram (e-lek″tro-fer′o-gram) [*electro-* + Gr. *pherein* to carry + *gramma* mark] see *electrophoretogram.*

electrophile (e-lek′tro-fīl) [*electro-* + Gr. *philein* to love] a reagent that is preferentially attracted to a site of low electron density in a substrate. The term is generally used to refer to a species that can accept an unshared pair of electrons (Lewis acid). Cf. *nucleophile.*

electrophoresis (e-lek″tro-fo-re′sis) [*electro-* + Gr. *phoros* bearing, carrying + *-ēsis* process] a laboratory technique used to separate mixtures of ionic solutes by the differences in their rates of migration in an applied electric field. It is used routinely to separate the protein fractions of serum, urine, or cerebrospinal fluid; to separate serum lipoproteins; to separate the lactate dehydrogenase and creatine kinase isoenzymes; and to detect hemoglobin variants. Electrophoresis is also used in conjunction with immunodiffusion to separate proteins and identify them by antigenic differences; see also *immunoelectrophoresis.*

In the most common procedures the sample is applied to a small spot on a solid support, such as cellulose acetate film, which is saturated with buffer solution. The support is placed in an electrophoresis apparatus, and high voltage is applied to the electrodes. Each ionic species in the sample migrates at a rate dependent on its net electric charge and the viscous drag produced by its motion through the solvent. Anions migrate toward the positive electrode (anode) and cations toward the negative electrode (cathode). Over time, the proteins in the sample separate into several fractions (electrophoretic bands), after which the support is removed and the bands fixed and stained to facilitate visualization. A scanning densitometer can then be used to quantitate the fractions. It produces a graph of the dye density in each fraction and integrates the area under each peak of the graph.

The drag forces on a molecule depend on its size and shape; the net charge depends both on the numbers of acidic and basic groups in the molecule and on the pH of the buffer. In proteins, the acidic side-chains of aspartic acid and glutamic acid residues are negatively charged at any pH above their pK, and the basic side-chains of lysine and arginine are positively charged at any pH below their pK of 10.5 and 12.5. In routine serum protein electrophoresis (SPE), a pH 8.6 buffer is used and all serum proteins have a net negative charge and migrate toward the anode.

Cellulose acetate and paper supports absorb hydroxyl ions from the buffer; thus, the buffer is positively charged relative to the medium and flows toward the cathode, sweeping the protein molecules of the sample along with it. This counterflow is called electroendosmosis or endosmosis. In SPE the most negatively charged fraction, prealbumin, migrates the farthest toward the anode, while the least negatively charged fraction, the gamma globulin, may be swept backward toward the anode. Agarose gel (AGE) is also used for SPE; it has the advantages that it does not cause electroendosmosis and has little affinity for proteins.

Both separation time and resolution are affected by the ionic strength of the buffer. As the ionic strength is increased, the migration rate decreases because the buffer ion field retards the migration of the sample components; resolution is increased, however.

Disc gel electrophoresis uses a gel support with a fine pore size and is, in effect, a combination of electrophoresis and gel-filtration chromatography. Using polyacrylamide gel, the serum proteins can be separated into 20 or more fractions, whereas routinely used media such as cellulose acetate or agarose produce only five to seven bands.

See also *lipoprotein assays, protein electrophoresis,* and the accompanying illustration.

electrophoretic (e-lek″tro-fo-ret′ik) pertaining to electrophoresis.

electrophoretic mobility (μ) the velocity at which an ion moves during electrophoresis divided by the applied field strength. It is customarily reported in mobility units, defined as 10^{-5} $cm^2/V{\cdot}s$.

electrophoretogram (e-lek″tro-fo-ret′o-gram) [*electro-* + Gr. *phoros* bearing + *gramma* mark] a developed (stained) electrophoresis strip showing the separated bands or the chart produced by a scanning densitometer from a developed strip. Also called *electropherogram.*

electrophysiology (e-lek″tro-fiz″e-ol′o-je) the study of the electric reactions of an organism; the science of physiology in its relation to electricity.

electropositive (e-lek″tro-poz′ĭ-tiv) 1. having low electronegativity.

2. having a positive electric charge.

electroretinogram (ERG) (e-lek″tro-ret′ĭ-no-gram″) [*electro-* + *retina* + Gr. *gramma* mark] the record obtained from electroretinography; usually the complex, extracellular electric potential recorded between an electrode placed on the cornea and a reference electrode on another part of the head. The ERG has two distinct components: a steady resting potential and a multiphasic transient potential produced in response to light. The transient potential reaches full development in the human at age 1 yr; typically, it consists of four principal waves: *a, b, c,* and *d.*

The *a* wave is a small, sharp, negative potential that reaches maximal development within about 15 msec of stimulus (light) onset and relates in part to photoreceptor processes of both the rods and cones. It is followed by a high-amplitude positive potential (*b* wave) that peaks 60–70 msec after stimulus onset and represents complex activity of the retinal bipolar layer. The response related to Müller cell activity alone is sometimes referred to as the *m* wave. The *c* wave, also electropositive, is produced by the pigmented epithelium of the retina in response to changes in extracellular potassium (K^+) resulting from photoreceptor activity. The *d* wave, not always prominent in the human ERG, is produced by cone receptors when a light stimulus is terminated.

As stimulus parameters (wavelength, intensity, duration, and pattern) are altered, the waveform characteristics of the ERG can be altered. In general, as the stimulus intensity increases, the amplitude of the ERG increases and the latency (time from stimulus onset to beginning of *a* wave) shortens. The amplitude of the *b* wave usually decreases with age.

See also *corneoretinal p.* under *potential* and *electroretinography.*

electroretinography (e-lek″tro-ret″ĭ-nog′rah-fe) [*electro-* + *retina* + Gr. *graphein* to record] the recording of the changes in electric potential from the retina following stimulation of the retina by light. There is no universal standard accepted procedure for recording the electroretinogram (ERG), and no single technique is useful in assessing all aspects of retinal function. Generally, an electrode is placed on the cornea and a reference electrode is placed on another part of the head. The potential difference between these electrodes is amplified and displayed on an oscilloscope or oscillograph that should represent uniformly all frequencies from 0 to 120 Hz, so that the response to light flashes or flickers of vari-

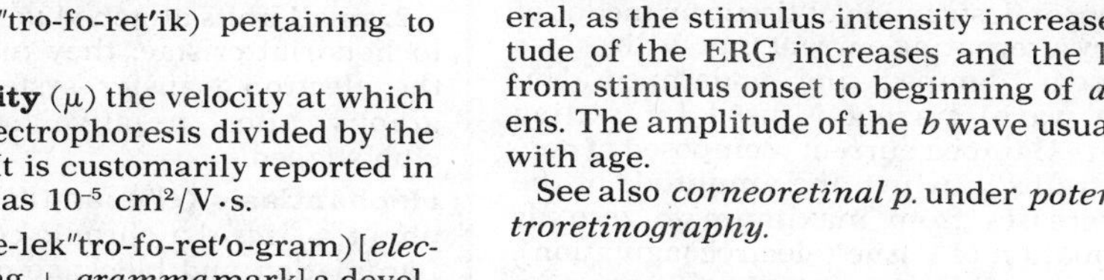

Electrophoresis. Cross section of a simple electrophoresis apparatus; E = electrodes; B = baffle system for minimizing diffusion of breakdown products of buffer; and C = cellulose acetate membrane on carrier. (From Raphael, S. S.: Lynch's Medical Laboratory Technology. 3rd ed. Philadelphia, W. B. Saunders Co., 1976.)

ous wavelengths, intensities, durations, frequencies, and patterns can be evaluated. The potentials are measured and plotted as recorded or are stored on magnetic tape for computer analysis.

Electroretinography is useful in the diagnosis of hereditary or acquired retinal degeneration, night blindness, and circulatory disturbances of the retina because of the characteristic electrical changes that may be found.

See also *electroretinogram* and *visual evoked p.* under *potential.*

electroscope (e-lek′tro-scōp) [*electro-* + Gr. *skopein* to examine] a device that measures electric charge, such as in a pocket dosimeter.

electrostatic (e-lek″tro-stat′ik) [*electro-* + Gr. *statikos* causing to stand or stop] pertaining to the forces and effects produced by stationary electric charges.

electrostatic unit (esu) the electrostatic centimeter-gram-second (cgs) unit of electric charge, defined as the magnitude of each of two identical charges that repel one another with a force of 1 dyne when separated by 1 centimeter. It is equal to 3.335635×10^{-10} coulomb (C) (which is 10 divided by the velocity of light in cm/s). Also called *franklin* and *statcoulomb.*

electrosurgery (e-lek″tro-sur′jer-e) the surgical removal, incision, or destruction of tissue by means of high-frequency alternating current that utilizes two types of current, damped and undamped. Undamped (sine wave) current is used for cutting (electrosection). Damped current (composed of successive wave trains in which the amplitude of the oscillation decreases from maximum to zero) is used for coagulation of tissue (electrocoagulation). The current is applied between a concentrating electrode (the electrosurgical or electrocautery pencil) and a dispersing electrode (the patient-grounding pad).

eleidin (el-e′ĭ-din) a substance related to keratin that is found in the stratum lucidum of the skin.

Elek test (el′ek) an in vitro immunodiffusion test for the detection of toxigenic strains of *Corynebacterium diphtheriae.* In the modified test currently used, the mixed primary culture is streaked on a specially prepared agar plate next to a strip of filter paper perfused with diphtheria antitoxin. The exotoxin produced by the bacteria forms a band of precipitation, with antitoxin diffusing from the filter paper.

element (el′ĕ-ment) [L. *elementum*] 1. a primary or irreducible part of something.

2. a chemical element, a pure substance that cannot be decomposed by chemical reactions; it consists of all the atoms with a given number of protons (and the same number of electrons). The number of neutrons and thus the mass of the atoms varies. Atoms with the same proton number but different neutron numbers are called isotopes. Each element has an atomic number (Z), (which is the number of protons), and an atomic weight (which is the average mass per atom expressed in arbitrary units in which the isotope carbon-12 has a mass of 12.000). No element with Z greater than 83 has a stable isotope, but uranium (92) and thorium (90) have half-lives on the order of the age of the earth; they and their decay products occur naturally.

Each element has unique chemical and physical properties determined by its electronic configuration. The electrons occupy orbitals (quantum states) with a maximum of two electrons (one spin-up and one spin-down) to an orbital. All the orbitals with the same energy constitute a shell. In the ground state, the lowest energy orbitals are occupied. A closed (full) shell of electrons has little effect on the properties of an element; the electrons in the incomplete outer shell (valence electrons) are responsible for the chemical bonding. The periodic table is an arrangement of the elements that shows the relationships by grouping the elements according to their valence electronic configurations.

elementary body (el″ĕ-men′tah-re) the extracellular infectious stage in the developmental cycle of *Chlamydia,* a genus of microorganisms that causes ocular, urogenital, and respiratory infections in humans.

elementary charge (e) the fundamental electric charge, 1.6022×10^{-19} C. All elementary particles except quarks have a charge that is an integral multiple of e; the electron is –e and the proton is +e.

elementary particle 1. any constituent of matter or energy that cannot be subdivided, e.g., a proton, neutron, electron, neutrino, or photon. All the particles of a type (e.g., all electrons) are identical; they have the same mass, charge, spin, magnetic moment, and other properties.

2. small units attached to the inner surface of mitochondrial cristae; they may contain enzymes of the electron transfer system. In electron micrographs after negative staining, they appear club-shaped.

elephantiasis (el″ĕ-fan-ti′ah-sis) [Gr. *elephas* elephant + *-iasis*] a chronic condition marked by inflammation and blockage of the lymph channels, which results in the accumulation of large volumes of fluid and hypertrophy of the skin and subcutaneous tissues. The disease chiefly affects the legs and genital area, causing them to enlarge massively. True elephantiasis is caused by the parasitic filarial worms *Wuchereria bancrofti* and *Brugia malayi,* although any disease that results in hypertrophy, enlargement, and skin thickening may also be called by this name. See also *filariasis.*

elimination reaction (e-lim″ĭ-na′shun) in organic chemistry, a reaction in which groups bound to carbon atoms are removed, generally increasing the degree of unsaturation of the substrate, e.g., NaOH + $CH_3CH_2Br \rightarrow CH_2{=}CH_2 + H_2O$ + NaBr. See also *addition reaction* and *substitution reaction.*

ELISA (acronym from *e*nzyme-*l*inked *i*mmuno-*s*orbent *a*ssay) a sensitive laboratory method used to detect the presence of either antigens or antibodies of interest in biologic samples. This method utilizes enzyme-labeled immunoreactants (antigen or antibody) and a solid-phase binding support (e.g., test tubes, beads, or microtiter plates). In various types of assay modifications, the amount of enzyme activity attached to the solid support after a suitable reaction time is proportional to the concentration of the analyte being measured. Nano- and picogram quantities of analyte can be detected, making this system as sensitive as most radioimmunoassays and much more sensitive than agglutination, hemagglutination, complement-fixation, and immunofluorescent techniques.

Some common enzymes used for labeling of the reactants include alkaline phosphatase, horseradish peroxidase, glucose oxidase, β-galactosidase, glucoamylase, and carbonic anhydrase. These enzymes are frequently used because of their high substrate turnover rate, ease of conjugation to the immunoreactant, low cost, and commercial availability. The products of the enzyme reaction are usually detected by photometry or fluorimetry. Labeling is performed by covalently linking the enzyme to the immunoreactant by use of glutaraldehyde, periodate, or dimaleimide as enzyme-protein coupling agents.

Three methods of antigen detection are commonly used, each with its own advantages and disadvantages. The selection of the appropriate method depends on characteristics of the test antigen and includes size, purity, chemical nature, and scarcity.

DIRECT COMPETITION. The solid phase is coated with antibody specific for the test antigen. Both sample and enzyme conjugated antigen are added to the reaction mixture, and competition for binding sites on the solid-phase antibody occurs. After incubation and washing, enzyme substrate is added. The enzyme attached to the solid phase catalyzes a chemical reaction that forms a colored product inversely proportional to the amount of antigen in the sample. Conversely, if the analyte is an immunoglobulin, an enzyme-labeled antibody and solid-phase bound antigen may be used. Also called competitive inhibition assay.

DOUBLE ANTIBODY (ANTIGEN) SANDWICH. Specific antibody is adsorbed onto the solid phase, sample is added, and antigen, if present, attaches to the bound antibody. Then, enzyme-labeled antibody is added and binds to the antigen, creating a "sandwich" of antigen between two antibodies. After washing, substrate addition, and incubation, the color production is directly proportional to the amount of antigen in the sample. Conversely, if the analyte is an antibody, enzyme-labeled antigen and solid-phase bound antigen may be used.

ANTIBODY INHIBITION. Sample is added to specific enzyme-labeled antibody. If present, antigen attaches to the antibody conjugate. This mixture, with reduced availability for subsequent attachment to a solid-phase antigen, is then added to the antigen bound to a solid phase. After incubation, washing and substrate addition, color formed during incubation is inversely proportional to the amount of antigen in the sample.

ELISA assays have the same problems as other immunoassays, particularly assurance of reagent specificity and construction of the calibration curve. A problem unique to ELISA is ensuring uniformity of the binding of the antigen or antibody to the solid support. ELISA has an advantage over RIA in that it avoids the handling of radioactive materials. It is also relatively simple to automate. As with any assay, positive and negative controls should be run each time and records of accurate quality control maintained.

ELISA may be used to evaluate the quantity of the antigens or antibodies associated with most infectious diseases. The method is most often applied to the diagnosis of viral diseases with reagents available for cytomegalovirus, measles, herpes, rubella, adenovirus, rotavirus, mumps, picornavirus, Epstein-Barr virus, and arbovirus. Nonviral applications of ELISA include *Mycoplasma pneumoniae* and *Legionella pneumophila,* as well as many parasite and fungal infections.

See also *enzyme assisted immunoassay technique* and *enzyme immunoassay.*

ALAN D. RINKER, M.S.

ellipse (ĕ-lips′) [Gr. *ēlleipsis* an omission, a falling short] a closed curve consisting of all points for which the sum of their distances from two fixed points (the foci) is a constant.

ellipsoid (ĕ-lip′soid) [*ellipse* + Gr. *eidos* form] a geometric solid having cross sections that are all ellipses or circles. See also the illustration accompanying *contour.*

ellipsoidal (ĕ″lip-soi′dal) having the shape of an ellipsoid. An ellipsoidal object has a circular outline when viewed along its major axis and an elliptical outline in other views. See also the illustration accompanying *contour.*

elliptical (ĕ-lip′tĭ-kal) having the shape of an ellipse.

elliptocyte (ĕ-lip′to-sīt) [*ellipse* + Gr. *kytos* hollow vessel] an oval or elliptical erythrocyte. It may be found in normal blood (less than 1 percent) and in increased numbers (up to 10 percent) in anemias, particularly anemias associated with leukemia, thalassemia, iron deficiency, and megaloblastic hematopoiesis. Elliptocytes in anemias may depart only slightly from the normal spherical shape or may have so exaggerated a ratio of long to short axis as to be pencil-like in shape (elliptocytes I–IV).

In hereditary elliptocytosis, the number of elliptocytes is in the range of 25–75 percent or higher. The oval shape is usually marked and tends to be uniform.

Also called *ovalocyte.* See also *hereditary e.* under *elliptocytosis.*

elliptocytosis (ĕ-lip″to-si-to′sis) [*elliptocyte* + *-osis* condition] the presence of red cells in the blood that are oval or elliptical in shape. Also called *ovalocytosis.*

hereditary e. (HE), a hereditary condition of poikilocytes, transmitted as an autosomal dominant trait, that is associated with varying degrees of hemolysis. In some families, the gene is linked with the Rh blood type. Elliptically shaped erythrocytes appear in the peripheral blood in large numbers; HE can be distinguished from other hematologic disorders by having at least 25 percent (often up to 50-90 percent) of such cells and by the absence of other types of red cell malformation.

Elliptocyte formation is apparently limited to red cell aging; marrow erythroblasts are normal in shape, and reticulocytes are not as oval as are the mature erythrocytes. The rapid decline in ATP and 2,3-DPG and the increase in sodium efflux seen in incubated cells suggest a defect in membrane permeability similar to that of hereditary spherocytosis.

Most affected individuals have no clinical manifestations; approximately 12 percent exhibit evidence of a chronic hemolytic state, although anemia, if present, is mild. Red cell life span is moderately shortened, but uncompensated hemolytic disease may show a red cell half-survival time as short as 5 da.

elongation (e″long-ga′shun) the growth of the peptide chain in translation. See also *translation.*

elongation factor a specific protein involved in ribosomal peptide chain elongation during protein synthesis. The second molecule of transfer RNA (tRNA), plus all succeeding molecules, is brought to the ribosome in combination with an elongation factor. This factor also binds guanosine triphosphate (GTP) during the process. Elongation involves at least one, and perhaps several, additional protein factors in eukaryotes. The enzymatic hydrolysis GTP→GDP + P_i causes release of the elongation factor, leaving tRNA and its amino acid loaded on the ribosome.

El Tor vibrio (el-tor′) a hemolytic biotype of *Vibrio cholerae,* first isolated from healthy pilgrims returning from Mecca through the quarantine station at El Tor, on the Sinai Peninsula. The organisms are pathogenic and are the causative agent of the pandemic of cholera that began in 1961 and spread throughout Asia and Africa during the following two decades. It is more resistant to chemical and physical agents than are the classic nonhemolytic strains.

eluate (el′u-āt) the substance separated out by elution.

eluent (e-lu′ent) a solvent or solution used in elution.

elute (e-lūt′) [L. *elutus,* from *eluere* to wash out] to remove adsorbed material from an adsorbent by the use of a solvent.

elution (e-lu′shun) 1. in chemistry, the separation of material by washing, as with a solvent that dissolves just one component.

2. in chromatography, the process of developing the chromatogram by passing the mobile phase (usually a liquid solvent) over the stationary phase (as in column chromatography).

3. the removal or release of a compound attached to some insoluble adsorbent.

4. the leakage or removal of a radiotracer that does not permanently bind to its intended site, e.g., elution of ^{51}Cr from chromium-tagged red cells, which introduces an error into red cell survival measurements by radiochromium.

5. the removal of antibodies adsorbed onto the erythrocyte surface. This procedure is performed for several reasons: to detect and identify the presence of a single antibody bound to the red cells of infants affected with hemolytic disease of the newborn, to detect and determine specificity of the antibodies responsible for transfusion reactions or for a positive antiglobulin test in acquired hemolytic anemia, to prepare nonspecific antibody for further testing, to prepare erythrocytes free of attached antibodies, and to demonstrate the presence of weak subgroups of the ABO system.

Two techniques are commonly employed, heat elution and ether elution. For both methods it is essential that all unadsorbed antibody be removed. Heat elution efficiently removes IgM antibodies; packed, washed red cells suspended in saline are constantly agitated while being incubated at 56°C, and are then centrifuged and the eluate tested. Ether elution efficiently removes IgG antibodies; packed, washed red cells are mixed with saline and ether. After elution is complete, the eluate is centrifuged and tested with the antiglobulin test. Recently, xylene has been found to give superior results.

elutriation (e-lu″tre-a′shun) [L. *elutriare* to wash out] the process of separating substances by pulverizing them and mixing them with water so that the heavier particles settle out.

em- (em) [Gr.] a prefix word element to denote in, e.g., empyema.

EMB abbrev. for eosin-methylene blue. See *eosin–methylene blue a.* under *agar.*

Embadomonas (em″bah-dom′o-nas) the former name for a genus of flagellates now called *Retortamonas.*

EMB agar abbrev. See *eosin–methylene blue a.* under *agar.*

Embden-Meyerhof pathway (em′den mi′er-hof) [C. G. *Embden,* German biochemist, 1874–1933; Otto Fritz *Meyerhof,* German biochemist, 1884–1951] a series of chemical reactions catalyzed by specific enzymes that convert glucose to pyruvate, yielding high-energy phosphate (e.g., ATP) in the process. The reactions occur in muscle and in many, but not all, microorganisms. Also known as *glycolysis.*

embedding (em-bed′ing) in histology, the process of surrounding and filling in the spaces of a tissue specimen with a supporting medium so that thin sections can be cut with a microtome for histologic examination. Paraffin wax is routinely used as the embedding medium, and the addition of synthetic polymers gives improved results. After dehydration and clearing, the tissue is submerged in two or three changes of melted wax for several hours, during which time the tissue becomes infiltrated (impregnated) with wax. The tissue is then placed in a mold filled with melted wax and rapidly cooled, a procedure called casting or blocking.

The ultrathin sections required for electron microscopy necessitate the embedding of the tissue specimens in plastic. Various combinations of epoxy resins, accelerators, and curing agents are used. The tissue blocks are hardened by allowing the plastic to polymerize in an oven for several hours. Plastic embedding in glycol-methacrylate may be used for the preparation of thin sections for certain light-microscopic studies.

See also *Carbowax* and *celloidin.*

embolism (em′bo-lizm) [L. *embolismus,* from Gr. *en-* in + *ballein* to throw] the sudden blockage of an artery resulting in the cessation or diminution of blood flow. The obstructing agent is usually a clot or foreign material that lodges in an arterial bifurcation or narrowing; this deprives the distal tissue of blood, which leads to ischemia. In addition to clots, fat globules, gas bubbles, atherosclerotic debris, tissue fragments, and clumps of bacteria may act as embolic agents. Cf. *thrombosis.*

air e., see *gas e.*

amniotic fluid e., an embolism of amniotic fluid, which may contain epithelial squames, lanugo hair, mucus, and other debris, that enters the vascular system during tumultuous labor by the forcing of fluid into uterine venous sinuses during uterine contractions. It is a potentially fatal maternal obstetric complication and is a cause of disseminated intravascular coagulation (DIC).

arterial e., an acute blockage of arterial blood flow due to the migration of an embolus; a frequent complication of heart disease. More than half of the emboli reach the lower extremities and may cause pain, numbness, weakness, pallor, and the collapse of superficial veins. The lesion may progress to necrosis and gangrene. Arteriography and ultrasound examination may be useful in diagnosis. If the embolic agent is a blood clot, heparin treatment may be useful; surgery may also be required.

bone marrow e., an uncommon form of embolism that involves the occlusion of small vessels by fat and hematopoietic cells of the marrow. The usual cause is traumatic injury that produces fracture of the long bones at sites containing abundant marrow. It is a complication of closed cardiac massage secondary to rib fracture. A few individuals develop the fat embolism syndrome (respiratory insufficiency, cerebral symptoms, and petechiae). Also called *fat e.*

cerebral e., the lodging in a cerebral artery of a clot or other material that originated at some other site; one of the major causes of cerebrovascular accidents (CVA). The occluding material may consist of blood clot, tumor, fat, air, or clumps of bacteria. Occlusion may result in cerebral infarction, causing a stroke. Symptoms usually develop rapidly with no previous warning, but there may be evidence of recent emboli to other organs. Computed tomography (CT), cerebral angiography, and brain scans may be useful in determining the diagnosis. In all cases an attempt must be made to determine the source of the emboli. See also *cerebrovascular accident.*

fat e., see *bone marrow e.*

gas e., a disorder characterized by the presence of gas bubbles in the blood. It may be caused by overinflation of the lungs with rupture of alveolar walls and pulmonary veins due to expanding pulmonary gas during reduction of surrounding pressure (as occurs in underwater diving ascents). This leads to loss of consciousness, possibly with other central nervous system manifestations. Another cause is the introduction of large amounts of air into the veins (as in intravenous procedures), which leads to inefficient heart pumping and heart failure. Also called *air e.*

massive e., the condition that occurs when a large blood clot has detached from its site of formation and attachment and travels with the blood flow, becoming lodged in a major vessel or vessels.

pulmonary e., the lodging of a clot or other foreign substance in a pulmonary artery, with obstruction of the blood supply to the lung parenchyma. About 75 percent of emboli arise in the deep leg veins. This condition is commonly seen in elderly, immobile patients. Clinical and laboratory manifestations are related to the size and location of the embolus, and include infarction and even death. Symptoms include sudden dyspnea, anxiety, and hyperventilation. There may be pulmonary hypertension, right ventricular failure, shock, and arterial hypoxia. Circulatory collapse and sudden death can occur with a large embolus.

Radiographs often appear normal, although pulmonary artery enlargement, pulmonary densities, or a small effusion may be visible. Electrocardiograms may reveal tachycardia, without other abnormalities. Perfusion scintiphotographs with technetium-99, inhalation tests (xenon-133), and pulmonary angiography can be valuable in establishing the diagnosis.

Also called pulmonary thromboembolism.

embolus (em′bo-lus), pl. *emboli* [Gr. *embolos* plug] a piece of matter, such as a clot, fat, atherosclerotic debris, tumor cells, or a bubble of gas, within a blood vessel. The material is carried along within the circulation until it lodges in a vessel, obstructing blood flow. This reduction or cessation of blood flow often results in an infarct of tissue supplied by the obstructed vessel in the affected organ. See also *embolism.*

embryo (em′bre-o) [Gr. *embryon*] 1. in plants, the elements of the seed that develops into a new individual.

2. in animals, those derivatives of the fertilized ovum that eventually become the offspring, during their period of most rapid development, i.e., after the long axis appears until all major structures are represented. In humans, the developing organism is an embryo from about the second week after fertilization to the end of the second intrauterine month; thereafter, it is termed a fetus.

embryology (em″bre-ol′o-je) [*embryo* + *-logy*] the science of the development of the individual. In mammals, it refers particularly to development during the intrauterine period. Morphologic development is an expression of genetic information in the nuclei of the gametes. The organized process of maturation of a particular part of the body is influenced by chemical activating agents or inductors that diffuse from adjacent tissues. Development may be affected by hormones, vitamins, nucleic acids, and other factors.

The process of differentiation of a tissue is accompanied by the development of new structural and biochemical properties of its component cells. Growth is achieved by an increase in the number of cells, by the formation of intercellular tissues, and to a limited degree by enlargement of some cells. Growth is normally limited by functional restraints, the mature form of the tissue being maintained through progressive replacement of lost cells from primitive precursors. More highly specialized cells are not replaceable.

Disturbances of the normal embryologic development of tissues may result in the emergence of anomalies, and tissues are particularly vulnerable in the early stages of their formation. Teratogenic agents include certain drugs, e.g., thalidomide, and organisms, e.g., rubella virus.

embryoma (em″bre-o′mah) [*embryo-* + Gr. *ōma* swelling] a general term used to describe tumors that recapitulate embryonic cells or tissues. See also *nephroblastoma* and *pulmonary blastoma.*

e. of kidney, see *nephroblastoma.*

embryonal (em′bre-o-nal) pertaining to the embryo.

embryonal cell carcinoma a malignant germ cell tumor whose cells are multipotential. See also *ovarian tumors* and *testicular tumor.*

embryonate (em′bre-o-nāt) 1. pertaining to or resembling an embryo.

2. containing an embryo.

3. impregnated; fecundated.

embryonic (em″bre-on′ik) of or pertaining to the embryo.

embryonic development the sequence of changes in form and structure that a developing individual undergoes during the intrauterine period. Fertilization of the ovum generally occurs in the lateral portion of the uterine tube, forming a diploid cell that then goes through a series of mitotic divisions (the process of cleavage). There is relatively little synthesis of cytoplasm, and the result is a ball of smaller cells, the blastocyst. As the number of cells increases, those at the periphery become arranged in a layer surrounding a central cavity into which an inner cell mass protrudes. The outer cells form the trophoblast, which later develops into the fetal membranes and placenta, while the inner cell mass forms the embryo proper.

The blastocyst implants in the prepared endometrium, usually high on the posterior wall of the uterus, at around 6 da following fertilization. Enzymes produced by the trophoblast aid its penetration, and it is completely immersed by the twelfth day. The trophoblast differentiates into an outer syncytial layer and an inner cytotrophoblastic layer and the inner cell mass forms a bilaminar embryonic disk composed of a layer of columnar ectodermal cells and a layer of cuboidal endodermal cells. An amniotic cavity appears between ectoderm and trophoblast.

Spaces within the syncytial layer of the trophoblast on the deep aspect of the embryo expand and communicate with maternal vessels, establishing the uteroplacental circulation. Cells from the inner aspect of the trophoblast proliferate as the extraembryonic mesoderm, and cavities within this mass of cells become confluent to create the extraembryonic coelom or chorionic cavity. Endodermal cells then form the (secondary) yolk sac that protrudes into the chorionic cavity. Mesodermal cells appear between ectoderm and endoderm and migrate laterally; by the seventeenth day the embryo is a trilaminar disk. With further growth, it folds so that its margins come to rim the umbilical opening, an elaborate system of placental villi develops, and the embryo becomes suspended within the chorionic cavity by a connecting stalk containing the umbilical vessels. (See the accompanying illustration.)

In the course of later development, the ectodermal layer forms the nervous system and eyes, anterior pituitary, epidermis and contiguous areas of mucosal epithelium, adnexal structures, and salivary glands. Endodermal derivatives include the epithelium of the alimentary and respiratory systems, liver, pancreas, thyroid, parathyroids, thymus, bladder, and prostate. The mesoderm forms the connective tissues, including blood and vessels, mesothelium, kidneys, and adrenal cortices.

embryonic hemoglobin one of the hemoglobins detectable only in the first 3 mo of fetal development. Embryonic hemoglobins are synthesized by the erythroid cells derived from the yolk sac and include Gower 1 ($\zeta_2\epsilon_2$), Gower 2 ($\alpha_2\epsilon_2$), and hemoglobin Portland ($\zeta_2\gamma_2$). See also *hemoglobin.*

embryoniform (em″bre-on′ĭ-form) resembling an embryo.

embryonization (em″bre-o-nĭ-za′shun) reversion to the embryonic form on the part of a tissue or cell.

emergency medical technician (EMT) (e-mer′-jen-se) [L. *emergere* to raise up] an individual trained to manage the emergency care of sick or injured persons during transport to a hospital. The EMT can administer injections and intravenous fluids, read electrocardiograms, and, under a physician's orders, perform defibrillation and other advanced life-support measures. Educational preparation involves completion of an approved program; graduates are certified by the states in which they work. An advanced EMT (EMT II) is also called a *paramedic.*

emergency procedure an established method for responding to an emergency. In the laboratory, such procedures are mandated by National Fire Protection Association regulations for controlling chemical spills, extinguishing clothing fires, actuating alarm systems, evacuating the laboratory, shutting down equipment, and implementing fire control operations by the public fire department or by an emergency control group within the organization.

emergency water a readily available piped supply of water for the emergency flushing of irritating, corrosive, or toxic chemicals from the face and body of laboratory personnel. It may be provided effectively through eyewash fountains, drench hoses,

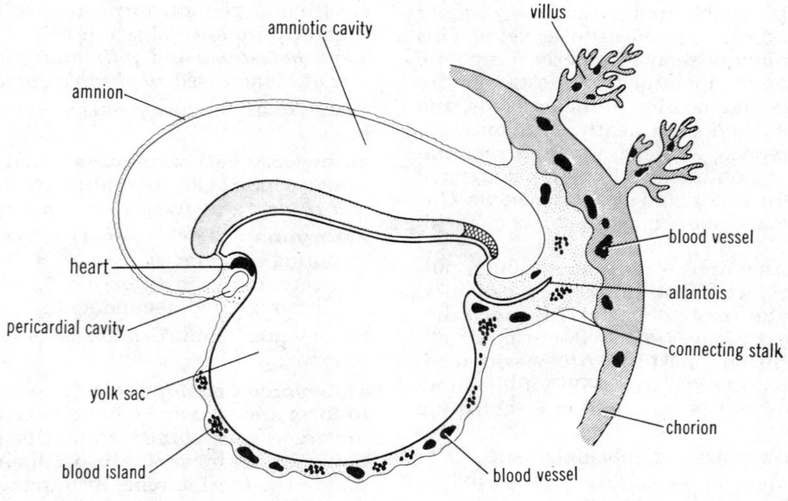

Embryonic development. Extraembryonic blood vessel formation in the villi, chorion, connecting stalk, and wall of the yolk sac in a presomite embryo at approximately 19 da. Note the angiogenetic cell clusters in relation to the prochordal (buccopharyngeal) plate. (From Langman, J.: Medical Embryology. 4th ed. Baltimore, Williams & Wilkins Co., 1981.)

and safety showers. The water must be of potable (drinkable) quality, readily available, and sufficient to provide for 15 min of flushing or longer.

Water is needed in clinical laboratories in two different types of emergency: water supply failure and chemical splash. JCAH (Joint Commission on the Accreditation of Hospitals) standards require hospitals to provide for emergency water supplies in case of failure of the supply, and hospital laboratories to provide emergency water for the flushing of chemicals from anyone who may be splashed. OSHA (Occupational Safety and Health Administration) standards and accepted safety practice also require that suitable facilities be provided for immediate emergency use by anyone who may be exposed to injurious chemicals. The recommended emergency treatment of chemical splashes in the eyes or on the face or body is *immediate* flushing with potable water for 15 min.

emesis (em′e-sis) [Gr. *emein* to vomit] see *vomiting.*

-emesis (em′ĕ-sis) [Gr. *emein* to vomit] a suffix word element to denote vomiting, e.g., hyperemesis.

emetine (em′ĕ-tēn) 6′,7′,10,11-tetramethoxyemetan, the principal alkaloid of ipecac, the ground roots of *Uragoga ipecacuanha;* M.W. 480.63. It is used as an antiamebic agent and inhibits protein synthesis.

EMF, emf abbrev. See *electromotive force.*

EMG abbrev. See *electromyography.*

-emia (e′me-ah) [Gr. *haima* blood + *-ia*] a suffix word element to denote blood condition, e.g., anemia.

eminence (em′ĭ-nens) a prominence or projection, especially one on the surface of a bone.

frontal e., a rounded prominence on either side of the frontal bone above the orbits, forming the most prominent portion of the forehead. Also called the frontal tuber.

hypothenar e., the fleshy eminence on the palm along the ulnar margin.

median e., a raised area on the tuber cinereum of the hypothalamus; continuous with the infundibulum. It gives rise to the capillaries of the hypothalamic-hypophyseal portal system and is considered to be a part of the neurohypophysis.

parietal e., a rounded prominence on each parietal bone projecting superiorly and laterally above the superior temporal line. Also called the parietal tuber.

thenar e., the mound on the palm at the base of the thumb formed by the abductor pollicis brevis, opponens pollicis, and flexor pollicis brevis.

emissary vein (em′ĭ-sa″re) [L. *emissarium* drain] a small vein that passes through a perforation in one of the cranial bones, providing a communication between the veins outside the bone and the venous sinuses within.

emission (e-mish′un) [L. *emissio* a sending out] any particle or radiation given off by a substance, such as a beta particle or a photon. A process that emits particles at one or more distinct, characteristic energies is called line emission, e.g., gamma radiation; one that emits particles with a range of energies is called continuous emission, e.g., beta radiation.

emission line a wavelength at which an atom, molecule, or ion emits a photon in a transition from an excited state to the ground state. See also *atomic absorption spectrometry* and *flame photometry.*

emission spectroscopy the spectrophotometric identification of metallic and semimetallic elements by their emission spectra when excited by a flame, arc, or spark. See also *flame photometry.*

emission spectrum the wavelength distribution of light emitted by a source, particularly the intensities of the various emission lines.

EMIT trademark for Enzyme Multiplied Immunoassay Technique. See under *enzyme assisted immunoassay technique.*

emitter (e-mit′er) 1. a radionuclide considered as a radiation source, e.g., a gamma emitter.

2. one of the terminals of a junction transistor or unijunction transistor.

emitter-coupled logic (ECL) the type of commercially available logic circuitry with the fastest switching speed. ECL gates are integrated circuits (ICs) containing several junction transistors operated in a nonsaturated condition. Cf. *complementary metal oxide semiconductor logic* and *transistor-transistor logic.*

emmetr/o (em′ĕ-tro) [Gr. *emmetros* in proper measure] a word element used in combining form to denote in due measure, e.g., emmetropia.

Emmonsia (ĕ-mon′se-ah) a former name for the genus *Chrysosporium.*

Emmonsiella (e-mon″se-el′ah) a genus of fungi of which the species *E. capsulata* is the perfect state of the fungus *Histoplasma capsulatum capsulatum* and *H. capsulatum duboisii.* Heterothallic and similar in morphology to the Ascomycetes, *E. capsulata* has eight ascospores, which are globose, hyaline, and smooth. *Emmonsiella* is considered to be the same genus as *Ajellomyces,* and it has been proposed that *E. capsulata* be placed in the genus *Ajellomyces* as *A. capsulatus.*

emperipolesis (em-per″ĭ-po-le′sis) [*em-* + Gr. *peripolēsis* a going about] penetration of and movement within a cell by another cell, as of a macrophage by a lymphocyte.

-emphraxis (em-frak′sis) [Gr.] a suffix word element to denote obstruction or blockage, e.g., salpingoemphraxis.

emphysema (em″fĭ-se′mah) [Gr. "an inflation"] a general term for the accumulation of air within a tissue. The term refers most often to pulmonary emphysema.

interstitial e., the escape of air into connective tissue of the lung, mediastinum, or subcutaneous region. The latter is generally termed subcutaneous emphysema. The condition results from a tear in the respiratory passages or alveoli, as from a chest wound or in pulmonary emphysema. Accumulation of air in the subcutaneous tissues may produce marked swelling and a distinctive crackling crepitation on pressure.

pulmonary e., a disorder of the lung characterized by the abnormal, permanent enlargement of air spaces distal to the terminal bronchiole, accompanied by destruction of their walls. Many patients with pulmonary emphysema also have chronic bronchitis. The increased resistance to air flow within the distal respiratory passages in most patients with emphysema contributes to the syndrome of chronic obstructive pulmonary disease.

At least three forms of emphysema within the lungs are recognized. In panlobular emphysema, alterations involve the entire pulmonary lobule, and the lungs are usually diffusely affected. In centrilobular emphysema, the destructive process is centered within the lobule while alveoli at the periphery are normal. The process is often diffuse within the lung and the basal segments may be more severely affected. Tractional emphysema is characterized by a focal dilation of the distal respiratory spaces adjacent to areas of chronic atelectasis or fibrosis. The term compensatory emphysema is sometimes applied to dilation of alveoli that occurs in response to loss of lung tissue as, for example, following surgical removal of a lobe. In pulmonary emphysema, confluence of the affected air spaces may produce large subpleural blebs or bullae.

The etiology of emphysema is unclear, but a number of factors probably contribute, including smoking and air pollution. Genetic factors also may be involved: alpha$_1$-antitrypsin deficiency has been correlated with severe panlobular emphysema. Symptoms are most severe with the panlobular form, but both centrilobular and panlobular forms may cause severe disability, respiratory failure, and death.

subcutaneous e., the presence of air or gas bubbles in the subcutaneous tissue, which may occur following surgical procedures.

empirical (em-pir′e-kal) [Gr. *empeirikos* experienced] based on experience; determined from experimental data as opposed to theory.

Empirin (em′pĭ-rin) trademark. See *acetylsalicylic acid.*

empyema (em″pi-e′mah) [Gr.] the collection of a purulent exudate within body cavities or hollow organs. It commonly occurs in the thoracic cavity (suppurative pleuritis) as a complication of a suppurative pulmonary infection, less frequently of lymphogenous or hematogenous spread from a distant infection. The infection is usually bacterial or mycotic. Gram stain and aerobic, anaerobic, and fungal cultures are necessary to identify the infecting organism. Thoracentesis may be performed to obtain material for culture.

subdural e., a suppurative lesion in the brain between the inner surface of the dura and the outer surface of the arachnoid. It is caused by pyogenic organisms that are seeded from the paranasal sinuses, a brain abscess, or the cerebrospinal fluid or that gain access during neurosurgical procedures. Persons affected experience headache, malaise, and fever, which eventually progress to focal or generalized neurologic disturbances that may include seizures, hemiplegia, aphasia, and coma. Examination of the CSF reveals increased pressure, raised white blood cell count, elevated protein, and normal glucose; the CSF is sterile. Diagnosis is made by cranial radiography, CT scan, and carotid arteriography.

EMT abbrev. See *emergency medical technician.*

emu abbrev. see *electromagnetic unit.*

emulsify (e-mul′sĭ-fi) to convert or be converted into an emulsion.

emulsion (e-mul′shun) [NL. *emulsio,* from *emulgere* to milk out] 1. a suspension of globules of one liquid in another, such as mayonnaise.

2. in photography, the photosensitive material on film, plates, or papers.

en- (en) [Gr. *en* within] a prefix word element to denote within, e.g., encystation.

ENA abbrev. See *extractable nuclear antigen.*

enamel (e-nam′el) [M.E. *enamelen,* from O.Fr. *esmail*] the white, translucent, hard substance that covers the crown of a tooth. It is composed primarily of inorganic substances (up to 96 percent by weight) and serves to protect the dentin of the tooth while providing a hard surface for chewing.

enamel organ the ectodermal part of the tooth bud that forms a cap over the dental papilla. Composed of epithelial cells, these organs differentiate to form the enamel of the tooth.

enantiobiosis (en-an″te-o-bi-o′sis) [Gr. *enantios* opposite + *bios* life] the condition in which two organisms are antagonistic toward each other's development. Cf. *symbiosis.*

enantiomer (en-an′te-o-mer) one of two compounds whose molecules are mirror images. See also *isomerism.*

enantiomerism (en-an″te-o-mer′izm) [Gr. *entanios* opposite + *meros* part] the relationship that exists between molecules that are mirror images (enantiomers); see under *isomerism.*

enantiomorph (en-an″te-o-morf′) see *enantiomer.*

enantiomorphism (en-an″te-o-morf′izm) [Gr. *enantios* opposite + *morphē* form] see *enantiomerism.*

en bloc (ahn blok′) [Fr.] in a lump; as a whole.

encapsulated (en-kap′su-lāt-ed) [*en-* + L. *capsula* little box] enclosed within a capsule.

encephal/o (en-sef′ah-lo) [Gr. *enkephalos* brain] a word element used in combining form to denote relationship to the brain, e.g., encephalitis.

encéphale isolé (en-sa-fal′ e-so-la′) an experimental preparation in which a mammal's neuraxis is transected at the first cervical segment, and blood pressure and respiration are artificially maintained. The electroencephalogram shows electrical activity associated with a normal sleep-wakefulness cycle.

encephalitis (en″sef-ah-li′tis), pl. *encephalitides* [*encephal-* + *-itis* inflammation] an inflammatory process that involves the cerebrum, brain stem, or cerebellum. It may be caused by infection with an arbovirus, herpes simplex virus, enterovirus, or adenovirus. It may also accompany an exanthematous disease such as measles or infectious mononucleosis, or may follow viral vaccination. Toxic forms also exist, with poisons or bacterial toxins causing the cerebral inflammation. Encephalitis due to arbovirus infection (St. Louis, eastern equine, western equine, and California encephalitis) is transmitted by infected mosquitos.

Brain tissue may be edematous and may have small hemorrhages. There usually are inflammatory infiltrates with mononuclear cells, as well as polymorphonuclear neutrophils, especially localized around small vessels. Neuronal changes are frequently found, and there may be proliferation of microglia. Various forms of inclusion bodies may be found in neurons or glial cells in viral encephalitis.

Clinically, encephalitis presents as an acute febrile illness occurring with malaise, stiff neck, sore throat, vomiting, stupor, or coma, and is often accompanied by other focal neurologic deficits. Encephalitis may be distinguished from aseptic meningitis by the clinical evidence of cerebral dysfunction. Acute viral encephalitis may have a fatal outcome, and a certain number of survivors will have residual neurologic deficits. The mortality rate and frequency of residual complications depend on the infecting virus.

Cerebrospinal fluid cell content, protein concentration, and pressure are typically elevated. Diagnosis can often be confirmed by demonstrating increasing antibody titers to the etiologic agent. The electroencephalogram usually shows diffuse slow activity and may be helpful in following the course of the disorder. In herpes simplex encephalitis, the findings may be more specific, often showing repetitive slow-wave complexes that may suggest the diagnosis. In many cases of presumed viral encephalitis, viral infection cannot be documented.

arthropod-borne virus e., a type of encephalitis in which the encephalitis-causing viruses are carried by mosquitoes and ticks. The prevalence varies by geographic locations; for example, in the Western Hemisphere the occurrence of eastern and western equine, St. Louis, Venezuelan, and California forms of encephalitis is frequent.

eastern equine e. (EEE), an acute type of group A arbovirus encephalitis that occurs along the Atlantic or Gulf Coast of the United States near freshwater hardwood swamps. Transmitted largely among wild birds by the *Culex melanura* mosquito, this disease is most often seen in children during late summer. The mortality rate for hospitalized patients with EEE is about 50 percent. There is an increase in CSF cells, protein concentration, and pressure levels. If patients survive EEE, their convalescence is slow and they are often left with severe residual deficits, such as mental disturbances, seizures, and focal motor or sensory abnormalities. In fatal cases, death occurs usually within 2 wk of the initial symptoms.

herpes simplex e., a type of encephalitis caused by the herpes simplex virus and occurring in individuals of all ages. It is usually caused by the type 1 herpes simplex virus whereas type 2 infections are often manifested as aseptic meningitis, or disseminated infection in neonates. Herpes encephalitis occurs sporadically. The disorder may range from mild to severe but is often fatal. Initial symptoms are those of any other acute encephalitis, but additional symptoms may subsequently indicate disproportionate involvement of the frontal and temporal lobes of the brain. The CSF contains an increased cell and protein content.

Diagnosis may be accomplished by brain biopsy or immunofluorescence of the inflammatory cells in the CSF. During the first 14 da of the illness, characteristic abnormalities may be found in the electroencephalogram (EEG), with periodic, repetitive slow waves occurring on a slow background, but this finding is not invariable. As the disease progresses, the interval between the complexes tends to shorten and the complexes may appear bilaterally. These EEG changes can be particularly helpful in suggesting the diagnosis.

lethargic e., a worldwide epidemic encephalitis that occurred between 1915 and 1926. One of the most destructive outbreaks of disease in recent times, lethargic encephalitis was marked by headache, malaise, increasing apathy, drowsiness, and ophthalmoplegia. Increased numbers of lymphocytes and an elevated protein concentration were often present in the CSF. The mortality rate was high. Many survivors had severe residual deficits, and a number developed a parkinsonian syndrome after several months or years. No etiologic agent or virus was ever isolated. Also called Economo's encephalitis.

western equine e. (WEE), a type of encephalitis that affects horses and humans, which is caused by group A arbovirus. In humans, infection may be inapparent or mild and denguelike, or occasionally it may occur as a severe encephalitis that may be fatal. Observed only in the western hemisphere, the virus is carried by small birds and mammals and is transferred to humans by the *Culex tarsalis* mosquito. The disease occurs in the summer and early fall and has a mortality rate of 10 percent. Besides the usual clinical manifestations of encephalitis, WEE has an incubation period of 5–10 da and a fever that does not last more than a week. It may cause spastic or flaccid paralysis in children.

encephalocele (en-sef′ah-lo-sēl) extracranial cerebral tissue, with a connection to the brain, that forms a mass, usually subcutaneous, on the bridge of the nose but occasionally inside the nose. Radiographs of the skull may demonstrate bony defects in the floor of the anterior cranial fossa.

encephalocystocele (en-sef″ah-lo-sis′to-sēl) [*encephalo-* + Gr. *kystis* sac, bladder + *kēlē* hernia] hernial protrusion of brain tissue distended by cerebrospinal fluid through a defect in the cranial vault. Also called hydrencephalocele.

encephalogram (en-sef′ah-lo-gram″) [*encephalo-* + Gr. *gramma* mark] an x-ray or gamma-ray radiograph of the brain.

encephalography (en-sef″ah-log′rah-fe) [*encephalo-* + Gr. *graphein* to write, record] x-ray or gamma-ray radiography of the brain.

encephalomeningocele (en-sef″ah-lo-mĕ-ning′go-sēl) [*encephalo-* + Gr. *mēninx* membrane + *kēlē* hernia] hernial protrusion of meninges, cerebrospinal fluid, and brain tissue through a cranial skeletal defect. Also called hydrocephalomeningocele.

encephalomyelitis (en-sef″ah-lo-mi″ĕ-li′tis) [*encephalo-* + Gr. *myelos* marrow + *-itis* inflammation] inflammation of both the brain and spinal cord. See also *encephalitis.*

postinfectious e., acute disseminated encephalomyelitis that follows a viral infection, such as measles, mumps, varicella, rubella, influenza, infectious mononucleosis, smallpox, and upper respiratory infections. A similar syndrome (postvaccinal encephalomyelitis) can occur following smallpox and other viral vaccinations. Neurologic complications, most commonly convulsions and deepening coma, may appear 4–18 da after the symptoms of viral infection.

encephalopathy (en-sef″ah-lop′ah-the) [*encephalo-* + Gr. *pathos* disease] a general term used to describe any disorder of cerebral function.

alcoholic e., see *Wernicke-Korsakoff syndrome.*

anoxic e., a condition resulting from an inadequate supply of oxygen to the brain, most frequently due to either cardiac or respiratory failure (e.g., from suffocation, carbon monoxide poisoning, myocardial infarction, circulatory collapse, shock, or diseases that paralyze the respiratory muscles). Mild hypoxia may merely affect judgment, attention, or muscle coordination, without lasting impairment. Severe cases, especially when the brain is deprived of oxygen for more than 10 min, may lead to total unawareness, unresponsiveness, and loss of all brain stem function (including spontaneous respiration). Depending on the degree of anoxia, the patient may die within several days or continue to survive in this comatose state with an isoelectric electroencephalogram (EEG), an irreversible condition commonly referred to as "brain death syndrome."

Diagnosis of anoxic encephalopathy depends on the clinical history and the finding of cardiorespiratory failure or evidence of intoxication (e.g., a cherry-red skin color following carbon monoxide poisoning).

Also called hypoxic encephalopathy.

hepatic e., a condition occurring secondarily to advanced disease of the liver, or in patients with portacaval shunts. It may also occur in the hyperammonemic syndromes of childhood, and in Reye's syndrome. Hepatic encephalopathy is marked by disturbances of consciousness, with confusion and drowsiness, that may progress to deep coma (hepatic coma), flapping tremor, and fetor hepaticus. Electroencephalographic (EEG) changes accompany the clinical progression of the disease. Theta and delta waves come to replace the alpha rhythm, and triphasic complexes (consisting of a large positive wave preceded and followed by small negative waves) occur as the disease progresses. The electroencephalogram decreases in amplitude and is interrupted by periods of electrocerebral silence during terminal stages of the disease. Also called portal-systemic encephalopathy.

hypercapnic e., brain dysfunction induced by chronic respiratory acidosis, commonly resulting from chronic emphysema or fibrosing lung disease. Headache, asterixis, confusion, drowsiness, and mental dullness may occur, culminating in extreme cases with coma. Papilledema sometimes occurs and may be mistakenly attributed to an intracranial structural lesion. The cerebrospinal fluid is under increased pressure in established cases. The Po_2 may exceed 75 mmHg and the arterial Po_2 may be less than 50 mmHg. Treatment is with forced ventilation; pulmonary infection, heart failure, and other complications or predisposing factors must also be treated actively.

hypertensive e., an acute condition in which severe hypertension is associated with headache, nausea, confusion, stupor, convulsions, and coma. Transient or persistent focal neurologic abnormalities, such as hemiparesis and hemisensory defects, may also occur.

Clinical examination reveals a diastolic blood pressure of 110–120 mmHg or more, and a retinopathy of grade 3–4. Laboratory tests commonly reveal an elevated cerebrospinal fluid pressure and CSF protein concentration. This condition represents a medical emergency for which antihypertensive therapy should be initiated immediately to prevent a fatal outcome.

hypoglycemic e., brain dysfunction resulting from a low blood glucose concentration (below 30 mg/100 ml). The most common causes are overdosage of insulin or an oral hypoglycemic drug; insulin production by an islet cell tumor; Reye's syndrome; acute liver damage of other cause; and glycogen storage disease in infancy. The sequence of symptoms ranges from nervousness, confusion, sweating, tremulousness, drowsiness, restlessness, air hunger, muscular spasms, to deepening coma. Prompt correction of the hypoglycemia is the treatment.

lead e., a degenerative condition of the brain, occurring most frequently in children, that is due to the ingestion of large amounts of lead. It is characterized by irritability, convulsions, aphasia, cortical blindness, mania, delirium, stupor, or coma and signs of increased intracranial pressure (vomiting, lethargy, and convulsions).

Presumptive diagnosis relies on the qualitative urinary coproporphyrin test (UCPT). Urinary lead determinations may be helpful in confirming the diagnosis; blood values may be normal.

See also *lead poisoning.*

uremic e., a progressive encephalopathy that may occur in individuals with renal failure and is characterized by confusion, stupor, twitches, and other symptoms, including fits. An encephalopathy may also complicate chronic hemodialysis.

Wernicke's e., see *Wernicke-Korsakoff syndrome.*

encephalotrigeminal syndrome (en-sef″ah-lo-tri-jem′ĭ-nal) [*encephalo-* + L. *trigeminus* threefold] see *Sturge-Weber syndrome.*

enchondroma (en″kon-dro′mah) [*en-* + Gr. *chondros* cartilage + *-oma* tumor] a benign cartilaginous neoplasm, arising within the medullary cavity of bone, that most commonly affects the small bones of the hand. Although the neoplasm is composed of hyaline cartilage, it often contains areas of calcification that are visible radiographically. Careful histologic examination is necessary to exclude chondrosarcoma.

Multiple enchondromas occur in enchondromatosis (Ollier's disease, dyschondroplasia), a hereditary disorder of skeletal development that results in joint deformity, retarded growth of long bones, knobby fingers, and pathologic fractures. The bones of the skull are rarely affected. Cartilaginous masses appear as radiolucent areas in radiographs, which also show bone expansion, linear lucent streaks, and thinning and ballooning of the cortex. Enchondromatosis tends to be unilateral and is associated with a high incidence of chondrosarcomatous transformation of preexisting enchondromas.

Multiple congenital enchondromas occur in the condition of multiple osteocartilaginous exostoses (chondrodysplasia, diaphyseal aclasis). This is a hereditary disorder in which approximately half the children of affected parents develop variable numbers of enchondromas. The regions of the knees, ankles, and shoulders are most often involved, and bowing and shortening of the extremities is characteristic. As in multiple enchondromas, the bones of the skull (formed by intramembranous ossification) are rarely affected. The basic defect may be one of glycosaminoglycan metabolism. The condition is also sometimes seen in patients with pseudohypoparathyroid syndrome. Chondrosarcomatous transformation at the site of an exostosis has been estimated to occur with a frequency as high as 10 percent.

Also called *chondroma.*

encoches frontales (ahn-kosh′fron-tal′) [Fr. "frontal notches"] a pattern of electrical activity recorded during wakefulness or sleep from the prefrontal regions of the brain in infants from about 35 wk of conception age to several weeks postterm. It consists of a biphasic sharp wave (negative-positive) followed by a slow wave and may be unilateral or bilateral. Also called *frontal sharp transients.*

encode (en-kōd′) to translate information into a particular coded form.

encoder (en-kōd′er) a digital-to-analog converter or

any other electronic device that produces coded outputs corresponding to digital inputs.

encoding (en-kōd′ing) the translation of information from one form to another (e.g., from analog to digital) without significant loss of information.

end/o (en′do) [Gr. *endon* within] a prefix word element to denote within, or an inward situation, e.g., endogenous, endoscopy.

end arborization the bushy, terminal branching of a nerve fiber.

endarteritis (end″ar-ter-i′tis) [*end-* + Gr. *artēria* artery + *-itis* inflammation] the inflammation of the innermost layer of arteries (tunica intima), seen in a variety of immunologic disorders. As the pathologic process tends to involve the entire thickness of the wall of smaller vessels, the term arteritis is more appropriate.

e. obliterans, the nonspecific response of small arteries to a variety of insults, which results in inflammation, fibrosis, and subsequent collapse and closure of the smaller branches.

end artery an artery that ends in fine branches that do not interconnect with one another.

end bulb of Krause (krow′zĕ) [Wilhelm Johann Friedrich *Krause,* German anatomist, 1833–1910] a small, bulbous sensory nerve ending, invested with a laminated connective tissue sheath, that is found in the skin, mucous membranes, conjunctiva, and cardiac muscle.

end-diastolic volume the volume of blood in each ventricle at the end of diastole, usually amounting to 120–130 ml in the normal heart.

endemic (en-dem′ik) [Gr. *endēmos* dwelling in a place] 1. present in a community at all times.

2. a disease of low morbidity that is constantly present in a human community but clinically recognizable in only a few individuals.

endemic hemoptysis see *paragonimiasis.*

endergonic reaction (end″er-gon′ik) [*end-* + Gr. *ergon* work] a chemical reaction for which ΔG (Gibbs free-energy change) is positive and which therefore does not proceed spontaneously. Only when this reaction is coupled to an exergonic reaction so that the overall reaction is exergonic (the total ΔG for the two reactions is negative) can the reaction proceed spontaneously.

end-expiration a point of zero airflow in the respiratory cycle that occurs at the end of a forced expiration to the residual volume.

end-inspiration a point of zero airflow in the respiratory cycle that normally occurs at the end of a maximal inspiration to total lung capacity position (maximal lung inflation).

endo- (en′do) [Gr. *endon* within] a prefix word element to denote within, e.g., endogenous.

endoamylase (en″do-am′ĭ-lās) α-amylase; see under *amylase.*

endobronchial (en″do-brong′ke-al) situated or occurring within a bronchus. Also called *intrabronchial.*

endocardial (en″do-kar′de-al) [*endo-* + Gr. *kardia* heart] 1. situated in or occurring within the heart.

2. pertaining to the endocardium.

endocarditis (en″do-kar-di′tis) [*endo-* + Gr. *kardia* heart + *-itis*] inflammation of the endocardium, caused by microbial infection in most cases, although noninfective forms can occur in other conditions such as systemic lupus erythematosus and rheumatoid arthritis.

Infective endocarditis can be clinically divided into two forms, acute and subacute; each has a distinct clinical course. In acute endocarditis, the infecting organism is extremely invasive, preexisting valvular damage is not usually present, metastatic foci are common, and the disease runs a comparatively brief and often fatal course. Conversely, subacute endocarditis is most commonly caused by streptococci of the enterococcus viridans groups, is associated with previous valvular damage, and may last for many months. Subacute endocarditis begins with a noninfectious lesion on the valve often caused by previous damage. Continued trauma causes the development of a sterile platelet-fibrin thrombus; if bacteremia is present, a subacute infective inflammatory process may develop on the thrombus sites.

Factors predisposing to infective endocarditis include active microbial infection, drug abuse (through unsterile parenteral inoculations), rheumatic valvular disease, congenital heart disease, degenerative heart disease, cardiac surgery, and the presence of prosthetic valves.

Laboratory diagnosis of the etiologic agent is made by multiple blood cultures.

acute infective e., a rapidly progressive infection of healthy or damaged heart valves and prosthetic implants that may lead to severe endocardial damage and valvular destruction. Foci of microorganisms colonize heart valves following severe bacteremias, surgical procedures, abscesses, sepsis, or injection of bacterially contaminated foreign materials. Staphylococci, streptococci, and gram-negative coliforms are the most common bacterial agents; organisms such as *Staphylococcus, Pseudomonas,* and *Candida* are frequently implicated in drug users. Severe infections with fever, chills, and multiple embolic episodes are common. Although blood cultures are necessary to confirm diagnosis, antimicrobial treatment should be immediately instituted. Metastatic abscess formation is a dangerous complication of this disease.

rheumatic e., see *rheumatic fever.*

subacute infective e., endocarditis characterized by colonization of the endocardium by bacteria, fungi, or other microbiologic agents, usually superimposed on preexisting rheumatic, valvular, or congenital heart disease. Following endocardial colonization, fibrin and platelet thrombi are deposited, forming friable masses of microorganisms and debris that can dislodge and embolize to other organs. Bacteremia, especially following respiratory infections, dental extractions, or contamination by medical instrumentation, often precipitates subacute infective endocarditis. Clinical findings include splenomegaly, splinter hemorrhages of the nail beds, hypertrophic osteoarthropathy, cardiac murmurs, and tachycardia. There may also be associated immune complex nephritis, cardiac or renal failure, or both. Hematuria, proteinuria, an increased erythrocyte sedimentation rate, and normochromic anemia are common clinical observations.

Enterococci and streptococci viridans are by far the most common etiologic agents. Constantly present in the mouth and throat, they can enter the blood stream after even minor trauma. Less often, nonhemolytic streptococci are the infectious agents.

When *Streptococcus faecalis* is the responsible agent, its source is usually an external wound or other trauma. Staphylococci and certain fungal species are less common etiologic agents; many other types of microorganisms have been implicated on occasion. Multiple blood cultures may be required to obtain more than one positive culture of the same organism. Echocardiography may be useful to locate large endocardial masses or vegetations.

verrucous e., a form of verrucous noninfective endocarditis seen in patients with systemic lupus erythematosus. It is characterized by the presence of sterile vegetations on the heart valves, chordae tendineae, or both. Histologically, the vegetations are composed of fibrin strands accompanied by infiltrates of polymorphonuclear leukocytes, lymphocytes, and histiocytes in the connective tissue of the affected structure. The lesions usually contain the characteristic "hematoxylin bodies," granular, basophilic clumps of cellular debris analogous to the bodies in LE cells in the bone marrow. Also called *Libman-Sacks endocarditis*. See also *systemic l. erythematosus* under *lupus*.

endocardium (en″do-kar′de-um) [L., from *endo-* + Gr. *kardia* heart] [NA], the endothelial cell lining of the chambers of the heart and the dense connective tissue layer beneath it.

endocervicitis (en″do-ser″vĭ-si′tis) [*endo-* + L. *cervix* neck + *-itis* inflammation] inflammation of the mucosa of the endocervical canal.

endocervix (en″do-ser′viks) [*endo-* + L. *cervix* neck] the mucosal lining of the cervical canal. The epithelium is a single layer of tall, mucus-forming cells that clothes the surface and extends into branching glands. It meets the squamous epithelium of the ectocervix at the external os and merges with the endometrium at the upper end of the canal. See also *uterus*.

endochondral bone see *cartilage bone*.

endocrine (en′do-krīn, en′do-krin) [*endo-* + Gr. *krinein* to separate] secreting internally; applied to organs and glands that secrete substances (hormones) released directly into the blood without the intervention of ducts.

endocrine cancer therapy treatment that changes the hormonal milieu of cancer patients with the objective of therapeutic benefit. It is used mainly for patients with cancers arising in hormone-dependent tissues, i.e., the breast, endometrium, and prostate. Such treatment may be ablative (removal of the organs responsible for the production or the release of critical hormones) or additive (administration of drugs that change the hormonal balance).

endocrine system the system of cells that form secretory products (hormones), which in most instances pass directly into the circulation for distribution. The endocrine system is a complex integrated series of cells designed for intercellular chemical communication. It includes the specifically named endocrine glands (pituitary, thyroid, parathyroid, adrenal, pancreatic islets), and scattered small clusters or isolated hormone-producing cells. Together with the nervous system, the endocrine system influences and coordinates many of the activities of the cells and tissues of the body. In general, rapid and local actions are effected through the nervous system, which releases neurotransmitter substances from axon terminations in the immediate vicinity of the target cell. Slower and more diffuse effects are produced by hormones. Certain hormones affect a local territory, as in the case of those conveyed by the hypothalamic-hypophyseal portal systems. For more information, see the specific endocrine glands and hormones; see also *diffuse neuroendocrine system*.

endocrinology (en″do-krĭ-nol′o-je) [*endo-* + Gr. *krinein* to separate + *-logy*] the study of the endocrine system, including regulation of those body processes that are hormonally controlled, and the study and management of patients suffering from endocrinologic disorders.

endocytosis (en″do-si-to′sis) [*endo-* + Gr. *kytos* hollow vessel + *-osis*] the engulfing of particles by a cell such as a macrophage. Part of the cell membrane surrounds the particle and is pinched off to form a vacuole. See also *phagocytosis* and *pinocytosis*. Cf. *exocytosis*.

endodeoxyribonuclease (en″do-de-ok″se-ri″bo-nu′kle-ās) a general name for many enzymes of the hydrolase class (EC 3.1.21–25) that catalyze the interior hydrolytic cleavage of polynucleotides in a strand of DNA. The enzymes are important in the metabolism and repair of deoxyribonucleic acids. See also *d. I* and *II* under *deoxyribonuclease* and *endonuclease*.

endoderm (en′do-derm) [*endo-* + Gr. *derma* skin] in the developing embryo, the innermost of the three primary germ layers; it remains chiefly as a sheet exposed on one surface throughout embryonic and fetal development. From it are differentiated the mouth, pharynx, gastrointestinal tract, liver, gallbladder, pancreas, and respiratory system. Also called *entoderm*. See also *embryo*.

endodermal (en″do-der′mal) pertaining to or derived from the endoderm.

endodermal sinus tumor a histologic variant of germ cell tumor in which the cells mimic, to varying degrees, the appearance of the fetal yolk sac. The histologic appearance may assume a reticular, festooned (containing Schiller-Duval bodies), polyvesicular, vitelline, or solid pattern. The tumor arises in the testes and ovaries, or it may be extragonadal, arising in the retroperitoneum or mediastinum. Most of those affected are children or young adults. Also called infantile [juvenile] embryonal carcinoma and *yolk sac tumor*.

Endodermophyton (en″do-der-mof′ĭ-ton) [*endo-* + Gr. *derma* skin + *phyton* a growth] the former name for a genus of fungi now called *Trichophyton;* see *Trichophyton*.

endoenzyme (en″do-en′zīm) an intracellular enzyme; one that is retained inside a cell and does not normally diffuse into the surrounding medium.

end of file (EOF) 1. a condition that occurs when the last record of a computer data file has been read. 2. a special control character that signals the end-of-file condition.

end of tape the end of the usable recording area of a magnetic tape.

end-of-tape marker a physical marker or bit pattern that signals the end-of-tape condition to the computer program or operator.

endogenote (en″do-je′nōt) in bacterial gene transfer (transduction, transformation, or conjugation), the entire genome of the recipient cell. See also *merozygote*. Cf. *exogenote* and *heterogenote*.

endogenous (en-doj′ĕ-nus) [*endo-* + Gr. *gennan* to produce] 1. growing from within. Cf. *exogenous.*

2. developing or originating within the organism, or arising from causes within the organism.

endogenous bacterium in bacterial disease, a normally benign bacterium that occurs as part of the normal microbial flora in humans but may become pathogenic when resistance is lowered by factors such as radiation, surgery, and antibiotic and steroid therapy. Cf. *exogenous bacterium.*

endogenous variable in a mathematical model, one of the dependent variables, the values of which are determined by the model. Cf. *exogenous variable.*

Endolimax (en″do-li′maks) [*endo-* + Gr. *leimax* a snail] a genus of amebas including species parasitic to humans and other mammals.

E. nana, a nonpathogenic parasite found in the human alimentary tract.

endolymph (en′do-limf) [*endo-* + L. *lympha* water] the viscous fluid, with an ionic composition resembling that of intracellular fluid, that is contained in and secreted by the membranous labyrinth of the inner ear. Also called liquor of Scarpa. Cf. *perilymph.*

endolymphatic sac (en″do-lim-fat′ik) a blind, membranous pouch at the end of the endolymphatic duct.

endometrial (en″do-me′tre-al) pertaining to the endometrium.

endometrial adenocarcinoma see under *uterine tumors.*

endometrial brush an instrument used for obtaining endometrial samples.

endometrial carcinoma a carcinoma arising from the glandular epithelium that lines the endometrial cavity.

Also called endometrioid adenocarcinoma. See also *adenoacanthoma* and *uterine tumors.*

endometrial cycle also called *ovarian cycle.* See under *menstrual cycle.*

endometrioma (en″do-me″tre-o′mah) [*endo-* + Gr. *metra* uterus + *-oma* tumor] endometriosis in an extrauterine location, forming a discrete mass. See also *endometriosis.*

endometriosis (en″do-me″tre-o′sis) [*endo-* + Gr. *metra* uterus + *-osis* condition] the occurrence of endometrial glands accompanied by endometrial stroma in abnormal locations. Common sites include the ovaries and pelvic peritoneum; less commonly, the colon, appendix, vagina, and umbilicus are involved. Within the myometrium, the condition is generally termed adenomyosis. Some degree of adenomyosis can be found in more than 10 percent of uteri that are examined histologically.

Ectopic endometrium usually responds to the ovarian hormones and undergoes cyclic menstrual changes with bleeding. Histologically, there is usually evidence of recent hemorrhage, accumulation of hemosiderin in macrophages, inflammation and fibrosis in the stroma surrounding foci of endometriosis. When there is extensive hemorrhage, blood-filled cysts may form, producing a clinically detectable mass (endometrioma), a finding particularly common in the ovaries.

The patient with extrauterine endometriosis may suffer from severe dysmenorrhea and pelvic pain. Extensive endometriosis involving the ovaries or fallopian tubes, or both, may render the patient infertile due to extensive tissue damage, fibrosis, and adhesions.

endometritis (en″do-mĕ-tri′tis) [*endo-* + Gr. *metra* uterus + *-itis* inflammation] an acute or chronic inflammation of the endometrium, usually due to bacterial infection. It may be caused by retained products of conception following delivery or abortion, by instrumentation, or by gonorrhea. Chills, fever, lower abdominal pain, and vaginal discharge are usually present.

Laboratory studies should include Gram stains and cultures of urine, blood, and endometrial specimens. Leukocytosis with a shift to the left is usually present; urinalysis is normal unless there is an associated urinary tract infection.

endometrium (en″do-me′tre-um), pl. *endometria* [L., from *endo-* + Gr. *metra* uterus] the mucosal lining of the uterus that rests on the myometrium. It is simple columnar epithelium, which forms branching glands supported by a modified connective tissue stroma. The endometrium undergoes a cyclic series of changes each menstrual cycle in response to hormonal stimulation. At the end of a cycle, if fertilization has not occurred, most of the endometrium is shed, leaving only a basal layer (lamina basalis) from which regeneration takes place. See also *uterus.*

endomitosis (en″do-mi-to′sis) chromosome division not followed by nuclear division, which doubles the chromosome number. Also called *endoreduplication.*

Endomyces (en″do-mi′sēz) [*endo-* + Gr. *mykēs* fungus] a genus of fungi, class Ascomycetes, of which the species *E. geotrichum* is the perfect stage of the fungus *Geotrichum candidum.*

endomysium (en″do-mis′e-um) [N.L., from *endo-* + Gr. *mys* muscle] the delicate sheath of fine reticular fibers that surrounds each muscle fiber.

endoneurium (en″do-nu′re-um) [N.L., from *endo-* + Gr. *neuron* nerve] the delicate, loose connective tissue sheath that surrounds individual nerve fibers.

endonuclease (en″do-nu′kle-ās) a general name for many enzymes (with varying specificity) of the hydrolase class (EC 3.1.21–31) that catalyze the hydrolytic cleavage of polynucleotides; examples are deoxyribonuclease, endodeoxyribonuclease, and endoribonuclease. Some members of this group are important in the metabolism and repair of DNA and RNA.

A specific class of deoxyribonucleases known as restriction endonucleases cleaves DNA at specific nucleotide sequences. These enzymes protect the cells from foreign DNA, but they do not act on the host DNA. They have been used extensively in DNA sequencing and recombinant DNA technology.

endoparasite (en″do-par′ah-sīt) [*endo-* + Gr. *parasitos* parasite] a parasite that inhabits the host's body. Cf. *ectoparasite.*

endopeptidase (en″do-pep′tĭ-dās) the trivial name for a group of peptidase enzymes (EC 3.4.21–24) that catalyze the hydrolysis of interior peptide bonds in polypeptide chains. For more information, see the specific endopeptidase, e.g., *cathepsin, chymotrypsin, thrombin,* and *trypsin.*

endophlebitis (en″do-flĕ-bi′tis) [*endo-* + Gr. *phleps* vein + *-itis* inflammation] inflammation of the internal coat (tunica intima) of a vein. One of the most common causes is the prolonged placement and use of intravenous infusion devices.

endophthalmitis (en″dof-thal-mi′tis) [*endo-* + Gr. *ophthalmos* eye + *-itis* inflammation] a suppurative inflammation of the eye, affecting the uveal tract and retina, which may extend to involve all coats of the eye (panophthalmitis). This disorder is due to ocular infection with pyogenic organisms, usually through trauma, hematogenous spread, or local extension. A granulomatous endophthalmitis, often mistaken for retinoblastoma, may be seen in children with toxocariasis. Those affected experience intense pain, rapid vision loss, swelling of the eyelid, and extensive eye destruction. Gram stain and cultures of the eye are essential for diagnosis and selection of appropriate antibiotics.

endoplasm (en′do-plazm) [*endo-* + Gr. *plasma* something formed] the central region of the cytoplasm of a cell. It is a sol containing vacuoles, granules, mitochondria, and endoplasmic reticulum. The organelles are moved about by cytoplasmic streaming. Cf. *ectoplasm.*

endoplasmic recticulum (ER, er) (en″do-plaz′mik) an organelle in the cytoplasm of eukaryotic cells, which consists of an interconnected system of tubes and flattened membranous sacs. It is classified as rough (granular) ER if it has attached ribosomes or as smooth (agranular) ER if it does not. Cells contain variable amounts of either or both types, depending on their function. Those engaged in the secretion of proteins contain an extensive system of rough ER. Proteins are synthesized on the attached ribosomes, are transported vectorially into the cisternae during synthesis, and are processed (proteolytically shortened and often glycosylated) within the cisternae. The proteins are transported to the Golgi apparatus for packaging for secretion. The ER membrane is a major site for lipid metabolism in the cell. Steroid-forming cells are rich in smooth ER.

See also *membrane, nuclear envelope,* and *ribosome.*

J. Kenneth Hoober, Ph.D.

endopolyploidy (en″do-pol′e-ploi″de) the occurrence of two, four, eight, etc., times the normal number of chromosomes, resulting from endomitosis.

endoreduplication (end) (en″do-re-du″plĭ-ka′shun) see *endomitosis.*

endoribonuclease (en″do-ri″bo-nu′kle-ās) a general name for several enzymes of the hydrolase class (EC 3.1.26, 27, 30, and 31) that catalyze the hydrolysis of interior nucleotide bonds in ribonucleic acids, forming mono- and oligonucleotides. See also *ribonuclease.*

endorphin (en-dor′fin) [acronym from *endo*genous mo*rphin*e-like substance] originally any opiate-like compound occurring in the brain (such compounds are now called opioid peptides). The term is now restricted to three peptides, α-, β-, and γ-endorphin, that have the same *N*-terminal sequence and are cleaved from β-lipotropin. β-Endorphin includes residues 61–91; α-endorphin, residues 61–76; and γ-endorphin, residues 61–77. β-Endorphin is found primarily in the pituitary gland, but lesser amounts are found in the hypothalamus and in other regions of the brain. It is involved in the modulation of pituitary hormone release and may also be involved in the processing of pain perceptions. See also *enkephalin.*

endorphin assays competitive binding assay using opiate-like radioligand, or bioassay using smooth muscle preparation. Such assays may be important in the evaluation of psychotic disorders; elevated levels have been reported in the CSF of schizophrenic and manic-depressive patients. The reference range of endorphin in CSF has been reported as 1–2.5 pmol/ml, using the competitive binding technique.

endoscope (en′do-skop) [*endo-* + Gr. *skopein* to examine] an instrument used for the examination of a hollow organ or body cavity. Most types are flexible tubes that use fiberoptic cables for the transmission of light to illuminate the tissues and to return the images to the eyepiece. Most types allow use of implements for obtaining biopsy specimens or for performing minor surgical procedures.

endoscopic retrograde cholangiopancreatography (en″do-skop′ik) see *ERCP.*

endoscopy (en-dos′ko-pe) the procedure by which a rigid or flexible tube is inserted into a viscus of the body to visualize surface structure; to localize, identify, and photograph pathologic alterations, and to obtain biopsy material. The introduction of fiberoptic instruments has greatly extended the range and convenience of the various procedures that fall within the broad category of endoscopy.

In the gastrointestinal tract, direct visualization of the intestine is possible down to the second portion of the duodenum by using a panendoscope, and as proximal as the cecum by using a colonoscope. Endoscopy of the esophagus, stomach, and duodenum (panendoscopy) can provide material for cytologic and histologic evaluation in more than 90 percent of cases, and is useful for localizing sites of upper gastrointestinal tract bleeding. Retrograde cannulation of the common bile duct or main pancreatic duct can be achieved by a skilled operator.

See also *bronchoscopy, colonoscopy, cystoscopy, laparoscopy,* and *mediastinoscopy.*

endosmosis (en″dos-mo′sis) [*endo-* + Gr. *ōsmos* impulsion] osmosis from without (the cell, vessel, or organ being described) to within. The term is sometimes used for any osmosis, as in electrophoresis. Cf. *exosmosis.*

endospore (en′do-spōr) [*endo-* + Gr. *sporos* seed] see *bacterial s.* under *spore.*

endosteum (en-dos′te-um) [*endo-* + Gr. *osteon* bone] the membrane that lines the marrow-containing medullary cavity of a bone.

endosulfan (en″do-sul′fan) a toxic chlorinated hydrocarbon insecticide, 1,2,3,4,7,7-hexachlorobicyclo[2.2.1]-2-heptene-5,6-bisoxymethylene sulfite. See also *chlorinated hydrocarbon pesticides.*

endothelioma (en″do-the″le-o′mah) [*endothelium* + *-oma*] a general term for a neoplasm that arises from endothelial cells.

endothelium (en″do-the′le-um), pl. *endothelia* [L., from *endo-* + Gr. *thēlē* nipple] a thin layer of squamous epithelial cells that lines the cavities of the heart and the blood and lymph vessels.

continuous e., endothelium in which no fenestrae or gaps are present.

discontinuous e., endothelium in which large gaps occur, allowing for the permeation of large particles or cells, as in the sinusoids of bone marrow.

fenestrated e., endothelium that contains a large number of pores (fenestrae), as in glomerular capillaries.

endothermic (en″do-ther′mik) [*endo-* + Gr. *thermē* heat] absorbing heat; denoting a chemical reaction during the progress of which there is absorption of heat. Cf. *exothermic.*

endothrix (en′do-thriks) [*endo-* + Gr. *thrix* hair] a fungal invasion with growth and formation of arthrospores, chiefly within the shaft of a hair. Fungi that cause endothrix infections include *Trichophyton tonsurans, T. violaceum, T. yaoundei, T. soundanense, T. gourvilii,* and *T. rubrum.* These fungal infections are Wood's lamp–negative. Cf. *ectothrix.*

endotoxemia (en″do-tok-se′me-ah) [*endo-* + L. *toxicum* poison + Gr. *haima* + *-ia*] the presence of endotoxin (lipopolysaccharides) in the blood. It occurs during gram-negative bacterial sepsis and may lead to shock. Cf. *endotoxin* and *septic shock.*

endotoxin (en″do-tok′sin) [*endo-* + L. *toxicum* poison] a complex lipopolysaccharide in the cell walls of gram-negative bacteria, which is released only when cell integrity is disturbed. Endotoxins are more heat-stable than the protein exotoxins, but they are less potent and less specific in their pharmacologic actions. They are also less antigenic and are not modified to toxoid formation by exposure to formaldehyde. The phospholipid fractions are responsible for toxicity, the polysaccharide moieties for antigenicity.

A phospholipid component known as lipid A is capable of producing numerous biologic effects, the most important of which are: (1) pyrogenicity, through release of endogenous pyrogen from polymorphonuclear leukocytes; (2) irreversible hemorrhagic shock syndrome, by mechanisms that are only partly understood and probably complex; and (3) altered resistance to bacterial infections, which is incompletely understood. Altered resistance to bacterial infections is peculiarly biphasic. Large doses of endotoxin depress resistance to infection and phagocytosis, but small doses enhance both. Animals given repeated injections of endotoxin become quite unresponsive, known as the state of tolerance, to these biologic effects.

See also *lipopolysaccharide.* Cf. *exotoxins.*

end-plate activity the spontaneous electrical activity that is recorded from a needle electrode inserted in the region of the muscle end-plate. End-plate activity may have either of two characteristic waveforms: the low amplitude, monophasic potentials commonly referred to as end-plate noise, or the biphasic spikes (end-plate spikes) that represent the propagated action potentials of muscle fibers excited by bursts of spontaneous activity in the nerve terminals. These sporadically occurring, biphasic (negative-positive) potentials have an amplitude of 100–300 μV and a duration of 2–5 msec.

end-plate noise the series of low-amplitude (10–40 μV), short-duration (0.5–1 msec), negative monophasic potentials recorded as normal spontaneous activity from a needle electrode inserted in the muscle end-plate region. The potentials occur in a dense, irregular, high-frequency discharge pattern. End-plate noise is thought to correspond to the extracellular recording of miniature end-plate potentials that are initiated by disruption of packets of acetylcholine by the electrode tip. Also called roar and seashell noise.

end-plate potential (EPP) a local, nonpropagated depolarization of the postsynaptic membrane of the neuromuscular junction. It is created by an influx of sodium ions generated by the release of acetylcholine (ACh) with the arrival of an impulse at the nerve terminal. The amplitude of the potential varies with the amount of ACh released. If the end-plate potential is of sufficient amplitude (threshold), an action potential is propagated along the muscle fiber membrane.

end point the stage of a titration at which chemically equivalent amounts of the reactants have been added and the titration is stopped. Also called *equivalence point.*

end product the final product in a chain of metabolic reactions or in the synthesis of a chemical compound in the laboratory.

endrin (en′drin) a chlorinated cyclodiene insecticide. See also *chlorinated hydrocarbon pesticides.*

end-stage kidney a term used to describe a kidney so badly damaged and scarred that the original underlying renal disease cannot be determined morphologically. A variety of diseases can produce this condition. See also *glomerulopathy* and *tubulointerstitial nephropathy.*

end-systolic volume the volume of blood that remains in each ventricle after ejection during systole, usually amounting to 50–60 ml in the normal heart.

end-tidal CO_2 tension the CO_2 tension in a sample of gas collected during the last portion of expiration, considered to be a good approximation of the CO_2 tension in mixed alveolar gas. It is normally equal to about 40 mmHg. As end-tidal CO_2 tension is also approximately equal to the P_{ACO_2} in a subject at rest, it can be used as an indicator of the level of alveolar ventilation.

-ene (ēn) a suffix word element in organic chemistry to denote the presence of a carbon-carbon double bond in the parent chain, e.g., propene (CH_3-$CH{=}CH_2$). A multiplying prefix denotes the number of double bonds, e.g., 1,3-butadiene ($CH_2{=}CH{-}CH{=}CH_2$). Cf. *-ane* and *-yne.*

enema (en′ĕ-mah) 1. the introduction of fluid into the rectum.

2. a fluid introduced into the rectum to promote the evacuation of feces, or as a means of administering nutrients or a radiographic contrast medium (e.g., barium).

barium e. (BE), the routine radiologic examination of the colon. The colon is thoroughly cleansed by restriction of the subject to a liquid diet for 24 hr, administration of a cathartic such as castor oil, bisacodyl, or senna, and administration of a cleansing enema.

Two different procedures are used. The opaque or full-column barium enema is performed by filling the small intestine with barium sulfate suspension under fluoroscopic control; spot films are made at intervals during filling, and films are made before and after evacuation of the enema. The double-contrast barium enema is performed by filling the colon with barium sulfate suspension up to the splenic flexure. The barium is then drained from the rectum, and 1800–2000 ml of air is instilled into the rectum, forcing the barium forward. The patient is rotated under radioscopic control so that the barium forms a thin, even coating of the entire colon. This method reveals fine detail and is useful in the diagnosis of ulcerative colitis, regional colitis, and polyps.

small intestine e., see under *gastrointestinal intubation.*

energy (*E*) (en′er-je) [Gr. *energeia*] a fundamental physical quantity that is conserved in all physical processes. Many different forms of energy have been given special names because they are separately conserved in some process or may be converted one into another in other processes, e.g., work, heat, mass, and kinetic energy. Energy and work are measured in joules, heat in joules or calories (1 cal = 4.18 J), and mass in kilograms.

binding e., that which holds the nucleus together; the difference in mass between an atomic nucleus and the mass of the protons and neutrons if separated.

bond e., the energy needed to break a chemical bond, specifically, the heat per mole absorbed in such a reaction at constant pressure, volume, and temperature (enthalpy per mole).

free e., see *free energy.*

kinetic e., the energy due to motion; at low velocities, given by the equation: $E = 1/2\ mv^2$, where m is mass and v is velocity.

potential e., the energy of a physical system that is solely a function of the positions of its parts.

energy resolution the range of energies recorded by a radiation detector responding to monoenergetic particles. It is usually measured as the full-width half-maximum (FWHM) counting rate, expressed as a percentage of the particle energy. It is routinely measured in quality control checks of scintillation cameras, rectilinear scanners, and gamma-well counters.

enflagellation (en-flaj″el-la′shun) the formation of flagella.

enhancement (en-hans′ment) the phenomenon of improved survival of tumor cells after immunization against the tumor cell antigens, a process that has been observed in laboratory animals. The protection may occur by a feedback inhibition of antibody response owing to antibody already present in the circulation, by the action of suppressor T cells, or by the coating of tumor cells by "blocking factor" antibodies, which prevents sensitized lymphocytes from killing the cells.

enkephalin (en-kef′ah-lin) [*encephalo-* + *-in*] either of two pentapeptides, methionine enkephalin (met-enkephalin) or leucine enkephalin (leu-enkephalin), that are opioid neurotransmitters in the central nervous system. They bind to the same cell surface receptors as do the opiates. Enkephalin-containing neurons are found in many places in the brain and in the dorsal gray matter of the spinal cord. The primary function of enkephalins in the spinal cord is believed to be modulation of pain perception. In the brain, their functions are unclear but are involved in sedation and elevation of the pain threshold. Receptors for enkephalins are involved in the production of euphoria by morphine. See also *endorphin.*

enol (e′nol) a compound that contains an alcohol or hydroxyl group attached to a double bond, a vinyl alcohol; these compounds usually exist as keto-enol tautomers:

enol form — keto form

In general (but not always), the enol form of a carbonyl compound is less stable than the keto form, with which it is in equilibrium. See also *tautomer.*

enolase (e′no-lās) an enzyme, 2-phospho-D-glycerate hydro-lyase (EC 4.2.1.11). It catalyzes the reaction 2-phospho-D-glycerate ⇄ phosphoenolpyruvate + H_2O, which is a part of the Embden-Meyerhof pathway of glucose metabolism.

en plaque (ahn plak′) [Fr.] possessing the form of a plaque or plate.

enrichment (en-rich′ment) the addition of nutrients. See also *enrichment m.* under *medium.*

enrichment culture a culture grown in an enrichment medium.

ENT abbrev. for ear, nose, and throat.

entamebiasis (en″tah-me-bi′ah-sis) [*Entamoeba* + *-iasis*] infection with *Entamoeba.*

Entamoeba (ent″ah-me′bah) [Gr. *entos* within + *amoeba*] a genus of amebas of which several species are intestinal parasites found in humans.

E. coli, a nonpathogenic ameba found in the human intestine. *E. coli* is frequently mistaken for *E. histolytica* because of similar morphology but it can be differentiated in the trophozoite and mature cystic stages by its lack of progressive motility in saline mounts or its characteristic nuclear morphology in iron-hematoxylin stain. *E. coli* has 1–8 nuclei; *E. histolytica,* 1–4.

E. gingivalis, a nonpathogenic oral human parasite, found worldwide, which lives in the gingival tissues surrounding the teeth. It can be contracted by close contact with an infected individual or through contaminated dishes. Diagnosis requires identification of the trophozoite stage from material taken from the gingival tissues.

E. histolytica, a small ameba (18–20 μ in diameter) recognized as the cause of amebic dysentery. This disease is found worldwide; its highest incidence is in tropical and subtropical areas. It is transmitted to humans through ingestion of cysts in food and water. Laboratory diagnosis includes microscopic examination of feces for trophozoites and cysts, and the indirect hemagglutination assay. See also *amebic d.* under *dysentery.*

enter/o (en′ter-o) [Gr. *enteron* intestine] a word element used in combining form to denote the intestines, e.g., enteropathy.

enteric (en′ter′ik) [Gr. *enterikos* intestinal] pertaining to the intestines.

enteric cytopathogenic human orphan virus see *echovirus.*

enteritis (en″ter-i′tis) [*enter-* + Gr. *-itis* inflammation] inflammation of the intestines, especially of the small intestine. Enteritis may be caused by bacteria and viruses, poisonous foods, bacterial or chemical substances, or excessive food or alcohol consumption. Regardless of the cause, it usually results in abdominal pain and irritation, nausea, vomiting, or diarrhea. Fecal cultures may aid in the identification of the etiologic agent in individuals with bacterial enteritis. See also *gastroenteritis.*

regional e., see *Crohn's disease.*

Enterobacter (en″ter-o-bak′ter) a genus of Enterobacteriaceae, which are gram-negative and rod-shaped. These bacteria are widely distributed in nature and occur in the intestinal tract of humans and animals. The genus is closely related to *Klebsiella* and *Serratia* but can be differentiated from them by biochemical tests. Organisms of the genus are frequently isolated from clinical cultures, although they are not usually the primary source of infection. The most commonly occurring species of the genus is *E. cloacae.* There are numerous reports of hospital outbreaks secondary to the contamination of medical devices with *Enterobacter.* See also *Enterobacteriaceae.*

Enterobacteriaceae (en″ter-o-bak-te″re-a′se-e) a family of interrelated gram-negative, nonsporeforming facultatively anaerobic bacilli that inhabit the large intestines of vertebrates. They are capable of growth on relatively simple media. Except for two genera, *Klebsiella* and *Shigella,* they are motile with peritrichous flagella. Glucose fermentation and nitrate reduction (with a few exceptions) are shared biochemical properties, as is the absence of indophenol oxidase. Some strains, especially virulent ones, possess pili. Enterobacteriaceae are also referred to as enteric bacilli; however, this term sometimes is meant to include the vibrios of the intestine, which are commonly present in fecal cultures. In fact, they belong to a different family (Vibrionaceae); their flagella are polar and they are oxidase positive.

CLASSIFICATION. Early dependence on cultural and biochemical behavior gave way in the 1940s and 1950s to antigenic analysis. Kauffman and White devised an elaborate scheme for the speciation of *Salmonella* that was based on differences in O and H antigens; this system was adopted widely and applied to other enterics as well. In recent years, DNA hybridization has clarified some of the previous confusion in the taxonomy of this complex family of bacteria and brought about a number of rearrangements, including the introduction of new genospecies and genera. Subtyping of certain species is also possible; e.g., bacteriophage typing identifies 72 subtypes of *Salmonella typhi* (an important epidemiologic tool) and colicin is used in typing of *Shigella sonnei.*

Most of the discoveries in bacterial genetics, including recombination, have been made with the Enterobacteriaceae, particularly *Escherichia coli* (see *bacterial g.* under *genetics*). The enormous mixed population of bacteria in the colon is in a continuous state of flux. Bacteriophages and plasmids are responsible for the rapid exchange of genetic material, which can occur even between different species of enteric bacilli. The practical consequence is a complex continuum of interrelated organisms that are very difficult to identify in the laboratory in order to provide the information needed for diagnosis, clinical management, and public health needs.

ECOLOGY. Most enteric bacilli are part of the normal flora of the intestine, the composition of which is quite stable despite the continuous introduction of new strains via the mouth. Enteric bacilli are also frequently present in cultures from extraintestinal sites, because they are regular inhabitants of the animal gut and therefore present in soil and water and on vegetation. Indeed, *E. coli* is the traditional index organism of fecal pollution of water supplies. Thus the presence of Enterobacteriaceae in small numbers in clinical specimens has by itself no etiologic significance. Except for a few primary pathogens, such as *S. typhi,* colonization and extensive multiplication on or in the tissues is a prerequisite for clinical infection. The ubiquitous distribution of enteric bacilli explains the frequency with which they are found in cultures from areas other than the intestine, such as the skin, surface membranes, and wounds. However, when encountered in specimens from the genitourinary tract, the origin most likely is the intestine. A few salmonellae, *S. typhi,* for example, and the *Shigella* are rarely encountered outside the human host.

VIRULENCE FACTORS. The harmful effects of endotoxin are diverse. There is a widely held opinion that some or most of these effects are related to hypersensitivity.

The production of exotoxin, in this case enterotoxin, seems to be a property of only certain strains of enteric bacilli. Best known are the enterotoxins of *E. coli* (known as ETEC), although the list of enterotoxigenic species continues to increase. The heat-labile toxin closely resembles cholera toxin. There is a possibility that neither this nor the heat-stable toxin is produced—or at least becomes manifest—unless pili are also present to aid in attachment to the small bowel mucosa. Apparently, these structures are responsible for the colonization and multiplication in the small intestine that must precede toxin production. The enteropathogenic strains of *E. coli* (called EPEC) may produce a different enterotoxin. In any event, the 15–16 serotypes classified as EPEC are not the same as those producing the heat-stable and heat-labile toxins.

Some enteric bacilli, particularly *E. coli* and *Shigella* species, can invade and multiply in the mucosa of the colon, producing a dysentery syndrome of pus and blood in a diarrheic stool. Indeed, they may be both enterotoxic and invasive. Among the shigellae, however, the primary pathogenicity factor is invasiveness.

CLINICAL INFECTION. Since the early days of clinical microbiology, the enteric bacilli have been among the most, if not the most, frequent group of bacteria cultured from clinical specimens. In recent years, however, the pattern has changed dramatically in developed countries as a result of improved sanitation, immunization, and antibiotic therapy. The typhoid and paratyphoid bacilli, *Shigella flexneri* and *S. sonnei,* so often responsible in the past for large outbreaks of disease, have been replaced by a variety of less well known Enterobacteriaceae species, some only recently recognized as having pathogenic potential—for example, *Edwardsiella agglomerans.* The rising importance of the opportunistic infections these organisms produce is a consequence of both host and parasite factors. The hardy nature of these bacteria (that is, their relatively high resistance to antibiotics, drying, and disinfectants) is a major factor, and their simple growth requirements enable them to multiply rapidly in liquids that do not support the growth of many other bacteria. On the host side are iatrogenic factors such as the reduction by antibiotics of the usual bacterial antagonism arising from activities of the normal flora, lower immunity levels from immunosuppressive drugs, and reduced resistance from surgical procedures and instrumentation. Thus, not only has the list of pathogenic Enterobacteriaceae species increased but so has the variety of clinical diseases they can produce; this trend is expected to continue.

The categorization of a particular species as nonpathogenic or pathogenic is often difficult. For example, *E. coli* is the predominant facultative commensal in the colon, yet it is the leading cause of urinary tract infection and a common incitant of infections in other parenteral regions of the body. Certain strains are enterotoxic, enteropathogenic, or enteroinvasive and cause important enteric disease.

IDENTIFICATION. Many culture media are available for primary isolation of the enteric bacilli from clinical specimens. There are four categories: general purpose, solid, and selective media, and enrichment broths. The general-purpose media, such as blood agar, support the growth of many types of bacteria, including those that are fastidious. The principal application to Enterobacteriaceae is culturing other than fecal specimens. Fecal specimens invariably contain a mixture of bacteria in large numbers; these are inoculated to solid media that differentiate and/or select among the various species of enteric bacilli. Differential plates, e.g., MacConkey agar, are designed primarily to distinguish between lactose fermenters and nonlactose fermenters. Inhibitory activity is limited. Selective media are much more inhibitory, so as to retard the growth of some enteric bacteria, but still allow the satisfactory growth of *Salmonella* and many *Shigella* strains. The differential quality can be retained, as it is in Hektoen enteric agar. Some laboratories add a highly selective medium such as bismuth sulfite agar, which is especially good for *Salmonella.* The enrichment broths not only select but also enable a few *Salmonella* organisms to multiply and be more easily detected when overnight growth is subcultured to differential and selective plates.

Colonies of possible importance on the primary plates are inoculated to a battery of media for initial screening. Three such agar media are triple sugar iron agar (TSIA), lysine-iron agar (LIA), and Christensen's urea. An oxidase test at this stage can sometimes avoid wasted effort. Nonfecal spcimens are often inoculated at the same time to appropriate media for citrate utilization, motility, and production of ornithine-decarboxylase and urease.

Serologic grouping of suspected *Salmonella* and *Shigella* isolates should be performed. The reagents are available commercially and the procedure is simple. With *Salmonella,* antisera for groups A, B, C, C_2, D, and E are sufficient. Vi antiserum is needed for biochemically suspect *S. typhi.* Commercial antisera are available for *Shigella* groups A–D. It is also advisable to include a polyvalent Alkalescens-Dispar group serum for these anaerogenic, nonmotile *E. coli* strains that resemble *Shigella* on TSIA.

A large number of gram-negative bacilli from both fecal and extraintestinal specimens, including blood, are typical with respect to one or more of the criteria in the above tables. For the details and interpretation of aforementioned methods and the handling of atypical organisms, standard manuals and books of clinical laboratory microbiology should be consulted.

ANTIBIOTIC SUSCEPTIBILITY. Strains from outside hospitals show the natural susceptibility-resistance patterns of the Enterobacteriaceae. Those recovered from hospitalized patients are more resistant, with the patterns reflecting the types of antimicrobial therapy current in each institution.

In general, enteric bacilli are susceptible to sulfonamides, tetracyclines, ampicillin, cephalosporins, and aminoglycosides. However, resistance to the beta-lactam group of antibiotics develops readily, and plasmid-mediated resistance is so frequent and unpredictable that all potentially important isolates should be tested with a battery of selected antimicrobials.

Automated kits for the rapid identification and susceptibility testing of Enterobacteriaceae are available commercially.

For more information, see the specific genera.

enterobiasis (en″ter-o-bi′ah-sis) an infection caused by nematodes of the genus *Enterobius.*

Enterobius (en″ter-o′be-us) [*entero-* + Gr. *bios* life] a genus of nematode worms of the super family Oxyuroidea.

E. vermicularis, a nematode, commonly known as pinworm or seatworm, that is found in the colon. The adult worms are spindle-shaped; the male is 2–5 mm long, and the female 8–13 mm long. Pinworm is common among children and has a cosmopolitan distribution. The eggs are transmitted via anus-to-mouth contact by finger contamination. Infection may cause itching. Diagnosis is based on the microscopic detection of eggs or worms in swabs (most commonly, the cellophane tape swab) from the perianal region.

enterocele (en′ter-o-sēl″) [*entero-* + Gr. *kēlē* hernia] a posterior vaginal hernia, usually developing after birth trauma and commonly seen in multiparous females. A frequent urge to defecate and a sense of rectal and vaginal fullness are common complaints. If a rectocele is present, the enterocele sac will lie above it. Lateral (erect) pelvic radiographs accompanying small bowel study can be used to show the presence of an enterocele. Cf. *rectocele.*

enterochromaffin (en″ter-o-kro-maf′in) a term applied to cells in the epithelium of the alimentary canal that are argentaffin-positive and stain with potassium dichromate. They include the serotonin-forming cells.

enterochromaffin cells scattered, usually solitary endocrine cells that are located in the epithelium of the stomach and intestine. Together with the endocrine cells of the pancreas, they are collectively referred to as the gastroenteropancreatic (GEP) endocrine system. With the exception of the insulin-forming beta cells of the pancreatic islets, the various GEP cell types (approximately 15 in number) may occur within the gut or pancreas. Immunoperoxidase studies have revealed that these cells produce a wide range of peptides and/or amines that function as hormones or neurotransmitters; they may be grouped within the APUD series of cells or be collectively designated as paraneurons.

By electron microscopy, the cells are usually solitary, resting on the basal lamina and rarely reaching the lumen. They contain dense-core granules of a size range seen in other polypeptide-forming endocrine cells (150–400 nm). In most instances the granules are spherical, but in certain cell types, particularly within the midgut, they are angular or pleomorphic; the functional significance of this variability is not understood. Only some of the secretory products of the enterochromaffin cells are known to act as circulating hormones. Conceivably, others could directly affect neighboring cells of the gastrointestinal mucosa, but this has not been proven.

enterochromaffin staining techniques to localize enterochromaffin cells. Sections are impregnated with silver and toned with gold chloride; unreduced silver is removed with sodium thiosulfate. The sections are counterstained with safranin and mounted. The enterochromaffin cells exhibit granules that are brown to black in color. Masson's argentaffin reaction and Gomori's methenamine-silver techniques stain these cells by a similar reaction.

enterococcus (en″ter-o-kok′us), pl. *enterococci* [*entero-* + Gr. *kokkos* berry] a term frequently used for *Streptococcus faecalis.* Enterococci are serologic group D streptococci, which are capable of growth in liquid media containing 6.5 percent sodium chloride. Normal inhabitants of the human intestinal tract, these organisms are an important cause of subacute infective endocarditis and urinary tract infections. They are troublesome because of their relatively high resistance to chemical agents, including antibiotics. The clinically less important species *S. faecium* and *S. durans* are also enterococci. See also *streptococcus.*

enterocolitis (en″ter-o-ko-li′tis) [*entero-* + Gr. *kolon* colon + *-itis* inflammation] inflammation of the small intestine and colon. See also *enteritis.*

acute necrotizing e., see *pseudomembranous e.*

neonatal necrotizing e., a disease of unknown etiology characterized by intestinal necrosis (usually of the ileum and proximal colon) that primarily affects premature infants in intensive care nurseries. An infection may be the contributory or precipitating cause (especially gram-negative aerobes), but the usefulness of antibiotics has not been demonstrated for prophylaxis or treatment except if sepsis is present. Formula feeding, intestinal ischemia, infant respiratory distress syndrome, congenital heart disease, and low birth weight are other factors that have been implicated in the pathogenesis of this syndrome. The mortality rate is 20–40 percent; death usually results from endotoxic shock.

pseudomembranous e., a serious disorder, with acute onset, that is characterized by the presence of necrotic plaques on the intestinal mucosa that coalesce to form a solid membrane over large portions of the intestines and colon. The raised, yellowish-white plaques are composed of necrotic debris, mucus, and fibrin. Pseudomembranous enterocolitis is most often seen in association with antibiotic therapy (especially clindamycin and lincomycin) or after intestinal surgery, although a small number of cases occur as a complication of diseases affecting the intestinal tract. *Staphylococcus aureus* and *Clostridium difficile* are the organisms most frequently isolated from fecal specimens from patients with this disease.

enterogastrone (en″ter-o-gas′trōn) [*entero-* + Gr. *gastēr* stomach + chal*one*] a term for a substance originating in the small intestine with the capacity to inhibit gastric acid secretion and emptying. It is believed to be released by fatty acid stimulation from the duodenum to enable more time for fat digestion. Several hormones, including secretin and cholecystokinin-pancreozymin (CCK-PZ), also have enterogastrone-like activity; whether enterogastrone exists as a hormonal substance separate from these established gastrointestinal hormones has not been determined.

enteroglucagon (en″ter-o-gloo′kah-gon) a glucagonlike polypeptide hormone found in the mucosa of the small intestine. It is released upon the absorption of fat and glucose in the intestine, and stimulates glycogenolysis. This material demonstrates immunologic cross-reactivity with antibodies to pancreatic alpha-cell glucagon, and has also been described as "gut glucagon" or as having "glucagon-like immunoreactivity" (GLI). The physiologic importance of GLI has not been established.

enterokinase (en″ter-o-ki′nās) see *enteropeptidase.*

Enteromonas (en″ter-o-mo′nas) a genus of flagellate protozoa.

E. hominis, a pear-shaped protozoan, measuring 4–10 μm by 3–6 μm, found in human intestines. It is nonpathogenic but has been identified in diarrheic stools. Infection is probably due to ingestion of cysts in food or drink.

enteropathy (en″ter-op′ah-the) [*entero-* + Gr. *pathos* disease] a general term used to describe any disease of the intestine.

gluten-sensitive e., see *celiac s.* under *sprue.*

protein-losing e., a condition characterized by the excessive loss of plasma proteins through leakage into the intestinal lumen. Causes include inflammation in the intestinal wall, lymphangiectasis, malignant tumors, and allergy. Those affected typically have hypoproteinemia.

enteropeptidase (en″ter-o-pep′tĭ-dās) an enzyme of the hydrolase class (EC 3.4.21.9) that catalyzes the cleavage of the Lys^6-Ile^7 bond in trypsinogen. It is secreted by the small intestine and is a highly specific protease, catalyzing the conversion of typsinogen to its active form, trypsin. Similar enzymes are found in many fungi. Formerly called *enterokinase.*

enterotoxigenic (en″ter-o-tok″sĭ-jen′ik) producing or containing a toxin specific for the cells of the intestinal mucosa.

enterotoxin (en″ter-o-tok′sin) [*entero-* + L. *toxicum* poison] an exotoxin specific for the cells of the intestinal mucosa, which produces violent vomiting and diarrhea. Enterotoxins produced by bacteria are the primary factors in food poisoning by *Staphylococcus aureus, Clostridium perfringens,* and *Bacillus cereus.* Enterotoxins produced by *Escherichia coli* and the cholera vibrios cause severe diarrhea. See also *exotoxins.*

enterovirus (en″ter-o-vi′rus) a single-stranded RNA virus belonging to the Picornaviridae family, which is primarily found in the enteric tract. Enteroviruses were originally divided into polioviruses, coxsackieviruses, and echoviruses on the basis of their culturing properties, antigenic relationships, host specificity, and pathologic effects. Because there were enteroviruses that could not be unambiguously classified, however, recently discovered organisms (agents 68–71 to date) are now simply called enteroviruses, and all subdivisions have been dropped. (The first 67 immunotypes are still subclassified according to the earlier tripart scheme.) Although most enterovirus infections are subclinical, the virus has been observed to cause encephalitis, meningitis, pneumonitis, bronchiolitis, and possibly gastroenteritis. See also *coxsackievirus, echovirus,* and *poliovirus.*

enterozoon (en″ter-o-zo′on), pl. *enterozoa* [*entero-* + Gr. *zōon* animal] any parasite species that infects the intestines.

enthalpy (*H*) (en′thal-pe) [*en-* + Gr. *thalpein* to warm] the sum of the internal energy (*E*) of a system in thermodynamic equilibrium and the product of its pressure (*p*) and its volume (*V*), i.e., $H = E + pV$. Also called *heat content*. See also *standard enthalpy of formation*.

enthalpy of reaction the enthalpy change that accompanies a chemical reaction (negative for exothermic reactions); the amount of heat that is liberated by the reaction and by the return of the products to the temperature and pressure of the reactants.

Entner-Doudoroff pathway (ent′ner doo′do-rof) a series of chemical reactions, catalyzed by specific enzymes, that converts glucose to pyruvate in bacteria by way of the intermediate compound 2-keto-3-deoxy-6-phosphogluconate; high-energy phosphate (ATP) is formed in the process. This is the major route of hexose metabolism in *Pseudomonas;* it is also used in *Escherichia coli* to utilize gluconate.

entoderm (en′to-derm) [Gr. *entos* within + *derma* skin] see *endoderm*.

Entoloma (en″to-lo′mah) a genus of fungi of which the species *E. lividum* causes mycetismus gastrointestinalis (mushroom poisoning). The onset of symptoms may occur within a few minutes and last up to 72 hr. Symptoms may include nausea, vomiting, diarrhea, water loss, electrolyte imbalance, dizziness, hallucination, and various cerebral manifestations.

entom/o (en′to-mo) [Gr. *entomon* insect] a word element used in combining form to denote relationship to an insect or insects, e.g., entomology.

Entomophthora (en″to-mof′thor-ah) [*entomo-* + Gr. *phthora* destruction, death] a genus of soil fungi of which the species *E. coronata* is the causative agent of rhinoentomophthoromycosis. *E. coronata* is pathogenic for several arthropods; in humans, it causes nasal polyps and palpable subcutaneous masses. Colony morphology appears folded, with white aerial mycelia. As growth continues, the lid of the dish becomes covered with conidia and the colony turns brown. Microscopically, large conidia are seen at the end of short conidiophores, and produce several hairlike appendages that give rise to secondary conidia.

entomophthoromycosis (en″to-mof″tho-ro-mi-ko′sis) [*Entomophthora* + Gr. *mykēs* fungus + *-osis* condition] a chronic granulomatous fungal disease involving the nasal mucosa or subcutaneous tissue. It includes two clinically distinct diseases: rhinoentomophthoromycosis and subcutaneous phycomycosis (basidiobolomycosis), which are caused by the etiologic agents *Entomophthora coronata* and *Basidiobolus haptosporus*, respectively.

entopic (en-top′ik) [*en-* + Gr. *topos* place] occurring in the proper place. Cf. *ectopic*.

entrapment neuropathy (en-trap′ment) see *entrapment n.* under *neuropathy*.

entropy (S) (en′tro-pe) [*en-* + Gr. *tropein* to turn] a thermodynamic quantity, defined by the formula $\Delta S = \Delta H/T$, where ΔS is the change in entropy during a reversible process at constant temperature, ΔH is enthalpy change, and T is absolute temperature. For any spontaneous change at constant temperature, the entropy of the universe (i.e., of a system plus its surroundings) must increase. Localized decreases in entropy can occur, but only because there is an increase in entropy somewhere else in the universe. Because entropy is proportional to the logarithm of the probability of the occurrence of a given thermodynamic state, it is said to be a measure of randomness or disorder (of that state). For example, diffusion proceeds spontaneously because the resulting state of the system is more random (and thus more likely) and is therefore associated with a higher entropy. In a chemical reaction (in the gas phase, for example), a state that has the atoms arranged into more individual molecular units is more random (and therefore more probable) and has the higher entropy.

Whether a reaction occurs spontaneously (i.e., has a free-energy change greater than zero; $-\Delta G$) or does not occur spontaneously depends both on the enthalpy change ΔH (which is related to changes in bond energies in going from reactants to products) and on the entropy term ($T\Delta S$); $\Delta G = \Delta H - T\Delta S$. Because only differences in entropy are physically significant, the zero point can be arbitrarily defined so that the entropy of all crystalline (regularly ordered) solids at absolute zero temperature is zero. The entropy change in the course of any reaction is equal to the sum of the entropies of the products minus the sum of those for the reactants.

enucleate (e-nu′kle-āt) [L. *enucleare*] 1. to remove whole and clean, as in removing an eyeball from its socket.

2. to remove the nucleus from a cell.

enucleated (e-nu′kle-āt″ed) 1. removed; said of an organ or tumor.

2. having no nucleus; said of a cell, such as a red blood cell.

Also called *anuclear* and *anucleated*.

enuresis (en″u-re′sis) [Gr. *enourein* to void urine] a clinical symptom characterized by uncontrollable urination while sleeping. Most children achieve bladder control by age 5–7 yr; beyond this age enuresis usually has an associated cause, such as overflow incontinence, neurogenic bladder, infection, congenital anomalies, and psychologic problems.

Culture and microscopic examination of the urine are performed to establish a diagnosis. If necessary, more complex tests may be utilized, including excretory urography, voiding cystourethrography, cystoscopy, urethroscopy, and urodynamic studies.

envelope (en′vĕ-lōp) 1. in virology, a lipoprotein membrane that surrounds the nucleocapsid of certain viruses. The envelope consists of an inner protein membrane and an outer lipoprotein complex. The lipoprotein complex is derived from the cytoplasmic membrane of the infected cell.

2. in bacteriology, the cell membrane together with the cell wall of a bacteria.

environment (en-vi′ron-ment) [Fr. *environner* to surround] the physical surroundings of some object, particularly the totality of all external factors and conditions that affect the development of an organism.

enzootic (en″zo-ot′ik) [*en-* + Gr. *zōon* animal] pertaining to a disease of low morbidity that is present in a certain animal community at all times, or one of high morbidity that is present in a small number of animals at all times. It is analogous to the term endemic in a human population. Cf. *epizootic*.

enzymatic (en″zi-mat′ik) relating to, caused by, or of the nature of an enzyme, e.g., an enzymatic reaction.

enzymatic digestion methods histochemical methods for the positive identification of a substance based on its susceptibility to enzymatic digestion. Parallel sections are prepared: a nonincubated group and a group incubated at physiologic pH and temperature with an enzyme that digests the substance. Both groups are then subjected to identical tissue processing and staining using a staining method specific for the substance. Tissue constituents that stain in the control sections but not in the enzyme-digested sections are identified as the substrate of the enzyme.

enzyme (en′zīm) [*en* + Gr. *zymē* leaven] a protein that acts as a catalyst. Like all catalysts, enzymes do not alter the direction of the reaction but only the rate at which it proceeds; they cannot alter the K_{eg} but do increase the reaction rate by lowering the activation energy. Unlike other catalysts, enzymes are highly specific: a given enzyme generally catalyzes a single type of reaction involving a few closely related molecules (its substrates). A large part of biochemistry is concerned with the study of enzymes and their physical and chemical properties, inasmuch as all physiologic functions (muscular contraction, energy utilization, hormone secretion, nerve conduction, and kidney excretion, for example) are based on the concerted activity of a number of enzymes.

All enzymes are proteins and consist of one or more associated peptide chains. They vary in size and shape, with molecular weights varying from 15,000 to over 1 million. The structure of enzymes has been examined in great detail, including the sequencing of amino acids and x-ray crystallographic studies. The sequence and native conformation for some enzymes, e.g., ribonuclease, have been established.

Enzymes range in complexity from single chains with no activators and no coenzymes, to associated groups of two or four peptide chains, to complexes of many enzymes and their associated activators and coenzymes. The structure of many enzymes is known in some detail, including the sequence of amino acids, the amino acids involved at the "active center," and details of configurational structure.

The rate of an enzyme-catalyzed reaction can be controlled by many mechanisms. Substrate concentration influences all reaction rates. Many important enzymes are controlled by allosteric regulation in which effector molecules (activators, inhibitors, and modulators) that bind at allosteric sites increase or decrease the enzymatic activity. Thus, the rates of different pathways are coordinated by feedback control. Some enzymes are controlled by phosphorylation. Addition of a phosphate group catalyzed by a protein kinase converts the enzyme from an inactive to an active form (or vice versa). An enzyme may also be controlled by genetic regulation; the synthesis of the enzyme is repressed or induced by control of the transcription process. Both phosphorylation and genetic regulation are involved in the mechanism of action of many hormones.

An enzyme molecule is absolutely stereospecific in regard to particular groupings on substrates undergoing transformation (e.g., D-lactate, not L-lactate, is the substrate for lactic dehydrogenase, LDH). Each enzyme has a unique spatial conformation, allowing it to bring together chemical groups on the same or different substrates into a particular spatial configuration that permits an interaction to occur with an appreciably lowered energy of activation. As is true for most proteins, enzymes are physically unstable and are easily denatured (with resultant loss of activity) by extremes of pH or temperature, mechanical energy, high concentrations of salts, organic solvents, and a variety of other chemicals.

NOMENCLATURE. For many years, enzymes were named by adding the suffix "-ase" to the name (or the stem of the name) of the substrate acted on (e.g., urease, phosphatase). Others were named on the basis of the kind of reaction catalyzed and product formed (citrate synthetase, succinic dehydrogenase, phosphoglucose mutase). Many of these remain as practical names of the enzymes. International scientific organizations, as a result of decisions made in 1956, 1972, and 1979, have systematized the nomenclature of enzymes. In this scheme, enzymes are divided into six classes according to the type of reaction catalyzed: (1) oxidoreductases, (2) transferases, (3) hydrolases, (4) lyases, (5) isomerases, and (6) ligases. Each class is further subdivided into subclasses and sub-subclasses, according to the specific substrates involved. A unique number code of four numbers, separated by periods, is assigned to each enzyme, the numbers representing the classes and subclass to which the enzyme belongs. The code number is preceded by the letters EC, standing for Enzyme Commission. Each enzyme is also given a unique systematic name, which includes both the name(s) of the substrate(s) acted on and the specific type of reaction involved. Because some of these names are rather long, a recommended common or practical name is also assigned. Once assigned to an enzyme the four-number codes are not to be changed, although in 1979 the numbers assigned to some proteases were replaced by new numbers, reflecting an improved classification of the many, very similar, proteases.

COMPOSITION. An enzyme may be a simple protein whose catalytic activity derives from the specific structure and configuration of the peptide chain (e.g., urease). Other enzymes require the addition or presence of some nonprotein cofactor before activity can be manifested. The protein moiety is referred to as the apoenzyme, and the nonprotein prosthetic group as a coenzyme (if it is an organic compound serving as a cosubstrate) or an activator (if it is some inorganic ion such as K^+, Mg^{2+}, Cl^-). Many of the B vitamin derivatives serve as coenzymes (e.g., thiamine pyrophosphate for carboxylase, and pyridoxal-5′-phosphate for transaminases). The combination of protein and cofactor is referred to as the holoenzyme. Activators apparently modify the configuraton of the enzyme, thus permitting or enhancing its activity; most, but not all, are obligate, i.e., absolutely necessary for activity. Many important metabolites serve as enzyme modulators, capable of either accelerating or inhibiting activity of some key enzymes, depending on their concentration in the reaction milieu. Cofactors are bound to the enzyme protein (apoenzyme), but usually can be removed by dialysis or by molecular sieve filtration.

Many proteases and peptidases are synthesized in the form of inactive precursors (zymogens, proenzymes); they are activated by scission of one or more small peptide fragments from the protein chain (e.g., chymotrypsinogen to chymotrypsin, procarboxypeptidase to carboxypeptidase). The activating agent is often a protease such as trypsin in the given examples or HCl in the case of pepsinogen.

INHIBITION. Some chemical agents (inhibitors) can reduce the rate of the enzyme-catalyzed reactions. Many inhibitors are competitive; i.e., they compete with one of the substrates or activators or coenzymes for the pertinent "active center" on the enzyme. Other agents are noncompetitive in that they do not bind at the "active center" but bind at some other area of the enzyme, creating a change in configuration and, as a result, a decrease in enzyme activity. Complete inactivation or decrease in activity may result from heavy metal ions reacting with free sulfhydryl groups on the enzyme or by oxidation of SH groups to disulfide bonds.

TEMPERATURE AND pH. As temperature is increased, the rate of enzyme-catalyzed reactions increases to an optimal or maximal value after which the rate falls rapidly to zero. The Q_{10} value (increase in activity for each 10°C increase in temperature) for such reactions varies from about 1.6 to 2.3. The temperature effect is the result of two phenomena: an increase in the chemical reaction rate with temperature, and the increased rate of enzyme denaturation and loss of catalytic activity. Most enzymes have a temperature optimum of about 37–42°C and are inactive at temperatures above 50–55°C. Each enzyme has a pH optimum; for most enzymes it is in the range of 6.8–7.5, but it may be as low as 1.5 (pepsin) or 4.9–6.0 (acid phosphatase), or as high as 10.4 (alkaline phosphatase). The pH effect reflects the fact that only one of the several different protonated (ionized) forms of the substrate may be acted on by the enzyme. The activity of the enzyme may also be a function of its degree of protonation.

KINETICS. An enzyme reaction occurs by the formation of a transitory complex of enzyme and substrate. This occurs at the "active center"; coenzymes and second substrates, if involved in the reaction, bind also in the vicinity of this active site. This enzyme-substrate complex, called the Michaelis-Menten complex, decomposes into enzyme and product (or products). This reaction can be written (in simplified form) as:

$$\underset{\text{free enzyme}}{E_f} + \underset{\text{substrate}}{S} \longrightarrow \underset{\text{enzyme-substrate complex}}{ES} \longrightarrow \underset{\text{free enzyme}}{E_f} + \underset{\text{product}}{P.}$$

The reaction velocity is related to the concentration of ES; hence, for a given quantity of enzyme, as S is increased, ES will increase and the velocity will increase. When all the enzyme is in the ES form, the enzyme is saturated with substrate (no free enzyme), and no further increase in rate is possible. A maximal velocity will have been reached. Maximal reaction rate is thus obtained only in the presence of excess substrate. A plot of reaction rate against substrate concentration gives a hyperbolic curve. If the substrate is constantly supplied at a fixed maximal level and the product concentration is kept near zero by removing it from the reaction, a steady-state condition is reached where the velocity (V) of the reaction is:

$$V = \frac{V_{max}\,S}{K_m + S}$$

This is the Michaelis-Menten equation, in which V_{max} is maximal velocity and S is substrate concentration. In this equation, K_m is the substrate concentration at which the velocity is half the maximal velocity: this is the Michaelis constant and may be determined experimentally. The value of K_m is a measure of the intensity of binding between enzyme and substrate, although it is not a true association constant. The maximal velocity (V_{max}) is a fixed quantity for a given enzyme under defined conditions. It is the maximal theoretical rate of reaction under conditions in which the active site of the enzyme is continually saturated with substrate, so that the rate of reaction depends only on the amount of enzyme present in a given solution. The kinetic analysis of enzymatic reactions involves the use of these two parameters (V_{max} and K_m) that describe the overall process of the reaction.

ASSAYS. Enzyme assays are measures of the activity of the enzyme. The actual quantity of an enzyme often cannot be measured, and this quantity may also include denatured inactive protein. Activity values are thus measures of the amount of enzyme in terms of the one property that differentiates it from all other proteins, its specific catalytic activity. Activity is expressed in units, which give the amount of reaction (substrate consumed or product formed) per unit time interval under prescribed experimental conditions. The change in substrate or product concentration can be measured by any convenient property or technique, such as spectrophotometry. Substrates are chosen so that the reaction rate may be measured by some convenient color change. Dehydrogenation reactions are easily measured by the change in the cosubstrate (coenzyme) concentration (nicotinamide adenine dinucleotide = NADH) measured at 340 nm.

Ideally, enzyme assays are performed when the rate is constant and independent of substrate and product concentration (zero-order reaction). This is not always possible, but an enzyme assay must be carefully designed so that the amount of enzyme present is the only limiting factor. The rate of reaction should be linear during the reaction period; continuous monitoring of the reaction (e.g., recorder trace) is the best technique, but multipoint assays over a short reaction time can be satisfactory. The generally accepted unit of enzyme activity is the International unit (U), defined as the amount of activity catalyzing the transformation of 1 micromole of substrate per minute (1 μmol/min); the catalytic concentration is expressed in units per liter (U/l). Before establishment of the International Unit, activities were given in terms of any convenient quantity unit (milligram, millimole) produced in any convenient time interval (1 hr, 30 min, 10 min).

CLINICAL SIGNIFICANCE. The use of enzymes in the diagnosis and treatment of disease is known as clinical enzymology. In a large hospital laboratory, enzyme assays may account for as much as 25–35 percent of the total workload, with 10–12 different enzymes being assayed routinely. Enzyme assays are important in clinical diagnosis because activity of some enzymes is markedly altered in the course of different disease processes. For example, in serum such change may be due to the increased release of enzymes from damaged tissue and sometimes may indicate the tissue of origin. The determination of individual isozymes and their relative amounts is often significant in this regard, as ratios differ among different tissues. More than 50 different enzymes have been identified in serum. The most common of these, with the disease processes of interest, are shown in the accompanying table.

Assays of enzyme activity in erythrocytes and leukocytes have been useful in the diagnosis of genetic disorders and some acquired systemic conditions. Measurements of enzyme concentrations are also carried out in other body fluids (such as gastrointestinal juices, cerebrospinal fluid, pleural fluid, and urine).

Of increasing importance are enzyme defects associated with genetic metabolic disorders. Many human metabolic defects have been traced to the absence of activity of a single specific enzyme. The loss may be caused by lack of enzyme synthesis or by production of a mutant protein unable to perform its regular function. More than 1000 genetically transmitted abnormalities are known, many involving defects in enzyme functions. Of particular interest in clinical diagnosis are those genetic abnormalities in which prenatal diagnosis may result in a decision to terminate pregnancy (β-*N*-acetyl-D-galactosaminidase in Tay-Sachs disease) and those in which neonatal diagnosis may determine prophylactic treatment and prevention of disability (UDPglucose-hexose-1-phosphate uridyltransferase in galactosemia).

For more information, see the specific enzymes and other related terms, such as *coenzyme, Hill equation, inhibitor, isozyme, kinetics, Lineweaver-Burk equation, Michaelis-Menten equation,* and the accompanying table.

enzyme analyzer an instrument that determines the enzyme activity in a specimen. A spectrophotometer measures the change in absorbance in the reaction mixture (sample with reagents) at regular intervals as the enzyme reaction proceeds. If the absorbance decreases or increases linearly with time (zero-order reaction), the activity is proportional to the rate of absorbance change. Most analyzers are designed to measure absorbance at 340 nm, which permits measurement of the appearance or disappearance of NADH (or NADPH). The analyzers may have adjustable temperature controls and mechanical devices to add reagents and samples automatically, and to process multiple specimens in sequence. Some analyzers have microcomputers that calculate the activity and reject measurements that do not have acceptable linearity or are otherwise unacceptable.

enzyme assays measurement of the quantity of some native enzyme present in a body fluid specimen. The actual mass or molar concentration is seldom measured because enzymes are present in low concentrations and in a matrix containing a large number of chemically similar proteins and other biochemicals. Enzymes are most conveniently measured in terms of their catalytic activity, which is expressed in activity units, such as International Units (U).

Many factors affect the rate of an enzyme-catalyzed reaction: (1) the enzyme should be present in its active, proper conformational form (not denatured); (2) all essential and nonessential activators

ENZYME. SERUM ENZYMES WITH DEMONSTRATED DISEASE ABNORMALITIES

	HEPATITIS	INFECTIOUS MONONUCLEOSIS	CIRRHOSIS	OBSTRUCTIVE JAUNDICE	HEART FAILURE	MYOCARDIAL INFARCTION	PROGRESSIVE MUSCULAR DYSTROPHY
Acid phosphatase	N	N	N	N	N	N	N
Alanine aminotransferase	+++	++	+	+	+	±	++
Alkaline phosphatase	+	+	+	+++	+	N	N
α-Amylase	N	N	N or –	N	N	N	N
Aspartate aminotransferase	+++	++	+	+	+	++	++
Cholinesterase	–	–	–	N or +	N or +		N
Creatine kinase	N		N	N	N	++	+++
Fructose bisphosphate aldolase	+++	+	+	N or +	+	++	++
Glucosephosphate isomerase	+++	++	+	+	+	++	+
γ-Glutamyl transferase	+		+	++	+		
Hydroxybutyrate dehydrogenase	+	+	±	±	+	+++	±
L-Iditol dehydrogenase	+++	+	+	N or +		N	N
Isocitrate dehydrogenase	+++	+	N or +	N or +	+	N	N
Lactate dehydrogenase	+	++	+	N or +	+	++	++
Leucine aminopeptidase	+	+++	+	+++	++	N	N
Lipase (triacylglycerol)	N	N	N	N	N	N	N
5′-Nucleotidase	+		+	+++			
Ornithine carbamoyl transferase	+++		+				

Note: Abnormality indicated by range of normal to marked increase: – indicates slight decrease; ± indicates slight increase or decrease; + indicates slight increase; ++ indicates moderate increase; +++ indicates marked increase; and N indicates no change.

should be present at optimal concentrations; (3) substrates and cosubstrates or cofactors should be present in excess; and (4) inhibitors of any type (competitive, non-competitive) must be absent or neutralized by appropriate reagents. Under such ideal conditions, the catalytic rate is governed only by the quantity (concentration) of enzyme present in the specimen.

Older methods for measuring enzyme activity utilized two-point assays (fixed reaction times). In these procedures, the enzyme-catalyzed reaction is permitted to proceed for a fixed time period; the quantity of substrate consumed (or product formed) in that time serves as a measure of enzyme activity.

Current techniques monitor the progress of the reaction continuously or at frequent intervals, either electronically or by the use of a recorder. This allows the analyst to confirm the linearity of the reaction and to select for calculation of the activity only those segments of the reaction rate curve that follow zero-order kinetics. Achievement of zero-order kinetics in some instances makes it necessary to remove the product of the reaction with a trapping agent or by adding an excess of another enzyme, which catalyzes the conversion of the product into a noninterfering material.

Enzyme assays may give erroneous results due to hemolysis, with the release of red cell enzymes into the serum; the inhibitory influences of anticoagulants, heavy metal ions, chromic acid, or detergents; or the denaturation of the enzyme by heat.

enzyme-assisted immunoassay technique a homogeneous (one-phase) enzyme-labeled immunoassay method used for the detection and quantitation of drugs, hormones, and metabolites, such as morphine, phenytoin, and cortisol, in body fluids. It is most often used to detect drugs of abuse or for the quantitative measurement of selected drugs in serum and plasma for therapeutic drug monitoring.

The clear specimen is mixed with the enzyme-labeled antigen (the drug or metabolite being assayed bonded covalently to an appropriate enzyme), a solution of antibodies specific for the drug or metabolite, and the substrate appropriate for the enzyme. In the absence of the suspected analyte in the specimen, the antigen (enzyme-labeled analyte) and antibody react, forming a complex that blocks the active center of the enzyme so that enzyme-substrate interaction is inhibited or prevented, and thus preventing any enzyme reaction.

If the material to be measured is present in the specimen, it will displace the enzyme-labeled material in proportion to the concentration of the analyte. The displaced enzyme-labeled material is then able to bind with substrate, permitting the enzyme reaction to take place. The extent of the reaction can be related to the concentration of the analyte (e.g., drug) by comparison with a standard curve. Lysozyme with bacterial cell suspension (as source of mucopolysaccharide) and alkaline phosphatase and *p*-nitrophenyl phosphate are examples of enzyme-substrate combinations in use. A widely utilized technique of this type is the enzyme-multiplied immunoassay technique (EMIT).

See also *ELISA.*

Enzyme Commission (EC) the International Commission on Enzymes, a committee established in 1956 by the International Union of Biochemistry (IUB) to standardize enzyme classification and nomenclature. First issued in 1961, the enzyme list is revised periodically.

enzyme demonstration methods histochemical methods for the localization of enzymes in tissue sections. This is accomplished by incubating the section at optimal pH and temperature for the enzyme in the presence of a natural or artificial substrate that enters into the enzyme-catalyzed reaction and forms a colored product localized at the enzyme site.

The tissue sections must be processed to preserve maximal enzyme activity and prevent enzyme movement. Cryostat or freeze-drying methods preserve enzyme activity, but soluble enzymes diffuse away from their in vivo site. For these, some form of mild fixation with cold formalin, alcohol, or acetone is necessary.

Several methods are used for capturing the reaction product at the enzyme site. A product such as orthophosphate may be precipitated as a salt (e.g., lead phosphate), which is then converted to a colored salt (e.g., black lead sulfide). In other methods, a product may immediately react with another compound to form a dye or colored product. For example, phosphatases and other esterases hydrolyze artificial naphthyl esters, releasing a naphthol, which can be coupled to a diazo compound to form an azo dye.

See also the specific enzyme.

enzyme immunoassays (EIA) see *nonradioisotopic i.* under *immunoassays.*

enzyme induction a mechanism of control of gene expression: the synthesis of an enzyme in response to a chemical signal. In bacteria, the genes coding for the enzymes involved in the metabolism of certain substrates are expressed only when the substrate is present. The genes are linked in an operon, which is transcribed to mRNA in response to the substrate. Similar mechanisms presumably operate in eukaryotes.

Steroid hormones also cause enzyme synthesis: the hormone binds to a cytoplasmic receptor protein and is carried to the nucleus, where it is believed to initiate transcription of specific genes.

negative control e. i., an induction control mechanism in which transcription continuously occurs in the absence of the repressor of the operon (the control element) and is turned off when the control element is present. An example is the lactose operon.

positive control e. i., an induction control mechanism in which transcription does not occur (or occurs only at low levels) until there is specific activation by a regulatory molecule. An example is the arabinose operon.

enzyme inhibition the effect produced by an inhibitor, an effector substance that combines with an enzyme and reduces its activity. There are three types of enzyme inhibition: competitive, noncompetitive, and uncompetitive (see the accompanying figure). These forms may be differentiated and identified by the changes in the Lineweaver-Burk plots as the inhibitor concentration is varied. A competitive inhibitor competes reversibly with the substrate for the active center of the enzyme, reducing the amount of bound enzyme and thus also the apparent values of K_m. At very high substrate concentrations, however, all the inhibitor is displaced and V_{max} remains unchanged. The Lineweaver-Burk equation for the inhibited enzyme reaction is: $(1/V) = (1/[S](K_m/V_{max})(1 + [I]/K_i) + (1/V_{max})$, where I is the inhibitor concentration and K_i is the binding constant for enzyme and inhibitor. The plots of $(1/V)$ vs. $(1/[S])$ for all inhibitor concentrations have the same y-intercept $(1/V_{max})$, but the slope increases with an increase in $[I]$ and the x-intercept approaches zero (0).

A noncompetitive inhibitor either binds irreversibly to the active center of the enzyme, thus reducing the quantity of catalytically active enzyme, or it binds at some remote locus on the enzyme by which the catalytic activity of the enzyme protein is reduced. The K_m is unchanged, but the V_{max} decreases with increase of $[I]$. When $(1/V)$ is plotted against $(1/[S])$, the x-intercept $(-1/K_m)$ is unchanged, but the y-intercept $(-1/V_{max})$ increases toward infinity.

In uncompetitive inhibition, both K_m and V_{max} change with increasing $[I]$. This form of inhibition is seen when the inhibitor binds to the substrate complex to form the ternary complex (ESI), which does not yield any product. In this case the plot of $(1/V)$ against $(1/[S])$ gives an x-intercept and a y-intercept that increase numerically with $[I]$, although the slope (K_m/V_{max}) is unchanged. In more complicated forms of inhibition, Lineweaver-Burk plots may not be linear, and K_m and V_{max} may not be easily evaluated.

enzyme-linked antibody test a method of antigen detection in which enzyme is chemically linked to an antibody. The antibody-enzyme complex is allowed to react with the antigen; the enzyme then is combined with its substrate, which permits detection of the antigen-antibody complex. Horseradish peroxidase and alkaline phosphatase are commonly used in this type of assay.

enzyme-multiplied immunoassay technique (EMIT) see under *enzyme-assisted immunoassay technique*.

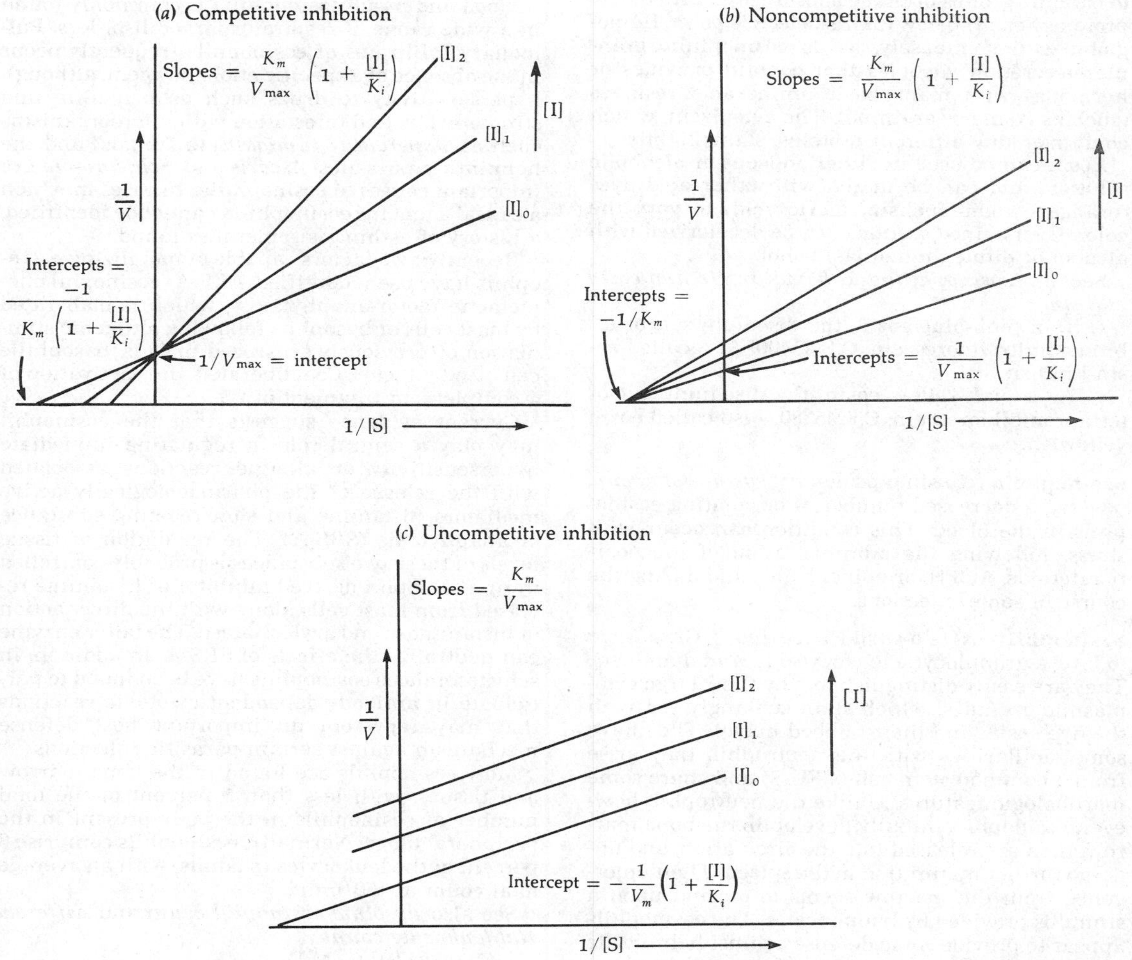

Enzyme inhibition. **Double reciprocal plots illustrating different types of inhibition of an enzymatic reaction: (*a*) Competitive inhibition; (*b*) noncompetitive inhibition; and (*c*) uncompetitive inhibition. K_m and V_{max} are estimated from the slopes and intercepts of the uninhibited reactions and K_i from the slopes and/or intercepts of the inhibited reactions. (From White, A., et al.: Principles of Biochemistry. 6th ed. New York, McGraw-Hill Book Co., 1978.)**

enzyme repression see *end-product r.* under *repression.*

EOG abbrev. See *electrooculogram.*

EOR abbrev. See *exclusive OR.*

eos abbrev. See *eosinophil.*

eosin/o (e-o-sin′o) [Gr. *ēōs* dawn] a word element used in combining form to denote rosy or dawn-colored, e.g., eosinophil.

eosin (e′o-sin) [Gr. *ēōs* dawn] any of several rose-colored acid dyes used as cytoplasmic stains in histology. These dyes are widely used as counterstains, not only in the routine hematoxylin and eosin (H and E) staining method, but also with other basic and metachromatic dyes. Eosin is a component of the Romanowsky stains used for staining blood cells and of the Papanicolaou stains used in exfoliative cytology.

Acid dyes have anionic dye molecules, which bind to cationic groups of tissue substances, particularly proteins at a pH below their isoelectric point. Hemoglobin stains intensely, as do eosinophilic granules—secretion vacuoles that contain enzymes or hormones with many basic amino acid residues (such as lysine or arginine). The cytoplasm, which contains many different proteins, stains lightly.

Eosin can be used in either aqueous or alcoholic solution, and can be mixed with other acid dyes (orange G, acid fuchsin, picric acid) to vary the color. Overstained sections can be decolorized with alcohol or dilute ammonia-alcohol.

See also *eosinophilic* and *hematoxylin and eosin staining.*

e. B, a pink-blue eosin, the disodium salt of dibromodinitrofluorescein; C.I. 45400. Also called eosin I bluish.

e. Y, a pink-yellow eosin, the disodium salt of tetrabromofluorescein; C.I. 45380. Also called eosin yellowish.

eosinopenia (e″o-sin″o-pe′ne-ah) [*eosino-* Gr. *penia* poverty] a decreased number of circulating eosinophils in the blood. This condition can occur with stress; following the administration of glucocorticosteroids, ACTH, or epinephrine; and during the course of some infections.

eosinophil (eos) (e″o-sin′o-fil) [*eosino-* + Gr. *philein* to love] a granulocytic leukocyte (12 μ in diameter). They are easily distinguishable by their large cytoplasmic granules, which stain strikingly red with the dye eosin, and their bilobed nuclei. They have some similarities with the neutrophil: they arise from a common stem cell (CFU-S) and share some morphologic features. Unlike the neutrophil, however, eosinophils initially develop in the bone marrow, then are released into the circulation, and undergo further maturation in the spleen. Their emergence from the marrow seems to depend upon a stimulus provided by lymphocytes. The eosinophils appear to provide some defense against helminthic parasites, and there is evidence that they phagocytize foreign particles and antigen-antibody complexes. Although their primary function is unclear, it appears to be related to their reactions with and response to endogenous substances including products from mast cells and lymphocytes, coagulation factors, complement, hormones, and kinins.

In tissues where the eosinophils fulfill their major function, they have a half-life up to 12 da. As eosinophils mature, they display acidophilic staining of their cytoplasmic granules, which do not contain lysozyme present in neutrophils but do have more peroxidase, arysulfatase, D-glucuronidase, β-glycerophosphatase, and arginine-rich basic protein than the neutrophil. Although they have phagocytic capability, this appears to be less efficient than that of other granulocytes. Like other phagocytic cells, eosinophils have Fc receptors capable of immune adherence for subsequent ingestion of immune complexes or engulfment and killing of microorganisms.

Eosinophils have traditionally been associated with IgE reaginic antibody-mediated reactions but are not limited to this type of response. Increased numbers of eosinophils (eosinophilia) can be manifested in the absence of raised serum IgE in a wide range of conditions, such as pulmonary disorders, polyarteritis nodosa, drug sensitivity, carcinomas, and Hodgkin's disease.

Blood and tissue eosinophilia is commonly found in a wide range of respiratory tract disorders. Pulmonary infiltrates of eosinophils frequently occur in the absence of a specific etiologic agent, although hypersensitivity to drugs such as penicillin and streptomycin, and infestation with microorganisms such as *Aspergillus fumigatus* (a fungus) and the helminthic parasites *Ascaris* and *Schistosoma* are important causes of eosinophilia. In cases in which a causal agent for eosinophilia cannot be identified, a history of asthma is sometimes found.

Recently, two factors capable of mobilizing eosinophils have been identified: ECF-A (eosinophil chemotactic factor-anaphylaxis), which is elaborated by mast cells or basophils following antigenic stimulation of previously sensitized mast or basophilic cells, and a factor, C5a, liberated after activation of a complement fragment of C5.

Current evidence suggests that the eosinophil may play a central role in regulating immediate hypersensitivity or allergic reactions associated with the release of the pharmacologically active mediators histamine and slow-reacting substance of anaphylaxis (SRS-A). The regulation of tissue levels of these two substances is probably controlled by an eosinophil-derived inhibitor of histamine released from mast cells along with the direct action of histaminase and arylsulfatase. The latter enzyme can neutralize the effects of SRS-A. In addition, in schistosomiasis eosinophils have been found to participate in antibody-dependent cytotoxic reactions that may represent an important host defense mechanism against certain parasitic infections.

Most eosinophils are found in the bone marrow and tissues, with less than 1 percent of the total number of eosinophils in the body present in the peripheral blood. Normally, eosinophils comprise 3 percent of the leukocytes in adults, with an average total count of 150/mm^3.

See also *absolute eosinophil count* and *differential leukocyte count.*

CHARLES PAVIA, M.D.

eosinophil chemotactic factor of anaphylaxis (ECF-A) one of two tetrapeptides—Val-Gly-Ser-Glu or Ala-Gly-Ser-Glu—that are preferential chemotactic attractants for eosinophils. These tetrapeptides are secreted from the granules of mast cells and perhaps basophils. They are responsible for enhancing the expression of complement receptors for C3b on eosinophils and enhancing antibody- and complement-dependent damage to some parasites by eosinophils. There is also intermediate-molecular-weight ECF (M.W. 1500–3000) secreted by the mast cells.

eosinophil count see *absolute eosinophil count* and *differential leukocyte count*.

eosinophilia (e″o-sin″o-fil′e-ah) [*eosino-* + Gr. *philein* to love] the formation and accumulation of an abnormally large number of eosinophils in the blood: eosinophil counts are characteristically greater than 450 cells/mm^3. Disorders in which eosinophil counts are elevated include parasitic infections, allergic disorders, a number of skin diseases, hypereosinophilic syndrome, certain gastrointestinal disorders, some neoplasms, and various hereditary disorders. Eosinophilia can also be produced by injections of histamine. Also called eosinophilic leukocytosis.

eosinophilic (e″o-sin″o-fil′ik) having an affinity for acidic dyes, such as eosin. The main eosinophilic substances are proteins that have an abundance of the basic amino acid residues, arginine, lysine, histidine, and hydroxylysine; these proteins cause the general eosinophilia of cytoplasm. Some proteins are intensely eosinophilic, e.g., hemoglobin and the acid hydrolase that are present in the eosinophilic granules characteristic of eosinophilic leukocytes. Also called *acidophilic*.

eosinophilic fasciitis an uncommon condition in which soft tissues of the extremities are thickened and infiltrated with lymphocytes, mainly eosinophils. Eosinophilia and hypergammaglobulinemia are present, and flexion deformities may be produced by contraction of the thickened fascia.

eosinophilic granule the largest of granulocytic granules, which are refractile and stain orange-red with eosin. The granules are primarily lysosomes containing lysosomal enzymes (acid phosphate, glycuronidase, cathepsins, ribonuclease, aryl phosphate, and others) and contain basic amino acids such as lysine and arginine. The peroxidase present is different from myeloperoxidase. With electron microscopy, eosinophilic granules may be seen to contain oblong or rhomboid crystals, with a periodicity in humans of about 3 nm. In tissues rich in eosinophils, Charcot-Leyden crystals may form; they may also be produced by squashing eosinophils between the slide and the coverslip.

eosinophilic granuloma see under *histiocytosis*.

eosinophilic index (EI) see *eosinophilia i.* under *squamous cell index*.

eosinophilic leukocyte see *eosinophil*.

eosinophil stimulation promoter (ESP) a lymphokine that affects the movement of eosinophils. This factor is produced by antigen-stimulated T cells. It is unrelated to eosinophil chemotactic factors (ECF); however, the relationship between ESP and chemotactic stimuli is unclear. The production of ESP is macrophage-dependent. See also *lymphokines*.

eosinotactic (e″o-sin″o-tak′tik) [*eosino-* + Gr. *taktikos* regulating] exhibiting an influence on eosinophilic cells, either repelling them (termed negatively eosinotactic) or attracting them (positively eosinotactic).

EPA abbrev. for eicosapentaenoic acid (see under *prostaglandin*), Environmental Protection Agency.

EPEC an acronym from *e*ntero*p*athogenic *Escherichia coli*. See *Enterobacteriaceae* and *E. coli* under *Escherichia*.

ependyma (ĕ-pen′dĭ-mah) [Gr. "upper garment"] a layer of closely packed cuboidal or columnar epithelial cells that line the ventricles of the brain and the central canal of the spinal cord.

ependymoma (ĕ-pen″dĭ-mo′mah) a neoplasm arising from the epithelial lining of the ventricular system of the brain or spinal cord. Ependymomas make up about 5 percent of intracranial gliomas, and the majority arise within the fourth ventricle. The incidence is slightly higher in children, especially in the first decade when the tumor is usually in the posterior fossa. Ependymomas make up more than 60 percent of gliomas of the spinal cord, and at least one-third involve the lower cord or filum terminale.

Ependymomas are usually well-demarcated benign tumors, but the prognosis can be poor because of the technical difficulty of complete removal. Local spread to extraneural tissue occasionally occurs, but distant metastases are unusual.

The histologic hallmarks of the ependymoma are the ependymal rosette, and cilia or their basal bodies (blepharoplasts) may be demonstrable by light or electron microscopy. Neoplastic ependymal cells are capable of developing cytoplasmic extensions containing glial filaments, and characteristically these processes encircle small vessels. Papillary formations, often accompanied by a mucinous stroma, are seen in the myxopapillary variant that occurs at the tip of the spinal cord. Histologic distinction between an ependymoma of the fourth ventricle and a subependymal astrocytoma may be difficult.

ephedrine (ĕ-fed′rin, ef′ĕ-drin) a drug used alone or in combination with other drugs for the alleviation of bronchial asthma. Its toxicity is low, although overdosage may cause anxiety and rapid heartbeat. Ephedrine is detected by thin-layer chromatography screening assays for basic drugs and by amphetamine assays.

epi- (ep′ĭ) [Gr. *epi* on] a prefix word element to denote above or upon, e.g., epigastric.

epicanthus (ep″ĭ-kan′thus) [*epi-* + Gr. *kanthos* canthus] the fold of skin that extends from the area between the eyebrow and the upper eyelid to the side of the nose. It is present as a normal physical characteristic in persons of certain races and sometimes occurs as a congenital anomaly in others. Also called epicanthic fold.

epicardium (ep″ĭ-kar′de-um) [N.L. from *epi-* + Gr. *kardia* heart] the inner layer of the serous pericardium that covers the heart and roots of the great vessels; the areolar connective tissue underlining its mesothelial cells blends with the interstitial tissue of the myocardium and contains the fat in which portions of the coronary vessels are embedded. Also called *visceral pericardium*. See also under *pericardium*.

epichlorohydrin (ep″ĭ-klo″ro-hi′drin) a toxic epoxide, 1-chloro-2,3-epoxypropane, used in the manufacture of epoxide resins (polymers); M.W. 92.53. It is highly irritating to all tissues; chronic exposure may cause kidney damage.

epicondyle (ep″ĭ-kon′dīl) [*epi-* + Gr. *kondylos* condyle] a projection or eminence on a bone situated above its condyle; it serves as a point for muscle attachment and does not participate in articulation.

epicondylitis (ep″ĭ-kon″dĭli′tis) [*epicondyle* + *-itis* inflammation] a common condition characterized by inflammation and pain in the lateral aspect of the elbow in the area of the common extensor insertion. The inflammation may be disabling in severe cases. It is due to repetitive strenuous wrist extension or pronation-supination against resistance, as in manual screwdriving or playing tennis.

Radiographs are generally negative, although occasional minute foci of calcification may be visible in the tendon fibers adjacent to the lateral epicondyle. Diagnosis is based on clinical examination and may be confirmed by injecting procaine into the affected area, which temporarily abolishes all signs and symptoms of the disorder.

Also called lateral humeral epicondylitis and *tennis elbow.*

epicranial aponeurosis (ep″ĭ-kra′ne-al) [*epi-* + Gr. *kranion* skull] see *g. aponeurotica* under *galea.*

epidemic (ep″ĭ-dem′ik) [Gr. *epidēmios* prevalent] 1. attacking many people in a region at the same time; widely diffused and rapidly spreading.

2. a disease of high morbidity, which is only occasionally present in the human community.

epidemiology (ep″ĭ-de″me-ol′o-je) [Gr. *epidēmios* prevalent + *-logy*] 1. the study of the factors determining the frequency and distribution of disease in a human population. An example is cancer epidemiology, which has become increasingly important in our society, i.e., the association of specific tumors with industrial or environmental carcinogens.

2. the field of medicine that deals with the determination of specific causes of localized outbreaks of infection, of toxic poisoning, or of any other disease of recognized origin. For example, infectious disease epidemiology may be concerned with determining the specific cause of a local outbreak of hepatitis.

epidermal (ep′ĭ-der″mal) pertaining to the epidermis.

epidermal inclusion cyst a dermal cyst, generally small and superficial, that is lined by stratified squamous epithelium and contains desquamated keratin. Also called keratinous cyst.

epidermal nevus see *epidermal n.* under *nevus.*

epidermis (ep″ĭ-der′mis), pl. *epidermides* [*epi-* + Gr. *derma* skin] [NA], the protective, outermost layer of the skin composed of stratified squamous epithelium. See also *skin.*

keratohyalin granule of e., a granule of keratohyalin as seen within an epidermal cell by light microscopy; these granules are prominent in the granular layer. The overlying cornified (horny) layer is formed by the fusion of aggregates of keratohyalin. See also *keratin.*

membrane-coating granule of e., an ovoid granule containing parallel lamellae found within epidermal cells. These granules are discharged into the extracellular space to promote cohesion of the epidermal cells. Through their content of phospholipid, they reduce permeability to water. Also called Odland body.

epidermoid (ep″ĭ-der′moid) [*epi-* + Gr. *derma* skin + *eidos* form, shape] resembling the cells of the epidermis.

epidermoid carcinoma see *squamous carcinoma.*

epidermolysin see *exfoliatin.*

Epidermophyton (ep″ĭ-der-mof′ĭ-ton) [*epi-* + Gr. *derma* skin + *phyton* plant] a genus of dermatophytic fungi that causes eczema marginatum of the crural region and dermatophytosis of the foot but does not infect hair. In cultures, colonies appear folded, suedelike, and olive or khaki; the underside of the colony ranges from colorless to brown. Microscopically, there are characteristic beaver tail–shaped macroaleuriospores, usually occurring in groups, which have smooth, thin walls.

E. floccosum, a species that attacks both skin and nails; a causative agent of tinea corporis, tinea cruris, tinea manus, and tinea pedis.

epididym/o (ep″-ĭ-did′ĭ-mo) [*epi-* + Gr. *didymos* testis] a word element used in combining form to denote the epididymis, e.g., epididymitis.

epididymis (ep″ĭ-did′ĭ-mis), pl. *epididymides* [*epi-* + Gr. *didymos* testis] the tubular structure attached to the testis by the efferent ductules in which the spermatozoa mature and are stored.

epididymitis (ep″ĭ-did″ĭ-mi′tis) [*epi-* + Gr. *didymos* testes + *-itis* inflammation] an acute or recurring inflammation of the epididymis, which may be unilateral or bilateral. It is usually found as a complication of bacterial urethritis or prostatitis, and can be a manifestation of gonorrhea or be of nonbacterial origin. Symptoms include fever, severe pain, swelling, and tenderness in the epididymis.

Urine culture and prostatic secretion culture usually reveal the causative organism.

See also *sexually transmitted diseases.*

epididymography (ep″ĭ-did″ĭ-mog′rah-fe) [*epi-* + Gr. *didymos* testes + *graphein* to record] radiologic examination of the epididymis to investigate conditions such as cysts, tumors, orchitis, or sterility. A water-soluble iodinated contrast medium is injected into the deferent ducts prior to radiologic examination of the epididymis. See also *epididymovesiculography.*

epididymovesiculography (ep″ĭ-did″ĭ-mo-vĕ-sik″-u-log′rah-fe) [*epi-* + Gr. *didymos* testes + L. *vesicula* small bladder + Gr. *graphein* to record] a positive contrast radiologic examination of the seminal ducts, which combines epididymography and vesiculography.

epidural (ep″ĭ-du′ral) [*epi-* + L. *dura* hard] situated on or outside the dura mater.

epidural space the space between the dura mater of the spinal cord and the walls of the vertebral canal. It contains loose connective tissue, fat, and venous plexuses.

epigastric region (ep″ĭ-gas′trik) [*epi-* + Gr. *gastēr* belly] 1. the upper middle region of the abdomen within the arch of the rib cage.

2. the region of the abdomen above the transpyloric plane and between the lateral sagittal planes, used in radiographic positioning (see the illustration accompanying *abdominal regions*).

epigastric zone the part of the abdomen above the transpyloric plane. It consists of the epigastric and left and right hypochondriac regions.

epigenesis (ep″ĭ-jen′ĕ-sis) [*epi-* + Gr. *genesis* origin] the development of an organism from an undifferentiated cell during which new cell lines, tissues, and structures arise by the process of differentiation. The theory of epigenesis was opposed in the early nineteenth century by the erroneous theory of preformation, which held that all the different structures preexist in miniature form in the fertilized egg.

epigenetics (ep″ĭ-jĕ-net′iks) the study of gene action, particularly the expression and regulation of genes.

epigenotype (ep″ĭ-je′no-tīp) the inherited potential to express a particular type of differentiation; the commitment to a pathway of development. In developing embryos, commitment to a particular pathway often occurs long before there is any overt expression of differentiated properties. Cf. *epiphenotype.*

epiglott/o (ep″ĭ-glot′o) [Gr. *epiglōttis*] a word element used in combining form to denote the epiglottis, e.g., epiglottitis.

epiglottis (ep″ĭ-glot′is) [*epi-* + Gr. *glōttis* glottis] the thin, leaflike lamella of elastic fibrocartilage located in front of the entrance to the larynx. It functions as a lid over the larynx to prevent food from entering the larynx and trachea on swallowing.

epiglottitis (ep″ĭ-glot-tī′tis) [*epiglottis* + *-itis* inflammation] inflammation of the epiglottis, which may be life-threatening by causing respiratory obstruction. Prompt clinical recognition is essential. This disease is most common in infants and young children but is also seen in adults. *Hemophilus influenzae* is a common causative organism.

epilepsia partialis continua (ep″ĭ-lep′se-ah) a restricted form of focal motor epilepsy characterized by continuous rhythmic clonic activity of a group of muscles in the face or part of a limb, without spread to other parts of the body. During an attack, the electroencephalogram may remain normal or may show focal spikes, sharp waves, and/or slow waves that originate in the cortical area associated with the muscle movement.

epilepsy (ep′ĭ-lep″se) [Gr. *epilēpsia* seizure] a disorder characterized by a tendency to recurrent seizures due to the paroxysmal discharge of cells within the central nervous system. The seizures may be manifest clinically by transient impairment or loss of consciousness, or by involuntary motor, sensory, or psychic phenomena. Epilepsy is a fairly common disorder, occurring in about 0.5 percent of the general population.

Several theories based on experimental findings have been proposed for the origin of the hypersynchronous neuronal discharges that are the pathophysiologic basis of the seizures. One hypothesis proposes that the discharges result from the failure of tonic inhibitory effects on the cerebral cortex, brain stem, and cerebellar systems on the afferent pathways. This results in excessive central bombardment by afferent signals. Other theories relate the development of seizures to neuronal membrane instability due to ionic imbalances, deficiencies in the inhibitory neurotransmitter γ-aminobutyric acid (GABA), or perturbations in the enzymes associated with adenosine triphosphate (ATP) production.

Epilepsy can be classified etiologically as idiopathic or symptomatic. Idiopathic epilepsy is of obscure origin but may have a genetic basis; a single dominant autosomal gene whose penetrance varies with age has been implicated in the inheritance of the abnormal electroencephalographic pattern that often accompanies this form of epilepsy. Epileptic attacks in individuals with idiopathic epilepsy may be triggered by hypoglycemia, hypocapnia, drowsiness, menstruation, or repetitive sensory stimuli. The phenotypic expression of this gene is represented by bilaterally synchronous spike and wave discharges on the electroencephalogram (EEG).

Symptomatic epilepsy is secondary to some other disorder, which may include birth trauma, metabolic and toxic processes (e.g., drug withdrawal), head injuries, tumors, intracranial infection, and vascular disorders. There is also evidence, however, that suggests the involvement of genetic factors in symptomatic epilepsy, for individuals with brain lesions are more likely to experience epileptic attacks when there is a family history of epilepsy.

Epilepsy can also be classified on the basis of seizure type and EEG as being primary or secondary generalized epilepsy, and partial (focal) epilepsy. The interictal EEG is often abnormal in epileptic individuals and is invaluable in establishing a diagnosis. However, abnormal "epileptiform" EEG patterns may also be recorded from individuals who have never experienced a seizure, and the diagnosis of epilepsy must therefore be made on clinical grounds.

A diagnosis of epilepsy may be suspected in persons having recurrent episodes of cerebral dysfunction. Evaluation will necessitate a complete history, physical and neurologic examinations, hematologic and biochemical screening tests (to exclude other possible causes of the seizures), an EEG, and often a CT scan (to exclude an underlying structural cause for the seizures).

See also *absence attack, activation, electroencephalography, periodic lateralized epileptiform discharge, seizures, s. epilepticus* under *status,* and *tonic-clonic attack.*

benign focal e., a form of idiopathic epilepsy that occurs in otherwise healthy children between the ages of 5 and 12 yr. The seizures are focal (usually hemifacial) during wakefulness and may become generalized during sleep. The EEG is characterized by unilateral or bilateral centrotemporal sharp waves occurring on a normal background. Most children become seizure-free in the later teenage years. Underlying focal pathologic alterations of the brain can rarely be found to account for the seizures. Also called *rolandic e.*

focal e., see *partial e.*

jacksonian e., a form of epilepsy characterized by seizures that arise from a discrete lesion of the frontal lobe, with particular involvement of the rolandic cortex. Jacksonian seizures usually begin with tonic contraction or rhythmic twitching of the fingers, hand, foot, or face on one side of the body. The involuntary muscle activity spreads (marches) from the area first affected to other ipsilateral body parts according to their representation in the cortex. Changes in the EEG during an attack may not be detected by surface electrodes.

Also called *jacksonian march* and *jacksonian motor seizure.* See also under *cortical e.*

myoclonus e., a form of familial epilepsy characterized by myoclonic and tonic-clonic (grand mal) attacks, dementia, and progressive cerebellar dysfunction. The interictal EEG is grossly abnormal and consists of bilaterally synchronous single and multiple spikes superimposed on a background of theta and delta activity. Spike discharges sometimes accompany the myoclonic jerking. Several varieties of myoclonus epilepsy have been described. Also called *progressive familial myoclonic e.*

partial e., a form of epilepsy characterized by partial, i.e., focal, seizures, which arise from a localized region of the brain and may then remain focal or secondarily become generalized. They are caused by a lesion or abnormality to a specific area of brain tissue. Such lesions may result from a variety of causes, including congenital maldevelopment, metabolic disorders, trauma, vascular disease, neoplasm, and infectious disease. Partial epileptic attacks can be provoked by hyperventilation, sleep, or sleep deprivation in some individuals.

The interictal EEG may show intermittent focal sharp waves or spikes, continuous or paroxysmal focal slow waves, or localized slow-wave and spike activity. Ictal EEG patterns may show no change from the interictal findings, or there may be local or diffuse discharges. Ictal discharges are often followed by transient low-voltage activity and then slow-wave activity that may have a localized distribution. The use of depth (implanted) electrode recording may be helpful in localizing the epileptogenic focus more precisely, when surgical removal of the focus is under consideration.

Formerly called *focal e.*

primary generalized e., a disorder characterized by seizures that are generalized from their onset—e.g., absences, tonic-clonic attacks, and bilateral myoclonus—and by a lack of neurologic or psychologic evidence of cerebral abnormality. The seizures usually begin in the first two decades of life, and no clear etiology for them can be established.

progressive familial myoclonic e., see *myoclonus e.*

psychomotor e., a form of partial (focal) epilepsy with particular involvement of either the cortical temporal lobe (temporal lobe epilepsy), amygdala and hippocampus, or cortical frontal lobe, and characterized clinically by the occurrence of complex partial seizures. The clinical manifestation of such seizures includes the temporary impairment of consciousness; muscle movements typified by chewing, smacking of the lips, stereotyped limb movements, or turning of the head; and cognitive or ideational disturbances, affective symptoms, illusions, and hallucinations. Hallucinations may be simple olfactory, gustatory, visual, or auditory, or may have a very complex content.

The interictal EEG in this disorder may show focal abnormalities, especially in the temporal or frontal region on one or both sides, and these may be provoked by hyperventilation, sleep, or sleep deprivation. The ictal EEG may be characterized by an initial transient desynchronization, followed by rhythmic activity of variable frequency, with or without associated sharp transients. After an attack, focal slow activity may persist for as long as several days.

See also under *cortical e.*

rolandic e., see *benign focal e.*

secondary generalized e., a disorder characterized by seizures (such as absences, tonic-clonic attacks, or bilateral myoclonus) that are generalized from their onset. The seizures are due to diffuse or multifocal cerebral lesions.

temporal lobe e., a form of epilepsy characterized by partial seizures arising in the temporal lobe.

epileptiform (ep″ĭ-lep′tĭ-form) [Gr. *epilēptikos* + L. *forma* shape] 1. resembling epilepsy.
2. occurring in severe or sudden paroxysms.

epileptiform pattern interictal electroencephalographic activity characterized by paroxysmal spike, polyspike, or sharp-wave discharges. This activity is often accompanied by slow waves and may be focal, multifocal, diffuse, unilateral, or bilateral. When bilateral, the activity may be synchronous or asynchronous and symmetric or asymmetric. Multifocal activity may result from one primary focus generating mirror foci in homologous contralateral brain tissue; a primary deep focus discharging to homologous regions of the cortex; or distinct foci discharging asynchronously. This pattern of EEG activity is commonly found in patients who have seizure disorders but have never experienced a seizure; conversely, it may not be present in the interictal record of epileptic patients. See also *epilepsy.*

epimer (ep′ĭ-mer) one of a pair of compounds that differ only in their configuration at one asymmetric carbon atom. If they have other asymmetric carbon atoms, they are not enantiomers (mirror images), but diastereoisomers. See also *isomerism.*

epimerase (ĕ-pim′er-ās) one of a subgroup of enzymes of the isomerase class (EC 5.1) that catalyzes the inversion of the configuration about an asymmetric atom, e.g., the conversion of ribulose-5-phosphate to xylulose-5-phosphate catalyzed by ribulose-5-phosphate-3-epimerase.

epimerization (ĕ″pĭ-mer″ĭ-za′shun) the inversion of the configuration at one (and only one) asymmetric atom (center of chirality) in a chemical compound that has several such atoms.

epimysium (ep″ĭ-mis′e-um) [N.L., from *epi-* + Gr. *mys* muscle] the tough, fibrous connective tissue sheath that envelops an entire muscle.

epinephrine (ep″ĭ-nef′rin) a hormone secreted by the adrenal medulla in response to splanchnic nerve stimulation, 3,4-dihydroxy-α-[(methylamino)-methyl]benzyl alcohol; M.W. 183.20. It is stored in chromaffin granules and is released predominantly in response to hypoglycemia, fear, anger, or stress. Epinephrine is a potent stimulator of the sympathetic nervous system. It also increases such metabolic activities as glycogenolysis in the liver (raising plasma glucose) and muscles and lipolysis in adipose tissue. Epinephrine is used pharmaceutically as a sympathomimetic and cardiac stimulant and to relax bronchial smooth muscles. It is the most effective drug for treatment of anaphylaxis.

The cardiovascular effects of circulating epinephrine resemble those of sympathetic adrenergic stimulation, varying with the relative proportion of alpha- and beta-adrenergic receptors in a particular vascular bed. In minute doses (0.1 μg/kg or less), epinephrine has a predominantly depressor effect owing to its action on the more sensitive $beta_2$-receptors of the blood vessels that supply the skeletal muscles. Larger doses produce a rise in blood pressure (particularly systolic arterial pressure) due to activation of the alpha receptors of the blood vessels that supply the skin, kidneys, and mucosa. Through its action on the $beta_1$-receptors present in the pacemaker cells, conducting tissue, and myocardium, epinephrine has a powerful positive chronotropic and inotropic effect on the heart, resulting in an increase in cardiac output.

Epinephrine is also a neurotransmitter in some specialized locations of the central nervous system. In general, the action of epinephrine is mediated by the presence of alpha or beta receptors on the effector cells, as it can stimulate both of these receptors. In some of the interactions with the receptor, epinephrine initiates a cascade of enzymatic reactions, involving cyclic AMP and Ca^{2+} as intracellular second messengers that are essential in the evolution of physiologic response.

Epinephrine is synthesized from tyrosine; dopa, dopamine, and norepinephrine are intermediates in this pathway. It is metabolized via two major pathways: O-methylation and *N*-deamination, the main urinary metabolites being metanephrine and vanillylmandelic acid (VMA). Plasma and urinary levels of epinephrine and its metabolites are useful in assessing the functional status of the adrenal medulla and in confirming the presence of pheochromocytoma. The reference range for epinephrine in plasma is 1.8–2.6 ng/ml.

Also called *adrenalin.* See also *catecholamine.*

epinephrine and norepinephrine assays see *catecholamine assays.*

epineurium (ep″ĭ-nu′re-um) [N.L., from *epi-* + Gr. *neuron* nerve] the connective tissue sheath that envelops an entire peripheral nerve.

epiphenotype (ep″i-fe′no-tīp) the actual expression of differentiated properties by a particular epigenotype. It is generally assumed that environmentally caused changes in the epiphenotype are due to regulatory effects on gene expression and, in some cases, to definite changes in RNA synthesis. Cf. *epigenotype.*

epiphyseal plate (ep″ĭ-fiz′e-al) the thin, cartilaginous disk between the epiphysis and diaphysis that, together with a transitional region of newly forming tissue (metaphysis), forms the growth zone of a growing long bone. The epiphyseal plate ossifies when the mature length of the bone is attained.

epiphysis (ĕ-pif′ĭ-sis), pl. *epiphyses* [Gr. "an ongrowth; excrescence"] 1. [NA], the end of a long bone, usually wider than the shaft, and either entirely cartilaginous or separated from the shaft by a cartilaginous disk.

2. the part of a bone formed from a secondary center of ossification, commonly found at the ends of long bones and the margins of flat bones.

epiphyte (ep′ĭ-fīt) [*epi-* + Gr. *phyton* plant] a plant or organism parasitic upon another plant or animal organism.

episi/o (ĕ-piz′e-o) [Gr. *epision* the region of the pubes] a word element used in combining form to denote the vulva, e.g., episiotomy.

episode (ep′i-sōd) a particular incident or event occurring in the course of a larger sequence of events.

episodic (ep″ĭ-sod′ik) proceeding as a series of episodes; discontinuous; irregular.

episomal (ep″ĭ-so′mal) pertaining to an episome.

episome (ep′ĭ-sōm) a term used to describe a plasmid or a virus that can replicate autonomously and can also integrate into the chromosome of bacteria.

epispadias (ep″ĭ-spa′de-as) [*epi-* + Gr. *spadōn* a rent] a congenital defect producing a gutterlike opening of the urethra on the upper surface of the penis.

epistasis (ĕ-pis′tah-sis) [*epi-* + Gr. *stasis* a standing] 1. a stoppage of a flow, secretion, or excretion.

2. a scum that forms on the surface of urine upon standing.

3. the interaction of genes at different loci, resulting in the masking of a character. For example, when two genes code for enzymes in the same synthesis pathway, the abnormal phenotype may occur when either gene is defective; the dihybrid ratio would be 9:7 instead of the 9:3:3:1 observed in mendelian inheritance.

epistatic (ep″ĭ-stat′ik) masking the expression or action of a nonallelic gene. Cf. *dominant* and *hypostatic.*

epitestosterone (ep″ĭ-tes-tos′tĕ-rōn) 17α-hydroxyandrost-4-en-3-one, a metabolite of androstenedione, which is formed by the action of 17α-hydroxysteroid dehydrogenase. Although some researchers have suggested that measurement of epitestosterone before and after stimulation of the ovary with gonadotropins may be useful in detecting primary ovarian failure or in confirming the ovarian stromal hyperfunction in polycystic ovary disease, the clinical importance of this metabolite has not been established.

epithelial (ep″ĭ-the′le-al) pertaining to or composed of epithelium.

epithelial cell one of the cells that make up an epithelium.

epithelial cell disease see under *glomerulopathy.*

epithelioid (ep″ĭ-the′le-oid) [*epithelium* + Gr. *eidos* form] resembling epithelium, as in the modified smooth muscle cells of the juxtaglomerular apparatus, the swollen fibroblast of skin during an allergic response, and histiocytes in a granulomatous reaction.

epithelioid nevus see *spindle n.* under *nevus.*

epithelioid sarcoma a malignant soft tissue tumor of undetermined histogenesis that commonly arises in the distal extremities; initially it pursues an indolent course, but ultimately, often after several recurrences, metastasizes to the regional nodes and lungs. The neoplastic cells are spherical to ovoid and occasionally elongated; they possess markedly eosinophilic cytoplasm that ultrastructurally contains large numbers of intermediate filaments and in some cases moderate numbers of mitochondria and lipid droplets. The tumor can readily be mistaken for squamous carcinoma, melanoma, or granulomatous inflammation.

epithelioma (ep″ĭ-the″le-o′mah) [*epithelium* + Gr. *ōma* swelling] a general term for an epithelial tumor that connotes a benign neoplasm, although it is sometimes loosely and incorrectly used as a synonym for carcinoma.

e. adenoides cysticum, see *trichoepithelioma.*
basal cell e., see *basal cell carcinoma.*
calcifying e. of Malherbe, see *pilomatrixoma.*

epitheliosis (ep′ĭ-the″le-o′sis) [*epithelium* + *-osis* condition] a benign epithelial proliferation of the breast that arises in small ducts and lobules. It is characterized by a solid or fenestrated but nonpapillomatous architecture, and cytologically by bland nuclei and a lack of atypical mitoses. Periductal inflammation and fibrosis may accompany the epithelial changes. This condition carries no increased risk of the development of breast carcinoma. See also *papillomatosis of breast.*

epithelium (ep″ĭ-the′le-um), pl. *epithelia* [N.L., from *epi-* + Gr. *thēlē* nipple] the tissue that covers a surface on or within the body. Different histologic types of epithelia are adapted for particular functional requirements. An epithelium is said to be simple when it is composed of a single layer of cells, and stratified when more than one cell layer is present. In addition, an epithelium is usually classified according to the shape of its component cells. Epithelia rest on and are supported by connective tissue, and the two are usually separated by a basal lamina.

The term squamous epithelium is often considered synonymous with a stratified squamous epithelium, as in the epidermis, but has a broader connotation to histologists, i.e., an epithelium is composed of cells that because of their shape and apposition have a scalelike appearance when seen in profile. A simple squamous epithelium lines blood vessels (endothelium) and serous cavities (mesothelium). Under certain circumstances, these cells may become plump rather than flattened; thus, cells of the postcapillary venules in the paracortical zone of lymph nodes are cuboidal, and exfoliated reactive mesothelial cells are spherical.

Stratified squamous epithelium covers the skin (epidermis) and the mucosal surfaces of the oropharynx, esophagus, anal canal, and vagina. Adjacent squamous cells are united by numerous desmosomes with tonofilaments inserted onto their attachment plaques. In the epidermis the cells form keratin, which accumulates in the cytoplasm. The deeper cells are round, but more superficial cells become flattened and lose their nuclei, and the surface of the epidermis is covered by a dense acellular band of keratin (horny layer).

There is no sharp distinction between epithelia composed of cuboidal and columnar cells, and a continuous spectrum of cell shape can be seen in the ducts of exocrine glands, such as the salivary glands and pancreas. Tall, slender columnar cells are seen to good advantage in the small intestine, where they illustrate the diversity that can be present within a single epithelium by an intermingling of absorptive, mucus-secreting, and endocrine cells. The apical surface of each absorptive cell is increased by the presence of many microvilli.

The epithelium lining the urinary passages is stratified, but the surface cells, unlike those of stratified squamous epithelium, do not become flattened and are therefore designated transitional epithelium.

Most of the respiratory passages are lined by ciliated, columnar cells with nuclei at different levels, and some cells do not reach the lumen. Respiratory epithelium is therefore a pseudostratified, ciliated, columnar epithelium.

epitope (ep′i-top) see *antigenic determinant.*

epizootic (ep″ĭ-zo-ot′ik) [*epi-* + Gr. *zōōn* animal] a term that refers to a disease of low morbidity that attacks many animals in a certain community at the same time, or one of high morbidity that is only occasionally present in an animal community. It is analogous to the term epidemic in a human population. Cf. *enzootic.*

EPN a highly toxic organothiophosphate insecticide and acaricide, *O*-ethyl *O-p*-nitrophenyl phenylphosphonothioate. See also *organophosphate compounds.*

epoch (ep′ok) in electroencephalography, an arbitrarily determined period of recording time.

Epon (e′pon) trademark for a series of epoxy resins.

eponychium (ep″o-nik′e-um) [*epi-* + Gr. *onyx* nail] 1. [NA], the narrow band of epidermis that extends from the nail wall onto the nail surface; commonly called the cuticle.

2. the horny fetal epidermis at the side of a future nail.

eponym (ep′o-nim) [Gr. *epōnymos* named after] a name or phrase formed from or including the name of one or more persons, e.g., Hodgkin's disease, von Hippel–Lindau disease.

epoophoron (ep″o-of′o-ron) [*epi-* + Gr. *ōophoron* ovary] [NA], a rudimentary structure situated in the lateral mesosalpinx and consisting of 10–15 short tubules that converge to end blindly at the ovary. A remnant of the mesonephric tubules, the epoophoron runs along the broad ligament parallel with the uterine tube. Also called *Rosenmüller's organ.*

epoxide (ep-ok′sīd) a functional group, an oxygen atom bound to two different carbon atoms in a three-membered ring, a cyclic ether. Some epoxides are trivially named as oxides, e.g., ethylene oxide (1,2-epoxyethane).

epoxy (ĕ-pok′se) 1. a prefix in IUPAC nomenclature designating the epoxide group, e.g., 1,2-epoxyethane. Cf. *epoxide.*

2. a polymer formed by the reaction of several monomers, one of which is an epoxide. Epoxy resins are used as bonding agents, embedding media, in paints, and as laboratory bench tops.

EPP abbrev. See *end-plate potential, equal pressure point.*

EPR abbrev. for electron paramagnetic resonance; see *electron spin resonance.*

EPROM abbrev. See *erasable programmable r.-o. m.* under *read-only memory.*

epsilon (E, ϵ) (ep′sĭ-lon) the fifth letter of the *Greek alphabet.*

Epstein-Barr virus (EBV) (ep′stīn bahr) [Michael Anthony *Epstein,* English physician, born 1921; Yvonne M. *Barr,* English virologist, 20th century] an enveloped double-stranded DNA virus that belongs to the Herpetoviridae family. EBV is the causative agent of infectious mononucleosis and is closely associated with Burkitt's lymphoma and nasopharyngeal carcinoma. It is ubiquitous and may be transmitted through saliva, via blood transfusions, and possibly by mosquitos. In healthy adults, 80–90 percent have antibody to EBV. If an individual is not infected during adolescence and later develops a primary infection with EBV, infectious mononucleosis results. After an initial EBV infection, neutralizing antibodies develop and life-long immunity usually protects from further exogenous reinfections. However, once infected, an individual remains a life-long carrier of the virus. EBV can survive in peripheral blood lymphocytes for years without producing disease.

Clinically, infectious mononucleosis presents as fever, malaise, lethargy, sore throat with exudate, enlarged lymph nodes in the neck, mild hepatitis, enlarged spleen, and sometimes maculopapular and blotchy skin rash. Although the disease lasts for approximately 2 wk, convalescence may take months. Characteristic of infectious mononucleosis are enlarged lymphocytes with atypical nuclei.

Burkitt's lymphoma in East Africa and nasopharyngeal carcinoma in South China are associated with EBV infection. Although there is no direct evidence that EBV causes these malignant diseases, a relationship is suggested because lymphocytes are transformed in vitro by EBV and antibodies to EBV are also present. Which additional factor leads to the progression of infectious mononucleosis to malignancy is still unknown. In the laboratory, EBV-transformed lymphoblastoid cell lines can be made to produce specific monoclonal antibody.

Epstein-Barr virus has several different antigens, which may be used to relate different diseases to EBV infections. Viral capsid antigens are prepared by acetone fixation of virus-infected lymphoblastoid cells and may be detected by immunofluorescence. All persons affected by acute-phase infectious mononucleosis have viral capsid antigens (VCA). The titer of antibody to VCA is maximal during the second week of this disease and then gradually decreases, remaining at a low level throughout life. Early antigen is prepared by acetone fixation of virus-superinfected nonproductive lymphoblasts. These early antigens disappear quickly after recovery from infectious mononucleosis. Early antigens are also associated with Burkitt's lymphoma and nasopharyngeal carcinoma, and may be detected by immunofluorescence.

Epstein-Barr nuclear antigen (EBNA) is found in lymphoblast cells that carry the EBV genome, as well as in biopsies of Burkitt's lymphoma and nasopharyngeal carcinoma. EBNA is detected by the anticomplement immunofluorescence technique.

See also *Burkitt's lymphoma* and *infectious mononucleosis.*

Epstein-Barr virus antibody assays tests for detecting and titering antibody directed against Epstein-Barr virus (EBV). The antibody can be directed against any of a number of the cell-associated viral antigens, including the EB virus capsid antigen (VCA), EB virus membrane antigen, EB nuclear antigen (EBNA), EB virus–induced early antigen, and various soluble antigens. Antibody against the cell-associated antigens is usually detected by means of indirect immunofluorescence, whereas antibody against soluble antigens is demonstrated using complement fixation and immunodiffusion. Virus neutralization tests have been developed for detecting antibody against EB virus.

Demonstration of antibodies to EBV is important (1) to determine the susceptibility or immunity to infectious mononucleosis; (2) to determine if the heterophil antibody-negative mononucleosis syndrome in an individual is due to EBV; (3) to determine if EBV can be implicated in a number of syndromes of unknown etiology (e.g., hepatitis, encephalitis, and hemolytic anemia) that have been associated with EBV infection; and (4) to facilitate epidemiologic analysis.

Antibodies to VCA are commonly detected using an indirect immunofluorescence test. The test uses the individual's serum and an EBV-infected producer lymphoid cell line as the substrate. VCA antibodies appear after the onset of infectious mononucleosis, and peak about the second week of the illness. Twenty percent of acutely infected individuals show a fourfold rise in titer between collection of the first and subsequent acute-phase titer. Anti-VCA titers decline to levels seen in 18- to 30-yr-old control blood donors after the illness and are associated with permanent immunity. Individuals with Burkitt's lymphoma or nasopharyngeal carcinoma also have high anti-VCA titers.

Antibodies against early antigens are detected with indirect immunofluorescence, using the patient's serum cell line as the substrate. Eighty percent of sera from newly infected persons have antibodies against the early antigen components. These antibodies are evidence of extensive, current, or very recent disease. Individuals with Burkitt's lymphoma, nasopharyngeal carcinoma, or chronic lymphocytic leukemia often have antibodies to early antigens.

Antibodies to EBNA are detected using a combination complement-fixation–immunofluorescence test. EB virus genome containing lymphoblastoid cell lines is used as the substrate. The test serum is added, followed by (after incubation and washing) fresh human serum lacking anti-EBV antibodies as a source of complement, and fluorescein-conjugated antihuman complement antibody. Antibodies to EBNA appear later in the infection (in the third or fourth week after onset of infectious mononucleosis) in a minority of patients. By 6 mo, all convalescent infectious mononucleosis patients have anti-EBNA antibody, which persists for life.

There are two types of tests for neutralizing antibodies against EBV. The first type detects the ability of serum to prevent the transformation of human leukocytes, or the induction of DNA synthesis in human umbilical cord lymphocytes by EBV. The second type measures the ability of serum to neutralize the induction of early antigen in nonproducer cell lines by Burkitt tumor virus. The presence of EBV-neutralizing antibody correlates with that of antibody to VCA but not with heterophil antibody. Neither height of titer nor time required for development of antibody against VCA or EBNA correlates with the severity or duration of infectious mononucleosis.

See also *heterophil antibody test.*

EP toxicity a regulatory term applied to chemical waste containing arsenic, barium, cadmium, lead, mercury, selenium, silver, or any one of six specific pesticides. Such chemicals may be classified as hazardous waste and be regulated by standards of the EPA/RCRA (Environmental Protection Agency/Resource Conservation and Recovery Act). If the concentrations of these pollutants meet or exceed the values listed in the RCRA standards, the waste is said to exhibit EP toxicity, and its disposal must meet regulations for hazardous waste.

epulis (ĕ-pu'lis), pl. *epulides* [Gr. *epoulis* a gumboil] a poorly defined term used clinically to connote a tumorlike lesion of the gingiva. Most are hyperplastic conditions. The congenital epulis of the newborn is a more specific entity, histologically comparable with granular cell tumors (myoblastomas) in other locations.

Eq abbrev. See *equivalent.*

equal pressure point (EPP) that point along the respiratory airways where the lateral intraluminal pressure equals the compressive pressure on the outer airway wall during a forced expiration. Transmural airway pressure is zero at this point.

It is only at points closer to (i.e., downstream from) the mouth than to the EPP—where the pressure surrounding the airway wall exceeds the intraluminal pressure—that dynamic airway compression (and thus flow limitation) can develop. With increasing expiratory effort (and thus increasing pleural pressure), the point of equal pressure is shifted (i.e., upstream) increasingly toward the alveoli, becoming fixed only when maximal flow is reached (the plateau of the isovolume pressure flow curve is achieved). Thus, at peak expiratory flow, any additional increase in pleural pressure serves only to increase the compression of segments downstream from the EPP. The driving pressure (the pressure head that results in expulsion of air from the terminal airway units to outside the body) of segments upstream from the EPP is essentially equal to the elastic recoil pressure of the lung.

Equanil (ek′wah-nil) trademark. See *meprobamate.*

equation (e-kwa′zhun) [L. *aequatio,* from *aequare* to make equal] a mathematical statement of the equality of two expressions, which are connected by the sign of equality, =.

chemical e., a symbolic expression representing a chemical reaction, e.g., $N_2 + 3\ H_2 \rightarrow 2\ NH_3$, which states that one molecule of nitrogen may react with three molecules of hydrogen to make two molecules of ammonia. An equation must always be balanced; i.e., each element must appear the same number of times on both sides. Double arrows ($\rightleftarrows$) are used to show reversible reactions.

equational division (e-kwa′zhun-al) the second meiotic division. See also *meiosis.*

equatorial (e″kwah-to′re-al) 1. pertaining to an equator; equidistant from the poles.

2. in chemistry, pertaining to the set of hydrogens (or substituents that replace them) or the bonds to these atoms in a cyclohexane ring that lies nearer to the "plane" of the ring than the other (axial) set. See also under *conformation.*

equatorial plate the central plane of a dividing cell, along which the centromeres of the chromosomes are located during metaphase. Also called *metaphase plate.*

equator of eyeball an imaginary line encircling the eyeball equidistant from the anterior and posterior poles, which divides the eye into anterior and posterior halves.

equilibration (e-kwil″ĭ-bra′shun) the achievement of a balance between opposing elements, forces, or reactions.

equilibrium (e″kwĭ-lib′re-um) [L. *aequus* equal + *libra* balance] a state of balance between opposing forces or reactions that does not change with time.

chemical e., the state of a system in which the sums of the chemical potentials of all the products and all the reactants are identical. The system has reached a minimum in free energy. The concentration or partial pressure of each chemical reaction component remains unchanged with time.

dynamic e., a system in which the concentration of a given component is constant because the rate of its formation is equal to the rate of its decomposition; the system, however, is not in thermodynamic equilibrium. Biologic systems are in a state of dynamic equilibrium determined by regulatory enzymes. Also called *steady state.*

physiologic e., a state of balance between material taken into the body and material discharged so that the amount in the body is constant.

radioactive e., a steady ratio of the amount of a radioisotope and the amount of its radioactive daughter. The activities of both decline with the parent's half-life.

secular e., a radioactive equilibrium in which the parent has a much longer half-life (by 10^4 times or more) than the daughter. At equilibrium the activities of both parent and daughter are the same.

thermal e., the state of a system in which all of its parts are at the same temperature.

thermodynamic e., the state of a system in mechanical, thermal, and chemical equilibrium. The free energy difference between parts of the system is zero ($\Delta G = 0$), and no useful work or further chemical change can occur.

transient e., a radioactive equilibrium in which the parent has roughly 10 times the half-life of the daughter. The daughter has the higher activity, e.g., the ^{99}Mo–^{99m}Tc generator, the source of ^{99m}Tc.

equilibrium constant (K) a constant that determines the concentrations of the reactants and products of a chemical reaction when it has reached a state of equilibrium. The equilibrium constant is equal to the product of the concentrations of the reaction products, each raised to a power equal to the coefficient of the product in the equation, divided by the product of the concentrations of the reactants, each raised to its coefficient. For example, for the reaction $2H_2 + O_2 \rightleftarrows 2H_2O$, $K = [H_2O]^2 / [H_2]^2[O_2]$.

The equilibrium constant varies with temperature and is related to the standard free energy change ($\Delta G°$) of a reaction by the equation $\Delta G° = RT \ln K$, where T is the absolute temperature and R is the gas constant.

In theoretical terms, K is defined by thermodynamic activities instead of by concentrations. The symbols K_c and K_p may be used to indicate equilibrium constants defined in terms of concentrations and partial pressures, respectively.

equipment (e-kwip′ment) the various devices and instruments that are used to perform some group of related tasks or functions.

equipotential (e″kwĭ-po-ten′shal) [L. *aequus* equal + *potentia* ability, power] 1. having equal power or capability, such as a pair of electrodes displaying the same voltage at a given time.

2. in electroencephalography, a term that is sometimes used to refer to a lack of electrocortical activity. See also *electrocerebral inactivity.*

equipotential line a line, real or imaginary, connecting points or electrodes that are simultaneously at the same potential difference (voltage) when compared with a common reference.

equivalence (e-kwiv′ah-lens) 1. a term used to describe the ratio of antigen-antibody concentration where maximal precipitation occurs. For this to occur, both antigen and antibody must be multivalent. Antibody-antigen equivalence is most often used in the description of a precipitin curve in the quantitative precipitin assay (antigen excess and antibody excess are terms describing situations of nonequivalence).

2. in logic, a relation that holds between a set of propositions when they are either all true or all false.

equivalence point see *end point.*

equivalence relation ($\sim$) in mathematics, a relation that is reflexive, symmetric, and transitive; that is, $x \sim x$; $x \sim y$ implies $y \sim x$; and $x \sim y$ and $y \sim z$ imply $x \sim z$.

equivalent (e-kwiv′ah-lent) [L. *aequivalens,* from *aequus* equal + *valere* to be worth] 1. equal in value, effect, power, force, or meaning.

2. in chemistry, equivalence of combining capacity; having the same valence. Equivalent amounts of two compounds will completely react with each other. In acid-base reactions, one equivalent of material will react with or give off 1 mol of protons; in oxidation-reduction reactions, the basis of equivalency is the gain or loss of 1 mol of electrons. In acid-base reactions, the equivalent weight of a reactant is calculated by dividing the molecular weight by the number of protons available and, in redox reactions, it is the molecular weight divided by the number of electrons per molecule involved in the reaction. Fe^{3+} is triequivalent as an acid (salt), but only monoequivalent as an oxidant.

3. (abbrev. Eq), the amount of substance in an equivalent weight of any chemical moiety; also called chemical equivalent.

ER abbrev. for emergency room, *endoplasmic reticulum, estrogen receptor.*

Er symbol for the chemical element *erbium.*

-er (er) a suffix word element to denote one who or that which performs a task or function, e.g., radiographer.

erase (ĕ-rās′) 1. to reset a computer storage device so that all bits are zero.

2. to destroy the recorded information on a magnetic tape by application of a high-frequency alternating magnetic field, which randomizes the tape magnetism.

erbium (Er) (er′be-um) [from Ytt*erby,* the Swedish town where the element was discovered] a soft, lustrous, silvery metallic element; atomic number 68; atomic weight 167.26; a 4f transition element (lanthanide or rare earth); oxidation state +3. See also *rare earth elements.*

Erb's disease (erbz) [Wilhelm Heinrich *Erb,* German neurologist, 1840–1921] limb-girdle muscular dystrophy. See *muscular dystrophy.*

Erb's point [W. H. *Erb*] the angle made by the clavicle and the posterolateral border of the sternocleidomastoid muscle, located 2–3 cm above the clavicle at the level of the sixth cervical vertebra. In motor nerve conduction studies, the nerve trunks contributing to the brachial plexus are best stimulated with electrodes placed at this site.

ERC abbrev. See *erythropoietin-responsive cell.*

ERCP [acronym from *e*ndoscopic *r*etrograde *c*holangio*p*ancreatography] a type of cholangiopancreatography used when neither oral nor intravenous cholecystography is possible because of impaired liver function or because of obstruction to the common bile duct. In this procedure, a small catheter is inserted through the papilla of Vater into either the common bile duct or the pancreatic duct under direct visual control, using a fiberoptic endoscope. A radiopaque constrast medium is then injected through the catheter to fill the biliary tree or pancreatic duct under fluoroscopic control.

erect (ĕ-rekt′) standing upright, such as the position of the trunk when standing or sitting.

erethism (er′ĕ-thizm) [Gr. *erethisma* stimulation] excessive irritability or sensitivity of the body parts, particularly the sex organs. It also refers to a psychic disturbance marked by irritability, shyness, fatigue, and depression, particularly as manifested in chronic mercurialism. See also *mercury.*

ERG abbrev. See *electroretinogram.*

erg/o (er′go) [Gr. *ergon* work] a word element used in combining form to denote work, e.g., adrenergic.

erg (erg) [Gr. *ergon* work] the centimeter-gram-second (cgs) unit of work, energy, or heat equal to 1 dyne-centimeter (dyn·cm) or 10^{-7} joule (J).

ergastoplasm (er-gas′to-plazm) [Gr. *ergasia* work + *plasma* something formed] rough endoplasmic reticulum. See also *cell.*

ergocalciferol (er″go-kal-sif′er-ol) [USP], vitamin D_2, 5,7-cholestadien-3β-ol, a fat-soluble vitamin that differs from vitamin D_3 (cholecalciferol) by having a double bond between C-22 and C-23 and a methyl group at C-24. It is produced by the ultraviolet irradiation of ergosterol, a steroid found in yeasts and fungi, and is the form of vitamin D found in enriched food products (bread and milk) and in many vitamin preparations. Ergosterol and cholecalciferol have equivalent potential antirachitic potency in humans. Also called *viosterol.*

ergoloid mesylates (er′go-loid) a 1:1:1 mixture of the methanesulfonate salts of three hydrogenated ergot alkaloids (dihydroergocristine, dihydroergocornine, and dihydroergocryptine). It is used for relief of signs and symptoms of idiopathic decline in mental capacity (including impairment of recent memory, confusion, and disorientation) in individuals over 60 yr old.

ergometer (er-gom′ĕ-ter) [*ergo-* + Gr. *metron* measure] an instrument used to record the work performed by a muscle or group of muscles. A bicycle ergometer records the work performed by an individual during pedal cycling.

ergonovine maleate (er″go-no′vēn) [USP], an alkaloid derived from ergot, used to prevent postpartum hemorrhage due to uterine atony by stimulation of uterine contractions. Adverse reactions include vomiting, high blood pressure, and ergotism (all occur rarely). Trademark, Ergotrate Maleate.

ergosterol (er-gos′tĕ-rol) an important provitamin D, ergosta-5,7,22-triene-3β-ol, found in yeast and plants. When irradiated with ultraviolet light, it is converted to ergocalciferol (vitamin D_2), a potent antirachitic substance.

ergot (er′got) [Fr., from L. *ergota*] the dried sclerotium (mass of hyphae) of *Claviceps purpurea,* a hard, thick-walled, blackish fungus that attacks rye (*Secale cereale*) and other grains. It contains alkaloids related to lysergic acid, some of which directly stimulate smooth muscle (e.g., arteries and the uterus); others block stimulation by epinephrine (alpha-adrenergic blockade) and thus produce vasoconstriction.

Acute ergot poisoning causes nausea, vomiting, diarrhea, confusion, dizziness, and coma. Chronic ergot poisoning (ergotism) produces gangrene of the extremities because of peripheral vasoconstriction. Another type of ergotism, characterized by spasms and convulsions, occurred in the past when contaminated rye was eaten by persons with dietary deficiencies. In the Middle Ages, ergotism was known as St. Anthony's fire.

ergotamine (er-got′ah-mēn) an alkaloid isolated from ergot. Ergotamine tartrate [USP] is used alone or in combination with vasoconstrictors or antiemetics for treatment of severe migraine. Daily use may cause habituation.

ergotamine tartrate (er-got′ah-mēn) [USP], an alkaloid derived from ergot, used for the treatment of migraine attacks. It stimulates the cranial arteries to constrict and causes alpha-adrenergic blockade. Adverse reactions include nausea, vomiting, irregular heart rate, numbness, tingling, and muscle pain. Chronic excessive use may cause ergotism; the total weekly dose should not exceed 10 tablets (10 mg). This agent is given orally or parenterally, either alone or in combination with caffeine (also a vasoconstrictor) and antiemetics. Trademarks, Gynergen, Ergomar.

ergothioneine (er″go-thi″o-ne′in) a histidinelike amino acid of unknown function found in the liver, in red blood cells, and (in abnormal amounts) in the urine of some cancer patients.

ergotism (er′got-izm) chronic ergot poisoning. See under *ergot.*

Erlenmeyer flask (ār′len-mi″er) [Emil Richard August Carl *Erlenmeyer,* German chemist, 1825–1909] a glass flask with a conical body, a broad flat base, and a narrow or wide neck.

Erlenmeyer flask-like pertaining to objects shaped like an Erlenmeyer flask. See also the illustration accompanying *contour.*

erogenous zone (ĕ-roj′ĕ-nus) any part of the body that when stimulated produces sexual desire, usually including the genitals, lips, anus, and breast.

erosion (ĕ-ro′zhun) [L. *erosio,* from *erodere* to eat out] 1. the process by which a substance is worn away.

2. a skin lesion characterized by a loss of all or part of the epidermis; it may be seen in association with any pruritic dermatitis. Treatment is aimed at preventing secondary bacterial infection.

ERPF abbrev. See *effective renal plasma flow.*

error (er′or) a defect in structure or function; a deviation. In statistics, two types of error are distinguished. Random errors are those caused by some random (chance-dependent) process that causes the measured values to be scattered about a central value. The response to random error is to use a sample size large enough to assure that the standard error of the mean (corresponding roughly to the precision of the measurement) is as small as required. Systematic error, in contrast, adds the same bias to every measured value. The scatter of the measured values is not affected, but the central value and thus the mean of the measured values has been shifted away from the "true" value (the difference between the two, corresponding to the *accuracy* of the measurement). Elimination of systematic error requires comparison of the measurements with some more accurate measurement, as occurs when a laboratory procedure is standardized by use of reference materials.

error detector the device in an automatic control system that generates the error signal, the measure of how far the system is out of control.

error rate the rate at which bits or characters of a transmission are incorrectly received.

eruption (e-rup′shun) [L. *eruptio* a breaking out] 1. the act of breaking out, appearing, or becoming visible, as eruption of the teeth.

2. Visible, efflorescence lesions of the skin due to disease, and marked by redness, prominence, or both; a rash. See also *exanthem.*

bullous e., an eruption of large blebs or blisters.

drug e., an eruption or a solitary cutaneous lesion caused by a drug taken internally. Also called drug rash.

fixed e., a circumscribed inflammatory skin lesion that recurs at the same site over a period of months or years; each attack lasts only a few days but leaves residual pigmentation, which is cumulative.

Kaposi's varicelliform e., a generalized and serious vesiculopustular eruption of viral origin, superimposed on a preexisting atopic dermatitis. It may be caused by the herpes simplex virus (eczema herpeticum) or vaccinia (eczema vaccinatum).

macular e., an eruption in the form of spots, due to hemorrhage, congestion, or increased or diminished pigmentation.

maculopapular e., an eruption consisting of both macules and papules; the term is sometimes used loosely when only one or the other is present.

polymorphous e., an eruption characterized by lesions in many different stages of evolution, from incipient through mature to healing.

polymorphous light e., a rather uniform skin eruption, although highly variable in different individuals, that occurs on the sun-exposed surfaces of the skin. This form is not attributable to photosensitizing applications or medications, or to systemic disease; it is typically initiated and aggravated by exposure to sunlight.

ERV abbrev. See *expiratory reserve volume.*

Erwinia (er-win′e-ah) [*Erwin* F. Smith, U.S. bacteriologist, 1854–1927] a genus of bacteria of the Enterobacteriaceae family. These bacteria are motile, gram-negative, facultatively anaerobic rods that are primarily plant pathogens and saprophytes; they may have been associated with a large epidemic of hospital-acquired septicemia due to contamination of intravenous solutions.

erysipelas (er″ĭ-sip′ĕ-las) [Gr. *erythros* red + *pella* skin] a febrile, rapidly spreading cutaneous infection, marked by erythema and edema, and caused mainly by beta-hemolytic group A and rarely by C or G streptococci. The disease begins without an obvious means of entry and most commonly appears on the face, but other parts of the body may also be affected. The lesions, marked by neutrophilic infiltration in the dermis and epidermis, spread in a maplike fashion; they are swollen, red, and hot to the touch. Streptococci can generally be recovered from edema fluid.

Erysipelothrix (er″ĭ-sip′ĕ-lo-thriks″) [*erysipelas* + Gr. *thrix* hair] a genus of gram-positive, nonmotile, rod-shaped filamentous organisms, of widespread occurrence as parasites in fish, sheep, poultry, and crustacea. It consists of a single species, *E. rhusiopathiae* (*insidiosa*), the cause of erysipelas in swine and an erysipeloid disease in humans that is characterized by spreading, painful skin eruptions on the fingers and hands following contact with infected fish, meats, hides, or bones.

erythem/o (er-ĭ-the′mo) [Gr. *erythēma* flush on the skin] a word element used in combining form to denote flushed redness, e.g., erythema.

erythema (er″ĭ-the′mah) [Gr. *erythēma* flush on the skin] pink-red appearance of the skin, due to increased arterial and capillary blood flow. It may result from heat, irritation, or inflammation from many causes.

e. ab igne, redness of the skin caused by exposure to radiant heat.

e. annulare, a type of erythema multiforme in which the areas of redness are ring shaped.

e. chronicum migrans (ECM), see under *Lyme disease.*

e. induratum, chronic, often ulcerating bluish-red cutaneous nodules, most commonly occurring on the calves. At one time, this lesion was thought to be a form of tuberculosis. This view has been abandoned, and the etiology is unknown at the present time. Nonspecific inflammation, granulomas, and necrosis are seen in the fat and lower dermis, and vasculitis is often present. See also *panniculitis.*

e. marginatum rheumaticum, an eruption associated with rheumatic endocarditis, characterized by red or bluish-red semicircles or rings over the abdomen, the sides of the thorax, and the back.

e. multiforme, a reaction pattern of the skin and mucous membranes in response to a variety of agents, including infectious organisms, e.g., herpes simplex virus and a variety of drugs. Vivid red lesions symmetrically distributed on the skin are characteristic, with blisters and erosions found on the buccal membranes. The local lesions are perivascular inflammatory infiltrates with endothelial changes in small vessels.

e. neonatorum, a diffuse redness of the skin of a newborn infant; it is usually temporary.

e. nodosum, a hypersensitivity vasculitis characterized by tender, pale red to blue nodules, which are accompanied by intense itching and burning. The lesions are transient, lasting for several weeks, and do not ulcerate; they may be associated with a variety of infectious diseases, and with use of drugs and oral contraceptives. See also *panniculitis.*

palmar e., redness of the palms, which occurs in certain diseases including cirrhosis of the liver, tuberculosis, and nutritional deficiencies; during pregnancy; and, rarely, as a hereditary condition.

toxic e., a generalized, diffuse erythematous eruption or a widespread erythematomacular eruption that occurs as a result of the administration of a drug; it may also be caused by bacterial toxins or other toxic substances.

erythrasma (er″ĭ-thraz′mah) [N.L., from Gr. *erythros* red] a chronic infection of the stratum corneum that results in brownish-red lesions or scaly patches involving major body folds and clefts of skin. It is caused by the bacterium *Corynebacterium minutissimum,* a common resident of skin.

erythremia (er″ĭ-thre′me-ah) [*erythro-* + Gr. *haima* blood + *-ia*] see *polycythemia vera.*

erythremic myelosis a poorly defined syndrome characterized by proliferation of erythropoietic cells in the bone marrow, producing megaloblastic erythroblasts. This megaloblastosis is not associated with vitamin B_{12} deficiency. The acute form exhibits disproportionately large numbers of immature erythroblasts and severe thrombocytopenia; if accompanied by proliferation of myelocytes, it merges with erythroleukemia. More common is the chronic form, in which the erythroblasts are more mature and the thrombocytopenia more moderate; this condition often leads to acute myelogenous leukemia.

Some authorities favor grouping this disorder with Di Guglielmo's syndrome.

See also *erythroleukemia* under *leukemia.*

erythritol (ĕ′rith′rĭ-tol) *meso*-1,2,3,4-butanetetrol, the sugar alcohol formed by reduction from erythrose.

erythrityl tetranitrate (ĕ-rith′rĭ-til) [USP], an organic nitrate used as a coronary vasodilator in the treatment of angina pectoris.

erythro- (ĕ-rith′ro) [Gr. *erythros* red] 1. a prefix word element to denote red, e.g., erythrocyte.

2. a prefix word element in organic chemistry to denote a stereoisomer having a structure similar to erythrose, e.g., D-*erythro*-2-deoxypentose (D-deoxyribose).

erythroblast (ĕ-rith′ro-blast) [*erythro-* + Gr. *blastos* germ] a generic term that includes all types of nucleated erythrocytes; see under *erythropoiesis.*

definitive e., in fetal development, a nucleated red cell formed extravascularly in the liver from about the sixth week of embryonic life, in contrast to the primitive (megaloblastic) erythroblasts formed by the yolk sac. Definitive erythroblasts are smaller than primitive ones, although they are still larger than mature erythrocytes. The nucleus is usually extruded from the cell before it enters the circulation.

erythroblastic (ĕ-rith″ro-blas′tik) of or relating to erythroblasts.

erythroblastic island a group of erythroid cells in the bone marrow that surround a centrally located reticulum cell occasionally referred to as a nurse cell. Although erythroblastic islands usually are disrupted during preparation of bone marrow smears, they can usually be seen in erythroid hyperplasia, as seen in hemolytic anemia and erythroleukemia.

The corona of erythroblasts surrounding the central reticulum cell are the same stage of maturation, but occasionally two concentric rings of erythroblasts are found, the outer one composed of more mature cells. The central reticulum cell probably transfers ferritin, and possibly other materials, to the surrounding erythroblasts. Conversely, nuclei extruded by mature erythroblasts may be phagocytosed by the central reticulum cells, the cytoplasmic extensions of which are in contact with all the peripheral erythroblasts.

erythroblastosis (ĕ-rith″ro-blas-to′sis) the presence of nucleated erythrocytes in the circulating blood. Normally present in small numbers, these erythrocytes are greatly increased in conditions that cause hemolysis, such as hemolytic anemia and hemolytic disease of the newborn.

e. fetalis, see *hemolytic disease of the newborn.*

e. neonatorum, see *hemolytic disease of the newborn.*

erythrocuprein (ĕ-rith″ro-koo′pre-in) see under *copper storage protein.*

erythrocytapheresis (ĕ-rith″ro-si″tah-fĕ-re′sis) [*erythrocyte* + Gr. *aphairesis* removal] a procedure that involves the withdrawal of blood, the separation and retention of red blood cells, and the retransfusion of the remainder into the donor.

erythrocyte (ĕ-rith′ro-sīt) [*erythro-* + Gr. *kytos* hollow vessel] the mature red blood cell. It is a nonnucleated biconcave disk, 6–8 μm in diameter, and pink or pinkish-gray when stained with Wright stain. Erythrocytes originate in the red bone marrow. Their average life span is 120 da; old or damaged cells are removed from the circulation by the bone marrow, spleen, and liver.

Red blood cells make up the great majority of cells (3.8–5.8 million/mm^3) found in the peripheral blood. Their vast surface area is important in the transport of oxygen from the lungs to the tissues because of the quick exchange of oxygen in both sites that occurs across the red cell surface. Erythrocytes owe their oxygen-carrying ability to hemoglobin, which contains iron and gives blood its red color. These blood cells are subject to many alterations in shape, size, staining properties, and structure in different disease processes.

Also called *red blood cell.* See also *blood cell count* and *erythropoiesis.*

erythrocyte antigens cell surface antigens of the red cell plasma membrane that determine blood group specificity. See also *blood groups.*

erythrocyte membrane an envelope that surrounds the erythrocyte. It is composed of inner and outer layers of phospholipids interspersed with proteins and glycoproteins. Of the major phospholipids present in the membrane, 80 percent of the phosphatidylethanolamine and 100 percent of the phosphatidylserine are contained within the inner layer, whereas 75 percent of the phosphatidylcholine and 80 percent of the sphingomyelin are in the outer layer where they are exposed to the plasma. Glycophorin A, which traverses the entire membrane and projects above it, carries the blood group antigens M and N.

The membrane must be able to undergo shape changes in the circulation and maintain its permeability, as well as provide sufficient surface area for cellular activity. Filaments formed by the protein spectrin are attached to the membrane and protrude into the cell. They are closely related to actin and are attached to the inner erythrocyte membrane by ankyrin.

Plasma anions, chloride, bicarbonate, and water can pass freely through the membrane, while sodium and potassium cations are actively regulated by an energy-dependent active ion transport system, the sodium-potassium pump. Sodium passively enters the cell and is actively pumped out, and potassium is actively pumped into the cell and passively diffuses out.

erythrocyte sedimentation rate (ESR) a laboratory test that determines the rate at which the erythrocytes in well-mixed venous blood fall to the bottom (sediment) of a test tube. The ESR is increased by factors that decrease the negative charge (zeta potential) on erythrocytes, which tends to keep them apart, or that increase rouleaux formation. The zeta potential is decreased by elevated fibrinogen and globulin levels; rouleaux formation is increased in patients with anemia and decreased in those with sickle cell disease and spherocytosis. Another influential factor involved is that macrocytes sediment more rapidly than normocytes, which in turn sediment more rapidly than microcytes. The ESR is markedly elevated in patients with monoclonal gammopathies and hyperfibrinogenemias and moderately elevated in those with rheumatoid arthritis, chronic inflammations, and neoplasia. See also *Westergren sedimentation rate method, Wintrobe sedimentation rate method,* and *zeta sedimentation ratio method.*

erythrocythemia (ĕ-rith″ro-si-the′me-ah) [*erythrocyte* + Gr. *haima* blood + *-ia*] an increase in the number of erythrocytes in the blood. Also called *erythrocytosis.*

erythrocytic (ĕ-rith″ro-sit′ik) pertaining to erythrocytes.

erythrocytic series the sequence of morphologically recognizable precursors of the erythrocyte: pronormoblast, basophilic normoblast, polychromatophilic normoblast, orthochromatic normoblast, and reticulocyte; see under *erythropoiesis.*

erythrocytophagy (ĕ-rith″ro-si-tof′ah-je) [*erythrocyte* + Gr. *phagein* to devour] see *erythrophagocytosis.*

erythrocytosis (ĕ-rith″ro-si-to′sis) [*erythrocyte* + *-osis* condition] an increase in the concentration of red cells in the peripheral blood measured by the red cell count, hemoglobin, or packed cell volume (PCV). It may be due to an actual increase in the total number of red cells (also referred to as the red cell mass and measured as milliliters of red cells per kilogram of body weight), or due to a reduction in the plasma volume.

absolute e., a condition marked by a true increase in the red cell mass (the total number of circulating erythrocytes). Once the diagnosis is established, this condition must be distinguished from polycythemia vera, in which leukocyte and platelet levels are also usually increased. Absolute erythrocytosis represents a chronic increase in the production of red cells arising from an inadequate oxygen supply to the tissues (secondary polycythemia), which stimulates erythropoietin production and thus promotes red cell production. It can be attributed to conditions such as decreased atmospheric oxygen pressure (see *mountain sickness*); impaired oxygenation of hemoglobin, as in pulmonary disease or hemoglobin M disease; congenital heart disease; hypoventilation syndromes; and abnormal hemoglobins with increased affinity for O_2. Cf. *polycythemia vera.*

relative e., an increase in erythrocyte count due to a decrease in the volume of plasma. This can occur through the loss of body fluids following extensive burns, persistent vomiting, or diarrhea. A chronic form of the disorder is referred to as Gaisböck's syndrome, benign or stress erythrocytosis, and benign, pseudo-, or spurious polycythemia. Affected individuals are predominantly mildly obese adult males. This form of erythrocytosis is believed to be caused by stress; laboratory results reflect a normal blood volume but decreased plasma volume. Also called pseudoerythrocytosis.

erythroderma (ĕ-rith″ro-der′mah) [*erythro-* + Gr. *derma* skin] a general term applied to several skin diseases characterized by an intense and widespread reddening of the skin and usually exfoliation.

erythrodextrin (ĕ-rith″ro-dek′strin) a dextrin, *e*-dextrin, a mixture of polyglucans containing relatively short chains of glucose units, which stain red with iodine. They are products of partial hydrolysis of starch.

erythrogenesis (ĕ-rith″ro-jen′ĕ-sis) [*erythro-* + Gr. *genesis* origin] the production of erythrocytes.

erythrogenic (ĕ-rith″ro-jen′ik) [*erythro-* + Gr. *gennan* to produce] 1. producing erythrocytes.

2. producing or causing erythema.

erythrogenic toxin a rash-producing toxin, specifically an exotoxin produced by certain strains of the group A streptococci that cause the rash occurring with scarlet fever. There are three immunologically distinct forms (types A, B, and C). When injected into the skin of susceptible children (Dick test), the toxin produces a localized erythematous reaction. Erythrogenic toxins are also produced by some group C and group D hemolytic streptococci and some staphylococci. See also *exotoxins.*

erythroid (er′ĭ-throid) [*erythro-* + Gr. *eidos* form] 1. of a red color; reddish.

2. pertaining to the developmental series of cells ending in erythrocytes.

erythrokinetics [*erythro-* + Gr. *kinētikos* of motion] the quantitative study of the in vivo production and destruction of erythrocytes, described by laboratory measurements of total red cell volume, rate of red cell production reflected by ferrokinetics studies, and red cell life span, which reflects the rate of destruction.

erythromycin (ĕ-rith″ro-mi′sin) a macrolide antibiotic consisting of a macrocyclic lactone ring attached to two sugar residues. Erythromycin inhibits protein synthesis in bacteria by preventing peptide chain elongation. The antibiotic binds to the 50S ribosomal subunit. Resistance to erythromycin results from decreased permeability, alteration of 50S ribosomal protein, or alteration of the 23S ribosomal RNA of the 50S subunit by methylation of adenine.

In vitro, erythromycin inhibits a variety of gram-positive organisms, *Neisseria* species, *Hemophilus influenzae, Bordetella pertussis,* treponemes, actinomycetes, mycoplasmas, chlamydiae, and rickettsiae. Whether erythromycin is bacteriostatic or bactericidal depends on the concentration used, the bacterial species, the phase of bacterial growth, and the bacterial inoculum density.

Activity of erythromycin against both gram-positive and gram-negative bacteria increases markedly as the pH is increased from 5.5 to 8.5.

See also *antibacterial agents* and *macrolides.*

erythromyeloblastic leukemia (ĕ-rith″ro-mi″ĕ-lo-blas′tik) see *erythroleukemia* under *leukemia.*

erythron (er′ĭ-thron) [Gr. *erythros* red] the circulating red cells in the blood, their precursors, and all the elements of the body concerned in their production.

erythrophagocytosis (ĕ-rith″ro-fag″o-si-to′sis) the engulfment or consumption of intact red cells by monocytes, polymorphonuclear neutrophils, or fixed macrophages of the reticuloendothelial system. It is primarily associated with pathologic processes, and suggests damage to the red cell membrane by complement-fixing antibodies, protozoa, bacteria, or chemical poisons. Erythrophagocytosis can be seen in peripheral blood smears or in bone marrow preparations. Erythrophagocytosis is not normally seen in routine bone marrow preparations, although normal red cells undergo erythrophagocytosis by bone marrow macrophages at the end of their lives. Also called *erythrocytophagy.*

erythroplasia of Queyrat (ĕ-rith″ro-pla′ze-ah) an outmoded term for squamous carcinoma in situ of the glans penis or vulva.

erythropoiesis (ĕ-rith″ro-poi-e′sis) [*erythro-* + Gr. *poiēsis* making] the formation of mature, nonnucleated, highly specialized red cells from primitive precursor cells in the bone marrow. Cell development passes through a series of morphologically recognizable stages.

Current classification of erythroblasts (nucleated red cells) divides the cell series into the pronormoblast and the basophilic, polychromatophilic, and orthochromic normoblasts. The pronormoblast (about 20 μm in diameter) is characterized by a large nucleus that occupies about 80 percent of the cell and a border of basophilic cytoplasm containing ferritin (which distinguishes the cell from the myeloblast). No hemoglobin is present in the pronormoblast, nor in the basophilic normoblast, a smaller cell that has slightly condensed chromatin and no visible nucleoli. Pink areas near the nucleus indicate the first appearance of hemoglobin in the polychromatophilic normoblast; the cell is also identified by clumps of deeply staining nuclear chromatin. When the cytoplasm contains a nearly complete concentration of hemoglobin, the cell is termed an orthochromic normoblast. At this stage the cell has shrunk to 8–12 μm in diameter, and the nucleus may exhibit bizarre shapes as the chromatin greatly condenses and the nucleus becomes reduced in size. Eventually the nucleus is extruded from the cell to be phagocytosed by macrophages in the marrow.

The irregular, polylobulated, nonnucleated cell that is formed is called a reticulocyte, the last stage before the formation of the mature red cell. It is somewhat larger than the final red cell and exhibits a characteristic precipitation of its ribosomal RNA into a network of aggregated clumps (reticulum), as demonstrated by supravital staining techniques. It remains in the marrow for 2–3 da and is then released into the circulation, where it assumes the characteristic biconcave disk of the circulatory erythrocyte.

Two stem cells committed to the red cell line have been demonstrated, CFU-E and BFU-E (see *stem cell*). Both are stimulated to proliferate and mature into the pronormoblast by the hormone erythropoietin (see *erythropoietin*), which probably binds to a receptor on the red cell membrane. Erythropoietin is produced by the kidneys in response to the level of tissue oxygenation: a decreased red cell population causes hypoxia that stimulates secretion of erythropoietin, which in turn stimulates erythropoiesis. The time involved in the maturation of the red cell from pronormoblast to its release as a reticulocyte into the circulating pool is variously estimated at 4–7 da. Erythropoiesis takes place in the liver and spleen in the human fetus and in some pathologic conditions (see *myeloid metaplasia*).

See also *normoblast* and *reticulocyte.*

ineffective e., the death of developing red cells (normoblasts to reticulocytes) in bone marrow during the process of maturation. As a consequence, relatively few reticulocytes reach the peripheral circulation, although there are normal and usually increased numbers of nucleated red cells in the marrow.

erythropoiesis stimulating factor a term used initially to indicate the substance, then incompletely characterized, responsible for stimulation of erythropoiesis; see *erythropoietin.*

erythropoietin (ĕ-rith″ro-poi′ĕ-tin) a nondialyzable, relatively thermostable alpha-globulin. It is a glycoprotein hormone, M.W. 46,000, composed of 70 percent protein and 30 percent carbohydrate (10.8 percent sialic acid). According to current research, erythropoietin is synthesized in the kidneys and released into the blood in response to hypoxia or anemia. Using anephric animals, it has been shown that erythropoietin is also synthesized in small quantities in the liver. Its most important action is to induce erythropoietin-responsive stem cells, primarily in bone marrow, to differentiate into developing erythrocytes and thereby regulate the rate of erythropoiesis.

The concentration of erythropoietin increases in response to a decrease in either the hemoglobin concentration in the blood or the degree of arterial hemoglobin saturation, or to an increase in the hemoglobin affinity for oxygen. Erythropoietin concentration falls when these conditions are reversed or when red blood cells are transfused into the patient. Increased erythropoietin concentration (ectopic production) may be found in association with certain neoplasms (pheochromocytoma, hepatocellular carcinoma, hemangioblastoma, renal cell carcinoma and uterine leiomyomas). Pathologic decreases are seen in polycythemia vera, certain renal diseases, chronic inflammation, and some secondary anemias.

Currently, the erythropoietin assay is based on the hemagglutination inhibition technique. The reference range is 7–36 milliimmunochemical units/ml of serum. The erythropoietin assay is helpful in distinguishing polycythemia vera (normal or low erythropoietin) from secondary polycythemia (increased erythropoietin). Also called *hemopoietin.*

erythropoietin-responsive cell (ERC) a committed stem cell, no longer pluripotential but committed to produce only cells of the erythroid lineage. ERCs include BFU-E (burst-forming unit–erythroid) and CFU-E (colony-forming unit–erythroid), the two erythroid progenitor cells that have been cultured. These cells precede the earliest recognizable erythroid cell, the pronormoblast, and are stimulated to differentiate by the hormone erythropoietin. See also *erythropoiesis* and *stem cell.*

erythrose (er′ĭ-thrōs, ĕ-rith′rōs) an aldotetrose, the epimer of threose.

erythrose 4-phosphate the 4-phosphate derivative of erythrose that is an important intermediate in the pentose shunt of glucose metabolism.

Es symbol for the chemical element *einsteinium.*

escape beats those beats that have escaped from the controlling influence of a pacemaker having a faster rate—usually the sinoatrial node. The escape occurs after an interval longer than the dominant cycle (i.e., during a pause); this allows time for a lower pacemaker to reach the threshold and fire.

Anything that provides a pause longer than the prevailing cycle may permit escape to occur, including the slow phase of sinus arrhythmia, sinoatrial block, atrioventricular block, and premature systoles or paroxysms of tachycardia that are followed by a pause. It represents a safety mechanism and therefore should not be suppressed.

Escherichia (esh″ĕ-rik′e-ah) [Theodor *Escherich,* German physician, 1857–1911] a genus of widely distributed gram-negative rod-shaped microorganisms of the family Enterobacteriaceae. A normal inhabitant of the intestinal tract and one of the "coliform group" of bacteria, it can be identified by specific biochemical and physiologic characteristics, as well as by its antigenic reactions. The genus consists of only one species, *E. coli.* See also *Enterobacteriaceae.*

E. coli, the single species of the genus, which is a common inhabitant of the large intestine. Usually not pathogenic, it is a potential pathogen elsewhere in the body, producing infections of the urinary tract, bacteremia, peritonitis, and neonatal meningitis. In some circumstances, it is pathogenic in the gastrointestinal tract, e.g., acute infant diarrhea, and "traveler's diarrhea." Public health laboratories routinely test for *E. coli* in water supplies as an indicator for fecal contamination. *E. coli* is one of the most widely studied of all organisms, and the knowledge gained from the studies has contributed to striking advances in bacterial and molecular genetics.

In recent years, strains of *E. coli* other than those belonging to the enteropathogenic serotypes of infant diarrhea have been isolated from adults with diarrhea. These have been shown to produce heat-labile and/or heat-stable enterotoxins resembling the enterotoxin of *Vibrio cholerae* (see *exotoxins*). In addition, certain serogroups can invade the epithelial cells of the large bowel, producing symptoms similar to those of shigellosis.

Esidrix (es′ĭ-driks) trademark for hydrochlorothiazide; see under *thiazide diuretics.*

-esis (e′sis) [Gr. *-ēsis*] a suffix word element to denote a state or condition, e.g., enuresis.

eso- (es′o) [Gr. *esō* within, inward] a prefix word element to denote inward, e.g., esophoria.

esophag/o (ĕ-sof′ah-go) [Gr. *oisophagos* esophagus] a word element used in combining form to denote the esophagus, e.g., esophagography.

esophageal (ĕ-sof″ah-je′al) pertaining to the esophagus.

esophageal manometry a diagnostic procedure performed to determine the effectiveness of esophageal impulses and to measure the pressure along various parts of the esophagus. The information obtained is useful in diagnosing disorders such as achalasia and progressive systemic sclerosis.

esophageal pressure measurement in pulmonary function tests, the recording of the pressure within a balloon that has been introduced into the midthoracic esophagus. In the procedure, the small, tubular, slightly inflated balloon, attached to the end of a catheter in communication with a pressure transducer, is swallowed and positioned in the intrathoracic esophagus. When changes in tidal volume are relatively small, the changes in intraesophageal pressure are a good estimate of changes in intrapleural pressure, a quantity that cannot be measured noninvasively. The simultaneous measurement of intrapleural (intraesophageal) pressure, airflow, and lung volume yields information regarding the mechanical properties of the lungs.

esophageal tumors neoplasms of the esophagus. Benign esophageal neoplasms are uncommon; most are of connective tissue origin, the majority leiomyomas. Usually single, they rarely occur multiply. Such neoplasms may occur anywhere in the esophagus but usually in the lower third; they may encircle the esophagus and constrict it. When intraluminal, these tumors elevate the mucosa as a sessile or pedunculated polyp. Less common benign mesenchymal esophageal neoplasms include lipomas and fibroepithelial polyps. Benign epithelial tumors (papillomas) of the esophagus are distinctly rare.

Malignant esophageal neoplasms are predominantly carcinomas, which have a peak incidence in the sixth and seventh decades; are more common in males than in females; and are epidemiologically linked to tobacco use, high alcohol consumption, and, in some populations, to foods contaminated with aflatoxins. The carcinoma can occur in any portion of the esophagus but is most frequently found in the middle and lower thirds, eventually producing constriction and obstruction. Extension is via submucosal lymphatics and direct invasion. The 5-yr survival rate is less than 5 percent.

Most esophageal carcinomas are squamous (epidermoid) carcinomas. The majority are well differentiated and show keratinization; the remainder are moderately and poorly differentiated variants that include the relatively uncommon small cell and spindle cell carcinomas. The latter may be difficult to distinguish from a sarcoma even with the aid of electron microscopy. An uncommon type of squamous carcinoma is the verrucous carcinoma, which is an exophytic, well-differentiated carcinoma with the potential of invading locally but rarely metastasizing. Primary adenocarcinoma of the esophagus is rare, generally resembles adenocarcinoma of the stomach, and is usually found in the lower third of the esophagus; it arises from esophageal glands or foci of ectopic gastric mucosa. Unusual forms of adenocarcinoma include mucoepidermoid carcinoma and adenoid cystic carcinoma.

Malignant mesenchymal tumors are quite rare in the esophagus; essentially all are leiomyosarcomas. They may occur at any level. In the absence of invasion, distinction of this tumor from a leiomyoma is based on the findings of cellular pleomorphism and the frequency of mitotic figures. Prognosis is largely a function of completeness of excision, as metastasis from leiomyosarcoma is rare. Miscellaneous malignant neoplasms of the esophagus include Paget's disease, malignant melanoma, malignant lymphoma, plasmacytoma, and carcinosarcoma.

Diagnosis of esophageal neoplasms is aided by radiologic examination, endoscopy and endoscopic biopsy, and esophageal washings or brushings for cytologic examination.

esophagitis (ĕ-sof″ah-ji′tis) [*esophag-* + *-itis* inflammation] an acute or chronic inflammation of the esophagus, which may be due to gastric reflux, corrosive substances, or infectious agents.

corrosive e., an acute, severe inflammation of the esophagus due to the ingestion of a caustic substance. It is most common in children who accidentally swallow such substances, but it also occurs as a result of suicide attempts. Strong acids and alkalis are among the chemicals most often implicated. The burned areas are edematous, inflamed, frequently necrotic, and may lead to perforation. The individual experiences severe substernal pain and burning, nausea, vomiting, and diarrhea. Endoscopy may be used to determine the extent of damage to the esophagus.

infectious e., an inflammation of the esophagus commonly due to overgrowth of *Candida albicans.* It is most frequently seen in immunosuppressed individuals or those suffering from chronic debilitating diseases. Pain and difficulty in swallowing may be present. Radiographs may show irregularities and ulceration in the esophagus.

reflux e., an inflammation of the esophagus characterized by substernal burning or pain that usually occurs after eating, difficulty in swallowing, hematemesis, and melena. The condition is caused by the reflux of gastric acid and pepsin. This may be due to an incompetent lower esophageal sphincter and is associated with hiatus hernia. Complications include esophageal stenosis and ulcer formation.

Diagnosis may be aided by esophageal pH monitoring, esophagoscopy, esophageal manometry, and the Bernstein test; radiographic studies may be useful in demonstrating a hiatus hernia.

esophagogastroduodenoscopy (ĕ-sof″ah-go-gas″-tro-du″o-dĕ-nos′ko-pe) [*esophago-* + Gr. *gastēr* stomach + *duodenum* + Gr. *skopein* to examine] endoscopic examination of the esophagus, stomach, and duodenum.

esophagogastroscopy (ĕ-sof″ah-go-gas-tros′ko-pe) [*esophago-* + Gr. *gastēr* stomach + *skopein* to examine] endoscopic examination of the esophagus and stomach.

esophagography (ĕ-sof″ah-gog′rah-fe) [*esophago-* + Gr. *graphein* to record] radiographic examination of the esophagus. Barium is generally used as a contrast medium.

esophagus (ĕ-sof′ah-gus) [Gr. *oisophagos,* from *oisein* to carry + *phagēma* food] [NA], the muscular epithelium-lined tube, approximately 25 cm long, that conveys food from the oropharynx to the stomach. It begins at the level of the lower border of the cricoid cartilage as a continuation of the pharynx, and runs down the posterior mediastinum on the vertebral bodies, curving in conformity with the shape of the spine. It deviates to the left as it exits from the thorax and passes through an opening in the diaphragm just anterior to the vertebral column at the level of the ninth or tenth thoracic vertebra, where it becomes continuous with the stomach. Structures that lie in front of the esophagus include the trachea, left bronchus, pericardium, and left atrium. The descending aorta is initially to its left and then passes behind it. It is separated on each side from the lungs by pleura. The vagus nerves run to it from plexuses at the roots of the lungs and ramify over its lower part. With endoscopy, the level of a lesion within the esophagus can be recorded by its distance from the incisor teeth: the commencement of the esophagus is approximately 15 cm from the teeth, and the gastroesophageal junction is at about 40 cm.

Much of the esophageal wall is made up of smooth muscle, with an admixture of striated muscle fibers in its upper half. The smooth muscle is arranged in inner circular and outer longitudinal layers. The circular smooth muscle is thickened at the upper and lower ends to form the upper and lower esophageal sphincters. Contraction of the circular muscle produces deep longitudinal grooves in the mucosa. The lining is stratified squamous epithelium, supported by a thin lamina propria and a relatively thick muscularis mucosae. The submucosa contains mucus-forming glands, and at the upper and lower ends there are similar glands within the lamina propria. The esophagus is of foregut derivation, and its lower portion is therefore supplied through a branch of the celiac artery that arises from the left gastric artery and ascends through the esophageal opening of the diaphragm. Small branches from the aorta supply the upper part.

The process of swallowing (deglutition) occurs in three stages and is normally initiated involuntarily, although one can of course swallow deliberately. The second and third stages of swallowing are completely involuntary. Muscular coordination of swallowing is synchronized by neurons in the floor of the fourth ventricle, and efferent fibers are conveyed by the ninth, tenth, and twelfth cranial nerves.

ESP abbrev. See *eosinophil stimulation promoter.*

ESR abbrev. See *electron spin resonance, erythrocyte sedimentation rate.*

essential oil see *volatile oil.*

ester (es′ter) any compound formally derived from an alcohol and an acid by the removal of water. Esters are named as if they were salts of the acid, e.g., methyl methanoate, CHO_2CH_3. The general formula is $RCOOR^1$. See also *functional group.*

esterase (es′ter-ās) any of a large group of enzymes of the class of hydrolases, EC 3.1, that hydrolyze ester bonds of a variety of esters, yielding an alcohol and the respective acid ion. Formerly, the term was applied to the enzyme carboxylesterase (EC 3.1.1.1). See also the particular esterases: *carboxylesterase, endonuclease, lipase, nucleotidase, phosphatase,* and *phosphodiesterase.*

esterase staining methods histochemical techniques for the localization of various esterases: lipases, nonspecific esterases, acetylcholinesterase, and pseudocholinesterase. The frozen-section, freeze-dry, or freeze-substitution technique is used to preserve enzyme activity. Sections are incubated at 37°C in a buffered solution containing an artificial substrate of the enzyme hydrolyzed by the enzyme to form a product that can be stained.

In Tween methods, the substrate is polysorbate (Tween), which yields a long-chain fatty acid on hydrolysis. Adding lead nitrate produces an insoluble lead soap, and adding ammonium sulfide produces dark brown deposits of lead sulfide. These methods are used for lipases but are not specific.

In thioacetic acid methods, the substrate is thioacetic acid (CH_3COSH), which, although not an ester, is attacked, liberating hydrogen sulfide. The H_2S reacts with lead nitrate in the substrate solution to yield lead sulfide. This method is used primarily for the cholinesterases.

In the indoxyl methods, the substrate is the acetyl or butyryl ester of indoxyl, which is hydrolyzed to free indoxyl, which in turn is oxidized by atmospheric oxygen to form indigo (C.I. 73000). This method is used for nonspecific esterases.

In the azo dye methods, the substrate is the acetate of α-naphthol, β-naphthol, or naphthol AS(2-hydroxy-2-naphthoic acid anilide), which is hydrolyzed to free naphthol, which in turn is azo-coupled to a diazonium salt, producing an azo dye. The naphthol AS methods produce more insoluble dyes. These methods are used for nonspecific esterases.

Enzyme activators or inhibitors, such as organophosphorus compounds that are cholinesterase inhibitors, can be used to increase the specificity of these methods.

esterification (ĕ-ster″ĭ-fi-ka′shun) the formation of an ester or ester linkage.

estetrol (E_4) (es′tĕ-trol) an estrogen that is produced in the fetus by the 15-α hydroxylation of estrogen precursors and/or estriol and found in the serum of pregnant females, in amniotic fluid, and in the urine of newborn infants. It has been suggested that the measurement of estetrol in maternal serum may be a better indicator than estriol for detecting fetal distress during the third trimester of pregnancy. See also *estriol.*

esthesi/o (es-the′ze-o) [Gr. *aisthēsis* perception, sensation] a word element used in combining form to denote feeling (nervous sensation), e.g., anesthesia.

esthesioneuroblastoma (es-the″ze-o-nu″ro-blas-to′mah) [*esthesio-* + Gr. *neuron* nerve + *blastos* germ + *ōma* swelling] a term that connotes a primitive neural tumor of sensory nerve-ending cells. The term is commonly used to refer to an olfactory neuroblastoma or olfactory neuroepithelioma. See also *olfactory n.* under *neuroblastoma.*

estimate (es′tĭ-māt) [L. *aestimare* to value, to estimate] 1. an approximate calculation or one based on incomplete data.

2. a statistic used to make a statement about the value of a population parameter based on the values of a random sample (a process called statistical estimation). Also called estimator.

biased e., a point estimate that is not unbiased.

consistent e., a statistic that converges to the parameter being estimated as the sample size increases; i.e., the sampling error can be made as small as desired by taking a large enough sample.

interval e., a statistical estimate that states with a specified level of confidence or probability that the parameter lies in a specified interval. See also *confidence interval* and *tolerance interval.* Cf. *point e.*

median unbiased e., a point estimate having a sampling distribution with a median equal to the parameter being estimated; for example, the sample median of an odd-sized sample is a median unbiased estimate of the population median.

point e., a statistical estimate that specifies a value for the parameter. Cf. *interval e.*

unbiased e., a point estimate having a sampling distribution with a mean equal to the parameter being estimated; for example, the sample mean and variance are unbiased estimates of the population mean and variance.

17β-estradiol (E_2) (es″trah-di′ol) a female steroid hormone, 3,17β-dihydroxyestra-1,3,5(10)-triene, the main estrogenic hormone secreted by the ovary; M.W. 272.37. It is synthesized by the aromatization of testosterone. The primary function of estradiol is to prepare the uterine mucosa for the progestational stage, which it accomplishes by inducing the proliferative growth of the endometrial mucosa, by enlarging the uterine glands, and by increasing vascularity. It also suppresses the production of follicle-stimulating hormone (FSH) and stimulates preovulatory luteinizing hormone (LH) release from the pituitary. Measurement of plasma 17β-estradiol is considered sufficient to evaluate the status of ovarian function. The plasma concentration of estradiol reaches its highest level a day before the LH surge and rises again when the corpus luteum is formed. Estradiol concentrations are frequently useful in evaluating a variety of menstrual dysfunctions, feminization in children, and estrogen-producing tumors. Estradiol may be elevated in gynecomastia and cirrhosis. It is often measured when exogenously administered gonadotropins are given to induce ovulation in order to reduce the incidence of multiple births and polycystic ovarian disease.

Reference ranges for estradiol (E_2) in plasma are: for adult males, 8–36 pg/ml; for adult females—follicular: 10–90, midcycle: 100–500, luteal: 50–240, and postmenopausal: 10–30.

Also called *dihydrofolliculin.*

estradiol assays various methods (gas-liquid chromatography, colorimetric, fluorometric) used to determine estrogens in plasma. The simplest and most suitable estradiol determination for clinical diagnostic purposes is the radioimmunoassay, using highly specific antisera against estradiol. However, for urinary estradiol measurements, some form of chromatography is still necessary for sample purification. The sensitivity of this method is in the range of picograms per milliliter.

estradiol receptor see *estrogen receptor.*

estramustine (es-trah-mus'tēn) a cancer chemotherapeutic drug; trademark, Emcyt. For more information, see *Appendix A.*

Estren-Dameshek anemia (es'tren dam'ĕ-shek) [Solomon *Estren,* U.S. physician, born 1918; William *Dameshek,* U.S. hematologist, 1900–1969] see *Estren-Dameshek a.* under *anemia.*

estriol (E_3) (es'tre-ol) estra-1,3,5(10)-triene-3,16α,-17β-triol, an estrogen produced by the metabolism of the active hormone estradiol in nonpregnant women; M.W. 288.37. It is less potent than estradiol. Estriol is the major estrogen in pregnancy, being synthesized directly in the placenta from 16α-hydroxy-dehydroepiandrosterone sulfate (16α-OH-DHEA-SO_4), a precursor supplied by the fetus.

Estriol measurements are primarily utilized to assess fetoplacental function in the third trimester of pregnancy, when rapid increases occur. Once estriol has been synthesized in the placenta from the fetal precursor (16α-OH-DHEA-SO_4), it passes into the maternal circulation and finally reaches the maternal liver, where it is conjugated as the glucuronide and sulfate. The latter substances are water-soluble and easily excreted by the kidneys.

Owing to the short half-life (20 min) of conjugated estriol, serial measurements (on a daily basis) of serum or a 24-hr urine collection are very useful in assessing fetoplacental distress in pregnancies associated with toxemia, hypertension, diabetes mellitus, preeclampsia, and cardiovascular disease. Sudden drops in estriol levels usually signal fetal jeopardy, but the overall patient history must be taken into account in making any clinical decision.

See also *estrogen.*

conjugated e., the estriol that has been conjugated in the liver in the form of a variety of glucuronides and sulfates. It is in this form that most of the estriol is excreted in the urine.

free e., see *unconjugated e.*

serum e., the levels of either total or unconjugated estriol in serum. Its measurement is generally preferred to the measurement of the urinary estriol concentration, because specimens are readily available and the problems and shortcomings of 24-hr urine collections are avoided.

total e., the summation of unconjugated estriol, estriol conjugated as the glucuronide and sulfate, and the estriol bound to plasma proteins, such as albumin, referring to either urine or serum specimens.

Reference ranges for estriol in urine are: at 28–32 wk of gestation, 7–25 mg/da; at 32–36 wk, 10–35; and at 36–40 wk, 15–55. Reference ranges for estriol in blood are: at 28–32 wk of gestation, 30–150 ng/ml; at 32–36 wk, 40–200; and at 36–40 wk, 50–400.

unconjugated e., the estriol that has not been conjugated as the glucuronide or sulfate. Because the unconjugated estriol is synthesized in the placenta from a fetal precursor and has not been metabolized by the maternal liver, maternal serum concentrations are thought to be a better indicator of fetoplacental function than total estriol. Reference ranges are: at 28–32 wk of gestation, 4–14 ng/ml; at 32–36 wk, 5–16; and at 36–40 wk, 6–25. Sometimes called *free estriol,* an imprecise term.

urinary e., the amount of estriol in a 24-hr urine specimen, composed almost entirely of glucuronide and sulfate conjugates. Because of difficulties in obtaining a 24-hr urine collection and because the maternal liver and kidneys contribute to the metabolism and excretion of estriol, the serum concentration reflects more accurately the function of the fetoplacental unit.

estriol assays radioimmunoassay (RIA) for serum or urinary estriol. The preferred measurement is serum estriol using antibody specific for unconjugated estriol. Total estriol can be determined by RIA following enzymatic hydrolysis of estriol conjugates.

estrogen (es'tro-jen) [N.L. *estrus* the recurrent period of ovulation and sexual receptiveness in female mammals + Gr. *gennan* to produce] the generic term for a group of steroid female sex hormones characterized by an aromatic ring. Their functions include promoting the development of the sexual organs and secondary sexual characteristics, regulating the menstrual cycle, and maintaining the proper uterine environment for the fetus during pregnancy. More than 30 estrogens have been identified, but only estriol, estrone, 2-hydroxyestrone (catechol estrogen), and estradiol are present in significant amounts in the serum or urine. Estradiol is the most potent of the estrogens; it is also the major estrogen in nonpregnancy states, whereas estriol is the most abundant estrogen during pregnancy.

Estrogens are secreted primarily by the ovarian follicles (in nonpregnancy states), by the placenta (in pregnancy states), and, to a lesser degree, by the testes and adrenals. Specific high-affinity cytoplasmic receptors for estrogens are found in the uterus, vagina, mammary glands, hypothalamus, and adenohypophysis. Interaction of an estrogen with cytoplasmic receptor forms a receptor-estrogen complex. This product binds to the nonhistone protein of the chromatin, which leads to the initiation of RNA and protein synthesis, resulting in biologic response. The 18-carbon parent hydrocarbon for all estrogens is estrone, which possesses an aromatic A ring. A ketone or hydroxy group at C17 and a phenolic hydroxy at C3 are essential for biologic activity. Estrogens circulate in blood either free or as glucuronides and sulfates. Most estrogens are excreted in the urine as the glucuronide and sulfate conjugates.

Acetate, cholesterol, progesterone, and testosterone (the male sex hormone) are precursors of estrogen biosynthesis. The regulation of estrogen levels is accomplished via a feedback mechanism involving the ovaries, hypothalamus, and adenohypophysis. A follicle-stimulating hormone/luteinizing hormone (FSH/LH)–releasing hormone that is synthesized and released by the hypothalamus aids in controlling FSH/LH secretion by the adenohypophysis, which in turn stimulates the ovaries to produce estrogens. There are two distinct estrogen peaks during the menstrual cycle, one occurring close to the LH peak and just before ovulation (ovulatory peak), and a second occurring 5–10 da after ovulation (luteal peak).

Serum estrogen levels are increased in individuals with certain types of ovarian and testicular tumors, and hyperovarianism, and are decreased in females with amenorrhea due to agenesis of the ovaries, primary ovarian malfunction, dysfunction of the pituitary, and aging (postmenopausal).

See also *estradiol, estriol,* and *estrone.*

estrogen assays tests to determine the concentration of estrogen in blood or urine, usually performed by radioimmunoassay. The measurement of estrogens in females during their reproductive life is important for evaluation of the functional status of the ovaries. Determination of total urinary excretion is preferred, as urine is the principal route of estrogen excretion.

Estrogens can be determined by fluorometric or colorimetric methods, although these are rapidly being replaced by RIA. When heated with sulfuric acid, they turn orange-yellow with an intense greenish fluorescence. The colorimetric assay is based on the Kober reaction, in which a specific pink color is formed only with estrogens. In the Brown modification of the Kober reaction (the most commonly used colorimetric method), the essential steps involve acid hydrolysis of the conjugated estrogens and several extraction and separation procedures before the Kober pink color is developed. The color complex can then be measured either colorimetrically or fluorometrically.

estrogen receptor (ER) a specific cytoplasmic protein, with high affinity and great specificity for estrogen, that is found in target tissue cells such as the uterus and breasts, and pituitary and hypothalamus glands. Estrogen (as well as other steroid hormones) enters target cells by passive diffusion through the plasma membrane. After hormone binding, the receptors undergo some kind of enzymatic or conformational change, referred to alternately as either activation or transformation. Following transformation, the steroid-receptor complex enters the nucleus by a process called translocation. Inside the nucleus, the transformed hormone-receptor complex is thought to interact directly with the genetic material by binding to specific regions of the target cell chromatin called acceptor sites, resulting in the formation of messenger RNA (mRNA). The new mRNA molecules are transported back to the cytoplasm where they direct the synthesis of specific proteins responsible for influencing certain biologic activities of the cell.

As estrogen influences metabolic responses in target cells that normally contain ER protein, a reduction in estrogen levels in the body would be expected to reduce the metabolic activity of cells containing ERs: this has been the rationale for the use of endocrine therapy in females with breast carcinoma. Approximately 30 percent of those with metastatic breast carcinoma obtain an objective remission after the use of various types of endocrine therapy directed at lowering the concentration of estrogen; such therapy includes oophorectomy, hypophysectomy, and adrenalectomy (ablative therapy), as well as the administration of antiestrogens and androgens (additive therapy).

Cytoplasmic ER is now routinely measured in samples of breast carcinoma after surgical removal of the tumor. Approximately 60–85 percent of patients have a positive ER, i.e., >3 femtomoles/mg of tumor cytosol protein. In such patients, 50–70 percent will show an objective remission in response to endocrine therapy.

False-negative results—in which the ER is negative but the patient responds to endocrine therapy—are observed when storage of the sample is not maintained at –70°C, when nonneoplastic tissue or only ER (negative) tissue is sampled, or when most of the cytoplasmic receptor sites are already saturated with endogenous estrogens, which is common in premenopausal females. False-positive results—in which the ER is positive and the patient does not respond to endocrine therapy—are more common than false-negative results. They occur when the tumor is predominantly ER-negative but a focus of ER-positive tumor has been sampled, and when nonneoplastic binding of estrogen occurs.

As progesterone receptor (PgR) synthesis seems to be estrogen-dependent, measurement of PgR activity appears to be a useful indicator of ER concentration. Patients with both ER- and PgR-positive tumors have a response rate of greater than 75 percent, whereas those with ER-positive and PgR-negative tumors have only a 30 percent response rate to endocrine therapy.

Also called *estradiol receptor.* See also *hormonal therapy* and *progesterone receptor.*

estrogen receptor assays methods for the measurement of estrogen receptor (ER) sites in cytosols utilizing radioactive estradiol as a tracer that binds specifically and with high affinity to the receptor protein. At low temperatures only unoccupied receptor sites bind the labeled estradiol, as elevated temperatures are required for the exchange of unlabeled bound ligand. If a labeled ligand with a known specific activity is used, the binding sites in tumor cytosols can be quantitated. Nonspecific binding can be evaluated by competitive inhibitions using a large excess of unlabeled diethylstilbestrol (DES), as this nonsteroidal analog binds to the receptor but not to sex hormone–binding globulin (SHBG) and other binding proteins. Therefore, only displaceable binding sites are considered to be ER sites.

The most reliable and reproducible methods for cytosol receptor assay appear to be either the multiple-point dextran-coated charcoal assay analyzed by Scatchard plot, or the sucrose gradient ultracentrifugation assay. These conventional assays measure only the receptor that is in the cytosol and not occupied by estradiol. In the charcoal assay, ERs are titrated to saturation with increasing concentrations of radioactive estradiol under equilibrium conditions with and without excess unlabeled DES. Separation of the tightly bound complexes from the unbound steroid is achieved by adsorption of the free labeled steroid onto dextran-coated charcoal. The resulting saturation curve is then analyzed by Scatchard plot to yield an estimate of the quantity and affinity of ERs. In the ultracentrifugation method, estimates are obtained of the quantity of ER present and of the size and shape of the estrogen-binding species. Because less tissue is required for this assay, only a single concentration of radioligand is used. Information derived from ER assays generally dictates the modality of treatments, and for this reason every effort must be made to minimize the possibility of assay error.

See also *estrogen receptor.*

estrone (E_1) (es′trōn) 1,3,5-estratrien-3-ol-17-one, an estrogen produced in the ovaries and testes (minor) from the peripheral conversion of androstenedione and from estradiol metabolism; M.W. 270.36. Estrone is a more potent estrogen than estriol but is less potent than estradiol. Most of the circulating estrone is in the form of the sulfate and, unlike estradiol, shows no midcycle peak or consistent pattern in the menstrual cycle. See also *estrogen*.

eta (H, η) (a′tah) the seventh letter of the *Greek alphabet*.

ETEC an acronym from *entero toxic* E*scherichia* c*oli;* see *Enterobacteriaceae* and *E. coli* under *Escherichia*.

ethacrynic acid (eth″ah-krin′ik) [USP], a very potent diuretic that acts in the kidneys by blocking the reabsorption of sodium in the ascending loop of Henle. It is used to treat hypertension and edema, particularly in patients who have not responded to other diuretics. Adverse effects are due to excessive diuresis; these include low blood volume and electrolyte imbalance, particularly potassium depletion. Close clinical supervision is necessary. Trademarks, Edecril, *Edecrin,* Hydroinedin, and others.

ethambutol (ĕ-tham′bu-tol) a synthetic agent that inhibits the growth of mycobacteria. The mechanism of action is unknown, but RNA synthesis is affected. Occasional resistant isolates occur. Ethambutol is often used in combination with other antituberculous drugs to prevent the emergence of resistant strains. Peripheral neuropathy is a potential adverse reaction. See also *antibacterial agents*.

ethane (eth′ān) a colorless, odorless gas, CH_3CH_3; M.W. 30.07. It is highly flammable (flammability limits in air, 3.0–12.5 percent). Natural gas is about 9 percent ethane. At very high concentrations, ethane is an asphyxiant.

ethanediol (eth″ān-di′ol) 1,2-ethanediol; see *ethylene glycol*.

ethanoic acid (eth″ah-no′ik) the systematic name for acetic acid, CH_3COOH.

ethanol (eth′ah-nol) a colorless, volatile liquid, CH_3CH_2OH, that is miscible with water, methanol, ether, acetone, and chloroform; M.W. 46.07. Several grades of ethanol are produced. Ordinary alcohol contains about 5 percent water, because when ethanol is distilled from water, an azeotrope boiling lower (78.15°C) than pure alcohol (78.3°C) comes over first. Absolute alcohol (anhydrous, greater than 99.9 percent C_2H_5OH) is prepared by removing the water by chemical means.

It is commonly used as the depressant recreational drug in alcoholic beverages, as a solvent in many laboratory procedures, as a solvent for drugs (a tincture), as a dehydrating agent in histology, and as a disinfectant. For industrial use, alcohol is denatured by adding an impurity so that it cannot be used as a beverage and therefore is not taxed.

Toxic symptoms, including nausea, vomiting, central nervous system depression, and impaired perception and coordination, occur at blood levels above 500 mg/l. Chronic use of ethanol may cause liver damage, and death may occur at levels above 4 g/l. The combination of ethanol and barbiturates is much more toxic than either alone.

Also called *alcohol* and *ethyl alcohol*. See also *cirrhosis* and *hepatitis*.

ethanolamine (eth″ah-nol′ah-mēn) 2-aminoethanol, a colorless, moderately viscous liquid with an ammoniacal odor, $NH_2 \cdot CH_2 \cdot CH_2OH$. It is contained in phosphatidylethanolamine and is derived metabolically by the decarboxylation of serine. The oleate is used as a sclerosing agent in the treatment of varicose veins.

ethanol assays 1. colorimetric methods. The simplest procedures use the reduction of orange-colored dichromate to the green chromic ion. This test is not specific because other alcohols and aldehydes interfere. This chemical reaction can be carried out on either blood or urine in microdiffusion (Conway) cells. Quantitative procedures measure the unreduced dichromate by titration with thiosulfate or by spectrophotometry.

2. enzymatic methods. Ethanol is oxidized to acetaldehyde by the enzyme alcohol dehydrogenase accompanied by the reduction of NAD to NADH. The absorbance of NADH at 340 nm is used to calculate the ethanol concentration. These procedures can be automated. Other alcohols may serve as a substrate for this enzyme and thus may interfere.

3. gas chromatography. Samples of body fluids may be injected directly into a gas chromatograph (see *alcohol assays*), or the volatile components may be first separated by diffusion into the airspace of a test tube (headspace technique).

4. determination by specific instruments. These so-called breath analyzers have also been used to analyze the alcohol content of breath, which is related to the blood alcohol concentration. Such instruments are mainly used by police departments.

ethanol gelation test a screening test for disseminated intravascular coagulation. This test detects the presence of fibrin monomers present in plasma by precipitating the monomers with ethyl alcohol, forming a gel or precipitate.

ethchlorvynol (eth-klōr′vĭ-nol) a yellow pungent liquid, used as a sleeping aid. Overdosage may result in coma; ingestion of an amount 10–100 times the therapeutic dose may be fatal. Chronic use causes dependence; the effect of sudden withdrawal is similar to that of withdrawal from barbiturates and alcohol. Trademark, *Placidyl*.

ethchlorvynol assays 1. colorimetric test. The sample is treated with trichloroacetic acid, and an aliquot of the supernatant is reacted with diphenylamine to form a pink product, which is measured spectrophotometrically at 510 nm.

2. gas chromatography. Ethchlorvynol is extracted into ethyl acetate or separated by the headspace procedure and quantitated by gas chromatography.

ethene (eth′ēn) the systematic name for *ethylene*.

ether (e′ther) 1. a compound formally derived by the elimination of water from two alcohol molecules. The general formula is R—O—R. Ethers have common names based on their derivation, e.g., dimethyl ether, methyl ethyl ether. IUPAC nomenclature considers the group R—O as an alkoxy group, e.g., methoxymethane, $CH_3—O—CH_3$. If the two alcohols are the same, the ether is called simple or symmetric; if they are not, it is called mixed, complex, or unsymmetric (see *functional group*).

2. [USP], diethyl ether. Formerly used by inhalation as a general anesthetic. Also called *ethyl ether*.

ether storage the storage of ethyl ether and solvents such as isopentane (2-methylbutane), substances that are extremely volatile, that have easily ignitable vapors, and for which special consideration must be given to their storage. These two solvents (as well as some others) have flash-point temperatures below the temperatures of most refrigerators and freezers and can generate explosive concentrations of vapor within refrigerators and other enclosed and unventilated spaces. Many explosions have been reported.

Small cans of ethyl ether can be safely stored on the bench, in cupboards, or in flammable liquid storage cabinets (which do not contain the sources of ignition present in ordinary refrigerators or cold rooms). Ethyl ether can also be safely stored in a flammable materials storage refrigerator or in an explosion-proof refrigerator or freezer. (Before purchasing a special refrigerator for storage of ether, isopentane, or solvents that also have low flash-point temperatures, alternatives to refrigerated storage should be considered carefully.) See also *explosion proof.*

ethics (eth′iks) [Gr. *ēthikos* ethical, from *ēthos* moral custom] the rules and principles of proper professional conduct, such as those promulgated by the professional societies and governmental agencies that elaborate the duties and obligations of the professional and the rights of patients and fellow practitioners.

ethinamate (ĕ-thin′ah-māt) [USP], a nonbarbiturate hypnotic, 1-ethynylcyclohexanol carbamate. Its effects are additive with those of alcohol and other central nervous system depressants. Overdosage produces respiratory depression similar to that caused by barbiturate poisoning. Chronic use in large dosages may lead to physical and psychic dependence.

ethinyl estradiol (eth′in-il es-trah-di′ol) a cancer chemotherapeutic drug. Trademark, Estinyl. For more information, see *Appendix A.*

Ethiodan (ĕ-thi′o-dan) trademark. See *iophendylate.*

ethiodized oil (ĕ-thi′o-dīz′d) [USP], a radiopaque contrast medium used in hysterosalpingography and lymphography. It consists of ethyl esters of iodinated fatty acids from poppyseed oil. Trademark, *Ethiodol.*

Ethiodol (ĕ-thi′o-dol) trademark. See *ethiodized oil.*

ethion (ĕ-thi′on) a highly toxic organothiophosphate ester, phosphorodithioic acid *S,S′*-methylene *O,O,O′,O′*-tetraethyl ester, used as an insecticide and miticide. See also *organophosphate compounds.*

ethionamide (ĕ-thi″on-am′īd) a synthetic derivative of isonicotinic acid that inhibits the growth of *Mycobacterium tuberculosis.* Because of frequent gastrointestinal intolerance, its use is limited to retreating drug-resistant tuberculosis. See also *antibacterial agents.*

ethionine (ĕ-thi′o-nēn) the ethyl homolog of methionine.

ethm/o (eth′mo) [Gr. *ēthmos* sieve] a word element used in combining form to denote a sieve, e.g., ethmoid.

ethmoid bone (eth′moid) an unpaired bone of the skull that lies in front of the sphenoid between the orbits. Much of its interior is occupied by communicating air sinuses. The ethmoid consists of a perpendicular plate that supports two lateral ethmoidal labyrinths. A perforated sheet of bone, the cribriform plate, joins each labyrinth to the upper part of the perpendicular plate. An olfactory bulb lies on the cribriform plate and receives olfactory nerves that pass through its perforations. The superior margin of the perpendicular plate of the ethmoid projects upward into the anterior cranial fossa as the crista galli.

ethoheptazine citrate (eth″o-hep′tah-zēn) an analgesic drug similar to meperidine in structure and action but less potent and of low abuse potential.

ethopropazine (eth″o-pro′pah-zēn) [USP], an antihistamine of the phenothiazine type with some anticholinergic and ganglion-blocking activity, used in the treatment of Parkinson's disease.

ethosuximide (eth″o-suk′sĭ-mīd) an anticonvulsant that is the drug of choice in the treatment of absence attacks (petit mal seizures). Its use in mixed seizure disorders must be supplemented by drugs effective against tonic-clonic attacks (grand mal seizures). Adverse reactions include nausea, vomiting, anorexia, central nervous system effects (drowsiness, dizziness, headache, lethargy, aggravation of previously existing behavioral disturbances), skin reactions, and hematopoietic abnormalities (leukopenia, thrombocytopenia, eosinophilia, agranulocytosis, pancytopenia, and aplastic anemia). Some fatalities resulting from bone marrow depression have occurred. Periodic blood counts should be performed during ethosuximide therapy. The serum ethosuximide concentration is monitored during therapy; the usual therapeutic level is 40–80 mg/l. Trademark, *Zarontin.*

ethosuximide assays 1. gas chromatography. Ethosuximide and the internal standard (α,α-dimethyl-β-succinamide) are extracted from serum with toluene; the toluene is extracted with ammonium hydroxide, which is acidified and extracted with methylene chloride. An *N*-butyl derivative is prepared by reaction with butyl iodide in *N,N*-dimethylacetamide. The derivative is quantitated by gas chromatography, utilizing a nonpolar stationary phase and a flame ionization detector.

2. EMIT homogeneous enzyme immunoassay for ethosuximide in serum.

3. high-pressure liquid chromatography (HPLC). After protein precipitation, the supernatant is chromatographed on a reverse-phase column.

ethoxy- (eth-ok′se) a prefix word element in organic chemistry to denote the ethoxy functional group (CH_3CH_2O—), e.g., ethoxypropane (ethyl propyl ether).

ethyl- (eth′il) [*ether* + Gr. *hylē* matter] a prefix in organic chemistry to denote the ethyl group (CH_3-CH_2—), e.g., 3-ethylpentane, $(C_2H_5)_3CH$. In certain radicofunctional names, ethyl is followed by a space, e.g., ethyl alcohol (ethanol) and ethyl acetate.

ethyl acetate a colorless, volatile, flammable liquid with a fruity odor, $CH_3COOC_2H_5$, used as a lacquer solvent; M.W. 88.10. It is chemically an ester and is moderately toxic by inhalation or skin absorption, producing drying of the skin and respiratory tract irritation.

ethyl alcohol see *ethanol.*

ethyl chloride a colorless gas, chloroethane; M.W. 64.52. It was formerly used as a topical anesthetic.

ethyl cyanide see *propanenitrile.*

ethylene (eth′ĭ-lēn) a colorless gas, $CH_2{=}CH_2$, which is somewhat lighter than air and has a slightly sweet taste and odor. It is used for inducing general anesthesia. Also called *ethene.*

ethylene chlorohydrin a volatile, colorless liquid, 2-chloroethanol; M.W. 80.52. Used in the synthesis of pesticides and as a solvent, it is highly toxic by skin absorption and penetrates rubber gloves; exposure may be fatal.

ethylenediaminetetraacetic acid (eth″il-ēn-di′-ah-mēn-tet″rah-ah-se′tik) see *EDTA*.

ethylene dibromide a dense, colorless, nonflammable liquid with the odor of chloroform, 1,2-dibromoethane, CH_2BrCH_2Br; M.W. 187.88. It is used as a scavenger in leaded gasoline and as a fumigant and solvent. Ethylene dibromide is toxic when ingested, inhaled, or absorbed through the skin, and can produce blisters, lung damage, and central nervous system depression; liver and kidney damage can result from chronic exposure.

ethylene dichloride see *1,2-dichloroethane.*

ethylene glycol the common name for 1,2-ethanediol, a colorless, viscous, hygroscopic liquid; M.W. 62.07. It is used commercially as a permanent antifreeze, as a paint and ink solvent, and in the manufacture of polyester. When an amount of 50–100 ml is ingested, signs of drunkenness may occur leading to stupor, coma, and death from respiratory arrest. Ethylene glycol is metabolized to oxalic acid through intermediate substances that can cause hypocalcemic tetany and acute renal failure with renal tubular deposition of oxylate crystals, even when less than an acute lethal dose is ingested.

ethylene glycol assays 1. colorimetric assay; oxidation with Schiff's reagent yields a product that absorbs light at 555 nm. This method can give blank values of 350 g/l, i.e., false positives.

2. gas chromatography using a polar column and flame ionization detector with propylene glycol as an internal standard. Blood, urine, or the supernatant from a tissue homogenate is chromatographed. Common volatile substances do not interfere.

ethylene glycol dinitrate a volatile liquid, $O_2NOCH_2CH_2ONO_2$, an explosive used in low-freezing dynamite; M.W. 152.06. It is toxic when inhaled or absorbed through the skin and produces methemoglobinemia and vasodilation, causing headache, hypotension, and palpitation.

ethylene oxide a colorless, water-soluble gas, 1,2-epoxyethane, the simplest epoxide; M.W. 44.05. It is a potent microbicidal chemical widely used for the gaseous disinfection of dry surfaces, as a fumigant for foodstuffs and textiles, and for the sterilization of heat-sensitive and other objects in hospitals. Ethylene oxide is highly irritating to eyes and mucous membranes. Potentially hazardous, it acts as an alkylating agent to inactivate proteins and is mutagenic for bacteria, plant seeds, and *Drosophila.*

ethyl ether see *ether.*

ethylidene dichloride (eth′il-ĭ-dēn) see *1,1-dichloroethane.*

ethyl iodophenylundecylate see *iophendylate.*

ethylmorphine hydrochloride (eth″il-mor′fēn) a narcotic analgesic also used as an antitussive and expectorant.

ethyne (eth′īn) the systematic name for *acetylene.*

eti/o (e′te-o) [Gr. *aitio* fundamental] 1. a word element used in combining form to denote cause, e.g., etiology.

2. in organic chemistry, a word element used in combining form to denote a chemical compound produced by degradation of the reference compound, e.g., etiocholanolone.

etiocholanolone (e″te-o-ko-lan′o-lōn) 3α-hydroxy-5β-androstan-17-one; M.W. 290.43. It is a primary metabolite of dehydroepiandrosterone and androstenedione, found in the urine of males (1.4–5.0 mg/d) and females (0.8–4.0 mg/d). Etiocholanolone is devoid of androgenic activity, but has pyrogenic properties.

etiocobalamine (e″te-o-ko-bal′ah-mēn) cobinamide dicyanide, vitamin B_{12p}, Factor B; M.W. 1042.17. This vitamin B_{12} factor is obtained by removal of nucleotide from cyanocobalamine by acid hydrolysis.

etiologic agent (e″te-o-loj′ik) the causative agent of a disease, e.g., the microorganism causing a specific infectious disease.

etiology (e″te-ol′o-je) [*etio-* + *-logy*] the causes of a disease, such as genetic factors, infection, toxin or trauma. Etiology is distinguished from pathogenesis, the physiologic and biochemical mechanisms by which the disease progresses. Cf. *pathogenesis.*

etoposide (ĕ-to-po′sīd) a cancer chemotherapeutic drug. For more information, see *Appendix A.*

Eu symbol for the chemical element *europium.*

eu- (u) [Gr. *eu* well] a prefix word element to denote good, well, or easily, e.g., euploid.

eubacteria (u″bak-te′re-ah) prokaryotic organisms with rigid walls that give the cells an unchanging form; motility, when present, is by means of flagella. These organisms should be distinguished from spirochetes and myxobacteria (gliding motility).

Eubacterium (u″bak-te′re-um) [*eu-* + Gr. *baktērion* little rod] a genus of bacteria of the family Propionibacteriaceae. The organisms are gram-positive, obligately anaerobic, nonsporulating rods. They are normal inhabitants of mammalian and human cavities and skin, occasionally causing infections of soft tissue.

eucalyptol (u″kah-lip′tol) a colorless, fragrant liquid obtained by the fractional distillation of eucalyptus oil, and used in cough syrups and expectorants.

eucalyptus oil (u″kah-lip′tus) [*eu-* + Gr. *kalyptos* covered] [NF], a volatile oil distilled with steam from the fresh leaf of *Eucalyptus globulus* and other species of *Eucalyptus.* It is used as a flavoring agent and as an expectorant, local antiseptic, and vermifuge.

eucaryote (u-kar′e-ōt) see *eukaryote.*

euchromatin (u-kro′mah-tin) [*eu-* + Gr. *chrōmatos* color + *-in*] areas of chromatin in the interphase nucleus where the chromosomes have uncoiled to the extent that they appear clear by light microscopy, in contrast to the denser heterochromatin. See also *heterochromatin.*

eugenol (u′jĕ-nol) [USP], 4-allyl-2-methoxyphenol, the chief constituent of clove oil; M.W. 164.20. It is also obtained from other natural sources and is used in dentistry as an antiseptic in the repair of cavities.

Euglena a genus of flagellated protozoa that has been extensively studied as representative of the class because of its large size. The organism has a delicate pellicle with spiral thickenings, beneath which a layer of contractile fibrils enables the protozoon to alter its shape. The cytoplasm contains green chloroplasts and a red pigmented eye spot with photoreceptors. A single, whiplike flagellum is attached to the mouth end of the organism near the eye spot, which aids in locomotion.

euglenoid movement (u-gle′noid) a wormlike movement characteristic of many flagellated protozoa and species of the genus *Euglena.* Expansion and contraction of the body, similar to muscle contraction, propels and directs the organism's movement.

euglobulin (u-glob′u-lin) [*eu-* + L. *globulus* globule] any globulin protein that is soluble in salt solution but not in water.

euglobulin lysis test a screening procedure that evaluates systemic fibrinolysis by measuring the time required for a clot to lyse that has been formed from the euglobulin fraction of plasma. The euglobulin fraction prepared by dilution and acid precipitation of plasma contains fibrinogen, clotting factors, fibrinolytic factors, and fibrinolytic activators, but is free of fibrinolytic inhibitors. The normal value for complete lysis of a clot formed by resuspension and subsequent clotting of the euglobulin fraction is 90 min to 6 hr. Lysis in less than 90 min indicates enhanced fibrinolytic activity.

eugonic (u-gon′ik) [*eu-* + Gr. *gonē* seed] growing luxuriantly; the term is used in reference to bacterial cultures, especially species of *Mycobacterium* that produce heavy growth on culture media. Cf. *dysgonic.*

eukaryon (u-kar′e-on) [*eu-* + *karyon* nucleus] 1. a highly organized nucleus surrounded by a nuclear membrane, characteristic of eukaryotes.

2. eukaryote.

eukaryosis (u″kar-e-o′sis) [*eu-* + Gr. *karyon* nucleus + *-osis*] the state of having a true nucleus, the nuclear material being surrounded by a membrane. Cf. *prokaryosis.*

eukaryote (u-kār′e-ōt) [*eu-* + Gr. *karyon* nucleus] an organism whose cells have a true nucleus, i.e., all organisms higher than bacteria (prokaryotes). The differences between eukaryotic and prokaryotic cells are many. Prokaryotes lack membrane-bounded intracellular organelles; eukaryotes have a nucleus bounded by two membranes (the nuclear envelope), as well as endoplasmic reticulum, the Golgi complex, mitochondria, chloroplasts, and lysosomes. The genetic material in prokaryotes is a single loop of double-stranded DNA; in eukaryotes, this material is a complex of double-stranded DNA and histones divided into several chromosomes. Furthermore, in eukaryotes the ribosomes are of the large 80S type, as opposed to the consistently smaller 70S ribosomes of prokaryotes. Eukaryotes also have more complex forms of cell divisions (mitosis and meiosis). See also *cell.*

eukaryotic (u-kar″e-ot′ik) pertaining to a eukaryon or a eukaryote.

Eulenburg's disease (oil′en-burgz) [Albert *Eulenburg,* German neurologist, 1840–1917] see *paramyotonia congenita.*

eumelanin (u-mel′ah-nin) [*eu-* + Gr. *melas* black] a black pigment found in skin and hair. See also *melanin.*

eumycotic mycetoma (u″mi-kot′ik) see under *mycetoma.*

eunuchoidism (u′nŭ-koi″dizm) [Gr. *eunouchos* a castrated person] a deficiency or absence of testicular hormone production, which results in retarded sexual development with persistence of prepubertal characteristics.

euphoria (u-fo′re-ah) [Gr. "the power of bearing easily"] bodily comfort; well-being; absence of pain or distress. In psychiatry, an abnormal or exaggerated sense of well-being particularly common in the manic state. Cf. *dysphoria.*

euploid (u′ploid) [*eu-* + Gr. *-ploos* a fold] referring to a chromosome number (and by extension to the nuclear DNA content) that is exactly one, two, three, or more times the gametic chromosome number.

euploidy (ū-ploi′de) the state of having an exact multiple of the haploid number of chromosomes.

eupnea (ūp-ne′ah) [*eu-* + Gr. *pnein* to breathe] the condition of normal respiration characterized by the coordinated, rhythmic repetition of alternating cycles of active inspiration and passive expiration.

europium (Eu) (u-ro′pe-um) [*Europe*] a soft, silvery, metallic element; atomic number 63; atomic weight 151.96; a 4f transition element (lanthanide or rare earth); oxidation states +2, +3, +4. See also *rare earth elements.*

eurythermal (u″re-ther′mal) [Gr. *eurys* broad, wide + *thermē* heat] in bacteriology, capable of good growth at 28°C, and also at 50°C and above.

eustachianography (u-sta″ke-ah-nog′rah-fe) [*eustachian* + Gr. *graphein* to examine] radiologic examination of the eustachian tubes and the tympanic cavity after the introduction of a water-soluble, iodinated contrast medium by reflux filling during swallowing or by injection through the tympanic membrane. It is used to detect strictures, polyps, and inflammation, and to demonstrate the patency of the eustachian tubes. Also called *tympanography.*

eustachian tube (u-sta′ke-an) [Bartolommeo *Eustachio,* Italian anatomist, 1524–1574] see *auditory tube.*

Eustrongylus (u-stron′jĭ-lus) a genus of nematode parasites of aquatic birds. The species *E. gigas* is now called *Dioctophyma renale.*

eutectic (u-tek′tik) [Gr. *eutēktos* easily melted or dissolved] 1. melting readily; pertaining to a eutectic mixture.

2. the mixture that has the composition indicated as a minimum on the plot of composition versus freezing point: thus, usually the mixture that melts at a lower temperature than any other mixture of the same ingredients in different proportion.

eutectic temperature the melting point of a eutectic mixture.

Eutriatoma (u″trĭ-at′o-mah) a genus of reduviid bugs of which several species are vectors of *Trypanosoma cruzi.* See also *Chagas' disease.*

Eutrombicula (u″trom-bik′u-lah) a genus of mites. See also *chigger.*

E. alfreddugési, the most common species of mites found in the United States that causes chiggers.

eutrophic (u-trof′ik) [*eu-* + Gr. *trophē* nutrition] 1. pertaining to a state of good nutrition.

2. rich in nutrients that promote the growth of particular organisms to the disadvantage of other organisms in the ecosystem, as in lakes with an overgrowth of aerobic photosynthetic organisms. Cf. *oligotrophic.*

eV abbrev. See *electron volt.*

evacuation (e-vak″u-a′shun) [L. *evacuatio,* from *e*

out + *vacuus* empty] withdrawal or removal of material from the body or from a physical system.

evacuation procedures formulated plans for the emergency evacuation of laboratories, which should include a definition of hazardous events for which evacuation may be needed; the conditions in which evacuation is necessary, the methods of alarm transmission, actions to be taken, exit routes, and assembly sites; procedures for accounting for all occupants of the emergency area; and signals for the end of the emergency. Such evacuation procedures should be considered for fires, explosions, spills, leaks, or releases of hazardous materials, and acts of nature such as tornadoes, hurricanes, and floods.

evaporation (e-vap″o-ra′shun) [L. *e* out + *vaporare* to steam] the conversion of a liquid or solid into vapor.

eventration (e″ven-tra′shun) [L. *eventratio* disembowelment, from *e* out + *venter* belly] 1. protrusion of the bowels from the abdomen.

2. removal of the abdominal viscera.

diaphragmatic e., an elevation or bulging of the diaphragm into the thorax. It is due to defective muscularization of the diaphragm in the region of the pleuroperitoneal hiatus.

eversion (e-ver′zhun) 1. a turning outward or inside out.

2. a radiographic position, used to demonstrate the ankle, in which the foot is rotated outward. Cf. *inversion.*

EVM abbrev. See *electronic voltmeter.*

evoked potential (e-vōkd′) a localized electric potential recorded from the brain or spinal cord in response to stimulation of the sensory organs or of some point along the ascending pathway from the sensory organs or within the central nervous system. Characteristics of the potential vary with recording location, stimulus modality and intensity, and level of consciousness or anesthesia.

brain stem auditory e. p. (BAEP), a potential that originates in the subcortical auditory pathways of the brain in response to acoustic stimuli. Because the potential is volume-conducted to the surface of the brain, it can be recorded from an electrode placed on the scalp at the vertex, with a reference electrode on the ear lobe. The electrical activity recorded in this way is filtered, amplified, averaged, and printed out by a plotter for further analysis.

The standard acoustic stimulus used to elicit the BAEP for diagnostic purposes in humans is a series of square-wave clicks (frequency, about 10/sec; amplitude, 60 dB above the individual's hearing threshold) presented to one ear via headphones. The auditory responses of the outer ear are masked by white noise of at least 40 db HL. An average response from several trials (each trial consisting of the averaged responses to 2000–4000 clicks) is recorded. The typical waveform occurring within 10 msec of a click consists of five peaks or waves, each wave representing the sequential activation of a portion of the brain stem auditory pathway.

As shown in the accompanying figure, wave I represents activation of the acoustic nerve (cranial nerve VIII). Wave II represents activation of the cochlear nuclei, and activation of the superior olivary nuclei may be represented by wave III. Waves IV and V may represent activation of the lateral lemnisci and inferior colliculi, respectively. Wave V is the most reliable aspect of the BAEP and is characterized by a positive deflection followed by a large, sharp negative one. In fact, however, the precise origin of these various waves is unclear, and the procedure is best regarded as a simplification without established validity at this time.

The latencies between the waves of the BAEP reflect the conduction velocity between components of the central auditory pathway. For example, wave I to wave III latency is a measure of conduction from the acoustic nerve to pontomedullary regions of the brain; wave III to V latency reflects conduction from pontomedullary regions to the midbrain. When stimulus phase, rate, and intensity are held constant, several nonneurologic factors affect wave amplitude and interwave latency. Interpeak latencies are prolonged by hypothermia (body temperature below 32°C), and in children under 2 yr of age; hyperthermia may have the opposite effect. Damage to the cochlea specifically increases wave I latency. The III–V and I–V latencies are shorter in females than in males, perhaps because of differences in anatomic distances within the auditory pathway.

The BAEP is not altered by most nonspecific central nervous system depressants and is preserved even when spontaneous electroencephalographic activity is absent, as in drug overdose. Because the BAEP is resistant to change in the presence of metabolic factors and drugs, persistence of the BAEP can be used to differentiate coma due to metabolic factors from that due to structural damage. The presence of the BAEP suggests the reversibility of the coma when cephalic reflexes and spontaneous respiration are absent and the electroencephalogram

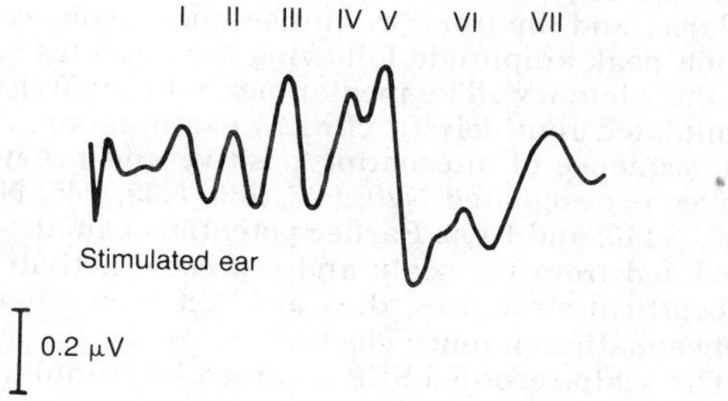

Brain stem auditory evoked potential. **Latency norms for young adults. In this diagram, two independent averages of 2048 responses from the same ear are superimposed to show intertrial reproducibility. (Modified from Stockard, J. J., et al: Nonpathologic factors influencing brainstem auditory evoked potentials. American Journal of EEG Technology *18*:177, 1978.)**

is isopotential. Conversely, the absence of all waves of the BAEP except wave I in these clinical circumstances suggests extensive structural brain stem damage and implies brain death.

An abnormal BAEP in the presence of a clinically identified lesion of the spinal cord or cerebrum suggests the presence of a multiplicity of lesions and supports a diagnosis of multiple sclerosis if this is likely on clinical grounds.

In the absence of clinical signs or radiologic abnormalities, BAEP abnormalities may indicate an infratentorial neoplasm such as an acoustic neuroma. With removal of the tumor and subsequent decompression of the nervous tissue, the BAEP pattern may reverse toward normal. Recently, the BAEP also has been employed in the screening of high-risk infants for sudden infant death syndrome (SIDS) and for hearing impairment.

Also called *auditory evoked potential.* See also *evoked potential.*

scalp-recorded somatosensory e. p., the SEP recorded between one of several electrodes placed on the scalp and a reference electrode placed on the ear, forehead, hand, knee, or some other remote site. The maximal amplitude SEP is usually obtained from the scalp electrode placed over the contralateral somatosensory cortex. The signal is amplified, averaged, and then plotted out with a printer or displayed on an oscilloscope.

The scalp-recorded SEP is characterized by a sequence of positive and negative waves, the latency and amplitude of which vary with the recording site and location of the stimulating electrodes. When comparable stimulus intensities and locations are used, the wave sequence is consistent over several recording sessions and is similar among individuals. The sequence of waves is identified by their polarity and the time (in milliseconds) required to reach peak amplitude following the stimulus (i.e., by their latency). The median nerve in the wrist is stimulated routinely in clinical examination, and the sequence of alternating positive and negative waves is designated N20, P25, P30, N35, P45, N55, P80, N140, and P190. Earlier potentials can also be recorded from the scalp and represent activity in subcortical structures; they are best seen when a noncephalic reference electrode is used.

The scalp-recorded SEP obtained by stimulation of a leg nerve at the knee consists of P34, N44, P55, N74, P98, N126, and P203 msec, respectively; see the accompanying illustration.

The conformation of the SEP depends on the integrity of large, rapidly conducting myelinated axons from joint and cutaneous receptors. The absence of the scalp-recorded SEP or changes in latency or amplitude can be used to locate lesions within the sensory conduction pathways. This is important in the diagnosis of multiple sclerosis, for the scalp-recorded SEP may be abnormal even when a sensory deficit cannot be demonstrated clinically.

When sensory deficits can be demonstrated, changes in the scalp-recorded SEP correspond to the nature and degree of the deficit. For example, if only the responses to pinprick and temperature are diminished, the scalp-recorded SEP is normal. With loss of joint position sense, the scalp-recorded SEP may be abnormal in amplitude and/or latency. With complete spinal cord lesions, no scalp-recorded SEP can be elicited from stimulation of nerves below the lesions. In general, lesions in the sensory pathway between the peripheral nerve and thalamus increase the latency of the scalp-recorded SEP, whereas with lesions of the cortex, the latency to onset of the SEP is normal but amplitude is reduced. Individuals with congenital indifference to pain have scalp-recorded SEPs within the normal range. Enhanced scalp-recorded SEPs can be recorded from certain individuals with myoclonus and epilepsy, those with hyperthyroidism, and children with late-infantile–onset ceroid lipofuscinosis.

The scalp-recorded SEP may be useful in determining the prognosis for recovery of the comatose person in the presence of an isoelectric electroencephalogram. The absence of the SEP correlates with the loss of both cephalic reflexes and intracranial circulation.

Also called cerebral somatosensory evoked potential.

somatosensory e. p. (SEP), a potential recorded from the spinal cord or the cerebral hemispheres

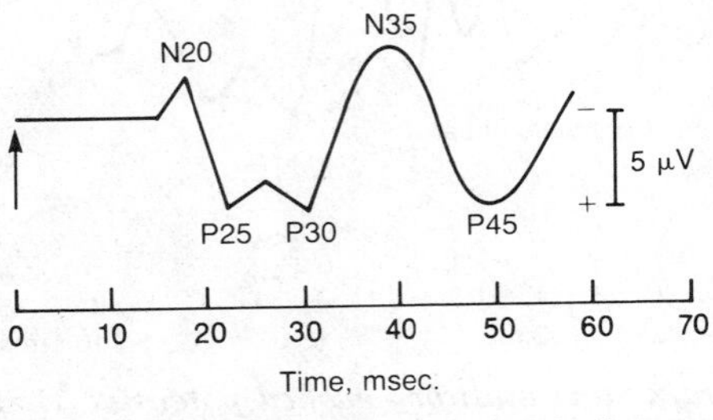

Scalp-recorded somatosensory evoked potential, Figure 1. SEP following medial nerve stimulation at the wrist (the W configuration). (Adapted from Giblin, D. R.: Somatosensory evoked potentials in healthy subjects and in patients with lesions of the nervous system. Annals of the New York Academy of Science *112*:93, 1964.)

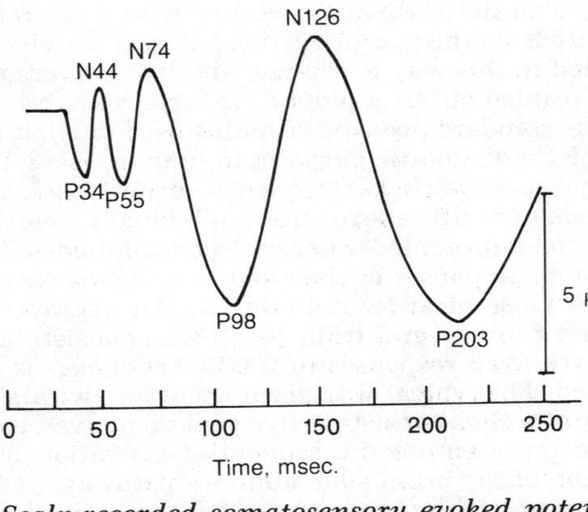

Scalp-recorded somatosensory evoked potential, Figure 2. SEP following lateral popliteal nerve stimulation at the knee. (Adapted from Tsumoto, T., et al.: Analysis of somatosensory evoked potentials to lateral popliteal nerve stimulation in man. Electroencephalography and Clinical Neurophysiology *33*:379, 1972.)

following electrical or mechanical stimulation of a cutaneous or mixed nerve in a limb.

The stimulation parameters for the nerve vary with the experimental or clinical situation. For mechanical stimulation, a brisk tap is delivered to the subject's fingernail or toenail. The quantification and reproducibility of this stimulus is difficult to control. For electrical stimulation, bipolar electrodes (cathode [–] proximal to anode [+]) are placed on or into the skin adjacent to an accessible peripheral nerve—median, radial, plantar, or sural nerve—or on a digit. Square wave pulses of 0.1 msec in duration and about three or four times the sensory threshold are commonly used to stimulate sensory axons in the peripheral nerves, at a rate of 1–2 Hz.

The characteristic waveform of the SEP varies with the recording site and with stimulation parameters. When these are held constant, the components of the SEP are similar among individuals. Deviation in latency or amplitude of the various wave components can be used clinically in the detection, diagnosis, and prognosis of lesions in the peripheral or central sensory conduction pathways of the nervous system.

spinal somatosensory e. p., the SEP recorded from electrodes placed on the skin over the spinal cord or from electrodes placed epidurally or intrathecally. The waveform of the spinal SEP varies with the type of electrode (depth or surface) and with the location on the spinal cord (cervical, thoracic, lumbar areas). Generally, the records obtained from depth electrodes are of higher amplitude and contain fewer electrical artifacts from muscle movements than those from surface electrodes. Depth electrodes, however, cause discomfort to the patient and are potentially hazardous, so in most clinical applications the spinal SEP is recorded from surface electrodes. The spinal SEP recorded from such electrodes following median nerve stimulation at the wrist of a normal adult human is characterized by a series of four negative (surface electrode relative to midfrontal reference electrode) waves of increasing amplitude. Each is designated by the mean latency (in milliseconds) of its peak from the stimulus: N9, N11, N13, and N14 (see the accompanying illustration). These waves of the spinal SEP reflect the conduction of sensory afferent impulses from the periphery, spinal ascending tracts, and brain; N9 is related to activity at the level of the brachial plexus, N11 to activity in the dorsal horn, and N13–14 to activity of the dorsal column nuclei and lemniscal system. The amplitude of the wave components may vary among individuals, but latencies deviate from the norm only in the presence of lesions within the nervous system. Changes in latency in the spinal SEP enable demonstration of nervous system abnormalities in the absence of clinical signs. Also called *cervical somatosensory evoked potential.*

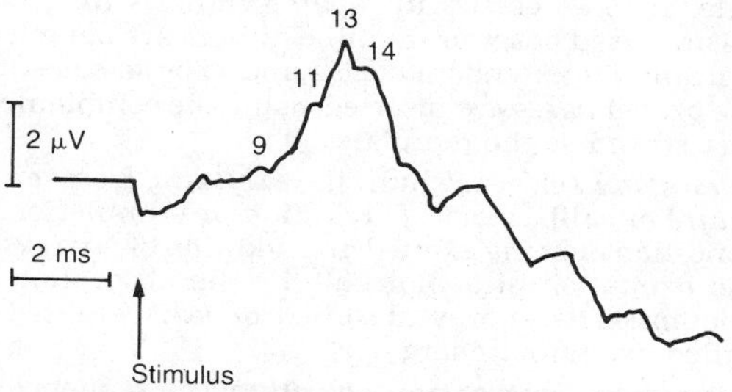

Spinal somatosensory evoked potential. The normal SEP from stimulation of the median nerve at the wrist. (From Matthews, W. B.: The cervical somatosensory evoked potential in diagnosis. *In* Aminoff, M. J. Electrodiagnosis in Clinical Neurology. New York, Churchill Livingstone, 1980.)

visual e. p. (VEP), an electric potential recorded from the occipital cerebral cortex in response to a visual stimulus. This potential represents the summated postsynaptic potentials on cortical cells from fibers projecting from the fovea of the retina, and therefore primarily reflects activity of the cone receptors. The latency of the waveform reflects the conduction velocity of the neural processes that project from the retina to the visual cortex.

For clinical testing of humans, an electrode is placed on the midline of the skull 1–2 cm above the inion. This electrode is referenced to an electrode placed in the midfrontal region or the vertex, or on the earlobe. Unpatterned (flash) or patterned (e.g., checkerboard) stimuli can be used to elicit the response. The potential difference between the recording electrodes is amplified, the response to a specified number of trials is averaged by a computer, and a permanent record of the result is then printed, using a plotter.

The characteristic waveform of the VEP varies with the nature, pattern, intensity, color, and frequency of the stimulus, as well as with the age of the individual, pupil size, and level of light adaptation of the eye. The peak latencies of the various waveform components are less affected by electrode placement and recording artifacts than their amplitudes, and therefore are a useful measure in assessing lesions of the anterior visual pathways resulting from optic neuritis, multiple sclerosis, tumors, and other disorders. Changes in visual evoked potentials may also accompany certain progressive neuronal diseases, including Tay-Sachs, Santavuori, Bielschowsky-Jansky, and Spielmeyer-Vogt diseases.

evolution (ev″o-lu′shun) [L. *evolutio,* from *e-* out + *volvere* to roll] any change in the genetic composition of a population over time, usually described in terms of the population frequencies of the alleles of different genes. Allelic frequencies change in response to four biologic processes: mutation, selection, genetic drift, and migration.

MUTATION. The very existence of allelic alternatives of a gene can be traced to permanent hereditary changes (mutations) in the genetic material. Any conversion of one allele into another by mutation results in a small change in the frequencies of the two allelic forms, but mutations are so rare (less than 0.0001 per gene per generation) that the resulting frequency changes are trivial. Mutation is primarily important in evolution as a mechanism for the generation of new variations.

SELECTION. Some genotypes are better adapted to their environmental circumstances than others. The more adaptive genotypes either have a greater probability of survival to reproductive age, or are more fertile once they reach that age than are less adaptive genotypes. Selection is the differential reproductive contribution of different genotypes and leads to an increase in the frequency of highly adaptive genotypes over time, thus improving the overall adaptiveness of the population. Because environmental circumstances differ from locality to locality, selection favors different genotypes in different populations. The resulting genetic divergence between populations of a single species is known as adaptive radiation.

GENETIC DRIFT. The progeny of one generation are a genetic sample of their parents from the previous generation. This genetic sampling process (reproduction) is subject to sampling error, and the genotypic frequencies of the progeny are generally different from those of their parents. This indeterminacy of allelic frequencies over time is called genetic drift; small populations are particularly susceptible to such drift. All populations experience genetic drift to some degree, and populations tend to diverge randomly over time.

MIGRATION. The physical exchange (migration) of individuals leads to genetic mixing of these populations. Allelic frequencies change as a consequence of the mixing, and gene flow (admixture) tends to reduce the frequency differences between populations. The real importance of migration as an evolutionary force is that it serves to weld the different populations of a single species together.

The evolution of a species is the net result of the variation generating aspects of mutation, the adaptive effects of selection, the random effects of genetic drift, and the cohesive effects of migration. The sum of many small allelic frequency changes (for different genes) is a substantial temporal change in the genetic composition of the population and the species.

Given sufficient time and genetic divergence, two populations may become so different that intermating either no longer occurs or yields no viable offspring. Once this level of genetic radiation has been reached, migration can no longer hold populations together genetically, and the populations have become different species. All living species have evolved from a smaller number of ancestral species, sharing a common genetic heritage. Thus, although the diversity of living organisms is very large, the whole of the biotic world shares a commonality of basic genetic and biochemical information. It is this commonality that allows scientists to extrapolate lessons learned from one organism to another with such facility; the details vary from one organism to another, but the essential principles are the same.

PETER SMOUSE, PH.D.

E wave abbrev. for expectancy wave. See *contingent negative variation.*

Ewing's tumor (u'ingz) [James *Ewing,* U.S. pathologist, 1866–1943] a malignant small cell tumor of bone, of unknown histogenesis. Most patients are under the age of 30. Any bone can be affected, but more than half of these tumors arise in the diaphysis or metaphysis of the long bones of the extremities. Local pain and swelling are the usual symptoms. In the long bones, concentric deposition of layers of subperiosteal bone may produce a distinctive onionskin pattern radiographically. Histologically, the tumor is composed of diffuse sheets of small round cells with uniform cell and nuclear profiles, scanty organelles, and lakes of cytoplasmic glycogen. Zones of necrosis and hemorrhage are common. The prognosis is poor, with a 5-yr survival of less than 20 percent, but improvements are being reported with combinations of radiotherapy and chemotherapy. A soft tissue neoplasm that is morphologically identical to Ewing's tumor of bone has been described.

ex- (eks) [L. *ex,* from Gr. *ex* out, away from] a prefix word element to denote out, away from, or without, e.g., excision.

exa- (E) (ek'sah) a prefix attached to International System (SI) units of measurement to make a unit equal to 1 quintillion of the basic units (10^{18} unit).

examination (ek-sam″ĭ-na'tion) [L. *examinare*] an inspection or investigation, especially as a means of diagnosing disease. The term is qualified according to the methods employed, e.g., physical examination, radiologic examination, cystoscopic examination.

exanthem (ek-san'them) [Gr. *exanthema,* from *exanthein* to break out] 1. a skin eruption.

2. a disease in which eruptions or eruptive fevers occur.

exanthem subitum a presumed viral disease of infants and children that is characterized by an irregular but persistent fever; it usually lasts 3 da, when it peaks and falls, and is followed by an eruptive rash on the trunk. Also called roseola infantum.

exchange (eks-chānj') the substitution of one thing for another. See also *exchange t.* under *transfusion* and *plasma exchange.*

exchangeable mass (eks-chānj'ah-b'l) the mass of a substance in a body compartment, as determined by isotope dilution. It is the activity of the tracer retained in the body (counts injected minus counts excreted) divided by the specific activity of the tracer in a sample (counts per unit mass or per mole of the tracee, the stable, naturally occurring isotope). To emphasize the assumptions behind the measurement, it is sometimes called apparent exchangeable mass.

exchange pairing the synapsis of homologous chromosomes during prophase of meiosis I, which is generally believed to allow genetic recombination (crossing over) to occur. See also *meiosis.*

excipient (ek-sip'e-ent) [L. *excipiens,* from *ex-* + *capere* to take] a more or less inert substance added to a drug preparation to give it the proper consistency or (for a pill) shape. Also called vehicle.

excision (ek-sizh'un) [L. *excisio,* from *ex-* + *caedere* to cut] 1. removal, as of an organ, by cutting.

2. the removal of nucleotides from a DNA molecule, such as occurs in repair synthesis in which mismatched bases or thymine dimers are cut out of a strand by an endonuclease and exonuclease and the proper bases are inserted, using the complementary strand as the template.

excitation (ek″si-ta'shun) [L. *excitatio,* from *ex* + *citare* to call] an act of irritation or stimulation; a condition of being excited; the addition of energy, as the excitation of a molecule by the absorption of photons. The energy absorbed or later emitted is called excitation energy.

excitation contraction coupling the sequence of events through which excitation of the surface membrane (sarcolemma) of a muscle fiber is linked to activation of the contractile process. In mammalian skeletal muscle, the steps involved in this process of electromechanical coupling can be summarized as follows: arrival of an action potential at the motor nerve end-plate triggers a depolarization of the sarcolemma (the muscle action potential) that is conducted in both directions along the membrane away from the end-plate. The action potential is conducted into the depths of the fiber along the sarcotubular system (the transverse tubules and the sarcoplasmic reticulum); depolarization of the lateral sacs of the sarcoplasmic reticulum causes release of calcium ions sequestered within. Binding of the calcium ions to the muscle regulatory protein troponin in turn leads to a change in position of the tropomyosin molecule (another regulatory protein). The molecule can no longer interfere sterically with binding of the cross-bridge heads of the myosin filament to sites on the actin filament. When this binding occurs, a sequential interaction of binding sites produces tension in the cross-bridge linkages formed between the actin and myosin filaments, leading to a sliding of the filaments past one another; the sarcomere (the contractile unit of skeletal muscle) thus shortens (i.e., contracts) slightly. The myosin molecule is detached from the actin by the energy provided from hydrolysis of adenosine triphosphate (ATP) bound to the myosin head. The head can then attach to the next binding site on the actin molecule, producing a new cycle of cross-bridge movement.

Each cross-bridge attaches and detaches many times as it moves along the actin filament during a single contraction. Active transport of calcium ions back into the sarcoplasmic reticulum lowers the level of calcium in the sarcoplasm, allowing troponin to again inhibit the attachment of myosin cross-bridge heads to the actin filament. The muscle can then relax.

See also *skeletal m.* under *muscle.*

excitation spectrum the spectrum of wavelengths at which a fluorescent compound absorbs light, followed by the emission of light at a different wavelength from that of the absorbed light.

excited state an energy level of a system that is higher than the lowest, stable level (the ground state). The system will decay to the ground state and emit the energy difference (excitation energy), usually in the form of one or more photons. Rotational or vibrational excited states of molecules emit infrared photons. Electronic excited states of atoms and molecules emit visible or x-ray photons or Auger electrons. The excited or metastable states of nuclides emit gamma rays and are indicated by the lower case letter m suffixed to the mass number, e.g., ^{99m}Tc.

exclusive OR (EOR or XOR) (eks-kloo′siv) a binary logical operation that is true if, and only if, one but not both of the arguments is true.

excoriation (eks-ko″re-a′shun) [L. *excoriare* to flay, from *ex-* + *corium* skin] a skin lesion appearing as a linear crusted area. It is caused by chronic scratching or picking, and is often found in association with atopic dermatitis. Biopsy of the skin may reveal evidence of the underlying disorder.

excretion (eks-kre′shun) [L. *excretio* sifting, sorting out] the process of removing metabolic waste and end products from the body. Examples are the removal of carbon dioxide via the lungs; the removal of nitrogenous waste, water, and ions by the kidneys, which are eliminated with the urine; and detoxification of drugs and toxins by the liver and their elimination in the bile.

execute (ek′sĕ-kūt) 1. to run a compiled or assembled computer program.

2. (abbrev. EXEC or XEQ), a job control language instruction to the operating system of a computer to run a particular program.

3. to carry out one computer instruction.

execution (ek″sĕ-ku′shun) the performance of a single machine-language instruction or of an entire computer program.

execution time 1. the time required to execute a single instruction, which often takes several machine cycles.

2. pertaining to events that occur while a program is being run, e.g., the assignment of variable values or dynamic storage allocation. Cf. *compile time.*

exergonic reaction (ek″ser-gon′ik) [*ex-* + Gr. *ergon* work] a chemical reaction for which ΔG (Gibbs free-energy change) is negative and free energy is released to the environment in converting reactants to products. The equilibrium constant (K'_{eq}) is greater than 1.0, and the reaction proceeds spontaneously.

exfoliatin (eks-fo″le-a′tin) [*ex-* + L. *folium* leaf] an exotoxin produced by some strains of *Staphylococcus aureus* (phage group II). It is heat-stable and acid-labile. Exfoliatin cleaves the stratum granulosum of the epidermis, causing exfoliative dermatitis, epidermal necrolysis, and impetigo (scalded skin syndrome) in infants and neonates. Also called *epidermolysin.* See also *exotoxins.*

exfoliation (eks-fo″le-a′shun) [L. *exfoliare* to strip of leaves] the falling off or shedding, as of epithelium, in layers or individual cells.

exhalation (eks″hah-la′shun) [L. *exhalatio,* from *ex-* + *halare* to breathe] the act of breathing out; see *expiration.*

exhale (eks-hāl′) [*ex-* + L. *halare* to breathe] to expel air from the lungs; to breathe out. See also *expire.*

exhaust system a system for removing room air and contaminants. The exhaust system for a clinical laboratory should be designed to protect personnel in the laboratory by capturing released contaminants, to provide the necessary air supply to the laboratory (by providing air to be exhausted) in a manner that does not interfere with the performance of laboratory hoods and local exhaust ventilation, to prevent the recirculation or spread of odors or potential contaminants, and to disperse the exhaust above the roof and away from air intake systems.

existence proof (eg-zis′tens) in mathematics, a proof that does not give an explicit method of solving a problem. It merely demonstrates that a solution must exist, because otherwise a contradiction would be implied. Cf. *constructive proof.*

exit 1. the portion of a means of egress that provides a protected way of travel to the exit discharge. An exit is required to be separated from all other spaces of the building or structure by fire-resistant construction and approved self-closing fire doors. In most multistory buildings, exits consist of enclosed stairwells.

2. the instruction or programing technique that leaves a loop in a computer program, or that terminates the program and returns control to the operating system (also called stop or end).

exit access the portion of a means of egress that

leads to an exit. In most buildings the corridors provide the exit access.

exit discharge the portion of a means of egress between the termination of an exit and a public way. The exit discharge may include yards, courts, open spaces, or other passageways from the exit to a public way.

exo- (ek′so) [Gr. *exō* outside] a prefix word element to denote outside or outward, e.g., exogenous.

exocellular (eks″o-sel′u-lar) external to the cell membrane, yet still attached, e.g., flagella, capsule.

exocervix (ek″so-ser′viks) [*exo-* + L. *cervix* neck] the region of the uterine cervix that is adjacent to the vagina, is external to the cervical canal, and is covered by stratified squamous epithelium.

exocrine (ek′so-krin) [*exo-* + Gr. *krinein* to separate] 1. secreting outwardly via a duct. Cf. *endocrine.*
2. denoting such a gland or its secretion.

exocytosis (eks″o-si-to′sis) [*exo-* + Gr. *kytos* hollow vessel + *-osis* condition] 1. the expulsion of material from the inside of a cell to the outside of that cell. This usually occurs by the combining membrane of a vacuole with the cell membrane; the resulting fused membranes reform the cell membrane with the material to be eliminated outside of the cell. Cf. *endocytosis.*
2. the process of leukocyte aggregation in the epidermis during the inflammatory process.

exodus (ek′sŏ-dus) [Gr. *exodos* a going out] the appearance of endometrial cells with small mononuclear phagocytes in cytologic preparations at the fifth day of the menstrual cycle or later.

exoenzyme (ek″so-en′zīm) an enzyme that acts outside the cell that secretes it.

exogenote (ek″so-je′nōt) in bacterial genetics, a bacterial chromosome fragment transferred in transduction or conjugation. See also *merozygote.* Cf. *endogenote* and *heterogenote.*

exogenous (eks-oj′ĕ-nus) [*exo-* + Gr. *gennan* to produce] 1. developed or originating outside an organism; caused by external factors.
2. growing by addition to the outer surface. Cf. *endogenous.*

exogenous bacterium in bacterial disease, a bacterium acquired from a source external to the body, usually the environment. Cf. *endogenous bacterium.*

exogenous variable in a mathematical model, one of the independent variables, the values of which are determined by observation, experiment, or other considerations outside the model. Cf. *endogenous variable.*

exon (ek′son) a coding sequence of DNA, i.e., a section of a chromosome that codes for the section of the final mRNA that is translated into a polypeptide sequence.

In eukaryotes, most genes are composed of exons separated by intervening sequences (introns) of DNA. The whole gene is transcribed as a precursor RNA. Then, in posttranscription processing, the introns are excised and the exons spliced together to make a final mRNA that is translated into a polypeptide sequence.

exonuclease (ek″so-nu′kle-ās) a general name for several enzymes of the hydrolase class (EC 3.1.11, 13, 14, 15, and 16) that catalyze the hydrolytic cleavage of single nucleotide residues from only the end of the deoxyribo- or ribopolynucleotide chains. These enzymes can be contrasted to endonucleases, which cleave polynucleotides at positions within the chain. They are important in the catabolism, maintenance, and repair of nucleic acids. These enzymes have been used in the sequence determination of polynucleotides. Exonuclease activity has also been found in the *Escherichia coli* DNA polymerase I, which catalyzes the addition of nucleotide units to the free 3′-hydroxyl terminus of the primer DNA chain. Examples are *exodeoxyribonuclease I* (EC 3.1.11.1), *ribonuclease II* (EC 3.1.13.1), and *spleen exonuclease* (EC 3.1.16.1).

exopeptidase (ek″so-pep′tĭ-dās) a general name for a proteolytic enzyme that catalyzes the hydrolysis of terminal peptide linkages in a polypeptide chain, thus releasing free amino acids. See also the specific enzyme, e.g., *aminopeptidase, carboxypeptidase,* and *prolidase.*

Exophiala (ek-sof″e-al′ah) a genus of dematiacious fungi whose species are often found in association with mycetoma, tinea nigra, and phaeohyphomycosis.

E. jeanselmei, a species that causes actinomycotic mycetoma (maduromycosis) of the extremities, which is characterized by small abscesses in the subcutaneous tissue. The infection can extend from bone to skin surface, where the orifice may have elevated collars of tissue. The colony morphology initially appears mucoid and dark; with time, a gray-black mycelium develops with a black pigment on the reverse side. Clinical diagnosis is made from mycotic culture and observation of black, worm-shaped grains in pus taken from draining fistulas.

exophthalmos (ek″sof-thal′mos) [*ex-* + Gr. *ophthalmos* eye] an abnormal degree of protrusion of the eyeball, seen in Graves' disease and to a mild degree in Cushing's syndrome and cirrhosis. It appears to be due to infiltration of the orbital soft tissues by inflammatory cells, fluid, and mucopolysaccharides. Persons affected have cell-mediated immunity to orbital antigens; it is postulated that thyroglobulin may bind to extraocular muscle and in turn bind antithyroglobulin antibodies, setting up an immunologic reaction. Usually the process is self-limiting. Severe progressive (malignant) exophthalmos occurs in approximately 2 percent of those with Graves' disease.

exophytic (ek″so-fit′ik) [*exo-* + Gr. *phyein* to grow] growing outward.

exophytic growth a protruding type of lesion that is elevated above the surface of the surrounding, uninvolved tissue.

exoribonuclease (ek″so-ri″bo-nu′kle-ās) a general name for several enzymes of the hydrolase class (EC 3.1.13, 14, 15, and 16) that catalyze the hydrolysis of terminal bonds of ribonucleic acid strands, yielding mononucleotides.

exosmosis (ek″sos-mo′sis) [*ex-* + Gr. *ōsmos* impulsion] osmosis from within (the cell, vessel, or organ being described) to without. Cf. *endosmosis.*

exostosis (ek″sos-to′sis) [*ex-* + Gr. *osteon* bone] an abnormal bony protuberance.

exothermic (ek″so-ther′mik) [*exo-* + Gr. *thermē* heat] giving up or producing heat, as a chemical reaction. Cf. *endothermic.*

exotoxins (ek″so-tok′sinz) [*exo-* + L. *toxicum* poison] toxic proteins excreted by gram-positive and gram-negative bacteria. Bacterial toxins are divided into two types: exotoxins, which are released by bacterial cells into body tissue, and endotoxins, which are present in the membranes of some gram-negative bacteria and are released only by cell lysis. Toxins play an important role in the pathogenicity of an organism. Exotoxins of bacteria such as *Corynebacterium diphtheriae, Clostridium tetani, C. botulinum,* and *Shigella dysenteriae* are among the most powerful poisons known.

The production of exotoxins enables an organism to produce disease without spreading or multiplying extensively, as organs and tissues can be affected at a distance from the site of infection. Some exotoxins exhibit specificity toward particular cell types or tissues and cause clinical signs and symptoms characteristic of damage to that tissue: e.g., neurotoxins, which affect cells of the central nervous system (botulinum toxin, tetanospasmin), and enterotoxins, which affect cells of the gastrointestinal tract. In contrast, other toxins such as diphtheria toxin appear to act on a number of different types of tissues and can produce a variety of pathologic effects.

PRINCIPAL EXOTOXINS. The most important exotoxins and the bacteria that produce them are described below, and their effects are listed in the accompanying table.

Bacillus anthracis. The primary target of anthrax toxin activity is still unknown. The anthrax exotoxin produces edema in guinea pigs or rabbits following subcutaneous injection and is lethal in mice following intravenous injection. Almost all *B. anthracis* strains produce toxin. In vitro, toxin production is dependent on cell density and the presence of bicarbonate ions. The toxin consists of three heat-labile, antigenically distinct components: edema factor (factor I), essential for edema production; protective antigen (factor II), which stimulates production of protective antibody; and lethal factor (factor III), essential for lethality. Factors I and II together are necessary for edema production, and factors II and III together are necessary for lethality.

Bacillus cereus. There are two clinical forms of self-limited *B. cereus* food poisoning: diarrheal and emetic, which are mediated by two different, heat-stable enterotoxins. The emetic (short-incubation) form has been associated with the ingestion of contaminated fried rice, and the diarrheal (long-incubation) form has been associated with meats and vegetables contaminated with preformed toxin.

Bordetella pertussis. B. pertussis produces a heat-labile toxin that is dermonecrotic in rabbits and lethal for mice. The toxin is released upon lysis of the bacterial cell. The toxin's role in the pathogenesis of whooping cough has not been well defined.

Clostridium botulinum. Botulinum toxin is an exotoxin produced by germinating spores and growing vegetative cells of *C. botulinum.* The thermolabile neurotoxin (inactivated in 10 min at 100°C) is not inactivated by gastric acid or proteolytic enzymes of the stomach and upper GI tract, but rather is absorbed from the GI tract into the blood stream, where it travels to neuromuscular junctions and to peripheral autonomic synapses. There, the toxin binds to the presynaptic terminals, blocking the release of the neurotransmitter acetylcholine from nerve endings. This results in a decrease of skeletal muscle function, which may progress to paralysis, respiratory failure, and cardiac arrest.

There are seven immunologically distinct forms of botulinum toxin (A–G). In the United States, type A neurotoxin causes 62 percent of all cases of botulism; type B, 28 percent; and type E, 10 percent. Types A and B are associated with uncooked meats or improperly canned vegetables, and type E with seafood. Infant botulism appears to be primarily due to types A and B neurotoxins.

Type A botulinum toxin is a protein (M.W. 900,000) consisting of a neurotoxin (M.W. 150,000), a hemagglutinin, and a nontoxic portion. With some toxin types, activation by a proteolytic enzyme is required. The binding of toxin to the nerve cell membrane receptor is partially susceptible to antitoxin inactivation. Once the toxin moves into the cell, it becomes resistant to inactivation by antitoxin.

In some strains, the production of botulinum toxin is dependent on the presence of a prophage. The toxin is one of the most potent biologic toxins known: 1 μg constitutes a lethal dose for 200,000 mice and may be close to the fatal human dose.

Botulinum toxin may be demonstrated in food, serum, feces, gastric contents, or vomitus in individuals with food-borne botulism, and in the feces or intestinal contents of infants with infant botulism. Honey containing *C. botulinum* spores has been implicated in some cases. Home-canned foods contaminated with spores have been implicated as a source of most outbreaks of botulism. Boiling of improperly processed or canned foods for at least 10 min destroys the toxin.

Clostridium difficile. The *C. difficile* organism produces an exotoxin that causes a severe, necrotizing disease of the large intestine called pseudomembranous colitis. The disease usually occurs in association with antibiotic therapy, although toxin has been detected in stools of patients without a previous antibiotic history. The protein toxin, which is heat-labile and acid-sensitive, causes severe colitis when injected into the cecum of hamsters. Neither its molecular structure nor its mode of action has been determined. The toxin may be detected in stool supernatants of persons with suspected pseudomembranous colitis by tissue culture or counterimmunoelectrophoresis.

Clostridium perfringens. A number of exotoxins active against tissues have been produced by *C. perfringens.* This organism is classified into five types (A–E) on the basis of neutralization of toxins by antisera. Type A is involved in most human disease. Alpha toxin is a lethal, necrotizing lecithinase (phospholipase C) that splits lecithin in cell membranes into phosphorylcholine and diglyceride. Alpha toxin has been associated with gas gangrene; it is hemolytic and causes widespread capillary damage. Other species of *Clostridium* that can cause gas gangrene produce toxins similar to those of *C. perfringens.*

C. perfringens type C has been implicated in enteritis necroticans, a severe necrotizing disease of the small intestine. The beta toxin appears to be a major pathogenic factor.

Certain strains of *C. perfringens* cause diarrheal disease, which is mediated by a heat-labile protein enterotoxin (M.W. 34,000), with type A accounting for most cases. Inadequately cooked and improperly stored meats serve as a source of *C. perfringens.* The

EXOTOXINS. EFFECTS OF EXOTOXIN-PRODUCING BACTERIA

ORGANISM	DISEASE	TOXIN	ACTIVITY
Bacillus			
B. anthracis	Anthrax	Anthrax	Lethal, edema-producing
B. cereus	Food poisoning	Two types of enterotoxin	Emetic or diarrheagenic
Bordetella pertussis	Whooping cough	Whooping cough	Lethal, dermonecrotic
Clostridium			
C. botulinum	Botulism	Botulinum (7 type-specific neurotoxins)	Paralytic
C. difficile	Pseudomembranous colitis	*C. difficile*	Necrotizing, diarrheagenic
C. perfringens	Gas gangrene	Alpha	Lecithinase, necrotizing, hemolytic
		Beta	Lethal, necrotizing
		Gamma	Lethal
		Delta	Lethal
		Epsilon	Lethal, necrotizing
		Eta	Lethal
		Iota	Lethal, necrotizing
		Theta	Lethal, hemolytic, cardiotoxic
		Kappa	Lethal, proteolytic (collagenase)
		Lambda	Proteolytic
		Mu	Hyaluronidase (spreading factor)
	Food poisoning	Enterotoxin	Diarrheagenic
	Enteritis necroticans	Beta	Lethal, necrotizing
C. tetani	Tetanus	Tetanospasmin	Lethal, neurotoxic (spastic)
		Tetanolysin	Hemolytic, cardiotoxic
Corynebacterium diphtheriae	Diphtheria	Diphtheria toxin (Shick toxin)	Lethal, dermonecrotic protein synthesis inhibition
Escherichia coli	Gastroenteritis	Enterotoxin	Diarrheagenic
Pseudomonas aeruginosa	Pyogenic infections	Exotoxin A	Lethal
Staphylococcus aureus	Pyogenic infections	Alpha hemolysin	Lethal, necrotizing, hemolytic
		Beta hemolysin	Lethal, leukocidic, hemolytic
		Gamma hemolysin	Necrotizing, hemolytic
		Delta hemolysin	Lethal, hemolytic, leukolytic
		Leukocidin	Leukocidic
	Exfoliative dermatitis	Exfoliatin	Epidermolytic
	Toxic shock syndrome	Not defined at present	Not defined at present
	Food poisoning	Enterotoxin	Emetic
Streptococcus pyogenes	Pyogenic infections	Streptolysin O	Lethal, cardiotoxic, hemolytic
		Streptolysin S	Lethal, hemolytic
	Scarlet fever	Erythrogenic toxin (Dick toxin)	Erythrogenic
Vibrio			
V. cholerae	Cholera	Enterotoxin (choleragen)	Diarrheagenic
V. parahemolyticus	Gastroenteritis	Enterotoxin	Diarrheagenic
Salmonella species	Gastroenteritis	Enterotoxin	Diarrheagenic
Shigella dysenteriae type 1 (Shiga)	Bacillary dysentery	Neurotoxin	Lethal, paralytic
Yersinia			
Y. enterocolitica	Gastroenteritis	Enterotoxin	Diarrheagenic
Y. pestis	Plague	Murine	Lethal

toxin is released in the intestine, inhibiting glucose transport and causing protein loss from the intestine. Gastrointestinal disease is self-limited.

Clostridium tetani. Tetanospasmin is a highly potent neurotoxin elaborated by germinating spores of *C. tetani.* The toxin is produced as a single polypeptide chain consisting of two subunits, alpha and beta. Although there are several different antigenic types of *C. tetani,* there is only one immunotype of tetanospasmin. It is this toxin that is responsible for the clinical manifestations of tetanus; thus, immunity to the disease is achieved only with antibody to the neurotoxin.

The toxin is produced in an infected wound but acts on the central nervous system. It is unclear whether tetanospasmin travels retrogradely along axons in the peripheral nerves or via the blood stream. Once the toxin reaches the spinal cord, it accumulates in the cell bodies and dendrites of motor neurons, migrates transsynaptically, and the beta-chain subunit of the toxin binds to a ganglioside on a synaptosome membrane. Tetanus toxoid when mixed with brain emulsion prevents tetanospasmin activity by inhibiting the binding of toxin to ganglioside.

Once bound, tetanospasmin prevents the release of the inhibitory transmitters glycine and GABA, which mediate the normal inhibitory regulation of spinal motor neurons. This results in the muscular spasms characteristic of tetanus. The alpha subunit has no known effect on enzymatic reactions within the nerve cells.

Tetanolysin, an oxygen-labile hemolysin, is not known to play a significant role in human disease.

Corynebacterium diphtheriae. Diphtheria toxin is produced by strains of *C. diphtheriae* infected with a temperate bacteriophage, the genome of which contains the *tox* gene, coding for the synthesis of diphtheria toxin. Toxin production by *C. diphtheriae* is regulated by the concentration of Fe^{++} ions. The exotoxin (M.W. 60,000) is secreted as a single polypeptide chain. Proteolysis and reduction of a disulfide bond results in separation into two fragments, A (M.W. 31,000), which has enzyme activity, and B (M.W. 38,000), which is essential for binding of fragment A to the membranes of susceptible cells. Fragment B also facilitates the entrance of fragment A into the cell, in which fragment A exerts its activity. Fragment A inhibits protein synthesis in eukaryotic cells by inactivating the elongation factor 2 required for translocation of polypeptidyl-tRNA from acceptor to donor site on the eukaryotic ribosome.

All laboratory isolates of *C. diphtheriae* are tested for toxin production by in vitro (Elek immunodiffusion) or in vivo (guinea pig lethality) tests. In vivo tests are more reliable, although not as rapid as the Elek test.

Escherichia coli. Some strains of *E. coli* possess a plasmid that codes for the production of an enterotoxin. Strains producing enterotoxin are responsible for diarrheal disease in developing countries, for traveler's diarrhea, and for outbreaks of diarrheal disease. There are two forms of enterotoxin: heat-stable and heat-labile. Strains may produce one or the other or both types of toxin. Heat-labile toxin is similar to cholera toxin in its mechanism of action in the intestine (i.e., stimulation of adenylcyclase and serologic specificity) (see *V. cholerae* below). Production of cyclic AMP is stimulated in cells of the small intestine, resulting in an outpouring of fluid containing ions into the intestinal lumen.

Heat-stable toxin has a smaller molecular weight (M.W. 4000–5000), is poorly antigenic, and stimulates guanyl cyclase. Illnesses due to heat-stable or heat-labile toxins do not appear to differ clinically. Heat-labile toxin may be asssayed by sensitive but expensive cell culture techniques (Y-1 adrenal or Chinese hamster ovary cells). Assay of heat-stable toxin is carried out by a rabbit ileal loop preparation or injection into the stomach of the infant mouse. Such techniques are not routinely performed in clinical microbiology laboratories.

Pseudomonas aeruginosa. Exotoxin A (M.W. 50,000–55,000) is a potent, heat-labile toxin produced by more than 87 percent of clinical isolates. It plays an important role in the pathogenesis of *P. aeruginosa* infections and is more potent than *P. aeruginosa* endotoxin. The LD_{50} of exotoxin A in mice is about 0.1 μg.

Exotoxin A inhibits protein synthesis by inactivating elongation factor 2, in a manner similar to that of diphtheria toxin (see *C. diphtheriae* above). Diphtheria toxin and exotoxin A appear to bind to different cell membrane receptors and are antigenically different. Like diphtheria toxin, iron concentrations regulate toxin production by the organism. Exotoxin A is produced as a single polypeptide chain and is subsequently cleaved by proteases to yield an enzymatically active molecule. The entire molecule is required for binding to susceptible cell membranes.

Salmonella Species. Salmonella species have been reported to produce enterotoxins, but additional study is required to define the mechanism of pathogenesis of disease caused by these species.

Shigella Species. Enteroinvasiveness is probably the major factor in the pathogenesis of shigellosis, and endotoxin also plays a role in bacillary dysentery. One species, *Shigella dysenteriae* type 1 (Shiga bacillus), produces a neurotoxin that causes paralysis and death in mice and rabbits. The toxin causes hemorrhages in the spinal cord of the rabbit, leading to edema, which exerts pressure on the nerves. It was found recently that a purified preparation was cytotoxic to various mammalian cells, and also that it exhibited enterotoxin activity.

Staphylococcus aureus. S. aureus produces four chemically and serologically distinct hemolysins —alpha, beta, gamma, and delta—differing in erythrocyte specificity and mechanism of action. Hemolysins may damage cells other than erythrocytes. Alpha hemolysin (M.W. 33,000) causes ion leakage from artificial membranes. It is dermonecrotic after local injection in laboratory animals and is lethal when given systemically. Beta-hemolysin sphingomyelinase C (M.W. 30,000) is cytotoxic for a variety of tissue cells. Leukocidin causes degranulation of polymorphonuclear leukocytes and macrophages.

Exfoliatin (epidermolytic toxin or epidermolysin) is produced, probably with plasmid gene control, by about 5 percent of *S. aureus* isolates, mostly of phage group II. It is a heat-stable protein (M.W. 24,000) and is responsible for exfoliative dermatitis, or scalded skin syndrome, particularly in very young infants. The toxin cleaves cells of the stratum granulosum of the epidermis.

About 50 percent of *S. aureus* strains produce one of five serologically distinct (A–E), heat-stable enterotoxins (M.W. 25,000–30,000). The toxins cause emesis, sensory emetic stimuli reaching the brain's vomiting center via the vagus and sympathetic nerves. The mechanism whereby diarrhea is produced has not been established. Enterotoxin B has been associated with pseudomembranous colitis.

Streptococcus pyogenes. S. pyogenes yields a number of extracellular products (see *Streptococcus*) including two distinct hemolysins, streptolysin S and streptolysin O. Oxygen-labile, immunogenic streptolysin O is produced by most strains of *S. pyogenes.* It is toxic to a variety of cell types, including erythrocytes, polymorphonuclear leukocytes, and platelets. Streptolysin O causes lysis of lysosomes in leukocyte fractions, and is cardiotoxic when injected intravenously into laboratory animals. Streptolysin S, like streptolysin O, damages the membranes of a variety of cell types.

Erythrogenic toxin is responsible for the rash of scarlet fever; strains producing the toxin are lysogenic. Three immunologically distinct forms exist. The mode of action of the toxin has not been well defined. The presence of protective antitoxin in the serum of patients can be determined by the Dick test.

Vibrio cholerae. Cholera toxin (choleragen) is a protein enterotoxin (M.W. 84,000) consisting of three subunits: B (M.W. 11,000), A1 (M.W. 24,000), and A2 (M.W. 5000). Each toxin molecule contains one each of the A subunits, connected by a disulfide bond, and five B subunits. The B subunits, collectively called choleragenoid, do not stimulate adenylcyclase but are responsible for binding to a cell membrane receptor, monosialoganglioside, G_{m1}. The A1 subunit is responsible for stimulation of the adenylcyclase system, located on the inner surface of the cell membrane, and subsequent hypersecretion of chloride and bicarbonate G_{m1} ions.

Cholera enterotoxin is closely related to the heat-labile enterotoxin of *E. coli.* Both bind to G_{m1} ganglioside, possess similar A1 subunits, and require NAD for adenylcyclase activation. Unlike the *E. coli* enterotoxin, however, the toxigenicity of *V. cholerae* is determined by a chromosomal, not a plasmid, gene. Cholera antitoxin neutralizes *E. coli*–labile toxin, but *E. coli* antitoxin does not neutralize cholera toxin.

V. cholerae non-O group 1 (formerly called noncholera vibrios or nonagglutinating vibrios) produce a disease similar to cholera by producing choleralike enterotoxins, whereas *V. parahemolyticus* produces a heat-stable enterotoxin that is hemolytic and cardiotoxic and that causes accumulation of fluid in the rabbit ileal loop.

Yersinia Species. Y. enterocolitica appears to produce a heat-stable enterotoxin. The exotoxin produced by *Y. pestis* is cardiotoxic in mice, but the significance of the toxin to human disease is unclear.

See also the specific genus and species entries for information relating to other characteristics of these exotoxins.

exp symbol. See *exponential function.*

expectancy (E) wave (ek-spek′tan-se) see *contingent negative variation.*

expectation (ek″spek-ta′shun) [L. *expectare,* from *ex-* + *spectare* to look at] the mean value of a random variable. See also *mean.*

experiment (ek-sper′ĭ-ment) [L. *experimentum* proof from experience] a scientific procedure performed to test a hypothesis, acquire new data, or to investigate the behavior of some natural processes.

expiration (ek″spĭ-ra′shun) [*ex-* + L. *spirare* to breathe] 1. death or termination.

2. the act of expelling air from the lungs, or breathing out; exhalation. The expiration that follows normal spontaneous inspiration is a passive process resulting from recoil of the elastic tissues of the lungs and thorax: the thoracic cage and lungs are returned to midposition, the pressure of the alveolar gas increases above atmospheric, and air flows outward along the resulting pressure gradient to the mouth.

In forced expiration, contraction of the expiratory muscles (abdominal and internal intercostal muscles) further decreases the intrathoracic volume to the residual volume level.

Cf. *inspiration.*

expiratory (ek-spi′rah-tor″e, eks′pĭ-rah-tor″e) pertaining to or occurring during expiration.

expiratory reserve volume (ERV) the maximal volume of gas that can be forcibly expelled after a normal tidal expiration (from any end-tidal expiratory level), normally amounting to 800–1200 ml in the young adult.

expire (ek-spīr′) 1. to breathe out; to exhale.

2. to die or terminate.

explode (eks-plōd′) [L. *explodere,* from *ex* out + *plaudere* to clap the hands] to release energy in an explosion; to cause an explosion to occur.

exploded view (eks-plōd′ed) in mechanical drawing or computer graphics, a drawing of a piece of equipment in which the parts are separated but have the same spatial relationship and orientation as in the assembled piece of equipment.

explosion (eks-plo′zhun) a chemical or nuclear reaction that releases a large amount of energy in a very short time, producing a high temperature and often a large volume of gas and a shock wave.

explosion-proof an inexact but commonly used term to describe an enclosure for electrical equipment especially constructed to fulfill three requirements: (1) it does not become hot enough to ignite surrounding gases or vapors, (2) it can withstand an internal explosion of flammable vapors or gases, and (3) it has joints to prevent the propagation of flame hot enough to ignite surrounding gases or vapors.

It should be noted that different gas and vapor-air mixtures vary considerably in their ignition temperatures, the pressures they develop during explosion, and the propagation of their flames through joints in equipment, conduit, and junction boxes, so that equipment that is explosion-proof for one material may not be for another. For example, a refrigerator that is explosion-proof for the storage of ethyl ether (equipment rated for hazardous locations containing Class 1, Group C atmospheres) is not safe or acceptable in acetylene or hydrogen atmospheres (Group A or B atmospheres).

The NFPA (National Fire Protection Association) does not require use of explosion-proof electrical equipment in laboratories that use chemicals. Under some conditions of extraordinary hazard (such as large-volume extraction or distillation operations), it may be necessary to classify a laboratory or a part thereof as a hazardous location for the purpose of designating suitable electrical installations. Such hazardous locations requiring classified electrical equipment (commonly referred to as explosion-proof) would be temperature-controlled storage compartments for flammable liquids and stirrer motors exposed to flammable concentrations of combustible vapors.

explosive (eks-plo′siv) [L. *explosus,* from *ex-* + *plaudere* to clap the hands] a substance that, on ignition by heat, impact, friction, or detonation, undergoes very rapid combustion and produces heat, forming gases that exert tremendous pressure as they expand. The term is used in codes and regulations to describe compounds designed to function by explosion, such as dynamite, mercury fulminate, and lead azide. Although a number of compounds used or produced in clinical laboratories can explode (e.g., magnesium perchlorate, picric acid, copper azide in drain lines, and flammable gases and vapors), use of the term is generally limited to commercial explosives.

explosive atmosphere air mixed with dust or inflammable gases or vapors in concentrations that are capable of exploding.

explosive limits see *flammable limits.*

explosive material as used in codes and regulations, a term that includes explosives (compounds designed to function by explosion), blasting agents, and propellants.

exponent (eks′po-nent) the power to which a number is raised; denoted by a superscript, e.g., x^2.

exponential decay (eks″po-nen′shal) the decay or damping out of some quantity that declines as an exponential function of the time.

exponential function the mathematical function describing a variable that changes at a rate equal to its value; denoted e^x or exp x. For example, the fraction of the original amount of radioisotope remaining after a period of time, t, is $e^{-\lambda t}$, where λ is the fraction disintegrating per unit time.

exposure (ek-spo′zhur) 1. the act of laying open, as in surgical exposure.

2. the condition or process of being subjected to something, such as infectious agents or radiation.

3. the projection of light or other radiation onto photographic materials.

4. photographic film that is exposed but not developed.

5. in photography, the length of time that film is exposed to light.

6. in radiography, the product of intensity of x-rays and the time the film is exposed (usually in milliampere-seconds, mAs).

7. the amount of radiation (in roentgens) at a certain point. Also called exposure dose.

exposure angle in body-section radiography, the angle through which the x-ray tube and film move during the exposure. See also *tomography.* Cf. *operative angle.*

exposure switch the switch on an x-ray apparatus that initiates a radiograph.

exposure values the settings that control radiographic density; kilovoltage (tube voltage), milliamperage (tube current), and exposure time. See also *tube-rating chart.*

expressivity (ek″spres-iv′ĭ-te) the extent to which a gene is expressed or is apparent in the phenotype. It is usually variable in dominant disorders. Cf. *penetrance.*

exsanguination (eks-sang″wĭ-na′shun) [*ex-* + L. *sanguis* blood] the loss or removal of much of the blood supply of an individual, leading to tissue hypoxia that may be life-threatening or fatal.

exsiccant (ek-sik′ant) 1. desiccant, an agent used to remove moisture.

2. an agent capable of depriving crystalline substances of their water of hydration.

exsiccate (ek′sĭ-kāt) [L. *exsiccare,* from *ex-* + *siccus* dry] the removal of moisture by a drying agent. Also called *desiccate;* see *desiccator.*

exsiccation (ek″sĭ-ka′shun) the act of drying; in chemistry, depriving a crystalline substance of its water for crystallization.

Extended Binary Coded Decimal Interchange Code see *EBCDIC.*

extension (ek-sten′shun) [L. *extensio*] the act of straightening a joint so that the angle made by the bones becomes less acute; the condition of having been extended. Cf. *flexion.*

extensor (ek-sten′sor) [L.] [NA], a general term for any muscle that extends a joint.

external (ek-ster′nal) [L. *externus* outside] pertaining to or located on the outside; affecting only the outside.

external ear the portion of the ear consisting of the outer appendage (auricle) and a narrow passage (external auditory meatus). The external ear channels and conducts sound waves from the exterior to the middle ear.

external occipital protuberance the protuberance at the center of the outer surface of the occipital bone found at the lower rear of the skull. The point of this protuberance is called the *inion.*

external rotation in referring to the humerus, the turning of the arm so that the palm faces first to the front and then to the outside, a radiographic position used to demonstrate the shoulder. Cf. *internal rotation.*

exteroceptor (ek″ster-o-sep′tor) a sensory nerve ending that receives information from the skin or mucous membranes. Cf. *interoceptor, proprioceptor,* and *receptor.*

extinction (ek-sting′shun) 1. in genetics, inhibition of the expression of differentiated properties in hybrid cells from differentiated and undifferentiated parental cells. See also *hybrid c.* under *cell.*

2. see *absorbance.*

extinction coefficient 1. that dilution of an antibody at which its specific activity is no longer manifest.

2. in spectrophotometry, an obsolete term for *absorptivity.*

extra- (ek′strah) [L. *extra* outside, above, beyond] a prefix word element to denote outside of, e.g., extracellular, or additional, e.g., extrasystole.

extracellular (ek″strah-sel′u-lar) outside the cell; external to the cell wall, e.g., extracellular enzymes.

extracellular fluid (ECF) the body fluids that are outside the cells of the body. They include the plasma, interstitial fluid, fluid in the gastrointestinal tract and potential spaces of the body, and the cerebrospinal and intraocular fluids. See *body flu-*

ids for compositional and volume data. See also *electrolyte balance and homeostasis.*

extracerebral potential (ek″strah-ser′ĕ-bral) in electroencephalography, any electric potential not originating from the brain. See also *artifact.*

extract [L. *extractum*] 1. (eks′trakt), a concentrated preparation obtained by removing the active constituents from a crude product or sample with a suitable solvent, evaporating all or nearly all the solvent, and adjusting the resulting mass to a prescribed standard.

2. (ek-strakt′), to withdraw or remove; to prepare an extract.

extractable nuclear antigen (ENA) (ek-strakt′-ah-b′l) a preparation of nucleic acid to which patients with mixed connective tissue disease (MCTD) show a high titer of antibody. These antibodies are usually detected by passive hemagglutination of ENA-coated red cells.

extraction (ek-strak′shun) [L. *extrahere* to draw out] 1. the process or act of pulling or drawing out.

2. the preparation of an extract.

3. in chemistry, a solvent extraction in which a mixture is treated with a solvent for the purpose of dissolving and removing one or more of the components of the mixture. The mixture to be extracted may be solid or liquid. Often the mixture is dissolved in one solvent; this solution is then treated with another solvent, which is immiscible with the first. The two solvents may be shaken together in a separatory funnel and then allowed to reseparate on standing.

4. the process of removing only substances that are of interest from a tissue or body fluid specimen by dissolving them in a solvent that is immiscible with the original solvent and other components of the sample.

extrafusal fiber (ek-strah-fu′zal) see *extrafusal fibers of m.* under *muscle.*

extrapolation (ek-strap″o-la′shun) the process of estimating a function beyond the region in which its values are known.

extrapyramidal tract (ek″strah-pĭ-ram′ĭ-dal) a functional rather than anatomic unit involved in motor activities, comprising the nuclei and fibers other than those of the pyramidal tract. These nuclei and fibers control and coordinate especially the postural, static, supporting, and locomotor mechanisms. The extrapyramidal tract consists of the corpus striatum, subthalamic nucleus, substantia nigra, and red nucleus, along with their interconnections to the recticular formation and cerebrum. Some anatomists also include the cerebellum and vestibular nuclei as part of the tract.

extrasystole (ek″strah-sis′to-le) see *premature contraction.*

extravasation (ek-strav″ah-sa′shun) [*extra-* + L. *vas* vessel + *-atio*] the escape or expulsion of a substance, such as blood or an infused solution, into an extravascular site. Cf. *intravasation.*

extremity (ek-strem′ĭ-te) 1. a distal or terminal portion.

2. an arm or leg.

extrinsic (ek-strin′sik) [L. *extrinsecus* situated on the outside] coming from or originating outside; having relation to parts outside the organ or limb in which found.

extrinsic factor the former name for *vitamin B_{12}.*

extrinsic pathway see under *coagulation pathways.*

extrude (ek-strōōd) [L. *extrudere* to drive out] to force out or to push through an opening.

exudate (eks′u-dāt) [L. *exsudare* to sweat out] an effusion of fluid into a serous cavity produced by damage, e.g., by neoplasm, infection, inflammation, trauma, involving the mesothelial lining of a cavity. In constrast to a transudate, it has a high content of protein and leukocytes. The recommended laboratory criteria for distinguishing transudates from exudates vary with the type of serous cavity. For more information, see *pericardial fluid, peritoneal fluid,* and *pleural fluid.* Cf. *transudate.*

exudation (eks″u-da′shun) the process of forming an exudate. See also *exudate.*

eye (i) [L. *oculus;* Gr. *ophthalmos*] one of the pair of organs that provide vision. The eyeball is almost spherical and is suspended within the orbit, which protects it from injury. It is rotated by the action of the extraocular or extrinsic muscles.

The eyeball is formed by three coats, or tunics, and their enclosed contents. The outer tunic consists of the sclera and cornea; the middle tunic is a vascular structure composed of the choroid, ciliary body, and iris; and the innermost tunic, the retina, contains the photoreceptors.

Enclosed within the coats of the eyeball are two chambers: the anterior chamber, which is between the cornea and the iris and lens, and the posterior chamber, which lies between the lens and iris and communicates with the anterior chamber through the pupil. Both contain clear liquid, the aqueous humor. The posterior four-fifths of the eyeball is occupied by the vitreous body, which is clear and jelly-like in consistency and is 99 percent water in composition. It is traversed by the hyaloid canal and adheres to the retina at the optic disk.

The sclera is made up of dense fibrous tissue that, when expanded by intraocular pressure, imparts the characteristic shape to the eye; 75 percent of the sclera's dry weight is collagen. Continuous with the sclera is the cornea, which makes up the anterior one-sixth of the eyeball and is the area through which light enters the eye. The cornea is more convex than the rest of the eyeball and is the major refractive structure in the eye. It possesses no blood vessels but is composed of five layers of cells in which free nerve endings are interspersed. Lining the sclera is the vascular choroid, whose highly pigmented epithelium serves to prevent scattering of light within the eye. The choroid is connected with the iris by the ciliary body, which suspends the crystalline lens and accounts for accommodation. The ciliary body consists of the internal ciliary processes and the external ciliary muscles. The ciliary processes are approximately 70 radially oriented folds, which interdigitate with the choroid at the ora serrata. The ciliary muscles are composed of radial and circular fibers, which function to alter the shape of the lens.

The iris is the colored circular structure in front of the lens, connected at its periphery with the ciliary body and separated from the cornea by the iridocorneal angle. It is covered anteriorly with epithelium and posteriorly with two layers of columnar pigmented cells that are continuous with the nonreceptive periphery of the retina. Its central aperture, the pupil, acts as an iris diaphragm for the lens by regulating the amount of light that enters the eye. The size of this aperture is controlled by the sphincter muscle that contracts the pupil, and radially arranged fibers of the dilator muscle that dilate it.

The lens of the eye is an encapsulated, biconvex, clear structure. It is composed of concentric layers of mesenchymal cells containing a small amount of fat. In the process of accommodation for near vision, tension of the ciliary muscle draws the choroid and the ciliary processes forward, thus slackening the suspensory ligament and easing tension on the capsule of the lens, which, being elastic, then becomes more convex.

The retina lies within the choroid, in contact with the vitreous body. Anteriorly it extends over the ciliary body to the iris. The optic and ciliary parts of the retina are separated by a scalloped border, the ora serrata.

At the posterior pole of the eyeball there is a small yellow spot, the macula lutea, within which a central depressed area, the fovea centralis, contains a high concentration of photoreceptors. Slightly nasal (approximately 3 mm) to the macula lutea is a small depression, the optic disk. This is the point of departure from the eye of the optic nerve fibers. As there are no photoreceptors at this point, it is called the "blind spot" of the eye.

Derived from the ectoderm of the neural tube, the retina is morphologically and functionally an extension of the central nervous system. Microscopically, as many as 10 layers can be distinguished within the retina. From within the eyeball toward its outside, these layers are the internal limiting lamina, nerve fiber layer, ganglion cell layer, internal plexiform layer, internal nuclear layer, external plexiform lamina, external nuclear lamina, external limiting lamina, receptor layer, and pigment cell layer. The last is contiguous with the choroid.

The retina contains the visual receptors of the eye, the rods and cones. The human retina has more than 1 million rods and at least 5 million cones. The fovea, which contains only cones, is the area of greatest visual acuity. The visual receptors converge onto approximately 1 million ganglion cells in the retina, whose axons form the optic nerve.

Within the eye, light strikes the retina and is absorbed by molecules of photosensitive substances. This results in a change in the permeability of the receptor to ions and in the production of an electrical signal, which proceeds through the various levels of the retina, eventually reaching the visual cortex. In the rods, this light-sensitive substance is rhodopsin. The cone cells are less sensitive than rod cells and operate under conditions of greater light intensity. There is more than one type of cone and photosensitive substance present. In conditions of low light intensity the pupil expands, and in the process of dark adaptation there is an enormous increase in the sensitivity of the rods.

For more information, see entries related to the eye, *color vision,* and *eye tumors.*

eye and face protection devices used to shield the eyes and faces of laboratory personnel from chemical splashes or flying particles. Such devices include safety glasses, cover goggles, and face shields. Standards promulgated by OSHA (Occupational Safety and Health Administration), based on the American National Standard for Occupational and Educational Eye and Face Protection, specify that "protective eye and face equipment shall be required where there is a reasonable probability of injury that can be prevented by such equipment. In such cases, employers shall make conveniently available a type of protector suitable for the work to be performed, and employees shall use such protectors." In addition to the requirements for occupational protection, many states have laws requiring eye and face protection for students engaged in laboratory activities.

Safety glasses that meet the requirements for occupational and educational eye protection, standards developed by ANSI (American National Standards Institute) have impact-resistant lenses at least 3.0 mm thick, and frames that are slow burning and specially designed to retain the lenses against impact. Glasses meeting FDA (Food and Drug Administration) requirements for all eyewear have significantly less impact resistance, and no specifications for the frames. Glasses provided for employees and students should exceed the minimum FDA requirements and should meet ANSI standards to comply with state laws and OSHA requirements.

eyebrow (i'brow) the prominent arches of skin surmounting the orbits, which support numerous short coarse hairs. Movement of the eyebrows is effected by fibers of the orbicularis oculi and occipitofrontalis muscles.

eyelash (i'lash) one of the series of short, thick, curved hairs that grows from the free edges of the eyelids, generally distributed in double or triple rows. The hairs on the upper lid are longer than those on the lower lid.

eyelid (i'lid) either of a pair of thin, movable folds that, when closed, protect the anterior surface of the eye. The upper lid is larger and more movable than the lower. Also called *palpebra.*

eyepiece (i'pēs) the system of lenses in a microscope that is nearest to the viewer's eye. It magnifies and focuses the virtual image produced by the objective. Also called *ocular.*

comparison e., an eyepiece that presents, as though in juxtaposition, the images of separate objects being transmitted through two different objectives.

compensated e., an eyepiece that corrects chromatic defects produced by the objective and gives a flatter field than other oculars. Such eyepieces are usually marked "Comp" or "K."

high eyepoint e., an eyepiece with an eyepoint higher than usual, which may be used by viewers wearing eyeglasses.

huygenian e., a microscope ocular composed of two simple lenses. Although it can be used with low-power achromat objectives, it introduces lateral color when used with high-power achromats or apochromats; compensating eyepieces are required with these objectives.

Ramsden e., an eyepiece composed of two compound lenses.

widefield e., an eyepiece that has a field of view that is wider than usual.

eyepoint (i'point) the point above a microscope eyepiece where the image is focused and where the eye should be positioned for viewing.

eye tumor localization a procedure in nuclear medicine used to differentiate benign from malignant tumors of the eye. Sodium phosphate P 32 is administered intravenously; the ^{32}P is taken up by the DNA and RNA of rapidly dividing cells. Because the ^{32}P is a pure beta emitter, special miniaturized Geiger-Müller probes are required; they are placed within 2–3 mm of the lesion (an incision of the conjunctiva is required for posterior lesions). Malignant tumors produce a count rate at least 60 percent in excess of that for normal tissue.

eye tumors neoplasms of the eye; retinoblastoma is the most common intraocular tumor in children, and melanoma is the most frequent in adults. Metastatic carcinoma, particularly from the lung and breast, may present as a tumor of the eye.

Retinoblastoma is a tumor of primitive retinal cells, which can be familial. It is usually discovered within the first 2 yr of life. There is bilateral involvement in at least 30 percent of affected children. The tumor cells are small, round, and compactly grouped; rosette formations are usually present. Invasion of the optic nerve is an unfavorable prognostic sign.

Most intraocular melanomas arise from pigmented cells of the choroid, and grow inward into the vitreous. They must be distinguished from benign nevi. Histologic evaluation is of some value in determining the prognosis: persons whose tumors are composed of spindle cells do better than those with epithelioid cell melanomas. The 5-yr survival rate for those with melanomas containing a mixture of cell types is roughly 50 percent.

eyewash equipment an emergency device for flushing chemicals from the eyes, which provides a controlled flow of clean water to both eyes simultaneously at a velocity that does not injure the eyes. Some eyewash devices are designed to flush the face and eyes simultaneously. Effective flushing requires that the entire conjunctival sac be irrigated. This is made difficult because the eye sac is obscured by the running water, and an irritated or injured eye has a tendency to close due to muscle spasm; thus, instruction on the need to hold the eyelids open during washing and practice in using eyewash devices are recommended before an actual emergency arises.

F

F symbol for *Fahrenheit; farad; Faraday constant;* fertility (see *F p.* under *pilus* and *F p.* under *plasmid*); the chemical element *fluorine; force;* fragment of an antibody, e.g., Fc; Helmholtz free energy; *inbreeding coefficient; phenylalanine* (in amino acid sequence structure of proteins); a ratio of variances (see under *F-test*).

f symbol for atomic orbital with angular momentum quantum number 3, *breathing frequency, femto-, frequency.*

FA abbrev. See *fatty acid, fluorescent-antibody technique.*

FAB abbrev. for formalin ammonium bromide. See under *fixative.*

Fab a fragment of IgG immunoglobulin involved with antigen binding. Enzymatic digestion of an IgG immunoglobulin by papain results in two Fab fragments and one Fc fragment.

F(ab′)$_2$ the antigen-binding fragment of an IgG immunoglobulin after digestion with the enzyme pepsin. F(ab′)$_2$ consists of two Fab molecules and small peptides (known as the hinge region), held together by inter-heavy-chain disulfide bonds. See also the accompanying illustration.

Fabry's disease (fah′brez) [Johannes *Fabry,* German dermatologist, 1860–1930] see *diffuse a.* under *angiokeratoma.*

face (fās) [L. *facies*] 1. the anterior, or ventral, aspect of the head from forehead to chin and from ear to ear, inclusively.

2. any presenting aspect or surface.

facial (fa′shal) [L. *facialis*] of or pertaining to the face.

facial artery a branch of the external carotid artery that hooks around the lower border of the mandible, then passes forward and upward across the face to the medial angle of the eye.

facial myiasis see *facial m.* under *myiasis.*

facial nerve cranial nerve VII; a mixed motor and sensory nerve. The motor root arises in the pons and leaves the skull through a canal in the temporal bone; in the parotid gland it divides into branches that fan out to supply the facial muscles. It also carries secretory fibers to the lacrimal and salivary glands. The sensory root contains taste fibers for tongue and palate, and the chorda tympani nerve, which is distributed through the lingual branch of the mandibular nerve. See also *cranial nerves.*

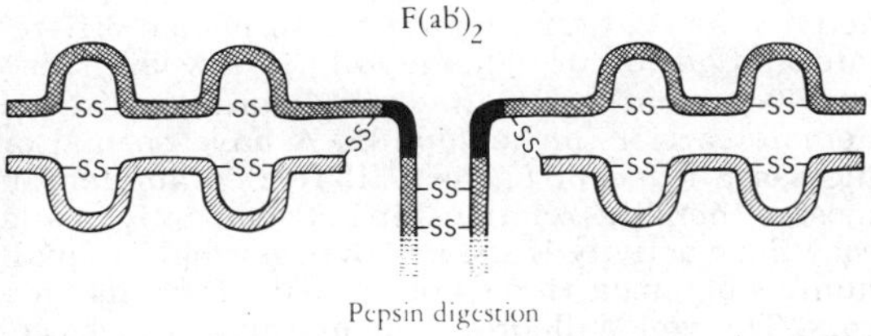

F(ab′)$_2$. Schematic representation of the degradation of IgG by pepsin. The Fc portion is hydrolyzed below the interchain disulfide bonds, leaving a single fragment with two combining sites intact, the F(ab′)$_2$. (From Bellanti, J. A.: Immunology II. Philadelphia, W. B. Saunders Co., 1978.)

facies (fa′she-ēz), pl. *facies* [L.] 1. a term used in anatomy to designate both the anterior or ventral aspect of the head from forehead to chin, and a specific surface of a body structure, part, or organ.

2. the expression or appearance of the face, especially as a diagnostic sign linked to certain diseases.

adenoid f., a characteristic facial appearance with dull expression and open mouth, seen in children with adenoidal hyperplasia that causes obstruction of the nasopharynx.

f. hepatica, a characteristic facial appearance that occurs in certain forms of chronic liver disorder. It is marked by a thin face, sallow complexion, and sunken eyeballs with yellow conjunctivae.

f. leontina, a characteristic, deeply furrowed, lionlike facial appearance associated with certain advanced cases of lepromatous leprosy. Also called leonine facies.

leprechaun f., a thin, hirsute face with full lips, as seen in Donohue's syndrome; see also *Donohue's syndrome.*

Parkinson's f., a characteristic facial appearance that is pathognomonic for certain forms of untreated Parkinson's disease. It is marked by a stolid, masklike face and infrequent blinking. Also called parkinsonian facies. See also *Parkinson's disease.*

facilitated diffusion a mechanism of transport across a membrane in which a specific interaction between the transported molecule and a membrane component is involved. The direction of net flux of the substance is down the electrochemical gradient, the direction typical of diffusion processes, and therefore a source of exogenous energy is not required. These processes are termed facilitated because the membrane component serves as a "carrier" to aid passage of the molecule across the membrane. Generally, the membrane component is a protein with highly specific binding properties. Facilitated diffusion has the following characteristics: it exhibits specificity for the transported substance, including stereospecificity; the rate of flux reaches a maximum when the concentration of the transported substance is sufficiently high to saturate the carrier; the same substance can be transported in both directions across the membrane; and, if two closely related substances are transported by the same carrier, the presence of the one will inhibit by competition the transport of the other. The major example of this type of transport is the flux of glucose from blood into cells. See also *active transport* and *diffusion.*

J. K. Hoober, Ph.D.

facio- (fa′she-o) [L. *facies* face] a word element used in combining form to denote relationships to the face, e.g., facioplasty.

factor (fak′tor) [L. "maker"] 1. a cause that contributes to the production of a specified effect.

2. an agent or chemical substance whose presence is required for normal health or for some process to occur, e.g., a coagulation factor, eosinophil chemotactic factor of anaphylaxis, corticotropin releasing factor.

3. in mathematics, one of the numbers multiplied together to obtain a product.

Factor I fibrinogen, a high-molecular-weight glycoprotein composed of three pairs of nonidentical polypeptide chains ($\alpha_2\ \beta_2\ \gamma_2$) held together by disulfide bonds. By hydrolyzing four specific arginyl-glycine bonds, thrombin cleaves two fibrinopeptides each from the α-chains and β-chains, forming soluble fibrin monomers that then polymerize to form an insoluble fibrin clot. The normal hemostatic concentration is 0.15–0.35 g/100 ml, with a metabolic half-life of 100–144 hr. Fibrinogen can be evaluated using a determination of thrombin time and/or quantitative fibrinogen methods. Replacement therapy is with plasma or cryoprecipitate. Fibrinogen concentrates are unavailable because they have a high hepatitis transmission rate.

Two disorders can result from a deficiency of this factor: afibrinogenemia and dysfibrinogenemia. Afibrinogenemia (or hypofibrinogenemia, a less serious form of the disease) can be acquired, as seen in disseminated intravascular coagulation, or in rare instances is transmitted as an autosomal recessive trait. Dysfibrinogenemia, a more common disorder, results from structurally abnormal fibrinogens, causing abnormal fibrin monomer polymerization and/or impaired cleavage by thrombin.

For more information on all the blood coagulation factors, see the accompanying table.

Factor II prothrombin, a glycoprotein that consists of a single polypeptide chain formed in the liver. It is vitamin K–dependent and is converted to thrombin by Factor Xa, a phospholipid surface (platelets), Ca^{++}, and Factor V. The normal plasma concentration is 150 μg/ml, a 100-fold excess over what is necessary for in vivo hemostasis. The metabolic half-life is 50–80 hr.

A deficiency of Factor II is extremely rare but, when present, results in the prolongation of the prothrombin time and the activated partial thromboplastin time. Replacement therapy is with plasma or prothrombin complex concentrate.

Factor III tissue factor, a lipoprotein present in the intima of the aorta, liver, brain, lung, kidneys, spleen, and plasma membrane of endothelial cells. When released into the circulatory system, it initiates the extrinsic pathway of blood coagulation by reacting with Factor VII and Ca^{++} to form Factor VIIa, and then activates Factor X to Xa. Factor Xa can increase Factor VIIa in turn 70-fold. A deficiency of this factor has never been reported. Also called *tissue thromboplastin.*

Factor IV calcium (Ca^{++}), a factor required in many phases of blood coagulation. For in vitro coagulation testing, Ca^{++} is removed from the blood sample to prevent clotting by the oxalate or citrate anticoagulants and is returned to the test system in the form of $CaCl_2$.

Factor V proaccelerin, a heat- and storage-labile glycoprotein synthesized in the liver. Factor V participates in the common pathway. It does not have enzymatic activity by itself, but rather it participates in prothrombin activation by binding Factor Xa to the platelet surface. It is stabilized by Ca^{++}, and loses activity in the presence of chelating agents. Its activity is increased severalfold by the presence of low levels of thrombin. Factor V has a half-life of 12–36 hr.

Inherited Factor V deficiency, in which bleeding is usually mild, is rare and leads to a hemorrhagic disorder known as Owren's disease or parahemophilia. Both the prothrombin time and activated partial thromboplastin time are prolonged. Replacement therapy is with fresh plasma. Also called *accelerator globulin* and *labile factor.*

Factor VI accelerin, an obsolete term previously used to designate the activated form of Factor V.

Factor VII proconvertin, a heat- and storage-stable serine protease, which participates in the extrinsic pathway. It is formed in the liver, is vitamin K–dependent, and is essential in the development of thromboplastin activity from a tissue source. Factor VIIa forms a complex with tissue thromboplastin and Ca^{++} and activates Factor X to Xa. The metabolic half-life is approximately 6 hr.

The hereditary deficiency of Factor VII (also called serum prothrombin conversion accelerator deficiency and stable factor deficiency), transmitted as an autosomal recessive trait, is rare. Bleeding in affected individuals is usually mild. The activated partial thromoplastin time is normal; the prothrombin time is prolonged. Replacement therapy is with plasma or prothrombin complex concentrates. Also called *autoprothrombin I, serum prothrombin conversion accelerator (SPCA) factor,* and *stable factor.*

Factor VIII antihemophilic factor, a glycoprotein (M.W. approximately 1.2 million). Its site of manufacture in the organism is unclear. Factor VIII participates in the intrinsic pathway by forming a complex with phospholipids (platelets), Ca^{++}, and Factor IXa, which enzymatically catalyzes the activation of Factor X. Low concentrations of thrombin increase the coagulant activity of Factor VIII several times over. Factor VIII is also required for normal platelet function, and is related to the ability of the platelets to adhere to the subendothelial surface of blood vessels, a property called von Willebrand factor (VWF factor), which is unaffected by thrombin.

Factor VIII has three measurable activities: coagulant, Factor VIII antigen, and von Willebrand factor (VIII_{VWF}). Coagulant activity is decreased in hemophilia A and may be decreased in von Willebrand's disease. The normal half-life of coagulant activity is 8–12 hr. Normal levels of Factor VIII–related antigen occur in hemophilia A; low levels (below 40 percent) occur in von Willebrand's disease. Female carriers of hemophilia A have normal or increased levels of Factor VIII–related antigen; in most of them the relationship between antigen and coagulant activity is greater than normal. A small number of noncarrier women also fall into this category. The von Willebrand factor enhances ristocetin-induced platelet agglutination.

The Factor VIII molecule comprises a high-molecular-weight fragment containing both antigenic activity and von Willebrand factor activity, and a small-molecular-weight (1×10^5) fragment containing coagulant activity.

Two genetically transmitted diseases are associated with a deficiency of Factor VIII: classical he-

FACTOR. BLOOD COAGULATION FACTORS

COMPONENT*	SYNONYMS	CLASSIFICATION	SITE OF SYNTHESIS
Factor I	Fibrinogen	Glycoprotein	Liver
Factor II	Prothrombin; thrombinogen prethrombin	Zymogen	Liver (vitamin K–dependent)
Factor III	Tissue thromboplastin; tissue factor		
Factor IV	Calcium ions		
Factor V	Proaccelerin; labile factor; plasma accelerator globulin	Cofactor	Liver and possibly endothelial cells
Factor VI	Not assigned		
Factor VII	Proconvertin; serum prothrombin conversion accelerator (SPCA); stable factor; autoprothrombin I	Zymogen	Liver (vitamin K–dependent)
Factor VIII	Antihemophilic globulin (AHG); antihemophilic factor (AHF); von Willebrand's factor; antihemophilic factor A	Cofactor	Endothelial cells
Factor IX	Plasma thromboplastin component (PTC); Christmas factor; antihemophilic factor B; autoprothrombin II; platelet cofactor II	Zymogen	Liver (vitamin K-dependent)
Factor X	Stuart-Prower factor; Stuart factor; autoprothrombin III	Zymogen	Liver (vitamin K–dependent)
Factor XI	Plasma thromboplastin antecedent (PTA); antihemophilic factor C	Zymogen	Liver
Factor XII	Hageman factor	Zymogen	Liver (?)
Factor XIII	Fibrin-stabilizing factor; fibrinase; Laki-Lorand factor; fibrinoligase	Zymogen	Liver or platelets or megakaryocytes
Fletcher factor	Prekallikrein	Zymogen	Liver (?)
Fitzgerald factor	Fitzgerald-Williams-Flaujeac factor; high-molecular-weight kininogen	Cofactor	Liver (?)

* The activated form of the clotting factor would be designated by an "a" attached to the roman numeral.

mophilia, the most common inherited coagulation factor deficiency (one in 25,000 individuals), which is transmitted as an X-linked recessive trait; and von Willebrand's disease (VW disease), also quite common, which is transmitted as an autosomal dominant trait.

The decreased coagulant activity results in a prolonged activated partial thromboplastin time but a normal prothrombin time. In very mild cases of either disease (when Factor VIII is greater than 25 percent), the aPTT may be normal. In von Willebrand's disease, Factor VIII levels may fluctuate, at times reaching normal levels.

Replacement therapy is with fresh frozen plasma, cryoprecipitated concentrate of plasma composed primarily of Factor VIII and fibrinogen, or commercial lyophilized Factor VIII concentrates. The activity of von Willebrand factor decreases with increased purification, resulting in the need for either fresh frozen plasma or cryoprecipitate for the treatment of individuals with von Willebrand's disease. When patients with VW disease are transfused with normal (or hemophilic) plasma, there is an increase in Factor VIII coagulant activity greater than the amount of activity infused; this activity persists longer than the half-life of Factor VIII. The half-life of transfused von Willebrand factor is quite short (3–4 hr). Stored plasma or whole blood has minimal Factor VIII activity. Also called *antihemophilic globulin* (*AHG*).

Factor VIII–crossed immunoelectrophoresis a two-dimensional or "crossed" immunoelectrophoretic technique that measures the integrity of the subunit and molecular weight structure of the Factor VIII–related antigen molecule. The test plasma is compared with normal, pooled Factor VIII–related antigen, with results reported as either normal or abnormal.

Factor VIII inhibitor the most common clotting factor inhibitor. Antibody to Factor VIII arises in 10 percent of individuals with classic hemophilia secondary to a prior transfusion. The Factor VIII inhibitor also arises spontaneously in otherwise normal postpartum females, in elderly individuals with underlying disease, and in those with autoimmune disorders such as lupus erythematosus. Also called *circulating anticoagulants.*

Factor VIII–related antigen test a "rocket" immunoelectrophoretic technique used to measure the concentration of the antigenic portion of the Factor VIII molecule for the diagnosis of von Willebrand's disease. Normal levels of Factor VIII–related antigen occur in hemophilia A; low levels (below 40 percent) occur in von Willebrand's disease. Female carriers of hemophilia A have normal or increased levels of Factor VIII–related antigen, which is statistically greater than their level of Factor VIII procoagulant activity.

Factor IX plasma thromboplastin component (PTC), a single-chain polypeptide synthesized in the liver. It participates in the intrinsic pathway and is vitamin K–dependent. Factor XIa, a serine protease itself, activates Factor IX to IXa. Factor IXa in the presence of Ca^{++}, phospholipid (platelets), and Factor VIII activates Factor X; molecular variants have been described. The biologic half-life of Factor IX is 20 hr.

A congenital deficiency of this factor, transmitted as an X-linked recessive trait, results in a hemorrhagic syndrome called hemophilia B or Christmas disease. Factor IX deficiency can also be acquired from severe liver disease and warfarin administration. Decreased coagulant activity results in a prolonged activated partial thromboplastin time and, in some cases, a prolonged prothrombin time, which is probably due to an inhibitory effect of abnormal Factor IX or activation of Factor X by Factor VIIa–tissue factor complex. Also called *antihemophilic factor B, autoprothrombin II,* and *Christmas factor.*

Factor X Stuart factor, a storage-stable, vitamin K–dependent serine protease synthesized in the liver. It consists of heavy and light chains joined by disulfide bonds with the activation of the factor resulting from the cleavage of an activation peptide from the heavy chain. There is considerable chemical homology between Factor IX, prothrombin, and Factor X. Factor X participates in the common pathway that is responsible for the conversion of prothrombin to thrombin, the reaction being greatly accelerated in the presence of Factor V, phospholipid, and Ca^{++}. The metabolic half-life of Factor X is 30–50 hr.

Factor X deficiency, transmitted as an autosomal recessive trait, exhibits mild bleeding tendencies; the deficiency can also be acquired in severe liver disease. Decreased coagulant activity results in a prolonged prothrombin time and activated partial thromboplastin time. Replacement therapy is with plasma or prothrombin complex concentrate. Also called *autoprothrombin III* and *Stuart-Prower factor.*

Factor Xa inhibitor see *a. III* under *antithrombin.*

Factor XI plasma thromboplastin antecedent (PTA), a serine protease probably synthesized in the liver, which participates in the intrinsic pathway. The factor consists of identical subunits joined by disulfide bonds, with activation associated with the hydrolysis of the peptide bonds. In its active form, Factor XI activates Factor IX in the presence of Ca^{++}. The half-life of Factor XI is 40–80 hr.

A congenital deficiency of this factor results in a systemic blood clotting defect called hemophilia C, or Rosenthal syndrome. Transmitted as a recessive trait, it occurs predominantly in Europeans of Jewish ancestry. Bleeding is usually mild and rarely spontaneous. Also called *antihemophilic factor C.*

Factor XII Hageman Factor, an enzyme whose conversion to its active form (Factor XIIa) by exposure to a foreign surface initiates the intrinsic pathway. Kallikrein, a plasma proteinase, can also activate Factor XII; this yields Factor XIIf fragments with the activation enhanced by high-molecular-weight kinogen (Fitzgerald factor). Once activated, Factor XII can activate Factor XI, convert prekallikrein (Fletcher factor) to kallikrein, and initiate the activation of the fibrinolytic system. The half-life of Factor XII is 52–60 hr.

A deficiency of Factor XII, inherited as an autosomal recessive trait, results in a prolonged activated partial thromboplastin time and a prolonged whole blood clotting time in glass, but no bleeding tendency. Also called glass factor, contact factor, or activation factor. See also *Fitzgerald factor, Fletcher factor,* and *Passavoy factor.*

Factor XIII fibrin-stabilizing factor (FSF), a tetrameric protein composed of two pairs of nonidentical polypeptide chains ($\alpha_2\beta_2$), which may be synthesized in the liver; it is found in plasma, platelets, and the placenta. Thrombin activates Factor XIII to Factor XIIIa; Factor XIIIa catalyzes the formation of linkages between glutamine side-chains in one fibrin monomer with a lysine side-chain in another, cross-linking the fibrin monomers and forming a fibrin clot that is insoluble and resistant to lysis. The half-life of Factor XIII is 100 hr. A single unit of blood or plasma is effective replacement therapy.

Deficiency of Factor XIII, transmitted as an autosomal recessive trait, is rare. It can produce a severe hemorrhagic tendency, accompanied by defective wound healing. All routine laboratory screening tests are normal. The solubility of the fibrin clot in urea or acetic acid must be determined. Normal clots are insoluble. Also called *Laki-Lorand factor.*

factor assays in hematology, the quantitative determination of the percentage concentration of individual clotting factors. The specific deficient clotting factor is determined by the failure of plasma deficient for that factor to correct a prolonged prothrombin time (PT) or activated partial thromboplastin time (aPTT). The PT or aPTT is determined on serial dilutions of normal plasma with the known deficient plasma. The percentage concentration is calculated by comparing a normal curve with aPTT or PT results obtained on serial dilutions. Inhibitors of specific factors can be quantitated by measuring the residual clotting factor after incubation of freshly drawn plasma, usually for 2 hr. Also called *coagulation factor assay.*

factor deficiency anemia see *factor deficiency a.* under *anemia.*

factorial (fak-tor'e-al) the product of all the positive integers less than or equal to a given integer; written $n!$ and spoken "n factorial." By definition, $0! = 1$; $5! = 5 \cdot 4 \cdot 3 \cdot 2 \cdot 1 = 120$.

facultative (fak'ul-ta"tiv) capable of adaptation to different conditions.

f. organisms, microorganisms, including the great majority of those of medical importance, which can grow in a wide range of oxygen tension by shifting from aerobic to anaerobic metabolism.

FAD abbrev. for the oxidized form of the redox coenzyme *flavin adenine dinucleotide.*

$FADH_2$ abbrev. for the reduced form of the redox coenzyme *flavin adenine dinucleotide.*

Fahrenheit (F) temperature scale (far'en-hīt) [Gabriel Daniel *Fahrenheit,* German physicist, 1686–1736] the customary scale of temperature on which water freezes at 32°F and boils at 212°F. See also *temperature.*

failure (fāl'yer) inability to perform.

failure rate in automatic data processing, the average number of units failing per unit time commonly expressed as the percentage of failures per thousand hours. See also *mean time between failures.*

faint (fānt) a temporary loss of consciousness resulting from a generalized lack of oxygen to the brain. It is often due to emotional or physical stresses and extremes. Also called *syncope.*

falciform (fal'sĭ-form) [L. *falx* sickle + *forma* form] shaped like a sickle.

fallopian tube (fal-lo'pe-an) [Gabriele *Falloppio* (*L. Fallopius*), *Italian anatomist, 1523–1562*] one of a pair of uterine tubes. The fallopian tubes are long, slender conduits that extend from the superior lateral angle of the uterus to the ovaries. Acting to transport ova from the ovaries to the uterus, the tubes are tipped by a funnel-shaped expansion, the infundibulum, which overhangs the ovaries. Fertilization usually occurs in the fallopian tube. Also called *oviduct* and *uterine tube.*

fallopian tube tumors neoplasms of the fallopian tubes. Primary adenocarcinoma of the fallopian tube is rare. More frequently, the tube is affected by the secondary spread of a tumor of the uterus or ipsilateral ovary. Tubal adenocarcinomas are usually papillary. If such tumors have extended to the peritoneum at the time of diagnosis, the prognosis is significantly worsened; overall 5-yr survival rates are less than 50 percent.

Adenomatoid tumors similar to those of the epididymis may occur in the fallopian tube. They are benign neoplasms of mesothelial origin. Rarely, the tube is the site of a mixed mesodermal sarcoma, teratoma, or smooth muscle tumor.

Fallot's tetralogy see *tetralogy of Fallot.*

false negative a test result that erroneously reports the absence of a disease or condition that is actually present. Cf. *false positive.*

false positive a test result that erroneously reports the presence of a disease or condition that is actually absent. Cf. *false negative.*

falx (falks), pl. *falces* [L. "sickle"] a sickle-shaped organ or structure.

f. of cerebellum, a sickle-shaped fold of dura mater that projects forward from the internal occipital crest toward the vermis of the cerebellum, partially separating the cerebellar hemispheres.

f. of cerebrum, a strong arched process of dura mater that extends into the longitudinal fissure between the two cerebral hemispheres. It is attached anteriorly to the crista galli of the ethmoid and fuses with the tentorium posteriorly.

inguinal f., see *conjoined t.* under *tendon.*

familial (fah-mil'e-al) [L. *familia* family] occurring in several members of the same family; transmitted in families, as by genetic or cultural inheritance.

family (fam'ĭ-le) 1. a group of genetically related individuals; in particular, parents and their children. See also *pedigree chart.*

2. a taxonomic classification (taxon) comprising one or more genera. Families are grouped into orders.

Fanconi's anemia [Guido *Fanconi,* Swiss pediatrician, b. 1882] see *aplastic a.* under *anemia.*

fan-in (fan'in) the number of inputs that can be connected to a logic device.

Fannia (fan'e-ah) a genus of flies. Two species, *F. canicularis* (the lesser house fly) and *F. scalaris* (the latrine fly), are known to cause intestinal and urinary myiasis in humans.

fan-out (fan'out) the number of other logic devices (from the same logic family, e.g., transistor-transistor logic) that can be driven by a logic device. When the fan-out is exceeded, the device cannot generate the required logic voltage levels.

farad (F) (far'ad) [Michael *Faraday,* English physicist, 1791–1867] the international System (SI) unit of electrical capacitance equal to 1 coulomb per volt (C/V). Capacitor values are usually given in microfarads, nanofarads, or picofarads.

faraday (far'ah-da) a unit of electric charge defined as the charge of 1 mole of electrons, which is equal to 96,487 coulombs (C).

Faraday constant (F) the charge per mole of electrons, 96,487 C/mol (C = coulombs).

Faraday effect the rotation of the plane of polarized light by solutions placed in a magnetic field. In the absence of the field, only asymmetric molecules cause optical rotation.

Faraday's law of electrolysis stated as: one faraday of electric charge is required to oxidize or reduce one equivalent of a chemical species.

Farber's disease (far′berz) see *Farber's lipogranulomatosis.*

Farber's lipogranulomatosis a disorder of sphingolipid metabolism, transmitted as an autosomal recessive trait, that is due to a relative or absolute deficiency of the enzyme ceramide trihexosidase and results in the accumulation of ceramide. This disorder appears in infants shortly after birth and is characterized by periarticular swelling of the joints, bone erosion, subcutaneous nodules, liver enlargement, and mental retardation. Affected organs may contain ceramide-filled macrophage foam cells, and the lipid content of the heart, lungs, liver, and spleen is increased. There is motor and mental retardation. Also called *Farber's disease.* See also *sphingolipidoses.*

farcy (far′se) the nodular abscesses observed in the skin, subcutaneous tissue, and lymphatics in chronic glanders. See also *glanders.*

farmer's lung (far′merz) a form of pulmonary hypersensitivity to a variety of plant antigens or spores and molds growing on stored grain, wood, or hay. Disease onset occurs acutely following recent exposure; those affected become severely ill, with cough, dyspnea, and fever. Histologically, there is interstitial pneumonitis with alveolar exudate. Several months may be required for recovery. A subsequent exposure will produce a more severe attack. See also *hypersensitivity p.* under *pneumonitis.*

Farrant's medium a water-soluble mounting medium with an index of refraction of 1.43, prepared by dissolving acacia in warm distilled water and adding glycerol.

fasci/o (fash′e-o) a word element used in combining form to denote fascia (fibrous membrane separating and enveloping muscle tissue), e.g., fasciotomy.

fascia (fash′e-ah), pl. *fasciae* [L. "band"] sheets of connective tissue formed by interlacing layers of collagen fibers with interspersed fibroblasts. Fascia is found throughout the body, where it defines compartments and tissue planes and invests the muscles and viscera.

deep f., dense, fibrous sheets of fascia that invest the skeletal muscles and subdivide some body compartments. The deep fascia is attached to the bones and joints, and forms sheets (retinacula) that bind down tendons at the wrists and ankles.

f. lata, the deep fascia of the thigh. It is thin medially, stronger over the popliteal fossa, and particularly strong on the lateral side of the thigh where it is thickened to form the iliotibial tract. Fascial sheets extend from its inner surface to the back of the femur as intermuscular septa.

f. occludens, the tight junction that seals adjacent epithelial cells at their luminal margins. Also called *zonula occludens.*

perirenal f., an extension of the transverse fascia that splits to enclose the kidney and adrenal gland in a perirenal fascial space (of Gerota).

renal f., condensed fibroareolar tissue that surrounds the kidney and perirenal fat. Also called Gerota's fascia or capsule.

superficial f., a continuous sheet of fascia that underlies the skin over the entire body and contains an admixture of fat in some areas. It is traversed by the vessels and nerves of the skin. The superficial fascia is particularly dense on the scalp, palms, and soles.

fascicle (fas′i-k′l) a small bundle or cluster, generally of nerve or muscle fibers.

fascicular (fah-sik′u-lar) pertaining to a fascicle; fasciculated.

fasciculated (fah-sik′u-lāt-ed) clustered together or occurring in bundles.

fasciculation (fah-sik″u-la′shun) the random, spontaneous contraction of a group of muscle fibers that are thought to compose the same individual motor unit. The twitching of the fibers is frequently visible through the skin.

f. potential, the electrical activity that occurs with fasciculation. Fasciculation potentials commonly occur singly, and less frequently as grouped discharges. Single fasciculation potentials, often sporadic in occurrence, can appear normally and are generally similar in dimension to a motor unit potential under voluntary control. Complex fasciculation potentials of the irregularly polyphasic type are seen in motor unit disorders; those of the iterative type (with a repetitive discharge pattern) can be seen in myokymia, in alkalotic states, and with incipient tetany. Characterization of the duration, amplitude, configuration, number of phases, and especially the frequency of discharge can be of diagnostic value in distinguishing the fasciculation potentials seen in various disorders from one another and from those which occur normally.

fasciculus (fah-sik′u-lus), pl. *fasciculi* [L., dim. of *fascis* bundle] [NA], a general term for a small bundle of nerves, muscles, or tendon fibers.

fasciitis (fash′e-i′tis) an inflammation of the fascia that spreads along the fascial planes, often leading to the separation of overlying skin from deeper structures. This condition may be due to infection, especially with mixed or clostridial populations, drug toxicities, malignancies, or overuse of a part.

eosinophilic f., a syndrome consisting of fascial inflammation, myositis, eosinophilia, and hypergammaglobulinemia, which results in a scleroderma-like condition. There is pain, swelling, and nonpitting induration of the extremities, which is often associated with physical exercise. The presence of eosinophilia in both blood and bone marrow is a key to diagnosis. This condition may respond well to corticosteroid therapy.

necrotizing f., an inflammation of fascia due to infection with group A streptococci, *Staphylococcus aureus,* facultative gram-negative rods, and mixed aerobic or anaerobic cultures. The infection may spread rapidly through deep fascial planes, with separation of the skin from deeper structures, as well as severe toxicity and high mortality.

nodular f., a pseudosarcomatous proliferation of fibroblasts, probably a response to trauma, that forms a firm nodule up to several centimeters in size, usually located in the upper arm and shoulder region. Other sites are less frequently involved. The lesion begins in the superficial fascia and generally extends into the subcutaneous fat. Histologically, plump, loosely arranged, and haphazardly oriented fibroblasts are present within a fibrous-to-myxoid stroma; they typically show mitotic activity. The importance of the lesion lies in its recognition, as it simulates a sarcoma.

Fasciola (fah-si′o-lah) [L. *fasciola* a band] a genus of flukes.

F. gigantica, the giant liver fluke, which inhabits the liver tissues and ducts of humans. It is geographically distributed throughout Africa and Asia, and occasionally infects humans. In Africa, the intermediate hosts are the snails of the species *Lymnaea natalensis,* whereas in Asia, *L. auricularia rufescens* and *L. acuminate* have been incriminated. *F. gigantica* can be differentiated from *F. hepatica* by its shape (it is more lanceolate) and by the size of its eggs (they are larger, measuring 160–190 μm long by 70–90 μm wide).

Human infection is caused by ingestion of aquatic vegetation bearing encysted metacercariae. Fever, eosinophilia, hepatomegaly, and an elevated erythrocyte sedimentation rate are common clinical characteristics. Laboratory diagnosis requires recovery and identification of eggs in the feces.

F. hepatica, the sheep liver fluke, which inhibits the bile ducts or liver parenchyma of humans. Predominantly a parasite of sheep (although humans are occasionally infected), *F. hepatica* is distributed throughout the world wherever sheep and the appropriate snail host are present.

The fluke is a large, brownish, flat parasite, measuring up to 30 mm long by 13 mm wide. The large eggs are operculated and light brown in color, measuring 130–150 μm long by 63–90 μm wide; they are undeveloped when deposited.

Human infection is caused by ingestion of aquatic vegetation (e.g., watercress) bearing encysted metacercariae. The parasites excyst in the intestine and migrate through the intestinal wall, finally reaching the bile ducts, where they mature. The undeveloped eggs are passed from humans or infected ruminants (especially sheep, horses, and goats) in the feces and must reach water or be kept moist to remain viable. After a developmental period the eggs hatch, and the miracidia attach and penetrate an appropriate snail host (e.g., species of *Lymnaea*).

Following development in the snail, free-living cercariae are liberated and encyst upon aquatic vegetation until they become metacercariae.

Clinical characteristics of infection include vomiting, coughing, and abdominal pain; diarrhea, fever, jaundice, and urticaria may be present. Eosinophilia, dysproteinemia, and hepatosplenomegaly are also common.

Laboratory diagnosis requires recovery and identification of large operculate eggs in the feces or from duodenal or biliary fluid. The eggs of *F. hepatica* resemble those of *Fasciolopsis buski* and should be differentiated. Infection with *F. hepatica* may also be diagnosed by complement-fixation and indirect hemagglutination tests.

fascioliasis (fas″e-o-li′ah-sis) an infection with flukes from the genus *Fasciola.*

fasciolopsiasis (fas″e-o-lop-si′ah-sis) an infection with flukes from the genus *Fasciolopsis.*

Fasciolopsis (fas″e-o-lop′sis) [L. *fasciola* a band + Gr. *opsis* appearance] a genus of trematode worms.

F. buski, a large intestinal fluke, ranging in size from 20 to 75 mm long and from 8 to 20 mm wide. Infection is common throughout Asia, the principal hosts being humans and pigs. Consumption of uncooked waterplants possessing metacercariae results in infection, causing inflammation and ulceration. Other symptoms include diarrhea, nausea, and vomiting.

Diagnosis is based on identification of the adult worm or eggs (130–140 mm long by 80–85 mm wide) in the feces. This may be difficult owing to the resemblance of the adult worm to *Fasciola hepatica.* Distinguishing characteristics of *F. buski* include lack of cephalic cone, unequal-sized suckers, and unbranched intestinal crura.

FASEB abbrev. See *Federation of American Societies for Experimental Biology.*

fast activity in electroencephalography, any electrical activity of frequency greater than 13 Hz.

fast green FCF a green acid dye; C.I. 42053. It is used in histology as a plasma stain and as a stain for collagen.

"fast" hemoglobins hemoglobins with electrophoretic mobility greater than Hb A at pH 8.6 in barbital buffer, such as Hb Bart's, Hb I, and Hb H.

fastidious (fas-tid′e-us) in bacteriology, referring to an organism with specific nutritional requirements.

fasting blood sugar the common term for a blood glucose determination in a fasting patient. See also *glucose.*

fat (fat) 1. adipose tissue, a white or yellowish tissue that forms soft pads between various organs of the body. It serves to smooth and round out body contours and as a reserve supply of energy.

2. see *triglyceride.*

subcutaneous f., the adipose tissue that is accumulated in the loose areolar tissue continuous with the dermis. It acts as a thermal insulator and facilitates movement of the skin. Variations in the distribution of subcutaneous fat over the body are related to sex, age, climate, and other factors.

fat absorption tests 1. chemical methods; determination of the fraction of an oral dose of fat in a standard diet (50–150 g/da) that is excreted rather than absorbed in the intestinal tract. For adults, the most reliable measurement is the total daily output of fat evaluated from a 3-da stool specimen collected while the patient is on a standard diet. An excretion of greater than 6 g/da in adults indicates steatorrhea. For infants and children, "percent coefficient of fat retention" (the difference between fecal fat and dietary fat expressed as a percentage of dietary fat) is used. The fat is extracted from the stool specimen by a lipid solvent and, after evaporation of the solvent, measured gravimetrically, or lipids are saponified to free fatty acids, which are measured by titration with standard alkali.

2. radioisotope methods. Radioisotope-labeled fat (triolein ^{131}I) or fatty acid (oleic acid ^{125}I) is ingested, and the absorption is determined by measuring the radioactivity in blood or stool. Although the differential absorption of the two agents has been used to distinguish between pancreatogenous and enterogenous steatorrhea, the results are unreliable.

fat assays 1. microscopic examination. A stool suspension is stained with Sudan III, Sudan IV, or oil red O. The number of fat droplets counted in a high-power microscope field serves as an index of steatorrhea. The top layer of a centrifuged urine specimen can be similarly examined for the presence of chyluria or lipiduria.

2. gravimetric method for fat in feces. A weighed dry stool specimen is extracted with petroleum ether, after which the extract is dried and weighed. Normal values by this method are less than 7 g/da for adults.

3. titrimetric method. An aliquot of urine or feces is dried and redissolved in ethanol. The lipids are saponified with strong potassium hydroxide solution, and fatty acids are precipitated by hydrochloric acid and then extracted into petroleum ether. The extract is dried and redissolved in ethanol, and the fatty acids are titrated with standard sodium hydroxide. The reference range for fecal fat by this method is less than 6.3 g/da.

4. electrical capacitance method. Lipids are extracted from feces or urine into chlorinated benzenes. The capacitance of the extract as compared with that of triolein standards is a measure of fat content.

fat depot (fat de′po, dep′o) [Fr. *dépôt,* from L. *depositum*] a site in the body in which large quantities of fat are stored as adipose tissue of subcutaneous tissue.

fat necrosis destruction of fat cells with an associated inflammatory response. In the subcutaneous tissues the condition is usually secondary to trauma. When the process involves the female breast, retraction of the overlying skin may simulate the changes produced by a carcinoma. Escape of pancreatic enzymes as a result of trauma or acute inflammation involving the pancreas will produce areas of fat necrosis within and around the organ, and if the enzymes are absorbed into the blood, they can give rise to focal fat necrosis in distant locations.

f. n. of the pancreas, the destruction of adipose tissue contiguous to the pancreas, occurring as a result of the leakage of potent pancreatic lipases. Often caused by blocked pancreatic ducts, it results in tissue inflammation and necrosis.

fat staining 1. diazo dye staining of unfixed frozen sections, the most frequently used method for demonstrating neutral fat (triacylglycerides) seen with fatty change of the heart, liver, and other organs and with fat embolism. Oil red O, Sudan III, and Sudan IV are commonly used, dissolved either in aqueous isopropyl alcohol or propylene glycol. Hematoxylin is used as a counterstain. Neutral fats are bright red and nuclei blue.

2. fluorescence microscopy after staining with phosphine, methylene blue, or 3,4-benzpyrene. These methods demonstrate all lipids.

3. osmium tetroxide staining, which stains black all compounds that contain double bonds. It is sometimes used as a stain for degenerating myelin. Also called *lipid staining.*

fatty (fat′e) pertaining to or characterized by fat.

fatty acid any straight- or branched-chain monocarboxylic acid. Fatty acids occur in nature only in small quantities in the free state; it occurs in abundance in ester or amide linkage in the lipids. There are three important structural properties associated with fatty acids: (1) they are mainly monocarboxylic acids, having a carboxyl group and a nonpolar, acylic, unbranched hydrocarbon chain; (2) they usually contain an even number of carbon atoms, although some with an odd number do occur; and (3) they may be saturated or may contain one (a monounsaturated fatty acid) or more (a polyunsaturated fatty acid) double bonds. The double bonds are usually all-*cis-,* and multiple double bonds are usually separated by a methylene group (i.e., $—CH{=}CH—CH_2—CH{=}CH—$). Some fatty acids with conjugated double bonds occur in plants.

essential f. a., unsaturated fatty acid that cannot be formed in the body and therefore must be provided by the diet. The most important are linoleic acid, linolenic acid, and arachidonic acid. Arachidonic acid can be formed in the body from dietary linoleic acid.

free f. a. (FFA), see *nonesterified f. a.*

nonesterified f. a. (NEFA), fatty acid in blood plasma that is not bound in the form of lipid esters. These substances constitute about 5 percent of the total quantity of fatty acids present in plasma and are primarily straight-chain saturated fatty acids, such as stearic acid and palmitic acid. They are transported in the plasma bound to albumin. The reference range for nonesterified fatty acid in plasma is 0.3–0.95 mmol/l. Also called *free f. a.* and *unesterified f. a.*

unesterified f. a. (UFA), see *nonesterified f. a.*

fatty acid assays the determination of plasma nonesterified fatty acids (NEFA). Fatty acids are extracted from acidified plasma or serum into an isopropanol-heptane mixture and titrated with sodium hydroxide solution, using thymol blue as the end-point indicator. Palmitic acid is used as the standard. See also *fat assays.*

fatty acid oxidation the utilization of fatty acids as fuel by combustion to carbon dioxide and water, which occurs in the mitochondria. The fatty acids may be derived from dietary fat or synthesized from other dietary components. The oxidation occurs in two stages: the first oxidation converts all the fatty acid carbons to acetyl coenzyme A (CoA), and then the acetyl-CoA is oxidized in the tricarboxylic acid cycle. Both stages contribute to the production of ATP by oxidative phosphorylation.

On entering the cell from the blood, fatty acids are first activated by conversion to acyl CoA compounds. These do not enter the mitochondrion as such but are transported across the inner mitochondrial membrane in the form of acyl carnitine. In the mitochondrial matrix the acyl CoA derivatives are reformed, releasing carnitine. There, these CoA derivatives are oxidized by a repeated sequence of four successive reactions (called β-oxidation) that shorten the fatty acid chain by two carbon atoms. The two carbon atoms are split off in the form of acetyl-CoA, which can enter the TCA cycle directly for oxidation to CO_2 and H_2O. The complete oxidation of one molecule of palmitic acid to CO_2 and H_2O yields about 129 ATP molecules. Of the total energy derived from complete combustion of palmitic acid, about 40 percent is stored in ATP and 60 percent is released as heat.

Two other types of fatty acid oxidation occur. In α-oxidation, a long-chain fatty acid is converted to a 2-hydroxy, then a 2-keto acid, and then by oxidative decarboxylation to a fatty acid with one less carbon atom. In ω-oxidation, medium- and long-chain fatty acids are converted to ω-hydroxy acids and then to α,ω-dicarboxylic acids. In both cases the product is further oxidized by β-oxidation. In addition, unsaturated fatty acids, or fats containing them, can be oxidized when in contact with air by a process referred to as autoxidation.

fatty acid profile separation, identification, and determination of the fatty acids present in serum lipids by gas chromatography. Lipids are saponified with potassium hydroxide, and the unsaponifiable lipids are removed by extraction with petroleum ether. The aqueous phase containing the saponified fatty acids is acidified, the precipitated fatty acids are extracted into petroleum ether, and the extract is dried. The fatty acids are then converted to methyl esters by reaction with diazomethane and chromatographed, using an ethylene glycol succinate or diethylene glycol succinate liquid phase and a flame ionization detector.

fatty acid synthesis the formation of fatty acid molecules from precursor acetyl CoA molecules obtained from the oxidation of carbohydrates or amino acids. This biosynthesis, the principal process of lipogenesis, occurs primarily in the liver in humans. The primary subcellular site of lipogenesis is the cytosol.

The synthesis of fatty acids from acetyl CoA is similar to fatty acid oxidation in reverse. The acyl group is lengthened by the successive additions of acetyl groups, producing 3-oxoacyl-CoA, followed by reduction to an acyl group with two additional carbons.

These reactions are catalyzed by two enzyme systems, acetyl CoA carboxylase and fatty acid synthetase (FAS). Each acetyl group that is added to the fatty acid chain is first converted to malonyl CoA by enzymatic carboxylation, a process regaining the vitamin biotin. The FAS of mammals and birds is a protein having two identical subunits, each catalyzing at least seven different reactions needed for the synthesis of the end product, palmitate. It is thus a multifunctional enzyme. In bacteria, each of the enzyme activities is on a separate and dissociable subunit.

The reduction of oxoacyl groups in the reductive synthesis of the fatty acid molecules uses NADPH as the reducing agent. The major sources of the cytosolic NADPH are pentose phosphate pathway dehydrogenases and cytosolic NADP-malate dehydrogenase reactions.

Oxidation of glucose or another appropriate substrate provides energy as ATP for fatty acid synthesis and pyruvate for acetyl CoA formation. The tricarboxylic acid cycle provides a means of getting acetyl CoA into the cytosol via the carrier molecule, citric acid, which is cleaved in the cytosol to acetyl CoA and oxalacetate.

Some fatty acids can be synthesized in mitochondria by reversal of the β-oxidation sequence. Chain elongation can occur in both mitochondria and cytosol, whereas chain desaturation can take place on the endoplasmic reticulum by action of mixed function oxidase enzymes.

The regulation of fatty acid synthesis is fairly complex. Substrate glucose must be plentiful, and insulin must be presented to the tissue. Acetyl CoA carboxylase, a key regulatory enzyme, is activated by cytosolic citric acid. The enzymes producing NADPH are inducible by high levels of substrate glucose and presentation of insulin. Glycolysis is also regulated by the level of cytosolic citrate.

fatty change a general term used to describe the accumulation of fat within parenchymal cells, especially of the liver, due to an imbalance between lipid storge and usage. Also called fatty degeneration or fatty metamorphosis.

fatty liver the diffuse intracellular accumulation of neutral triglycerides in hepatocytes in sufficient amounts to be visible by light microscopy. This acquired change is not characteristically associated with any biochemical abnormalities and may be apparent as mild hepatomegaly only on physical examination. There are many etiologies, including industrial chemicals (carbon tetrachloride and yellow phosphorus), ethanol, drugs (corticosteroids and large doses of tetracycline), protein malnutrition, diabetes mellitus, pregnancy, and small intestine bypass surgery. A fatty liver is almost always clinically nonsignificant and is potentially reversible after the underlying cause is corrected. Diagnosis is accomplished by percutaneous needle biopsy and histologic frozen section preparation of the tissue with a fat-staining dye (e.g., Sudan III or oil red O). Also called *steatosis.*

fatty meal in radiology, a meal containing foods high in fat content, such as eggs, butter, and cream, given to cause the emptying of the gallbladder during cholecystography. When the fats reach the duodenum, they stimulate secretion of the hormone cholecystokinin, which in turn stimulates the contraction of the gallbladder. Maximal contraction occurs about 40 min after ingestion. Commercial preparations, flavored vegetable oil, and water emulsions are often used. See also *cholagogue* and *cholecystagogue.*

fatty oil see *fixed oil.*

fauces (faw'sēz) [L. pl. of *faux* "a gorge, narrow pass"] the throat; the passage from the mouth to the pharynx, including the walls and the orifice.

favism (fa'vism) [It. *fava* bean] an acute hemolytic anemia acquired as a result of contact with the fava bean or plant. This disease occurs only in those individuals who possess a genetic defect leading to a deficiency in the enzyme glucose-6-phosphate dehydrogenase. However, not all members of a family with the defect are necessarily sensitive to the bean, and an additional defect may be involved, possibly in glucuronide formation.

favus one of the most disfiguring fungal diseases; a clinical term for a severe form of dermatophytosis or ringworm of the scalp, the classical feature of which is the development of scutula. The infection starts in the hair follicle and forms yellowish, cup-shaped scutula or crusts consisting of mycelium and epidermal debris. Hair follicles are destroyed and baldness ensues. The fungi most commonly involved are *Trichophyton schoenleinii, T. violaceum,* and *Microsporum gypseum.* However, scalp infection with these fungi does not always result in favus. Three levels of severity are seen: mild, with redness of the scalp and no hair loss; intermediate, with the formation of scutula and the loss of hair; and severe, with extensive loss of hair and atrophy of skin. Clinical severity is probably due more to host factors such as hygiene level or innate susceptibility than it is to the type of etiologic agent.

Diagnosis is made by observation of scutula and fungal mycelia in the horny layer of the scalp, only a mild inflammatory response, and a history of similar infections in other members of the family. Also called *tinea favosa.*

F body a fluorescent body that can be seen in male

cells; it represents staining of the distal end of the human Y chromosome. In interphase cells and spermatozoa, it can be seen by fluorescence microscopy with quinacrine mustard dihydrochloride, and the number of Y chromosomes can be counted.

FBS abbrev. for fasting blood sugar.

5-FC abbrev. See *5-fluorocytosine.*

Fc a crystallizable fragment of the IgG immunoglobulin, which is produced by enzymic digestion of IgG by papain.

F^- cell a bacterial cell lacking an F plasmid that serves as a genetic recipient (female) by receptor cells in conjugation. F^- cells must be viable for successful F plasmid transfer from F^+ cells (donor males); $F^- \times F^-$ crosses are sterile. Cf. *F^+ cell.* See also *conjugation, F p.* under *pilus,* and *F p.* under *plasmid.*

F^+ cell a bacterial cell that serves as a genetic donor (male) in conjugation owing to the presence of an F plasmid and an F pilus. F^+ cells transfer the F plasmid to F^- cells (recipient females) with high frequency; $F^+ \times F^+$ crosses have low fertility. Cf. *F^- cell.* See also *conjugation, F p.* under *pilus,* and *F p.* under *plasmid.*

FDA abbrev. See *Food and Drug Administration.*

***F* distribution** the probability distribution of the statistic $F = (x^2/n)/(y^2/d)$, where x^2 has the chi-squared distribution with n degrees of freedom and y^2 has the chi-squared distribution with d degrees of freedom. The reciprocal $1/F$ has the F distribution produced by exchanging the degrees of freedom in the numerator and denominator. The upper α percentile point is written $F_{\alpha,n,d}$; $P(F > F_{\alpha,n,d}) = \alpha$. The lower α percentile point is $F_{1-\alpha,n,d} = 1/F_{\alpha,d,n}$. For n greater than 1 there is a mode at $(n-2)d/(d+2)n$; for n equal to 1, the probability density becomes infinite at $F = 0$.

If s_1^2 and s_2^2 are sample variances of samples of size n and d from normally distributed populations with variances σ_1^2 and σ_2^2, then the variable $(s_1^2/s_2^2)/(\sigma_1^2/\sigma_2^2)$ has the F distribution with $n-1$ degrees of freedom in the numerator and $d-1$ degrees of freedom in the denominator, and $(s_1^2/s_2^2)/F_{\alpha/2,n-1,d-1} < (\sigma_1^2/\sigma_2^2) < (s_1^2/s_2^2)F_{\alpha/2,d-1,n-1}$ is a $100(1-\alpha)$ percent confidence interval for the ratio of the two variances.

The null hypothesis $\sigma_1 = \sigma_2$ is rejected, and the two-sided alternative $\sigma_1 \neq \sigma_2$ is accepted at the significance level α if s_1^2/s_2^2 exceeds $F_{\alpha/2,n-1,d-1}$ or if s_2^2/s_1^2 exceeds $F_{\alpha/2,d-1,n-1}$. The one-sided alternative $\sigma_1 > \sigma_2$ is accepted if s_1^2/s_2^2 exceeds $F_{\alpha,n-1,d-1}$.

See also *analysis of variance.*

FDNB abbrev. for 1-fluoro-2,4-dinitrobenzene reagent. See under *amino acid assays.*

F donor a cell that donates F factor in bacterial conjugation. See also *conjugation, F p.* under *pilus,* and *F p.* under *plasmid.*

FDP abbrev. See *fibrin (fibrinogen) degradation products.*

F-duction the transfer of an F′ plasmid from an F^+ cell (donor) to an F^- cell (recipient) in bacterial conjugation. See also *F′ p.* under *plasmid.*

Fe [L. *ferrum*] the symbol for the chemical element *iron.*

Fe^{2+} abbrev. See *ferrous.*

Fe^{3+} abbrev. See *ferric.*

$F_{E_{CO_2}}$ the fractional concentration of CO_2 in a sample of expired gas.

$F_{E_{O_2}}$ the fractional concentration of oxygen in a sample of expired gas.

febrile (feb′ril) [L. *febrilis*] pertaining to or characterized by a fever; feverish. See also *fever.*

febrile agglutination tests a battery of bacterial agglutination tests to detect serum antibodies in patients with certain types of febrile illness. The usual antigens include suspensions of killed *Salmonella, Brucella,* and *Proteus* species and *Francisella tularensis.*

Serial dilutions of serum are tested with standardized antigens and, if possible, with the specific organism isolated from the patient. A fourfold increase in titer during the course of the illness is significant. The test with standardized antigens is not highly specific; titers may be elevated in hyperglobulinemic conditions such as chronic liver disease. Febrile agglutination tests should not be used as a substitute for the direct cultural demonstration of the infecting microorganism.

fecal (fe′kal) pertaining to or of the nature of feces.

feces (fe′sēz) [L. *faeces,* pl. of *faex* refuse] the excrement discharged from the intestines, consisting of bacteria, cells exfoliated from the intestines, secretions (primarily those of the liver), and food residue.

Federation of American Societies for Experimental Biology (FASEB) a professional organization of investigators in biology and pathology.

feedback (fēd-bak) 1. the return of part of the output of an amplifier or other electronic device to the input. Feedback can be either positive or negative. Positive feedback accentuates distortions and noise, whereas negative feedback (of opposite sign to the input) reduces distortion and noise.

2. in metabolic systems, the return of information to an earlier stage of process where it exerts control, such as end-product inhibition of a synthesis pathway. In simplified terms, the feedback system may be described as one in which the degrees of function of two variables, *A* and *B,* are interdependent. When *A* is directly proportional to *B* (i.e., when *B* increases, and *A* also increases), the relationship is described as positive feedback; whereas if *A* is inversely proportional to *B* (i.e., when *B* increases, and *A* decreases), a negative feedback exists. In the positive feedback mechanism, the initiating stimulus causes more of the same; unless this is a part of an overall control system terminating in a negative feedback, it does not lead to a steady state but to an uncontrolled process. Negative feedback reduces or opposes changes in the output of a system and thus is a cardinal feature for the maintenance of homeostasis in the living system.

feedback loop the closed loop in a feedback circuit around which part of the input passes through the amplifier and back through the feedback transfer component to the amplifier input.

FEF abbrev. See *forced expiratory flow.*

Fehling's solution (fa′lingz) [Herman Christian von *Fehling,* German chemist, 1812–1885] a solution of copper(II) sulfate, sodium hydroxide, and potassium tartrate. The $CuSO_4$ and alkaline tartrate are prepared separately and mixed just before use. Solutes with reducing properties such as sugars (glucose) reduce the copper, forming a yellow to red-orange precipitate of copper(I) oxide.

felon (fel′on) see *whitlow.*

Felton phenomenon (fel′tun) the induction of immunologic unresponsiveness in mice caused by the injection of large amounts of polysaccharide from the bacterium pneumococcus.

Felty's syndrome (fel′tēz) [A. R. *Felty,* American physician, born 1895] a complex of symptoms including rheumatoid (chronic) polyarthritis, fever, and anemia, with splenomegaly, leukopenia, thrombocytopenia, leg ulcers, and neuropathy. This hypersplenic disorder is of unknown cause.

female (fe′māl) [L. *femella,* dim. of *femina* woman] 1. pertaining to the sex that produces ova.
2. an individual of this sex.
3. pertaining to a connector that has a slot or receptacle into which the corresponding (male) connector fits.

female carrier a female who is heterozygous for an X-linked recessive allele and thus is not affected by the trait but may pass the trait on to offspring.

female hormones a class of steroid hormones produced by the female, responsible for secondary sex characteristics and for regulating the growth and development of the genital tract. The primary types of female hormones are the estrogenic hormones (e.g., estradiol) and the progestational hormones (e.g., progesterone). For more information, see the specific hormone. Cf. *male hormones.*

feminization (fem″ĭ-nĭ-za′shun) 1. the normal induction of female sex characteristics.
2. the development of female secondary sex characteristics in a male. See also *testicular feminization syndrome.*

feminizing tumor adrenal adenoma and carcinomas of the type associated with adrenogenital syndrome. It may rarely produce isosexual precocity in females before puberty and feminization in males, with gynecomastia, loss of libido, and sometimes a diminution in the size of the penis. Urinary estrogens and 17-ketosteroids are commonly elevated.

femor/o (fem′o-ro) a word element used in combining form to denote the femur (thigh bone), e.g., femoral.

femoral (fem′or-al) [L. *femoralis*] pertaining to the femur or to the thigh.

femoral artery the continuation of the external iliac artery that begins behind the inguinal ligament, runs down the front and medial sides of the thigh, and passes through the opening in the adductor magnus, where it becomes the popliteal artery.

femoral canal the fascia-lined tunnel in the middle third of the thigh that contains the femoral vessels. It is partially enclosed by the adductor muscles and roofed over by the sartorius. The space allows for expansion of the femoral vein and is the route taken by a femoral hernia. Also called adductor canal or subsartorial canal.

femoral nerve a nerve formed in the lumbar plexus by branches from the second, third, and fourth lumbar nerves. It descends through psoas major and passes behind the inguinal ligament to supply thigh muscles, including the quadriceps, and innervate skin on the front of the thigh and medial side of the leg and foot.

femoral puncture a method to obtain a blood sample from a femoral vessel when it is not possible to use one of the normal venipuncture sites. The sample is extracted from below the inguinal ligament.

femoral vein the continuation of the popliteal vein that commences at the opening in the adductor magnus and ends at the inguinal ligament by becoming the external iliac vein.

femto- (f) (fem′to) [Danish *femten* fifteen] a prefix attached to International System (SI) units to make a unit that is one-quadrillionth of the basic unit (10^{-15} unit).

femtoliter (fl) (fem″to-le′ter) a unit of volume equal to one-quadrillionth of a liter (10^{-15} l). In hematology, it is the recommended unit for expressing the erythrocyte index mean corpuscular volume (MCV) and is equal to the formerly used measure, the cubic micron.

femtometer (fm) (fem′to-me″ter) a unit of length equal to one-quadrillionth of a meter (10^{-15} m). Also called *fermi.*

femtomole (fmol) (fem′to-mōl″) a unit of substance amount equal to one-quadrillionth of a mole (10^{-15} mol).

femur (fe′mur), pl. *femora* [L.] the bone of the thigh. It is the longest and heaviest bone in the body and is thickly covered with muscles. Its upper end includes the head, which articulates with the acetabulum, a supporting neck, and two protuberances, the greater and lesser trochanters. The posterior border of the shaft of the femur forms a roughened ridge, the linea aspera. The lower end of the bone is made up of two large condyles with a shared articular surface for tibia and patella in the knee joint.

fenac a toxic herbicide, (2,3,6-trichlorophenyl)acetic acid.

fenestra (fĕ-nes′trah), pl. *fenestrae* [L. "window"] 1. [NA], a general term for an opening or open area.
2. an opening in a bandage or cast, or in the blade of a forceps.
f. cochleae, see *round window.*
f. vestibuli, see *oval window.*

fenestrated (fen′es-trāt″ed) pierced with one or more openings.

fennel oil [USP], a volatile oil distilled with steam from the dried, ripe fruit of *Foeniculum vulgare;* used as a flavoring agent for pharmaceuticals and as a carminative.

fenoprofen calcium (fen-o-pro′fen) an antiinflammatory analgesic and antipyretic nonsteroidal drug used for symptomatic relief in rheumatoid arthritis and osteoarthritis. It is an arylacetic acid derivative similar to ibuprofen and naproxen. The most common side-effects are gastrointestinal intolerance (dyspepsia, nausea), headache, somnolence, and tinnitus. Trademark, Nalfon.

fentanyl citrate (fen′tah-nil) a short-acting narcotic analgesic, with actions similar to morphine and meperidine, used as a preanesthetic and, in combination with droperidol (a butyrophenone major tranquilizer), as a neuroleptanalgesic (an agent that produces stupor and total analgesia). Adverse reactions are those of narcotics, such as bradycardia, and respiratory depression, which is reversed by narcotic antagonists. Trademark, *Sublimaze.*

feral (fer′al) [L. *feralis*] 1. wild or savage.
2. pertaining to animals living in the wild after escape from domestication.

ferment (fer-ment′) [L. *fermentare* to cause to rise

or ferment] to carry out fermentation, especially the decomposition of carbohydrates.

fermentation (fer″men-ta′shun) 1. the energy-yielding enzymatic decomposition of organic substrates, primarily carbohydrates, in the absence of oxygen.

2. the microbial conversion of sugars to particular products in anaerobic cultures. The best known is the fermentation of glucose by certain yeasts, producing ethanol and CO_2. The ability of different microorganisms to ferment various sugars is valuable clinically in their identification, particularly in the case of Enterobacteriaceae and other gram-negative bacteria.

3. in industrial usage, the large-scale processes catalyzed by microbes producing commercially valuable products such as ethanol, organic solvents, and vitamins, extending even to strongly aerobic processes used in antibiotic production.

mixed acid f., anaerobic decomposition by a bacterial culture that results in the formation of several acids (e.g., acetic, lactic, succinic, and formic) instead of a single acid (e.g., lactic) as a product of metabolism of sugars. This type of fermentation produces a positive reaction to the methyl red test, a reaction used in the identification of *Enterobacteriaceae.*

fermentation test a test formerly used for the detection of some types of sugars. The unknown is added to a buffered solution of baker's yeast; the evolution of carbon dioxide bubbles indicates the presence of a fermentable carbohydrate such as glucose or fructose. These can be differentiated from galactose and other unfermentable sugars. The test is also used in microbiology to aid in identification of species by differences in the types of carbohydrates fermented.

fermi [Enrico *Fermi,* Italian physicist, 1901–1954; winner of the Nobel Prize for Physics in 1938] see *femtometer.*

fermium (Fm) (fer′me-um) [Enrico *Fermi*] a synthetic, metallic radioactive element; atomic number 100; most stable isotope, Fm-257 (half-life, 100.5 da); a 5f transition element (actinide element); oxidation states +2, +3.

ferning (fern′ing) the appearance of branched, crystalline structures resembling ferns. It occurs in a dried specimen of cervical mucus and indicates the presence of estrogen. Also called fern phenomenon.

ferredoxin (fer″ĕ-dok′sin) one of a fairly large group of iron-sulfide proteins found in microorganisms and in animals. See also *iron-sulfide protein.*

ferric (Fe^{3+} or Fe(III)) (fer′ik) [L. *ferrum*] containing iron in the plus-three oxidation state.

ferric chloride a black-brown solid, iron(III) chloride; M.W. 162.21. It is very hygroscopic, readily absorbing water in air to form the hexahydrate; or it is a yellow-orange deliquescent crystalline solid, ferric chloride hydrate, $FeCl_3 \cdot 6H_2O$. Ferric chloride is acidic in aqueous solutions and is a corrosive skin and tissue irritant.

ferric chloride test a nonspecific colorimetric test used to detect a variety of substances in urine. Addition of an acidic solution of ferric chloride to the specimen results in the formation of colored products with a number of metabolites; examples are phenylpyruvic acid (transient blue), homogentisic acid (blue), and bilirubin (colors from blue to green to red), melanogens (black), acetoacetic acid (red to red-brown), and phenothiazines and salicylates (purple to pink).

ferric ferricyanide reduction test a histochemical test for the demonstration of reducing substances. Formalin-fixed paraffin sections are stained in a freshly prepared ferric ferricyanide solution. Reducing substances reduce Fe^{3+} to Fe^{2+}, which then forms insoluble ferrous ferricyanide (Turnbull blue). Chromaffin, enterochromaffin, melanin, lipofuscin thyroid colloid, and substances containing sulfhydryl groups (keratin and keratohyalin) stain dark blue. Also called *Schmorl reaction.*

ferric ferrocyanide see *Prussian blue.*

ferricyanide (fer″e-si′ah-nid) a coordinate complex anion, with a valence of –3, containing a ferric (Fe^{3+}) ion linked to six cyanide (CN^-) ions. It is a weak oxidizing agent in alkaline solution; i.e., it can oxidize D-glucose and other hexoses to form a mixture of products, while it is reduced to a ferrocyanide ion. Several nonspecific methods for assaying blood glucose are based on this reaction. In these procedures, the yellow ferricyanide ion is reduced to the colorless ferrocyanide ion (reverse colorimetry):

$$Fe^{3+}(CN)_6{}^{3-} \xrightarrow[\text{glucose}]{+e^-} Fe^{2+}(CN)_6{}^{4-}$$

ferrihemoglobin (fer″e-he′mo-glo″bin) see *methemoglobin.*

ferrimagnetic (fer″ĭ-mag-net′ik) pertaining to materials, such as ferrite, in which the intrinsic magnetic moments of neighboring dissimilar atoms are antiparallel (but of different sizes so that they do not cancel) throughout microscopic domains. The large-scale properties are similar to those of ferromagnetism.

ferrite (fer′īt) any of several multiple oxides of iron and other elements that are ferrimagnetic. They are used for cores of inductors and transformers, for magnetic core computer memories, for the oxide coating on magnetic tape, and as electrical insulators.

ferritin (fer′ĭ-tin) a metalloprotein, iron-apoferritin complex; a chief form in which iron is stored and yet most readily available in the body; M.W. 465,000. Ferritin is composed of 24 identical or nearly identical polypeptides, M.W. 18,500, which form a protein spherical shell. The iron content of ferritin constitutes about 25 percent of the total mass, and the iron is present as micelles of hydrated ferric oxide–phosphate complexes, adhering to the inner spherical surface of apoferritin. Ferritin is colorless, is finely dispersed, and may aggregate into microscopically identifiable siderotic granules present in the cytoplasm of immature red blood cells. Small amounts of ferritin are also found in the plasma; this quantity is directly related to the stored ferritin in reticuloendothelial and parenchymal cells. Accordingly, hypotransferrinemia is found in iron deficiency states and hypertransferrinemia in some iron storage diseases (e.g., essential hemochromatosis). Plasma ferritin concentrations are determined by radioimmunoassay. See also *apoferritin.*

ferritin-coupled antibody the combined form of ferritin (an iron-containing protein) with antibody. Because ferritin is highly electron dense, the electron microscope can be used to localize antigen-antibody complexes in fixed tissue.

ferrochelatase (fer″ro-ke′la-tās) a mitochondrial enzyme of the lyase class (protoheme ferro-lyase, EC 4.99.1.1) that catalyzes the incorporation of iron (Fe^{2+}) into protoporphyrin to form protoheme: protoporphyrin + iron(II) ⇄ protoheme + 2 H^+. A deficiency of this enzyme has been observed in erythropoietic protoporphyria, an autosomal dominant trait with variable penetrance and expressivity, and in variegate porphyria, also inherited as an autosomal dominant trait. See also *porphyria.*

ferrocyanide (fer″o-si′ah-nīd) a coordinate complex anion with a valence of –4, in which a ferrous (Fe^{2+}) ion is coordinately linked to six cyanide (CN^-) groups. It is formed by the reduction of the ferricyanide ion, as for example in some methods for blood glucose determination. See also *ferricyanide.*

ferrokinetic (fer″ro-ki-net′ik) pertaining to the turnover or rate of change of iron in the body.

ferrokinetics study a procedure in nuclear medicine that uses ^{59}Fe as a tracer to follow the metabolism of iron in the body over a 3-wk period. Ferrous citrate Fe 59 is injected after incubation with the patient's blood. The plasma protein transferrin carries the iron to the marrow, where it is bound into hemoglobin in newly formed red blood cells. The radioactivity of both the red blood cells and plasma is counted in blood samples; the radioactivity of the marrow (in the sacrum), heart, spleen, and liver is determined by external counting.

A plot is made of the variation of organ activities over time. The blood sample counts are used to determine several indices: (1) plasma iron clearance, the half-time for reduction of plasma activity; (2) daily percentage of red cell incorporation, the fraction of the injected iron in the red cells; (3) plasma iron turnover rate, the rate (in milligrams per day) at which iron is removed from the plasma; and (4) red cell iron turnover rate, the rate (in milligrams per day) at which iron is incorporated in red cells. See also *red cell survival test.*

ferromagnetic (fer″ro-mag-net′ik) pertaining to materials, such as iron, nickel, cobalt, and certain alloys, in which the intrinsic magnetic moments of the atoms (due to the spins of unpaired electrons) are coherent. Throughout regions 1–100 μm in diameter, called domains, all the atomic magnetic moments are aligned. In unmagnetized material the magnetizations of the domains are randomly directed. The domains aligned with an applied magnetic field grow as the field strength is increased, until the saturation magnetization is reached when all the atomic magnetic moments are aligned. When the applied field is removed, some remanence magnetization remains; an opposing field (the coercive field) is required for removing all magnetization. Ferromagnetic susceptibilities can be as high as 10^6. Above a certain temperature, the Curie point, such materials become paramagnetic and their susceptibility is inversely proportional to the difference between the temperature and the Curie point.

ferrous (Fe^{2+} or Fe(II)) (fer′us) containing iron in the plus-two oxidation state.

ferrous citrate Fe 59 a radiopharmaceutical. See also *ferrokinetics study* and *iron-59.*

ferrous ferricyanide see *Turnbull blue.*

ferroxidase (fer-ok′si-dās) an enzyme of the oxidoreductase class (EC 1.16.3.1) that catalyzes the reaction 4 iron(II) + 4 H^+ + O_2 ⇄ 4 iron(III) + 2 H_2O. It is a copper-containing protein commonly known as *ceruloplasmin.*

ferruginous (fer-u′jĭ-nus) [L. *ferruginosus; ferrugo* iron rust] containing iron.

ferruginous micelles the nonferritin aggregates of iron in the mitochondria of pathologic normoblasts.

fertile (fer′til) [L. *fertilis*] fruitful; capable of producing offspring.

fertility (fer-til′ĭ-te) the capacity to conceive or to induce conception.

fertility factor see *F p.* under *plasmid.*

fertility inhibition the mechanism by which the transfer operon of plasmid transfer is regulated. Fertility-inhibition (fin) genes repress the operon by not allowing formation of F pili. Fin^- mutants derepress the operon by forming F pili in all or most cells. See also *p. transfer* under *plasmid.*

fertilization (fer′tĭ-lĭ-za′shun) the process involving the fusion of male and female gametes and the combination of their genetic information to form a potential individual. It occurs in a complex sequence and involves release of gametes, their transportation to the fertilization site, gamete maturation, acrosome reaction, sperm penetration, fusion of egg and sperm pronuclei, egg activation, cortical reaction, egg engulfment of sperm, completion of meiosis, fusion of haploid nuclei, and initiation of the development of the fertilized egg.

Release and Transport of the Gametes to the Fertilization Site. The process of gametogenesis results in the formation of the sperm and egg, which are usually produced by two separate individuals.

In animals that have external fertilization, the male and female gametes are deposited in the same area at approximately the same time. The gametes come together (usually by random collision), and as the sperm approaches the egg a sticky, gelatinous coat surrounding the egg (cumulus oophorus) traps the sperm.

In animals that have internal fertilization, the male and female gametes travel to specific locations to meet. In mammals, the oocyte is normally transported from the ovary into the oviduct by fluid flow and the fimbria structure of the uterus. Fertilization usually occurs in the ampulla of the oviduct, although abdominal pregnancies occur if a suitable place for the placenta is found. The oocyte can be fertilized for only about 24 hr after release. Sperm and seminal fluid are deposited either into the vagina (in humans) or into the uterus, the volume varying with the species. The sperm reach the ampulla rapidly (in 30 min in humans). The combined effect of the estrogen released by the female, the oxytocin released by the female at orgasm, and the prostaglandins present in the semen stimulates the muscle contraction and cervical changes that aid in the sperm's penetration of the uterus. In the human male, of the several hundred million sperm released in one ejaculate, only a few hundred sperm survive to reach the ampulla; they have the capability of fertilization for only about 48 hr.

Final Maturation of the Gametes. The male and female gametes continue to mature; capacitation of the sperm (a sequence of events that is not well understood) is one of the continuing developments. This process, which takes 5–6 hr in humans, must occur prior to the acrosome reaction; normally it occurs in the female reproductive tract. In vitro, capacitation can be induced in a saline solution.

The Acrosome Reaction and Penetration of the Sperm. This reaction involves the opening of the acrosome vessel of the sperm and the release of its contents. The sperm's plasma membrane fuses to the acrosome membrane in the sperm head and acrosomal enzymes are released; these probably help to form a passageway through the cumulus oophorus and zona pellucida surrounding the egg. The spermatozoan nucleus then enters the egg. (The plasma membrane does not.)

The acrosomal enzymes released from the sperm play an important role in the fusion and passageway formation processes. Among the enzymes are hyaluronidase (which is responsible for penetration through the cumulus oophorus) and acrosin (a protease that penetrates through the zona pellucida).

Fusion of Egg and Sperm Pronuclei. After the sperm nucleus has entered the egg, the male and female pronuclei enlarge and fuse to form a single zygote nucleus. DNA replication usually is initiated at this point.

Egg Activation and the Cortical Reaction. The egg's response to the penetration of the sperm is the beginning of embryonic development. Within seconds after fusion of the gamete plasma membranes, the membrane potential of the egg has changed to prevent the entrance of more than one sperm (polyspermy). Initially, the inside of the egg is slightly negatively charged, becoming slightly positively charged after sperm contact.

In the cortical reaction of sea urchins, the cortical granules (small membrane-bound vesicles) under the plasma membrane fuse with the membrane. As they release their contents into the space between the plasma membrane and the inner vitelline membrane, all sperm other than the one responsible for fertilization detach from the egg's surface. The vitelline membrane fills with fluid and becomes the fertilization membrane. The contents of the cortical granules include vitelline delaminase (a protease), which breaks the bonds between the vitelline and plasma membranes; a glycoprotein, which draws water into the vitelline layer; a factor to harden the fertilization layer; and hyalin, a structural protein. Collectively the contents effect complete blockage to polyspermy. It is believed that related events occur with the mammalian egg.

Engulfment of the Sperm. By the time the fertilization membrane is formed, the entire head of the fertilizing sperm is engulfed by the cytoplasm of the egg.

Completion of Meiosis by Oocyte. In most animals, the oocyte nucleus does not complete meiosis until after the sperm nucleus has completely entered the cytoplasm of the egg. Formation of new polar bodies (haploid meiotic daughter cells with virtually no cytoplasm) is one of the earliest signs of successful fertilization.

Conditions for in vitro fertilization can be achieved for many animals. Greater success is obtained with oocytes that have been removed after ovulation. When sperm that have undergone capacitation are added to these mature oocytes, fertilization occurs, followed by embryonic development.

See also *androgenesis, gametogenesis, gynogenesis,* and *parthenogenesis.*

FET abbrev. See *field effect t.* under *transistor.*

fetal (fe′tal) of or pertaining to a fetus, or to the in utero development that occurs after the embryonic period.

fetal antigen a tumor-associated antigen that is normally found in fetal tissue but not in normal adult tissue. Fetal antigens may reappear in those individuals who develop a neoplastic disease. Carcinoembryonic antigen and alpha-fetoprotein are two examples of fetal antigens.

fetal circulation the movement of blood through the vascular system of the fetus and placenta. In order that the fetal blood may be directed through the placenta for purposes of oxygenation and nutrition, certain anatomic modifications are necessary.

Blood reaches the fetus from the placenta via the umbilical vein. This oxygenated blood enters the ductus venosus, a large vessel that arises at the juncture of the portal and umbilical veins. Any blood that has passed through the liver joins with blood from the ductus venosus in the inferior vena cava. The valve of the latter directs this blood through the foramen ovale in the interatrial septum directly into the left atrium. The blood then passes through the left atrioventricular valve into the left ventricle and then into the aorta, from which it is distributed primarily to the heart muscle itself, the head, and the upper extremities.

Blood that has circulated throughout the upper body returns to the heart via the superior vena cava and is directed into the right atrium and on into the right ventricle. From there, this unoxygenated blood is pumped into the pulmonary trunk. At the juncture of the right and left pulmonary arteries, the ductus arteriosus connects directly with the descending aorta.

The blood flow through fetal lungs is minimal; the pressure exerted by the unexpanded lungs and the resulting hypoxia of the surrounding tissue result in high vascular resistance in the pulmonary arteries, causing the blood to flow directly through the ductus arteriosus and into the aorta. This blood, mixed with a small quantity from the left ventricle, flows to the viscera and lower extremities, but most of it is carried by the paired umbilical arteries directly to the placenta.

Dramatic changes in the circulatory system result at birth: loss of the placental circulation doubles the systemic vascular resistance while the pulmonary resistance drops drastically with lung inflation. The equalization of pressures between the two atria caused by the drop in flow from the inferior vena cava and the increased flow in the pulmonary vein causes closure of the valve-like foramen ovale.

As oxygenated blood flows at fairly high pressure through the aorta, it flows back through the ductus arteriosus toward the pulmonary trunk, which at this stage has a much lower resistance. The high oxygen tension in the blood causes vasoconstriction of the ductus arteriosus and thereby functional closure, which may also be influenced by nervous innervation. Anatomic occlusion through fibrosis takes several months.

Within hours of birth, strong muscular contractions in the wall of the ductus venosus result in its closure, and the circulation of blood through the liver increases.

See also the accompanying diagrams of the human circulation before and after birth.

fetal hemoglobin (Hb F) a major form of hemoglobin (Hb) found in fetal blood. It contains two alpha-

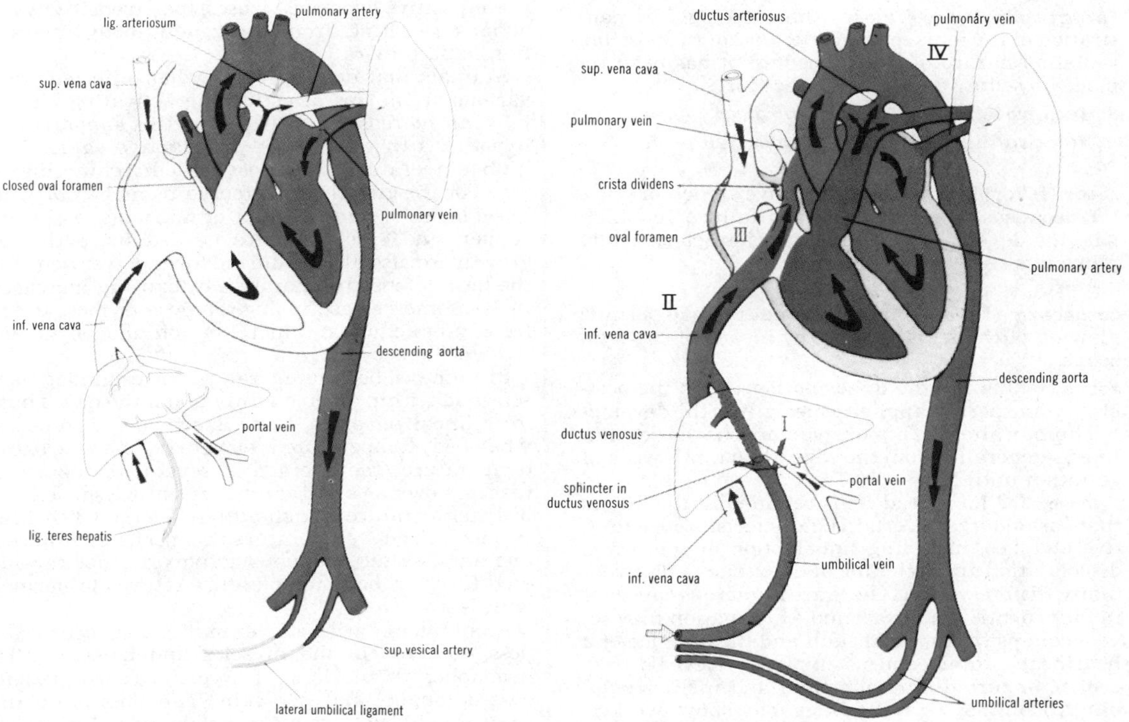

Fetal circulation. Left, Plan of the human circulation before birth. Arrows indicate the direction of the blood flow. *Right,* Plan of the human circulation after birth. Note the changes occurring as a result of the beginning of respiration and the interruption of the placental blood flow. (From Langman, J.: Medical Embryology. 4th ed. Baltimore, Williams & Wilkins Co., 1981.)

and two gamma-globin chains ($\alpha_2{}^A\gamma_2{}^A$). Hb F can be quantitated by the alkali denaturation technique; the distribution of fetal hemoglobin in red blood cells can be measured using the acid elution technique.

The level of Hb F is abnormally elevated in some hemoglobinopathies, and in certain types of thalassemia, leukemia, and aplastic anemia.

Also called *hemoglobin F.* See also *hemoglobin.*

fetal hemoglobin tests 1. the alkali denaturation test, used to quantitate fetal hemoglobin. It is based on the knowledge that fetal hemoglobins are more resistant to alkali denaturation than are other hemoglobins. The hemolysate is mixed with sodium hydroxide; after the addition of half-saturated ammonium sulfate, the denatured hemoglobin is filtered. The absorbance of the supernatant solution at 540 nm reflects the fetal hemoglobin concentration of the blood. The percent Hb F concentration is calculated as the ratio of the absorbance of the treated and untreated tubes times 100.

The reference value for adult blood is less than 2.5 percent. Elevated levels (72.5 percent) are seen in congenital hemolytic anemia, hypoplastic anemia, acute and chronic leukemia, myelopthisic anemia, untreated pernicious anemia, and carcinoma, as well as the β-thalassemia trait. Markedly elevated levels (greater than 15 percent) are seen in homozygous β-thalassemia and hereditary persistence of fetal hemoglobin.

2. differential staining, a technique used to determine the distribution of fetal hemoglobin in erythrocytes. Hemoglobin A (Hb A) and its variants are eluted from fixed erythrocytes in a smear by a citric acid–disodium phosphate buffer at pH 3.3, leaving hemoglobin F (Hb F) within the cell. After staining with eosin, cells containing Hb F stain pink, whereas those containing Hb A appear as ghost cells. In most conditions with acquired elevation of Hb F (aplastic anemia, and hemoglobinopathies including thalassemia and sideroblastic anemia), the distribution of Hb F in red cells is heterogeneous.

Persistence of high fetal hemoglobin generally is manifested by a uniform distribution of Hb F in all red cells, with 25 percent Hb F in each red cell in hereditary persistence of fetal hemoglobin (HPFH) of the Negro type, and 15 percent Hb F in the Greek form. However, some types of low level (3 percent) congenital HPFH have been described with a heterogeneous distribution of Hb F. This technique can also be used to detect fetal red blood cells in the maternal blood system. Also called *acid elution test, Betke-Kleihauer test,* and *Betke stain.*

fetal membrane the amnion and chorion, which

fuse to enclose the fluid-filled amniotic cavity within which the embryo is suspended. See also *amnion* and *chorion.*

α_1-fetoglobulin see *alpha$_1$-fetoprotein.*

fetography (fe-tog'rah-fe) the radiologic demonstration of the fetus in utero. Because of the possible radiation hazard of this procedure, it has been replaced by ultrasonographic procedures.

α_1-fetoprotein see *alpha$_1$-fetoprotein.*

α_1-fetoprotein assays see *alpha$_1$-fetoprotein assays.*

fetor (fe'tor) [L.] a foul or offensive stench or odor.

f. hepaticus, a symptom of liver failure, in which patients develop a peculiar and characteristically pungent sweet-sour breath odor.

f. oris, see *halitosis.*

fetoscopy (fe-tos'ko-pe) a procedure that permits viewing of the fetus in utero by means of the fetoscope.

fetus (fet'tus) [L.] the unborn offspring in the postembryonic period; applied especially to the developing human after the major structures have been outlined—generally, from the seventh to ninth week of gestation until birth.

macerated f., a dead fetus retained in the uterus that has undergone certain characteristic degenerative changes, including liquefaction of the brain, discoloration and softening of the tissues, and, eventually, disintegration. There are numerous causes of in utero death. An ultrasound examination may reveal collapse of the fetal skull and the absence of a heartbeat; amniocentesis typically reveals red, brown, or turbid amniotic fluid and methemoglobin. Abdominal x-ray findings may show overlapping of skull bones, malpositioning of the fetus, exaggerated curvature of the fetal spine, and fetal gas. Treatment involves induction of labor with monitoring of the maternal fibrinogen level.

Feulgen reaction (foil'gen) [Robert *Feulgen,* German physiologic chemist, 1884–1955] a specific histochemical identification for DNA. Mild acid hydrolysis (usually a few minutes in normal hydrochloric acid at 60°C) removes the purine bases and opens the furanose ring of 2-deoxyribose to expose an aldehyde group. Other 2-deoxy-sugars also react, but ordinary aldoses, e.g., glucose, ribose, and xylose, do not. The aldehyde group reacts with Schiff reagent to produce a deep red–purple stain. RNA is Feulgen-negative. Glutaraldehyde and Bouin's fixative should not be used. Also called Feulgen-Schiff reaction.

Feulgen stain a technique for the demonstration of DNA using the Feulgen reaction.

FEV abbrev. See *forced expiratory volume.*

FEV-1 abbrev. for the forced expiration volume over the first second of expiration. See *forced expiratory volume.*

fever (fēver) [L. *febris*] an elevation above normal in the thermoregulatory set point around which body temperature is adjusted. This elevation does not represent a failure of the temperature regulating system, because the heat loss (vasodilation, sweating) and heat conservation (vasoconstriction, shivering) mechanisms remain intact: the temperature of a febrile individual will return to the previously elevated level following warming or cooling of the body. Fever results when an activating agent induces the production of pyrogenic proteins (endogenous pyrogens) by immunologically active phagocytic cells (see *pyrogen*). Activators of fever include endotoxins, the lipopolysaccharide component of the cell wall of gram-negative bacteria; gram-positive bacteria; viruses; hypersensitivity reactions resulting from antigen-antibody interactions; and tumors.

Animals that develop fever when infected with various organisms affecting the activating agents have an increased survival rate; this supports the hypothesis that fever has an adaptive value. The high temperature of the host has a direct inhibitory effect on the growth of microorganisms. Circulating blood levels of minerals and/or nutrients (e.g., iron, copper, and zinc) that are needed for pathogen growth are also altered during fever. Fever benefits the host defense mechanisms by causing increases in lysosome release of hydrolytic enzymes, interferon production, and mobility and phagocytic activity of leukocytes.

In humans, body temperature varies among persons and within a person throughout the day. Thus, for clinical purposes, fever is considered to occur when body temperature is elevated 1°–2° above basal temperature (the average of several temperature readings over a period of time) and always when the body temperature is higher than 37.7°C (100°F). Elevations in body temperature that occur in children and adults after strenuous activity are not considered fever, as body temperature returns to normal with rest.

An individual with a fever may experience weakness, soreness in the muscles and bones, chills, headache, thirst, loss of appetite, constipation, coated tongue, and dry skin. The pulse rate increases 8–10 beats/min for each degree of increase in temperature. With high and sudden onset of fever in children, delirium and convulsions may occur.

Clinical management of an individual with fever includes detection and elimination of the primary cause whenever possible. Fluids are administered orally or intravenously to prevent dehydration. Small feedings of high-calorie, high-protein liquids are recommended to combat fatigue. In some cases it may be necessary to lower the body temperature by administering antipyretic drugs (e.g., aspirin, sodium salicylate) or by sponging the body with tepid water or alcohol.

In addition to mammals, several species of birds, reptiles, amphibians, and fish develop fever in response to such activators as gram-negative bacteria.

See also *febrile s.* under *seizure* and *set point.* Cf. *hyperthermia* and *hypothermia.*

FF abbrev. See *flip-flop.*

FFA abbrev. for free fatty acids. See *nonesterified f. a.* under *fatty acids.*

F factor abbrev. for fertility factor. See *F p. under plasmid.*

FFP abbrev. for fresh frozen plasma.

$F_{I_{CO_2}}$ the fractional concentration of CO_2 in a sample of inspired gas.

$F_{I_{O_2}}$ the fractional concentration of oxygen in a sample of inspired gas.

fiber (fi'ber) a threadlike structure, usually one large enough to be seen with the light microscope. A nerve fiber (neuron) is a single cell with a long process (axon). A muscle fiber is a multinucleated cell that contains many component myofibrils, each made up of a large number of myofilaments. The term collagen fiber generally refers to the elongated strands of connective tissue visible with the light microscope, each composed of large numbers of collagen fibrils, which in turn are formed by the orderly aggregation of tropocollagen filaments. See also *fibril, filament,* and *muscle.*

fiber density 1. the number of nerve or muscle fibers in a given unit area of tissue.

2. in single-fiber electromyography, the mean number of discharges that meet the acceptance criteria for single-fiber action potentials. It is calculated on the basis of a systematic search utilizing random electrode insertions, and can be used to determine the number of fibers per unit area that belong to the same motor unit. A mean fiber density of 1.55 is found in the pickup zone (usually a hemisphere with a diameter of 250–350 μ) of an electrode inserted in the extensor digitorum communis muscle. Fiber density increases with age and with the process of reinnervation.

fiberoptic pertaining to the transmission of light through thin fibers of glass or plastic, called light pipes.

fiberoptics (fi″ber-op′tiks) the transmission of an image along flexible bundles of coated parallel glass or plastic fibers that propagate light by internal reflections. Bundles of light pipes are capable of transmitting images, electronic signals coded as light pulses, or light for measurement by a photometer.

fiber spectrum the range of fiber diameters within a peripheral nerve, which gives an indication of the range of conduction velocities of that nerve.

fibr/o (fi′bro) [L. *fibra* fiber] a word element used in combining form to denote fibers or fibrous tissue, e.g., myofibrosis.

fibril (fi′bril) [L. *fibrilla*] a threadlike structure considerably smaller than the fiber of which it is a component part. Fibrils are generally visible only at high magnification with the light microscope, or when the electron microscope is used. Examples are myofibril and collagen fibril. See also *fiber* and *filament.*

fibrillar (fi′brĭ-lar) pertaining to fibrils.

fibrillated (fi′brĭ-lāt-ed) made up of fibrils.

fibrillation (fi-brĭ-la′shun) 1. a form of cardiac arrhythmia characterized by a rapid, chaotic, uncoordinated sequence of activation of atrial or ventricular contraction. An adequate force of ejection cannot be produced, and pumping of blood by the affected heart chamber stops completely. Fibrillation may be an expression of reentrant activity (circus movement), in which the wave of depolarization travels around the myocardium in a continuous erratic loop, or it may be provoked by irritable ectopic foci that are the result of damage to the myocardium.

2. a local, involuntary skeletal muscle contraction, not visible grossly, that is the result of spontaneous activity in an individual muscle fiber. In electromyography, the term is used loosely as a synonym for the preferred term *fibrillation potential.*

atrial f., the rapid, disorganized contraction of the atrial myocardium. It may be diagnosed by the following electrocardiographic features: a rapid atrial rate of 350–600/min, the absence of the P wave, and the presence of characteristic fibrillatory (f) waves in the baseline. Also, ventricular depolarization is completely irregular. Despite loss of atrial function, the heart can continue to pump with 70–95 percent efficiency. Thus, atrial fibrillation may be present and well tolerated for years, especially if the ventricular rate is nearly normal. This relatively common condition accompanies rheumatic, primary myocardial, and arteriosclerotic heart disease.

f. potential, the electrical activity recorded from an individual muscle fiber undergoing spontaneous contractions that are invisible through the skin. Each action potential recorded from a single fibrillating fiber consists of a biphasic or triphasic spike with an initial positive deflection. The spikes are of relatively low amplitude (usually 20–300 μV) and short duration (less than 5 msec), and occur with regular or irregular rhythm at a frequency of 1–50 Hz. When heard over a loudspeaker, the potentials emit a characteristic short, high-pitched, repetitive clicking sound.

Fibrillation potentials can be provoked by needle electrode movement or may occur spontaneously in denervation and certain myopathic disorders. Because these potentials are seen in a variety of diseases, they are no longer considered to be pathognomonic of any single disorder.

ventricular f., a catastrophic form of cardiac arrhythmia, usually the cause of sudden cardiac death. If this ineffective, rapid, irregular sequence of ventricular activation is not immediately converted to an effective sinus rhythm (by direct-current electrical shock), death invariably ensues. The QRS complex and T wave are completely absent from the electrocardiogram during ventricular fibrillation, and characteristic low amplitude waves in the baseline are seen. Ventricular fibrillation can be provoked by electrocution, pronounced electrolyte imbalances, severe hypothermia, and myocardial infarction and ischemia.

fibrin (fi′brin) the insoluble protein formed from fibrinogen by the proteolytic action of thrombin during the normal clotting of blood. Thrombin proteolysis of fibrinogen causes the release of fibrinopeptides A and B and the formation of the fibrin monomers. The fibrin monomers aggregate, forming a soluble fibrin clot. The clot is finally stabilized by the action of Factor XIII, forming the intermolecularly highly cross-linked, insoluble fibrin clot.

fibrin/o (fi′brĭ-no) a word element used in combining form to denote fibrin or the threads of a clot, e.g., fibrinolysis.

fibrin (fibrinogen) degradation products (FDP) the breakdown products of fibrin and fibrinogen that result from activation of the fibrinolytic system. They are found in the serum of individuals with disseminated intravascular coagulation (DIC), in primary fibrinolysis, and in the urine of renal transplant patients. Four fragments are formed—X (M.W. 270,000), Y (M.W. 15,000), D (M.W. 90,000), and E (M.W. 30,000–50,000)—which act as anticoagulants, interfering with the polymerization of the fibrin monomer or by inhibiting the action of thrombin on fibrinogen. The largest fragment, X, reacts slowly with thrombin to form an abnormal fibrin clot, whereas fragments Y, D, and E act as strong inhibitors to various stages of the clotting sequence.

Screening methods for FDP include the protamine gelation and the ethanol gelation tests. FDP can be quantitated using the staphylococcal clumping test, the red cell hemagglutination inhibition technique, or a commercially prepared kit that uses antibody-coated latex particles.

fibrin (fibrinogen) degradation products methods methods used to quantitate the concentration of fibrin (fibrinogen) degradation products.

latex agglutination test, an immunologic technique that detects the presence of FDP. Serum obtained from whole blood or urine treated with thrombin and a fibrinolytic inhibitor (soybean trypsin inhibitor) is reacted with latex particles that have been coated with antibody to human fibrinogen fragments D and E, and then observed for agglutination. Elevated levels are found in any process that activates the fibrinolytic system. Normal levels are 2–8 μg/ml.

staphylococcal clumping test, an immunologic technique that detects the presence of FDP. Serum obtained from whole blood treated with thrombin and the fibrinolytic inhibitor ε-aminocaproic acid (EACA) or trypsin inhibitor is mixed with a suspension of *Staphylococcus aureus,* Newman D_2C, coagulase negative, and observed for clumping. Normal levels are 0–8 μg/ml of fibrinogen equivalents. Elevated levels are found in any process that activates the fibrinolytic system.

tanned red cell hemagglutination inhibition test, the most sensitive immunologic technique for detecting FDP. Fibrinogen-coated, tanned erythrocytes are agglutinated by dilute antifibrinogen antiserum. In the presence of FDP, prior adsorption of antifibrinogen antiserum with an affected individual's serum interferes with this reaction. As little as 5 μg/ml of fibrinogen or degradation products can be detected with this method. Levels of > 25 μg/ml are associated with abnormal bleeding.

fibrin monomer (fi′brin mon′o-mer) the altered fibrinogen molecule that results when thrombin cleaves fibrinopeptide A and B from two of the three paired chains of the fibrinogen molecule. Fibrin monomers polymerize to form an insoluble fibrin clot. See also *fibrin.*

fibrinogen (fi-brin′o-jen) [*fibrin* + Gr. *gennan* to produce] 1. see *Factor I.*

2. [USP], a sterile compound derived from normal human plasma and dried from the frozen state; used to increase the coagulability of blood.

fibrinogen I 125 a radiopharmaceutical used in the detection of deep-vein thrombosis of the legs. The labeled fibrinogen is incorporated into blood clots.

fibrinogenic (fi″brĭ-no-jen′ik) producing or causing the formation of fibrin.

fibrinogen method a quantitative procedure for determining the amount of fibrinogen in a plasma sample. A measured amount of thrombin is added to plasma; the clotting time is noted and compared with clotting times of plasmas containing known amounts of fibrinogen. From this information, the amount of fibrinogen in the unknown sample is determined. Reference ranges are 150–400 g/100 ml.

fibrinogenolysis (fi″brin-o-jĕ-nol′ĭ-sis) [*fibrinogen* + Gr. *lysis* dissolution] the proteolytic destruction or inactivation of fibrinogen in the blood, a result of the activation of plasmin. Fibrinogenolysis clinically resembles disseminated intravascular coagulation (DIC) and is activated by similar mechanisms.

fibrinogenopenia (fi-brin″o-jen″o-pe′ne-ah) an abnormally low concentration of fibrinogen in the blood due to a congenital deficiency of fibrinogen, primary fibrinolysis (fibrinogenolysis), and fibrinolysis secondary to disseminated intravascular coagulation (DIC) or (acquired) defective production of fibrinogen in liver disease. See also *disseminated intravascular coagulation.*

fibrinogenous (fi″brĭ-noj′ĕ-nus) caused by fibrin; resulting from the formation of fibrin.

fibrinogen titer test a method used to estimate the blood level of fibrinogen. Thrombin is added to serial dilutions of an individual's plasma; the fibrinogen titer is the highest plasma dilution in which a visible fibrin clot will form. Clot formation in a 1:32 dilution indicates that normal levels of fibrinogen needed for hemostasis are present (fibrinogen concentration greater than 100 mg/100 ml). A reduction in titer indicates low or abnormal fibrinogen. Heparin and fibrin degradation products will produce a falsely low titer.

fibrinoid (fi′brĭ-noid) [*fibrin* + Gr. *eidos* form] a term used in histology to denote a homogeneous, eosinophilic substance that stains like fibrin but which is probably homogenized collagen or ground substance. It is found in degenerating connective tissue, in rheumatic nodules, and in many other pathologic processes.

fibrinokinase (fi″bri-no-ki′nās) an undesirable synonym for plasmin activator that is extracted from a tissue source.

fibrinolysin (fi″bri-nol′ĭ-sin) see *plasmin.*

fibrinolysis (fi″brĭ-nol′ĭ-sis) [*fibrin* + Gr. *lysis* dissolution] the enzymatic dissolution of fibrin that results from the activation of plasminogen to plasmin. Although the identity of the circulating plasminogen activator is not fully understood, known activators include kallikrein (and thus indirectly Factor XIIa), urokinase (found normally in urine), and streptokinase. Both urokinase and streptokinase have been used therapeutically on an experimental basis for dissolution of in vivo clots. Hereditary abnormalities of plasminogen have been reported with an immunologically normal amount of plasminogen but abnormal fibrinolysis. Fibrinolysis occurs rarely as a primary disorder and is usually secondary to disseminated intravascular coagulation (DIC).

fibrinolytic (fi″brĭ-no-lit′ik) pertaining to or causing fibrinolysis.

fibrinopenia (fi″brĭ-no-pe′ne-ah) [*fibrin* + Gr. *penia* poverty] a deficiency of fibrinogen in the blood. See also *fibrinogenopenia.*

fibrinopeptide (fi″brĭ-no-pep′tīd) one of the two acidic polypeptide fragments, fibrinopeptide A and B, accounting for 3 percent of the weight of fibrinogen. They are released in pairs and sequentially from the terminal ends of the alpha and beta chains of fibrinogen by the proteolytic action of thrombin.

fibrin plate lysis a measure of fibrinolytic activity. Active plasmin, and available plasmin obtained through plasminogen activation with streptokinase, can be measured by applying the samples to a fibrin-agarose gel substrate, and then examining the gel for lysis after incubation. This procedure has largely been replaced by the casein hydrolysis test for research purposes and the euglobulin lysis test in clinical practice.

fibrin-stabilizing factor (FSF) see *Factor XIII.*

fibrin-stabilizing factor test a test that demonstrates the activity of Factor XIII (fibrin-stabilizing factor). Plasma is recalcified and allowed to clot. Subsequently the clot is suspended in 5 mol/l of urea that disrupts the hydrophobic bonds. In the absence of Factor XIII, covalent bonds are not formed between the fibrin monomers, and the clot will dissolve in less than 24 hr.

fibrin staining 1. a normal technique for the demonstration of acidophilic substances. Fibrin stains pink with eosin and stains with other plasma stains, such as picrofuchsin or light green SF. It stains blue to purple with phosphotungstic acid hematoxylin (PTAH) and is PAS-positive (periodic acid–Schiff). See also *fibrinoid.*

2. see *Gram-Weigert stain.*

fibroadenoma (fi″bro-ad″e-no′mah) [*fibro-* + Gr. *aden* gland + *-oma* tumor] a benign tumor containing fibrous and glandular neoplastic elements.

f. of the breast, a benign tumor of breast tissue in which glands and stroma are present in varying proportions. It is not encapsulated but is sharply demarcated from surrounding normal breast tissue. It is the most common breast tumor in younger women. More than 10 percent of females with a fibroadenoma have or will develop multiple lesions. The tumor may grow more rapidly during pregnancy. Malignant change in a fibroadenoma of the breast is extremely rare. Simple surgical excision of a fibroadenoma is the correct treatment. Cf. *cystosarcoma phyllodes.*

fibroblast (fi′bro-blast) [*fibro* + Gr. *blastos* germ] a spindle-shaped connective tissue cell, derived from mesenchyme, that is involved in the production of extracellular materials (ground substance) and collagen and elastic fibrils. Fibroblasts are active during wound repair, contributing to the formation of granulation tissue and the contraction of the wound (myofibroblasts).

fibroblastic (fi″bro-blas′tik) pertaining to fibroblasts or their proliferation.

fibrocartilage (fi″bro-kar′tĭ-lij) white, fibrous cartilage that serves as a cushion or buffer. It consists of dense bundles of collagen, with small scattered groups of chondrocytes between the bundles, surrounded by cartilaginous matrix. Fibrocartilage is usually seen as a disk between articulating bones.

fibrocystic disease of breast see *cystic disease of breast.*

fibroelastic (fi″bro-e-las′tik) composed of fibrous and elastic tissue.

fibroelastosis (fi″bro-e″las-to′sis) a proliferation of fibroblasts with the formation of collagen and elastic fibers. The term commonly refers to involvement of the subendocardial connective tissue.

endocardial f., a rare disease of unknown cause, characterized by a focal or diffuse fibroelastic thickening of the endocardial walls. It occurs primarily in infants and young children, possibly with a genetic link. Grossly, there is an opaque thickening of the heart walls, particularly the left ventricle. The heart is often enlarged and dilated. Histologically, there is a marked increase of the collagenous and elastic fibers that run parallel to the surface. In affected infants there is often a sudden onset of cardiac failure, which may be delayed even to adulthood, when congestive heart failure is common.

fibroepithelial polyp a polypoid lesion of the skin or a mucosal surface, in which a connective tissue core is covered by nonneoplastic epithelium. Generally, the term is applied to cutaneous lesions, and the epithelial covering is stratified squamous in type.

fibroepithelioma a variant of basal cell carcinoma in which slender sheets and cords of cells branch within the dermis. Although it is typically indolent, it can progress into an infiltrating carcinoma.

fibroid (fi′broid) [*fibro-* + Gr. *eidos* form] 1. having a fibrous structure.

2. See *uterine l.* under *leiomyoma.*

fibroma (fi-bro′mah) [*fibro-* + Gr. *-oma* tumor] a benign tumor of fibroblasts. Fibromas are relatively uncommon and can be difficult to distinguish histologically from a fibromatosis.

chondromyxoid f., a benign localized tumor of bone that contains chondroid and myxoid elements in varying proportions; 75 percent occur in bones of the lower limb, particularly the tibia, and most patients are between the ages of 10 and 30 yr. The tumor may recur following curettage, and local excision of the entire lesion is preferable.

nonossifying f., a bone lesion that occurs in the long bones of the extremities and is seen in young people. Multiple lesions may be present, each forming a well-circumscribed lucent opacity surrounded by a rim of sclerotic bone on x-ray. These are benign lesions and most are asymptomatic, but occasionally one is responsible for a pathologic fracture. Typically, they are metaphyseal in location; histologically, they appear to fall within the broad group of fibrous histiocytomas by virtue of their fibroblast-like cells arranged in a storiform pattern with admixed pleomorphic cells and vacuolated macrophages. Treatment is by curettage. Also called fibrous cortical defect.

odontogenic f., a myxoma of the jaw in which there is increased fibrous stroma and odontogenic epithelial rests.

ossifying f., a benign fibroosseous lesion that commonly occurs in the jaws and frequently in long bones. Small spicules of bone with a peripheral layer of osteoblasts lie within a fibrous stroma. The lesion usually grows slowly but tends to recur after curettage.

fibromatosis (fi″bro-mah-to′sis) [*fibro-* + Gr. *-oma* tumor + *-osis* condition] a group of soft tissue lesions produced by a proliferation of fibroblasts. They are histologically benign, but some, such as the so-called desmoid tumor, can aggressively infiltrate adjacent tissues. Consequently, they are difficult to eradicate surgically and recurrences are common; they should nevertheless be treated as conservatively as possible.

The following conditions are generally included among the fibromatoses: plantar and palmar fibromatosis (Dupuytren's contracture), penile fibromatosis, retroperitoneal and mediastinal fibrosis, and aggressive fibromatoses (abdominal and extraabdominal desmoids). Fibromatoses occurring mainly in infants and children include: congenital generalized fibromatosis, sternomastoid tumor, digital fibrous tumors, juvenile aponeurotic fibroma, hereditary gingival fibroma, and fibrosis hyalinica multiplex juvenilis.

gingival f., a rare hereditary condition in which the gums become thickened by the proliferation of fibrous tissue. It may be present at birth but more frequently develops as the deciduous teeth erupt, and the teeth may become submerged or even buried by the fibrous overgrowth. Surgical excision of the gingival tissue is the only treatment. See also *gingival h.* under *hypertrophy.*

fibromyoma a leiomyoma containing a considerable admixture of fibrous connective tissue. See also *leiomyoma.*

fibromyositis (fi″bro-mi″o-si′tis) [*fibro-* + Gr. *mys* muscle + *-itis*] inflammation of fibromuscular tissue; a term used to describe a group of ill-defined nonspecific disorders that lack a detectable pathologic change. This condition frequently involves joints, joint capsules, muscles, and adjacent structures, and leads to pain, stiff joints, and tenderness. Fibromyositis is seen most commonly in the lower back, shoulders, and neck, and may be initiated by trauma, exposure to cold and dampness, and psychogenic factors. Diagnosis is established by exclusion of other possible causes. The condition usually resolves spontaneously within several days and may respond favorably to heat and massage.

fibronectin (fi″bro-nek′tin) a major fibroblast surface-associated glycoprotein that has been isolated in either monomeric or dimeric form; M.W. 220,000. It has been shown to be identical to cold insoluble globulin.

fibroplasia (fi″bro-pla′se-ah) the formation of fibrous tissue, as in response to trauma or injury. Also called *desmoplasia* and *fibrosis.*

retrolental f., an ocular condition found in premature infants, characterized by vascular proliferation and, often, leakage. It leads to detachment of the retina, arrested eye growth, and blindness. The cause has been associated with the use of abnormally high oxygen concentrations in caring for premature infants. When this association was discovered and corrected, the disease virtually disappeared. Also called retinopathy of the premature.

fibros/o (fi-bro′so) a word element used in combining form to denote fibrous tissue, e.g., fibrositis.

fibrosarcoma (fi″bro-sar-ko′mah) [*fibro-* + Gr. *sarx* flesh + *-oma* tumor] the malignant tumor of fibroblasts. Fibrosarcomas can arise almost anywhere in the body, but the majority involve the limbs and limb girdles. A well-differentiated fibrosarcoma may be histologically indistinguishable from an aggressive fibromatosis, and fibrosarcomas are frequently confused with other sarcomas by light microscopy; ultrastructural confirmation of the cell type in doubtful cases is therefore useful. Fibrosarcomas infiltrate surrounding tissues and may be difficult to eradicate surgically. They tend to recur and the more malignant tumors may metastasize. See also *dermatofibrosarcoma protuberans, fibromatosis, histiocytoma,* and *soft tissue tumors.*

fibrosis (fi-bro′sis) [*fibro-* + Gr. *-osis* condition] the formation of fibrous tissue, as in the wound healing response to trauma or injury. See also *desmoplasia* and *fibroplasia.*

cystic f., see *cystic fibrosis.*

diffuse interstitial f., see *pulmonary f.*

endomyocardial f., a condition affecting the heart muscle, which is characterized by progressive fibrosis and hyalinization of the endocardium and subendocardial myocardium of the inflow tracts of both ventricles. The etiology is unknown, but environmental factors are suspected. Most common in Africa, it is usually seen in children and young adults. The involvement of the mitral and tricuspid valves may lead to regurgitation. As the disease progresses, cardiac output decreases and congestive heart failure develops. Physical examination may reveal ascites and edema. Response to treatment is poor. X-rays, electrocardiograms, and cardiac catheterization are useful in diagnosis.

hepatic f., the presence of excess fibrous tissue in the liver, caused by the consolidation of preexisting, or the active production of new collagenous fibers. Hepatic fibrosis may be the result of hepatic injury with regeneration and remodeling (see *cirrhosis*), or it may occur in congenital or acquired forms without liver cell damage.

Congenital hepatic fibrosis is a variant of polycystic disease of the liver. This condition, transmitted as an autosomal recessive trait, is often associated with renal cysts. Such livers contain excess mature portal and periportal connective tissue that interferes with portal venous blood flow, producing portal hypertension.

Acquired hepatic fibrosis may be seen in idiopathic portal hypertension; portal areas and portal vein branches display variable increases in connective tissue. It may also occur as a result of schistosomiasis. There is a delayed hypersensitivity reaction to the ova of the parasite, resulting in an increased deposition of portal connective tissue. Portal hypertension, varices, and hepatomegaly are commonly seen without evidence of hepatocellular injury and regeneration.

Diagnosis of any form of hepatic fibrosis relies on the clinical picture and histologic examination of a liver biopsy. Stains that are specific for connective tissue (e.g., aniline blue or trichrome stains) may aid in the identification.

mediastinal f., progressive fibrosis in the mediastinum, comparable and sometimes associated with retroperitoneal fibrosis. In some patients it follows an infectious process. The symptoms are variable, but a superior vena caval syndrome may be produced.

pulmonary f., a term used to refer to the deposition of fibrous tissue within the lungs. It is a general term in its origin, being applicable to the localized fibrosis of tuberculosis and other infections, but in current usage pulmonary fibrosis is a shortened form of diffuse interstitial pulmonary fibrosis and is a specific response to a number of toxic agents or processes. This response is characterized by a progressive and diffuse deposition of fibrous tissue within alveolar walls, accompanying or following an active interstitial and/or alveolar inflammatory process. The causes are many, some of them obscure and as yet unidentified, and include inhaled toxic substances, immune disorders involving the deposition of immune complexes within the alveolar septa, diffuse granulomatous disorders such as sarcoidosis, and the late sequelae of the adult respiratory distress syndrome (ARDS).

Also called cryptogenic fibrosing alveolitis (a British term), desquamative interstitial pneumonitis (DIP), diffuse interstitial fibrosis, and usual interstitial pneumonitis (UIP).

retroperitoneal f., proliferation of fibrous tissue in the lower retroperitoneum to form a plaque that envelops and compresses anatomic structures in this region. Most patients are between 40 and 60 yr. The most serious effect is produced by compression of the ureters, resulting in hydronephrosis and elevation of the serum levels of BUN and creatinine.

Ureteral obstruction and dilation may be identified by intravenous pyelography. Corticosteroid therapy may be helpful; however, surgical intervention to relieve the obstruction is often required. Frequently, the cause of the condition is not determined, but an association with the antiserotonin drug methysergide, used in the treatment of migraine headache, has been reported.

fibrotic (fi-brot′ik) pertaining to or characterized by fibrosis.

fibrous (fi′brus) composed of or containing fibers.

fibrous dysplasia a bone lesion in which irregular plates of immature bone replace the normal bone. The process may affect one bone or it may be a multiple one; in the latter condition, the patient may manifest cutaneous café au lait spots and various endocrine disorders (Albright's syndrome).

fibrous histiocytoma a benign soft tissue neoplasm in which there is a proliferation of spindle cells that typically form a storiform (radiating) pattern. Varying numbers of larger cells, some of them bizarre or multinucleated, or vacuolated xanthomatous cells are intermingled with the groups of spindle cells. The lesion may be viewed as the benign counterpart of the malignant fibrous histiocytoma. A variant with often considerable mitotic activity has been described in the skin, and designated atypical fibrous xanthoma; reportedly, it does not metastasize. The nature of the proliferating cell in the fibrous histioctyomas is controversial, and fibroblasts, histiocytes, or some intermediate form (facultative fibroblasts) have been suggested. Ultrastructurally, many cells resemble fibroblasts but show more of a tendency toward lipid production. Probably a cell of mesenchymal origin with varying morphologic expression is involved.

atypical f. h., a skin lesion, usually seen on an exposed area in older individuals, which is composed of fibroblasts, pleomorphic cells with irregular or multiple nuclei, and vacuolated cells. Mitotic activity may cause the pathologist concern but there are only occasional reports of metastases. Also called atypical fibroxanthoma.

malignant f. h., a soft tissue sarcoma characterized histologically by a storiform arrangement of spindle cells with varying numbers of interspersed, large, bizarre or multinucleated cells. The cell of origin is probably mesenchymal with variable expression toward the fibroblast or fat cell, and the tumor overlaps with fibrosarcoma and liposarcoma. It is the most common soft tissue malignancy in older people. Myxoid and angiomatoid forms have been described.

fibrous proteins a broad class of proteins constituted of one or more polypeptide chains or groups of such chains; they are elongated, very asymmetric molecules whose length may be 10 or more times their diameter. The polypeptide chains may be coiled and may be cross-linked by disulfide bonds and by hydrogen bonds. See also *protein.* Cf. *globular proteins.*

fibrous thyroiditis see *invasive fibrous t.* under *thyroiditis.*

fibul/o (fib′u-lo) a word element used in combining form to denote the fibula, e.g., fibular.

fibula (fib′u-lah) [L. "buckle"] [NA], the more lateral of the two bones of the leg between the knee and ankle joints. The fibula is a slender bone largely covered by muscle. It articulates above and below with the tibia; in addition, its lower end has a facet for the talus and projects as the lateral malleolus.

ficin (fi′sin) [L *ficus* fig] an enzyme of the hydrolase class (EC 3.4.22.3). It is a thiol proteinase able to attack a wide range of protein substrates. There is some preference for peptide bonds involving neutral, alkyl amino acids. Ficin is prepared from the sap of fig trees (*Ficus*), and is used in blood banks to enzymatically treat red cells to remove sialic acid residues from the cell membranes. This treatment lowers the zeta potential of the cells and allows some otherwise nonagglutinating antibodies to agglutinate saline suspended cells. The treatment may enhance reactions in some antigenic systems, notably the Kidd and Rh systems. Alternately, some antigens are destroyed; e.g., Duffy.

Fick's law (fik) [Adolph Eugen *Fick,* German physiologist, 1829–1901] stated as: the rate of diffusion is proportional to the concentration gradient.

Fick principle a concept that allows the measurement of blood flow through an organ by indirect measurement using a diffusable indicator, either a dye or a radioisotope tracer. The rate of accumulation or consumption of the indicator in the organ, divided by the difference of the indicator concentrations in the blood flowing into and out of the organ, is equal to the blood flow rate. This is a consequence of conservation of the indicator. Originally, the cardiac output is the oxygen consumption rate divided by the difference in oxygen concentrations in pulmonary arterial and venous blood.

FID abbrev. for flame ionization detector. See under *gas chromatography.*

field (fēld) 1. an area or open space, such as an operative field or the visual field.

2. a range of specialization in knowledge, study, or occupation.

3. a physical quantity that varies throughout space rather than being localized at a single point, such as an electromagnetic field, gravitational field, or radiation field.

4. in computer programming, an area of an input/output record or a computer word that contains one data item.

f. of microscope, the area of a specimen that can be seen through a microscope at one time. A high-power field is that area visible under the high-power objective; a low-power field is that visible under low power.

f. of view, the area seen by a camera that should appear on a photograph.

FIGLU see *formiminoglutamic acid.*

filament (fil′ah-ment) [L. *filamentum*] 1. the threadlike component of fibrils, visible only with the electron microscope. Examples are myofilament and tropocollagen filament. Cf. *fiber* and *fibril.*

2. in bacteriology, a greatly elongated bacillus due to a delay or failure of cleavage during growth.

filamentous (fil-ah-men′tus) being composed of long, threadlike structures; said of rod-shaped bacteria that grow in long threads.

Filaria (fĭ-la′re-ah) [L. *filum* thread] the former genus for members of the superfamily Filarioidea.

F. bancrofti, see *W. bancrofti* under *Wuchereria.*

F. demarquayi, see *M. ozzardi* under *Mansonella.*
F. loa, see *L. loa* under *Loa.*
F. medinensis, see *D. medinensis* under *Dracunculus.*
F. ozzardi, see *M. ozzardi* under *Mansonella.*
F. sanguinis, see *D. immitis* under *Dirofilaria.*
F. tucumana, see *M. ozzardi* under *Mansonella.*
F. volvulus, see *O. volvulus* under *Onchocerca.*

filaria (fi-la're-ah), pl. *filariae.* a nematode worm of the superfamily Filarioidea. See also the accompanying illustration.

filariasis (fil"ah-ri'ah-sis) a human infection with filarial nematodes, most commonly *Wuchereria, Brugia, Dipetalonema, Mansonella, Loa,* and *Onchocerca.* This disease is transmitted by the bite of a mosquito (*Culex, Aedes,* and *Mansonia*), a midge (*Culicoides*), a tabanid (*Chrysops*), or a black fly (*Simulium*). With the larval invasion of lymph nodes and blood vessels, a chronic insidious infection results of variable manifestation, with some degress of progressive lymphedema and inflammation, particularly in the lower extremities and the external genitalia. Adult worms live in the lymph nodes, microfilariae in the blood. As adult worms die, fibrinoid necrosis, eosinophilic infiltration, granuloma formation, and fibrosis occur. In severely infected individuals, lymphatic obstruction may lead to elephantiasis, with resultant massive enlargement of the affected parts.

Filariasis can be detected by complement-fixation tests, bentonite flocculation, and indirect hemagglutination tests.

See also *Bancroft's filariasis, elephantiasis,* and *Malayan filariasis.*

Bancroft's f., see *Bancroft's filariasis.*
Malayan f., see *Malayan filariasis.*

filaricide (fĭ-lar'i-sīd) any chemical or agent that kills filariae.

Filarioidea (fĭ-lar"e-oi'de-ah) a superfamily of tissue-inhabiting nematodes such as filarial worms and trichina worms. The adult worms are threadlike; the female lays eggs that develop into microfilariae (prelarvae). The microfilariae are ingested by blood-sucking insects, develop in this host, and return to humans as the final host through infected insects. Filariae that infect humans include *Wuchereria, Onchocerca, Brugia,* and *Loa.*

file (fīl) 1. an area of computer storage, particularly on a disk or on magnetic tape, that is assigned to one user or set of data; the information stored there.

2. an instrument with a finely serrated surface used for reducing or smoothing hard substances (e.g., metal, bone) or the materials used in dental restorations.

file maintenance a data-processing operation that consists of updating a computer file.

file management the operating system facilities that support the definition of computer files and information storage and retrieval using these files.

filiform (fil'ĭ-form, fi'lĭ-form) [L. *filum* thread + *forma* form] slender; threadlike.

filling defect a space-occupying mass in the lumen of a hollow organ, which appears on a positive-contrast radiograph as an area of decreased density.

film (film) 1. a thin layer or coating.

2. a thin sheet of plastic coated with a light-sensitive emulsion, used to make photographs or radiographs.

no-screen f., x-ray film with an emulsion that has a faster film speed than plain film and is more sensitive to x-rays than to light. Because it has more detail and contrast than plain films, it is used in cardboard holders to produce radiographs of thin parts.

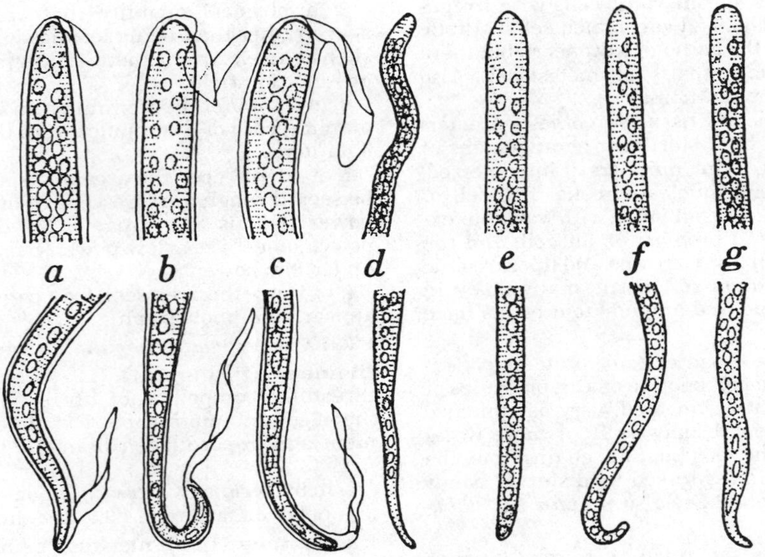

Filaria. Differential characteristics of the anterior and posterior ends of microfilariae found in humans: *a, Wuchereria bancrofti; b, Brugia malayi; c, Loa loa; d, Onchocerca volvulus; e, Dipetalonema perstans; f, Dipetalonema streptocerca;* and *g, Mansonella ozzardi.* (From Faust, E. C., et al.: Craig and Faust's Clinical Parasitology. 8th ed. Philadelphia, Lea & Febiger, 1970.)

plain f., x-ray film designed to be used in x-ray cassettes, thus having an emulsion more sensitive to the ultraviolet light produced by the intensifying screens. It also is generally used in cardboard holders in place of no-screen film in radiography of the extremities. Also called regular film and screen film.

rapid processing (RP) f., x-ray film designed for use with rapid automatic processing equipment. See also *automatic f. p.* under *film processing.*

x-ray f., 1. photographic film used for making radiographs. It usually is coated with emulsion on both sides. See also *no-screen f.* and *plain f.*

2. a radiograph. Also called *view.*

film badge a personal radiation-monitoring device that measures an individual's exposure to beta-, gamma-, and x-radiation. It consists of a piece of photographic film, a light-opaque holder, and various filters that absorb some radiation so that different areas of the film show the cumulative exposure to different energies of radiation.

film base the plastic film on which the emulsion of a photographic film is coated.

film density calibration a quality control check for a rectilinear scanner. It ensures that variations in the observed count rate are accurately recorded by proportional changes in the film density (darkness) of the photograph.

film holder a device to hold x-ray film while it is being exposed. It seals out light and has a sheet of lead foil behind the film that absorbs backscatter. Cardboard film holders are one type; the other is aluminum cassettes, which also have intensifying screens that decrease patient exposure, improve detail, and sandwich the film.

film processing a series of chemical reactions that make the latent image on exposed photographic film visible and permanent. In the first step, development, the exposed silver halide grains in the film emulsion are reduced to metallic silver by the developer, a solution of hydroquinone (the reducing agent) and other chemicals. (In manual processing, the film is then washed in a water bath and an acid stop bath to completely neutralize the developer.) In the next step, fixation, all undeveloped silver halide grains are dissolved by the sodium thiosulfate in the fixer, and the emulsion is hardened and preserved by other chemicals. In the last step, the film is washed and dried.

automatic f. p., the mechanical processing of x-ray film. The processor has three baths: developer, fixer, and wash bath. A system of rollers carries the film through the baths and dryer. The baths are continuously agitated and chemicals added, as they are used up by the development and fixation. The whole process takes 3–6 min; a rapid processor (RP) takes about 90 sec.

film speed the amount of response or blackening of a photographic film to a given amount of light exposure.

Filobasidiella (fi″lo-bah-sid″i-el′ah) a genus of perfect fungi of the class Basidiomycetes. It includes species that are the sexual phase of the genus *Cryptococcus.*

F. bacillisporus, the perfect state for *Cryptococcus neoformans* serotypes B and C.

F. neoformans, the perfect state for *Cryptococcus neoformans* serotypes A and D.

filter (fil′ter) [L. *filtrum*] 1. a device that strains suspended solids out of a liquid.

2. an element of an optical system that absorbs part of the light. Most filters selectively pass certain wavelengths. In x-ray equipment, filters are metal plates, usually aluminum, that absorb soft x-rays before they reach the patient. High-voltage therapeutic x-rays require tin, copper, or lead filters.

3. an electronic circuit that preferentially passes signals of certain frequencies.

added f., an aluminum plate that is inserted into the filter slot of the x-ray tube to remove soft x-rays and thus improve contrast. A minimum of 2 mm of added filter is used in making diagnostic radiographs. Each additional millimeter of filtration requires an increase of the kilovoltage by 2–4 kVp to maintain the same density.

bacterial f., a filter used to remove bacteria from a solution. The maximal pore diameter is 1 nm. Various types have been developed, such as asbestos (Seitz), diatomaceous earth (Berkefeld), porcelain (Selas), sintered glass (Corning), or nitrocellulose (Millipore); they are used for sterilization of solutions that do not tolerate heat treatment. The last-named type can also be used to obtain viable counts, as bacterial colonies develop on the surface when the used filter is placed on a solid culture medium.

barrier f., in a fluorescence microscope, a filter that passes only light in the visible range, thus preventing damage to the eye from the ultraviolet light source.

Berkefeld f., a bacterial filter made of infusorial earth, available in three pore sizes: V (*viel,* or coarse), N (normal), and W (*wenig,* or fine). Most bacteria are removed by the V filter, all are usually removed by the N, and the W is used for exceedingly small organisms.

blocking f., see under *interference f.*

Centriflo f., trademark for an ultrafilter that can sieve out molecules with a molecular weight as low as 20,000; it is used for protein concentration.

Chamberland f., a bacterial filter cylinder made of unglazed porcelain, available in several graded porosities.

collodion f., a type of synthetic cellulose nitrate filter that has pore sizes so uniform that they can be used to measure the size of viruses.

exciter f., a filter in a fluorescence microscope that passes only the wavelength that excites fluorescent dye or other material.

gelatin f., an optical filter that consists of a layer of gelatin containing an organic dye sandwiched between two glass plates. Also called *Wratten f.*

Gelman f., trademark for cellulose triacetate filters that are approximately 150 μm thick; they are supplied in pore sizes of 0.2–5 μm. Physical and optical properties are similar to those of the Millipore filter. See also *membrane filter techniques.*

HEPA f., a filter designed to remove particles 0.3 μm in size or larger from an air stream. HEPA filters should be used in laboratory exhaust systems to remove highly infectious or radioactive materials before the exhaust is discharged to the atmosphere (according to National Fire Protection Association regulation NFPA 56C-1980). They are also used in biological safety cabinets in which air is recirculated to reduce contamination of cultures and media. (Pharmacy departments often use HEPA filters in special air supply systems that blow filtered air out across solutions or materials needing protection from contamination. Use of such laminar flow systems does not protect laboratory personnel if air flows toward them.)

Because HEPA filters may become damaged during shipping and installation, which may allow air to bypass the filters, biological safety cabinets that depend on the performance of the filter system to protect laboratory personnel must be regularly tested after cabinet and filter installation.

high-pass f., in electronics, a filter that passes all frequencies above a certain cutoff frequency while attenuating lower frequencies.

inherent f., the oil between an x-ray tube and the port in its shield. It is equivalent to a 0.5-mm aluminum added filter.

interference f., an optical filter that consists of a dielectric spacer (such as magnesium fluorite) sandwiched between two semitransparent metal films. Interference filters can have an extremely narrow bandpass—8 nm or less.

Light rays are reflected back and forth between the films many times before leaving the dielectric. If the thickness of the dielectric is a multiple of half the wavelength of the light, rays reflected a different number of times constructively interfere. Light of other wavelengths is removed by destructive interference. Only one of the transmitted harmonics is used; the others are absorbed by glass-blocking filters—one that absorbs higher wavelengths and one that absorbs lower wavelengths.

A multilayer interference filter consists of 5–25 layers of alternating high- and low-refractive index layers of dielectric. Light rays are reflected at the interference between layers; as with single-layer filters, only harmonics of twice the layer thickness are transmitted.

low-pass f., in electronics, a filter that passes all frequencies below a certain cutoff frequency while attenuating higher frequencies.

membrane f., a filter made of a thin membrane film of cellulose used for removing particulate matter and microorganisms from water and liquid solutions. It exists in a range of defined pore sizes. Examples are Gradecol and Millipore filters.

microaggregate f., a filter with pore sizes of 20–40 μm, used to remove leukocytes and particulate debris from donor blood prior to transfusion.

Millipore f., trademark for cellulose acetate filters that are approximately 130 ± 10 μm thick; they are supplied in pore sizes of 8 μm to 10 nm. The 5 μm-pore size is recommended for cytologic use. See also *membrane filter techniques.*

Nuclepore f., trademark for polycarbonate filters that are μm thick; they are supplied in pore sizes of 0.1–8 μm. The filters are colorless, transparent membranes with two refractive indices, 1.585 and 1.623 (or 1.584 and 1.616), with uniform cylindrical pores. See also *membrane filter techniques.*

Seitz f., a disposable asbestos pad made to fit a special apparatus; used for filtering out microorganisms.

Thoraeus f., an x-ray filter used primarily in deep therapy. The beam passes through a layer of tin, then copper, then aluminum. The layers absorb the softer x-rays of the beam and also the secondary rays produced in preceding layers. In supervoltage therapy, a lead filter precedes the Thoraeus filter.

Wratten f., see *gelatin f.*

filterable (fil′ter-ah-b′l) small enough to pass through a bacterial filter; said of viruses and subcellular units. The term also is often used more precisely in terms of the maximal pore size of the filter employed.

filter capacitor a large capacitor used in the filter of a power supply. It is connected in parallel with the load so that it provides a low-impedance path for any alternating current component (ripple), and therefore smooths the direct current passing through the load.

filtering (fil′ter-ing) in electronics, the processing of a signal to remove noise by reducing frequency components at frequencies other than the signal frequency, or the processing of the output of a direct current power supply to remove alternating current components.

filter paper a special paper made for use as a filter in a funnel or for use as a support medium in chromatography or electrophoresis.

filter photometer see *colorimeter.*

filtrate (fil′trāt) a liquid that has passed through a filter.

filtration (fil-tra′shun) the process of passing something through a filter or trapping something in a filter. It is applied to either the separation of particulate matter or the separation of high molecular mass compounds from the remaining smaller molecules that pass readily through the filter.

filum terminale (fi′lum ter-mi-na′lē), pl. *fila terminalia* [L.] a thin, threadlike projection of fibrous connective tissue that extends from the caudal tip of the spinal cord, the conus medullaris, to the dorsal aspect of the first coccygeal vertebra. Approximately 20 cm long, the filum is continuous with the pia mater of the spinal cord proximally and blends into the periosteum of the first coccygeal segment distally. The extensive subarachnoid space surrounding the filum is the preferred site for spinal puncture.

fimbria (fim′bre-ah) [L. *fimbriae* (pl.) a fringe] 1. a fringe, border, or edge; fringelike structure, as on the free end of the fallopian tube.

2. one of the minute filamentous appendages of certain bacteria, consisting of a protein (pilin). They are shorter and thinner than flagella. Also called *pilus.*

ovarian f., a single fimbria of the infundibulum of the uterine tube, longer than the rest, which is attached to the tubal ends of the ovaries.

fimbriated (fim′bre-āt-ed) fringed.

finder (find′er) a device on a microscope that facilitates the finding of some object in the field.

fine structure 1. see *ultrastructure.*

2. in atomic spectroscopy, a splitting of spectral lines caused by spin-orbit coupling.

finger (fing′ger) any one of the five digits of the hand.

finite (fi′nīt) [L. *finitus* limited] bounded or limited; in mathematics, contained within some definite interval (not infinite), i.e., in absolute value, less than some specifiable value.

fire (fīr) a chemical process releasing heat and light that requires fuel, oxidizer, ignition energy, and a flame chain reaction. In a laboratory, the fuel for a fire may be present if flammable liquids are handled in open containers at temperatures above their flash-point temperatures; if the oxidizer is present in atmospheric oxygen; and if the ignition energy is present in flames, heating elements, lighted smoking material, or static electricity. See also *combustible liquid, combustion, fire extinguishing, fire prevention, flammable liquid, flash-point temperature,* and *ventilation.*

fire ant an aggressive ant of the order Hymenoptera that attacks humans; commonly found in the southeastern United States. Its sting is painful and results in clusters of pustules. Two types of reactions to the sting can occur, local and systemic. The local reaction is thought to be caused by a necrotizing toxin, solenamine; the systemic reactions are allergic. Diagnosis requires a histopathologic examination of a 72-hr-old pustule. Also called *Solenopsis saevissima richteri.*

fire area an area of a building separated from the remainder of the building by construction with a fire resistance of at least 1 hr and having all communicating openings properly protected by an assembly with a fire resistance rating of at least 1 hr. A fire area has walls that extend to the bottom of the floor above (not stopping at a suspended ceiling), and all openings between the area and the rest of the building have labeled fire doors. Storage limits for flammable and combustible liquids are based on the quantities within separate fire areas. See also *fire door* and *flammable liquid storage limits.*

fire blanket a blanket intended for use in smothering the flames of a clothing fire. It should be noted that fire blankets can be very hazardous if people whose clothing is on fire go to the fire blanket, particularly if they run, which will fan the flames; if they use the blanket in a standing position, which will allow flames and smoke to rise to the face; or if they keep the blanket wrapped around them, which will prevent cooling of burned material and thereby increase the severity of burn injuries. To discourage laboratory personnel from running when on fire and using fire blankets unsafely, some authorities now use the term shock blankets and encourage their use only in the first-aid treatment of shock. For recommended action in case of fire, see *clothing fires.*

fire detection system an automatic system for detecting and signaling the presence of one or more products of combustion, such as heat, infrared or ultraviolet radiation, ionized particles of combustion, rate of temperature rise, or smoke. It makes possible a quick response so that corrective measures may be taken and the fire extinguished. Automatic fire extinguishing systems are preferred if the hazards are severe or if valuable equipment and specimens need to be protected, because such systems provide both fire detection and initial extinguishment.

fire door a door designed to protect an opening and limit the spread of fire into an exit or between two fire areas. A fire door is part of an assembly that includes hinges, frames, closer, and latch. Fire doors and fire-rated assemblies have been tested for resistance to fire by exposure for a specified length of time (e.g., 1 hr, 3 hr). Doors that meet the test standards are labeled with the fire endurance rating of the door and the name of the testing laboratory that performed the tests and lists the doors, such as Underwriters Laboratories or Factory Mutual Laboratories.

Fire doors on clinical laboratories may be held open by electromagnetic holdopens, which are released in case of power failure, actuation of the fire alarm system, or actuation of a fire detection system.

Fire doors on laboratories and stairwells should have the maximal allowable area of wired glass view panel, to minimize collision of personnel using the doors. One-hour fire doors are permitted to have up to 100 $in.^2$ of wired glass in a view panel; such wired glass must be 0.25-in. minimal thickness with wires running in two directions. (It may be possible to retrofit some existing fire doors with wired glass view panels without destroying their fire resistance).

fire extinguishing the quenching of fire by use of equipment or extinguishing agents that remove the supply of fuel, exclude the oxidizer, cool the fuel below its ignition temperature, or suppress the flame chain reaction.

Removal of the supply of fuel can be accomplished by means such as shutoff valves on flammable gas supplies, or by use of special foam extinguishing agents that form an aqueous film to suppress the solvent vapors. Exclusion of the oxidizer can be accomplished by blanketing with carbon dioxide to exclude atmospheric oxygen. Cooling of the fuel below its ignition temperature is usually done by applying water to cool burning combustible materials or liquids. Suppression of the flame chain reaction can be accomplished by dry chemical extinguishing agents, such as potassium bicarbonate or monoammonium phosphate, or by halogenated extinguishing agents, such as Halon 1301 or Halon 1211.

See also *fire-extinguishing system* and *fire prevention.*

fire-extinguishing system an automatic system in which fire is detected and an extinguishing agent is released automatically when predetermined conditions are reached. The most common and least expensive is a sprinkler system in which water is released in a fine cooling spray at each sprinkler head, being activated by the heat generated by a fire. If a water flow alarm is included in the piping to the sprinkler heads, the system can also serve as a fire detection system. Sprinkler systems are suitable even for electronic equipment and computers, according to manufacturers and fire protection consultants. The systems release water only when heat from a fire is great enough to melt the fusible plug that normally blocks water flow. The cooling effect of the water minimizes the spread of fire and damage to equipment. Automatic sprinkler systems may be used alone or as a backup for a special system.

Also available are special automatic fire-extinguishing systems that delay release of the extinguishing agent until fire is detected by two detectors, or that allow for manual action. Special extinguishing agents include carbon dioxide, dry chemicals, and halogens.

See also *sprinkler system.*

fire load the amount of combustibles present in an area, usually calculated in weight of combustible material per square foot.

fire prevention the control of factors necessary for fire. Control of fuel availability may be accomplished by ventilating the handling of flammable liquids, limiting sizes of glass containers, using safety cans whenever possible, and limiting quantities of flammable and combustible materials exposed to fire. The limiting of oxidizer availability may include special inerting procedures (such as filling an anerobic incubator with nitrogen or carbon dioxide) and storage of strong oxidizers such as sulfuric, nitric, and perchloric acid separate from combustible liquids such as acetic acid. Limiting of ignition sources may include no-smoking regulations, a system for controlling any welding or other "hot work" in the laboratory, and special electric equipment that is classified for hazardous locations (so-called explosion-proof equipment), or equipment that is enclosed, purged, and pressurized to exclude flammable vapors.

fire-rated assembly a fire door and its hinges, frame, closer, latch, and wired glass panel. Fire doors and their entire assembly have been tested for resistance to fire by exposure for a specified length of time (e.g., 1- and 3-hr periods). See also *fire door.*

fire-resistant construction building construction that is expected to withstand fire and to function even when exposed to fire. Fire-resistance tests generally require walls and floors to withstand a standard fire test for a specified time and to continue to support their loads without collapse, and also to prevent the passage of heat or flame sufficient to ignite materials on the other side of the wall or floor. Codes may require certain construction to have specified minimal fire-resistance ratings, such as 1 hr for laboratory walls and floors.

firing rate the frequency at which action potentials are repeated, usually expressed in impulses per second (Hertz).

firmware in a computer, microprograms—small programs that the computer uses to perform some instructions.

first arch syndromes a variable pattern of congenital malformations that results from abnormalities of the various components of the first pharyngeal arch. Examples include Goldenhar's syndrome, hemifacial microsomia, *Pierre Robin developmental field complex,* and *Treacher Collins syndrome.*

first-order reaction a chemical reaction whose rate equation involves the substrate (A) at an exponential power of one, the number of molecules of (A) participating in the reaction. The rate of change of the concentration of (A) is proportional to the concentration of (A) remaining. See also *kinetics.*

Fischer projection (fish'er) [Emil Herman *Fischer,* German chemist, 1852–1919] a two-dimensional representation used to specify the absolute spatial con-

Fischer projection, Figure 1. Projections shown are one enantiomer of 1-bromo-1-chloroethane and two views of wedge projection. (From Ternay, A. L., Jr.: Contemporary Organic Chemistry. 2nd ed. Philadelphia, W. B. Saunders Co., 1976.)

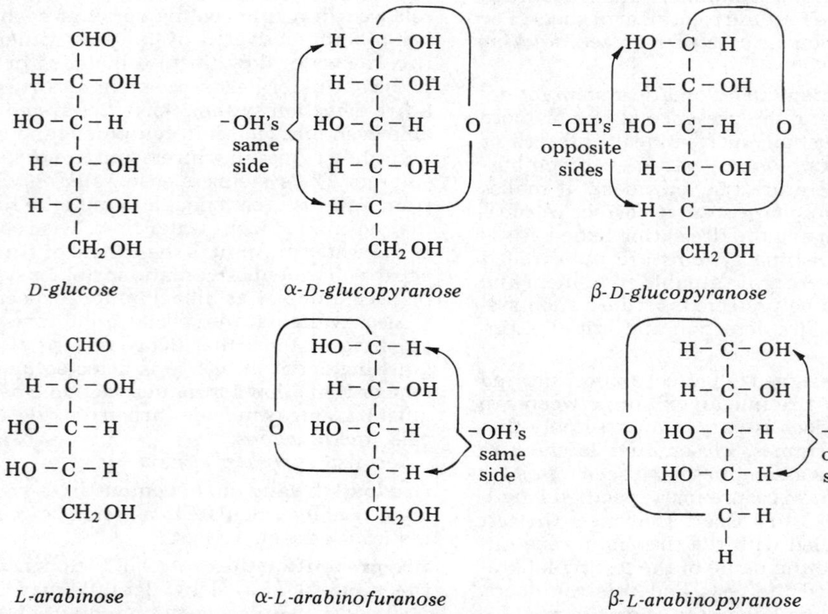

Fischer projection, Figure 2. Illustrations of Fischer projection for specifying molecular configurations. (From Banks, J. E.: Naming Organic Compounds. 2nd ed. Philadelphia, W. B. Saunders Co., 1976.)

figuration of an organic compound. Each carbon atom is shown with its four bonds at right angles. The substituents to the right and left of the carbon are actually in front of the page, and those above and below are behind the page. Interchanging any two substituents in a Fischer projection reverses the absolute configuration of a chiral center.

For the open-chain forms of sugars, the carbon backbone runs vertically, with the lowest numbered carbon (the end closest to the carbonyl group) at the top. For the cyclic form, the potential carbonyl carbon is shown at the top with its upper bond bent around to the ring oxygen at the side. In both forms, if the hydroxyl group of the highest numbered chiral carbon is on the right, the molecule has the D configuration; otherwise it is L.

See also Figures 1 and 2 and *isomerism.*

Fisher's exact test (fish′erz) a statistical hypothesis test of independence or homogeneity for 2 × 2 contingency tables. The null hypothesis is that the two classifications are independent. The conditional probability of the observed frequencies given the row and column totals is $c_1!c_2!r_1!r_2!/n!a_{11}!a_{12}!a_{21}!a_{22}!$, where a_{ij} is the observed frequency in row *i*, column *j*; $r_i = a_{i1} + a_{i2}$ is the total for row *i*; $c_j = a_{1j} + a_{2j}$ is the total for column *j*; $n = c_1 + c_2 = r_1 + r_2$ is the sample size; and ! is the factorial function. If a_{11} is the smallest observed frequency, the one-tailed significance level (α) is calculated by adding these probabilities for the value of a_{11} actually observed and each smaller value down to and including zero. (Each number subtracted from a_{11} is also added to a_{12} and a_{21} and subtracted from a_{22} to maintain the observed row and column totals.)

This test, unlike the chi-squared test, uses an exact significance level and is always preferred for 2 × 2 tables, unless the computation required exceeds the available capability. However, when the expected values in all four cells of the table exceed five, the chi-squared test yields a close approximation to the Fisher exact test. Note that the chi-squared test yields a two-tailed P value and would be halved for comparison with the exact procedure.

fission (fish′un) 1. the act of splitting.

2. a form of asexual reproduction of unicellular organisms in which they divide into two new, independent cells.

3. the splitting of an atomic nucleus into two nuclei and several neutrons. Energy is released as kinetic energy of the fission products and as gamma rays. Some nuclides, such as ^{235}U, can decay by spontaneous fission. Fission can also be induced by a neutron striking the nucleus; this is the process that occurs in a reactor or atomic bomb.

fissure (fish′ūr) [L. *fissura*] a cleft or groove. Also called *sulcus.*

inferior orbital f., a cleft in the posterolateral wall of the orbit through which pass the maxillary and zygomatic nerves. The fissure is bounded by the greater wing of the sphenoid, the maxilla, and the orbital process of the palatine bone.

fistula (fis′tu-lah), pl. *fistulas, fistulae* [L. "tube"] any abnormal connection between two internal structures, or any abnormal passageway from an internal structure to the external surface of the body. Fistulas are often tunnel-shaped or tube-like. They may occur congenitally, or be induced by therapy (e.g., radiation), trauma (e.g., childbirth), or disease (e.g., malignant tumors and infections). The more common sites for fistulas are between the vagina and rectum, the vagina and bladder, and the bladder and rectum. Cf. *sinus.*

arteriovenous f., an abnormal passage between an artery and a vein. Cf. *arteriovenous a.* under *anastomosis.*

branchial f., an abnormal passage that results from failure of the branchial clefts to fuse. It opens on the surface of the neck close to the anterior border of the sternomastoid muscle and usually communicates interiorly with a lateral cervical (branchial cleft) cyst. Rarely, an internal branchial fistula opens into the pharynx in the tonsillar region.

thyroglossal f., a fistula formed through connection of a persistent thyroglossal duct with the skin, usually from rupture of a thyroglossal duct cyst.

FITC abbrev. See *f. isothiocyanate* under *fluorescein.*

Fite's method a staining method for acid-fast organisms such as lepra bacilli. Tissue sections are deparaffinized in a 2:1 solution of xylene and peanut oil, which preserves the acid-fastness sometimes lost in normal processing. The sections are then stained with Ziehl-Neelsen carbolfuchsin and methylene blue. See also *acid-fast staining methods.*

fitness (f) (fit′nes) in genetics, the relative ability of an organism (or of its genes considered separately) to pass on genes to the next generation; the ratio of the average number of progeny produced by organisms with a particular genotype to the average number of progeny produced by those with the normal genotype. See also *natural s.* under *selection.*

"fitter" cell theory a theoretical mechanism of epithelial cancer formation. Normally, only basal cells can divide; the remaining cells differentiate and are eventually cast off from the epithelial surface—they are "mortal." Mutations occasionally produce epithelial cells that can divide, even after migrating from the basal layer. Such a mutant is "fitter" than the surrounding mortal cells; it will produce a clone that grows faster than the mortal cell population. A mutant clone may have unstable genetic material; this will cause further mutations, which may produce a clone that is not restricted by the normal laws of growth, i.e., a cancer.

Fitzgerald factor a high-molecular-weight kininogen, one of the plasma substrates for kallikrein and a precursor of bradykinin, which may be required for the interaction of Factors XII and XI; the deficiency is described as Fitzgerald trait.

fix (fiks) 1. to preserve tissues using a fixative.

2. to determine a position; a determined position.

3. to preserve a photographic print by placing it in a fixer.

fixation (fik-sa′shun) [L. *fixatio*] 1. in film processing, the removal of undeveloped silver salts from the emulsion by the fixer, producing light areas on the negative.

2. in histology, the immersion of a tissue specimen in a fixative solution. See also *fixative.*

3. in psychiatry, the persistence of libidinal or aggressive attachment to an object of infancy or childhood, which renders related parts of the personality

unable to progress through the normal phases of development.

secondary f., the use of a second type of fixative immediately following the first fixation in order to improve demonstration of substances not optimally fixed by a primary fixative; for example, the use of a dichromate after formalin fixation makes phospholipids insoluble in neural tissues.

fixation artifact a feature that occurs as a consequence of the procedure of fixation. Cf. *artifact.*

fixative (fik′sah-tiv) a solution, often containing several chemicals, into which histologic specimens are placed in order to prevent autolysis and maintain the cells as closely as possible to their living state in morphology and localization of chemical constituents. The time required varies with the fixative but should be rapid to minimize autolytic change. Fixed tissues are hardened and rendered resistant to distortion during subsequent dehydration, clearing, and embedding in paraffin or plastic.

The primary effect of a fixative is to denature proteins. The tissue component to be demonstrated determines the choice of fixative, as different fixatives react with different cellular constituents. For light microscopy, the routinely used fixatives contain either formalin, alcohol, picric acid, mercuric chloride, potassium dichromate, or various combinations of these chemicals. Osmium tetroxide, glutaraldehyde, and paraformaldehyde are used for electron microscopy.

The fixatives most frequently used are solutions that contain formalin. Formaldehyde gas is irritating and requires a well-ventilated working area. Formalin is relatively unreactive but does form links (methylene bridges) between the denatured proteins. Unless buffered, the formic acid contained in formalin will react with blood to form a dark brown pigment (acid hematin or "formalin pigment"), which may be removed from tissue sections with ammonia or picric acid solutions.

A common formalin fixative is 10 percent buffered neutral formalin. Some special-purpose formalin fixatives are formalin ammonium bromide (FAB), which is used before gold or silver staining of nerve cells, and alcoholic formalin, which is used to fix sputum.

Chromates are used in combination with other fixatives and as primary fixatives to produce the chromaffin reaction in pheochromocytomas and to render phospholipids insoluble. Orth's solution is composed of potassium dichromate and concentrated (37–40 percent) formalin.

Mercuric salts react with the carboxyl and thiol groups of proteins. They are used in several fixatives and enhance staining of nuclei and connective tissue, although they leave granular mercury deposits. These granules can be removed from the tissue section prior to staining with an alcoholic iodine solution. B5 is a fixative composed of $HgCl_2$ and $NaC_2H_3O_2$ in water, with concentrated (37–40 percent) formalin added before use. Two mercuric salt fixatives contain a solution of $K_2Cr_2O_7$ and of $HgCl_2$ in water; to obtain Zenker's fluid, glacial acetic acid is added before use; to obtain Helly's fluid, concentrated (37–40 percent) formalin is added before use.

Picric acid reacts with proteins to form picrates. Picric acid fixatives are particularly good for the demonstration of glycogen but are poor for red blood cells or for DNA. One picric acid fixative, Bouin's fluid, is composed of a saturated solution of picric acid in water, concentrated formalin, and glacial acetic acid. Another, Gendre's fixative, is composed of a saturated solution of picric acid in 95 percent ethanol, concentrated formalin, and glacial acetic acid.

Ethanol, methanol, and acetone are used when enzymes are to be demonstrated, although they cause distortion of shapes, dissolve away lipids, and cause polarization (the movement of cytoplasm to one side of cells) unless very cold temperatures are employed. Carnoy's fixative (pure ethanol, chloroform, and glacial acetic acid) is a rapidly acting fixative used for thin slices of tissue. It preserves glycogen well.

Paraformaldehyde is used in buffered solutions at 4 percent strength. Before use, sodium hydroxide is added to depolymerize the paraformaldelhyde to formalin, which is free of the methanol and formic acid contained in commercial formalin. Glutaraldehyde is a dialdehyde that works like formalin but forms more cross-links, and thus gives better fixation.

Osmium tetroxide is very reactive; it gels proteins by bridge formation and forms diester linkages with unsaturated double bonds of lipids. It also fixes minute structures very well and stains tissue components gray-to-black in proportion to the number of reactive groups. This fixative is generally used in solutions buffered with barbital, phosphate, or collidine buffers. Osmium tetroxide is often used following fixation in buffered glutaraldehyde or paraformaldehyde and rinsing in the buffer, a procedure called double fixation. The vapors of osmium tetroxide are highly irritating; it should be used under a fume hood, and plastic gloves and eye protectors should be worn.

Fluid specimens are best processed immediately or refrigerated if a delay occurs. The addition of an equal volume of 50 percent ethanol is sometimes suggested.

coating f., a solution applied to cytologic smears, which fixes the specimen and also protects it during transit to the laboratory. It must be removed before staining by immersing the slide in ethyl alcohol.

The most commonly used coating fixatives are aerosol sprays, e.g., Spray-cyte and Cytospray. (Some hair sprays containing little oil may also be used.) These generally contain ethyl or isopropyl alcohol as the fixative and polyethylene or polypropylene glycol as the coating agent. A liquid substitute is 5 g of polyethylene glycol 1540 (Carbowax) added to 100 ml of 95 percent ethyl alcohol (or of 1:1 ethyl alcohol-ether); a few drops are applied to each slide.

fixed oil an oil that does not evaporate on warming. Such oils, consisting of a mixture of fatty acids and their esters, are classified as solid (chiefly stearin), semisolid (chiefly palmitin), and liquid (chiefly olein). Fixed oils are also classified as drying, semidrying, and nondrying, depending on their tendency to solidify when exposed in a thin film to air. Also called *expressed oil* and *fatty oil.*

fixed-point variable in computing, a storage location used to represent a number with a specified number of digits on each side of the radix point. In most high-level languages, the only allowed fixed-point variables are integers; PL/1, however, allows both binary and decimal fractional fixed-point variables. Cf. *floating-point variable.*

fixed sediment method see under *cell block preparation.*

fixer (fiks'er) a solution used in developing photographic film; it finishes development of the latent image and hardens it. Fixer is sometimes incorrectly called hypo. See also *film processing.*

fixing time the time a photograph is in the fixer. It should be twice the clearing time—the time that it takes the fixer to remove all unexposed silver halide. See also *film processing.*

fl abbrev. See *femtoliter.*

flaccid (flak'sid, flas'id) [L. *flaccidus*] weak, lax, and soft; flabby; without tone.

flag (flag) in a computer, a variable or register used to indicate the status of a peripheral device or program step. A flag with two possible states is often said to be raised or lowered rather than on or off.

flagellar (flah-jel'ar) of or relating to a flagellum.

flagellin (flah-jel'in) the protein occurring in the flagella of bacteria. It is similar in structure to keratin, myosin, and fibrinogen; antibody to it is specific. Flagellin-induced agglutination by specific antibody immobilizes the organism, the basis of the *Treponema pallidum* immobilization test for syphilis.

flagellum (flah-jel'um), pl. *flagella* [L. "whip"] a long, mobile, whiplike projection from the free surface of a cell that serves as a locomotor organelle. In eukaryotic cells, flagella consist of a bundle of nine fibrils surrounding two central fibrils. They are also common to prokaryotic cells. The long, fine, and hairlike flagellum of bacterial cells originates on a basal body on the plasma membrane and is made up of tightly wound strands in helix formation that contain a single kind of protein subunit—flagellin. The flagella may be peritrichous (around the entire surface) or polar (either at one or both ends). Polar distribution may be monotrichous (a single flagellum), lophotrichous (two or more at one end), or amphitrichous (tufts at each end).

flame (flām) 1. the luminous, irregular appearance usually accompanying combustion caused by the light emitted from energetically excited chemical species, or an appearance resembling it.

2. to render an object sterile by exposure to a flame.

flame background see *background interference.*

flame cell 1. one of the flagellate cells at the termination of the collecting tubules of the excretory system of flatworms and nemerteans; so-called because the beating of the flagella suggests a flickering flame. Also called *protonephridium* and *solanocyte.*

2. an abnormal plasmacyte that has a pyrinophilic cytoplasm and reflects the active synthesis of immunoglobin. The peripheral cytoplasm stains a distinct reddish or bright red color with Wright stain, which gives the cell its characteristic appearance.

flame intensity zones the zones of a flame, which differ in temperature, luminosity, and the combustion processes occurring in them. A flame with a low oxidant/fuel ratio is luminous yellow throughout owing to incandescent particles of unburned carbon. With a higher ratio, the flame is clear blue with clearly visible inner and outer cones. Primary combustion occurs at the inner cone; secondary combustion (oxidation of hydrogen and carbon monoxide formed in the inner zone) occurs at the outer cone. No combustion occurs in the intermediate zone between the cones, which is the hottest part of the flame.

flame ionization detector (FID) see under *gas chromatography.*

flame photometer an instrument for performing flame photometry. It consists of a burner that produces flame temperatures with a range between 1800°C (natural gas–air flame) and 3100°C (acetylene–oxygen flame); an aspirator and atomizer, in which the sample is drawn up a capillary tube and dispersed into a mist of small droplets by a jet of gas and sprayed into the flame; a narrow bandpass monochromator, which uses a grating, prism, or filter to isolate the emission lines used for measurement; and a detector system, usually a photomultiplier tube or photocell.

In single-beam (direct-reading) instruments, there is only one set of optics, with the sample concentration determined by a comparison of readings with those produced by standard solutions. In double-beam (internal standard) instruments, there are two sets of optics, and the sample concentration is determined by the readings at two separate wavelengths, corresponding to emission lines of the analyte and internal standard.

flame photometry an analytic method, more precisely called flame emission photometry, for determining some metal ions, usually sodium, potassium, and lithium. The sample is aspirated into a flame, and the thermally excited atoms emit light of characteristic wavelengths (resonance line). The intensity of the light emitted at one of these emission lines is a measure of the amount of the element present.

Flame photometry is subject to a variety of instabilities and interferences that must be controlled. The emission intensity fluctuates with variations in droplet size or gas flow to the burner. In instruments using filters to isolate the emitted wavelengths, there may be spectral interference due to more than one emission line falling within the bandwidth of the filter. The filter serves to correct for the continuous emission of the flame background and to eliminate emissions from other atoms. At higher sample concentrations, self-absorption (absorption of emitted radiation by other nonexcited atoms of the same element) produces a nonlinearity in the relation between concentration and emission. Mutual excitation (the transfer of ionization energy from one element to another) causes the emission to vary with the concentration of other readily excited metals in the sample. In particular, potassium emission increases with sodium concentration. This kind of atom-atom interaction is sometimes referred to as cation interference or ionization interference.

Anion interference is due to the presence of acids and salts furnishing anions that form high-melting compounds with the analyte so that it is not completely dissociated into free atoms in the flame. Calcium emission, especially, is depressed by the presence of phosphate and aluminate. Anion interference can be eliminated at times and in part by adding an agent that forms an easily decomposed complex with the analyte (EDTA chelate with calcium), or by forming an insoluble precipitate of the interfering ion.

In the internal standard method, a reference element such as lithium or cesium is added to specimens and standards, and the concentration is determined from the ratio of the emission intensities of the analyte and the internal standard. This serves two functions: variations in the flame or in atomization of the sample are compensated for by simulataneous measurement of both elements, and the internal standard can also serve as a radiation buffer. Because of its high concentration, which is identical in specimens and standards, it produces a large mutual excitation effect on the analyte, which swamps the effect produced by other metals in the sample.

The logarithm of the emission ratio is approximately equal to a constant plus the logarithm of the concentration of the analyte over some range of concentrations. For some metals emission is directly proportional to concentration, e.g., Na, K. In practice, the formula used is $E_{Na}/E_{Li} \times F - C =$ Na concentration, where E_{Na} and E_{Li} are the emission readings for the sodium and lithium lines, F is a calibration (slope) adjustment, and C is the offset of the calibration curve from zero. A calibration curve can be used outside the linear region.

See also *sodium and potassium assays.*

flammability (flam″ah-bil′ĭ-te) a measure of the ease of ignition, intensity of burning, and rate of flamespread.

flammable (flam′ah-b′l) [L. *flammare* to catch fire] a combustible material that ignites very easily, burns intensely, or has a rapid rate of flamespread. Flammable solids include fine dusts, spontaneously igniting materials, and materials with low ignition points. Flammable gases form explosive mixtures with air. Oxygen, fluorine, and chlorine, which support combustion, are themselves nonflammable. The term flammable is used in preference to the term inflammable to avoid confusion caused by the prefix *in-* (which in some words indicates the negative). Cf. *combustible, noncombustible,* and *nonflammable.*

flammable concentration the concentration in air (expressed as a volume percentage) of a combustible gas, vapor, or liquid. Consideration of the actual flammable concentration that is or may be present in the vicinity of ignition sources is important, because the mere presence of a flammable vapor is not a fire hazard unless the concentration approaches the lower flammable limit of the vapor. For example, if ventilation is sufficient to prevent accumulation of significant quantities of vapor-air mixtures in a concentration over one-fourth of the lower flammable limit, it is considered adequate for the prevention of fire and explosion (National Fire Protection Association regulation 30-1981).

flammable gas any gas that, according to the NFPA (National Fire Protection Association), will burn in the normal concentrations of oxygen in the air. Each flammable gas burns only within a certain range of gas-air mixtures—the flammable range between the lower and upper flammable limits—and each gas has an ignition temperature at which the combustion reaction is initiated. Also called *combustible gas.*

flammable limits the extreme concentration limits of a combustible substance in air or other oxidizing atmosphere through which a flame will propagate. Vapor-air mixtures below the lower flammable limit or lower explosive limit (LEL) will burn if they reach an ignition source, but the flame will not propagate or travel away from the source of ignition in a flash fire or explosion. Vapor-air mixtures above the upper flammable limit will be too rich to burn. If the combustion of a flammable mixture of vapor in air is confined, the resulting pressure buildup may cause an explosion.

Flammable limits commonly reported are for mixtures of the combustible in air with the normal concentration of oxygen. In oxygen-enriched atmospheres, ignition will occur at lower temperatures and the upper flammable limit is increased.

Also called *explosion limits.*

flammable liquid a liquid (such as alcohol, acetone, ether, and xylene) with a flash point below 37.8°C (100°F) and a vapor pressure not exceeding 2068.6 mmHg (40 psia) at 37.8°C (100°F). Flammable liquids produce flammable concentrations of vapor if exposed or spilled at temperatures above their flash point.

Flammable liquids are Class I liquids and have the following subclassification. Class IA: flash-point temperatures below 22.8°C (73°F) and a boiling point below 37.8°C; examples include ethyl ether, isopentane, and some petroleum ethers. Class IB: flash-point temperatures below 22.8°C and a boiling point at or above 37.8°C; examples include acetone, ethyl alcohol, methanol, and toluene. Class IC: flash-point temperatures at or above 22.8°C without consideration of boiling point.

The safe dispensing of flammable liquids requires ventilation, control of ignition sources, fire protection, and provision for spill prevention. Ventilation is needed to prevent the accumulation of flammable concentrations of vapors and the excess exposure of workers to toxic or irritating vapors. In laboratories in health-related institutions, dispensation from bulk stock containers of flammable and combustible liquids should be done in a separate room or in a laboratory hood. If vapors from the transfer of small quantities of flammable liquids are not controlled by general dilution ventilation in the laboratory, local exhaust ventilation may be needed. Ignition control includes provision for bonding metal containers, provision of adequate humidity to control static electricity, and prohibition of smoking and open flames in any area in which there may be flammable concentrations of vapor.

Also called Class I liquid. See also *container size limitation, fire prevention, flammable liquid storage cabinet,* and *storage limits.*

flammable liquid storage cabinet a cabinet for the storage of flammable and combustible liquids constructed in accordance with the requirements in the NFPA (National Fire Protection Association) Flammable and Combustible Liquids Code. Such cabinets provide some reduction in fire hazard and an allowable increase of quantities permitted within a fire area.

Suitable storage cabinets insulate the interior of the cabinet so that exposure to a standard fire (1000°F at 5 min and 1300°F at 10 min) will not raise the interior to a temperature in excess of 325°F (which is slightly below the ignition temperatures of paper and ethyl ether). The cabinets are commercially available in double-walled metal and in 1-in.–thick plywood of exterior grade; tests have shown that the plywood cabinets provide better insulation than the metal cabinets.

National codes do not require storage cabinets to be ventilated, even though metal cabinets have provision for connections to a narrow-diameter ventilation system. Ventilation may be desirable, however, if containers within the cabinets release vapors that are corrosive, toxic, or malodorous. As there are no ignition sources within storage cabinets, flammable vapors within the cabinet do not present a hazard.

flammable liquid storage limits regulatory and accreditation standards for laboratories that limit the quantities of flammable and combustible liquids that may be present within a laboratory, and the quantities that may be outside safety cans, outside storage cabinets or storage rooms, on open shelves, in apparatus, or in ordinary laboratory cabinets and cupboards.

The National Fire Protection Association in its 1973 regulations (NFPA 56C-1973) allows a maximum of 10 gal (37.85 l) of flammable and combustible liquids (Classes I, II, and IIIA) outside an approved storage cabinet in a single fire area, and limits fire areas to a maximum of 5000 ft^2 (464.4 m^2). In 1980, the size restriction for hospital laboratories was discontinued and the limits for flammable and combustible liquids outside approved storage cabinets was changed to 10 gal/5000 ft^2 (37.85 l/464.4 m^2).

The Joint Commission on Accreditation of Hospitals (JCAH) has adopted the same standards as the NFPA. The maximal storage limit permitted by the College of American Pathologists, however, is smaller: CAP accreditation standards for clinical laboratories have limited the amount of flammable liquids in a laboratory to a maximum of 5 gal.

NFPA regulation 45-1981 applies to clinical laboratories not located within a hospital building containing four or more patients incapable of self-preservation in case of fire. Quantity limits in this regulation are based on occupancy, fire resistance, and areas; quantities allowable on open shelves may be approximately doubled if half is kept in safety cans or storage cabinets, and may be approximately doubled again if the laboratory has a sprinkler system or is provided with some other automatic fire-extinguishing system.

flammable liquid storage room a specially constructed fire-resistant room that may be built within a hospital or laboratory building for the storage of up to 5000 gal of flammable and combustible liquids. National Fire Protection Association regulations (NFPA 56C-1980) require that a hospital regularly maintain a reserve storage capacity of flammable and combustible liquids in excess of 300 gal (1135.5 l) and have available at least one approved storage room.

The requirements for an approved storage room vary, depending on the location of the room within the building, quantities to be stored, sizes of containers, and classes of liquids, but generally they include the following: construction separating the storage room from the hospital or laboratory building that has a fire-resistance classification of 1 or 2 hr, ventilation that will prevent the accumulation of flammable concentrations of vapors, wiring that is appropriate to the hazards, and room design that will prevent spills and firefighting water from flowing from the storage room into the rest of the building.

flammable material storage refrigerator refrigerated cold storage without any ignition sources within the storage compartment. This design eliminates the hazard of explosion within the refrigerator if a flammable concentration of vapors is produced by evaporation within the compartment.

flank (flank) the part of the body below the ribs and above the iliac crest.

flashcard (flash′kard) a device used to mark radiographs. Identifying information is typed on a card and transferred photographically to an unexposed corner of the film, which was covered by a lead strip while the radiograph was made.

flash-point temperature the minimal temperature at which a liquid gives off vapor in a concentration sufficient to form an ignitable mixture with air near the surface of the liquid. The flash-point temperature of a liquid corresponds to the lowest temperature at which the vapor pressure of the liquid is sufficient to produce a vapor-air mixture at the lower flammable limit. In simple terms, the spill of a liquid at any temperature above its flash point will produce a flammable concentration of vapor in the vicinity of the spill and the possibility of a flash fire or explosion. Flash-point temperatures are lower than boiling points and ignition temperatures.

Flash-point temperature is the most important criterion of the relative hazard of flammable and combustible liquids; other criteria include ignition temperature, flammable range, rate of evaporation, and burning characteristics.

Flammable mixtures can be generated at temperatures far below the flash-point temperature of a liquid if the pressure is reduced or if the material is sprayed, foamed, or dispersed over a matrix (such as cloth or other porous surface) so that the surface-to-mass ratio is increased.

See also *combustible liquid, flammable limits,* and *flammable liquid.*

flask a container, such as a narrow-necked vessel of glass for holding liquid.

flat (flat) 1. lying in one plane; having an even surface.

2. having little or no resonance.

flat bone a bone whose thickness is slight, sometimes consisting of only a thin layer of compact bone, or of two layers with intervening spongy bone and marrow. It is usually bent or curved, rather than flat.

flat substrate method a method used in autoradiography for electron miscroscopy. Sections are placed on microscope grids previously attached to glass slides. The grids remain attached to the slides during exposure and processing. See also *autoradiography.*

flatulence (flat′u-lens) [L. *flatulentia*] a normal occurrence in humans that consists of the passage of gas through the rectum. Excessive flatulence may be due to the swallowing of a large amount of air (aerophagia) or to the formation of large amounts of gas by intestinal bacteria. Foods such as beans and cabbage have large amounts of undigestible polysaccharides and are easily converted to gaseous products by the bacteria. Treatment is directed at decreasing the consumption of such foods and decreasing those habits that cause excess aerophagia. Also called *gas.*

flatworm (flat′werm) a common name for members of the phylum Platyhelminthes. See also *worm.*

flav/o [L. *flavus* yellow] a word element used in combining form to denote yellow, e.g., flavin, flavivirus.

flavin (fla′vin) [L. *flavus* yellow] any of a group of pigments containing the isoalloxazine nucleus, such as riboflavin, which is a constituent of several flavoproteins. These proteins contain flavin mononucleotide (FMN) or flavine adenine dinucleotide (FAD) attached in covalent linkages. FMN and FAD act as prosthetic groups for a large number of enzymes of the oxidoreductase class, which catalyze electron transfers (oxidation-reduction) reactions. The electrons are transferred as hydrogen atoms, changing the coenzyme from the oxidized form (FAD or FMN) to the reduced form ($FADH_2$ or $FMNH_2$). There is also a half-reduced form (FADH or FMNH), a stable semiquinone free radical, which can go to either the oxidized or the reduced form in a one-electron transfer. The oxidized forms of flavins are yellow with an intense green fluorescence. Riboflavin is a water-soluble vitamin and is widely distributed throughout plant and animal life. See also *riboflavin.*

flavin adenine dinucleotide (FAD) a coenzyme that is a condensation product of riboflavin 5′-phosphate (FMN) and adenosine 5′-phosphate (AMP). It forms the prosthetic group of certain oxidoreductases, including succinate dehydrogenase, D-amino acid oxidase, and electron-transferring flavoproteins. See also *flavin.*

flavin mononucleotide (FMN) riboflavin 5′-phosphate, a coenzyme that forms the prosthetic group in certain oxidoreductases including NADH dehydrogenase. See also *flavin.*

Flavobacterium (fla″vo-bak-te′re-um) [L. *flavus* yellow + Gr. *bakterion* a small rod] a genus of gram-negative, rod-shaped bacilli, usually oxidative but sometimes fermentative. The organisms are oxidase positive, are usually nonmotile, form a yellow pigment, and produce indole after a 48-hr incubation. They occur widely in soil and water, and are opportunistic pathogens in humans.

F. meningosepticum, a species that is an important cause of nosocomial infections. It can produce meningitis and septicemia with a high fatality rate in both newborn and premature infants. In adults, it is the source of a milder postoperative bacteremia.

flavoprotein (fla″vo-pro′te-in) a conjugated protein in which the prosthetic group, sometimes covalently bound, contains a flavin. See also *riboflavin.*

flaxseed oil (flaks′sēd) see *linseed oil.*

flea (fle) a small, wingless insect of the order Siphonaptera, ectoparasitic on birds and mammals. Most species measure 1.5-4.0 mm long and have mouthparts of the piercing-sucking type. Fleas are known vectors of diease, such as bubonic plague, murine typhus, and rickettsial disease, and their bites can cause dermatitis. See also the accompanying illustration.

Fletcher factor (flech′er) a prekallikrein whose active form (kallikrein) probably enhances the function of already activated Hageman factor (Factor XII). The deficiency described as Fletcher trait is not associated with bleeding; the activated partial thromboplastin time is prolonged, but it becomes progressively shortened upon incubation with kaolin. Fletcher trait plasma has defective fibrinolysis, chemotactic activity, kinin generation, and esterase activity. See also *Factor XII.*

flex (fleks) [L. *flexus* bent] to bend or put in a state of flexion.

flexion (flek′shun) [L. *flexio*] the act of bending a joint so that the angle made by the bones becomes

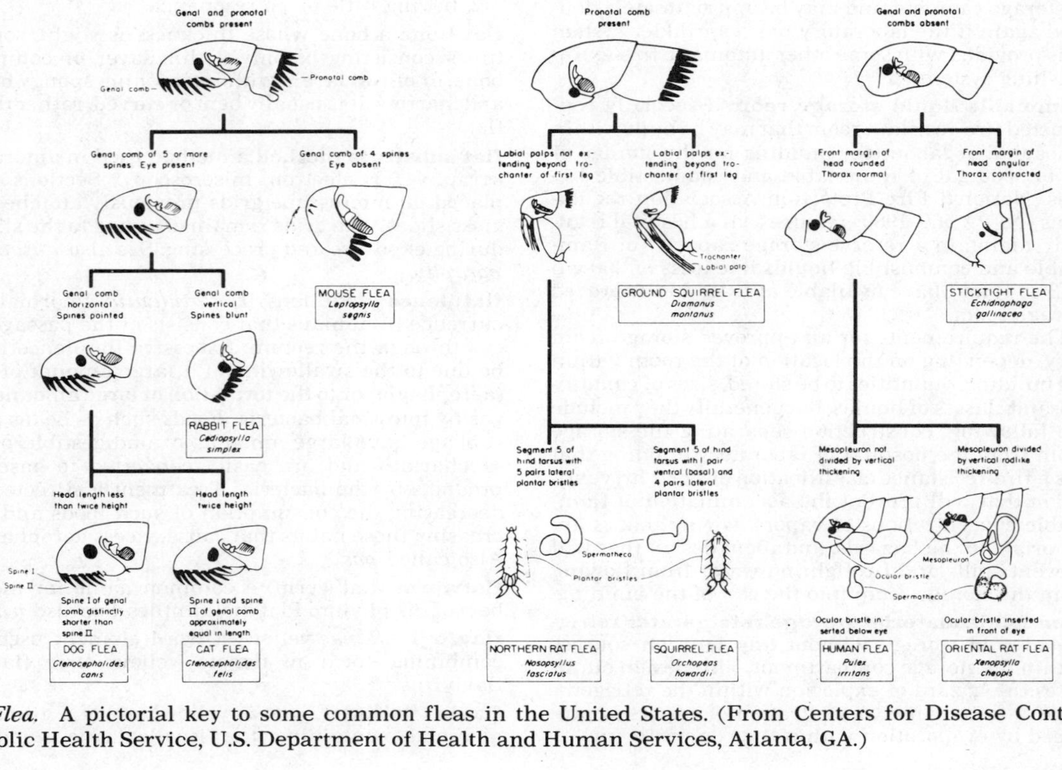

Flea. A pictorial key to some common fleas in the United States. (From Centers for Disease Control, Public Health Service, U.S. Department of Health and Human Services, Atlanta, GA.)

more acute; the condition of having been so bent. Cf. *extension.*

Flexner's bacillus (fleks'nerz) [Simon *Flexner,* American pathologist, 1863–1946] see *S. flexneri* under *Shigella.*

flexor (flek'sor) [L.] a muscle that flexes or bends a joint.

flexure (flek'sher) a bending; a bent portion of a structure of an organ.

flint glass a highly refractive glass in which calcium has been replaced in large part by lead; used for lenses and prisms and in the manufacture of cut glass.

flip-flop (FF) an electronic logic circuit that may be used for data storage, counting, frequency division, or many other purposes. A simple flip-flop called a toggle has one input and one output; the output is complemented each time the input changes from 0 to 1 and does not change otherwise. Thus, the output changes from 0 to 1 every second time the input does.

A counter can be made of a chain of N flip-flops, with the outputs of one connected to the input of the next. This system can count 2^N input transitions: the outputs give an N-bit binary number equal to the number of input pulses, with the first flip-flop's output being the least significant bit. More complex flip-flops may have more than one input and may provide both the output and its complement, and the output may be a more complex function of the inputs. Some commonly available flip-flop families are called D-type, R/S, and J-K.

flipped LDH see under *lactate dehydrogenase isoenzyme determination.*

floating-point variable in computing, a storage location used to represent a number with a specified number of significant figures. Part of the location contains the mantissa (m), a sign, and a series of digits with the radix point at the left, which thus represents a fraction of less than 1; the rest of the location contains the exponent (e), a signed integer. The represented number is $m \cdot b^e$ where b is the base of the number system (usually 2 or 16). To retain the maximal number of significant figures, the result of each arithmetic operation is normalized; i.e., the exponent is adjusted so that the first digit of the mantissa is nonzero. If the result of an operation would have an exponent greater than is allowed, an overflow error condition occurs; too large a negative exponent produces an underflow error condition or a zero result, depending on the programming. In FORTRAN and ALGOL, floating-point variables are called real variables. Cf. *fixed-point variables.*

floc (flok) small masses formed in a fluid through coagulation, agglomeration, or biochemical reaction of the fine suspended particles in a colloidal sol.

floccose (flok'ōs) [L. *floccosus* full of flocks of wool] woolly; said of a bacterial growth appearing like tufts of wool.

flocculation test a group of diagnostic tests of liver function that detect qualitative and quantitative changes in the plasma protein fractions. Numerous tests have been used; all have some value in differentiating hepatitis or cirrhosis from obstructive jaundice, but all are now obsolete and have been largely replaced by more specific tests. See also *cephalin-cholesterol flocculation test, thymol turbidity test,* and *zinc sulfate turbidity test.*

flocculus (flok'u-lus), pl. *flocculi* [L. "tuft"] [NA], a small oval structure on the ventral aspect of each cerebellar hemisphere. Attached to the cerebellum by its peduncle, this slightly crenated structure is situated below the point of entrance of the vestibulocochlear (VIII) nerve into the brain stem, and is crossed by fine branches of the glossopharyngeal (IX) and vagus (X) nerves as they pass to the jugular foramen.

flood plate (flud) a plate for bacterial culture prepared by flooding the surface of an agar culture medium with a liquid inoculum and withdrawing the excess with a sterile pipet.

flood source a disk-shaped radiation source that is placed over the collimator of a scintillation camera. It provides an even gamma-ray illumination over the field of view for calibration checks.

floppy disk a small, inexpensive, flexible computer disk. See also *disk.*

flora (flo'rah) [L. *Flora,* the goddess of flowers] the plant life present in or characteristic of a specific location; it may be discernible with the unaided eye (macroflora) or only with the aid of a microscope (microflora). See also *normal flora.*

Florence flask (flor'ens) a laboratory flask with a spherical body and a cylindrical neck. Some have a flattened base.

Florisil trademark for a selective adsorbent made of magnesia-silica gel, commonly used as an adsorbent in the measurement of steroids by competitive protein-binding assays. Florisil adsorbs to the unbound steroids and thus allows its separation from the bound fraction.

flotation (flo-ta'shun) a technique first introduced in 1906 to isolate microscopic parasites from the stool. The suspending medium used is heavier than the parasites, so they rise to the top where they can be collected. Care should be taken in choosing a medium that does not cause shrinkage of specimen. The most common utilization of this technique is for the collection of hookworm eggs.

flotation bath a pan of distilled water heated to 38°C on which cut tissue sections are floated. The ribbon of sections is placed on the bath and the sections are separated with dissecting needles. When the sections have flattened they are picked up on slides and dried.

flotation rate the velocity at which a substance rises in the liquid medium in a centrifuge tube divided by the applied relative centrifugal force. It is measured in Svedberg flotation units (S_f) equal to 10^{-13} sec. Cf. *sedimentation rate.*

flotation techniques cytologic methods for separating cancer cells from a fluid specimen, such as blood or hemorrhagic fluid, using the difference in the specific gravities of the various types of cells (red blood cells have an average specific gravity [sp. gr.] of about 1.094; leukocytes, 1.065; cancer cells, 1.056; and platelets, 1.032).

A fluid such as silicone 702 (sp. gr., 1.075) or 20 percent albumin (sp. gr., 1.054) is placed in the bottom of a centrifuge tube. Polyvinylpyrrolidone and a wetting agent are mixed with the specimen to prevent agglutination of the cells and to keep the platelets and cellular debris in suspension; the specimen is carefully layered over the silicone or albumin without mixing. After centrifugation, the heavier red cells have sunk to the bottom, and the lighter lymphocytes and cancer cells are floating in a layer on top of the silicone or albumin. This layer is removed and saponin added to hemolyze any remaining red cells; the layer is then fixed in buffered neutral formalin and concentrated by Millipore filtration. Ficoll (cross-linked sucrose polymer) and diatrizoate solutions have also been used in place of silicone.

flow (flo) 1. the continuous bulk movement of a fluid.

2. the amount of fluid moving through an organ or part in a specified time. See also *effective renal plasma flow.*

flow chart a diagram representing a process such as a computer program. Each procedural step is framed with a specific shape representing the type of operation (e.g., arithmetic, decision, input-output). The boxes are connected with arrows indicating the sequence of operations. Templates with flow-chart symbols are available; see the accompanying illustration.

flow cytometry see under *cytometry.*

flow meter a device that indicates the flow rate of a fluid in a pipe, e.g., the gas supply of a gas chromatograph or the fuel supply of a flame photometer.

flow-volume curve a curve that relates the instantaneous expiratory airflow reached during a forced vital capacity maneuver to the lung volume at which the particular flow occurs. Instantaneous volumetric flow ($\dot{V}_{max}$) in liters per second is plotted on the *y* axis and the expired volume in liters or percentage of vital capacity (VC) on the *x* axis.

maximal expiratory f.-v. c. (MEFV), a curve relating to the maximal instantaneous expiratory airflow reached during a forced expiration over the full range (from the total lung capacity to the residual volume) of the vital capacity (VC) to the simultaneous value of lung volume (expressed as a percentage of VC). The flow increases rapidly to a peak obtained at 80 percent of the VC and then steadily declines to zero as the residual volume is reached. An effort-dependent portion of the curve (above 75 percent of VC) reflects the force-velocity relationship of the expiratory muscles. Below 75 percent of the VC, flow is effort-independent, reflecting the maximal expiratory flow possible at specific lung volumes. Additional increases in effort will not increase the flow any further. The maximal forced expiratory flow obtained at particular lung volumes can also be plotted against simultaneous values of transpulmonary pressure in order to generate isovolume pressure flow curves.

An important use of the maximal expiratory flow-volume curve is to establish the presence of airflow limitation (reflected as a marked reduction in the slope of the curve) in individuals with chronic obstructive lung disease.

See also the accompanying illustration.

floxuridine (floks-ur'ĭ-dēn) a cancer chemotherapeutic drug. For more information, see *Appendix A.*

flu (floo) a popular name for *influenza.*

fluctuation (fluk″tu-a'shun) 1. a variation, especially a random one, as about a fixed value or mass.

2. a wavelike motion, as of a fluid in a cavity of the body after succussion.

flucytosine (floo-si'to-sēn) an oral antifungal agent, a fluorinated pyrimidine (5-fluorocytosine), used in the treatment of serious infections due to

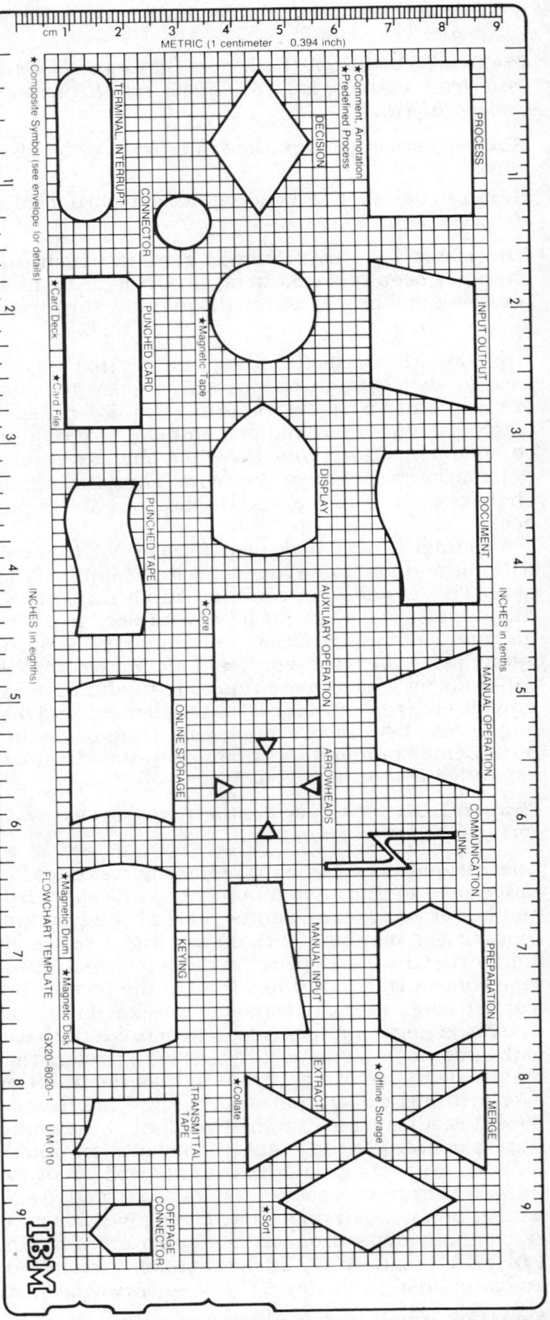

Flow chart symbols. Common flow chart symbols represented on a template. (Courtesy of IBM.)

Candida or *Cryptococcus* organisms. Because flucytosine can cause bone marrow depression, frequent monitoring of liver function and hematopoiesis is necessary during therapy. It is often used in combination with amphotericin B for the synergistic effect and for the prevention of emerging flucytosine-resistant fungal strains.

fluid (floo'id) [L. *fluidus,* from *fluere* to flow] 1. any substance in which the molecules can move past one another without the formation of fracture

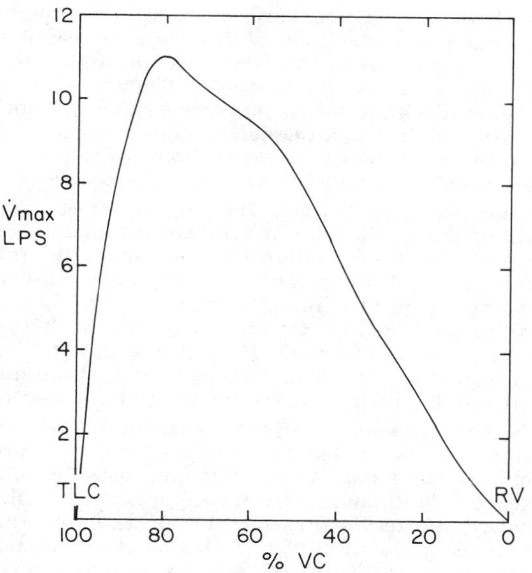

Maximal expiratory flow-volume curve. Diagram shows normal curve. (From Bates, D. V., et al.: Respiratory Function in Disease. 2nd ed. Philadelphia, W. B. Saunders Co., 1971.)

planes, i.e., any liquid or gas and some amorphous solids such as wax or glass.

2. flowing freely.

fluid balance and homeostasis the ability to maintain the amount of body fluid at a fairly constant equilibrium despite stress. Depending on their location, body fluids are described as intracellular or extracellular. They are composed principally of water, plus electrolytes, proteins, and other substances. A complex system of controls that keeps the amount of fluid and electrolytes in the body at a fairly constant level involves both hormones and regulatory organs such as the skin, kidneys, heart, and digestive system. When loss of fluids or electrolytes occurs during stress or disease, these controls quickly act to bring the concentrations of fluids and electrolytes back to normal.

Approximately two-thirds of the total body water is in the form of intracellular fluid, the remaining one-third being extracellular fluid. Of the extracellular fluid, about one-fourth is plasma and three-fourths is interstitial fluid. For example, in a male weighing 70 kg, 60 percent of his weight (42 kg or 42 l) is water, 40 percent (28 l) is intracellular fluid, 5 percent (3.5 l) is plasma, and 15 percent (10.5 l) is interstitial fluid. Both intracellular and extracellular fluids contain electrolytes. Na^+, Cl^-, and HCO_3^- are the principal ions in the extracellular fluid, and K^+, Mg^+, Ca^{++}, and organic anions are predominant in the intracellular fluid.

VOLUME DEPLETION. Most problems of fluid imbalance concern the extracellular fluid. Clinically, this is seen as volume excess or depletion. Volume depletion occurs when a person has abnormal losses of extracellular fluid, such as losses through the gut produced by diarrhea, vomiting, or nasogastric suction; through the urine, resulting from the use of diuretics, or in renal disease; or through sequestration of fluid (making it essentially inaccessible to the body) in the interstitial space. The last occurs in cases of severe burns, trauma, pancreatitis, or peritonitis. In each instance, failure to replace the lost fluid, either orally or intravenously, results in volume depletion. Clinical signs include a postural change in blood pressure, decreased skin turgor, decreased urine output, and, in severe cases, lethargy.

Laboratory studies show an increased packed red blood cell volume, increased plasma protein level, increased urine specific gravity, and increased blood urea nitrogen (BUN) out of proportion to a change in creatinine. The serum sodium remains normal in the absence of other problems. Treatment consists of fluid replacement with isotonic saline. In severe cases, a central venous pressure catheter may be used to estimate the extent of fluid losses and to guide replacement therapy.

VOLUME EXCESS. This state occurs when there is renal retention of sodium and consequent retention of extracellular fluids, as observed in congestive heart failure, cirrhosis, and nephrosis. (In these diseases, the perceived arterial volume is probably decreased, causing the kidney to respond as if the body fluid were depleted, thus retaining more salt and water.) The clinical signs include edema, weight gain, pulmonary congestion, and distended neck veins. There are no significant changes in laboratory values caused by volume excess alone. Treatment consists of correcting the underlying disease and giving medications to increase the excretion of sodium and water.

FLUID BALANCE. Consideration of fluid balance is important in selecting solutions for intravenous use in patients who temporarily have no oral intake, such as postoperative patients or those with severe injuries. A normal person loses about 2 l/da of fluid through urine output, and undergoes an insensible loss through the skin and lungs. When intravenous therapy is used, these losses should be replaced by giving a solution of dextrose and water with appropriate concentrations of electrolytes. In stress or injury the body's fluid losses may be higher than normal; in kidney failure they may be much lower than normal. A careful record of the patient's intake and output is used to assess daily replacement needs so that fluid balance may be maintained.

See also *acid-base balance* and *electrolyte balance and homeostasis.*

NANETTE SMITH, M.D.

fluid level the interface between a body fluid and air. On a radiograph taken with the central ray directed horizontally, it appears as a sharp line between the radiolucent air above and the fluid, which has intermediate density, below.

fluke (flook) a worm in the class Trematoda. Most flukes are leaflike and flat, and range in length from a few millimeters to several centimeters. Flukes have been found to infect human intestines, blood, liver, and lungs. Infection is common in individuals in Asia owing to a high consumption rate of contaminated water, vegetation, and aquatic animals. See also *worm.*

fluor (floo′or) [L. "a flux"] a material having the property of fluorescence.

fluor/o (floor′o) 1. a prefix word element to denote fluorescence, e.g., fluoroscope.

2. a prefix word element in organic chemistry to denote the presence of fluorine as a substituent, e.g., fluoromethane (CH_3F).

fluorescein (floo″o-res′e-in) an acid fluorochrome

dye; C.I. 45350. Fluorescein is an orange-red crystalline powder having a bright yellow-green fluorescence in alkaline solutions. It is used in histology as a fluorescent stain; acetone or ethanol is used for fixation because formalin and other fixatives induce fluorescence.

f. isothiocyanate (FITC), the isothiocyanate derivative of fluorescein. It reacts with acidic and basic side-chains of proteins. This provides a stable, fluorescent label for the protein. The maximal fluorescence at pH 8.0 is about one-third that of free fluorescein. The fluorescence is quenched in acidic solution. See also *immunofluorescence techniques.*

f. mercuric acetate, a specific histochemical reagent for the detection of disulfide (—S—S—) or mercapto (—S—H) groups.

f. sodium, [USP], the disodium salt of fluorescein used in ophthalmologic examinations. A solution is applied to the cornea that stains abrasions, ulcers, or foreign bodies a green color.

fluorescence (floo″o-res′ens, floor-es′ens) the emission of electromagnetic radiation by a substance after the absorption of energy in some form (e.g., the emission of light of one color [wavelength] when a substance is excited by irradiation with light of a different wavelength). Fluorescence is sometimes distinguished from phosphorescence in having a lifetime of less than 10 msec after the excitation ceases. See also *Stokes shift.*

fluorescence immunoassays see *nonradioisotopic i.* under *immunoassays.*

fluorescence microscopy highly sensitive microscopic technique for the demonstration of naturally fluorescent materials (such as nucleic acids, lipids, or steroid hormones), slide specimens stained with fluorescent dyes, or fluorescent-labeled antibodies. Uses in the clinical laboratory include the identification and localization of many proteins, including immunoglobulin; microorganisms; and the binding sites of various substances (e.g., hormones and neurotransmitters) in body tissue. See also *fluorescent m.* under *microscope* and *immunofluorescence techniques.*

fluorescent (floo″o-res′ent) exhibiting fluorescence.

fluorescent antibody (FA) technique see *immunofluorescence techniques.*

fluorescent dye see *fluorochrome.*

fluorescent material a material that fluoresces readily when excited by ultraviolet light, x-rays, an electron beam, or other energy sources.

fluorescent scan an image made using the characteristic fluorescent x-rays emitted by atoms in the body when they are excited by an external source. A modified rectilinear scanner is used for thyroid imaging. Gamma rays at 60 KeV excite the naturally occurring iodine, so that the iodine emits 28-KeV-x-rays.

fluorescent staining the coloration of tissues with a fluorescent dye. See also *fluorescent m.* under *microscope* and *immunofluorescence techniques.*

fluorescent treponemal antibody absorption (FTA-ABS) test a serologic assay that detects specific antibodies to *Treponema pallidum,* the etiologic agent of syphilis. The organism, grown in a rabbit, is placed on a slide with the patient's serum. If the test is positive, an antigen-antibody reaction occurs, and the bound antibody may be detected with fluoresceinated antihuman gamma-globulin antibody. The specificity of this test is increased by absorbing the serum with nonvirulent treponemes to remove nonspecific reactivity. The test, which is highly sensitive, detects 90 percent of cases of primary syphilis and almost all secondary or more advanced cases. Once an individual has a positive FTA-ABS, it usually remains positive for life.

fluoride (F^-) (floo′rīd, floor′īd) the negatively charged ion of fluorine or a salt containing this ion. Small amounts (less than 1 mg) of various fluoride salts are applied topically to the teeth as a rinse, in toothpaste, or in drinking water (about 0.7 mg/l) to resist tooth decay. Chronic ingestion of higher amounts causes fluorosis. Fluoride occurs in rat and ant poison, phosphate fertilizer, and aluminum ores, and is used in many industrial processes.

fluoride assays 1. hydrogen fluoride is liberated from a sample of blood, urine, or tissue by sulfuric or perchloric acid. A qualitative test uses the color reagent lanthanum alizarin Complexone, a blue color indicates the presence of fluoride. A quantitative test traps the hydrogen fluoride by diffusion into solid sodium hydroxide, which is then dissolved with the color reagent. The absorbance of the sample at 620 nm is compared with that of a standard.

2. a fluoride-specific electrode is used to measure directly the fluoride concentration of urine.

fluoride number (FN) the percentage inhibition of plasma pseudocholinesterase (CHS) activity by a fluoride concentration of 5×10^{-5} mol/l.

The actual degree of inhibition seen varies with the substrate used to measure the CHS activity. Using propionyl thiocholine (PTC), the percent inhibition observed for the $E_1^uE_1^u$ (normal), $E_1^uE_1^f$ (heterozygous) and $E_1^fE_1^f$ (homozygous) genotypes is about 79, 68, and 60, respectively.

See also *cholinesterase assays, dibucaine number,* and *pseudocholinesterase deficiency.*

fluorine (F) (floo′ŏ-rēn) [Fr., from L. *fluor* a fluorine-containing mineral] a pale yellow, violently reactive, gaseous element, moleular form F_2; atomic number 9; atomic weight 18.9984; Group VII of the periodic table (the halogens); oxidation number –1. It is the most electronegative element; elemental fluorine is highly toxic, corrosive, and flammable. See also *fluoride.*

fluorine 18 (^{18}F, F-18) an isotope of fluorine that decays to stable oxygen 18 with a half-life of 110 min. The decay modes are: positron beta decay (97 percent) and electron capture (3 percent). The $^{18}F^-$ ion is bone seeking and has been used for bone scans. It has the advantages of high bone-to-background ratio and low absorbed dose. Its disadvantages are its expense, because it must be produced in a cyclotron or reactor just before use, and the 511-KeV photons, which require use of a rectilinear scanner or positron camera. Fluorine 18 has been almost totally replaced by ^{99m}Tc radiopharmaceuticals, such as ^{99m}Tc-medronate, for bone scanning.

fluoroacetamide a highly toxic rat poison and insecticide; M.W. 77.06. Also called 1081. See also *fluoroacetate assays.*

fluoroacetate assays gas chromatography. Fluoroacetate and its amide may be extracted into ether and the methyl ester formed. This is then detected by gas-liquid chromatography, using two different columns.

fluorocarbon (floo″or-o-kar′bon) any fluorine-substituted hydrocarbon, such as the polymer Teflon. Sometimes the term refers to the fluorocarbon aerosols that have the trademark Freon. Freon-12, dichlorodifluoromethane, for example, is used as a refrigerant and as an aerosol propellant. Fluorocarbon toxicities range from nontoxic to highly toxic. They are irritating; high concentrations are narcotic and may be fatal. Also called *chlorofluorocarbon.*

fluorocarbon assays gas-liquid chromatography, with electron capture detector. The fluorocarbons either are extracted into hexane, or are separated by head space diffusion.

fluorochrome (floo′or-o-krōm) a compound that has the property of absorbing light of one wavelength and emitting light of another. Steroids, porphyrins, and nucleic acids are naturally occurring fluorochromes. Fluorochromes such as rhodamine and fluorescein conjugated to antibodies are used in clinical laboratories for the detection and localization of antigens.

Fluorescein isothiocyanate (FITC) is a fluorescein compound that readily binds covalently to proteins at an alkaline pH through ϵ-amino residues of lysine and terminal amino groups. Its absorption maximum is 490–495 nm; it emits a characteristic green color at 517 nm. Tetramethyl rhodamine isothiocyanate has an absorption maximum at 550 nm and a maximal red emission (red) at 580 nm.

The brightness of fluorescence observed with the fluorescent microscope depends on the efficiency with which the dye converts incident light into fluorescent light, the concentration of dye in the tissue specimen, and the intensity of the exciting (absorbed) radiation.

5-fluorocytosine (5-FC) an antifungal agent effective against certain yeasts. It is considered as a first choice in treating *Cryptococcus neoformans* in meningitis, especially when combined with amphotericin B. Administered orally, 5-fluorocytosine is also effective against most *Candida* species and *Torulopsis glabrata.* Resistance may develop, however, after prolonged treatment. Several types of resistant organisms have been reported to be deficient in permease, in cytosine deaminase, or in uridine monophosphate pyrophosphorylase. 5-FC has proved effective not only against yeast infections, but against chromomycosis.

fluorometer (floo″or-om′ĕ-ter) an instrument for performing fluorometry. It consists of an ultraviolet light source, such as a mercury vapor lamp; a primary filter that removes visible light from the exciting beam; a sample cuvet (glass for exciting wavelengths above 320 nm, otherwise quartz); a secondary filter that removes scattered UV from the beam, leaving the cuvet at right angles to the exciting beam; and a photomultiplier tube detector. Spectrofluorometers have xenon arc sources, which emit a continuous spectrum, and grating monochromators, which are used to select the excitation and emission wavelengths.

fluorometry (floo″or-om′ĕ-tre) an analytic method for determining fluorescent compounds (e.g., porphyrins, catecholamines, quinidine, procainamide, calcium, magnesium, salicylate, tyrosine, phenylalanine). The sample is placed in a beam of ultraviolet light, and fluorescent compounds are excited, emitting visible light. The fluorescence intensity at a specific wavelength is proportional to the concentration of the fluorescent compound.

In contrast to visible-UV absorption spectrophotometry, fluorometric methods generally have 100–10,000 times more sensitivity, with detection limits below 1 pg/l, and have a greater range of linearity (for some substances, the emission is proportional to the concentration over a range of five orders of magnitude. They are also more specific; nonfluorescent substances cannot interfere. However, fluorometric methods do have three major sources of measurement error: interference by fluorescent compounds, such as drugs; quenching of the fluorescence by other compounds in the sample that absorb at the same wavelength; and sensitivity of the fluorescence process to environmental factors, such as temperature, pH, and solvent.

fluoroscope (floo′ŏ-ro-skōp) a device for x-ray examination. The x-rays that have passed through the patient strike a screen covered with a phosphor, such as zinc sulfide, which then emits yellow-green light. The viscera can be seen in motion. Some fluoroscopes use electronic image intensification and form the image on a television screen; this procedure eliminates irradiation of the operator and provides a clearer image than that seen on a fluoroscope screen.

fluoroscopic screen the viewing screen used in fluoroscopy. It consists of a layer of zinc sulfide phospor coated on a sheet of plastic that is sealed between a protective radiolucent cover on the tube side and leaded glass on the viewing side. The light generated by the phosphor is a greenish-yellow color (about 530 nm) in the region of the eye's maximal sensitivity. The leaded glass partially protects the operator from x-rays.

fluoroscopy (floo″or-os′ko-pe) examination by means of a fluoroscope. Also called *radioscopy.*

fluorosis (flū″o-ro′sis) a condition caused by excessive chronic ingestion of fluoride. Daily ingestion of more than about 1 mg causes mottled teeth (dental fluorosis), and of more than 25 mg may cause bone degeneration, stiffness, and pain (skeletal or chronic fluorosis).

fluorouracil (floo″ro-ūr′ah-sil) [USP], 5-fluorouracil (5-FU), a cytotoxic drug used as a cancer chemotherapeutic drug. It is an antimetabolite of uracil that blocks the demethylation of dUMP to dTMP and interferes with DNA synthesis. Trademark, Adrucil. For more information, see *Appendix A.*

fluoxymesterone (floo-ok″sĭ-mes′tĕ-rōn) a cancer chemotherapeutic drug; trademark, Halotestin. For more information, see *Appendix A.*

fluphenazine (floo-fen′ah-zēn) a piperazine-type phenothiazine tranquilizer used in the management of psychotic disorders. See also *phenothiazine tranquilizers.* Trademarks, *Permitil* and *Prolixin.*

f. enanthate, [USP], the salt of fluphenazine used for injection.

f. hydrochloride, [USP], the salt of fluphenazine, used for both oral and intramuscular administration.

flurazepam hydrochloride (floor-az′ĕ-pam) a benzodiazepine drug used as a sleeping pill. See also *benzodiazepine.* Trademark, *Dalmane.*

flutter (flut′er) a rapid vibration or pulsation.

atrial f., a cardiac arrhythmia in which the atrial contractions are rapid (200–350/min) and regular. It is thought to be caused by a circus movement pathway of impulse conduction around the atria. Because of the long refractory period of the atrioventricular (A-V) node, not all of the atrial impulses are conducted to the ventricles, and a 2:1 A-V block is generally present. The typical electrocardiographic features of atrial flutter are the fast atrial rate, a ventricular rate of about 150 beats/min (when a 2:1 A-V ratio is present), high-amplitude flutter of F waves in leads II, III, and aV_f, and a regular saw tooth pattern in the baseline.

Atrial flutter is commonly associated with conditions such as rheumatic heart disease, conditions leading to dilation of the atria, or primary myocardial disease.

Direct-current cardioversion is used to convert the flutter to a normal sinus rhythm in the frequent instances in which the condition proves resistant to treatment with antiarrhythmic drugs such as digitalis or quinidine.

ventricular f., a highly unstable pattern of ventricular arrhythmia, characterized by a regular ventricular rate in excess of 200 beats/min, the presence of prominent sinusoidal waves in the electrocardiogram, and severe impairment of cardiovascular function. It tends to revert spontaneously to a normal sinus rhythm or to convert to ventricular fibrillation.

flux (fluks) [L. *fluxus*] 1. an excessive flow or discharge.

2. a borax-containing substance that maintains the cleanliness of metals to be united and facilitates the easy flow and attachment of solder.

fly (flī) a two-winged insect of the order Diptera. The fly is the largest group of arthropods, which serve as vectors for human pathogens.

fruit f., see *Drosophila.*

tsetse f., see *Glossina.*

Fm symbol for the chemical element *fermium.*

fm abbrev. See *femtometer.*

FMN abbrev. See *flavin mononucleotide.*

fmol abbrev. See *femtomole.*

FN abbrev. See *fluoride number.*

***f* number** a numerical expression of the relative aperture of a camera lens, obtained by dividing the focal length of the lens by the diameter of the diaphragm opening as seen through the front lens elements. All lenses, regardless of their focal length, produce optical images of the same brightness when set at a particular *f* number.

foam (fōm) a dispersion of a gas in a liquid or solid. Liquid foam usually requires a foaming agent, such as detergent, for stability.

foam cell a cell, usually a macrophage with a vaculated appearance due to the presence of complex lipids in the cytoplasm. Because such a cell is seen prominently in xanthomas, it has been termed a *xanthoma cell.*

foam stability test a rapid test for measuring the presence of adequate quantities of lung surfactant in amniotic fluid. It is based on the formation of a stable foam after shaking amniotic fluid in the presence of ethanol. More precise tests are available; see *lecithin/sphingomyelin ratio.* Also called shake test.

FOCAL (fo'kal) [acronym from *fo*rmula *cal*culation] a high-level computer language similar to BASIC, which is used in an interactive time-sharing environment. The interpreter runs either whole programs or single statements so that the system can be used like a computer or calculator.

focal (fo'kal) pertaining to or occupying a focus; in pathology, localized in a specific part of the body.

focal distance see *focal length.*

focal epilepsy see *partial e.* under *epilepsy.*

focal-film distance the distance between the focal spot, where the x-rays orignate, and the x-ray film.

focal length in a simple lens, the distance from the front of the lens to the point where an image of the light source is formed; in a compound lens, the distance from a point between the component lenses to the image. Also called *focal distance.*

focal plane in an optical system, the plane through the focal point perpendicular to the optical axis. A converging collimator on a gamma camera or scintillation detector creates a focal point toward which all the collimator holes converge. Images of objects in the focal plane are better resolved and less blurred. With electronic circuitry, devices such as the multiplane tomographic scanner move the sharply resolved plane to depths other than the natural focal plane of the collimator. Cf. *focusing c.* under *collimator.*

focal plane tomography radiography or gamma photography in which those objects above and below the focal plane appear blurred while those in the focal plane are sharply focused. In gamma photgraphy, the blurring is due to the focusing effect of the collimator. In radiography, both the x-ray tube and the film are moved during the exposure so that only objects in the focal plane cast their images on a single point on the film, while the other images move and are blurred. Also called *laminagraphy, planigraphy,* and *stratigraphy.* Cf. *computed tomography.*

focal segmental glomerulosclerosis see under *glomerulopathy.*

focal spot the area of an x-ray tube cathode from which the x-rays radiate; called the actual or electronic focal spot. The projection perpendicular to the central ray, which is its apparent area from the position of the film, is called the effective or the optical spot.

focal zone (FZ) the region above and below the focal plane in which an object is adequately focused. Also called *depth of field.*

focus (fo'kus), pl. *foci* [L. "fire-place"] 1. in an optical system, a point toward which rays of light converge or away from which rays diverge.

2. to move a lens in an optical system in order to make a sharp image.

3. in electroencephalography, a restricted region of scalp or brain tissue that displays a particular pattern of electrical activity. The pattern, identified by wave amplitude, frequency, and/or phase reversal, may be either normal or abnormal.

4. in pathology, a region of interest or one undergoing a localized pathologic process.

conjugate f., the point of convergence of rays diverging from a point after being refracted by a lens.

principal f., the point of convergence of parallel rays after being refracted by a lens.

focusing (fo'kus-ing) the act of converging at a point.

fog (fog) generalized cloudiness in a photograph,

especially a radiograph, caused by exposure of the film to light or radiation before development, by improper development, or by use of film that is too old.

folate (fo′lāt) a salt, ester, or anion of folic acid.

folate reductase (fo′lāt re-duk′tās) see *tetrahydrofolate dehydrogenase.*

fold (fōld) a thin, recurved margin or doubling. Also called *plica.*

aryepiglottic f., a fold of mucous membrane that stretches between the side of the epiglottis and the apex of the arytenoid cartilage.

circular f.'s of intestine, large, permanent folds that project into the lumen of the bowel. They retard the passage of food and provide an increased surface for absorption. Also called *plicae circulares* and valves of Kerckring.

epicanthic f., see *epicanthus.*

ileocecal fold, a fold of peritoneum attached to the ileum above, cecum laterally, and appendix or its mesentery below.

folded-cell index see under *squamous cell index.*

folic acid (FA) a water-soluble vitamin; M.W. 441.40. Chemically it is a pteroylmonoglutamate, and the structure consists of three residues, namely, pteridine, *p*-aminobenzoic acid, and L-glutamic acid. The major dietary sources of folic acid include leafy vegetables, eggs, milk, yeast, liver, whole-grain cereals, and fruits. It is also synthesized by intestinal microorganisms. In most dietary sources folate occurs as pteroyl*poly*glutamates; these are hydrolyzed to pteroyl*mono*glutamate by the enzyme conjugase.

Folate is absorbed by the proximal jejunal cells. In these cells, folate is reduced (5,6,7,8-tetrahydrofolate, FH_4) and converted to its transportable form, N^5-methyl-5,6,7,8-tetrahydrofolate (N^5-methyl-FH_4). N^5-Methyl-FH_4 is transported in the plasma to tissues for utilization. In these tissues, N^5-methyl-FH_4 is reconverted to FH_4, the primary acceptor and carrier of single carbon units, —CHO, —CH_2-, and —CH=NH. This reconversion process is coupled to the conversion of homocysteine to methionine, catalyzed by an enzyme dependent on a coenzyme of vitamin B_{12}. Thus, a deficiency of vitamin B_{12} produces, in effect, a deficiency of folic acid, which explains the observation that a deficiency in either produces indistinguishable hematologic complications.

As indicated, folate coenzymes function as carriers of single-carbon units and play a vital role in the metabolism of nucleotides (biosynthesis of purines, thymine) and amino acids (interconversion of serine to glycine, catabolism of histidine). Folate deficiency initially affects all tissues with a high degree of cell multiplication, namely, red blood cells, platelets, leukocytes, and intestinal epithelial cells. The most characteristic features of folate deficiency are megaloblastic anemia, hypersegmentation of neutrophils, and, in advanced cases, leukopenia and thrombocytopenia.

Folate in the form of N^5-methyl-FH_4 is stored in the liver; it takes about 3–6 mo to develop anemia with a folate-deficient diet. Deficiencies in folate can arise from a variety of causes: nutritional folate deficiency, defective absorption of folate (e.g., malabsorption syndromes, blind-loop syndrome, tropical and nontropical sprue, long-term use of anticoagulants and of oral contraceptives in some women), increased requirement of folate not met by regular intake (e.g., pregnancy, increased cell proliferation as seen in some hematopoietic and hemolytic processes, neoplasms), inadequate utilization of folate (e.g., biochemical lesions in the interconversion of folate coenzymes, folate antagonists such as methotrexate in the therapy of malignant neoplasms, alcoholism), and liver disease. In the methotrexate therapy of neoplastic diseases, particularly with high doses, the deficiency of folate, which leads to myelosuppression, can be ameliorated by administration of N^5-formyl-FH_4 (leucovorin) after the drug therapy. The antibacterial action of sulfonamides is due to its inhibition of folate synthesis in susceptible organisms. Sulfonamides are structural analogs (antimetabolite) of *p*-aminobenzoic acid, a constituent of folate.

The recommended daily dietary allowance for folate is 400 mg to provide an estimated minimal daily requirement of 50 μg. However, it should be noted that growth, pregnancy, lactation, and certain drugs increase the demands for folate.

In clinical chemistry, folic acid or folate refers to *pteroylglutamic acid* and its structurally related derivatives.

N. V. BHAGAVAN, PH.D.

folic acid anemia see *folic acid (folate deficiency) a.* under *anemia.*

folic acid assays 1. microbiologic assays using *Lactobacillus casei* as the test organism with folic acid as standards. This organism responds to FA and most of the FH_4 derivatives. Reference ranges for serum are 3–25 ng/ml; for RBC folate 180–850 ng/ml of packed cells. These methods are time-consuming, require very careful technique, and are subject to various interferences.

2. competitive protein-binding methods using a folate-binding protein in bovine milk (lactoglobulin fraction). Serum folate and its derivative compete with added ^{125}I-labeled folate for binding sites on the binding protein. By comparing radioactivity of the bound fraction of the unknowns with that of folate standards, serum folate concentrations can be calculated. Reference ranges are: for serum, 2–15 ng/ml; for RBC folate, 150–450 ng/ml of packed cells. This method has largely replaced microbiologic assays.

3. an indirect assay, measurement of the amount of formiminoglutamic acid (FIGLU) in the urine. FIGLU is an intermediate in the conversion of histidine to glutamate with the conversion of FIGLU to glutamate requiring FH_4. If FH_4 is deficient or absent, FIGLU accumulates and is found in increased levels in the urine. Reference ranges are: after a 15-g histidine loading, normal FIGLU output is 1–15 mg/8–hr period, or <35 mg/d; ranges over 50 mg/d (up to 1000 mg/d) indicate folic acid deficiency. See also *formiminoglutamic acid.*

Folin-Ciocalteu reagent an analytic reagent, golden yellow in color, constituted of a phospho-tungsto-molybdic acid complex. It is used to detect and quantitate phenols and some other aromatic ring structures, such as indole and imidazole, or compounds containing such groups as tyrosine and proteins (fibrinogen). The reagent is reduced to a deep blue color that is measured spectrophotometrically at 670 nm.

folinic acid N_5-formyltetrahydrofolic acid, the formyl derivative and active form of folic acid. Folinic acid was first recognized as the growth factor for *Leuconostoc citrovorum* and called citrovorum factor. It is administered parenterally for treatment of megaloblastic anemia due to folic acid deficiency caused by poor nutrition or by the administration of very high doses of folic acid antagonists, which block folate reduction and are used in the treatment of some malignancies. Also called *citrovorum factor, leucovorin*, and *N_5-formyl FH_4*. See also *leucovorin calcium*.

folium of cerebellum (fo'le-um), pl. *folia* one of the many long, narrow, curved folds of gray matter on the surface of the cerebellum. Separated by grooves or fissures, these small gyri in the cortex give the cerebellum its laminated appearance and increase its surface area up to seven times.

follicle (fol'lĭ-k'l) 1. a sac or pouchlike depression or cavity.
2. see *hair follicle*.
3. see *lymph nodule*.
4. see *ovarian follicle*.
nabothian f., see *nabothian cyst*.

follicle-stimulating hormone (FSH, hFSH) a hormone secreted by the anterior pituitary under the control of a gonadotropin-releasing hormone (LH-releasing hormone) secreted by the hypothalamus. FSH, a glycoprotein (M.W. 30,000) with alpha and beta subunits, binds to specific receptors on the plasma membrane of its target cells, activating adenylate cyclase, leading to an increase in cyclic AMP. It stimulates the development of gonadal tissues that secrete steroid hormones and is essential for fertility. FSH stimulates the ovarian follicles for ovulation in females and spermatogenesis in males. The control of FSH is effected by a negative feedback mechanism of the steroid hormones on the hypothalamus and/or anterior pituitary.

FSH is increased in primary gonadal failure, ovarian or testicular agenesis, Klinefelter's syndrome, and FSH-secreting tumors. Decreased concentrations are seen in panhypopituitarism, hypogonadotropic hypogonadism, anorexia nervosa, and cancer of the testes, ovaries, or adrenals; in prepubertal children; and with estrogen administration.

Reference ranges for FSH in serum are: for males, 4–25 mIU/ml; for females—follicular phase, 5–30; midcycle peak, 15–90; luteal phase, 5–18; menopausal phase, 50–250.

See also *glycoprotein hormones*.

follicle-stimulating hormone assays methods for the quantitation of serum or urinary levels of FSH: (1) mouse uterine weight assay, (2) rat ovarian augmentation reaction assay, and (3) radioimmunoassay. Of all the methods described, RIA permits direct and routine quantitation of hFSH in serum, plasma, and urine, and provides an accurate, reproducible, rapid, and specific assay that generally is many times more sensitive than most other assay systems.

follicle-stimulating hormone–releasing hormone (FSH-RH) see *gonadotropin hormone–releasing hormone*.

follicul/o (fo-lik'u-lo) a word element used in combining form to denote a follicle or small sac, e.g., follicular.

follicular (fo-lik'u-lar) [L. *follicularis*] of or pertaining to a follicle or follicles.

follicular carcinoma a carcinoma of thyroid follicular cells. In the well-differentiated tumors, follicles are formed. Infrequently, a more solid follicular carcinoma behaves aggressively in a manner comparable with anaplastic thyroid carcinomas. Most differentiated carcinomas of thyroid follicular cells contain both follicular and papillary arrangements of the tumor cells. The tumor may show uptake of radioactive iodine. Metastases are common, particularly to regional lymph nodes, bone, and lungs.

follicular center the lighter central zone of a lymphoid follicle, as seen by light microscopy. It represents the site of B-cell differentiation and the high-level production of antibodies. The cells are larger and have more cytoplasm than do the surrounding small lymphocytes. Cell types identified in normal follicular centers are cleaved cells (small and large), noncleaved cells (small and large), histiocytes, and dendritic reticulum cells. The cleaved and noncleaved cells form a basis for classification of B-cell lymphomas. Also called *germinal center*. See also *lymph node* and *lymphoma*.

folliculitis (fŏ-lik"u-li'tis) an inflammation of follicles, usually the hair follicles.

fomite (fo'mīt) an object, such as a book, article of clothing, or eating utensil, which is not in itself harmful but which may harbor pathogenic microorganisms and thus serve as a vehicle of transmission of infection.

Fonsecaea (fon-se-se'ah) a genus of Fungi Imperfecti belonging to the family Dematiaceae; it contains species that are the causative agents of chromoblastomycosis. The colonies are slow-growing, velvety or woolly, and olive-to-black in color. Isolates are extremely polymorphic.

F. compactum, a soil-inhabiting fungus that is an etiologic agent for chromomycosis. The colony morphology of this organism is folded, brittle, olive-to-black in color, and develops a black fuzz with age. Microscopically, the conidiophores are compact and the spores are ovoid. Also called *Phialophora compactum*.

F. dermatitidis, a soil-inhabiting fungus that occasionally can cause chromomycosis. *F. dermatitidis* has two colony types—a glistening, yeastlike colony and an olive-gray, fuzzy mycelial form. Microscopically, the yeastlike colony shows budding, yeastlike cells; the mycelial form shows conidiophores with several spores and phialides. Also called *Phialophora dermatitidis*.

F. jeanselmei, see *P. jeanselmei* under *Phialophora*.

F. pedrosoi, a fungus that causes chromomycosis, a dermatitis usually confined to the lower extremities. This fungus is usually introduced into the tissue by trauma. The colony morphology is variable but is most often gray-black in color and fluffy with radiations. Microscopically, there are three types of sporulations: *Cladosporium* type, *Phialophora* type, and *Rhinocladiella* (*Acrotheca*) type.

Fontana-Masson staining method an ammoniacal silver nitrate stain for argentaffin material used in the diagnosis of melanomas, pheochromocytomas, and carcinoid tumors. Paraffin sections fixed in formalin or Bouin's fluid are stained in ammoniacal silver nitrate solution, then toned in gold chloride solution, fixed in sodium thiosulfate solution (hypo), and counterstained in safranine, eosin, or nuclear fast red. Melanin and argentaffin granules are stained black; carcinoid granules are stained brown.

Fontana's spaces (fon-tah'nahz) [Felice *Fontana,* Italian naturalist and physiologist, 1720–1805] spaces of the iridocorneal angle. These spaces, located between the trabeculae of the sinus venosus and the pectinate ligament, communicate between the anterior chamber and sinus venosus, permitting aqueous humor to reach the lumen of the sinus.

fontanelle (fon"tah-nel') [Fr., dim. of *fontaine* spring, filter] an unossified space in the skull of the fetus and newborn, located at the angles of the parietal bones and palpable as a soft area. The anterior fontanelle is bounded by the two halves of the frontal bone and the parietal bones, and is diamond-shaped. The posterior fontanelle is bounded by the parietal bones and the occipital bone, and is triangular. The two are united by the sagittal suture. The position of the fetal head during labor can be determined by palpation of the fontanelles. As ossification of the skull bones is completed, the fontanelles close, the posterior shortly after birth and the anterior by the end of the second year.

Food and Drug Administration (FDA) an agency of the United States government that regulates the manufacture, testing, and labeling of all drugs. It requires that all drugs be proved both safe and effective, when used as recommended, before they are approved for marketing.

food poisoning an acute gastroenteritis or neurologic syndrome that results from the ingestion of food contaminated with pathogenic microorganisms or the products (toxins) of microorganisms, as well as poisonous chemicals. The most common type of food poisoning is bacterial; this form may be self-limiting, but certain cases may be life-threatening and can be effectively treated only if the etiologic agent is identified.

The ingestion of preformed toxin in food may involve *Staphylococcus aureus, Bacillus cereus,* or *Clostridium botulinum.* If food contains certain living bacteria that, when ingested, can infect the intestinal tract and elaborate a toxin, food poisoning will result, but with a longer incubation period than for preformed toxin. Bacteria responsible for this type of food poisoning are *C. perfringens,* enterotoxigenic *Escherichia coli,* and *Vibrio cholera. Shigella* species and invasive *E. coli* may cause a food-borne gastroenteritis by direct tissue invasion. There are some bacteria that cause food poisoning by a combination of tissue invasion and toxin production. These include *Vibrio parahemolyticus, Yersinia enterocolitica,* and sometimes *Salmonella* and *Shigella* species. Chemical food poisoning may involve heavy metals, mercury, or chemically toxic food such as mushrooms.

TABLE 1. **Food Poisoning Syndromes: Primarily Gastrointestinal Symptoms**

AGENT	FOODS	INCUBATION PERIOD	CLINICAL PRESENTATION AND DURATION OF ILLNESS	DIAGNOSIS	THERAPY	PREVENTION
A. Upper Gastrointestinal Symptoms Predominate						
Bacterial						
Staph. aureus enterotoxin (heat-stable)	Meats, cream, desserts (high protein)	1–6 hours	Nausea, vomiting, watery diarrhea; fever uncommon; duration 12–24 hours	(a) Coagulase (+) *Staph. aureus* in vomitus, feces, food (>10^5 organisms per gram) (b) Toxin in food (RIA, gel precipitation)	Supportive	Avoid temperatures of 8–45 C for food, food handler contamination
Bacillus cereus toxin (heat-stable)	Fried rice	1–6 hours	Vomiting, abdominal cramps, occasional diarrhea; duration <12 hours	Food with >10^5 organisms per gram	Supportive	Avoid reheated rice
Heavy metals						
Zinc, copper, tin, cadmium	Acid beverages (pH 5) in metallic containers, tubing, nitrate-containing foods	5 minutes–2 hours	Nausea, vomiting, cramps, headache, diarrhea (zinc, tin); duration 2–24 hours	Clinical syndrome, metal in food or beverage	Supportive	Prolonged storage of acid beverages in metal containers or tubing should be avoided
Protozoan						
Anisakiasis (eosinophilic gastritis)	Raw fish	Days–months	Abdominal pain, intestinal obstruction, heme (+) stool, eosinophilia	Gastroscopy	(a) Remove larvae via gastroscopy (b) Surgery	(a) "Gut" fish and refrigerate prior to use (b) Thorough cooking
B. Lower Gastrointestinal Symptoms Predominate, No Fecal Leukocytes						
Bacterial						
Clostridium perfringens enterotoxin (heat-labile) release in gut	Meats, gravies, poultry, fish	8–16 hours	Watery diarrhea, cramps, nausea (30–50%); duration 24 hours	(a) Food and stool for *C. perfringens* (>10^5/gm) (+) (b) Enterotoxin in stool (CIEP) (c) Rise in serum antibody to enterotoxin	Supportive	Eat or store food rapidly after preparation; 15–50 C permits growth
Bacillus cereus enterotoxin (heat-labile) release in gut	Raw meats, vegetables, dried foods	8–16 hours	Watery diarrhea, nausea, cramps; fever rare; duration 48 hours	(a) Stool (+) for *B. cereus* (b) Enterotoxin activity in stool, food (rabbit ileal loop)	Supportive	Avoid prolonged warming of food
Enterotoxigenic *Escherichia coli* (heat-labile and heat-stable enterotoxins; LT and ST)	Water-borne; salads, raw vegetables	1–4 days	Travel history, watery diarrhea, fever in children, nausea, vomiting, muscle ache; duration 1–5 days	Enterotoxin assay LT:tissue culture (CHO or Yl adrenal) or immunoassay ST:suckling mouse	Supportive (oral glucose electrolyte solutions—bismuth subsalicylate)	Avoid incriminated foods, water Doxycycline 100 mg/day (most strains) Bismuth subsalicylate

TABLE 1. Food Poisoning Syndromes: Primarily Gastrointestinal Symptoms (*Continued*)

AGENT	FOODS	INCUBATION PERIOD	CLINICAL PRESENTATION AND DURATION OF ILLNESS	DIAGNOSIS	THERAPY	PREVENTION
Vibrio cholerae enterotoxin secreted in small intestine	Water-borne; contaminated foods, Gulf region shellfish	24–72 hours	Travel history, achlorhydria, explosive and painless watery diarrhea, hypovolemia, acidosis	(a) Rapidly motile comma-shaped bacteria on dark field of stool (b) TCBS culture of stool	(a) Oral electrolyte solutions; 3.5 gm NaCl, 2.5 gm $NaHCO_3$, 1.5 gm KCL, 20 gm glucose in 1 liter H_2O (b) IV replacement (c) Tetracycline 10 mg/kg PO q6H × 2 days if sensitive	Avoid infected water; vaccine for travel to endangered area (60–80% efficacy × 3–6 months)
Protozoan						
Entamoeba histolytica	Water-borne; fecal contamination of foods	2–7 days	Gradual onset diarrhea (dysentery-like), abdominal pain, fever 30%; can be chronic	(a) Stool exam, trichrome stain for trophozoite (b) Indirect hemagglutination (CDC) (+) 80–90% (c) Proctoscopy, scraping of ulcers	Metronidazole, 750 mg PO tid × 10 days (if shorter duration of therapy, follow with diloxanide furoate* 500 mg PO tid × 10 days (CDC)	Adequate sanitation
Giardia lamblia	Water-borne (Rocky Mountains) (Leningrad)		Travel history, persistent diarrhea, malabsorption, abdominal bloating, nausea	(a) Stool exam × 3 (b) Enterotest (examine duodenal contents)	Quinacrine, 100 mg PO tid × 10 days	Sanitation; avoid surface water
C. Lower Gastrointestinal Symptoms Predominate, Fecal Leukocytes Present						
Bacterial						
Salmonella (enterotoxin effect and invasion)	Poultry, beef, ice cream; marijuana	6–48 hours	Diarrhea (watery or dysentery-like), fever, cramps, hypovolemia; duration 2–7 days	(a) Stool culture (b) Positive blood cultures rare	(a) Supportive (b) Avoid antibiotics (don't alter course, prolong carrier state) unless systemic syndrome (enteric fever, chronic bacteremia, abscess)	(a) Adequate cooking and refrigeration (b) Identify carriers (c) Isolate active cases
Salmonella typhi (typhoid fever) (also *S. paratyphi*, *S. schottmülleri*, *S. hirschfeldii*—paratyphoid fever)	Fecal contamination; water, milk	10–14 days	Travel history, fever, malaise, headache, chills, constipation or diarrhea, cough, sore throat, rose spots, hepatosplenomegaly; duration 3–4 weeks	(a) (+) Blood culture (1st week) (+) stool culture not definitive (b) Serology (Widal 50% rise) (c) Leukocytosis, ↑ SGOT, ↑ LDH, monocytes in stool	(a) Chloramphenicol, 50 mg/kg/day PO, divided 4 doses × 4 days; if resistant, ampicillin, 100 mg/kg/day PO or IV qid × 14 days, or trimethoprim-sulfamethoxazole, 2–4 (80/400 mg) tablets PO q 12 h × 14 days (b) Avoid antipyretics (c) Supportive (d) Monitor Hct, stools for blood	(a) As above (b) Immunization increases infective dose of bacteria
Shigella enterotoxin and invasion	Potato, egg salads; fecal contamination, water-borne	36–72 hours	Fever, abdominal cramping, watery diarrhea followed by bloody mucoid stools, nausea, vomiting; duration, average 7 days	(a) Abundant fecal leukocytes (b) Stool culture on selective media	(a) Supportive (b) Ampicillin, 50 mg/kg/day in 4 divided doses PO × 5–6 days; if resistant, trimethoprim + sulfamethoxazole, 2 (80/400 mg) tablets PO q 12h × 5 days	(a) Adequate sanitation (b) Hand washing (c) Isolate active cases
Vibrio parahemolyticus enterotoxin (heat-labile) + invasion	Bivalve mollusks, crabs, raw saltwater fish (Japan); untreated seawater	12–24 hours	Explosive watery diarrhea, cramps, nausea, headache, fever 20% or dysentery, abdominal pain; duration up to 10 days	Culture stool, food (TCBS media) (Kanagawa, hemolysin (+) stain in stool)	(a) Supportive (b) If dysentery or prolonged illness, ampicillin, 100 mg/kg/day PO or IV qid × 5–7 days, or tetracycline, 500 mg PO qid × 5–7 days	(a) Proper cooking of seafood (b) Rapid refrigeration
Yersinia enterocolitica	Milk, ice cream, meat, mussels; water-borne	16–48 hours	Fever, diarrhea, abdominal pain, mesenteric adenitis, arthritis, erythema nodosum; duration 1–3 weeks	(a) Stool culture (b) Blood culture (c) Serology	Supportive unless septicemia; then gentamicin, 5 mg/kg/day IV, or chloramphenicol, 50 mg/kg/day PO or IV	None specific
Invasive *Escherichia coli*	Cheese, meats	24–72 hours	Dysentery, fever, malaise, myalgia, abdominal cramps	Sereny test	Supportive	None specific
Non-0-1 *V. cholerae* ("*noncholera vibrio*")	Seafood, water-borne	24 hours	Travel, diarrhea, abdominal cramps, nausea, vomiting, fever (58%), biliary disease	Stool culture on TCBS agar	(a) Supportive (b) Antibiotic—ampicillin, 100 mg/kg/day PO or IV qid 7–14 days, if sensitive organism	Proper cooking of seafood
Campylobacter fetus spp. jejuni	Water-borne; poultry, raw milk, farm animal, canine exposure; ?garden vegetables	72 hours	Bloody diarrhea, cramps, fever, vomiting; duration 1–4 days; relapse common	(a) Special stool culture in selective media, reduced pO_2 at 42 C (b) Blood culture	(a) Supportive (b) Erythromycin, 500 mg PO qid × 7 days (longer therapy if bacteremic syndrome develops)	Avoid raw milk, farm animal contamination

*Investigational drug. Available from Center for Disease Control, Atlanta, Georgia.

From Conn, H. F.: Current Therapy 1981. Philadelphia, W. B. Saunders Co., 1981.

TABLE 2. **Food Poisoning Syndromes: Gastrointestinal Plus Neurologic Symptoms**

AGENT	FOODS	INCUBATION PERIOD	CLINICAL PRESENTATION AND DURATION OF ILLNESS	DIAGNOSIS	THERAPY	PREVENTION
			A. Without Paresthesias			
Bacterial						
Clostridium botulinum neurotoxin (A, B, E, heat-labile) ingestion	Low acid home-canned vegetables, fruits; < 10% of cases from commercial foods – vichyssoise, peppers, beef stew, mullet	18–36 hours	Nausea, vomiting, diarrhea (25%), followed by constipation and descending symmetrical motor weakness (cranial nerves initially); duration weeks–months	(a) Presence of toxin and *C. botulinum* in food and stool (mouse test with antisera) (b) Electromyography, facilitation of action potential with repetitive stimuli	(a) Respiratory support, tracheostomy if needed (b) Emetics/cathartics to remove unabsorbed toxin (c) Botulinal antitoxin if severe case (20% side effects, R/O horse serum allergy) (d) ? Guanidine hydrochloride, 35 mg/kg/day PO, improves eye/limb weakness only (e) Report CDC: 404-329-3753 or 404-329-3644 (nights, weekends)	(a) pH < 4.5 home-canned foods (b) Boil prior to ingestion (c) Store food < 10 C (d) Nitrites are inhibitory
Clostridium botulinum, infants: neurotoxin released in gut	Honey, ?soil, dust		Age 2–26 weeks, constipation, poor feeding, descending motor paralysis (weak cry, "floppy baby"), 20% respiratory arrest; duration weeks–months	Clinical picture plus above	(a) Supportive (b) Antitoxin not required for recovery (c) Guanidine no longer recommended	Unknown
Chemical						
Organic phosphates (insecticides), cholinesterase inhibitors	Sugar, flour, bread, cereals, pastries	15 minutes–2 hours	Parasympathetic hyperactivity, cramps, nausea, vomiting, diarrhea, blurred vision, urinary/fecal incontinence, respiratory failure; 30% fatality	Clinical presentation plus low red cell and plasma cholinesterase levels	(a) Gastric lavage (b) Atropine, 0.4 mg IV q6h as needed (c) Pralidoxime, 1 gram IV, can be repeated × 1	Avoid insecticide use close to harvest
Solanine (potato poisoning)	Potato "eyes," sprouts, skin	7–19 hours	Abdominal pain, vomiting, diarrhea, fever, confusion, hallucinations, visual alterations; duration 1–2 days	(a) Clinical presentation (b) Solanine dose > 25 mg in food	Supportive	(a) Toxin water soluble, removed by boiling (b) If eating > 1 lb potatoes, peel and boil
			B. With Paresthesias			
Fish toxins						
Scromboid (histamine, saurine)	Tuna, mackerel bonito, skipjack	5 minutes–1 hour	Histamine reaction, cramps, nausea, vomiting, diarrhea, flushing, oral burning, paresthesias, urticaria, bronchospasm, pruritus; duration hours	Histamine in fish > 100 mg/100 grams	(a) Antihistamines (b) Emetic and cathartic (c) Treat bronchospasm, epinephrine or aminophylline	(a) Avoid storage of fish at 20–30 C (68–86 F) (b) Avoid fish with bitter, peppery taste
Puffer fish tetrodotoxin (heat-stable)	Puffer fish	10–45 minutes	Paresthesias of lip, tongue, and extremities; nausea, vomiting, cramps, loss of proprioception, flaccid paralysis, respiratory failure; 40–50% mortality	Tetrodotoxin bioassay (food)	(a) Supportive (b) Emetic and enemas	Avoid puffer fish served in Japan
Ciguatera fish ciguatoxin (heat-stable)	400 species: barracuda, red snapper, larger fish; 90% Hawaii or Florida	1–6 hours	Abdominal cramps, nausea, vomiting, watery diarrhea, paresthesias of lips and tongue, metallic taste, dry mouth, visual disturbance, transient blindness, sensation of loose and painful teeth, reversal of hot-cold sensation, hypotension, respiratory paralysis; duration days; residual years	(a) Bioassay for toxin (b) RIA toxin assay in food	(a) Supportive (b) Enemas (c) Analgesics (d) Atropine, 0.4 mg IV q6h, for CNS and GI manifestations	(a) Avoid fish liver, intestine, ovary ingestion (b) Clean fish immediately
Neurotoxic shellfish *Gymnodinium breve* (dinoflagellate), heat-stable toxins (red tide)	Oysters, clams, mussels (Gulf coast)	5 minutes–4 hours	Paresthesias of mouth and lips, reversal of hot-cold sensation, no paralysis, nausea, vomiting, diarrhea; can get respiratory syndrome; duration hours–days	Toxin in food	Supportive	Avoid possible contaminated bivalves
Paralytic shellfish *Gonyaulax catenella* (Pacific coast), *Gonyaulax tamarensis* (Atlantic coast), saxitoxin and other neurotoxins (heat-stable), red tide (summer, fall)	Oysters, clams, mussels, scallops	5 minutes–4 hours, dose-dependent	Paresthesias of mouth and lips, paralysis, respiratory insufficiency (first 12 hours), nausea, vomiting, diarrhea; duration hours–days	(a) Mouse bioassay of toxin in food (b) Dinoflagellates in seawater	(a) Cathartic, gastric lavage (b) Supportive	(a) Mollusks can be toxic without red tide (b) Avoid possible contaminated bivalves
Chemical						
Monosodium-L-glutamate	Wonton soup (absorption increased when stomach empty)	1 hour	Paresthesias; burning of neck, chest, arms; chest pain, headache, flushing, lacrimation, nausea, cramps, thirst; duration hours	MSG in food (> 4 grams total dose)	None needed	Susceptible individuals should avoid MSG, especially on empty stomach

From Conn, H. F.: Current Therapy 1981. Philadelphia, W. B. Saunders Co., 1981.

TABLE 3. **Food Poisoning Syndromes: Gastrointestinal Plus Other Systemic Diseases**

AGENT	FOODS	INCUBATION PERIOD	CLINICAL PRESENTATION AND DURATION OF ILLNESS	DIAGNOSIS	THERAPY	PREVENTION
Mushroom poisoning						
Muscarine	Inocybe, clitocybe species	<2 hours	Parasympathetic hyperactivity, salivation, diarrhea, diaphoresis, bradycardia, bronchospasm; duration 24 hours	Mushroom identification	(a) Atropine, 0.4 mg IV q6h, as needed (b) Supportive	Use commercial mushrooms only
Disulfiram-like	*Coprinus atramentuis* plus/minus alcoholic beverages up to 48 hours after mushroom ingestion	<2 hours	Nausea, vomiting, flushing, palpitations, tachycardia; duration 24 hours	As above	Supportive	As above
General gastrointestinal irritants	Many species	<2 hours	Nausea, vomiting, cramps, diarrhea	As above	Supportive	As above
Amatoxins, phallotoxins	*Amanita phalloides, Amanita virosa, Amanita verna, Galerina autumnalis, Galerina marginata, Galerina venenata*	6–24 hours	Abdominal cramps, watery diarrhea for 24 hours, then hepatic and/or renal failure–hypoglycemia, metabolic acidosis, cardiomyopathy; 30% mortality; duration days	(a) As above (b) Renal/hepatic abnormalities	Supportive, including dialysis and metabolic correction; consider thiocitic acid (experimental)	As above
Gyromitrin	Helvella species	6–24 hours	Cramps, diarrhea, followed by hepatic failure	Identify mushroom	Supportive	As above
Parasite						
Trichinosis	Pork, bear	1 week	Often asymptomatic; intestinal phase – malaise, anorexia, cramps, vomiting; muscle invasion – bilateral orbital edema, myalgias, fever, urticaria for 1–3 weeks, then convalescence, fatigue, listlessness; duration 3–10 weeks	(a) Deltoid or gastrocnemius muscle biopsy (b) Serology (c) Eosinophilia increased LDH, CPK	95% spontaneous recovery (a) Thiabendazole, 25 mg/kg bid × 5 days in early stages (b) Prednisone up to 60 mg PO qd for <2 weeks to treat severe symptoms	(a) Freeze food (b) Cook pork to internal temperature > 70 C (c) Use cuts of pork <6″ thick
Viral						
Hepatitis A	Mollusks, salads, cole slaw, sandwiches; waterborne	14–49 days	Fever, malaise, headache, anorexia, nausea, vomiting, then hepatomegaly, jaundice; duration 3–24 weeks	(a) Elevated SGOT, bilirubin (b) Hepatitis A particle in stool by IEM (c) Anti-hepatitis A (fourfold rise) in serum	Supportive	(a) Human immune globulin (0.02 ml/kg IM) if known contaminated ingestion within 6 weeks and asymptomatic or travel to endemic area (b) Isolation of cases (c) Handwashing (d) Eliminate primate spread

From Conn, H. F.: Current Therapy 1981. Philadelphia, W. B. Saunders Co., 1981.

TABLE 4. **Food Poisoning Syndromes: Neurologic Symptoms Alone**

AGENT	FOODS	INCUBATION PERIOD	CLINICAL PRESENTATION AND DURATION OF ILLNESS	DIAGNOSIS	THERAPY	PREVENTION
Mushroom						
Ibotenic acid, muscimol	*Amanita muscaria, Amanita pantherina*	1–2 hours	Confusion, restlessness, visual disturbance; duration 24 hours	Mushroom identification	(a) Supportive (b) Physostigmine, 1 mg IV, for anticholinergic symptoms	Use commercial mushrooms only
Psilocybin, psilocin	Psilocybe species	<2 hours	Psychotic reaction, hallucinations; duration 12 hours	Mushroom identification	Supportive	As above
Chemical						
Alkyl mercury	Pork, grain, fish, shellfish	<2 hours or chronic exposure	Ataxia, agitation, visual impairment, hyperreflexia, coma; duration months	Increased mercury in food, serum, hair	(a) Supportive (b) Dimercaprol (BAL), 0.5 mg/kg IM q4h × 2 days; q12h × 1 day; qd × 5–10 days	Avoid alkyl mercury–treated grain or animal feed

From Conn, H. F.: Current Therapy 1981. Philadelphia, W. B. Saunders Co., 1981.

The clinical management of food poisoning involves clinical and laboratory diagnosis, supportive and antitoxin therapy, and epidemiologic control. Food poisoning syndromes may be divided into seven types: (1) upper gastrointestinal symptoms predominating, (2) lower GI symptoms predominating with no fecal leukocytes present, (3) lower GI symptoms predominating with fecal leukocytes present, (4) GI plus neurologic symptoms without paresthesias, (5) GI plus neurologic symptoms with paresthesias, (6) GI plus other systemic disease, and (7) neurologic symptoms alone. In the accompanying tables, these types of food poisoning list the types of food commonly contaminated, the incubation period, clinical symptoms, diagnosis, therapy, and prevention.

foot (foot), pl. *feet* [L. *pes*] the distal portion of the vertebrate leg on which one stands and walks.

foot-and-mouth disease a disease that occurs predominantly in cloven-hooved animals owing to infection with a picornavirus. It rarely affects humans, although infection may occur after contact with tissue or body fluids of diseased animals.

There is a short incubation period and febrile illness with vesicular lesions appearing on the palms, soles, and oropharyngeal membranes. No therapy is effective and the disease is self-limited.

foot process 1. a terminal expansion of an astrocytic process, usually investing the blood vessels and the ependymal and pial surfaces of the central nervous system. Also called end feet.

2. a short extension of cytoplasm from an epithelial cell (podocyte) of a renal glomerulus that attaches to the basement membrane. The slender clefts between adjacent foot processes constitute filtration slits.

Foot's reticulin method a procedure for staining reticulin in tissue sections using potassium permanganate oxidation, silver impregnation with Foot's silver oxide solution, reduction to metallic silver with formalin, and gold toning. See also *reticulin staining.*

foramen (fo-ra′men), pl. *foramina* [L.] [NA], a general term for a natural opening or passage.

epiploic f. of Winslow, the aperture through which the lesser sac of the peritoneum communicates with the greater sac. Also called *aditus of lesser sac of the peritoneum.*

intervertebral f., an opening, bounded by the pedicles of adjacent vertebrae, that transmits a spinal nerve and contains its dorsal root ganglion.

jugular f., a large opening between the occipital and petrous temporal bones. It transmits the inferior petrosal sinus; the glossopharyngeal, vagus, and accessory nerves; and the internal jugular vein.

f. lacerum, a short, wide canal that extends from the exterior of the skull base to the middle cranial fossa. The carotid canal opens into its upper end.

f. magnum, the large opening in the floor of the posterior cranial fossa through which the brain becomes continuous with the spinal cord.

f. of Monro, the foramen that connects each lateral ventricle of the brain with the third ventricle.

nutrient f., a passage in a bone through which the nutrient artery passes.

obturator f., a wide opening in the hip bone below the acetabulum. The obturator membrane attaches to its margins and closes it, except at the point where the obturator nerve and vessels leave the pelvis.

optic f., the canal in the lesser wing of the sphenoid bone at the back of the orbit through which the optic nerve passes.

oval f. of heart, a large oblique opening in the fetal interatrial septum that allows blood to pass from the right to the left atrium but not in the opposite direction. It usually closes shortly after birth. Also called foramen ovale.

oval f. of skull, an opening in the base of the skull at the posterior margin of the greater wing of the sphenoid that transmits the mandibular division of the trigeminal nerve.

primary interventricular f., in the developing embryo, a connection between the two ventricles of the heart, present by the fourth week of fetal development and normally closed in the seventh week by expansion of the endocardial cushions.

f. rotundum, a round opening that pierces the greater wing of the sphenoid immediately below and posterior to the medial end of the superior orbital fissure. It conducts the maxillary division of the trigeminal nerve.

f. spinosum, a short canal in the floor of the cranial cavity that transmits the middle meningeal vessels. It is located posterolateral to the oval foramen.

stylomastoid f., an opening behind the root of the styloid process. It transmits the facial nerve.

zygomaticofacial f., the opening that pierces the zygomatic bone near the orbital border through which the zygomaticofacial nerve passes.

zygomaticotemporal f., the opening that pierces the lateral surface of the zygomatic bone through which the zygomaticotemporal nerve passes.

Forbes-Albright syndrome (forbz al′brīt) a syndrome unassociated with pregnancy that is characterized by excessive lactation and the absence of the menstrual cycle. The etiology is unknown, but the disorder is possibly due to a chromophobic pituitary tumor. Urinalysis shows low levels of gonadotropins, and radiographs may reveal enlargement of the sella turcica. Cf. *Chiari-Frommel syndrome.*

Forbes' disease a hereditary disease, transmitted as an autosomal recessive trait, in which there is a deficiency of amylo-1,6-glucosidase, the debranching enzyme. Glycogen cannot be degraded beyond branch points and is stored abnormally, thus affecting the heart, liver, kidneys, and skeletal muscles. Hepatomegaly, hypoglycemia, acidosis, and stunted growth may also occur. Also called Cori's disease, glycogenosis storage disease III, and *limit dextrinosis.* See also *glycogenoses.*

force (F) (fōrs) [L. *fortis* strong] the influence, such as gravity, that causes an object to accelerate; usually measured in unit of newtons. It is equivalent to pressure times area or energy gradient.

forced expiratory flow (FEF) the maximal instantaneous volumetric airflow rate achieved at a stated lung volume, expressed as a percentage of the vital capacity (VC), during the performance of a forced expiratory vital capacity maneuver. For example, FEF_{25} is the forced expiratory flow after 25 percent of the VC has been expelled and 75 percent of the VC is still in the lungs, FEF_{50} is the forced expiratory flow at 50 percent of the VC, and FEF_{75} is the maximal flow generated when 75 percent of the VC has been exhaled and 25 percent remains within the lungs. Forced expiratory flow can also be expressed as the mean flow over a specified interval of volume (percentage of VC), such as FEF_{25-75}.

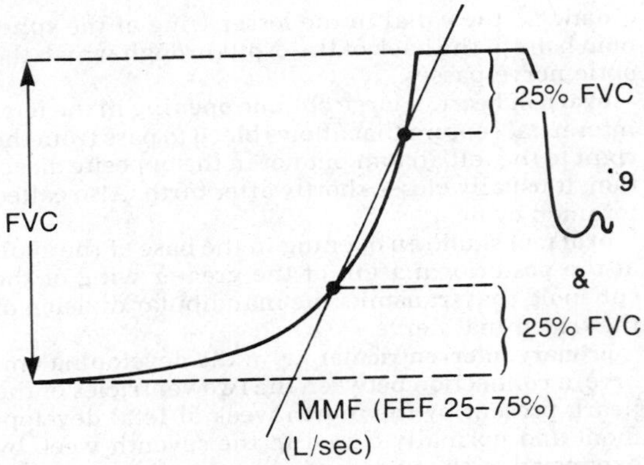

Forced expiratory flow. Flow rate, 25% FVC. (Adapted from Halsted, J. A., and Halsted, C. H.: The Laboratory in Clinical Medicine. 2nd ed. Philadelphia, W. B. Saunders Co., 1981.)

See also *maximal expiratory f.-v. c.* under *flow-volume curve* and the accompanying illustration.

forced expiratory volume (FEV) a test of pulmonary mechanical function based on the measurement with a spirometer of the volume of a single, maximally fast expiration, starting from an inspiration to the total lung capacity. The volume forcibly exhaled in the first second after the start of the expiration (the FEV–1 sec) is an important and frequently used measure of lung function, reflecting both a volume capacity of the lungs and the speed with which air can be exhaled. The FEV–1 can be expressed in either of two ways: (1) as a percentage of the expected FEV–1 for a normal individual of the same age, height, and sex; or (2) as a percentage of the individual's *own* total FEV (vital capacity). The latter is expressed as FEV–1/FVC × 100 and is usually greater than 75 percent. If this percentage falls below the predicted normal value, the presence of some obstructive disease is indicated.

forced vital capacity (FVC) the total volume of gas (expressed in liters or milliliters) that can be rapidly and forcefully exhaled following a maximal inspiration. It is equal to the vital capacity in normal subjects without airway obstruction.

forceps (for'seps) [L.] 1. an instrument having two jaws and handles resembling pliers or tongs. It is used in surgical operations for compressing or grasping tissues and for handling sterile dressings; in the chemistry laboratory, it is used for grasping objects too hot to handle.

2. an anatomic structure shaped like a forceps, e.g., the terminal fibers of the corpus callosum.

Fordyce's disease (for'dīs-es) [John Addison *Fordyce,* New York dermatologist, 1858–1925] the presence of normal sebaceous glands inside the oral cavity: a common condition. The painless, yellow pinpoint elevations that result may vary in number and are of no pathologic significance. Also called Fordyce's granules.

forearm (fōr'arm) the part of the upper limb of the body between the elbow and wrist.

forefinger the index finger.

foregut a portion of the yolk sac included within the embryo as a result of headfold formation. The foregut gives rise to the pharynx, lungs, esophagus, stomach, liver, and part of the duodenum and pancreas.

forehead the part of the face above the eyes.

foreign body any object from outside the body that becomes lodged in a tissue or body cavity and cannot be readily absorbed or removed by physiologic processes.

foreign body localization the determination of the exact site of a foreign body by radiography or radioscopy. This procedure consists of two groups of methods: right-angle and parallax.

The right-angle methods use two exactly perpendicular projections, usually anteroposterior (or posteroanterior) and lateral. The position of the foreign body in the frontal plane is determined from the first projection, and the position in the medial plane from the second. Points directly anterior (or posterior) and lateral to the foreign body are marked on the patient's skin. When the foreign body is to be surgically removed, the patient is adjusted to the position for surgery and not moved while the biplane projections are made. Oblique views may also be taken (usually under radioscopic control) to demonstrate whether the foreign body is lodged in or separated from particular tissues.

The parallax methods use only a single projection and calculate the depth of the foreign body from the amount that its image shifts as the tube is moved. A radiopaque marker is placed against the patient's skin in the transverse plane containing the foreign body, and is adjusted up or down until both the marker and the foreign body show the same amount of motion as the radioscopic tube and fluorescent screen (or image intensifier) are moved back and forth. This is the radioscopic method of choice when it is contraindicated to turn the patient for right-angle views.

In the single-film triangulation technique, a double exposure (using half the exposure time for each exposure) is made with a measured tube shift between exposures. The foreign body–film distance is then calculated as the focal-film distance multiplied by the image-shift distance divided by the sum of the image-shift and tube-shift distances. This is subtracted from the skin-film distance to give the exact depth of the foreign body beneath the skin.

In the fixed-angle technique, which is more precise than the parallax method, the beam is collimated to thin fan by a narrow slit. The tube is moved so that first one edge of the beam and then the other intersect the foreign body; the positions are marked on the radioscopic screen, which remains stationary. The distance between the foreign body and the screen is proportional to the image-shift distance, and the proportionality constant is determined from the image shift of a test object. For localization of foreign bodies in the eye, see *Pfeiffer-Comberg method* and *Sweet method.*

forensic (fo-ren'zik) [L. *forēnsis* relating to the market place] pertaining to or applied in legal proceedings.

forensic medicine the application of medical knowledge and biomedical science to questions of law, such as those concerning the causes of death, definition of death, results of injuries, effects of violent crimes, effects of toxic agents, and implications of biologic materials found as evidence in a criminal investigation.

foreskin (fōr'skin) the prepuce of the penis.

forespore (fōr′spōr) the precursor of an endospore in a bacterial cell, seen as a slightly refractive area at one end of the cell.

formaldehyde (fōr-mal′dĕ-hīd) a colorless, flammable gas with a choking, suffocating odor, HCHO; M.W. 30.03. It is very soluble in water and polymerizes readily. Formaldehyde is highly toxic; concentrations above 2 ppm are irritating to the eyes and respiratory tract, producing tearing, coughing, and burning sensations. It is also a potent skin sensitizer. Also called *methanal.* See also *formalin.*

formaldehyde-induced fluorescence method a technique for demonstrating biogenic amines in tissue sections and touch preparations. Slides are desiccated, incubated at 80°C over paraformaldehyde powder, mounted in a low fluorescent medium, and examined by fluorescent microscopy. Biogenic amines show a green-yellow fluorescence.

Control slides incubated at 80°C without exposure to the formaldehyde vapor show any autofluorescent background.

formalin a solution of formaldehyde gas, HCHO, in water, used as a disinfectant and in histology as a tissue fixative. A saturated solution contains about 400 g/1 and is often called full-strength or 100 percent formalin; 10 percent formalin contains about 40 g/1. Commercial formalin usually contains 15 percent methanol to reduce paraformaldehyde formation. Formaldehyde gas is very irritating to mucous membranes. On storage, HCHO in the formalin oxidizes to formic acid. See also *fixative.*

alcoholic f., see under *fixative.*

f. ammonium bromide (FAB), see under *fixative.*

buffered neutral f., see under *fixative.*

formalin-ether sedimentation method a technique that concentrates protozoan cysts, helminths, larvae, and the eggs of most intestinal parasites for detection and identification. It is also used for the detection in stools of fatty substances that can interfere with the zinc sulfate centrifugal flotation technique. This method is not recommended for detection of trophozoites. Recently, ethyl acetate has been recommended as a substitute for ether, being less flammable and less hazardous as a lipid solvent.

formalin pigment in histology, a dark-brown granular pigment formed by the action of acidic (pH below 5.6) formalin fixatives on hemoglobin. It is birefringent and iron negative. The pigment can be removed from tissue sections by treatment with 1 percent solutions of ammonia water in 70 percent ethanol (Kardasewitsch's method), ammonia water in a 1:1 mixture of acetone and 3 percent hydrogen peroxide (Lillie's method), or saturated alcoholic picric acid. No pigment is formed when buffered neutral formalin fixation is used. Also called *acid formaldehyde hematin.*

format (for′mat) 1. a part of a computer program that specifies the form and arrangement of input or output data.

2. the form of input or output data.

forme (fōrm), pl. *formes* [Fr.] form or appearance, as in the description of a disease.

f. fruste, (pl. *formes frustes*), an atypical form of a disease or disorder. The term is most often used to describe mild or incomplete expression of the symptoms or pathology of a given disease. Dominantly inherited disorders frequently present as formes frustes because of the variable expressivity of the gene.

f. tardive, a description applied to a disease occurring at a stage in life that is later than expected. It is often used to describe childhood or adolescent diseases that first appear in adulthood.

formic acid the simplest carboxylic acid, HCOOH, methanoic acid.

formiminoglutamic acid (FIGLU) an intermediate compound in the catabolism of histidine. FIGLU is converted to glutamate by the enzyme FIGLU transferase, which utilizes a folate coenzyme in the reaction: *N*-formiminoglutamate + tetrahydrofolate (FH_4) → N^5-formimino FH_4 + glutamate. A deficiency of folic acid can therefore lead to an accumulation of FIGLU, which eventually is excreted in the urine. In a suspected folate-deficient individual, the presence of abnormal quantities of FIGLU after oral administration of histidine confirms the folate deficiency.

Although more sensitive radioisotopic assays using folate binders for the measurement of plasma folate are available, a FIGLU test is useful in elucidating the uncommon forms of megaloblastic anemia that are due to defects in the interconversion of various folate coenzyme forms. Under these conditions, a positive FIGLU test is found despite high levels of plasma folate levels. It should be noted that individuals with vitamin B_{12} deficiency may exhibit a similar pattern, because vitamin B_{12} is required in the formation of the initial folate coenzyme, FH_4, required in the intermediary metabolism of purines, pyrimidines, and amino acids. This possibility can be eliminated, however, by measuring serum B_{12}. See also *folic acid, folic acid assays.*

formula (fōr′mu-lah), pl. *formulas, formulae* [L., dim. of *forma* form] 1. a specific statement of a procedure to be followed for obtaining a desired result, such as the procedure for preparing a medicine.

2. a representation of a chemical entity that uses chemical symbols to represent the atoms, subscripts to show the number of atoms of an element, and other devices to show the bonding or spatial arrangement. Formulas can be divided into five types: (1) the empirical formula or constitutional formula, which indicates the relative number of atoms of each element, e.g., CH_2O, a carbohydrate, and CH, ethyne or benzene; (2) the molecular formula, which indicates the number of atoms of each element present in an entity, e.g., $C_6H_{12}O_6$—a hexose, C_2H_2—ethyne, C_6H_6—benzene, CH_3—a methyl group, or NH_4^+ ammonium ion; (3) the structural formula, which indicates how the atoms are bonded together—usually by using one, two, or three lines to indicate a single, double, or triple bond (see *ethyne* and *benzene* in the accompanying illustration)— occasionally, only atoms other than carbon and hydrogen and the bonds between carbon atoms are shown and a circle inside the hexagonal structure is sometimes used to show an aromatic ring (see *benzene* and *adenine* in the accompanying illustration); (4) the generic formula, which indicates the composition of a class of compounds by using variable subscripts or the letter R to represent any hydrocarbon group, e.g., C_nH_{n+2}—a saturated hydrocarbon, R—O—R′—an ether, or RNH_2—an amine; and (5) the spatial formula, which shows the positions of the atoms in space, e.g., the Fischer or Haworth formulas for sugars (see under *isomerism*).

formulary (fōr′mu-lār″e) a collection of formulas for drug preparations. See also *National Formulary.*

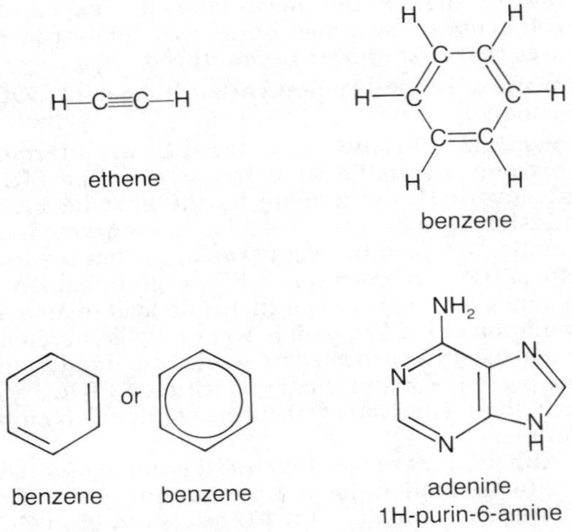

Formula. (From Banks, J. E.: Naming Organic Compounds. 2nd ed. Philadelphia, W. B. Saunders Co., 1976.)

formyl- (for′mil, for′mēl) a prefix word element used in organic chemistry to denote the formyl group (—CHO), e.g., 4-formylbenzoic acid ($HOOCC_6H_4CHO$).

***N*₅-formyl FH₄** see *folinic acid.*

***N*-formyl methionine** (fōr′mil mĕ-thi′o-nin) [L. *formic* + Gr. *hylē* matter] an amino acid derivative; used to begin the synthesis of polypeptide chains in prokaryotic cells and in the mitochondria and chloroplasts of eukaryotic cells. See also *protein synthesis* and *translation.*

fornix (for′niks), pl. *fornices* [L. "arch"] [NA], a general term for an archlike structure or the vaultlike space created by such a structure.

f. of cerebrum, an arched fiber tract that lies below the corpus callosum. Its two lateral halves unite in the median plane, forming the body of the fornix, and separate in front as the anterior columns and behind as the posterior columns. Most of the fibers of the fornix convey olfactory impressions.

conjunctival f., the cul-de-sacs that are formed by reflection of the conjunctiva from the upper and lower lids onto the eyeball. The superior conjunctival fornix receives the openings of the ducts of the lacrimal gland.

f. of vagina, the arched recess between the uterine cervix and vagina.

FORTRAN [acronym from *for*mula *tran*slation] a very widely used high-level computer language similar to mathematical notation and to the BASIC language. FORTRAN compilers are available for all computers except the smaller microcomputers. Scientific and mathematical programs usually compile and run faster if they are written in FORTRAN rather than in other high-level languages.

forward bias a voltage across a diode or *p-n* junction that causes conduction. The *p*-terminal is positive with respect to the *n*-terminal. Cf. *reverse bias.*

fosfomycin an antibiotic of no clinical value but important in bacteriologic research because of its role in the study of the permeability of the outer membranes of bacteria. It is an analog of *p*-enolpyruvate in muramate synthesis. Also called phosphoromycin. See also *antibacterial agents.*

fossa (fos′sah), pl. *fossae* [L.] [NA], a general term for a hollow or depressed area.

cranial f., a hollowed-out area in the floor of the cranial cavity. There are three cranial fossae: anterior, middle, and posterior. The frontal lobes rest on the anterior cranial fossa; the temporal lobes and pituitary occupy the middle cranial fossa; and the cerebellum, pons, and medulla lie in the posterior cranial fossa.

cubital f., see *antecubital space.*

ischiorectal f., a wedge-shaped space deep to the skin of the perineum. It lies lateral to the levator ani muscle, contains a pad of fat, and is traversed by smaller vessels and nerves.

oval f. of heart, a shallow, oval depression on the lower part of the septum in the right atrium.

pterygoid f., a cuneiform interval that separates the lateral and medial pterygoid plates of the pterygoid process of the sphenoid bone.

pyriform f., a small recess on each side of the laryngeal orifice that separates the aryepiglottic fold from the thyroid cartilage and thyrohyoid membrane.

temporal f., the anatomic region between the zygomatic arch and temporal fascia laterally and the skull medially.

founder effect the result of a small number of individuals leaving one large population to form a community. If among these individuals' genotypes there is a rare recessive allele, the frequency of the allele will be higher in the community than in the parent population, and the effect of genetic drift will be greater. See also *evolution.*

fourchette (foor-shet′) [Fr. "a fork-shaped object"] a fold of skin in virginal females that joins the posterior ends of the labia minora behind the vaginal orifice.

Fourier analysis (foo′ryā) [Baron Jean Baptiste Joseph *Fourier,* French mathematician and physicist, 1768–1830] the process of representing a waveform or mathematical function as a superposition (sum) of the average (direct-current) level and sine and cosine waves of various frequencies. This is the mathematical equivalent to the representation of a complex sound as a combination of pure tones, as is done by the ear.

A periodic waveform with frequency f can be represented by a Fourier series, which contains sine and cosine waves only at the fundamental frequency and higher harmonics (at frequencies nf, where n is a whole number). Any function can be represented by a Fourier transform, which contains sine and cosine waves of all frequencies. It is a complex-valued function of frequency; the real part gives the amplitude of the cosine component as a function of frequency, and the imaginary part gives the sine component.

A periodic function that is sampled at N points evenly spaced in each period is represented by its finite Fourier transform, which contains components only at the N frequencies $0, f, 2f, \ldots, (N-1)f$, because the higher harmonics are equal to one of these components at the sampled data points.

Fourier analysis is used in electronics to describe the effects of linear devices, such as filters and amplifiers, that attenuate or boost each frequency component by a fixed gain that does not depend on the other frequency components present. The finite Fourier transform is also used in computed tomography. Also called harmonic analysis and spectrum analysis.

four locus one of the two major human histocompatibility loci located close together on the same chromosome, of significance in transplantation immunology. Also called HLA-2 or B locus.

fourteen- and six-Hz positive burst in electroencephalography, a burst of waves at about 14 and/or 6 Hz seen usually in the posterior temporal area during sleep and most commonly occurring in children and young adults. The sharp components of the waves generally are electrically positive relative to other regions. They are best demonstrated using a unipolar montage over the posterior temporal region of the skull and an earlobe reference electrode. The clinical significance of this pattern is controversial.

fovea (fo′ve-ah), pl. *foveae* [L.] [NA], a general term for a small pit in the surface of a structure or organ.

central f. of retina, a small depression at the center of the macula of the retina. See also *macula lutea of retina.*

foveate (fo′ve-āt) [L. *foveatus*] pitted.

foveola (fo-ve′o-lah), pl. *foveolae* [L., dim. of *fovea*] [NA], an extremely small pit or depression.

Fowler's solution (fow′lerz) [Thomas *Fowler,* English physician, 1736–1801] see *potassium arsenite solution.*

F pilus see *F p.* under *pilus.*

FPN reagent a water solution of perchloric acid, nitric acid, and ferric chloride, which is used as a color reagent. It reacts with phenothiazines to form a product that is blue, purple, or red in color.

Fr symbol for the chemical element *francium, franklin.*

fraction (frak′shun) in chemistry, one of the separable constituents of a mixture.

fractionation (frak″shun-a′shun) 1. in radiation therapy, the administration of the total dose in parts timed at intervals.

2. in chemistry, the separation of a mixture or solution of two or more solutes into its component substances, as by distillation, crystallization, or chromatography.

fracture (frak′chur) [L. *fractura,* from *frangere* to break] the breaking of a part (especially a bone) that leads to changes in shape, function, and continuity. Most fractures are due to applied stress and trauma, although disease processes may predispose to fracture. Fractures are classified into many types, including complete or incomplete (greenstick); closed, with intact overlying tissue, or open (compound); and comminuted, with bone splintering. There are also congenital fractures, which can occur to the fetus in utero. The speed of healing and the perfection of repair depend on the extent of the fracture and its location, and the age and general health of the individual.

fragility (frah-jil′ĭ-te) the susceptibility or lack of resistance to factors capable of causing disruption, injury, or breakage.

capillary f., the susceptibility of capillaries to breakage and extravasation of red cells under conditions of increased stress. Increased fragility may be found in platelet disorders, infectious diseases, renal failure, scurvy, and diabetes. See also *tourniquet test.*

erythrocyte f., the susceptibility of erythrocytes to hemolysis when exposed to increasingly hypotonic saline solutions (osmotic fragility) or when subjected to mechanical trauma (mechanical fragility).

mechanical f., see under *erythrocyte f.*

osmotic f., see under *erythrocyte f.*

fragillograph (frah-jĭl′ō-grăf″) [L. *fragilitas* fragility + Gr. *graphein* to write or record] an instrument for the automated measurement of red cell fragility, consisting of a cuvet, the sides of which consist of a dialyzing membrane. Red cells diluted in a solution of sodium chloride are placed in the cuvet, which is surrounded by distilled water. As the salt concentration in the cuvet decreases, the degree of lysis of the red cells is recorded as a fragility curve. The first derivative of the curve is also recorded.

fragment (frag′ment) one of the small pieces into which a larger entity has been broken.

fragmentation (frag″men-ta′shun) 1. a division into fragments.

2. a form of reproduction seen in organisms such as flatworms in which the body of the parent may break into several pieces, each piece then developing into a whole organism.

fragment D a fibrin degradation product of fragments X and Y; M.W. approximately 90,000. See also *fibrin (fibrinogen) degradation products.*

fragment E a degradation product of fragment Y, the smallest of the fibrin degradation products; M.W. 30,000–50,000. See also *fibrin (fibrinogen) degradation products.*

fragment X the first and largest fibrin degradation product; M.W. approximately 280,000. See also *fibrin (fibrinogen) degradation products.*

fragment Y one of the fibrin degradation products of fragment X; M.W. approximately 155,000. See also *fibrin (fibrinogen) degradation products.*

frame (frām) a structure, usually rigid, designed for giving support or for immobilizing a part.

frame shift mutation a loss or gain of a base pair in DNA, which causes all the codons to be misread from that point forward.

Francisella (fran-sĭ-sel′ah) [Edward *Francis,* American bacteriologist] a genus of very small, aerobic, nonmotile, gram-negative coccobacilli, found in water and in many animals.

F.* (*Pasteurella*) *tularensis, the causative organism of human tularemia, usually transmitted by direct contact with the tissues of infected rabbits but also from the bites of flies or ticks. The organism is extremely virulent. It can be identified by specific fluorescent antibody stains of smears, or by a slide-agglutination test with specific antiserum. See also *tularemia.*

Francis skin test a test for the presence of antibody bound to pneumococci, in which pneumococcal polysaccharide capsular material is injected into the skin. A positive test results in an immediate hypersensitivity wheal-and-flare reaction.

francium (Fr) (fran′se-um) [from *France*] a radioactive element; atomic number 87; most stable isotope, Fr-223 (half-life, 21.8 min); Group I of the periodic table (the alkali metals); oxidation state +1. It is the most electropositive element.

franklin (Fr) (frangk′lin) [Benjamin *Franklin,*

American statesman and scientist, 1706–1790] the unit of electric charge in the electrostatic centimeter-gram-second (cgs) system of units, equal to 3.335635×10^{-10} coulomb (C). Also called *electrostatic unit* and statcoulomb.

Franklin's disease a rare form of proliferative plasma cell dysfunction marked by the overproduction of Fc fragments of gamma heavy chains. There are lymphadenopathy, hepatomegaly, and splenomegaly, and a strong suggestion of a predisposition to lymphoma, with a pleomorphic infiltrate including lymphocytes and plasma cells; skeletal involvement is uncommon.

Most patients with Franklin's disease have hypoalbuminemia with a normal total serum protein level. Immunoelectrophoresis of serum and urine reveals a precipitin arc with anti-IgG and anti-Fc serum. No light chains are found in the urine. Also called gamma heavy-chain disease.

Frank-Starling mechanism see *Starling's law of the heart.*

FRC abbrev. See *functional residual capacity.*

freckle (frek″l) a brownish, pigmented spot on the skin. Freckles are due to the discrete accumulation of melanin as a result of sunlight acting on clusters of melanocytes that have higher than normal tyrosinase activity. Also called ephelis.

free electron an electron not bound to an atom, which therefore is accelerated exactly in proportion to the applied electric and magnetic fields. See also *conduction electron.*

free energy either of two thermodynamic quantities: the Helmholtz free energy ($A = E - TS$) or the Gibbs free energy ($G = H - TS = E + PV - TS$), where E is internal energy, T is absolute temperature, S is entropy, P is pressure, H is enthalpy, and V is volume. The change in free energy, ΔG, is a measure of the tendency of a reaction at constant pressure to proceed spontaneously; ΔA is used for reactions at constant volume. In chemistry, an unspecified free energy is G.

free fatty acids (FFA) fatty acids that are not covalently linked in ester or amide linkage to other molecules. They are found chiefly in blood plasma in low concentrations but may also occur in very small quantities in some tissues. In plasma, they are noncovalently bound to proteins, chiefly to albumin. Also called *nonesterified fatty acids* (NEFA) and *unesterified fatty acids* (UFA).

free radical an atom or molecule that has one or more unpaired electrons and thus may be very reactive (though some free radicals are stable).

free thyroxine index (FT_4 index) see under *triiodothyronine resin uptake test.*

freeze-clamp a device for instantaneously stopping metabolic reactions in a perfused organ of a small animal. It consists of a pair of tongs with metallic blocks that serve as jaws; they are chilled in liquid nitrogen and then closed over the organ to freeze it. The instantaneous freezing allows measurement of small quantities of metabolites.

freeze-cleave method see *freeze-fracture-etch method.*

freeze-drying 1. in histology, a method of tissue preparation in which small tissue specimens are quick frozen (quenched) at about –150°C. Water is sublimed from the frozen tissue in a high vacuum, after which paraffin or Carbowax is infiltrated into the tissue. Chemical changes to the tissue are minimized because there is no exposure to fixing, dehydrating, or clearing agents. Because this method is expensive and time-consuming, it is used primarily as a research technique.

2. in biochemistry, a freezing and dehydration procedure used to preserve proteins, enzymes, cell fractions, blood, etc., for study or for the preparation of commercial products. It prevents the heat denaturation of proteins. In bacteriology, the procedure is used for preserving viruses and bacteria. Also called *lyophilization.*

freeze-etch method see *freeze-fracture-etch method.*

freeze-fracture-etch method a technique for preparing electron microscope specimens. After optimal glutaraldehyde fixation, the tissue is rinsed, infiltrated with glycerol, and quick frozen at –160°C. The frozen block is split in two (fractured), and the cellular structures are exposed by subliming away the water under high vacuum. A replica is made of the fracture face, prepared by depositing a layer of platinum, which is studied using the transmission electron microscope. This method is used particularly to demonstrate cell membranes and surfaces. Also called *freeze-cleave method* and *freeze-etch method.*

freeze-substitution in histology, a method of tissue preparation in which specimens are quick frozen (quenched) at about –150°C. The tissue is then fixed in alcohol or acetone fixatives at a temperature of –20°C or below. This is followed by routine processing. An alternate freeze-substitution method uses frozen section cutting of the quenched tissue. The sections are dehydrated in acetone at –70°C, then mounted on slides and stained.

freezing point the temperature, at a specified pressure, at which the solid and liquid phases of a substance are in equilibrium. The term is used when referring to the liquid phase; when referring to the solid, the term melting point is used.

freezing point depression osmometer an instrument that measures the number of solute particles per liter of water by the freezing point depression method. Also called *cryoscope.* See *osmometer.*

Frei test (frī) [Wilhelm *Frei,* dermatologist, 1885–1943] an intracutaneous skin test for the diagnosis of lymphogranuloma venereum, a sexually transmitted disease. Originally, the test was performed using heated pus from a human lymphogranulomatous lymph node; the antigen now used is a partially purified suspension of *Chlamydiae* grown in yolk sac. A test is indicative of a delayed hypersensitivity reaction to *Chlamydiae* antigen when a red indurated papule greater than 6 mm in diameter appears within 48 hr. An individual will be skin-test positive 2–3 wk after infection and will remain so for life. See also *lymphogranuloma venereum.*

frenulum (fren′-u-lum), pl. *frenula* [L., dim. of *fraenum* a small bridle] [NA], a general term for a small fold of integument or mucous membrane that checks, curbs, or limits the movements of an organ or part.

f. of clitoris, the joining, below the clitoris, of the two medial folds of the labium minus.

lingual f., the small vertical band of mucous membrane that attaches the tongue to the floor of the mouth.

Freon trademark for a group of compounds. See *fluorocarbon.*

frequency (f, ν) (fre′kwen-se) 1. the number of occurrences or cycles per unit time, usually measured in units of hertz (Hz) and also cycles per second (cps).

2. the fraction of a population that has some particular characteristic, e.g., gene frequency.

angular f. (ω), the frequency multiplied by 2π: $\omega = 2\pi f$.

frequency distribution see *density function.*

frequency polygon a graph of grouped statistical data obtained by plotting a point above the midpoint of each class interval at a height equal to the class frequency and connecting adjacent points with straight lines. Cf. *histogram.*

Fresnel fringe an overfocus halo used in the correction of astigmatism in the transmission electron microscope.

Fresnel zone plate a type of coded aperture used in coded aperture imaging; it is a series of concentric open rings that allows entry of gamma rays to the gamma camera, alternating with rings of lead shielding in a "bull's-eye" pattern.

Freund's complete adjuvant a water-and-oil suspension of killed tubercle or (*Mycobacterium butyricum*) bacilli, usually added to an antigen in the aqueous phase for the purpose of increasing the immune response to that antigen. Freund's incomplete ajuvant lacks the mycobacteria.

Freund's incomplete adjuvant a water-and-oil suspension, usually added to an antigen in the aqueous phase for the purpose of increasing the immune response to that antigen.

friable (fri′ah-bl) [L. *friabilis* breakable into small pieces] easily crumbled or broken into small pieces, such as bacterial or fungal colonies on damaged heart valves, which then detach and spread microbes throughout the body.

friction (frik′shun) [L. *frictio*] the rubbing of one surface against another surface or of a fluid flowing past a solid surface. The force produced by the rubbing of two flat surfaces is proportional to the force pressing the surfaces together. The proportionality constant depends on the nature of the surfaces and is termed the coefficient of friction.

Friedländer's bacillus (frēd′len-derz) [Carl *Friedländer,* German pathologist, 1847–1887] see *K. pneumoniae* under *Klebsiella.*

Friedländer's pneumonia [Carl *Friedländer*] see *Klebsiella p.* under *pneumonia.*

Friedreich's ataxia (frēd′riks ah-tak′se-ah) [Nikolaus *Friedreich,* Heidelberg physician, 1825–1882] see *Friedreich's a.* under *ataxia.*

frons (fronz) [L. "the front, forepart"] [NA], the forehead.

frontal (frun′tal) [L. *frontalis*] 1. pertaining to the forehead.

2. pertaining to a radiographic projection in which the frontal plane is perpendicular to the central ray, i.e., either an anteroposterior or posteroanterior projection. See also *Corbin technique.*

frontal bone the shell-like unpaired cranial bone in the front of the skull above the orbits and nasal cavity.

frontal lobe the anterior portion of a cerebral hemisphere. Bordered posteriorly by the central sulcus, the frontal lobe comprises the precentral, superior frontal, middle frontal, and inferior frontal gyri.

frontal plane see *coronal plane.*

frontal sharp transients see *encoches frontales.*

front-end processor a minicomputer that functions as a data concentrator. It accepts data from low-speed peripheral units (such as teletypes and CRT terminals), performs routine processing of the data (such as translating from one character code to another), and passes the data to a large mainframe computer that runs the user programs.

frostbite (frost′bit) damage and injury to tissues from exposure to freezing cold temperatures. The effects may be local (usually affecting the extremities) or systemic. Cell injury may be direct, due to high intracellular salt concentrations that occur during the formation and melting of ice crystals, or it may be indirect, due to the ischemia that results from impairment of the microcirculation. Severe frostbite can lead to cell death, necrosis, and gangrene of the involved tissue. See also *hypothermia.*

frozen red blood cells red blood cells suspended in glycerol and frozen at –65°C or below. Red cells prepared in this manner may be stored for 3 yr, thus permitting the stockpiling of rare blood types or cells for autologous transfusion. Before use, the cells are thawed in a warm-water bath and deglycerolized. After thawing, the cells must be used within 24 hr.

frozen section method a histologic technique in which tissue specimens are frozen and cut into sections with a cryostat or freezing microtome. The sections then are immediately mounted on a slide and stained. Because sections can be prepared in just a few minutes, this method is routinely used for the rapid diagnosis of biopsy specimens. Toluidine blue, polychrome methylene blue, or hematoxylin and eosin (H and E) staining is routinely used. (The H and E stain requires a short fixation in formalin or acetone.) The frozen section technique is also used for the demonstration of enzymes and of fats, which are dissolved by solvents used in other methods and for fluorescent microscopy.

fructofuranose (fruk″to-fur′rah-nōs) fructose in its hemiketal furanose ring form. In solution, the furanose form is in equilibrium with the pyranose and the open chain forms. See also *furanose.*

β-D-fructofuranosidase (fruk″to-fu-ra′no-sĭ-dās) an enzyme of the hydrolase class (β-D-fructofuranoside fructohydrolase, EC 3.2.1.26) that catalyzes the reaction sucrose = glucose + fructose. It also catalyzes the hydrolysis of the terminal β-D-fructofuranoside residues in β-D-fructofuranosides. The enzyme occurs in the brush border of the intestinal mucosa and is important for sucrose utilization. A congenital deficiency of the enzyme, transmitted as an autosomal recessive trait, results in various degrees of sucrose intolerance called disaccharidase deficiency. Also called fructosidase, invertase.

fructokinase (fruk″to-ki′nās) an enzyme of the transferase class (ATP:D-fructose-6-phosphotransferase, EC 2.7.1.4) that catalyzes the reaction ATP + D-fructose ⇄ ADP + D-fructose 6-phosphate. This enzyme is not to be confused with ketohexokinase, EC 2.7.1.3 (ATP:D-fructose 1-phosphotransferase), which was formerly called fructokinase. It is this latter enzyme that is deficient in a genetic disorder called essential fructosuria, a benign asymptomatic condition characterized by fructose in the urine.

fructopyranose (fruk″to-pi′rah-nōs) fructose in its hemiketal pyranose ring form. In solution, the pyranose form is in equilibrium with the furanose and the open chain forms. See also *pyranose.*

fructose (fruk′tōs) [L. *fructus* fruit] a 2-ketohexose isomer of glucose. The naturally occurring isomer, D-fructose, is found in honey and sweet fruits and as a component of the disaccharide, D-sucrose (table sugar). Fructose is the main carbohydrate fuel in semen and is also important for fetal nourishment in many mammals. Inulin, occurring in artichokes, is a polyfructosan. Metabolism involves phosphorylation to fructose-1-phosphate, followed by aldolase splitting to glyceraldehyde and dihydroxyacetone-phosphate. These products then enter either the glycolytic or biosynthetic pathways. Genetic defects in fructose metabolism cause essential fructosuria, fructose intolerance, and fructose-induced hypoglycemia. The D-fructose is also called *levulose.* See also *glucose.*

fructose assay Seliwanoff's test. Fructose yields a positive red color with the Seliwanoff reagent. Hot hydrochloric acid converts fructose to hydroxymethylfurfural, which links with resorcinol to produce a red-colored compound. Fructose does not react with glucose oxidase tests (Clinistix) and can be identified by paper chromatography.

fructose-1,6-bisphosphate (fruk′tōs bis-fos′fāt) see *fructose diphosphate.*

fructose-bisphosphate aldolase (fruk′tos bis′-fos-fāt al′do-lās) an enzyme of the lyase class (D-fructose-1,6-bisphosphate D-glyceraldehyde-3-phosphate-lyase, EC 4.1.2.13) that catalyzes the hydrolysis of the reaction D-fructose 1,6-bisphosphate ⇄ dihydroxyacetone phosphate + D-glyceraldehyde 3-phosphate. Also called *aldolase.*

fructose diphosphate (fruk′tos di′fos-fāt) a key intermediate in cellular glycolysis. Its formation is the committed step of the glycolytic sequence. Also called *fructose-1,6-bisphosphate.*

fructose intolerance (fruk′tōs in-tol′er-ans) [L. *fructus* fruit + *in* not + *tolerare* to bear] a rare hereditary disorder of metabolism, transmitted as an autosomal recessive trait, that involves deficient activity of the hepatic enzyme fructose-1-phosphate aldolase, and is manifest in infants soon after the introduction of fructose into the diet. It is characterized by hypoglycemia and its clinical manifestations, which are also associated with various other symptoms, including fructosuria, fructosemia, anorexia, vomiting, failure to thrive, jaundice, hepatomegaly, and an aversion to fructose-containing foods. Aminoaciduria and albuminuria also occur. If the condition is left untreated, death may occur. See also *essential f.* under *fructosuria.*

fructosemia (fruk″to-se′me-ah) the presence of fructose in the blood; seen in fructose intolerance. Also called *levulosemia.* See also *fructose intolerance.*

fructose 6-phosphate the Neuberg ester; it can enter the glycolytic, glycogen synthesis, pentose phosphate, and glucuronic acid synthesis pathways.

fructose test colorimetric tests for the presence of fructose in urine. Fructose yields an orange-red color with the Seliwanoff reagent. In this test, hot hydrochloric acid converts fructose to hydroxymethylfurfural, which reacts with resorcinol to produce a red-colored compound. Fructose gives a negative reaction in glucose oxidase tests (e.g., Clinistix), but it reacts weakly with *o*-toluidine. Fructose can be separated and positively identified by use of paper or thin-layer chromatography procedures, employing appropriate staining agents.

fructosuria (fruk″to-su′re-ah) [*fructose* + Gr. *ouron* urine + *-ia*] the presence of fructose in the urine; seen in essential fructosuria, in fructose intolerance, and occasionally after the ingestion of large amounts of fructose.

essential f., a benign, asymptomatic hereditary disorder of carbohydrate metabolism caused by a deficiency in the activity of the hepatic enzyme ketohexokinase. It is transmitted as an autosomal recessive trait; the only manifestations are occasional fructosemia and fructosuria. See also *fructokinase* and *fructose intolerance.*

fructosyl (fruk′to-sil) a radical derived from or relating to fructose.

FSF abbrev. for fibrin-stabilizing factor. See *Factor XIII.*

FSH abbrev. See *follicle-stimulating hormone.*

FSH-RH abbrev. for follicle-stimulating hormone–releasing hormone. See *gonadotropin hormone–releasing hormone.*

FT_3 abbrev. for free triiodothyronine. See under *triiodothyronine assays.*

FT_3 index abbrev. for free triiodothyronine index. See under *triiodothyronine assays.*

FT_4 abbrev. for free (unbound) thyroxine. See *free t.* under *thyroxine.*

FT_4 index abbrev. for free thyroxine index. See under *thyroxine assays* and *triiodothyronine resin uptake test.*

FTA-ABS test see *fluorescent treponemal antibody absorption test.*

FTI abbrev. for free thyroxine index. See under *thyroxine assays* and *triiodothyronine resin uptake test.*

FTT abbrev. for failure to thrive.

FU abbrev. See *fluorouracil.*

fuchsin (fook′sin) [from the pink, red, or purple flower *fuchsia,* after Leonard *Fuchs,* German botanist, 1501–1566] any of several triphenylmethane dyes that are red to purple in color.

acid f., an acid dye, a trisulfonic acid derivative of rosaniline; C.I. 42685.

basic f., a mixture of the triphenylmethane dyes rosaniline (C.I. 42510), pararosaniline (C.I. 42500), and magenta II.

carbol f., an alcoholic solution of basic fuchsin and phenol used in staining acid-fast bacteria.

new f., a basic dye, trimethylpararosaniline; C.I. 42520.

L-fucose (fu′kōs) a deoxymonosaccharide, 6-deoxy-L-galactose; L-fucose is unusual in that it is formed metabolically from a D-hexose in which carbon-6 is a methyl group. It occurs in a number of mucopolysaccharides and mucoproteins, including the blood group polysaccharides.

α-L-fucosidase (fu-ko′sĭ-dās″) an enzyme of the hydrolase class (α-L-fucoside fucohydrolase, EC 3.2.1.51) that catalyzes the reaction α-L-fucoside + H_2O ⇄ an alcohol + L-fucose. The enzyme is important in mucopolysaccharide lipid metabolism. A genetic deficiency of the enzyme, transmitted as an autosomal recessive trait, results in the accumulation of fucose-containing sphingolipids, oligosaccharides, and polysaccharides in cells (fucosidosis).

fucosidosis (fu″ko-sĭ-do′sis) a lysosomal storage disorder, transmitted as an autosomal recessive trait, characterized by a deficient enzymatic activity of fucosidase, resulting in the accumulation of fucose in the cells. The disease is classified as one of the mucolipidoses and manifests itself with progressive cerebral degeneration, muscle weakness, an enlarged heart, thick skin, and profuse sweating. See also *mucolipidosis.*

fugacity (fu-gas′ĭ-te) a thermodynamic quantity used to indicate the extent to which a real gas deviates from ideal gas behavior. For ideal gases (real gases at very low pressures), fugacity, f, equals pressure, P. The ratio, f/P, is the activity coefficient.

Fujiwara reaction the reaction of pyridine with halogenated hydrocarbons under alkaline conditions to form a red complex. See also *halogenated hydrocarbon assays.*

full scale pertaining to the maximal value that can be indicated by the readout (e.g., meter or digital readout) of a measuring device set to a particular range.

full-width half-maximum (FWHM) a measure of resolution; the width of a peak on a graph at half the maximal height. The term is used to describe energy resolution or the spatial resolution of a gamma detector.

fumagillin (fu″mah-jil′in) an antibiotic produced by *Aspergillus fumigatus.* Although ineffective against bacteria or fungi, fumagillin is a potent amebicide and is useful in the treatment of amebic dysentery. See also *antibacterial agents.*

fumarase (fu′mah-rās) see *fumarate hydratase.*

fumarate hydratase (fu′ma-rāt hi′drah-tās) an enzyme of the lyase class (L-malate hydro-lyase, EC 4.2.1.2) that catalyzes the reaction L-malate ⇄ fumarate + H_2O. It is one of the reactions in the citric acid cycle of cellular fuel combustion. Also called *fumarase.*

fumaric acid (fu″mar′ik) an unsaturated dibasic acid, HOOC·CH:CH·COOH, *trans*-2-butenedioic acid (maleic acid is the *cis*-isomer); an intermediate compound of the tricarboxylic acid cycle.

fume hood see *laboratory hood.*

fumigation (fu″mĭ-ga′shun) [L. *fumus* smoke, vapor] the exposure of an area or object to a gas or vapor, usually to disinfect or purify it.

function (funk′shun) [L. *functio* a performance] 1. the special, normal, or proper action of any part or organ.

2. in mathematics, a rule or relation that assigns to each member of some set exactly one member of another set. The set on which the function is defined is called the domain; the set of values of the function is called the range. The value of a function, f, assigned to the element, x, is usually denoted $f(x)$.

3. a computer subprogram in a high-level language, such as FORTRAN or BASIC, that evaluates a mathematical function and is called by using the function name in an expression.

functional (funk′shun-al) 1. of or pertaining to a function.

2. usable, workable.

3. affecting the functions of an entity but not the structure; the term is used in medicine to denote disturbances of function that have no apparent organic cause.

functional group the group of atoms in an organic compound that gives it its characteristic chemical properties and determines its name, e.g., the hydroxy group of an alcohol, the carbonyl (oxo) group of an aldehyde or ketone, the carboxyl group of a carboxylic acid, or the amino group of an amine. See also the accompanying table.

functional residual capacity (FRC) the volume of gas that remains in the lungs at the resting end-tidal respiratory position, when the inspiratory muscles and lungs are in a relaxed state. It is the sum of the expiratory reserve and the residual volumes and is equal to 1800–2400 ml in the normal young adult. Without this residual air remaining in the alveoli between each breath, the alveoli would be unstable and would tend to collapse, and the gas exchange would fluctuate markedly with each respiratory cycle.

fundal (fun′dal) pertaining to a fundus, especially to the bulge upward and to the left of the cardia in the stomach.

fundus (fun′dus), pl. *fundi* [L.] [NA], the bottom or base of an organ or the part farthest from the mouth of a hollow organ.

fungal (fung′gal) pertaining to or caused by a fungus.

fungicidal (fun″jĭ-si′dal) [*fungus* + L. *caedare* to kill] destroying fungus.

fungicide (fun′ji-sīd) see *antifungal agent.*

fungiform (fun′jĭ-form) shaped like a fungus or mushroom.

Fungi Imperfecti (fun′ji im″per-fek′ti) [L., pl.] one of the four classes of true fungi characterized by the lack of demonstration of a sexual stage. Fungi Imperfecti are classified by their asexual spores (thallospores and conidia), and some are pathogenic. Also called *Deuteromycetes.*

fungi staining techniques to demonstrate the capsules, mycelia, and spores of fungi; many methods are available for staining. Gram stain, Giemsa stain, and some acid-fast stains all demonstrate the presence of fungi in tissues. Chromic acid–Schiff methods are commonly used for fungi, the chromic acid helping to reduce background staining. See also *Gridley stain.*

Fungizone trademark. See *amphotericin B.*

fungus (fung′gus), pl. *fungi* [L.] a general term for a type of organism that is eukaryotic and thallus-forming and requires an external carbon source, as they lack both chlorophyll and chemolithotrophic machinery. Fungi may exist as saprophytes or parasites, invading nonliving organic substances of living organisms (e.g., humans). The reproduction of fungi involves spores, which may be produced sexually or asexually. The single cell form of fungi is known as a yeast, whereas the multinuclear filamentous form is a mold. Fungi are classified according to their sexual structures (if present). Most fungi known as pathogenic to humans belong to the subphylum Deuteromycotina, the Fungi Imperfecti. Each fungus contains a nucleus with a nuclear membrane, endoplasmic reticulum, Golgi apparatus, and mitochondria, and thus is considered eu-

NAME	STRUCTURAL FORMULA	CONDENSED FORMULA	NATURE OF R, X*
Acetal	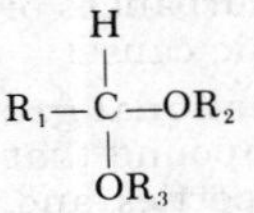		$R_1 = B$; $R_2, R_3 = A$
Acyl halide	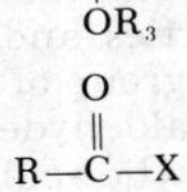	RCOX	R = B; X = halogen
Acyl peroxide	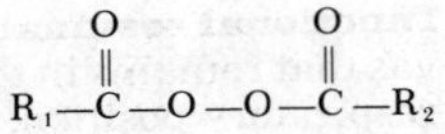	$(RCO_2)_2$	$R_1, R_2 = B$
Alcohol	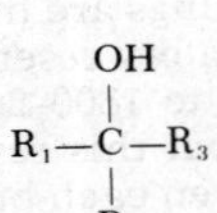	ROH	$R_1, R_2, R_3 = B$
Aldehyde	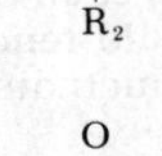	RCHO	R = B
Alkene	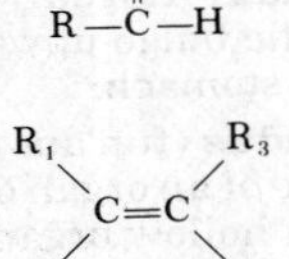		R = B
Alkyl peroxide	$R_1—O—O—R_2$	ROOR	$R_1, R_2 = A$
Alkyne	$R_1—C{\equiv}C—R_2$		$R_1, R_2 = B$
Amide	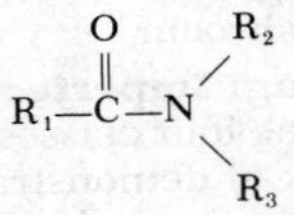	$RCONR_2$	$R_1, R_2, R_3 = B$
Amine	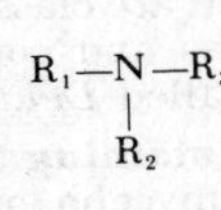	R_3N	$R_1, R_2, R_3 = B$
Azide	R—N=N≡N	RN_3	R = A
Carboxylic acid	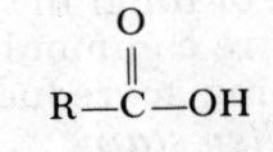	RCO_2H	R=B
Carboxylic acid anhydride	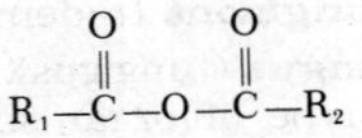	$(RCO)_2O$	$R_1, R_2, R_3 = B$
Cyanide	See *Nitrile*		
Disulfide	$R_1—S—S—R_2$	RSSR	$R_1, R_2 = A$
Enol	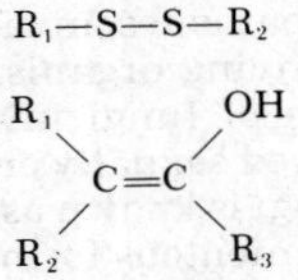		$R_1, R_2, R_3 = B$
Ester	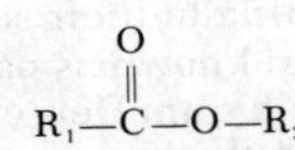	RCO_2R	$R_1 = B$; $R_2 = A$

NAME	STRUCTURAL FORMULA	CONDENSED FORMULA	NATURE OF R, X*
Ether	R_1—O—R_2	ROR or R_2O	$R_1, R_2 = A$
Hemiacetal	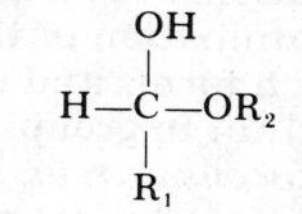		$R_1 = B; R_2 = A$
Hemiketal	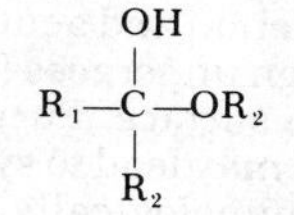		$R_1, R_2, R_3 = A$
Hydroperoxide	R—O—O—H	RO_2H	R = A
Imine	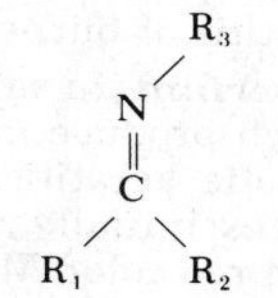	$R_2C = NR$	$R_1, R_2, R_3 = B$
Isocyanate	R—N=C=O	RNCO	R = A
Ketal	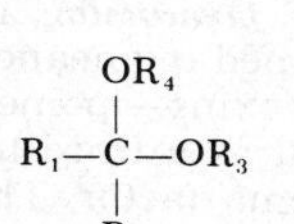	$R_2C(OR)_2$	$R_1, R_2, R_3, R_4 = A$
Ketone	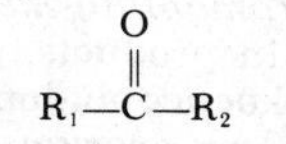	R_2CO	$R_1, R_2 = A$
Lactone	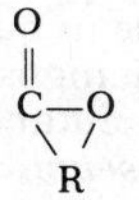		R = A, cyclic ester
Mercaptan	see *Thiol*		
Nitrile	R—C≡N	RCN	R = A
Peracid	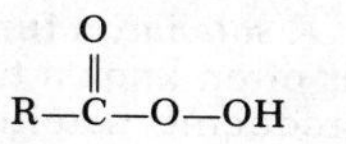	RCO_3H	R = B
Perester	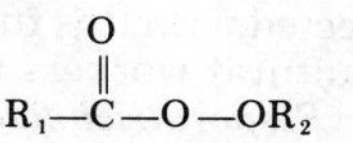	RCO_3R	$R_1 = B; R_2 = A$
Phenol	ArOH		Ar = aryl
Sulfide	R_1—S—R_2	R_2S or RSR	$R_1, R_2 = A$
Sulfonic acid	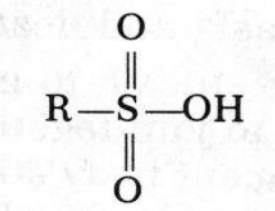	RSO_3H	R = A
Thioester	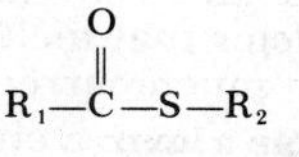	RCOSR	$R_1 = B; R_2 = A$
Thiol	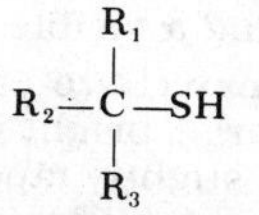	RSH	$R_1, R_2, R_3 = B$

* A stands for alkyl or aryl; B stands for alkyl or aryl or hydrogen.
Courtesy of Norbert W. Tietz, Ph.D.

karyotic. The rigid cell wall is composed of polysaccharides, protein lipids, and sterols. The main structural features of fungal cell wall polysaccharides include chitin (chains of *N*-acetyl-D-glucosamine linked by β-1-4 glycosidic bonds) and glucans (polymers of glucose in either α- or β-glycosidic bonding).

funnel (fun′el) a vessel used for filtering or to aid in pouring into a narrow-mouthed container, often a conic hollow structure with a narrow opening at the apex. Among those commonly used in chemistry and pharmacy are: the ordinary filtering funnel, made of glass or plastic and used with a filter paper; and the Büchner funnel, made of porcelain or glass, which has a perforated plate sealed into the funnel and is used for suction filtration.

funnel chest a congenital defect characterized by a reduced distance between the xiphoid and the vertebrae, with posterior displacement of the body of the sternum, and deformity of the costal cartilages. When the condition is marked, there is interference with cardiac or respiratory function. Symptoms of limited cardiopulmonary function are compounded by cosmetic and psychologic problems. Corrective cosmetic surgery is often indicated. Also called *pectus excavatum.*

FUO abbrev. for fever of unknown origin.

furan (fu′ran, fu-ran′) a heterocyclic compound, CH:CH·CH:CH, formed from wood tar. It is a colorless liquid that is insoluble in water and soluble in alcohol and in ether.

furanose (fu′rah-nōs) a sugar in which the hemiacetal or hemiketal ring contains five atoms; ribose and fructose in their cyclic forms are furanoses. The name derives from the relationship to furan, C_4H_4O, which has a five-membered ring composed of four carbon atoms and an oxygen atom. Cf. *pyranose.*

furanoside (fu-ran′nōs-īd) a glycoside of a furanose sugar.

furazolidone (fu″rah-zol′ĭ-dōn) a synthetic antibiotic used as an oral antibacterial and antiprotozoan drug in the treatment of bacterial enteritis and giardial intestinal infections. See also *antibacterial agents* and *nitrofuran.*

furc/o (fur′ko) a word element used in combining form to denote forking or branching, e.g., bifurcate.

furcal (fur′kal) [L. *furca* fork] forked; shaped like a fork.

furcate (fur′kāt) [L. *furca* fork] forked; branched like a fork.

furfural (fur′fu-ral) an aromatic compound, CH:CH·CH:C·CHO, formed from the distillation of
└——O——┘
such materials as bran or sawdust. It is formed as a dehydration product of pentoses, and condenses with various phenols to form colored products that are the basis of a number of color tests for sugars. It causes convulsions in animals.

furfural reagent a solution of furfural in ethanol (100 ml/l), used as a color reagent. It reacts with meprobamate and other carbamates to form a purple-black color.

furosemide (fu-ro′sĕ-mīd) [USP], a potent diuretic that acts primarily by blocking the reabsorption of sodium in not only the proximal and distal tubules but also the loop of Henle in the kidney. It is used to treat hypertension, pulmonary edema, edema due to congestive heart failure, cirrhosis of the liver, and kidney disease. Adverse effects are due to rapid or excessive diuresis and include low blood volume and electrolyte imbalance, particularly potassium depletion. Trademark, *Lasix.*

furuncle (fu′rung-k′l) [L. *furunculus* boil] a focal inflammation of the skin and subcutaneous tissue, which forms and exudes pus. Furuncles may occur singly or in groups and are usually caused by *Staphylococcus aureus.* Bacteria enter through a hair follicle, penetrate, and form an area of local tissue destruction and acute inflammation. The center of the lesion undergoes liquefaction and drains toward the skin surface. Furuncles cause pain and discomfort and may lead to systemic infections in debilitated or immunologically compromised hosts. See also *folliculitis.*

fusariomycosis a fungal infection with organisms of the genus *Fusarium,* which may cause mycotic keratitis of burned skin.

Fusarium (fu-sa′re-um) a genus of fungi, some of which produce mycotoxins and/or are involved in mycotic keratitis. *Fusarium* is a rapidly growing fungus; initially white and fluffy, with time it develops a red color. Microscopically, short branched hyphae with conidiophores and fusoid multiseptate macroconidia are seen.

F. javanicum, a fungus that produces mycotoxins termed ipomeanols. This fungus produces two hepatotoxins—ipomeamarone and ipomeamaronal, as well as a third toxin, 4-ipomeand, known as lung edema factor. The effect of these toxins is severe pulmonary interstitial edema.

F. moniliforme, a fungus that, when growing on grain products, produces a mycotoxin that causes leukoencephalomalacia in animals.

F. oxysporum, a fungus that may cause mycotic keratitis in burn patients. The fungal mycelia have been demonstrated in the crusts and debris of burned cutaneous tissue.

F. roseum, a fungus that produces a mycotoxin when growing on grain used for flour. When ingested, this toxin produces a syndrome known as "drunken bread eater." The fungus is also isolated from burned skin.

F. solanae, a fungus that produces mycotic keratitis often known to infect the cornea of the eye and producing satellite lesions. Most individuals infected with this fungus have been identified as agricultural workers from southern Florida.

F. sporotrichoides, a fungus that produces the mycotoxin fusariogenin when grown in grain under certain conditions. If this toxin is ingested, alimentary aleukia results, characterized by necrotic rashes on the skin, leukopenia, vertigo, and gangrenous lesions; eventually the condition can produce aphasia and death.

fuse (fuz) 1. to melt.

2. to join together, as the abnormal coherence of adjacent body structures.

3. an electrical circuit element containing a conductor that melts and breaks the connection when too much current is drawn.

fuse alarm a circuit that indicates a blown fuse by giving a visible or audible signal.

fuseau (fĕ-zo′), pl. *fuseaux* [Fr.] a fungal spore that is large, bright in color, multiseptate, thick-walled, and slightly tapered; a spindle-shaped fungal spore like a fusoid macronconidium of dermatophytes.

fusiform (fu′zĭ-form) [L. *fusus* spindle + *forma*

form] spindle-shaped; in bateriology, applied to a bacillus that is tapered at both ends.

fusion (fu'zhun) [L. *fusio*] 1. melting; the change from the solid to the liquid state.

2. a nuclear reaction combining two nuclei into one and releasing other particles and large amounts of energy, e.g., the reaction occurring in the hydrogen bomb.

3. the operative process of joining individual parts, such as bone or nerve.

-fusion (fu'zhun) a suffix word element to denote pouring, e.g., transfusion.

Fusobacterium (fu"zo-bak-te're-um) [L. *fusus* spindle + Gr. *bakterion* a small rod] a genus of gram-negative, nonsporulating, anaerobic, rod-shaped bacteria; one of the family of Bacteroidaceae. The organisms are found in the cavities of humans and animals; some species are pathogenic, especially *F. necrophorum*, occurring in purulent or gangrenous infections. Two species, *F. nucleatum* and *F. necrophorum*, are frequently found in the mouth and upper respiratory tract in the absence of disease.

F. necrophorum, the species most often associated with one-time frequent membranous tonsillitis (Vincent's angina). It occasionally causes virulent disseminated infection.

F. nucleatum, the type of species of the genus, and one of the gram-negative anaerobic bacilli most commonly recovered from clinical infections of the respiratory tract.

fusospirillosis see *fusopirochetosis.*

fusospirochetosis (fu"zo-spi"ro-ke-to'sis) a condition characterized by ulcerative lesions of the mucous membranes, especially the mouth, often caused by fusospirochetes, in combination with other bacteria.

When the lesions are oral, they appear as painful superficial or deep ulcers rimmed by edema and inflammatory cells. The gingival margins and gums are involved. In susceptible hosts, fusospirochetes may also attack genital areas, the lungs, and the pharynx and tonsillar areas.

Also called *fusospirillosis, trench mouth,* and Vincent's angina.

fuzz see *glycocalyx.*

fuzzy coat see *glycocalyx.*

FVC abbrev. See *forced vital capacity.*

F wave a compound muscle action potential with a longer latency and smaller amplitude than the direct motor response (M wave), evoked by supramaximal stimulation of a motor nerve. The amplitude and latency are more variable than the M wave of the same muscle, and the latency increases as the stimulation site is moved farther away from the spinal cord.

The F wave, which occurs in all motor neurons, is thought to involve the recurrent discharge of alpha motor neurons that are activated antidromically by peripheral nerve stimulation; the impulses return from the spinal cord via orthodromic conduction along the same neurons and initiate the muscle action potential.

F waves can be of particular clinical value in the evaluation of the proximal conduction velocity of a peripheral nerve (e.g., Guillain-Barré syndrome or radiculopathy).

Cf. *H wave.*

FWHM abbrev. See *full-width half-maximum.*

FZ abbrev. See *focal zone.*

G

G symbol for *conductance, gauss,* Gibbs free energy, *giga-, glycine, guanosine.*

G1 abbrev. for Grid 1. See *input terminal 1.*

G2 abbrev. for Grid 2. See *input terminal 2.*

g symbol for *gram,* the standard acceleration due to gravity, 9.80665 m/s^2.

Γ the Greek capital letter *gamma.*

γ the Greek lower case letter *gamma;* symbol for: (1) photon; (2) the heavy chain of IgG; (3) in an aliphatic compound, the carbon separated from the carboxyl group by two other carbon atoms; (4) one of the hemoglobin monomers in fetal hemoglobin; (5) microgram (obsolete symbol).

γ- the designator for a constituent of the gamma–plasma protein fraction, e.g., γ-globulin.

Ga symbol for the chemical element *gallium.*

GABA abbrev. See *γ-aminobutyric acid.*

gadfly (gad'fli) see *Tabanus.*

gadolinium (GD) (gad"o-lin'e-um) [from the mineral *gadolinite*] a lustrous, silvery-white metallic element; atomic number 64; atomic weight 157.25; a 4f transition element (a lanthanide or rare earth element); oxidation state +3. See also *rare earth elements.*

Gaffkya (gaf'ke-ah) [George Theodor August *Gaffky,* German bacteriologist, 1850–1918] a genus name, no longer recognized, for anaerobic, gram-positive cocci. These organisms are now classified as peptococci.

gain (gān) an increase in amount or value; the increase in the size of a signal produced by an amplifier, usually the ratio of output to input.

galact/o (gah-lak'to) [Gr. *gala, galaktos* milk] a word used in combining form to denote relationship to milk, e.g., galactocele, galactosemia.

galactan (gah-lak'tan) a polymer of galactose; agar is a well-known example.

galactic (gah-lak'tik) 1. pertaining to milk. 2. promoting the flow of milk.

galactitol (gah-lak'tĭ-tol) a derivative of galactose, in which the carbonyl functional group on C-1 is reduced to an alcohol functional group. In the disease galactosemia, galactitol can accumulate in the lens of the eye and result in the formation of cataracts. See also *galactose.*

galactocele (gah-lak'to-sēl) [*galacto-* + Gr. *kēlē* tumor] the cystic dilation of a mammary duct that occurs some weeks after termination of nursing in a lactating breast. It forms a firm but movable cystic swelling toward the center of the breast that contains inspissated milk. The contents of the cyst should be aspirated to prevent secondary infection.

galactocerebroside (gah-lak"to-ser'ĕ-bro-sīd) a ceramide monosaccharide. It functions usually as structural material and occurs most abundantly in the myelin sheath of nerves. Upon hydrolysis, galactocerebrosides yield one molecule each of sphingosine, fatty acid, and D-galactose. The D-galactose (a hexose) is linked to ceramide in β-glycosidic linkage. See also *cerebroside.*

galactocerebroside β-galactosidase see *galactosylceramidase.*

galactokinase (gah-lak"to-ki'nās) an enzyme of the transferase class (ATP:D-galactose-1-phosphotransferase, EC 2.7.1.6) that catalyzes the reaction ATP + D-galactose ⇄ ADP + α-D-galactose-1-phosphate. D-Galactosamine can also serve as PO_4 acceptor. This is the first reaction in the metabolism of galactose to glucose. Galactokinase deficiency is occasionally encountered, causing galactosuria on ingestion of galactose or lactose. The inborn metabolic disease galactosemia is caused by the absence of another liver enzyme. See also *galactosemia.*

galactolipid (gah-lak"to-lip'id) a lipid that contains galactose as a part of its molecules; examples are the galactosyl cerebrosides, the galactosyl diglycerides, and the sulfatides (cerebroside sulfates). The compounds all occur in myelin. Also called *galactolipin.*

galactolipin (gah-lak"to-lip'in) see *galactolipid.*

galactorrhea (gah-lak"to-re'ah) [*galacto-* + Gr. *rhoia* flow] a general term used to describe the inappropriate, excessive, or persistent flow of milk irrespective of nursing, which is usually due to increased levels of prolactin. Galactorrhea may occur in association with amenorrhea after pregnancy (Chiari-Frommel syndrome) or with a pituitary chromophobe adenoma (Forbes-Albright syndrome). It may also be associated with hypothyroidism, ingestion of phenothiazine drugs, ectopic production of prolactin by a neoplasm, and central nervous system disease.

Diagnostic testing should include CT scan and skull roentgenogram and radiograph to rule out a brain tumor, and thyroid function testing to rule out hypothyroidism. Treatment involves removal of any source of excess prolactin and correction of underlying defects.

See also *Chiari-Frommel syndrome* and *Forbes-Albright syndrome.*

galactosamine (gah-lak"to-sam'in) an amino sugar (2-amino-2-deoxy-α-D-galactose), a hexosamine. Sometimes it occurs as a structural carbohydrate but more often as the *N*-acetyl derivative. It is present in glycoproteins, mucoproteins, and glycosaminoglycans. See also *galactose.*

galactose (gah-lak'tōs) an aldohexose monosaccharide, an optical isomer of glucose that is obtained from lactose (milk sugar) by the action of the enzyme lactase, or by hydrolysis with a mineral acid. It is a white crystalline substance and resembles glucose in most of its properties, although it is less soluble, is less sweet, and forms mucic acid when oxidized with nitric acid. D-Galactose is also found in brain cerebrosides, in raffinose of the sugar beet, and in many gums and seaweeds; L-galactose is contained in flaxseed mucilage. Galactose is metabolized by a series of reactions that cause a net conversion of galactose to glucose-1-phosphate, which then enters degradative or biosynthetic pathways. A hereditary defect in the metabolism of galactose gives rise to the condition of galactosemia. See also *glucose.*

galactose assay the galactose oxidase method, which is analogous to the determination of glucose by glucose oxidase. Galactose in urine can also be determined by thin-layer chromatography.

galactosemia (gah-lak″to-se′me-ah) an inborn error of galactose metabolism most often caused by a deficiency of the enzyme UDPglucose-hexose-1-phosphate uridylyltransferase. A small number of cases are caused by galactokinase deficiency. The resulting accumulation of galactose-1-phosphate and/or galactitol can cause cataracts, liver failure, and mental retardation. The disease can be detected by assay for the enzyme in the red blood cells. Treatment consists of complete avoidance of all foods containing galactose, in either its free or combined forms. See also *UDPglucose-hexose-1-phosphate uridylyltransferase.*

galactose tolerance test a rarely used test of liver function that measures the ability of the liver to convert galactose to glucose. The blood galactose level is measured 1 hr after administration of an oral (40 g) or intravenous (0.5 g/kg) dose of galactose. Because of the great reserve functional capacity of the liver, the test is not very sensitive and is seldom carried out.

β-D-galactosidase (gah-lak″to-si′dās) a nonspecific enzyme of the hydrolase class (β-D-galactoside galactohydrolase, EC 3.2.1.23) that hydrolytically splits off the terminal nonreducing residues in β-D-galactosides and also hydrolyzes lactose to D-galactose and D-glucose. It is present in most cells and is differentiated from a specific galactosidase, called lactase, found in the intestinal brush border. GM_1 gangliosidosis (GM_1 β-galactosidase) and Krabbe's leukodystrophy (galactosylceramide β-galactosidase) arise from an inborn deficiency of different β-D-galactosidases. See also *lactase* and *lipidoses.*

galactoside (gah-lak′to-sīd) a glycoside that contains galactose.

galactosuria (gah-lak″to-su′re-ah) [*galactose* + Gr. *ouron* urine + *-ia*] the presence of galactose in the urine.

galactosylceramidase (gah-lak′to-sēl-ser-am′ĭ-dās) an enzyme of the hydrolase class (EC 3.2.1.46) that catalyzes the reaction D-galactosyl-*N*-acylsphingosine + H_2O ⇄ D-galactose + *N*-acylsphingosine. A genetic deficiency of the enzyme causes the accumulation of galactosylceramides in the brain, resulting in progressive cerebral deterioration, a condition known as Krabbe's leukodystrophy. Also called *cerebroside β-galactosidase, galactosylceramide β-galactosidase,* and *galactosylceramide β-galactosyl-hydrolase.*

galactosylceramide β-galactosyl-hydrolase see *galactosylceramidase.*

galacturia (gal″ak-tu′re-ah) [*galact-* + Gr. *ouron* urine + *-ia*] an obsolete term for the discharge of urine that is milklike in appearance; see also *chyluria.*

gale (gahl) [Fr.] see *scabies.*

galea (ga′le-ah) [L.] [NA], a general term for a helmet or helmetlike structure.

g. aponeurotica, a fibromuscular sheet that covers the upper part of the skull. It extends from the highest nuchal line of the occipital bone forward to the frontal bellies of the occipitofrontal muscle; laterally, it extends over the temporal fascia to the zygomatic arches. The galea aponeurotica adheres to the skin through the superficial fascia. Also called *epicranial aponeurosis.*

Galerina (gal″er-e′nah) a genus of small mushrooms. *G. venerata* produces a toxin that creates symptoms similar to amanitine poisoning. The toxin initially affects the liver by inhibiting enzymes of carbohydrate, fat, and protein metabolism.

gall (gawl) [L. *galla*] see *bile.*

gallbladder (gawl′blad-der) a pear-shaped hollow organ on the undersurface of the liver, approximately 10 cm long and 3 cm at its widest, with a capacity of 50 ml. Its lower end (fundus) lies against the anterior abdominal wall, whereas the narrow upper end (neck) is continuous with the cystic duct. The gallbladder stores bile and, by absorbing water and some inorganic ions, concentrates it. The stimulus for the release of bile from the gallbladder is hormonal, principally the gastrointestinal peptide cholecystokinin. The mucosa of the gallbladder is lined by a single layer of simple columnar epithelium; some mucus glands are present in the lamina propria. There is no muscularis mucosae. In its relaxed state the mucosa forms elongated folds or rugae. Invaginations of the surface epithelium form the so-called Rokitansky-Aschoff sinuses that can extend through the muscularis.

Gall body a lymphocyte vacuole composed partly of lipids; it is best demonstrated by phase microscopy.

gallium (Ga) (gal′e-um) [L. *Gallia* Gaul, France] a silvery-white liquid (m.p., 29.771°C) metallic element; atomic number 31; atomic weight 69.72; Group III of the periodic table; oxidation states 0, +1, +2, +3. Its compounds with Group V elements (phosphorus, antimony, and arsenic) are used as semiconductors. This metal has been proposed as a temperature standard (gallium cell, obtainable from the National Bureau of Standards) in enzyme work, inasmuch as its melting point is very near to 30°C, the recommended temperature for measurement of enzyme activity in clinical laboratories.

gallium-67 (^{67}Ga, Ga 67) a radionuclide with a half-life of 78 hr that decays by electron capture and emits gamma rays at 93, 184, 296, and 388 KeV; it must be produced in a cyclotron. The two most common uses are for localizing tumors and hidden abscesses. When injected in ionic form, as ^{67}Ga-citrate, it is preferentially concentrated in some tumors and by polymorphonuclear leukocytes accumulating in a region of abscess or inflammation. It is not entirely specific for malignancy or abscess. See also *gallium scan.*

gallium citrate Ga 67 the gallium salt used as a radiopharmaceutical.

gallium scan a procedure in nuclear medicine for imaging the whole body or certain areas of interest following injection of gallium citrate Ga 67. It is used for the localization and staging of some neoplasms, particularly Hodgkin's disease and non-Hodgkin's lymphomas, hepatoma, and various adenocarcinomas, and for the localization of occult abscesses.

Activity is also seen in normal bones, liver, mediastinum, nasopharynx, and secreting exocrine glands. Because gallium is excreted by the colon, cleansing enemas are necessary prior to the scan to reduce background activity. Tumor scans are made 48–72 hr after injection, abscess scans after 6–24 hr.

gallocyanin (gal″o-si′ah-nin) a blue oxazin mordant dye; C.I. 51030. Gallocyanin forms blue lakes with chromium ions and blue-black lakes with iron. Chrome alum gallocyanin is used as a stain for Nissl substance.

gallstone (gawl′stōn) a calculus formed in the biliary tract. Most are found in the gallbladder, but occasionally stone formation occurs in a major intra- or extrahepatic bile duct. See also *calculus* and *cholelithiasis.*

galvanic (gal-van′ik) [Luigi *Galvani,* Italian physician and physiologist, 1737–1798] pertaining to galvanism.

galvanic cell an electrochemical cell that produces electric power.

galvanism (gal′vah-nizm) 1. galvanic electricity; unidirectional electric current derived from a chemical battery.

2. the therapeutic use of direct current.

galvanometer (gal″vah-nom′e-ter) an instrument for measuring or indicating electric current by movements of a magnetic needle or a coil in a magnetic field. Some do not measure in specific units and are used only to indicate the presence of current.

gam/o- (gam′o) [Gr. *gamos* marriage] a combining form to denote relationship to marriage or sexual union, e.g., gamogenesis.

Gambian trypanosomiasis (gam′be-an tri-pan″-o-so-mi′ah-sis) see *African t.* under *trypanosomiasis.*

gamet/o (gam′ĕ-to) [Gr. *gametē* wife, *gametēs* husband] a word element used in combining form to denote a gamete, e.g., microgametocyte.

gamete (gam′ēt) [Gr. *gametē* wife, *gametēs* husband] 1. a haploid germ cell, either a spermatozoon or an ovum; loosely, a synonym for gametocyte. See also *fertilization* and *gametogenesis.*

2. in parasitology, the term for the malarial parasite during its sexual development in the intestine of a mosquito. The male (microgamete) and female (macrogamete) form a zygote upon fertilization, which develops into an oocyst.

gametocide (gam′ĕ-to-sīd″) an agent capable of destroying gametes or gametocytes.

gametocyte (gah-mēt′o-sīt) [Gr. *gametē* wife, *gametēs* husband + *kytos* hollow vessel] 1. a cell that produces gametes; an oocyte or spermatocyte.

2. the sexual stage of the malarial parasite, which may produce gametes when taken into the mosquito.

gametogenesis (gam″ĕ-to-jen′ĕ-sis) [*gameto-* + Gr. *genesis* production] the developmental process that forms the mature egg or sperm. It is important for maintaining the continuity of germ plasm between generations as well as for providing the oportunity for genetic recombination (see *meiosis*). Early in embryogenesis, uncommitted cells are "set aside"; these become the primordial germ cells. This occurs in the yolk sac of the embryo, and from there they migrate through the dorsal hindgut to the gonadal ridges. It is at this stage that the development of eggs diverges from the development of sperm.

TESTIS. In the presence of a Y chromosome or male-inducing genes, tubules begin to form in the developing gonad, with the germ cells penetrating deep into the mesenchyme of this developing organ. It is possible that histocompatibility Y (H-Y) antigen is the male inducing substance responsible for this developmental pathway. Although the male gonads grow rapidly at this very early state of embryogenesis (the second month of human development), testicular development then becomes quite slow, with only small changes other than a general increase in number of cells and tubules occurring before puberty. At puberty the germ cells change in appearance and move to the basement membrane of the spermatogenic tubule. Here they are separated by the Sertoli cells (the supporting cells for developing sperm) from the more luminal part of the tubule in which spermatogenesis will occur.

The spermatogonia divide by mitosis, but cytokinesis is incomplete, which leaves the dividing spermatogonia joined by intercellular bridges. The dividing spermatogonia are pushed away from the basement membrane and pass across the blood-testes barrier, the barrier (similar to the blood-brain barrier) formed by the tight junctions joining the Sertoli cells. Mitotic divisions result in a syncytium of up to 64 interconnected early spermatocytes, which then enter prophase of meiosis I.

It is at about this time that the X chromosome of the male is apparently inactivated (see *Lyon hypothesis*). Prophase of meiosis I is an active period of RNA and protein synthesis, and the spermatocyte becomes quite large. After meiosis I is completed, meiosis II rapidly follows and results in early spermatids still interconnected by intracellular bridges. These "indifferent cells" give rise to sperm via a complex developmental pathway. The perinuclear Golgi apparatus gives rise to the acrosomal cap, while at the opposite end of the nucleus the centriole forms the sperm flagellum. Gradually the nucleus is condensed, and the characteristic sperm shape results. Much of this development may occur with new RNA and protein synthesis, which continues after meiosis. The apparent lack of haploid gene expression may be largely due to the passage of proteins and RNA between cells, which the intercellular bridges permit. When the sperm has finally developed its mature shape, it is released into the lumen of the spermatogenic tubule. However, the sperm at this stage is not ready to fertilize an egg, and sperm maturation continues as it is transported through the epididymis and vas deferens.

OVARY. Initially, the ovary does not show a degree of development comparable to that of the testis at the same stage; the germ cells remain at the surface. However, the development of the ovary soon overtakes that of the testes, with the germ cells undergoing many mitoses. The maximal number of germ cells is reached at the fifth month of human pregnancy when mitosis ceases and the germ cells start developing as oocytes. No oocytes are produced after this time, and there is a huge loss of oocytes before birth. These oocytes constitute the lifetime supply for the individual. They enter prophase of meiosis while still in the fetus (in utero). It is probably at about this time that the previously inactivated X chromosome is reactivated. The oocytes reach the diplotene stage of meiosis shortly before birth, and although this is a "resting phase" the oocyte is very active synthetically. Ribosomes are probably stored in preparation for the first divisions of the embryo, and some messenger RNA also is probably stored for early embryogenesis. This resting state of the oocyte is terminated only shortly before ovulation. In the human female, the first oocyte to develop resumes meiosis at puberty, whereas the last to develop may not do so until age 45–50—a 30-yr difference in age between the two. This aging of the meiotic apparatus may be a frequent cause of nondisjunction, which leads to the high incidence of chromosomal aberrations, especially that of Down's syndrome in the offspring of older females.

Oogenesis occurs while the egg is surrounded by granulosa cells, which seem to play a role similar to that played by Sertoli cells in the development of sperm. For instance, the zona pellucida may consist of proteins contributed by granulosa cells as well as by the oocytes. With the elevation of FSH during each reproductive cycle, a "crop" of oocytes is stimulated to develop further to become eggs. However, as this development occurs, most of these degenerate. Finally, when the luteinizing hormone surge occurs, one oocyte reenters meiosis. Prophase of meiosis I is completed and the first polar body extruded, after which the egg rests at metaphase II. Ovulation occurs, and if the egg is fertilized, meiosis resumes with the second polar body being extruded.

It is perhaps worth noting some of the dissimilarities between oogenesis and spermatogenesis. During oogenesis, all the mitoses, which increase the number of eggs, have occurred before birth. If the ovary is exposed to radiation or chemicals that kill oocytes, they will be deficient in number. In contrast, during spermatogenesis mitosis is continued throughout the life of the individual, with continuous regeneration of spermatocytes. In the human female, usually only one egg per cycle is ovulated. This egg contains a very large store of proteins and nucleic acids in preparation for the early development of the embryo. In males, millions of sperms a day are produced, but only one will fertilize an egg, contributing a haploid genome—and probably nothing else—to the embryo. During oogenesis, both X chromosomes are active, whereas during spermatogenesis probably no X chromosome is active. Finally, in oogenesis the meiotic divisions are the final event, being completed only at the end of the differentiation pathway. In contrast, most of the differentiation that constitutes spermatogenesis occurs after meiosis. Thus, there is a possibility of haploid gene expression during spermatogenesis.

gamma (Γ, γ) (gam′ah) the third letter of the *Greek alphabet.*

gamma-aminobutyric acid see *γ-aminobutyric acid.*

gamma camera a device that images gamma radiation; see also *scintillation camera.*

gamma globulin (GG) a class of serum proteins that migrates during electrophoresis to a zone designated as gamma. These molecules are highly positively charged and consequently move toward the cathode (cationic). Most immunoglobulins and antibodies are gamma globulins.

gamma heavy chain disease see under *heavy chain disease.*

gammaphoto an image of the gamma rays emitted by a radioisotope, usually one made by a scintillation camera, which shows the distribution of the isotope in the patient.

gamma ray a photon emitted by a radionuclide, the same as an x-ray except that it is more energetic. The emission process, called isomeric transition, leaves the nuclide with the same mass number and atomic number; it may immediately follow alpha or beta decay. Two 511-KeV-gamma rays result from the annihilation of an electron and a positron following positron beta decay. Gamma rays penetrate the human body with only moderate absorption. In the most common use, a gamma-emitting radioisotope tracer is administered to a patient and localizes in one organ or structure. The radioactivity is measured over a period of time (an uptake test), or an image is made of the distribution of activity with a scintillation camera. Most gamma-ray detectors use NaI(Tl) crystals, which produce luminescent photons when struck by gamma rays, and photomultiplier tubes, which produce an electrical current proportional to this light pulse. Gamma-ray sources must be shielded—usually by lead—to protect personnel from radiation exposure.

gamma-ray spectrum 1. the characteristic energies at which a radionuclide emits gamma rays and the percentages that are emitted at each energy.

2. the response of a physical detector to these gamma rays: the peaks are broadened and additional peaks representing physical processes in the detector are introduced.

gamma spectrometer see *pulse height analyzer.*

gamma spectrometry see under *gamma-well counter.*

gamma streptococcus any species of *Streptococcus* that produces gamma hemolysis. See also *Streptococcus.*

gamma-well counter an instrument for measuring the gamma radiation emitted by a test-tube sample. Test tubes fit into a well in an NaI(Tl) crystal, which rests on a photomultiplier tube. The whole device is surrounded by a lead shield that blocks background radiation. Gamma rays cause the crystal to scintillate, and the photomultiplier tube converts each light pulse to an electrical pulse that has an amplitude (height) proportional to the gamma-ray energy. One or more discriminators (pulse-height analyzers) accept and pass to a counter only those pulses in a certain preset energy range (window). Because gamma rays are emitted at one or more characteristic energies for each radioisotope, radiation from different isotopes can be counted separately; this is sometimes called gamma spectrometry.

gammopathy (gam-op′ah-the) an immunoproliferative disorder that involves cells that usually synthesize and secrete immunoglobulins. The proliferation may be monoclonal, in that only one class of heavy chain or one type of light chain is produced in excess, or polyclonal, when there is a heterogeneous increase in immunoglobulins, which suggests the involvement of multiple cell lines. Examples of the former type include multiple myeloma, macroglobulinemia, and heavy-chain disease. A transition is possible from polyclonal to monoclonal gammopathy.

monoclonal g., a heterogeneous group of immunologic diseases in which a single clone of lymphoid cells produces a monoclonal immunoglobulin that may be detected in serum or urine. Examples of monoclonal gammopathies include multiple myeloma, Waldenström's macroglobulinemia, amyloidosis, heavy-chain disease, and chronic lymphocytic leukemia. The monoclonal immunoglobulin produced in this type of lymphoreticular disorder may also be called paraprotein, M protein, or myeloma protein. Clinically, monoclonal gammopathies result in increased plasma levels and increased total IgG levels due to an increase in IgG synthesis. Immunoelectrophoresis can be used to determine what type of immunoglobulin is produced in these diseases.

polyclonal g., a type of gammopathy resulting in a heterogeneous increase in immunolglobins that involves more than one cell line. Usually, three major classes of immunoglobulins and both types of light chains are involved. Examples of diseases associated with polyclonal gammopathies include Hodgkin's disease, rheumatoid arthritis, lupus erythematosus, cirrhosis of the liver, tuberculosis, leishmaniasis, certain lymphomas, metastatic carcinoma, and lymphoblastic lymphadenopathy.

Gamna-Gandy bodies brown or yellow pigmented nodules seen in certain instances of enlarged spleen. They are organizing foci of hemosiderin deposition in perifollicular locations, and indicate splenic congestion. Also called *siderotic nodules.*

gangli/o (gang'gle, gang'gle-o) [Gr. *ganglion* knot] a word element used in combining form to denote a ganglion, e.g., ganglioneuroma.

ganglion (gang'gle-on), pl. *ganglia, ganglions* [Gr. "knot"] 1. a knot or knotlike mass.

2. [NA], a general term to designate a collection of uni- or multipolar nerve cell bodies located outside the central nervous system.

3. a benign cystic tumor arising by focal mucinous degeneration of a synovium or tendon, as in the wrist.

autonomic g., a cluster of multipolar nerve cell bodies outside the central nervous system, at which autonomic nerves synapse before reaching their destination.

celiac g., the largest autonomic ganglion in the body. It lies on the crus of the diaphragm, embedded in the celiac plexus. The greater and lesser splanchnic nerves end in the celiac ganglion; a large number of branches leave it for the aorta and its branches and the viscera.

ciliary g., a minute ganglion that lies behind the eyeball to the lateral side of the optic nerve. It receives and distributes motor fibers from the oculomotor nerve for the ciliary muscle and sphincter muscle of the pupil, sensory fibers for the interior of the eyeball, and sympathetic fibers for the blood vessels of the eyeball.

g. of Corti, see *spiral g.*

dorsal root g., see *spinal g.*

gasserian g., see *trigeminal g.*

geniculate g., the sensory ganglion of the facial nerve. Peripheral branches of the ganglion cells run in the chorda tympani nerve to the anterior part of the tongue, and in the greater superficial petrosal nerve for the palate.

inferior g. of vagus, a reddish, cylindrical swelling of the vagus nerve distal to its exit through the jugular foramen. The ganglion, which contains only sensory afferent fibers, is made up of unipolar neurons. The ganglion makes contact with the hypoglossal nerve, the superior cervical ganglion of the sympathetic trunk, and a loop between the first and second cervical nerves. Also called the *nodose g.*

nodose g., see *inferior g. of vagus.*

otic g., a minute ganglion on the mandibular division of the trigeminal nerve. It lies on the medial pterygoid branch close to its origin from the main trunk of the mandibular nerve, between it and the tensor palati muscle. It connects with the chorda tympani and nerve of the pterygoid canal, and gives passage to motor fibers for the tensor palati and tensor tympani muscles. The only fibers that relay within the ganglion are parasympathetic secretory fibers received from the glossopharyngeal nerve and distributed by the auriculotemporal nerve to the parotid gland.

pterygopalatine g., a large parasympathetic ganglion situated in the pterygopalatine fossa beneath the maxillary nerve. Preganglionic fibers enter the ganglion from the facial nerve via the petrosal nerve and the nerve of the pterygopalatine canal. Postganglionic fibers leave the ganglion and travel with the maxillary nerve before branching off to the lacrimal, nasal, and palatine glands. Also called *sphenopalatine g.*

semilunar g., see *trigeminal g.*

sphenopalatine g., see *pterygopalatine g.*

spinal g., the ganglion found on the dorsal root of each spinal nerve, composed of the unipolar nerve cell bodies of the sensory neurons of the nerve. Also called *dorsal root g.*

spiral g., a sensory ganglion of the cochlear nerve, situated in the spiral canal of the modiolus, that contains mostly bipolar neurons. Two classes of cells are derived from the ganglion: type I cells, which send large myelinated fibers peripherally to the hair cells in the organ of Corti and centrally as part of the olivocochlear complex; and type II cells, which are small and unmyelinated and appear to direct their fibers only peripherally to the organ of Corti. Also called *g. of Corti.*

trigeminal g., the sensory ganglion of the fifth cranial nerve. It overlies the foramen lacerum and is mostly enclosed in a cave of the dura mater. The ophthalmic, maxillary, and mandibular divisions of the trigeminal nerve arise in the ganglion. Also called *gasserian g.* and *semilunar g.*

ganglion blocker a drug that blocks the transmission of nerve impulses at synapses of the autonomic ganglia. See also *cholinergic receptors.*

ganglioneuroblastoma (gang"gle-o-nu"ro-blas-to'mah) [Gr. *ganglion* knot + *neuron* nerve + *blastos* germ + *-oma* tumor] a tumor composed of a mixture of neuroblastomatous and ganglion cell elements. It evolves through maturation of a neuroblastoma, and histologically consists of ganglion cells in varying stages of development, together with groups of neuroblasts. Ultrastructurally, the maturing cells have longer processes than the neuroblasts, with many microtubules but generally sparse dense-core granules. In some individuals, ganglioneuroblastomas mature to become benign ganglioneuromas, but in others death occurs from metastasizing neuroblastoma. The overall prognosis is distinctly more favorable (roughly a 60 percent 3-yr survival rate) than that for neuroblastoma (less than a 10 percent 3-yr survival rate).

ganglioneuroma (gang"gle-o-nu-ro'mah) [Gr. *ganglion* knot + *neuron* nerve + *-oma* tumor] a benign tumor of elements of the sympathetic nervous system, composed of groups of ganglion cells and bundles of nerve fibers. It may occur in the adrenal gland, retroperitoneum, or posterior mediastinum. It is cured by excision but must always be examined carefully for the presence of neuroblasts (ganglioneuroblastoma). See also *ganglioneuroblastoma* and *neuroblastoma.*

ganglionic (gang″gle-on′ik) pertaining to a ganglion.

ganglioside (gang′gle-o-sīd) a general designation for a class of glycolipids that are relatively abundant in the brain but also are present in other tissues. Structurally, these sphingolipids are ceramide oligosaccharides containing at least one residue of *N*-acetylneuraminic acid (sialic acid) in addition to other sugar residues, i.e., glucose, galactose, and *N*-acetylgalactose.

gangliosidosis (gang″gle-o-si-do′sis), pl. *gangliosidoses* a term used to describe metabolic lipid storage diseases, especially Tay-Sachs disease and generalized gangliosidosis. These diseases are characterized by an accumulation of gangliosides (sphingolipids) in tissues owing to the genetic lack of an enzyme needed for their metabolism. The accumulation of these lipids in cells of the central nervous system leads to mental retardation and other neurologic defects. See also *sphingolipidoses.*

G_{M1} g. see *generalized g.*

G_{M2} g. see *Tay-Sachs disease.*

generalized g., a rare metabolic disease, transmitted as an autosomal recessive trait, that is characterized by the lack of the enzyme G_{M1} ganglioside β-galactosidase. This enzyme deficiency leads to the accumulation of a sphingolipid (ganglioside G_{M1}) in the tissues, particularly those of the nervous system. It occurs early in life usually before age 2 yr., producing mental retardation, enlargement of the liver, skeletal deformities, and cherry-red retinal spots. Diagnositc tests are now available to assay for the disease antenatally. Also called G_{M1} *gangliosidosis.* See also *sphingolipidoses.*

gangosa (gang-go′sah) [Sp. "muffled voice"] an ulcerative lesion that occurs in the later stages of the disease yaws. The ulceration and inflammation are destructive and are particularly common around the nose and mouth. Gangosa may also be seen in leprosy and leishmaniasis. Also called rhinopharyngitis mutilans.

gangrene (gang′grēn) [Gr. *gangraina* an eating sore] the death and subsequent necrosis of body tissues, most often associated with ischemia, that is due to loss of blood supply, infection, and bacterial putrefaction. The extremities are frequently the site of gangrene, although internal organs can also be involved. There is pain, offensive smell, and color change in the affected tissues.

dry g., gangrene that is associated with the slow, chronic deprivation of blood to an affected tissue. Bacterial involvement is not prominent, and the pattern of necrosis is coagulative, resulting in dry, shriveled tissue. It is seen only in the extremities and is most often associated with systemic disease (e.g., diabetes mellitus, arteriosclerosis).

gas g., gangrene that is associated with infection with any of a large group of gram-positive exotoxic anaerobic bacteria, especially *Clostridium.* The spores of infectious agents are introduced into wounds where they start a rapidly spreading, necrotizing inflammation aided by a large variety of toxic enzymes, including fibrolysin, hyaluronidase, lecithinase, and collagenase.

Diagnosis is confirmed by the finding of spores and abundant large, gram-positive rods in smears of exudates and by anaerobic culture. Copious gas production and rapid tissue necrosis are observed. Surgery or use of hyperbaric oxygen therapy may be indicated.

Cf. *myonecrosis* and *clostridial m.* under *myositis.*

moist g., gangrene that is predominantly characterized by liquefaction necrosis. It is associated with an abrupt stoppage of blood flow and local severe edema. Causes include burns, freezing, severe crushing trauma, clots, and physical blockage. This type of gangrene is rapid and is associated with the presence of toxins.

gangrenous (gan′grĕ-nus) pertaining to or of the nature of gangrene.

Ganser's syndrome (gan′serz) [Sigbert Joseph Maria *Ganser,* Dresden psychiatrist, 1853–1931] a syndrome of disturbed consciousness manifested by hallucinations, lapses of memory, and absurd acts and replies to questions. Also called acute hallucinatory mania.

Gantrisin (gan′trĭ-sin) trademark. See *sulfisoxazole.*

gap (gap) an unoccupied interval in time; an opening or hiatus.

GAPD abbrev. See *glyceraldehyde-phosphate dehydrogenase.*

gap junction see *nexus.*

garbage collection in computer programming, the process of finding usable storage space. With some dynamic storage allocation techniques, such as those used with SNOBOL and LISP, memory for new variables (strings or lists) is assigned as needed and marked as free when no longer needed. When the available memory has been used up, a housekeeping routine called a garbage collector makes a list of the free storage areas for allocation to new variables.

garbage in, garbage out (GIGO) an aphorism that succinctly reminds a computer user, who thinks the computer has made a mistake, that almost certainly the problem is a human error by keypuncher, computer operator, or programmer. The computer has correctly processed the data, operator actions, and program (garbage), producing valid output (garbage).

Gardner's syndrome (gard′nerz) [Eldon J. *Gardner*] a condition, transmitted as an autosomal dominant trait, that is characterized by the occurrence of multiple adenomas (with a high rate of malignant degeneration) of the large, and less frequently the small, intestine. The polyps may not be detected until adult life. Various soft tissue abnormalities are associated with the syndrome, including abnormal dentition, skeletal osteomas and exostoses, lipomas, fibromatoses, and cutaneous cysts.

gargoylism (gar′goil-izm) see *Hurler's syndrome.*

gas (gas) 1. a state of matter at a temperature sufficiently high, relative to the energy of bonding between molecules, that molecules are not held together and instead fill the available space. Cf. *liquid, plasma,* and *solid.*

2. any matter in the gaseous state.

3. see *flatulence.*

gas amplification the ratio of the number of ion pairs collected at the electrodes to the number produced by the radiation in an ion-collection radiation detector, such as a proportional counter or a Geiger-Müller counter. The primary ion pairs are accelerated by the electrode voltage, collide with gas molecules, and, if their kinetic energy is above 35 eV, produce secondary ion pairs. The gain can be as high as 10^6.

gas chromatograph (gas kro-mat′o-graf) an instrument for performing gas chromatography.

gas chromatography (GC) (gas kro″mah-tog′-rah-fe) a chromatographic technology used to separate and quantitate mixtures of volatile substances or materials that can be transformed into volatile derivatives. GC is used both for screening procedures and for quantitative assays with a relatively high degree of precision, specificity, and sensitivity.

PRINCIPLES OF OPERATION. A minute sample (1–10 μl) is vaporized and swept along by an inert gas (nitrogen or helium) through a column packed with a suitable sorbent. In gas-liquid chromatography (GLC), the sorbent is a nonvolatile liquid, such as silicone oil or a polyglycol, that is thinly coated on a finely divided inert solid support such as diatomaceous earth. In gas-solid chromatography (GSC), however, the sorbent is a solid (e.g., a porous polymer). As the molecules pass through the column, they transfer many times between the moving phase (the carrier gas) and the stationary phase (the sorbent). The components with a greater affinity for the sorbent stay longer in the stationary phase and have a longer retention in the column; those with weaker affinity move faster along the column and leave the column sooner. At the exit end of the column, the gas mixture is passed through a detector that is sensitive to changes in composition of the gas stream. The detector signal activates a chart recorder to trace a graph (chromatogram), with the specimen components appearing as a series of separate peaks on the graph. The area under the peaks is proportional to the amount of the components producing the peaks.

Although the retention times (on the column) depend on the nature of the sorbent, the carrier gas flow rate, and the column temperature, retention times can be used to identify the sample components under specified operating conditions. This is usually accomplished by a simultaneous assay of standard substances selected according to the nature of the specific kinds or classes of compounds being separated by the column. Retention times of the peaks can be compared with the relative position of the standard and used for qualitative analysis; areas under the peaks are used for quantitation.

ASSAYS. A stationary phase is selected for its ability to separate the compounds of interest into well-resolved peaks. Nonpolar stationary phases separate compounds of similar nature on the basis of boiling point differences, the retention time increasing with boiling point. Highly polar stationary phases separate compounds primarily on the basis of polarity, the retention time increasing with polarity. With moderately polar stationary phases, both mechanisms are operative.

The temperature of operation chosen is a compromise. A higher temperature speeds up the analysis, but may cause chemical decomposition of the sample components or of the liquid sorbent. High temperature may also cause "bleeding" of the liquid phase (evaporation and loss from the column). Temperature programming, a linear increase of the column temperature at a preset rate, permits good resolution of the most volatile components at low column temperatures without producing an excessively long wait for the high boiling components.

Many compounds are not volatile enough or are too unstable to withstand thermal decomposition. In the case of such compounds, suitable derivatives are formed, which are more volatile and/or stable; such derivatives can usually be prepared by silylation, alkylation, or esterification.

In quantitative assays, a known amount of an internal standard is added to the specimen to be analyzed and to the reference solutions of the compounds of interest. The internal standard should be chemically similar to the analytes, e.g., an experimental drug of the same family that has the same recovery efficiency in any steps in the specimen preparation and that produces comparable detector response. The specimen concentration is expressed by the formula: $C_x = C_r \cdot R_x / R_r$, where C_x and C_r are the concentrations in the specimens and reference solution, and R_x and R_r are the ratios of the peak areas of the internal standard and the analyte in chromatograms of the specimen mixture and the reference solution. When the chromatograph recorder is not equipped with an integrator, peak heights may be used in place of peak areas, although this is less accurate.

GAS CHROMATOGRAPH. In the gas chromatograph, the gas supply and flow regulator maintain a constant flow rate through the system despite changes in temperature. The gas flows first through the sample injection system. By use of a microliter syringe, the sample is injected through a self-sealing silicone rubber septum into a heated metal block. The sample vaporizes instantly and is carried into the column. The temperatures of the injection system, column, and detector are independently maintained by three separate heaters and temperature controls. The detector signal is boosted by a high-impedance amplifier, an electrometer, before it is transmitted to the chart recorder.

DETECTORS. The four most widely used types of detector are thermal conductivity, flame ionization, electron capture, and nitrogen-phosphorus flame ionization detectors.

In the thermal conductivity (TC) detector, the column eluent flows past a heated wire, the temperature of which varies in proportion to the amount of substance flowing by in the carrier gas. The temperature determines the resistance of the wire and thus the detector output. The TC detector is not sufficiently sensitive to be used in most clinical applications.

The flame ionization (FI) detector is the most widely used type because it has adequate sensitivity (nanogram quantities) and because of its ability to detect most compounds. The sample eluent is burned in a hydrogen-oxygen flame and the ions produced are collected by a small loop electrode. The amplified current is sent to a recorder for display.

The electron capture (EC) detector is far more sensitive (picogram quantities) than the two types mentioned above but detects only compounds with a strong affinity for electrons. In practice, its use is limited to the detection of compounds containing halogens or those that can form halogen derivatives.

The nitrogen-phosphorus (NP) detector (alkali flame detector) is similar to the flame ionization detector except that ions of an alkali metal (e.g., rubidium) are introduced into the flame. This increases the ionization of compounds containing nitrogen or phosphorus and permits the detection of picogram quantities of organonitrogen and organophosphorus compounds.

GAS CHROMATOGRAPHY–MASS SPECTROMETRY (GC-MS). In this system the conventional detector is replaced by a mass spectrometer, which positively identifies the sample component in each peak by its fragmentation pattern. GC-MS is used in some toxicology laboratories. It is most useful in analyses that must identify a great number of compounds, as in drug screening, pesticide analysis, and forensic toxicology.

Also called *vapor-phase chromatography.* See also *mass spectrometer.* Cf. *high-pressure liquid chromatography.*

gas constant (R) the proportionality constant of the gas law; the energy per degree of temperature of 1 mole of an ideal gas: 0.0821 L·atm/mol·K, or 62.36 L·torr/mol·K, or 8.314 J/mol·K, or 1.987 cal/mol·K.

gaseous (gas′e-us, gash′us)) of the nature of a gas.

gas law stated as: the product of the pressure (P) and the volume (V) of an ideal gas is proportional to the product of the number of moles of the gas (n) and the absolute temperature (T). The proportionality constant (R) is called the gas constant. The formula is $PV = nRT$. The gas law is an approximation that assumes there are no interactions between molecules except elastic collisions. Thus, it is only approximately true for a real gas and is accurate only at temperatures well above the boiling point. Also called *ideal gas law.* Cf. *gas constant.*

gas-liquid chromatography (GLC) see under *gas chromatography.*

gasoline (gas′o-lēn) a mixture of low-molecular-weight hydrocarbons used as motor fuel. It contains primarily 4–12 carbon branched-chain alkanes but also appreciable concentrations of cycloalkanes, alkenes, and aromatic hydrocarbons. Gasoline is highly flammable, with explosive limits in air 1.3–6.0 percent by volume.

Ingestion produces vomiting, vertigo, headache, giddiness, confusion, and stupor. Aspiration produces bronchitis or pneumonia and may cause cardiac arrest or respiratory paralysis. Leaded gasoline contains tetraethyl lead, which can produce lead poisoning.

gasometry (gas-om′e-tre) [*gas* + Gr. *metron* measure] the determination of the amount of gas present in a mixture by releasing the gas from the solution and measuring the volume of gas. This technique was formerly used for measuring respiratory gases.

gasping (gasp′ing) a series of inspiratory efforts that are brief, convulsive, and usually maximal with an abrupt cessation. The individual gasps may occur rhythmically or irregularly.

gas-solid chromatography (GSC) see under *gas chromatography.*

gas sterilizer an instrument that utilizes ethylene oxide gas for sterilization.

gas storage limits limitations on the storage of flammable compressed gases within the laboratory, which should be minimized to reduce delivery traffic and to minimize hazards in case of fire. Standards for laboratories set by the National Fire Protection Association attempt to set realistic and workable limitations on the sizes and quantities of flammable gases stored within a laboratory work area, as well as to provide guidance on alternate locations and piping systems. See also *compressed gas storage.*

gaster (gas′ter) [Gr. *gastēr* stomach] the stomach.

Gasteromycetes (gas″ter-o-mi-se′-tēz) [Gr. *gastēr* + *mykēs* fungus] a type of Basidiomycete with spores developing from cavities within the fruit body. The Gasteromycetes contain bipolar species (multiple alleles at the mating type locus).

Gasterophilus (gas″ter-of′ĭ-lus) [Gr. *gastēr* + *philein* to love] a genus of flies. The larval stage of some species is parasitic in humans; the most common, *G. hemorrhoidalis, G. intestinalis,* and *G. nasalis,* burrow into the skin, causing swelling and itching.

gastr/o (gas′tro) [Gr. *gastēr*] a word element used in combining form to denote the stomach, e.g., gastritis.

gastric (gas′trik) [L. *gastricus*; Gr. *gastēr*] pertaining to, affecting, or originating in the stomach.

gastric artery, left one of the three terminal branches of the celiac artery. It ascends to the esophageal opening in the diaphragm, then courses down the lesser curvature of the stomach to anastomose with the right gastric branch of the hepatic artery.

gastric function tests a group of measurements of the secretion of hydrochloric acid by the stomach. The tests are performed in cases of suspected pernicious anemia, duodenal or stomal ulcer, or Zollinger-Ellison syndrome.

Following a 12-hr fast and 24-hr withholding of medications that influence gastric secretions (antacids, anticholinergics, alcohol, reserpine, adrenergic blockers, adrenocorticosteroids), the patient is intubated through the mouth or nose. After the tip of the tube is adjusted (under fluoroscopic control) so that it lies at the most dependent point of the stomach, the gastric residue is aspirated and subjected to qualitative and quantitative examination (blood, lactic or butyric acid, pH).

In the determination of basal secretion, the patient is at rest and is not exposed to stimuli that influence gastric secretion, particularly the sight or odor of food, or to psychologic stimuli that produce fear, anger, or depression. In the determination of maximal secretion, the patient is given a dose of pentagastrin or betazole (Histalog) sufficient to produce maximal gastric stimulation.

The stomach is continuously aspirated in both tests, and the aspirate is divided into samples collected over successive 15-min intervals. For each 15-min specimen the volume (in milliliters), pH, and titratable acidity (in millimoles per liter) are measured, and the acid output (in millimoles per hour) is calculated as the product of the volume and the acidity divided by the time interval.

The pH is determined using a pH meter. The titratable acidity is the number of millimoles of sodium hydroxide added per liter of stomach content needed to raise the pH to 7.0 (some authorities prefer pH 7.4 as the end point). Another concept commonly used is that of "free acid," the titratable acidity using pH 3.0 or 3.5 as the end point.

The basal acid output (BAO) is defined as the average acid output during four consecutive 15-min intervals. The maximal acid output (MAO) is defined as the average acid output during four consecutive 15-min intervals following administration of the gastric stimulant. The peak acid output (PAO) is defined as the acid output per hour calculated on the basis of the two consecutive 15-min intervals following administration of the gastric stimulant during which the acid output is highest. When betazole is used as the gastric stimulant, the peak output often occurs in the second hour of the test.

Intermediate values of acid output are not pathognomonic; there is a wide overlap of the ranges of normal and abnormal values. Anacidity (pH above 6.0 during basal and maximal secretion) occurs in almost all cases of pernicious anemia and in some cases of advanced gastric carcinoma. Hypersecretion is characteristic of Zollinger-Ellison syndrome. A BAO greater than 60 percent of the MAO or PAO strongly suggests the presence of the disorder; a BAO/MAO ratio greater than 40 percent is also suggestive of the syndrome.

The reference values for BAO and MAO vary with the technique and definition of acidity used. An MAO or PAO of 40 mmol/hr is rarely seen in normal individuals but occurs in about 40 percent of males with gastric ulcers. Acid output of females is about 50–70 percent that of males. The values decline with age.

See also *anacidity* and *insulin hypoglycemia test.*

gastric inhibitory polypeptide (GIP) a gastrointestinal polypeptide hormone, consisting of 43 amino acids; M.W. 5105. It is found in the mucosa of the duodenum and jejunum. Release of GIP is promoted by the presence of glucose or fat in the duodenum. GIP acts to stimulate the release of insulin from the pancreas, and inhibits gastric acid secretion and motility.

gastric lavage (gas′trik lah-vahzh′) see *gastric l.* under *lavage.*

gastric myiasis (gas′trik mi-a′sis) see *gastric m.* under *myiasis.*

gastric parietography (gas′trik pah-ri″e-tog′rahfe) the radiologic examination of the stomach wall after introduction of gas both around (in the peritoneal space) and inside the stomach.

gastric residue examination the examination of gastric residue, the contents of the stomach aspirated following a 12-hr fast. The residue has a volume that is normally 20–100 ml (usually less than 50 ml); is colorless or opalescent; and has a faintly pungent, sour odor. The volume may be increased by delayed emptying (as in pyloric obstruction), which often is also associated with the presence of food particles; by the regurgitation of material from the duodenum, which is also indicated by a green or yellow coloration of the residue and the presence of bilirubin (as confirmed by reagent strip test); or by increased secretion, as in duodenal ulcer or Zollinger-Ellison syndrome.

A small amount of blood may normally be present in the residue from the intubation procedure; a large amount of blood may indicate a gastric lesion such as gastric carcinoma, peptic ulcer, or gastritis, or it may have come from the mouth, nasopharynx, or lungs. In an acid-secreting stomach, blood has a brown, granular, "coffee-grounds" appearance due to the formation of hematin. The presence of blood is confirmed by the *o*-toluidine or guaic reagent strip tests.

See also *gastric function tests.*

gastrin (gas′trin) a polypeptide hormone consisting of 17 amino acids; M.W. 2100. This hormone is produced and stored primarily by the G cells of the antral mucosa, and also by the D cells in the pancreas and intestinal mucosa. The release of gastrin into the blood stream is promoted by vagal stimulation initiated by smell, taste, and chewing; stimulation of local reflexes (in addition to vagal reflexes) caused by distention of the stomach; or by a direct effect due to the presence of substances such as peptides, amino acids, alcohol, and calcium in the stomach.

Gastrin stimulates the parietal cells to secrete HCl, promotes the secretion of pepsinogen, and increases pancreatic HCO_3^- and hepatic bile output. The ability of gastrin to stimulate secretion of HCl by the parietal cells appears to be mediated by histamine. Gastrin also increases gastric and intestinal motility. Along with other gastrointestinal hormones, gastrin directly stimulates insulin secretion. The secretion of gastrin is inhibited by means of a negative feedback process by H^+ released in response to a protein meal. Gastric fluid at pH 1 brings about maximal suppression, and at about pH 2.5, 80 percent suppression.

Two types of gastrin exist, gastrin I and gastrin II; the latter contains sulfated tyrosine in position 12. Only the C-terminal tetrapeptide residue of the gastrin molecule is responsible for all its physiologic action. Based on that knowledge, a number of gastrin analogs (e.g., pentagastrin) have been sythesized.

The determination of gastrin in the serum of fasting patients is important in the evaluation of normal gastric function and also in the case of individuals with Zollinger-Ellison (Z-E) syndrome or in those with pernicious anemia, in whom elevated values of gastrin are observed. Radioimmunoassay is the method of choice for the determination of serum gastrin.

Reference values for serum gastrin are less than 100 pg/ml, whereas in persons with Z-E this value can rise as high as 60,000 pg/ml. Other causes of fasting hypergastrinemia include gastric ulcer diseases, antral G-cell hyperplasia, surgical resection or diseases of the kidneys (gastrin is catabolized in the kidneys), short-bowel syndrome, and pyloric obstruction with gastric distention vagatomy unaccompanied by gastric resection. In some complex cases of hypergastrinemia, the response of serum gastrin to calcium infusion, secretin infusion, or a standard meal may be of value in the diagnosis.

gastrin assay radioimmunoassay for serum gastrin in the fasting patient. A variety of techniques have evolved. With most antibodies used for RIA of gastrin, there is detectable cross-reactivity with cholecystokinin-pancreozymin (CCK-PZ). With antibodies against human gastrin I or crude tissue gastrin, immunologic cross-reactivity with CCK-PZ is minimal and does not significantly interfere with RIA measurement of gastrin. This method replaces old bioassay methods.

gastrinoma (gas″trin-o′mah) see *pancreatic islet neoplasm.*

gastritis (gas-tri′tis) [*gastr-* + *-itis* inflammation] a common inflammation of the lining of the stomach. Gastritis occurs in a number of forms (acute, chronic, toxic) and is caused by a variety of agents (such as harsh foods, infection, and drugs). Severe stress secondary to burns, sepsis, trauma, or surgery may also cause gastritis.

acute g., an acute, usually transient, mucosal inflammation of the stomach lining. The causes are many, including drugs (especially aspirin), excessive alcohol, smoking, uremia, infections, toxins and poisons, shock, stress and irritating agents.

There may be pain, bleeding, distress, nausea, and vomiting. Symptoms may spread to other areas of the intestinal tract. Diagnosis is confirmed by early gastroscopy and biopsy.

chronic g., a long-term inflammation of the lining of the stomach, which often leads to atrophy of the gastric glands and subsequently to hypochlorhydria. Either the fundal or antral area or patchy areas of each may be affected. Fundal gland gastritis is found with high frequency in autoimmune pernicious anemia. Stress, excessive alcohol consumption, hiatal hernia, and ulcers may also be involved in the etiology of chronic gastritis. Diagnosis is commonly confirmed by gastroscopy and biopsy.

giant hypertrophic g., see *Ménétrier's disease.*

phlegmonous g., a rare condition characterized by an acute bacterial infection of the stomach wall. The etiologic agent most frequently is streptococci, although staphylococci, pneumococci, and *Escherichia coli* may be implicated. Affected individuals have a painful abdomen, purulent peritonitis, ascites, nausea, and vomiting. Serum amylase levels are normal. This disease may occur as a complication of systemic infection, ulcer, cancer, chronic alcoholism, or surgical manipulations. Antibiotic treatment should be followed by laparotomy, with drainage or removal of the involved stomach areas. Without surgery, this disease very often is fatal.

gastrocele (gas′tro sēl) [*gastro-* + Gr. *kēlē* hernia] the hernial protrusion of the stomach or of a gastric pouch.

gastrodisciasis (gas″tro-dis-ki′ah-sis) infection with *Gastrodiscoides hominis.*

Gastrodiscoides (gas″tro-dis-koi′dēz) [*gastro-* + Gr. *diskos* disk + *eidos* form] a genus of trematodes that are parasitic in the intestinal tract of humans. Also called *Gastrodiscus.*

G. hominis, a trematode that is pyriform-shaped, reddish-orange in color, and 5–14 mm in length. Its geographic distribution includes India, Vietnam, and the Philippines. *G. hominis* is found in the cecum and colon; the eggs are ovoid and immature when passed, measuring 150 μm long by 65 μm wide. Also called *Gastrodiscus hominis.*

Gastrodiscus (gas″tro-dis′kus) see *Gastrodiscoides.*

G. hominis, see *G. hominis* under *Gastrodiscoides.*

gastroduodenal (gas″tro-du″o-de′nal) pertaining to or communicating with the stomach and duodenum, as in a gastroduodenal fistula.

gastroduodenoscopy (gas″tro-du″o-dĕ-nos″ko-pe) [*gastro-* + *duodenum* + Gr. *skopein* to examine] the endoscopic examination of the stomach and duodenum. In this procedure the gastroscope is either passed through the esophagus or, if performed during surgery, through an incision in the gastric wall.

gastroenteric (gas″tro-en-ter′ik) [*gastro-* + Gr. *enteron* intestine] pertaining to the stomach and intestine.

gastroenteritis (gas″tro-en″tĕ-ri′tis) [*gastro-* + *enteritis*] an acute inflammation of the lining of the stomach and intestines, characterized by anorexia, nausea, diarrhea, vomiting, abdominal pain, and weakness. Gastroenteritis can have many causes, including bacterial infections or toxins from organisms such as *Escherichia coli, Staphylococcus aereus,* and *Salmonella,* as well as viral infections, protozoan infections, consumption of irritating food and drink, allergies, and psychologic factors such as anger, stress, and fear.

Stool examination and culture may prove useful in the diagnosis of bacterial infection; eosinophilia may help in indicating the possibility of parasitic infection. Sigmoidoscopy, food cultures, and agglutination tests all may be useful in determining the etiologic agent.

gastroenterologist (gas″tro-en″ter-ol′o-jist) a physician who specializes in the treatment of disorders of the stomach and intestines. He or she is commonly an expert in the use of endoscopic techniques such as proctoscopy and gastroscopy for diagnosis and treatment.

gastroenterology (gas″tro-en″ter-ol′o-je) [*gastro-* + Gr. *enteron* intestine + *-logy*] the study of diseases of the stomach and intestines, and their diagnosis and treatment.

gastroenteropancreatic (GEP) endocrine system see under *enterochromaffin cells.*

Gastrografin (gas″tro-graf′in) trademark. See under *diatrizoate.*

gastrointestinal (GI) (gas″tro-in-tes′tĭ-nal) [*gastro-* + *intestinal*] pertaining to the stomach and intestine.

gastrointestinal blood loss test a nuclear medicine procedure for determining blood loss into the GI tract. ^{51}Cr-labeled red blood cells are given intravenously. The amount excreted in the stool in 3 da is compared to the average of the blood concentrations on the first and last days. This gives the blood loss, expressed in milliliters per 72 hr.

gastrointestinal motility study a series of films made following a routine GI series, which demonstrate the peristaltic function of the GI tract. The gastric motility showing the emptying of the stomach is demonstrated by serial films after ingestion of the contrast medium. Motility of the large intestine is demonstrated by films taken 24, 48, and 72 hr after ingestion. Mixtures of food and barium are more physiologic tests of intestinal motility.

gastrointestinal protein loss test a nuclear medicine procedure for determining the loss of plasma proteins into the GI tract. A radioisotope-labeled protein is given intravenously. The amount excreted in the stool in 4 da is compared to the amount injected, or the daily excretion is compared to the serum concentration at the start of the collection period. ^{51}Cr-albumin is the most commonly used tracer; ^{131}I-polyvinylpyrrolidone and ^{59}Fe-iron-dextran are also used. The three tracers give similar, but not equivalent, results.

gastrointestinal series (GI series) the radiologic examination of the esophagus, stomach, and duodenum (an upper GI series) and, when indicated, of the small and large intestines; it is used to detect lesions of these organs. Barium sulfate is the routine contrast medium, but water-soluble iodinated media such as diatrizoate are used when barium is contraindicated, as in cases of perforation.

The patient is prepared so that the stomach and colon are empty. A suspension of the contrast medium, the test meal, is ingested, and its progress is followed by fluoroscopy and spot-film radiography of the patient from several angles in both erect and recumbent positions.

For the stomach, the double-contrast technique is also used; the barium coats the mucosa, and negative contrast is provided by the gastric air bubble or by carbonation or gas-emitting powders added to the test meal. Films of the small intestine are usually made after a delay of 1–2 hr; films of the large intestine after a delay of 24–48 hr.

gastrointestinal tract the system of the body concerned with the ingestion and absorption of food. It comprises the alimentary canal and its accessory glands. In the embryo, these accessory glands develop as outpouchings of the primitive digestive tube and remain in contact with the gut by their ducts, through which secretions are passed into the gut lumen. The alimentary canal commences at the mouth and terminates at the anus; uncoiled, it would be more than 6 m long.

The alimentary canal comprises the oral cavity, pharynx, esophagus, stomach, small intestine (duodenum, jejunum, ileum), large intestine or colon (which includes the sigmoid and rectum), and anal canal. Each of these segments has its own particular morphologic features and activities, but there are basic histologic similarities. The epithelial lining of the GI tract is supported by a layer of connective tissue termed the lamina propria, which in turn lies on a thin sheet of muscle, the muscularis mucosae. These three structures are collectively referred to as the mucosa. An underlying layer of connective tissue, the submucosa, contains vessels and nerves and is surrounded by the muscular coat. Some areas of the gut are partially clothed by a thin layer of connective tissue covered by mesothelium, the serosa.

The primitive digestive tube grows in length much more rapidly than does the developing embryo, and part of it herniates temporarily through the umbilical opening. This part, termed the midgut, separates the foregut from the hindgut. Three main arteries supply each of these segments: the artery to the foregut is the celiac; to the midgut, the superior mesenteric; and to the hindgut, the inferior mesenteric. Branches of these vessels supply the mature derivatives of these segments of the developing alimentary canal. Through its branches, the celiac artery conveys blood to the esophagus, stomach, and proximal duodenum together with the liver, gallbladder, pancreas, and spleen. Extending from the point of entry of the common bile duct down to the proximal two-thirds of the transverse colon, the midgut is supplied by the superior mesenteric artery, whereas the distal colon is supplied by the inferior mesenteric. As the midgut returns to the abdomen, it undergoes a counterclockwise rotation, which accounts for the anatomic locations of its various parts. Portions of the gut lie on the posterior wall covered by peritoneum. Throughout most of its length, however, the gut is suspended by the mesentery, mesocolon, and omentum, sheets of loose connective tissue covered with peritoneum through which the blood vessels run.

In the digestive process, when food is taken into the oral cavity, it is broken down by mastication through the chewing actions of the teeth and the movements of the tongue. Firmer foods are softened by the secretions of the salivary glands, and carbohydrates are broken down by ptyalin, an enzyme in the saliva. Saliva is produced by the three paired major salivary glands (parotid, submandibular, and sublingual) and by many small aggregates of salivary tissue, the minor salivary glands, which are located in the submucosal connective tissue of the lips, cheeks, and palate. Food is then passed down the esophagus by the act of swallowing (deglutition).

The esophagus is a muscular tube lying on the posterior wall of the thoracic cavity close to the midline. Like the oropharynx, it is lined by stratified squamous epithelium. Most of its muscle is smooth muscle arranged in an inner circular and outer longitudinal layer, but the upper portion is also enveloped in skeletal muscle that is continuous with that of the pharynx. At the lower end of the esophagus, at the level of the diaphragm, a functional sphincter relaxes to allow food to pass into the stomach.

The stomach, the widest portion of the alimentary canal, is suspended across the upper abdomen by a fold of peritoneum (the lesser omentum) and is flattened so that it has an anterior and posterior wall that meet at borders termed the curvatures (greater and lesser) of the stomach. Because the stomach bulges more toward the left, the greater curvature is longer than the lesser curvature. Several anatomic regions of the stomach are given names for descriptive purposes. The area close to the esophagus is the cardia, and the bulge upward and to the left of the cardia is the fundus. The major portion of the stomach is its body, which leads into the pyloric antrum and canal. Between the stomach and duodenum, there is a thickening of the smooth muscle, the pyloric sphincter. The mucosa of the stomach is thrown into a series of more or less longitudinal folds termed rugae; its surface area is further increased by the presence of many tubelike glands into which the epithelium is continuous. The epithelial cells of the stomach form the components of the gastric juice, including hydrochloric acid and the protein-digesting enzyme pepsin, together with mucin that serves to protect the surface of the stomach from the action of the acidic gastric juice. The smooth muscle in the gastric wall is arranged in three concentric layers.

The duodenum is a C-shaped structure approximately 25 cm long, lying on the posterior abdominal wall. It is the proximal part of the small intestine and connects the stomach with the jejunum. Food enters the duodenum through the pyloric sphincter and is then exposed to the secretions of the liver (bile), exocrine pancreas, and gland cells of the duodenal wall. Like the rest of the small intestine, the duodenal mucosa has projections and invaginations. The former are the intestinal villi, and the tubelike pockets between villi are the crypts of Lieberkühn. The duodenum is unique in possessing submucosal glands (Brunner's glands) that form an alkaline secretion that neutralizes the acidity of the gastric juice. The duodenum is continuous with the jejunum, and the jejunum and ileum make up most of the length of the small intestine. The jejunum and ileum are suspended within the peritoneal cavity by the mesentery, which contains branches of the superior mesenteric artery, and their free surface is covered by peritoneum. The mucosa has numerous villi and crypts, and the smooth muscle is arranged in well-defined circular and longitudinal layers. The simple columnar epithelium of the small intestine is arranged in microvilli composed of mucin-forming (goblet) cells and a vast number of absorptive cells. The stroma of the microvilli of the small intestine contains a rich network of capillaries and lymphatics.

In the lower right corner of the abdomen, on its posterior wall, the ileum connects with the large intestine through the ileocecal valve. The cecum is a blind pouch below the level of the ileocecal valve, with the vermiform appendix attached to its tip. The ascending colon runs up the right side of the abdomen on its posterior wall and bends below the liver (the hepatic flexure) to become the transverse colon, which is slung across the abdomen suspended by mesocolon. Close to the spleen, the transverse colon makes a sharp bend (the splenic flexure) to become the descending colon. The gut again becomes suspended by mesocolon as the sigmoid colon loops into the pelvis, then expands into the rectum, which lies in front of the sacrum and becomes the short anal canal. The colonic mucosa has numerous crypts but no villi, and most of its cells, particularly in its distal portion, are mucin-forming goblet cells. In the colon, much of the water is absorbed from the gut contents.

Motility of the alimentary canal is achieved by the rhythmic contractions of the smooth muscle in its walls, controlled by the action of the vagus nerves, which form a rich plexus in the submucosa and between the circular and longitudinal muscle layers. In the large intestine, the longitudinal muscle is limited to three bands, the teniae coli, which meet at the base of the appendix. The secretory activities of the GI tract are controlled by hormones produced by cells in the wall of the tract and in the pancreatic islets.

The GI tract can be evaluated clinically by radiologic studies, including contrast examinations with barium. Much of the upper and lower portions of the tract can be visualized by endoscopy, and biopsies can be obtained from as low as the duodenum and as high as the cecum. Analysis of specimens of gastric juice, duodenal secretions, or stool can provide information on secretory functions of cells in the alimentary canal and its accessory glands.

See also the accompanying illustration.

gastroscope (gas′tro-skōp) [*gastro-* + Gr. *skopein* to examine] an endoscope for examining the interior of the stomach.

gastroscopic (gas″tro-skop′ik) pertaining to gastroscopy or the gastroscope.

gastroscopy (gas-tros′ko-pe) the endoscopic examination of the interior of the stomach.

gastrula (gas′troo-lah) the early embryonic stage that follows formation of the blastula. The simplest type consists of two layers, the ectoderm and the mesentoderm, and two cavities, one lying between the ectoderm and entoderm and the other, formed by invagination, lying within the entoderm and having an opening called the blastopore.

gastrulation (gas″troo-la′shun) the process by which a blastula becomes a gastrula or, in forms without a true blastula, the process by which three germ cell layers are acquired.

gate (gāt) 1. a digital electronic circuit that performs a logical operation. Its output is on only when its inputs satisfy some logical relation (e.g., OR, AND, NAND). Also called *logic circuit.* See also the illustration under *schematic.*

2. one of the terminals of a field effect transistor, a silicon-controlled rectifier, or a silicon-controlled switch to which a control signal is applied.

3. an electronic circuit that passes a signal or pulse only when a signal (the gate pulse, normally a square wave) is present at a second input.

gating (gāt′ing) the selection of electrical signals by a gate circuit, which passes signals only when a control signal, the gate pulse, is present, or which passes only signals with certain characteristics, such as a pulse height.

Gaucher cell (go-sha′) [Phillipe Charles Ernest *Gaucher,* French physician, 1854-1918] a large macrophage and storage cell characteristic of Gaucher's disease, which has accumulated glucocerebroside owing to a congenital defect in the enzyme glucosylceramidase. Pseudo-Gaucher cells result in the absence of the enzyme deficiency when an overload of cerebroside or related compounds is phagocytosed by macrophages in chronic granulocytic leukemia (CGL) or thalassemia. The overload of cerebrosides is probably due to massive cell destruction. With the electron microscope, Gaucher cells contain within lysosomes tubular structures with a diameter of approximately 30 nm, in which 8-nm filaments with a spiral arrangement are present.

Gaucher cells are round or polyhedral and 20–80 μm in diameter; they are filled with characteristic lamellar, arcuate, or whorl-like lipid inclusions separated by blue-stained cytoplasm, giving a wrinkled, tissue-paper appearance to the cell. Those features serve to distinguish Gaucher cells from the cells of other lipid storage disorders.

See also *Gaucher's disease.*

Gaucher's disease [Phillipe Charles Ernest *Gaucher*] a familial disorder, transmitted as an autosomal recessive trait, due to a relative or absolute deficient activity of the enzyme glucosylceramidase (glucocerebrosidase). It is manifested in three forms: (1) a chronic adult type; (2) an acute infantile neuronopathic type, resulting in neurologic deterioration or early death; and (3) a subacute neuronopathic disorder. It is characterized by the accumulation of glucocerebroside-laden histiocytes (Gaucher cells) throughout the body, especially marked in the spleen, liver, and bone marrow; hepatosplenomegaly; pigmentation of the skin; and, in some cases, life-threatening thrombocytopenia. Total serum acid phosphatase is elevated in some patients. See also *sphingolipidoses.*

gauge (gāj) 1. a standard scale of measurement.

2. a measuring device, such as a catheter gauge.

gauss (G) (gows) [Johann Karl Friedrich *Gauss,* German mathematician, physicist, and astronomer, 1777–1855] the electromagnetic centimeter-gram-second (cgs) unit of magnetic induction (magnetic flux density or magnetization, defined as 1 maxwell per square centimeter (1 Mx/cm^2), which is equal to 10^{-4} tesla (T). Also called abtesla.

gaussian distribution (gow′shun) see *density function* and *normal distribution.*

gavage (gah-vahzh′) [Fr. "cramming"] 1. forced feeding, especially through a tube passed into the stomach.

2. the therapeutic use of a very full diet; superalimentation.

GAW abbrev. See *airway conductance.*

Gay-Lussac's law (ga″lū-sahks′) [Joseph Louis *Gay-Lussac,* French naturalist, 1778–1850] see *Charles' law.*

G-banding [from *G*iemsa banding] see under *chromosome banding.*

GC abbrev. See *gas chromatography, gonococcus.*

GC value the ratio of the amount of guanine (G) +

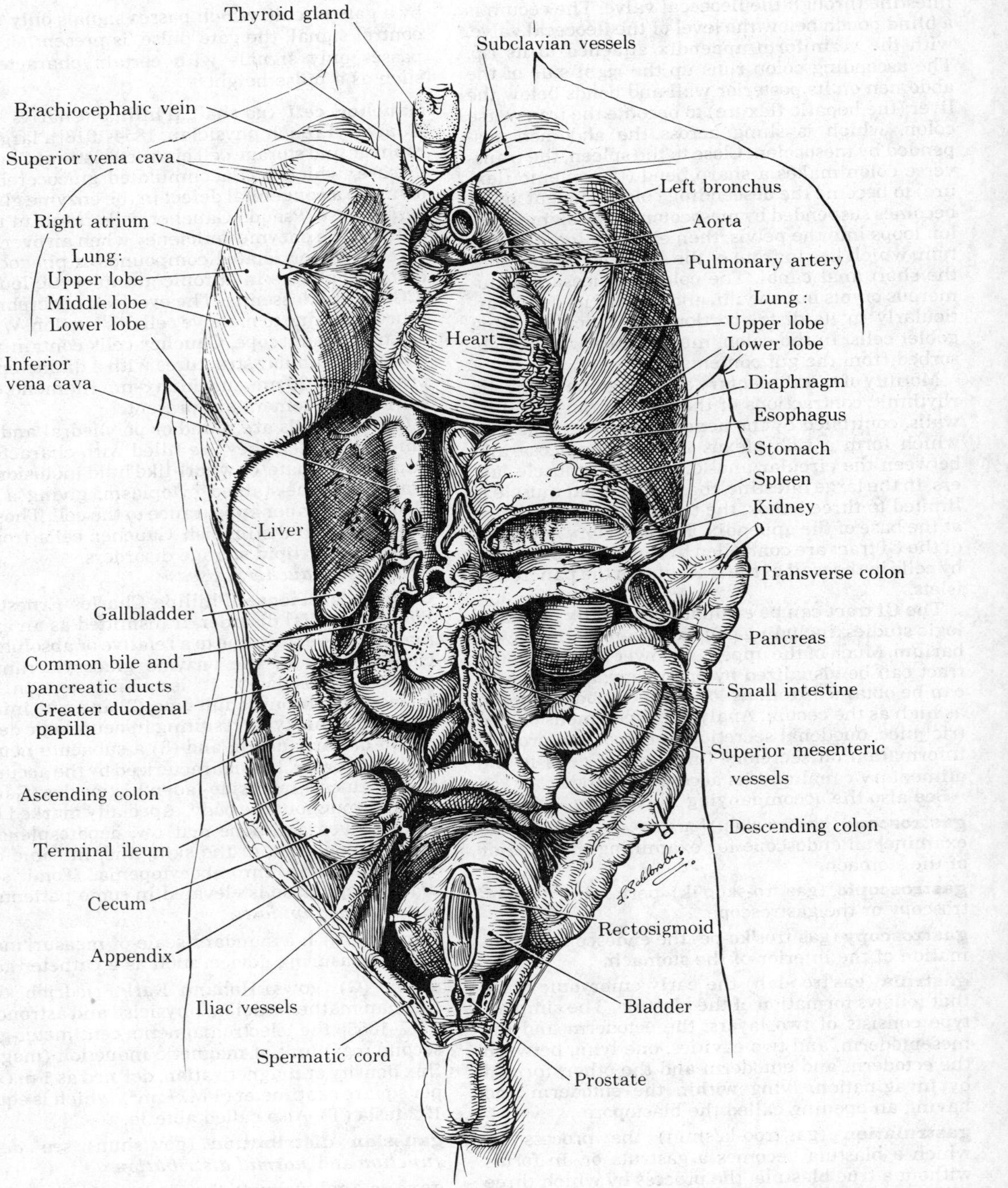

Gastrointestinal tract. The GI tract including thoracic and abdominal viscera. (From Dorland's Illustrated Medical Dictionary. 26th ed. Philadelphia, W. B. Saunders Co., 1981.)

cytosine (C) divided by the amount of adenine (A) + thymine (T) + guanine + cytosine in a sample of deoxyribonucleic acid, usually expressed as mole percent of G + C. In bacteriology, the GC value is quite constant for a given species and is a valuable criterion in bacterial classification. It has a range of about 22-75 percent for bacterial DNA. Also called GC ratio. See also *AT/GC ratio.*

Gd symbol for the chemical element *gadolinium.*

GDP abbrev. See *guanosine diphosphate.*

GDP-L-fucose guanosine diphosphate-L-fucose, a fucose donor molecule for the synthesis of mucopolysaccharides and mucoproteins, including the blood group polysaccharides.

GDP-D-mannose guanosine diphosphate-D-mannose, a mannose donor molecule for the synthesis of glycoprotein side-chains.

Ge symbol for the chemical element *germanium.*

Geiger-Müller (GM) counter (gi'ger mil'er) a radiation detector used primarily as an area survey meter or as a beta-particle detector. It cannot distinguish different types or energies of particles, nor can it record particles received within a period (the resolving time, about 100–500 μs) after the entry of another particle. Above 10,000 cpm, a considerable fraction of the radioactivity is not recorded. All alpha- or beta-particles are detected at low counting rates if they are energetic enough to penetrate the tube wall, a thin mica window. Less than 2 percent of gamma photons are registered. Also called Geiger counter.

gel (jel) a colloidal state in which the molecules of the dispersed phase form a three-dimensional structure in the continuous phase. For example, a warm, dilute (2 percent) solution of gelatin (a protein mixture) forms, on cooling, a stiff gel in which the molecules of the continuous phase are trapped in the holes of a "brush-heap"-like structure of the gelatin. In this case, gelation is reversible, i.e., on heating the gel reverts to a sol.

gelatin (jel'ah-tin) [L. *gelatina,* from *gelare* to congeal] [USP], a product obtained by the partial hydrolysis of collagen derived from the skin, white connective tissue, and bones of animals. Gelatin is a heterogeneous mixture of proteins of large molecular weight. It does not occur naturally, and it dries to colorless or slightly yellow sheets that can absorb 10–15 times their weight of water to form a solution or a more or less solid gel, depending on the temperature. Gelatin is deficient in tryptophan and low in several other amino acids, and thus is not a good nutritional source of protein. It is used as a suspending agent and pharmaceutically in the manufacture of capsules and suppositories. Gelatin has also been suggested for intravenous use as a plasma substitute and as an adjuvant protein food.

gelatinous (je-lat'ĭ-nus) [L. *gelatinosus*] like jelly or having the characteristics of softened gelatin.

gelatin slide adhesive pharmaceutical gelatin added to the flotation bath (5 g/100 ml) to make the tissue sections adhere to the slides. When gelatin is used, albuminized slides are unnecessary.

gelation (jĕ-la'shun) the conversion of a sol into a gel.

gel-filtration chromatography see under *chromatography.*

gel-permeation chromatography see under *chromatography.*

gem (from *gem*inal) a prefix word element in organic chemistry to denote a compound having two substituent groups bonded to the same carbon.

***gem*-diol** (gem-di'ōl) [L. *gemini* twins] an alcohol having two hydroxyl groups on the same carbon atom.

geminal (gem'ĭ-nal) pertaining to organic compounds having two substituent groups bonded to the same carbon atom. Cf. *vicinal.*

geminate (jem'ĭ-nāt) [L. *geminatus*] paired; occurring in pairs; coupled.

gemistocyte (jem-is'to-sīt) [Gr. *gemistos* laden, full + *-cyte*] a plump, rounded fibrillary astrocyte. Characterized by abundant homogeneous cytoplasm and an eccentrically placed nucleus, gemistocytes are formed in response to injury to the central nervous system, such as an infarct. Gemistocytes are also seen in some differentiated astrocytomas.

gemistocytic (jem-is"to-si'tik) composed of large, round cells; a term applied to certain astrocytomas.

gemistocytic tumor see under *central nervous system tumors.*

gemma (jem'ah) [L. "bud"] 1. a budlike body or structure.

2. a chlamydospore, especially of a zygomycete.

gemmation (jĕ-ma'shun) [L. *gemmare* to bud] reproduction by budding.

gemmule (jem'ūl) [L. *gemmula* dim. of *gemma* bud] 1. one of the many small protrusions found on the dendrites of most nerve cells, which are sites of synaptic contact. Also called spine.

2. a bud that forms by the extension of one area of a cell wall during cellular reproduction (e.g., chlamydospore formation in fungi).

gen/o (jen'o) [Gr. *gennan* to produce] a word element used in combining form to denote producing or beginning, e.g., genome.

-gen (jen') [Gr. *gennan*] a suffix word element to denote an agent or product of the word element, e.g., pathogen.

Gendre's fluid a picric acid fixative; see under *fixative.*

gene 1. in classical genetics, the fundamental unit of heredity that carries a single mendelian trait. It can be defined operationally by its ability to mutate and to undergo recombination.

2. in molecular genetics, the genetic information that specifies the amino acid sequence of a single polypeptide chain or the nucleotide sequence of a functional RNA (rRNA or tRNA). In both eukaryotic and prokaryotic cells and in most viruses this information is coded in the base sequence of chromosomal DNA; in some viruses the genetic material is RNA.

Genes can be divided into structural genes, which code for enzymes, structural proteins, and functional RNAs, and regulatory genes, which are involved in the control of gene expression. In eukaryotic organisms the coding sequences (introns) of a gene can be interrupted by noncoding sequences (exons), which are removed from the mRNA transcript of a gene before it is translated. Eukaryotic cells also have a large amount of DNA that has no known function.

The smallest unit of mutation (a muton) or of recombination (a recon) is a single base pair. A gene is equivalent to a cistron, the smallest unit that can be detected by the cis-trans test, which determines whether two mutations are located on the same functional unit. This differs from the classical concept of the gene, which was the smallest unit of function and at the same time the smallest unit of mutation and recombination.

See also *chromosome* and *genetic code.* For more information, see the specific gene.

major g., a gene that produces a marked phenotypic effect as opposed to its modifying genes, which are nonallelic genes that influence the expressivity of the major gene.

modifying g., see under *major g.* Also called *modifier.*

gene cloning see *cloning.*

gene dosage the number of copies of a given gene that are present in a cell or in all the cells of an individual.

gene flow the redistribution of alleles between large populations, resulting in a gradual change in gene frequency. Also called *migration.* See also *evolution.*

gene frequency the fraction of loci (two per individual in a population) that have a particular allele.

gene library a collection of cloned gene fragments that probably contains the whole genome of a particular organism (repetitive sequences especially are rapidly lost during the amplification process).

gene pool the totality of the genes possessed by all the members of a population that will reproduce.

generalization (gen″er-al-i-za′shun) in electroencephalography, the propagation of a particular pattern of electrical activity (or waveform) from a limited region to all regions of the head. Also called spread.

general radiation see *bremsstrahlung.*

generation (jen″e-ra′shun) [L. *generatio*] 1. the act or process of reproduction.

2. a class composed of all individuals removed by the same number of successive ancestors from a common predecessor, or occupying positions on the same level in a genealogic chart.

spontaneous g., abiogenesis; the discredited concept of the development of living organisms from nonliving matter.

generation time (GT) the time required for all components of a cell culture to multiply by two; $G_1 + S + G_2 + M$(meiosis) phases of the cell cycle. Also called *doubling time.* See also *cell cycle* and *neoplastic growth.*

generative (jen′ĕ-ra″tiv) pertaining to reproduction.

generator (gen′er-a″tor) 1. any device that produces electricity from mechanical energy.

2. the circuitry composed of transformers and rectifiers that produces high-voltage direct current for an x-ray tube.

3. a system for the production of short-lived radionuclide pharmaceuticals, the most commonly used being ^{99m}Tc and ^{113m}In. The desired nuclide is continuously produced by decay of its long-lived parent. When a dose is wanted, it is separated from the parent by chromatography, solvent extraction, or other means, and is then used before most of it can decay. Also called *cow.*

generic (jĕ-ner′ik) [L. *genus, generis* kind] 1. pertaining to a genus.

2. applicable to or referring to all members of a genus, class, group, or kind.

3. nonproprietary (e.g., in case of drugs), not referring to trademark. See also *generic name.*

generic name 1. in chemistry, a name for a group of similar compounds, e.g., acid, salt, protein, ketone, aromatic compound.

2. in pharmacology, a short coined name, usually a contraction of the systematic chemical nomenclature, given to a drug by an official body: a United States Adopted Name (USAN), a British Approved Name (BAN), or an International Nonproprietary Name (INN). The generic name may be used to describe or prescribe the drug without regard to the manufacture. Also called approved name or public name.

-genesis (jen′ĕ-sis) [Gr. *genesis* production, generation] a suffix word element to denote producing or the condition of forming, e.g., carcinogenesis.

gene splicing the in vitro insertion of one DNA sequence into another DNA molecule; the basis of recombinant DNA technology. Genes are spliced into bacterial replicons and then cloned in bacterial cells. Both the replicon (plasmid of phage DNA) and the gene to be inserted are cleaved at specific sites by a restriction endonuclease that produces cohesive termini at the cleavage site. The complementary ends are then reannealed, and some of the products are recombinant replicons having a segment of foreign DNA spliced into the plasmid of phage DNA. The annealed products are covalently sealed by the enzyme polynucleotide ligase. Alternatively, appropriate nucleotide "tails" may be added to DNA to allow annealing.

genetic (je-net′ik) 1. pertaining to development, or to birth or origin.

2. inherited.

genetic code the manner in which DNA or RNA represents information for polypeptide chains. There are four kinds of nucleotide bases in DNA: two purines, C (cytosine) and G (guanine), and two pyrimidines, A (adenine) and T (thymine); RNA has the same bases except that U (uracil) replaces thymine. The genetic code is read in groups of three nucleotides called codons, each of which specifies a single amino acid. There are 64 possible codons and only 20 amino acids, so the code is degenerate and more than one codon can translate into the same amino acid. The degeneracy arises in two ways: first, some amino acids have several tRNAs with different anticodons; second, there is an imprecision called "wobble" in the pairing of the third base of the anticodon so that one tRNA can recognize several different codons.

Translation of a polypeptide chain begins with the initiation codon AUG; it begins with the chain with *N*-formylmethionine (in prokaryotes) or methionine (in eukaryotes). The termination codons are UAG, UAA, and UGA; they stop translation. They are also called nonsense codons because they do not code for any amino acid.

Transcription involves making a strand of mRNA from a strand of DNA. Complementary bases pair: C pairs with G, but the A of the DNA pairs to an RNA U, so that the RNA single strand contains no thymine.

Translation involves making a polypeptide chain from the mRNA strand translating the sequence of mRNA codons into a sequence of amino acids. Each amino acid is aligned for insertion in the growing polypeptide chain by a tRNA molecule that reads an mRNA codon by binding to it with a complementary three-base sequence called the anticodon.

Mistakes in pairing of the bases are called copy errors and can appear in DNA replication or transcription. A transitional copy error is the pairing of one purine base (e.g., adenine) with the complementary pyrimidine of the other purine (e.g., guanine) or of one pyrimidine (e.g., thymine) with the other pyrimidine (e.g., cytosine). A transversional copy error exchanges a purine for a pyrimidine, or a pyrimidine for a purine. When they occur during DNA replication, they are mutations.

A deletion or an insertion occurs when a nucleotide base is dropped or added, respectively, from the chain. Such deletions or insertions affect codons beyond the one carrying the mutation because these changes shift the reading-frame; that is, the basis are divided into groups of three (codons) starting at the wrong point. When a mutation results in a different amino acid appearing in a particular protein, it is called a missense mutation. A nonsense mutation occurs when a mutant codon is a termination codon that stops translation of the rest of the chain prematurely.

The genetic code is nearly universal: even nonsense codons appear to be universal in both prokaryotes and eukaryotes, although some differences in the code have been detected in mitochondrial DNA. This universality, however, does not mean that DNA base ratios are similar for genes specifying similar proteins. The fact that the code is degenerate enables many bases to be changed by mutation in a sequence of mRNA, but this mRNA could still produce the same amino acid sequence.

See also *mutation, nucleic acids, protein synthesis, wobble hypothesis,* and the accompanying table.

genetic counseling see *genetic screening.*

genetic drift the changes in gene frequencies that result from random events, e.g., from the migration of individuals from a large population to a small population. The gene frequencies in the small population are not representative of the parent population. See also *evolution* and *founder effect.*

genetic engineering see *bacterial g.* under *genetics* and *cloning.*

genetic map 1. the location of mutations along the length of a chromosome, as determined by recombination experiments. The unit of length is the centimorgan (cMo), one cross-over per 100 meioses.

2. the sequence of base pairs along the DNA of a chromosome, a technique rapidly being applied to humans.

genetic mapping the determination of the location of genes on chromosomes. A number of different techniques are employed, and the map distance may be the actual physical distance or an indirect measure, such as cross-over frequency or time.

LINKAGE ANALYSIS. This category includes the oldest group of mapping methods. Pedigree analysis of two-factor and three-factor crosses is used to map the genes in terms of cross-over frequencies. The distance between genes is specified in terms of the map unit or centimorgan (cMo). Two genes are separated by a distance of *n* centimorgans (map units) if there is an *n* percent frequency of cross-overs between them. For short distances the cross-over frequency is equal to the recombination frequency, whereas for longer distances there are an appreciable number of multiple cross-overs, and the recombination frequency underestimates the map distance.

For very long distances there are many cross-overs between the genes, the recombination frequency is 50 percent, and the genes are unlinked. Genes on the same chromosome are referred to as syntenic genes. Synteny can be demonstrated even when the genes are too far apart to show linkage, by showing that both are linked to genes between them or by other methods, such as somatic cell genetics.

The simplest type of linkage analysis is the analysis of a double-backcross mating. This is a two-fac-

GENETIC CODE

1ST BASE	2ND BASE: *U*	*C*	*A*	*G*	3RD BASE
U	UUU Phe	UCU Ser	UAU Tyr	UGU Cys	U
	UUC Phe	UCC Ser	UAC Tyr	UGC Cys	C
	UUA Leu	UCA Ser	UAA Nonsense	UGA Nonsense	A
	UUG Leu	UCG Ser	UAG Nonsense	UGG Trp	G
C	CUU Leu	CCU Pro	CAU His	CGU Arg	U
	CUC Leu	CCC Pro	CAC His	CGC Arg	C
	CUA Leu	CCA Pro	CAA Gln	CGA Arg	A
	CUG Leu	CCG Pro	CAG Gln	CGG Arg	G
A	AUU Ile	ACU Thr	AAU Asn	AGU Ser	U
	AUC Ile	ACC Thr	AAC Asn	AGC Ser	C
	AUA Ile	ACA Thr	AAA Lys	AGA Arg	A
	AUG Met	ACG Thr	AAG Lys	AGG Arg	G
	AUG F-Met				
G	GUU Val	GCU Ala	GAU Asp	GGU Gly	U
	GUC Val	GCC Ala	GAC Asp	GGC Gly	C
	GUA Val	GCA Ala	GAA Glu	GGA Gly	A
	GUG Val	GCG Ala	GAG Glu	GGG Gly	G

From DeRobertis, E. D. P., and DeRobertis, E. M. F., Jr.: Cell and Molecular Biology, 7th ed. Philadelphia, W. B. Saunders Co., 1980, p. 469.

tor cross in which one parent is doubly heterozygous and the other is doubly homozygous for the recessive alleles. If the heterozygous parent has the genotype AB/ab (both dominant alleles on the same chromosome), the genes are said to be "linked in coupling" or to have the "cis configuration." In the other case (Ab/aB—dominant alleles on homologous chromosomes), the genes are said to be "linked in repulsion" or to have the "trans configuration." If the parental genes have the cis configuration, offspring that inherit only one of the dominant alleles are recombinants. If the configuration is trans, those that inherit both or none are the recombinants.

Deletion Mapping. When a particular chromosomal aberration involving deletion is associated with the loss of a phenotypic character, it can be inferred that the gene is located in the deleted region.

Duplication Mapping. In some cases, a chromosomal aberration involving a duplication or a trisomy can produce an alteration in phenotype, such as an enzyme activity that is 150 percent of normal. It can then be inferred that the gene is in the duplicated region.

Somatic Cell Genetics. Using the techniques of somatic cell hybridization, human-rodent hybrid cells can be formed. The hybrid cells express genes on chromosomes of both species, and the analogous human and rodent proteins can be identified by protein electrophoresis. In cultured hybrid cell lines, human chromosomes are preferentially lost from the hybrids. Because the human chromosomes can be identified by standard cytogenetic techniques, it is possible to assign a gene to a chromosome by determining that the gene product is produced only by hybrid clones possessing a specific chromosome.

In Situ dna Hybridization. When pure messenger RNA for a particular gene or the cloned gene can be isolated, it can be radioactively labeled. When the double-stranded DNA is denatured, the strands separate and can reanneal with the labeled probe, forming DNA-RNA or DNA-DNA hybrids. The segment of the chromosome to which the probe is complementary is identified by autoradiography.

Transduction and F-duction Mapping. Transfer of genetic material in bacteria involving transducing phages or conjugative plasmids proceeds at a constant rate. By examining which genetic markers are transferred when the mating is artificially interrupted, it can be determined how far genes are apart in terms of the time required to transfer the genetic material that lies between them.

DNA Sequencing. Recently, technology has been developed that allows DNA segments of moderate size to be completely sequenced. When the amino acid sequence of a particular protein is known, the DNA sequence that codes for it can be located.

Genetic Maps. The human genome has been well mapped by linkage analysis, somatic cell genetics, and other methods, and about 100 markers have been assigned to specific loci. The X chromosome has been well mapped by pedigree analysis of two-point and three-point crosses. The bacterium *Escherichia coli* has been almost completely mapped using both F-duction mapping and linkage analysis of recombinants. The first organism for which the entire DNA sequence has been determined is the coliphage ϕX174, a small single-stranded DNA virus. Surprisingly, it was found to have overlapping genes with reading frames that are out of phase.

genetic marker a gene that has alleles which are all expressed in the phenotype (i.e., are codominant) and which can be used to study inheritance in families and in populations. The various blood group systems and serum or red blood cell proteins that can easily be detected by electrophoresis or immunodiffusion are commonly used as markers.

genetic regulation the molecular mechanisms that control gene expression. These include controls that operate at every stage of protein determination: transcription of DNA, posttranscriptional processing of mRNA, translation of mRNA, and posttranslational modification of proteins. The genome of an organism contains DNA sequences of several different types, including structural genes, which specify the amino acid sequences of enzymes and structural proteins or the nucleotide sequences of ribosomal RNAs or transfer RNAs; and regulatory genes and signals, which code for regulatory proteins, and control the initiation and termination of transcription or provide binding sites for regulatory molecules.

In prokaryotes, the basic mechanism of regulation is described by the Jacob-Monod model exemplified by the lac operon in *Escherichia coli*. The length of DNA transcribed into mRNA at one time is called an operon. It begins with a promoter, the binding site for RNA polymerase, which is followed by an operator, the binding site for a regulatory protein, which in turn is followed by a sequence of structural genes. When the regulatory molecule is bound to the operator, transcription is blocked. In inducible systems the repressor (or aporepressor) binds to the operator in its native conformation. When a specific allosteric effector (inducer) is present, it binds to the aporepressor, which undergoes a conformational change so that it does not bind to the operator, and transcription of the operon can begin. This is termed negative control. In end-product repression the repressor does not bind to the operator in its native conformation, but it does when it is bound to an effector molecule (a corepressor). This is termed positive control.

Eukaryotic DNA is contained in chromosomes, which are chromatin complexes of DNA, RNA, and proteins. Chromosomes, single pieces of double-stranded DNA wound around spheres of basic proteins called histones, consist of structures with the appearance of strings of beads (nucleosomes). The acidic proteins complexed with DNA (nonhistone chromosomal [NHC] proteins) and the histone (H1) that is not bound in nucleosomes may have functions in genetic regulation. Chromatin is a less efficient template than is naked DNA. Specific NHC proteins may serve to activate transcriptions.

Posttranscriptional control of gene expression in eukaryotes involves RNA processing. Initially, transcribed RNA contains extra nucleotides that are later removed. Ribosomal RNA precursors are also cut into several shorter segments, and transfer RNA precursors are processed by enzymatic modification of bases. Messenger RNA starts as a primary transcript. This is modified by addition of a cap at the 5′ end and a polyA tail at the 3′ end, forming heterogenous nuclear RNA (hnRNA). The introns are then removed by special enzymes that splice the exons together, forming mature cytoplasmic mRNA.

There are message-specific controls that affect translational steps in the production of functional gene products. Populations of mRNA that differ in the ability to compete for translational initiation factors represent a control mechanism. The competitive mRNAs are translated at different rates. Autogenous control, a message-specific translational control, is demonstrated by the effect of iron on the synthesis of ferritin, the iron-binding protein of the liver. If iron is not present, ferritin is not synthesized. When iron is added to the system, the production of ferritin is increased without synthesis of new mRNA.

Translational control (tc) RNA, a special class of RNA recently hypothesized, is reported as two types: one type, found in a particular initiation factor, inhibits the translation of heterologous messages; the other type affects the availability of message for translation.

Masked messages are located in the cytoplasm of unfertilized eggs in different animals; they are inactive and unavailable to the translational machinery of the cell. The message becomes available at fertilization; tcRNA may have a role in controlling message translation.

The half-life of mRNA can determine the number of times that message is translated. Messenger RNAs have different stabilities as the state of the cell changes and as they are selectively stabilized and degraded.

Many proteins must undergo posttranslational modification to become functional. Alterations such as cleavage, modification of amino acids, or the addition of prosthetic groups are common. The formation of functional molecules may occur in a single step or in a cascade reaction requiring a number of consecutive steps.

Cellular specialization is a result of differential gene expression. There are three possible mechanisms by which genetic alteration may play a role in cellular differentiation. The genes needed for specialized functions may be increased in numbers in differentiated cells when large amounts of product are required, a process called gene amplification. Also, as development proceeds, the genes for the cell may be removed from the chromosome or be permanently inactivated.

See also *gene, genetic code, RNA processing, transcription,* and *translation.*

genetics (jĕ-net′iks) [Gr. *gennan* to produce] the study of genes and heredity and their effect on the structure and functioning of living organisms.

bacterial g., the study of the heredity of bacteria. The physical basis for inheritance is the gene, DNA that is about 1000 nucleotides in length. The genetic information of a gene is coded by the sequence of nucleotides. The total genetic make-up, or genotype, determines the phenotype of a microorganism—its morphology, physiology, and biochemistry. In *Escherichia coli,* a typical bacterium, there is enough DNA for about 5000 genes, whereas in a human cell there is enough for about 4×10^6 genes.

Generally, DNA genetic code is transcribed into one messenger RNA (mRNA), which, in turn, is translated into one protein or enzyme, a process accomplished in the following manner: A word of the DNA genetic code consists of a triplet of any of the four nucleotides: guanosine (G), cytidine (C), adenosine (A), or thymidine (T). A gene consists of 300–400 such code words (about 1000 nucleotides). The genetic code of a gene is transcribed into an mRNA as a complementary copy that follows certain base pair rules: G is transcribed as C, and vice versa; A is transcribed as uracil (U), and vice versa (U generally replaces mRNA). The mRNA is translated into a protein at sites on the ribosome. Translation requires transfer RNA (tRNA), the adaptor molecule, which bridges mRNA and amino acids. At one end of tRNA is the anticodon, which is complementary (G↔C; U↔A rules) to the codon on the mRNA. On the other end is a specific amino acid of that particular tRNA. As the mRNA moves along the ribosome, amino acids are positioned according to the sequence of the code along the mRNA, and a protein molecule is assembled by peptide binding. (See also *deoxyribonucleic acid, genetic code, ribonucleic acid, transcription,* and *translation.*)

Based on the estimated number of proteins and enzymes required for existence and replication, there is more DNA per bacterial cell than is needed. One explanation for the extra DNA is that some genes are found in multiple codes, although the reason for this redundancy of genes is not clearly understood. Another explanation is that there are segments of DNA that do not code for proteins or enzymes. These DNA segments (about the size of a gene) are part of the regulatory apparatus for controlling the expression of structural genes, i.e., genes that code for proteins or enzymes. The best example of genetic control is the regulation of the lactose operon of *E. coli.*

A set of structural genes under unit control is called an operon. The lactose operon consists of three structural genes that account for lactose utilization. Adjacent to them is a segment of DNA, termed an operator. The operator acts as the on-off switch to coordinate transcription of the three structural genes. Somewhat distant from the operator is a regulator that codes for a protein, termed a repressor. The repressor is an allosteric protein that has dual affinity—in this case for the operator and lactose. The repressor attaches to the operator and prevents transcription of the lactose operon. In the presence of a sufficient amount of lactose, the repressor binds to the lactose. As a consequence, the repressor detaches from the operator, allowing the lactose operon to be transcribed. The active component of transcription is the DNA-dependent RNA polymerase. It attaches to a region of DNA called the promoter, which is next to the operator. The promoter determines the rate at which transcription proceeds. (See also *genetic regulation.*)

The lactose operon is an example of an inducible enzyme system, in that the operon is induced by the presence of lactose to be transcribed. A repressible enzyme system, such as in the biosynthesis of an amino acid, is controlled in a similar way. The main difference between enzyme induction and repression is the nature of the repressor. In a biosynthetic pathway, the repressor is not active unless it binds to an end product of the pathway. Transcription of an operon for amino acid biosynthesis is normally "on," until a sufficient amount of the amino acid activates the repressor to stop transcription.

Genes, operons, regulators, operators, and promoters are located along a threadlike structure, the chromosome. The bacterial chromosome is a single molecule of double-stranded DNA. Replication of the chromosome is regulated by a complex interplay of genes and DNA polymerases. A unit of DNA replication, such as a chromosome, is called a replicon. When nonchromosomal units of DNA are present in bacteria, e.g., plasmids, they constitute their own replicon, which may replicate independently of the chromosomal replicon. (See also *DNA synthesis.*)

Duplication of double-stranded DNA follows this scheme: The double-stranded DNA starts to separate while new strands of DNA are synthesized as complementary copies of the old, with adenosine (A) paired with thymidine (T), guanosine (G) paired with cytidine (C), and vice versa. Each daughter cell receives an old and new strand of DNA, and hence an identical set of genes. An important exception to the inheritance of identical genetic information by daughter cells occurs when one cell in the line of descendants mutates.

MUTATION. Mutation is a change in the nucleotide sequence of a gene, independent of genetic recombination. (See also *mutation.*) Mutation rates are low, on the order of one mutation event per 10^6 cell doublings. However, in any large population (10^6 or greater) there are mutations affecting the antigenicity or virulence or biochemical reactions of bacteria. For example, the latter type of mutations probably accounts for the wide range of biochemical types of species that have evolved in the family Enterobacteriaceae. Mutations are also significant in the emergence of antibiotic-resistant bacteria as a result of the use of antibiotics; antibiotics favor the outgrowth of resistant mutants from a large susceptible population.

Mutations occur spontaneously, i.e., during normal growth conditions. However, their frequency of occurrence can be increased by the use of physical agents such as x-rays, or chemical agents such as nitrogen mustard. These mutagenic agents have one common characteristic—they directly or indirectly affect DNA.

The genetics of microorganisms, like that of higher forms of life, depends on the availability of mutants. As a result of the use of mutagenic agents, a variety of mutants of bacteria have become available for studying the nature of a gene, its replication, and its regulation. The availability of many mutants has made possible studies on the special feature of gene transfer between bacteria, which in turn has led to the discovery of plasmids and the advent of genetic engineering. See also *mutagenicity test.*

GENE TRANSFER. The transfer of genes between bacteria usually results in general recombination. This phenomenon first requires pairing of homologous DNA between the transferred DNA and the recipient's chromosome. Next, there is an exchange between the homologous regions. This crossing-over event requires a complex series of endo- and exonucleases and DNA repair mechanisms. Another type of genetic interaction resulting from the transfer of genes is additive recombination. In this type of recombination, genetic elements such as plasmids and chromosomes integrate to form composite molecules. General recombination is limited to members of the same or closely related species. Additive recombination can occur even between members of different species.

The transfer of genes between bacteria occurs via three processes: transformation, conjugation, and transduction.

1. Transformation is the transfer of free, naked DNA from one bacterium to another. DNA is extracted from a bacterial culture by any of several routine methods and mixed with living bacteria. The recipient bacteria must be in the state of competency for the irreversible uptake of DNA, the nature of which is not completely understood. With some bacterial strains, competency occurs during certain stages in the growth cycle of a culture; with others, competency is associated with a soluble surface protein or even structural proteins, pili. After the DNA enters the recipient cell, it undergoes general recombination with the chromosome of the recipient bacterium.

Transformation occurs in many species of bacteria. A relatively recent discovery was the use of Ca^{++} to make *E. coli* strain K12 competent for transformation. This was one of the technologic breakthroughs of genetic engineering.

2. Conjugation (mating) is a process of gene transfer that requires physical contact between the participating pairs of bacteria. The following information is based on the mating system of *E. coli* strain K12: There are distinct donor and recipient strains. Contact is due to a sex pilus. The production of this pilus and the ability to transfer genes are determined by a fertility (F) factor in the donor. The F factor is a member of a group of genetic elements called plasmids. Donors that carry the F factor as a replicon independent of the chromosome replicon are called F^+. The F factor can insert into and excise from the chromosome as a rare event (about once per 10^6 generations). Donors with the inserted F factor are called Hfr. Donors in which the F factor excises from the chromosome are called F' (F-prime). During this excision process, one, two, or several chromosomal genes are carried along and become a part of the F replicon. The F factor with chromosomal genes is called an F genote. The recipient, called F^-, lacks the F factor.

In an $F^+ \times F^-$ mating, the pilus makes contact with the recipient. This triggers replications of the F replicon for transfer to the recipient, converting the recipient to an F^+. In an $F' \times F^-$ mating, the pilus contact triggers replicative transfer of the F genote to the recipient, which now becomes an F'. This mating is often referred to as sexduction of F-duction. In an Hfr $\times$ F^- mating, the chromosome behaves as if it is part of the F replicon. The pilus contact triggers replication of the chromosome for transfer in an oriented linear fashion, with the F factor destined to go over last. Usually, though not always, the transfer spontaneously stops and only about one-third of the chromosome is transferred. The recipient remains F^-.

The F factor has an affinity for many loci on the host chromosome. This generates different Hfr donor strains. Each Hfr strain transfers different lead genes, resulting in a high frequency of general recombination for those genes in the recipient, when compared with that for the distal genes. Many matings using different Hfr donors demonstrated that there is an orderly, linear linkage of genes and that this genetic map has neither beginning nor end. This discovery indicated that the chromosome is actually circular, and this has been confirmed by autoradiography.

F factor–mediated conjugation also occurs in *Salmonella typhimurium.* Conjugation in other species, such as *Vibrio cholerae* and *Pseudomonas aeruginosa,* is mediated by other sex factors. Conjugation has not been described in as many species of bacteria as has transformation or transduction.

3. Transduction is the process of gene transfer between bacteria that is commonly found in a variety of gram-positive and gram-negative bacteria. This process starts with the infections of a bacterium with a phage (bacterial virus). During the course of phage replication, bacterial DNA is incorporated into some phage particles in place of phage DNA. After replication is completed, the phage population consists of a mixture of complete phage particles and transducing phage particles, i.e., those that contain bacterial DNA. Any bacterial gene or set of closely linked genes or operons can be transferred to another bacterium of the same species, a process called generalized transduction (for more information on specialized transduction, as well as on the phenomenon of lysogeny, see under *bacteriophage g.*).

PLASMIDS. Plasmids are additional, nonessential genetic elements found in bacteria. They are circular, double-stranded molecules of DNA, ranging in size from about 3×10^6 to 1×10^8 daltons, compared with a size of about 3×10^9 for the chromosome. They are their own replicons. When plasmids integrate into the chromosome, they become part of the chromosomal replicon. In this respect, they resemble the prophages of some temperate phages. Plasmids can transfer from one host to another by transformation, conjugation, or transduction.

Often, during replication, plasmids are not equally distributed to the daughter cells, resulting in the spontaneous loss of plasmids. Maintenance of a plasmid-containing population depends on selection of the host cells that exhibit properties determined by genes of the plasmid, e.g., resistance to antibiotics. Loss of plasmids ("curing") is often enhanced by treating plasmid-containing cultures with ultraviolet light or acridine dyes.

Some plasmids confer recognizable properties to the host. For example, the F factor is a sex factor plasmid that confers mating ability upon the host. It is unique among plasmids in that it has a relatively high affinity for the host chromosome. For a time, this characteristic was considered important enough to put the F factor into a separate category of genetic elements, i.e., episomes.

Bacteriocinogenic factors are plasmids that carry genes coding for the production of bacteriocins. These are soluble proteins or structural proteins or protein-containing materials that are lethal for other bacteria, usually of the same species. This type of plasmid is widely found in gram-negative and gram-positive bacteria.

R factors are plasmids that code for resistance to single or multiple (as many as eight) antibiotics. Resistance is due to alteration of cell wall permeability or to production of enzymes. There are enzymes that acetylate or phosphorylate antibiotics, thereby inactivating them. The penicillinase and cephalosporinase of some plasmids destroy the beta-lactam ring of penicillin and cephalosporin. The general term beta lactamase is used for penicillin- or cephalosporin-destroying enzymes.

R factors are widespread among enteric bacilli (*E. coli, Shigella, Salmonella*) and other gram-negative bacteria. Among gram-positive bacteria, the beta-lactamase plasmid of *Staphylococcus* is well known. Most of the *S. aureus* isolates from a hospital environment, which are resistant to penicillin, carry a beta-lactamase plasmid. This plasmid of *Staphylococcus* can be transferred by transduction, whereas R factors of the enteric bacilli are transferred by transformation, conjugation, or transduction.

There have been outbreaks of dysentery, typhoid fever, and cholera due to bacteria that carry R factors, conferring multiple drug resistance to the etiologic agent. Strains of *Neisseria gonorrhoeae* are emerging that carry a beta-lactamase plasmid; such strains cause gonorrhea that is refractory to routine penicillin therapy.

There are several reasons why R factors are so widespread. The use of antibiotics in clinical situations and in animal feeds selectively favors outgrowth of R factor–carrying strains of bacteria. Also, transmission of R factors can occur among *E. coli, Shigella, Salmonella,* and *Pasteurella* species. For example, an *E. coli* strain carrying a multiple drug resistance R factor can transmit that resistance to *Salmonella typhi.*

TRANSPOSABLE GENETIC ELEMENTS: These are distinct units of DNA (double-stranded) in bacterial chromosomes, plasmids, or phage that are found at a particular genetic locus but that, on DNA replication, can be found at another genetic locus. Translocation of these DNA units does occur within a replicon or between replicons (chromosomes ⇄ plasmids ⇄ prophages). Identical transposable genetic elements are found in different species of bacteria. This is taken as evidence that these elements can cross species barriers. Identical transposable genetic elements are found even in bacteria and phages. There are two types of transposable elements, insertion sequences (IS) and transposons.

IS elements are small pieces of DNA, of about 800–1400 nucleotide sequences (M.W. $2.8–4.9 \times 10^5$). There are at least five different IS elements, with classification based on DNA sequence homology as determined by DNA hybridization and electron microscopy (heteroduplex analysis). IS elements can switch on or off the transcription of an adjacent gene or operon. This switching can, for instance, account for phase variation of *Salmonella.*

IS elements account for additive recombination. The unique affinity of the F factor for the host chromosome is explained by the existence of homologous IS elements in both replicons. A similar site-specific DNA homology explains the insertion of prophage into the host chromosome (see under *bacteriophage g.*), although the enzymology of site-specific recombination remains to be elucidated.

Transposons are antibiotic resistance genes bounded by IS elements, and thus are larger than IS elements. Transposons can translocate within a plasmid and into a chromosome of even prophage.

GENETIC ENGINEERING: There are restriction endonucleases that recognize unique nucleotide sequences and cleave DNA at that unique site. Specific cleavage due to any one restriction endonuclease occurs without regard to the source of DNA. Under appropriate conditions and with DNA ligase, cleaved DNA fragments can be reannealed. Cleavage of R factor and human DNA by a particular restriction endonuclease, and an annealing of these heterologous DNA fragments, results in the formation of DNA chimera. The chimera can be transformed into competent (Ca^{++}-treated) *E. coli* strain K12. The chimera can also be packaged into a phage and transferred into a host via the process of transduction. The host with a chimera can be selected from the population on the basis of its R factor–mediated resistance to antibiotics. In this manner, human genes—actually, any genes—can be cloned in bacteria.

By means of such technology, the genes for interferon, insulin, and somatostatin have been cloned in *E. coli.* There is usually the problem of foreign gene expression (transcription → translation) in bacteria. Once this problem is solved (perhaps with a different solution for each gene), these products as well as others can be mass produced in cultures of bacteria.

See also *molecular c.* under *cloning* and *genetic regulation.*

LEONARD J. ZUBRZYCKI, PH.D.

bacteriophage g., the study of heredity of bacterial viruses. The physical basis for phage inheritance is the gene. A phage gene is double- or single-stranded DNA or single-stranded RNA, depending on the phage type. The number of genes per complete phage particle is determined by its size, i.e., from 2 genes in small phages to about 170 genes in large phages.

For most phage genes, the one gene–one protein concept holds true (see under *bacterial g.*). In some small phages, however, the middle part of one gene is transcribed as the beginning of another. This allows a genome with apparently enough nucleic acid to code for only two proteins to be transcribed into a messenger RNA (mRNA) that is translated into three proteins. This concept of overlapping genes is being applied to genetic studies of higher forms of life such as bacteria and mammalian cells.

Like bacteria, phages are haploid. Their genes, operons, regulators, and promoters are located along a single chromosome. Duplication of double-stranded DNA occurs by the same scheme as occurs in bacteria. Duplication of single-stranded DNA and RNA, which constitute the genes of some phages, follows a variation of this simple scheme. Either way, each daughter phage particle receives an identical set of genes, except in the case of mutation.

There are many types of phage mutants. Some affect the structural proteins of a phage and others the regulatory proteins. When two mutants of the same phage type simultaneously infect a host, the chromosomes of both mutants replicate and also undergo general recombination. The genetic map of phage, i.e., the order in which genes are aligned along the chromosome, can be deduced by studying the progeny of such simultaneous infections. For some of the best-studied phages, e.g., T_4, the genetic map is a circle.

The first step in a phage infection is adsorption to a receptor site on the bacterial surface. This surface interaction is very specific and is the basis for the phage-typing schemes that divide a bacterial species, e.g., *Staphylococcus aureus,* into many groups or phage types and thus provide important epidemiologic information. Only the phage nucleic acid gets into the host; the head protein (capsid) remains on the outside. Replication of phage nucleic acid, the synthesis of capsids, and their assembly into a complete phage are accompanied by death and lysis of the host. Lysis is accompanied by the release of 50–100 or even 1000 phage particles within an hour or somewhat longer, depending on the phage. Phages that exist in this manner are called virulent phages. Others, called temperate phages, can replicate in an inconspicuous as well as lethal manner.

LYSOGENY. Temperate phages can lyse or lysogenize a host. When they lysogenize, they are reduced to a prophage state (only DNA), which replicates with the host. Lysogeny is restricted to double-stranded DNA phages. The prophages of some temperate phages just exist as dormant entities within, and replicate in synchrony with, the host. Other prophages form composite molecules with the host chromosome. The most widely studied temperate phage, lambda, is of the latter type.

The DNA of lambda is a linear, double-stranded DNA molecule. When it enters the host, e.g., *Escherichia coli* strain K12, the DNA circulizes. Lambda DNA has a unique small sequence of nucleotides that is homologous to a specific site of the host chromosome. This site is between the genes for galactose utilization and biotin synthesis. The circular phage molecule inserts at this site as an additional linear stretch of DNA within the host chromosome. The genetic map of this prophage is a circular permutation of the genetic map of the vegetative (or self-replicating) phage particle. The prophage now replicates as part of the host chromosomal replicon.

A consequence of lysogeny is immunity. Immunity is due to a phage gene that codes for a repressor. The repressor is a protein that interacts with the appropriate operator of the prophage to inhibit prophage replication other than its replication as part of the host chromosomal replicon. The repressor also inhibits superinfection by phage of the same type. In other words, *E. coli* strain K12 lysogenized by lambda is immune to a lytic infection by lambda phage. The phage adsorbs to the lysogenic host and injects its DNA, but vegetative replication is prevented. Immunity is specific; i.e., a host bacterium lysogenic for one kind of phage is immune to that phage but is not immune to another kind of phage.

Spontaneously, prophage can initiate a lytic cycle of growth. This occurs at a frequency (usually very low) that varies with the prophage. Ultraviolet light can induce a lytic cycle for some prophages; in the case of lambda, UV light can induce a lytic cycle in about 100 percent of lysogenized bacteria.

Lysis of lysogeny is determined by a complex interplay among repressor proteins, transcription initiation proteins, and the specific operators for these proteins. The protein products of the *c* genes (I, II, III) are important for lysogeny and immunity, as are the protein products of the *N, O, cro* genes for lysis. There are also specific phage genes for integration and others for excision of lambda DNA into and out of the host chromosome, and lambda excision is the best model for an understanding of specialized transduction.

SPECIALIZED TRANSDUCING PHAGE. When lambda prophage excises from the host chromosome, the adjacent galactose (or biotin) genes are excised along with lambda DNA, some of which is left behind. These excised host genes become part of the lambda replicon, which now replicates vegetatively. This part-host and part-phage DNA is packaged into a capsid that constitutes the specialized transducing particle. In the case of lambda, the transducing particle transfers only the galactose (or biotin) genes to another host. Such a particle is usually defective in that it cannot initiate vegetative replication in a recipient host. The nature of a phage infection is so overwhelming that lysis in a portion of a host population results in a mixture of complete phage and specialized tranducing particles. This ensures a simultaneous infection of some members of the remaining population by complete and specialized transducing particles. Simultaneous infection bypasses the immune system, which takes a period of time to set up. This situation results in the replication of the defective specialized transducing particle by the following mechanism: As the complete phage replicates, it provides the missing vital function of the defective phage. For example, if the defective phage genome lacks the genes for a vital, transcription-initiating protein, the complete phage genome codes for this vital protein, which can be used for replicating both genomes.

Different excision events result in specialized transducing particles that contain different proportions of host chromosomal and phage DNA. Some specialized transducing particles are not defective—lambda biotin, for example—because the vital portion of the phage genome is intact. There are specialized transducing phages other than lambda. The characteristic common to all is the ability to transfer a particular gene or set of closely linked genes between members of a strain or species of bacteria.

GENERALIZED TRANSDUCING PHAGE. Some temperate phages (actually their prophages) have a low or nondetectable affinity for the host chromosome. During a lytic cycle of replication, any section of the host chromosome roughly equivalent in size to that of the phage genome is packaged into the phage capsid. In any population of such phages, there is a mixture of complete and defective phage particles. The defective particles contain little, if any, phage DNA, and so cannot be propagated even with the help of a complete phage genome.

What characterizes generalized transducing phages is the ability to transfer any gene or set of closely linked genes between members of a strain or species of bacteria. Typical are the phage P1, whose hosts are strains of *E. coli* and *Shigella,* and the phage P22, whose hosts are strains of *Salmonella typhimurium.* These generalized transducing phages have been helpful in constructing the genetic maps of *E. coli* strain K12 and *S. typhimurium.*

LYSOGENIC CONVERSION. Infection of some bacteria by particular temperate phages results in profound changes in the host. Toxin production by *Corynebacterium diphtheriae* is due to the *tox* gene of the beta prophage. The production of erythrogenic toxin by strains of *Streptococcus pyogenes* and toxins by some strains of *Clostridium botulinum* depends on the presence of specific prophages in these strains. Antigenic changes of some *Salmonella* species are due to the alternating presence and absence of specific prophages. When these hosts lose the prophages, which can happen spontaneously, the properties conferred by the phage genes are lost.

Experiments have shown that a prophage can become defective through mutation. Such prophages do not self-replicate. However, when the prophage causes the host to produce a toxin or certain antigens, the properties conferred remain, even though the defective prophage is difficult to detect. In such situations, one might assume erroneously that those properties are due to bacterial genes and not phage genes. Discoveries such as this encourage speculation that, in mammalian host-virus associations, undetectable provirus genes cause cancer.

LEONARD J. ZUBRZYCKI, PH.D.

behavior g., the study of the genetics of behavioral traits. In humans it is mostly limited to quantitative and correlative studies because of the complexity of human behavior. Experimental studies in animals are more tractable.

biochemical g., the study of the fundamental relationships between genes, protein, and metabolism. Alterations in the nucleic acid sequences of genes may cause the synthesis of an altered peptide sequence that can result in abnormal phenotypes. Biochemical genetics also deals with human biochemical (metabolic) disorders and pharmacogenetics.

developmental g., the study of gene expression during the development of an organism through its life cycle: gametogenesis, fertilization, embryogenesis, and maturation. Aging and injury repair may also involve similar mechanisms.

immunogenetics, the study of the genetics of transplantation and tissue rejection (mainly in mice), histocompatibility loci, immunologic response, immunoglobulin structure, and immunosuppression.

mathematical g., the statistical analysis of probabilities of genetic transmission, genetic ratios (ascertainment and inheritance), and hypothesis testing.

medical g., the study of the causes and inheritance of genetic disorders. It is significant in various fields of clinical medicine: an estimated one-third of all pediatric hospital admissions involve genetic disorders. Applications in obstetrics include the prenatal diagnosis of certain genetic defects and improvement of prenatal conditions. In adult medicine, diseases such as cancer of the breast in females, coronary heart disease, hypertension, and diabetes mellitus have been found to have predisposing genetic components; preventive medical techniques aimed at such components can sometimes slow or prevent the disease.

mendelian g., the study of the inheritance of unit characters. The laws of Mendel (unit inheritance, segregation, and independent assortment) are the basis for modern genetics.

molecular g., the study of gene expression and its regulation centered around the role of DNA as a template for RNA synthesis (transcription) and the role of mRNA in determining the amino acid sequence of proteins (translation). DNA is the carrier of genetic information; the flow of the information is always from nucleic acids (DNA or RNA) to proteins, never the reverse.

population g., the study of the distribution of genes in populations and how the frequencies of genes and genotypes are maintained and/or changed.

somatic cell g., the study of genetic phenomena in cultured somatic cells. The range of somatic cell genetics is broad, encompassing the expression of mutant cells in culture; gene mapping; the study of differentiated function and malignancy; and the factors controlling differentiation in culture, cloning, and hybridization. Somatic cells have demanding nutritional requirements, and most cell lines are short-lived. Occasionally, cell lines become established and continue growth indefinitely; such cell lines are usually of malignant origin.

There are many advantages to the study of genetic disorders in cell culture rather than in live patients;

cell lines can be used for experimental procedures that might raise problems if attempted in the living. Cultured cells can also be used to investigate metabolic disorders and in prenatal diagnosis of genetic defects.

The development of culturing techniques has allowed the expression of differentiated properties in culture. There are two major classes of differentiated cells that can be grown well in culture. The first are cells derived from malignant tumors that express differentiated properties in the intact animal and continue to do so when placed in culture. Such cells are less demanding in their growth requirements than normal cells and generally are more capable of becoming permanent cell lines. The second class of cells are those derived from normal tissue. The behavior of these cells differs from tissue to tissue. Normal cells usually do not become permanent cell lines. Examples of normal cells grown in culture include the heart muscle, lens, liver, and pituitary cells, as well as melanocytes and myoblasts.

Media for the growth of somatic cells are based on poorly defined additives, such as serum or embryo extract, but can still be defined as permissive (culture conditions that support the expression of differentiated properties) and nonpermissive (culture conditions that do not support differentiation). For instance, under permissive conditions, some myoblast cells form multinucleate myotubes, whereas others do not fuse but line up end to end or pile up on each other. If cultures are grown as monolayers, contact inhibition tends to suppress the expression of differentiation. Under clonal conditions, where each colony develops without contact with other cells, cells can frequently express differentiated properties.

See also *cell culture, cell line, cellular h.* under *hybridization, cloning, genetic mapping,* and *hybrid c.* under *cell.*

genetic screening the search in a population for individuals with inherited disease and/or those at high risk of having offspring with serious genetic disorders. Genetic screening programs represent a new concept in medical care aimed at prevention. There are three principal types of genetic screening: (1) for the identification of individuals possessing a genotype already associated with a disease that requires rapid medical management, in order to prevent permanent neurologic damage or death (e.g., newborn screening); (2) for the identification of persons at high risk for genetic disease in their descendants, so that prior identification of marriages at high risk can offer reproductive options (heterozygote or carrier screening); and (3) for the identification of genotypes that may produce variations not specifically known to be associated with disease, but where the collection of epidemiologic data can be used to study the prevalence of genetic variants in defined populations (i.e., genetic screening for research). In current usage, the term genetic screening is used to refer to all three types.

Newborn Screening. For a select group of inborn errors of metabolism, newborn screening provides the opportunity for primary prevention of mental retardation and/or fulminating neonatal death by the rapid start of therapy. Neonatal screening for hyperphenylalaninemia is the prototype for genetic screening for inborn errors of metabolism. In 1962 the impetus for a demonstration newborn screening program came from the realization that a diet low in phenylalanine, if started during the first weeks of life, could prevent the neurologic damage associated with classic phenylketonuria (PKU). The concurrent development of an accurate assay for blood phenylalanine led to a successful pilot program. At present, newborn screening for PKU is mandatory in most states.

For mass screening to be effective, detection techniques should be simple, economical, and automated. To detect abnormal phenylalanine metabolites, many laboratories use the Guthrie bacterial inhibition assay (GBIA), a microbiologic test based on an inhibition of bacterial growth. A mutant strain of *Bacillus subtilis* (ATCC 6051) cannot grow in a minimum culture medium with β-2-thienylalanine. The inhibition is prevented by the presence of phenylalanine, phenylpyruvic acid, and phenyllactic acid. The McCaman and Robins fluorometric assay and chromatographic procedures, either on paper or thin-layer plates, are also accepted test procedures.

When a newborn is still in the hospital nursery (average age, 4 da) and has ingested normal amounts of a regular formula, a small amount of capillary blood is obtained, usually by heel puncture, and placed on a disk of absorbent filter paper. A blood level of more than 4 mg/100 ml is considered positive. All borderline and positive tests should be repeated immediately. A second positive test result should be confirmed by a quantitative determination of phenylalanine concentration in a plasma or serum sample and an enzyme assay to establish a precise biochemical diagnosis (see *aminoacidopathy*).

In some states, newborn screening programs have been enlarged to include additional inborn errors of metabolism such as maple syrup urine disease, homocystinuria, galactosemia, and adenosine deaminase deficiency, or related endocrine disorders such as hypothyroidism. These disorders were selected because they meet the primary objective of newborn screening—to prevent or minimize irreversible damage by prompt institution of therapy.

There are additional types of genetic disease that will benefit from early identification—the genetically determined drug and food intolerances, and disorders in which early diagnosis and treatment can significantly assist in clinical management. Sickle cell disease is in the latter category. Electrophoresis for sickle cell disease, hemoglobin C, and other abnormal hemoglobin variants has been instituted in some states, and the pilot research projects show a low rate of false-negatives and false-positives. As part of comprehensive programs that include monitored follow-up of positive tests, precise biochemical diagnosis, genetic counseling, and pediatric treatment facilities, the genetic screening of newborns will become an increasingly important neonatal diagnostic procedure.

Heterozygote Screening. Heterozygote screening, or screening for carriers of genes that cause autosomal recessive disease, provides the opportunity for the prospective prevention of mendelian inherited disorders by identifying high-risk couples even before birth of an affected child. Unfortunately, a tragic index case is usually the first indication that both parents are heterozygous for a serious metabolic disease. If it were possible to identify parents as carriers of a particular mutant gene, and therefore at a 25 percent risk of occurrence at each pregnancy when both parents are carriers, it would permit the choice of a therapeutic abortion in monitored pregnancies if the fetus were affected.

One of the sphingolipidoses, Tay-Sachs disease, was the subject of the first successful public heterozygote screening program. The elucidation of the basic enzyme defect, a deficiency of hexosaminidase A, and the automation of methods for its quantification established the methodology for mass screening. The effectiveness of the program was based on four factors, which have since become guidelines for mass heterozygote screening: (1) The disease occurs predominantly in a defined population—Tay-Sachs disease has a carrier rate of 1 in 30 individuals of Ashkenazi Jewish ancestry, compared with 1 in 300 in non-Jewish individuals. (2) The heterozygous state can be simply, accurately, and inexpensively determined from an easily available biologic material, a serum assay of hexosaminidase A. (3) Prenatal diagnosis early in pregnancy is available. Couples at risk for Tay-Sachs disease, identified through carrier screening, can monitor each pregnancy by amniocentesis at approximately the sixteenth week of gestation. Families can then choose to have only unaffected offspring. (4) A research pilot program with community participation and a strong educational component should precede public screening. In one successful screening project, Tay-Sachs disease carrier screening was offered to the public after 14 mo of planning. All aspects of the project were evaluated for error, and ongoing follow-up studies are part of the continuing mass screening program now available in 60 cities throughout the world.

Although the first two criteria also apply to sickle cell anemia carrier screening, the third criterion was not met when screening was begun, and the fourth was frequently not met. Thus, initial screening efforts were usually unsuccessful.

MURIEL GLUCKSON, M.S.

-genic (jen′ik) [Gr. *gennan* to produce] a suffix word element to denote producing, or produced by or in, e.g., immunogenic.

geniculate (jĕ-nik′u-lāt) [L. *geniculatus*] 1. bent, like a knee.
2. pertaining to the knee.

geniculum (jĕ-nik′u-lum), pl. *genicula* [L., dim. of *genu*] [NA], a general term to designate a sharp, kneelike bend in a small structure or organ, such as a nerve.

genin (jen′in) see *aglycone.*

genital (jen′ĭ-tal) [L. *genitalis* belonging to birth] pertaining to reproduction or to the organs of reproduction.

genitalia (jen″ĭ-ta′le-ah) [L., pl.] the reproductive organs.

genitofemoral (jen″ĭ-to-fem′or-al) pertaining to the genital and femoral regions.

genitofemoral nerve a nerve that arises from the first and second lumbar nerves in the lumbar plexus and descends, piercing the psoas major, to cross behind the ureter and divide somewhere above the inguinal ligament into genital and femoral branches. The genital branch enters the inguinal canal through the deep ring to supply the cremaster in the male and labium majus in the female. The femoral branch passes behind the inguinal ligament to enter the femoral sheath, where it lies lateral to the femoral artery, and supplies skin over the upper part of the femoral triangle.

genitourinary (jen″ĭ-to-u′rĭ-nar-e) pertaining to the genital and urinary organs.

genitourinary myiasis see *genitourinary m.* under *myiasis.*

genome (je′nōm) [*gene* + chromos*ome*] all the genes of a gamete; a haploid set of chromosomes.

genotype (jen′o-tīp) [*geno-* + Gr. *typos* type] the genetic make-up of an individual as distinguished from its phenotype.

genotypic (jen″o-ti′pik) pertaining to or expressive of the genotype.

gentamicin (jen″tah-mi′sin) one of the aminoglycoside antibiotics produced by a fungi of the genus *Micromonospora.* It consists of three closely related compounds containing a 2-deoxystreptamine linked to saccharide units. It is a broad-spectrum, relatively toxic antibiotic that is effective against many gram-positive and most gram-negative organisms. Gentamicin is used topically for skin infections and for systemic infections—especially those due to gram-positive cocci and *Pseudomonas.* See also *aminoglycoside* and *antibacterial agents.*

gentian violet (jen′shun) [USP], a mixture of *N*-hexamethyl-*N*-pentamethyl and *N*-tetramethyl-pararosaniline chlorides. It has been used as a topical antiinfective and as an internal anthelmintic. Also called *methylrosaniline chloride.* Cf. *crystal violet* and *methyl violet.*

gentiobiase (jen″tĭ-o-bi′ās) see *β-D-glucosidase.*

genus (je′nus), pl. *genera* [L.] a taxon, or category of classification of organisms, that is contained in a family and that contains one or more species. The scientific binomial nomenclature of an organism gives the genus (capitalized) and species (lower case), e.g., *Homo sapiens, Staphylococcus aureus,* or *Escherichia coli.*

geo- (je′o) [Gr. *gē* earth] a word element used in combining form to denote relationship to the earth or to soil, e.g., geobiology.

Geodermatophilus (je″o-der″mah-tof′ĭ-lus) [*geo-* + *dermatophilus*] a genus of bacteria of the family Dermatophilaceae, of the order Actinomycetales. Isolated from soil samples, the organism is similar to the pathogenic *Dermatophilus,* although it is less filamentous and is not virulent for animals. The genus contains a single species, *G. obscurus.*

geographic pathology an aspect of epidemiology that is concerned with the linking of specific diseases with specific locations to gain better insight into such contributing factors as causes and vectors. Geographic pathology analysis has been particularly valuable in emphasizing environmental factors in the etiology of cancer. See also *epidemiology.*

geometric efficiency (G) a measure of the collecting ability of gamma rays of a collimator; the fraction of photons emitted by a 1-cm² area in the field of view that is received by the detector. It is expressed as $G = A_O A_D / 4\pi T^2$, where A_O is the hole area on the front face, A_D is the hole area on the detector face, and T is the thickness of the collimator. The effective geometric efficiency, (G_O), is $A_O G / A_D$, where A_O is the area of the object being viewed and A_D is the area of the field of view at the object distance.

geometric isomerism a type of stereoisomerism due to restricted rotation about double bonds or in fused ring systems. Geometric isomers are diastereoisomers that are not optical isomers. See also *isomerism.*

geometric mean the *n*th root of the product of *n* numbers. It is less affected by extremes than is the arithmetic mean.

geophagia (je-o-fa′je-ah) [*geo-* + Gr. *phagein* to eat] the ingestion of earth or clay. Such a practice may often accompany iron deficiency and contribute to its cause by interfering with iron absorption. See also *pica.*

geophilic (je″o-fil′ik) [Gr. *gē* earth + *philein* to love] characterized by an affinity for soil, as in microorganisms that live in soil, such as the terricolous human dermatophytes *Microsporum gypseum, Trichophyton ajelloi,* and *T. terestre.*

geotrichosis (je″o-trik-o′sis) a rare, opportunistic fungal infection of oral, intestinal, bronchial, or pulmonary tissues caused by *Geotrichum candidum.* It is most often involved in a mixed infection. Laboratory diagnosis is made by demonstration of characteristic arthrospores in the sputum and by isolation of this fungus. At present there are no serologic procedures for diagnosing this disease.

Geotrichum (je-ot′rĭ-kum) a genus of yeastlike Fungi Imperfecti that produces conidia by fragmentation of hyphae.

G. candidum, a fungus that is the causative agent of geotrichosis. This fungus grows at room temperature as a dry, white colony. Microscopically, it has hyphae with rectangular-shaped arthrospores that seem to germinate at one end by a germ tube. No carbohydrates are fermented, and only glucose and galactose show assimilation.

G. immite, see *C. immitis* under *Coccidioides.*

geotropism (je-ot′ro-pizm) [*geo-* + *tropos* a turning] growth or movement influenced by gravity.

GEP abbrev. for *gastroenteropancreatic endocrine system.* See under *enterochromaffin cells.*

ger/o (jer′o) [Gr. *gēras* old age] a word element used in combining form to denote old age, e.g., geriatric.

geranyl diphosphate (je′ran-il di-fos′fāt) a diprenyl (C-10, having carbons of two isoprene units) compound that is a biosynthetic precursor of cholesterol and of many other polyisoprenoidal compounds in nature.

geranyl geranyl diphosphate a tetra- or polyprenyl (C-20, having carbons of four isoprene units) compound that is a biosynthetic precursor of many naturally occurring polyisoprenoidal compounds not including cholesterol.

geriatric (jer″e-at′rik) [Gr. *gēras* old age + *iatrikē* surgery, medicine] pertaining to the treatment of the elderly.

geriatrician (jer″e-ah-trish′an) a specialist in geriatrics.

geriatrics (jer″e-at′riks) the branch of medicine that treats all problems peculiar to old age, including senescence and senility.

germ/o (jer′mo) [L. *germen* germ] a word element used in combining form to denote sprout or seed, e.g., germinal vesicle.

germ (jerm) [L. *germen* germ] 1. a pathogenic microorganism.

2. a living substance that is capable of developing into an organ, part, or organism as a whole; a primordium.

germanium (Ge) (jer-ma′ne-um) [L. *Germānia* Germany] a grayish-white semiconducting element; atomic number 32; atomic weight 72.59; group IV of the periodic table; oxidation states +2, +4. It is used industrially in alloys and as doped single crystals in semiconductor electronic devices.

German measles see *rubella.*

germ cell either an ovum or a spermatozoon.

germ cell tumor a neoplasm that arises from the primordial cells of the male or female gonad. See also *ovarian tumors* and *testicular tumor.*

germicide (jer′mĭ-sīd) [*germ-* + L. *caedere* to kill] a chemical agent that destroys pathogenic microorganisms rapidly and in a useful way.

germinal (jer′mĭ-nal) [L. *germinalis*] pertaining to a germ cell, or the primitive stage of development.

germinal center see *follicular center.*

germinal vesicle the nucleus of an unripe ovum.

germinoblast (jer′mĭ-no-blast″) a term, used particularly in the European literature, for a follicular center B lymphocyte. According to Lennert, it is a cell with a round nucleus, fine chromatin, multiple nucleoli, and basophilic cytoplasm, and it coexists with germinocytes, cells having larger and lighter nuclei, no apparent nucleoli, and sparse cytoplasm. "Large pyrinophilic cells" are immunoblasts, and the B-cell lymphomas are germinoblastomas or germinoblastic sarcomas. The Lukes-Collins terminology for follicular center cells and the lymphomas derived from them is more logical, is immunologically and clinically relevant, and avoids possible confusion with germ cell tumors.

germinoma (jer″mĭ-no′mah) a neoplasm that arises in germ cell tissue. See also *dysgerminoma* and *seminoma.*

pineal g., a misnomer for an intracranial, extragonadal germ cell tumor that usually occurs in the vicinity of the pineal gland. The histologic spectrum of germ cell tumors, including teratomas, has been described in this location.

germ layers the three primary layers of cells—ectoderm, mesoderm, and entoderm—formed in the early embryo. It is from these layers that the organs and tissues of the body are formed. See also *early embryonic development.*

germ tube a short projection developing on many types of germinating fungal spores that elongate into hyphae. The production of germ tubes by *Candida albicans* and *C. stellatoidea* when incubated in certain proteinaceous media is a characteristic used to differentiate these species from other yeasts.

geroderma (jer″o-der′mah) [*gero-* + Gr. *derma* skin] age-associated changes that give the outward appearance of old age. Such changes are primarily confined to the skin, which becomes wrinkled and less elastic. Atrophy and wrinkling of the genitals is also observed in this condition. The term may also be applied to any lesion that gives the appearance of old age. Also called gerodermia.

geront/o (jer-on′to) [Gr. *gerōn, gerontos* old man] a word element used in combining form to denote old age, e.g., gerontology.

gerontologist (jer″on-tol′o-jist) a physician who treats diseases of old age, or a physician who specializes in gerontology.

gerontology (jer″on-tol′o-je) the science that deals with the study of old age, an area that has become increasingly important in recent years owing to the increasing life span of humans.

gestagen (jes′tah-jen) any hormone with progestational activity, progesterone being the most important.

gestation (jes-ta′shun) [L. *gestatio,* from *gestare* to bear] the period of development of the young in viviparous animals, from the time of fertilization of the ovum until birth. See also *pregnancy.*

gestosis (jes-to′sis) any of the possible toxic conditions suffered by the mother during pregnancy. The term often refers to toxemia of pregnancy or eclampsia. See also *eclampsia* and *t. of pregnancy* under *toxemia.*

GeV abbrev. See *giga electron volt.*

g factor the ratio of the magnetic moment of a particle to the Bohr magneton (μ_B).

GFR abbrev. See *glomerular filtration rate.*

GG abbrev. See *gamma globulin.*

GGT abbrev. See *γ-glutamyltransferase.*

GH abbrev. See *growth hormone.*

ghost cell an abnormally shaped, anucleated cell characteristic of squamous lung cancer. The cytoplasm produces an abundance of keratin, which obscures the nucleus and gives the cell a very sharp outline. The cytoplasm is given a brilliant orange or yellow color by Papanicolaou stain. When a cytologic diagnosis of malignancy has been established, these cells indicate a keratinizing squamous carcinoma pattern.

GH-RIH abbrev. See *growth hormone–release-inhibiting hormone.*

GHz abbrev. See *gigahertz.*

GI abbrev. See *gastrointestinal.*

giant cell 1. any very large cell.

2. any of the large, multinucleated cells formed by fusion, or by nuclear division without cytoplasmic division, of histiocytes.

foreign body g. c., a multinucleated large cell formed by fusion of macrophages; it is seen in tissues as part of an inflammatory response, particularly a chronic reaction to the presence of foreign material, such as sutures. See also granulomatous inflammation under *inflammation.*

Langhans g. c., a type of multinucleated giant cell. See *multinucleated g. c.*

multinucleated g. c., a multinucleated cell that arises from the fusion of macrophages as part of the process of chronic granulomatous inflammation. The nuclei may be clumped at the center or one pole (Touton giant cell), or arranged in a complete or partial ring at the cell periphery (Langhans giant cell). Either type may be seen in immune- and nonimmune-related granulomas. See also *granuloma* and *granulomatous i.* under *inflammation.*

Touton g. c., a type of multinucleated giant cell. See *multinucleated g. c.*

tumor g. c., a large cell occurring in a tumor, particularly one with extensive cytoplasm and a large irregular nucleus, or with multiple nuclei. Cells with this appearance are characteristic of malignant fibrous histiocytomas, but may be seen in a wide range of neoplasms, particularly following radiation therapy.

giant cell thyroiditis see *subacute t.* under *thyroiditis.*

giant cell tumor a neoplasm containing many large, multinucleated cells. Several types are recognized in particular anatomic locations.

g. c. t. of bone, a tumor of bone composed of plump, ovoid, or elongated cells with numerous uniformly interspersed, osteoclastlike multinucleated cells. It comprises about 4 percent of all tumors arising within bone. Most of those afflicted are between the ages of 20 and 50 yr. The most common sites are the long bones of the extremities, particularly the region of the knee and the distal radius; the small bones of the hands and feet are rarely affected. In the axial skeleton, the sacrum may be involved. The tumor arises in the epiphysis of a long bone, spreads to the metaphysis, may erode the cortex, and extends to adjacent soft tissues. Most giant cell tumors of bone are benign, but there are some reports that as many as 20 percent exhibit malignant behavior.

Radiographic findings are not specific but should suggest the diagnosis. Biopsy is necessary for confirmation, and caution is necessary in assessing the histology, as similar giant cells are ubiquitous in reactive as well as neoplastic bone lesions. Treatment may require local resection of the involved segment of bone. Metastases are rarely present at the time of surgery, but some malignant giant cell bone tumors subsequently give rise to distant spread.

g. c. t. of lung, a bronchogenic carcinoma in which large, pleomorphic, and often multinucleated cells are present. In many instances, differentiated areas of the neoplasm show squamous or adenocarcinomatous features, but some do not and must be viewed as anaplastic forms of large cell undifferentiated lung carcinoma.

malignant g. c. t. of soft parts, a malignant soft tissue tumor characterized by the presence of numerous osteoclast-like giant cells. It tends to occur in the lower extremities; deeply located tumors in the thigh may metastasize to the lungs and have a 5-yr survival rate of approximately 20 percent. This tumor is probably a variant of malignant fibrous histiocytoma.

g. c. t. of tendon sheath, a lesion that arises from the sheath of a tendon, commonly on the flexor surface of the hand or foot. It is rarely larger than 3 cm and is benign, but it may erode adjacent bone and tends to recur if incompletely excised. Histologically, it contains numerous osteoclastlike giant cells surrounded by plump or elongated cells. Mitotic figures may be numerous, leading the unwary into making an erroneous diagnosis of sarcoma. Although this tumor is regarded by some as a reactive process, others consider it to be a benign neoplasm related to the fibrous histiocytomas. Also called nodular tenosynovitis.

giant hairy nevus see *giant hairy n.* under *nevus.*

giant neutrophilia a benign hereditary disorder, transmitted as an autosomal dominant trait. It is characterized by enlarged neutrophil hypersegmentation, with 6–10 lobes, a volume twice normal, and a mean diameter of 16.9 μm (normal, 12–15 μm). This unusual morphologic abnormality of neutrophils apparently does not interfere with their function. Also called hereditary hypersegmentation of neutrophils.

Giardia (je-ar′de-ah) [Alfred *Giard,* biologist in Paris, 1846–1908] a genus of flagellate protozoa that is parasitic in human intestines. Most species are nonpathogenic, although they may cause diarrhea.

G. lamblia, a pear-shaped flagellate found in human intestines. The infection is usually caused by ingestion of cysts in food and water; however, *G. lamblia* can be transmitted through sexual contact. Laboratory diagnosis requires microscopic examination of feces for trophozoites and cysts.

giardiasis (ji″ar-di′ah-sis) a common infection caused by *Giardia lamblia,* an intestinal flagellate of worldwide distribution. Acute or chronic diarrhea, malabsorption syndrome, and weight loss may occur.

Human infection is caused by the ingestion of cysts from contaminated food or water. Several outbreaks of giardiasis have been traced to *Giardia* cysts from tap water and from the stools of beavers who were trapped in city reservoirs.

The pathogenesis *G. lamblia* is poorly understood. Some workers believe that the cysts are excysted in the duodenum and that the trophozoites multiply rapidly and cover the intestinal epithelium wall, thereby preventing normal absorption. Others believe that a synergistic relationship between enterobacteria or fungi and *G. lamblia* may be the cause of malabsorption.

With the aid of the scanning electron microscope, workers have shown that the repeated attachment and detachment of the flagellate by its sucking disk injures the mucosal cell. This irritation and damage can compromise the function of important enzymes (e.g., lactase, sucrase, and leucynaphthylamidase) and the absorption of vitamin B_{12}.

Many infections with *Giardia* may be asymptomatic. However, a small percentage of cases present a wide range of symptoms, including nonspecific gastrointestinal discomfort, mild-to-profuse diarrhea, and weight loss. The infection is more common in children than in adults, particularly those associated with various hypogammaglobulinemic disorders. Infected travelers returning from endemic areas (Mexico, South and Southeast Asia, West and Central Africa, and western South America) may have severe symptoms. Giardiasis can also be a sexually transmitted disease, especially among homosexual populations.

Laboratory diagnosis requires the identification of trophozoites and/or cysts in the intestinal contents. In some cases, cysts are found in formed stools, and trophozoites may be present in unformed stools. Wet mount preparations can by used by cysts and trophozoites. Concentration methods may be used to demonstrate the cysts (the trophozoites are destroyed by concentration). Often the clinical characteristics still suggest giardiasis although the stool specimens are negative. In these patients, examination of duodenal drainage fluid is indicated and may demonstrate motile trophozoites.

G. lamblia cysts are distinguished by their oval shape, four nuclei, axis style, and internal flagella. The trophozoites are pear shaped and possess two nuclei, numerous flagella, and an axis style.

Also called *giardiasis dysentery.*

Giemsa stain (gēm′sah) [Gustav *Giemsa,* German bacteriologist and chemist, 1867–1948] a Romanowski-type stain used to stain peripheral blood smears for differential counting, for staining thick blood smears for malarial parasites and protozoa, for use in the G-banding chromosome staining technique in karyotyping, and for demonstrating *Chlamydia* and *Dermatophilus* species. It contains the basic dyes methylene blue, azure A, and azure B (tetra-, tri-, and dimethylthionine) and the acid dye eosin. It is available commercially in mixtures certified by the Biological Stain Commission.

Giemsa stain is dissolved in 1:1 methanol-glycerol and diluted 50:1 with buffer solution before use. For blood, pH 6.5 is used; for chromosome banding, pH 6.8; for malaria parasites, pH 7–7.2.

When stained, the erythrocytes appear pinkish-orange, nuclei of leukocytes are purplish-blue, cytoplasm is ivory or pale blue, neutrophilic granules are beige or faintly violet-pink (depending on small changes in the pH), eosinophilic granules are orange-red, basophilic granules are dark blue to purple, platelet granules are dark lilac, and malaria parasites have sky-blue cytoplasm and red-purple chromatin. These colors can vary even when the same dye lot is used.

Gierke's disease (gēr′kēz) [Edgar Otto Konrad von *Gierke,* German pathologist, 1877–1945] see *von Gierke's disease.*

GIF abbrev. for growth hormone–inhibiting factor. See *growth hormone–release-inhibiting hormone.*

giga- (G) (jig′ah, gig′ah) [Gr. *gigas* giant] a prefix word element attached to International System (SI) units of measurement to denote a unit that is equal to 1 billion of the base unit (10^9 unit).

giga electron volt (GeV) a unit of energy equal to 1 billion electron volts (10^9 eV). Formerly called *billion electron volts* (BeV).

gigahertz (GHz) (jig′ah-herts, gig′ah-herts) a unit of frequency equal to 1 billion Hertz (10^9 Hz).

gigant/o (ji-gan′to) [Gr. *gigas, giantos* giant] a word element used in combining form to denote huge, e.g., gigantomastia.

gigantism (ji-gan′tizm; ji′gan-tizm) [Gr. *gigas* giant] a condition involving abnormal increases in bone length and width, characterized by height exceeding 200 cm in the adult male or 3 SD above the mean in children. The condition is due to a benign eosinophilic adenoma, resulting in hypersecretion of the pituitary growth hormone before closure of the epiphyses. It may be associated with childhood acromegaly. There may also be soft tissue disorders, peripheral neuropathy, myopathy, arthropathy, and generalized pituitary insufficiency.

When measured by radioimmunoassay, concentrations of serum growth hormone may exceed 10 ng/ml and are not suppressed during the glucose tolerance test. X-rays, CT scans, and polytomography may be useful in the determination of a pituitary adenoma, especially when there is an associated enlargement and erosion of the sella turcica. Treatment may require supervoltage irradiation of the pituitary, although cryohypophysectomy or surgical hypophysectomy is more commonly used. See also *acromegaly.*

gigantomastia (ji-gan″to-mas′te-ah) extreme enlargement of one or both breasts, most frequently occuring in the female. It can be due to a variety of causes, including tumor, mastitis, and cystic hyperplasia.

GIGO abbrev. See *garbage in, garbage out.*

gigohm (GΩ) (jig′ōm) [*giga-* + *ohm*] a unit of electrical resistance equal to 1 billion ohms (10^9 Ω).

GIH abbrev. for growth-inhibiting hormone. See *growth hormone–release-inhibiting hormone.*

Gilbert's syndrome see *h. I* under *hyperbilirubinemia.*

Gilchrist's disease [Thomas Caspar *Gilchrist,* American dermatologist, 1862–1927] see *blastomycosis.*

Gilles de la Tourette's syndrome (zhēl-dĕ-lah-toor-etz′) [Georges *Gilles de la Tourette,* French physician, 1857–1904] see *Tourette's disease.*

Gimenez stain a method used for staining *Rickettsia* and *Chlamydia* organisms. A thin smear is air dried and treated with carbolfuchsin in phosphate buffer (pH 7.45), washed with water, and counterstained with malachite green or fast green; elementary bodies stain red against a greenish background.

gingiv/o (jin′jĭ-vo) [L. *gingiva* gum] a word element used in combining form to denote gums, e.g., gingivitis.

gingiva (jin-ji′vah, jin′jĭ-vah) [L. "gum of the mouth"] the layer of soft tissues that covers the alveolar processes of the mandible and maxillae. It is fibrous but vascular and is covered with stratified squamous epithelium. The marginal gingiva surrounds the neck of each tooth like a collar and its epithelium is heavily keratinized. The remainder of the gingiva is usually referred to as the attached gingiva; it is firmly bound to the bone of the alveolar processes and has relatively little keratin. Also called *gum.*

gingival (jin-jĭ-val, jin-ji′val) pertaining to the gingiva.

gingivitis (jin″jĭ-vi′tis) [*gingiva* + *-itis*] an inflammatory lesion confined to the papillary and marginal gingiva. Symptoms include bleeding, erythema, and alterations in tissue contour (usually enlargement). The major etiologic factor is bacterial plaque. It is thought to be the first stage of periodontal disease. The types most frequently encountered include plaque-associated, hormonal, drug-induced, and acute necrotizing ulcerative gingivitis. Treatment involves elimination or control of the microorganisms.

gingivosis (jin″jĭ-vo′sis) [*gingivo-* + *-osis*] the chronic state of gingival inflammation. This particular condition is marked by the signs of gingivitis (i.e., redness, pain, bleeding), as well as by the sloughing off of the papillary epithelium and mucous membranes.

gingivostomatitis (jin″jĭ-vo-sto″mah-ti′tis) [gingivo- + Gr. *stoma* mouth + *-itis* inflammation] the inflammation of the gingiva that extends beyond the gums to the oral mucosa.

herpetic g., an infection of the oral mucosa (including the gingiva) by the herpes simplex virus, which is characterized by the formation of multiple vesicles and painful ulcers.

necrotizing ulcerative g., an inflammatory condition of the gums that causes painful ulcers and necrosis while progressively destroying the underlying tissues. The condition, which is limited to the interdental papillae and free gingival margins, is marked by foul mouth odor, increased salivation, and bleeding. It is thought that factors such as poor health, stress, and poor nutrition predispose to the combined infection by several bacterial species, especially spirochetes and fusiforms. Also called *Vincent's stomatitis.* See also *fusospirochetosis.*

GIP abbrev. See *gastric inhibitory polypeptide.*

GI series see *gastrointestinal series.*

gitalin (jit′ah-lin) a digitalis glycoside that occurs as a white crystalline powder; it is obtained from the plant *Digitalis purpurea.* Gitalin is a mixture of the pure glycosides digitoxin, gitoxin, and gitaloxin, and traces of other glycosides and aglycones. Trademark, Gitaligin. See also *digitalis glycosides.*

gitaloxin (jit″ah-loks′in) a pure digitalis glycoside obtained from the plant *Digitalis purpurea.*

gitoxin (ji-tok′sin) a pure digitalis glycoside obtained from *Digitalis purpura.* It also occurs in *D. lanata.*

gitterzell a globular microglial cell, which is formed as the result of phagocytic activity by a normal microglial cell and seen in various pathologic processes in the brain and spinal cord. Also called compound granular corpuscle.

glabella (glah-bel′ah) [L. *glaber* smooth, i.e., without hair] 1. the region above the nasion (the intersection of the frontal and two nasal bones), between the superciliary arches.

2. the most prominent point in the midsagittal plane between the eyebrows; used as an anthropometric landmark.

glabelloalveolar line (glah-bel″o-al-ve′o-lar) the line passing through the glabella and the alveolar point, the line in the midsagittal plane that touches the front of the skull at the brow and beneath the nose. It is used in radiographic positioning.

glabellomeatal line (glah-bel″o-me-a′tal) the line passing through the glabella and the auricular point, that is, between the midpoint of the brow ridge and the center of the opening of the ear (the external auditory meatus). It is used in radiographic positioning.

glabrous (gla′brus) [L. *glaber* smooth] smooth and bare; free of hair.

glacial (gla′shal) [L. *glacialis*] resembling ice; solid.

glacial acetic acid [USP], a clear, colorless liquid that is at least 99.4 percent acetic acid and has a vinegar odor; beause it freezes at 16.7°C, it is sometimes solid at room temperature.

gland (gland) [L. *glans* acorn] a single cell or an organized aggregate of many cells whose function is the elaboration of a specific secretion. In exocrine glands, the secretion is conveyed to its site of activity by ducts. In endocrine glands, the secretion (a hormone) diffuses from the cell into an adjacent thin-walled blood vessel.

Most secretions of gland cells are proteins, and their molecules are formed by ribosomes on the cisternae of the endoplasmic reticulum, then transported to the Golgi complex where they are invested by a unit membrane to form a secretory granule. The granules may accumulate in the cytoplasm, but on receipt of an appropriate stimulus, they leave the cell by exocytosis. The formation of steroid hormones is less well understood, but the smooth endoplasmic reticulum that is plentiful within the cells bears some of the enzymes involved in their synthesis; the hormones do not form electron-dense aggregates in the cytoplasm.

An example of a monocellular gland is the goblet cell, many of which are located in the epithelium of the intestine. Mucin accumulates in the apical cytoplasm before it is released into the lumen of the duct. The exocrine cells that form the saliva are organized into three pairs of major salivary glands and many, much smaller minor salivary glands. Exocrine gland cells form acini in which the cells surround a small lumen that is in continuity with a fine duct. The larger the gland, the more extensive and elaborate the tributaries of the duct system. Expression of secretion from the acini of exocrine glands is effected by the contraction of myoepithelial cells located between the basal lamina and the base of the cells. Cytoplasmic extensions of the myoepithelial cells interweave around the periphery of the acinus and their contraction squeezes secretion into the duct.

Monocellular endocrine units are present in the epithelium of the respiratory and alimentary passages. The cells may not reach the lumen but are in contact with the basal lamina. An example is the serotonin-forming argentaffin cell. In the larger endocrine glands, the cells may form groups as in the pituitary anterior lobe and adrenal medulla, cords as in the adrenal cortex, or storage follicles as in the thyroid gland. In every instance, the groups of cells lie immediately adjacent to thin-walled and often fenestrated venous sinusoids.

For more information, see the specific gland.

glanders (glan′derz) [L. *malleus*] an infectious disease of horses, mules, and donkeys, which may be transmitted to humans. It is caused by the nonmotile, gram-negative, aerobic bacillus *Pseudomonas mallei.* Glanders may occur in an acute febrile form, a chronic indolent form, or a relapsing form. The disease is seen in individuals in Asia, Africa, and South America; because of control measures, it has now been eradicated in the United States.

The acute disease is characterized by nasal cellulitis and septal necrosis, with pharyngeal ulceration, and cutaneous cellulitis, ulceration, and abscess formation. There is fever, malaise, chills, and nausea. The organism may spread along lymphatics. Chronic glanders may lead to chronic draining abscesses of the skin, hepatosplenomegaly, and chronic granulomas. Pulmonary involvement is common.

Diagnosis is based on demonstration of complement-fixing antibodies, organism recovery, or positive mallein skin tests.

Also called *farcy.*

glandular (glan′du-lar) pertaining to or of the nature of a gland.

glandular epithelium the epithelial cells of glands. In simple tubular glands, the cells are usually cuboidal. In the acini of exocrine glands such as the pancreas, the cells surround a small acinar lumen and have a narrow apex and a broader base so that they resemble the slices of a pie in cross section. In the glandular epithelium of endocrine organs, the cells are cuboidal and pass their secretion through the base of the cell into an adjacent capillary or sinusoid.

glans (glanz), pl. *glandes*[L. "acorn"] [NA], a general term for a small, rounded mass or glandlike body.

g. clitoris, a small, rounded tubercule of spongy, erectile tissue situated at the free extremity of the clitoris.

g. penis, a caplike conical enlargement at the distal extremity of the corpus spongiosum. The glans forms a concave surface into which the corpora cavernosa insert, and projects over the margins of the body of the penis to form the corona.

Glanzmann's thrombasthenia (glahnz′manz) [Edward *Glanzmann,* Swiss pediatrician, 1887–1959] see *thrombasthenia.*

glass (glas) [L. *vitrum*] 1. a hard, brittle, amorphous (noncrystalline) solid made of fused silica and various metallic oxides, silicates, and carbonates. Untinted glass can transmit more than 95 percent of visible light.

2. a container made of glass.

3. an amorphous solid that is reversibly changed to a liquid on heating.

borosilicate g., a type of strong, heat-resistant glass that contains at least 5 percent boric oxide; used in laboratory glassware.

cover g., a thin glass plate on a glass slide used to cover an object.

heat-resistant g., 1. low-alkali, borosilicate glass; made from silica and boric oxide, it has high resistance to heat, corrosion, and thermal shock. Trademarks, *Pyrex* and Kimax.

2. pure silica glass; it can withstand higher heat and chemical corrosion than can borosilicate glass. Trademark, Vycor.

3. chemically strengthened alumina-silicate glass; it is six times stronger than borosilicate glass. Trademark, Corex.

low-actinic g., glass that is tinted to absorb light in the range of 300–500 nm in order to protect light-sensitive contents, e.g., bilirubin.

optical g., glass having uniformity of refractive index (RI) and light dispersion used to make lenses and prisms. Types of optical glass include crown (calcium containing, low RI), flint (lead containing, high RI), and fluorite (high dispersion).

glass-bead retention method see *Salzman method.*

glass-ceramic a material having the composition of glass but with crystalline structure. Because of its high heat and corrosion resistance, it is used to make laboratory bench tops, hot plates, and heat exchangers.

glass fiber filter a filter composed entirely of borosilicate fibers, which gives a combination of fine retention and extremely rapid filtering speed. It is used especially for the filtration of heavy viscous solutions or gels.

glassy (glas′e) like glass; hyaline.

glassy cell carcinoma a carcinoma of the uterine cervix that is characterized by the presence of large tumor cells with a filmy, hazy-appearing cytoplasm that is granular and vacuolated. These cells have large nuclei with large, prominent nucleoli, which must not be mistaken for inclusions of herpesvirus in Papanicolaou stains.

glassy membrane 1. the basal lamina surrounding the theca interna of some atretic (degenerated) ovarian follicles, which becomes thicker and more nearly transparent in the degenerative process.

2. the basal lamina separating the external root sheath of a hair follicle from the underlying connective tissue.

3. see *Bruch's membrane* (of the eye).

glauc/o (glaw′ko) a word element used in combining form to denote gray, e.g., glaucoma.

glaucoma (glaw-ko′mah) [Gr. *glaukōma* opacity of

the lens] a group of diseases of the eye that share the pathogenic mechanism of increasing the intraocular pressure to a level sufficient to damage tissue, especially the optic nerve; they are the leading cause of adult blindness. Pressure of aqueous humor builds up within the eye either because its outflow at several possible points is obstructed, or less commonly because it is produced at an excessively rapid rate. If untreated, the condition can lead to visual field defects and eventually to blindness. It affects more than 2 percent of those over 40 and may be more common in persons with diabetes mellitus.

angle closure g., an acute, painful glaucoma marked by a sudden increase in intraocular pressure caused by blockage by the iris of the outflow channels in the angle. This condition may be of secondary or primary origin, the primary form being due to a genetic anatomic variation of the eye characterized by a shallow anterior chamber and a narrow angle. Also called narrow angle glaucoma.

congenital g., a developmental defect in the architecture of the eye so that the flow of aqueous humor is impaired or prevented, which leads to increasing intraocular pressure and glaucoma.

infantile g., congenital glaucoma that is fully developed at birth or in the first years of life. The eyes are enlarged, with hazy corneas.

open angle g., glaucoma in which the intraocular pressure is elevated owing to an outflow obstruction caused by degeneration of the nearby efferent channels, the trabecular network, or Schlemm's canal. It can occur as a primary or secondary condition. Also called simple glaucoma and chronic glaucoma.

primary g., genetically determined glaucoma. Primary glaucoma can be further divided into angle closure and open angle forms.

secondary g., glaucoma secondary to another ocular disorder such as tumor, inflammation, or trauma. It can be further divided into angle closure and open angle forms.

GLC abbrev. for gas-liquid chromatography. See under *gas chromatography.*

glenoid cavity (gle′noid kav′ĭ-te) [Gr. *glēnē* socket + *eidos* form] a depression or socket in the superior lateral angle of the scapula that serves as the articular surface for the head of the humerus.

gli/o (gli′o) [Gr. *glia* glue] a word element used in combining form to denote glue or neuroglial tissue, e.g., glioma.

glia (gli′ah) [Gr. "glue"] see *neuroglia.*

gliadin (gli′ah-din) a principal protein of wheat. See under *gluten.*

glial (gli′al) of or pertaining to the neuroglia.

glioblast (gli′o-blast) [*glio-* + Gr. *blastos* germ] any of the embryonic epithelial cells developed about the neural tube, which become transformed into neuroglial or ependymal cells. Also called *spongioblast.*

glioblastoma (gli″o-blas-to′mah) a general term used to describe a grade III–IV malignant astrocytoma. See also *central nervous system tumors.*

g. multiforme, a term for an astrocytoma, grade III–IV, that reflects the aggressive behavior and cellular pleomorphism of these neoplasms. See also *astrocytoma.*

glioma (gli-o′mah) [*glio-* + *-oma*] a tumor of neuroglial cells (the supporting cells of the central nervous system). Gliomas include astrocytomas, oligodendrogliomas, and ependymomas.

Glisson's capsule (glis′unz) [Francis *Glisson,* English physician and anatomist, 1597–1677, one of the founders of the Royal Society] a sheath of areolar connective tissue that surrounds the vessels and ducts through the hepatic portal canals. It is continuous with the fibrous capsule of the liver.

Gln abbrev. See *glutamine.*

globin (glo′bin) any member of a group of globulin proteins similar to those polypeptides occurring in hemoglobin and myoglobin. Globins are tetramers in hemoglobin and monomers in myoglobin, and are synthesized on the ribosomes in the cytoplasm of the erythroblast and reticulocyte. They are bound to the heme moiety by the iron in the heme and by the negative charges on the porphyrin ring.

-globin (glo′bin) a suffix word element to denote protein, e.g., hemoglobin.

globose (glo′bōs) [L. *globus* a ball] globe shaped, spherical.

globoside (glob′o-sid) the predominant glycolipid in erythrocyte membranes. The general composition is ceramide-$(\text{glucose})_m$-$(\text{galactose})_n$-(N-acetylhexosamine$)_p$. Globoside is a component only of plasma membranes and has been isolated from the kidney and leukocytes; it may be present in the plasma membranes of other cells.

globular (glob′u-lar) 1. like a globe or globule. 2. composed of globules.

globular protein a class of proteins that are soluble in water, usually in the presence of salts. The molecules are spheroidal or ellipsoidal in shape when in solution. The class encompasses a large variety of protein types, such as albumins, globulins, and basic proteins, and includes all known enzymes, oxygen-transport proteins, and protein hormones. The globular shape is in part held together by the large array of hydrogen bonds existing within the molecule. In addition, internally placed aliphatic and aromatic R groups form hydrophobic bonds to further support the spherical structure. Internally located electrostatic bonds also stabilize the shape.

The surface of the protein molecule is mainly hydrophilic and many polar groups, including both cationic and anionic R groups of amino acids, are hydrated and in contact with a layer of water molecules (bound water) surrounding the protein. This water layer also helps support the globular structure. The surface of each protein has a net electrical charge, the polarity of which depends on the pH of the buffered solvent and on the kind and number of proton-binding groups.

globule (glob′ūl) [L. *globulus* globule] a small spherical mass or body.

globulin (glob′u-lin) [L. *globulus* globule] an operational definition for a large group of proteins; included are those proteins insoluble in pure water, those soluble in solutions containing salt in low concentrations (0.10–0.50 mol/l), and those insoluble in solutions containing salt at high concentrations (1.7–3.5 mol/l). The actual solubility range for any globulin depends on the kind of salt (ionic strength) used, the actual protein structure, and the solvent dielectric strength. The definition has been of most relevance in the study of plasma proteins. By use of electrophoresis, globulins are further separated into α-, β-, and γ-globulins, and even into subfractions of these subclasses. Each group or subgroup may include many individual specific proteins.

-globulin (glob′u-lin) a suffix word element to denote protein, e.g., gamma globulin.

α_1-globulin see *alpha₁-globulin.*

globus (glo′bus), pl. *globi* [L.] 1. [NA], a general term denoting a large spherical mass.

2. a subjective sensation, as of a lump or mass, e.g., *g. hystericus.*

g. hystericus, the subjective sensation of a lump in the throat, a condition frequently seen in patients with hysterical conversion symptoms.

g. pallidus, [NA], the small, pale, medial portion of the lentiform nucleus, separated from the putamen by the external medullary lamina. It is the main efferent center of the basal ganglia and may be damaged in various conditions, including Parkinson's disease, resulting in disordered regulation of motor function.

glomangioma (glo-man″je-o′mah) [*glomus* + Gr. *angeion* vessel + *ōma* tumor] see *glomus tumor.*

glomera aortica (glom′er-ah a-or′tĭ-kah) [L., *glomera,* pl. of *glomus* a ball + *aortica*] [NA], see *aortic bodies.*

glomerul/o (glo-mer′u-lo) a word element used in combining form to denote the glomerulus, e.g., glomerulonephritis.

glomerular (glo-mer′u-lar) pertaining to or of the nature of a glomerulus. The term is used most frequently to refer to the renal glomerulus.

glomerular basal lamina the basement membrane of the renal corpuscle. Relatively thick (approximately 330 nm), it is thought to act as a selective filter, allowing the passage of water and small molecules while excluding large molecules and red blood cells.

glomerular filtration the process by which blood plasma diffuses across the glomerular capillary membrane of the kidney into Bowman's capsule. During this process, the effective filtration pressure is equal to the blood pressure in the glomerulus minus the pressure opposing filtration, i.e., the osmotic pressure of the plasma proteins. The glomerular filtrate normally contains no cells and almost no protein (about 0.03 g/dl). The concentration of electrolytes and other small solutes in the filtrate is the same as in plasma, except that chloride and bicarbonate are about 5 percent higher in order to balance the excess of positive protein ions in the filtrate.

Damage to the glomerular membrane can allow the passage of plasma proteins in the urine; the extent of proteinuria depends on the degree of glomerular damage; see also *glomerulopathy.*

glomerular filtration rate (GFR) the rate at which a given compound passes through the glomeruli per time unit (generally per minute). If such a compound is not reabsorbed or excreted by the tubules, the amount of compound found in the urine per unit time is a measure of the GFR. Inulin fulfills these requirements and thus the inulin clearance test is used as a measure of the GFR.

As inulin clearance tests are not commonly performed in clinical laboratories, the endogenous creatinine clearance test serves as a substitute, although values are slightly lower. The average GFR is 125 ml/min. The clearance rate in a normal individual is related to body surface area. Values are therefore corrected by multiplying with the factor: 1.73/A, where 1.73 is the average body surface and A is the patient's body surface area in square meters. The GFR can also be obtained by measuring the clearance of radioiostope-labeled compounds such as ^{125}I-iothalamate and ^{131}I-diatrizoate. See also *creatinine clearance.* Cf. *inulin clearance.*

glomerulitis (glo-mer″u-li′tis) [*glomerul-* + *-itis* inflammation] an inflammation of the renal glomeruli. See also *glomerulopathy.*

glomerulonephritis (glo-mer″u-lo-nĕ-fri′tis) [*glomerulo-* + Gr. *nephros* kidney + *-itis* inflammation] see *glomerulopathy.*

acute g., a glomerulopathy of rapid onset associated with an excellent prognosis. See also under *glomerulopathy.*

antibasement membrane g., see under *glomerulopathy.*

chronic g., a glomerulopathy of insidious onset, which leads to renal failure. Scarring damage of the kidney is so severe that the original process cannot be determined morphologically.

diffuse g., see under *glomerulopathy.*

focal g., see under *glomerulopathy.*

membranous-proliferative g., see under *glomerulopathy.*

mesangial proliferative g., see under *glomerulopathy.*

postinfectious g., see under *glomerulopathy.*

rapidly progressive g., see under *glomerulopathy.*

glomerulopathy (glo-mer″u-lop′ah-the) [*glomerulo-* + Gr. *pathos* disease] the general term used to describe diseases affecting the renal glomeruli. Individuals with a glomerulopathy may present with the nephrotic syndrome, nephritis (hematuria, hypertension, and varying degrees of renal failure), a combination of the nephrotic syndrome and nephritis, or hematuria and/or proteinuria. The forms of glomerulopathies most frequently associated with the nephrotic syndrome include membranous nephropathy, epithelial cell disease, focal segmental glomerulosclerosis, diabetic glomerulosclerosis, and amyloid deposition. Most proliferative glomerulopathies are associated with nephritis and/or hematuria. Persons with mesangiocapillary glomerulopathy frequently have both nephritis and the nephrotic syndrome.

A glomerulopathy may result from a disease process limited to the kidneys or may be part of a multisystem disease. Conversely, a single morphologic type of glomerulopathy (e.g., crescentic glomerulopathy) may be caused by a large number of different diseases, and a single systemic disease process (e.g., lupus erythematosus) may cause many different types of morphologic lesions. For example, mesangial proliferative glomerulopathy with mesangial IgA and/or IgG deposits may be the glomerular manifestation of Henoch-Schönlein syndrome. (When an identical morphologic and immunologic disease process is limited to the kidneys, it is known as IgA or Berger's nephropathy.) There are many entities that result in crescentic glomerulopathy, including antibasement membrane glomerulopathy, idiopathic crescentic glomerulopathy, and postinfectious glomerulopathy, as well as a number of systemic diseases such as Wegener's granulomatosis, Henoch-Schönlein syndrome, and lupus erythematosus. Although most examples of membranous nephropathy are of the idiopathic type, a minority are associated with known antigens. Epithelial cell disease and focal glomerulosclerosis apparently are processes in which only the kidney is involved.

CLASSIFICATION. The classification of the glomerulopathies is based on morphologic changes due to the response of the affected glomeruli to injury. In the case of immunologic insult, the classification is also based on the pattern of immunofluorescence and the location of immune complexes as determined by electron microscopy. Frequently, light microscopy, immunofluorescence, and electron microscopy are all needed to classify a glomerulopathy accurately. A morphologic classification of glomerulopathies is presented in the accompanying table. Some of the terms used to describe the distribution of glomerular disease employed in the diagnostic categories include focal, meaning that some but not all glomeruli are affected; diffuse, meaning that all or nearly all of the glomeruli are affected; segmental, meaning that only affected portions of an individual glomerulus are involved; and global, meaning that the entire glomerulus is involved.

The proliferative glomerulopathies are characterized by an increase in the number of glomerular cells. Inflammatory cells may also be present. The subcategories are defined by types of cells proliferating and the extent of cellular proliferation, as well as by the type and location of immune complexes. Inflammation and necrosis are frequent findings in proliferative glomerulopathies. Diffuse, generalized proliferative glomerulopathy almost always results from trapping of circulating immune complexes in the glomeruli following an infection in another site, usually streptococcal pharyngitis. The deposits can be demonstrated by immunofluorescent and ultrastructural techniques. When 80 percent or more of the glomeruli reveal florid parietal epithelial proliferation filling or partially filling Bowman's space, the term crescentic glomerulopathy is used. Focal and segmental proliferation is a common and often nonspecific response of the glomerulus to injury. Such changes may be associated with a wide variety of renal and systemic diseases.

Mesangial proliferation (mesangial proliferative glomerulopathy) is also a common response to a wide variety of different injuries. When associated with IgA and/or IgG in the mesangium without evidence of systemic disease, the term IgA or Berger's glomerulopathy is used; when IgM is the globulin in the mesangium, the process is labeled mesangial proliferative glomerulopathy with IgM. When mesangial proliferation is associated with IgA or

GLOMERULOPATHY. MORPHOLOGIC CLASSIFICATION BASED ON LIGHT MICROSCOPY, ELECTRON MICROSCOPY, AND IMMUNOFLUORESCENCE

CATEGORY	DESCRIPTION
I	Proliferative glomerulopathies (with and without inflammation)
	A. Diffuse generalized (almost always postinfectious etiology)
	B. Crescentic
	C. Focal and segmental
	D. Mesangial proliferative
	With IgA
	With IgM
	E. Mesangiocapillary (membranoproliferative)
	Type I
	Type II
	Type III
II	Membranous glomerulopathy
	A. Idiopathic
	B. Secondary
III	Epithelial cell disease (minimal lesion, lipoid nephrosis)
IV	Focal segmental glomerulosclerosis
V	Changes in capillary wall in the absence of deposits
	A. Diabetic glomerulopathy
	B. Familial and hereditary nephropathies
VI	Deposition of immunoglobulins secondary to abnormal production or configuration
	A. Myeloma and light-chain diseases
	B. Amyloid
	C. Cryoglobulinemia
VII	Chronic glomerulopathy and end-stage renal disease

Courtesy of Richard L. Kempson, M.D.

IgG in the mesangium with systemic disease, i.e., vasculitis, the term Henoch-Schönlein syndrome is used.

Mesangiocapillary glomerulopathy (membranoproliferative glomerulopathy) is characterized by mesangial cell proliferation and interposition of mesangial cell cytoplasm along the capillary basement membranes. The subcategories of this entity are based on the distribution of immune complexes and protein in the glomeruli. Type I is characterized by subendothelial immune complex deposits, type II by dense protein deposits within the basement membrane, and type III by subepithelial deposits.

Membranous glomerulopathy is defined as the presence of regular, small subepithelial deposits of immune complexes around the capillary basement membranes unassociated with significant cellular proliferation. Epithelial cell disease is not associated with immune complexes and the glomerulus is normal by light microscopy. Ultrastructurally, there is almost total epithelial cell process obliteration. Focal segmental glomerulosclerosis features focal sclerotic glomerular lesions containing IgM.

DIAGNOSIS. Almost all glomerulopathies are associated with morphologic changes in the glomeruli, which can be recognized by using light or electron microscopic techniques. Morphologically similar glomerulopathies, with some exceptions, have similar outcomes and similar responses to therapy; hence, renal biopsy is a useful diagnostic technique. Most, but not all, glomerulopathies result from immunologic injury during which immunoglobulins are deposited in the affected glomeruli. It is possible to detect these immunoglobulins in tissue sections. Almost all of the immune-mediated human glomerulopathies result from one of two types of immunologic injury: glomerular deposition of circulating immune complexes formed elsewhere (immune complex glomerulopathy), or host antibodies reacting against constituents of the glomerular basement membranes or against antigens trapped in the basement membranes (antibasement membrane glomerulopathy). Immune complexes may be demonstrated by immunofluorescent techniques as granular or bumpy deposits in the glomeruli, whereas antibodies against antigens in the basement membrane are distributed in a smooth linear pattern. In addition, immunofluorescent techniques can be used to determine the localization of immune complexes whether in the mesangium, the capillary basement membranes, or both. Examination of renal tissue using the electron microscope also reveals the location of immune complexes because the complexes stain with electron-dense heavy metals such as lead and uranium. Electron microscopy may also be used to detect morphologic alterations that cannot be resolved with the light microscope.

Also called *glomerulonephritis.*

RICHARD KEMPSON, M.D.

glomerulosclerosis (glo-mer″u-lo-skle-ro′sis) [*glomerulo-* + Gr. *sklēros* hard + *-osis* condition] see *glomerulopathy.*

glomerulus (glo-mer′u-lus), pl. *glomeruli* [L., dim. of *glomus* ball] a general term used to denote a tuft or cluster, usually of blood vessels or nerve fibers; used alone to designate one of the glomeruli of the kidney. See also *kidney.*

glomus (glo′mus), pl. *glomera* [L. "a ball"] [NA], a small arteriovenous shunt, commonly located in the skin but also found in deeper structures, which is concerned with temperature regulation. The anastomotic channel (Sucquet-Hoyer canal) is lined by modified smooth muscle (glomus) cells. See also *glomus tumor.*

glomera aortica, see *aortic bodies.*

g. caroticum, see *carotid body.*

g. coccygeum, a small, irregular mass of arteriovenous anastomoses adjacent to the apex of the coccyx.

g. intravagale, see *intravagal p.* under *paraganglion.*

glomus tumor a tumor arising from modified smooth muscle cells in the wall of an arteriovenous shunt (Sucquet-Hoyer canal) found principally in the skin, where it functions in temperature regulation. Glomus tumors are almost always benign. They form small nodules that are often exquisitely tender. The tips of the fingers are the commonest location, but other parts of the skin, and deeper structures such as the stomach, may also be involved. Occasionally, multiple glomus tumors and familial cases are reported. Also called *glomangioma.*

gloss/o (glos′o) [Gr. *glōssa* tongue] a word element used in combining form to denote tongue, e.g., glossitis.

glossal (glos′al) pertaining to the tongue; lingual.

Glossina (glos-si′nah) a genus of biting flies. It includes species of tsetse flies (e.g., *G. morsitans, G. pallidipes,* and *G. palpalis*) that transmit the organisms *Trypanosoma gambiense,* the cause of sleeping sickness, and *T. rhodesiense,* the cause of Rhodesian trypanosomiasis.

glossitis (glo-si′tis) [*gloss-* + *-itis*] any inflammation of the tongue. Glossitis is commonly encountered in states of malnutrition such as pellagra, in which the normal growth and replacement of mucosal cells is limited. Redness and a smooth, irritated tongue surface are seen.

glossopharyngeal (glos″o-fah-rin′je-al) [*gloss-* + *pharynx*] pertaining to the tongue and pharynx or to the cranial nerve (IX) of that name.

glossopharyngeal nerve cranial nerve IX; mainly a sensory nerve to the pharynx, posterior tongue (including taste), and middle ear. It also carries motor fibers to the stylopharyngeus muscle and secretory fibers to the parotid gland. The motor fibers arise in the medulla. The sensory ganglia are in the jugular foramen. The nerve leaves the cranial cavity through the jugular foramen and descends through the neck between the internal jugular vein and the internal carotid artery, then curves forward under the submandibular gland and breaks up into its terminal branches. See also *cranial nerves.*

glottal (glot′al) pertaining to the glottis.

glottis (glot′is), pl. *glottides* [L. *glōttis*] [NA], the vocal apparatus of the larynx, consisting of the vocal folds and cords and the opening between them (rima glottidis).

glow modulator tube an electronic device that produces a light pulse proportional to the current pulse input. It is used in some rectilinear scanners as the light source in the photorecorder.

Glu abbrev. See *glutamic acid.*

gluc/o (gloo′ko) [Gr. *gleukos* sweetness] a word element used in combining form to denote sweetness, and more specifically a relationship to glucose, e.g., glucocorticosteroids and gluconeogenesis.

glucagon (gloo'kah-gon) a polypeptide hormone consisting of 29 amino acids; M.W. 3485. The glucagon hormone is secreted by the alpha cells of the islets of Langerhans in the pancreas in response to hypoglycemia, beta-adrenergic compounds, and amino acids. Glucagon acts to elevate glucose levels in blood by promoting glycogenolysis in the liver via activation of hepatic adenylate cyclase. Other actions of glucagon consist of the breakdown of protein and lipids. In general, the function of glucagon is to mobilize stored fuels and make them available for needy tissues. In addition to its action on hepatic glycogenolysis, glucagon also stimulates gluconeogenesis and ketogenesis. In general, the actions of insulin and glucagon are antagonistic, and thus fuel homeostasis is achieved by a precise coordination of the secretion of these two hormones.

Another hormone also produced by a different pancreatic islet cell (D-cells), somatostatin, inhibits the secretion of both insulin and glucagon. Glucagon's secretion is inhibited by insulin, whereas glucagon stimulates both the secretion of insulin and somatostatin. Thus, an interplay between these three hormones elaborated between the neighboring cells of the islets and the regulation achieved by each other's secretion effects the eventual metabolism of fuels.

A neoplasm of islet alpha cells known as glucagonoma, which may be more likely to be malignant than insulinomas and which occurs most frequently in postmenopausal females, has clinical features that include glucose intolerance, an erythematous and eczematous dermatitis, glossitis, stomatitis, vaginitis, and unexplained weight loss. Laboratory findings, in addition to pronounced fasting hyperglucagonemia with hyperglycemia, may include anemia, hypoproteinemia, hypoaminoacidemia, and hypolipidemia. It should be noted that glucagonomas (as other islet tumors) may secrete multiple hormones.

Other causes of mild hyperglucagonemia are diabetes mellitus, burn injury, acute trauma, bacteremia, cirrhosis, renal failure, and Cushing's syndrome. Glucagon deficiency may occur in idiopathic alpha-cell deficiency and chronic pancreatitis, leading to hypoglycemia. Plasma glucagon concentration can be measured by radioimmunoassay (RIA).

Glucagon is used clinically in the treatment of hypoglycemia and also as a diagnostic test for some types of glycogen storage disease, insulinomas, growth hormone deficiency, and pheochromocytoma.

Also called *hyperglycemic-glycogenolytic factor* (HGF).

N. V. BHAGAVAN, PH.D.

glucagon for injection [USP], a lyophilized preparation of glucagon dissolved in diluting solution. It is used, by injection, for the treatment of severe hypoglycemic states in diabetic patients and during insulin shock therapy. One milliliter of the prepared solution contains 1 unit (1 mg) of pure glucagon; the diluent is water at the proper pH, containing glycerol (1.6 percent) and phenol (0.2 percent preservative). Glucagon acts only on liver glycogen, and carbohydrate is given orally to restore liver glycogen.

glucagonoma (glu"kah-gon-o'mah) a tumor of the pancreatic islets that forms glucagon. The hormone is usually elevated in the serum, and can be demonstrated in sections of the tumor immunocytochemically. Most of the component cells are A cells. More than half of the tumors are malignant. Clinically, the patient typically has mild diabetes and a distinctive skin rash (migratory necrolytic erythema), and may be anemic and have diarrhea. The clinical spectrum is not precise since more than one hormone is frequently produced in addition to the glucagon. See also *pancreatic tumors.*

glucan (gloo'kan) a homopolymer of glucose. Examples include glycogen, a storage polymer of glucose in animals; starch, the storage carbohydrate of plants; cellulose, occurring mainly in plants as a structural component; and dextrans, which are gelatinous polymers that coat some bacteria.

1,4-α-glucan branching enzyme an enzyme of the transferase class (EC 2.4.1.18) that catalyzes the transfer of a segment of the amylose chain to a primary hydroxyl group in a glucan chain, resulting in a new branch in a glycogen molecule (glycogen branching enzyme) or amylopectin molecule (amylopectin branching enzyme). A genetic deficiency, transmitted as an autosomal recessive trait, occurs in type IV glycogen storage disease (amylopectinosis, Andersen's disease). The clinical symptoms include hepatosplenomegaly, ascites, cirrhosis, and liver failure. Diagnosis is made by measuring leukocyte branching enzyme activity. Also called *branching enzyme* and *Q enzyme.*

D-glucaric acid (gloo-kar'ik) see *saccharic acid.*

glucitol see *sorbitol.*

glucocerebrosidase (gloo"ko-ser"ě-bro-si'dās) see *glucosylceramidase.*

glucocerebroside (gloo"ko-ser'ě-bro-sīd") a ceramide monosaccharide (a glucosyl derivative of ceramide). It accumulates in the tissues in Gaucher's disease as a breakdown product of ceramide-oligosaccharides. See also *galactocerebroside.*

glucocorticoid (gloo"ko-kor'ti-koid) a hormone, produced by the adrenals, that has distinct effects on carbohydrate metabolism including the promotion of gluconeogenesis, liver glycogen deposition, and elevation of blood glucose concentrations. These hormones also accelerate the breakdown of protein such as albumin, and inhibit amino acid uptake and protein synthesis by many extrahepatic tissues. In supraphysiologic amounts, glucocorticoids inhibit the inflammatory and allergic reactions of naturally occurring steroids. Only cortisol, cortisone, corticosterone, and 11-dehydrocorticosterone have appreciable glucocorticoid activity, and of these cortisol is the most potent. See also *cortisol.*

glucofuranose (gloo"ko-fu'rah-nōs) the furanose form of glucose in which the molecule has a 5-membered ring.

glucogenesis (gloo"ko-jen'ě-sis) the formation of glucose from other metabolites. If the source is glycogen, the process is called glycogenolysis, which occurs in the liver. If the sources are amino acids, fatty acids, and pyruvic and other oxo-acids, the process is referred to as gluconeogenesis and requires energy. Other intermediary products of glycolysis such as fructose-6-phosphate can also give glucose directly.

glucogenic (gloo″ko-jen′ik) giving rise to or producing glucose, either through gluconeogenesis or glycogenolysis.

glucokinase (gloo″ko-ki′nās) an enzyme of the transferase class (ATP: D-glucose-6-phosphotransferase, EC 2.7.1.2) that catalyzes the reaction ATP + D-glucose ⇄ ADP + D-glucose-6-phosphate. Under physiologic conditions the reaction favors the production of D-glucose-6-phosphate. This enzyme is one of a group of enzymes involved in the regulation of the blood glucose concentration.

gluconeogenesis (gloo″ko-ne″o-jen′ĕ-sis) the formation of glucose from noncarbohydrate sources such as lactate, amino acids, and glycerol.

gluconeogenetic (gloo″ko-ne″o-jĕ-net′ik) pertaining to or involved in gluconeogenesis.

glucopyranose (gloo″ko-pi′rah-nōs) the pyranose form of glucose in which C-1 and C-5 are joined by a hemiacetal linkage to form a six-membered (pyran) ring.

glucosamine (gloo″ko-sam′ēn) an amino sugar (2-amino-2-deoxy-α-D-glucose), a hexosamine, that sometimes occurs as a structural carbohydrate, although the *N*-acetyl derivative is more commonly found. It is obtained from mucin and chitin by hydrolysis.

***N*-acetyl g.,** the structural unit of chitin, a polysaccharide of arthropods, beetles, and some fungi. It is found in mucoproteins and mucopolysaccharides. See also *glucose.*

glucose (gloo′kōs) [Gr. *gleukos* sweetness; *glykys* sweet] a monosaccharide, an aldohexose, a reducing sugar; it is a main source of energy for living organisms. Glucose occurs naturally in the free state in fruits and other parts of plants; it is combined in glucosides, in many di- and oligosaccharides, in the polysaccharides cellulose and starch, and in glycogen. In therapy it is used in intravenous fluids as a nutrient.

Naturally occurring sugars (including glucose) are mostly of the D-configuration, but can also exist as α-, β-, or mixed α- and β-anomers.

The assignment of D or L to the enantiomers of glucose depends on the configuration at C-5. If it is the same as D-glyceraldehyde, it is labeled D or DG. L or LG is used to specify the relationship to L-glyceraldehyde.

At equilibrium in aqueous solution, glucose exists as a mixture of two anomeric cyclic forms and the open-chain form. In the open-chain form, glucose has an aldehyde group and five hydroxyl groups with a total of four chiral centers. In the cyclic form, the C-5 hydroxyl group has reacted with the aldehyde group to form a cyclic hemiacetal with an additional chiral center. Thus, in the cyclic form, glucose exists as two stereoisomers (anomers), one in which the hemiacetal hydroxyl is in the plane of the ring (an equatorial substituent) designated as the α-anomer, and the other in which that hydroxyl is perpendicular to the ring (an axial substituent) designated as the β-anomer. To indicate the formation of a six-membered ring, glucose in its cyclic form can be named glucopyranose. The equilibrium mixture contains about 64 percent of the β-anomer, about 36 percent of the α-anomer, and only 0.024 percent of the open-chain form in neutral solution. It is the open-chain aldehyde that acts as reducing agent; thus, glucose is a reducing sugar (as are other sugars that are hemiacetals or hemiketals). If a single anomer is dissolved in water, the optical rotation changes from that of the pure anomer to that of the mixture as equilibrium is established. This is an example of the phenomenon of mutarotation. The illustration accompanying *isomerism* shows the Fischer projections of the open chain forms of D- and L-glucose, the Fischer and Haworth projections of α- and β-D-glucose, and the conformational representation of the latter.

Formerly called blood sugar, dextrose, and grape sugar. See also *anomer, isomerism,* and *mutarotation.*

renal threshold for g., the plasma glucose concentration above which glucose cannot be reabsorbed by the renal tubules and thus appears in the urine, i.e., at a concentration of approximately 180 (150–190) mg/dl.

glucose assays 1. hexokinase methods. Hexokinase enzymatically catalyzes the phosphorylation of glucose by ATP to form glucose-6-phosphate (G-6-P). In the indicator reaction, a second enzyme, glucose-6-phosphate dehydrogenase (G-6-PD), is used to catalyze the oxidation of G-6-P by NADP to form NADPH in direct proportion to the amount of glucose originally present. NADPH production is measured photometrically at 340 nm. The procedure is highly specific and capable of high accuracy and precision. It can be used directly with serum without deproteinization. The hexokinase method has been accepted as a reference procedure.

2. glucose oxidase method. In this enzymatic method, the enzyme glucose oxidase (GO) catalyzes the reaction of glucose to gluconic acid by molecular oxygen, with formation of hydrogen peroxide (H_2O_2). In one version of this procedure, the oxygen consumed in this reaction is measured with an oxygen electrode, and the decrease in PO_2 is used as a measure of glucose concentration. In most other versions of the GO procedure, peroxidase transfers oxygen from the H_2O_2 formed to an organic chromogen to form a colored product, which is measured photometrically. *o*-Toluidine and *o*-dianisidine have been used as oxygen acceptors. The GO acts only on β-D-glucose, and thus the reaction mixture should contain a D-glucose racemase to convert the α-D-glucose to the beta form. Alternatively, the H_2O_2 formed in the GO reaction can also be measured by a hydrogen-peroxide electrode.

The GO procedures are also fairly specific; however, in the peroxidase coupled procedure, oxygen acceptors such as ascorbic acid and urates may interfere if present in higher than normal concentrations.

3. *o*-toluidine methods. Glucose and other aldoses and ketoses condense with aromatic amines to form a colored product, which can be measured colorimetrically. *o*-Toluidine is the agent most commonly used. Other sugars react also but give products with much less color intensity, with the exception of D-galactose, which is more reactive than glucose. Saccharoids do not react or interfere with the reagent.

4. reduction methods. Procedures based on the reduction of metallic ions such as Cu^{2+} or ferricyanide were once popular, but their use has been discontinued owing to lack of specificity. The only copper reduction method still in use is that for the semiquantitative determination of reducing substances

in urine (Clinitest). This test is retained mainly because of its convenience and its ability to screen for the presence of other reducing sugars in urine. More specific qualitative tests for the detection of glucose in urine involve the GO reaction (e.g. Clinistix, Tes-Tape). The quantitative determination of glucose in urine can be carried out with the above-mentioned hexokinase techniques or the GO method based on oxygen consumption.

glucose metabolism an essential process for the maintenance of life in humans and most organisms. Normally, glucose is the only carbohydrate (CHO)x found in significant amounts in body fluids; its oxidation can produce a significant fraction of the energy required by the cells of the body. In fact, in normal circumstances there is an absolute requirement for glucose as the metabolic fuel for both brain cells and red blood cells. Glucose may participate in all three aspects of metabolism: anabolic, intermediate, and catabolic. It can follow the three metabolic pathways of glycolysis, glycogenesis, and the pentose-phosphate shunt. By being transformed into appropriate products, it can provide carbon skeletons for the synthesis of proteins, lipids, other carbohydrates, and heteropolysaccharides.

Normal fasting plasma glucose concentrations in humans may have a range of 65–105 mg/dl (3.6–5.9 mmol/l). If for any reason plasma levels rise to above normal (hyperglycemia), hormonal mechanisms act to remove glucose from blood and deposit it in liver and muscle cells as glycogen for later use, and in adipose tissue as triacylglycerol. Similarly, a fall in plasma glucose (hypoglycemia) is counteracted by a release of glucose from the liver by glycogenolysis or by synthesis de novo from amino acids (gluconeogenesis).

In glycolysis, glucose is converted to a series of phosphorylated six- and three-carbon intermediates, which eventually yields 2 mol of pyruvate (a three-carbon intermediate), 2 mol of NADH (reducing equivalents oxidized in the electron transport system of mitochondria), and 2 mol of ATP (stored biochemical energy) per mol of glucose. Pyruvate may be processed along a number of varied metabolic pathways: reduction to lactate, oxidation to produce energy via the tricarboxylic pathway (producing 36 mol of ATP), synthesis of fatty acids via acetyl CoA, and conversion to some of the nonessential amino acids.

Glucose is also metabolized through the pentose-phosphate shunt (10 percent in humans and up to 40 percent in other organisms based on cell specialization) via a series of three-, five-, and seven-carbon phosphorylated sugars. Every mole of glucose produces 6 mol of CO_2 and 12 mol of NADPH, which is essential for many synthetic reactions (such as fatty acid synthesis). The by-products of this pathway provide ribose phosphate for nucleic acid synthesis.

Glucose in excess of needs is converted into a highly branched polyglucan (glycogen) and stored in liver and muscle cells by a synthetase system. When the energy of glucose is needed, the glycogen is phosphorylized to glucose-6-phosphate by a different enzyme system involving an allosteric phosphorylase.

Glucose homeostasis in humans is under complex control by a number of regulating mechanisms including hormones, allosteric enzymes, and humoral agents. Among the hormones affecting glucose metabolism are insulin, glucagon, thyroxine, somatostatin, cortisol, and epinephrine. The main disease group involving a breakdown in glucose homeostasis is diabetes mellitus, reflecting in part a diminished output of insulin or a diminished number of functioning insulin receptors on cells.

glucose oxidase (gloo′kōs ok′sĭ-dās) an enzyme of the oxidoreductase class (β-D-glucose:oxygen 1-oxidoreductase, EC 1.1.3.4) that catalyzes the reaction β-D-glucose + O_2 ⇄ D-glucono-δ-lactone + H_2O_2. The lactone may be further hydrolyzed to D-gluconic acid. The enzyme is a flavoprotein, highly specific for β-D-glucose. It is used in the clinical laboratory in the determination of "true" glucose.

glucose-6-phosphatase (gloo′kōs fos′fah-tās″) an enzyme of the hydrolase class (D-glucose-6-phosphate phosphohydrolase, ED 3.1.3.9) that catalyzes the reaction D-glucose-6-phosphate + H_2O ⇄ D-glucose + orthophosphate. Some preparations can act as a pyrophosphatase and others have transphosphatase activity. The enzyme is widely distributed in many animal tissues (e.g., liver, kidneys, intestinal mucosa) but is absent in vertebrate muscle. It occurs embedded in the lipids associated with endoplasmic reticulum, and its presence is used as an identifying marker for this organelle. The enzyme is defective or absent in type I glycogen storage disease (von Gierke's disease).

glucose-1-phosphate (gloo′kōs fos′fāt) an important intermediate in carbohydrate metabolism, $CH_2OH(CHOH)_4CHOPO_3^{2-}$. It is important for glycogen synthesis and breakdown, the metabolism of galactose, and the uronic acid pathway.

glucose-6-phosphate (G-6-P) the first compound, $CHO(CHOH)_4CH_2OPO_3^{2-}$, formed in the metabolism of glucose when glucose enters a cell. It is formed from glucose and ATP by the action of a kinase. It is an important junction compound in glucose metabolic pathways.

glucose-6-phosphate dehydrogenase (GPD, G-6-PD) (gloo′kōs fos′fāt de-hi′dro-jen-ās) an enzyme of the oxidoreductase class (D-glucose-6-phosphate:$NADP^+$ 1-oxidoreductase, EC 1.1.1.49) that catalyzes the reaction D-glucose-6-phosphate + $NADP^+$ ⇄ 6-phospho-D-glucono-δ-lactone + NADPH + H^+. The reaction is the first step in the pentose-phosphate shunt of glucose utilization, producing NADPH for synthetic reactions and pentose phosphates for nucleotide synthesis. Some 200 biochemical variants of the red blood cell enzyme have been described.

Activity of G-6-PD in erythrocytes increases in pernicious anemia, Werlhof's disease, hyperthyroidism, viral hepatitis, myelogenous leukemia, and in serum after myocardial infarction. Several forms of genetic deficiencies of the enzyme are recognized, affecting some black males, people of Chinese origin, and Sephardic Jews and other persons of Mediterranean origin. G-6-PD deficiencies cause a severe hemolytic crisis when those affected are treated with antimalarial or sulfonamide drugs or with some nonsulfonamide antibacterial agents on ingestion of a naturally occurring compound found in fava beans (favism). Hemolytic crisis can also occur when the stress of other illness is present.

G-6-PD is often used as an indicator enzyme in the activity measurement of other enzymes (e.g., creatine kinase) or substrates (e.g., glucose); it is determined by spectrophotometric measurement of the NADPH formed.

Also called *hexosephosphate dehydrogenase* and Zwischenferment.

glucose-6-phosphate dehydrogenase deficiency a genetic disorder, transmitted as an X-linked trait, in which deficiency of the red cell enzyme (in various polymorphic forms) is the basis for various anemias. These include favism, primaquine sensitivity and other drug-sensitive hemolytic anemias, anemia and jaundice in the newborn, and chronic nonspherocytic hemolytic anemia. The enzyme is important for the maintenance of cellular concentrations of reduced nucleotide, NADPH. See also *primaquine sensitivity.*

glucose-6-phosphate dehydrogenase tests 1. fluorescent spot test. Whole blood is mixed with G-6-P, NADP, saponin, and buffer (pH 7.8), incubated for 10–30 min, and spotted on filter paper. Spots of control blood or normal specimens fluoresce brightly (owing to NADPH); G-6-PD–deficient blood does not.

2. dye reduction test. Hemolyzed blood is incubated with G-6-P, NADP, and buffer, as well as the dye brillant crescent blue, which is reduced to a colorless form by NADPH. The time required to decolorize the solution is inversely proportional to the G-6-PD activity. This test is specific for G-6-PD deficiency but is not sensitive enough to detect heterozygotes.

3. ascorbate cyanide test. Aerated whole blood (EDTA, ACD, or heparin anticoagulant) is incubated at 37°C with ascorbate and cyanide. Ascorbate is oxidized in the presence of oxyhemoglobin, producing hydrogen peroxide. Because catalase is inhibited by cyanide, the H_2O_2 must be reduced by NADPH-dependent glutathione peroxidase. With G-6-PD–deficient blood, insufficient NADPH is produced and hemoglobin is oxidatively denatured by H_2O_2, forming a brown pigment in 1–4 hr.

4. quantitative assay for G-6-PD activity. In most assays, the activity of 6-phosphogluconate dehydrogenase (6-PGD), which catalyzes the next step in the hexose monophosphate pathway and also produces NADPH, is also determined, along with the true G-6-PD activity. The NADPH formed is quantitated spectrophotometrically at 340 nm or fluorometrically with excitation at 340 nm and emission at 460 nm. The combined activity of G-6-PD and 6-PGD is determined by incubating hemolyzed blood with NADP, G-6-P, and 6-phosphogluconate (6-GP) at pH 7.5 and 30°C; the G-6-PD activity is determined using a reaction mixture that is identical except that no G-6-P is added. The difference between the rates of NADPH formation in the two reactions gives the G-6-PD activity; the rate of NADPH formation in the second reaction gives the 6-PG-D activity.

5. see *Heinz body test.*

glucosephosphate isomerase (GPI) (gloo′kōs-fos′fāt i-som′er-ās) an enzyme of the isomerase class (D-glucose-6-phosphate ketolisomerase, EC 5.3.1.9) that catalyzes the reaction D-glucose 6-phosphate ⇄ D-fructose 6-phosphate. The reaction is an early step in glucose metabolism. The normal enzyme resolves into three electrophoretic bands with reports of mutations affecting enzyme activity and electrophoretic mobility. An increased serum activity of the enzyme has been used as an indicator of metastatic carcinoma and as a monitor in therapy. Decreased red cell enzyme activity is seen in hereditary nonspherocytic hemolytic anemia. Also called *hexosephosphate isomerase.*

glucosephosphate isomerase assays fructose-6-phosphate (F-6-P) is used as substrate and the isomerase reaction is coupled with the glucose-6-phosphate dehydrogenase (G-6-PD) reaction. The glucose-6-phosphate (G-6-P) formed in the first reaction is oxidized to 6-phosphogluconic acid, and the extent of the reaction is measured by the increase in the amount of NADPH. In an older method using G-6-P as substrate, the F-6-P formed is measured by some variant of the Selivanoff reaction (color formation with resorcinol).

glucosephosphate isomerase deficiency a hereditary red cell enzyme deficiency seen in association with hereditary nonspherocytic hemolytic anemia. It is second in prevalence to phosphokinase deficiency among Embden-Meyerhof pathway enzymes. A deficiency of GPI has been demonstrated in leukocytes, platelets, and tissues, but is not accompanied by functional impairment. Hepatic glycogen stores may be increased because of the diversion of glucose metabolism toward glycogen synthesis. Some patients may be improved by splenectomy.

glucose tolerance test a test used to measure the response of the body to a challenge load of glucose. It is used to aid in the diagnosis of diabetes mellitus, although today it is believed that the test is rarely useful except in pregnant patients suspected of having the disease. When a standard dose of glucose (e.g., 100 g) is given orally to a nondiabetic healthy individual, the ingested glucose is rapidly absorbed, and the rising blood glucose level stimulates the pancreatic beta cells to secrete insulin. This causes glucose to leave the blood and to enter muscle and hepatic cells, thus limiting the rise of blood glucose to approximately 60 percent above the fasting level, with a peak concentration 30–60 min after the glucose load. Fasting levels are reached at about 2.5–3 hr. In diabetic patients, the peak concentration of glucose is much higher and may not be reached until 2–3 hr after the glucose load, followed by a prolonged decrease in blood glucose concentration. The test is sensitive, perhaps too sensitive, but lacks specificity; diminished carbohydrate tolerance is encountered in many otherwise healthy elderly persons and is seen in patients with diminished hypothyroid, pituitary, or adrenocortical function, as well as after stress. False-negative results may be seen with gastrointestinal malabsorption.

Many test protocols have been developed over the years. In the most accepted protocol, for 3 da prior to the test, the patient is placed on a diet containing at least 250 g of carbohydrate. In the morning after an overnight fast, the patient is given 100 g (or 1.75 g/kg of body weight) of glucose orally, and blood specimens are collected before and 1, 2, and 3 hr after ingestion of the glucose. In some protocols, specimens are also collected at 30 and 90 min. A variety of criteria have been proposed for the diagnosis of diabetes, but have now been replaced by the following: (1) the fasting glucose concentration must be at least 140 mg/dl, and at least two of the specimens collected after the glucose load must exceed 200 mg/dl; (2) the 2-hr specimen must exceed 200 mg/dl.

The 2-hr postprandial glucose tolerance test is used to screen for diabetes mellitus. A plasma glucose concentration above 200 mg/dl obtained 2 hr after ingestion of either 100 g of glucose or a meal containing 100 g of carbohydrates is suggestive of the disease and warrants further evaluation. See also the accompanying table.

α-D-glucosidase (gloo-ko′sĭ-dās) an enzyme of the hydrolase class (α-1,4-glucosidase, EC 3.2.1.20) that catalyzes the hydrolysis of terminal, nonreducing 1,4-α-glucoside linkages in oligosaccharides with the release of α-glucose. The enzyme is defective or absent in type II glycogen storage disease (Pompe's disease), a hereditary disease transmitted as an autosomal recessive trait. Also called *maltase.* See also *disaccharidase deficiency.*

β-D-glucosidase a lysosomal enzyme of the hydrolase class (β-D-glucoside glucohydrolase, EC 3.2.1.21) that catalyzes the hydrolysis of terminal, nonreducing β-D-glucose residues with release of β-D-glucose. Also called *cellobiase* (although this may be a specific β-D-glucosidase).

glucoside (gloo′ko-sīd) a glycoside in which the sugar constituent is glucose.

glucosuria (gloo″ko-su′re-ah) [*glucose* + Gr. *ouron* urine + *-ia*] the presence of D-glucose in the urine at concentrations above the average normal concentration of 20–30 mg/dl. Also called *dextrosuria.*

glucosyl (gloo′ko-sil) a glucose radical.

glucosylceramidase (gloo″ko-sil-ser-am′ĭ-dās) an enzyme of the hydrolase class (EC 3.2.1.45) that catalyzes the reaction D-glucosyl-*N*-acylsphingosine + H_2O ⇄ D-glucose + *N*-acylsphingosine. A genetic deficiency of the enzyme causes the accumulation of glucosylceramide, especially in the spleen and liver, resulting in severe neurologic disorders (Gaucher's disease). Also called *cerebroside β-glucosidase* and *glucocerebrosidase.*

glucosylceramidase assays determination of the glucosylceramidase activity in fetal cells cultured from amniotic fluid, biopsy specimens, peripheral blood leukocytes, or cultured skin fibroblasts. ^{14}Carbon-labeled glucocerebroside or β-D-glucopyranosides of chromogenic or fluorescent phenols are used as substrates. A chromogenic substrate used is 2-hexadecanolamino-4-nitrophenyl-β-D-glucopyranoside, which is hydrolyzed by the enzyme to a yellow product that is measured spectrophotmetrically. A fluorogenic substrate is 4-methylumbelliferyl-β-D-glucopyranoside. The leukocyte assay requires the more sensitive radiometric or fluorometric assays, and the activity varies with the differential count because most of the enzyme activity is in neutrophils. Cultured skin fibroblasts are preferred for assays because they contain higher enzyme activity, and the cells are stable to freezing so that they can be stored or transported over long distances. These assays are performed in the diagnosis of Gaucher's disease.

glucuronate (gloo″ku-ron′āt) the anion of glucuronic acid. See also *glucuronic acid.*

glucuronic acid (gloo″ku-ron′ik) a uronic acid formed by the oxidation of the primary alcohol group at C-6 of glucose to form a carboxyl. Glucuronic acid residues are found in mucopolysaccharides, glycoproteins, and proteoglycans. Many phenols, alcohols (including sterols), and bilirubin are converted in the liver to more soluble glucuronic acid conjugates (glucuronides). This will metabolically inactivate and/or detoxify these compounds and aid in their excretion.

β-D-glucuronidase (gloo″ku-ron′ĭ-dās) an enzyme of the hydrolase class (β-D-glucuronide) glucuronosohydrolase. EC 3.2.1.31) that catalyzes the reaction β-D-glucuronide + H_2O = an alcohol + D-glucuronate. Present in most tissues, it is abundant in the liver. The enzyme is used for the hydrolysis of urinary steroid hormones, which are largely excreted as glucuronic acid conjugates. The hydrolysis is a preliminary step in the assay of steroid hormones in urine. A genetic deficiency of the enzyme, transmitted as an autosomal recessive trait, is found in mucopolysaccharidosis VII (MPS VII).

β-D-glucuronidase deficiency a rare genetic disorder of more than one allelic form, transmitted as an autosomal recessive trait, that is characterized by abnormal mucopolysaccharide metabolism,

GLUCOSE TOLERANCE TEST. VARIOUS CRITERIA FOR THE STANDARD ORAL GLUCOSE TOLERANCE TEST

	HOUR	WHOLE BLOOD*	PLASMA*	POINTS
Wilkerson Point System	0	110	130	1
	1	170	195	½
	2	120	140	½
	3	110	130	1

Values equal to or more than those listed are given points as shown. Two points or more are judged diagnostic of diabetes.

	HOUR	WHOLE BLOOD*	PLASMA*	POINTS
Fajans-Conn Criteria	1	160	185	
	1½	140	165	
	2	120	140	

All levels must be equal to or greater than values shown at the times specified to make a diagnosis of diabetes. Criteria apply to ambulatory individuals under the age of 50.

University Group Diabetes Program

The subject is judged diabetic if the sum of values obtained at 0, 1, 2, and 3 hours equals 500 or more for whole blood, or 600 or more for plasma.

* Values for whole blood or plasma are given in milligrams per 100 milliliters.

From Tietz, N. W.: Fundamentals of Clinical Chemistry. 2nd ed. Philadelphia, W.B. Saunders Co., 1979, p. 252.

leading to progressive mental deterioration, splenic and hepatic enlargement, and dysostosis multiplex. It is due to a deficiency of the enzyme β-D-glucuronidase and leads to the increased excretion of dermatan sulfate (chondroitin sulfate B) in the urine. Prenatal diagnosis is feasible, and lymphocytes of affected individuals possess characteristic inclusion bodies. Also called mucopolysaccharidosis VII (MPS VII) and *Sly syndrome.* See also *mucopolysaccharidoses.*

glucuronide (gloo″ku-ron′īd) any glycosidic compound of glucuronic acid. Many important biochemicals such as phenols, alcohols, sterols, and carboxylic acids are transformed in the liver into inactive and water-soluble glucuronides. This is an important pathway by which many drugs and poisons are detoxified and converted for ease of excretion.

glucuronyl-transferase see *UDP-glucuronate:bilirubin-glucuronosyltransferase.*

glutamate (gloo′tah-māt) a salt of glutamic acid.

glutamate decarboxylase (gloo′tah-māt de″kar-bok′sĭ-lās) an enzyme of the lyase class (L-glutamate-1-carboxy-lyase, EC 4.1.1.15) that catalyzes the reaction L-glutamate ⇄ 4-aminobutyrate + CO_2. The enzyme contains pyridoxal phosphate as a coenzyme and is found in some synapses. The reaction produces 4-aminobutyrate in the synaptic vesicles, which acts as a neurotransmitter in promoting the transfer of Cl^- across the synaptic membranes. These synapses are inhibitory, making larger stimulations necessary for the transmission of nervous impulses.

glutamate dehydrogenase (gloo′tah-māt de-hi′dro-jen-ās) a group of enzymes of the oxidoreductase class (L-glutamate:NAD^+ or $NADP^+$ oxidoreductase (deaminating), EC 1.4.1.2–4). They catalyze the reaction L-glutamate + H_2O + NAD^+ (or $NADP^+$) ⇄ 2-oxoglutarate + NH_3+NADH (or NADPH). The enzyme is present in the mitochondria of most tissues and plays an important role in the regulation of glutamate and ammonium balance in the cell.

glutamate-pyruvate transaminase (GPT) see *alanine aminotransferase.*

glutamate semialdehyde (gloo′tah-māt sem″e-al′dĕ-hīd) an intermediate in the enzymatic interconversion of ornithine and glutamate and in proline catabolism.

glutamic acid (Glu or E) (gloo′tah-mik) [from *glutamine*] 2-aminopentanedioic acid, $HOOC(CH_2)_2CH(NH_2)COOH$; a naturally occurring, nonessential amino acid; M.W. 147.13. It serves as a constituent of proteins and is an important nitrogen donor in transamination reactions. Glutamic acid is a precursor in the biosynthesis of the amino acids ornithine, arginine, proline, hydroxyproline, and glutamine, and is a precursor of glutathione and of γ-aminobutyric acid. It can form α-ketoglutaric acid to replenish the tricarboxylic acid cycle intermediates, and can function as an ammonia carrier by forming glutamine. Glutamic acid is a constituent of many proteins. Its source is from diet proteins and biosynthesis, mainly from α-ketoglutarate. See also under *amino acids.*

glutamic-oxaloacetic transaminase (GOT) see *aspartate aminotransferase.*

glutaminase (gloo-tam′ĭ-nās) an enzyme of the hydrolase class (L-glutamine amidohydrolase, EC 3.5.1.2) that catalyzes the reaction L-glutamine + H_2O ⇄ L-glutamate + NH_3. This enzyme occurs in the kidneys and small intestine.

glutamine (Gin or Q) (gloo′tah-mēn) [*gluten* + *amine*] 2-aminoglutaramic acid, 2-amino-4-carbamoylbutanoic acid, a monoamide of glutamic acid, $HOOCCH(NH_2)(CH_2)_2CONH_2$, a naturally occurring, nonessential amino acid; M.W. 146.15. It occurs as a constituent of proteins, serves as an ammonia transport molecule, and acts as a nitrogen donor molecule for purine and pyrimidine base biosyntheses. Its sources are dietary protein and, more important, biosynthesis from glutamic acid. See also under *amino acids.*

glutaminyl (gloo-tam′ĭ-nil) the acyl radical derived from or relating to glutamine.

glutaminyl-peptide-γ-glutamyltransferase (glo-o-tam′ĭ-nil pep′tīd gloo′tah-mil trans′fer-ās) an enzyme of the transferase class (EC 2.3.2.13) that catalyzes the formation of intra- and intermolecular covalent bonds between fibrin units in the course of blood clotting. The enzyme circulates in the blood as the inactive form, protransglutaminase. Also called *transglutaminase.*

glutamyl (gloo′tah-mil) the acyl radical derived from or relating to glutamic acid.

γ-glutamyltransferase (GGT) (gloo″tah-mil-trans′fer-ās) an enzyme of the transferase class ((5-glutamyl)-peptide:amino acid 5-glutamyltransferase, EC 2.3.2.2) that transfers a terminal γ-glutamyl group from peptides or similar compounds to some acceptor. It appears to be associated with the transfer of amino acids across cell membranes. It occurs in all cells, primarily in the cell membrane. Increased activity in serum occurs in any and all forms of liver disease, i.e., hepatocellular disease, biliary obstruction (highest values), cholangitis, malignancies, fatty liver, alcoholic cirrhosis, and cystic fibrosis. Furthermore, increases in activity are seen in alcoholics and persons on drug therapy. Enzyme activity is determined with γ-glutamyl-*p*-nitroanilide (GGPNA) as a substrate, measuring the formation of *p*-nitroaniline at 405 nm. Reference ranges for γ-glutamyl transferase are: for males, 9–50 U/l; and for females, 8–40U/l.

Also called *glutamyl transpeptidase.*

γ-glutamyltransferase assays determinations of GGT activity in serum using the peptide analog γ-glutamyl-*p*-nitroanilide (GGPNA) or its carboxylated derivative as the substrate and glycylglycine as the γ-glutamyl residue acceptor. The transpeptidation reaction yields the transfer product γ-glutamylglycylglycine and the donor residue *p*-nitroaniline, which is measured by its absorbance at 405 nm. A substrate blank is used to correct for nonenzymatic hydrolysis of GGPNA.

γ-glutamyl transfer cycle a mechanism postulated for the transport of amino acids into cells. Glutathione reacts with the incoming amino acid at the cell membrane, producing the γ-glutamyl amino acid derivative and the byproduct cysteinylglycine in a reaction catalyzed by the membrane-bound enzyme γ-glutamyltransferase. In the cytosol, the γ-glutamyl amino acid derivative is hydrolyzed to produce the free amino acid. The glutamic acid and the other split products of glutathione are recombined to regenerate glutathione. This cyclic process for the translocation of a given amino acid requires the participation of six enzymes and three ATP molecules.

glutamyl transpeptidase see *γ-glutamyltransferase.*

glutaraldehyde (gloo″tah-ral′dĕ-hīd) 1,5-pentanedial, $CHO(CH_2)_3CHO$, used as a histologic fixative; see under *fixative.*

glutaric acid a dicarboxylic acid, $COOH(CH_2)_3COOH$, obtained by oxidation of cyclopentanone.

glutathione (gloo″tah-thi′ōn) [*glutamic* acid + Gr. *theion* sulfur] a tripeptide, γ-glutamylcysteinylglycine (GSH), present in animal and plant tissues. It can exist in reduced (GSH) or oxidized (GSSG) forms, and has several functions: (1) in disulfide exchange, e.g., the formation of disulfide bridges in proinsulin by reaction of two sulfhydryl groups with GSSG; (2) in transport of amino acids into cells by the γ-glutamyl transfer cycle; (3) in preventing oxidative damage to erythrocytes by reducing the accumulation of methemoglobin and hydrogen peroxide; (4) in association with glucose-6-phosphate dehydrogenase and in the maintenance of erythrocyte integrity; (5) in brain metabolism; and (6) in a variety of oxidation-reduction systems in tissues.

glutathione peroxidase (gloo″tah-thi′ōn pĕr-ok′sĭ-dās) an enzyme of the oxidoreductase class (glutathione : hydrogen - peroxide oxidoreductase, EC 1.11.1.9) that catalyzes the reaction 2 glutathione + H_2O_2 ⇄ oxidized glutathione + 2 H_2O. The reaction serves to remove dangerous levels of hydrogen peroxide within the cell. The enzyme is a seleno-protein (it contains selenium). Deficiency of the enzyme is associated with neonatal jaundice.

glutathione reductase (gloo″tah-thi′ōn re-duk′tās) an oxidoreductase enzyme (NAD(P)H:oxidized-glutathione oxidoreductase, EC 1.6.4.2) that catalyzes the reaction: NAD(P)H + oxidized glutathione ⇄ $NAD(P)^+$ + 2 glutathione. It is a flavoprotein requiring FAD as a coenzyme and is found in erythrocytes. Stimulation of the enzyme in erythrocytes by added FAD is used as an assay of the nutritional status of riboflavin in humans. The enzyme is important in minimizing the accumulation of methemoglobin in erythrocytes, and in the clinical diagnosis of anemia and cyanosis.

glutathione reductase assays 1. screening procedure. Oxidized glutathione (GSSG) and NADPH are reacted with hemolyzed blood to produce reduced glutathione (GSH) and $NADP^+$. The decrease of fluorescence with time, due to NADH oxidation, is a function of the enzyme activity in the sample. The fluorescence is observed on spots of reaction mixture dried on filter paper, examined under ultraviolet light, and compared with similarly treated deficient control blood.

2. spectrophotometry. Hemolyzed blood is reacted with GSSG and NADPH. The glutathione reductase activity is determined from the rate of decrease in the absorbance at 340 nm caused by oxidation of NADPH to $NADP^+$. One reported normal range is 6.3–39.0 U/10^9 erythrocytes.

glutathione reductase deficiency a genetic defect, transmitted as an autosomal dominant trait, that can result in erythrocyte hemolysis upon administration of a variety of agents in affected individuals. See also *primaquine sensitivity.*

glutathione stability test a screening test useful in the differential diagnosis of a hemolytic process. The test establishes the presence of red blood cells with a significantly reduced stability when incubated in the presence of acetylphenylhydrazine. This instability derives from low levels of reduced glutathione (GSH) due to the deficiency of glucose-6-phosphate dehydrogenase (G-6-PD) activity. The absence of this activity prevents the reduction of $NADP^+$ to NADPH, which is needed to keep GSH in the reduced state. As a result, cell wall integrity cannot be maintained and the cells lyse. Normal cells respond similarly to such a procedure but much less dramatically. The test is nonspecific, complicated, and difficult to perform properly, and hence is infrequently carried out.

GSH levels in normal cells, before and after incubation with acetylphenylhydrazine, are about 60–65 mg of GSH/dl. For a person with affected, hemolysis-sensitive cells, the preincubation GSH level is slightly less than normal, whereas after a 2 hr incubation the GSH concentration drops to about 10 mg of GSH/dl. Abnormal results with the test are seen also in 6-phosphogluconic dehydrogenase deficiency, and perhaps on occasion with GSH-peroxidase and GSH-reductase deficiencies. The test is negative in cases of deficiencies of the many other red cell enzymes. Normal results are seen in hereditary spherocytosis, pyruvate kinase (PK) deficiency, hexokinase (HK) deficiency, and triosephosphate isomerase deficiency.

glutathione synthetase (GSH synthetase) (gloo″-tah-thi′ōn sin′thĕ-tās) an enzyme of the ligase class (EC 6.3.2.3) that catalyzes the reaction ATP + γ-L-glutamyl-L-cysteine + glycine ⇄ ADP + orthophosphate + glutathione. GSH synthetase is one of the enzymes concerned in the synthesis of glutathione to replace that consumed in transferring amino acids into cells across membranes. It is important in the maintenance of red blood cell integrity. A rare genetic deficiency of the enzyme in erythrocytes is associated with a nonspherocytic hemolytic anemia and favism. The cells of affected individuals are extremely sensitive to primaquine.

gluteal (gloo′te-al) [Gr. *gloutos* buttock] pertaining to the buttocks.

gluteal region the region that overlies the gluteal muscles; the buttock.

gluten (gloo′ten) [L. "glue"] a protein of wheat and other grains; a mixture of gliadin and glutenin, the principal endosperm proteins. Celiac disease may be alleviated when gluten is removed from the diet.

glutenin (gloo′tĕ-nin) a principal endosperm protein of wheat. See under *gluten.*

gluten-sensitive enteropathy see *celiac s.* under *sprue.*

glutethimide (gloo-teth′ĭ-mīd) [NF], a drug structurally similar to the barbiturates that is used as a sleeping pill and sedative. Large overdoses (10 g, 20–40 pills) may cause coma and respiratory and circulatory failure. The drug is absorbed erratically and little is excreted in urine, most being metabolized by the liver. Chronic use may lead to dependence; withdrawal causes severe reactions. Trademark, *Doriden.*

glutethimide assays the determination of glutethimide in blood or urine. As a very weak acid, glutethimide is extracted into chloroform, dichloromethane, or petroleum ether, which may be washed with strong base and then with acid to remove interfering substances. Glutethimide is found in the neutral fraction. The evaporate of the extract is dissolved in ethanol, and potassium hydroxide is added. This hydrolyzes the glutethimide, resulting in a decrease of the ultraviolet absorbance at 235 nm. The decrease over 10 min is compared with that of a reference solution. Quantitation may instead be performed by gas chromatography, using a nonpolar stationary phase and a flame ionization detector. This procedure can detect 2 mg/l in blood; it can also detect the two primary metabolites. See also *barbiturate assays* for a colorimetric test.

glutin (gloo′tin) 1. a sticky substance from glutenin: gluten-casein.
2. gelatin in its soft, dissolved state.

glutinous (gloo′tĭ-nus) [L. *glutinosus*] sticky; adhesive.

Gly abbrev. See *glycine.*

glyc/o (gli′ko) [Gr. *glykys* sweet] a word element used in combining form to denote sugar or carbohydrate, e.g., glycoproteins.

glycan (gli′kan) see *polysaccharide.*

glyceraldehyde (glis″er-al′de-hīd) 2,3-dihydroxypropanal; glyceric aldehyde; α,β-dihydroxypropionaldehyde. It is obtained from the mild oxidation of glycerol and exists in two stereoisomeric forms. Glyceraldehyde is the simplest aldose and its D- and L- forms are used as the configurational reference standard for carbohydrates. See also *glucose.*

glyceraldehyde 3-phosphate (glis″er-al′de-hīd fos′fāt) an ester formed by the 3-hydroxyl group of glyceraldehyde and phosphoric acid, the 3-phosphate derivative of glyceraldehyde. It is an important intermediate of the pentose shunt of glucose metabolism, as well as of the Embden-Meyerhof pathway of glycolysis. See also *triose phosphate.*

glyceraldehyde-phosphate dehydrogenase (GAPD) (glis″er-al′de-hīd fos′fāt de-hi′dro-jen-ās) an enzyme of the oxidoreductase class (D-glyceraldehyde-3-phosphate:NAD$^+$ oxidoreductase (phosphorylating), EC 1.2.1.12) that catalyzes the reaction D-glyceraldehyde 3-phosphate + orthophosphate + NAD$^+$ $\rightleftarrows$ 3-phospho-D-glyceroyl phosphate + NADH + H$^+$. The reaction is a critical energy-yielding step in the Embden-Meyerhof scheme of carbohydrate metabolism. A genetic deficiency of the enzyme, transmitted as an autosomal dominant trait, may be associated with some anemias. In hypophosphatemia, this reaction (especially in erythrocytes) is severely compromised, leading to the decreased production of 2,3-diphosphoglycerate (DPG) and adenosine triphosphate (ATP) and affecting oxygen delivery to the tissues. Also called *triose phosphate dehydrogenase.*

glyceride (glis′er-īd) any ester of glycerol, an acyl glycerol. Neutral fats are triglycerides (triacylglycerols).

glycerin (glis′er-in) [L. *glycerinum*] see *glycerol.*

glycerin method a method for preserving unstained cytologic smears during mailing to the laboratory. The smears are fixed in 95 percent ethanol, covered with glycerin and another glass slide, and wrapped in wax paper. If available, spray coating fixatives are preferred.

glycerol (glis′er-ol) 1,2,3-propanetriol, CH_2OH-$CHOHCH_2OH$, a clear, colorless, odorless, oily liquid with a sweet taste; M.W. 92.09. Used industrially as a solvent, humectant, plasticizer, emollient, and sweetener, glycerol is hygroscopic and soluble in both water and alcohol. It is a component of neutral fats (triacylglycerols) and of phosphatides and cardiolipin. Also called *glycerin.*

glycerol gelatin medium a water-soluble mounting medium, with a refraction index of 1.40–1.47. The medium is prepared by dissolving gelatin in hot distilled water and mixing with glycerol dissolved in distilled water to which thimerosal (Merthiolate) or thymol is added as a preservative. It is melted at 55–60°C for use, and sets on cooling. This medium causes bleeding of basic dyes.

glycerolize (glis′er-o-līz) to treat with or preserve in glycerol, as in the agitation of red blood cells with glycerol solution so that the glycerol diffuses into the cells before they are frozen to protect the red cells against freezing injury.

glycerophosphate (glis″er-o-fos′fāt) 1. any salt of glycerophosphoric acid.
2. L-α-glycerophosphate or *sn*-glycero-3-phosphate, an important biologic intermediate formed from dihydroxyacetonephosphate by L-α-glycerophosphate dehydrogenase and NADH. This intermediate serves in a shuttle for electrons from cytosol into mitochondria. It is also a substrate for synthesis of phosphatidic acid, which is a key intermediate in the synthesis of triglycerides and a number of important phosphoglycerides in the body.

glycerophosphatide (glis″er-o-fos′fah-tīd) one of a group of compounds that contain residues of diacylglycerol and phosphoric acids. Some of these compounds also may contain another residue that may or may not have nitrogen, e.g., choline, ethanolamine, serine, and inositol. Glycerophosphatides are often referred to as phospholipids and are important constituents of cellular membranes. See also *phosphatidylcholine, phosphatidylethanolamine, phosphatidylinositol,* and *phosphatidylserine.*

glyceryl (glis′er-il) the mono-, di-, or trivalent alkyl radical formed by the removal of hydroxyl groups from 1, 2, or 3 of the carbons of glycerol. Examples are alkyl glyceryl ether, glyceryl chloride, or glyceryl acetate (the preferred name of which is acetyl glycerol).

glyceryl ether lipids lipids that may be visualized as being formed by an ether linkage between a long-chain (saturated or unsaturated) alcohol and one hydroxyl group of glycerol, and with fatty acids esterified at the other two hydroxyl groups. Such lipids have been isolated from a variety of tissues including human neoplasms and bovine erythrocytes.

glycine (Gly or G) (gli′sēn) [Gr. *gleukos* sweetness] aminoacetic acid; H_2NCH_2COOH, a naturally occurring, nonessential amino acid; M.W. 75.07. It is a component of many proteins and other compounds, composing about one-third of the amino acids of collagen and elastin. Glycine functions as a conjugating agent and in nervous tissue as a neurotransmitter. It supplies one-carbon groups and nitrogen atoms for biosynthetic functions. See also under *amino acids.*

glycinemia (gli″sĭ-ne′me-ah) [*glycine* + Gr. *haima* blood + *-ia*] see *hyperglycinemia.*

glycinuria (gli″sĭ-nu′re-ah) [*glycine* + Gr. *ouron* urine + *-ia*] see *hyperglycinuria.*

glycobiarsol (gli″ko-bi-ar′sol) [USP], an organic bismuth compound formerly used to treat amebic colitis.

glycocalyx (gli″ko-kal′iks) a glycoprotein or mucoprotein coat that covers some free cell surfaces so thickly that it can be seen with a light microscope when periodic acid–Schiff (PAS) staining is used. The thickness and exact chemical composition vary from one cell type to another. Antigenic characteristics unique for specific cells and tissues are associated with the chemistry of this cell component. Also called *cell coat.*

glycochenodeoxycholate (gli″ko-ke′no-de-ok-se-ko′lāt) a bile salt, the salt or dissociated form of the glycine conjugate of chenodeoxycholic acid. In the conjugate, the carboxyl group of chenodeoxycholic acid, a bile acid, and the amino group of glycine are joined by an amide linkage. See also *chenodeoxycholic acid.*

glycochenodeoxycholic acid (gli″ko-ke′no-de-ok-se-ko′lic) *N*-chenodeoxycholoyl glycine, the amide conjugate of chenodeoxycholic acid with glycine. It is a major component of the bile of many species.

glycocholate (gli″ko-kōl-āt) the anion of glycocholic acid. Used with the name of the cation, as in sodium glycocholate, it describes a salt; used with the name of the parent alcohol, as in methylglycocholate, it describes an ester.

glycocholic acid (gli″ko-kol′lik) the glycine conjugate of cholic acid; the amide formed by the combination of the carboxyl group of cholic acid with the amino group of glycine. In the weakly basic bile fluid, this acid is converted to a salt. See also *cholate* and *glycocholate.*

glycodeoxycholic acid (gli″ko-de-ok-se-ko′lik) a bile acid conjugate in which the carboxyl group of deoxycholic acid and the amino group of glycine are joined by an amide linkage. It is formed in the liver from deoxycholic acid (produced in the gut by the bacterial dehydroxylation of cholic acid) and returned via the enterohepatic circulation.

glycogen/o (gli′ko-jen′o) a word element used in combining form to denote glycogen, e.g., glycogenolysis.

glycogen (gli′ko-jen) [*glyco-* + Gr. *gennan* to produce] a highly branched polyglucan, the chief carbohydrate storage material in animals. This polysaccharide acts as a reservoir of glucose residues for use as a fuel and a precursor of other metabolites. It is formed and stored primarily in the liver and in muscles, being depolymerized via glucose-1-phosphate to glucose-6-phosphate and glucose to be utilized or liberated as needed. Glycogen consists of short chains of glucose residues joined by α-(1→4) linkage, with branches joined by α-(1→6) linkage after every 8–12 glucose residues. The longer branched sequences occur at the periphery. The branches prevent any helix formation, and the result is a treelike structure.

A number of glycogen storage diseases are known in which glycogen may accumulate pathologically in one or more tissues. These diseases typically result from a defect in or absence of any enzyme involved in either the synthesis or the degradation of glycogen.

See also *glycogenoses.*

hepatic g., glycogen stored in the liver.

tissue g., glycogen stored in tissues other than the liver, especially in muscle.

glycogen branching enzyme see *1,4-α-glucan branching enzyme.*

glycogen digestion a control procedure used in glycogen staining. Control slides are processed normally except that before staining they are incubated for 30–60 min at 20–37°C in a solution of malt diastase (containing the enzyme α-amylase). Structures stained in the test slides but not in the controls contain glycogen.

glycogenesis (gli″ko-jen′ĕ-sis) [*glyco-* + Gr. *genesis*] 1. the formation or synthesis of glycogen from sugars, as opposed to glyconeogenesis, the formation of glycogen from amino acids or fats.

2. the production of sugar in the general sense.

glycogenic (gli″ko-jen′ik) pertaining to, characterized by, or promoting glycogenesis. The glycogenic amino acids are alanine, arginine, asparagine, aspartic acid, cysteine, glutamic acid, glutamine, histidine, hydroxyproline, isoleucine, methionine, ornithine, proline, serine, threonine, tryptophan, and valine.

glycogenolysis (gli″ko-jĕ-nol′ĭ-sis) [*glycogen* + Gr. *lysis* dissolution] the enzymatic breakdown of glycogen to glucose-1-phosphate and glucose. This process serves to convert glucose from its storage form, glycogen, particularly in liver, to forms usable for energy production or for support of blood glucose. In skeletal muscle tissue, which contains about two-thirds of all glycogen in the body, the breakdown products of glycogen do not yield glucose because of the absence of a requisite phosphatase (glucose-6-phosphatase). Thus, muscle glycogen is used primarily to supply energy needs of the muscle. Glycogenolysis in both liver and muscle is under careful regulation.

glycogenolytic (gli″ko-jen″o-lit′ik) pertaining to or promoting glycogenolysis.

glycogenoses (gli″ko-jĕ-no′ses) a group of rare inherited storage disorders each due to the specific deficiency of an enzyme essential to the degradation of glycogen, the main form in which carbohydrate is stored in the body. Glycogen is a branched-chain polysaccharide stored primarily in liver and muscles. It has a multibranched, treelike structure and is a polymer made up of only one type of residue, α-D-glucose. The usual end-to-end linkage of most glucose residues occurs between carbon atoms 1 and 4 (α-1,4 linkage). The branching links, however, are formed by α-1,6-glucosidic bonds. Approximately 50 percent of the molecule consists of free-end outer chains, 7–10 glucosyl units in length. During normal metabolic activity, glycogen molecules are constantly degraded and resynthesized according to the body's immediate requirements.

About nine different disorders of glycogen synthesis and breakdown have been described and the specific enzyme defect identified. In 1952 the first specific enzyme defect in an inborn error of metabolism was demonstrated. This was deficiency of glucose-6-phosphatase in a patient with a hepatic form of glycogen storage disease. As additional enzyme studies were performed on tissues from patients with glycogen storage diseases, it became clear that a variety of enzymes are involved in glycogen synthesis or degradation, and that an enzyme concerned with a particular step may not be the same in all tissues. For example, the cleavage of the α-1,4 bonds in the outer chains of the glycogen molecule is catalyzed by a different phosphorylase enzyme in muscle and in the liver, even though the end product is the formation of glucose-1-phosphate. A mutation either may affect the muscle phosphorylase enzyme, limiting only glycogen storage to muscle tissue (McArdle's disease—Cori type V), or may create blockage in liver phosphorylase with hepatic storage of glycogen (Hers' disease—Cori type VI). Although synthesis can still take place, accumulation occurs because degradation cannot proceed further than the step normally catalyzed by the deficient enzyme.

Precise diagnosis of the type of glycogen storage disease depends on liver and/or muscle biopsy and appropriate biochemical assays. In the hepatic forms, the diagnosis is suggested by failure to grow, hepatomegaly, and a tendency to develop fasting hypoglycemia. The primary clinical features of the glycogenoses that affect muscle glycogen are easy fatigability, muscle weakness, and stiffness.

Treatment by frequent feedings (nighttime pharyngeal drip of 10 percent glucose) ameliorates the symptoms in types I and III, which improve with age, whereas types II and IV are uniformly fatal.

See also the accompanying table.

MURIEL GLUCKSON, M.S.

glycogen phosphorylase (gli′ko-jen fos-for′ĭ-lās) an enzyme of the transferase class (1,4-α-D-glucan:orthophosphate α-D-glucosyltransferase, EC 2.4.1.1) that catalyzes the degradation of glycogen in the reaction $(1,4\text{-}\alpha\text{-D-glucosyl})_n$ + orthophosphate ⇄ $(1,4\text{-}\alpha\text{-D-glucosyl})_{n-1}$ + α-D-glucose-1-phosphate. In mammalian muscle, the enzyme exists in active form (phosphorylase a, phosphorylase P) or inactive form (phosphorylase b, phosphorylase H). Reactions of the enzyme are of major importance in liberating glucose or glucose-1-phosphate from glycogen stores of liver or muscle to be used for energy and for maintaining blood glucose. A genetic deficiency of the enzyme, transmitted as an autosomal recessive trait, is found in type V and type VI glycogen storage disease. See also *phosphorylase.*

glycogen staining the histologic demonstration of glycogen using the periodic acid–Schiff (PAS) technique or Best's carmine stain. Glycogen is best preserved in ice-cold fixatives with a high alcohol content; Gendre's fixative, Carnoy's fixative, Bouin's fluid, alcoholic formalin, or acetic acid–alcohol-formalin (5:85:10) may be used.

The PAS reaction with a control digested with diastase is the method of choice. Hematoxylin is used as a counterstain. Glycogen stains magenta with PAS or red with Best's carmine; the nuclei stain blue. See also *Best's carmine stain, fixative, glycogen digestion,* and *periodic acid–Schiff reaction.*

glycogen storage diseases see *glycogenoses.*

glycogen (starch) synthase (sin-thās) an enzyme (UDPglucose:glycogen 4-α-D-glucosyl transferase, EC 2.4.1.11) that acts during glycogen synthesis to catalyze the transfer of glucose residues in the activated state from UDP-glucose to the nonreducing ends of a glycogen primer molecule to form glucan chains. The synthetase, a highly regulated allosteric enzyme, is regulated in concert with glycogen phosphorylase so that the breakdown and synthesis of glycogen will not occur together in an energy-depleting futile cycle. The synthetase can be phosphorylated to an inactive D form (dependent) by the cyclic AMP–dependent enzyme protein kinase. This form becomes active in the presence of glucose-6-phosphate (G-6-P). The D form can be converted to an active I (independent) form by a phosphatase enzyme that cleaves the phosphate group from the D form of the synthetase protein. The I form is not activated by G-6-P.

glycogen synthesis (gli′ko-jen sin′thĕ-sis) the overall process by which glycogen is synthesized from primer molecules and glucose. Almost all body cells synthesize some glycogen, but the liver and muscles are the principal sites of storage.

The primer molecule may be a polyglucose (a partially degraded glycogen molecule) or an oligoglucosaccharide (small glucose polymer) of at least four residues. Glycogen is made by adding one glucosyl residue at a time to a glycogen primer mol-

GLYCOGENOSES

SYNDROME	ENZYME DEFECT	GLYCOGEN STRUCTURE	MODE OF INHERITANCE*
Glycogen storage disease I (von Gierke's)	Glucose-6-phosphatase	Normal	AR
Glycogen storage disease II (Pompe's)	α-D-Glucosidase (α -1,4-glucosidase; lysosomal	Normal	AR
Glycogen storage disease III (Forbes')	Amylo-1,6-glucosidase	Abnormal—short outer chains	AR
Glycogen storage disease IV (Andersen's)	1,4-α-Glucan branching enzyme (amylo-(1,4-1,6)-transglucosidase)	Abnormal—long chains with few branch points	AR
Glycogen storage disease V (McArdle's)	Phosphorylase (muscle)	Normal	AR
Glycogen storage disease VI (Hers')	Phosphorylase (liver)	Normal	AR
Glycogen storage disease VII	Phosphofructokinase (muscle)	Normal	AR
Glycogen storage disease VII	Phosphorylase kinase (liver)	Normal	X-Linked
Glycogen synthetase deficiency	Glycogen synthetase	Normal but decreased levels in liver	AR

* AR = autosomal recessive.

ecule, creating long linear chains of glucose residues (amylose chains) that are then rearranged to make additional branch points. The glucose donor molecule for synthesis is uridine diphosphate glucose (UDP-glucose), which is derived from glucose-6-phosphate. The amylose chains are extended by the enzyme glycogen synthetase, which catalyzes the addition of glucose units from UDP-glucose to the primer in $\alpha(1\rightarrow4)$glycosidic linkage.

The formation of new branch points involves the enzymatic removal of the last seven terminal residues of an amylose chain followed by the attachment of one end of the seven-residue stub in $\alpha(1\rightarrow6)$-glycosidic linkage to an amylose chain at a glucosyl unit that is at least four glucosyl units from an existing branch point. The branching enzyme is 1,4-α-glucan branching enzyme.

Glycogen synthesis is a highly regulated process that is closely interlocked with the regulation of glycogen breakdown so that the two processes do not occur simultaneously, which would result in waste of the energy required for synthesis. The regulation of glycogen metabolism in the liver differs somewhat from that in muscle. The primary control is at the level of the activities of glycogen synthetase and glycogen phosphorylase. These activities are regulated hormonally by insulin, glucagon, and epinephrine. Adrenocortical hormones and thyroxine also affect glycogen synthesis. Phosphorylation or dephosphorylation of several key enzymes is involved in the control. Metabolites such as AMP, Ca^{2+} ions, glucose-6-phosphate, and glycogen affect the activities of these enzymes.

A number of important hereditary disorders of glycogen metabolism are known, which lead in many cases to excessive accumulation of glycogen at a variety of organ sites; see also *glycogenoses.*

glycol (gli′kol) the trivial name for any aliphatic dihydric alcohol, such as ethylene glycol, $HOCH_2$-CH_2OH. The systematic name is diol, e.g., 1,2-ethanediol.

glycolipid (gli″ko-lip′id) a lipid that contains carbohydrate groups, usually glucose, galactose, *N*-acetylated sugars, *N*-acetyl neuraminate, inositol, or others. The carbohydrate moiety is attached to ceramide or, in some cases, to diacylglycerol. It can range from a single monosaccharide residue to complex branched structures with several such residues or their derivatives.

glycolipid staining histologic methods for the demonstration of glycolipids, e.g., the gangliosides and cerebrosides that accumulate in lipid storage diseases such as Gaucher's disease. Because these substances contain a hexose, they are stained by the periodic acid–Schiff (PAS) technique. They can be differentiated from other PAS-positive diastase-labile substances because they also are stained by fat stains.

glycolithocholic acid (gli″ko-lith″o-ko′lik) a bile acid conjugate in which the carboxyl group of lithocholic acid and the amino group of glycine are joined by an amide linkage. It is formed in the liver from lithocholic acid (produced in the gut by the bacterial dehydroxylation of chenodeoxycholic acid) and returned via the enterohepatic circulation.

glycol methacrylate 2-hydroxymethyl methacrylate ($CH_2{=}C(CH_3)COOH_2CH_2OH$), which polymerizes in the presence of ultraviolet light and catalysts to form an acrylic resin. Glycol methacrylate resin is used in histology as an embedding medium for cutting thin plastic sections in light microscopy.

glycolysis (gli-kol′ĭ-sis) [*glyco-* + Gr. *lysis* solution] often known as fermentation; literally, the splitting of glucose into smaller fragments. Glycolysis is nothing more than the Embden-Meyerhof pathway (named after two biochemists who completed the elucidation of glycolytic reactions in the 1930s) for the conversion of glucose residues to pyruvate, with the added action of lactate dehydrogenase to form lactate from pyruvate. By this series of reactions, 1 mol of glucose yields 2 mol of lactate, anaerobically, with the concomitant transformation of energy as ATP. Glycolysis occurs in the cytosol of the cell, whereas subsequent aerobic oxidation of pyruvate occurs in the mitochondria.

glycolytic (gli″ko-lit′ik) pertaining to, characterized by, or promoting glycolysis.

glycone (gli′kōn) 1. the carbohydrate portion of glycoside.

2. a glycerol suppository.

glyconeogenesis (gli″ko-ne″o-jen′ĕ-sis) [*glyco-* + Gr. *neos* new + *gennan* to produce] the formation or synthesis of glycogen from amino acids or fats.

glycopeptide (gli″ko-pep′tīd) any of a class of peptides that contain carbohydrates, i.e., that are covalently linked to carbohydrates, including the amino sugars or neuraminic acids.

glycophorin (gli″ko-fo′rin) a membrane protein, the main glycoprotein of the red blood cell, which traverses the cell membrane. It consists of a single peptide chain, linked covalently at the *N*-terminal end to some 125 sugar residues, exposed to the outside of the cell. Glycophorin carries many blood group substances as well as receptors for viruses, hemagglutinins, and other materials.

glycoprotein (gli″ko-pro′tēn) 1. a substance containing proteins covalently linked to carbohydrates. The carbohydrate usually consists of branched heterooligosaccharides attached by *O*-glycosidic linkages with the hydroxyl group of serine or threonine or by *N*-glycosidic linkage to the asparagine side-chain of proteins.

The monosaccharides commonly occurring in the oligosaccharide moieties of mammalian glycoproteins are fucose, galactose, *N*-acetylglucosamine, *N*-acetylgalactosamine, mannose, and sialic acids (usually *N*-acetylneuraminate in humans). Other monosaccharides occur in proteoglycans. The carbohydrate content of glycoproteins varies from only a few carbohydrate chains to many chains, making up half of the glycoprotein molecule.

Glycoproteins occur in extracellular fluids (all the plasma proteins except albumin are glycoproteins), in the ground substance of cartilage, and in the basement membrane and surface coat of epithelium. They also occur in membrane proteins, e.g., ABH red cell antigens and some hormone receptors. Intracellularly, glycoproteins are usually localized in lysosomes. The gonadotropic and thyroid-stimulating hormones are examples of glycoproteins, as are some enzymes, antibodies, and structural proteins.

See also *mucopolysaccharide* and *proteoglycan.*

2. a covalently linked carbohydrate and protein in which the carbohydrate component is not an acid mucopolysaccharide. Cf. *mucoprotein.*

glycoprotein hormones a group of structurally similar glycoproteins, most likely descended from a common precursor by biochemical evolution, which includes the thyroid-stimulating hormone (TSH), follicle-stimulating hormone (FSH), and luteinizing hormone (LH)—all of which are synthesized in the pituitary—and the human chorionic gonadotropic hormone (hCG) of the placenta. Each of these hormones is composed of two polypeptide chains, designated alpha and beta. The carbohydrate content, consisting of fucose, mannose, galactose, glucosamine, and galactosamine, comprises 15–31 percent of the total molecular weight. The alpha chains are very similar, if not identical, for all four hormones. The beta chains are different, however, and confer hormonal specificity on the molecule.

The immunologic specificity also resides in the beta chain. Those antibodies that are elicited to intact glycoprotein hormones cross react with the other hormones because of the common alpha subunit. It became possible, once this structure-function relationship was understood, to elicit antibodies only against the beta subunit; the net result was a more specific antibody and a more specific assay, e.g., the beta subunit assay for hCG. This has aided in the early determination of pregnancy by eliminating cross reactivity with LH, which produces false-positive results.

glycoprotein staining a stain for demonstrating the presence of glycoproteins, such as mucins, gonadotropic and thyroid-stimulating hormones, and serum mucoproteins. The most commonly employed technique is the periodic acid–Schiff (PAS), for which glycoproteins are positive.

glycopyrrolate (gli″ko-pi′ro-lāt) a quaternary ammonium compound and anticholinergic drug that acts by blocking muscarinic receptors and thus reduces gastric, bronchial, tracheal, and other secretions. It is used as a premedication in anesthesia and as an adjunct in the management of peptic ulcers. Adverse reactions include dry mouth, blurred vision, urinary retention, and tachycardia. Also called *glycopyrronium bromide.*

glycopyrronium bromide (gli″ko-pi-ro′ne-um) see *glycopyrrolate.*

glycosaminoglycan (gli″kōs-ah-mēn″o-gli′kan) one of a group of linear heteropolysaccharides (chondroitin sulfate, dermatan sulfate, keratan sulfate, heparan sulfate, heparin, and hyaluronic acid) that contain hexosamines and occur both as components of proteoglycans and as free compounds. The disaccharide repeating unit contains a hexuronic acid (except for keratan sulfate, which contains galactose) and an *N*-acetylhexosamine sulfate (except in hyaluronic acid, which contains *N*-acetylglucosamine). Each disaccharide repeating unit of all glycosaminoglycans, except hyaluronic acid and keratan sulfate, contains both a carboxyl (—COOH) and an acid sulfate (—SO_3H) residue. Hyaluronic acid contains only a —COOH residue and keratan sulfate a —SO_3H residue per repeating unit. In water solutions at physiologic pH, all glycosaminoglycans have many negative charges, producing electrostatic repulsion. This causes the molecules to spread out through a large volume of solvent, forming a highly viscous fluid. Formerly called *mucopolysaccharide,* a name still common in clinical usage. See also *mucoprotein, proteoglycan,* and the specific glycosaminoglycan.

glycosaminolipid (gli″kōs-am″ĭ-no-lip′id) any of a class of lipids that contain amino sugars. See also *glycolipid.*

glycosidase (gli′ko-sĭ-dās) any one of a large group of enzymes of the hydrolase class (EC 3.2) that attack glycosidic linkages; these enzymes are now classified according to the glycosyl group present in the compound. Some glycosidases act as transglycosidases. See also *galactosidase* and *glucosidase.*

glycoside (gli′ko-sid) a compound formed by the condensation of a furanose or pyranose at the anomeric carbon with a second molecule. Typically, the resulting compound is an acetal, although nitrogen glycosides and phosphate ester glycosides are also known. It is convertible by hydrolytic cleavage into sugar and a nonsugar component (aglycone), and is named specifically for the sugar contained, e.g., glucoside (glucose), pentoside (pentose), and fructoside (fructose).

cardiac g., any one of a group of steroid glycosides occurring in certain plants (e.g., *Digitalis*) that have a characteristic action on the heart. At very low doses these glycosides may be used to regulate heart action; at high doses they are very toxic. Examples are digitonin and ouabain.

cyanophoric g., a glycoside that, on hydrolysis, yields hydrocyanic acid, e.g., amygdalin.

sterol g., a phytosterolin; a glycoside found in plants and formed by the condensation of a sugar (like glucose) and a sterol (like sitosterol).

glycosphingolipid (gli″ko-sfing″o-lip′id) a group that includes several classes of lipids that are derivatives of ceramide, including cerebrosides, ceramide oligosaccharides, and gangliosides. Structurally, the molecules are ceramide linked glycosidically through the number one hydroxyl group of sphingosine to either a monosaccharide or an oligosaccharide. Fairly abundant in the brain and spinal cord, they also occur in small amounts in other tissues, e.g., globoside (a ceramide oligosaccharide) of the red blood cell membranes.

glycosuria (gli″ko-su′re-ah) [*glyco-* + Gr. *ouron* urine + *-ia*] the presence of glucose in the urine in concentrations above the normal.

glycosylated hemoglobin hemoglobin A_{1c}. See *Hb* A_{1a}, A_{1b}, and A_{1c} under *hemoglobin.*

glycosyl ceramide see *cerebroside.*

glycosyltransferase (gli″ko-sil-trans′fer-ās) a subclass (EC 2.4) of the transferase class of enzymes, consisting of those that catalyze the transfer of a glycosyl group from one compound to another, i.e., the transfer of a sugar from an oligosaccharide or a high-energy compound to another carbohydrate molecule. Clinically important enzymes of the group include phosphorylase and purine-nucleotide phosphorylase.

glycyl (gli′sil) the acyl radical derived from or relating to glycine.

Glycyphagus (gli-sif′ah-gus) [Gr. *glykys* sweet + *phagein* to eat] a genus of mites. The most common species, *G. domesticus,* causes grocers' itch. These mites get on the hands and migrate under the skin, causing the itching. If swallowed in food, they can be identified by microscopic examination of the feces or urine. Also called food mite.

GM abbrev. See *Geiger-Müller counter.*

gm abbrev. See *gram.*

Gm allotype see *Gm marker.*

Gm marker an allotype marker found on the heavy chains of IgG that indicates inherited differences on these human immunoglobulins.

GMP abbrev. See *guanosine-5-phosphate.*

3′:5′-GMP abbrev. for guanosine 3′:5′-cyclic phosphate. See *cyclic guanosine monophosphate.*

GN abbrev. See *gram negative.*

gnath/o (nath′o) [Gr. *gnathos* jaw] a word element used in combining form to denote jaw, e.g., gnathodynia.

Gnathostoma (nath-os′to-mah) [*gnatho-* + Gr. *stoma* mouth] a genus of nematode worms, several species of which are parasitic in humans. The most common species, *G. spinigerum,* causes a creeping disease in which the parasite produces abscesses underneath the skin.

gnathostomiasis (nath″o-sto-mi′ah-sis) infection with the nematode *Gnathostoma.*

GN broth see *GN (gram-negative) b.* under *broth.*

gnos/o (no′so) [Gr. *gnōsis* knowledge] a word element used in combining form to denote knowledge, e.g., diagnosis.

gnotobiota (no″to-bi-o′tah) [Gr. *gnotos* known + *biota* the flora and fauna of a region] the specifically and entirely known microfauna and microflora of animals reared espcially for use in the laboratory.

gnotobiote (no″to-bi′ōt) an animal reared especially for use in the laboratory, the specific microfauna and microflora of which are known in their entirety.

gnotobiotic (no″to-bi-ot′ik) pertaining to a gnotobiote or to gnotobiotics. See also *axenic.*

gnotobiotics (no″to-bi-ot′iks) the science of rearing animals, the specific microflora and microfauna of which are known in their entirety, especially for use in the laboratory.

gnotophoresis (no″to-for′ĕ-sis) [Gr. *gnotos* known + *phōresis* a carrying] the state of existence of an organism bearing one or more known species in intimate contact with it and bearing no other demonstrable viable microorganisms.

GnRH abbrev. See *gonadotropin hormone–releasing hormone.*

GΩ abbrev. See *gigohm.*

goblet cell a mucus-secreting epithelial cell with a large apical globule of mucin that gives the cell a goblet-shaped appearance. These cells are numerous in the large intestine and are also present in other mucosal epithelia, including the respiratory passages and the conjunctiva.

goiter (goi′ter) 1. enlargement of the thyroid gland. 2. a clinical term used for any visible or palpable enlargement of the thyroid gland.

colloid g., see *endemic g.*

congenital g., see *dyshormonogenic g.* and *endemic g.*

dyshormonogenic g., a goiter caused by an inbred error of metabolism, with a familial pattern of inheritance characterized by different groups of defects along the pathway of thyroid hormone synthesis related to deficiencies of specific enzyme systems. When the defect is severe, hypothyroidism with goiter (congenital goiter) and even cretinism may occur. If the defect is not severe, the goiter may not appear until adult life. Also called congenital goiter and familial goiter.

endemic g., a form of simple goiter that occurs in individuals living in geographic areas where the iodine content of soil and water is low. It can be prevented by the addition of adequate iodine to the diet, usually in the form of iodized salt. Enlarged thyroid in children in endemic areas is largely due to vascular and follicular cell hyperplasia in association with a small store of colloid (parenchymatous goiter). Congenital goiter of the endemic type occurs in infants in association with dwarfism, hypothyroidism, and mental retardation (cretinism) as a result of severe iodine deficiency in the mother during pregnancy. In adults, the enlargement is due to massive storage of colloid (colloid goiter), which can be diffuse (diffuse colloid goiter) or nodular (nodular colloid goiter).

lymphadenoid g., see *chronic t.* under *thyroiditis.*

nodular toxic g., see *Plummer's disease.*

parenchymatous g., see *endemic g.*

simple g., a noninflammatory, nonneoplastic, diffuse or nodular enlargement of the thyroid gland without hyperthyroidism. It includes the morphologic variants of endemic and sporadic goiter.

sporadic diffuse g., a benign, diffuse thyroid enlargement of moderate size, usually occurring in adolescent, young adult, and pregnant females. The thyroid follicles containing increased stores of colloid become uniformly enlarged. Some instances may represent mild cases of endemic goiter in those with suboptimal iodine intake. In affected patients with a normal iodine intake, the etiology is unknown. Involution usually occurs spontaneously. Also called adolescent goiter, diffuse colloid goiter, and simple colloid goiter.

sporadic nodular g., the most common type of thyroid enlargement seen in the United States. It is of unknown etiology and is characterized by a well-defined nodule or nodules affecting part of one or both lobes of the thyroid. The histologic features of the individual nodule are identical with those seen in nodules of endemic nodular goiter. The major clinical concern is to differentiate the solitary nodule of nodular goiter from thyroid carcinoma. Also called nodular hyperplasia.

gold (Au) (gōld) [A. S.; L. *aurum*] a yellow metallic element; atomic number 79; atomic weight 196.967; a 5d transition element; common oxidation states +1 and +3. It normally is present in the body only in trace amounts. Therapeutically, radioactive colloidal Au is used as an antineoplastic, and organic gold compounds are used to treat arthritis. Toxic effects commonly involve the skin and mucous membranes; more rarely observed are kidney or liver inflammations or blood disorders.

gold-198 (^{198}Au, Au 198) a radioisotope of gold, with a half-life of 2.7 da. It emits 411-KeV gamma rays, as well as beta-decay and internal-conversion electrons. Because of the electron emission, patients receive a much higher radiation dose from ^{198}Au than from pure gamma emitters; thus, ^{198}Au has been replaced in clinical use by pure gamma emitters (e.g., ^{99m}Tc) for imaging and by the pure beta emitter ^{32}P for radiation therapy.

gold assays atomic absorption spectrophotometry at 242.8 nm, using a gold hollow-cathode lamp; either serum or urine specimens may be used.

Goldblatt kidney (gōld′blat) [Harry *Goldblatt,*

Cleveland physician, born 1891] a kidney with a partially obstructed renal artery. When this lesion is experimentally produced, renal ischemia occurs, leading to systemic hypertension. This is thought to occur through the mediation of the renin-angiotensin-aldosterone system. Although this pathophysiology of hypertension has been established experimentally, the contribution of renal ischemia and the renin cascade to human hypertension is yet to be defined.

gold chloride a crystalline solid, yellow to red in color, $AuCl_3$, used in histology for gold toning in silver impregnation methods and in gold impregnation methods. See also *Cajal's gold-sublimate method* and *gold toning.*

gold chloride reagent a 1:1 mixture of 20 percent trichloroacetic acid and 0.25 percent gold chloride ($AuCl_3$). It is used as a reagent in spot tests for phenothiazines (indicated by a red color) and bromides (indicated by a brown color).

Goldflam's disease (gōlt′flahmz) see *myasthenia gravis.*

Goldman-Offner reference see *average potential reference.*

gold thioglucose see *aurothioglucose.*

gold toning a step in most histologic silver impregnation procedures. The sections are placed in a yellow gold–chloride solution after they have been impregnated using silver nitrate or ammoniacal silver solutions and the silver oxide has been reduced to metallic silver using formalin or hydroquinone solutions. This replaces the silver with gold and changes the background stain from yellow to pale gray. Gold-toned sections are more transparent and counterstain better.

Golgi complex (gol′je) [Camillo *Golgi,* Italian histologist, 1843–1926; co-winner, with Sangiago Ramón y Cajal, of the Nobel Prize for medicine and physiology in 1926 in recognition of their work on the structure of the nervous system] an organelle found in most cells that functions in secretion and glycoprotein synthesis; sometimes called just "the Golgi." It consists of saccules (flat, fenestrated vesicles) composed of unit membrane and arrayed in stacks of three to eight. The saccule closest to the nucleus is called the forming (proximal) face; that closest to the cell membrane is called the maturing (mature, maturation, or distal) face. Usually, all saccules are bowl shaped, with the concave face toward the cell membrane. The forming face is created by absorption of intermediate (transfer, or transport) vesicles budded off from the endoplasmic reticulum. A saccule's membrane is derived from the membranes of many intermediate vesicles, and its lumen is filled with their contents. Condensing vacuoles bud off from the maturing face, eventually consuming it, and move to the cell membrane. The membrane of condensing vacuoles is added to the cell membrane and the contents are secreted (exocytosis). The carbohydrate side-chains of glycoproteins are added in the saccules by sugar transferases. In thin section, the Golgi complex appears to consist of many isolated stacks of saccules, but high-voltage electron microscopy has shown that these actually are cuts through one stack running through the cell like a pile of ribbons. Also called Golgi body.

Golgi tendon organ a sensory receptor located within the tendons of muscles, where it serves to regulate muscle tension by responding to regular contractions and particularly to excessive stretching (inverse stretch reflex). It consists of a ramification of the terminal nerve branches close to the muscle tendon junction. Also called *musculotendinous organ.*

Gomori's method for chromaffin (go-mor′rez) [George *Gomori,* Hungarian-American histochemist, 1904–1957] a modification of Mallory's collagen stain using first azocarmine G and then aniline blue and quinoline yellow or orange G. Chromaffin granules stain purple-red; alpha cells of the pancreas, some cells of the anterior pituitary, neutrophils, and myelocytes stain similarly.

Gomori's trichrome stain a one-solution trichrome mixture used in histology as a connective tissue stain. Following nuclear staining with iron hematoxylin, sections are washed and counterstained with trichrome solution, which contains chromotrope 2R, light green SF yellowish, phosphotungstic acid, and glacial acetic acid. Muscle fibers appear red, collagen stains green, and nuclei appear blue to black.

gon/o (gon′o) [Gr. *gonē* seed] a word element used in combining form to denote seed or semen, e.g., gonocyte.

gonad/o (go′nad-o) [L. *gonas,* from Gr. *gonē* seed] a word element used in combining form to denote the sex glands, e.g., gonadogenesis.

gonad (go′nad, gon′ad) a gamete-producing gland; an ovary or testis.

gonadal (go′nad-al) pertaining to a gonad.

gonadal dysgenesis see *Turner's syndrome.*

gonadal stromal tumors a group of neoplasms of the ovary or testis that arise from specialized stromal cells. See also *granulosa–theca cell tumors* and *Sertoli-Leydig cell tumors.*

gonadotropic (gon″ah-do-trōp′ik) [*gonado-* + Gr. *tropos* a turning] stimulating the gonads; applied to hormones of the anterior pituitary, which influence the gonads.

gonadotropin (gon″ah-do-tro′pin) a hormone that acts primarily on the gonads. The anterior pituitary secretes two gonadotropins: follicle-stimulating hormone (FSH), which stimulates follicular development in the ovaries and gametogenesis in the testes; and luteinizing hormone (LH), which acts primarily in promoting luteinization of the ovaries and Leydig cell function of the testes. The serum values of both gonadotropins are low during infancy and then have a twofold increase, becoming pulsatile at the time of puberty.

In the adult female, the menstrual cycle is divided by a midcycle surge of both LH and FSH into follicular and luteinizing phases. Some disorders in the hypothalamic-pituitary-gonadal axis cause changes in gonadotropin plasma levels, determination of which is used to ascertain the etiology of gonadal dysfunction in males and females.

See also *follicle-stimulating hormone, luteinizing hormone,* and the accompanying illustration.

gonadotropin hormone–releasing hormone (GnRH) a hypothalamic peptide hormone that directly induces the release of luteinizing hormone (LH) and follicle-stimulating hormone (FSH) from the anterior pituitary; this action is mediated through the elevation of intracellular cAMP. It is a

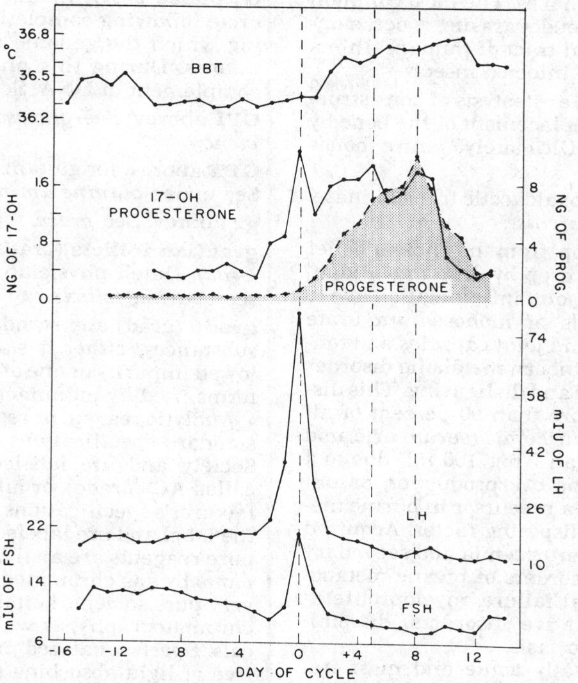

Gonadotropin. Mean daily plasma follicle-stimulating hormone, luteinizing hormone, progesterone, and 17α-OH progesterone concentrations and basal body temperatures during 16 presumptively ovulatory cycles from 15 young females. (Adapted from Ross, G. T., et al.: Pituitary and gonadal hormones in women during spontaneous and induced ovulatory cycles. Recent Progress In Hormone Research *26*: 1–62, 1970.)

decapeptide whose *N*-terminal amino acid is pyroglutamic acid and whose carboxy terminal has a substituted amide group. This hormone is used clinically to differentiate between hypothalamic and pituitary dysfunction and to induce ovulation in patients with hypothalamic amenorrhea. Also called *follicle-stimulating hormone–releasing hormone* (*FSH-RH*), *luteinizing hormone/follicle-stimulating hormone–releasing hormone* (*LH/FSH-RH*), and *luteinizing hormone–releasing hormone* (*LH-RH*).

Gongylonema (gon″jĭ-lo-ne′mah) [Gr. *gongylos* round + *nēma* thread] a genus of nematode worms. The species *G. pulchrum* is found in the mouths of humans and causes local irritation. Laboratory diagnosis requires microscopic identification.

gonion (go′ne-on), pl. *gonia* [Gr. *gōnia* angle] the protruding point at the lower rear of the lower jaw, the apex of the exterior angle of the mandible; used as an anatomic landmark.

gonococcus (GC), pl. *gonococci*. see *N. gonorrhoeae* under *Neisseria.*

gonorrhea (gon″o-re′ah) [gono- + *rhein* flow] a contagious genitourinary infection with the gram-negative coccus *Neisseria gonorrhoeae.* The gonococcus attacks the genital and urinary mucous membranes, causing inflammation and pus formation. In the female, the infection may be asymptomatic but if left untreated may lead to salpingitis, oophoritis, and ovarian abscesses. In both sexes, there may be a bacteremia, with arthritis and, rarely, meningitis or endocarditis. During delivery, an infected mother's gonococcal infection may be transmitted to the infant during its passage through the birth canal. The resulting contamination of the eyes, if untreated, will lead to blindness. See also *N. gonorrhoeae* under *Neisseria.*

gonorrheal (gon″o-re′al) of or pertaining to gonorrhea.

Goodell's sign (good′elz) [William *Goodell,* American gynecologist, 1829–1894] a sign resulting from the systematic changes associated with pregnancy that occur in the female reproductive tract. The cervix, uterus, and vagina soften because of the hormonal stimulation that is effected by the developing fetus.

goodness of fit the degree to which a set of statistical data supports a specified probability model in the sense that the observed data do not represent an unlikely occurrence, under the assumption that the model holds, i.e., is valid.

Goodpasture's syndrome (good-pas′churz) [Ernest William *Goodpasture,* American pathologist, 1886–1960] a rare disease, primarily occurring in young males, that is characterized by a rapid, necrotizing glomerulonephritis and by pneumonitis that is predominantly hemorrhagic. The lung and kidney lesions are thought to be a result of antiglomerular basement membrane antibodies. There is hemoptysis and progressive renal failure with a high mortality.

Good's syndrome an immunodeficiency syndrome that consists of thymoma, hypogammaglobulinemia, and pure red cell aplasia. The condition is exceedingly rare.

Gordius (gor′de-us) [Gordian knot] a genus of worms of the class Gordiacea, also known as the horsehair worms or hair snakes. The most common species, *G. aquaticus,* a pseudoparasite, is occasionally found in the intestinal tract of humans. Infection is due to ingestion of infected insects.

Gorham's disease massive osteolysis of bony structures, with a progessive replacement of the bone by vascular fibrous tissue. Ultimately, entire bones may undergo resorption.

Got abbrev. for glutamic-oxaloacetic transaminase. See *aspartate aminotransferase.*

gout (gowt) [L. *gutta* a drop, from the ancient belief that a harmful agent fell drop by drop into a joint] acute recurrent attacks of joint inflammation due to the deposition of crystals of monosodium urate monohydrate in and around joint capsules and tendons. Primary gout is an inborn metabolic disorder that is potentially chronic and disfiguring. This disease may be familial; more than 90 percent of all cases are in males. Hyperuricemia (serum uric acid concentrations greater than 7 mg/100 ml) due to a genetic defect causing the overproduction or underexcretion of uric acid (a precursor in purine metabolism) is a major predisposing factor. Acquired conditions leading to hyperuricemia and secondary gout include acquired disorders of purine metabolism, lactic acidosis, renal failure, myeloproliferative and lymphoproliferative disorders, disseminated carcinoma, and psoriasis.

Initial attacks are usually acute and most frequently affect the metatarsophalangeal joint of one big toe. The crystals may be deposited as aggregates (tophi), triggering a foreign body immune response; they also may be deposited in subcutaneous tissues, cartilage, bone, and kidneys. Following deposition, the crystals are phagocytized by polymorphonuclear cells, leading to actue inflammation. Pain, swelling, redness, and heat are the primary signs. Early attacks usually last several days. Without control, subsequent attacks may occur up to several times a year, leading to erosive joint disease and enlarging tophi. Chronic gout predisposes to the formation of urinary calculi at an incidence far greater than that found in the general population.

Diagnosis is most often suspected on the basis of clinical evaluation. Also, serum urate concentrations exceed 7.5 mg/100 ml in the majority of cases. Monosodium urate monohydrate crystals are demonstrable in synovial fluid, either floating free or within phagocytes. The crystals are negatively birefringent on polarized light examination. Radiographs reveal punched-out lesions in the subchondral bone of peripheral joints. An elevated erythrocyte sedimentation rate (ESR) and white blood cell count may be seen. For the first several attacks, colchicine is the drug of choice. Anti-inflammatory drugs may also be required.

gouty (gow'te) affected with or of the nature of gout.

G-6-P abbrev. See *glucose-6-phosphate.*

GPD abbrev. See *glucose-6-phosphate dehydrogenase.*

G-6-PD abbrev. See *glucose-6-phosphate dehydrogenase.*

G_0 phase a term used to indicate cells that leave the mitotic cycle to become quiescent. See also *cell cycle.*

G_1 phase presynthetic gap; the phase of the cell cycle prior to DNA synthesis. During this phase the cell has a single complement of DNA. See also *cell cycle.*

G_2 phase postsynthetic gap; the phase of the cell cycle following completion of DNA synthesis (during which the genome is replicated) and prior to mitosis. During this phase the cell has a double complement of DNA. See also *cell cyle.*

GPI abbrev. See *glucosephosphate isomerase deficiency.*

GPT abbrev. for glutamate pyruvate transaminase. See under *alanine aminotransferase.*

gr abbrev. See *grain.*

graafian follicle (graf'e-an) [Reijnier (Regner) *de Graaf,* Dutch physician and anatomist, 1641–1673] see *ovarian follicle.*

grade (grād) any standard of purity for chemical substances, either a standard specification of allowed impurity or one of several general descriptive terms used by manufacturers.

Analytic reagent or reagent grade chemicals meet standard specifications of the American Chemical Society and are labeled AR or ACS (sometimes called ACS grade), or alternatively meet the manufacturer's specifications, which are usually given on the label and are labeled AR. Chromatographically pure reagents are analyzed for absence of contaminants by gas chromatography. This group includes very pure solvents suitable for high-pressure liquid chromatography, as well as highly pure biochemicals. Spectroanalyzed or spectrograde solvents are free of light-absorbing substances and are used in spectrophotometry.

USP (U.S. Pharmacopeia) and NF (National Formulary) grades are standards for drugs and chemicals used in drug preparations. Only impurities affecting health are limited; the chemical purity is incidental.

Other grades of chemicals are not uniform in designation and are unsuitable for the most precise work. Among these are chemically pure grade (labeled CP) and highest purity grade. Less pure grades are called purified, practical, or pure grade. The lowest purity grades are called technical or commercial grade and are limited to use in manufacturing.

-grade (grād) [L. *gredi* to go] a suffix word element used to denote go, e.g., anterograde.

gradient (gra'de-ent) the rate of change of a variable along a specified direction, or the vector composed of the rate of change in all three directions.

graduate (grad'u-āt) [L. *graduatus*] a measuring vessel marked by a series of lines representing increments of volume.

graduated cylinder a common item of laboratory volumetric glassware: a glass cylinder with a flanged bottom and open top, usually with a lip for pouring and having graduated markings indicating the volume of fluid contained.

graft (graft) 1. any tissue or organ for implantation or transplantation.

2. to implant or transplant such tissue.

allogeneic g., a graft between individuals of the same species but of different genotype. Also called *allograft, homograft,* and *homologous graft.*

autologous g., a graft of tissue from one site on the body to a different site on the same body. Also called *autochthonous graft, autogeneic graft, autograft,* and *autoplast.*

heterologous g., a graft of tissue between individuals of different species and, therefore, of different genotype. Also called *heterogeneic graft, heterograft, xenogeneic graft,* and *xenograft.*

isogeneic g., a tissue or organ for implantation or transplantation that has a genotype identical to that of the recipient. Also called *isograft, syngeneic graft,* and *syngraft.*

graft rejection host rejection of a graft of tissue or organ, frequently due to immunologic incompatibility. See also *histocompatibility* and *HLA complex.*

first-set g.r., an immunologic incompatibility between graft and host. A hyperacute rejection results in an immediate inflammatory response because of the presence of preformed antibody. An acute rejection occurs after 6 da of graft introduction and results in a loss of function for the transplanted tissue or organ. Chronic rejection involves a progressive loss of function for the graft.

second-set g.r., an immunologic rejection of a graft by a host that is already immune to antigens in the graft tissue. This condition is usually due to previous exposure to that graft. A second-set graft rejection is immunologically more rapid than a first-set graft rejection.

graft-versus-host (GVH) disease, reaction the acute, hyperacute, or chronic attack of foreign histoincompatible cells on host tissues. Such a response necessitates the presence of (1) histoincompatibility between graft and recipient cells, (2) immunocompetent graft cells, and (3) immunoincompetent recipient cells. The GVH reaction may result from the infusion of blood or blood products containing viable lymphocytes or from the transplantation of fetal thymus, fetal liver, or bone marrow. Reaction onset occurs 7–30 da after introduction of the incompatible lymphocytes. Once the reaction has begun, little can be done to modify its course, and it is usually fatal in immunodeficient individuals.

In the acute form of the reaction, there is a maculopapular rash, frequently mistaken for a viral or allergic rash, that eventually begins to scale. Other symptoms include diarrhea, hepatosplenomegaly, jaundice, cardiac irregularity, irritability, and pulmonary infiltration. The patient's susceptibility to infection is enhanced.

The hyperacute form also begins with a maculopapular rash, but it progresses to a form that resembles toxic epidermal necrolysis, usually with accompanying severe diarrhea. Other symptoms resemble the acute form. Death occurs shortly after the reaction begins.

The chronic form is usually the result of maternal-fetal transfusion or bone marrow transplantation. The clinical features may range from slightly to markedly abnormal. Chronic desquamation of the skin is present. Hepatosplenomegaly and lymphadenopathy may occur, as may chronic diarrhea and failure to thrive. Secondary infections are a complication. Biopsy of the skin or lymph nodes shows histiocytic infiltration; this may lead to the misdiagnosis of Letterer-Siwe disease, although GVH patients have severe immunodeficiency, in contrast to Letterer-Siwe patients. Chronic GVH disease may also be confused with acrodermatitis enteropathica.

Diagnosis of GVH disease is suggested when an immunocompromised patient who received potentially immunocompetent cells 7–30 da prior to the onset of symptoms develops these symptoms; diagnosis may be confirmed by demonstration of sex or HLA chimerism. There is no adequate treatment. Immunosuppressive therapy, such as administration of corticosteroids or antilymphocyte globulin, further compromises the patient without controlling the disease. Prevention of the reaction is the only viable alternative; thus, any patient, especially an infant, suspected of having cellular immunodeficiency should receive only blood products that have been treated with 3000–6000 R to destroy immunocompetent lymphocytes.

Graham-Cole test see *oral c.* under *cholecystography.*

Graham's law (gra'amz) [Thomas *Graham,* English chemist, 1805–1869] stated as: the relative rates of the diffusion of gases vary inversely with the square root of their densities.

grain (grān) [L. *granum*] 1. the discrete unit of a photographic image; a small particle of metallic silver.

2. any small particle, such as a single silver halide crystal in a photographic emulsion or a phosphor crystal in an x-ray intensifying screen.

3. (abbrev. gr), a unit of mass in the obsolete apothecaries' and avoirdupois systems equal to 0.0648 g.

grain count halving time a measure of the turnover time of a labeled cell compartment, i.e., the time taken by the radioactive label to drop to 50 percent of its initial value, as determined by the average grain count over cell nuclei in radioautographs.

graininess (gra'ne-ness) the mottled appearance of a photographic image due to the finite size of the grains of metallic silver. Graininess is increased with faster films or longer development.

grain itch see under *predaceous mites.*

grain itch mite see under *Pyemotes.*

gram (g) (gram) [Fr. *gramma*] an International System (SI) unit of mass defined as one-thousandth of a kilogram, which is the base unit; about 0.035 oz. Note that an alternate abbreviation "gm" is not preferred and is never used with prefixes or with other units, for example, with abbreviations such as mg and g/cm^3.

-gram (gram) [Gr. *gramma* that which is written; a mark] a suffix word element used to denote a recording, graphic output, or radiograph, e.g., program, cardiogram.

gramicidin (gram″ĭ-si'din) a polypeptide antibiotic produced by *Bacillus brevis,* one of the principal components of tyrothricin. It is a mixture of several open chain and cyclic peptides each about 15 amino acids long. It is too toxic for systemic use but is used in topical preparations, often in combination with other antibiotics. Gramicidin acts by increasing the permeability of the plasma membrane. See also *antibacterial agents.*

Gram's iodine (gramz) [Hans Christian Joachim *Gram,* Danish physician, 1853–1938] a strong iodine solution containing iodine and potassium iodide dissolved in water.

gram negative (gram neg'ah-tiv) [Hans Christian Joachim *Gram*] losing the primary stain or decolorized by alcohol in Gram's method of staining; a primary characteristic of certain microorganisms. The Gram stain reaction of an organism is based primarily on the cell wall structure. The gram-negative cell wall is composed of a thin layer of electron-dense peptidoglycan (about 1 nm) that is surrounded by an outer membrane of lipoprotein and lipopolysaccharide. As the outer membrane is permeable to small molecules but less permeable to hydrophobic or amphipathic molecules, gram-negative organisms are thus less susceptible to antibiotics. Examples of gram-negative organisms include the enterics, *Neisseria, Hemophilus,* and *Pseudomonas.* See also *Gram stain.* Cf. *gram positive.*

gram positive (gram poz'ĭ-tiv) [H.C.J. *Gram*] retaining the primary stain or resisting decolorization by alcohol in Gram's method of staining; a primary characteristic of certain microorganisms. The Gram stain reaction of an organism is based primarily on the cell wall structure. The gram-positive cell wall is composed of a thick layer of electron-dense peptidoglycan (20–80 nm) with attached teichoic acids. Gram-positive organisms are sensitive to antibiotics such as penicillin, erythromycin, and vancomycin. Examples of such organisms include *Streptococcus, Staphylococcus, Corynebacterium,* and *Clostridium.* See also *Gram stain.* Cf. *gram negative.*

Gram stain (gram) [H.C.J. *Gram*] the standard staining procedure for the visualization and primary classification of bacteria. This procedure differentiates bacteria into two groups termed gram-positive and gram-negative organisms.

The bacterial cells are fixed to the slide by heat or methanol and stained with a basic dye (e.g., crystal violet) that stains all bacteria. The slides are then treated with an iodine-Kl mixture (Gram's iodine) and a mordant that fixes the primary stain, and then washed either with acetone or 95 percent ethyl alcohol, or with a mixture of alcohol-acetone, to decolorize gram-negative cells. Next, they are counterstained with a dye of a different color (e.g., safranin). Gram-positive organisms retain the original violet stain (purple), whereas gram-negative organisms lose the original color when the organic solvent is added, and show the counterstain color (pink, if safranin is used).

The difference in Gram stain reaction between bacteria is based on differences in cell wall structure between gram-positive and gram-negative organisms. The cell wall of gram-positive bacteria is thick (20–80 nm), consisting of peptidoglycan and an inner cell membrane. The reason why gram-positive bacteria are not decolorized has not been clearly defined. Nonviable gram-positive bacteria may stain as gram-negative cells. The cell wall of gram-negative bacteria consists of an inner cell membrane, a very thin peptidoglycan layer (1 nm), and an outer membrane. The solubility of the outer membrane to the organic solvent used in the decolorizing step may partially explain the loss of the primary stain from the bacterial cell.

APPLICATIONS. Gram stains may be used for the preliminary identification of certain bacterial types observed in direct examination of specimens or in smears made from cultures. The morphology in liquid media is usually more representative of the bacterium's true morphology than that on solid media.

A direct gram-stained smear from the specimen is an inexpensive and rapid procedure that often provides early presumptive diagnosis and aids in antibiotic selection when used in combination with clinical findings. Purulent portions of specimens should be chosen for both culture and smears. Gram stains of specimens should be examined first under low power (×100) for the presence of epithelial cells and/or leukocytes and then under oil (×970). Nuclei of properly stained cells should appear dark pink to red in color and the cytoplasm pink. If the cytoplasm or nucleus is purple (i.e., not decolorized sufficiently), the oil may be blotted and the slide immersed in xylene to remove excess oil. The slide may then be restained, starting at the decolorization step. Slides that have been overdecolorized may also be restained.

When reporting the results of direct specimen smears, it is important to note the presence or absence of leukocytes and/or epithelial cells. The presence of leukocytes is consistent with an inflammatory process; the presence of epithelial cells suggests contamination with normal flora that makes interpretation of culture results difficult. Bacteria should be reported semiquantitatively (e.g., rare, scattered, moderate, many) so that the clinician knows which bacterial types predominate. The presence of intracellular bacteria is suggestive of an active infectious process. Bacterial morphology, the source of the specimen, and the suspected diagnosis may suggest the identity of certain types of bacteria; for example, gram-positive cocci are probably staphylococci if the patient has osteomyelitis, tiny gram-negative bacilli may suggest *Hemophilus influenzae* in a patient with pneumonia, and gram-positive branching filaments in exudate are consistent with the diagnosis of nocardiosis in an immunocompromised host. It is important that the laboratory so indicate when several morphologic types are present, because this suggests mixed infections, which suggests the need for combined antibiotic therapy.

Direct smears also serve as an aid in the selection of isolation media. The same morphologic types of bacteria observed in a gram-stained smear should be present in the corresponding cultures. Failure to recover such types may reveal deficiencies in the collection, transport, or handling of specimens, or it may be due to defective culture media or improper incubation procedures. For example, fastidious, slow-growing organisms that require prolonged incubation may be present. Squamous epithelial cells suggest contamination with normal flora and questionable culture results. The value of direct gram-stained smears varies with the nature of the specimen.

SPINAL FLUID. Gram stains of spinal fluid can be of great assistance in the rapid diagnosis of bacterial meningitis if many bacteria are present in the spinal fluid. Previous antibiotic treatment may reduce the number of cells, particularly in culture. Smears of spinal fluid must be interpreted cautiously, however, because staining artifacts may resemble organisms; either overdecolorizing or underdecolorizing slides is a frequent pitfall that leads to incorrect interpretation.

SPUTUM. Gram stains are especially important for determining if a sputum specimen is likely to be representative of the lower respiratory tract. Specimens contaminated with throat flora yield false-positive cultures, and specimens with many squamous epithelial cells are generally considered unacceptable. An unsatisfactory specimen should be repeated at once. Examination of gram-stained smears may be helpful in establishing a tentative diagnosis of staphylococcal, pneumococcal, *Hemophilus,* meningococcal, or gram-negative bacterial pneumonia, especially when large numbers of organisms with typical morphology are seen in conjunction with polymorphonuclear (PMN) leukocytes.

URINE. A direct gram-stained smear of urine (one drop of uncentrifuged urine) is a useful screening device to distinguish urinary tract infection from contamination. In 80 percent of urinary infections, one or more bacterial cells per oil immersion field (more than 10^5 bacteria per milliliter) are found, usually accompanied by at least one PMN leukocyte per field. Generally, no bacteria or leukocytes are seen when fewer than 10^4 bacteria per milliliter are present. If squamous epithelial cells and normal mixed vaginal flora are present, there is contamination with normal flora, and the specimen must be repeated. A positive gram-stained smear followed by a negative culture suggests one of the following: a specimen mix-up, use of a "hot loop" in plating the urine, the presence of a fastidious aerobe or anaerobe (the latter is a very rare cause of urinary tract infection), or effective antibiotic therapy prior to culturing.

CERVICAL AND URETHRAL SPECIMENS. Direct Gram stains can be very useful with cervical and urethral specimens. Classically, in acute gonorrhea, gram-negative, kidney bean–shaped diplococci with polymorphonuclear leukocytes are observed. In males there is a high correlation (98 percent) between results with Gram stain and a confirmed diagnosis of gonorrhea. Gonococcal urethritis can be diagnosed in males with approximately 95 percent sensitivity and nearly 100 percent specificity by Gram stain. The absence of gram-negative diplococci correlates highly with the failure to recover *Neisseria gonorrhoeae* in culture and with the final diagnosis of nongonococcal urethritis. In females, the sensitivity of endocervical smear examination is only about 60 percent. However, if gram-negative intracellular diplococci and polymorphonuclear leukocytes are found in a specimen from a female with symptoms of pelvic inflammatory disease, a presumptive diagnosis is justified, pending culture results. Conversely, if epithelial cells and mixed flora are present, vaginal contamination is indicated and, although intracellular gram-negative cocci may be observed, the diagnosis of gonorrhea can be neither supported nor refuted by Gram stain. For both males and females, when large numbers of organisms of different morphologic type are present, the specificity of the smear is decreased, as other organisms may mimic the morphology of the gonococcus. In such instances, culture is necessary.

In Gram stains from genital specimens, *Trichomonas vaginalis* can be observed as a gram-negative, pear-shaped organism (15–18 μm long by 5–15 μm wide). The organisms are smaller than epithelial cells but larger than leukocytes. The cytoplasm is lacy in appearance, with deeply stained edges. The nucleus appears elongated and almond shaped. Flagella and an axostyle may be seen.

ANAEROBIC CULTURES. Because the usual primary incubation period is 48 hr rather than 24 hr for anaerobic cultures, utilization of direct Gram stains is even more important: the presence of bacteria and their morphology seen on a Gram stain can avoid a 2-da delay in the selection of rational antibiotic therapy. The Gram stain also permits a comparison of the growth on aerobic and anaerobic plates, which serves as a guide to the need for further incubation. The presence of bacteria on the direct smear, but no growth aerobically after 48 hr, may indicate either the presence of a fastidious, slow-growing anaerobe or a quality control problem with specimen transport or the culturing technique. When a number of different organisms are observed by Gram stain in conjunction with polymorphonuclear leukocytes or proteinaceous, necrotic debris (polymicrobic infections), multiple antibiotic therapy is indicated. The presence of epithelial cells suggests specimen inadequacy and contamination with normal flora.

Some anaerobes have a fairly consistant morphologic appearance in gram-stained smears.

1. Among gram-negative bacilli, *Bacteroides fragilis* are typically pleomorphic rods with rounded ends and bipolar staining (shaped like a safety pin); *B. melaninogenicus* are typically small coccobacilli; and *Fusobacterium* species typically have tapered ends, with some species very pleomorphic.
2. Thick, gram-positive rods with large capsules and rather square ends, but an absence of visible spores, is typical of *Clostridum perfringens*, which is the primary agent of gas gangrene and accounts for about half of the clostridial isolates in the laboratory. Other clostridial species may have a similar appearance but sporulate more readily, or they may instead appear either as delicate, thin rods, often without spores, or as weakly gram-positive or even gram-negative cells.
3. Thin, pleomorphic gram-positive bacilli—often in short chains and showing occasional bifurcated forms—may possibly be *Actinomyces* and *Bifidobacterium* species, although other gram-positive, nonspore-forming anaerobic bacilli also have this appearance.

Gram-positive anaerobic cocci cannot be differentiated from facultative cocci by Gram stain alone.

STOOLS. In cases of acute enteritis, a gram-stained smear may occasionally be helpful by suggesting early presumptive diagnosis. For example, the presence of leukocytes, in association with small, curved, gram-negative rods and a suppressed normal flora, suggests *Campylobacter* enteritis. In staphylococcal enterocolitis, the Gram stain may show leukocytes and many gram-positive cocci in clusters. Such a diagnosis must, of course, be supported by culture. Direct examination of stools for the presence of leukocytes allows characterization of patients with diarrhea. There is a close correlation between the presence of fecal leukocytes and the isolation of enteric pathogens. Information regarding leukocyte types present (polymorphonuclear versus mononuclear versus none) is best obtained not with the Gram stain but by use of methylene blue wet preparations.

OTHER CLINICAL USES. Gram stains may also pick up etiologic agents that would be missed by routine culture. For instance, *Strongyloides stercoralis* larvae or ova may be observed in the tracheal aspirates of patients with hyperinfestation. In cases of suspected Vincent's angina, leukocytes, spirochetes, and fusiform bacilli may be observed in smears from the throats of infected patients. Gram stains of throat or mouth scrapings may also be helpful when a *Candida* infection is being considered. Invasion by *Candida* species is characterized by the presence of leukocytes, yeast cells, and pseudohyphae; the latter suggest such invasion if the specimen was transported to the laboratory immediately and handled promptly. Pseudohyphae may develop in a specimen that has been stored for long periods at room temperature. Gram stains of several sites that show budding yeasts with pseudohyphae as well as leukocytes yield early data regarding possible disseminated disease, especially in immunosuppressed patients.

Reports of the results of Gram stains of positive blood cultures should include the arrangement of cells (e.g., chains, clusters, diphtheroids). A Gram stain of the buffy coat of a blood culture specimen may be useful in life-threatening situations. Gram stains of colonies in primary culture on solid media are needed when colony identity is uncertain.

Also called Gram's stain.

Gram-Weigert stain (gram-wi′gert) [H.C.J. *Gram;* Karl *Weigert,* German pathologist, 1845–1904] a stain for fibrin and bacteria. Paraffin sections are deparaffinized, hydrated, and stained first in lithium carmine (or basic fuchsin), then in crystal violet, mordanted in Gram's iodine, and differentiated in (1:1) aniline-xylene.

Fibrin and gram-positive bacteria stain blue-black to violet; nuclei are red (magenta if basic fuchsin is used). Collagen and keratin stain a lighter violet than does fibrin.

grand mal attack (grahn mahl) [Fr. "big illness"] former name for *tonic-clonic attack.*

Granger method (grān′jer) [Amedee *Granger,* American radiologist, 1879–1939] 1. a radiologic procedure using the Granger face rest (with an opening for the nose) to obtain particular views of the sinuses or sella turcica. The face mask and cassette are placed on an angle block; the patient's face rests on the mask, which makes the glabelloalveolar line parallel to the angle block. Granger's 23° position is used for radiography of the frontal, anterior ethmoidal, and maxillary sinuses. The angle block is tilted 23° toward the feet, and the central ray projects vertically in the plane, touching the infraorbital margins. Granger's 107° position is used for the sphenoidal, posterior ethmoidal, and maxillary sinuses. The angle block is tilted 17° toward the head, and the central ray projects vertically in the plane, touching the floor of the external acoustic meatuses. In another position used for an anterior view of the sella turcica, the angle block is tilted 17° toward the head, and the central ray projects through the glabella at an angle of 10° toward the head.

2. a radiologic procedure using Granger's mastoid localizer for obtaining a lateral projection of the mastoid processes. The localizer immobilizes the head and centers the mastoid; it rests on an angle block tilted 15° toward the feet and 13° toward the face. The central ray is vertical.

granul/o (gran′u-lo) [L. *granulum* granule] a word element used in combining form to denote granules, e.g., granulocyte.

granular (gran′u-lar) [L. *granularis*] composed of or marked by the presence of granules.

granular cell tumor a relatively uncommon and usually benign neoplasm that can occur almost anywhere in the body. It is so named because of a granular appearance of the tumor cells by light microscopy: this is due to the presence of many lysosomes. Initially the tumor was called granular cell myoblastoma, but ultrastructural studies have excluded the possibility of muscle cell origin. The histogenesis is still uncertain, but Schwann cell derivation is favored. Granular cell tumors are only rarely malignant, although they can be multiple. Simple excision is usually curative.

granular endoplasmic reticulum see under *endoplasmic reticulum.*

granular leukocyte see *granulocyte.*

granular pneumocyte see *type II pneumocyte* under *alveolar cell.*

granulation (gran″u-la′shun) [L. *granulatio*] 1. the subdivision of hard or metallic substances into small particles.

2. the process of formation of cytoplasmic granules.

granulation tissue tissue characteristic of healing inflammation, composed of proliferating myofibroblasts and small blood vessels with chronic inflammatory cells in a loose mixture. It forms the pink, soft, edematous tissue that appears on the surface of healing wounds.

granule (gran′ūl) [L. *granulum*] 1. in microscopy, a small, round, heavily stained region in a cell. Ultrastructurally, many granules have an electron-dense care and a limiting membrane. See also *metachromatic granule.*

2. the insoluble, nonmembranous particles found in the cytoplasm of blood cells. In myeloid cells, the granules are distinguished by their staining characteristics, each type having an affinity for either acid or basic stain. Primary azurophilic granules, secondary neutrophilic granules of neutrophils, eosinophilic granules of eosinophils, azurophilic granules of monocytes, and, probably, basophilic granules of basophils are lysosomes that stain their characteristic colors with Wright stain. Erythrocytes may contain siderocytic granules that stain blue with Perls' Prussian blue stain. For more information, see the specific granule.

granules of developing neutrophils the granules present at different stages of neutrophil maturation. Myeloblasts contain reaction products for peroxidase in the rough endoplasmic reticulum (RER), perinuclear cisterna, and Golgi cisternae; they may also contain a few azurophilic (peroxidase-positive) granules, which are approximately 500 nm in diameter. Promyelocytes have numerous azurophilic granules; these contain, in addition to myeloperoxidase, lysosomal acid hydrolases, proteases (elastase and cathepsin), cationic bacterial protein, acid mucosubstances, and lysozyme. The other two-thirds of neutrophil lysozyme is associated with the secondary specific granules developing in myelocytes.

A hiatal cell contains only the primary peroxidase-positive azurophilic granules but not the reaction products in the Golgi and RER, which indicates that production of the azurophilic granules has ceased. In the myelocyte stage, the smaller secondary "specific granules" are produced; they are peroxidase negative and contain lactoferrin, which has some antimicrobial activity, probably the result of its ability to chelate iron. The contents of both primary and secondary granules are discharged into phagocytic vacuoles that surround ingested bacteria, where the various antibacterial substances become effective. Degranulation accompanies effective phagocytosis, as can be observed by phase microscopy, as well as electron microscopic studies. The azurophilic granules appear reddish-purple, owing to metachromatic staining in Wright-Giemsa smears only in the early stages (promyelocytes), whereas they appear as violet granules in myelocytes. The secondary granules are at the limit of resolution with the light microscope; they are not individually visible but impart a beige or pink color to the cytoplasm.

On separation of granules, alkaline phosphatase is associated with specific granules in some species (rabbit) and with the lighter membrane fraction in humans.

Although the azurophilic granules are no longer produced in later (myelocyte) stages of maturation, they persist, are identifiable by their peroxidase reaction, and are halved in number with each myelocytic division.

See also *azurophilic granule.*

granulocyte (gran′u-lo-sīt″) [*granulo-* + Gr. *kytos* hollow vessel] any cell that contains granules, especially polymorphonuclear neutrophils. Also called *granular leukocyte.* See also *basophil, eosinophil,* and *polymorphonuclear neutrophil.*

granulocyte concentrate a concentrated suspension of granulocytes collected by leukapheresis. A single unit of concentrate should contain at least 1×10^{10} granulocytes; if possible, it should be obtained from blood relatives of the patient to reduce the incidence of alloimmunization. Granulocyte concentrates are indicated for patients with transient severe neutropenia ($<$ 500 granulocytes/mm^3), sepsis, and an inadequate response to antibiotics.

granulocytic (gran″u-lo-sit′ik) pertaining to or of the nature of granulocytes.

granulocytic series one of the white blood cell series that develops in the bone marrow and passes into the circulation, and then into the tissues where the cells perform their function.

There are seven stages of maturation, designated M_1 through M_7: myeloblast (M_1), promyelocyte (M_2), myelocyte (M_3 and M_4), metamyelocyte (M_5), band form (M_6), and polymorphonuclear neutrophil (M_7). Stages M_1–M_4 undergo amplification and maturation; after this point the cells (M_5–M_7) are no longer capable of division and simply mature.

There are three parallel cell lines in the granulocytic series (neutrophils, eosinophils, and basophils), which can be distinguished beginning with the promyelocyte or myelocyte stages. Classification of these cells is based on nuclear characteristics and the type and number of granules as seen in Giemsa- or Wright-stained smears. All granulocytes produce azurophilic granules during their early maturation. In the myelocyte stage, only "specific granules" are produced, which are neutrophilic, eosinophilic, or basophilic; these granules are also called secondary granules, in contrast to the primary or azurophilic granules.

The neutrophilic series is the most prominent of the granulocytic series; eosinophils and basophils normally represent 0.5–3.0 percent of the white cells in the peripheral blood, whereas neutrophils represent 40–70 percent. Thus, the neutrophilic series is implied if the granulocytic series is discussed without further specification.

granulocytopenia (gran″u-lo-si″to-pe′ne-ah) [*granulocyte* + Gr. *penia* poverty] a symptom complex characterized by the reduction of neutrophilic polymorphonuclear leukocytes in peripheral blood below 1500/mm^3. Levels of 500–1000/mm^3 carry increased risk of infection; levels below 500/mm^3 virtually always are followed by bacterial infection unless suitable precautions are taken. The most common cause of granulocytopenia is drugs. Certain drugs induce granulocytopenia in a small but definite number of users, and any drug can occasionally cause granulocytopenia on an idiosyncratic basis in susceptible individuals. In both circumstances, the drug suppresses granulocytopoiesis in the marrow. Another cause is severe gram-negative infection (sepsis). A transient form may occur during the onset of many infectious diseases.

In rare instances, granulocytopenia may be due to peripheral destruction of leukocytes by antibodies directed against the cells themselves or by antibodies directed against a drug-modified cell surface of the leukocytes. It may also be caused by the attachment of drug-antibody complexes to the leukocytes and their destruction by complement. Peripheral destruction of leukocytes (often associated with red cell and platelet destruction) may be caused by hypersplenism. Finally, congenital granulocytopenias have been described and include cyclic neutropenia, myelokathexis, and other rare syndromes. The severe form is called *agranulocytosis.* See also *hypersplenism* and *neutropenia.*

granulocytopoiesis (gran″u-lo-si″to-poi-e′sis) [*granulocyte* + Gr. *poiein* to make] the production and maturation in the bone marrow of the cells in the granulocytic series. See also *granulocytic series.*

granulocytopoietic (gran″u-lo-si″to-poi-et′ik) stimulating granulocytopoiesis.

granulogenesis (gran″u-lo-jen′ĕ-sis) [*granulo-* + Gr. *genesis* production] the formation of granules.

granuloma (gran″u-lo′mah) [*granulo-* + Gr. *ōma* tumor] a nodular aggregate of macrophages and lymphocytes involved in organized phagocytic and immune activities, accompanied by fibroblasts producing collagen tissue. It represents a major site of cell-mediated immune response in chronic granulomatous inflammation.

The distinctive cell types found in many granulomas, epithelioid cells and giant cells, are both derived from macrophages. The epithelioid cell is a differentiated macrophage that is so named because it exhibits a strong cytologic resemblance to certain epithelial cells. In the process of transformation from an undifferentiated macrophage, the epithelioid cell loses the property of phagocytosis but retains the capacity by the process of pinocytosis to take up subcellular-size particles of foreign material. Larger fragments of foreign material, including microorganisms, are ingested by phagocytic macrophages for degradation by lysosomal digestion. Fragments too large to be engulfed by a single cell are surrounded by several macrophages that then fuse into a single cell. This process results in the formation of a multinucleated giant cell. In the multinucleated giant cell, the nuclei may be either clumped in the center or at one pole (the Touton giant cell) or arranged in a complete or partial ring at the cell periphery (the Langhans giant cell). Either type may be seen in both immune and nonimmune-related granulomas.

When the immune system is involved in chronic granulomatous inflammation, antigen-sensitized T lymphocytes are stimulated to proliferate in the thymus-dependent areas of lymph nodes and the spleen, giving rise to circulating effector T lymphocytes. On subsequent contact with the original antigen, the effector lymphocytes respond by the release of various lymphokines (chemical mediators of cell-mediated immunity), which are responsible for the attraction of macrophages to the granuloma (chemotactic factor), their immobilization within the granuloma (macrophage migration inhibiting factor), the activation of some macrophages, and, where appropriate, enhancement of their cytocidal activities toward invasive microbes and neoplastic cells (macrophage activating factor) and the transformation of some macrophages into epithelioid cells. The development of epithelioid cells appears to be part of a cell-mediated immune reaction: neonatal thymectomy greatly reduces the granulomatous reaction to schistosome eggs, whereas in intact animals the tissue lesion includes a large epithelioid cell element.

The role of the lymphocyte in promoting the killing of phagocytized microorganisms by macrophages is dramatically demonstrated in *Mycobacterium leprae* infections. In the lepromatous form of leprosy, granulomas are devoid of lymphocytes and, in their absence, the mycobacteria are free to thrive and multiply in the unactivated macrophages that have phagocytized them. In contrast, lymphocytes are abundant in granulomas in the tuberculous form of leprosy, leading to activation of the resident macrophages and effective killing of the phagocytized microorganisms.

In chronic granulomatous inflammation induced by nonantigenic foreign material, there is no sensitization of T lymphocytes, nor are they attracted to granulomas. In the absence of T lymphocytes, lymphokines are not released to effect the transformation of macrophages into epithelioid cells. Therefore, granulomas induced by nonantigenic foreign material are characterized by a predominance of macrophages and multinucleated giant cells with a conspicuous absence of lymphocytes and epithelioid cells.

The final event in the development of the granuloma is a mesenchymal host response. In both immune- and nonimmune-related granulomatous inflammation, the phagocytic process results in the secretion of neutral proteases with elastinolytic, collagenolytic, proteoglycan-degrading, and plasminogen-activating functions leading to local tissue destruction and eventually to fibrosis. In some forms of foreign body granuloma (for example, silicosis), reaction to the foreign material causes the death of the macrophage that ingests it, resulting in the release of lysozymes that produce local tissue necrosis as well as the attraction of new macrophages to repeat the cycle. This process ultimately produces extensive fibrosis of the granuloma and surrounding tissues.

In the infectious form of granulomatous inflammation, when the level of cell-mediated immunity is adequate to destroy the microorganisms, the healing process is accompanied by the laying down of collagen fibers within the granuloma and around its periphery, effectively walling off and isolating any remaining organisms from the rest of the body. In this instance, the fibrosis benefits the host, whereas in certain forms of foreign body granulomatous inflammation (such as pulmonary silicosis), the reactive fibrosis eventually becomes a major component of the disease process.

g. annulare, a collection of hard, reddish nodules thought to represent chronic granulomatous inflammation caused by an unknown agent. These eruptions occur on the skin of children and young adults, particularly on the hands, feet, neck, and buttocks, forming a circular pattern or ring. Histologically, the lesions are characterized by focal degeneration of collagen, fibrosis, and a reactive infiltrate of palisaded histiocytes.

beryllium g., a local noncaseating granulomatous reaction to the presence of beryllium in the lungs or skin. These lesions resemble sarcoid lesions and often progress to fibrosis and hyalinization. See also *berylliosis* and *granulomatous i.* under *inflammation.*

giant cell reparative g., a nonneoplastic lesion limited to the jaws, which is believed to be a reactive response. It is characterized by a loose fibrous stroma that is richly vascular and contains multinucleated giant cells thought to arise in response to hemorrhage. The majority (> 75 percent) occur in children and young adults and are twice as common in males as in females. The differential diagnosis includes the brown tumor of hyperparathyroidism, true giant cell tumor, osteosarcoma, and other fibroosseous lesions containing giant cells.

g. inguinale, a chronic, ulcerative granulomatous disease associated with conditions of inadequate cleanliness and poverty. It occurs in the genital or anal regions, beginning as a nodule and spreading to other areas of the abdomen. There is some suggestion that this disease may be sexually transmitted. It is caused by the gram-negative coccobacillus *Calymmatobacterium granulomatis* (formerly *Donovania granulomatis*), which does not grow on ordinary laboratory media, simple or complex, but instead grows in special media and egg yolk sacs.

Diagnosis is based on the presence of the organism (Donovan bodies) in tissue smears stained by the Wright stain or in biopsy material. The organism is most often identified within macrophages. Fibrosis and elephantiasis may occur as the infection progresses.

lethal midline g., a clinical syndrome characterized by destructive lesions of the upper respiratory tract including the nose, midface, nasopharynx, palate, and sinuses. It includes at least three pathologic conditions: Wegener's granulomatosis, malignant lymphoma (usually of large cell type), and polymorphic reticulosis.

lipoid g., a granuloma arising as part of a granulomatous response to exogenous or endogenous lipid.

mineral oil g., a foreign-body granulomatous reaction elicited by the presence of mineral oil in body tissues. The oil may be aspirated into the lungs when taken as a dietary contaminant or self-medication, or absorbed from the gastrointestinal tract and accumulated in the abdominal lymph nodes and spleen.

multifocal eosinophilic g., see *localized h.* under *histiocytosis.*

plasma cell g., a postinflammatory lesion that contains a polymorphous infiltrate of inflammatory cells including abundant plasma cells with Russell bodies and lipid-containing histiocytes. Such lesions are seen in the lungs as solitary large nodules, especially in younger adults, and also in the soft tissues of the mouth. In both sites the lesion must be differentiated from an extramedullary plasmacytoma. Also called inflammatory pseudotumor.

pyogenic g., a solitary elevated or pedunculated

cherry-red skin nodule that appears congested and bleeds when traumatized. It is composed of granulation tissue that arises in the skin (commonly the fingers or face) or oral cavity (frequently in association with pregnancy). It grows rapidly and may involute spontaneously, leaving a small focus of fibrosis; satellite foci sometimes develop. This lesion is thought to be a reparative process in response to trauma or nonspecific infection, but it must be differentiated from a vascular neoplasm.

swimming pool g., a benign, self-healing granulomatous lesion at the site of trauma and injury. It is most often seen in wounds sustained in swimming pools, owing to infection with *Mycobacterium balnei*, an organism that survives in that aqueous environment.

unifocal eosinophilic g., see *localized h.* under *histiocytosis.*

granulomatous (gran″u-lom′ah-tus) composed of or containing granulomas.

granulomatous thyroiditis see *subacute t.* under *thyroiditis.*

granulopenia (gran″u-lo-pe′ne-ah) [*granulo-* + Gr. *penia* poverty] see *granulocytopenia.*

granulophthisis (gran″u-lo-thi′sis) [*granulo-* + Gr. *phthisis* wasting] the degeneration or destruction of granulopoietic tissue.

granulopoiesis (gran″u-lo-poi-e′sis) [*granulocyte* + Gr. *poiein* to make] the formation of granulocytes; used incorrectly for *granulocytopoiesis.*

granulopoietic (gran″u-lo-poi-et′ik) pertaining to or concerned with the formation of granulocytes.

granulopoietin (gran″u-lo-poi-e′tin) an undefined substance thought to stimulate the development of granulocytes.

granulosa cell (gran″u-lo′sah) the specialized ovarian stromal cell type that forms the granulosa cell layer surrounding the ovarian follicle. After ovulation these cells enlarge, accumulate lipid, and are transformed into pale-staining polygonal lutein cells, a process called luteinization. Granulosa-lutein cells make up the bulk of the corpus luteum. See also *theca cell.*

granulosa cell tumor (gran″u-lo′sah) an ovarian neoplasm arising from the epithelial cells that surround the developing hair follicle. See also *granulosa–theca cell tumor.*

granulosa–theca cell tumor ovarian stromal cell neoplasms that exhibit, to varying degrees, differentiation toward granulosa or thecal cells or both. Most tumors in this category produce estrogen, and in the 5 percent of patients of prepubertal age, precocious puberty may be produced. Older females tend to develop endometrial hyperplasia.

These tumors display an extensive range of histology.

A relatively pure granulosa cell tumor can vary considerably in size and may be solid or contain cystic areas. In most instances the cells resemble those of the normal granulosa layer that surrounds the developing follicle, forming sheets of uniform round cells in which rosette formation or Call-Exner bodies may be present. Theca cell admixtures introduce a spindle cell component into these tumors. Approximately 10 percent of granulosa cell tumors are malignant. Prognosis depends on the extent of the tumor when treatment is initiated. See also *ovarian tumors* and *thecoma.*

graph (graf) [Gr. *graphein* to write or record] a diagram or curve representing varying relationships between sets of data.

-graph (graf) [Gr. *graphein*] a suffix word element to denote an instrument for writing or recording, e.g., spectrograph, electrocardiograph.

graphic (graf′ik) written or drawn; pertaining to the representation of data by diagrams.

graphic analysis the examination of the relationship between sets of data by the use of graphs.

graphics (grah′fiks) in data processing or data communications, the ability to process pictorial information (as distinct from textual information).

graphic terminal a computer input/output device used for graphic display. See also *computer graphics.*

graph tablet a computer input device that senses the position (x and y coordinates) of a stylus or cursor while it is used to draw or trace a figure on a graphic tablet. Also called graphic digitizer.

-graphy (graf′e) [Gr. *graphein* to write, record] a suffix word element to denote the process of recording, e.g., electroencephalography.

grating (gra′ting) a device for dispersing light into a spectrum, used in the monochromators of spectrophotometers. It consists of a series of ruled grooves on a reflecting surface. Light rays reflected from different grooves interfere constructively if the difference in path length is a multiple of the wavelength; otherwise, destructive interference occurs and the waves cancel. Because the path length difference depends on the angle of reflection, each wavelength is reflected at a different angle.

The dispersed spectrum falls on a narrow slit that passes only a small region of the spectrum—about 1–10 nm wide.

replica g., a grating made by casting from a master grating. It consists of an aluminized coating on an epoxy resin base.

Graves' disease (grāvz) [Robert James *Graves,* Irish physician, 1797–1853] a disorder characterized by hyperthyroidism, ocular changes, and skin lesions. Graves' disease is most common in females aged 20–40 yr. There is a diffusely enlarged thyroid, accompanied by ocular changes (such as exophthalmos, lid lag, and diplopia) and raised, thickened skin over the dorsum of the legs and feet (pretibial myxedema). The hyperthyroid state results in weight loss, tremor, emotional instability, intolerance to heat, diarrhea, and cardiac arrhythmias or failure. This condition is thought to be caused by serum IgG immunoglobulins, which bind to thyroid tissue and stimulate increased hormone production. Diagnosis is confirmed by elevated concentrations of serum T_3 and T_4 and increased resin T_3 uptake (RT_3U), free T_4 index (FT_4I), and radioactive iodine uptake (RAIU).

Treatment includes the administration of chemical agents to block thyroid hormone production or the destruction of thyroid tissue either surgically or with radioactive iodine. Glucocorticoids administered systemically are helpful in alleviating the associated ocular changes and may be applied topically for treatment of the skin lesions.

Also called *Basedow's disease* and *Parry's disease.*

gravid/o (grav′ĭ-do) [L. *gravida* heavy, loaded] a word element used in combining form to denote pregnancy, e.g., gravidity.

gravid (grav′id) pregnant.

gravimetric pertaining to measurement by weight; performed by weight, as a gravimetric method.

gravitation (grav″ĭ-ta′shun) a force that interacts with all matter proportionally to its mass.

gravity (grav′ĭ-te) [L. *gravitas*] 1. weight, the force of attraction of all masses by the earth.

2. (abbrev. *g,*) a unit of acceleration, 9.80665 m/sec^2, used to express the relative centrifugal force (RCF) of centrifuges.

Gravlee jet wash a procedure for irrigating the endometrial cavity under negative pressure, used to procure cells for cytologic study. Using an instrument composed of a double polyethylene tube, one tube is attached to a reservoir of fluid (e.g., saline) and the other to a syringe. The tip of the double tube is inserted into the endometrial cavity. Aspiration by means of the syringe creates negative pressure and draws fluid from the reservoir. The fluid bathes the endometrium and is aspirated into the syringe. The fluid containing the endometrial sample can then be studied cytologically. Also called *negative pressure lavage.*

Grawitz's granules (grah′vits-ez) [Paul Albert *Grawitz,* pathologist in Greifswald, 1850-1932] minute granules that produce the characteristic stippling seen in the red blood cells of persons with lead poisoning. The granules possess a coarse basophilic granulation best demonstrated by modification of the methylene blue stain. This lesion, although not diagnostic of lead poisoning, is nonetheless highly suggestive of the condition.

Grawitz's tumor see *hypernephroma.*

gray (Gy) (gra) the proposed new International System (SI) unit of absorbed radiation dose, the transfer of 1 joule of energy per kilogram of absorber (1 J/kg). One gray equals 100 rads.

gray matter the gray tissue of the central nervous system. It is composed of the cell bodies, initial axon segments, glial cells, dendritic arborizations, and terminals of the nervous elements within the CNS. In the brain it is predominantly located peripherally, whereas in the spinal cord it is surrounded by white matter.

gray-patch ringworm a common ectothrix fungal infection seen in children, which is caused by *Microsporum canis* and *M. audouinii.* The infection progresses from a small erythematous papule around the hair shaft to an inflammatory ring form involving the scalp and hair.

gray platelet syndrome a rare platelet function disorder in which platelets almost completely lack granules and stain a peculiar gray color in a Wright-stained peripheral blood smear. Biochemical studies report a decreased concentration of platelet ATP and extractable phosphatides. Response to ADP, epinephrine, and collagen is normal, as is platelet factor 3 (PF_3) activity.

gray ramus see under *ramus communicans.*

gray scale a representation of numbers by shades of gray so that the optical density of the gray is proportional to the number. It is used to represent computer-processed pictures in computed tomography, scintillation photography, and ultrasonography.

Greek alphabet the letters of the Greek alphabet (see table), commonly used in science as specific symbols or to designate an element in a sequence: α, the first; β, the second; γ, the third; and so forth.

GREEK ALPHABET

CAPITAL	SMALL LETTER	NAME	TRANS-LITERATION
Α	α	alpha	a
Β	β	beta	b
Γ	γ	gamma	g
Δ	δ	delta	d
Ε	ϵ	epsilon	e
Ζ	ζ	zeta	z
Η	η	eta	ē
Θ	θ,ϑ	theta	th
Ι	ι	iota	i
Κ	κ	kappa	k
Λ	λ	lambda	l
Μ	μ	mu	m
Ν	ν	nu	n
Ξ	ξ	xi	x
Ο	ο	omicron	o
Π	π	pi	p
Ρ	ρ	rho	r
Σ	σ, ς	sigma	s
Τ	τ	tau	t
Υ	υ	upsilon	y
Φ	φ,ϕ	phi	ph
Χ	χ	chi	ch
Ψ	ψ	psi	ps
Ω	ω	omega	ō

From Dorland's Illustrated Medical Dictionary. 26th ed. Philadelphia, W. B. Saunders Co., 1981, p. xviii.

In an old system of chemical nomenclature (whose names for familiar compounds are still in use), the Greek letters denote the positions of substituent groups. For many aliphatic compounds, the Greek letter locants are not the same as the numeric IUPAC locants, because in the old system the numbering starts with the carbon atom next to the principal functional group, whereas in the IUPAC system the numbering starts with the first carbon atom in the chain. If the principal functional group contains a carbon atom (e.g., a carboxyl or aldehyde), the Greek letter locants are one less than the numeric locants (e.g., an α-amino carboxylic acid is a 2-amino acid; γ-amino butyric acid is 4-aminobutanoic acid).

The plasma protein electrophoretic bands are named in order of decreasing electrophoretic mobility, prealbumin, albumin, α_1, α_2, β_1, β_2, and γ-globulin. The different polypeptide chains or monomeric units that compose a protein are usually designated by Greek letters (e.g., hemoglobin $A_1 = \alpha_2\beta_2$). Greek letters are also used to differentiate allotropic forms of a chemical element and to identify different forms of related compounds having the same trivial name, e.g., α-, β-, and γ-tocopherol. See also the entries for the individual letters (alphabetized according to their transliterations) and the names of the letters (e.g., *alpha*).

green (grēn) [A.S. *grēne*] a spectral color that corresponds to the perceived hue of monochromatic light having a wavelength between 492 and 577 nm (i.e., between blue and yellow).

grenz (grenz) [Ger. *Grenze* boundary] a boundary or limiting zone.

grenz rays low-energy x-rays with energies of about 10 KeV.

grid (grid) 1. in radiology, a device that reduces the fogging of a radiographic image by scattered x-rays. It is composed of thin lead strips separated by spaces of radiolucent material. The primary x-rays are parallel (or nearly parallel) to the lead strips and can pass between them, but most of the secondary x-rays, which originate from scattering in the object, will be absorbed by the lead strips.

2. a lattice of equally spaced vertical and horizontal lines used for plotting a graph.

3. any of the electrodes in a vacuum tube that control the flow of current in the tube.

4. a fine-mesh grid usually made from copper, which is used to support the ultrathin tissue sections used in transmission electron microscopy.

aligned g., a grid having all the lead strips aligned so that x-rays diverging from a point (the grid focus) will be parallel to the lead strips.

If the focal spot of the x-ray tube is at the grid focus, the grid lines will be very thin, and less of the primary ray will be absorbed than with a parallel grid. If the central ray is at an angle to the grid, or the focal-film distance is not optimum, the grid lines will be wider; this is called off-distance, off-center, or off-level cutoff. Also called *focused g.* Cf. *parallel g.*

Bucky-Potter g., a grid that is an integral part of an x-ray table, which moves during the exposure so that no grid lines show on the film. Its motion is controlled by the exposure timer.

crossed g., a grid composed of two superimposed parallel grids having lead strips at right angles to each other. It absorbs more secondary x-rays than other grids but cannot be used with an angled central ray without excessive cutoff.

focused g., see *aligned g.*

g. index, a measure of the fraction of primary x-rays blocked by a particular grid, defined as the number by which the nongrid exposure (milliampere-seconds) must be multiplied to obtain the proper exposure with the grid.

g. lines, the shadows cast on a radiograph by the lead strips of a grid.

parallel g., a grid having all the lead strips parallel so that the grid lines increase in width toward the edges of the film. Cf. *aligned g.*

g. ratio, the ratio of the height of the lead strips in a grid to the distance separating them. The grid ratio is proportional to film contrast and absorption of scattered radiation and inversely proportional to radiographic density.

Grid 1 see *input terminal 1.*

Grid 2 see *input terminal 2.*

Gridley stain (grid'le) a stain used for fungi in tissue sections. It utilizes chromic acid as an oxidizer, Coleman's Feulgen reagent with a sulfurous acid rinse, aldehyde-fuchsin stain, alcohol rinse, and metanil yellow as a counterstain. Mycelium and yeasts stain blue in color, conidia rose to purple, and the background yellow.

Grimelius' argyrophil method (grim-ēl'e-us) a silver impregnation method for the demonstration of various granule-containing cells such as APUD cells. Slides are incubated at 37°C in a buffered silver nitrate solution and reduced in a hydroquinone and sodium sulfite solution at 45°C. Sections may be reincubated and redeveloped if the original reaction is weak. Reactive cell granules appear black.

grip (grip) [Fr. *grippe*] an old term for influenza; also called grippe.

griseofulvin (gris"e-o-ful'vin) an oral antibiotic from *Penicillium griseofulvum* and *P. janezewskii.* It is active against almost all dermatophytes, as well as many other fungi, but is not active against bacteria and most yeasts. Griseofulvin binds to RNA, where it interferes with nucleic acid synthesis and mitosis. It has been established that griseofulvin is active only against growing cells, which indicates primary involvement of microtubular changes in the drug's mechanism of action.

Grocott-Gomori methenamine-silver method (gro'kot go-mor'e) a method for demonstrating fungi in tissue. Sections are chromated in chromic acid and then rinsed in sodium bisulfite to remove excess chromic acid. They are then placed in a hot (58°C) methenamine–silver nitrate solution to impregnate the fungi with silver. After they are washed, the sections are toned in gold chloride and any remaining unreduced silver is removed with sodium thiosulfate. The sections are then counterstained briefly with light green and mounted. Fungal capsules and walls appear black; mycelia, rose; mucins, taupe to gray; and the background, pale green.

groin (groin) [M.E. *grynde*] the junctional region between the abdomen and the thigh.

gross (grōs) [L. *grossus* rough] coarse or large; large enough to be visible to the naked eye.

ground (ground) 1. a low-resistance connection between an electrical device and the earth or another large conducting body. In electrodiagnosis, the subject is connected to a ground to eliminate the occurrence of extrinsic signals (particularly of power line frequency) that might prove hazardous or create interference with the electrical potentials being monitored.

2. the point in an electrical circuit considered to be at zero volts whether grounded or not, usually the chassis of an eletronic instrument. If not grounded, the circuit is said to be floating.

grounded (groun'ded) connected to an electrical ground.

ground glass denoting a filmy, hazy appearance, as in radiographs of a lung containing excess fluid, the cytoplasm of certain tumor cells, or nonneoplastic cells infected by a virus.

ground glass hepatocyte see under *hepatitis.*

groundnut oil see *peanut oil.*

ground state the lowest energy state of a physical system. From another state (an excited state), a system such as an atom or nuclide will undergo a transition to the ground state by emitting energy. The ground state is stable.

ground substance the acellular amorphous matrix in which cells are embedded. Particularly associated with connective tissue, it is a viscous gel with a high proportion of water, and its proteoglycan molecules occupy extensive domains. The proteoglycans are anions and bind cations, including the dyes colloidal iron, Alcian blue, toluidine blue, and crystal violet.

grouping (groo'ping) the aggregation of raw statistical data into classes to simplify the data analysis or to construct a histogram.

growing point (grō′ing point) the point on a DNA strand at which replication occurs. See also *nucleic acid.*

growth (grōth) 1. an increase in the protoplasmic mass of a tissue or organism, frequently equated with cellular proliferation, but which can occur irrespective of cell division. Growth is the quantitative increase of a living system that results from anabolism in excess of catabolism. Cf. *differentiation.*

2. the proliferation of cells as in a bacterial culture.

growth fraction the number of cells cycling in a cell population divided by the total number of cells in the population. See also *cell cycle.*

growth hormone (GH, hGH) a polypeptide hormone consisting of 191 amino acids, synthesized and released by the anterior pituitary; M.W. 21,500. GH stimulates overall protein synthesis, accompanied by a decrease in blood levels of amino acids and urea; it has a lipolytic effect on adipose tissues, increasing serum-free fatty acids and affecting carbohydrate metabolism. GH antagonizes the effects of insulin in muscle and increases glycogen synthesis in the liver, probably through a gluconeogenic effect. It also enhances electrolyte metabolism (mainly calcium) and mimics some effects of prolactin, e.g., stimulation of the mammary glands and lactogenesis. GH stimulates production of somatomedins from the liver and kidneys, which themselves have some properties of GH. The release of GH is under hypothalamic control. Growth hormone–releasing hormone exerts a positive control, whereas growth hormone–release-inhibiting hormone inhibits GH release.

Reference ranges for GH in plasma (determined by RIA) are: for newborns, 15–40 ng/ml; and for adults, 1–5. A decreased level of GH is found in dwarfism, and an increased level is found in gigantism and acromegaly. GH can be demonstrated in tissue sections by immunoperoxidase methods. Also called *somatotropin.*

growth hormone–release-inhibiting hormone (GH-RIH) an inhibitory peptide consisting of 14 amino acids. First isolated from sheep hypothalamic extracts, this hormone has been shown to inhibit the release of the growth hormone. It has also been found in the D cells of the pancreas and stomach. Also called growth hormone–inhibiting factor (GIF), growth-inhibiting hormone (GIH), and *somatostatin.*

growth hormone–releasing factor (GHRF) a hypothalamic factor that promotes the release of the growth hormone. Its structure and exact physiologic role are not yet clear.

GRS abbrev. See *β-glucuronidase.*

GSC abbrev. for gas-solid chromatography. See under *gas chromatography.*

GSD abbrev. See *genetically significant d.* under *dose.*

GSH abbrev. for reduced glutathione. See under *glutathione.*

GSSG abbrev. for oxidized glutathione. See under *glutathione.*

GSW abbrev. for gunshot wound.

GT abbrev. See *generation time.*

GTP abbrev. See *guanosine triphosphate.*

GU abbrev. See *gastric ulcer* (under *ulcer*), *genitourinary.*

guaiac (gwī′ăk) a resin from the wood of *Guajacum officinale* L. and *G. sanctum* L. (Zygophyllaceae), trees native to Haiti and the Dominican Republic. It contains α- and β-guaiaconic acid, guaiacic acid, vanillin, and other chemicals. Guaiac is brown to green in color, and is insoluble in water but soluble in many organic solvents. It is used as a reagent in tests for occult blood in feces.

guanase (gwan′ās) see *guanine deaminase.*

guanethidine (gwan-eth′ĭ-dēn) an antiadrenergic drug used to treat high blood pressure in combination with thiazide diuretics and possibly other antiadrenergics when they are not effective by themselves. Guanethidine acts by depleting norepinephrine from the peripheral sympathetic nervous system and interfering with its release from the nerves. Adverse reactions include dizziness from low blood pressure when standing, and diarrhea. It cannot be used with MAO inhibitors, and many psychoactive drugs reduce its effect. Guanethidine may be identified by TLC screening assays for basic drugs; it stains with iodoplatinate.

g. sulfate [USP], the sulfate salt of guanethidine. Trademark, *Ismelin.*

guanidinium group (gwan″ĭ-di′ne-um) the substituent derived from the guanidinium ion $NH_2C(=NH_2^+)NH_2$ by replacing a hydrogen on one of the NH_2 groups by another substituent. This group is present in the amino acid arginine.

guanidino-aminovaleric acid (gwan″ĭ-din-o ahme″no-va-le′rik) see *arginine.*

guanine (gwan′in) a white crystalline base, 2-amino-6-oxypurine, $C_5H_5N_5O$, found in animal and plant tissues as a purine base constituent of both classes of nucleic acids (DNA and RNA). It is present in the guanylyl compounds: guanosine, guanosine monophosphate (GMP), guanosine diphosphate (GDP), guanosine triphosphate (GTP), and cyclic GMP. Cytosine is its complementary base in a DNA double strand or in transcription of RNA from a DNA template. Guanine may be found as a free base in body fluids.

guanine deaminase (GR) (gwan′in de-am′ĭ-nās) an enzyme of the hydrolase class (guanine aminohydrolase, EC 3.5.4.3) that catalyzes the reaction guanine + $H_2O \rightleftarrows$ xanthine + NH_3. Serum levels of the enzyme are markedly elevated in acute hepatitis. Also called *guanase.*

guanine deaminase assays measurement of guanine deaminase activity in serum. The specimen is incubated with buffered guanine for 1 hr at 37°C, the reaction is stopped with perchloric acid, and the amount of deaminated guanine is determined by measuring the decrease in absorbance at 245 nm. The reference range for guanine deaminase in serum is 0–3 U/l.

guanosine (G) (gwan′o-sēn) a nucleoside, guanine riboside, $C_{10}H_{13}O_5N_5$. It is a compound that occurs on biosynthetic pathways from guanine to guanine nucleotides, and on degradative pathways from guanine nucleotides to uric acid. The synthesis of riboflavin by green plants, most bacteria, and fungi utilizes a phosphorylated derivative of guanosine as a substrate.

guanosine 3′:5′-cyclic phosphate (3′:5′-GMP) see *cyclic guanosine monophosphate.*

guanosine diphosphate (GDP) (gwan′o-sēn di-fos′fāt) a compound that has both a product and a precursor relationship with guanosine triphosphate (GTP). Formed hydrolytically from GTP, it can, by substrate level phosphorylation in the citric acid cycle, be converted to GTP. As with GTP, GDP is involved in many metabolic reactions.

guanosine monophosphate (GMP) (gwan′o-sēn mon″o-fos′fāt) see *guanosine-5′-phosphate.*

guanosine-5′-phosphate (GMP) (gwan′o-sēn fos′-fāt) a mononucleotide formed from guanine, ribose, and phosphoric acid. Also called *guanosine monophosphate* and *guanylic acid.* See also under *nucleotide.*

guanosine triphosphate (GTP) (gwan′o-sēn tri-fos′fāt) an energy-rich compound analogous to adenosine triphosphate (ATP). It is involved in numerous metabolic reactions including fatty acid and amino acid metabolism, gluconeogenesis, lipid and protein synthesis, and capping of messenger RNA, and as a phosphate donor.

guanylic acid (gwan-ĭ′lic) see *guanosine-5′-phosphate.*

guanylyl (gwan′ĭ-lil) a name for guanylic acid when it is being named as a substituent on some parent group or as an ester.

guarding a barrier or enclosure provided to prevent the inadvertent contact or entanglement of workers and/or their clothing with machinery and electrical circuits. Guarding on some laboratory equipment consists of interlocking mechanisms such as a centrifuge cover that cannot be opened until rotation has stopped; others have cages or enclosures that cover moving shafts and pulleys and belts. Guarding of laboratory equipment and machines should be assessed to assure personnel protection and compliance with standards set by the Occupational Safety and Health Administration. Also called machine guarding.

Guarnieri's bodies (gwar″ne-er′ēz) [Giuseppe *Guarnieri,* Italian physician, 1856–1918] small inclusion bodies within the cells of tissues affected by smallpox or vaccinia.

Guillain-Barré syndrome (ge-yan′ bar-ra′) [Georges *Guillain,* French neurologist, 1876–1961; Jean Alexander *Barré,* French neurologist, born 1880] a rare demyelinating disease of the peripheral nervous system that is thought to have an autoimmune etiology. The disease is usually characterized by acute weakness, areflexia, and mild sensory loss. The cerebrospinal fluid (CSF) may initially be normal, but CSF protein increases as the disease progresses; there is usually no increase in the number of leukocytes. Although most cases resolve completely, some patients are left with permanent weakness due to axonal degeneration. Also called *acute idiopathic polyneuritis,* acute inflammatory polyradiculoneuropathy, and postinfectious polyneuritis.

guinea pig (gin′e pig) a small rodent, *Cavia cobaya,* native to South America. It is popular as a domestic pet and is widely used in laboratories for experimental and biologic research work.

guinea worm infection see *dracunculiasis.*

Gull's disease (gulz) [William Withey *Gull,* English physician, 1816–1890] hypothyroidism due to thyroid atrophy, often resulting in systemic myxedema. See also *hypothyroidism* and *myxedema.*

gum (gum) [L. *gummi*] 1. a mucilaginous excretion from various plants; a polysaccharide that, on hydrolysis, yields hexoses, pentoses, and uronic acids.
2. see *gingiva.*

gum arabic (gum ăr′ah-bik) see *acacia.*

gum karaya (gum kar′a-ah) a gum extracted from species of *Sterculia,* used as a bulk laxative.

gumma (gum′ah), pl. *gummas, gummata* [L. *gummi* gum] a localized reaction in tertiary syphilis thought to be due to hypersensitivity to the causative spirochete or its products. The lesions may range in size from microscopic to several centimeters in diameter. Histologically, there is a central area of caseous necrosis surrounded by mononuclear cells, histiocytes, epithelioid cells, occasionally giant cells, and perivasculitis. They may occur in any tissue or organ site. The organism *Treponema pallidum* is rarely found in gummatous lesions.

gustin (gus′tin) a polypeptide of saliva that is high in histidine (8 percent) and contains two zinc atoms; M.W. 27,000. Gustin is closely related if not identical to nerve growth factor. The presence of this protein, perhaps as a source of zinc, appears to be necessary for the normal development of taste buds.

gut (gut) 1. the intestine or bowel.
2. the primitive digestive tube, consisting of the fore-, mid-, and hindgut.

Guthrie bacterial inhibition assay (GBIA) a test used in the screening of newborns for phenylketonuria (PKU). See under *genetic screening.*

GVH abbrev. for graft-versus-host. See *graft-versus-host disease, reaction.*

Gy abbrev. See *gray.*

Gymnodinium (jim″no-din′e-um) a genus of protozoa. Many species have colored chromatophores, which cause a red tide when these protozoa are present in large numbers in fresh, salt, or brackish waters. This red tide is suspected of killing many fish and invertebrates.

GYN abbrev. See *gynecology.*

gyn/o (gi′no) [Gr. *gynē* woman] a word element used in combining form to denote woman or female, e.g., gynopathy.

gynandroblastoma (jĭ-nan″dro-blas-to′mah) a rare ovarian neoplasm in which there is a blending of granulosa-theca cells and hilus cell elements. Hormonal activity is predominantly masculinizing. See also *ovarian tumors.*

gynec/o (gi′nĕ-ko) [Gr. *gynē, gynaikos* woman] a word element used in combining form to denote woman or female, e.g., gynecology.

gynecoid (gi′ne-koid) [Gr. *gynē* woman + *eidos* form] a term used to describe the typical female pelvis, which is heart shaped, with a more or less round pelvic inlet and thin bones—a pattern found in approximately 44 percent of all females. Cf. *android.*

gynecologic (gi″nĕ-ko-log′ik) pertaining to or affecting the female reproductive tract.

gynecologist (gi″nĕ-kol′o-jist) a physician who specializes in the practice of gynecology.

gynecology (GYN) (gi″nĕ-kol′o-je) the branch of medicine that deals with disorders and diseases of the female genital tract and reproductive system.

gynecomastia (gi″nĕ-ko-mas′te-ah) [*gyneco-* + Gr. *mastos* breast] the enlargement of the male breast, most often seen as a normal variant in adolescence. It is due to actual or relative estrogen increases or to the increased sensitivity of the male breast to estrogens. Marked degrees of breast enlargement in adolescence or in later life may be due to treatment with exogenous estrogen compounds, cirrhosis, endocrine disorders of puberty, and estrogen-producing tumors, including choriocarcinomas, pituitary adenomas, and estrogen-secreting tumors of the adrenal. Histologically, this condition is characterized by ductal epithelial hyperplasia and periductal stromal edema.

gynogenesis (gi″no-jen′ĕ-sis) [*gyno-* + Gr. *genesis* production] the situation in which the male pronucleus stimulates egg development but makes no contribution to the resulting individual. Consequently, the eggs develop without releasing the second polar body, and form diploid individuals (e.g., some fish species). In mammals, the development of such a "fertilized egg" can result in normal individuals (this is accomplished experimentally by removing the male pronucleus with a micropipet). See also *fertilization.* Cf. *androgenesis.*

gyrate (ji′rāt) [L. *gyratus* turned round] twisted in a ring or spiral shape.

gyration (ji-ra′shun) revolution in a circle or circles.

gyrus (ji′rus), pl. *gyri* [L.; Gr. *gyros* ring or circle] [NA], a tortuous convolution of the surface of the brain, which is produced by infolding of the cortex.

H

H symbol for *enthalpy, henry, Hounsfield unit,* the chemical element *hydrogen, magnetic field strength.*

H_0 abbrev. See *null hypothesis.*

H_1 abbrev. See *alternative hypothesis.*

h symbol for *hecto-,* height, *hour,* Planck's constant, the secondary constriction of a chromosome.

habenula (hah-ben′u-lah), pl. *habenulae* [L., dim. of *habena*] [NA], a small nodal eminence on the dorsomedial aspect of the thalamus immediately rostral to the posterior commissure. Receiving afferents from the amygdaloid complex via the stria medullaris thalami and from the hippocampal formation via the fornix, the habenula is an integrative point for olfactory, visceral, and somatic afferent pathways. The habenula mediates such activities as gastric and intestinal secretion, mastication, and swallowing. It has also been implicated in thermoregulation.

Haber's halforisms [S. L. *Haber,* American pathologist, born 1934] a list of faintly amusing dictums relating to circumstances that cause inaccuracy, delay, or loss of laboratory results.

habituation (hah-bit″u-a′shun) 1. the gradual adaptation to a stimulus or the environment; the formation of a habit.

2. a drug dependence, especially one not characterized by tolerance and physical dependence. See also *drug d.* under *dependence.*

habitus (hab′ĭ-tus) [L. "habit"] a body type or physique; the general structure or form of the body. The position, size, and tonus of the internal organs are correlated with the habitus.

asthenic h., a very slender body type having a narrow, shallow thorax. Most of the internal organs are located at a lower position than in the other body types.

hypersthenic h., a massive body type having a broad, deep thorax. Most of the internal organs are located at a higher position than in the other body types.

hyposthenic h., an intermediate body type between the sthenic and asthenic types.

sthenic h., the predominant or average body type.

Haemadipsa (he″mah-dip′sah) [Gr. *haima* blood + *dipsa* thirst] a genus of land leeches (blood-sucking annelids).

Haemagogus (hem″ah-go′gus) [*haima* + Gr. *agōgos* leading] a genus of mosquitoes that includes the species that transmits jungle yellow fever in tropical Central and South America.

Haemaphysalis (hem″ah-fis′ah-lis) [*haima* + Gr. *physallis* bubble] a genus of ticks, several species of which are transmitters of human disease.

H. concinna, one of the transmitters of *Rickettsia sibirica,* which causes Siberian or North Asian tick typhus.

H. spinigera, one of the principal transmitters of the Kyasanur Forest disease virus in Indian forest workers.

Haemophilus (he-mof′ĭ-lus) see *Hemophilus.*

Haemosporidia (he″mo-spo-rid′e-ah) [*haemo-* + Gr. *sporos* seed] an order of sporozoa that are parasites of the red blood cells of vertebrates. It includes the families Plasmodiidae, Haemoproteidae, and Leucocytozoidae.

Hafnia (haf′ne-ah) [L. *Hafnia* old name for Copenhagen] a genus of bacteria of the family Enterobacteriaceae, consisting of motile, gram-negative, facultatively anaerobic rods. The organisms are very similar to those of the genus *Enterobacter* and are sometimes classified as *Enterobacter hafnia;* the preferred terminology now is *Hafnia alvei.* See also *Enterobacteriaceae.*

H. alvei, a species found in the feces of humans and animals, as well as in soil, water, and dairy products. It is similar to *Enterobacter* in biochemical reactions but produces an alkaline reaction in triple sugar iron agar.

hafnium (Hf) (haf′ne-um) [L. *Hafnia* Copenhagen] a lustrous, ductile metallic element very similar in properties to zirconium; atomic number 72; atomic weight 178.49; a 5d transition element; oxidation states 0, +1, +3, +4 (the most common). It has low toxicity. Hafnium is utilized in the production of nuclear reactor control rods.

Hageman factor see *Factor XII.*

Hailey-Hailey disease see *benign familial p.* under *pemphigus.*

hair (hār) [L. *pilus;* Gr. *thrix*] a long, slender filament. The term especially refers to the filamentous appendages of the skin and to the aggregate formed by these skin filaments. Hairs are fibers of modified keratin, each having a shaft and root. Within the dermis the hair is surrounded by the cells of the hair follicle.

anagen h., a hair that is actively growing; the germinal matrix in the hair bulb is synthesizing new hair.

club h., a hair that has ceased growing. The root is surrounded by a keratinized bulbous enlargement, and the hair may easily be plucked from the follicle. Also called *telogen h.*

lanugo h., very fine hair growing all over the body of the fetus; it is most prominent during the middle of fetal life and is normally lost before birth.

telogen h., see *club h.*

terminal h., the coarse hair growing on various areas of the body in the adult; it represents the final stage of hair development.

hair analysis the analysis of hair for various elements, especially trace elements and toxic metals, which is most often performed by atomic absorption spectrophotometry.

hair cells sensory cells with hairlike projections found in the organ of Corti and the semicircular canals. These cells respond to movement, either vibrations or acceleration, that displaces the hairs.

hair follicle a funnel-shaped invagination in the skin that supports the root of the hair. The follicle penetrates the dermis and, in some cases, the subcutaneous tissues. The ducts of one or more sebaceous glands open into each follicle.

hairpin loop an RNA molecule transcribed from

DNA palindromes with the ability to fold back on itself and form a double strand. RNA of this sort is found in the nuclei of eukaryotic cells and in the cloverleaf configuration of tRNA molecules. See also *palindrome.*

Haldane effect (hawl′dān) [John Scott *Haldane,* English physiologist, 1860–1936] the effect of an increasing (or decreasing) O_2 saturation of hemoglobin on the CO_2-binding capacity of the blood. In the lungs, as increasingly more O_2 binds to hemoglobin, the hemoglobin becomes a stronger acid, resulting in the displacement of CO_2 from the hemoglobin. At the tissue level the opposite effect occurs, with O_2 leaving hemoglobin and encouraging CO_2 combination. The Haldane effect is an important factor in CO_2 transport, as it acts to almost double the amount of CO_2 that can be removed from the blood in the lungs, as well as that taken up by hemoglobin in the tissue capillaries.

Haldol (hal′dol) trademark. See *haloperidol.*

half-axial see *semiaxial.*

half-bandwidth the range of wavelengths in which the transmittance of an optical filter is greater than half the peak value. Also called *bandpass.*

half-cell half of an electrochemical cell, i.e., one electrode and the surrounding solution.

half-life ($t_{\frac{1}{2}}$) the time during which one-half of a substance will be converted to a product or eliminated by a process, e.g., a chemical reaction, radioactive decay, or biologic elimination.

biologic h., the time during which half of some substance will be eliminated by biologic processes, e.g., the removal of a radiotracer from the body by kidney filtration or from a particular organ by circulation, or the removal of a drug or toxin by the kidneys or by its metabolic transformation to an inactive substance.

physical h., the time during which an amount of radiostope will decay to one-half the original amount. Each radionuclide has its own characteristic half-life.

halforisms (hal′for-ismz) see *Haber's halforisms.*

half-reaction either the oxidation half or the reduction half of a complete oxidation-reduction reaction; any oxidation-reduction reaction can be thought of as the sum of these two half-reactions. In electrochemical reactions, the oxidation half-reaction takes place at the anode, the reduction half-reaction at the cathode.

half-value layer (HVL or hvl) the thickness of a material that will absorb or scatter one-half of the x-rays or gamma rays that enter it. It varies with the photon energy of the radiation. In radiation safety, HVL is used to measure shielding thickness. In radiology, it is used to describe filters and to measure the quality of a therapeutic x-ray beam by the HVL of an aluminum, copper, or lead filter in the beam.

half-wave potential see under *polarography.*

halide (hal′īd) a halogen anion (e.g., Cl^-), a compound containing this ion, or an organic compound containing a covalently bonded halogen atom. See also *halogen.*

Hallervorden-Spatz disease a rare hereditary disease in which pigmented material accumulates in certain areas of the basal ganglia, notably the globus pallidus and substantia nigra, with progressive degeneration of neurons. Symptoms usually appear when the patient is young, and include abnormal muscle tone, involuntary movements, indistinct speech, and progressive intellectual impairment, leading to increasing generalized rigidity and death. Wilson's disease should be considered in the differential diagnosis.

Hall's method a histologic method for bile pigments. Formalin-fixed paraffin sections are oxidized in Fouchet's ferric chloride reagent and counterstained in van Gieson's picrofuchsin. Bile pigments are various shades of green; collagen, bright red; and muscle, yellow.

hallucination (hal-lu″sĭ-na′shun) [L. *hallucinatio;* Gr. *aylein* to wander in the mind] a sensory perception that does not correspond to any external stimulus.

hallucinatory (hah-lu′sĭ-nah-to″re) characterized by hallucinations.

hallucinogen (hah-loo′sĭ-no-jen″) any of a large group of illegal recreational drugs that produce heightened sensations, synesthesia, alteration of body image, hallucinations, delusions, depersonalization, and the attachment of significance to trivial objects. In susceptible individuals, acute anxiety reactions may occur; rarely, persistent psychotic states are precipitated. In some individuals there are spontaneous recurrences, called flashbacks, of hallucinations or altered perceptions.

Many hallucinogens are structurally related to the neurotransmitter serotonin. Among these are the indole compounds lysergic acid diethylamide (LSD), ibogaine, and harmaline, and the tryptamine derivatives *N,N*-dimethyltryptamine (DMT), psilocybin, and psilocin. Other hallucinogens include mescaline (a phenylethylamine), tetrahydrocannabinol (Δ^9-THC, a dibenzopyran), phencyclidine (PCP), and the psychomimetic amphetamines 2,5-dimethoxy-4-methylamphetamine (DOM, STP), 3,4-methylenedioxyamphetamine (MDA), and *p*-methoxyamphetamine (PAM).

hallucinogenic (hah-lu″sĭ-no-jen′ik) producing hallucinations.

hallux (hal′uks), pl. *halluces* [L.] [NA], the great toe, or first digit, of the foot.

halo- (hal′o) [Gr. *hals* salt] 1. a prefix word element to denote a relationship to salt.

2. a prefix word element in microbiology used to denote a microorganism with an unusual salt requirement; e.g., *Halobacterium* requires a high salt concentration for growth.

3. a prefix word element in organic chemistry used to denote a halogen as a substituent in a halogenated hydrocarbon, e.g., haloalkane.

halogen (hal′o-jen) [*halo-* + Gr. *gennan* to produce] a group VII element: fluorine, chlorine, bromine, iodine, or astatine.

halogenated (hal′o-jĕ-na″ted) 1. having halogen atoms, as in halogenated hydrocarbon; produced by halogenation.

2. treated with a halogen, e.g., halogenated water.

halogenated hydrocarbon assays 1. microdiffusion assay. Volatile halohydrocarbons, such as chloroform, carbon tetrachloride, trichloroethane, and chloral hydrate, are absorbed by toluene in a microdiffusion cell. Pyridine and sodium hydroxide solution are added to the toluene, which is then boiled. A red color indicates a halohydrocarbon. By comparison of the absorbance at 530 nm with that of reference samples, quantitative results accurate to within 10 percent may be obtained.

2. see *head space analysis.*

halogenation (hal″o-je-nā′shun) the addition or substitution of a halogen atom or atoms into a compound.

halo nevus see *halo n.* under *nevus.*

Halon system an automatic fire extinguishing system that uses a halogenated hydrocarbon or Halon compound as the extinguishing agent, e.g., Halon 1301 (bromotrifluoromethane) and Halon 1211 (bromochlorodifluoromethane). Although these systems do have some advantages, they are costly and the halogenated compounds are toxic.

haloperidol (hah″lo-per′ĭ-dol) [NF], a major tranquilizer in the butyrophenone group used to treat mental disorders, particularly schizophrenia, and Gilles de la Tourette's syndrome. It is a dopamine blocker and may cause extrapyramidal, parkinson-like reactions of loss of coordination. Prolonged use may cause tardive dyskinesia. Trademark, *Haldol.*

haloperidol assays determination of haloperidol in urine using gas chromatography. Haloperidol is extracted from the specimen at pH 8–9 into chloroform and chromatographed using a silicone stationary phase and a flame ionization detector with chlorpheniramine as the internal standard.

halophile (hal″o-fīl) [*halo-* + Gr. *philein* to love] a microorganism that requires a concentration of NaCl for growth greater than that found in the usual laboratory media or in physiologic saline (0.85 percent).

haloprogin (hah″lo-pro′jin) an antifungal agent, 3-iodo-2-propynyl-2,4,5-trichlorophenyl ether; an inhibitory substance to most etiologic agents of dermatophyte infection as well as to *Candida.* Haloprogin is applied only topically.

halothane (hal′o-thān) [USP], a colorless, volatile liquid, 2-bromo-2-chloro-1,1,1-trifluoroethane. It is used as an inhalation anesthetic.

halothane assay determination of halothane in blood using gas chromatography. Halothane is extracted into benzene and chromatographed using a detergent stationary phase and an electron capture detector.

halzoun (hal′zun) a disease found in individuals in Syria and Lebanon caused by eating inadequately cooked food containing third-stage larvae of the family Linguatulidae; it inhabits the pharyngeal mucous membrane of humans and blocks the airways. It was once thought to be caused by *Fasciola hepatica.*

hamamelis water (ham″ah-me′lis) see *witch hazel.*

hamart/o (ham′ar-to) [Gr. *hamartia* defect, sin] a word element used in combining form to denote relationship to a defect, e.g., hamartoma.

hamartia (ham-ar′she-ah) [Gr. "defect"] a term used to describe defective tissue combination in embryogenesis and development.

hamartoma (ham″ar-to′mah) [*hamarto-* + *-oma*] a benign, tumorlike focal overgrowth of mature cells or tissues normally present within an organ. Although these cells are identical to the mature cells found in the remainder of the organ, they do not reproduce its characteristic architecture.

hamatum (hah-ma′tum) [L. "hooked"] a wedge-shaped carpal bone with a hooklike process on the distal part of its palmar surface. It articulates with the fifth metacarpal, pisiform, and capitate bones. Also called hamate.

Hamman's disease (ham′anz) [Louis *Hamman,* American physician, 1877–1946] interstitial emphysema due to alveolar rupture, which causes the escape of air into the connective tissue stroma of the lung, mediastinum, and, at times, subcutaneous tissue.

Hamman-Rich syndrome (ham′an rich) [Louis *Hamman;* Arnold Rice *Rich,* American pathologist, born 1893] see *diffuse interstitial f.* under *fibrosis.*

hamster (ham′ster) a small, ratlike rodent, native to Europe and Asia, having large cheek pouches and a short tail. It is popular as a domestic pet and is used extensively in laboratories for experimental and biological research work.

hamstring (ham′string) see *hamstring t.* under *tendon.*

Ham's test (hamz) [Thomas Hale *Ham,* U.S. physician, b. 1905] see *acidified serum test.*

hamular (ham′u-lar) shaped like a hook.

hamulus (ham′u-lus), pl. *hamuli* [L. "little hook"] [NA], a general term used to denote a hook-shaped process.

hand (hand) [L. *manus*] the part of the upper limb distal to the forearm, composed of the carpals, metacarpals, and phalanges.

H and D curve [after *Hurter* and *Driffield*] a graph, supplied with x-ray films, that shows their exposure response. It is a plot of optical density (absorbance) versus log relative exposure, the logarithm of the x-ray energy to which the film is exposed. Also called *characteristic curve.*

H and E staining abbrev. See *hematoxylin and eosin staining.*

H and P abbrev. for history and physical.

Hand-Schüller-Christian disease (hand shil′er kris′chan) [Alfred *Hand;* Artur *Schüller;* Henry A. *Christian*] see *systemic h.* under *histiocytosis.*

HANE abbrev. for hereditary angioneurotic edema. See *angioneurotic e.* under *edema.*

Hanes equation see under *Lineweaver-Burke equation.*

hanging drop a procedure used to determine motility in a microorganism. After a drop of liquid culture is placed on a coverslip, a slide with a hollowed-out depression or one fitted with a plastic ring is pressed onto the coverslip, inverted, and examined under a microscope. Swimming motions in a direction opposite to brownian movement indicate a motile organism.

Hanker-Yates reagent a reagent used to react with horseradish peroxidase (HRP), which forms an osmiophilic colored reaction product permitting visualization of the exogenous tracer. The reagent, consisting of *p*-phenylenediamine and pyrocatechol, couples with HRP to form a deep blue melaninlike compound. This reagent reacts more rapidly than 3,3-diaminobenzidine, which has classically been used for HRP studies; it also has the advantage of being noncarcinogenic and not deeply staining red blood cells.

Hansen's disease (han′sunz) [Gerhard Henrik Ar-mauer *Hansen,* Norwegian physician, 1841–1912] see *leprosy* and *M. leprae* under *Mycobacterium.*

H antigen [Ger. *Hauch* film] 1. a bacterial flagellar antigen used in the serologic classification of certain enteric bacteria, especially *Salmonella.* The designation H was introduced by Weil and Felix in 1917 to describe the film formed by swarming of highly motile *Proteus* bacilli on moist agar, which resembles the mist caused by breathing on glass. Later, H was associated with the flagellar antigen of this type and other types of bacteria. Agglutination of bacteria possessing H flagellar antigen with H antiserum forms a light, fluffy precipitate. See also *O antigen.*

2. a nonwater-soluble glycolipid with antigenic activity determined by galactose plus fucose configuration without *N*-acetylgalactosamine (A antigen) or an additional galactose (B antigen) found on the erythrocyte membrane. When controlled by the A and B genes, H antigen acts as the substrate for the production of A and B antigen. As A and B genes are absent in type O individuals, they have large quantity of H antigen. See also *H gene, H substance,* and *secretor groups.*

HAPC abbrev. See *hospital-acquired penetration contact.*

hapl/o (hap′lo) [Gr. *haploos* simple, single] a word element used in combining form to denote simple or single, e.g., haploid.

haploid (hap′loid) [*haplo-* + Gr. *eidos* form] referring to the chromosome number in the germ cell after the second reduction mitosis.

haploid number the number of chromosomes in a gamete, 23 in humans; the number of groups of homologous chromosomes in polyploid cells.

haploidy (hap′loi-de) the state of being haploid.

Haplorchis (hap-lor′kis) a genus of small trematodes that are occasionally parasitic in the intestines of humans and other vertebrates.

haplosomic (hap″lo-so′mik) see *monosomic.*

haplotype (hap′lo-tip) 1. a group of genes so closely linked that they are rarely recombined during meiosis. The haplotype on each homologous chromosome is therefore inherited from a single grandparent; the term is most frequently used in immunogenetics.

2. all the genes of a gamete or the half of an individual's genes that are contributed by one parent.

hapt/o (hap′to) a word element used in combining form to denote relationship to touch, grasping, or combining, e.g., haptoglobin.

hapten (hap′ten) that region of an antigenic molecule which by itself is incapable of inducing the formation of antibodies (nonimmunogenic), but which can react specifically with antibodies (antigenic). Haptens usually are small, chemically defined groups, such as the dinitrophenyl (DNP) group.

haptoglobin (Hp) (hap″to-glo′bin) a plasma glycoprotein, containing about 20 percent carbohydrate, that migrates electrophoretically with the $alpha_2$ band. It is produced primarily by hepatocytes and is the principal defense against the loss of body iron from intravascular hemolysis. Haptoglobin irreversibly binds to free hemoglobin, forming a complex too large to pass through the glomerular membrane for excretion. The complex is removed from circulation by reticuloendothelial cells and the iron is recycled.

As with immunoglobulins, each haptoglobin monomer contains four polypeptide chains: two light (α) chains and two heavy (β) chains. Haptoglobin is polymorphic, there being two different allelic forms of alpha chains (α^1 and α^2). Thus, there are three different phenotypic haptoglobins: type 1-1, with two α^1 chains; type 2-2, with two α^2 chains; and type 1-2, with one of each. Type 1-1 is monomeric (M.W. 8500) but types 1-2 and 2-2 occur in several polymeric forms with molecular weights up to 1 million.

Serum haptoglobin concentrations (measured directly or in terms of hemoglobin bound) are greatly increased when there is extensive tissue damage or necrosis. Extensive hemolysis, as well as extensive liver damage, lowers haptoglobin levels. Neonates generally have no haptoglobin unless they have acquired an infection in utero. The synthesis of haptoglobin begins a few days or weeks after birth.

The reference range for plasma haptoglobin in adults is 40–180 mg/dl (hemoglobin bound). The absolute values for serum haptoglobin are 100–300 mg/dl. About 4 percent of blacks and a lesser proportion of Caucasians have no haptoglobin (congenital ahaptoglobinemia); the mechanism of iron conservation in these individuals is unknown.

haptoglobin assays 1. column chromatography. Hemoglobin (Hb) is added to the serum and the hemoglobin-haptoglobin complex (Hb-Hp) is isolated by using cross-linked dextran gel (Sephadex) filtration. The bound hemoglobin concentration is determined by its absorbance at 415 nm.

2. electrophoresis. Free Hb is separated from Hb-Hp electrophoretically. At pH 7.0, Hb migrates toward the anode but Hb-Hp toward the cathode. The complex is quantitated by using staining and densitometry, or by elution and colorimetry using the peroxidase reaction.

3. immunologic methods. Radial immunodiffusion (RID), immunoelectrophoresis, and nephelometry have been used. Because of the different molecular sizes of the haptoglobin variants, RID requires a knowledge of the haptoglobin phenotype.

Harada's syndrome [E. *Harada,* Japanese ophthalmologist] a disease, with possibly a viral etiology, that is characterized by inflammation and uveomeningitis. It is associated with transient or permanent deafness or blindness, and occasionally with brief alopecia, vitiligo, and poliosis.

hardcopy computer printout on paper, as opposed to a CRT terminal display or storage on magnetic tape or magnetic disk. Hardcopy is considered to be a backup method of storing data that is independent of the computer system.

hardness (hard′ness) 1. the concentration in water of calcium carbonate or sulfate (which forms an insoluble curd with soaps).

2. the properties of x-rays related to penetrability and wavelength. Hard x-rays have high-energy photons; soft x-rays have lower-energy photons.

3. the resistance of a material to indentation or abrasion. Hardness of materials is measured using several arbitrary scales. Two such scales are the Rockwell scale, based on the indentation produced by a steel ball pressed on the material by a prescribed force, and the Mohs scale, based on the ability of one material to scratch another.

hardware (hard′wār) in a computer, the physical equipment in particular, as opposed to software (programs) and firmware (microprograms).

Hardy-Weinberg law stated as: in an infinite population, the gene frequencies and genotype frequencies at a particular locus will remain constant if there is random mating and no appreciable mutation or selection. If there are only two alleles (*A* and *a*), with gene frequencies *p* and $q = 1-p$, respectively, then the genotype frequencies are p^2 (for *AA*), $2pq$(*Aa*), and q^2 (*aa*). This is called the Hardy-Weinberg equilibrium because these genotype frequencies will be approached after several generations, even if the population is established with different genotype frequencies.

harelip (hār′lip) see *cleft lip.*

Hargraves cell (har′grāvs) see *lupus erythematosus cell.*

Harleco synthetic resin (HSR) trademark for a synthetic resin mounting medium used in histology, which has an index of refraction ranging from 1.5202 (60 percent xylene solution) to 1.5390 (the solid). It is a polymer of β-pinene.

harmaline (har′mah-lēn) a CNS stimulant and hallucinogen, the principal psychoactive alkaloid isolated from seeds of *Peganum harmala.* It also acts as a parasympathomimetic agent and as a monoamine oxidase (MAO) inhibitor.

harmine (har′mēn) a stimulant, hallucinogenic drug isolated from seeds of *Peganum harmala.* See also the related drug *harmaline.*

harmonic (har-mon′ik) 1. in accoustics, pertaining to a sound having a frequency that is an integral multiple of a reference sound (the fundamental). By extension, it refers to any wave, such as an electronic signal, with a frequency that is a multiple of the fundamental.

2. in physics, pertaining to sinusoidal motion.

Hartmannella (hart″man-el′ah) a genus of free-living, soil-inhabiting amebae, often classified together with *Acanthamoeba* as H-A or hartmannellid amebas. These two closely related genera are similar in appearance to the ameboid stage of *Naegleria* but have no flagellate stage. *Hartmannella* probably does not produce infection in humans, but *Acanthamoeba* does. The species *H. hyalina,* a coprozoic ameba, has been identified in human feces.

Hartnup disease (hart′nup) a rare genetic disorder in the metabolism of alpha–amino acids, transmitted as an autosomal recessive trait, that results in a variety of pathologic changes, many of which are the same as those seen in pellagra. There is impaired renal and intestinal transport of neutral amino acids, with subsequent defects in the conversion of tryptophan to nicotinic acid. Large amounts of 3-indoleacetic acid and indoleacetyl glutamine are excreted in the urine. There are pellagra-like skin and CNS lesions, along with cerebellar ataxia, nystagmus, and sometimes dementia, which can be prevented by nicotinamide therapy and a high-protein diet. See also *aminoacidopathies* and *pellagra.*

Harvard criteria of irreversible coma a series of guidelines for determining whether brain death has occurred. As originally proposed in 1968 by an ad hoc committee of the Harvard Medical School, these criteria require that: (1) the patient's body temperature is greater than 90°F (32°C); (2) drugs that depress the central nervous system (e.g., barbiturates) are absent from the body; (3) the patient is totally unreceptive and unresponsive to externally applied stimuli; (4) the patient is unable to breathe or move spontaneously; (5) corneal, pupillary, pharyngeal, ocular, blink, and stretch (tendon) reflexes are absent; and (6) the electroencephalogram is isoelectric when recorded under conditions of maximal sensitivity of the recording equipment. All the above conditions must persist for 24 hr.

Guidelines for establishing brain death, which have been published by a number of different organizations, are continually being revised as new technologies are developed. See also *brain death syndrome* and *electrocerebral inactivity.*

harvest mite see *Trombicula.*

Hashimoto's disease (hash″ĭ-mo′tōz) [Hakaru *Hashimoto,* Japanese surgeon, 1881–1934] see *chronic t.* under *thyroiditis.*

Hassall's corpuscles (has′alz) [Arthur Hill *Hassall,* English chemist and physician, 1817–1894] concentric, tightly wound bodies of the thymic medulla. Derived from epithelial cells, these bodies are centrally hyalinized. They are found during fetal development and increase in number during thymic involution.

haustrum (hows′trum), pl. *haustra* [L. *haustor* drawer] [NA], a term to denote a recess, as in the spaces between the outpouchings of the colonic wall.

HAV abbrev. See *h. A v.* under *hepatitis virus.*

Haverhill fever (ha′ver-il) [from *Haverhill,* Mass., where an epidemic occurred in 1925] a disease caused by *Streptobacillus moniliformis.* Although identical to rat-bite fever, it is transmitted through infected food or milk rather than through the bite of a rodent. Cf. *rate-bite fever.*

haversian canal (ha-ver′shan) [C. *Havers,* English physician and anatomist, 1650–1702] a branching channel found at the core of a haversian system in bone, through which blood vessels, lymph vessels, and nerves pass.

haversian system [C. *Havers*] the basic structural unit of bone, consisting of concentrically arranged lamellae surrounding a central haversian canal.

Hawaii agent a virus that causes acute infectious nonbacterial gastroenteritis in adults and children. This virus has not yet been classified but is probably either echovirus, group A coxsackievirus, or reovirus.

Haworth formula [Walter Norman *Haworth,* British chemist, 1883–1950] a convention used to represent the structure of a cyclic compound (usually having a five- or six-membered ring). In this convention, the ring is shown as a planar ring (though, in fact, the real compound generally is not planar) nearly perpendicular to the plane of the paper; the substituents on the ring are shown at the ends of lines projecting vertically from the ring plane. It is most often used to represent the ring structures of pyranoses and furanoses; see the accompanying illustration. Haworth projections of these sugars are always drawn with the anomeric carbon (the potential carbonyl carbon) to the right and the oxygen bridge to the rear (the three bonds in the front are sometimes indicated with heavy lines). For α-D or β-L configurations, the hydroxyl group of the anomeric carbon is below the ring, and for β-D or α-L configurations, it is above the ring. The Haworth

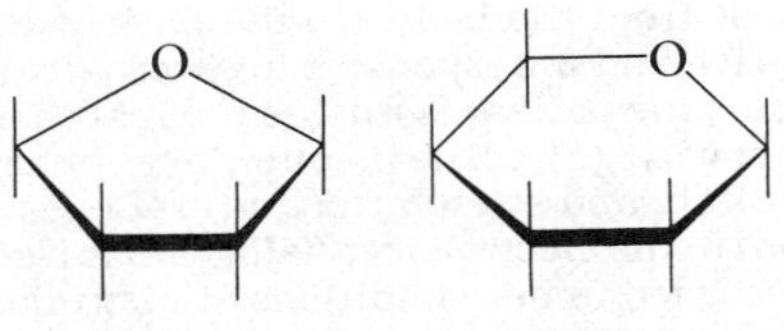

Haworth formula. Formula for furanose and pyranose. (From Ternay, A. L., Jr.: Contemporary Organic Chemistry. 2nd ed. Philadelphia, W. B. Saunders Co., 1976.)

formula does not represent the true conformation (chair or boat) of pyranose rings; for this purpose perspective drawings are required. See also *isomerism.*

hay fever see *allergic r.* under *rhinitis.*

Haygarth's nodes (ha'garths) [John *Haygarth,* English physician, 1740–1827] joint swellings that are characteristic of, and associated with, rheumatoid arthritis.

hazard (haz'ard) a condition or activity that presents a potential for injury, illness, or property damage. See also *hazardous chemicals, hazardous materials,* and *hazardous substances;* while generally referring to the same entities, each term is separately defined below.

hazard identification in a laboratory safety program, the determination of hazards and the institution of a system of labels and signs to alert and inform people about identified hazards. For example, all doors leading to laboratories in hospitals should be marked with the multicolored diamond emblem described by the National Fire Protection Association (NFPA 704), with numerical coding to indicate the relative hazards of chemicals intended to be used within the area (according to NFPA 56C-1980). The hazard identification system gives (from left to right in the sections of the diamond) the relative health hazards from a spill or contact with rated chemicals, the relative fire hazard, and the relative instability or reactivity of the chemical; e.g., the number 4 indicates extreme hazards, 3 is severe, 2 is moderate, 1 is minor, and 0 indicates hazards that are not unusual.

As an illustration, a laboratory containing bottles of acetone, ethyl ether, picric acid (wet with 13 percent water), sodium hydroxide, sulfuric acid, and xylene, would have hazards ratings as shown in the accompanying table. If the ethyl ether was in a new 5-lb can and the picric acid was in a new 5-lb bottle, the combined rating for the laboratory would use the numbers assigned by the NFPA committee for the concentrated material. In this case, the combined hazard rating for the laboratory would be the highest degree of hazard in each category, or 3 – 4 – 4 – ₩. If the ethyl ether was in a single, new quarter-pound can stored in a flammable liquid storage cabinet, the degree of hazard for the fire hazard of ether could be reduced. If the picric acid was in a single, new 1-lb bottle, or if it consisted solely of a saturated solution of picric acid in water, the fire and instability-reactivity hazards of the picric acid would be much less and the hazard rating could be reduced. In this case, the combined hazard rating would be 3 – 3 – 3 – ₩, or perhaps 3 – 3 – 2 – ₩.

The symbol ₩ indicates the possible hazard of using water on the concentrated material in a small container or closed vessel. According to NFPA 49-1975, Hazardous Chemicals Data, the symbol ₩ does not mean that it would be unsafe or inappropriate to use water to keep containers of such material cool or to flush such materials away if they are spilled or splashed.

According to NFPA 45-1981, entrances to laboratories, storage areas, and associated facilities should have signs warning emergency personnel of unusual or severe hazards such as unstable chemicals, water-reactive chemicals, and pathogenic materials. That regulation also calls for content identification and precautionary information on all containers of hazardous chemicals, except those being used in experiments or ongoing tests. Storage cabinets and other storage facilities should also be appropriately marked.

Containers used for storage of peroxidizable compounds or materials that become hazardous upon prolonged storage are to be dated when opened and retention limited to a maximum of 6 mo after opening, unless measures are taken to remove the peroxides.

hazardous chemicals a term used to refer to those chemicals that pose potential danger to health and safety because of their inherent properties. Chemicals are considered hazardous if they are irritating, corrosive, toxic, flammable, capable of producing combustible vapors at temperatures below 93.4°C (200°F), pyrophoric, water reactive, unstable, reactive, or capable of rapid release of energy or explosive decomposition. National Fire Protection Association regulation 45-1981 defines hazardous chem-

HAZARD IDENTIFICATION. HAZARD RATINGS OF SOME COMMON LABORATORY CHEMICALS

CHEMICAL	EMERGENCY HEALTH HAZARD	FIRE HAZARD	INSTABILITY-REACTIVITY	OTHER
Acetone	1	3	0	
Ethyl ether	2	4	1	
Picric acid	1	4	4	
Sodium hydroxide	3	0	0	
Sulfuric acid	3	0	2	₩*
Xylene	2	3	0	

*See text.

icals as any with hazard degree ratings of 2, 3 or 4, according to the hazard rating system in NFPA 704-1975.

hazardous concentration a concentration of material that may be hazardous, e.g., a combustible vapor-air mixture in the flammable range, or an airborne concentration of a toxic substance above the permissible exposure limit for the substance.

hazardous materials a term used to refer to those materials that pose potential dangers to health and safety because of their inherent properties. Hazardous materials are likely to be subject to regulations concerning handling, packaging, labeling, shipping, waste disposal, monitoring, licensing, or recordkeeping. For example, the Nuclear Regulatory Commission has established regulations for radioactive materials, and the Department of Transportation has regulations regarding hazardous materials such as poisons, irritants, corrosives, explosives, flammable materials, oxidizers, radioactive materials, etiologic agents, compressed gases, and materials that are dangerous when wet.

hazardous materials labeling see *labeling of hazardous materials.*

hazardous substances a term used to refer to those substances that pose potential danger to health and safety because of their inherent properties. For example, the Consumer Product Safety Commission under the Federal Substances Labeling Act regulates compressed gases or substances that are irritating, corrosive, toxic or extremely toxic, flammable or extremely flammable, or that have other properties which may adversely affect users of products intended or liable to be used in households.

hazardous waste a term used to refer to those waste materials that pose potential danger. Specific examples include materials that can cause injury during their removal from the laboratory or the building; materials that can damage the sewage disposal system or the personnel who service the sewage disposal system; materials that can pollute the atmosphere, biosphere, or water supply; or materials that can injure anyone at the disposal site at the time of disposal or later.

The Environmental Protection Agency (EPA) has defined hazardous waste as waste identified and listed as acute hazardous waste or toxic waste, or waste that exhibits the characteristics of ignitability, corrosivity, EP toxicity, or reactivity. Hazardous waste regulations adopted by the EPA define the responsibilities of those who generate hazardous waste, as well as those who transport it and those who own and operate hazardous waste treatment, storage, and disposal facilities.

The accountability of the agencies or institutions generating hazardous wastes in amounts or concentrations that are regulated are divided between those who produce the wastes and those who manage removal of the wastes. Laboratory personnel who produce hazardous waste have three major responsibilities: (1) to identify wastes that are hazardous according to regulations; (2) to properly tag such waste before it is removed; and (3) to keep a record of any test result, waste analysis, or other information used to identify a waste as hazardous. Personnel who manage hazardous waste removal have four major responsibilities: (1) to prepare manifests for the wastes and to arrange for shipments via registered transporters to appropriate disposal facilities; (2) to follow up on any shipment if the manifest is not returned within an allotted time; (3) to file all manifest records and submit yearly reports; and (4) to retain the hazardous waste tags (prepared by the producer) as part of the recordkeeping and verification system.

See also *corrosivity, ignitability, EP toxicity, reactivity,* and *toxic waste.*

acute h. w., the term used by the EPA (Environmental Protection Agency) to identify specific commercial chemical products and their containers and spill residues if and when they are discarded or are intended to be discarded. The chemicals, which include compounds such as acrolein, carbon disulfide, cyanides, osmium tetroxide, pesticides, sodium azide, and sodium cyanide, are listed in the 1980 regulations adopted under the Resource Conservation and Recovery Act.

hazard symbol a symbol that warns of a specific hazard. Those that may be encountered in the clinical laboratory include the biohazard symbol, the chemical hazard identification symbol used by National Fire Protection Association, and the hazard symbols on shipping labels required by the Department of Transportation.

HB abbrev. for hepatitis B. See *hepatitis.*

Hb abbrev. for *hemoglobin.* The different types of hemoglobin are identified by capital letters, e.g., Hb A, Hb M, Hb S. Two or more hemoglobins with the same electrophoretic mobility are distinguished by the geographic area of discovery added as a subscript, e.g., Hb D_{Punjab}, Hb $D_{St.\ Louis}$. New hemoglobins are assigned common names, usually representing the laboratory, hospital, or city in which they were discovered, e.g., Hb Bethesda, Hb Richmond. They are also given a scientific name that indicates the substitution and variant chain.

H band [Ger. *heller* lighter] the region of a sarcomere that contains only myosin filaments. See also *skeletal m.* under *muscle.*

Hb Bart's abbrev. See *Bart's hemoglobin.*

HBcAg abbrev. See *h. B core a.* under *hepatitis antigen.*

Hb CO abbrev. See *carboxyhemoglobin.*

α-HBD abbrev. for α-hydroxybutyrate dehydrogenase. See under *lactate dehydrogenase.*

HBE abbrev. See *His bundle electrogram.*

HBeAg abbrev. See *h. B e a.* under *hepatitis antigen.*

Hb F abbrev. See *fetal hemoglobin.*

Hb O_2 abbrev. See *oxyhemoglobin.*

HBsAg abbrev. See *h. B surface a.* under *hepatitis antigen.*

HBV abbrev. See *h. B v.* under *hepatitis virus.*

hCG abbrev. for human chorionic gonadotropin. See *chorionic gonadotropin, human.*

hCG-α subunit abbrev. See *c.g.-alpha subunit* under *chorionic gonadotropin.*

hCG-β subunit abbrev. See *c.g.-beta subunit* under *chorionic gonadotropin.*

HCl abbrev. See *hydrogen chloride.*

hCS abbrev. for human chorionic somatomammotropin. See *chorionic somatomammotropin.*

HCT, Hct abbrev. See *hematocrit.*

HD abbrev. for Hodgkin's disease. See *malignant l.* under *lymphoma.*

HDL abbrev. for high-density lipoprotein. See *high-density l.* under *lipoprotein.*

HDN abbrev. See *hemolytic disease of the newborn.*

He symbol for the chemical element *helium.*

head (hed) [L. *caput;* Gr. *kephalē*] 1. the upper, anterior, or proximal extremity of an organism, especially the part containing the brain and sense organs.

2. the expanded end of a structure, e.g., head of pancreas, head of caudate nucleus.

headache (hed′āk) a general term for aches and pains in the head. In clinical usage, the term is applied to unpleasant sensations of the cranial vault characterized by dull, aching, constant or throbbing pain, or tightness and pressure. The intensity, location, duration, degree of incapacity rendered by the pain, and associated symptoms (e.g., nausea and vomiting) all vary with the specific cause and among individuals.

Headache is a symptom rather than a disease and is one of the most frequent discomforts in human experience. The differential diagnosis is often difficult, for headache can accompany the tensions or fatigue incidental to everyday life, or it can relate to biologic or environmental events such as onset of menstruation, hypoglycemia, changes in environmental temperature or pressure, or exposure to such air pollutants as carbon monoxide, lead, or nitrates. However, headache can also be a primary symptom of more serious disease, including brain tumor, meningitis, and subdural hematoma.

There are several mechanisms by which headache is produced. As the brain parenchyma, ependyma, pia mater, and parts of the dura mater are insensitive to pain, headache pain has its origin in other intra- and extracranial structures that are sensitive to pain. These include the skin; the subcutaneous tissue and muscles of the skull; the delicate structures of the eyes, ears, and nasal cavities; and both intra- and extracranial vessels. Traction or inflammation of any of these structures, vascular dilation and spasm, or excessive muscle contraction will result in the pain of headache. Sensory stimuli from these structures are conveyed to the sensory perceptive areas of the central nervous system (thalamus and cortex) by the first three cervical nerves, as well as by cranial nerves V, IX, and X (the trigeminal, glossopharyngeal, and vagus nerves, respectively). The trigeminal nerve conveys sensory information from structures above the tentorium in the anterior and middle regions of the skull, whereas the cervical nerves and cranial nerves IX and X convey information from below the tentorium and posterior skull. The pain from intracranial disease is sensed as being in the part of the skull supplied by these nerves (i.e., it is referred); tenderness of the scalp often accompanies the pain.

Severe headache of recent origin or a change in pattern of a preexisting headache may require extensive clinical, laboratory, and radiologic evaluation so that a specific cause can be identified and treated. Often, no specific cause can be found and treatment is then symptomatic.

Also called *cephalgia.*

cluster h., a headache characterized by severe, constant (nonthrobbing) pain around one eye. It is of sudden onset (usually occurring within 2–3 hr of falling asleep) and lasts for 1–2 hr. These headaches occur in "clusters"; that is, they recur nightly for several weeks or months and then may not recur for years. The pain is often accompanied by ipsilateral lacrimation and nasal congestion, followed by rhinorrhea and facial flushing. The disorder is more frequent in males than in females and tends to recur during periods of stress or overwork. This headache is usually treated with ergotamine alkaloids, indomethacin, propranolol, or histamine desensitization. Also called *histamine headache, Horton's syndrome, migrainous neuralgia,* and *paroxysmal nocturnal cephalgia.* See also *vascular h.*

inflammatory h., a headache caused by an inflammatory lesion, e.g., of the meninges, cranial vessels (arteritis), or nasal sinuses (sinusitis). Its nature and clinical accompaniments depend on the underlying disease. Treatment is directed at the causal conditions.

migraine h., a headache characterized by recurrent throbbing pain, sometimes restricted to one side, with or without associated visual, psychologic, or gastrointestinal symptoms. Such headache afflicts about 5 percent of the population, is more common in females than in males, and can begin at any age. Classic migraine is preceded by an aura, e.g., disturbances of vision, weakness, dizziness, confusion, or numbness and tingling of the lips, face, and hands. The headache itself may be accompanied by sleep disturbances, nausea, and vomiting; it is often restricted to one side of the head and can last for up to several days at a time. In contrast, common migraine is not accompanied by an aura; the headache may be generalized.

The electroencephalogram of migrainous patients may show nonspecific slowing both during and between attacks. Arteriographic and blood flow studies indicate arterial constriction and decreased cerebral circulation early in the attack, whereas vasodilation and excessive pulsation of branches of the external carotid artery occur as the headache begins.

The specific cause of migraine is not known but may be multifactorial. An increased sensitivity to vasoactive substances (norepinephrine, epinephrine, and serotonin) has been held to lead to vasospasm in susceptible individuals (humoral-amine theory of migraine). However, a heat-stable polypeptide related to the kinins in activity (neurokinin) can be aspirated from tissue on the side of the headache; when this is injected at another site, it causes increased capillary permeability and pain. Attacks often cease during pregnancy, suggesting a role for hormonal factors, and in some instances the attacks can be linked with certain items of diet. Finally, there may be a genetic component for susceptibility to migraine, as a high proportion of the sufferers give a family history of the disorder.

Treatment for migraine consists of prophylaxis and management of the acute attack. Prophylactic treatment is aimed at reducing the severity and frequency of the headache. Generally, the total health and life style of the patient are considered, including the relative amounts of rest and exercise obtained, any use of addictive drugs (including alcohol and tobacco), and the patient's ability to cope with anxiety. Frequently, the elimination of certain foods from the diet—those containing the vasoactive substances tyramine, nitrate, and monosodium glutamate, as occur in ripened cheese, processed meats, and chocolate—proves therapeutically helpful. Substances may be prescribed that reduce vasospasm of the cephalic vessels, e.g., ergot alkaloids, mild analgesics, aspirin, or acetaminophen. Pharmacotherapy for the acute attack is designed to relieve pain, reduce associated nausea and vomiting, relieve anxiety, and reduce central vasomotor reactivity.

See also *vascular h.*

muscle contraction h., a headache caused by vigorous contraction of the head and neck muscles. It is characterized by dull, steady pain that progresses in intensity throughout the day. The pain is bilaterally distributed over the head and may be accompanied by soreness of the neck muscles. The duration is variable, from a day to weeks to months. This type of headache is one of the leading causes of chronic and recurrent headache and is often precipitated by anxiety, depression, or emotional conflict.

Treatment includes resolution or management of the emotional conflict, local heat and massage, analgesics, and—in some instances—biofeedback (conscious relaxation).

tension h., a headache that is gradual in onset with either diffuse bilateral distribution over the cranium or occipitonuchal localization. It may consist of a tightness or pressure, or of waves of aching pain. It is usually present continuously throughout the day and night, and can persist for weeks. Tension headaches are frequent during middle life and coincide with periods of anxiety or depression. Simple analgesics are usually ineffective in relieving the pain. Treatment techniques may include massage and conscious relaxation, local anesthesia, development of methods for coping with the stress, and/or the administration of anxiety-relieving drugs.

traction h., a headache that results from displacement of one or more of the pain-sensitive structures in the head by a lesion, such as a tumor, abscess, or subdural hematoma, or by changes in intracranial pressure.

traumatic h., a headache caused by a blow to the skull; it may develop immediately after a head injury. In addition, however, headache is often a conspicuous feature of the posttraumatic syndrome, developing some time after the injury itself. It may also follow a postinjury subdural hematoma, but this is usually accompanied by a disturbance of consciousness and by focal neurologic signs. See also *traction h.*

vascular h., a headache caused by abnormal vasodilation and characterized by pain that is acute in onset and throbbing in quality. Migraine and cluster headaches are two common types. Vascular headaches are associated with changes in circulating levels of such vasoactive substances as norepinephrine, serotonin (5-hydroxytryptamine), prostaglandins, bradykinin, and histamine. Cranial vasodilation can also accompany systemic infection, fever, hypertension, metabolic disturbances, drug abuse, and ingestion of foods rich in tyramine, monosodium glutamate, and nitrates.

Treatment with ergot alkaloids is most commonly prescribed, but other agents, including 5-hydroxytryptamine antagonists, β-adrenergic blocking agents, clonidine, and drugs that influence monoamine metabolism, are also effective.

See also *cluster h.* and *migraine h.*

head space analysis (for volatile organic substances) a method for assaying organic volatile substances by gas chromatography. A sample of blood or another body fluid is placed in a vial with a rubber septum cap and warmed to 40–60°C. A sample is drawn from the air in the vial (head space) with a syringe and injected into the gas chromatograph. A flame ionization detector may be used or, for greater sensitivity with halogenated hydrocarbons, an electron capture detector.

heal (hēl) 1. to become healthy; to return to a normal, healthy condition.

2. the act of restoring an individual to health.

healing (hēl′ing) the restoration or attempt at restoration of tissue structure by the proliferation of fibroblasts and formation of connective tissue. Accompanying this process is the body's attempt to restore the functional elements of the organ involved: for example, the proliferation of liver cells and the fibrous repair of liver damage, or the formation of bridging skin over scar tissue uniting an injury of the skin. Some organs, most notably central nervous tissue and the heart, are unable to reform any functional tissue in the area of injury and can only fill the area with scar tissue.

The healing of a cutaneous wound is in many respects a model for healing elsewhere in the body. Initially the defect is partially or wholly filled with clotted blood, forming a scab. An inflammatory reaction occurs in the surrounding tissue, with neutrophils predominating. Epidermal cells begin to undergo mitosis and reepithelialize the area immediately below the clot within 48 hr. Macrophages replace the neutrophils on about the third day, destroying and removing necrotic cells and clotted blood. At this point, proliferation of fibroblasts occurs and capillaries begin to invade the area. This vascularization soon fills the fibrous tissue and remains until fibroblasts have laid down collagen fibers to fill the wound. Over a period of several months the area is transformed into an acellular, avascular, collagenous scar with considerable mechanical strength.

See also *union.*

health (helth) the absence of disease or mental or physical impairment. Health is more broadly defined by some authorities, such as the World Health Organization, as a state of optimal physical, mental, and social well-being.

health physics monitoring, shielding, and disposal procedures designed to safeguard personnel from harmful exposure to radiation.

healthy (hel′the) pertaining to or promoting health.

hearing (hēr′ing) [L. *auditus*] the sense by which sounds are perceived.

heart the muscular organ in the thorax that, by its contractions, propels blood through the vessels of the body. It is enclosed in a fibroserous sac (the pericardium) in the mediastinum and, like the vessels of the body, is lined by endothelium (the endocardium). The heart has four chambers: right and left atria, and right and left ventricles. Functionally, the right atrium and ventricle constitute the right side of the heart, propelling blood through the pulmonary circulation. The left atrium and ventricle are responsible for the systemic circulation of blood through the rest of the body.

The walls of the chambers of the heart are composed of cardiac muscle fibers, and constitute the myocardium. Muscle cells of the heart are capable of spontaneous contraction, but their rate of activity is controlled by sympathetic (acceleratory) and parasympathetic (inhibitory) nerves. Contraction of

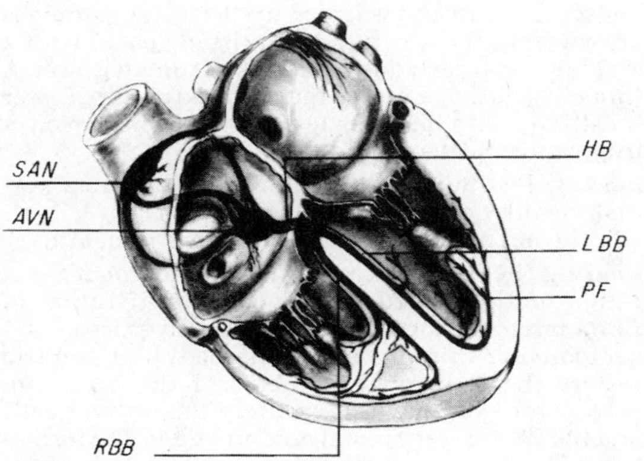

Heart, Figure 1. Diagram of the conduction system of the heart. SAN = sinoatrial node; AVN = atrioventricular node; HB = bundle of His; LBB = left bundle branch; RBB = right bundle branch; and PF = Purkinje fiber. (From Braunwald, E.: Heart Disease. Philadelphia, W. B. Saunders Co., 1980.)

the myocardium is coordinated by a system of conducting fibers, the neuromyocardium. The forward direction of the flow of blood is maintained by valves between the atria and ventricles, and at the outflow points of the ventricles. The normal function of the myocardium depends on an efficient arterial blood supply provided through the coronary arteries, which arise where the aorta begins.

The shape of the heart is roughly that of a blunt cone. The apex, formed by the left ventricle, points forward and to the left. The atria form the base of the heart at the upper part of the back wall. The portion of the heart seen from the front is mainly the ventricles, but a tip of each atrium (its auricle) projects forward above the ventricles. The margins of the four chambers of the heart are indicated on its surface by grooves, some of which contain vessels. The atrioventricular groove encircles the heart between the atria and ventricles, whereas the interventricular groove demarcates the surface of the ventricles. The apex of the heart is opposite the fifth left intercostal space, 8–9 cm from the midline.

Venous blood from the upper and lower parts of the body reaches the heart by means of the superior and inferior venae cavae, which enter the right atrium. This chamber also receives most of the venous return from the myocardium. When the right atrium contracts, blood is forced through the right atrioventricular (tricuspid) valve into the right ventricle, the upper part of which is funnel shaped (the infundibulum), leading to the pulmonary valve with its three semilunar cusps. The right ventricle forces blood through the pulmonary circulation, which returns to the heart to enter the left atrium. The left atrioventricular (mitral) valve has two cusps; blood passes through it to reach the left ventricle. The left ventricle is the most powerful of the four chambers, and its wall is normally three times as thick as that of the right ventricle. It is continuous with the aorta through the aortic valve.

The atrioventricular valves have thin cusps covered by endocardium; they are attached at their free border by slender fibrous cords (chordae tendineae) to the papillary muscles that project from the ventricular wall. The three cusps of the aortic and pulmonary valves do not have chordae tendineae and are protected against inversion by their pocketlike construction.

The coronary arterial system supplies the myocardium through branches of the right and left coronary arteries, which arise at the base of the aorta. A system of veins collects the blood from the myocardium and returns it to the chambers of the heart, principally the right atrium.

Contraction of the chambers of the heart is synchronized by a conducting system within the myocardium that is composed of modified cardiac muscle cells. Contraction begins at the sinoatrial node, a slender structure about 1 cm long in the wall of the right atrium. This is the pacemaker of the heart; it fires off impulses at regular intervals, the rate of activity normally being influenced by the superimposed effects of the autonomic nerves to the heart. Impulses spread throughout the atria from one heart muscle cell to the next, although there are certain preferential pathways that speed its passage and coordinate a trial contraction. Ventricular contraction is initiated by the atrioventricular node, which is located near the tricuspid valve; from it, a bundle of conducting tissue (the atrioventricular bundle) runs down the septum, and its branches ramify through the walls of the ventricles. The atrioventricular bundle is frequently termed the bundle of His, and its fine branches are the Purkinje network.

See also *cardiac m.* under *muscle, pacemaker,* and the accompanying illustrations.

heart attack see *myocardial infarction.*

heart block see *atrioventricular block.*

heart disease see *atherosclerotic heart disease.*

heart failure a condition of diverse etiology and pathogenesis, in which the heart is unable to pump sufficient blood to meet the metabolic needs of the body. It may develop because of the presence of intrinsic cardiac pathology that affects the performance of the myocardium, or because of an inability of the heart to compensate for overloading such as that resulting from hypertension or valve dysfunction. An increased hemodynamic burden placed on the heart may be a volume load, as in aortic insufficiency, or a pressure load, as from aortic stenosis. Volume overloads produce dilation of the heart followed by hypertrophy, whereas pressure overloads typically produce hypertrophy, dilation developing only late in the course of the disease. Both dilation and hypertrophy occur in primary myocardial disorders. The heart is better able to respond to a volume overload and may be able to adjust to a sustained overload when an acute overload of similar magnitude would induce failure. A consequence of heart failure is a rise in venous pressure that produces congestion in the pulmonary or systemic circulations, or both. A consequence of heart failure is a rise in venous pressure that produces congestion in the pulmonary or systemic circulations, or both. See also *congestive heart failure.*

acute h. f., heart failure of sudden onset, as may occur following myocardial infarction.

backward h. f., the accumulation of blood within the venous system proximal to a failing ventricle. The distinction between backward and forward heart failure is not clinically important.

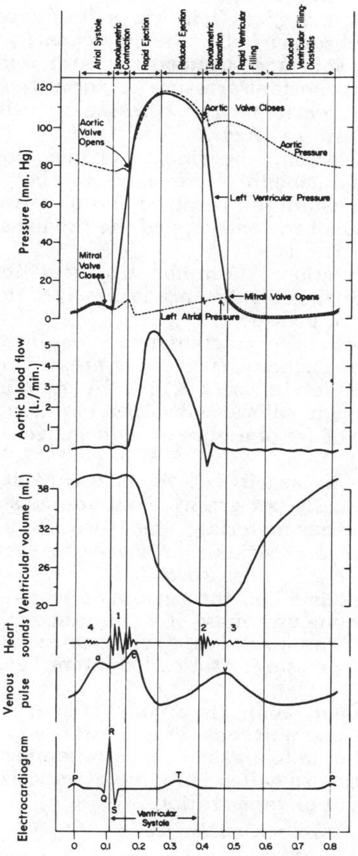

Heart, Figure 2. Events of the cardiac cycle. A complete cardiac cycle in the dog, showing left atrial, aortic, and left ventricular pressure pulses correlated in time with aortic flow, ventricular volume, heart sounds, venous pulse, and electrocardiogram. (From Berne, R. M., and Levy, M. N.: Cardiovascular Physiology. 3rd ed. St. Louis, C. V. Mosby Co., 1977.)

chronic h. f., heart failure of long duration, i.e., persisting for months or years.

congestive h. f., venous and tissue congestion associated with inadequate cardiac function. The clinical findings may indicate both systemic and pulmonary congestion if both ventricles are impaired.

forward h. f., the consequences of decreased cardiac output, with inadequate filling of the arterial system.

high-output h. f., a form of heart failure in which the cardiac output is in the normal or high-normal range but is inadequate to meet increased metabolic needs of the body.

left-sided h. f., a form of heart failure in which the clinical manifestations are due to inadequate performance of the left ventricle. Pulmonary congestion and edema result and may cause dyspnea, orthopnea, cough, and wheezing.

low-output h. f., a more common form of heart failure than high-output heart failure, in which the cardiac output is in the low-normal range or is below normal and is insufficient to meet the needs of the tissues. The condition is seen with myocardial disease, hypertension, and valvular disease.

right-sided h. f., a form of heart failure in which the clinical consequences result from inadequate function of the right ventricle. It may develop acutely with pulmonary embolism and more gradually with severe, chronic lung diseases; the most common cause, however, is left-sided heart failure.

heart failure cell an alveolar macrophage that has ingested hemosiderin. Its presence is indicative of hemorrhages into the pulmonary parenchyma. The hemosiderin-containing granules in the cytoplasm can be demonstrated by use of one of the iron stains.

heart-lung machine an apparatus that provides mechanical circulatory support during open-heart surgery, bypassing the heart to facilitate surgery on the organ. The basic function of the machine is to oxygenate the body's venous supply of blood and then pump it back into the arterial system. The machine also provides intracardiac suction, filtration, and temperature control.

COMPONENTS. Some of the more important components of these machines include pumps, oxygenators, temperature regulators, and filters. Most heart-lung machines use a roller pump, which pushes the blood through the machine's flexible tubing by means of rollers. There are three types of oxygenators used: (1) In the most common type, the bubble oxygenator, gas (97 percent oxygen, 3 percent carbon dioxide) is bubbled into the blood. After gas exchange occurs, the bubbles are burst and released by silicone antifoaming compounds. (2) In the second type, the film oxygenator, exchange takes place at the blood-gas interface formed by a thin film of blood on a rotating disk or stationary screen. (3) In the third type, the membrane oxygenator, exchange occurs through a semipermeable membrane. A heat exchanger is used to control the temperature of the returned blood and the patient's body temperature, and filters are employed in the circuit to remove gas bubbles, platelet aggregates, fibrin, particles from calcified aortic and mitral valves, and other debris.

PROCEDURE. The system is initially filled with sterile water, dextrose, electrolytes, and albumin. The hemodilution produced by water with the patient's blood reduces both sludging in the capillaries and renal damage. Extracorporeal circulation is initiated by fully heparinizing the patient before inserting various catheters. An arterial return catheter is usually inserted in the aorta or one of its branches; venous uptake catheters are inserted in the superior and inferior vena cavae; and a catheter is inserted through the right superior pulmonary vein into the left ventricle, through which blood is aspirated and sent to the oxygenator.

At the conclusion of surgery, after the patient has been withdrawn from extracorporeal perfusion, the contents of the heart-lung machine are slowly reinfused into the patient.

The procedure is not without possible serious complications, which include aortic dissection from arterial cannulation, and air embolism from the open heart or open oxygenator. Also, there is always some damage to the platelets, red cells, and white cells as well as denaturation of plasma proteins.

Commonly, the patient experiences moderate fever for several days following the operation.

heart rate the number of contractions of the ventricles per unit of time, standardly recorded in beats per minute.

heart tumors neoplasms of the heart. Metastatic tumors may involve the heart, either by direct extension of a mediastinal neoplasm, or through blood-borne metastases. Bronchogenic carcinoma, lymphomas, and melanomas are the most common secondary tumors involving the heart.

Primary cardiac neoplasms are rare. The most common is the benign myxoma, which usually forms a polypoid lesion within an atrium, where it may interfere with the passage of blood by obstructing a valve orifice. Spindle and stellate cells are loosely arranged in a myxoid stroma that contains many small vessels. Occasionally, an organizing thrombus is mistakenly interpreted as a cardiac myxoma.

Cardiac rhabdomyomas are rare lesions, often multiple, that are viewed by some as hamartomas rather than as true neoplasms. Most occur in infants in association with the tuberous sclerosis complex.

Various other benign mesenchymal tumors occurring in the heart are rarely reported; they include angiomas and lipomas. The histogenesis of the so-called mesothelioma of the atrioventricular node is controversial.

Sarcomas arising within the heart are also uncommon, and only some can be classified. They include angiosarcomas and rhabdomyosarcomas.

heartworm (hart'werm) See *D. immitis* under *Dirofilaria.*

heat (*Q*) (hēt) [L. *calor;* Gr. *thermē*] a form of energy that is the kinetic energy of the random motion of molecules and atoms (including the rotation and vibration of molecules). Heat can be produced by the conversion of other kinds of energy, such as mechanical work, into heat. It can be transferred by three processes: conduction, the flow of heat through stationary matter; convection, the flow of heat carried by the movement of matter; and radiation, the flow of heat carried across space by thermal (blackbody) electromagnetic radiation. The International System (SI) unit of heat, work, and energy is the joule (J); in chemistry, the calorie (cal), which equals 4.185 J, is commonly used to measure heat. See also *temperature* and *thermodynamics.*

h. capacity (*C*), the amount of heat required to raise the temperature of a system or substance by 1 K (1°C). The customary units are calories per kelvin (cal/K^{-1}). See also *molar h. capacity* and *specific h. capacity.*

h. of combustion, the amount of heat liberated by the complete oxidation of a unit mass or of 1 mol of a substance at constant volume or constant pressure.

h. of formation, see *standard enthalpy of formation.*

h. of fusion, the amount of heat absorbed by 1 mol or one unit mass of a substance in changing from a solid to a liquid at constant temperature and pressure. Also called latent heat of fusion.

latent h., the amount of heat absorbed or liberated in a change of state (e.g., melting or evaporation) of 1 mol or one unit mass of a substance at constant temperature and pressure. The latent heat associated with a particular change of state is called the *h. of fusion, h. of sublimation,* or *h. of vaporization.*

molar h. capacity (*C*), the heat capacity per mole of a pure substance as measured for a temperature change at constant pressure (C_p) or at constant volume (C_v), customarily expressed in calories per mole-kelvin (cal/mol·K).

h. of reaction, the amount of heat liberated or absorbed during the occurrence of a chemical reaction at constant temperature and pressure, i.e., the difference of the enthalpy of the products and that of the reactants.

h. of solution, the amount of heat liberated or absorbed when a substance is dissolved in a solvent at constant pressure.

specific h., a contraction for and equivalent to specific heat capacity, (usually expressed in calories per gram-kelvin, cal/g·K) i.e. the quantity of heat (expressed in calories) absorbed in raising the temperature of 1 g of a pure or homogeneous material 1°C (1 K).

specific h. capacity (*c*), the heat capacity per unit mass (usually per gram) of a pure substance or a homogeneous material as measured for a temperature change at constant pressure (c_p) or at constant volume (c_v). See also *specific h.*

h. of sublimation, the amount of heat absorbed by 1 mol or one unit mass of a substance in changing directly from a solid to a gas at constant temperature and pressure. Also called latent heat of sublimation.

h. of vaporization, the amount of heat absorbed by 1 mol or one unit mass of a substance in changing from a liquid to a gas at constant temperature and pressure. Also called enthalpy of vaporization and latent heat of vaporization.

heat content see *enthalpy.*

heat precipitation test a test used to demonstrate unstable hemoglobins. A hemolysate is prepared from washed red cells and incubated in a phosphate buffer at 50°C. The percentage of unstable hemoglobin precipitated during the incubation is then calculated; normally it is less than 1 percent.

heat sink 1. in thermodynamics, a region where heat is absorbed.

2. in electronics, a device that absorbs and dissipates heat, such as the aluminum base with cooling fins on which a power transistor is mounted, or the alligator clip temporarily attached to a wire between a heat-sensitive device and a connection being soldered.

heat stroke (hēt strōk) see *systemic h.* under *hyperthermia.*

heat unit (HU) a convenient unit used to specify the ability of an x-ray tube to dissipate heat. It is the product of the kilovoltage, milliamperage, and exposure time (in seconds) for an exposure, e.g., 60 kV × 100 mA × 0.25 sec = 1500 HU. Each tube has a specified heat-dissipation rating (in heat units per minute) used to determine whether a rapid sequence of exposures can be made without damage to the tube.

heavy chain a polypeptide that is a structural component of an immunoglobulin molecule; M.W. 55,000. Each immunoglobulin molecule has two identical heavy chains that have approximately twice the number of amino acids that light chains have.

heavy-chain disease a rare form of monoclonal

gammopathy that results in the presence of monoclonal proteins (predominantly Fc fragments) in the serum and urine. The protein possesses the antigenic determinants of the parent immunoglobulin's heavy chain but not the light chain. The Fd portion of the heavy chain appears to be deleted in the monoclonal heavy chains. There is lymphocyte and/or plasma cell proliferation in the intestinal mucosa and mesenteric lymph nodes, so that the disease more closely resembles malignant lymphocytic lymphoma than multiple myeloma. Osteolytic lesions are not observed.

There are three classes of heavy-chain disease: (1) Gamma heavy-chain disease, IgG, occurs in the elderly, with lymphadenopathy and liver and spleen enlargement. There is a diffuse infiltrate of plasma cells and lymphocytes, mixed with eosinophils. Gamma heavy chains and a globulin fragment resembling a gamma Fc piece are found in the serum or urine on immunoelectrophoresis with monoclonal antiserum. (2) Alpha heavy-chain disease, IgA, occurs primarily in children, with massive infiltration of the lamina propria of the gut with plasma cells and histiocytes. There is a marked increase in alpha heavy chains in the serum. (3) Mu heavy-chain disease, IgM, is seen in chronic lymphocytic leukemia, with liver enlargement, spleen enlargement, and plasma cell infiltration of the marrow. Antiserum shows an increase in mu heavy chains.

See also *Franklin's disease.*

heavy metals a term used to refer to the relatively heavy metallic elements or their ions, such as antimony, arsenic, bismuth, iron, lead, and mercury. Most of these metals and especially their ions are highly toxic, even if present at a low concentration. For more information on toxicity and assay methods, see the specific metal.

heavy particle therapy irradiation of some part of a patient by a beam (of protons, neutrons, or other nuclides) that is produced by a particle accelerator, linear accelerator, cyclotron, or synchrotron. The beam deposits most of its energy at one particular depth called the Bragg peak. Tissues near the skin are exposed to about one-fourth as much radiation damage as those at the Bragg peak; deeper tissues receive almost no radiation. This method has been used to treat acromegaly and some types of Cushing's syndrome.

Heberden's nodes (he′ber-denz) [William *Heberden*, English physician, 1710–1801] nodes that occur in osteoarthritis and affect the terminal interphalangeal joints. These small, hard nodules are more common in females and may be genetically determined.

hecto- (h) (hek′to) [Fr., from Gr. *hekaton* one hundred] a prefix attached to units of measurement to make a unit that is equal to 100 of the basic units.

hectogram (hek′to-gram) a unit of mass equal to 100 g (10^2 g).

hectometer (hm) (hek′to-me″ter, hek-tom′ĕ-ter) a unit of length equal to 100 meters (10^2 m).

heel (hēl) the hindmost part of the foot.

heel effect a variation in the x-ray intensity (which increases toward the cathode end of the x-ray tube) over the width of the beam; the effect is negligible in modern equipment.

Heerfordt's disease (hār′forts) [Christian Frederick *Heerfordt*, Danish ophthalmologist] a form of sarcoidosis characterized by facial paralysis, with uveal inflammation and enlargement of the parotid gland. It is most frequently seen in persons in their late teens, and in black females. The parotid glands become bilaterally swollen, firm, and nodular; the facial paralysis may be bilateral.

Hegar's sign (ha′garz) [Alfred *Hegar*, gynecologist in Freiburg, 1830–1914] softening of the lower uterus, detectable around the sixth week of pregnancy by bimanual examination.

Heidenhain's azan stain (hi′den-hīnz) [Rudolf Peter *Heidenhain*, German physiologist, 1834–1897] a histologic stain for connective tissue. Paraffin sections are stained with azocarmine B or azocarmine G, differentiated in aniline-alcohol, mordanted in phosphotungstic acid, and stained with aniline blue–orange G. Nuclei, neuroglia, erythrocytes, and osteocytes stain red; muscle, yellow to red; and mucin, collagen, and reticulin, blue. Also called *azan stain*. See also *Mallory's collagen stain*.

Heinz bodies (hīntz) [Robert *Heinz*, German pathologist, 1865–1924] intracellular inclusions usually attached to the red cell membrane, which increase the fragility of the cell. Heinz bodies are 0.3–2 μm in diameter and consist of denatured hemoglobin. They occur in thalassemia, primarily in nucleated red blood cells in the bone marrow; in α-thalassemia after splenectomy as single inclusions (distinct from the diffuse stippling of presplenectomy H-hemoglobin when stained with brilliant cresyl blue or new methylene blue); in enzymopathies of the hexose monophosphate shunt, such as glucose-6-phosphate dehydrogenase deficiency after ingestion of primaquine or other drugs precipitating hemolysis; after administration of phenylhydrazine, chlorates, and other drugs; in some hemoglobinopathies with unstable hemoglobins (e.g., Köln and Zürich); and generally after splenectomy.

Cells with Heinz bodies may assume a teardrop shape, and the bodies may be removed as red cells pass through the cords of the spleen with the subsequent formation of spherocytes.

Heinz bodies are demonstrated by supravital staining with crystal violet, which stains the bodies purple but does not stain the reticulocytes. They are also seen after supravital staining with new methylene blue or other reticulocyte stains staining less clearly than the "reticulum," and also by phase microscopy.

Heinz-body hemolytic anemia [Robert *Heinz*] see *unstable hemoglobin disease* under *anemia*.

Heinz body test [Robert *Heinz*] a screening for glucose-6-phosphate dehydrogenase (G-6-PD) deficiency. Acetylphenylhydrazine is added both to a test blood specimen and to a control blood specimen. After incubation at 37°C for 2 and 4 hr, the treated blood specimens are examined for cells with five or more Heinz bodies; the control should have less than 30 percent such cells. A value above 45 percent in the test specimen indicates G-6-PD deficiency or the presence of some other defect resulting in deficiency of reduced glutathione. Glutathione is required to protect hemoglobin from oxidative denaturation by some chemical agents and to maintain the integrity of an unstable hemoglobin. The test is sensitive to changes in oxygen tension and hematocrit, and has been largely superseded by more specific methods.

Heister's valve (hīs′terz) [Lorenz *Heister*, German anatomist, 1683–1758] see *spiral v.* under *valve.*

Hektoen enteric agar (hek′tōn) [Ludvig Hektoen, Chicago pathologist, 1863–1951] see *Hecktoen enteric a.* under *agar.*

HeLa cells (he′lah) [acronym from *He*nrietta *La*cks, the patient from whose cervical carcinoma the parent carcinoma cells were isolated in 1951 by Dr. George O. Gey at Johns Hopkins Hospital] aneuploid, epithelial-like cells that represent the first continuously cultured human carcinoma. They are used in experimental studies of life processes, including viruses, at the cellular level. These cells possess the qualities of cancerous cells, including loss of anchorage dependence in culture; they are often used in the examination of chemotherapeutic drug metabolism.

Heleidae (hĕ-le′ĭ-de) a family of flies of the suborder Nematocerca in the order Diptera. Several genera, including *Culicoides, Leptoconops,* and *Lasiohelea,* have species that are parasitic in humans and transmitters of various diseases. Also called Ceratopogonidae, *no-see-ums,* and *punkies.*

helenine (hel′ĕ-nēn) an antiviral agent, a ribonucleoprotein, produced by *Penicillium funiculosum.* This agent inhibits the growth of poliovirus 2 and echovirus 9 in cell culture.

helic/o (hel′ĭ-ko) [Gr. *helix* coil] a word element used in combining form to denote relationship to a coil or snail, e.g., helical.

helical (hel′ĭ-kal) shaped like a helix.

helicotrema (hel″ĭ-ko-tre′mah) [*helico-* + Gr. *trēma* hole] [NA], the passage of the ear that connects the scala tympani and scala vestibuli at the apex of the cochlea.

helium (He) (he′le-um) [Gr. *hēlios* the sun, where it was first discovered by spectroscopy] a colorless, odorless, inert, gaseous element; atomic number 2; atomic weight 4.0026; Group 0 of the periodic table (the noble gases); only known oxidation state 0 (no compounds). Helium is used as an inert atmosphere, as a cryogenic coolant (b.p., 4.2°K), as a radiolucent contrast medium, and [USP] as a diluent and vehicle for the administration of oxygen, anesthetics, and other gases.

A helium-4 nucleus emitted in radioactive decay is called an alpha particle.

helix (he′liks) [Gr. "snail," "coil"] 1. the curve made by a point both revolving around an axis and traveling along it with a constant speed; the shape of a spiral staircase. Several biologic macromolecules have helical structure; see under *deoxyribonucleic acid* and *protein.*

2. the superior and posterior free margin of the pinna of the ear.

helle Zellen [Gr. "clear cell"] large, clear cells, of unknown significance, that are occasionally present in the endometrial surface epithelium during the proliferative phase.

Helly's fluid a mercuric chloride-dichromate fixative; see under *fixative.*

helmet cell see *schiztocyte.*

helminth (hel′minth) [Gr. *helmins* worm] a parasitic worm; the term includes trematodes (flukes), cestodes (tapeworms), and nematodes (pinworms, hookworms, roundworms, and filariae). For more information, see the accompanying illustration and the specific type of worm.

helminthemesis (hel″min-them′ĕ-sis) [Gr. *helmins* + *emesis* vomiting] the vomiting of worms.

helminthiasis (hel″min-thi′ah-sis) a general term used to describe infection with worms; see also *helminthic disease.*

helminthic (hel-min′thik) pertaining to or caused by parasitic worms.

helminthic disease any disease caused by the infection of worms, including the classes Nematoda (roundworms), Trematoda (flukes), and Cestoda (tapeworms). Helminthic infections occur worldwide but the majority are concentrated in the tropics. Many of the parasites require special temperature conditions, whereas others need a particular vertebrate or invertebrate host or insect for the completion of their life cycle.

Among the class Nematoda, the medically important species of roundworms include *Ascaris lumbricoides,* the hookworms *Ancylostoma duodenale* and *Necator americanus, Strongyloides stercoralis* (threadworm), *Trichuris trichiura* (whipworm), and *Enterobius vermicularis* (pinworm).

Common tapeworms of the class Cestoda include *Hymenolepis nana* (dwarf tapeworm), *Taenia saginata* (beef tapeworm), *T. solium* (pork tapeworm), and *Diphyllobothrium latum* (fish tapeworm).

The most common Trematoda infections include the intestinal flukes *Fasciolopsis buski* and *Echinostoma ilocanum; Fasciola hepatica* (sheep liver fluke); *Paragonimus westermani* (Oriental lung fluke); the blood flukes *Schistosoma japonicum, S. mansoni,* and *S. haematobium; Clonorchis sinensis* (Oriental liver fluke); *Opisthorchis felineus;* and *O. viverrini.*

helminth identification procedures various methods and techniques used to preserve, concentrate, and identify helminths in the feces. If a stool cannot be examined within 3 hr, the specimen can be fixed in merthiolate-iodine-formalin (MIF) or 10 percent formalin, which will preserve the helminth eggs for some months.

When a specimen is being examined, the first phase is to concentrate the helminth's eggs by separating them from the bulk fecal material; this can be done by utilizing the differences in specific gravity. The three most common concentrating methods are the formalin-ether sedimentation method (the eggs being heavier than the suspending liquid, they collect in the bottom); the acid-sodium sulfate-triton-NE-ether concentration-AMS method (uses centrifugation to collect eggs); and the zinc sulfate flotation method (uses heavy liquid so that the eggs float to the top). The last technique usually gives best separation results but is not recommended for trematode or broad fish tapeworm eggs.

Following concentration, identification of helminths can be made through various techniques. Intestinal nematodes are generally fixed and examined with alcohol and glycine or alcohol-formalin-acetic acid (AFA). Glacial acetic acid is useful for killing and clearing nematodes for microscopic examination. Formalin usually is not recommended as a fixative because of its hardening properties, but a dilute solution is an excellent fixative for adult *Ascaris.* Pinworm eggs usually do not appear in the feces and are most easily diagnosed by the Scotch-tape method. Both cestodes and trematodes are generally fixed in AFA solution and stain well in Semichon's acetic carmine, Delafield's hematoxylin, or Alum cochineal (Trematodes only).

Evaluation of the therapy in progress with infections, especially hookworm, can be made by monitoring the egg count of several specimens using the Stoll dilution method, the Beaver direct smear method, the McMaster helminth technique, and the Kato thick smear technique.

Some of the blood and tissue-dwelling nematodes that cause filariasis and trichinosis can be diagnosed from blood samples by immunodiagnostic tests. For filariasis, complement-fixation (CF), bentonite flocculation (BF), and indirect hemagglutination (IH) tests are performed. For trichinosis, intradermal (ID), CF, BF, IH, latex (L), indirect fluorescent antibody (IFA), and precipitin (P) tests are used.

helminthism (hel′min-thizm) the presence of worms in the body.

helminthology (hel″min-thol′o-je) [Gr. *helmins* + *logos* word, reason] the science or study of parasitic worms.

Helminthosporium (hel-min′tho-spo″re-um) a common dematiacious fungus of the soil and of plants, which can be isolated from the skin and sputum of humans. It is usually considered a saprophytic fungus; on rare occasions it may cause pulmonary disease.

Helophilus (hĕ-lof′ĭ-lus) a genus of flies in the family Syrphidae. When food contaminated with eggs is ingested, nasal or intestinal myiasis can result.

helper T lymphocyte see *helper T l.* under *lymphocyte.*

hem/o (he′mo) [Gr. *haima, haimatos* blood] a word element used in combining form to denote blood, e.g., hemoglobin.

hemacytometer (he″mah-si-tom′ĕ-ter) a counting chamber for blood cells. The instrument consists of a glass block with a depression of definite depth, the floor of which is ruled off into squares. Blood cells are counted with the aid of a microscope in the known volume between the ruled squares and the coverglass. Also called *hemocytometer.* See also *blood cell count.*

hemagglutination (hem″ah-gloo″tĭ-na′shun) the clumping together of erythrocytes in the presence of specific antibody, certain virus particles (e.g., influenza virus, mumps virus), or substances such as high-molecular-weight dextrans. Hemagglutination is a basic technique widely used in blood banking, serology, and immunology for antibody detection. It is a simple, inexpensive and very sensitive method.

hemagglutination inhibition a semiquantitative method for detecting small amounts of soluble antigen in serum or other body fluids. The antigen to be assayed is preincubated with specific antibody, and then antigen-coated erythrocytes are added. In the presence of high amounts of antigen in the specimen, the specific antibody is neutralized and thus no reaction occurs after addition of the erythrocytes. If the amount of antigen in the specimen is low, the specific antibody is neutralized, and thus reacts with the antigen coated to erythrocytes (agglutination). This assay is useful in detecting HBsAg in hepatitis and blood clotting Factor VIII in individuals with hemophilia. See also the accompanying illustration.

hemagglutinin (hem″ah-gloo′tĭ-nin) [*hem-* + *agglutinin*] 1. a surface component of many viruses that possesses an intrinsic property of combining with certain receptors on the surface of red cells to cause hemagglutination, e.g., a rod-shaped glycoprotein located on the surface of an influenza virus. Hemagglutinin may also bind to host cell receptors and facilitate the disease process by aiding in the attachment of virus to the epithelial cells that line the respiratory tract. See also *influenza virus.*

2. an antibody that agglutinates red blood cells. Hemagglutinins may require a specific environment such as 0.85 percent sodium chloride, hydrophilic colloids (albumin, fibrinogen), or treatment with proteolytic enzymes.

autologous h., an antibody that acts with red blood cells of the same organism.

cold h., an antibody that acts at temperatures lower than 37°C with greater affinity than at 37°C. The thermal amplitude of cold agglutinin expresses the relationship of temperature to its optimal activity.

heterologous h., an antibody that acts with red blood cells of individuals of other species.

homologous h., an antibody that acts with red blood cells of other individuals of the same species.

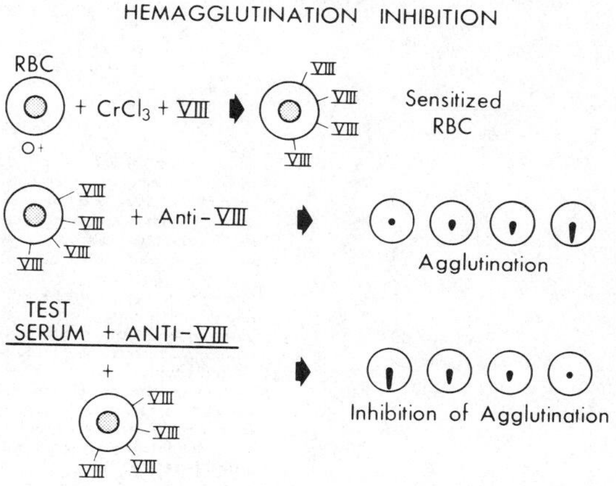

Hemagglutination inhibition. Human O+ red blood cells (RBC) are conjugated with coagulation Factor VIII antigen by chromic chloride. The sensitized red blood cells are reacted with specific antibody to Factor VIII and are agglutinated. In the well of a V-shaped microtiter plate, agglutinated red blood cells appear as discrete dots. Nonagglutinated cells form a streak when the plate is incubated at a 45° angle. Agglutination of sensitized red blood cells can be inhibited by the presence of homologous Factor VIII antigen present in the test serum. With decreasing amounts of serum added to the test, the specific antibody agglutinates sensitized cells and forms a dot in the microtiter well. A semiquantitative estimation of the amount or titer of antigen in a test serum can be made in this way. (From Fudenberg, H. H., et al.: Basic & Clinical Immunology. 2nd ed. Los Altos, CA, Lange Medical Publications, 1976.)

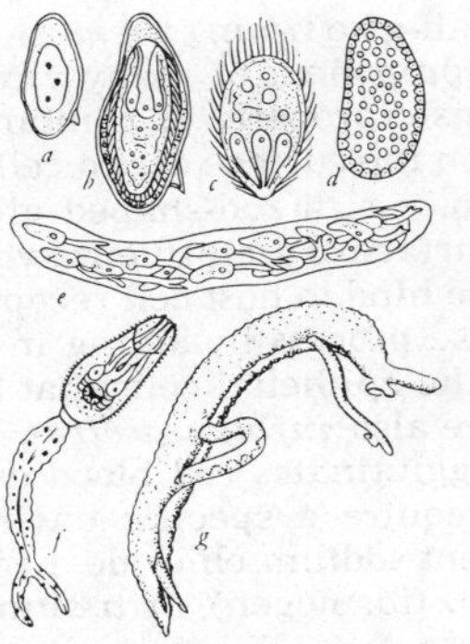

No. 302. Schistosoma mansoni. Life cycle from snail (intermediate host, *c–e*) to man (final host, which the cercariae [*f*] enter via the skin). *a* Freshly laid egg from a vein. *b* Excreted egg with miracidium. *c* Miracidium. *d* Young mother sporocyst with germ masses. *e* Older daughter sporocyst with cercariae. *f* Cercaria. *g* Adult male and female flukes from a rectal vein. (Different magnifications; after PIEKARSKI, 1954.)

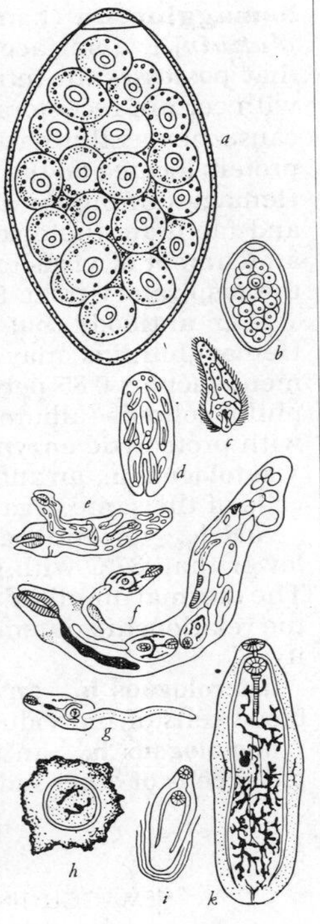

No. 304. Fasciolopsis buski. a Egg, showing oöcyte in upper half. (After LOOSS, 1905.) *b–k* Life cycle from snail (1st intermediate host, *b–f*), through red caltrop (*Trapa natans*, 2nd intermediate host, *h*) to man (final host, *h–k*). *b* Immature egg as laid. *c* Free-swimming miracidium. *d* Sporocyst with rediae. *e* Mother redia containing daughter rediae. *f* Daughter redia with cercariae. *g* Free-swimming cercaria. *h* Metacercaria. *i* Metacercaria escaping from cyst in intestine. *k* Adult fluke. (Different magnifications; after PIEKARSKI, 1954.)

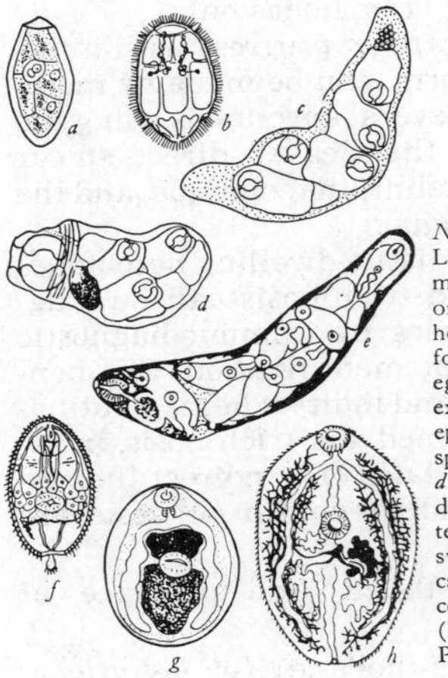

No. 308. Paragonimus westermani. Life cycle from snail (1st intermediate host, *b–e*), through crab or crayfish (2nd intermediate host, *f* and *g*) to man (final host for adult worm, *h*). *a* Immature egg as laid. *b* Miracidium (only excretory system and ciliated epithelial cells shown). *c* Mature sporocyst with mother rediae. *d* Mature mother redia with daughter rediae. *e* Mature daughter redia with cercariae. *f* Free-swimming ('microcercarial') cercaria after leaving snail. *g* Metacercaria from crab. *h* Adult fluke. (Different magnifications; after PIEKARSKI, 1954.)

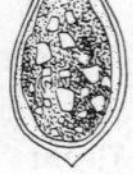

No. 310. Clonorchis sinensis. Right: egg, ∼400 ×; below: schematic arrangement of organs, 4×. (After PIEKARSKI, 1954.)

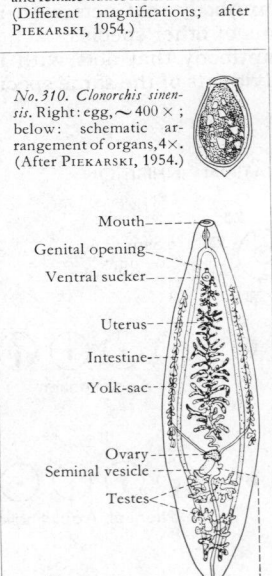

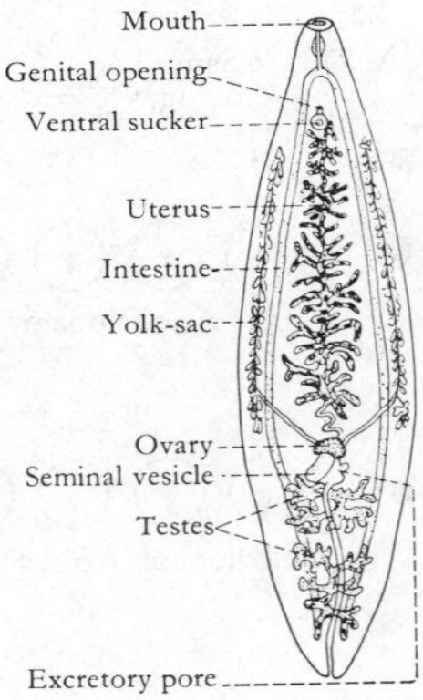

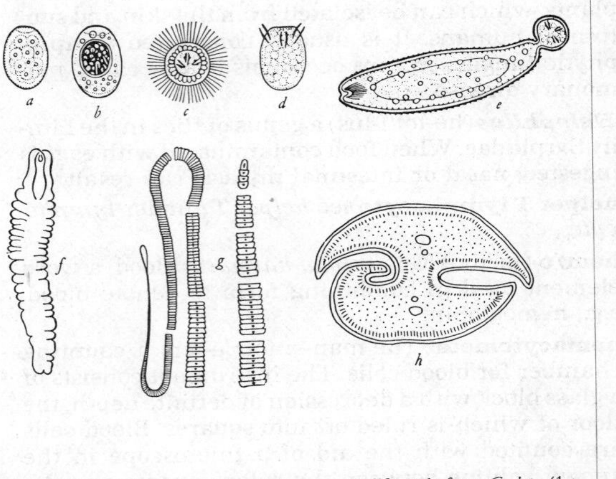

No. 313. Diphyllobothrium latum. Diagrammatic life cycle from *Cyclops* (1st intermediate host, *c* to *e*) through fish (2nd intermediate host with plerocercoid, *f*) to man (final host). *a* Freshly laid egg. *b* Egg with developing coracidium. *c* Free-swimming coracidium. *d* Six-hooked larva from coracidium, as seen in *Cyclops*. *e* Mature procercoid. *f* Plerocercoid, invasive larva with two pseudobothria. *g* Adult tapeworm. *h* Section through head. (Different magnifications; *a* to *g* after PIEKARSKI, 1954, *h* after BRAUN.)

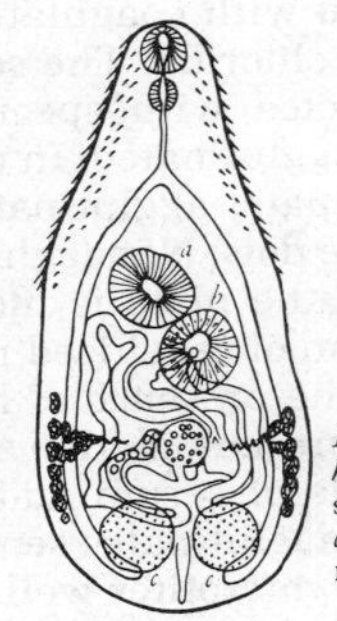

No. 312. Heterophyes heterophyes. a Ventral sucker. *b* Genital 'sucker'. *c* Two testes. (After PIEKARSKI, 1954.)

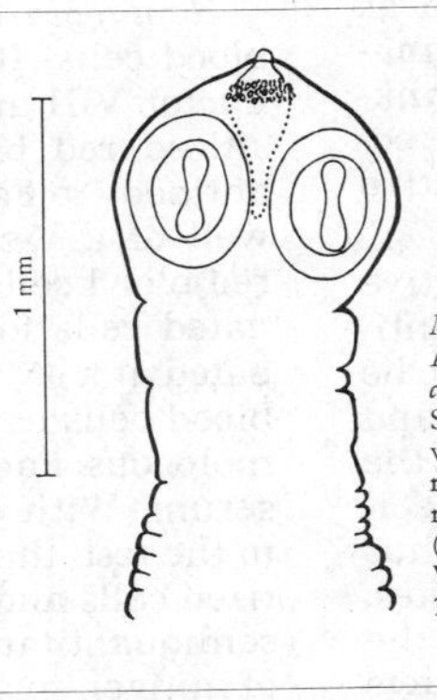

No. 315. Dipylidium caninum. Scolex of worm with retracted rostellum. (After WITENBERG, 1932.)

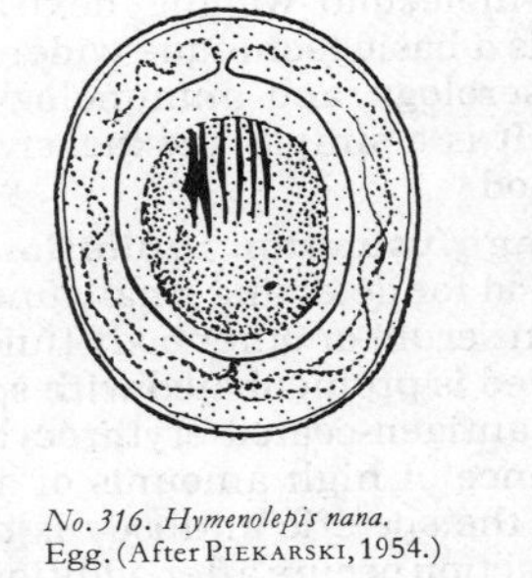

No. 316. Hymenolepis nana. Egg. (After PIEKARSKI, 1954.)

Helminth. Representative helminthic genera and species. (From Baer, J. G., et al.: Pathogenic Organisms and Infectious Diseases. Basle, Switzerland, Ciba-Geigy Ltd., 1971.)

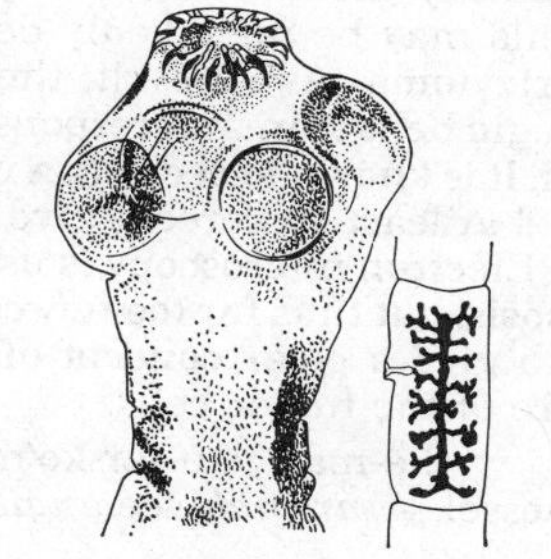

No. 317. Taenia solium. Left: head. (After SZIDAT and WIGAND, 1934.) Right: tapeworm segments with branching uterus containing eggs. (After RIBBERT-HAMPERL, 1944.)

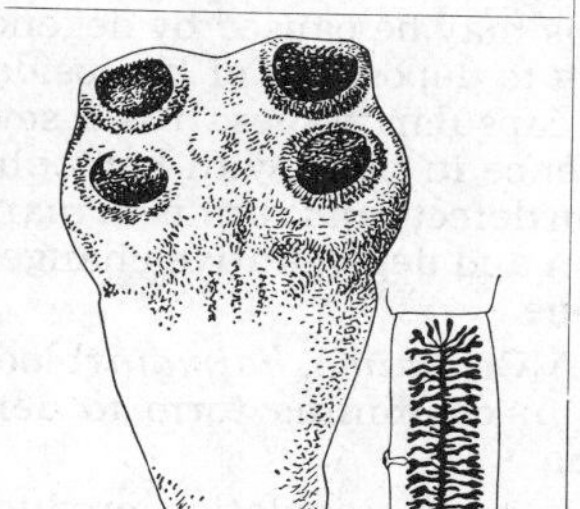

No. 318. Taenia saginata. Left: head. (After SZIDAT and WIGAND, 1934.) Right: tapeworm segments with branching uterus containing eggs. (After RIBBERT-HAMPERL, 1944.)

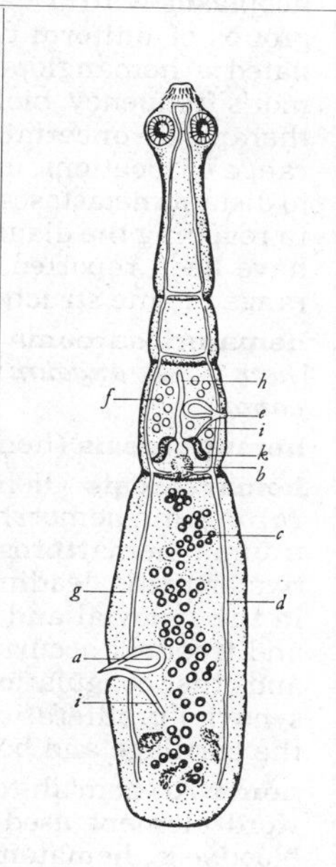

No. 320. Echinococcus granulosus. Adult worm in gut of dog. *a* Cirrus-sac. *b* Yolk-sac. Eggs. *d* Excretory canal. *e* Genital orifice. *f* Testes. *g* Mature segment. *h* Uterus. *i* Vagina. *k* Ovary. (After PIEKARSKI, 1954.)

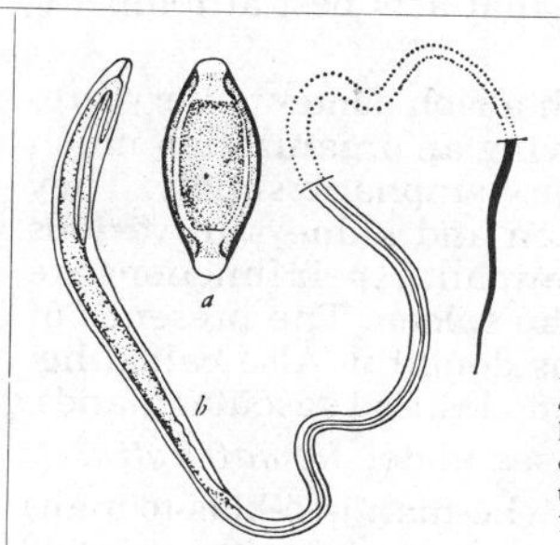

No. 322. Trichuris trichiura. *a* Egg. *b* Complete worm. The head is at the slender end; the dotted section lies in the intestinal mucosa. (After FAUST, 1930.)

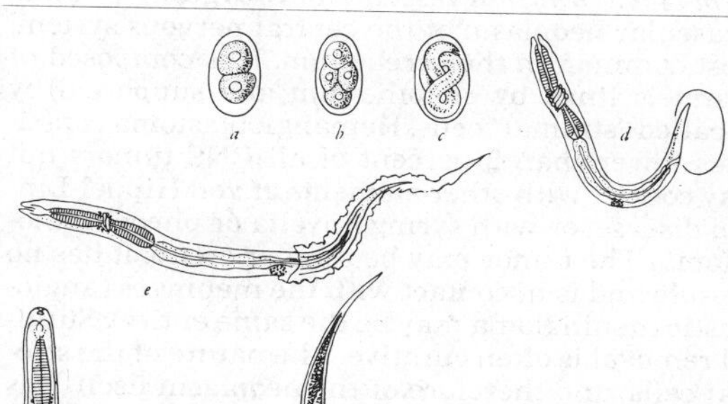

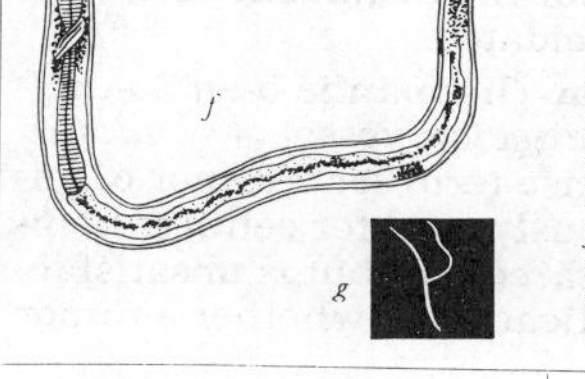

No. 324. Ancylostoma duodenale. Life cycle. *a, b* Two- and four-celled eggs as excreted. *c* Egg containing larva. *d* Rhabditiform larva in process of hatching. *e* Molting of rhabditiform larva. *f* Sheathed filariform larva (infective form). *g* Position during copulation. (Different magnifications; after PIEKARSKI, 1954.)

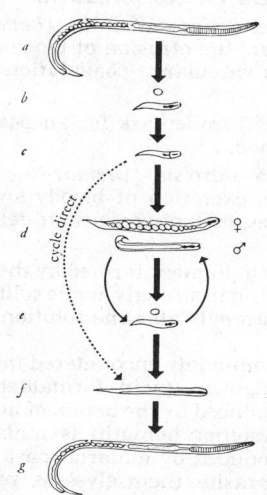

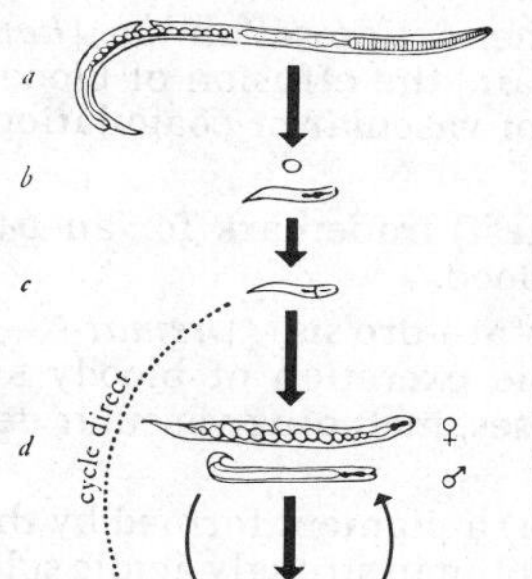

No. 327. Strongyloides stercoralis. Life cycle. *a* Parthenogenetic female (in intestinal mucosa). *b* Egg and rhabditiform larva (in faeces). *c* Rhabditiform larva (free-living). *d* Bisexual generation (free-living). *e* Egg and rhabditiform larva (free-living). *f* Filariform larva. *g* Parthenogenetic female (in intestinal mucosa). *a–g* Indirect or bisexual development. *a, b, c, f, g* Direct or parthenogenetic development (auto-infestation by penetration of filariform larvae in the skin of the anal region. (After PIEKARSKI, 1954.)

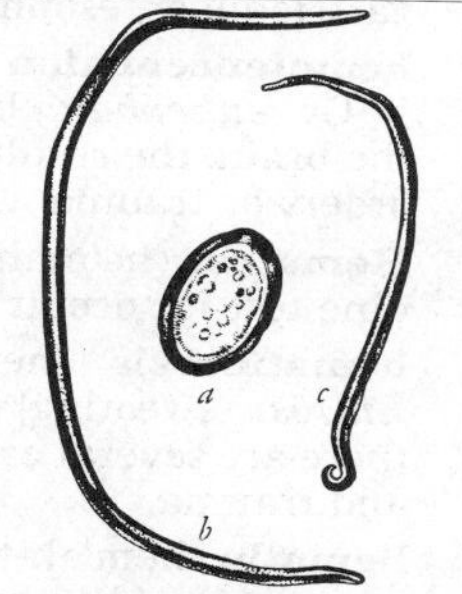

No. 328. Ascaris lumbricoides. *a* Egg (external appearance). *b* Female worm. *c* Male worm. (After SZIDAT and WIGAND.)

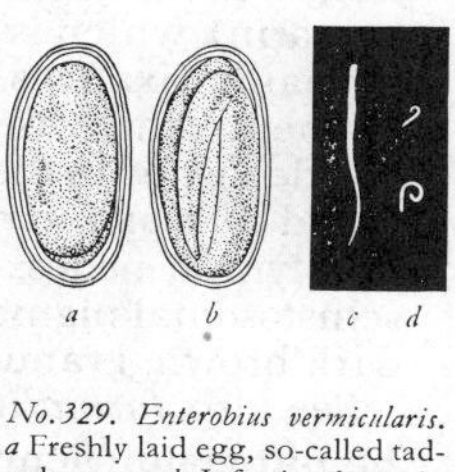

No. 329. Enterobius vermicularis. *a* Freshly laid egg, so-called tadpole stage. *b* Infective larva in egg capsule. *c, d* Mature worms, natural size, female (*c*) and males (*d*). (*a, b* After PIEKARSKI, 1954; *c, d* after RIBBERT-HAMPERL, 1944.)

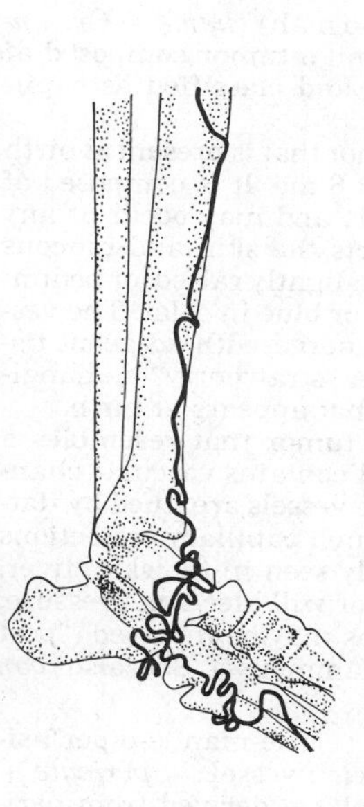

No. 331. Dracunculus medinensis. X-ray photograph of worm injected with contrast medium. (After BOTREAU-ROUSSEL.)

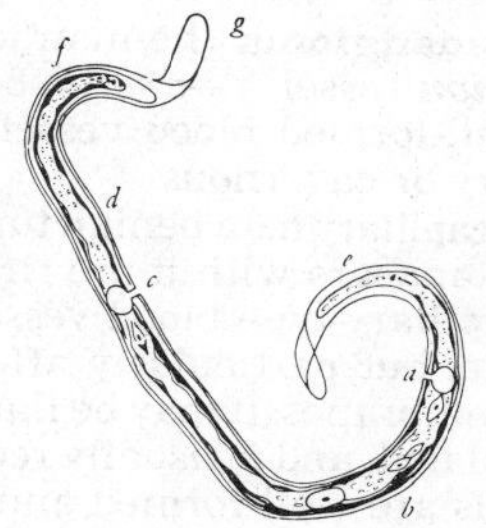

No. 334. Loa loa. Sheathed microfilaria. *a* Anus. *b* Intestine. *c* Excretory pore. *d* Nerve ring. *e* Tail end. *f* Head end. *g* Sheath. (After PIEKARSKI, 1954.)

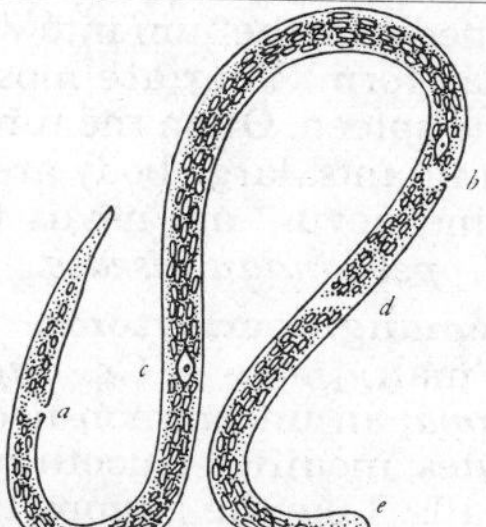

No. 335. Oncocerca volvulus. Microfilaria without sheath. *a* Anal pore. *b* Excretory pore. *c* Genital cell. *d* Nerve ring. *e* Head end. (After FAUST, 1930.)

warm h., an antibody that acts best at temperatures around 37°C.

hemal nodes nodes with a rich content of erythrocytes within sinuses, having an organization much like a lymph node but no lymphatic supply. They are found near the spleen and kidneys in various mammals, especially ruminants; their functions are probably like those of the spleen. The presence of such nodes in humans is doubtful. Also called hemal glands, hemolymph nodes, and vascular glands.

hemalum (hem-al′um) see under *hematoxylin.*

hemangioblastoma (hĕ-man″je-o-blas-to′mah) [*hem-* + Gr. *angeion* vessel + *blastos* germ + *-oma*] a vascular neoplasm of the central nervous system, most common in the cerebellum. It is composed of channels lined by endothelium and supported by so-called "stromal" cells. Hemangioblastoma constitutes fewer than 2 percent of all CNS tumors but may coexist with other elements of von Hippel-Lindau disease, or with syringomyelia or pheochromocytoma. The tumor may be solid or cystic; it has no capsule and is in contact with the meninges (angioblastic meningioma may be the same entity). Surgical removal is often curative. The nature of the stromal cells, and therefore of the neoplasm itself, has not been adequately elucidated.

hemangioendothelioma (hĕ-man″je-o-en″do-the″-le-o′mah) [*hem-* + Gr. *angeion* vessel + *endothelium* + *-oma*] an imprecise term for a tumor of endothelial cells. It is variously used for cellular hemangiomas and for angiosarcomas, but is unsatisfactory as it provides no indication of whether a tumor is benign or malignant.

hemangioma (hĕ-man″je-o′mah) [*hem-* + Gr. *angeion* vessel + *-oma*] a benign tumor composed of well-formed blood vessels and classified as capillary or cavernous.

capillary h., a benign tumor that is present at birth or appears within the first 6 mo. It is composed of capillary-type blood vessels and may occur at any site, but particularly affects the skin and mucous membranes. It may be flat, slightly raised, or pedunculated, and is usually red or blue in color. The vessels are well formed and merge with adjacent tissues; there is no capsule. A "strawberry" hemangioma is a common lesion that appears at birth.

cavernous h., a benign tumor that resembles a capillary hemangioma but contains vascular channels of large diameter. The vessels are lined by flattened endothelium into which papillary projections may form. They are mostly seen in the skin, liver, and spleen. Often the tumor will bleed on pressure. In infants, large body areas may be involved ("port wine nevus" or "nevus flammeus"). See also *von Hippel-Lindau disease.*

hemangiopericytoma (hĕ-man″je-o-per″ĭ-si-to′mah) [*hem-* + Gr. *angeion* vessel + *pericyte* + *-oma*] an uncommon neoplasm derived from pericytes, modified smooth muscle cells of blood vessel walls. Like the glomus tumor, the cells have some smooth muscle features, but the two are different neoplasms. Hemangiopericytoma cells are elongated and often present a crescentic profile: they are compactly grouped in the stroma between channels of a rich capillary network; this relationship and vascular pattern can be well demonstrated by a reticulin stain. The branching vessels present a staghornlike configuration.

The tumor is overdiagnosed, inasmuch as any neoplasm with a capillary meshwork enveloping groups of uniform cells may be mistakenly designated a hemangiopericytoma. As a result, the tumor's frequency, biologic behavior, and response to therapy are uncertain. It is known to occur in a wide range of locations, and at least 10 percent give rise to distant metastases. Electron microscopy is useful in reaching the diagnosis, but thus far too few cases have been reported to give a clear concept of the range of fine structure of the tumor cells.

hemangiosarcoma (hĕ-man″je-o-sar-ko′mah) [*hem-* + Gr. *angeion* vessel + *sarcoma*] see *angiosarcoma.*

hemapheresis (hem″ah-fer′ĕ-sis) see *pheresis.*

hemarthrosis (hem″ar-thro′sis) [*hem-* + Gr. *arthron* joint] hemorrhage into a joint. Usually due to trauma, hemarthrosis may be caused by degenerative arthritis, leading to deposition of hemosiderin in the synovial and capsular tissues. It is a severe and frequent occurrence in those with hemophilia and other coagulation defects and results in marked synovial proliferation and degenerative changes in the cartilage and bone.

hemat/o (hem′ah-to) [Gr. *haima, haimatos* blood] a word element used in combining form to denote blood, e.g., hematoma.

hematein (hem″ah-te′in) the oxidation product of the dye hematoxylin, which is the form actually used in most hematoxylin staining procedures. See also *hematoxylin.*

hematemesis (hem″ah-tem′ĕ-sis) [*hemat-* + Gr. *emesis* vomiting] the vomiting of blood, often due to gastric ulcer, esophageal varices, or gastritis.

hematencephalon (hem″at-en-sef′ah-lon) [*hemato-* + Gr. *enkephalos* brain] the effusion of blood into the brain, the result of vascular or coagulation disorders or trauma.

Hematest (he′mah-test) trademark for an *o*-toluidine test for occult blood.

hematidrosis (hem″at-i-dro′sis) [*hemat-* + Gr. *hidrōsis* sweating] the excretion of bloody sweat; there are several causes, including vascular defects and trauma.

hematin (hem′ah-tin) a pigment formed by the denaturation of hemoglobin in strongly acidic solution (acid hematin) or in strongly alkaline solution (alkaline hematin).

The hematin most commonly encountered in histology is formalin pigment (acid formaldehyde hematin), which is produced by the action of acidic formalin fixatives. Another hematin is malarial pigment, which is produced by malarial parasites and deposited in the parasites themselves, as well as in red cells and in macrophages in the liver, spleen, and lymph nodes. A third hematin is the similar schistosomal pigment. All these pigments consist of dark brown, granular, microcrystalline material.

See also *formalin pigment.*

hematocele (hem′ah-to-sēl″) [*hemato-* + Gr. *kēlē* tumor] the accumulation of blood within the body's cavities, especially the tunica vaginalis of the testis. It is uncommon, occurring after trauma or torsion of the vascular supply to the testes, with resulting hemorrhage into the cavity. Vascular abnormalities, bleeding tendencies, and neoplastic invasion are also possible causes. The hematocele does not transilluminate.

hematochezia (hem″ah-to-ke′ze-ah) [*hemato-* + Gr.

chezein to go to stool] the passage of bright red blood through the rectum. The source of hemorrhage is usually the colon, rectum, or anus, although depending on transit time other sites may also be involved. Maternal blood swallowed by the newborn during the birth process will be passed bright red. When blood remains in the gut for longer than 8 hr, it becomes brown and its passage is know as melena. Vascular diseases, ulcers, colitis, neoplasms, and coagulation disorders are the most frequent causes of hematochezia.

Laboratory tests should include measurements of clotting functions and platelet and white blood cell counts. Radiographic studies may be helpful. The Apt test is indicated in the newborn.

See also *melena.*

hematoclasis (hĕm″ah-tŏk′lah-sis) [*hemato-* + Gr. *klasis* broken, in pieces] the breaking up and phagocytosis of erythrocytes by phagocytic cells after ingestion, the normal fate of senescent red cells.

hematoclastic (hem″ah-to-klas′tik) pertaining to hematoclasis.

hematocrit (HCT, Hct) (he-mat′o-krit) [*hemato-* + Gr. *krinein* to separate] the volume of red cells expressed as a percentage of the volume of whole blood in a sample. It is determined by subjecting properly anticoagulated and well-mixed blood to centrifugal force sufficient to pack the cells into the smallest volume possible.

The hematocrit may be determined by the macromethod of Wintrobe, which utilizes Wintrobe hematocrit tubes and moderate-speed centrifugation in any standard laboratory centrifuge; or by the micromethod, which utilizes capillary hematocrit tubes and high-speed centrifugation in specialized small centrifuges designed for that purpose. Reference ranges are: for males, 39.8–52.2 ml/100 ml of blood; and for females, 34.9–46.9. A low hematocrit indicates anemia, whereas an elevated hematocrit indicates polycythemia.

Also called *packed cell volume* (PCV). See also *blood cell count* and *blood volume measurements.*

large vessel h. (LVH), the hematocrit measured from a sample of blood obtained from a large vessel, usually the antecubital vein. The total body hematocrit (TBH) generally is 0.92 of the LVH as determined from isotopic measurements of red cell mass and plasma volume. See also *total body h.*

mean circulatory h., see *total body h.*

total body h. (TBH), the mean hematocrit of all vessels, defined as the total red cell volume divided by the sum of the total red cell volume and plasma volume. It is measured using labeled red cells and iodinated albumin. The ratio of TBH to the large vessel hematocrit (LVH) is approximately 0.92 and, when applied to the red cell volume calculated from a measured plasma volume, equals the total red cell volume measured with labeled red cells.

hematoidin (hem-ah-toid′en) [*hemato-* + Gr. *eidos* form] a pigment that is chemically similar to bile pigments but found as golden yellow, orange, or reddish-brown crystals at sites of old hemorrhage or infarction. See also under *bilirubin demonstration in tissue.*

hematologist (hem″ah-tol′o-jist) a specialist in the study of blood and its disorders.

hematology (hem″ah-tol′o-je) [*hemato-* + *logy*] the branch of medicine that deals with the study of the blood and its components.

hematolysis (hem″ah-tol′ĭ-sis) [*hemato-* + Gr. *lysis* dissolution] see *hemolysis.*

hematoma (he″mah-to′mah) [*hemato-* + Gr. *-oma* tumor] a collection of extravasted, usually clotted, blood that has been localized within a tissue or cavity. Hematomas may occur at almost any site in the body. Small hematomas such as bruises are often insignificant, with gradual absorption and removal of the blood from the site. Hematomas within the enclosed space of the cranium, however, are always serious, as they place pressure on the brain. Secondary infection of hematomas can also occur. In large muscles, hematoma formation may lead to development of myositis ossificans.

epidural h., a clot of extravasated blood that usually forms as a result of skull fracture, with laceration of the middle meningeal artery and vein. These lesions place pressure on the brain and, as they enlarge, can impair brain function and lead to cerebral herniation and death. Usually some time elapses between injury and onset of coma. These clots are readily recognized by CT scan or angiography. Surgical intervention may be urgent and life-saving. Also called extradural hematoma.

subdural h., a clot of extravasated blood that forms in the subdural space as a result of head injury owing to tearing of bridging veins that drain the cerebral cortex. These lesions may be classified as acute or chronic, depending on their time-course. Headache and mental changes are common manifestations; focal deficits such as a hemiparesis are less conspicuous. CT scans and arteriography are the most helpful laboratory tests for diagnosis. Surgical intervention is usually indicated.

hematopoiesis (hem″ah-to-poi-e′sis) [*hemato-* + Gr. *poiein* to make] the formation and development of blood cells. See also *erythropoiesis, granulocytopoiesis, lymphocyte, stem cell,* and *thrombocytopoiesis.*

extramedullary h., the formation and development of blood cells outside the bone marrow, as in the spleen, liver, and lymph nodes. See also *myeloid metaplasia.*

hematopoietic (hem″ah-to-poi-et′ik) [*hemato-* + Gr. *poiein* to make] 1. pertaining to or affecting the formation of blood cells.

2. an agent that promotes the formation of blood cells.

hematopoietic stem cell see *stem cell.*

hematopoietic tissue organs or tissues in which blood cell production occurs. Embryonic and fetal hematopoiesis occurs initially outside the embryo in the mesenchyme of the yolk sac in blood islands. At the sixth week of development, hematopoiesis begins in the liver, which then becomes the major blood-producing organ of early and midfetal life; the spleen and lymph nodes also have a minor role. In the latter half of fetal life, the bone marrow becomes more important as a site of blood cell production, and the role of the liver diminishes.

Shortly after birth, hematopoiesis in the liver ceases, and the bone marrow becomes the only site of production of erythrocytes, granulocytes, and platelets. Lymphocytes continue to be produced both in the marrow and in the secondary lymphoid organs.

At birth, the total marrow space is occupied by active hematopoietic (red) marrow. Later in childhood, only the flat bones (skull, vertebrae, thoracic cage, shoulder, and pelvis) and the proximal parts of the long bones (femora and humeri) remain as sites of blood formation.

hematopoietin (hem″ah-to-poi′e-tin) an obsolete term for erythropoietin; see *erythropoietin.*

hematoside (hem′ah-to-sīd″) a sphingoglycolipid, NeuAc(2→3)Gal(1→4)Glc-Cer. It occurs in the erythrocyte stroma and in the brain and spleen.

hematoxylin (hem″ah-tok′sĭ-lin) a natural dye extracted from the logwood tree, *Haematoxylon campechianum,* a member of the pea family. In histology, the various hematoxylin formulas are the most commonly used nuclear stains, with hematoxylin staining followed by eosin counterstaining being the routine stain; see *hematoxylin and eosin (H and E) staining.*

Hematoxylin is a yellow-orange crystalline solid, oxidized in solution to form hematein, the active dye. The oxidation may be accomplished by exposure to air for several weeks (called ripening) or by adding an oxidizing agent to the formulation; mercuric oxide (HgO), sodium iodate ($NaIO_3$), or potassium permanganate ($KMNO_4$) is commonly used.

Hematein is always used with a mordant, a trivalent metal ion. It forms a blue lake with aluminum and chromium(III) salts and a blue-black lake with iron(III) salts. Most formulas use an alum, potassium alum, $K_2SO_4 \cdot Al_2(SO_4)_3 \cdot 24H_2O$; ammonium alum, $(NH_4)_2 \cdot Al_2(SO_4)_3 \cdot 24H_2O$; iron alum, $Fe_2(SO_4)_3 \cdot (NH_4)_2SO_4 \cdot 24H_2O$; or chrome alum, $K_2SO_4 \cdot Cr_2(SO_4)_3 \cdot 24H_2O$. Other ions can be used as mordants, and hematoxylin is used without a mordant to detect metals in tissue. Lead stains dark gray-blue and copper clear blue.

Hematoxylin is usually employed as a regressive stain. Sections are overstained and then differentiated (or decolorized) in dilute acid alcohol, which dissolves the dye and mordant, selectively removing it from cell constituents that weakly bind it. Oxidizing agents, which bleach the dye, or excess mordant, which forms a soluble lake, are also used as differentiators.

Formulations that contain potassium alum are made acidic so that aluminum hydroxide does not precipitate out of solution. After differentiation, sections must be placed in mild base (tap water or dilute lithium carbonate) so that the insoluble dye lake can form, a process called blueing.

The hematein-mordant complex is a basic stain, and stains acid (basophilic) tissue components, such as nucleic acids (in nuclear chromatin, nucleoli, and endoplasmic reticulum). It also stains sulfated proteoglycans (mucopolysaccharides), such as heparin (in mast cells and basophilic leukocytes) and chondroitin sulfate (in cartilage). Alum hematoxylin is also called *hemalum.* See also *phosphotungstic acid hematoxylin.*

Harris' alum h., the most commonly used hematoxylin stain; used as a regressive stain. A solution of hematoxylin in absolute alcohol is combined with distilled water containing ammonium alum and then boiled. Mercuric oxide is added, and when the solution turns deep purple, it is rapidly cooled.

Heidenhain's iron h., a technique in which sections are mordanted in aqueous iron alum for several hours, overstained in ripened alcoholic hematoxylin, and differentiated in the iron alum mordant. Eosin or van Gieson's stain may be used as a counterstain.

Lillie's h., a progressive hematoxylin stain containing hematoxylin, ammonium alum, and sodium iodate dissolved in distilled water and glycerol.

Mayer's h., a progressive hematoxylin stain containing hematoxylin, sodium iodate, ammonium or potassium alum, citric acid, and chloral hydrate (as a preservative) dissolved in distilled water. Also called Mayer's hemalum.

Weigert's iron h., a progressive hematoxylin stain made by combining equal volumes of one stock solution (hematoxylin in absolute ethanol) with another (ferric chloride, concentrated hydrochloric acid, and distilled water) just before use.

hematoxylin and eosin (H and E) staining the routine method of histologic staining. Tissue sections are deparaffinized and brought to water. Mercury deposits can be removed by immersion in alcoholic iodine if mercuric fixatives have been used and the iodine bleached and rinsed out. The sections are placed in an alum hematoxylin (e.g., Harris') until they are overstained, and are then differentiated in acid alcohol until the nuclei are properly stained. Finally, the sections are blued in dilute lithium carbonate, counterstained in eosin, cleared in xylene, and mounted. Cell nuclei stain blue; cartilage, bone, and calcium, a darker and browner blue; mucin, light blue; and keratin, dark blue. Cytoplasm stains varying shades of pale pink, whereas muscle fibers, red blood cells, and eosinophil granules stain bright red.

hematoxylin body a globular mass of nuclear material that stains bluish-purple with hematoxylin, and which is a diagnostic factor in lupus erythematosus. Hematoxylin bodies have been found in many tissues.

hematuria (hem″ah-tu′re-ah) [*hemat-* + Gr. *ouron* urine + *-ia*] the presence of blood in the urine; a serious clinical finding that requires immediate diagnostic evaluation. The more common causes of hematuria include hematologic and vascular disorders, glomerular disease, urinary tract infections, tumors, trauma, and calculi. Microscopic examination of urine sediment for red blood cells or casts, along with urine tests for free hemoglobin or myoglobulin, is important for documenting the presence of hematuria and establishing its etiology.

heme (hēm) ferroprotoporphyrin IX; M.W. 619; the prosthetic group of hemoglobin and myoglobin, but also present in catalase and some cytochromes and peroxidases.

hemi- (hem′e) [Gr. *hēmi-* half] a prefix word element to denote half, e.g., hemisphere.

hemiacetal (hem″e-as′ĕ-tal) a derivative formed by a combination of aldehyde with an alcohol. In the sugars, hemiacetal formation is internal, resulting in pyranoses and furanoses. In general, hemiacetals are easily hydrolyzed back to the original aldehyde and alcohol. See also *furanose* and *pyranose.*

hemianopia (hem″e-ah-no′pe-ah) [*hemi-* + *an-* neg. + Gr. *ōpē* vision + *-ia*] blindness in one-half of the visual field. The cause is usually a lesion along the optic pathway, which may be due to trauma, vascular disease, or tumor. Also called hemianopsia.

hemiblock (hem′e-blok) the interruption of cardiac impulse transmission in either of the two main systems of fascicles of the left bundle branch. QRS complexes are increased slightly in duration but usually are still within normal limits.

left anterior h., blockage of the excitation wave in

the left anterior superior fascicle, which delays activation of the upper anterior free wall of the ventricle. This condition manifests itself as a left axis deviation, often –30° to –60°. The QRS is only slightly longer and usually remains within normal limits (<0.12). This condition may be masked or mimicked by an infarction.

left posterior h., an interruption of impulse transmission in the posterior fascicles of the left bundle branch. Associated with widespread left ventricular disease, this relatively uncommon condition results in dramatic right axis deviation. The Q is small or absent in leads X, V_5, and V_6. Left posterior hemiblock can mask anterior infarction.

hemic (he′mik) pertaining to blood.

hemidesmosome (hem″e-des′mo-sōm) see *hemidesmosome* under *desmosome.*

hemiglobin (HiHb) (he″mĭ-glo′bin) see *methemoglobin.*

hemin (he′min) [Gr. *haima* blood] Fe(III) porphyrin, the oxidized form of heme. It serves as a precursor of the prosthetic groups of respiratory enzymes and is a growth factor (Factor X) provided by blood for certain species of *Hemophilus.*

hemiparesis (hem″e-par′e-sis) [*hemi-* + *paresis*] muscular weakness affecting one side of the body.

hemiplegia (hem″e-ple′je-ah) [*hemi-* + Gr. *plēgē* stroke] the paralysis of an arm, leg, and sometimes the face on one side of the body, often due to pathologic involvement of the corticospinal tract originating from the opposite cerebral hemisphere.

hemisphere (hem′ĭ-sfēr) [*hemi-* + Gr. *sphaira* a ball or globe] half of any spherical or roughly spherical structure or organ, as in the hemispheres of the brain. It is demarcated by passing a plane through the poles or along the equator.

cerebellar h., the paired lateral portions of the cerebellum, which are connected by the vermis.

cerebral h., one of the two large, convoluted portions of the cerebrum.

hemizygous (hem″e-zi′gus) normally, a property of genes on the single X chromosome of males. As there is only one copy of the gene, the allele must be expressed and will also be passed on to each daughter. Genes on other chromosomes have two homologous copies, which may be heterozygous (different) or homozygous (identical). Genes on the monosomic part of a chromosome in a partial monosomy (e.g., 5p-) are also hemizygous. Cf. *heterozygous* and *homozygous.*

hemoagglutination (he″mo-ah-glu″tin-a′shun) see *hemagglutination.*

hemochromatosis (he″mo-kro″mah-to′sis) a rare disease of iron metabolism that results in the deposition of iron in the parenchyma of organs such as the liver, pancreas, heart, and pituitary, with subsequent tissue necrosis and fibrosis. Several forms of this disorder have been characterized, including primary idiopathic hemochromatosis, erythropoietic hemochromatosis, and hemochromatosis following chronic liver disease, chronic excessive iron ingestion, or chronic transfusion therapy. Regardless of the cause, the disease rarely appears before age 20 yr and is associated with a bronze skin pigmentation, diabetes mellitus, impairment of heart and liver function, joint disease, and hypogonadism. Liver and spleen enlargement, jaundice, loss of libido, and weight loss may also be seen.

Diagnosis is based on clinical signs and a combined increase in serum iron concentration, saturation percentage of transferrin, and serum ferritin. Abnormal results indicate the need for a liver biopsy to measure the extent of iron deposition and tissue damage. Because it has been suggested that primary idiopathic hemochromatosis is associated with certain HLA antigens and may be transmitted as an autosomal recessive trait, diagnosis of this disease requires that the other family members be examined for it.

Also called *bronze diabetes.*

hemocystinuria (hem″o-sis″tĭ-nu′re-ah) the excretion of excessive amounts of methionine and homocystine in the urine.

hemocytoblast (he″mo-si′to-blast) [*hemo-* + Gr. *kytos* hollow vessel + *blastos* germ] a bone marrow stem cell, believed by early morphologists to be morphologically an identifiable immature bone marrow cell. It is now realized that such identification in marrow smears is not possible; however, the term is of historical interest as it foreshadowed the existence of the totipotent hematopoietic stem cell as postulated by the early investigators of the marrow. See also *stem cell.*

hemocytometer (he″mo-si″tom′e-ter) see *hemacytometer.*

hemodialysis (he″mo-di-al′ĭ-sis) the technique used to remove toxic substances from the blood, e.g., low-molecular-weight compounds, electrolytes in excess, and toxins present in the blood when the kidneys cannot adequately clear these components. It relies on the diffusion of substances down a concentration gradient, across a semipermeable dialysis membrane, and into a chemically prepared bath of dialysis fluid. For example, if there is an excess of potassium in the blood, it can be cleared by allowing the blood to contact a dialysis fluid that is low in potassium across the membrane. According to osmotic principles, the potassium flows across the membrane from fluids of high concentration (blood) to fluids of low concentration (dialysis fluid), effectively lowering the blood concentration. There are two commonly used techiques of hemodialysis: extracorporeal hemodialysis, which utilizes synthetic membranes, and peritoneal hemodialysis, which utilizes the membranes that line the peritoneal cavity. Although these techniques are most commonly used in cases of renal failure, they may also be employed to remove toxins, poisons, and life-threatening excesses of total body water.

Extracorporeal hemodialysis usually requires implantation of an arterial venous cannula (shunt). Blood is removed from the cannula and passed over a synthetic membrane. At the membrane, the blood is free to dialyze with a fluid bath adjusted to proper flow rates (200–500 ml/min) and composed of electrolytes, alkali equivalents, and glucose in concentrations appropriate to the patient's condition. The patient usually also requires heparin anticoagulation therapy.

In those with acute renal failure, hemodialysis treatment can reduce blood urea nitrogen (BUN) and creatinine by about 50 percent, and can correct metabolic acidosis and hyperkalemia; it usually requires 4–6 hr to complete. Persons with chronic renal failure usually require regular maintenance hemodialysis, which may be performed at home, in limited care facilities, or at medical centers. Such dialysis usually requires three 8-hr sessions weekly. Long-term maintenance hemodialysis may be associated with anemia, peripheral neuropathy, muscle cramps, myocardial infarctions, cerebral edema and ischemia, and infections.

Peritoneal hemodialysis, dialysis through the peritoneum, is a more simple technique to perform, requiring placement of a catheter into the peritoneal space. The fluid bath is then instilled into the space, and dialysis occurs across the peritoneal membrane. Following variable exposure time (20–60 min), the fluid is removed. This process may require repeated exposures, with instillation of the fluid bath at 1–2 l/hr for 24–48 hr. The characterization and the efficiency of peritoneal hemodialysis are still being evaluated. At present its use is limited, owing to the long time necessary to reduce the BUN and creatinine to satisfactory levels.

See also *renal failure.*

hemodialyzer (he″mo-di′ah-liz″er) an apparatus used to perform hemodialysis, which employs a semipermeable cellophane membrane to remove noxious substances from the blood to dialysis fluid, an osmotically balanced solution of electrolytes and glucose in water.

In the procedure, heparinized blood from the patient enters a tubing pump and flows through the dialyzer on one side of the membrane past the dialysis fluid on the other side, flowing in the opposite direction. Waste products and excess ions diffuse across the membrane and are eliminated with the dialysate, and the blood is returned to the patient after passing through a bubble detector. Three basic types of hemodialyzers are currently available, employing designs of parallel-plates, coils, or hollow fibers. A newer technique now under clinical evaluation is hemofiltration, which removes the plasma water with the undesirable constituents from the blood by rapid ultrafiltration. A reconstituting solution is then added either before or after the blood flows through the dialyzer.

hemofiltration (he″mo-fil-tra′shun) see under *hemodialyzer.*

hemoflagellate (he″mo-flaj′ĕ-lāt) any blood-dwelling flagellate protozoan. Two genera with species parasitic in humans are *Trypanosoma* and *Leishmania.*

hemofuscin (he″mo-fūs′in) [*hemo-* + L. *fuscus* brown] see *lipofuscin.*

hemoglobin (Hb) (he′mo-glo″bin) the allosteric protein in the blood that is responsible for the transport of O_2, CO_2, and H^+. It is composed of four polypeptide chains containing over 100 amino acids, each linked to a heme prosthetic group and having the property of reversible oxygenation. The iron of the heme group is responsible for the reaction with oxygen. The chains are designated alpha, beta, gamma, and delta, with normal adult hemoglobin containing two alpha and two non-alpha (beta, delta, or gamma) chains.

The primary structure of human hemoglobin subunits consists of amino acids in linear sequence: the alpha chain contains 141 amino acids, and the other three contain 146 amino acids. In about 75 percent of hemoglobin, the secondary structure (the spatial relationship between adjacent residues along the chain) is in the form of an alpha helix. It is interrupted at specific locations in the hemoglobin subunit by segments that lack helical conformation, allowing the chain to bend. The tertiary structure (i.e., the configuration of a protein subunit in three-dimensional space) and the quaternary structure (i.e., the spatial relationship of each of the four subunits of hemoglobin to each other) result in a tetrahedral arrangement with a twofold axis of symmetry. This conformation is oxygen-dependent, within which two alternate configurations correspond to the oxy- and deoxyhemoglobin configuration of the molecule. In the oxyhemoglobin configuration, oxygen affinity is high, whereas in the latter configuration it is low.

The hemoglobin molecule functions as an important component of the body's buffer system. The imidazole group of its histidine residues acts as proton acceptors, having a dissociation constant in the physiologic range of blood. Hemoglobin thus has a high buffer capacity (about 53 mmol/l) over the normal range of blood pH, which helps to minimize changes in blood pH that occur as O_2 is loaded and CO_2 released in the lungs, and in the opposite process in the tissues.

Hemoglobin is degraded primarily in the macrophages of the reticuloendothelial system following phagocytosis of senescent erythrocytes. The protoporphyrin ring of heme is cleaved to produce biliverdin, which is reduced to unconjugated bilirubin. The bilirubin is conjugated in the liver and excreted in the bile, where it is further reduced to urobilinogen by anaerobic bacteria in the colon. In the process, carbon monoxide (CO) is produced, and iron is released and transported to the marrow to be reincorporated.

Plasma hemoglobin refers to that small amount of hemoglobin released into the plasma as a result of the breakdown of erythrocytes. Because the removal of the hemoglobin from the plasma is rapid, any increase is indicative of acute intravascular hemolysis. Reference values for carefully collected samples are less than 2.5 mg/dl.

Hemoglobin is first detected in the embryonic state. The embryonic hemoglobins—Gower-1 ($\zeta_2\epsilon_2$), Gower-2 ($\alpha_2\epsilon_2$), and hemoglobin Portland ($\zeta_2\gamma_2$)—are detectable only in the first 3 mo of fetal development and are synthesized by the erythroid cells derived from the yolk sac. The appearance of fetal hemoglobin, Hb F ($\alpha_2\gamma_2$), coincides with the shift of erythropoiesis from the yolk sac to the liver and spleen.

The normal adult hemoglobins, Hb A ($\alpha_2\beta_2$) and Hb A_2 ($\alpha_2\delta_2$), are normally the predominant hemoglobins present after the first year of life when the hemoglobin is synthesized by erythroid precursors in the bone marrow during the 6- to 8-da period of erythroid cell differentiation. The switchover mechanism from fetal to adult hemoglobin is unknown.

The different types of hemoglobin are determined by the specific combinations of the four chains, with the number of chains indicated by subscript numbers, e.g., Hb F ($\alpha_2\gamma_2$) and Hb A ($\alpha_2\beta_2$). Many hemoglobins with differing electrophoretic mobilities and characteristics have been reported and include Hb S, C, D, E, H, Bart's, and others.

Because refined biochemical techniques have led to the discovery of additional hemoglobins, certain standards for nomenclature have been devised. The hemoglobin electrophoretic mobility is designated by a capital letter; if two or more hemoglobins have the same mobility, the geographic area of discovery is indicated as a subscript, for example, Hb $M_{Saskatoon}$ (Hb M_S) and Hb $M_{Milwaukee}$ (Hb M_M). To restrict the increasing use of capital letters, new hemoglobins are named simply for the city, hospital, or laboratory in which they were discovered (e.g., Hb Norfolk). When known, the number and name of each amino acid substitution in each polypeptide in the molecule should be indicated by the appropriate subscript numeral.

Abnormal hemoglobins can be caused by point mutations in the amino acid sequence, as in Hb S; by differences in chain association, as in the thalassemias; or by gene crossover, as in Hb Lepore. For more information on abnormal hemoglobins, see *hemoglobinopathy* and *thalassemia*.

The method of choice for quantitative hemoglobin determination is the cyanomethemoglobin method. Hemoglobin electrophoresis in various mediums and buffer systems is used to separate, identify, and quantitate hemoglobin components.

Hb A, Hb A_1 ($\alpha_2{}^A\beta_2{}^A$), the major component (96–98 percent) of normal adult hemoglobin. Cellulose acetate electrophoresis at an alkaline pH (8.6–9.2) is used routinely to identify and quantitate hemoglobin A. See also *adult hemoglobin*.

Hb A_{1a}, Hb A_{1b}, Hb A_{1c}, glycosylated forms of hemoglobin that can be separated from the main hemoglobin fractions HbA_1 and HbA_2 by zone electrophoresis at an alkaline pH (where they appear as a smear running anodal to Hb A), by cation exchange column chromatography, or by high-performance liquid chromatography (HPLC). Only the last technique permits isolation and quantitation of the Hb-A_{1c} fraction apart from the minor HbA_{1a} and HbA_{1b} forms. With the simpler methods, the three fractions are measured and reported as a group. In normal individuals, the values for the three fractions are: 1.8, 0.8, and 3.5–6.0 percent of total hemoglobin, respectively, for the A_{1a}, A_{1b}, and A_{1c} fractions; or 5.5–7.5 for the three combined. The fractions obtained by column chromatography may be measured colorimetrically using 5-hydroxymethylfurfural and thiobarbituric acid.

Hb A_{1c} is Hb A with a glucose moiety on the *N*-terminal valine of the beta chain. This hemoglobin variant is formed by the slow, nonenzymatic glycosylation of hemoglobin throughout the 120-da the Hb A_{1c} life span of the erythrocyte. The reaction rate is proportional to the blood glucose concentration, and thus the Hb A_{1c} concentration reflects the average blood glucose level over the previous several weeks. In individuals with uncontrolled diabetes mellitus the Hb A_{1c} concentration may be three to four times higher than normal. This increased concentration also correlates well with glucose intolerance. With good diabetic control, the Hb A_{1c} concentration returns to the normal range, permitting Hb A_{1c} assays to be used to assess diabetic control.

Hb C, the second most common abnormal hemoglobin variant caused by a point mutation in the amino acid sequence, $\alpha_2\beta_2{}^{6\ Glu \rightarrow Lys}$. See also hemoglobin C–beta thalassemia under *thalassemia* and hemoglobin C disease under *hemoglobinopathy*.

Hb Constant Spring (Hb CS), an abnormal hemoglobin composed of two normal beta chains and two elongated alpha chains. See also *thalassemia*.

Hb D, an abnormal hemoglobin variant that is caused by a point mutation in the amino acid sequence. Migration at alkaline pH is identical to that of Hb S. See also hemoglobin D disease under *hemoglobinopathy*.

Hb E, the third most prevalent abnormal hemoglobin caused by a point mutation in the amino acid sequence $\alpha_2\beta_2{}^{26\ Glu \rightarrow Lys}$. See also hemoglobin E–beta thalassemia under *thalassemia* and hemoglobin E disease under *hemoglobinopathy*.

Hb F, the major form of hemoglobin found in fetal blood, $\alpha_2{}^A\gamma_2{}^A$. Hb F can best be identified by electrophoretic techniques. It can be quantitated by the alkali denaturation technique; the distribution of Hb F in individual red blood cells can be determined by the acid elution technique. See also *embryonic hemoglobin, fetal hemoglobin,* and *fetal hemoglobin tests*.

Hb H, an abnormal hemoglobin composed of four normal beta chains. See also hemoglobin H disease under *hemoglobinopathy*.

Hb Lepore, an abnormal hemoglobin that has two normal alpha chains associated with two chains resulting from the fusion of beta- and delta-chain segments. See also *thalassemia*.

Hb M, any of several variants having amino acid substitutions either in the alpha or beta chains and all associated with methemoglobinemia. See also hemoglobin M disease under *hemoglobinopathy* and *methemoglobinemia*.

Hb S, the most common abnormal hemoglobin, caused by a point mutation in the amino acid sequence, in which valine replaces glutamic acid at position six of the beta chain. See also both hemoglobin S-C disease and sickle cell anemia under *hemoglobinopathy*.

hemoglobin assays 1. colorimetric method used to determine the concentration of hemoglobin in blood. The standard method of hemoglobinometry (by international agreement) is the (hemiglobincyanide, HiCN) cyanmethemoglobin method. A sample of blood is diluted in Drabkin's solution, which lyses red cells and quantitatively converts all forms of hemoglobin except sulfhemoglobin to HiCN. The absorbance of HiCN at 540 nm is proportional to its concentration. The method is standarized by comparison with cyanmethemoglobin standards (e.g., those certified by the American College of Pathologists). This method is used both manually and by automated cell-counting devices, which also produce the red cell indices mean corpuscular hemoglobin (MCH) and mean corpuscular hemoglobin concentration (MCHC). Reference ranges for blood hemoglobin are: for adult males, 13.5–18.0 g/dl (2.09–2.79 mmol/l); and for adult females, 12.0–16.0 (1.86–2.48).

2. test for free hemoglobin in plasma. The test is based on the absorbance measurement of a serum sample (diluted with sodium bicarbonate) at 380, 415, and 450 nm against a bicarbonate solution as reference. The reading at 415 nm (absorption peak for hemoglobin) is a measure of the hemoglobin concentration, whereas the readings at 380 and 450 nm correct for backround absorbance (Allen correction). A factor converts absorbance values into the hemoglobin concentration. Therefore: Hb(mg/dl) = $A_{415} - (A_{380} + A_{450})/2 \times 16.6 \times$ dilution factor.

Samples containing a high concentration of bilirubin require a special correction involving absorbance readings of a serum dilution with saline at 415, 450, 560, and 575 nm.

hemoglobinated (he″mo-glo′bin-āt-ed) containing hemoglobin.

hemoglobin demonstration in tissue 1. the Lepehne-Pickworth method for hemoglobin peroxidase. Frozen sections fixed in buffered neutral formalin are incubated at 37°C in a solution of benzidine and nitroprusside, then washed and placed in 3 percent hydrogen peroxide. Hemoglobin and other heme proteins act as peroxidases, catalyzing the coupled reduction of peroxide and oxidation of benzidine to a colored product. Hemoglobin, myoglobin, and other peroxidases are stained deep blue to black in color. It should be noted that benzidine is carcinogenic.

2. the Lison-Dunn leuko patent blue method for hemoglobin peroxidase. Paraffin sections are stained in leuko patent blue peroxide reagent (the stock solution contains patent blue V, powdered zinc, and glacial acetic acid in water, which is boiled until colorless; the working solution contains acetic acid and 3 percent hydrogen peroxide in 10 ml of the stock solution). Hemoglobin stains dark blue–green.

hemoglobin electrophoresis see *electrophoresis* and *hemoglobin identification.*

hemoglobinemia (he″mo-glo″bĭ-ne′me-ah) [*hemoglobin* + Gr. *haima* blood + *-ia*] the presence of hemoglobin in the plasma of the blood. Only traces normally are present, probably because a few erythrocytes are always lysed, even during careful collection of blood (about 0.5–2.5 mg/dl with special precautions in collection).

hemoglobin identification any of a number of methods by which normal and abnormal human hemoglobins are distinguished. The commonly used procedures involve electrophoresis at various pH levels and on a variety of support media.

The most commonly used techniques for hemoglobin identification are electrophoresis on cellulose acetate at pH 8.6 and electrophoresis in agar gel at pH 6.2. Other electrophoresis media that are occasionally employed to identify abnormal hemoglobin variants include potato starch gel, paper, agarose, and polyacrylamide gel. A recent technique, isoelectric focusing, is also being used to identify hemoglobin variants.

CELLULOSE ACETATE ELECTROPHORESIS. In this simple and convenient technique for identifying hemoglobins, the hemoglobins migrate according to their net charge from cathode (negative side) to anode (positive side). They do so in the following order: Hb C (A_2, E, and O_A); Hb N and Hb S (D_2 and G); Hb F, Hb A, and Hb K; and Hb H, Hb I, and Hb J. To further identify hemoglobin variants with similar mobilities, electrophoresis in several media and at different pH is utilized.

AGAR GEL ELECTROPHORESIS. This technique, at pH 6.2, is used to aid the identification of hemoglobin variants E, D, G, and O_A; Hb F and Hb A are also clearly separated in this medium. Proceeding from the anode, the hemoglobin migrate to the following positions: C, S, A, and F. Hemoglobins A_2, E, G, D, and A have similar mobilities in this medium. This technique is commonly used to screen newborns for hemoglobinopathies (Hb S, Hb AS, Hb C, and Hb AC).

ISOELECTRIC FOCUSING IN POLYACRYLAMIDE GEL. See under *isoelectric focusing* and *isoelectric point.*

See also *electrophoresis.*

hemoglobinometer (he″mo-glo″bĭ-nom′e-ter) [*hemoglobin* + Gr. *metron* measure] an instrument for measuring hemoglobin in the blood by spectrophotometry using the 540-nm absorption maximum of cyanmethemoglobin. The procedure is done after a suitable reagent, which hemolyzes red cells and converts all hemoglobins except sulfhemoglobin (including methemoglobin) to cyanmethemoglobin, has been added to the specimen of whole blood.

hemoglobinometry (he″mo-glo″bĭ-nom′ĕ-tre) the measurement of the hemoglobin of the blood. See also *hemoglobinometer.*

hemoglobinopathy (he″mo-glo″bĭ-nop′ah-the) [*hemoglobin* + Gr. *pathos* disease] one of several types of a hematologic disorder that is caused by an alteration in the normal molecular structure of hemoglobin, which results in a characteristic complex of clinical and laboratory abnormalities. The specific features of these hemoglobin abnormalities are related to variation of the composite globin polypeptide chains (designated α, β, γ, δ), to changes or substitutions in the sequential arrangement of the amino acids constituting these chains, or to their deletion from their appropriate place in the molecule.

In the first few years after discovery of the molecular basis of sickle cell disease (i.e., the abnormal structure of Hb S), additional abnormal hemoglobins were described, and letters of the alphabet beginning with the letter C were assigned to distinguish them from normal hemoglobin (Hb A) and Hb S. Hb M was reserved for hemoglobins that result in methomoglobinemia. When hemoglobins with the physical characteristics of previously described hemoglobins were discovered, they were assigned the same letter, with a subscript indicating the geographic location in which the particular hemoglobin was first discovered, e.g., Hb $M_{Saskatoon}$.

Full characterization of the structural abnormality of hemoglobins is achieved by indicating the amino acid substitution in the globin chain or chains involved e.g., Hb S is $\alpha_2\beta_2{}^{6\ Glu\rightarrow Val}$ and the Hb G $_{Norfolk}$ is $\alpha_2{}^{85Asp\rightarrow Asm}\beta_2$. The number indicates the position of the substituted amino acid in the chain.

Clinically significant hemoglobinopathies include sickle cell diseases (sickle cell anemia, sickle cell–hemoglobin D disease, sickle cell–hemoglobin C disease, and sickle cell–beta thalassemia), hemoglobin D disease, hemoglobin E disease, hemoglobin C disease, hemoglobin M disorders, unstable hemoglobin disorders, polycythemia-producing hemoglobins, and the thalassemias. Many more abnormal hemoglobins exist but are rare (see *thalassemia.*).

SICKLE CELL ANEMIA. This form of sickle cell disease is due to the homozygous inheritance of the gene for Hb S. The major clinical manifestations include chronic hemolytic anemia, impairment of growth and development with increased susceptibility to infection, vasoocclusive or painful "crisis" and organ damage due to microvasoocclusive events, leg ulcers, and renal impairment. Sickle cell–hemoglobin C disease and other variants are clinically much milder. Hb S is the most common abnormal hemoglobin and is caused by a point mutation in the amino acid sequence, where valine replaces glutamic acid at position six of the beta chain, giving the hemoglobin a positive charge. Accordingly, with cellulose acetate electrophoresis at an alkaline pH, Hb S migrates slowly to the same position as Hb D and Hb G. It can be distinguished from these other hemoglobin variants by using citrate agar electrophoresis at an acid pH (6.0–6.5). It is also distinguished from Hb D and Hb G by a positive sickle cell test (Sickledex).

Hb S is freely soluble when fully oxygenated but polymerizes on deoxygenation to form "tactoids," rigid crystals that deform the red cell and give it the characteristic sickle shape. In this condition the red cells—in sickle cell disease but not in the sickle cell trait—are readily trapped in small blood vessels. This accounts for manifestations such as splenic infarcts, leg ulcers, aseptic necrosis of bone, and renal disease. The sickled erythrocyte is extremely fragile and has a shortened survival.

The homozygous state, Hb SS, results in a chronic anemia and is usually life-shortening, although a small proportion of affected individuals may have a life span that is normal or close to normal. The disorder manifests itself in sickling crises, vasoocclusive disease of bones, renal impairment, and complications due to infections.

Sickle cells are seen in small-to-moderate numbers in peripheral blood smears of affected individuals. Howell-Jolly bodies are seen in older children and adults, owing to asplenia secondary to infarction of the spleen. The marrow shows normoblastic hyperplasia and increased storage iron. Provided there have been no recent transfusions, electrophoresis indicates no Hb A. (Both alleles for the beta chain are affected, imparting the amino acid substitution to all beta chains produced.) On electrophoresis, hemoglobin values are 80–95 percent for Hb S, 2–20 percent for Hb F, and normal for Hb A_2. The fetal hemoglobin is distributed unevenly among the red cells.

SICKLE CELL TRAIT. Hb AS, sickle cell trait, is due to the heterozygous inheritance of Hb A and Hb S, and is present in about 10 percent of all blacks in the United States. Under normal circumstances no clinical sign of disease occurs. The trait confers protection from falciparum malaria, which accounts for its major distribution in central Africa. Blood smears appear normal, but deoxygenated supravital (wet) preparations of fresh blood shows sickling. On electrophoresis, hemoglobin values are 55–65 percent for Hb A, 35–45 percent for Hb S, less than 2 percent for Hb F, and normal for Hb A_2.

HEMOGLOBIN S-C DISEASE. This form of sickle cell anemia, $\alpha_2\beta_2{}^{6\ \mathrm{Val}}$, $\alpha_2\beta_2{}^{6\ \mathrm{Lys}}$, is the most common genetic variant. It is clinically milder than Hb SS disease and has fewer complications when it occurs in childhood. Sometimes individuals are clinically asymptomatic into adulthood, being diagnosed when a routine screening smear shows target cells, rare irreversibly sickled cells, and a relative degree of reticulocytosis (3–10 percent). The disorder is inherited in a double, abnormal homozygous manner, with one parent contributing a sickle hemoglobin gene and the other parent a gene for Hb C. The red cells contain a mixture of Hb S and Hb C.

SICKLE CELL HEMOGLOBIN D_{Punjab} DISEASE. This form, $\alpha_2\beta_2{}^{6\ \mathrm{Val}}$, $\alpha_2\beta_2{}^{121\ \mathrm{Glu}}$, is a severe hemolytic anemia, though it is somewhat milder than Hb SS disease. On cellulose acetate electrophoresis at alkaline pH, Hb D_{Punjab} migrates with Hb S, although it can be distinguished from Hb S on citrate agar electrophoresis at acid pH. Hb D_{Punjab} is suspected in heterozygotes when a negative sickle test occurs, yet an Hb component is evident at the S position. Sickle cell Hb D_{Punjab} is inherited in a double, abnormal homozygous manner, with one parent contributing a sickle hemoglobin gene and the other parent a gene for Hb D_{Punjab}.

SICKLE CELL–BETA THALASSEMIA. See under *thalassemia.*

Hb S–HEREDITARY PERSISTENCE OF FETAL HEMOGLOBIN (S-HPFH). See *hereditary persistence of fetal hemoglobin.*

HEMOGLOBIN C DISEASE. This disorder is due to the homozygous inheritance of the gene for Hb C. The second abnormal hemoglobin to be discovered, Hb C is the second most common hemoglobin disorder and is found primarily among blacks. It is caused by a point mutation in the amino acid sequence, in which lysine replaces glutamic acid at position six of the beta chains, $\alpha_2\beta_2{}^{6\ \mathrm{Glu}\rightarrow\mathrm{Lys}}$, thus giving the hemoglobin a relatively high positive charge. Accordingly, on zone electrophoresis at an alkaline pH, Hb C migrates slowly to the same position as Hb A_2, Hb E, and Hb O. It can be separated from Hb A_2 by column chromatography, and from the other hemoglobin variants by citrate agar electrophoresis at an acid pH (6.0–6.5). The oxygen saturation curve of Hb C is normal, but whole blood oxygen affinity is reduced, presumably owing to an increased mean corpuscular hemoglobin concentration (MCHC).

The homozygous state, Hb CC, produces a hemolytic anemia that is mild to moderate, with hemoglobin levels from 8–12 g/100 ml. The majority of red cells on peripheral blood smear are target cells. Homozygous Hb C cells form intracellular crystals when suspended in a hypertonic medium.

The heterozygous state, Hb AC, hemoglobin C trait, is unimportant clinically. Double heterozygosity for Hb S and Hb C presents a disease of moderate severity (see *Hb S-C disease,* above).

HEMOGLOBIN D DISEASE. This form is due to the homozygous inheritance of the gene for Hb D. The abnormal hemoglobin exists in several molecular forms, the most common being Hb D_{Punjab}, $\alpha_2\beta_2{}^{121\ \mathrm{Glu}\rightarrow\mathrm{Gln}}$.

All D hemoglobins involve the substitution of a neutrally charged amino acid for a negatively charged residue or the substitution of a positively charged amino acid for a negatively charged residue, which results in an increase in positive charge. Accordingly, on zone electrophoresis at an alkaline pH, Hb D migrates at a rate identical to that of Hb S, although it can be differentiated from Hb S on agar gel electrophoresis at an acid pH. None of the variants sickle, nor do they have a positive solubility test.

Homozygosity for Hb D (Hb DD) is rare. Anemia and splenomegaly are absent, osmotic fragility is decreased, and oxygen affinity is higher than normal. Hemoglobin values and red cell indices are generally within normal limits, with 95 percent Hb D and normal Hb A_2 levels seen on electrophoresis. Double heterozygosity for Hb D and beta thalassemia result in a mild anemia with minimal hemolysis.

HEMOGLOBIN E DISEASE. This form is due to the homozygous inheritance of the gene for Hb E. Hb E, $\alpha_2\beta_2{}^{26\ \mathrm{Glu}\rightarrow\mathrm{Lys}}$, is the third most prevalent abnormal hemoglobin in the world, occurring primarily in Orientals. On zone electrophoresis at an alkaline pH, Hb E migrates at a rate identical to that of Hb A_2, Hb O_{Arab}, and Hb C. On citrate agar electrophoresis at an acid pH, Hb E migrates with Hb A but does not migrate with Hb O_{Arab} and Hb C. The hemoglobin is somewhat unstable when subjected to oxidative stress. The whole blood oxygen dissociation curves demonstrate a slight shift to the right.

The homozygous state, Hb EE, is associated with microcytosis, target cell formation, and a mild hemolytic anemia. The heterozygous state, Hb AE or Hb E trait, is commonly encountered and demonstrates no hematologic abnormalities. Double heterozygosity for Hb E and beta thalassemia results in an anemia of much greater severity than Hb EE.

HEMOGLOBIN CONSTANT SPRING. See under *thalassemia.*

HEMOGLOBIN H DISEASE. This form is due to the production of Hb H, a tetramer composed of four normal beta chains. It is seen in some individuals with alpha thalassemia; see also under *thalassemia.*

HEMOGLOBIN M DISEASE. Hemoglobin M (Hb M) arises from an amino acid substitution in an area of the globin molecule that stabilizes heme iron in the ferric (oxidized) form. Such a substitution results in methemoglobin formation and cyanosis. In four of the five known Hb M forms, the amino acid substitutions are tyrosine for histidine, either in the alpha or beta chains. Hb M can be identified by spectral abnormalities and hemoglobin electrophoresis on agar gel at pH 7.1 after hemolysate has been oxidized by potassium ferricyanide; this demonstrates a brown band that migrates slightly on the anodal side of hemoglobin A. Hb M is inherited as an autosomal dominant trait. See also *methemoglobinemia.*

UNSTABLE HEMOGLOBIN DISEASE. Another group of hemoglobinopathies is characterized by the presence of unstable hemoglobins. The latter are structural variants of Hb A; they undergo denaturation within the red cell, which results in irreversible precipitation and the formation of insoluble inclusions (Heinz bodies). Anemias caused by unstable hemoglobins are designated as unstable hemoglobin hemolytic anemias.

Unstable hemoglobins are transmitted as a autosomal dominant trait. The Heinz bodies are selectively removed in the spleen; prior to splenectomy they may not be discernible without the presence of oxidative stress. Because of the low gene frequency, a homozygous state must be a rare event and is probably incompatible with life. However, Heinz body anemia may be quite mild or moderately severe, depending on the variant.

Of the approximately 70 known hemoglobin variants that cause unstable hemoglobin hemolytic anemias, most are beta-chain mutants; only about 8 are alpha-chain mutants. A single gamma mutation has been described, but owing to the gradual disappearance of the associated neonatal jaundice it may be overlooked. Many substitutions are neutral, with their electrophoretic mobility indicative of Hb A.

Most variants demonstrate some degree of variability in oxygen affinity, although in some cases it may be normal. Variants exhibiting decreased oxygen affinity tend to have lower hemoglobin levels. In some patients, Heinz body formation to any marked degree may occur only after drug injection. In vitro Heinz body formation that is absent prior to splenectomy may be demonstrable on incubation.

HEMOGLOBINOPATHIES WITH ABNORMAL OXYGEN BINDING. These occur as an erythrocytosis in patients with increased oxygen affinity and a reduction in oxygen unloading, and as an anemia in patients with decreased oxygen affinity (Hb Kansas). As a general rule, clinical manifestations are minor, although cyanosis might occur in variants with decreased oxygen affinity.

hemoglobinorrhea (he″mo-glo″bĭ-no-re′ah) [*hemoglobin* + Gr. *rhoia* flow] the escape of hemoglobin from the blood vessels.

hemoglobinuria (he″mo-glo″bĭ-nu′re-ah) [*hemoglobin* + Gr. *ouron* urine + *-ia*] the presence of free hemoglobin in the urine, often due to intravascular hemolysis.

epidemic h., a fatal disease of newborn infants. In addition to severe hemoglobinuria it is characterized by jaundice, cyanosis, polyuria, collapse, and convulsions. Also called Winckel's disease.

malarial h., see *blackwater fever.*

paroxysmal nocturnal h., see *paroxysmal nocturnal hemoglobinuria.*

toxic h., hemoglobinuria associated with exposure to poisons or other toxic agents.

hemogram (he′mo-gram) [*hemo-* + Gr. *gramma* a writing] a record or graph of a differential blood cell count.

hemolymph (he′mo-limf) [*hemo-* + *lymph*] the bloodlike nutrient fluid of certain invertebrates.

hemolymph heteroagglutinin an agglutinin extracted from the hemolymph of the horseshoe crab *Limulus,* which is used to agglutinate red blood cells in cell separation methods.

hemolysate (he-mol′ĭ-sāt) the product of red cell hemolysis. Hemolysates, which are used for analysis of hemoglobin and to study erythrocytic enzymes, are prepared with distilled water, toluene, and other reagents that promote lysis of the cell membrane.

hemolysin (he-mol′ĭ-sin) [*hemo-* + Gr. *lysis* dissolution] an antibody or any other substance that liberates hemoglobin from red blood cells by interrupting their structural integrity. Hemolysins may be naturally present in the body, or may be formed as a result of injections of foreign red cells.

The hemolysin formed by the injection of blood from the same species is called isolysin or isohemolysin; that formed by the injection from another species, a heterolysin; and that which destroys cells of the animal's own body, an autolysin. Hemolysins are also produced by a variety of microorganisms (see *exotoxins.*).

hemolysis (he-mol′ĭ-sis) [*hemo-* + Gr. *lysis* dissolution] 1. the liberation of hemoglobin from red cells.

2. the premature destruction of erythrocytes in "hemolytic" anemia, i.e., anemia due to defective red cells with a shortened life span. Usually, the life span must be shortened by more than 50 percent to be classified as a hemolytic anemia, although lesser degrees of shortening of the red cell life span occur in a variety of other anemias.

The main causes of hemolytic anemia are hemoglobinopathies (structurally abnormal hemoglobins or the disproportionate production of alpha and beta chains, as in thalassemias); enzymopathies (pyruvate kinase, hexose kinase, glucose-6-phosphate dehydrogenase deficiency, and others); red cell membrane defects (hereditary spherocytosis, stomatocytosis, pyropoikilocytosis, "spur cell anemia in liver disease," and other lipid abnormalities of the membrane); paroxysmal nocturnal hemoglobinuria; and milieu defects (both iso- and autoantibodies, bacterial toxins, heavy metals, disseminated intravascular coagulation, mechanical destruction due to vascular prostheses, and vasculitis or microangiopathic anemia).

alpha h., a zone of hemolysis surrounding a colony of microorganisms, most often streptococci, on a blood agar medium. Typically, there is a clear zone of completely hemolyzed erythrocytes surrounding an inner zone of incomplete hemolysis, and a green discoloration of the colonies.

beta h., a zone of complete hemolysis surrounding a colony of microorganisms on a blood agar medium.

colloid osmotic h., hemolysis that occurs after a cell has reached its maximal volume (spherocyte) and the osmotic gradient is further increased. The erythrocyte acts as an osmometer, concentrating K^+ as its main osmotically active solute and regulating its own volume by varying the K^+ content. A slow but constant leak of K^+ from the cell into the plasma is normally just matched by the active transport of K^+ into the cell by a membrane-bound cation pump. (Na^+ ions are transported from the cell by a similar mechanism.) If the pump fails or is overwhelmed by the increased passage of cations into the cell, it equalizes osmotic pressure by allowing water into the cell, thus increasing the cell volume. This increase is limited by the surface area of the cell: when the cell reaches its maximal volume, it assumes the shape of a sphere. A further increase in water content results in hemolysis. Colloid osmotic hemolysis also occurs in solutions of low osmolarity. This is the basis of the osmotic fragility test.

extravascular h., red cell death mediated by macrophages in the reticuloendothelial system (phagocytosis). This is the normal mechanism of red cell death due to senescence. In hemolytic anemia, red cells are removed by this process, or are initially hemolyzed within the circulation with the liberation of hemoglobin and the stroma of lysed cells subsequently removed by the reticuloendothelial system (RES). See also *intravascular h.*

extrinsic h., the shortening of the life span of a red blood cell owing to changes outside the cell such as those produced by toxins, antibodies, or mechanical damage.

gamma h., referring to the absence of hemolysis around a colony of streptococci on a blood agar plate. Such organisms are known as nonhemolytic streptococci.

immune h., the lysis by complement of erythrocytes sensitized as a consequence of interaction with specific antibody to the erythrocytes.

intramedullary h., hemolysis of the erythrocyte within the bone marrow. See also *ineffective e.* under *ertyhropoiesis.*

intravascular h., lysis of the red cell membrane, usually due to the action of complement on red cells coated with antibody. The cell is destroyed before it can be removed from the circulation by the reticuloendothelial system (RES), resulting in the liberation of free hemoglobin into the plasma.

osmotic h., the leakage of hemoglobin from red cells due to exposure to a hypotonic solution (i.e., a solution containing less than physiologic quantities of NaC1—0.9 percent). Lesser degrees of osmotic swelling that do not sustain loss of hemoglobin are reversible.

passive h., the lysis of erythrocytes on which antigen has been absorbed in the presence of complement and antiserum to that antigen.

traumatic h., hemolysis attributed to physical trauma to the red cell, seen in intravascular coagulation, cardiac valvular disease and prosthesis, exposure to vegetable poisons (e.g., fava bean) and animal poisons (e.g., snake venom, spider toxins), and in the presence of infectious agents (e.g., *Plasmodium falciparum* and *Mycoplasma pneumoniae*).

hemolysis interference in colorimetric assays, erroneous results due to the presence of hemoglobin in the specimen, which may interfere either in the reaction producing the color or in the actual measurement of color intensity.

hemolytic (he″mo-lit′ik) pertaining to, characterized by, or producing hemolysis.

hemolytic anemia see *hemolytic a.* under *anemia.*

hemolytic disease of the newborn (HDN) a hemolytic anemia seen in the newborn. It is caused by the transfer across the placenta of maternal blood group antibodies that are capable of destroying fetal red blood cells. The condition is most commonly due to RH_o(D) or ABO incompatibility, approximately 2 percent of cases being attributed to minor blood group incompatibilities, including Kell, E, Lutheran, C, and others.

Clinical symptoms range in severity and include anemia, jaundice, pallor, and hepatosplenomegaly. The jaundice is usually absent at birth because of the ability of the placenta to remove and transport bilirubin, but it rises rapidly after birth if the hemolytic process is severe. A great majority (90 percent) of severely affected newborns suffer from Rh_o(D) incompatibility, the most grave cases resulting in hydrops fetalis; ABO incompatibility usually causes only a mild anemia.

Unlike Rh_o(D) isoimmune hemolytic anemia, which requires prior immunization (either by previous pregnancy or transfusion), ABO incompatibility frequently occurs in first-born infants of mothers with no transfusion or sensitization history. ABO incompatibility usually has no effect on subsequent pregnancies. To prevent Rh_o(D) sensitization, anti-Rh_o(D) antibody (RhoGAM) is administered to all nonimmunized Rh-negative mothers within 72 hr of delivery of each Rh-positive infant.

ABO incompatibility is characterized by spherocytosis, reticulocytosis, and usually mild anemia; the direct Coombs' test is usually only weakly positive. Rh_o(D) incompatibility is associated with erythroblastemia, reticulocytosis, and moderate-to-severe anemia; the direct Coombs' test is strongly positive.

The treatment of choice for severely affected infants is exchange transfusion, which removes the unconjugated bilirubin, anitbody to the infant's red cell, and sensitized red cells, thereby decreasing the source of the excess bilirubin production. Phototherapy is used to further reduce bilirubin levels in the serum in order to prevent kernicterus.

Also called *erythroblastosis fetalis, erythroblastosis neonatorum,* and *isoimmune hemolytic anemia.*

hemolyzable (he″mo-liz′ah-b′l) capable of undergoing hemolysis.

hemolyze (he′mo-liz) to undergo hemolysis. See also *hemolysis.*

hemopericardium (he″mo-per″ĭ-kar′de-um) the effusion of pure blood into the pericardial sac.

hemoperitoneum (he″mo-per″ĭ-to-ne′um) an effusion of blood into the peritoneal cavity. This condition is most often seen in association with trauma and malignant disease.

hemopexin (he″mo-pek′sin) a serum protein (M.W. 57,000) that serves as a specific scavenger protein for trapping hemin; it is released from lysed erythrocytes and minimizes the loss of hemin iron through the kidneys.

hemophil (he′mo-fil) a microorganism that grows best on media containing hemoglobin, e.g., *Haemophilus* species.

hemophilia (he″mo-fil′e-ah) [*hemo* + Gr. *philein* to love + *-ia*] a group of congenital disorders of coagulation, which characteristically involve a defect of a single coagulation protein. The transmission of these diseases is genetically determined. In several types of hemophilia, the coagulation protein is present in the blood in a normal concentration but is functionally defective. Individuals with hemophilia usually do not display massive bleeding; rather, hemorrhage is delayed and occurs as a prolonged oozing or trickling following minor trauma or surgery. Hematomas in deep subcutaneous or intramuscular layers are common. Joint deformities, gastrointestinal bleeding, and hematuria are a result of repeated hemorrhage and may lead to ankylosis or permanent nerve damage with muscle atrophy. The extent and frequency of bleeding episodes are variable, depending on the type of hemophilia. Generally, individuals with hemophilia are advised to avoid contact sports and hazardous occupations. Prophylactic measures should be observed in hemophiliacs before surgery (including tooth extractions).

Hemophilia was once considered a hopeless disease, with most of those severely affected dying before adulthood. However, medical research has now enabled hemophiliacs to live relatively normal lives with longer life expectancies owing to the improved ability to transfuse various clotting factors.

h. A, classic hemophilia, transmitted as a sex-linked recessive trait, which is the most common hereditary coagulation disorder, affecting approximately 1 in 25,000 individuals. The severity of the disorder is directly related to the deficiency of Factor VIII, which may be mild, moderate, or severe. It is characterized by hemarthrosis and soft tissue hemorrhage. The bleeding time and prothrombin time are normal, whereas the activated partial thromboplastin time (aPTT) is usually prolonged. The aPTT can be corrected by the addition of adsorbed plasma. Replacement therapy or prophylaxis is with fresh frozen plasma, cryoprecipitated concentrate of plasma, or commercial lyophilized Factor VIII concentrates.

h. B, a hereditary bleeding disorder, transmitted as a sex-linked recessive trait, which is due to a deficiency of Factor IX. This disease is clinically indistinguishable from classic hemophilia, hemophilia A. Its severity is directly related to the concentration of Factor IX with multiple subtypes whose classificiation is dependent on laboratory results. Both the bleeding time and the prothrombin time are usually normal. The activated partial thromboplastin time (aPTT) is prolonged but can be corrected by the addition of aged serum. Replacement therapy is with commercial concentrate of prothrombin complex factor or with plasma. Also called *Christmas disease* and *hereditary plasma thromboplastin component (PTC) deficiency.*

h. B Leyden, a variant of Factor IX deficiency, characterized by a decreased level of Factor IX activity and a corresponding decrease of Factor IX–related antigen. The clinical manifestations diminish with increasing age and are associated with an increase in the level of Factor IX.

h. Bm, a variant of Factor IX deficiency, characterized by the prolongation of the prothrombin time when performed with ox-brain thromboplastin; this is because of the competitive inhibition of the reaction between Factor VII and the ox-brain tissue thromboplastin by the abnormal analog to Factor IX. Materials that antigenically cross react (CRM) with Factor IX have been found in the plasma of most Bm-variant patients.

h. C, a rare inherited coagulation factor deficiency, transmitted as an autosomal incompletely recessive trait, which is due to a deficiency of Factor XI. It occurs primarily in persons of Jewish ancestry. The bleeding is usually mild; spontaneous bleeding is rare. The bleeding and prothrombin times are normal; the activated partial thromboplastin time (aPTT) is prolonged but can be corrected with the addition of either adsorbed plasma or aged serum. Also called *plasma thromboplastin antecedent (PTA) deficiency* and *Rosenthal's syndrome.*

hemophiliac (he″mo-fil′e-ak) an individual affected with hemophilia.

hemophilic (he-mo-fil′ik) 1. pertaining to or characterized by hemophilia.

2. having an affinity for blood; living or growing especially well in the presence of blood.

hemophilic factor A see *Factor VIII.*

Hemophilus (he-mof′ĭ-lus) a genus of microorganisms characterized by minute gram-negative rods or coccobacilli, often filamentous. They are nonmotile, nonsporulating, hemophilic aerobes that require either one or both growth factors (Factor X, which can be replaced by hematin, or Factor V, which can be replaced by nicotinamide adenine dinucleoside) provided by blood. These organisms are normal inhabitants of the upper respiratory tract but may become primary or secondary pathogens. The type species is *H. influenzae,* one of the three leading causes of bacterial meningitis.

H. aegyptius, a species that produces purulent conjunctivitis in humans and is very similar to *H. influenzae.* It requires coagulation Factors X and V for growth. Also known as *Koch-Weeks bacillus.*

H. ducreyi, a species that causes soft chancres or chancroids on the genitals. Gram-stained smears from lesions show small gram-negative coccobacilli in pairs and short chains. *H. ducreyi* requires coagulation Factor X for growth but not Factor V. See also *chancroid* and *sexually transmitted diseases.*

H. hemolyticus, a nonpathogenic species. It requires both Factors X and V for growth; the hemolytic colonies are easily mistaken for those of *Streptococcus pyogenes.*

H. influenzae, a prevalent pathogenic species, the most common cause of bacterial meningitis in children, in whom it also causes potentially fatal epiglottitis and obstructive laryngitis. In adults, pathogenicity usually occurs as a secondary infection of the upper respiratory tract following a viral influenza. It requires Factors X and V for growth, and is nonhemolytic. Positive identification depends on serologic typing or immunofluorescence procedures. See also *pneumonia.*

H. parainfluenzae, a species that is part of the normal oral flora but occasionally causes bacterial endocarditis.

hemophthalmia (he″mof-thal′me-ah) [*hemo-* + Gr. *ophthalmos* eye] the leakage of blood from the vascular spaces into the eye. Causes include trauma and vascular and coagulation disorders.

hemopneumopericardium (he″mo-nu″mōper″ĭ-kar′de-um) the effusion into, and collection of, both blood and air within the pericardial sac.

hemopneumothorax (he″mo-nu″mo-tho′raks) the effusion of both blood and air into the pleural cavity.

hemoprotein (he″mo-pro′tēn) a conjugated protein that contains heme as the prosthetic group. Among the hemoproteins are hemoglobin, myoglobin, cytochrome, and catalase.

hemoptysis (he-mop′tĭ-sis) [*hemo-* + *ptyein* to spit] the spitting up or coughing of blood from respiratory tract bleeding. The hemorrhage may arise anywhere from the major vessels to the capillaries in either the bronchial or pulmonary circulation. There are many causes, most of which are associated with inflammation; bronchitis and bronchiectasis are frequently implicated. Other causes include pulmonary infection (especially with tuberculosis or aspergillosis organisms), bronchogenic carcinoma, trauma, pulmonary embolism and infarct, congestive heart failure, pulmonary hypertension, aneurysms, and clotting abnormalities.

The source of blood is an important diagnostic criterion. The hemoptysis must be differentiated from hematemesis and from blood originating from the nose, mouth, or nasopharynx. The amount and location of the bleeding should also be determined. Bleeding of more than several ounces of bright red blood suggests massive hemorrhage, but fatal pulmonary bleeding is rare. History, physical examination, and chest x-ray are essential preliminary steps in determining the etiology of this disorder. Lung scans, angiography, and endoscopic examinations may also be required. The prognosis is determined by both the amount and the underlying cause of the hemorrhage.

parasitic h., an infection of the lung by flukes of the genus *Paragonimus.* Also called pulmonary distomiasis, endemic hemoptysis, and Oriental lung fluke disease. See also *P. westermani* under *Paragonimus.*

hemorrhage (hem′or-ij) [*hemo-* + Gr. *rhēgnynai* to burst forth] the escape of blood from the vascular system, either into surrounding tissues or into the environment. Hemorrhage may occur as a result of mechanical trauma, infection with tissue necrosis, rupture of vessels due to congenital or acquired weaknesses in the vessels, high blood pressure, defects in hemostasis, or a combination of the above. Hemorrhage may result in anemia, decreased blood volume, and shock or death, depending on the rate of blood loss and the cardiovascular adaptive potential of the patient.

hemorrhagic (hem″o-raj′ik) pertaining to or characterized by hemorrhage.

hemorrhagic disease of the newborn a hemorrhagic syndrome occurring between the second and seventh days of life; it is due to a deficiency of vitamin K–dependent clotting factors. With an incidence rate of 0.1–1.0 percent of live births and a fatality rate of 5–30 percent of untreated cases, it is most often seen in breast-fed infants because of the lower vitamin K content of human milk compared with cow's milk.

The disorder begins precipitously with spontaneous bleeding, the hemostatic defect being characterized by a prolonged prothrombin time, a normal platelet count, and normal fibrinogen levels. Prophylaxis and treatment is with vitamin K; because the fully developed syndrome is slow to respond, fresh plasma transfusions may be necessary as an emergency measure.

hemorrhoid (hem′o-roid) the enlargement of a portion of the venous hemorrhoidal plexus in the mucosal membrane in the region of the rectum. These lesions typically cause pain, itching, and bleeding. They may also result from increased hydrostatic pressure in the venous system (as in pregnancy), straining at stools, or systemic disease.

external h., a varicosity of the inferior hemorrhoidal veins under anal skin, which leads to pain and swelling around the anal sphincter.

internal h., a varicosity of the superior and middle hemorrhoidal veins under the anal mucosa. Pain is not a frequent complaint, but bright red blood in the stool may occur.

hemosiderin (he″mo-sid′er-in) [*hemo-* + *sidēros* iron] iron-containing granules found mainly in the cytoplasm of the liver, spleen, and bone marrow cells. These microscopically visible granules appear to be composed of a complex of ferric ions [Fe(III)] associated with hydroxide ion (OH^-), various polysaccharides, and proteins. They may be aggregates of ferritin material, with a greater concentration of Fe(III)(35–37 percent), and accumulate when iron intake is greater than can be stored in the liver as ferritin. The disintegration of renal tubular cells may liberate hemosiderin into the urine.

hemosiderin staining the Prussian blue reaction for ferric iron (see under *iron-positive pigment demonstration*). Buffered neutral formalin must be used as the fixative because hemosiderin is dissolved by acids.

hemosiderinuria (he″mo-sid″er-in-u′re-ah) the presence of hemosiderin in the urine, due to iron overload, abnormal iron metabolism, and, most commonly, hemolysis.

hemosiderinuria test a procedure that involves the microscopic examination of urine sediment. Hemosiderin occurs as coarse brown granules, which are stained blue by potassium ferrocyanide.

hemosiderosis (he″mo-sid″er-o′sis) [*hemo-*| *Gr. sidēros* iron + *-osis* condition] a relative or absolute increase in the amount of stored iron (often aggregates of ferritin micelles) in the body. Hemosiderosis may occur in specific organs (e.g., idiopathic pulmonary hemosiderosis or paroxysmal nocturnal hemoglobinuria), or it may be generalized throughout the body. It may be due to localized hemorrhage, infarct, or congestion of an organ (localized), specific metabolic defect, or iron overload. The condition may also be seen in mitral stenosis, Goodpasture's syndrome, chronic hemolysis, pyridoxine deficiency, and lead poisoning, following repeated transfusions, and after administration of parenteral iron dextrans and oral iron. Hemosiderin deposition causes little, if any, tissue injury (cf. *hemochromatosis*). Hemosiderosis is a morphologic finding and does not require therapy unless it progresses to hemochromatosis. Also called *siderosis.*

idiopathic pulmonary h., a rare disease of unknown etiology characterized by chronic and recurrent extravasation of blood into pulmonary tissue, which results in low-grade inflammation, fibrosis, and hemosiderin-filled pulmonary macrophages. It primarily affects children and young adults and causes hemoptysis, dyspnea, pulmonary infiltrates, and microcytic hypochromic anemia with iron deficiency. The pulmonary hemorrhage may range from mild to severe and leads to prominent fibrosis and degeneration of alveolar epithelial cells.

The disease may pursue an erratic course with remissions and exacerbations; progressive forms usually lead to impaired respiratory function and cardiac failure. This disorder is distinguished from Goodpasture's syndrome by its lack of renal involvement. Therapy is symptomatic and supportive. Death may occur as a result of massive pulmonary hemorrhage.

Hemosporidia (he″mo-spo-rid′e-ah) see *Haemosporidia.*

hemostasis (he″mo-sta′sis, he-mos′tah-sis) [*hemo-* + Gr. *stasis* halt] 1. the arrest of bleeding, either by the physiologic properties of vasoconstriction and coagulation or by surgical means.

2. the stagnation or arrest of blood flow through any vessel or to an anatomic area.

hemostat (he′mo-stat) 1. a small surgical clamp for constricting a blood vessel.

2. an agent that checks hemorrhage when applied to a bleeding point.

hemostatic (he″mo-stat′ik) [*hemo-* + Gr. *statikos* standing] 1. pertaining to the arrest of blood flow that has physiologic, pathologic, or surgical causes.

2. an agent that arrests the flow of the blood.

hemothorax (he″mo-tho′raks) [*hemo-* + Gr. *thōrax* chest] the effusion into, and collection of, blood within the pleural cavity.

hemozoin (he″mo-zo′in) the pigment found in malarial parasites. It consists of insoluble ferriprotoporphyrin polymers, which enable the parasites to sequester in a benign form. In chronic cases this pigment collects in tissues (e.g., in the spleen), giving the organ a color that is gray to black in appearance.

HEMPAS abbrev. for hereditary erythroblastic multinuclearity with a positive acidified serum; see *congenital dyserythropoietic a.* under *anemia.*

Henderson-Hasselbalch equation (hen′der-son has′el-balk) [Lawrence Joseph *Henderson*, Boston chemist, 1878–1942; Karl A. *Hasselbalch*, Copenhagen scientist, 1874–1962] a rearrangement of the definition of the dissociation constant, used to calculate the pH of a buffer solution:

$$\mathrm{pH} = \mathrm{p}K'_a + \log \frac{[\mathrm{A}^-]}{[\mathrm{HA}^-]}$$

where $\mathrm{p}K_a$ is the negative logarithm of the dissociation (equilibrium) constant of the acid, A^- is the activity (which, in dilute solutions, is approximately equal to the concentration of the acid anion or, more precisely, conjugate base) and HA is the activity concentration of the undissociated acid.

Henle's loop (hen′lēz) [Friedrich Gustav Jakob *Henle*, German anatomist, 1809–1885] a U-shaped portion of the renal tubule between the proximal convoluted and distal convoluted tubules. This medullary portion of the nephron is divided into thin and thick segments. See also *nephron.*

Henoch-Schönlein syndrome (hen-ōk-shān-lin) [Edouard Heinrich *Henoch*, German pediatrician, 1820–1910; J. L. *Schönlein*, German pediatrician, 1793–1864] an acute or chronic inflammation of the small vessels of the skin (arms and trunk), joints (knees and ankles), and gastrointestinal and renal systems, which primarily affects the young. This purpura is nonthrombocytopenic and may be associated with erythema and urticaria. There is blood effusion into joints and hand pain, often with hematuria and acute glomerulitis. The condition is thought to be a hypersensitivity reaction of unknown cause.

Laboratory findings may show anemia, leukocytosis, and a rapid sedimentation rate, but for the most part they are normal. Immunologic findings vary, but circulating IgA immune complexes are often found.

Also called *anaphylactoid purpura* and Henoch-Schönlein purpura.

henry (H) (hen′re) [Joseph *Henry*, American physicist, 1797–1878] the International System (SI) unit of inductance equal to 1 volt-second per ampere (1 V·s/A).

Henry's law (hen′rēz) [William *Henry*, English chemist, 1774–1836] stated as: the solubility of a gas in a liquid is proportional to the partial pressure of the gas in contact with the liquid. The law does not hold for gases that combine chemically with the liquid, and holds exactly only for ideal solutions (where there is no association between any compounds in the system).

Henschen position one of three positions used to obtain semiaxial lateral projections of the mastoid process and petrous regions of temporal bones. The patient is prone or erect with the median sagittal plane of the head parallel to the film, and the central ray is directed through the external auditory meatus, at an angle of 15° toward the feet (25° in the Schüller position, 35° in the Lysholm position).

All three positions demonstrate the mastoid cells, mastoid antrum, external and internal auditory meatuses, and tegmen tympani (the roof of the middle ear). This position is also particularly used to demonstrate acoustic nerve tumors; the Lysholm position to demonstrate the labyrinth and the carotid canal; and the Schüller position to demonstrate the dural sinuses and the mastoid emissary vein.

Hensen's node (hen′senz) [Victor *Hensen*, German anatomist and physiologist, 1835–1924] in the developing embryo, the knob formed at the forward end of the primary streak, indicating the immediate source of the cells of the notochord.

HEPA filter [acronym from *h*igh *e*fficiency *p*articulate *a*ir] see *HEPA f.* under *filter.*

heparan-*N*-sulfatase see *heparitinsulphate lyase.*

heparan sulfate (hep′ah-ran sul′fāt) a mucopolysaccharide (glycosaminoglycan), a constituent of connective tissues, that consists of alternating residues of uronic acid and glucosamine. The uronic acid position may be occupied by glucuronic, L-iduronic, or sulfated L-iduronic acid residues; the glucosamine residue may be acetylated on the amino nitrogen group or it may be sulfated on the amino nitrogen or hydroxyl group. The catabolism of these mucopolysaccharides is accomplished by lysosomal acid hydrolases, and the deficiency of one or more of these enzymes leads to a variety of disorders collectively known as mucopolysaccharidoses. See also *mucopolysaccharidoses.*

heparin (hep′ah-rin) a complicated heteropolysaccharide, structurally similar to heparan sulfate, except that it has more sulfate groups and its glucosamine residues are not acetylated. Heparin is not a constituent of connective tissues; it occurs within the metachromatic granules in mast cells, especially those in the liver, lungs, and skin. It functions to activate lipoprotein lipase.

Heparin inhibits the clotting of blood by activating antithrombin III; heparin sodium is widely used as an anticoagulant in the management of patients with myocardial infarctions and strokes to help prevent further clot formation, during surgery to prevent pulmonary embolism (the dissemination of clots to the lung), to prevent blood clot obstruction in patients with indwelling catheters, in surgery requiring extracorporeal circulation, and for exchange or neonatal transfusions. Heparin is not currently used for storing red cells for transfusion.

In small quantities, heparin has no significant effect on many laboratory determinations and is commonly used as an anticoagulant for blood samples in clinical laboratories.

heparin cofactor see *a. III* under *antithrombin.*

heparinize (hep′er-ĭ-nīz″) to treat with heparin in order to inhibit the clotting of blood.

heparitinsulphate lyase (hep′ah-rih-tin-sul′fāt li′ās) an enzyme of the lyase class (heparin-sulphate lyase, EC 4.2.2.8) that catalyzes the elimination of sulfate in heparin sulfate by acting on the linkages between *N*-acetamido-2-deoxy-D-glucose and uronate. A genetic deficiency of the enzyme, transmitted as an autosomal recessive trait, results in the accumulation of heparan sulfate in tissue with resulting excretion in urine; the condition is known as mucopolysaccharidosis III A (Sanfilippo's syndrome A). Also called *heparan-N-sulfatase.*

hepat/o (hep′ah-to) [Gr. *hēpar, hēpatos* liver] a word element used in combining form to denote liver, e.g., hepatocyte.

hepatic (hĕ-pat′ik) [L. *hepaticus;* Gr. *hēpatikos*] pertaining to the liver.

hepatic artery one of the three terminal branches of the celiac artery. It ascends to the liver in the free edge of the lesser omentum in company with the portal vein and common bile duct, gives off the cystic artery to the gallbladder, and enters the liver at the porta hepatis.

hepatic cords plates or sheets of liver cells radiating from a central vein and separated by venous sinusoids in the liver lobules.

hepatic encephalopathy see *hepatic e.* under *encephalopathy.*

hepatic portal see *p. hepatis* under *porta.*

hepatitis (hep″ah-ti′tis), pl. *hepatitides* [*hepat-* + *-itis*] an inflammation of the liver. The term is more generally used to refer to the clinical, laboratory, and/or histologic effects of liver injury, whether or not inflammation is present. Most cases are the result of damage to the liver cells (hepatocytes). Some hepatocytes are affected much more severely than others, and a certain proportion are irreversibly injured. In nonfatal cases the lost hepatocytes are usually replaced by the regeneration of new cells. Hepatic failure occurs when the number of liver cells destroyed is so great that too few remain to maintain basic liver function; in such cases, the term fulminant hepatitis is applied.

Hepatitis can be caused by viruses, bacteria, fungi, parasites, drugs, toxins, and physical agents such as heat, hyperthermia, and radiation, as well as many other agents. Because hepatitis is a generic term, whenever possible it should be qualified with an etiologic modifier, such as viral hepatitis, mononucleosis (EB virus) hepatitis, alcoholic hepatitis, and radiation hepatitis. Although many viruses may cause hepatitis, the terms viral hepatitis and acute viral hepatitis are generally reserved for cases caused by specific hepatotropic virsues. Some cases of hepatitis are idiopathic: no etiology is identified. Hepatitis occurring in neonates is termed neonatal hepatitis. When multinucleate liver cells are prominent, the lesion is often designated neonatal giant cell hepatitis.

The signs and symptoms of most forms of hepatitis reflect either the edema and the inflammation of the organ as a whole (tender enlarged liver, right upper quadrant pain) or the effects of hepatocyte injury and altered function (anorexia, malaise, jaundice, dark urine, and, in severe cases, hemorrhagic phenomena due to decreased synthesis of clotting factors and hepatic encephalopathy). (For differentiating characteristics of hepatitis A and B, see the accompanying table.)

The common changes in serum biochemistry in individuals with hepatitis are the result of altered hepatocyte function (e.g., hyperbilirubinemia) and the release of cytoplasmic enzymes into the circulation from injured or dying hepatocytes. The two serum enzymes most commonly measured are serum glutamic oxaloacetic transaminase (SGOT) and serum glutamic pyruvic transaminase (SGPT). The quantity of the enzymes in the circulation rises shortly after liver cell injury. Alkaline phosphatase, an enzyme found in high concentrations in the biliary tree, is also released into the serum in hepatitis, but the levels are rarely as high as those seen in diseases that primarily affect the biliary tract.

Morphologic changes that occur in the liver vary with the cause of hepatitis. In general, the hepatocytes show nonspecific evidence of injury, with cell swelling (called ballooning degeneration when severe) and necrosis—either as shrunken eosinophilic bodies (acidophil bodies) or as small cytoplasmic fragments of ruptured hepatocytes.

Chronic excessive intake of alcoholic beverages may be associated with the development of alcoholic hepatitis. The hepatocyte damage is most severe around the central vein, where there is cell swelling, fatty change, infiltrate of polymorphonuclear leukocytes, and pericellular scarring. A characteristic feature of alcoholic hepatitis is the presence of pink-red intracellular masses known as Mallory's alcoholic hyaline.

The hepatotropic viruses include hepatitis A, hepatitis B, and hepatitis non-A–non-B. These viruses primarily affect the liver, and produce generally similar clinical syndromes and morphologic alterations in the liver.

HEPATITIS A. Formerly known as infectious hepatitis, this form is the cause of most epidemic outbreaks of hepatitis in the normal population. The agent is passed by the fecal-oral route; there is an incubation period of 2–6 wk. Most of those affected

HEPATITIS. DIFFERENTIATING CHARACTERISTICS OF HEPATITIS TYPES A AND B

PROPERTY	TYPE A	TYPE B
Usual transmission	Fecal-oral	Parenteral inoculation†
Characteristic incubation period*	15-40 days	60-160 days
Type of onset	Acute	Insidious
Fever > 38°C	Common	Uncommon
Seasonal incidence	Autumn and winter	Year-round
Age incidence	Commonest in children and young adults	All ages; commonest in adults
Size of virus	27 nm	42 nm
Viruses in feces	Incubation period and acute phase	Not demonstrated
Virus in blood	Incubation period and acute phase	Incubation period and acute phase; may persist for years
Appearance of HBsAg	Absent	30-50 days after infection
Detection of HBsAg		Blood (less often in feces, urine, semen, bile)
Duration of HBsAg		60 days to years
Prophylactic value of γ-globulin	Good	Good if titer of anti-HBsAg is high

* Considerable overlapping in the duration of incubation periods for types A and B has been noted in volunteers as well as in patients during epidemics, i.e., as long as 85 days for type A hepatitis and as short as 20 days for type B hepatitis.

† Parenteral injection is probably not the predominant mode of transmission in developing countries where the means of spread is unknown.

From Davis, B. T., et al.: Microbiology. 3rd ed. Hagerstown, MD, Harper & Row, 1980, p. 1224.

have subclinical, or anicteric, hepatitis. The vast majority recover without sequelae, although (rarely) massive hepatic necrosis and acute hepatic failure occur (fulminant viral hepatitis) and are associated with a high mortality rate. Previous infection by hepatitis A can be determined by the finding of specific antibody to hepatitis A in an individual's serum.

HEPATITIS B. Formerly known as serum hepatitis and posttransfusion hepatitis, this form commonly follows parenteral exposure to an infected individual, although other modes of transmission are known to occur. The incubation period is 1–6 mo. As with hepatitis A, subclinical (anicteric) infections are common, but unlike hepatitis A there is a significant risk of the development of chronic hepatitis. Antigens to various components of the hepatitis B virion have been identified: hepatitis B surface antigen (HBsAG), also called Australia antigen because it was first identified in an Australian aborigine, and core antigen (HGcAg). Corresponding antibodies in these antigens have also been detected. Hepatitis e antigen (HBeAg) is also associated with hepatitis B virus. Patients who have recovered from hepatitis B infection usually have specific antibodies to the hepatitis B antigens present in their serum. Some individuals, called chronic carriers, are unable to clear the hepatitis B antigens from their system, and surface, core, or e antigens (or combinations thereof) may be found in their serum. See the accompanying figure.

HEPATITIS NON-A–NON-B. A group of patients has been identified with the clinical syndrome of acute viral hepatitis but without the serologic markers (either antigens or antibodies) of hepatitis A or B. At least one other agent is suspected to be the cause of viral hepatitis in these circumstances. Until there is full characterization of the agent(s), the noncommittal term hepatitis non-A–non-B is recommended.

VIRAL HEPATITIS. The histologic features of acute viral hepatitis, whether the result of A, B, or non-A–non-B viruses, are characteristic but nonspecific. There is a portal infiltrate of mononuclear inflammatory cells. The hepatocytes show variations in size and shape, with ballooning degeneration and occasional acidophil bodies. There is apparent loss of organization of the cells in the lobule, a feature termed lobular disarray. In severe cases of acute viral hepatitis, there may be necrosis of entire groups of liver cells (confluent necrosis). When such necrosis connects portal tracts and/or central veins, the term bridging necrosis is used. Bridging necrosis is most significant when it extends between portal tracts and central veins (as opposed to central vein to central vein or portal tract to portal tract bridging), since in such cases the potential for permanent alteration of normal hepatic architecture is greatest.

Cases of viral hepatitis that are associated with clinical and histologic evidence of a significant degree of cholestasis are termed cholestatic viral hepatitis.

CHRONIC HEPATITIS. This form is said to be present when hepatocyte injury has persisted more than 6 mo. Like hepatitis, the term chronic hepatitis does not imply a specific etiology: it may be idiopathic or caused by viruses (especially hepatitis B and hepatitis non-A–non-B), drugs, or metabolic diseases such as Wilson's disease.

Most patients with chronic hepatitis may be placed into one or two prognostic groups on the basis of the changes seen on a liver biopsy. Chronic persistent hepatitis (CPH) defines a lesion with a relatively favorable prognosis and more indolent

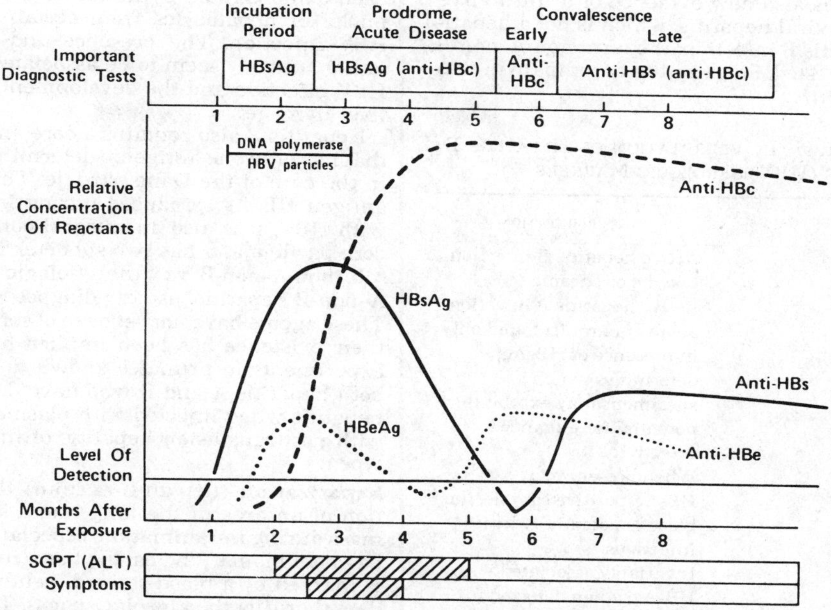

Hepatitis. Serologic and clinical patterns observed during acute hepatitis B virus infection. (From Lennette, E. H., et al.: Manual of Clinical Microbiology. 3rd ed. Washington, DC, American Society for Microbiology, 1980.)

clinical course. Patients with this lesion show portal tract inflammation and, histologically, relatively minor degrees of liver cell injury with correspondingly mild biochemical abnormalities. Chronic active hepatitis, also known as chronic aggressive hepatitis (CAH), implies an unfavorable prognosis. Those affected show evidence of more severe ongoing liver injury biochemically and histologically than in CPH. The histologically common hallmark of CAH is piecemeal necrosis—extension of inflammatory cells and fibrous tissue from the portal tracts into the lobules, with loss of the liver cells and destruction of the "limiting plate" boundary between the portal tract and the adjacent liver cells. As in acute viral hepatitis, bridging necrosis occurs in CAH and is an unfavorable prognostic sign.

A few patients with a clinical diagnosis of chronic hepatitis have changes that predominantly affect the liver lobule. The histologic picture resembles acute viral hepatitis, yet by definition the patients have chronic hepatitis. In such cases, the term chronic lobular hepatitis (CLH) or unresolved hepatitis has been applied. The prognosis of CLH is thought to be relatively good.

Patients with chronic hepatitis caused by chronic hepatitis B infection often have hepatocytes with an eccentric nucleus and a homogeneous "ground-glass" cytoplasm. Such ground-glass hepatocytes stain positively with aldehyde fuchsin and have been found to contain large amounts of hepatitis B surface antigen. The ground-glass appearance is due to the proliferation of smooth endoplasmic reticulum associated with the surface antigen.

THOMAS V. COLBY, M.D.

hepatitis antigen a part of the hepatitis B virus particle.

h. B core a. (HBcAg), the core of the hepatitis virus particle. It is 27 nm in diameter and is located in the nuclei of hepatocytes in patients with viral hepatitis. Antibodies to HBcAg are present in many patients with chronic hepatitis. Also called *core antigen.*

h. B e a. (HBeAg), an antigen produced during the initial infection with hepatitis B virus. Also called hepatitis B early antigen.

h. B surface a. (HBsAg), the envelope of the hepatitis virus particle. It is 22 nm in diameter and is found in the body fluids of patients with hepatitis B viral infection. Detection of this antigen by radioimmunoassay is commonly used as a diagnostic test for hepatitis B.

hepatitis B surface antigen tests tests performed on donor blood to determine if hepatitis B surface antigen (HBsAg) is present in the serum, including radioimmunoassay (RIA), which is the most sensitive; enzyme-linked immunosorbent assay (ELISA), which has the advantage of not requiring isotopes; and reversed passive hemagglutination (RPHA).

In addition to these commonly employed techniques, certain latex agglutination tests are acceptable and occasionally utilized. False-positive results occasionally occur, and all positive findings should be confirmed by another procedure if possible. Units of blood found to be reactive by any of these methods are unacceptable for transfusion, and the donor must be permanently rejected as a blood donor. The donor of the unit must be notified of the results of the test.

See also *immunoperoxidase technique* for hepatitis B antigen demonstration.

hepatitis virus one of the viruses that attacks the liver and causes hepatitis—infectious hepatitis (hepatitis A virus) and serum hepatitis (hepatitis B virus). There is also new evidence of a third virus that produces viral hepatitis, which is not a hepatitis A or hepatitis B infection; the term non-A–non-B has been suggested. See also the accompanying table and *hepatitis.*

HEPATITIS VIRUS. INTERPRETATION OF HEPATITIS B VIRUS (HBV) SEROLOGIC MARKERS

POSITIVE TEST	INTERPRETATION
HBsAg (surface antigen)	Active hepatitis B infection, acute or chronic
HBeAg[a]	Active hepatitis B infection, acute or chronic; found only in presence of HBsAg; determines which specimens may exhibit the potential for enhanced infectivity
Anti-HBe	When present in a HBsAg-positive sample, the blood is potentially less infectious
Anti-HBc	Invariably associated with HBsAg; when detected in the absence of HBsAg and anti-HBs, a presumptive diagnosis of active HBV infection, acute or chronic, can be entertained
Anti-HBs (± anti-HBc)	Specifies immunity against reinfection with HBV

[a] Other HBV serologic markers that may be present at the same time include HBV (Dane) particles observable by electron microscopy. By disrupting the virions, HBcAg and viral DNA polymerase can be measured. From Lennette, E. H., et al.: Manual of Clinical Microbiology. 3rd ed. Washington, DC, American Society for Microbiology, 1980, p. 919.

h. A v. (HAV), a nonenveloped, icosahedral, single-stranded RNA virus, 27 nm in diameter, that belongs to the family Picornaviridae. Both full and empty particles are seen by electron microscopy. It is stable in ether and to a pH of 3.0. Its properties resemble those of an enterovirus. Three major polypeptides are associated with the RNA. HAV multiplies in the cytoplasm of infected cells.

h. B v. (HBV), a hepatotropic virus that is microbiologically unrelated to hepatitis A virus (HAV). A double-stranded DNA virus, it exists in three distinct forms: (1) a spherical particle 22 nm in diameter; (2) a filamentous form 22 nm wide by 50–250 nm long; and (3) a Dane particle, the least common, 42 nm in diameter, which represents the virion, contains an outer layer and core (27-nm nucleocapsid), and is infectious. Antigenically, HBV is more complex than HAV. Hepatitis B surface antigen (HBsAg) was formerly called Australia Ag (Au Ag) and hepatitis-associated Ag. One antigenic (a) specificity is common to all HBsAg. Because there are also two sets of subimmunotypes that are mutually exclusive (d or y and w or r), there are thus four possible subtypes of HBsAg: adw, ayw, adr, and ayr. The predominant subtype in North America is adw, followed by ayw.

A new HBsAg-associated delta antigen (δ Ag) has been demonstrated by immunofluorescence in the nuclei of hepatocytes from certain patients with HBV infection. The presence and persistence of anti-δ antibody seem to be associated with chronic HBV infection and the development of progressive liver damage.

Hepatitis B also contains a core antigen (HBcAg) that has only one antigenic determinant; it is found in the core of the Dane particle. There is an early antigen HBeAg, produced during initial infection with HBV; it is also an integral component of the core particle and has two subdeterminants.

h. non-A–non-B v., the etiologic agent of non-A–non-B hepatitis, usually diagnosed by exclusion. These agents have not yet been observed physically; their existence has been implied by transmission experiments to primates known to be immune to both hepatitis A and B who have developed active hepatitis when injected with plasma from patients with posttransfusion hepatitis of the non-A–non-B type.

hepatization (hep″ah-ti-za′shun) the transformation of an area of the lung into a solid "liverlike" mass during inflammation, especially as seen in lobar pneumonia. The early phase, red hepatization, is marked by a blood-stained, neutrophil-rich exudate that fills the alveolar spaces. The later phase, gray hepatization, is characterized by an accumulation of fibrinopurulent exudate.

hepatoblastoma (hep″ah-to-blas-to′mah) [*hepato-* + Gr. *blastos* germ + *-oma*] a tumor of liver cell origin occurring mainly in infants. The cells are like small hepatocytes that vary in their degree of maturity and form solid masses, sheets, ribbons, and rosettes. The tumor stroma may contain primitive mesenchymal cells, and foci of bone or cartilage. Extramedullary hematopoiesis may be present. This tumor has been described in association with various congenital anomalies but not with cirrhosis. Its behavior is aggressive, frequently producing metastases to the lymph nodes and lungs.

hepatocele (he-pat′o-sēl) [*hepato-* + Gr. *kēlē* hernia] a hernial protrusion of the liver beyond the boundaries of its normal framework.

hepatocellular (hep″ah-to-sel′u-lar) pertaining to the cells of the liver (hepatocytes) or to an agent or process affecting the cells of the liver.

hepatocellular carcinoma see *liver cell carcinoma.*

hepatocholangitis (hep″ah-to-ko″lan-ji′tis) inflammation involving both the liver and the bile ducts.

hepatocuprein (hep″ah-to-koo′prin) see under *copper storage protein.*

hepatocyte (hep′ah-to-sīt) a parenchymal liver cell.

hepatolenticular (hep″ah-to-len-tik′u-lar) pertaining to the liver and the lenticular nucleus.

h. degeneration, see *Wilson's disease.*

hepatoma see *liver cell carcinoma.*

hepatomegaly (hep″ah-to-meg′ah-le) a general term that describes enlargement of the liver.

hepatopancreatic (hep″ah-to-pan″kre-at′ik) pertaining to the liver and pancreas.

hepatorenal (hep″ah-to-re′nal) pertaining to the liver and kidneys.

hepatorenal glycogenosis type I glycogen storage disease. See *glycogen storage disease.*

hepatorenal syndrome an involved and poorly understood complex in which renal failure follows an episode of liver failure, such as in cirrhosis or prolonged obstructive jaundice. The kidneys demonstrate no visible pathologic alterations; rather, they seem to experience a failure due in part to decreased renal perfusion, marked hyperaldosteronism, and decreased plasma volume. This condition is marked by a hypovolemia and a tendency to hemorrhage, leading to severe morbidity and high mortality.

hepatosplenomegaly (hep″ah-to-sple″no-meg′ah-le) [*hepato-* + Gr. *splēn* spleen + *megas* big] a general term that describes the enlargement of both the liver and the spleen.

hepta, hept (hep′tah) [Gr. *hepta* seven] a word element used in combining form to denote seven, e.g., heptachromic.

heptachlor a chlorinated cyclodiene insecticide. See also *chlorinated hydrocarbon pesticides.*

heptachlor epoxide a metabolite of heptachlor. The epoxide persists in body fat longer than the parent compound.

heptane (hep′tān) 1. a colorless, volatile, flammable liquid, *n*-heptane, $CH_3(CH_2)_5CH_3$, used as a solvent; M.W. 100.20. It is moderately toxic and a respiratory tract irritant; high concentrations are narcotic.

2. any seven-carbon alkane.

herbicide (her′bĭ-sid) [L. *herba* herb + *caedare* to kill] a pesticide used to destroy weeds.

hereditary (he-red′ĭ-ter-e) [L. *hereditarius*] genetically transferred from parent to offspring.

hereditary erythroblastic multinuclearity with a positive acidified serum (HEMPAS) see *congenital dyserythropoietic a.* under *anemia.*

hereditary persistence of fetal hemoglobin (HPFH) a genetically transmitted hematologic disorder characterized by the continued production of hemoglobin F in large amounts into adult life. Significant anemia, hemolysis, or ineffective erythropoiesis is absent. The red cells may be normal or mildly aniso-, poikilo-, and/or microcytic. The condition can be confused with β-thalassemia.

HPFH syndromes have been divided into two categories. In the pancellular syndromes, both heterozygotes and homozygotes have Hb F in all their red cells, although in some instances the distribution of Hb F may not be uniform. Heterozygotes have 25–30 percent Hb F, whereas homozygotes have 100 percent. The homozygotes have mild thalassemic symptoms. The condition appears to be similar to $\delta\beta$-thalassemia, in which the homozygotes also have 100 percent Hb F. However, in $\delta\beta$-thalassemia, Hb F is variably distributed, with many cells having very little Hb F. Further, the red cells are hypochromic and microcytic in heterozygote $\delta\beta$-thalassemia, but appear normal in heterozygotes of HPFH. Apparently, in $\delta\beta$-thalassemia, α-globin synthesis in the perinatal period is markedly suppressed, which leads to a greater deficiency of globin synthesis.

In heterocellular HPFH, both heterozygotes and homozygotes lack Hb F in some of their red cells. The mutations leading to both pancellular and heterocellular HPFH are linked to the genes for β- and δ-globin synthesis. A Swiss form with 1–3 percent Hb F and a British form with about 20 percent Hb F have been described.

The differential staining technique is useful in diagnosing the disorder (see *fetal hemoglobin tests*).

hereditary plasmathromboplastin component (PTC) deficiency see *h. B* under *hemophilia.*

hereditary spherocytosis see *hereditary spherocytosis* under *anemia.*

heredity (he-red′ĭ-te) [L. *hereditas*] the inheritance by offspring of genes from their parents and also of the traits produced by the genes.

hermaphrodite (her-maf′ro-dīt) [Gr. *hermaphroditos* a person with attributes of both sexes] an individual exhibiting hermaphroditism.

hermaphroditism (her-maf′ro-di-tizm″) a rare developmental condition in which there is the presence of histologically recognizable ovarian and testicular tissue within the same person. Sexual structures and secondary sex characteristics may show any combination of male- or femaleness. About half the affected individuals have a 46,XX karyotype and 25 percent 46,XY karyotype, the remainder being mosaics. The condition is also called true hermaphroditism to distinguish it from the various types of pseudohermaphroditism.

Hermetia (her-me′she-ah) a genus of flies of the family Stratiomyidae.

H. illucens, the soldier fly. This species of larvae develops in decaying fruits and vegetables and when ingested causes intestinal myiasis in humans.

hermetic (her-met′ik) [L. *hermeticus*] impervious to air; airtight.

hermetic seal (her-met′ik) [for the Egyptian god Toth, called *Hermes trimegistos* by the Greeks, who invented a magic seal to make vessels airtight] an airtight seal.

herni/o (her′ne-o) [L.] a word element used in combining form to denote hernia, e.g., herniorrhaphy.

hernia (her′ne-ah) [L.] the protrusion of a loop or segment of tissue through an abnormal opening in the surrounding tisues.

diaphragmatic h., a congenital malformation that results from defective formation and/or fusion of the pleuroperitoneal membranes that normally close the pericardioperitoneal canals—there is no separation of the pleural and peritoneal cavities. The defect is usually unilateral, occurring more often on the left side than on the right. Occasionally, the stomach, spleen, and part of the liver herniate into the thoracic cavity. The abdominal viscera enter the pleural cavity, pushing the heart anteriorly and compressing the lungs, which are often hypoplastic. Respiration is difficult and feeding may be a problem; the newborn dies shortly after birth.

The occurrence of diaphragmatic hernia is 1 in 2200 births. Although little is known of the cause, experimental evidence in mice suggests that diets lacking in vitamin A produce diaphragmatic defects in offspring. Treatment requires immediate reduction of the hernia and surgical closure of the defect.

Also called congenital diaphragmatic hernia of Bochdalek.

epigastric h., a protrusion of abdominal tissues or organs through the midline of the anterior abdominal wall above the umbilicus. More common in males, such hernias may affect 3–5 percent of the population.

esophageal h., a congenital malformation that results from shortness of the esophagus. The upper part of the stomach may be in the thorax and constricted at the level of the diaphragm.

femoral h., a protrusion of abdominal tissues through the femoral canal. Because it can extend upward to lie above the inguinal ligament, this hernia must be differentiated from an inguinal hernia. Femoral hernias may be irreducible and may become strangulated.

hiatal h., a condition, either congenital or acquired, in which part of the stomach protrudes above the diaphragm. Most individuals are asymptomatic; however, gastric reflux, chest pain, strangulation of the hernia, or gastrointestinal bleeding may be associated with the condition. X-rays are used for diagnosis; when the condition is uncomplicated, no treatment is required.

incarcerated h., a hernia in which the herniated organs do not return to their normal position, either spontaneously or with manual pressure. This is often a result of herniation through a narrow opening. Also called *irreducible h.*

inguinal h., a hernia into the inguinal canal. In the indirect form, the herniated tissue, commonly a loop of intestine, leaves the peritoneal cavity through the deep (internal) inguinal ring. In the direct form, the posterior wall of the inguinal canal is breached by the herniating tissue.

irreducible h., see *incarcerated h.*

h. of Morgagni, a congenital malformation that results in a hernia located between the sternal and sternocostal portions of the diaphragm. The intestinal loops may enter the chest. Treatment requires surgical correction, as the defect can lead to incarceration. Also called *retrosternal h.*

peritoneal h., a hernia in which tissues lie between the parietal peritoneum and the fascia of the transversalis muscle of the abdominal wall.

retrocolic h., a congenital malformation that results in the entrapment of portions of the small intestinal loops behind the mesocolon. Such hernias are due to an unusually long mesentery.

retrosternal h., see *h. of Morgagni.*

Richter's h., an incomplete herniation of a loop of bowel so that at no point along this loop is the full circumference of the bowel protruded. This term may also imply strangulation or incarceration of the protruded segment.

strangulated h., a hernia in which the blood supply to the herniated tissues is compromised, often resulting in gangrenous necrosis.

umbilical h., a protrusion of abdominal contents through a defect in the abdominal wall at the navel. A defect of varying size, it contains the umbilical vessels present at birth, and normally constricts and is ablated during the first 2 yr. In adults, such a hernia may indicate increased abdominal pressure from masses, fluid, or obesity.

hernial (her′ne-al) pertaining to a hernia.

hernial sac the layer or layers of tissue that enclose a herniated structure.

herniated (her′ne-āt″ed) protruding like a hernia; enclosed in a hernia.

heroin (her′o-in) [an old trademark] diacetylmorphine, an opiate with effects similar to those of morphine except that it produces less nausea and more euphoria. Any use or production of heroin is illegal in the United States. The toxic effects are the same as those of morphine; overdose deaths due to pulmonary edema also occur but may be caused by adulterants in street drugs.

Heroin is metabolized to monoacetylmorphine and morphine, and excreted as morphineglucuronide; all can be detected by morphine assays.

herpangina (herp″an-ji′nah) [*herpes* + *angina*] a pharyngitis caused by either group A or group B coxsackieviruses or echoviruses. It is characterized by small gray vesicles and ulcers on the mucous membranes of the throat. This disease occurs in the summer, usually affecting children under 3 yr of age. The incubation period is short (3–5 da), at which time there is an abrupt rise in temperature (up to 104°F), which lasts for 3 da. Virologic diagnosis is made by isolation of the virus from either stool or throat and by an increase in serum complement fixing or neutralizing antibodies. Also called *vesicular pharyngitis.*

herpes (her′pēz) [L.; Gr. *herpēs*] any inflammatory skin disease caused by herpesvirus. The most common herpes infection is a gingivostomatitis, which is characterized by small vesicles of the skin and mucous membrances of the oral cavity that collapse and ulcerate. Other primary herpesvirus infections are rhinitis, keratoconjunctivitis, herpetic whitlow, genital herpes, and meningoencephalitis.

h. corneae, a herpesvirus infection of the cornea.

h. febrilis, a herpes simplex virus infection of the lips or the nares. Also called *cold sores* and *fever blisters.*

h. genitalis, a herpes simplex virus infection of the genital area. It is one of the most common types of venereal disease. Symptoms in the female are more severe than in the male, but all vesicular lesions are self-limiting. Herpes genitalis at term in a pregnant patient can lead to severe generalized infection of the neonate.

herpesvirus (her″pēz-vi′rus) [L.; Gr. *herpēs* + L. *virus*] a large group of intranuclear, double-stranded DNA viruses that are remarkably capable of establishing a latent infection many years after a primary infection. The herpesvirus group is responsible for such diseases as fever blister and keratoconjunctivitis (herpes simplex virus type 1), venereal disease (herpes simplex virus type 2), chickenpox (varicella), and shingles (herpes zoster, caused by varicella–herpes zoster virus), cytomegalic inclusion disease (cytomegalovirus), and infectious mononucleosis (Epstein-Barr virus).

The herpes virion has an icosahedral capsid with 162 capsomers and has two additional protein coats. The nucleic acid (M.W. 100 million) has significant amounts of guanine and cytosine. as the virus replicates, it modifies the host cell nuclear membrane, replacing host protein with viral protein but using host lipid and carbohydrate. This may or may not result in the virus being enveloped with a lipoprotein coat. Herpesvirus buds from the nucleus where it matures, and it exits from the cell in a type of reverse phagocytosis. This virus is capable of passing from cell to cell without releasing free viral particles, and can thereby remain protected from any antibodies present in serum.

A herpesvirus becomes latent when viral DNA becomes inserted into host DNA. As the cell replicates, so does the viral DNA. The latent virus is confined to sensory nerve ganglia, usually in the trigeminal region. A latent herpesvirus may be activated by such stimuli as stress due to fever, irradiation, sunburn, immunosuppression, menstruation, pituitary or adrenal hormones, allergic reactions, or trauma. Partial activation of latent herpesvirus is associated with malignancy in such cases as herpes simplex type 2 and carcinoma of the cervix.

See also *cytomegalovirus* and *Epstein-Barr virus.*

CLINICAL DISEASE. Herpes simplex virus has two serotypes: 1 and 2. Herpes simplex 1 infections are usually acquired during childhood and remain for life. Often, the initial infection is subclinical. After latency and eventual reactivation, the virus multiplies and travels down a nerve fiber to the epidermis, where infection causes a crop of vesicles to break out at mucocutaneous junctions of the lips or nose. These fever blisters usually last for several days and are self-limiting. Herpes simplex type 1 is also the etiologic agent for gingivostomatitis, vesicular pharyngitis and tonsillitis, keratoconjunctivitis, and meningoencephalitis. In exposed individuals who have a chronic eczema, the virus may extensively invade the skin and cause the severe febrile disease eczema herpeticum.

Herpes simplex type 2 is the cause of a major venereal disease in which vesicles and small ulcers appear on the cervix, vagina, and perineum of the female and the penis of the male. If the female has an active herpes infection (vulvovaginitis) at the time of birth, the infant will most likely become infected. Genital herpes is usually transmitted by sexual contact. During the first 20 wk of pregnancy, herpes simplex type 2 infection presents a high risk of spontaneous abortion; after 32 wk the probability of neonatal infection, possibly resulting in microencephaly, retinal dysphasia, or brain damage, is extremely high. Vulvovaginitis with herpes simplex type 2 is associated with carcinoma of the cervix, in that 80 percent of patients with this carcinoma have antibodies to herpes simplex type 2.

Aseptic meningitis caused by herpes simplex type 2 is prevalent in young adults. The course of this disease is benign and self-limiting in contrast to an acute form of necrotic encephalitis caused by type 1. Herpes simplex type 2 can easily be isolated; type 1 can rarely be isolated from spinal fluids.

Varicella (chickenpox), caused by a herpesvirus, is one of the four most common viral diseases of childhood. Varicella virus infects the nonimmune individual, gaining entry through the respiratory tract. Fever develops after an incubation period of 2–3 wk. One day after onset of the fever, a papular skin rash appears, which progresses from a ballooning of the prickle cells of the skin to pustules, and then to scales; unlike smallpox, however, all stages of the skin lesion may be seen simultaneously. The skin rash remains on the trunk of the body and may not necessarily appear on the face and limbs. In the adult, chickenpox may be complicated by pneumonitis and encephalitis. Neonates may be infected with varicella virus transplacentally. This virus may also become latent in the dorsal root gainglion or the cranial nerve ganglion.

Herpes zoster virus is physically and immunologically indistinguishable from varicella virus. It causes shingles, a recurrent varicella infection in older people. In this infection the latent virus becomes activated, travels down sensory nerve fibers, and produces a sudden onset of pain and tenderness accompanied by a mild fever and malaise. Vesicular lesions appear on the trunk and face unilaterally. Herpes zoster may affect 1 percent of the population annually.

LABORATORY DIAGNOSIS. Herpes simplex infections may be diagnosed by observing scrapings from the base of the vesicle microscopically. Multinuclear giant cells with intranuclear eosinophilic inclusion bodies are indicative of herpes simplex. During the early stages of infection, the virus may also be isolated from vesicular fluid, saliva, and throat or vaginal swabs, and cultured on human fetal fibroblasts or human or rabbit kidney cell lines. Cytopathic changes are observed after 48 hr. Herpesvirus also kills infant mice and, when injected into embryonic eggs, causes pock formation on the chorioallantoic membrane. Serologically, a rise in antibody titer to herpes virus from the onset of disease to 3 wk later in convalescence is indicative of infection. Usually, the complement-fixation test is used to detect antigens to herpes simplex virus, although this test cannot distinguish between types 1 and 2. Indirect immunofluorescence can also be used to detect herpes simplex antibodies. To distinguish type 1 from type 2 herpes simplex, the indirect hemagglutination inhibition test or indirect immunofluorescence is used.

Laboratory diagnosis of varicella and herpes zoster is made by microscopic examination of giant cells from a lesion and observation of inclusion bodies. In addition, the virus may be cultured similarly to herpes simplex virus. Serologically, varicella–herpes zoster antibodies may be detected by the complement-fixation test or by fluorescence microscopy of antibody against membrane antigen, the FAMA test. The FAMA test determines the clinical diagnosis of infection as well as the susceptibility to varicella. Human lung embryonic fibroblasts are infected with varicella–herpes zoster and later combined with serially diluted test serum. After incubation, centrifugation, removal of supernatant, and washing, fluorescence-labeled antihuman globulin is added. A ring of fluorescence is observed. Two controls should be used for the FAMA test: uninfected fibroblasts as a negative control, and positive varicella–herpes zoster serum as a positive control.

TREATMENT. Herpes simplex lesions are self-limiting; however, cytosine arabinoside, 5-iodo-2′-deoxyuridine (IUDR), or adenine arabinoside in the form of eyedrops has been shown to be therapeutic for keratoconjunctivitis. Varicella–herpes zoster may be treated topically with 5–40 percent iododeoxyuridine in dimethyl sulfoxide.

Herpetomonas (her″pĕ-tom′o-nas) [Gr. *herpeton* creeper + *monas* monad] a genus of flagellate protozoa of the family Trypanosomatidae, parasitic in sandflies of the genus *Phlebotomus.* The life cycle consists of four morphologic stages: amastigote, promastigote, epimastigote, and one stage similar to the trypomastigote.

H. donovani, see *L. donovani* under *Leishmania.*
H. furunculosa, see *L. tropica* under *Leishmania.*
H. tropica, see *L. tropica* under *Leishmania.*

Herring bodies (her′ing) [Percy Theodore *Herring,* English physiologist, born 1872] vesicles containing secretory hormones, found in axons in the neurohypophysis of the pituitary gland. The hormones are synthesized in the cell bodies of secretory neurons located in the hypothalamus. They can be stained with Gomori's chrome-alum-hematoxylin method.

herringbone (her′ĭng-bōn) having a pattern of rows of slanted parallel lines; the direction of the slant alternates with each row, as in the intersecting fascicles of a well-differentiated fibrosarcoma.

Hers' disease (herz) [H. G. *Hers,* French pathologist] a hereditary disorder, transmitted as an autosomal recessive trait, characterized by the abnormal synthesis and deposition of glycogen in the liver. The disease is due to a relative or absolute deficiency of the enzyme liver phosphorylase. This may lead to hepatomegaly, increased susceptibility to infection, and bleeding tendencies. The spleen is normal, as are levels of glucose and lipids. Mild acidosis and hypoglycemia may also occur. Diagnosis may be accomplished by assaying enzyme levels in liver biopsies or in leukocytes. Also called glycogen storage disease (VI) of liver. See also *glycogenoses.*

hertz (Hz) (herts) [Heinrich *Hertz,* German physicist, 1857–1894] the International system (SI) unit of frequency equal to one reciprocal second (s^{-1}), i.e., one period of the oscillation per second. Formerly called cycle per second (cps).

Herxheimer's spiral (herks'hīm-erz) [Karl *Herxheimer,* German dermatologist, 1861–1944] a small twisted coil of mucus seen in gynecologic cytologic smears.

HES abbrev. See *hydroxyethyl starch.*

hetastarch (het'ah-starch) an artificial, colloid plasma volume expander, hydroxyethyl starch, used in treatment of shock and postoperative hypovolemia, and as a cryoprotective agent for preserving erythrocytes. Some 20–25 percent of the free hydroxyls of either amylose or amylopectin are reacted with ethylchlorhydrin to give—O—CH_2-CH_2OH groups. See also *plasma volume expander.*

heter/o [Gr. *heteros* other] a word element used in combining form to denote other or relationship to another, e.g., heterozygous.

heterauxesis (het"er-awk-se'sis) [*heter-* + Gr. *auxēsis* growth] see *allometry.*

heterecious (het"er-e'shus) [*heter-* + Gr. *oikia* house] see *metoxenous.*

heteroagglutinin (het"er-o-ah-gloo'tĭ-nin) any agglutinin produced by one species that reacts with cells or other particulate antigens of a different species.

heteroagglutination (het"er-o-ah-gloo"tĭ-na'shun) the clumping of particulate antigens (on cells or adsorbed on inert carrier particles) of one species by agglutinins from organisms of another species.

heteroallele (het"er-o-ah-lēl') one of several mutations that differ from the normal protein by mutations at different base pairs. Mutations at the same site are called homoalleles or eualleles. Cf. *homoallele.*

heteroantibody (het"er-o-an"tĭ-bod'e) an antibody produced by an organism of one species that is specific for antigens produced by another species.

heteroantigen (het"er-o-an'tĭ-jen) an antigen originating in a different species from that of the antibody producer.

heteroatom (het"er-o-at'om) any atom except carbon with a ring-shaped chemical nucleus.

Heterobilharzia (het"er-o-bil-har'ze-ah) a genus of schistosomes. The cercariae of *H. americana* cause dermatitis in humans.

heteroblastic (het"er-o-blas'tik) [*hetero-* + Gr. *blastos* germ] having origin in different types of tissue.

heterobrachial inversion a pericentric chromosome inversion; see under *inversion.*

heterochromatin (het"er-o-kro'mah-tin) chromosomal material that remains tightly coiled during interphase, so that it can be stained and viewed with a light microscope. See also *Barr body.* Cf. *euchromatin.*

constitutive h., the chromatin in regions of chromosomes that are invariably heterochromatic, located near the centromere and telomere and in the distal end of the long arm of the human Y chromosome. It contains highly repetitive sequences of DNA that are genetically inactive, and serves as a structural element of the chromosome.

facultative h., the chromatin in regions of chromosomes that become heterochromatic in some cells or tissues; e.g., one entire X chromosome, except for a small part of the short arm, is heterochromatic in all but some embryonic cells and oocytes.

heterochthonous (het"er-ok'tho-nus) [*hetero-* + Gr. *chthōn* a particular land or country] 1. originating in a region other than that in which it is found, as in a disease contracted in a foreign country.

2. exogenous. Cf. *autochthonous.*

heterocycle (het"er-o-sīk'l) [*hetero-* + Gr. *kyklos* circle] a compound that is heterocyclic in structure.

heterocyclic (het"er-o-sīk'lik) having or pertaining to a cyclic structure (some of the atoms in the compound form a ring) that includes one or more atoms other than carbon in the ring.

heterocyclic compound an organic compound that has at least one ring, at least one member of which is an atom other than carbon, often nitrogen, oxygen, or sulfur—for example, purine, pyrimidine, thiophene, or furan.

heterocytotropic (het"er-o-si"to-trop'ik) [*hetero-* + *cyto-* + Gr. *tropos* a turning] having an affinity for cells of different species.

heterocytotropic antibody antibody capable of passively sensitizing the tissues of other species lacking that antibody. For example, rabbit IgG antibodies may passively sensitize guinea pig skin, resulting in local passive cutaneous anaphylaxis (PCA).

Heterodera (het"er-od'er-ah) a genus of nematodes. The species *H. radicicola* is parasitic in many edible plants. When these infected plants are ingested by humans, the eggs and larvae may be found in the feces. The eggs (82–120 μ long by 24–43 μ wide) are elongate-ovoidal in shape, with rounded ends and thin shells. Care should be taken in identification to avoid confusion with infertile *Ascaris* or with hookworm eggs. Also called *Meloidogyne javanica.*

heteroduplex (het"er-o-doo'pleks) a molecule formed by annealing two heterologous DNA strands. Where the strands are homologous, they form segments of double-stranded DNA; nonhomologous segments form single-stranded loops or tails.

heterodyne (het"er-o-dīn') pertaining to the mixing of two alternating current signals so that signals are produced at the sum and difference frequencies.

heterofermentation (het"er-o-fer"men-ta'shun) fermentation producing more than one major product.

heterogametic sex the sex which produces gametes differing for the sex chromosomes and thus which determines the sex of the offspring; in humans, the male sex. Cf. *homogametic sex.*

heterogeneic (het"er-o-jen-e'ik) [*hetero-* + *gennan*

to produce] in transplantation biology, denoting individuals or tissues from individuals of different species.

heterogeneic graft see *heterologous g.* under *graft.*

heterogeneous (het″er-o-je′ne-us) [*hetero-* + *genos* kind] consisting of dissimilar elements or ingredients.

heterogeneous nuclear RNA (hnRNA) the probable precursor of messenger RNA (mRNA), so named because its size distribution is heterogeneous and its location is strictly nuclear; no base sequences have been found in cytoplasmic mRNA that are not also represented in hnRNA from the same cell. The half-life of hnRNA is about 1500 sec; at least 80 percent of this RNA is degraded in the nucleus and never reaches the cytoplasm. Some of this must represent degradation, but as hnRNA molecules are precursors of mRNA molecules, a substantial number of nucleotides are removed during processing, removing introns and leaving exons. Heterogeneous nuclear RNA molecules are estimated to be 5–15 kb in length, with very few in the upper range; mRNA molecules, however, are usually less than 1.2 kb long and few exceed 4 kb.

Synthesis of both hnRNA and mRNA shows the same drug sensitivity: inhibition by high concentrations of actinomycin D and low concentrations of α-amanitin. Therefore, hnRNA and mRNA appear to be transcribed by RNA polymerase II.

Some hnRNA molecules contain polyA sequences at their 3′ ends similar to those found on many cytoplasmic mRNA molecules.

See also *ribonucleic acid* and *RNA processing.*

heterogeneous nucleation 1. the crystallization from a metastable solution in vitro by adding a seed crystal or by scratching the wall of the beaker.

2. the formation of bone around the "crystalline" fibers of the collagen matrix; these fibers act as a nucleation catalyst for the transformation of calcium and phosphate in solution in the tissue fluids into the solid-phase mineral deposits.

heterogenote (het′er-o-je″nōt) in bacterial genetics, a merozygote in which the corresponding alleles at a specific locus of the diploid region of the genome are different. See also *merozygote.* Cf. *homogenote.*

heterogony (het″er-og′ŏ-ne) [*hetero-* + *gonos* procreation] see *allometry* and *alternation of generations.*

heterograft (het′er-o-graft) see *heterologous g.* under *graft.*

heterokaryon (het″er-o-kar′e-on) [*hetero-* + Gr. *karyon* nucleus] 1. in fungi, a cell that contains two or more nuclei of different genetic constitutions. The nuclei divide separately when the cell divides.

2. in somatic cell genetics, the state when two cells have fused but their nuclei have not yet fused (the cell becomes a synkaryon when the nuclei fuse).

heterolactic (het″er-o-lak′tik) bacterial fermentation that produces large quantities of lactic acid along with acetic acid, ethanol, and CO_2.

heterologous (het″er-ol′o-gus) [*hetero-* + Gr. *logos* due relation, proportion] 1. composed of tissue not normal to the part.

2. see *xenogeneic.*

heterologous graft see *heterologous g. under graft.*

heterolysosome (het″er-o-li′so-sōm) see *heterophagic vacuole.*

heterolytic (het″er-o-lit′ik) [*hetero-* + Gr. *lysis* dissolution] 1. the destruction of cells of one species by a lysin produced by a different species of cells.

2. in organic chemistry, the severing of a covalent bond involving a carbon atom to produce two oppositely charged fragments ($A{:}B \rightarrow A^+ + {:}B^-$).

heterolytic cleavage (het″er-o-lit′ik klēv′ij) the process of breaking a single covalent bond in such a way that one fragment retains both electrons of the bond, producing ions in the process.

heteromorphic (het″er-o-mor′fik) [*hetero-* + Gr. *morphē* form] in genetics, pertaining to synaptic chromosomes that differ in size, form, or structure.

heteromorphic bivalent a bivalent composed of two chromosomes that are structually different and have matching genes along only part of their lengths, e.g., the XY bivalent or one that has an aberrant chromosome. Cf. *homomorphic bivalent.*

heteromorphic chromosomes see *homologous c.'s* under *chromosome.*

heterophagic (het″er-of′ah-jik) pertaining to heterophagy.

heterophagic vacuole a digestive vacuole formed in the cytoplasm when primary lysosomes fuse with a membrane-bound sac of phagocytosed material (phagocytic vacuole). Also called *heterophagosome* and *heterolysosome.* See also *phagolysosome* and *secondary lysosome.*

heterophagosome (het″er-o-fag′o-sōm) see *heterophagic vacuole.*

heterophagy (het″er-of′ah-je) [*hetero-* + Gr. *phagein* to eat] the process by which cells dispose of phagocytosed material. Primary lysosomes fuse with the membrane-bound sac and discharge their lytic enzymes into it. Material that cannot be completely digested may persist in the cytoplasm as a residual body or be ejected from the cell. See also *lysosome.*

heterophil (het′er-o-fil″) [*hetero-* + Gr. *philein* to live] a cell analogous to polymorphonuclear neutrophils (PMN) in humans. Heterophil granules differ in size and staining reaction according to species. In the rabbit and guinea pig, the granules have a predilection for acid dyes and superficially resemble eosinophils, hence the designation of the cells as "pseudoeosinophilic." Also called *heterophilic leukocyte.*

heterophil antibody an antibody that can interact with heterogeneic (a variety of phylogenetically unrelated species) antigens. This type of antibody may be involved in those disease processes in which a heterophil antibody synthesized against a nonhuman antigen can react with human tissue; for example, in rheumatic heart disease, an antibody produced against a bacterium also reacts with human heart tissue. Heterophil antibodies may be a useful tool in laboratory diagnosis, as is the case with infectious mononucleosis. The antibody produced in this disease, caused by Epstein-Barr virus (EBV), reacts with sheep erythrocytes. It is not known whether a heterotypic antigen on EBV causes its formation.

heterophil antibody test a test for infectious mononucleosis, in which the titer of antibodies to erythrocytes rises during the progression of the disease. Serial dilutions of the patient's serum are added to washed suspensions of erythrocytes in a series of test tubes and incubated. The greatest dilution that agglutinates the erythrocytes is noted. The heterophil antibody cannot be absorbed with guinea pig kidney but can be by ox red cells (a property used to increase the specificity of the test). These properties differentiate it from Forssman antibody, another agglutinin of red blood cells. The antibodies appear in 85–90 percent of adolescents and young adults with infectious mononucleosis, but rarely in children. The titer reaches significant levels during the first week of illness, and peaks in 2–3 wk. The height of the titer has no correlation with the severity of the disease. Commercially available tests use erythrocytes from a variety of species. See also *infectious mononucleosis* and *Paul-Bunnell test.*

heterophilic (het″er-o-fil′ik) 1. having an affinity for other antigens or antibodies besides the one for which it is specific.

2. staining with a type of stain other than the usual one.

heterophilic leukocyte see *heterophil.*

Heterophyes (het″er-of′ĭ-ēz) [*hetero-* + Gr. *phyē* stature] a genus of minute flukes that are parasitic in the small intestines of humans. They are commonly found in Egypt, Japan, southern Korea, Taiwan, central and southern China, the Philippines, and western India. *H. heterophyes* is the most common species. Infection is caused by ingestion of uncooked contaminated fish.

Diagnosis requires identification of eggs found in the feces. They are small (29 by 16 μm), light brown, ovoid, and operculate. Care should be taken to differentiate them from other heterophyid trematodes.

heterophyiasis (het″er-o-fi-i′ah-sis) infected with flukes of the genus *Heterophyes.*

heteroploid (het′er-o-ploid″) 1. pertaining to heteroploidy.

2. an individual or cell with an abnormal number of chromosomes.

heteroploidy (het′er-o-ploi″de) the state of having an abnormal number of chromosomes.

heteropolymer (het″er-o-pol′ĭ-mer) [*hetero-* + *poly-* + Gr. *meros* part] a polymer formed from monomer units that are not all the same, e.g., a protein or a complex polysaccharide. See also *polymer.*

heteropolysaccharide (het″er-o-pol″e-sak′ah-rīd) any polysaccharide macromolecule that contains two or more different sugars.

heteropyknotic (het″er-o-pik-not′ik) referring to chromosomal regions that are more (positively heteropyknotic) or less (negatively heteropyknotic) tightly coiled than most of the chromosomal material of a cell. These differences are detected by the degree of staining with Giemsa or other chromosomal stains. Cf. *isopyknotic.*

heteroscedasticity (het″er-o-ske″das-tis′ĭ-te) the property of having unequal variances. Cf. *homoscedasticity.*

heterosexual (het″er-o-seks′u-al) [*hetero-* + L. *sexualis*] 1. pertaining to the opposite sex; directed toward a person of the opposite sex; the opposite of homosexual.

2. one who is sexually attracted to persons of the opposite sex.

heterosis (het″er-o′sis) [Gr. *heterōsis* alternation] hybrid vigor, the greater vigor as measured by the growth, survival, and fertility exhibited by the hybrid crosses between two inbred strains. The mechanism of heterosis is an increase in heterozygosity. The hybrid usually has fewer genes that are homozygous for deleterious alleles than does either parent, but direct positive effects are also present.

heterosomal pertaining to a heterosome.

heterosomal aberration see *interchromosomal aberration.*

heterosome (het″er-o-sōm) one of a group of heteromorphic chromosomes. Cf. *autosome.*

heterothallism (het″er-o-thal′izm) a mating system of perfect fungi that requires the fusion of nuclei derived from different mating strains to produce a sexual spore. Because different mating strains are required, this process results in genetic heterogeneity. Cf. *homothallism.*

heterotopic (het″er-o-top′ik) occurring at an abnormal place or on the wrong part of the body.

heterotopic graft a tissue transplant from one location in the body to another location. Cf. *orthotopic graft.*

heterotroph (het′er-o-trōf) feeding on others; an organism, such as an animal or microorganism, that requires carbon in organic compounds found in plants or other animals for food and energy. Also called *chemoheterotroph* and *organotroph.* See also *photoheterotroph.* Cf. *autotroph.*

heterotrophic (het″er-o-trōf′ik) pertaining to heterotrophs.

heterozygote (het″er-o-zi′gōt) an individual that is heterozygous for a particular gene.

manifesting h., a female heterozygous for an X-linked trait, in whom the trait is expressed about as severely as in a hemizygous male due to X inactivation. See also *Lyon hypothesis.*

heterozygous (het″er-o-zi′gus) in genetics, having two different alleles of a particular gene and therefore the ability to pass either allele onto an offspring. A heterozygous individual will have characteristics produced by the dominant allele, or by both together if they are codominant. Cf. *hemizygous* and *homozygous.*

HETP abbrev. for height equivalent to a theoretical plate. See under *theoretical plate.*

heuristic (hu-ris′tik) [Gr. *heuriskein* to find out] useful in discovery or exploration but not having a mathematical proof; the term is used to describe an argument or solution to a problem that is plausible but lacks logical rigor.

h. method, a problem-solving approach in which there is no predetermined formula for obtaining a solution. The heuristic approach is exploratory in that a variety of different methods, in combination or sequence, may be brought to bear on a problem and, after each step in the process, an evaluation is made of the progress toward a solution. Cf. *algorithm.*

hex/a (hek′sa) [Gr. *hex* six] a word element used in combining form to denote six, e.g., hexose.

hexachlorobenzene (hek″sah-klor″o-ben′zēn) a white crystalline solid, C_6Cl_6, used as a fungicide; M.W. 284.40. Poisoning due to chronic ingestion has resulted in cases of porphyria cutanea tarda. Hexachlorobenzene should not be confused with benzene hexachloride (BHC), $C_6H_6Cl_6$.

1,2,3,4,5,6-hexachlorocyclohexane (HCH) a highly toxic insecticide. Some isomers are nerve poisons that can cause convulsions; others are central nervous system depressants. Also called *ben-*

zene hexachloride (BHC). See also *chlorinated hydrocarbon pesticide assays* and *lindane.*

hexachlorophene (hek″sah-klo′ro-fēn) an antibacterial substance used in emulsion with detergents for skin cleaning before surgery. It should not be used on infants or on wounds or burns because of the central nervous system effects it causes when absorbed. If swallowed, hexachlorophene can cause convulsions, shock, and death. Trademark for hexachlorophene detergent emulsion, pHisoHex.

hexachlorophene assay performed by extraction from blood into a mixture of ethanol and ether. An acetyl derivative is formed by reaction with acetic anhydride and pyridine in benzene. The derivative is analyzed by gas chromatography using an electron capture detector and a nonpolar stationary phase. Concentrations as low as 5 mg/l can be detected.

hexadecimal (hek″sah-des′ĭ-mal) pertaining to the base 16 number system that is used in computers. The 16 hexadecimal digits are usually represented by the symbols: 0, 1, 2, 3, 4, 5, 6, 7, 8, 9, A, B, C, D, E, F. See also *number system.*

hexamer (heks′ah-mer) 1. a polymer molecule composed of six monomers.

2. a capsomer having six structural subunits.

hexamethonium bromide (hek″sah-mĕ-tho′ne-um) $[(CH_3)_3N^+—(CH_2)_6-N^+(CH_3)_3]\cdot 2Br^-$, a quaternary ammonium compound that produces ganglion blocking by occupying receptor sites and by stabilizing the postsynaptic membranes against the action of acetylcholine.

hexamethylenetetramine (hek″sah-meth″il-ēn-tet′rah-mēn) see *methenamine.*

hexamethyl-melamine (hek″sah-meth″il mel′ah-mēn) a cancer chemotherapeutic drug. For more information, see *Appendix A.*

hexamethylpararosanilin (hek″sah-meth″il-par″-ah-ro-san′ĭ-lin) see *crystal violet.*

hexane (hek′sān) 1. a colorless, volatile, flammable liquid with a faint odor, *n*-hexane, $CH_3(CH_2)_4CH_3$, used as a solvent; M.W. 86.17. It is a component of gasoline and petroleum ether. Hexane is moderately toxic, an upper respiratory tract irritant, and a narcotic at high concentrations.

2. any six-carbon alkane.

hexanoic acid (hek″san-o′ik) see *caproic acid.*

hexavalent (hek″sah-va′lent) see *sexivalent.*

hexobarbital (hek″so-bar′bĭ-tal) [NF], a short acting 1,5,5 trisubstituted barbiturate used to produce sedation before and after anesthesia.

hexokinase (HK) (hek″so-ki′nās) an enzyme of the transferase class (ATP:D-hexose-6-phosphotransferase, EC 2.7.1.1) that catalyzes the reaction ATP + D-hexose ⇄ ADP + D-hexose-6-phosphate. Mannose, fructose, and glucosamine can serve as PO_4 acceptors; inosine triphosphate may also serve as a PO_4 donor. Isoenzyme forms of the enzyme exist. Hexokinase occurs in the brain and liver and catalyzes the first step in the metabolism of glucose. Because of its analytic specificity, the hexokinase reaction is used for the clinical laboratory determination of glucose in body fluids.

hexosamine (heks″ōs-am″in) a nitrogenous sugar in which an amino group replaces a hydroxyl group.

hexosaminidase (hek″sos-ah-min′i-dās) an enzyme of the hydrolase class (2-acetamido-2-deoxy-β-D-galactoside acetamidodeoxygalactohydrolase, EC 3.2.1.53) having two isoenzymes, A and B, which catalyze the removal of β-*N*-acetylgalactosamine residues from G_{M2}-ganglioside. Deficiencies or partial deficiencies of one or both isoenzymes are responsible for the various G_{M2}-gangliosidoses. The recommended name is *β-N-acetyl-D-galatosaminidase.*

h. A., an isoenzyme of hexosaminidase. A deficiency in the enzyme, occurring especially in Jewish populations, is the cause of Tay-Sachs disease, which results in progressive blindness and degeneration of the central nervous system in affected children. The disease is identified by an absence of this enzyme in the amniotic fluid cells of the unborn fetus. Carriers of the trait have lowered cell levels of this enzyme, permitting screening of suspected populations and genetic counseling of carriers thus identified.

hexose (hek′sōs) a monosaccharide containing six carbon atoms.

h. diphosphate, a diester of a hexose with phosphoric acid, e.g., fructose-1,6-bisphosphate. Also called *hexose bisphosphate.*

h. monophosphate, see *hexosephosphate.*

hexose monophosphate shunt (hek″sōs mon″o-fos′fāt) see *pentose phosphate pathway.*

hexosephosphate (hek″sōs-fos′fāt) an ester of a hexose with phosphoric acid, e.g., glucose-6-phosphate, glucose-1-phosphate, and fructose-6-phosphate.

hexosephosphate dehydrogenase (hek″sōs-fos′fāt de-hi′dro-jen-ās) see *glucose-6-phosphate dehydrogenase.*

hexosephosphate isomerase (hek″sōs-fos′fāt i-som′er-ās) see *glucosephosphate isomerase.*

hexose-1-phosphate uridyltransferase (hek′sōs fos′fāt u″ri-dil-trans′fer-ās) see *UDPglucose-hexose-1-phosphate uridylyltransferase.*

hexosephosphoric esters (hek″sōs-fos-fōr′ik) the four esters involved in the chemical processes of muscle contraction and the fermentation of glucose by yeast: the Cori ester (glucose-1-phosphate), the Harden-Young ester (fructofuranose bisphosphate), the Neuberg ester (fructose-6-phosphate), and the Robison ester (glucose-6-phosphate).

hexuronate (hek″su-ron′āt) the anion of a hexuronic acid.

hexuronic acid (hek″su-ron′ik) a member of the class of tetrahydroxy aldehyde acids obtained from the aldohexose sugars by oxidation of the C-6 hydroxyl group to a carboxylic acid; glucuronic acid and iduronic acid are examples.

hexylresorcinol (hek″sil-rĕ-zor′sĭ-nol) [NF], 4-hexyl-1,3-dihydroxybenzene, existing as white crystals and soluble in ether, chloroform, acetone, alcohol, and vegetable oils. Hexylresorcinol is used as a topical skin antiseptic and as an agent for the treatment of intestinal roundworms and trematodes.

Hf symbol for the chemical element *hafnium.*

Hfr mutant abbrev. See *high-frequency recombination mutant.*

hFSH abbrev. for human follicle-stimulating hormone. See *follicle-stimulating hormone.*

Hg [L. *hydrargyrum,* from Gr. *hydrarguros* "silver water"] symbol for the chemical element *mercury.*

H gene a gene that produces a fucosal transferase.

It has two alleles, H and the rare amorph h. Individuals homozygous for h allele lack the transferase and cannot attach fucose to galactose on the precursor substance, and H substance cannot be produced. This results in the O_h or Bombay blood type.

HGF abbrev. for hyperglycemic-glycogenolytic factor. See under *glucagon.*

hGH abbrev. for human growth hormone. See *growth hormone.*

HHT 12-L-hydroxy-5,8,10-heptadecatrienoic acid, a product of the nonenzymatic breakdown of prostaglandin H_2, which has no apparent biologic activity.

5-HIAA abbrev. See *5-hydroxyindole acetic acid.*

hiatus (hi-a'tus) [L.] [NA], a gap, cleft, or opening in a structure or organ.

hibernoma (hi"ber-no'mah) a tumor of brown fat cells. It is rare, is usually benign, and occurs in the soft tissues of the axilla or upper back. See also *brown fat.*

Hickey position (hik'e) a radiographic position used to obtain posterior tangential views of the mastoid tips. The patient is supine, with the head resting on the film cassette on a caudally inclined 15°-angle block and rotated so that the median sagittal plane makes a 55°angle with the horizontal. The central ray is directed vertically through the anterior border of the mastoid process on the upper side.

HiCN abbrev. See *cyanomethemoglobin.*

hidr/o (hid'ro) [Gr. *hidrōs* sweat] a word element used in combining form to denote sweat, e.g., hidrocystoma.

hidradenitis (hi"drad-ĕ-ni'tis) [*hidro-* + Gr. *adēn* gland + *-itis* inflammation] the inflammation of an apocrine sweat gland, often due to staphylococci. It has a tendency to recur and heals in a scarring manner.

h. suppurativa, a recurrent suppurative infection of the apocrine sweat glands, often in the area of the axillae or groin. Commonly, there is occlusion of the ducts, with bacterial infection (often staphylococcal) and inflammation. These lesions are slow to drain and heal, and often scar.

hidradenoma (hi"drad-ĕ-no'mah) [*hidro-* + *adenoma*] a tumor of apocrine gland cells, occurring most commonly in the vulva. It is composed of elaborate glandular and papillary structures supported by a delicate connective tissue stroma. It is benign but can readily be mistaken for an adenocarcinoma.

hidrocystoma (hid"ro-sis-to'mah) [*hidro-* + *cystoma*] a retention cyst in an apocrine gland.

high-altitude acclimatization the adaptive mechanisms that are triggered by, and result in an increased tolerance to, the chronic hypoxic stress (decreased in Po_2 of the ambient air) present at high altitudes. The physiologic effects of the lower O_2 availability are felt during rest and activity between altitudes of 6500 and 9840 ft (2000–3000 m), becoming increasingly severe with higher elevations. Limits to human tolerance are reached at about 33,000 ft (8545 m).

Initial exposure to high altitude commonly causes a varying group of symptoms (headache, dyspnea, insomnia, lethargy, decreased mental proficiency, nausea and, when severe, chest rales, cyanosis, and cerebral edema), known collectively as acute mountain sickness. In individuals lacking the ability to acclimatize, these symptoms do not diminish within several days or weeks but persist as chronic mountain sickness (Monge's disease).

The physiologic, biochemical, and anatomic adaptations that occur on both a short- and a long-term basis (some of which may occur during growth and development in the highland native) are directed toward increasing the pulmonary ventilation, the diffusing gradient of O_2 at the lungs and systemic tissues, the oxygen-carrying capacity of the blood, the lung volume, and the effectiveness of the utilization of available O_2 at tissues.

After initial exposure to high altitude, minute ventilation may reach a value 65 percent above that at sea level. This hyperventilatory response, mediated by hypoxic stimulation of the arterial chemoreceptors, leads to a nonadaptive decrease in alveolar, arterial, and cerebrospinal fluid (CSF) Pco_2; if uncompensated for, this results in respiratory alkalosis. With several days to weeks of exposure, a further increase in ventilation (up to three to seven times the sea level value) and decrease in Pco_2 occur. In addition, the ventilatory response to a given level of alveolar Pco_2 is augmented. This initial ventilatory acclimatization of the high-altitude sojourner is thought to be a consequence of the following sequence of physiologic events: There is an initial exposure to hypoxia, which induces a peripheral chemoreceptor-mediated increase in ventilation, which results in decreased arterial and CSF Pco_2. The pH of the CSF consequently increases, stimulating an active transport of HCO_3^- out of the CSF (which acts to decrease CSF pH) and partially inhibiting the extent of peripheral chemoreflex-induced hyperventilation. Within 7–10 da, the CSF pH is restored to sea level values, ceasing inhibition of the peripheral chemoreceptor drive and thus allowing for a further increase in ventilation. Because the CSF [HCO_3^-] is low, the ventilatory response mediated by the central chemoreceptors will exhibit an increased sensitivity at any given level of CSF pH. The changes in ventilation and Pa_{CO_2} with high altitude thus increase as a function of the time of exposure, as well as with the height of ascent above sea level.

high-density lipoprotein see *high-density l.* under *lipoprotein.*

high-energy phosphate any phosphate compound having one or more energy-rich phosphate bonds that on hydrolysis have a standard free-energy change ($\Delta G°$) between –5000 and –13000 cal/mol (21,000–54,400 J/mol).

Classes of such compounds include phosphoric acid anhydrides, phosphoric esters of enols, and phosphamic acid derivatives (R—NH—PO_3H). Examples of such compounds are acetyladenylate, phosphoenolpyruvate, cyclic AMP and cyclic GMP, ATP (inner and terminal bonds), phosphocreatine, 1,3-diphosphoglycerate, and acetyl phosphate.

high-frequency (bizarre) discharge the series of polyphasic muscle action potentials, of as yet uncertain physiologic origin, that begins spontaneously or after electrode movement or voluntary muscle contraction. The potentials have a constant amplitude (in the range of 100 μV–1 mV) and configuration and discharge at a uniform frequency of 5–100 Hz. Their onset and cessation are abrupt. This complex, repetitive discharge is nonspecific and may occur in individuals with chronic partial denervation, muscular dystrophy, or polymyositis. See also the accompanying illustration.

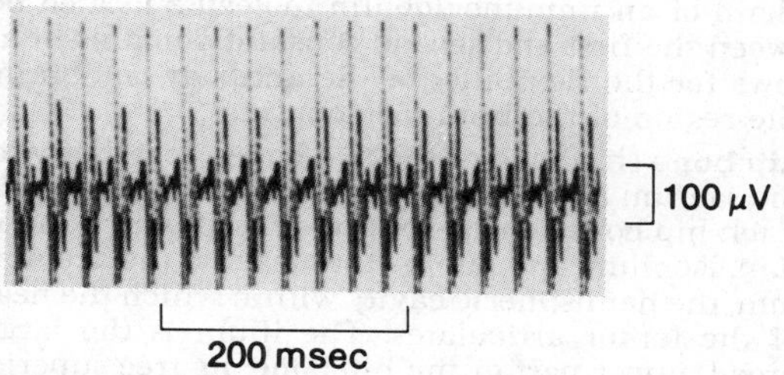

High-frequency (bizarre) discharge. Spontaneous, high-frequency discharge of action potentials in a partially denervated muscle. (From Aminoff, M. J.: Electromyography in Clinical Practice. Menlo Park, CA, Addison-Wesley Publishing Co., 1978.)

high-frequency recombination (Hfr) mutant an F+ cell in which the F plasmid has become integrated into the bacterial chromosome so that, in conjugation, transfer of the initiating segment of the plasmid is followed by the chromosome. Recombination with such mutants is increased 1000-fold. See also *conjugation* and *F p.* under *plasmid.*

high level the more positive of the two output levels of a digital logic circuit.

high-level language a computer language such as BASIC, FORTRAN, OR PL/I, in which programs can be written. The programs are processed by another program, either a compiler or an interpreter, which gives machine language instructions to the computers that carry out the programmed procedure.

Highman's Congo red technique a diazo dye staining technique in which the dye attaches to amyloid fibers parallel to their plane of orientation, thus giving a green birefringence in polarized light. Sections are stained in an alcoholic Congo red solution, differentiated in potassium hydroxide, and counterstained with alum hematoxylin. Amyloid appears pink to red and, in polarized light, exhibits the diagnostic green birefringence and dichroism.

Highman's method for amyloid a technique for staining amyloid that employs either crystal violet or methyl violet dye. Sections are initially stained in Weigert's iron hematoxylin and, after washing, are restained in methyl violet (or crystal violet). Amyloid appears reddish-purple; the nuclei, blue to black. Thick (12-μm) sections stained by this technique permit demonstration of minute quantities of amyloid.

high-order pertaining to the most significant digit, bit, or byte of a computer word or register.

high-pressure liquid chromatography (HPLC) a chromatographic technology used to separate and quantitate mixtures of substances in solution. It is particularly useful in pharmacology and toxicology, where its versatility and precision make it the most suitable method of assay for most organic compounds.

PRINCIPLES OF OPERATION. The sample is injected into a moving stream of solvent, which flows through a column and detector. The passage through the column separates the sample compounds by one of four different methods: adsorption, partition, ion exchange, or size exclusion. Water-soluble ionic compounds are best separated by ion-exchange or normal-phase partition. Water-insoluble nonpolar compounds are best separated by adsorption or reversed-phase partition. Non-ionic polar compounds are separated by partition or adsorption. Size exclusion is effective only when there are very large differences between the molecular weights and sizes of the components. The solvent is pumped through the system at a controlled pressure, which can be varied between 500 and 5000 psi.

ELUTION MODES. In isocratic elution, the composition of the solvent remains constant during the analysis. This may produce long retention times and decrease the sensitivity for some sample components. In gradient elution, the composition of the solvent is continuously varied during the analysis. In flow programming, the flow rate is increased continuously during the analysis. The latter two methods speed up multicomponent analyses, but they cannot be used with some detectors and may decrease the clarity and efficiency of separation.

DETECTORS. The most widely used detectors are fixed wavelength or variable wavelength ultraviolet-visible photometers. The variable wavelength photometers have good specificity and sensitivity, and can detect nanogram quantities of most substances. Fluorometers have a high sensitivity for fluorescent compounds. Electrochemical detectors have very high sensitivity for compounds that can undergo oxidation-reduction reactions. They measure the sample concentration either by amperometry or by polarography. The refractive index detector is widely used in exclusion chromatography but is less sensitive than ultraviolet detectors.

ASSAYS. HPLC is used for the separation and quantitation of steroid hormones; pesticides and other ecologic poisons; toxic and carcinogenic compounds in drinking water; drugs (especially for drug abuse or drug overdose analysis); and also for the study of the metabolism of carcinogens and drugs. In a typical assay procedure, the substances of interest (analytes) are coassayed with an internal standard, a substance of the same chemical class having the same recovery efficiency in the extraction steps of the specimen preparation and comparable separation and detection characteristics. With the particular column and elution method used for the assay, the elution times relative to the internal standard characterize the compounds and are used to identify them. The peak areas relative to the internal standard are proportional to their concentration in the sample and are used to quantitate them.

Also called high-performance liquid chromatography. See also *chromatography.* Cf. *gas chromatography.*

high voltage pertaining to the circuit in a piece of electrical equipment that has the highest operating voltage (about 300 V in vacuum tube amplifiers, 10 kV in cathode ray tube [CRT] displays, and 100 kV in diagnostic x-ray machines).

high-voltage transformer a transformer that steps up the power line voltage to that required for the high-voltage circuit. In x-ray equipment, it steps up 230 V to about 150 kVp and is immersed in oil, which provides electrical insulation while conducting heat.

HiHb abbrev. for hemiglobin. See *methemoglobin.*

Hill equation a modification of the Michaelis-Menten equation used originally to describe the binding of oxygen to hemoglobin and later to describe the cooperativity among the catalytic sites of an allosteric enzyme. It is not theoretically rigorous but does provide a good empirical description.

For the case of a multimeric enzyme in which the binding of the substrate to one active site changes the conformation and influences the substrate affinity at the other active sites, the Hill equation is $\log (v/(V_{max} - v)) = n_H \log [S] - \log K$, where v is the reaction velocity, V_{max} is the maximal reaction velocity, [S] is the substrate concentration, K is a constant analogous to the Michaelis constant, and n_H is the Hill coefficient. For $n_H = 1$, the logarithmic form of the Michaelis-Menten equation, there is no cooperativity. For $n_H < 0$, there is negative cooperativity; binding of substrate reduces the affinity at other sites. For $n_H > 0$, there is positive cooperativity; binding of the substrate increases the affinity at other sites. In this case, the usual Michaelis-Menton plot of v against [S] is sigmoidal (S shaped) rather than hyperbolic. The value of n_H does not exceed the number of sites at which the substrate can be bound (usually the number of subunits of the allosteric enzyme).

For the case of hemoglobin, a tetrameric transport protein that can bind four oxygen (O_2) molecules, each molecule bound facilitating the binding of the next, the Hill equation is $\log (So_2/(1 - So_2)) = n_H(\log Po_2 - \log P_{50})$, where Po_2 is the partial pressure of oxygen, So_2 is the oxygen saturation (the bound oxygen expressed as a fraction of the capacity of four molecules of O_2 per molecule of hemoglobin), and P_{50} is the Po_2 at half saturation (at $So_2 = 0.5$). A plot of logit So_2 against log Po_2 is a straight line with a slope n_H, which for hemoglobin is 2.7 ± 0.2.

See also *Michaelis-Menten equation.*

hilum (hi'lum), pl. *hila* [L.] see *hilus.*

hilus (hi'lus,), pl. *hili* [L. "a small thing"] [NA], a general term for a depression or pit at the site in an organ where vessels and nerves enter. It is often used alone to designate the hilus of the kidney or lung. Also called *hilum.*

hilus cells cells that are morphologically identical with testicular Leydig cells (vestiges of the provisional male-directed gonad), located in the hilus of the ovary and the mesovarium, which secrete androgenic steroids. They represent the cell of origin of hilus cell tumors of the ovary, and one cell constituent of virilizing ovarian androblastoma and some types of gonadoblastoma. See also *ovarian tumors.*

Hind II a restriction endonuclease from *Hemophilus influenzae* that hydrolyzes double-stranded DNA between the pyrimidine-purine site of the sequence GTPyrPuAC and the purine-pyrimidine site of the palindromic complement. See also *restriction endonuclease.*

Hind III a restriction endonuclease from *Hemophilus influenzae* that hydrolyzes double-stranded DNA between the AA of the sequence AAGCTT and the AA site of the palindromic complement. See also *restriction endonuclease.*

hindbrain (hīnd'brān) see *rhombencephalon.*

hindgut (hīnd'gut) that part of the embryonic elementary canal caudal to the umbilical opening. It is supplied by the inferior mesenteric artery. The hindgut gives rise to the distal transverse colon, descending colon, sigmoid, and rectum.

hinge region an amino acid sequence in the heavy chain of an immunoglobulin molecule located between the first and second constant domains. It allows for the flexibility of the antibody combining site region of the immunoglobulin.

hip bone (hip) one of the two bones, together with the sacrum and coccyx, that form the pelvic girdle. Each hip bone consists of three fused parts—the ilium, ischium, and pubis—that meet at the acetabulum, the hemispheric cavity within which the head of the femur articulates. The ilium is the large, broad, upper part of the hip bone; its free superior margin forms the iliac crest. The pubis and ischium enclose the obturator foramen, and the right and left pubes meet at the pubic symphysis. The thickened posterior part of the ischium that bears the weight when sitting is the ischial tuberosity. Also called *innominate bone.*

hip joint the ball and socket synovial joint between the head of the femur and the acetabulum of the pelvis.

Hippelates (hip″ĕ-la'tēz) a genus of insects of the order Diptera, family Chloropidae. These flies, known as the eye gnats, are small, measure 0.5–2.5 mm in length, and feed off sebaceous secretions, blood, or pus. Several species are known transmitters of human disease such as conjunctivitis and yaws, especially in the United States, Mexico, Haiti, and Jamacia.

Hippel's disease (hip'elz) see *von Hippel's disease.*

Hippeutis (hi-pu'tis) a genus of mollusks that may serve as hosts for *Fasciolopsis buski* (a fluke) throughout China, North Vietnam, and Taiwan.

hippocampus (hip″o-kam'pus) [Gr. *hippokampos* sea horse] [NA], in the brain, an elongated, curved swelling in the floor of the inferior horn of the lateral ventricle. Consisting of the dentate gyrus and the horn of Ammon, it resembles a sea horse when viewed in coronal section. Afferent information reaches the hippocampus primarily from the entorhinal cortex and subicular regions, with some afferent fibers arising from the cingulate gyrus, septal nuclei, and reticular formation. All efferent information leaves the hippocampus via the fornix.

Hippuran I 131 (hip'u-ran) see under *iodohippurate.*

hippuric acid (hĭ-pu'rik) [Gr. *hippos* horse + *ouron* urine] C_6H_5—CO—NH—CH_2—COOH, a crystallizable acid primarily found in the urine of domestic animals, but also in human urine. Because it is formed in the liver, its rate of excretion after oral administration of benzoic acid was formerly employed as a liver function test. Also called *benzoylaminocetic acid, benzoylglycine,* and *urobenzoic acid.*

hippuric acid excretion test an obsolete test to measure the conjugating ability of the liver.

Hipputope (hip'u-tōp) see under *iodohippurate.*

Hirschsprung's disease (hirsh'sproongz) [Harald *Hirschsprung,* Danish physician, 1830–1916] see *aganglionic m.* under megacolon.

hirsutism (her'sūt-izm) excessive hairiness, especially in females. This condition may be diffuse or localized and congenital or acquired. It is often due to genetic and hormonal factors and occasionally may be the first sign of a neoplastic disease. Some therapeutic treatments, including steroid drugs, may also induce hirsutism.

Hirudinea (hir″u-din′e-ah) a class of leeches that includes the genera *Haementeria, Hirudo, Hirudinaria, Haemadipsa, Limnatis, Macrobdella,* and *Haemopis.*

Hirudo (hĭ-roo′do), pl. *hirudines* [L. "leech"] a genus of leeches of the class Hirudinea.

H. aegyptiaca, see *Limnatis.*

His abbrev. See *histidine.*

His bundle [Wilhelm *His,* Jr., Swiss physician, 1863–1934] see *atrioventricular bundle.*

His bundle electrocardiography [Wilhelm *His,* Jr.] an intracardiac technique used to record the electrical events of the right atrium atrioventricular (A-V) node and His bundle, areas of the heart that are silent on electrocardiograms recorded from body surface leads.

A J-shaped catheter with three ring electrodes at its tip is passed through the femoral vein and advanced to a position in proximity to the tricuspid valve. The three bipolar intracardiac electrograms obtained are displayed on an oscilloscope simultaneously with the tracings from three or more standard electrocardiographic leads and recorded. Waves of depolorization, consisting of A (atrial depolarization), H (His bundle depolarization), and V deflections (depolarization of the ventricular septum), are characteristically seen. The measurement of the various intervals between these deflections, the P-A, A-H, and H-V intervals, can be of value in determining the site, extent, and mechanism of (and thus the appropriate therapy for) a particular conduction defect or arrhythmia. See also the accompanying illustration.

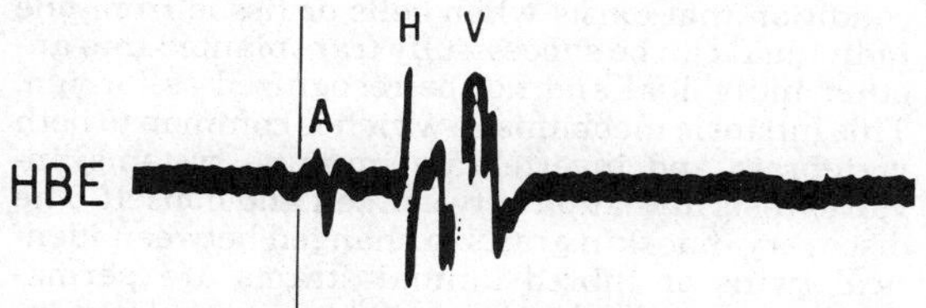

His bundle electrocardiography. His bundle bipolar electrogram (HBE); A, atrial depolarization; H, depolarization of the His bundle; and V, depolarization of the upper ventricular septum. The P-A interval represents intraatrial conduction time (upper to lower atrium); A-H represents atrioventricular nodal conduction; H-V represents the His-Purkinje conduction time; and the thin vertical line indicates the onset of atrial activation. (Adapted from Braunwald, E., Heart Disease. Philadelphia, W. B. Saunders Co., 1980.)

His bundle electrogram (HBE) [Wilhelm *His,* Jr.] a record of the electrical activity obtained from intracardiac electrodes positioned in the vicinity of the septum above and below the tricuspid valve. See also *His bundle electrocardiography.*

hist/o (his′to) [Gr. *histos* web, tissue] a word element used in combining form to denote tissue, e.g., histology.

histadyl (his′tah-dil) the acyl radical derived from or relating to histidine.

Histalog (his′tah-log) trademark. See *betazole hydrochloride.*

histamine (his′tah-mēn) an amine, β-imidazolylethylamine, formed by decarboxylation of histidine and occurring in many plants, bacteria, and mammalian tissues; M.W. 111.15. Histamine is synthesized and secreted mainly by mast cells of the tissues and circulating basophils. It is a powerful vasodilator, dilating the terminal arterioles, increasing capillary permeability, and causing a drop in blood pressure. It also causes constriction of bronchial smooth muscles of the lungs. Histamine is also synthesized and secreted by certain types of gastric mucosal cells as well as other tissue cells (histaminocytes). In the stomach it is the final common mediator of gastric HCl secretion. Histamine generally increases glandular secretion (e.g., sweat, adrenal, salivary, and bronchial secretions), and is also implicated as one of many mediators of immediate hypersensitivity.

The various actions of histamine are due to the presence of two types of receptors, H_1 and H_2, in the target cells. The contraction of smooth muscle in various organs (gut, bronchi) is mediated by H_1 receptors, and the conventional antihistamine drugs such a diphenhydramine and pyrilamine are H_1-receptor antagonists used in the management of various allergic disorders. The secretion of hydrochloric acid by the stomach and an increase in heart rate are mediated by H_2-receptors; these actions are antagonized by H_2-receptor blockers, e.g., cimetidine, metiamide. The H_2-receptor blockers have been useful in the control of gastric acid secretion and are thus helpful in the treatment of gastric ulcers. Histamine is metabolized rapidly in the liver, and its two main metabolites—methylimidazolacetic acid and imidazolacetic acid–riboside—are secreted in the urine.

histamine headache see *cluster h.* under *headache.*

histi/o (his′te-o) [Gr. *histion,* diminutive of histos web, tissue] a word element used in combining form to denote tissue, e.g., histiocyte.

histidase (his′tĭs-dās) see *L*-histidine ammonia-lyase.

histidinase (his′tĭ-dĭ-nās) see *L-histidine ammonia-lyase.*

histidine (His) (his′tĭ-dēn) 2-amino-3-(4-imidazolyl)propanoic acid, $(C_3H_3N_2)CH_2CH(NH_2)COOH$, a naturally occurring amino acid that is nonessential for adults but essential for optimal growth in infants; M.W. 155.16. Present in proteins, it is involved in conformational changes of hemoglobin when binding oxygen (Bohr effect), and in forming cross-links in collagen. Substances formed from it are carnosine, formiminoglutamate (FIGLU), histamine, urocanate, and one-carbon groups. Blood levels are elevated in histidinemia. Its source is from dietary protein. See also under *amino acids.*

L-histidine ammonia-lyase (his′tĭ-dēn ah-mo′ne-ah li′ās) an enzyme of the lyase class (EC 4.3.1.3) that catalyzes the reaction L-histidine ⇄ urocanate + NH_3. A genetic deficiency of the enzyme, transmitted as an autosomal recessive trait, causes histidinemia. Also called *histidase, histidinase,* and *histidine α-deaminase.*

histidine α-deaminase (his′tĭ-dēn de-am′ĭ-nās) see *L*-histidine ammonia-lyase.

histidinemia (his″tĭ-dĭ-ne′me-ah) a hereditary metabolic disorder, transmitted genetically as an autosomal recessive trait, which results in excessive amounts of histidine in the blood and the urine. It is thought to be due to abnormal or deficient histidinase (L-histidine ammonia-lyase) activity. Affected patients may be normal, be mentally retarded, and/or have abnormal speech development. See also *aminoacidopathy*.

histidinuria (his″tĭ-dĭ-nu′re-ah) the presence of excess histidine in the urine due to various disorders that affect the normal metabolism of histidine. See also *aminoacidopathy* and *histidinemia*.

histiocyte (his′te-o-sīt″) [*histio-* + Gr. *kytos* hollow vessel] see under *macrophage*.

histiocytic (his″te-o-sit′ik) pertaining to histiocytes.

histiocytic lymphoma a malignant lymphoma in which the proliferating cells are transformed B lymphocytes. Formerly called reticulum cell sarcoma, and currently also called large cell lymphoma. See also *malignant l.* under *lymphoma*.

histiocytic medullary reticulosis a subleukemic form of monocytic leukemia characterized by extreme hyperplasia of the histiocytes. It is a severe and fatal disease with generalized node enlargement, hepatosplenomegaly, and severe anemia; reticulocytosis is moderate. Phagocytosis of erythrocytes, granulocytes, and platelets by abnormal histiocytic elements, primarily in the bone marrow, is diagnostic. Also called histiocytic leukemia, malignant histiocytosis, and medullary histiocytosis.

histiocytoma (his″te-o-si-to′mah) [*histiocyte* + *-oma*] a lesion formed by a proliferation of histiocytes. It is a localized form of chronic inflammation. Also used synonymously but incorrectly with *dermatofibroma*.

histiocytosis (his″te-o-si-to′sis) one of a group of diseases characterized by a proliferation of histiocytes that contain cytoplasmic Langerhans' granules. These cells are probably a specific family of histiocytes concerned with skin surveillance, as the epidermal Langerhans' cell is of similar appearance. They have been shown to possess IgA surface receptors.

Three clinical entities are recognized. They may be grouped as localized (eosinophilic granuloma) and systemic (Hand-Schüller-Christian disease, Letterer-Siwe disease). In 1953, Lichtenstein suggested the term histiocytosis X to indicate the similar histopathology of the three disorders; other terms used have included reticuloendotheliosis, proliferative histiocytosis, and differentiated histiocytosis.

localized h., eosinophilic granuloma, a localized form of histiocytosis that frequently involves bone but may affect soft tissues. In bone it is usually solitary and is most common in the third and fourth decades. It forms a circumscribed lytic lesion, and biopsy shows a proliferation of histiocytes with eosinophils. The histiocytes have folded or indented nuclei and contain Langerhans' granules in varying numbers. A solitary bone lesion can be treated by curettage or radiation, but close follow-up is necessary because of the possibility that it may be part of a more widespread process.

The condition may occur in the soft tissues or lungs; those affected are usually young adults. A lung lesion may appear localized on x-ray, but when a diffuse infiltrate is present the term pulmonary histiocytosis is more appropriate, because extensive lung involvement indicates a poor prognosis. Biopsy is necessary to establish the diagnosis and distinguish the lesion from nonspecific chronic inflammatory processes. The possibility that an apparently solitary lesion is part of a more widespread process must always be investigated.

malignant h., see *histiocytic medullary reticulosis*.

systemic h., the form of histiocytosis that includes two recognized disseminated forms, Hand-Schüller-Christian disease and Letterer-Siwe disease. Each has a broad spectrum of clinical expression, and they cannot be clearly separated. Involvement of the region of the base of the skull has been associated with Hand-Schüller-Christian disease, producing lytic lesions in the skull bones, diabetes insipidus, and exophthalmos. The course is generally more prolonged than in the typical case of Letterer-Siwe disease, in which an infant has a hemorrhagic rash, lymphadenopathy, and hepatosplenomegaly, and the disease progresses rapidly. The more extensive the systemic histiocytosis, the poorer the prognosis, and the older the patient, the better the chance of recovery. Histologic sections of involved areas show a proliferation of histiocytes, but eosinophils are often fewer than in the solitary bone lesions. Langerhans' granules can usually be identified within the cytoplasm of the histiocytes by electron microscopy.

histochemistry (his″to-kem′is-tre) the study of the chemical composition of cells and tissues; the localization of a particular compound in cells or tissue as demonstrated by specific stains or autoradiography.

Histoclad (his′to-klad) trademark for a synthetic resin mounting medium used in histology. It has an index of refraction of 1.54 (as a solid).

histocompatibility (his″to-kom-pat″ĭ-bil′ĭ-te) the condition that exists when cells or tissue from one individual can be successfully transplanted into another individual and not be recognized as foreign. This intrinsic mechanism, which is common to both vertebrate and invertebrate immune systems, involves discrimination between self and nonself. The discovery that skin grafts exchanged between identical twins or inbred animal strains are permanently accepted, whereas grafts from unrelated individuals or outbred animal populations are readily destroyed, has demonstrated that the compatibility of grafted tissue is genetically determined.

The acceptance or rejection of transplanted tissue is dependent on the presence or absence of specific transplantation antigens. Recipient lymphocytes that recognize foreign histocompatibility antigens present on donor tissue grafts are induced to clonally expand a population of immune effector cells that produce cytotoxic T cells and antibodies capable of interacting with the alien transplantation antigens and destroying the graft. Transplantation antigens that induce the strongest responses are coded for by a cluster of genes referred to as the major histocompatibility complex (MHC). In mammals, the MHC is the most polymorphic gene complex yet defined. This polymorphism results both from a number of different histocompatibility loci and from a large number of different alleles at each locus. This complex is termed HLA in humans and the H-2 locus in the mouse.

The development of increasing numbers of inbred strains of mice has provided a plethora of information about the major histocompatibility complex and has proved a valuable tool for genetic investigation. Histocompatibility alleles are codominant, and their products, transplantation antigens, can be individually demonstrated in the F_1 progeny of two different inbred mouse strains. Grafts from syngeneic (genetically identical) animals are always accepted. Inbred homozygous parental grafts are also accepted when transplanted to their F_1 progeny, as the immune system of the F_1 animals recognizes no foreign antigens on the parental tissue. Grafts from F_1 animals to either parent, however, evoke strong rejection responses directed against the complement of histocompatibility antigens inherited from the other parental strain and present on the F_1 tissue.

Although the gene products of the major histocompatibility complex provide the strongest barrier to the successful transplantation of tissue, they represent a minority of the total number of histocompatibility loci present in most species. Non-MHC histocompatibility loci code for antigenic determinants referred to as minor or weak transplantation antigens. These antigens do not induce rapid immunologic rejection responses, and grafted tissue histocompatible at the MHC but incompatible for minor loci is generally successful initially. In the absence of immunosuppressive drug therapy, however, MHC identical transplants may undergo a prolonged chronic rejection. Skin grafts exchanged between mice identical at the H-2 locus but differing at minor loci may survive for up to 200 da. The larger the immunogenetic disparity between donor and recipient with respect to weak histocompatibility loci, the greater the variation in graft survival time. Minor histocompatibility antigens cannot be categorized with respect to individual potency, but it appears that they can work synergistically. Survival time for grafts incompatible at two minor histocompatibility loci may be significantly shorter than those differing by only one or the other alone. This synergistic effect may also account for the extreme potency of the MHC gene products in inducing rapid graft rejection. Mouse skin grafts differing by only one H-2 antigenic specificity survive longer than those differing by two or more.

The number of histocompatibility loci present in mice of a given species can be estimated from an assay known as the F_2 test. If parental strains differ by two unlinked histocompatibility loci, 56 percent (nine-sixteenths) of their F_2 offspring should accept grafts from one of the parental strains. This F_2 population developed from inbred strains would also be susceptible to the growth of a parental strain tumor. The proportion of susceptible animals to tumor growth would be equal to $(3/4)^n$. The exponential n is equal to the number of histocompatibility loci at which the parental strains differ. Experimental evidence indicates that certain inbred mouse strains may differ by as many as 32 histocompatibility genes.

A notable exception to the rule that syngeneic grafts are always accepted is found in certain strains of mice when grafts from males transplanted to females of the same strain do not take, whereas similar grafts from female-to-male animals experience no rejection episodes. As the only genetic difference between male and female members of the same inbred strain is that male animals possess a Y chromosome and females do not, the location of a minor histocompatibility locus was mapped to the Y chromosome and termed H-Y. Cells from XXY males immunized normal females to normal isologous male spleen cells, but cells from XO females did not. These experiments indicate that the Y histocompatibility factor results from the presence of a Y chromosome and not from the absence of a second X chromosome. Grafts from castrated males to normal females showed increased survival times, suggesting that, although the synthesis of a Y-linked minor histocompatibility antigen is determined by the Y chromosome, its antigenicity may be influenced by male hormones.

See also *alloantigen, allograft, major histocompatibility complex*, and *transplantation.*

GARY FAGIN, B.S.

histocompatibility antigen an alloantigen present on the surface of a nucleated cell that is responsible for the cell being recognized as foreign and rejected by a genetically different individual. See also *histocompatibility.*

major h. a., an antigen coded for by the major histocompatibility complex responsible for rapid graft rejection between allogeneic individuals.

minor h. a., an antigen coded for by the minor histocompatibility complex responsible for slow graft rejection between individuals who are genetically homologous at the major histocompatibility complex but heterologous at the minor complex.

histodifferentiation (his″to-dif″er-en″she-a′shun) the acquisition by specialized cell types of their specific characteristics.

histogenesis (his″to-jen′ĕ-sis) [*histo-* + Gr. *genesis* production] 1. in embryology, the process by which the cells of the germ layers differentiate into the specialized cell types that compose the various tissues. Cf. *morphogenesis.*

2. in oncology, the development of a tumor from a prototypic cell.

histogram (his′to-gram) [*histo-* + Gr. *gramma* a drawing, picture] a bar graph that shows the frequency distribution of a statistical sample. The range of the measured values is divided into equal intervals, with bar drawn intervals having a height proportional to the number of items in that interval. See also the accompanying illustration.

histogram mode a method of computer storage of data from a scintillation camera. A sequence of images or frames having preprogrammed duration is stored for later analysis. The framing rate cannot be altered after the study. Also called frame or dynamic mode. Cf. *list mode.*

histologic (his″to-log′ik) pertaining to tissue.

histologic grading see *tumor grading.*

histologic technician a technician trained in histopathologic techniques used to prepare tissue specimens for microscopic examination and diagnosis. Educational preparation involves completion of an accredited 1-yr program and/or on-the-job training under the supervision of a pathologist. Certification is provided by several agencies. Those certified by the Board of Registry of the American Society of Clinical Pathologists are designated HT(ASCP), Histologic Technician.

histologist (his-tol′o-jist) a specialist in histology, generally connoting a technician who processes tissue specimens for light microscopy.

histology (his-tol′o-je) [*histo-* + *-logy*] the microscopic study of the structure of cells and tissues. The techniques of dehydrating, clearing, embedding,

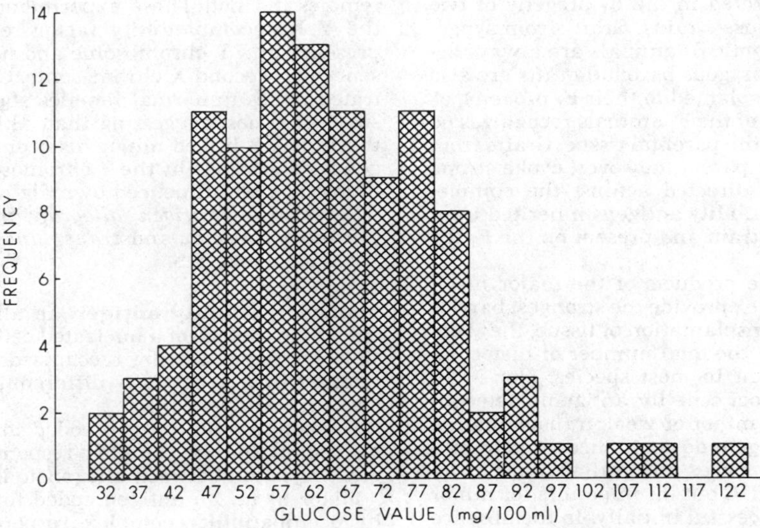

Histogram. Graph shows 105 blood glucose values from newborn infants. The values along the horizontal axis represent the midpoints of the intervals; the limits of the intervals extend from 2.5 mg/100 ml below the midpoint to 2.5 mg/100 ml above it. (From Tietz, N. W.: Fundamentals of Clinical Chemistry. 2nd ed. Philadelphia, W. B. Saunders Co., 1976.)

and staining prepare tissues for light microscopic examination; the techniques of cell culture and transparent chambers allow the study of living tissue.

histolysis (his-tol′i-sis) [*histo-* + Gr. *lyein* to loosen] the breaking down of tissue.

histolytic (his′to-lit′ik) pertaining to, characterized by, or causing histolysis.

histone (his′tōn) a major protein (M.W. 11,000–21,000) of the protein component of chromatin, a nucleoprotein. These basic proteins are bound to DNA by ionic linkages. Histones are relatively small proteins that contain a high proportion of amino acids with cationic side-chains (lysyl and arginyl residues); histones are therefore isoelectric in basic solutions. Blood treated with histone coagulates with difficulty. Histone has been found in the urine of individuals with leukemia and febrile conditions. See also *nucleoprotein.*

histopathology (his″to-pah-thol′o-je) the histologic study of diseased tissues.

Histoplasma (his″to-plaz′mah) a genus of imperfect fungi of the family Moniliaceae, order Moniliales. *Histoplasma* is a dimorphic fungus that is the etiologic agent of histoplasmosis. Below 35°C, *Histoplasma* grows as a mycelial fungus that is white to brown in color; at 37°C, it forms small, budding yeast cells. There are three medically significant species: *H. capsulatum capsulatum,* which causes histoplasmosis; *H. capsulatum duboisii,* which causes an African variety of histoplasmosis; and *H. farciminosum* (formerly called *Blastomyces farciminosus, Leishmania farciminosum,* and *Zymonema farciminosum*), the cause of lymphangitis epizootica. *H. farciminosum* differs from *H. capsulatum capsulatum* and *H. capsulatum duboisii* in having smooth macroaleuriospores in its saprophytic stage. *H. capsulatum capsulatum* and *H. capsulatum duboisii* share a single teleomorph, *Emmonsiella capsulata* (*Ajellomyces capsulatum*).

See also *histoplasmosis* and the accompanying illustration.

***Histoplasma* antibody assays** tests to detect antibodies against the fungus *Histoplasma.* The most widely used assay is a complement-fixation test. The antigens used are killed yeast-form cells of *Histoplasma* or histoplasmin, which is a soluble culture filtrate antigen from the mycelial stage. Antibodies are usually demonstrable by the time symptoms of histoplasmosis appear. Titers of antiyeast antibodies usually appear first, with antihistoplasmin titers rising later in the course of the disease and predominating in chronic cases. A titer of 1:8 to either antigen is presumptive evidence of infection; a titer of 1:32 or greater is highly indicative but not conclusive, as false-positive reactions may occur. A fourfold change in titer in either direction is most indicative of the progression or regression of disease. The complement-fixation test is positive in more than 90 percent of histoplasmosis cases. Cross reactions may occur in specimens from those individuals with blastomycosis, coccidioidomycosis, and other fungal infections.

Other tests used to detect *Histoplasma* antibodies are immunodiffusion and counterelectrophoresis, both of which use histoplasmin as the antigen. Of the six precipitin bands that form in positive tests, two are useful diagnostically. The h band is not influenced by skin testing and is found in cases of active histoplasmosis. The m band varies with skin test reactivity; it is found in cases of acute and chronic histoplasmosis and in normal individuals sensitized through skin testing. The m precipitin is found in 70 percent of proven histoplasmosis cases; the h precipitin in about 10 percent. If an individual

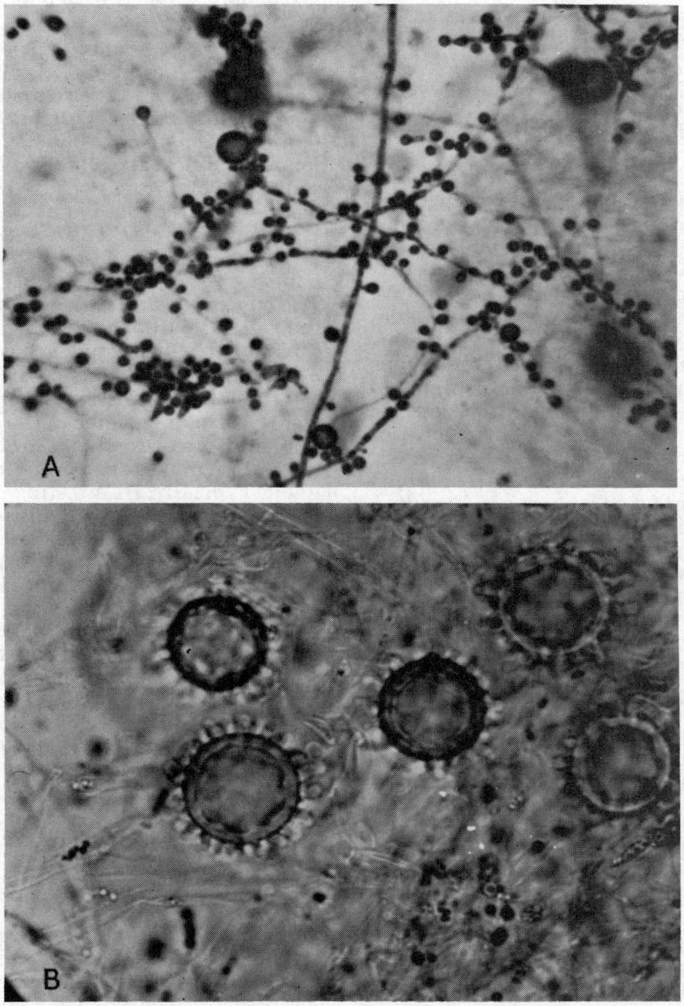

Histoplasma. Micrographs show *H. capsulatum* conidia and macroconidia from Sabouraud's glucose agar. *A,* Small, smooth conidia, round to pyriform in shape; ×600. *B,* Large, thick-walled, round tuberculate macroconidia; ×1150. (From Conant, N. F., et al.: Manual of Clinical Mycology. 3rd ed. Philadelphia, W. B. Saunders Co., 1971.)

has not had a recent histoplasmin skin test, the m band may be an indication of early disease, as it appears first and is present longer than the h band. The presence of both m and h precipitins is highly suggestive of active histoplasmosis. Another precipitin, y, may be indicative of acute histoplasmosis, particularly when m and h bands are not present.

The latex agglutination test, which is performed with latex beads coated with histoplasmin, may also be used to detect *Histoplasma* antibodies. It is excellent for the early detection of acute histoplasmosis but is usually negative in chronic cases. Titers of 1:32 or greater are considered significant. As false-positive results can occur, this test should be confirmed with the complement-fixation or immunodiffusion test. Skin testing may have a profound effect on any serologic tests for *Histoplasma* antibodies from sensitized individuals. Therefore, persons with suspected active histoplasmosis should not be skin-tested prior to the serologic testing. If the individual has been skin-tested, the specimen should be taken 2-3 da after the test, as antibodies resulting from the test would not form that soon.

histoplasmin (his″to-plaz′min) soluble growth products of the fungus *Histoplasma capsulatum capsulatum* when grown in the mycelial stage on synthetic medium. Histoplasmin is used in vitro to stimulate antibody response in the complement-fixation test for histoplasmosis. It can also be injected intradermally; past or active infection is indicated by an area of induration 5 mm or larger that appears within 24–48 hr.

histoplasmosis (his″to-plaz-mo′sis) a systemic fungal infection caused by *Histoplasma capsulatum capsulatum.* The organism is a dimorphic fungus with a yeast and a hyphal phase, and lives in the soil, especially that contaminated by chicken, bat, or bird dung. Spores from the soil are inhaled and spread through the pulmonary lymphatics to the blood via the thoracic duct. Histoplasmosis most often affects very young, very old, and debilitated individuals. The disease is found worldwide, although it is more common in tropical climates. In the United States, it is common in the valley of the Mississippi River and its tributaries.

A primary infection with *H. capsulatum capsulatum* is usually asymptomatic, but it sometimes causes an upper respiratory tract infection, which is known as the primary acute form of histoplasmosis. This form presents as a cough, hoarseness, chest pain, hemoptysis, and cyanosis, with fever, chills, and malaise. The lung involvement is a bilateral, diffuse, miliary type, with local lymphadenopathy. As a sequela to primary histoplasmosis, coin lesions may develop in the lungs, or lesions indistinguishable from reinfection with pulmonary tuberculosis may be seen. A progressive disseminated form of histoplasmosis is rare but serious. Respiratory symptoms are few, but there is fever, an enlarged liver and spleen, anemia, and leukopenia. Finally, a chronic cavitary form of histoplasmosis may develop into a tuberculosis-like disease.

Diagnosis is made with a combination of history and physical examination and delayed hypersensitivity skin testing. A rise in complement-fixing antibodies to *Histoplasma* antigens is confirmatory. With disseminated histoplasmosis, urine and blood cultures may be positive, and organ biopsies stained with periodic acid–Schiff (PAS) may show the fungus histologically. Primary histoplasmosis is usually left untreated. If the disease increases in severity, amphotericin B is currently the drug of choice.

An African variety of histoplasmosis due to the organism *H. capsulatum duboisii* is also known to occur and is also probably acquired by respiratory exposure to the organism in soil. Unlike the ordinary form of histoplasmosis, this variation rarely involves the lung and is characterized by yeast cells within giant cells. It may be clinically divided into two categories: (1) that producing cutaneous, subcutaneous and bone lesions; and (2) that producing dissemination with multiple lesions.

historadiography (his″to-ra″de-og′rah-fe) x-ray photography of microscopic sections of tissues, particularly bone sections. When x-rays, which are strongly absorbed by calcium, are used, the concentration of calcium at each point can be measured by densitometry.

histotechnologist (his″to-tek-nol′o-jist) an allied health professional skilled in the theory and practice of histopathologic laboratory procedures. Educational preparation typically involves extensive experience and continuing education beyond that required for a histologic technician; such technologists are certified by the Board of Registry of the American Society of Clinical Pathologists and are designated HTL(ASCP), Histotechnologist.

histotechnology (his″to-tek-nol′o-je) [*histo-* + *technology*] tissue-processing technique, including fixation, dehydration, embedding, sectioning, routine and special staining, mounting, decalcification, and frozen section techniques—all procedures used in preparing histologic specimens for examination by a pathologist or for scientific study.

hives (hīvz) see *urticaria.*

HK abbrev. See *hexokinase.*

HLA abbrev. for *human leukocyte antigen.* See under *HLA complex.*

HLA complex human leukocyte antigen complex, the major histocompatibility complex in humans and the principal genetic system controlling transplantation antigens. This highly polymorphic system is responsible for the cell membrane antigens found on almost all cells of the body. Residing on the short arm of chromosome 6, there are at least four distinct loci for these genes, which are designated HLA-A, B, C, and D. The antigenic products of these genes are glycoproteins, which are the determinants for recognition and rejection of foreign grafts. The glycoproteins span the cell membrane, with their major portion extending beyond it. From continuous cell culture studies it is evident that they are permanent constituents of the membrane.

Antibodies against these antigens are obtained from pregnant females and transfusion recipients. Pure antisera are difficult to obtain, and cross-reactivity often makes determination of a phenotype difficult. Typically, HLA testing is performed by incubating lymphocytes with antisera and complement. If the antibody recognizes the HLA antigen on the membrane, cellular death occurs. The NIH standard technique follows the rationale. Other methods of HLA typing include the mixed lymphocyte culture (MLC) technique and the primed lymphocyte typing (PLT) technique. For the MLC technique, a population of lymphocytes is treated with mitomycin C or x-irradiation to prevent their responding to a second population of potential recipient cells. If incompatible, the lymphocytes from the potential recipient respond with an increase in nuclear volume, cell division, and the assumption of a primitive appearance. Cells responding in this way will halt this reaction if incubated together for an extended period. In the PLT method, these "primed" lymphocytes that are no longer responding can be stimulated again if a new population of cells with the same HLA antigen is placed in the culture. The response in the PLT technique is much more rapid than in the MLC technique. Lymphocytotoxicity is the primary technique for HLA-A, B, and C antigens. HLA-D antigens are defined with the MLC and PLT techniques, and are employed in the selection of compatible transplant donors.

HLA antigens have proved extremely important in organ transplants, and care should be exercised to achieve a match between donor and recipient. Further applications of the HLA complex include a role in platelet and granulocyte transfusions, paternity testing, and anthropologic studies. There has also been a strong correlation demonstrated between HLA antigens and different diseases.

hLH abbrev. for human luteinizing hormone. See *luteinizing hormone.*

hm abbrev. See *hectometer.*

HMD abbrev. for hyaline membrane disease. See *infant respiratory distress syndrome.*

hnRNA abbrev. See *heterogeneous nuclear RNA.*

Ho symbol for the chemical element *holmium.*

hobnail cell (hob′nāl) a descriptive term for a type of cell seen in some ovarian adenocarcinomas. It has an expanded apical portion formed through expansion of the cytoplasm above the level of the surrounding epithelial surface.

Hodgkin's disease (hoj′kinz) [Thomas *Hodgkin,* English physician, 1798–1866] see *malignant l.* under *lymphoma.*

hof [Ger. "court"] the cytoplasm of a cell that occupies the space created by an indentation in the nucleus.

Hofbauer cells (hof′bow-er) [J. Isfred Isidore *Hofbauer,* American gynecologist, born 1878] large, vacuolated cells in the stroma of the chorionic villi that are found in greatest numbers in the early placenta. They resemble macrophages and are believed to serve in the remodeling of the stroma during placental growth.

Hoffmann reflex (hof′man) [Johann *Hoffmann,* Heidelberg neurologist, 1857–1919] see *H reflex.*

hol/o (hol′o) [Gr. *holos* entire] a word element used in combining form to denote entire or whole, e.g., holoenzyme.

holandric (hol-an′drik) [*holo-* + Gr. *anēr, andros* man] pertaining to the putative inheritance of genes on the Y chromosome: they are passed from each father to all of his sons and to none of his daughters.

hole (hōl) a vacant electron quantum state in a crystal, which is produced by the thermal transfer of an electron to a higher state or by a *p*-type of impurity atom (one with one less valence electron) in the lattice. Holes appear to move through the lattice in response to applied electric fields as electrons are transferred from atom to atom. In a *p*-type semiconductor, holes are the majority current carriers.

Hollander test (hol′an-der) see *insulin hypoglycemia test.*

Hollerith code (hol′ĕ-rith) the 12-bit character code used with punched cards. Each character is represented by a column on the punched card, where a hole is punched in as many as 3 of the 12 rows.

Hollerith punched card see *punched card.*

Holmes' alkaline buffer (hōmz) an alkaline buffer, pH 7.4–9.0, consisting of varying proportions of boric acid (H_3BO_3) and borax ($Na_2B_4O_7 \cdot 10\ H_2O$). It is frequently used in stains with silver salts. Also called *boric acid borax buffer.*

Holmes' method a histologic staining method for axons. Formalin-fixed paraffin sections are placed in a silver nitrate solution for 2–12 hr and then in an impregnating solution containing silver nitrate, boric acid borax buffer, and pyridine overnight at 37°C. The silver is reduced in hydroquinone, and the sections are toned with gold chloride. Axons are black against a gray background.

holmium (Ho) (hol′me-um) [N.L. *Holmia* Stockholm] a lustrous, silvery metallic element; atomic number 67; atomic weight 164.9304; a 4f transition element (lanthanide or rare earth); oxidation state +3. See also *rare earth elements.*

holocrine (hol′o-krīn) [*holo-* + Gr. *krinein* to separate] wholly secretory; denoting that type of exocrine secretion in which entire cells and their accumulated secretory granules form the product of the gland. Cf. *apocrine* and *merocrine.*

holoenzyme (hol″o-en′zīm) the catalytically active compound formed by combination of an apoenzyme and its appropriate coenzyme.

Holophyra coli (hol-of′ir-ah ko′le) see *B. coli* under *Balantidium.*

holotype (hol′o-tīp) the type culture of a species of microorganism as designated in the original description of the genus.

Holter ECG recording (hol′ter) see *ambulatory e.* under *electrocardiography.*

Holzer's method a histologic staining method for neuroglia. Formalin-fixed frozen or paraffin sections are immersed in dilute alcoholic phosphomolybdic acid and then in a 4:1 chloroform-ethanol mixture until they become translucent. They are then stained with crystal violet, rinsed in potassium bromide solution, and differentiated in an aniline-chloroform-ammonia mixture. Glial fibers stain deep violet against a pale violet background.

homatropine (ho-mah′tro-pēn) a semisynthetic anticholinergic drug, the mandelic acid ester of tropine.

h. hydrobromide, [USP], a salt used as a mydriatic.

h. methylbromide, [USP], a salt used as a mydriatic and in treating gastrointestinal spasm.

home/o (ho′me-o) [Gr. *homoios* like, resembling, always the same, unchanging] a word element used in combining form to denote sameness, unchanging, or constant, e.g., homeostasis.

homeostasis (ho″me-o-sta′sis) [*homeo-* + Gr. *stasis* standing] the tendency in biologic systems to maintain relatively constant conditions in the internal environment. It is achieved by a system of control mechanisms activated by negative feedback. Through homeostatic mechanisms the body maintains, for example, the body temperature, pH, hormonal concentrations, and osmotic pressure within physiologic limits, and thus a cellular environment is maintained within the normal range that sustains life.

immunologic h., the normal state of the adult animal in which it produces antibodies or develops cell-mediated immunity to foreign antigens but not to its own antigens.

homeostatic (ho″me-o-stat′ik) pertaining to homestasis.

homo- [Gr. *homos* same] 1. a word element used in combining form to denote sameness, e.g., homology. 2. a prefix word element in chemistry to denote the addition of one CH_2 group to a compound, e.g., cysteine and homocysteine.

homoallele (ho″mo-ah-lēl′) one of several mutations that differ from the normal protein by mutations at the same base pair. Also called *euallele.* Cf. *heteroallele.*

homobiotin (ho″mo-bi′o-tin) a homologue of biotin that acts as a biotin antagonist and that has an additional CH_2 group in the side-chain.

homobrachial inversion (ho″mo-bra′ke-al) [*homo-* + L. *brachialis,* from *brachium* arm] a paracentric chromosome inversion. See also under *inversion.*

homocarnosine (ho″mo-kar′no-sēn) a dipeptide, α-aminobutyryl histidine, that is present in human brain tissue.

homocysteine (ho″mo-sis-te′in) an α-amino acid, $HS(CH_2)_2CHNH_2COOH$, resulting from the demethylation of methionine via adenosylmethionine and utilized to synthesize cysteine. A genetic deficiency of the enzyme cystathionine-β-synthase blocks the conversion of homocysteine to cystathionine and leads to elevated plasma levels of homocysteine and methionine and the condition of homocystinuria. Vitamin B_6 deficiency can also cause homocystinuria because both cystathionine-β-synthase and the next enzyme in the pathway, cystathionine-γ-lyase, are pyridoxal phosphate enzymes. Homocysteine is not a constituent of proteins. See also *homocystinuria.*

homocystine (ho″mo-sis′tin) the disulfide derivative of homocysteine, $[-S(CH_2)_2CH(NH_2)COOH]_2$. Homocystine is homologous with cystine. It is associated with an inborn error of metabolism, homocystinuria, which is characterized by deficiency of cystathionine- β-synthase and excretion of homocystine in urine.

homocystinuria (ho″mo-sis″tin-u′re-ah) a group of disorders of homocystine metabolism, most of which are thought to be transmitted as autosomal recessive traits, and which are due to the relative or absolute deficiencies of enzymes responsible for sulfur-containing amino acid metabolism. Those affected have increased levels of homocystine in the blood and urine. Homocystinurias represent the second most common form of aminoacidopathy (1 in every 200,000 live births).

Three biochemically and clinically distinct forms of this disease are known. The first and most common form is due to the deficiency of the liver enzyme cystathionine β-synthase, resulting in increased concentrations of methionine, homocystine, and other sulfur-containing amino acids in the body fluids. Affected individuals develop symptoms and signs after birth, the most common of which is dislocation of the ocular lenses by age 3 yr. Other common signs include mental retardation and motor seizures in approximately 50 percent of patients, osteoporosis and skeletal deformities, arterial and venous thromboemboli (due to increased platelet adhesion), and defective formation of collagen and connective tissue. The ectopic lens formation may suggest a diagnosis of Marfan's syndrome. In this form of homocytinuria, daily urinary excretion of homocystine may exceed 300 mg/da as determined by the cyanide-nitroprusside test, and blood levels of methionine are markedly elevated. Diagnosis may be confirmed by demonstration of deficient cystathionine β-synthase activity in cultured lymphocytes or fibroblasts. Treatment requires early detection and the feeding of a methionine-restricted, cystine-supplemented diet. In approximately half of the cases, massive doses of pyridoxine have produced both biochemical and clinical signs of improvement. Carrier detection and in utero screening are possible.

The second form of homocystinuria is due to a deficiency of 5,10-methylenetetrahydrofolate reductase. In this form, concentrations of methionine in body fluids are normal or decreased, and homocystine levels are increased. Cerebral atrophy and retardation, seizures, behavior changes, and weakness are common. Treatment with folate supplements may offer clinical improvement.

The third form is due to a defect in the synthesis of methylcobalamin, a vitamin B_{12} coenzyme required by methyltetrahydrofolate:homocystine methyltransferase. Homocystinuria, hypomethioninemia, and methylmalonic aciduria are seen. Measurement of serum cobalamin absorption can help to distinguish this disorder from pernicious anemia. Treatment with cobalamin supplements may be beneficial.

See also *aminoacidopathies.*

homocystinuria tests see the ntiroprusside test under *cystinuria tests.*

homocytotropic antibody (ho″mo-si″to-trop′ik) [*homo-* + *cyto-* + Gr. *tropos* a turning] antibody capable of sensitizing cells of an animal of the same species. The term usually refers to IgE antibody, which attaches to mast cells and basophils.

homofermentation (ho″mo-fer″men-ta′shun) fermentation that produces one major product, primarily lactic acid, by way of the Embden-Meyerhof-Parnas pathway.

homogametic sex the sex that produces gametes all having the same sex chromosome; in humans, the female sex. Cf. *heterogametic sex.*

homogenate (ho-moj′ĕ-nāt) a material subjected to homogenization, such as tissue that is finely shredded and mixed (broken cell preparation).

homogeneity (ho″mo-jĕ-ne′ĭ-te) the state or quality of being homogeneous.

homogeneous (ho″mo-je′ne-us) [*homo-* + Gr. *genos* kind] 1. consisting of or composed of similar elements or ingredients; of a uniform quality or consistency throughout.

2. in chemistry, the term used to describe the chemical constitution of a pure compound or element. A quantity of a pure compound that has the same molecules or ions throughout its structure is homogeneous; a mixture of several compounds is described as heterogeneous.

3. also used loosely to describe a mixture of several compounds that are uniformly dispersed in each other. Homogenized milk is a mixture in which very small fat particles are uniformly dispersed throughout an aqueous medium.

4. having the same radiographic density throughout.

homogeneous immersion the employment in microscopy of a liquid of nearly the same refractive index as the cover glass.

homogenize (ho-moj′ĕ-nīz) to render homogeneous, of uniform quality or consistency throughout.

homogenote (ho′mo-je″nōt) in bacterial genetics, a merozygote in which the corresponding alleles at a specific locus of the diploid region of the genome are identical. See also *merozygote.* Cf. *heterogenote.*

homogentisate 1,2-dioxygenase (ho″mo-jen′tĭ-sāt di-ok′sĕ-jen″ās) an enzyme of the oxidoreductase class (homogentisate:oxygen 1,2-oxidoreductase [decyclizing], EC 1.13.11.5) that catalyzes the reaction homogentisate + O_2 ⇄ 4-maleylacetoacetate. A genetic deficiency of the enzyme causes alkaptonuria, a rare but well-recognized metabolic disease characterized by an accumulation of homogentisic acid in urine, as evidenced by the darkening of the urine on standing. Also called *homogentisate oxidase* and homogentisicase.

homogentisate oxidase (ho″mo-jen′tĭ-sāt ok′sĭ-dās) see *homogentisate 1,2-dioxygenase.*

homogentisic acid (HGA) (ho″mo-jen″tĭ′sic) 2,5-dihydroxyphenylacetic acid, an intermediate in the metabolism of phenylalanine and tyrosine. It is formed by the oxidation of *p*-hydroxyphenylpyruvate, and is oxidized by homogentisate 1,2-dioxygenase to 4-maleylacetoacetate. The absence of this enzyme leads to the rare, genetically derived disease of alkaptonuria or homogentisuria, which results in the excretion of HGA in the urine. Oxidized HGA also accumulates in the tissues, causing pigmentation referred to as ochronosis. See also *alkaptonuria* and *alkaptonuria tests.*

homograft (ho′mo-graft) see *allogeneic g.* under *graft.*

homolactic (ho″mo-lak′tik) bacterial fermentation that produces lactic acid by way of the Embden-Meyerhof-Parnas pathway.

homologous (ho-mol′o-gus) [Gr. *homologos* agreeing, correspondent] 1. having a similar appearance, function, or structure; corresponding in value or structure.

2. pertaining to homologous chromosomes, homologous organs or structures, a homologous series of chemical compounds, etc.

Cf. *analogous.*

homologous chromosomes a matched pair of chromosomes that have the same genes (possibly different alleles) arranged in the same physical order. The normal human chromosome complement consists of 22 homologous pairs of autosomes and two sex chromosomes. In females, the sex chromosomes are both X chromosomes and are homologous. Males have an X and a Y chromosome, which are homologous only in a region at the end of their short arms. During the zygotene stage of meiosis I, homologous chromosomes pair (synapse) in a point-for-point association; X and Y chromosomes synapse in the homologous region. One of each pair of homologous chromosomes is donated by each parent.

homologous graft see *allogeneic g.* under *graft.*

homologous series a series of organic compounds, each having one more CH_2 group than the last, e.g., methanol, ethanol, 1-propanol. There is usually a regular change in a property such as boiling point or solubility as the series progresses, although the first members of the series may be an exception to this rule.

homologous structures structures that have a common evolutionary origin, although they do not necessarily have the same function or appearance, e.g., the arms of humans and the wings of birds. Cf. *analogous structures.*

homologue (hom′o-log) a homologous chromosome or structure. Cf. *analog.*

homology (ho-mol′o-je) [Gr. *homologia* agreement] the quality of being homologous; the morphologic similarity of corresponding parts, which may be used for different functions; a structural relatedness due to descent from a common form.

homolytic (ho-mo-lit′ik) 1. destruction of cells by a lysin produced by the same type of cells.

2. in organic chemistry, the decomposition of a chemical compound involving a carbon atom in a manner to produce fragments each with one electron (e.g., $A{:}B \rightarrow A\cdot + \cdot B$).

homolytic cleavage (ho-mo-lĭt′ik klēv′ij) the process of breaking a single covalent bond in such a way that each fragment retains one electron of the bond, producing free radicals in the process.

homomorphic (ho-mo-mor′fik) [*homo-* + Gr. *morphē form*] in genetics, pertaining to chromosomes of similar size and form that pair during synapsis of the first meiotic division.

homomorphic bivalent a bivalent composed of homologous chromosomes. Cf. *heteromorphic bivalent.*

homopolymer (ho″mo-pol′ĭ-mer) a polymer formed from monomer units that are all the same, e.g., glycogen (polyglucose). See also *polymer.*

homoscedasticity (ho″mo-ske″das-tis′ĭ-te) the property of having equal variances. An assumption of homoscedasticity underlies most analysis of variance and regression statistical procedures. Cf. *heteroscedasticity.*

homosexuality (ho″mo-seks″u-al′ĭ-te) [*homo-* + *sexuality*] sexual attraction toward those of the same sex. See also *lesbianism.*

homosomal (ho-mo-so′mal) pertaining to events occurring within one chromosome.

homosomal aberration see *intrachromosomal aberration.*

homothallism (ho″mo-thal′izm) a mating system of perfect fungi in which a nucleus from within the same thallus fuses with another nucleus of that thallus, resulting in the formation of spores. The process favors genetic homogeneity. Cf. *heterothallism.*

homovanillic acid (HVA) (3-methoxy,4-hydroxyphenyl) acetic acid, the final metabolite of dopamine (a catecholamine); M.W. 182.17. HVA is formed from dopamine by an *O*-methylation and oxidative deamination and is excreted in free form in the urine.

Urinary measurements of HVA are more often used, owing to the difficulty in determining concentrations in the blood. Urinary HVA can be elevated in malignant pheochromocytoma, neuroblastoma, and ganglioneuroma. The reference value for HVA is up to 15 mg/da.

See also *catecholamines* and *dopamine.*

homozygote (ho″mo-zi′gōt) [*homo-* + *zygote*] an individual that is homozygous for a particular gene.

homozygous (ho″mo-zi′gus) in genetics, having two identical alleles of a particular gene. A homozygous individual has the characteristics produced by the allele, even if it is recessive, and will pass it on to all offspring. Cf. *hemizygous* and *heterozygous.*

homunculus (ho-munk′u-lus) [L. "a little man"] a diagrammatic representation of the areas of the cortex that are involved with the innervation of respective regions of the body. The relative size of these cortical areas reflects the degree of innervation rather than the size of the region.

hone (hōn) an abrasive surface used to sharpen knives.

automatic h., a motor-driven device having a plate-glass hone that is used to sharpen microtome knives.

honing (ho′ning) in histology, the sharpening of microtome knives using abrasives such as a carborundum hone, or a water suspension of corundum or diamantine spread on a glass plate.

hood see *laboratory hood* and *ventilation.*

Hooke's law (hooks) [Robert *Hooke,* English physicist, 1635–1703] stated as: the force acting on a perfectly elastic body is directly proportional to the resulting displacement (change in length or volume) of the structure from an equilibrium position as long as the elastic limit is not exceeded. This relationship is important in respiratory physiology, as it holds true for normally functioning lungs.

hookworm (hook′werm) a parasitic nematode. Hookworm disease is an infection of the small intestine by *Necator americanus*, the New World hookworm, and *Ancylostoma duodenale*, the Old World hookworm (see the accompanying illustration). *N. americanus* (females measuring 9–11 by 0.35 mm, males 5–9 by 0.30 mm) is common throughout North and South America in underdeveloped areas, where as *A. duodenale* (females measuring 10–13 by 0.60 mm, males 8–11 by 0.45 mm) is found in Europe, the Mediterranean region, the west coast of South America, and regions of India and China. There also are other kinds of hookworms from canines or felines, which cause creeping eruption of human skin (cutaneous larva migrans).

The infective filariform larvae enter humans by penetration of the skin, usually through the feet. At this stage, especially with infection by *N. americanus,* the larvae may cause a local dermatitis, "ground" or "dew itch," that develops into blisters. The larvae migrate to the lungs through the blood, then to the trachea where they are swallowed, and finally, as adult worms, localize in the small intestines, feeding off their host and causing a significant blood loss.

Laboratory diagnosis requires identification of the eggs in the feces by direct smears. Distinction between the eggs of *N. americanus* (64–76 by 35–40 μm) and *A. duodenale* (56–60 by 35–40 μm) is not essential, but if possible differentiation should be made between rhabditiform larvae or *Strongyloides* and hookworms by a stained smear. The stools should be examined by some concentrating method such as the formalin-ether sedimentation method or AMS or zinc sulfate techniques. The Stoll dilution and the Beaver direct smear techniques are useful quantitative egg-counting procedures for determining the worm burden.

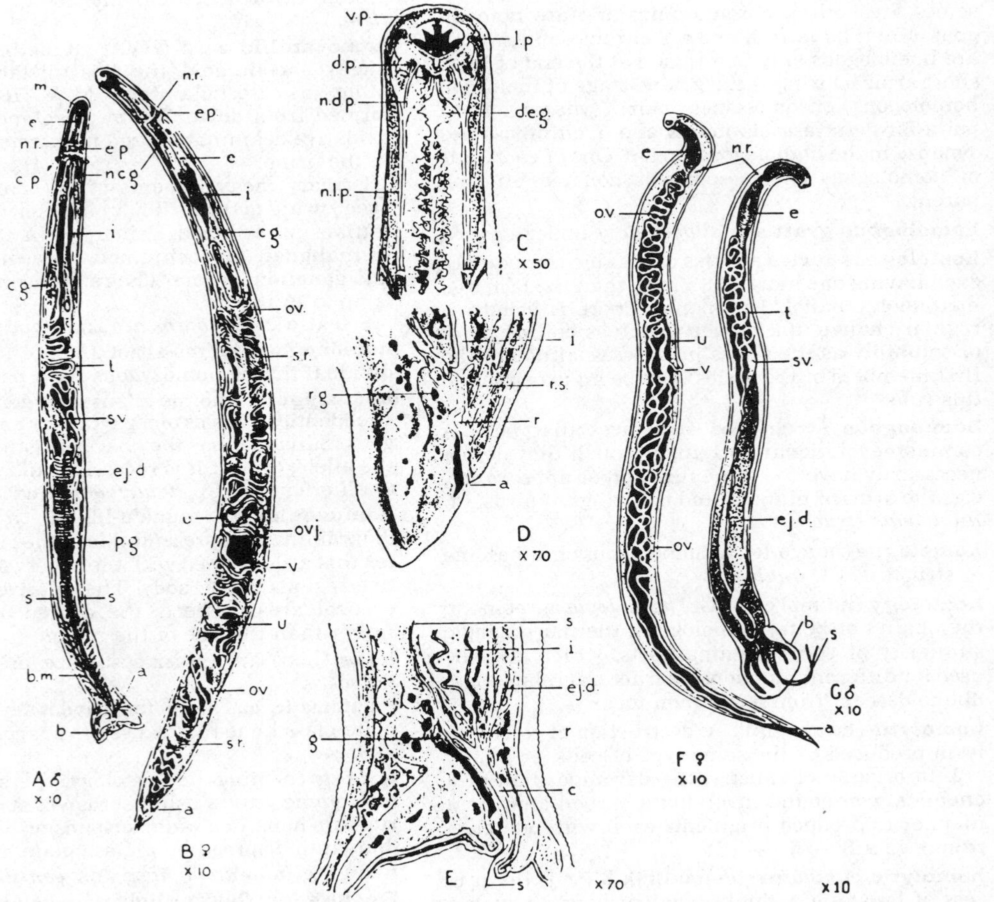

Hookworm. Important hookworms that inhabit humans. *A,* Adult male *Ancylostoma duodenale* from ventral side; *B,* young adult female *A. duodenale* from right side; *C,* anterior end of *A. duodenale* from dorsal side; *D,* longitudinal section through end of female *A. duodenale,* somewhat diagrammatic; *E,* longitudinal section through end of male *A. duodenale,* not quite median; *F,* female *Necator americanus; G,* male *N. americanus.* Lower case letters: a indicates anus; b, bursa; b.m., bursal muscles; c, cloaca; c.g., cervical gland; c.p., cervical papilla; d.e.g., dorsal esophageal gland; d.p., dorsal papilla; e, esophagus; e.p., excretory pore; n.d.p., nerve of dorsal papilla; n.l.p., nerve of lateral papilla; n.r., nerve ring; ov, ovary; ovj., ovejector; p.g., prostatic glands; r, rectum; r.g., rectal ganglion; r.s., rectal sphincter; s, spicules; s.r., seminal receptacle; s.v., seminal vesicle; t, testis; u, uterus; v, vulva; v.p., ventral papilla. (From Joklik, W.: Zinsser Microbiology. 16th ed. New York, Appleton-Century-Crofts, 1976.)

horizontal (hor″ĭ-zon′tal) level, parallel to the horizon. Cf. *vertical.*

hordeolum (hor-de′o-lum) [L. "barleycorn"] see *sty.*

horizontal plane see *transverse plane.*

horizontal ray pertaining to a radiographic projection in which the central ray is horizontal. It is used to demonstrate fluid levels, which appear as well-defined lines of demarcation, and in double-contrast arthrography to permit the opaque medium to drain to the lower part of the joint, leaving a thin coating on the upper part.

Hormodendrum (hor″mo-den′drum) 1. a former genus of Fungi Imperfecti; most saprophytic species are now placed in the genera *Cladosporium* and *Fonsecaea.*

2. a mode of asexual sporulation currently referred to as the "Cladosporium-type."

H. algeriensis, see *F. pedrosoi* under *Fonsecaea.*

H. compactum, see *F. compactum* under *Fonsecaea.*

H. japonicum, see *F. pedrosoi* under *Fonsecaea.*

H. pedrosoi, see *F. pedrosoi* under *Fonsecaea.*

H. rossicum, see *F. pedrosoi* under *Fonsecaea.*

hormonal (hor′mo-nal) pertaining to or of the nature of a hormone.

hormonal therapy a type of cancer treatment that uses the manipulation of steroid hormones to inhibit the growth of hormonally responsive neoplasms.

Steroid hormones are molecules that normally influence a wide variety of cellular functions in body tissues. Their biochemical effects are thought to be mediated by specific cytosol receptor proteins. Each type of receptor binds avidly and reversibly but preferentially to a species of steroid; for example, estradiol binds best to the estrogen receptor.

Steroid hormones are lipophilic and freely traverse most cell membranes. In the appropriate tissues, they enter the cell, bind to the receptor, undergo a conformational change, and are translocated to the nucleus. It is there that these complexes interact with nuclear DNA, which results in the synthesis of messenger RNA and proteins, the biochemical consequences of the hormones' action.

Evaluation of hormone receptors (i.e., whether one has increased estrogen receptors (ER^+) or decreased estrogen receptors (ER^-)) has demonstrated their clinical value in treatment of patients with breast cancer. Roughly 50 percent of patients with increased ER in their breast cancers seem to have a lower postoperative recurrence rate than their ER^- counterparts. For those with disseminated breast cancer about 60 percent of ER^+ individuals respond favorably to hormone therapy, whereas only 5 percent of ER^- individuals benefit similarly. However, ER levels have not proved to be of value in predicting tumor response to radiation or chemotherapy.

Steroid hormone receptors (corticoid, androgen, and progesterone, as well as estrogen) have been demonstrated in many types of malignancies, including melanomas, lymphomas, leukemias, and carcinomas of the breast (in both males and females), endometrium, ovaries, liver, gastrointestinal tract, and kidneys. However, at present the utility of receptor measurement has been firmly documented only for breast cancer.

Breast and prostate cancer are the two tumors most commonly treated by hormonal therapy. This approach to therapy is based on animal studies demonstrating the effects of steroid hormones (usually maturing or antagonistic) on corresponding end organs or tumors of these end organs. The classic example is the involutional effects of estrogen on the normal prostate and the similar antitumor effect on prostate cancer. Furthermore, the sequential use of hormones has proved useful for cancer patients. A good antitumor response (i.e., long duration with low toxicity) is predictive of a good second response to a different hormone therapy, and so forth.

The rationale of hormonal therapy is to change the hormonal milieu of the host to inhibit tumor growth. This can be done by addition (administration of exogenous hormones) or ablation (surgical removal of endocrine glands or administration of antihormones). The clinical utility and major toxicity of these treatments are summarized in the accompanying table.

MICHAEL A. FRIEDMAN, M.D.

hormone (hor′mōn) [Gr. *hormaein* to set in motion, spur on] a chemical substance that is produced in the body by an organ or the cells of an organ, which has a specific regulatory effect on the activity of a particular organ. Originally, the term was applied to substances secreted by various endocrine glands and transported in the blood stream to the target organ on which their effect was produced; later it was applied to various substances not produced by special glands but having similar action. For more information, see the specific hormone.

hormone demonstration in tissue see under *immunoperoxidase technique.*

hormone receptor a unique protein of a target tissue for the specific binding of hormones. Receptor sites may exist on the plasma membrane of the cell, in the cytosol, in the nucleus, on the endoplasmic reticulum, or in the Golgi apparatus.

horn (horn) [L. *cornu*] a pointed projection such as the paired processes on the head of various animals; any structure resembling a horn in shape.

h. of Ammon, an integral part of the hippocampus that is continuous with the dentate gyrus. The horn is a laminar structure with at least six sublayers containing a variety of inhibitory and excitatory neurons. See also *hippocampus.*

anterior h. of spinal cord, the ventrally projecting column of gray matter, resembling a horn in transverse section, that extends the length of the spinal cord. This short, broad projection of neuronal cell bodies does not reach the surface of the spinal cord. Also called ventral horn.

cutaneous h., a projection of varying size and shape formed through hyperkeratosis and seen in actinic keratosis.

lateral h. of spinal cord, a small projection of gray matter that extends laterally from the columns of gray matter in the thoracic and upper lumbar regions of the spinal cord.

h.'s of lateral ventricle, the three curved projections—anterior, posterior, and inferior—of the lateral ventricles of the brain, which contain cerebrospinal fluid. The anterior horns enter the frontal lobe, passing forward, laterally, and slightly downward on each side of the septum pellucidum. The rostral border of the anterior horn is the posterior

HORMONAL THERAPY. CLINICAL UTILITY AND ACCOMPANYING TOXICITY OF HORMONAL TREATMENTS

HORMONAL TREATMENT	PRIMARY ANTITUMOR INDICATION	MAJOR TOXICITY
Corticosteroids	Acute lymphoblastic leukemia Chronic lymphocytic leukemia Myeloma Lymphoma Breast	Elevated calcium, decreased potassium, glucose intolerance, fluid retention, catabolic musculoskeletal osteoporosis, GI bleeding
Adrenalectomy	Breast Prostate	Corticoid replacement necessary
Estrogens	Prostate Breast (postmenopausal)	Thromboemboli, fluid retention, elevated calcium
Antiestrogens (oophorectomy or medical)	Breast (premenopausal)	--
Androgens	Breast Renal	Fluid retention, elevated calcium
Orchidectomy	Prostate	--
Progesterone	Endometrium Breast Renal	Fluid retention, elevated calcium
Hypophysectomy	Breast Prostate	Thyroid and corticoid replacement necessary

Courtesy of Michael A. Friedman, M.D.

surface of the genu of the corpus callosum; the floor of the horn is the surface of the caudate nucleus. The posterior horns curve backward and medially into the occipital lobe. These slightly asymmetric and phylogenetically recent horns, which are bounded laterally and above by the tapetum of the corpus callosum, are found in anthropoids. The inferior horn is the largest of the three, and curves around the posterior thalamus to traverse the temporal lobe. It is bounded by the tapetum above and the hippocampus and collateral eminence below.

posterior h. of spinal cord, the long, narrow column of spinal gray matter projecting dorsolaterally almost to the surface of the spinal cord and running along its length. It is primarily concerned with afferent connections. Also called dorsal horn.

Horner's syndrome (hor′nerz) [Johann Friedrich *Horner,* Swiss ophthalmologist, 1831–1886] pupil constriction, ptosis, and ipsilateral facial anhidrosis due to a lesion involving the sympathetic fibers to the eye at any point along their course.

horror autotoxicus (hor′or aw″to-tok′sĭ-kus) [L. "fear of self-poisoning"] a concept first proposed in the 19th century, and now accepted, which suggests that immunity can distinguish self- from nonself-antigens and that individuals are somehow protected against autoimmunity.

horsefly see *Tabanus.*

Horsley-Clarke apparatus (hors′lē klark) [Sir Victor Alexander Haden *Horsley,* English surgeon, 1857–1916] see *stereotactic instrument.*

Horton's syndrome see *cluster h.* under *headache.*

hospital (hos′pĭ-tal) an institution that provides medical and surgical treatment, care of the sick and injured, and training of physicians and other health care personnel.

hospital-acquired penetration contact (HAPC) any exposure to infectious materials through breaks in the skin sustained during hospital work or job-related activities, as from needles, broken glass, slides, coverglasses, paper cuts, and computer cards. See also *biohazard.*

host (hōst) [L. *hospes*] 1. an animal or plant that provides physical protection and nourishment for another organism (parasite). Various types of relationships are possible: in some protozoa and helminths with complex life cycles, development depends on not only one, but two and sometimes more hosts.

2. the recipient of an organism or other tissue transplanted from another organism (the donor).

accidental h., a host that harbors a parasite that usually is not parasitic to that species.

alternate h., the species in which larval stages of the parasites develop. Also called intermediate host and secondary host.

definitive h., a host in which sexual reproduction occurs. Also called final host and primary host.

intermediate h., the host in which a parasite passes its larval or nonsexual stage.

paratenic h., a species that acts as a substitute intermediate host of a parasite, acquiring the parasite by ingesting the original host.

h. of predilection, the preferred host of the parasite.

reservoir h., a species that serves as a host for the parasite and a source from which other species may acquire the parasite.

transfer h., a host that serves until the definitive host is reached, yet is not a necessaary component of the parasite's life cycle.

host-parasite relationship see under *bacterial pathogenicity.*

host response the reaction of the tissues of an individual to a foreign element, as by the recruitment of antibodies or inflammatory cells. See also *immune response* and *inflammation.*

hot (hot) 1. characterized by high temperature.

2. containing dangerous radioactive material; dangerously radioactive.

hot antigen suicide the inhibition of specific lymphocyte functions by radioiodinated antigens. Antigen is labeled with ^{131}I radioisotope and incubated in vivo or in vitro with lymphocytes. This allows the attachment of antigen to lymphocyte, resulting in lymphocyte radiolysis.

Hotchkiss-McManus PAS technique a technique for demonstrating fungi in tissue sections or smears. It employs the standard periodic acid–Schiff (PAS) technique and is counterstained with Harris' hematoxylin. Fungal capsules and walls appear purple-red.

hot lesion in gamma-ray photography or scanning, a lesion that takes up more radionuclide tracer than does the surrounding tissue, which causes it to appear brighter in the picture. A hot lesion is more easily detected than the reverse situation, a cold lesion. Brain and bone scans are examined primarily for hot lesions. Cf. *cold lesion.*

Hounsfield unit (H) the unit of attenuation used for CT scans. Water has an attenuation of 0 H; air, – 1000 H; and compact bone. + 1000 H. Some systems use these values divided by two. Also called *CT number.*

hour (h, hr) (owr) a unit of time equal to 60 min or 3600 sec.

housekeeping (hous′kēp″ing) in computer programming, pertaining to operations or routines that are not dictated by the logic of the algorithm, but on the contrary are peculiar to the implementation of the algorithm using a particular computer or programming language. Examples are allocating storage, setting flags and counters, buffering and formatting input and output, and declaration of data types.

Howell-Jolly body (how′el zho-le′) [William Henry *Howell,* American physiologist, 1860–1945; Justin Marie Jules *Jolly,* French histologist, 1860–1953] a small, round, or oval inclusion body that is 1 μm in diameter and purple or violet in color. Howell-Jolly bodies, formed from red cell nuclear fragments, are found in erythrocytes, reticulocytes, and normoblasts. They appear regularly after splenectomy and in megaloblastic anemias, and sometimes in severe hemolytic anemias.

Howship's lacuna (how′ships) [John *Howship,* English surgeon, 1781–1841] a pit or groove containing an osteoclast and found in a developing bone that is undergoing resorption.

Hp abbrev. See *haptoglobin.*

hpf abbrev. for high-power field (microscope).

HPFH abbrev. See *hereditary persistence of fetal hemoglobin.*

hPL abbrev. See *human placental lactogen.*

HPLC abbrev. See *high-pressure liquid chromatography.*

H. P. Wright method see under *platelet adhesiveness test.*

hr abbrev. See *hour.*

H reflex an electrically induced spinal reflex, generally considered to be monosynaptic in nature. It is initiated by a submaximal stimulus that excites only the spindle afferent (I-a) fibers from a muscle. In the spinal cord, these afferent neurons make a monosynaptic connection with and activate the alpha motor neurons to the muscle, resulting in the compound muscle action potential known as the H wave.

A useful clinical application of an H-reflex study is in the diagnosis of unilaterial S-1 radiculopathy; elicitation of the H wave can also be of use in studies of proximal nerve conduction in conditions such as Guillain-Barré syndrome.

See also *H wave.*

HS abbrev. See *hereditary spherocytosis* under *anemia.*

HSA abbrev. See *hypersomnia–sleep apnea syndrome.*

H spike the deflection in the His bundle electrogram that is the result of depolarization of the His bundle.

HSR abbrev. See *Harleco synthetic resin.*

H substance a glycolipid on cell membranes or a glycoprotein in secretions having the same sugar-sugar linkages defining the H-antigenic identity. A and B genes of the ABO blood group system utilize H substance as the substrate for the production of A and B antigens. See also *blood groups.*

5-HT abbrev. for 5-hydroxytryptamine. See *serotonin.*

hTSH abbrev. for human thyroid-stimulating hormone. See *thyroid-stimulating hormone.*

HU abbrev. See *heat unit.*

Hucker-Conn crystal violet solution a mixture of crystal violet dissolved in 95 percent ethanol and ammonium oxalate that is dissolved in water. This solution is used in the Gram-Weigert stain for bacteria and fibrin.

hue (hu) [A.S. *hēo*] perceived color. See also under *color vision.*

hum (hum) electrical noise at a frequency of 60 Hz, 120 Hz, or higher harmonics; it is due to coupling between the power line and signal circuitry.

human (hu′man) an individual, male or female, belonging to the species *Homo sapiens.*

human chorionic gonadotropin (hCG) see *chorionic gonadotropin, human.*

human chorionic somatomammotropin (hCS) see *placental lactogen, human.*

human engineering the design of machines so that people can easily use them, diagnose breakdowns, and repair them, as opposed to engineering that only considers efficient mechanical performance.

human pituitary gonadotropin (hPG) see *pituitary gonadotropin.*

human placental lactogen (hPL) see *placental lactogen, human.*

humectant (hu-mek′tant) [L. *humectus,* from *humectare* to be moist] 1. a substance that absorbs water and is used to keep something moist.

2. moistening.

3. a substance that promotes retention of moisture.

humer/o (hu′mer-o) a word element used in combining form to denote the humerus (the upper arm bone), e.g., humeral.

humerus (hu′mer-us), pl. *humeri* [L.] [NA], the long bone of the upper arm. Its expanded upper end articulates with the scapula to form the shoulder joint. Its lower end forms the elbow joint with the radius and ulna. Named prominences include the greater and lesser tuberosities at the upper end of the bone and the deltoid tuberosity at the midshaft level. The lower end is flattened and bears two articular facets, the capitulum for the radius and the trochlea for the ulna.

humor (hu′mor), pl. *humors, humores* [L. "a liquid"] a fluid or semifluid substance; used in anatomic nomenclature to designate certain fluid materials in the body, e.g., aqueous humor.

aqueous h., the fluid that fills the eyeball; the metabolic avenue for the avascular tissues of the lens and cornea. The aqueous humor is responsible for interocular pressure, and thus for the optical dimensions of the eyeball.

vitreous h., see *vitreous body.*

humoral (hu′mor-al) pertaining to molecules in solution in body fluids, particularly antibodies and complement.

humoral immunity a major component of the immune system that pertains to the production and presence of immune molecules (antibody and complement) in body fluids. Its functions are interrelated with the other major component of the immune system, cellular immunity. See also *cell-mediated immunity* and *immunity.*

Hunner's cystitis, ulcer (hun′erz) [Guy LeRoy *Hunner*, American surgeon, born 1868] a condition in which a severe interstitial cystitis is associated with extensive ulceration of the urinary bladder.

Hunter's canal (hunt′erz) [John *Hunter*, Scottish anatomist and surgeon, 1728–1793] an intermuscular tunnel in the medial aspect of the middle third of the thigh, which contains the femoral vessels and saphenous nerve. It is bounded by the vastus medialis and the adductors longus and magnus, and is covered by the sartorius. Also called adductor canal or subsartorial canal.

Hunter-Schreger lines alternating light and dark zones, differing in degree of calcification, that cross the enamel of a tooth radially from the dentin to the surface.

Hunter's syndrome (hunt′erz) a genetic disorder, transmitted primarily as an X-linked recessive trait or arising spontaneously, that varies in severity and leads to abnormalities in mucopolysaccharide metabolism. It is due to relative or absolute deficiencies of iduronate sulfatase. Affected individuals possess grotesque features, joint stiffness, and slow progressive mental deterioration. Cardiac and circulatory abnormalities and deafness are also common, but corneal clouding is not observed. Expected survival time varies according to the severity of the disease. The urinary excretion of heparan sulfate, and often dermatan sulfate, is increased.

This disease may be diagnosed prenatally (with cultured and cloned amniotic fluid cells) and postnatally (in serum and cultured fibroblasts) by demonstrating deficiencies of iduronate sulfatase.

Also called mucopolysaccharidosis II (MPS II). See also *mucopolysaccharidoses.*

Huntington's chorea (hunt′ing-tunz) [George *Huntington*, American physician, 1850–1916] see *Huntington's c.* under *chorea.*

Hurler's syndrome (hoor′lerz) [Gertrud *Hurler*, Austrian pediatrician] a genetic disorder, transmitted as an autosomal recessive trait, that is characterized by abnormalities of mucopolysaccharide metabolism. It is due to relative or absolute deficiencies of the enzyme α-L-iduronidase, which results in excessive accumulation of intracellular mucopolysaccharides. Cells of the nervous system, endocrine glands, liver, bones, and heart are most frequently affected, leading to skeletal abnormalities; spleen and liver enlargement; corneal opacity; and progressive, severe mental retardation. Large amounts of dermatan sulfate and heparan sulfate are excreted in the urine. Circulating lymphocytes often contain metachromatic granules (Reilly bodies). Radiographic abnormalities include defects of the skull, vertebrae, limbs, and heart. Although normal at birth, the affected infant begins to display abnormalities (usually within the first year) that progress in severity; death usually occurs before age 10 yr.

Prenatal diagnosis is possible by culturing amniotic cells and demonstrating the enzyme deficiency. Postnatal diagnosis is based on enzyme studies.

Also called gargoylism and mucopolysaccharidosis I H (MPS I H). See also *mucopolysaccharidoses.*

Hürthle cell (her′tel) [Karl W. *Hürthle*, German histologist, 1860–1945] a metaplastic thyroid follicular epithelial cell characterized by strongly eosinophilic cytoplasm due to the presence of abundant mitochondria. See also *chronic t.* under *thyroiditis.*

Hürthle cell tumor a tumor of the thyroid follicular cells in which a marked proliferation of mitochondria has occurred. The cells appear strikingly eosinophilic by light microscopy. This type of transformation is uncommon in the normal gland, but occurs with some frequency in follicular cell adenomas and carcinomas. It has no prognostic significance.

Hutchinson-Gilford disease (huch′in-sun gil′-ford) [Sir Jonathan *Hutchinson;* Hastings *Gilford*, English physician, 1861–1941] see *progeria.*

Hutchinson's teeth (huch′in-sunz) [Sir Jonathan *Hutchinson*, English surgeon, 1828–1913] a childhood manifestation of congenital syphilis that results in abnormal tooth development. Central incisors are notched and widely spaced, and "mulberry molars" with poor caps are formed.

Hutchinson's triad [Sir Jonathan *Hutchinson*] three childhood manifestations of congenital syphilis: diffuse keratitis, labyrinthine disease, and Hutchinson's teeth.

huygenian eyepiece (hi-gen′e-an) [named for Christian *Huygens*, Dutch physicist, 1629–1695] a microscope ocular composed of two simple lenses. See also under *eyepiece.*

HVA abbrev. See *homovanillic acid.*

H-V interval the conduction time through the His-Purkinje system of the heart, usually equal to 30–55 msec in the healthy adult. It is measured from the onset of the first His bundle (H) spike on the His bundle electrogram to the onset of ventricular depolarization as viewed from surface or intracardiac electrocardiographic leads.

HVL abbrev. See *half-value layer.*

H wave a compound muscle action potential of consistent configuration and latency (approximately 30 msec) that is smaller in amplitude and longer in latency than the direct motor response (M wave). It is almost exclusively elicited from muscles (particularly those of the calf) innervated by the tibial nerve and S-1 roots by application of electrical stimuli of submaximal intensity. A supramaximal stimulus (sufficient to evoke an M wave of maximal amplitude) suppresses the H wave. Cf. *F wave.*

hyal/o (hi′al-o) [Gr. *hyalos* glass] a word element used in combining form to denote a resemblance to glass, e.g., hyaline.

hyalin (hi′ah-lin) [Gr. *hyalos* glass] a histologic term used in the description of the condensation and aggregation of protein, regardless of the chemical nature. The most common causes of hyalinization in humans are aging and chronic injury. The condensation material is derived from collagenous connective tissue.

hyaline (hi′ah-līn) [Gr. *hyalos* glass] glassy and transparent.

hyaline arteriolosclerosis see under *arteriosclerosis.*

hyaline body see *colloid body.*

hyaline cartilage semitransparent, opalescent cartilage characteristic of tracheal, nasal, costal, and articular cartilages.

hyaline membrane 1. homogenous and eosinophilic material that lines alveoli, alveolar ducts, and bronchioles in individuals with diffuse alveolar damage associated with a variety of related clinical syndromes. At the ultrastructural level, hyaline membranes are composed of cytoplasmic and nuclear debris from sloughed cells, which is admixed with fibrin. See also *infant respiratory distress syndrome.*

2. a membrane between the outer root sheath and the inner fibrous layer of a hair follicle.

hyaline membrane disease (HMD) see *infant respiratory distress syndrome.*

hyaloid (hi′ah-loid) [*hyal-* + Gr. *eidos* form] resembling glass.

hyaloid canal a channel that runs through the vitreous body of the eye from the optic disk to the center of the posterior surface of the lens in the fetus. This canal transmits the hyaloid artery.

hyalomere (hi′ah-lo-mēr″) [*hyalo-* + Gr. *meros* part] the pale, agranular peripheral zone that surrounds platelets.

hyaloplasm (hi′ah-lo-plazm″) [*hyalo-* + Gr. *plasma* anything formed] the ground substance of cell cytoplasm, as opposed to organelles and other structures.

hyaluronate (hi″ah-lu′ro-nāt) the polyanion form of hyaluronic acid, probably qualifying as a proteoglycan because it contains a small amount of protein (1–2 percent by weight); M.W. 1–3 million. The bulk of the molecule is composed of a long heteropolysaccharide chain containing 5000 carbohydrate residues. The chain contains alternating residues of D-glucuronate and *N*-acetyl-D-glucosamine, linked β,1→3, with disaccharide units that are linked β,1→4.

The high viscosity of hyaluronate contributes to its serving as an effective lubricant of joints, as well as being a resilient buffer against mechanical damage. Thus, it is an important constituent of the synovial fluid in joints. It is also present in arterial walls and umbilical cords, and in a variety of other connective tissues.

hyaluronic acid (hi″ah-lu-ron′ik) a glycosaminoglycan mucopolysaccharide that forms the backbone of proteoglycan aggregates and is found in cartilage, skin, blood vessel walls, the umbilical cord, synovial fluid, and vitreous humor.

The repeating unit of the polysaccharide chain is a disaccharide of D-glucuronic acid and *N*-acetyl-D-glucosamine joined by 1,4-linkage. The molecule is a straight chain about 5000 residues long; M.W. 1–3 million. In water solution, because of repulsion between the anionic groups, the molecules extend throughout a very large volume and form a highly viscous fluid.

hyaluronidase (hi″ah-lu-ron′ĭ-dās) enzymes of the hydrolase class, hyaluronoglucosaminidase (hyaluronate 4-glycanohydrolase, EC 3.2.1.35) and hyaluronoglucuronidase (hyaluronate 3-glycanohydrolase, EC 3.2.1.36). These enzymes catalyze the hydrolysis of hyaluronate to 2-acetamido-2-deoxy-β-D-glucose (2-glucosamine) and β-D-glucuronate residues. They hydrolyze chondroitin, chondroitin 4- and 6-sulfates, dermatan, and hyaluronic acid. The hyaluronidases are extracellular enzymes secreted by testicular tissue, the spleen, and many gram-positive bacteria, including staphylococci and streptococci. The ability of these cocci to lyse the ground substance of connective tissue is thought to be related to their pathogenicity. Also called *invasin,* mucinase, and *spreading factor.*

hyaluronidase digestion a technique employed in histochemistry to remove hyaluronic acid and chondroitin sulfate from tissue sections. Hyaluronidase is available from extracts of mammalian testes and certain bacterial culture filtrates (e.g., streptococci and *Clostridium perfringens*). Testicular hyaluronidase hydrolyzes both hyaluronic acid and chondroitin sulfates A and B, whereas bacterial hyaluronidase is specific for hyaluronic acid. Following treatment with the enzyme, the test sections and control sections are stained with Alcian blue pH 2.5 and examined for metachromasia.

hyaluronoglucosaminidase (hi″ah-lu-ron″o-glu″-ko-să-min′ĭ-dās) an enzyme of the hydrolase class (hyaluronate 4-glycanohydrolase, EC 3.2.1.35) that catalyzes the hydrolysis of 1,4-linkages between 2-acetamido-2-deoxy-β-D-glucose and D-glucuronate residues. See also *hyaluronidase.*

hyaluronoglucuronidase (hi″ah-lu-ron″o-glu″ku-ron′ĭ-dās) an enzyme of the hydrolase class (hyaluronate 3-glycanohydrolase, EC 3.2.1.36) that catalyzes the hydrolysis of 1,3-linkages between 2-acetamido-2-deoxy-D-glucose and β-D-glucuronate residues in hyaluronate. See also *hyaluronidase.*

H-Y antigen a membrane-bound antigen that is believed to promote the testicular differentiation specified by a structural gene, coded for or regulated by the Y chromosome. This is a histocompatibility antigen present in all tissues of the normal male, although only the gonadal cells are thought to have specific receptors for it. Development of the testes is believed to require the presence of the H-Y antigen. Karyotypic (XY) males are usually externally phenotypic females in the absence of the antigen. Sex-reversed (Sxr) XX females develop testes and male secondary sex characteristics without an apparent Y chromosome when their cells contain the antigen. See also *sex determination* and *sex-reversed m.* under *mutation.*

hybrid (hi′brid) an animal or plant produced by intercrossing parents that are unrelated or that are of two different species.

hybrid cell a cell formed by the fusion of whole cells or cell parts of different genotypes. The growth of hybrid cells usually requires selective media that will not support the multiplication of either parent but only the multiplication of hybrids that contain genes from both parents; an example is hypoxanthine-aminopterin-thymidine (HAT) medium. Initially, at least, hybrid cells contain most of the chromosomes of both parents, but as clones are produced, certain chromosomes are preferentially lost.

Properties expressed by the hybrid cells may include: (1) the equal expression of genes from both parents (codominance); (2) the inhibition of expression of differentiated properties in hybrids from differentiated and undifferentiated cells (extinction); and (3) the activation of genes from an undifferentiated cell, which results from its hybridization with a differentiate cell (cross activation).

See also *cellular h.* under *hybridization.*

hybridization (hi″brid-ĭ-za′shun) a procedure in which nucleic acids are denatured and reannealed. Homologous sequences form hybrid double helices.

DNA:DNA hybridization may be used to determine the sequence complexity of genomes (see *cot value*). DNA:RNA hybridization is used to determine the number of repetitions in the genome of the particular gene from which the RNA was transcribed (DNA excess) or the complexity of an RNA population (RNA excess; see *crot value*).

cellular h., the formation of viable hybrid cells by fusion of whole cells or cell parts of different phenotypes. The information provided is useful in analyzing the cellular differentiation of dominant or recessive phenotypes and the possible mechanisms for the resulting phenotypic behavior. Hybridization techniques include: (1) fusion of two complete cells to form a hybrid "sum" of the parentals (heterokaryon); (2) formation of a viable cell with cytoplasm (cytoplast) from one parent and nucleus (minicell) from another; (3) fusion of an enucleated cell with a complete cell of a different type (cybrids); and (4) the addition of a few chromosomes from one cell to another by fusion of a microcell with a normal cell. Cellular hybridization was originally discovered in mixed cultures of established cell lines as a spontaneous phenomenon. See also *hybrid c.* under *cell.*

competition h., a DNA-RNA hybridization technique used to determine the tissue specificity of RNA; it involves examination of how effectively an unlabeled RNA preparation competes with a known amount of radioisotopically labeled RNA for specific sites on a known amount of denatured DNA. If the two RNAs are sequentially similar, increasing the concentration of unlabeled RNA decreases the amount of labeled RNA that is hybridized, because the unlabeled RNA competes for complementary sites. If the sequences of the labeled RNA are very different from those of the unlabeled RNA, there is no competition for DNA sites, and the amount of unlabeled RNA is inconsequential. See also *DNA-RNA h.*

cross h., hybridization of radiolabeled nucleic acid probe sequence to another nucleic acid sequence that is not perfectly complementary.

DNA-DNA h., see *DNA renaturation.*

DNA-RNA h., a hybridization technique used to examine the specificity of transcription in animal tissues, bacteriophage, and bacteria. RNA is isolated directly from the source, or chromatin preparations are transcribed from RNA polymerase in vitro. Double-stranded DNA is then heated, which causes the strands to separate. The DNA is cooled rapidly to prevent renaturation, and single-stranded RNA is added. Double helices of DNA-RNA hybrids form in addition to the original DNA-DNA helices.

The formation of the hybrid can be detected in several ways, the simplest of which entails the use of filters that trap the helices but allow passage of single-stranded RNA. Hybridization can also be measured by assaying the amount of DNA resistant to a nuclease that degrades single-stranded DNA.

See also *DNA renaturation.*

RNA-RNA h., the formation of a duplex from the single-stranded superprevalent mRNA sequences and RNA from certain DNA sequences never expressed as cytoplasmic mRNA. It has been suggested as a possible control element in RNA processing.

saturation h., a type of DNA-RNA hybridization used to determine how many sites in a limited amount of DNA can be hybridized by RNA under saturation conditions in order to determine the complexity of the RNA population. Also called RNA-excess hybridization. See also *DNA-RNA h.*

hybridoma (hi″brĭ-do-mah) a cell culture consisting of a clone of fused (hybrid) cells of different kinds, e.g., mouse lymphocytes and rat myeloma cells. A spleen cell that produces antibody against a specific antigenic determinant may be rendered "immortal" by fusing it with a tumor cell, with the aid of a surface-altering agent such as polyethylene glycol. The resulting hybrid proliferates into a clone of cells that produce homogeneous monoclonal antibody of a single specificity. See also the accompanying illustration.

hybrid orbital a wavefunction that approximately describes the localization of an electron in a molecule. It is a linear combination of atomic orbitals (LCAO). A carbon atom with four single bonds has four sp^3 hybrid orbitals, formed from one s and three p atomic orbitals.

hydantoin (hi-dan′to-in) 1. 2,4-imidazolidinedione. 2. any of several anticonvulsant drugs containing a hydantoin ring.

See also *mephenytoin* and *phenytoin.*

hydatid (hi′dah-tid) [L. *hydatis* a drop of water] 1. any cystlike structure. 2. a hydatid cyst, the larval stage in the life cycle of *Echinococcus granulosus,* which may form single or multiple unilocular cysts in human infections (called unilocular hydatid disease); see the accompanying illustration. The adult tapeworm is parasitic in the intestines of dogs and cannot develop in humans. Human infection is acquired through the ingestion of eggs, which hatch in the small intestine. The liberated larvae are then carried throughout the body, localizing in the liver and lungs. Unilocular hydatid disease is of worldwide distribution, with a large percentage found in sheep-raising regions.

There are many diagnostic tests for the disease, including intradermal, precipitin, complement-fixation, bentonite flocculation, latex slide agglutination, whole-scolex complement-fixation, fluores-

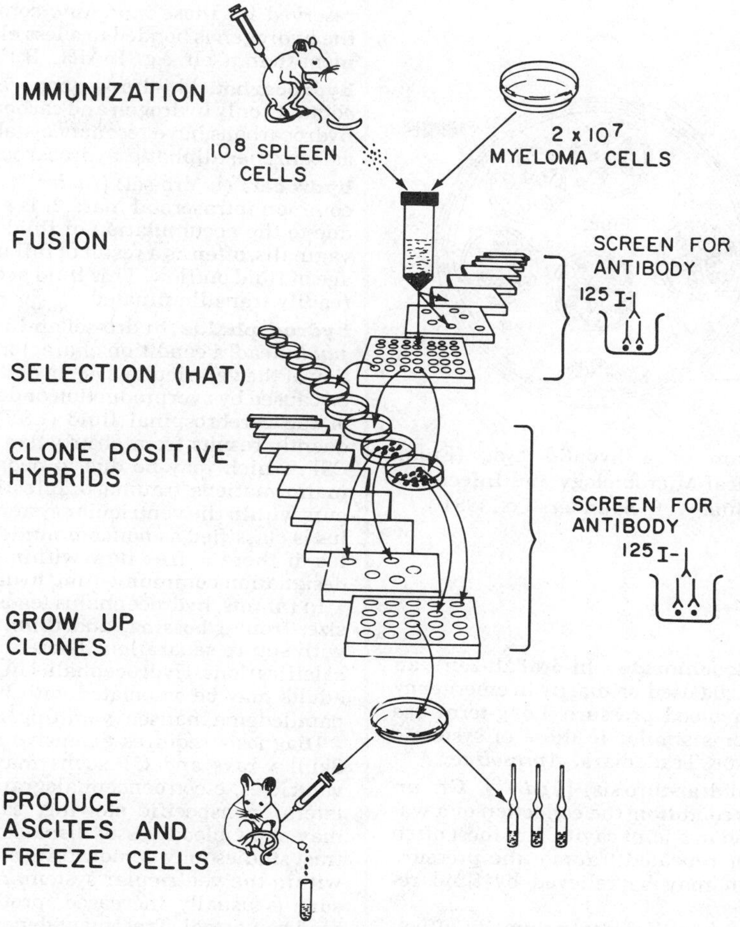

Hybridoma. A schematic diagram of a technique used in producing hybridomas. (From Yelton, S., et al.: Hybridomas and monoclonal antibodies. Laboratory Management *19*(1):19-24, 1981.)

cent-antibody, and indirect hemagglutination tests, the last-named being the most valuable. Results of serology are generally good with active infection but poor with dead cysts. X-ray examination is also helpful; cysts in the liver and lungs have a cannon-ball shape on the films. If puncture is performed, diagnosis may be made by examination of hooklets or scoleces, or both, in the hydatid fluid.

alveolar h. disease, a disease caused by the larval stage of *Echinococcus multilocularis,* which invades the affected organ and destroys the host's tissue. *E. multilocularis* is found primarily in the Northern Hemisphere. The adult tapeworm measures 1.2–3.7 mm in length and is parasitic in foxes, dogs, and cats. Human infection occurs in the same way as in unilocular hydatid disease, except that the larvae form aggregates of small cysts that proliferate by budding. The liver is the primary organ of involvement. This parasitic infection may be confused with hepatocarcinoma, as the tissue destruction resembles a malignant tumor and may even form metastases.

Because the disease resembles carcinoma of the liver, diagnosis requires histologic examination of a biopsy specimen. Radioisotopic scanning is also useful in noncalcified hepatic cysts. Serologic tests are the same as for *E. granulosus* infection.

hydatidiform (hi″dah-tid′ĭ-form) resembling a hydatid or cystlike structure.

h. mole, an intrauterine lesion that develops from an aberration in normal pregnancy, in which there is abnormal proliferation of placental tissues to produce a mass of small cystic vesicles. Histologically, these are avascular placental villi with varying degrees of trophoblast proliferation.

In the United States, the incidence of hydatidiform mole is approximately 1 in 2000 pregnancies; it is more commonly seen in older females. Serum and urinary chorionic gonadotropin concentrations are elevated. Approximately 15 percent of hydatidiform moles become locally invasive (chorioadenoma destruens), and 5 percent evolve into the highly malignant choriocarcinoma.

hydatidosis (hi″dah-tĭ-do′sis) infection with *Echinococcus,* hydatid disease.

hydatiduria (hi″dah-tĭ-du′re-ah) the presence of hydatid material in the urine.

hydr/o (hi′dro) [Gr. *hydōr* water] a prefix word element used generally to denote relationship to water (e.g., hydrolysis), to fluids (e.g., hydrostatic), or to hydrogen (e.g., hydrocarbon), and specifically to denote a compound formed by the (conceptual) addition of hydrogen at double bonds, e.g., tetrahydrofolic acid.

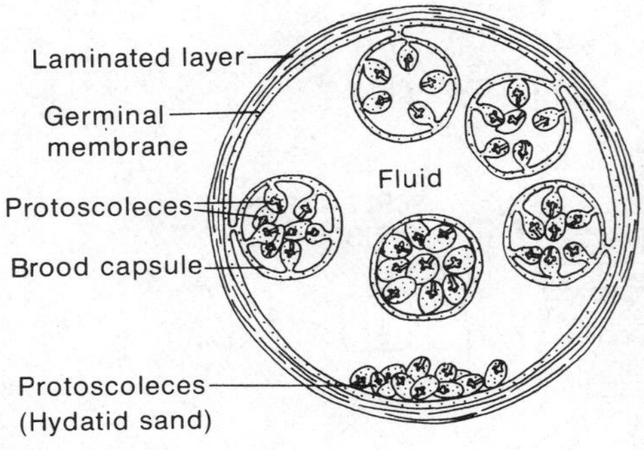

Hydatid. Diagram of a hydatid cyst. (From Braude, A. I.: Medical Microbiology and Infectious Disease. Philadelphia, W. B. Saunders Co., 1981.)

hydralazine hydrochloride (hi-dral′ah-zēn) an antihypertensive drug used primarily in emergency situations to lower blood pressure. Long-term use may cause symptoms similar to those of systemic lupus erythematosus. Trademark, *Apresoline.*

hydrarthrosis (hi″drar-thro′sis) [*hydr-* + Gr. *arthron* joint + *-osis* condition] the collection of a watery, serous effusion in a joint cavity. It is most often caused by acute or repeated trauma; the pressure and resulting pain may be relieved by fluid removal.

intermittent h., a rare disorder, primarily affecting young females, that is characterized by periodic effusions of fluid into the joints, particularly the knee. The cause of this disorder is unknown but may precede the development of rheumatoid arthritis.

hydratase (hi′drah-tās) see *hydro-lyase.*

hydrate (hi′drāt) [*hydr-* + *-ate*] the association of water and another compound in a definite proportion as a crystalline solid. The water is called water of crystallization and is indicated in formulas by a centered dot followed by an indication of the number of water molecules, e.g., $CuSO_4 \cdot 5H_2O$.

hydrated (hi′drāt-ed) combined with water; forming a hydrate.

hydrated alumina see *aluminum hydroxide.*

hydration (hi-dra′shun) 1. the act of combining or causing to combine with water.

2. the reaction of a compound with water to form a hydrate.

3. the sorption of water by a substance, as in the hydration of cellulose.

hydrazine (hi′drah-zēn) a colorless, gaseous diamine, $H_2N \cdot NH_2$; also, any member of a group of its substitution derivatives. Also called *diamide* and *diamine.*

hydrencephalocele (hi″dren-sef′ah-lo-sēl″) see *encephalocystocele.*

hydride (hi′drīd) [Gr. *hydōr* water] any compound of hydrogen with another element. The term is often reserved for those inorganic compounds in which the hydrogen is bonded to a less electronegative element than itself, e.g., $LiAlH_4$, B_2H_6, and $HMn(CO)_5$.

hydrocarbon (hi-dro-kar′bon) a compound that contains only hydrogen and carbon atoms. Aromatic hydrocarbons have resonance-stabilized rings, such as benzene; aliphatic hydrocarbons do not.

hydrocele (hi′dro-sēl) [*hydro-* + Gr. *kēlē* tumor] a common intrascrotal mass. It is a painless swelling due to the accumulation of fluid within the tunica vaginalis, often as a result of inflammation or blockage of fluid outflow. This fluid accumulation can be readily transilluminated.

hydrocephalus (hi″dro-sef′ah-lus) [*hydro-* + Gr. *kephalē* head] a condition characterized by the distention of the ventricular system of the brain. This may be caused by overproduction or defective absorption of the cerebrospinal fluid (CSF), but it most frequently results from obstruction of the flow of the CSF, which may be due to neoplasms, congenital malformations, trauma, or infection. If the block occurs within the ventricular system, the hydrocephalus is classified as noncommunicating hydrocephalus; if there is free flow within the ventricles, the designation communicating hydrocephalus is used.

In infants, hydrocephalus leads to increased head size, frontal bossing, and thinning of skull bones with suture separation. There may be intracranial calcifications. Hydrocephalus in older children and adults may be associated with headache, diplopia, papilledema, nausea, vomiting, and blurred vision.

Diagnosis requires extensive neurologic studies. Skull x-rays and CT scans may reveal distended ventricles, electroencephalography may reveal bilateral nonspecific slowing, carotid angiography may show blood vessel displacement, and air contrast studies may demonstrate an obstructive lesion within the ventricular system. Although CSF pressure is usually increased, protein concentrations may be normal. Treatment depends on the etiology; establishment of a ventricular shunt may lower the pressure, relieve any obstruction, and alleviate symptoms.

h. ex vacuo, the compensatory enlargement of the ventricular system of the brain due to severe brain atrophy. The cerebrospinal fluid is produced and absorbed normally. This condition is most frequently associated with Alzheimer's disease and Pick's disease.

normal pressure h., a condition characterized by the gradual impairment of intellectual function, coupled with the development of gait disturbance and urinary incontinence. Computed tomography reveals ventricular enlargement without cortical atrophy. Cerebrospinal fluid (CSF) pressure during lumbar puncture is normal. Pneumoencephalography shows dilated ventricles. Isotope cisternography reveals a pathologic reflux of CFS into the ventricles with delayed cortical subarachnoid filling. The electroencephalogram (EEG) demonstrates generalized theta activity in mild cases and diffuse delta activity in severe cases.

This condition may occur following meningitis, encephalitis, subarachnoid hemorrhage, or head trauma, or it may have no obvious cause. In all cases, however, there is some abnormality of the subarachnoid spaces over the cerebral hemispheres, resulting in a block to the normal circulation and absorption of CSF. There may be improvement after introduction of a ventriculoatrial or ventriculoperitoneal shunt to bypass the obstruction to the circulation and absorption of CSF.

hydrochloric acid (hi″dro-klor′ik) an aqueous solution of hydrogen chloride (HCl); a colorless, fuming liquid with a pungent odor, which may be tinted yellow by impurities. It is a strong mineral acid: a solution of 1.0 mol/l has a pH of 0.10; 0.1 mol/l, a pH of 1.10; 0.01 mol/l, a pH of 2.02; 0.001 mol/l, a pH of 3.02; and 0.0001 mol/l, a pH of 4.01. Commercial concentrated hydrochloric acid is about 38 percent HCl by weight. A constant boiling azeotrope (b.p. 108.58°C) contains 20.22 percent HCl.

Concentrated solutions can produce severe burns of the skin or, when ingested, of the mouth, throat, and stomach. Burns of the eyes may cause permanent damage. Inhalation of hydrogen chloride fumes produces coughing, choking, and respiratory tract inflammation.

The acidity of the stomach content is produced by hydrochloric acid secreted by the parietal cells of the gastric mucosa. This secretion is stimulated by the hormone gastrin. The parietal cells secrete a solution containing 155 mmol/l of HCl and 7 mmol/l of KCl by means of active transport involving carbonic anhydrase and an ATPase electrolyte pump (not the sodium-potassium pump that maintains the cellular electrolyte levels). The hydrogen ion concentration of the secretion is about a million times that of plasma.

See also *alkaline tide* and *gastric function tests.*

hydrochlorothiazide (hi″dro-klo″ro-thi′ah-zīd) [USP], see under *thiazide diuretics.* Trademarks, *Esidrix, Hydrodiuril,* and *Oretic.*

hydrocodone (hi″dro-ko′dōn) a synthetic codeine derivative used as hydrocodone bitartrate [USP] in a variety of proprietary cough and cold preparations; its abuse potential is between that of codeine and morphine. Also called *dihydrocodeinone.*

hydrocortisone (hi″dro-kor′tĭ-sōn) the nonproprietary drug name for *cortisol.*

hydrocyanic acid (hi″dro-si-an′ik) see *hydrogen cyanide.*

hydrocytosis (hi″dro-si-to′sis) the increased water content of erythrocytes. This condition is caused by the greatly increased permeability to cations with the accumulation of sodium and water in excess of the potassium loss.

Hydrodiuril (hi″dro-di′u-ril) trademark for hydrochlorothiazide; see under *thiazide diuretics.*

hydroflumethiazide (hi″dro-floo″mĕ-thi′ah-zīd) [NF], see under *thiazide diuretics.*

hydrofluoric acid (hi″dro-floor′ik) an aqueous solution of hydrogen fluoride gas, an extremely corrosive acid used to etch glass. It can produce severe burns. See also *hydrogen fluoride.*

hydrogen (H) (hi′dro-jen) [*hydro-* + Gr. *gennan* to produce] a colorless, odorless gaseous element; molecular form H_2; atomic number 1; atomic weight 1.0079; Group I of the periodic table; oxidation states +1, −1 (in hydrides). Hydrogen is the most abundant element in the universe and is the fuel for hydrogen fusion, which heats the stars. On earth it occurs primarily in water and organic compounds. Hydrogen gas is just about one-fourteenth as dense as air and is highly flammable. It is used as a fuel (an oxyhydrogen torch can produce a 2800°C flame), in the synthesis of organic compounds (hydrogenation), and as a cryogenic coolant (b.p., 20.4°K).

The hydrogen ion concentration, $[H^+]$, commonly expressed in terms of pH ($-\log_{10}[H^+]$), determines the acidity or alkalinity of a solution. In aqueous solutions, the hydrogen ions are actually in the form of H_3O^+, $H_5O_2^+$, or $H_7O_3^+$. A molecule or ion (e.g., HF, hydrofluoric acid) that can donate a hydrogen ion (proton) is called a protonic (or Bronsted-Lowry) acid. The molecule remaining after the proton is removed (e.g., F^-) is called the conjugate base of the acid and is a Bronsted-Lowry base (a proton acceptor). An acid-base reaction is the equilibrium between an acid and base and the conjugate base and acid; for example, HF (acid) + H_2O (base) $\rightleftarrows$ F^- (conjugate base) + H_3O^+ (conjugate acid). Three isotopes of hydrogen are known and are often referred to by special names: *protium* (^1H), *deuterium* (^2H), and *tritium* (^3H).

See also *acid* and *pH.*

hydrogenase (hi″droj′en-ās) a group of enzymes of the oxidoreductase class that catalyze the oxidation of H_2 to H^+. Included are those using NAD^+ or $NADP^+$ as acceptor (EC 1.12.1), e.g., hydrogen:NAD^+ oxidoreductase, EC 1.12.1.2, $H_2 + NAD^+ = H^+ + NADH$; those using a cytochrome as acceptor (EC 1.12.2), e.g., hydrogen:ferricytochrome c_3 oxidoreductase, EC 1.12.2.1, H_2 + 2 ferricytochrome c_3 = 2 H^+ + ferrocytochrome c_3; and those using H^+ as acceptor (EC 1.18.3), e.g., ferredoxin:H^+ oxidoreductase, EC 1.18.3.1, 2 reduced ferredoxin + H^+ = 2 oxidized ferredoxin + H_2, in which molecular hydrogen is used for the reduction of a variety of substances.

hydrogenate (hi′dro-jen-āt″) to cause to combine with hydrogen; to reduce with hydrogen. Sometimes a distinction is made between hydrogenation (addition of H_2 to a double or triple bond) and hydrogenolysis (cleavage of a single bond by reaction with H_2).

hydrogenation (hi″dro-jen-a′shun) a chemical reaction in which hydrogen is added to a compound, particularly one in which hydrogen is added to a double or triple bond. See also *hydrogenate.*

hydrogen chloride a colorless, corrosive, nonflammable gas, HCl, with a sharp, pungent odor; M.W. 36.47. See also *hydrochloric acid.*

hydrogen cyanide an extremely toxic, colorless liquid or gas with a characteristic almond odor (b.p., 25.6°C) produced by the reaction of cyanides with acids. It is used as a fumigant. Also called *hydrocyanic acid.* See also *cyanide.*

hydrogen fluoride a colorless gas, HF, used as a fluorinating reagent; M.W. 20.01. It is extremely toxic and corrosive, being capable of producing severe burns of the eyes, skin, and mucous membranes, which may not be noticed for several hours. See also *hydrofluoric acid.*

hydrogen ion concentration the molar concentration of hydrogen ions in a solution. In dilute solutions, $[H^+]$ is related to pH by the equation pH = $-\log_{10}[H^+]$. For example, the reference interval for blood pH, 7.35–7.45, is equivalent to a hydrogen ion concentration of 44–35 nmol/l. See also *pH.*

hydrogenolysis (hi″dro-jen-ol′ĭ-sis) the cleavage of single bonds in organic compounds as the result of treatment with hydrogen. See also *hydrogenate.*

hydrogen peroxide a colorless liquid, HOOH, that is soluble in water and ethanol; M.W. 34.02. It is a strong oxidizing agent; 30 percent aqueous hydrogen peroxide solutions are used industrially or in laboratory applications as a disinfectant or bleach. Stabilizers are usually added to hydrogen peroxide solutions to inhibit the spontaneous decomposition: $2H_2O_2 \rightarrow 2H_2O + O_2$.

In histotechnology, hydrogen peroxide solution is used as a bleach for melanin and as a reagent in peroxidase staining methods and in immunoperoxidase procedures.

h. p. solution, 1. [USP], a 3 percent aqueous solution of hydrogen peroxide used as a topical antiinfective.

2. a 30 percent aqueous solution used industrially or in laboratory applications as an oxidizing agent.

hydrogen sulfide a colorless gas with the foul odor of rotten eggs, H_2S, which is flammable and highly toxic; M.W. 34.08. Hydrogen sulfide is formed as a waste product in some industrial processes, such as the refining of high-sulfur oil, and by the decay of organic matter.

Hydrogen sulfide is produced in certain bacterial cultures by the reduction of sulfate. The reaction causes the formation of black ferrous sulfide along the stab line in a triple sugar iron agar culture, and is used in preliminary screening for enteric bacilli. *Arizona, Citrobacter, Edwardsiella,* most species of *Salmonella,* and certain species of *Proteus* produce H_2S; other Enterobacteriaceae are generally negative.

In humans, hydrogen sulfide acts like cyanide in producing, at high concentrations, immediate death from respiratory failure by the inhibition of cytochrome oxidase. As the acuity of smell is inhibited at H_2S concentrations above 150 ppm, there may be no warning of the danger. Low concentrations produce conjunctivitis (with corneal scarring in severe cases), headache, dizziness, nausea, diarrhea, lassitude, and loss of weight.

hydrolase (hi′dro-lās) one of the six main classes of enzymes (EC 3), consisting of those that catalyze the hydrolytic cleavage of various bonds with the addition of water. Clinically and physiologically important hydrolases are phosphatases, glycosidases, esterases, lipases, proteinases, peptidases, and nucleotidases.

hydro-lyase (hi″dro-li′ās) a subclass of enzymes of the hydrolase class (EC 4.2.1) that catalyzes the breakage of a carbon-oxygen bond by elimination of water, leading to the formation of an unsaturated product. Also called *dehydratase* and *hydratase.*

hydrolysis (hi-drol′ĭ-sis) the splitting of a compound into fragments by the addition of water, the hydroxyl group being incorporated in one fragment and the hydrogen atom in the other, such as the enzymatic breakdown of a protein, polysaccharide, or nucleic acid into monomers.

hydrolytic pertaining to, characterized by, or promoting hydrolysis.

hydrolyze (hi′dro-līz) to subject to hydrolysis.

hydromeningocele (hi″dro-mĕ-ning′go-sēl) [*hydro-* + Gr. *mēninx* membrane + *kēlē* hernia] see *meningocele.*

hydrometer (hi-drom′ĕ-ter) [*hydro-* + Gr. *metron* measure] a device used to measure the density or specific gravity of a liquid; usually, a weighted glass rod that indicates the density by the depth at which it floats in the liquid. The density is read from a scale attached to the rod.

hydromorphone hydrochloride (hi″dro-mor′fōn) a morphine derivative used as a narcotic or analgesic. Like morphine, it is addicting, but it is 5–10 times more toxic: an oral dose of 10–100 mg may be fatal in adults; smaller doses cause stupor or coma. It can be detected in urine by thin-layer chromatography procedures. Also called *dihydromorphinone hydrochloride.* Trademarks, *Dilaudid* and *Hymorphan.*

hydromyelia (hi″dro-mi-e′le-ah) a swelling of the central canal of the spinal cord. See also *syringomyelia.*

hydronephrosis (hi″dro-nĕ-fro′sis) [*hydro-* + Gr. *nephros* kidney] a condition characterized by gross dilation of the renal pelvis and calices with urine, caused by an obstruction of the urinary tract. Initially only the renal tubules are affected, but 2–3 wk later irreversible defects may be seen in the glomeruli.

Untreated bilateral hydronephrosis may result in complete renal failure. Unilateral hydronephrosis, however, can also be destructive, as a long time may elapse before diagnosis if the other (healthy) kidney is compensating. The most common symptom is pain. Diagnosis is established by radiographic studies, including intravenous urography.

hydronium ion (hi-dro′ne-um) the hydrated proton, H_3O^+; the form in which the proton (hydrogen ion, H^+) exists in aqueous solution. It is a combination of H^+ and H_2O, the positive charged proton being bound or attracted to the lone pair of orbital electrons on the oxygen atom.

hydropericardium (hi″dro-per″ĭ-kar′de-um) [*hydro-* + Gr. *peri* around + *kardia* heart] an accumulation of an excessive amount of low-gravity serous transudate in the pericardial cavity. Volumes may reach 500 ml or more; the severity of the condition depends on the rate of the buildup. This condition may occur in chronic congestive heart failure, liver and kidney diseases, and hypoproteinemic states.

hydroperitoneum (hi″dro-per″ĭ-to-ne′um) [*hydro-* + Gr. *peritoneum* stretch around] see *ascites.*

hydroperoxide (hi″dro-pĕ-rok′sīd) an organic compound with the general formula R—O—OH, in which R is an aliphatic and/or aromatic group.

hydrophilic (hi″dro-fil′ik) [*hydro-* + Gr. *philein* to love] readily binding or absorbing water, as in a hydrophilic gel. A hydrophilic compound is soluble in water. A hydrophilic group, such as the carboxyl, hydroxyl, and amino groups of amino acids, may bind water on the exterior of proteins and membranes. See also *hydrophilic gel, hydrophobic,* and *hygroscopic.*

hydrophilic gel a colloidal material that can absorb and bind large quantities of water and still retain firm or semifirm solid form, e.g., food gelatin. Many homo- and heteropolysaccharides and proteins behave as hydrophilic gels; others can absorb sufficient water to form solutions (sols). The materials used for molecular exclusion chromatography (gel filtrations) consist of beads of inert, highly hydrated polymeric materials; examples are Sephadex (cross-linked dextran), polyacrylamide, and agarose (polygalactans).

hydrophobia (hi″dro-fo′be-ah) [*hydro-* + Gr. *phobos* fear + *-ia*] see *rabies.*

hydrophobic (hi″dro-fo′bik) 1. pertaining to or affected with hydrophobia (rabies).

2. insoluble in water, e.g., fats, oils, and waxes. The term is also used to refer to parts of a molecule,

e.g., the alkyl groups of amino acids or triglycerides, which are pushed to the interior of proteins or membranes to be away from water; the term hydrophobic bond is used to describe this interaction between alkyl groups. Cf. *hydrophilic.*

hydrophobic gel a gel consisting of porous beads of hydrophobic materials such as methylated Sephadex, polystyrene, and cross-linked polymethacrylate, suspended in an appropriate water-insoluble organic solvent. Such gels are used to separate water-insoluble compounds by gel-filtration chromatography. The most important application is separation of lipids, triglycerides, fatty acids, and glycerophosphatides. See also *hydrophilic gel* and *Sephadex.*

hydrophthalmos (hi″drof-thal′mos) [*hydro-* + Gr. *ophthalmos* eye] a form of primary glaucoma in which the eyeball becomes distended with aqueous humor because of a congenital malformation at the angle of the anterior chamber that prevents its normal drainage. It is an early childhood disease, found at birth or in early infancy. The accumulation of fluid distends the eyeball and causes atrophy of the cornea and ciliary apparatus.

hydropneumatosis (hi″dro-nu″mah-to′sis) [*hydro-* + Gr. *pneumatōsis* inflation] the accumulation of gas and fluid within tissues.

hydropneumopericardium (hi″dro-nu″mo-per″ĭ-kar′de-um) [*hydro-* + Gr. *pneuma* air + *peri* around + *kardia* heart] an accumulation of watery fluid in the pericardial cavity.

hydropneumoperitoneum (hi″dro-nu″mo-per″ĭ-to-ne′um) [*hydro-* + Gr. *pneuma* + *peritoneum*] the presence of both air and low-density, protein-poor transudate in the peritoneal cavity. This can be caused by the edema of systemic metabolic disturbances or of local circulatory obstructions, often with trauma.

hydropneumothorax (hi″dro-nu″mo-tho′raks) [*hydro* + Gr. *pneuma* air + *thorax* chest] the accumulation of both air and protein-poor, low-density serous fluid within the pleural cavity.

hydrops (hi′drops) [L.; Gr. *hydrōps*] a condition in which there is accumulation of watery or serous fluids in the body tissues or cavities.

h. fetalis, the general accumulation of fluid within fetal tissues, as may be seen in severe hemolytic disease of the newborn and α-thalassemia gene-1 (Hb Bart's) disease.

hydroquinone (hi″dro-kwin′ōn) 1. a white crystalline solid, 1,4-benzenediol, used in photography as a film developer. It is toxic if ingested: 1 g produces convulsions, 5 g may cause death. See also *film processing.*

2. [USP], used in ointments as a skin bleach and depigmenting agent.

3. any aromatic diol that can be oxidized to form a quinone. See also *quinone.*

hydrostatic (hi″dro-stat′ik) [*hydro-* + Gr. *statikos* standing] pertaining to a liquid in a state of equilibrium or to the pressure exerted by a stationary fluid.

Hydrotaea (hi″dro-te′ah) a genus of flies. One species, *H. meteorica,* is known to attack human eyes and nostrils.

hydrothorax (hi″dro-tho′raks) [*hydro-* + Gr. *thorax* chest] an abnormal accumulation of serous fluid within the pleural cavity. The collection of such fluid may have a number of causes, including venous obstruction and systemic disorders such as chronic congestive heart and renal failure. Measurement of the fluid's specific gravity may be used to differentiate between a transudate, which is secondary to heart or renal failure, and an exudate, which is caused by infection or neoplasia, or has some other etiology. See also *pleural fluid examination.*

hydrotympanum (hi″dro-tim′pah-num) a collection of serous fluid within the tympanum, or middle ear. This condition may have a number of causes, including trauma and metabolic disorders.

hydroxide (hi-drox′sīd) an ionic compound that contains a hydroxide ion.

hydroxide ion the anion, OH^-, formed by the ionization of water or other compounds containing this ion. The generic term hydroxide may be applied to compounds that contain this ion, as, for example, metal hydroxide.

hydroxocobalamin (hi-drok″so-ko-bal′ah-min) vitamin B_{12b}, an analog of cyanocobalamin, in which the cyanide ion is replaced with a hydroxyl group. It is used in the therapy of megaloblastic anemias. See also *cyanocobalamin* and *vitamin B_{12}.*

hydroxy- (hi-drok′se) a chemical prefix indicating the presence of a hydroxyl group.

D-3-hydroxyacyl coenzyme A (hi-drok′se-as′il ko-en′zīm) an intermediate formed by action of enoyl CoA hydratase on a $\Delta^{2,3}$-enoyl CoA molecule. The D-3-isomer must be isomerized to the L-3-isomer before beta oxidation can proceed.

L-3-hydroxyacyl coenzyme A an intermediate formed during the beta oxidation of long-chain acyl CoA molecules.

hydroxyamphetamine hydrobromide (hi-drok″-se-am-fet′ah-mēn) [NF], a sympathomimetic amine used as a mydriatic, decongestant, and vasoconstrictor.

hydroxyapatite (hi-drok″se-ap′ah-tīt) a crystalline mineral that is the major constituent of tooth enamel and bone. It is primarily $Ca_{10}(PO_4)_6(OH)_2$, but it also contains carbonate, magnesium, citrate, and fluoride ions. Also called *apatite.*

hydroxybenzene (hi-drok″se-ben′zēn) see *phenol.*

***p*-hydroxybenzoic acid** (hi-drok″se-ben-zo′ik) a colorless crystalline solid, $HO—C_6H_4—COOH$; M.W. 138.13. It is used as a chemical intermediate in the synthesis of dyes and drugs and as a food preservative. *p*-Hydroxybenzoic acid is a metabolite of some drugs and appears as the free acid or in conjugated form in urine.

α-hydroxybutyrate dehydrogenase (HBD) (hi-drok″se-bu′tĭ-rāt de-hi-droj′en-ās) a term used to identify the serum enzyme that catalyzes the oxidation of α-hydroxybutyrate. HBD activity is believed to be due to certain lactate dehydrogenase (LD) isoenzymes, primarily LD-1 and LD-2; determination of HBD activity has therefore been advocated as a measure of the increase in LD-1 activity following myocardial infarction. Today this test has largely been replaced by creatine kinase and LD isoenzyme determinations. See also *lactate dehydrogenase.*

3-hydroxybutyrate dehydrogenase an enzyme of the oxidoreductase class (D-3-hydroxybutyrate: NAD^+ oxidoreductase, EC 1.1.1.30) that catalyzes the reaction D-3-hydroxybutyrate + $NAD^+ \rightleftarrows$ acetoacetate + NADH + H^+. The reaction is important in the oxidation of fatty acids in the liver. Also called β-hydroxybutyrate dehydrogenase. See also *ketone body formation.*

α-hydroxybutyrate dehydrogenase assays the determination of HBD activity by methodology similar to that used for measuring lactate dehydrogenase (LD). HBD reversibly catalyzes the reduction of α-ketobutyrate by NADH to form α-hydroxybutyrate and NAD^+. The decrease in absorbance of 340 nm is a measure of the enzyme activity.

The reference range for serum HBD in adults depends on the procedure used; it has been reported as 60–150 U/l at 30°C for the reverse reaction. For clinical purposes, the measurement of LD-1 by electrophoresis is more useful and is therefore preferred.

β-hydroxybutyric acid (BHBA) (hi-drok″se-bu′tĭ-rik) see under *ketone bodies.*

hydroxychloroquine sulfate (hi-drok″se-klo′ro-kwin) [USP], one of the 4-aminoquinoline group of antimalarial drugs; also used to treat skin lesions of discoid lupus erythematosus (DLE) and to treat rheumatoid arthritis. Prolonged use may cause retinopathy; overdose may cause convulsions or cardiac or respiratory failure. It may be identified by thin-layer chromatography screening for basic drugs.

17-hydroxycorticosteroids (17-OHCS) (hi-drok″se-kor″tĭ-ko-ster′oidz) a group of steroid hormones characterized by a hydroxyl group substituted at C-17 with or without oxygen at C-11. They are formed in the adrenal cortex by the action of 17-hydroxylase. Such hormones include cortisol and cortisone, 11-deoxycortisol, and their tetrahydro derivatives. The excretion of 17-OHCS in urine is an index of the functional status of the adrenal cortex, as well as the rate of cortisol metabolism. The plasma concentration of 17-OHCS is a direct index of the amount of cortisol to which the body's tissues are exposed.

The determination of urinary total 17-OHCS is a valuable indirect indicator of the secretory rate of cortisol, as these hormones are the primary urinary products of cortisol. Increased concentrations in urine occur in Cushing's disease, pregnancy, obesity, pancreatitis, and various extreme stresses. Decreased concentrations occur in Addison's disease and pituitary hypofunction. The measurement of urinary 17-OHCS is also used in dynamic testing procedures involving suppression (e.g., dexamethasone) and stimulation (e.g., ACTH), which aid in the diagnosis of clinical conditions related to hypo- and hyperfunction of the adrenal cortex and to alterations in the pituitary-adrenal axis.

The reference ranges for the 17-ketogenic steroid method are: for children up to 1 yr, < 1 mg/da; for children 1–10 yr, 2.3–3.8; for adult males, 5–23; and for adult females, 3–15. Reference ranges for the Porter-Silber method are: for males, 3–10 mg/da; for females, 2–8.

17-hydroxycorticosteroids assays 1. colorimetric determination of urinary 17-OHCS after they are oxidized by sodium bismuthate ($NaBiO_3$) to 17-ketosteroids, which then can be assayed colorimetrically using the Zimmerman reaction. (The steroids detected with this procedure are referred to as the 17-ketogenic steroids.) The procedure includes the sodium borohydride ($NaBH_4$) reduction to convert 17-hydroxy-20-keto-21-deoxysteroids (e.g., 17-hydroxyprogesterone) to C_{20}-hydroxysteroids, which then can also be oxidized by sodium bismuthate along with direct metabolites of cortisol (e.g., tetrahydrocortisol) originally present in the specimen. The $NaBH_4$ reduction also serves to exclude 17-ketosteroids in the specimen from being assayed, because they are converted to C_{19} 17-hydroxysteroids, which are not reoxidized by sodium bismuthate and thus do not undergo the Zimmerman reaction.

2. colorimetric determination of urinary or plasma corticosteroids using the Porter-Silber reaction based on the formation of a yellow pigment by reaction with phenylhydrazine.

3. determination of plasma 17-OHCS using sulfuric acid–induced fluorescence after extraction of cortisol and corticosterone with dichloromethane.

17-hydroxycorticosterone (hi-drok″se-kor″tĭ-ko-ster′ōn) see *cortisol.*

18-hydroxycorticosterone the immediate precursor to aldosterone; M.W. 362.47. 18-Hydroxycorticosterone possesses no mineralocorticoid activity and is a marker for the late synthesis of aldosterone. It is metabolized from corticosterone in the zona glomerulosa of the adrenal cortex via hydroxylation of a methyl group at position C-18. A deficiency of the 18-hydroxylase enzyme that catalyzes the conversion of corticosterone to aldosterone causes the impaired production of aldosterone.

The patients are salt losers but do not develop adrenal hyperplasia or virilization. Concentrations of 18-hydroxycorticosterone are more elevated in primary aldosteronism than in hyperplasia; this is usually reflected in an early morning sample after overnight recumbency.

See also *aldosterone* and *corticosterone.*

hydroxyethyl starch (HES) (hi-drok″se-eth′il)) a synthetic analog of starch given to leukapheresis donors to promote rouleaux formation and to facilitate the separation of red blood cells from granulocytes.

5-hydroxyindoleacetic acid (5-HIAA) (hi-drok″-se-in″dōl-a-se′tik) a metabolite of serotonin formed by oxidative deamination. 5-HIAA is excreted in the urine primarily in the free form, but a small amount is present in the conjugated form as a sulfate ester.

Under normal circumstances, the serotonin–5-HIAA pathway accounts for about 1 percent of the metabolism of tryptophan, but in patients with carcinoid tumors (argentaffinomas) as much as 60 percent of tryptophan may be metabolized via this pathway, leading to significant elevations in urinary–5-HIAA concentrations. Increased urinary concentrations are also observed in patients with Hartnup's disease or nontropical sprue, and in those receiving reserpine treatment. Decreased amounts are sometimes found in patients with radical resection of the gastrointestinal tract, renal insufficiency, phenylketonuria, and some tumors. The reference range is 2–8 mg/da.

See also *serotonin.*

5-hydroxyindoleacetic acid assay 1. qualitative tests. The qualitative screening test is based on the development of a color that is purple to deep blue upon the addition of 1-nitroso-2-naphthol and nitrous acid to urine, followed by extraction of other interfering chromogens with ethylene dichloride. This simple screening test is adequate for most cases of carcinoid tumors where excretion rates of 5-HIAA are high. However, for early diagnosis, when tumors are small and have not metastasized, the more sensitive and specific quantitative test is required. The sensitivity of the qualitative test is about 25–30 mg/da (1.7–2.0 mg/dl or 0.089–0.10 mmol/l).

2. quantitative test. The quantitative assay is specific for 5-HIAA and involves pretreatment of the urine with dinitrophenylhydrazine to react with interfering keto acids and removal of indoleacetic acid by chloroform extraction. The 5-HIAA is then isolated by solvent extraction (e.g., ether) and reacted with 1-nitroso-2-naphthol and nitrous acid as in the qualitative method. The absorbance at 540 nm, compared with the absorbance of a pure standard, is used as the basis for quantitation. The normal excretion rate for urinary 5-HIAA ranges from 2–8 mg/da (11–42 μmol/da). Excretions exceeding 350 mg/da are often observed in patients with carcinoid tumors. 5-HIAA may also be determined chromatographically.

See also *serotonin assay.*

hydroxyl (hi-drok′sil) the univalent radical OH.

hydroxylase (hi-drok′sĭ-lās) any of a subgroup of enzymes (EC 1.14) of the oxidoreductase class, which catalyze the coupled oxidation of two hydrogen donors with incorporation of oxygen from O_2 into one of the donors. Hydroxylases of clinical importance are those that act on steroids to synthesize cortisol and corticosterone, and those that act on the aromatic rings in phenylalanine, tyrosine, and tryptophan metabolism. Also called *dioxygenase* and *monooxygenase.* See also *steroid-21-hydroxylase.*

hydroxyl group (hi-drok′sil) an organic functional group, —OH, a hydrogen bonded to an oxygen bonded to a carbon. A compound that has one hydroxyl group attached to an aliphatic carbon atom is called an alcohol. If the hydroxyl group is bonded to an aromatic ring, the compound is called a phenol. See also *hydroxide ion.*

***o*-hydroxyphenylacetic acid** (hi′drok″se-fen′il-ah-se″tik) a minor metabolite of phenylalanine, $HOC_6H_4CH_2COOH$, formed by oxidative decarboxylation of phenylpyruvate, followed by orthohydroxylation. In phenylketonuria, it is one of the abnormal metabolites found in urine.

***p*-hydroxyphenyllactic acid** (hi-drok″se-fen″il-lak′tik) a metabolite of tyrosine that appears in the urine of premature infants or in normal newborns fed tyrosine. The metabolite is due to the low activity of *p*-hydroxyphenylpyruvate dioxygenase in fetal liver. It also accumulates in hereditary tyrosinemia (a deficiency of *p*-hydroxyphenylpyruvate dioxygenase) and in ascorbic acid deficiency (scurvy). Trace amounts are found in the urine of infants with phenylketonuria.

***p*-hydroxyphenylpyruvate dioxygenase** (hi-drok″se-fen′il-pi″roo-vāt di-ok′se-jen-ās) an enzyme of the oxidoreductase class (4-hydroxyphenylpyruvate:oxygen oxidoreductase [hydroxylating, decarboxylating], EC 1.13.11.27), that catalyzes the reaction 4-hydroxyphenylpyruvate + $O_2 \rightleftharpoons$ homogentisate + CO_2. A deficiency of this enzyme is the cause of hereditary tyrosinemia, a well-recognized biochemical disease that is marked by a rise in serum and urinary tyrosine, and an increased excretion of *p*-hydroxyphenylpyruvate and other related metabolites in the urine. Also called *p-hydroxyphenylpyruvate oxidase.*

***p*-hydroxyphenylpyruvate oxidase** see *p-hydroxyphenylpyruvate dioxygenase.*

***p*-hydroxyphenylpyruvic acid** (hi-drok″se-fen″il-pi-roo′vik) a normal constituent of wine in low amounts. The excretion of this compound is greatly increased in neonatal and hereditary tyrosinemia (owing to deficiency of the enzyme *p*-hydroxyphenylpyruvic acid dioxygenase), in tyrosinosis (owing to deficiency of the enzyme tyrosine α-ketoglutarate aminotransferase), and in ascorbic acid deficiency. See also *p-hydroxyphenyllactic acid.*

17α-hydroxyprogesterone (17α-OHP, 17-OHP) hi-drok″se-pro-jes′ter-ōn) 4-pregnen-17α-ol-3,20-dione, a progestational steroid, with minor androgenic activity, that is produced in the adrenal cortex (major source) and testes; M.W. 330.45. Its biosynthesis occurs by an enzyme-catalyzed (17α-hydroxylase) hydroxylation at the C-17 position of progesterone. In turn, it is directly metabolized to 11-deoxycortisol, 21-deoxycortisol, 17-hydroxypregnanolone, or androstenedione. Owing to a lack of 21-β-hydroxylase (major cause) and/or 11-β-hydroxylase (minor cause), serum concentrations of 17-OHP are elevated in congenital adrenal hyperplasia.

As the disease is inherited, elevations of 17-OHP can be detected in newborns either in blood from the umbilical cord or in a plasma specimen, so that glucocorticoid replacement can be initiated. Elevated concentrations of 17-OHP are sometimes found in association with certain tumors and during pregnancy.

Reference values for 17-OHP are: for adult males, less than 1 ng/ml; for adult females, 0.1–3.3; and for children, up to 0.5.

See also *congenital adrenal h.* under *hyperplasia* and *pregnanetriol.*

hydroxyprogesterone caproate a cancer chemotherapeutic drug; trademark, Delalutin. For more information, see *Appendix A.*

hydroxyproline (Hyp) (hi-drok″se-pro′lēn) a substance that occurs in blood and urine in three forms: free Hyp, Hyp combined in peptides, and Hyp in proteins. In urine it is mainly (90 percent) in the peptide form. In serum, five fractions can be separated by gel filtration or Sephadex 200. The lower-molecular-weight forms are unimolecular or small peptide complexes, but the largest fraction (80 percent) is bound to protein and can be precipitated with tricarboxylic acids along with the associated proteins. This portion is referred to as hypro-protein. The nature of this protein is not clear. Collagen is the only human protein in tissues and urine that contains appreciable amounts of hydroxyproline.

hydroxyproline assays in urine, used as a measure of collagen turnover. Most urinary Hyp is derived from collagen, and only very small amounts are derived from other tissues. Thus, increased output reflects diseases involving connective tissue and bone, and active bone growth in children; depressed output reflects failure of collagen to develop. Dietary intake of gelatin must be eliminated for several days to avoid false elevated values. Most methods involve oxidation of Hyp to a chromogen, which produces a red color with Ehrlich's reagent (*p*-dimethylaminobenzaldehyde). See also *collagen assays.*

hydroxyproline index a calculated parameter useful in evaluating the extent of certain forms of endocrine disease. The Hyp index is defined as the ratio of Hyp output to creatinine output times the patient's weight in kilograms. When endocrine disease is present, increased levels of thyroxine, parathormone, or growth hormone in serum are accompanied by increased urinary Hyp output. High levels are also found inconsistently in some diseases of the connective tissue. In children, the more rapid and variable growth rate is paralleled by a much higher and more variable Hyp excretion. The Hyp index has been used as a test of growth when assessing the response of malnourished assessing to treatment.

hydroxyprolinemia (hi-drok″se-pro″lin-e′me-ah) a hereditary condition, transmitted as an autosomal recessive trait, that is characterized by defective metabolism of the amino acid hydroxyproline, with excesses of hydroxyproline in the serum and urine. Clinical features include thrombocytopenia, microscopic hematuria, and mental retardation. Cases have been described with no clinical abnormalities other than hydroxyproline excesses. The deficient enzyme is probably hydroxyproline oxidase. Also called hyperhydroxyprolinemia. See also *aminoacidopathy.*

hydroxyproline oxidase (hi-drok″se-pro′lēn ok′sĭ-dās) see *4-oxoproline reductase.*

hydroxyprolinuria (hi-drok″se-pro″lēn-u′re-ah) the excretion of hydroxyproline in the urine. This occurs as part of the syndrome of hydroxyprolinemia, which is probably caused by the deficiency of hydroxyproline oxidase. Another type of hydroxyprolinuria, called iminoglycinuria, has been observed in one patient and is probably due to a defect in the renal transport of proline, hydroxyproline, and glycine.

hydroxystilbamidine isethionate (hi-drok″se-stil-bam′ĭ-dēn is″eth-i′o-nāt) [USP], an aromatic diamidine that has antifungal activity against *Blastomyces dermatitidis* and occasionally against *Nocardia asteroides.* It is toxic to the liver and kidneys and has been largely replaced by amphotericin B.

5-hydroxytryptamine (5-HT) (hi-drok″se-trip′-tah-mēn) see *serotonin.*

hydroxyurea (hi-drok″se-ur-e′ah) a cancer chemotherapeutic drug; trademark, Hydrea. For more information, see *Appendix A.*

hydroxyzine (hi-drok′sĭ-zēn) a drug that acts as a central nervous system depressant and muscle relaxant. It is used as a minor tranquilizer and is available as h. hydrochloride [NF] or h. palmoate [NF]. Toxic effects include dryness of the mouth, drowsiness, and involuntary motor activity. It may be identified by thin-layer chromatography screening for basic drugs. Trademarks, *Atarax* and *Vistaril.*

hygro- (hi″gro) [Gr. *hygros* moist] a word element used in combining form to denote moist or a relationship to moisture, e.g., hygrometer.

hygroma, pl. *hygromas* or *hygromata* [*hygro-* + Gr. *-oma* tumor] a cystic space, sac, or bursal area filled with accumulated fluid.

cystic h., a large cystic lymphangioma in the lower neck. It may extend beneath the clavicle into the upper mediastinum.

hygrometer (hi-grom′ĕ-ter) [*hygro-* + Gr. *metron* measure] an instrument that measures atmospheric relative humidity or some other parameter of the amount of moisture in a gas.

hygrophilous (hi″gro-fil′us) preferring a moist condition.

hygroscopic (hi″gro-skop′ik) taking up and retaining water from the air or any medium, like silica gel, calcium chloride, or zinc chloride. Such a substance, used as a drying agent, is called a desiccant. Cf. *deliquescent.*

Hygroton (hi′gro-ton) trademark for chlorthalidone; see under *thiazide diuretics.*

hymen (hi′men) [Gr. *hymēn* membrane] [NA], a thin fold of mucous membrane that partially or wholly occludes the external vaginal orifice.

imperforate h., a hymen that completely closes the vaginal orifice.

hymenolepiasis (hi″mĕ-no-lep-i′ah-sis) infection with tapeworms of the genus *Hymenolepis.*

Hymenolepididae (hi″men-o-lep′ĭ-di-de) a family of tapeworms to which the genus *Hymenolepis* belongs. Several species of this genus are parasitic in humans and are medically important.

Hymenolepis (hi″mĕ-nol′ĕ-pis) [Gr. *hymēn* membrane + *lepis* rind] a genus of tapeworms, of which several species are parasitic in humans.

H. diminuta, a large tapeworm measuring 20–60 cm long. Of cosmopolitan distribution in the rat and mouse (its intermediate host), *H. diminuta* is found in humans throughout Europe, Russia, Africa, Japan, and the Americas. Human infection is caused by the ingestion of contaminated insects, fleas, cockroaches, and mealworms, often found in grains and cereals. Those infected are usually asymptomatic but, in cases of massive infection, symptoms may include dizziness, abdominal pain, diarrhea, and convulsions.

Diagnosis requires identification of the eggs found in the feces. The eggs are spherical, measuring 60–86 μ, with a transparent yellowish shell and a six-hooked oncosphere within an inner envelope. Sometimes this envelope may have polar thickening, although never polar filaments as *H. nana* eggs have.

Also called *rat tapeworm* and *Taenia diminuta.*

H. nana, a small tapeworm measuring 25–40 mm long. It has a cosmopolitan distribution, but the largest percentage of those infected live in warm climates. *H. nana* is the only human tapeworm that does not utilize an intermediate host but can be transmitted by rodents. The eggs, measuring 30–47 μ, are ingested and hatch in the small intestine; the developing larvae grow into adult worms.

Diagnosis requires identification of eggs in the feces. The eggs are broadly ovoid and have a thin, smooth outer shell and a clear area between the shell and inner envelope. They have a six-hooked embryo in an enclosed inner envelope with a number of filaments attached to each of the two polar thickenings of the inner envelope.

Also called dwarf tapeworm, *Taenia murina,* and *T. nana.*

Hymenomycetes (hi″mĕ-no-mi-se′tēz) [Gr. *hymēn* membrane + *myketes* fungus] a series of fungi in the class Basidiomycetes. These fungi contain multiple alleles so that only thalli with different alleles are compatible, which results in dikaryotic mycelia.

Hymorphan (hi′mor-fan) trademark. See *hydromorphone hydrochloride.*

hyoid (hi′oid) [Gr. *hyoeides* U-shaped] 1. shaped like the Greek lower case letter upsilon (υ).

2. pertaining to the hyoid bone.

hyoid bone a U-shaped bone that lies in the front of

the neck and is therefore part of the axial skeleton, although it does not articulate with any other bone. It consists of a body with two posterior projections (the greater horns) and two small, pointed upward projections (the lesser horns).

hyoid region the region of the front of the neck that overlies the hyoid bone.

hyoscine (hi'o-sin) [L. *hyoscina*] see *scopolamine.*

hyoscyamine (hi"o-si'ah-mēn) *l*-hyoscyamine, an alkaloid extracted from plants of the family Solanaceae (*dl*-hyoscyamine is atropine), used as an anticholinergic and antispasmodic.

h. hydrobromine, [NF], a salt of hyoscyamine, with similar uses.

h. sulfate, [NF], a salt of hyoscyamine, with similar uses.

Hyp abbrev. See *hydroxyproline.*

Hypaque (hi'pāk) trademark. See under *diatrizoate.*

hyper- (hi'per) [Gr. *hyper* above] a prefix word element to denote above, beyond, or excessive, e.g., hyperplasia.

hyperacidity (hi'per-ah-sid'ĭ-te) increased acidity, as in the excessive secretion of hydrochloric acid by the gastric mucosa.

hyperactivity (hi"per-ak-tiv'ĭ-te) 1. abnormal activity on the part of an individual.

2. in children a disorder manifested by constant motion, restlessness, irritability, and a short concentration span; it usually abates in adolescence.

hyperacute (hi"per-ah-kūt') extremely acute.

hyperadrenalism (hi"per-ah-dren'al-izm) a group of disorders characterized by an abnormal increase in the secretions of the adrenal glands, most often of the adrenal cortex. The term is often used to refer to the overproduction of cortisol. The most common causes are adrenocortical hyperplasia, benign and malignant adrenal cortical neoplasms, and hypothalamic-pituitary dysfunction. The clinical symptoms may overlap, but three general syndromes may be described by the type of adrenocortical hormone that is overproduced. Excess production of the principal glucocorticoid, cortisol, results in Cushing's syndrome; excess production of the principal mineralocorticoid, aldosterone, results in hyperaldosteronism; and excess production of adrenal androgens results in adrenal virilism. Also called *hyperadrenocorticism.* See also *Cushing's syndrome, hyperaldosteronism,* and *adrenal v.* under *virilization.*

hyperadrenocorticism (hi"per-ah-dre"no-kor'tĭ-sizm) see *hyperadrenalism.*

hyper-β-alaninemia a disorder of alanine metabolism, thought to be transmitted as an autosomal recessive trait, that may be due to an absolute or relative deficiency of the enzyme β-alanine:α-ketoglutarate aminotransferase. Those affected show increased concentrations of β-alanine, β-amino-isobutyric acid, and taurine in the blood and urine. Metabolic acidosis, ataxia, and mental and physical retardation may result. Also called β-alaninemia. See also *alaninemia* and *aminoacidopathy.*

hyperaldosteronemia (hi"per-al"do-ster-ōn-e'meah) [*hyper-* + *aldosterone* + Gr. *haima* blood + *-ia*] an abnormally elevated concentration of aldosterone in the blood; see *hyperaldosteronism.*

hyperaldosteronism (hi"per-al"do-ster'ōn-izm) a form of hyperadrenalism in which the principal adrenal cortex mineralocorticord, aldosterone, is abnormally overproduced and hypersecreted.

primary h., hyperaldosteronism due to an adenoma, carcinoma, or hyperplasia of the glomerulosa cells of the adrenal cortex. Affected individuals most frequently demonstrate hypertension (usually benign), muscular weakness, tetany, polyuria, and polydipsia. Edema is rarely present.

Laboratory findings include decreased potassium and increased sodium levels in the plasma, and associated alkalosis. Kidney damage is frequent (proteinuria, urinary calculi, and decreased concentration ability), and the resultant low specific gravity of the produced urine cannot be reversed by vasopressin. Urinary and plasma concentrations of aldosterone are increased, whereas plasma renin levels are decreased. Electrocardiographic changes are seen, owing to the associated hypertension and hypokalemia. Adrenal neoplasms are usually too small to be visible on radiographs but may be seen with adrenal angiography or ^{131}I-19-iodocholesterol scanning. Direct plasma assays for aldosterone are still experimental.

Diagnosis is based on the failure of aldosterone suppression by sodium loading and on the failure of several hours of upright positioning to increase plasma renin concentrations. Furthermore, persons affected with primary hyperaldosteronism undergo a complete reversal of the associated symptoms after 4–8 wk of spironolactone administration. Treatment requires surgical removal of the adrenal neoplasms.

Also called *Conn's syndrome.*

secondary h., a condition marked by the presence of abnormally high amounts of aldosterone in the blood secondary to increases in renin-angiotensin, as seen in renal ischemia, edematous states, and renin-producing neoplasms. There is potassium deficiency in the blood often associated with alkalosis, along with excesses of potassium in the urine and sodium in the blood.

hyperalgesia (hi"per-al-je'ze-ah) [*hyper-* + Gr. *algēsis* pain + *-ia*] increased sensibility to pain.

hyperalgesic (hi"per-al-je'sik) pertaining to or characterized by hyperalgesia.

hyperalimentation (hi"per-al"ĭ-men-ta'shun) 1. the ingestion or administration of a greater than customary amount of nutrients.

2. the parenteral administration of nutrients through a catheter inserted into a large central vein. It is used for the temporary correction of the nutritional depletion most often caused by malabsorption or other intestinal disease (as occurs in Crohn's disease, malabsorption syndrome, or ulcerative colitis) until the gastrointestinal dysfunction can be corrected by drug treatment or by surgery.

If the major problem is malabsorption without obstruction, normal feeding may be continued during hyperalimentation; otherwise, the patient receives all nutrients intravenously. The most common complications of the procedure are infection from contamination of the catheter or nutrient solution; febrile reaction associated with the rate of flow; electrolyte imbalances; and hyperglycemic, hyperosmolar, or nonketotic coma.

The nutrient mixture varies according to the patient's needs, but a typical solution contains 165 g of anhydrous dextrose plus 860 ml of 5 percent dextrose in a 5 percent protein hydrolysate solution with electrolytes (such as sodium, potassium, magnesium, iron, calcium, phosphate) and vitamins (such as K_1, B_{12}, and folic acid) may also be added. Each liter contains 1000 kcal and 42 g of protein, which is the correct ratio for protein synthesis and anabolism. Normally, 2–3 l/da are administered to adults. The maximal fluid administration is 4 l/da; therefore, a more concentrated solution, obtained by adding glucose or fat emulsion, is used for patients with severe burns or trauma, who need more calories. Hyperalimentation solutions are hypertonic but are rapidly diluted in the large venous blood flow.

During hyperalimentation, vital signs are checked frequently and laboratory tests are performed periodically. The most closely watched measurements are blood and urine glucose, serum electrolytes, blood urea nitrogen, acid-base status, and urine acetone, specific gravity, and volume.

Patients who cannot resume enteral feeding but are free of disease can be maintained indefinitely with hyperalimentation at home, receiving infusions during sleep five to seven nights a week. This is also called home parenteral nutrition (HPN), and is used, for example, to maintain patients with short bowel syndrome (SBS), the result of surgical resection of so much of the small intestine that food cannot be adequately absorbed.

Also called intravenous hyperalimentation, parenteral hyperalimentation, intravenous alimentation, total parenteral alimentation (TPA), and total parenteral nutrition (TPN).

hyperaminoacidemia (hi″per-am″ĭ-no-as″ĭ-de′me-ah) a concentration of amino acid in the blood above normal levels, often named by the specific amino acid involved, e.g., hyperglycinemia, hypervalinemia. See also *aminoacidopathy.*

hyperaminoaciduria (hi″per-am″ĭ-no-as″ĭ-du′re-ah) a concentration of amino acid in the urine above normal levels secondary to disorders of amino acid metabolism. See also *aminoacidopathy.*

hyperammonemia (hi″per-am″mo-ne′me-ah) [*hyper* + *ammonia* + Gr. *haima* blood + *-ia*] an abnormally high concentration of ammonia in the blood. It usually occurs as the result of altered ammonia metabolism secondary to severe hepatic disease. When ammonia can no longer be metabolized adequately in the liver, blood concentrations rise, producing toxic effects, particularly in the brain. Two congenital forms of this condition occur, owing to the deficiency of two different enzymes.

h.I, see *ornithine carbamoyltransferase deficiency.*

h.II, see *carbamoyl-phosphate synthetase I deficiency.*

hyperamylasemia (hi″per-am″ĭ-lās-e′me-ah) [*hyper-* + *amylase* + Gr. *haima* blood + *-ia*] the presence of increased concentrations of amylase in the blood, which occurs in patients with pancreatitis, gall bladder and biliary duct disease, and certain other diseases such as mumps, salpingitis, intestinal disorders, macroamylasemia, and rarely in serous ovarian and some lung tumors.

hyperamylasuria (hi″per-am″ĭ-lās-u′re-ah) [*hyper-* + *amylase* + Gr. *ouron* urine + *-ia*] the presence of increased amounts of amylase in the urine, which occurs in (1) those disorders in which the plasma amylase is elevated in the presence of normal renal function (except in macroamylasemia), and (2) in some conditions in which reabsorption of amylase in the renal tubules is competitively inhibited (e.g., pancreatitis, burns). A 2-hr urine amylase test can be used to diagnose these disorders but is no longer recommended.

hyperbaric (hi″per-bār′ik) [*hyper-* + Gr. *baros* weight] characterized by greater than normal pressure or weight; the term is applied to gases under greater than atmospheric pressure (e.g., hyperbaric oxygenation) or to a solution of greater specific gravity than a reference solution of the same components.

hyperbaric oxygenation the administration of pure oxygen at greater than normal atmospheric pressures in special chambers designed for this purpose. Hyperbaric oxygenation can increase oxygen transport above normal levels; at an atmospheric pressure of 3 ATA, dissolved oxygen increases to about 6 ml of oxygen per 100 ml of blood, causing the Po_2 to rise to 2000 mmHg. This technique has only limited clinical applications and is accompanied by some risk to the patient. Appropriate uses include conditions that cause acute tissue hypoxia, such as cyanide or carbon monoxide poisoning, circumstances in which gas bubbles form in tissue, such as decompression sickness and air embolism, and clostridial myonecrosis.

hyperbilirubinemia (hi″per-bil″ĭ-roo″bĭ-ne′me-ah) [*hyper-* + *bilirubin* + Gr. *haima* blood + *-ia*] an abnormal increase in the amount of bilirubin in the blood. This condition occurs during disorders of the liver or biliary tract, or with the excessive destruction of erythrocytes. Deposition of excess bilirubin in the skin results in jaundice. See also *Crigler-Najjar syndrome, jaundice,* and *Rotor syndrome.*

h. I, a benign, relatively common, and frequently familial subclinical form of hyperbilirubinemia that is caused by reduced rates of hepatic uptake and conjugation of bilirubin. In familial cases, it is transmitted as an autosomal dominant trait. Characteristically, liver function tests are normal except for an elevated serum level of unconjugated bilirubin. Liver biopsies reveal no specific pathologic alteration except for increased amounts of lipofuscin in hepatic cells. Therapy is not indicated and the prognosis is excellent. Also called *Gilbert's syndrome.*

h. II, a chronic idiopathic jaundice, transmitted as an autosomal recessive trait, that affects the hepatic excretory function. The resulting increase in conjugated bilirubin in serum is caused by a defect in transport of conjugated bilirubin into the bile canaliculi. The hyperbilirubinemia is of fluctuating severity, liver function tests are variably affected, and bilirubinuria is generally observed. There is sometimes hepatomegaly, but the liver characteristically contains a dark gray or green-black pigment that appears dark brown under the microscope. The condition is generally harmless. Also called *Dubin-Johnson syndrome.*

conjugated h., type III, a form of conjugated hyperbilirubinemia presumably distinct from the Rotor type or the Dubin-Johnson form. A primary defect in bilirubin storage or hepatic uptake is postulated.

hyperbola (hi-per′bo-lă) [N.L., from Gr. *huperbolē* a throwing beyond] a plane curve, having two branches, that is the locus of points for which the difference of the distances to two fixed points, the foci, is a constant. In rectangular coordinates, the equation of a hyperbola with foci on the *x* axis is $(x/a)^2 - (y/b)^2 = 1$.

hyperbradykinism (hi″per-brad″ĕ-ki′nin-izm) a syndrome of orthostatic hypotension characterized by high plasma levels of bradykinin and the dilation of blood vessels in the legs, which results in reduced venous return. In such cases, standing often causes a fall in systolic blood pressure, an increase in heart rate and diastolic pressure, and a purplish discoloration and ecchymoses on the legs. It can occur in a familial form.

hypercalcemia (hi″per-kal-se′me-ah) [*hyper-* + *calcium* + Gr. *haima* blood + *-ia*] an abnormal increase in the concentration of calcium in serum (>8.5–10.5 mg/dl; ionized, 4.25–5.25 mg/dl). Primary hyperparathyroidism and various malignant neoplasms are responsible for more than 80 percent of all hypercalcemia; other causes include hyperthyroidism, vitamin D intoxication, immobilization, milk-alkali syndrome, sarcoidosis, thiazide diuretics, and elevated concentrations of plasma proteins. Approximately 10 percent of all diagnosed hypercalcemia is due to artifacts, such as contamination of laboratory glassware or cork stoppers, and venous stasis during blood removal. The ability of primary and metastatic neoplasms to produce parathyroid hormone and osteolytic factors ectopically and to invade bone directly are recognized as causes of hypercalcemia.

Hypercalcemia is characterized by nausea, anorexia, vomiting, depression, fatigability, muscle weakness, and constipation. Renal concentrating mechanisms may be impaired, resulting in polyuria and nocturia. Severe hypercalcemia (>12 mg/dl) should be considered a medical emergency, as coma, delirium, and death may result. Prolonged hypercalcemia may lead to renal damage, azotemia, myopathic disorders, and the precipitation of calcium salts and stones in the parenchyma of the kidneys, bladder, and viscera. Q-T intervals may be shortened on electrocardiographic examination. Serum calcium concentrations above 18 mg/dl frequently are fatal.

Elevated serum calcium and low serum phosphate concentrations suggest primary hyperparathyroidism or ectopic parathyroid hormone production. Hypercalcemia in association with metabolic alkalosis suggests milk-alkali syndrome. The combination of anemia and azotemia with hypercalcemia suggests the diagnosis of multiple myeloma.

See also *hyperparathyroidism.*

idiopathic infantile h., a syndrome found in infants that is thought to be associated with excess vitamin D intake or hypersensitivity. Serum calcium levels are elevated, and vomiting, weakness, lethargy, mental abnormalities, and polyuria are present. Abnormalities of the skeleton (increased density) and teeth (incomplete formation), as well as renal disorders, are also observed.

hypercalciuria (hi″per-kal″se-u′re-ah) [*hyper-* + *calcium* + Gr. *ouron* urine + *-ia*] an excess of urinary calcium.

hypercapnia (hi″per-kap′ne-ah) [*hyper-* + Gr. *kapnos* smoke + *-ia*] an abnormal increase in the pressure of carbon dioxide in the blood (increased P_{CO_2}). This condition often results from respiratory disorders that impair gas exchange and give rise specifically to alveolar hypoventilation; it can lead to respiratory acidosis. The pressure of carbon dioxide in the blood is measured during arterial blood gas analysis. Also called *hypercarbia.*

hypercapnic (hi″per-kap′nik) pertaining to or characterized by hypercapnia.

hypercapnic acidosis see *respiratory acidosis.*

hypercarbia (hi″per-kar′be-ah) see *hypercapnia.*

hypercellular (hi″per-sel′u-lar) pertaining to or characterized by an increased number of cells.

hypercellularity (hi″per-sel″u-lar′ĭ-te) an increase in the number of cells in a tissue. Hypercellularity may be normal in certain circumstances, for example, the increased number of cells seen in the breast lobule during lactation. See also *hyperplasia.*

hyperchloremia (hi-per-klo-re′me-ah) [*hyper-* + *chloride* + Gr. *haima* blood + *-ia*] a concentration of chloride in the blood above normal levels, sometimes ocurring in renal or renal tubular acidosis, in Fanconi's syndrome, and following the administration of carbonic anhydrase–inhibiting drugs (e.g., acetazolamide).

hyperchloremic (hi″per-klo-re′mik) pertaining to or characterized by hyperchloremia.

hypercholesterinemia (hi″per-ko-les″-ter-in-e′me-ah) see *hypercholesterolemia.*

hypercholesterolemia (hi″per-ko-les″ter-ol-e′me-ah) [*hyper-* + *cholesterol* + Gr. *haima* blood + *-ia*] abnormal increases in the amount of cholesterol in the plasma. This condition is thought to be due to environmental, genetic, or dietary factors, and is associated with coronary heart disease, xanthomas, and pancreatitis.

familial h., see under *hyperlipoproteinemia.*

hyperchromasia (hi″per-kro-ma′se-ah) see *hyperchromatism.*

hyperchromatic (hi″per-kro-mat′ik) 1. staining more intensely than is normal.
2. pertaining to or marked by hyperchromatism.

hyperchromatism (hi″per-kro′mah-tizm) excessive pigmentation or staining.

hyperchromia (hi″per-kro′me-ah) see *hyperchromatism.*

hyperchromic (hi″per-kro′mik) highly or excessively stained or colored.

hyperchromic shift a shift in the absorption band of a chromophore resulting in an increase of absorbance.

hypercoagulability (hi″per-ko-ag″u-lah-bil′ĭ-te) the state of being more readily coagulated than normal, leading to thrombosis. It is important that hypercoagulability be distinguished from the defibrination syndromes associated with disseminated intravascular coagulation (DIC) that are due to the sudden entry into the circulation of thromboplastic material, to activation of intrinsic clotting by endothelial damage, or to gram-negative endotoxins found in infections. Although the initiation of intravascular coagulation may be considered a stage of hypercoagulation, DIC usually induces fibrinolysis, and the end result is hemorrhage rather than thrombosis.

hypercoagulable (hi″per-ko-ag′u-lah-bl) characterized by abnormally increased coagulability.

hypercorticism (hi″per-kor′tĭ-sizm) the abnormal overproduction of any adrenal cortex hormone, hyperadrenocorticism (e.g., Cushing's syndrome).

hypercortisolism (hi″per-kor′tĭ-sōl″izm) see *Cushing's syndrome.*

hyperdiploid (hi″per-dip′loid) having a chromosome number greater than the diploid number (in humans, more than 46).

hyperdipsia (hi″per-dip′se-ah) [*hyper-* + Gr. *dipsa* thirst + *-ia*] excessive drinking of water, which may be due to habitual drinking of beverages such as beer or to great thirst, or may be secondary to hypovolemia or serum hyperosmolality. See also *polydipsia.*

hyperdiuresis (hi″per-di″u-re′sis) [*hyper-* + Gr. *diourein* to urinate] the excessive passage of urine. This condition may be attributable to renal dysfunction and diabetes insipidus. Hormonal abnormalities may also be contributory.

hyperechoic (hi″per-ĕ-ko′ik) in ultrasonography, pertaining to material that produces more or larger echoes than normal for the surrounding medium.

hyperemesis (hi″per-em′e-sis) [*hyper-* + Gr. *emesis* vomiting] frequent and excessive vomiting. Possible causes of this condition include gastrointestinal obstruction, increased intracranial pressure, psychogenic factors, ingestion of toxic substances, and infections.

h. gravidarum, a condition occurring during pregnancy that is characterized by persistent, excessive vomiting to the point of dehydration, acidosis, weight loss, and, possibly, avitaminosis; it occurs in 0.2 percent of all pregnant females. Complications may include jaundice, which indicates secondary liver damage, and hemorrhagic retinitis.

Laboratory studies show evidence of dehydration, including elevated concentrations of blood urea nitrogen (BUN), sodium, chloride, and potassium, as well as decreased serum proteins and alkali reserves, and hemoconcentration. Small amounts of protein and ketone bodies in a concentrated urine are also present.

hyperemia (hi″per-e′me-ah) [*hyper-* + Gr. *haima* blood + *-ia*] a localized increase of blood volume due to the dilation of small blood vessels, leading to the congestion of affected tissues with blood. Active hyperemia is due to increased arterial inflow to the tissue, as seen during exercise or at an inflammatory site. Passive hyperemia occurs in response to diminished venous outflow in conditions such as heart failure or obstructive venous disease.

hyperemic (hi″per-e′mik) marked by hyperemia.

hyperesthesia (hi″per-es-the′ze-ah) [*hyper-* + Gr. *aisthēsis* sensation + *-ia*] increased sensitivity to cutaneous stimulation.

hyperextension (hi″per-ek-sten′shun) the extension of a limb or a part of the body beyond its normal range of motion, often causing damage to the joint.

hyperflexion (hi″per-flek′shun) the forcible overflexion of an extremity.

hypergammaglobulinemia (hi″per-gam″ah-glob″-u-lĭ-ne′me-ah) an excess of gamma globulins in blood.

monoclonal h., an excess of gamma globulins or immunoglobulins produced by a single clone of cells. Only one class of heavy chain and one type of light chain are present.

polyclonal h., an excess of gamma globulins or immunoglobulins produced by various cells with different heavy-chain classes or different types of light chains.

hyperglycemia (hi″per-gli-se′me-ah) [*hyper-* + Gr. *glykys* sweet + *haima* blood + *-ia*] the presence of above-normal amounts of glucose in the blood. Such a condition results most commonly from insulin deficiencies in idiopathic diabetes mellitus, along with increased glucose in the urine. Other causes of hyperglycemia include disorders of the pancreas and islets of Langerhans, endocrine hyperfunction disorders, nervous system disease, and certain drugs.

hyperglycemic (hi″per-gli-se′mik) pertaining to, characterized by, or causing hyperglycemia.

hyperglycemic glycogenolytic factor (HGF) see *glucagon.*

hyperglycinemia (hi″per-gli″sĭ-ne′me-ah) [*hyper-* + *glycine* + Gr. *haima* blood + *-ia*] a group of hereditary disorders of glycine metabolism that are characterized by excessive glycine in the blood and urine. Also called *glycinemia.* For more information, see the individual diseases and *aminoacidopathy.*

ketotic h., see *β-ketothiolase deficiency, methylmalonic acidemia,* and *propionic acidemia.*

nonketotic h., a disorder of glycine metabolism, thought to be transmitted as an autosomal recessive trait, that is characterized by a defect in the glycine breakdown pathway, possibly involving the enzyme glycine decarboxylase. As a result, there are increased levels of glycine in the blood, leading to renal "spillover" into the urine and resulting in hyperglycinuria. Severe central nervous system depression is evident soon after birth in those affected, as well as convulsions, generalized hypotonia, seizures, hyperactivity, and areflexia. Also called type II hyperglycinemia. See also *aminoacidopathy.*

hyperglycinuria (hi″per-gli″sĭ-nu′re-ah) [*hyper-* + *glycine* + Gr. *ouron* urine + *-ia*] a hereditary condition in which there is an excess of glycine in the urine. Two types are known. One is iminoglycinuria, in which there is a urinary excess of glycine plus the imino acids proline and hydroxyproline, which share a renal tubular resorptive mechanism with glycine; this form is transmitted as an autosomal recessive trait. The other is glucoglycinuria, in which there is renal glycosuria and hyperglycinuria without the increased secretion of other amino acids; it is transmitted as a very rare autosomal dominant trait. Also called *glycinuria.*

hypergonadism (hi″per-go′nad-izm) a condition marked by the excessive production of androgenic hormones, which leads to precocious puberty and sexual development in the child, but little if any morphologic or functional change in the adult. Primary causes are functioning testicular tumors. Tumors in the region of the third ventricle producing abnormal levels of gonadotropins cause secondary hypergonadism. Plasma testosterone and urinary 17-ketosteroids are measured in diagnosis.

hyperimmune (hi″per-im-mūn′) having large quantities of specific antibodies in the serum from repeated immunization or infection.

hyperimmunity (hi″per-ĭ-mu′nĭ-te) a high degree of immunity.

hyperimmunization (hi″per-im″u-nĭ-za′shun) the practice of establishing a heightened state of actively acquired immunity by the administration of repeated doses of antigen, often used in allergy desensitization, or of passively acquired immunity by the injection of hyperimmune gamma globulin.

hyperinflation (hi″per-in-fla′shun) an excessive inflation or expansion. Overinflation of the lungs occurs in emphysematous or asthmatic individuals because the severe expiratory obstruction present in these disorders leads to incomplete alveolar emptying and a large increase in the functional residual capacity.

hyperinsulinemia (hi″per-in″su-lĭ-ne′me-ah) [*hyper-* + *insulin* + Gr. *haima* blood + *-ia*] the presence of an excessive and inappropriate amount of insulin in the blood. This occurs in insulinomas, which are tumors of the pancreatic islet cells, and in some forms of obesity. It has also been observed in pregnancy, particularly during the third trimester. When adiposity is reduced, blood insulin concentrations often return to normal.

hyperinsulinism (hi″per-in′su-lin-izm″) 1. secretion of above-normal amounts of insulin by the pancreas, which most often results in hypoglycemia. This excess of insulin in the blood may be due to a functional disturbance of the pancreas or to an insulin-producing beta-cell tumor of the pancreas. The hypoglycemia in such disorders is promptly relieved by glucose administration.

2. the insulin shock observed after administration of excessive amounts of insulin.

hyperkalemia (hi″per-kah-le′me-ah) an abormally high concentration of potassium in the serum. Defective renal excretion, increased dietary intake, and Addison's disease may lead to this condition. Cardiac changes, including electrographic T-wave elevation, widening of the QRS complex, and lengthening of the P-R interval, may be noted. Diarrhea and muscle weakness leading to paralysis are also seen. In vivo causes must be differentiated from increases in potassium that are due to improper specimens, e.g., those with hemolysis or those that have been in contact with erythrocytes for too long a time. Also called *hyperpotassemia.* See also *electrolyte balance and homeostasis.*

hyperkeratosis (hi″per-ker″ah-to′sis) [*hyper-* + Gr. *keras* horn + *-osis* condition] an increase in the thickness of the stratum corneum of stratified squamous epithelium. It commonly occurs on the skin, but may also be seen on mucosal surfaces, including the mouth, larynx, vulva, and cornea, in response to increased intake of vitamin A or irritation.

epidermolytic h., a type of degenerative change involving the epidermis, in which the cells tend to accumulate excessive keratin and the intercellular spaces are widened. In light microscopic sections, the acantholytic tendency is exaggerated by shrinkage artifact. It is seen in a number of skin disorders, including the dominant form of congenital ichthyosiform erythroderma, and is sometimes termed granular degeneration.

hyperlipemia (hi″per-li-pe′me-ah) [*hyper-* + Gr. *lipos* fat + *haima* blood + *-ia*] see *hyperlipidemia.*

hyperlipidemia (hi″per-lĭ-pĭ-de′me-ah) an abnormally high amount of lipids in the blood. This condition is subject to dietary and hereditary influences, and is related to lipoprotein levels. Also called *hyperlipemia.* See also *hyperlipoproteinemia.*

carbohydrate-induced h., see under *hyperlipoproteinemia* (type IV).

fat-induced h., see under *hyperlipoproteinemia* (type I).

hyperlipoproteinemia (hi″per-lip″o-pro″tēn-e′me-ah) [*hyper-* + *lipoprotein* + Gr. *haima* blood + *-ia*] an excess of lipoproteins in the blood; a large group of disorders characterized by elevations in the plasma levels of lipoproteins secondary to an inability to metabolize dietary or endogenous lipids successfully or the overproduction of endogenous lipids, or both. The hyperlipoproteinemias are often accompanied by excessive lipid deposition in the tissues, which result in accelerated atherosclerosis, xanthomas, and hepatosplenomegaly.

Dietary fats are taken up in the intestine and complexed with apoproteins to produce chylomicrons—large lipoprotein particles that travel through the lymphatic system into the systemic circulation. When brought to adipose or muscle tissue, chylomicrons are acted on by the tissue lipoprotein lipase, an enzyme that hydrolyzes triglycerides in these complexes, leaving the chylomicron remnants to return via the circulation to the liver. The triglycerides are taken up and stored in adipose tissue or are used in energy-releasing processes in the muscle tissue. The liver itself can produce triglycerides from stored carbohydrates, later secreting these bound to protein. These complexes of protein and lipid are called very-low-density lipoprotein (VLDL). These can then provide triglycerides to muscle and adipose tissue in the absence of dietary lipids. Once acted on by tissue lipoprotein lipase, the resulting lipoprotein particles with diminished triglyceride content are called low-density lipoprotein (LDL).

There are five major types of hyperlipoproteinemia, some of which are genetic. Patterns of serum lipid excess identical or similar to these familial disorders are also found in individuals with no definite family history of hyperlipopoteinemia. Environmental factors (dietary intake of fats plus obesity, diabetes, and alcohol consumption) also play a major role in both groups of people.

Type I hyperlipoproteinemia is a rare disorder, transmitted as an autosomal recessive trait, in which there is an absence of the tissue lipoprotein lipase, resulting in an inability of the adipose and muscle tissues to free triglycerides from chylomicrons. After a fatty meal, the plasma triglyceride levels of affected individuals may climb above 2000 mg/dl. The triglycerides are deposited in the skin, producing cutaneous xanthomas, or are taken up by histiocytes in the liver, spleen, or bone marrow, resulting in hepatosplenomegaly. The high triglyceride levels may also be associated with a fulminant pancreatitis.

Type II hyperlipoproteinemia is characterized by the elevation of plasma LDL levels (type IIa) owing to a lack of a cellular LDL receptor or to a different LDL receptor in all tissues. The inability of the body tissues to absorb the cholesterol-laden LDL is thought to be accompanied by increased production of LDL on the part of the liver, which fails to sense the increased plasma levels. Individuals may be homozygous for the defective LDL receptor gene with plasma cholesterol levels $\geq$ 500–600 mg/dl in childhood, or heterozygous, with cholesterol levels averaging 300–400 mg/dl and appearing sometime after childhood. Both groups have accelerated atherosclerosis, with myocardial infarction and ischemic peripheral vascular disease occurring at a much earlier age (earliest in homozygotes) than in the general population. An almost pathognomonic sign of the type II disorder is the formation of xanthomas in the tendons. One in 10 heterozygotes has elevated triglyceride levels type IIb (increased VLDL), as well as hypercholesterolemia. Also called *familial hypercholesterolemia.*

Type III hyperlipoproteinemia can be an inherited disorder in which abnormal lipoproteins, intermediate density lipoproteins (IDL), are found. Atherosclerosis and xanthoma formation occur, the latter often erupting in the palm or palmar creases of the fingers. Xanthomas in these patients may reach extremely large size (> 8 cm in diameter). The clinical presentation of this disorder is rapid and severe, resulting in early myocardial infarction, peripheral vascular disease, and strokes. There is a high frequency of concurrent affliction with diabetes, hypothyroidism, and obesity, as these disorders are associated with high triglyceride levels or slow metabolic turnover of lipids.

Types IV and V hyperlipoproteinemias occur in the disorder known as familial hypertriglyceridemia. This disorder, transmitted as an autosomal dominant trait, produces elevated VLDL through an unknown metabolic defect, and so yields high serum triglyceride levels (type IV). In some individuals, the use of estrogens or the development of diabetes mellitus or hypothyroidism may be associated with a substantial rise in VLDL and chylomicron-like lipoproteins (type V). Those with a predominantly type IV pattern show accelerated coronary and peripheral vascular disease; those with type V develop hepatosplenomegaly and are also predisposed to pancreatitis.

Several other disorders can produce the patterns of serum lipoprotein excess similar to those produced by these inheritable conditions. Lupus erythematosus may result in a type I hyperlipoproteinemia, and malignancies that produce immunoglobulins (e.g., multiple myeloma) may result in a type III or type IV hyperlipoproteinemia. Stress may produce a pattern similar to type IV hyperlipoproteinemia, and liver tumors may produce increased amounts of endogenous cholesterol, resulting in a type IIa pattern.

A useful diagnostic tool in the confirmation of hyperlipoproteinemia is lipoprotein electrophoresis, which separates serum lipids into their respective fractions: VLDL, LDL, and chylomicrons. In the type III disorder, VLDL and the chylomicron remnants form a wide band intermediate in electrophoretic position between VLDL and LDL fractions. The simple observation of serum overnight refrigerated storage produces several phenotypes, as shown in the accompanying figure. A creamy white layer floating on the serum (crosshatching) is typical of those patterns with elevated chylomicrons or chylomicron-like lipoproteins, whereas increased serum turbidity (stippling) is produced by elevated VLDL or LDL fractions.

PAUL JURKOWSKI, M.D.

hyperlucency (hi″per-loo′sen-se) increased radiolucency; having a greater penetrability by x-rays.

h. of bone, a term used in diagnostic radiology to describe decreased density, indicative of either osteoporosis or osteomalacia, when the exact condition is unknown.

hyperlysinemia (hi″per-li″sin-e′me-ah) [*hyper-* + *lysine* + Gr. *haima* blood + *-ia*] a group of disorders of lysine metabolism, all thought to be transmitted as autosomal traits, that are primarily associated with the increased concentration of lysine or its metabolites in the blood. The most frequently occurring hyperlysinemias are hyperlysinemia types I and II, saccharopinuria, hydroxylysinemia, pipecolic acidemia, and α-ketoadipic aciduria. The most common clinical feature associated with these disorders is mental retardation. Also called *lysemia.* See also *aminoacidopathy* and *saccharopinuria.*

h. type I, a disorder of lysine metabolism, transmitted as an autosomal recessive trait, that is due to a relative or absolute deficiency of the enzyme lysine:αketoglutarate reductase. Those affected have increased levels of lysine and homoarginine in the blood and urine. Central nervous system dysfunction with variable mental retardation, ammonia intoxication, hypotonia, vomiting, and coma may occur. Attacks of hyperlysinemia may follow ingestion of high-protein meals; diets low in lysine may be helpful. Also called *lysine intolerance* and periodic hyperlysinemia. See also *aminoacidopathy.*

h. type II, a disorder of lysine metabolism, transmitted as an autosomal recessive trait, that is due to an unknown enzyme deficiency. Those affected may show increased levels of lysine in the blood and variable degrees of central nervous system disturbances and muscle weakness. Also called persistent hyperlysinemia. See also *aminoacidopathy.*

hypermature (hi″per-mah-tūr′) past the stage of normal maturity.

hypermelanosis (hi″per-mel″ah-no′sis) [*hyper-* + Gr. *melas* black + *-osis* condition] excessive deposition of melanin in the skin, which can be due to a variety of causes. Cf. *hypomelanism.*

hypermenorrhea (hi″per-men″o-re′ah) [*hyper-* + Gr. *mēn* month + *rhein* to flow] a relative increase in the duration and/or quantity of the menstrual flow, ocurring at normal cycle intervals, that is frequently associated with anovulation. Clinical evaluation of this condition is important.

hypernatremia (hi″per-na-tre′me-ah) [*hyper-* + L. *natron* sodium + Gr. *haima* blood + *-ia*] an abnormal condition characterized by a concentration of serum sodium (Na^+) above the normal range of 136–145 mmol/l (310–340 mg/dl, as Na^+). This condition generally results from a loss of body fluids that contain more water than Na^+, followed by inadequate intake of water. The causes of hypernatremia are associated with either renal or extrarenal factors. Renal disturbances include decreased pituitary secretion of ADH (antidiuretic hormone) or renal insensitivity to ADH (both constituting diabetes insipidus), osmotic diuresis, hypercalcemia, and hypokalemia. Extrarenal disturbances include excessive sweating, diarrhea, disorders of the thirst mechanism, and grossly excessive sodium intake with inadequate intake of water.

Symptoms of hypernatremia are primarily central nervous system dysfunctions, including confusion, seizures, neuron and muscle excitability, and coma. Urine may be of low volume and highly concentrated. Weight loss, rapid heart rates, low blood pressure, increased blood urea nitrogen (BUN) due to deficient kidney perfusion, and elevated serum K^+ may occur. This disorder may be dangerous in infants, producing gastroenteritis and severe diar-

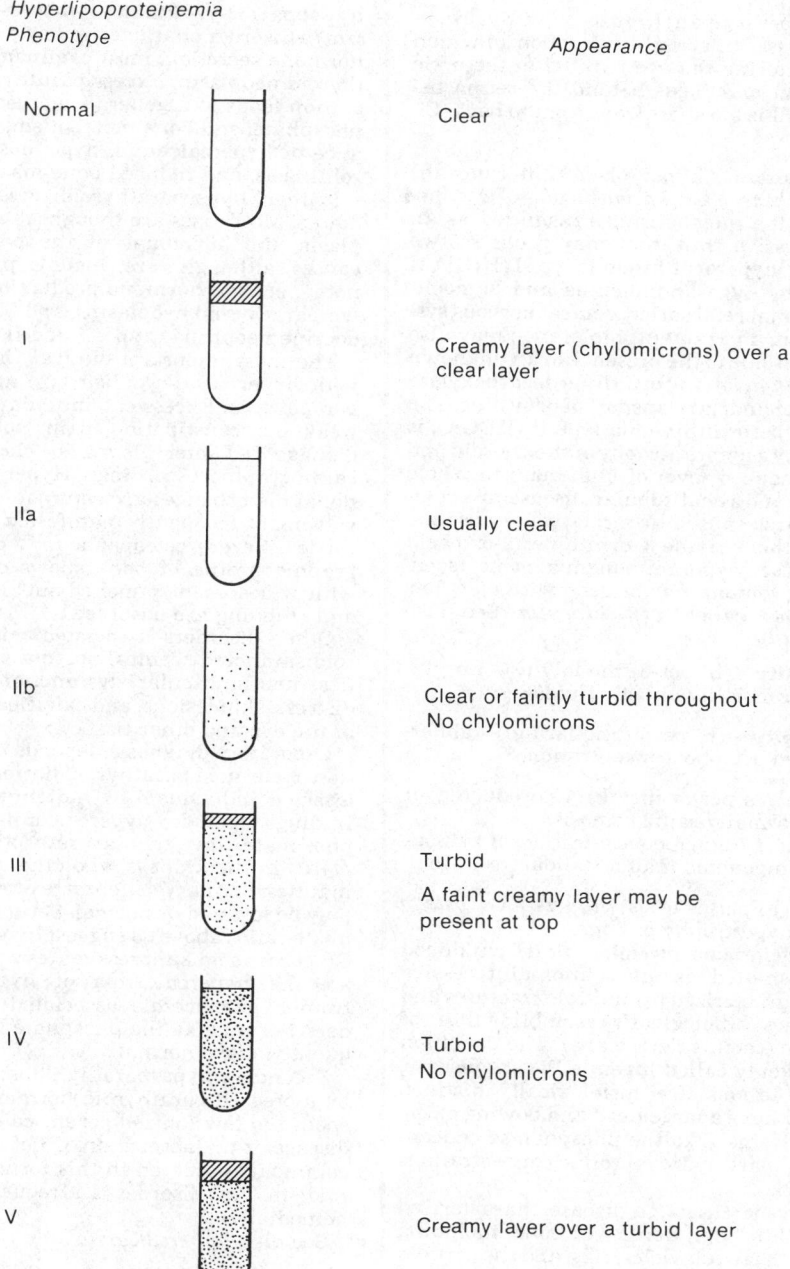

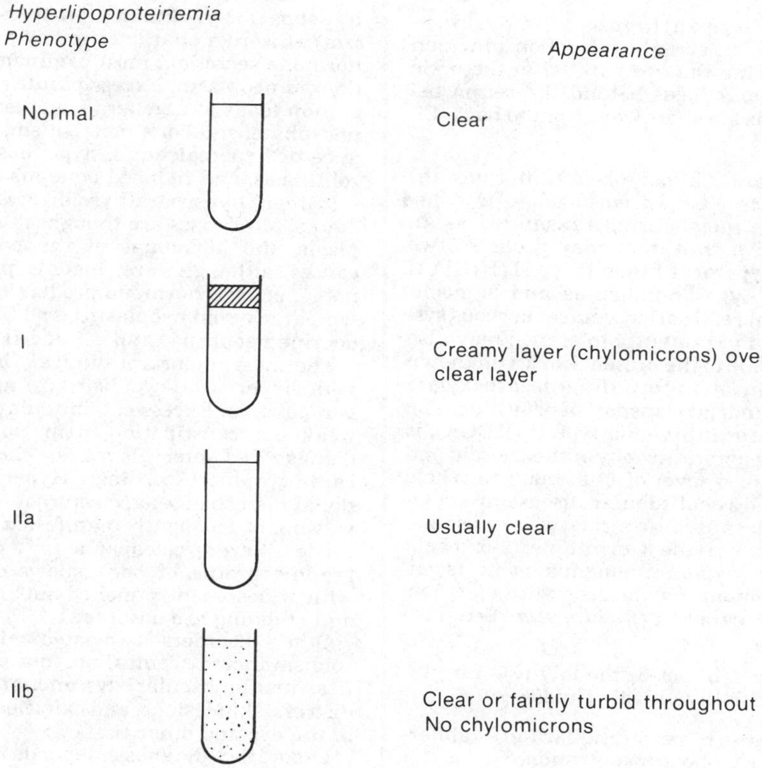

Hyperlipoproteinemia. Typical appearance of serum after standing at 4°C for 18 hr. The hatched portion indicates the creamy layer of chylomicrons; the speckled portion indicates the turbid layer associated with increased pre-β lipoprotein. (From Tietz, N. W.: Fundamentals of Clinical Chemistry. 2nd ed. Philadelphia, W. B. Saunders Co., 1976.)

rhea. Hypernatremia is treated by replacing body water and, if necessary, electrolytes.

See also *electrolyte balance and homeostasis.*

hypernephroma (hi″per-ne-fro′mah) [*hyper-* + Gr. *nephros* kidney + *-oma*] a widely used misnomer for adenocarcinoma of the renal cortex (renal cell adenocarcinoma or renal carcinoma). The term arose because of the misconception that the tumor so designated had its origin in adrenal rests in the renal cortex. Although histogenetically incorrect, the term persists because of its long usage, but is used more in verbal than in written medical communication. See also *renal tumors.*

hyperopia (hi″per-o′pe-ah) [*hyper-* + Gr. *ōps* eye + *-ia*] farsightedness; an error of refraction in which rays of light entering the eye parallel to the optic axis are brought to a focus behind the retina because the eyeball is too short from front to back. Cf. *myopia*.

hyperornithinemia (hi″per-or-nĭ″thin-e′me-ah) [*hyper-* + *ornithine* + Gr. *haima* blood + *-ia*] a disorder of ornithine metabolism, transmitted as an autosomal recessive trait, that may occur in two forms. The first, hyperornithinemia type I (HHH), is characterized by hyperammonemia and homocitrullinemia; mental retardation, central nervous system dysfunction, and protein intolerance may also be seen. Type I is due to the presence of an unknown enzyme, possibly involving ornithine decarboxylase or altered mitochondrial transport of ornithine. The second type, hyperornithinemia type II (HOGA), is characterized by a gyrate atrophy of the choroid and retina and a reduced level of glutamate in whole blood. Hepatic and renal tubular disease are common. This form is caused by a relative or absolute deficiency of the enzyme L-ornithine: 2-oxo-acid aminotransferase; hyperammonemia is not seen. Variable improvement may be seen with diets low in protein. Also called *ornithinemia*. See also *aminoacidopathy*.

hyperosmolality (hi″per-oz″mo-lal′ĭ-te) an increase in the osmolality of body fluids.

hyperosmolarity (hi″per-oz″mo-lar′ĭ-te) abnormally increased osmolar concentration.

hyperosmotic (hi″per-oz-mot′ik) 1. producing or caused by abnormally rapid osmosis.

2. containing a higher concentration of osmotically active components than a standard solution.

hyperostosis (hi″per-os″to′sis) [*hyper-* + Gr. *osteon* bone + *-osis*] hypertrophy of bone.

h. corticalis deformans juvenilis, a rare childhood disorder, transmitted as an autosomal recessive trait, that is characterized by multiple fractures and bone deformities radiologically resembling those of Paget's disease (osteitis deformans). The condition is often mistakenly called juvenile Paget's disease, although the lesions are histologically distinct. Those affected have a large head and bowing of the extremities. Plasma alkaline phosphatase concentrations and urinary hydroxyproline concentrations are increased.

h. corticalis generalisata, a disease characterized by an abnormally high density of bone, including that in the skull, jaw, clavicles, ribs, and the cortices of the bones of the arms and legs. The changes in bone formation may cause increased pressure on the nerves, especially those exiting the skull, and result in losses of vision and hearing and paralysis of the facial muscles. The increased bone is of normal histologic structure, and alkaline phosphatase levels are elevated. Also called van Buchem's syndrome.

hyperoxaluria (hi″per-ok″sah-lu′re-ah) the excretion of large amounts of oxalic acid in the urine, often causing the formation of kidney stones. Both genetic and environmental causes are known. Also called *oxaluria*.

primary o., see *oxalosis*.

hyperparathyroidism (hi″per-par″ah-thi′roid-izm) a disorder characterized by excess parathyroid hormone secretion, most commonly due to a parathyroid neoplasm. Excess parathyroid hormone secretion leads to a generalized disorder of calcium, phosphate, and bone metabolism, with the appearance of hypercalcemia, hypophosphatemia, nephrolithiasis, and reduced bone mass.

Primary hyperparathyroidism is most common in adults. Most cases are thought to arise from hyperplasia and adenomas of the parathyroid. Other causes, although rare, include parathyroid carcinoma, ectopic hormone production by a variety of nonparathyroid neoplasms, and MEN (multiple endocrine neoplasia), types I and II.

The most important clinical findings associated with hyperparathryoidism are attributable to hypercalcemia. Excess calcium may produce nausea, weakness, constipation, pain, polyuria, and renal damage. Q-T intervals may be shortened in electrocardiographic recordings. Hypertension and emotional disturbances are common. There is bone involvement, frequently manifested as osteitis fibrosis cystica. Severe osteopenia may occur. The radiographic profile of bone shows decreased density with widespread "punched-out" lesions. Joint pain and clubbing are observed.

Other disorders associated with hyperparathyroidism include central nervous system abnormalities, neuromuscular dysfunction, gastrointestinal distress, skin lesions, and calcification of the cornea of the eye and other tissues.

Laboratory diagnosis depends on the demonstration of elevated parathyroid hormone in the blood of affected individuals by radioimmunoassay. Other findings include hypercalcemia, reduced blood phosphate, low tubular resorption of phosphate (TRP) in the kidneys, and other electrolyte abnormalities. Urinary calcium excretion is high, but may be lowered or normal. Serum chloride to phosphate ratios above 33 suggest hyperparathyroidism. Glucocorticoid suppression tests help to differentiate the hypercalcemia of hyperparathyroidism from hypercalcemia associated with other disorders. Serum alkaline phosphate levels also are frequently above normal.

Secondary hyperparathyroidism is characterized by increased parathyroid hormone secretion in response to low ionized serum calcium due to renal disease or malabsorption. Chief cell hyperplasia is commonly observed in this form of hyperparathyroidism. This disorder is a frequent complication of hemodialysis.

See also *hypercalcemia*.

hyperphenylalaninemia (hi″per-fen″il-al″ah-nĭ-ne′me-ah) [*hyper-* + *phenylalanine* + Gr. *haima* blood + *-ia*] one of a group of metabolic disorders characterized by the deficient enzymatic conversion of phenylalanine to tyrosine, and result in the accumulation of phenylalanine in the plasma. These genetic diseases, transmitted as autosomal recessive traits, result in the partial or complete deficiency in enzymes or cofactors that are essential in the normal breakdown of phenylalanine. The most common disorder of this group is phenylketonuria (PKU).

Benign persistent hyperphenylalaninemia is characterized by elevations of the plasma phenylalanine levels, but generally not exceeding concentrations of 16 mg/dl. Mental and physical development in these individuals is normal without dietary restriction. Transient phenylketonuria occurs when the phenotypical characteristics and biochemical abnormalities of phenylketonuria spontaneously remit during infancy or childhood, and the plasma phenylalanine concentrations become normal or nearly normal without dietary restriction. The mechanism of this remission is unknown. In mild atypical phenylketonuria, individuals have an increased tolerance for phenylalanine and can consume up to 2 g in the diet. A partial liver enzyme deficiency has been suggested.

"Lethal" hyperphenylalaninemia is seen in those children who fail to develop normally despite phenylketonuria dietary management. These patients also show abnormally decreased capacities to synthesize serotonin and L-dopa. Many develop seizure disorders and die before age 5 yr. A deficiency of dihydropteridine reductase, a cofactor in the conversion of phenylalanine to tyrosine, has been documented as the cause. This cofactor may be assayed in skin fibroblast cultures. It is of practical importance to distinguish lethal hyperphenylalaninemia from classical phenylketonuria. These diseases differ both in the response to therapeutic management and in the eventual prognosis.

See also *aminoacidopathy* and *phenylketonuria.*

hyperphosphatasia (hi″per-fos″fah-ta′ze-ah) abnormally elevated plasma concentrations of alkaline phosphatase.

hyperphosphatemia (hi″per-fos″fah-te′me-ah) [*hyper-* + *phosphate* + Gr. *haima* blood + -ia] an abnormal condition characterized by an excess of phosphates in the blood. Normal fasting serum concentrations of phosphates, measured as inorganic phosphorus, are 1–1.5 mmol/l (3–4.5 mg/dl) in adults and higher in children. Causes of hyperphosphatemia include excessive growth hormone (acromegaly), hypoparathyroidism or pseudohypoparathyroidism (both associated with low calcium), renal insufficiency or acute failure, excessive phosphate intake, and hypervitaminosis D. Acute increases in phosphate levels are frequently associated with a decrease in serum calcium and a reduction in serum bicarbonate. The symptoms associated with this disorder are usually secondary to the disease process that initiated the hyperphosphatemia. See also *electrolyte balance and homeostasis.*

hyperphosphaturia (hi″per-fos″fah-tu′re-ah) [*hyper-* + *phosphate* + Gr. *ouron* urine + *-ia*] an abnormal condition characterized by an excess of phosphorus in the urine (> 0.9–1.3 g/24 hr). One of the causes may be a dietary intake of an excess of phosphorus-containing foods.

hyperpigmentation (hi″per-pig″men-ta′shun) a general term for skin disorders in which there is an increased concentration of melanin, e.g., ephelides, lentigines, café au lait spots, or pigmented nevi. Occasionally, generalized hyperpigmentation may be related to endocrine, nutritional, metabolic, chemical, or toxic factors.

hyperpituitarism (hi″per-pĭ-tu′ĭ-tah-rizm″) a condition characterized by the abnormally increased synthesis and secretion of hormones of the anterior pituitary. Most often, only prolactin, growth hormone, or adrenocorticotropic hormone (ACTH) are increased. The most frequent cause is a functioning pituitary adenoma.

Hypersecretion of prolactin is the most common form of hyperpituitarism. Affected females may experience galactorrhea, amenorrhea, decreased libido, hirsutism, or decreased estrogens. In males this condition leads to hypogonadism, decreased libido, or infertility. Hypersecretion of ACTH in hyperpituitarism leads to Cushing's disease, with loss of the normal diurnal rhythm of fluctuation of ACTH and cortisol plasma levels. Hypersecretion of growth hormone results in gigantism in children and acromegaly in adults.

Laboratory determinations reveal increased serum prolactin (> 100–150 ng/ml). Prolactin response to the administration of thyrotropin-releasing factor (TRF) or chlorpromazine is blunted. X-rays, CT scans, and polytomography may be useful in demonstrating pituitary neoplasms. Visual field disturbances also may occasionally be present.

See also *acromegaly, Cushing's disease,* and *gigantism.*

hyperplasia (hi″per-pla′ze-ah) [*hyper-* + Gr. *plasis* formation + *-ia*] a cellular overgrowth; a controlled proliferation of cells in excess of normal that is irreversible when the inciting stimulus is removed. Hyperplasia is characterized by an increase in the number of cells per unit volume of tissue. This state can be brought about by an increase in the rate of cell proliferation, an increase in the number of cells in the replicating pool, or the prolonged life span of the involved cells. The stimulus for hyperplasia may be acute injury (e.g., epidermal hyperplasia occurring in a healing wound of the skin), chronic irritation (e.g., epithelial hyperplasia of the buccal mucosa produced by irritation from poorly fitted dentures), and prolonged excessive hormonal stimulation (e.g., adrenal cortical hyperplasia following increased stimulation by elevated secretions of pituitary adrenocorticotropic hormone). Some forms of hormonally-induced hyperplasia are physiologic; e.g., increased glandular proliferation in the female breast during puberty and pregnancy. Compensatory hyperplasia is another form of physiologic hyperplasia in which the volume of the remaining tissue or organ increases to maintain a normal level of physiologic function when a portion of that tissue or organ is lost; e.g., the increase in the size of the remaining kidney following surgical removal of the opposite kidney.

The cells participating in hyperplastic proliferation usually remain relatively normal in size, shape, and function. In some cellular proliferations, however, abnormal cytologic features may be present (see *atypical h.*). These findings are thought to indicate that there is a continuum from hyperplasia to malignancy, with the degree of cytologic and architectural atypia representing the extent of progression along this continuum. Although there is some evidence to support this hypothesis, it is by no means established.

adenomatous h., a form of hyperplasia in which glands exhibit budding and branching. Most frequently the term is used to describe such changes in the endometrium, but it may be applied to other organs as well.

atypical h., hyperplasia in which either cytologic or architectural abnormalities, or both, are present. The degree of severity of the atypia in this form of hyperplasia ranges from mild alterations, in which there is minimal deviation from that of normal glandular epithelium, to severe alterations that merge at the other end of the spectrum with well-differentiated malignancy. The term is applied to hyperplastic proliferations associated with morphologic alterations in a variety of tissues and sites in the body.

benign prostatic h., a common disorder of the prostate that occurs with increasing frequency and severity after middle age. It is characterized by benign proliferation of the prostatic glands, fibromuscular stroma, or both. The lateral lobes are involved most frequently; the posterior lobe, rarely.

Through encroachment on the prostatic urethra, hyperplasia of the prostate produces varying degrees of obstruction to urinary flow. The more common symptoms are frequency, urgency, and hesitancy of urination and incomplete voiding of the bladder. Complications of prolonged obstruction of urine flow include urinary tract infections and azotemia. Diagnosis and evaluation are aided by prostatic palpation, excretory urography, cystoscopy, and, when indicated, biopsy.

congenital adrenal h., a group of disorders characterized by enzymatic deficiencies in the biosynthesis of the adrenal hormones. Clinical presentation depends on both the specific enzyme that is absent and the age at which the deficiency is expressed.

Six enzyme defects in the adrenal have been characterized. (1) A deficiency of 20α-hydroxylase results in the decreased synthesis of all adrenal steroids, leading to adrenal insufficiency and ambiguous genital development in males. (2) A deficiency of 3β-hydroxysteroid dehydrogenase results in the deficient excretion of corticoids and aldosterone and the increased excretion of dehydroepiandrosterone, leading to ambiguous genital development in infants of both sexes, adrenal insufficiency, and increased urinary 17-ketosteroids. (3) A deficiency of 17α-hydroxylase results in the deficient production of cortisol, aldosterone, and total body androgens and estrogens. There is an overproduction of corticosterone and 11-deoxycorticosterone (DOC). As a result, there are compensatory increases in the secretion of adrenocorticotropin (ACTH) and gonadotropin, accompanied by hypertension, alkalosis, and retarded sexual development. (4) The most common adrenal enzyme deficiency, 21-hydroxylase, results in the deficient production of both cortisol and aldosterone, and a concomitant increase in ACTH concentrations, leading to adrenal hyperplasia and the excessive elaboration of adrenal androgens. If this enzymatic defect is severe, there may be salt wasting, hypotension, shock, and prerenal azotemia. Virilism occurs as a result of the overproduction of adrenal androgens. The female fetus undergoes masculinization (fusion of labioscrotal folds, clitoral enlargement), whereas the male fetus undergoes relatively normal development. If the disorder is not treated, females grow rapidly, become muscular, and display male patterns of hair growth (hirsutism) and voice deepening. Males undergo precocious puberty. Diagnosis is accomplished by demonstration of increased urinary pregnanetriol and easy suppression of pregnanetriol and 17-ketosteroids by administration of glucocorticoids. This enzyme is linked to the HLA locus. (5) Deficiency of 11β-hydroxylase results in the deficient production of corticoids and aldosterone, and the overproduction of DOC and 11-deoxycortisol. High circulating concentrations of ACTH cause adrenal hyperplasia, with the resultant elaboration of excessive adrenal androgens. The clinical symptoms of this defect are virilism and hypertension. The excesses of 17-ketosteroid may diagnostically be suppressed by administration of glucocorticoids. (6) Deficiency of 18-hydroxysteroid dehydrogenase leads to the deficient production of aldosterone and the increased elaboration of corticosterone. The result is excessive sodium loss, dehydration, and hypotension.

Diagnosis of these disorders relies on clinical presentation and laboratory determination of excessive or diminished adrenal hormone precursors or products. Treatment usually requires replacement of adrenal hormones. Plastic surgery may be necessary to correct the development of abnormal sex characteristics. See also *adrenogenital syndrome* and *virilism.*

cystic h., a form of glandular hyperplasia in which the hyperplastic glands are large and cystically dilated, and generally show scant evidence of atypia. This variant of hyperplasia is common in the endometrium where, in its pure form, it is thought to carry a low risk for transformation to adenocarcinoma. See also *adenomatous h.*

endometrial h., hyperplasia of the endometrial lining of the uterus; a process that occurs in response to prolonged and continuous estrogenic stimulation unopposed by progesterone stimulation. Endometrial hyperplasia may be cystic, characterized by large, cystically dilated glands unaccompanied by atypia; adenomatous, characterized by budding and branched glands with intervening stroma that may exhibit a spectrum of architectual and cytologic atypia; or mixed, containing both cystic and adenomatous components.

In its pure form, cystic endometrial hyperplasia is thought to carry little or no risk of transformation to endometrial adenocarcinoma, whereas adenomatous endometrial hyperplasia is thought to carry an increased risk of transformation to endometrial adenocarcinoma—a risk that increases with the severity of the cytologic and architectural atypia of the hyperplasia.

glandular h., an abnormally increased amount of glandular tissue (increased volume of glands, increased number of glands per unit area, or both). Glandular hyperplasias may exhibit a wide range of combinations of architectural disarray, epithelial cell stratification, and cytologic alteration representing a spectrum from no atypia to markedly severe atypia. See also *adenomatous h.* and *cystic h.*

nodular mesothelial h., discrete foci of reactive mesothelial cells that may exhibit a papillary configuration, and that produce small and often multiple nodules. They must be differentiated cytologically and histologically from mesothelioma.

wasserhelle h., a form of parathyroid gland hyperplasia characterized by a diffuse proliferation of water-clear cells arranged in solid masses and acini. These cells appear to have an empty cytoplasm at the light microscopic level, but with electron microscopy the cytoplasm is seen to contain many spherical membrane-limited vacuoles and secretory granules. This cell type is not seen in the normal parathyroid gland. The wasserhelle cells of the normal parathyroid gland are glycogen-rich cells that lack the ultrastructural appearance of the cells of water-clear-cell hyperplasia. When water-clear-cell hyperplasia is present, it manifests its presence by hyperparathyroidism, accounting for 2–4 percent of all cases of this condition. Also called water-clear-cell hyperplasia. See also *hyperparathyroidism.* Cf. *wasserhelle cell.*

hyperplastic (hi″per-plas′tik) pertaining to or characterized by hyperplasia.

hyperploid (hi′per-ploid) having more than the typical number of chromosomes, as in Down's syndrome. Cf. *hypoploid.*

hyperploidy (hi″per-ploi′de) the state of being hyperploid.

hyperpnea (hi″perp-ne′ah) [*hyper-* + Gr. *pnoia* breath] a general term denoting an increase in depth of breathing, which may or may not be accompanied by an increase in the respiratory rate, without implication of any subjective sensation of the increased respiratory effort. A maximal hyperpnea occurs during strenuous exercise.

hyperpneic (hi″perp-ne′ik) pertaining to or characterized by hyperpnea.

hyperpolarization (hi″per-po″lar-ĭ-za′shun) an increase in the size of the transmembrane potential of an excitable cell. In a hyperpolarized cell, the interior becomes more negative than it is under normal resting conditions. Cf. *depolarization.*

hyperpotassemia (hi″per-pot″ah-se′me-ah) [*hyper-* + *potassium* + Gr. *haima* blood + *-ia*] see *hyperkalemia.*

hyperprolactinemia the abnormal increase in circulating prolactin concentration in the blood. Females affected with this condition display amenorrhea, galactorrhea, and decreased estrogens and libido. Affected males may develop gynecomastia, often with hypogonadism. Causes of hyperprolactinemia include functional hypothalamic disorders (e.g., Chiari-Frommel syndrome), autonomous prolactin production (e.g., pituitary chromophobe adenoma), endogenous metabolic disorders (e.g., acromegaly, hypothyroidism, and chronic renal failure), and chlorpromazine therapy (antipsychosis therapy). Prolactin levels are transiently increased in women following vigorous exercise.

Diagnosis is based on radioimmunoassay of prolactin. Concentrations of > 100–150 ng/ml usually indicate a functional pituitary adenoma. See also *prolactin.*

hyperprolinemia (hi″per-pro″lĭ-ne′me-ah) [*hyper-* + *proline* + Gr. *haima* blood + *-ia*] a disorder of imino acid metabolism, transmitted as an autosomal recessive trait, that is characterized by an excess of proline in the body fluids. The aminoaciduria includes hydroxyproline and glycine as well as a proline, as a common renal tubular active transport mechanism is shared.

There are two types of hyperprolinemia. The Type I defect involves the enzyme proline oxidase, which oxidizes proline to pyrroline carboxylate. Although mental retardation does not occur, renal abnormalities may be produced with this form. The Type II defect involves the enzyme Δ′-pyrroline-5-carboxylic acid dehydrogenase. Mental retardation may variably occur, and renal abnormalities and seizures are seen with this form. Also called *prolinemia.* See also *aminoacidopathy.*

hyperproteinemia (hi″per-pro″tēn-e′me-ah) [*hyper-* + *protein* + Gr. *haima* blood + *-ia*] an abnormally increased concentration of protein in the blood. See also *hyperlipoproteinemia.*

hyperpyretic (hi″per-pi-ret′ik) pertaining to, exhibiting, or causing hyperpyrexia.

hyperpyrexia (hi″per-pi-rek′se-ah) [*hyper-* + Gr. *pyressein* to be feverish] a highly elevated body temperature. See also *hyperthemia.*

hyperreflexia (hi″per-re-flek′se-ah) exaggeration of reflexes.

autonomic h., a condition associated with lesions above the outflow of the splanchic nerves and characterized by paroxysmal hypertension, bradycardia, and severe headache probably due to the sudden release of catecholamines by stimulation of the splanchnic nerves.

hypersarcosinemia (hi″per-sar″ko-sēn-e′me-ah) a hereditary condition, transmitted as an autosomal recessive trait, that is characterized by mild mental retardation and motor disability. The biochemical lesion is in the enzyme sarcosine dehydrogenase, and results in increased levels of sarcosine in the blood and urine. Also called *sarcosinemia.*

hypersegmentation (hi″per-seg″men-ta′shun) the appearance of being divided into multiple segments or lobes.

hereditary h. of neutrophils, a benign hereditary condition characterized by the presence of polymorphonuclear neutrophils with more lobes than are normal. See also *polymorphonuclear neutrophil.*

hypersensitive (hi″per-sen′sĭ-tiv) 1. abnormally increased sensitivity.

2. highly reactive to the application of or exposure to specific allergens in quantities that would be innocuous to normal individuals.

hypersensitivity (hi″per-sen′sĭ-tiv″ĭ-te) see *delayed hypersensitivity* and *immediate hypersensitivity.*

hypersomnia (hi″per-som′ne-ah) [*hyper-* + L. *somnus* sleep] uncontrolled drowsiness; pathologically excessive sleep. This disturbance is characteristic of individuals with encephalitis lethargica, trypanosomiasis, and brain tumors or other lesions involving the diencephalon (particularly the posterior hypothalamus). Hypersomnia may also occur in servere myxedema. See also *hypersomnia–sleep apnea syndrome* and *Kleine-Levin syndrome.*

hypersomnia–sleep apnea (HSA) syndrome a syndrome that occurs most frequently in obese middle-aged males and is characterized by excessive daytime sleepiness, recurring apnea during sleep, and loud intermittent snoring. It is associated with systemic hypertension, cardiac arrhythmias, erythremia, pulmonary hypertension, cardiac hypertrophy, and cerebral and myocardial infarction.

Sleep apneas rarely occur in normal middle-aged persons but may occur as frequently as 200 times in a 6-to 8-hr sleep period in those with HSA. During these apneas the heart rate may alter to such an extent that therapeutic intervention is necessary. During sleep, the airway of many HSA patients is functionally obstructed at the velopharyngeal sphincter in the oral pharynx; the only proved treatment for this is a tracheostomy that allows the obstruction to be bypassed.

hypersplenism (hi″per-splen′izm) a condition characterized by enlargement of the spleen, with some degree of pancytopenia despite the presence of hyperactive bone marrow. The most common cause is congestive splenomegaly secondary to cirrhosis of the liver and portal hypertension, but a variety of other conditions also may contribute: e.g., thrombosis, vascular stenosis, other vascular deformities such as aneurysm of the splenic artery, and cysts.

Hypersplenism may also accompany primary disorders such as infiltrative diseases (Gaucher's disease and Niemann-Pick disease), lymphoproliferative diseases (leukemias and lymphomas), inflammatory diseases (infectious mononucleosis and tuberculosis), and congenital hemolytic anemias. Individuals affected with hypersplenism may experience sudden hematemesis and gastrointestinal bleeding. Fever, pain, abdominal fullness, and purpura may also be seen.

Laboratory findings include decreased white blood cell and platelet counts, the result of pooling and sequestration. Anemias (normocytic or normochromic) may be mild and may be accompanied by an increased reticulocyte count. Granulocytes may undergo a shift to the left. The ^{51}Cr red cell life span is decreased. A variety of other tests may be indicated to determine the primary disease that leads to hypersplenism, and treatment should be selected to relieve the primary disorder. In certain cases, splenectomy may be advised.

hypersplenosis (hi″per-splen-o′sis) see under *spleen.*

hypertelorism (hi″per-te′lor-izm) [*hyper-* + Gr. *tēlouros* distant] a congenital malformation that results in abnormal distance between two paired organs; usually applied to the eyes.

ocular h., a congenital malformation of the cranial bones that results in wide-set eyes. It may be associated with mental deficiency, brachycephaly, and a depressed nasal bridge. Ocular hypertelorism is a characteristic of many syndromes, including acrocephalosyndactyly, otopalataldigital syndrome, and craniofacial dysostosis.

hypertension (hi″per-ten′shun) [*hyper-* + *tension*] a common and significant cardiovascular disorder characterized by elevations in the systemic arterial blood pressure. Persons with hypertension have a greater risk of developing cerebrovascular disease with transient ischemic attacks and stroke, and cardiovascular disease including atherosclerosis, coronary artery disease, heart failure, kidney failure, and retinopathy (damage to the vasculature of the eye).

Blood pressures recorded from a population constitute a continuum of values. Although increased risk of cardiovascular dysfunction accompanies any elevation in blood pressure, the degree of hypertension can be classified depending on the pressure elevation. In adults, resting systolic pressures of less than 140 mmHg and diastolic pressures of less than 90 mmHg are considered normal; blood pressures greater than 165/95 (systolic/diastolic) are said to be hypertensive. Individuals with pressures frequently between normal and hypertensive levels are classed as borderline hypertensives and are considered to be more likely to develop hypertension. Diastolic pressures of 90–104 mmHg constitute class I or mild hypertension; 105–119 mmHg, class II or moderate hypertension; and 120 mmHg or greater, class III or severe hypertension.

Blood pressure is determined by the balance of cardiac output (the amount of blood pumped by the heart) and total peripheral resistance (the total resistance to flow of all the blood vessels). Changes in these two parameters are continuously being made within the body to maintain blood pressure at the normal level. About 30 percent of borderline hypertensives show an elevated cardiac output; in 70 percent of these individuals and in patients with established hypertension, however, the cardiac output is normal and the total peripheral resistance is elevated owing to constriction of the blood vessels. Despite considerable research, no single cause for the elevated peripheral resistance in essential hypertension has been found. Many factors may be involved, including changes in the blood pressure control center in the central nervous system, elevations in blood volume, humoral changes, changes in nervous stimulation of the heart and blood vessels, and increased sensitivity of the blood vessels to nervous or humoral stimulation. In the clinical evaluation of suspected hypertension, both diastolic and systolic pressures are recorded, but diagnosis and therapy are based primarily on the diastolic levels. This is largely because the benefits of and goals for treating systolic pressure elevations have not been well established. Also, systolic pressure tends to increase throughout life as vascular compliance decreases (increased vessel wall stiffness). Exceptions to this general rule include individuals younger than 35 yr who exhibit systolic pressures above 150 mmHg or those over 60 yr with systolic pressures above 180 mmHg.

Hypertension is one of the most important health problems in the United States, affecting an estimated 20 percent of the adult population. In addition, as screening programs become more widespread, hypertension in children is becoming recognized as a significant problem. In 80–90 percent of cases, the exact cause of the rise in blood pressure is unknown; the disease is called essential hypertension or primary hypertension. Although essential hypertension is not curable in the normal sense, the blood pressure can usually be controlled and reduced to normal or near-normal levels with an appropriate treatment regimen. With good blood pressure control, the risks and complications of the disease are also significantly reduced. In the remaining 10–20 percent of cases, the hypertension has a specific cause and is usually the result of renal or endocrine problems such as obstruction of kidney blood flow (renal hypertension), coarctation of the aorta (coarctation hypertension), an aldosterone secretory tumor (primary aldosteronism), or a catecholamine-secreting tumor (pheochromocytoma). Secondary hypertension is often correctable with surgical or medical treatment. A common type of secondary hypertension is seen in females taking oral contraceptives. The blood pressure usually returns to normal after the medication is stopped.

Certain groups of peoples are at greater risk for developing hypertension. The disease is more prevalent in blacks and is more common in males than in females. A genetic component may predispose individuals to develop hypertension, as the incidence of hypertension is greater in those with a familial history of the disease. Other risk factors include obesity, diabetes mellitus, cigarette smoking, high salt intake, lack of regular exercise, and lipid abnormalities.

Diagnosis of a patient with documented hypertension begins with a thorough history and physical examination. A major goal is to try to distinguish those individuals with secondary hypertension necessitating specific treatment from the vast majority with essential hypertension. The medical history should include any previous history of high blood pressure and its treatment, diabetes mellitus, cardiac or renal disease, and stroke, as well as the use of birth control pills or other hormones. Any familial history of cardiovascular disease should be determined. Cardiovascular risk factors such as cigarette smoking, high salt intake, and lack of regular exercise should also be part of the history.

The physical examination should include two or more blood pressure determinations; funduscopic examination of the eyes; auscultation of the lungs and heart; examination of the neck for bruits and distended veins, examination of the abdomen for kidney enlargement or bruits, aortic dilation; and examination of the extremities for edema, peripheral pulses, and any neurologic deficits associated with stroke. Appropriate laboratory tests include hematocrit; urinalysis for protein, blood, and glucose and creatinine, or blood urea nitrogen (BUN) to assess renal function; plasma sodium and potassium to check for hyperaldosteronism and to establish a baseline before diuretic therapy is begun; and an electrocardiogram to assess cardiac function. Other tests often include a chest x-ray to assess heart size; fasting blood sugar to rule out diabetes mellitus; serum cholesterol to help evaluate the risk of cardiovascular disease; and uric acid to rule out gout, as uric acid levels may rise with diuretic therapy. If the screening examination suggests secondary hypertension, more specific laboratory tests may be indicated, depending on the suspected diagnosis: for example, evaluation of renal circulation and various tests of endocrine function. In most cases, essential hypertension is the diagnosis.

In mild cases of essential hypertension, initial treatment may consist of weight reduction, salt restriction, exercise, or relaxation techniques. If these changes are insufficient, or if a more severe blood pressure elevation exists, medications are employed. A diuretic is often the first drug chosen. If this is not successful, adrenergic blocking medications are often used. These drugs act both in the CNS and peripherally to decrease nervous stimulation of the heart and blood vessels, thereby reducing cardiac output and peripheral vascular resistance. In some instances a direct vasodilator drug is added to cause additional decreased peripheral vascular resistance; in resistant cases an angiotensin-converting enzyme inhibitor may be used. A variety of diuretics and adrenergic blockers are available, and in almost all cases of essential hypertension good blood pressure control can be obtained with minimal side-effects. This is important, as hypertension is usually asymptomatic and many patients, because they feel well, stop taking a medication whose side-effects are significant. Thus, an effective treatment regimen provides good control of blood pressure and allows an individual with hypertension to greatly reduce the risks of morbidity and mortality associated with this common disease.

essential h., see *idiopathic h.*

idiopathic h., hypertension of unknown origin. Also called *essential* or primary hypertension.

malignant h., severe systemic hypertension characterized by a rise in systemic blood pressure to levels of 200/140 mmHg or higher. Such a pressure rise may occur early in the development of hypertension or after a long period of less severe hypertension, and is not necessarily a logical progression of the disease. The greatly elevated blood pressure produces necrotic changes that weaken the blood vessel walls, primarily in the small arteries and arterioles. The vessels of the brain, eyes, and kidneys are particularly sensitive to such changes, and resulting effects include brain dysfunction (hypertensive encephalopathy) brain hemorrhage (stroke), impaired vision due to papilledema, and acute renal failure. The elevated blood pressure also increases the workload of the left ventricle, which, if uncorrected, causes hypertrophy and even left heart failure. Plasma renin activity levels are elevated secondary to kidney damage, and in turn elevate aldosterone secretion, which further elevates the blood pressure.

Treatment of malignant hypertension is essential; if the condition is prolonged, death usually results from heart failure, cerebral hemorrhage, or renal failure. The aim of treatment is to reverse the rapid rise in blood pressure, a situation often termed hypertensive crisis. Direct vasodilators or agents that inhibit neurally mediated vasoconstriction are often administered intravenously or intramuscularly, followed by a combination of oral antihypertensive drugs.

mineralocorticoid h., systemic hypertension due to elevated levels of mineralocorticoids. This type is rare, accounting for less than 1 percent of the hypertension reported. The most common cause is an adrenal tumor that produces excessive amounts of aldosterone (primary aldosteronism); the aldosterone stimulates increased salt and water reabsorption by the kidney, producing a volume-dependent hypertension. Less often, adrenal hyperplasia or a tumor secretes large amounts of desoxycorticosterone or related compounds, which produce the same effects as elevated aldosterone levels. Elevations in blood pressure with this type of hypertension are generally mild. A similar type of volume-dependent hypertension can occur in Cushing's syndrome, as excessive levels of glucocorticoids can exert mineralocorticoid-like activity.

Treatment generally involves surgical removal of the tumor. If the patient's condition precludes surgery, treatment with an aldosterone antagonist such as spironolactone is sometimes effective in increasing salt and water loss, thus decreasing blood pressure.

paroxysmal h., hypertension of any origin that is characterized by hypertensive periods separated by periods of normotension. The hypertensive periods may be precipitated by stress in susceptible individuals or by intermittent catecholamine secretion from an adrenal medullary tumor (pheochromocytoma), or may have less obvious causes. Borderline hypertensives often show such periods of elevated pressure interspersed with periods of normal pressure.

portal h., elevated blood pressure in the hepatic portal circulation. Such rises in pressure frequently result from impairment of the circulation through the liver due to various forms of cirrhosis. Infrequently, the portal circulation is impaired by an embolism in the portal vein or by compression of the portal vein by a tumor or bile duct infection. Elevation of portal blood pressure may also have extrahepatic causes, such as congestive heart failure, which elevate venous pressure.

The elevated hepatic pressure causes increased filtration of fluid from capillaries of the liver and intestine, and the subsequent accumulation of the fluid (ascites) in the abdomen. As liver function decreases, hypoalbuminemia develops, further impairing the reabsorption of fluid at the capillaries.

Elevated plasma levels of vasopressin and aldosterone enhance fluid and salt retention to replace the fluid lost from the vascular system, although this enhances the hypoalbuminemia.

pulmonary h., abnormally elevated blood pressure in the pulmonary circulation, in which normal pulmonary artery pressure has a mean of 12–16 mmHg and a systolic pressure of 18–25 mmHg. Pulmonary hypertension is said to exist if the mean pressure rises above 20 mmHg and the systolic pressure above 30 mmHg. In the great majority of cases the elevated pulmonary pressure has a demonstrable cause and is termed secondary hypertension. If no cause is demonstrable, the condition is termed primary pulmonary hypertension (although the terms idiopathic hypertension and essential hypertension are also used).

Secondary pulmonary hypertension is due largely to cardiac or pulmonary disorders that impede blood flow through the pulmonary vascular bed. Venous drainage of the pulmonary vascular bed can be decreased by congenital pulmonary vein stenosis, pulmonary venoocclusive disease, or cardiac dysfunction such as mitral value disease or left ventricular failure. Decreased flow through the pulmonary vascular bed can also be produced by constriction of the pulmonary vessels, as seen in several parenchymal diseases including chronic obstructive pulmonary disease, or by several pulmonary artery vascular disorders. Pulmonary thromboembolism can also increase the flow impedance. Environmental factors, such as living at high altitude and smoking, also contribute to pulmonary hypertension. The cause of primary pulmonary hypertension is unknown, but a genetic factor may be involved, as differences in vessel reactivity and vessel wall morphology have been reported in individuals with this disease. Treatment of secondary pulmonary hypertension aims at correction of the primary disease process causing the hypertension. In primary pulmonary hypertension, pulmonary vasodilators may be effective, although they do not appear actually to reverse the disease process. Anticoagulants are widely used, both as a prophylaxis against thromboembolism and because recurrent pulmonary embolism has been reported in many cases thought to be primary pulmonary hypertension.

renal h., systemic hypertension due to renal disease, most commonly renal parenchymal disease. It is the second most common type of secondary hypertension, affecting 2–5 percent of the hypertensive population. Onset may be rapid in cases of ureteral obstruction, vascular obstruction by emboli, acute glomerulonephritis, or acute oliguric renal failure; a more gradual onset may be seen in chronic glomerulonephritis, chronic pyelonephritis, or diabetic nephropathy. Major causes appear to be blood volume expansion due to decreased salt and water excretion, or activation of the renin-angiotensin system by the impaired renal blood flow. In cases of renal insufficiency, the volume expansion component may be more important, although plasma renin activity can also be elevated. In disease processes in which renal insufficiency is not pronounced, the renin-angiotensin system may be the major causative agent.

Treatment of renal hypertension depends on the specific disease process causing the elevated blood pressure. In cases of ureteral occlusion or vascular emboli, elimination of the occlusion usually reverses the hypertension. In cases of renal insufficiency, careful attention to diet, including reduced salt intake, and diuretic treatment may be effective. In more resistant cases involving activation of the renin-angiotensin system, an adrenergic blocking agent is often effective. In a small minority of patients, bilateral nephrectomy may be the only means of reversing the hypertension.

renovascular h., systemic hypertension due to renal artery obstruction. The most common causes of obstruction are atherosclerosis, fibroplastic disease, aneurysms, and embolism. This form of hypertension affects 2 percent of the hypertensive population; blacks have a lower incidence than Caucasians. Despite the greater incidence of vascular disease in diabetics, they are not more susceptible to atherosclerotic renal artery stenosis than nondiabetics.

The disease is most often seen as obstruction of one renal artery. The resulting renal ischemia causes renin release, leading to vasoconstriction by elevated activity of the renin-angiotensin system. With time, salt and water retention also occurs owing to the stimulation of aldosterone secretion by the renin-angiotensin system. On a chronic basis, renin levels fall in about one-third of the cases, yet the hypertension remains, which suggests more complex mechanisms than direct vasoconstriction and aldosterone-induced volume expansion.

Medical therapy with diuretics, beta-adrenergic blockers, vasodilators, and possibly an angiotensin-converting enzyme inhibitor is effective in controlling the hypertension and preventing further renal impairment in most patients. In those whose hypertension cannot be effectively controlled medically, surgery to correct the stenosed renal artery is indicated. In rare instances, removal of the stenosed kidney is necessary.

GREGORY A. STEPHENS, PH.D.

hypertensive (hi″per-ten′siv) 1. characterized by or causing increased pressure or tension, as in abnormally elevated blood pressure.

2. a person with abnormally elevated blood pressure.

hyperthecosis (hi″per-the-ko′sis) hyperplasia with excessive luteinization of the cells of the inner stromal layer (the theca interna) of the ovary. It may be associated with hirsutism and amenorrhea.

hyperthelia (hi″per-the′le-ah) [*hyper-* + Gr. *thēlē* nipple] a developmental abnormality in either sex, leading to the presence of an excessive number of nipples.

hyperthermia (hi″per-ther′me-ah) [*hyper-* + Gr. *thermē* heat + *-ia*] abnormally high body temperatures. Hyperthermia may result from prolonged, vigorous exercise or may be due to systemic disorders, infections, or therapeutic management. Cf. *hypothermia.*

systemic h., hyperthermia occurring after long exposure to exogenous heat or failure to dissipate endogenous heat; body temperatures may rise to greater than 42°C. When this occurs, there may be generalized vasodilation and reduction of effective blood volume. The pulse quickens and the heart dilates, resulting in reduced cardiac efficiency; respiration increases, becomes irregular, and, if severe enough, ceases. The electroencephalogram may be reversibly depressed. There may be pooling of blood with hypoxic cell injury and increases in blood potassium. Death may follow from a combination of factors. Also called *heat stroke* and heat prostration.

hyperthyroidism (hi″per-thi′roi-dizm) an abnormal increase in the activity of the thyroid gland, leading to the excess production of the thyroid hormones. It occurs most frequently in middle-aged females. Hyperthyroidism is most commonly part of a syndrome referred to as Graves' disease, which includes exophthalmos, goiter, and pretibial myxedema, although the cause of hyperthyroidism in the syndrome is unclear. Other causes of hyperthyroidism include a nodular toxic goiter, thyroid carcinomas, trophoblastic tumors such as choriocarcinoma of the testes and hydatidiform mole, ovarian neoplasms, and pituitary adenomas.

A variety of associated clinical manifestations may be observed, including tachycardia, goiter, nervousness, weakness, weight loss, heat intolerance, loose stools, warm thin skin, tremor, and bruit or thrill over the thyroid.

The diagnosis of hyperthyroidism may be suggested by the history and clinical picture, and confirmed by laboratory evaluations. T_4 levels are increased. Thyroidal radioiodine and radio–T_3 uptakes are increased. Decreases in thyroid-stimulating hormone (TSH) combined with an elevation of long-acting thyroid stimulator (LATS) and other thyroid-stimulating immunoglobulins (TSI) may be seen in Graves' disease, along with a nonsuppressible thyroid.

Other laboratory findings include elevated basal metabolic rate (BMR), urinary creatine, calcium, and phosphate; decreased serum cholesterol and potassium; and postprandial glycosuria. X-rays may reveal thyroid enlargement and diffuse bony changes, frequently present in the hands (acropathy). The electrocardiogram shows major changes in P and T waves, often associated with tachycardia and atrial fibrillation. Therapy is directed at decreasing the hormone production of the thyroid. Antithyroid drugs, radioiodine, and surgery may play a role in the treatment.

Also called *thyrotoxicosis*. See also *Graves' disease*.

hypertonia (hi″per-to′ne-ah) [hyper- + Gr. *tonos* tension + *-ia*] increased resistance of muscle tissue to passive stretching. Spasticity and rigidity are important forms of hypertonia. The former is associated with corticospinal tract dysfunction and the latter with abnormalities in the basal ganglia and its connections.

hypertonic (hi″per-ton′ik) having a higher osmotic concentration of solutes than is present in blood. Cells lose water by osmosis when exposed to a hypertonic solution. Cf. *hypotonic*.

hypertrichosis (hi″per-trik-o′sis) [*hyper* + Gr. *thrix* hair + *-osis*] the excessive growth of hair, often secondary to masculinization in the female. It can be induced by drugs or genetically determined. Cf. *hirsutism*.

hypertriglyceridemia (hi″per-tri-glis″er-ĭ-de′me-ah) [*hyper-* + *triglyceride* + Gr. *haima* blood + *-ia*] an excess amount of triglycerides ciculating in the blood. Inherited forms of this disorder occur in the hyperlipoproteinemias (types I and IV).

hypertrophic (hi″per-trof′ik) pertaining to or marked by hypertrophy.

hypertrophy (hi-per′tro-fe) [*hyper-* + Gr. *trophē* nutrition] the enlargement of an organ or tissue due to an increase in the size of its cells. Hypertrophy may occur as a physiologic or pathologic response to environmental or hormonal stimuli. Cf. *hyperplasia*.

gingival h., enlargement and overgrowth of the gum tissue, which may occur in response to the prolonged intake of phenytoin (Dilantin, diphenylhydantoin). Barbiturates may induce a similar but less severe response.

ventricular h., enlargement of the myocardium of a ventricle due to enlargement of individual myocardial cells in response to a stimulus to increase cardiac output. Other causes of this condition include hypertension, valvular disease, occlusive coronary artery disease, and intense athletic training.

hypertyrosinemia, Oregon type cytosol tyrosine α-ketoglutarate aminotransferase deficiency, in which elevated serum tyrosine concentrations are caused by a deficiency of the soluble fraction of hepatic aminotransferase. Clinical features include mental retardation, palmar and plantar keratosis, and sometimes corneal dystrophy. Unlike *p*-hydroxypyruvate oxidase deficiency, renal and hepatic function are normal. See also *tyrosinemia*.

hyperuremia (hi″per-u-re′me-ah) [*hyper-* + Gr. *ouron* urine + *haima* blood + *-ia*] a condition characterized by an increased concentration of urea (blood urea nitrogen) in serum, secondary to a variety of disease conditions. See also *azotemia*.

hyperuricemia (hi″per-u″rĭ-se′me-ah) [*hyper-* + *uric* acid + Gr. *haima* blood + *-ia*] an excess of uric acid in the blood; see *uricemia*.

hyperuricuria (hi″per-u″rik-u′re-ah) [*hyper-* + *uric* acid + Gr. *ouron* urine + *-ia*] an excess of uric acid in the urine.

hypervalinemia (hi″per-val″ĭ-ne′me-ah) [*hyper-* + *valine* + Gr. *haima* blood + *-ia*] a disorder of valine metabolism, thought to be transmitted as an autosomal recessive trait, that is due to a relative or absolute deficiency of the enzyme valine aminotransferase (valine transaminase). Increases in blood or urine levels of valine, but not ketoacids, are seen. Affected infants may show mental and physical retardation, protein intolerance, central nervous system dysfunctions, vomiting, and blindness. This condition may improve through use of a valine-restricted diet. Also called *valinemia*. See also *aminoacidopathy*.

hyperventilation (hi″per-ven″tĭ-la′shun) increased rate and depth of respiration, generally resulting in increased or excessive exchange of air between the lungs and external environment, leading to a reduction in alveolar and arterial tension. This state is most often seen in anxiety states or in relation to emotional stress, although it may also result from drug toxicity or neurologic disorders. Compensation hyperventilation is seen in individuals with acidosis.

Hyperventilation is used as an activation procedure for provoking electroencephalographic abnormalities. The patient is asked to breathe deeply at a rate of 15–20 breaths/min for about 3–4 min. The electroencephalogram (EEG) is recorded during this period and for 2 min after hyperventilation has been discontinued. The fall in arterial carbon dioxide concentration initiates cerebral vasoconstriction; it is this change in cerebral blood flow that may cause changes in the electrical activity of the brain.

Such changes are more pronounced in children and are enhanced in both adults and children by hypoglycemia. Typically, normal EEG activity is replaced by a slow buildup of bilaterally synchronous theta activity followed by delta activity. Persistence of the response for an excessive period, i.e., for more than about 30 sec after overbreathing has ceased, is regarded as abnormal, as is an asymmetric response.

Hyperventilation may evoke or enhance EEG abnormalities in individuals with cerebrovascular disease or neoplasms. In those with epilepsy, bilaterally symmetric spike and wave discharges can be provoked, and focal abnormalities may be enhanced. In children suspected of having absence attacks (petit mal epilepsy), hyperventilation is a particularly valuable means of provoking characteristic 3-Hz spike and slow-wave discharges.

h. syndrome, a pattern of rapid, irregular breathing, characterized by intermittent deep, sighing respirations, that is commonly precipitated by emotional stress in individuals with varying forms of anxiety neuroses. The hyperventilation may lead to respiratory alkalosis, a tightness of the chest and feeling of suffocation, dizziness without actual syncope, numbness of the hands and feet, and occasionally even tetany (as evidenced by carpopedal spasm). The diagnosis of hyperventilation syndrome is supported by the presence of hypocarbia associated with the above symptoms.

hypervitaminosis (hi″per-vi″tah-mĭ-no′sis) a condition associated with the excessive administration of vitamins. It is a particular problem with certain fat-soluble vitamins (A, D, and E) not readily cleared by the body and with vitamin K in newborn infants.

h. A, a condition acutely characterized by bone remodeling, headaches, nausea, and diarrhea. Skin desquamation often occurs also following a toxic dose of vitamin A. Chronic hypervitaminosis A may lead to increased intracranial pressure, skin disorders, loss of hair, skeletal deformities, and psychiatric side-effects. High doses of vitamin A are potentially teratogenic.

h. D, a condition caused by the excessive ingestion of vitamin D and characterized by hypercalcemia, hypercalciuria, and often metastatic calcification. Renal toxicity and renal stones may also occur.

h. K, a condition produced by the administration of large doses of vitamin K to infants, particularly premature infants. It may be associated with hyperbilirubinemia, hemolytic anemia, hepatomegaly, and, in severe cases, death.

hypervolemia (hi″per-vo-le′me-ah) [*hyper-* + *volume* + Gr. *haima* blood + *-ia*] an abnormal increase in the intravascular volume. Causes of this disorder include renal dysfunction and electrolyte imbalances. Chronic hypervolemia may lead to hypertension.

hypesthesia (hip″es-the′ze-ah) [*hypo-* + Gr. *aisthēsis* sensation + *-ia*] decreased sensitivity to cutaneous stimuli. Also called hypoesthesia.

hypha (hi′fah), pl. *hyphae* [L.] a fungal filament that develops from the growth of a germinating spore. It is the fundamental element of a mycelium.

hypn/o (hip′no) [Gr. *hypnos* sleep] a word element used in combining form to denote sleep, e.g., hypnotic.

hypnagogic (hip″nah-goj′ik) [*hypno-* + Gr. *agōgos* leading] 1. producing sleep.

2. occurring just before sleep; said of hallucinations that occur just as one is falling asleep

hypnagogic hypersynchrony in electroencephalography, a pattern of electrical activity characterized by runs or bursts of high-amplitude rhythm having a frequency of 2–5 Hz. This pattern occurs at age 4–6 mo during the early stages of sleep (drowsiness), is maximally expressed at age 3–5 yr, and can persist until age 12 or 13.

hypnotic (hip-not′ik) [Gr. *hypnōtikos* sleepy, causing sleep] 1. inducing sleep.

2. a drug that acts to induce sleep; a central nervous system (CNS) depressant prescribed in the treatment of insomnia. The most commonly prescribed hypnotic is the benzodiazepine compound flurazepam (Dalmane), which has less potential for producing tolerance and physical dependence than other hypnotics (barbiturates, chloral hydrate, triclofos, methaqualone, methyprylon) and no potential for suicidal overdosage. Hypnotics and other CNS depressants such as alcohol, antianxiety drugs, and opiates have additive effects and are dangerous when taken concurrently. Cf. *sedative.*

hypo (hi′po) a conventional term for hypodermic injection or syringe (see *hypodermic n.* under *needle*), or for photographic fixer (by contraction of hyposulfite, an obsolete term for sodium thiosulfate).

hypo- (hi′po) [Gr. *hypo* under] 1. a prefix word element to denote under or beneath, or deficient or abnormally decreased; e.g., hypochromia.

2. a prefix word element in inorganic chemistry to denote a compound, usually an oxo acid or its salt, in which the central oxygen atom has its lowest oxidation state in a series of similar compounds, e.g., hypoboric acid ($H_2B_2O_4$), hypochlorous acid ($HClO$), or sodium hypochlorite ($NaClO$).

hypoacidity (hi″po-ah-sid′ĭ-te) deficiency of acid; lack of normal acidity.

hypoadrenalism (hi″po-ah-dre′nal-izm) see *hypoadrenocorticism.*

hypoadrenocorticism (hi″po-ah-dre″no-kor′tĭ-sizm) a group of disorders characterized by the abnormally decreased and often inadequate secretion of adrenocortical steroid hormones. It usually refers to decreased glucocorticoid concentrations, although hypoadrenocorticism may be used to describe conditions that cause decreased levels of mineralocorticoids and adrenal androgens. The cause of this disorder may be broadly divided into two categories: primary (Addison's disease or acute adrenal crisis), in which there is insufficient hormone elaboration due to a defect within the adrenal glands, and secondary, in which there is secondary failure due to a primary falure in the elaboration of adrenocorticotropic hormone (ACTH).

Also called *adrenocortical insufficiency* and *hypoadrenalism.* For more information, see the specific syndrome.

primary h., the abnormally diminished and often insufficient synthesis or secretion of adrenal steroid hormones, due to an adrenal lesion and existing in acute or chronic forms.

Acute primary hypoadrenocorticism is a medical emergency caused by a sudden lack of adrenal steroid hormones, which results in inadequate plasma concentrations. This condition may arise from a variety of conditions, including exacerbation of chronic primary hypoadrenocorticism (Addison's disease), trauma, stress, surgery, overwhelming bacteremia, adrenalectomy, pituitary necrosis, and cessation of long-term adrenal steroid therapy. Affected individuals display headache, nausea, vomiting, abdominal pain, and fever. Hypotension, cyanosis, and a positive Rogoff's sign may be noted.

Laboratory tests reveal eosinophilia, decreased blood glucose and sodium concentrations, and increased concentrations of serum urea nitrogen, potassium, and calcium. The blood cortisol concentrations are depressed, leading to increases in serum adrenocorticotropic hormone (ACTH) levels. Also called *acute adrenal insufficiency* and *adrenal crisis.* See also *Waterhouse-Friderichsen syndrome.*

Chronic primary hypoadrenocorticism is the establishment of slow and insidious deficiencies of adrenal steroid hormones. It may primarily affect the glucocorticoids, the mineralocorticoids (see *hypoaldosteronism*), or both. In the past, it was frequently due to adrenal tuberculosis; today most cases are considered to be idiopathic or possibly due to autoimmune disorders. Rarely is it caused by metastatic carcinoma, fungal diseases of the adrenals, amyloidosis, or hemochromatosis. This disorder is characterized by weakness, anorexia, nausea and vomiting, gastrointestinal dysfunction, and mental changes. There may be changes in the patterns of hair distribution, as well as hyperpigmentation and creases of the mucous membranes, nipples, and skin. Hypotension (arterial BP 80/50 or less), lymphoid hyperplasia, and a decreased heart size are also common.

Laboratory findings include elevated lymphocyte and eosinophil counts, neutropenia, and hemoconcentration. Serum concentrations of sodium and chloride are reduced; potassium and blood urea nitrogen levels are elevated. Hypercalcemia and low fasting blood glucose are common. Concentrations of urinary 17-ketosteroids and 17-hydroxycorticosteroids are depressed, as is blood cortisol ($< 5\ \mu g/dl$) when drawn in the morning. X-ray examination may reveal adrenal calcification. The diagnosis of Addison's disease may require measurement of plasma cortisol response to ACTH stimulation, water excretion tests, or a radioimmunoassay of plasma ACTH. Characteristically, the electrocardiographic picture reveals low voltage and prolonged P-R and Q-T intervals. Electroencephalograms demonstrate a slowed discharge, especially in the alpha range.

Also called *Addison's disease.*

secondary h., a deficiency of adrenocortical function due to pituitary adrenocorticotropic hormone (ACTH) deficiency. It may result from excessive glucocorticoid administration or from panhypopituitarism. Those affected may experience signs and symptoms similar to those seen in primary hypoadrenocorticism (Addison's disease), but characteristically there is no hyperpigmentation. Diagnosis is based on demonstration of the presence of hypoadrenocorticism, with low plasma concentrations of ACTH determined by radioimmunoassay.

hypoalbuminemia (hi″po-al-bu″min-e′me-ah) [*hypo-* + *albumin* + Gr. *haima* blood + *-ia*] an abnormally low serum albumin concentration, which can be due to malnutrition, to a diminished capacity of the liver to synthesize albumin, as in cirrhosis or hepatitis; or to abnormal losses of albumin with massive proteinuria, as in nephrotic syndrome or blood loss in such conditions as hepatic schistosomiasis or portal hypertension. Hypoalbuminemia with sufficiently lowered colloidal osmotic pressure can lead to the secondary complication of dependent edema and ascites through increased fluid transudation from capillaries.

hypoaldosteronism (hi″po-al″do-ster′ōn-izm) the abnormally decreased synthesis or secretion of mineralocorticoids, most frequently aldosterone. Isolated aldosterone deficiencies may occur with hyporeninism, protracted heparin therapy, pretectal lesions of the brain stem, and aldosterone-secreting neoplasms. Most frequently it is found in adults with renal failure due to diabetic nephropathy. This disorder is characterized by low plasma renin and low aldosterone concentrations that fail to rise during sodium restriction. Aldosterone concentrations also fail to rise following adrenocorticotropic hormone (ACTH) administration, but cortisol secretion rises normally. Hyperkalemia is also observed.

hypobaric (hi″po-bār′ik) [*hypo-* + Gr. *baros* weight] below normal pressure.

hypobetalipoproteinemia (hi″po-ba″tah-lip″o-pro″tēn-e′me-ah) [*hypo-* + *beta lipoprotein* + Gr. *haima* blood + *-ia*] a rare genetic disorder, transmitted as an autosomal dominant trait, that is characterized by reduced serum concentrations of beta lipoproteins (also known as low-density lipoproteins, LDLs). Serum lipids are reduced, and plasma cholesterol concentrations have a range of 70–120 mg/dl. Fat absorption is unimpaired, and although some cases of acanthocytosis have been reported, there are usually no clinical signs or symptoms. No treatment is required. The homozygous state of this rare gene causes a more severe form of the disorder. See also *hypolipoproteinemia.*

hypocalcemia (hi″po-kal-se′me-ah) [*hypo-* + *calcium* + Gr. *haima* blood + *-ia*] the abnormally low concentration of calcium in serum (plasma). The decrease in concentration may involve either the ionic or protein-bound calcium fraction, or a combination of both. Causes for this condition include hypoparathyroidism, renal diseases associated with proteinuria, and failure of the kidneys to form 1,25-dihydroxycholecalciferol (1,25-OHD_3). Vitamin D deficiency, which is generally associated with concurrent malabsorption of calcium as well as acute hemorrhagic pancreatitis, also leads to hypocalcemia. Significant decreases in the ionized calcium fraction lead to tetany, spasms, and neuromuscular derangements.

hypocapnia (hi″po-kap′ne-ah) [*hypo-* + Gr. *kapnos* smoke + *-ia*] an abnormally low pressure of carbon dioxide gas (low arterial P_{CO_2}) in the blood. Hypocapnia is always caused by increased alveolar ventilation (forced, mechanical): either as a primary response to a stimulus (such as high altitude), resulting in respiratory alkalosis; or as a secondary response to a primary metabolic disorder (such as diabetic ketoacidosis), in which the hypocapnia becomes a secondary, compensating force that ameliorates the acidosis.

hypocapnic (hi″po-kap′nik) pertaining to or characterized by hypocapnia.

hypocarbia (hi″po-kar′be-ah) see *hypocapnia.*

hypocellular (hi″po-sel′u-lar) pertaining to or characterized by a decreased number of cells.

hypocellularity (hi″po-sel″u-lar′ĭ-te) abnormally

low numbers of cells present within a particular tissue or organ. This condition can have a number of causes, including necrosis (when cells are destroyed) or fibrosis (when cells are replaced by fibrous tissue).

hypochlorhydria (hi″po-klor-hi′dre-ah) [*hypo-* + Gr. *chlōros* green + *hydōr* water + *-ia*] a condition characterized by decreased secretion of "free" hydrochloric acid. In the basal state, secretion may be nil (pH of gastric fluid, $>$ 3.5), but some acid is produced after maximal stimulation. See also *gastric function tests.* Cf. *achlorhydria.*

hypochlorite (hi″po-klo′rīt) [*hypo-* + Gr. *chlōros* green] a salt of hypochlorous acid, HOCl; the hypochlorite ion (OCl^-). Hypochlorite solutions are good oxidizing agents, and are used as sanitizing and antiseptic agents in the food service and dairy industries (e.g., sodium hypochlorite and calcium hypochlorite).

hypocholesterolemia (hi″po-ko-les″ter-o-le′me-ah) [*hypo-* + *cholesterol* + Gr. *haima* blood + *-ia*] abnormally low concentrations of total cholesterol in the blood. This condition may be seen in individuals in the hyperthyroid state and in those with elevated estrogen concentrations. Cholesterol values are usually in the range of low-normal to low. Significant decreases are seen in advanced hepatitis owing to hepatic necrosis and resultant decreased synthesis. Individuals with an absence or deficiency of high-density lipoprotein (HDL) and low-density lipoprotein (LDL) also show low cholesterol values.

hypochondriac (hi″po-kon′dre-ak) [*hypo-* + Gr. *chondros* cartilage (of the rib cage)] 1. pertaining to the hypochondriac region or to hypochondriasis.
2. a person with hypochondriasis.

hypochondriac region 1. the upper lateral region of the abdomen on either side, lying above the subcostal plane and lateral to a vertical plane passing through the midinguinal point and the ninth costal cartilage near its tip. Also called *hypochondrium.*
2. a region above the transpyloric plane and to the outside of a lateral sagittal plane; used in radiographic positioning. See illustration under *abdominal regions.*

hypochondriasis (hi″po-kon-dri′ah-sis) [so-called because the hypochondrium, and especially the spleen, was supposed to be the cause of the disorder] pathologic concern about one's health. Also called hypochondria.

hypochondrium (hi″po-kon′dre-um), pl. *hypochondria.* see *hypochondriac region.*

hypochromatism (hi″po-kro′mah-tizm) [*hypo-* + Gr. *chrōma* color] abnormally deficient pigmentation.

hypochromia (hi″po-kro′me-ah) [*hypo-* + Gr. *chrōma* color + *-ia*] an abnormal decrease in staining intensity. The term is most commonly used in the laboratory to describe weakly stained erythrocytes containing decreased concentrations of hemoglobin.

hypochromic (hi″po-kro′mik) pertaining to or marked by hypochromia.

hypochromic anemia see *hypochromic a.* under *anemia.*

hypochromic shift a shift in the absorption band characteristic of a chromophore, resulting in a decrease in absorbance.

hypodermic (hi″po-der′mik) [*hypo-* + Gr. *derma* skin] applied or administered beneath the skin, as in the subcutaneous or intramuscular injection of drugs.

hypodiploid (hi″po-dip′loid) having a chromosome number less than the diploid number (in humans, less than 46).

hypoechoic (hi″po-ĕ-ko′ik) in ultrasonography, pertaining to material that produces fewer or smaller echoes than is normal for the surrounding medium.

hypofibrinogenemia (hi″po-fi-brin″o-jĕ-ne′me-ah) an abnormally low concentration of fibrinogen in the blood. Hypofibrinogenemia is a rare condition that is inherited as an autosomal recessive trait (afibrinogenemia is probably the homozygous expression of the same trait), and is usually of no clinical significance. Serum fibrinogen concentrations sufficiently low to cause abnormal bleeding are most frequently encountered secondary to acquired conditions such as disseminated intravascular coagulation (DIC) or extracorporeal circulation with insufficient heparinization, owing to the rapid utilization of fibrinogen in the formation of clots. See also *afibrinogenemia* and *dysfibrinogenemia.*

hypogammaglobulinemia (hi″po-gam″ah-glob″-u-lĭ-ne′me-ah) [*hypo-* + *gamma globulin* + Gr. *haima* blood + *-ia*] a congenital or acquired absence or severe depression of one or more gamma globulins that results in an increased susceptibility to the infectious diseases that immunoglobulin-associated mechanisms usually defend against. Among the congenital disorders, distinct types have been identified: (1) X-linked hypogammaglobulinemia (Bruton's disease); (2) selective absence of IgA, or of IgA and IgG, or of subclass of IgG (such as IgC, IgG_2); (3) transient hypogammaglobulinemia of infancy; (4) acquired hypogammaglobulinemia (possibly congenital "late onset"); and (5) severe combined immunodeficiency (Swiss-type hypogammaglobulinemia). Related immunodeficiency diseases involving defects in cellular thymus-dependent immunity with normal IgG levels include: (1) congenital thymic aplasia (DiGeorge's syndrome), (2) Wiskott-Aldrich syndrome (with low IgM and normal IgG and IgA), and (3) hereditary ataxia telangiectasia (with low IgA). For defects of the complement system, see *complement.*

Swiss-type h., hypogammaglobulinemia, transmitted either as an X-linked or autosomal recessive trait, in which infants lack B and T cells, as well as plasma cells characteristic of X-linked and other hypogammaglobulinemias. Infections begin within 2–3 mo of birth—after maternal protection has subsided—and death usually occurs within 2 yr. Therapy with bone marrow transplants is still experimental. Also called *alymphocytosis, combined immunodeficiency,* and *thymic alymphoplasia.*

X-linked h., hereditary hypogammaglobulinemia, transmitted as an X-linked recessive trait, that affects only males. The serum concentration of IgG is less than 100 mg/ml, with undetectable concentrations of IgA, IgM, IgD, and IgE. The thymus gland and cell-mediated immunity are normal, but the few B cells present function poorly or not at all. Plasma cells are lacking or few. Clinical manifestations develop after age 9 mo, previous protection from increased susceptibility to infection being due to the transference of maternal antibodies during pregnancy. Complications include collagen-vascular disease, such as arthritis and, occasionally, fatal dermatomyositis. Prolonged survival and well-being are achieved by repeated injections of gamma globulin. Also called *Bruton's disease.*

hypogastric (hi″po-gas′trik) [*hypo-* + Gr. *gastēr* stomach] pertaining to the hypogastrium.

hypogastric region 1. the lower region of the abdomen below the level of the anterior iliac spines. Also called *hypogastrium* and *pubic region.*

2. the region of the abdomen below the transtubercular plane and between the lateral sagittal planes; used in radiographic positioning. See illustration under *abdominal regions.*

hypogastric zone the part of the abdomen below the transtubercular plane. It consists of the hypogastric (pubic) and left and right iliac (inguinal) regions.

hypogastrium (hi″po-gas′tre-um) see *hypogastric region.*

hypoglossal (hi″po-glos′al) [*hypo-* + Gr. *glōssa* tongue] 1. beneath the tongue.

2. pertaining to the XIIth cranial nerve.

hypoglossal nerve cranial nerve XII; the motor nerve to the muscles of the tongue. It arises in the medulla, leaves the cranial cavity through the anterior condylar canal, descends in the neck between the internal carotid artery and internal jugular vein, and then runs forward through the submandibular region to reach the tongue. See also *cranial nerves.*

hypoglycemia (hi″po-gli-se′me-ah) [*hypo-* + Gr. *glykys* sweet + *haima* blood + *-ia*] a decrease in blood sugar, or glucose, sufficient to deprive the central nervous system—a concentration below 40 mg/dl of blood. Two forms of hypoglycemia can be distinguished: that in the fed state and that in the fasting state.

Hypoglycemia in the fed state, occurring after the ingestion of food, involves an increase in the production of insulin by the pancreas and a decrease in the production of glucose in the liver. Normally, glucose production is later resumed to maintain the blood glucose at a normal level during a nonfed state. In the condition of hypoglycemia, however, the return to glucose production in the liver is delayed, which results in a decreased concentration of blood glucose.

Fasting hypoglycemia is characterized by clinical hypoglycemia occurring after a missed meal, and is often the result of an inability to release sufficient glucose into the blood stream from the body's stores. Insufficiency of adrenal glucocorticoids, pituitary hormone deficiencies (e.g., growth hormone), glycogen storage diseases, and severe liver disease produce fasting hypoglycemia through this mechanism. This form is also found in individuals with insulin-secreting beta-cell adenomas of the pancreas. Alcoholic excess and tumors of the retroperitoneal space may also produce episodes of fasting hypoglycemia, in each case through mechanisms not well understood.

Clinically, hypoglycemia is characterized by preciptous tachycardia, weakness, anxiety, nervousness, tremulousness, and hunger; consciousness is almost always preserved. Treatment may involve control of the duration, frequency, and content of food intake. A diet high in protein and low in carbohydrates may reduce the condition, as low carbohydrates do not cause the overproduction of insulin. Anticholinergic drugs are also useful. See also *glucose tolerance test.* Cf. *hyperglycemia.*

hypoglycemic (hi″po-gli-se′mik) pertaining to, characterized by, or producing hypoglycemia.

oral h. agents, synthetic drugs that lower the concentration of glucose in the body. Currently, sulfonylureas are used, including chlorpropamide (Diabinese), tolbutamide (Orinase), tolazamide (Tolinase), and acetohexamide (Dymelor). These drugs, which stimulate the synthesis and release of insulin from the beta cells of the islets of Langerhans, are used to treat individuals with noninsulin-dependent diabetes mellitus (NIDDM). They have no hypoglycemic effect in individuals with insulin-dependent diabetes mellitus (IDDM), who have nonfunctional beta cells that cannot produce insulin. Although it is thought that these drugs should not be used as a substitute for adherence to a strict diet, they have proved effective in the treatment of patients who have stable NIDDM that is not controllable by diet alone and who prefer not to take insulin.

hypogonadism (hi″po-go′nad-izm) decreased functional activity of the gonads, resulting in diminished sexual development and secondary sex characteristics when there is loss of interstitial cell function with decreased or absent production of male sex hormones. Seminiferous tubule hypofunction of sperm production may be associated with impaired hormone production. Measurement of serum and urinary gonadotropins is used to distinguish primary and secondary hypogonadism.

hypokalemia (hi″po-kah-le′me-ah) [*hypo-* + L. *kalium* potassium + Gr. *haima* blood + *-ia*] abnormally low levels of potassium in the blood. There are a variety of causes, including inadequate intake, excessive loss (vomiting, diarrhea, renal dysfunction), and adrenocortical hyperactivity. It results in regressive changes of muscle that are particularly severe in the heart, where myofibrillar change and necrosis is observed. Severe cases are associated with cardiac arrhythmias and sometimes cardiac arrest. Also called *hypopotassemia.* See also *electrolyte balance and homeostasis.*

hypokalemic (hi″po-kal-e′mik) pertaining to or characterized by hypokalemia.

h. nephropathy, severe potassium deficiency leading to impairment of renal concentrating mechanisms. There is development of large vacuoles in the cytoplasm of the proximal convoluted tubules, as well as polyuria and nocturia. Although the lesions are reversible, residual fibrosis is sometimes seen.

hypoleydigism (hi″po-li′dig-izm) abnormally low secretions of Leydig cells. This results in a diminished amount of circulating androgens and in a regression of secondary sex characteristics.

hypolipoproteinemia (hi″po-lip″o-pro″te-in-e′me-ah) [*hypo-* + *lipoprotein* + Gr. *haima* blood + *-ia*] the relative or absolute deficiency of lipoproteins in the blood. Primary hypolipoproteinemias are a group of rare familial disorders characterized by the abnormal reductions of serum lipoprotein concentrations. Different conditions may affect beta lipoproteins (hypobetalipoproteinemias, abetalipoproteinemia), alpha lipoproteins (Tangier disease), or the enzyme lecithin-cholesterol acyltransferase (lecithin-cholesterol acyltransferase deficiency). Hypolipoproteinemias may also occur secondary to a number of systemic disorders, including malabsorption, malnutrition, anemia, and hyperthyroidism. For more information on primary hypolipoproteinemias, see the individual disorder.

hypomagnesemia (hi″po-mag″nĕ-se′me-ah) [*hypo-* + *magnesium* + Gr. *haima* blood + *-ia*] an abnormally low magnesium content of the blood plasma, manifested chiefly by neuromuscular irritability. It is observed in many disorders or clinical situations, e.g.: steatorrhea and other gastrointestinal diseases, associated with gastrointestinal fluid loss; acute diabetic ketoacidosis with insulin treatment; alcoholism and alcoholic cirrhosis; thyrotoxicosis; hyperaldosteronism; hypo- and hyperparathyroidism; following starvation and postsurgical trauma; with intravenous fluid replacement; excessive lactation; in infants with protein-calorie malnutrition (kwashiorkor); some renal diseases (e.g., glomerulonephritis, pyelonephritis, renal tubular acidosis); hypercalcemic states associated with malignant osteolytic metastases; and congestive heart failure after diuresis with mercurials, ethacrynic acid, and furosemide. Some cases are idiopathic.

hypomenorrhea (hi″po-men″o-re′ah) [*hypo-* + Gr. *mēn* month + *rhein* to flow] a diminished quantity of menstrual flow, usually of no clinical significance.

hyponatremia (hi″po-nah-tre′me-ah) [*hypo-* + L. *natrium* sodium + Gr. *haima* blood + *-ia*] the condition of salt depletion that leads to an abnormally low concentration of sodium in the circulating plasma and extracellular fluids. It is seen in diabetes insipidus, polyuria, renal tubular disease, and Addison's disease, and as a result of sodium loss in diarrhea. See also *electrolyte balance and homeostasis.*

hyponatruria (hy″po-nah-tru′re-ah) [*hypo-* + L. *natrium* sodium + Gr. *ouron* urine + *-ia*] abnormally low concentrations of sodium in the urine.

hyponychium (hi″po-nik′e-um) [*hypo-* + Gr. *onyx* nail] [NA], the boundary between the nail bed and the distal portion of the epidermis of the phalanx.

hypoparathyroidism (hi″po-par″ah-thi′roid-izm) a condition due to the insufficient secretion of parathyroid hormone, which leads to metabolic abnormalities characterized by hypocalcemia and hyperphosphatemia. Most frequently, it occurs after the accidental removal of or damage to the parathyroids during thyroidectomy or surgery for parathyroid neoplasms. Rarely, the condition may occur transiently in children or idiopathically, especially in association with magnesium deficiency.

Affected individuals most often experience tetany as a result of the neuromuscular hyperexcitability present in calcium deficiency. Cramps, convulsions, dyspnea, photophobia, lethargy, and personality changes may also occur. Skin, bone, and reflexes may be altered, and there is an increased incidence of fungal infections. Physical examination reveals a positive Chvostek's sign (facial contraction following pressure on the facial nerve near the angle of the jaw) and a positive Trousseau's phenomenon (carpal spasm following application of an inflated blood pressure cuff to the upper arm).

Laboratory tests reveal a serum calcium concentration in the latent tetany (7–8 mg/dl) or overt tetany (<7 mg/dl) range. Serum phosphate concentrations are elevated, whereas urinary phosphate and calcium concentrations are low to absent. Alkaline phosphatase and creatinine clearance are both normal. Radioimmunoassay of parathyroid hormone reveals decreased to absent concentrations. X-rays may reveal basal ganglia calcification, increased bone density, and soft tissue calcification. There may be an increased sensitivity to galvanic current, producing muscle contraction (Erb's sign). Electrocardiograms may show dysrhythmias and a prolonged Q-T interval. Cataracts may occur and may be visible on slit lamp examination. Treatment of the hypocalcemia involves administration of calcium and active vitamin D monitored by 24-hr urine calcium determinations.

See also *hypocalcemia* and *tetany.*

hypophosphatasia (hi″po-fos″fah-ta′ze-ah) [*hypo-* + *phosphatase* + *-ia*] a genetic inborn error of metabolism characterized by a deficiency of serum alkaline phosphatase, leading to abnormalities of bone mineralization. The disease is most severe in infants and is often fatal. The radiologic picture is similar to that for rickets. Phosphoethanolamine and phosphocholine are excreted in the urine. In adults there is tooth loss and osteomalacia.

hypophosphatemia (hi″po-fos″fah-te′me-ah) [*hypo-* + *phosphate* + Gr. *haima* blood + *-ia*] an abnormal condition characterized by a lower than normal concentration of phosphates in the blood. Normal fasting serum concentrations of phosphates, measured as inorganic phorphorus, are 1–1.5 mmol/l (3–4.5 mg/dl in adults, higher in children). Causes of this disorder include decreased supply or absorption or increased loss of phosphate (as in hyperparathyroidism, hyperthyroidism, and renal tubular defects), electrolyte abnormalities (as in hypercalcemia and hypomagnesemia), respiratory alkalosis, uncontrolled diabetes mellitus, and chronic alcoholism. Chronic hypophosphatemia may lead to anorexia, bone resorption, hemorrhage, rhabdomyolysis, and abnormalities of the central nervous system, including confusion, seizures, and coma. Treatment is directed toward increasing serum phosphate concentrations without causing hypocalcemia. See also *electrolyte balance and homeostasis.*

familial h., a sex-linked, dominantly inherited disorder of phosphate metabolism, which may be associated with vitamin D–resistant rickets, renal tubular defects, dwarfism, and poorly defined metabolic abnormalities related to vitamin D.

hypophosphaturia (hi″po-fos″fah-tu′re-ah) [*hypo-* + *phosphate* + Gr. *ouron* urine + *-ia*] an abnormal condition characterized by a decrease of phosphorus in the urine (<0.9–1.3 g/24 hr), as seen in hypoparathyroidism.

hypophyseal (hi″po-fiz′e-al) pertaining to the pituitary gland.

hypophysiotropic (hi″po-fiz″e-o-trop′ik) acting on the hypophysis, as in hypophysiotropic hormones.

hypophysis (hi-pof′ĭ-sis) [*hypo-* + Gr. *phyein* to grow] the hypophysis cerebri or pituitary gland: a pea-sized body suspended beneath the brain and encased within a cavity in the sphenoid bone, the sella turcica (see the accompanying illustration). Hormones formed by the gland influence many activities of other endocrine glands and various body functions. The gland's secretory activities are in turn governed by hypothalamic influences.

The pituitary is derived from two embryologic sources. A small diverticulum in the roof of the primitive oral cavity (Rathke's pouch) grows upward toward the developing brain and loses its con-

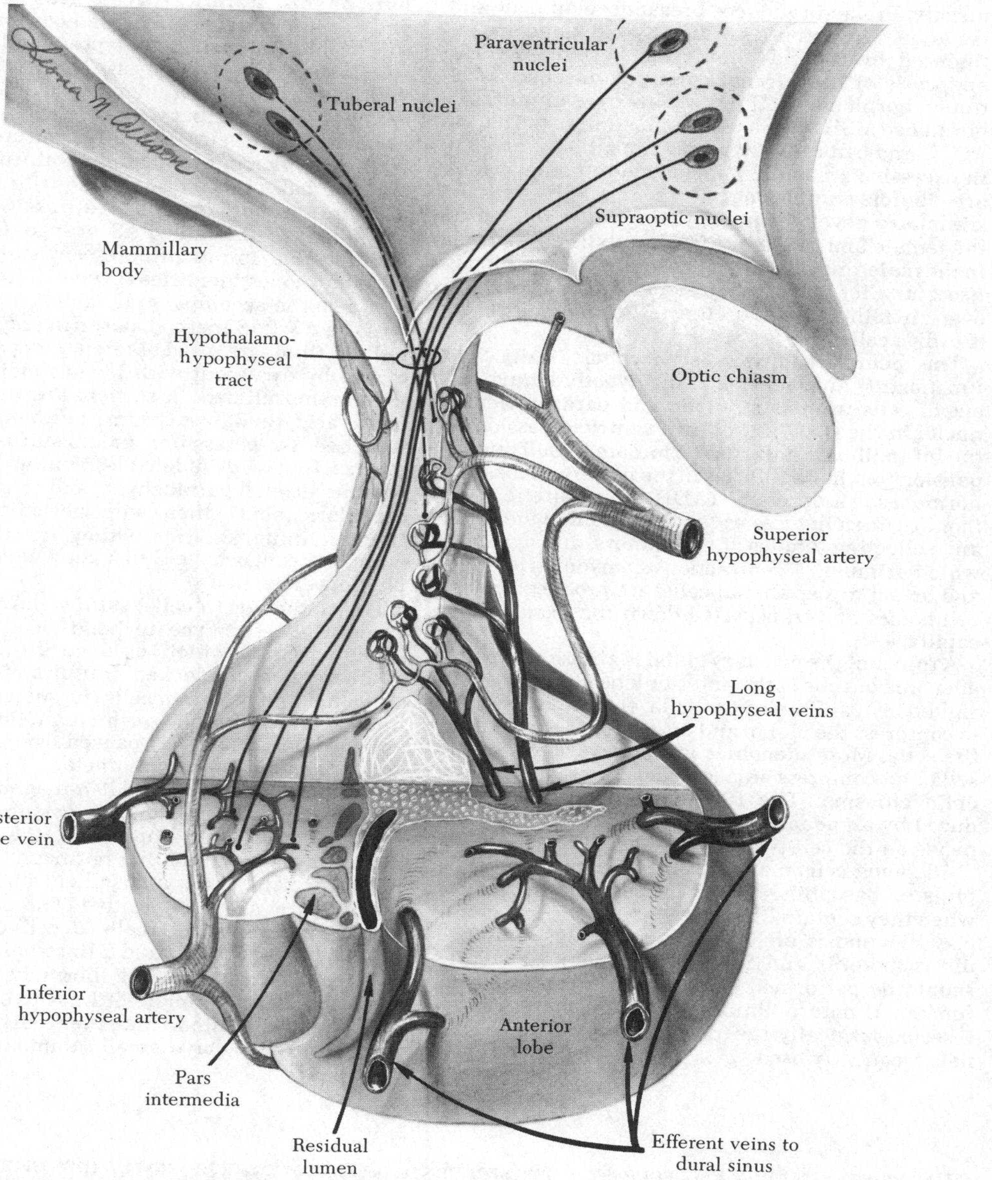

Hypophysis. Diagram illustrating the principal vascular and nervous relations. (From Leeson, C. R., and Leeson, T. S.: Histology. 4th ed. Philadelphia, W. B. Saunders Co., 1981.)

nection with the oral cavity. It comes in contact with a downgrowth from the diencephalon, the infundibulum. Cells from both sources proliferate; those from Rathke's pouch form the adenohypophysis, which includes the anterior lobe, while the infundibulum forms the posterior lobe that retains its connection to the hypothalamus through the infundibular stalk.

The anterior lobe is composed of compact groups of polygonal cells in a rich network of sinusoids. Elaborate histologic staining procedures, immunocytochemistry, and electron microscopy have delineated at least six cell types that can be related to the production of one or more of the anterior pituitary hormones. Ultrastructurally, all the cells contain electron-dense cytoplasmic granules varying in size and number. The largest occur in resting prolactin-forming cells, whereas the smallest form a single layer beneath the cell membrane of thyrotrophs. Hormone secretion by cells of the anterior pituitary is controlled by hypothalamic releasing and inhibiting factors that reach the gland via vessels of the hypothalamohypophyseal portal system.

Growth hormone (STH, somatotropic hormone) from the anterior lobe of the pituitary stimulates the growth of the body, and its deficiency results in dwarfism. Hypersecretion before the epiphyses are fused causes giantism, and in adults produces acromegaly. Prolactin induces breast development and lactation. The activities of the thyroid gland are influenced by thyroid-stimulating hormone (TSH), and those of the adrenal cortex by adrenocorticotropic hormone (ACTH). Melanocyte-stimulating hormone (MSH) has a molecule similar to that of ACTH and can cause hyperpigmentation if present in excessive amounts. The gonadotropic hormones are follicle-stimulating hormone (FSH), which stimulates development of the ovarium follicle in the female and the seminiferous tubule epithelium in the male, and luteinizing hormone (LH), which is necessary for normal hormonal function by the ovarian follicle cells or the testicular interstitial (Leydig) cells.

The neurohypophysis is morphologically and functionally an extension of the hypothalamus. Axons of cells in the supraoptic and paraventricular nuclei in the floor of the third ventricle pass down the infundibular stalk and terminate in bulbous expansions on the capillaries in the posterior lobe. The hormones vasopressin (ADH, antidiuretic hormone), which induces water absorption in the distal and collecting tubules of the kidneys, and oxytocin, which stimulates contraction of myometrial cells and breast myoepithelial cells, are produced by the cell bodies and transported down the axons to the capillaries.

A tumor of the pituitary gland is almost always an adenoma of cells of the anterior lobe. Because of the rigid bony confines of the sella, the tumor is likely to compress the gland, and often erodes the walls of the sella. Most adenomas grow upward out of the sella and compress adjacent structures, such as the optic chiasma. The functional disturbance produced by an adenoma of the anterior pituitary depends on the cell type and its degree of activity.

Adenoma cells may stain histologically as acidophils or basophils, or may appear chromophobic when they contain little stored secretion, but such a classification is of little clinical value; combined ultrastructural and immunocytochemical studies should be performed on a tumor to determine its functional nature. Pituitary adenomas are usually resected surgically; the transsphenoidal approach is now frequently used.

hypophysis staining procedures histochemical and immunohistochemical methods for identifying the various functional cell types found in the anterior lobe of the hypophysis. Originally, the cells were classified as chromophils or chromophobes, on the basis of whether they stained with hematoxylin and eosin or azure-eosin. The chromophils were further divided into acidophils (stained red with eosin) and basophils (stained blue with hematoxylin or azure). A more complicated classification based on aldehyde-thionine-PAS-orange G (AT-PAS) staining and immunofluorescent staining of specific hormones identifies seven different cell types (see also the accompanying table).

In the AT-PAS method, paraffin sections fixed in Helly's fluid are used. Mercury deposits are removed by treatment with Lugol's iodine and then sodium thiosulfate. The sections are oxidized in sulfuric acid and potassium permanganate, and bleached in potassium metabisulfite. They are stained first with aldehyde-thionine (thionine, 70 percent alcohol, paraldehyde, and concentrated hydrochloric acid), then with periodic acid–Schiff (PAS) staining, and finally they are counterstained with 2 percent orange G in 5 percent aqueous phosphotungstic acid.

The acidophils (α cells) stain yellow-orange with orange G. These can be further divided into GH cells (somatotrophs), which produce growth hormone and have densely packed granules 350–450 nm in diameter, and prolactin cells (mammotrophs, lactotrophs, or luteotrophs), which produce prolactin and have large, sparsely packed irregular granules greater than 550 nm in diameter.

The basophils stain reddish-magenta with PAS staining, blue with aldehyde-thionine, or purple with both. Being glycoproteins, the trophic hormones thyroid-stimulating hormone (TSH), luteinizing hormone (LH), and follicle-stimulating hormone (FSH) are PAS-positive. The adrenocorticotropic hormone (ACTH) cells (β_1 cells or corticolipotrophs) produce ACTH and β-lipotropin, a precursor of melanocyte-stimulating hormone (MSH), and have abundant, strongly PAS-positive granules approximately 360 nm in diameter. TSH cells (β_2 cells or thyrotrophs) have small, abundant, dark blue

HYPOPHYSIS STAINING PROCEDURES. CORRESPONDENCE OF IMMUNOCYTOCHEMICALLY IDENTIFIED FUNCTIONAL CELL TYPES IN THE HUMAN PARS DISTALIS WITH THOSE DIFFERENTIATED BY TINCTORIAL MEANS

FUNCTIONAL NOMENCLATURE	ROMEIS-EZRIN GREEK-LETTER NOMENCLATURE	CLASSICAL NOMENCLATURE
Somatotrophs or GH cells	α	Acidophils
Lactotrophs or prolactin cells (resting)	?	
Lactotrophs or prolactin cells (pregnancy, lactation)	η	
Cortico-lipotrophs or ACTH/LPH cells	β_1	Basophils
Thyrotrophs, or TSH cells	β_2, γ	
Gonadotrophs, or FSH/LH cells	δ, γ?	
Poorly granulated cells of all varieties	Chromophobes	Chromophobes
Follicular cells	Chromophobes	

From Weiss, L., and Greep, R. O.: Histology. 4th ed. New York, McGraw-Hill Book Co., 1977, p. 1047.

granules less than 150 nm in diameter. LH cells (δ_1 cells or LH gonadotrophs) have discrete blue-purple granules; FSH cells (γ_2 cells or FSH gonadotrophs) have bright red granules; in both, the granules are 200–250 nm in diameter. ACTH cells (β_3 cells or corticotrophs) have faintly PAS-positive cytoplasm and relatively few blue-purple granules 100–250 nm in diameter. The chromophobes are considered to be degranulated chromophils.

Immunohistochemical methods such as Sternberger's peroxidase antiperoxidase (PAP) technique utilizes specific antisera to the hormones to demonstrate the cell type by the hormone present.

hypopigmentation (hi″po-pig″men-ta′shun) decreased melanin concentration, which usually occurs as localized dermal lesions, as in the ovoid lesions found on the trunk and limbs of many newborns affected with tuberous sclerosis. It must be differentiated from depigmentation by means of a Wood's lamp, which shows depigmented areas as a striking ivory white.

hypopituitarism (hi″po-pĭ-tu′ĭ-tar-izm) a condition characterized by the deficient production or secretion of the pituitary hormones. It may affect the posterior pituitary, leading primarily to a deficiency of vasopressin that results in diabetes insipidus. More commonly, however, it affects the anterior pituitary, causing a deficiency of one or more of the pituitary hormones, including prolactin, growth hormone, gonadotropins, thyrotropin, and adrenocorticotropic hormone (ACTH). Deficiency of all pituitary hormones (Simmonds' disease or panhypopituitarism) primarily affects the gonads, thyroid, and adrenal cortex, and interferes with glucose metabolism.

Anterior pituitary insufficiency in adults is most commonly due to a chromophobe adenoma. Other causes include craniopharyngioma, metastatic carcinoma (especially from the breast), aneurysm of the internal carotid artery, granulomas (sarcoid, fungi, and tuberculosis), head irradiation, trauma, and postpartum necrosis (Sheehan's syndrome). Affected individuals are generally weak with thin, cool, and pale skin; they have decreased resistance to cold, stress, and fasting, and display pubic and axillary hair loss. Low blood pressure, orthostatic hypotension, and slow pulse are also common. Prolactin deficiency may result in the absence of lactation in postpartum females, whereas growth hormone deficiency may lead to dwarfism in children, with delayed sexual development and hypoglycemia. Deficiency of gonadotropins may cause the delayed appearance of secondary sex characteristics, amenorrhea, and sexual dysfunction. Deficient thyrotropin may lead to secondary hypothyroidism, whereas ACTH deficiency results in hypoadrenocorticism.

Laboratory findings may include low concentrations of ACTH, thyroid-stimulating hormone (TSH), luteinizing hormone (LH), and follicle-stimulating hormone (FSH), as determined by radioimmunoassay. Growth hormone concentrations as determined by immunochemical methods are shown to be reduced and unresponsive to insulin, arginine, or levodopa. Plasma concentrations of estrogen and testosterone are reduced, as are urinary and serum gonadotropins. The metyrapone stimulation test shows limited pituitary reserve. T_4 is reduced, and anemia is common. Radioactive iodine uptake is low, as are urinary levels of 17-ketosteroids and 17-hydroxycorticosteroids; all three increase in response to exogenous TSH and ACTH. Fasting blood glucose is low, and the glucose tolerance curve is flat. The insulin tolerance test reveals marked insulin sensitivity. New techniques that measure FH, LH, and TSH concentrations following administration of synthesized LH- and TSH-releasing hormones aid in differentiating among hypothalamic, pituitary, and end-organ lesions. X-rays, CT scans, and polytomography may be useful in demonstrating pituitary neoplasms and expanding lesions. Bitemporal hemianopia may be present if the pituitary lesion extends to involve the optic chiasma.

hypoplasia (hi″po-pla′ze-ah) [*hypo-* + Gr. *plasis* formation + *-ia*] the condition in which a tissue or organ fails to develop to its normal state or size, such as a congenital malformation due to the failure of the anlage of an organ to grow to its normal size. It differs from the condition of aplasia, in which there is a complete lack of development. Also called hypoplasty. Cf. *aplasia.*

hypoplastic (hi″po-plas′tik) characterized by incomplete development.

hypoploid (hi′po-ploid) having fewer than the typical number of chromosomes (46 in humans), a condition that is almost always lethal. Cf. *hyperploid.*

hypoploidy (hi″po-ploi′de) the state of being hypoploid.

hypopotassemia (hi″po-po″tah-se′me-ah) [*hypo-* + *potassium* + Gr. *haima* blood + *-ia*] see *hypokalemia.*

hypoproteinemia (hi″po-pro″tēn-e′me-ah) an abnormally low serum protein concentation, usually seen secondary to renal disease. Severe hypoproteinemia in the absence of starvation is almost always indicative of massive proteinuria.

hypoprothrombinemia (hi″po-pro-throm″bĭ-ne′me-ah) a rare, congenital deficiency of prothrombin (coagulation Factor II deficiency), transmitted as an autosomal recessive trait, that usually causes relatively mild bleeding problems. The prothrombin time and activated partial thromboplastin time are moderately prolonged. Cf. *dysprothrombinemia.*

hyporeflexia (hi″po-re-flek′se-ah) diminution or depression of the reflexes.

hyposensitivity (hi″po-sens″ĭ-tiv′ĭ-te) decreased immunologic sensitivity to a specific antigen (allergen).

hyposensitization (hi″po-sen″sĭ-tĭ-za′shun) desensitization; in the treatment of allergy, the repeated administration of allergen until sufficient nonreaginic antibody is formed and a relative state of tolerance produced.

hypospadias (hi″po-spa′de-as) [*hypo-* + Gr. *spadōn* a rent] a developmental abnormality that results in malformation of the urethral groove in the male, so that the urethral canal opens on the ventral surface of the penis. This condition is associated with a high incidence of other genital abnormalities and may prevent normal ejaculation and insemination.

female h., a developmental malformation in the female that results in the opening of the urethra into the vagina.

hyposplenism (hi″po-splen′izm) absent or reduced splenic function, usually due to surgical removal, congenital aplasia, tumor replacements, or splenic vascular accident. Erythrocyte abnormalities (the presence of inclusion bodies, nucleated erythrocytes, or target cells) are a common consequence. Hyposplenism is associated with increased risk of bacterial sepsis, particularly that due to pneumococcus.

hyposthenuria (hi″pos-thĕ-nu′re-ah) [*hypo-* + Gr. *sthenos* strength + *ouron* urine + *-ia*] the formation and excretion of urine of low specific gravity.

hypotension (hi″po-ten′shun) reduced blood pressure, which has both acute and chronic forms. Hypotension may be a serious situation that leads to a decreased perfusion of tissues (shock), or it may be a chronic nonpathologic state.

Acute hypotension, which leads to shock, is life-threatening. Possible causes include hypovolemia with fluid loss or sequestration, cardiac abnormalities (myocardial infarcts and arrhythmias), obstruction to blood flow, and neuropathic conditions.

Chronic hypotension, in which the systolic pressure is in the range of 85–110 mmHg, may be a normal conditon (in which case it is associated with a greater life expectancy). It may occur with myocardial diseases, obstruction to blood flow, drug toxicity, adrenal insufficiency, malnutrition, cachexia, and a variety of neurologic abnormalities. Chronic low blood pressure may be asymptomatic or may produce lethargy, weakness, easy tiring, dizziness, and syncope; treatment is most frequently directed at the underlying cause.

See also *shock.*

orthostatic h., an excessive fall in blood pressure that occurs on assuming an upright posture. Orthostatic hypotension is most commonly caused by drugs that block autonomic reflexes, including antihypertensive drugs, ganglionic blockers, α-adrenergic blockers, monoamine oxidase inhibitors, and tricyclic antidepressants. Other causes include prolonged recumbency, sympathectomy, reduction in blood volume, and neuropathic disorders of the autonomic, peripheral, or central nervous system.

Those affected may experience lightheadedness, confusion, blurred vision, syncope, or seizures on standing. Diagnosis is based on clinical information, and treatment is directed at the underlying cause.

Also called postural hypotension.

hypotensive (hi″po-ten′siv) 1. characterized by or causing reduced tension or pressure.

2. a person with abnormally low blood pressure.

hypothalamic (hi″po-thah-lam′ik) of or involving the hypothalamus.

hypothalamohypophyseal tract (hi″po-thal″am-o-hi″po-fiz′e-al) the bundle of nerves formed by axons of neurons in the supraoptic and paraventricular nuclei of the hypothalamus that extend down the pituitary stalk and terminate on capillaries in the posterior lobe of the pituitary. The hormones of the posterior lobe are transported down their axoplasm.

hypothalamus (hi″po-thal′ah-mus) [*hypo-* + Gr. *thalamos* inner chamber] [NA], that portion of the diencephalon that forms the anterior floor and lower lateral wall of the third ventricle. It includes the optic chiasma, tuber cinereum, neurohypophysis, and mamillary bodies. Each lateral half is composed of a medial portion, in which there are many nuclei, and a lateral portion, which mainly consists of nerve fibers. Afferent fibers reach the hypothalamus from the cerebral cortex, basal ganglia, and thalamus. It has numerous efferent pathways including descending fibers that enter the midbrain, and the hypothalamo-hypophyseal outflows. The hypothalamus is basically a coordinating center for the control of visceral endocrine and many somatic functions.

hypothenar (hi-poth′ĕ-nar) [*hypo-* + Gr. *thenar* palm] 1. [NA], the region of the palm along the bases of the fingers on the ulnar side.

2. relating to the hypothenar region.

hypothenar eminence (hi-poth′ĕ-nar) [*hypo-* + Gr. *thenar* palm] the elevation close to the ulnar border of the palm produced by the three short muscles to the little finger.

hypothermia (hi″po-ther′me-ah) [*hypo-* + Gr. *thermē* heat + *-ia*] an abnormal decrease in body temperature. Hypothermia may occur accidentally with unprotected exposure to cold; it may be secondary to acute illness; or it may be therapeutically induced as a means of reducing the body's metabolism and its demand for oxygen, especially during surgical procedures. Accidental hypothermia is a medical emergency and may have a fatal outcome if untreated.

Hypothermia produces transient and reversible electrocerebral inactivity. A rectal temperature of above 32°C (90°F) is therefore necessary before the electroencephalogram can be used to establish brain death.

accidental h., the uncontrolled lowering of the core body temperature to below 35°C (95°F), as a result of prolonged exposure (atmospheric or immersion) to extreme cold. Acute alcoholism can increase the risk of hypothermia. The heart is most sensitive to cooling, and ventricular fibrillation and asystole may occur at body temperatures between 21° and 24°C (70°–75°F). Mental confusion and cyanosis are early signs of this disorder. Dehydration and abnormal electrocardiographic readings are common. Metabolic acidosis, pneumonia, and renal failure are also seen.

Under certain conditions, individuals exposed to cold water may undergo a phenomenon known as the mammalian diving reflex, with the diversion of blood from the extremities to the cardiopulmonary and cerebral circulatory tract. Heart rates may drop to 6–8 beats/min. This reflex is strongest in young, healthy individuals, and cases have been recorded in which persons without detectable pulse or respiration have been revived without significant body damage after immersion in cold water for periods longer than 30 min.

acute illness h., acute hypothermia seen in individuals with systemic disorders, including congestive heart failure, uremia, hypoglycemia, diabetes mellitus, acute respiratory failure, and drug overdoses. Many patients are elderly and may exhibit body temperatures of 33.3°–34.4°C (92°–94°F). Metabolic acidosis and coma are frequently seen, and cardiac arrhythmias may result. This disorder is thought to result from failure of thermoregulation. Affected individuals respond well to gradual rewarming. Prevention of acute illness hypothermia is dependent on treatment of the underlying systemic disease.

hypothesis (hi-poth′ĕ-sis) [*hypo-* + Gr. *thesis* a setting down] a supposition that appears to explain observed phenomena and is assumed as a basis of reasoning and experimentation. See also *theory.*

hypothesis testing a statistical procedure for determining whether a set of observations as sample data is consistent with the particular hypothesis being tested, which is called the null hypothesis (H_0). The null hypothesis is so-named because in most cases it states that some effect, such as difference of population means or a dependence between variables, does not exist. The null hypothesis determines the sampling distribution of a test statistic T, which is calculated from the data. The result of the test is a decision to reject H_0 if the value of T is unusual, i.e., if it falls in a specified area called the critical region. For the test to be consistent, any value in the critical region must be less likely under H_0 than any value outside the critical region. The probability α of T falling in the critical region when H_0 is true can be determined because H_0 specifies the sampling distribution of T. This probability α is called the significance level (or α level) of the test: it is the probability of rejecting H_0 when it is in fact true (a Type I error).

When H_0 is rejected, an alternate hypothesis (H_1) is accepted. For the test to be consistent, each value of T in the critical region must be more likely under H_1 than under H_0. The probability β of T falling outside the critical region when H_0 is false can be determined from the sampling distribution of T under H_1; it is the probability β of accepting H_0 when it is in fact false (a Type II error). The probability $1 - \beta$ of accepting H_1 when it is true is called the power of the test. When more than one sampling distribution of T (simple alternative) is consistent with H_1, there may be a different power for each simple alternative. One test is considered to be better than another if it is more powerful (at a given α level) for all simple alternatives.

In practice, no decision is actually made, and hypothesis testing is used only as a standard frame of reference for discussion of the data; usually, a P value is reported. This is the lowest α level at which the null hypothesis can be rejected on the basis of the data at hand; the P value is the probability of observing a set of data at least as inconsistent with H_0, if H_0 were true. A P value below 0.05 (sometimes below 0.01) is regarded as significant as a rough guideline, but the actual significance depends on the relative importance of Type I and Type II errors to each user of the data.

See also *one-tailed test* and *two-tailed test*. For examples, see under *analysis of variance, chi-squared test,* and *t distribution.*

hypothyroid (hi″po-thi′roid) marked by or due to hypothyroidism.

hypothyroidism (hi″po-thi′roi-dizm) an abnormal decrease in the activity of the thyroid gland, resulting in the deficient secretion of thyroid hormones. This condition may occur as primary hypothyroidism due to intrinsic disorders of the thyroid or as secondary hypothyroidism due to a deficiency of pituitary thyroid-stimulating hormone (TSH) or hypothalamic thyrotropin-releasing factor (TRF). Hypothyroidism may be congenital in infants (cretinism) and acquired in children (juvenile hypothyroidism) and adults. When severe, it causes myxedema.

In infants, congenital hypothyroidism may be due to the failure of thyroid development or to the failure of hormone synthesis or secretion. The gland may be absent, or may be large and goitrous. Acquired hypothyroidism may be due to infection or surgery, or may have unknown causes. Children affected with either form have cool and dry skin, puffy extremities, and a characteristic body appearance. The heart rate and body temperature are low. There is delayed physical and mental development, characteristically leading to dwarfism. Sexual development is delayed but eventually occurs. Most affected individuals have anemia.

Laboratory tests reveal depressed T_4(D) (T_4-competitive protein binding) activity, usually less than 3 μg/100 ml. Serum T_4 is decreased. Radioimmunoassays of TSH reveal elevated concentrations. Other findings include a depressed basal metabolic rate (BMR), increased serum cholesterol, increases in aspartate aminotransferase, lactate dehydrogenase, and creatine kinase enzymes, and elevated uric acid. X-ray examination reveals delayed skeletal maturation, and electrocardiograms show a decreased rate and voltage.

In adults, primary thyroid deficiency may result from surgical removal of the thyroid, radioactive iodine therapy, ingestion of goitrogens, or inflammatory processes. Some cases follow x-ray therapy to the neck, but most are due to thyroid atrophy from unknown cause. Secondary thyroid deficiency may follow pituitary deficiency or destruction, or hypothalamic dysfunction.

Affected individuals may exhibit signs and symptoms ranging from mild to severe (myxedema). Early effects of hypothyroidism include intolerance to cold, weakness, lethargy, constipation, dry skin, and nervousness. Hair may become sparse, coarse, and brittle. There is pallor, poor muscle turgor, and delayed deep reflexes. As this conditon progresses, there may be personality changes, peripheral edema, muscle cramps, dyspnea, menstrual changes, and anginal pain. Physical findings include skin and eyelid puffiness, thinning of outer halves of the eyelids, thickening of the tongue, hard pitting edema, joint effusion, and cardiac enlargement.

Laboratory tests reveal decreased serum T_4, T_3-U (T_3 resin uptake), and thyroidal radioactive iodine uptake (RAIU). Radioimmunoassay of TSH shows increased concentrations. Serum cholesterol and total serum protein are elevated. Macrocytic anemia is also common. The electrocardiogram shows decreased amplitude and flattened or inverted T waves. Patients may show dramatic recovery following administration of thyroid hormone.

See also *cretinism* and *myxedema.*

hypotonic (hi″po-ton′ik) [*hypo-* + Gr. *tonikos,* from *tonos* tension] having a lower osmotic concentration of solutes than is present in blood. Cells gain water by osmosis when exposed to a hypotonic solution. Cf. *hypertonic.*

hypotriploid (hi″po-trip′loid) having an aneuploid chromosome number close to but less than the triploid chromosome number.

hypoventilation (hi″po-ven″tĭ-la′shun) a reduction in ventilation below levels adequate to meet the body's metabolic requirements for O_2 and for the removal of CO_2. It is the result of either a reduction in absolute minute ventilation, or of a reduction in alveolar ventilation (the volume of air that reaches the gas-exchanging regions of the lungs each minute, equal to total minute ventilation minus the physiologic dead space) in the face of a normal or even elevated total minute ventilation (the volume of air breathed in or out of the lungs each minute).

When minute ventilation is reduced, an elevation of arterial P_{CO_2} and hypercapnic respiratory failure ensue. Arterial hypoxemia during breathing of room air is an inevitable consequence of hypoventilation, whatever the underlying cause.

Inadequate alveolar ventilation in the presence of an increased total minute ventilation implies the presence of an abnormally large physiologic dead space (the volume of each inspiration that does not undergo gaseous exchange with the pulmonary capillary blood) that leads to wasted ventilation. This condition results from various intrinsic lung disorders such as obstructive emphysema and pulmonary vascular disease. Hypercapneic respiratory failure secondary to a reduction in total minute ventilation may result from respiratory center depression (by drugs or as the result of head injury), neuromuscular disorders (e.g., poliomyelitis, cervical spinal cord injuries, Guillain-Barré syndrome, myasthenia gravis), and thoracic cage abnormalities and injuries (e.g., flail chest, ankylosing spondylitis, pectus excavatum, kyphoscoliosis).

Oxygen enrichment can provide a normal or even excess arterial oxygen tension during periods of severe hypoventilation.

hypovitaminosis (hi″po-vi″tah-mĭ-no′sis) a state in which there is a deficiency of an essential vitamin. Its severity and effects are dependent on the nature of the vitamin deficit.

h. A., a condition due to a deficiency of vitamin A, usually caused by low dietary intake, by diseases that affect the intestinal absorption and conversion of carotene to vitamin A, by infectious disease in chronically malnourished children, or by lowered levels of transport protein due to protein deficiency. Sufficiently low levels cause conjunctival and corneal degeneration and dry skin. Loss of night vision due to failure of rhodopsin regeneration is generally the earliest symptom; it can progress to xerophthalmia, Bitot's spots and corneal erosion, and, eventually, keratomalacia if left untreated. Treatment consists of vitamin A administration and correction of the underlying disorder.

hypovolemia (hi″po-vo-le′me-ah) [*hypo-* + *volume* + Gr. *haima* blood + *-ia*] an abnormal decrease in the intravascular volume. Normal blood volume in males is 52–83 ml/kg and for females, 50–75. The causes of hypovolemia can be classified into two general categories: external causes, which include hemorrhage, burns, and gastrointestinal disorders such as vomiting and diarrhea; and internal causes, which include exudative disorders such as ascites and peritonitis, and traumatic injuries producing hemorrhage. A reduction in blood volume of 10 percent may be asymptomatic, whereas a 15–25 percent reduction usually leads to tachycardia, tachypnea, pallor, and cerebral effects. Losses above these levels result in hypovolemic shock. Generally, any blood loss that causes a reduction of more than 50 percent of intravascular volume is fatal. See also *hypovolemic s.* under *shock.*

hypovolemic (hi″po-vo-le′mik) pertaining to or characterized by hypovolemia.

hypoxanthine (hi″po-zan′thēn) 6-oxypurine, a purine base, $C_5H_4N_4O$, being an intermediate product of uric acid sythesis. It is formed from adenylic acid and is itself a precursor of xanthine. The much greater solubility in serum and urine of hypoxanthine than uric acid provides the rationale for treating gout with allopurinol, a structural analog compound of hypoxanthine. This compound competitively inhibits the degradation of hypoxanthine to uric acid; the hypoxanthine is excreted more readily than is the less soluble uric acid.

hypoxanthine guanine phosphoribosyltransferase see *hypoxanthine phosphoribosyltransferase.*

hypoxanthine phosphoribosyltransferase (hi″-po-zan′thēn fos″fo-ri″bo-sil-trans′fer-ās) an enzyme of the transferase class (IMP:pyrophosphate phosphoribosyltransferase, EC 2.4.2.8) that catalyzes the reaction inosine 5′-monophosphate (IMP) + pyrophosphate ⇄ hypoxanthine + 5-phospho-α-D-ribose-1-disphosphate (PRPP). Guanosine-5′-phosphate (GMP) can replace IMP, with guanine as the product instead of hypoxanthine. The reverse reaction acts as a salvage mechanism for conserving preformed purines. A hereditary deficiency, Lesch-Nyhan syndrome, transmitted as an X-linked trait, results in some neurologic manifestations and hyperuricemia as a consequence of the increased accumulation of PRPP. The enzyme deficiency has been demonstrated in liver, kidney, and brain tissues and in skin fibroblasts, erythrocytes, and leukocytes of those affected. Also called *hypoxanthine guanine phosphoribosyltransferase.*

hypoxemia (hi″pok-se′me-ah) [*hypo-* + *oxygen* + Gr. *haima* blood + *-ia*] a reduction in the oxygen tension or oxygen-carrying capacity of hemoglobin in arterial blood. The term should be contrasted with anoxemia, which indicates the absence of oxygen in arterial blood or oxygen present in amounts less than those required for life.

hypoxia (hi-pok′se-ah) a lack or deficiency of oxygen at the tissue level; a reduction in the tissue oxygen tension below a critical level. Hypoxia can be caused by any of the multitudinous physiologic and anatomic factors that contribute to the following conditions: the inadequate oxygenation of the lungs, an alveolocapillary diffusion barrier, a ventilation-perfusion imbalance, the inadequate circulatory transport of oxygen, an increase in tissue oxygen demand, or an impaired capability of the tissue to utilize the available oxygen.

Four general types of hypoxia (anemic, histotoxic, hypoxic, and ischemic) are commonly differentiated on the basis of these causative factors. The sypmtoms of a generalized hypoxia may include depression and aberration in mental activity that can culminate in coma, tachycardia, systemic hypotension (sometimes hypertension when the hypoxia is severe and sympathetic nervous system stimulation occurs), pulmonary hypertension, hyperventilation, tissue acidosis, respiratory alkalosis, anorexia, nausea, and vomiting. The respiratory mechanism is more sensitive to changes in P_{CO_2} during some forms of hypoxia. Respiratory minute volume is greater (both the depth and rate of breathing increase) at any given level of increased P_{CO_2} when the alveolar P_{O_2} has been lowered. This increased sensitivity of the chemoreceptor reflexes is of adaptive value in restoring adequate oxygen delivery.

Oxygen therapy is of great value in treating the many forms of hypoxic hypoxia, and in treating anemic hypoxia, particularly when oxygen under increased atmospheric pressure is used.

Cf. *anoxia.*

anemic h., the hypoxia that occurs when arterial

Po_2 is at normal levels, but the capacity of the blood to transport the oxygen is reduced owing to a deficiency in the concentration of hemoglobin or red blood cells or to an abnormality in the hemoglobin affinity for oxygen.

histotoxic h., a lack of oxygen at the cellular level that occurs despite a normal arterial Po_2. It is caused by an increased tissue demand for oxygen (strenuous exercise), by tissue edema (when the length of the diffusion pathway from capillary to cell is increased), or by factors that lead to an inhibition of cellular enzymes (particularly cytochrome oxidase in cyanide poisoning). Also called cytotoxic hypoxia.

hypoxic h., the hypoxia that results from inadequate oxygenation of arterial blood leaving the heart and lungs. It is caused by an extrinsic or disease factor that leads to a deficiency of oxygen in the inspired air, hypoventilation, an imbalance in alveolar ventilation in relation to the pulmonary capillary blood flow, an alveolocapillary diffusion block, or to shunts within the heart and lungs. Also called *anoxic anoxia.*

ischemic h., the hypoxia that is caused by a general or local circulatory deficiency. Although arterial oxygen tension and hemoglobin concentration are at normal levels, the reduced blood flow results in inadequate oxygen delivery to the tissues. Ischemic hypoxia can cause damage to major organs during shock, damage to the lungs during prolonged circulatory collapse, and/or congestive heart failure when the cardiac output is severely reduced. Also caled stagnant hypoxia.

hypoxic (hi-pok′sik) pertaining to or characterized by hypoxia.

hypro-protein (hip″ro-pro′tēn) see *hydroxyproline.*

hypsarrhythmia (hip″sah -rith′me-ah) [Gr. *hypsi* high + *arrhythmos* unrhythmic + *-ia*] in electroencephalography, an abnormal pattern of electrical activity, occurring in infants and young children, that consists of high-voltage, arrhythmic, synchronous slow waves with superimposed multifocal sharp wave and spike discharges. This pattern usually reflects a diffuse insult to the developing brain and is frequently associated with the clinical syndrome of infantile spasms.

hypsochrome (hip′so-krōm) [Gr. *hypsi* high + *chrōma* color] an atom or group whose introduction into a compound shifts the compound's absorption maximum to a shorter wavelength.

hypsochromic shift (hip″-so-kro″mik) a shift in the absorption peak of a chromophore to a shorter wavelength.

hyster/o (his′ter-o) [Gr. *hystera* uterus] a prefix word element to denote the uterus, e.g., hysterosalpingography.

hysterectomy (his″ter-ek′to-me) [*hystero-* + Gr. *ektomē*] surgical removal of all or part of the uterus.

hysteresis (his″tĕ-re′sis) [Gr. *hysterēsis* a lagging behind] the failure of coincidence of two associated phenomena, or the influence of the direction of change from a previously held value of an independent variable on the subsequent value of a dependent variable. In respiratory physiology, volume hysteresis is seen when the deflationary limb of a pressure-volume curve of the lungs falls far to the left of the immediately preceding inflationary limb.

hysteresis loop a curve that shows two values of a dependent variable for each value of the independent variable: one when the independent variable is increasing, and one when it is decreasing.

hysteria (his-tēr′e-ah) [*hyster-* + *-ia*] 1. a psychoneurosis, the symptoms of which are based on conversion of anxiety into physical symptoms. Symptoms may include hyperesthesia, pain and tenderness, choking sensation, dimming of vision, paralysis, tonic spasms, convulsions, vasomotor disturbances, hallucinations, and catalepsy. There are no consistent or characteristic changes in the electroencephalogram. Also called conversion reaction.

2. a state characterized by lack of control over acts and emotions.

hysterosalpingography (his″ter-o-sal″ping-gog′rah-fe) [*hystero-* + Gr. *salpinx* tube + *graphein* to record] a radiographic examination of the uterus and uterine tubes after injection of a contrast medium (such as diatrizoate or acetrizoate), using a uterine catheter. Also called *uterosalpingography.*

Hz abbrev. See *hertz.*

I

I symbol for electric current, *inosine, intensity,* the chemical element *iodine, ionic strength,* moment of inertia.

i symbol for *isochromosome.*

ι the Greek lower case letter *iota.*

-ia (e'ah) a suffix word element to denote a condition or process, e.g., leukemia.

Ia antigen abbrev. for immune response gene–associated antigen; antigen controlled by Ir genes and found on various tissues, on the surface of most lymphocytes, and on macrophages. Ia antigens on macrophage may act as receptors for a soluble T-lymphocyte factor, which would provide a mechanism for T lymphocyte–B lymphocyte cooperation in the process of antibody production.

IAP abbrev. See *International Academy of Pathology.*

-iasis (i'ah-sis) a suffix word element to denote a condition, e.g., choledocholithiasis.

iatro- (i'at-ro) [Gr. *iatros* physician] a word element used in combining form to denote relationship to a physician or to medicine, e.g., iatrogenic.

iatrogenic (i-at″ro-jen'ik) [*iatro-* + Gr. *gennan* to produce] resulting from the actions of the physician. The term most often refers to infections that are acquired by the patient during the course of treatment by a physician or surgeon.

iatrogenic anemia see *iatrogenic a.* under *anemia.*

iatrotherapy (i″at-ro-ther'ah-pe) the placebo effect; a therapeutic effect produced by the doctor-patient relationship, not by a specific drug or surgical treatment.

-iatry [Gr. *iatreia*] a suffix word element to denote medical treatment, e.g., psychiatry.

I band [from *isotropic*] the region of a sarcomere that contains only actin filaments. See also *skeletal m.* under *muscle.*

IBF abbrev. See *immunoglobulin-binding factor.*

ibuprofen (i-bu'pro-fen) an analgesic and antipyretic nonsteroidal antiinflammatory drug (NSAID), used for symptomatic relief in rheumatoid arthritis and osteoarthritis. Like other NSAIDS, ibuprofen acts by inhibiting the synthesis of mediators of the inflammatory response, such as prostaglandins and kinins. It is an arylacetic acid derivative similar to naproxen, ketoprofen, and fenoprofen. The most common side-effects are gastrointestinal intolerance (nausea, heartburn), dizziness, itching, and skin rashes. Trademark, *Motrin.*

IC abbrev. See *inspiratory capacity, integrated circuit.*

-ic (ik) 1. a suffix word element to denote pertaining to or characterized by, e.g., analgesic.

2. a suffix word element used in inorganic chemistry to denote the higher of the two most common oxidation states of a metal cation, e.g., ferric ion, the trivial name for iron(III) ion, or of an oxo acid, e.g., sulfuric acid. Cf. *-ous.*

ICD abbrev. See *isocitrate dehydrogenase.*

ice (is) the solid form of water, which melts at 0°C at 1 atm.

ice point the temperature (273.15 K) at which a mixture of pure ice and air-saturated water is in equilibrium at a pressure of 1 atm, the freezing point of water. Cf. *triple point.*

ICG abbrev. See *indocyanine green.*

ICG excretion test see under *dye excretion tests.*

ichthy/o (ik'the-o) [Gr. *ichthys* fish] a word element used in combining form to denote a relationship to fish or a scalelike appearance.

ichthyosarcotoxism (ik″the-o-sar″ko-tok'sizm) [*ichthyo-* + Gr. *sarkos* flesh + *toxikon* poison] intoxication resulting from the ingestion of poisonous fish, excluding ordinary bacterial food poisoning. Symptoms range from minor gastrointestinal distress to severe neurologic disorders.

ichthyosis (ik″the-o'sis) [*ichthyo-* + *-osis* condition] a general term used to refer to a variety of skin disorders that are characterized by roughness, scaliness, and dryness. Several forms are recognized that differ in their pattern of inheritance but have in common excessive keratin production (hyperkeratosis).

i. congenita, a congenital disorder of the skin characterized by diffuse hyperkeratosis with the formation of extensive horny scales.

i. hystrix, a rare disorder that affects the epidermis and is marked by hyperkeratosis and brown, linear, verrucoid ridges or horny knobs.

i. uteri, a disorder that affects the uterine cavity, causing the endometrium to undergo metaplasia from a glandular to a squamous epithelium.

icosahedral symmetry (i-ko″sah-he'dral) a type of symmetry displayed by many viruses that is based on the fact that the assembly of the protein subunits (capsomers) causes the capsid of the virus to be at a state of minimal energy. An icosahedron is a regular polyhedron with 20 triangular faces and 12 corners; it also has axes of two-, three-, and fivefold rotational symmetry passing through the edges, faces, and corners, respectively. Thus, an icosahedron is referred to as a solid with a 5:3:2 rotational symmetry (see the accompanying illustration). The number and arrangement of capsomers in an icosahedral capsid can be found according to certain geometric formulas and is sometimes used in identifying various viruses.

ICSH abbrev. for interstitial cell–stimulating hormone. See *luteinizing hormone.*

ICSP abbrev. See *International Council of Societies of Pathology.*

ictal (ik'tal) [L. *ictus* stroke] pertaining to or characterized by ictus.

icter/o [L. *icturus*; Gr. *ikteros*] a word element used in combining form to denote affected with or pertaining to jaundice.

icteric (ik-ter'ik) pertaining to or characterized by jaundice.

icterogenic (ik″ter-o-jen'ik) causing or capable of causing jaundice.

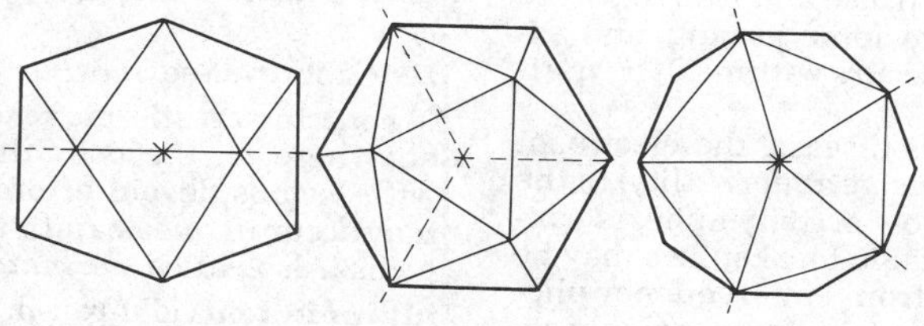

Icosahedral symmetry. Regular icosahedron viewed along twofold (*A*), threefold (*B*), and fivefold (*C*) axes. (From Fenner, F. J., and White, D. O.: Medical Virology. 2nd ed. New York, Academic Press, 1976.)

icterogenic spirochetosis see *leptospiral j.* under *jaundice.*

icterus (ik′ter-us) [L.; Gr. *ikteros*] jaundice; a sign of one of a number of different diseases and disorders of the liver, gallbladder, and bile metabolism, or of hemolysis. See also *jaundice.*

congenital familial i., see *hereditary spherocytosis* under *anemia.*

i. gravis, a severe condition in newborn infants that is due to hemolytic anemia and usually associated with maternal incompatibility with fetal erythrocyte antigens, i.e., ABO or Rh blood group incompatibility. There is severe anemia and pallor accompanying an obvious jaundice, with liver and spleen enlargement and extramedullary erythropoiesis. Also called icterus gravis neonatorum. See also *kernicterus.*

i. neonatorum, the jaundice sometimes seen in newborns.

icterus index a measure, now obsolete, of the degree of icterus in a serum or plasma specimen; the absorbance in the yellow, at 460 nm is compared with that of a standard potassium dichromate solution.

icterus interference in colorimetric assays, erroneous results due to the presence of the yellow bilirubin pigment in the specimen.

ictus (ik′tus), pl. *ictus* [L. "stroke"] a seizure, stroke, blow, or sudden attack of any sort.

ICU abbrev. for intensive care unit.

ID abbrev. for identification, *iditol dehydrogenase, infectious disease,* inside diameter, *intradermal.*

ID_{50} abbrev. See *median infectious d.* under *dose.*

id (id) [Gr. *idios* own, peculiar] 1. a skin eruption that occurs as an allergic reaction to an agent causing primary lesions elsewhere.

2. Freud's term for the psychologic components present at birth, the instincts and instinctual drives that are striving for expression.

-id (id) [Gr. *eidos* form, shape] a suffix word element to denote resembling or having the shape of, e.g., dermatophytid.

-ide (id) [from *oxide,* from Fr. *acide* acid] a suffix word element in inorganic chemistry to denote (1) monatomic anions, e.g., bromide, hydride, sulfide; or (2) certain polyatomic anions, e.g., cyanide, hydroxide. The suffix is also used in naming some compounds related to these ions, as in the class of organic thioethers called sulfides and the halogenated hydrocarbons, the halides.

ideal gas (i-de′al) a theoretical model for gases, which assumes that they consist of point particles that interact only by elastic collision and that there are no attractive forces between them. For such a gas, the ideal gas law holds exactly at any temperature or pressure.

ideal gas law see *gas law.*

identifier (i-den′tĭ-fi″er) in a computer system, a code that uniquely identifies a file, program, data block, record, or other groups of data. A character string identifier is usually referred to as the [program, data set, or file] name.

identity (i-den′tĭ-te) a term that describes a reaction pattern of precipitin lines resulting from the double diffusion of antibody and antigen in agar. An identity type of reaction results in a complete fusion of the precipitin lines when the two antigen wells contain a single antigen and the antibody well contains antibody to that single antigen. See also *Ouchterlony immunodiffusion.*

identity pattern see under *Ouchterlony immunodiffusion.*

idi/o (id′e-o) [Gr. *idios* own, peculiar] a word element used in combining form to denote own, self, or individual, e.g., idiopathic.

idiocy (id′e-o-se) severe mental retardation. See also *mental retardation.*

amaurotic familial i., a class of rare, neuronal lipid storage diseases due to enzymatic defects of lipid metabolism that result in sphingolipid accumulation in the brain. There is progressive deterioration of the cerebromacular area, leading to dementia, blindness, spasticity, and, invariably, death. Large nerve cells of many areas are distended with gangliosides or lipofuscin. Lipid-containing macrophages also are frequently seen. Age of onset determines the classification of the diseases in this group as Bielschowsky-Jansky syndrome (late infantile), Spielmeyer-Vogt syndrome (juvenile), or Kufs' disease (adult). For more information, see the specific disease.

juvenile amaurotic familial i., a genetic disorder, transmitted as an autosomal recessive trait, that is characterized by cerebroretinal degeneration leading to progressive blindness and mental deterioration. This syndrome is considered to be the juvenile form of amaurotic familial idiocy, usually manifesting itself by ages 5–6 yr. The ocular lesions affect retinal rods, cones, and ganglion cells. There is optic atrophy, loss of foveal reflex, threadlike retinal vessels, and red-purple discoloration in the area of macular degeneration, leading to eventual blindness. Cerebral lesions are diffuse and lead to severe dementia, convulsions, myoclonic jerking, and advancing weakness. Death occurs within 10–15 yr after onset of symptoms.

During the course of this disease, the electroencephalogram shows progressive abnormality. In the early stages, generalized slow activity appears continuously or in bursts; sporadic focal spikes may be present. Potentials evoked from low-frequency photic stimuli appear as large single or polyphasic spikes. As the disease progresses, spike and wave complexes appear on a background dominated by theta or delta activity. This background activity becomes slower and irregular in the later stages of the disease while the spike complexes are reduced.

Also called *Batten's disease,* Batten-Spielmeyer-Vogt syndrome, and *Spielmeyer-Vogt syndrome.* See also *amaurotic familial i.*

mongolian i., the former name for Down's syndrome; see *Down's syndrome.*

idiogram (id′e-o-gram″) [*idio-* + *-gram*] a diagrammatic representation of a karyotype that shows the shape of each chromosome and the bands observed when a particular staining method is used. It is usually prepared by cutting up a photographic print of a well-spread nucleus and then arranging the cut-out chromosomes in order.

idiopathic (id″e-o-path′ik) occurring without known cause. The term usually refers to those diseases whose cause is unknown. For diseases or conditions beginning with this adjective, see the noun.

idiosyncrasy (id″e-o-sing′krah-se) [*idio-* + Gr. *synkrasis* mixture] an unusual or abnormal sensitivity of an individual to a therapeutic agent or process (e.g., drugs or anesthesia).

idiotype (id′e-o-tīp) an antigen, or group of antigens, that represents the antigenic component of the antibody-combining site of an antibody molecule. This antigen is unique to each antibody or myeloma protein. Also called idiotypic antigenic determinant.

idioventricular rhythm (id″e-o-ven-trik′u-lar) a broad term used to refer to heart rhythm in which the natural pacemaker is in the ventricle. The rate is usually slow, below 50 (or 60) beats/min.

iditol (i′dĭ-tol) a hexahydric alcohol, CH_2OH-$(CHOH)_4CH_2OH$.

iditol dehydrogenase (ID) (i″dĭ-tol de-hi′dro-jen-ās) an enzyme of the oxidoreductase class (EC 1.1.1.14) that catalyzes the reaction L-iditol + NAD^+ ⇄ L-sorbose + NADH. It also acts on D-sorbitol, giving D-fructose. The enzyme occurs in significant quantities only in the liver, with very small amounts also present in the prostate and kidneys. Increased activity in serum strongly suggests parenchymal liver cell damage, most frequently due to acute hepatitis, or to carbon tetrachloride poisoning or other forms of acute hepatic necrosis. Also called *polyol dehydrogenase* and *sorbitol dehydrogenase.*

iditol dehydrogenase assays determination of the serum ID activity using the forward reaction (sorbitol + NAD → fructose + $NADH_2$) at pH 8.5–9.5 or the reverse reaction at pH 6.0–7.5. Either reaction may be quantitated spectrophotometrically by measuring the change in absorption at 340 nm due to NADH formation.

IDL abbrev. See *intermediate-density l.* under *lipoprotein.*

ID-MS abbrev. See *isotope dilution–mass spectrometry.*

IDP abbrev. See *inosine diphosphate.*

id reaction an allergic reaction to a fungal infection anywhere on the body distal to the infected site, with lesions devoid of organisms. The id reaction may occur in tinea capitis and, less commonly, tinea pedis. Also called *dermatophytid reaction.*

iduronic acid (id′u-ron-ik) a substance occurring as the L-compound that is structurally equivalent to the 5-epimer of D-glucuronic acid. It is found in proteoglycans such as dermatan sulfate and heparin.

iduronic sulfatase (id′u-ron-ik sul′fah-tās) an enzyme that catalyzes the hydrolysis of the iduronic-sulfate bond in dermatan sulfate and heparan sulfate. The reaction is important in the metabolism of mucopolysaccharides. A genetic deficiency of the enzyme, transmitted as an X-recessive or autosomal recessive trait, leads to the accumulation of dermatan or heparan sulfates in tissue and results in their excretion in the urine, a condition known as mucopolysaccharidosis (MPS) II (Hunter's syndrome). Also called *L-sulfoiduronate sulfatase.*

L-iduronidase (id″u-ron′ĭ-dās) an enzyme of the lyase class (EC 3.2.1.76) that catalyzes the hydrolysis of α-L-iduronosidic linkages in desulfated dermatan. The enzyme is important in the metabolism of mucopolysaccharides. A genetic deficiency of the enzyme, transmitted as an autosomal recessive trait, leads to the accumulation of dermatan sulfate and heparan sulfate in cells, with resulting excretion in urine. The disorder is known as mucopolysaccharidosis (MPS) I (Hurler and Scheie syndromes).

IEEE (i trip′l e) abbrev. See *Institute of Electrical and Electronic Engineers.*

iff in mathematical proofs, an abbreviation of "if and only if." A iff B means B is a necessary and sufficient condition for A. See also *necessary condition* and *sufficient condition.*

ifosfamide (i-fos′fah-mīd) a cancer chemotherapeutic drug; trademark, Cyfos. For more information, see *Appendix A.*

Ig abbrev. for immunoglobulin of any of the five classes: IgA, IgD, IgE, IgG, or IgM; see *immunoglobulin.*

IgA nephropathy see *Berger's disease.*

IGFET abbrev. for insulated gate field effect transistor. See *metal oxide semiconductor field effect t.* under *transistor.*

ignitability degree of combustibility; the term is used by the Environmental Protection Agency to identify the degree of combustibility that defines whether a waste will be regulated as hazardous under the Resource Conservation and Recovery Act.

Flammable liquids and Class II combustible liquids (i.e., those with a flash-point temperature less than 60°C (140°F) are classified as hazardous wastes, with the exception of alcohol-water solutions containing less than 24 percent alcohol by volume. Other wastes included in this category are: flammable compressed gases; oxidizers as defined by Department of Transportation standards; and solids capable of causing fire through friction, absorption of moisture, or spontaneous chemical changes, and that burn so vigorously and persistently when ignited that the fire creates a hazard.

ignition point (ig-nĭ′shun) [L. *ignis* fire] the lowest temperature required to cause a substance to burn in the absence of a spark.

ignition source control the control of ignition sources so that they are not in the vicinity of combustible or flammable materials, so that they are protected from combustible materials reaching them, or so that flame cannot propagate even if vapors or gases reach an ignition source: an important part of a fire prevention program. Ignition sources include open flames; lighted tobacco; welding and cutting procedures; heating elements and other hot surfaces; frictional heat; radiant heat; spontaneous ignition; heat-producing chemical reactions; lighting; and static, electrical, and mechanical sparks.

Methods for controlling ignition sources may include designation of No Smoking areas, employment of special electrical equipment, and prohibition of the use of flames or other heat-producing activities when or where flammables are in use.

Electrical equipment that must be used when flammable vapors or gases are present can be specially purchased as "explosion-proof" or intrinsically safe for the specific condition, or regular equipment can be enclosed and ventilated or purged to prevent flammable vapors or gases from reaching the ignition source.

Another method used in the laboratory to prevent ignition of flammable gases is use of a gas to which sufficient inert gas has been added to prevent formation of a flammable mixture of gases. For example, hydrogen used for anaerobic incubation chambers is provided in a dilute mixture with an inerting gas so that the combination is not flammable.

ignition temperature the minimum temperature to which a substance (vapor or gas) in air must be heated to initiate self-sustained combustion. Ignition temperatures vary with pressure, concentration of a vapor-air mixture, size of space containing the ignitible mixture, and other factors.

IHSS abbrev. See *idiopathic hypertrophic s. s.* under *subaortic stenosis.*

IL 1 abbrev. See *interleukin 1.*

IL 2 abbrev. See *interleukin 2.*

Ile abbrev. See *isoleucine.*

ile/o (il′e-o) [L. *ileum*] a word element used in combining form to denote the ileum (the third part of the small intestine), e.g., ileostomy.

ileal (il′e-al) pertaining to the ileum.

ileitis (il″e-i′tis) a general term used to describe the inflammation of the distal portion of the small intestine, the ileum. The potential causes are many, including infection, autoimmunity, irritation (especially drug-related), and metabolic and absorption disorders.

terminal i., an idiopathic inflammation of the ileum, also known as Crohn's disease or regional enteritis. See also *Crohn's disease.*

ileocecal (il″e-o-se′kal) pertaining to the ileum and cecum, as in the ileocecal valve, which connects the small and large intestines.

ileocolitis (il″e-o-ko-li′tis) an inflammation of the ileum and colon.

ileum (il′e-um) [L.] [NA], the distal segment of the small intestine. Approximately 3.5 m long, it is suspended over its entire length by mesentery and terminates at the ileocecal valve in the right lower quadrant of the abdomen where the large intestine begins. The ileum is of midgut derivation, and the location of the apex of the embryologic midgut loop is approximately 1 m from the end of the ileum (when a Meckel's diverticulum is present, it is located at this point).

The structure of the ileum is basically similar to that of the jejunum (for minor differences, see under *jejunum*). Its principal function is absorption, which is facilitated by the movements of its wall and by the vast surface area produced by the villi with their covering of epithelial cells, each with many surface microvilli. Concentric contractions of the small bowel occur at short intervals so that segments are formed, and conductive contractions are superimposed on these rhythmic segmenting contractions to move the contents in a distal direction (peristalsis). The ileum is invaginated into the cecum at the ileocecal valve. This valve regulates the passage of material from the lumen of the ileum into the large bowel and prevents reflux of the bacteria-laden colonic contents.

Hormones formed by enterochromaffin cells within the musosa influence the movements of the small bowel and stomach and the contractions of the gallbladder smooth muscle, and regulate secretion by the epithelial cells of the GI tract and pancreas. Absorption is highly selective. Water and solutes are rapidly absorbed in the proximal small bowel through hypothetical pores in the cell membrane. Electrolytes may be passively absorbed in the jejunum, but in the ileum and colon active mucosal transport occurs. Glucose can be absorbed by the intestine against a concentration gradient, which occurs more rapidly in the jejunum. Proteins are mainly digested in the duodenum and jejunum by the action of the pancreatic enzymes and are absorbed as amino acids in the jejunum and ileum. Triglycerides are hydrolyzed to bi- and monoglycerides and some glycerol, which are then reesterified in the epithelial cell cytoplasm and packaged with a fine protein coat as chylomicrons. They traverse the lateral cell membrane, and from the intercellular space pass through the basal lamina and enter the lymphatics. Most fat absorption takes place in the duodenum and upper jejunum. Fat-soluble vitamins are probably absorbed in a similar manner to fat. The absorption of vitamin B_{12} occurs in the terminal ileum, mediated by the glycoprotein intrinsic factor formed in the stomach.

Aggregates of lymphoid tissue are found throughout the intestines, but in the ileum they form grossly visible ovoid bodies, Peyer's patches, in the lamina propria and submucosa, particularly on the antimesenteric aspect. They are a major component of the gut-associated lymphoid tissue.

ileus (il′e-us) [L.; Gr. *eileos*, from *eilein* to roll up] an obstruction of the intestines, especially the ileum.

adynamic i., an intestinal obstruction due to paralysis of the musculature of part or all of the intestinal tract. This condition is most often seen in association with peritonitis. Also called paralytic ileus.

gallstone i., a rare condition in which gallstones erode through an inflammed gallbladder, enter the intestine through fistulas, and obstruct it by impacting at narrow points.

mechanical i., ileus that is most often the result of peritoneal adhesions or incarcerated hernias in adults and intussusception in children. Symptoms include colicky abdominal pain, severe constipation, and vomiting. Abdominal distention develops;

the lower the obstruction is, the greater is the degree of distention. Dehydration may lead to prerenal azotemia, acidosis or alkalosis, and hemoconcentration. Complications include necrosis of the intestinal wall, which increases the mortality rate. Radiographs of the abdomen show multiple loops of bowel filled with gas, which does not show progression in repeat films. Treatment may be both supportive and surgical.

meconium i., see *m. ileus* under *meconium.*

spastic i., ileus due to the consistent contraction of the muscles of the intestine or a bowel segment, often the result of neurologic disorders.

i. subparta, ileus due to pressure exerted by the enlarging gravid uterus on the pelvic colon of the pregnant female.

ili/o (il′e-o) [L. *ilium*] a word element used in combining form to denote the ilium, e.g., iliac.

iliac (il″e-ak) [L. *iliacus*] pertaining to the ilium and certain structures in its immediate vicinity, notably the iliac arteries, veins, and lymph nodes.

iliac artery, common one of the paired terminal branches of the abdominal aorta. Each divides into an internal and an external iliac artery.

iliac artery, external one of the two terminal branches of the common iliac artery. It arises in front of the sacroiliac joint and descends obliquely to enter the thigh behind the inguinal ligament, becoming the femoral artery.

iliac artery, internal the artery that arises from the common iliac artery in front of the sacroiliac joint and descends to the greater sciatic foramen; there it divides into an anterior branch, which continues to the ischial spine, and a posterior branch, which leaves the pelvis through the greater sciatic foramen.

iliac region 1. a region on the left or right side of the hypogastric (pubic) region.

2. a region of the abdomen below the transtubercular plane and to the outside of a lateral sagittal plane, used in radiographic positioning. Also called *inguinal region.* See illustration accompanying *abdominal regions.*

iliac vein, common the vein formed in front of the sacroiliac joint by the union of the external and internal iliac veins. It passes obliquely upward to meet its fellow from the opposite side; together they form the inferior vena cava on the right side of the fifth lumbar vertebral body.

iliac vein, external the continuation of the femoral vein. It begins behind the inguinal ligament and ends in front of the sacroiliac joint, where it meets the internal iliac vein; together they form the common iliac vein.

iliac vein, internal the vein that arises near the greater sciatic foramen and ascends with the internal iliac artery to meet the external iliac vein in front of the sacroiliac joint; together they form the common iliac vein.

ilium (il′e-um), pl. *ilia* [L.] one of the three conjoined parts of the hip bone. Its lower end is continuous with the ischium and pubis, and forms approximately two-fifths of the acetabulum. Its upper border is the iliac crest whose ends form the useful anatomic landmarks, the anterior and posterior iliac spines.

ill-defined diffuse or nebulous. In radiology, the term is used to refer to lung lesions characterized by diffuse, homogeneous radiographic shadows with poor lateral demarcation. In pathology, the term denotes lesions that macro- or microscopically have poorly circumscribed borders.

illuminance (ĭ-lu′mĭ-nans) see *illumination.*

illumination (ĭ-lu″mĭ-na′shun) [L. *illuminatio*] 1. the lighting up of a part, cavity, organ, or object for inspection.

2. the luminous flux (light intensity) per unit area falling on a surface; the unit of illumination is the lux (lx). Also called *illuminance.*

3. in microscopy, the casting of light, which is focused by the condenser from the light source (illuminant or illuminator) onto the object. There are two widely used methods of critical illumination. In the Nelson method, the image of the light source (lamp filament) is sharply focused in the object plane by the substage condenser. In the Köhler method (Köhler illumination), the image of the light source is focused on the back lens of the substage condenser by a lamp condenser, and the substage condenser sharply focuses the image of the lamp condenser in the object plane; also called *critical illumination.*

IM abbrev. for intramuscularly (by intramuscular injection).

im- a prefix word element used in chemistry to denote the bivalent group =NH.

image (im′ij) [L. *imago*] 1. a mental picture or conception.

2. a picture or representation of an object made by processing the radiant energy reflected or emitted by the object or transmitted through it, such as an optical image focused by a lens.

image intensification a technique used in fluoroscopy in which the x-ray image is electronically amplified, thereby greatly reducing the necessary radiation dose to the patient.

imaginary number (ĭ-maj′ĭ-nar″e) a complex number with a real part equal to zero. See also *complex number.*

imaging (im′ah-jing) 1. the production of an image.

2. any method of producing diagnostic images, such as radiography, computed tomography, ultrasonography, or scintiphotography.

imbibition (im″bĭ-bish′in) [L. *imbibere* to drink] 1. the act of imbibing.

2. the absorption of a liquid into the microscopic pores of a solid such as cellulose.

3. the absorption of a solvent by a gel.

4. the absorption of dye by gelatin, as in the dye-transfer process.

imidazolepyruvic acid (im″id-az″ōl-pi-roo′vik) the α-keto acid corresponding to the α-amino acid histidine; it is the histidine metabolite excreted in the urine of individuals affected with histidinemia.

imide (im′īd) a cyclic amide formed from a dicarboxylic acid, e.g., phthalimide or succinimide.

imine (ĭ-mēn′) a chemical compound containing the imino group (=NH), e.g., ethanimine (CH_3-CH=NH). When the hydrogen on the nitrogen is replaced by a nonacyl group, the compound is a substituted imine.

imino- (ĭ-mēn′o) a prefix word element in organic chemistry to denote either the imino group (=NH) as a substituent, e.g., 2-iminoethanol (HN=$CHCH_2$-

OH), or the disubstituted nitrogen in amines when naming compounds of symmetrical structure, e.g., iminodiacetic acid, $HN(CH_2CO_2H)_2$.

imino acid any carboxylic acid that also contains the imino group.

iminoacidopathies (ĭ-me″no-as″ĭ-dop′ah-thēz) see *hydroxyprolinemia* and *hyperprolinemia.*

imipramine (ĭ-mip′rah-mēn) the generic name for a derivative of the tricyclic compound dibenzazepine, which is used as an antidepressant. See also *tricyclic antidepressant.* Trademark for imipramine hydrochloride, Tofranil.

imipramine and desipramine assays 1. colorimetric assays. Imipramine and desipramine can be detected by the green oxidation product that is formed by reaction with Forrest reagent, or by the blue product that is formed by reaction with cerium(IV) sulfate and which absorbs at 620 nm.

2. fluorometric assays. Imipramine and desipramine can be determined by fluorometry with excitation at 290 nm and emission at 415 nm.

3. chromatography. Imipramine and desipramine can be separated and quantitated using gas chromatography with a nitrogen, electron capture, or mass fragmentography detector, or by using high-pressure liquid chromatography (HPLC).

immature (im″ah-tūr′) unripe or not fully developed. Examples of immature cells are basal cells of squamous epithelium and reserve cells of columnar epithelium.

immature pattern in electroencephalography, a pattern of electrical activity recorded from a subject that is normally recorded from subjects who are younger or at a lesser stage of development.

immediate hypersensitivity the immediate response of a host to an antigen to which it has previously been exposed. The onset of the response is often within seconds and usually occurs within the first few hours of exposure. It is usually mediated by specific "reaginic" IgE antibody with binding of antigen to IgE on mast cells. The mast cells degranulate and release the mediators histamine, SRS-A (slow-reacting substance of anaphylaxis), and ECF-A (eosinophil chemotactic factor of anaphylaxis). Immediate hypersensitivity to a particular antigen or allergen is usually tested by determining whether there is evidence of an IgE-mediated response to (1) skin testing, (2) food challenge, (3) bronchial provocation, or (4) the RAST (radioallergosorbent test) procedure. (See also the accompanying illustration.)

For mast cell degranulation to occur, two IgE molecules must be bridged by the antigen or anti-IgE antibody. Bridging of two IgE molecules initiates the changes that lead to an influx of Ca^{2+}. Two methyltransferases are supposedly involved in the conversion of a phosphatidylethanolamine to phosphatidylcholine. This conversion is associated with the Ca^{2+} influx. Cyclic adenosine monophosphate (cAMP) and cyclic guanosine monophosphate (cGMP) are also involved in the regulation of degranulation. An increase in cAMP is associated with a decrease in degranulation. Theophylline and β-adrenergic agonists act to increase cAMP, thus inhibiting histamine release. Theophylline acts to inhibit cAMP metabolism by a phosphodiesterase, while β-agonists increase production of cAMP by adenylate cyclase.

Histamine and ECF-A are preformed in mast cell granules, whereas SRS-A is newly synthesized. Histamine vasodilates and increases capillary permeability, thereby causing angioedema and urticaria. It is rapidly metabolized in vivo by histaminase and histamine methyltransferase. ECF-A is a low-molecular-weight peptide that is a selective chemoattractant for eosinophils; it will attract neutrophils but only at higher concentrations. SRS-A is a low-molecular-weight sulfur-containing metabolite of arachidonic acid recently characterized as leukotriene C. It is formed by the lipoxygenase pathway of arachidonic acid metabolism and is inactivated by arylsulfatases. SRS-A is not preformed and accumulates on IgE activation. It has effects on vascular permeability and on bronchial smooth muscle, causing bronchospasm.

Of the tests used to determine whether there is evidence of an IgE-mediated response, skin testing correlates well with significant sensitization. Prick or scratch testing is usually used for initial testing in suspected cases of significant sensitization, followed by intradermal skin tests with higher dilutions of the allergen. Without significant skin test reactivity it is unlikely that there is significant sensitization. Food challenge to confirm the history is used in individuals with immediate hypersensitivity responses to ingested foods. Bronchial provocation involves inhalation challenges with increasing concentrations of antigens to see whether a particu-

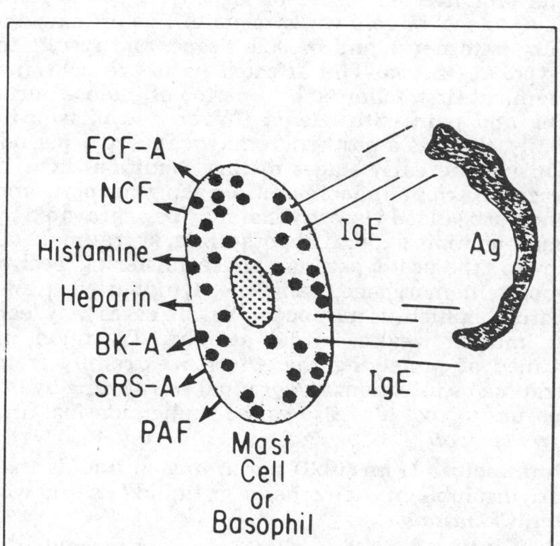

Immediate hypersensitivity. Interaction of antigen with two adjacent IgE molecules attached to Fc receptors on a basophil or mast cell, resulting in the release (or generation and release) of seven known primary mediators of IgE-mediated hypersensitivity reactions. Degranulation occurs concomitantly. ECF-A = eosinophilic chemotactic factor of anaphylaxis; NCF = neutrophil chemotactic factor; BK-A = basophil kallikrein of anaphylaxis; SRS-A = slow-reacting substance of anaphylaxis; and PAF = platelet activating factor. (From Bierman, C. W., and Pearlman, D. S.: Allergic Diseases of Infancy, Childhood, and Adolescence. Philadelphia, W. B. Saunders Co., 1980.)

lar antigen to which there is skin sensitivity also produces bronchospasm on challenge. The RAST procedure involves taking a disk or solid support, binding a particular antigen to it, and then taking test sera to see whether there is any IgE present that will bind to the support. A radioactive anti-IgE antibody is then added and will bind only to bound IgE. The counts bound will give a measure of the specific IgE present against the particular antigen bound to the disk. Correlation of the clinical history of an immediate hypersensitivity state with these tests is often imprecise, and considerable expertise by allergists is needed for their correct interpretation.

See also *anaphylaxis, atopy,* and *IgE.* Cf. *delayed hypersensitivity.*

GERALD B. KOLSKI, M.D., PH.D.

immersion (ĭ-mer′shun) [L. *immersio*] 1. the placing or plunging of a body into a fluid.

2. in microscopy, the placement of a liquid between the cover glass and the objective lens. An immersion objective requires a liquid with a particular refractive index; the higher the refractive index, the more light is transmitted and the better the resolution.

oil i., the use of an immersion medium having a high refractive index. Various organic oils and liquids are used.

water i., the use of water (refractive index, l.33) as the immersion medium.

immersion syndrome a disorder characterized by the prolonged exposure of an extremity (hand or foot) to cool or cold water or mud. The primary injury is to nerve and muscle tissue, and results in hypoxic trauma. The affected parts are cold and numb at first, followed by a period of intense burning and pain with edema (hyperemic phase); finally, there is a posthyperemic or recovery period. During the early stages of this condition there is vasoconstriction, decreased oxygen transport, and increased blood viscosity that may be aggravated by malnutrition, general hypothermia, or trauma. Following the posthyperemic phase, blistering, ecchymoses, hemorrhage, gangrene, lymphangitis, and thrombophlebitis may occur. Severe cases may lead to muscle weakness and atrophy. Treatment is aimed at protecting the affected extremity from trauma or infection, and gradual rewarming by exposure to cool air. Also called immersion foot and *trench foot.*

immiscible (ĭ-mis′ĭ-b′l) pertaining to liquids that are insoluble in each other, e.g., liquid fats and water. Cf. *miscible.*

immobile (ĭ-mo′bil) unable to move, or incapable of being moved.

immobility (im″mo-bil′ĭ-te) the state of being immovable.

immobilization (im-mo″bil-ĭ-za′shun) [L. *in* not + *mobilis* movable] the process of rendering immovable, as by a cast or splint. In radiology, immobilization refers to procedures taken to reduce voluntary or involuntary movement during the exposure of radiographs; for example, in abdominal radiography, compression is applied evenly over the abdomen using an air-filled bag and compression band to reduce movement of the viscera.

immobilized enzyme (im-mo′bil-īz′d) a preparation of an enzyme that is chemically covalently bonded to an insoluble particulate adsorbent material such as cellulose or agarose. In this form enzymes are used as recoverable reagents. Commercial preparations are available for use in batch processes and in continuous flow assay systems.

immotile (ĭ-mo′til, ĭ-mōt′l, ĭ-mo′tīl) the absence of the quality or state of being motile; a lack of contractility.

immotile cilia syndrome a hereditary defect in cilia motility thought to be due to the absence or deformity of microtubular dynein arms. This abnormality leads to persistent respiratory infections, especially in the sinuses and bronchi, and to infertility. It is sometimes associated with situs inversus, when it is known as Kartagener's syndrome.

immotility (im″mo-til′ĭ-te) the state of being immotile.

immun/o (im′u-no) [L. *immunitas* security, safety] a word element used in combining form to denote safety or protection, usually involving the body's immune response, e.g., immunogenic.

immune (ĭ-mūn′) [L. *immunis* free, exempt] the relative resistance of the host to reinfection by a given microorganism due to the production of humoral antibodies or the development of cellular immunity, or both. In a broader context, the term refers to the ability of a host to respond to a foreign antigen of any type.

immune adherence a function of the complement system, which is associated with the fixation of C3b to the cell surface for the purpose of enhancing phagocytosis. The immune adherence phenomenon applies to an in vitro assay for the determination of the presence of antigen by visualizing the agglutination of erythrocytes. Microorganisms can adhere to the surface of any cell that has a C3b receptor and then aggregate; C3b receptors have been found on human erythrocytes, B lymphocytes, neutrophils, monocytes, macrophages, and platelets.

immune complex the product of the interaction of antibody with antigen. Normally, immune complexes are formed during an immune response. They have a positive role in the clearance of foreign antigens and a negative role in immune complex diseases. Also called *antigen-antibody complexes.*

immune complex diseases a group of immunologic disorders, occurring in chronic and acute forms, that stem from the deposition of immune complexes in tissue and the resulting inflammatory response. According to the Gell and Coombs classification of immune mechanisms in tissue damage, immune complex diseases are type III (Arthus-type) reactions. The pathogenesis of immune complex diseases involves the formation of antigen-antibody complexes, followed by the fixation of complement to the complexes and the release of active complement components. This results in an accumulation of polymorphonuclear leukocytes and the release of lysosomal enzymes in an inflammatory site.

Most often, immune complex diseases are chronic, with continued tissue damage and deposition of fibrin. The immune complexes themselves are dynamic, and the ratio of antigen to antibody is constantly changing; when the ratio is in antigen excess, the immune complex disease is more severe. Examples of immune complex diseases include bacterial infections that cause acute poststreptococcal glomerulonephritis or subacute bacterial endocarditis, viral infections, parasitic infections, disseminated malignancy, autoimmune disorders, and drug reactions (serum sickness).

immune complex glomerulopathy see under *glomerulopathy.*

immune complex nephropathy see under *tubulointerstitial nephropathy.*

immune elimination the period of accelerated degradation of antigen (e.g., foreign gamma globulin) that is a consequence of its removal and destruction by antibodies. The term also refers to a technique for determining an antibody response that is performed by measuring the rate of removal of the labeled antigen from the circulation in an immunized animal. Also called *immune clearance.*

immune response the response of a host to a foreign antigen, which may be either primary or secondary. The primary response occurs with the initial exposure and production of circulating antibodies of the IgM class followed by IgG antibodies. If the antigen exposure has occurred at a mucosal surface, such as the gastrointestinal or respiratory tract, secretory IgA antibodies may be elicited. The secondary response occurs with a second or subsequent exposure to an antigen to which the host has previously been exposed.

With the primary response, sensitized lymphocytes specific for the antigen are produced. Both B and T cells with memory for the specific antigen can be elicited. The production of antibody or cell-mediated immunity is dependent on the type of antigen, dose, and mode of exposure. There is a lag in antibody production of 1 wk after initial exposure to an antigen. Delayed hypersensitivity responses take approximately 2 wk to detect.

The secondary response is associated with a more rapid onset of the immune response. Because of prior exposure to the antigen, there are sensitized lymphocytes (memory cells) that are primed to respond to that particular antigen and do so immediately. The primary response selects cells with a high affinity for the antigen; then, with a second exposure, these cells proliferate and some differentiate into the cells that produce antibody (plasma cells) or mediate cellular immunity.

Immunization is an example of how the primary and secondary responses are utilized. The host is immunized with an attenuated or inactive agent to produce committed memory cell lymphocytes. It is hoped that on exposure to the wild infectious agent or toxin these committed cells will produce a rapid secondary immune response and prevent severe infection. Occasionally, however, because of an inadequate primary response to the immunizing agent, there is not a sufficient population of committed cells, and infection occurs. With wild infections the infection is usually significant enough to produce a good primary response, whereas immunization with inactivated or attenuated agents may not.

See also *delayed hypersensitivity, immunity, immunization,* and *lymphocyte.*

GERALD B. KOLSKI, M.D., PH.D.

immune response genes those genes that control the immune response to specific antigens or to a group of similar antigens. The ability to generate an immune response is usually an autosomal dominant trait. Immune response genes may have either of two effects on the immune response: their presence can determine the ability to respond to a given antigen (whereas their absence can result in an inability to respond) or they can control the level of response to an antigen in a regulatory manner.

Immune response genes may be divided into two categories: histocompatibility-linked immune response genes, which are associated with the major histocompatibility complex, and immunoglobulin allotype–linked immune response genes, which determine the structure of the immunoglobulin receptor on B lymphocytes.

Also called *Ir genes.*

immune surveillance a theory suggesting that the immune system is constantly monitoring the body against neoplastic growths, destroying newly arising tumor cells as a result of their antigenic foreignness to the host. This theory postulates that malignant transformations are common and that it is the continuous action of the immune system that suppresses the transformations.

immune system the complex network of cells and circulating components responsible for the body's reactions to substances recognized as foreign. The cellular components include macrophages and lymphocytes; the circulating components include the products of the cells, i.e., antibodies and lymphokines. Genetics plays an important role in the immune system, as genes control the degree of an immune response to a particular substance and the expression of cell surface molecules that are important in cellular interactions. See also *cell-mediated immunity, immune response,* and *immunity.*

immunity (ĭ-mu'nĭ-te) [L. *immunitas*] the ability of a host to defend itself against foreign antigens. Immunity may be divided into local, humoral, and cellular immunity processes.

LOCAL IMMUNITY PROCESS. Local immunity can be mediated by nonspecific and specific factors in host defense. Nonspecific factors include the skin and mucous membranes. The skin acts as a barrier that prevents penetration of organisms into underlying tissues. The barrier is mechanical; its disruption (such as in lacerations and burns) leads to an increased risk of infection. In the mucous membrane of the respiratory, genitourinary, and gastrointestinal tracts, the mucus produced forms a barrier against infection; in the respiratory tract it combines with the ciliated epithelium to prevent penetration of organisms deeper into the respiratory tract.

In this type of response, specific regional immunologic factors are important. They include tissue macrophages (alveolar, peritoneal, Langerhans' cells, etc.) locally to prevent dissemination, regional lymph nodes, and (in the respiratory, genitourinary, and GI tracts) secretory antibodies (i.e., secretory IgA) and leukocytes from the circulating pool, which are also available through the local vasculature for local immunity.

HUMORAL IMMUNITY PROCESS. Humoral immunity involves the noncellular arm of immunity that is available to prevent dissemination of the foreign antigen. It is composed of antibodies and the complement system. The antibodies are specific against the antigen, but their production is dependent on host exposure to the antigen. The primary immune response to the antigen involves production of specific antibodies by B lymphocytes and plasma cells, which usually takes about 7 da. If the host has had previous exposure to the antigen, a more rapid secondary immune response occurs with rapid antibody production. Unlike the antibody system, the complement system is not specific. The interaction of the first component of complement with antigen-antibody complexes leads to the activation of the classical pathway, whereas the alternate pathway may be activated without antibody by some antigens. This is probably one of the primitive nonspecific factors for eliminating some organisms. Interaction of antibody and complement thus amplifies the immune response by producing chemotactic factor anaphylatoxin and eventually lysis of microorganisms.

CELLULAR IMMUNITY PROCESS. The cellular immune response can be divided into the nonspecific and specific responses. The nonspecific cellular response includes the polymorphonuclear leukocytes, eosinophils, and monocyte-macrophages that interact with antigen. These cells utilize receptors for the Fc portion of immunoglobin and C3b receptors as stimulants for phagocytosis. The cellular response involves antigen-specific T lymphocytes. As with antibody-mediated immunity, cell-mediated immunity involves a primary and secondary immune response. The primary immune response entails initial exposure to an antigen and sensitization of the appropriate cells. The secondary response involves the interaction of an antigen with the appropriately sensitized lymphocytes on subsequent exposure. Delayed hypersensitivity skin tests are measures of the ability of the host to mount a secondary response to antigens to which it has previously been exposed.

On antigen exposure, sensitized T lymphocytes produce lymphokines (e.g., migratory inhibiting factor, MIF) that activate and mobilize macrophages to the area. In addition, the T cell produces factors that stimulate other lymphocytes to proliferate, with some becoming cytotoxic. A soluble factor–transfer factor is produced and may also transfer specific immunity to other T lymphocytes. The T lymphocytes can also secrete interferon and toxins called lymphotoxins. The cell-mediated response thus involves T lymphocytes, macrophages, cytotoxic lymphocytes, and toxins working in conjunction to control the foreign antigen. Cell-mediated immunity is important in resistance against viruses, fungi, and intracellular bacterial infections; it is also of consequence in self-identification, transplant rejection, and neoplastic surveillance.

TYPES OF IMMUNITY. Certain individuals, species, or races may have an inherent ability to resist certain infections despite a lack of previous exposure to an agent. This natural immunity explains why some diseases affect different animal species but not humans, and vice versa.

Immunity to most other infectious agents is acquired by previous exposure, a process called active immunity, which involves the response to the active infectious agent or modified vaccine derived from the agent. Memory cells are thus generated for subsequent infections. Occasionally it is necessary to give an individual immune material to help fight infections, a procedure called passive immunity. The most common form of this involves immune serum for tetanus toxoid, hepatitis A and B, and herpes zoster virus.

See also *antigen, complement, delayed hypersensitivity, immune response, lymphocyte,* and *macrophage.*

GERALD B. KOLSKI, M.D., PH.D.

immunity substance see *repressor.*

immunization (im″u-ni-za′shun) the process by which specific foreign antigens are introduced into a host deliberately to produce a specific protective immune response. In most cases, the purpose of the immunization is to produce a primary antibody response that leads to sensitized lymphocytes that are present for a secondary immune response on reintroduction of the antigen. Immunization is important both clinically and experimentally.

In clinical situations, active immunization with viral or bacterial antigens is important in preventing severe infection or disease from the specific agent immunized against. With viruses, the immunization involves either killed or live attenuated viruses. Measles, mumps, and rubella are common childhood illnesses for which live, attenuated viral vaccines are available for immunization. Polio immunization also involves live attenuated virus, but it is given orally to produce secretory antibodies in the gastrointestinal tract for this enteric virus.

Bacterial immunization involves live attenuated bacteria, inactivated soluble products from the bacteria, or killed bacteria. The most common agents used for immunization are the inactivated toxins (called toxoids) of diphtheria and tetanus and killed *Bordetella pertussis.* There are a number of other agents used for immunization in endemic areas, including BCG, which is the live dried bacillus Calmette-Guérin strain of *Mycobacterium tuberculosis* var. *bovis.*

In experimental situations, immunization usually involves the injection of antigen for the purpose of eliciting a primary antibody response. The mode and timing of the immunization injections can affect the type of immune response. For example, antigen can be presented in a form that enhances a particular response. Adjuvants also enhance the immune response and are often added to the antigen preparations. Complete Freund's adjuvant (CFA) is a preparation of killed mycobacteria commonly used with mineral oil and emulsifier in antigen injections, although it is not given to humans because of granuloma formation. Other adjuvants include *Corynebacterium parvum* and *B. pertussis.* Alum, potassium aluminum sulfate, and aluminum hydroxide have also been used as adjuvants, especially in eliciting an IgE response from weanling animals.

Because IgM is the first antibody formed in a primary response, immunization with frequent injections of an antigen over an interval of 1–2 wk will elicit a high titer of IgM antibodies. This is the method by which antibody is made against sheep red blood cells for complement studies. The various methods of immunization are very numerous; they are based on factors that include: (1) the animal to be immunized; (2) the type of response desired (i.e., IgM, IgG, IgE, T-dependent); (3) the antigen to be used; and (4) the immune status of the animal. These factors determine the choice of adjuvant, the route of administration (i.e., subcutaneous, intravenous, oral), the timing of the injections, and the concentration of antigen to be used.

Passive immunization involves the introduction of an antibody into a host for the purpose of giving immediate protection. The antibody or antiserum given is usually against a microorganism or toxin to which the host has not been exposed. The most commonly used is tetanus toxoid antiserum. The protection of the individual is only for the time that sufficient antibody remains in the system—usually 4–6 wk. New methods of infusing large amounts of antibody intravenously have been developed for clinical purposes.

See also *vaccination.*

GERALD B. KOLSKI, M.D., PH.D.

immunoassay (im″u-no-as′sa) the measurement of antigen-antibody interaction, utilizing such procedures as immunofluorescent techniques, radioimmunoassay, and nonradioisotopic immunoassay.

nonradioisotopic i., the detection of a primary antigen-antibody reaction through light-scattering properties of immune complexes or through the use of marker molecules attached to constituents of the immune reaction.

LIGHT-SCATTERING IMMUNOASSAYS. The light-scattering assays involve the detection of antigen-antibody complex formation in an immune reaction by changes in turbidity or light scattering in a fluid medium.

Turbidimetric immunoassays measure light absorption by immune complexes consisting of antigen-antibody particles and are probably most useful when measuring dense concentrations of particles.

Nephelometric immunoassays measure light reflected at an angle from a light source illuminating immune complexes formed in an antigen-antibody reaction. The nephelometric assays are most useful when used to measure low concentrations of immune reactants. These assays are divided into two types, direct and indirect. Direct assays measure the reaction between antibody and a complete antigen. Indirect assays are based on the interaction of antibody, an incomplete antigen (hapten) coupled to a high-molecular-weight protein, together called a developer antigen, and hapten from a sample under assay (analyte). A popular application of the indirect nephelometric assay is the nephelometric inhibition assay (NIA), which uses small quantities of analyte to reduce significantly the reaction between antibody and developer antigen. The reduction of light scattering by antibody and developer antigen is proportional to the concentration of the hapten under assay; the sensitivity of this reaction is such that extremely small quantities of analyte may be quantitated in serum or other fluids.

Latex particles may also be used in light-scattering assays, coating antigen or antibody on latex, with amplification of light scattering by aggregations of latex particles bound into antigen-antibody complexes. The detection of particle aggregation may be accomplished by electron particle sizing or by visual means.

FLUORESCENCE IMMUNOASSAYS. Fluorescent compounds absorb light, emitting a second wavelength that may be detected visually or through use of specialized instrumentation. Fluorescence immunoassays are carried out by conjugating fluorescent compounds to antibodies and then detecting the presence of fluorescence in antigen-antibody reactions. Such compounds in common use include fluorescein and rhodamine.

Microscopically, antigen specifically bound to the labeled antibody can be detected by the presence of fluorescence when viewed against a dark background. Antigen in fixed tissue sections or cell suspensions may be detected by fluorescence immunomicroscopy.

Microscopes used for immunomicroscopy are simply modified standard light microscopes. Filter systems placed in the beam of the fluorescence light source select an optimal wavelength for excitation of fluorescent label bound to antigen. A barrier filter is then used to limit light viewed through the objective of the microscope to the fluorescent light emitted by the antigen-antibody complex. For direct immunofluorescence, fluorescent antibody is attached directly to the antigen under assay. Amplification of fluorescence emanating from antigen-antibody complexes may be achieved through indirect immunofluorescence assay.

The indirect immunofluorescence assay first applies an unlabeled antibody to an antigen. Subsequently, a second fluorescent antibody specific for the unlabled immunoglobulin is allowed to react with the antigen-antibody complex. Multiple labeled antibodies attach to a single unlabeled immunoglobulin molecule, thus amplifying fluorescence emission by an immune complex beyond that of the direct method. The indirect assay is convenient for the detection of the presence of serum antibody to a known antigen.

Several other microscopic methods have been designed for the detection of unknown antigens (or antibody) by fluorescence microscopy, including fluorescence inhibition assays, in which the presence of an unknown antibody specific for a substrate antigen is used to inhibit the attachment of a fluorescein-labeled antibody specific for the antigen.

Heterogeneous and homogeneous fluorescence immunoassays (see below) are generally dependent on sophisticated instrumentation such as laser optics and photomultipliers. These assays are quite useful for measurements of small haptenic antigens such as drugs at low concentration. Heterogeneous assays require a separation step to isolate bound antigen-antibody from free antigen, whereas homogeneous assays do not require a separation phase, and an indicator molecule is modulated upon antigen-antibody reaction. Modulation of the indicator provides a measure of the concentration of reactants. These assays are manipulated to provide optimal conditions for the detection of very small concentrations of analyte and may be sensitive from 10^{-10}–10^{-15} mol/l.

FLUORESCENCE IMMUNOASSAYS

Fluorescence microscopy
Heterogeneous enzyme immunoassay
- Solid-phase antigen assay
- Solid-phase antibody assay

Homogeneous enzyme immunoassay
- Antibody quenching
- Fluorescence polarization
- Internal reflection spectroscopy
- Fluorescence excitation transfer
- Fluorescence protection

In the heterogeneous tests, a solid phase is measured for separated fluorescent analyte following the antigen-antibody reaction. Heterogeneous fluorescence tests may be designed to be: (1) competitive, with labeled and unlabeled haptens competing for limited antibody bound to a solid matrix; (2) indirect, first with reaction of an antigen with a solid-phase antibody, and then, upon separation of bound antigen, with a second fluorescent antibody; or (3) fluoroimmunometric, with reaction of antigen and fluorescent antibody (measurement of analyte follows addition of an excess solid-phase antigen).

Different homogeneous assays allow detection of an antigen-antibody reaction based on any of several different principles. (1) Antibodies to certain fluorescent-labeled antigens quench emitted fluorescence. Measurement of quenching denotes a primary antigen-antibody reaction. (2) Increased polarization of a fluorescence-labeled hapten may take place on combination with an antibody; polarization of hapten-antibody complex is then proportional to the level of unknown antigen (or antibody) added to mixtures of fluorescent antigen and antibody constituents. (3) Internal reflection spectroscopy measures the fluorescence of a labeled antibody bound to antigen absorbed onto a quartz plate (part *A* in the accompanying illustration). Only fluorescent molecules at the quartz surface are measured, by photometry. Free antigen placed in solution adjacent to the quartz reduces fluorescence at the quartz surface, providing a measure of antigen concentration within the fluid phase. (4) Fluorescence excitation transfer employs two labels, a donor fluorescer attached to an antigen, and an acceptor, or quencher, attached to an antibody. The combination of antigen and antibody quenches the fluorescent emission of the antigen. The direct antigen-labeled method uses an unlabeled analyte to abate quenching, providing measure of the unknown analyte. In the indirect antigen-labeled method, separate portions of the specific antibody molecule are labeled with fluorescer and quencher. Donor and acceptor antibody molecules, reacting in close proximity over multivalent antigenic determinants, provide a basis for energy transfer between

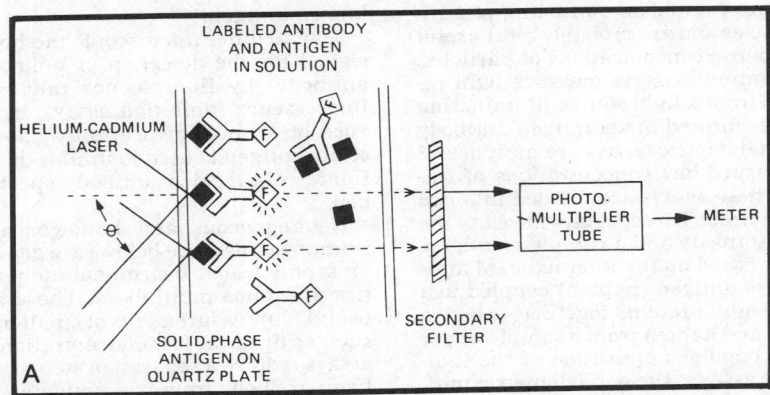

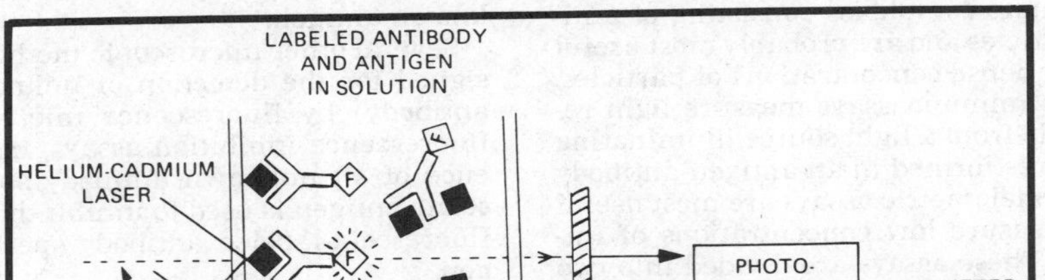

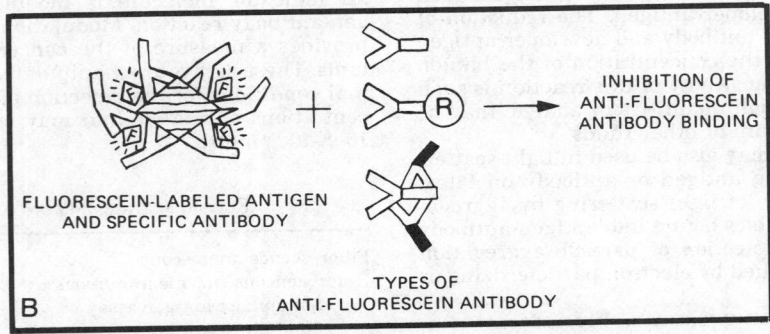

Nonradioisotopic immunoassay. *A*, Homogeneous fluorescence immunoassay by internal reflection spectroscopy. The fluorescence of the surface of the quartz plate is measured by internal reflection so that only the antigen-labeled antibody reaction on the surface is measured. Labeled antibody free in solution is not activated. *B*, Homogeneous fluorescence protection immunoassay. The antigen is labeled with fluorescein. When the labeled antigen is reacted with specific antibody to the antigen, the complex formed inhibits the binding of antifluorescein antibody. The antifluorescein antibody will quench the fluorescence of the labeled antigen when the antibody binds with fluorescein. Different types of antifluorescein antibody may be used. However, because of the mechanism of inhibition by steric hindrance, the antifluorescein antibody labeled with rhodamine or coupled with another antibody to form a larger molecule is more effective in the assay procedure. The method may be used to measure antigen or antibody. (From Nakamura, R. M., and Vito, W. R.: Nonradioisotopic immunoassay for therapeutic drug monitoring. Laboratory Medicine *11*:807–817, 1980.)

Nonradioisotopic Immunoassay. Enzymes in Immunoassays

Assay	Enzyme
Heterogeneous EIA	Horseradish peroxidase
	Alkaline phosphatase
	Glucose oxidase
	β-D-Galactosidase
Homogeneous EIA	Lysozyme
	Malate dehydrogenase
	Glucose-6-phosphate dehydrogenase

Courtesy of W. S. Nichols, M.D., and R. M. Nakamura, M.D.

donor and acceptor and quenching of antibody fluorescence. (5) Fluorescence protection immunoassay involves fluorescence-labeled antigen and separate antibodies to fluorescent label and antigen (part *B* in the accompanying illustration). Specific antibody to antigen, when forming antigen-antibody complexes, sterically prevents attachment of antibody to fluorescent label, thus protecting the reaction from inhibitory combination of label with its corresponding antibody and providing a means for measuring the analyte.

Enzyme Immunoassays (EIAs). EIAs are assays using catalyzing properties of enzymes for the detection of immunologic reactions. Enzyme-labeled antibodies or antigens are reacted with ligand, and introduction of enzyme substrate with detection of catabolic products denotes the presence of an antigen-antibody reaction. EIAs are divided into heterogeneous and homogeneous assays, the principles of which are similar to those of the fluorescent immunoassays.

Heterogeneous EIAs require a separation step involving solid-phase antibody or antigen, and usually a second enzyme-labeled antibody for identification of separated antigen-antibody complex. Homogeneous assays include enzyme-labeled hapten assays wherein active enzyme-hapten conjugates are modulated on binding of hapten-specific antibody to the complex. Free hapten added to the inactive complex competes for antibody-binding sites, releasing active enzyme with detection of catabolites equated to the presence of the analyte. (See also *ELISA* and *enzyme-assisted immunoassay technique.*)

Enzyme assays involving light microscopic observation of catabolites (color change) are popular and are similar to immunofluoresence microscopic assays. Several enzymes are currently available for the EIAs, as shown in the accompanying table.

Chemoluminescence Assays. Chemoluminescence depends on a process that releases light as a result of oxidative chemical reactions. Bioluminescence is chemoluminescence arising from living organisms. Homogeneous and heterogeneous chemoluminescent assays exist utilizing chemoluminescence as an indicator for antigen-antibody reactions. Following immune reaction of constituents bearing a chemoluminescent label, the analyte is detected by measuring light emitted from the chemoluminigenic label on addition of reaction substrates.

Aminophthalylhydrazides such as isoluminal are efficient light emitters when bound to proteins and other compounds serving as labeled ligands. After reaction, the amount of label in a free state is quantitated using H_2O_2 and metal activator for light production and qualification of the analyte.

W. S. Nichols, M.D.
R. M. Nakamura, M.D.

radioisotopic i., see *radioimmunoassay.*

immunobiology (im″u-no-bi-ol′o-je) the branch of immunology concerned with the biologic interactions of the immune system with infectious diseases, the growth and development of immune cells, and any involvement that the immune system has with other cells of the body.

immunoblast (im″u-no-blast′) a large lymphoid cell (15–25 μm in diameter) formed as a result of the transformation of a small lymphocyte. The process can be induced in vitro by various mitogens and in vivo by antigenic stimulation. Formerly called activated reticulum cell, atypical mononuclear histocyte, pyrinophilic cell, and reticular lymphoblast. See also *immunoblastic l.* under *lymphadenopathy* and *lymph node.*

immunoblastic sarcoma a variant of large cell lymphoma in which varying degrees of plasmacytoid transformation occur within the proliferating transformed lymphocytes. See also *sarcoma.*

immunochemistry (im″u-no-kem′is-tre) the branch of immunology concerned with the chemical substances and reactions of the immune system, the specific study of antigens and antibodies, and their interactions with one another.

immunocompetence (im″u-no-kom′pĕ-tens) the ability to mount a normal immune response.

immunocompromised (im″u-no-kom′pro-mīz′d) having an attenuated immune response, often caused by the administration of immunosuppressive drugs but also by irradiation, by malnutrition, and by some pathologic processes (e.g., neoplasia).

immunocyte (im″u-no-sīt′) any lymphoid cell that is able to specifically react with antigen and/or elaborate immunologic cell products. Also called *immunologically competent cell.*

immunocytoadherence (im″u-no-si″to-ad-hēr′ens) a method for detecting those cells that have immunoglobulin on their surfaces. Erythrocytes coated with specific antigens form rosettes with the cells containing immunoglobulin. To identify the cells with bound immunoglobulin, the rosettes can be separated from the rest of the cell population by centrifugation. Once separated, the cells can be stained and characterized.

immunodeficiency (im″u-no-de-fish′en-se) an impairment of the immune response that refers to one of the following mechanisms: (1) the first-order defenses of the body (skin, mucous membranes), (2) phagocytic activity, (3) inflammation, (4) the complement system, (5) the antibody defense system, or (6) cell-mediated immunity. It results in impaired resistance to infections and probably to tumors. When more than one mechanism is involved, for example, B-cell– and T-cell–mediated immunity, the disorder is known as a combined immunodeficiency.

immunodeficiency diseases a general term for those conditions resulting from the functional impairment of components of the immune system. This may include deficiency or malfunction of a cell

IMMUNODEFICIENCY DISEASES. CLASSIFICATION OF IMMUNODEFICIENCY DISORDERS

I. Antibody (B cell) immunodeficiency diseases
- X-linked hypogammaglobulinemia (congenital hypogammaglobulinemia)
- Transient hypogammaglobulinemia of infancy
- Common, variable, unclassifiable immunodeficiency (acquired hypogammaglobulinemia)
- Immunodeficiency with hyper-IgM
- Selective IgA deficiency
- Selective IgM deficiency
- Selective deficiency of IgG subclasses

II. Cellular (T cell) immunodeficiency diseases
- Congenital thymic aplasia (DiGeorge syndrome)
- Chronic mucocutaneous candidiasis (with or without endocrinopathy)

III. Combined antibody-mediated (B cell) and cell-mediated (T cell) immunodeficiency diseases
- Severe combined immunodeficiency diseases (autosomal recessive, X-linked, sporadic)
- Cellular immunodeficiency with abnormal immunoglobulin synthesis (Nezelof's syndrome)
- Immunodeficiency with ataxia-telangiectasia
- Immunodeficiency with eczema and thrombocytopenia (Wiskott-Aldrich syndrome)
- Immunodeficiency with thymoma
- Immunodeficiency with short-limbed dwarfism
- Immunodeficiency with enzyme deficiency
- Episodic lymphopenia with lymphotoxin
- GVH disease

IV. Phagocytic dysfunction
- Chronic granulomatous disease
- Glucose-6-phosphate dehydrogenase deficiency
- Myeloperoxidase deficiency
- Chédiak-Higashi syndrome
- Job's syndrome
- Tuftsin deficiency
- "Lazy leukocyte syndrome"
- Elevated IgE, defective chemotaxis, eczema, and recurrent infections

V. Complement abnormalities and immunodeficiency diseases
- C1q, C1r, and C1s deficiency
- C2 deficiency
- C3 deficiency (type I, type II)
- C4 deficiency
- C5 dysfunction, C5 deficiency
- C6 deficiency
- C7 deficiency
- C8 deficiency

From Fudenberg, H. H., et al.: Basic & Clinical Immunology. 3rd ed. Los Altos, CA, Lange Medical Publications, 1981, p. 410.

population (e.g., phagocytic cells, subpopulations of lymphocytes), lack of an antibody response, or complement abnormality. For more information, see the accompanying table, the specific immunodeficiency disease, and *immunity.*

immunodepression (im″u-no-de-presh′un) see *immunosuppression.*

immunodiffusion (im″u-no-dĭ-fu′zhun) the diffusion of antigen and antibody in a gel medium until both combine and form a precipitate. Various techniques of immunodiffusion include the double diffusion test (Oudin test) and the single diffusion test (Ouchterlony test).

immunodominance (im″u-no-dom′ĭ-nans) that property of an antigenic determinant, or part of an antigenic determinant, that causes it to be responsible for the major portion of binding energy between antigen and antibody. An immunodominant antigen is the antigen responsible for the strongest immune response when given to a host in combination with other antigens or antigenic determinants.

immunoelectrophoresis (ĭ-mu″no-e-lek″tro-fo-re′sis) a type of electrophoresis that combines zone electrophoresis with antigen-antibody reactions in gel. Immunoelectrophoresis is a two-step process whereby serum proteins are electrophoretically separated, after which specific antisera are added and allowed to diffuse through the agar. Precipitin bands form where antigen-antibody concentrations are in equivalence (see *precipitin curve*). Because the electrophoresis agar is mostly buffer, serum is quickly separated into albumin, α_1-, α_2-, β-, and γ-globulins. (See the accompanying illustration.)

After electrophoresis of the serum, a new area of agar with a linear trough is added to the electrophoresis plate. The trough runs along the direction of electrophoretic separation. Antibodies diffuse linearly from the trough, and antigens diffuse radially from their electrophoretic placement. These two types of diffusion combine to form precipitates in the shape of ellipsoid arcs.

Immunoelectrophoresis can detect characteristic abnormalities of paraproteins in serum as well as in urine or other body fluids. This procedure can determine the exact heavy-chain class or light-chain type of paraprotein. Immunoelectrophoresis can also distinguish polyclonal from monoclonal gammaglobulinemias. Immunodeficiencies and myelomas may be diagnosed with this procedure.

counter i., see *counterimmunoelectrophoresis.*

radio-i., a combination of radioautography and immunoelectrophoresis that allows the detection of radiolabeled antigens. Proteins or immunoglobulins should be prelabeled with ^3H or ^{14}C amino acids during biosynthesis. Immunoelectrophoresis is performed, and the plate is overlaid with high-speed x-ray film. With this method, radiolabeled antigens can be compared with nonradiolabeled antigens by staining the precipitation lines. This procedure is used for research investigation of paraproteinemias.

reverse i., see *counterimmunoelectrophoresis.*

rocket i., a type of immunoelectrophoresis that quantitates antigens other than immunoglobulins. Antiserum is fixed onto agar so that it will not migrate; then, different samples of antigen are placed into wells. The antigens are electrophoresed into the antiserum, and precipitin bands form at the zones of equivalence (see *precipitin curve*). This precipitation occurs along lateral margins as the antigen advances. The antigen concentration decreases as precipitate forms and eventually diminishes to a point. The resultant pattern resembles a rocket. (See also the accompanying illustration.)

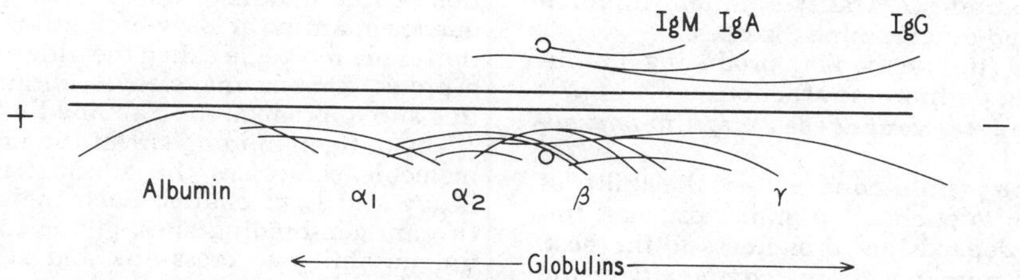

Immunoelectrophoresis. Diagrammatic representation of an immunoelectrophoretic pattern. Purified preparations of human IgM, IgA, and IgG are placed in the upper well; whole human serum in the lower well. Each protein on electrophoresis moves from the well according to its characteristic mobility under the conditions employed. After electrophoresis, antibody prepared against human serum is placed in the trough and the pattern of precipitation between each protein and its specific antibody develops. (From Freeman, B. A.: Burrows' Textbook of Microbiology. 21st ed. Philadelphia, W. B. Saunders Co., 1979.)

The total distance the antigen has migrated or the total area under the resultant curve is linearly proportional to the quantity of antigen. This system can detect proteins at concentrations higher than 0.5 μg/ml.

Also called *Laurell technique* and one-dimensional single electroimmunodiffusion.

two-dimensional i., a variation of immunoelectrophoretic technique used for quantitation purposes. The normal technique of electrophoresis is completed, and the resultant separated components are electrophoresed a second time at a 90° angle to the first run. Precipitant arcs containing antigen-antibody complexes then form.

immunofixation electrophoresis (im″u-no-fik-sa′shun) a technique in which the antigen in an antigen-antibody system is immobilized following electrophoresis. This technique, which gives higher resolution than chemical precipitation, permits identification of a specific macromolecule.

A sample of antigen is electrophoresed on a thin agarose gel, as in standard protein electrophoresis.

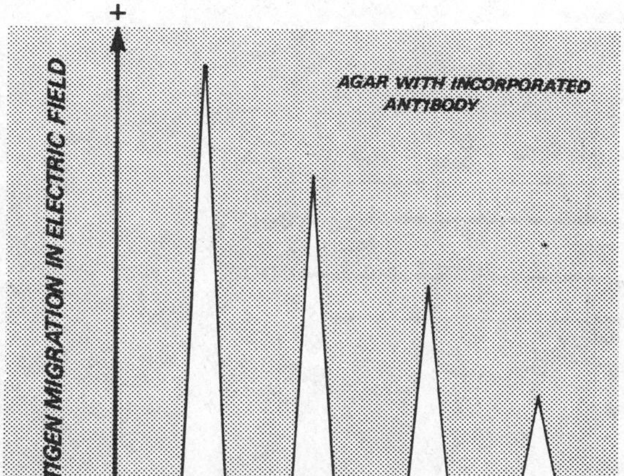

Rocket immunoelectrophoresis. (From Fudenberg, H. H., et al.: Basic & Clinical Immunology. 3rd ed. Los Altos, CA, Lange Medical Publications, 1980.)

Following separation, cellulose acetate saturated with antibody is laid over the gel to allow formation of an antigen-antibody complex that fixes the antigen. The gel may then be washed and stained for identification.

immunofluorescence techniques (im″u-no-floo″-o-res′ens) an immunologic technique that employs the use of antibodies conjugated to fluorochromes—chemicals that fluoresce when excited by short-wave light such as ultraviolet light. The fluorochromes commonly used are fluorescein and rhodamine.

For immunofluorescence, an antiserum to the antigen to be detected is produced in a heterologous species. The direct method (direct immunofluorescence) utilizes a fluorochrome conjugated to an antibody, which is added directly to a tissue or cell suspension for the detection of a specific antigen.

The indirect method (indirect immunofluorescence) permits detection of an antigen with a non-fluorochrome-conjugated antibody, a technique commonly used in the clinical laboratory. The method is an adaptation of the antiglobulin reaction (Coombs' test) or double antibody technique. The unconjugated antibody is incubated with a tissue section or cell suspension and then overlaid with a fluorochrome-conjugated antiimmune globulin that reacts with the antibody in the initial immune complex, forming what is referred to as a sandwich. The indirect method eliminates the need to purify and conjugate antibodies to an individual antigen, and because more than one antiimmune globulin molecule can react with each molecule of the unconjugated antibody, the fluorescence produced is greater than can be achieved with the direct method. Indirect immunofluorescence is commonly used to detect serum antibodies and immune complexes in tissues and to identify microorganisms in specimens from patients with infectious diseases.

Also called *fluorescent antibody technique.* See also *fluorescence microscopy, fluorochrome,* and *nonradioisotopic i.* under *immunoassay.*

immunogen (im′u-no-jen) any substance capable of generating an immune reaction, in contrast to any substance that binds to an antibody (i.e., an antigen). Cf. *antigen.*

immunogenetics (im″u-no-jĕ-net′iks) the study of the genetics of antigens, antibodies, and their interactions, encompassing blood groups and blood group incompatibilities, transplantation, immune deficiencies, and autoimmune diseases.

immunogenic (im″u-no-jen′ik) producing immunity; generating an immune reaction.

immunogenic determinant see *antigenic determinant.*

immunogenicity (im″u-no-jĕ-nis′ĭ-te) the ability of an immunogen to elicit an immune response. Immunogenicity depends on foreignness to the host, the size of the immunogen, the complexity of the immunogen molecular structure, the length of time it remains in the host, and its ability to reach certain immunocompetent cells in order to generate immunity. See also *antigen.*

immunoglobulin (Ig) (im″u-no-glob′u-lin) an extremely heterogeneous group of glycoproteins found in serum, with the unique ability to combine specifically with a wide spectrum of unrelated molecules, commonly called antigens, that may be proteins, carbohydrates, lipids, nucleic acids, or other chemicals. Immunoglobulins may be native or foreign to the host. Normally, immunoglobulins function as part of an animal's defense mechanism against invading pathogens, but under certain circumstances they may be induced to antigens derived from the host.

All immunoglobulins have a common structure consisting of four polypeptide chains. Two of the chains are called heavy or H chains (M.W. 50,000–70,000), whereas the other two are called light or L chains (M.W. 25,000). These are joined by disulfide bonds to form a four-chain basic structure, as shown in the accompanying illustration. The amino terminal of each chain is responsible for binding to antigens and structurally shows a high degree of variability, hence its name, the variable region. The remainder of the chain is similar from molecule to molecule and is called the constant portion. At the middle of the H chain is a distinct sequence of amino acids, which forms a flexible portion of the molecule called the hinge region. Papain, a proteolytic enzyme, cleaves immunoglobulins at this site to produce the Fab and Fc fragments.

The antigen-binding site of the immunoglobulin molecule comprises the amino terminals of the heavy and light chains. Each molecule possesses two antigen-binding sites, giving the molecule its unique ability to cross-link and agglutinate antigens.

The light chains, which are common to all immunoglobulins, are either of the kappa or lambda type. Approximately 65 percent of immunoglobulins have kappa and 35 percent have lambda light chains. There are five major groups of heavy chains, which determine the class (isotype) and the biologic function of the molecule:

Immunoglobulin G (IgG) (M.W. 150,000) is present in the highest concentration and has a sedimentation coefficient (S value) of 7. It has the longest half-life in the serum of any of the immunoglobulins, fixes complement, and can cross the placenta. Its physiologic functions include neutralizing toxins and viruses, agglutinating antigens, opsonizing antigens to facilitate phagocytosis, and lysing bacteria with the aid of complement. IgG is capable of forming circulating immune complexes that can cause injury to the host (e.g., Arthus reaction, serum sickness, glomerulonephritis, and some types of vasculitis).

Immunoglobulin A (IgA) (M.W. 350,000) is found in serum and in secretions such as tears, milk, and those of the intestinal lumen. It is frequently found as a dimer, with both subunits joined by a J chain. When present in secretions, the enzymatically vulnerable regions are protected by a polypeptide called the secretory component. IgA mediates agglutination and the neutralization of toxins and

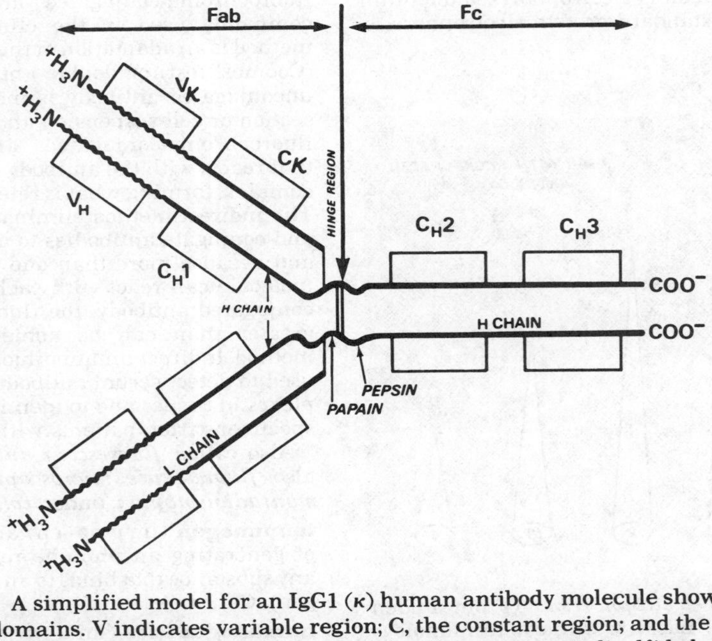

Immunoglobulin. A simplified model for an IgG1 (κ) human antibody molecule showing the four-chain basic structure and domains. V indicates variable region; C, the constant region; and the vertical arrow, the hinge region. Thick lines represent H and L chains; and thin lines represent disulfide bonds. (From Fudenberg, H. H., et al.: Basic & Clinical Immunology. 3rd ed. Los Altos, CA, Lange Medical Publications, 1980.)

IMMUNOGLOBULIN, TABLE 1. PROPERTIES OF HUMAN IMMUNOGLOBULIN CHAINS

DESIGNATION	H CHAINS					L CHAINS		SECRETORY COMPONENT	J CHAIN
	γ	α	μ	δ	υ	κ	λ	SC	J
Classes in which chains occur	IgG	IgA	IgM	IgD	IgE	All classes	All classes	IgA	IgA, IgM
Subclasses or subtypes	1,2,3,4	1,2	1,2	. . .	. . .	. . .	1,2,3,4	. . .	. . .
Allotypic variants	Gm(1)-(25)	A2m(1), (2)	. . .	. . .	. . .	Km(1)-(3)†	. . .	. . .	. . .
Molecular weight (approximate)	50,000*	55,000	70,000	62,000	70,000	23,000	23,000	70,000	15,000
V region subgroups	V_HI - V_HIV					$V_\kappa I$-$V_\kappa IV$	$V_\lambda I$-$V_\lambda VI$		
Carbohydrate (average percentage)	4	10	15	18	18	O	O	16	8
Number of oligosaccharides	1	2 or 3	5	?	5	O	O	?	1

*60,000 for γ3.
†Formerly Inv(1)-(3).
From Fudenberg, H. H., et al. Basic & Clinical Immunology. 3rd ed. Los Altos, CA, Lange Medical Publications, 1980, p. 31.

may fix complement through the alternate pathway.

Immunoglobulin M (IgM) (M.W. 900,000) consists of five polymerized subunits joined by a J chain. IgM fixes complement, is an efficient agglutinator, serves as an antigen receptor on B lymphocytes, and has a sedimentation coefficient of 19S. It is the oldest Ig from an evolutionary standpoint.

Immunoglobulin D (IgD) is found on the surface of B lymphocytes; along with IgM, it serves mainly as an antigen receptor.

Immunoglobulin E (IgE) is unique in that it is usually present in the lowest concentration; it has reaginic activity (i.e., it binds to mast cells and basophils, and mediates antigen-triggered release of vasoactive amines responsible for allergic reactions such as anaphylaxis).

Many of the classes of immunoglobulins are subdivided into subclasses with minor structural and functional differences.

In several diseases, immunoglobulins may be either absent or present in low levels. Levels of all classes are low in the congenital immunodeficiencies, such as X-linked hypogammaglobulinemia and severe combined immunodeficiency, and are variably depressed in ataxia-telangiectasia. Selective deficiencies of just one class of Ig may also occur, selective IgA deficiency being the most common. Acquired Ig deficiencies may also arise in a number of diseases, including lymphoreticular malignancies, thymoma, and protein-losing diseases. Immunoglobulin deficiencies are best evaluated by quantitative immunoglobulin measurement, usually done by radial immunodiffusion, which measures IgG, IgM, IgA, and IgD; quantitation of IgE requires the more sensitive technique of radioimmunoassay. Serum protein electrophoresis detects only severe hypogammaglobulinemia, not the selective immunodeficiencies. Immunoelectrophoresis provides rapid, semiquanititative estimates of IgG, IgM, and IgA, but is not sensitive below 30 mg/dl.

The abnormal overproduction of a single Ig is seen in diseases such as multiple myeloma, Waldenström's macroglobulinemia, and benign monoclonal gammopathy. Multiple myeloma may produce a monoclonal antibody of any Ig class, whereas Waldenström's macroglobulinemia produces a monoclonal IgM. These entities are detected by serum protein electrophoresis, which shows a characteristic spike representing the abnormal protein. Immunoelectrophoresis is useful for evaluating which class is in excess and the monoclonality of the abnormal protein.

Also called *antibody* and *gamma globulin.* See also *autoantibody* and Tables 1–3.

BRUCE RICHARDSON, M.D., PH.D

immunoglobulin-binding factor (IBF) a factor that inhibits primary and secondary immune responses in vitro. It is probably a soluble Fc receptor of suppressor T lymphocytes.

immunoglobulin class a subdivision of immunoglobulins based on differences in the Fc portion of the heavy chains. In humans there are five antigenically distinct classes of immunoglobulins: IgA, IgD, IgE, IgG, and IgM. See also *immunoglobulin.*

immunoglobulin subclass a subdivision of immunoglobulin classes based on structural and antigenic differences in the heavy chains. Immunoglobulin subclasses differ in the number of interchain disulfide bonds and in their biologic properties. For example, human IgG may be divided into four subclasses, IgA into two.

immunohematology (ĭ-mu″no-hem″ah-tol′o-je) the branch of hematology that studies antigen-antibody reactions and analogous phenomena as they relate to the pathogenesis and clinical manifestations of blood disorders. The term is generally used synonymously with blood banking in clinical usage.

immunohistochemical (im″u-no-his″to-kem′ĭ-kal) pertaining to the application of antigen-antibody interactions to histochemical techniques.

See also *immunohistochemical techniques.*

IMMUNOGLOBULIN, TABLE 2. BIOLOGIC ACTIVITIES OF THE FIVE CLASSES OF HUMAN ANTIBODIES AS SEEN FROM THE VIEWPOINT OF THE ANTIBODY PRODUCED

CLASS OF ANTIBODY	BENEFICIAL ACTIVITIES	INJURIOUS ACTIVITIES
IgG	Toxin neutralizing Agglutinating Opsonizing Bacteriolytic (with aid of complement system)	Antigen-IgG antibody complexes are capable of mediating tissue injury; e.g., Arthus reaction, serum sickness
IgM	Toxin neutralizing Agglutinating Bacteriolytic (with aid of complement system) Antigen receptor on B lymphocytes	Same as above
IgA	Toxin neutralizing Agglutinating ? Opsonizing	?
IgD	Antigen receptor on B lymphocytes	?
IgE	Mediate changes in vascular permeability	Local and systemic immediate hypersensitivity or anaphylactic reactions

From Benacerraf, B., and Unange, E.: Textbook of Immunology. Baltimore, Williams & Wilkins Co., 1979, p. 50.

immunohistochemical techniques assays for determining the location of antigen in tissue, using specific antibody that has been labeled with a compound that allows visualization. The antibody is incubated with slices of tissue on a slide to produce complexes with a specific antigen. From observation of the location of the bound antibody, the location of the corresponding antigen in the tissue can then be determined. The various immunohistochemical techniques include immunofluorescence, enzyme-linked antibody test with horseradish peroxidase, enzyme-linked immunosorbent assay (ELISA), immunoperoxidase technique, ferritin-coupled antibody methods, and autoradiography. For more information see the specific immunohistochemical technique and *nonradioisotpic i.* under *immunoassay.*

immunologic (im″u-no-loj′ik) pertaining to immunology.

immunologically competent cell see *immunocyte.*

immunologic enhancement the phenomenon of improved survival of tumor cells after immunization against the tumor cell antigens, a process that has been observed in laboratory animals. The protection may occur by a feedback inhibition of antibody response due to antibody already present in the circulation, by the action of suppressor T cells, or by the coating of tumor cells by "blocking factor" antibodies, which prevents sensitized lymphocytes from killing the cells.

immunologic unresponsiveness the lack of ability to mount an immune response to an antigen.

IMMUNOGLOBULIN, TABLE 3. CHARACTERISTICS OF HUMAN IMMUNOGLOBULINS

CHARACTERISTIC	IMMUNOGLOBULIN				
	IgG	IgA	IgM	IgD	IgE
Molecular weight	150,000	150,000-350,000	900,000	180,000	190,000
Sedimentation coefficient ($S_{20,w}$)	7	7 (9-15)	19	7	8
Carbohydrate (approx. %)	3	7	12	12	12
Biologic survival (plasma T—1/2 da)	21	6	5	3	2
Placental transfer	+	–	–	–	–
Activation of classical complement system	+	–	+	–	–
Serum concentration (mg/100 ml)	1,100	250	100	3	.01

From Benacerraf, B., and Unange, E.: Textbook of Immunology. Baltimore, Williams & Wilkins Co., 1979, p. 50.

This may occur naturally (tolerance to self-antigens), be artificially induced (induced tolerance), or be the result of a pathologic process (immunosuppressive diseases. See also *immunosuppression* and *tolerance.*

immunologist (im″u-nol′o-jist) a person who makes a special study of immunology.

immunology (im″u-nol′o-je) the study of the factors involved in the response of a host to a specific challenge with a foreign antigen. This medical specialty involves an assessment of factors nonspecific in the host defense, as well as those factors specific to the antigen with which the host is challenged. The study of the immune response takes into account the noncellular or humoral elements and the cellular elements of immunity. Immunology involves the study of both normal and abnormal immune function. The latter includes immunodeficiency states, autoimmune diseases, and hypersensitivity disorders, particulary allergy.

immunoparalysis (im″u-no-pah-ral′ĭ-sis) the induction of immunosuppression by a given antigen. The properties of an antigen that confer immunoparalytic activity include molecular size and configuration, route and timing of antigen injection, and fragmentation of the antigen. Two closely related antigens can cause antigenic competition, resulting in immunoparalysis. See also *tolerance.*

immunopathogenesis (im″u-no-path″o-jen′ĕ-sis) the development of disease due to immunologic disorders; pathology arising from or altered or affected by a cellular or humoral immune response or the products of an immune reaction. Examples include the interstitial deposition of immune complexes in tubulointerstitial nephropathy and their deposition in glomeruli in systemic lupus erythematosus.

immunopathology (im″u-no-pah-thol′o-je) 1. an area of biomedical science concerned with the study of immune reactions associated with disease, which may or may not result in a harmful clinical disorder.

2. the structural and functional manifestations associated with immune responses to disease.

immunoperoxidase technique (im″u-no-pĕ-rok′-sĭ-dās) a method of histologic staining that combines excellent morphologic detail with specific immunologic identification of tissue or cellular antigens. It is, in essence, a labeled antibody method, strictly analogous to immunofluorescence techniques. The end result is a colored reaction product produced by the enzymatic action of a horseradish peroxidase label that is employed in lieu of a fluorescent compound. The immunoperoxidase technique has, however, certain advantages over immunofluorescence methods, making it particularly suitable for use in diagnostic surgical pathology: it is applicable to fixed paraffin sections, retrospective studies are possible on tissue stored as paraffin blocks, the stained product is visible by ordinary light microscopy, and the morphologic detail is excellent.

APPLICATIONS. The immunoperoxidase method is of value to the surgical pathologist in the identification of a variety of normal and abnormal cells and tissues that are not readily distinguishable by morphology alone. For example, it is possible to identify a poorly differentiated metastatic tumor as being of prostatic origin on the basis of a positive immunoperoxidase stain, using antibody to the prostate-specific isoenzyme of acid phosphatase or an antibody to prostate-specific epithelial antigen; both these antisera stain prostatic epithelium but not other epithelial cells.

Another use of the immunoperoxidase method is in the assessment of the functional activity of endocrine cells. For example, until recently the standard method of assessing the hormone production of normal pituitary glands or of pituitary adenomas involved a series of histochemical stains (periodic acid–Schiff, orange G, tetrachrome, etc.), giving staining patterns that were believed to correlate with production of the various pituitary hormones. Immunoperoxidase staining has revealed that such correlations are tenuous, and today the only way to assess pituitary function in a tissue section is to perform an immunohistologic stain. Similarly, to assess thyroid function in tissue sections or the extent of function of parafollicular C cells in the thyroid, it is necessary to perform immunohistologic stains using antisera to thyroglobulin and calcitonin, respectively. Other applications include the demonstration of an abnormal distribution or number of cells in a lesion, demonstration of a loss of normal tissue antigens in a neoplasm, detection of oncofetal antigens in a neoplasm, identification of microorganisms, and detection of antibodies. Many of the antigens demonstrable in tissue sections by immunoperoxidase techniques are listed in Table 1. Numerous other antigens have been demonstrated for the purposes of research and investigation but as yet have little significance for the surgical pathologist.

TECHNIQUE. The immunoperoxidase technique utilizes the specificity of an antibody in the detection of the corresponding antigen within a tissue section or other cell preparation. The first stage, therefore, involves the addition of a specific antibody that binds to the antigen; however, because antibody molecules cannot be directly visualized, they must be labeled in some way to render their localization directly visible with the microscope. The different ways of attaching the label (horseradish peroxidase plus chromogen) compose the different variations of the immunoperoxidase method (as shown in the accompanying illustration). The final step is to reveal the sites of localization of the peroxidase-labeled antibody by the addition of a chromogenic substrate system (Table 2) to produce a colored reaction product visible by light microscopy.

CHOICE OF METHOD. Of the methods illustrated in the figure, the peroxidase-antiperoxidase (PAP) method and a modified biotin-avidin (avidin-biotin–conjugate) method are the most sensitive. The PAP method is most widely employed in studies using rabbit or goat antisera (requiring the use of rabbit or goat PAP, respectively). In utilizing monoclonal hybridoma–derived primary antibodies (mouse immunoglobulin), either a mouse PAP system or the avidin-biotin–conjugate system is preferred. In some circumstances, however, the direct or indirect conjugate methods prove entirely satisfactory if sufficient amounts of high-quality antibody are available for the preparation of conjugates.

TISSUES EMPLOYED. The immunoperoxidase method can be used to demonstrate antigens in cell smears or imprints, frozen sections, fixed paraffin sections, and electron microscopic material. It can also be employed for demonstrating cell surface antigens on living cells in suspension. This method is

Immunoperoxidase Technique, Table 1. Immunohistologic Staining Patterns in Surgical Pathology

Identification and Research Pertaining To:	Antisera Versus:
Plasma cells, plasma cell precursors, and B lymphocytes; myeloma, B-cell lymphomas	Light chain (κ, λ) Heavy chain (γ, α, μ, δ) J chain
Granulocytes, granulocytic proliferations	Lysozyme (muramidase) Lactoferrin
Histiocytes, histiocytic proliferations	Lysozyme (muramidase) α-1-Antitrypsin
Erythroid precursors, erythroblastic proliferations	Hemoglobins A, F
Iron containing cells, iron balance	Transferrin, ferritin
Embryonic colon and other endodermal derivatives; colonic neoplasms	Carcinoembryonic antigen Secretory piece
Epithelial proliferation and neoplasia of lacrimal and salivary glands	Lysozyme (muramidase) Lactoferrin Salivary duct epithelium
Paneth cells	Lysozyme (muramidase)
Central nervous system, glial cells	Glial fibrillary acidic protein
Placental trophoblast, trophoblastic elements in germ cell tumors	Human chorionic gonadotropin Pregnancy specific beta-1 glycoprotein Placental lactogen
Liver cells, particularly fetal liver, regenerating liver, and hepatocellular neoplasms	α-Fetoprotein α-1-Antitrypsin
Liver biopsy specimens in cirrhosis and suspected α-1-antitrypsin deficiency	α-1-Antitrypsin
Ovarian and testicular endocrine elements, germ cell tumors, endodermal sinus tumors, gonadal stromal cell tumors	Human chorionic gonadotropin α-Fetoprotein Hemoglobin G Testosterone Estradiol
Parathyroid cells; parathyroid hyperplasia and neoplasia	Parathormone
Thyroid parafollicular C cells; medullary cell carcinoma of thyroid	Calcitonin
Thyroid epithelial cells; thyroid adenoma and thyroid carcinoma	Thyroglobulin
Pancreatic islet tissue; islet cell function, islet cell adenoma and carcinoma; pancreatitis	Insulin Glucagon Somatostatin Gastrin
Gastrointestinal tract "hormone" secreting cells	Gastrin Vasoactive intestinal polypeptide
Anterior pituitary function, hyperplasia, and adenoma	ACTH Growth hormone Thyroid-stimulating hormone Follicle-stimulating hormone Luteinizing hormone

IMMUNOPEROXIDASE TECHNIQUE, TABLE 1. (*Continued*)

Identification and Research Pertaining To:	Antisera Versus:
"Ectopic" hormone production	ACTH Calcitonin Human chorionic gonadotropin
Prostatic epithelium; prostatic hyperplasia and carcinoma	Prostatic epithelial antigen Prostatic acid phosphatase
Breast epithelium; breast neoplasms	Human chorionic gonadotropin Pregnancy specific beta-1 glycoprotein Estradiol-estrogen receptor Mammary epithelial membrane antigen (MEMA 70) Transferrin Carcinoembryonic antigen Insulin
Mesenchymal cells and corresponding neoplasms	Factor VIII antigen Myoglobin
Inflammatory tissue, fibrin, blood clot; hyaline membrane disease; basement membranes	Fibrin Fibronectin
Hepatitis B surface antigen, hepatitis and cirrhosis	Hepatitis B surface antigen
Herpes virus infected cells	Herpes virus antigen
Other viruses	Foot and mouth disease virus Rabies virus Sendai virus Pneumonia virus of mice Buffalo pox virus Measles

Adapted from Taylor, C. R., and Kledzik, G.: Immunohistologic techniques in surgical pathology—a spectrum of "new" special stains. Human Pathology *12*:594-595, 1981.

IMMUNOPEROXIDASE TECHNIQUE, TABLE 2. HORSERADISH PEROXIDASE–SUBSTRATE CHROMOGEN SYSTEMS

Chromogen	Color	Comment
Diaminobenzidine tetrahydrochloride	Brown	Alcohol-fast; possible carcinogen
3-Amino-9-ethyl carbazole	Red	Alcohol-soluble
4-Chloro-1-naphthol	Blue-black	Alcohol-soluble
Hanker-Yates reagent	Brown	Alcohol-fast
Alpha-naphthol pyronin	Red	Alcohol-soluble

Note: H_2O_2 is the substrate and is prepared in solution with the chromogen.
Courtesy of Clive R. Taylor, M.D.

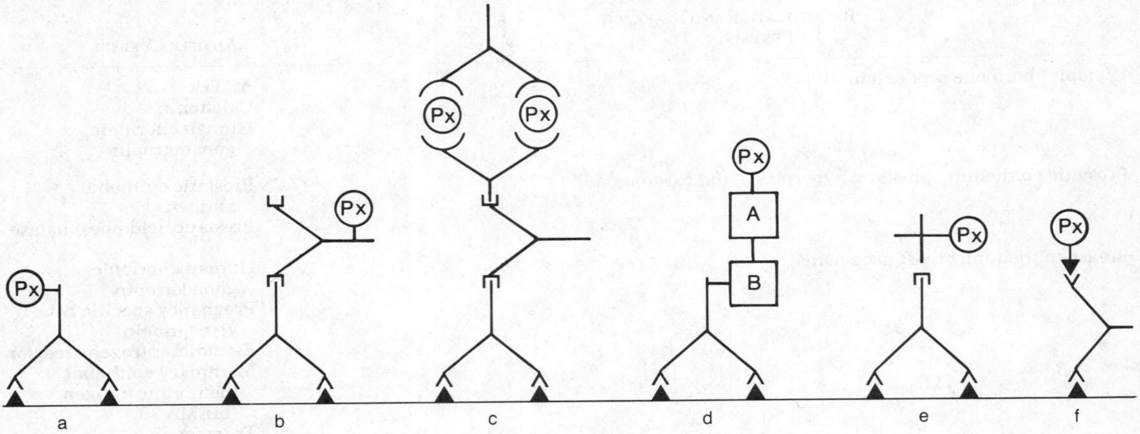

Immunoperoxidase technique. The major methods are: *a*, direct conjugate; *b*, indirect conjugate; *c*, PAP (peroxidase-antiperoxidase); *d*, biotin-avidin-peroxidase (including avidin-biotin-complex method); *e*, protein A–peroxidase conjugate; and *f*, labeled antigen method. (Courtesy of Clive R. Taylor, M.D., and Gary Kledzik, Ph.D.)

most widely used in formalin-paraffin sections and in electron microscopic studies, for in these areas its advantages over other labeled antibody methods are most important.

Fixation and processing may alter and destroy antigens. Different antigens survive formalin fixation to a useful degree; other antigens, particulary those present in small amounts on cell surfaces, fare less well (e.g., lymphocytic T–cell surface antigen) and are best revealed in frozen sections following brief (10-sec) fixation in acetone.

SOURCE OF REAGENTS. Many commercial companies market antibodies of interest to the surgical pathologist. Several companies sell peroxidase-conjugated antibodies for performing the indirect conjugate method, or PAP reagent for the peroxidase-antiperoxidase method. In all these instances, the user must first perform a series of titrations to select the optimal concentration of primary antibody and any other antibodies employed.

More recently, immunoperoxidase kits have been introduced that contain all the antibodies and reagents necessary for the successful performance of an immunoperoxidase stain against a wide range of antigens (Table 1). All kits currently available are based on the PAP system.

CONTROLS. In immunohistologic studies, orthodox controls attempting to assess the specificity of antibodies in solution by immunodiffusion are of limited value, as such methods are not particulary sensitive and as the tissues contain enormous numbers of antigens not readily detectable by diffusion methods. In immunohistology two types of so-called negative controls are employed: one consists of sections of the test tissue in which the immunoperoxidase stain is performed without the primary antibody (preferably substituting preimmune serum), whereas the other involves the completion of the immunoperoxidase stain on a tissue section known to lack the antigen in question. By contrast, a positive control involves the performance of the immunoperoxidase stain on a tissue section known (from independent studies) to contain the antigen in question. Positive and negative controls should be performed in parallel with staining of the test section. In many instances, a section contains intrinsic biologic controls; for example, in staining a suspected medullary (C–cell) carcinoma of the thyroid for calcitonin, any residual normal thyroid will contain normal parafollicular (C) cells, which should be positive for calcitonin (positive control), whereas the thyroid follicular epithelium, stromal cells, blood vessels, etc., should show no staining (negative control).

FUTURE DEVELOPMENTS. The availability of new high-quality conventional antibodies and monoclonal (hybridoma) antibodies has vastly extended the range of usefulness of immunoperoxidase techniques in the past 5 yr. The introduction of simple kits puts the technique within reach of all. It seems certain that immunoperoxidase techniques will form a standard part of surgical pathology practice in the mid-1980s and will occupy an important position in research and for investigative purposes.

CLIVE R. TAYLOR, M.D.

immunopotency (im″u-no-po′ten-se) the ability of an antigen to be immunogenic and thus stimulate the production of specific antibody.

immunopotentiation (im″u-no-po-ten″she-a′shun) enhancement of the immune response by the use of adjuvants to increase the rate, intensity, or length of response. Potentiation can enhance both cellular and humoral responses to a wide variety of antigens or to a specific antigen. General adjuvants include water and oil emulsions (Freund's adjuvant); synthetic polynucleotides (e.g., poly A·U); hormones, drugs, and cyclic nucleotides; endotoxins; and allogeneically stimulated T lymphocytes. Specific potentiators include transfer factor and immunogenic RNA. See also *poly A·U* and *transfer factor.*

immunoprecipitation (im″u-no-pre-sip-ĭ-ta′shun) precipitation that results from the combination of antigen with specific antibody. For precipitation to take place, both the antigen and the antibody must be divalent. The amount of precipitation formed depends on the ratio of antigen to antibody. Immunoprecipitation is a common method of demonstrating antigen-antibody reactions in the laboratory. See also *immunodiffusion* and *precipitin curve.*

immunoprophylaxis (im″u-no-pro″fĭ-lak′sis) the use of vaccines or therapeutic antisera to prevent disease. A significant example of immunoprophylaxis is the prevention of viral diseases. See also *immunization* and *vaccination.*

immunoradiometry (im″u-no-ra″de-om′ĕ-tre) a radioimmunoassay procedure that uses radioactively labeled antibody rather than antigen. See also *radioimmunoassay.*

immunosorbent (im″u-no-sor′bent) a substance attached to an antigen in such a manner that the antigen can adsorb homologous antibodies and then be separated from the remaining solution. See also *ELISA.*

immunostimulant (im″u-no-stim′u-lant) an agent, such as transfer factor, thymus extracts, or immune RNA, that stimulates an immune response through action on a target cell of the immune system.

immunostimulation (im″u-no-stim″u-la′shun) enhancement of the immune system by adjuvants or other chemicals for the purpose of increasing tumor-specific immune responses or defense against infections. Because cancer, as well as cancer chemotherapy and radiotherapy, causes immunosuppression, immunostimulation is sometimes used in its treatment. A common immunostimulant is bacille Calmette-Guérin (BCG).

immunosuppressant (im″u-no-su-pres′ant) an agent that induces immunosuppression.

immunosuppression (im″u-no-su-presh′un) suppression of the immune response, which can be of a natural and beneficial (e.g., tolerance to self-antigens) or pathologic (e.g., chronic infectious disease or lymphoreticular neoplasias) origin. Immunosuppression can also be artificially induced by the administration of antigen, antibody, antilymphocytic antisera, cytotoxic drugs, or radiation doses; clinical uses include allergy desensitization, the prevention of maternal Rh(D) sensitization, and the prevention of tissue graft or organ transplant rejection. Also called *immunodepression.* See also *tolerance.*

immunotherapy (ĭ-mu″no-ther′ah-pe) the use of immunologic approaches in the therapy of human neoplastic disease. Human immune responses to tumors have been observed in both the cellular and the humoral immune systems. Within the cellular immune system, the primary operant cells appear to be the lymphoid cells, including macrophages, T lymphocytes, and non–T lymphocytes. These cellular populations function in a cell-mediated reaction to the tumor cell population, which includes specific antitumor cytolytic properties. Both cytotoxic and tumor growth inhibition properties have been observed in individuals with neuroblastomas, malignant melanomas, and sarcomas, as well as carcinomas of the colon, breast, cervix, and testis. Humoral immunity also plays a role in the human response to tumors. Antibodies capable of reacting with tumor cells are produced in many systems, and include cytotoxic antibodies and specific "arming" antibody complexes. However, antitumor antibodies are not thought to play a major role in the inhibition of human tumor growth.

IMP abbrev. See *inosine-5′-phosphate.*

impaction (im-pak′shun) [L. *impactio*] the condition of being firmly lodged or retained in a body part, as in bone fragments from a fracture wedged together so that neither can move, or a tooth confined within the jaw.

fecal i., a collection of putty-like or hardened feces in the rectum or sigmoid colon.

impalpable (im-pal′pah-b′l) [L. *in* not + *palpare* to feel] not detectable by touch.

impedance (*Z*) (im-pe′dans) 1. mechanical opposition to physical action.

2. the relation between voltage and current in an electrical system; composed of resistance and reactance, which are considered to be vector quantities operating at right angles to each other. It is expressed by the formula $Z = R + iX$, where Z is the impedance, R is the resistance, X is the reactance, and $i = \sqrt{-1}$. Resistance appears in all electrical systems, whereas reactance appears only when voltage and current vary with time; the latter has the effect of creating a difference in phase between voltage and current.

For a voltage expressed as $E\cos(2\pi ft)$, the current is $I\cos(2\pi ft + \theta)$ and $E/I = |Z|$ where $|Z|$ is the magnitude of the vector impedance, f is the frequency of the sinusoidal voltage, t is time (in seconds), and θ is the phase angle due to impedance.

3. the analog of electrical impedance, e.g., acoustic impedance.

electrode i., the opposition to the flow of an alternating current across the interface between a stimulating or recording electrode and the surface with which it is in contact, expressed in ohms. It relates inversely to the area of the electrode and varies with the frequency of the stimulus or recorded electrical activity. Cf. *electrode r.* under *resistance.*

imperforate (im-per′fo-rāt) [L. *imperforatus*] abnormally closed or covered; not open.

i. anus, a congenital malformation of the hindgut in which the anal canal is closed by a persisting membrane or, in more serious cases, by a thick layer of fibrous tissue.

impermeable (im-per′me-ah-b′l) [L. *in* not + *per* through + *meare* to move] not permeable; not permitting passage, e.g., of fluid.

impetigo (im″pĕ-ti′go) [L.] a common superficial skin infection most often caused by staphylococcal or streptococcal organisms. The characteristic lesion of this infection is an erosive vesicle that ruptures, becoming covered with a honey-colored crust. The disease is most common in infants, children, and adults having low resistance, and is contagious by direct spread.

bullous i., see under *scalded skin syndrome.*

implantation (im″plan-ta′shun) [L. *in* into + *plantare* to set] 1. the embedding of the fertilized ovum in the uterine lining.

2. the insertion of an organ or tissue such as skin, nerve, or tendon into the body. The term also refers to placement of medication or artificial devices such as a pacemaker within the tissues.

implantation site the site on the inner surface of the uterine wall where the developing embryo attaches. Normally, this is the posterior wall close to the fundus.

impotence (im′po-tens) [L. *in* not + *potentia* power] the inability of a sexually aroused male to establish and maintain an erection sufficient to culminate in sexual intercourse. Most often impotence is due to emotional disturbances, but it may also result from diseases of the sacral spinal cord or from diabetic polyneuritis and other endocrine disorders.

imprecision (im-pre-sĭ′shun) in clinical chemistry, an indication of the random error of measurement, often expressed as the standard deviation or coefficient of variation of a series of repeated measurements. The other sufficient statistics—the mean value and number of trials—should be specified along with the analytic method and the type of variation, for example, between laboratory or day-to-day. Cf. *precision.*

impregnation (im″preg-na′shun) [L. *impregnatio*] 1. the act of fecundation or of rendering pregnant.

2. in histology, the process of infiltrating a wax or plastic embedding medium into tissue specimens. Also called *infiltration.* See also *embedding.*

3. in histology, a staining procedure in which heavy metal (usually silver) salts are precipitated in cellular components, as opposed to true staining in which an organic dye is chemically bound to some cellular substance.

impulse (im′puls) [L. *impulsus* impelled] 1. a force, push, or thrust.

2. a sudden urge or desire.

3. in physics, the integral of a force over a time interval, which is the change in momentum produced by the force on an unconstrained object.

4. in physics and electronics, a pulse of infinitesimal duration but finite effect. Many physical systems or electronic circuits can be conveniently described in terms of their response to a unit impulse.

impulse sealing the sealing of plastic materials by applying a short pulse of intense heat and then rapid cooling. The technique is used in pathology for storing specimens in plastic tubing.

impurity 1. a contaminant, an unwanted substance present in a small amount in an otherwise pure substance or specified mixture of substances.

2. in solid-state physics, an element diffused throughout a crystalline semiconductor to alter its electrical properties. See also *extrinsic s.* under *semiconductor.*

IMViC tests [acronym from *i*ndole, *m*ethyl red, *V*oges-Proskauer, *c*itrate] a series of metabolic tests, including indole, methyl red, Voges-Proskauer, and citrate, used as standard procedure to distinguish *Escherichia coli* from *Enterobacter* organisms. The IMViC formula for *E. coli* is + + − −, for *Enterobacter aerogenes* and *E. cloacae,* − − + +. For more information, see the specific test.

In symbol for the chemical element *indium.*

in- (in) [L. *in* not, in, into] a prefix word element to denote not or in, e.g., inactivate, incision.

-in a suffix word element in organic chemistry to denote what were once termed neutral substances (i.e., not alkaloids), as in protein, globulin, etc. For some compounds, such as the amino acids, this ending has become *-ine.*

inactivation (in-ak″tĭ-va′shun) the destruction of biologic activity, as of an enzyme, microorganism, or virus.

inadequacy (in-ad′ĕ-kwah-se) [L. *in* not + *adaequare* to make equal] the inability to perform an allotted function; insufficiency; incompetence.

Inapsine (in-ap′sēn) trademark. See *droperidol.*

inborn error of metabolism a congenital biochemical disorder that is caused by a specific genetic defect in the function or structure of a protein molecule. The term was first used in 1908 to describe the genetic diseases alkaptonuria, albinism, cystinuria, and pentosuria. Later, genetic research established the one gene–one enzyme concept, the theory that a single gene mutation alters a cell's ability to perform a single chemical reaction. The term inborn error has since been expanded to include the malfunction of proteins of transport and binding, so that now the concept is more properly stated as one cistron–one polypeptide, the concept that a single gene mutation alters the formation or structure of a single polypeptide chain, thus affecting a metabolic reaction or process. Extensive investigation of the inborn errors of metabolism has been conducted to determine the therapy and diagnosis of the disease processes, as well as to establish the biochemical and genetic causes of the diseases.

Inborn errors, which have been described for all types of proteins, involve three main types:

1. Errors Due to Specific Enzyme Deficiency. The largest and most thoroughly investigated, this class consists of errors involving the loss of an enzyme function caused by a lack of synthesis or by the production of a mutant, nonfunctional protein. Examples include disorders of carbohydrate metabolism (glycogenoses, hemolytic anemia), lipid metabolism (sphingolipidoses, mucolipidoses), amino acid and organic acid metabolism (aminoacidopathies), purine and pyrimidine metabolism (gout, hemolytic anemia), collagen and mucopolysaccharide metabolism (mucopolysaccharidoses), steroid metabolism (adrenal hyperplasia), porphyrin and bilirubin metabolism (porphyria), and miscellaneous disorders such as acatalasia and acid phosphatase deficiency.

2. Errors Due to Defects in Membrane Structural Components. These are errors involving the transport of specific compounds across membranes or the binding of hormones or proteins to specific membrane receptors (cystinuria, type II hypercholesterolemia).

3. Errors Due to Defects in Circulating Proteins. These are errors involving the proteins of the blood, and include errors of transport proteins (lipoproteins), defects in hormones (insulin), defects in coagulation proteins (Factors I–XII), defects affecting the immune system (hypogammaglobulinemia), and defects in inhibitor proteins (angioneurotic edema).

For more information, see the specific conditions.

inbreeding (in′brēd-ing) the mating of closely related individuals. Offspring of such individuals are said to be inbred. Because with inbreeding there is an increased risk of producing individuals homozygous for recessive traits, marriages between closely related individuals are restricted in many societies. See also *consanguinity.*

inbreeding coefficient (F) the probability that both alleles of any particular gene in an individual are descended from a single gene in a common ancestor of both parents; also, the proportion of genetic loci at which the individual is homozygous.

incidence (in′sĭ-dens) [L. *incidere* (*in* + *cadere*) to occur, to happen] an expression of the rate at which a certain event occurs, as in the number of new cases of a specific disease arising during a certain period. See also *incidence r.* under *rate.* Cf. *prevalence.*

incident light (in′sĭ-dent) the direct light that falls on a surface.

incineration (in-sin″ĕ-ra′shun) the process of burning to ashes; cremation.

inclusion (in-klu′zhun) [L. *inclusio*] the act or condition of being enclosed, or something enclosed, such as a cytoplasmic inclusion.

cytoplasmic i., a distinct, often temporary body in the cytoplasm of cells. Depending on its size, it may be visible by light or electron microscopy. Cf. *organelle.*

inclusion body an intracellular mass of viral material. It may be an accumulation of virions, unassembled viral components, or "scars." There may be more than one present in the nucleus (e.g., adenovirus), the cytoplasm (e.g., rabiesvirus Negri bodies), or both (e.g., measles). The term also refers to an intracytoplasmic microcolony of chlamydiae made up of replicating noninfectious or mature infectious particles, eventually resulting in lysis of the infected cell. The presence of either viral or chlamydial inclusion bodies aids in the diagnosis of infections.

inclusive OR (in-klu′siv) see *OR.*

incompatibility (in″kom-pat″ĭ-bil′ĭ-te) 1. in immunology and serology, a mismatch between donor and recipient. Antibodies present in the recipient's serum are directed against antigens in the donor product, or antibodies or sensitized lymphocytes present in donor blood are directed against the recipient's cells. Such a mismatch may result in a transfusion reaction in which, for example, donor blood is hemolyzed, or in the rejection of a donor organ (e.g., kidney) by HLA antibodies or lymphocytes produced by the donor.

2. in plasmid genetics, the existence of plasmids with the same repressor specificity and usually extensive DNA homology. Incompatibility in a cell line results in the loss of all plasmid types except one in the absence of strong selection for each type. See also *plasmid.*

incomplete antibody (in-kom-plēt′) 1. an antibody that combines with antigen without producing an observable reaction (i.e., without precipitation). When such antibodies are present in the serum of individuals with asthma, hay fever, eczema, and similar allergic diseases, they are called reagins.

2. IgG anti-Rh antibody, which does not agglutinate Rh-positive erythrocytes in normal physiologic saline owing to the low density of Rh antigen sites on erythrocytes, but which in the presence of antihuman globulin (Coombs serum) or high-molecular-weight media (e.g., albumin) causes red cell clumping.

Also called saline inactive antibody.

incomplete dominance see *semidominance.*

incontinence (in-kon′tĭ-nens) [L. *incontinentia*] the inability to control excretory functions such as defecation (fecal incontinence) or urination (urinary incontinence).

fecal i., the failure of voluntary control of the anal sphincters, with the involuntary passage of feces and flatus. it may be due to nervous or muscular disorders resulting from disease or trauma; it may also be due to severe and acute emotional stress.

urinary i., a clinical symptom characterized by the involuntary passing of urine from the bladder. Causes may include neurogenic bladder, pelvic surgery, congenital anomalies, psychologic problems, and inflammation due to infection, cancer, or catheters. In postmenopausal females, lack of estrogen may lead to stress incontinence brought on by any action that increases abdominal pressure. If the urethra is obstructed and urine accumulates, overflow or paradoxical incontinence may result.

To diagnose the cause of incontinence, culture and microscopic examination of the urine are routinely performed. If diagnosis cannot be confirmed, more complex tests may be made, including excretory urography, voiding cystourethrography, cystoscopy, urethroscopy, and urodynamic studies.

increment (in′krĕ-ment) [L. *incrementum*] an addition or increase in the amount by which a given quantity or value is increased.

incrementing response (in″krĕ-ment′ing) in electromyography, the progressive increase in the amplitude of successive responses (M waves) when utilizing supramaximal stimuli of the motor nerve. During high-frequency (10–50 Hz) stimulation of a motor nerve, the increment in amplitude may amount to as much as 40 percent in normal subjects. Cf. *decrementing response.*

incubate (in′ku-bāt) [L. *incubare* to lie in or on; to watch over jealously] 1. to place in an optimal situation for development, as by provision of the proper temperature and humidity for the growth of living cells such as ova, microorganisms, or tissue cells.

2. to maintain a culture or a reaction mixture at a fixed temperature.

3. material that has been incubated.

incubation (in″ku-ba′shun) [L. *incubatio*] 1. the induction of development. Cf. *decubation.*

2. the development of the embryo in the eggs of oviparous animals.

3. the development of microorganisms or other cells in an appropriate media under specified temperature conditions. The temperature is usually maintained in a thermostatically controlled chamber or water bath. Other factors such as humidity, light, and CO_2 may also be controlled for optimal growth conditions.

incubation period the time between exposure to, or establishment of, microorganisms in or on a host's tissues and the first appearance of clinical symptoms due to that infection. The period is variable but reasonably consistent for a given organism and disease.

incubator (in′ku-ba-ter) 1. an apparatus for maintaning a premature infant in an environment of proper temperature and humidity.

2. an apparatus for maintaining a constant and suitable temperature for the development of eggs, cultures of microorganisms, or other living cells.

incus (ing′kus) [L. "anvil"] [NA], the middle of the three auditory ossicles.

IND abbrev. for investigative new drug, the subject of a form called Notice of Claimed Investigational Exemption for a New Drug. This form is filed with the Food and Drug Administration (FDA) before the clinical trials of either a new drug or a new use of a marketed drug can proceed. It describes the composition and manufacture of the drug, the results of tests on laboratory animals, and the protocol of the investigation.

independence (in″de-pen′dens) 1. in mathematics,

a relation between equations that holds when none is a linear combination of the rest.

2. in statistics, a relation between events that holds when the probability of any one is not affected by the occurrence of the rest. See also *probability.*

independent assortment (in″de-pen′dent) see *independent a.* under *assortment.*

independent variable 1. in mathematics, the argument of a function, e.g., x in $y = f(x)$.

2. in statistics, a variable used to predict another random variable whose distribution depends on the level or value of the independent variable. The independent variable may be stochastic (random) or fixed by the experimental design. See also *linear regression.*

Inderal (in′der-al) trademark. See *propranolol hydrochloride.*

index (in′deks) [L. forefinger, pointer] 1. (pl. *indices*), the forefinger, the second digit of the hand.

2. (pl. *indices*), in mathematics, a subscript or superscript that indicates a particular element of a set, such as a coordinate of a vector or a term of a series.

3. (pl. *indexes*), a list of references arranged in alphabetical order, such as the index of a book or the *Index Medicus.*

4. (pl. *indexes*), a dimensionless quantity, such as an index of refraction, specifying the magnitude of some physical effect. An index is usually defined as the ratio of two quantities having the same dimensions.

index case 1. see *propositus.*

2. in epidemiology of contagious disease, the first case of an outbreak of a disease.

Index Medicus a publication of the U.S. National Library of Medicine that indexes, by subject and author, most of the world's scientific literature relevant to medicine.

index of refraction (n) the ratio c/v, where c is the velocity of light in a vacuum and v is the velocity of light in a material. It varies with the wavelength of the light and with the density of the material. The index of refraction at a specified temperature, wavelength, and pressure (1 atm) is used for the identification of materials. The temperature (in degrees Celsius) is indicated by a superscript and the wavelength (in nanometers) by a subscript (D indicates the D line of sodium), e.g., n_D^{20} or n_{550}^{25}. Also called *refractive index.*

index register a special-purpose register in a computer's central processor. The contents of an index register are used to form the address of data in the computer's memory.

India ink mount (in′de-a) a solution used for microscopic detection of the capsule surrounding the fungus *Cryptococcus.* Occasionally, carbon particles in the ink may be repelled by white cells, leaving a fuzzy, halo-type appearance around the cells. Therefore, recognition of a sharply demarcated capsule, as well as cell wall, intracellular granules, and budding yeast cells, is essential in order to avoid errors.

Indian file (in′de-an) a single-file arrangement of cells.

indican (in′dĭ-kan) 1. plant indican, a yellow indoxyl glycoside from plants that yields indigo. On hydrolysis it yields β-D-glucose and indoxyl.

2. potassium indoxyl sulfate, which is formed in the intestine by the decomposition of tryptophan, and then absorbed, conjugated, and excreted in the urine.

indican tests the detection of indican in urine by the addition of acidic ferric chloride reagent (0.2 percent w/v, $FeCl_3$), which decomposes indican and oxidizes the indoxyl to indigo blue. This dye is extracted from the aqueous layer into chloroform; a deep violet-to-blue color in the chloroform layer indicates a positive test result. Normal human urine gives no color or turns a faint blue.

indicator (in′dĭ-ka″ter) [L.] an organic compound (often dye) that indicates the presence of some substance or its concentration by a change in color. The color changes occur when the acid form of the indicator changes into the ionic (or salt) form. The appearance, disappearance, or change of the color is sometimes used to determine the end point of a titration or to approximate the pH of a solution.

indicator organism a microorganism used to monitor a specific process, e.g., the spore strips used to monitor autoclaves.

indicator tube a glass tube containing a specific solid chemical that changes color to indicate the presence of specific compounds in air being drawn through the tube. It is commonly used to detect alcohol in exhaled air, or to detect or identify different types of air pollutants after a measured volume of air has been passed through the tube.

indigenous (in-dij′ĕ-nus) [L. *indigenus*] native to a particular place or country; not exotic.

indigenous bacterium a bacterial species that is routinely encountered on superficial tissues such as skin and mucous membranes as part of the normal flora; a commensal. Also called autochthonous bacterium. See also *normal flora.*

indigestion (in″dĭ-jes′chun) irregular digestion that produces vague discomfort, including nausea, heartburn, and belching. The cause may be stress, improper eating habits, or irritating foods. Indigestion may also accompany influenza, food poisoning, allergies, and inflammations of the gastrointestinal tract.

indirect (in″dĭ-rekt′) [L. *indirectus*] 1. not immediate or straight; oblique.

2. acting through an intermediary agent.

indirect addressing a method for specifying the location of data in a computer memory. The indirect address points to a location containing not the data but the true address of the data.

indirect agglutination a method used to detect antibodies to soluble antigens. Antigens are passively attached to inert particles or erythrocytes. The addition of antiserum specific for the test antigen will agglutinate the particles (latex agglutination) or erythrocytes (hemagglutination). Also called *passive agglutination.*

indirect transport see under *active transport.*

indium (In) (in′de-um) [L. *indicum* indigo, from a blue spectral line] a soft, bluish-white, ductile metallic element; atomic number 49; atomic weight 114.82; Group III of the periodic table; oxidation states +1, +3. Indium is used industrially in alloys as a semiconductor.

indium-111 (^{111}In, In 111) a cyclotron-produced radionuclide used primarily for cisternography. Indium-111 has a half-life of 2.8 da; it decays by electron capture and immediately emits 173- and

247-keV gamma rays, which make good images with either a scintillation camera or a rectilinear scanner.

indium In 111 pentetic acid a radiopharmaceutical, a chelate of ^{111}In with pentetic acid (DTPA). It is the agent of choice for radionuclide cisternography because its half-life of 2.8 da is suitable for 24- to 48-hr delayed scans. Also called indium-111-DTPA.

indium-113m (^{113m}In, In 113m) a generator-produced radionuclide used as an alternative to ^{99m}Tc for blood pool, brain, and liver scans. Indium-113m has a half-life of 1.7 hr; it decays by isomeric transition, emitting a 393-keV photon too energetic for scintillation camera use but suitable for the rectilinear scanner.

indium In 113m colloid a radiopharmaceutical; colloidal particles of insoluble indium hydroxide formed from the generator eluate by raising the pH above 4.0. It now is rarely used for the scanning of the liver, spleen, bone marrow, and lungs. By the addition of ferric chloride to the generator eluate and by carefully controlling the pH, particles of various sizes can be formed. Also called indium In 113m iron hydroxide colloid.

indium In 113m pentetic acid a radiopharmaceutical used in brain scanning, a pentetic acid (DTPA) chelate of indium-113m prepared from the generator eluate by use of a sterile reagent kit. Also called indium-113m-DTPA.

Indocin (in′do-sin) trademark. See *indomethacin.*

indocyanine green (ICG) (in″do-si′ah-nēn) a tricarbocyanine dye occurring as a crystalline powder (dark green, blue, black, or olive-brown in color), which has been used in determinations of blood volume and cardiac output, and in the evaluation of liver function, where it has largely replaced Bromsulphalein. See also *dye excretion test.* Trademark, Cardio-Green.

indole (in′dōl) a heterocyclic compound, 2,3-benzopyrrole; M.W. 117.14. Indole is obtained from coal tar and is also produced by the bacterial decomposition of tryptophan in the intestines. It has an intense fecal odor. The indole test is used in differentiating the enteric bacteria. In a positive reaction, the enzyme tryptophanase produced by the test organism catalyzes both the deamination and decarboxylation of tryptophan present in the medium and converts it to indole. The indole is detected by reaction with *p*-dimethylaminobenzaldehyde (Kovac's reagent) in the acid medium, forming a red color. See also *IMViC tests.*

indoleacetic acid (5 OH IAA) (in″dōl-ă-se′tik) a metabolite of tryptophan that appears in the urine of mammals as indoleaceturic acid. It is formed by conjugation with glycine. A possible precursor is tryptamine, formed in the large intestine by the bacterial decarboxylation of tryptophan. Indoleacetic acid and indolelactic acid are excreted in increased amounts in the urine of individuals with phenylketonuria.

indoleaceturia (in″dōl-as″ĕ-tu′re-ah) the presence of indoleacetic acid in the urine. A small amount of both 3- and 5-hydroxyindoleacetic acids is excreted by healthy individuals. Excessive amounts of 5-hydroxyindoleacetic acid, the urinary metabolite of serotonin, may be excreted when carcinoid tumors are present. Ingestion of serotonin-containing foods (tomatoes, plums, bananas) increases the excretion of 5-hydroxyindoleacetic acid. See also *5-hydroxyindoleacetic acid.*

indoleaceturic acid (in″dōl-a-set′u-rik) the glycine conjugate of indoleacetic acid.

indolelactic acid (in″dōl-lak′tik) a metabolite of tryptophan that is excreted in increased amounts in the urine of individuals with phenylketonuria.

indoluria (in″dōl-u′re-ah) [*indole* + Gr. *ouron* urine + *-ia*] the presence of indole in the urine.

indomethacin (in″do-meth′ah-sin) [NF], an antiinflammatory, antipyretic, and analgesic nonsteroidal drug, an indole derivative that inhibits the synthesis of prostaglandin. It is used for the treatment of gouty arthritis, rheumatoid arthritis, osteoarthritis, and ankylosing spondylitis. Headache, dizziness, nausea, and gastrointestinal disturbances are commonly occurring side-effects; psychic disturbances such as vertigo and depression also arise. Blood levels of indomethacin are increased by the concurrent use of salicylates or probenicid. Indomethacin also may potentiate an anticoagulant effect, which is reflected in an increased prothrombin time. Trademark, Indocin.

indophenol (cytochrome oxidase) test (in″do-fe′nol) a test that differentiates members of Enterobacteriaceae from nonpigmented strains of *Pseudomonas* and other oxidase-positive, gram-negative bacilli. In a positive test, cytochrome oxidase in the bacterial culture acts as a catalyst to couple dimethyl-*p*-phenylenediamine with alpha-naphthol, forming a bright blue product, indophenol blue.

indoxyl (in-dok′sil) [Gr. *indikon* indigo + *oxys* sharp] an oxidation product of indole, $C_6H_4 \cdot C$-(OH):CH·NH, formed in the intestines from indoleacetic acid, a metabolite of tryptophan. It is excreted in the urine as indican (potassium indoxyl sulfate).

indoxyl sulfate (in-dok′sil sul′fāt) see *indican.*

indoxyluria (in″dok-sil-u′re-ah) [*indoxyl* + Gr. *ouron* urine + *-ia*] the presence of an excess of indoxyl in the urine, mostly as sulfate or glucuronide.

induce (in-dūs′) [L. *inducere* to lead in] to cause or to bring about.

inducer (in-dūs′er) something that induces. In molecular genetics, the term refers to a molecule that causes a cell or organism to produce large amounts of the enzymes involved in their metabolism. For instance, the inducer may bind with a repressor; this inactivates the repressor so that it cannot bind to the operator site and prevent transcription of the operon. Also called *activator.* See also *enzyme induction* and *operon.*

inducible (in-dūs′ĭ-b′l) capable of being induced. See also *induction.*

inductance (in-duk′tans) [L.] the opposition of an inductor or coil to a change in electric current; the voltage across the inductor divided by the rate of change of current. The unit of inductance is the henry.

induction (in-duk′shun) [L. *inductio* to lead in] 1. the act or process of inducing or causing to occur.

2. in embryology, the influence of an organizer (evocator) on the differentiation of adjacent cells or on the development of an embryo.

3. in enzymology, the process of increasing the amount or activity of an enzyme by the presence of an inducer, which acts by suppressing a repressor

and liberating an operator gene (operon) for enzyme production.

4. in microbiology, the change from probacteriophage to vegetative phage, which occurs spontaneously or as a result of physical or chemical agents.

5. in physics, the appearance of an electric current or of magnetic properties in a body because of the presence of another electric current or magnetic field nearby. See also *magnetic induction.*

inductor (in-duck′ter) an electrical circuit component that is a small electromagnet. Its property of resisting changes in current is called inductance. Also called *choke* and *coil.*

induration (in″du-ra′shun) [L. *induratio*] 1. the process or quality of becoming hard and firm.

2. an abnormally hard spot or place.

industrial poison see *industrial p.* under *poison.*

-ine (in, ēn) 1. a suffix word element to denote pertaining to, similar to, or derived from, e.g., crystalline, bovine; or to denote an abstract noun, e.g., medicine.

2. a suffix word element in chemistry to denote certain classes of substances: halogens, e.g., fluorine; hydrogen compounds with group V elements, e.g., phosphine, arsine, and stibine; some alkaloids, e.g., codeine; some organic nitrogenous bases, e.g., purine; and amino acids, e.g., glycine. See also *-in.*

inert (in-ert′) [L. *iners* inactive] having no action; not reacting chemically, as the inert gases; helium, neon, argon, krypton, xenon, and radon. This term is understood in a relative sense, for nothing is completely inert chemically under all conditions. For example, N_2 and CO_2 are often used to provide an inert atmosphere for chemical reaction, but both are reactive under the proper conditions. Inert gases such as helium and neon now are usually called "the noble gases" because, although they are quite stable under most conditions, they do react with some compounds.

inertia (in-er′she-ah) [L.] 1. inactivity, the inability to move spontaneously.

2. the physical property of an object that resists acceleration; equivalent to the mass of the object.

in extremis (in ek-stre′mis) [L. "at the end"] at the point of death.

infantile (in′fan-tīl) possessing the qualities of an infant; relating to infants.

infantile paralysis see *poliomyelitis.*

infantile spasms a type of massive myoclonus occuring in infants and young children. Such myoclonic spasms may result from any severe, diffuse, developmental, or acquired encephalopathy that occurs in the first year or so of life, or they may develop without recognizable cause in a previously healthy child. Developmental delay, mental impairment, and a variety of neurologic deficits may be associated. The electroencephalogram typically—but not always—shows a hypsarrhythmic pattern, and a variety of other abnormalities (such as suppression-burst or focal spike activity) may be encountered. Infantile spasms sometimes respond dramatically to treatment with adrenocorticotropic hormone (ACTH). Also called *salaam attacks.*

infantilism (in-fan′tĭ-lizm) the retention of the characteristics of childhood into adult life. Intelligence, stature, and reproductive organs may fail to develop, retaining their immature patterns. The cause often is abnormal endocrine function or specific nutrient deficiency such as zinc deficiency.

infant respiratory distress syndrome (IRDS) a respiratory distress syndrome, appearing shortly (6–8 hr) after birth, that is associated with the initial ventilation of lungs that lack adequate surfactant stores. (The surfactant, a lipoprotein mixture secreted by type II alveolar cells, reduces the surface tension of the fluids that line the alveoli, thus minimizing the tendency of alveoli to collapse.) Deficiency of surfactant leads to instability and atelectasis of the smaller air spaces, preventing the formation of a functional residual capacity. The consequent uneven distribution of ventilation and perfusion of hypoventilated (atelectatic) air spaces results in inadequate gas exchange and respiratory distress. A characteristic layer of eosinophilic material called a hyaline membrane, which is composed largely of fibrin and cellular debris derived from necrotic alveolar lining cells, is found adherent to the walls of alveoli, alveolar ducts, and respiratory bronchioles upon postmortem examination of affected lungs.

Premature infants are especially susceptible to the development of IRDS. Precipitous delivery (especially by cesarean section without prior labor) necessitated by perinatal asphyxia, maternal hemorrhage, or diabetes is another important predisposing factor.

The etiology of IRDS is still unknown. A well-documented and well-accepted theory is that the lungs of premature infants may not have reached a stage of development at which surfactant synthesis is sufficient to meet postnatal demands. The inadequate alveolar inflation that results initiates sequelae that lead to congestion of the alveolar capillaries and an exudation and transudation of plasma proteins and fluids. Other theories hold that the condition is aggravated by an initial pulmonary vasoconstriction, by an increased permeability of the alveolar wall, or by hypotension.

Classic clinical signs of the respiratory difficulty associated with IRDS include tachypnea, dyspnea, inspiratory subcostal and substernal retraction, expiratory grunting (representing an attempt to prolong inspiration), generally poor or harsh breathing sounds, and, in more severe cases, cyanosis. Right-to-left shunts, systemic hypotension and inadequate peripheral perfusion, metabolic and respiratory acidosis, hyperkalemia, and hyperbilirubinemia are also seen.

Pulmonary function tests reveal a reduction in pulmonary compliance, tidal volume, functional residual capacity, and crying vital capacity. Blood gas analysis shows an increased P_{CO_2} and often severely depressed P_{O_2} consistent with a picture of alveolar hypoventilation and hypoxemia. Characteristic radiologic findings are a diffuse reticulogranularity throughout the parenchyma of both lungs and an air bronchogram.

Treatment at the onset of the 3- to 5-da clinical course of the disease is mainly supportive: correction of acidosis, maintenance of body temperature and nutritional status, and alleviation of hypotensive shock, if necessary, by blood transfusion. An inspired air mixture sufficient to maintian arterial P_{O_2} at 50–70 mmHg, often in combination with assisted or controlled ventilation, is used to correct the hypoxemia.

If the conditon is untreated, death usually ensues

within 72 hr. In treated infants, complications such as pneumonia or pulmonary or intracranial hemorrhage may lead to death at a later date.

Also called *hyaline membrane disease* and idiopathic respiratory distress syndrome of infants. See also *surfactant.*

infarct (in′farkt) [L. *infarctus*] a local area of cell death within a tissue due to the blockage of normal blood supply of that area. The arterial blockage may be caused by occlusion (preventing oxygenated blood from reaching the tissue) or venous blockage (preventing blood outflow). Infarcts are most commonly due to a thrombus or an embolus.

infarction (in-fark′shun) [L. *infarcire* to stuff in] the process of forming an infarct; an infarct.

cerebral i., the destruction of cerebral tissue owing to a disturbance of the blood supply to the brain. The affected individual suffers neurologic impairment proportional to the extent and location of the infarction. See also *cerebrovascular accident.*

intestinal i., acute ischemic necrosis of intestinal tissue. This type of infarction is a serious and frequently fatal condition that arises from the occlusion of a vessel or vessels that supply the affected segment of intestine, or hypoxia without vascular occlusion. The mortality rate is 60–70 percent in patients with massive bowel infarction.

Occlusive infarction due to thrombi or thromboemboli involving branches of the mesenteric artery or vein usually arises in association with advanced arteriosclerosis, but may also be due to systemic arteritis, disorders leading to hypercoagulability, trauma, and compression of vessels by tumor.

Nonocclusive infarction characteristically occurs in conditions that compromise the delivery of oxygenated blood to the bowels, e.g., hypotension, congestive heart failure, or systemic hypoxia.

myocardial i., see *myocardial infarction.*

pulmonary i., a hemorrhagic necrosis of a localized area of the pulmonary parenchyma, with an overlying pleural inflammation; it may be a consequence of a reduction in or the total obstruction of the pulmonary arterial blood supply to that area. Pulmonary infarction is frequently a major complication of pulmonary embolism; the latter occurs when a dislodged thrombus (commonly detached from a site of origin in the deep leg veins or right heart) or nonthrombotic matter (such as air, fat, tumor) impacts in the pulmonary vascular bed. This lodging of emboli in the pulmonary vasculature may compromise the circulation downstream from the site of mechanical obstruction, causing local ischemic areas and often leading to pulmonary infarction.

The exact mechanism underlying formation of a pulmonary infarction is not well understood. Pulmonary embolism does not invariably lead to pulmonary infarction, nor does the size of the occluded vessel always correlate well with the subsequent size of an infarct. It is recognized, however, that infarction seems to occur with greatest frequency in a lung that is infected, congested, hypoventilated, or otherwise predisposed to circulatory stasis. It may be that the factors that normally sustain the lung following embolization (augmentation of the circulation through collaterals or distal anastomoses with the bronchial arterial circulation) are delayed in onset or are of no benefit in the presence of these other underlying conditions.

An infarcted area of the pulmonary parenchyma is hemorrhagic and airless, appearing after the first day as wedge-shaped or humped shadows on radiographs. The infarct may be accompanied by a variable amount of pleural effusion, atelectasis, and edema of surrounding areas. Clinical manifestations of pulmonary infarction include cough, hemoptysis, pleuritic chest pain, fever, moderately severe dyspnea, tachycardia, pleural friction rub, and elevated leukocyte count and serum LDH and bilirubin concentrations. These physical and radiographic signs usually clear within several weeks.

See also *pulmonary e.* under *embolism.*

renal i., ischemic necrosis of renal tissue due to vascular occlusions in the major or minor renal arteries or veins. As is true of most organ infarctions, arterial occlusion is more likely to cause renal infarction than is venous occlusion. Renal infarction can lead to systemic hypertension, loss of renal function, and, occasionally, death. Oliguric renal failure may occur in individuals with solitary kidneys or compromised renal function. Infarction following renal vein thrombosis may produce a nephrotic syndrome. Diagnosis must usually be confirmed by angiographic studies.

infect (in-fekt′) [L. *inficio* dip into, corrupt] to produce infection.

infection (in-fek′shun) the multiplication of microorganisms in or on body tissues, producing cellular injury. The infection may remain localized, subclinical, and temporary if the body's defense mechanisms are effective enough. Local infections may persist and spread by extension to become an acute, subacute, or chronic clinical infection or disease state. Local infections may also become systemic when the microorganisms gain access to the lymphatic or vascular systems of the body.

airborne i., an infection that is contracted by inhalation of microorganisms or spores suspended in air on water droplets or dust particles. Microorganisms are often rendered airborne as a result of a sneeze or cough. Cf. *droplet nuclei.*

colonization i., an infection characterized by the attachment and subsequent growth of the invading microorganism on or within tissue.

inapparent i., an infection with no clinical symptoms that is unnoticed by the affected individual.

nosocomial i., see *nosocomial infection.*

pyogenic i., an infection caused by pus-producing microorganisms, commonly species of *Staphylococcus* and *Streptococcus.* The most numerous cells responding immunologically to a pyogenic infection are the polymorphonuclear leukocytes.

infectious (in-fek′shus) capable of being transmitted from one host to another.

infectious agent a microorganism capable of causing infection in humans, animals, or plants. See also *biohazard.*

infectious disease a disease that is caused by a microorganism. The etiologic agent may be a bacterium, virus, fungus, or animal parasite. It may be acquired from another host or arise from the host's own indigenous microflora.

Modern medicine has had a great impact on infectious disease. Improved treatment has resulted from increased knowledge of pathogens and disease mechanisms and the development of new antimicrobial drugs. However, problems have been caused by increased occasions for compromising the patient's immune status, by the expanded use of catheterization (resulting in additional portals of entry for microorganisms), and by an increased opportunity for the misuse of antimicrobial therapy.

infectious hepatitis see under *hepatitis.*

infectious mononucleosis (in-fek′shus mon″o-nu″-kle-o′sis) a usually self-limiting disease caused by the Epstein-Barr virus (EBV) and characterized by fever, membranous pharyngitis, lymphocyte proliferation, lymph node and splenic enlargement, and the presence of atypical lymphocytes in the blood. Hepatitis and encephalomeningitis are potential complications. It is most frequently a disease of young adulthood, is spread by saliva transfer and possibly other modes, and gives rise to a variety of immune reactions, including the development of a transient heterophile and a persistent EBV antibody response.

Although infectious mononucleosis is a self-limiting disease, laboratory diagnosis is important to distinguish it from similar but more serious diseases. Infectious mononucleosis may be confused with diphtheria, pharyngitis, Vincent's angina, lymphadenitis with scarlet fever, hepatitis, or pertussis. Currently, the most effective method of laboratory diagnosis is serologic. All individuals with infectious mononucleosis produce heterophile antibodies, which have an affinity for related antigens located on sheep and beef red blood cells. Heterophile antibodies produced in those with infectious mononucleosis must be distinguished from Forssman heterophile antibodies that are present in almost all human sera.

The presumptive heterophile test, an agglutination test to determine the total amount of heterophile antibody present, involves a serial dilution of serum in saline, followed by the addition of 2 percent sheep red blood cells. This mixture remains undisturbed for 2 hr at room temperature and is observed for agglutination. A titer of 1:56 or greater is indicative of the need for further testing to differentiate Forssman antibodies.

Another procedure, the Davidsohn differential test, involves two procedures—adsorption and titration. Antigen from guinea pig kidney tissue will adsorb the Forssman and serum sickness heterophile antibodies if present. Beef red blood cell antigen will adsorb infectious mononucleosis and serum sickness heterophile antibodies if present. If antigens are adsorbed, there is a loss in the serum's ability to agglutinate sheep red blood cells. A comparison of the agglutination titers indicates which antibody is present.

The Monospot test is a rapid specific test for heterophile antibodies due to infectious mononucleosis. It involves two stages, adsorption of sera with guinea pig kidney and beef erythrocytes, followed by reaction with horse red blood cells. The guinea pig kidney contains the Forssman antigen but not the antigen of infectious mononucleosis. The beef red blood cells contain heterophile antigen to infectious mononucleosis but not the Forssman antigen. Horse red blood cells, rather than sheep red blood cells, are used as indicators. The entire test is performed on a glass slide, and agglutination occurs within minutes. If the guinea pig kidney adsorbed serum agglutinates horse red blood cells, the test is positive for infectious mononucleosis.

Also called *Pfeiffer's disease.* See also *Epstein-Barr virus.*

infectious wastes waste material consisting of clinical specimens or cultures containing, or having the potential to contain, microorganisms capable of causing disease in humans. Waste materials should be placed into waterproof bags and their contents clearly labeled. Infectious material must be rendered harmless by decontamination before being discarded. Written procedures must be established for the proper disposal of infectious wastes.

infective (in-fek′tiv) infectious; pertaining to or characterized by the presence of microbial pathogens or their products. Cf. *antiinfective.*

infectivity (in″fek-tiv′ĭ-te) referring to the level of infectiousness, or the ability of a microorganism to spread from a source to a host.

inferior (in-fēr′e-or) [L. "lower"] situated below or directed downward.

inferosuperior (in″fer-o-su-pe′re-or) pertaining to a radiographic projection in which the central ray passes through the part from bottom to top (not necessarily in a vertical direction).

infertility (in″fer-til′ĭ-te) [L. *in* not + *fertilis* fruitful, prolific] sterility: in the male, the inability either to inseminate or of his sperm to fertilize ova; in the female, the inability to conceive during the course of unprotected coitus for at least 1 yr. Physical and pelvic examination of the female and physical examination of the male should be performed, with emphasis on the genital and rectal examinations. A full medical and sexual history is also obtained. Diagnostic testing to determine the cause of the infertility in both partners may be aided by semen analysis, hysterosalpingography, tubal insufflation, vaginal smears, endometrial biopsy, testicular biopsy, culdoscopy, and analysis of the sex chromosomes.

infestation (in-fes-ta′shun) the attack or subsistence of ticks, mites, or insects on the skin and appendages. The term is also used to describe helminthic invasion of organs and tissues. Infestation differs from bacterial and viral infections in that the animal parasites are larger and do not multiply within the body; they are usually acquired periodically over a long course of time. Cf. *infection.*

infiltrate (in-fil′trāt) 1. to penetrate the interstices of a tissue or substance.

2. any material deposited by infiltration.

infiltration (in″fil-tra′shun) 1. the accumulation in a tissue or in cells of substances not present in the healthy state (e.g., neoplastic cells in invasive cancer), or the accumulation of excessive amounts of substances. It also refers to the material so accumulated.

2. in histology, the process of infiltrating a wax or plastic embedding medium into tissue specimens. Also called *impregnation.* See also *embedding.*

infinite (in′fĭ-nit) [L. *in* not + *finitus* finite] unbounded, unlimited, or immeasurable; in mathematics, capable of assuming arbitrarily large values or (of a set) containing more elements than any integer.

infinitesimal (in″fĭ-nĭ-tes′ĭ-mal) in mathematics, capable of assuming arbitrarily small values.

infinity (∞) (in-fin′ĭ-te) 1. in mathematics, the limit of a sequence or integral that has no finite limit and that exceeds arbitrarily large positive values (a limit of $+\infty$) or negative values (a limit of $-\infty$).

2. in computer programming, a value larger than

the largest number that can be expressed in the number storage system in use.

3. any distance from a camera lens at which objects are in focus while objects at great distances are also in focus.

inflammable (in-flam′ah-b′l) [L. *inflammare* to ignite] easily ignited and rapidly burning. The term flammable is now used for better clarity to describe such hazardous materials in the laboratory. See also *flammable.*

inflammation (in″flah-ma′shun) [L. *inflammatio; inflammare*] the process by which reaction to injury occurs within the tissues of the body. The outcome of this process depends on the nature and severity of the injury and on the body's capacity to respond. The result can be complete tissue restoration, destruction, or scarring, or it can be combinations of these results.

Injury can be produced by both replicating and nonreplicating agents. Viruses, rickettsiae, bacteria, fungi, and parasites are microorganisms making up the replicating category. Chemical agents such as acids, bases, and proteolytic enzymes, and physical agents such as irradiation, heat and cold, and trauma constitute nonreplicating agents.

The inflammatory process is characterized by a complex interplay of vascular, humoral, and cellular factors, and can be further defined in two broad categories: acute and chronic inflammation.

ACUTE INFLAMMATION. The acute inflammatory process is basically exudative; i.e., the elements of which it consists arise from the circulating blood and exude into the tissues. This form of inflammation is characterized by the classic signs of redness, heat, swelling, pain, and loss of function. These signs are primarily the result of vascular changes, alterations in blood flow, and permeability of blood vessels. If the injury is not severe, an arteriolar dilation occurs and blood flow is increased, producing heat and redness. If the injury is more severe, vessel destruction can occur and thrombosis and coagulation necrosis may increase the extent of tissue destruction.

An alteration in vascular permeability leads to an extravasation of plasma through the blood vessel walls into the extravascular space, forming edema or swelling. These changes occur because of the release of chemical mediators (see below), some of which, such as bradykinin, cause pain. Extravasations of higher protein content (specific gravity, > 1.018) are considered exudates rather than transudates and may be defined as serous, fibrinous, or sanguineous, depending on their content. Although different patterns of vascular leakage have been described, it is primarily the postcapillary venules that respond to the chemical mediators of inflammation. The capillary bed may also be involved, usually as the result of direct injury and disruption.

The primary leukocyte in acute inflammation is the polymorphonuclear leukocyte or neutrophil. These motile, circulating, nonreplicating cells appear early in an area of acute inflammation. Initially they marginate along the inner vascular wall and then emigrate through the vessel wall between endothelial cells into the injured tissues. This is a directed movement brought about by the release of chemical mediators, a chemotaxis. Cells of the mononuclear phagocyte series derived from circulating monocytes also are present early in acute inflammation: the longer the inflammation persists, the greater are the numbers of these cells.

Neutrophils and particularly mononuclear phagocytes have the capacity to phagocytize foreign substances, destroy certain microorganisms, and degrade and digest foreign materials. Aiding in phagocytosis are substances called opsonins, which enhance adherence to the cell surface. Common opsonins are gamma globulin and complement; neutrophils and mononuclear phagocytes have Fc and C3b receptors on their surface.

The processes of cellular digestion involve a burst of energy, a fall in pH, and activation of enzyme systems. The release of lysosomal enzymes from storage granules and vesicles into the phagocyte vacuole, the phagosome, forms a secondary lysosome or phagolysosome within which these digestive processes occur. The formation of hydrogen peroxide from peroxidases, lysozymes, and cationic proteins contributes to destruction of the microorganisms. At times phagocytosis is incomplete and proteolytic enzymes are released external to the cell, causing tissue destruction, primarily because of collagenase and elastase activities. Cellular motility, phagocytosis, and degranulation all involve membrane movement of the cell, which is dependent on the cellular microskeleton composed of microtubules and microfilaments.

Many chemical mediators have been described that have the capacity to cause chemotaxis and alterations in blood flow and vascular permeability. These substances can be derived from cells either circulating or in tissues and from plasma constituents. Histamine and 5-hydroxytryptamine are released from mast cells in tissues and from basophils and platelets in the circulating blood. Products of arachidonic acid metabolism, prostaglandins, endoperoxides, thromboxanes, and leukotrienes are released from both inflammatory cells and damaged tissues. Substances are derived primarily from plasma through three interrelated systems: the formation of kinins, blood coagulation, and complement. Each of these involves protein-protein interactions and activation of enzyme sequences.

The orchestration of mediators derived from the circulation and tissues is not completely understood, but histamine, kinins, and prostaglandins are of primary importance in producing alterations in vascular permeability, and complement activation in chemotaxis. The extracellular release of collagenase and elastase further contributes to tissue damage.

Various inhibitors of these systems are present in the circulation and include: the inhibitor of C1 esterase, α_2-macroglobulins, and α_1-antitrypsin. Granules of the eosinophilic leukocyte contain antihistaminases and substances capable of degrading leukotrienes. One function of these cells is therefore the curtailment of inflammation initiated by the release of granules from mast cells.

Mononuclear phagocytes increase in number as the agents producing acute inflammation persist. These cells are the primary reacting cells if the stimulus is bland, such as particulate substances in tattoos. These cells not only are avid phagocytes but also have a secretory capacity. Activated macrophages have enhanced capacities and can secrete profibrinolytic substances, collagenases, elastases, and various factors that cause fibroblasts and blood vessels to proliferate.

Subacute inflammation is a poorly defined term for the type of inflammation that displays characteristics of both acute inflammation and chronic inflammation.

CHRONIC INFLAMMATION. This process occurs if the agents producing inflammation persist. It is both an exudation and a cellular proliferation, comprising both the cells involved in immune mechanisms and cells of the repair process. A persistence of inflammation can occur for a variety of reasons: because of persistence of the inflammatory agent, necrosis of tissues, foreign bodies, poor blood supply, or the development of an immunologic response.

The primary cells of chronic inflammation are lymphocytes and plasma cells. In certain forms of inflammation, lymphocytes are the initial and major responding cells. This is true in viral infections and delayed hypersensitivity responses. Mononuclear phagocytes are also a feature of chronic inflammation. Granulomatous inflammation is a form of chronic inflammation characterized by a predominance of mononuclear phagocytes.

Compared with acute inflammation, little is known of the chemical mediation of chronic inflammation. Lymphokines, including interferon, antibodies secreted locally by plasma cells, and secretions of macrophages are undoubtedly important. The types and the relative frequencies of the various types of lymphocytes present may also be critical. Our understanding of how the proportion of B and T lymphocytes (helper, cytotoxic, and suppressor T cells, and K cells) interact in tissues is poor.

Depending on the stimulus, the cells of immunity and repair occur simultaneously in varying numbers. If tissue destruction is present, the cells of the repair process eventually appear. These include proliferating fibroblasts and endothelial cells, together making up granulation tissue. As fibroblasts lay down increasing amounts of collagen, a scar tissue is formed. In long-standing inflammatory processes such as in abscesses and ulcers, changes of both acute exudative and chronic inflammation with scarring can be seen together.

Although the inflammatory process is basically a protective one, at times it is the inflammatory process itself that is primarily responsible for tissue destruction. This is particularly true in hypersensitivity responses in which the stimulus often is not damaging of tissues, but the immune inflammatory response is damaging. A component of hypersensitivity leading to tissue destruction is found in diseases produced by microorganisms such as tuberculosis and in those immune inflammations in which the process is directed against the individual's own tissues, an autoimmune response.

GRANULOMATOUS INFLAMMATION. The granulomatous inflammation process is a form of chronic inflammation characterized by granuloma formation. Tuberculosis, leprosy, certain fungal and bacterial diseases, schistosomiasis, sarcoidosis, and foreign body reactions are all forms of granulomatous inflammation. The process is thought to be dependent on a functioning T-cell–mediated immune system; see also *granuloma.*

EDWARD L. HOWES, M.D.

inflammatory carcinoma see under *breast neoplasms.*

inflation (in-fla'shun) [L. *in* into + *flare* to blow] distention with air, gas, or a fluid.

influenza (in"flu-en'zah) [Ital. "influenza"] an acute viral infection of the respiratory tract, which may occur as an isolated case, epidemic, or pandemic. Influenza is a disabling disease and is not usually fatal in a healthy individual. However, debilitated persons or the very young or very old are susceptible to secondary bacterial superinfections, which place them in greater danger. The disease is caused by the specific influenza virus, of which there are three antigenic types, designated A, B, and C.

Clinically, influenza may present as an uncomplicated infection or a more severe pneumonia. Uncomplicated influenza appears with a sudden onset after a 2- to 3-da incubation period following exposure. Malaise and chills are followed by headache, fever, diffuse myalgia, and possibly sore throat. Within the first day of onset of symptoms, the patient's temperature can rise to 102°F (39°C). Acute illness lasts 3–5 da, at which time a scratchy throat, dry cough, and nasal obstruction are common. After the acute illness, the principal symptoms may subside but the patient is fatigued.

Bronchopulmonary influenza, a more severe state of influenza, involves the lower respiratory tract also and causes a stronger cough and chest pain. This disease usually lasts 3 wk. Primary influenza viral pneumonia affects older individuals or cardiac patients. The progression of this type of influenza is rapid (36 hr) and the interstitial exchange of air is difficult, resulting in irregular breathing and cyanosis. Antibiotic therapy does not help and the prognosis is poor.

Of all respiratory tract infections caused by viruses, influenza uniquely predisposes individuals to secondary bacterial infections. The most common bacteria involved are *Staphylococcus aureus, Streptococcus pneumoniae,* and *Hemophilus influenzae.* Postinfluenzal bacterial pneumonia appears during recovery and improvement as a sudden onset of chills, fever, and chest pain. The cough is productive with a bloody sputum; antibiotic therapy is necessary. Treatment before identification of the bacterium involved should be a pencillinase-resistant semisynthetic penicillin derivative, as many *S. aureus* strains are resistant to penicillin G. The great pandemic of 1918, which was responsible for 20 million deaths, was associated with secondary bacterial pneumonias.

Laboratory diagnosis may be performed by viral culture into embryonated eggs or Rhesus monkey kidney cells. Serologically, the hemagglutination inhibition assay may be used to detect antibodies to viral surface antigens. Diagnosis of influenza depends on a fourfold increase in the hemagglutination inhibition titer from acute serum to convalescent serum. Also, complement-fixing antibody to the soluble (S) antigen is present within 9 da of infection and is an indicator of current infection.

Prevention of influenza through vaccination is difficult because of antigenic drifts and shifts. However, by the use of genetic engineering, it is possible to produce hybrid vaccines for mass vaccination programs in a relatively short time, as demonstrated by the United States' national program for vaccination against swine influenza virus in 1976. Amantadine hydrochloride has been shown to be effective in treating influenza A_2. Only when there is a secondary bacterial infection should antibiotics be used.

Also called flu and grip.

influenza virus the etiologic agent of influenza. Influenza virus belongs to the myxovirus group of viruses. It is pleomorphic, either spherical or filamentous in form, and is about 100 μ in diameter. Its nucleocapsid has a helical symmetry. Projecting from the envelope that surrounds the virus is a rod-shaped glycoprotein polymer called hemagglutinin. The hemagglutinin binds to receptors on red blood cells and on the epithelial cells that line the respiratory tract.

Also projecting from the envelope is a spike-shaped glycoprotein polymer called neuraminidase, an enzyme that cleaves host cell receptors to release the virus. Neuraminidase does not affect the binding of virus to host cells but is responsible for the release of free, viable viral particles that can infect other cells. The nucleic acid of the influenza virus is single-stranded RNA, which is divided into seven separate segments. Once the virus has gained access to the inside of a host cell, viral transcriptase transcribes mRNA, which leads to the synthesis of cellular RNA. Finally, viral proteins and RNA are assembled to make a new virus.

Influenza virus is divided into three antigenic types, A, B, and C, on the basis of their capsid antigens. Within these groups, the influenza virus may be serologically typed further on the basis of its neuraminidase and hemagglutinin. The standard form of nomenclature is: (1) the antigenic type (A, B, or C), (2) the location of identification, (3) the year of isolation, and (4) the surface antigens hemagglutinin and neuraminidase. Antigenic shifts may occur where there is a change in one part of one of the surface antigens, usually hemagglutinin. Antigenic drifts may also occur where there is a minor shift within a single type of surface antigen. Because of these antigenic changes associated with the nucleic acid being segmented into seven pieces, changes in the antigenic structure of influenza virus are common. This explains why immunity to one type of influenza is not helpful against other antigenic variations.

Influenza virus may be transmitted through the air from one human to another. When an infected individual sneezes or coughs, droplets containing viruses are expelled, and these can be inhaled by others in close proximity. Depending on their size, the droplets may travel into the respiratory tract. There, the viral hemagglutinin enables the virus to attach to epithelial cells. If the virus is not removed by respiratory cilia or IgA, it will multiply and cause inflammation. New virus will be released by the viral neuraminidase and infect other cells.

information (in″for-ma′shun) 1. meaningful, nonrandom data; the content of a message.

2. in information theory, a measure of the information content of a message, defined as the negative logarithm of its probability of selection. Usually, base-2 logarithms are used; then the units of information are bits. When all messages are equally likely, the information is the negative logarithm of the number of possible messages. For example, in computers a byte can have any of 256 different values and requires eight bits of storage; in DNA each position along a strand can have any one of four different bases and therefore contains two bits of information; a codon (three bases) contains six bits of information. Information is the negative of entropy, as defined in statistical physics, and so is sometimes called negentropy.

information retrieval the processes by which the specific item desired is searched for and recovered from a large computer data base.

information theory a mathematical theory, used in communications and statistics, that deals with the transmission of messages over communication channels affected with random noise and with error-correcting codes that permit the maximal possible rate of transmission for a specified noise level and error rate.

infra- (in′frah) [L. *infra* beneath] a prefix word element to denote below or inferior to, e.g., infrasonic.

infraaxillary (in″frah-ak′sĭ-lar″e) below the axilla.

infraaxillary region (in″frah-ak′sĭ-lar″e) the region below the axillary region.

infraclavicular (in″frah-klah-vik′u-lar) beneath the clavicle.

infraclavicular region the region of the front of the chest immediately below the clavicle.

infracostal (in″frah-kos′tal) see *subcostal.*

infracostal line see *subcostal line.*

inframammary (in″frah-mam′ah-re) below the mammary gland.

inframammary region the region of the front of the chest that extends from the mammary region down to the level of the lower end of the body of the sternum.

infraorbital (in″frah-or′bĭ-tal) lying under or on the floor of the orbit.

infraorbital line the line that passes across the lowest points of the bony ridges beneath both eyes (the inferior margins of the orbits), used in radiographic positioning.

infraorbital region the region on either side of the face below the eye and lateral to the nose.

infraorbitomeatal line (in″frah-or″bĭ-to-me-a′tal) the line passing through the bony ridge beneath the eye (infraorbital margin) and the center of the opening of the ear (external auditory meatus), used in radiographic positioning.

infrared (IR) (in-frah-red′) pertaining to electromagnetic radiation with wavelengths between 770 and 12,000 nm. It is absorbed by molecules, changing their vibration or rotation, and is felt as heat.

infrared CO_2 analyzer an instrument that is used to continuously monitor the CO_2 concentration in a sample of respiratory gas. The analysis of CO_2 concentration is based on the principle that molecules of CO_2 absorb energy from a specific portion of the infrared spectrum. It is commonly used in exercise physiology, pulmonary function tests, animal research, patient intensive care, and the monitoring of anesthetized patients.

infrared spectroscopy the measurement of the extent to which a substance absorbs infrared radiation as a function of the wavelength frequency or energy of that radiation. (The term usually refers to infrared absorption spectroscopy, although infrared emission spectroscopy is also possible.) When a substance absorbs infrared radiation, vibrational motion is excited. Because individual functional groups may absorb at characteristic group frequencies, infrared spectroscopy plays an important role in structure determination. It is also used as a criterion for purity and in the quantitative analysis of mixtures.

infrascapular (in″frah-skap′u-lar) beneath the scapula.

infrascapular line the horizontal line on the surface of the back at the level of the inferior angles of the scapulae, used in radiographic positioning.

infrascapular region the region of either side of the back that extends from the inferior angle of the scapular region down to the twelfth rib.

infraspinous (in″frah-spi′nus) beneath the spine of the scapula.

infundibulum (in″fun-dib′u-lum), pl. *infundibula* [L. "funnel"] [NA], a general term used to designate a funnel-shaped passage.

i. of heart, see *c. arteriosus* under *conus.*

i. of hypophysis, an embryologic downgrowth from the floor of the developing fourth ventricle that develops into the stalk and posterior lobe of the pituitary gland. See also *hypophysis.*

i. of uterine tube, the expanded outer end of the uterine tube that opens into the peritoneal cavity near the ovary.

infusion (in-fu′zhun) 1. [L. *infusio;* from *in* into + *fundere* to pour], the steeping of a substance in water to obtain its soluble principles. See also *culture media.*

2. [L. *infusum,* gen. *infusi*], a solution obtained by steeping a substance in water.

3. the therapeutic introduction by gravity of a fluid other than blood into a vein, e.g., saline. Cf. *injection, instillation,* and *insufflation.*

ingestion (in-jes′chun) the taking into the stomach of food, drugs, foreign bodies, or poisons. Conventionally, ingestion refers to the entry of substances into the stomach by swallowing; technically, however, it also includes entry via gastrostomy or nasogastric tube.

inguin/o (ing′gwĭ-no) [L. *inguen* groin] a word element used in combining form to denote the groin, e.g., inguinofemoral.

inguinal canal a channel that extends from the superficial to the deep inguinal ring parallel to and above the inguinal ligament. It gives passage to the spermatic cord in the male, the round ligament in the female, and the ilioinguinal nerve in both sexes.

inguinal region (ing′gwĭ-nal) [L. *inguinalis*] 1. a region on the left or right side of the pubic or hypogastric region.

2. a region of the abdomen below the transtubercular plane and to the outside of a lateral sagittal plane, used in radiographic positioning.

Also called *iliac region.* See illustration under *abdominal regions.*

inguinal ring an aperture in one of the layers of the abdominal wall through which the spermatic cord or round ligament passes.

deep i. r., an oval opening, located in the fascia transversalis between the symphysis pubis and anterior superior spine of the ilium, which serves as a safety valve to disperse pressure when the intraabdominal pressure is raised.

superficial i. r., a cleft in the aponeurosis of the external oblique muscle lateral to the pubic crest. It is a larger structure in males than in females, and the spermatic cord passes through it. In females it encloses the round ligament of the uterus.

INH abbrev. for isonicotinic acid hydrazide. See *isoniazid.*

inhalation (in″hah-la′shun) [L. *inhalatio*] 1. the drawing into the lungs of air, mists, vapors, and suspended particulates by breathing.

2. a drug that is inhaled as a vapor or as a nebulized mist, now more often referred to as an inhaled aerosol.

inhalation therapy the former name for *respiratory therapy.*

inherent (in-hēr′ent) [L. *inhaerens* sticking fast] implanted by nature; intrinsic; innate.

inherent filter see *inherent f.* under *filter.*

inheritance (in-her′ĭ-tans) 1. the transmission from parents to offspring of genetically influenced traits, characteristics, or diseases.

2. the traits that are inherited. See also *character.*

autosomal dominant i., the mendelian inheritance of an autosomal dominant trait. For a rare genetic defect, the usual pattern of inheritance is the mating of an affected heterozygote Aa with a normal homozygote aa. On the average, 50 percent of the children are normal (aa) and 50 percent abnormal (Aa).

Autosomal dominant inheritance is recognized by the following criteria: the trait is transmitted to half the children of each affected individual; unaffected individuals do not transmit the trait, so the trait appears in an unbroken sequence of generations with no skips; and males and females are equally likely to have and to transmit the trait. Many dominant traits are not fully penetrant, so the ideal pattern may not be apparent.

autosomal recessive i., the mendelian inheritance of an autosomal recessive trait. For a rare genetic defect, the usual pattern of inheritance is the mating of two normal carriers (Aa). On the average, 25 percent of the children are normal (AA), 50 percent are carriers (Aa), and the other 25 percent are affected with the trait (aa).

Autosomal recessive inheritance is recognized by the following criteria: usually only siblings are affected, not their parents or offspring. The recurrence risk (of the defect occurring in a sibling of an affected child of unaffected parents) is 25 percent, with males and females equally likely to have and to transmit the trait. Parental consanguinity increases the likelihood of the appearance of an autosomal recessive trait.

codominant i., the pattern of mendelian inheritance observed when both allelic genes are expressed in the heterozygote. An example is the ABO blood group; type AB individuals produce both A and B red cell antigens. Also called *intermediate i.*

cytoplasmic i., see *extrachromosomal i.*

extrachromosomal i., the inheritance of traits controlled by genes located on the DNA of cytoplasmic organelles (in humans, mitochondria). Being transmitted in the mitochondria of the ooplasm, the extrachromosomal genes are inherited entirely from the mother. Extrachromosomal inheritance is nonmendelian. The many mitochondria of a cell may not be genetically identical nor are they evenly distributed to daughter cells in cell division. Also called *cytoplasmic i.* and *maternal i.*

intermediate i., see *codominant i.*

maternal i., see *extrachromosomal i.*

mendelian i., the pattern of inheritance according to Mendel's laws, exhibited by independent genetic traits controlled by single genes. In the simplest case of a single autosomal gene with two alleles A (dominant) and a (recessive), there are three genotypes: AA, aa (homozygotes), and Aa (heterozygote); and two phenotypes: the dominant trait (exhibited by AA and Aa) and the recessive trait (exhibited by aa).

In a mating of two known genotypes wx and yz, the four possible combinations of one gene from each parent (wy, wz, xy, and xz) occur with equal frequency in the progeny.

In Mendel's original experiments, two pure strains, AA and aa, were crossed, producing progeny (the F_1 generation) all of which had genotype Aa and the dominant phenotype. Then the Aa hybrids were crossed, producing progeny (the F_2 generation) in which the genotypes AA, Aa, and aa occurred in a 1:2:1 ratio and the dominant and recessive traits in a 3:1 ratio.

In crossing pure strains for two traits, AABB and aabb, which produces a dihybrid F_1 generation AaBb, and in crossing the hybrids, Mendel also observed that the characters assorted independently, producing in the F_2 generation the phenotype ratios AB:Ab:aB:ab of 9:3:3:1. This independent assortment is now known to occur only when the two genes are on different chromosomes (not linked).

See also *Mendel's laws.*

multifactorial i., a term used to describe the etiology of a number of diseases that cluster in families. Environmental factors, random factors, major genes, and polygenes each contribute to the pathogenesis.

polygenic i., the inheritance pattern of a polygenic character; a continuously variable phenotype character that is controlled by the combined effects of many genes, e.g., total fingerprint ridge count. If the effects of the genes are additive and roughly the same size, the correlation of the trait in two relatives as measured by the correlation coefficient is equal to their coefficient of relationship (the fraction of genes they have inherited from common ancestors), e.g., one for monozygotic twins, one-half for other siblings or for a parent and child, etc. Thus, the average value of the character in offspring is halfway between the average of the parents. The actual observed values show that if the midparent value is far above or below the population mean, the offspring value will tend to the mean (regression on the mean), a phenomenon explained by interactions between genes and the environment. Also called *quantitative i.* See also *multifactorial i.* and *quasicontinuous i.*

quantitative i., see *polygenic i.*

quasicontinuous i., the multifactorial inheritance of a trait, such as infantile pyloric stenosis, in which there is an underlying continuous variation but no expression of the trait unless some threshold value is exceeded. In many such traits, the threshold is higher in one sex than in the other; the recurrence risk is therefore higher if the propositus is of the less susceptible sex (and is likely to have a more extreme underlying variation).

X-linked dominant i., the mendelian inheritance of an X-linked dominant trait, such as familial hypophosphatemia. Having only one X chromosome, males are either normal (genotype X_a Y) or affected hemizygotes (genotype X_A Y).

All progeny of an affected male and a normal female will be affected, the sons being X_A Y and the daughters X_A X_a, whereas in the progeny of an affected female X_A X_a heterozygote and a normal male, on the average half the children of either sex will be affected and half normal. These will be the usual mating types for a rare genetic defect. All progeny of an affected female homozygote will be affected.

X-linked dominant inheritance is demonstrated only in the progeny of affected males; in the progeny of affected females, the pattern of inheritance is the same as for autosomal dominant inheritance. Males are affected with the frequency P with which the gene occurs in the population. The ratio of affected females to affected males is $2 - P$ to 1 or about 2:1 for rare traits.

X-linked recessive i., the mendelian inheritance of an X-linked recessive trait, such as hemophilia A. Males are either normal (genotype X_A Y) or affected (genotype X_a Y) hemizygotes.

In the progeny of an affected male and a normal female, all sons will be normal (X_A Y) and all daughters will be carriers (X_A X_a heterozygotes), whereas in the progeny of a carrier female with a normal male, on the average half the daughters will be normal (X_A X_A) and half carriers (X_A X_a), and half the sons will be normal (X_A Y) and half affected (X_a Y). For a rare trait these will be the common inheritance patterns.

X-linked recessive inheritance is recognized by the following criteria: there is a much higher incidence of the trait in males (being affected with the frequency P with which the gene occurs (by the Hardy-Weinberg law), whereas females are affected with frequency P^2); an affected father never transmits the trait to his son but transmits the trait through all his daughters (who are carriers) to half of their sons; and affected males are related through females.

inhibit (in-hib′it) to retard, arrest, or restrain.

inhibition (in″hĭ-bish′un) [L. *inhibere* to restrain; *in* in + *habere* to have] the arrest or restraint of a process or function. See also *enzyme.*

inhibitor (in-hib′ĭ-tor) any substance that interferes with a chemical reaction, growth, or other biologic activity, e.g., a negative activator or catalyst (a substance that reduces the rate of a chemical reaction), an enzyme inhibitor (a substance that reduces the activity of an enzyme), or a biologic antagonist (which inhibits the growth of microorganisms or tissue cultures).

α_1-inhibitor see *alpha$_1$-globulin.*

inhibitor assay a test for Factor VIII inhibitor. Serial dilutions of the abnormal plasma together with normal plasma are incubated for 2 hr and the residual amount of Factor VIII measured. A reduction to 50 percent of the amount of Factor VIII in the normal plasma is 1 Bethesda unit. Similar methodology can be used for measurements of other specific inhibitors.

inion (in′e-on) [Gr. "the back of the head"] [NA], the point of the external occipital protuberance, the point in the midsagittal plane at the lower rear of the skull, used as an anatomic landmark.

initialization (ĭ-nish″al-ĭ-za′shun) a part of a computer program that sets the starting values of such things as counters, variables, and pointers, either before entering a loop or at the beginning of a subroutine.

initiation (ĭ-nish″e-a′shun) [L. *initialis,* from *initium* beginning] 1. the beginning of protein synthesis, involving messenger RNA (mRNA) codons, aminoacyl transfer RNA (tRNA) anticodons, initiation factors, and *N*-formyl methione in prokaryotes and methionine in eukaryotes. The codon that signals initiation is AUG. See also *start codon* and *translation.*

2. the beginning of RNA synthesis. In prokaryotes, it involves promoter recognition, the sigma factor (σ) of the core polymerase, and binding sites for RNA polymerase. See also *transcription.*

initiation codon see *start codon.*

initiation factor a complex of specific proteins involved in the beginning of synthesis of a polypeptide on a ribosomal messenger RNA (mRNA) complex. Initiator transfer RNA (tRNA), carrying a methionyl (or *N*-formyl methionyl) group, a molecule of guanosine triphosphate (GTP), and the initiation factors, forms a complex that fits on a particular location on a light ribosomal subunit. Enzymatic hydrolysis of GTP → GDP + P_i results in a conformational change in the initiation factor, its release, and binding of a heavy ribosomal subunit to form a complete ribosome with attached methionyl (or *N*-formyl methionyl) tRNA.

injection (in-jek′shun) [L. *injectio,* from *in* into + *jacere* to throw] 1. the introduction of a fluid into a part, as into the subcutaneous tissues, the vascular tree, or an organ, usually by means of a syringe or other device connected to a hollow needle. Cf. *infusion.*

2. the solution so administered; in pharmacy, a solution of a medicinal substance suitable for an injection.

3. the condition of being injected; congested.

innervation (in″er-va′shun) [L. *in* into + *nervus* nerve] the distribution or supply of nerves to a part of the body, a particular tissue, or a cell.

double i., the innervation of a part of the body by two kinds of nerve fibers, e.g., sympathetic and parasympathetic.

reciprocal i., the balanced innervation of the muscles around a joint, so that when a particular muscle is excited its antagonist is inhibited.

innidiation (ĭ-nid″e-a′shun) [L. *in* into + *nidus* nest] the growth and development of cells in an area to which they have gained access through metastatic spread.

innominate (ĭ-nom′ĭ-nāt) [L. *innominatus,* from *in* not + *nomen* name] nameless; not having a name. The term is applied to certain structures better identified by their descriptive names, as in the innominate (brachiocephalic) artery and the innominate (hip) bone.

Innovar (in′o-var) trademark for a narcoleptoanalgesic that is a combination of *droperidol* and *fentanyl citrate.*

inochondritis (in″o-kon-dri′tis) [*ino-* + Gr. *chondros* cartilage + *-itis* inflammation] an inflammation of a fibrocartilage, often due to trauma or injury.

inoculate (ĭ-nok′u-lāt) [L. *in* into + *oculus* bud] to introduce microbial material or tissue cells on or into a medium for the purpose of multiplication and differentiation.

inoculation (ĭ-nok″u-la′shun) [L. *inoculatio*] the introduction of microbial material or tissue cells on or into a medium for the purpose of multiplication and differentiation.

Microorganisms are placed on solid media (e.g., agar, tissue) or into liquid media (e.g., nutrient broth, serum). Tissue cells are inoculated into chemically defined basal media fortified with serum, embryo extract, and/or conditioned medium (medium in which cells have been previously grown but not to the point of nutrient exhaustion). Tissue culture vessels are occasionally lined with collagen or gelatin.

Attenuated and inactive infectious agents can be inoculated into living organisms for the purpose of examining immune response, and to induce antibody formation and specific cellular responses in order to establish resistance to an infectious disease.

See also *vaccination.*

inoculum (ĭ-nok′u-lum), pl. *inocula* [L.] the material used to inoculate a medium. Microorganisms are commonly introduced on a metal needle, loop, or cotton swab. Liquid cultures and tissue cells are transferred in larger volume by pipet or syringe.

inorganic (in″or-gan′ik) [L. *in* not + *organicus* organic] 1. not involving living organisms.

2. pertaining to matter that is not part of and was not produced by living organisms.

3. the chemistry of all the elements (including carbon) and their compounds except the large class of carbon compounds called hydrocarbons and their derivatives. The borderline between organic and inorganic chemistry is not clear; organometallic compounds, for example, belong to both areas.

inorganic acid an acid that contains no carbon atoms, e.g., HNO_3.

inorganic phosphate (P_i) (in″or-gan′ik fos′fāt) any salt of phosphoric acid (orthophosphoric acid); H_3PO_4; it includes the several forms of partly or fully ionized species of phosphoric acids, ubiquitously and abundantly present in biologic materials. In mammals, the P_i is present primarily in the extracellular fluid in the form of HPO_4^{2-} and $H_2PO_4^-$, in the ratio of approximately 4:1 at a pH of approximately 7.40. This ratio may change to as much as 1:100 at a pH of 4.5, which may be observed in urine. Also called inorganic orthophosphate.

inorganic pyrophosphatase an enzyme of the hydrolase class (EC 3.6.1.1) that catalyzes the reaction pyrophosphate (PP_i) + H_2O ⇄ 2 orthophosphate (P_i). The enzyme occurs widely in body tissues and functions in the regulation of endogenous pyrophosphate concentration. Alkaline phosphatase (EC 3.1.3.1) possesses pyrophosphatase activity at about pH 7.4, and it is possible that pyrophosphatase activity in some tissues may be identical with the phosphatase activity.

inorganic pyrophosphate (PP_i) (in″or-gan′ik pi″ro-fos′fāt) any salt of pyrophosphoric acid ($H_4P_2O_7$). The most abundant ionic form at pH 7.4 is $HP_2O_7^{3-}$. PP_i is formed in numerous reactions involving ATP as a substrate and in which AMP + PP_i are ultimately formed.

inosine (I) (in′o-sin) a nucleoside, hypoxanthine riboside, $C_{10}H_{12}N_4O_5$, a crystalline compound obtainable by the hydrolysis of inosine-5′-phosphate or the deamination of adenosine. It is an intermediate in the pathway by which purine derivatives are converted and also in the purine salvage cycle. The compound is present in meat extracts and sugar beets.

inosine diphosphate (IDP) (in′o-sin di-fos′fāt) a compound that has both a product and a precursor relationship with inosine triphosphate (ITP). It is formed hydrolytically from ITP.

inosine monophosphate (in′o-sin mon″o-fos′fāt) see *inosine-5′-phosphate.*

inosine-5′-phosphate (IMP) (in′o-sin fos′fāt) a mononucleotide formed from hypoxanthine, ribose, and phosphoric acid. It is a deamination product of adenylic acid on the pathway to uric acid. It is also found in tissues and in some nucleic acids, and occurs as an intermediate in the de novo synthesis of the purine nucleotides AMP and GMP. Also called *inosine monophosphate* and *inosinic acid.* See also under *nucleotide.*

inosine phosphorylase (IP) (in′o-sin fos-for′ĭ-lās) see *purine nucleoside phosphorylase.*

inosine triphosphate (ITP) (in′o-sin tri-fos′fāt) an energy-rich compound analogous to adenosine triphosphate that is involved in metabolic reactions.

inosinic acid (in″o-si′nik) see *inosine-5′-phosphate.*

inositol (in-o′sĭ-tol) hexahydroxycyclohexane; M.W. 180.16. Inositol is a crystalline sugarlike substance that is widely distributed in plant and animal cells and occurs as phytic acid in corn. It is a member of the vitamin B complex and serves as an essential growth factor for fibroblasts, some cell cultures, yeasts, some animals, and various microorganisms. It is active as a lipotropic agent.

inositol hexaphosphate (in-o′sĭ-tol hek″sa-fos′fāt) see *phytic acid.*

inotropic (in″o-trop′ik) [*ino-* + Gr. *tropos* a turning] affecting the force or energy of muscular contractions. An increase in the strength of contraction is a positive inotropic effect; for example, a positive inotropic agent working on the heart increases the strength of contraction of the heart. A decrease in the strength of contraction is a negative inotropic effect.

inpatient (in′pa-shent) a patient who is hospitalized.

input (in′put) 1. any information fed into a computer or the process of feeding this information.

2. an electrical signal that is fed into an electrical circuit or the terminals across which this signal is applied.

Cf. *output.*

input/output (I/O) referring to the transfer of data between a computer and its peripherals (such as printers, keyboards, mass storage). I/O operations usually are relatively time-consuming.

input terminal 1 the input terminal of the differential amplifier of an electroencephalograph that, when electronegative relative to the other input terminal, produces an upward deflection of the recording pen. Formerly called *black lead* and *Grid 1.*

input terminal 2 the input terminal of the differential amplifier of an electroencephalograph that, when electronegative relative to the other input terminal, produces a downward deflection of the recording pen. Formerly called *Grid 2* and *white lead.*

inquiry (in-kwir′e) in automatic data processing, a request for the retrieval of an item of information entered into a computer by a user at a terminal.

inscription (in-skrip′shun) [L. *inscriptio,* from *in* upon + *scribere* to write] see under *prescription.*

insecticide (in-sek′tĭ-sīd) [L. *insectum* insect + *caedere* to kill] a pesticide used to kill or control insects. See also *pesticide.*

insertion (in-ser′shun) [L. *insertio,* from *in* into + *serere to join*] 1. the act of implanting, or the condition of being implanted.

2. a place of attachment, as of muscle to bone.

3. see *insertional translocation.*

parasol i., a form of insertion of the umbilical cord to the placenta, in which the vessels of the cord separate before they join the placenta and simulate the ribs of a parasol.

velamentous i., attachment of the umbilical cord directly to the fetal membranes. See also *placenta.*

insertional activity (in-ser′shun-al) the burst of electrical activity (injury potentials) produced by the mechanical activation of the muscle cell membrane that occurs with insertion or movement of a needle electrode. In normal muscle, insertional activity generally ends abruptly when the movement is ceased. Insertional activity that is reduced, absent, or prolonged, or that is accompanied by fibrillation potentials or positive sharp waves, is characteristic of a variety of neuromuscular disorders.

insertional translocation a chromosomal aberration in which a broken piece of one chromosome is inserted between portions of nonhomologous chromosomes. This requires three chromosome breaks and subsequent repairs.

insertion sequence a type of transposable element that inactivates the gene in which it is inserted. Insertion sequences (700–1400 base pairs) are smaller than transposons and are flanked by short (five to nine bases) direct repeats of host sequences. See also *bacterial g.* under *genetics, transposable element,* and *transposon.*

in situ (in si′tu) [L.] in the natural or normal place; confined to the site of origin without invasion of neighboring tissues.

insol (in-sol′) abbrev. See *insoluble.*

insoluble (insol) (in-sol′u-b′l) [L. *insolubilis, from in* not + *solvere* to dissolve] not soluble in a given solvent. There is no quantitative definition of the limit at which a substance is considered insoluble. In organic chemistry, a substance that has a solubility of less than 3 g in 100 g of solvent may be considered insoluble; in toxicology, the limit is at less than one part in 10,000 parts of solvent.

insomnia (in-som′ne-ah) [L. *in* not + *somnus* sleep + *-ia*] a group of disorders characterized by difficulty in initiating and/or maintaining sleep. The normal organization of sleep stages is disrupted, and there may be abnormal associated electroencephalographic patterns, including spindles occurring during rapid eye movement (REM) sleep, rapid eye movements during Stage 2 sleep, and alpha-delta sleep patterns during non-REM sleep.

Insomnia is a frequent complaint of individuals with psychiatric disorders, including anxiety, depression, mania, and psychoses. Primary insomnia occurs in those who do not display symptoms of psychiatric or other medical disorders but who experience unrestful sleep consisting of low arousal threshold, decreased REM sleep, and increased Stage 2 sleep. Treatment may include the prescription of drugs, the type (hypnotic or barbiturate) and dosage depending on the form of insomnia.

insonation (in″so-na′shun) the application of sound or ultrasound to an object.

inspiration (in′spĭ-ra′shun) [L. *inspirare,* from *in* in + *spirare* to breathe] the act of drawing air into the lungs, or breathing in. During a quiet spontaneous inspiration (tidal volume), descending impulses from the medullary inspiratory center (via the phrenic and intercostal nerves) excite the diaphragm and external intercostal muscles to contract. Descent of the convex (when quiescent) diaphragm on contraction increases the vertical dimension of the thoracic cavity. Contraction of the external intercostal muscles increases the anteroposterior and transverse diameters of the thoracic cage. Intrathoracic volume is thus increased by enlargement in three dimensions. As intrathoracic volume increases with expansion of the thoracic cage, the intimate contact between the parietal pleura lining the thorax and the visceral pleura covering the lungs allows for a decrease in intrapleural pressure to a more subatmospheric value (from –2.5 to – 6 torr), expansion of the lungs (the alveoli, alveolar ducts, and bronchioles), and, as the alveolar gas expands, a decrease in its pressure to subatmospheric values (Boyle's law). Air (at atmospheric pressure) flows into the respiratory passages down the pressure gradient thus created. At the end of inspiration, airflow ceases as intraalveolar pressure equalizes with atmospheric pressure.

During the initial stages of an inspiration from residual volume in the standing position, more of the inspired volume goes to the apices than to the bases of the lungs (owing to gravitational forces, transpulmonary pressure is higher in the apices and airway diameter is greater relative to the bases). The lung bases fill preferentially late in the inspiratory effort.

During a forced inspiration (in which minute volume is increased to a minimum of 50–100 l/min), the auxiliary inspiratory muscles (the posterior neck and back muscles; the sternocleidomastoid, mylohyoid, alae nasi, digastric, levator palatini, and platysma; and the cheek, tongue, and laryngeal muscles) aid in inspiration by further enlarging the thorax and/or reducing the resistance to airflow. Maximal contraction of all the inspiratory muscles can decrease intrapleural pressure to a subatmospheric value of as much as –60 to –100 torr.

Cf. *expiration.*

inspiratory (in-spi′rah-to″re) pertaining to or occurring during inspiration.

inspiratory capacity (IC) the volume of gas (3600 ml in the healthy young adult male) that can be forcibly inspired, beginning at the resting and end-expiratory level, and distending the lungs to the maximal degree. It is equal to the sum of the tidal and inspiratory reserve volumes.

inspiratory reserve volume (IRV) the additional volume of gas that can be forcibly inspired from any end-tidal inspiratory position; it usually amounts to 3000 ml in the normal young adult male.

inspire (in-spīr′) to draw air into the lungs; to breathe in; to inhale.

inspissated (in-spis′āt-ed) [L. *inspissatus,* from *in* intensive + *spissare* to thicken] to make thick and viscous. The term often refers to body fluids that become dried, viscid, and less fluid, often plugging a duct or gland.

inspissation (in″spis-sa′shun) [L. *inspissatio*] the process of thickening by the evaporation of vaporizable fluid.

instability (in″stah-bil′ĭ-te) 1. an undesired oscillation of the output of a control system or amplifier caused by excessive positive feedback.

2. an undesired drift in the characteristics of an electronic component or instrument that is not related to operating conditions.

instillation (in″stil-la′shun) [L. *instillatio,* from *in* into + *stillare* to drop] the dropping of a liquid into a cavity, as into the eye.

Institute of Electrical and Electronic Engineers (IEEE) a professional organization for the advancement of electronics, electrical engineering, and related branches of science and technology.

instruction (in-struk′shun) a code, stored in memory, that tells a computer what operation to perform and the location of the operands. See also *machine language.*

instruction set a computer's repertoire of instructions: all the operations that the computer hardware can carry out in the execution of a single instruction.

instrument (in′stroo-ment) [L. *instrumentum* implement, tool] any tool, device, or appliance, particularly any electronic device used to measure or control a process.

instrumentation (in″stroo-men-ta′shun) the use of instruments; work performed by instruments. The term includes equipment or devices that automatically perform some measurement or control process or indicate the results of measurements. See also *blood cell count automation, clinical chemistry automation, cytometry, differential leukocyte count automation, microbiology automation,* and *radioimmunoassay automation.*

insufficiency (in″sŭ-fish′en-se) [L. *insufficientia,* from *in* not + *sufficiens* sufficient] a condition in which an organ is not able to fulfill its innate physiologic role; a functional inability.

aortic i., see *aortic regurgitation.*

circulatory i., the inability of the circulatory system to perform its physiologic role. The defect may be in the heart (cardiac), coronary vessels (coronary), valves of the heart, or valves of the veins. In the valves of the heart, this condition leads to blood backflow (regurgitation); in the valves of the veins, it leads to edema.

mitral i., see *mitral regurgitation.*

respiratory i., the condition in which the respiratory system is unable to meet the demands placed on it. The causes are varied and include injury, disease (such as pneumonia and emphysema), and increased physical activity.

tricuspid i., see *tricuspid regurgitation.*

velopharyngeal i., defective speech, seen in cleft palate or muscular dysfunction, that results from the failure of velopharyngeal closure. Also called palatopharyngeal incompetence.

insufflation (in″sŭ-fla′shun) [L. *in* into + *sufflatio* a blowing up] 1. the introduction of air or gas into a body cavity.

2. a finely powdered solid or atomized liquid drug introduced into the respiratory passages as an aerosol.

perirenal i., the introduction of a gas directly into the perirenal space in order to delineate the kidney and adrenal gland on the side of the injection.

presacral i., the introduction of a gas into the retroperitoneal space by way of the presacral space in order to delineate both kidneys and adrenals.

retroperitoneal gas i., see *presacral i.*

insula (in′su-lah), pl. *insulae* [L. "island"] [NA], a pyramidal elevation on the lateral surface of each cerebral hemisphere. In the intact brain it is hidden from view by the overlapping walls of the lateral sulcus.

insulator (in′su-la″tor) a material having a high electrical or thermal resistance, which is used to prevent the flow of electricity, e.g., glass, or heat.

insulin (in′su-lin) [L. *insula* island (of the pancreas) + *-in*] a protein hormone consisting of 51 amino acids in two chains linked by disulfide bridges; M.W. 5734. It is produced and secreted by the beta cells of the pancreatic islets of Langerhans. The messenger RNA for insulin directs the synthesis of a larger-molecular-weight peptide containing 101 amino acids (pre-proinsulin) which is subsequently cleaved to 84 amino acids to form a substance referred to as proinsulin. The proinsulin contains the A and B chains of insulin linked by a 33–amino acid connecting peptide (C peptide). The connecting peptide is cleaved in the beta cell and released into the circulation together with insulin in equimolar proportions. The connecting peptide has no known biologic function, but it does provide a useful index of insulin secretion in those in whom insulin cannot be measured by immunoassay techniques owing to the presence of antibodies (e.g., most type I diabetics, who are treated with heterologous insulins). The insulins used to treat patients with diabetes are presently obtained from cows and pigs. Procedures that utilize recombinant DNA methodology may provide human insulin for treatment in the near future.

Insulin is involved in the control of carbohydrate metabolism and the maintenance of the blood level of glucose. Elevation of blood glucose levels directly stimulates the release of insulin within a minute; amino acids and fatty acids can also stimulate its release, but only in the presence of glucose. Insulin has an immediate hypoglycemic action, promoting glucose transport into muscle and adipose tissue. In addition, insulin promotes the transport of other monosaccharides, amino acids, nucleosides, potassium, calcium, and inorganic phosphate ions. Insulin also increases glycogenesis, glycogen storage, fatty acid synthesis, and protein synthesis. It directly stimulates the RNA-mediated synthesis of key glycolytic enzymes (e.g., glucokinase) and suppresses the synthesis of gluconeogenic enzymes.

The insufficiency or inefficient utilization of insulin is known as diabetes mellitus; a lack of insulin characterizes juvenile diabetes. Hyperglycemia accompanies both situations.

Reference ranges for insulin (assayed by radio-immunoassay) in plasma are 5–37 μU/ml. See also *diabetes*.

insulin hypoglycemia test a test performed 3–6 mo after vagotomy to confirm the completeness of the nerve division. After a 2-hr determination of basal gastric secretion, a dosage of insulin sufficient to produce hypoglycemia is administered; the gastric secretion is measured for 2 hr (at 15-min intervals) and the blood glucose level is measured at 30-min intervals.

The test is invalid if the blood glucose does not fall below 45 mg/dl. Incomplete vagotomy is suggested by an acid output in the postinsulin 2-hr period that exceeds the output in the basal 2-hr period by 0.5 mmol or by a total acid output greater than 2 mmol/hr.

Also called *Hollander test.* For determination of acid output, see under *gastric function tests.*

insulinlike activity, nonsuppressible (NSILA-s) a polypeptide material that is synthesized and released by nonpancreatic tumors. It does not cross react with antibodies produced against insulin. NSILA-s behaves like insulin in that it binds to insulin receptors, making it measurable by the insulin radioreceptor assay.

insulinoma (in″su-lin-o′mah) a tumor of the beta cells of the pancreatic islets, rarely located outside the pancreas. The cells form insulin, and the patient may suffer from clinical hypoglycemia. Blood glucose levels are below 50 mg/dl, and the symptoms are relieved by administration of glucose. About 10 percent of beta cell tumors metastasize, generally to the liver. The primary tumor may be small and is multicentric: arteriography can be useful in preoperative localization, but when the symptoms are classic, the radioimmunoassay is positive, and no tumor is detectable at surgery, a subtotal pancreatectomy should be performed. See also *pancreatic tumors.*

integral (in′tĕ-gral) 1. an indefinite integral of a function $f(x)$; a function $F(x)$ (symbolized $\int f(x)dx$) whose derivative is $f(x)$. Any function $F(x) + C$, where C is a constant, is also an indefinite integral of $f(x)$.

2. a definite integral of $f(x)$; a number (symbolized $\int_a^b f(x)dx$) equal to $F(b) - F(a)$, where $F(x) = \int f(x)dx$; a and b are called the lower and upper limits of integration.

The definite integral gives the product of the average value of the function between the limits of integration and the distance between the limits; this is equivalent to the area between the graph of $f(x)$ and the x-axis.

Cf. *derivative.*

integral proteins see under *cell membrane.*

integrate (in′tĕ-grāt) to make whole by bringing together the various parts; to unify or unite.

integrated circuit (IC) (in′tĕ-grāt″ed ser′kit) an electronic circuit contained on a minute slab of silicon crystal called a chip. The different electronic components, such as transistors, resistors, and connectors, are made by depositing layers of oxide and various impurities on the silicon chip. The large-scale integration (LSI) process produces chips with thousands of components, such as microprocessors.

integration (in″tĕ-gra′shun) 1. the combining of parts or processes into a harmonious whole.

2. in physiology, anabolism, the building up of tissues.

3. in mathematics, the process of obtaining an integral.

4. in genetics, the process by which genetic material is inserted into the genome.

integrator (in′te-gra″tor) 1. an electrical or mechanical device attached to a chart recorder (as on a gas chromatograph or a densitometer) that measures the area under the peaks on the graph by indicating each unit of area.

2. an electronic circuit that produces an output

waveform approximately the integral of the input waveform, such as a triangular output for a square wave input. A circuit diagram and explanation may be found under *differentiator.*

integument (in-teg′u-ment) [L. *integumentum,* from *in* on + *tegere* to cover] the covering or investment of the body, the skin. It includes the hair, nails, and skin glands.

intelligence (in-tel′ĭ-jens) [L. *intelligere* to understand] the ability to comprehend or understand.

intelligent terminal (in-tel′ĭ-jent) a minicomputer or microcomputer that is used both as a stand-alone small computer and as a remote batch terminal of a large computer system. Also called *smart terminal.*

intelligibility (in-tel″ĭ-jĕ-bil′ĭ-te) the percentage of words that are correctly understood by the listener in an auditory test or in a communication. The intelligibility of words in normal sentences is about 15 percent higher than the intelligibility of isolated words. The term articulation is used for the percentage of correctly understood nonsense syllables.

intensification factor (in-ten″sĭ-fĭ-ka′shun) [L. *intensus* intense + *facere* to make] in radiology, the ratio of the optical densities obtained with a particular film, object, and exposure factor when an intensifying screen is (and is not) being used. Cf. *screen speed.*

intensifying screen (in-ten′sĭ-fi″ing) a flexible sheet coated with phosphors that glows when struck with x-rays. These sheets are placed on each side of the film in a cassette. The film exposure is 10–60 times that which would be caused by the x-rays alone. This lowers the amount of the patient's exposure to radiation and shortens exposure times, which reduces blurring caused by patient motion.

intensity (in-ten′sĭ-te) [L. *intensus* intense, from *in* on + *tendere* to stretch] 1. a high degree of energy, tension, or activity.

2. (abbrev. I), the amount of some physical property, such as electric field intensity or radiation intensity.

3. the power per unit area carried by a wave across a surface, expressed in $J/S \cdot m^2$, for radiation, $rad/s \cdot m^2$, for light, $cd/s \cdot m^2$. Only when the relative intensity is important is the detected or generated power called the intensity, as in a spectrophotometer. For x-rays, the milliamperage may be referred to as intensity if the kilovoltage is not being changed.

inter- (in′ter) [L. *inter* between] a prefix word element to denote between, e.g, interalveolar.

interaction (in″ter-ak′shun) the process of two or more things acting on or with each other.

interaction of radiation with matter the various scattering and absorption processes undergone by particles of ionizing radiation; alpha particles (helium-4 nuclei), electrons (beta particles), photons (x-rays and gamma rays), and positrons.

The primary interactions of alpha particles are Rutherford scattering, ionization, and excitation. Rutherford scattering is the elastic scattering of the alpha particle by the electric field of an atomic nucleus. Some of the particle kinetic energy is transferred to the nucleus and adds heat to the material. Scattering by the electric field of atomic electrons is inelastic; the atom is excited (an electron moves to a higher orbital) or ionized (an electron is entirely removed). In some cases the ejected electron receives enough kinetic energy to create more ion pairs (and is then called a delta ray). The range of alpha particles is roughly proportional to their energy and is inversely proportional to the density of the absorbing material: 3–9 cm in air or 3–9 μm in water or soft tissue for the 3- to 9-MeV particles that are emitted by alpha decays. The specific ionization produced is about 5000 ion pairs per millimeter of air or per micrometer of soft tissue.

Electrons and positrons interact with atoms by the same processes as do alpha particles; the effects are different, however, because of the electron's much smaller mass. In the Rutherford scattering, an appreciable amount of the energy is emitted as bremsstrahlung, which is emitted by all accelerated charges; it consists of x-rays at all energies up to the electron's initial energy. The bremsstrahlung spectrum has a single peak somewhat below the maximal energy. About 1 percent of the electron energy is emitted as bremsstrahlung, whereas 99 percent goes to heating the material. There is less ionization and excitation than with alpha particles. The specific ionization is only about 10–200 ion pairs per millimeter of air. The range is about 10 m in air or 1 mm in soft tissue. Positrons undergo exactly the same processes as do electrons, but after they are stopped, they are annihilated; the positron and an electron are converted to two 511-keV gamma rays emitted simultaneously in opposite directions.

Photons undergo three important processes. In water or soft tissue, the photoelectric effect predominates below about 50 keV, the Compton effect predominates from 50 keV to 15 MeV, and pair production predominates above 15 MeV.

In the photoelectric effect, the photon is absorbed by an atom and an electron is ejected. When an electron drops from a higher orbital to the vacated orbital, a visible, ultraviolet, or x-ray photon is emitted with an energy that is the difference of the energies of the two orbitals. (Atoms ionized or excited by alpha particles or electrons also undergo the same process, but electrons are not ejected from the lowest orbitals and x-rays are not emitted.) The specific ionization produced by this process is only one tenth to one hundredth of that produced by electrons.

Photoelectric absorption is roughly proportional to $(Z/E)^3$, where Z is the atomic number of the atom and E is the photon energy. Thus, the calcium and phosphorus atoms have about 12 times the absorbance of oxygen atoms in water and soft tissue, the iodine and barium atoms in x-ray contrast media have about 290 and 340 times the absorbance, and lead atoms 1000 times the absorbance.

The exact relation is more complicated. A photon can ionize an atom only by removing an electron with a lower binding energy than the photon energy. As the photon energy increases, there is a large jump in absorption at the binding energy of an atomic energy level. This jump is called the K (L, etc.) absorption edge for the K (L, etc.) level. Above and below the absorption edge, the absorption falls off as the third power of the energy.

Compton scattering is the elastic scattering of a photon by a free electron (or by a valence electron with a binding energy that is negligible compared with that of the photon). Only a fraction of the photon energy is transferred to the electron. The Compton scattering is roughly independent of Z and inversely proportional to E.

Pair production is the conversion of a photon to an electron-positron pair by interaction with the strong electric field near a nucleus. The photon energy must be above 1.02 MeV, the rest energy (mass) of the created particles. Energy in excess of 1.02 MeV is converted to kinetic energy of the particles. The pair production absorption is roughly proportional to $Z \times E$.

interactive processing (in″ter-ak′tiv) the execution of a computer program with interaction between the program and the user. As specified by the program, the computer displays questions or intermediate data on the screen of the user's terminal and waits for a response, which the program uses as input. (In a time-sharing system, other programs are run simultaneously.)

inter-alpha-globulin (in′ter al′fah glob′u-lin) thyroxine binding globulin that has an electrophoretic mobility between that of $alpha_1$- and $alpha_2$-globulins. The term is no longer widely used. See also *thyroxine-binding globulin.*

interband (in″ter-band′) the region between two bands of a chromosome.

intercalary (in-ter′kah-ler″e) [L. *intercalarius,* from *inter-* + *calare* to call] inserted or placed between; interposed.

intercalary deletion see under *deletion.*

intercalate (in-ter′kah-lāt) to insert between.

intercalated disk (in-ter″kah-la′ted) a junctional complex at which the cells of cardiac muscle are attached end to end. See also *muscle.*

intercalated duct the slender initial portion of a duct situated between the acinus and the secretory duct.

intercellular situated or occurring outside of or between cells. Cf. *intracellular.*

intercellular bridge a misnomer for the attachment sites between cells of stratified squamous epithelium, so-called because of an illusion of cytoplasmic continuity at the light microscope level. Ultrastructural examination confirms that these strands between adjacent cells are formed by protrusions of cytoplasm united by desmosomes.

intercellular canaliculus (kan″ah-lik′u-lus) a canal that connects the side of an epithelial cell with a duct or lumen of the organ. See also *bile canaliculus.*

intercellular cement a hypothetical substance formerly thought to glue epithelial cells together. See also *cell j.* under *junction.*

interchange (in′ter-chānj) see *interchromosomal aberration.*

interchromosomal aberration (in″ter-kro″mo-so′mal) the exchange of segments between nonhomologous chromosomes; a reciprocal translocation. Also called *heterosomal aberration* and *interchange.* Cf. *intrachromosomal aberration.*

intercostal (in″ter-kos′tal) [*inter-* + L. *costa* rib] situated between the ribs.

intercristal (in″ter-kris′tal) [*inter-* + L. *crista* ridge] between two crests.

intercristal space the space enclosed within the inner membrane of a mitochondrion. It contains the mitochondrial matrix. Cf. *intramembranous space.*

interelectrode distance (in″ter-e-lek′trōd) [*inter-* + Gr. *ēlektron* amber + *hodos* way] in electrophysiology, the distance between a pair of electrodes.

interface (in′ter-fās) 1. in chemistry, the surface that separates two phases of a heterogeneous system, as between a liquid and a gas or between two immiscible liquids.

2. in a computer, the connection or connections between two subsystems, or a special circuit required to change data from one form to another at such a connection.

interfacial canal (in″ter-fāsh′e-al) an intercellular space between epithelial cells. See also *mesothelium.*

interference (in″ter-fēr′ens) [*inter-* + L. *ferire* to strike] 1. the interaction of two waves such as light or sound. Where the waves are in phase, the amplitude is combined; where they are out of phase, they cancel each other.

2. the collision of the depolarization waves from two different pacemakers in the heart, which produces fusion beats.

3. see *chemical interference.*

constructive i., interference between two coherent waves that are in phase so that the amplitudes add, as occurs when a beam of light is split and recombined and the path length difference is a multiple of the wavelength.

destructive i., interference between two coherent waves that are out of phase so that they cancel each other.

interference filter 1. an optical filter that removes wavelengths of light by utilizing interference phenomena instead of scattering or absorption. See also *interference m.* under *microscope.*

2. a filter that stops interference from entering a receiver through its power line, or one that stops unwanted carrier signals in the tuned circuits of the receiver itself.

interference pattern a pattern of electrical activity that can be recorded from a muscle during maximal voluntary contraction. The number of activated motor units, which fire asynchronously, is so great that individual potentials overlap and cannot be identified.

In the normal situation, when a full interference pattern occurs, the baseline of the recording is continuously disrupted by the overlapping potentials. In disorders affecting the motor neuron, the density of the interference pattern can be reduced to such a degree that some individual motor unit potentials can be seen. If this reduction is significant enough to allow identification of each potential, the recorded electrical activity is referred to as discrete. This parameter should be specified, as the interference pattern varies with the forces of the voluntary contraction.

interferon (in″ter-fēr′on) a class of proteins that inhibits viral multiplication. It was discovered in 1957 by Isaacs and Lindemann, who infected chick embryo cells with inactivated influenza virus and found that, free of virus, the supernatant fluid protected fresh chick embryo cells from infection with influenza virus. Interferon was initially considered important only for its antiviral activity. It was described as a protein produced and released by essentially *all* viral infected cells but protecting only the cells of the species from which it was derived. Thus, there is human interferon, chicken interferon, and so forth; the interferon derived from each of these species protects their own cells against infection with all viruses. There are some exceptions—human interferon does protect the cells of some other mammalian species.

It has since been found that cells are coded to produce many species of interferons, and the family of interferons has a far broader range of activity than just antiviral action. Although the various interferon species differ in their antigenicity and molecular weight, all have a similar range of biologic activity, with some significant quantitative differences. The family of interferons not only inhibits viral replication but also the growth of some neoplastic cells.

In addition, interferon has an important regulatory role in the immune response that is apparently directed toward enhancing cellular immunity rather than the production of more antibody. Immune interferon affects the immune response in opposite ways: it suppresses B lymphocytes, the producers of antibody; conversely, it stimulates the activity of T lymphocytes and monocytes, and the cytotoxicity of natural killer (NK) cells. NK cells are normally present in the blood and spleen; their exact cellular lineage is not known, as they have properties of both lymphocytes and monocytes. The interferons are unusually potent compounds, for as few as 15–20 molecules effect biologic changes in cells.

Procedure Assay. When dilute suspensions of virus particles are added to a sheet of susceptible cells, they settle as isolated particles and grow and destroy cells, leaving readily detected, isolated, clear areas called plaques. The addition of interferon to a sheet of cells before virus is added inhibits viral replication, and the number of plaques is reduced.

A unit of interferon is defined as the highest dilution of interferon in a specific preparation that effects a 50 percent reduction in the number of plaques. Thus, if an interferon preparation is diluted out to a 10^{-6} dilution and reduces the number of plaques by half, the interferon preparation is said to have 10^{6} units of interferon per milligram or 10^{12} units per kilogram. The preparations of human leukocyte interferon used in clinical studies (see below) had a concentration of approximately 10^{6} units/mg. Purified interferon has a titer of 10^{8}–10^{9} units/ml. The availability of purified interferon made by recombinant DNA procedure should give adequate supplies of interferon containing 10^{9} units/mg.

Production of Human Interferon. Interferons are classified as Type 1 or Type 2, based on the cell source and the stimulus used to activate the cell to make interferon. Type 1 interferon obtained from viral activated human leukocytes and diploid fibroblasts was used in the studies summarized herein. Type 2 interferon, immune interferon, has not been used in any clinical studies.

Leukocytes, obtained from transfusion blood, are treated with an RNA virus to activate the interferon genes; a double-stranded RNA made during viral replication is a powerful interferon gene activator. On the basis of variations in antigenicity and molecular weight (M.W. 16,000–21,000), a dozen different interferon species have been obtained from human leukocytes. All the species have the same biologic activities but vary in their potency. The precise cells producing interferon in the leukocyte suspensions have not been identified, although T cells and NK cells are likely candidates. Because of the difficulty in preparing interferon from human cells, only a small number of individuals have been treated with the drug.

A second source of interferon for therapeutic use is diploid human fibroblast cells. An RNA virus is used to stimulate interferon production. Synthetic chemicals can also be used as activators of interferon, such as a polynucleotide, the double-stranded polyribosinic acid–polyribocytidylic acid, which apparently mimics the double-stranded structure of RNA that appears during replication of an RNA virus. Leukocyte and fibroblast interferon, although differing antigenically, are similar in their biologic activity.

Unlike leukocyte and fibroblast interferon, immune interferon is not produced for therapeutic purposes. It appears naturally in the body following stimulation of cells of the immune system by foreign proteins. Type 2 immune interferon is 10–100 times more potent than Type 1 interferon in the regulation of the immune response.

A definitive understanding of the role of interferon in the treatment of viral infections and tumors awaits the availability of interferon produced by the recombinant DNA techniques. It is anticipated that supplies produced by these techniques will be adequate and the cost will be less than 1 percent of that of human leukocyte interferon. For producing recombinant DNA interferon, various species of human interferon are being introduced into DNA plasmids of the bacterium *Escherichia coli* or yeast cells. The microbes, particularly yeast, can be grown in large quantities, allowing determination of the most potent of human interferon species that can be used in humans.

Mode of Action. Antiviral action is the aspect of interferon that has been studied most extensively. Interferon itself is not the agent that effects the biologic changes in the cell. It functions instead as an inducer, activating a second gene that produces the protein(s) that inhibit(s) viral replication. Several proposed mechanisms for the inhibitory action of the interferon system have been described: inhibition of uncoating of the virus, inhibition of assembly of viral proteins, and inhibition of viral transcription or translation of viral messenger RNA. However, the most conclusive data indicate that interferon stimulates the production of enzymes activating an endonuclease that destroys viral messenger RNA (mRNA). A protein kinase that inhibits translation of viral mRNA has also been observed. It is suggested that the production by a virus of a molecule apparently alien to the normal cell activates cell enzymes designed to destroy these foreign molecules.

DNA viruses are also inhibited by interferon but are not known to produce double-stranded RNA during their cellular replication. However, a double-stranded DNA has been extracted from cells infected with DNA virus (vaccinia virus), suggesting that there is a double-stranded phase in the replication of some DNA viruses. Little is known about how immune interferon inhibits replication of tumor cells or exerts a regulatory action on the immune system. Like all interferons, it stimulates the cell to produce proteins. Little is known concerning the more detailed enzymatic events that result in changes in the target cells.

Interferon has an inhibitory effect on the growth of tumors in culture and, to varying degrees, of tumors in the body. What is not clear is whether interferon has a direct action on tumors and/or stimulates effector cells, such as NK cells, that in turn destroy tumors. It has been observed that in the case of a virus infection due to vaccinia virus, interferon did not directly inhibit viral replication in culture, but when injected into monkeys, it inhibited the development of the vaccinia skin lesions.

Studies show that interferon can activate NK cells, which then inhibit tumor growth. Nude mice (genetically deficient and hairless) do not produce T lymphocytes, which are cells that have been considered essential in protection against tumors. However, nude mice that have a high concentration of NK cells show no increase in susceptibility to tumors over that of normal mice. The moderate tumoricidal action of NK cells is greatly stimulated by the action of interferon produced in the body. If antibody directed against interferon is administered to nude mice with a slow-growing tumor, neutralization of interferon action results, and there is rapid growth and spread of the tumor.

The sensitivity of tumor cells to the action of interferon varies considerably. Thus, in Burkitt's lymphoma, which is associated with a viral infection, tumor cells are inhibited in cell culture by 1 unit of interferon. An ovarian carcinoma, not known to be virus related, requires 300 units of interferon to inhibit in culture.

Interferon may be toxic to normal cells. In high concentrations, interferon can inhibit the growth of bone marrow cells, platelets, and leukocytes, and inhibits the regeneration of liver cells in mice. The extent of interferon toxicity will be determined only when the concentration needed to achieve its maximal therapeutic effectiveness is known. Such studies remain to be completed.

Clinical Treatment. Interferon is produced by the body during the course of viral infections. It probably plays an important role in resistance to viral replication. Thus, antibody against interferon given to mice infected with the virus of murine hepatitis causes a marked increase in severity of the infection. The effect of additional amounts of interferon given for therapeutic purposes remains to be determined.

In certain viral infections, some notable effects have been observed. Interferon treatment of human chronic hepatitis reduced the number of viral particles found in the blood of the patient, though cure was not achieved. In studies of herpes zoster, interferon hastened the healing and reduced pain. A response has also been observed in disseminated varicella. Interferon treatment given to monkeys before infection with rabies virus prevented the disease. A prophylactic effect of interferon can be expected for many viral infections.

Very few tumors have been treated with either human leukocyte or fibroblast interferon, and those few were treated perhaps in inadequate doses; yet there have been a few promising results. For example, in laryngeal papilloma, a virus-induced benign tumor, treatment has resulted in dramatic regression of the tumor but unfortunately with later recurrence. Burkitt's African lymphoma, associated with a herpesvirus, is highly susceptible in culture to interferon. There are reports that nasopharyngeal carcinoma, also associated with a herpesvirus and osteogenic sarcoma, responded well clinically to treatment with interferon. In other cases, the therapeutic effect on tumor growth has been minimal or modest. The data obtained to date suggest that tumors induced by viruses may respond unusually well to treatment with interferon. A better assessment of the therapeutic effectiveness of interferon awaits adequate supplies of the compound to enable completion of the necessary clinical studies.

Morton Klein, Ph.D.

interkinesis (in″ter-ki-ne′sis) [*inter-* + Gr. *kinēsis* motion] the brief interphase between the two meiotic cell divisions. Unlike the interphase between mitotic divisions, no DNA replication occurs.

interleukin 1 (IL 1) a factor produced by activated macrophages (and thus a monokine, rather than a lymphokine); M.W. 12,000–16,000. It was originally defined by its ability to enhance thymocyte proliferation, either alone or in conjunction with T-cell mitogens (concanavalin A or phytohemagglutinin). IL 1 can also enhance the in vitro antisheep red blood cell plaque-forming cell response of normal spleen cell cultures and T-cell depleted cell cultures, and generate alloantigen-specific cytotoxic T cells. Formerly called blastogenic factor (BF), lymphocyte activating factor (LAF), and mitogenic factor (MF).

interleukin 2 (IL 2) a factor produced by T cells after stimulation by a mitogen such as concanavalin A; M.W. 35,000 in the murine system, M.W. 15,000 in the rat and human systems. Biologically, IL 2 is similar to IL 1 in that it has the ability to enhance the thymocyte mitogenic response, to generate cytotoxic T cells, and to enhance the antibody response to erythrocytes. IL 2 is distinguished by its ability to maintain the continuous proliferation of activated T lymphocytes in culture. Formerly called T-cell growth factor.

intermediary metabolism (in″ter-me′de-ār″e) the various chemical reactions involved in the conversion of dietary nutrients such as sugars, amino acids, fatty acids, and mineral elements into storage molecules such as triglycerides, glycogen, and proteins; into a large array of reaction intermediates such as glycoproteins, heteropolysaccharides, and phospholipids; or into special function molecules such as hormones, nucleotides, and vitamins.

The term intermediary metabolism is used to refer to those biochemical reactions occurring in cells by which the many biochemical intermediates are formed and/or transformed into other products necessary for life. Glycolysis, for example, produces glucose-6-phosphate, which can be transformed into ribose, glucuronate, glycerol, pyruvate, oxoglutarate, glutamate, ascorbic acid, etc. To produce the large number of intermediates requires intertwined metabolic pathways, all carefully regulated by allosteric enzymes and hormones. Futhermore, the intermediate reactions need to be coupled with catabolic reactions to obtain energy to drive the individual synthetic or transformation reactions.

In contrast to intermediary metabolism, catabolic metabolism refers to energy-forming reactions and the formation of waste products, whereas anabolic metabolism is concerned with synthesizing structural units and essential enzymes, nucleic acids, and high-energy compounds.

intermediate (in″ter-me′de-āt) [*inter-* + L. *medius* middle] 1. between two extremes; in radiology, between radiolucent and radiopaque—for example, the penetrability of muscle and connective tissue, blood, and cartilage.

2. a substance formed in a chemical process that is essential to the formation of the end product of the process.

intermediate-density lipoprotein (IDL) see *intermediate-density l.* under *lipoprotein.*

intermediate sleep see *s. stages* under *sleep.*

intermittent (in″ter-mit′ent) [L. *intermittens,* from *inter* between + *mittere* to send] occurring at separated intervals; having periods of cessation of activity.

intermittent claudication see *intermittent c.* under *claudication.*

intermittent positive pressure breathing (IPPB) see *intermittent p. p. b.* under *positive pressure breathing.*

internal (in-ter′nal) [L. *internus* inside] pertaining to or located on the inside; affecting the inside.

internal capsule a broad band of white fibers bent laterally that separate the lentiform nucleus laterally from the head of the caudate nucleus, the dorsal thalamus, and the tail of the caudate nucleus medially. It consists of an anterior limb, a genu, a posterior limb, and retrolentiform and sublentiform parts. It carries both afferent and efferent fibers and connects the cortex with the brain stem.

internal conversion a type of radioactive decay in which a metastable state of a nuclide transfers energy to an orbital electron (a conversion electron) in returning to the ground state. Unlike beta electrons, conversion electrons are emitted at a few discrete energies.

internal medicine the branch of medicine that deals especially with the diagnosis and treatment of diseases and disorders of the internal structures of the body.

internal rotation in referring to the humerus, the turning of the arm so that the palm faces first to the rear and then to the outside, a radiographic position used to demonstrate the shoulder. Cf. *external rotation.*

internal standard in analytic procedures, a chemical compound that is added in known amounts to a specimen and carried through all steps of the procedure to provide an accurate quantitation, despite variations in the recovery efficiency of the individual procedural steps. The internal standard is similar chemically and structurally to the substance being assayed. The same percentage of both analyte and internal standard is recovered at each step, because of their similar chemical and physical properties.

The original concentration of the analyte in the specimen is determined from the known concentration of the internal standard in the specimen and the measured relative concentrations of the two in the extract. This technique is frequently used in gas chromatography and high-pressure liquid chromatography.

International Academy of Pathology (IAP) a professional organization of pathologists.

International Council of Societies of Pathology (ICSP) a professional organization of pathologists.

International Society for Clinical Laboratory Technology (ISCLT) a professional organization of clinical laboratory technicians.

International System (SI) a coherent system of measuring units, comprising seven independent base units, other coherent units derived from products and quotients of the base units, and prefixes used to form multiples and submultiples of these units. It is officially known as the International System of Units (*le Système International d'Unités* in French) and is abbreviated SI in all languages. The SI units were recommended in 1960 by the General Conference on Weights and Measures. They consist of seven base units, coherent derived units, supplemental units, and multiplicative prefixes (see the accompanying tables).

The prefixes are used to provide units of convenient size, e.g., 1 mm = 10^{-3} m = 0.001 m. The symbols for multiplicative units are regularly formed by combining the symbols for the prefix and the unit. Except for the centimeter, only the prefixes for powers of three are normally used, which permits any measurement to be expressed using a value between 1 and 1000. Only one prefix can be attached to a unit. The former practice of combining prefixes is no longer necessary; e.g., millimicro has been replaced by nano, and micromicro by pico.

When units are raised to a power, the power applies to the prefix as well, e.g., $mm^3 = 10^{-9} m^3$. When units are combined in products or quotients, only one unit (the first) should have a prefix; e.g., kg/l is preferred to g/ml. It should be noted that kilogram is a special case: it is a base unit even though it has a prefix, and kg/kg is preferred to g/g.

Because of its widespread use and convenient size, one noncoherent unit, the liter (l), defined as a cubic decimeter ($dm^3 = 10^{-3} m^3$), has been retained for use with SI units. Concentrations are commonly expressed in kilograms per liter or moles per liter.

When new units are proposed, they are formed as coherent units and are products or quotients of the base unit without conversion factors. For example, a new unit of catalytic activity, the katal (kat)—equal to 1 mol/s—has been proposed. Although it has not yet been accepted, it may replace the International Unit of enzyme activity, a noncoherent unit equal to 1 μmol/min.

In SI, temperature is no longer a peculiar property measured in degrees: absolute temperature is measured in kelvins and no degree symbol is used. However, the degree symbol is still properly used with customary (Celsius) temperature, for example, 0°C = 273.16 K.

In clinical chemistry and hematology, the transition to the use of SI units is still taking place. It has been recommended that all concentrations of single chemical species, such as glucose or chloride, be expressed in moles per liter and that concentrations of indeterminate mixtures, e.g., protein or 17-ketosteroids, be expressed in kilograms per liter instead of grams per 100 ml, which formerly prevailed.

At present, non-SI units to measure pressure (millimeters of mercury, mmHg), enzyme activity (the International Unit, U), and osmolality (the osmole, Osm) are being retained.

International 10–20 System a system for the placement of electrodes on the scalp for recording the electroencephalogram. Placement is determined by taking 10 or 20 percent of the total distances between a given pair of skull refernce points. There are only a few reference points, namely, nasion, inion, and right and left preauricular points. The system is designed to ensure that the interelec-

INTERNATIONAL SYSTEM, TABLE 1. SI UNITS

QUANTITY	UNIT	SYMBOL	PRONUNCIATION	DERIVATION
Base Units				
length	meter	m	me'ter	
mass	kilogram	kg	kil'o-gram	
time	second	s	sek'und	
electric current	ampere	A	am'pēr	
temperature	kelvin	K	kel'vin	
luminous intensity	candela	cd	kan-del'ah	
amount of substance	mole	mol	mōl	
Supplementary Units				
plane angle	radian	rad	ra'de-an	
solid angle	steradian	sr	stĕ-ra'de-an	
Derived Units				
force	newton	N	noo'ton	$kg \cdot m/s^2$
pressure	pascal	Pa	pas'kal	N/m^2
energy, work	joule	J	jōōl	Nm
power	watt	W	wot	J/s
electric charge	coulomb	C	koo'lom	A·s
electric potential	volt	V	vōlt	J/C
electric capacitance	farad	F	far'ad	C/V
electric resistance	ohm	Ω	ōm	V/A
electric conductance	siemens	S	se'menz	Ω^{-1}
magnetic flux	weber	Wb	web'er	V·s
magnetic flux density	tesla	T	tes'la	Wb/m^2
inductance	henry	H	hen're	Wb/A
frequency	hertz	Hz	herts	s^{-1}
luminous flux	lumen	lm	loo'men	cd·sr
illumination	lux	lx	luks	lm/m^2
temperature	degree celsius	°C	sel'ze-us	K–273.15
radioactivity	becquerel	Bq	bek-rel'	s^{-1}
absorbed dose	gray	Gy	gra	J/kg
absorbed dose equivalent	sievert	Sv	se'vert	J/kg

From Miller, B. F., and Keane, C. B.: Encyclopedia and Dictionary of Medicine, Nursing, and Allied Health. 3rd ed. Philadelphia, W. B. Saunders Co., 1983, p. 1023.

INTERNATIONAL SYSTEM, TABLE 2. PREFIXES FOR SI UNITS

MULTIPLICATION FACTOR	PREFIX	SYMBOL	PRONUNCIATION
1 000 000 000 000 000 000 = 10^{18}	exa	E	ek'sah
1 000 000 000 000 000 = 10^{15}	peta	P	pet'ah
1 000 000 000 000 = 10^{12}	tera	T	ter'ah
1 000 000 000 = 10^{9}	giga	G	jig'ah
1 000 000 = 10^{6}	mega	M	meg'ah
1 000 = 10^{3}	kilo	k	kil'o
100 = 10^{2}	hecto	h	hek'to
10 = 10	deka	dk	dek'ah
0.1 = 10^{-1}	deci	d	des'ĭ
0.01 = 10^{-2}	centi	c	sen'tĭ
0.001 = 10^{-3}	milli	m	mil'ĭ
0.000 001 = 10^{-6}	micro	μ	mi'kro
0.000 000 001 = 10^{-9}	nano	n	nan'o
0.000 000 000 001 = 10^{-12}	pico	p	pi'ko
0.000 000 000 000 001 = 10^{-15}	femto	f	fem'to
0.000 000 000 000 000 001 = 10^{-18}	atto	a	at'to

From Miller, B. F., and Keane, C. B.: Encyclopedia and Dictionary of Medicine, Nursing, and Allied Health. 3rd ed. Philadelphia, W. B. Saunders Co., 1983, p. 1023.

trode distances are equal along any anteroposterior or transverse line and that coverage of the convexity of the cerebral hemispheres is fairly comprehensive. See also the accompanying illustration.

International Union of Pure and Applied Chemistry (IUPAC) a professional association that promulgates standards for chemical nomenclature and terminology.

International Unit 1. (abbrev. U), the unit of enzyme activity proposed by the International Union of Biochemistry in 1964. Specifically, it is the amount of enzyme that catalyzes the conversion of 1 μmol of substrate or coenzyme per minute under the specified conditions (temperature, pH, substrate concentration) of the assay method. Also called *unit.* See also *katal.*

2. (abbrev. IU), any of several arbitrary units that have been adopted by an international body to express the quantity of certain vitamins (A, C, D, and thiamine hydrochloride), hormones (androgens, chorionic gonadotropin, estradiol benzoate, estrone, insulin, progesterone, and prolactin), and drugs (digitalis, penicillin).

interneuron (in″ter-nu′ron) [*inter-* + Gr. *neuron* nerve] any neuron in a chain of neurons that is situated between the primary afferent (sensory) neuron and the final motor neuron. The term also refers to any neuron whose processes are entirely confined within a specific area, as within the olfactory lobe, and which synapse with neurons extending into that area. Also called intercalated neuron.

inhibitory i., an internuncial neuron that partially or completely arrests the activity of a neuron upon which it synapses; examples include Renshaw cells, cerebellar basket cells, and Purkinje cells.

internodal (in″ter-no′dal) [*inter-* + L. *nodus* knot] between two nodes, particularly the distance on an axon between two consecutive nodes of Ranvier or the portions of the conducting system of the heart between the sinoatrial and atrioventricular nodes.

internodal tracts pathways of conducting Purkinje myocytes and ordinary cardiac myocytes that conduct impulses more rapidly than normal cardiac muscle from the sinoatrial node to the atrioventricular node. There appear to be three tracts—the anterior, posterior, and middle—connecting the two nodes.

internode (in′ter-nōd) the segment of an axon between two nodes of Ranvier; see under *myelin sheath.*

interoceptor (in″ter-o-sep′tor) a sensory nerve ending that receives information from the internal organs. Cf. *exteroceptor, proprioceptor,* and *receptor.*

interocular distance (in″ter-ok′u-lar) [*inter-* + L. *ocularis* from *oculus* eye] the distance between the two eyes, generally used in reference to the interpupillary distance.

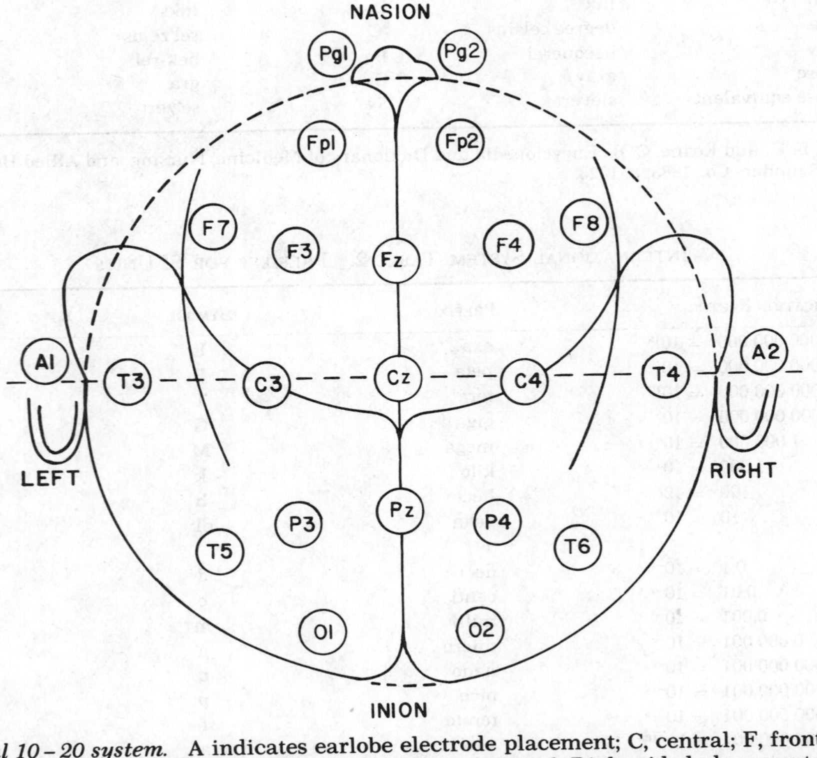

International 10–20 system. A indicates earlobe electrode placement; C, central; F, frontal; Fp, frontal polar; P, parietal; Pg, nasopharyngeal; T, temporal; and O, occipital. Right-sided placements are indicated by even numbers, left-sided placements by odd numbers, and midline placements by Z. (From Aminoff, M. J.: Electrodiagnosis in Clinical Neurology. New York, Churchill Livingstone, 1980.)

interorbital (in″ter-or′bĭ-tal) [*inter-* + L. *orbita* orbit] situated between the orbits.

interorbital line see *interpupillary line.*

interosseous (in″ter-os′e-us) [L. *interosseus,* from *inter-* + *os* bone] between bones.

interperiod line (in″ter-per′e-od) [*inter-* + Gr. *peri* around + *hodos* way] see under *myelin sheath.*

interphase (in′ter-fāz) [*inter-* + Gr. *phasis* an appearance] the period between successive mitoses. See also *cell cycle.* Cf. *interkinesis.*

interpolation (in-ter″po-la′shun) the process of estimating the intermediate values of a function from the values given at a discrete set of points. The simplest type is linear interpolation, in which the intermediate values are given by the straight line graph between adjacent points. Other methods of interpolation usually involve fitting a higher-order polynomial through several consecutive data points.

interpreter (in-ter′pre-ter) a computer program that, like a compiler, enables a program written in a high-level language to be run on a computer. However, it does not translate the program into machine language to be run at a later time; instead, it reads the program and immediately performs the specified operations. With a small program that does few calculations, an interpreter will run fast and do more error checking, if much calculation is to be done or the program is to be run many times, the interpreter will run far slower than a compiled program. For example, WATFIV is a FORTRAN interpreter and most implementations of BASIC are interpreters.

interproximal (in″ter-prok′sĭ-mal) [*inter-* + L. *proximus* next] between adjoining surfaces, as in the space between adjacent teeth.

interproximal projection the common bite-wing dental x-rays; see under *dental radiography.*

interpupillary (in″ter-pu′pĭ-lar″e) [*inter-* + L. *pupilla* girl] between the pupils.

interpupillary distance the distance between the centers of the pupils of the two eyes when both are looking in the same direction.

interpupillary line the line passing through the middle of both eyes, i.e., through the inner canthi or through the inner margins of the orbits; used in radiographic positioning. Also called *interorbital line.*

interrupt (in″ter-rupt′) [L. *interruptus; inter-* + *ruptus* broken] a break in the normal execution of a program due to an error (e.g., division by zero) or the need to attend to an I/O device. Control is transferred to the supervisor program.

interscapular (in″ter-skap′u-lar) [*inter-* + L. *scapula* shoulder blade] situated between the scapulae.

interscapular region the region of the back between the scapulae.

intersexuality (in″ter-sek″su-al′ĭ-te) the varying degrees of intermediate determination between male and female gonadal sex. See also *hermaphroditism, pseudohermaphroditism,* and *sex determination.*

interspinal (in-ter-spi′nal) [*inter-* + L. *spina* a spine or thorn] between two spinous processes.

interspinal line the line on the anterior surface of the abdomen that passes through the anterior superior iliac spines.

interstice (in-ter′stis) [L. *interstitium*] a small interval, space, or gap in a tissue or structure.

interstitial (in″ter-stish′al) [L. *interstitialis; inter* + *sistere* to set] situated between parts or in the interspaces between the cells of a tissue.

interstitial cell of Leydig see *Leydig cell.*

interstitial cell–stimulating hormone (ICSH) a luteinizing hormone, so-called because it also stimulates the Leydig (interstitial) cells of the testes; see under *luteinizing hormone.*

interstitial deletion see under *deletion.*

interstitial fluid that body fluid situated or occurring outside body cells and between parts or in the interspaces of a tissue. The blood plasma is not included in this fluid compartment. See *body fluids* for compositional and volume data.

interstitial growth growth by the addition of material throughout a structure. Only nonrigid material, such as cartilage, can grow in this way. Cf. *appositional growth.*

interstitial nephritis see under *tubulointerstitial nephropathy.*

interstitial nephropathy see under *tubulointerstitial nephropathy.*

interstitium (in″ter-stish′ĭ-um) [L.] 1. a small interval, space, or gap in a tissue or structure. 2. interstitial tissue.

intertrigo (in″ter-tri′go) [*inter-* + L. *terere* to rub] a skin rash and erythematous eruption that occurs on surfaces of the body that rub against other surfaces (e.g., folds of the groin, the axillae, and beneath pendulous breasts). Intertrigo, most common in the obese and those with diabetes mellitus, is due to a variety of agents, including friction, chafing, and bacteria; it is especially prevalent in warm, moist climates. The condition may lead to itching, maceration, and even erosion.

intertubercular (in″ter-tu-ber′ku-lar) between tubercles.

intertubercular plane see *transtubercular plane.*

interval (in′ter-val) [*inter-* + L. *vallum* rampart] the space between two objects or parts; the lapse of time between two events.

interval estimate see *confidence interval.*

interval scale a numerical scale having the property that the variable is a linear function of the quantity measured, i.e., the zero point is arbitrary. See also *scale.*

intervening sequence (in″ter-ven′ing) see *intron.*

interventional radiology the growing body of interventional procedures controlled by fluoroscopy, which are performed by the radiologist. This new radiology subspecialty includes numerous therapeutic procedures such as reduction of intussusception by barium enema, angioplasty of thrombosed arteries, therapeutic occlusion of bleeding vessels, removal of stones from the biliary and urinary tracts, percutaneous transhepatic placement of biliary drainage catheters, and drainage of abscesses. Intracardiac and intravascular defects can be occluded, and installation of antibiotics or chemotherapy through indwelling catheters is feasible. Such procedures entail clinical judgment, technical skill, and knowledge of complications and the ability to avoid them on the part of the radiologist before, during, and after the procedure. The rapid growth of interventional radiology may be attributed to the great versatility of fluoroscopic image-intensifying systems and the addition of television. A large variety of new catheters and other instruments have been developed by radiologists for these techniques.

intervertebral (in″ter-ver′tĕ-bral) [*inter-* + L. *vertebra*] situated between two contiguous vertebrae.

intervertebral disk a fibrocartilagenous disk located between the bodies of adjacent vertebrae. Its outer part is composed of dense fibrous cartilage (the annulus fibrosus). The central portion (the nucleus pulposus) is relatively soft and can herniate and compress a spinal nerve. The presence of the intervertebral disks confers flexibility and resilience on the vertebral column.

A ruptured, or herniated disk, is a major cause of low back pain, the herniation occurring as the result of forces producing or extending radial and circumferential tears in the annulus fibrosis of the intervertebral disk. At some point these tears may coalesce to allow protrusion of all or part of the nucleus pulposis through the annulus. Most commonly, it protrudes posterolaterally and impinges on the laterally placed nerve roots of the spinal cord, usually in the lumbosacral region.

There is severe back pain that is aggravated by sneezing, coughing, or straining with bowel movements, and is relieved by lying on the back. The ability to bend forward is limited, and there may be signs of nerve root impingement. The pain often radiates down the back of the thigh and leg, areas innervated by the sciatic nerve (L4, L5, S1). With prolonged compression, weakness, fasciculations and atrophy of the involved musculature may be seen, as well as sensory loss in the affected dermatome.

Less common forms of disk rupture may produce pain in the chest similar to angina in its distribution. If there is degeneration of the posterior longitudinal ligament, a lumbar disk may protrude directly posteriorly, pressing on several (sacral) nerve roots simultaneously, to produce a distinctive pattern of bilateral nerve root symptoms in several sacral dermatomes and myotomes.

Diagnosis rests on clinical examination, although radiographic studies may be necessary to rule out spinal canal tumors or simple muscle strains. Plain films of the lumbar spine may show evidence of decreased density in or narrowing of the disk region or of erosion of vertebral end-plates (producing Shmorl's nodes). Computed tomography may permit direct imaging of a herniated disk. In some patients, however, dye or air contrast myelography or visualization of the disk itself (through diskography, the injection of the disk with contrast material) is necessary to confirm the diagnosis. This latter procedure not only allows visualization of the disk, it may also reproduce, because of increased pressure on the disk, the symptoms described by the patient.

See also *low back pain.*

intestinal (in-tes′tĭ-nal) [L. *intestinalis*] pertaining to the intestine.

intestinal flora see under *normal flora.*

intestinal lymphangiectasia (in-tes′tĭ-nal lim-fan″je-ek-ta′ze-ah) a disorder, usually affecting children and young adults, that is characterized by dilation of the intestinal lymphatic system, particularly the lacteals, which results in a protein-losing enteropathy. Symptoms include massive edema, mild intermittent diarrhea, and occasional chylous effusions and ascites.

Peroral jejunal biopsy shows dilation of lymphatics, which can distort the villous architecture. Radioisotope studies can be used to demonstrate protein loss. Laboratory tests show markedly decreased serum albumin, ceruloplasmin, and transferrin, decreased immunoglobulins (IgA, IgM, and IgG), and lymphocytopenia. Steatorrhea can occur, but D-xylose excretion is normal.

intestinal myiasis see *intestinal m.* under *myiasis.*

intestinal obstruction a condition in which transit of the intestinal contents is blocked. Causes are generally mechanical, such as hernia, adhesions, volvulus, foreign bodies, intussusception, inflammation, and tumors. See also *ileus.*

intestinal villi projections of the mucous membrane of the small intestine. These highly vascular structures expand the surface area of the small intestine.

intestine (in-tes′tin) [L. *intestinus* inward, internal; Gr. *enteron*] that portion of the alimentary canal extending from the pyloric opening of the stomach to the anus. It is a long, coiled membranous tube that consists of the highly convoluted small intestine and the straighter large intestine. Also called *bowel.* See also *gastrointestinal tract.*

large i., [NA], the distal portion of the alimentary canal, between the small intestine and the anus. The major function of the large intestine is the absorption of water and electrolytes, although food products are also absorbed in the proximal colon. As in the small bowel, movements of the colon are produced by contraction of the smooth muscle in its wall, and are both segmental and propulsive. The entire length can be examined radiologically (barium enema) or endoscopically (colonoscopy).

The colon constitutes most of the large intestine. It commences in the right iliac fossa as the blind-ending cecum and continues up the right side of the abdomen on its posterior wall as the ascending colon. A sharp bend, the right colic or hepatic flexure, leads to the transverse colon, which arches across the abdomen suspended by the transverse mesocolon. The transverse colon becomes the descending colon at the left colic or splenic flexure, just below the spleen. The descending colon runs down the left posterior wall and, at about the level of the left anterior superior iliac spine, curves medially to become the sigmoid colon, which varies considerably in length but typically hangs down into the pelvis as a loop suspended by mesocolon. It is continuous with the rectum. The colon becomes narrower in its distal portion. The transverse and sigmoid colons are completely covered by peritoneum, but the transverse colon has two lines of peritoneal attachment, from the transverse mesocolon and the greater omentum, whereas the sigmoid colon has only one, its mesocolon.

Histologically, the large intestine has the same layers as the small bowel; however, the mucosa has crypts but no villi. Most of the epithelial cells are mucus-forming goblet cells, but there are many interspersed enterochromaffin cells throughout its entire length, most of them serotonin-producing. The outer layer of smooth muscle is longitudinally oriented, as in the small intestine, but is gathered to form three discrete bands, the teniae coli, with only a thin layer of longitudinal muscle between them. Small peritoneal pouches filled with fat protrude between the teniae and are called appendices epiploicae. Contraction of the teniae produces a puckering of the colon.

Being of both mid- and hindgut derivation, the large bowel receives its blood from both the superior and inferior mesenteric arteries. The two segments meet at the junction of the middle and distal thirds of the transverse colon, and the arterial supply of this junctional region is occasionally precarious. Also called *colon* and large bowel.

small i., the proximal portion of the intestine, extending from the pylorus to the cecum. Also called small bowel. See also *duodenum, jejunum,* and *ileum.*

intima (in′tĭ-mah) [L.] [NA], a general term denoting an innermost structure, used alone to designate the tunica intima of blood vessels.

intimal cell (in′tĭ-mal) an endothelial cell lining the lumen of blood vessels.

intolerance (in-tol′er-ans) [L. *in* not + *tolerare* to bear] an inability to withstand or consume. In particular, the term is used to refer to an individual's sensitivity to a drug so that the drug's normal effects are brought about by a dosage that is less than what is normally indicated—an abnormal reaction called idiosyncrasy. Cf. *tolerance.*

intoxication (in-tok″sĭ-ka′shun) [L. *in* intensive + Gr. *toxikon* poison] 1. poisoning; the state of being poisoned.

2. the condition produced by excessive consumption of alcohol or an overdose of drugs.

intr/o (in′tro) [L. *intro* within] a word element used in combining form to denote into or within, e.g., introgastric.

intra- (in′trah) [L. *intra* within] a prefix word element to denote within, e.g., intravenous.

intraarterial (in″trah-ar-te′re-al) [*intra-* + L.; Gr. *artēria*] within an artery or arteries.

intraarticular (in″trah-ar-tik′u-lar) [*intra-* + L. *articulus* joint] within a joint.

intrabronchial (in″trah-brong′ke-al) [*intra-* + L. *bronchialis,* from Gr. *bronchos* windpipe] see *endobronchial.*

intracellular (in″trah-sel′u-lar,) [*intra-* + L. *cellula* cell] situated or occurring within a cell or cells.

intracellular fluid that fluid situated or occurring within a cell or cells; see *body fluids* for compositional and volume data. See also *electrolyte balance and homeostasis.*

intrachange (in′tra-chānj) see *intrachromosomal aberration.*

intrachromosomal aberration (in″tra-kro″mo-so′-mal) the movement of a segment from one place to another on the same chromosome. Also called *chromosomal aberration* and *intrachange.* Cf. *interchromosomal aberration.*

intracranial (in″trah-kra′ne-al) [*intra-* + L. *cranialis,* from *cranium* head] situated within the cranium.

intracristal space (in″trah-kris′tal) [*intra-* + L. *crista* ridge] see *intramembranous space.*

intradermal (in″trah-der′mal) [*intra-* + Gr. *derma* skin] within the dermis.

intradermal test a skin test or dermal sensitivity reaction used to diagnose infectious and allergic diseases. The test consists of an intradermal antigen injection in one forearm and a control injection in the other forearm. If a reaction occurs on the antigen-injected arm, the test is positive and the patient has antibodies present against the antigen. See also *delayed h.* and *immediate h.* under *hypersensitivity.*

intraductal (in″trah-duk′tal) [*intra-* + L. *ductus,* from *ducere* to lead] situated or occurring within the duct of a gland.

intradural (in″trah-du′ral) [*intra-* + L. *dura* hard] within or beneath the dura.

intragastric (in″trah-gas′trik) [*intra-* + L. *gastricus,* from Gr. *gastēr* stomach] situated or occurring within the stomach.

intraluminal (in″trah-lu′mĭ-nal) [*intra-* + L. *lumina* light] within the lumen of a tube, as of a blood vessel.

intramembranous (in″trah-mem′brah-nus) within a membrane.

intramembranous space the space between the inner and outer membranes of a mitochondrion. Also called *intracristal space.* Cf. *intercristal space.*

intraocular (in″trah-ok′u-lar) [*intra* + L. *oculus* eye] within the eye.

intraocular pressure (IOP) the pressure exerted by the fluids within the eye against its tunics, which acts to keep the eyeball distended. In the normal individual (as measured by tonometry) it averages approximately 16 mmHg, but it may be altered in pathologic conditions such as glaucoma, in which it is increased. Normally, intraocular pressure is regulated at an almost constant value by a mechanism that involves changes in the resistance of the outflow of aqueous humor from the anterior chamber to Schlemm's canal.

intraoral (in″trah-or′al) [*intra-* + L. *oralis* pertaining to the mouth] within the mouth; pertaining to a radiograph made with the film held inside the mouth or between the teeth. See also *dental radiography.*

intraorbital (in″trah-or′bĭ-tal) [*intra-* + L. *orbita* orbit] within the orbit.

intraosseous (in″trah-os′e-us) [*intra-* + L. *osseus,* from *os* bone] within a bone.

intraperitoneal (in″trah-per″ĭ-to-ne′al) [intra- + L.; Gr. *peritonaion* from *per* around + *teinein* to stretch] within the peritoneal cavity.

intraperitoneal gas air introduced into the peritoneal cavity by a rupture of the abdominal viscera, usually detected in an erect position. It is also demonstrated radiographically by placing the patient in the left lateral decubitus position so that the gas will rise and be trapped under the right half of the diaphragm (a procedure that takes 10–20 min). The intraperitoneal gas is not superimposed on the gas in the stomach and can be demonstrated in an anterior or posterior view of the abdomen.

intrapleural (in″trah-ploor′al) [*intra-* + Gr. *pleura* rib, side] within the pleural cavity.

intrapleural pressure (Ppl) the pressure (relative to atmospheric) in the potential space between the visceral and parietal pleurae. Intrapleural pressure becomes more subatmospheric during each inspiration. The gravity-dependent gradient in intrapleural pressure down the vertical axis of the lung (values at the apex are 7 cm of H_2O more negative than at the base) is in part responsible for the regional subdivision of lung volume, or the proportional expansion of different lung regions at different volumes.

intrapulmonary (in″trah-pul′mo-ner″e) [*intra-* + L. *pulmonarius,* from *pulmonis* lung] situated in the substance of the lung.

intrauterine (in″trah-u′ter-in) [*intra-* + L. *uterinus* pertaining to the uterus] within the uterus.

intravasation (in-trav″ah-za′shun) the entrance of foreign material into a blood vessel. Cf. *extravasation.*

intravenous (IV) (in″trah-ve′nus) [*intra-* + L. *venosus,* from *vena* vein] within a vein or veins.

intraventricular (in″trah-ven-trik′u-lar) [*intra-* + L. *ventriculus,* dim. of *venter* belly] within a ventricle.

intraventricular pressure in the heart, the pressure within the right or left ventricle. Left and right intraventricular pressures have average systolic values of about 120 and 25 mmHg, respectively. Both intraventricular pressures fall to near-zero values during diastole. In the brain, the term refers to the pressure of the cerebrospinal fluid within the ventricles. It is increased when there is obstruction in the circulation of this fluid. See also *cerebrospinal fluid* and *hydrocephalus.*

intrinsic (in-trin′sik) [L. *intrinsecus* situated on the inside] situated entirely within or being exclusively associated with a part; inherent.

intrinsic factor a glycoprotein secreted by the parietal cells of the gastric mucosa. It is necessary for the absorption of vitamin B_{12} (cyanocobalamin, the extrinsic factor) from the gastrointestinal tract. Two molecules of cobalamin are bound to each molecule of intrinsic factor. Cf. *extrinsic factor.*

intrinsic pathway see under *coagulation pathways.*

introitus (in-troi′tus) an opening, especially the opening into the vagina.

intron (in′tron) an intervening sequence of DNA between coding sequences (exons). Also called *intervening sequence.* See also *exon.*

intubate (in′tu-bāt) to treat by intubation.

intubation (in″tu-ba′shun) [L. *in* into + *tuba* tube] the process of inserting a tube into a body canal or hollow organ, such as the trachea or stomach. Gastric intubation is performed for gastric lavage, to remove specimens for gastric function tests, or to provide nourishment (tube feeding). Endotracheal intubation (via the mouth or nose) is performed to provide a patent airway, to administer oxygen, and to remove airway secretions (by suctioning).

gastrointestinal i., the insertion of a tube, via the nose and stomach, into the duodenum, where a balloon at the end is inflated and carried by peristalsis into the small intestine. This procedure is performed therapeutically to relieve distention or obstruction of the small bowel. In radiology, it is performed to introduce a contrast medium, usually barium sulfate suspension, to demonstrate either a particular obstruction or the whole small intestine. The same result may be accomplished in a retrograde fashion from the colon.

rapid duodenal i., a method used in hypotonic duodenography and in radiologic examination of the small intestine. In this procedure, the duodenum is intubated under fluoroscopic control, using a flexible guidewire to insert the tube.

intussusception (in″tus-sus-sep′shun) [L. *intus* within + *suscipere* to receive] the telescoping or invagination of a part of the intestinal tract into a neighboring (usually distal) segment. It is most common in the young and may lead to intestinal obstruction. In the adult, the prolapse is often associated with the presence of a tumor.

inulin (in′u-lin) a polyfructan, composed of β-D-fructofuranose units, which is found in some plant tubers (e.g., dahlia, artichoke, sweet potato). It is relatively resistant to hydrolysis in the intestines and thus is an unimportant source of fructose. As inulin is readily filtered through the glomeruli without being reabsorbed by the tubules, it is used in a diagnostic test (inulin clearance) to measure the glomerular filtration rate.

inulin clearance the procedure for determining the glomerular filtration rate that is generally accepted as being the most accurate. It is used predominantly in research, and rarely in clinical studies because of the requirement for continuous infusion of inulin to maintain a constant plasma concentration during the procedure. It has been established that inulin is not metabolized nor is it absorbed or secreted by the tubules. The average clearance value is about 125 ml/min for males and 115 ml/min for females, although clearance decreases with age. See also *creatinine clearance* and *glomerular filtration rate.*

in utero (in u′ter-o) [L.] in the uterus.

inv abbrev. See *inversion.*

in vacuo (in vak′u-o) [L.] in a vacuum.

invagination (in-vaj″ĭ-na′shun) [L. *invaginatio,* from *in* within + *vagina* sheath] the infolding or insertion of a structure within itself or another structure.

invasin (in-va′zin) see *hyaluronidase.*

invasion (in-va′zhun) [L. *invasio; in* into + *vadere* to go] 1. the attack or onset of a disease.

2. the simple, harmless entrance of bacteria into the body, or their deposition in the tissues, as distinguished from infection.

3. the extension of a neoplasm into adjacent normal tissues. The mechanism of invasion is obscure; factors thought to play a part in the process include: (1) the physical pressure exerted by the progressive proliferation of tumor cells; (2) the loss of mutual adhesiveness between malignant cells; and (3) the production of collagenases that destroy connective tissue, thus permitting the intermingling of neoplastic tissue with normal connective tissue. See also *metastasis* and *neoplasm.*

invasive (in-va′siv) 1. having the quality of invasiveness, as in a malignant tumor.

2. in diagnostic medicine, a technique that involves the insertion of an instrument or foreign material into the body.

invasiveness (in-va′siv-nes) 1. the ability of a pathogenic microorganism to enter and spread throughout the tissues of the body.

2. the ability to infiltrate and actively destroy surrounding tissue, said of malignant neoplasms.

inverse-square law (in′verz skwār) stated as: the intensity of any broadcast radiation (e.g., light or gamma rays) decreases as the square of the distance. For example, at twice the distance there is one-fourth the intensity, and at three times the distance there is one-ninth. This does not apply to focused beams like those from a laser.

inversion (in-ver′zhun) 1. a turning inward, inside out, or upside down.

2. a radiographic position used to demonstrate the ankle, in which the foot is rotated inward. Cf. *eversion.*

3. (abbrev. inv), in genetics, a chromosomal aberration in which a chromosome section is reversed by breakage and healing. A pericentric inversion includes the centromere in the reversed portion; a paracentric inversion does not. With crossing over in pericentric inversions, only a portion of the gametes will be normal after meiosis; the rest will contain duplication deficiencies.

4. an obsolete term for the enzymatic hydrolysis of polysaccharides.

5. a symmetry operation in which an object is reflected through a point; that is, each point of the object is moved to an equidistant point on the opposite side of the point of inversion.

invertase (in-ver′tās) see *β-D-fructofuranosidase.*

inverted repeat (in-ver′ted) see *palindrome.*

inverter (in-ver′ter) an electronic logic circuit whose output is the logical complement of its input: if the input is "false" the output is "true," otherwise the output is "false." Also called *NOT gate.*

in vitro (in ve′tro) [L. "within glass"] referring to a process, test, or procedure in which something is measured or observed outside a living organism after extraction from the organism. Cf. *in vivo.*

in vivo (in ve′vo) [L. "within the living body"] referring to a process, test, or procedure in which something is measured or observed in a living organism. Cf. *in vitro.*

involucrum (in″vo-lu′krum) 1. the covering of a part.

2. in osteomyelitis, referring to new bone produced by the periosteum around a sequestrum.

involuntary (in-vol′un-ter″e) [L. *involuntarius,* from *in* against + *voluntas* will] performed independently of the will.

involuntary muscle see *nonstriated muscle.*

involution (in″vo-lu′shun) [L. *involutio,* from *in* into + *volvere* to roll] 1. a rolling or turning inward over a rim.

2. one of the movements involved in gastrulation of many types of animals.

3. a retrograde change, applied to a lessening of the size of a tissue caused by a reduction in the number of cells without degeneration.

4. the retrograde changes in the uterus that result in a return to normal size after delivery.

involution form an abnormally shaped bacterial cell that occurs in an old culture or one cultured under unfavorable conditions, such as the presence of an antibiotic substance.

I/O abbrev. See *input/output.*

iocetamic acid (i″o-sĭ-tam′ik) a radiopaque contrast medium used in cholecystography. Trademark, *Cholebrine.*

iod/o (i-o′do) [Gr. *iōdēs* violetlike; *ion* a violet + *eidos* form] 1. a prefix word element to denote the presence of iodine.

2. a prefix word element in organic chemistry to denote compounds in which iodine is present as a substituent, e.g., iodomethane (CH_3I).

iodamide meglumine (i-o′dah-mīd meg′lu-mēn) a water-soluble iodinated radiopaque contrast medium used for intravenous excretory urography. Trademark, *Renovue.*

Iodamoeba (i″o-dah-me′bah) a genus of amebas that is parasitic in human intestines. *I. buetschlii* is generally regarded as a nonpathogenic species, which is of worldwide distribution, although less commonly found than is *Entamoeba coli* or *Endolimax nana. I. buetschlii* is transmitted to humans by ingestion of viable cysts in fecally contaminated food. Diagnosis requires identification of glycogen vacuoles in iodine-stained fecal films or nuclear structure and glycogen vacuoles in hematoxylin-stained fecal films.

iodate (i′o-dāt) a salt of iodic acid; a compound containing the iodate ion IO_3^-.

I/O device [from *i*nput/*o*utput] any device such as the computer console, card reader, card reader-punch, printer, or CRT terminal used to transfer information to or from a computer.

iodic acid (i-o′dik) a colorless or white crystalline solid, HIO_3; M.W. 175.93. A moderately strong acid, it is a strong eye and skin irritant.

iodide (i′o-dīd) 1. an organic compound containing iodine.

2. the −1 ion of iodine (I^-).

iodide assays 1. spot test. After precipitation of proteins, gold chloride reagent is added to the filtrate. A brown color indicates iodide or bromide.

2. titration. Potassium hydroxide is added to a blood sample, which is then ashed in a nickel crucible. The resulting potassium iodide is extracted into ethanol, oxidized to iodine, and distilled into weak acid; after conversion to iodic acid, the iodine is determined by titration with thiosulfate, using starch as the indicator. These tests have little application in clinical chemistry.

iodine (I) (i′o-dīn) [Gr. *ioeides* violet-colored] a violet-black, crystalline, solid, nonmetallic element that sublimes, giving off pungent, irritating, violet vapor; molecular form I_2; atomic number 53, atomic weight 126.904; Group VII of the periodic table (the halogens); common oxidation states −1, +1, +5, +7. Solutions of I_2 in nonpolar solvents are also violet. Iodine is the least reactive of the naturally occurring halogens. It is an essential nutrient that circulates in the blood, from which it is trapped by the thyroid gland. Iodine reacts in the presence of a peroxidase to iodinate tyrosyl residues of the protein thyroglobulin, which is then converted into two hormones, thyroxine (T_4) and triiodothyronine (T_3).

butanol-extractable i. (BEI), see under *thyroxine assays.*

protein-bound i. (PBI), all plasma iodine bound to protein, particularly that contained in those fractions of the hormones triiodothyronine (T_3) and thyroxine (T_4), that are bound to their carrier proteins. In some thyroidal disorders it may also include follicular iodine. Measurement of protein-bound iodine has been largely replaced by the measurement of thyroxine; see under *thyroxine assays.*

i. solution, strong, [USP], a concentrated dark-brown solution of potassium iodide and iodine in pure water, used for the oral administration of iodine. Solutions of iodine are also used as a histologic stain (e.g., for Verhoeff's stain of elastic tissue) and, in diluted form, to stain protozoan cysts. More commonly called *Lugol's solution.*

tincture of i., [USP], a red-brown solution containing iodine and sodium iodide in aqueous alcohol, used as an antiseptic on the skin.

iodine-123 (^{123}I, I 123) a cyclotron-produced radionuclide with a half-life of 13.3 hr. It decays by electron capture to ^{123m}Te, emitting photons at 159 and 27.5 keV that can be used for efficient imaging with both the rectilinear scanner and scintillation camera. The radiation dose to the thyroid is very low, less than one-tenth of that from ^{131}I. Because of the short half-life, ^{123}I is expensive and not readily available.

iodine-125 (^{125}I, I 125) a radionuclide with a half-life of 60 da. It decays by electron capture to ^{125m}Te, emitting very low–energy photons at 27.5 and 35.4 keV that require special equipment for scanning. Because of the low photon energy, ^{125}I can be used only for scanning of superficial organs such as the thyroid, or for in vitro procedures. The radiation dose to the thyroid is only slightly lower than that from ^{131}I because of the long half-life. ^{125}I is the most widely used radionuclide for radioimmunoassay procedures.

iodine-131 (^{131}I, I 131) a radionuclide with a half-life of 8.05 da. It undergoes beta decay to ^{131m}Xe, emitting a 364-keV photon that can be imaged by a rectilinear scanner. The beta emission causes high patient irradiation. Other gamma emissions cause some loss of resolution as the result of septal penetration. A scintillation camera can also be used, although the sensitivity is low: only one-fourth of the photons are detected. Because of their low cost and long shelf life, ^{131}I radiopharmaceuticals are widely used.

iodine-131-6β-iodomethyl-19-norcholesterol (i′o-dīn i-o″do-meth′il nor″ko-les′ter-ol) an investigational drug used in adrenal scanning. Like iodocholesterol I 131, it is taken up by the adrenal cortex and by adrenocortical adenomas, but not by adrenocortical carcinomas.

iodine-131 therapy the administration of a large dose of radioactive ^{131}I as iodide, which accumulates in the thyroid gland for the purpose of destroying some or all of the thyroid tissue by radiation. A dose of about 3500 rads is given for hyperthyroidism as an alternative to drug therapy or surgical partial thyroidectomy. Following surgery for thyroid carcinoma, ^{131}I is sometimes administered to ablate any remaining thyroid tissue. Doses 20–50 times larger than those used for hyperthyroidism are used to treat metastatic follicular thyroid carcinoma.

iodine-131 uptake tests see under *thyroid uptake tests.*

iodine escape peak a peak in the gamma-ray spectrum as observed by using an NaI crystal detector that is 28 keV below a real gamma-ray photopeak. Some of the gamma rays cause an iodine atom to emit a secondary x-ray that escapes from the crystal so that only part of the energy is absorbed and measured. The term is also used to refer to a peak produced at 28 keV when the secondary x-ray does not escape and is also detected.

iodine staining a staining method used to demonstrate protozoan cysts in wet mounts of fecal specimens; diluted Lugol's iodine should be used. If properly stained, the glycogen of the cyst stains reddish-brown, the cytoplasm yellow, and the more refractile nucleus a lighter yellow. Iodine is also used to stain a variety of carbohydrates (e.g., starch, amyloid, cellulose, and glycogen); Gram's iodine is used in the Gram stain for bacteria. See also *Gram stain.*

iodipamide (i″o-dip′ah-mīd) a water-soluble, iodinated, radiopaque contrast medium used in intravenous cholangiography and cholecystography and in hysterosalpingography.

iodipamide meglumine [USP], trademark, *Cholografin.*

iodized oil (i′o-dīzd) [NF], an iodine addition product of vegetable oil, used as a radiopaque medium in radiography of the uterus and uterine tubes.

iodobismuthate (i-o″do-bis′muth-āt) a solution containing bismuth subnitrate, potassium iodide, and acetic acid, used as a spray reagent in thin-layer chromatography. It is used after an iodoplatinate spray to detect basic drugs such as morphine and codeine. Also called *Dragendorff's Solution.*

iodochlorhydroxyquin (i-o″do-klor″hi-drok′se-kwin) [NF], an antifungal and antibacterial agent applied topically in the treatment of vaginal *Trichomonas* infections and in various forms of atopic dermatitis and infections of the skin. Trademark, Vioform.

iodocholesterol I 131 (i-o″do-ko-les′ter-ol) a radiopharmaceutical, ^{131}I-19-iodocholesterol, used in adrenal scanning. Like cholesterol, a precursor of adrenocorticosteroids, it is taken up by the adrenal cortex and by adrenocortical adenomas, but not by adrenal cortex carcinomas.

5-iododeoxyuridine (IUDR, IDUR) (i-o″do-de-ok″-se-u′rĭ-dēn) an antiviral agent that is an analog of pyrimidine nucleoside. IUDR is most commonly used to treat keratoconjunctivitis caused by herpes simplex virus. However, this antiviral agent has not been proved safe and effective in eradicating the herpesviruses systemically. IUDR acts by replacing thymine during viral DNA synthesis, resulting in both replication and transcription errors. See also *antiviral agent.*

iodohippurate (i-o″do-hip′u-rāt) a radiographic contrast medium. Also called *orthoiodohippurate.*

sodium i. I 131, [USP], a radioisotope-labeled compound that is excreted by the kidneys by both glomerular filtration and tubular secretion. It is used to measure renal plasma flow and to make renograms. Trademarks, *Hippuran I 131* and *Hipputope.*

iodophor (i-o′do-fōr) a complex of iodine bound with a detergent carrier, which provides available free iodine at an effective but nonirritating concentration. It is used as a skin disinfectant.

iodoplatinate (i″o-do-plat′ĭ-nāt) an aqueous solution of potassium iodide and either platinum chloride or chloroplatinic acid, which is used as a spray reagent in thin-layer chromatography. It reacts with nitrogen-containing compounds such as opiates, phenothiazines, and benzodiazepines, forming a product that is blue to purple in color.

iodopsin (i″o-dop′sin) [*iodo-* + Gr. *opsis* vision] a photosensitive violet retinal pigment, found in the retinal cones of some animals, that is important for color vision. The function of this pigment appears to be similar to that of rhodopsin. Measurements of the spectra in single human cones before and after bleaching reveal that there are three different pigments, each present in individual cones. Corrected absorption maxima for the three are 430 nm (blue), 540 nm (green), and 575 nm (red); these are in accord with expectations from the trichromatic theory. The chromophore in all iodopsins is 11-*cis*-retinal; visual perception involves the conversion of 11-*cis* to the all-*trans* isomer. The different types of hereditary color blindness are due to deficiencies of particular opsins, affecting the appropriate iodopsins. See also *rhodopsin.*

iodopyracet (i-o″do-pi′rah-set) [NF], a radiopaque contrast medium that is used for intravenous urography or for retrograde pyelography. Trademark, Diodrast.

ion/o (i′on-o) [Gr. *iōn* going] a word element used in combining form to denote ions or charged particles, e.g., ionic.

ion (i′on) [Gr.] a charged atom or molecule. Anions are negative ions; cations are positive ions. Zwitterions have both positive and negative charges on different parts of the molecule, e.g., $NH^{+}_{3}\cdot CH_2\cdot COO^{-}$, the glycine zwitterion.

ion counter see *ionization chamber.*

ion-exchange chromatography chromatography using an ion-exchange resin as the stationary phase; see under *chromatography.*

ion-exchange resin an insoluble granular material that can remove ions selectively from solution by exchanging them for similar ions bound to the material. Such resins are constituted of a polymer of high molecular weight, to which many charged functional groups are covalently attached. These charged groups can bind specific groups of ions. The cation-exchange resins contain sulfonate, carboxylate, or phenolate groups, and bind or exchange cations; anion-exchange resins contain tertiary- or quaternary-ammonium groups, and bind anions. These resins are used to isolate or separate amino acids and other charged metabolites in mixtures, to separate proteins in mixtures, and to remove mineral salts from water (water conditioning, preparing purified water).

ionic (i-on′ik) pertaining to an ion or ions. See also *ionic b.* under *bond.*

ionic charge the electric charge on an ion. It is indicated in chemical formulas by a right upper index, e.g., Fe^{2+}, or in chemical names of positive ions by a roman numeral, e.g., iron(II).

ionic strength a measure of the attraction between ions and their surrounding ionic atmospheres. It is defined as one-half the sum of all terms, obtained by multiplying the molar concentration of each ionic species by the square of its electrical charge (valence), and is used to calculate activity coefficients. The term is often employed to specify the concentration of buffer solutions when these are used in electrophoretic and similar work in which the presence of ions of multiple unit charge may affect the movement of other ionic species in an electrical field.

ionization (i″on-i-za′shun) the process of becoming ionized.

specific i. (s), the number of ion pairs per unit path length created by a charged (alpha, beta, or position) particle moving through soft tissue. See also *linear energy transfer.*

ionization chamber a device for measuring radiation by the number of ion pairs that the radiation causes in a gas-filled chamber, particularly one that does not use gas amplification. Most ionization chambers detect only gamma rays or gamma and beta rays. The current flowing through the gas between two electrodes is proportional to the density of ion pairs, as the applied voltage is too low to cause secondary ionization. A different detection method is the pocket dosimeter, in which ions are drawn to the charged plates of an electrometer. This process reduces the charge and voltage on the electrometer and indicates the radiation.

ionization constant see *dissociation constant.*

ionization interference in flame photometry, a nonlinear relationship between emission intensity and concentration due to differences in the degree to which the element being measured is ionized. It occurs because of the ionization equilibrium that exists with other ionizable metals in the specimen.

ionize (i′on-iz) to form ions. There are a variety of mechanisms by which a neutral compound can yield ions or become an ion. For example, ionic compounds (such as sodium chloride, $Na^{+}\ Cl^{-}$) separate into free ions when they are melted or dissolved in a polar solvent in which attraction between the solvent and ions is greater than that between the ions themselves. The presence of a strong electric field or the impact of high-energy radiation, such as x-rays and alpha, beta, and gamma rays, may eject electrons from molecules (or atoms), leaving ions as residues. The addition of an acid or base to a water solution of a second acid or base, by binding protons, may free conjugate bases or acids as free ions.

ionizing radiation the electromagnetic radiation (gamma rays and x-rays) and particles that have enough energy to remove electrons from atoms and thereby produce ions (charged atoms).

X-rays and gamma rays are short-wavelength electromagnetic radiation. They are physically indistinguishable and are identified by their source. Gamma rays are produced by the radioactive decay of atoms; x-rays are produced by the rapid acceleration or deceleration of charged particles and by transitions between electronic shells in atoms.

Ionizing particles include high-speed electrons (beta particles), protons, and neutrons, alpha particles, and many more exotic particles. Sources include the radioactive decay of nuclei (both natural and created), secondary particle showers due to cosmic radiation from outer space, fission and fusion reactions, and particle accelerators for scientific research and radiation therapy.

Ionization can cause molecular and cellular damage by both direct and indirect means. For example, a direct "hit" on a DNA molecule can cause a break in an interatomic bond that is not repaired before cell division. Because a large fraction of the substance of cells consists of water, this type of direct damage is not as probable as indirect damage, which proceeds by the ionization of water and the subsequent chemical production of highly reactive free radicals. It is the free radicals that produce the damage, rather than the ionizing radiation (see *radiation effects*).

The biologic effectiveness of a given radiation dose depends on the type of radiation. Radiation (e.g., neutrons) that produces a high-ionization density is much more damaging (per unit dose) than low-ionization density radiation (e.g., x-rays).

ARTHUR E. BURGESS, PH.D.

ionophore (i-on′o-fōr″) any of a class of compounds, usually cyclic, that have the ability to bind inorganic cations for transport across membrane barriers, thus increasing the permeability of the membrane for specific ions. Several chemical classes of antibiotics are active as ionophores, e.g., valinomycin, gramicidin, nonactin, nigericin, and monensin. See also *electron transport inhibitors.*

ion pair a pair of oppositely charged ions held together by coulombic (electrostatic) attraction without formation of a covalent bond. Experimentally, an ion pair behaves as one unit in determining conductivity, kinetic behavior, osmotic properties, etc. When the ions are not held together, they are termed free ions.

iontophoresis (i-on″to-fo-re′sis) the introduction of soluble ions into body tissues by means of an electric current, often for therapeutic purposes. One application of this technique is the introduction of pilocarpine into the skin to induce sweating in the sweat test. Also called ion therapy and iontotherapy.

IOP abbrev. See *intraocular pressure.*

iopanoic acid (i″o-pan-o′ik) [USP], a radiopaque contrast medium used in oral cholecystography. It is a cream-colored, water-insoluble solid. The liver excretes the glucuronide salt, which is stored in the gallbladder. Trademark, *Telepaque.*

iophendylate (i″o-fen′dĭ-lāt) [USP], an oily, radiopaque contrast medium used in myelography. Trademarks, *Ethiodan* and *Pantopaque.*

iota (I, ι) (i-o′tah) the ninth letter of the *Greek alphabet.*

iothalamate (i-o thal′ah-māt) a radiopaque contrast medium used in urography and angiography. It is a water-soluble triiodobenzene derivative.

i. meglumine, [USP], trademark, *Conray.*
i. sodium, [USP], trademark, *Conray.*

IP abbrev. for *inosine phosphorylase.* See *purine nucleoside phosphorylase.*

IPC a toxic carbamate herbicide, *N*-phenyl isopropyl carbamate. Also called propham.

ipodate (i′po-dāt) a radiopaque contrast medium used in cholecystography. It is a water-soluble triiodobenzene derivative.

i. calcium, [USP], trademark, *Oragrafin.*
i. sodium, [USP], trademark, *Oragrafin.*

IPPB abbrev. See *intermittent p. p. b.* under *positive pressure breathing.*

iproniazid (i″pro-ni′ah-zid) a monoamine oxidase (MAO) inhibitor similar to isoniazid but more toxic. It is presently not used therapeutically.

ipsilateral (ip″sĭ-lat′er-al) [L. *ipse* self + *latus* side] on or affecting the same side. Cf. *contralateral.*

IR abbrev. See *infrared.*

Ir symbol for the chemical element *iridium.*

IR drop the voltage drop across a resistor that is produced by a current, given by Ohm's law, $V = IR$, where V is the voltage, I is the current, and R is the resistance.

IRDS abbrev. See *infant respiratory distress syndrome.*

Ir genes see *immune response genes.*

irid/o, ir/o (ir′id-o, ir′o) [Gr. *iris, iridos* rainbow, colored circle] a word element used in combining form to denote the iris (the colored portion of the eye), e.g., iridology, iritis.

iridium (Ir) (ĭ-rid′e-um, i-rid′e-um) [L. *iris* rainbow, from the tints of its salts] a hard, silvery-white metallic element of the platinum group; atomic number 77; atomic weight 192.22; a 5d transition element; oxidation states +1 through +6 (+1, +3, and +4 are most common).

Iridium is the densest element (based on a calculated density of 22.65). Platinum-iridium alloy is extremely hard and corrosion resistant; it is used for electrodes and to make the primary standards of mass and length. Iridium has low toxicity.

iridocapsulitis (ir″ĭ-do-kap″su-li′tis) [*irido-* + L. *capsula* a little box + Gr. *-itis* inflammation] an inflammation of the iris and the capsule of the lens.

iridocyclitis (ir″ĭ-do-si-kli′tis) [*irido-* + Gr. *kyklos* circle + *-itis* inflammation] an inflammation of the iris and ciliary body. The inflammatory pattern is often of the chronic, nongranulomatous type and may develop secondary to various primary infections such as tuberculosis and syphilis.

heterochromic i., an inflammation of the iris and the ciliary body, which is most often unilateral and low grade and which leads to depigmentation of the affected iris. Also called heterochromic uveitis.

iridokeratitis (ir″ĭ-do-ker″ah-ti′tis) [*irido-* + Gr. *keras* horn, cornea + *-itis* inflammation] an inflammation of the iris and cornea.

iris (i′ris), pl. *irides* [Gr. "rainbow," "halo"] 1. the circular, contractile colored diaphragm that lies between the cornea and lens of the eye. Its periphery is continuous with the ciliary body, and the central aperture forms the pupil. The iris contains smooth muscle fibers and its posterior surface is covered with pigmented epithelial cells. The smooth muscle is arranged circularly (sphincter muscle of the pupil) and radially (dilator muscle of the pupil).

2. the rhizome of *Iris versicolor,* formerly considered a purgative, emetic, and diuretic.

iritis (i-ri′tis) [*iris* + *-itis* inflammation] an inflammation of the iris. The clinical symptoms include a deep aching pain, photophobia, tearing, and blurring of vision. Onset of symptoms is usually gradual, with no accompanying discharge. The pupil becomes small and irregular, the pupillary reflex is sluggish, and the iris may become discolored. The infection usually remains confined to the affected eye. Atropine-induced dilation of the pupil is suggested to prevent synechiae (adhesion of the iris to the cornea or lens) formation. See also *anterior u.* under *uveitis.*

iron (Fe) (i′ern) [A.S. *iren;* L. *ferrum*] a soft, gray, ductile, magnetic, metallic element found as oxides and salts in certain minerals, in nearly all soils, and in mineral water; atomic number 26; atomic weight 56.847; a 3d transition element; oxidation states +2 and +3 (common), and +1, +4, and +6 (rare). Iron is an essential constituent of hemoglobin, the cytochromes, and other components of the respiratory enzyme systems. The chief function of these chemicals is in the transport of oxygen to tissues (hemoglobin) and in cellular oxidation mechanisms. Iron is also in ferritin and may be bound to transferrin. It is used to increase the synthesis of hemoglobin in anemia. The compounds of iron are used as astringents and styptics. Reference ranges for serum total nonhemoglobin iron in serum are: for newborns, 100–250 μg/dl; for infants, 40–100; for children, 50–120; for adult males, 60–150; for adult females, 50–130; and for the elderly, 40–80.

iron 59 (^{59}Fe, Fe 59) a radionuclide with a half-life of 45 da. It emits both beta and gamma rays. The 1.1-MeV and 1.3-MeV gamma rays are used for detection, but the energy is too high for imaging.

iron assays 1. colorimetry. Serum iron is almost entirely bound to the transport protein transferrin in the iron(III) form, which is liberated by the addition of an acid buffer (pH 1.9) and reduced to iron(II) with asorbic acid, hydrazine, or thioglycollic acid. A chromogen such as α,α′-dipyridyl 2,2′,2″-tripyridine (2,6-dipyridylpyridine), bathophenanthroline (1,4-diphenyl-1,10-phenanthroline), TPTZ (2,4,6-tripyridyl-*s*-triazine), or Ferrozine [3(2-pyridyl)-5,6*bis*(4-phenylsulfonic acid)-1,2,4-triazine] is added; the iron concentration is proportional to the absorbance of the iron-chromogen complex measured with a filter photometer. This method can also be used to measure total iron in tissues, foods, or whole blood (this is a referee method for hemoglobin, which is 0.347 percent iron) after the sample has been digested in acid or ashed in a muffle furnance and dissolved. (As a further isolation step, the iron may be precipitated as hydroxide, then redissolved.)

2. atomic absorption flame spectrophotometry. Proteins and hemoglobin iron are removed from the serum sample to avoid matrix effects and interference by precipitation with hot trichloroacetic acid and centrifugation; alternately, the iron may be reduced, complexed with bathophenanthroline, and extracted into methyl isobutyl ketone. The iron is determined by its atomic absorption at 248.3 nm.

iron-binding capacity a measure of the amount of iron that is bound to apotransferrin, the plasma carrier protein. This protein is usually 25–30 percent saturated, representing the serum iron content. The amount of additional iron that can be bound to apotransferrin, expressed in milligrams per deciliter (mg/dl), is called the unsaturated (or latent) iron-binding capacity (UIBC or LIBC). Both values together represent the total iron-binding capacity of serum (serum iron + UIBC = TIBC). Another useful relation between these values is the percentage of saturation, which is expressed as serum iron/TIBC × 100. This is usually a better index of iron stores than is serum iron alone. The accompanying table shows some changes in these parameters under various clinical conditions.

total i.-b. c. (TIBC), a measure of the amount of iron that can be bound by serum transferrin. Excess iron is added to serum until all apotransferrin has been saturated with iron; the excess iron is removed by resin or adsorbent, and the remaining iron represents the TIBC.

This iron can be determined by two types of methods. The first is measurement by atomic absorption, either directly or after chelating the iron and extraction of the complex. The second method involves colorimetry. Such procedures involve dissociation of the iron-protein complex, precipitation of the protein (in most methods), reduction of all iron to the Fe^{2+} form, and reacting the reduced (free) iron with agents such as α,α′-dipyridyl, *o*-phenanthroline, or bathophenanthroline. The absorption of the iron complex is directly proportional to the amount of iron. TIBC may also be determined by measuring serum iron and then the unsaturated iron-binding capacity (UIBC). TIBC then is equal to the sum of these two values.

unsaturated i.-b. c. (UIBC), a method to measure the amount of additional iron above that already present in the serum that could be bound by apotransferrin. A known excess amount of iron is added to serum to saturate all apotransferrin. The Fe-transferrin complex is precipitated, and the excess iron present in the supernatant is determined. The UIBC = [iron added] – [excess iron measured]. Also called latent iron-binding capacity.

iron clearance see under *ferrokinetics study.*

iron deficiency anemia see *iron deficiency a.* under *anemia.*

iron lung see *Drinker r.* under *respirator.*

iron-positive pigment demonstration 1. the Prussian blue reaction for ferric iron in hemosiderin and other iron-positive pigments in tissues. The ferric ion reacts with potassium ferrocyanide, $K_4Fe(CN)_6$, to form ferric ferrocyanide, $Fe_4(Fe(CN)_6)_3$ (Prussian blue). Also called *Perls' reaction.*

2. treatment of sections with fresh, unoxidized solutions of hematoxylin without mordant. Ferric iron oxidizes the dye and forms a blue-black lake with it.

3. the Turnbull blue reaction for ferrous iron. The ferrous ion reacts with potassium ferricyanide, $K_2Fe(CN)_6$, to form ferrous ferricyanide, $Fe_3(Fe(CN)_6)_2$ (Turnbull blue).

4. the Quinke-Tirmann-Schmelzer method for ferric and ferrous iron. Treatment with ammonium sulfide converts both Fe^{2+} and Fe^{3+} to ferrous sulfide, which is then demonstrated with the Turnbull blue reaction.

iron storage disease see *hemochromatosis.*

iron-sulfide protein one of a group of nonheme iron proteins. These proteins contain iron-sulfur centers in which iron is coordinately linked to the

IRON-BINDING CAPACITY. SERUM IRON, TIBC, AND PERCENT SATURATION IN VARIOUS CONDITIONS

	SERUM FE	TIBC	SATURATION
NORMAL	60-150 (μg/dl)	280-380 (μg/dl)	20-50 (%)
Iron deficiency	↓	↑	↓
Chronic infections	↓	↓	↓
Malignancy	↓	↓	↓
Menstruation	↓	N	↓
Iron poisoning	↑	↓	↑
Hemolytic anemia	↑	N, ↓	↑
Hemochromatosis	↑	N, ↓	↑
Pyridoxine deficiency	↑	N	↑
Late pregnancy	↓	↑	↓
Oral contraceptives	N, ↑	↑	N
Viral hepatitis	↑	↑	N, ↑
Nephrosis	↓	↓	↑
Kwashiorkor	↓	↓	↑
Thalassemia	↑	↓	↑

↓ = decrease; ↑ = increase; N = normal; TIBC = total iron binding capacity.

Modified from Henry, J. B.: Clinical Diagnosis and Management. 16th ed. Philadelphia, W. B. Saunders Co., 1979, p. 296.

sulfur of cysteine side-chains. This molecular arrangement is found in the proteins of the electron-transfer systems of mitochondria, chloroplasts, bacterial plasma-membrane vesicles, the membrane of the endoplasmic reticulum, and a relatively small group of soluble enzymes. Characteristically, these proteins exhibit absorption in the visible region of the spectrum and, when reduced, give rise to a distinct electron spin resonance spectrum with a peak at $g = 1.94$.

irradiation (ir-ra″de-a′shun) [L. *in* into + *radiare* to shine forth] 1. exposure to ionizing radiation or ultraviolet light.

2. the spread of nerve impulses from one region of the nervous system to another.

irreversible (ir″re-ver′si-b′l) that which cannot be reversed.

irreversibly sickled cell (ISC) any erythrocyte that remains sickled on reoxygenation, even though the interior structure of the oxyhemoglobin S is not in the gel state. The membrane has undergone irreversible deformation, probably owing to a depletion of ATP. These ISCs are seen in oxygenated capillary blood films from individuals suffering from sickle cell anemia. Recent investigations suggest that the rigidity of ISCs is reversible in vitro by lowering their mean corpuscular hemoglobin concentration (MCHC).

irrigation (ir″ĭ-ga′shun) [L. *irrigatio,* from *in* into + *irigare* to carry water] 1. washing by a stream of water or other fluid. See also *lavage.*

2. a liquid used for irrigation.

irritability (ir″ĭ-tah-bil′ĭ-te) [L. *irritabilitas,* from *irritare* to tease] 1. abnormal responsiveness to slight stimuli.

2. the ability of living organisms to respond to stimuli.

irritable bowel syndrome (ir′ĭ-tah-b′l bow′el) a functional disorder of the large and small intestines that is characterized by abdominal pain, altered bowel habits (constipation and/or diarrhea), hypersecretion of colonic mucus, dyspeptic symptoms, and an absence of detectable organic disease. It is the most common gastrointestinal disorder encountered in clinical practice and is thought to be either a reaction to emotional conflict or depression in susceptible individuals.

Physical examination is within normal limits, possibly excepting tenderness of the colon on palpation. Laboratory test results are normal. Diagnosis is based on clinical history and exclusion of organic intestinal disease.

Also called adaptive colitis, *mucoenteritis, mucous colitis,* nervous colon, *spastic colitis,* and spastic colon.

IRV abbrev. See *inspiratory reserve volume.*

ISC abbrev. See *irreversibly sickled cell.*

isch/o (is′ko) [Gr. *ischein* to suppress] a word element used in combining form to denote holding back, e.g., ischuria.

ischemia (is-ke′me-ah) [*isch-* + Gr. *haima* blood] the reduction or abolition of the blood supply to a tissue. This results in deficiency of available oxygen and nutrients and may lead to cell death. The causes include thrombosis, embolism, vessel disease, spasm, and physical compression. The extent and severity of ischemia depend on the speed of development, the degree of blockage and of collateral circulation, and the vulnerability of the affected organ. See also *infarct.*

myocardial i., a condition caused by a deficiency in the blood flow and oxygen supply to the myocardium, which produces the clinical syndrome of angina pectoris. An increase in heart rate, systolic pressure, or cardiac contractility may induce the condition. Coronary arteriosclerotic heart disease, aortic stenosis, and aortic insufficiency, among other disorders, may be underlying conditions. ECG testing, radiography, echocardiography, exercise stress testing, thallium and technetium scanning, cardiac catheterization, and coronary angiography may all be useful in diagnosing the underlying disease. See also *angina pectoris* and *myocardial infarction.*

ischemic (is-kem′ik) pertaining to or affected with ischemia.

ischi/o (is′ke-o) [Gr. *ischion* hip] a word element used in combining form to denote the ischium (hip bone), e.g., ischialgia.

ischium (is′ke-um), pl. *ischia* [L.; Gr. *ischion*] the part of the hip bone that fuses with the pubis and ilium, forming part of the acetabulum. The ischial ramus fuses with the pubis to complete the obturator foramen.

ISCLT abbrev. See *International Society for Clinical Laboratory Technology.*

ISE abbrev. See *ion-selective e.* under *electrode.*

islet (i′let) a cluster of cells or an isolated piece of tissue.

islets of Langerhans (i′lets lahng′er-hanz) [Paul *Langerhans,* German pathologist, 1847–1888] clusters of endocrine cells that are distributed throughout the pancreas. They vary in size up to groups of a few hundred cells and are more numerous in the tail of the organ. Like other endocrine tissues, they have a rich capillary network. Using electron microscopy, three morphologic cell types have been described in the human pancreas. The A (alpha) cells make up about 20 percent of the total in an islet and contain spherical dense-core granules; they are known to form glucagon and may also produce gastrin. B (beta) cells make up more than 70 percent of the islet cells, have granules with crystalline cores, and form insulin. D (delta) cells with spherical granules smaller than those of the A cells have been described, and immunocytochemical studies suggest that they may form somatostatin. See also *pancreatic islet stains.*

Ismelin (is′me-lin) trademark for the sulfate salt of guanethidine. See *guanethidine.*

iso- (i′so) [Gr. *isos* equal] 1. a prefix word element to denote equal, alike, or the same. In immunology, it indicates genetic identity (as in an isograft) or the existence of alternate forms in the same population (as in isoantigen).

2. a prefix used in chemistry to denote a structural isomer. In trivial names of alkanes, iso- indicates a one-carbon branch next to the end of the chain; e.g., isohexane is 2-methylpentane. An isoalkyl group has its free valence at the opposite end of the chain from the branch, i.e., a substituent with two methyl groups at the end of an otherwise straight chain; for example, isohexyl is 4-methylpentyl.

isoagglutinin (i″so-ah-gloo′tĭ-nin) an agglutinin that acts on cells of members of the same species.

isoallele (i″so-ah-lēl′) an allele that cannot be distinguished from the normal one by its phenotypic effect. It can be identified only with special tests or when combined in a heterozygote with a mutant allele.

isoallelism the presence of more than one kind of normal allele at a locus.

isoantibody (i″so-an′tĭ-bod″e) a term used primarily in blood banking and immunohematology to designate an antibody produced by one individual that reacts with antigens of another individual of the same species. Also called *alloantibody* in clinical and basic immunology.

isoantigen (i″so-an′ti-jen) an antigen that exists in alternate (allelic) forms in a species and which is coded for at the same gene locus in that species. It induces an immune response when one form is transferred to species members who lack that form. This might occur in a tissue graft or blood transfusion. The blood group antigens are an example. Also called *alloantigen* in clinical and basic immunology.

isobar (i′so-bar) [*iso-* + Gr. *baros* weight] one of several nuclides that have the same atomic mass number but different atomic numbers, e.g., ^{99}Mo and its decay product ^{99m}Tc. Cf. *isotope.*

isobaric (i″so-bār′ik) 1. having equal weights or exerting equal pressure.

2. having equal specific gravity, as in isobaric solutions of an anesthetic solution having the same specific gravity as cerebrospinal fluid.

isobutyl- (i″so-būt′l) a prefix word element in organic chemistry to denote the 2-methylpropyl group,—$CH_2CH(CH_3)_2$, e.g., isobutyl alcohol and isobutylamine.

isobutyl alcohol a colorless, flammable liquid, 2-methyl-1-propanol, $(CH_3)_2CHCH_2OH$; M.W. 74.12. It is used as a solvent and is a strong irritant to the skin and respiratory tract.

isobutyric acid an acid, $(CH_3)_2CH{\cdot}COOH$, 2-methylpropanoic acid, found in the urine. It probably is produced as a metabolite of valine.

isocarboxazid (i″so-kar-bok′sah-zid) [NF], an antidepressant; trademark, Marplan. See under *monoamine oxidase inhibitors.*

isochromatid break (i″so-kro-mat′id) a chromosomal aberration in which both sister chromatids break at the same point and fuse to form a dicentric chromatid and an acentric fragment.

isochromosome (i″so-kro′mo-sōm) an aberrant chromosome that has identical arms. It is formed when the centromere divides improperly during mitotic anaphase. One isochromosome receives both short arms from a chromatid; another receives both long arms.

isochronal (i-sok′ro-nal) isochronous.

isochronal rhythm the type of motion exhibited by the cilia of some epithelial tissues in which all the cilia beat in unison. Cf. *metachronal rhythm.*

isochronous (i-sok′ro-nus) [*iso-* + Gr. *chronos* time] having the same frequency or time of occurrence.

isocitrate (i″so-cĭ′trāt) a salt or ester of isocitric acid.

isocitrate dehydrogenase (NAD^+ or $NADP^+$) (ICD) (i″so-cĭ′trāt de-hi′dro-jen-ās) *threo*-D_s-isocitrate:NAD^+ or $NADP^+$ oxidoreductase (decarboxylating), an enzyme of the oxidoreductase class that catalyzes the reaction: *threo*-D_s-isocitrate + $NAD(P)^+$ = α-ketoglutarate (2-oxoglutarate) + CO_2 + NAD(P)H + H^+. The reaction is an oxidative decarboxylation. The enzyme requiring NAD^+ (EC 1.1.1.41) occurs in cell mitochondria, and its reaction is of key importance in the function and regulation of the citric acid cycle. The enzyme requiring $NADP^+$ (EC 1.1.1.42) is soluble and occurs in serum (serum ICD). It functions mainly in auxiliary biosynthetic pathways; however, as it is predominantly present in liver tissue, its assay is clinically important in the early detection of liver disease.

An elevated ICD in serum is seen in viral hepatitis, infectious mononucleosis, and biliary tract inflammations. Certain drugs (alcohol, *p*-aminosalicylic acid) increase ICD activity. The ICD activity in serum is assayed by continuously monitoring (at 340 nm) the NADPH formed in the reaction. The reference range for isocitrate dehydrogenase, at 30°C, is 1.2–7.0 U/l.

isocitrate dehydrogenase ($NADP^+$) assays the quantitation of enzyme activity by measuring the increase in absorbance due to NADPH production upon the appropriate incubation of serum (or another appropriate specimen) with buffered isocitrate and NADP. The conventional unit of enzyme activity (Wolfson and Williams-Ashman) is the number of nanomoles of NADPH formed per milliliter of serum per hour at a specified temperature. Using 25°C, the normal range is 50–260 W,W-A units, which is equivalent to 1.2–7.0 U/l at 30°C. The distribution is skewed toward higher values. Newborn infants have a range of 125–490 W,W-A units, which is equivalent to 3–12 U/l at 30°C.

isocitric acid (i″so-sit′rik) 1-hydroxy-1,2,3-propane-tricarboxylic acid, $CHOH(COOH){\cdot}CH(COOH){\cdot}CH_2(COOH)$, an isomer of citric acid. It is an intermediate compound of the tricarboxylic acid cycle.

isocyanate (i″so-si′ah-nāt) an organic compound containing the —N=C=O group. See also *functional group.*

isodesmosine (i″so-des′mo-sēn) an *N*-heterocyclic ring structure formed as a result of cross-linking in elastin. It differs from desmosine in the positions of attachment of the four lysyl side-chain carbons to the heterocyclic ring. See also *elastin.*

isodose (i′so-dōs) in radiation therapy, a radiation dose equal to that administered to another body part. An isodose curve on a drawing connects points receiving isodoses.

isoelectric (i″so-e-lek′trik) showing no variation in electrical potential. The term is usually applied to a molecule that carries an equal number of positive and negative charges or to a pair of electrodes having the same voltage at a given instant in time.

isoelectric focusing a special type of electrophoresis. A pH gradient is established along the support medium (gel), and each protein in the sample migrates to the point where the pH equals its isoelectric point. The pH gradient is caused by ampholytes added to the gel, which migrate in the electrophoresis current when one end of the gel is immersed in acid and the other in base. Isoelectric focusing in polyacrylamide gel is used to detect abnormal hemoglobins. The relative order of hemoglobins and myoglobin seen after isoelectric focusing, beginning at the acidic anodal end, is myoglobin, Hb A, Hb S, and Hb C.

isoelectric point (pI, pH_I) the pH at which a molecule (usually an amino acid or protein) has no net charge and will not move in an electric field (e.g., at pH 6.02, alanine has the structure H_3N^+—CH_2—CO_2^-).

isoenzyme (i″so-en′zīm) one of a group of related enzymes catalyzing the same reaction but having different molecular structures, and characterized by varying physical, biochemical, and immunologic properties. Some are multiunit proteins, with the individual isoenzymes varying in the proportion of the individual, but related, subunits (see *lactate dehydrogenase*). Because the proportions of the different isoenzyme forms may vary between tissues, identification of these patterns in serum can be used clinically to indicate the tissue of origin. Isoenzymes of alkaline phosphatase, creatine kinase, and lactate dehydrogenase are important in clinical differential diagnosis. Also called *isozyme.*

isogamy (i-sog′ah-me) [*iso-* + Gr. *gamos* marriage] a reproductive process, occurring in protozoa, that consists of the union of two cells or gametes of the same size and structure.

isogeneic (i″so-jĕ-nĕ′ik) see *syngeneic.*

isogeneic graft see *isogeneic g.* under *graft.*

isograft (i′so-graft) see *isogeneic g.* under *graft.*

isohydric shift (i″so-hi′drik) the series of chemical reactions that allows the carbon dioxide from metabolic processes to be transported in the blood without causing a change in pH. The carbon dioxide produced by cellular respiration dissolves in the plasma, diffuses into erythrocytes, and is there converted to carbonic acid by the enzyme carbonic anhydrase. The H_2CO_3 dissociates into HCO_3^- and H^+ ions. Concurrently, the release of oxygen from hemoglobin forms deoxygenated hemoglobin, which is a weaker acid than oxyhemoglobin (the Bohr effect) and thus binds additional hydrogen ions. Deoxygenated hemoglobin also binds more carbon dioxide by forming carbamino (—$NHCOO^-$) groups. The organic and inorganic phosphates in the red blood cells also buffer some of the hydrogen ions formed from H_2CO_3. See also *buffer system* and *chloride shift.*

isoimmune (i″so-i-mūn′) specifically immune to an isoantigen.

isoimmune hemolytic anemia see *hemolytic disease of the newborn.*

isoimmunization (i″so-im″u-nĭ-za′shun) the development of antibodies in response to antigens from genetically dissimilar individuals of the same species. See also *isoantigen.*

isolate (i′so-lāt) 1. to separate from other persons, materials, or objects.

2. in microbiology, to obtain from a source such as a clinical specimen a pure strain that may have been part of a mixed primary culture.

3. a population that has been obtained by isolation (such as bacteria or other cells obtained in pure culture), or a group of individuals prevented by geographic, ecologic, or social barriers from interbreeding with others of their kind, and thus differentiated by the accumulation of new characteristics.

isolation (i″so-la′shun) 1. the process of isolating, or the state of being isolated.

2. the physiologic separation of a part, as by tissue culture or by interposition of inert material.

3. the chemical extraction of an unknown substance in pure form from a tissue.

4. the separation from contact with others of patients having a communicable disease.

5. the successive propagation of a growth of microorganisms until a pure culture is obtained.

isoleucine (Ile or I) (i″so-lu′sēn) 2-amino-3-methylpentanoic acid, $CH_3CH_2CH(CH_3)CH(NH_2)COOH$, a naturally occurring amino acid; M.W. 131.17. Isoleucine serves as a component of protein molecules; its source is dietary proteins. See also under *amino acids.*

isoleucyl (i″so-loo′sil) the acyl radical derived from or relating to isoleucine.

isomaltase (i″so-mawl′tās) see *oligo-1,6-glucosidase.*

isomer (i′so-mer) [*iso-* + Gr. *meros* part] 1. a metastable excited state of a nuclide that decays by isomeric transition.

2. see under *isomerism.*

isomerase (i-som′er-ās) a major class of enzymes (EC 5). These enzymes catalyze intramolecular rearrangements or isomerization reactions that do not involve a net change in the concentration of compounds other than the substrate, e.g., the interconversion of aldoses and ketoses, the racemization about an optically active atom, cis-trans isomerization, and intramolecular transfer of PO_4 groups. The class includes enzymes variously known as racemase, epimerase, and mutase. Clinically important examples are *hexosephosphate isomerase* (EC 5.3.1.9) and *ribulosephosphate-3-epimerase* (EC 5.1.3.1).

isomeric (i″so-mer′ik) see under *isomerism.*

isomeric transition a type of radioactive decay in which an excited, metastable state of a nuclide undergoes a transition to the ground state and emits a gamma ray. An example is the decay of ^{99m}Tc to ^{99}Tc with the emission of a 140-keV gamma ray.

isomerism (i-som′ĕ-rizm) a relationship between two or more different chemical compounds having the same molecular formula but different structures and properties. The compounds are isomers (of each other) and are isomeric (to each other). There are many types of isomerism that describe the particular way in which the isomers differ. These fall into two large groups: structural isomerism (also called constitutional and position isomerism) and stereoisomerism (also called configurational, stereochemical, and spatial isomerism).

Structural isomers (Fig. 1) differ by having their atoms bonded in different sequences, and differ in their structural formulas and chemical properties. Tautomers, which are in chemical equilibrium and freely change from one form to the other, are a special class of structural isomers. The equilibrium process is called tautomerism. Stereoisomers differ not in the order in which the atoms are attached but in the spatial positions of the atoms; a spatial formula is necessary to distinguish them. These can be subdivided into two groups: enantiomers and diastereomers (which are further subdivided into optical and geometric isomers, as discussed below). Enantiomers (antipodes, enantiomorphs) are a pair of stereoisomers (and are therefore nonidentical or nonsuperimposable) that have a mirror image relationship. Diastereoisomers are stereoisomers that do not have a mirror image relationship.

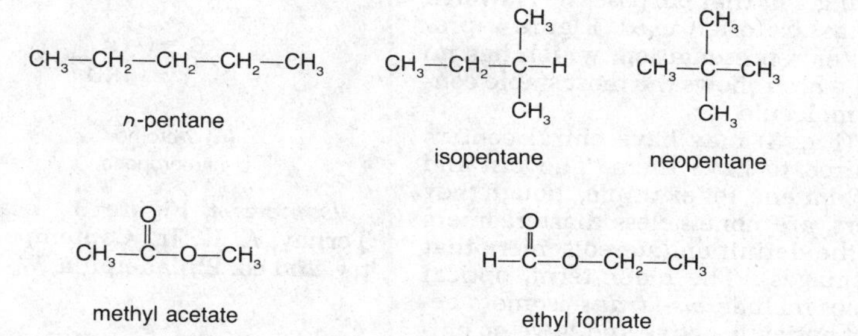

Isomerism, Figure 1. Structural (constitutional) isomers. (From Ternay, A. L., Jr.: Contemporary Organic Chemistry. 2nd ed. Philadelphia, W. B. Saunders Co., 1976.)

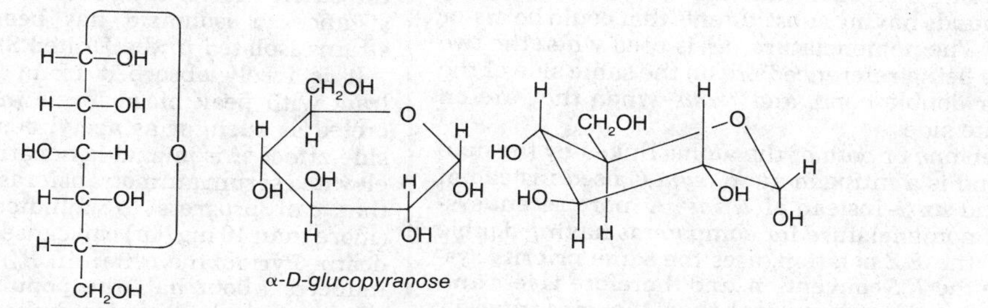

Isomerism, Figure 2. *A,* Fischer, *B,* Haworth, and *C,* perspective formulas of α-D-glucopyranose. (From Banks, J. E.: Naming Organic Compounds. 2nd ed. Philadelphia, W. B. Saunders Co., 1976.)

A molecule that cannot be superimposed on its mirror image is said to be chiral. Chirality is the property of handedness (as in a right or left hand) that a chiral molecule possesses. A molecule with a single asymmetric carbon (one with four different groups attached) is chiral. A molecule can be chiral even though it lacks an asymmetric carbon atom (a chiral carbon or chiral center), and molecules with more than one asymmetric carbon can be achiral (not chiral). Certain fundamental symmetry properties determine whether a molecule is chiral. Chiral molecules have the property of being optically active; that is, they can rotate the plane of polarization of a polarized light beam (optical rotation).

Each member of a pair of enantiomers is chiral and therefore is optically active. Enantiomers have identical properties in an achiral environment. However, they do form different products when they react with another chiral molecule, and they do behave differently in polarized light. One enantiomer will rotate the plane of polarization by an angle α in one direction; the other enantiomer will rotate it by an angle α in the other direction. The direction of rotation, the optical rotation, is designated as (+) (formerly *d*-, or dextro, to the right) or (–) (formerly *l*-, or levo, to the left). A racemic form (also racemic modification or *dl* pair), an equimolar mixture of a pair of enantiomers, is designated (±) (formerly *dl*) and is optically inactive.

There are two nomenclature conventions currently used to designate the absolute configuration of chiral centers, the D,L system and the *R,S* system. A particular stereoisomer with one chiral center is designated as D if it has the same configuration as D-(+)-glyceraldehyde, and L if it has the opposite configuration. In sugars, by convention, the configuration of the highest numbered chiral center is used for the assignment of D or L; the designations D_g or L_g are sometimes used to specify the relationship to glyceraldehyde. In amino acids the configuration of the lowest numbered chiral carbon is used and the reference standard is serine; the designations D_s and L_s are thus sometimes used for amino acid.

The *R,S* convention is a more systematic and general system than the D,L convention. To assign *R* or *S* to the configuration of a particular chiral atom, the groups attached to it are assigned a priority based on the following rules: Functional groups are ranked giving highest priority to the highest atomic mass of the atom to which the bond is attached; an unshared electron pair ranks lowest. If these first atoms are the same, then second atoms (those bonded to the first) are compared and taken in order of priority. Multiple bonds are treated as though they had duplicate or triplicate single bonds. Now, with the lowest ranking group pointing away from the viewer, the affix *R*- is used if the other three groups are arranged in order of decreasing rank in a clockwise direction; the affix *S*- is used for those arranged counterclockwise.

There are several conventions in use for representing in two dimensions on paper the three-dimensional spatial arrangements of atoms in a real molecule with chiral atoms; the Fischer projection formulas are one such convention. In them, horizontal bonds are understood to extend out the plane of the paper toward the viewer, and vertical bonds are understood to extend behind the plane away from the viewer. For the cyclic form of sugars, the Fischer projection formulas show the configurations at each of the chiral centers, but they do not show the shape of the ring. For that purpose the Haworth projection formulas are often used. Figure 2 provides an even better representation, which has no special name and which shows the most stable conformation of the molecule.

Diastereomers (Fig. 3) may have chiral centers but are not required to have them. The *cis-* and *trans-*isomers of 2-butene, for example, though they lack chiral centers, are nonetheless diastereomers because they fit the definition (stereoisomers that are not mirror images). The older term, optical isomerism, does not include *cis-/trans-* isomers because they are not optically active and have no chiral centers. Instead, they are, in the older classification, placed in a separate category called geometric isomerism, a category that also includes some ring compounds having substitutents that could be *cis-*or *trans-*. The nomenclature *cis-* is used when the two groups being referenced are on the same side of the ring or double bond, and *trans-* when they are on opposite sides.

When one or both of the atoms linked by the double bond is a nitrogen atom, *syn-* is used instead of *cis-*, and *anti-* instead of *trans-*. A more recent system of nomenclature for compounds having double bonds, the *E,Z* notation, uses the same priority system as the *R,S* convention, and therefore is less ambiguous and more general than the *cis-/trans-* or *syn-/anti-*conventions. In it, all the groups attached to the double bonds are assigned a priority. If the highest priority groups at each end of the double bond are on the same side, the *Z* (for the German word *zusammen*, meaning together) assignment is made. If they are on opposite sides, the *E* (for *entgegen*, meaning across) assignment is made. Diastereomers have different chemical and physical properties.

Conformational isomers (single-bond torsional isomers, conformers) are stereoisomers that have not been included in this discussion; they are isomers that can be readily interconverted at room temperature by rotation about a single bond. Under normal conditions, conformational isomers cannot be separated and isolated from one another.

See also *anomer, conformation, Fischer projection,* and *Haworth formula.*

JOSEPH W. WILSON, PH.D.

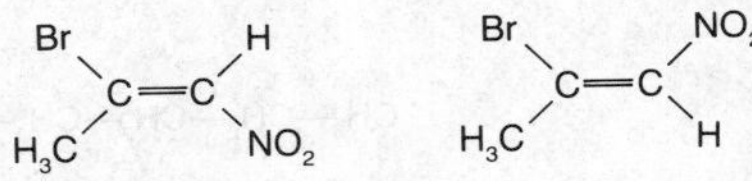

Isomerism, Figure 3. Diastereoisomers. (From Ternay, A. L., Jr.: Contemporary Organic Chemistry. 2nd ed. Philadelphia, W. B. Saunders Co., 1976.)

isomerization (i-som″er-ĭ-za′shun) a chemical reaction in which the principal product is isomeric with the principal reactant.

isometric (i″so-met′rik) [*iso-* + Gr. *metron* measure] maintaining a constant measure or length; with reference to a skeletal muscle contraction, the development of tension or force at a constant muscle length. Cf. *isotonic.*

isoniazid (i″so-ni′ah-zid) a synthetic antimycobacterial agent chemically related to nicotine, 4-pyridinecarboxylic acid, or isonicotinic acid hydrazide (INH). It is bactericidal against growing *Mycobacterium tuberculosis* and acts on intracellular as well as extracellular organisms by inhibiting mycolic acid synthesis. The exact mechanism of killing has not been defined.

Isoniazid is the drug of choice in the treatment of tuberculosis and for prophylaxis in individuals who are recently negative to positive tuberculin skin test converters. For therapy the drug is used in conjunction with other "first-line" or primary drugs such as rifampin, streptomycin, or ethambutol to prevent the emergence of drug-resistant mycobacteria. Resistance to isoniazid has been reported among strains isolated in the United States.

It is freely absorbed from the gastrointestinal tract with peak blood levels in 1–3 hr, and is excreted as such, or as acetyl derivative. A common side-effect of isoniazid is hepatitis accompanied by elevated serum aminotransferase levels, a condition that can progress to jaundice. Large overdoses (more than 10 mg/kg) can cause coma, seizures, and death. Pyridoxine (vitamin B_6) deficiency may be induced. About half the population lacks the enzyme to acetylate isoniazid; these slow inactivators may incur more toxic effects than do rapid inactivators.

See also *antibacterial agents.*

isoniazid assays spectrophotometry. Isoniazid is extracted into polar solvents from alkalinized serum. Reaction with *trans*-cinnamaldehyde produces a product that can be measured by its absorption at 340 nm.

isoniazid phenotype test a procedure to determine slow acetylators of isoniazid. A urine sample is taken 6 hr after administration of isoniazid; the fraction that has been excreted in acetylated form is determined spectrophotometrically. Slow inactivators will have acetylated less that 70 percent. Glucose, vitamin B_6, and some drugs interfere.

isonicotinic acid hydrazide (INH) (i″so-nik″o-tēn′ik hi′drah-zīd) see *isoniazid.*

isoosmotic (i″so-oz-mot′ik) see *isosmotic.*

Isopaque (i″so-pāk′) trademark. See under *metrizoate.*

Δ²-isopentenyl diphosphate (i″so-pen′tēn-il di-fos′fāt) see *dimethylallyl diphosphate.*

Δ³-isopentenyl diphosphate the general donor of prenyl groups for the synthesis of all polyprenyl compounds.

isopentyl- (i″so-pen′til) a prefix word element in organic chemistry to denote the 3-methylbutyl group, $—CH_2CH_2CH(CH_3)_2$, e.g., isopentylamine, isopentyl alcohol. Cf. *n-pentyl-* and *neopentyl-.*

isopleth (i′so-pleth) 1. a line, cutting the scales of a nomogram, that gives the associated values of the variables.

2. a line on a graph that represents the points conveying the corresponding values of the dependent and independent variables.

3. a graph that shows the occurrence or frequency of a phenomenon or parameter as a function of two variables.

isoprene (i′so-prēn) 2-methyl-1,3-butadiene,

$CH_2{=}C(CH_3)CH{=}CH_2$. The isoprene unit, the basic building unit of terpenes and terpenoid compounds, has the same carbon skeleton as isoprene.

isoprenoid (i″so-prēn′oid) a compound that can be considered to be structurally formed by linking of isoprene (C_5H_8) units together. Many polyprenyl compounds occur in nature: ubiquinone side-chain carotenes, rubber, steroids, and the cyclic terpenoid compounds of camphor, pinene, limonene, and many others.

isopropamide iodide (i″so-pro′pah-mīd) [NF], an anticholinergic drug, which has a quaternary ammonium group and primarily acts on the ganglia. It is used in the treatment of irritable bowel syndrome, spastic colon, and mucous colitis. Adverse reactions include dry mouth, urinary retention, constipation, blurred vision, and tachycardia.

isopropanol (i″so-pro′pah-nōl) isopropyl alcohol, 2-propanol, $CH_3CHOHCH_3$; a transparent, volatile, colorless liquid used as a rubbing compound and antiseptic, as well as to denature ethyl alcohol; M.W. 60.09. Ingestion or inhalation of the vapors causes nausea, vomiting, and dizziness; a larger amount can be fatal. In the chemical laboratory it is used to extract and dissolve lipids, and similarly in histology it is used as a solubilizer for fat stains and as a dehydrating agent.

isopropanol assays methods for the measurement of isopropanol in the blood or urine. Colorimetric and enzymatic methods for the determination of ethanol are nonspecific and also respond to methanol and isopropanol. Isopropanol can be quantitated using the head space method with gas chromatography. See also *ethanol assays* and *head space analysis.*

isopropyl- (i″so-pro′pil) a prefix word element in organic chemistry to denote the 1-methylethyl group, $—CH(CH_3)_2$, e.g., isopropylamine, isopropyl alcohol. Cf. *n-propyl-.*

isoproterenol (i″so-pro-ter′ĕ-nol) an adrenergic drug, a sympathomimetic amine similar to epinephrine but acting primarily on the β-adrenergic receptors. It has an inotropic effect on the myocardium, increasing the cardiac output; it also acts to relax the smooth muscle of the bronchioles and the gastrointestinal tract. Isoproterenol is used in the treatment of bronchial asthma, shock, cardiac and respiratory arrest, and ventricular tachycardias and arrhythmias. Adverse reactions include tremors, nervousness, palpitation, tachycardia, and headache.

i. hydrochloride, [USP], a salt administered orally, parenterally, and by inhalation.

i. sulfate, [NF], a salt administered by inhalation as a bronchodilator.

isopyknic (i″so-pik′nik) [*iso-* + Gr. *pyknos* thick] having equal density; in centrifugation, the term refers to the density of both sample and solvent.

isopyknotic (i″so-pik-not′ik) [*iso-* + Gr. *pyknōsis* condensation] referring to chromosomal regions that are as tightly coiled as most of the chromosomal material of a cell. Cf. *heteropyknotic.*

isosbestic point (i″so-sbes′tik) in ultraviolet-visible spectroscopy, any wavelength at which two solutions of equal concentration have equal absorbances.

isosexual (i″so-seks′u-al) [*iso-* + L. *sexualis*] a general term used to describe developmental trends toward the same gender; in females, a isosexual characteristics include enlargement of the breasts and broadening of the hips.

isosmotic (i″sos-mot′ik) having the same osmotic pressure or osmolality. Also called *isoosmotic.*

isosorbide dinitrate (i″so-sor′bīd di-ni′trāt) an organic nitrate compound used as a coronary vasodilator for the treatment of angina pectoris.

Isospora (i-sos′po-rah) [*iso-* + Gr. *sporos* spore] a genus of sporozoan parasites found in birds, reptiles, amphibians, and, occasionally, humans. The species *I. belli* and *I. hominis* are both mild pathogenic parasites of the human small intestine with worldwide distribution; they are particularly found in warm climates. Infection is caused by the ingestion of fecally contaminated food with oocysts.

For *I. belli,* diagnosis requires identification in the feces of unstained immature oocysts: they are ovoid and elongated, measuring 30 by 12 μm.

The oocysts have also been found in duodenal fluid. *I. hominis* can be distinguished from *I. belli* by the mature oocysts found in the feces and by the absence of oocyst wall.

I. hominis, is no longer considered to be one of *Isospora* but rather represents the sexual stages of two species of *Sarcocystis: S. fusiformis* (from cattle) and *S. miescheriana* (from swine).

isothermal (i″so-ther′mal) [*iso-* + Gr. *thermē* heat] having or being held at a constant temperature or the same temperature.

isotone (i′so-tōn) one of several nuclides having the same number of neutrons in their nuclei. Cf. *isobar* and *isotope.*

isotonic (i″so-ton′ik) [*iso-* + Gr. *tonos* tone]

1. having the same osmotic pressure as blood or the intracellular fluids of a cell or tissue. Cells bathed in an isotonic solution do not gain or lose water by osmosis.

2. maintaining or possessing a constant or equal tension, especially with reference to a skeletal muscle contraction during which the muscle shortens to lift a constant load and is therefore under a constant tension. Cf. *isometric.*

isotope (i′so-tōp) [*iso-* + Gr. *topos* place] one of several nuclides that have the same atomic number but different atomic mass numbers, e.g., ^{12}C (stable) and ^{14}C (radioactive). Isotopes are species of the same chemical element. Cf. *isobar.*

isotope dilution–mass spectrometry (ID-MS) a special form of mass spectrometry in which an isotope is added as a form of internal standard. It is capable of high accuracy and precision and is thus used as a definitive method against which reference methods are compared. A known quantity of an isotopically labeled form of the unknown (analyte) is added to the sample, which is then analyzed in the mass spectrometer. The ratio of the naturally occurring isotopes relative to the added labeled isotope gives the concentration of the unknown, generally to within about 0.1 percent of the "true" value.

isotropic (i″so-trop′ik) [*iso-* + Gr. *tropos* a turning] having equal properties in all directions; having rotational symmetry.

isovaleric acid (i′so-vah-ler″ik) a branched chain fatty acid, 3-methylbutenoic acid, ($CH_3CH(CH_3)$-CH_2COOH), occurring as an intermediate in the metabolism of leucine.

isovaleric acidemia a disorder of leucine metabolism, transmitted as an autosomal recessive trait, that is due to a relative or absolute deficiency of the enzyme isovaleryl CoA dehydrogenase. This leads to increased levels of isovaleric acid and isovalerylglycine in the blood and urine. Affected infants have vomiting, severe metabolic acidosis, a variable degree of mental retardation, and a characteristic body odor similar to that of sweaty feet. Neonatal death is common. This condition may be treated with variable success by the feeding of low-protein (especially low-leucine) diets. In utero detection of this condition is considered feasible. See also *aminoacidopathy.*

isovaleryl-CoA dehydrogenase an enzyme of the oxidoreductase class (isovaleryl-CoA: (acceptor) oxidoreductase, EC 1.3.99.10) that catalyzes the reaction isovaleryl-CoA + acceptor ⇄ 3-methylcrotonoyl-CoA + reduced acceptor, which is a step in the metabolism of leucine. A deficiency of this enzyme is the cause of isovaleric acidemia.

isovolume pressure flow curve (IVPF) a curve that relates the expiratory airflow as a specific lung volume is reached (commonly a specific percentage of the vital capacity) to the simultaneous value of transpulmonary pressure. IVPF curves can be plotted from simultaneous airflow, lung volume, and intrathoracic pressure measurements made during the performance of a series of forced expiratory vital capacity maneuvers of graded effort. Each curve demonstrates the effects of an increasing driving pressure (the difference between alveolar and mouth pressures) on the expiratory flow at a constant lung volume.

At lung volumes near the total lung capacity (when the lung is approximately 70–95 percent inflated), the expiratory flow continues to increase as the expiratory effort becomes more vigorous (and thus the driving pressure increases). At smaller lung volumes, the flow rate plateaus, or reaches a maximum, despite further increases in the driving pressure. This maximal airflow for a given lung volume is reached because airway resistance increases (owing to dynamic compression of the intrathoracic airways) proportionately with any increase in driving pressure.

See also the accompanying illustration.

isoxsuprine hydrochloride (i-sok'su-prēn) [NF], a sympathomimetic amine that produces peripheral vasodilation and is used to alleviate symptoms of cerebral vascular insufficiency or peripheral vascular disease. Adverse reactions include palpitation, tachycardia, hypotension, and vomiting.

isozyme (i'so-zīm) see *isoenzyme.*

-ist (ist) [L. *-ista;* Gr. *-istēs*] a suffix word element to denote a specialist, e.g., nephrologist, neurologist.

isthmus (is'mus), pl. *isthmi* [Gr. *isthmos*] [NA], a general term to designate a narrow connecting structure or region between two larger bodies or parts.

i. of fauces, the constricted segment between the cavity of the mouth and the pharynx. It is bounded above by the soft palate, laterally by the palatoglossal arches, and below by the tongue. Also called *oropharyngeal isthmus.*

i. of thyroid gland, the narrow band of tissue that connects the lower parts of the lobes of the thyroid gland.

itch (ich) pruritus; an unpleasant skin sensation that provokes a scratching or rubbing response. Generalized itching may be a symptom of skin disorders, fungal and parasitic infections, response to stress, drug reactions, blood disorders, or malignant neoplasms.

-ite (īt) 1. a suffix word element to denote a segment or constituent of a body or of a part of a body.

2. a suffix word element to denote a mineral, e.g., fluorite.

3. a suffix word element used in organic chemistry to denote the anion (or ester) of an oxo acid in which the central atom has the lower of the two common oxidation states, e.g., sulfite, the common name for thioxosulfate (SO_3^{2-}).

iteration (it"er-a'shun) [L. *iteratio,* from *iterum* again] 1. the repetition of a sequence of steps in a computer program or algorithm. Also called *looping.*

2. each of the passages through a loop in a computer program.

iterative process (it'er-ah-tiv) a calculation performed by repeating a sequence of steps. Each iteration uses the result of the previous iteration to produce a new result that is nearer to the desired answer. The process ceases when the error is within acceptable limits.

-itis (i'tis,), pl. *-itides*[*-itis,* a feminine adjectival termination agreeing with Gr. *nosos* disease (understood) — e.g., neuritis = Gr. *hē neuritis nosos* inflammatory disease of the nerves] a suffix word element to denote inflammation, e.g., nephritis.

ITP abbrev. See *idiopathic thrombocytopenic purpura* and *inosine triphosphate.*

IU abbrev. See *International Unit.*

IUB abbrev. for International Union of Biochemistry. See under *Enzyme Commission.*

IUDR abbrev. See *5-iododeoxyuridine.*

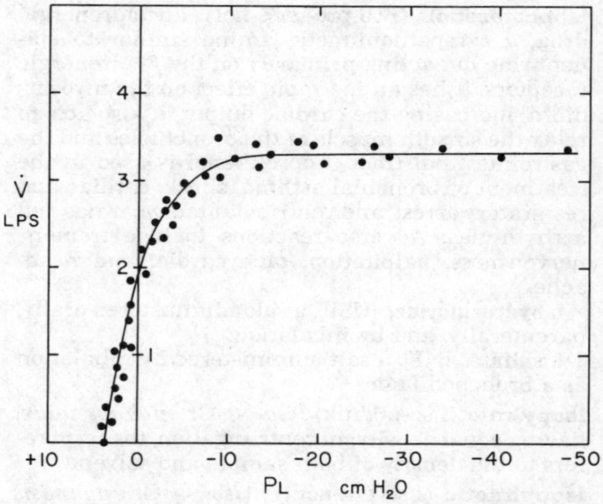

Isovolume pressure flow curve. An example of the isovolume pressure flow curve obtained in a normal subject at 33 percent vital capacity. These curves are obtained by plotting the flows as the subject passes through a specific lung volume against the simultaneous values of transpulmonary pressure. (From Bates, D. V., et al.: Respiratory Function in Disease. 2nd ed. Philadelphia, W. B. Saunders Co., 1971.)

-ium (e′um) a suffix word element used in many chemical elements, e.g., barium, and in many cases to denote a cation, e.g., methylcarbenium perchlorate ($CH_3{}^+ClO_4{}^-$) and pyridinium chloride.

IUPAC (u′pak) abbrev. See *International Union of Pure and Applied Chemistry.*

IV abbrev. See *intravenous.*

IVP abbrev. for intravenous pyelography. See under *urography.*

IVPF abbrev. See *isovolume pressure flow curve.*

IVU abbrev. for intravenous urography. See under *urography.*

Ixodes (iks-o′dēz) [Gr. *ixōdēs* sticky, from *ixos* bird-lime] a genus of hard ticks, several species of which are parasitic in humans: *I. cavipalpus* is an African tick that infests monkeys and humans (children); *I. frequens* is a tick commonly implicated in human infestation in Japan, and *I. pacificus* is a deer or cattle tick that occasionally bites humans and is thought to transmit tularemia. Another species, *I. scapularis,* is common in the eastern United States; called the black-legged tick, it causes a painful bite in humans.

ixodiasis (iks″o-di′ah-sis) any condition or lesion caused by tick bites; being infested with ticks.

ixodic (ik-sod′ik) caused by ticks.

-ize (īz) [Gr. *-izō*] a suffix word element to denote a specific action or treatment, e.g., adrenalectomize.

J

J symbol for *joule,* the unit for energy and heat.

jacksonian march (jak-so′ne-an) [John Hughlings *Jackson,* London neurologist, 1835–1911] see *jacksonian e.* under *epilepsy.*

jacksonian motor seizure [John Hughlings *Jackson*] see *jacksonian e.* under *epilepsy.*

Jacobson's organ (ja′kub-sunz) [Ludwig Levin *Jacobson,* Danish anatomist, 1783–1843] a short rudimentary canal lined with olfactorylike epithelium, which opens blindly into the nasal septum. This structure is vestigial in humans, but in other mammals it appears to have a chemosensory function. Also called vomeronasal organ.

Jaffe reaction (jaf′e) [Max *Jaffe,* German biochemist, 1841–1911] see under *creatinine assays.*

Janeway lesion (jān′wa) [Theodore Caldwell *Janeway,* American physician, 1872–1917] a small hemorrhagic macular lesion infrequently found on the soles and palms in bacterial endocarditis. Also called Janeway's spots.

Janus green B (jan′us) a basic axo dye; C.I. 11050. It is used as a supravital stain.

Jarisch-Herxheimer reaction (yah′rish herks′-hīm-er) [Adolf *Jarisch,* Austrian dermatologist, 1850–1902; Karl *Herxheimer,* German dermatologist, 1861–1944] an immunologic complication characterized by fever, headache, myalgia (muscle pain), and increased discomfort from preexisting skin lesions that can occur a few hours after antibiotic treatment of secondary syphilis, borreliosis, brucellosis, and typhoid fever.

The Jarisch-Herxheimer reaction is a common complication of syphilis treatment, occurring in nearly half the patients treated, but it is much less frequent in other diseases. It is thought to result from the release of antigens from killed microorganisms; the intensity of the reaction is probably related to the amount of local inflammation present before treatment.

jaundice (jawn′dis) [Fr. *jaunisse,* from *jaune* yellow] a state characterized by the yellow-green discoloration of the skin and mucous membranes and of the whites of the eyes (sclerae) owing to the accumulation of bilirubin. Hyperbilirubinemia (greater than 2–3 mg/dl) is due either to an increase in bilirubin formation or to a decrease in its excretion. Jaundice is symptomatic of a number of diseases, including hepatic disease (cirrhosis, hepatitis, functional disorders), gallstones, gallbladder disorders, hemolytic disorders, and biochemical abnormalities. See also *bilirubin, bilirubin assays, cirrhosis,* and *hepatitis.*

acholuric j., jaundice caused by elevations in unconjugated bilirubin concentrations—albumin-bound bilirubin is insoluble and cannot be filtered by the renal glomerulus into the urine. Acholuric jaundice is usually due to hemolysis. See also *erythroblastosis fetalis* and *hemolytic j.*

acute febrile j., jaundice associated with infectious hepatitis. Also called acute infectious jaundice.

cholestatic j., jaundice due to the inhibition of bile flow and secretion, with the resultant accumulation of bile pigments in the blood. Usually there is conjugated hyperbilirubinemia due to either intrahepatic or extrahepatic obstruction.

hemolytic j., jaundice associated with the hemolytic anemias. The increases in erythrocyte breakdown increase the breakdown of hemoglobin, and bilirubin levels rise. There is an unconjugated hyperbilirubinemia and an acholuric jaundice. There may be an increase in gallstones associated with chronic hemolytic jaundice in the adult. Excess free unconjugated bilirubin in the neonate may lead to bilirubin deposition in neural tissue and brain damage. Also called hematogenous jaundice. See also *hemolytic a.* under *anemia.* Cf. *nonhemolytic j.*

hepatocellular j., jaundice due to liver cell death or injury, as in exposure to hepatotoxic agents.

leptospiral j., jaundice associated with severe leptospirosis or Weil's disease. See also *Weil's disease.*

nonhemolytic j., jaundice due to abnormalities in the metabolism or excretion of bilirubin, as opposed to its excessive production. Cf. *hemolytic j.*

obstructive j., jaundice due to the obstruction of the flow of bile at any point along the biliary tree. The obstruction may be due to mechanical blockage, as with stones or neoplasm, or to inflammatory change.

JCAH abbrev. See *Joint Commission on Accreditation of Hospitals.*

J chain a polypeptide chain normally present in polymeric IgA and IgM; M.W. 15,000. The in vivo function of the J chain is to induce the polymerization of monomeric IgA and IgM. There are two known polymeric IgA myelomas that lack J chains, which indicates that J chains are not an essential prerequisite for IgA polymerization. However, the concentration of intracellular J chains influences the ratio of polymeric to monomeric immunoglobulins. In polymeric immunoglobulins, individual monomers are linked through disulfide bonds in such a manner that each polymeric immunoglobulin has only one J chain, regardless of the number of monomers involved. See also *immunoglobulin.*

jejun/o (jĕ-joo′no) [L. *jejunum* empty] a word element used in combining form to denote the jejunum (the second part of the small intestine), e.g., jejunostomy.

jejunitis (jĕ″joo-ni′tis) an inflammation of the jejunum. It either is caused by a specific agent such as bacteria or fungi, or occurs as part of a systemic disorder. See also *enteritis.*

jejunoileitis (jĕ-joo″no-il″e-i′tis) an inflammation of both the jejunum and ileum. See also *enteritis.*

jejunum (jĕ-joo′num) [L. "empty"] [NA], the second of the three segments of the small intestine. It commences at the duodenojejunal flexure and merges imperceptibly with the ileum. Together the jejunum and ileum are approximately 6 m long, the jejunum making up the proximal two-fifths of the total length. The small intestine is suspended by the mesentery, a reflection of peritoneum whose base runs diagonally across the posterior abdominal wall from the upper left to the lower right, following the line of the superior mesenteric artery. Branches of the artery, tributaries of the portal vein, and lymphatics radiate with the mesentery, supported by a thin layer of fibroadipose tissue. The jejunum and ileum form coils that occupy much of the abdominal cavity; those of the jejunum are mainly above and to the left of the ileal loops.

The wall of the jejunum contains the same coats as the duodenum and ileum, differing from them only in degree. Compared with the ileum, the jejunum has larger villi, more mesenteric fat, a thicker and more vascular wall, more closely spaced circular mucosal folds (plicae), and fewer and smaller Peyer's patches. It is also of wider caliber.

Jendrassick-Grof method see under *bilirubin assays.*

JFET abbrev. See *junction field effect t.* under *transistor.*

jigger (jig'ger) a common name for *Tunga penetrans,* also known as the burrowing flea, sand flea, or chigoe. Gravid female fleas burrow into the skin and lay eggs, causing lesions that itch and become inflamed. The fleas are usually removed surgically.

jitter (jit'ter) in single-fiber electromyography, the variability in the time interval between the consecutive discharges of muscle action potentials of two fibers from the same motor unit. The jitter, usually equal to 10–30 μsec, is caused by inconsistencies in the synaptic delays at the two myoneural junctions. High jitter values are usually seen in patients with abnormal neuromuscular transmission (e.g., myasthenia gravis).

Job's syndrome (jōbz) a rare genetic disorder of neutrophils that is characterized by abnormal or absent chemotactic responses. This defect leads to repeated staphylococcal abscesses and eczema. High serum levels of IgE are also characteristic.

jock itch see *tinea cruris.*

joint (joint) [L. *junctio* a joining, connection] the junction between two or more skeletal components. Joints are of three basic types: fibrous or fixed, cartilaginous or "slightly movable," and synovial or "freely moving."

cartilaginous j., a slightly movable joint in which the bony elements are connected by cartilaginous tissue.

fibrous j., a fixed or minimally movable articulation either between bones joined by fibrous connective tissue or in sutures. Also called *synarthrosis.*

intervertebral j.'s, the joints between the vertebrae from the second cervical to the first sacral. They are of two types: cartilaginous joints, which articulate the vertebral bodies, and synovial joints, articulations between the vertebral arches.

synovial j., a freely movable articulation, with the bony elements surrounded by an articular capsule and movement occurring over viscous synovial fluid. Also called *diarthrosis.*

Joint Commission on Accreditation of Hospitals (JCAH) a professional health organization responsible for hospital accreditation.

joint scan a scintillation camera scan of a joint of the body. It is a nonspecific procedure that shows areas of active inflammation, such as occur in rheumatoid arthritis, gouty arthritis, infectious arthritis, and osteoarthritis. A variety of imaging agents, usually labeled with technetium-99m, are used, including pertechnetate, serum albumin, and the phosphate bone agents (pyrophosphate, polyphosphate, and diphosphonate).

Jolly test (yo'lē) [Friedrich *Jolly,* German neurologist, 1844–1904] a method by which a stimulating current is applied to a motor nerve and the evoked muscle contraction is recorded. The modern technique for detection of conduction defects through the recording of the M waves elicited by repeated supramaximal stimuli to a motor nerve has replaced this test in clinical electromyography.

Jones' method (jonz) a histologic staining method for demonstrating glomerular basement membranes. Paraffin sections are oxidized in periodic acid and placed in a freshly prepared methenamine-silver solution buffered at pH 8.2 at 60°C until the background is stained an even yellow-brown. They then are toned with gold chloride, fixed with thiosulfate, and counterstained with hematoxylin and eosin. Basement membrane and reticulum fibers stain black; nuclei stain blue; cytoplasm, collagen, and connective tissue stain pink to orange.

Jones-Mote reaction (jōnz mōt) a type of delayed hypersensitivity that results in maximal inflammation within 24 hr after cutaneous challenge with an antigen to which the individual has been previously sensitized. This reaction may be induced by immunization with proteins in incomplete Freund's adjuvant. The resultant antigen-antibody complexes are in antibody excess. Histologically, the Jones-Mote reaction is characterized by a predominantly basophil infiltrate, the remaining cells being lymphocytes.

joule (J) (jo͞ol, joul) [James Prescott *Joule,* English physicist, 1818–1899] the International system (SI) unit of energy, work, or heat defined as the work produced by a force of 1 newton acting through a distance of 1 meter (1 N·m).

Joule's Law (jo͞olz) [James Prescott *Joule*] stated as: the electrical energy (in watts) dissipated as heat in a resistor is equal to the product of the resistance (in ohms) and the square of the current (in amperes).

joystick (joi'stik) a small rod that controls the position of an indicator dot or cursor on a computer CRT display. It can be used to specify regions of interest in CT or radionuclide scans. The motion of the stick is translated into X-Y coordinates, which are then used by the computer to position the indicator.

J point a reference point immediately following the QRS complex at the very beginning of the ST segment. It is the point of zero current flow in the normal resting electrocardiogram, at which time the spreading wave of depolarization has activated all areas of the heart.

jugular (jug'u-lar) [L. *jugularis; jugulum* neck] 1. pertaining to the neck.

2. a jugular vein.

jugular vein one of the system of paired veins that returns blood to the heart from the head and neck.

external j.v., the vein that drains blood from the face and scalp and runs down the side of the neck superficial to the sternomastoid to about the middle of the clavicle, where it pierces the deep fascia and terminates in the subclavian vein.

internal j. v., the vein that receives blood from the brain and exits the cranial cavity through the jugular foramen. It runs down through the neck in the carotid sheath, receiving tributaries from the face and neck, and meets the subclavian to form the brachiocephalic vein.

jump (jump) in a digital computer, an instruction that permits a change in the normal sequential execution of instructions. See also *conditional jump* and *unconditional jump.*

jumping gene (jump'ing) a gene located on a transposable element.

junction (junk'shun) an area or surface where two different organs or types of tissue are in contact. See also *joint.*

gap j., see *nexus.*

tight j., see *zonula occludens.*

junctional (junk'shun-al) pertaining to a junction.

junctional automaticity the capacity of the atrioventricular (AV) node region (junction) to act as an ectopic pacemaker and maintain or control the ventricular rate.

junctional complex a group of associated cell junctions that unites cells of a simple columnar epithelium at their luminal ends, such as in the epithelium of the small intestine. It comprises a zonula occludens, zonula adherens, and desmosome, and is called a terminal bar in light microscopy.

junctional escape the occurrence of one or more escape beats initiated in the atrioventricular (AV) node region (junction). See also *escape beats.*

junctional rhythm the rhythm established by the atrioventricular (AV) node region (junction) acting as an ectopic pacemaker. The rate is usually about 50 beats/min.

junctional tachycardia rapid action of the heart consisting of two types: paroxysmal junctional tachycardia (similar to paroxysmal supraventricular tachycardia), in which the rate is 120–220 beats/min; and nonparoxysmal junctional tachycardia or accelerated junctional rhythm, in which the rate is 60–120 beats/min.

junction potential the voltage across a liquid-liquid junction in a electrolytic cell. To reduce measurement error, the junction potential must be kept as low as possible and must be reproducible.

jungle fever (jun'g'l) see *malaria.*

juniper oil (joo'nĭ-per) a volatile oil used to preserve catgut sutures and formerly as a diuretic. It is distilled with steam from the dried, ripe fruit of *Juniperus communis.*

justify (jus'tĭ-fi) to align in a field of an input or output record. A character string that begins in the leftmost position, as is usual with words and phrases, is left-justified. A character string that ends in the rightmost position, as is usual with numbers, is right-justified.

juxta- (juks'ta) [L. *juxta* near, close by] a prefix word element to denote near or adjoining, e.g., juxtaposition.

juxtaglomerular (juks"tah-glo-mer'u-lar) [*juxta-* + *glomerulus*] pertaining to the cells of the juxtaglomerular apparatus or complex.

juxtaglomerular apparatus a complex located at the vascular pole of a renal glomerulus in which the enzyme renin is produced. The apparatus comprises cells in the afferent and efferent arterioles (which contain secretory granules or juxtaglomerular granules demonstrable with special stains by light microscopy or by electron microscopy), the macula densa of the distal convoluted tubule, and a small amount of intervening connective tissue. Renin is secreted in response to a drop in the volume of extracellular fluid (ECF); the resulting action of aldosterone on the distal tubules causes sodium retention and leads to an increase in ECF volume.

juxtaglomerular granules secretory granules found in the juxtaglomerular cells. They can be demonstrated using Bowie's stain. This stain is made by adding 1 percent aqueous ethyl violet to 1 percent aqueous Biebrich scarlet until the neutralization end point is reached (where the color changes from red to violet), filtering out and drying the precipitate, dissolving it in 95 percent ethanol, and diluting with 20 percent ethanol just before use.

Mercury deposits are removed from paraffin sections of tissues fixed in Helly's fluid by treatment with iodine and thiosulfate. Slides are then mordanted in potassium dichromate, stained in Bowie's stain, blotted, dipped in acetone, and differentiated in a 1:1 mixture of xylene and clove oil (or alternately, in 100 percent ethanol) until the sections are red or magenta.

Juxtaglomerular granules and elastic tissue stain purple; tubular epithelial cell cytoplasm and collagen, orange to red; and mitochondria, magenta.

juxtanuclear (juks-ta-nu'kle-ar) close to or adjoining the nucleus of a cell.

juxtaposition (juks"tah-po-zish'un) [*juxta-* + L. *positio* place] the placement of things in proximity or near by.

juxtapulmonary-capillary receptor (J receptor) any of the deflation receptors, innervated by unmyelinated vagal afferents, found in the interstitial tissue between the alveoli and pulmonary capillaries. Stimulation of the receptors is implicated in the tachypnea that can accompany pulmonary capillary congestion, hypertension, and edema.

K

K symbol for, in computer technology, the number 1024 (e.g., 62K core memory); *equilibrium constant; kelvin; lysine;* the chemical element *potassium* (kalium).

K_a symbol for acid *ionization constant.*

K_b symbol for *base ionization constant.*

K_d symbol for *dissociation constant.*

K_{sp} symbol for *solubility product.*

k symbol for the Boltzmann constant, *kilo-*.

κ the lower case form of the Greek letter *kappa;* symbol for one of the two immunoglobulin light chains.

kabure (kah-boo′re) a skin disease commonly found in Japan. It is believed to be caused by the cercariae of *Schistosoma japonica,* which burrow into the skin.

Kahler's disease (kah′lerz) [Otto *Kahler,* Austrian physician, 1849–1893] see *multiple m.* under *myeloma.*

Kahn test (kan) [Reuben Leon *Kahn,* American bacterioloist, born 1887] a flocculation test once widely used for the diagnosis of syphilis. An individual's serum is mixed with a cardiolipin extract of beef heart. Agglutination is positive for syphilis. The Kahn test detects nontreponemal antibodies or reagin and is less specific than those that detect treponemal antibodies.

kal/i (ka′le) a word element used in combining form to denote potassium, e.g., kaliuresis.

kala-azar (kah′lah ah-zar′) [Hindi "black fever"] an infection caused by the presence of *Leishmania donovani,* a round or ovoid parasite measuring 2–5 μm in diameter. Kala-azar has wide geographic distribution; it is prevalent in various parts of India (Assam and Bengal), North China, areas of the Soviet Union (Transcaucasia), the border countries of the Mediterranean, Ethiopia, the Sudan, parts of West Africa, and throughout South America. The strains responsible for the Eurasian and American kala-azar are sometimes referred to as *L. infantum* and *L. chagasi.*

L. donovani passes through only two stages in its life cycle—amastigote (leishmanial) and promastigote (leptomonad)—and requires vertebrate (i.e., human) and invertebrate (i.e., insect) hosts, respectively. Infection is transmitted by a sandfly of the genus *Phlebotomus,* except for the American kala-azar, which is transmitted by genus *Lutzomyia.* The parasite, in the promastigote stage, is transferred to a new host when the infected insect is feeding. After an incubation period (2 wks to 18 mo), the parasites spread to the viscera via the blood stream, where they proliferate and parasitize the cells of the reticuloendothelial system in the spleen, liver, bone marrow, and lymph nodes. The liver and spleen are usually enlarged, and the affected individual may have chills, fever, and vomiting. The serum proteins usually show an enormous rise in IgG globulins, but this rise does not appear to be protective.

Laboratory diagnosis requires identification of *L. donovani* in stained smears of spleen or bone marrow tissue or lymphatic nodes, by blood cultures on NNN medium (Novy, MacNeal and Nicolle's), or by hamster inoculation. Sternal puncture is preferred, as it is less hazardous than splenic and liver puncture and is positive in approximately 80 percent of cases. Inoculation of blood on NNN medium shows promastigotes within 1–4 wk in positive cases; cultures should be kept 2 mo before they are considered negative. The buffy coat films, formol-gel test, and complement-fixation tests are considered useful. The Montenegro skin test is positive in treated cases but not in active cases.

Two groups of compounds are used to treat kala-azar: pentavalent organic antimonials and aromatic diamidines. In the first group, sodium antimony gluconate is preferred; the toxic effects are rare and the drug can be administered intravenously and intramuscularly. This drug should be protected from light to prevent the formation of hepatotoxic compounds. In India a 6-da dosage is sufficient, but in Africa treatment should continue for at least 30 da. Pentamidine and amphotericin B are the preferred alternate drugs when sodium antimony gluconate is ineffective; they are also used for initial treatment in the Sudan, where most cases are resistant in antimonials. Patients treated successfully with antimony compounds may still develop cutaneous lesions called leishmanoids, a post-kala–azar dermal leishmaniasis resembling lepromatous leprosy. This dermal form, which contains amastigotes, is important in maintaining the transmission cycle. Also called black sickness, *dumdum fever,* ponos, splenic anemia of infants, tropical splenomegaly, and *visceral leishmaniasis.*

kalium (ka′le-um) [L.] modern Latin for *potassium.*

kallidin (kal′ĭ-dĭn) a decapeptide, composed of bradykinin with an *N*-terminal lysine added, which is liberated by the action of kallikrein from kininogen (an alpha$_2$-globulin). Kallidin has actions similar to those of bradykinin and is a kinin type of peptide. See also *bradykinin* and *kinin.*

kallikrein (kal″ĭ-kre′in) an enzyme of the hydrolase class (EC 3.4.21.8). It belongs to the kinin system and cleaves kininogen to produce bradykinin.

kallikrein system see under *kinin system.*

Kanagawa phenomenon (ka′na-gah″wa) see *V. parahaemolyticus* under *Vibrio.*

kanamycin (kan″ah-mi′sin) one of the aminoglycoside antibiotics. Produced by *Streptomyces kanamyceticus* and first isolated in Japan, kanamycin is chemically similar to streptomycin and neomycin. Like streptomycin, it is effective against many gram-positive and most gram-negative organisms; it is more effective than streptomycin against gram-positive cocci, and drug resistance is less frequent. Kanamycin is used primarily in the treatment of infections due to gram-negative organisms such as *Klebsiella pneumoniae* and *Enterobacter* species, and for systemic or urinary tract infections caused by enteric bacilli. It is often used in combination with other drugs because of its toxicity and the development of resistant mutants. See also *aminoglycosides* and *antibacterial agents.*

Kaposi's sarcoma (kap'o-sēz) [Moritz *Kaposi* (Moritz Kaposi Kohn), Austrian dermatologist, 1837–1902] a malignant neoplasm related to angiosarcoma, first described by Kaposi as idiopathic hemorrhagic sarcoma. Typically, nodular skin lesions occur on the distal extremities, especially the feet and ankles, and progress proximally. Histologically, the lesions are composed of thin-walled vessels and spindle cells, forming nodules within the dermis; the spindle cells resemble fibroblasts but are actually primitive mesenchymal cells with vasoformative potential, as can be demonstrated ultrastructurally or by immunoperoxidase staining for Factor VIII–related antigen. In about 10 percent of all those affected, lesions with similar histology are present in lymph nodes or viscera such as the stomach. Kaposi's sarcoma is common in some areas of eastern Europe and Africa, where it tends to affect children and where a higher incidence of visceral involvement is observed.

In 1981, a serious outbreak of Kaposi's sarcoma occurred among male homosexuals in a number of geographic areas of the United States. Although the pathogenesis and mode of transmittal have not been identified, compromise of the immune system is suspected. Kaposi's sarcoma occurring in patients with acquired immune deficiency syndrome (AIDS) produces a higher rate of mortality than occurs in the classic form of the disease described above.

See also *acquired immune deficiency syndrome.*

kappa (K, κ) (kap'ah) the tenth letter of the *Greek alphabet.*

kappa chain one type of light chain of human immunoglobulins. In IgG, 60 percent of the molecules have kappa chains and 40 percent have lambda light chains. See also *immunoglobulin.*

kappa rhythm in electroencephalography, a rhythm of alpha or theta frequency recorded from the temporal areas of the scalp in mentally active subjects. There is controversy as to the origin of this rhythm, particularly regarding whether it is cerebral in origin or relates to fine lateral eye movements.

Karnofsky Scale (kar-nof'ske) a rating of the performance status of a patient with a malignant neoplasm, which describes and quantifies the impact that a malignancy has on the patient's daily life style (see the accompanying table). Any change in the scale conveys information about improvement or deterioration during the treatment program.

Kartagener's syndrome [Manes *Kartagener*, Swiss physician, born 1897] see under *immotile cilia syndrome.*

kary/o (kar'e-o) [Gr. *karyon* nucleus, or nut] a word

Karnofsky Scale. Criteria of Performance Status

Criterion	Rating	Performance Status
Able to carry on normal activity; no special care is needed	100	Normal; no complaints; no evidence of disease
	90	Able to carry on normal activity; minor signs or symptoms of disease
	80	Normal activity with effort; some signs or symptoms of disease
Unable to work; able to live at home and care for most personal needs; a varying amount of asistance is needed	70	Cares for self; unable to carry on normal activity or to do active work
	60	Requires occasional assistance but is able to care for most of needs
	50	Requires considerable assistance and frequent medical care
Unable to care for self; requires equivalent of institutional or hospital care; disease may be progressing rapidly	40	Disabled; requires special care and assistance
	30	Severely disabled; hospitalization is indicated although death not imminent
	20	Very sick; hospitalization necessary; active supportive treatment is necessary
	10	Moribund; fatal processes progressing rapidly
	0	Dead

element used in combining form to denote the nucleus, e.g., karyocyte.

karyocyte (kar′e-o-sīt) a nucleated cell.

karyogamy (kar″e-og′ah-me) [*karyo-* + Gr. *gamos* marriage] the fusion of the nuclei of gametes after fertilization.

karyokinesis (kar″e-o-ki-ne′sis) [*karyo-* + Gr. *kinesis* motion] the division of the cell nucleus in a cell division, as opposed to the division of the cytoplasm (cytokinesis). See also *cytokinesis.*

karyolysis (kar″e-ol′ĭ-sis, kar″e-o-ly′sis) [*karyo* + Gr. *lysis* dissolution] a manifestation of cell death, characterized by dispersal of the nucleus due to its slow disintegration.

karyon (kar′e-on) [Gr.] the nucleus of a cell.

karyoplast (kar′e-o-plast) see *minicell.*

karyopyknotic index (KI) see *squamous cell index.*

karyorrhectic (kar″e-o-rek′tik) pertaining to, characterized by, or causing karyorrhexis.

karyorrhexis (kar″e-o-rek′sis) [*karyo-* + *rhēxis* a breaking] a necrotic process in which the nucleus of a cell breaks up into fragments that are usually small and round and may vary in size. Cf. *karyolysis.*

karyotype (kar′e-o-tip) the character of a cell as determined by the nature of the chromosomes in the nucleus of that cell. In a eukaryotic (nucleated) organism, the chromosomes are most frequently studied when the cell is in the metaphase of mitosis (the middle stage of somatic or body cell division), the stage at which the chromosomes reach their greatest condensation and appear as identifiably discrete entities. Each species (kind of organism) has its own characteristic chromosome number and morphology in every somatic cell. Karyotypes are the systematic display of all the chromosomes in a single somatic cell. When a sufficient number of karyotypes from one individual are studied, the chromosome constitution of that individual is ascertained. When the karyotypes of a number of normal individuals of a species are compared and shown to be identical, the definitive chromosome complement of that species is established. The diagrammatic representation of the established karyotype of a species is called the ideogram.

The normal diploid chromosome number of an organism is indicated by the symbol $2n$. The gametes have half the diploid number of chromosomes (a haploid set), which is indicated by n. The normal human karyotype is a complete diploid set ($2n = 46$) of mitotic chromosomes, which consists of 22 pairs of autosomes (nonsex chromosomes) and 2 sex chromosomes (two X chromosomes in the female and one X and one Y chromosome in the male). The chromosomes of a matching pair (the homologous chromosomes) in the diploid complement contain two copies (alleles) of every specific gene. The presence of multiple sets of chromosomes in a cell is a condition called polyploidy. In humans, polyploidy such as tetraploidy ($4n$) occurs normally in certain liver cells. Triploid ($3n$) human fetuses have been observed but do not usually survive to full term. Deviation of one or more chromosomes from the normal chromosome number (euploidy) of a species is called aneuploidy. Trisomy describes the state of having an extra chromosome; for example, individuals with Down's syndrome (trisomy 21 syndrome) have an extra chromosome per cell. If a chromosome is missing from the diploid set, the individual is said to be monosomic for that particular chromosome.

The accompanying illustration shows the karyotype of a normal human male; the chromosomes have been stained by the Giemsa banding technique. Morphologic identification is based on the relative size of the chromosomes, their arm ratio, and certain secondary morphologic features. Individual human chromosomes can now be identified

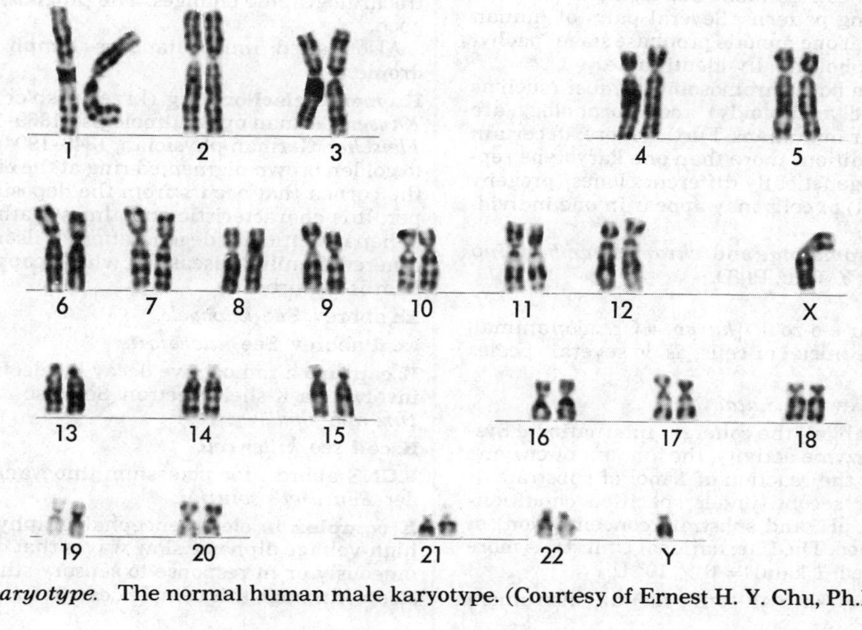

Karyotype. The normal human male karyotype. (Courtesy of Ernest H. Y. Chu, Ph.D.)

after staining with various banding techniques. By international convention, the human chromosome pairs are numbered and arranged in descending order of length. The mean relative length of the longest human chromosome (number 1) is 9.1 percent of the total autosomal (nonsex chromosome) length, whereas that of the shortest (chromosome 21) is 1.7 percent. Chromosome 22 is actually longer (mean relative length, 1.8 percent) than chromosome 21. However, because the chromosome that in the trisomic state causes Down's syndrome has long been called 21 in the scientific literature, it was thought impractical and confusing to reverse the numbers.

Chromosomes 1 and 3 are metacentric with a centromere in the middle of the chromosome, giving a chromosome-arm ratio of about 1:1. Chromosome 2 is on the borderline between metacentric and submetacentric, whereas chromosomes 4 and 5 represent the subtelocentric type. Chromosomes 6–12, including the X, are submetacentric. Chromosomes 16, 19, and 20 are metacentric, and chromosomes 17 and 18 are submetacentric with distinguishable size and arm-ratio difference. Chromosomes 13–15, 21, and 22 are acrocentric, usually displaying satellites (small euchromatin regions distal to the secondary constriction on the short arms). The secondary constrictions on these chromosomes are the locations of multiple genes for ribosomal RNA. The size of both short arms and satellites of these chromosomes can vary among different individuals.

Chromosomes 1, 9, and 16 sometimes show fuzzy regions next to the centromere on the long arms and can be recognized on this basis. These are the locations of repetitious short sequences of DNA. The Y chromosome usually assumes an easily recognizable morphology (the ruffled appearance of the short arm and the tightly paired sister chromatids of the long arm). The normal human Y varies markedly in length from person to person.

Karyotypes of human meiotic chromosomes, usually at one stage of meiotic prophase (diakinesis) or at first meiotic metaphase, have also been constructed. Individual bivalents (pairs of homologous chromosomes) can be identified by their size and various banding patterns. Several pairs of human chromosomes at one meiotic prophase stage (pachytene) are morphologically identifiable.

Variations in both chromosome number (such as polyploidy and aneuploidy) and morphology are known to occur in humans. Furthermore, in certain abnormal conditions more than one karyotype representing cytogenetically different clones (progeny of a single cell) of cells may appear in one individual.

See also *chromosome* and *chromosome banding.*

ERNEST H. Y. CHU, PH.D.

karyozoic (kar″e-o-zo′ik) [*karyo-* + Gr. *zōon* animal] inhabiting the nuclei of cells, as do several species of protozoa.

kat (kat) abbrev. See *katal.*

katal (kat) (kah′tal) the coherent International System unit of enzyme activity, the amount of enzyme that catalyzes the reaction of 1 mol of substrate or coenzyme per second under specified conditions (temperature, pH, and substrate concentration) of an assay method. The International Unit (U) is more commonly used; 1 katal $= 6 \times 10^7$ U.

katharometer (kath″ah-rom′e-ter) an instrument used for the electrometric measurement of the basal metabolic rate. It measures the concentration of gases by recording the current changes that occur in a Wheatstone bridge when the gas being measured is allowed to conduct heat from a hot arm of the bridge, thus changing the electrical resistance of the arm. The gas being measured (sample gas) has been diluted in a reference gas. Another arm of the Wheatstone bridge assumes an electrical resistance that is inversely proportional to the thermal conductivity of the undiluted reference gas: any difference in the thermal conductivities of the reference and sample gas thus unbalances the Wheatstone bridge to an extent that is directly proportional to the difference in conductivities and is related to the percentage of the sample in the reference gas. The degree of unbalance of the bridge is measured with a high-impedance potentiometer or a galvanometer.

Kato thick smear technique (ka′to) a technique used for the fecal examination of helminth eggs. The sample (approximately 50 mg) is placed on a glass slide, covered with a pretreated cellophane strip (soaked in a glycerin solution), and pressed to form a film. After drying at room temperature, the slide is examined for the presence of parasite eggs.

Kauffman-White classification (kawf′man whīt) a scheme for the serologic identification of species of *Salmonella* by classification of their reactions to O, H, and Vi antisera. See also *Enterobacteriaceae* and *Salmonella.*

Kawasaki disease a multisystem disease of unknown etiology, primarily affecting children (2 mo to 9 yr), that is characterized by a prodromal fever, conjunctivitis, and cervical adenopathy. Within several weeks there is a progression of symptoms to include cracked lips, strawberry tongue, macular erythematous rash, and desquamation of the fingers and toes. Extremity edema and coronary artery angiitis, with the risk of coronary artery thrombosis, may also occur.

Laboratory tests reveal an increase in C-reactive protein, peripheral leukocytosis, and thrombocytosis. Myocardial involvement is also seen with electrocardiographic changes. The prognosis is usually good.

Also called mucocutaneous lymph node syndrome.

Kayser-Fleischer ring (ki′zer flīsh′er) [Bernhard *Kayser,* German ophthalmologist, 1869–1954; Bruno *Fleischer,* German physician, 1848–1904] a greenish to golden brown pigmented ring at the outer edge of the cornea that occurs from the deposition of copper. It is characteristic and almost pathognomonic of hepatolenticular degeneration (Wilson's disease), a heredofamilial disease in which copper metabolism is disturbed.

kc abbrev. See *kilocycle.*

kcal abbrev. See *kilocalorie.*

K capture a radioactive decay by electron capture involving a K-shell electron. See also *electron capture* and *shell.*

K cell see *killer cell.*

KCNS abbrev. for potassium thiocyanate. See under *Benedict's solution.*

K complex in electroencephalography, a burst of high-voltage diphasic slow waves that occurs spontaneously or in response to sensory stimuli during sleep. Although this complex can be induced by sensory stimuli of any modality, auditory stimuli evoke the K complex most readily. It is frequently associated with a sleep spindle. The K complex has its origin in the depolarization of cortical pyramidal cells by nonspecific thalamic inputs. Recorded maximally from the vertex of the skull, the complex is characteristic of Stage 2 or 3 of sleep. Asymmetry of K complexes may indicate the presence of a structural cerebral lesion, and it may be difficult to evoke complexes in patients with Alzheimer's disease.

kedani mite (kĕ-dah′ne) see *Trombicula.*

Keflex (kef′leks) trademark. See *cephalexin.*

Kell blood group system see under *blood groups.*

keloid (ke′loid) [Gr. *kēlē* tumor + *eidos* form] the exuberant production of collagen within a scar, seen more commonly in black individuals. Keloids may recur following excision.

kelvin (K) (kel′vin) [William Thompson, Lord *Kelvin,* British physicist, 1824–1907] the International System unit of absolute temperature defined as 1/273.16 of the absolute temperature of the triple point of water. The kelvin is the same magnitude as the degree Celsius used for customary temperature. Temperatures are converted from the Kelvin to the Celsius scales by adding 273.16. Formerly called degree Kelvin.

Kelvin temperature scale [Lord *Kelvin*] the scale of absolute temperature that has units the same size as the degree Celsius. See also *temperature.*

Kemadrin (kem′ah-drin) trademark. See *procyclidine hydrochloride.*

kerasin (ker′ah-sin) a cerebroside found chiefly in the brain. It is composed of a hexose (galactose) and a fatty acid (lignoceric acid). Its concentration in the body tissues is elevated in certain sphingolipidoses. See also *sphingolipidoses.*

kerat/o (ker′ah-to) [Gr. *keras* horn, cornea] a word element used in combining form to denote horny, hard, or cornea, e.g., keratogenesis, keratocyte.

keratan sulfate (ker′ah-tan) a mucopolysaccharide (glycosaminoglycan) that contains alternating residues of D-galactose and *N*-acetyl-D-glucosamine 6-sulfate. There are two different forms, varying in the carbohydrate content of their attached oligosaccharide units. Keratan sulfate I, which is found in the cornea, is attached to the protein core of proteoglycans by a covalent linkage between *N*-acetylglucosamine and asparagine; keratan sulfate II is attached by a linkage between N-acetylgalactosamine and serine or threonine.

keratin (ker′ah-tin) an insoluble fibrous protein that is the principal constituent of epidermis, hair, nails, and the organic matrix of tooth enamel. Keratin fibers are composed of bundles of fibrils; each fibril is composed of three polypeptide chains (each a right-handed α-helix) twisted in a left-handed helix. The fibers are embedded in a matrix made from polypeptide chains rich in cysteine. As the keratinocyte moves toward the skin surface, these chains are linked by disulfide bridges forming a dense, interlocking network that fills the cell, which loses its internal structure. The polypeptides forming the fibers are referred to as α-keratins; those forming the matrix, keratohyalins.

keratinization (ker″ah-tin″ĭ-za′shun) an accumulation of keratin in the cytoplasm of squamous epithelial cells of the skin.

keratinize (ker′ah-tin-īz) to make, or become, keratinous.

keratinocyte (ker″ah-tin′o-sīt) a cell that synthesizes keratin; see also *keratin.*

keratinous (ke-rat′ĭ-nus) containing or resembling keratin; horny.

keratin staining techniques to demonstrate the presence of keratin in various tissues, e.g., the skin, hair, and nails.

The Ayoub-Shklar method is a modified connective tissue stain. Sections are first stained in acid fuchsin and immediately transferred to aniline blue–orange G solution. Sections are differentiated in ethanol and mounted. Keratin appears bright red; connective tissue, deep blue; and prekeratin, orange.

Dane's method for keratin involves initial staining in Mayer's hemotoxylin followed by blueing in tap water. Sections are consecutively stained in phloxine, alcian blue, and orange G solutions. Keratin and prekeratin appear orange to red; acid mucopolysaccharides, blue; and nuclei, brown.

keratitis (ker′ah-ti′tis) an inflammation of the cornea, commonly caused by microbial infection or trauma. Clinical signs and symptoms include moderate-to-severe pain, blurred vision, and ciliary injection. See also *keratoconjunctivitis.*

keratoacanthoma (ker″ah-to-ak″an-tho′mah) a skin lesion, usually occurring on the head, neck, or upper extremity, that grows rapidly to form a nodule with a central, keratin-filled crater. Eventually it involutes, leaving a small focus of scarring. Keratoacanthoma may be distinguished from squamous carcinoma by its rapid evolution and, in histologic sections, by the absence of infiltration at its base.

keratoconjunctivitis (ker″ah-to-kon-junk″tĭ-vi′tis) an inflammation of the cornea and conjunctiva.

keratocyte (ker′ah-to-sit) [*kerato-* + Gr. *kytos* cell] 1. an erythrocyte having one (or rarely two) notches on its circumference when seen in smears. The resulting projections take on the appearance of spicules (horns). The formation of keratocytes results from the interaction of the erythrocytes with fibrin strands. The erythrocyte wraps itself around the fibrin strand, and part of the opposing portions of the membrane fuse. When the blood flow releases the cell, the fused portions form a pseudovacuole (prekeratocytic stage). This vacuole later ruptures, leaving the characteristic notch.

Keratocytes are found whenever deposition of fibrin strands occurs in the circulation, as in disseminated microangiopathic hemolytic anemia, some cases of glomerular nephritis, renal transplant rejection, and cavernous hemangiomas, and sometimes after insertion of a cardiac valve prosthesis.

2. a finely branching, flat fibroblast that is interposed between the corneal lamellae. The branching offsets of these cells appear to communicate with one another although they do not form a syncytium.

keratohyalin (ker″ah-to-hi′ah-lin) aggregates of keratin in squamous cells, seen best in the granular layer of the epidermis.

keratohyalin granule see *keratohyalin granule of the e.* under *epidermis.*

keratomalacia the softening and necrosis of the cornea that is associated with vitamin A deficiency. See also *h. A* under *hypovitaminosis.*

keratosis (ker″ah-to′sis) [*kerato-* + Gr. *-osis* condition] a condition characterized by the formation of a growth of horny tissue. Certain types of keratosis, such as actinic or solar keratosis, are premalignant lesions.

actinic k., a common lesion of the skin of older, fair-complexioned persons, caused by prolonged exposure to sunlight. The face, forearms, and dorsal aspects of the hands are the usual sites. The lesions are erythematous and often multiple, and may show hyperkeratosis, varying degrees of atrophy of the epidermis with atypical basal cells, or more severe abnormalities that merge with the histologic picture of squamous cell carcinoma. Probably 20 percent of individuals with actinic keratosis eventually develop cutaneous squamous carcinoma. The underlying dermis shows varying degrees of collagen degeneration, elastosis, and infiltration by chronic inflammatory cells. Also called *solar k.*

arsenical k., a skin condition that develops following treatment with arsenic salts, which once were widely employed for the treatment of arthritis, asthma, and psoriasis. Hard, discrete wartlike keratoses appear on the palms and soles of individuals treated with arsenic years previously. A few lesions undergo malignant transformation to basal or squamous carcinomas.

k. follicularis, a slowly progressive skin eruption most commonly inherited as an autosomal dominant trait, although many cases arise through mutations. Small, uniform, reddish papules form on the hair-bearing areas of the skin. The face generally is affected first, and lesions extend to the upper chest and extremities. The oral mucosa sometimes is also involved. With coalescence of the lesions, crusted, greasy areas, or occasionally hyperkeratotic elevated lesions are formed. Histologically, suprabasal clefts form in the epidermis and enlarge to produce lacunae within which detached acantholytic cells are present, and into which fingerlike papillae covered by a single layer of basal cells (villi) project. More superficially in the epidermis, dyskeratosis results in the formation of the so-called *corps ronds,* cells in which accumulation of keratin has caused compression atrophy of the nucleus and where acantholytic loss of cohesion creates a clear halo around the cell. Treatment is symptomatic. Also called *Darier's disease.*

k. pilaris, a common disorder of keratinization in which the pores of hair follicles become blocked by horny plugs. Although the cause is unknown, the disorder is considered benign and is chiefly a cosmetic problem. The lesions present as multiple, minute, pointed papules on the arms, thighs, and buttocks. This disorder is more prevalent in cold weather.

seborrheic k., a common skin lesion that forms an elevated, sharply demarcated brownish plaque, often with a roughened, wartlike surface. Frequently multiple, these lesions are usually found on the face of older person, but can also be seen on the trunk or on the extremities apart from the palms or soles. Sections show varying degrees of hyperkeratosis, acanthosis, and papillomatosis. Typically the base of a lesion is in the same plane as that of adjacent normal epidermis, but fingerlike tracts of epidermal cells may extend down into underlying dermis. Pseudohorn cysts produced by invaginations of the thickened horny layer are often present. The lesion is benign, but when inflamed or cut tangentially may be mistaken by the pathologist for a basal or squamous carcinoma, and when heavily pigmented may be mistaken clinically for a melanoma.

solar k., see *actinic k.*

kerion (ke're-on) [Gr. *kērion* honeycomb] a boggy, circumscribed area of swelling caused by a massive inflammatory infiltrate. It is often seen in dermatophyte infections of the scalp.

kernicterus (ker-nik'ter-us) [Ger. "nuclear jaundice"] a condition in which high levels of bilirubin in the blood are associated with widespread destructive changes of the brain and severe central nervous system symptoms. It is characterized by deep yellow staining of the basal ganglia, hippocampal cortex, cerebellum, and subthalamic nuclei, which is due to the ability of unconjugated bilirubin to cross the blood-brain barrier.

Unconjugated bilirubin levels begin to rise after birth, and levels as low as 8–10 mg/100 ml can be associated with kernicterus in premature infants or in infants who suffer from hypoxia. Full-term infants who have levels of 20 mg/100 ml are thought to be at risk. Kernicterus has been a common sequela of icterus gravis neonatorum in the past. Treatment includes exchange transfusion therapy and phototherapy.

Also called *bilirubin encephalopathy.* See also *hemolytic disease of the newborn.*

ketal (ke'tal) the functional group having the general formula $(RO)_2CR_2$ (all of the R groups can be different). A ketal in general can be formed by reacting a ketone with at least two equivalents of an alcohol in the presence of an acid catalyst. Water must be removed to force the reaction to completion.

ketamine hydrochloride (ke'tah-mēn) [NF], a nonbarbiturate, rapid-acting anesthetic that produces a "dissociative anesthesia" characterized by profound analgesia, normal muscle tone, and light sleep. It is used for minor surgical procedures not requiring skeletal muscle relaxation, for induction of anesthesia, and to supplement other anesthetics. Some patients may experience emergence reactions varying from pleasant dreams to hallucinations, confusion, and delirium.

ketimine (ke'tĭ-mēn) an imine derived from a ketone; i.e., the carbon of the carbon-nitrogen double bond has no hydrogen attached to it. See also *imine* and *Schiff base.*

keto- (ke'to) a prefix word element used in organic chemistry to denote possession or presence of the carbonyl group, $>C{=}O$, as in keto acids (β-ketobutyric acid). It is equivalent to the preferred prefix, "oxo," as in 2-oxobutanoic acid. In the expression "keto sugar," the prefix refers to the hemi-ketal structure in monosaccharides such as D-fructose.

keto acid an organic (carboxylic) acid containing one or more oxo (C=O) groups, e.g., β-ketobutyric acid ($CH_3C{=}OCH_2COOH$), α-oxoglutaric acid ($COOHCH_2CH_2C{=}OCOOH$), and pyruvic acid.

ketoacidosis (ke"to-ah"sĭ-do'sis) a condition characterized by the presence of so-called ketone bodies (β-hydroxybutyric acid, acetoacetic acid, and acetone) in the blood owing to their increased production. Ketoacidosis occurs in starvation, in chronic alcoholism, and most commonly in untreated diabetes mellitus. The condition may be preceded by 24–48 hr of polydipsia and polyuria, and may progress to mental stupor and neurologic coma.

The disorder is due to increased adipose tissue

lipolysis and hepatic ketogenesis as a result of increased glucagon levels in the presence of insulin insufficiency. Ketone bodies may be present in the urine in concentrations of greater than 10–13 mmol/l. Fatigue, nausea, vomiting, and hypotension may be seen. A fruity odor to the breath may be present, owing to the presence of acetone.

Laboratory findings in patients with ketoacidosis include massive (4+) glycosuria, hyperglycemia, marked ketonuria, and ketonemia; lowered blood pH and plasma bicarbonate are also frequently observed. There is a substantially increased anion gap. Magnesium and total body potassium may be decreased, whereas serum potassium is slightly increased. Lipidemia may also be present. Therapy is concentrated on slow administration of insulin, replacement of fluids and electrolytes, and correction of potassium and phosphate concentrations.

Also called ketosis. See also *d. mellitus* under *diabetes.*

ketoaciduria (ke″to-as″ĭ-du′re-ah) see *ketonuria.*

ketoconazole (ke″to-ko′nah-zōl) a newer broad-spectrum, oral antifungal agent used to treat systemic fungal infections and chronic mucocutaneous candidiasis. It is active in vitro against *Candida* species, dermatophytes (*Trichophyton* species, *Microsporum* species, *Epidermophyton floccosum*), *Blastomyces dermatitidis, Histoplasma capsulatum, Malassezia furfur, Coccidioides immitis,* and *Cryptococcus neoformans.* Ketoconazole is an imidazole compound that probably acts by impairing the synthesis of ergosterol, a component of fungal cell membranes. It is less toxic and better tolerated than amphotericin B. Recent reports, however, have raised concern regarding hormonal disturbances (e.g., development of gynecomastia) in ketoconazole-treated patients.

ketogenesis (ke″to-jen′e-sis) [*ketone* + Gr. *genesis* production] the production of ketone bodies; see *ketone body formation.*

ketogenic (ke″to-jen′ik) forming or capable of being converted into ketone bodies, namely acetoacetate, β-hydroxybutyrate, and acetone. Fatty acids, some of the amino acids (leucine, isoleucine, lysine, phenylalanine, tyrosine), and ethanol are ketogenic.

17-ketogenic steroids assays see *17-hydroxycorticosteroids assays.*

α-ketoglutarate (ke″to-gloo′tah-rāt) a salt or anion of α-ketoglutaric acid.

α-ketoglutarate dehydrogenase see *oxoglutarate dehydrogenase.*

β-ketoglutaric acid (ke″to-gloo-tah′rik) see *2-oxoglutaric acid.*

keto group a carbonyl group bonded to two carbon atoms, as in a ketone.

ketohexokinase (ke″to-hek″so-ki′nās) an enzyme of the transferase class (ATP:D-fructose-1-phosphotransferase, EC 2.7.1.3) that catalyzes the reaction ATP + D-fructose ⇄ ADP + D-fructose-1-phosphate. A genetic deficiency of this enzyme results in essential fructosuria. Ketohexokinase was formerly called fructokinase, which is now used to refer to ATP:D-fructose-6-phosphotransferase, EC 2.7.1.4.

ketohexose (ke″to-hek′sōs) a hexose that contains a ketone group. Cf. *aldohexose.*

ketone (ke′tōn) an organic compound containing a carbonyl (or oxo) group (a carbon atom double bonded to an oxygen) attached to two other carbon atoms, e.g., $CH_3COC_2H_5$, 2-butanone or methyl ethyl ketone. A carbonyl group bonded to a hydrogen and a carbon is called an aldehyde.

ketone bodies the products of incomplete fat metabolism in conditions when the body is using fatty acids as a principal source of metabolic energy (e.g., starvation) or insufficient intracellular carbohydrate metabolism (e.g., diabetes mellitus). They consist of the substances acetone, acetoacetic acid (AcAcOH), and β-hydroxybutyric acid (BHBA). AcAcOH is formed first, 80 percent being then reduced to BHBA by a dehydrogenase. A smaller fraction is decarboxylated to acetone. AcAcOH is also produced in the metabolism of the ketogenic amino acids. Excessive accumulation of these bodies results in ketosis. In untreated diabetes mellitus, ketone bodies can be found in large quantities in blood and urine. AcAcOH and BHBA are also commonly called 3-oxobutyric acid (β-ketobutyric acid) and 3-hydroxybutyric acid (D-3-hydroxybutyrate), respectively.

ketone bodies tests 1. semiquantitative tests. The Acetest tablets and Ketostix strips are based on the nitroprusside (Rothera) reaction. The test is most sensitive for acetoacetate (AcAcOH), less so for acetone, and does not react at all with β-hydroxybutyrate (BHBA). As reagent strips for ketone bodies are known to deteriorate when exposed to air, Acetest tablets, which do not decompose as readily, are preferred by many laboratories. In Gerhardt's test, ferric chloride reacts with AcAcOH to give a red color. If the specimen is first heated, AcAcOH decomposes and evaporates, and thus no color reaction occurs. This also allows detection of interference from salicylates and antipyrine, which react with the same reagent. The presence of BHBA can be confirmed by first boiling the specimen to eliminate AcAcOH and acetone and then oxidizing BHBA with peroxide or dichromate to AcAcOH, which then reacts with the reagent. Qualitative and semiquantitative tests are designed to give negative results with specimens from healthy persons. The limit of sensitivity is 5–10 mg/dl (as AcAcOH).

2. quantitative tests. The most common and convenient method is gas chromatography, although precise quantitation is seldom needed in clinical work. Reference values for plasma acetone are 0.3–2.0 mg/dl; for acetone plus acetoacetic acid, 0.5–3.0.

ketone body formation the mitochondrial synthesis of acetoacetate and β-hydroxybutyrate from acetyl CoA, which occurs primarily in the liver, but also in the kidneys. This provides an alternate mechanism for the oxidation of the acetyl CoA groups derived from fatty acid oxidation, because the ketone bodies can be exported and utilized in other tissues for energy.

Acetoacetyl CoA is formed from two molecules of acetyl CoA by acetoacetyl-CoA thiolase. A third molecule of acetyl CoA can then react with the acetoacetyl CoA, catalyzed by hydroxymethylglutaryl CoA synthase to produce 3-hydroxy-3-methyl-glutaryl-CoA (HMG-CoA) and HSCoA. The HMG-CoA is then cleaved at a different point by an irreversible reaction to yield free acetoacetate and acetyl CoA. A part of the acetoacetate formed is converted by a mitochondrial β-hydroxybutyrate dehydrogenase to β-hydroxybutyrate.

ketone body utilization the oxidation of acetoacetate and β-hydroxybutyrate to carbon dioxide and water for the production of energy in the form of ATP, which occurs in the cardiac and skeletal muscles, brain, testes, and kidneys. The mitochondria of these tissues have a β-hydroxybutyrate dehydrogenase catalyzing the conversion of this compound to acetoacetate.

Another enzyme, acetoacetate-succinyl-CoA transferase, catalyzes the transfer of coenzyme A from succinyl CoA to acetoacetate. The acetoacetyl CoA formed undergoes thiolytic cleavage to produce two molecules of acetyl CoA, which can be metabolized in the tricarboxylic acid cycle to produce energy.

ketonemia (ke″to-ne′me-ah) [*ketone* + Gr. *haima* blood + *-ia*] an excess of ketone bodies (acetone, acetoacetate, and β-hydroxybutyrate) in the blood seen in starvation and uncontrolled diabetes mellitus with acidosis.

ketonuria (ke″to-nu′re-ah) [*ketone* + Gr. *ouron* urine + *-ia*] the presence of ketone bodies (acetone, acetoacetate, and β-hydroxbutyrate) in the urine, as occurs in uncontrolled diabetes mellitus, starvation, and certain metabolic disorders. Also called *ketoaciduria.*

ketopentose (ke″to-pen′tōs) a pentose that contains a ketone group. Cf. *aldopentose.*

ketoprofen (ke″to-pro′fen) a nonsteroidal antiinflammatory drug similar to ibuprofen, fenoprofen, and naproxen.

ketose (ke′tōs) any monosaccharide, e.g., fructose, having a ketone group (>C=O) in the open-chain form. Ketoses usually exist in the cyclic hemiacetal form, the result of a reversible intramolecular reaction between the ketone group and a hydroxyl group in the same molecule. Cf. *aldose.*

ketosis (ke-to′sis) see *ketoacidosis.*

17-ketosteroid (ke″to-ster′oid) a group of steroids possessing a ketone group at position C17 of the steroid nucleus. The major 17-ketosteroids include androsterone, epiandrosterone, etiocholanolone, dehydroepiandrosterone, 11-keto- and 11-β-hydroxyandrosterone, and 11-keto- and 11-β-hydroxyetiocholanolone. In the female, precursors for 17-ketosteroids are produced primarily by the adrenal cortex, whereas in the male, the testes contribute about one third of the total amount. For this reason, 17-ketosteroid concentrations in males are a summation of testicular and adrenocortical activity, and in females primarily a reflection of adrenocortical activity. Determinations of 17-ketosteroids are useful as a screening test for the diagnosis of adrenal or gonadal disease; they are not a good index of androgen production, however, and plasma testosterone values should be utilized for that purpose. Most of the 17-ketosteroids found in urine are in the form of glucuronides and sulfates.

Increased concentrations are observed in adrenocortical carcinoma, adrenal adenoma, adrenal hyperplasia, testicular tumors, pregnancy, hirsutism, treatment with adrenocorticotropic hormone (ACTH), and severe stress. Decreased values are seen in Addison's disease, Simmonds' disease, panhypopituitarism, female hypogonadism, castrated or eunuchoid males, and occasionally in myxedema and anorexia nervosa.

Reference ranges for 17-ketosteroids in urine are: for females, 6–15 mg/da; and for males, 8–20.

17-ketosteroid assays colorimetry. The quantitative determination of the 17-ketosteroids is based on the Zimmerman reaction, in which *m*-dinitrobenzene reacts with the steroids in alcoholic alkali to produce a reddish-purple color with maximal absorption at 520 nm. As 17-ketosteroids are excreted as water-soluble conjugates of glucoronic acid and sulfuric acid, they are acid hydrolyzed, extracted, and alkali washed before being determined. 17-Ketosteroids can also be determined and fractionated by gas-liquid chromatography.

Ketostix (ke′to-stiks) trademark. See under *ketone bodies tests.*

β-ketothiolase (ke″to-thi′o-lās) see *acetyl-CoA acyltransferase.*

β-ketothiolase deficiency a rare disorder of isoleucine metabolism, transmitted as an autosomal recessive trait, that is characterized by a deficiency of the enzyme acetyl-CoA acyltransferase (β-ketothiolase) and results in recurrent severe metabolic acidosis. Ketosis and hyperglycinemia may also occur. The urine contains large amounts of α-methylacetoacetic acid. Those affected may have retarded physical and mental development. A low-protein diet is helpful in reducing the frequency of acute episodes. Also called hyperglycinemia with ketoacidosis and leukopenia, and *α-methylacetoaceticaciduria.* See also *aminoacidopathies.*

ketotic (ke-tot′ik) pertaining to, characterized by, or causing ketosis.

ketotransferase (ke″to-trans′fer-ās) see *transketolase.*

ketotriose (ke″to-tri′ōs) a monosaccharide with a ketonic functional group and three carbon atoms; dihydroxyacetone is the only example.

keV abbrev. See *kilo electron volt.*

key (ke) 1. in computer programming, a field in a data record that uniquely identifies a record. Usually, only the keys are used for identification when a file is sorted or searched.

2. in taxonomy, a means of identifying the taxon (the family, genus, or species) to which an unknown organism belongs by the presence or absence in the organism of certain key characters.

The most common type of key is a dichotomous key, which gives the user a series of two-way choices each of which leads either to another choice or to a classification of the organism. A multiple-entry key (also called a random-access key, or polyclave) allows the user to select the characters used for the identification. The user selects enough characters (possibly including many-valued or continuous characters) for the unknown organism to be identified by a computer program or other device as used in the method of numerical taxonomy.

A natural key uses the evolutionary tree of the taxa as the decision tree for the key. Because the characters with evolutionary significance are sometimes difficult to identify, natural keys are useful only as synopses of the system of classification. For identification, artificial keys, which distinguish taxa by their more obvious characters, are used. A partial key is one that does not distinguish every pair of taxa; some unknown organisms can be placed only within groups of several similar taxa.

keyboard the keys on a typewriter or the similar keys on a computer console or CRT terminal that are used to communicate with the computer.

key punch a machine with a keyboard similar to that of a typewriter, which is used to punch data into cards for computer input.

kg abbrev. See *kilogram.*

kHz abbrev. See *kilohertz.*

KI symbol for *karyopyknotic index* (see under *squamous cell index*), *potassium iodide.*

Kidd blood group system see under *blood groups.*

kidney (kid'ne) [L. *ren;* Gr. *nephros*] the paired organ that is the functional unit of the urinary system. The kidneys filter the blood, excreting various substances in the urine, and play an important role in fluid and electrolyte balance and maintenance of blood pressure. They are retroperitoneal and each is bean shaped, measuring roughly 12.5 cm from upper to lower pole; the left kidney is slightly higher than the right. Each kidney is invested in a connective tissue capsule surrounded by perinephric fat. The concave aspect of each kidney faces medially and gives passage to the renal artery conveying blood from the aorta, and the renal vein returning blood to the inferior vena cava. Urine leaves the kidney through the calyceal system, passing into the funnel-shaped renal pelvis, which is continuous with the ureter.

The kidney (see the accompanying illustration) is composed of a large number of individual functional units, the nephrons; there are at least 1 million in each kidney. A nephron consists of a slender, partially coiled tube (renal tubule) that is continuous at its distal end with a collecting duct. It has a blind expanded proximal end (renal corpuscle) into which a tuft of capillaries (glomerulus) is invaginated. The glomeruli are located in the outer zone of the kidney, which is grossly evident as the cortex. Much of each renal tubule lies in the more central medulla, and the collecting tubules converge on pyramidal projections of the medulla, each of which is clothed by a lesser calyx.

Arterial blood enters the hilum of the kidney through the renal artery. Its main branches radiate outward toward the junction of cortex and medulla, where lateral branches run in the plane of the corticomedullary junction and give off vessels that pass outward toward the capsule. A small arteriole reaches each renal corpuscle, where it forms a glomerular tuft of capillaries that invaginates the blind end of the nephron (commonly called Bowman's capsule); the capillaries become intimately invested by the reflected layer of Bowman's capsule. A stalk of supporting (mesangial) cells forms a core for the glomerular capillaries. Blood leaves the capillaries through an efferent arteriole, then flows over the renal tubule as a further plexus of capillaries before reaching a tributary of the renal vein. The afferent and efferent arterioles of a glomerulus lie side by side at its vascular pole.

Within a glomerulus, the capillary loops are sepa-

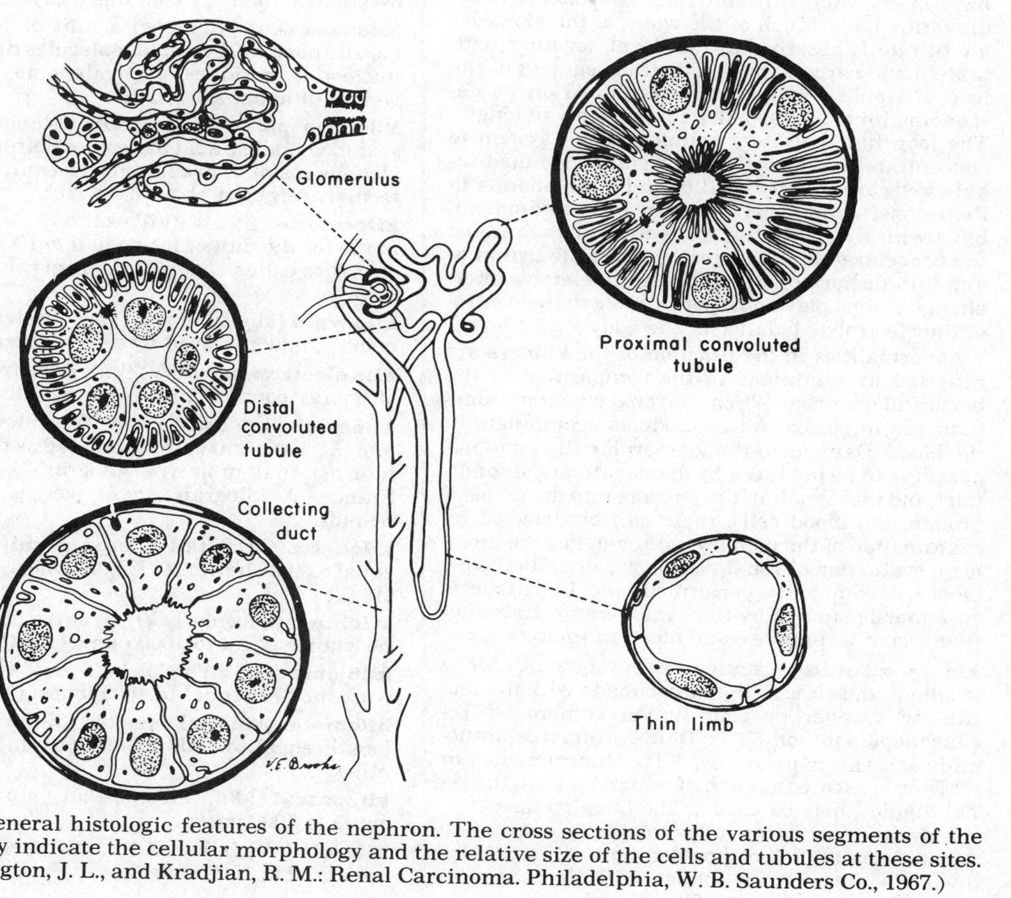

Kidney. General histologic features of the nephron. The cross sections of the various segments of the tubule roughly indicate the cellular morphology and the relative size of the cells and tubules at these sites. (From Bennington, J. L., and Kradjian, R. M.: Renal Carcinoma. Philadelphia, W. B. Saunders Co., 1967.)

rated from the epithelial cells of the reflected layers of Bowman's capsule by the fused basal laminae of the epithelial and endothelial cells. The epithelial cells are of elaborate construction. They have long cytoplasmic extensions that run along the capillary surface and make contact with the basal lamina through a large number of short foot processes (hence the term podocyte for the epithelial cell). The capillaries have a fenestrated endothelium; the filtration barrier in the glomerulus is consequently formed by the clefts between adjacent podocyte foot processes, the basal lamina, and the fenestrated capillary endothelium. Fluid and molecules from the blood that pass through this barrier enter the lumen of the nephron and flow down the renal tubule.

Each renal tubule consists of a proximal coiled (convoluted) portion, a hairpinlike loop (of Henle) that extends down into the medulla, and a distal convoluted tubule that approximates to the glomerulus and is continuous with a collecting tubule. Many of the loops of Henle have a portion with a thin wall, commonly termed the thin segment. A modified part of the distal tubule, called the macula densa, is composed of slender, closely packed cells; together with the adjacent afferent and efferent arterioles of the glomerulus and the intervening mesangium, it forms the juxtaglomerular complex.

Fluid and molecules that enter the lumen of the renal tubule are exposed to the actions of the tubule cells. In the proximal convoluted tubule, the cells have many microvilli and extensive lateral interdigitating folds. Much of the water of the glomerular filtrate is absorbed at this level, together with protein and carbohydrate. The thin segment of the loop of Henle is principally positioned on its descending limb, and it varies considerably in length. The loop functions as a countercurrent system to concentrate the urine. In the distal convoluted tubule, cells are slightly smaller and less elaborate in their construction than those of the proximal tubule; with the collecting ducts they further adjust the concentration of the urine under the action of antidiuretic hormone, and through a selective interchange of ions play an important role in the control of the electrolyte balance of the body.

Abnormalities in the function of the kidneys are reflected in alterations in the composition of the blood and the urine. When the renal excretory functions are impaired, waste products accumulate in the blood. Damage to the glomerular filtration apparatus can be produced by many pathologic conditions and may result in the passage into the urine of protein and blood cells; these can be detected by examination of the urinary sediment. For the histologic evaluation of renal pathology, a percutaneous biopsy is commonly performed, and the tissue is customarily studied by light microscopy, immunofluorescent techniques, and electron microscopy.

kidney scanning 1. static imaging showing kidney locations and sizes. They can be made with the rectilinear scanner or scintillation camera. ^{99m}Tc-Glucoheptonate or ^{99m}Tc-DMSA (dimercaptosuccinic acid) or, more rarely, ^{197}Hg-chlormerodrin or ^{99m}Tc-iron ascorbate, each of which binds to the renal tubules, may be used as the imaging agent.

2. dynamic scanning following the progress of an agent, usually ^{131}I orthoiodohippurate or ^{99m}Tc-Sn-DPTA, through the kidney. This demonstrates renal perfusion and filtration. See also *effective renal plasma flow, glomerular filtration rate, radionuclide c.* under *cystography, renogram,* and *residual urine volume measurement.*

Kienböck's disease (kēn-bek) [Robert *Kienböck,* Austrian roentgenologist, 1871–1953] see under *osteochondritis juvenilis.*

kieselguhr (ke'sel-gōōr) [Ger. *Kiesel* pebble + *Guhr* loose earth deposited by water] see *diatomaceous earth.*

killer cell a cell belonging to the lymphoid cell group that is the effector cell of antibody-dependent cell-mediated cytotoxicity (ADCC); it may interact with IgG-coated target cells and cause lysis without the involvement of the complement system. These cells have high-affinity Fc receptors for the Fc portion of antigen-bound immunoglobulin. They appear to be lymphocytic, nonphagocytic, nonadherent cells that may be low-affinity T cells, or null cells. They act directly on foreign target cells or through soluble mediators called lymphotoxins. Killer cells are distinct from killer T lymphocytes. Also called *K cell.* See also *lymphocyte.* Cf. *natural killer cell.*

kilo (k) (kil'o) [Fr., from Gr. *chilioi* thousand] 1. (symbol k), a prefix word element attached to International System (SI) units of measurement to denote a unit 1000 times as large; e.g., 1 kilovolt (kV) equals 1000 volts (V).

2. (symbol K), a prefix word element in computer science to denote multiplication by 1024 (2^{10}); e.g., a 64-kilobyte memory contains 65,536 bytes.

kilobase (kb) (kil'o-bās) a unit of length of single-stranded nucleic acid molecules defined as 1000 nucleotide residues, equivalent to a molecular weight of about 3.3×10^5.

kilobase pair (kbp) a unit of length of double-stranded nucleic acid molecules defined as 1000 nucleotide residues in each strand, equivalent to a molecular weight of about 6.6×10^5.

kilocalorie (kcal) (kil'o-kal"o-re) the preferred name for the unit of heat equal to 1000 calories (10^3 cal). Also called *Calorie,* kilogram calorie, and large calorie.

kilocycle (kc) (kil'o-si"k'l) an obsolete unit of frequency, now replaced by the *kilohertz.*

kilo electron volt (keV) (kil'o e-lek'tron volt) a unit of energy equal to 1000 electron volts (10^3 eV).

kilogram (kg) (kil'o-gram) the International System (SI) base unit of mass defined as the mass of the international prototype kilogram kept at Sèvres, France. A kilogram mass weighs about 2.2046 pounds.

kilohertz (kHz) (kil'o-herts) a unit of frequency equal to 1000 hertz (10^3 Hz). Formerly called kilocycle (kc).

kilohm (kΩ, formerly k) (kil'ōm) a unit of electrical resistance equal to 1000 ohms (10^3 Ω).

kilojoule (kJ) (kil'o-jōōl, kil'o-joul) a unit of energy, work, or heat equal to 1000 joules (10^3 J).

kilometer (km) (kil'o-me"ter, kil-om'ĕ-ter) a unit of length equal to 1000 meters (10^3 m), about 0.6214 miles.

kilopascal (kPa) (kil'o-pas-kal") a unit of pressure equal to 1000 pascals.

kilovolt (kV) (kil'o-vōlt) a unit of electrical potential equal to 1000 volts.

kilovoltage (kil″o-vol′taj) the electrical potential in kilovolts applied across an x-ray tube. The kilovoltage controls the maximum energy and penetrability of the x-rays produced.

kilovolt-ampere (kVA) (kil′o-vōlt am′pēr) a unit of apparent power in alternating current circuits, equal in magnitude to 1 kilowatt.

kilowatt (kW) (kil′o-wot) a unit of power equal to 1000 watts (10^3 W).

kilowatt-hour (kW-hr) a unit of energy or work equal to 3600 kilojoules, the energy produced in 1 hour at a constant rate of 1 kilowatt.

Kimex trademark. See *heat-resistant g.* under *glass.*

Kimmelstiel-Wilson disease (kim′el-stēl wil′son) [Paul *Kimmelstiel,* German pathologist in the United States, born 1900; Clifford *Wilson,* English physician, born 1906] diabetic glomerulopathy; a histopathologic pattern of glomerular disease considered to be almost pathognomonic of diabetes mellitus. Approximately 15–30 percent of long-term diabetics develop this type of glomerular lesion, which takes the form of rounded and often laminated hyaline masses situated in the centrolobular region of the glomerulus with compression or, occasionally, aneurysmal dilation of the surrounding capillaries. One or several lobules in the individual glomerulus may be involved, as may any number of glomeruli in the kidney. The nodules are PAS-positive; ultrastructurally, they have the same appearance as the mesangial matrix. Nodular glomerulosclerosis occurring in persons with diabetes mellitus is not, as was originally suggested, invariably associated with the nephrotic syndrome with hypertension (a clinical triad known as the Kimmelstiel-Wilson syndrome), but it is reasonably well correlated with severe renal dysfunction. Also called K-W lesion and nodular glomerulosclerosis. See also *glomerulopathy.*

kin (kin) 1. kindred.

2. genetically related.

kinase (ki′nās) 1. a nonsystematic name applied to an enzyme of the phosphotransferase subclass (EC 2.7) that catalyzes the transfer of a phosphate group from a donor (ATP or GTP) to an acceptor. The acceptor may be an alcohol group (EC 2.7.1), a carboxyl (acyl) group (EC 2.7.2), a nitrogenous group (EC 2.7.3), or another phosphate group (EC 2.7.4). Also called phosphotransferase and transphosphorylase.

2. a nonsystematic name applied to an activating enzyme that converts an inactive or precursor form of an enzyme to its active form (e.g., *enterokinase, staphylokinase*).

kindred (kin′dred) a group of genetically related individuals.

kinesi/o (ki-ne′se-o) [Gr. *kinēsis* movement] a word element used in combining form to denote movement, e.g., kinesitherapy.

kinet/o (kī-ne′to) [Gr. *kinētos* movable] a word element used in combining form to denote movable, e.g., kinetoscopy.

kinetics (kĭ-net′iks, ki-net′iks) [Gr. *kinētikos* pertaining to or causing motion] 1. in physics, the study of motion.

2. in medicine, the study of the turnover of some factor (e.g., red blood cells—erythrokinetics; leukocytes—leukokinetics; iron—ferrokinetics). The rate of production, clearance, or destruction and the duration of life span are usually determined.

3. in chemistry, the study of the rate at which a reaction proceeds and of the reaction mechanism, the intermediate steps constituting the overall reaction. The reaction rate is the rate of change of the concentrations of a reactant or product expressed in moles per liter per second (mol/l·sec). It varies with temperature, and the presence (or absence) of catalysts, and the concentration of one or more products or other molecular species. When these conditions are fixed, it is equal to the rate constant for the reaction multiplied by the product of the concentrations of the reactants, with each concentration raised to a specific power. For a one-step reaction, this power is equal to the number of molecules of each reactant. The sum of the powers for all of the reactants is called the reaction order. Other variables, such as pressure or optical rotation, may be used in defining rate.

A first-order reaction has the chemical equation $A \rightarrow$ products, the rate equation rate $= k[A]$, and the concentration equation $[A] = [A]_0 e^{-kt}$, where k is the rate constant, and $[A]_0$ is the concentration at time $t = 0$. A second-order reaction has the equations: $A + A \rightarrow$ products, or $A + B \rightarrow$ products. A zero-order reaction is independent of concentration, rate $= k$ and $[A] = [A]_0{}^{-kt}$. In this case, the enzyme is completely saturated with substrate, and the rate depends only on the concentration of the catalyst.

The overall rate equation for a reaction that has intermediate steps may have a fractional reaction order.

kinetochore (ki-ne′to-kōr) [*kineto-* + Gr. *chora* spare] see *centromere.*

kinetoplast (ki-ne′to-plast) [*kineto-* + Gr. *plassein* to form] an accessory body, sometimes called a micronucleus, that has been found in the order Kinetoplastorida of the phylum Protozoa. Originally described as a strongly eosinophilic granule at the base of the flagellum in cells stained with Romanowsky-type stains, the kinetoplast is now known to be an enlarged and specialized region of a mitochondrion containing a large amount of DNA.

kinetosome (ki-ne′to-sōm) [*kineto-* + Gr. *sōma* body] the basal body of a cilium or flagellum.

Kinevac trademark. See *sincalide.*

kingdom (king′dum) [A.S. *cyningdom*] in biology, a major category into which living material is classified. Primary categories are the animal kingdom (motile, nonphotosynthetic organisms) and the plant kingdom (nonmotile, photosynthetic organisms). A third kingdom, the Protista, includes all single-celled organisms and multicelled organisms of primitive differentiation.

Kingella (king-el′la) [E. O. *King,* American bacteriologist] a recently created genus of bacteria that consists of gram-negative, facultatively anaerobic rods that ferment glucose, are catalase negative and oxidase positive, and are nonmotile. Their natural habitat is the human oropharynx.

K. denitrificans, a species isolated from throat specimens. It is not pathogenic but is important because it may be mistakenly identified as *Neisseria gonorrhoeae* owing to the common characteristics of growth on Thayer-Martin medium, colony morphology, and reactions to oxidase and carbohydrate. *K. denitrificans* reduces nitrate, however, which differentiates it from the nitrate-negative *N. gonorrhoeae.*

K. kingae, a species composed of short rods with squared ends that occur in pairs and short chains. They are gram negative but have a tendency to retain stain. Colonies on blood agar produce a zone of clear, beta-like hemolysis. They are maltose positive, but urease and indole negative. This species contains strains pathogenic for humans, and they have been isolated from blood, bone, and joint specimens.

kinin (ki′nin) the generic name for a group of endogenous peptides that act on the blood vessels, smooth muscles, and nociceptive nerve endings. Examples include *bradykinin* and *kallidin.*

kinin system (ki′nin) a series of enzyme reactions resulting in the formation of bradykinin, which produces slow contractions of smooth muscle. The kinin system can also cause chemotaxis, dilation of peripheral arterioles, and increased capillary permeability. This system is initated by the activation of coagulation Factor XII (Hageman factor).

The kinin system interacts with the immune system in two ways: (1) C1 esterase inhibitor of the complement system inhibits the formation of bradykinin; and (2) kallikrein, an intermediate enzyme in the kinin system, is directly chemotactic for polymorphonuclear leukocytes.

kinocilium (ki″no-sil′e-um), pl. *kinocilia.* a nonmotile cilium found on the hair cells of the semicircular canals of the ear. It is so called to distinguish it from the many stereocilia (long microvilli) on these cells.

Kinyoun carbol fuchsin stain a stain for acid-fast bacteria. A smear is air dried, heat fixed, and then treated with carbol fuchsin solution. The slide is washed with water, decolorized with HCl alcohol, and finally counterstained with methylene blue. Acid-fast organisms retain the original stain and appear red against a blue background. The demonstration of acid-fast organisms is presumptive evidence of *Mycobacterium.* See also under *mycobacterium.*

Kirchoff's laws (Kir′kofs) [Gustav Robert *Kirchoff,* German physicist, 1824–1887] stated as: (1) the sum of the instantaneous currents flowing into a junction of an electrical circuit is equal to the sum of the instantaneous currents flowing out of the junction; also called Kirchoff's current law or Kirchoff's first law. (2) the algebraic sum of the instantaneous voltage drops and voltage sources around a closed circuit in an electrical network is zero; also called Kirchoff's voltage law or Kirchoff's second law.

kit (kit) a commercially prepared collection of reagents, pharmaceuticals, and associated equipment used to perform an assay, test, or diagnostic procedure. It is purchased as a unit and should contain instructions for use and calibration; there should also be information on the precision, accuracy, and specificity of the test, as well as the purity, the stability, and the expiration date for the reagents.

Examples include clinical chemistry kits, which contain prepared reagents and, often, disposable pipets and cuvets; radioimmunoassay (RIA) kits, which contain a prepared antibody reagent and radioisotope-labeled antigen reagent for assay of a particular antigen (usually a drug or hormone); radiopharmaceutical kits which are necessary for the preparation (immediately before use) of agents containing short-lived nuclides, such as technetium ^{99m}Tc; and generator kits, which produce a sterile, nonpyrogenic eluate of the nuclide (^{99m}Tc is produced as pertechnetate). For some uses, the eluate is combined with another kit pharmaceutical using sterile technique to produce the required agent (e.g., technetium Tc 99m serum albumin).

kJ abbrev. See *kilojoule.*

Kjeldahl's method (kel′dahlz) [Johan Gustav Christoffer *Kjeldahl,* Danish chemist, 1849–1900] a method for the determination of organic nitrogen. The procedure is most often used to quantitate urinary or fecal nitrogen and to establish values for protein standards. The specimen is boiled in concentrated sulfuric acid containing a catalyst (e.g., copper sulfate, mercuric sulfate, or selenium dioxide) and potassium sulfate, which raises the boiling point. This step, the Kjeldahl digestion, converts (oxidizes) organic carbon, hydrogen, sulfur, and phosphorus to inorganic oxides, and converts organic nitrogen to ammonium ions; these ions are converted to ammonia. On the addition of alkali, the ammonia is distilled into acid and quantitated by back titration of the excess acid with standard base. See also *nonprotein nitrogen assays* and *protein assays.*

Klebsiella (kleb″se-el′lah) [Theodor Albrecht Edwin *Klebs,* German physician, 1834–1913] a genus of micro-organisms of the family Enterobacteriaceae; small, gram-negative, facultatively anerobic rods that are widely distributed in nature and are frequently found in the intestinal tract. Usually harmless, these organisms are a primary cause of gram-negative bacteremia occurring as urninary and pulmonary infections in hospitalized patients. They are distinguished as being nonmotile and orithine decarboxylase negative. Most strains can be typed serologically. See also *Enterobacteriaceae.*

K. oxytoca, a species similar to *K. pneumoniae,* except that it is indole positive and may or may not liquefy gelatin.

K. ozaenae, a species that causes ozena, a chronic inflammatory disease of the upper respiratory tract; it is rarely encountered elsewhere. Unlike *K. pneumoniae,* it is Voges-Proskauer and malonate negative.

K. pneumoniae, the type species and the most important human pathogen of the genus. Encapsulated and the second most frequent cause of acute bacterial pneumonia, *K. pneumoniae* is urease, Voges-Proskauer, and malonate positive. Also called *Friedländer's bacillus.* See also *pneumonia.*

K. rhinoscleromatis, a species that causes and is found only in rhinoscleroma, a destructive granuloma of the nose and pharynx. It is urease negative, malonate variable, methyl red positive, and Voges-Proskauer negative.

Klebs-Löffler bacillus (klebz′ lerf′ler) [T. A. E. *Klebs,* 1834-1913, and Friedrich A. J. *Löffler,* 1852-1915, German bacteriologists] see *C. diphtheriae* under *Corynebacterium.*

Kleine-Levin syndrome (klīn lĕ′vin) [Willi *Kleine,* German neuropsychiatrist; Max *Levin,* U.S. neurologist] a syndrome, more common in males than females, that is characterized by periodic hypersomnia lasting for several days and accompanied by compulsive overeating. Onset is usually in adolescence and attacks may occur two or three times a year. Also called period hypersomnia.

Klenow fragment a fragment of DNA polymerase I, obtained by proteolytic cleavage, that lacks the 5′→3′ exonuclease activity. It is used in recombinant DNA technology for double-stranding single-strand DNA.

Klinefelter's syndrome [Harry Fitch *Klinefelter*, Jr., American physician, born 1912] an abnormality of the sex chromosome resulting from the nondisjunction of the XY chromosomes. The sexual karyotype is XXY, but there are several variants of the syndrome, including XXYY, XXXY, and XXXXY. Individuals are phenotypic males with small testes that lack germ cells. Secondary sex characteristics usually are poorly developed, gynecomastia may appear, and many of those affected are tall and eunuchoid with subnormal intelligence.

Development prior to puberty is generally normal, although some degree of testicular degeneration occurs in early adulthood. About 15 percent of those with Klinefelter's syndrome are mosaics, XY/XXY being the most common form.

See also *sex determination*.

Klippel-Feil syndrome (klĭ-pel′fīl) [Maurice *Klippel*, French neurologist, 1858–1942; André *Feil*, French physician, born 1884] a grouping of congenital malformations that results in extreme shortness of the neck owing to the absence or fusion of cervical vertebrae. Also called *brevicollis*.

km abbrev. See *kilometer*.

knee (ne) 1. the site of articulation between the thigh (femur) and leg (tibia).

2. any structure bent like a knee.

knee cap see *patella*.

knee jerk a monosynaptic stretch reflex that involves the quadriceps femoris muscle. When the patellar tendon is tapped, the fibers of the attached muscle are stretched. The stretch elicits a reflex contraction of the muscle that results in an abrupt extension of the lower leg from a flexed position. The reflex is elicited clinically to determine the extent to which function is normal in all components of the reflex arc.

knee joint the compound synovial joint formed by the articular surfaces of the patella, the femoral condyles, and the upper end of the tibia.

knife (nif) a cutting instrument such as a surgical scalpel or a microtome knife. See also *honing* and *microtome*.

knizocyte a nondiscoid erythrocyte with two or more concavities. The diameter of the cell is decreased, with the hemoglobin forming a band across the center of the cell. Knizocytes are difficult to distinguish on Giemsa-stained blood smears because of their pale appearance. The mechanics of knizocyte formation in vivo are unknown. Knizocytes are associated with hemolytic anemias, particularly with acquired hemolytic anemias due to autoimmune or isoimmune antibodies.

knot (not) 1. an intertwining of the ends or parts of one or more threads, sutures, or strips of cloth so they cannot be easily separated.

2. in anatomy, a small, knoblike swelling.

syncytial k.'s, protuberances of syncytium along the free surfaces of chorionic villi. They appear to aid in maintenance of the epithelial plate.

Knott's technique a concentration technique for the detection and identification of microfilariae, which hemolyzes the red blood cells and then concentrates the leukocytes and microfilariae. In this procedure, blood obtained by venipuncture is mixed with formalin and centrifuged. The supernatant is discarded, and thick films are prepared from the sediment. When dry, the films are stained with either Wright or Giemsa stain and examined for microfilariae.

KΩ abbrev. See *kilohm*.

Koch's postulates (kōks) [Robert *Koch*, German bacteriologist, 1843–1910, discoverer of tubercle bacillus; winner of the Nobel Prize for medicine, 1905] a four-part set of criteria, all of which must be fulfilled to establish a given microorganism as the etiologic agent of a given disease: (1) the organism is observed in all cases of the disease; (2) it can be isolated in pure culture or artificial media; (3) innoculation of this culture produces a similar disease in animals used experimentally; and (4) the organism can be recovered from lesions in these animals. Some etiologic agents do not meet all of these postulates as set forth in the 1870s.

Koch-Weeks bacillus (kōk wēks) [Robert *Koch;* John Elmer *Weeks,* New York ophthalmologist, 1853–1949] see *H. aegyptius* under *Hemophilus*.

Köhler's disease (ka′lerz) [Alban *Köhler*, German physician, 1874–1947] see under *osteochondritis juvenilis*.

Köhler illumination [Alban *Köhler*] see under *illumination*.

Kohn's one-step staining technic see *chlorazol black E stain*.

KOH test see *potassium hydroxide test*.

koil/o (koi′lo) [Gr. *koilos* hollow] a word element used in combining form to denote hollow or concave, e.g., koilonychia.

koilocytotic (koi″lo-si-tot′ik) [*koilo-* + *cytosis*] pertaining to hollow or concave cells.

koilocytotic atypia a lesion in which the cells have a perinuclear clear zone or cavitation and nuclear abnormalities. The change has been observed in dysplasia and in condyloma acuminatum. With electron microscopy, viral particles of the type found in the papova group have been identified in cells with koilocytotic atypia in condyloma acuminatum.

koilonychia (koi″lo-nik′e-ah) [*koilo-* + Gr. *onyx* nail + *-ia*] dystrophy of the fingernails, sometimes associated with iron deficiency anemia. The nails become thin and concave and have raised edges.

Koplik's spots (kop′liks) [Henry *Koplik*, American pediatrician, 1858–1927] tiny white spots that occur on the buccal mucosa during the prodromal stage of measles. They are usually found lateral to the molar teeth and centered on small red areolae of injected mucosa.

Korsakoff's syndrome (kor-sak′ofs) [Sergei Sergeevich *Korsakoff*, Russian neurologist, 1854–1900] see under *Wernicke-Korsakoff syndrome*.

Kovats index see *retention index*.

kPa abbrev. See *kilopascal*.

Kr symbol of the chemical element *krypton*.

Krabbe's disease (krab′ēz) [Knud H. *Krabbe*, Danish neurologist, 1885–1961] a fatal genetic disease of sphingolipid metabolism, transmitted as an autosomal recessive trait, that is due to a relative or absolute deficiency of the enzyme galactocerebroside β-galactosidase, and results in the accumulation of galactocerebrosides. It occurs early in infancy, before age 6 mo, and is characterized by progressive mental retardation, paralysis, blindness, deafness, and pseudobulbar palsy. Globoid cells, large multinucleate histiocytes stuffed with accumulated products, are seen around blood vessels in the white matter of the central nervous system. The disease invariably leads to death, usually within 1 yr. No therapy is available. Prenatal diagnosis may be made from cells in amniotic fluid. Also called galactosylceramide lipidosis and globoid leukodystrophy. See also *sphingolipidoses.*

kraurosis (kraw-ro'sis) [Gr. *krauros* brittle] a dried, shriveled condition of a part, especially of the vulva.

kraurosis vulvae (kraw-ro'sis) [Gr. *krauros* brittle] an atrophic condition of the vulva that is accompanied by hyperkeratosis and varying degrees of epithelial atypia. Rarely, squamous carcinoma develops in sites of preexisting kraurosis vulvae. In addition to the epithelial changes, histologic sections show edema of the superficial dermis and an underlying band of inflammatory cells. Also called lichen sclerosus et atrophicus.

Krebs' cycle (krebz) [Sir Hans Adolf *Krebs,* German biochemist in England, born 1900; co-winner, with F. A. Lipmann, of the Nobel Prize for medicine and physiology in 1953 for discovery of the tricarboxylic acid cycle] see *tricarboxylic acid cycle.*

Krebs-Henseleit cycle [Sir Hans Adolf *Krebs;* K. *Henseleit,* German internist, b.1907] see *urea cycle.*

Krukenberg's tumor (kroo'ken-bergz) [Friedrich Ernst *Krukenberg,* German pathologist, born 1871] a term for a metastatic, mucin-forming adenocarcinoma within the ovary. The tumor cells have a signet-ring appearance, and the primary tumor is frequently located in the stomach. See also *ovarian tumors.*

krypton (Kr) (krip'ton) [Gr. *kryptos* hidden] a colorless, odorless, gaseous element; atomic number 36; atomic weight 83.80, oxidation state +2 (in krypton difluoride, which is unstable at room temperature). It is used in lasers and as an inert atmosphere in fluorescent lights.

krypton-85 a gaseous nuclide with a half-life of 10.6 yr that emits both beta and gamma rays. Because of its high photon energy (511 keV) and long half-life, it is no longer used; ^{133}Xe is now preferred.

KUB abbrev. for the radiographic examination of the kidneys, ureters, and bladder. This procedure is usually performed before urography.

Kufs' disease (ko͞ovs) [H. *Kufs,* German neurologist, 1871–1955] the late juvenile or adult form of amaurotic familial idiocy, occurring between ages 15 and 26 yr, and characterized by cerebellar and ganglial abnormalities, It differs from the other types of amaurotic familial idiocy in that there are no retinal disorders. Also, unlike Tay-Sachs disease, this disorder shows no racial predilection. See also *amaurotic familial i.* under *idiocy* and *Tay-Sachs disease.*

Kupffer cell (koop'fer) [Karl Wilhelm von *Kupffer,* German anatomist, 1829–1902] a large, stellate, fixed macrophage attached to the endothelium of the hepatic sinusoids. These cells, which are part of the reticuloendothelial system, are highly phagocytic. See also *monohistiocytic series.*

kurtosis (kur-to'sis) any measure of the degree to which a probability distribution is concentrated in a single peak. A distribution with a sharp, narrow peak (relative to the normal distribution) is termed leptokurtic; one with a broad, flat peak is termed platykurtic.

kuru (koo'roo) a subacute spongiform encephalopathy that has been attributed to a chronic viral infection that occurs in individuals in New Guinea. The onset of this disease is insidious, but cerebellar ataxia and various motor disturbances subsequently lead to death within a few months. The cerebrospinal fluid is normal. There is no known treatment. The etiologic agent of kuru has been transmitted from the human brain to the brain of certain primates and has produced a syndrome similar to kuru. See also *slow viruses.*

Kussmaul respiration (koos'mowl) [Adolf *Kussmaul,* German physician, 1822–1902] the rapid, deep breathing caused by stimulation of the medullary respiratory center during severe metabolic acidosis; it is commonly seen in diabetic ketoacidosis. Also called air hunger and Kussmaul-Kien respiration.

kV abbrev. See *kilovolt.*

kVA abbrev. See *kilovolt-ampere.*

Kveim test [M.A. *Kveim,* Norwegian physician, b.1892] the intracutaneous injection of antigen prepared from human sarcoid tissue (lymph nodes or spleen). A red-purple papule that increases in size, and on biopsy resembles the tuberculoid granulomas of sarcoidosis, is considered to indicate a positive reaction; it appears about 1 wk after administration of the antigen.

kVp abbrev for kilovolts peak, the kilovoltage used in making an x-ray film. See also *peak kilovoltage.*

kW abbrev. See *kilowatt.*

kwashiorkor (kwash-e-or'kor) [from Gia dialect of Ghana, "the disease the first child gets when the second is on the way"] a nutritional deficiency syndrome seen most frequently in children older than age 2 yr. It results from inadequate protein intake, with a low or normal caloric intake. Kwashiorkor is prevalent in economically depressed areas of Africa, Asia, southern Europe, and Central and South America where diets are deficient in high-quality protein and probably in many minerals and vitamins.

Clinical signs include a generalized pitting edema, ascites, growth failure, apathy, skin rash, desquamation and pigment changes, ulcers, loss of hair, liver enlargement, anorexia, and diarrhea. Systemic involvement includes decreased mass and function of the heart and kidneys; decreased blood volume, hematocrit, and serum albumin concentration; atrophy of the pancreas and intestines; decreased immunologic resistance; slow wound healing; and abnormal temperature regulation.

Diagnostic tests include a 24-hr urinary creatinine excretion/body weight ratio, a sensitive and practical indicator of protein metabolism, which is decreased in kwashiorkor. Other tests include measurement of the excretion of 3-methylhistidine, serum albumin and transferrin levels, and packed cell volume. Plasma cortisol is increased, T_3 is decreased, and reverse T_3 may be increased. Heart size is decreased on echocardiography, and cardiac output is diminished. Sagittal radiographs of the arms show decreased muscle size and bulk. Treatment consists of the gradual feeding of high-quality protein (milk, eggs, and meat). The extent of recovery depends on the severity of the disease.

Also called malignant or protein malnutrition. Cf. *marasmus*.

kW-hr abbrev. See *kilowatt-hour*.

Kyasanur Forest disease [from the *Kyasanur Forest* in India] a tick-borne flavivirus disease that occurs geographically in the Mysore state of India; it is maintained in this small, rural region by the circular infection of wild and domestic vertebrates, especially monkeys and rodents, and ticks of the genus *Haemaphysalis*. Humans living in wooded farmland run the highest risk of infection.

Clinical manifestations include the sudden onset of fever, headache, muscle pain, and gastrointestinal disturbances, followed in 4–5 da by mild bronchopneumonia with slight hemorrhaging of the bronchi and intestinal tract and the formation of petechiae. In the second week, recurrent fever accompanied by meningitis and/or encephalitis may arise. Kyasanur Forest disease is rarely fatal and no permanent sequelae have been reported.

Diagnosis is based on identification of the virus in serum by complement-fixation or neutralization techniques. Isolation of the virus by inoculation of serum into various tissue culture cell lines and intracerebrally into suckling mice is also diagnostic. Treatment is symptomatic.

kypho/o (ki'fo) [Gr. *kyphos* a hump] a word element used in combining form to denote humpback, a convex prominence of the thoracic spine, e.g., kyphosis.

kyphoscoliosis (ki"fo-sko"le-o'sis) [*kypho-* + *scoliosis*, from Gr. skoliōsis curvation] a skeletal and thoracic deformity that is the result of curvature of the spinal column in both the lateral (scoliosis) and anteroposterior (kyphosis) planes. Approximately 70–80 percent of the cases are of unknown etiology; the remainder occur secondary to neuromuscular weakness, Pott's disease, rickets, or intrinsic disease of the spine.

In more advanced cases, deformation of the ribs and intrathoracic structures can lead to a significant reduction in lung volumes and in ventilatory flow rates, and to a disturbance in the ventilation/perfusion ratio. The resultant respiratory insufficiency leads to chronic hypoxia and hypercapnia, severe dypsnea on exertion, and polycythemia, and may eventually lead to cor pulmonale.

Orthopedic surgery can stabilize the deformed spine in adolescents and children. In adults, once the more severe secondary complications (cor pulmonale) have set in, the prognosis is generally poor.

kyphosis (ki-fo'sis) [Gr. *kyphōsis* humpback] an abnormality of thoracic spine so that when viewed from the side the spine displays an increased convexity. This condition may result from abnormal development or disorders of bone development. Cf. *lordosis* and *scoliosis*.

L

L symbol for angular momentum; *inductance; Lambert;* left; *leucine; liter* (in the United States, sometimes used instead of l to distinguish the symbol from the number 1, although SI system recommends using lower case L); lower.

L- a stereodescriptor used to specify one of the two enantiomorphic forms of optically active organic compounds, particularly carbohydrates and amino acids. The L- enantiomers of sugars have the same configuration at the asymmetric carbon atom most distant from the carbonyl function as does L-glyceraldehyde. The mirror image of the L- compound is labeled D-. The enantiomers of amino acids have the same configuration at the α-carbon atom as does L-serine. If two or more asymmetric atoms are present, the prefixes L_g and L_s are used to denote whether the configuration being specified relates to glyceraldehyde or to serine, e.g., threonine = (L_s;D_g)2-amino,3-hydroxybutanoic acid. In the new, more general *R,S* system of specifying configuration, L-isomers have the *S* configuration, and threonine is (2*S*;3*R*)-2-amino,3-hydroxybutyric acid.

L_g- see under L-.

L_s- see under L-.

l symbol for *length, liter* in the SI system (in the United States L is sometimes used to distinguish the symbol from the number 1).

***l*-** the chemical prefix used to designate a levorotatory compound; now commonly replaced by (–)-.

Λ the Greek capital letter *lambda.*

λ the Greek lower case letter *lambda;* symbol for: (1) wavelength (obsolete), (2) decay constant, (3) one of the two forms of immunoglobulin light chain, (4) microliter (obsolete).

La symbol for the chemical element *lanthanum.*

label (la'b'l) 1. something that identifies; an identifying mark, tag, etc.

2. in nuclear medicine, a radioisotope attached to another substance so that the distribution of the substance in the body can be detected by the emitted radiation.

3. in a computer program, a symbolic name used to refer to (i.e., represent) the address of an instruction or storage location in an assembly language program or a statement in some high-level languages (e.g., PL/I).

labeling index (LI) the number of cells in S phase in a cell population divided by the total number of cells in the population. See also *cell cycle.*

labeling of hazardous materials labeling with content identification and precautionary information; it should be provided on all original and subsequent containers of hazardous chemicals, although this is required by only a few governmental jurisdictions. Precautionary labeling is provided by many chemical manufacturers, even in the absence of any federal requirement. Such labeling follows the American National Standards Institute wording developed by the Chemical Manufacturers Association (formerly Manufacturing Chemists Association). Hazardous materials such as hazardous wastes must comply with regulations established by the Department of Transportation for the labeling, as well as for packaging, placarding of vehicles, and preparation of shipping papers.

label variable in high-level computer languages, a variable that can be assigned the value of the label of a step in the program.

labi/o (la'be-o) [L. *labium* lip] a word element used in combining form to denote lips, e.g., labial.

labile (la'bīl) [L. *labilis* unstable, from *labi* to glide] unstable or easily changed, as by heat or oxidation.

labile factor see *Factor V.*

labium (la'be-um), pl. *labia* [L.] a fleshy border or edge; used in anatomic nomenclature as a general term to designate such a structure, especially the labium major and labium minor of the vulva.

labor (la'bor) [L. "work"] the function of the female organism by which the product of conception is expelled from the uterus through the vagina to the outside world. The process of labor takes place in three stages: (1) opening or dilation of the cervix uteri; (2) passage of the fetus through the birth canal, or vagina; and (3) separation and expulsion of the placenta.

Following the onset of labor, urinalysis and hematocrit/hemoglobin determinations should also be carried out. It is necessary to examine the urine for albuminuria (found elevated in association with preeclampsia/eclampsia) and glucosuria (found elevated in association with maternal diabetes mellitus); the hematocrit/hemoglobin determination is necessary to rule out anemia. If not previously determined, the blood type, including Rh typing, status of maternal immunity to rubella, and serologic reactivity for syphilis, should be performed.

Labor is believed to be triggered by the release of oxytocin after a fall in the levels of other hormones. Oxytocin, which is stored in the posterior lobe of the pituitary gland, is normally released at the end of pregnancy and stimulates contraction of the uterine muscles. Labor may be induced electively or nonelectively through the intravenous administration of oxytocin. Elective induction can be performed when the fetus is known to be mature; nonelective induction is performed when there are conditions present such as prolonged rupture of the membranes and maternal diabetes. In cases of fetal death, the intraamniotic injection of saline or prostaglandin $F_{2\alpha}$ is used to induce labor.

Advances in technology permit electronic monitoring (internally and externally) of the pressure of uterine contractions during labor; electrodes placed on the fetus can monitor the fetal heart rate (via electrocardiogram) in cases in which fetal hypoxia is suspected. Fetal scalp pH determination is also useful in confirming the diagnosis.

Also called *parturition.*

laboratory (lab'o-rah-to"re) [L. *laboratorium* workshop] a place equipped for performing experimental work or pursuing investigative procedures for the preparation and testing (analysis) of drugs, chemicals, equipment, etc. A clinical laboratory is that part of a hospital or clinic in which specimens of tissues or body fluids are analyzed.

controlled access l., facilities in which the personnel have specific training in the handling of pathogenic agents and are supervised by competent scientists. Access is limited by the supervisor when experiments are being conducted. Hospital microbiology laboratories are examples of this type of facility.

restricted access l., facilities to which access is strictly controlled by the laboratory supervisor. Because of experiments involving hazardous infectious agents, the laboratory is either in a separate building or in a controlled area completely isolated from all other areas of the building.

laboratory hood an enclosure to confine and exhaust materials that may be flammable, irritating, corrosive, toxic, infectious (or potentially so), or otherwise noxious. Laboratory hoods are intended to remove vapors, gases, mists, aerosols, and other particulate material, as well as fumes.

A typical laboratory hood has one open face, which may be provided with an adjustable sash for additional enclosure of equipment or operations that release contaminants harmful to laboratory personnel or equipment.

Effective performance of laboratory hoods depends partly on the design and maintenance of the entire ventilation system, and partly on the use of laboratory techniques that recognize the limitations of laboratory hoods. Laboratory hoods are not designed either to capture contaminants generated outside the hood enclosure or to capture contaminants released at velocities higher than the face velocity of the hood. Contaminants generated within a hood can easily be blown out of the hood by interfering drafts or air currents from air supply system louvers, cooling fans in the laboratory, traffic in front of the hood, or opened windows.

Hoods are generally more effective in containing contaminants and exhausting them from the laboratory and the building if the face opening at the front of the hood can be kept as small as possible consistent with the work in the hood, if exhaust openings at the back of the hood can be kept open and unobstructed, and if the release of contaminants can be as far toward the back of the hood as possible to avoid interference from cross-currents at the front. Laboratory standards developed by the National Fire Protection Association include many specific requirements for hoods, including prohibition of recirculation of the air exhausted from laboratory hoods.

Also called *fume hood.*

face velocity of l. h., the linear velocity of air entering a laboratory hood at the front or face of the hood. Although not a definitive measure of hood performance because eddies and cross-currents in the air resulting from traffic and air-supply louvers may cause interference, measurement of hood face velocities over a period of time can be useful in assessing needs for system maintenance or upgrading.

labyrinth (lab'ĭ-rinth) [Gr. *labyrinthos*] a system of tortuous canals and cavities within the petrous part of the temporal bone. See also *ear.*

bony l., a series of three cavities hollowed out of the petrous part of the temporal bone; consisting of the vestibule, semicircular canals, and cochlea, these cavities are lined with periosteum and filled with a clear liquid, the perilymph.

membranous l., a system of ducts within the bony labyrinth of the internal ear; filled with endolymph, it includes the utricle and saccule in the vestibule, the semicircular ducts within the semicircular canals, and the cochlear duct in the cochlea. Branches of the vestibulocochlear nerve are distributed throughout its walls.

lac (lak), pl. *lacta* [L.] milk.

laceration (las"er-a'shun) [L. *laceratio,* from *lacer* torn, maimed] 1. the act of tearing.
2. a torn, ragged wound.

Lacis see *extraglomerular m.* under *mesangium.*

lac operon (lak op'er-on) an operon in *Escherichia coli* that contains three structural genes (beta-galactosidase, beta-galactosidase transport protein, and beta-galactosidase transacetylase) involved in the metabolism of lactose. It has been extensively studied as a model for bacterial genetic regulation. See also *bacterial g.* under *genetics.*

lacrim/o (lak'rĭ-mo) [L. *lacrima* tear] a word element used in combining form to denote tear or tear duct, e.g., lacrimal.

lacrimal (lak'rĭ-mal) [L. *lacrimalis*] pertaining to the tears.

lacrimal apparatus the lacrimal gland and its associated ducts, the lacrimal canaliculi, lacrimal sac, and nasolacrimal duct. These structures are involved in the production of tears and their distribution to the conjunctiva.

lacrimal bone one of the paired, small, thin bones that form part of the medial wall of each orbit.

lacrimal canaliculus see *lacrimal d.* under *duct.*

lacrimal gland the tear gland; a serous gland situated at the superior lateral angle of the orbit. Divided into a larger orbital and a smaller palpebral part, the lacrimal glands secrete tears that are isotonic with blood plasma and contain lysozyme, which has bactericidal properties. The lacrimal secretion bathes the conjunctival surface and drains into the nasolacrimal sac.

lact/o (lak'to) [L. *lac, lactis* milk] a word element used in combining form to denote milk, e.g., lactoglobulin.

α-lactalbumin (lak"tal-bu'min) a soluble protein only found in milk. It is used as a standard for evaluating the nutritional value of proteins, being readily digestible and of good amino acid composition. α-Lactalbumin in the mammary gland interacts with a membrane–bound galactosyltransferase to form the enzyme lactose synthetase, which is needed to synthesize lactose. The α-lactalbumin alters the specificity of galactosyltransferase so that glucose, otherwise very weakly active, becomes a good acceptor substrate for the galactose.

β-lactamase (lak'tah-mās) see *penicillinase.*

Lactarius (lak-ta're-us) a genus of fungus, including both edible and poisonous species, that often causes mycetismus gastrointestinalis (mushroom poisoning).

lactase (lak'tās) an enzyme (β-D-galactosidase, EC 3.2.1.23) that catalyzes the hydrolysis of lactose to galactose and glucose. It is one of the *disaccharidases.* See also *β-D-galactosidase.*

lactase deficiency either a rare congenital disorder or a common maturational phenomenon in which there is a lack of disaccharidase lactase activity in the brush border of cells of the intestinal mucosa. Normally, human infants have high concentrations of lactase, which begins to decline during the first 4–5 yr of life; in most of the world's populations (e.g., most blacks and Indians, and Orientals) these levels are virtually absent by early adult life. Ingestion of significant amounts of lactose may cause bloating, cramps, and flatulence with failure to hydrolyze and absorb intestinal sugars, which leads to osmotic diuresis and diarrhea.

Diagnosis of lactase deficiency is based on the presence of acidic (pH <6.0) stools and a flat lactose oral tolerance test, and is confirmed by demonstration of deficient lactase activity in intestinal mucosal cells obtained in a biopsy. The rare disorder of congenital lactase deficiency and the normal loss of lactase that occurs with age should be differentiated from secondary lactase deficiencies, which may be found in any intestinal disorder in which there is damage to the mucosal brush border. Although there is no treatment for lactase deficiency, symptomatic relief may be obtained by avoiding all lactose-containing food products.

See also *disaccharidase deficiency* and *lactose intolerance.*

lactate (lak'tāt) 1. any salt or ester of lactic acid. See also *lactic acid* and *lactic acid assays.*

2. to secrete milk.

lactate dehydrogenase (LD, LDH) (lak'tāt de-hi'-dro-jen-ās) a hydrogen transfer enzyme of the oxidoreductase class (lactate:NAD^+ oxidoreductase, EC 1.1.1.27) that catalyzes the reaction L-lactate + $NAD^+ \rightleftharpoons$ pyruvate + NADH + H^+. The enzyme also reduces α-hydroxybutyrate (this is referred to as α-hydroxybutyrate dehydrogenase, α-HBD activity). The enzyme occurs in the cytoplasm of the cells of almost all body tissues. Activity in some tissues may be as much as five hundred–fold greater than that in serum; thus, an increased serum activity of LD occurs as a result of leakage from damaged cell tissue. Serum HBD activity is thought to be a measure of the activity of the LD_1 and LD_2 isoenzymes.

lactate dehydrogenase assays 1. spectrophotometric methods for determining LD activity in serum, cerebrospinal fluid (CSF), or other body fluids. The rate of increase or decrease in absorbance at 340 nm due to either NADH formation or to utilization, respectively, is monitored. Procedures use either the forward (lactate + NAD→pyruvate + NADH) or backward (reverse) reaction catalyzed by LD. Continuous monitoring procedures are commonly used.

2. fluorometric methods based on measuring the fluorescence of NADH or the fluorescence of an addition product of NAD^+ formed with methyl ethyl ketone.

3. colorimetric methods. Dyes such as 2,6-dichloroindophenol or various tetrazolium salts, which are colorless until reduced by NADH, can be used with the forward reaction. Pyruvate reacted with 2,4-dinitrophenylhydrazine, which forms a golden brown phenylhydrazone at alkaline pH, can be used with the backward reaction. Colorimetric procedures are inferior in terms of precision and accuracy to continuous monitoring methods.

4. determination of heat-stable LD activity: the activity of lactate dehydrogenase in muscle (LDM) tissue after 15–60 min of heat treatment at 60°C as compared with the activity of untreated specimens. This method is used for estimating the amount of myocardial isoenzymes, primarily the heat-stable LD_1, but electrophoretic LD isoenzyme separation is preferred.

5. α-hydroxybutyrate dehydrogenase assay, which measures LD_1 and, to a lesser extent, LD_2. See under *α-hydroxybutyrate dehydrogenase assays.*

lactate dehydrogenase isoenzymes the isoenzymes of lactate dehydrogenase; LD is a tetramer containing M (muscle) and H (heart) subunits; it exists as five distinct isoenzymes: LD_1 (HHHH), which is found mainly in cardiac muscle, erythrocytes, and the kidneys; LD_2 (MHHH) and LD_3 (MMHH), which are found in the lungs; LD_4 (MMMH), which occurs in small amounts in the liver; and LD_5 (MMMM), which is found in the liver and skeletal muscle. All isoenzymes are also found in varying amounts in a variety of other tissues.

After a myocardial infarct or a severe ischemic episode, LD_1 is released into the circulation. It can be detected in serum within 12–24 hr, reaches a peak in 3–4 da, and returns to normal after 5–14 da. LD_2 is normally present in serum in higher amounts than LD_1 (when the amount of LD_1 rises and surpasses the amount of LD_2 in the serum, the resulting pattern is termed flipped LDH or flipped LD_1/LD_2 ratio). LD and CK isoenzymes are frequently used in conjunction to assess myocardial damage. CK-MB has higher sensitivity, flipped LD_1/LD_2 ratio has a higher specificity, and both together have very high predictive value. This enables more accurate diagnosis than does assessment by electrocardiogram (ECG) alone or ECG with total CK, LD, and aspartate aminotransferase (AST) levels. Usually, three samples are drawn over a 2- to 3-da period.

LD_1 is increased in renal infarction and myocarditis; LD_2 and LD_3 are increased in pulmonary infarction; and all of these are increased in myocardial infarction, various anemias, and certain malignancies. LD_4 abnormalities are noted in malignancies, and LD_5 is increased in hepatitis, cirrhosis, extrahepatic obstruction, congestive heart failure, infectious mononucleosis, and malignancy. Unusual LD isoenzyme patterns are frequently observed in neoplastic disorders.

Reference ranges differ with the support medium used, with the following values being an example for cellulose acetate electrophoresis: LD_1, 15–29 percent; LD_2, 28–45; LD_3, 16–27; LD_4, 5–15; and LD_5, 3–12.

See also *creatine kinase isoenzymes.*

lactate dehydrogenase isoenzymes determination 1. electrophoretic separation at alkaline pH (8.6), usually on cellulose acetate or agarose, to separate the individual LD isoenzymes. The bands are visualized utilizing the lactate-to-pyruvate reaction. The NADH formed reduces a tetrazolium salt to a deeply colored formazan dye that can be quantitated by densitometry.

2. separation by adsorption on anion exchange resin, followed by elution with solutions of varying pH and salt concentration.

lactation (lak-ta'shun) [L. *lactatio,* from *lactare* to suckle] the secretion of milk by the breasts; the process by which a female, usually postpartum, is able to provide nourishment in the form of milk to the newborn infant.

Lactation appears to be regulated by hormones. The rising concentrations of estrogen, progesterone, human chorionic gonadotropin (hCG), and prolactin throughout pregnancy stimulate the growth of glandular and ductal breast tissue. After delivery, the hormonal levels fall rapidly; however, prolactin levels temporarily and rapidly rise throughout the lactation period when stimulated by sucking, which indicates that high levels of prolactin are necessary for lactation to begin. Prolactin also serves to suppress ovulation. Oxytocin, also released after the sucking stimulus, forces the myoepithelial cells of the breast to contract and let the milk out through the nipple.

In the first few days after delivery, sucking stimulates the production of colostrum, a yellowish, alkaline fluid that contains antibodies against bacteria and viruses. Within 3–4 da, the mother's breasts become engorged and milk can be expressed from the nipples.

Breast milk enhances the infant's ability to resist infection because it is rich in macrophages, iron-binding protein (lactoferrin), and lysozyme. Free taurine, lower levels of sulfated amino acids, and higher levels of polyunsaturated fatty acids make breast milk nutritionally superior to cow's milk and infant formula.

The intake of drugs should be carefully watched during lactation, as most drugs are excreted in the breast milk and may affect the amount of milk produced. For example, atropine and oral contraceptives decrease the milk supply and can be harmful to the infant; and heroin, lead, mercury, certain anticoagulants, and cathartics are excreted readily in breast milk and are harmful to the fetus.

Ingestion of a generous normal diet with supplemental fluids is usually adequate maternal nutrition. Hormone administration prior to breast engorgement usually prevents lactation if the mother opts not to breastfeed her child.

lacteal (lak′te-al) [L. *lacteus* milky] 1. pertaining to milk.

2. a lymphatic vessel in the intestinal villi that transports chylomicrons in the form of a fluid called chyle. Lacteals are so named because of the white, milky appearance of the chyle.

lactescence (lak-tes′ens) [L. *lactescere* to become milky] resemblance to milk; milkiness. The term is generally used to refer to serum (plasma) specimens that are turbid owing to the presence of lipid globules.

lactic (lak′tik) pertaining to milk.

lactic acid 2-hydroxypropanoic acid, CH_3CHOH-$COOH$; M.W. 90.08. L-Lactic acid occurs in body tissues and body fluids in the anionic form known as lactate; the D form is produced by certain bacteria; and the DL racemic mixture occurs in sour milk, in the stomach, and in fermentation products such as sauerkraut and silage. Lactate is an end product of anaerobic glucose metabolism. It can be synthesized by most tissues in the body; however, the skin, muscles, erythrocytes, brain, and intestinal mucosa are most active in its production. It is estimated that under basal conditions these tissues produce about 1300 mmol/da; 60 and 30 percent of this is reconverted to glucose in the liver and the kidneys, respectively.

Under certain circumstances, lactate synthesis may increase severalfold, which also increases the liver's capacity to metabolize it. Values of up to 17 mmol/l in blood are common after exertion. Abnormal, persistent elevations of lactate are known as lactic acidoses.

Reference ranges for lactic acid in whole blood are: venous, 0.5-2.2 mmol/l; and arterial, 0.5-1.6.

lactic acid assays enzymatic methods commonly utilized for measuring blood lactate. Special collection procedures are needed to prevent changes in the lactate concentration during and following drawing of the specimen. The patient should be fasting and at complete rest. Under these conditions, venous and arterial concentrations are virtually identical. Blood should be collected in a syringe and deproteinized immediately. Plasma kept at 25°C is also satisfactory if collected in tubes containing sodium fluoride and potassium oxalate, and if the plasma is separated from the cells within 15 min of collection.

In the presence of NAD^+, lactate dehydrogenase oxidizes lactate to pyruvate. The NADH formed in the reaction is measured spectrophotometrically at 340 nm and is a measure of the lactate concentration. At a pH of 9.0–9.6, in the presence of hydrazine to trap pyruvate and of excess NAD^+, the equilibrium of the reaction can be shifted to the right with quantitative production of NADH.

Other methods of assay, such as gas chromatography and colorimetry, are also available.

lactic acid bacteria a group of several genera (*Streptococcus, Leuconostoc, Pediococcus, Lactobacillus*) of bacteria that are facultative anaerobes and catalase negative, requiring various B vitamins and amino acids as growth factors. Some occur widely as normal flora of the human body (lactobacilli and streptococci) in the nasopharynx, intestinal tract, and vagina. These include several important human pathogens of the genus *Streptococcus.*

lactic acidosis (lak′tik as″ĭ-do′sis) a condition characterized by the accumulation of excess lactic acid in the blood, sometimes due to the increased production of lactic acid by the tissues, as in tissue hypoxia. Similarly, this condition may be due to the diminished removal of lactic acid by the liver, as in hepatic failure. It may also be associated with cardiac decompensation, respiratory failure, systemic infection, infarctions, leukemia, and metastatic disease. Sudden and severe lactic acidosis may be encountered in those with glycogen storage disorders. It has also been reported to occur following the administration of phenformin (an oral hypoglycemic agent) for the treatment of diabetes mellitus. Individuals with lactic acidosis initially show hyperventilation, which is followed by mental confusion and coma.

Laboratory findings include low plasma bicarbonate and pH (acidosis), a high anion gap, lack of ketosis, and hyperphosphatemia. Plasma values for lactic acid from promptly chilled and separated blood may increase to 7–30 times the normal value of 1 mmol/l. The normal plasma lactate to pyruvate ratio of 10:1 is greatly exceeded. Alkalinization therapy is required immediately to raise the blood pH to greater than 7.2.

See also *lactic acid* and *lactic acid assays.*

Lactobacillaceae (lak″to-bas″il-la′se-e) a family of gram-positive, rod-shaped bacteria whose principal genera are *Lactobacillus, Listeria,* and *Erysipelothrix.* They have complex organic nutritional requirements and are highly saccharolytic, with the production of large amounts of lactic acid.

Lactobacillus (lak″to-bah-sil′lus) [*lacto-* + L. *bacillus* small rod] the single genus of the family Lactobacillaceae, occurring as large, gram-positive, anaerobic or microaerophilic bacilli. They are long, slender rods or pleomorphic in shape, nonspore forming, and nonmotile. These organisms occur widely in nature and are normally encountered in the mouth, vagina, and intestinal tract of humans. At one time they were associated with the formation of dental caries, but are now thought to have a minor role, if any. The organisms produce lactic acid as the principal end product of carbohydrate fermentation; they are involved in the production of foods such as cheese, yogurt, and sauerkraut, and of silage.

lactoferrin (lak′to-fer″in) a protein that binds two molecules of iron; M.W. 77,000. It is found in the granules of polymorphonuclear leukocytes and in milk, and may contribute to their antimicrobial activity by making iron unavailable to organisms.

lactoglobulin (lak″to-glob′u-lin) β-lactoglobulin, the principal protein of cow's whey, amounting to about 50–60 percent of bovine whey protein.

immune l., the antibody (immunoglobulin) that occurs in the colostrum of animals.

lactone (lak′tōn) a cyclic organic compound in which the chain is closed by ester formation between a carboxyl and a hydroxyl group in the same molecule.

lactoperoxidase radioiodination a type of radioiodination method that utilizes the enzyme lactoperoxidase to catalyze iodine attachment to proteins as a marker for determining the presence of specific substances. Lactoperoxidase catalyzes the reaction of hydrogen peroxide to water and hydrogen. In immunology, because this technique selectively identifies only surface proteins in a complex molecular aggregate, it is useful in the study of antigen-antibody complexes on the surface of lymphocytes.

lactophenol cotton blue (lak″to-fe′nol) a solution used as a stain in mycology. It consists of phenol crystals, glycerol, lactic acid, and distilled water, to which cotton blue or crystal violet is added after heating.

lactose (lak′tōs) [L. *saccharum lactis*] [USP], a heterodisaccharide that contains residues of D-galactose and D-glucose (*O*-β-D-galactopyranosyl-[1→4]-β-D-glucopyranoside). Lactose is a reducing disaccharide, as it contains a free anomeric carbon atom on the glucose residue. It is synthesized by the secretory cells of the mammary gland during lactation and is thus a sugar present in milk. Lactose is used as a tablet and capsule diluent, as an osmotic laxative and diuretic, and in infant feeding formulas. It is not tolerated well by many humans once they are weaned, owing to reduced intestinal lactase activity. Also called milk sugar.

lactose intolerance a normal developmental phenomenon in almost all Oriental, black, and Mediterranean peoples, with loss of lactase function between the ages of 5 and 10 yr. It may also occur as an extremely rare congenital deficiency of the enzyme lactase apparent soon after birth, producing diarrhea, vomiting, and failure to thrive. It may be fatal if untreated, but removal of lactose from the diet results in disappearance of symptoms. See also *disaccharidase deficiency, lactase,* and *lactase deficiency.*

lactose tests 1. screening test. Lactose may be present when qualitative copper reduction tests indicate the presence of a reducing sugar that is not glucose as confirmed by reagent strips based on the glucose oxidase reaction.

2. qualitative methylamine test. The specimen is treated with methylamine hydrochloride and NaOH and heated at 56°C for 30 min. Lactose (and other reducing disaccharides) give a red color.

3. Rubner's test. A urine specimen is shaken with lead acetate and filtered. The filtrate is then boiled, treated with concentrated ammonia, and reheated. Lactose forms a red solution and eventually a red precipitate.

4. definitive identification by use of chromatography. Disaccharides move slowly on paper or thin-layer chromatography plates; they thus are easily separated from pentoses and hexoses, and can be identified by their position and color after application of appropriate stains.

lactose tolerance test a functional test for small bowel mucosal lactase deficiency. On the first day of the test, a glucose tolerance test is performed to determine the patient's normal glucose absorption and tolerance; on the second day, the test is repeated with 100 g of lactose substituted for glucose. If lactase activity is normal, the lactose is split to yield glucose and galactose, and the tolerance curve is similar to that in the glucose test. A flat tolerance curve after lactose administration with a rise not exceeding 20 mg/dl over the fasting level indicates lactase deficiency.

lactosuria (lak″to-su′re-ah) [*lactose* + Gr. *ouron* urine + *-ia*] the presence of lactose in the urine, found in females during lactation and occasionally toward the end of pregnancy.

lactosyl ceramide (lak-to′sil ser′ah-mīd) see *ceramide lactoside.*

lactulose (lak′tū-lōs) a synthetic disaccharide, 4-*O*-β-D-galactopyranosyl-D-fructofuranose, used in the treatment of fulminant hepatic failure and as a laxative. Because lactulose cannot be digested, colonic bacteria metabolize it to lactic acid, which removes ammonia from the blood and reduces the degree of hepatic encephalopathy. Lactulose also increases the water content of the stool

lacuna (lah-ku′nah), pl. *lacunae* [L.] 1. a small pit or hollow cavity.

2. [NA], in anatomy, a general term used to indicate a hollow compartment within or between cells or tissues. Also called *lake.*

lacunar (lah-ku′nar) pertaining to or containing lacunae; of the nature of a lacuna.

lacunar cell a large cell, considered to be a variant of the Sternberg-Reed cell, characterized by one or several irregular or hyperlobulated nuclei, and a surrounding space or lacuna produced through shrinkage induced by formalin fixation. It is seen in the nodular sclerosing form of Hodgkin's disease.

Laennec's cirrhosis (la″en-neks′) [René Théophile Hyacinthe *Laennec,* French physician, 1781–1826] a form of cirrhosis associated with chronic alcoholism. See also *cirrhosis.*

Lafora's bodies (lah-fo′rahz) [Gonzalo Rodriguez *Lafora,* Spanish physician, born 1887] homogeneous or concentric round cytoplasmic inclusions found in central nervous system neurons, particularly in myoclonus epilepsy. They have been reported to contain an acid mucopolysaccharide. Also called Lafora's amyloid inclusions.

lag (lag) 1. the difference in time between two related events, such as a stimulus and response or the input and output of a circuit. Also called *lag time.*

2. the amount by which one periodic electrical waveform trails behind another, expressed in terms of phase angle. Also called *phase lag.*

3. see *lag p.* under *phase.*

Lagochilascaris (lag″o-ki-las′kah-ris) a genus of nematodes. The species *L. minor* has been recovered from subcutaneous abscesses of humans in Trinidad and Surinam. The adult male worms measure 9 mm long by 0.4 mm wide; the adult females, 15 mm by 0.5 mm. The eggs are globose and thick shelled, and measure 65 μ in diameter.

lag phase see *lag p.* under *phase.*

lag time see *lag.*

lake (lāk) 1. the separation of hemoglobin from erythrocytes.

2. [L. *lacus* lake, basin], a circumscribed collection of fluid in a hollow or depressed area. See also *lacuna.*

3. [Fr. *laque* lake (pigment), lacquer], in histochemistry, an insoluble complex that consists of a dye and a mordant, which binds the dye to the tissue components.

Laki-Lorand factor (LLF) see *Factor XIII.*

Lamarckian theory (la-mark′e-an) [Jean Baptiste Pierre Antoine Monet de *Lamarck,* French naturalist, 1744–1829] a theory of evolution proposed by Lamarck in 1809, now remembered for one element of the theory: the idea that the adaptations an organism makes to its environment during its life can be inherited by its offspring and that the accumulation of these acquired adaptive traits explains how species become adapted to their environments. Since acceptance of Darwin's theory, it is held that genetic change is random, not adaptive, and that species become adapted by natural selection. For contrast, these two points of view are sometimes termed Lamarckism and Darwinism. The basic doctrine of Lamarckism is usually phrased "the inheritance of acquired characteristics."

lambda (Λ, λ) (lam′dah) the eleventh letter of the *Greek alphabet.*

lambda chain one type of light chain of human immunoglobulins. Lambda chains are distinguished from the other type of light chain (kappa) by the amino acid sequence of the constant region of the light chain in the immunoglobulin molecule. Lambda light chains may be divided into four subtypes based on amino acid sequence homology. See also *immunoglobulin.*

lambda wave in electroencephalography, a sharp wave recorded in the occipital region of the head in awake subjects during visual exploration that is mainly positive in relation to other brain areas. Its amplitude is usually less than 50 μV. Lambda waves are related in time to saccadic eye movements, and waves of similar form are sometimes recorded during nonrapid eye movement (non-REM) sleep. These waves can be recorded in healthy infants during the first few months of life. They have no diagnostic significance.

lambdoid wave (lam′doid) [Gr. *lambda* + *eidos* form, lambda shaped] see *positive occipital sharp transient of sleep.*

lambert (L) (lam′bert) [Johann Heinrich *Lambert,* German mathematician and physicist, 1728–1777] a unit of luminance (photometric brightness) defined as $1/\pi$ candela per square centimeter.

Lambert's canal (lam′berts) [Edward H. *Lambert,* U.S. physician] one of the epithelium-lined collateral channels between distal segments of the bronchiolar tree (especially the preterminal bronchioles) and alveoli. These structures provide a direct route for the passage of air from the bronchioles to the alveoli.

Lambert's law [Johann Heinrich *Lambert*] see *Beer's law.*

lambliasis (lam-bli′ah-sis) [from Vilem Dusan *Lambl,* Bohemian physician, 1824–1895] infection with *Giardia lamblia.*

lamella (lah-mel′ah), pl. *lamellae* [L. dim of *lamina*] 1. a thin leaf or plate, as of bone.

2. a medicated disk or wafer, prepared from gelatin, glycerin, and distilled water, that contains a small quantity of an alkaloid to be inserted under the eyelid.

lamin/o (lam′ĭ-no) [L. *lamina* layer] a word element used in combining form to denote lamina (a thin, flat plate or layer), e.g., laminectomy.

lamina (lam′ĭ-nah), pl. *laminae.* 1. [L.] a thin, flat plate or layer.

2. [NA], in anatomy, a general term used to indicate a plate or layer of a composite structure. See also *layer* and *stratum.*

l. propria, a layer of vascular loose connective tissue that supports the epithelium and basement membrane of a mucosal surface.

laminagraphy (lam″ĭ-nag′rah-fe) [*lamina* + Gr. *graphein* to record] a type of body-section radiography. See under *tomography.*

laminar (lam′ĭ-nar) [L. *laminaris*] made up of or arranged in laminae.

laminar flow burner a burner used in an atomic absorption spectrophotometer that atomizes the sample into fine droplets and then burns it using a wide flame, which makes a longer light absorption path.

laminated (lam′ĭ-nāt″ed) composed of thin layers or laminae.

lamp (lamp) an apparatus for furnishing heat or light.

hollow cathode l., the light source used in an atomic absorption spectrophotometer, a neon or argon discharge tube with a cathode made from the metal to be analyzed. When the lamp is turned on, metal atoms sputter off the cathode, and the emission spectrum of the metal is added to the red glow of the neon (or purple of the argon). Each metal analyzed requires its own specific hollow cathode lamp.

mercury-vapor l., a lamp that produces light by an electric arc in an ionized mercury-vapor atmosphere. It emits bluish-green light primarily in the ultraviolet region (254 nm). Mercury-vapor lamps are widely used in hospitals, animal rooms, and inoculating areas in clinical laboratories to reduce airborne infection; they are also used in photometry.

tungsten l., a tungsten-filament incandescent lamp with a glass envelope. At an operating temperature of 2600–3000 K, the maximal emission is at 1100 nm in the near-infrared range; only 15 percent of the emission is visible light.

tungsten halogen l., a tungsten-filament incandescent lamp with a quartz envelope and a halogen (usually iodine) atmosphere. It has a higher operating temperature than other tungsten lamps and emits primarily in the visible and near-ultraviolet range.

lampbrush chromosome a type of chromosome found in oocytes of many animals and, briefly, in spermatocytes of at least some animals during the diplonema period of meiosis. Extending out from the chromosome (a bivalent) are loops of DNA on which transcription of messenger RNA occurs, permitting the synthesis of yolk proteins.

lanatoside C (lah-nat′o-sīd) a digitalis glycoside that occurs as a white crystalline powder and is extracted from the plant *Digitalis lanata.* It consists of the aglycone digoxigenin, two digitoxose sugar residues, one acetyldigitoxose residue, and one glucose residue. Lanatoside C is administered orally but only traces are absorbed; it is metabolized by intestinal bacteria to acetyldigoxin and digoxin, which are absorbed. The total absorption of glycosides is 40–65 percent. Trademark, Cedilanid. See also *digitalis glycosides.*

Lancefield grouping (lans′fēld) [Rebecca Craighill *Lancefield,* New York bacteriologist, 1895–1981] a serologic classification of β-hemolytic streptococci based on precipitin reactions with antiserum of carbohydrate components (C substance) of the bacteria. Immunologic groups are designated by the letters A through O. See also *Streptococcus.*

lanceolate (lan′se-o-lāt) shaped like a lance.

lancet (lan′set) [L. *lancea* lance] a small, pointed, two-edged surgical knife that is also used for skin punctures to collect blood for microanalysis.

lancet fluke see *Dicrocoelium.*

Landouzy-Dejerine disease (lan-doo′ze deh″-zher-ēn′) [Louis Theophile Joseph *Landouzy,* French physician, 1845–1917; Joseph Jules *Dejerine,* French neurologist, 1849–1917] facioscapulohumeral muscular dystrophy; see *muscular dystrophy.*

Langerhans' cell (lang′er-hanz) [Paul *Langerhans,* German pathologist, 1847–1888] a dendritic epidermal cell that contains distinctive, disk-shaped, cytoplasmic granules (Langerhans' granules). The cells are members of a family of histiocytes that possess IgA surface receptors. See also *histiocytosis.*

Langerhans' granule [Paul *Langerhans*] one of the racquet-shaped organelles found in the cytoplasm of the epidermal Langerhans' cell. Identical granules are present in the cells of the histiocytosis X spectrum of disorders. The function of the Langerhans' granule is not known, but it is frequently seen in continuity with the plasma membrane; the possibility that it might act as an endocytotic organelle has been suggested.

Langhans' layer [Theodor *Langhans,* German pathologist, 1839–1915] see *cytotrophoblast.*

language (lang′gwij) in computing, a system of rules for writing instructions to a computer. There are four levels of computer languages: in machine language, the instructions are binary codes specifying operations; in assembly language, the operations are specified symbolically; in high-level languages such as FORTRAN, the instructions are statements specifying many operations; and in job control languages, the instructions specify which programs, data sets, and input/output (I/O devices) are to be used.

Lanoxin (lah-nok′sin) trademark. See *digoxin.*

lanthanide (lan′thah-nīd) the chemical element lanthanum (atomic number 57) or one of the succeeding 4f transition elements (atomic numbers 58–71); originally, it included only the elements following lanthanum. The term is used both as noun and adjective. Formerly called *lanthanoid.* See also *rare earth elements.*

lanthanoid (lan′thah-noid) see *lanthanide.*

lanthanum (La) (lan′thah-num) [Gr. *lanthanein* to be concealed] a malleable, ductile, white metallic element; atomic number 57; atomic weight 138.9055; a 5d transition element; oxidation states 0, +3. See also *rare earth elements.*

lanugo (lah-nu′go) [L.] [NA], in the developing embryo, the first generation of dense fetal hair. It covers the body as a soft, downy coat and is shed before or shortly after birth.

LAO abbrev. See *left anterior oblique.*

LAP abbrev. See *leucine aminopeptidase, leukocyte alkaline phosphatase.*

lapar/o (lap′ah-ro) [Gr. *lapara* flank] a word element used in combining form to denote the loin, flank, or abdominal wall, e.g., laparotomy.

laparoscope (lap′ah-ro-skōp″) an endoscope used for inspection of the peritoneal cavity.

laparoscopy (lap″ah-ros′ko-pe) [*laparo-* + Gr. *skopein* to examine] a procedure performed to examine the abdominal contents with a fiberoptic light source. It requires the use of anesthesia and operating room facilities, but it gives a better view of pelvic contents than does culdoscopy. Cauterization and sectioning of the fallopian tubes with use of a laparoscope is an accepted method of female sterilization.

laparotomy (lap″ah-rot′o-me) [*laparo-* + Gr. *tomē* a cutting] an exploratory surgical incision made through any part of the abdominal wall into the peritoneal cavity. Also called celiotomy.

lapinization (lap″in-ĭ-za′shun) [Fr. *lapin* rabbit] a method of producing a virus vaccine by attenuating the virus through passage in rabbits. Several passages in rabbits modify the virus so that it loses virulence to the original host.

Laplace's law [Pierre-Simon *Laplace,* French mathematician and astronomer, 1749–1827] stated as: the transmural pressure difference (ΔP) at each point on a curved surface varies directly with the tension (T) and inversely with the radius of curvature (R); the equation representing this relationship is $\Delta P = 2T/R$ (for a sphere) or $\Delta P = T/R$ (for a cylinder). See also *pulmonary surfactant.*

large intestine see *large i.* under *intestine.*

large-scale integration (LSI) semiconductor manufacturing technology that produces integrated circuits with tens of thousands of components on a single silicon wafer (chip), such as microprocessors and computer memories.

larva (lar′vah), pl. *larvae* [L.] an independent, immature stage in the life cycle of an animal. It is unlike the adult stage and the animal must undergo changes in form and size to become an adult.

larva migrans (lar′vah mi′grans) human infections with the larvae of nematode parasites of lower animals. Larva migrans may be either cutaneous or visceral, depending on the body area affected and the parasite species found.

Cutaneous larva migrans is commonly caused by

the filariform larvae of the dog and cat hookworm (e.g., *Ancylostoma braziliense*). In humans, the larvae are unable to proceed farther than the cutaneous layers in the region of penetration. The larvae migrate a distance of from several millimeters to a few centimeters a day, producing serpiginous tunnels in the stratum germinativum of the skin. Erythema and purpura make the eruptions visible, in addition to elevations of the skin. The most common symptom is intense itching. Secondary infections may complicate the disease. Also called *creeping eruption.*

Visceral larva migrans is commonly caused by the larvae of *Toxocara canis,* the common roundworm of dogs, although the roundworm of cats, *T. cati,* and many other animal parasites are also potentially capable of producing this infection. *T. canis* is cosmopolitan in distribution. It appears to cause little difficulty for the dogs as a normal host; its life cycle resembles that of *Ascaris lumbricoides* in humans. However, when a person becomes an accidental and abnormal host through ingestion of the embryonated eggs, the eggs hatch in the intestine, and the larvae penetrate into the mucosa and the circulation and continue to migrate aimlessly, chiefly to the liver. The worst consequence of these migrating larvae is their fortuitous entry into the myocardium or the central nervous system, where they may cause myocarditis or encephalitis, or their entry into the eyes, where they may cause a retinal granuloma that clinically resembles retinoblastoma. The larvae remain immature and die in the tissues, where they provoke a marked inflammatory response. The infection is more common in children, especially those with a history of pica, than in adults, and is characterized by a persistent high eosinophilia, leukocytosis, hypergammaglobulinemia, and hepatomegaly.

The clinical and laboratory findings are generally nonspecific. Diagnostic confirmation is usually based on demonstration of the larvae in biopsy or autopsy specimens. There is no specific therapy, but corticosteroids seem to attenuate the inflammation. Thiabendazole and diethylcarbamazine are used with some success.

laryng/o (lah-ring'go) [Gr. *larynx* larynx] a word element used in combining form to denote the larynx e.g., laryngoplegia.

laryngeal (lah-rin'je-al) pertaining to the larynx.

laryngeal nerve a nerve arising from the inferior ganglion of the vagus. It receives a branch from the superior cervical ganglion of the sympathetic trunk and divides into internal and external branches. The internal branch provides sensory innervation to the mucous membranes of the larynx down to the level of the vocal folds, and also transmits muscle spindle afferents and stretch receptor fibers from the larynx. The (smaller) external branch supplies the inferior constrictor of the pharynx and the cricothyroid muscle.

recurrent l. n., a branch of the vagus nerve that innervates all the intrinsic muscles of the larynx except the cricothyroid, and supplies the mucous membrane of the esophagus and trachea. The right branch exits the right vagus nerve ventral to the right subclavian artery, and the left branch splits off from the left vagus nerve near the aortic arch. Both nerves ascend along the esophageotracheal groove. Damage to the nerve may be caused by an aneurysm or tumor, or may occur during thyroid surgery.

laryngeal nodule (lah-rin'je-al nod'ūl) one of the small, circumscribed condensations of hyaline material that characteristically develops at the junction of the anterior and middle third of the free edges of the true vocal cords. These structures are caused by vocal cord trauma and abuse, and result in hoarseness; they are characterized histologically by vascular ectasia and by mucoid degeneration of the stroma with cyst formation and focal amyloid-like deposits. Also called *singer's nodules.*

laryngismus stridulus (lar"in-jiz'mus strid'u-lus) [L.; Gr. *laryngismos* a whooping] a condition marked by the sudden, spasmodic closure of the larynx, which is followed by crowing inspiration and the development of cyanosis. The condition is associated with laryngeal inflammation and vitamin D deficiency rickets. Usually, the larynx opens within seconds. Also called pseudocroup.

laryngitis (lar"in-ji'tis) an acute or chronic inflammation of the larynx. Acute inflammations may be due to localized bacterial or viral infections or be associated with systemic disease (e.g., influenza, measles, diphtheria) or inhalation of an irritant. The laryngeal mucosa may become red and swollen, and there may be pain, cough, hoarseness, and other changes in the voice. If edema is marked, dyspnea may result. This disease is commonly associated with infections of the nose, pharynx, or trachea.

Chronic laryngitis may be due to repeated acute inflammations of the larynx, abuse of the vocal cords, chronic sinus and throat infections, chronic exposure to irritants, tuberculosis, or syphilis. Chronic hoarseness, cough, and the production of thick mucous secretions may occur; in severe cases, ulcerations may result. Chest x-rays may be used to check for tuberculosis; a serologic test to check for syphilis; and biopsies if carcinoma is suspected.

Systemic antibiotics are useful in the treatment of bacterial inflammation. Exposure to irritants should be avoided and the voice should be rested.

laryngography (lar"ing-gog'rah-fe) [*laryngo-* + Gr. *graphein* to record] the radiographic examination of the larynx and laryngopharynx. Contrast is provided by the air in the pharynx or by an iodized oil, such as Dionosil, with which the larynx is coated. Also called *laryngopharyngography.*

laryngopharyngography (lah-ring"go-fah"rin-gog'rah-fe) see *laryngography.*

laryngoscope (lah-ring'go-skōp) see under *laryngoscopy.*

laryngoscopy (lar"ing-gos'ko-pe) [*laryngo-* + Gr. *skopein* to examine] a clinical technique that facilitates the visual examination of the larynx. A laryngoscope, a hollow or fiberoptic endoscope containing a light source, transmits a magnified image of the larynx through a system of lenses and mirrors.

Laryngoscopy is often used to assess the integrity and mobility of the vocal cords, especially in response to unexplained voice changes. This procedure may reveal the presence of neoplastic or other lesions. Samples of sputum and biopsies may also be obtained by using brushes or forceps attached to the laryngoscope. Laryngoscopy is also used to facilitate the passage of an endotracheal tube.

laryngotracheitis (lah-ring"go-tra"ke-i'tis) inflammation of the larynx and trachea.

laryngotracheobronchitis (lah-ring″go-tra″ke-o-brong-ki′tis) see under *croup.*

larynx (lar′inks), pl. *larynges*[Gr. "the upper part of the windpipe"] [NA], the organ of voice, located in the lower neck. It communicates above with the pharynx through the laryngeal inlet, and below is continuous with the trachea. It is overlapped by the sternomastoid muscles, and lies between the carotid sheaths, behind the thyroid, and in front of the pharynx. Patency of the larynx is maintained by a series of cartilages within its wall, including the thyroid cartilage that forms the laryngeal prominence in the front of the lower neck, the cricoid cartilage, and the leaf-shaped epiglottis. These and smaller cartilages articulate with one another and are covered by membranes and the intrinsic muscles of the larynx.

The laryngeal inlet communicates with the laryngeal part of the pharynx and is bounded in front by the epiglottis and around the rest of its rim by folds of mucosa. The piriform fossa is a small space in the pharynx that separates the side of the laryngeal inlet from the thyroid lamina and thyrohyoid membrane. The upper part of the larynx is termed its vestibule.

Mucosa lines the larynx; the epithelium is mostly respiratory in type, although some stratified squamous epithelium with a few taste buds is found on the epiglottis. Within the larynx, there are two pairs of opposed folds. The upper pair are the vestibular folds or false cords, blunt ridges of mucosa raised up by the underlying vestibular ligament. The lower folds are the vocal or true cords, which have sharp edges; the sounds of the voice are produced by alterations in the shape and apposition of these edges as expired air rushes past them. Stratified squamous epithelium covers the vocal folds and is tightly bound to an underlying elastic ligament that in turn is supported by muscle: because of the sparse blood vessels, the vocal folds appear white. The cricothyroid and several other muscles modify the tension of the vocal folds. Sounds of speech are recognized by the relative temporal variations among their frequency components. The precise frequencies are less significant than the relations among them, and these relative frequencies elicit responses from the cells of the auditory cortex.

The innervation of the mucosa lining the larynx is by fibers of the internal laryngeal nerve above the level of the vocal fold and by the recurrent laryngeal nerve below this level. The intrinsic muscles are also supplied by the recurrent laryngeal nerve, with the exception of the cricothyroid, which receives its innervation through the external laryngeal nerve.

ventricle of l., a recess in the lateral wall of the larynx, located between the vocal and ventricular folds.

laser (la′zer) [acronym from *l*ight *a*mplification by *s*timulated *e*mission of *r*adiation] a device that produces an intense, nondiverging, monochromatic beam of light. It is a perfect light source for spectrophotometry, although the expense involved has limited it to special applications. Pulsed lasers can deliver intense energy in a brief pulse (about a nanosecond) into a very small area and have been used in a number of surgical procedures, e.g., in the surgical welding of detached retinas.

Lash's casein hydrolysate-serum medium a culture medium for *Trichomonas,* especially *T. vaginalis.* Agar slants of casamino acids, sugars, sodium lactate, and salts with a layer of beef blood serum are inoculated with vaginal specimens; after incubation at 37.5°C for 24–48 hr, they can be examined for growth.

Lasiohelea (las″e-o-he′le-ah) a genus of flies of the family Heleidae.

Lasix (la′siks) trademark. See *furosemide.*

Lassa fever a viral disease primarily found in individuals in central West Africa. It is transmitted to humans by contact with rodent (*Mastomys natalensis*) excrement, and spread by interpersonal contact. Infections are characterized by fever, headache, myalgia, chills, and malaise. Later, pharyngitis, lymphadenopathy, vomiting, and shock may occur; the mortality is high.

Laboratory tests reveal leukopenia, proteinuria, and increases in serum enzymes (serum glutamic-oxaloacetic transaminase, creatine kinase, and lactate dehydrogenase). Chest x-rays may reveal pneumonitis and pleural effusion, and electrocardiographic changes are seen. Diagnosis is made by staining conjunctival or throat scrapings or various secretions with fluorescent anti-Lassa antiserum. Serologic tests and virus isolation from blood, throat, or urine may also be required.

lassitude (las′ĭ-tūd) [L. *lassitudo* weariness] the feeling of weakness or exhaustion.

latency (la′ten-se) the interval between the time of application of a stimulus to a point along a nerve (which can be marked on the cathode-ray screen as the stimulus artifact) and the onset of the resulting deflection of the compound muscle (motor latency) or sensory nerve (sensory latency) action potential. It corresponds to the time taken in the fastest conducting fibers for the wave of depolarization to pass from the stimulation site to the recording electrodes positioned at more distant points on the muscle or nerve. Also called *conduction time* or latent period.

distal l., the time it takes for the fastest conducted impulse to travel from a point of stimulus application to the active recording electrode. Distal motor latencies measured from a stimulus site closest to the muscle may be prolonged in peripheral neuropathies. Also called *terminal l.* Cf. *proximal l.*

proximal l., the latent period measured from a site of stimulation farthest from the recording electrodes. Cf. *distal l.*

residual l., the time difference between the distal latency of a muscle action potential that is actually observed and the predicted distal latency that is based on the conduction velocity recorded from a segment of nerve proximal to the stimulating electrode. This discrepancy between the measured and expected values of the distal motor latency can be accounted for by the decreased conduction velocity of the fine terminal branches of the nerve fibers, the synaptic delay at the neuromuscular junction, and the time taken for volume conduction of the potential change to the pickup zone of the surface recording electrodes.

terminal l., see *distal l.*

latent (la′tent) [L. *latens* hidden] concealed; not manifest; potential.

latent image the invisible image on a photographic film that has been exposed but not yet developed.

later/o (lat′er-o) [L. *latus* side] a word element used in combining form to denote side, e.g., lateroabdominal.

lateral (lat′er-al) [L. *lateralis*] 1. farther from the median plane of the body or a structure.

2. on one side of the median plane.

3. in radiology, referring to a view or projection in which the beam goes through the patient from side to side.

lateral abdominal region a region of the abdomen on either side of the umbilical region. Cf. *lumbar region.* See illustration under *abdominal regions.*

lateral geniculate body a small, ovoid mass situated on the inferior aspect of the thalamus ventral to the medial geniculate body and covered by a portion of the temporal lobe. Presenting a highly organized laminar appearance, the six layers of the lateral geniculate correspond to retinotopic projections from both eyes. Layers one, four, and six receive input from the contralateral retina; layers two, three, and five, from the ipsilateral retina. There does not appear to be any integration between laminae, only between the neurons within a layer. Efferent fibers from the lateral geniculate radiate retinotopically to the occipital visual cortex.

lateralized (lat″er-a-lizd) in electroencephalography, a term used to describe any pattern of electrical activity that is recorded primarily from either the right or the left side of the head.

lateral sagittal plane a sagittal (vertical anteroposterior) plane that passes midway between the midsagittal (median) plane and the anterior superior iliac spine (the forward projection of the top of the hipbone). It divides the left (or right) hypochondriac, lumbar, and iliac regions of the abdomen from the epigastric, umbilical, and hypogastric regions, respectively. See also *Addison's planes.* Cf. *midclavicular line.*

late replicating X chromosome the inactive X chromosome in female mammalian cells (or any of the inactive X chromosomes in cells with an abnormal complement of X chromosomes—only one X is active). Autoradiography using labeled thymidine shows that the inactive X replicates later in the cell cycle than the active X and the autosomes. The late replicating chromosome is not present in normal males and is at the periphery of the nucleus, where it is seen (as the Barr body) by use of light microscopy. It is known to be the inactive X by studies in hybrids, such as the mule, in which the horse and donkey Xs are distinguishable, and certain X-linked gene products, such as glucose-6-phospate dehydrogenase, can be distinguished. See also *Lyon hypothesis.*

late response any evoked compound muscle action potential with a latent period longer than that of the M wave. See also *F wave* and *H wave.*

lateromedial (lat″er-o-me′de-al) 1. pertaining to a radiographic projection in which the central ray passes through a part (e.g., elbow, ankle, breast) from the lateral side to the medial side.

2. a projection of the sternum in which the patient lies supine on the cassette and the central ray is centered on the sternum, inclining laterally at 12°–22°, so that the shadows of the spine and sternum are separated.

latex (la′teks) [L. "fluid"] 1. a white viscous fluid obtained from plants. It contains suspended microscopic globules of natural rubber.

2. similar synthetic materials, such as polystyrene, styrene-butadiene rubber, neoprene, and polyvinyl chloride.

latex agglutination test see *latex fixation test.*

latex fixation test a type of antigen-antibody agglutination test in which soluble antigens are absorbed to latex particles and then mixed with specific antibody. Agglutination of the coated latex particles is indicative of specific antigen-antibody interaction.

The latex fixation test is most commonly used as an assay for rheumatoid factor in individuals with rheumatoid arthritis. The rheumatoid factor is an IgM molecule, which specifically reacts with a 7S IgG molecule. In this assay, 7S IgG is absorbed with latex particles and then reacted with the patient's specimen to determine the presence of rheumatoid factor (IgM). In reversed agglutination, antibody is placed on particles and agglutinated by test antigens. Also called *latex agglutination test.* See also *chorionic gonadotropin assays* and *fibrin (fibrinogen) degradation products methods.*

lathyrism (lath′ĭ-rizm) a pathologic condition resulting from ingestion of the seeds of leguminous plants of the genus *Lathyrus,* which includes many kinds of peas. It is characterized by spastic paraplegia, pain, hyperesthesia, paresthesia, defective skeletal development, and urinary excretion of large amounts of hydroxyproline-containing peptides. The peas contain β-aminopropionitrile; this irreversibly inhibits the copper-containing amine oxidase of plasma and the lysyl oxidases of bone and connective tissue, which produce cross-links between tropocollagen molecules.

latitude (lat′ĭtūd) in radiography, the variation or error in contrast and exposure within which visibility of detail acceptable for diagnosis is maintained. Some film types have more latitude than others. Increasing the contrast decreases the latitude.

Latrodectus (lat″ro-dek′tus) [L. *latro* robber + Gr. *daknein* to bite] a genus of spiders, family Theridae, of which the species *L. mactans* is the black-widow spider. Found in the United States and parts of Central and South America, *L. mactans* is one of the few species of spiders capable of producing severe envenomation in humans. These spiders are coal black with orange or red markings; the females can be identified by the red hourglass-shaped marking on the underside of their abdomen. The males are about 6.25 mm in length; the females, 12.5 mm.

The venom is a nonhemolytic neurotoxin. Although the bite may not be noticeable at first, within a few minutes to several hours a sharp pain develops at the site of the bite. Muscle pain, spasms, and rigidity occur, especially in areas of the abdomen, thorax, and back; nausea, vomiting, profuse sweating, and shock may also occur.

L. bishopi, a species common to southern Florida.

L. geometricus, a species found in California and southern Florida, and throughout Africa.

L. mactans, the black widow spider, a species common to the United States. Its bite can cause severe symptoms and may result in death.

LATS abbrev. See *long-acting thyroid stimulator.*

LATS-p abbrev. See *LATS protector.*

LATS protector (LATS-p) an antibody present in about 90 percent of patients affected with Graves' disease; in vitro it prevents the inactivation of LATS by thyroid tissue fractions. LATS-p can also directly stimulate the thyroid gland.

lattice (lat′is) the system of points describing the arrangement of atoms or molecules in a crystal; usually called space lattice, sometimes called crystal lattice.

Laurell technique (lor′el) see *rocket i.* under *immunoelectrophoresis.*

Laurence-Moon-Biedl syndrome [John Zachariah *Laurence*, British ophthalmologist, 1829–1870; R.C. *Moon*, U.S. ophthalmologist, 1844–1914; Arthur *Biedl*, Prague endocrinologist, 1869–1933] an inherited condition, transmitted as an autosomal recessive trait, that is characterized by obesity, mental deficiency, hypogenitalism, polydactyly, and retinitis pigmentosa. Also called Laurence-Moon syndrome and Laurence-Moon-Bardet-Biedl syndrome.

lauric acid (law′rik) a saturated fatty acid, $CH_3(CH_2)_{10}COOH$, from laurel seed oil, coconut oil, and milk fat.

lavage (lah-vahzh′) [Fr.] the act or process of washing out, flooding, or irrigating a body organ or cavity (e.g., stomach).

bronchopulmonary l., the introduction of a saline-based solution into a segment, lobe, or whole lung through a bronchoscope or a divided tracheobronchial catheter to wash out or retrieve alveolar fluid. In the case of alveolar proteinosis, the lavaging process can be therapeutic, with a goal of improved alveolar function. More recently, the process has been used diagnostically to harvest and identify alveolar cells participating in an active alveolitis. During the procedure, ventilation and gas exchange are maintained through the opposing channel of a double-lumen divided tracheal catheter. In the case of bronchoscopy, the lavage is limited to the segment or lobe into which the tip of the scope has been wedged.

gastric l., 1. the clinical procedure performed to wash out noncorrosive poisons and drugs from the stomach. A large-bore gastric lavage tube is inserted and copious amounts of water, physiologic saline, or antidotes are pumped into the stomach. The stomach contents may be removed by gravity, siphon, or syringe. The process is repeated until the washings return free of poison or drug. For comatose patients who have ingested antidepressant drugs, gastric lavage is usually preceded by the insertion of a cuffed tracheal tube to avoid aspiration of the washings. Sodium carbonate should not be included in the lavage fluid, because it increases the absorption of certain poisons (salicylates) and may encourage pulmonary aspiration.

2. a technique to obtain gastric epithelial cells for cytologic examination. The lavage is performed using saline, and the collected fluid is spun down to produce a pellet of cells. These are smeared on microscope slides, which are then immersed in a fixative; 95 percent ethanol is satisfactory for most purposes, but if the preparation appears bloody, Carnoy's solution may be used to hemolyze the erythrocytes. The fixed smears are stained using the Papanicolaou or other cytologic stains.

peritoneal l., a diagnostic procedure to detect intraabdominal bleeding following blunt trauma. It is best performed on conscious, cooperative patients. A sterile plastic catheter is introduced into the peritoneal cavity through an incision in the midline between the umbilicus and the pubic symphysis. A dialysis solution (1 l) of normal saline or lactated Ringer's solution is slowly infused into the peritoneum over the course of 10–15 min. An empty infusion bottle is placed below the patient, and the lavage fluid is collected by gravity. If the fluid is deeply tinged red with a hematocrit of greater than 1 percent, the diagnosis of significant intraabdominal hemorrhage can reliably be made.

law (law) a general rule or principle that describes a natural phenomenon, e.g., Beer's law, which is used in spectrophotometry. For more information, see the specific law.

lawn plate a solid culture medium plate inoculated by swab or with a liquid inoculum to produce a uniform, confluent growth of microorganisms.

law of mass action stated as: in a reversible reaction, the rates of the forward and reverse reactions are proportional to the concentrations of the reacting substances. At equilibrium, the rates of the forward and reverse reactions are equal, and the ratio of the rate constants for the reverse and forward reactions k_r/k_f is called the equilibrium constant K_{eq}: $k_r/k_f = K_{eq} = [C][D]/[A][B]$, where [C] and [D] are the concentrations of the products, and [A] and [B] are the concentrations of the reactants.

Law position a radiographic position used to obtain a lateral projection of the mastoid process and petrous portion of the temporal bone. The median sagittal plane is parallel to the film, which is centered to a localization point 1 in. posterior to the external auditory meatus. The central ray is directed at angles of 15° toward the feet and 15° toward the face.

This position demonstrates the mastoid cells, the sigmoid sinus and mastoid emissary vein, the internal and external acoustic meatuses, and the tegmen tympani (the roof of the middle ear). Other Law projections are inferosuperior oblique projections of the facial bones and of the paranasal sinuses.

lawrencium (Lr, formerly Lw) (law-ren′se-um) [Ernest Orlando *Lawrence*, American physicist, 1901–1958; winner of the Nobel Prize for physics in 1939 and the inventor of the cyclotron] a synthetic, metallic radioactive element; atomic number 103; most stable isotope, Lr-260 (half-life, 3 min); a 5f transition element (actinide element); oxidation state +3.

layer (la′er) a sheetlike mass of tissue of nearly uniform thickness, several of which may be superimposed, one above the other. Also called *lamina* and *stratum.*

lazy leukocyte syndrome an immunologic disease of children in which the migratory capacity of neutrophil leukocytes is defective. There is no increase in peripheral blood neutrophils when an individual is injected with stimulatory epinephrine or endotoxin. Children affected with this syndrome are unusually susceptible to bacterial infections.

LCAT abbrev. See *lecithin-cholesterol acyltransferase.*

L chain abbrev. See *light chain.*

LD abbrev. for *lactate dehydrogenase*, lethal dose.

LD_{50} abbrev. See *lethal d., median*, under *dose.*

LDH abbrev. See *lactate dehydrogenase.*

LDL abbrev. See *low-density l.* under *lipoprotein.*

LE abbrev. See *l. erythematosus* under *lupus.*

leaching (lēch′ing) the extraction of the soluble

components of a mixture by washing. Also called *lixiviation.*

lead (lēd) 1. a pair of wires attached to an electronic component.

2. in cardiography, the specific electrode placements customarily used to record the heart's electrical activity from different spatial perspectives on the body surface, and the electrocardiographic record obtained from that specific placement.

l. I, see under *standard limb l.*

l. II, see under *standard limb l.*

l. III, see under *standard limb l.*

augmented limb l., a unipolar lead system used in electrocardiography in which the exploring electrode is placed on one of the three limbs, and the Wilson reference electrode is altered by elimination of the connection to the central terminal of the limb on which the recording electrode is positioned. This modification of the unipolar system increases the amplitudes of the resulting ECG deflections 50 percent above those recorded by ordinary unipolar limb leads. The augmented leads are designated according to whether the exploring electrode is placed on the right arm (aV_r), left arm (aV_l), or left leg (aV_f). Also called augmented unipolar limb lead, *Goldberger l.,* and *unipolar limb l.*

bipolar l., a lead used in electrocardiography from which the changes in potential difference between the positive and negative electrodes (positioned in separate locations on the body surface) are recorded. The standard limb leads (I, II, and III), which are commonly used for cardiac monitoring, are bipolar leads. Cf. *unipolar l.*

bipolar limb l., see *standard limb l.*

Goldberger l., see *augmented limb l.*

limb l., a lead used in electrocardiography derived from electrodes positioned on the right arm, left arm, and left leg. See also *augmented limb l.* and *standard limb l.*

precordial l., a lead used in electrocardiography in which the exploring electrode is placed on the chest wall. A precordial lead may be a bipolar or a unipolar lead.

standard limb l., a bipolar lead connecting two limbs. Electrodes are placed on the right arm (R), left arm (L), and left leg (F). The potential difference between R(−) and L(+) is recorded from lead I; lead II records the difference in electrical potential between R(−) and F(+); and lead III is a record of the potential difference between L(−) and F(+). Each lead forms one axis of a triaxial reference system represented by the Einthoven triangle. Also called *bipolar limb l.*

unipolar l., a lead system used in electrocardiography that consists of a positive exploring electrode and a reference electrode that is formed by connecting each limb lead to a common negative pole through a 50,000-Ω resistance (the Wilson central terminal). The result is the recording of a local unipolar voltage that is contrasted with a relatively unchanging (and approximately zero) one. The unipolar exploring electrode may be placed anywhere on or in the body. Six standard positions on the anterior chest wall are designated V1, V2, V3, V4, V5, and V6. Other locations may be explored, e.g., V7, V8, V3R (V3 position on the right), and VE (unipolar esophageal lead).

VR, VL, and VF are unipolar limb leads recording potential variations of the right arm, left arm, and left leg. These have largely been replaced by the augmented unipolar limb leads aV_r, aV_l, and aV_f. See also *augmented limb l.* Cf. *bipolar l.*

unipolar chest l., see under *unipolar l.*

unipolar limb l., see *augmented limb l.*

V l., see under *unipolar l.*

Wilson l., see under *unipolar l.*

lead (Pb) (led) [A. S.; L. *plumbum*] a soft grayish-blue metal; atomic number 82; atomic weight 207.19; Group IV of the periodic table; oxidation states +2, +4. Because lead is very dense and efficiently absorbs radiation, it is used to make shielding devices such as lead aprons, gloves, gonad shields, and syringe shields, and radiation imaging devices such as collimators and grids.

Lead and lead compounds are highly toxic when ingested; they occur in paints, ceramic glazes, and leaded gasoline, and in industrial processes. Toxic effects include gastrointestinal distress, colic, pain in the joints, and encephalopathy (headache, drowsiness, stupor, convulsions, and coma) that may have a fatal outcome. Chronic low-grade exposure to lead dust or fumes may cause anemia, colic, and a peripheral neuropathy.

Normal individuals have less than 50 μg/dl of lead in whole blood; more than 100 μg/dl indicates probable toxicity, even in the absence of noticeable symptoms. Urinary excretion is less than 80 μg/da.

lead apron an apron used to protect physicians, technicians, and patients from unnecessary exposure to radiation during radiologic and nuclear medicine procedures. Usually the apron contains 0.25–0.5 mm of lead having a reduction factor of two or four for x-rays.

lead assays 1. colorimetric procedure. Organic matter is removed from a blood or urine sample by digestion with acid and oxidizing agents. Interfering metal ions are removed by extractions at controlled pH or by chelation. A red complex of lead and dithizone is formed. The color intensity at 505 nm is read spectrophotometrically and compared with a standard and a blank. The relative error of this method is about 10 percent.

2. atomic absorption spectrophotometry. Lead can be isolated from samples by solvent extraction of lead chelates; this requires 5 ml of blood. Samples as small as 1 μl may be used with flameless atomic absorption spectrometry. The relative error is about 5 percent. All glass and plastic ware used must be acid washed to remove lead contamination, or must be tested for freedom from lead.

Because lead interferes with heme synthesis, assays of the precursor compounds coproporphyrin, protoporphyrin, and δ-aminolevulinic acid or of the enzyme δ-aminolevulinate dehydratase can be used as screening tests for lead exposure. Red blood cell protoporphyrin is the most sensitive.

The provocative chelation or mobilization test is a measure of urinary lead after administration of edetate calcium disodium, which chelates lead and increases its excretion. More than 1 μg of lead per mg of edetate administered indicates an increased body content in lead.

See also *δ-aminolevulinate dehydratase assays, δ-aminolevulinic acid assays,* and *porphyrin assays.*

lead demonstration in tissue histologic methods for the localization of lead in tissue sections. Paraffin sections are stained in a fresh, unoxidized hematoxylin solution without mordant. Lead is stained dark grayish–blue to black. In other methods, lead salts are converted to black lead sulfide by treatment with hydrogen sulfide solution or to yellow lead chromate by treatment with acidic potassium chromate solution.

lead fixatives histologic fixatives containing lead, which precipitate proteins. The most commonly used are Lillie's alcoholic lead nitrate formalin (lead nitrate, formalin, water, and ethanol) and lead subacetate (lead subacetate in water or formalin with enough acetic acid added to dissolve the precipitate of lead carbonate; this fixative must be protected from air because it absorbs CO_2). Lead fixatives are used primarily for the preservation of acid mucopolysaccharides and for the demonstration of mast cells.

leading (lē'ding) in gas chromatography, the phenomenon exhibited by a peak that has gradual rise and sharp fall, which is caused by overloading the column.

lead x-ray peak a peak in a gamma-ray spectrum recorded with a scintillation detector that has a lead collimator or lead shielding. This 77-keV peak is due to secondary characteristic x-rays produced by gamma rays absorbed in the lead.

learning (ler'ning) a relatively long-lasting adaptive behavioral change that occurs as a result of experience.

learning disorder a general term used to describe the condition in which the intellectual performance of children is significantly less than their potential. No single etiology is known; however, five times more males than females are affected, and 5–15 percent of all children in the United States are identified as having such a problem. Symptoms include hyperactivity, emotional lability, and motor incoordination. Medical, educational, sensory, and psychologic evaluations may be useful in identifying the cause of the disorder.

least (lēst) lowest or smallest.

least significant bit (LSB) the least significant digit of a binary number.

least significant digit (LSD) 1. the rightmost significant digit in a number. See also *significant digits.*

2. the low-order digit in a computer word or register. For fixed-point numbers, the digit in the one's place. Cf. *most significant digit.*

least squares regression a method for fitting a mathematically defined function to a set of data, often used in linear regression. The unspecified constants in the function are calculated to minimize the squared deviations of the observations from the function. See also *linear regression.*

Leber's optic atrophy (la'berz) [Theodor *Leber,* German ophthalmologist, 1840–1917] a genetic disorder that is characterized by progressive bilateral atrophy of the optic nerve. Most frequently, it occurs in adult males; it may be associated with a defect of the motor pathways of the cerebellum. Leber's optic atrophy leads to a rapid loss of vision and permanent central blindness. Also called Leber's disease.

LE cell abbrev. See *lupus erythematosus cell.*

LE cell test the formation of LE cells in vitro. The term was formerly used to denote a test for systemic lupus erythematosus. Due to the lack of sensitivity and specificity of this test, it has been superseded by other serologic tests, e.g., for antinuclear and anti-DNA antibody. See also *lupus erythematosus cell.*

lecithin (les'ĭ-thin) [Gr. *lekithos* yolk of egg] see *phosphatidylcholine.*

lecithinase (les'ĭ-thin-ās) a generic name for enzymes that split various bonds in phosphatidyl glycerols (phospholipids). These enzymes are differentiated by the letters A, B, C, and D, for example, lecithinase A (which is phosphatide 2-acylhydrolase, EC 3.1.1.4). Also called *phospholipase.*

lecithinase A see *p. A_2* under *phospholipase.*

lecithinase B see *lysophospholipase.*

lecithinase C an enzyme of the hydrolase class (phospholipase C, phosphatidylcholine cholinephosphohydrolase, EC 3.1.4.3) that catalyzes the reaction phosphatidylcholine (lecithin) + $H_2O \rightleftharpoons$ 1,2-diacylglycerol + choline phosphate. The enzyme is the active principle in the lethal, necrotizing, and hemolytic exotoxins of some species of *Clostridium,* and its presence is a means of differentiating species within the genus. Lecithinase C is identified by the presence of an opaque halo around bacterial colonies on egg yolk medium. Also called *Clostridium welchii* α-toxin and *phospholipase C.*

lecithin–cholesterol acyltransferase (LCAT) (les'ĭ-thin ko-les'ter-ol as"il-trans'fer-ās) an enzyme of the transferase class (EC 2.3.1.43) that catalyzes the reaction lecithin + cholesterol $\rightleftharpoons$ 1-acylglycerophosphocholine + cholesterol ester. The enzyme occurs in the blood; a genetic deficiency leads to a defect in lipid metabolism. Also called *phosphatidylcholine-cholesterol acyltransferase.*

lecithin–cholesterol acyltransferase deficiency a genetic disorder, transmitted as an autosomal recessive trait, that is characterized by a relative or absolute deficiency of the enzyme lecithin–cholesterol acyltransferase (LCAT), the enzyme that catalyzes the transfer of a fatty acid from lecithin to cholesterol to form a cholesterol ester. As a result, unesterified cholesterol, phospholipids, and triglycerides accumulate in the blood. The onset of this disorder occurs in young adulthood; there may be hemolytic anemia, liver and kidney failure, vascular degeneration, and lens opacities. Electrophoresis and ultracentrifugation reveal abnormal structures of all lipoproteins. There is no treatment and the prognosis is poor. Also called familial LCAT deficiency and *Norum's disease.*

lecithin-sphingomyelin (L/S) ratio a diagnostic test used to evaluate fetal lung maturity. Prior to the thirty-fourth week of gestation, the concentration of the phospholipids lecithin and sphingomyelin in amniotic fluid are approximately equal. After this time, there is a marked increase in lecithin synthesis, and the L/S ratio increases to greater than 2 at term.

Delivery of a low-weight (premature) fetus, whose amniotic fluid lecithin concentration is less than 1.25 mg/dl (lecithin phosphorus of less than 0.050 mg/dl or L/S ratio of less than 2.0), is contraindicated, as the infant will probably develop respiratory distress or hyaline membrane disease. An L/S ratio of more than 2.0 indicates adequate fetal lung maturity and suggests that development of respiratory distress after delivery is not probable.

The L/S ratio is most often determined by

one-dimensional thin-layer chromatography and identification of the phospholipids by charring with sulfuric acid or by colorimetric tests. Newer techniques indicate that two-dimensional chromatography is preferred, as it eliminates the false high-lecithin values caused by poorly separated phosphatidylinositol, which may be observed in the same location as lecithin. See also *surfactant.*

lecithin-sphingomyelin ratio determination thin-layer chromatography using silica gel plates. The plates may be developed with one of several solvent mixtures, e.g., a 65:25:4 mixture of chloroform, methanol, and water. The developed plates are sprayed with sulfuric acid and charred; the ratio of the areas of lecithin and sphingomyelin is determined by densitometry and compared with spots obtained with individual lecithin and sphingomyelin standards or a 3:1 mixture of lecithin and sphingomyelin.

Amniotic fluid samples are prepared by centrifuging the amniotic fluid to remove cell debris. The supernatant is then mixed with an equal volume of methanol and extracted with twice its volume of chloroform. After separation, the chloroform layer is removed and evaporated, and the residue is dissolved in acetone, which is then spotted on the silica plates.

lectin (lek′tin) an extract made from mollusks and the seeds of certain plants that has the ability to agglutinate red blood cells. Some lectins possess the ability to react with specific red cell antigens.

lectotype (lek′to-tīp) a type culture taken from a group of microorganisms for which the original investigator did not designate a type.

LED abbrev. See *light-emitting diode.*

leech (lēch) [L. *hirudo*] any annelids of the class Hirudinea. Most leeches of medical importance are of the blood-sucking species of the genera *Hirudo, Poecilobdella, Dinobdella,* and *Limnatis,* and are found in fresh water or are terrestrial. Aquatic leeches are found in temperate and tropical areas, whereas land leeches are distributed only in subtropical and tropical regions. Leech bites cause extensive blood loss, and in addition the lesions frequently become infected.

Lee-White clotting test see *whole blood clotting time.*

left anterior oblique (LAO) in radiology, pertaining to a view with the left anterior aspect of the patient closest to the film and an obliquity of 45° unless otherwise stated.

left axis deviation in electrocardiography, deviation of the mean QRS vector in the frontal plane to a direction more negative than −30°; seen in left ventricular hypertrophy, left anterior hemiblock, left bundle branch block, and diaphragmatic myocardial infarction.

left posterior oblique (LPO) in radiology, pertaining to a view with the left posterior aspect of the patient closest to the film and an obliquity of 45° unless otherwise stated.

left ventricular ejection time (LVET) see under *systolic time interval.*

left ventricular hypertrophy the increase in mass of the left ventricle, independent of natural growth, which is due to enlargement of its constituent cells.

legal age the age of majority, which differs from state to state.

Legg-Calvé-Perthes disease (leg kal-va′ per′tēz) [Arthur Thornton *Legg,* Boston surgeon, 1874–1939; Jacques *Calvé,* French orthopedist, 1875–1954; Georg Clemens *Perthes,* German surgeon, 1869–1927] see under *osteochondritis juvenilis.*

Legionella (le″jun-el′ah) [L. *legio* army] a bacterial genus, first recognized after its isolation and identification as the cause of a 1976 outbreak of pneumonia that became known as Legionnaires' disease. Legionellae are aerobic, motile, pleomorphic, gram-negative bacilli with a uniquely high content of branched fatty acids. Primary isolation was at first very difficult, requiring guinea pig passage to chick embryos, but once adapted to artificial media the organisms grow readily on media containing L-cysteine and iron.

The original species was named *L. pneumophila.* At present six additional species are generally accepted, and others will undoubtedly be established from a collection of isolates referred to as LLO (*Legionella*-like organisms). *L. micdadei* is the designation of the "Pittsburgh pneumonia agent"; *L. dumoffii, L. bozemanii, L. gormanii, L. longbeachae,* and *L. jordanis* are the five other species. All but the last-named were isolated from pneumonia patients, and *L. gormanii* is now known to cause human infection.

The evidence is strong that the normal habitat of *Legionella* is the environment, probably soil. All but *L. bozemanii* have been found in cooling-tower water, river banks, or a similar environmental location. Noteworthy is the isolation of *L. micdadei* from nebulizers of respiratory therapy equipment. Members of this genus have now been reported from many areas of the world.

L. pneumophila, a species of microorganisms of the genus *Legionella,* family Legionellaceae, occurring as thin, gram-negative, pleomorphic rods. In 1976, this organism was discovered to be the causative organism of Legionnaires' disease. It is aerobic, forming slow-growing colonies on charcoal yeast extract agar. The organism can be cultured in and isolated from inoculated guinea pigs and embryonated hen eggs. *L. pneumophila* is difficult to demonstrate in tissue specimens by Gram stain but is easily seen by the Dieterle silver impregnation method. Laboratory identification can also be made by direct fluorescent antibody test of the acute and convalescent sera. Erythromycin is the drug of choice.

legionellosis (le″jun-el-o′sis) disease caused by infection with *Legionella pneumophila,* including Legionnaires' disease and Pontiac fever. See also *Legionella, Legionnaires' disease,* and *Pontiac fever.*

lei/o (li′o) [Gr. *leios* smooth] a word element used in combining form to denote smooth, e.g., leiomyoma.

leiomy/o (li-o-mi′o) [*leios* + Gr. *mys* muscle] a word element used in combining form to denote smooth muscle, e.g., leiomyosarcoma.

leiomyoblastoma (li″o-mi″o-blas-to′mah) a term coined to designate a smooth muscle tumor, particularly of the stomach, that differs histologically from a typical leiomyoma in having bizarre cytologic features—frequently an "epithelioid" transformation of its cells and scanty or absent evidence of smooth muscle origin at the ultrastructural level. The term is unsatisfactory, as it leaves unanswered the question of whether a particular neoplasm is benign or malignant.

leiomyoma (li″o-mi-o′mah) a benign tumor of smooth muscle cells. It can occur virtually anywhere in the body but is most common in the uterus. Typically, leiomyomas are well-circumscribed lesions with a whitish cut surface that has a whorled appearance. Histologic sections show intersecting bundles of spindle cells similar to those of normal smooth muscle; ultrastructurally, smooth muscle myofilaments are generally evident. Degenerative changes can occur toward the center of a large leiomyoma and should not be mistaken for malignant transformation, which is an uncommon event. Distinction between a cellular leiomyoma and a low-grade leiomyosarcoma may be difficult. Occasionally, a uterine leiomyoma that appears benign histologically metastasizes throughout the peritoneal cavity or to the lungs.

uterine l., the most common tumor of the uterus. At least one leiomyoma is present in more than 20 percent of adult uteri, although most are asymptomatic. The tumors vary greatly in size from tiny nodules to occasional large masses and are usually multiple. Those located in the superficial myometrium can become pedunculated and protrude into the peritoneal or endometrial cavities. Multiple large leiomyomas can greatly distort the size and shape of the uterus, cause uterine bleeding, or interfere with implantation or delivery. Various forms of degeneration occur in uterine leiomyomas, generally toward the center of a large tumor as a result of impaired blood supply. Sarcomatous degeneration is uncommon.

The cause of uterine leiomyomas remains poorly understood, although the influence of ovarian hormones is often invoked.

Also called *fibroid.*

leiomyosarcoma (li″o-mi″o-sar-ko′mah) a malignant neoplasm of smooth muscle cells. Leiomyosarcomas can occur in many locations but are most common in the deeper tissues of the thigh, uterus, gastrointestinal tract, and retroperitoneum; infrequently they arise from a large artery or vein. Superficial leiomyosarcomas are uncommon. Some uterine leiomyosarcomas arise from a preexisting leiomyoma. In children, the genitourinary tract, especially the bladder and prostate, may be involved.

The gross appearance is not distinctive. The tumors vary greatly in size and may appear encapsulated but rarely are. Most leiomyosarcomas are fairly firm, are white or tan, and may have a whorled appearance on cut surface. Areas of hemorrhage and necrosis are common in the larger neoplasms.

Well-differentiated tumors are composed of cells that are similar to those of normal smooth muscle but are generally plumper and have more hyperchromatic nuclei. Typically they form intersecting fascicles. Light microscopy reveals that there is little collagen in most leiomyosarcomas, in contrast to some fibrosarcomas. Pleomorphic cells are seen in poorly differentiated forms. Histologic differentiation of a leiomyosarcoma from a cellular leiomyoma is based on the finding of specified numbers of mitotic figures in the former. It may be difficult to distinguish a leiomyosarcoma from other sarcomas if the tumor is not well differentiated, and electron microscopy can be useful in demonstrating smooth muscle myofilaments and other features of the tumor cells.

Some smooth muscle tumors that arise from the GI tract depart from the typical histologic appearance and show varying degrees of so-called epithelioid transformation by light microscopy, associated with a loss of smooth muscle characteristics at the ultrastructural level. A similar type of change may be seen in smooth muscle tumors in the uterus and other locations.

Assessment of the prognosis of a leiomyosarcoma on the basis of the histologic appearance is precarious. Some well-differentiated uterine tumors that are thought to be benign subsequently metastasize.

The behavior of a malignant smooth muscle tumor is unpredictable but local recurrence is frequent and liver or lung metastases may develop. In children, leiomyosarcomas of the prostate and bladder are usually aggressive neoplasms.

Leishman-Donovan bodies (lēsh′man don′o-van) the nonflagellated intracellular form of *Leishmania donovani,* which appears as small, round, or oval bodies in reticuloendothelial cells of the spleen and liver in kala-azar. The cytoplasm and cell membrane of these organisms may be visible by Giemsa stain, but the nucleus and kinetoplast together are distinctive. The term is also used to refer to similar forms of *L. tropica* and *Trypanosoma cruzi.*

Leishmania (lēsh-ma′ne-ah) [Sir William Boog *Leishman,* English army surgeon, 1865-1926] a genus of flagellate protozoa of worldwide distribution, several species of which are parasitic in humans. These species have only two stages in their life cycle—amastigote and promastigote stages—and require vertebrate (i.e., human) and invertebrate (i.e., insect) hosts. Phlebotomine sandflies are known transmitters of *Leishmania.*

L. braziliensis, a species widely distributed throughout Central and South America (except Chile and Argentina) and parasitic in humans, dogs, monkeys, and rodents—that causes American or mucocutaneous leishmaniasis. Three subspecies of *L. braziliensis* have been differentiated: *L. b. braziliensis, L. b. guyanensis,* and *L. b. panamensis. L. braziliensis* is morphologically identical to *L. tropica* and *L. donovani* and lives in tissue cells and endothelial cells of the skin and mucous membranes of the nose, mouth, and pharynx. It is transmitted by the sandflies of the genera *Lutzomyia* and *Psychodopygus* and causes cutaneous lesions similar to those produced by *L. tropica,* as well as ulceration of tissues that gradually produces gross deformity in the nose and pharynx.

Diagnosis requires identification of the genus in material from the ulcer by Giemsa or Wright stain or by cultures on Novy, MacNeal and Nicolle (NNN) medium. However, isolation of the organism is difficult, even by hamster inoculation. Serologic tests, such as the Montenegro skin test, are helpful, being positive several months after initial onset of the infection. Recently, the indirect fluorescent antibody test with an amastigote antigen has also been used with some success.

L. caninum, see *L. donovani.*

L. donovani, the parasite that causes the Old World visceral leishmaniasis, or kala-azar, in Africa, Asia, and Europe. *L. donovani* is a round or ovoid parasite, measuring 2–5 μm in diameter, which infects humans, dogs, cats, and rodents. Sixty percent of infected humans are between ages 10 and 20 yr. Infection is transmitted by sandflies of the genus *Phlebotomus.* The parasite multiplies in macrophages, which are liberated in the blood stream, and then lodges in the viscera, where it proliferates and destroys the cells of the spleen, liver, bone marrow, and other centers of the reticuloendothelial system. For unknown reasons, a small percentage of patients who recover from visceral leishmaniasis develop a late syndrome called postkala-azar dermal leishmanoid.

Diagnosis requires identification of the genus in smears of spleen or bone marrow tissue, lymphatic juices, or buffy coat films. Serum concentration of gamma globulin is greatly increased in patients with kala-azar, and there is a reversal of the A/G ratio. Other tests used are blood cultures on Novy, MacNeal and Nicolle (NNN) medium and the formol gel test, complement-fixation test, and Montenegro skin test.

Also called *Herpetomonas donovani, L. caninum,* and *L. infantum.* See also *kala-azar.*

L. infantum, a name given to the parasite of infantile visceral leishmaniasis, or kala-azar, of the Old World. Of those infected, 80–90 percent are younger than 10 yr. *L. infantum* has various members of the *Canidae* as reservoir hosts. There is no general agreement yet on whether *L. infantum* is *L. donovani,* or if it should be a separate, specific species. See also *L. donovani.*

L. nilotica, see *L. tropica.*

L. peruviana, a species parasitic in humans and dogs that causes the cutaneous leishmaniasis known as *uta* in Peru. It is endemic on the western slopes of the Peruvian Andes and the Argentinian highlands.

L. tropica, a species causing the Old World cutaneous leishmaniasis, which occurs in two main forms: *L. tropica* var. *major,* seen in dry, semidesert rural areas of Central Asia and the Middle East, where rodents constitute the reservoir; and *L. tropica* var. *minor,* an urban form found in large cities and maintained by reservoirs in humans and dogs. Cutaneous leishmaniasis is also found in North Africa, the dry sub-Saharan area of West Africa, and the highland area of Ethiopia and Kenya (where the name *L. aethiopica* is preferred).

Human infection is transmitted by the infected sandfly of the genus *Phlebotomus.* The organism is introduced into the skin, causing ulceration and necrosis as it subsequently invades the reticuloendothelial cells and lymphoid tissue. The flagellate is found in the amastigote form in human infections, and the promastigote form in insects and in biologic culture. *L. tropica* is morphologically identical to *L. donovani,* which causes visceral leishmaniasis.

Diagnosis requires microscopic examination of material from the sore or ulcer with Giemsa or Wright stain. Lymphoid material can be inoculated onto Novy, MacNeal and Nicolle (NNN) medium, with penicillin to control bacterial contamination and incubation. If promastigote forms are recovered, the diagnosis is positive.

Also called *Helcosoma tropicum, Herpetomonas furunculosa, H. tropica,* and *L. nilotica.*

leishmaniasis (lēsh″mah-ni′ah-sis) a disease caused by the presence of *Leishmania,* a genus of flagellate protozoa. Infection is transmitted by sandflies of the genera *Phlebotomus* and *Lutzomyia.*

American l., see *mucocutaneous l.*

cutaneous l., a condition due to the presence of *Leishmania tropica,* which causes a chronic ulcerative granuloma (Oriental sore) found mostly on the extremities. This form of leishmaniasis is prevalent in tropic and subtropical regions. See also *L. tropica* under *Leishmania.*

mucocutaneous l., an infection caused by the presence of *Leishmania braziliensis.* A primary cutaneous lesion spreads to the mucous membranes of the mouth, nose, and pharynx. This infection is commonly found in Central and South America. Also called *American l.* See also *L. braziliensis.*

leishmanicidal (lēsh″man-ĭ-si′dal) any chemical or material that is destructive to the genus *Leishmania.*

-lemma (lem′ah) [Gr. "rind"] a suffix word element to denote a cell membrane, as in plasmalemma.

lemniscus (lem-nis′kus), pl. *lemnisci* [L.; Gr. *lēmniskos* filler] 1. a ribbon or band.

2. [NA], in anatomy, a general term currently used to designate a band or bundle of fibers in the central nervous system.

lemon oil (lem′un) [USP], the volatile oil, obtained by expression from the fresh peel of the fruit *Citrus limon,* which is used as a flavoring agent.

Lendrum's inclusion body stain (len′drums) [A.C. *Lendrum,* Scottish pathologist, 20th Century] a histologic method for staining acidophilic inclusion bodies. Paraffin sections are stained first in Mayer's hematoxylin and then in phloxine solution (a solution of phloxine B and calcium chloride) and differentiated in a saturated solution of tartrazine in Cellosolve. Inclusion bodies stain red, nuclei blue, and the background yellow.

length (l) (length) 1. physical distance or spatial extension. The International System (SI) unit of length is the meter (m).

2. the longest dimension of an object or the distance from end to end.

Lennox-Gastaut syndrome [William Gordon *Lennox,* American neurologist, born 1884; Henri *Gastaut,* French neurologist] a form of secondary generalized epilepsy characterized by slow spike and slow waves on the electroencephalogram and, clinically, by mental retardation, abnormalities on neurologic examination, and a mixed seizure disorder with tonic, akinetic, atypical absence, and tonic-clonic seizures that are often refractory to anticonvulsant drugs. This syndrome can result from static (e.g., anoxic) or progressive (e.g., Batten's disease) encephalopathies. Onset of seizures is usually between ages 6 mo and 3 yr but can be delayed until the second decade. Prognosis for normal intellectual development is poor when seizures begin before age 2 yr or when the electrical activity of the brain at any time shows a spike-wave pattern having a frequency of less than 1.5 Hz.

lens (lenz) [L. "lentil"] 1. a piece of glass or other transparent substance that is used to focus light by refraction, as in a microscope or eyeglasses.

2. [NA], the transparent biconvex structure in the eye, situated between the posterior chamber and the vitreous body, that focuses light on the retina. Its shape adjusts according to its distance from the object through the action of the ciliary muscle, a phenomenon known as accommodation.

lenticular (len-tik′u-lar) [L. *lenticularis,* from *lenticula,* dim. of *lens*] pertaining to or shaped like a lens.

lenticular nucleus part of the corpus striatum that is shaped like a biconvex lens. It includes the putamen and globus pallidus and lies lateral to the internal capsule.

lenticular proteins proteins of the eye lens; several (e.g., α-, β-, and γ-crystallin) have been characterized. They can undergo changes during the aging process, resulting in opacity.

lentigo (len-ti′go), pl. *lentigines* [L. "freckle"] a small (1–5 mm), flat or slightly elevated brown spot on the skin or mucous membrane whose color is due to the increased deposition of melanin. The borders of the spot are well demarcated. Histologically, hyperplasia of melanocytes, elongation of the rete ridges, and hyperpigmentation of the epidermis are seen. A lentigo may evolve into compound or intradermal forms. Also called acquired melanocytic nevus.

malignant l., an intraepidermal form of malignant melanoma that occurs in older individuals, usually on exposed areas such as the hands and face. Progression to an invasive malignant melanoma, which occurs in about one-third of the cases, usually does not take place until the lesion has grown to the size of 4–6 cm and has been present for 5 yr, or frequently longer. Also called *melanotic freckle of Hutchinson.* See also *malignant m.* under *melanoma.*

Lentivirinae a subfamily of Retroviridae that consists of maedi/visna slow viruses of sheep. See also *Retroviridae.*

lepra cell (lep′rah) [Gr. *lepros* scaly] a macrophage found in the lesions of lepromatous (progressive) leprosy. Lepra cells have a foamy cytoplasm and contain many acid-fast bacilli, which stain poorly.

lepromin (lep′ro-min) a heat-treated extract, consisting of homogenized lepromatous nodules containing many *Mycobacterium leprae,* that is used in the skin test for leprosy.

lepromin skin test an immunologic assay using the antigen lepromin to determine the state of tissue resistance to *Mycobacterium leprae.* After intradermal injection, a delayed-type (24–48 hr) inflammatory reaction is observed in tuberculoid leprosy but not in lepromatous leprosy. This test is not diagnostic for leprosy, although it is useful for assessing the prognosis of the disease. A negative lepromin test in an individual known to have leprosy indicates a progression of the disease to the lepromatous stage, unless it is properly treated with chemotherapy. The lepromin antigen is not specific and can cross react with other mycobacterial antigens as well as with certain bacteria.

leprosarium (lep″ro-sa′re-um) [L.] a hospital or colony for the treatment and isolation of leprosy patients. The national leprosarium of the United States is in Carville, Louisiana.

leprosy (lep′ro-se) [Gr. *lepros* scaly, scabby, rough] a chronic infectious disease involving the skin, peripheral nerves, eyes, mucous membranes, and many other organ sites. The etiologic agent of leprosy is the acid-fast bacterium *Mycobacterium leprae.* The most probable mode of transmission is the respiratory route, although direct skin contact is also considered possible. Leprosy is a contagious disease, although not all people are susceptible; most who are have a defective cell-mediated immunity to *M. leprae.*

There are three degrees of clinical manifestation of leprosy: tuberculoid disease, lepromatous disease, and dimorphous or borderline leprosy. The tuberculoid disease type of leprosy, the least severe form, is characterized by very few lesions with only the local cutaneous and peripheral nerves enlarged. The most severe form, lepromatous leprosy, is characterized by the involvement of any combination of the following: organs, skin, nerves, testicles, and respiratory tract. There are large erythematous macules that become plaquelike, or generalized papular and nodular lesions, or multiple, firm, waxy nodules with loss of body hair. Dimorphous, or borderline, leprosy is characterized by a clinical picture that is of intermediate severity and shows features of both tuberculoid and lepromatous leprosy. Individuals with this form of leprosy may eventually develop a clinical picture more consistent with a pure lepromatous or pure tuberculoid leprosy form.

Leprosy is diagnosed by clinical observation of the skin lesions, and sensory loss, and by microbiologic analysis of the lesions. *M. leprae* stains acid-fast but has not been cultured in vitro. Serologically, the skin test may be used to determine the immune status toward *M. leprae.* The treatment of choice for leprosy is administration of dapsone for a period ranging from 1 to 10 yr. depending on the stage of the disease.

lept/o (lep′to) [Gr. *leptos* slender] a word element used in combining form to denote slender, thin, or delicate, e.g., leptodactyly, leptomeninges.

Leptoconops (lep″to-ko′nops) a genus of bloodsucking flies of the family Heleidae.

leptocyte (lep′to-sīt) [*lepto-* + Gr. *kytos* cell] an erythrocyte with an increased ratio of surface to volume. It can be classified as macro-, micro-, or normal in size. The cell is thinner and paler than normal erythrocytes and has a colorless center. Leptocytes frequently have a shallow cup shape; when cup depth increases, they are classified as codocytes, which become target cells in smears. This abnormality can be attributed to a lack of hemoglobin, as seen in iron deficiency anemia and thalassemia; to reduced amounts of water (desiccytes); or to an increase in the cell membrane, as seen in retention icterus. Cf. *torocyte.*

leptocytosis (lep″to-si-to′sis) the presence of leptocytes in the blood.

leptokurtic (lep″to-kur′tik) pertaining to a probability distribution with a sharp, narrow peak. See also *kurtosis.*

leptomonad (lep″to-mo′nad) [*lepto-* + Gr. *monas* unit] 1. a term used to describe a promastigote stage in the life cycle of protozoa of the family Trypanosomatidae.

2. pertaining to the genus *Leptomonas.*

Leptomonas (lep″to-mo′nas) a genus of protozoa parasitic in the digestive tract of insects. These organisms have an elongated body with a nucleus near the center and a single anterior flagellum arising from a kinetosome close to the kinetoplast. They lose the flagellum during their life cycle, assuming a round amastigote (leishmanial) form and becoming cysts. Their life cycle is completed when these cysts are ingested by the next host; they escape, grow a new flagellum, and develop to adult forms.

leptonema (lep″to-ne′mah) [*lepto-* + Gr. *nēma* thread] see *leptotene.*

Leptopsylla (lep″to-sil′ah) a genus of fleas, a known transmitter of the plague. The most common species, *L. segnis* (also called *Ctenopsyllus segnis* and *L. musculi*), is parasitic in mice and rats.

Leptosphaeria (lep'to-sfē"re-ah) a genus of loculoascomycete fungi capable of causing maduromycosis. *Leptosphaeria* produce black grains that aggregate, grow in diameter with age, and become hollow. In culture, this fungus forms a colony that is gray to brown in color. Ascocarps are produced, in which each ascus usually contains eight ascospores. There are two medically recognized species, *L. senegalensis* and *L. tompkinsii.* See also *mycetoma.*

Leptospira (lep"to-spi'rah) [*lepto-* + Gr. *spira* coil] a genus of microorganisms of the family Spirochaetaceae, order Spriochaetales. Visible by darkfield microscopy, they consist of single, finely coiled, motile, aerobic cells with hooked ends. They are mostly pathogenic, causing acute febrile systemic disease that is usually acquired from contact with water contaminated with the urine of infected rodents, livestock, or domestic animals. Laboratory diagnosis is most often based on microscopic agglutination tests; serologic typing and a fluorescent antibody procedure can also be used. See also *leptospirosis* and *spirochete.*

L. interrogans, the type species of the genus causing human disease. Formerly called *Leptospira icterohaemorrhagiae* and *Spirochaeta icterohaemorrhagiae.*

leptospirosis (lep"to-spi-ro'sis) infection caused by any of the spiral organisms of the genus *Leptospira,* most often through contact with infected animals. Human infection causes a disease lasting 1–2 wk, during which time the causative organism can be found in the blood and urine.

leptotene (lep'to-tēn) [*lepto-* + Gr. *tainia* ribbon] the first stage of prophase in meiosis during which the chromosomes first become visible. Also called *leptonema.* See also *meiosis.*

Leptotrichia (lep'to-tri"she-ah) [lepto- + Gr. *thricis* hair] a genus of anaerobic microorganisms of the family Bacteroidaceae, consisting of straight or slightly curved, nonmotile, gram-negative rods that occur in pairs or long filaments. The species *L. buccalis,* a natural inhabitant of the oral cavity, is not pathogenic, although it may be found in clinical material from oral or urogenital infections.

Leptus (lep'tus) [L.] a name for a larval form in the life cycle of mites of the genus *Trombicula* and the subgenus *Eutrombicula.*

lesbianism (lez'be-ah-nizm) [Gr. *Lesbios* of Lesbos, the home of the poetess Sappho and her followers] female homosexuality.

Lesch-Nyhan syndrome (lesh ni'han) [Michael *Lesch,* American physician, born 1939; William L. *Nyhan,* Jr., American physician, born 1926] a rare, dramatic cause of hyperuricemia due to a hereditary deficiency. It is caused by a mutation in the X-linked recessive gene for the purine-base, salvage enzyme hypoxanthine guanine phosphoribosyltransferase (HGPRT), which converts hypoxanthine and guanine to inosine 5'phosphate and guanosine 5'phosphate. Features of the syndrome include mental retardation, spastic cerebral palsy, choreoathetosis, uric acid urinary stones, self-destructive biting of fingers and lips, and other aggressive and bizarre behavior. The enzyme deficiency can be demonstrated prenatally by studies on fibroblasts obtained by amniocentesis before the twentieth week, thus allowing therapeutic abortion.

lesion (le'zhun) [L. *laesio,* from *ladere* to hurt] any wound, trauma, pathologic change, or loss of function.

LET abbrev. See *linear energy transfer.*

lethal (le'thal) [L. *lethalis,* from *lethum* death] 1. deadly, fatal.

2. in genetics, a mutant gene or chromosome abnormality that causes the premature death of the organism. A dominant lethal kills every mutant; a recessive lethal kills only when it is homozygous. A gene that causes sterility is sometimes also called lethal because it cannot be inherited.

lethal equivalent a recessive lethal gene carried in the heterozygous state; an equivalent combination of recessive semilethals. The lethal equivalent value is the sum of the probabilities that each semilethal has of causing death when homozygous. The average human is estimated to carry three to five lethal equivalents.

lethargy (leth'ar-je) [Gr. *lēthargia* drowsiness] a general term used to describe a condition of indifference and drowsiness.

Letterer-Siwe disease (let'er-er si'we) [Erich *Letterer,* German physician, born 1895; Sture August *Siwe,* German physician, born 1897] see *systemic h.* under *histiocytosis.*

leu abbrev. See *leucine.*

leucine (leu or L) (lu'sēn) [Gr. *leukos* white] 2-amino-4-methylpentanoic acid, a naturally occurring essential amino acid, $(CH_3)_2CHCH_2CH(NH_2)$-COOH; M.W. 131.17. It serves as a component of protein molecules; its source is from dietary proteins. See also under *amino acids.*

leucine aminopeptidase (LAP) (lu'sēn ah-me"-no-pep'tĭ-dās) an enzyme of the hydrolase class (α-aminoacylpeptide hydrolase [cytosol], EC 3.4.11.1) that catalyzes the hydrolysis of small peptides at the *N*-terminal end to form the *N*-terminal amino acid plus a peptide. It is an exoenzyme of broad specificity, never attacking an internal peptide bond, and preferentially attacking peptides containing aliphatic amino acids such as leucyl-glycyl-glycine. LAP can be isolated from the kidneys but is present in many tissues.

LAP in serum has been measured with leucyl-β-naphthylamide or leucyl-*p*-nitroanilide as substrates, but these substrates may measure a different enzyme, an arylaminopeptidase, insofar as the former enzyme is only weakly active toward these two substrates. Serum LAP (arylaminopeptidase) is often elevated in conditions involving pathology in the region of the common duct, such as acute pancreatitis, pancreatic carcinoma, liver disease, and infectious mononucleosis.

See also *aminopeptidase (cytosol).*

leucofuchsin (loo"ko-fook'sin) see under *Schiff reagent.*

leucovorin (loo"ko-vo'rin) see *folinic acid.*

leucovorin calcium the generic drug name for the calcium salt of folinic acid, an active metabolite of folic acid. Folinic acid circumvents the metabolic block produced by folic acid antagonists (such as methotrexate) and is used as an antidote to these drugs. It is also used to treat megaloblastic anemia due to folate deficiency.

leucyl (loo′sil) the acyl radical derived from or relating to leucine.

leuk/o (loo′ko) [Gr. *leukos* white] a word element used in combining form to denote white or colorless, e.g., leukocyte.

leukapheresis (loo″kah-fĕ-re′sis) [*leuko-* + Gr. *aphairesis* removal] an experimental procedure in which leukocytes and sometimes platelets are separated from donor whole blood by centrifugation or reversible fiber adhesion. The leukocyte-poor and platelet-poor red blood cells and plasma are continuously or intermittently (depending on the type of centrifugation used) returned to the donor throughout the procedure. This type of pheresis involves some risk to the patient, and its efficacy has not been firmly established.

leukemia (loo-ke′me-ah) [*leuko-* + Gr. *haima* blood + *-ia*] a progressive, malignant disease of the blood-forming organs that is characterized by the abnormal proliferation of the precursors of one type of leukocyte (lymphocytes, granulocytes, or monocytes). Both peripheral and bone marrow blood cells are changed qualitatively and quantitatively. The leukemias are classified according to the course of illness (acute or chronic), the cell type involved (such as lymphocytic or granulocytic), and, within a given cell line, the stage of maturation (such as myeloblastic or promyelocytic).

Diagnosis combines clinical observation with cytologic studies of the blood and bone marrow. Further cytochemical and histochemical studies may be needed to establish a differential diagnosis.

The incidence of leukemia has increased three- to sixfold over the past 20 yr, with an even distribution between acute and chronic leukemias. The exact etiology of leukemia is unclear, but the effects of viruses, ionizing radiation, chemical agents, and genetic predisposition are all suspect. The disease occurs more often in males than in females. Certain categories of people are at high risk for developing leukemia: (1) the identical twin of a leukemic individual; (2) some persons with acquired hematologic disorders, including polycythemia vera; (3) those with congenital syndromes associated with chromosomal abnormalities, including Down's syndrome, Bloom's syndrome, and Fanconi's anemia; (4) those who have been accidentally exposed to excessive radiation (nuclear weapon–testing or nuclear accidents); and (5) physicians and scientists exposed to excessive amounts of radiation.

In the acute leukemias, large numbers of abnormal cells (blast forms) saturate the bone marrow and eventually spill over into the blood (the presence of leukemic cells in the blood is indicative of advanced disease). As these cells accumulate in the bone marrow, they produce quantitative and qualitative changes in the normal cells of the bone marrow and cause the secondary change commonly seen in leukemias: a decrease in the production of erythrocytes, granulocytes, and platelets. This decrease in normal cellular elements leads to the common complications of the disease, including anemia, infection, and hemorrhage. Death, rarely attributed to cellular proliferation alone, usually results from either (1) the accumulation of leukemic cells in the bone marrow, which interferes with normal hematopoiesis; (2) the production and release into the circulation of senescent leukemic cells that contain abnormal quantities of active enzymes, intracellular electrolytes, and nucleic acid metabolites; or (3) the infiltration of extramedullary leukemic cells.

Acute leukemias are more severe than chronic leukemias. Clinical symptoms of acute leukemia include an abrupt onset of pallor and anemia. The infiltration of leukemic cells may cause lymphadenopathy, splenomegaly, hepatomegaly, and bone and joint pain. Hemorrhage caused by a decrease in the number of thrombocytes due to leukemic replacement of the marrow and/or therapy, infection attributed to a compromised immune system and caused by decreased leukocyte production from leukemic replacement and/or therapy, and disseminated intravascular coagulation (DIC) can be life-threatening. The development of platelet and coagulation factor concentrates to treat hemorrhage, and broad-spectrum antibiotics to fight infection, has provided a means of treatment that can sustain or at least prolong the lives of patients with acute leukemia.

The acute leukemias are divided into four prognostically significant categories: (1) acute lymphocytic leukemia (ALL), encountered primarily in children and young adults; (2) acute myelogenous leukemia (AML), found primarily in adults; (3) acute promyelocytic leukemia, encountered primarily in adults; and (4) acute monocytic leukemia, found primarily in children and young adults.

Treatment of the acute leukemias includes blood transfusions, the addition of platelet concentrates, chemotherapy, analgesics, and, occasionally, radiation or immunotherapy. If complications arise, specific treatments are then added. The goal of chemotherapy is to kill all leukemic cells; successful chemotherapy involves consolidation, remission, and maintenance.

Unlike the acute leukemias, the chronic leukemias appear insidiously. They are often discovered only upon a routine physical examination, with the patient complaining of low-grade fevers, night sweats, weight loss, weakness, and easy fatigability. By this time, lymphadenopathy, splenomegaly, and hepatomegaly are present. The peripheral white cell count may be subnormal but most often is markedly elevated into the hundreds of thousands (50,000–500,000 cells/mm^3 of blood).

The chronic leukemias are divided into two subgroups: (1) chronic myelogenous leukemia (CML); and (2) chronic lymphocytic leukemia (CLL). In CLL the predominant cells are mature lymphocytes, although some immature cells are not uncommon; in CML, the predominant cells are neutrophils and metamyelocytes (with increased numbers of immature forms also found). In both forms, the number of platelets is depressed, although it may be elevated in the early stages of CML.

Chronic leukemias progress slowly; without treatment, survival times of 2–3 yr are common. Therapy, which includes irradiation and a wide variety of chemotherapeutic agents (alkylating agents, antimetabolites, purine antagonists, and pyrimidine antagonists), may induce remission for 2–5 yr in CML and for 10–15 yr in CLL.

acute lymphocytic l. (ALL), a neoplastic disorder of acute onset, typified by the abnormal proliferation of lymphocytes and lymphoblasts of the hematopoietic organs (bone marrow, liver, spleen). It is primarily a malignant disease of children, although the incidence increases again in later life. Clinically, generalized lymphadenopathy, splenomegaly, and hepatomegaly are common, and preleukemic symptoms are rare.

Diagnosis is made from examination of a peripheral blood smear and bone marrow aspirate. Cytochemical and histochemical studies may be required for confirmation. The leukocyte count is usually elevated (100,000 cells/mm^3 of blood), with the number of lymphocytic cells increased and granulocytic and erythroid cells decreased. The bone marrow is saturated with younger varieties of circulating lymphocytes (lymphoblasts). The disorder must be differentiated from infectious mononucleosis, toxoplasmosis, and cytomegalovirus infection.

There are three morphologic patterns: L1, a T-cell disorder characterized by a homogeneous population of convoluted lymphocytes and frequently associated with the T-cell mediastinal lymphoma of childhood; L2, a heterogeneous cell population that shares the characteristics of L1 and L3 cells; and L3, a homogeneous population of large cells (three to four times the size of small lymphocytes).

Approximately 5 percent of individuals with ALL possess abnormal lymphocytes with receptors to sheep erythrocytes. These lymphocytes form rosettes in the absence of antibody or complement and are lysed by anti–T-cell antibody. Abnormal lymphocytes with B-cell receptors are rare. Most cases of ALL are not associated with markers for either B or T cells and are designated "null" cell leukemias.

Therapy includes treatment with chemical agents and irradiation directed to eliminate leukemic cells from the hematopoietic tissues and residual foci in the central nervous system.

A common complication of ALL is central nervous system leukemia (CNS-L, meningeal leukemia). It is attributed to the presence of the leukemic cells in the CNS and can be caused by the seeding of leukemic cells into the meninges during relapse or the slow entrance of chemotherapeutic drugs into the CNS. To prevent this complication, cranial irradiation and the intrathecal injection of chemotherapeutic agents are utilized.

The prognosis for ALL has improved, but about 50 percent of those affected succumb either to therapy or to relapse.

Also called acute undifferentiated leukemia and lymphoblastic leukemia.

acute megakaryoblastic l. (AMegL), a very rarely observed type of acute myelogenous leukemia characterized by the proliferation of megakaryocytic blast forms in the bone marrow. Because it is difficult to differentiate blast forms by normal staining techniques, AMegL may occur more frequently than is now reported. When morphologically identifiable, the cells are frequently micromegakaryocytes, have low nuclear ploidy, and stain with usual megakaryocytic stains. Symptoms are typical of acute myelogenous leukemia. AMegL may present as a terminal event in myelofibrosis or chronic myelogenous leukemia.

acute myelogenous l. (AML), a neoplastic disorder of acute onset; it is the most common leukemia seen in infants but is primarily a disease of adults. AML is occasionally attributed to past exposure to radiation, chemicals, genetic disorders, and chronic acquired hematologic disorders, most notably polycythemia vera and chronic myelogenous leukemia. Frequently there is a long preleukemic phase, and chemotherapy is discouragingly ineffective.

Different varieties are recognized and are described by the cellular elements involved: (1) AML is characterized by the replacement of normal bone marrow elements by immature, undifferentiated granulocytic cells (also called acute granulocytic leukemia, AGL). (2) Acute monomyelocytic leukemia is characterized by the replacement of normal bone marrow elements with leukemic cells that possess features of both myeloblasts and monoblasts. (3) Erythroleukemia is a rare leukemia characterized by the proliferation in the bone marrow of abnormal, often multinucleated erythroblasts and the accompanying hyperplasia of the granulocytic series. (4) Promyelocytic leukemia is characterized by the replacement of normal bone marrow elements with a predominance of promyelocytes that contain abnormal granules. It is a distinct variety because of the high incidence of disseminated intravascular coagulation associated with the disorder. (5) Smoldering leukemia is a leukemia that progresses very slowly in the early stages, with the bone marrow containing no more than 20–30 percent of the abnormal myeloblasts or promyelocytes.

The principal clinical features of AML (anemia, hemorrhage, and infection) are attributed to bone marrow dysfunction, which develops from the proliferation of an abnormal clone of cells. These cells accumulate over time and eventually lead to marrow replacement by primitive and ineffectual, rather than mature and functional, cells.

Diagnosis is made by the examination of the blood and bone marrow, which demonstrates the presence of abnormal numbers of immature cells. These cells may resemble dysplastic myeloblasts, normoblasts, promyelocytes, or monoblasts; mixed cell types do exist. An additional diagnostic aid in differentiating AML from acute lymphocytic leukemia is the presence of Auer rods, red strands of precipitated lysozyme found in the cytoplasm of immature granulocytes. These rods are not seen in lymphoblasts. Also, by cytochemical special studies, most leukemic myeloblasts are myeloperoxidase, Sudan black, and α-naphthol AS-D chloroacetate esterase positive.

The prognosis for survival without therapy is 2–5 mo. Therapy with cytosine arabinoside (ara-C) and daunorubicin (DNR) when used together has prolonged survival to 1–2 yr after diagnosis in about 60 percent of patients; other chemotherapeutic agents also are used.

chronic lymphocytic l. (CLL), a neoplastic disorder typified by the accumulation rather than the proliferation of small mature lymphocytes in the peripheral blood and bone marrow; blast cells comprise less than 5 percent of the lymphoid cells. It is primarily a disease of older adults (two-thirds of those affected are over 60) and is rare in children. The clinical course is variable; in some instances, significant symptoms take years to develop. Lymphadenopathy and splenomegaly are common, and the patient complains of anorexia, fatigue, weight loss, and sweats.

Diagnosis is easily made from examination of the peripheral blood smear and bone marrow aspirate. The total absolute lymphocyte count is elevated (10,000–150,000/mm^3 of blood), and the cell population is homogeneous. It appears to be monoclonal in origin, with most cells derived from B lymphocytes and possessing identical immunoglobulins.

Therapy includes treatment with alkylating agents and adrenoglucocorticoids. It is aimed at controlling and relieving symptoms and improving anemia, thrombocytopenia, and granulocytopenia rather than attaining complete remission. The median life expectancy is 5 yr.

Other neoplastic disorders associated with the proliferation of abnormal lymphocytes in addition to CLL include Waldenström's macroglobulinemia, Sézary syndrome, and hairy cell leukemia.

chronic myelocytic l. (CML), see *chronic myelogenous l.*

chronic myelogenous l. (CML), a neoplastic disease of insidious onset caused by the abnormal expansion of the granulocytic pool in the bone marrow, spilling over into the peripheral blood and spleen. Occasionally seen in adolescents, it is predominantly a disease of the middle-aged.

CML is attributed to the leukemogenic effects of ionizing radiation, alkylating agents, and other biologically active chemicals, and is characterized by a specific chromosomal abnormality, the Philadelphia chromosome (Ph^1). This chromosome is present in about 90 percent of those with CML. Ph^1 is characterized by the deletion of part of the long arm of one of the G chromosomes (chromosome 22) and the translocation from chromosome 22 to chromosome 9. Laboratory and physical findings in Ph^1-positive and Ph^1-negative individuals are similar, but those who are Ph^1-negative suffer from a more aggressive disease and have a poorer prognosis.

The clinical and laboratory findings show the result of an increase in myeloid cells. The earliest symptoms include malaise, fatigue, lack of exercise tolerance, pallor, and weight loss. The spleen and liver become enlarged, and increased sternal tenderness is present. Production of red cells and platelets is usually decreased, but returns to normal and even excess production after effective therapy. The differential count of peripheral blood is similar to that obtained from normal bone marrow. Cells are present at all stages of maturation, with a predominance of more mature cells. These cells have a greatly reduced content of alkaline phosphatase—a feature common to CML and an important factor in distinguishing this disorder from the leukemoid reactions.

Treatment with radiation or chemotherapy is initially very successful. Eventually, the disease progresses to a blastic phase (blast crisis) after 2–5 yr. Response to treatment decreases, and death usually results from fever, infection, hemorrhage, and/or organ infiltration with the leukemic cells.

Also called *chronic granulocytic leukemia, chronic myelocytic leukemia,* and *neutrophilic leukemia.*

erythroleukemia (EL), an acute or chronic myeloproliferative disorder characterized by the presence of neoplastic erythroid cells as well as neoplastic myeloid cells. The disorder is considered to be a subgroup of acute myelogenous leukemia because of the mixed cell population, which probably arises from the same stem cell precursor. It occurs in all age groups but is rare in childhood.

The presence of the megaloblastoid erythroblast, commonly found with B_{12} or folate deficiency, is a characteristic of the disorder; in erythroleukemia, B_{12} levels are normal. The bone marrow is hypercellular and demonstrates erythroid hyperplasia. Erythroblasts as well as immature myeloid cells are often present in the peripheral blood, but reticulocytosis is uncommon. As the disease progresses, myeloid cells predominate, and the end stage of the disease resembles acute myelogenous leukemia. Erythrokinetic studies demonstrate a rapid iron clearance but abnormal iron utilization and ineffective erythropoiesis. Clinically, anemia (usually normochromic, normocytic), malaise, weakness, fever, purpura, hemorrhage, and susceptibility to infection are common.

It is important but sometimes difficult to distinguish this disorder from atypical megaloblastic anemia, severe hemolysis (acquired hemolytic anemia), metastatic carcinoma, and the other myeloproliferative disorders.

Treatment with chemotherapeutic drugs found to be effective against acute granulocytic leukemia (such as cytosine-arabinoside and daunorubicin) has been utilized but with limited success. Owing to the insidious nature of the disorder, survival times are difficult to determine but are estimated to have a range of 2–23 mo.

Also called *DiGuglielmo syndrome, erythromyeloblastic leukemia,* and *erythremic myelosis.*

hairy cell l., a form of chronic leukemia characterized by a proliferation of "hairy cells" that resemble large lymphocytes and are so named because of delicate surface projections of their plasma membranes. On peripheral blood smears, the cells possess a slightly basophilic cytoplasm with irregular, convoluted borders. The origin of these cells is currently controversial. Typically, the onset is insidious. Patients present with massive splenic enlargement, neutropenia, anemia, and thrombocytopenia. The spleen and bone marrow are infiltrated by the same hairy cells that appear in the blood. The cells may contain a tartrate-resistant isoenzyme of acid phosphatase and, in a minority of cases, cytoplasmic inclusions referred to as ribosomal-lamellar complexes. The prognosis for hairy cell leukemia is better than for most acute leukemias. Splenectomy without chemotherapy is advised as initial therapy. Also called *leukemic reticuloendotheliosis.*

monocytic l. (A MonoL), an acute leukemia characterized by the proliferation of abnormal and immature monocytes (promonocytes and monoblasts) in the bone marrow and peripheral blood. Symptoms are similar to those found in other leukemias and include malaise, fatigue, and lack of exercise tolerance. In addition the gums become hyperplastic and inflamed, and there is a high incidence of skin lesions and CNS involvement. It is primarily a disease of children and young adults but occurs in all age groups.

Diagnosis is established on the basis of cytochemical and histochemical studies; in monocytic leukemia the abnormal cells resemble monocytes but give a negative reaction to peroxidase stain, indicating that the cells are not myeloid in origin. The cells are also Sudan and chloroacetate negative.

The use of multichemical therapeutic agents, effective in the treatment of acute myelogenous leukemia, offers a slightly improved prognosis.

Also called *monoblastic leukemia* and *Schilling leukemia.* See also *histiocytic medullary reticulosis.*

monomyelocytic l. (AMML), an acute leukemia characterized by a prolonged preleukemic phase and the presence of both neoplastic monocytic and myelocytic cells in the bone marrow and peripheral blood. AMML is usually classified as a subvariety of acute myelogenous leukemia (AML), and symptoms resemble those seen in AML including fatigue, a tendency for spontaneous bleeding, and recurrent infections.

Clinically, muramidase levels are extremely elevated; in cytochemical studies the monocytic cells often give a positive peroxidase reaction, indicating that they are myeloid in origin. The cells are also sudanophilic, as well as myeloperoxidase and chloroacetate esterase positive.

AMML is treated with drugs useful in the treatment of AML, such as cytosine arabinoside, daunorubicin, and thioguanine. Survival after diagnosis has a range of 3–12 mo.

Formerly called *Naegeli leukemia.* See also *acute myelogenous l.*

promyelocytic l. (A ProL), a subvariety of acute myelogenous leukemia in which the predominant cells are neoplastic promyelocytes rather than myeloblasts. It is often associated with disseminated intravascular coagulation and is primarily found in adults. Also called *progranulocytic leukemia.*

stem cell l., a highly acute leukemia characterized by the appearance in the blood of extremely immature forms, resembling the precursor stem cells of the bone marrow. Cytochemically, these cells possess none of the characteristics of either the myeloid or lymphoid series. Because of the acuteness of the disorder, death occurs within a few months. Also called *blast cell leukemia.*

leukemic (loo-ke′mik) pertaining to or affected by leukemia.

leukemic reticuloendotheliosis (loo-ke′mik rĕ-tik″u-lo-en″do-the-le-o′sis) see *hairy cell l.* under *leukemia.*

leukemogenesis (loo-ke″mo-jen′ĕ-sis) the induction of neoplastic hematopoietic growth. Many theories of etiology have been proposed, including viruses, chemicals, and ionizing radiation, as well as host genetic factors such as chromosome abnormalities.

leukemoid reaction the abnormal proliferation of peripheral blood cellular elements resembling leukemia but actually having other causes. The common characteristic is leukocytosis with immaturity of one or more cell lines. The reaction can be attributed to severe viral infections, an inflammatory reaction, or the growth and infiltration of metastatic neoplasms.

The cytochemical stain leukocyte alkaline phosphatase (LAP) is useful in differentiating the leukemoid reaction from leukemia: the LAP is characteristically high in cells of a leukemoid reaction, and low in those of acute myelogenous leukemia.

leukocidin (loo″ko-si′din) [*leuko-* + L. *caedere* to kill] a substance that is toxic to leukocytes; specifically, an exotoxin produced by some pathogenic staphylococci and streptococci that destroys leukocytes by lysis of the cytoplasmic granules and is partially responsible for the pathogenicity of the organisms. Monocytes as well as macrophages may be injured. Nonlethal concentrations inhibit leukocyte mobility. Both the S and O hemolysins of streptococci have leukotoxic properties. See also *exotoxins.*

leukocyte (loo′ko-sīt) [*leuko-* + Gr. *kytos* cell] the white blood cell, the body's primary defense against infection. There are 5000–10,000 leukocytes per cubic millimeter of blood, and they consist of three types: (1) granulocytes (neutrophils, eosinophils, and basophils), which can phagocytose bacteria; (2) monocytes, which phagocytose cellular debris and interact with lymphocytes in the processing of antigens in the immune reaction; and (3) lymphocytes, which participate in humoral (B lymphocyte) and cell-mediated (T lymphocyte) immunity.

Of the various types of leukocytes, neutrophils are the most numerous, forming 40–70 percent of the total number of white blood cells; lymphocytes form 20–40 percent, and monocytes, 2–8 percent. Granulocytes and monocytes originate in the bone marrow, whereas lymphocytes are formed in the lymphoid tissue (the spleen, Peyer's patches of the small bowel, and lymph nodes).

For more information, see the specific leukocyte.

Also called *white blood cell* (*WBC*). See also *blood cell count, bone marrow count,* and *differential leukocyte count.*

basophilic l., see *basophil.*

eosinophilic l., see *eosinophil.*

granular l., see *granulocyte.*

heterophilic l., see *heterophil.*

mast l., an undesirable designation for the circulating blood basophil, which is morphologically and histiogenetically different from the tissue mast cell.

neutrophilic l., see *neutrophil.*

polymorphonuclear l., see *polymorphonuclear neutrophil.*

transitional l., see *monocyte.*

Türk's irritation l., a lymphocyte with increased basophilia.

leukocyte alkaline phosphatase (LAP) a phosphomonoesterase with an optimal pH of 10, which is found in the cytoplasmic granules of normal neutrophils and their precursors. LAP levels are markedly lowered in chronic myelogenous leukemia (CML) and are raised toward normal levels during remission. Low levels are seen in a variety of conditions in addition to CML, including paroxysmal nocturnal hemoglobinuria, idiopathic thrombocytic purpura, infectious mononucleosis, and aplastic anemia. LAP levels may be elevated by the administration of corticosteroids. See also *alkaline phosphatase.*

leukocyte alkaline phosphatase methods methods for specific histochemical staining of LAP and scoring the results. Fresh blood smears are incubated with an aromatic phosphate, which is hydrolyzed by LAP and coupled to a diazonium salt to form a colored azo dye. The sections are counterstained with hematoxylin to stain the nuclei, and then examined. On a scale of 0–4, which ranges from no staining (0) to most of the cytoplasm filled with stain (4), 100 neutrophils are examined and scored. The normal range depends on the specifics of the technique.

leukocyte inhibitory factor (LIF) a protease produced by sensitized lymphocytes that inhibits the migration of polymorphonuclear leukocytes; M.W. 68,000. LIF is a heat-stable protein that is inactivated by the enzyme chymotrypsin and is resistant to the enzyme neuraminidase. To assay for LIF, polymorphonuclear leukocytes are observed for their ability to migrate in capillary tubes in a 24-hr period.

leukocyte-poor red blood cells red blood cells with at least 70 percent of the leukocytes removed. This component is indicated for individuals who experience severe, febrile, nonhemolytic transfusion reactions.

Removal of the leukocytes can be effected by centrifugation or saline washing techniques and is most effective on whole blood that has been stored for at least 6–10 da.

leukocytic (loo″ko-sit′ik) pertaining to leukocytes.

leukocytoblast (loo″ko-si′to-blast) [*leukocyte* + Gr. *blastos* germ] an obsolete term for an immature leukocyte.

leukocytogenesis (loo″ko-si′to-jen′ĕ-sis) [*leukocyte* + Gr. *genesis* production] an obsolete term for the formation of leukocytes; see *granulocytopoiesis.*

leukoderma (loo″ko-der′mah) [*leuko-* + Gr. *derma* skin] an acquired localized absence of pigment in the skin.

leukodystrophy (loo″ko-dis′tro-fe) [*leuko-* + L. *dystrophia,* from Gr. *dys-* abnormal + *trephein* to nourish] a general term used to describe heredofamilial defects of myelin formation and breakdown, usually due to congenital enzyme defects. The white matter is affected and the disease most frequently is progressive, terminating in death. There is no available therapy.

globoid l., see *Krabbe's disease.*

metachromatic l., a genetically determined disorder of sphingolipid metabolism, transmitted as an autosomal recessive trait, which is characterized by the abnormal breakdown of myelin. Those affected have a relative or absolute deficiency of the enzyme arylsulfatase A (cerebroside sulfatase), which leads to the accumulation of metachromatic staining lipids (sulfatides, cerebroside sulfates, galactosylsulfatide, or other lipids with a galactosyl-3-sulfate moiety). These lipids are primarily deposited in the white matter of the central nervous system, peripheral nerves, kidneys, spleen, and liver. Myelin is abnormally metabolized, leading to the progressive impairment of motor function, and to dementia, visual impairment, dysphagia, and a bedridden state; nerve conduction velocity is decreased and there is deposition of sulfatide material in free spaces or within macrophages. In the early stages of the disease the electroencephalogram may appear normal even though neurologic abnormalities are present, but eventually high-amplitude irregular slow activity dominates the record. The disease usually begins around age 2–3 yr and may be fatal by age 10, but variants are described with onset in late childhood or in adult life.

Diagnosis is based on peripheral nerve conduction velocity tests, nerve biopsy, and measurement of arylsulfatase A in the urine (decreased in this disease). A definitive diagnosis is made by establishing the near-absence of arylsulfatase A in leukocytes. Both carrier detection and prenatal diagnosis are now feasible.

Also called *sulfatide lipidosis.* See also *sphingolipidoses.*

leukoencephalopathy (loo″ko-en-sef″ah-lop′ahthe) any of a group of diseases characterized primarily by pathologic involvement of white matter of the central nervous system.

progressive multifocal l., a rare, demyelinating disease of the central nervous system that usually develops in immunosuppressed individuals, those with chronic neoplastic disease (especially of the reticuloendothelial system), and those with chronic granulomatous disorders. Dementia and disturbances of motor function, vision, sensation, and speech are the typical clinical manifestations. The JC and SV40 viruses have been implicated in the etiology of the disorder. The cerebrospinal fluid shows little abnormality and the electroencephalogram shows nonspecific slowing. No therapy is known; the disorder follows a subacute progressive course to death.

leukoerythroblastic (loo″ko-ĕ-rith″ro-blas′tik) pertaining to leukoerythroblasts.

leukoerythroblastic anemia see *leukoerythroblastic a.* under *anemia.*

leukoerythroblastosis (loo″ko-ĕ-rith″ro-blas-to′sis) see *leukoerythroblastic a.* under *anemia.*

leukokinin (loo″ko-ki′nin) a gamma-globulin moiety that coats polymorphonuclear leukocytes and is capable of stimulating phagocytosis as demonstrated in vitro. The biologic activity depends on a single small peptide in the leukokinin molecule called tuftsin. See also *tuftsin.*

leukoma (loo-ko′mah) [Gr. *leukōma* whiteness] a white, dense opacity of the cornea.

leukopenia (loo″ko-pe′ne-ah) a reduction in the total number of leukocytes in the blood, the usual criterion being fewer than 4000 per mm^3. It usually reflects neutropenia, although lymphocyte, monocyte, eosinophil, or basophil counts may also be reduced.

leukoplakia (loo″ko-pla′ke-ah) [*leuko-* + Gr. *plax* plate + *-ia*] a condition of an epithelium marked by the development of white, thickened patches due to the abnormal formation of keratin (hyperkeratosis), which may be due to any of a number of causes.

leukopoietin (loo″ko-poi-e′tin) a substance thought to stimulate leukocyte development. It has not yet been isolated.

leukorrhea (lu″ko-re′ah) [*leuko-* + Gr. *rhoia* flow] an abnormal, often white, nonbloody discharge from the vagina, which may be associated with itching, odor, vaginismus, and painful coitus. It is a common gynecologic complaint of all age groups. The most frequent cause is infection in the lower reproductive tract, which can be due to *Candida albicans, Trichomonas vaginalis, Hemophilus vaginalis,* gonococci, or other microorganisms, as well as neoplasms, estrogen depletion or stimulation, and foreign bodies. A complete history should be obtained, and physical examination and bacteriologic, cytologic, and microscopic studies of the discharge performed, to identify the specific cause. A Pap smear is necessary to rule out malignancy.

Leukosporidium a basidiospore-forming yeast that belongs to the family Sporobolomycetaceae of the order Ustilaginales. The species *L. neoformans* was proposed as being the perfect stage of *Cryptococcus neoformans.*

leukotriene (loo″ko-tri′ēn) a group of biologically active substances, originally found in leukocytes, that cause bronchial and other smooth muscle contraction. Leukotrienes are formed by the action of lipoxygenase on arachidonic acid to form 5-hydroperoxyarachidonic acid, the ultimate precursor of all other leukotrienes. After rearrangement to an epoxide derivative, it is enzymatically converted to a glutathione conjugate, which is also called leukotriene C. The latter compound can be metabolized by γ-glutamyltransferase into a corresponding cysteinylglycine derivative, or leukotriene D. It is currently believed that a slow-reacting substance of anaphylaxis (SRSA), which is released from mast cells after antigenic challenge, is composed of leukotrienes C and D. See also *immediate hypersensitivity, inflammation,* and *slow-reacting substance of anaphylaxis.*

l. A (LTA), 5-*trans*-5,6-oxido-7,9-*trans*-11,14-*cis*-eicosatetraenoic acid, an unstable leukotriene derived from arachidonic acid. It serves as a precursor of all other leukotrienes, including slow-reacting substance of anaphylaxis. LTA is found in the lungs of asthmatic individuals, in leukocytes, and in sensitized mast cells.

l. B (LTB), 5,12-dihydroxy-6,8,10,14-eicosatetraenoic acid, a leukotriene formed enzymatically from leukotriene A. It is found mainly in leukocytes.

l. C (LTC), 5-hydroxy-6-glutathionyl-7,9-*trans*-11,14-*cis*-eicosatetraenoic acid, a leukotriene produced in the lungs of asthmatic individuals, in leukocytes, and in antigen-challenged mast cells. It contracts bronchial smooth muscle and guinea pig ileum. LTC is part of slow-reacting substance of anaphylaxis, which is released in various immediate hypersensitivity reactions.

l. D (LTD), 5-hydroxy-6-cysteinyl-glycine-7,9-*trans*-11,14-*cis*-eicosatetraenoic acid, the most potent leukotriene and a component of slow-reacting substance of anaphylaxis. LTD is formed from LTC by the action of the enzyme γ-glutamyltransferase.

lev/o (le′vo) [L. *laevus* left] a word element used in combining form to denote left or to the left, e.g., levocardia.

Levaditi's method (lev″ah-de′tēz) [Constantin *Levaditi,* Rumanian bacteriologist in Paris, 1874–1928] a histologic staining procedure for spirochetes. Tissue blocks are fixed in formalin, impregnated in 2 percent silver nitrate solution for 4 da at 37°C, developed in a reducing solution (pyrogallol and formalin) for 2 da, dehydrated, cleared in cedar oil, embedded in paraffin, sectioned, and mounted. Spirochetes stain black; the background, yellow-brown.

levallorphan tartrate (lev″al-lor′fan) [USP], a narcotic antagonist used to treat respiratory depression caused by narcotic overdosage. It acts by competitive inhibition of opiates. It may add to the respiratory depression produced by other drugs such as barbiturates, and it causes withdrawal symptoms when given to narcotics addicts. High dosages may produce hallucinations or disorientation.

levamphetamine (le″vam-fet′ah-mēn) the optical isomer of amphetamine that has the lesser central nervous system stimulating effect. See also *amphetamine* and *amphetamine assays.* Cf. *dextroamphetamine.*

levan (lev′an) polyfructosan; a homopolymer of fructose residues in β-2,6 linkages, formed from sucrose by certain bacteria (e.g., strains of *Bacillus* and *Streptococcus*). It is a constituent of dental plaque.

levarterenol bitartrate (lev″ar-tĕ-re′nol bi-tar′trāt) [USP], the generic drug name for the naturally occurring neurotransmitter norepinephrine. It is used to treat severe hypotension by stimulating the heart and constricting the blood vessels.

levator (le-va′tor), pl. *levatores* [L. *levare* to raise] [NA], any muscle that raises or elevates the structure or organ into which it inserts.

levo- a prefix word element in chemistry to denote a levorotatory compound, e.g., levodopa.

levodopa (le″vo-do′pah) see under *dopa.*

levorotatory (le″vo-ro′tah-to-re) [*levo-* + L. *rotare* to turn] pertaining to an optically active compound with a negative optical rotation, i.e., rotation to the left or counterclockwise as the observer looks toward the beam of polarized light.

levorphanol tartrate (le-vor′fah-nōl tar′trāt) [NF], a potent synthetic narcotic analgesic that produces the same degree of analgesia as morphine with less gastrointestinal intolerance. It can produce physical dependence. Respiratory depression due to overdosage can be reversed by levallorphan.

levothyroxine sodium (le″vo-thi-rok′sēn) [USP], the generic drug name for the natural thyroid hormone thyroxine (T_4), used for replacement therapy in hypothyroidism.

levulose (lev′u-lōs) [L. *laevus* left + *-ose*] see under *fructose.*

Lewis acid (lu′is) [Gilbert N. *Lewis,* American chemist, 1875–1946] an electron-pair acceptor; any molecule or ion that contains an atom that can form a coordinate covalent bond with an unshared electron pair of an atom in another molecule or ion (a Lewis base or electron-pair donor).

The Lewis acid concept is a generalization of the Brönsted-Lowry acid (proton donor) concept. A proton (hydrogen ion) is a Lewis acid because an electron pair gives it a complete valence shell. Many other compounds, however, such as boron trifluoride (BF_3), contain an atom (B in BF_3) that needs two electrons to complete its valence shell and are also Lewis acids, for example, $BF_3 + NH_3 \rightarrow F_3BNH_3$.

Also called *electrophile.* See also *coordination compound.*

Lewis base [Gilbert N. *Lewis*] an electron-pair donor. This is equivalent to a Brönsted-Lowry base (a proton acceptor). Also called *nucleophile.*

Lewis blood group see under *blood groups.*

Lewy body an eosinophilic hyaline body composed of compact aggregations of fibrillary material located in the cytoplasm of pigmented neurons. Lewy bodies are a frequent finding in the substantia nigra and locus ceruleus in idiopathic Parkinson's disease, but occasionally are found in asymptomatic patients.

Leydig cell (li′dig) [Franz von *Leydig,* German anatomist, 1821–1908] a polyhedral cell arranged in clusters in the interstices between the seminiferous tubules of the testes. Under the influence of the hypophyseal gonadotropic hormone, LH, these cells synthesize and secrete the androgenic steroid hormones, principally testosterone. In humans, Leydig cells contain prominent cytoplasmic crystals (of Reinke), and possess a conspicuous Golgi complex and extensive smooth endoplasmic reticulum characteristic of steroid-secreting cells. Also called *interstitial cell of Leydig.* See also *testis.*

Leydig cell tumor [Franz von *Leydig*] a tumor of the Leydig or interstitial cells of the testis. The tumor is usually benign but may be associated with signs of hyperfunction such as gynecomastia. Also called interstitial cell tumor. See also *Sertoli-Leydig cell tumors.*

L-form a transitional phase variant of certain bacteria, distinguished by a defective or absent cell wall. L-forms can replicate as small, filterable elements in suitable hypertonic media. Penicillin, which impairs cell wall synthesis, induces the formation of L-phase bacteria. The role of L-forms in pathogenicity is uncertain, but they are recovered from cases of pyelonephritis and endocarditis. See also *L-phase variant, protoplast,* and *spheroplast.*

LGV abbrev. See *lymphogranuloma venereum.*

LH abbrev. See *luteinizing hormone.*

LH-RH abbrev. for luteinizing hormone–releasing hormone. See *gonadotropin–releasing hormone.*

LI abbrev. See *labeling index.*

Li symbol for the chemical element *lithium.*

LIBC abbrev. for latent iron-binding capacity. See under *iron-binding capacity tests.*

libido (lĭ-be′do), pl. *libidines* [L.] 1. sexual desire.

2. in psychiatry, energy derived from the instinctual drives, some of which is available for use by the conscious mind and some of which exists in various forms of repression. Many of the symptoms of psychopathology have been related to the denial of libidinal desires.

Libman-Sacks endocarditis (lib′man saks) [Emanuel *Libman,* New York physician, 1872–1946; Benjamin *Sacks,* New York physician, 1873–1939] see *verrucous e.* under *endocarditis.*

library in a computer, a collection of data sets and programs available for general use, such as compilers and programs used in frequently performed operations.

Librium (lib′re-um) trademark. See *c. hydrochloride* under *chlordiazepoxide.*

lichen (li′ken) [Gr. *leichēn* a tree-moss] 1. a plant consisting of a symbiotic association of an alga and a fungus, usually a green or blue-green alga and an ascomycete.

2. any of a variety of papular skin diseases in which the lesions resemble lichens growing on rocks.

l. planus, a common subacute or chronic dermatosis characterized by itchy, violet-colored, cutaneous, flat papules with a predilection for the flexor surfaces of the extremities and the genital and oral mucosae. The histologic appearance of lichen planus lesions includes hyperkeratosis, accentuation of the granular layer, acanthosis, degeneration of the basilar layer, and an infiltrate of chronic inflammatory cells in the upper dermis. The cause is unknown, but some cases have been associated with use of drugs such as chloroquine or quinacrine, or with exposure to chemicals such as color film developers. The condition usually resolves spontaneously after several years. Squamous cell carcinoma develops at the site of persistent oral lesions in 1–4 percent of cases.

l. sclerosus et atrophicus, a disorder characterized by the presence of numerous small, flat-topped white macules or slightly raised papules, which may coalesce to form white patches that may be indurated. The condition affects females more frequently than males and usually occurs after middle age. In both sexes the genital area is the site most frequently involved. Histologically, the lesion is characterized by hyperkeratosis, epithelial atrophy with degeneration of the basal layer, homogenization of dermal collagen, and chronic inflammatory cells that form a bandlike infiltrate in the middermis.

l. simplex chronicus, a chronic condition of the skin associated with persistent itching of pigmented, thickened, furrowed (lichenified) skin. The disorder may arise spontaneously or following contact dermatitis. Hereditary disposition and local trauma are also suspected factors. It is most common on the neck, wrists, forearms, and thighs. An "itch-scratch" cycle tends to extend this disease. Also called localized neurodermatitis and *Vidal's disease.*

lichenoid (li′ken-oid) [*lichen* + Gr. *eidos* form] resembling lichen.

lid (lid) 1. a covering for a hollow receptacle.

2. see *eyelid.*

lidocaine (li′do-kān) [USP], a white or yellow crystalline powder that is insoluble in water but soluble in nonpolar organic liquids; is similar in chemistry and action to cocaine, procaine, and dibucaine; and is used as a local anesthetic and to treat ventricular arrhythmias, primarily during heart surgery or after a myocardial infarction. Adverse reactions include drowsiness, tremors, convulsions, and cardiac or respiratory arrest.

l. hydrochloride, [USP], the salt used in aqueous solution for injection.

lidocaine assays 1. gas chromatography. Lidocaine can be extracted from alkalinized serum into ether or can be absorbed on charcoal and eluted with chloroform. A gas chromatograph with a flame ionization detector and nonpolar silicone column may be used. The lidocaine peak height or area is compared with that of an internal standard (such as tetracaine or mepivacaine); the relative error is about 5 percent.

2. EMIT, a homogenous enzyme immunoassay used for the therapeutic drug monitoring of lidocaine serum levels.

Liebermann-Burchard reaction (le′ber-mahn bur-shahrd′) [Leo von Szentlorincz *Liebermann,* Hungarian physician, 1852–1926; H. *Burchard,* German chemist, 19th century] a chromogenic reaction used in the spectrophotometric determination of cholesterol. The reaction takes place in an anhydrous medium. The solvent may be acetic acid or chloroform; the reagent consists of acetic anhydride and concentrated sulfuric acid. When these are added to a solution of cholesterol, a green or blue-green color is formed, possibly owing to the formation of cholestapolyenes. The reaction mechanism is still not fully elucidated.

lien (li′en) [L.] [NA], the spleen.

LIF abbrev. See *leukocyte inhibitory factor.*

life (lif) [M.E. *lif* (L. *vita;* Gr. *bios* or *zōe*)] 1. the aggregate of vital phenomena; the principle that endows organized beings with certain powers and functions not associated with inorganic matter. Generally, living things share, in varying degree, the characteristics of organization, irritability, movement, growth, reproduction, and adaptation.

2. the length of time that an instrument is technologically or economically useful. See also *economic life* and *technologic life.*

3. the length of time that a substance is present in a biologic system or that a radioactive element continues to decay. See also *half-life.*

life table a table presenting the results of a clinical trial in which the subjects enter and leave the study at different times. Each subject has a clearly defined starting point (e.g., beginning of treatment) and end point (e.g., relapse). For each time interval (e.g., each year after the starting point), the table provides the number of subjects remaining under the study at the beginning of the interval, the number reaching their end point during the interval, and the number leaving the study during the interval without reaching their end point. The technique derives from the method long used by actuaries to compute expected length of life at specified ages from census data and mortality counts. See also *survival curve.*

ligament/o (lig-ah-men′to) [L. *ligamentum,* from *ligare* to tie, bind] a word element used in combining form to denote ligament, e.g., ligamentous.

ligament (lig′ah-ment) 1. a cord, band, or sheet of dense fibrous tissue connecting anatomic structures such as bones or cartilage.

2. a fold or reflection of peritoneum.

3. the cordlike remnant of certain fetal structures that have lost their original lumen.

alar l.'s, a pair of connective tissue bands that connect the top of the odontoid process of the second cervical (axis) vertebra to the medial sides of the condyles of the occipital bone.

annular l., a circular band that encircles the greater part of the head of the radius, securing its articulation with the radial notch of the ulna.

arcuate l.'s, two tendinous bands (lateral and medial) by which the diaphragm is attached to the posterior body wall on each side of the midline. The lateral arcuate ligament arches across the quadratus lumborum from the twelfth rib to the first lumbar transverse process. The medial arcuate ligament crosses the psoas muscle from the first lumbar transverse process to the body of the second lumbar vertebra.

arteriosum l., [NA], a short, thick, fibromuscular cord that extends from the left pulmonary artery to the arch of the aorta. It is the remnant of the ductus arteriosus.

broad l., the fold of peritoneum on each side of the uterus that extends to the pelvic sidewall. The uterine tube lies within its free edge, and the ovary is attached to its upper surface. It also contains the round ligament of the uterus as well as the uterine and ovarian vessels and nerves.

capsular l., a connective tissue sleeve, lined by synovial membrane, that links bones at a synovial joint.

check l.'s, slender bands of connective tissue that connect the sheaths of the lateral and medial rectus muscles of the eyeball to the wall of the orbit.

conoid l., part of the ligament that connects the clavicle with the coracoid process of the scapula, restraining the backward movement of the clavicle. See also *trapezoid l.*

coronary l., a reflection of peritoneum between the upper surface of the liver and the overlying diaphragm.

cruciate l.'s, two ligaments: (1) Cruciate ligaments of the knee joint consist of two ligaments, anterior and posterior, that connect the upper surface of the tibia with the femoral condyles. They cross one another like the limbs of a letter X. The anterior ligament is tense in extension, whereas the posterior ligament is tense when the knee is flexed. (2) Cruciate ligament of the occipitoaxial articulation consists of a pair of intersecting ligaments through which the second cervical (axis) vertebra is connected with the base of the skull. The transverse band extends between the lateral masses of the first cervical (atlas) vertebra, holding the odontoid process of the axis against the anterior arch of the atlas. The longitudinal component is formed by bands that extend from the back of the body of the axis to the occipital bone at the anterior lip of the foramen magnum.

deltoid l., a strong ligament on the medial side of the ankle joint. It is attached anteriorly to the medial malleolus and expands distally to attach to the navicular tuberosity, os calcis, and talus.

denticulate l.'s, pointed processes of the pia mater that penetrate the arachnoid to attach to the dura. They suspend the spinal cord.

falciform l., a triangular fold of peritoneum that binds the anterior surface of the liver to the anterior abdominal wall. The ligamentum teres lies in its free edge.

flaval l.'s, paired, slender, elastic sheets that connect the laminae of two adjacent vertebrae.

gastrophrenic l., a fold of peritoneum that extends from the fundus of the stomach near the esophagus to the diaphragm.

gastrosplenic l., a fold of peritoneum that extends from the left side of the fundus of the stomach to the hilum of the spleen.

iliolumbar l., a strong band of connective tissue that radiates from the fifth lumbar transverse process to the iliac crest.

inguinal l., a strong ligament formed by the recurved lower border of the external oblique muscle of the anterior abdominal wall. It extends from the anterior superior iliac spine to the pubic tubercle, marking the boundary between abdomen and thigh.

intraarticular l., a ligament that stretches across a joint between articulating bones. Examples are the cruciate ligaments of the knee and the ligament of the femoral head.

ischiofemoral l., the thickened part of the capsule of the hip joint that passes from the ischium upward and laterally over the neck of the femur.

middle umbilical l., a fibrous cord, the remnant of the urachus, that extends from the bladder to the umbilicus, forming the median umbilical fold.

nuchal l., a strong ligamentous band at the back of the neck, attached above to the external occipital crest and by its anterior border to the cervical spines. Its posterior border is a free edge that gives origin to several muscles. Also called *ligamentum nuchae.*

patellar l., the central and main portion of the tendon of insertion of the quadriceps femoris muscle. It extends from the back of the patella to the tubercle of the tibia.

pectinate l.'s, posterior fibers of the cornea that radiate into the iris and enclose the spaces of the iridocorneal angle.

pectineal l., a triangular expansion from the medial part of the inguinal ligament, attached to the pectineal line of the pubic bone in front of the conjoined tendon.

pulmonary l., a fold of pleura that extends downward from the root of the lung.

round l.'s, two ligaments: (1) Round ligament of the liver is a fibrous remnant of the fetal umbilical vein. It runs in the free edge of the falciform ligament from the umbilicus to the lower border of the liver, then continues backward to the porta hepatis to join the left branch of the portal vein. Also called *ligamentum teres.* (2) Round ligament of the uterus is a connective tissue cord that attaches to the anterolateral aspect of the uterus near the uterine tube and runs along the lower border of the broad ligament to the deep inguinal ring. It traverses the inguinal canal and descends to insert into the skin of the labium majus and adjacent fascia.

spring l., the plantar calcaneonavicular ligament. It is attached to the anterior margin of the sustentaculum tali and to the plantar surface of the navicular. Broad and thick, it supports the head of the talus, and the deltoid ligament is attached to its medial edge.

suspensory l., a thin, membranous sheet on which the eyeball rests.

trapezoid l., a ligament that, with the conoid ligament, forms the coracoclavicular ligament that binds the clavicle to the coracoid process of the scapula. The trapezoid portion restrains the forward movement of the clavicle.

triangular l.'s, two folds of peritoneum (right and left) that connect the upper surface of the liver to the diaphragm.

umbilical l.'s, two ligaments: (1) Median umbilical ligament is a fibrous cord that extends from the apex of the bladder to the umbilicus. It is the vestige of the fetal urachus. (2) Lateral umbilical ligament is a fibrous remnant of part of the umbilical artery and extends from the upper part of the bladder to the umbilicus.

ligament of Treitz see under *duodenum.*

ligamentum (lig"ah-men'tum), pl. *ligamenta* [L. "a bandage"] a ligament; a band of tissue that connects bones or supports viscera.

l. arteriosum, the fibrous remnant of the fetal ductus arteriosus. It extends from the left pulmonary artery to the arch of the aorta; the left recurrent laryngeal nerve hooks around it.

l. nuchae, see *nuchal l.* under *ligament.*

l. teres, see *round l.'s* under *ligament.*

l. venosum, a slender, fibrous cord, a remnant of the fetal ductus venosus, that extends from the left branch of the portal vein to the inferior vena cava at the point of entrance of the left hepatic vein.

ligand (li'gand, lig'and) [L. *ligare* to tie or bind] a molecule, ion, or atom that is bound to the central atom (usually a metal atom) of a coordination compound or chelate. An example is the porphyrin ring that binds the iron ion in hemoglobin.

ligandin (li'gan-din) [L. *ligare*] a liver protein that has been assigned a role in organic ion transport into the liver. It also functions as the enzyme glutathione *S*-transferase B, rendering a number of compounds (which are foreign to living cells) water soluble and less toxic for excretion by the kidneys.

ligase (li'gās) one of a class of enzymes (EC 6) that catalyze the formation of a bond between two substrate molecules, which is coupled to the cleavage of a pyrophosphate bond in ATP or other energy donor. The bonds formed are often high-energy bonds. The class includes enzymes also named as synthetases. Clinically important enzymes of the class include glutathione synthetase (EC 6.3.2.3), argininosuccinate synthetase (EC 6.3.4.5), carbamoyl-phosphate synthetase (EC 6.3.4.16), and polydeoxyribonucleotide synthetase (EC 6.5.1.1, 2).

ligate (li'gāt) to tie or bind with a ligature.

ligature (lig'ah-chūr) [L. *ligatura* a bond] a thread used to tie a blood vessel or other part in order to constrict it.

light (līt) the electromagnetic radiation, particularly visible light, which has wavelengths between 390 and 770 nm and stimulates the retina of the eye.

light chain a structural subunit of the immunoglobulin; M.W. 23,000. A light chain is a polypeptide, and each monomeric immunoglobulin molecule has two light chains. There are two antigenic types of light chains, kappa and lambda; a given immunoglobulin molecule contains either kappa or lambda light chains, but never both. In multiple myeloma, the Bence Jones proteins found in serum or urine are light chains. Also called *L chain.* See also *immunoglobulin.*

light-emitting diode (LED) a semiconductor device used in the glowing type of readout seen on calculators and other digital equipment.

light green SF yellowish an acid triphenylmethane dye, primarily used as a counterstain for cytoplasm, as in Papanicolaou's stain; C.I. 42095. Also called light green.

light microscope a microscope that uses light waves as the illuminating source. See also under *microscope.*

light pen a computer input device used with a cathode-ray tube. When the tip is placed against the screen, it communicates its position to the computer; the program can then follow the pen as it draws lines or marks areas of the screen.

light pipe a flexible transparent plastic rod that transmits light from one end to the other by internal reflection. It is used in some scintillation cameras to carry light from the detectors to the photomultipliers.

light-scattering immunoassays see *nonradioisotopic i.* under *immunoassays.*

lignoceric acid (lig'no-se-rik) *n*-tetracosanic acid, a saturated acid with 24 carbon atoms present as a constituent of brain sphingolipids.

ligroin (lig'ro-in) a petroleum distillation fraction used as an organic solvent. The term usually refers to the higher boiling fractions of these low-molecular-weight hydrocarbon mixtures. Normal or low-boiling ligroin has a boiling range of 65°–74°C; high-boiling ligroin, 100°–115°C. It is occasionally classified as a petroleum ether but is sometimes distinguished from petroleum ether because of its boiling range. See also *petroleum ether.*

Lillie's allochrome method (lil'ēs) [Ralph Dougall *Lillie,* U.S. pathologist, 20th century] a histologic staining procedure useful for differentiating connective tissues. Sections are oxidized with periodic acid and reacted with Schiff reagent. To block the periodic acid–Schiff (PAS) reaction of collagen and reticulum, the sections are treated with sodium metabisulfite. They are stained with iron hematoxylin and counterstained with picromethyl blue: collagen and reticulum appear bright blue, with the basement membranes, lens capsules, suspensory ligaments, and Descemet's membranes deep red.

limb (lim) one of the paired appendages of the body used in grasping or locomotion; in humans, an arm or a leg with all its component parts.

limbic (lim'bik) pertaining to a limbus, or margin; forming a border around.

limbic system a group of structures in the brain associated with olfaction, autonomic functions, and certain emotional and behavioral states. The system is generally considered to include the olfactory bulbs and tracts, the hippocampus, the dentate and cingulate gyri, the amygdaloid complex, areas of the septum, and parts of the thalamus and hypothalamus.

limbus (lim′bus), pl. *limbi* [L.] [NA], a general term for a border, hem, or fringe. The term is often used alone to designate the limbus of the cornea, which is the point of junction between the sclera and the cornea of the eye.

limit (lim′it) [L. *limes* boundary] 1. a boundary or threshold.

2. in mathematics, the value that a sequence approaches as the number of terms increases.

limit check in clinical chemistry, a quality control check that may be performed by a laboratory computer. It is used to identify test results that fall outside predetermined limits. Also called *alert check.*

limit dextrin the end product of hydrolysis of branched-chain polyglucans by amylase, consisting of the polyglucan skeleton containing 1–6 glucosidic bonds with one or two glucose stubs. See also *ϕ-dextrin.*

limit dextrinosis see *Forbes' disease.*

limit of resolution see *resolving power.*

Limnatis (lim-na′tis) a genus of leeches. The most common species, *L. nilotica*, an aquatic leech, is found in North Africa, middle Europe, and the Near East. Infection in humans is acquired from drinking infested water. The leeches become lodged in the nasal passages, larynx, and pharynx, and occasionally in the upper digestive tract; they may cause anemia and asphyxia when present in large numbers. Also called *Hirudo aegyptiaca.*

limp (limp) 1. weak, flaccid.

2. a walk that favors one side, usually due to weakness or immobility of part of the favored leg.

Limulus test (lim′u-lus) [*Limulus* a genus of king crabs and the type genus of Limulidae] see under *pyrogen.*

lincomycin (lin″ko-mi′sin) a macrolide antibiotic, produced by *Streptomyces lincolnensis,* that consists of an amino acid linked to an amino sugar. By chemical modification of the lincomycin molecule, clindamycin is derived from lincomycin. Lincomycin inhibits protein synthesis by binding to the 50S subunit of the bacterial ribosome. A consequence of binding of lincomycin is the dissociation of ribosomes into 50S and 30S subunits. Bacterial resistance can be achieved through alterations in the ribosomal binding site.

In general, both lincomycin and clindamycin are active at clinically achievable concentrations against a variety of gram-positive organisms, with the exception of enterococci. Clindamycin is active in vitro against clinically significant anaerobic bacteria, especially *Bacteroides fragilis.* The Enterobacteriaceae and some strains of the anaerobic *Peptococcus* species and nonperfringens *Clostridium* species are resistant to clindamycin. Because of the higher activity and absorption properties of clindamycin compared with lincomycin, clindamycin is favored for clinical usage.

Clinical indications include *B. fragilis* infections outside the central nervous system and as an alternative to penicillin for treatment of *C. perfringens* infections. Clindamycin has been associated with the development of pseudomembranous colitis caused by the toxigenic *C. difficile.*

See also *antibacterial agents* and *macrolides.*

lindane (lin′dān) [USP], an insecticide, the gamma isomer of hexachlorocyclohexane, used medically to treat infestations with mites (scabies) or with lice. It is a nerve poison in large doses, causing loss of coordination, tremors, convulsions, and circulatory failure. See also *chlorinated hydrocarbon pesticide assays.*

Lindau's disease (lin′dowz) [Arvid *Lindau*, Swedish pathologist, born 1892] cerebral hemangioblastomas associated with von Hippel-Lindau disease. See also *von Hippel–Lindau disease.*

Lindau–von Hippel disease (lin′dow von hip′el) [Arvid *Lindau*; Eugen *von Hippel*, German ophthalmologist, 1867–1939] see *von Hippel–Lindau disease.*

line (līn) [L. *linea*] 1. a mark, stripe, or streak; often an imaginary line connecting different anatomic landmarks. Also called *linea.*

2. pertaining to an electrical power line, as in line voltage (115 or 230 VAC).

3. a one-dimensional curve.

Nélaton's l., a line drawn from the anterior superior spine of the ilium to the most prominent part of the tuberosity of the ischium.

semilunar l., the groove in the external abdominal wall that extends from the top of the ninth costal cartilage to the pubic tubercle, along the lateral margin of the rectus abdominis muscle.

linea (lin′e-ah), pl. *lineae* [L.] 1. a stripe, streak, mark, or narrow ridge.

2. [NA], in anatomy, a general term used to designate a streak or long narrow mark on the surface of some structure.

l. alba, [NA], the tendinous band running vertically along the entire length of the anterior abdominal wall in the midline between the two rectus muscles. It provides a relatively bloodless site for a surgical incision. Also called *white line.*

linear (lin′e-ar) [L. *linearis*] pertaining to or resembling a line. See also the illustration under *contour.*

linear accelerator a device used in radiation therapy (e.g., in treatment of deep-seated tumors) to obtain megavoltage x-rays of 1–2 MeV. The machine accelerates particles (usually electrons) to high energy in a straight line (to avoid synchrotron radiation); the high voltages are produced when the high-energy electron beam strikes the target. See also *radiation therapy equipment.*

linear attenuation coefficient the fraction of an x-ray or gamma-ray beam that is absorbed or scattered by a unit thickness of material, such as shielding. It depends on the photon energy and the density and composition of the shielding. If μ is the attenuation and x is the shielding thickness, then the fraction that passes the shielding is $e^{-\mu x}$. The quantity, $0.693/\mu$, is called the half-value layer, the thickness of shielding that absorbs half the radiation. Also called linear absorption coefficient when scattering is not considered.

linear energy transfer (LET) the amount of energy per unit pathlength absorbed by soft tissue from charged particles (alpha, beta, or positrons). It is equal to the specific ionization (s) multiplied by 30 eV and is approximately proportional to the square of the charge on the particle divided by the square of its speed. This energy transfer constitutes the radiation dose to a patient.

linear equation 1. a mathematical equation in two variables x and y: $y = mx + b$. The constants m and b are often called the slope and the y-intercept.

2. an n-dimensional linear equation: $y = b + m_1x_1 + m_2x_2 + \cdot\cdot\cdot + m_nx_n$.

linear focus the shape of the electronic focal spot in an x-ray tube, a rectangle about three times as long as it is wide. Because the beam is emitted from the target at an angle of 15°–20°, the optical focal spot is approximately square.

linearity (lin″e-ar′ĭ-te) a straight-line relationship between two quantities, in which a change in one causes a proportional change in the other; the ability of an amplifier or detector to produce an output linearly related to an input.

linearity check one of the quality control procedures in clinical laboratories. It acts to verify that a scintillation camera produces (without distortion) an image of a bar phantom having parallel straight lines, and to verify that the energy window setting of a pulse height analyzer is proportional to the detected gamma-ray photon energy.

linear regression a statistical procedure for fitting a straight line to data consisting of n paired values (X_i, Y_i), where each value Y_i is an observation on a random variable associated with a value X_i. X is not treated as a random variable; the analysis is conditional on the given values of X. Y is called the dependent variable; X, the independent variable. The standard method is to fit the line $Y = a + bX$ so as to minimize the total squared deviation $\Sigma_i(Y_i - a - bX_i)^2$ of the observed values of Y from the values predicted by the regression line. This is called a least-squares fit. See also *least squares regression.*

The least-squares estimates are given by the formulas: $b = \Sigma_i(X_i - \mu_X)(Y_i - Y)/n\sigma_X{}^2$ and $a = Y - b\mu_X$, where $Y = \Sigma_i Y_i/n$ is the sample mean of the Y values and $\mu_X = \Sigma_i X_i/n$ and $\sigma_X{}^2 = \Sigma_i(X_i - \mu_X)^2/n$ are the mean and variance of the X values.

If the conditional distribution of Y given X is the normal distribution with mean $\mu_Y + \beta(X - \mu_X)$ and standard deviation $\sigma_{Y \cdot X}$ (independent of X), then Y estimates μ_Y, b estimates β, and $s_{YX}{}^2 = \Sigma_i(Y_i - Y - b(X - \mu_X))^2/(n-2)$ estimates $\sigma_{Y \cdot X}{}^2$ ($s_{Y \cdot X}$ is called the standard error of estimate).

The statistics Y and b have independent normal distributions with standard deviations $\sigma_{X \cdot Y}/\sqrt{n}$ and $\sigma_{X \cdot Y}/\sigma_X\sqrt{n}$. Both are independent of $(n - 2)\cdot s_{Y \cdot X}{}^2/\sigma_{Y \cdot X}{}^2$, which has the chi-squared distribution with $n - 2$ degrees of freedom.

Therefore, $(Y - \mu_Y)/(s_{Y \cdot X}/\sqrt{n})$ and $(b - \beta)/(s_{Y \cdot X}/\sigma_X\sqrt{n})$ have the t distribution with $n - 2$ degrees of freedom, and $\overline{Y} \pm (s_{Y \cdot X}/\sqrt{n})t_{\alpha/2, n-2}$ and $b \pm (s_{Y \cdot X}/\sigma_X\sqrt{n})t_{\alpha/2, n-2}$ are the 100 $(1 - \alpha)$ percent confidence limits for μ_X and β, where $t_{\alpha/2, n-2}$ is the upper $\alpha/2$ percentile of the t distribution with $n - 2$ degrees of freedom. The null hypothesis that $\beta = \beta_0$ can be rejected and the alternative $\beta \neq \beta_0$ accepted at the α level of significance if this confidence interval does not contain β_0.

The variance of $\overline{Y} + b(X_0 - \mu_X)$ is $(\sigma_{Y \cdot X}{}^2/n) \cdot (1 + (X_0 - \mu X)^2/\sigma_X{}^2)$, where X_0 is arbitrary. The variance of any future observation of Y will be $\sigma_{Y \cdot X}{}^2$. A confidence interval for $\mu_Y + \beta(X_0 - \mu_X)$, the ordinate at X_0 of the true regression line, has the limits $\overline{Y} + b(X_0 - \mu_X) \pm kt_{\alpha/2, n-2}$, where $k^2 = (s_{Y \cdot X}{}^2/n) \cdot (1 + (X_0 - \mu_X)^2/\sigma_X{}^2)$.

If $2F_{\alpha/2, n-2}$ (the upper percent point of the F distribution with 2 degrees of freedom in the numerator and $n-2$ degrees of freedom in the denominator) is used instead of $t_{\alpha\,2, n-1}$, this produces a confidence interval for the whole regression line. There is a 100 $(1 - \alpha)$ percent probability that $\mu_Y + \beta X_0$ lies within the confidence limits for every value of X_0. This is a Scheffé interval; see under *analysis of variance.*

line filter an electrical filter inserted in the power line of an electrical instrument to block out high-frequency, high-voltage noise by filtering out frequencies above the 60-Hz line frequency.

line focus in an x-ray tube, the point where the electron beam strikes the anode, producing x-rays. Its projection in the direction of the central ray is foreshortened to a small area, the optical focal spot.

line number a number that identifies a statement in a FORTRAN or BASIC program and is used to refer to the statement.

line printer a computer output device that prints text a whole line at a time. Conventional high-speed line printers print more than 3000 lines/min. Cf. *typewriter terminal.*

line spectrum an absorption or emission spectrum in which radiation is absorbed or emitted only at discrete frequencies corresponding to a transition between quantum states. An example is atomic absorption spectrophotometry.

line-spread function a measure of the spatial resolution of a scintillation camera or rectilinear scanner; the response of the detector to a line source (e.g., a catheter filled with radioactive solution) as a function of the distance from the image's center.

Lineweaver-Burk equation [Hans *Lineweaver,* U.S. chemist, born 1907; Dean *Burk,* U.S. chemist, born 1904] a form of the Michaelis-Menten equation in which reciprocals of both sides are equated to give the linear form, $1/V = (K_m/V_{max})(1/[S]) + 1/V_{max}$, where V is the reaction velocity, [S] is the substrate concentration, and K_m is the Michaelis-Menten constant. A plot of $1/V$ (the Y coordinate) as a function of 1/[S] (the X coordinate) is a straight line from which V_{max}, the maximal velocity, can be determined from the y-intercept ($= 1/V_{max}$) and K_m, which measures the enzyme-substrate affinity, can be determined from the x-intercept ($= -1/K_m$). Several other linearized forms of the Michaelis-Menten equation have been derived: $([S]/V) = (1/V_{max})[S] + (K_m/V_{max})$ (Hanes Plot), and $(V) = (-V/[S])(K_m) + (V_{max})$ (Eadie-Hofstee Plot). These equations make it possible to calculate K_m values from experimental data and are useful in the study of enzyme activation and inhibition. Graphs of these equations are shown in the accompanying illustration. See also *enzyme inhibition* and *Michaelis-Menten equation.*

lingu/o (ling′gwo) [L. *lingua* tongue] a word element used in combining form to denote tongue, e.g., linguodental.

lingua (ling′gwah), pl. *linguae* [L. "tongue"] see *tongue.*

lingual (ling′gwal) [L. *lingualis*] pertaining to or toward the tongue.

lingual artery a branch of the external carotid artery that supplies the tongue.

lingual nerve a sensory nerve arising from the posterior trunk of the mandibular nerve, which receives fibers of the chorda tympani nerve and supplies the mucous membrane of the anterior tongue, floor of the mouth, and mandibular gums. The lingual nerve descends medial to the ramus of the mandible, proceeds forward along its medial surface, and passes to the tongue. In addition to its

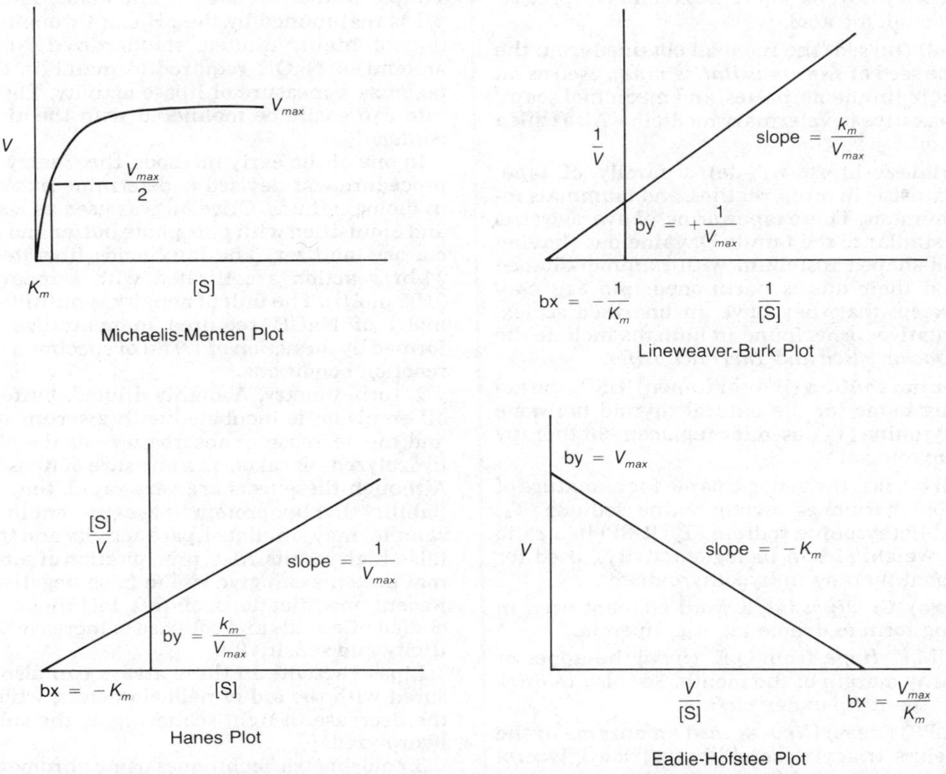

Lineweaver-Burk equation. Linearized forms of the Michaelis-Menten equation, including the Lineweaver-Burk equation. (Courtesy of Norbert W. Tietz, Ph.D.)

role as a sensory nerve, the lingual nerve carries postganglionic fibers from the submandibular ganglion to the sublingual and anterior lingual glands.

Linguatula (ling-gwat′u-lah) a genus of tongueworms. The adult forms live in the respiratory tract of vertebrates, sometimes including humans. The larval forms inhabit the digestive tract and lungs. Halzoun, a Syrian disease, is sometimes found in association.

L. serrata, a species whose adult forms are parasitic in the respiratory tracts of dogs. Infection in humans is acquired by ingestion of larvae from the nasal discharges of infested animals. The larvae hatch and bore through the intestinal wall, where they become encysted in the viscera. *L. serrata* is also known to invade the eyes and cause visual damage.

linguatuliasis (ling-gwat″u-li′ah-sis) infection with *Linguatula.*

Linguatulidae (lin-gwah-tu′lĭ-de) a family of endoparasitic arthropods (known as tongueworms or linguatulids) of the order Porocephalida, class Pentastomida. Their body is elongate or tonguelike, some species having a ringed or annulated body. Linguatulids lack external appendages and have two pairs of hooks near the mouth. Adult forms inhabit the respiratory tract of vertebrates, and encysted larvae are found in the viscera of humans.

lingula (ling′gu-lah), pl. *lingulae* [L., dim. of *lingua*] [NA], a general term for a small, tonguelike structure.

linitis (lĭ-ni′tis) [Gr. *linon* thread + *-itis*] an inflammation of the gastric wall.

l. plastica, an uncommon variety of gastric (or rarely, colonic) adenocarcinoma that infiltrates all layers of the gut wall and incites a desmoplastic response. The stomach or intestinal wall becomes diffusely thickened and loses its pliability.

linkage (ling′kij) 1. the associated inheritance of two genes on the same chromosome; the distance between the loci of two such genes, as measured by the recombination frequency. Cf. *synteny.*

2. a covalent chemical bond.

linkage map a genetic map that shows the order of the known genes on a chromosome and the distances between them as measured in centimorgans, the number of cross-overs per 100 meioses.

linoleate (lin-o′le-āt) the anion of linoleic acid. See also *linoleic acid.*

linoleic acid (lin″o-lā′ic) [L. *linum* flax + *oleum* oil] an essential fatty acid, a major component of many vegetable oils, e.g., cottonseed, soybean, peanut, corn, sunflower seed, and linseed oil, in which it occurs as a glyceride. Also called *cis*-9,*cis*-12-octadecadienoic acid.

linolenic acid (lin″o-len′ik) a triply unsaturated essential fatty acid from linseed and other vegetable oils.

α-linolenic a., the linolenic acid of plant oils, 9,12,15-octadecatrienoic acid.

γ-linolenic a., 6,9,12-octadecatrienoic acid, which occurs in animal tissues. It is formed from linolenic acid by a dehydrogenation reaction and is a precursor of arachidonic acid.

linseed oil (lin′sēd) the fixed oil obtained from the dried, ripe seed of *Linum usitatissimum;* used as an emollient in liniments, pastes, and medicinal soaps, and as a laxative in veterinary medicine. Also called *flaxseed oil.*

Linstowiidae (lin-sto-wi′ĭ-de) a family of tapeworms parasitic in birds, reptiles, and mammals including humans. These tapeworms, of average size, are very similar to the family Davaineidae (having a cushion-shaped rostellum with hammer-shaped hooks and their uterus partitioned into egg capsules), except that they have an unarmed scolex. Representative forms found in humans include the genera *Oochoristica* and *Inermicapsifer.*

liothyronine sodium (li″o-thi′ro-nēn) [USP], the generic drug name for the natural thyroid hormone triiodothyronine (T_3), used for replacement therapy in hypothyroidism.

liotrix (li′o-triks) the generic name for a mixture of the thyroid hormones levothyroxine sodium (T_4) [USP] and liothyronine sodium (T_3) [USP] in a ratio of 4:1 by weight (1:1 in biologic activity), used for replacement therapy in hypothyroidism.

lip/o (lip′o) [Gr. *lipos* fat] a word element used in combining form to denote fat, e.g., lipemia.

lip (lip) [M.E. *lippe,* from O.E. *lippa*] the upper or lower fleshy margin of the mouth. See also *labium.*

hare l., see *c. lip* under *cleft.*

lipase (LPS) (lipās) [*lipo-* + *-ase*] an enzyme of the esterase class, triacylglycerol lipase (triacylglycerol acylhydrolase, EC 3.1.1.3), that catalyzes the reaction triacylglycerol + $H_2O \rightleftarrows$ diacylglycerol + a fatty acid anion. The enzyme acts on the substrate-water interface in emulsions, and hydrolysis occurs primarily at positions 1 and 3. Lipase is primarily produced in and secreted by the pancreas, and acts in the small intestine to break down fats to free fatty acids and mono- or diglycerides before absorption by the intestinal mucosa. There is also a lipase that is secreted by the gastric mucosa. Serum lipase is increased in acute pancreatitis and obstruction of the pancreatic duct. Also called *pancreatic lipase* and *steapsin.*

lipase assays 1. titrimetric method. Lipase activity in serum or other fluids is determined by the amount of free fatty acid liberated from a purified olive oil emulsion buffered at pH 8.0 by serum in 3 hr at 37°C. After the lipase is denatured with ethanol, the liberated fatty acids are determined by titration with sodium hydroxide, using pH 10.5 as the end point. The end point is detected either potentiometrically with a pH meter or with the aid of thymolphthalein as the indicator. The lipase activity is determined from the difference between NaOH added in titrating the reaction mixture after the incubation period and that added in titrating a blank containing substrate and buffer with serum added at the end of the incubation period. The Tietz-Fiereck unit of activity is the quantity of lipase in 1.0 ml of serum that liberates 50 μmol of fatty acids under these test conditions (1.0 Tietz-Fiereck unit/ml equals 280 U/l).

An advanced technique based on a similar principle utilizes a pH stat. This test is significantly faster and more sensitive. In this approach, a diluted olive oil or triolein emulsion is incubated with serum sample in the presence of bile acids. The reaction pH is maintained by the pH stat through the addition of highly diluted, standardized NaOH. The amount of NaOH required to maintain the pH is taken as a measure of lipase activity. The reaction rate can easily be monitored with the aid of a recorder.

In one of the early methods, the Cherry-Crandall procedure was devised to determine lipase activity in biologic fluids. Olive oil was used as a substrate, and emulsified with phosphate buffer and gum acacia as stabilizer. The fatty acids liberated after a 24-hr reaction are titrated with standard NaOH (0.05 mol/l). The unit of activity is milliliters of 0.05 mol/l of NaOH required to neutralize the acid formed by the action of 1.0 ml of specimen under the reaction conditions.

2. turbidimetry. A highly diluted, buffered olive oil emulsion is incubated with a serum specimen, and the decrease in absorbance—as the olive oil is hydrolyzed—is taken as a measure of lipase activity. Although these tests are very rapid, they have the liability that lipoprotein lipase (present in the same sample) may simulate lipase activity and thus cause false-high results. Also, precipitation of some abnormal proteins can give rise to false-negative results. Recent modifications of this technique have included bile acids and colipase to increase both specificity and sensitivity.

Lipase activity in these assays can also be measured with the aid of nephelometers, which detect the decrease in light scattering as the substrate is hydrolyzed.

3. colorimetric techniques using chromogenic water-soluble substrates. Although such assays have also been proposed, they measure esterase activity and thus should not be used for measurements of lipase activity.

lipedema (lip″ĕ-de′mah) [*lipo-* + *edema,* from Gr. *oidēma* swelling] an accumulation of excess fat and associated fluid in the subcutaneous tissues.

lipemia (lĭ-pe′me-ah) [*lipo-* + Gr. *haima* blood + *-ia*] abnormally high concentrations of fat or lipid in the blood. See also *hyperlipidemia.*

absorptive l., a transient increase in the amount of blood lipids that transiently follows the ingestion of fat. Also called alimentary lipemia.

l. retinalis, the milky appearance of the veins and arteries of the retina accompanying high levels of lipids in blood.

lipid (lip′id) any of a group of organic substances that are insoluble in water but soluble in alcohol, ether, chloroform, and other fat solvents, and which have a greasy feel. The lipids, which are easily stored in the body, serve as a source of fuel and are an important constituent of cell structures. As used in the United States, the term includes fatty acids, neutral fats, waxes, steroids, phosphatides, and cerebrosides.

lipid assays the determination of total lipids (the sum of all classes of lipids that can be readily extracted from serum or other specimens), now obsolete because of its limited clinical usefulness. The reference range for total serum lipids is 400–700 mg/dl.

Methods used for the determination of total lipids are based on (1) turbidimetry; (2) extraction into an organic solvent and quantitation by weighing, titration, or microoxidation; (3) the sulfophosphovanillin reaction (measurement of a pink product formed when unsaturated lipids are oxidized with sulfuric acid and then reacted with vanillin in phosphoric acid); and (4) the summation method (totaling the values of the various lipid classes determined by separate assays). For more information, see *cholesterol assays, fatty acid assays, lipoprotein assays, phospholipid assays,* and *triglyceride assays.*

lipid embolism the sudden blocking of some blood vessels, caused by lipid particles entering the circulation, usually as a result of some extensive trauma such as multiple fractures of the long bones. These emboli are composed chiefly of triglyceride globules. The occurrence of lipid emboli can cause brain damage, pulmonary damage, pneumonia, and bone necrosis. A warning of the possible presence of emboli is the appearance of increased amounts of urinary triglycerides.

lipidemia (lip″ĭ-de′me-ah) [*lipid* + Gr. *haima* blood + *-ia*] see *hyperlipidemia* and *lipemia.*

lipidosis (lip″ĭ-do′sis) see *lipid storage disease.*

lipid pigments a variety of pigments having lipid characteristics, some of which also contain protein or iron. The most important is lipofuscin, which occurs in cells undergoing slow, regressive change. It is formed in lysosomes and is the product of oxidation and polymerization of the membrane lipids of autophagocytosed organelles. Lipofuscin is seen as a pigment that is yellow to brown in color, occurring in basophilic granules. Lipofuscin that is acid-fast and autofluorescent (greenish-yellow in frozen sections, brownish-yellow in paraffin sections) but Schmorl negative is called ceroid.

Lipochromes are carotenoids, fat-soluble pigments that impart a yellowish-red color to fat when large quantities of carotenes are present in the diet.

lipid stains see *fat stains.*

lipid storage disease the term for a group of disorders of cellular lipid metabolism that involves the abnormal accumulation of lipids. Also called *lipidosis.* See also *mucolipidoses* and *sphingolipidoses.*

lipid transport the movement of lipids throughout the body via the blood stream. The normally insoluble lipids are transported in the form of soluble complexes with specific plasma proteins. See also *lipoprotein.*

lipid transport disorder the term for a group of disorders of lipid metabolism characterized by abnormal levels or types of lipoprotein in the blood. These disorders can cause serious disease in infancy or childhood, but more commonly cause illness and a shortened life span owing to damage to the arterial vascular system. For more information, see the specific disorder (e.g., *abetalipoproteinemia, cholesterol ester storage disease, hyperlipoproteinemia, hypolipoproteinemia, lipoprotein lipase deficiency, Tangier disease, lecithin-cholestorol acyltransferase deficiency*), and *Wolman's disease.*

lipiduria (lip″ĭ-du′re-ah) [*lipid* + Gr. *ouron* urine + *-ia*] the presence of lipids in the urine. Fat globules or lipid emboli can enter the urine as a result of damage to the kidney (degenerative tubular disease, nephrotic syndrome, renal infarction, damage due to kidney stones). Cf. *chyluria.*

Lipiodol (lip-i′o-dol) trademark. See *iodized oil.*

lipoblastomatosis (lip″o-blas″to-mah-to′sis) a nodular proliferation, invariably benign, of fetal-like fat cells, which occurs in young children. It is a rare entity and is seldom seen in children older than age 3 yr.

lipochrome (lip′o-krōm) [Gr. *lipos* fat + *chrōma* color] any fat-soluble pigment, similar to carotene, that imparts a yellow, yellow-orange, or orange-red color to lipid-containing tissues. Among such pigments are the carotenes, lycopene, and xanthophyll. These are synthesized by plants, and, on ingestion, are dissolved or incorporated into animal fats or fatty tissue. It is lipochrome that imparts the yellow color to the corpus luteum, egg yolk, and yellow corn kernels. Also called carotenoids and lipofuscin. See also *carotenoid* and *lipofuscin.*

lipodystrophy (lip″o-dis′tro-fe) [*lipo-* + Gr. *dystrophis* dystrophy] a general term used to describe any abnormality in the metabolism of fat.

intestinal l., see *Whipple's disease.*

lipofuscin (lip″o-fus′sin) [*lipo-* + L. *fuscus* brown] a brown, granular, iron-negative pigment found particularly in muscle, heart, liver, and nerve cells. It is a product of cellular wear and tear that accumulates in lysosomes with age. Also called *hemofuscin* and sometimes *lipochrome,* although the latter term is usually reserved for carotenoid pigments. See also *lipid pigments.*

lipofuscinosis (lip″o-fu″sin-o′sis) a general term used to describe disorders of lipofuscin metabolism.

neuronal ceroid l., a group of metabolic diseases of unknown biochemical etiology, thought to have a genetic component and transmitted as autosomal recessive traits, that are characterized by central nervous system degeneration and optic nerve atrophy. As a group, the diseases generally appear in infancy or childhood. The clinical signs are extremely variable, including seizures, myoclonic jerks, mental retardation, macular degeneration, and retinitis pigmentosa. In a number of tissues (e.g., the liver, white blood cells, and muscle), curvilinear bodies (electron-dense deposits) may be seen by electron microscopy. This stored material has been labeled ceroid or lipofuscin. There is no known treatment.

lipogenesis (lip″o-jen′ĕ-sis) [*lipo-* + Gr. *genesis* production, generation] the formation of fat; the transformation of nonfat food materials into body fat.

lipogenic (lip″o-jen′ik) 1. forming, producing, or generating fat.
2. caused by or resulting from fat.

lipogranulomatosis (lip″o-gran″u-lo-mah-to′sis) see *Farber's lipogranulomatosis.*

lipoic acid (lip′o-ik) see *thioctic acid.*

lipolysis (lĭ-pol′ĭ-sis) [*lipo-* + Gr. *lysis* dissolution] the breakdown of fat and the release of fatty acids from fat cells into the blood. Also called *adipolysis.*

lipolysis regulation the hormone-mediated regulation of lipolysis occurring in adipose cells. The first messengers (thyroid-stimulating hormone, glucagon, epinephrine, norepinephrine, and adrenocorticotropic hormone) have a stimulatory effect on the membrane enzyme adenylate cyclase in the adipocyte. This enzyme catalyzes formation of the second messenger cAMP within the cell. Insulin, prostaglandin E_1, and nicotinic acid are inhibitors of cAMP production. Methylxanthines and thyroid hormone potentiate the action of cAMP by inhibiting its breakdown by a phosphodiesterase. cAMP has a stimulatory effect on protein kinase, which activates adipolytic lipase to an active phosphorylated form. The active form of the adipolytic lipase can again be converted to the inactive form by dephosphorylation by a phosphatase. Growth hormone promotes the synthesis of the adipolytic lipase. The activated adipolytic lipase catalyzes lipolysis of adipose triglycerides to free fatty acids and glycerol.

lipolytic (lip″o-lit′ik) pertaining to, characterized by, or causing lipolysis, the breakdown of fats; adipolytic.

lipoma (lĭ-po′mah) [*lipo-* + *-oma*] a common benign neoplasm that usually appears in middle age and is most often found in the subcutaneous tissues of the neck and trunk, although it may occur anywhere that fat is present. Most lipomas are small, poorly delimited, and thinly encapsulated; they have the histologic appearance of mature adipose tissue, occasionally mixed with fibrous elements or a proliferation of small vessels (angiolipoma). Aside from their cosmetic effect, lipomas rarely have clinical significance. Spindle cell, pleomorphic, intramuscular, and infiltrating variants occur.

lipomatosis (lip″o-mah-to′sis) a disorder in which abnormal deposits of mature fat occur in various locations, including the pelvis.

lipophilic (lip″o-fil′ik) [*lipo-* + Gr. *philein* to love + *-ic*] miscible with or attracted to lipids; soluble in lipids or capable of dissolving or absorbing lipids.

lipoprotein (lĭp″o-pro′tēn) a compound or complex of lipids and proteins linked together by a variety of bonds (hydrophobic, ionic). The major classes recognized are: chylomicrons, and very-low-density (VLDL), low-density (LDL), and high-density (HDL) lipoproteins. They serve to transport the otherwise insoluble lipids, such as triglycerides, cholesterol, and cholesterol esters in plasma, from the intestinal tract and liver to a variety of tissue sites. Other lipoprotein types are known in other tissue sites. See also *chylomicron.*

high-density l. (HDL), a combination (chemical complex) of lipids and proteins having a hydrated density of 1.063–1.21 g/ml. HDL is synthesized in the liver and the intestine. The main component of HDL is apoprotein (approximately 50 percent); phospholipids and cholesterol are the main lipid components. Electrophoretically, HDL migrates with the alpha-globulin band. These lipoproteins are involved in the turnover of tissue cholesterol and in the transport of excess cholesterol to the liver where it is metabolized to bile acids, which are eventually excreted.

HDL plays an intimate role in the conversion of VLDL to LDL. HDL has been subfractionated into three density classes, HDL_1 (1.050–1.063 g/ml), HDL_2 (1.063–1.120 g/ml), and HDL_3 (1.120–1.210 g/ml). The major proteins are apoA-I and apoA-II. The ratios of these two proteins vary within each HDL subspecies. Minor apoproteins are apoC, apoD, and apoE. Recent epidemiologic studies have shown a negative correlation between serum HDL cholesterol and premature coronary heart disease.

intermediate-density l. (IDL), a subclass of lipoproteins present in plasma, with a density between that of VLDL and LDL (1.009–1.015 g/ml). This class of lipoproteins is formed in plasma following the action of lipoprotein lipase on chylomicrons and VLDL. Cholesterol and phospholipids are the lipids present in the greatest amount; electrophoretically, IDL migrate with the beta-globulin fraction.

low-density l. (LDL), a combination or complex of lipids and proteins present in blood plasma, of the hydrated density class 1.019–1.063 g/ml. To a large extent it appears that LDL is derived from VLDL. The major apoprotein of LDL is apo-B, and the major lipid is cholesteryl linoleate. In the pathogenesis of atherosclerosis, one of the risk factors is an elevated level of LDL. Also called beta-lipoprotein (as these lipoproteins migrate electrophoretically with the beta-globulin fraction).

very-low-density l. (VLDL), a class of lipoproteins present in plasma, with a density of 0.95–1.006 g/ml. It plays a major role in the transport of triglycerides from the intestinal tract and liver to adipose tissues and muscles. The lipid component present in highest concentration is triglyceride (about 50 percent), and the apoproteins present are B, C, and some E. In electrophoresis, it migrates with the pre-beta fraction.

lipoprotein assays 1. electrophoretic technique. The preferred support media are agarose gel, agar gel, starch gel, and paper. After separation of the protein fractions, the lipid-associated proteins are visualized by staining with lipophilic stains. Four bands may be visualized: chylomicrons, at the point of application; a fraction in the beta-globulin zone (beta-lipoproteins); the fastest moving fraction (alpha-lipoprotein), which migrates with the alpha-globulins; and the pre-beta fraction, which moves slightly faster than the beta-lipoproteins. The fractions are quantitated spectrophotometrically with the aid of densitometers measuring the dye bound to the lipoproteins. Normal sera show only alpha- and beta-lipoprotein bands in the ratio of 1:3; chylomicrons, pre-beta, and increased beta bands are found in sera associated with lipid transport abnormalities.

2. ultracentrifugation. Lipoproteins are separated by virtue of differences in their density. Salt is added to the specimen to increase the density of the medium to 1.063 g/ml. The same or similar four classes as mentioned above can be separated and differentiated by their Svedberg flotation values (S_f). The HDL (high-density lipoproteins) sediment; the other fractions form lipid bands in the upper portion of the medium (i.e., LDL, low-density lipoprotein; VLDL, very-low-density lipoprotein; and chylomicrons). These bands are quantitated photometrically in the centrifuge. The HDL, LDL, and VLDL correspond to the alpha, beta, and pre-beta fractions measured electrophoretically.

3. chemical precipitation. Some fractions, e.g., LDL, can be precipitated by reagents such as heparin and manganous ion; the soluble lipoproteins (HDL) are measured (either as lipoproteins or HDL cholesterol), and the precipitated fraction (LDL) is obtained by calculations. This approach is used primarily to measure particular lipids (cholesterol, triglycerides) in the fractions.

4. assay of apolipoproteins. The protein chains of lipoproteins are freed from associated lipids, and the individual classes of apoproteins are identified electrophoretically or by immunochemical techniques.

lipoprotein chylomicron see under *chylomicron.*

lipoprotein lipase (lip″o-pro′te-in lĭ′pās) an enzyme (or group of enzymes) of the hydrolase class, triacylglycero-protein acylhydrolase (EC 3.1.1.34), that catalyzes the reaction protein-bound triacylglycerol + H_2O ⇌ protein-bound diacylglycerol +

fatty acid anion. The enzymes occur in liver, muscle, adipose, and capillary tissue, and hydrolyze triglycerides present in chylomicrons and low-density lipoproteins to form free fatty acids (for storage or transport) and smaller-sized lipoproteins. The adipose tissue enzyme is hormone activated; the plasma enzyme is membrane bound and released by injected heparin and activated by apoprotein C-II; it is inhibited by apoprotein CIII. A genetic deficiency of the plasma enzyme causes a severe lipidemia, leading to pancreatic inflammation and lipid deposits in the skin. Also called clearing factor lipase.

lipoprotein lipase deficiency a genetic defect, transmitted as an autosomal recessive trait, that results from a deficiency or alteration of activity of the enzyme lipoprotein lipase. Occurring in children and young adults, the disease is characterized by abdominal pains, excess chylomicrons in the blood, and, frequently, bouts of pancreatitis.

lipoprotein-X (Lp-X) an abnormal lipoprotein occurring in individuals with obstructive jaundice (either intra- or extrahepatic) and in those who lack the enzyme lecithin:cholesterol acyltransferase (LCAT). Lp-X has a flotation rate and electrophoretic mobility that places it among the low-density lipoproteins. It contains about 65 percent lecithin, 30 percent cholesterol, and 5 percent protein (apolipoprotein C and albumin).

liposarcoma (lip″o-sar-ko′mah) [*lipo-* + *sarcoma*] a malignant soft tissue neoplasm composed of lipogenic cells. Most sarcomas of this type capable of forming metastases are deeply located in the thigh or retroperitoneum of adults and typically are large tumors. In contrast, although superficial tumors of fat cells may display atypical histology, they rarely metastasize. Roughly one-third of liposarcomas are well-differentiated tumors that tend to recur but metastasize only when dedifferentiated areas are present. One-third of liposarcomas are composed of small, round-to-elongated cells loosely arranged within a myxoid stroma (myxoid liposarcoma), which are more common in the thigh than the retroperitoneum and which may give rise to metastases. One-third of liposarcomas are pleomorphic liposarcomas, which are aggressive tumors that have some histologic overlap with malignant fibrous histiocytoma. See also *malignant f. h.* under *fibrous histiocytoma.*

liposome (lip′o-sōm) [*lipo-* + Gr. *sōma* body] a vesicle formed by the homogenization (emulsification) of phospholipids in dilute salt solutions. Most are uniform-sized spheres of lipid bilayers that can be isolated from the suspending solution as a clear, separate phase. Liposomes are the prototypes of membrane-bound biologic structures.

lipotropic (lip″o-trop′ik) [*lipo-* + Gr. *rophē* a turning] 1. acting in lipid metabolism by hastening the removal of or decreasing the deposit of fat in the liver resulting from choline deficiency or a deficiency of other methyl group donors.

2. referring to an agent that has such effects. See under *betaine.*

lipping (lip′ing) the formation of small osteophytes at the margins of the articular surfaces of bones, as occurs in osteoarthrosis. Also called bone spur formation.

liquefaction (lik″wĕ-fak′shun) [L. *liquefactio,* from *liquere* to flow + *facere* to make] the conversion of a substance into a liquid form; the temperature at which conversion occurs is the liquefaction temperature.

liquefactive (lik″wĕ-fak′tiv) pertaining to, characterized by, or causing liquefaction.

liquefactive degeneration a type of necrosis characterized by tissue softening and the conversion of solid tissue into liquid. It is due to the autolysis and heterolysis of cells, which is accompanied by the release and activation of powerful hydrolytic enzymes. The condition is characteristic of areas of brain infarction and focal bacterial lesions, especially those due to coagulase-positive staphylococci, beta-hemolytic streptococci, and *Escherichia coli.*

liquid (lik′wid) [L. *liquidus,* from *liquere* to flow] 1. flowing readily; neither solid nor gaseous.

2. a state of matter in which the atoms or molecules move about freely but are held closely packed together by strong intermolecular forces. A liquid thus has a definite volume, takes the shape of a container, is almost incompressible, and may have a free upper surface.

liquid crystal a viscous organic liquid that changes its optical properties with small changes in temperature or with the application of an electric field. It is used to make the type of digital readout that uses reflected light.

liquid-liquid chromatography see under *chromatography.*

liquid-liquid junction potential see *diffusion potential.*

liquid scintillation counter a radiation detector used primarily for measuring low-energy beta emission from isotopes such as carbon-14 and tritium. Because many beta particles would be absorbed in any substance between the sample and scintillator, the sample is dissolved or suspended in toluene that contains fluors. (Substances insoluble in toluene can be dissolved with the aid of solubilizers.) Beta particles are absorbed by the toluene. The absorbed energy is transferred to a molecule of a primary fluor, which emits a visible photon that can be detected by a photomultiplier.

Any interference with the energy transfer is called quenching. Chemical quenching is due to impurities that absorb energy from the excited solvent molecules. Color quenching is due to photon-absorbing impurities. The quenching can be corrected by one of three methods. For internal standardization, a known amount of a nonquenching standard beta emitter is added to the sample; the efficiency with which the standard is counted is used to correct the unknown counts. External standardization, a second method, is similar, but the known activity consists of gamma rays from an external source. A third method uses the ratio of high-energy light pulses to low-energy light pulses; the correction is determined from a standard curve of counting efficiency versus channels ratio.

liquid scintillator a scintillator used in a liquid scintillation counter, usually an organic compound dissolved in toluene. See also *POP* and *POPOP.*

Lison-Dunn method see under *hemoglobin demonstration in tissue.*

LISP (lisp) [acronym from *Lis*t *P*rocessing Language] a high-level computer language for list processing in which all data and programs are in the form of list structures.

LISS abbrev. for low–ionic-strength medium test. See under *antibody detection.*

lissencephaly (lis″sen-sef′ah-le) a congenital malformation in which there is a lack of the normal convolutions and dense gliosis of the cerebral cortex. Symptoms include seizures and retardation. Death occurs in utero or soon after birth. Also called *agyria.*

list (list) 1. an instruction to a compiler or assembler to print out a listing of the source program along with error messages, symbol tables, storage requirements, and related information.

2. a data structure defined as a string of zero or more items (referred to as atoms) of a specified type of data. See also *list structure.*

Listeria (lis-ter′e-ah) [Lord Joseph *Lister,* English surgeon, 1827–1912] a genus of microorganisms that closely resembles the Corynebacteriaceae family. These organisms are composed of small, gram-positive, motile rods that sometimes grow in chains and that have a tendency to form palisades. *L. monocytogenes,* named for its striking monocytic action in blood, is ubiquitous and is transmitted by healthy animal and human carriers; it produces meningoencephalitis, meningitis, perinatal septicemia, and other acute and chronic disorders in humans. The organism is frequently confused with *Corynebacterium* diphtheroids, *Erysipelothrix,* and *Enterococcus;* positive identification depends on careful evaluation of cultural and biochemical characteristics, including fermentation reactions with trehalose, salicin, and mannitol.

listeriosis (lis-ter″e-o′sis) an infection with *Listeria monocytogenes,* which may occur in the fetus, newborn, or adult. In utero infections occur transplacentally and most frequently result in abortions, stillbirths, and premature birth; infections acquired during birth may result in acute illness with cardiorespiratory distress, diarrhea, and vomiting, and the appearance of meningitis within 4 wk. In adults, infection can occur in both healthy and immunosuppressed individuals, and produces meningitis, endocarditis, and disseminated granulomatous lesions. Diagnosis is established following acute culture of blood, cerebrospinal fluid, or discharges from affected areas. Treatment requires penicillin or other appropriate antibiotics.

listing (lis′ting) a printout of items, as of the text of a computer program.

list mode a method of computer storage of data from a scintillation camera. The position and the time of each detected photon are stored, a procedure allowing the most flexible analysis. The data may be used to make a sequence of images having any specified framing rate. Curves can be obtained of the activity of various regions of interest plotted versus time. Cf. *histogram mode.*

list structure a data structure defined as a string of zero or more items and list structures. This definition is inherently recursive; a list structure can contain itself as an item.

liter (l, L) (le′ter) [Fr. *litre*] a noncoherent unit of volume, used with the International System (SI), that is defined as one-thousandth of a cubic meter (10^{-3} m^3, 1 dm^3). The official abbreviation is l, which is used standing alone and with prefixes, e.g., ml, dl; however, because the letter l can be confused with the number 1, especially in typescript, the abbreviation L is sometimes used for liter: for example, g/L and mol/L. The official spelling, litre, is rarely used in the United States.

literal (lit′er-al) a constant specified in a computer program in a form that requires no conversion, e.g., a character string.

lith/o (lith′o) [Gr. *lithos* stone] a word element used in combining form to denote stone or calculus, e.g., litholysis.

lithic acid (lith′ik) see *uric acid.*

lithium (Li) (lith′e-um) [N.L.; L. *lithia* from Gr. *litheia* fine stone or marble] a silvery-white metallic element; atomic number 3; atomic weight 6.939; Group I of the periodic table (the alkali metals); oxidation state +1. Lithium does not occur naturally in the body; when administered, it is distributed between both extra- and intracellular fluids, unlike Na^+ and K^+. Lithium interferes with sodium transport and neurotransmitter metabolism in the nerves.

Lithium salts are administered to manic patients to diminish the intensity of manic episodes. The therapeutic serum concentration range of lithium is 0.5–1.5 mmol/l. Mild toxic effects, nausea, muscular weakness, and lack of coordination are observed at levels ranging from therapeutic to 2 mmol/l. Severe toxic effects, including coma and convulsions, are observed at higher concentrations. Cyclic AMP–mediated processes, which are regulated by peptide hormones, also seem to be inhibited by lithium (e.g., lithium-induced diabetes insipidus). Lithium should be monitored frequently.

l. carbonate, a white crystalline salt, Li_2CO_3. It is used in medicine for treating manic patients and in histology for blueing hematoxylin-stained slides and as a component of ammoniacal silver solutions.

l. citrate, the citric acid salt of lithium, which is used to treat manic patients.

lithium assays emission flame photometry or atomic absorption spectrophotometry. A suitably diluted serum sample is aspirated into the photometer flame; the light energy emitted or absorbed, respectively, at 670.8 nm is measured; and the results are compared with results obtained with an appropriate standard solution. In some procedures, serum proteins are removed or ion enhancement is corrected for by addition of physiologic concentrations of sodium to the standard and blank solutions. Potassium or cesium may be used as an internal standard.

lithium-drifted detector a gamma-ray and charged particle radiation detector that uses a silicon or germanium crystal doped with lithium ions. It has much better energy resolution than sodium iodide crystals but not as much sensitivity. See under *solid-state radiation detector.*

lithocholate (lith″o-ko′lat) [*litho-* + *cholate,* from Gr. *cholē* bile] any salt, ester, or dissociated form of lithocholic acid. See also *glycocholate* and *lithocholic acid.*

lithocholic acid (lith″o-ko′lic) 3α-hydroxy-5β-cholan-24-oic acid. It is formed by bacterial action in the gut by 7-dehydroxylation of chenodeoxycholic acid. Most of the lithocholic acid is lost in the feces. A small amount, however, undergoes enterohepatic circulation. Among the bile acids, lithocholic acid is relatively toxic to the liver (and other cells) and may play a role in the pathogenesis of liver disease after biliary stasis.

lithotroph (lith′o-trōf) [*litho-* + Gr. *trophē* nutrition] see *autotroph.*

litmus (lit′mus) [Old Norse *litmosi* dye-moss] an amphoteric pigment that is prepared from the lichen *Roccella tinctoria* and consists principally of a polymer of 7-hydroxy-2-phenoxazone. It is widely used as a pH indicator, with a pH range of 4.5 (red)–8.3 (blue).

litre (le′ter) [Fr.] see *liter.*

Little's disease (lit′elz) [William John *Little,* English physician, 1810–1894] see *cerebral p. syndromes* under *palsy.*

littoral cell a macrophage attached to the lining of the vascular sinusoids of the spleen, bone marrow, liver, and lymph nodes (sinus histiocyte). The term littoral cell is given a broader connotation by some histologists who use it as a synonym for the fenestrated endothelial cells of the sinusoids.

liver (liv′er) [L. *jecur;* Gr. *hēpar*] the large accessory organ of the gastrointestinal tract that lies in the right upper abdomen, tucked under the diaphragm. The liver develops from the distal foregut and weighs roughly 1500 g in the adult. Peritoneum covers most of its surface, and is reflected onto the anterior abdominal wall as the falciform ligament and onto the lesser curvature of the stomach as the lesser omentum. The liver has two lobes (the right larger than the left), although there are no external markings precisely indicating the separation. A cleft on the undersurface of the liver, the porta hepatis, is the site at which three important structures enter or leave the organ: the hepatic artery, which brings blood from the celiac artery; the portal vein, which carries venous blood from the abdominal alimentary canal; and the common bile duct, formed by the union of the right and left hepatic ducts in the porta, through which bile leaves the liver. A short side branch of the common bile duct, the cystic duct, leads to the gallbladder beneath the right lobe. The common bile duct enters the second part of the duodenum with the main pancreatic duct.

Despite the diversity of the liver's functions, its parenchymal cells, called hepatocytes, are of a single type. They are arranged in sheets one cell thick, which curve and branch to produce a spongelike structure that is tunneled by slender sinusoids. In a histologic section, connective tissue investing the vessels and bile ducts subdivides the hepatocytes into lobules that are roughly hexagonal. The branches of the hepatic artery, portal vein, and bile duct, with their surrounding connective tissue, constitute portal tracts or triads. Within a lobule, the sinusoids are arranged radially and converge on a small central vein, a tributary of the main hepatic veins that empty into the inferior vena cava. Arterial blood and portal venous blood from vessels in the portal tracts enter the sinusoids and percolate through them to the central vein. Mixing of hepatic arterial and portal venous blood thus occurs within the sinusoids; if the presinusoidal sphincters of arterioles within the portal tracts are damaged, arterial pressures can be transmitted to the portal circulation. Although the hepatic artery carries only one-fifth of the liver's blood supply, it conveys half of the oxygen; thus, the central zones of the lobules are particularly vulnerable in anoxic conditions. Elevated venous pressure in the systemic circulation, as from a failing heart, is transmitted first to the central veins of the liver lobules.

Interchange between the blood within the sinusoids and the hepatocytes takes place across the attenuated and fenestrated endothelium of the sinusoid and a slender space of Disse into which microvilli of the hepatocytes project. Mononuclear phagocytes (Kupffer cells) are attached to the inner surface of the sinusoids.

The liver has many functions, including the metabolism of carbohydrates, fats, proteins, and vitamins; the detoxication of drugs; and the formation and excretion of bile. Bile passes to the periphery of a lobule through slender canaliculi, which are mere separations of the adjacent cell membranes of two hepatocytes, and enters small bile ductules within the portal tracts.

liver cell carcinoma a malignant neoplasm of hepatocytes, often associated with cirrhosis. It is particularly common in some areas of Africa. The tumor cells vary in their degree of differentiation, and distinction from a metastatic carcinoma may be difficult on biopsy. The cells may be solidly grouped or may form sheets and cords that line the sinusoidal channels. Bile formation is sometimes demonstrable, and most liver cell carcinomas form alpha$_1$-fetoprotein. Vascular invasion is common, with the development of lung metastases, although regional lymph node involvement and intraabdominal extension also occur. The prognosis is worse in tumors that arise in cirrhotic livers. Also called *hepatocellular carcinoma* and *hepatoma.*

liver scan a radionuclide scan using either a scintillation camera or a rectilinear scanner. Static images of the liver, which show its size and position and lesions larger than about 2 cm, are obtained using technetium Tc 99m sulfur colloid. Intravenously injected colloidal particles are ingested by the reticuloendothelial (RES) cells in the liver and spleen. Those areas containing fewer or no RES cells then appear as cold spots on the image. Intravenously injected HIDA and related compounds are cleared by the hepatocytes of the liver and excreted in bile. A scan with these materials shows some of the same features as the sulfur colloid scan in the liver, but does not show the spleen. In addition, it may reveal total obstruction of the common bile duct or the cystic duct to the gallbladder if either is present. The latter is a useful aid to the diagnosis of acute cholecystitis. See also *cholangiography; cholecystography; selective a.* under *arteriography;* and *ultrasonography.*

liver spots see *tinea versicolor.*

lixiviation (liks″iv-e-a′shun) [L. *lixivia* lye] the separation of soluble from insoluble matter by dissolving out the soluble matter and drawing off the solution. Also called *leaching.*

L layer the outer membrane layer of the cell wall of a gram-negative bacterium.

lm abbrev. See *lumen.*

Loa (lo′ah) [a native word in Angola, West Africa] a genus of tissue-inhabiting nematodes that is parasitic in humans.

L. loa, a species of threadlike worms, found in West and Central Africa, that causes loiasis. The males measure 30–34 mm in length, and the females average 59–70 mm. Both are filiform, semitransparent, and bluntly tapered at each end. The parasite is acquired through the bite of infected tabanid flies of the genus *Chrysops.* The larvae, which are approximately 2 mm long, mature slowly in the subcutaneous tissues. Adult worms migrate through the subcutaneous tissues, causing a temporary inflammation known as fugitive or calabar swelling.

Laboratory diagnosis requires identification of the microfilariae in thick smears from peripheral blood or in fluid from the fugitive or calabar swelling. The microfilariae can be concentrated by Knott's modified survey method or a filter technique. *L. loa* should be differentiated from other sheathed microfilariae (*Wuchereria bancrofti* and *Brugia malayi*); it is characterized by a tapering tail and the position of its caudal nuclei, diurnal periodicity, and a larger body nucleus that stains less deeply. Immunologic tests, such as the indirect fluorescent antibody test with *Dipetalonema viteae* antigen, have been found useful. Certain filarial worms can be made visible in humans by use of a simple fluorescent method after the administration of tetracycline.

Also called *eye worm, Filaria lacrymalis, F. oculi, F. subconjunctivalis,* and *microfilaria diurna.* See also *loiasis.*

load (lōd) 1. any burden or resistance, particularly the electrical power drawn from a power or signal source, the power consumed by the burden on a machine, or the weight supported by a structure. The term also refers to the resistor drag or weight causing the burden.

2. an above-normal body content of some substance, particularly water, salt, or carbohydrate. A below-normal content is a negative load, and the process of inducing this load is called loading.

3. the transfer of data from a computer memory to a register for processing, or the instruction causing this transfer.

4. to move a compiled or assembled program into memory for execution. The program that does this is called a loader.

load factor the fraction of the time an item of equipment is in use. See also *queuing theory.*

lob/o (lo'bo) [L. *lobus,* from Gr. *lobos* lobe] a word element used in combining form to denote lobe, e.g., lobular.

lobar (lo'bar) pertaining to or affecting a lobe.

lobate (lo'bāt) [L. *lobatus*] having or divided into lobes.

lobe (lōb) 1. a more or less well defined portion of an organ. Lobes may be demarcated by fissures, sulci, or connective tissue.

2. one of the main divisions of the crown of a tooth, developmentally representing a center of calcification.

lobeline (lo'be-lēn) the principal alkaloid extracted from the herb *Lobelia inflata.* Lobeline was formerly used as an analeptic and is currently used in antismoking preparations. It is similar to nicotine but less potent.

lobomycosis (lo"bo-mi-ko'sis) a chronic, localized subcutaneous fungal disease caused by the fungus *Loboa loboi.* This disease begins with an initial infection through trauma to the skin and is characterized by small, hard, painless nodules that resemble keloids.

lobster claw deformity a developmental anomaly in which deep clefts are present in the middle of the hand or foot, and the fingers and toes demonstrate varying degrees of syndactyly.

lobular (lob'u-lar) [L. *lobularis*] of or pertaining to a small lobe.

lobular carcinoma a form of carcinoma of the breast in which the cells arise from the breast lobules; when invasive, the cells tend to infiltrate in a single-file pattern. Bilateral involvement is more frequent than with duct cell breast cancers. See also *breast tumors.*

local (lo'kal) [L. *localis*] restricted to an area or region; not general.

local immunity see under *immunity.*

localization (lo"kah-lĭ-za'shun) 1. the determination of the site or particular area where some process, object, or lesion is found. See also *foreign body localization.*

2. restriction to a limited area.

locant (lo'kant) a symbol (usually a number but sometimes a letter) in a systematic chemical name that indicates the position in the parent compound of a substituent group, a multiple bond, or the functional group; the carbon atoms of an unbranched chain or ring are numbered consecutively. The carbon atom in the functional group or to which the functional group is attached is numbered 1 for terminal functional groups. The locant of a multiple bond is the lower numbered atom in the bond. For example, 4-fluoro-2-butenal is $CH_2F{-}CH{=}CH{-}CHO$.

location (lo-ka'shun) in statistics, the property of a population measured by the mean or median, either of which is called a location parameter.

lockjaw (lok'jaw) see *tetanus.*

locus (lo'kus), pl. *loci* [L.] 1. [NA], a general term for a site in the body.

2. the place on a chromosome occupied by a particular gene or its alleles.

Löffler's coagulated serum medium (lef'lerz) [Friederich August Johannes *Löffler,* German bacteriologist, 1852–1915] see *Löffler's coagulated serum m.* under *medium.*

Löffler's endocarditis [Wilhelm *Löffler,* Swiss physician, born 1887] fibroplastic endocarditis associated with persistent and profound eosinophilia. The cardiac involvement is thought to be a consequence of prolonged exposure to products released from the eosinophils. The eosinophilic myocarditis of the primary stage progresses toward a fibroplastic thickening of the endocardium, and mural thrombi. Among the most prominent clinical manifestations of Löffler's endocarditis are congestive heart failure and systemic embolism.

Löffler's syndrome [Wilhelm *Löffler*] a benign, self-limited form of pulmonary eosinophilia that results in little or no permanent tissue damage. The clinical manifestations include a low-grade fever, weight loss, general malaise, and, most important, the presence of transient, focal pulmonary infiltrates due to a peripheral eosinophilia. It may be attributed to a type I allergic reaction to causative agents such as parasitic helminths, chemicals such as nickel carbonyl, and drugs such as sulfonamides, chlorpropamide, and *p*-aminosalicylic acid.

log (log) 1. a comprehensive record of work done, such as a daily record of all specimens received and tests performed by a laboratory, or a permanent record of all calibration work and/or maintenance checks executed in the laboratory as a whole or relating to a given instrument.

2. abbrev. for logarithm (base 10).

log/o (log′o) [Gr. *logos* word, reasoned speech] a word element used in combining form to denote words or speech, e.g., logopathy.

logarithm (log′ah-rith″m) the inverse function of exponentiation. If $x = b^y$, then $y = \log_b x$ (y equals the logarithm of x to the base b); b is a fixed constant. Base 10 logarithms are called common or briggsian logarithms; an unspecified base is normally 10. Base e logarithms are called natural or naperian logarithms and often are denoted $\ln x$ instead of $\log_e x$.

logarithmic (log″ah-rith′mik) pertaining to a logarithm.

logarithmic curve the graph of the function $y = \log cx$, where c is a constant.

logarithmic phase see *logarithmic p.* under *phase.*

logic (loj′ik) 1. the study of reasoning, particularly of methods by which valid conclusions can be drawn from stated propositions.

2. the branch of mathematics that deals with logical inference, in which propositions and relations are represented by mathematical symbols, and proofs are stated using rigorous formal mathematics. Also called *symbolic logic.*

3. in electronics, circuitry designed to perform logical operations. See also *complementary metal oxide semiconductor logic, emitter-coupled logic, logic circuit,* and *transistor-transistor logic.*

logical (loj′ik-al) pertaining or referring to logic.

logical function 1. the result of a logical operation considered as a function of its operands.

2. see *logic element.*

logical instruction a machine-language instruction for a digital computer in which a logical operation (such as AND, OR, exclusive OR) is applied to the corresponding bits of two words to produce each bit of the result.

logical operation a mathematical or computer language operation that operates on two-valued (true or false) logical variables. The basic logical operators are AND, OR, and NOT. NOT operates on one variable, changing true to false and vice versa. AND and OR are binary operators. The result of an AND is true only if both operands are true; the result of an OR is true only if either operand is true. NAND and NOR are short for the combined operations NOT-AND (i.e., AND followed by NOT) and NOT-OR. EXCLUSIVE-OR, usually available only in assembly language, produces a true result if either operand is true (but not both).

logical variable in computer languages, such as FORTRAN and PL/1, a variable that can have either a true or a false value. In ALGOL, these are called boolean variables. See also *logical operation.*

logic circuit an electronic circuit that performs a logical operation. It may have more than two inputs; for example, one type, called AND gate, produces an output only if all of its inputs are on. See also *gate.*

logic device see *logic element.*

logic diagram a diagram of electronic logic circuitry that shows the various symbolic logic elements (gates) and their interconnections but not the electronic components in the gates. See also *logical operation.*

logic element an electronic device that performs a logical operation. Also called *gate.*

logit (loj′it) a function; $\text{logit}(x) = [\log x/(1-x)]$, sometimes used to transform data relating the fraction of material reacted to the concentration of one of the reactants, so that a linear function of the latter is obtained. The blood oxygen dissociation curve (relating the percentage of hemoglobin that is oxygenated as a function of the Po_2) and radioimmunoassay standardization curves are examples in which the logit transformation is useful.

lognormal distribution (log-nor′mal) in statistics, a probability distribution; the logarithm of a lognormal variable has the normal distribution. This distribution is sometimes used for determining reference intervals; the usual statistical procedures are used on the logarithms of the raw data.

-logy (lo′je) [Gr. *logos* word, reasoned speech] a suffix word element to denote the science or study of, e.g., hematology.

loiasis (lo-i′ah-sis) a form of filariasis that is due to infection with the filarial nematode *Loa loa.* Transmitted to humans by the bite of deerflies of the genus *Chrysops,* this disease is found in individuals in Central and West Africa. Adult worms mature within 12 mo and migrate subcutaneously, often producing transient local swellings (calabar swellings) due to severe immunologic reactions. Migration may occur subconjunctivally, resulting in irritation, lacrimation, and a foreign-body sensation.

Laboratory examination reveals eosinophilia and a positive complement-fixation test; diagnosis may be confirmed by demonstration of blood microfilaria or adult worms in the tissue swellings. The prognosis is good following treatment with diethylcarbamazine.

See also *L. loa* under *Loa.*

lomustine (lo-mus′tēn) a cancer chemotherapeutic drug. For more information, see *Appendix A.*

London force the intermolecular attraction due to the electrostatic force between temporary dipoles in molecules. The motion of the electrons produces a fluctuating dipole moment, and the temporary dipole field of a molecule induces parallel dipoles in nearby molecules. Also called dispersion force. See also *van der Waals forces.*

long-acting thyroid stimulator (LATS) an IgG immunoglobulin that is demonstrable in the majority of those with Graves' disease. LATS activity was originally defined by a bioassay in which injection of the patient's serum into mice produces a release of thyroid hormones, peaking at about 16 hr, as opposed to the 2-hr peak produced by thyroid-stimulating hormone (TSH). This action is presumably caused by binding of these immunoglobulins at the TSH receptor sites of the thyroid gland. Recently, radioreceptor assay has been used to demonstrate IgG that competitively inhibits the binding of radiolabeled bovine TSH to human TSH receptor sites. The assay for LATS has now been replaced by *thyroid-stimulating immunoglobulins* (TSI).

long-acting thyroid-stimulator hormone assay 1. bioassay in which the patient's serum is injected into mice; a prolonged release of thyroid hormones indicates the presence of LATS.

2. LATS has more recently been determined im-

munologically; LATS is an autoantibody (IgG) formed against a thyroid protein and mimics most actions of thyrotropin. Thirty-five percent of patients with Graves' disease and some patients with Hashimoto's disease have detectable levels of LATS; in normal individuals, none is detected.

long bone a bone having a longitudinal axis of considerable length, that consists of a shaft (the diaphysis) and an expanded portion (the epiphysis) at each end, which is usually articular; any of the long bones of the limbs.

longitudinal (lon″jĭ-too′dĭ-nal) [L. *longitude* length] lengthwise; parallel to the long axis of the body or a body part.

loop (lo͞op) 1. a turn, curve, or bend in a cord, fiber, or tubular structure. See also *ansa*.

2. a sequence of statements in a computer program that are executed repeatedly, either a fixed number of times that have been set before entry into the loop or until some termination condition is satisfied.

3. in microbiology, a device consisting of a long, narrow shank that holds a short wire formed into a loop at the free end. It is used for the inoculation of bacterial cultures. The standard loop has an inside diameter of 4 mm.

looping (loop′ing) see *iteration*.

lophotrichous (lo-fot′rĭ-kus) [Gr. *lophos* crest + *thrix* hair] a term used to describe a rod-shaped bacterial cell having a tuft of flagella at one or both ends. See also *flagellum*.

lorazepam (lor-ah′ze-pam) a benzodiazepine compound, similar to diazepam, that is used as an antianxiety drug. Adverse reactions include sedation, weakness, and dizziness. It potentiates the effects of alcohol, barbiturates, and other central nervous system depressants and can produce tolerance with long-term use. Withdrawal symptoms are similar to those of alcohol or barbiturate withdrawal. Trademark, *Ativan*.

lord/o (lor′do) [Gr. *lordos* bent backward] a word element used in combining form to denote swayback or curve, e.g., lordosis.

lordosis (lor-do′sis) [Gr. "a bending backward"] 1. a curvature of the spine that is concave toward the rear, resulting from either the normal curvature of the cervical and lumbar regions or an abnormally increased concavity, particularly in the lumbar region (hollow back). Cf. *kyphosis* and *scoliosis*.

2. the increase in the posterior concavity of the spine that occurs in bending backward.

lordotic (lor-dot′ik) pertaining to lordosis.

lordotic view a semiaxial posterior or anterior radiographic view of the lungs and mediastinum. It is obtained using a horizontal central ray, with the patient leaning backward at an angle of approximately 45°. Both views demonstrate interlobular effusions; the posterior view demonstrates the lung apices also, and is also called the *apical lordotic view*.

lot (lot) a batch of manufactured materials, such as chemical reagents or electronic components, which have been manufactured either in one production run from homogeneous raw materials or in several production runs and have been subjected to uniform quality control testing. The items of a lot are marked with an identifying lot number. For reagent-grade chemicals, aliquots of each lot are analyzed, and the actual amount of each impurity is reported on the label.

louse (lows), pl. *lice* [L. *pediculus*] a general term that encompasses various parasitic insects. Lice are small, wingless insects that are parasitic in humans. The biting lice, order Mallophaga, are found on birds and other mammals but rarely on humans. The sucking lice, order Anoplura, include the family Pediculidae, which is parasitic in humans.

Lice are known vectors of relapsing fever, typhus, and trench fever. They occur worldwide, especially in cooler climates where wool clothing is worn.

See also *pediculosis*.

body l., see *P. humanus corporis* under *Pediculus*.
crab l., see *P. pubis* under *Phthirus*.
head l., see *P. humanus capitis* under *Pediculus*.
pubic l., see *P. pubis* under *Phthirus*.

lousiness (lows′e-nes) pertaining to an environment where lice exist. See also *typhus*.

low back pain pain in the lower back, frequently due to osteoarthritis. Other causes include a ruptured intervertebral disk, congenital bony defects, trauma, infection, tumor, and back strain due to pregnancy, obesity, or strenuous work. It is not always possible to determine the precise cause of the pain.

X-rays should include oblique films to show the intervertebral facet joints. Depending on the clinical context, other investigations may be necessary, including analysis of spinal fluid to detect infection, computed tomography of the spine, and myelography to localize a compressive lesion when surgery or radiation therapy is contemplated. Treatment depends on the underlying cause.

Also called *lumbago*.

Low-Beer position a position used for radiography of the petrous portion of the temporal bone. See under *parietotemporal projections*.

low-density lipoprotein see *low-density l.* under *lipoprotein*.

Lowenstein-Jensen medium (LJM) [Ernst *Löwenstein*, Vienna pathologist, born 1878] see *Löwenstein-Jensen m.* under *medium*.

Lowe's syndrome (lōz) [Charles Upton *Lowe*, American pediatrician, born 1921] see *oculocerebrorenal syndrome*.

low level the more negative of the two output levels of a digital logic circuit.

low-level language a computer language in which the programmer directly specifies each machine language instruction of the program. Also called assembly language.

low order pertaining to the least significant digit, bit, or byte of a computer word or register.

loxapine (loks′ah-pēn) a dibenzoxazepine major tranquilizer used in the management of psychotic disorders. It is chemically unrelated to phenothiazine, thioxanthene, or butyrophenone major tranquilizers; however, its action and side-effects are similar. Adverse reactions include drowsiness, dizziness, confusion, and extrapyramidal effects such as restlessness, parkinsonism, and dyskinesia. Persistent tardive dyskinesia may also appear during or after long-term therapy.

l. hydrochloride, the salt of loxapine used in oral concentrate solutions.

l. succinate, the salt of loxapine used in capsules.

Loxosceles (loks-os′sĕ-lez) [NL., from Gr. *loxos*

slanting + *skelos* leg] a genus of six-eyed spiders of the family Loxoscelidae, distributed throughout the temperate and tropical zones of the world. The spiders are nocturnal; they inhabit basements and caves, and may also be found beneath stones and the bark of trees.

L. laeta, the brown spider, which causes loxoscelism in individuals in the central region of South America. The bite is followed by a painful erythematous vesicle and progresses to a gangrenous slough of the affected area.

L. reclusa, the brown recluse spider, which causes loxoscelism in individuals in North America. The bite causes stinging and mild-to-severe pain, resulting in a blister and ulceration; it may evoke a systemic reaction in children.

L-phase variant a variant phase of certain bacteria induced by penicillin or high salt concentration. It exists in spherical form with a defective or absent cell wall, yet is capable of growth and multiplication. Often stable but sometimes able to revert to the normal bacterial cell, such cells may be responsible for latency in infectious disease. The terms L-phase variants and L-phase of bacteria have been used interchangeably with the designation L-forms.

LPO abbrev. See *left posterior oblique.*

LPS abbrev. See *lipase.*

Lp-X abbrev. See *lipoprotein-X.*

Lr symbol for the chemical element *lawrencium.*

LSD abbrev. See *least significant digit* and *lysergic acid diethylamide.*

LSH abbrev. See *lymphocyte-stimulating hormone.*

LSI abbrev. See *large-scale integration.*

L/S ratio abbrev. See *lecithin/sphingomyelin ratio.*

LT abbrev. See *lymphotoxin.*

LTA abbrev. See *l. A* under *leukotriene.*

LTB abbrev. See *l. B* under *leukotriene.*

LTC abbrev. See *l. C* under *leukotriene.*

LTD abbrev. See *l. D* under *leukotriene.*

LTH abbrev. See *luteotropic hormone.*

Lu symbol for the chemical element *lutetium.*

luc/o (loo′ko) [L. *lux* light] a word element used in combining form to denote light or transparency, e.g., lucotherapy.

lucent (loo′sent) [L. *lucens,* from *lucere* to shine] translucent or radiolucent; used in radiology to designate lesions of the lungs or other parts that are characterized by a greater than normal amount of air or fat.

Lucilia (loo-sil′e-ah) a genus of greenbottle flies of widespread distribution. Larvae of the species *L. caesar* (the gold fly) and *L. sericata* (also called *Phaenicia sericata*) have been found in cutaneous, intestinal, and genitourinary myiasis.

Ludwig's angina (lood′vigz) [Wilhelm Friedrich von *Ludwig,* German surgeon, 1790–1865] a diffuse cellulitis of the submandibular space, floor of the mouth, connective tissue, fascia, and muscles, but usually not of the glandular structures of the neck. A characteristic manifestation of the disease is gangrene with serosanguineous, putrid infiltration but little or no frank pus. Spread of the cellulitis is by continuity rather than by lymphatics. Bilateral involvement commonly occurs; embarrassment of the airway is one of the serious complications. Anaerobes are often the causal agents and may or may not involve group A streptococci.

Lugol's solution (loo-golz′) [Jean Guillaume Auguste *Lugol,* French physician, 1786–1851] see *i. solution, strong,* under *iodine.*

lumb/o (lum′bo) [L. *lumbus* loin] a world element used in combining form to denote the lower back or loins, e.g., lumbocolostomy.

lumbago (lum-ba′go) see *low back pain.*

lumbar (lum′bar) pertaining to the loins, the part of the back between the thorax and the pelvis.

lumbarization (lum″ber-ĭ-za′shun) a congenital malformation in which the first segment of the sacrum is not fused with the second but coalesces with the transverse processes of the fifth lumbar vertebra. Thus, the result is an extra vertebra and only four segments to the sacrum.

lumbar plexus (lum′ber plek′sus) see *lumbar p.* under *plexus.*

lumbar puncture a procedure performed to sample the cerebrospinal fluid (CSF) for diagnostic studies, to inject radiopaque dyes, or to inject medications intrathecally. It is performed by passing a needle in the midline between the spines of the third and fourth (or fourth and fifth) lumbar vertebrae into the lumbar subarachnoid space. CSF may be removed and analyzed to yield information about a variety of neoplastic, infective, inflammatory, degenerative, traumatic, or vascular conditions affecting the central nervous system or meninges.

Subarachnoid hemorrhage produces a bloody CSF, which must be differentiated from that due to local trauma in performing the lumbar puncture; the degree of xanthochromia provides a rough index of the length of time the red cells have been in the fluid. Characteristic gamma-globulin profiles in the CSF may support a clinical diagnosis of multiple sclerosis. Purulent meningitis causes a CSF with increased protein and white cell content, decreased glucose concentration, and elevated pressure. Cytology, culture, and serology of the CSF may also provide diagnostic information about conditions such as metastatic meningeal carcinoma, various types of nonpurulent or chronic meningitis, neurosyphilis, the various encephalitides, and a number of other conditions.

Lumbar puncture may also be used to administer anesthetic agents in spinal anesthesia. Antibiotics and chemotherapeutic agents may be introduced into the CSF to treat CNS infections and malignancies. In these cases, an amount of CSF is withdrawn that is equal to the amount of drug to be administered.

This procedure is relatively simple but should never be performed if evidence of increased intracranial pressure is present unless it is essential for diagnosis and special precautions are taken, as it may lead to fatal complications. Other relative contraindications may include nearby local infections, septicemia, and coagulation disorders, depending on the circumstances. Headache, dizziness, and nausea are common and usually short-lived sequelae of an otherwise uncomplicated lumbar puncture.

Also called *spinal puncture.* See also *cerebrospinal fluid assays.* Cf. *cisternal puncture.*

lumbar region 1. a region of the back between the

rib cage and the pelvis and to one side of the vertebral column.

2. a region of the abdomen below the transpyloric plane, above the transtubercular plane, and to the outside of a lateral sagittal plane, i.e., on either side of the umbilical region; used in radiographic positioning. Also called *lateral abdominal region.* See illustration under *abdominal regions.*

lumbosacral (lum″bo-sa′kral) pertaining to the loins and sacrum.

lumbosacral plexus a term applied to the combined lumbar and sacral nerve plexuses.

lumbricosis (lum″brĭ-ko′sis) being infected with lumbrici (ascarides). See also *ascariasis.*

lumbricus (lum-bri′kus), pl. *lumbrici* [L. "earthworm"] 1. the ascaris, a worm of the genus *Ascaris* (a large intestinal nematode parasite). See also *ascariasis.*

2. an earthworm.

lumen (loo′men) [L. "light"] 1. (pl. *lumina*), the cavity or channel within a tube or tubular organ, such as an artery or the intestine.

2. (abbrev. lm; pl. *lumens*), the International System (SI) unit of luminous flux equal to 1 candela-steradian (cd·sr).

luminal (loo′mĭ-nal) pertaining to the lumen of a hollow organ or structure.

luminescence (loo″mĭ-nes′ens) the emission of light due to a nonthermal process such as a chemical reaction or the absorption of ionizing radiation.

luminescent (loo″mĭ-nes′ent) able to exhibit luminescence.

luminophore (loo′mĭ-no-fōr″) [L. *lumen* light + Gr. *phoros* bearing] the part of a compound that absorbs and emits photons and thus makes the compound luminescent.

luminous (loo′mĭ-nus) emitting or reflecting light; glowing with light.

luminous flux the radiant power per unit time falling on a surface, measured according to response of the human eye to the light. It is measured in units of lumens (lm).

luminous flux density the luminous flux per unit area falling on a surface; measured in units of lux (lx). Also called *illuminance.*

luminous intensity the luminous flux falling on a surface divided by the solid angle that the surface subtends; measured in units of candelas (cd).

lunate (loo′nāt) [L. *lunatus* crescent-shaped, from *luna* moon] moon-shaped or crescentic.

lunate bone one of the carpal bones. It lies between the scaphoid and triquetrum, and articulates with the radius and with other carpal bones.

lung (lung) [L. *pulmo;* Gr. *pneumōn* or *pleumōn*] the organ of respiration; either of the paired organs that effect the aeration of the blood. Exchange of oxygen and carbon dioxide between the inspired air and the blood takes place in the alveoli of the lungs.

The lungs develop from the lung bud, an outpouching of the ventral wall of the foregut, that migrates into the surrounding mesoderm and bifurcates, growing to form the right and left lungs. Fissures subdivide the lungs into lobes that attach at the root or hilum on the mediastinal surface of the lung where the bronchi and vessels enter. Each lung has an oblique fissure that forms upper and lower lobes; the right lung also has a transverse fissure that creates an additional middle lobe. The lungs are covered over most of their surface by a serous membrane, the pleura, with its visceral layer intimately investing the lung surface and extending into the fissures. The negative pressure within the pleural space causes the lung to expand with movements of the chest wall and diaphragm. Expiration is normally passive, the elasticity of the lung causing it to resume its resting size and shape.

Air reaches the alveoli by traversing the tubular respiratory passages. The main bronchi are formed by the bifurcation of the trachea, and progressively smaller subdivisions of the bronchial tree lead ultimately to the alveoli. The wall of a bronchus is reinforced by small plates of cartilage. Respiratory passages that are smaller than 1 mm in diameter no longer have cartilage in their walls and are called bronchioles. There are roughly 16 subdivisions of the bronchial passages within the conducting zone, which ends at the terminal bronchioles (diameter, approximately 0.5 mm). The subdivisions of the terminal bronchioles are the respiratory bronchioles, which give rise to alveolar ducts, alveolar sacs, and alveoli. As a few alveoli open directly off the walls of the respiratory bronchioles, the functional zone of the lung commences at the respiratory bronchioles (respiratory zone). A terminal bronchiole with its peripheral ramifications is therefore a functional unit and is called a pulmonary lobule. The cross-sectional diameter of the respiratory passages expands rapidly at the level of the terminal bronchioles, and movement of air within the respiratory zone is by diffusion. The bronchopulmonary segments are roughly fourth-order branches of the bronchial tree with their distal subdivisions. There are 10 segments in the right lung and 8 in the left, but intersegmental flow of air probably can occur and there are no obvious connective tissue septa separating the segments.

An alveolus is a small outpouching of an alveolar sac, connected to its neighbors through small pores (pores of Kohn). Between adjacent alveoli, the thin septum contains collagen and elastic fibrils, some macrophages, a few fibroblasts, and a dense network of capillaries. Each alveolus is lined by cells with markedly attenuated cytoplasm, the type-1 pneumocytes, but also contains a few type-2 pneumocytes, spherical cells that form the surface tension–reducing material, surfactant. A basal lamina separates the alveolar lining cells from septal capillaries, and the gas diffusion barrier therefore consists of the thin epithelium of the type-1 pneumocyte, the fused basal laminae of the alveolar lining cell and septal capillary, and the endothelium of the capillary. Through this barrier, oxygen from the inspired air reaches the erythrocytes in the alveolar capillaries, and carbon dioxide is eliminated from the blood into the alveoli.

Although the lungs can be expanded voluntarily under cerebral control, respiration is normally under control of the pons and medulla. Respiration is influenced by the oxygen content of the blood, which is monitored by the carotid and aortic bodies, but the basic control stimulus is the concentration of hydrogen ions in the blood as sensed by a chemosensitive area in the ventral medulla.

Respiratory function can be evaluated by blood gas analysis, noninvasive pulmonary studies, bronchoscopy, and bronchography. Cytologic examinations are performed on sputum and bronchial washings and brushings. Biopsies can be obtained through a bronchoscope or by percutaneous fine needle aspiration. When the clinical situation warrants, an open lung biopsy can provide tissue for light and electron microscopy, microbiology, and other studies. Some pulmonary diseases cause the accumulation of fluid within the pleural cavity that can be withdrawn and examined cytologically and chemically. See also *lung tumors, pleural fluid,* and *pleural fluid examination.*

lung fluke a parasitic worm that infests the lungs. In humans, the trematode *Paragonimus westermani* causes lung fluke disease.

lung scan see *pulmonary perfusion scan.*

lung tumors neoplasms of the lung. The great majority of pulmonary neoplasms arise from the epithelium of the respiratory passages or associated mucous glands; primary mesenchymal neoplasms of the lung are uncommon. Most pathologists subclassify carcinomas of the lung into four types: adenocarcinoma, squamous carcinoma, and undifferentiated large cell and undifferentiated small cell carcinoma. Carcinoid tumors form a separate group, and are distinct from the infrequent bronchial gland mucoepidermoid and adenoid cystic tumors. Histologic diagnosis of a lung tumor is based on study of cytologic smears of sputum, bronchial washings, or brushings; bronchoscopic biopsy; fine-needle aspiration biopsy; cytologic examination of pleural effusions; or biopsy or resection at thoracotomy. In some instances, the diagnosis is based on a study of cells in a metastatic site such as a scalene lymph node in a patient who clinically and radiologically has a primary lung tumor.

The extent of the disease at the time of diagnosis is determined by accumulation of information from a number of staging procedures, including the physical examination, radiologic studies and scans, bronchoscopy, and mediastinoscopy, and after surgery, from the report of the pathologist. Clinical staging allows some estimate of prognosis and is helpful in selecting therapy. The stage may be revised during or after treatment. Nomenclature for staging (see *tumor staging*) is commonly used.

A basic subdivision of pulmonary carcinomas into small cell undifferentiated carcinoma (30 percent) and other types (nonsmall cell tumors) (70 percent of lung cancers) is clinically relevant, as the small cell carcinoma differs from the others in its mode of spread and response to chemotherapy. Ectopic hormone production can be associated with nonsmall cell lung cancers, but is seen more often with small cell cancers. ACTH and calcitonin are the most common hormonal polypeptides formed by these tumors, and their production may be used to monitor response to therapy.

In the United States, some 30 percent of carcinomas of the lung are adenocarcinomas, an incidence that seems to be increasing at the expense of squamous cell tumors. The majority of adenocarcinomas form peripheral masses that are not clearly related to bronchi. There may be evidence of some prior pathologic process in the involved area of the lung such as chronic pneumonitis with fibrosis or bronchiectasis. If the tumor reaches the pleura, histologic distinction from a mesothelioma may become a problem. Diagnosis of an adenocarcinoma of the lung by cytology or bronchoscopy is made less frequently than with more centrally located cancers. The degree of differentiation is determined by assessing the extent of gland formation and mucin production.

A small number of peripheral adenocarcinomas are composed of tall columnar cells that spread over the existing alveolar framework, form papillary structures, and display ultrastructural features of cells of the distal respiratory passages, notably the nonciliated bronchiolar (Clara) cell. They are termed bronchiolar, alveolar cell, or bronchiolo-alveolar cell carcinomas. Precision in the recognition of the bronchiolar variant of lung adenocarcinoma is difficult by light microscopy alone.

Squamous carcinoma currently makes up in excess of 30 percent of cancers of the lung in the United States. More than two-thirds are centrally located and involve a bronchus. Almost 50 percent of superior sulcus (Pancoast) tumors are squamous in type. The degree of histologic differentiation of a bronchogenic squamous cancer has some prognostic value, although not as great as clinical staging. Regional lymph node metastases are principally seen with the larger tumors. Because of their usually central location and continuity with the bronchial tree, a positive diagnosis is frequently made from sputum cytology. Eighty percent show mixtures of keratinizing and nonkeratinizing cells. Mixtures of squamous and adenocarcinomas are relatively common among lung tumors, but usually one component clearly predominates. Metastases involving the liver, bones, or adrenal glands are seen in roughly one-quarter of patients with squamous carcinoma of the lung examined at autopsy.

Adenocarcinomas and squamous carcinomas of the lung may dedifferentiate; that is, they may progressively lose their distinctive morphologic features and become indistinguishable. A point is reached at which differentiating features can no longer be detected; the tumor is then termed an undifferentiated large cell carcinoma. In some, a minor degree of differentiation can be found by electron microscopy. Approximately 15 percent of cancers of the lung fall into the undifferentiated large cell category. The cells are larger and have some cytologic differences from those of most small cell lung cancers, but occasionally a tumor cannot be confidently placed in either category; e.g., it is made up of a mixture of the two cell types, or it represents a transitional form. The behavior of adenocarcinoma appears to parallel that of undifferentiated large cell carcinoma.

Small cell cancers of the lung are composed of round or elongated cells with scanty cytoplasm, generally forming diffuse sheets with frequent zones of necrosis. More than 70 percent are located in the vicinity of the hilum, but a bronchus may not be involved, and cytologic or bronchoscopic diagnosis may not be possible. Most small cell cancers have spread beyond the lung at the time of diagnosis, and consequently the prognosis is even poorer than for those with nonsmall cell tumors. Limited success is, however, being achieved with combination forms of chemotherapy and radiation. Clinical staging is usually confined to dividing the patients into those with limited and those with extensive disease, respectively. In limited disease, the tumor is confined to one hemithorax including ipsilateral supraclavicular lymph nodes; all other patients are considered to have extensive disease.

Most endocrine tumors occurring in the lungs are collectively designated as carcinoid tumors, despite

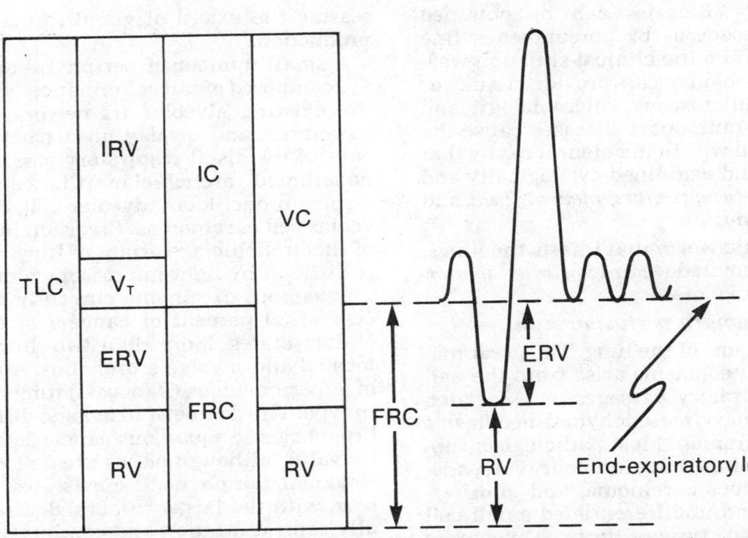

Lung volume subdivisions. Diagram of the components of lung volume: VC, vital capacity; RV, residual volume; FRC, functional residual capacity; V_T, tidal volume; ERV, expiratory reserve volume; IRV, inspiratory reserve volume; and IC, inspiratory capacity. (From Halsted, J. H., and Halsted, C. H.: The Laboratory in Clinical Medicine. 2nd ed.: Philadelphia, W. B. Saunders Co., 1981.)

the fact that immunocytochemical studies may fail to demonstrate serotonin within the cells (see also *carcinoid tumor*). Ultrastructurally, these tumors contain dense-core cytoplasmic granules 200–400 nm in diameter. Dense-core granules may also be found in some small cell lung cancers, but they are smaller and fewer in number than those of the typical carcinoid tumor. It is rarely possible to predict the course of a carcinoid tumor from its histology, but it should be regarded as having the potential for aggressive behavior and even metastasis. Small nests of cells similar to those seen in a carcinoid tumor may be encountered in the lungs, which have been designated as tumorlets.

In the United States, it is estimated that, if the trend continues, there will be nearly 300,000 new cases in the year 2000. Lung cancer is responsible for one-third of the cancer deaths in males. The gravity of the situation is increased by the poor prognosis associated with the disease, and by limited advances in therapy. Overall, males with lung cancer have a 5-yr survival rate of less than 30 percent when the diagnosis is made while the tumor is still localized; this figure falls below 10 percent when extension beyond the lung has occurred. As fewer than one patient in four is diagnosed at an early stage of the disease, the current outlook for patients with lung cancer is dismal. Screening programs applied to the general population have some value in detecting early cases, but they cannot economically be used on a large scale and are usually restricted to high-risk patients such as older males who have been heavy smokers. The increased likelihood of lung cancer incurred by cigarette smoking has been clearly documented, but other etiologic factors are not as well defined. An association with asbestos exposure has been shown, and a potent synergistic effect between asbestos and cigarette smoking in lung cancer has been reported.

lung volume subdivisions the various static parameters that comprise the total amount of gas in the lungs after a maximal inspiration. These include the tidal, inspiratory and expiratory reserve, and residual volume, and the vital, functional residual, and inspiratory capacities. A negative correlation exists between these static volumes and age, and a positive correlation with height. Measurement of the subdivisions of lung volume is a basic method still used to assess the status of pulmonary function. For more information, see the accompanying illustration and the specific subdivision terms.

lupus (loo′pus) [L. "wolf" or "pike"] a term originally referring only to localized destruction or degeneration of the skin as a result of any of a number of diseases. It is now commonly synonymous with *discoid* or *systemic l. erythematosus*.

discoid l. erythematosus (DLE), a skin disorder characterized by flat red lesions that scale and flake, leaving deep scars. Often the hair follicles are plugged, and atrophy of the skin occurs with loss or alteration of the hair. Dilated capillaries may be seen in these areas. DLE progresses to systemic lupus erythematosus in a small number of individuals.

Diagnosis is made on the basis of lesion appearance and from biopsies of the involved skin; there are essentially no diagnostic laboratory tests.

l. erythematosus (LE), an inflammatory disease encountered in one of two forms: the systemic, disseminated form or the discoid form.

systemic l. erythematosus (SLE), a disorder, primarily affecting women aged 20–40 yr, that is characterized by inflammation usually involving several organ systems. Most commonly, the disease manifests itself by skin lesions, including rashes, and by joint pain affecting several joints bilaterally. Other abnormalities may include decreased white cell, red cell, and platelet counts, and vascular inflammation of pericardial and pleural tissues and inflammation of the kidneys. At least 50 percent of those affected with SLE have central nervous system involvement, which arises from direct inflammation of the cerebral vessels or from the hypertension often found in these individuals. Widespread infarction of cerebral tissue may also be found, and SLE may present clinically as a seizure disorder or a psychiatric disturbance. Although the kidneys are involved in only 40 percent of SLE patients, the resultant decrease in kidney function is the major cause of death in severe SLE.

The disease is thought to be caused by the formation of antibodies against the body's own tissue and the subsequent trapping of antigen-antibody complexes in the capillaries of the affected organs. SLE usually arises spontaneously. However, it may be induced by certain drugs, most commonly by hydralazine and procainamide, and is usually reversible upon discontinuance of the drug. Viral infections in individuals genetically predisposed to the disease are thought to be an important etiologic factor.

Laboratory diagnosis, in addition to the abnormal blood counts, includes positive test results for the presence of antinuclear antibodies (ANA), antidouble-stranded DNA antibodies, increases in serum gamma globulins above 1.5 g/100 ml, a decrease in the levels of serum complement components C3 and C4, and an erythrocyte sedimentation rate above 20 ml/hr. Also, microscopic examination of blood smears or bone marrow may reveal neutrophils with eosinophilic, homogeneous, and round cytoplasmic inclusions. Such cells are called LE cells (see *lupus erythematosus cell*). Urinalysis may show abnormalities in those with kidney involvement, and studies showing deterioration of renal function also correlate with this complication. Histologic examination of the skin reveals a pattern similar to that of SLE.

Although there is no cure for this form of lupus, steroids and immunosuppressive drugs are often helpful in controlling its course, and 90 percent of those affected currently survive more than 10 yr.

lupus erythematosus cell (LE cell) a polymorphonuclear leukocyte found in the bone marrow and peripheral blood of SLE patients and characterized by the presence of a homogeneous, cytoplasmic mass which results from the reaction of the 7S IgG antibody with deoxyribonucleoprotein (DNA) and complement in the nucleus of damaged leukocytes. The mass is extruded from the cell and is then ingested by a polymorphonuclear leukocyte. LE cells are also found in diseases such as rheumatoid arthritis, scleroderma, and polydermatomyositis. Also called *Hargrave cell*. Cf. *tart cell*.

lupus erythematosus inhibitor a circulating anticoagulant that arises spontaneously in 5–10 percent of patients with lupus erythematosus. The inhibitor has the properties of an IgG immunoglobulin, and can be directed against Factors VIII or IX, or the Factor Xa-V-phospholipid complex. Usually it does not cause bleeding.

Luschka's ducts (lush′kahz) [Hubert von *Luschka*, German anatomist, 1820–1875] bile ducts located along the hepatic surface of the gallbladder that open directly into the liver.

luteal (loo′te-al) pertaining to or produced by the corpus luteum.

lutein (loo′te-in) [L. *luteus* yellow] a yellow pigment found in the corpus luteum, in fat cells, and in the yolk of eggs.

lutein cells the large, pale, polyhedral cells of the corpus luteum, which form progesterone and some estradiol.

luteinization (loo″te-in″ĭ-za′shun) the process by which, after ovulation, the ovarian follicle is transformed into the corpus luteum.

luteinizing hormone (LH, hLH) a gonadotropin, a glycoprotein; M.W. approximately 40,000. LH is released from the anterior pituitary and acts on the gonads. In the female, LH stimulates the graafian follicle, the corpora lutea, and ovulation. LH promotes steroidogenesis in the corpus luteum by stimulating the conversion of cholesterol to pregnenolone, and has a similar influence on the male, in whom it stimulates testosterone production by the interstitial Leydig cells. Reference ranges for luteinizing hormone in plasma are: for children aged 10–14 yr, 4–20 mIU/l; for adult males, 6–23; and for adult females: follicular phase—5–30, midcycle peak—75–150, luteal phase—5–40, and menopausal—30–200. Also called *interstitial cell–stimulating hormone*. See also *gonadotropin*.

luteinizing hormone assays assays for luteinizing hormone, generally performed with the radioimmunoassay technique. Increased concentrations of LH in the plasma of females are found in primary amenorrhea (due to ovarian failure), pituitary or hypothalamic tumors, ovariectomy, premature menopause, ovarian agenesis, polycystic ovarian disease, secondary amenorrhea (due to pituitary failure), hypophysectomy, and after administration of oral contraceptives, estrogen, or testosterone. Factors causing increased LH concentrations in males include primary testicular failure, seminiferous tubule dysgenesis (Klinefelter's syndrome), anorchia, and testicular feminizing syndrome; factors causing decreased concentrations include secondary testicular failure (due to pituitary failure), testosterone administration, and hypophysectomy.

luteinizing hormone–releasing hormone (LH-RH) see *gonadotropin-releasing hormone*.

Lutembacher's syndrome (loo′tem-bak″erz) [René *Lutembacher*, French physician, born 1884] the relatively rare combination of a congenital atrial septal defect and acquired (generally as the result of rheumatic valvulitis) mitral stenosis. The condition occurs more frequently in adults than in children and is usually seen in females.

Although the atrial septal defect exerts an ameliorating effect on the mitral stenosis (by causing a lowering of the pressures in the left atrium and pulmonary venous system, and a left-to-right shunt), the mitral stenosis exacerbates the hemodynamic consequences of the septal defect.

Electrocardiography, echocardiography, and radiography are among the diagnostic techniques successfully used to reveal the hemodynamic disturbances characteristic of the syndrome. Lutembacher's syndrome is usually amenable to surgical repair.

luteotropic (loo″te-o-trōp′ik) [L. *luteus* yellow + Gr. *trophē* nourish] stimulating the formation of the corpus luteum.

luteotropic hormone (LTH) a hormone that stimulates the formation of the corpus luteum and is identical to prolactin. Also called *luteotropin.* See also *prolactin.*

luteotropin (loo″te-o-tro′pin) see *luteotropic hormone.*

lutetium (Lu) (loo-te′she-um) [L. *Lutetia* pre-Roman Paris, France] a soft, ductile, silvery metallic element; atomic number 71: atomic weight 174.97; a 4f transition element (lanthanide or rare earth element); oxidation state 0, +3. See also *rare earth elements.*

Lutheran blood group system see under *blood groups.*

lux (lx) (luks) [L. "light"] the International System (SI) unit of illuminance or luminous flux density, equal to 1 lumen per square meter (lm/m^2).

luxation (luk-sa′shun) [L. *luxatio,* from *luxus* dislocated] dislocation.

Luxol fast blue trademark for a group of dyes that are used in histology as stains for complex lipids, particularly for myelin. They have a marked affinity for phospholipids, lecithin, and cephalin. Luxol fast blue AR, ARN, and G are diarylguanidine salts of sulfonated polyazo dyes; Luxol fast blue MBSN is a copper phthalocyanin.

LVH abbrev. See *large vessel h.* under *hematocrit.*

Lw formerly the symbol for the chemical element *lawrencium* (Lr).

lx abbrev. see *lux.*

lyase (li′ās)) any of a class of enzymes (EC 4) consisting of those that reversibly cleave C—C, C—O, C—N, and other bonds without hydrolysis or oxidation-reduction, yielding two units, one or both of which contain a double-bonded carbon. Clinically important enzymes of the class include aldolase (ALD) (EC 4.1.2.13), δ-aminolevulinate dehydratase (EC 4.2.1.24), and ornithine decarboxylase (EC 4.1.1.17). The class includes enzymes also called decarboxylase, aldolase, synthase, hydrase, dehydratase, deaminase, and nucleotide cyclase.

lye (li) 1. an alkaline solution obtained from the leaching of wood ashes.

2. a strong alkaline solution that contains potassium hydroxide or sodium hydroxide, used in the household and in industry.

lye stricture (li strik′tūr) a decrease in size of the lumen of the esophagus that may develop years after the ingestion of lye and is identified by dysphagia and a history of lye ingestion. Because these strictures are associated with a greatly increased risk of carcinoma of the esophagus, radiographic studies, endoscopy, and exfoliative cytology should be performed periodically.

Lymantria (li-man′tre-ah) a genus of caterpillars. The species *L. monacha* (the Nun moth), which possesses poisonous hairs, is found throughout Europe.

Lyme disease (līm) an illness of uncertain etiology; so named because it was originally found in Lyme, Connecticut. It is manifested typically by erythema chronicum migrans (ECM), a distinctive, expanding, annular, erythematous skin lesion, and recurrent bouts of arthritis or arthralgia. Although ECM and joint abnormalities sometimes occur independently, they are thought to be part of a single disease process caused by a penicillin-sensitive infectious agent transmitted by *Ixodes* species ticks. Aseptic meningitis, encephalitis, cranial or spinal neuropathies (especially unilateral or bilateral Bell's palsy), and cardiac abnormalities are present in a minority of cases, and chronic arthritis has been reported as an infrequent residual outcome.

Lymnaea (lim-ne′ah) [Gr. *limnaios* of the marsh] a genus of snails, several species of which serve as an intermediate host for numerous flukes (e.g., *Fasciola hepatica*).

lymph/o (lim′fo) [L. *lympha* water] a word element used in combining form to denote lymph, e.g., lymphangiogram.

lymph (limf) a yellowish, slightly basic fluid derived from tissue fluid. Lymph is collected from peripheral tissues throughout the body and is carried in lymph vessels to the circulatory system via the thoracic duct and the right lymphatic duct. While filtering through the lymph nodes, the fluid receives macrophages, lymphocytes, and immunoglobulins. The lacteals of the small intestine add chyle (lipid) to the lymph, imparting to it an opalescent quality.

lymphaden/o (lim-fad′ĕ-no) [*lymph-* + Gr. *adēn* gland] a word element used in combining form to denote lymph gland, e.g., lymphadenitis.

lymphadenitis (lim-fad″ĕ-ni′tis) [*lymphaden-* + *-itis*] an inflammation of one or more lymph nodes, which can be caused by any pathogen. Usually the inflammation is due to a primary focus of infection elsewhere (especially that from streptococci and staphylococci). Symptoms may include tenderness and node enlargement, inflammation of the overlying skin, and inhibition of motion of adjacent structures; systemic symptoms may or may not be present. Lymph node aspiration, incision, or biopsy may be needed to determine the cause.

lymphadenopathy (lim-fad″ĕ-nop′ah-the) [*lymphadeno-* + Gr. *pathos* disease] a general term used to describe any disease of the lymph nodes.

dermatopathic l., lymph node involvement occurring in association with a skin condition, which results in the presence of lipid, and melanin within nodal histiocytes.

immunoblastic l., a condition in which immunoblasts of varying degrees of maturity dominate the histology of the lymph node; usually associated with systemic symptoms. Although the process is not definitely neoplastic, the condition occasionally progresses to immunoblastic sarcoma. Also called angioimmunoblastic lymphadenopathy.

lipogranulomatous l., a reactive process to lipid material in a lymph node. A similar process may occur in the spleen.

secondary l., lymph node enlargement occurring as part of a systemic disease process other than the lymphoreticular disorders.

sinus histiocytosis with massive l., a condition in which there is a proliferation within markedly enlarged lymph nodes of phagocytosing histiocytes, accumulated within dilated sinusoids. Most of the ingested cells are lymphocytes. The condition appears to be benign, and its etiology is not known. Also called *Rosai-Dorfman disease.*

lymphangi/o (lim-fan′je-o) [*lymph-* + Gr. *angeion* vessel] a word element used in combining form to denote lymph vessels, e.g., lymphangitis.

lymphangiectasis (lim-fan″je-ek′tah-sis) [*lymphangi-* + Gr. *ektasis* distention] the diffuse swelling of part of a limb, which results from marked dilation of the superficial lymphatics.

lymphangiogram (lim-fan″je-o-gram) a radiograph of the lymph vessels.

lymphangiography (lim-fan″je-og′rah-fe) [*lymphangio-* + Gr. *graphein* to write, record] the imaging of the lymph vessels after injection of an x-ray contrast medium or a radioisotope tracer. See also *lymphography.*

lymphangioma (lim-fan″je-o′mah) a benign neoplasm of lymphatic endothelial cells. The component channels are often small, but they can be cavernous, as in the cystic hygroma. Most lymphangiomas occur in the superficial tissues of the head and neck, but deeper tumors are occasionally encountered within the trunk. Some lymphangiomas are present at birth; they tend to enlarge with the growth of the individual. When there is smooth muscle in the wall of the channels, the tumor is termed a lymphangiomyoma. See also *cystic h.* under *hygroma* and *lymphangiomatosis.*

lymphangiomatosis (lim-fan″je-o-mah-to′sis) a rare disorder characterized by proliferation of lymphatic channels containing excessive smooth muscle within their walls. The retroperitoneal and mediastinal lymphatics are usually involved; similar changes are seen in the lymph nodes and in some patients within the lungs. Patients are typically females in their reproductive years. Some cases are associated with tuberous sclerosis, but lymphangiomatosis alone does not appear to be a familial condition. Pulmonary involvement is associated with progressive development of respiratory insufficiency, leading to death after one to several years.

lymphangiosarcoma (lim-fan″je-o-sar-ko′mah) [*lymphangio-* + *sarco-* + *-oma*] a malignant neoplasm of lymphatic endothelial cells seen in various locations including a lymphedematous extremity, such as the arm following radical breast surgery with lymph node dissection. Histologically, it generally is not possible to distinguish between a tumor of endothelial cells of blood vessels from one of lymphatic vessels. The separation of lymphangiosarcoma from angiosarcoma is largely an academic distinction, as treatment and prognosis are the same. See also *angiosarcoma.*

lymphangitis (lim″fan-ji′tis) [*lymphangi-* + *-itis*] an acute or chronic inflammation of the lymphatic vessels. Group A β-hemolytic streptococci are the most common etiologic agents, although any organism can be causative. Painful subcutaneous red streaks, corresponding to inflamed lymphatic vessels, fever, malaise, anorexia, cellulitis, and bacteremia may occur. In acute lymphangitis, there is leukocytosis with a shift to the left. Culture and sensitivities of wound exudates or blood cultures are used to determine the causative organism. Chronic lymphangitis leads to thrombosis and fibrosis of the lymphatics, resulting in a firm cord under the skin and altered lymph drainage from the involved site.

lymphatic (lim-fat′ik) [L. *lymphaticus*] 1. pertaining to lymph.

2. a lymphatic vessel, one vessel of the system of capillaries, collecting vessels, and trunks that collect lymph from the tissues and carry it to the blood.

lymphatic tissue, diffuse see *diffuse lymphatic tissue.*

lymphedema (lim″fe-de′mah) [*lymph-* + *edema*] a progressive nonpitting edema of subcutaneous tissues that does not respond to elevation of the affected part. It is always due to an obstruction within the lymphatic system.

Primary lymphedema most frequently occurs in females and is caused by developmental abnormalities in the lymphatic system. Initially the tissue is soft but it may become firm and nonpitting. The condition may be bilateral. Also called *Milroy's disease.*

Secondary lymphedema has an extralymphatic cause. Prostate cancer in males and lymphoma in females that lead to lymphatic obstruction are the most common causes. Lymphangiograms may help demonstrate the point of obstruction.

lymph node (limf nōd) a discrete, encapsulated aggregate of lymphoid tissue. A lymph node is a reniform body ranging in size from 1 mm to more than 1 cm; some reactive nodes are even larger. Lymph nodes are located within the course of the lymphatic vessels that convey lymph from the peripheral tissues to the large veins in the lower part of the neck. The nodes are one component of the lymphoid tissue of the body, which includes similar cells in the spleen, bone marrow, thymus, wall of the gastrointestinal tract, and other tissues. Lymph nodes filter the lymph, removing organisms and other particulate material that are phagocytosed by macrophages within the node. Lymph nodes are a site of formation of new lymphocytes, of maturation of lymphocytes to plasma cells, and of antibody production.

The connective tissue framework of a lymph node consists of the enveloping capsule and a series of branching trabeculae that extend from the inner surface of the capsule toward the hilum. Delicate strands of reticular connective tissue further subdivide the node into a vast number of compartments and channels. The channels are sinuses, the largest of which is located immediately subjacent to the capsule (peripheral or subcapsular sinus). Afferent lymph vessels pierce the capsule, and carry lymph into the subcapsular sinus from whence it percolates through small sinuses in the direction of the hilum, where efferent lymph vessels carry it away from the node.

The tissue within a lymph node is organized into a cortex and medulla. The cortex can be further subdivided into the outer cortex, which contains B cells and lymphoid follicles, and an inner cortex (paracortex), which is the T-cell zone of the node. Blood vessels enter the node at the hilum, and arterioles reach the cortex through the trabeculae where they form a capillary plexus. In the paracortical zone, the postcapillary venules have cuboidal endothelial cells, and many circulating lymphocytes enter the lymph node through these venules. The medulla is a B-cell compartment. It is occupied by converging lymph and blood vessels, and contains many plasma cells in addition to small lymphocytes and macrophages.

The typical appearance of a lymph node is that of a reactive structure with variable numbers of lymphoid follicles in the outer cortex. The relative prominence of the elements of the node depends on the antigenic stimulus. The appearance of the follicles is indicative of the response of the lymph node to antigenic stimulation. Cells within the germinal center of the follicle are lymphocytes undergoing a sequence of morphologic and functional transformation. Cells in the germinal center are larger than those in the surrounding mantle zone, some of the nuclei are indented (cleaved), the nuclear chromatin is fine and dispersed, and nucleoli are prominent. In addition to the lymphocytes, the lymph node parenchyma contains cells termed dendritic reticular cells. They have long, slender processes insinuated between the lymphocytes, and are believed to function in the trapping of antigen. Many of the macrophages within a lymph node are adherent to the inner surface of the sinuses (littoral cells), where their presence creates turbulence in the flow of the lymph, facilitating the phagocytic activities of the cells.

Particular care should be exercised in procuring and processing lymph nodes for histologic examination. The biopsied node must be representative of the pathologic process, and the largest accessible node should therefore be excised with its capsule intact, sliced thinly, and fixed promptly in 10 percent buffered formalin for paraffin embedding. When indicated, a small portion can be separately fixed in buffered glutaraldehyde for electron microscopy; tissue may also be provided for microbiologic studies and for cell marker and other hematologic procedures. Imprints prepared from a fresh-cut surface of the node are helpful in some cases; they can be fixed in 95 percent alcohol and stained with hematoxylin and eosin, or air-dried for Wright's stain.

See also the accompanying illustration.

germinal center of l. n., a group of transforming

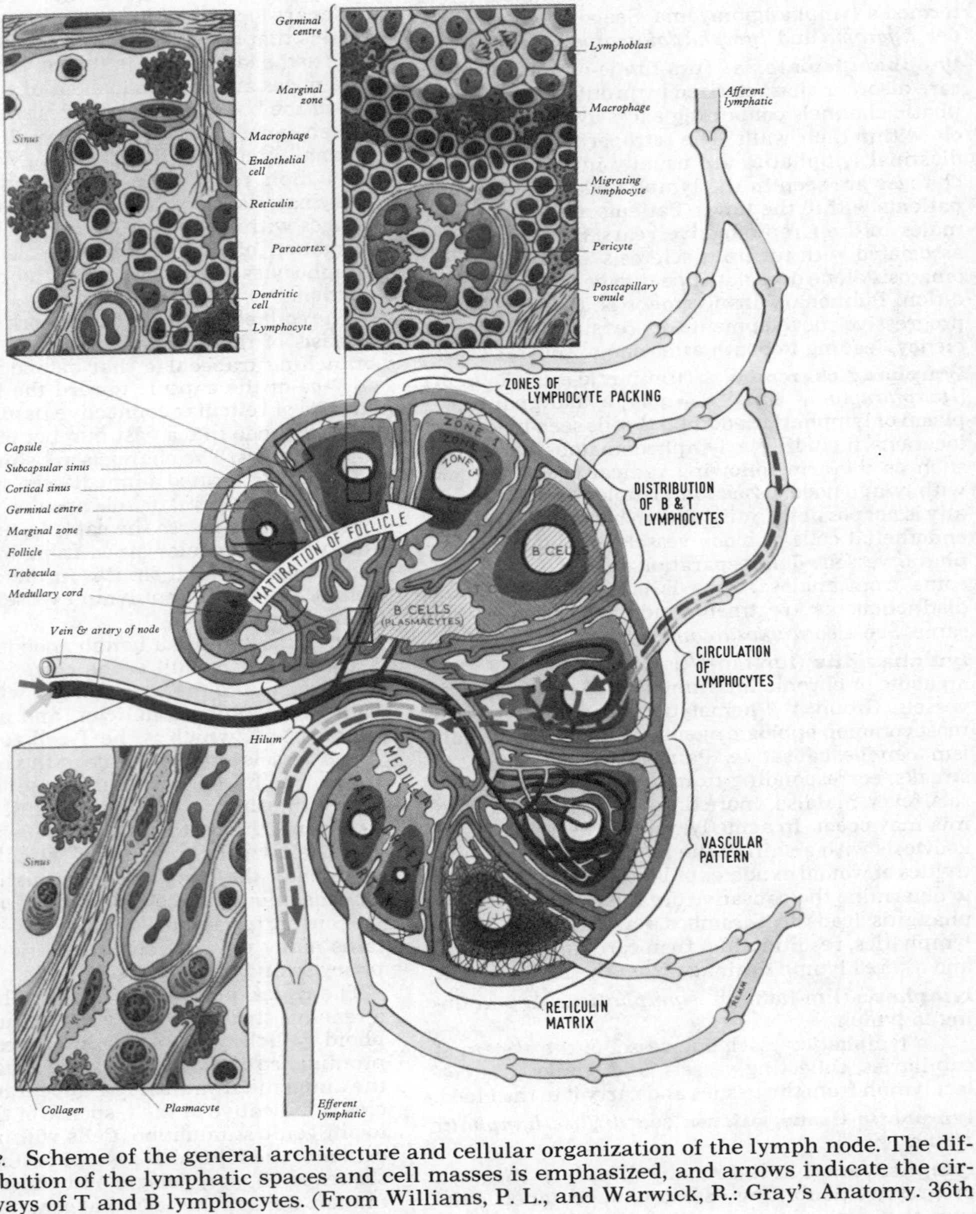

Lymph node. Scheme of the general architecture and cellular organization of the lymph node. The differential distribution of the lymphatic spaces and cell masses is emphasized, and arrows indicate the circulatory pathways of T and B lymphocytes. (From Williams, P. L., and Warwick, R.: Gray's Anatomy. 36th ed. Philadelphia, W. B. Saunders Co., 1980.)

lymphocytes in the cortical zone of a reactive node that appear in response to antigenic stimulation of B lymphocytes. A morphologic sequence of transformation of these cells forms the basis for the Lukes-Collins classification of B-cell lymphomas. The germinal center is surrounded by a mantle zone of small lymphocytes, and together they constitute a secondary lymphoid follicle. See also *lymphoma.*

lymphoblast (lim'fo-blast) [*lympho-* + Gr. *blastos* germ] an immature "blast cell" of the lymphoid cell line, which normally matures into a lymphocyte. The lymphoblast is characterized by a nucleus with loosely packed euchromatin and a large nucleolus, and cytoplasm with numerous polyribosomes. Lymphoblasts measure 15–30 μm in diameter. In the presence of a foreign antigen, lymphoblasts become numerous in the lymph nodes and eventually differentiate into B and T lymphocytes.

lymphoblastic (lim"fo-blas'tik) pertaining to a lymphoblast.

lymphoblastosis (lim"fo-blas-to'sis) an excess of lymphoblasts in the blood.

lymphocyte (lim'fo-sīt) [*lympho-* + *-cyte*] a mononuclear leukocyte whose primary function is concerned with the immune response; it is involved with antibody production, immunologic memory, and cell-mediated immunity. Lymphocytes arise from the bone marrow from a lymphoblast stage, enter the blood circulation, and continuously pass through lymphoid and connective tissue, especially the cortex of lymph nodes and the white pulp of the spleen. They differentiate into two major classes, B and T, depending on inductive events at the location of maturation.

Lymphocytes account for 20–35 percent of the circulating white cells in the blood and are second in abundance to neutrophils in the peripheral blood. Their approximate normal concentration ranges from an average of 7.0 cells $\times$ $10^3/\mu g$ at age 1 yr to 3.5 cells at age 6 and 2.5 cells at age 21.

Lymphocytes are small, round cells, 10 μm in diameter, that have a large, round, and sometimes indented nucleus; they are slightly larger than erythrocytes. The cytoplasm appears pale blue when stained with hematoxylin and eosin; densely distributed chromatin may be seen in the nucleus. Although lymphocytes have no specific granules, a few azurophilic granules are occasionally present.

See also the accompanying illustration.

B l., bone marrow–derived lymphocyte, a thymus-independent cell that migrates to the tissues without passing through or being influenced by the thymus. These cells play a major role in humoral immunity; on stimulation by antigen they mature into plasma cells that synthesize humoral antibody.

The B lymphocyte was defined in the chicken and is derived from cells that migrate through the bursa of Fabricius in these animals. In humans it is derived in embryonic life from fetal liver and subsequently from the bone marrow. The bursal equivalent in mammals is unidentified. (The T lymphocyte is also derived from the bone marrow but matures and differentiates in the thymus.)

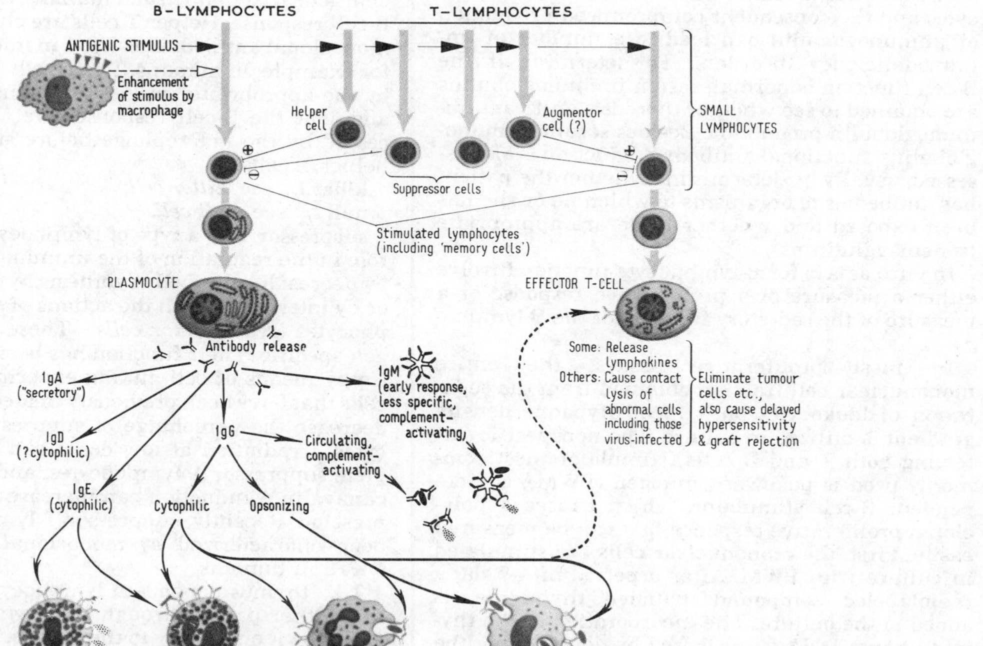

Lymphocyte. Diagram of the origins and functions of the various subclasses of lymphocyte, including the role of antibodies in activating antigens and in initiating defensive activities in other classes of cell. (From Williams, P. L., and Warwick, R.: Gray's Anatomy. 36th ed. Philadelphia, W. B. Saunders Co., 1980.)

B cells are found throughout the body in the lymph nodes, spleen, bone marrow, and blood. They constitute approximately 15–20 percent of all circulating lymphocytes. In the lymph nodes, the B cells are localized primarily in follicles and germinal centers. They recirculate by leaving lymph nodes through endothelial venules, returning via afferent lymphatics. There are both short-lived and long-lived memory B cells.

The B lymphocyte passes through several differentiation steps before becoming an antibody-producing cell. Initial differentiation involves a large proliferating cell without surface immunoglobulin. Cytoplasmic IgM is the first immunoglobulin product noticed in the pre-B cell, which is followed by differentiation into a lymphocyte containing monomeric surface IgM. Other immunoglobulins appear on the surface, notably IgD, IgA, and IgG; all may be present at one time. The plasma cell formed on terminal differentiation has only one type of immunoglobulin, which it secretes. In addition to surface immunoglobulin, there are also complement receptors on the more differentiated B cells. These receptors are used in counting and separating the B cells. Sheep red blood cells that have been sensitized with antibody and then activated with the early classic complement components are designated EAC. B cells will form rosettes with the EAC, and the number of EAC rosettes is used as a measure of B-cell numbers.

For B-cell differentiation and activation to take place, interaction with macrophages and usually T lymphocytes must occur (see *macrophage*). The final stages of B-cell differentiation are also driven by specific antigen.

CLINICAL DISEASE. The malfunction of B lymphocytes and the consequent compromised production of immunoglobulin can lead to a number of immunodeficiency disorders. To determine if the B-cell function is normal, serum immunoglobulins are obtained to see whether there is significant immunoglobulin production. Besides serum immunoglobulins, functional antibody production is also assessed, usually by determining whether the patient has antibodies to organisms to which he or she has been exposed and whether there are appropriate isohemagglutinins.

In vitro assays for B-lymphocyte function involve either a measure of a proliferative response or a measure of the secretory function of the B lymphocytes.

In most proliferative assays, the entire mononuclear cell fraction obtained from the separation of leukocytes on a Ficoll-Hypaque density gradient is utilized in culture. The nonspecific (affecting both T and B cells) stimulator most commonly used is pokeweed mitogen (PWM), a T-dependent B-cell stimulator, which causes a polyclonal proliferative response that can be measured easily. First, the mononuclear cells are stimulated in culture with PWM. After a period of 4–7 da, a radiolabeled compound, tritiated thymidine, is added to the culture. The incorporation of the thymidine into DNA is measured by determining the radioactivity. This indicates the level of DNA synthesis and thus blastogenesis. In humans, another T-dependent mitogen is endotoxin. *Nocardia* water-soluble mitogen, Epstein-Barr virus, and staphylococcal protein A are T-dependent B-cell mitogens.

B-cell function involves the appropriate production of antibody to an antigenic stimulus. However, methods that can detect the small quantities of immunoglobulin secreted in vitro by an antigenic stimulus are not readily available; for this reason, polyclonal activation is often used, as with PWM. Even using PWM, however, very sensitive methods have been developed to determine secreted immunoglobulins:

1. Solid-phase quantitative radioimmunoassay (RIA). One solid-phase RIA takes advantage of the fact that secreted proteins strongly adhere to plastic microtiter plates. The adsorbed protein is then quantitated using an appropriately labeled antibody against the desired immunoglobulin. As a standard curve must be generated to determine any unknown, appropriate standards must be available.

2. Reverse hemolytic plaque-forming cells. Reverse hemolytic plaque assays utilize the coupling of anti-Ig antibodies Fab with staphylococcal protein A to sheep red blood cells. The cells are suspended along with the lymphocytes in a semisolid medium. After incubation, the secreted Ab binds to coupled anti-Ig Fab. An appropriate antisera and complement lyses the red blood cells that have bound the secreted immunoglobulin, and a plaque forms around the secreting cell.

3. Incorporation of radiolabeled amino acids into newly synthesized immunoglobulin molecules. This method has also been used to measure secreted Ab. Appropriate antisera are necessary to react with newly synthesized immunoglobulin to quantify the precipitable counts.

Also called *B cell.*

helper T l., a population of T cells, which can be characterized in mice and humans, that enhances a B-cell response. Helper T cells are characterized by monoclonal antibodies as Lyt-1 in mice and $OKT4^+$, for example, in humans. These cells are stimulated by the appropriate antigen to produce factors that augment the B-cell response; the antigen is processed by the macrophage before stimulating the helper T cells.

killer l., see *killer cell.*

null l., see *null cell.*

suppressor T l., a type of lymphocyte that plays a role in the regulation of the immune system, either by decreasing antibody synthesis by B lymphocytes or by interfering with the actions of effector T lymphocytes (see *effector cells*). These cells are antigen-specific. Their function has been studied in vitro by means of cell-mixing experiments utilizing cells that have been previously treated to increase or decrease the percentage of suppressor T lymphocytes. Irradiation at low doses can selectively deplete suppressor T lymphocytes, and previous concanavalin A induction can increase the T-cell suppression. Recently, suppressor T lymphocytes have been characterized by monoclonal antibodies as OKT8 in humans.

T l., thymus-dependent lymphocyte; lymphocyte that either passes through the thymus or is influenced by it on its way to the tissues. T lymphocytes can suppress or assist the stimulation of antibody production in B lymphocytes in the presence of antigen, and can kill such cells as tumor and transplant tissue cells. Several subsets of T lymphocytes are recognized on the basis of surface markers and function.

T lymphocytes arise in bone marrow, differentiate in the thymus, and finally migrate to the lymph nodes and spleen. Differentiation in the thymus appears to be dependent on thymic epithelial-derived humoral factors (i.e., thymosin, thymopoietin, etc.). Most T cells actually die in the thymus. On migrating to the secondary lymphoid organs (e.g., lymph nodes, spleen, blood), T cells are available for cell-mediated immunity. Unlike the B cell, the T cell does not have intact surface immunoglobulin, but it may have a portion of an immunoglobulin molecule as an antigenic binding protein on its surface. The T cell does not have a C3b receptor and does not form EAC rosettes, but it does aggregate with sheep red blood cells without previous sensitization: this capability has been used to measure T-cell numbers and for experimental T-cell separation. The T-cell population has been studied extensively in mice and has been found to have various subclasses. There are also cells in humans that enhance a B-cell response (T-helper cells) and others that inhibit the response (T-suppressor cells). These subpopulations of T lymphocytes appear to play a regulatory role on B-cell response. After antigen processing by the macrophages, various T-lymphocyte populations interact with the macrophages. The T cells then augment or inhibit the response of the B cells to the antigen. In addition to affecting the B-cell response, T lymphocytes also act as cytotoxic cells. They can act directly on foreign target cells or through soluble mediators called lymphotoxins. There are other soluble mediators, called lymphokines, which are secreted; they activate and localize monocyte-macrophages to the area. The most well studied of the lymphokines is macrophage activation factor (MAF).

The most reliable test for determination of normal T-cell function is delayed hypersensitivity skin testing. If the test is positive, cellular-mediated immunity is intact. Other tests, in vitro lymphocyte stimulation tests, may also be performed; these tests use plant lectins (e.g., phytohemagglutinin, PHA; and concanavalin A, Con A) that act as mitogens or nonspecific stimulators of lymphocyte transformation. In vitro, PHA and Con A stimulate T lymphocytes to transform into lymphoblasts. Incorporation of tritiated thymidine occurs as the cells differentiate. The incorporation of a radioactive label is used as a measure of blastogenesis.

Lymphocyte subpopulations can be characterized and separated by a number of methods. The usual procedure involves initially separating the mononuclear cells from the granulocytes and erythrocytes by centrifugation using Ficoll-Hypaque density gradients. The mononuclear cell layer contains monocytes and lymphocytes. The monocytes may be removed from the lymphocytes by adherence or by iron carbonyl treatment, followed by separation of the cells that contain iron by use of a magnet or by their density characteristics. Adherence to nylon wool columns also removes some lymphocytes (predominantly B lymphocytes); this is not appropriate if both T and B cells are desired. T lymphocytes preferentially aggregate with sheep erythrocytes; they can be separated by aggregation and subsequent density gradient separation. Following this, the red cells can be removed by preferential lysis. Depletion of different lymphocyte subsets may then be achieved using the monoclonal antibodies against the appropriate subset followed by complement.

Also called *T cell.*

GERALD B. KOLSKI, M.D., PH.D.

lymphocyte-stimulating hormone (LSH) one of two substances (LSHh, M.W. 15,000; LSHr, M.W. 80,000) isolated from calf thymus. Both can cause lymphocytopoiesis by producing an increase in antibody titers and the number of plaque-forming cells.

lymphocytic (lim″fo-sit′ik) pertaining to lymphocytes.

lymphocytic choriomeningitis (LCM) a type of aseptic meningitis caused by arenavirus, an RNA virus transmitted by contamination with excreta of the common house mouse or pet hamster. Usually, only adults are affected by this disease, most often in the winter when mice move indoors, increasing human contact. The symptoms include fever, headache, stiff neck, and lymphocytic cerebrospinal fluid (CSF) pleocytosis. The infection is biphasic with an initial influenza-type illness, followed by a meningeal phase. Leukopenia and thrombocytopenia frequently develop. Recovery usually occurs within 14 da.

Acute LCM appears to be a result of cell-mediated immune injury by sensitized lymphocytes; viral infection by itself is relatively innocuous and long-lasting (a type of slow disease). Virus may be present in blood, urine, or CSF specimens, which can be cultured with the inoculation of suckling mice or guinea pigs. Clinical diagnosis of LCM, however, is usually based on determination of antibody development; virus isolation is rarely attempted.

lymphocytic series the white cell series composed of the lymphoblast, large lymphocyte, and small lymphocyte. The series arises from a stem cell in the bone marrow (and thymus), which gives rise to a lymphoblast and, in turn, to the large and small lymphocytes. The small lymphocytes are then also capable of transforming into other cells. Unlike other white cells, lymphocytes are capable of leaving and reentering the peripheral blood. This is intrinsic to their functional properties in the immune response and allows a large number of cells to be exposed to antigens.

The life span of a lymphocyte is variable and, because of its wandering nature, difficult to determine. One-third of the circulating lymphocytes live 10–20 da, whereas the rest may live many months to several years.

Lymphocytes disappear through transformation into other cells in response to antigenic stimulation, are lost in the digestive tract and lungs, or are phagocytized at the end of their life span by histiocytes (macrophages).

See also *lymphoblast* and *lymphocyte.*

lymphocytic thyroiditis see *chronic t.* under *thyroiditis.*

lymphocytoblast (lim″fo-si′to-blast) see *lymphoblast.*

lymphocytolysis (lim″fo-si-tol′e-sis) [*lymphocyte* + Gr. *lysis* dissolving, loosening] an in vitro assay for cellular immunity, which is an extension of the mixed lymphocyte culture assay. The target population of lymphocytes is used to sensitize the allogeneic lymphocytes. Also called cell-mediated lympholysis (CML). See also *mixed lymphocyte culture.*

lymphocytoma cutis (lim″fo-si-to′ma ku′tis) [*lymphocyte* + *-oma*] see *pseudolymphoma of Spiegler-Fendt.*

lymphocytopenia (lim″fo-si″to-pe′ne-ah) [*lymphocyte-* + Gr. *penia* poverty] a reduction in the number of lymphocytes in the blood.

lymphocytopoiesis (lim″fo-si″to-poi-e′sis) [*lymphocyte* + Gr. *poiein* to make] the production of lymphocytes.

lymphocytorrhexis (lim″fo-si″to-rek′sis) [*lymphocyte* + Gr. *rhēxis* rupture] the rupture or bursting of lymphocytes.

lymphocytosis (lim″fo-si-to′sis) [*lymphocyte* + *-osis*] an excess of normal lymphocytes in the blood or in an effusion.

acute infectious l., an acute, benign, infectious disease of children that is characterized by an excess of normal small lymphocytes in the blood without lymphadenopathy or splenomegaly, with varying degrees of clinical expression and constitutional response. Also called Carl Smith disease.

lymphocytotoxicity (lim″fo-si″to-tok-sis′ĭ-te) the quality or capability of lysing lymphocytes, as in procedures in which lymphocytes having a specific cell surface antigen are lysed when incubated with antiserum and complement. Also called leukocytotoxicity.

lymphocytotoxin (lim″fo-si″to-tok′sin) a toxin that has a specific destructive action on lymphocytes.

lymphoepithelioma (lim″fo-epi″ĭ-the″le-o′mah) a nonkeratinizing squamous carcinoma arising from the epithelium of the nasopharynx or tonsil. The tumor cells are admixed with varying numbers of lymphocytes, and in primary location or cervical node metastasis can closely resemble histologically a large cell lymphoma or Hodgkin's disease. Electron microscopy may be necessary to identify the tumor as carcinoma.

lymphogranuloma venereum (LGV) (lim″fo-gran″u-lo′mah ve-ne′re-um) a contagious venereal disease, with both acute and chronic forms, that is caused by the obligate intracellular bacterium *Chlamydia trachomatis.* Found primarily in individuals in warm climates, the disease is transmitted only through sexual contact.

Following infection, a small vesicle forms at the area of inoculation 1–4 wk later. This lesion heals spontaneously within a few days and may go unnoticed. Regional lymphadenopathy is usually the first clinical symptom to be detected. The inguinal nodes in males and the perirectal nodes in females become matted and painful. Eventually, mutiple sinuses develop to drain the purulent material. During active lymphadenitis, the individual may have a fever, headache, joint pain, and nausea. If untreated, this chronic inflammatory process may lead to fibrosis; in addition, the *Chlamydia* may become disseminated to involve the central nervous system and cause lymphatic obstruction.

Lymphogranuloma venereum is diagnosed by clinical observation, microscopic examination of the purulent material, skin testing, and serologic methods. Because *Chlamydia* are intracellular obligates, they must be propagated in living tissue such as the yolk sac of embryonated egg in cell culture (e.g., iododeoxyuridine-treated McCoy cells). Infected tissue may be stained with Macchiavello or Giemsa stain or iodine and examined for intracytoplasmic inclusions. The skin test, known as the Frei test, uses an antigen of killed *Chlamydia* from yolk sac culture. Individuals who test positively 2–3 wk after infection remain so for life. *Chlamydia* may also be diagnosed serologically using a complement-fixation test or by direct immunofluorescence.

See also *Chlamydia.*

lymphography (lim-fog′rah-fe) [*lympho-* + Gr. *graphein* to unite, record] the imaging of the lymph nodes and vessels to detect pathologic processes such as the presence and extent of lymphomas. Ethiodized oil is injected into the lymphatics of the feet or hands. X-ray films taken a few hours later show the vessels; those taken about 24 hr later show the nodes. Scintillation imaging employing gold, technetium, or indium radiocolloids has also been used, although the resolution is not as good.

lymphoid leukocyte a term occasionally used when the observer is uncertain whether the cell in question is a lymphocyte. The modern tendency is to avoid the term.

lymphoid stem cell a cell believed by early morphologists to be an identifiable pluripotential bone marrow stem cell.

lymphokines (lim′fo-kinz) [*lympho-* + Gr. *kinēsis* movement] soluble factors released during cell-mediated immunity, or the delayed hypersensitivity reaction by sensitized lymphocytes when the latter are incubated with antigen. Generally, lymphokine production is one of the numerous manifestations of lymphocyte activation. It may be induced by the specific antigenic stimulation of lymphocytes derived from sensitized animals and by the nonspecific stimulation of lymphocytes from nonsensitized animals. After appropriate stimulation, both T and B lymphocytes can be induced to produce lymphokines in vitro for relatively brief intervals.

Lymphokines are neither immunoglobulins nor immunogloblulin fragments and probably do not possess structural homology to any known immunoglobulin sequence. A high proportion of the factors studied are protein or glycoprotein molecules (M.W. 50,000–100,000), several are peptides (M.W. 10,000–25,000), and rare molecules are larger proteins (M.W. greater than 100,000). Usually, these molecules are not preformed cellular components and are not present in appreciable amounts in resting immunocompetent cells. Lymphokines are normally synthesized and released as the result of stimulation by agents interacting with membrane receptors. Thus, they differ from mediators of anaphylaxis, which are stored in granule-bound form, and from enzymes of phagocytes, which are extruded as the result of stimulation.

Most lymphokines were discovered, defined, and assayed by a specific biologic activity on a target cell, usually under in vitro conditions. Although lymphokines are antigen induced, the vast majority do not have specific antigen-binding sites, do not exhibit specificity for the inducing antigen, and do not require antigen to perform their function. However, several factors are involved in the afferent arm of the immune response (cell cooperation and suppressor factors) and show antigen specificity; the term lymphokine may not strictly apply to these antigen-specific factors.

Various lymphokines appear to affect their target cells by reacting with specific membrane receptors,

LYMPHOKINES. BIOLOGIC EFFECTS OF LYMPHOKINES AND OTHER CYTOKINES

FACTORS	TARGET CELLS
Migration inhibition factor (MIF)	Macrophages
Macrophage agglutination factor (MAggF)	Macrophages
Macrophage chemotactic factor (MCF)	Macrophages
Macrophage activation factor (MAF)	Macrophages
Specific macrophage arming factor (SMAF)	Macrophages
Interleukin 1 (IL 1)	Lymphocytes
Interleukin 2 (IL 2)	Lymphocytes
T-cell replacing factor (TRF)	Lymphocytes
Soluble immune response suppressor (SIRS)	Lymphocytes
Antigen-specific helper factor	Lymphocytes (macrophages)
Antigen-specific suppressor factor	Lymphocytes
Leukocyte-inhibitory factor (LIF)	Polymorphonuclear neutrophils
Chemotactic factor: PMN	Polymorphonuclear neutrophils
Eosinophil chemotactic factor of anaphylaxis (ECF-A)	Eosinophils
Eosinophil stimulation promoter (ESP)	Eosinophils
Basophil chemotactic factor (BCF)	Basophils
Lymphotoxin (LT)	Other cells
Proliferation inhibitory factor (PIF)	Other cells
Cloning inhibitory factor (CIF)	Other cells
Interferon	Other cells
Tumor necrosis factor (TNF)	Tumor cells
Colony-stimulating factor (CSF)	Hemopoietic cells
Osteoclast-activating factor (OAF)	Osteoclasts
Immunoglobulin-binding factor (IBF)	Immunoglobulin
Skin reactive factor (SRF)	In vivo effects

although such receptors are not demonstrated for most lymphokines. These receptors contain sugars as an essential component. It has been suggested that lymphokines interact with their target cell via two binding sites—one governing target cell recognition, the second responsible for the specificity of the biologic effect. There is no evidence so far for the penetration of lymphokines into the interior of the cell or for a direct effect of lymphokines on an intracellular structure. The basic mechanism of the action of lymphokines can best be shown by analogy with glycoprotein hormones in that there is (1) binding to a specific membrane receptor, (2) delivery of a secondary messenger, and (3) an intracellular biochemical sequence causing the specific lymphokine effect.

Although lymphokines act directly on target cells (and not by means of other known mediators such as complement components, coagulation factors, or mediators of acute allergic reactions), this does not mean that lymphokines in complex in vivo situations act in isolation from other mediators.

Lymphokines do not appear to be enzymes. This holds true for all lymphokines, with the exception of the polymorphonuclear leukocyte migration inhibitory factor, which may act as an esterase. Lymphokines affect a wide range of cell types, including lymphocytes; macrophages; neutrophil, basophil and eosinophil polymorphonuclear leukocytes; thymocytes and bone marrow cells; fibroblasts; lymphoid cell lines; osteoclasts; and endothelial cells. Some lymphokines apparently affect cell-free substances such as immunoglobulin, complement components, and coagulation factors.

Recently, various lymphokines have been found to be similar in action and chemical characteristics. Attempts have therefore been made to revise the nomenclature of these molecules on a unified basis.

It must be emphasized that, although lymphokines are normally studied as free molecules in solution (usually represented by a cell culture supernatant), it is quite possible that their normal mode of action in the intact animal is at a short range from the producing cell and occasionally occurs while they are still attached to the membrane of their cell of origin.

See also the accompanying table and *cell-mediated immunity, delayed hypersensitivity, lymphocyte,* and *macrophage.*

ALAN SOLINGER, M.D.

lymphoma (lim-fo'mah) [*lymph-* + Gr. *ōma* swelling] a general term applied to any neoplastic disorder of the lymphoid tissue, including Hodgkin's disease.

extranodal l., a lymphoma arising in tissues other than the hemopoietic and lymphoid tissues.

Lennert's l., a rare form of malignant lymphoma characterized by a high content of epithelioid histiocytes. It was initially believed to be a peculiar form of Hodgkin's disease. Those affected are usually older adults who present with cervical lymphadenopathy, splenomegaly, and, less frequently, hepatomegaly. The involved tissues are replaced by a polymorphous infiltrate containing many T lymphocytes and poorly defined clusters of epithelioid histiocytes. Reed-Sternberg cells are sparse or absent. The clinical course is variable, with rapid progression in some patients. The precise nature of

Lennert's lymphoma is controversial, but it does appear to constitute a distinct clinicopathologic entity within the non-Hodgkin's lymphomas.

malignant, a solid neoplasm derived from cells of the lymphoreticular system. Malignant lymphomas may be limited to a single anatomic site, particularly lymph nodes, but they may also arise from the spleen, tonsillar tissue of Waldeyer's ring, lymphoid tissues of the gastrointestinal tract, and, in 15–25 percent of all cases, from sites outside the usual lymphoid-containing organs (extranodal lymphomas). Dissemination may occur by involvement of the bone marrow and peripheral blood, at which time the lymphoma may be indistinguishable from leukemia. The basic distinction between lymphomas and leukemia depends on the anatomic distribution of disease and its presentation, and on the evolution of the neoplastic process.

Lymphomas are divided into two major clinicopathologic groups, Hodgkin's disease and the non-Hodgkin's lymphomas. Hodgkin's disease is manifested primarily by lymph node enlargement and may remain localized to one site for a variable length of time. It tends to spread in a predictable manner, involving contiguous lymph node groups and organs. The anatomic distribution of lesions in patients with untreated Hodgkin's disease differs considerably from that found in the non-Hodgkin's lymphomas. For example, studies show a relatively low percentage of involvement of the mesenteric nodes and bone marrow as compared with many non-Hodgkin's lymphomas; in contrast, Hodgkin's disease has a higher incidence of mediastinal lymph node involvement.

HODGKIN'S DISEASE. The diagnosis of Hodgkin's disease is made primarily on the basis of histopathologic changes, and depends on the identification of the Reed-Sternberg cell. Currently thought to be of macrophage/histiocytic lineage, the cell is classically binucleated; the nuclei appear mirror imaged, with large, acidophilic, inclusionlike nucleoli, and are surrounded by a clear perinuclear halo. The recognition of Reed-Sternberg cells is mandatory in the initial diagnosis of Hodgkin's disease, provided that these cells are present in an appropriate stromal environment, which varies depending on the subclassification. Currently, the Rye modification of the Lukes and Butler classification is used. The classification (see below) depends on the number of lymphocytes, which ranges from many (lymphocytic predominance) to a form in which lymphocytes are rare but Reed-Sternberg cells are remarkably increased (lymphocytic depletion); the mixed cellularity type falls between these two types. The nodular sclerosing type is separate and forms the largest category of Hodgkin's disease. In this form, the lymphoid tissue is divided into nodules by proliferating bands of collagen; Reed-Sternberg cells and variants (lacunar cells) may lie within clear spaces within the lymphoid nodules.

RYE CLASSIFICATION OF HODGKIN'S DISEASE*

Lymphocytic predominance
Nodular sclerosis
Mixed cellularity
Lymphocytic depletion

*Classification modified from Lukes and Butler.

The pathologic subtypes of Hodgkin's disease historically are predictable in their clinical behavior. The nodular sclerosing type is found typically in

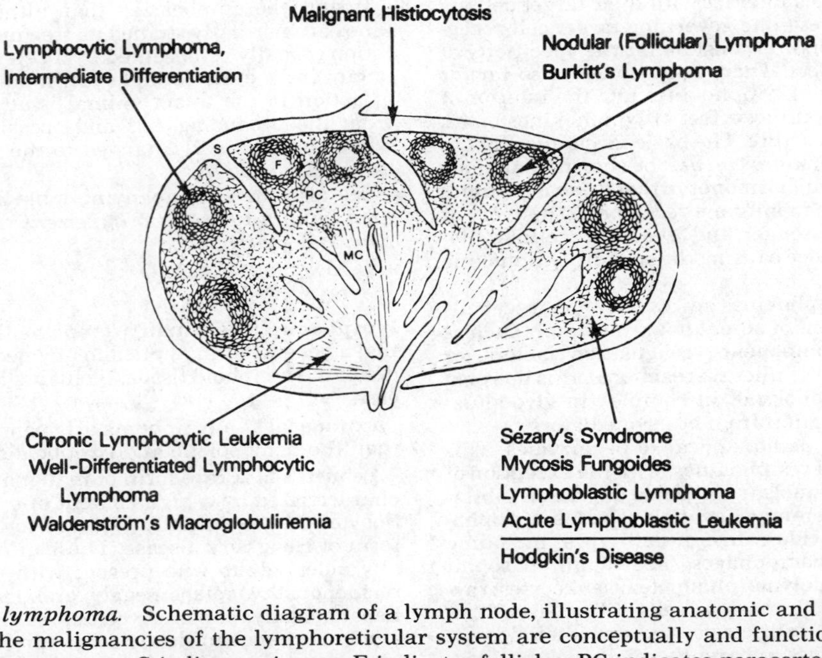

Malignant lymphoma. Schematic diagram of a lymph node, illustrating anatomic and functional compartments. The malignancies of the lymphoreticular system are conceptually and functionally related to the above compartments. S indicates sinuses, F indicates follicles, PC indicates paracortex, and MC indicates medullary cords. (From Mann, R. B., et al.: Malignant lymphomas. American Journal of Pathology *94*:159, 1979.)

Malignant Lymphoma. Working Formulation of Non-Hodgkin's Lymphomas for Clinical Usage

Grade	Lymphoma Type
Low	Malignant lymphoma, small lymphocytic
	Malignant lymphoma, follicular, predominantly small cleaved cell
	Malignant lymphoma, follicular, mixed small cleaved and large cell
Intermediate	Malignant lymphoma, follicular, predominantly large cell
	Malignant lymphoma, diffuse, small cleaved cell
	Malignant lymphoma, diffuse, mixed small and large cell
	Malignant lymphoma, diffuse, large cell
High	Malignant lymphoma, large cell, immunoblastic
	Malignant lymphoma, lymphoblastic
	Malignant lymphoma, small noncleaved cell
Miscellaneous	Composite malignant lymphoma
	Mycosis fungoides
	Extramedullary plasmacytoma
	Unclassifiable
	Other

Courtesy of Jerome S. Burke, M.D.

young females, with a predilection for the mediastinum, including both the lymph nodes and thymus. Such patients generally have a good prognosis. The lymphocytic predominance form represents about 5 percent of all cases of Hodgkin's disease, is found mainly in children, and has a good prognosis. Conversely, the lymphocytic depletion form has a bad prognosis, and patients often have bulky disease with widespread involvement. The mixed cellularity form falls between the nodular sclerosing type and lymphocyte depletion form in prognosis. Under modern therapeutic regimens employing both radiation therapy and combination chemotherapy, the subtypes of Hodgkin's disease are losing their importance in terms of prognosis. The clinical stage of the disease (extent and symptomatology) is the paramount indicator for prognosis and type of therapy.

Non-Hodgkin's Lymphomas. The non-Hodgkin's lymphomas represent a diverse clinical and pathologic group of neoplasms, most of which arise from lymphocytes in various degrees of transformation. The nomenclature and classification of non-Hodgkin's lymphomas have been the subject of controversy, but the classification in the accompanying table has been proposed to serve as a correlation between the numerous schemes. The formulation divides lymphomas into three prognostic groups, designated as low, intermediate, or high grade, which imply the virulence or degree of malignancy. For each prognostic category, there are several histopathologic types based both on the identification of the predominant cell type and the architectural pattern, diffuse or follicular (nodular). For example, individuals with follicular lymphomas have a significantly longer survival than those with the diffuse counterpart, but within the follicular lymphomas the lymphomas composed of larger cells have a worse prognosis. Paradoxically, despite their favorable prognosis, follicular lymphomas show a tendency for early wide dissemination to many sites—including bone marrow, which is reported to be involved in as many as 60 percent of these cases. It has recently been demonstrated that all lymphomas with a follicular pattern, regardless of cell type, are derived from lymphocytes originating in the follicular or germinal center (B lymphocytes).

The majority of diffuse lymphomas also are derived predominantly from B lymphocytes. The diffuse large cell lymphomas, for example, originate from both bone marrow–derived and follicular center cell B lymphocytes, as well as thymic-processed (T) lymphocytes. Regardless of origin, this form of lymphoma frequently presents in extranodal sites, and despite apparent localized disease has an aggressive clinical course and prognosis. Malignant lymphomas in children are different; the working formulation is not strictly applicable. Follicular lymphomas of any type are virtually nonexistent in children and adolescents, as is the small lymphocytic type. The childhood non-Hodgkin's lymphomas are characterized by cells that have primitive cytologic features with a high mitotic index, rapid growth, and a high incidence of mediastinal and extranodal presentations. The lymphoblastic type, for example, commonly presents with mediastinal masses and displays a tendency for early marrow and peripheral blood involvement, at which time the lymphoma is indistinguishable from acute lymphocytic leukemia. In contrast, the small, noncleaved variety of lymphoma, which is equally common in children, has a tendency for extranodal presentations such as GI tract or jaw, and a lesser tendency for leukemic manifestations.

As with Hodgkin's disease, modern therapy employing radiation and chemotherapy, and more accurate procedures for staging the extent of disease, have blurred the natural history of many clinicopathologic subtypes of non-Hodgkin's lymphomas.

Jerome S. Burke, M.D.

nodular l., another name for follicular lymphoma; see under *malignant l.*

lymphomatoid papulosis (lim-fo′mah-toid pap-u-lo′sis) a nodular skin lesion formed by a cellular infiltrate of lymphocytes, many with irregular nuclear profiles. Mycosis fungoides may be simulated histologically, but the lesions are transient and involute spontaneously.

lymphoproliferative disorders a general term for the group of malignant neoplasms arising from the lymphoreticular system (histiocytic, lymphocytic, and plasmacytic). Cells giving rise to these neoplasms are related by a common multipotential, primitive lymphoreticular cell. Normal lymphoreticular cells are present in most tissues of the body but are particularly concentrated in such extramedullary locations as the lymph nodes, spleen, tonsils, thymus, liver, and submucosa of the bronchial and GI tracts. Lymphoreticular cells are also present in varying degrees in the bone marrow.

Examples of neoplasms comprising the group of lymphoproliferative disorders include the lymphocytic, histiocytic, and monocytic leukemias; multiple myeloma and plasmacytoma; Hodgkin's disease; all forms of lymphocytic lymphoma; and immunosecretory disorders associated with monoclonal gammopathy, e.g., Waldenström's macroglobulinemia.

An interrelationship is thought to exist with tumors that comprise myeloproliferative disorders.

Also called lymphoproliferative disease. See also *leukemia, lymphoma,* and *plasma cell dyscrasias.* Cf. *lymphoreticular disorders.*

lymphoreticular (lim″fo-rĕ-tik′u-lar) pertaining to the reticuloendothelial cells of the lymph nodes.

lymphoreticular disorders a condition characterized by the proliferation of lymphocytes or lymphoid tissues that are either benign, e.g., lymphocytosis or lymphoid hyperplasia, or malignant, e.g., acute and chronic lymphocytic leukemia, multiple myeloma, Waldenström's macroglobulinemia, and nonHodgkin's lymphomas. Cf. *lymphoproliferative disorder.*

lymphoreticular system the channels and nodes of the lymphatic system, which, through the activities of their component cells, are involved in the production of cells for blood and lymph, in effecting the immune response, and in phagocytosis.

lymphotoxin (LT) (lim″fo-tok′sin) a lymphocyte-effector molecule that manifests direct cell lysis; it consists of four classes: (1) LT complex (M.W. $>$200,000), (2) alpha (α) LT (M.W. 70,000–90,000), (3) beta (β) LT (M.W. 35,000–50,000), and (4) gamma (γ) LT (M.W. 10,000–20,000). It appears that only activated lymphoid cells can release LT in vitro. Lymphotoxins are nonspecific in their action on cells.

Lyon hypothesis (li′on) [Mary L. *Lyon*, British geneticist] the theory that only one of the two X chromosomes in females is active in humans and other mammals; the other is condensed as sex chromatin. The inactivation occurs in every cell during embryonic development, and all descendants of a cell have the same X (maternal or paternal) inactivated. A portion of the short arm remains active on the inactive X. The X-linked recessive genes on the active chromosome are expressed even if they are heterozygous. During oogenesis, the inactive X is reactivated so that products of both Xs are represented in the mammalian egg. Interestingly, there is a growing body of evidence that the single male X is inactivated during spermatogenesis (see *gametogenesis*). Also called the single active X theory of dosage compensation. See also *X chromosome.*

lyonization (li″on-ĭ-za′shun) [after Mary L. *Lyon*] the phenomenon that X chromosomes in excess of one in a cell are inactivated. See also *Lyon hypothesis.*

lyophilization (li-of″ĭ-lĭ-za′shun) [Gr. *lyein* to loosen, dissolve + Gr. *philein* to love] a method of removing water from a substance (e.g., biologic substances such as blood plasma or serum, antibiotics, or coffee solutions). The substance is frozen rapidly and then placed in a high vacuum in which the ice sublimes and is removed. Because the conditions are mild, the substance (minus the water) is left stable and undamaged. Also called *freeze drying.*

lyophilize (li-of′ĭ-līz) to subject to lyophilization.

Lyponyssus (li″po-nis′us) a genus of mites that occasionally infest humans.

Lys abbrev. See *lysine.*

lysate (li′sāt) the material formed by the lysis of cells. In microbiology, these soluble or finely dispersed cell constituents can be separated from any residual intact cells by, for example, centrifugation.

lyse (līz) 1. to cause or produce disintegration of a compound, substance, or cell.

2. to undergo lysis.

lysemia (li-se′me-ah) see *hyperlysinemia.*

Lysenkoism (li-seng′ko-iz″um) [Trofim Denisovich *Lysenko*, Russian biologist, born 1898] the doctrine of the inheritance of acquired characteristics, established in the Soviet Union as official dogma between 1932 and 1965. It conflicted with darwinian evolution and mendelian and molecular genetics. See also *lamarckian theory.*

lysergic acid diethylamide (LSD) (li-sur′jik as′id di″eth-il-am′īd) a synthetic hallucinogenic drug prepared from ergot alkaloids, which produces mood changes, sensory distortions, hallucinations, delusions, synesthesia, and depersonalization. Anxiety attacks or acute panic reactions occur in some users. LSD use may precipitate a persistent psychotic state. Some persons, especially chronic users, may experience flashbacks—recurrences of the hallucinogenic state triggered by stress or drug use. There is no solid evidence that LSD is a teratogen or mutagen, although this has been the subject of much discussion.

lysergic acid diethylamide assays ultraviolet fluorescence. LSD can be identified on sugar cubes, paper, and other media by its characteristic blue fluorescence under ultraviolet light. After extraction at pH 8.5–9 into an organic solvent, LSD can be quantitated spectrofluorometrically using excitation at 335 nm and fluorescence at 435 nm. The sample and extract must be protected from light and heat, which decompose LSD. In biologic specimens, LSD can be quantitatively measured by immunoassay techniques.

Lysholm position [E. *Lysholm*, Swedish radiologist, 1892–1947] 1. a radiologic position used to obtain a semilateral projection of the mastoid process and petrous portion of the temporal bone. See under *Henschen position.*

2. a position used in radiography of the petrous portions. See *parietotemporal projections.*

3. a position used for an axiolateral projection of the cranial base.

lysin (li′sin) [Gr. *lyein* to dissolve] an antibody or other entity that has the power to cause the rupture of cells. See also *bacteriolysin* and *hemolysin.*

lysine (Lys or K) (li′sēn) 2,6-diaminohexanoic acid, $H_2N(CH_2)_4CH(NH_2)COOH$, a naturally occurring, essential amino acid present in many dietary proteins; M.W. 146.19. It is an important functional residue serving as a binder for biotin, lipoic acid, pyridoxal phosphate, and retinal moieties in enzymes. Lysine is also involved in cross-linking in collagen, fibrin, and keratin. See also under *amino acids.*

lysine dehydrogenase an enzyme of the oxidoreductase class (L-lysine:NAD$^+$ oxidoreductase, EC 1.4.1.15) that catalyzes the reaction lysine + NAD$^+$ ⇄ 1-didehydro-piperidine-2-carboxylate + NH_3 + NADH. A genetic deficiency of the enzyme is the cause of congenital lysine intolerance.

lysine intolerance see *hyperlysinemia type I.*

lysine ketoglutarate reductase see *saccharopine dehydrogenase.*

L-lysine:NAD$^+$ oxidoreductase see under *lysine dehydrogenase.*

lysine-2-oxoglutaryl reductase see *lysine ketoglutarate reductase.*

lysing (lī′sing) pertaining to lysis.

lysing agent in automated blood cell counting, a solution added to whole blood to lyse red cells. It is usually isotonic saline that contains saponin.

lysis (li′sis) [Gr. "dissolution; a loosing, setting free, releasing"] 1. the destruction of a cell, such as by the enzymatic digestion of the cell membrane or by the action of a lysin.

2. the enzymatic decomposition of a compound into smaller compounds, e.g., glycolysis.

3. the abatement of the symptoms of a disease.

-lysis a suffix word element to denote breakdown, separation, or destruction, e.g., glycolysis, cytolysis.

lyso- (li′so) a word element used in combining form to denote lysis or dissolution, e.g., lysosome.

lysochrome (li″so-krōm′) [*lyso-* + Gr. *chrōma* color] a dye that is soluble in fats and oils.

lysogeny (li-soj′e-ne) [*lyso-* + *-geny,* from Gr. *genesis* generation] the hereditary ability of certain bacteria to produce virions. Most viruses are virulent, as they usually kill the cells they infect. However, certain viruses (temperate viruses) have more subtle effects on cells. Such viruses frequently are agents of heredity rather than of disease. Their genetic material can become integrated into the bacterial host genome, duplicated along with the host genetic material, and transferred from one bacterium to another. The bacteria infected by the temperate phage appear normal but have the hereditary ability to produce phage; they are referred to as lysogenic. Lysogenic bacteria may exhibit characteristics not displayed by the corresponding nonlysogenic strain. For example, virulent *Corynebacterium diphtheriae* produces toxin only in the presence of a lysogenic phage within the organism.

Although cells of a lysogenic strain rarely produce virus, every cell has the potential. Lysogeny can thus be considered a genetic trait of a bacterial strain. Ordinarily this trait is not expressed; when it is, it results in lysis of the bacterial cell.

Lysogenization is generally encouraged by suboptimal growth conditions and/or the presence of certain inhibitors of protein synthesis, such as chloramphenicol.

See also *transduction.*

lysolecithin (li″so-les′ĭ-thin) see under *lysophosphatide.*

lysophosphatidate (li″so-fos′fah-tīd-āt) a salt or anion form of lysophosphatidic acid. See also *lysophosphatide.*

lysophosphatide (li″so-fos′fah-tīd) a phosphatide from which one molecule of fatty acid has been split off, as by the action of an enzyme present in cobra venom. Examples include lysophosphatidic acid, lysolecithin (or lysophosphatidyl choline), and lysophosphatidylethanolamine.

lysophosphatidyl choline (li″so-fos-fat′ĭ-dil ko′lēn) see under *lysophosphatide.*

lysophosphatidylethanolamine (li″so-fos-fat″ĭ-dil-eth″ah-nol-am′ēn) see under *lysophosphatide.*

lysophospholipase (li″so-fos″fo-lip′ās) an enzyme of the hydrolase class (EC 3.1.1.5) that catalyzes the reaction lysolecithin + H_2O ⇄ phosphatidylcholine + fatty acid anion. The reaction is important in the metabolism of dietary phospholipids. Also called *lecithinase B* and *phospholipase B.*

lysosomal (li″so-so′mal) of or pertaining to a lysosome.

lysosomal storage disease the term for a group of diseases that result from inherited deficiencies of certain lysosomal enzymes, the most important of which are glycogenosis II, some of the sphingolipidoses, mucolipidoses, and mucopolysaccharidoses. They are characterized by the intracellular accumulation in various organs of unmetabolized substrate proximal to an enzyme block in one of the steps of the cell's intermediary metabolism. Cf. *glycogenoses, mucolipidoses, mucopolysaccharidoses,* and *sphingolipidoses.*

lysosome (li′so-sōm) [*lyso-* + Gr. *sōma* body] a cytoplasmic organelle that consists of a membrane-bound sac of lytic enzymes. The enzymes are formed by ribosomes of the endoplasmic reticulum, and the limiting membrane is added at the Golgi complex to form a primary lysosome. Material to be digested, whether from within the cell or phagocytosed, is enclosed within a membrane, and primary lysosomes then fuse with this sac and discharge their enzymes into it, forming a secondary lysosome. Material that cannot be completely digested persists in the cell as a residual body or is discharged into the extracellular space. See also *autophagy, Chédiak-Higashi disease, heterophagy,* and *lysosomal storage disease.*

lysostaphin (li-so-staf′in) a peptidase enzyme that attacks the pentaglycine bridges in the cell wall of *Staphylococcus aureus,* producing wall-deficient L-phase variants. It is an exoenzyme produced by certain other strains of *Staphylococcus* microorganisms.

lysozyme (li′so-zīm) [*lyso-* + Gr. *zyme* leaven] an enzyme of the hydrolase class, mucopeptide *N*-acetylmuramoylhydrolase (EC 3.2.1.17), that catalyzes the hydrolysis of mucopolysaccharide or mucopeptide; M.W. 14000. Lysozyme is an intracellular bacteriolytic enzyme produced by granulocytes and monocytes but not lymphocytes. It is found in low concentrations in human milk, tears, saliva, and serum. Moderate elevations of serum lysozyme levels have been reported in patients with tuberculosis, sarcoidosis, Crohn's disease, and myeloproliferative disorders. Marked increases in serum and urine levels have been found in those with monomyelocytic leukemia. Lysozyme found in the serum of normal individuals and patients with myeloproliferative disorders is derived primarily from the degradation of granulocytes. The elevated levels in those with granulomatous inflammation are due to liberation from tissue macrophages and histiocytes; in those with monocytic leukemia, the levels are due to liberation from leukemic monocytic cells.

Lysozyme is thought to play a role in modulating neutrophil function, as well as enhancing molecular and structural damage to certain gram-negative bacteria by antibody and complement.

Also called mucopeptide glycohydrolase and *muramidase.*

lysozyme assays 1. turbidimetry. The decrease of turbidity of a suspension of *Micrococcus lysodeikticus* when incubated with a serum or urine specimen is measured at 540, 640, or 645 nm and related to the lysozyme concentration by means of a calibration curve. The reference range is 2.8–8.0 mg/l for serum and 0–2 mg/l for urine.

2. the lysoplate method is an agar diffusion assay. The serum or urine specimen diffuses into an agar gel plate containing *M. lysodeikticus.* The radius of the zone cleared of bacteria is proportional to the log of the enzyme concentration.

3. immunoelectrophoresis using antibody-containing agarose gel.

4. immunoassay, using a human lysozyme-bacteriophage conjugate.

5. viscometry, using the decrease in viscosity of a suspension of *M. lysodeikticus* produced by the mucolytic activity of the enyzme.

lysyl (li′syl) the acyl radical derived from or relating to lysine.

-lytic (lit′ik) [Gr. *lysis* dissolution] a suffix word element to denote destruction, e.g., hemolytic.

M

M symbol for *mega-, methionine, molar* (not recommended in the SI system), *monocyte.*

α_2M see *alpha$_2$-macroglobulin.*

m symbol for *mass,* sample mean, *median, meter, milli-.*

m- abbrev. See *meta-.*

μ the Greek lower case letter *mu;* symbol for: (1) *micro-,* (2) *mean,* (3) *linear attenuation coefficient,* (4) the heavy chain of IgM, (5) chemical potential, (6) *permeability* (μ_0, permeability of vacuum), (7) *magnetic moment* (μ_B, Bohr magneton; μ_N, nuclear magneton), (8) *micrometer* (formerly micron).

mA abbrev. for *milliampere* or, in radiology, *milliamperage.*

μA abbrev. See *microampere.*

MAA abbrev. for macroaggregated albumin. See *aggregated a.* under *albumin.*

macaque (mă-kahk′) [Fr.] a member of Old World monkeys, belonging to genus *Macaca.* These animals are frequently used for physiologic research.

MacCallum's patch a lesion of the wall (mural) of the endocardium associated with rheumatic fever. It forms a gray, ridged, furrowed thickening on the posterior wall of the left atrium just above the posterior leaflet of the mitral valve.

Macchiavello stain (mah″ke-ah-vel′o) a method used for staining *Chlamydia.* A heat-fixed smear is treated with basic fuchsin, washed, then treated with citric acid, washed, and counterstained with methylene blue; elementary bodies stain red against a blue background.

MacConkey agar (mah-kon′ke) [Alfred Theodore *MacConkey,* English bacteriologist, 1861–1931] see *MacConkey a.* under *agar.*

maceration (mas″er-a′shun) [L. *macerare* to soften] 1. the softening of a solid by soaking. In histology, the softening of a tissue by soaking, especially in acids, until the connective tissue fibers are so dissolved that the tissue components can be teased apart.

2. the softening of tissues after death by autolysis.

Machado-Guerreiro test a complement-fixation test for the diagnosis of Chagas' disease, which uses antigen from *Trypanosoma cruzi.* Positive results are obtained in 95 percent of cases. Occasionally, cross reactions occur with mucocutaneous leishmaniasis, but the clinical characteristics of the two diseases are so different that an incorrect diagnosis is rare.

machine (mah-shēn′) [L. *machina*] 1. any device that transmits applied forces (as a lever) or converts heat or mechanical energy into motion (as a motor).

2. in automatic data processing, pertaining to hardware rather than software, as in machine language.

machine error a computer error due to a failure in the hardware as opposed to one in the software (bug).

machine language the instruction set of a computer, which is the final form of all computer programs after processing by an assembler, compiler, or interpreter.

macro- (mak′ro) [Gr. *makros* large, long] a prefix word element to denote large, e.g., macroglossia.

macroaggregate (mak″ro-ag′re-gāt) an unusually large mass of aggregated particles of a substance.

macroamylase (mak″ro-am′ĭ-lās) [*macro-* + Gr. *amylon* starch + *-ase*] a homogeneous molecular complex in which normal serum amylase may be bound to a variety of specific binding proteins, probably immunoglobulins; M.W. 200,000. Such a complex is too large in size for renal clearance, so it accumulates in the blood, causing increases in plasma amylase activity that may be six- to eightfold above normal.

Although it is not correlated with any specific disease state, the presence of macroamylase may be suspected in cases of hyperamylasemia when urinary amylase levels are low or are not increased in proportion to the observed serum levels. The presence of macroamylase may be confirmed by measuring the ratio of amylase clearance to creatinine clearance, which will be extremely low.

macroamylasemia (mak″ro-am″il-ah-se′me-ah) [*macro-* + *amylase* + Gr. *haima* blood + *-ia*] a condition characterized by the presence of macroamylase in the blood. See also *amylase* and *macroamylase.*

Macrobdella (mak″rob′del-ah) a genus of fresh water leeches. Its most common species, *M. decora,* the American leech, is found throughout the United States and Canada.

macrocephaly (mak″ro-sef′ah-le) [*macro-* + Gr. *kephalē* head] an abnormally enlarged head. This condition occurs in association with a brain weighing more than 1800 g and does not as such indicate mental deficit. When it results from an abnormal increase in cranial contents such as in hydrocephalus, hemorrhage, or tumor, evidence of brain dysfunction may be expected. One form, known as Sotos' syndrome, occurs with macrosomia.

macroconidium (mak″ro-ko-nid′e-um), pl. *macroconidia* [*macro-* + NL *conidium,* from Gr. *konis* dust] a large multicellular conidium that is multinucler and contains two or more septa.

macrocyte (mak′ro-sīt) [*macro-* + *-cyte,* from Gr. *kytos* hollow vessel] a large erythrocyte (having a volume greater than 100 μm^3) with an increased hemoglobin content. In stress erythropoiesis the production of erythropoietin is increased and results in early release of erythrocytes and accelerated hemoglobin synthesis in the normoblast, causing formation of macronormoblasts and macroreticulocytes. There is some remodeling of the resulting macrocytes (such as loss of membrane), and they are short-lived, but as a rule in stress erythropoiesis a sufficient number persist to elevate the mean corpuscular volume (MCV).

Macrocytes are found in association with hemolytic anemia and hyperthyroidism and in those recovering from acute hemorrhage, and are also observed in erythroblastosis fetalis. Macrocytes can be caused by the altered permeability of the erythrocyte membranes, which can lead to hydrocytosis.

Although the term macrocyte is usually reserved for the abnormally large red cell, it is sometimes used to denote large cells of other series, e.g., macrocytic platelets.

See also *macrothrombocyte* and *megalocyte.*

macrocythemia (mak″ro-si-the′me-ah) [*macrocyte* + Gr. *haima* blood + *-ia*] see *macrocytosis.*

macrocytic (mak″ro-sit′ik) pertaining to the formation of abnormally large erythrocytes.

macrocytic anemia (mak″ro-sit′ik) see *macrocytic a.* under *anemia.*

macrocytosis (mak″ro-si-to′sis) a condition in which the erythrocytes are larger than normal. Also called *macrocythemia.*

macrogamete (mak″ro-gam′et) [*macro-* + Gr. *gametē* wife] the larger of two conjugants, usually considered as equivalent to the ovum or female gamete. In the malarial parasite, it becomes fertilized by a microgamete (the mature male microgametocyte) in the mosquito, forming a zygote upon fertilization, which develops into an oocyst.

macrogametocyte (mak″ro-gah-me′to-sit) [*macro-* + Gr. *gametē* wife + *kytos* hollow vessel] the sexually immature female form as in the malarial parasite in the red blood cells of humans. It is this stage that is transferred to the mosquito.

macroglia (mak-rog′le-ah) [*macro-* + Gr. *glia* glue] the large nonneural cells of the central nervous system, including the astrocytes, oligodendrocytes, and glioblasts. The macroglia provide support and nutrition for the nervous tissue, lay down myelin, act as electrical insulators, and provide a framework for neurons to follow during development.

macroglobulin (mak″ro-glob′u-lin) a plasma protein with a high molecular weight, such as alpha$_2$-macroglobulin or the monoclonal IgM immunoglobulin produced in Waldenström's macroglobulinemia.

α_2-macroglobulin see *alpha$_2$-macroglobulin.*

macroglobulin assays tests to detect macroglobulins (IGM) in serum. The most commonly used and informative is zone electrophoresis. If macroglobulins are present, an electrophoretically restricted protein spike occurs in the gamma-globulin region of the electrophoretogram. Because the trailing edge of immunoglobulins extends into the beta and sometimes the alpha regions, spikes in these regions may be indicative of macroglobulins. Confirmation of the IGM nature depends on immunoelectrophoresis.

macroglobulinemia (mak″ro-glob″u-lin-e′me-ah) [*macroglobulin* + Gr. *haima* blood + *-ia*] a condition characterized by excessive macroglobulin in the blood; see *Waldenström's macroglobulinemia.*

macroglossia (mak″ro-glos′e-ah) [*macro-* + Gr. *glōssa* tongue + *-ia*] an uncommon congenital malfunction that results in an excessively large tongue owing to generalized hypertrophy; it may be associated with specific syndromes, e.g., Beckwith-Wiedemann syndrome.

macrognathia (mak″ro-na′the-ah) [*macro-* + Gr. *gnathos* jaw + *-ia*] overdevelopment of the jaw.

macrohomology (mak″ro-ho-mol′o-je) in microbiology, the similarity of the map order of homologous genes in related species, used to demonstrate close relationships between different genera, e.g., *Escherichia* and *Shigella.* Cf. *microhomology.*

macrolides (mak′ro-lids) a group of antibiotics produced by actinomycetes and distinguished by the presence of a large lactone ring linked to a sugar in a glycosidic linkage. These antibiotics are effective against gram-positive bacteria, although they also inhibit growth in some gram-negative bacteria; their action is due to the inhibition of protein synthesis. They can be given orally and are useful in cases of allergy to penicillin. Drug-resistant mutants are known to arise during treatment. Erythromycin is the most important of the group, which also includes *carbomycin, oleandomycin,* and *triacetyloleandomycin.* See also *antibacterial agents.*

macromethod (mak′ro-meth″od) a chemical method in which the quantity of a substance to be analyzed is such that the procedure can be performed with the customary laboratory equipment. The classification is relative: frequently, methods utilizing at least a 0.1-ml quantity of specimen are classified as macroprocedures, and those using less as microprocedures. Cf. *micromethod.*

macromethod of Wintrobe see under *hematocrit.*

macromolecular (mak″ro-mo-lek′u-lar) having large molecules; pertaining to macromolecules.

macromolecule (mak″ro-mol′ĕ-kūl) any very large molecule having a polymeric chain structure, such as proteins, polysaccharides, and other natural and synthetic polymers. These range in molecular weight from about 10^5 for a typical protein to about 10^{11} for the DNA in a human chromosome.

macronucleus (mak″ro-nu′kle-us) [*macro-* + L. *nucleus,* dim. of *nux* nut] the larger of two types of nuclei found in the cell of ciliate protozoa. The macronucleus is necessary for vegetative reproduction in the life cycle and not for sexual reproduction. Also called *trophic nucleus* and *trophonucleus.* Cf. *micronucleus.*

macrophage (mak′ro-fāj) [*macro-* + Gr. *phagein* to eat] a large cell (10–20 μ in diameter) derived from the circulating monocyte, which arises in the bone marrow. It has a significant role in both nonspecific and specific immune responses. The roles associated with the tissue to which the macrophage has migrated are outlined in Table 1. The macrophage arises from the differentiation sequence of stem cell → promonocyte → monocyte → macrophage (see also *monohistiocytic series*).

ISOLATION OF MONOCYTE-MACROPHAGE. Human monocytes are isolated in the mononuclear cell

MACROPHAGE, TABLE 1. TYPES OF MACROPHAGE AND ASSOCIATED TISSUE

TYPE	TISSUE
Alveolar macrophage	Lower respiratory tract
Peritoneal macrophage	Peritoneum
Kupffer cell	Liver
Reticuloendothelial cell	Spleen, bone marrow
Microglial cell	Central nervous system
Langerhans' cell	Skin
Free and fixed macrophages	Lymph nodes

Courtesy of Gerald B. Kolski, M.D., Ph.D.

fraction from human peripheral blood by Ficoll-Hypaque buoyant density centrifugation, continuous albumin gradients, or Percoll gradients. During Ficoll-Hypaque centrifugation, the mononuclear cell layer is present at the interface between the Ficoll-Hypaque and the isolating medium; the granulocytes and erythrocytes are in the pellet. The monocytes can then be separated from the lymphocytes by adherence to glass, plastic, or fibronectin; the adherent cells are predominantly monocytes. The monocytes present can be determined by nonspecific esterase staining. As monocytes are maintained in culture (usually in an essential medium with supplemental serum), they take on macrophage characteristics.

Human peritoneal macrophages and pulmonary alveolar macrophages can be conveniently isolated from ascitic fluid and bronchopulmonary lavage, respectively. They can be further separated by the previous steps of Ficoll-Hypaque centrifugation and adherence. Macrophages produce lysosomal enzymes, complement components, and more superoxide earlier in culture than do monocytes.

MACROPHAGE ACTIVITY. Macrophages have lysosomal enzymes in nonspecific granules and can secrete the products shown in Table 2. The macrophage has a ruffled membrane with receptors for the Fc portion of immunoglobulin, a C3b receptor for the activated fragment of the third component of complement, a C5a receptor (the anaphylatoxin derived from C5), and a receptor for formyl-methionyleucylphenylalanine (f-MLP, a synthetic chemoattractant). These receptors are important in mediating some of the functional reactions of the macrophage. The functions of the macrophage can be separated into those nonspecific functions important in host defense—chemotaxis, phagocytosis, and ingestion and killing—and the specific function of antigen processing.

The nonspecific role of macrophages begins with

MACROPHAGE, TABLE 2. SECRETORY PRODUCTS OF MONONUCLEAR PHAGOCYTES

ENZYMES
- Lysozyme
- Neutral proteases
  - Plasminogen activator
  - Collagenase
  - Elastase
  - Angiotensin-convertase
- Acid hydrolases
  - Proteases
  - Lipases
  - (deoxy)Ribonucleases
  - Phosphatases
  - Glycosidases
  - Sulfatases
- Arginase

COMPLEMENT COMPONENTS
- C1
- C4
- C2
- C3
- C5
- Factor B
- Factor D
- Properdin
- C3b inactivator
- β1H

ENZYME INHIBITORS
- Plasmin inhibitors
- α_2-Macroglobulin

BINDING PROTEINS
- Transferrin
- Transcobalamin II
- Fibronectin

NUCLEOSIDES AND METABOLITES
- Thymidine
- Uracil
- Uric acid

ENDOGENOUS PYROGENS

REACTIVE METABOLITES OF OXYGEN
- Superoxide
- Hydrogen peroxide
- Hydroxyl radical
- Singlet oxygen (?)

BIOACTIVE LIPIDS
- Arachidonate metabolites
  - Prostaglandin E_2
  - 6-keto-Prostaglandin $F_{1\alpha}$ (from prostacyclin)
  - Thromboxane
  - Leukotriene
  - Hydroxy-eicosatetraeneoic acids (including slow-reacting substance of anaphylaxis)
- Platelet-activating factors

FACTOR CHEMOTACTIC FOR NEUTROPHILS

FACTORS REGULATING SYNTHESIS OF PROTEINS BY OTHER CELLS
- Hepatocytes
  - Serum amyloid A
  - Haptoglobin
- Synovial-lining cells
  - Collagenase

FACTORS PROMOTING REPLICATION OF:
- Lymphocytes (lymphocyte-activating factors)
- Myeloid precursors (colony-stimulating factors)
- Erythroid precursors
- Fibroblasts
- Microvasculature

FACTORS INHIBITING REPLICATION OF:
- Lymphocytes
- Tumor cells
- Viruses (interferon)
- *Listeria monocytogenes*

From Nathan, C.F., et al.: The macrophage as an effector cell. Reprinted by permission of the New England Journal of Medicine, *303*: 622, 1980.

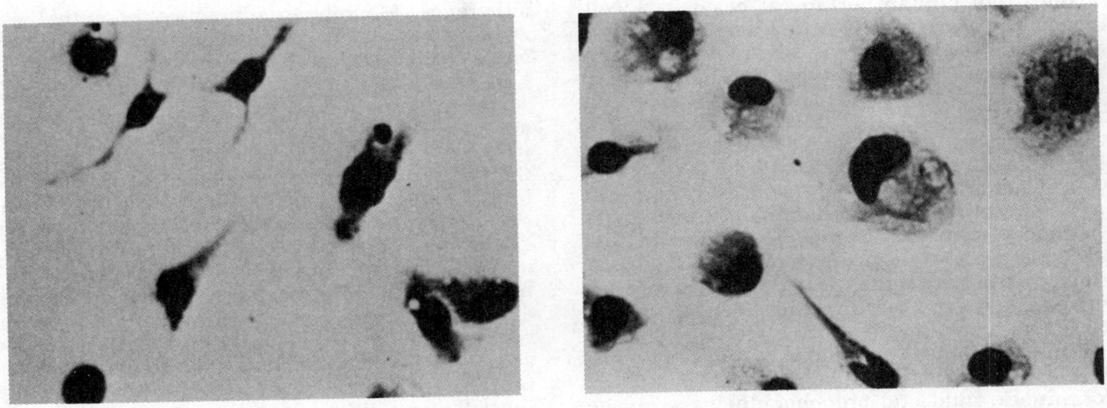

Macrophage. Normal and activated macrophages. *Left,* Normal macrophages, which are large mononuclear cells with cytoplasmic granules and vacuoles, indented or multiple nuclei, and spreading borders. *Right,* Activated macrophages, which are larger, have more granules and vacuoles, spread more on glass, and have an increased capacity to kill microorganisms. (×160.) (From Wing, E. J., and Remington J. S.: Cell-mediated immunity and its role in resistance to infection. Western Journal of Medicine *126*:14, 1977.)

MACROPHAGE, TABLE 3. PROPERTIES OF ACTIVATED MACROPHAGES COMPARED TO NORMAL MACROPHAGES

Increased size and spreading
Increased ruffled membrane activity
Increased adherence to glass
Increased glucose utilization through the hexose monophosphate shunt
Increased carrier-mediated transport of glucose and amino acids
Increased membrane enzyme adenylate cyclase and increased cytoplasmic enzyme lactate dehydrogenase
Production and release of collagenase
Increased production of plasminogen activator and prostaglandins
Increased Ca^{2+} influx
Increase in cGMP
Increase in the number of cytoplasmic granules
Increased phagocytosis of some particles (IgG-coated particles) but not others (aggregated hemoglobin)
Phagocytosis of C3b-coated particles
Increased pinocytosis
Enhanced bacterial killing
Tumor inhibition and killing

From Fudenberg, H. H., et al.: Basic & Clinical Immunology. 3rd ed. Los Altos, CA, Lange Medical Publications, 1980, p. 135.

chemotaxis, in which there is directional movement of the macrophage to a chemoattractant stimulus. This may involve C5a, f-MLP, or macrophage inhibition factor (MIF). After arriving at the site of stimulation, the macrophage is activated and can phagocytize appropriately opsonized particles. Antibody bound to antigen can interact with the Fc receptor as an opsonin, or particles with the activated complement fragment C3b on the surface can interact with the C3b receptor and be engulfed. The opsonized particles are ingested into a vacuole, the vacuole then fuses with lysosomal granules, and the lysosomal enzymes (which work to digest the ingested particle) are discharged into the vacuole. (See also the accompanying illustration and Table 3.)

In addition to these phagocytic functions, the macrophage also acts as an antigen processor and is necessary for T- and B-lymphocyte activation. The antigen is processed and presented in some form to the lymphocytes; this presentation involves a histocompatibility gene product (called the Ia surface antigen in mice and related to HLA-D antigen in humans) and ensures histocompatible lymphocyte and macrophage interactions.

Macrophage function can be enhanced experimentally by previous treatment with specific agents such as bacille Calmette-Guérin (BCG), *Listeria monocytogenes,* or *Corynebacterium parvum.* These "activated macrophages" appear to function better in terms of both phagocytosis and killing of bacteria and general cytotoxicity. There is enhanced metabolism and increased lysosomal enzyme release, adherence, and complement synthesis. Some of these functions are also increased in macrophages elicited in large numbers by various other agents, including casein, mineral oil, thioglycollate broth, and starch. These macrophages are designated elicited macrophages and are commonly used in experimental studies of laboratory animals in which larger numbers of macrophages are necessary.

ASSAYS FOR MACROPHAGE ACTIVITY. There are several methods of assay to determine macrophage activity.

1. Phagocytosis by macrophages. This can be determined in two ways. In the first, C3b- or IgG-coated erythrocytes labeled with ^{51}Cr can be phagocytized, the cells washed and lysed, and the radioactivity measured. Counts from the lysed cells are a measure of the phagocytosed erythrocytes. C3b- or immunoglobulin IgG–coated erythrocytes can also be stained and counted to measure phagocytosis. In the second, zymosan (*Candida* cell walls) can be opsonized with serum and then incubated with

cells. The amount of phagocytosis can be further determined by gamma counting if radioactively labeled zymosan is used, or by staining and counting if nonradioactively labeled zymosan is used.

2. Killing. Killing for bacteria or fungi can be determined by incubating the organism with the cells in various ratios. After incubation, the bacteria or fungi in the supernatant can be plated and colonies counted, as well as those viable organisms obtained from the cells after lysis. In a similar manner, viral permissivity can be determined by incubating virus and cells. After incubation, the plaque-forming units present in the supernatant and lysate can be determined.

3. Cytotoxicity. For tumor cells, cytotoxicity can be determined by using ^{51}Cr-labeled target cells, which are usually virus-transformed cell lines, and macrophages or monocytes as the effector cells. Various target to effector cell ratios are used.

4. Chemotaxis. This can be determined using migration through a filter to a chemoattractant (Boyden chamber method) or migration under agarose. In the latter method, wells are punched in the agarose and attractant and cells put into the different wells. Cell migration toward the attractant is measured by watching the directional movement toward the chemoattractant and comparing it with that of the controls.

GERALD B. KOLSKI, M.D., PH.D.

macrophage activation factor (MAF) a type of lymphokine released from a sensitized lymphocyte, which results in the activation and differentiation of a macrophage for the purpose of clearing foreign material (bacteria) from the body. Physically, MAF is indistinguishable from migration inhibition factor (MIF). See also *lymphokines.* Cf. *migration inhibition factor.*

macrophage agglutination factor (MAggF) a lymphokine found in antigen- or mitogen-induced lymph node cell supernatants, presumably elaborated by T cells. It causes the visible agglutination of peritoneal macrophages onto the walls of culture tubes and may have an important role in delayed hypersensitivity.

macrophage chemotactic factor (MCF) a factor that enhances migration of monocytes/macrophages in the direction of an increasing concentration gradient. MCF activities have been described in human, murine, rat, and chicken systems. This factor is the putative mediator responsible for attracting mononuclear cells to the site of local immune responses in vivo. MCF is also found in graft-versus-host reactions, which suggests that it may play an important role in the pathogenesis of the inflammatory reaction.

macrophage migration inhibition factor see *migration inhibition factor.*

macroreticulocyte (mak″ro-rĕ-tik′u-lo-sīt″) [*macro-* + L. *reticulum* small net + Gr. *kytos* hollow vessel] see *stress r.* under *reticulocyte.*

macroscopic (mak″ro-skop′ik) [*macro-* + Gr. *skopien* to view] visible with the unaided eye.

macrosomia (mak″ro-so′me-ah) see *gigantism.*

macrostomia (mak″ro-sto′me-ah) [*macro-* + Gr. *stoma* mouth + *-ia*] the failure of the fetal mouth slit to reduce normally, resulting in an abnormally large mouth opening.

macrothrombocyte (mak″ro-throm′bo-sīt) [*macro-* + Gr. *thrombos* clot + *kytos* hollow vessel] a giant platelet commonly seen in leukemias and hematopoietic dysplasia. Macrothrombocytes may be associated with giant granules and abnormalities of other cellular organelles.

macula (mak′u-lah), pl. maculae [L. "a spot"] 1. a localized stain, spot, or plaquelike thickening, distinguishable by color or some other feature from its surroundings.

2. a small, discolored area of various sizes and shapes that is even with the surface of the skin. Also called *macule.*

acoustic m., small oval thickenings of the wall of the utricle and saccule that contain sensory receptors of the vestibular apparatus (hair cells) innervated by the vestibular branch of the acoustic (auditory) nerve. See also *ear.*

m. adherens, see *desmosome.*

m. densa, a specialized zone of the distal renal tubule that participates, together with the afferent and efferent glomerular arterioles, in the formation of the juxtaglomerular apparatus. See also *juxtaglomerular apparatus.*

m. occludens, see *zonula occludens.*

m. retinae, an irregular, yellowish depression on the retina at the posterior pole of the eye, lateral to and slightly below the optic disk. It is the site of maximal visual acuity in the retina.

macular (mak′u-lar) 1. pertaining to or characterized by maculae.

2. pertaining to the macula of the retina.

macular degeneration any of several genetic disorders characterized by degenerative changes in the macula of the retina.

macule (mak′ūl) [L.] a general term used to describe any flat, discolored spot on the skin, having a diameter of less than 10 mm. See also *macula.*

maculopapular (mak″u-lo-pap′u-lar) combining the elements of macular and papular lesions. Such rashes have areas of circumscribed discoloration and small, solid lesions elevated above the plane of the skin. Viral, bacterial, fungal, and parasitic infections lead to maculopapular exanthemas. The location, duration, extent, and size of the lesions may be helpful in diagnosis.

Madura foot see under *mycetoma.*

Madurella (mad″u-rel′ah) a genus of imperfect fungi of the family Dematiaceae that can be the etiologic agent of eumycotic mycetoma (maduromycosis). *Madurella* produces black grains that are spherical or oval and can aggregate and grow. There are two medically important species, *M. mycetomi* and *M. grisea,* which grow best at 37°C and 30°C, respectively. See also *mycetoma.*

maduromycetoma (ma-door″o-mi-sĕ-to′mah) see under *mycetoma.*

maduromycotic mycetoma (ma-door″o-mi-kot′ik) see under *mycetoma.*

MAF abbrev. See *macrophage activation factor.*

Maffucci's syndrome (mah-fu′chēz) [Angelo *Maffucci,* Italian physician, 1845–1903] a rare, congenital, nonhereditary disease characterized by the appearance of multiple enchondromas of bone and cavernous hemangiomas of the skin. Individuals with this syndrome have an increased incidence of chondrosarcoma. See also *enchondroma.*

magaldrate (mag′al-drāt) [USP], aluminum magnesium hydroxide monohydrate, $AlMg_2(OH)_7 \cdot H_2O$, used as a gastric antacid.

magenta (mah-jen′tah) [after *Magenta,* Italy] 1. any of several dyes, red to purple in color, more commonly called *fuchsin.*

2. the characteristic color of these dyes.

acid m., acid fuchsin; C.I. 42685.

basic m., basic fuchsin.

m. I, rosaniline (methylpararosaniline).

m. II, triaminoditolyphenylmethane chloride, a component of basic fuchsin.

m. III, new fuchsin (trimethylpararosaniline); C.I. 42520.

m. O, pararosaniline; C.I. 42500.

MAggF abbrev. See *macrophage agglutination factor.*

maggot (mag′ot) the soft-bodied larva in the life cycle of an insect. The species *Phaenicia sericata* (the greenbottle fly) and *Phormia regina* (the blackbottle fly) were formerly used to treat osteomyelitis and other pus-forming infections. Maggots usually attack only diseased tissue, and secrete allantoin (a white crystallizable substance) thought to promote epithelial formation in wounds.

Congo floor m., the larva of *Auchmeromyia luteola,* found in tropical Africa. Living in the ground during the day, these maggots emerge at night and produce wounds when sucking the blood of their hosts (which include humans).

rat-tail m., the maggot of the genera *Eristalis* and *Helophilus* of the family Syrphidae (hoverflies), which have been found in human intestines and nasal passages. Infection is caused by drinking contaminated water (e.g., foul water in ditches or puddles).

magnesia (mag-ne′zhe-ah) [the name of a district of ancient Lydia] magnesium oxide, which combines with water to form magnesium hydroxide (milk of magnesia). It has been used therapeutically as an antacid ingredient.

milk of m., [USP], a suspension of 7.0–8.5 percent magnesium hydroxide, used as an antacid and cathartic.

magnesium (Mg) (mag-ne′ze-um) [L. from *magnesia*] a light, silvery, metallic element; atomic number 12; atomic weight 24.312; group II of the periodic table (the alkaline earths); oxidation state +2. Magnesium is an essential dietary mineral; the average intake is about 5 mg/kg/da, equivalent to about 14 and 12 mmol/da for adult males and females, respectively. The recommended daily allowance for pregnant or lactating females is 19 mmol.

About 21 g (880 mmol) is present in the body; about 35 percent in the cells, 64 percent in the bones, and only 1 percent in the extracellular fluid, the serum level being 0.7–1.1 mmol/l. Magnesium is involved as activator in the ATP phosphate transfer reactions and in many other biochemical phenomena. Deficiency is usually due to malabsorption or excessive loss, and primarily affects the nervous system, causing muscular weakness, tremor, vertigo, cardiac arrhythmia, tetany, and sudden convulsive seizures.

Inhalation of magnesium metal fumes in industry may result in metal fume fever.

m. hydroxide, [USP], a white powder, $Mg(OH)_2$; M.W. 58.34. It is used medicinally as a gastric antacid.

m. oxide, [USP], a fine white powder, MgO; M.W. 40.32. It is used as a gastric antacid and dietary magnesium supplement. Also called *magnesia.*

m. trisilicate, [USP], a slightly hygroscopic powder, $Mg_2Si_3O_4$, used medicinally as a gastric antacid.

magnesium ammonium phosphate see *ammonium magnesium p.* under *phosphate.*

magnesium assays 1. atomic absorption spectrophotometry. This procedure, using the 285.2-nm emission line (magnesium hollow cathode lamp), provides the most accurate and reliable method for assay of magnesium in body fluids. Interfering phosphate ions are bound with lanthanum or strontium salts ($LaCl_3$, $SrCl_2$). Depending on the method, specimens may or may not be deproteinized with trichloroacetic acid.

2. titan yellow spectrophotometric procedure. After deproteinization, the specimen is treated with an alkaline solution of titan yellow (Clayton yellow, thiazole yellow G), with the formation of a red "lake" resulting from the adsorption of the dye by colloidal particles of magnesium hydroxide. Polyvinyl alcohol is added to stablize the $Mg(OH)_2$ sol particles. The absorbance of the red complex at 540 nm is approximately proportional to the concentration of Mg^{2+}. The method, although relatively simple, has limited accuracy ($\pm$10–15 percent).

3. fluorometry. Magnesium forms a chelate complex with 8-hydroxyquinoline-5-sulfonic acid, which fluoresces at 510 nm in acid solution after activation at 380–410 nm. The procedure is rarely used today.

4. colorimetry. Magnesium forms a colored complex with methylthymol blue (MTB), which is measured at 600 nm. Ethylene bis(oxyethylenenitrilo) tetraacetic acid (a chelating agent) is added to minimize interference by calcium, which also can react with MTB. The method correlates well with the method that employs atomic absorption spectrophotometry.

magnet (mag′net) [L. *magnes,* from Gr. *Magnētis lithos,* stone of Magnesia, an ancient city in Asia Minor] 1. a piece of material such as iron in which the magnetic moments of the atoms are aligned to produce a net magnetic field.

2. an electromagnet, a coil of wire that produces a magnetic field when current is flowing through the wire.

magnetic (mag-net′ik) [L. *magneticus*] pertaining to the magnetic field or to a magnet. See also *diamagnetic, ferrimagnetic, ferromagnetic,* and *paramagnetic.*

magnetic core memory a computer memory in which each bit of information is represented by the direction of magnetization (clockwise or counterclockwise) of a magnetic core (a small ferrite ring). Core memories have now been replaced by semiconductor memories in which the information is represented by the state of a logic circuit.

magnetic field see *magnetic field strength* and *magnetic induction.*

magnetic field strength (**H**) a vector quantity used to describe the magnetic field in a magnetized material. The magnetic induction (**B**) is proportional to the sum of the magnetization (**M**) and the magnetic field strength: $\mathbf{B} = \mu_0 (\mathbf{H} + \mathbf{M})$, where μ_0

is the permeability of vacuum. In International System (SI) units, the magnetic field strength at the center of a coil of wire is equal to the product of the current in the wire and the number of turns per meter of length, and is measured in amperes per meter (A/m). Another unit of magnetic field strength is the oersted (Oe). The magnetic induction in the coil depends on the magnetic susceptibility of the material. Also called magnetic field intensity and magnetizing field.

magnetic flux (Φ) the integral over a surface of the normal component of the magnetic induction. The voltage produced in a loop of wire is equal to the negative of the rate of change of the magnetic flux through any surface bounded by the loop: $V = -d\Phi/dt$. The International System (SI) unit of magnetic flux is the weber (Wb), which is equal to 1 volt-second (V·s). Another commonly used unit of magnetic flux is the maxwell (Mx).

magnetic induction (**B**) a vector quantity that measures the magnitude of the magnetic field. The force (**F**) exerted on a moving charged particle by the magnetic field is equal to the particle charge (q) times the vector product of the particle velocity (**v**) and the magnetic induction (**B**): $\mathbf{F} = q(\mathbf{v} \times \mathbf{B})$. The International System (SI) unit of magnetic induction is the tesla (T), which is equal to 1 weber per square meter (Wb/m^2). Another commonly used unit of magnetic induction is the gauss (G). Also called magnetic field and magnetic flux density.

magnetic moment (**m** or μ) a vector quantity that measures the strength of a magnetic dipole, such as a magnet, an elementary particle, or a current loop. The potential energy (E) of the dipole in an applied magnetic field (**B**) is equal to the negative of the scalar product of the magnetic moment and the magnetic field: $E = -\mathbf{m}\cdot\mathbf{B}$.

The magnetic moment of a planar current loop is equal to the product of the current and the area bounded by the loop. In International system (SI) units, magnetic moment is measured in ampere-square meters ($A\cdot m^2$) or joules per tesla (J/T). Two convenience units, the Bohr magneton (μ_B), and the nuclear magneton (μ_N), are used for atoms and molecules. The magnetic moment of the proton is 2.793 μ_N, of the neutron −1.913 μ_N, and of the electron 1.00115966 μ_B. The magnetic moment produced by the orbital motion of an electron in an atom is $n\mu_B$, where n is a nonnegative integer. The intrinsic magnetic moment of an atom or free radical is due to the magnetic moment produced by unpaired electrons.

Also called magnetic dipole moment.

magnetic susceptibility (χ_m) in paramagnetic and diamagnetic materials, the ratio of the magnetization (**M**) to the magnetic field strength (**H**). In ferromagnetic and ferrimagnetic materials, the term refers to the ratio of the magnetization produced in unmagnetized material by a small applied field to the applied magnetic field strength: $\mathbf{M} = \chi_m\mathbf{H}$. The magnetic susceptibility and permeability (μ) are related to the equation $\mu = \mu_0(1 + \chi_m)$, where μ_0 is the permeability of vacuum.

magnetic tape a plastic tape coated with iron oxide, used to record information in audio, videotape, and computer recorders.

magnetization (mag″net-ĭ-za′shun) 1. the process of making a substance magnetic.

2. (symbol **M**), the magnetic moment per unit volume of a substance.

magnification (mag″nĭ-fĭ-ka′shun) [L. *magnificatio,* from *magnus* great + *facere* to make] 1. the process of making something appear larger, as by using a microscope.

2. apparent increase in size, as in a substance viewed under a microscope, and particularly the ratio of the size of the image to the size of the real object. The useful magnification of a microscope is limited by resolution: for a light microscope, it is about 2000 times; for a transmission electron microscope, about 500,000. The magnification can be indicated by a multiplication sign—1000×.

The degree of enlargement of an x-ray image is usually expressed as percentage magnification, which is the object-film distance divided by the difference between the focal-film and object-film distances. Magnification causes some blurring of the image. In nuclear medicine, some magnification is provided by use of a pinhole collimator or a converging collimator.

Cf. *minification.*

magnify (mag′nĭ-fi) [L. *magnificare,* from *magnificus* noble, splendid] to cause to appear larger by the use of lenses or suitable mirrors.

main (mān) [A.S.; Fr.] 1. hand.

2. principal or most important.

main frame the central processing unit of a digital computer.

maintenance (mān′te-nans) the procedures used in repairing an instrument or other item of equipment or in keeping it in serviceable condition (preventive maintenance, which includes routine servicing and modification).

Majocchi's disease (mah-yok′ēz) [Domenico *Majocchi,* Italian dermatologist, 1849–1929] a rare disease characterized by a symmetric purpuric eruption that usually develops on the lower extremities. The initial lesions may coalesce in a patterned form; they also may rupture or become thrombosed or hemorrhagic, producing pigmented areas. Histologically, there may be vasculitis in the upper corium, hyalinization of blood vessels, and inflammatory ion. Central necrosis, atrophy, and loss of hair may result. Also called *purpura annularis telangiectodes.*

major (ma′jer) large; of more importance.

major dense line see under *myelin sheath.*

major histocompatibility complex (MHC) a series of alloantigens on the surface of nucleated cells that are responsible for allograft rejection. These alloantigens are similar to erythrocyte alloantigens that provoke the production of hemolytic antibodies. Histocompatibility systems include all antigenic systems that effect the rejection phenomena. Histocompatibility antigens represent a unique model of polymorphism for studying the complexity of systems that possess many alleles. These antigens are practically ubiquitous. Genes that control them are codominant (i.e., each antigen is expressed when the allele is present in the genome). Study of histocompatibility has found numerous clinical applications, particularly in the selection of the best donor for organ grafts or, more recently, in the study of the genetic basis of some diseases.

The major histocompatibility complexes of various species have been described: human (HL-A), chimpanzee (ChL-A), rhesus monkey (RHL-A), dog (DL-A), pig (SL-A), rabbit (RbH-1), rat (RtH-1), chicken (B), and mouse (H-2). As the most studied species is the mouse, most of the characteristics of the MHC have been worked out in this model system, analogies then being drawn to other species. The following points have been elucidated:

1. When transplanted across MHC differences, skin and other tissue grafts are rejected by an acute process in less than 3 wk; skin grafts transplanted across minor histocompatibility loci differences are usually rejected in more than 3 wk, often by a chronic process lasting many days; and some grafts are not rejected at all. Grafts of other tissues may completely overcome the minor loci barrier. With an MHC difference, second-set grafts are often rejected as white grafts, whereas this type of rejection is very rare with a minor locus difference.
2. The MHC is extremely complex genetically, consisting of perhaps several hundred loci.
3. The MHC is extremely polymorphic genetically and probably can exist in several different forms.
4. The MHC is intimately associated with genes controlling the immune response to a variety of antigens.
5. The MHC is strongly involved in the mixed lymphocyte and graft-versus-host reactions.
6. The number of lymphocytes capable of reacting to MHC antigens in mixed lymphocyte culture or in graft-versus-host reaction is substantially higher than the number of lymphocytes capable of reacting with antigens controlled by the minor histocompatibility loci.
7. Preimmunization of the donor against the antigens of the host increases graft-versus-host reactivity, if the donor and host differ in minor loci, but does not substantially alter the reaction if the donor and host differ in the MHC.
8. Immunization across the MHC barrier induces both cellular and humoral immunity.
9. The MHC is involved in physiologic cooperation between macrophages, T cells, and B cells.
10. It is much more difficult to induce tolerance to antigens controlled by the MHC than to those controlled by the minor histocompatibility loci.
11. The immune response to MHC antigens is more difficult to control by immunosuppression than the response to minor histocompatibility loci.

See also *alloantigen, histocompatibility,* and *transplantation.*

ALAN SOLINGER, M.D.

major tranquilizer see *antipsychotic drug.*

mal- (mal) [Fr.; L. *malum* ill] a prefix word element to denote bad, e.g., malaise.

malabsorption (mal″ab-sorp′shun) impaired absorption. Most commonly this term refers to decreased nutrient absorption in the intestine.

malabsorption syndrome a group of disorders characterized by the markedly impaired digestion of nutrients, their absorption from the intestinal tract, or both, which leads to their consequent loss in the stool. Common to all diseases of malabsorption irrespective of etiology are the symptoms of weight loss (due to wastage of dietary calories) and diarrhea (due to the stimulus of malabsorbed bile acids or fatty acids on the colon, resulting in increased colonic secretion of water and electrolytes). The disorders of malabsorption may be grouped into those primarily of maldigestion, those of decreased absorption by the small intestine, and those with mixed features; see also the accompanying table.

malachite green a basic triphenylmethane dye; C.I. 42000. It has been used as a stain for bacteria and as a bacteriostatic agent.

malacia (mal-la′she-ah, mah-la′se-ah) [Gr. *malakia* softness] the abnormal softening of a part or tissue occurring in a disease process.

-malacia a suffix word element to denote softening, e.g., osteomalacia.

malaco- (mal′ah-ko) [Gr. *malakos* soft] a prefix word element to denote a condition of abnormal softness, e.g., malacoplakia.

malacoplakia (mal″ah-ko-pla′ke-ah) [*malaco-* + Gr. *plax* plaque] an uncommon disorder associated with chronic bacterial infection, usually seen in the urinary tract, in which inflammatory cells accumulate within the subepithelial connective tissue. Most of the inflammatory cells are histiocytes; some contain spherical cytoplasmic bodies in which salts of calcium and iron are deposited in an aggregate of phospholipid membranes, concentrically oriented and formed from lysosomal action (Michaelis-Gutmann bodies). Malacoplakia is rarely fatal. Also called malakoplakia.

maladie de Roger (mal″ah-de′ duh ro-zhā) [Fr.] see *Roger's disease.*

malaise (mal-āz′) [Fr.] a general symptom described as a vague feeling of uneasiness or of being unwell; general bodily discomfort. It is often a sign of infection or disease.

malar (ma′lar) [L. *mala* cheek] pertaining to the cheek or cheek bone.

malaria (mah-la′re-ah) [It. "bad air"] an infectious febrile disease caused by protozoa of the genus *Plasmodium* that are transmitted by infected mosquitoes of the genus *Anopheles.* In the acute form, the disease is characterized by fever, anemia, splenomegaly, chills, and sweating. The fever, chills, and sweating occur at intervals, depending on the time required for a new generation of parasites to develop in the body. Following the primary attack, the disease has a tendency to become chronic, with occasional relapses.

Malarial infections are distributed throughout the temperate and tropical regions of the world. There are four *Plasmodium* species that occur in humans, each with many strains: *P. vivax,* the most common cause of the infection, has a wider distribution than the other types; *P. falciparum* is predominantly found throughout the tropics; *P. malariae,* although rare, is observed in temperate and subtropic areas; and *P. ovale* is relatively uncommon, most cases being found in Africa with a less frequent incidence in Asia, Europe, and South America.

The life cycle of the plasmodium parasite consists of two phases: an exogenous sexual phase (sporogony) in mosquitoes and an endogenous asexual phase (schizogony) in humans.

When the female mosquito bites an infected individual, she ingests blood containing mature sexual forms (male and female) called gametocytes. The male cell (microgametocyte) matures by extending flagellumlike structures containing nuclear chromatin that eventually become detached to form microgametes. The female cell (macrogametocyte)

MALABSORPTION SYNDROME. CLASSIFICATION OF INTESTINAL MALABSORPTION SYNDROMES

	PHYSIOLOGIC PATHOLOGY	CLINICAL FEATURES
Diseases of Maldigestion		
Gastric resection with gastrojejunostomy	Decreased pancreatic stimulation because of duodenal bypass. Poor mixing of food, bile, pancreatic enzymes. Decreased intrinsic factor. Bacterial stasis in afferent loop	Weight loss, moderate steatorrhea, anemia (combination of iron, B_{12} malabsorption, folate deficiency)
Pancreatic insufficiency (chronic pancreatitis, pancreatic carcinoma, pancreatic resection, cystic fibrosis)	Reduced intraluminal pancreatic enzyme activity with maldigestion of lipid and protein	History of abdominal pain followed by weight loss. Marked steatorrhea, azotorrhea. Also frequent glucose intolerance (70% in pancreatic insufficiency)
Short gut syndrome. Postsurgical resection or bypass. Crohn's enteritis	Loss of ileal absorbing surface leads to reduced bile salt pool size and reduced vitamin B_{12}	Weight loss, steatorrhea. Abnormal Schilling test, low D-xylose absorption
Bacterial overgrowth syndrome (surgical strictures, blind loops, enteric fistulas, multiple jejunal diverticula, scleroderma)	Overgrowth of intraluminal bacteria in jejunum, especially anaerobic organisms, to greater than 10^6/ml, results in deconjugation of bile salts, decreased effective bile salt pool size; also bacterial utilization of vitamin B_{12}	Weight loss, steatorrhea. Abnormal Schilling test, low D-xylose absorption
Zollinger-Ellison syndrome	Hyperacidity in duodenum inactivates pancreatic enzymes	Ulcer diathesis, steatorrhea
Lactose intolerance	Deficiency of intestinal lactase results in high concentrations of intraluminal lactose with osmotic diarrhea	Affects 70% of U.S. blacks and probably all other noncaucasian races. Varied degrees of diarrhea and cramps after ingestion of lactose-containing foods. Positive lactose tolerance test, decreased intestinal lactase
Diseases of Mucosal Malabsorption		
Celiac disease (gluten-sensitive enteropathy)	Toxic response to a gluten fraction by surface epithelium results in destruction of absorbing surface	Weight loss, diarrhea, bloating, anemia (low folate, iron), osteomalacia, steatorrhea, azotorrhea, low D-xylose absorption. Flat intestinal biopsy. Responds to gluten restriction
Tropical sprue	Unknown toxic factor results in mucosal inflammation, partial villous atrophy	Weight loss, diarrhea, anemia, (low folate, B_{12}). Steatorrhea. Low D-xylose absorption, abnormal Schilling test. Typical but nonspecific biopsy change
Whipple's disease	Bacterial invasion of intestinal mucosa	Arthritis, hyperpigmentation, lymphadenopathy, serious effusions, fever, weight loss. Steatorrhea, azotorrhea, diagnostic biopsy
Certain parasitic diseases (giardiasis strongyloides, coccidiosis, capillariasis)	Damage to or invasion of surface mucosa	Diarrhea, weight loss, steatorrhea. Organism may be seen on jejunal biopsy or recovered in stool
Immunoglobulinopathy	Decreased local gut defenses, lymphoid hyperplasia, lymphopenia	Frequent association with giardiasis. Hypogammaglobulinemia or isolated IgA deficiency. Diagnostic or typical biopsy changes

From Halsted, C.H., and Halsted, J.A., The Laboratory in Clinical Medicine. 2nd ed. Philadelphia, W.B. Saunders Co., 1981, p. 230.

matures into a macrogamete, and when the microgamete fertilizes the macrogamete, a zygote is formed. The active zygote (then called an ookinete) becomes elongated and motile. This organism breaks through the wall of the mosquito's stomach, lodging in the outer layer to become an oocyst. Maturation of the oocyst results in the production of slender, threadlike sporozoites. These motile sporozoites are liberated from the ruptured oocyst and migrate through the mosquito's body. Those that become lodged in the salivary glands may be introduced into humans while the mosquito is feeding.

Within the human body, the sporozoites are cleared from the blood system within 40 min and invade the parenchymal cells of the liver (the exoerythrocytic stage). In the liver, the parasites undergo asexual development, resulting in schizonts. After maturation of the schizonts (the process of schizogony), merozoites are liberated from the schizonts and invade the circulation, initiating the erythrocytic stage. During the erythrocytic stage, the infected red blood cells reproduce merozoites through the stages of trophozoites (ring stage) and schizonts; the time required to complete the cycle determines the periodicity of the chills, fever, and sweating.

Following several generations of merozoites, some develop into male and female cells (microgametocytes and macrogametocytes, respectively). Continuation of the cycle is dependent on ingestion of the gametocytes by a mosquito. In the relapsing malarias (*P. vivax, P. malariae,* and *P. ovale*), merozoites from the circulation can reenter the hepatocytes, but in *P. falciparum* malaria there is no secondary invasion of hepatocytes, and thus relapses do not occur.

The most characteristic features of malaria are periodic fever, splenomegaly, anemia, and leukopenia. All four types of malarial infection show the typical paroxysms, chills, fever, and sweating stages. In between the paroxysms, the individual feels healthy and appears normal.

Many individuals exhibit a partially acquired immunity (premunition) following infection. This is thought to occur because the parasitized cells are sensitized by antibodies, and the individual is protected by phagocytosis and digestion of the parasitized red blood cells by the macrophages. A degree of immunity to *P. falciparum* is conferred upon individuals with deficiencies of glucose-6-phosphate dehydrogenase and the sickle cell anemia trait. In addition, it has been shown that blacks with the FyFy genotype are refractory to infection by *P. vivax.*

Laboratory diagnosis requires demonstration and identification of malarial parasites in peripheral blood films. The most commonly used methods are Giemsa thin films or stained thick blood films (the latter method is considered superior). Definitive diagnosis depends on the presence of the parasite in conjunction with the clinical symptoms. Serologic tests may occasionally be of value in helping to diagnose long-standing, low-level infections with relapsing malaria.

Antimalarial drugs can be used to treat the clinical attack, prevent relapses, suppress the clinical manifestations of the disease, and/or act as a sporontocidal agent (preventing transmission by vector). Chloroquine is the drug of choice in treating acute malaria, attacking the erythrocytic forms of the parasite. Infection with chloroquine-resistant *P. falciparum,* however, should be treated with pyrimethamine-sulfadoxine or quinine. A renewed interest in malarial vaccines has occurred because of the persistence of malarial infection and the continuing development of resistant strains. The culture methods established in vitro may provide a means for future vaccine production and the testing of antimalarial drugs.

Also called *ague, jungle fever,* and *paludism.* For more information on the individual species, see *Plasmodium.*

malariacidal (mah-lār″e-ah-si′dal) [*malaria* + L. *caedere* to kill] an agent that destroys the malarial parasite; plasmodicidal (destructive to plasmodia).

Malassezia (mal″ah-se′ze-ah) [Louis Charles *Malassez,* physiologist in Paris, 1842–1909] a genus of fungi that causes tinea versicolor. The two genera *Malassezia* and *Pityrosporum* are synonymous (see *Pityrosporum*).

M. furfur, see *P. orbiculare* under *Pityrosporum.*

malate (ma′lāt) any salt of malic acid.

malate dehydrogenase (MD, MDH) (ma′lāt de-hi′-dro-jen-ās) an enzyme of the oxidoreductase class (EC 1.1.1.37) that catalyzes the reaction L-malate + $NAD^+ \rightleftarrows$ oxaloacetate + NADH. The enzyme occurs both in the mitochondria and in the cytosol. The reaction is important in the citric acid cycle. It participates in the malate-aspartate shuttle, which permits the electrons of cytosolic NADH to reduce mitochondrial NAD^+. Increased enzyme levels in the serum have been observed in cases of myocardial infarction, hepatic necrosis, megaloblastic anemia, and neoplastic disease.

malathion (mal″ah-thi′on) a moderately toxic insecticide and miticide, *O,O*-dimethyl dithiophosphate of diethyl mercaptosuccinate. See also *organophosphate compounds.*

Malayan filariasis a condition caused by the presence of the filarial parasite *Brugia malayi* in the lymphatics, lymph nodes, or connective tissues of humans. Malayan filariasis is distributed throughout Malaya, India, New Guinea, Thailand, Vietnam, and parts of China, Korea, and Japan.

Laboratory diagnosis of the parasite requires demonstration of microfilariae in the blood. As *B. malayi* filariae usually have a nocturnal periodicity, the best time to draw blood is between 10 PM and 2 AM. Fresh wet preparations of blood should be examined, as well as thick and thin blood films stained with Field's rapid stain method (thick films), Leishman stain method (thin films), Giemsa stain, or hematoxylin to differentiate morphologic features. Serologic tests such as the indirect hemagglutination and flocculation tests, using *Dirofilaria immitis* extracts as antigen, are used, but they demonstrate only the presence of the filarial group, not the species. Diethylcarbamazine (Hetrazan) is the drug of choice.

See also *elephantiasis.* Cf. *Bancroft's filariasis.*

Malayan pit viper venom see under *thrombolytic agents.*

male (māl) [Old Fr. from L. *masculus*] 1. pertaining to the sex that produces small motile gametes (spermatozoa).

2. an individual of this sex.

3. pertaining to a connector that fits into a corresponding (female) connector.

male hormones a class of 19-carbon steroid hormones that have androgenic activity. The principal male hormone is testosterone. Other notable male hormones are dihydrotestosterone, androstenediol, and androstanediol. See also *androgen.* Cf. *female hormones.*

malformation (mal″for-ma′shun) [*mal-* + L. *formatio* a forming] a congenital anomaly of an organ structure that occurs during embryogenesis. Malformations are usually considered to have intrinsic causes, although they are potentially caused by chemical or viral teratogens introduced from outside the embryo. See also *agenesis, aplasia,* and *hypoplasia.*

congenital m., structural abnormalities of development that are evident at birth. They may be inherited or due to environmental factors that affect the developing fetus in utero. Cf. *inherited m.*

inherited m., disorders that are wholly genetically determined and may or may not be evident at birth.

malfunction (mal-funk′shun) a failure to function normally.

malic acid (mah′lik) a hydroxysuccinic acid, $COOH \cdot CH_2CHOH \cdot COOH$, found in unripe and sour apples and in many fruits. It is an intermediate of the tricarboxylic acid cycle, and is also involved in the metabolism of some amino acids. Small amounts are found in blood and urine.

malignancy (mah-lig′nan-se) [L. *malignare* to act maliciously] 1. the quality or property of being malignant.

2. a malignant tumor.

malignant (mah-lig′nant) [L. *malignans* acting maliciously] an abstract concept referring to the tendency to become progressively worse and to result in death. In reference to neoplasms, the term denotes the properties of invasiveness and metastasis. Other features that help define the concept of malignancy include cellular aneuploidy, altered regulation of cell proliferation, altered cell kinetics, abnormal chromosome complement, misprogrammed gene function, nonspecific metabolic pathways and isoenzyme patterns, ectopic hormone production, loss of isoantigens, and transplant stability. See also *metastasis* and *neoplasia.* Cf. *benign.*

malleolus (mal-le′o-lus), pl. *malleoli* [L., dim. of *malleus* hammer] [NA], the general term for a rounded process, such as the protuberance on either side of the ankle joint.

lateral m. of fibula, the lower end of the fibula, which forms the prominence on the lateral side of the ankle. Its medial surface articulates with the talus.

medial m. of tibia, the distal projection on the lower end of the tibia, which forms the prominence on the medial side of the ankle. Its lateral surface articulates with the talus.

Malleomyces (mal″e-o-mi′sēz) [L. *malleus* glanders + Gr. *mykēs* fungus] the former name for a genus of pseudomonads, e.g., *Pseudomonas* (*Malleomyces*) *mallei* and *P.* (*Malleomyces*) *pseudomallei.*

M. malleomyces, the former name for the bacterium *Pseudomonas mallei.* See P. *mallei* under *Pseudomonas.*

malleus (mal′e-us) [L. "hammer"] [NA], the largest of the three auditory ossicles, which is attached by its lateral end to the tympanic membrane and medially to the incus.

Mallophaga (mal-of′ah-gah) [Gr. *mallos* wool + *phagein* to eat] an order of biting lice found primarily on birds but occasionally on humans and other mammals. These lice measure 1–10 mm in length and have mouthparts of the chewing type. The order includes the medically important genera *Damalinia, Felicola, Heterodoxus,* and *Trichodectes.* Cf. *Anoplura.*

Mallory bodies (mal′o-re) [Frank Burr *Mallory,* pathologist in Boston, 1862–1941] rounded or irregular masses of hyaline acidophilic material (alcoholic hyalin) that develop near the nuclei of damaged liver cells, as in alcoholic cirrhosis. They are well stained by acid fuchsin, eosin, or Mallory's phosphotungstic acid–hematoxylin (PTAH) or hemalum-phloxine stains.

Mallory's collagen stain [Frank Burr *Mallory*] a histologic method for demonstrating connective tissue, which has also proved useful in hypophyseal cell differentiation. Paraffin sections fixed in Zenker's fluid are hydrated and placed in iodine followed by sodium thiosulfate to remove mercury deposits. Sections are initially stained in aqueous acid fuchsin and transferred directly into a solution of aniline blue, orange G, and phosphotungstic acid. Nuclei and alpha cells stain red; collagen, ground substance, mucin, amyloid, and beta cells stain various shades of blue; and erythrocytes and myelin stain yellow. See also *Gomori's method for chromaffin* and *Heidenhain's azan stain.*

Mallory-Weiss syndrome [G. Kenneth *Mallory,* U.S. pathologist, born 1900; Soma *Weiss,* U.S. internist, 1898–1942] a condition characterized by massive, acute hemorrhage from the upper gastrointestinal region. It is due to a longitudinal tear in the gastric mucosa near the gastroesophageal junction, usually following prolonged vomiting and retching. The majority of affected patients are alcoholics. Diagnosis is based on patient history, esophagogastroscopy, and selective angiography.

malnutrition (mal″nu-trish′un) [*mal-* + L. *nutritio,* from *nutrio* to suckle or nourish] any disorder of nutrition, which may be due to an unbalanced or insufficient diet or to the defective assimilation or utilization of foods.

malignant m., see *kwashiorkor.*

protein m., see *kwashiorkor.*

malocclusion (mal″o-kloo′zhun) a disorder characterized by malpositioning and abnormal contact of the maxillary and mandibular teeth, and which may interfere with mastication. Most frequently, the cause is developmental, such as an excess number of teeth, but malocclusion can also be acquired. X-rays of the facial bones, skull, and teeth, as well as models of the teeth, are used in diagnosis. Therapy is aimed at preventing dental and periodontal disease and at improving mastication and speaking.

malonic acid (mal-on′ik) a crystalline dibasic acid, $COOH \cdot CH_2 \cdot COOH$, formed by oxidizing malic acid with chromium trioxide and used in the manufacture of barbiturates. Malonic semialdehyde is formed in mammalian tissues from the degradation of β-alanine.

malonyl coenzyme A (mal′o-nil) the CoA thioester, $HOOCCH_2COSCoA$, of malonic acid. It is the first product synthesized from acetyl CoA in the sequence of reactions leading to long-chain fatty acid formation. The reaction that leads to the formation of malonyl CoA from acetyl CoA is a biotin-dependent carboxylation and is the rate-controlling step in fatty acid synthesis.

malposition (mal″po-zish′un) [*mal-* + L. *positio* placement] a general term used to describe abnormal positioning of a part of the body.

malpractice (mal-prak′tis) [*mal-* + L. *practicare,* from Gr. *praktikos* practical from *prassein* to practice] a term usually referring to poor or improper medical treatment, especially that resulting in harm to the patient. One of the major areas of concern in malpractice suits today concerns the issue of informed consent: the right of patients to understand the methods involved in, risks of, and alternatives to medical procedures they are to undergo.

malrotation (mal″ro-ta′shun) [*mal-* + L. *rotatio,*

from *rotare* to turn] abnormal or pathologic rotation, as of the gastrointestinal tract.

malrotation of the bowel a group of developmental disorders in which the intestines fail to achieve their normal adult position and orientation. The normal intestinal rotation may fail to occur, may occur partially, or may occur in the reverse of normal direction. Complications include intestinal obstruction, ulceration, and malabsorption. The disorder is diagnosed by barium enema, and upper GI and small bowel radiologic examinations.

Malta fever (mawl'tah) see *brucellosis.*

malt agar (mawlt) a growth medium for fungal yeast cells and for the production of ascospores from the yeast cells. The medium consists of malt extract, agar, and water. Yeasts are streaked onto the prepared malt agar and incubated at room temperature for 24–48 hr.

maltase (mawl'tās) see *α-D*-glucosidase.

maltose (mawl'tōs) *O*-α-D-glucopyranosyl-(1→4)-D-glucopyranose, a disaccharide. Maltose is a white crystalline sugar formed when starch is hydrolyzed by amylase, and is used as a nutrient and sweetener. Also called malt sugar.

maltosuria (mawl"to-su're-ah) the presence of maltose in the urine. It has been reported to occur along with glucose in the urine of some diabetic individuals.

mamillary (mam'ĭ-ler"e) [L. *mamilla,* dim. of *mamma*] pertaining to or resembling a nipple.

mamillary bodies a pair of small, white, hemispherical masses of brain tissue situated in the interpeduncular fossa just rostral to the posterior perforated substance. Although enclosed by white fibers from the fornix, they are part of the hypothalamus.

mamillary line a vertical line passing through the center of a nipple. Also called *midclavicular line* and *nipple line.* Cf. *mammary line.*

mamm/o (mam'o) [L. *mamma* the mother's breast] a word element used in combining form to denote breast, e.g., mammography.

mammal (mam'al) an individual belonging to the class Mammalia. A mammal is a homeothermic vertebrate possessing the characteristics of seven cervical vertebrae, body hair and of mammary glands for milk production.

mammalgia (mah-mal'je-ah) see *mastodynia.*

Mammalia (mah-ma'le-ah) [NL., from *mammalis* of the breast] the biologic taxonomic class that comprises mammals.

mammalian (mah-ma'le-en) of or pertaining to a mammal.

mammary (mam'er-e) [L. *mammarius*] pertaining to the mamma, or breast.

mammary duct ectasia an inflammatory disorder of the mammary ducts that usually first affects the subareolar ducts and spreads to smaller ducts throughout the breast. It is characterized by periductal fibrosis and duct dilation. Also called *periductal mastitis.*

mammary dysplasia an imprecise and confusing term for nonmalignant diseases of the breast. It carries a connotation of precancerous change of unspecified type and severity. The term mammary dysphoria has no communicative value for pathologists or clinicians.

mammary gland see *breast.*

mammary line the horizontal line that intersects the nipples. Cf. *mamillary line.*

mammary region the region of the front of the chest that overlies and surrounds the breasts.

mammography (mam-og'rah-fe) [*mammo-* + Gr. *graphein* to write, record] a technique of soft tissue radiography to produce images of the mammary gland. Most methods in current use employ x-rays of relatively low kilovoltage that enhance small tissue density differences. The resultant image is recorded either on x-ray film (film mammography) or on selenium-coated plates (xeroradiography).

Specialized radiographic equipment with generators capable of repeated exposures in the range of 25–35 kV and an x-ray tube with a molybdenum anode that produces x-rays of optimal energy are required to record maximal breast tissue detail on standard x-ray film. High-resolution film is packaged in specialized cassettes containing intensifying screens that closely contact the film. The film image is thus created by the radiation-induced luminescence of these screens to provide high-quality mammograms at the lowest possible radiation dose. The most efficient of these systems delivers a radiation dose to the breast comparable with that of a routine chest x-ray.

Optimal exposure of the selenium-coated plate for xeroradiography requires a radiation dose several times in excess of that required for film-screen mammography. Increased filtration of the x-ray beam using additional layers of aluminum is commonly utilized to reduce radiation dosage to the breast. Dosage to the midplane of the breast, however, remains 4–10 times greater with this technique than with film-screen mammography.

With either the film or xerographic modes of breast imaging, one can obtain standard views in the craniocaudal and mediolateral positions. For both of these views, a compression device is applied to the breast, flattening the organ to more uniform thickness and minimizing the object-film distance. The craniocaudal view is obtained with the patient sitting, with the vertical x-ray beam entering the superior aspect of the breast and exiting inferiorly to expose the image receptor. The mediolateral projection can be obtained with the patient sitting or lying on her side, with the vertical x-ray beam entering the inner surface of the breast and exiting laterally.

Although film-screen mammography and xeromammography are the methods of breast radiography in most common use, experimental mammography using CT scanners and ultrasound techniques is currently being investigated.

At present, mammography is performed almost exclusively for the detection of breast cancer. This technique has enabled physicians to discover approximately one-third of breast cancers before they grow large enough to form a clinically palpable lump. Preliminary studies indicate that these preclinical cancers detected by mammography have a lower rate of local spread and a higher potential for cure than those detected clinically.

This important tool in early cancer detection aroused controversy in 1976 when it was suggested that the level of radiation associated with mammography might result in an increased frequency of breast cancer among those screened. Subsequent improvements in film-sceen combinations and x-ray beam filtration have reduced the radiation dose delivered to the individual in most applications.

Current assessment of the risk-benefit of mammography strongly supports the benefits to be derived from early breast cancer detection; with modern, low-radiation dose techniques. These benefits are widely considered to substantially outweigh the radiation risk.

A 1980 statement issued by the American Cancer Society recommends baseline mammography for all women between the ages of 35 and 40, to be followed by annual mammograms after the age of 50. Between the ages of 40 and 50, the frequency of mammographic examination should depend on individual risk factors for the development of breast cancer, and other variables to be evaluated by the patient and her physician.

Also called *mastography.*

F. R. MARGOLIN, M.D.

mammotropic (mam″o-trop′ik) [*mammo-* + Gr. *tropikos* inclined] having affinity for or a stimulating effect on the mammary gland.

mammotropin (mah-mot′ro-pin) see *prolactin.*

manchette (man-chet′) [Fr. "a cuff"] a small, cylindric structure, composed of microtubules, that forms at the caudal pole of the nucleus during spermiogenesis. Also called caudal sheath.

Mandelin's reagent a solution of ammonium vanadate (NH_4VO_3) in sulfuric acid, used in color tests for alkaloids.

mandible (man′dĭ-b′l) the bone of the lower jaw, the body of which is curved like a horseshoe. Flattened rami project upward from the posterior ends of the body, each bearing a coronoid and a coracoid process. The latter participates in the temporomandibular joint.

mandibul/o (man-dib′u-lo) [L. *mandibula* mandible] a word element used in combining form to denote the lower jawbone, e.g., mandibular.

mandibular nerve (man-dib′u-lar) the largest branch of the trigeminal nerve. It supplies the skin of the lower face and temporal region, the muscles of mastication, the teeth and gums of the mandible, and the anterior tongue. The nerve has a large sensory root and a smaller motor root. The sensory root emerges from the semilunar ganglion and passes through the foramen ovale; the motor root passes below the ganglion and unites with the sensory root just beyond the foramen ovale. The nerve divides into anterior and posterior trunks. The anterior trunk branches into a sensory component, the buccal nerve, and a motor component consisting of the masseteric, deep temporal, and lateral temporal nerves. The posterior trunk is primarily sensory and divides into the lingual, auriculotemporal, and inferior alveolar nerves.

mandibulofacial dysostosis (man-dib″u-lo-fa′shal dis″os-to′sis) see *Treacher Collins syndrome.*

manganese (Mn) (man′gah-nēs) [L. *manganum, manganesium*] a metallic element resembling iron; atomic number 25; atomic weight 54.938; a 3d transition element; oxidation states +1 through +7 (+2, +4, +7 are common). It is an essential mineral nutrient; about 0.2 mmol is normally present in the body, where it is a cofactor for several enzymes. Deficiency has not yet been encountered in humans.

Industrial workers, particularly those involved in manganese mining and smelting, may be exposed to toxic doses. Inhalation of manganese dust can cause manganese pneumonitis; chronic exposure can cause a degeneration of the central nervous system that is clinically similar to parkinsonism.

manganese assays spectrophotometry. The specimen is digested in strong acids, and all of the manganese is oxidized with lead dioxide (PbO_2) or sodium bismuthate ($NaBiO_3$) to permanganate (MnO_4^-). The concentration is proportional to the absorbance at 420 nm. Specimen quantities as small as 0.1 μg/g can be determined with 10 percent reproducibility. Improved sensitivity and precision can be obtained with atomic absorption spectrophotometry using flameless techniques.

manganic (man-gan′ik) pertaining to the manganese(III) ion, Mn^{3+}, as in manganic oxide, Mn_2O_3.

manganism (man′gah-nizm) chronic manganese poisoning; see under *manganese.*

manganous (man′gah-nus) pertaining to the manganese(II) ion, Mn^{2+}, as in manganous oxide, MnO.

mania (ma′ne-ah) [Gr. "madness"] 1. a word element used as a suffix to denote obsessive preoccupation with something, e.g., dipsomania.

2. a mental disorder characterized by extreme mental excitement, elation, agitation, pressure of speech, and increased motor activity. See also *manic-depressive illness.*

acute hallucinatory m., see *Ganser's syndrome.*

manic-depressive illness (man″ik de-pres′iv) a disorder of affect (mood), which may be characterized by cyclic and often recurring mood changes, resulting in periods of depression and/or elation that are beyond the range of normal mood swings. The depressive phase is marked by a loss of interest in living, sadness, withdrawal, and feelings of guilt; the manic phase (which may or may not occur) is marked by elation, pressure of speech, and increased motor activity. The disorder may have a genetic basis, and neurochemical imbalances involving the biogenic amines may be a prime precipitating factor in causation.

mannans (man′anz) a polymer composed of protein and two polysaccharide moieties differing in their structure and mode of attachment to the peptide. The first polysaccharide contains mannose ($C_6H_{12}O_6$) in α-1,6 linkages, with α-1,2 and α-1,3 branches; the second polysaccharide consists of rather short mannooligosaccharides. It is found in the cell walls of fungi, especially yeasts.

mannitol (man′ĭ-tol) [USP], a sugar alcohol, derived from mannose, $HO(CH_2OH)_4CH_2OH$; M.W. 182.19. Found in many plant materials and exudates, mannitol is obtained from seaweed and by hydrogenation of invert sugar. The ability to utilize mannitol is used in the identification of strains of bacteria, e.g., *Escherichia coli, Salmonella,* and *Streptococcus.*

Mannitol is used as an osmotic diuretic, which is nontoxic, not metabolized, and excreted entirely by glomerular filtration. It is administered by intravenous infusion; this increases the osmotic pressure in the blood and the renal tubules, causing a reduction in the reabsorption of sodium and water and drawing water away from the cerebrospinal and intraocular fluids. Mannitol diuresis is used to increase the excretion of drugs in cases of poisoning and to reduce intraocular and intracranial pressure. It is contraindicated when renal function is impaired.

mannose (man′ōs) a monosaccharide, an aldohexose sugar that is an epimer of glucose. It is used in the biosynthesis of fucose and neuraminates. Mannose is present in some glycoproteins and contributes to the disease mannosidosis.

α-D-mannosidase (man′o-sĭ-dās) an enzyme of the hydrolase class (α-D-mannoside mannohydrolase, EC 3.2.1.24) that catalyzes the hydrolysis of terminal nonreducing α-D-mannose residues in α-D-mannosides. A rare genetic deficiency of the enzyme causes mannosidosis.

mannosidosis (man″o-sĭ-do′sis), pl. *mannosidoses.* an inborn error of metabolism characterized by a deficiency of lysosomal α-D-mannosidase, which is involved in metabolism of the oligosaccharide moieties of glycoproteins. There is lysosomal storage and excess urinary excretion of oligosaccharides, and cultured leukocytes and fibroblasts are deficient in acid α-D-mannosidase. The severe form of mannosidosis has symptoms similar to those in mucopolysaccharidoses; in a mild form, mental retardation and hearing deficit are the predominant symptoms. See also *lysosomal storage disease.*

Mann-Whitney rank sum statistic see under *rank sum test.*

manometer (mah-nom′ĕ-ter) [Gr. *manos* thin + *metron* measure] a device to measure pressure, usually having a U-shaped tube filled with liquid, as in a sphygmomanometer.

manometry (mah-nom′ĕ-tre) the measurement of pressure with a manometer.

Mansonella (man″so-nel′ah) a genus of filarial nematodes.

M. ozzardi, a filarial nematode parasitic in humans that causes a mild allergic reaction and edema. *Mansonella* infections are found in Central and South America, and sometimes in the West Indies. The principal intermediate hosts are gnats of the genus *Culicoides.* Adult filariae inhabit the mesentery or visceral adipose tissue; unsheathed microfilariae are found in the blood at all times, having a thick, pointed tail without nuclei.

Laboratory diagnosis requires identification of the microfilariae in the blood by fresh wet preparations and stained thick (Field's rapid stain method) and thin (Leishman stain method) blood films. Giemsa and hemotoxylin stains are also useful in differentiating morphologic features.

Also called *Filaria demarquayi, F. ozzardi* and *F. tucumana.*

mansonelliasis (man″so-nel-i′ah-sis) infection with *Mansonella ozzardi.*

Mansonia (man-so′ne-ah) [Sir Patrick *Manson*] a genus of mosquitoes. Several species are known transmitters of *Brugia malayi,* the parasite that causes Malayan filariasis, and *Wuchereria bancrofti,* which causes Bancroft's filariasis. The species *M. metallica* is a vector of the virus that causes West Nile fever, a condition found distributed throughout Africa, the Middle East, South Asia, and southern Europe.

Mansonioides (man-so″ne-oi′dēz) [Sir Patrick *Manson*] a subgenus of *Mansonia.* The species *M. annulifera* is the principal transmitter of *Brugia malayi* in India.

mantle (man′t′l) [L. *mantellum* cloak] an enveloping cover or layer.

m. of lymphoid follicle, the peripheral zone of small lymphocytes that surrounds the germinal center.

Mantoux test (man-too′) [Charles *Mantoux,* French physician, 1877–1947] an intracutaneous test for delayed hypersensitivity to the tubercle bacillus *Mycobacterium tuberculosis.* Solutions of purified protein derivative of tuberculin (0.1 ml of 1:10,000 or 1:100 dilution) are injected into the skin; 10 mm or more of induration indicates a positive reaction. The higher concentration should be used only in persons suspected of having active tuberculosis who fail to react to the first low dose and may be anergic.

manual input the entry of data into a computer by the operator, as opposed to input from another machine.

manubrium (mah-nu′bre-um), pl. *manubria* [L.] [NA], a general term for a handlelike structure or part; used alone to designate the manubrium sterni.

m. sterni, [NA], the widest, thickest, and uppermost of the three parts of the sternum. It articulates with the clavicles and the first two costal cartilages.

MAO abbrev. for *maximal acid output,* monoamine oxidase (see under *amine oxidase* [*flavin-containing*]).

map (map′) a two-dimensional graphic representation of arrangement in space.

fate m., a plan of the blastula or early gastrula stage that shows areas of prospective significance in normal development.

genetic m., a map of the location of genes on a chromosome. See also *genetic map.*

memory m., a diagram used to indicate specifically assigned areas in a digital computer's memory.

maple syrup urine disease a hereditary aminoacidopathy, transmitted as an autosomal recessive trait, in which there is deficient decarboxylation of branched-chain α-ketoacids derived from valine, leucine, isoleucine, and alloisoleucine. These amino acids and ketoacids increase in the blood and urine. The disease is characterized by mental retardation, toxic encephalopathy, and an odor of maple syrup in urine. Unless diagnosed and treated, it is usually fatal in weeks or months. Also called *branched-chain aminoaciduria, branched-chain ketoaciduria,* and leucinosis. See also *aminoacidopathy.*

maprotiline (mah-pro′tĭ-lēn) a tetracyclic antidepressant with actions and side-effects similar to those of the tricyclic antidepressants. It is believed to act by inhibiting the reuptake of the neurotransmitter norepinephrine at central synapses. Whereas most tricyclic antidepressants also inhibit the reuptake of serotonin, maprotiline does not.

map unit see *centimorgan.*

marantic (mah-ran′tik) [Gr. *marantikos* wasting away] a general term used to describe protein-calorie malnutrition that is characterized by wasting of muscle, loss of body fat, and growth retardation.

marasmus (mah-raz′mus) [Gr. *marasmos* a dying away] a malnutrition state most often due to a relatively inadequate intake of all nutrients. It is common in the young and leads to retardation of growth, atrophy of muscle and other tissue, and skin changes without edema. Diarrhea, systemic disease, and any cause of prolonged negative energy balance may also lead to marasmus. See also *kwashiorkor.*

marble bone disease see *osteopetrosis.*

Marburg agent (mar′berg) [from *Marburg,* West Germany] a type of rhabdovirus that causes Marburg virus disease. This virus has a bizarre, filamentous, tubelike appearance with regular surface projections.

Marburg virus disease an acute febrile condition caused by the Marburg agent, a virus. The disease is characterized by an abrupt onset of headache, myalgia, rash, and hemorrhagic manifestations. The incubation period is 5–9 da, with fever of 39.4°–40°C (103°–104°F). A watery diarrhea develops 1–3 da after onset, and leukocytopenia and thrombocytopenia are usually present. Virus has been directly observed by electron microscopy in tissues from the liver, lungs, and spleen, and in in vitro cell cultures. Its filamentous shape, occasional branching, and extreme length are unique and characteristic of this disease.

Marchiafava-Bignami disease (mar″ke-ah-fah′-vah bēn-yah-′me) [Ettore *Marchiafava,* Italian pathologist, 1847–1935; Amico *Bignami,* Italian pathologist, 1862–1929] a rare disorder, usually occurring in middle-aged male alcoholics, that is characterized by agitation, confusion, emotional disturbances, hallucinations, memory disturbances, seizures, and/or progressive dementia, usually leading to stupor and coma. The clinical picture is extremely variable, however, and may be masked by the features of alcoholic intoxication or withdrawal. The disorder has a variable course, but complete recovery is rare. Pathologically, there is symmetric, progressive demyelination of the corpus callosum and, less consistently, of other structures.

Marchiafava-Micheli syndrome [Ettore *Marchiafava;* F. *Micheli,* Italian physician, 1872–1936] see *paroxysmal nocturnal hemoglobinuria.*

Marfan's syndrome (mar-fahnz) [Bernard-Jean Antonin *Marfan,* French pediatrician, 1858–1942] a generalized disorder of connective tissue, transmitted as an autosomal dominant trait with variable expression. The metabolic defect is unknown. Marfan's syndrome is diagnosed on clinical grounds, including increased long bone length, cardiovascular abnormalities, and lens dislocation. There is no specific test to detect this syndrome.

margin (mar″jin) [L. *margo, marginis*] an edge or border, such as the boundary of an organ or other anatomic structure.

Marie's ataxia (mah-rēz′) [Pierre *Marie,* French physician, 1853–1940] see under *spinocerebellar degeneration.*

Marie's disease [Pierre *Marie*] see *acromegaly.*

marijuana (mar″ĭ-hwah′nah) [Mexican Spanish] the hemp plant *Cannabis sativa* or the dried flower tops and leaves of this plant, which are smoked to produce euphoria. See also *C. sativa* under *Cannabis* and *tetrahydrocannabinol.*

marker (mark′er) 1. something used as a mark or indicator.

2. a cell surface molecule, or, rarely, an intracellular molecule that can be detected by an immunologic reaction using a tagged antibody. Antibodies labeled with fluorochrome or enzymes are commonly used to detect these antigens using standard immunohistochemical methods. Some examples of clinically useful immunologic markers are the Leu series markers on leukocytes detected with monoclonal antibodies, surface immunoglobulins on B lymphocytes, and terminal deoxynucleotidyl transferase present in the nuclei of primitive lymphocytes. See also *genetic marker* and *tumor markers.*

fecal m., a substance such as carmine, that is ingested to mark the beginning and end of fecal collection periods.

marker chromosome an abnormal chromosome often observed in precancerous or cancerous cells. The abnormality may be in the size or shape of the chromosome; for example, very long marker chromosomes that distort the cell nucleus are observed in cancer cells from carcinoma in situ of the uterine cervix. Hyperchromasia of cancer cells may relate to an increase in the constitutive (C banding) heterochromatin in certain marker chromosomes.

marker rescue a method of locating genetic markers on a genetic map from restriction endonuclease fragments. A purified, wild-type DNA fragment is transfected into a cell infected with a mutant phage. Wild-type progeny are produced by recombination if the DNA fragment overlaps the mutation. See also *genetic mapping.*

mark sense reader a computer input device that reads pencil marks placed in outlined areas on a card or sheet of paper, such as a standardized test answer sheet.

Maroteaux-Lamy syndrome a rare genetic disorder, transmitted as an autosomal recessive trait, that is characterized by abnormal mucopolysaccharide metabolism, leading to severe skeletal deformities, corneal clouding, and dwarfing of the trunk. Radiologically, there are defects of the metaphyses and epiphyses, and of the vertebrae. Inclusions are found in both the lymphocytes and neutrophils. This disease has been linked to deficiencies of *N*-acetylgalactosamine-4-sulfatase (arylsulfatase B), and leads to increased urinary excretion of dermatan sulfate (chondroitin sulfate B).

Prenatal diagnosis of this disease is possible. Intelligence is normal, but death frequently occurs before age 30 yr.

Also called mucopolysaccharidosis VI (MPS VI). See also *mucopolysaccharidoses.*

Marquis reagent a solution of formaldehyde in sulfuric acid used in color tests for morphine, other alkaloids, and aromatic hydrocarbons.

marrow (mar′o) see *bone marrow.*

Martin-Gruber anastomosis the crossing over of fibers from the median to the ulnar nerve in the forearm. As 15–20 percent of the general population have this anomalous neural communication, it presents a possible source of error in diagnostic investigations utilizing nerve conduction studies.

Existence of the anastomosis can be detected by comparison of the amplitudes of the potentials evoked by stimulation of the ulnar nerve at the wrist and the elbow: in the presence of the anastomosis, the amplitude of the evoked potential is greater when stimulated from the wrist.

Martin-Lester agar see *Martin-Lester a.* under *agar.*

mA-s abbrev. See *milliampere-second.*

masculine (mas′ku-lin) [L. *masculinus*] pertaining

to the male sex, or to primary or secondary male sex characters.

masculinization (mas″ku-lin-ĭ-za′shun) the normal development of male sex characteristics in the male and the abnormal development of secondary male characteristics in the female. See also *virilization.*

masculinovoblastoma (mas″ku-lin-o″vo-blas-to′-mah) a rare, usually benign tumor of the ovaries that elaborates 17-ketosteroids and may cause masculinization. The origin of the tumor cells is uncertain. Also called lipid (lipoid) cell tumor.

masked message an mRNA sequence that is bound tightly to its macromolecule and is unavailable for translation. These messages are located in the cytoplasm of the unfertilized egg and in very early embryos of some species, becoming active in translation only after fertilization. In the unfertilized egg, the masked message exists as stable ribonucleprotein (RNP) particles. Also called informosome. See also *ribonucleoprotein (RNP) complex.*

mass (mas) [L. *massa*] 1. a lump or body made up of covering particles.

2. (abbrev. m), the quantity of matter in an object, the strength of the interaction between the object and a gravitational field. The International System (SI) unit of mass is the kilogram. The atomic mass unit (amu) or dalton (1.6604×10^{-27} kg) is used for atomic and molecular weights. The mass of an elementary particle is often measured, in electron volts, by the energy released in its annihilation (e.g., the mass of an electron is 511 keV).

mass action law stated as: the rate of a homogeneous chemical reaction at constant temperature is proportional to the concentrations of the reacting substances. See also *kinetics.*

mass attenuation coefficient the linear attenuation coefficient divided by the density of the absorbing material.

mass concentration the mass of solute per unit volume of solution; preferred units include kilograms per liter (kg/l), grams per liter (g/l), and milligrams per liter (mg/l).

mass fragmentography (mas frag″men-tog′rah-fe) a form of mass spectrometry (MS) dealing with the identification and sometimes the quantitation of the sample components by study of their mass spectra (the masses and amounts of the fragments produced by an ionizing electron beam), frequently after separation of the sample components by gas chromatography. In mass fragmentography, a single-ion monitoring device is generally used. See also *gas chromatography* and *mass spectrometer.*

mass memory a random-access computer peripheral storage medium capable of storing large amounts of data, e.g., disk or drum.

mass number (A) the number of nucleons (protons and neutrons in a nuclide), which is approximately the mass in daltons. The mass number specifies an isotope, e.g., the 131 in iodine-131 (^{131}I or I 131).

Masson's trichrome method a histologic staining method for connective tissue. Formalin-fixed paraffin sections are deparaffinized, mordanted in Bouin's fluid, and stained: (1) with iron hematoxylin; (2) with Biebrich scarlet and acid fuchsin or with ponceau 2R and acid fuchsin; and (3) following mordanting in phosphomolybdic and phosphotungstic acids, with aniline blue or with light green. Nuclei stain blue-black; muscle, cytoplasm, keratin, and intercellular fibers stain red; and collagen stains blue (with aniline blue) or green (with light green).

mass spectrograph a device similar to a mass spectrometer, except that the sorted ion beams are recorded by sensitizing a photographic plate.

mass spectrometer an analytic instrument that can be used to provide accurate information about the molecular mass and structure of complex molecules present in microgram quantities in simple or complex matrix materials. When coupled with techniques permitting separation of mixture components (e.g., gas chromatography), such information may be obtained with a high degree of reliability.

The components of the specimen must be ionized; for this purpose, liquids are volatilized and passed through an electron beam, and solids are vaporized and ionized by a high-power electric spark. The ions are then accelerated by a variable electrostatic field and deflected along a circular path by a constant magnetic field. The radius of the path is inversely proportional to the velocity of the ion and to its charge/mass ratio (e/m). The accelerating field is scanned over a range of voltages. At each voltage, ions with a specific e/m value are deflected to the collector electrode and their location recorded. The scan thus produces an ion-mass spectrum, i.e., a graph of the number of ions detected versus their position as determined by e/m value.

The mass spectrum includes not only the parent (base) ions (singly and multiply ionized molecules from the sample) but also dissociation fragments produced from the base by the ionization process. Every chemical compound has a unique pattern of breakdown because cleavage usually occurs at a few weak bonds. Thus, the mass spectrum of a compound serves as a molecular fingerprint, providing data on the kind, size, and stability of structural groups in the parent molecule.

See also under *gas chromatography.*

mass spectrometry analysis using the mass spectrometer to identify and quantitate substances in a sample by their mass-fragment spectrum.

mass storage a computer peripheral storage medium capable of storing large amounts of data, e.g., disk, drum, or tape.

mast/o (mas′to) [Gr. *mastos* breast] a word element used in combining form to denote breast, .g., mastitis.

mast cell a round cell found in loose connective tissue that is morphologically similar to the basophil of the blood. In immediate hypersensitivity responses, the mast cells release their content of heparin, histamine, slow-reacting substance of anaphylaxis, and eosinophil chemotactic factor of anaphylaxis. The release is IgE dependent and is inhibited by drugs such as theophylline and isoproterenol, which increase the mast cell's cyclic AMP. See also *immediate hypersensitivity.*

mast cell disease a collection of disorders characterized by the accumulation of excessive aggregates of connective tissue mast cells in the skin and occasionally in other organs; the cause is unknown. The symptoms relate to the release of biologically active mediators (e.g., histamine) by mast cells and to the disruption of organ structure by mast cell infiltrates.

Mast cell disease may occur in several forms. It is noted most commonly in children and affects only the skin (urticaria pigmentosa). This form of mast cell disease becomes less severe as the patient reaches adulthood, disappearing completely in half of those affected. In infants with this disease, there may be a large, solitary, nodular collection of mast cells, referred to as a mastocytoma. Palpating such a lesion may lead to colic, flushing, and pronounced local edema. Mast cell disease may also occur in a diffuse form, systemic mastocytosis. Both the skin and noncutaneous organs, especially the bones, liver, spleen, and gastrointestinal tract, may be involved.

Diagnosis of mast cell disease requires biopsy of the affected tissue (see *mast cell staining* for a summary of stains used to demonstrate mast cell granules). The diagnosis of systemic mast cell disease may also be aided by bone films, which reveal alternating areas of decreased density and sclerosis. Laboratory tests may also reveal anemia, leukopenia, thrombocytopenia, and elevation of blood, tissue, and urine histamine concentrations. There is no known effective treatment for the systemic form of the disease.

Also called *mastocytosis.*

mast cell staining histologic methods for the demonstration of mast cells. Formalin is generally used for fixation. Many different mast cell stains have been used. All are used because they react with the acid mucopolysaccharide in the granules. Among the more commonly used stains are aldehyde-fuchsin (mast cell granules stain purple-violet), Giemsa stain (rusty red), and toluidine blue (granules exhibit gamma metachromasia and stain purple-red to pink).

mast cell tumor a solitary tumor of the skin composed of mast cells occurring in the absence of systemic mast cell disease. A common skin tumor in dogs, it is occasionally seen in cats and cows, and in humans, in whom the histopathologic distinction of a mass cell tumor from a lymphoma involving the skin may be difficult. Diagnosis is aided by use of a stain to demonstrate mucopolysaccharide in the cytoplasmic granules (see *mast cell staining*). Also called *mastocytoma.*

mastectomy (mas-tek′to-me) [*mast-* + Gr. *ektomē* excision] the surgical removal of breast and surrounding tissue, a procedure used to treat breast cancer or, rarely, other disorders. The classic radical mastectomy involves removal of the breast, pectoral muscles, and axillary nodes, and may also include removal of the internal mammary nodes (extended radical mastectomy). A modified radical mastectomy spares the pectoral muscles. A simple mastectomy and wide local excision removes only the soft tissue of the breast.

master file (mas′ter) a computer file that is used as an authoritative and relatively permanent source of data.

Master two-step test [Arthur M. *Master,* American physician, born 1895] a dynamic exercise stress test in which the exercise performed is of a fixed duration and specific (submaximal) intensity. The patient repeatedly ascends and descends a two-step stair (each step is 9 in. high) during a 1.5-min interval, with the total number of ascents predetermined from standard tables on the basis of age, weight, and sex. The double Master test is conducted over 3 min, with twice the number of ascents.

The supine 12-lead electrocardiogram is recorded immediately prior to the test. Leads I, II, V_4, and V_6 are recorded immediately subsequent to and at 2-, 4-, 6-, and 10-min intervals after the test. A flat S-T segment displacement of at least 1 mm (O.1 mV) in any lead is considered to be a positive indication of myocardial ischemia.

Although the Master two-step test has been successfully used to detect subclinical coronary artery disease, it sometimes does not provide enough stress to the heart to be of significant clinical value. It is also less safe than modern treadmill or bicycle exercise tests, as there is no monitoring during the exercise to detect ischemia or serious arrhythmias.

mastication (mas″ti-ka′shun) [L. *masticare* to chew] the process of chewing food in preparation for swallowing and digestion.

Mastigophora (mas″tĭ-gof′o-rah) [Gr. *mastix* whip + *pherein* to bear] a superclass of Protozoa, including all species that possess one or more flagella throughout most of their life cycle and a simple, centrally located nucleus. This subphylum includes the classes Phytomastigophorea and Zoomastigophorea, the latter having several genera that are parasitic in humans (e.g., *Enteromonas, Giardia, Trichomonas, Leishmania,* and *Trypanosoma*).

mastigophorous (mas″tĭ-gof′o-rus) of or pertaining to the superclass Mastigophora.

mastigote (mas′tĭ-gōt) any member of the superclass Mastigophora.

mastitis (mas-ti′tis) [*mast-* + *-itis*] inflammation of the breast, which may have a variety of causes such as mycotic and bacterial infections. Granulomatous inflammation may occur without identifiable etiology. Perforated cysts produce both acute and chronic reactions. Puberty mastitis may occur in young girls; it is marked by pain, swelling, and nipple discharge, and most often disappears spontaneously. Puerperal mastitis is a breast inflammation that occurs following several weeks of nursing; it is characterized by pain, swelling, and abscess formation, and most often is due to infections with *Staphylococcus aureus.* Other types of breast inflammation may be due to systemic infection and disease, as seen in mumps and tuberculosis.

chronic cystic m., see *cystic disease of breast.*

mast leukocyte an obsolete term for the circulating blood basophil, which is distinct from the tissue mast cell. See also *basophil* and *mast cell.*

mastocytoma (mas″to-si-to′mah) see *mast cell tumor.*

mastocytosis (mas″to-si-to′sis) see *mast cell disease.*

mastodynia (mas″to-din′e-ah) [*masto-* + Gr. *odynē* pain] a pain in the breast. Its causes include onset of puberty, menstruation, pregnancy, hematoma, inflammation, cysts, and late carcinoma of the breast. Also called *mammalgia.*

mastography (mas-tog′rah-fe) [*masto-* + Gr. *graphein* to write] see *mammography.*

mastoid/o (mas-toi′do) [Gr. *mastos* breast + *eidos* form] a word element used in combining form to denote the mastoid process, e.g., mastoiditis.

mastoid (mas′toid) [Gr. *mastos* breast + *eidos* form] 1. breast shaped.

2. the mastoid process of the temporal bone.

mastoiditis (mas″toi-di′tis) an inflammation of the mastoid antrum and cells. Acute mastoiditis usually follows acute otitis media, may occur after pyogenic infections, and results in pain, suppuration, and hearing loss. There may be radiologic evidence of bone destruction. Chronic mastoiditis most often follows chronic otitis media; if it occurs in infancy, mastoid cellular structure may fail to develop. Cholesteatomas resulting from squamous cell ingrowth and desquamation of keratin may occur.

mastopathy (mas-top′ah-the) [*masto-* + Gr. *pathos* disease] an imprecise term with no generally accepted definition for nonmalignant abnormalities of the breast.

Mastophora (mas-tof′o-rah) a genus of spiders of the family Araneidae. One species occurring in South America, *M. gasteracanthoides,* is the venomous, orb-weaving, cat-headed spider, whose bites cause necrotic spots; seen especially among vineyard workers.

material safety data sheet a form for providing information on the safety and health hazards of a particular material. Such data are required in federal laboratories (per Federal Standard 313) and in laboratories in states and cities that have adopted regulations requiring employers to inform their employees of the hazards of the materials with which they work.

mathematical logic see under *logic.*

mating (māt′ing) [Ger. *mat* companion] 1. the pairing of male and female to accomplish reproduction.

2. in bacterial genetics, the form of conjugation requiring contact between a donor (male) and a recipient (female) cell, apparently by means of F pili. Recombinants develop in the recipient as a result of gene transfer.

assortative m., nonrandom mating in which the genotypes of individuals are correlated with their mating. If similar parents mate more frequently than would be expected by chance, this is positive assortative mating; if they mate less frequently, it is negative assortative mating.

consanguineous m., mating between individuals with a common ancestor within several generations; this tends to increase the proportion of homozygotic gene loci in the population above chance frequencies.

matrix (ma′triks), pl. *matrices* [L.] 1. the groundwork on which anything is cast, or the basic material from which a structure develops.

2. the extracellular substance or stroma of a tissue.

3. in histology, the light-staining region surrounding denser components, e.g., mitochondrial matrix, cytoplasmic matrix.

4. in mathematics and computer technology, a two-dimensional array of numbers, represented by rows and columns of data items. See also *array, subscripted variable,* and *vector.*

Matrix Reference Materials see under *reference materials.*

matt (mat) a term applied to the morphology of bacterial colonies that are dull and slightly granular but not rough. The term was first used by British microbiologists for colonies, usually those of hemolytic streptococci, that have a ground-glass appearance when seen by reflected light.

matter (mat′er) 1. any substance that possesses mass and is composed of atoms; elementary particles that have mass, as opposed to those (e.g., photons and neutrinos) that are massless.

2. pus.

maturation (mach″u-ra′shun) [L. *maturatio* ripening, from *maturus* ripe] 1. the stage or process of becoming mature or fully developed; the attainment of full intellectual and emotional, physiologic, or morphologic development.

2. in biology, a type of cell division that halves the chromosome number; see also *meiosis.*

maturation index (MI) see under *squamous cell index.*

Maurer's dots (mow′rerz) [Georg *Maurer,* German physician in Sumatra, 20th century] irregular dots or clefts in erythrocytes infected with *Plasmodium falciparum* that stain red with Leishman's stain. Also called Maurer's clefts.

May-Grünwald stain (ma′ grēn′wald) a Romanowsky stain for blood cells, consisting of a neutral alcoholic mixture of methylene blue and eosin.

maxill/o (mak′sil-o) a word element used in combining form to denote the upper jaw, or upper jawbone, e.g., maxillitis.

maxilla (mak-sil′ah), pl. *maxillos* or *maxillae* [L.] [NA], one of the paired skull bones that together form the upper jaw. Each maxilla has a body and zygomatic, frontal, alveolar, and palatine processes. See also *mandible.*

maxillary (mak′sĭ-ler″e) [L. *maxillaris*] pertaining to the maxilla.

maxillary artery a terminal branch of the external carotid artery. It emerges from the parotid gland and runs forward to the pterygopalatine fossa. It is distributed to the upper and lower jaws, including the muscles of mastication, and to the nose.

maxillary nerve the second division of cranial nerve V (trigeminal). It arises from the trigeminal ganglion, gives off a small branch to the dura, then runs forward in the wall of the cavernous sinus and leaves the cranial cavity through the foramen rotundum. Traversing the upper parts of the pterygo-palatine and infratemporal fossae, it passes through the infraorbital fissure where it becomes the infraorbital nerve.

The maxillary nerve is purely sensory. Through its spheno-palatine, zygomatic, superior alveolar, and infraorbital branches, it innervates mucosa in the oral cavity, maxillary sinus, and nasal cavity, and the skin of the midanterior face and cheek. Secretory fibers for the lacrimal gland, carried to the spheno-palatine ganglion in the greater superficial petrosal nerve, reach the gland in the zygomatic branch of the maxillary nerve.

maximal (mak′sĭ-mal) the greatest possible, allowable, or appreciable.

maximal acid output (MAO) the rate of acid secretion (millimoles of titratable acidity per hour) by the stomach after maximal stimulation by pentagastrin or betazole (Histalog). Specifically, it refers to the amount secreted in the first hour after the stimulant has been administered. See also *gastric function tests.*

maximal breathing capacity (MBC) see *maximal voluntary ventilation.*

maximal expiratory flow rate (MEFR) the velocity of forceful expiration of a given volume of expired gas from a maximal inspiration (the forced expiratory flow, 200–1200 l/min). It is commonly measured in liters per minute over the first liter (after discarding the first 200 ml). The normal range in the young adult is 400–600 l/min.

maximal expiratory flow volume (MEFV) see *maximal expiratory f. v. c.* under *flow volume curve.*

maximal midexpiratory flow rate (MMFR) a clinical test of pulmonary function, based on measurement of the average velocity of forceful exhalation over the middle half of the total expired volume, starting from a full inspiration. It is equivalent to the forced expiratory flow (in liters per second) at 25–75 (FEF_{25-75}), where 25 and 75 represent percentages of the forced expiratory volume and indicate that the average flow was recorded between these two values.

maximal voluntary ventilation (MVV) the greatest volume of gas that can be voluntarily exchanged per minute by rapid and deep breathing, commonly measured over an interval of 12–15 sec; in the young male, it normally amounts to 150–170 l/min. Evaluation of the results of this test of pulmonary function is complicated by the fact that it is a measure of motivation and physical strength and endurance, as well as of airway resistance. Also called *maximal breathing capacity* (MBC).

maximum (mak′sĭ-mum), pl. *maxima* [L. "greatest"] 1. the greatest possible effect or quantity.

2. in mathematics, the largest value assumed by a function, or, loosely speaking, the argument for which it assumes this value, e.g., an absorption maximum of a chemical compound. Cf. *minimum.*

3. the acme of a disease or process.

maximum impurities reagents see under *reagent grade.*

maxwell (Mx) (maks′wel) [James Clerk *Maxwell,* British physicist, 1831–1879] the electromagnetic centimeter-gram-second (cgs) unit of magnetic flux equal to 10^{-8} weber (Wb) or 10 nWb. Also called abweber.

Mayer's acid alum hematoxylin stain (ma′erz) [Paul *Mayer,* German histologist, 1848–1923] a general histologic stain for nuclei and chromatin. The stain is progressive and does not require differentiation in acid alcohol. It is generally used in combination with eosin and can also be used as a counterstain.

Mayer position a radiographic position used to obtain a half-axial oblique view of the petrous portions of the temporal bone. In the original method, the median sagittal plane makes a 45° angle with the film, and the central ray is directed through the dependent external auditory meatus at an angle of 45° toward the feet. This view demonstrates the external auditory meatus; the tympanic cavity, antrum, and attic; the aditus; and the ossicles. Because this view is difficult to duplicate, many modifications of head rotation (15°–45°) and central ray angulation (25°–45°) are used.

mayfly (ma′fli) an insect of the order Ephemeroptera. The species *Hexagenia bilineata* (also called lake fly) formerly inhabited the shores of Lake Erie in large numbers. Breathing of fragments of the cast skins of these insects were found to cause allergic reactions in some people, leading to severe asthma. Few cases are reported now, owing to changes in ecological conditions that have reduced their numbers. Artificial replicas are frequently prepared from natural materials as an integral item in the paraphernalia used for the acquisition of certain piscene species, notably *Salmo gordinarii,* by the technique referred to as angling.

May-Hegglin body an inclusion body consisting of blue staining material and resembling Döhle bodies. It is primarily found in neutrophils and eosinophils but may be present in any leukocyte. These structures are commonly seen in platelets in May-Hegglin anomaly, a condition transmitted as an autosomal dominant trait and associated with a morphologic platelet abnormality, and occasionally in thrombocytopenia. Usually there is no significant bleeding disorder.

mazoplasia (ma″zo-pla′se-ah) [Gr. *mazos* breast + *plassein* to form] an imprecise term, used vaguely to denote some form of degenerative or hyperplastic alteration in mammary lobules. It has no specific histologic connotation.

Mazzotti test a procedure for the detection of microfilariae of the filarial parasite *Onchocerca volvulus.* This test is used when microfilariae cannot be identified by skin biopsy, scarification, or aspiration of a subcutaneous nodule because of their low number. The test consists of ingesting 50 mg of diethylcarbamazine. In positive cases, the patient will have a pruritic skin reaction within 24 hr.

MB abbrev. for the isoenzyme of creatine kinase that contains one M and one B subunit. See under *creatine kinase.*

M band see under *paraprotein.*

mbar abbrev. See *millibar.*

μ-bar abbrev. See *microbar.*

MBC abbrev. for maximal breathing capacity (see under *maximal voluntary ventilation*), minimal bactericidal concentration (see under *minimal lethal concentration*).

MBK abbrev. See *methyl butyl ketone.*

MBP abbrev. See *myelin basic protein.*

Mc abbrev. See *megacycle.*

mC abbrev. See *millicoulomb.*

μC abbrev. See *microcoulomb.*

McArdle's disease (mak-ar′d′lz) [B. *McArdle,* English neurologist, 20th century] a hereditary disorder, transmitted as an autosomal recessive trait, that is characterized by abnormal glycogen metabolism due to a deficiency of the enzyme myophosphorylase. There is muscle weakness and contracture on exercise, which may be associated with myoglobinuria. Symptoms occur in adolescence and are slowly progressive.

Diagnosis is based on demonstration of the enzyme deficiency in a biopsy of skeletal muscle, and is suggested by the lack of increased blood lactate during ischemic muscle exercise. The disease can also be diagnosed by nuclear magnetic resonance spectroscopy. Also called glycogen storage disease type V and myophosphorylase deficiency. See also *glycogenoses.*

MCD abbrev. See *mean of consecutive differences.*

MCF abbrev. See *macrophage chemotactic factor.*

MCH abbrev. See *mean corpuscular hemoglobin* and *red cell indices.*

MCHC abbrev. See *mean corpuscular hemoglobin concentration* and *red cell indices.*

mCi abbrev. See *millicurie.*

μCi abbrev. See *microcurie.*

mCi-hr abbrev. See *millicurie-hour.*

μCi-hr abbrev. See *microcurie-hour.*

McLeod phenotype (mak-lowd′) the red cell phenotype exhibited by those rare individuals who have Kell blood group antigens so weak that they are not demonstrated by normal techniques.

McMaster technique an egg-counting method used to determine the worm burden from fecal specimens. This method is most useful in evaluating hookworm, *Ascaris,* and *Trichuris* infections. The procedure requires the use of a McMaster egg-count slide; it is a simple and accurate technique, and is used for routine examination.

After a 2-g sample of fresh feces is suspended in a saturated salt solution and mixed well, the chambers of a McMaster counting slide are filled and covered with a glass coverslip. Any eggs present will float to the top of the suspension after a few minutes and attach to the coverslip. Two chambers are counted under a low-magnification microscope and averaged; four separate counts should be made, and the average number should not vary more than 25 percent.

M colony abbrev. See *mucoid c.* under *colony.*

M component [from myeloma or macroglobulinemia] a high concentration of a structurally homogeneous plasma protein, either monoclonal immunoglobulins or monoclonal heavy or light chains; found in most plasma cell dyscrasias. Also called *M protein.*

MCTD abbrev. See *mixed connective tissue disease.*

MCV abbrev. See *mean corpuscular volume* and *red cell indices.*

MD abbrev. See *malate dehydrogenase.*

M.D. abbrev. for Doctor of Medicine (L. *Medicinae Doctor*), the degree conferred on graduates of colleges of medicine.

Md symbol for the chemical element *mendelevium.*

MDA abbrev. and street name for *3,4-methylenedioxyamphetamine.*

MDH abbrev. See *malate dehydrogenase.*

2 ME abbrev. See *2-mercaptoethanol.*

mean (mēn) [from L. *medius* middle] 1. an average, the value between two extremes.

2. in statistics, the expectation or average value. The expectation of a random variable X is the mean (symbol μ) of the probability distribution of X, defined for a discrete distribution by $\mu = \Sigma_x x p_x$ and for a continuous distribution by $\mu = \int x f(x) dx$; μ is often referred to as the population mean. The sample mean (symbol $\overline{X}$) is defined by $\overline{X} = \Sigma_k X_k / n$, where n is the sample size and the X_k are the sample observations. The sample mean is a statistic with a probability distribution having mean μ and variance σ^2/n, where μ is the population mean and σ^2 is the population variance (if μ and σ are defined). Cf. *median.*

arithmetic m., the sum of a group of numbers divided by the number in the group, e.g., $(A + B)/2$.

geometric m., the nth root of the product of n numbers. Equivalently, it is the antilog of the arithmetic mean of the logarithms of n numbers, e.g., $\sqrt{A \times B}$.

trimmed m., the sample mean calculated after the k largest and k smallest values are discarded, $(X_{(k+1)} + X_{(k+2)} + \ldots + X_{(n-k)})/(n-2k)$, where n is the sample size and $X_{(m)}$ in the mth smallest sample observation. When the distribution of X is symmetric, the trimmed mean is an unbiased estimator of the population mean, and is less influenced by extreme values than is the sample mean.

windsorized m., the sample mean calculated after the k largest and k smallest values are replaced by the most extreme values that are retained, $[(k+1)X_{(k+1)} + X_{(k+2)} + \ldots + X_{(n-k-1)} + (k+1)X_{(n-k)}]/n$, where n is the sample size and $X_{(m)}$ *is the* m th smallest sample observation. It has the desirable properties of the trimmed mean; in addition, the middle $n - 2k - 2$ sample values influence the windsorized mean in the same way they influence the regular sample mean. Cf. *trimmed m.*

mean arterial pressure see under *arterial pressure.*

mean cell threshold (MCT) in the operation of a Coulter counter, the relative change in the measured mean cell volume (MCV) value for a one-division change in the lower threshold setting.

mean corpuscular hemoglobin (MCH) a quantitative measure of hemoglobin per red cell, determined by dividing the hemoglobin concentration in 1000 ml of blood by the number of erythrocytes per cubic millimeter of blood:

$$\text{MCH} = \frac{\text{hemoglobin g/1000 ml blood}}{\text{red cell count (millions/mm}^3)}.$$

The reference range is 26.4–34.0 pg. See also *red cell indices.*

mean corpuscular hemoglobin concentration (MCHC) a quantitative measure of the concentration of hemoglobin in grams per milliliter (g/100 ml) of red cells. It is determined either by multiplying the amount of hemoglobin per 100 ml of blood by 100 and dividing it by the packed cell volume, or by multiplying the red blood cells (RBC) (in millions) by the MCV (divided by 1000):

$$\text{MCHC} = \frac{\text{hemoglobin g/100 ml} \times 100}{\text{packed cell volume (percent)}} \quad \text{or}$$

$$\text{MCHC} = \frac{\text{hemoglobin g/100 ml} \times 1000}{\text{MCV} \times \text{RBC (in millions)}}$$

The reference range is 31.5–35.8 percent. See also *red cell indices.*

mean corpuscular volume (MCV) a quantitative measure of the average volume of individual red cells expressed in cubic micrometers or femtoliters. The MCV is determined by dividing the packed cell volume by the red cell count per cubic millimeter of blood:

$$\text{MCV} = \frac{\text{volume of packed erythrocytes/1000 ml blood}}{\text{red cell count (millions/mm)}}.$$

The reference range is 80.5–100.0 μm^3. See also *red cell indices.*

mean deviation the average absolute deviation of a set of measurements from their arithmetic mean; a rarely used measure of the variation among a set of measurements.

mean effective life in nuclear medicine, the average length of time until an administered radionuclide either decays or is excreted: 1.44 times the effective half-life.

mean life in nuclear medicine, the average length of time until an atom of a radioisotope decays: the reciprocal of the number of disintegrations per unit time, 1.44 times the half-life.

mean of consecutive differences (MCD) a technique used in single-fiber electromyography as a qualitative expression of the jitter. It is the mean value of the interpotential interval time differences of 50–200 consecutive discharges. See also *jitter.*

mean square deviation in statistics, the average squared deviation of a random variable from a defined value. When the value is the mean of the squared variable, the mean squared deviation corresponds to the variance.

mean time between failures (MTBF) a measure of the reliability of a piece of equipment, the average time that elapses between the time when the device is put into service after a repair and the time when it breaks down again.

measles (me'zelz) an extremely contagious viral infection characterized by a maculopapular rash, conjunctivitis, and inflammation of the respiratory tract. Measles is a common disease among children but may also involve nonimmune individuals of any age. The peak season for infection is late winter to early spring.

The etiologic agent of measles is a paramyxovirus that has a single-stranded, nonsegmented RNA with its own transcriptase. This virus is enveloped with a loose lipoprotein coat and contains hemagglutinin and hemolysin. Unlike other paramyxoviruses, the measles virus lacks neuramidase; it is released from infected cells by budding. There is only one antigenic type of measles virus, and immunity is lifelong. The virus may be grown in tissue cultures of primate kidney or chick embryo cells.

Clinical symptoms begin after an 11-da incubation period. The virus enters the respiratory tract as droplet nuclei and multiplies in the epithelial cells of the respiratory tract. Infection spreads through the reticuloendothelial system, producing lymphoid hyperplasia, frequently accompanied by characteristic Warthin-Finkeldey giant cells. After the incubation period, fever, malaise, myalgia, and headache appear, followed by conjunctivitis with exudate in the conjunctival sac. Coughing and sneezing follow this prodromal stage. The characteristic measles rash first appears on the buccal mucosa of the inside of the cheek. Small red lesions with bluish-white centers, known as Koplik's spots, may be seen inside the mouth on the third and fourth days of the prodromal period. Finally, a cutaneous rash appears on the head, spreading down the trunk and to the extremities. The lesions of the rash are slightly elevated, last for 5 da. and are probably due to a hypersensitivity reaction of the virus and the immune system. Fever peaks at 39.5°C.

Although measles usually is a benign disease, very young and very old individuals may develop complications; the most common are secondary bacterial infections in the form of otitis media, pneumonia, or laryngitis. A rare, fatal giant-cell pneumonia may occur, often without a rash, in immunocompromised children. Rarely, subacute sclerosing panencephalitis may develop years after an initial measles infection. In recent years an atypical form of measles has also been observed in children who received killed measles vaccine and who years later were exposed to wild measles virus.

Diagnosis is most often made by clinical observation. Measles must be differentiated from rubella, scarlet fever, infectious mononucleosis, secondary syphilis, drug eruptions, and infections due to other viruses. Laboratory identification may be useful for an early accurate diagnosis. During the prodromal stage, nasal mucus may be stained and observed for multinucleated (Warthin-Finkeldey) giant cells that react with specific fluorescent antibody. Measles virus may be isolated from the nose, throat, eyes, or blood. Cytopathic changes will occur in a week in human fetal kidney or monkey kidney cells.

The treatment of measles is nonspecific and, after onset of the infection, only the symptoms may be treated. Antimicrobial therapy is useful only if there is reason to expect a secondary bacterial infection as a complication. Vaccination has been highly effective for the prevention of measles. The current measles vaccine is an attenuated live virus, which causes immunity through infection. Only one dose is required for protective immunization; it should be given after the age of 1 yr.

Also called *morbilli* and *rubeola.* See also *paramyxovirus* and *rubella* (German measles).

measly (me'zle) containing cysticerci, a larval form of tapeworm. See also *cysticercus.*

measure (mezh'er) [L. *mensurare*] 1. to make a measurement.

2. a scale used in measuring, e.g., a meter rule or graduated cylinder.

3. a reference standard of measurement, such as the standard kilogram.

measurement (mezh'er-ment) the determination of the dimension, quantity, or capacity of some substance, or the property of a system, for example, of the cardiac output of a patient or of the concentration of calcium in serum. In clinical chemistry, a measurement is specified by system (e.g., serum), component (glucose), kind of quantity (substance concentration), value, and unit (e.g., millimoles per liter, mmol/l).

meatus (me-a'tus), pl. *meatus* [L. "a way, path, course"] 1. an opening or passage.

2. [NA], in anatomy, a general term for an opening or passageway in the body.

external auditory m., the passage from the concha to the tympanic membrane of the ear. The lateral third is cartilaginous; the remainder has rigid bony walls.

internal acoustic m., a short passage in the petrous portion of the temporal bone that transmits the vestibulocochlear, intermediate, and facial nerves and the labyrinthine vessels.

urinary m., the external orifice of the urethra through which urine and semen are discharged.

mebutamate (mĕ-bu'tah-māt) a drug, chemically related to meprobamate, that acts as a central nervous system depressant, tranquilizer, and sedative. It has been used as a centrally acting antihypertensive agent.

mecamylamine hydrochloride (mek"ah-mil'ah-min) [USP], a ganglionic blocking drug used to treat severe hypertension.

mechanical (mĕ-kan'ĭ-kal) [Gr. *mēchanikos*] 1. pertaining to or accomplished by machines or tools.
2. performed by means of some artificial mechanism.

mechanical ileus see *mechanical i.* under *ileus.*

mechanical ventilation the use of mechanical means (usually a ventilator, an automatic cycling machine) to assist in or provide all of the ventilation of the lungs. In most cases, a positive pressure is applied to the airways to inflate the lungs with an adequate volume of gas during inspiration. The inspiration can be triggered solely by the ventilator (controlled mechanical ventilation) or, when possible, the patient's own inspiratory effort can be used to trigger the machine (patient-cycled ventilation). Expiration is passive, but in some instances (e.g., conditions such as pulmonary edema, increased lung compliance, or vascular congestion), it may be desirable to raise artificially the intrapulmonary pressure at the end of expiration (i.e., apply positive end-expiratory pressure) to prevent alveolar collapse.

To initiate mechanical ventilation using positive pressure, the ventilator outflow is delivered to the patient via an airtight face mask (particularly in emergency use) or an endotracheal or tracheostomy tube. The ventilator is initially adjusted to deliver a large tidal volume (10–15 mg/kg of body weight) at a respiratory rate of 10–12 breaths/min. The hypocapnia and respiratory alkalosis that may result can usually be eliminated by increasing the dead space of the breathing circuit or by adding CO_2 at a controlled partial pressure to the inspired air, or by adjusting the minute ventilation downward. An O_2 concentration just sufficient to maintain 90 percent saturation of arterial hemoglobin should be used to ventilate the patient to avoid oxygen toxicity.

Mechanical ventilation can also be provided by using a negative-pressure breathing apparatus such as the body respirator (e.g., Drinker respirator, or iron lung). The patient's entire body below the neck (or in some models, just the anterior chest) is encased in an airtight plastic or metal tank into which a negative pressure is clinically applied. The negative pressure enlarges the thorax and decreases intraalveolar pressure to subatmospheric values so that ambient air can flow down a pressure gradient into the lungs.

Criteria generally used to establish the need for mechanical ventilation are: the presence of apnea, a Pa_{O_2} less than 60 mmHg (despite the use of mask oxygenation, bronchodilators, or physiotherapy), an alveolar-arterial Po_2 difference greater than 400 mmHg, a shunt fraction greater than 30–40 percent, a respiratory rate greater than 35 breaths/min, and a tidal volume less than 4 ml/kg of body weight.

See also *positive end-expiratory pressure, positive pressure breathing,* and *ventilator.*

mechanism (mek'ah-nizm) [Gr. *mēchanē machine*] 1. a machine or machinelike structure.
2. the process by which some effect occurs. An example is a chemical reaction mechanism, which specifies the intermediate steps of an overall reaction.

mechlorethamine (mĕ-klor-eth'ah-mēn) a cancer chemotherapeutic drug; trademark, Mustargen. For more information, see *Appendix A.*

mecillinam (mĕ-sil'ĭ-nam) see *penicillins.*

Mecistocirrhus (me-sis"to-sir'us) a genus of nematodes, of which the species *M. digitatus* is parasitic in humans. Also called *Strongylus gibsoni.*

Meckel's cartilage (mek'elz) [Johann Friedrich *Meckel* (the younger; grandson of J. F. *Meckel,* the elder), anatomist in Halle, 1781–1833] in the developing embryo, the ventral portion of the cartilage of the first branchial arch that develops into the malleus, the sphenomandibular and anterior malleolar ligaments, and the distal portion of the mandible.

Meckel's diverticulum [Johann Friedrich *Meckel* the younger] see *Meckel's d.* under *diverticulum.*

meclizine hydrochloride (mek'lĭ-zēn) [USP], an antihistamine with only weak anticholinergic properties, used to control the vertigo, dizziness, nausea, and vomiting of motion sickness. Adverse reactions typical of antihistamines occur (e.g., drowsiness, dryness of the mouth). Meclizine has been shown by animal studies to be teratogenic and should not be used by females who are or may become pregnant.

meconium (mĕ-ko'ne-um) [L.; Gr. *mēkōnion*] a dark-green, mucus-like material in the intestine of the full-term infant that is composed of intestinal secretions and the contents of amniotic fluid. This substance constitutes the first stools of an infant and should be passed within the first 24 hr of life.

m. ileus, intestinal obstruction in infants due to abnormally thick, very tenacious, adherent meconium at the level of the ileum, and often extending into the colon. This disorder is almost always an early manifestation of cystic fibrosis. Loops of the intestine become distended, leading to volvulus and often to intestinal infarction. Diagnosis is dependent on clinical evidence of intestinal obstruction, and the demonstration of squamous cells in the meconium. Histologic sections of the bowel reveal an increase in both the number and size of the goblet cells. See also *cystic fibrosis.*

m. plug syndrome, a condition of infants characterized by intestinal obstruction with thick, rubbery, inspissated meconium. This substance can fill the entire colon and cause intestinal distention and vomiting. A barium enema will demonstrate the plug. Often this syndrome may be associated with a left colon of narrow caliber. Also called neonatal small left colon syndrome.

MEDAC syndrome [acronym from *m*ultiple *e*ndocrine *d*eficiency–*A*ddison's disease–*c*andidiasis] a juvenile familial endocrinopathy, transmitted most frequently as an autosomal recessive trait, that is characterized by mucocutaneous candidiasis occurring during the first 6 yr of life and by hypoparathyroidism and hypoadrenocorticism between yrs 9 and 12. Circulating tissue-specific antibodies to the adrenal gland and parathyroid are often found. The candidiasis is associated with hypergammaglobulinemia and IgA deficiency. Also called HAM syndrome (an acronym from *h*ypoparathyroidism–*A*ddison's disease–*m*ucocutaneous candidiasis) and hypoadrenocorticism-hypoparathyroidism-candidiasis.

medi/o (me'de-o) [L. *medius* middle] a word element used in combining form to denote middle, e.g., mediocarpal.

medial (me'de-al) [L. *medialis*] pertaining to the middle; closer to the median plane or midline of a body or structure; pertaining to the middle of three layers.

medial geniculate body an ovoid mass of gray

matter on the inferior aspect of the thalamus adjacent to the pulvinar and lateral to the superior colliculus. It does not present a highly organized internal structure: fibers received in the medial geniculate are relayed from both inferior colliculi or come directly from the ipsilateral lateral lemniscus via the inferior brachium. The medial geniculate projects out to the auditory cortex areas of the temporal lobe, anterior transverse, and superior temporal gyri.

median (me′de-an) [L. *medianus*] 1. pertaining to a plane that divides a body or structure into halves.

2. in statistics, the middle value. A median of the probability distribution of a random variable X(also called the population median) is any point (m) for which the probabilities $P(X \leq m)$ and $P(X \geq m)$ are at least one-half. The median may be a unique point, or every point in some interval $a \leq m \leq b$ may be a median [necessarily $P(a < X < b) = 0$]. For a random sample with an odd sample size, $2n + 1$, the sample median is the middle value $X_{(n+1)}$ of the ordered sample values $X_{(1)} \leq X_{(2)} \leq \ldots \leq X_{(2n+1)}$. For a sample with an even sample size, the sample median $2n$ is usually defined as the average of the two middle values $(X_{(n)} + X_{(n+1)})/2$. With this choice, the sample median is an unbiased estimator of the median of a symmetric distribution. As the sample size increases, the sample median converges to the unique population median or to the interval of population medians.

median nerve a nerve formed by the union of roots from the medial and lateral cords of the brachial plexus on the lateral side of the axillary artery. It descends through the arm, over the elbow joint, down the front of the forearm, and passes behind the flexor retinaculum to reach the palm, where it breaks up into terminal branches for the lateral three and one-half digits. An important branch, the anterior interosseous nerve, leaves the posterior surface of the main trunk in the proximal forearm to supply a number of the forearm muscles and the wrist joint.

mediastinitis (me″de-as″tĭ-ni′tis) an inflammation of the mediastinum, most often due to infection with pyogenic organisms. Acute infections are most frequently due to esophageal perforation. Diagnosis may be confirmed by contrast x-ray or endoscopic procedures. Chronic mediastinitis and fibrosis result from granulomatous inflammation. Radiographic findings include right paratracheal or anterior mediastinal masses; calcification may also be present.

mediastinoscopy (me″de-as″tĭ-nos′ko-pe) the endoscopic examination of the paratracheal and occasionally the hilar mediastinum, using a metal tube with a lighted bore, a mediastinoscope, which is inserted via a supra- or parasternal approach into the mediastinum. Mediastinoscopy permits biopsy of paratracheal and carinal lymph nodes and is used primarily for the diagnosis and staging of lung cancers, but it is also of use for the biopsy diagnosis of other diseases involving the mediastinum.

mediastinum (me″de-as-ti′num), pl. *mediastina*[L.] the central region of the thoracic cavity, bounded laterally by the pleural cavities. It is classically divided into the anterior mediastinum in front of the pericardium, the middle mediastinum within the pericardium, the posterior mediastinum between the pericardium and the vertebral column, and the superior mediastinum above a plane passing through the sternal angle and the fourth intervertebral disk.

A more clinically relevant subdivision into three compartments is achieved by including the portion of the superior mediastinum that is posterior to the posterior border of the pericardium in the posterior mediastinum, and the remainder of the superior mediastinum with the anterior mediastinum as the anterosuperior mediastinum. The middle mediastinum remains as defined. Thus, the anterosuperior mediastinum contains the thymus gland, the arch of the aorta with its major branches, and the trachea; the posterior mediastinum contains the esophagus, the descending aorta, the azygos system of veins, vagus nerves, and sympathetic chains, and the thoracic duct.

Medicaid (med′ĭ-kād) a federal health program under the Social Security Administration that pays for medical care rendered to eligible needy persons.

medical (med′ĭ-kal) pertaining to medicine or to the treatment of diseases; pertaining to medicine as opposed to surgery.

Medical Internal Radiation Dose (MIRD) 1. a Committee of the Society of Nuclear Medicine.

2. a standard method promulgated by this committee for estimating the radiation doses absrbed by the various organs from an administered dose of a radiopharmaceutical.

3. a standard notation for the quantities used in this method.

See also *dose estimate.*

medical laboratory technician a technician skilled in performing clinical laboratory tests. Educational preparation may involve completion of an accredited associate degree program and/or on-the-job training. Personnel certified by the American Society of Clinical Pathologists are designated MLT(ASCP), Medical Laboratory Technician; those certified by the National Certification Agency for Medical Laboratory Personnel are designated CLT(NCA), Clinical Laboratory Technician.

medical technologist an allied health professional skilled in both the theory and practice of clinical laboratory procedures that provide data which physicians use to determine the presence, extent, and cause of disease. The medical technologist can perform complex laboratory procedures, recognize errors or physiologic conditions that invalidate test results, carry out quality control procedures, and implement new procedures. Specialty areas in which a medical technologist may work include clinical chemistry, hematology, blood banking, immunology, immunohematology, bacteriology, serology, mycology, parasitology, and histology. Educational preparation usually involves completion of an accredited baccalaureate degree program. Examinations for certification are conducted by several groups: designation of certification includes MT(ASCP), Medical Technologist, from the Board of Registry of the American Society of Clinical Pathologists; and CS(NCA), Clinical Laboratory Scientist, from the National Certification Agency for Medical Laboratory Personnel.

Medicare (med′ĭ-kār) a federal health program under the Social Security Administration that helps individuals with the costs of health care for the aged.

medication (med″ĭ-ka′shun) [L. *medicatio*] 1. a medicine or drug.
2. the administration of a medicine or drug.

medicine (med′ĭ-sin) [L. *medicina*] 1. any drug or remedy.
2. the art and science of the diagnosis and treatment of disease and the maintenance of health.
3. the treatment of disease by nonsurgical means.

medina infection (mĕ-de′nah) [from *Médine,* Mali] see *dracunculiasis.*

mediolateral (me″de-o-lat′er-al) [*medio-* + L. *lateralis* lateral] pertaining to the middle and one side.

mediolateral projection a projection used in mammography. The patient is in the semilateral position with the breast supported by the film holder and the breast and nipple extended in profile. The central ray projects vertically.

medionecrosis (me″de-o-nĕ-kro′sis) see *medial n.* under *necrosis.*

m. of aorta, see *Erdheim's cystic medial n.* under *necrosis.*

Mediterranean anemia see under *thalassemia.*

Mediterranean fever a generalized infection caused by species of *Brucella;* see *brucellosis.*

familial M. f., a genetic disease of unknown etiology, transmitted as an autosomal recessive trait, that is characterized by fever and inflammation of the pleura or peritoneum, skin lesions, and arthritis; amyloidosis may also be seen. Although there is no specific diagnostic test, white blood cell and erythrocyte sedimentation rate counts are elevated; plasma fibrinogen, serum haptoglobin, ceruloplasmin, and C-reactive proteins may also be elevated during the recurrent periodic attacks. Also called familial paroxysmal polyserositis.

medium (me′de-um), pl. *mediums, media* [L. "middle"] 1. the pabulum in or on which microorganisms or tissue cells are cultured. See also *culture media.*
2. a preparation used in treating histologic specimens, e.g., a mounting medium.
3. a substance that transmits impulses.

chopped meat m., see *chopped meat b.* under *broth.*

contrast m., see *contrast medium.*

differential m., a culture medium, usually solid, that reveals the presence of two or more similar microorganisms by differences in the appearance of their colonies. Such a medium may or may not be selective also.

enrichment m., a basal culture medium that is supplemented with a specific nutrient (e.g., serum, blood) to promote the growth of a particular organism. Further enhancement can sometimes be obtained by incorporating a chemical that selectively inhibits the growth of competing organisms.

Löffler's coagulated serum m., an aerobic solid medium used for the isolation of *Corynebacterium diphtheriae.*

Lowenstein-Jensen m., a solid egg medium used for the primary isolation of mycobacteria. See also *mycobacteria.*

nutrient m., a culture medium to which certain nutrient materials have been added.

oxidation-fermentation (OF) m., a tubed medium designed primarily to detect microorganisms that utilize carbohydrates oxidatively rather than fermentatively. Glucose solution is added to the sterilized basal semi-solid medium to a final concentration of 1 percent. One of two such tubes, which has been stab-inoculated, is overlaid with sterile oil. Acid production in the open tube indicates the oxidative utilization of glucose; in both tubes it indicates fermentation; and no acid reaction at all indicates that the organism has failed to use glucose by either method. OF medium is particularly useful in the identification of pseudomonads.

Petragnani m., a solid egg medium used for culturing mycobacteria. See also *mycobacteria.*

selective m., see under *culture media.*

thioglycollate m., a rich culture medium used for isolating and culturing anaerobic bacteria; it also grows a wide variety of aerobic and facultative species. Thioglycollate medium is a good general-utility medium for clinical bacteriology.

transport m., see under *clinical bacteriologic specimens.*

medium-chain triglycerides oil (MCT) a dietary supplement consisting of triacyl glycerols that contains primarily (more than 90 percent) octanoic and decanoic acid. It benefits those individuals, such as very small premature infants, who cannot efficiently absorb and digest normal (long-chain) fats. It is contraindicated for those with cirrhosis of the liver, as coma may result from ingestion.

medium-scale integration (MSI) integrated circuit technology in which individual chips contain as many as 100 logic elements (gates). Cf. *large-scale integration.*

MEDLARS (med′larz) [acronym from *MED*ical *L*iterature *A*nalysis and *R*etrieval *S*ystem] a computerized bibliographic retrieval system of the National Library of Medicine from which the publication *Index Medicus* is produced.

MEDLINE (med′lin) [acronym from *MED*LARS on-*line*] a computerized bibliographic retrieval system for medically related publications that is an on-line segment of MEDLARS.

medroxyprogesterone (mĕ-drok″se-pro-jes′tĕ-rōn) a cancer chemotherapeutic drug; trademark, Provera. For more information, see *Appendix A.*

medull/o (mĕ-dul′o) a word element used in combining form to denote medulla (the internal section of an organ), e.g., medullary.

medulla (mĕ-dul′ah), pl. *medullae* [L.] [NA], a general term for the inmost portion of an organ or structure.

m. of bone, the soft material filling the cavities of the bones. It is composed of a meshwork of connective tissue, fat, and bone marrow.

m. of lymph node, the inner area of a lymph node, surrounded by cortex except at the hilus. The cells and connective tissue trabeculae form branching cords.

m. oblongata, [NA], the piriform-shaped caudal portion of the brain stem that extends from the pons rostrally to the first cervical nerve at the level of the atlas, where it is continuous with the spinal cord. The upper open portion contains the fourth ventricle and is covered dorsally by the cerebellum. The lower closed region has a central canal and resembles the spinal cord. The medulla transmits ascending and descending impulses and contains centers for controlling respiration, circulation, and other autonomic and sensory functions.

renal m., the inner portion of kidney, made up of the renal pyramids. It is composed of the loops of Henle, vasa recta, and collecting tubules.

spinal m., see *spinal cord.*

suprarenal m., the inner, reddish-brown part of a suprarenal gland. It synthesizes, stores, and releases catecholamines.

medullary (med′u-lār″e) [L. *medullaris*] pertaining to the marrow or to any medulla; resembling marrow.

medullary carcinoma of thyroid a carcinoma of the calcitonin-forming C cells. The tumor cells contain dense-core granules visible by electron microscopy. Amyloid is frequently present in the stroma. Calcitonin levels in the serum may be markedly elevated.

medullary cavity the central cylindric space in the diaphysis of long bones. It is lined with endosteum and communicates freely with the intratrabecular spaces at each end.

medullary cystic disease a common renal disease of unknown etiology, characterized by cystic dilation of the terminal collecting ducts and tips of the renal papillae. Nonhereditary and usually bilateral, this condition is usually benign, although secondary complications including renal calculi and infection can develop and lead to renal failure.

Medullary cystic disease is often discovered radiographically as an incidental finding. Diagnosis is made by use of intravenous urography. Therapy is based on treatment of any developing complications.

Also called *medullary sponge kidney.*

medullary reticulosis see *histiocytic medullary reticulosis.*

medullary sponge kidney see *medullary cystic disease.*

medullary velum a thin sheet of white matter that forms part of the roof of the fourth ventricle of the brain. The superior part stretches between the superior cerebellar peduncles and extends from the inferior colliculi to the vermis. The inferior portion consists of two thin sheets, one on each side of the nodule, and extends into the fourth ventricle to form part of its lateral walls.

medulloepithelioma (mĕ-dul″o-ep″ĭ-the″le-o′mah) 1. a rare intracerebral tumor that arises from embryonic elements in early life. It has a distinctive papillary and tubular pattern that simulates a metastatic, well-differentiated adenocarcinoma. The tumor grows rapidly, tends to recur following therapy, and has been known to metastasize beyond the central nervous system.

2. a synonym for a ciliary body tumor; the very rare type occurring in young children is also known as diktyoma.

MEFR abbrev. See *maximal expiratory flow rate.*

MEFV abbrev. See *maximal expiratory f.-v.c.* under *flow-volume curve.*

mega- (meg′ah) [Gr. *megas* big, great] 1. a prefix word element to denote great size or enlargement.

2. (abbrev. M), a prefix word element attached to International System (SI) units to make a unit that is equal to 1 million of the basic units (10^6 unit).

megacolon (meg″ah-ko′lon) a condition characterized by dilation and distention of the colon, usually with very infrequent or absent bowel movements. A number of different forms are known and all age groups may be affected.

acquired m., chronic constipation and distention of the colon that has a number of causes including infectious disease, neurologic disorders, and narcotic drugs. This condition may be associated with impaired or normal ganglionic innervation.

aganglionic m., a congenital disorder caused by the absence of the growth of ganglion cells into the plexuses of the distal colon. This results in the blockage of fecal transit and severe dilation of the colon. X-ray examination (with barium) is a useful diagnostic aid, and rectal mucosal biopsies permit examination for the presence of ganglion cells. Also called congenital megacolon and *Hirschsprung's disease.*

chronic idiopathic m., a psychogenic disorder characterized by severe and recurrent constipation with bowel distention, in association with normal anatomic features. X-ray examination reveals distention without narrowing, and rectal mucosal biopsies are normal for ganglion cells.

toxic m., a life-threatening complication of ulcerative colitis and occasionally of a number of infectious diseases affecting the colon. It is characterized by large areas of mucosal necrosis and inflammation extending to the muscular coat, and by systemic toxicity. There is high fever, electrolyte imbalances, tachycardia, leukocytosis, and profuse diarrhea. This complication is often preceded by vigorous use of cathartics or enemas or the excessive use of antimotility drugs. X-ray examination reveals an enlarged and distended colon.

megacycle (Mc) (meg′ah-si″k′l) an obsolete unit of frequency, now replaced by the *megahertz.*

megaelectron volt (MeV) (meg″ah-e-lek′tron) a unit of energy equal to 1 million electron volts (10^6 eV). Formerly called million electron volts.

megaesophagus (meg″ah-ĕ-sof′ah-gus) see under *cardiospasm.*

megahertz (MHz) (meg′ah-hertz) a unit of frequency equal to 1 million hertz (10^6 Hz). Formerly called *megacycle* (Mc).

megakaryocyte (meg″ah-kar′e-o-sīt) [*mega-* + Gr. *karyon* nucleus + *-cyte*] a giant polyploid cell found only in the bone marrow; it is 30–100 μ in diameter and ordinarily produces 1000–3000 platelets. Megakaryocytic maturation involves a series of nuclear replications within a common cytoplasm, resulting in 4–16 lobed nuclei, an elaboration of specific granules in the cytoplasm, the cytoplasmic demarcation into platelet subunits, and the release of platelets into the circulation through marrow sinusoids.

megakaryocytic leukemia see *megakaryocytic l.* under *leukemia.*

megakaryocytopoiesis (meg″ah-kar″e-o-si″to-poi-e′sis) [*megakaryocyte* + Gr. *poiesis* a making] the formation of megakaryocytes in the bone marrow; see also *thrombocytopoiesis.*

megal/o (meg′ah-lo) [Gr. *megas, megale,* big, great] a combining word element used to signify abnormally big or large, e.g., megalomania. See also words beginning *mega-.*

megalencephaly (meg″al-en-sef′ah-le) hypertrophy of the brain. This condition may be seen in individuals with exceptional intelligence or mental retardation and is not associated with any functional abnormality. In this condition, the brain may weigh up to 1800 g. Diagnosis can be made only after CT scan or air studies of the brain structure. Also called macrencephaly.

megaloblast (meg′ah-lo-blast″) [*megalo-* + Gr. *blas-*

tos germ] a large, nucleated, immature progenitor of the abnormal erythrocyte, the megalocyte. Megaloblasts arise in vitamin B_{12} and folic acid deficiencies and may be associated with leukemia or refractory anemia. They are characterized by asynchrony of maturation of the nucleus and cytoplasm; the hemoglobinization of the cytoplasm progresses to a stage corresponding to that of the reticulocyte, while the nucleus remains relatively immature and resembles that seen in a pronormoblast. The mechanism of formation is related to the inhibition of DNA synthesis and mitosis occurring during hemoglobin synthesis. Thus, the megaloblast corresponds to the normoblast of normal red cell maturation series and is correspondingly classified as basophilic, polychromatic, and orthochromatic. Like the megalocyte, the megaloblast is elliptic in shape.

megaloblastic (meg″ah-lo-blas′tik) relating to megaloblasts.

megaloblastic anemia see *megaloblastic a.* under *anemia.*

megaloblastoid (meg″ah-lo-blas′toid) resembling a megaloblast.

megalocyte (meg′ah-lo-sīt) [*megalo-* + *-cyte*] a large erythrocyte, usually oval in shape, that is the anucleate end stage of megaloblastic erythropoiesis; the mean corpuscular hemoglobin (MCH) and mean corpuscular volume (MCV) are increased. Its oval shape readily distinguishes it from a macrocyte (although this may not be true for individual cells). For positive identification, megaloblasts must be demonstrated in the bone marrow. Megalocytes are found in vitamin B_{12} and folic acid deficiencies, as well as in refractory anemia. In both types of vitamin deficiency, megalocytosis is usually associated with marked anisocytosis: many microcytes and abnormally shaped cells are present in addition to the characteristic megalocytes. See also *macrocyte* and *megaloblast.*

Megalopyge (meg″ah-lo-pij′e) a genus of hairy moths whose larvae (caterpillars) have stinging hairs. In some cases, the species *M. lanata* has caused dermatosis from contact with the poison hairs; *M. opercularis* (the puss caterpillar) produces a burning and stinging sensation following introduction of the poison substance into the skin.

megaloureter (meg″ah-lo-u-re′ter) a condition characterized by massive unilateral or bilateral dilation of the ureter in which obstruction and reflux are not evident. This lesion may be associated with congenital anomalies of the kidney, especially polycystic disease.

-megaly (meg′ah-le) [Gr. *megaleios* magnificant, *megale* great] a suffix word element to denote enlargement of the structure signified by the root to which it is attached, e.g., splenomegaly.

Megaselia (meg″ah-se′le-ah) a genus of flies, several species of which cause myiasis in humans.

megavolt (MV) (meg′ah-vōlt) a unit of electric potential (voltage) equal to 1 million volts (10^6 V).

megavoltage (meg″ah-vol′tij) pertaining to x-ray radiation therapy using photon energies above 1 MeV, used for treatment of deep-seated neoplasms. See also *radiation therapy equipment.*

megestrol acetate (mĕ-jes′trōl) a cancer chemotherapeutic drug; trademark, Megace. For more information, see *Appendix A.*

meglumine (meg′lu-mēn) [USP], a synthetic organic base, methylglucamine, that is combined with several triiodobenzoic acid derivatives in radiographic contrast media. These media are somewhat less toxic, less radiopaque, and more soluble than salts having inorganic anions (e.g., sodium).

megohm (MΩ, formerly M) (meg′ōm) [*mega-* + *ohm*] a unit of electrical resistance equal to 1 million ohms (10^6 Ω).

mei/o (mi′o) [Gr. *meiōn* smaller] a word element used in combining form to denote a decrease in size or number, e.g., meiosis.

meibomian cyst (mi-bo′me-an) [Heinrich *Meibom,* German anatomist, 1638–1700] see *chalazion.*

meibomian glands [Heinrich *Meibom*] the sebaceous glands found in the tarsal plates of the eyelid. They secrete an oily substance that seals the lid margins when the eyes are closed and prevent an overflow of tears when the eyes are open.

Meigs' syndrome (megz) [Joe Vincent *Meigs,* American surgeon, 1892–1963] the association of hydrothorax, and ascites, with an ovarian fibroma or other pelvic neoplasm.

meiocyte (mi′o-sīt) a cell that can undergo meiosis, e.g., an oocyte or primary spermatocyte. Also called *auxocyte.*

meiosis (mi-o′sis) [Gr. *meiosis* diminution] the process by which the chromosomes are separated during the formation of sex cells and their number reduced from the diploid to the haploid number. Meiosis involves two divisions of the nucleus following a single replication of the somatic chromosomes. It is a special type of cell division found in organisms in which there is sexual reproduction. Meiosis is a mechanism for distributing the genes between gametes, enabling their recombination and random segregation. It is in this process that genetic variation is produced. The meiotic divisions follow a standard scheme during which two successive divisions of the chromosomes occur:

FIRST MEIOTIC DIVISION. The first represents a reductional division in which homologous pairs of chromosomes are separated into daughter cells without duplication; i.e., their number is reduced to one-half. The fairly lengthy meiotic prophase I has been subdivided into five stages: leptotene (leptonema), zygotene (zygonema), pachytene (pachyonema), diplotene (diplonema), and diakinesis.

Prophase I—Leptotene. This is the first meiotic stage that differs from the previous interphase. There is an increase in nuclear volume and, despite the fact that DNA duplication has already taken place (in interphase) and that they have two chromatids, the leptotene chromosomes appear single rather than double. There are beadlike structures called chromomeres along their lengths. In some plants the chromosomes are clumped to one side of the nucleus (synizesis). In many insects they appear polarized, with their ends drawn together toward the portion of the nuclear membrane close to the centriole. The chromosomes become progressively shorter during the entire meiotic prophase.

Prophase I—Zygotene. The homologous chromosomes become aligned and undergo pairing in a process called synapsis. This pairing is highly specific and occurs between all homologous chromosome sections even if they are present on different nonhomologous chromosomes. It may occur because of the synaptonemal complex (a protein structure visible by electron microscope that is always found between homologues). After a transfer of a section of one chromosome to a nonhomologous chromosome (a translocation), the homologous exchanged material still pairs. Similarly, if the order of the chromosome material is inverted on two homologous chromosomes (an inversion), a loop will be formed between the two chromosomes so that tight pairing is preserved. A deletion in one chromosome causes the extra material in the homologous chromosome also to make a loop to keep the specific pairing.

During zygotene, previously unreplicated DNA is synthesized. This Z-DNA is rich in GC bases; it may represent repair synthesis.

Prophase I—Pachytene. This represents the stage of progressive shortening and coiling of the chromosomes. By middle pachytene, zygotene pairing has been completed. Each pair of homologous chromosomes is held in close longitudinal union, forming a unit called a bivalent or tetrad that contains four chromatids. Chromatids of the homologues can exchange segments (i.e., recombine). Transverse breaks are thought to occur at the chromatids followed by interchange and final fusion of the chromatid segments.

Protein synthesis seems essential to maintain chromosome pairing during pachytene. If protein synthesis is inhibited at late zygotene, the chromosome pairs fall apart and are not reconstituted. During pachytene, there is also a DNA synthesis of a smaller magnitude than that of zygotene. This P-DNA synthesis is apparently related to the process of recombination.

Prophase I—Diplotene. The intimately paired chromosomes repel each other and begin to separate. This separation is not complete, as the homologous chromosomes remain connected by actual physical crossover points called chiasmata. With a few exceptions, chiasmata are found in all plants and animals, and in many organisms their position and number seem to be constant for particular chromosomes.

Prophase I—Diakinesis. At diakinesis, coiling and contraction of the chromosomes become accentuated. The bivalents are more evenly spaced in the nucleus and migrate close to the nuclear membrane. The chiasmata move to the ends of the chromosome, a process formerly called terminalization. During the latter part of the stage, the nuclear membrane and nucleolus disappear.

Metaphase I. The chromosomes are the most condensed and appear smooth in outline. With the nuclear membrane gone, the spindle microtubules attach to the centromeres of the chromosomes. Each homologue is attached to one of the poles by the homologous centromere, and the two sister chromatids behave as a functional unit. The chromosomes become arranged at the equator, still attached at their ends by chiasmata while the centromeres are pulled toward the poles.

Anaphase I. The centromeres of the chromosomes move to their respective poles as the chiasmata separate. Anaphase chromosomes show different shapes, depending on the position of the centromeres.

Telophase I. Chromosomes may persist for some time in a condensed state. In most cases, once the homologues reach the spindle poles, a nuclear membrane is formed around them and the chromosomes pass into a short interphase before the second meiotic division begins. A nucleolus does not usually reform.

SECOND MEIOTIC DIVISION. The second meiotic division results in an equational division in which the sister chromatids are separated and four haploid cells are produced.

Interphase II. The length of the interphase may vary, but no DNA replication occurs during interphase II, whether the period is long or short.

Prophase II. If the chromosomes have uncoiled since telophase I, prophase II will be characterized by condensation of the chromosomes, and if the chromosomes were already condensed from telophase I, prophase II will be very short. A spindle apparatus begins to form in later prophase II at each of the two poles, and the nuclear envelope disintegrates.

Metaphase II. Chromosomes become arranged at the equatorial plate. Microtubules attach to each chromosome so that the sister chromatids are connected to opposite poles.

Anaphase II. Sister chromatids separate and go to opposite poles. Thus, at the end of anaphase II one complete haploid set of chromosomes has aggregated at each pole.

Telophase II. Nuclear envelopes form around each haploid set of chromosomes. The chromosomes uncoil and become diffuse as the nucleoli reform within each nucleus.

In the human female, the primary female germ cells appear in the human embryo in the wall of the yolk sac at about 20 da. At the end of the third month, the oogonia enter meiosis, which is arrested at diplotene until sexual maturity. The second meiotic division occurs only with fertilization. Most oocytes degenerate, and only about 400 survive to menarche.

In the human male, the primary gonocytes become incorporated into seminiferous tubules. Meiosis starts at puberty and ends in old age.

See also the accompanying illustration. Cf. *gametogenesis* and *mitosis.*

meiotic (mi-ot′ik) pertaining to meiosis.

Meissner's plexus (mīs′nerz) [Georg *Meissner,* German pathologist, 1829–1905] see *submucosal p.* under *plexus.*

MEK abbrev. See *methyl ethyl ketone.*

melan/o (mel′ah-no) [Gr. *melas* black] a word element used in combining form to denote black, e.g., melanoblast.

melancholia (mel″an-ko′le-ah) [*melano-* + Gr. *cholē* bile + *-ia*] an emotional illness similar to the depressive phase of manic-depressive illness. It is characterized by insomnia, depression, and an extreme sense of worthlessness, feelings that interfere with normal physical and mental activities. Melancholia affects three times more females than males.

melanin (mel′ah-nin) [Gr. *melas* black] a complex polymer, amorphous pigment that is usually dark in color and is synthesized in melanocytes. Melanocytes, which secrete melanin-containing organelles known as melanosomes, are found in the skin, dermis, dermal-epidermal junction, hair bulb, mucous membranes, mesentery, nervous system (pia arachnoid), internal ear, and eye (uveal tract and retinal pigment epithelium). In the skin, keratinocytes are the cells that deposit melanin, which they acquire by phagocytosis of melanosomes. Each melanocyte supplies melanosomes for about 30–40 keratino-

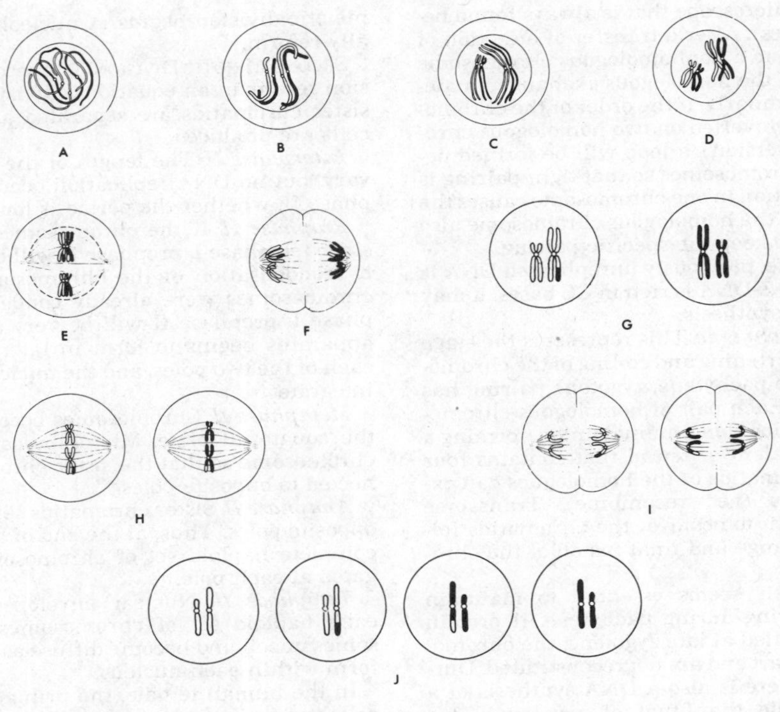

Meiosis. Only 2 of the 23 human chromosome pairs are shown, the chromosomes from one parent in black, from the other parent in outline. First Meiotic Division: *A, leptotene*—first appearance of chromosomes as thin threads; *B, zygotene*—pairing (synapsis) of chromosomes; *C, pachytene*—chromosomal thickening and shortening, the individual chromatids becoming visible; *D, diplotene;*—longitudinal separation of chromatids, the centromere remaining intact and a chiasma being formed (note: prophase includes steps *A–D* plus diakinesis, which is not shown; *E, metaphase*—movement of chromosomes into the equatorial plane; *F, anaphase*—separation of pairs, one member going to each pole; *G, telophase*—cell division, each of the two daughter cells being haploid. Second Meiotic Division: *prophase* (not shown)—chromosomes become visible; *H, metaphase*—movement of chromosomes into equatorial plane; *I, anaphase*—division of centromeres, the chromatids going to opposite poles; *J, telophase*—cell division, each daughter cell being diploid. (From Thompson, J. S., and Thompson, M. W.: Genetics in Medicine. 3rd ed. Philadelphia, W. B. Saunders Co., 1980.)

cytes, and this group of cells forms an epidermal melanin unit. The steps in the synthesis of melanin consist of the hydroxylation of tyrosine to form 3,4-dihydroxyphenylalanine (DOPA) followed by oxidation to DOPA-quinone (both steps catalyzed by the copper-containing enzyme tyrosinase), further oxidation, cyclization, and polymerization. The latter steps presumably occur by a non-enzymatic process. In the presence of zinc, which is found in high concentrations in the melanosomes, melanin is complexed with a melanosome protein via quinone-amino or quinone-sulfhydryl linkages to give rise to eumelanin, the final black pigment. Pheomelanin, the yellow-red pigment, is also synthesized starting from DOPA-quinone by an alternate pathway.

The major function of melanin may reside in its ability to protect the cells against the damaging effect of ionizing and ultraviolet radiation (sun screen). Exposure to this radiation enhances synthesis of melanin.

A heterogeneous group of heritable disorders of hypomelanosis is known as albinism. A biochemical lesion in some forms of albinism is due to tyrosinase deficiency. Other defects that can give rise to albinism may be due to the presence of inhibitors of tyrosinase, melanocyte deficiency, or melanocyte membrane defects.

melanin bleaching methods various methods in which tissue sections are immersed in a strong oxidizing agent to remove melanin pigment before staining. The most commonly used bleaches are 10 percent hydrogen peroxide for 24 hr and 0.25 percent potassium permanganate for 1–4 hr.

melanin staining methods Lillie's ferrous iron uptake method. Paraffin sections are hydrated and placed first in ferrous sulfate solution, then in potassium ferricyanide–acetic acid solution, and then are counterstained with van Gieson's picrofuchsin. Melanin chelates ferrous iron, which reacts with ferricyanide to form Turnbull blue and stains the melanin dark green. Melanin may also be stained using the argentaffin reaction or the Schmorl reaction. See also *ferric ferricyanide reduction test* and *Fontana-Masson staining method.*

melanin tests see *melanogen tests.*

melanoblast (mel′ah-no-blast″, mĕ-lan′o-blast) [*melano-* + Gr. *blastos* germ] a cell originating from the neural crest that differentiates into a melanocyte.

melanocyte (mel′ah-no-sīt, mĕ-lan′o-sīt) a cell that forms the pigment melanin. Most melanocytes are located in the basal layer of the epidermis, but some occur in the soft tissues. Melanin is deposited within membrane-bound vacuoles on a framework of protein, the premelanosome, to form a mature melanosome. Melanocytes are dendritic cells whose cytoplasmic extensions interweave between the epidermal cells. Melanosomes are transferred via the dendritic processes to the cytoplasm of the basal and squamous cells. See also *melanoma.*

melanocyte-stimulating hormone (MSH) a polypeptide hormone, secreted by the middle lobe of the pituitary. It occurs in two forms: α-MSH, which contains 13 amino acids that are almost identical to the first 13 amino acids of adrenocorticotropic hormone (ACTH), and β-MSH, which contains 22 amino acids and has 8 amino acids common to both α-MSH and ACTH. α-MSH also has some corticotropic activity, whereas ACTH has 1 percent of MSH activity. Hypothalamic peptides regulate both the release and the inhibition of release of MSH (see *melanocyte-stimulating hormone–release-inhibiting hormone* and *melanocyte-stimulating hormone–releasing hormone*).

Knowledge of the exact physiologic role of MSH in humans is lacking. In amphibia, however, MSH causes blackening of the skin by dispersal of black pigment present in the melanophore cells. This effect of MSH in amphibia is reversed by melatonin, causing a lightening of the skin color. Melatonin (*N*-acetyl-5-methoxytryptamine) is formed in the pineal gland. In addition, β-MSH has been shown to increase intracellular levels of cAMP, tyrosinase activity, and melanin content in mouse melanoma cells. Release of MSH and ACTH is stimulated in Addison's disease, causing pigmentation of the skin. This condition can be treated by hydrocortisone and cortisone, which inhibit the secretion of MSH and ACTH.

Also called *melanophore-stimulating hormone.*

melanocyte-stimulating hormone-releasing hormone (MRH) a peptide hormone (in all probability, a fragment of the oxytocin molecule) that is secreted from the hypothalamus. It acts to stimulate the release of MSH from the pituitary. Also called melanocyte-stimulating hormone–releasing factor (MRF).

melanocyte-stimulating hormone-release-inhibiting hormone (MRIH) a tripeptide hormone composed of proline, leucine, and glycinamide. It is secreted by the hypothalamus, which acts to inhibit the release of MSH from the pituitary. Also called melanocyte-stimulating hormone–inhibiting factor (MIF).

melanocytic (mel″ah-no-sit′ik) pertaining to melanocytes.

melanocytic nevus (mel″ah-no-sit′ik) see *melanocytic n.* under *nevus.*

melanodermatitis (mel″ah-no-der″mah-ti′tis) the inflammation of the skin associated with increased deposits of melanin.

melanogen (mĕ-lan′o-jen) [*melano-* + Gr. *gennan* to produce] a colorless chromogen that darkens on exposure to air and sunlight, being converted to the brown-black melanin. It may occur in the urine in certain diseases. Melanogens possibly are derivatives of orthoquinone, dopa, and indole-5,6-quinone. See also *melanuria.*

melanogen tests colorimetric tests for urinary melanogens, including the ferric chloride, Thormählen, and ammoniacal silver nitrate tests. Acidic ferric chloride solution added to urine produces a rapid color change to dark brown if melanogens are present. In the Thormählen test, melanogens in urine turn a color that is greenish-blue and bluish-black on the addition of fresh sodium nitroferricyanide solution followed by NaOH solution, cooling, and acidification with acetic acid. Normal urines give an olive or brownish-green color. Silver nitrate added to urine containing melanogens followed by the addition of ammonia produces darkening due to formation of both melanin and colloidal silver. In contrast, homogentisic acid in urine darkens the silver solution rapidly, even before the addition of ammonia.

melanoglossia (mel″ah-no-glos′e-ah) [*melano-* + Gr. *glōssa* tongue] a disorder characterized by the increased deposition of melanin on the surface of the tongue, forming black patches.

Melanoides (mel″ah-noid′ez) a genus of snails; *M. tuberculate* is the species in which the miracidium (first-stage larva) of the Chinese liver fluke, *Clonorchis sinensis,* develops.

melanoma (mel″ah-no′mah) [*melano-* + *-oma*] a term frequently used to refer to malignant melanoma; see *malignant m.*

acral lentiginous m., a primary melanoma of the volar or subungual skin that has a radial growth phase similar to that of mucosal melanomas; it is distinguishable from lentigo maligna melanoma and superficial spreading melanoma. Atypical spindle-shaped melanocytes with prominent dendrites extend diffusely along the dermal-epidermal junction, junctional nesting and infiltration of the granular layer are minimal, and fascicles of cells infiltrating the dermis are typically associated with a desmoplastic reaction.

amelanotic m., a melanoma whose cells do not contain demonstrable pigment by light microscopy or histochemistry. Premelanosomes may nevertheless be identified by electron microscopy.

desmoplastic m., a primary melanoma composed of fascicles of spindle-shaped cells associated with a dense, fibrous stroma.

juvenile m., an older term for a benign spindle or epithelioid melanocytic nevus (Spitz nevus). The term is misleading and should be abandoned.

lentigo maligna m., a cutaneous melanoma that begins as a circumscribed pigmented macular lesion (lentigo maligna or malignant freckle of Hutchinson), and enlarges slowly by lateral growth before dermal invasion occurs. It is most common on the face of elderly persons.

malignant m., a malignant neoplasm of melanocytes, the pigment-producing cells found in the skin, eyes, and mucous membranes. Malignant melanoma represents about 2 percent of all cancers and occurs more frequently on exposed areas of the skin. The risk of developing malignant melanoma increases with the lightness of an individual's skin pigmentation and with increasing exposure to the sun's rays. Malignant melanoma of cutaneous surfaces is almost unknown in blacks, but its frequency in the eyes, mucosa, and perianal area is about the same for both blacks and Caucasians. The incidence of malignant melanoma of the skin in light-skinned individuals appears to have increased in recent years in all countries in which the disease has been studied.

Cutaneous malignant melanoma has a number of recognizable forms (Table 1), the three most common of which are superficial spreading malignant melanoma (SSM), constituting approximately 70 percent of cutaneous melanomas; nodular melanoma (NOD), approximately 15 percent; and lentigo maligna melanoma (LMM), approximately 10 percent. SSM (formerly called premalignant melanosis and pagetoid melanoma) is characterized by a period of radial growth of atypical melanocytes in the epidermis and papillary dermis, associated in most instances with a lymphocytic cellular host response. Occasionally this response is associated with partial or complete regression of the radial growth phase. Deeply invasive growth, so-called vertical growth, is superimposed on the radial phase. The overall survival rate at 5 yr for patients with SSM is approximately 70 percent. NOD is characterized by direct invasion of neoplastic melanocytes into the dermis with a long period of radial growth, and its overall survival rate at 5 yr is approximately 60 percent. LLM is characterized by a slowly evolving pigmented macule, usually in the sun-exposed skin of the elderly. The noninvasive lesion shows intraepidermal neoplastic transformation, usually without appreciable host response. Deep invasion of this tumor is a late occurrence. LMM appears to be less aggressive than either SSM or NOD. In general a period of 5–50 yr is necessary for LLM to evolve, and invasion does not necessarily lead to distant metastases. The overall survival rate at 5 yr approaches 95 percent.

The prognosis for patients with SSM and NOD has been shown to be related to the depth of tumor invasion at the time of surgical excision. The depth of invasion can be assessed histopathologically according to the level of involvement of anatomic structures of the skin and by actual measurement of the thickness of tumor in millimeters, which is referred to as the microstage (see the accompanying illustration and Table 2). In assessing the prognosis for those with melanoma, the main factors to consider are tumor thickness and level of invasion; however, additional factors of known prognostic importance include the frequency of mitotic figures and the presence of vascular invasion and probably also the presence or absence of cellular and mesenchymal host responses. From these factors a melanoma may be classified as being of low, intermediate, or high risk; lesions showing regression, lesions altered by partial biopsy, and LMM are classified as of indeterminant risk.

LOW-RISK PRIMARY TUMORS. Tumors less than 0.76 mm in vertical thickness are considered to be of low risk. Generally, these are level II in invasion and are considered to be still in the radial growth phase. They are usually associated with cellular host response. The 5-yr prognosis is 98–100 percent survival with conservative therapy.

INTERMEDIATE-RISK PRIMARY TUMORS. Tumors with a vertical thickness of 0.76–1.50 mm are thought to be of intermediate risk. In general, tumors less than 1 mm thick seem to be associated with an excellent 5-yr prognosis. Almost 95 percent of patients with such tumors survive with conservative therapy.

HIGH-RISK PRIMARY TUMORS. Tumors more than 1.50 mm in vertical thickness are considered to be of high risk. With increasing thickness there is increasing risk, both of spread to regional draining lymph nodes and of systemic dissemination. Survival for patients with these tumors ranges from 50–60 percent to as little as 15–20 percent for those with deeply invasive tumors.

INDETERMINANT-RISK PRIMARY TUMORS. Currently classified as indeterminant in risk because of their unpredictable biologic behavior are low-risk tumors with a vertical thickness of less than 1 mm and significant areas of regression. Melanomas arising in lentigo maligna (also called Hutchinson's melanotic freckle) are also considered indeterminant in risk, as are tumors partially removed by biopsy and tumors for which there is insufficient tissue for evaluation. Histiogenic types of melanoma other than SSM and NOD are not currently evaluated by the microstage technique.

Special problems related to malignant melanoma include the evaluation of those neoplasms that arise in special locations (mucosal surfaces, uveal tract, and subungual or plantar sites), as well as those that arise in large, congenital melanocytic nevi. Many of these rather rare forms of melanoma show aggressive clinical behavior.

RICHARD W. SAGEBIEL, M.D.

MALIGNANT MELANOMA, TABLE 1. CLASSIFICATION OF MALIGNANT MELANOMA

	Form
I	Superficial spreading melanoma (SSM)
II	Nodular melanoma (NOD)
III	Lentigo maligna melanoma (LMM)
VI	Unclassified (including verrucous, spindle, and small nevoid variants)
V	Arising in congenital giant hairy nevus
VI	Arising in blue nevus
VII	Ocular malignant melanoma
VIII	Acral-lentiginous melanoma (volar, subungual)
IX	Mucous membrane melanoma (oral, vaginal, anal)
X	Malignant melanoma without demonstrable primary tumor
XI	Malignant melanoma arising in visceral site

Courtesy of Richard W. Sagebiel, M.D.

nodular m., a primary melanoma in which a radial growth phase is not evident. Clinically, it forms an elevated lesion. A variant of nodular melanoma with a polypoid configuration is particularly aggressive.

superficial spreading m., a cutaneous melanoma that extends by radial expansion, forming a flat, irregular lesion with varying degrees of pigmentation and depigmentation. With spread, the surface becomes roughened, and a vertical growth phase develops.

melanophage (mel′ah-no-fāj″) a histiocyte that contains phagocytosed melanosomes.

melanophore (mel′ah-no-fōr″) [*melano-* + Gr. *phoros* bearing] a melanin-containing cell. In lower

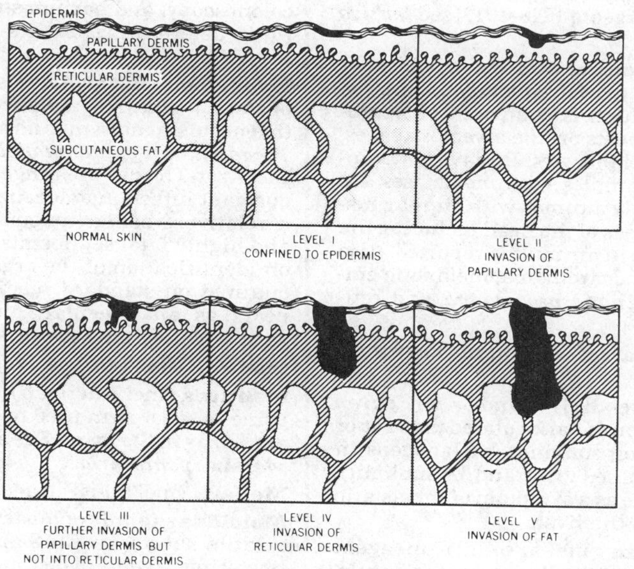

Malignant melanoma. Depth of invasion in localized (stage I) melanoma, in which a progressively worse prognosis is associated with increasing invasion of the skin and subcutaneous tissues. (From Horton, J., and Hill, G. J.: Clinical Oncology. Philadelphia, W. B. Saunders Co., 1977.)

vertebrates this term is usually reserved for such cells, and in humans for the pigment-containing cells of the iris and choroid.

melanophore-stimulating hormone (MSH) see *melanocyte-stimulating hormone.*

melanoplakia (mel″ah-no-pla′ke-ah) [*melano-* + Gr. *plax* plate + *-ia*] a disorder characterized by the increased deposition of melanin on the mucous membranes of the mouth, creating darkened patches.

melanosarcoma (mel″ah-no-sar-ko′mah) see *malignant m.* under *melanoma.*

melanosis (mel″ah-no′sis) [*melan-* + *-osis*] any condition in which there is abnormal brown or black pigmentation of the tissues or organs.

melanosis coli brown-black discoloration of the mucosa of the large intestine, which may involve a segment or the entire colon. Histologic sections show pigment granules within macrophages in the lamina propria, and the pigment shows features of lipofuscin. The condition does not give rise to symptoms and has not been proven to be associated with the development of other pathologic conditions, including carcinoma.

melanosome (mel′ah-no-sōm″) a membrane-bound cytoplasmic body in a melanocyte, within which melanin is deposited on a protein framework called the premelanosome.

melanotic (mel″ah-not′ik) pertaining to or characterized by the presence of melanin.

melanotic freckle of Hutchinson [Sir Jonathan

MALIGNANT MELANOMA, TABLE 2. MICROSTAGE OF MALIGNANT MELANOMA

LEVEL OF INVASION		THICKNESS	RISK
Intraepidermal	I	< 0.76 mm	Low-risk primary tumors
Papillary dermis	II Thin		
	II Thick	0.76–1.5 mm	Intermediate-risk primary tumors
	III Thin		
Junction of papillary and reticular dermis			
	III Thick	>1.5 mm	High-risk primary tumors
Reticular dermis/ subcutaneous fat	IV		
	V		

Courtesy of Richard W. Sagebiel, M.D.

Hutchinson, English surgeon, 1828–1913] see *lentigo maligna*.

melanotic neuroectodermal tumor a neoplasm of the anterior jaw, seen most frequently in infants younger than 6 mo, which is composed of neuroblasts that form solid sheets or line alveolar spaces, as well as groups of melanocytes. It may grow rapidly, but malignant examples with metastases are uncommon. Occasionally a tumor with similar histology involves other areas of the head including the brain, and rarely a case in an adult is reported. Also called congenital melanocarcinoma, melanotic epithelial odontoma, *melanotic progonoma*, and retinal anlage tumor.

melanotic progonoma see *melanotic neuroectodermal tumor*.

melanuria (mel″an-u′re-ah) [*melano-* + Gr. *ouron* urine + *-ia*] the excretion of dark-colored urine or of urine that turns dark on standing (melanogens in urine darken when exposed to air and/or sunlight). This condition can arise as a symptom of metastatic melanomas, usually in the liver.

melarsonyl potassium (mel-ar′so-nil) an agent used to treat infection with *Trypanosoma gambiense*. Trademark, Mel W.

melarsoprol (mel-ar′so-prōl) an organic arsenical agent used intravenously to treat late stages of infection with *Trypanosoma gambiense* and *T. rhodesiense*. Trademark, Mel B.

melasma (mĕ-laz′mah) [Gr. *melas* black] a circumscribed hyperpigmentation of body surfaces, most often affecting the forehead, cheeks, chin, and lips. There are areas of blotchy brown macules, which may coalesce to form the "mask of pregnancy" seen on pregnant females. The condition may also occur in females taking oral contraceptives, or in otherwise normal males and females. Although this condition is thought to be due to progesteronal effects, the hormonal levels, including melanocyte-stimulating hormone (MSH), are normal. Also called *chloasma*.

melatonin (mel″ah-to′nin) a hormone, *N*-acetyl-5-methoxy serotonin; M.W. 232.27. Melatonin is secreted from the pineal body; it lightens the color of the melanocytes in the skin of the frog and blocks the action of melanocyte-stimulating hormone (MSH) and adrenocorticotropic hormone (ACTH). This hormone is biosynthesized from serotonin by the action of *N*-acetyl transferase, followed by *O*-methylation. It is primarily metabolized in the liver, where it is hydroxylated and then conjugated with glucuronic or sulfuric acid and excreted into the urine. Release of melatonin is increased during lightening of the environment, which is mediated by adrenergic stimulation of the pineal body. The pineal hormones, such as melatonin, can exert other effects on the body, as indicated by experiments with pinealectomized rats.

melena (mel′ĕ-nah) [Gr. *melas* black] the darkening of stools due to the presence of blood. This condition reflects gastrointestinal bleeding at any point between the mouth and the colon. The source of the bleeding is usually above the ligament of Treitz. The dark color is due to the oxidation of heme by intestinal and bacterial enzymes, and takes 8 hr to form. Between 50 and 100 ml of blood per day will produce melena. Tests are available for the detection of occult blood in the stool. Hematologic tests, colonoscopy, and barium studies may also be helpful in determining the site and cause of the bleeding.

melioidosis (me″le-oi-do′sis) [Gr. *melis* a distemper of asses + *eidos* resemblance] a glanderslike disease that occurs in humans and animals and is caused by *Pseudomonas pseudomallei*. It is endemic in Southeast Asia. The disease ranges from an asymptomatic dormant infection to localized abscess formation to a relatively benign pneumonia or overwhelming and highly fatal septicemia. The diagnosis is based on identification of the organism, which is readily cultured on standard media; when stained, it appears as an irregular, bipolar-stained organism with a "safety pin" appearance.

melitose (mel′ĭ-tōs) see *raffinose*.

melituria (mel″ĭ-tu′re-ah) [Gr. *meli* honey + *ouron* urine + *-ia*] a term used to describe the presence of any sugar in the urine. See also *fructosuria, glucosuria,* and *pentosuria*.

Mellaril (mel′ah-ril) trademark. See *thioridazine*.

Meloidae a family of blister beetles that contain the volatile substance cantharidin, a rubefacient and blistering agent. The species *Lytta vesicatoria* ("Spanish fly") has been used commercially to obtain cantharidin for use as a diuretic or aphrodisiac.

When the blister beetles are crushed on the skin, their body fluids are discharged, forming blisters involving the outer layers of the skin. Internal doses of cantharidin are toxic, causing gastrointestinal irritation, nausea, vomiting, diarrhea, cramps, and, occasionally, collapse.

melphalan (mel′fah-lan) [USP], the phenylalanine derivative of nitrogen mustard, an alkylating agent used as a cancer chemotherapeutic drug. Trademark, Alkeran. For more information, see *Appendix A*.

melting point (m. p.) the temperature at which the solid and liquid phases of a pure substance are in equilibrium.

membrane (mem′brān) 1. a thin, continuous, sheetlike structure that surrounds cells and organelles. Cellular membranes are composed primarily of lipids and proteins. The matrix of the membrane is a bilayer of amphipathic lipid molecules, with nonpolar groups in the interior and polar groups on the surfaces. Proteins are embedded to varying degrees within the bilayer.

2. a term used to describe a thin layer of specialized tissue that divides a space or organ, lines a cavity, or covers a surface.

For more information, see the specific membrane; see also *endoplasmic reticulum* and *nuclear envelope*.

membrane bone any bone that develops directly within mesenchyme, in contrast to cartilage bone.

membrane component of diffusion (D_M) the portion of the total diffusion capacity of the lungs that is concerned with diffusion across the alveolocapillary membrane. It depends on the area (A) and thickness (y) of the membrane, and on the membrane diffusion coefficient (d) of the measured gas, as represented by the following equation: $D_M = Ad/y$. It amounts to about 70 ml of O_2/min/torr in the healthy adult.

membrane filter see *membrane f.* under *filter*.

membrane filter techniques methods for isolating cells for cytologic examination by filtration from fluid specimens. Two types of filters with 5-μm pores are commonly used: cellulose acetate filters, which are opaque, white, 140-μm–thick membranes; and polycarbonate filters, which are transparent, clear, 10-μm–thick membranes.

Unfixed fluids are used, as certain forms of fixation produce protein coagulation that clogs filter pores. After filtration of a specimen, the filters are removed and stained using conventional cytologic stains. Cellulose acetate filters are cleared in xylene and mounted on slides using a mounting medium with the same refractive index as the filter. Polycarbonate filters are placed on glass slides, dissolved in chloroform either before or after staining, and mounted with a conventional mounting medium.

membrane instability any tendency toward spontaneous depolarization of a nerve or muscle cell membrane subsequent to the voluntary activation or mechanical stimulation of the membrane.

membranelle (mem″brah-nel′) a small membrane composed of numerous short threads or cilia (which perform the function of locomotion) that covers the whole body of ciliates.

membrane potential the potential produced by a difference in ionic concentrations across a semipermeable membrane. When there is a difference in the concentration of nondiffusible ions, the equilibrium distribution of the diffusible ions will also be unequal. At equilibrium, the total ionic charge (anions plus cations) is zero on both sides, and the ratio of the concentrations on both sides of the membrane is determined for each diffusible ion from the membrane potential by using the Nernst equation. Also called *Donnan potential.*

membrane protein a protein that occurs in association with a membrane (e.g., cell membrane or endoplasmic reticulum). Such proteins have a hydrophobic part embedded in the membrane lipid core and a hydrophilic part exposed on one or both sides of the membrane. They provide structural support to the membrane, transport molecules across the membrane, and serve as cell surface antigens or hormone and transmitter receptors.

Membrane proteins are sometimes divided into two subtypes, peripheral and integral proteins. Peripheral proteins (or extrinsic proteins) are separated from the membrane by mild treatment with chelating agents or high-ionic-strength solutions, and are usually soluble in neutral aqueous solution free of lipids. Integral proteins (or intrinsic proteins) are separated from the membrane only by detergents or organic solvents, and are insoluble or aggregated with lipids in neutral aqueous solutions.

membrane transport see *active transport, facilitated diffusion,* and *passive transport.*

membranoproliferative glomerulopathy (mem″brah-no-pro-lif′er-ah-tiv) see under *glomerulopathy.*

membranous (mem′brah-nus) [L. *membranosus*] pertaining to or consisting of membranes.

membranous glomerulopathy (mem′brah-nus) see under *glomerulopathy.*

memory (mem′o-re) [L. *memoria*] 1. that mental faculty by which sensations, impressions, and ideas are recalled.

2. in a computer, an electronic device that stores numbers, characters, and program instructions. The term refers particularly to the main high-speed storage of a computer (usually composed of integrated circuits), as opposed to bulk storage devices (magnetic disks or tapes).

men/o (men′o) [Gr. *mēn* month; *mēniaia* the menses] a word element used in combining form to denote a relationship to the process of menstruation, e.g., menorrhagia.

menadiol (men″ah-di′ol) 2-methyl-1,4-naphthohydroquinone, an analog of vitamin K.

menadione (men″ah-di′ōn) see *vitamin* K_3.

menaquinone (men″ah-kwin′ōn) see *vitamin* K_2.

menarche (mĕ-nar′ke) [*men-* + Gr. *archē* beginning] the onset of the menstrual cycle in the adolescent female, which presently occurs at a mean age of 12.6 yr. Ordinarily, the menarche is preceded by development of the breasts and pubic hair. Menarche may be absent or delayed for a number of reasons, including the presence of Turner's syndrome and Addison's disease; however, delayed menarche beyond ages 14–15 is usually only a result of genetic factors. Cf. *amenorrhea.*

mendelevium (Md) (men″dĕ-le′ve-um) [Dimitri Ivanovitch *Mendeléeff,* Russian chemist, 1834–1907; inventor of the periodic table of the elements] a metallic, synthetic, radioactive element; atomic number 101; most stable isotope, Md-258 (half-life, 56 da); a 5f transition element (actinide element); oxidation states +2, +3.

Mendel's laws (men′delz) [Gregor Johann *Mendel,* Austrian monk and naturalist, 1822–1884] 1. the law of segregation. Inherited traits are controlled by discrete factors (genes), with each individual inheriting two forms (alleles) of a gene, one from each parent. The alleles are segregated into different gametes during meiosis and are passed to different offspring. This law is now known to hold only for autosomal, monogenic traits in diploid organisms.

2. the law of independent assortment. The alleles corresponding to different traits are distributed to the gametes independent of one another. This law is now known to apply not to genes but to chromosomes: genes on different chromosomes assort independently, whereas those on the same chromosome can be linked (if they are very distant, they may still segregate independently).

See also *mendelian i.* under *inheritance.*

Ménétrier's disease (mān″a-tre-āz′) [Pierre *Ménétrier,* French physician, 1859–1935] a rare form of gastric mucosal hyperplasia, of unknown etiology, that produces giant rugal hypertrophy of the stomach (chronic hypertrophic gastritis). Mucous cells replace the parietal and chief cells in the gastric glands, and the gastric juice contains little acid. The disease may be associated with protein loss of a degree sufficient to cause edema. The large gastric folds can be demonstrated by radiologic studies, but biopsy is necessary to differentiate the condition from lymphoma and carcinoma.

Menghini needle a needle used to obtain liver biopsies.

Ménière's disease (men″e-ārz′) [Prosper *Ménière,* French physician, 1799–1862] a disease of the inner ear characterized by recurrent aural vertigo, associated with progressive, unilateral hearing loss and tinnitus. The disease is seen most frequently in middle-aged adults and has no known cause. The caloric test displays an altered labyrinthine response, and audiometric tests suggest a nerve-type of hearing loss. Pathologically, there is dilation of the endolymphatic system. Treatment of acute attacks of vertigo is by bed rest and antihistamine drugs. Sedatives may help to reduce anxiety between attacks, and a low-salt diet may have some prophylactic value. Surgical treatment may be necessary for patients with disabling symptoms.

mening/o (mĕ-ning′go) [Gr. *mēninx* membrane] a work element used in combining form to denote the meninges (the membranes around the brain and spinal cord), e.g., meningococcemia.

meningeal (mĕ-nin′je-al) pertaining to the meninges.

meninges (me-nin′jēs) [Gr., pl. of *mēninx* membrane] [NA], the three membranous layers that envelop the brain and spinal cord: the dura mater, pia mater, and arachnoid.

meningi/o (mĕ-nin′je-o) a word element used in combining form to denote the meninges, e.g., meningioma.

meningioma (mĕ-nin″je-o′mah) [*meningi-* + *-oma* tumor] a tumor of meningeal cells, particularly those of the arachnoid. It is a common tumor, accounting for roughly 15 percent of intracranial and 25 percent of spinal neoplasms. Most cases occur in adults. The tumors are typically well demarcated from adjacent brain, but some grow diffusely, forming a dense plaque. A range of histologic appearances can be seen, but the cells are often elongated and may form whorls. Psammoma bodies are common, and some tumors are very vascular. The vast majority of meningiomas are benign, but they may nevertheless infiltrate adjacent tissues. Extracranial and extraspinal meningiomas are uncommon. Symptoms and signs depend on the location of the lesion. Surgical removal of the tumor, if accessible, is usually curative.

meningismus (men″in-jis′mus) signs and symptoms suggestive of meningitis in the presence of a totally normal central nervous system examination and normal cerebrospinal fluid findings. The condition is found most frequently in young children with infections such as pneumonia and shigellosis.

meningitis (men″in-ji′tis), pl. *meningitides* [*meningo-* + *-itis* inflammation] an inflammation of the arachnoid and pia mater. It may be caused by infection of these meninges and the intervening cerebrospinal fluid with a bacterium, virus, parasite, or fungus. The inflammation generally leads to headache, neck stiffness, and signs of meningeal irritation. Movement of the neck, particularly forward flexion, involves pain; thus, the individual maintains a rigid neck posture. Diagnosis involves analysis of CSF, which is obtained by lumbar puncture (see also *cerebrospinal fluid culture*). Treatment depends on the etiologic agent.

amebic m., a form of meningoencephalitis caused by the presence of amebas of the genera *Naegleria* (especially *N. fowleri*) and *Acanthamoeba*. Infection caused by *Naegleria* species is usually acute in nature and is associated with swimming or bathing in waters containing these amebas. By contrast, *Acanthamoeba* infections are usually more chronic and are not associated with any known mode of transmission. However, hematogenous dissemination has been reported, with appearance of the *Acanthamoeba* organisms in skin, eyes, and other organs. The disorder is characterized by an acute, febrile meningoencephalitis, with signs of cerebral and meningeal involvement.

Laboratory diagnosis requires demonstration of these organisms in the CSF by light or phase microscopy. The finding of amebas in CSF and the efforts to grow them in culture from pathogenic specimens have been more successful in *Naegleria* infections than in those involving *Acanthamoeba* species. The CSF may show a variable increase in cell content (mainly polymorphs), and some red cells may also be present; glucose concentrations may be normal or reduced, while protein concentration is increased. Treatment requires intravenous and intrathecal amphotericin B and miconazole, as well as oral rifampin, but the outcome is usually fatal.

Also called primary amebic meningoencephalitis.

aseptic m., an inflammation of the meninges that is characterized clinically by fever, headache, neck stiffness, and signs of meningeal infection, and by a CSF having an increased cell count (mainly mononuclear), normal concentration of glucose, normal or slightly increased protein concentration, and the absence of bacteria in direct smears and cultures. Aseptic meningitis is most often due to viral infection, but there are numerous other causes, including infection with mycobacteria, spirochetes, fungi, and protozoa. It can also be secondary to noninfectious conditions such as neoplastic invasion, reactions to intrathecal injections, lead poisoning, vaccination (allergic) reactions, and sarcoidosis.

bacterial m., an inflammation of the meninges caused by a bacterial infection. The type of bacterium most frequently isolated from the CSF of infected individuals differs with age: newborns are usually infected with *Escherichia coli*, other gram-negative bacilli, or group B streptococci; children younger than 15 yr with *Hemophilus influenza* type b or *Neisseria meningitidis;* and adults with *Streptococcus pneumoniae* or *N. meningitidis.* Epidemic outbreaks, which occur in environments similar to military camps, are usually caused by *N. meningitidis.* Recurring chronic cases are most often due to *S. pneumoniae.* These bacteria usually gain entry to the CSF as a result of bacteremia, upper respiratory tract infections, nasopharyngeal infections, abscesses, or a head injury. Once in the CSF, the bacteria multiply and produce a purulent exudate.

Clinically, there is an abrupt onset of headache, nausea, neck stiffness and pain, and confusion; as the disease progresses, confusion, stupor or loss of consciousness may occur. A rash may be present in individuals infected with *N. meningitidis.* If the cranial nerves become involved, there may be ocular palsies, facial weakness, or hearing loss. Seizures and focal cerebral deficits may also occur. Bacterial meningitis is a medical emergency requiring prompt treatment if sequelae such as mental retardation are to be avoided.

Laboratory diagnosis of bacterial meningitis involves examination of the CSF. At lumbar puncture, the CSF pressure may be increased to 200–300 mm of H_2O. A CSF cell count of 100–10,000 cells/mm^3 with a predominance of polymorphonuclear leukocytes is suggestive of bacterial meningitis. The CSF glucose concentration is often decreased (<40 mg/dl), whereas the protein concentration is increased (<100 mg/dl), and an abnormal amount of lactic dehydrogenase is present. The CSF should be centrifuged and the sediment Gram stained, as this may permit identification of the causal organism. Culture of the CSF to identify the responsible bacteria and antimicrobial susceptibility testing of the organism are essential for proper diagnosis and treatment. Cultures of the blood and nasopharynx may also be helpful.

***Candida* m.**, meningitis due to infection with *Candida albicans*. See also *mycotic m.*

cryptoccoccal m., a type of meningitis that may be fulminant or indolent and is caused by an infection with *Cryptococcus neoformans*. The most notable symptoms include headache, blurred vision, confusion, depression, and inappropriate behavior. The pathologic findings are of a granulomatous meningitis, but granulomas and cysts may also be found within the brain.

Investigations reveal a CSF with an elevated cell count (mostly lymphocytes) and protein concentration, and a decreased glucose concentration. An India ink stain of centrifuged CSF may reveal budding yeast cells surrounded by a capsule. The organism can be isolated on mycologic media, and cryptococcal antigens can be detected serologically. Treatment is with amphotericin B.

See also *Cryptococcus*.

mycotic m., meningitis caused by a fungal infection. It is most commonly caused by the *Cryptococcus* organism; however, *Candida, Coccidioides, Mucor, Actinomyces,* and *Aspergillus* are also potential pathogens. Amphotericin B is the chemotherapy of choice.

subacute m., a form of meningitis that evolves slowly over a period of several weeks. It may be caused by systemic fungal infections, tuberculosis, neoplasms, syphilis, and sarcoidosis. Meningeal involvement by neoplasms is often associated with acute lymphoblastic leukemia, gliomas, and metastatic carcinoma.

The history of previous or current illness is useful for diagnosis. The CSF shows an increased cell count primarily consisting of lymphocytes, as well as low glucose concentration and a high protein concentration. Microbiologic and histologic analyses of the CSF may indicate the etiologic agent.

syphilitic m., meningitis caused by the spirochete *Treponema pallidum*, the etiologic agent of syphilis. All forms of neurosyphilis begin with a meningitis, but the latter is often asymptomatic. However, it does sometimes lead to headache, vomiting, malaise, irritability, stiff neck, cranial nerve palsies, and convulsions either early in the infection or during a secondary relapse that is accompanied by a rash. This disease rarely lasts more than 1 mo. Increased cranial pressure and hydrocephalus can develop. The later manifestations of neurosyphilis are essentially the sequelae of a chronic syphilitic meningitis.

Laboratory studies show an increased cell count composed predominantly of mononuclear cells, an elevated protein concentration, and a normal glucose concentration. Syphilis can be detected by serologic analysis of the CSF with either the VDRL test or the FTA-ABS test.

See also *syphilis*.

tuberculous m., an inflammation of the meninges due to an infection with *Mycobacterium tuberculosis*. An extension of miliary tuberculosis, tuberculous meningitis is a serious and often fatal disease. When the *M. tuberculosis* organism enters the subarachnoid space, an immune response causes inflammation, production of an exudate, and eventually hydrocephalus. Clinically, there may be headache, lassitude, confusion, stiff neck, fever, oculomotor palsies, other cranial nerve abnormalities, and signs of meningeal irritations. There is usually evidence of active tuberculosis elsewhere, most often in the lungs.

Laboratory investigation shows a CSF with an elevated cell count (predominantly consisting of mononuclear cells), a low glucose concentration, and elevated protein concentration. Acid-fast staining and mycobacterial culture can identify the organism. There is usually a fatal outcome within 2 mo of onset, unless treatment is instituted with antituberculous drugs promptly.

See also *mycobacteria*.

viral m., a benign, self-limiting form of meningitis caused by a virus. The coxsackieviruses and echoviruses (enterovirus) are the most common agents, although poliovirus, mumps virus, herpes simplex viruses including Epstein-Barr virus, arboviruses, and lymphocytic choriomeningitis virus, may also be implicated.

The initial location of viral replication depends on the portal of entry. After the initial growth period, the virus enters the blood stream and eventually penetrates the blood-brain barrier into the CSF. Clinically, there is headache, fever, nuchal rigidity with full flexion, malaise, sore throat, and nausea, which can last for several weeks. A rash is sometimes present, especially if the etiologic agent is an enterovirus.

Laboratory evaluation involves an analysis of the CSF and blood. The blood cell count is often normal; however, the CSF examination usually demonstrates an increase in mononuclear cells. The CSF glucose concentration is normal, but the CSF protein concentration is increased. In all instances it is important to exclude tuberculous meningitis, fungal meningitis, brain abscesses, and encephalitis. Viruses can sometimes be identified by isolation techniques, as well as by serology, if acute and convalescent sera are available: a fourfold rise in antibody titer is indicative of infection. Owing to a lack of antiviral chemotherapy, treatment involves supportive therapy, bed rest, pain relief, and control of fever.

meningocele (mĕ-ning′go-sēl) [*meningo-* + Gr. *kēlē* hernia] a developmental abnormality that consists of a herniation of the meninges, in the form of a protruding sac, through a spina bifida. The spinal cord and nerve roots are unaffected. When a meningocele becomes filled with cerebrospinal fluid, it is known as a hydromeningocele.

meningocerebritis (mĕ-ning″go-ser″ĕ-bri′tis) [*meningo-* + L. *cerebrum* brain + *-itis*] see *meningoencephalitis*.

meningococcemia (mĕ-ning″go-kok-se′me-ah) [*meningo-* + Gr. *kokkos* berry, grain + *haima* blood + *-ia*] septicemia due to the presence of meningococci (*Neisseria meningitidis*) in the blood. See also *septicemia*.

meningococcus (mĕ-ning″go-kok′us), pl. *meningococci* [*meningo-* + Gr. *kokkos* berry, grain] see *N. meningitidis* under *Neisseria*.

meningoencephalitis (mĕ-ning″go-en-sef″ah-li′tis) [*meningo-* + Gr. *enkephalos* brain + *-itis*] an inflammation of the brain and its meninges. This condition may be due to viral, bacterial, fungal, or parasitic infection. See also *amebic m.* under *meningitis.*

meningoencephalomyelitis (mĕ-ning″go-en-sef″-ah-lo-mi″ĕ-li′tis) [*meningo-* + Gr. *enkephalos* brain + *myelos* marrow + *-itis*] inflammation of the meninges, brain, and spinal cord.

meningoencephalopathy (mĕ-ning″go-en-sef″ah-lop′ah-the) [*meningo-* + Gr. *enkephalos* brain + *-pathy*] disease of the cerebral meninges and brain.

carcinomatous m., metastatic carcinoma that affects the cerebral meninges and brain. Neurologic signs are variable and may include headache, confusion, and focal deficits. Laboratory findings may include elevation of lymphocyte counts and protein in the cerebrospinal fluid (CSF), sometimes with a concomitant decrease in the fluid sugar concentration. Neoplastic cells may be identified in stained sections of filtered CSF.

meningomyelitis (mĕ-ning″go-mi″ĕ-li′tis) [*meningo-* + Gr. *myelos* marrow + *-itis*] an inflammation of the spinal cord and its meninges. This condition may be seen in various bacterial, fungal, and parasitic infections.

meningomyelocele (mĕ-ning″go-mi′ĕ-lo-sēl″) [*meningo-* + Gr. *myelos* marrow + *kēlē* hernia] the herniation of spinal cord and overlying meninges through a defect in the vertebral column. When the hernial protrusion is saclike and becomes filled with cerebrospinal fluid, it is known as a hydromyelomeningocele.

meningomyeloradiculitis (mĕ-ning″go-mi″ĕ-lo-rah-dik″u-li′tis) [*meningo-* + Gr. *myelos* marrow + L. *radiculus* radicle + *-itis*] an inflammation of the meninges and spinal nerve root, with spinal cord involvement. If the spinal cord is not involved, the term meningoradiculitis is used.

meniscus (mĕ-nis′kus), pl. *menisci* [Gr. *mēniskos* crescent] 1. the curved surface of a liquid in a tube, caused by surface tension. In a pipet or buret, the reading is made at the bottom of a concave meniscus (as with water) or the top of a convex one (as with mercury).

2. [NA], a general term for the *semilunar cartilage.*

Menkes' syndrome [John H *Menkes,* U.S. pediatric neurologist, born 1928] a rare inherited disease, transmitted as an X-linked recessive trait, that is characterized by deficient intestinal copper absorption. Serum copper and ceruloplasmin levels are decreased in affected infants. Symptoms develop in the neonatal period. There may be hypothermia, poor feeding, seizures, progressive cerebral degeneration, retarded growth, and brittle hair. In affected infants, the electroencephalogram is characterized by high-voltage multifocal sharp waves, and background activity may be intermittently diminished in amplitude. The intravenous (but not oral) administration of copper may restore normal serum levels of copper and ceruloplasmin. Also called kinky hair syndrome.

menolipsis (men″o-lip′sis) a temporary cessation of menstruation, which may have a number of causes including hormone imbalances, ovarian disorders, marked nutritional deprivation, and psychogenic factors. See also *amenorrhea.*

menometrorrhagia (men″o-met″ro-ra′je-ah) menstrual uterine bleeding that is abnormal in frequency, duration, and amount. Its causes are similar to those of metrorrhagia.

menopause (men′o-pawz) [*meno-* + Gr. *pausis* cessation] the period in a female's life during which normal menstrual cycles cease. It occurs naturally between ages 45 and 55, or may be induced earlier artificially as a result of surgery or irradiation to the ovaries. Premature menopause (before age 40) is more common in females with infectious or surgical disorders of the genital tract. Symptoms may include menstrual irregularity that is followed by amenorrhea, hot flashes, nervousness, weight gain, painful breasts, dyspareunia, and an increase or decrease in libido. Osteoporosis, atrophic vaginitis, vulvitis, and, in severe cases, psychosis may also occur.

Laboratory studies show elevated serum and urinary follicle-stimulating hormone (FSH) and luteinizing hormone (LH) concentrations; vaginal smears show evidence of diminished estrogen. Estrogen replacement therapy may be necessary for those with severe symptoms.

menorrhagia (men″o-ra′je-ah) [*meno-* + Gr. *rhēgnynai* to burst forth] excessive uterine bleeding coupled with normal cycle length. The causes include polyps, benign and malignant tumors, infections, and inflammations. Aside from these local disorders, a bleeding diathesis, such as leukemia, and abnormal pregnancies must be considered as possible causes.

menostasis (me-nos′tah-sis) a suppression or cessation of menstruation during the reproductive period of a female's life for reasons unassociated with pregnancy or menopause. See also *amenorrhea.*

menses (men′sēz) [L.; pl. of *mensis* month] see *menstruation.*

menstrual (men′stroo-al) [L. *menstrualis*] pertaining to the menses.

menstrual cycle the female sexual cycle; the term is used to designate the cyclic changes in the endometrium that occur as a result of corresponding changes in the rates of secretion of ovarian female sex hormones and pituitary gonadotropins. The cycle can vary in length; most are between 25 and 30 da (average, 28 da), but cycles as short as 20 da or as long as 45 da can occur in normal females.

The changes in the ovaries during the menstrual cycle (ovarian cycle) are controlled by the gonadotropic hormones, follicle-stimulating hormone (FSH), and luteinizing hormone (LH), which are released by the pituitary in response to gonadotropin hormone–releasing hormone (GnRH) from the hypothalamus. Gonadotropin levels rise at the beginning of the cycle, LH at the onset of menstruation, and FSH about 2 da before menstruation. The rise in FSH levels causes the growth of about 20 ovarian follicles and the proliferation of granulosa cells, which secrete progesterone, and theca cells, which secrete estrogens. After about 1 wk of growth, one of the follicles outgrows all the others, which then undergo atresia. The intrafollicular concentrations of estrogen and progesterone are generally high in the follicle that will ovulate.

At the midpoint of the cycle, the level of LH increases by a factor of 6–10 and the level of FSH by a factor of 2. Although estrogens have a negative feedback effect on gonadotropin release during the rest of the menstrual cycle, the feedback effect on the hypothalamus becomes positive at the very high estrogen levels reached at this point, causing a rapid surge in the LH and FSH levels.

Ovulation occurs about 18 hr later; the mechanism of ovulation is still obscure. After expulsion of the ovum, the follicle undergoes luteinization induced by LH, and becomes the corpus luteum. The luteal cells secrete large amounts of progesterone and lesser amounts of estrogens, which cause a decrease in LH and FSH secretion through negative feedback. Unless pregnancy occurs, the corpus luteum degenerates 14 $\pm$ 2 da after ovulation. This ends the feedback suppression of FSH and LH secretion and starts a new cycle. If pregnancy occurs, human chorionic gonadotropin (hCG) is secreted by the syncytiotrophoblastic cells of the blastocyst; hCG binds to receptors for LH and prolongs the functional activity of the corpus luteum.

In the proliferative phase before ovulation, estrogens secreted by the ovaries cause the stromal and epithelial cells of the endometrium to proliferate rapidly, accompanied by growth of the endometrial glands and blood vessels in the endometrium. In the secretory phase after ovulation, progesterone secreted by the ovaries causes development of the endometrial glands and the secretion of large amounts of stored nutrients for the dividing blastocyst before the development of the placenta, if pregnancy occurs. At the end of the cycle the endometrium has a thickness of 4–6 mm. The large decrease in the secretion of estrogens and progesterone at the end of the cycle causes involution of the endometrium. The blood vessels become vasospastic, and the superficial layers of the endometrium undergo necrosis and are desquamated. Necrosis of blood vessels opens vascular channels with resultant menstrual bleeding. The blood and desquamated tissue are expelled by uterine contractions.

The hormone levels also have effects on vaginal squamous epithelial cells. Maturation of the squamous epithelium is induced by estrogens and is at a maximum at the time of ovulation. This makes it possible to estimate the time of ovulation from a vaginal smear.

Also called *ovarian cycle.* See also *squamous cell index* and the accompanying illustration.

menstruate (men'stroo-āt) [L. *menstruare*] to discharge blood and desquamated endometrium during menstruation.

menstruation (men"stroo-a'shun) the periodic discharge through the vagina of blood and necrotic epithelial debris from the sloughed endometrium of the nonpregnant uterus; the culmination of the menstrual cycle. Menstruation occurs approximately every 28 da in females from the time of puberty to menopause, except during pregnancy. Generally, the flow lasts 3–6 da. Also called *menses.*

MEN syndrome [acronym from *m*ultiple *e*ndocrine *n*eoplasia] a complex of several distinct genetic disorders, transmitted as autosomal dominant traits, that are characterized by multiple endocrine gland dysfunction (hyper- or hypofunction) due to the presence of multiple endocrine tumors. The pathogenesis is unclear; the disorders may result from aberrant control of cellular proliferation in affected endocrine organs, or from faulty differentiation and regulation of cells derived from the neural crest. The range of clinical symptoms encountered in the syndromes is vast and diagnosis is difficult. The majority of endocrine neoplasms that commonly occur are benign adenomas, although some are malignant. Formerly called MEA (multiple endocrine adenomatosis) syndrome.

MEN I, multiple endocrine neoplasia, type I, a dominantly inherited syndrome characterized by tumors or hyperplasia of the pituitary, adrenal cortex, parathyroid, and islet cells of the pancreas; the thyroid may also be involved. Adenomas of two or more of these endocrine glands are present. Symptoms, which may develop at any age, depend on the glands affected but may include peptic ulceration and gastric hypersecretion, hypoglycemia, hypercalcemia with impaired renal function, and pituitary dysfunction. Although many endocrine neoplasms in this syndrome are benign, pancreatic and adrenal cortical tumors may be malignant. Also called *Wermer syndrome.*

MEN II, multiple endocrine neoplasia, type II, a

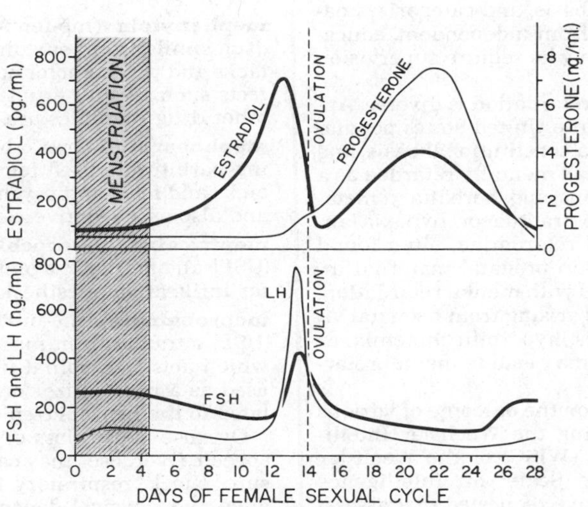

Menstrual cycle. Plasma concentrations of the gonadotropins and ovarian hormones during the normal female sexual cycle. (From Guyton, A. C.: Textbook of Medical Physiology. 6th ed. Philadelphia, W. B. Saunders Co., 1981.)

syndrome characterized by pheochromocytoma and medullary thyroid carcinoma: in about 50 percent of those affected, there is also parathyroid hyperplasia or adenoma. This syndrome, transmitted as an autosomal dominant trait, may occur at any age. In contrast to MEN I, peptic ulceration and pancreatic islet cell tumors are not seen.

The neoplasms of this condition are responsible for serum calcitonin elevations and catecholamine excess. Other tumors associated with MEN II include gliomas, glioblastomas, and meningiomas. Also called *Sipple's syndrome. See also medullary carcinoma of thyroid* and *pheochromocytoma.*

MEN III (or IIb), multiple endocrine neoplasia, type III or IIb, a dominantly inherited syndrome characterized by the presence of medullary thyroid carcinoma and pheochromocytoma, with multiple mucocutaneous neurofibromas. This variation of MEN II is associated with a higher frequency of malignant endocrine neoplasms. Also called *mucosal neuroma syndrome.*

mental (men'tal) 1. [L. *mens* mind] pertaining to the mind; psychic.
2. [L. *mentum* chin] pertaining to the chin.

mental point the most forward point of the chin in the midsagittal plane, the apex of the mental protuberance; used as an anatomic landmark. Also called *pogonion.*

mental region the region of the chin.

mental retardation disturbed intellectual functioning that relates to abnormal development from any of a number of causes. Although technically defined as an intelligence quotient (IQ) below 85 points, mental retardation is a vague term for an entity that usually is first noted in childhood or adolescence and that depends on social and cultural norms (which fluctuate with time). Formerly, systems of classification of the mentally retarded included such terms as moron, imbecile, and idiot, but these have now been abandoned. Newer systems avoid such labels and categorize individuals on a scale ranging from mild to profound retardation, depending on their IQ. Another classification scheme has a functional basis, and categorizes patients on a scale ranging from independent, educable, and trainable to those who require supervision all or most of the time.

The etiology of mental retardation is diverse. Approximately 3 percent of the United States population is mildly retarded on a constitutional basis, and approximately 15 percent is mentally retarded as a result of genetic conditions and hereditary metabolic disorders. Perinatal trauma or hypoxia/anoxia can produce mental retardation, often found with cerebral palsy. Certain prenatal maternal infections are also associated with mental retardation. Finally, encephalopathies arising from neonatal viral or bacterial meningitis, hyperbilirubinemia, or maternal toxin ingestion may lead to mental retardation.

Diagnosis usually rests on the outcome of various intelligence tests, including the Wechsler Intelligence Scale for Children (WISC) or the Wechsler Preschool and Primary Scale of Intelligence (WPPSI). Some authors have requested that assessments of social adaptability and emotional adjustment be linked to these early estimates of intelligence, as mental retardation may cause delays in emotional development and social adaptation.

Retarded children may benefit from special education, which can lead to greater independence. Severely affected individuals may never be able to care for themselves, however, and may then require institutionalized care. Certain types of mental retardation—particularly those due to metabolic disorders or maternal infection—can be prevented by appropriate prenatal care of pregnant females and by proper care of the newborn.

menthol (men'thol) [USP], 5-methyl-2-isopropylcyclohexanol, a crystalline solid with a peppermint taste and odor; used topically as an anesthetic and antipruritic and in nasal sprays and inhalers.

Menzies' method a staining technique for the striations in cardiac and skeletal muscle. Sections are stained in bromphenol blue and differentiated in dilute acetic acid. The sections are then briefly blued in Scott's tap water substitute and mounted. Cardiac and skeletal muscle stain deep blue, and when viewed with oil immersion the muscle striation can be clearly seen.

meparfynol (mĕ-par'fĭ-nōl) 3-methyl-1-pentyn-3-ol, an acrid-tasting liquid that has been used as a sedative, hypnotic, and anticonvulsant.

mepazine acetate (mep'ah-zēn) a phenothiazine derivative formerly used as a major tranquilizer and antiemetic.

meperidine hydrochloride (mĕ-per'ĭ-dēn) [USP], a synthetic analgesic with effects very similar to those of morphine except that the analgesic effect is only about one-tenth as strong. The potential for abuse and addiction and the withdrawal syndrome are also similar to those of morphine; its use is controlled by federal narcotics laws. Meperidine can be detected by screening assays for basic drugs. Tradename, *Demerol.*

mephenesin (mĕ-fen'ĕ-sin) a synthetic central nervous system depressant drug used as a skeletal muscle relaxant. It acts by depressing the basal ganglia, brain stem, and spinal synapses.

mephentermine sulfate (mĕ-fen'ter-mēn) a sympathomimetic amine used as a nasal decongestant and pressor.

mephenytoin (mĕ-fen'ĭ-to-in) an anticonvulsant drug similar to phenytoin, used for tonic-clonic attacks and psychomotor epilepsy. Because of side-effects such as skin eruptions and blood dyscrasias, other drug therapies are preferred.

mephobarbital (mef"o-bar'bĭ-tal) [NF], a long-acting barbiturate used for control of tonic-clonic attacks and focal and psychomotor epileptic seizures, and also as a sedative. See also *barbiturate.*

mepivicaine hydrochloride (mĕ-piv'ah-kān) [USP], an anesthetic agent similar to lidocaine, used for infiltration anesthesia and for nerve block.

meprobamate (mĕ-pro'bah-māt, mep"ro-bam'āt) [USP], a tranquilizer, muscle relaxant, and sedative; which acts as a spinal interneuron blocker and is used as a tranquilizer or sleeping aid. It is not related to the benzodiazepines.

Overuse causes loss of coordination and slurred speech. Overdoses may cause coma, low blood pressure, shock, respiratory failure, and death. Tolerance and physical dependence occur, and sudden withdrawal may cause vomiting, tremors, confusion, and, occasionally, convulsions. Therapeutic blood levels are 5–20 μg/ml; blood levels of 50–200 μg/ml can cause stupor, coma, and even fatalities.

Meprobamate is more dangerous when combined with other central nervous system depressants, and driving after mixing meprobamate and alcohol is especially discouraged. Trademarks include *Equanil* and *Miltown.*

meprobamate assays 1. thin-layer chromatography. Meprobamate, a neutral compound, is extracted into organic solvents. After separation, furfural is used as the spray reagent; a black spot may indicate meprobamate.

2. colorimetry. After extraction from basic solution, meprobamate is reacted with acetic acid–acetone reagent, *p*-dimethylaminobenzaldehyde reagent, and antimony trichloride acetic anhydride reagent. A red-violet compound is formed, the concentration of which is determined by the absorbance at 550 nm. Any other carbamate (e.g., carbromal or carisoprodol) will interfere.

3. gas chromatography. A methylated silicone column and flame ionization detector method is employed, with *p*-dimethylaminobenzaldehyde as the internal standard. Concentrations as low as 2 μg/ml can be detected, and the relative error is less than 2 percent.

mEq abbrev. See *milliequivalent.*

mer/o (mer′o) [Gr. *meros* part] a word element used in combining form to denote part or partial, e.g., merodiastolic.

M/E ratio see *myeloid/erythroid ratio.*

mercaptan (mer-kap′tan) [L. *mercurium captans* seizing or combining with mercury] the trivial name for a thiol, a compound containing the —SH functional group.

mercapto- (mer-kap′to) a prefix word element used to name the —SH group when it must be treated as a substituent in polyfunctional compounds, e.g., 2-mercaptoethanol ($HSCH_2CH_2OH$).

mercaptoacetic acid (mer-kap″to-ah-se′tik)) see *thioglycolic acid.*

2-mercaptoethanol (2 ME) (mer-kap″to-eth′ah-nol) a foul-smelling sulfhydryl chemical compound ($HSCH_2CH_2OH$) used to differentiate between IgM and IgG antibodies. Treatment of IgM antibodies results both in the breakage of their disulfide bonds and in the loss of agglutinating ability, thus permitting demonstration of remaining IgG antibodies in a mixture.

β-mercaptoethylamine (mer-kap″to-eth″il-am′ēn) a residue present in coenzyme A, which provides the sulfhydryl group for thioester linkage with acyl compounds. Also called *thioethanolamine.*

mercaptomerin sodium (mer-kap″to-mer′in) [USP], an organic, mercury-containing diuretic that must be injected; it is used when other diuretics are ineffective. Toxic effects are due to excessive diuresis or to mercury poisoning.

mercaptopurine (6-MP) (mer-kap″to-pu′rēn) [USP], 6-mercaptopurine, a structural analog of hypoxanthine. In the body it is converted to thioinosinic acid, which inhibits purine biosynthesis and the interconversion of purines. Its overall effect is the inhibition of DNA, RNA, and eventually protein synthesis. It is particularly effective against rapidly growing cells. Thus, it is primarily effective in the treatment of rapidly dividing cancer cells, namely, acute leukemias. Mercaptopurine and other purine analogs with antiproliferative action may also be used as immunosuppressive agents in the treatment of autoimmune diseases.

The drug is well absorbed from the gastrointestinal tract and is rapidly inactivated by xanthine oxidase to 6-thiouric acid. However, the inactivation may be inhibited by the concurrent administration of allopurinol, a xanthine oxidase inhibitor, achieving higher plasma concentrations of the cytotoxic agent.

Trademark, Purinethol. For more information, see *Appendix A.*

The toxicity of mercaptopurine is primarily of bone marrow depression. Other toxic factors include anorexia, nausea, vomiting, and jaundice.

mercurial (mer-ku′re-al) [L. *mercurialis*] 1. pertaining to mercury.

2. a drug containing mercury.

mercurialism (mer-ku′re-al-izm″) mercury poisoning; see under *mercury.*

mercuric (mer-ku′ric) pertaining to the mercury(II) ion, Hg^{2+}, as in mercuric chloride, $HgCl_2$.

mercuric fixative a histologic fixative that contains mercuric salts, usually mercuric chloride. See also under *fixatives.*

mercurous (mer′ku-rus) pertaining to the mercury(I) ion, Hg^{+}, as in mercurous chloride (calomel), Hg_2Cl_2.

mercury (Hg) (mer′ku-re) [L. *mercurius*] a silvery, very dense, liquid metallic element that is slightly volatile at room temperature; atomic number 80; atomic weight 200.59; a 5d transition element; oxidation states +1, +2. It can form Hg(I) and Hg(II) ions. It has no known metabolic function. Mercury, all its soluble inorganic compounds, and most of its organic compounds are highly toxic by skin absorption, ingestion, or inhalation of vapor. It acts by binding to the sulfhydryl groups of proteins, and thus denatures and inactivates enzymes; it is excreted through the kidney and colon.

Mercurials were formerly used medically for several conditions but now are used only as topical antiseptics and diuretics; because of their toxicity, however, they are not the first choice. Mercury amalgams are used in dentistry.

Mercury is widely used in industry. Acute poisoning (now rare) causes severe gastrointestinal irritation, kidney damage, and skin lesions. Chronic poisoning, called mercurialism, was once common among mercury miners, smelters, and hatters who used mercury nitrate to make felt. The symptoms are inflammation of the mouth, "hatters' shakes"—tremors due to brain damage, and erethism or irritability accompanied by anxiety and shyness. Workers exposed to organic mercurials may develop skin lesions.

The urinary excretion of mercury does not correlate well with toxic effects, yet is the best available measurement; individuals with no exposure to mercury excrete less than 5 μg/l; workers exposed to the recommended threshold of 50 $\mu g/m^3$ may excrete up to 150 μg/l.

See also *acrodynia* and *methyl mercury.*

mercury assays 1. Reinsch test. The sample is acidified with one-fifth of its volume of concentrated HCl; metallic copper is added as a coil or foil, and warmed. Heavy metals are reduced and deposited on the metallic copper strip. The mercury is distinguished by its silvery appearance and is confirmed by the salmon-pink color of mercury iodide when the deposit is reacted with cuprous iodide.

2. spectrophotometry. The sample is oxidized, the oxidizing agents removed, and a mercury-dithizone chelate formed. The concentration is proportional to the absorbance at 490 nm.

3. cold vapor atomic absorption spectrophotometry. The sample is digested in acid. The mercury is reduced to the free metal with stannous chloride; the Hg is then volatilized by bubbling air first through the sample, next through a dryer, and finally into the light path of the spectrophotometer. The peak reading is compared with a standard curve made by analyzing reference solutions. As little as 6 ng can be detected; there is 100 percent recovery from the sample.

mercury-197 (^{197}Hg, Hg 197) a cyclotron-produced radionuclide, with a half-life of 65 hr, that decays by electron capture to gold-197m, emitting 77-KeV gamma rays. See also *chlormerodrin mercury 197.*

mercury-203 (^{203}Hg, Hg 203) a reactor-produced radionuclide, with a half-life of 47 da, that undergoes beta decay to thallium-203 m, emitting 279-keV gamma rays. Because of the high radiation dose to the patient from ^{203}Hg, ^{197}Hg is now used instead.

merethoxylline (mer″ĕ-thok′sĭ-lēn) an organic, mercury-containing diuretic that must be injected and is used when other diuretics are ineffective. Toxic effects are due to excessive diuresis or to mercury poisoning.

m. procaine, the procaine sale of merethoxylline; when injected intramuscularly in combination with theophylline, it stabilizes and promotes absorption.

merge (merj) in automated data processing, the production of a single sorted sequence or file from two or more sorted sequences. For example, a computer program that reads *n* magnetic tapes and transfers all the data to one output tape in sorted order is called an *n*-way merge.

Merkel cell (mer′kel) [Friedrich Sigmund *Merkel,* German anatomist, 1845–1919] a dendritic cell found in the base of the epidermis and some squamous mucosal surfaces such as the oral cavity. The cytoplasm contains many small, dense-core granules concentrated within the dendritic processes. It is connected synaptically to a sensory axon (Merkel's corpuscle) and functions as a tactile receptor of low sensitivity. Merkel cells are believed to be the cell of origin of the cutaneous neuroendocrine carcinoma (Merkel cell tumor).

Merkel cell tumor [F. S. *Merkel*] a cutaneous neuroendocrine carcinoma believed to be derived from the Merkel cell of the epidermis. It forms a nodular lesion on the sun-exposed skin in older adults and initially tends to spread to regional lymph nodes. The ultrastructural features of the tumor cells are similar to those of neuroendocrine carcinomas in other locations, including dendritic cytoplasmic processes that contain accumulations of small (under 200 nm), dense-core granules.

Merkel's corpuscle [F. S. *Merkel*] a slow-adapting cutaneous mechanoreceptor, formed by a disk of nerve endings in the superficial dermis, that synapses with a specialized dendritic cell in the basal epidermis, the Merkel cell.

mermithid (mer′mĭ-thid) a member of the family Mermithidae.

Mermithidae (mer-mith′ĭ-de) a family of nematodes (including the cabbage snakes) of the superfamily Mermithoidea. These are long, opaque worms with a pointed anterior end. A few rare cases of human infection have been reported, believed to be caused by the accidental ingestion of food or water contaminated with larvae.

Mermithoidea (mer″mith-oi′de-ah) a superfamily of nematodes of the class Aphasmidia, including the family Mermithidae (cabbage snakes).

merocrine (mer′o-krin) [*mero-* + Gr. *krinein* to separate] partly secretory; denoting that type of exocrine glandular secretion in which the secretory granules leave by exocytosis, allowing the secretory cell to remain intact. Cf. *apocrine* and *holocrine.*

merogony (mĕ-rog′o-ne) [*mero-* + Gr. *gonos* procreation] 1. the incomplete development of a damaged ovum.

2. a type of cell division seen in sporozoan protozoa, in which the nucleus divides more than once before the cytoplasm separates.

meromelia (mer″o-me′le-ah) [*mero-* + Gr. *melos* limb + *-ia*] the congenital malformation that results in the attachment of the hands and feet to the trunk by only small, irregularly shaped bones.

meromyarial (mer″o-mi-a′re-al) [*mero-* + Gr. *mys* muscle] designating the type of muscle bands in nematodes that lack circular muscles. The muscle bands of these worms consist of a single layer of longitudinal, nonstriated muscle cells with MIC processes that extend into the body. In a cross section, the meromyarial type consists of only two cells in each quadrant, whereas the polymyarial type has numerous cells in each quadrant. Two genera of the meromyarial type are *Enterobius* and *Ancylostoma.*

merozoite (mer″o-zo′it) [*mero-* + Gr. *zōon* animal] a form liberated from the mature schizont in the exoerythrocytic and erythrocytic schizogony in the human cycle of the malarial plasmodium. Following the exoerythrocytic cycle in the parenchymal cells in the liver, merozoites penetrate the red blood cells, complete the erythrocytic cycle, and are liberated again to reinfect erythrocytes. After several generations, merozoites spontaneously develop into male and female sex cells. Further development of these gametocytes is dependent on their ingestion by a mosquito.

merozoite antigens species-specific antigens on the exerythrocytic form of the malarial parasite, which induce the formation of protective antibodies, primarily IgG and IgM, in the host. The immune response is not complement-dependent.

merozygote (mer″o-zi′gōt) [*mero-* + Gr. *zygōtos* yoked together] the partially diploid bacterial cell that results from the transfer of part of the genome from one bacterium to another by the process of transduction or by conjugation. The transferred fragment (the exogenote) coexists with the genome (the endogenote) of the recipient to form a transient merozygote. The process of genetic transformation by naked DNA also results in formation of a merozygote.

Merthiolate (mer-thi′o-lāt) trademark. See *thimerosal.*

mes- (mes) [Gr. *mesos* middle] a prefix word element to denote middle.

mesangial (mes-an′je-al) of or pertaining to the mesangium.

mesangial proliferative glomerulopathy see under *glomerulopathy.*

mesangiocapillary glomerulopathy (mes-an″je-o-kap′ĭ-lar″e) see under *glomerulopathy.*

mesangium (mes-an′je-um) [*mes-* + Gr. *angeion* vessel] the intercapillary supporting structure of the renal glomerulus. It consists of specialized mesangial cells embedded within a mesangial matrix, and lies in intimate contact with the foot processes of the podocytes and the fenestrated epithelium of the glomerular capillaries. The cells have the ability to contract and are actively phagocytic. Inflammatory cells and macromolecules can traverse or temporarily reside within the mesangium, and their presence may elicit hypertrophy or proliferation of the mesangial cells. Immune complexes can be deposited within the mesangium, and their recognition with immunocytochemical procedures or electron microscopy can be of diagnostic value.

extraglomerular m., a cushion of granule-containing cells, continuous with the intraglomerular mesangium, which surrounds the afferent and efferent arterioles of a glomerulus; it forms part of the juxtaglomerular apparatus. Also called *Lacis.*

mesaxon (mes-ak′son) [*mes-* + Gr. *axōn* axis] the line of invagination of the plasma membrane of a Schwann cell encircling an axon in an unmyelinated nerve.

mescal (mes-kahl′) [Mex.] see *peyote.*

mescaline (mes′kah-lēn, mes′kah-lin) a hallucinogenic drug, 3,4,5-trimethoxyphenylethylamine, isolated from the flowering heads of the peyote cactus (mescal buttons); M.W. 211.25. It produces vivid visual hallucinations and sensory distortions, but can also cause anxiety, hyperreflexia, and tremor. See also *peyote.*

mesencephalitis (mes″en-sef″ah-li′tis) [*mes-* + Gr. *enkephalos* brain + *-itis*] inflammation of the mesencephalon or midbrain.

mesencephalon (mes″en-sef′ah-lon) [*mes-* + Gr. *enkephalos* brain] 1. [NA], the part of the brain developed from the intermediate of the three primary vesicles of the embryonic neural tube. It includes the tectum and cerebral peduncles, possesses varied reflex activities, and contributes significantly to the reticular system. Also called *midbrain.*

2. in the developing embryo, the middle of the three primary brain vesicles situated between the prosencephalon and the rhombencephalon.

mesenchymal (mĕ-seng′kĭ-mal) pertaining to the mesenchyme.

mesenchyme (mes′eng-kīm) [*mes-* + Gr. *enchyma* infusion] the embryonic connective tissue derived from the mesoderm that later becomes the connective tissue and vessels of the body.

mesenchymoma (mes″en-ki-mo′mah) [*mesenchyma* + *-oma* tumor] a term applied to a soft tissue neoplasm that contains primitive mesenchymal cells differentiating into more than one type of soft tissue. The tumor may be benign or malignant. True mesenchymomas are uncommon neoplasms, and most of the recorded cases have involved the lower extremities.

mesenteric (mes″en-ter′ik) [Gr. *mesenterikos*] pertaining to the mesentery.

mesenteric artery an artery conveying blood from the abdominal aorta to the intestines.

inferior m. a., the artery of the hindgut. It arises from the front of the abdominal aorta about 3 cm above the bifurcation, runs downward into the left sigmoid mesocolon, and continues into the pelvis as the superior rectal artery. It supplies the distal transverse colon, descending colon, sigmoid colon, and rectum.

superior m. a., the artery of the midgut. It arises from the front of the abdominal aorta about 1 cm below the celiac artery, descends in front of the uncinate process of the pancreas, and runs in the root of the mesentery to the terminal ileum. Its branches supply the distal duodenum, jejunum, ileum, cecum, ascending colon, and proximal transverse colon.

mesenteric vascular occlusion a condition characterized by severe, diffuse abdominal pain, occasional associated nausea, vomiting, and diarrhea, and a lack of findings on physical examination early in the course of the disease. As the disorder progresses, abdominal distention, shock, and generalized peritonitis result and can lead to death if untreated. It most often occurs in older individuals; an increased incidence has also been noted with the use of oral contraceptives. The occlusion may be arterial when due to a generalized atherosclerotic disease usually associated with preexisting abdominal angina, or it may be venous when due to thrombosis, occurring frequently in association with portal hypertension, trauma, and abdominal sepsis.

Laboratory studies show leukocytosis, slightly elevated serum amylase, and elevated inorganic phosphate. Diagnosis is aided by abdominal x-rays, barium x-rays, and mesenteric arteriography. The present mortality rate is 45 percent.

mesenteric vein a vein carrying blood from the intestines to the portal vein.

inferior m. v., the vein that drains blood from the distal colon. It runs up the left posterior abdominal wall to end in the splenic vein.

superior m. v., the vein that drains blood from the small intestine and proximal colon. It ascends in the root of the mesentery on the right of the superior mesenteric artery and joins the splenic vein behind the neck of the pancreas to form the portal vein.

mesentery (mes′en-ter″e) [Gr. *mesenterion,* from *meson* between, among + *enteron* intestine] that portion of the peritoneum that encloses and suspends the small intestine, its blood vessels, nerves, and lymphatics, on the dorsal body wall.

mesiodistal plane (me″ze-o-dis′tal) a plane passing through the mesial and distal surfaces of a tooth that is tangential to the dental arch.

mesion (me′se-on) the plane that divides the body into right and left symmetric halves. Also called medial plane, median plane, *meson,* and *midsagittal plane.*

meso- (mes′o) [Gr. *mesos* middle] 1. a prefix word element to denote "middle," either situated in the middle or intermediate.

2. a prefix word element used in organic chemistry to denote an isomer (in a set of configurational isomers that include some chiral compounds) that is not chiral and is therefore optically inactive (i.e., has no effect on polarized light) because it is identical with its mirror image, as in *meso*-2,3-dibromobutane. An optically inactive compound like 1,2-dibromoethane, which has no optically active isomers, is not considered a *meso* form (or compound).

mesoappendix (mes″o-ah-pen′diks) [*meso* + *appendix*] [NA], the peritoneal fold that attaches the appendix to the mesentery of the ileum.

mesoblast (mes′o-blast) [*meso-* + *blastos* germ] see mesoderm.

mesoblastic nephroma (mes″o-blas′tik nĕ-fro′mah) a stromal renal neoplasm, almost invariably congenital and unilateral, that is composed of fibroblasts and smooth muscle cells of various degrees of differentiation. In the well-differentiated form it is benign; in less differentiated forms it may rarely recur. Poorly differentiated forms merge histologically with the sarcomatous form of nephroblastoma. Some authorities view this tumor as a stromal hamartoma; others regard it as a variably differentiated form of nephroblastoma. See also *renal tumors.*

Mesocestoides (mes″o-ses-toi′dēz) a genus of tapeworms of the family Mesocestoididae. The larvae have been found in dogs, cats, mice, and other vertebrates. A few cases have been reported of the adult form, which parasitizes human intestines. Infection is believed to be acquired from eating improperly cooked meat from animals infected with larvae (plerocercoid type).

Mesocestoididae (mes″o-ses-toi′di-de) a family of tapeworms of the order Cyclophyllidea, including the genus *Mesocestoides.*

mesocolon (mes″o-ko′lon) [*meso-* + Gr. *kolon* colon] [NA], the process of the peritoneum by which the transverse or sigmoid colon is attached to the posterior abdominal wall.

sigmoid m., the peritoneal fold that attaches the sigmoid colon to the pelvic wall.

transverse m., the broad peritoneal fold that connects the transverse colon to the posterior abdominal wall.

meso compound a chemical compound, such as *meso*-tartaric acid, that contains asymmetric carbon atoms but is nonetheless superimposable on its mirror image and is consequently achiral and optically inactive. The term also refers to any optically inactive isomer in a set of stereoisomers that contains some optically active isomers.

mesoderm (mes′o-derm) [*meso-* + Gr. *derma* skin] in the developing embryo, the middle of the three primary germ layers. From it are differentiated the skeletal muscles, kidneys, serous membranes, heart and vessels, spleen, suprarenal cortex, connective tissue, cartilage, bone, and blood. Also called *mesoblast.* See also the accompanying illustration and *embryo.*

mesodermal (mes″o-der′mal) pertaining to or derived from the mesoderm.

mesogastric region (mes″o-gas′trik) [*meso-* + Gr.

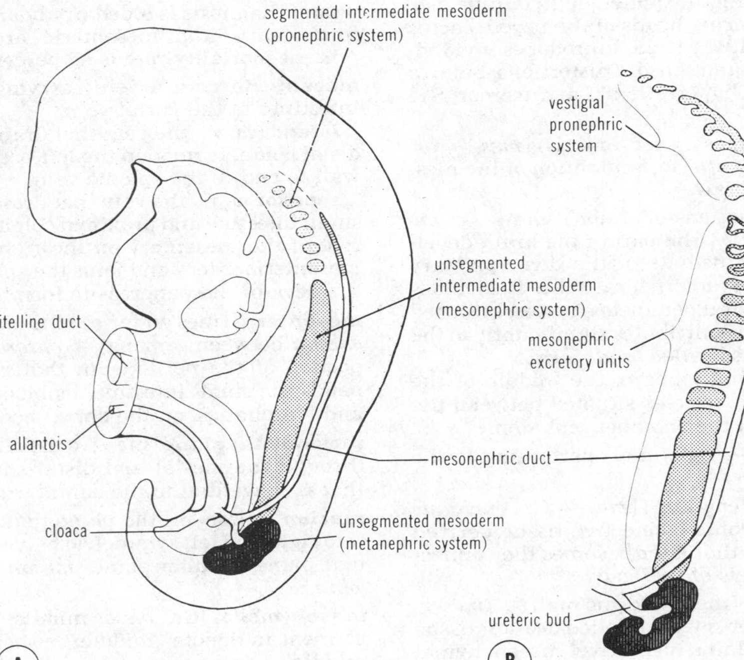

Mesoderm. A, Schematic diagram showing the relation of the intermediate mesoderm of the pronephric, mesonephric, and metanephric systems. In the cervical and upper thoracic regions, the intermediate mesoderm is segmented; in the lower thoracic, lumbar, and sacral regions, it forms a solid, unsegmented mass of tissue, the nephrogenic cord. Note the longitudinal collecting duct, initially formed by the pronephros but later taken over by the mesonephros. *B,* Schematic representation of the excretory tubules of the pronephric and mesonephric systems in a 5-week old embryo. The ureteric bud penetrates the metanephric tissue. Note the remnant of the pronephric excretory tubules and longitudinal collecting duct. (From Langman, J.: Medical Embryology. 4th ed. Baltimore, Williams & Wilkins Co., 1981.)

gastēr belly] the central region of the abdomen below the epigastric region and above the hypogastric region. See illustration under *abdominal regions.* Cf. *umbilical region.*

mesogastric zone see *umbilical zone.*

Mesogastropoda (mes″o-gas-trop′ŏ-dah) [*meso-* + Gr. *gastēr* stomach + *pous* foot] an order of snails of the class Gastropoda, including the subfamily Hydrobiinae, which contains the species *Oncomelania hupensis,* one of the principal hosts of *Schistosoma japonicum* in China.

mesometrium (mes″o-me′tre-um) [*meso-* + Gr. *mētra* uterus] [NA], the portion of the broad ligament below the mesovarium composed of layers of peritoneum that separate to enclose the uterus.

meson (mes′on, me′zon) 1. see *mesion.*
2. an elementary particle composed of a quark and an antiquark, e.g., the pion.

mesonephric (mes″o-nef′rik) pertaining to the mesonephros.

mesonephric duct (mes″o-nef′rik) see *mesonephric d.* under *duct.*

mesonephric remnant a small, cystic structure, frequently multiple, formed from persisting nests of mesonephric duct cells; it is found particularly in the stroma of the uterine cervix.

mesonephroma (mes″o-ne-fro′mah) [*mesonephros* + *-oma* tumor] an outmoded term originally used to describe two different tumors, the endodermal sinus tumor and clear cell adenocarcinoma of mesothelial origin. It is now recognized that neither is derived from a mesonephros and that the two terms are clinically and biologically distinct.

mesonephros (mes″o-nef′ros), pl. *mesonephroi* [*meso-* + Gr. *nephros* kidney] [NA], the second of the three kidney systems that develop in the embryo, preceded by the pronephros and followed by the metanephros, the permanent kidney. It is an ovoid mass formed of tubules that connect with a longitudinal collecting duct, the mesonephric or wolffian duct. Some of the lowest (caudal) tubules may persist as vestigial remnants attached to the testis or ovary, which is developing alongside the mesonephros. In the female, the mesonephric duct may disappear completely or persist as small remnants. In the male, the duct forms the vas deferens. Also called *wolffian body.* See also the accompanying illustration.

mesophile (mes′o-fil) [*meso-* + Gr. *philein* to love] an organism that grows best at temperatures between 30° and 45°C. Mammal-loving mesophiles have a temperature optimum of 39°–44°C. Cf. *psychrophile* and *thermophile.*

mesoridazine besylate (mes″o-rid′ah-zēn) a piperidine-type phenothiazine major tranquilizer used in the management of psychotic disorders and other psychiatric conditions. See also *phenothiazine tranquilizers.* Trademark, *Serentil.*

mesosalpinx (mes″o-sal′pinks) [*meso-* + Gr. *salpinx* tube] [NA], the portion of the broad ligament between the uterine tube and the mesovarium; the uterine tube is enclosed in its free border.

mesosome (mes′o-sōm) [*meso-* + Gr. *sōma* body] an irregular, convoluted invagination of the cytoplasmic membrane of certain gram-positive and gram-negative bacteria. Various mesosomes have functions in cell division, in secretion, and in electron transport of the organism. Also called plasmalemmosome.

mesothelioma (mes″o-the″le-o′mah) [*mesothelium* + *-oma* tumor] a neoplasm that originates from the serosal tissues lining the pleural, pericardial, and peritoneal cavities and covering the tunica vagina-

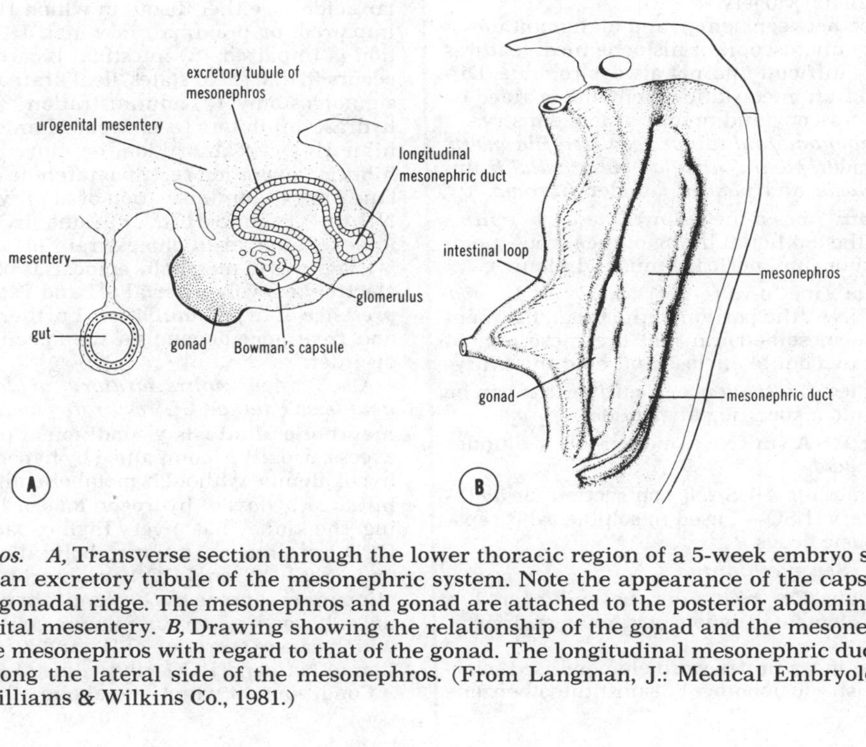

Mesonephros. *A,* Transverse section through the lower thoracic region of a 5-week embryo showing the formation of an excretory tubule of the mesonephric system. Note the appearance of the capsule of Bowman and the gonadal ridge. The mesonephros and gonad are attached to the posterior abdominal wall by a broad urogenital mesentery. *B,* Drawing showing the relationship of the gonad and the mesonephros. Note the size of the mesonephros with regard to that of the gonad. The longitudinal mesonephric duct (Wolffian duct) runs along the lateral side of the mesonephros. (From Langman, J.: Medical Embryology. 4th ed. Baltimore, Williams & Wilkins Co., 1981.)

lis. Both benign and malignant mesotheliomas are recognized.

Benign mesotheliomas are rare, noninvasive, and localized neoplastic lesions of the serosa. They are predominantly epithelial, although they often show transitions to fibrous components. Pure fibrous localized nodules of the pleura or peritoneum without epithelial differentiation are regarded as fibrous mesotheliomas by some authorities, and noncommittally as localized fibrous tumors by others.

Malignant mesotheliomas are also rare in the general population but have been reported as occurring in 5–10 percent of asbestos workers, with an average latent period of 20–40 yr after initial exposure. More than 80 percent of those with malignant mesothelioma have a history of exposure to asbestos, and are found to have asbestos bodies in their lungs and other body tissues with a frequency statistically greater than in nonexposed individuals.

Grossly, malignant mesotheliomas are typically diffuse, producing extensive involvement of serosal surfaces at the site of origin. They frequently invade and seed adjacent organs and structures, but metastasize infrequently. The usual cause of death is related to complications from the presence of the primary tumor. In most reported series, the median survival time for patients with malignant mesothelioma is 4–12 mo following the diagnosis. Prognosis for the most part is influenced by the tumor stage at the time of treatment.

The histologic pattern seen in malignant mesothelioma may resemble that of the surface epithelium of the normal serosa (epithelial mesothelioma, 50 percent of cases), the mesenchymal cells of the subsurface of the serosa (fibrous or sarcomatoid mesothelioma, 20 percent of cases), or a mixture of these two types (30 percent of cases). Those arising in the peritoneum are predominantly epithelial, whereas those arising in the pleura are predominantly fibrous. The prognosis is thought to be best for the epithelial variety.

Distinction between benign and malignant mesotheliomas by microscopic or histochemical features is extremely difficult and not always reliable. Differentiation from metastatic carcinoma is aided by electron microscopy and mucin histochemistry.

See also *adenomatoid tumor, localized fibrous tumor of p.* under *pleura, nodular mesothelial h.* under *hyperplasia,* and *pleural f.* under *fibroma.*

mesothelium (mes″o-the′le-um) [*meso-* + *epithelium*] [NA], the epithelial lining of the serous membranes (peritoneum, pericardium, and pleura).

mesovarium (mes″o-va′re-um) [*meso-* + L. *ovarium* ovary] [NA], the portion of the broad ligament between the mesometrium and the mesosalpinx, which is drawn out to enclose and hold the ovary.

message (mes′ĭj) a sequence of mRNA that can be translated into a specific polypeptide.

messenger RNA (mRNA) (mes′en-jer) see under *ribonucleic acid.*

mesylate (mes′ĭ-lāt) [USAN], contraction for methanesulfonate, CH_3SO_3—, used in soluble salt preparations of basic drugs.

Met abbrev. See *methionine.*

meta- (met′ah) [Gr. *meta* after, beyond, over] 1. a prefix word element to denote next, change, or near, e.g., metastasis.

2. (abbrev. *m-*), a prefix word element used in organic chemistry to denote a 1,3-substituted benzene (e.g., *meta*-xylene, 1,3-dimethylbenzene). See also the illustration accompanying *ortho-*.

3. a prefix word element used in inorganic chemistry to denote the less hydrated acid or its salt. Cf. *ortho-* and *para-*.

metabiosis (met″ah-bi-o′sis) [*meta-* + Gr. *biosis* way of life] the dependence of one organism on another for its physical protection and nourishment, without injury to its host. Also called *commensalism.*

metabolic (met″ah-bol′ik) [Gr. *metabolikos* changeable] pertaining to or of the nature of metabolism.

metabolic acidosis a condition in which an individual is acidotic due to a primary HCO_3^- deficit caused either by increased production or decreased excretion of acids or by loss of base. A compensating respiratory response of hyperventilation lowers the Pa_{CO_2} and thus tends to raise the blood pH. In severe metabolic acidosis, the Pa_{CO_2} can drop as much as 12–15 mmHg but the associated loss in carbonic acid cannot raise the pH to normal (7.4).

There are many causes of metabolic acidosis, which can be grouped on the basis of whether the anion gap is increased or normal. The anion gap, $[Na^+] - ([Cl^-] + [HCO_3^-])$, is equal to the concentration in milliequivalents per liter of the unmeasured anions minus the concentration of the unmeasured cations.

An increased anion gap is usually associated with metabolic acidosis and can occur in three types of conditions: (1) reduced excretion of acids in renal failure; (2) increased production of acidic metabolites in diabetic ketoacidosis or lactic acidosis; and (3) ingestion of poisons having acidic metabolites, e.g., salicylates, methanol, ethylene glycol, or paraldehyde.

Metabolic acidosis with a normal anion gap if $[Cl^-]$ increases to offset the decline in $[HCO_3^-]$; this type is called hyperchloremic metabolic acidosis and can occur in several different conditions: (1) renal tubular acidosis, either distal, in which H^+ excretion is impaired, or proximal, in which HCO_3^- reabsorption is impaired; (2) intestinal bicarbonate loss, as occurs in diarrheal states, ileal drainage, and ureterosigmoidostomy; (3) administration of carbonic anhydrase inhibitors (e.g., acetazolamide), which inhibit HCO_3^- reabsorption, or diuretics, which inhibit H^+ excretion (e.g., triamterene or spironolactone); or (4) administration of acidifying salts (e.g., NH_4Cl, arginine HCl, or lysine HCl) or the anion-exchange resin cholestyramine.

Diagnosis of metabolic acidosis is based on serum electrolyte levels, arterial pH and Pa_{CO_2}, and on the presence of hyperventilation. Further classification and treatment depend on the specific underlying disorder.

Also called *nonrespiratory acidosis.* See also *acid-base balance.* Cf. *respiratory acidosis.*

metabolic alkalosis a condition of primary HCO_3^- excess, usually accompanied by hypochloremia and hypokalemia. Although metabolic alkalosis can be initiated by loss of hydrogen ions or by alkali loading, the kidney has a very high capacity to excrete HCO_3^-; maintenance of metabolic alkalosis requires an increase in renal HCO_3^- reabsorption or regeneration in response to hypovolemia, hyperkalemia, renal salt wasting, or mineralocorticoid excess, any of which causes secretion of H^+ and K^+ and reabsorption of Na^+ and HCO_3^- in the distal tubules.

Conditions in which metabolic alkalosis can occur include (1) loss of gastric acid due to prolonged vomiting or nasogastric suction; (2) potassium depletion as seen in Cushing's syndrome, administration of ACTH or adrenocortical hormones, and aldosteronism; (3) Bartler's syndrome; (4) Liddle's syndrome; (5) excessive natriuresis caused by high-ceiling diuretics (e.g., furosemide or ethacrynic acid); and (6) posthypercapnic metabolic alkalosis during recovery from respiratory acidosis and hypercapnia.

Respiratory compensation for metabolic alkalosis is necessarily incomplete because excessive hypoventilation would cause hypoxia; the Pa_{CO_2} therefore rarely exceeds 55 mmHg.

Also called *nonrespiratory alkalosis.* See also *acid-base balance.* Cf. *respiratory alkalosis.*

metabolic bone disease a general term that covers a diverse group of disorders in which there are either focal or general abnormalities in the resorption and deposition of bony tissue; it includes osteoporosis, rickets and osteomalacia, osteitis deformans, and related conditions. All forms may be associated with an increased tendency to fracture and/or to bony deformities. Bone consists of cells (osteocytes, osteoblasts, and osteoclasts); an organic matrix consisting of a dense mat of collagen fibers embedded in a ground substance of proteoglycans; and minerals deposited in the organic matrix, the principal mineral being hydroxyapatite, a salt of calcium and phosphate. This combination of collagen and minerals results in great tensile and compressional strength.

Bone is in a constant stage of change. While parts of bone are being resorbed by the osteoclasts, new bone is being laid down by the osteoblasts in concert with osteocytes. Many details of the physiology of bone formation and repair are unknown, but calcium and phosphorus metabolism and their hormonal control mechanisms are important factors. Calcium is moved from or to the bones in order to maintain normal plasma calcium levels. Decreased plasma calcium causes the release of parathyroid hormone (PTH), which has three effects: increased bone resorption due to osteoclast activation, increased renal tubular calcium resorption, and conversion of vitamin D_3 to its active form (1,25-OH-D_3), which increases intestinal absorption of calcium. Elevated serum calcium causes the release of calcitonin, which decreases bone resorption by inhibiting osteoclasts and preventing their formation from progenitor cells.

Osteoporosis, a reduction in bone density below the level required for mechanical support, is the most common form of metabolic bone disease. On microscopic examination, the bone appears normal except that there is not enough of it; that is, there is less volume of bony tissue per unit volume of a specific bone. Osteoporosis is a diverse group of disorders. The etiology of the most common form, primary (postmenopausal, senile) osteoporosis, is unknown. Because it eventually develops in a large percentage of postmenopausal females, one theory holds that it is related to a lack of estrogens. This relationship is not clearly established, however, and estrogen therapy does not reverse the osteopenia. Another theory holds that the condition is due to a deficient calcium intake, yet many patients have a higher than normal calcium intake. Serum levels of calcium, phosphorus, and PTH are usually normal. Osteoporosis can also occur secondary to endocrine abnormalities including hyperthyroidism, Cushing's syndrome, chronic administration of corticosteroids, acromegaly, hyperparathyroidism, and hypogonadism. It is a feature of several genetic disorders including homocystinuria, osteogenesis imperfecta, Marfan's syndrome, and Ehlers-Danlos syndrome. In addition, it commonly occurs with immobilization, malabsorption syndrome, chronic administration of heparin, adult hypophosphatasia, and neoplasms involving bone cancer.

Osteomalacia is a condition in which bone is inadequately mineralized; the collagen matrix may be present but is not adequately calcified. This condition can result from disorders of phosphate or vitamin D metabolism. The pediatric counterpart of osteomalacia, rickets, results in deformities in the bones of growing children. In osteomalacia or rickets, serum levels of calcium or phosphorus may be low.

Osteitis deformans (Paget's disease of bone) is a common form of metabolic bone abnormality in older individuals. It is characterized by rapid and abnormal bone turnover, generally resulting in overproduction of bone with diminished structural integrity. The etiology is unknown but viral factors have been implicated.

Metabolic bone diseases generally can be differentiated with the aid of relevant laboratory tests and radiologic studies of bone. When an abnormality of bone metabolism cannot be defined by laboratory and radiologic studies, a bone biopsy can provide a definitive diagnosis based on quantitative determinations, including static measurements, i.e., the proportions of trabecular bone (resting), forming bone (covered by osteoid), or resorbing (showing Howship's lacunae), and dynamic measurements such as the distance between tetracycline-labeled mineralization fronts after timed double tetracycline labeling (mean mineralization rate).

For more information, see specific types of metabolic bone disease.

NANETTE SMITH, M.D.
ALLAN PONT, M.D.

metabolic pathway a chain of enzymatic reactions, each link producing a product that is a substrate in the next link. A pathway may produce energy (e.g., the citric acid cycle) or some structural product (e.g., fatty acid or glycogen).

metabolic pool the amount of a particular compound present in an organism and available to participate in metabolic processes, there being a dynamic equilibrium between the quantity leaving the pool and that entering the pool. The pool may be only a part of the total amount of substance in the body—that portion entering/leaving at reasonably rapid rates; other portions may not be involved, or only at very slow rates, as is true for much of the calcium pool. The term also refers to a group of compounds available to participate in some process, e.g., extracellular pool.

metabolism (mĕ-tab′o-lizm) [Gr. *metaballein* to turn about, change, alter] the sum of all the physical and chemical processes by which living organisms grow and maintain themselves, which can be divided into anabolism (the synthesis of complex materials) and catabolism (the breakdown of complex materials producing energy).

aerobic m., the process of cellular respiration by which food molecules are broken down and oxidized to intermediates, and ultimately to carbon dioxide and water, with the production of energy for the maintenance of life processes.

anaerobic m., the process by which food molecules are broken down in cells without using oxygen; carbon dioxide may or may not be produced. The energy produced is under 8 percent of that produced aerobically. In humans, this process is called glycolysis, and produces lactate. In microorganisms, it is called fermentation; an example is the production of ethanol and CO_2 by yeast.

basal m., the energy consumed by the body at complete rest. See also *basal metabolic rate assays.*

inborn errors of m., see *inborn errors of metabolism.*

intermediary m., See *intermediary metabolism.*

metabolite (me-tab′o-lit) a chemical compound that is formed by, or participates in, a metabolic process.

metabolizable (mĕ-tab′o-liz″ah-b′l) able to be used in the body's metabolism, as in food; able to be broken down or altered by metabolism into physiologically inert materials, as in detoxification.

metacarp/o (met-ah-kar′po) [*meta-* + Gr. *karpos* wrist] a word element used in combining form to denote metacarpals (the hand bones), e.g., metacarpectomy.

metacarpus (met″ah-kar′pus), pl. *metacarpi* [N.L., from Gr. *metakarpion*] [NA], the five metacarpal bones. They are numbered from lateral to medial as one through five. Each is a miniature long bone, articulating proximally with carpal bones and distally with the bases of the proximal phalanges.

metacentric (met″ah-sen′trik) [*meta-* + Gr. *kentrikos* of the center] pertaining to a mitotic chromosome having the centromere in the middle so that the arms are approximately equal in length. Cf. *submetacentric, subtelocentric,* and *telocentric.*

metacercaria (met″ah-ser-ka′re-ah), pl. *metacercariae* [*meta-* + Gr. *kerkos* tail] the encysted resting or maturing stage in the life cycle of a trematode. The free-living aquatic form, or cercaria (which cannot feed), liberates its tail and becomes a metacercaria when an appropriate host (either mollusks, fish, or vegetation) is found. Infection in humans is caused by the ingestion of contaminated vegetation or improperly cooked mollusks or fish.

metachromasia (met″ah-kro-ma′ze-ah) [*meta-* + Gr. *chrōma* color] the exhibition of metachromatic staining by a tissue component.

alpha m., the staining of tissue components in the orthochromatic (usual) color of the dye, e.g., blue for toluidine blue staining.

beta m., the staining of tissue a color that is intermediate between orthochromatic and metachromatic colors, e.g., violet for toluidine blue staining.

gamma m., the staining of tissue components in the metachromatic color of the dye, e.g., red for toluidine blue staining.

metachromatic (met″ah-kro-mat′ik) in histochemistry, pertaining to the staining of a tissue component with a dyestuff, resulting in a dye-tissue complex with an absorption spectrum sufficiently different from that of the dye itself and from most of its dye-tissue complexes to give a marked contrast in color. Cf. *orthochromatic.*

metachromatic dye a basic aniline dye that stains various tissue and cell components in colors different from those of the staining solution. The mechanism of the metachromasia exhibited by acid mucopolysaccharides is that the acid dye–binding sites are close enough together along the mucopolysaccharide molecule for the bound dye molecules to polymerize and change color.

Commonly used dyes of this type are toluidine blue, the azures, methylene blue, thionin, Bismarck brown, and the safranins. The red color exhibited by amyloid when stained by methyl violet, crystal violet, or ethyl green is due to a different mechanism.

metachromatic granule in bacteriology, a granular inclusion in bacterial cytoplasm that stains differently from the surrounding material, appearing bluish-purple when stained with methylene blue dye. It is a morphologic feature of *Corynebacterium diphtheriae.* Also called *Babès-Ernst granules.* See also *metachromasia* and *volutin.*

metachromatic leukodystrophy see *metachromatic l.* under *leukodystrophy.*

metachronal rhythm (mĕ-tak′ro-nal) a type of motion exhibited by the cilia of some epithelial tissues in which the beating of the cilia is coordinated as a wave traveling along the surface. This motion propels mucus or fluid along the free surface of the organ. Cf. *isochronal rhythm.*

metachronous (mĕ-tak′ro-nus) [*meta-* + Gr. *chronos* time] occurring at different times.

metagenesis (met″ah-jen′ĕ-sis) [*meta-* + Gr. *genesis* production] see *alternation of generations.*

metagonimiasis (met″ah-go″nĭ-mi′ah-sis) the condition caused by the presence of *Metagonimus yokogawai,* a small trematode found in the intestines of humans. *M. yokogawai* is considered the most common heterophyid fluke in humans in the Far East.

Metagonimus (met″ah-gon′ĭ-mus) [*meta-* + Gr. *gonimos* productive] a genus of digenetic trematodes or flukes, of which the species *M. yokogawai* is parasitic in humans.

M. yokogawai, a species of small trematodes (flukes), distributed throughout China, Japan, Russia, Spain, and the Balkan states, that is parasitic in human intestines. *M. yokogawai* is less than 3 mm in length; its embryonated eggs measure 26–28 μm long by 15–17 μm wide and are indistinguishable from those of *Heterophyes heterophyes.* The eggs are ingested by snails (intermediate hosts) in which the parasite develops and produces free-living cercariae that encyst (metacercariae) on aquatic plants. Infection is acquired from ingestion of contaminated fish that have been improperly cooked.

Diagnosis is difficult, as it requires identification from the feces of eggs that are identical to *H. heterophyes* and are similar to *Clonorchis sinensis* in shape. Specific diagnosis can be made from the examination of evacuated flukes.

metal (met″l) [L. *metallum;* Gr. *metallon*] 1. a crystalline solid that has high thermal and electrical conductivity, malleability, ductility, and luster. These characteristics are due to the metallic bonding of the valence electrons, which are not localized near individual atoms but instead move freely throughout the crystal lattice.

2. Any one of the group of chemical elements that form metallic crystals near room temperature, e.g., calcium, silver, and mercury. Cf. *nonmetal* and *semiconductor.*

alkali m., a common name for any of the chemical

elements (except hydrogen, a nonmetal) in group I of the periodic table, i.e., lithium, sodium, potassium, rubidium, cesium, and francium.

alkaline earth m., a common name for any of the chemical elements in group II of the periodic table, i.e., beryllium, magnesium, calcium, strontium, barium, and radium.

metaldehyde (met-al′de-hīd) a polymer of acetaldehyde, $(CH_3CHO)_n$, where *n* is four to six. A white crystalline solid that decomposes on heating to form acetaldehyde, metaldehyde is highly flammable. It is used as a fuel and as a slug and snail poison. This substance is a strong skin and respiratory tract irritant that, when ingested, can produce vomiting, diarrhea, fever, convulsions, and coma.

metallic (mĕ-tal′ik) pertaining to or composed of metals.

metalloenzyme (mĕ-tal″o-en′zīm) an enzyme containing tightly bound metal atoms as an integral part of its structure, e.g., carboxypeptidase and the cytochromes. Their presence is essential for enzymatic activity.

metalloflavoprotein (mĕ-tal″o-fla″vo-pro′te-in) any metalloprotein that functions as a dehydrogenase, catalyzing the oxidation of a substrate by a mechanism that involves the reduction of a prosthetic group; a derivative of riboflavin. An example is xanthine oxidase.

metalloprotein (mĕ-tal″o-pro′te-in) a protein that has one or more metal atoms or ions as prosthetic groups. The metal may be held by the functional groups of the amino acids that are part of the protein chain, or by special prosthetic groups such as the porphyrin ring of hemoglobin.

metamyelocyte (met″ah-mi′ĕ-lo-sīt″) [*meta-* + Gr. *myelos* marrow + *kytos* hollow vessel] the stage of granulocytic maturation that follows the myelocyte and precedes the polymorphonuclear neutrophil; it is designated as M_5. It is normally found only in the bone marrow.

On smears, the nucleus is kidney shaped and has a clumped, dense, coarse chromatin pattern. The cytoplasm is slightly acidophilic and contains both primary and secondary (eosinophilic, basophilic, or neutrophilic) granules. It is at this stage of cell development that locomotion begins.

See also *granulocytic series.*

metanephrine (met″ah-nef′rin) α-(methylaminomethyl) vanillyl alcohol (3-*O*-methylepinephrine), a metabolite of epinephrine that is excreted in the urine and formed in some tissues, e.g., the liver. Also called 3-methoxyepinephrine.

metanephrine assays methods for the determination of total metanephrines in urine. The colorimetric method is widely used. After acid hydrolysis, metanephrines are adsorbed on a weakly acidic, cation-exchange resin, eluted with dilute ammonium hydroxide solution, oxidized to vanillin by reaction with periodate, and quantitated by spectrophotometry at 360 nm. Fluorometric, gas chromatographic, and high-pressure liquid chromatographic methods have also been described.

metanephros (met″ah-nef′ros), pl. *metanephroi* [*meta-* + Gr. *nephros* kidney] the embryonic precursor of the permanent kidney; it develops from the mesonephric duct and the nephrogenic cords. Phylogenetically, it occurs later and develops more caudally than the mesonephros or the pronephros. Cf. *mesonephros.*

metanil yellow (met′ah-nil) a yellow monoazo dye; C.I. 13065. It is frequently used as a counterstain in periodic acid–Schiff (PAS) techniques or other acid-Schiff procedures such as in Gridley's stain for fungi.

metaphase (met′ah-fāz) the second phase of cell division, during which the chromosomes are arranged on the equatorial plate of the spindle. See also *meiosis* and *mitosis.*

m. chromosome, a chromosome at metaphase, when it is maximally contracted and easiest to use for chromosome identification.

m. plate, the equatorial plate; see under *mitosis.*

metaphosphoric acid (met″ah-fos-for′ik) see under *phosphoric acid.*

metaphysis (me-taf′ĭ-sis), pl. *metaphyses* [*meta-* + Gr. *phyein* to grow] the wider part at the extremity of the diaphysis of a long bone, adjacent to the epiphyseal disk. During development it contains the growth zone and consists of spongy bone; in adult life it is continuous with the epiphysis.

metaplasia (met″ah-pla′ze-ah) [*meta-* + Gr. *plasis* molding + *-ia*] the substitution of one adult cell type for another cell type. This change is thought to be reversible and to result from some type of stress. Such adaptive substitution may be seen in the respiratory tract of chronic smokers, where it results in the substitution of squamous cells for mucus-secreting columnar ciliated epithelium. The process reflects aberrant basal cell differentiation.

metaplastic (met″ah-plas′tik) pertaining to metaplasia.

metaraminol bitartrate (met″ah-ram′ĭ-nol) [USP], a sympathomimetic amine, which acts primarily on the α-adrenergic receptors, has a positive inotropic effect on the heart, and also produces peripheral vasoconstriction. It is used in the treatment of acute hypotension due to spinal anesthesia, hemorrhage, drug reactions, surgical complications, or shock. Adverse reactions include severe hypertension, which may cause pulmonary edema, arrhythmias, or cardiac arrest.

metarubricyte (met″ah-roo′brĭ-sīt) see *orthochromatic n.* under *normoblast.*

metastable state (met′ah-sta″b'l) an excited energy state of a nuclide that exists for an appreciable period of time before decaying by isomeric transition and emitting a gamma ray. It is indicated by an "m" after the mass number of the nuclide, e.g., ^{99m}Tc.

metastasis (mĕ-tas′tah-sis) [N.L., from Gr. *methistanai* to change] the discontinuous extension of a malignant neoplasm; the process by which malignant cells are disseminated from the tumor of origin (primary tumor) to form a new growth (secondary tumor) at a distant site.

Metastasis involves the liberation of malignant cells from the primary tumor; their subsequent transportation, generally via lymphatics to lymph nodes or blood vessels to tissues supplied by the vessels; their eventual arrest or deposition at distant sites; and under circumstances favorable to the tumor, their growth into a metastatic tumor.

See also *neoplasia.*

metastasize (mĕ-tas′tah-sīz) the process of forming metastases.

metastatic (met″ah-stat′ik) pertaining to metastasis or to metastases.

metatarsus (met″ah-tar′sus) [*meta-* + Gr. *tarsos* tarsus] the five bones that form the skeleton of the anterior half of the foot. The bones are numbered one through five from medial to lateral. Each metatarsal is a miniature long bone with a shaft and two ends. The proximal ends articulate with the tarsal bones through the cuneiforms and cuboid, and the distal ends articulate with the proximal phalanges.

metaxalone (me-taks′ah-lōn) a central nervous system (spinal interneurons) depressant, used as a skeletal muscle relaxant.

metaxeny (me-tak′sĕ-ne) see *metoxeny.*

metazoa (met″ah-zo′ah), pl. of *metazoon* [*meta-* + Gr. *zōa* animals] all multicellular animals whose cells differentiate to form tissues; all animals except protozoa.

metazoan (met″ah-zo′an) 1. pertaining to the metazoa.

2. a metazoon.

metencephalon (met″en-sef′ah-lon) [*meta-* + Gr. *enkephalos* brain] [NA], the part of the brain, composed of the cerebellum and pons, that develops from the anterior rhombencephalon.

meter (me′ter) [Gr. *metron* measure, Fr. *mètre*] 1. (abbrev. m), the International System (SI) unit of length defined as 1,650,763.73 wavelengths of the orange emission line of krypton 86, about 39.37 in. or 1.094 yd. Note that the official spelling, metre, is rarely used in the United States.

2. a measuring device or apparatus.

3. in electronics, an indicator, particularly one with a dial and pointer as opposed to a digital readout.

-meter (me′ter) a suffix word element to denote measure, e.g., spectrophotometer.

meter-kilogram-second (mks) system a coherent system of measuring units in which the meter, kilogram, and second are the base units. See also *International System.*

methacycline (meth″ah-si′klēn) a tetracycline antibiotic produced by a *Streptomyces* species that, like other tetracyclines, exhibits a broad antimicrobial spectrum. See also *antibacterial agents* and *tetracyclines.*

methadone (meth′ah-don) a synthetic opiate with action similar to that of morphine and heroin except that withdrawal is more prolonged and less severe. It is used for relief of severe pain, for heroin detoxification, and as a heroin substitute for addicts (methadone maintenance). Methadone use is controlled by the federal narcotics laws. As with other opiates, methadone is addicting, although it produces less euphoria. Overdoses may cause respiratory depression, stupor, coma, or death; narcotic antagonists block the respiratory depression, but also precipitate acute withdrawal syndrome in addicts.

Addicts on methadone maintenance generally have a urine concentration of less than 50 μg/ml.

m. hydrochloride, [USP], a soluble salt, the usual form of the drug.

methadone assays 1. spectrophotometry. Methadone and its metabolites are extracted into hexane at pH 9–12 and then into ceric sulfate–sulfuric acid. This is then refluxed until both compounds are oxidized to benzophenone and the concentration determined from the absorbance at 247 nm.

2. gas chromatography. This involves the use of a nonpolar silicone column and flame ionization detector. The drug is extracted from alkalinized blood samples (to which an internal standard has been added) into an organic solvent and then back into acid. After alkalinization, it is reextracted into an organic solvent and concentrated by evaporation before it is injected into the gas chromatograph. The peak height ratio of the unknown to the internal standard is compared with that for reference samples. Methadone and its metabolites are detected separately.

3. immunoassay. This involves either the EMIT or radioimmunoassay techniques, for which kits are commercially available.

methamphetamine (meth″am-fet′ah-mēn) the *N*-methyl derivative of amphetamine. It has a greater stimulating effect on the central nervous system and also a greater potential for abuse than does amphetamine. See also *amphetamine.*

m. hydrochloride, [USP], a soluble salt, the usual form of the drug.

methanal (meth′ah-nal) see *formaldehyde.*

methane (meth′ān) a colorless, odorless, flammable gas, CH_4; the principal component of natural gas. It is nontoxic but is an explosion hazard when mixed with air.

methanol (meth′ah-nol) [USP], a clear, colorless, flammable liquid alcohol, CH_3OH, with a characteristic odor. It is highly polar and miscible in other polar liquids, such as water or other alcohols. Methanol is used as a solvent for paints and varnishes, and is found in antifreeze and in solid canned fuel (Sterno), and may be contained in some moonshine whiskey.

Methanol is highly toxic; it is metabolized in the body to formaldehyde and formate by the enzyme alcohol dehydrogenase. These metabolites cause severe acidosis and can damage the optic nerve, causing blindness. Other symptoms are similar to those of ethanol poisoning.

A methanol blood level of 80 mg/dl is life-threatening. The lethal dose is usually 2–8 oz (60–240 ml), although doses as small as 8 ml have caused death.

Also called *methyl alcohol* and wood alcohol.

methanol assays 1. in a blood specimen or protein-free filtrate of blood, plasma, or serum, the methanol is oxidized to formaldehyde by permanganate. The formaldehyde is then reacted with chromotropic acid, producing a purple compound.

The oxidation step is not quantitative, and the color reaction may produce a false-positive result. Quantitative procedures have been established with this method using an unoxidized sample as a reference and reagent blank controls. Measurement is by spectrophotometry.

Heparin and EDTA interfere; oxalate should be used as the blood anticoagulant.

2. a diluted blood sample may be injected into a gas chromatograph. The peak areas for the specimen and standards are compared, and give the methanol concentration to within 3.0 mg/dl.

methapyrilene (meth″ah-pīr′ĭ-lēn) a histamine antagonist that also has some sedative effect. It is used for treatment of some allergic diseases and in some sedative preparations; it is contraindicated in individuals taking MAO inhibitors.

m. hydrochloride, [USP], a salt for oral or parenteral use.

methaqualone (mĕ-thah′kwah-lōn) [USP], a hypnotic drug, a quinazoline derivative unrelated to the barbiturates, used as a sedative and sleeping aid. It is a widely abused drug and its use is controlled by federal narcotics laws. Withdrawal symptoms include headache, nausea, abdominal cramps, and convulsions.

Acute overdosage may result in delirium and convulsions followed by coma and death. Alcohol and other central nervous system depressants potentiate the effects. Serum concentrations higher than 8 μg/ml usually produce coma. Death has been caused by a dose of 8 g (50 tablets); most fatalities occur when methaqualone is mixed with alcohol. Trademarks, *Quaalude* and *Sopor.*

methaqualone assays 1. spectrophotometry. Methaqualone is separated from its metabolites by extraction from alkalinized serum into *n*-hexane and then into strong acid. The ultraviolet spectra in hexane and in acid are characteristic; the absorbance maximum at 235 nm (in acid) is used for quantitation. Recovery is about 50 percent, the relative error about 10 percent.

2. gas chromatography involving a moderately nonpolar column and flame ionization detector. Extraction and reextraction into hexane recovers about 95 percent of added methaqualone. Butobarbituric acid has been used as an internal standard; the peak height ratio for the sample is compared with a standard curve prepared by measuring reference solutions. The coefficient of variation is about 3 percent.

metharbital (mĕ-thar′bĭ-tal) [USP], a barbiturate used to control tonic-clonic and absence attacks and myoclonic epileptic seizures. See also *barbiturate.*

methemalbumin (met″hem-al-bu′min) a 1:1 stoichiometric complex of hemin (oxidized hemoglobin) and albumin that forms when hemopexin is depleted, as in intravascular hemolysis. When new hemopexin is formed, it removes hemin from albumin, forming a complex that is cleared by the liver.

methemalbumin assays 1. the Schumm test, a semiqualitative test for methemalbumin in plasma. Ammonium sulfide is added, forming a complex with methemalbumin with an absorption maximum at 558 nm that can be detected spectrophotometrically.

2. serum protein electrophoresis. Any hemoglobin migrating in the albumin band indicates methemalbumin.

metheme (met′hēm) a catabolic product of hemoglobin in which the heme iron is in the Fe(III) state. Formerly called protohemin IX.

methemoglobin (met-he″mo-glo′bin) hemoglobin with iron in the ferric (Fe^{3+}) state, in contrast to the bulk of hemoglobin iron, which is in the ferrous (Fe^{2+}) state both in its oxygenated and deoxygenated forms. Methemoglobin is unable to carry oxygen and is therefore valueless as a respiratory protein.

Methemoglobin gives the blood a brown color, producing visible cyanosis when the concentration exceeds 1.5 g/100 ml. In normal blood, 1 percent of the total circulating hemoglobin is normally converted to the ferric state each day, with a balance maintained between spontaneous methemoglobin formation and reconversion to deoxyhemoglobin by the methemoglobin reductase system.

If normal hemoglobin A is oxidized to methemoglobin, the absorption spectrum has peaks at 502 and 632 nm and a valley at 600 nm at pH 7.0. The test that quantitates methemoglobin concentration utilizes this absorption spectrum by measuring the disappearance of the absorption band in the 630-nm range upon the addition of cyanide. The reference value is 0.5–3.0 percent of total hemoglobin.

Also called *ferrihemoglobin* and *hemiglobin.* See also *methemoglobinemia.*

methemoglobinemia (met″he-mo-glo″bĭ-ne′meah) [*methemoglobin* + Gr. *haima* blood + *-ia*] the presence of increased amounts of methemoglobin in blood, which renders the hemoglobin incapable of binding oxygen at physiologic partial pressures and may cause cyanosis. The condition may result from a defect or absence of the enzyme NADH methemoglobin reductase (cytochrome b_5 reductase) or from an abnormality in the hemoglobin molecule (hemoglobin M disease) that causes it to structurally favor the assumption of the oxidized (ferri) form of hemoglobin. It is more commonly induced by certain drugs or chemicals. In normal individuals, about 3 percent of the circulating hemoglobin is oxidized to methemoglobin each day.

congenital m., various forms of methemoglobinemia transmitted as autosomal recessive traits. Congenital methemoglobinemia is usually due to a deficiency of the NADH-diaphorase system, which is responsible for the reconversion of methemoglobin to hemoglobin; less commonly, it is due to an abnormal hemoglobin (Hb M). See also hemoglobin M disease under *hemoglobinopathy.*

toxic m., a chemically or drug-induced disorder that is caused by nitro or amino derivatives of benzene, nitrates, or aniline dyes. The causative agent either facilitates the oxidation of hemoglobin by molecular oxygen or directly oxidizes hemoglobin so that iron remains in the ferric form and cannot reversibly bind oxygen.

methemoglobin reductase (met″he-mo-glo′bin re-duk′tās) see *cytochrome b_5 reductase.*

methenamine (meth-en′ah-mēn) [USP], a tricyclo compound hydrolyzed in acid to ammonia and formaldehyde. It is used in the treatment of urinary tract infections when administered in conjunction with compounds to acidify the urine; the formaldehyde acts as a nonspecific antibacterial. See also *antibacterial agents.*

m. hippurate, the salt with hippuric acid, which also has an antibacterial action and aids in the acidification of urine.

m. mandelate, the salt with mandelic acid, which also has an antibacterial action and aids in the acidification of urine.

m. silver, a solution of methenamine and silver nitrate. It is used in many histologic techniques, as it is reduced by aldehyde in an alkaline solution.

methicillin (meth″ĭ-sil′in) one of the early semisynthetic penicillins. It is resistant to inactivation by penicillinase and is used as an antibiotic against penicillin-resistant staphylococci. It is acid labile and must be given intramuscularly or intravenously. Methicillin can give rise to drug-resistant mutant organisms, causing hospital-acquired infections of resistant staphylococci. See also *antibacterial agents* and *penicillins.*

methimazole (meth-im′ah-zōl) [USP], a thioamide drug that inhibits the synthesis of thyroid hormones; used for the treatment of hyperthyroidism. A rare adverse reaction is its interference with the formation of blood cells, causing agranulocytosis. If this occurs, drug therapy is stopped and alternate modalities (surgery, radioactive iodine) are used. Thioamides interfere with thyroid function tests.

methiodal sodium (mĕ-thi′o-dal) [USP], sodium iodomethanesulfonate, a water-soluble radiopaque contrast medium used in retrograde pyelography. Trademark, *Skiodan.*

methionine (Met or M) (mĕ-thi′o-nēn) 2-amino-4-methylthiobutanoic acid, $CH_3SCH_2CH_2CH(NH_2)$-COOH, a naturally occurring essential amino acid present in proteins; M.W. 149.21. As a methyl donor, methionine has lipotropic action. It can be formed by the methylation of its own metabolite, homocysteine. *N*-Formyl-methionine functions in the first step of the translation process in protein synthesis. It is obtained in the diet from proteins. See also under *amino acids.*

methionine malabsorption syndrome a rare hereditary disorder, transmitted as an autosomal recessive trait. Affected individuals have white hair, hyperpnea, convulsions, and mental retardation. Their urine has a unique odor, as of an oasthouse (a building for drying hops) or of burnt sugar. A number of α-ketoacids appear in the urine, and α-hydroxybutyric acid is in excess in the urine after methionine loading. Also called *oasthouse urine disease* and *Smith-Strang disease.* See also *aminoacidopathies.*

methionine synthase see *tetrahydropteroylglutamate methyltransferase.*

methionyl (mĕ-thi′o-nil) the acyl radical derived from or relating to methionine.

methisazone (mĕ-this′ah-zōn) see *antiviral agent.*

methixene hydrochloride (mĕ-thiks′ēn) an anticholinergic drug similar to atropine but somewhat milder in effect. It is used as a smooth muscle relaxant and to decrease the motility of the gastrointestinal tract in individuals with gastric or duodenal ulcer, gastroenteritis, irritable bowel, or pylorospasm.

methocarbamol (meth″o-kar′bah-mol) [USP], a central nervous system depressant drug used as a muscle relaxant. It may be administered intravenously, intramuscularly, or orally. Major adverse responses include lightheadedness, drowsiness, nausea, mental confusion, and allergic reactions.

methocycline (meth″o-si′klēn) see *tetracyclines.*

method (meth′ud) [Gr. *methodos*] a systematic procedure, which may involve following a specified protocol, for treating a disease or performing an operation or a laboratory test. A method is based on the scientific principles involved in the procedure, e.g., a particular chemical reaction used for a test in clinical chemistry and not on a specific technology. Cf. *technology.*

analytic m., in analytic chemistry, a procedure for performing an analytic measurement, involving written instructions describing in detail the procedural steps, the reagent preparation, and the equipment and apparatus needed.

definitive m., an analytic method having negligible inaccuracy.

field m., an analytic method developed for the routine determination of analytes in biologic and control materials. Such tests are clinically useful, but the accuracy and precision of field methods (often called routine methods) are limited by considerations of cost, ease of performance, and practicality. See also *definitive m.* and *reference m.*

reference m., an analytic method with thoroughly documented accuracy, precision, and low susceptibility to interfering substances, as established by comparison with a definitive method. Reference methods are used in the development and evaluation of field (routine) methods or commercial kit procedures.

special reference m., an analytic method that has the accuracy and precision of a reference method but for which there are no definitive methods or primary reference materials.

methodology (meth″ŏ-dol′o-je) the various general methods and procedures of a scientific discipline.

methohexital sodium (meth″o-hek′sĭ-tal) [USP], an ultrashort-acting barbiturate used as an injected general anesthetic. See also *barbiturate.*

methotrexate (meth″o-trek′sāt) a folic acid antagonist used in the treatment of severe psoriasis and as a cancer chemotherapeutic drug. Methotrexate acts as a competitive inhibitor of the enzyme dihydrofolate reductase, blocking the conversion of dihydrofolate to tetrahydrofolate. The synthesis of deoxythymidine monophosphate (dTMP) from deoxyuridine monophosphate (dUMP) requires 5,10-methylenetetrahydrofolate as a methyl donor and tetrahydrofolate as a reducing agent: methotrexate blocks DNA synthesis by stopping the synthesis of thymidine nucleotides.

For some highly malignant tumors, methotrexate has been administered in a very high dosage and followed by leucovorin rescue. Leucovorin (5-formyltetrahydrofolate) circumvents the metabolic block and permits DNA synthesis to resume. Neoplastic cells do not absorb leucovorin as readily as normal cells; thus, the normal cells are rescued while neoplastic cells continue to be killed by the methotrexate.

Trademark, Mexate. For more information, see *Appendix A.*

methotrimeprazine (meth″o-tri-mep′rah-zēn) [USP], a phenothiazine derivative chemically related to the tricyclic antidepressants; a central nervous system depressant used as an analgesic and preanesthetic medication. The drug is administered by intramuscular injection; its side-effects include orthostatic hypertension and pain at the injection site. The overall effects of the drug are additive with other CNS depressants.

methoxamine hydrochloride (mĕ-thok′sah-mēn) [USP], a sympathomimetic amine that acts on the alpha-adrenergic receptors and causes vasoconstriction. It is used to reverse a drop in blood pressure during administration of general anesthesia. High dosages may cause severe headache or vomiting, or may have cardiac effects.

methoxy- (mĕ-thok′se) a prefix word element used in organic chemistry to denote the methoxy functional group (CH_3O—), e.g., methoxyethane (ethyl methyl ether).

***p*-methoxyamphetamine** (PMA) (mĕ-thok″se-am-fet′ah-min) a psychotomimetic amphetamine, an illicit hallucinogen that is stronger than mescaline or 3,4-methylenedioxyamphetamine (DOM). Toxic effects include hypertension, hyperthermia, dysphoria, and respiratory depression. Overdose deaths have occurred. In fatal cases, concentrations greater than 0.3 μg/ml in blood and 6 μg/ml in urine have been observed.

***p*-methoxyamphetamine assays** gas chromatography. PMA is extracted from an alkalinized sample into an organic solvent; after acetylation, it is identified by its characteristic retention times using two different column packings (one nonpolar, the other moderately polar). The peak heights are compared with those of PMA reference solutions. A flame ionization detector is used.

methoxychlor (mĕ-thok′se-klor) the generic name for an insecticide similar to DDT that is less toxic to mammals.

methoxyflurane (mĕ-thok″se-floo′rān) [USP], a chlorofluoro-substituted ether, $CH_3OCF_2CHCl_2$; a liquid with a fruity smell; an inhalation anesthetic used primarily for the maintenance of anesthesia. Overdosage may cause cardiac arrest. A rare adverse reaction is liver damage.

methoxyphenamine hydrochloride (mĕ-thok″se-fen′ah-mēn) [USP], a sympathomimetic amine used as a bronchodilator and decongestant. It has little vasopressor effect.

methoxypromazine maleate (mĕ-thok″se-pro′mah-zēn) a phenothiazine compound formerly used as a major tranquilizer.

methscopolamine (meth″sko-pol′ah-mēn) the *N*-methyl derivative of scopolamine, a quaternary ammonium ion used as an anticholinergic and antispasmodic.

m. bromide, [USP], a salt of methscopolamine used in antispasmodic preparations.

m. nitrate, a salt of methscopolamine used in antispasmodic preparations.

methsuximide (meth-suk′sĭ-mīd) [USP], an anticonvulsant drug similar to ethosuximide, used to treat absence attacks (petit mal epilepsy) when other drugs are not effective.

methyclothiazide (meth″ĭ-klo-thi′ah-zīd) see under *thiazide diuretics.*

methyl (meth′il) [Gr. *methy* wine + *hylē* wood] referring to the methyl group, CH_3—; used alone in trivial names, e.g., methyl alcohol, methyl ketone; used as a prefix in systematic names, e.g., 2-methylpropane.

***N*-methylacetamide** (meth″il-ah-set′ah-mīd) a metabolite of *N,N*-dimethylacetamide. See also *N-methylformamide and N-methylacetamide assays.*

methyl acetate (meth′il as′ĕ-tāt) a colorless, volatile, highly flammable liquid with a pleasant odor, CH_3COOCH_3, used in paint remover and as a lacquer solvent; M.W. 74.08. It is moderately toxic when inhaled, producing respiratory tract irritation and, at high concentrations, narcosis.

α-**methylacetoaceticaciduria** (meth″il-ah-se″to-ah-se″tik-as-ĭ-dur′e-ah) see *β-ketothiolase deficiency* and *α-methyl-β-hydroxybutyric aciduria.*

methylation (meth-ĭ-la′shun) 1. treatment with reagent to introduce a methyl group into a compound.

2. in histology, esterification of carboxyl groups and removal of sulfate groups to reduce basophilia and abolish metachromasia.

methylbenzene (meth″il-ben′zēn) see *toluene.*

methyl bromide (meth′il bro′mīd) bromomethane, a colorless, dense, nonflammable gas with a burning taste and the odor of chloroform, CH_3Br; M.W. 94.95. Methyl bromide is used as an insect fumigant. It is highly toxic when ingested, inhaled, or absorbed through the skin and can produce narcosis, pulmonary edema, central nervous system depression, and kidney damage.

methyl butyl ketone (MBK) (meth′il bu′til ke′tōn) a colorless, moderately flammable liquid, 2-hexanone, $CH_3(CH_2)_3COCH_3$; M.W. 100.16. Used as a solvent, MBK is an irritant to the eyes, nose, and throat and, with chronic exposure, has produced peripheral neuropathy.

methyl chloroform (meth′il klo′ro-form) see *1,1,1-trichloroethane.*

β-**methylcrotonylglycinuria** (meth″il-kro″ton-il-gli″sin-ur′e-ah) a disorder of leucine metabolism, transmitted as an autosomal dominant trait, that is due to a relative or absolute deficiency of the enzyme β-methylcrotonyl-CoA carboxylase. Increased levels of β-methylcrotonylglycine and β-hydroxyisovaleric acid are seen in the urine. Those affected may show mental retardation and central nervous system dysfunction, muscle atrophy, metabolic acidosis, vomiting, and a urine odor similar to that of a tomcat. Carrier detection in this disorder is possible. Those affected may respond to controlled leucine intake or to large doses of biotin therapy. Also called β-hydroxyisovaleric aciduria. See also *aminoacidopathies.*

methyl demeton (meth′il dem′ĕ-ton) a highly toxic organothiophosphate insecticide, a mixture of phosphorothioic acid *O,O*-dimethyl *O*-[2-(ethylthio)-ethyl] ester and *O,O*-dimethyl *S*-[2-(ethylthio)ethyl] phosphorothioate. See also *organophosphate compounds.*

methyldopa (meth″il-do′pah) [USP], a drug that is converted in the body to a derivative of the neurotransmitter norepinephrine. It serves as a false neurotransmitter, reducing blood pressure and heart rate, and is used to treat hypertension. Adverse reactions include transient sedation, liver disorders, red cell sensitization (indicated by a positive Coombs' test), and hemolytic anemia. Also called alphamethyldopa. Trademark, *Aldomet.*

methyldopate hydrochloride (meth″il-do′pāt) [USP], the ethyl ester hydrochloride, used for injection in hypertensive emergencies.

methylene (meth″ĭ-lēn) 1. the trivial name for the substituent group —CH_2—.

2. the unstable neutral intermediate, CH_2:, which is a carbene.

m. chloride, a moderately toxic industrial solvent, CH_2Cl_2, formerly used as an inhalation anesthetic. Also called *dichloromethane* and *methylene dichloride.*

m. dichloride, see *m. chloride.*

methylene blue a metachromatic thiazine dye, methylthionine chloride; C.I. 52015. It is used in histology in Mallory's phloxine methylene blue stain as a metachromatic connective tissue stain, as a bacterial stain, and as an indicator of oxidation-reduction potential (Eh).

[USP], used in medicine as a reducing agent for the treatment of methemoglobinemia and as a urinary tract antiseptic. Administered intravenously, it reduces methemoglobin to hemoglobin. It has been given orally for nephritis, pyelitis, and cystitis.

polychrome m. b., a metachromatic dye formed by the oxidation of methylene blue. Methylene blue easily undergoes oxidative demethylation, which forms azures, and oxidative deamination, which forms thiazoles. The polychroming of methylene occurs without added oxidizers in a hot, mildly alkaline aqueous solution. The resulting mixture of dyes is used as a connective tissue stain and in the Romanowsky stains (Wright stain, Leishman stain) used for blood cells. Nuclei and basophilic substances stain blue; cartilage matrix, mucin, and mast cell granules stain reddish-violet.

3,4-methylenedioxyamphetamine (MDA) (meth″ĭ-lēn-di-ok″se-am-fet′ah-mēn) an amphetamine derivative that is an illegal and often abused drug. It causes central nervous system stimulation and hallucinations; overdoses may produce convulsions and death. Blood concentrations of 2.5–2.7 μg/ml have been reported as causing fatalities.

3,4-methylenedioxyamphetamine assays MDA is extracted from alkalinized specimens into chloroform and then into acid. It is identified by its characteristic ultraviolet spectrum, having peaks at 285 and 234 nm. The presence of MDA may be confirmed by gas chromatography of the acetylated derivative.

methylergonovine maleate (meth″il-er″go-no′vēn mal′e-āt) [USP], a semisynthetic ergot alkaloid used to prevent postpartum hemorrhage due to uterine atony by stimulation of uterine contractions. Adverse reactions include vomiting, transient high blood pressure (especially when it is administered intravenously), dizziness, headache, and ringing in the ears. Trademark, Methergine.

methyl ethyl ketone (MEK) (meth′il eth′il ke′tōn) a colorless, flammable liquid with the odor of acetone, 2-butanone, $CH_3COC_2H_5$; M.W. 72.10. It is a commonly used solvent. Concentrations in air of 2–10 percent are explosive. Vapors are irritating to the eyes and respiratory tract.

***N*-methylformamide** (meth″il-for′mah-mīd) a metabolite of *N,N*-dimethylformamide.

***N*-methylformamide and *N*-methylacetamide assays** the determination of the urine concentration of *N*-methylformamide (MMF) and *N*-methylacetamide (MMAC), metabolites of the toxic organic solvents *N,N*-dimethylformamide (DMF) and *N,N*-dimethylacetamide (DMAC). A urine sample may be injected directly into a gas chromatograph equipped with a flame ionization detector and a column consisting of either an adsorbent (porous polymer) or polar absorbent (polyethylene glycol) stationary phase. The MMF or MMAC concentration is proportional to the peak area on the chromatogram. An extraction step using cellulose column chromatography may be performed before the gas chromatography. The column is washed with a low concentration (3.5 percent) of methanol in dichloromethane, and the MMF and MMAC are eluted with a higher concentration (10 percent).

methyl green a green basic triphenylmethane dye, *N*-heptamethylpararosaniline; C.I. 42585.

methyl green–pyronine stain any of a number of variations of the original Pappenheim method for demonstration of DNA and RNA. DNA (chromatin) is stained blue to blue-green by methyl green. RNA—in nucleoli, Nissl bodies, and the cytoplasm (ribosomes) of cells that have a high rate of protein synthesis—is stained pink-red to purple-red by pyronine. This stain is particularly used to detect plasma cells, which have pyroninophilic cytoplasm. Also called *Pappenheim stain.*

α-methyl-β-hydroxybutyric acid 2-methyl-3-hydroxybutyric acid, an intermediate in the metabolism of isoleucine.

α-methyl-β-hydroxybutyric aciduria a disorder of valine and isoleucine metabolism, transmitted as an autosomal recessive trait, that is characterized by mental retardation, central nervous system dysfunction, ammonia intoxication, and episodes of vomiting and metabolic acidosis in infancy. This condition is thought to be due to a relative or absolute deficiency of α-methylacetoacetyl-CoA ketothiolase (β-ketothiolase). As a result, α-methyl-β-hydroxybutyric and α-methylacetoacetic acids are excreted in the urine. Carrier and prenatal detection are considered possible, and affected individuals may benefit from decreased intake of protein, especially isoleucine. Also called *α-methylacetoacetic-aciduria.* See also *aminoacidopathy.*

methyl isobutyl ketone (MIBK) (meth′il i″so-bu′til ke′tōn) a colorless liquid with a pleasant odor, 4-methyl-2-pentanone, $(CH_3)_2CHCH_2COCH_3$; M.W. 100.16. Its use is as a solvent for paints, varnishes, gums, and resins, and in the chemical laboratory to extract heavy metal chelates prior to analysis by atomic absorption spectrophotometry. MIBK is highly flammable (explosive limits in air, 1.4–7.5 percent) and moderately toxic by ingestion or inhalation, causing headache, nausea, vomiting, and irritation of the eyes and upper respiratory tract.

methylmalonic acid (meth″il-mah-lon′ik) an intermediate, $COOH\text{-}CH(CH_3)COOH$, in the catabolism of valine, isoleucine, and propionic acid. A carboxylase converts propionyl-CoA to (*R*)-methylmalonyl-CoA, which is then racemized to the (*S*)-methylmalonyl-CoA. The latter is converted to succinic-CoA by a cobalamin-enzyme, methylmalonyl-CoA mutase. If the enzyme is absent or vitamin B_{12} intake is deficient (pernicious anemia), the mutase reaction cannot proceed and methylmalonic acid accumulates, giving rise to one type of methylmalonic aciduria. Methylmalonic acid in urine may also increase in cases of deficiency of the (*S*)-(*R*) racemase and of the enzyme needed to form adenosyl cobalamin, the coenzyme for the mutase reaction.

methylmalonic acidemia a condition of elevated levels of methylmalonic acid in the serum and urine, transmitted as an autosomal recessive trait, that results from one of several genetic defects. One of the defects is methylmalonyl-CoA mutase deficiency; two abnormalities are vitamin B_{12}–responsive and are due to the defective synthesis of adenosylcobalamin.

Symptoms include repeated bouts of vomiting, acidosis, ketosis, high serum and urine methylmalonic acid, high serum glycine, developmental retardation, and intolerance to protein. Methylmalonic acid is derived metabolically in large part from branched-chain amino acids. The reason for the high serum glycine is not well understood. The vitamin B_{12}–responsive form may respond to megavitamin B_{12} therapy.

See also *aminoacidopathy.*

methylmalonic aciduria a hereditary condition that leads to elevated methylmalonic acid in the urine. See also *methylmalonic acidemia.*

methylmalonyl-CoA decarboxylase (meth″il-mah-lon′il de″kar-bok′sĭ-lās) see *propionyl-CoA carboxylase.*

***S*-methylmalonyl-CoA mutase** an enzyme of the isomerase class (methylmalonyl-CoA CoA-carbonylmutase; EC 5.4.99.2) that catalyzes the reaction *S*-methylmalonyl-CoA ⇄ succinyl-CoA. A deficiency of this enzyme causes methylmalonyl aciduria.

methylmercaptan (meth″il-mer-kap′tan) a gas, methyl hydrosulfide, $CH_3 \cdot SH$, formed in the intestines by the decomposition of proteins. Methylmercaptan is believed to impart distinct odors to the urine (similar to that noticed after eating asparagus) and to the breath (the characteristic odor of fetor hepaticus).

methyl mercury dimethylmercury, $(CH_3)_2Hg$; a highly toxic substance produced along with other alkyl mercury compounds from inorganic mercury pollution by the action of bacteria. It is concentrated as it travels up the food chain, and fish from contaminated waters contain especially high amounts. When it is ingested by humans, toxic symptoms include mental disturbance, ataxia, tremor, and disturbances of gait and speech.

methylmorphine (meth″il-mor′fēn) see *codeine.*

***N*′-methylnicotinamide** (meth″il-nik″o-tin′ahmid) the major metabolite of niacin, produced by the irreversible methylation of niacin in the liver. The reaction involves the enzymatic (by methyl transferase) transferral of a methyl group from *S*-adenosyl methionine. *N*′-Methylnicotinamide is then secreted into the urine by the tubules of the kidneys. See also *niacin.*

methyl orange a pH indicator with a pH range of 3.0 (red)–4.4 (orange-yellow).

methylparaben (meth″il-par′a-ben) [USP], a colorless crystalline solid with a burning taste, methyl *p*-hydroxbenzoate, $HOC_6H_4COOCH_3$; M.W. 152.14. It is used as a food additive and pharmaceutic aid to retard fungal growth.

methyl parathion (meth′il par″ah-thi′on) a highly toxic organothiophosphate insecticide, *O,O*-dimethyl *O-p*-nitrophenyl thiophosphate. See also *organophosphate compounds.*

methylphenidate (meth″il-fen′ĭ-dāt) [USP], a central nervous system stimulant with actions similar to those of amphetamine, used as methylphenidate hydrochloride [USP] to treat cases of minimal brain dysfunction or hyperactivity in children. Overdoses cause nervousness, insomnia, and excessive stimulation; symptoms include agitation, tremors, hallucinations, cardiac arrhythmia, convulsions, and coma.

methylphenidate assays gas chromatography using a silicone column having intermediate polarity and a flame ionization detector. Methylphenidate is separated from its metabolite, ritalinic acid, by extraction from urine at pH 11 into chloroform, and the ritalinic acid is converted to methylphenidate. The concentration of both extracts is then determined by comparing the peak height ratio of the sample and internal standard (diphenhydramine) with that of reference solutions.

methylprednisolone (meth″il-pred-nis′o-lōn) [USP], a synthetic antiinflammatory corticosteroid (6α-methylprednisolone), a potent glucocorticoid with little mineralocorticoid activity. See also *corticosteroid.*

methyl red a diazo-type acid-base indicator (pK'_a 5.3), with a pH range of 4.4 (red)–6.0 (yellow).

methyl red test in microbiology, the use of a methyl red solution to indicate the pH of a bacterial culture grown in a buffered glucose-peptone broth. In a positive reaction the culture is sufficiently acidic to allow the methyl red reagent to remain red. This basic metabolic test is used for identification of *Escherichia coli* and its differentiation from other organisms of the *Enterobacter* group. See also *IMViC tests.*

methylrosaniline chloride (meth″il-ro-zan′ĭ-lēn) see *gentian violet.*

methyl salicylate (meth′il sa-lis′ah-lāt) [USP], a pain reliever chemically related to aspirin that is used in lotions or ointments. It is an oily liquid with a characteristic odor and taste. This substance may cause serious accidental salicylate poisoning if ingested by a child. Also called oil of wintergreen.

methylthiouracil (meth″il-thi″o-u′rah-sil) [USP], a thyroid inhibitor; see the similar drug *propylthiouracil.*

methyltransferase (meth″il-trans′fer-ās) a subsubgroup (EC 2.1.1) of the transferase class of enzymes, consisting of those that catalyze the transfer of a methyl group from one compound to another. Also called *transmethylase.*

methyl violet a basic dye, a mixture of *N*-tetramethyl-, *N*-pentamethyl-, and *N*-hexamethylpararosaniline; C.I. 42535. See also *triphenylmethane dyes.* Cf. *crystal violet* and *gentian violet.*

methyprylon (meth″ĭ-pri′lon) [USP], a nonbarbiturate hypnotic; a derivative of piperidine, used as a sleeping pill. The dependency and the withdrawal syndromes are similar to those for barbiturates. Overdoses may cause coma, respiratory depression, and death. Blood concentrations above 30 μg/ml may produce coma; therapeutic doses produce a concentration of about 0.5 μg/ml.

methyprylon assays 1. colorimetry. After extraction from alkalinized specimen into chloroform, a blue product is formed by reaction with Folin-Ciocalteau reagent. The concentration is determined by the absorbance at 600 nm, as compared with that of reference solutions processed the same way.

2. gas chromatography using a silicone column having intermediate polarity and a flame ionization detector. Extraction is as in the first method. The concentration is determined by the ratio of height of the methyprylon peak to that of the internal standard (phenmetrazine), as compared with reference solutions processed the same way.

methysergide malate (meth″ĭ-ser′jid) [USP], a lysergic acid derivative that is an antagonist of the neurotransmitter serotonin. It is used to reduce the intensity and frequency of vascular headaches (migraine attacks). Because prolonged use occasionally causes retroperitoneal fibrosis and fibrosis of the pleura, heart, and lungs, its use is restricted to severe cases.

metocurine iodide (met″o-ku′rēn) [USP], a nondepolarizing neuromuscular blocking drug, dimethyl tubocurarine iodide, used to produce relaxation of the skeletal muscles during surgery and also during electroconvulsive therapy. Adverse reactions, primarily respiratory depression, are due to excessive muscle relaxation. A cholinesterase inhibitor such as neostigmine or edrophonium is administered to antagonize the relaxant effect or to assist recovery.

metoprolol tartrate (mĕ-to'pro-lōl) a selective $beta_1$-adrenergic blocking drug used to treat hypertension. Blockade of $beta_1$-adrenergic receptors reduces blood pressure, cardiac output, and heart rate. Bronchial constriction, a $beta_2$ effect, is produced only at higher dosages. Adverse reactions include precipitation of heart failure, bradycardia, hypotension, hypoglycemia, and, rarely, bronchospasm. Trademark, Lopressor.

metoxenous (mĕ-tok'sĕ-nus) [*meta-* + Gr. *xenos* host] in parasitology, requiring two hosts for completion of the life cycle. Also called *heterecious.*

metoxeny (mĕ-tok'sĕ-ne) the condition of being metoxenous.

metr/o (me'tro) [Gr. *metra* uterus] a word element used in combining form to denote uterus, e.g., metrocystosis.

metraterm (me'trah-term) [*metra-* + L. *terminus* boundary] the terminal opening of the uterus in several tapeworms of the family Diphyllobothriidae.

metre (me'ter) [Fr., from Gr. *metron* measure] see *meter.*

metri/o (me'tre-o) [Gr. *metra* womb] a word element used in combining form to denote uterus, e.g., metritis.

metric data (met'rik) quantitative statistical data. The data points or observations have numerical values, as with physical measurements, so that counts, sums, differences, and averages of series of values must also have meaning.

metric system a system of weights and measures based on a standard unit of length, the meter. The gram is defined as the mass of 1 cm^3 of water and the liter as the volume of 1 kg of water. The novel feature of the metric system as devised was that all auxiliary units were constructed by adding prefixes to these base units, which multiplied or divided them by a power of 10, thus making conversion factors unnecessary.

For scientific usage, the meter, gram, and liter have been more precisely defined, and new units have been added for measuring chemical and physical properties. The latest addition to the metric system is the International System (SI) of units. See also *International System.*

metritis (mĕ-tri'tis) [*metro-* + *-itis* inflammation] an inflammation of the uterus, often due to infection following miscarriage or the retention of conception products. See also *endometritis* and *myometritis.*

metrizamide (mĕ-trĭz'ah-mīd) a non-ionic, water-soluble, iodinated radiopaque contrast medium used in myelography and computed tomography of the brain; it is introduced into the spinal or intracranial subarachnoid space. Trademark, Amipaque.

metrizoate (met-rĭ-zo'āt) a radiopaque contrast medium used in urography and angiography. It is a water-soluble triiodobenzene derivative. Trademark for meglumine, sodium, calcium, and magnesium metrizoate, *Isopaque.*

metrocele (me'tro-sēl) [*metro-* + Gr. *kēlē* hernia] a herniation of the uterus, with or without the prolapse of the vagina. Metrocele may have a variety of causes, such as trauma, or may occur as a complication of pregnancy and labor.

metromalacia (me"tro-mah-la'she-ah) [*metro-* + Gr. *malakia* softness] an abnormal softening of the uterus. Also called metromalacoma.

metronidazole (me"tro-ni'dah-zōl) [USP], a nitroimidazole derivative used against amebic dysentery, giardiasis, and *Trichomonas* infections. It has clinical and in vitro activity against most obligate anaerobic bacteria. During treatment, patients should avoid alcohol, as the drug may produce a reaction like that of disulfiram (flushing, abdominal cramps, headache, and vomiting). The drug may also reduce the number of white blood cells. It is carcinogenic in rats and mice and mutagenic in bacteria, and generally should not be used by pregnant females.

metronidazole assays gas chromatography using a nonpolar column and a flame ionization detector. Metronidazole is extracted from alkalinized plasma into dichloromethane, silylated, and the concentration determined by comparing peak height ratios of the sample and reference solutions.

metrorrhagia (me"tro-ra'je-ah) [*metro-* + Gr. *rhēgnynai* to burst out] menstrual bleeding, usually normal in amount, that occurs at irregular intervals during the menstrual cycle. Common causes include endometrial carcinoma, cervical erosions and tumors, ovulation bleeding, and estrogen therapy that is inappropriate.

-metry (mĕ'tre) [Gr. *metrein* to measure] a suffix word element to denote measurement, e.g., spectrophotometry.

metyrapone (mĕ-tēr'ah-pōn) [USP], a drug, 2-methyl-1,2-di-3-pyridyl-1-propanone, that selectively inhibits the action of 11 β-hydroxylase, which converts 11-deoxycortisol to cortisol. Metyrapone is used as a diagnostic aid in testing pituitary-adrenal reserve. Trademark, Metopirone.

metyrapone stimulation test a test of the reserve capacity of the pituitary to release adrenocorticotropic hormone (ACTH). Metyrapone selectively inhibits the action of 11 β-hydroxylase, which converts 11-deoxycortisol (compound S) to cortisol. As compound S is not an effective inhibitor of the pituitary feedback mechanism, the pituitary releases more ACTH, which in turn results in adrenal cortical secretion of more 11-deoxycorticosteroids.

In persons affected with Cushing's syndrome, those with adrenal hyperplasia respond vigorously to metyrapone, whereas those with adrenal tumors do not. Conditions in which cortisol inhibition is not expected to result in a compensatory increase in ACTH secretion, such as panhypopituitarism, show no response to oral administration of metyrapone as evaluated by pre- and postplasma levels of compound S and urinary 17-ketogenic steroids.

MeV abbrev. See *megaelectron volt.*

mevalonate (mĕ-val'o-nāt) 3-methyl-3,5-dihydroxy valerate, a precursor of squalene, cholesterol, and coenzyme Q in plants and animals, of carotenoids and rubber in plants, and of carotenoids and polyisoprenol constituents of the membrane of microorganisms.

mevinphos (mev'in-fos") a highly toxic organophosphate insecticide, 3-hydroxycrotonic acid methyl ester dimethyl phosphate. See also *organophosphate compounds.*

Meyenburg's complex (mi′en-boorgz) see *von Meyenburg's complex.*

Meynet's nodes (ma-nāz′) [Paul Claude Hyacinthe *Meynet,* French physician, 1831–1892] nodules that occur in rheumatic conditions and in joint capsules and tendons. They are most commonly encountered in children.

mezlocillin (mez″lo-sil′in) see *penicillins.*

mF abbrev. See *millifarad.*

μF abbrev. See *microfarad.*

Mg symbol for the chemical element *magnesium.*

mg abbrev. See *milligram.*

μg abbrev. See *microgram.*

mH abbrev. See *millihenry.*

μH abbrev. See *microhenry.*

MHC abbrev. See *major histocompatibility complex.*

mho (mo) [*ohm* spelled backwards] a unit of electrical conductance, admittance, and susceptibility equal to 1 reciprocal ohm ($1\Omega^{-1}$).

MHz abbrev. See *megahertz.*

MI abbrev. for maturation index (see under *squamous cell index*), *mitotic index, myocardial infarction.*

mi/o (mi′o) [Gr. *meiōn* smaller] a word element used in combining form to denote small or less than, e.g., mionectic. See also *mei/o.*

MIBK abbrev. See *methyl isobutyl ketone.*

MIC abbrev. See *minimal inhibitory concentration.*

micelle (mi-sel′, mi′sel) generally, any colloidal particle of a colloidal suspension, frequently consisting of spherical or laminar aggregates of surface active molecules. The term usually refers to the colloidal aggregates of surface active agents such as soaps and synthetic detergents. The component molecules are amphipathic, with the hydrophilic portions of the molecules forming the surface of the micelle and interacting there with water molecules, and the hydrophobic portions of the molecules associating together in the interior of the micelle and extruding water. The latter, however, are capable of associating with nonpolar molecules. The molecules of the micelle are associated in an ordered spatial arrangement.

Mixed micelles are formed in the small bowel during fat digestion and absorption. Bile salts form micelles with the fatty acids and monoglycerides liberated at the surface of fat emulsion droplets by the action of pancreatic lipase. These micelles represent a triple complex of bile salts, monoglycerides, and fatty acids.

Michaelis-Gutmann bodies see *malacoplakia.*

Michaelis-Menten equation an equation that describes the rate of a reaction catalyzed by an enzyme (E) involving a single substrate (S) and product (P),

$$E + S \underset{k_{-1}}{\overset{k_1}{\rightleftarrows}} ES \xrightarrow{k_2} E + P,$$

under steady-state experimental conditions. It is assumed that the rate of the reverse reaction (P→S) is negligible compared with that of the forward reaction (S→P), and that the concentration of the intermediate complex, ES, remains constant. k_1, k_{-1}, and k_2 are reaction rate constants.

The Michaelis-Menten equation is $V = V_{max}[S] / (K_m + [S])$, where V is the initial reaction velocity occurring when E and S are freshly mixed, [S] is the substrate concentration, and *x*m and K_m are two parameters that characterize each combination of enzyme x substrate. V_{max} is the maximal velocity possible, the theoretic velocity limit, which is obtained when all the enzyme molecules are saturated with substrate. K_m, the Michaelis constant, is a measure of enzyme-substrate affinity (binding) and is equal to the concentration of substrate at which $V = 1/2(V_{max})$.

The plot of V as a function of [S] at constant enzyme concentration has the form of a hyperbola. When [S] is in large excess (e.g., $[S] > 100 \times K_m$), V approaches V_{max}. Under conditions of excess S, when $V = V_{max}$, V is proportional to total enzyme concentration and is independent of [S].

See also *Hill equation, Lineweaver-Burk equation,* and the accompanying illustration.

miconazole (mi-kon′ah-zol) a β-substituted 1-phenethylimidazole derivative with a broad spectrum of antifungal and antibacterial activity, applied topically for treatment of vulvovaginal candidiasis. It is administered intravenously in treatment of the severe systemic fungal infections coccidioidomycosis, candidiasis, paracoccidioidomycosis, and cryptococcal meningitis. However, its short half-life requires that it be administered frequently, and its poor penetration into the cerebrospinal fluid has necessitated intrathecal therapy for fungal meningitis. Common adverse reactions include itching and burning in topical use, and phlebitis, itching and rash, nausea and vomiting, and fever in internal use. Trademark, *Monistat.*

micro- (mi′kro) [Gr. *mikros* small] 1. a prefix word element to denote small, e.g., microscope.

2. (abbrev. μ), a prefix word element attached to International System (SI) units that indicates one-millionth of the basic unit; e.g., a micrometer (μm) is 10^{-6} meters (m).

microabscess (mi″kro-ab′ses) a very small abscess of the size detectable with the aid of a microscope.

microaerophile (mi″kro-a′er-o-fīl) [*micro-* + Gr. *aēr* air + *philein* to love] a microaerophilic microorganism.

microaerophilic (mi″kro-a′er-o-fil″ik) growing best in only a small amount of atmospheric oxygen.

microaleuriospore (mi″kro-ah-lu′re-o-spōr) a small, unicellular aleuriospore.

microampere (μA) (mi″kro-am′pēr) a unit of electric current equal to one-millionth of an ampere (10^{-6} A).

microaneurysm (mi″kro-an′u-rizm) a minute aneurysm that occurs as an outpouching of capillaries, most commonly in the retina. These lesions may be accompanied by hemorrhage and edema. They appear as cherry-red spots in the retina as a common manifestation of long-standing diabetes mellitus (10–20 yr in duration). Microaneurysms may also occur in other locations during thrombotic purpura.

microangiopathic (mi″kro-an″je-o-path′ik) pertaining to or characterized by microangiopathy.

microangiopathic hemolytic anemia see *microangiopathic hemolytic a.* under *anemia.*

microangiopathy (mi″kro-an″je-op′ah-the) [*micro-* + Gr. *angeion* vessel + *pathos* disease] a disorder or disease of small blood vessels, a condition most com-

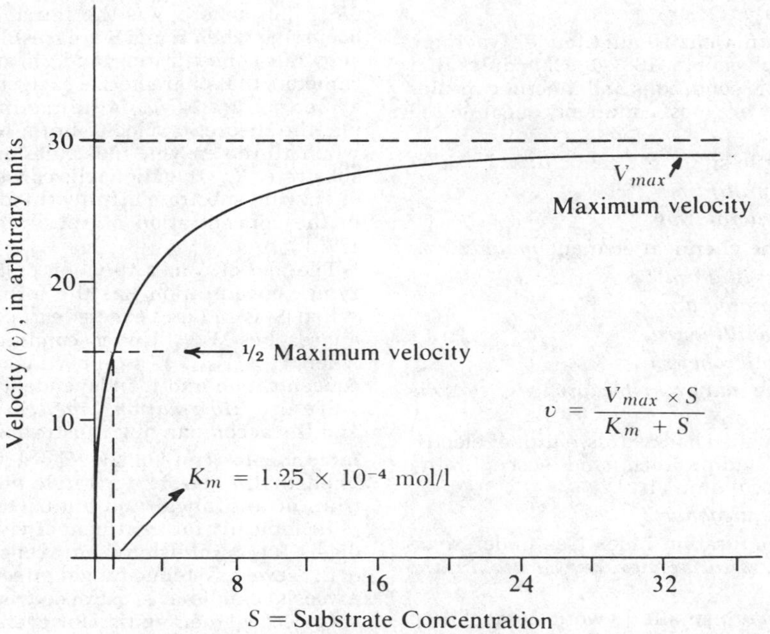

Michaelis-Menten equation. The Michaelis-Menten curve relating enzyme reaction velocity (rate) to substrate concentration. The value of K_m is given by the substrate concentration at which one-half the maximum velocity is obtained. (From Tietz, N. W.: Fundamentals of Clinical Chemistry. 2nd ed. Philadelphia, W. B. Saunders Co., 1976.)

monly seen in diabetes. Thrombotic microangiopathy, characterized by the formation of minute thrombi within small vessels, is also seen in thrombotic purpura. See also *d. mellitus* under *diabetes* and *purpura.*

microbar (μbar) (mi′kro-bar) the centimeter-gram-second (cgs) unit of pressure equal to 1 dyne per square centimeter (1 dyn/cm²), or 10^{-6} bar, or 0.1 pascal (Pa).

microbe (mi′krōb) [*micro-* + Gr. *bios* life] a microscopic organism. The term is applied to bacteria, protozoa, viruses, fungi, and rickettsiae.

microbial (mi-kro′be-al) pertaining to or of the nature of a microbe.

microbioassay (mi″kro-bi″o-as′a) the determination of minute quantities of active substances of a nutrient or other factor by a biologic method.

microbiologic (mi″kro-bi″o-loj′ik) pertaining to microbiology.

microbiologic assay the determination of the active power of a nutrient or other factor by noting its effect on the growth of a microorganism, as compared with the effect of a standard preparation.

microbiologist (mi″kro-bi-ol′o-jist) a scientist who specializes in microbiology.

microbiology (mi″kro-bi-ol′o-je) [*micro-* + Gr. *bios* life + *-logy*] the science that deals with the study of microorganisms, including bacteria, fungi, viruses, rickettsiae, and protozoa. Cf. *bacteriology.*

microbiology automation the use of automated equipment in the microbiology laboratory to detect primary growth from specimens, to test susceptibility to antimicrobial agents, or to identify microorganisms in pure culture. Although automation developed more slowly in clinical microbiology than in chemistry or hematology, semi- to fully automated procedures are rapidly becoming available. They are particularly applicable to susceptibility testing, because this is primarily a simple titration procedure and is the most frequently performed test in the microbiology laboratory. An increasing number of devices are capable of procedures involving both susceptibility and identification.

Detection of Bacterial Growth. Equipment has been designed for three methods (radiometric, impedance, turbidometric) used to detect the presence of bacterial growth in specimens from the body.

1. *Radiometric Devices.* The Bactec (Johnson Laboratories) is a semiautomated instrument developed originally as a rapid procedure for blood cultures. The culture medium contains radioactively labeled substrate(s) that, when metabolized by growing organisms, release(s) $^{14}CO_2$. The Bactec is generally regarded as a screening procedure to be employed with other blood culture methods. Bactec instruments are also used for detecting *Mycobacterium tuberculosis* in digested and concentrated sputum specimens, for susceptibility testing of *M. tuberculosis,* and for identifying *Neisseria* species.

2. *Impedance Devices.* This equipment involves a system for detecting bacterial growth in blood cultures and urine by measuring variances in electrical impedance. The Bactometer system (Bactomatic) is based on the fact that electrical conduction or resistance to the flow of alternating current through a broth medium is changed if microbial

cells and their metabolic by-products are present. Electrodes are used to monitor the conductivity.

3. *Turbidometric Devices.* Developed initially for the National Aeronautics and Space Administration (NASA) for the detection of life forms in outer space, the Automicrobic System (AMS) (Vitek Systems) now has clinical applications that include the detection of bacteria in urine cultures, susceptibility testing, and identification of gram-negative bacilli and yeasts. The system for detecting bacteria in urine uses a plastic card with several microchambers containing selective culture media. Inoculation of the microchambers with the test organism is automatic, as is the measurement of turbidity changes. The results appear as printouts within 6–12 hr. The AMS is applicable to both high- and low-volume laboratories.

SUSCEPTIBILITY TESTING AND IDENTIFICATION. Several broth microdilution methods are available for mimimal inhibitory concentration (MIC) determinations. Microtiter trays containing antibiotics and antibiotic concentrations may be prepared to fit individual specifications by using automated microtiter systems such as the MIC-2000 (Dynatech Laboratories) or Anderson-Pasco (Pasco Laboratories) systems. Antibiotic dilutions are prepared in large volumes and distributed to microtiter trays by the instrument. Many trays are prepared at the same time and frozen for later use. The trays may include wells containing media for the purpose of organism identification.

Some equipment utilizes commercially prepared frozen trays; two examples are the Micro-Media (Micro-Media Systems) and the Microscan (American Scientific Products) systems. Both supply trays with wells containing dilutions of antimicrobial agents and media for identification of gram-negative bacilli (the trays must be stored in a freezer). In both systems, all wells are simultaneously inoculated using a plastic seed trough and a plastic lid fitted with pegs corresponding to microdilution tray wells. The Micro-Media system offers a low-cost minicomputer into which MIC data and biochemical results are entered; it automatically prints the results and identifies the isolate based on biochemical data and the antibiogram. The Microscan system offers the autoSCAN, an instrument for automatic reading of the microdilution trays and for interpretation of the susceptibility results.

There are also commercial systems that offer freeze-dried antibiotic dilutions; these include the Sensititre (Gibco Diagnostic Laboratories) and the Sceptor (Baltimore Biological Laboratories) systems, both of which have an automated inoculator.

Another system, the API 3600 S (Analytab Products), measures the turbidity in each well of a rotor containing antibiotics and automatically categorizes the results as "sensitive," "intermediate," or "resistant."

Bacterial growth by forward light scattering can be measured by the Autobac system (General Diagnostics), the first semiautomated instrument marketed for susceptibility testing. It consists of a shaking incubator and a photometer that measures light scattered at a fixed angle (35°). In this procedure, antimicrobial agents are eluted from disks placed into broth in a multichambered plastic test cuvet, and the cuvet is inoculated with the test organism. As light scattering is very sensitive to variations in cell size or in suspending medium, both the broth used for the inoculum preparation and the cuvet must be optically clear. The inoculum standardization and susceptibility end points are determined by light-scattering readings. The instrument calculates a light-scattering index (LSI) for each drug in the test cuvet. "Sensitive," "intermediate," and "resistant" results can be obtained approximately 3–5 hr after inoculation. The instrument can also perform MIC testing and be used for the rapid screening of urine cultures for bacterial growth.

Another turbidometric system, the MS-2 (Abbott Laboratories), monitors the growth of an organism in the presence and absence of antibiotics by measuring the optical density. It consists of a disk dispenser-sealer, an analysis module, and a series of light-emitting diodes that measure the optical density in the cuvet at 5-min intervals. The data are stored in a computer that analyzes the growth curves and compares the antibiotic curves with the control curves. Results can usually be obtained in about 4 hr and are automatically printed as "sensitive," "intermediate," or "resistant." MIC values appear as printouts when the test organism is an "intermediate." The MS-2 also provides for the identification of Enterobacteriaceae and for the rapid screening of urine cultures for bacterial growth.

The Automicrobic System (AMS) mentioned above can measure antibiotic susceptibilities as well as bacterial growth; it can produce reliable results with gram-negative bacilli and enterococci in 4–8 hr. This multipurpose device can also be applied to the identification of gram-negative bacilli and yeasts.

All the above instruments and systems have undergone extensive evaluation by collaborative studies in selected laboratories. Some have been approved by the U.S. Food and Drug Administration.

For the application of instrumentation and automated systems to the identification of bacteria and yeasts, see *microbiology identification systems.*

microbiology identification systems those manual and automated commercially packaged micromethod systems that contain differential culture media for the identification of Enterobacteriaceae and other gram-negative bacilli (including nonglucose-fermenting species), anaerobic bacteria, and yeasts. The principal advantages in utilizing such prepared systems are the savings in time and labor realized by the inoculation of many tests at one time. In addition, packaged dehydrated systems have an extended shelf life, and the compact ones save storage space. Many of these systems provide computer-based biotype numbering programs that facilitate microorganism identification. The manufacturers generally provide ample directions and guidance for their use. Among the more commonly available systems are the following:

GRAM-NEGATIVE BACILLI. Micromethod systems were first developed to identify Enterobacteriaceae, and a number of useful devices are now on the market. One such system, the API 20E (Analytab Products), currently includes 9 carbohydrate fermentation tests and 11 other biochemical tests. It consists of a plastic strip with 20 microtubes, each containing dehydrated substrates. The procedure involves placing into each microtube a suspension of organisms that has been prepared by placing one bacterial colony in saline; the strip is then incubated overnight at 37°C. A rapid 5-hr procedure is also available. The API test results can be converted into a biotype number from which identification is made by means of a computer-based "analytical profile index," API. Modifications of the procedure and use of supplementry tests allow the user to identify commonly isolated nonglucose-fermenting gram-negative bacilli as well.

Another system, the Entero-set 20 system (Fisher Diagnostics), currently permits 10 carbohydrate utilization/fermentation and 10 other types of substrate tests to be performed. It consists of a series of chambers containing pieces of reagent-impregnated filter paper; in the procedure the strip is simply inoculated with test organisms and incubated at 37°C. A biotype number profile register is available.

In the Enterotube II system (Roche Diagnostics), a self-contained, compartmentalized plastic tube containing conventional media, the profile is composed of six oxidation-fermentation tests including gas production, and seven other biochemical tests. Inoculation is by means of a wire that touches a bacterial colony and then is pulled through all the chambers. The results are converted into a biotype number from which an identification may be made using a profile register. There is also an OXI/FERM tube that resembles the Enterotube II but contains the media used for identification of gram-negative nonglucose-fermenting bacilli.

A rapid procedure to identify Enterobacteriaceae, requiring only a 4-hr incubation period, is possible by means of the Micro-ID system (General Diagnostics). This consists of a rigid plastic tray with 15 chambers, each containing reagent-impregnated detection disks; inoculated trays are incubated at 37°C. A computer-assisted code book is available.

Two microtitration systems consisting of microdilution trays that contain test media for the identification of Enterobacteriaceae and other gram-negative bacilli, including nonglucose fermenters, are the Micro-Media (Micro-Media Systems) and Microscan (American Scientific Products) systems. Biochemical tests may be performed in combination with antibiotic broth dilution tests. In both systems, the prepared inoculum is poured into a sterile plastic seed trough. The lid of the trough, which contains plastic pegs that are immersed in the inoculum, is lowered into each well of the microdilution tray simultaneously. Results with the Microscan trays may be read and interpreted by an automated instrument (autoSCAN) after a 24-hr incubation period; an instrument is also available to interpret results with the Micro-Media trays. Instruments that allow the manufacture of plates to the user's own specifications are commercially available (e.g., the MIC-2000, Dynatech Laboratories; and the Anderson-Pasco, Pasco Laboratories).

Unlike other identification systems, the Minitek (Baltimore Biological Laboratories) allows the user flexibility in the choice of tests; more than 30 different substrate disks are available. In the Minitek system, reagent-impregnated disks are placed into a plastic incubation plate containing several wells to which a broth suspension is added, and the plate is incubated at 37°C. Biotype numbers can be assembled from the battery of biochemical tests if desired, and a computer-based system can be added for automated identification of Enterobacteriaceae and other gram-negative bacilli, including nonfermenters.

Another system for the identification of Enterobacteriaceae, the R/B system (Flow Laboratories), consists of two constricted tubes containing media for determination of phenylalanine deaminase, lactose and two fermentations with gas production, four other biochemical reactions, and motility. "Expander" tubes may be added to detect citrate utilization, DNase production, and four fermentations. A computer code book is available.

Two other systems are the Enteric-Tek (Flow Laboratories), which consists of a circular plate containing 11 independent wells, and the N/F (Flow Laboratories), an identification system for nonfermenters, which consists of a two-tube screen for identifying *Pseudomonas aeruginosa, P. putida,* and *P. fluorescens,* and a plate containing wells for determining 14 different biochemical parameters (Uni-N/F-Tek plate). Computer code books are available for both the Enteric-Tek and nonfermenter identification systems.

A replicator system that simultaneously inoculates up to 36 test isolates onto the surface of plated media is the Repliscan (Cathra International). It determines 16 biochemical and antimicrobial susceptibility reactions for the identification of Enterobacteriaceae. After incubation overnight, reactions are visually interpreted and electronically transmitted to a computer terminal that processes the information.

Automated systems that facilitate identification of Enterobacteriaceae include the AMS (Vitek Systems) and the MS-2 (Abbott Laboratories); see also *microbiology automation.* The AMS system contains a plastic card with 26 biochemical tests in a series of microwells, which, after inoculation, is placed in a reader incubator. Readings are monitored by the computer module, and results are printed automatically after 8 hr. The MS-2 identification cuvet contains 17 lyophilized biochemical substrates. The results are read by the computerized system and can generally be obtained within 5 hr.

Nonglucose-fermenting Bacteria. Several of the systems described above (API 20E, OXI/FERM, Minitek, Flow N/F) can be used to identify nonglucose-fermenting bacteria. All identify *Acinetobacter* species and *P. aeruginosa* adequately, but problems have been encountered with other species of nonfermenting bacilli.

Anaerobes. Several microsystems are available, including the API 20A system (Analytab Products) and the Minitek system (Baltimore Biological Laboratories). Both provide numerical codes and computer-based interpretation of the codes. The API 20A micromethod consists of a plastic strip with 20 microtubes, each containing dehydrated substrates. A suspension of colonies in a specified broth medium is prepared and inoculated into each microtube, and the inoculated strips are incubated anaerobically at 37°C. The system allows identification of most anaerobes in 24 hr. The procedure is simple, but there are some special cautions: (1) positive esculin hydrolysis must be verified by lack of fluorescence using an ultraviolet light of 365-nm wavelength; (2) the catalase reagent (H_2O_2) must be added after the strip has been exposed to air for 30 min; and (3) certain anaerobes, particularly the clostridia, may reduce the pH indicator in fermentation media, necessitating the addition of fresh indicator. A numerical code can be rapidly derived from the results obtained, and the computer-based API consulted for identification.

The Minitek system, which utilizes paper disks

impregnated with biochemicals, has 11 fermentation tests and 4 others. The system provides flexibility in that additional disks, e.g., gelatin hydrolysis, may be added. The disks are dispensed onto a plastic plate with wells into which a broth suspension prepared in a specified medium, is placed, and the trays are incubated anaerobically for 48 hr. The indicator is phenol red, and fresh indicator is added to facilitate the reading of reactions. A numerical coding system and computer-assisted interpretations are provided with the system.

Both the API 20A and Minitek systems have been well evaluated. Additional determinations may be performed with each system, such as morphology, reactions on egg yolk agar, activity in litmus milk, or gas-liquid chromatography profiles.

A packaged method for the presumptive identification of anaerobes is the Anaerobe-Tek plate system (Flow Laboratories). Its plate has a series of wells containing media for the determination of 15 reactions. An optional numerical coding system is available.

YEASTS. Two packaged systems are currently available for yeast identification. The API 20C (Analytab Products) is a miniaturized Wickerham test that tests for the assimilation of 19 carbohydrates. It consists of a strip with a series of microtubes that contain dehydrated substrates. The strip is inoculated, using a suspension of the yeast in a basal medium, and incubated at 30°C. The final reading is made at 72 hr, and the assimilation results interpreted using an API. The system is used in conjunction with observation of microscopic morphology of the growth on a separate plate of corn meal agar.

The Uni-Yeast-Tek system (Flow Laboratories) is used for the determination of morphology and for 9 biochemical or assimilation tests. Its series of wells utilizes corn meal agar as the medium. Incubation is at 30°C, and final results are recorded in 72 hr.

Yeast identification can also be made with an Automicrobic system (Vitek Systems).

MISCELLANEOUS SYSTEMS. Rapid identification of streptococci, including enterococci, nonenterococci, and pneumococci, can be made by means of an API system. There are also rapid procedures for the identification of *Neisseria* species, e.g., the Minitek system (Baltimore Biological Laboratories), which utilizes substrate-impregnated disks, and the Bactec system (Johnston Laboratories), which utilizes a radiometric method (see *microbiology automation*).

microbiotic (mi″kro-bi-ot′ik) pertaining to the microbiota, or to microscopic living organisms.

microbody (mi″kro-bod′e) see *peroxisome.*

microburet (mi″kro-bu-ret′) [*micro-* + Fr. *burette* cruet] a buret with capacity of 10 ml or less, often constructed like a syringe.

microcell (mi′kro-sel) a micronuclei of a mammalian cell surrounded by a thin ring of cytoplasm. See also *cellular h.* under *hybridization.*

microcephaly (mi″kro-sef′ah-le) [*micro-* + Gr. *kephalē* head] a head size more than three standard deviations below the norm, occurring in association with a defect in the growth of the brain as a whole. Many instances are unexplained, but congenital rubella, toxoplasmosis, syphilis, and hereditary factors may be causative. Skull x-rays, lumbar puncture, and serologic studies are useful in detecting infection. No treatment is available; however, correct diagnosis is necessary for future genetic counseling. It is a part of many genetic syndromes.

microchemistry (mi″kro-kem′is-tre) [*micro-* + *chemistry*] the branch of chemistry using small quantities of substances. Most typically, the term is used in clinical chemistry for reactions requiring 100 μl of specimen or less.

microchromosome (mi″kro-kro′mo-sōm) a tiny dumbbell-shaped chromatin structure often found in cells from childhood tumors, especially neuroblastomas. There may be several or many of these structures in a single metaphase plate. Also called double-minute chromosome or minute chromosome.

microcirculation (mi″kro-sir″ku-la′shun) the flow of blood in the microvasculature (arterioles, capillaries, and venules).

Micrococcaceae (mi″kro-kok-ka′se-e) [*micro-* + Gr. *kokkos* berry] a family of gram-positive, coccoid bacteria, consisting of aerobic or facultatively anaerobic organisms that divide primarily in more than one plane to form clusters. It includes three genera, *Micrococcus, Staphylococcus,* and *Planococcus.*

Micrococcus (mi″kro-kok′us) a genus of microorganisms of the family Micrococcaceae, consisting of spherical, gram-positive cells that usually occur in irregular masses. Saprophytic and nonpathogenic forms are found in soil, water, dust, and dairy products, and occasionally in clinical specimens. They are distinguished from *Staphylococcus* by being rather strict aerobes and by failing to ferment (although oxidizing) glucose.

microcolony (mi′kro-kol″o-ne) a colony of bacteria visible only under a low-power microscope.

microcomputer (mi″kro-kom-pu′ter) a general-purpose digital computer that uses a microprocessor for its arithmetic and control unit. Generally, only limited subsets of high-level programming languages are available.

microconidium (mi″kro-ko-nid′e-um), pl. *microconidia.* a small, unicellular conidium.

microcoulomb (μC) (mi″kro-koo′lom) a unit of electric charge equal to one-millionth of a coulomb (10^{-6} C).

microcrystalline (mi″kro-kris′tal-in) composed of minute crystals.

microcurie (μCi) (mi″kro-ku′re) a unit of radioactivity equal to one-millionth of a curie (10^{-6} Ci).

microcurie-hour (μCi-hr) (mi′kro-ku″re owr)) a unit of cumulated activity equal to one-millionth of a curie-hour.

microcyte (mi′kro-sīt) [*micro-* + Gr. *kytos* hollow vessel] an erythrocyte with reduced volume. Although the term is usually reserved for an abnormally small erythrocyte, it occasionally is also used to designate other abnormally small cells, e.g., "microcytic" platelets.

microcythemia (mi″kro-si-the′me-ah) [*microcyte* + Gr. *haima* blood + *-ia*] see *microcytosis.*

microcytic anemia (mi″kro-sit′ik) see *microcytic a.* under *anemia.*

microcytosis (mi″kro-si-to′sis) a condition in which the erythrocytes are smaller than normal. Also called *microcythemia.*

microdensitometer (mi″kro-den″sĭ-tom′ĕ-ter) a

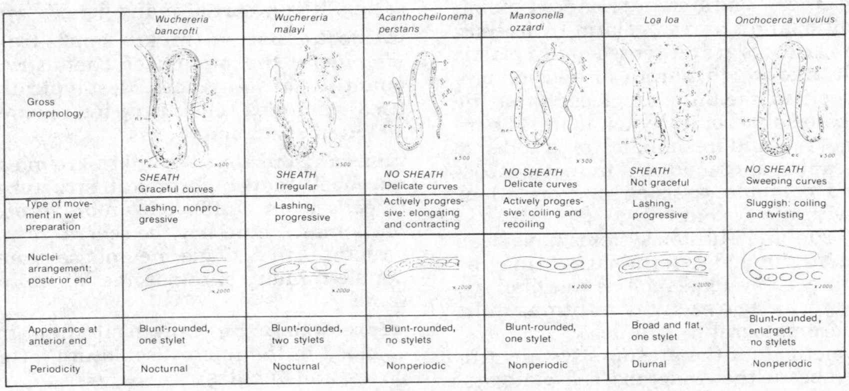

	Wuchereria bancrofti	*Wuchereria malayi*	*Acanthocheilonema perstans*	*Mansonella ozzardi*	*Loa loa*	*Onchocerca volvulus*
Gross morphology	×500 SHEATH Graceful curves	×500 SHEATH Irregular	×500 NO SHEATH Delicate curves	×500 NO SHEATH Delicate curves	×500 SHEATH Not graceful	×500 NO SHEATH Sweeping curves
Type of movement in wet preparation	Lashing, nonprogressive	Lashing, progressive	Actively progressive: elongating and contracting	Actively progressive: coiling and recoiling	Lashing, progressive	Sluggish: coiling and twisting
Nuclei arrangement: posterior end	×2000	×2000	×2000	×2000	×2000	×2000
Appearance at anterior end	Blunt-rounded, one stylet	Blunt-rounded, two stylets	Blunt-rounded, no stylets	Blunt-rounded, one stylet	Broad and flat, one stylet	Blunt-rounded, enlarged, no stylets
Periodicity	Nocturnal	Nocturnal	Nonperiodic	Nonperiodic	Diurnal	Nonperiodic

Microfilaria. Essential features of the microfilariae. *A,* anal pore; *e.c.,* excretory cell; *e.p.,* excretory pore; and g_1, g_2, g_3, and g_4, first, second, third, and fourth genital cells. (From Raphael, S. S.: Lynch's Medical Laboratory Technology. 3rd ed. Philadelphia, W. B. Saunders Co., 1976.)

high-sensitivity densitometer used to detect variations in film optical density too faint to be detected by the human eye.

microdiffusion analysis a method of separating volatile substances from a biologic specimen. The most common type of microdiffusion apparatus is the Conway cell, a cylindric dish having a second, smaller cylindric dish fixed in the center.

In this procedure, the sample and any reagents needed to free the volatile substance are placed in the outer well. A solvent that has a high affinity for the volatile substance (or a reagent that will react with the volatile substance) is placed in the inner well, and a glass lid, covered with sealant, is placed on the cell. The volatile substance will evaporate into the air in the cell and then be dissolved, bound, or otherwise trapped by the substance in the inner well.

In some procedures, the reagent in the inner well identifies the volatile substance by undergoing a color change on reaction with it. In other procedures, however, the volatile substance is identified by further tests, such as chromatography or spectrophotometry.

microdrepanocytic (mi″kro-drep″ah-no-sit′ik) containing microcytic and drepanocytic elements, as in sickle cell–thalassemia disease.

microelectrophoresis (mi″kro-e-lek″tro-fo-re′sis) electrophoresis in which the motion of particles is directly observed by light microscopy.

microfarad (μF) (mi″kro-far′ad) a unit of electrical capacitance equal to one-millionth of a farad (10^{-6} F).

microfibril (mi″kro-fi′bril) one of the small protein filaments (about 11 nm in diameter) found in elastic fibers. These filaments are embedded in an amorphous protein substance, elastin.

microfiche (mi′kro-fēsh) a sheet of microfilm, usually 4 × 6 in. (10 × 15 cm), that contains microimages of printed matter.

microfilament (mi″kro-fil′ah-ment) a type of contractile filament found in most cells. Formed of actin, it is about 5 nm in diameter. Microfilaments support and move cell membranes and compose the contractile ring during mitosis. Cf. *tonofilament.*

microfilaremia (mi″kro-fil″ah-re′me-ah) the presence of microfilariae in the blood.

microfilaria (mi″kro-fi-la′re-ah) the embryo of the filarial worms (superfamily Filarioidea), which circulates in the blood or subcutaneous tissues, depending on the species. These embryos uncoil and become delicate, snakelike organisms. If the egg membrane remains intact, it is considered "sheathed"; if the membrane ruptures, however, an "unsheathed" microfilaria is set free. Other diagnostic characteristics include the arrangement of nuclei, their presence or absence at the tail tip, and body curves (whether graceful or irregular); see also the accompanying illustration. Various filariae that infect humans include *Wuchereria, Brugia, Mansonella, Loa, Dipetalonema,* and *Onchocerca.*

Laboratory diagnosis of filariasis consists of detecting the microfilariae in the blood by wet preparations and thick and thin blood films appropriately stained. Chances of detection may be increased by use of the filtration method. As the microfilariae of *Onchocerca* are rarely found in the blood, they are detected by aspiration of the nodules or by microscopic examination of skin shavings.

See also the accompanying table.

microfilariasis being infected with microfilariae.

microfilm (mi′kro-film) fine-grain photographic film, usually 16, 35, 70, or 105 mm, used to record microimages of printed matter.

microflora (mi″kro-flo′rah) the entire population of microorganisms present in or characteristic of a specific location. See also *normal flora.*

microgamete (mi″kro-gam′ēt) [*micro-* + Gr. *gametēs* spouse] the smaller of two conjugate gametes, regarded as the male, that is actively motile and fertilizes the macrogamete (female gamete) in anisogamy, e.g., in the sexual cycle of the malarial plasmodium.

microgametocyte (mi″kro-gah-me′to-sīt) [*micro-* + Gr. *gametēs* spouse + *kytos* hollow vessel] a cell, or immature sexual form of the male gamete, that produces microgametes by nuclear division. An example of this process is the maturation of the malarial microgametocyte in the mosquito by the extension of slender filaments of nuclear chromatin, which detach to form motile microgametes.

MICROFILARIA. TABLE OF MICROFILARIAE

Filariid	Disease	Distribution	Vectors	Microfilariae: *Sheath*	*Tail Nuclei*	*Periodicity**
Wuchereria bancrofti	Bancroftian and Malayan filariasis:	Worldwide 41°N to 28°S	Culicidae (mosquitos)	+	Not to tip	Nocturnal or nonperiodic
Brugia malayi	lymphangitis, hydrocele, elephantiasis	Oriental region to Japan	Culicidae (mosquitos)	+	Two distinct	Nocturnal or subperiodic
Loa loa	Loiasis; Calabar swellings; conjunctival worms	Western and Central Africa	*Chrysops,* deer fly, mango fly	+	Extend to tip	Diurnal
Onchocerca volvulus	Onchocerciasis: skin nodules, blindness, dermatitis	Africa, Central and South America	*Simulium,* buffalo gnat, black fly	–	Not to tip	Nonperiodic in skin fluids.
Dipetalonema (or *Acanthocheilonema*) *perstans*	Dipetalonemiasis or acanthocheilonemiasis (minor disturbances)	Africa and South America	*Culicoides,* biting midge	–	Extend to tip	Nocturnal or diurnal or nonperiodic
Dipetalonema streptocerca	Usually nonpathogenic	Western and Central Africa	*Culicoides*	–	Extend to tip	In skin only
Mansonella ozzardi	Ozzard's mansonelliasis (benign), occasionally hydrocele	Central and South America	*Culicoides*	–	Not to tip	Nonperiodic

* Microfilariae are found in peripheral blood (in blood smear) only at night (nocturnal periodicity), largely at night or during crepuscular hours (subperiodicity), largely during daylight hours (diurnal periodicity), or without clear distinction (nonperiodic). Periodicity appears to be correlated with the bloodsucking habits of the chief vector insect in the particular area of transmission of the filaria.
From Jawetz, E., et al.: Review of Medical Microbiology. 12th ed. Los Altos, CA, Lange Medical Publications, 1976, p. 512.

microglioma (mi″kro-gli-o′mah) [*micro-* + Gr. *glia* glue + *ōma* a swelling] a tumor composed of microglial cells and their presumed precursors, cells of the reticuloendothelial system called reticulum cells that are distributed in the meningeal and perivascular spaces. Also called microgliomatosis, perivascular sarcoma, and reticulum cell sarcoma (of CNS).

microglobulin (mi″kro-glob′u-lin) a plasma globulin of low molecular weight.

β_2-microglobulin see *beta₂-microglobulin.*

microglossia (mi″kro-glos′e-ah) [*micro-* + Gr. *glōssa* tongue + *-ia*] a rare congenital malformation that results in an abnormally small tongue. The defect is usually associated with micrognathia.

micrognathia (mi″kro-na′the-ah) [*micro-* + Gr. *gnathos* jaw + *-ia*] underdevelopment of the jaw.

microgram (μg) (mi′kro-gram) a unit of mass equal to one-millionth of a gram (10^{-6} g, 10^{-9} kg).

micrograph (mi′kro-graf) [*micro-* + Gr. *graphein* to write] the photograph of a minute object or specimen (such as tissues) as seen through a microscope. Also called *photomicrograph.*

microhematocrit (mi″kro-he-mat′o-krit) a hematocrit obtained using a small specimen of blood in a capillary tube.

microhenry (μH) (mi′kro-hen″re) a unit of inductance equal to one-millionth of a henry (10^{-6} H).

microhm (μΩ) (mi′krōm) a unit of electrical resistance equal to one-millionth of an ohm (10^{-6} Ω).

microhomology (mi″kro-ho-mol′o-je) in microbiology, the similarity of the DNA sequence of homologous genes in related species, as demonstrated by DNA sequencing or by DNA hybridization methods. Microhomology is the most reliable basis for bacterial classification. There is also high correlation between the presence of large common nucleotide sequences and the capacity of two strains for genetic recombination. Cf. *macrohomology.*

microincineration (mi″kro-in-sin″er-a′shun) the incineration of minute specimens of tissue or other substances to identify the elements that remain in the ash.

microinfarct (mi″kro-in′farkt) an infarct due to the obstruction of an arteriole or capillary.

microinjection (mi″kro-in-jek′shun) the infusion of very small amounts of fluid or drugs into animals or humans.

microinjector (mi″kro-in-jek′tor) an instrument for infusion of very small amounts of fluid or drugs into animals or humans.

microinvasion (mi″kro-in-va′zhun) the microscopic (i.e., limited) extension (invasion) of malignant cells from a carcinoma in situ into the underlying stroma.

microinvasive carcinoma (mi″cro-in-va′siv) a term generally used for an in situ carcinoma of the uterine cervix that exhibits limited extension (invasion) into the underlying stroma, and the depth of penetration does not exceed 5 mm (some limit use of the term to tumors with invasion less than 3 mm and others to less than 2 mm).

microliter (μl) (mi'kro-le"ter) a unit of volume equal to one-millionth of a liter (10^{-6} l, 10^{-9} m^3, 1 mm^3).

microlithiasis (mi"kro-lĭ-thi'ah-sis) [*micro-* + Gr. *lithos* stone + *-iasis*] the formation of minute mineralized concretions within the parenchymal substance of an organ.

micromelia (mi"kro-me'le-ah) [*micro-* + Gr. *melos* limb + *-ia*] the congenital malformation that results in abnormally short limbs with all bone segments present.

micrometer 1. (mi'kro-me"ter) (μm) one-millionth of a meter (10^{-6} m, 10^{-3} mm)

2. (mi-krom'ĕ-ter) any of the ruled measuring scales, or instruments containing them, that are used in micrometry.

micromethod (mi"kro-meth'od) a chemical method in which the quantity of a substance (specimen) to be analyzed is much smaller than that used in customary methods (e.g., less than 100 mg or less than 100 μl). For very small quantities, the term ultramicromethod is often used.

micrometry (mi-krom'ĕ-tre) [*micro-* + Gr. *metron* measure] the measurement of small objects using a microscope. A micrometer eyepiece superimposes a ruled scale on the image. The size of each scale division is previously determined from the image of a ruled (a stage micrometer) that has accurately calibrated divisions. Photomicrographs of an object and stage micrometer at the same magnification can be compared by measuring with a ruler.

micromicro- (μμ) (mi"kro-mi'kro) a prefix word element formerly attached to units of measurement to denote a unit that was one-trillionth of the basic unit, e.g., micromicrofarad (μμF); see *pico-*.

micromole (μmol) (mi'kro-mōl) a unit of amount of substance equal to one-millionth of a mole (10^{-6} mol).

Micromonosporaceae (mi"kro-mo-nos"po-ra'se-e) [*micro-* + Gr. *monos* single + *spores* seed + *aceae* family] a family of microorganisms of the order Actinomycetales, consisting of gram-positive, spore-forming, generally aerobic organisms that tend to grow slowly and form branching filaments. The family contains six genera, two of which (*Micropolyspora* and *Thermoactinomyces*) contain the organisms responsible for the disease called farmer's lung.

micron (mi'kron), (μ), pl. *microns, micra* [Gr. *mikron* a little] the former term for a micrometer, 10^{-6} m.

micronucleus (mi"kro-nu'kle-us), pl. *micronuclei* [*micro-* + L. *nucleus*, dim. of *nux* nut] 1. the smaller "germ line" nucleus as distinct from the vegetative macronucleus found in ciliates.

2. a nuclear membrane-bound chromosome or small group of chromosomes induced by disrupting the mitotic spindle in a mammalian cell. See also *cellular h.* under *hybridization.*

microorganism (mi"kro-or'gan-izm) a microscopic organism. Those of medical interest are bacteria, rickettsiae, viruses, fungi, and protozoa.

microphthalmia (mi"krof-thal'me-ah) [*micro-* + Gr. *ophthalmos* eye + *-ia*] a congenital malformation that results in an abnormally small eye due to the abnormal development of the optic vesicle into the optic cup. Microphthalmia can occur as part of a hereditary condition or can result from intrauterine infections such as rubella, cytomegalovirus, or syphilis.

micropipet (mi"kro-pi-pet') a pipet for handling small quantities of liquids (up to 0.1 ml).

Micropolyspora (mi"kro-pol"e-spo'ra) [*micro-* + Gr. *poly* many + *sporos* seed] a genus of microorganisms of the family Micromonosporaceae, order Actinomycetales. One of the actinomycetes, the genus consists of gram-positive organisms occurring in branching filaments and forming a mycelium that produces spores.

M. faeni, a species that forms substrate and aerial mycelium and colonies that change from colorless to orange to brown, bearing short chains of spores. The organism is thermophilic and is the principal cause of farmer's lung. Formerly called *Thermopolyspora polyspora.*

micropredation (mi"kro-pre-da'shun) the derivation by an organism of elements required for its existence without causing injury to its host.

micropredator (mi"kro-pred'ah-tor) [*micro-* + L. *praedator* a plunderer, pillager] an organism that derives its nourishments from another organism, usually larger than itself, without causing injury to that organism.

microprobe (mi'kro-prōb) 1. a minute probe, such as that used in microsurgery.

2. an instrument used to perform the chemical analysis of a microscopic specimen. In the procedure, an electron beam is focused on an area about 1 μm in diameter, and the characteristic x-rays emitted are analyzed by an x-ray spectrometer. The x-ray spectrum and the intensity of the spectral lines are used to quantitate the elements present. See also *analytical e. m.* under *electron microscope.*

microprocessor (mi"kro-pros'es-or) a general-purpose digital computer on a single integrated circuit chip. It is the basic component of microcomputers and "smart" microprocessor-controlled instruments.

microprogram (mi"kro-pro'gram) a program that performs complicated operations in response to one instruction. Microprograms are changed only by the manufacturer and appear to the user as part of the hardware.

micropyle (mi'kro-pīl) [*micro-* + Gr. *pylē* gate] the small opening through which the spermatozoon, the mature male germ cell, enters the ovum in sporozoa and arthropods.

microroentgen (μR) (mi"kro-rent'gen) a unit of exposure dose of x-rays or gamma rays equal to one-millionth of a roentgen (10^{-6} R).

microscope (mi'kro-skōp) [*micro-* + Gr. *skopein* to view] an instrument that provides an enlarged and detailed image of small structures. The light or optical microscope consists of a frame or body that supports the magnifying tube with its lenses, the specimen stage, a condenser to focus light on the specimen, and the source of illumination.

The magnifying tube usually has two compound lenses to magnify the image: an ocular (paired on binocular instruments) and an objective (multiple on most instruments, with as many as five objectives of different powers mounted on a rotating turret). Most oculars provide a magnification of 10× or 15×, and a wide-angle ocular provides an expanded field of view. Objectives range in power from 2.5× to 100× on most microscopes; the highest-power objectives require the use of immersion oil between specimen and lens. Magnification is the product of the powers of objective and ocular, unless an additional lens is located in the tube of the microscope, in which case the magnification is the product of the powers of all three lenses. In photomicrography, in which a camera is positioned above an ocular, some correction for tube length is necessary.

The specimen is usually laid on a glass slide positioned on the microscope stage; it can be held in position by clamps and moved in a horizontal plane by mechanical controls, although most surgical pathologists do this by hand. The condenser is located between the stage and the source of illumination, which is generally a tungsten or halogen bulb.

See also the accompanying illustration.

binocular m., a microscope having two oculars.

color-contrast m., a microscope similar to a darkfield microscope, except that the background is one color and the object another. Also called Rheinberg microscope.

comparison m.'s, two matched microscopes, the eyepieces of which are replaced by a comparison eyepiece that produces a split image with half the field of view from each microscope, allowing the side-by-side comparison of objects.

compound m., a microscope having both objective and ocular lenses. Cf. *simple m.*

darkfield m., a microscope that illuminates the object only from oblique angles, so that it appears bright against a dark background. It is used on unstained specimens and is the preferred method of identifying spirochetes. Also called *darkground m.*

darkground m., see *darkfield m.*

electron m., see *electron microscope.*

fluorescent m., a modified light microscope in which light that has been absorbed by the specimen and reemitted at another wavelength is transmitted through the eyepiece. Appropriate filters are used to select the correct wavelength of incoming beam (excitation filter) to excite the fluorescent compound and to remove the unwanted incident wavelengths from the fluorescent light emitted by the specimen (barrier filter). The light sources most often employed in fluorescent microscopy are halogen-quartz lamps, mercury arcs, and xenon arcs.

Fluorescent microscopy employing epi-illumination (vertical illuminator and dichroic mirror), in which the excitation beam is focused directly on the specimen through the lens objective, offers a number of advantages over fluorescence microscopy using transmitted illumination.

Some biologic molecules that are naturally fluorescent, such as vitamin A, can be studied with fluorescence microscopy, but the technique is more commonly used with fluorescent dyes (e.g., quinacrine, used in karyotyping, or isothiocyanates, used to label antibodies to particular microorganisms).

See also *immunofluorescence techniques.*

infrared m., a microscope in which radiation of

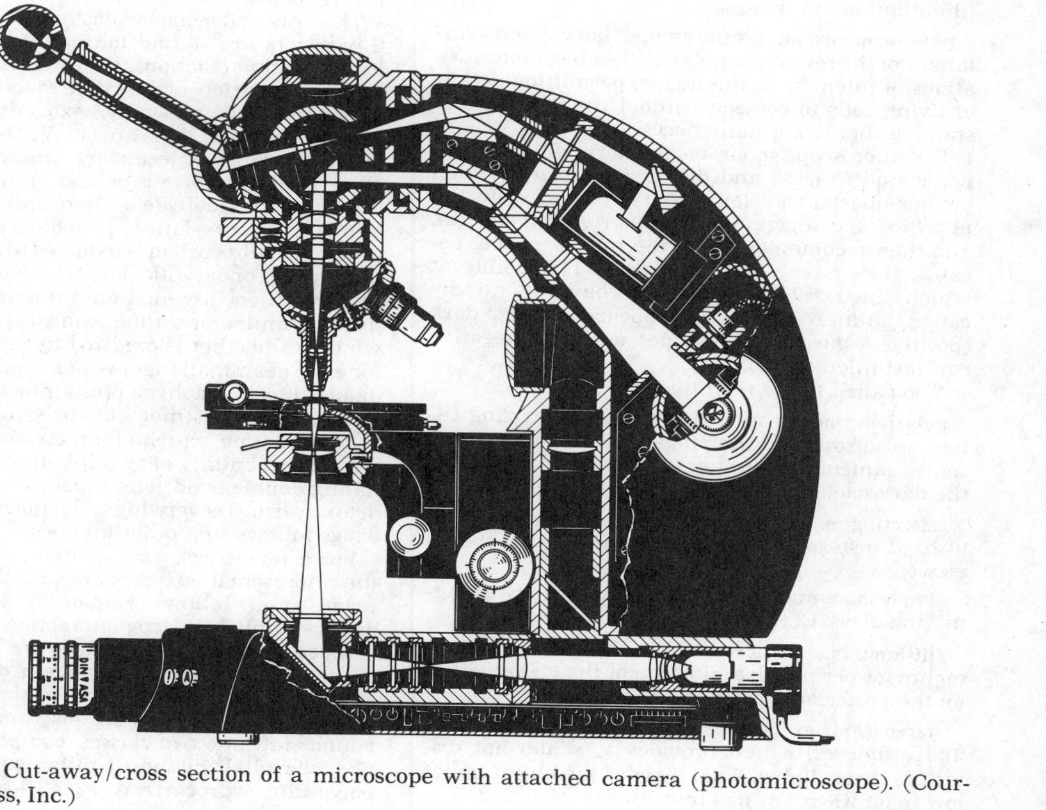

Microscope. Cut-away/cross section of a microscope with attached camera (photomicroscope). (Courtesy of Carl Zeiss, Inc.)

800 mμ or longer wavelength is used as the image-forming energy.

integrating m., a microscope in which a special mechanical stage permits recording of the sizes of the components of the specimen.

interference m., a microscope that converts optical path differences in the object to intensity differences in the image. This is accomplished by interference between light that passes through the object and light that passes through an empty region of the slide. The image produced is similar but superior to that in a phase-contrast microscope.

laser m., a microscope in which a laser beam is utilized to vaporize a minute area of tissue, as in a biopsy specimen, which is then subjected to emission spectrography.

light m., a microscope in which the specimen is viewed under visible light. Also called optical microscope.

Nomarski m., an interference microscope that produces a relief image of a reflecting surface. The image is produced by interference between a reference beam and a light beam reflected from the surface, and is not affected by variations in the refractive index of the surface.

operating m., a microscope employed in the performance of delicate surgical procedures, as in operations on the middle ear, on blood vessels, or in some operations on a vocal cord.

Oto-Microscope, trademark for an operating microscope especially devised to improve visualization of the surgical field in operations on the ear, providing both magnification of the structures and illumination of the area.

phase-contrast m., a microscope that converts variations of the refractive index in the object into variations of intensity in the image, permitting details of living cells to be seen without the fixation and staining that is normally necessary.

The microscope separates the normally superimposed undiffracted and diffracted images (which are one-quarter wavelength out of phase), shifts the phase of one image another quarter wavelength, and then recombines them; the images cancel because they have opposite phases. The points at which the refractive index is changing rapidly cause the most diffraction, appearing either dark (positive contrast microscope) or light (negative contrast microscope).

Also called phase microscope.

polarizing m., a microscope with polarizing filters; anisotropic (or birefringent) materials, such as some filaments and proteins, appear to glow against the dark background.

reflecting m., a microscope in which mirrors are utilized instead of lenses to form the image that is viewed.

simple m., a microscope with only one lens; a magnifying glass. Cf. *compound m.*

slit-lamp m., a microscope in which a special attachment permits examination of the endothelium on the posterior surface of the cornea.

stereoscopic m., a microscope with two objectives and eyepieces, which provides a (somewhat distorted) three-dimensional view of the object under low magnification (less than 40×).

trinocular m., a microscope in which a third eyepiece is used for photomicrography or for other uses.

ultraviolet m., a microscope that uses ultraviolet light. It requires quartz lenses and photographic imaging because of the damaging effect ultraviolet light can have on the eyes. Although resolution is better than with visible light microscopes, the primary benefit of this type of microscope is the localization of nucleic acids and some proteins by their characteristic ultraviolet absorption.

x-ray m., a microscope in which a beam of x-rays is used instead of light, the image usually being reproduced on film.

microscopic (mi″kro-skop′ik) 1. too small to be seen with the unaided eye.

2. pertaining to a microscope.

microscopy (mi-kros′ko-pe) [*micro-* + Gr. *skopein* to examine] 1. the use of a microscope.

2. the techniques involved in microscopic observations.

microsecond (μs, μsec) (mi′kro-sek″und) a unit of time equal to one-millionth of a second (10^{-6} sec).

microsomal antibodies see *thyroid microsomal antibodies.*

microsomal enzyme system a group of enzymes located primarily in the smooth endoplasmic reticulum of the liver but also in the kidneys and gastrointestinal epithelium. The enzymes are isolated in microsomes produced by fractionation of liver homogenates. The major component is a group of mixed-function oxidases that require NADPH and O_2. The terminal enzymes in the microsomal enzyme system are cytochrome P_{450} and cytochrome P_{450} reductase.

The only endogenous substances metabolized by this system are steroid hormones, which undergo hydroxylation reactions. However, the system is involved in a variety of oxidative reactions that detoxify many drugs and other exogenous substances. Among these reactions are (1) *N*-, *O*-, and *S*-dealkylation, in which a secondary amine ether or thioether is split to form a primary amine, alcohol, or thiol plus an aldehyde or ketone; (2) aromatic and aliphatic hydroxylation, in which an aromatic or aliphatic hydrocarbon is oxidized to a phenol or primary or secondary alcohol; (3) *N*-oxidation, an *N*-hydroxylation in which an amine is oxidized to a hydroxylamine or amine oxide; (4) *S*-oxidation, in which a thioether is oxidized to a sulfoxide or sulfone; (5) deamination, in which a primary amine is oxidized to an aldehyde plus ammonia; (6) desulfuration, in which a thiol is oxidized to an alcohol; and (7) epoxidation, in which an epoxide is formed by electrophilic attack of an aliphatic or aromatic resonating double bond. The capacity of this system to detoxify drugs is very high; the inactivation of most drugs follows first-order kinetics.

For a few drugs, e.g., phenytoin and dicumarol, the microsomal enzymes are rate-limiting and the inactivation follows zero-order kinetics. These drugs exhibit drug-drug interaction due to substrate competition. Many substances are potent inducers of the microsomal enzyme system, causing proliferation of the endoplasmic reticulum and increased synthesis of microsomal enzymes. These compounds fall into two classes: compounds similar to phenobarbital and those similar to the carcinogenic polycyclic hydrocarbons, e.g., 3,4-benzpyrene. Significant decreases of the plasma half-life of many drugs inactivated by microsomal enzymes can be caused by exposure to other drugs (e.g., phenobarbital or warfarin) or to xenobiotics in cigarette smoke or to chlorinated hydrocarbon pesticides.

Another important group of microsomal enzymes are the glucuronyltransferases, which catalyze the formation of glucuronide conjugates of many phenols, alcohols, and carboxylic acids, with UDP-glucuronate serving as the donor. The glucuronides are rapidly excreted in the urine and bile. The conjugates of certain drugs excreted by this mechanism can be hydrolyzed by β-glucuronidases in the intestines, allowing the free drug to be reabsorbed and thus prolonging a drug's half-life.

microsomal thyroid antibody see *antithyroid antibody.*

microsome (mi'kro-sōm) [*micro-* + Gr. *sōma* body] a small, membrane-bound vesicle experimentally produced by the disruption of cells. Microsomes are formed from fragments of endoplasmic reticulum and are separated from other cell debris by centrifugation. The microsomes contain the microsomal enzymes, which are embedded in the membrane of the endoplasmic reticulum and cannot be removed without losing their activity.

microsphere (mi-kro-sfēr') see under *spherocyte.*

microspore (mi'kro-spōr) [*micro-* + Gr. *sporos* seed] 1. the smaller of two types of spores produced by certain fungi and protozoa.

2. the smaller of the spores produced by heterosporous plants, from which the male gametophyte develops, e.g., pollen of seed plants.

Microsporum (mi-kros'po-rum) [*micro-* + Gr. *sporos* seed] a genus of fungi that is dermatophytic and may be the etiologic agent of ringworm (tinea barbae, tinea capitis, tinea corporis, or tinea favosa). It can invade hair follicles with an ectothrix type of infection. This fungus is characterized by macroaleuriospores (macroconidia), which are two- to several-celled, fusiform, and spindle-shaped with a rough, thickened cell wall, and microaleuriospores (microconidia), which are one-celled, sessile, clavate, and stalked. See also the various *tineas.*

microstomia (mi"kro-sto'me-ah) [*micro-* + Gr. *stoma* mouth + *-ia*] the condition of having an abnormally small mouth opening.

microtome (mi'kro-tōm) [*micro-* + Gr. *tomē* a cut] an instrument used to cut thin sections of tissue for histologic study; it is a steel, glass, or diamond knife held by clamps at the correct cutting angle. Sections are cut as the tissue, embedded in a block of paraffin, celloidin, or plastic, is moved past the fixed knife edge.

cold m., a standard rotary microtome, mounted in a refrigerated case, which is held at a very low temperature (about –20°C) for cutting frozen sections. An antiroll device, a plastic plate positioned parallel to the knife surface to keep the section from curling, is attached to the knife. See also *cryostat.*

freezing m., a microtome with the block mounted on a chuck into which liquid carbon dioxide is piped, thereby freezing the tissue block. The knife is moved back and forth as the chuck is raised to cut succeeding sections.

rocker m., a microtome on which the block is mounted on a rocker arm that moves past the knife. It performs like a rotary microtome, except that the sections are slightly curved.

rotary m., the type of microtome commonly used for cutting paraffin sections. A cut is made by each turn of a flywheel.

sliding m., the type of microtome used for cutting celloidin sections and large sections. Sections are cut as a sledge holding the block is pushed past the knife.

microtome knife any of the devices with a thin, sharpened edge used to cut histologic sections. The knives typically are made of metal, glass, or diamond.

Wedge-shaped metal knives with a wedge angle of 15° are most commonly used in light microscopy. When sharpened, these knives present a cutting edge with a circle of radius of 0.25 μm and can cut sections as thin as 3 μm.

Glass and diamond knives are used for cutting the ultrathin sections necessary for electron microscopy. Knives can be made of any type of glass, but hardened plate glass 0.7 cm thick is preferred. A trough filled with water or a water-acetone mixture is fixed to the glass or diamond knife so that thin sections can float away from the cutting surface. Diamond knives are generally used for high-volume sectioning or for cutting especially hard specimens; they are available commercially and are expensive, but with careful use they can provide long service, and sharpening is generally possible.

microtubule (mi"kro-tu'būl) a cylindric structure, 20–27 nm in diameter, found in many types of cells. It is composed of protein subunits about 4 nm in diameter called tubulin.

Microtubules make up part of the cytoskeleton, holding the shape of some cells, such as platelets. Mitotic spindle fibers are microtubules, and the fibrils of a cilium are modified microtubules. Microtubules are also found in the processes of neurons, where they are believed to facilitate axoplasmic transport.

microunit (mi'kro-u"nit) 1. (symbol μU), a unit of enzyme activity equal to one-millionth of an International Unit (10^{-6} U).

2. (symbol μIU), a unit of biologic activity equal to one-millionth of an International Unit.

microvilli (mi"kro-vil'i) [pl. of *microvillus* a tuft of hair] the protrusions from the free surface of many epithelial cells, which increase the surface area of the cell membrane and thus the efficiency of absorption. They are about 80–90 nm in diameter and 0.5–1 μm long. The thousands of microvilli covering the surface of a cell are called the brush (or striated) border. See also *stereocilia.*

microvolt (μV) (mi'kro-vōlt) a unit of electric potential (voltage) equal to one-millionth of a volt (10^{-6} V).

microwatt (μW) (mi'kro-wot) a unit of power equal to one-millionth of a watt (10^{-6} W).

microwave (mi'kro-wāv) pertaining to radio (electromagnetic) waves in the frequency range of 1–100 GHz (about 1–1000 mm in wavelength).

Micrurus (mi-kroo'rus) a genus of venomous snakes of which the species *M. fulvius* is the coral snake; see also *snakebite.*

micturate (mik'tu-rāt) see *urinate.*

micturition (mik"tu-rish"un) [L. *micturire* to urinate] see *urination.*

midaxillary line the vertical line that passes through the center of the armpit midway between the anterior and posterior axillary lines. Also called *axillary line*.

midbody (mid′bod-e) 1. a mass of granules developed in the equatorial region of the spindle during the anaphase of mitosis.

2. the middle region of the trunk.

midbrain (mid′brān) see *mesencephalon*.

midcapacity (mid″kah-pas′ĭ-te) the volume of the lungs that is ventilated under resting conditions. It is equal to half the tidal volume plus the functional residual capacity.

midclavicular line (mid″klah-vik′u-lar) a vertical line passing through the midpoint of one of the clavicles; alternatively, a mamillary line. See also *lateral sagittal plane*.

midcoronal plane (mid″ko-ro′nal) the vertical plane passing through the middle of the body from side to side (perpendicular to the midsagittal plane) and thus passing through the coronal suture of the skull.

Middlebrook 7H10 agar (mid″l-bruk) [G. *Middlebrook*, U.S. pathologist, born 1915] see *Middlebrook 7H10 a.* under *agar*.

middle ear see *tympanic cavity*.

middle lobe syndrome a form of chronic atelectasis of the right lung characterized by infection and collapse of the middle lobe of the lung due to bronchial compression and obstruction, often by enlarged surrounding lymph nodes. This condition is diagnosed by chest radiography and physical findings; bronchoscopy and bronchography may be necessary to rule out tumors and foreign bodies. A severe, nonproductive cough may be present, and a diminished lung capacity is seen.

midge (mij) a small, delicate insect of the order Diptera, family Ceratopogonidae. Several species give painful bites; some species of the genus *Culicoides* are blood suckers and known intermediate hosts of certain filarial worms that are parasitic in humans. See also *gnat*.

midgut (mid′gut) 1. in the developing embryo, a region that opens into the yolk sac between the foregut and the hindgut.

2. the developmental intestinal loop of the embryo, at approximately the sixth week, which later produces the distal duodenum, jejunum, ileum, and ascending and transverse colon.

midposition (mid″po-zĭ′shun) the position of the lungs and chest wall at end-tidal expiration, or at functional residual capacity.

midsagittal plane (mid-saj′ĭ-tal) the vertical plane passing from front to back through the middle of the body. Also called median plane and median sagittal plane.

midsternal line (mid-ster′nal) the line that passes down the middle of the sternum from the suprasternal notch to the xiphoid.

midsystolic click-murmur syndrome see *mitral valve prolapse syndrome*.

Miescheria (me-she′re-ah) [Johann Friedrich *Miescher*, Swiss pathologist, 1811–1887] see *Sarcocystis*.

MIF abbrev. for melanocyte-stimulating hormone–inhibiting factor (see *melanocyte-stimulating hormone–release-inhibiting hormone*); *migration inhibition factor*.

migraine (mi′grān) [Fr., from Gr. *hēmikrania* pain on one side of the head] see *migraine h.* under *headache*.

migrainous neuralgia see *cluster h.* under *headache*.

migration (mi-gra′shun) [L. *migratio*, from *migrare* to migrate] 1. a mass movement of animals or plants; see *gene flow*.

2. the movement of leukocytes through the intact walls of blood vessels. Also called *diapedesis*.

3. the bulk movement of charged particles in electrophoresis.

4. the movement of symptoms from site to site.

migration inhibition factor (MIF) a type of lymphokine that is released from a sensitized lymphocyte after contact with antigen that prevents the migration of macrophage; M.W. 25,000. MIF is produced 4–6 hr after a lymphocyte is stimulated by antigen, and can continue to be secreted for up to 4 da as long as antigenic stimulation is present. MIF alters the membrane of a macrophage so that several macrophages aggregate; this aggregation is thought to prevent cellular motility. Also called *macrophage migration inhibition factor*. See also *lymphokines*. Cf. *macrophage activation factor*.

Mikulicz's syndrome (mik′u-lich″ez) [Johann von *Mikulicz*-Radecki, Polish surgeon, 1850–1905] a chronic, benign, and usually painless swelling of the parotid, salivary, and lacrimal glands. It is often accompanied by chronic lymphocytic infiltration. The cause of this syndrome is unknown, but it is seen in association with Sjögren's syndrome, tuberculosis, sarcoidosis, lupus, leukemia, and lymphoma.

miliaria (mil″e-a′re-ah) [L. *milium* millet] a skin eruption due to blockage of the sweat glands.

m. profunda, a form of miliaria in which the sweat is trapped in the middermis, producing nonpruritic inflammatory papules.

m. rubra, a form of miliaria in which the sweat escapes into the epidermis, producing redness and itching. Also called prickly heat.

miliary (mil′e-er″e) [L. *miliaris* like a millet seed] resembling millet seeds. This term is often used to describe a form of acute tuberculosis in which the causative organisms are seeded to various organs through the blood, forming minute, millet seed–like tubercles in many organs. See also *tuberculosis*.

milium (mil′e-um), pl. *milia* [L. "millet seed"] small, white, spheroidal nodules that usually occur in the skin of the face. They are masses of lamellated keratin and sebaceous material, often seen in association with hair follicles. Also called *whitehead*.

milk (milk) [L. *lac*] 1. a nutrient fluid produced by the mammary glands of many animals for nourishment of the young.

2. a liquid (emulsion or suspension) that resembles the secretion of the mammary gland.

milk alkali syndrome a syndrome characterized by the excessive ingestion of milk products, antacids with calcium, or other absorbable alkali, leading to a systemic alkalosis. Blood calcium levels are raised and urinary calcium levels are lowered. Alkalosis contributes to the deposition of calcium in abnormal locations, including the kidneys, with resultant renal failure. This syndrome may disappear after milk and alkali intake is withdrawn.

milkers' nodules hard, circumscribed nodules on

the hands of persons who milk cows affected with cowpox.

milk-leg iliofemoral thrombosis, a condition characterized by an increase in the number and adhesiveness of platelets and by increases in the levels of several clotting factors, often encountered in the period after labor. This venous thrombus may be diagnosed by venography, ultrasound, and plethysmography. Also called phlegmasia alba dolens (painful white leg). See also *thrombosis.*

Milkman's syndrome (milk′manz) [Louis Arthur *Milkman*, American roentgenologist, 1895–1951] a generalized bone disease that is a special form of osteomalacia. This disorder is characterized by multiple, bilateral, symmetric stripes of absorption in various long and flat bones. X-rays reveal pseudofractures that represent shadows of calluses near arterial vessels that traverse and erode the soft skeleton. See also *osteomalacia.*

milli- (m) (mil′ĭ) [Fr. *mille* thousand] a prefix word element attached to units of measurement to denote a unit that is one-thousandth of the basic unit (10^{-3} unit).

milliammeter (mil″e-am′ĕ-ter) an ammeter for measuring current in milliamperes, i.e., current less than 1 ampere. See also *volt-ohm-milliammeter.*

milliamperage (mil″e-am′per-ij) the current supplied to an instrument, as, for example to an x-ray tube, measured in milliamperes (mA). This controls the quantity of x-rays produced; the penetrability is controlled by the kilovoltage and the filters.

milliampere (mA) (mil″e-am′pēr) [Fr.] a unit of electric current equal to one-thousandth of an ampere.

milliampere-second (mA-s) in radiology, a measure of relative exposure; the product of the milliamperage of the x-ray beam and the exposure time.

millibar (mbar) (mil′ĭ-bar) a unit of pressure equal to one-thousandth of a bar, or 0.1 kilopascal (kPa), or 100 newtons per square meter.

millicoulomb (mC) (mil″ĭ-koo′lom) a unit of electric charge equal to one-thousandth of a coulomb (10^{-3} C).

millicurie (mCi) (mil″ĭ-ku′re) a unit of radioactivity equal to one-thousandth of a curie (10^{-3} Ci).

millicurie-hour (mCi-hr) (mil″ĭ-ku′re-owr″) a unit of cumulated activity equal to one-thousandth of a curie-hour.

milliequivalent (mEq) (mil″ĭ-e-kwiv′ah-lent) a unit of amount of substance equal to one-thousandth of an equivalent.

millifarad (mF) (mil″ĭ-far′ad) a unit of electrical capacitance equal to one-thousandth of a farad (10^{-3} F).

milligram (mg) (mil′ĭ-gram) a unit of mass equal to one-thousandth of a gram (10^{-3} g, 10^{-6} kg).

millihenry (mH) (mil′ĭ-hen″re) a unit of inductance equal to one-thousandth of a henry (10^{-3} H).

millilambert (mL) (mil″ĭ-lam′bert) a unit of luminance (photometric brightness) equal to one-thousandth of a lambert (10^{-3} L).

milliliter (ml) (mil′ĭ-le″ter) a unit of volume equal to one-thousandth of a liter (10^{-3} l, 10^{-6} m^3, 1 cm^3).

millimeter (mm) (mil′ĭ-me″ter) a unit of length equal to one-thousandth of a meter (10^{-3} m), about 0.03937 in.

millimeter of mercury (mmHg) a unit of pressure, 133.32239 pascal (Pa), equal to the pressure exerted by a 1-mm column of mercury under standard conditions. This unit is commonly used for measurements of pressure in medicine, e.g., partial pressure of carbon dioxide and blood pressure, although recommendations have been made that the SI unit, the pascal, be used.

millimicro- (mμ) (mil″ĭ-mi′kro) a prefix word element formerly attached to units of measurement to denote a unit that was one-billionth of the basic unit, e.g., millimicrofarad (mμF); see *nano-.*

millimole (mmol) (mil′ĭ-mōl) a unit of amount of substance equal to one-thousandth of a mole (10^{-3} mol).

milliosmole (mOsm) (mil″ĭ-os′mōl) a unit of amount of substance equal to one-thousandth of an osmole (10^{-3} Osm).

millirad (mrad) (mil′ĭ-rad) a unit of absorbed dose of ionizing radiation equal to one-thousandth of a rad (10^{-3} rad).

millirem (mrem) (mil′ĭ-rem) a unit of absorbed dose of ionizing radiation equal to one-thousandth of a rem (10^{-3} rem).

milliroentgen (mR) (mil′ĭ-rent″gen) a unit of exposure dose of x-rays or gamma rays equal to one-thousandth of a roentgen (10^{-3} R).

milliroentgens per milliampere-second a unit used to measure the radiation dose to the patient per unit of x-ray exposure for a specified combination of kilovoltage, tube type, and focal-skin distance.

millisecond (ms, msec) (mil″ĭ-sek′ond) a unit of time equal to one-thousandth of a second (10^{-3} sec).

milliunit (mil′ĭ-u″nit) 1. (symbol mU), a unit of enzyme activity equal to one-thousandth of an International Unit (10^{-3} U).

2. (symbol mIU), a unit of biologic activity equal to one-thousandth of an International Unit.

millivolt (mV) (mil′ĭ-vōlt) a unit of electric potential (voltage) equal to one-thousandth of a volt (10^{-3} V).

milliwatt (mW) (mil′ĭ-wat) a unit of power equal to one-thousandth of a watt (10^{-3} W).

Millon's reagent (mil′onz) [Auguste N.E. *Millon*, French chemist, 1812–1867] a solution of mercuric nitrate and nitric acid. It reacts with various phenols and phenolic acids (such as tyrosine) to give a color that is red or orange. Because most proteins contain tyrosine, the Millon reaction is a useful method to detect proteins. See also under *tyrosine assays.*

Milroy's disease (mil′royz) [William Forsyth *Milroy*, American physician, 1855–1942] a hereditary, essential lymphedema that occurs at birth and affects primarily the lower extremities. It is thought to be due to faulty lymph vessel development, resulting in lymph outflow obstruction and accumulation. Diagnosis may be aided by lymphangiography. See also *lymphedema.*

Miltown (mil′town) trademark. See *meprobamate.*

-mimetic (mi-met′ik) [Gr. *mimētikos* imitative] a suffix word element to denote mimic or copy, e.g., sympathomimetic.

min (min) abbrev. See *minute.*

Minamata disease (min″ah-mah′tah) [from *Minamata* Bay, Japan] the name for a neurologic disorder that affected many individuals who ingested aklyl mercury from Minamata Bay in Japan. The victims of this poisoning suffered severe mental impairment and often death; most had consumed seafood contaminated with mercury from the bay.

mince (mins) 1. a preparation of fresh tissue used for in vitro metabolic studies, consisting of whole and broken cells. The mince is prepared by chopping a small piece of tissue or organ with a sharp blade.

2. to chop up into very small pieces.

mineral (min′er-al) [L. *minerale*] 1. in chemistry, an imprecise term that denotes an inorganic substance (element, compound, mixture) that originates in the earth's crust or atmosphere. The term is also sometimes used inexactly to describe organic substances supposedly from nonliving sources, as in mineral oil.

2. in nutrition, an elemental essential nutrient. For the recommended daily allowance, see the accompanying table.

mineralization (min″er-al-ĭ-za′shun) the introduction of minerals into a structure, as in the normal mineralization of bones and teeth or the pathologic mineralization of tissues, e.g., dystrophic calcification and metastatic calcification.

mineral nutrients a number of elements considered essential in the diet. These are sometimes divided into the bulk minerals (macronutrients), present in the human body in large amounts (several moles) in bone (calcium, phosphorus, and magnesium) and as electrolytes (sodium, chloride, potassium, and magnesium); and the trace elements or prosthetic minerals, present in small amounts (millimoles or micromoles) in metalloproteins (iron, zinc, copper, manganese, iodine, cobalt, molybdenum, selenium, and chromium). Fluorine is another trace element essential to the development of teeth and bones. Other elements that may be required at extremely low concentrations are nickel, silicon, vanadium, and tin. For more information, see also the specific elements.

mineralocorticoid (min″er-al-o-kor′tĭ-koid) a corticosteroid hormone that is particularly effective in causing the retention of sodium and the loss of potassium in the body. All the corticosteroids, with the exception of the androgens, have this action, aldosterone being the most potent.

mineral oil [USP], a mixture of liquid hydrocarbons obtained from petroleum, with a specific gravity of 0.860–0.905, used as a levigating agent. It is also used as a lubricant, laxative, and vehicle for drugs. Also called heavy liquid petrolatum, liquid paraffin, liquidum petrolatum, and white mineral oil.

light m. o., [USP], a mixture of hydrocarbons obtained from petroleum, with a specific gravity of 0.818–0.880, used as a vehicle for drugs and also as a laxative. Also called light liquid paraffin, light liquid petrolatum, and light white mineral oil.

minicell (min′e-sel) 1. a nucleus surrounded by a thin ring of cytoplasm. Also called *karyoplast.* See also *cellular h.* under *hybridization.*

MINERAL. RECOMMENDED DAILY ALLOWANCES OF COMMON MINERALS

	Age	Weight (kg)	Height (cm)	Energy Yield (MJ)	Protein N (mmol)	Retinol Equiv. (μmol)	Calciferol Equiv. (nmol)	Tocopherol Equiv. (μmol)	Ascorbate (μmol)
Infants	0-6 mo	6	60	0.49/kg	23/kg	1.5	25	9	200
	6-12 mo	9	71	0.45/kg	23/kg	1.4	25	12	200
Children	1-3 yr	13	86	5.5	260	1.4	25	16	230
	4-6	20	110	7.5	340	1.8	25	16	230
	7-10	30	135	10.0	400	2.4	25	21	230
Men	11-14	44	158	11.7	500	3.5	25	28	260
	15-18	61	172	12.5	620	3.5	25	28	260
	19-22	67	172	12.5	620	3.5	25	35	260
	23-50	70	172	11.3	640	3.5		35	260
	51+	70	172	10.0	640	3.5		35	260
Women	11-14	44	155	10.0	500	2.8	25	23	260
	15-18	54	162	8.8	550	2.8	25	26	260
	19-22	58	162	8.8	530	2.8	25	28	260
	23-50	58	162	8.4	530	2.8		28	260
	51+	58	162	7.5	530	2.8		28	260
	Pregnant			+1.2	+340	3.5	25	35	340
	Lactating			+2.1	+230	4.2	25	35	450

Notes: In converting allowances made by the Food and Nutrition Board of the National Academy of Sciences to a molar basis, the increments between ages used by the Board have been translated to the closest molar increment. That is, an increase of 10 mg of a nutrient might be converted to the nearest 0.05-mmol increase. The Board's estimate for the protein allowance is on the basis of proteins with a 75 percent efficiency of utilization. The fat-soluble vitamin allowances have been translated to equivalent moles of retinol, calciferol, and α-tocopherol. The Board regards β-carotenes to be 1/6 as effective as retinol in providing vitamin A activity on a weight basis. Those carotenes in which only one-half of the molecule yield retinol are 1/12 as effective per unit weight. The nicotinate allowance is calculated on the basis of 1 μmol of nicotinate being equivalent to 36 μmol of tryptophan. The folate allowance is determined on the basis of a microbiologic assay of the foods, and less than one-quarter of the stated amounts given as pure folate will be equally effective.

2. a portion of the bacterial cell with no chromosomes, formed by septation near the tip of filaments.

minicomputer (min″e-kom-pu′ter) a general-purpose digital computer of medium size; often dedicated to one use, such as image processing for a CT scanner or scintillation camera. This is the size of computer commonly used as a laboratory computer.

minification (min″i-fĭ-ka′shun) the reduction of the size of an image relative to the size of the real object. In nuclear medicine, diverging collimators can be used to reduce the size of large organs to the detector size. Cf. *magnification.*

minimal bactericidal concentration (MBC) see *minimal lethal concentration.*

minimal inhibitory concentration (MIC) the lowest concentration of a given antibiotic that inhibits the growth of a specific organism. See also *antibacterial agent susceptibility testing.*

minimal lethal concentration (MLC) the lowest concentration of a given antibiotic that kills a specific organism. Also called *minimal bactericidal concentration.* See also *antibacterial agent susceptibility testing.*

minimum (min′i-mum), pl. *minima* [L. "smallest"] 1. the least possible effect or quantity or the lowest detectable limit.

2. in mathematics, the smallest value assumed by a function. Cf. *maximum.*

Minipress (min′e-pres) trademark. See *prazosin hydrochloride.*

minocycline (mĭ-no-si′klēn) a broad-spectrum tetracycline antibiotic used for prophylaxis against meningococcal meningitis. See also *antibacterial agents* and *tetracyclines.*

minor (mi′nor) smaller, or of less importance.

minor histocompatibility complex a number of genetic loci that code for the cell surface antigens responsible for slow rejection of grafts between individuals differing genetically at these loci but not at the major histocompatibility complex. The more loci that are different, the faster is the graft rejection. See also *histocompatibility, major histocompatibility complex,* and *transplantation.*

minor tranquilizer see *antianxiety drug.*

minoxidil (mĭ-noks′ĭ-dil) a powerful antihypertensive drug used for management of hypertension that is unresponsive to other drugs. It is a direct-acting peripheral vasodilator. Side-effects include fluid and sodium retention; pericardial effusion; increased heart rate; and the abnormal growth, thickening, and darkening of fine body hair. Trademark, Loniten.

minute (min′it) 1. (abbrev. min), a unit of time equal to 60 sec.

2. (symbol ′), a unit of angular measurement equal to one-sixtieth of a degree of arc.

miracidium (mi-rah-sid′e-um), pl. *miracidia* [Gr. *meirakidion* a boy, lad, stripling] the first-stage ciliated larva of digenetic trematodes or flukes, which requires further development in the body of a snail.

MIRD abbrev. See *Medical Internal Radiation Dose.*

Mirex trademark for a highly toxic chlorinated hydrocarbon insecticide, 1,1a,2,2a,3,3a,4,5,5,5a,5b,6-do-

MINERAL. (*Continued*)

FOLATE (*μmol*)	NICOTINATE EQUIV. (*μmol*)	RIBOFLAVIN (*μmol*)	THIAMINE (*μmol*)	PYRIDOXINE (*μmol*)	COBALAMIN (*nmol*)	CALCIUM (*mmol*)	PHOSPHATE (*mmol*)	IODINE (*μmol*)	IRON (*mmol*)	MAGNESIUM (*mmol*)	ZINC (*mmol*)
0.1	40	1.1	1.0	2.1	0.2	9	7.7	0.3	0.18	2.5	0.05
0.1	65	1.6	1.7	2.5	0.2	13.5	13	0.35	0.27	3.0	0.08
0.2	75	2.1	2.3	3.5	0.7	20	26	0.5	0.27	6.0	0.15
0.5	100	2.9	3.0	5.5	1.1	20	26	0.65	0.18	8.5	0.15
0.7	130	3.0	4.0	7	1.5	20	26	0.85	0.18	10.5	0.15
0.7	145	4.0	4.7	9.5	2.2	30	39	1.0	0.32	14.5	0.25
0.7	165	4.8	5.0	12	2.2	30	39	1.2	0.32	17.0	0.25
0.7	165	4.8	5.0	12	2.2	20	26	1.1	0.18	14.5	0.25
0.7	145	4.3	4.7	12	2.2	20	26	1.0	0.18	14.5	0.25
0.7	130	4.0	4.0	12	2.2	20	26	0.9	0.18	14.5	0.25
0.7	130	3.5	4.0	9.5	2.2	30	39	0.9	0.32	12.5	0.25
0.7	115	3.7	3.7	12	2.2	30	39	0.9	0.32	12.5	0.25
0.7	115	3.7	3.7	12	2.2	20	26	0.8	0.32	12.5	0.25
0.7	105	3.2	3.3	12	2.2	20	26	0.8	0.32	12.5	0.25
0.7	100	2.9	3.3	12	2.2	20	26	0.65	0.18	12.5	0.25
1.8	+20	+0.8	+1.0	15	3.0	30	39	1.0	0.32+	19.0	0.30
1.4	+35	+1.3	+1.0	15	3.0	30	39	1.2	0.29	19.0	0.40

The stated protein nitrogen allowance may be converted to grams of "protein" by multiplying by 0.0875. The fat-soluble vitamin allowances may be converted to International Units by multiplying by the following conversion factors: I.U. vitamin A = μmoles retinol × 950, I.U. vitamin D = nmoles calciferol × 16, I.U. vitamin E = μmoles tocopherol × 1.6.

The molar allowances for the other vitamins and the minerals can be converted to a weight basis by multiplying by the molecular weights: ascorbate = 176, folate = 441, riboflavin = 376, thiamine = 301, pyridoxine = 170, cobalamin = 1.355, calcium = 40, phosphate = 31 (as P), iodine = 127, iron = 55.6, magnesium = 24, zinc = 65.4.

Modified from McGilvery, R. W.: Biochemistry: A Functional Approach. Philadelphia, W. B. Saunders Co., 1979, pp. 822–823.

decachlorooctahydro-1,3,4-metheno-1*H*-cyclobuta-[*cd*]pentalene. It has been used to control the fire ant, but its use is now restricted. See also *chlorinated hydrocarbon pesticides.*

mirror (mir′or) [Fr. *miroir*] a polished surface that reflects sufficient light to yield images of objects in front of it.

mirror focus in electroencephalography, spike activity originally arising in a particular area of one cerebral hemisphere that can also be recorded in the homologous area of the contralateral hemisphere. This pattern is seen frequently in the interseizure recording from individuals with cortical epilepsy, particularly with discharges arising in the frontal or temporal lobes.

The amplitude of the mirrored activity may be equal to or smaller than that of the primary focus. The mirrored activity, which may initially result from activation of the commissural connections between the cerebral hemispheres or from activation of subcortical structures, may eventually become autonomous.

miscibility (mis″ĭ-bil′ĭ-te) the degree to which one substance is miscible in another; the concentration of a saturated solution. Also called *solubility.*

miscible (mis′ĭ-b′l) pertaining to solid, liquids, or gases that are soluble in each other. Cf. *immiscible.*

infinitely m., miscible in all proportions, as are all gas-gas solutions and some liquid-liquid (e.g., ethanol-water) and solid-solid (e.g., copper-nickel) solutions.

partially m., miscible only to a certain extent, the limit of miscibility. Within some range of proportions, a mixture of two partially miscible liquids shaken together will separate into two phases. each a saturated solution of one in the other.

mist (mist) 1. a large mass of water vapor at or just above the ground, like a fog but less dense.

2. a suspension of colloidal particles of water, other liquids, or microparticulates in air or some other gas. It may be made using some form of atomizer, or it may be formed in the atmosphere. Some mists persist; others settle out slowly. Mists of toxic chemicals, such as sulfuric acid, constitute an air pollution hazard.

3. a thin film of moisture condensed on a surface, such as a film or fine droplets on cuvets, lenses, etc.

mistranslation (mis″trans-la′shun) during protein synthesis, the insertion of an incorrect amino acid into a growing polypeptide chain. It may be a random effect due to environmental factors, or it may be caused by a mutation in a tRNA or aminoacyl-tRNA synthetase.

MIT abbrev. See *monoiodotyrosine.*

mit/o (mi′to) [Gr. *mitos* thread] a word element used in combining form to denote threadlike or a relationship to thread, e.g., mitochondria.

mite (mit) any arthropod of the order Acarina, except the ticks. The mites are minute, with either a transparent or semitransparent body, and are parasitic on humans. Many produce various skin irritations (ascariasis). See also the accompanying illustration.

mithramycin (mith″rah-mi′sin) [USP], an antineoplastic antibiotic produced by *Streptomyces plicatus,* used as a cancer chemotherapeutic drug. It binds to DNA and inhibits the synthesis of RNA associated with malignancy. Trademark, Mithracin. For more information, see *Appendix A.*

miticidal (mi″tĭ-si′dal) an agent destructive to mites.

miticide (mi′tĭ-sid) any chemical that kills or is destructive to mites.

mitochondria (mi″to-kon′dre-ah, mit″o-kon′dre-ah), pl. of *mitochondrion* [*mito-* + Gr. *chondrion* granule] organelles found in the cytoplasm of most eukaryotic cells. Each is composed of two concentric membranes, the inner forming a series of folds that partially subdivide the interior (matrix) into communicating compartments. They are ovoid or elongated and contain a small amount of DNA; they increase in number by a process of fission. Their numbers vary according to the metabolic requirements of the cell type.

Energy, stored in the high-energy phosphate bond of ATP, is produced in the mitochondria by the process of oxidative phosphorylation in which NADH, formed in the enzymatic degradation of carbohydrates, fatty acids, and other substances, is oxidized by O_2 coupled with the formation of ATP. Approximately half the energy content of food is not stored but is lost as heat. ATP is transported into the cytosol, where it is used to drive metabolic and biosynthetic processes, maintain membrane potentials, and produce motion. Many other metabolic processes, such as the tricarboxylic acid cycle and fatty acid oxidation, also occur in the mitochondria. Mitochondria are visible by light microscopy but are seen best with the transmission electron microscope.

mitochondrial antibody (mi″to-kon′dre-al) see *antimitochondrial antibody.*

mitochondrial myopathy a heterogeneous group of congenital myopathies, transmitted in an unknown manner, with one common feature: numerous enlarged and abnormally shaped mitochondria in the muscle fibers. The mitochondria often contain dense cristae and paracrystalline inclusions. Similar changes can be seen in many unrelated skeletal muscle disorders such as poliomyositis, thyrotoxic myopathies, and spiral muscular atrophy. Also called mitochondria-lipid-glycogen disease, skeletal muscle disease with abnormal mitochondria, and sudanophilic mitochondrial disease. See also *congenital m.* under *myopathy.*

mitogen (mi′to-jen) a substance that stimulates cells to undergo mitosis. In immunology, mitogens are used to induce lymphocyte proliferation in tests of lymphocytic function. In cytogenetics, mitogens are used in preparing cell cultures for chromosome studies. See also *concanavalin A, phytohemagglutinin,* and *pokeweed mitogen.*

mitomycin (mi″to-mi′sin) an antitumor antibiotic produced by *Streptomyces caespitosus* used as a cancer chemotherapeutic drug. It cross-links with DNA by binding to two sites, one on each of the complementary DNA strands. The formation of covalent cross-links in the DNA molecule prevents separation of the complementary strands, thus inhibiting DNA replication. Bacteria treated with mitomycin exhibit inhibition of cell division. Because it is highly toxic, mitomycin is not frequently used clinically. Trademark, Mutamycin. See also *antibacterial agents* and *Appendix A.*

mitosis (mi-to′sis), pl. *mitoses* a type of cell division in eukaryotes that produces an even distribution of the essential hereditary components by allowing cytoplasmic division (cytokinesis) as well as nuclear

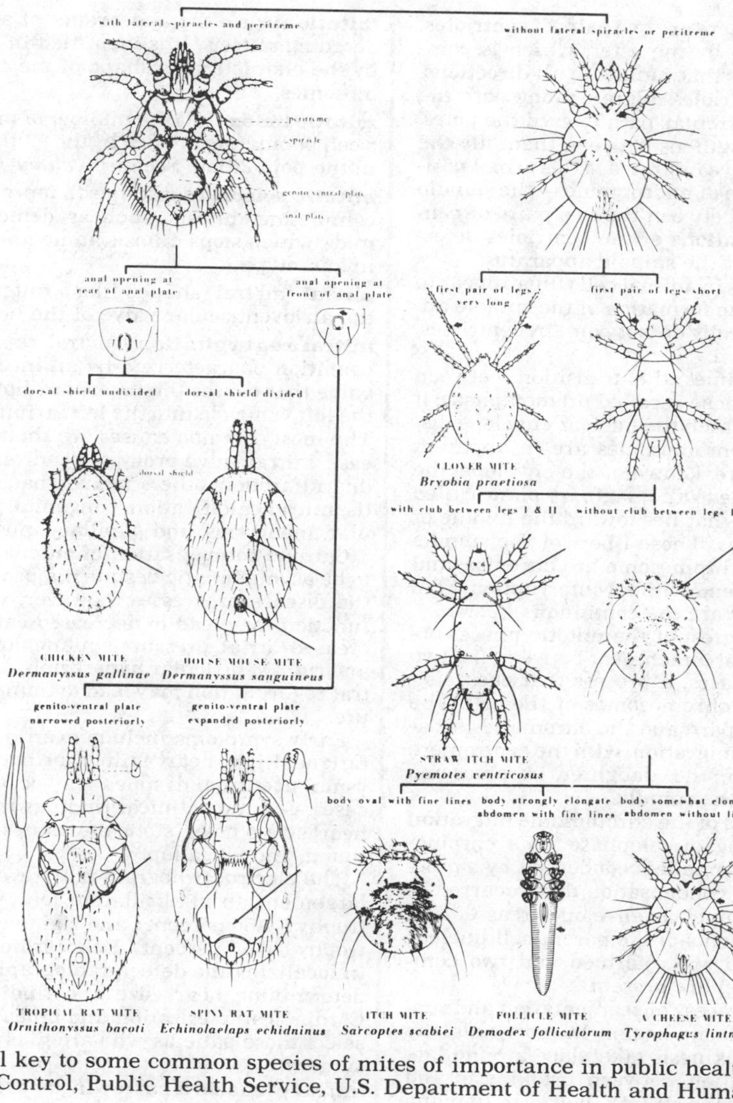

Mite. Pictorial key to some common species of mites of importance in public health. (Courtesy of Centers for Disease Control, Public Health Service, U.S. Department of Health and Human Services, Atlanta, Georgia.)

division. It is convenient when describing mitosis to divide the process into four phases: prophase, metaphase, anaphase, and telophase. The interphase period is between successive mitoses. Mitosis, however, does not actually occur in discrete steps but is a continuous process, and it is not always clear when one stage ends and another begins.

INTERPHASE. This is the period between successive cell divisions associated with growth and preparation for mitosis, when most DNA, RNA, and protein synthesis required for cell division occurs. On the basis of cell division in cultured mammalian cells, interphase has been divided into three stages: G_1 (first gap), S (synthesis), and G_2 (second gap). DNA synthesis and the general mass increase of the cell occur during all three stages. The G_1 stage normally lasts about 10 hr, S about 8 hr. and G_2 about 5 hr; in cultured or rapidly dividing cells, mitosis and cytokinesis together take from about 30 min (mouse spleen cells) to 180 min (grasshopper neuroblasts). The replication of DNA and the synthesis of histone proteins result in the duplication of the chromatin strands, which are not contracted (except for heterochromatin) and are not visible under the light microscope. The nucleus shows little internal differentiation at this time.

PROPHASE. The nuclear chromatin begins to condense by coiling and folding to a point where it becomes visible under the microscope as threadlike structures. Each chromosome appears to consist of two longitudinally parallel sister chromatid strands that are attached at a specific point by the centromere. Also within the nucleus, the nucleoli are reduced in size and finally disintegrate by the end of prophase as the nuclear envelope breaks down. At the same time in the cytoplasm, the spindle apparatus, a system of microtubules, is most conspicuous. The formation of the spindle apparatus in animal cells and in plant cells with motile germ cells is apparently directed by centrioles.

In early prophase there are two pairs of centrioles, each one surrounded by the aster, which is composed of microtubules that radiate in all directions. The two pairs of centrioles migrate along with the asters, describing a circular path toward the poles, while the spindle lengthens between them. By the time the centrioles have migrated to their final positions, there is a system of microtubules—the spindle apparatus—running between the two pairs of centrioles. The final positions of the centrioles determine the two poles of the spindle apparatus.

Although centrioles in animal cells thus appear to direct in some way the formation of the spindle apparatus, most plant cells do not contain centrioles, and asters do not form.

METAPHASE. Sometimes the transition between prophase and metaphase is called prometaphase; it is a short period in which the nuclear envelope disintegrates and the chromosomes are in apparent disorder. After the breakdown of the envelope, the chromosomes migrate to an imaginary plane called the metaphase plate that lies toward the middle of the spindle apparatus. Those fibers of the spindle that connect to the chromosome are chromosomal fibers; those that extend without interruption from one pole to the other are the continuous fibers.

ANAPHASE. The shortest of the mitotic phases occurs when the mutual attachment between the two sister chromatids ceases, a process that occurs simultaneously in all chromosomes of the cell. The centromeres move apart, and the chromatids separate and begin their migration, with the centromere leading the rest of the daughter chromosome toward the poles of the spindle.

TELOPHASE. The end of the chromosome migration marks the beginning of telophase. The chromosomes uncoil and become less condensed by a process that reverses the condensation that occurred in prophase. The new nuclear envelopes reassemble, possibly from fragments of the parent cell nuclear membrane. Nucleoli are reformed and two complete daughter nuclei are present.

Cytokinesis, the process of segmentation and separation of the cytoplasm, begins. In most cells, the initial events of cytokinesis take place around late anaphase. Coordination between cytokinesis and mitosis does not occur in all cells, however. In many insects, for example, the development of fertilized eggs proceeds by repeated nuclear division until several thousand nuclei are formed; then, multiple cytokinesis encloses each nucleus in a separate cell. Most frequently, when cytokinesis is coordinated with nuclear division, the equatorial region of animal cells constricts and deepens into a furrow that divides the cell roughly in half.

See also cell cycle and the accompanying illustration. Cf. *meiosis.*

three-part m., a result of the failure of some chromosomes to join in the movement of other chromosomes during mitosis. A number of chromosomes remain at both poles of the spindle while the majority form the metaphase plate. Also called tripolar mitosis.

mitotane (mi′to-tān) a cancer chemotherapeutic drug; trademark, Lysodren. For more information, see *Appendix A.*

mitotic (mi-tot′ik) pertaining to mitosis.

mitotic cycle the life cycle of a cell between mitoses. See also *cell cycle.*

mitotic figure the appearance of a cell that is undergoing mitosis. It is identified in a tissue section by the characteristic shape of the condensed chromosomes.

mitotic index (MI) the number of mitotic figures in a cell population divided by the total number of cells in the population. See also *cell cycle.*

mitotic poison a substance that prevents cells from completing mitosis, such as demecolcine (Colcemid), which stops mitosis at metaphase and is used in karyotyping.

mitral (mi′tral) shaped like a miter, beveled, as in the atrioventricular valve of the heart.

mitral regurgitation (mi′tral re-gur″ji-ta′shun) a condition characterized by an incompetent mitral valve that causes the backward flow of blood from the left ventricle into the left atrium during systole. The most common causes are rheumatic heart disease, mitral valve prolapse syndrome, and myocardial infarction; others include bacterial endocarditis, mitral calcification, congenital defects, ventricular aneurysms, and papillary muscle rupture.

Cardiac compensation often enables individuals to be asymptomatic despite major regurgitation. As the disease progresses, however, ventricular malfunction may lead to decreased cardiac output, increased atrial pressure, pulmonary hypertension, and right ventricular hypertrophy. Acute severe mitral regurgitation may lead to immediate heart failure.

Early symptoms include exertional dyspnea and fatigue. Right heart failure, orthopnea, and paroxysmal nocturnal dyspnea may occur in very severe cases. Common clinical findings include increased heart size, a holosystolic murmur, split second heart sound, and S3 gallop.

The electrocardiogram may reveal left atrial enlargement, atrial fibrillation, left ventricular hypertrophy (± 50 percent), and right ventricular hypertrophy (± 15 percent). Echocardiography is useful in localizing the defect; radiographs are helpful in determining heart size and finding calcification. Cardiac catheterization and cineangiography help select those patients who are likely to benefit from surgery.

mitral stenosis a narrowing of the orifice between the left atrium and ventricle. It usually occurs as a sequel to rheumatic fever, and occurs in about 40 percent of all individuals with rheumatic heart disease. Onset of symptoms usually occurs in adulthood after a latent period averaging 12 yr. About two-thirds of those affected are female. There may be fibrosis and thickening of the cusps of the mitral valve, shortening and thickening of the chordae tendineae, and deposition of calcium in the valve. In long-standing disease, the valve orifice may become severely narrowed, increasing the left atrial pressure and causing pulmonary hypertension and right heart hypertrophy. Consequences of progressive mitral stenosis include dyspnea, pulmonary edema, atrial arrhythmias, hemoptysis, cyanosis, and right ventricular failure.

On auscultation, the first heart sound is often loud. After the second sound there is often a third sound, the opening snap. This is followed by a low-pitched diastolic rumble produced by turbulent flow through the stenotic orifice. The diastolic murmur shows late diastolic accentuation with atrial contraction. The interval between closure of the

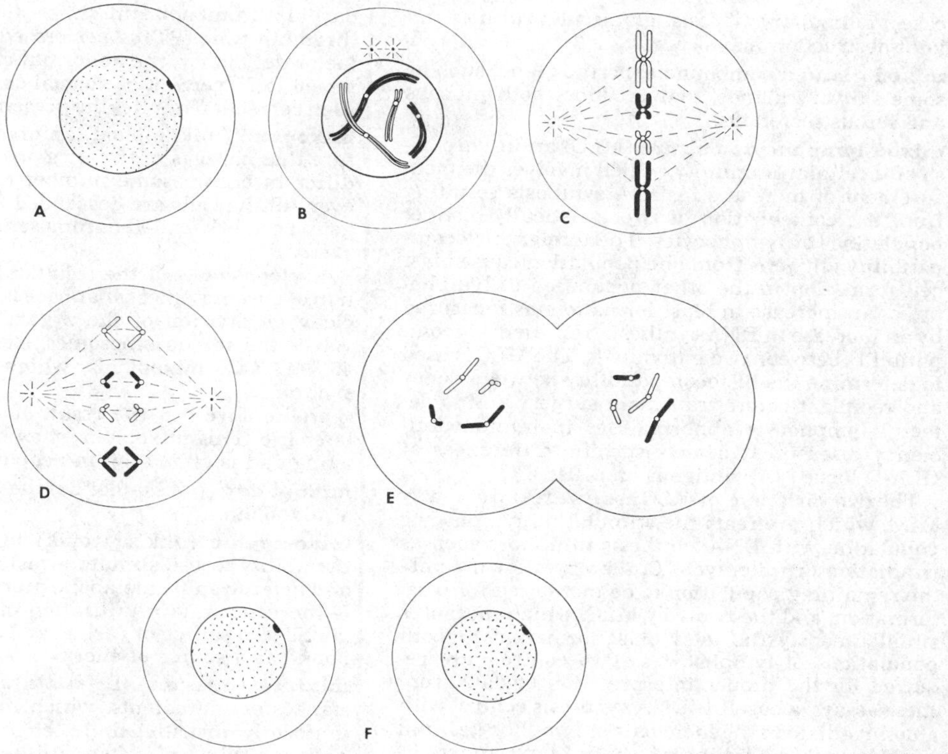

Mitosis. Only two chromosome pairs are shown. Chromosomes from one parent are shown in outline; chromosomes from the other parent, in black. *A,* interphase; *B,* prophase; *C,* metaphase; *D,* anaphase; *E,* telophase; and *F,* interphase. (From Thompson, J. S., and Thompson, M. W.: Genetics in Medicine. 3rd ed. Philadelphia, W. B. Saunders Co., 1980.)

aortic valve and the opening snap of the mitral valve (A_2-OS interval) is longer in individuals with mild mitral stenosis.

Findings indicative of the diagnosis are readily seen by phonocardiography. Echocardiography is the most sensitive noninvasive diagnostic tool; calcification and thickening of the anterior and posterior leaflets and reduced separation of the leaflets during diastole can usually be seen. Cardiac catheterization may be employed to objectively evaluate the mitral orifice area prior to surgical intervention.

congenital m. s., an anomalous narrowing or stricture of the left atrioventricular (mitral) valve orifice sometimes occurring in newborns.

mitral valve see *mitral v.* under *valve.*

mitral valve prolapse syndrome a condition in which the valve cusps of the mitral valve are everted into the left atrium during ventricular systole. It is one of the most common of the cardiac valvular abnormalities, occurring in 5–10 percent of the population. Most affected individuals are asymptomatic; the severity of symptoms relates to the degree of regurgitation and the concomitant reduction in cardiac reserve. Mitral valve prolapse is associated with many conditions, including Marfan's syndrome and other connective tissue and congenital disorders. Often the valve cusps exhibit a myxomatous proliferation.

Diagnosis is initially made by auscultation. A pronounced midsystolic click with or without a systolic murmur indicates the presence of the condition, which may be confirmed by echocardiography. In severe cases, the patient may experience palpitations and diminished cardiac reserve. Therapy ranges from observation to treating associated arrhythmias with drugs to surgical correction.

Also called Barlow's syndrome, floppy valve syndrome, and *midsystolic click-murmur syndrome.*

mIU abbrev. for milli-International Unit. See *milliunit.*

μIU abbrev. for micro-International Unit. See *microunit.*

mixed (mikst) affecting various parts at once; showing two or more different characteristics.

mixed connective tissue disease (MCTD) a syndrome having the clinical features of systemic sclerosis, systemic lupus erythematosus, and polymyositis. Characteristic serologic abnormalities are a positive antinuclear antibody (ANA) test and a high titer of antibodies to extractable ribonucleoprotein (anti-RNP antibodies). Anti-DNA and anti-Sm antibodies are usually absent. Rheumatoid factor, elevated erythrocyte sedimentation rate (ESR), and hypergammaglobulinemia are usually present. Those affected usually have polyarthritis, Raynaud's syndrome, swollen hands, and myopathy. In severe cases, pulmonary fibrosis, glomerulonephitis, and joint destruction may occur.

mixed gland a compound exocrine gland, such as some salivary glands, that produces both mucous and serous secretions.

mixed lymphocyte culture (MLC) an in vitro assay for cellular immunity, which involves the measurement of increases in DNA synthesis resulting from the coincubation of two genetically distinct populations of lymphocytes. The foreign histocompatibility antigens from one population cause blast cell formation in the other population of lymphocytes. An increase in blast formation, as measured by an increase in DNA synthesis, represents incompatibility between two individuals. The MLC is used to determine the histocompatibility between donor and recipient before transplant surgery and to detect T-lymphocyte abnormalities in immunodeficiency diseases. It detects specific differences at HLA-D locus [(IA)] antigens on cells.

The two variations of MLC assays are the one-way MLC, which pretreats the stimulating lymphocyte population with DNA synthesis inhibitors such as irradiation or mitomycin C, thereby allowing only the remaining population to be monitored for blast formation; and the two-way MLC, which measures simultaneously the total blast formation in both populations of lymphocytes. Two controls are required for the proper interpretation of data from these assays: a baseline DNA synthesis control with a nonirradiated syngeneic pair of lymphocytes, and a DNA synthesis inhibition control with an irradiated allogeneic pair of lymphocytes.

Also called *mixed lymphocyte reaction.*

mixed lymphocyte reaction (MLR) see *mixed lymphocyte culture.*

mixed tumor a tumor with a heterogeneous cell population. The term is customarily applied to a characteristic tumor of salivary gland origin that shows differentiation toward both duct and myoepithelial cells. Both benign and malignant forms are recognized, although the former is far more common. Benign mixed tumors that are incompletely excised may recur. Histologically, mixed tumors are characterized by glandular elements forming cords and solid sheets set within a myxoid matrix in which areas of cartilaginous differentiation generally are also present. A benign mixed tumor of the salivary gland is also called a pleomorphic adenoma.

mixed venous blood blood composed of venous blood from the heart and from all the peripheral tissues in proportion to their contribution to the venous return. Mixed venous blood is best collected from the main pulmonary artery.

mixed venous P_{CO_2} (Pv_{CO_2}) the partial pressure of carbon dioxide in mixed venous blood, approximately equal to 38–56 mmHg in the healthy individual at rest at sea level.

mixed venous P_{O_2} (Pv_{O_2}) the partial pressure of oxygen in a sample of mixed venous blood, approximately equal to 20–60 mmHg in the healthy subject at rest at sea level.

mixing test a test to distinguish between a clotting factor deficiency and an inhibitor of coagulation. It is used when an inhibitor is suspected of being present. Normal plasma is mixed with an equal amount of the patient's abnormal plasma, and an activated partial thromboplastin time (aPTT) and/or prothrombin time (PT) is performed. In the case of a factor deficiency, the abnormal clotting test is corrected to 75 percent of normal or better. Failure of such correction implies the presence of an inhibitor.

mixoploid (miks′o-ploid) an organism or cell culture that consists of two or more cell lineages that differ in chromosome number or structure. However, all the cells are descended from the same zygote. Formerly called chromosome mosaic. Cf. *chimera.*

developmental m., the result of incorrect segregation of chromosomes (anaphase lag) during an early cleavage division of the zygote. This usually involves the sex chromosomes, e.g., 45,X/46,XX and 45,X/47,XXX mixoploids, which exhibit Turner's syndrome.

proliferative m., the result of a mitotic error in later life. This mixoploidy may be associated with aging and is often seen in neoplasia.

mixoploidy (miks′o-ploi″de) the condition of being a mixoploid.

mixotrophic (mik″so-trof′ik) in microorganisms, the ability to use simultaneously both autotrophic and heterotrophic metabolic processes. An example is the concomitant utilization of an organic compound as a source of carbon and an inorganic compound as a source of energy.

mixture (miks′tur) [L. *mixtura*] a blend of substances or ingredients, which may or may not be uniformly distributed. In chemistry, a mixture, such as a solution, is distinguished from a pure substance, i.e., an element or compound.

mks system abbrev. See *meter-kilogram-second system.*

mL abbrev. See *millilambert.*

ml abbrev. See *milliliter.*

μl abbrev. See *microliter.*

MLC abbrev. See *minimal lethal concentration, mixed lymphocyte culture.*

MLD abbrev. See *minimal lethal d.* under *dose.*

M line a darker line in the center of the H band of a sarcomere. See also *myofibril* and *skeletal m.* under *muscle.*

MLR abbrev. for mixed lymphocyte reaction. See *mixed lymphocyte culture.*

MM abbrev. for the isoenzyme of creatine kinase that contains two M subunits. See under *creatine kinase.*

mm abbrev. See *millimeter.*

μm abbrev. See *micrometer.*

μμ abbrev. See *micromicro.*

MMFR abbrev. See *maximal midexpiratory flow rate.*

mmHg abbrev. See *millimeter of mercury.*

M-mode echo see under *echocardiography.*

mmol abbrev. See *millimole.*

μmol abbrev. See *micromole.*

Mn symbol for the chemical element *manganese.*

mnemonic (ne-mon′ik) [Gr. *mnēmonikos* pertaining to memory] 1. pertaining to or promoting recollection or memory.

2. any device, such as a formula or jingle, used as a memory aid.

mnemonic code the code employed to specify operations in a computer assembly language. It uses letter codes resembling the operation names, such as ST or STO for store. The instruction set and mnemonic code are unique to each family of computers.

MNS blood group see under *blood groups.*

Mo symbol for the chemical element *molybdenum.*

MΩ abbrev. See *megohm.*

μΩ abbrev. See *microhm.*

mobile (mo′bil) capable of moving or being moved.

mobile genes structurally and genetically discrete segments of DNA that have the ability to move around among the chromosomes and the extrachromosomal DNA molecules of bacteria and higher organisms.

mobile unit (mo′b′l) a piece of equipment, such as an x-ray machine or scintillation camera, that can be moved, as to an operating room or patient's bedside.

mobility (mo-bil′i-te) [L. *mobilitas*] 1. the quality or state of being mobile; the capacity of facility of movement or movability. Cf. *motility.*

2. referring to the freedom of movement of a charged particle in an applied electrical field.

3. a measure of the rate at which a solid is deformed under stress after the yield point has been exceeded.

mobilization (mo″bĭ-lĭ-za′shun) the rendering of a fixed part or substance movable.

mobilization test see under *lead assays.*

Möbius' disease (me′be-oos) [Paul Julius *Möbius,* German neurologist, 1853–1907] congenital, bilateral facial weakness, often associated with convergent strabismus. The disorder overlaps with other central nervous system disorders. Its cause is unknown.

modal (mō′dal) pertaining to a mode. The modal number in a sample is the one most frequently observed.

mode (mōd) in statistics, a measure of central tendency referring either to a maximal point of the probability density, or to the most frequently occurring value in a sample.

modem (mo′dem) [acronym from *mo*dulator/*de*-*m*odulator] a device that converts digital information from a computer or peripheral device into an audio-frequency signal that can be transmitted over a telephone line (modulation); it also converts received audio signals to digital information (demodulation).

An acoustically coupled low-speed modem that uses regular telephone lines can transmit 300 bits/sec, whereas high-speed modems using leased high-speed telephone lines can transmit up to 50,000 bits/sec.

moderator (mod′er-a-tor) 1. a substance or structure that reduces excessive or extreme movements or reactions.

2. an intermediary.

moderator band a muscular bridge between the interventricular septum and the base of the anterior papillary muscle at the apical end of the heart, which conveys the Purkinje fibers of the right limb of the atrioventricular bundle.

modifier (mod′ĭ-fi-er) 1. something that alters or changes.

2. in genetics, a gene that influences the expressivity of another gene. Also called modifying gene; see under *gene.*

modiolus (mo-di′o-lus) [L. "nave," "hub"] [NA], the conical, central pillar of spongy bone that forms an axis about which the bony canal of the cochlea makes its spiral turns.

modular (moj′u-lar, mod′u-lar) composed of modules.

modulate (moj′u-lāt, mod′u-lāt) to encode a signal on a waveform (the carrier wave) by varying the wave amplitude, frequency, or phase.

modulation (moj″u-la′shun, mod″u-la′shun) [L. *modulare* to measure] 1. the process of adapting to an environment; regulation.

2. changes in the appearance or rate of growth of cultured cells; the term is usually used in reference to the effects of environmental agents.

3. in electronics, the alteration of a signal to impose information on it.

modulation transfer function (MTF) a description of the resolution of an imaging system such as a scintillation camera or CT scanner. It indicates how responsive the system is to each spatial frequency in the object. If the object has a sinusoidally varying activity (density for CT) with amplitude A_0 and frequency *f,* and if the detector records the (smaller) amplitude *A,* then the MTF at that frequency, MTF(f), is A/A_0. Any detector has the best response at zero frequency, an even, gray image. The decline in response at high frequencies measures to what extent sharp edges are blurred and fine lines are washed out. Also called *detector transfer function.*

module (moj′ūl, mod′ūl) 1. a component or group of components that form a unit designed to be readily interchangeable (e.g., laboratory bench work of different configurations that fit into a given space) or replaceable (e.g., a circuit board in an instrument that, when defective, can be exchanged for an identical board).

2. a part of a computer program that can be separately compiled, link edited, and loaded.

modulus (moj′u-lus, mod′u-lus) [L. "standard of measure"] 1. a specified positive integer used as a divisor. The remainder of an integer *d* when divided by the integer *m* is written *d* mod *m.* Two integers, *i* and *j,* are said to be congruent modulus (or modulo) *m,* when $i \bmod m = j \bmod m$.

2. the capacity of a computer register or word, e.g., 2^n for an *n* bit register.

3. the absolute value of a complex number.

moiety (moi′ĕ-te) [Fr. *moitié,* from L. *medietas, medius* middle] any equal part, a half; also, any part or portion. In chemistry, the term also refers to an indefinite part of a complex molecule defined only in the context in which it is used, e.g., the protein portion of a lipoprotein molecule is referred to as a protein moiety.

mol (mol) symbol for *mole,* the International System (SI) unit.

molal (mo′lal) a unit for expressing the concentration of a solution; the number of moles of solute per kilogram of solvent. A molal solution is the same as a one-molal solution; a half-molal aqueous solution (0.5 molal) has 0.5 moles of solute per kilogram of water (abbrev. 0.5 mol/kg H_2O). Cf. *molar* and *normal.*

molality (mo-lal′ĭ-te) the mass fraction of a solution

expressed in moles of solute per kilogram of solvent. See also *molal.* Cf. *molarity* and *normality.*

molar (mo'lar) 1. pertaining to a mole of a substance, such as a molar volume, molar mass, or molar absorptivity, i.e., the quantity of some property associated with a mole of the substance.

2. a measure of the concentration of a solute, expressed as the number of moles of solute per liter of solution (symbol M), e.g., 0.25 M = 0.25 moles per liter (mol/l). The latter notation is used in the SI system, and the symbol M is discouraged.

3. a type of tooth, which is used for grinding food and which acts as a major jaw support in the dental arch. See also *tooth.*

molar absorptivity see *molar a.* under *absorptivity.*

molarity (mo-lar'ĭ-te) the substance concentration of a solution expressed in moles of solute per liter of solution (mol/l). See also *molar.* Cf. *molality* and *normality.*

molar weight the mass of 1 mol of a substance. The molar weight of a chemical compound has the value of the molecular weight of the compound and the unit gram (g).

mold (mōld) 1. a general term for filamentous fungi that appear as either a fuzzy, powdery, woolly, velvety, or relatively smooth colony. Some of the common molds are *Mucor, Penicillium, Rhizopus,* and *Aspergillus.*

2. in histology, a paper, plastic, or metal form used to orient and embed tissue in a medium suitable for sectioning.

mole (mōl) [F. *mole,* from L. *mola,* mill, cake (after Gr. *mylē*)] 1. (abbrev. mol), the International System unit for amount of substance; 6.022×10^{23} (Avogadro's number) of identical particles, i.e., atoms, molecules, ions, electrons, or other particles. In clinical chemistry, the use of moles is now preferred to grams or equivalents for reporting results of clinical measurements.

2. a fleshy mass or tumor formed in the uterus by the degeneration or abortive development of an ovum. See also *h. mole* under *hydatidiform.*

3. a pigmented fleshy growth; a term loosely applied to any blemish of the skin. See also *nevus.*

Breus' m., a malformation of the ovum consisting of tuberous subchorional hematoma of the decidua. Also called hematomole.

hydatidiform m., see *h. mole* under *hydatidiform.*

invasive m., see *chorioadenoma destruens.*

molecular (mo-lek'u-lar) of, pertaining to, or composed of molecules.

molecular biology the study of the molecules in living organisms, the reactions they undergo, how these reactions are controlled, and how molecules are assembled into larger structures such as membranes and fibers.

molecular exclusion chromatography see under *chromatography.*

molecular mass see *molecular weight.*

molecular sieve a fairly broad spectrum of materials used to separate molecules primarily on the basis of their size. Such materials include aluminosilicate substances, clays, feldspars, zeolites, and a variety of gels. Molecular sieving is most often used in laboratory medicine to remove salts from proteins and to separate proteins on the basis of their size.

In the procedure, a sieving or screening action occurs, permitting the separation of small molecules from large ones. The small molecules penetrate a network of uniform pores in the sieve material, enter the cavities, and are adsorbed on the interior surfaces. Larger molecules not penetrating the pores pass through the sieve quite rapidly. A number of gels are used for determining the molecular weight of proteins by a technique called gel filtration.

A wide variety of molecular sieves have uses in many fields of technology: to dry gases and liquids; for selective molecular separations based on size and polar properties; as ion-exchangers, catalysts, and chemical carriers; and in gas chromatography and in the petroleum industry to remove normal paraffins from distillates.

molecular sieve chromatography see under *chromatography.*

molecular weight (M.W.) the sum of the atomic weights of the elements of a chemical compound, each multiplied by the number of atoms of that element in the molecule. It is the average mass of a molecule relative to the mass of the carbon isotope ^{12}C, which is assigned the value of exactly 12. The term is imprecise (the term "weight" referring to gravitational force, not quantity of matter); a better term would be relative molecular mass, but the use of molecular weight is firmly established and generally accepted. Also called *molecular mass.* See also *atomic weight* and *molar weight.*

molecule (mol'ĕ-kūl) [L. *molecula* little mass] the smallest unit of a substance that still retains all of its chemical properties. The simplest molecules (e.g., neon) have only one atom; most molecules have more than one atom held together by covalent or polar covalent bonds.

mole fraction the ratio of the number of particles (or moles) of one component of a mixture to the total number of particles (or moles) of all the components.

molindone hydrochloride (mo-lin'dōn) a major tranquilizer, a dihydroindolone derivative, used in the management of psychotic disorders. Although chemically unrelated to the phenothiazine, thioxanthene, or butyrophenone major tranquilizers, its actions and side-effects (including drowsiness, restlessness, parkinsonism, and other extrapyramidal reactions) are similar. See also *phenothiazine tranquilizers.* Trademark, Moban.

Moll's gland (molz) [Jacob Antonius *Moll,* Dutch ophthalmologist, 1832–1914] a modified apocrine gland located in the eyelid.

Mollicutes (mol"ĭ-ku'tēz) [L. *mollis* soft + *cutis* skin] a class of bacterialike microorganisms within the mycoplasmas. It has been subdivided into a genus requiring sterols for growth (*Mycoplasma*) and another that does not (*Acholeplasma*). See also *mycoplasma.*

mollusc (mol'usk) see *mollusk.*

Mollusca (mŏ-lus'kah) [L., from *molluscus* soft] a phylum of invertebrates that usually have an exoskeleton (such as a shell). Examples include the snail, slug, mussel, oyster, clam, octopus, nautilus, squid, and cuttlefish.

molluscum (mŏ-lus'kum) [L. *molluscus* soft] a general term used to describe any disease that results in the formation of soft, rounded papules in the skin.

When used alone, it refers to molluscum contagiosum.

m. contagiosum, an infectious disease of ubiquitous distribution and protracted course, occurring primarily in children, that is caused by a virus of the pox group. The virus induces hyperplasia and degeneration of the epithelium of the skin and mucous membranes, with the formation of rounded, dome-shaped, waxy, umbilicated papules that exude a cheesy material. Transmission is by direct contact with the lesions, through sexual intercourse, or through fomites. The diagnosis of this viral disease may be made histologically through the presence of characteristic, large, cytoplasmic, viral inclusions (molluscum bodies) in the infected epithelial cells.

mollusk (mol'usk) any organism belonging to the phylum Mollusca.

molybdenum (Mo) (mo-lib'dĕ-num) [Gr. *molybdos* lead] a hard, silvery-white, metallic element; atomic number 42; atomic weight 95.94; a 4d transition element; oxidation states +2 through +6. It is an essential nutrient for plants and animals, being a cofactor for several oxidases and for bacterial nitrogen-fixing enzymes. Molybdenum is used in fertilizer and to make alloy steel. Deficiency disease and toxicity are unknown in humans.

molybdic (mo-lib'dik) an improper reference to molybdenum(VI), Mo^{6+}.

molybdous (mo-lib'dus) an improper reference to molybdenum(IV), Mo^{4+}.

momentum (*p*) (mo-men'tum) [L.] a physical quantity, the product of the mass and the velocity of a moving object.

mon/o (mon'o) [Gr. *monos* single] a word element used in combining form to denote one or single, e.g., monocyte.

monad (mo'nad, mon'ad) [Gr. *monas* a unit] 1. a single-celled protozoon or coccus.

2. a monovalent radical or element.

3. in genetics, one of the four single chromosomes that make up a bivalent (tetrad) during meiosis.

monamide (mon-am'id, mon-am'id) an amide that contains only one amide group.

monarthritis (mon"ar-thri'tis) [*mono-* + Gr. *arthron* joint + *-itis*] an inflammation of a single joint, as in trauma or a localized infection.

Mönckeberg's arteriosclerosis (menk'e-bergz) [Johann Georg *Mönckeberg,* German pathologist, 1877–1925] see *Mönckeberg's a.* under *arteriosclerosis.*

Mondor's disease (mon'dorz) [Henri *Mondor,* French surgeon, 1885–1962] a thrombophlebitis, often of unknown cause, that involves the superficial veins of the chest, most specifically the thoracoepigastric vein. This condition produces pain, warmth, and induration along the anterolateral chest wall; the thrombosed cords of the veins involved may be palpable.

Monge's disease see under *mountain sickness.*

mongolism (mon'go-lizm) [from *Mongol,* a member of one of the chief ethnologic divisions of Asiatic peoples] the former name for *Down's syndrome.*

moniliform (mo-nil'ĭ-form) [L. *monile* necklace + *forma* form] shaped like a necklace or string of beads.

Moniliformis (mo-nil"ĭ-for'mis) a genus of worms of the phylum Acanthocephala. The species *M. moniliformis* is a facultative parasite in humans; beetles and cockroaches serve as intermediate hosts. The adult worms (males measuring 4–5 cm long; females, 10–27 cm) have a chalky or creamy-white color and an elongated shape. The eggs are ellipsoidal and measure 85–118 μ by 40–52 μ.

Infection is acquired by ingestion of infected insects, which causes diarrhea, gastrointestinal pain, and exhaustion. Laboratory diagnosis requires identification of the eggs in feces.

moniliid (mo-nil'e-id) a secondary, sterile, vascular, or papular skin lesion caused by an immunologic response to *Candida* elsewhere in the body. Also called levurid or *candidid.* See also *candidiasis.*

monitor (mon'ĭ-tor) [L. "one who reminds," from *monere* to remind, admonish] 1. to check constantly on a state or condition, as on the vital signs of a patient under anesthesia and undergoing surgery, or as in the continuous recording of exposure to radiation.

2. a device used in monitoring, such as a cardiac monitor or pocket dosimeter.

monoallelic (mon"o-ah-le'lik) in genetics, having all of the alleles the same at a given locus; used only in referring to polyploids. Cf. *homozygous.*

monoamine (mon"o-am'ēn) an amine that contains only one amino group.

monoamine oxidase (MAO) (mon"o-am'ēn ok'sĭ-dās) see *amine oxidase (flavin-containing).*

monoamine oxidase inhibitors a group of drugs that inactivate the enzyme monoamine oxidase (MAO), which breaks down the biogenic amines such as serotonin and the neurotransmitters epinephrine, norepinephrine, and dopamine. MAO inhibitors may cause a hypertensive crisis when taken in combination with tricyclic antidepressants, with sympathomimetic substances such as amphetamine and methyldopa, and with tyramine, which is present in many foods. These inhibitors may potentiate central nervous system depressants, causing hypotension, and may also alter liver function.

MAO inhibitors are generally used to treat individuals not responding to other drugs. MAO inhibitors such as isocarboxazid, tranylcypromine, and phenelzine are used to treat depression, and pargyline to treat hypertension. They are rapidly metabolized and may not be detected with basic drug screening procedures.

monoaminodicarboxylic acid an acid that contains one amino group and two carboxyl groups in the molecule, e.g., glutamic acid.

monoaminomonocarboxylic acid an acid that contains one amino group and one carboxyl group in the molecule, e.g., alanine.

monobasic acid an acid that contains only one replaceable hydrogen atom, e.g., HCl.

monoblast (mon'o-blast) [*mono-* + Gr. *blastos* germ] the cell that is the precursor of the mature monocyte; see *monohistiocytic series.*

monoblastic leukemia (mon"o-blas'tik) see *monocytic l.* under *leukemia.*

monocentric (mon"o-sen'trik) in genetics, referring to a chromosome having the normal single centromere. Cf. *acentric* and *dicentric.*

monochromatic (mon″o-kro-mat′ik) [*mono-* + Gr. *chrōma* color] pertaining to light that has only one color, i.e., light that is restricted to a narrow bandwidth like that produced by a monochromator.

monochromator (mon″o-kro′ma-tor) a device that produces monochromatic light by reducing the unwanted wavelengths found in a light source. This is usually either a colored filter, or the combination of a diffraction grating or a prism that disperses the light into a spectrum and a slit that passes only part of the spectrum.

monoclonal (mon″o-klōn′al) derived from a single cell; pertaining to a single clone.

monoclonal antibodies immunochemically identical antibodies produced by a clone of plasma cells. Monoclonal antibodies are now being produced commercially using hybridomas. Because all the antigen-binding sites of monoclonal antibodies are identical, immunoassays using monoclonal antibodies are often superior in specificity and reproducibility to those using polyclonal antibodies, which are produced by the traditional method of antigenic challenge to an animal.

monoclonal band see under *paraprotein.*

monoclonal gammopathy a heterogeneous group of immunologic diseases in which a single clone of lymphoid cells produces a monoclonal immunoglobulin that may be detected in serum or urine. Examples of monoclonal gammopathies include multiple myeloma, Waldenström's macroglobulinemia, amyloidosis, heavy-chain disease, and chronic lymphocytic leukemia. The monoclonal immunoglobulin produced in this type of lymphoreticular disorder may also be called paraprotein, M protein, or myeloma protein. For example, monoclonal gammopathies result in increased plasma levels and increased total IgG levels due to an increase in IgG synthesis.

Laboratory diagnosis involves hematologic tests, routine clinical chemistry tests, a hemostatic profile, radiologic examination, and immunologic tests. Immunologically, serum protein electrophoresis is used to screen for increases in immunoglobulin levels. Immunoelectrophoresis can determine the type of IgG paraprotein that is produced by this disease, i.e., whether it is monoclonal and, if it is, of what class: IgG, IgA, IgD, IgE, or IgM.

See also *paraproteinemia.*

monoclonal immunoglobulin the structurally homogeneous immunoglobulin produced by a single clone of plasma cells.

monocyte (M) (mon′o-sit) [*mono-* + Gr. *kytos* hollow vessel] an actively phagocytic cell, formed in the bone marrow, that is capable of phagocytizing bacteria, viruses, antibody-antigen complexes, inorganic substances, and erythrocytes. Monocytes are known to transform into macrophages and multinucleated giant cells. The precursor cell of the monocyte has not been identified but may be a reticulum cell, which then develops into a pronormoblast and promonocyte.

Monocytes occur in various sizes. On peripheral blood smears, the large monocyte (30–40 μm in diameter) has a large, centrally or eccentrically located nucleus that is either irregular, kidney shaped, or multilobed. The chromatin pattern is lacelike or reticular. Nucleoli are always present but may be obscured by perinuclear chromatin. The cytoplasm has the appearance of ground glass; it is grayish-blue with fine, pink-purple granules. Vacuoles and azurophilic granules are commonly seen.

The small monocyte (20–30 μm in diameter) has a round or oval nucleus; a nucleolus generally is not visible. The cytoplasm is blue-gray and contains a few azurophilic granules. It is possible to confuse this cell with a large lymphocyte.

Cytochemically, the monocyte is weakly peroxidase-positive. It also reacts with α-naphthyl butyrate in a nonspecific esterase reaction, in contrast to the specific esterase reaction of neutrophilic "specific" granules. A monocyte produces and excretes lysozyme and fixes immunoglobulins on its membrane.

Formerly called hyaline leukocyte, *mononuclear leukocyte,* and transitional leukocyte. See also *macrophage* and *monohistiocytic series.*

monocytic (mon″o-sit′ik) characterized by or of the nature of monocytes.

monocytic leukemia see *monocytic l.* under *leukemia.*

monocytopenia (mon″o-si″to-pe′ne-ah) [*monocyte* + Gr. *penia* poverty] a lack of monocytes in the blood.

monocytopoiesis (mon″o-si″to-poi-e′sis) [*monocyte* + Gr. *poiein* to make] the production of monocytes.

monocytosis (mon″o-si-to′sis) an increase in the proportion of monocytes in the blood.

monoenoic fatty acid (mon′o-ēn″o-ik) a fatty acid with a single carbon-carbon double bond in the molecule, e.g., oleic and palmitoleic acids.

monoglyceride (mon″o-glis′er-īd) monoacylglycerol, a monoester of one molecule of fatty acid with one molecule of glycerol. After emulsification with bile salts, the dietary triglycerides are converted primarily to β-monoglycerides (2-monoacylglycerol) by the action of pancreatic lipase, which is then absorbed into the mucosal cells. Cf. *diglyceride.*

monohistiocytic series (mon″o-his″te-o-sit′ik) the phagocytic cell series that includes monocytes, alveolar macrophages, peritoneal macrophages, Kupffer cells, and the free and fixed macrophages of the bone marrow. The primary functions of these cells are to defend against microorganisms, remove dead and dying cells and cellular debris, and interact immunologically with lymphoid cells. They are also capable of ingesting inorganic compounds.

These cells arise in the bone marrow (probably from reticulum cells that develop into monoblasts and promonocytes), enter the blood as monoblasts, and, upon inflammatory stimulus, move by diapedesis into the tissues and develop into a large macrophage. Both monocytes and histiocytes can be readily transformed into macrophages.

Cells of this series are also called *mononuclear phagocytes.* See also *inflammation, macrophage,* and *monocyte.*

monohydric (mon″o-hi′drik) containing one atom of replaceable hydrogen.

monohydric alcohol an alcohol containing only one hydroxy group.

monoiodotyrosine (MIT) (mon″o-i-o″do-ti′ro-sēn) a precursor of triiodothyronine (T_3). It accounts for 17–28 percent of the total iodine in the thyroid gland, yet possesses no biologic activity. MIT is formed by an iodination at position 3 of the tyrosine residue on the thyroglobulin molecule in the thyroid follicular cell. One diiodotyrosine (DIT) and one

MIT molecule undergo oxidative condensation to form T_3, which is eventually cleaved by a thyroglobulin protease to release free T_3. MIT is subsequently deiodinated and the iodide recycled back into the iodide pool. Although MIT is present in small amounts in the serum, it is not normally measured. See also *diiodotyrosine* and *triiodothyronine*.

monolayer (mon″o-la′er) a monomolecular film; a layer of material one molecule thick.

monomer (mon′o-mer) a molecule that can be combined with other molecules to form a polymer; the repeating unit of a polymer. For example, proteins are made up of amino acid monomers.

monomeric (mon″o-mer′ik) [*mono-* + Gr. *meros* part] pertaining to a monomer; consisting of a single part, not polymeric.

monomorphic (mon″o-mor′fik) [*mono-* + Gr. *morphē* form] existing in only one form; maintaining the same form throughout all stages of development, as in certain protozoa and insects. Cf. *polymorphic*.

monomorphism (mon″o-mor′fizm) the quality or condition of being monomorphic.

monomyelocytic leukemia (mon″o-mi″ĕ-lo-sit′ik) see *monomyelocytic l.* under *leukemia*.

monomyositis (mon″o-mi″o-si′tis) [*mono-* + Gr. *myos* of muscle + *-itis*] an inflammation of a single muscle, which may follow trauma, overuse, localized infection, or other causes.

Mononchus (mon-ong′kus) a genus of nematodes found in fresh water or moist soil. Several cases have been reported in which these organisms have been found in human urine but they are not considered true parasites.

mononeuritis (mon″o-nu-ri′tis) [*mono-* + Gr. *neuron* nerve + *itis*] the inflammation of a single nerve, with pain and weakness in the affected area. When a disease or disease process affects a single nerve, it is referred to as a mononeuropathy.

m. multiplex, abnormal function in more than one nerve. The affected nerves are usually remote from each other, and involvement is usually asymmetric. Nerve involvement may be complete from outset, or progressive. Pain, weakness, and paresthesias are seen in the affected area. The etiology may be inflammatory (e.g., sarcoidosis, periarteritis nodosa) or angiopathic (e.g., diabetes mellitus). Nerve conduction studies and, in many cases, nerve and muscle biopsy help to establish the diagnosis.

mononeuropathy (mon″o-nu-rop′ah-the) [*mono-* + Gr. *neuron* nerve + *pathos* disease] a condition in which a single nerve is functionally impaired. The most common cause is nerve compression, but tumor, infection, or hemorrhage may also cause mononeuropathies. Electromyography and nerve conduction velocity tests are most helpful. See also *mononeuritis*.

mononuclear (mon″o-nu′kle-ar) [*mono-* + L. *nucleus*, dim. of *nux* nut] 1. having but one nucleus; mononucleate; uninucleate.

2. a cell having a single nucleus, especially a monocyte of the blood or tissues.

mononuclear phagocytes see *monohistiocytic series*.

mononuclear phagocyte system the term used to denote collectively the various phagocytic cells of the body, which are numerous in certain locations, notably in the lymph nodes; the sinusoids of the spleen, liver, and bone marrow; and the peripheral blood (monocytes). Polymorphonuclear leukocytes are not included. Formerly called *reticuloendothelial system*.

mononucleate (mon″o-nu′kle-āt) having a single nucleus; mononuclear.

mononucleosis (mon″o-nu″kle-o′sis) see *infectious mononucleosis*.

mononucleotide (mon″o-nu′kle-o-tīd″) a phosphoric acid ester of a nucleoside occurring either free (e.g., adenylic acid) or as a constituent of nucleic acids, which can be released on hydrolysis. It is composed of phosphoric acid linked to ribose (deoxyriboside) at carbon 3 or carbon 5, the pentose being linked to a purine or a pyrimidine at carbon 1. See also *nucleotide*.

monooxygenase (mon″o-ok′sĭ-jĕ-nās″) an enzyme of the oxidoreductase class that catalyzes the incorporation of one atom of oxygen from molecular O_2 into a substrate. It may act with a single hydrogen donor (EC 1.13.12), or it may require the presence of a second hydrogen donor in a coupled reaction (EC 1.14).

monophosphate (mon″o-fos′fāt) a salt containing a single PO_3^{3-} ion.

monoplegia (mon″o-ple′je-ah) [*mono-* + Gr. *plēgē* stroke] a general term used to describe complete paralysis of a single limb.

monoploid (mon′o-ploid) having the basic chromosome number of the polyploid series; in referring to humans, the term haploid is synonymous and is preferred.

monopolar (mon″o-po′lar) pertaining to the use of a single electrode in electrosurgery, electrocardiography, or electromyography, with the ground or with a second distant electrode serving as the second terminal or reference electrode.

monosaccharide (mon″o-sak′ah-rīd) a term used to classify the simple sugars that cannot be hydrolyzed to a simpler unit (as opposed to disaccharides, for example, which can be hydrolyzed to two monosaccharides). Monosaccharides are classified as trioses, tetroses, pentoses, hexoses, and so on, if they contain three, four, five, six, or more carbon atoms, respectively. Monosaccharides containing an aldehyde group are called aldoses; those containing a keto group are called ketoses.

monosodium glutamate (mon″o-so′de-um gloo′tah-māt) a salt of glutamic acid used as a seasoning in food. Its use affects some people who are sensitive to the salt, producing the "Chinese restaurant syndrome," which includes severe headaches, numbness, palpitations, and other neurologic disturbances due to glutamate concentrations considerably higher than those normally present in food.

monosome (mon′o-sōm) 1. the single chromosome of a homologous pair in a monosomic individual.

2. a messenger RNA molecule that has only one ribosome bound to it. Cf. *polysome*.

monosomic (mon″o-so′mik) pertaining to or characterized by monosomy.

monosomy (mon′o-so″me) the condition of having one chromosome less than the normal diploid complement. In humans, monosomy of the autosomes is lethal; only 45,X monosomy (Turner's syndrome) is observed in liveborns.

monospecific (mon″o-spĕ-sif′ik) having an effect only on a particular kind of cell or tissue, or reacting with a single antigen, as a monospecific antiserum.

monospermy (mon″o-sper′me) [*mono-* + Gr. *sperma* seed] the normal process of fertilization by only one sperm. Cf. *dispermy.*

Monosporium (mon″o-spo′re-um) [N.L., from *mono-* + Gr. *spora* seed] the incorrect name for a genus of fungi, correct name *Scedosporium. S. apiospermum* is the anamorph (asexual stage) of *Petriellidium boydii* (*Allescheria boydii*). See also *Petriellidium.*

Monospot test (mon′o-spot) see under *infectious mononucleosis.*

monotrichous (mon″o-trī′kus) [*mono-* + Gr. *thrix* hair] a term used to describe a bacterial cell or other unicellular organism having a single polar flagellum. See also *flagellum.*

monounsaturated (mon″o-un-sach′ĕ-ra″tėd) containing one double carbon-carbon bond, as in a monounsaturated fatty acid.

monovalent (mon″o-va′lent) 1. in chemistry, having a valence of 1. Also called *univalent.*

2. in immunology, pertaining to an antibody or antiserum that is specific for one antigen. Cf. *multivalent.*

monozygotic (mon″o-zi-got′ik) pertaining to or derived from one egg (zygote), as in identical twins. Cf. *dizygotic.*

mons (monz), pl. *montes* [L. "mountain"] [NA], a general term for an elevation or eminence.

m. pubis, [NA], the rounded eminence over the symphysis pubis, formed by a thickening of the subcutaneous adipose tissue. At the onset of puberty, it becomes covered with hair.

montage (mon-taj′) [Fr.] 1. an artwork made up from many, usually overlapping, pictures or designs.

2. the arrangement used to display simultaneously the potential differences between several pairs of electrodes in the electroencephalographic record. By convention, recordings from the right side of the scalp are commonly displayed above those from the left side, and recordings from anterior regions precede those from posterior regions. See also *International 10–20.*

average reference m., montage to display the potential difference between individual electrodes placed on the scalp and the average potential of all or many scalp electrodes. The average potential is obtained by joining the scalp electrodes to a common point through high resistors. For display purposes, the individual scalp electrode is connected to input terminal 1 and the average potential to input terminal 2. Also called *common reference.*

bipolar m., montage to display the potential difference between pairs of electrodes, no electrode being common to all derivations. Electrodes usually are equally spaced and placed on the scalp in an anteroposterior or transverse plane. The most anterior or right-hand electrode is connected to input terminal 1. With simultaneous recordings from two rows of electrodes at right angles to each other using linked bipolar derivations, abnormalities can be localized by identifying the electrode at which the pen deflections reverse in polarity or phase.

longitudinal bipolar m., montage with derivations from pairs of electrodes placed in longitudinal, usually anteroposterior, arrays on the scalp. See also *bipolar m.*

referential m., montage used to display the potential difference between pairs of electrodes when one electrode is placed on the scalp and the other (reference) electrode is placed at a relatively neutral point, often the ear, nose, chin, or neck, and is common to multiple derivations. The scalp electrode is connected to input terminal 1 and the reference electrode to input terminal 2. By using this technique, abnormalities in the electroencephalogram are identified on the basis of amplitude. Also called *common reference,* monopolar montage, and unipolar montage.

triangular bipolar m., montage consisting of derivations from pairs of electrodes among a group of three electrodes placed on the scalp in the form of a triangle.

Monte Carlo method (mon′tē kar′lō) a technique that produces an approximation to the solution of a mathematical problem by random sampling methods. For example, the relative area of an irregular contour within a larger contour can be estimated by the random placement of points in the larger contour and the calculation of the proportion that falls in the inner contour. The method is used in statistics to estimate a random sampling distribution when the distribution cannot be derived mathematically.

Monteggia's fracture (mon-tej′ahz) [Giovanni Battista *Monteggia,* Italian surgeon, 1762–1815] a fracture of the ulna in the proximal half of the shaft, located near the junction of the middle and upper thirds. This fracture is often accompanied by dislocation of the radial head.

MOPP abbrev. for Mustargen, Oncovin, procarbazine, and prednisone, a major established cancer chemotherapy drug regimen. For more information, see the specific drug (listed under its generic name) and *Appendix A.*

Morax-Axenfeld bacillus (mōr′aks ak′sen-felt″) [Victor *Morax,* Swiss ophthalmologist, 1866–1935; Theodor *Axenfeld,* German ophthalmologist, 1867–1930] see *M. lacunata* under *Moraxella.*

Moraxella (mo″rak-sel′ah) [from V. *Morax*] a genus of bacteria of the family Neisseriaceae, consisting of gram-negative rods that are often coccoid in shape. Similar to *Acinetobacter,* they are oxidase-positive, strictly aerobic, and highly susceptible to penicillin, but do not utilize carbohydrates. *Moraxella* organisms are found as parasites, most commonly on the mucous membranes, and may cause conjunctivitis and corneal infections.

M. lacunata, a species that causes conjunctivitis and corneal infections in humans. Also called *Morax-Axenfeld bacillus.*

M. lwoffi, see *Acinetobacter calcoaceticus lwoffi.*

morbidity (mor-bid′ĭ-te) [L. *morbidus* sick] 1. pertaining to, afflicted with, or causing disease; diseased.

2. a term used to describe the ratio of sick to healthy people in the community.

morbilli (mor-bil′i) [L.] see *measles.*

mordant (mor′dant) [L. *mordere* to bite] a substance whose physicochemical structure aids in attaching a dye or stain to histologic specimens. Usually a metallic salt, the mordant forms a complex with the dye and intensifies the reaction with the tissue.

Morgagni's nodules nodules of the aortic valve cusps.

morgan (mo) (mor′gan) [from Thomas Hunt *Morgan,* American biologist, 1866–1945, winner of the Nobel Prize for Medicine in 1933] a unit of relative distance on a genetic map, the frequency with which cross-overs occur between two genes. The centimorgan (percentage of cross-overs) is most frequently used.

Morganella [from T. H. *Morgan*] a genus of gram-negative, rod-shaped bacteria belonging to the Enterobacteriaceae family and the Proteeae tribe. The three genera—*Proteus, Providencia,* and *Morganella*—are related biochemically, serologically, morphologically, and through DNA hybridization studies.

There is only one species in the *Morganella* genus, *M. morganii* (formerly called *Proteus morganii*). This bacterium is identified in the microbiology laboratory by the following characteristics: an IMViC reaction of ++−−; and by being positive for urea, ornithine decarboxylase, and phenylalanine deaminase, and negative for H_2S (on triple sugar iron agar).

See also *Enterobacteriaceae.*

morning sickness nausea and vomiting of unknown cause, associated with the early stages of pregnancy. This disorder is most common in the fifth and sixth weeks of pregnancy and usually abates after the fourteenth or sixteenth weeks. Severe vomiting (hyperemesis gravidarum) may lead to hemoconcentration, decreased serum proteins and alkali, and elevations of blood urea nitrogen and serum sodium, chloride, and potassium. Retinal bleeding and detachment may also occur.

moron (mo′ron) [Gr. *mōros* stupid] a term formerly used to denote a person with an IQ in the range of 50–70. See also *mental retardation.*

morph/o (mor′fo) [Gr. *morphē* form] a word element used in combining form to denote shape or form, e.g., morphogenesis.

morphea (mor-fe′ah) a benign, circumscribed sclerosis characterized by connective tissue replacement of the skin and sometimes the subcutaneous tissue. Oval, firm, reddish plaques appear and evolve to white or yellow lesions with lilac-colored borders. There is no visceral or organ involvement in this localized form of scleroderma. Also called *circumscribed scleroderma.*

morphine (mor′fēn) [Fr., from L. *Morpheus,* a god characterized by Ovid as causing dreams in which a human being appears] the major phenanthrene alkaloid (constituting about 10 percent) of powdered opium; consisting of bitter-tasting, colorless, shining crystals. It is a central nervous system analgesic that reduces an individual's reaction to pain; produces euphoria, lethargy, and sleep; reduces anxiety; and depresses respiration and the cough reflex. Its side-effects include nausea and vomiting.

Doses greater than 100 mg may cause death due to respiratory failure. The morphine antagonist naloxone blocks the drug action but will precipitate withdrawal syndrome in addicts.

Morphine is highly addictive. Addicts can build considerable tolerance to the drug (use of up to 5 g/da has been observed). Withdrawal symptoms include cramps, diarrhea, chills, and tremors. Blood concentrations higher than 10 μg/dl are frequently fatal.

morphine assays 1. spectrofluorimetry. Morphine is extracted from biologic specimens with organic solvents at pH 9.4 (in urine specimens, morphine glucuronide is first cleaved by acid hydrolysis). A fluorophor is formed when morphine is heated under pressure after treatment with concentrated H_2SO_4 and NH_4OH. The emission is measured at 420 nm, using an excitation wavelength of 392 nm.

2. immunoassay. Morphine can be determined by EMIT homogeneous enzyme immunoassay or radioimmunoassay (RIA).

3. thin-layer chromatography. In TLC drug-screening tests, morphine can be detected with Marquis reagent (2 percent formaldehyde in sulfuric acid), giving a purple product, or with iodoplatinate, giving a product blue-to-purple in color.

4. gas chromatography. An acetylated derivative is prepared by reaction of the extracted morphine with acetic anhydride in pyridine, and quantitated by GC using nalorphine as the internal standard.

morphodifferentiation (mor″fo-dif″er-en″she-a′shun) the arrangement of cells, a process that occurs during morphogenesis.

morphogenesis (mor″fo-jen′ĕ-sis) [*morpho-* + Gr. *gennen* to produce] in embryology, the part of the development process by means of which the shapes of the body and organs are produced. It includes processes such as cell migration and aggregation, localized cell growth or degeneration, and the splitting and folding of tissue layers. Cf. *histogenesis.*

morphology (mor-fol′o-je) [*morpho-* + *-logy*] the study of the forms and structures of organisms.

morphometry (mor-fom′ĕ-tre) the technique or process for quantifying morphologic data. The term is generally applied to the quantitative analysis of histologic sections, specifically, measurement of the length, surface area, volume, and shapes of tissue structures, and the numbers of structures in a given area or volume of tissue.

Morquio's syndrome (mor-ke′ōz) [Louis *Morquio,* pediatrician in Montevideo, Uruguay, 1867–1935] a genetic disorder, transmitted as an autosomal recessive trait, that is characterized by abnormal glycosaminoglycan metabolism, leading to skeletal deformities, corneal clouding, and aortic regurgitation. Radiologic examination reveals osteoporosis, platyspondyly, and vertebral disorders. Intelligence levels are normal, but death frequently occurs in the second decade.

There are probably two forms of this disease, Morquio A (characterized by a relative or absolute deficiency of galactosamine-6-sulfate sulfatase) and Morquio B (characterized by a deficiency of β-galactosidase). Keratan sulfate is excreted in the urine in both forms and is diagnostic of the disorder. Assays for prenatal diagnosis are still in developmental stages.

Also called chondroosteodystrophy, Morquio-Brailsford syndrome, and mucopolysaccharidosis IV (MPS IV). See also *mucopolysaccharidoses.*

mort/o (mor′to) [L. *mors* death] a word element used in combining form to denote death, e.g., mortician.

mortality (mor-tal′ĭ-te) [L. *mortalitas,* from *mortalis* mortal] pertaining to or describing the condition of being dead. The term also refers to the death rate, as in the ratio of deaths due to a disease as compared with the total number of cases of that disease. See also *mortality r.* under *rate.*

Mortierella (mor″te-ah-rel′ah) a genus of fungi occasionally involved in zygomycosis. This fungus is characterized by a sporangium that lacks a columella; the sporangium is directly attached to the tapered sporangiophore. Small, one-celled conidia (stylospores) are present.

Morton's disease (mor′tunz) [Thomas George *Morton,* Philadelphia surgeon, 1835–1903] a condition characterized by unilateral pain and paresthesia in the interdigital webbing between the third and fourth toes, thought to be due to repeated nerve trauma and a resulting neuroma. Also called Morton's foot, metatarsalgia, neuroma, and toe; and plantar neuroma. See also *neuroma.*

morula (mor′u-lah) [L. *morus* mulberry] a solid ball of blastomeres formed by the cleavage of a fertilized ovum in mammals.

morular (mor′u-lar) 1. pertaining to a morula.

2. resembling a mulberry.

morule (mor′ool) a term used to describe a form of epithelial metaplasia in the endometrium, characterized by round-to-ovoid aggregates of bland epithelial cells with indistinct cell membranes. It is often found oriented around or projecting into gland lumens. When confluent or associated with necrosis, this process may be confused with a poorly differentiated carcinoma.

mosaic (mo-za′ik) [Gr. *mouseios* of the Muses] 1. a pattern made of numerous small pieces fitted together.

2. in genetics, an organism or cell culture that consists of two or more cell lineages, either a mixoploid or a chimera.

mosaic pattern an abnormal architectural pattern in formed bone seen in osteitis deformans (Paget's disease of bone).

MOSFET abbrev. See *metal oxide semiconductor field effect t.* under *transistor.*

mOsm abbrev. See *milliosmole.*

mosquito (mos-ke′to), pl. *mosquitoes* [Sp. "little fly"] a bloodsucking winged insect, belonging to the genera *Aedes, Anopheles,* or *Culex.* Several species are known transmitters of diseases such as malaria, yellow fever, and filariasis. For more information, see the specific disease and the accompanying illustration.

mosquitocidal (mos-ke″to-si′dal) destructive to mosquitoes.

mosquitocide (mos-ke′to-sid) [*mosquito* + L. *caedere* to kill] any chemical that kills or is destructive to mosquitoes.

most significant bit (MSB) the most significant digit of a binary number.

most significant digit (MSD) 1. the leftmost significant digit (leftmost nonzero digit) in a number. See also *significant digits.*

2. the high-order digit in a computer word or register. For an *n* digit register, the digit representing 10^{n-1} (or 2^{n-1}). Cf. *least significant digit.*

mother (muth′er) [L. *mater*] the female parent; also, something from which another thing is derived, as in a mother cell.

motile (mo′til, mōt′l, mo′tīl) having spontaneous but not conscious or volitional movement.

motility (mo-til′ĭ-te) 1. the quality or state of being motile; contractility. Cf. *mobility.*

2. in microbiology, the ability of an organism to move in the medium. Motility is determined by microscopic examination of wet-mount preparations, or by the ability of the organisms to spread in a special semisolid agar culture medium. In bacteria, motility is associated with the presence of flagella.

gastrointestinal m., the movement of the gastrointestinal tract and its contents; the peristaltic smooth muscle contractions of the esophagus, stomach, small intestine, and colon, and the intraluminal pressure exerted on ingested food. Conditions associated with altered GI motility include pyloric stenosis, intestinal obstruction, ileus, and constipation.

motion (mo′shun) 1. any movement.

2. movement of the bowels; defecation.

3. a movement that causes blurring on a radiograph, such as a heartbeat or active movement by the patient.

4. in physics, the continuous change of position with time.

laws of m., the physical laws governing the motion of bodies, such as Newton's second law of motion (which states that the acceleration of a body is equal to the applied force divided by its mass) or Einstein's special and general theories of relativity.

motion sickness a functional disorder characterized by nausea, vomiting, and dizziness. It is caused by linear, vertical, or angular motion; air-, car-, train-, swing- and seasickness are all specific forms. Excessive stimulation of the semicircular canals of the inner ear, in combination with visual stimuli, is thought to be a provoking factor; a variety of emotional and physical factors are also believed to be contributory.

motoneuron (mo″to-nu′ron) see *motor neuron.*

motor (mo′tor) [L.] 1. a muscle, nerve, or center that effects or produces movement.

2. a device that converts heat or electrical energy into mechanical energy (motion).

motor end-plate the region of contact between a motor nerve and a skeletal muscle fiber. Also called myoneural junction. See also *skeletal m.* under *muscle.*

motor neuron an efferent neuron that conducts motor impulses. Also called *motoneuron.*

lower m. n.'s, peripheral neurons whose cell bodies lie in the ventral gray columns of the spinal cord and whose terminations are on skeletal muscle fibers.

upper m. n.'s., neurons in the cerebral cortex that conduct impulses from the motor cortex to motor nuclei of the cranial nerves or to the ventral gray columns of the spinal cord.

motor neuron diseases (mo′tor nu′ron) a group of diseases characterized by progressive muscular atrophy, weakness, and wasting due to the involvement of lower motor neurons. The causative agents are generally unknown. Diseases in this category include amyotrophic lateral sclerosis, progressive bulbar palsy, and the spinal muscular and peroneal muscular atrophies. For more information, see the specific motor neuron disease.

motor point in clinical electromyography, a point on the skin where electrical stimulation of low voltage and short duration elicits contraction of a specific muscle.

motor unit the subdivision of centrally controlled skeletal muscle function, consisting of an anterior horn cell, its axon, the terminal arborizations, neu-

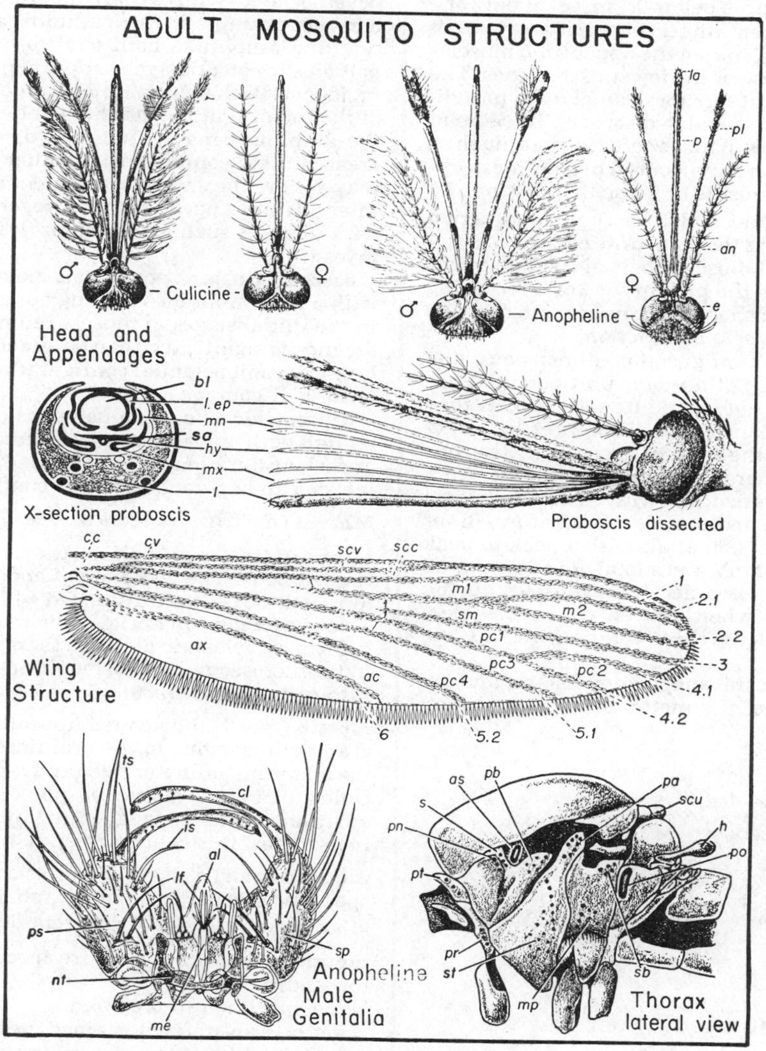

Mosquito. Drawings showing various adult mosquito structures: *ac,* anal cell; *al,* anal lobe; *an,* antenna; *as,* anterior thoracic spiracle; *ax,* axillary cell; *bl,* blood canal; *cc,* costal cell; *cl,* clasper; *cv,* costal vein; *e,* eye; *h,* halter; *hy,* hypopharynx; *is,* internal spine; *l,* labium; *la,* labellum; *lep,* labrum-epipharynx; *lf,* leaflets of mesosome; *m1, 2,* marginal cells by number; *me,* mesosome; *mn,* mandible; *mp,* mesepimeral bristles (lower); *mx,* maxilla; *nt,* ninth tergite; *p,* proboscis; *pa,* prealar bristles; *pb,* postspiracular bristles; *pc1,2,* posterior cells by number; *pl,* palpus; *pn,* pronotal bristles; *po,* posterior thoracic spiracle; *pr,* proternal bristles; *ps,* parabasal spines; *pt,* prothoracic bristles; *s,* spiracular bristles; *sa,* salivary canal; *sb,* subalar bristles (upper mesepimerals); *scc,* subcostal cell; *scu,* scutellum; *scv,* subcostal vein; *sm,* submarginal cell; *sp,* side piece; *st,* sternopleural bristles; *ts,* terminal spine of clasper; and *1, 2.1, 2.2, 3, 4.1, 4.2, 5.1, 5.2, 6,* longitudinal veins by number. (From Hunter, G. W., III, et al.: Tropical Medicine. 5th ed. Philadelphia, W. B. Saunders Co., 1976.)

romuscular junctions, and the many muscle fibers that the axon innervates. A descending impulse of threshold magnitude produces simultaneous contraction of all muscle fibers in the unit. The muscle fibers of a single unit are scattered diffusely among the fibers of other units, but all fibers of a single unit possess common histochemical and contractile properties.

Motor units of a certain muscle vary with respect to the innervation ratio or the total number of fibers innervated per total number of axons. The mean innervation ratio of all skeletal muscle fibers is 150, but in muscles capable of fine, graded movement, it may be as low as 2. In the major limb muscles, the ratio may be as high as 2000.

m. u. territory, 1. the region of a skeletal muscle over which the fibers of a motor unit are spatially dispersed.

2. the area of a muscle from which any recorded electrical activity reflects the compound action po-

tential (with a rise time below 0.5 msec) of only one motor unit. The motor unit territory has an approximate diameter of 5–7 mm in the upper limb muscles and 7–10 mm in those of the lower extremities. The size of the motor unit territory can change in individuals with neuromuscular disorders. In cases of neurogenic weakness, it may increase by as much as 40 percent; reduction may occur in myopathic disorders such as polymyositis or muscular dystrophy.

motor unit potential (MUP) a compound action potential that reflects the composite electrical activity of the individual muscle fibers of a single motor unit that are within the pickup zone of a recording electrode. This electrical activity is related to the force of skeletal muscle contraction.

The parameters (configuration, dimensions, and recruitment pattern) of a motor unit potential are relatively constant but should be specified, as they may vary in accordance with differences in the recording site, with the type of recording electrode and recording apparatus, with the muscle from which they are recorded, and with other physiologic factors such as age and muscle temperature. Bi- or triphasic motor unit potentials with a peak-to-peak amplitude of 0.2–3.0 mV and a total duration of 2–15 msec are normally recorded from muscles during voluntary activity when concentric needle electrodes are used (see also the accompanying illustration).

Abnormalities in the shape, dimensions, and recruitment pattern of the motor unit potential may be associated with certain neuromuscular disorders. For example, in myopathic disorders, the duration and amplitude both tend to be reduced, and polyphasic potentials may appear with an increased incidence. With neuropathic disorders, the duration of the motor unit potential may be increased while the amplitude may be normal, diminished, or increased. Late components (smaller potentials that may follow the motor unit potential after a brief interval) can appear with neurogenic disorders or with diseases such as muscular dystrophy or polymyositis.

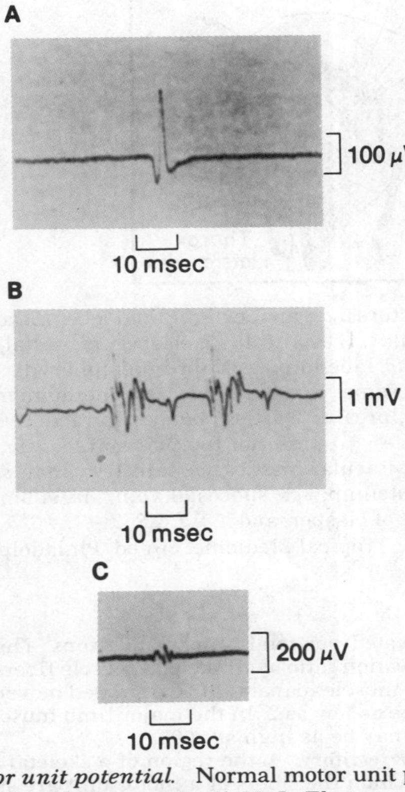

Motor unit potential. Normal motor unit potential. (Adapted from Aminoff, M. J.: Electromyography in Clinical Practice. Menlo Park, CA, Addison-Wesley Publishing Co., 1978.)

nascent m. u. p., a polyphasic motor unit potential with a low amplitude and long duration that is seen in the initial stages of muscle reinnervation. As no diagnostic significance can be attached to a particular motor unit potential configuration, the use of the term is discouraged.

neuropathic m. u. p., a polyphasic motor unit potential with an abnormally increased amplitude and a long duration. No particular diagnostic significance can be attached to this configuration.

Motrin (mo'trin) trademark. See *ibuprofen.*

Mott cell (mot) a plasma cell that is the origin of the Russell body. The cisternae of endoplasmic reticulum in these cells are distended with stored proteinaceous secretory material. This material coalesces to form cytoplasmic globules that, when viewed by light microscopy, are eosinophilic and hyalinized. Also called *thesaurocyte.* See also *Russell body.*

mottle (mot''l) the spotted appearance of a photographic image due to the graininess of the film or the quantum nature of light and x-rays; the latter is called quantum mottle or photon mottle. When quantum mottle is exaggerated by x-ray intensifying screens, it is called screen mottle.

mottled (mot'l'd) having a multicolored pattern of spots and streaks; in a radiograph, having a pattern of spots and streaks of different densities.

mount (mownt) 1. to prepare specimens and slides for study.

2. a specimen so prepared.

wet m., an unfixed, stained, or unstained specimen placed in water on a microscope slide for examination.

mountain sickness disturbances that result from poor physiologic adjustment to high altitudes. Acute mountain sickness, seen at altitudes greater than 2000 m, is characterized by headache, nausea, inactivity, dyspnea, and cyanosis. Later, visual and auditory disturbances may occur, with insomnia, weight loss, and tachycardia. Subacute mountain sickness, experienced at altitudes greater than 4500 m, may exhibit similar symptoms. Chronic mountain sickness (Monge's disease) is characterized by chronic alveolar hypoventilation, hypoxemia, polycythemia, and evidence of right heart enlargement. In all cases, a return to lower altitudes relieves the disorder.

mountant (mownt'ant) see *mounting medium.*

mounting (mownt'ing) in histology, the process of impregnating stained tissue sections with a mounting medium, which protects the tissue and dyes from deterioration and improves the visibility of the tissue components. In permanent mounting, the stained sections are dehydrated and cleared; enough resinous mounting medium is then placed on the section to fill the area under the coverglass.

Some preparations, such as fat stains and metachromatic stains, are dissolved or altered by xylene; semipermanent mounting in a water-soluble medium is used for them, and the sections can be made more permanent by sealing the edges of the coverglass with paraffin wax, nail varnish, or plastic cement.

mounting medium a clear substance placed between the coverglass and microscope slide that permeates the spaces of a tissue section. Its index of refraction should be close to that of glass (1.518) and different from that of the unstained tissue components (1.530–1.540) so that the tissue components are visible.

Permanent mounting media include natural resins, which are no longer used because they are acidic and cause the fading of stains—e.g., Canada balsam; and synthetic resins, which are neutral and do not cause fading—e.g., Permount, Harleco Synthetic Resin (HSR), and Histoclad.

Water-soluble media contain acacia (gum arabic), sugars, or glycerol, which raise the refractive index, and may also contain salts, which control the pH of the medium to prevent bleeding or fading of the dyes. These include Apathy's gum syrup medium, Farrant's medium, glycerol gelatin medium, and the commercially prepared media Paragon, Clearcol, and Abopon.

Water, glycerol, and mineral oil are also used as temporary mounting media.

Also called *mountant.* For more information, see the specific medium.

mouse (mows) a small rodent used extensively in laboratory experimental studies. In its natural habitat, the mouse serves as the natural reservoir for *Rickettsia akari,* the cause of rickettsialpox.

mouth (mowth) [L. *os, oris*] an opening or aperture; generally used to refer to the proximal orifice of the alimentary canal, or the oral cavity. Also called *os.*

Movat's pentachrome method a histologic staining method for connective tissue using five different stains. Formalin-fixed paraffin sections are stained first with Alcian blue 8GX, which is converted to an insoluble pigment by immersion in alkaline alcohol, and then successively in resorcin-fuchsin, Weigert's iron hematoxylin, Woodstain Scarlet N.S.–acid fuchsin, and, after mordanting in phosphotungstic acid and dehydrating in alcohol, alcoholic Safran du Gatinais (Woodstain Scarlet N.S. and Safran du Gatinais are proprietary dyes). Nuclei stain black, elastic fibers purple to black, collagen and reticulin yellow, ground substance blue to blue-green, fibrinoid intense red, and muscle red.

movement (mo͞ov′ment) an act of moving; motion. For more information, see the specific type of movement.

movement artifact see under *artifact.*

6-MP abbrev. See *mercaptopurine.*

m. p. abbrev. See *melting point.*

MPD abbrev. See *maximal permissible d.* under *dose.*

M phase the phase of mitosis. See also *cell cycle.*

M protein see *M component.*

MPS abbrev. See *mucopolysaccharide.*

MPS storage diseases I-VII see *mucopolysaccharidoses.*

mR abbrev. See *milliroentgen.*

μR abbrev. See *microroentgen.*

mrad abbrev. See *millirad.*

mrem abbrev. See *millirem.*

MRF abbrev. for melanocyte-stimulating hormone–releasing factor. See *melanocyte-stimulating hormone–releasing hormone.*

MRH abbrev. See *melanocyte-stimulating hormone–releasing hormone.*

MRIH abbrev. See *melanocyte-stimulating hormone–release-inhibiting hormone.*

mRNA abbrev. for messenger ribonucleic acid. See under *ribonucleic acid.*

MS abbrev. See *multiple s.* under *sclerosis.*

ms abbrev. See *millisecond.*

μs abbrev. See *microsecond.*

msec abbrev. See *millisecond.*

μsec abbrev. See *microsecond.*

MSH abbrev. See *melanocyte-stimulating hormone.*

MT abbrev. See *medical technologist.*

MTBF abbrev. See *mean time between failures.*

MTF abbrev. See *modulation transfer function.*

mU abbrev. see *milliunit.*

μU abbrev. See *microunit.*

mu (M, μ) (mu, moo) the twelfth letter of the *Greek alphabet.*

mμ abbrev. See *millimicro.*

muc/o (mu′ko) [L. *mucus*] a word element used in combining form to denote mucus, e.g., mucocutaneous.

mu-chain disease a rare type of monoclonal gammopathy in which the serum paraprotein consists of mu-type heavy chains of (IgM) immunoglobulins. Mu-chain disease results in chronic lymphocytic leukemia and hepatosplenomegaly. See also *monoclonal gammopathy.*

mucicarmine stain (mu″sĭ-kar′min) a specific stain for mucin prepared by heating carmine, aluminum hydroxide, and anhydrous aluminum chloride, and by adding 50 percent ethyl alcohol (stock solution diluted in 4–10 parts of distilled water immediately before use). Only mucus and the capsules of cryptococcus are stained red. Sections usually are also stained with hematoxylin for nuclei.

mucigen (mu′sĭ-jen) [*muc-* + Gr. *gennan* to produce] the glycoproteins in a secretory vacuole of a mucous cell, which become mucus after secretion.

mucin (mu′sin) 1. mucosubstance occurring in epithelial tissue, the substance of mucus. It is a highly viscous fluid composed of hydrated glycoproteins. In histochemistry, mucins are divided into neutral mucins, which are PAS-positive and not stained by Alcian blue; sialomucins, which are alcianophilic at pH 2.5 but not at pH 1.0 and are digested by sialidase; and sulfomucins, which are alcianophilic at pH 1.0. See also *mucigen, mucopolysaccharide,* and *mucopolysaccharide staining.*

2. any mucoprotein or mucopolysaccharide.

mucin clot test a test of the degree of polymerization of synovial fluid hyaluronate. A few drops of synovial fluid are added to a few milliliters of 5 percent acetic acid and allowed to stand for several minutes. A normal result (reported as "good") is indicated by the formation of a firm clot surrounded by a clear solution. A soft clot surrounded by a slightly turbid solution is reported as "fair," whereas a crumbly clot surrounded by a turbid solution that shreds when shaken is reported as "poor." When no clot forms, the test is reported as "very poor." Abnormal results occur in many inflammatory conditions, such as gouty and rheumatoid arthritis. Also called *Ropes test.*

mucinosis (mu″sĭ-no′sis) a disorder characterized by abnormal deposits of mucin in the skin. This condition is seen most frequently in association with the myxedema of hypothyroidism. See also *myxedema.*

mucin test test for excess urinary mucins in which urine is filtered and 33 percent acetic acid added dropwise under controlled conditions. Mucins are indicated by the appearance of opalescence, which is stable to the further addition of acetic acid, whereas other urinary proteins dissolve in the excess acid.

mucocele (mu′ko-sēl) [*muco-* + Gr. *kēlē* tumor] the dilation of an organ, gland, or duct with mucous secretions. Mucoceles are known to occur in the appendix, gallbladder, oral cavity, and nasal sinuses; the mucinous substances accumulate and cause inflammation and progressive cystic dilation.

mucocutaneous (mu″ko-ku-ta′ne-us) [*muco-* + *cutaneous*] pertaining to or affecting mucus membrane and skin.

mucoenteritis (mu″ko-en″ter-i′tis) see *irritable bowel syndrome.*

mucoepidermoid (mu″ko-ep″ĭ-der′moid) a general term used to describe a variable mixture of mucus-secreting cells and squamous epithelial cells.

mucoepidermoid carcinoma a malignant neoplasm formed by an admixture of epidermoid and mucin-forming cells in varying proportions. Most arise in salivary glands, but occasionally one is found in the bronchial tree. Although most tumors are of a low-grade malignancy, local recurrence is common, and the more aggressive tumors may give rise to regional lymph node metastases. The nests of cells show a transition from peripheral layers with epidermoid features to central, mucin-forming cells that frequently border an acinar lumen. The behavior of a mucoepidermoid carcinoma cannot be accurately predicted from its histology, but it is better with low-grade tumors in which mucin production and cystic change are evident by light microscopy.

mucoid (mu′koid) [*mucus* + Gr. *eidos* form] resembling mucus or mucin.

Mucolexx trademark for a fluid used as a mucoliquefying preservative for thick, mucoid cytology specimens.

mucolipidosis (mu″ko-lip″ĭ-do′sis), pl. *mucolipidoses* any inborn error of metabolism in which both glycosaminoglycans (GAGs) and sphingolipids accumulate in lysosomes, causing neurologic symptoms. They are distinguished from mucopolysaccharidoses in that there is no excess excretion of GAGs in the urine. Four diseases are named as mucolipidoses: mucolipidosis I (ML I, isolated neuraminidase deficiency), mucolipidosis II (I-cell disease), mucolipidosis III (a mild form of ML II), and mucolipidosis IV. The first three have symptoms similar to those of Hurler's syndrome. ML IV is marked by corneal clouding and psychomotor retardation. Several other storage diseases, such as G_{M1}-gangliosidosis, also fit the definition of a mucolipidosis. For more information, see also the accompanying table.

mucopeptide (mu″ko-pep′tīd) see *peptidoglycan.*

mucopolysaccharidase (mu″ko-pol″e-sak′ah-rī-dās) a group of enzymes that catalyze the hydrolysis of various types of mucopolysaccharides. Specific examples are α-L-iduronohydrolase, β-D-glucuronidase, and α-*N*-acetyl-D-glucosaminidase. In microbiology, it is a general term for several enzymes secreted by bacterial cells that catalyze the breakdown of cell wall constituents. See also *hyaluronidase, lysozyme,* and *neuraminidase.*

mucopolysaccharide (MPS) (mu″ko-pol″e-sak′-

MUCOLIPIDOSES

Condition	Biochemical Defect	Abnormal Metabolite*	Mode of Inheritance†
Mucolipidosis I	Neuraminidase	Sialic acid oligosaccharides (U)	AR
Mucolipidosis II	Deficiency of lysosomal acid hydrolases	Excess acid hydrolases (S)	AR
Mucolipidosis III	Deficiency of lysosomal acid hydrolases	Elevated acid hydrolases (S)	AR
Mucolipidosis IV	Unknown	Ganglioside and mucopolysaccharide accumulation (skin fibroblast cultures)	AR
Aspartylglucosaminuria	Deficiency of lysosomal β-aspartylacetylglucosaminidase	2-Acetamido-1-(β′-1-aspartamido)-1,2-dideoxyglucose (U)	AR
Fucosidosis	Deficiency of α-L-fucosidase	Fucose-rich glycolipids, glycoproteins, and mucopolysaccharides (T)	AR
Mannosidosis	Deficiency of lysosomal α-mannosidase	Mannose-containing oligosaccharides (U)	AR

* Serum = serum; U = urine; T = tissue.
† AR = autosomal recessive.

ah-rīd) 1. a mucosubstance occurring in the ground substance of connective tissue. Chemically, these polysaccharides are classed as glycosaminoglycans, heteropolysaccharides containing hexosamine sulfates, and hexoseuronic acids. They are associated with a protein component (mucoprotein) in aggregates called proteoglycans. See also *glycosaminoglycans.*

2. any polysaccharide with a high amino sugar content. They are divided into acid mucopolysaccharides (glycosaminoglycans) and neutral mucopolysaccharides, such as chitin.

mucopolysaccharide staining any of a number of histochemical staining procedures used to detect mucopolysaccharides in tissue. Some of the more common techniques employed include the periodic acid–Schiff (PAS) reaction, which demonstrates the presence of aldehyde groups after oxidation with periodic acid; the metachromasia demonstration using toluidine blue or Alcian blue at various pHs; aldehyde-fuchsin stain to visualize acid groups; and diamine methods oxidized with ferric chloride, which utilize isomers of diamine to differentiate between types of mucopolysaccharides.

The use of various blocking techniques (e.g., acetylation, saponification, sulfation, and methylation), as well as alteration by enzymatic digestion (e.g., hyaluronidase and sialidase) coupled with the staining procedures, permits more complete discrimination among various mucopolysaccharide substances.

mucopolysaccharide storage disease see *mucopolysaccharidoses.*

mucopolysaccharide tests 1. toluidine blue spot test. This is a screening test for the presence of acid mucopolysaccharides such as dermatan sulfate and heparan sulfate in the urine of patients with Hurler's syndrome and some other hereditary mucopolysaccharidoses. Separate 5-, 10-, and 25-μl spots of urine specimen and normal urine control, as well as 5μl of chondroitin sulfate standard solution, are applied to a piece of filter paper and the spots dried. The paper is then dipped into toluidine blue solution. Acid mucopolysaccharide stains purple, which can be easily seen against a blue background; the normal urine spot is blue. Alcian blue has also been used instead of toluidine blue.

2. turbidity test, a screening test. The surfactant cetylpyridinium chloride or cetyltrimethylammonium bromide produces a turbidity in a urine specimen containing acid mucopolysaccharides.

3. acid albumin turbidity test, a screening test. Albumin is added to dialyzed, buffered urine at an acid pH. Turbidity indicates the presence of acid mucopolysaccharides. Under appropriately standardized conditions, this method can be semiquantitative.

4. electrophoresis, a quantitative method. A concentrated urine specimen is subjected to electrophoresis, and mucopolysaccharides are quantitated by densitometry after acridine orange staining.

5. quantitative analysis. Mucopolysaccharides are precipitated with cetyltrimethylammonium bromide and are quantitated by determination of uronic acid in the redissolved precipitate.

mucopolysaccharidoses (mu″ko-pol″e-sak″ah-rĭ-do′sēz) a group of inherited progressive storage diseases characterized by excess excretion in the urine of mucopolysaccharide sulfates called glycosaminoglycans (GAGs) and the intralysosomal storage of products of partial MPS degradation. The GAGs are among the primary constituents of the extracellular matrix synthesized by connective tissue cells. Those affected have widespread deformities of many organs and tissues due to excessive storage and slow turnover of GAGs.

Lysosomes are organelles within the cell responsible for the digestion of large, complex macromolecules. They contain enzymes (catabolic hydrolases) that have an irreversible lytic action and are most active in an acid pH of 1.0–5.0. A genetic alteration in a specific lysosomal enzyme, which inactivates the enzyme, will cause an accumulation of the substrate of that enzyme in the lysosomes. The clinical manifestations of lysosomal storage disorders, of which the mucopolysaccharidoses are one major category, depend on the nature of the stored material and the function of the tissue. The biochemical identification of all the principal clinical mucopolysaccharidoses has been accomplished. Many of the enzyme deficiencies were elucidated as a direct result of the discovery of individual protein "corrective factors" in fibroblast cultures of patients with different MPS storage diseases. Complementation, or the intercellular exchange of corrective factors in vitro, could reduce or prevent the accumulation of GAGs among different forms of the disorders. Quite unexpectedly, the Hurler (MPS I H) and the Scheie (MPS I S) syndromes were demonstrated to be allelic mutations, and patients with an intermediate phenotype are believed to be compound heterozygotes with one MPS I H allele and one MPS I S. The accompanying table correlates early names of the syndromes with current nomenclature, delineates the enzyme defect, and identifies the clinical findings and modes of inheritance.

When clinical and radiographic evidence suggests an MPS storage disease, a urinary screening test is the start of the laboratory documentation of the disorder. The specific MPS excreted can be determined by thin-layer or ion-exchange chromatography. The abnormal accumulation of $^{35}SO_4$-labeled GAG, which can be corrected by in vitro complementation, is the test of choice for confirming mucopolysaccharidoses; an enzyme assay of cultured fibroblasts and/or leukocytes is required for the identification of an individual syndrome. Although no treatment is yet available, accurate enzyme identification is important for the purposes of genetic counseling and supportive therapy. Most mucopolysaccharidoses can be diagnosed prenatally using enzyme assays on cultured amniotic fluid cells.

For more information, see the specific MPS storage disease.

MURIEL GLUCKSON, M.S.

mucoprotein (mu″ko-pro′te-in) a carbohydrate-containing protein found in mucous secretions that has carbohydrate contents of between 4–6 and 30 percent. The carbohydrate component contains aminoglycans but no uronic acids, and hence no mucopolysaccharides (glycosaminoglycans). In contrast to mucoproteins, glycoproteins contain less than 4 percent carbohydrates, and proteoglycans contain 35–95 percent mucopolysaccharides strung along a protein polypeptide chain. Cf. *glycoprotein.*

mucoprotein assays colorimetric method. Most serum proteins are precipitated with perchloric acid; mucoproteins remain in the filtrate and are then precipitated with phosphotungstic acid, washed free of nonprotein nitrogen, dissolved in aqueous sodium carbonate, and reacted with the Folin-Ciocalteau phenol reagent. The blue color produced is compared with that produced by a standard tyrosine solution, using 0.042 g of tyrosine as equivalent to 1.0 g of mucoproteins. The reference range for mucoprotein in serum is 75–135 mg/dl. See also *uromucoid assays.*

mucopurulent (mu″ko-pu′roo-lent) containing both mucus and pus.

Mucor (mu′kor) [L.] a genus of zygomycete fungi that belongs to the family Mucoraceae, order Mucorales, and is an etiologic agent of mucormycosis. The fungus is characterized by branched sporangiophores arising from the mycelium. No stolons or rhizoids are present, in contrast to *Absidia* and *Rhizopus.* Medically important species include *M. ramosissimus, M. pusillus, M. javanicus, M. racemosus,* and *M. spinosus.* See also *Absidia, mucormycosis,* and *Rhizopus.*

mucormycosis (mu″kor-mi-ko′sis) a fungal infection caused by species of *Absidia, Mucor, Rhizopus, Cunninghamella,* and *Mortierella,* which are members of order Mucorales, subclass Zygomycetes, class Phycomycetes. Mucormycosis is grouped with entomophthoromycosis (Entomophthorales is the other order in Zygomycetes) as a zygomycosis, and because the human pathogens are usually zygomycetes, this name is preferred to the broader term phycomycosis. The terms subcutaneous phycomycosis and deep phycomycosis, however, are still commonly used to refer to infection by these organisms.

Infection by the first three genera named above is characterized by fulminating lesions of the orbital tissues and nasal sinuses, invasion of the blood vessels with formation of emboli, pulmonary lesions, and gastrointestinal ulcers. This kind of mycosis is most commonly associated with diabetes mellitus and other diseases that result in a state of acidosis. The *Cunninghamella* species, isolated from cancer patients, can cause pneumonia and dissemination, whereas *Mortierella* species, although rarely causing human infections, have been isolated from indolent skin ulcers. Species of *Absidia, Mucor, Rhizopus,* and *Mortierella* are also important agents of abortion in cattle and swine.

Clinical Diagnosis. The clinical diseases of mucormycosis are varied and depend on the type of preexisting disease present.

1. Rhinocerebral Mucormycosis. The most common of the mucormycoses, this form generally begins in the paranasal sinuses and extends rapidly to the orbit, palate, and turbinates. Ulceration and perforation of the palate is an important feature, and thrombosis of nasal vessels leads to the discharge of black necrotic material. Extension to the brain (particularly the frontal lobes) with multiple cerebral infarctions may occur and have fatal results.

2. Thoracic Mucormycosis. Associated with pulmonary involvement in patients with leukemia and lymphoma, this form has symptoms including a nonspecific bronchitis and lobar pneumonia. Direct invasion of pulmonary arteries results in the familiar triad of thrombosis, infarction, and necrosis. During the sudden onset of this disease, pain, pleural friction, and bloody sputum are found.

3. Gastrointestinal Mucormycosis. This form is most often associated with undernourished individuals with metabolic imbalances, but also with other diseases such as kwashiorkor, amebic colitis, and typhoid. It commonly produces ulceration of the alimentary tract, peritonitis, and infarction.

4. Cutaneous Lesions. This form involves infections acquired nosocomially and is associated with debilitated or burn patients. The granulomatous and abscessed lesions contain nonseptate hyphae of the infecting fungus. Tissue reaction is often minimal, even when the fungus is present in quantity. However, if an infarction does occur owing to systemic infection, there usually is severe inflammation in the area of the infarct.

Laboratory Diagnosis. The ubiquity of these fungi in the environment as contaminants often brings them to the attention of the laboratory worker. However, continuous isolation of these species from pus, sputum, nasal discharge, or significant isolates from cerebrospinal fluid, blood, or other tissue biopsy, should be regarded as serious.

Except for *Mortierella,* all species are rapidly

Mucopolysaccharidoses

Type	Enzyme Defect	Abnormal Urinary Metabolite	Mode of Iheritance*
IH (Hurler)	α-L-Iduronidase	Dermatan sulfate, heparan sulfate	AR
IS (Scheie)	α-L-Iduronidase	Dermatan sulfate, heparan sulfate	AR
IHS (Hurler-Scheie)	α-L-Iduronidase	Dermatan sulfate, heparan sulfate	AR
II (Hunter), severe	Iduronate sulfatase	Dermatan sulfate, heparan sulfate	X-Linked recessive
II (Hunter), mild	Iduronate sulfatase	Dermatan sulfate, heparan sulfate	X-Linked recessive
IIIA (Sanfilippo)	Heparitinsulphate lyase (heparan-*N*-sulfatase)	Heparan sulfate	AR
IIIB (Sanfilippo)	α-*N*-Acetyl-D-glucosaminidase	Heparan sulfate	AR
IVA (Morquio)	Galactosamine-6-sulfatase	Keratan sulfate, chondroitin sulfate	AR
IVB (Morquio)	β-Galactosidase	Keratan sulfate, chondroitin sulfate	AR
VI (Maroteaux-Lamy)	Arylsulfatase B (*N*-acetylgalactosamine sulfatase)	Dermatan sulfate	AR
VII (Sly)	β-Glucuronidase	Dermatan sulfate, heparan sulfate	AR

* AR = autosomal recessive.

growing fungi and can be cultured onto most routine media, especially on glucose-peptone or malt agar that contains chloramphenicol; the possibility of contaminants should be kept in mind. There are no serologic diagnostic procedures. However, a rapid presumptive diagnosis can be made by the use of phase-contrast microscopy to detect the characteristic hyphae on a wet-mount preparation from exudates. The broad, uneven, nonseptate, cenocytic hyphae seen in the histopathology of infected tissues are also diagnostic.

mucosa (mu-ko′sah) [L. "mucus"] see *mucous membrane.*

mucosal (mu-ko′sal) pertaining to the mucous membrane.

mucosal neuroma syndrome see *MEN III* under *MEN syndrome.*

mucosubstance (mu″ko-sub′stans) a general term referring to both mucopolysaccharide and mucin.

mucous (mu′kus) [L. *mucosus*] pertaining to, resembling, or secreting mucus.

mucous colitis (mu′kus ko-li′tis) see *irritable bowel syndrome.*

mucous gland a gland that secretes mucus. Such structures range from unicellular glands, the goblet cells of the intestinal and respiratory tracts, to multicellular glands, in which the mucous cells are below the epithelial surface and are connected to it by ducts. Some glands are entirely mucus secreting, whereas others are mixed, elaborating both serous and mucous secretions.

mucous membrane a mucous tunic or coat: the mucous membrane lining of various tubular structures. It comprises the epithelium, basement membrane, lamina propria mucosae, and lamina muscularis mucosae. Also called *mucosa.*

mucoviscidosis (mu″ko-vis″ĭ-do′sis) see *cystic fibrosis.*

mucus (mu′kus) [L.] a slimy, protective coating on many free surfaces of the body, secreted by mucus-forming (goblet) cells. See also *mucin.*

Mueller-Hinton agar see *Mueller-Hinton a.* under *agar.*

müllerian duct (mil-ĕ′re-an) [from Johannes Peter *Müller,* German physiologist, 1801–1858; one of the most distinguished physiologists of Germany and the founder of scientific medicine in that country] see *müllerian d.* under *duct.*

Müller's maneuver (mil′erz) [Johannes Peter *Müller*] a maximal inspiratory effort against a resistance (a closed glottis or airway). This maneuver lowers intrapulmonary (to as low as –60 to –100 torr) and intrathoracic pressures, resulting in an accumulation of blood in the intrathoracic vasculature. It can be used during fluoroscopic examination to aid in the recognition of esophageal varices and in the discrimination of vascular from nonvascular structures.

multi- (mul′ti, mul′tĭ) [L. *multus* many, much] a word element used in combining form to denote many or much, e.g., multicellular.

multicellular (mul″tĭ-sel-u-lar) [*multi-* + L. *cellula* cell] 1. composed of many cells.
2. containing many hollow spaces.

Multiceps (mul′tĭ-seps) a genus of tapeworms of the family Taeniidae. The larval stages of the species *M. multiceps* (the gid worm) and *M. serialis* are occasionally parasitic in humans, and cause cenurosis (gid).

multichannel analyzer (MCA) (mul″tĭ-chan″l) 1. an electronic device that classifies the signal pulses received according to their peak voltage and counts the number in each pulse-height range. Some scintillation cameras have an MCA that records the photopeak of the radionuclide being used. This is used to set the energy window controls.
2. any analytic device that simultaneously analyzes one sample for multiple constituents.

multifactorial (mul″ti-fak-tor′e-al) 1. pertaining to or arising from the influence of several factors.
2. in genetics, influenced by multiple genes and/or environmental factors. See *multifactorial i.* under *inheritance.*

multifocal (mul″tĭ-fo′kal) arising from or pertaining to many foci.

multiformatter (mul″tĭ-for′mat-er) a device that records the output from a scintillation camera or its computer store onto film. With electronic circuitry it performs instantaneous enlargement, minification, or projection of the image onto different parts of the oscilloscope screen in a preprogrammed mode if necessary. This allows ouput of many images from a patient study, either dynamic or static, onto a single film.

multigravida (mul″tĭ-grav′ĭ-dah) [*multi-* + L. *gravida* pregnant] a female who is pregnant for the third time or more. Also called *plurigravida.*

multilamellar body (mul″tĭ-lah-mel′ar) [*multi-* + L. *lamella,* dim. of *lamina* thin, flat plate] a membrane-bound body found in the type II pneumocyte, which represents the precursor form of pulmonary surfactant. It is composed of concentric whorls of phospholipid membranes. Also called *cytosome* and *lamellar body.*

multilobar (mul″tĭ-lo′bar) having multiple lobes.

multilobular (mul″tĭ-lob′u-lar) [*multi-* + L. *lobulus* lobule] having multiple lobes.

multilocular (mul″tĭ-lok′u-lar) [*multi-* + L. *loculus* cell] having many cells or compartments, e.g., a multilocular cyst. Cf. *unilocular.*

multilocular cystic kidney see under *renal tumors.*

multimeter (mul″tĭ-me′ter) see *volt-ohm-milliammeter.*

multipara (mul-tip′ah-rah) [*multi-* + L. *parere* to bring forth] a female who has had two or more pregnancies resulting in viable offspring. Also called *pluripara.*

multiplane tomographic scanner (mul′tĭ-plān to″mo-graf′ik skan′er) a nuclear medicine imaging device that uses the technologies of both the rectilinear scanner and scintillation camera to produce scans in 12 planes simultaneously—6 from each probe. Its operation is similar to that of the dual-probe rectilinear scanner, except that each probe contains a photomultiplier tube array and detects the position at which each count is received like a scintillation camera. From the position of the detector head, the position of the event in the detector, and the properties of the focusing collimator, the electronic circuitry determines the path of the gamma ray and plots a point in each of the six planes seen by one probe that corresponds to the intersection of the gamma ray and the readout plane. Each image is similar to a conventional rectilinear scan: the image of the distribution of radioactivity in the readout plane is in sharp focus, but the image of planes above and below is blurred; the blurring is proportional to the distance from the readout plane.

multiple (mul′tĭ-p′l) [L. *multiplex*] more than one; occurring in various parts of the body at once.

multiple access the simultaneous use of a computer system by several users at remote terminals.

multiple adenoma see *multiple p.* under *polyp.*

multiple endocrine adenomatosis see *MEN syndrome.*

multiple endocrine neoplasia see *MEN syndrome.*

multiple event curve a dose-response curve relating biologic response to radiation dose that falls off at low doses faster than a linear response. Such curves provide evidence for the multiple-hit theory, which holds that the sensitive target (presumably DNA) in the cell must be hit more than once for a biologic effect to occur.

multiple myeloma a progressive and usually fatal malignant neoplastic proliferation of a single clone of plasma cells, which leads to the overproduction of a single type of intact immunoglobin (IgG, IgA, IgD, or IgE) or Bence Jones protein (a dimer of two identical κ or λ light chains. The incidence of this disease has increased to the point at which it represents nearly 10 percent of all hematologic neoplasms. Persons over age 40 are most commonly affected. The initial symptoms may be infection, anemia, or bone pain. Osteolytic lesions are due to neoplastic replacement of bone and usually involve the skull or vertebrae. Spontaneous fractures and abnormalities of bone shape may occur, and hypercalcemia may follow bone destruction. Renal damage, weakness, weight loss, and recurrent infection (especially pneumonia) complete the clinical picture.

Laboratory tests reveal an anemia that is normochromic and normocytic. Reductions in white blood cell and platelet counts may occur as the disease progresses. Rouleaux formation is very common, the erythrocyte sedimentation rate (ESR) is markedly elevated, and hemolysis is increased. Serum globulin concentrations may exceed 10 g/dl. Protein electrophoresis reveals a sharp monoclonal spike with γ-electrophoretic mobility in the presence of IgG; β in the presence of IgA; β to γ in the presence of IgD, IgE, or free heavy chains; and α_2 to γ in the presence of light chains. An IgG peak is seen in about 50 percent of those affected and an IgA peak in 25 percent. Electrophoresis of urine shows a monoclonal κ or λ peak in about 40 percent of all patients. Those patients who hypersecrete only free monoclonal light chains tend to have an associated hypogammaglobulinemia. Cryoglobulins may also be increased.

Bone marrow aspiration and biopsy reveal increased numbers of plasma cells (often more than 20 percent of the total). They may be large, bizarre, or multinucleated, and form diffuse sheets. Bone radiographs reveal typical punched-out lesions and diffuse osteoporosis without bone replacement, whereas bone scans are often normal (as are serum alkaline phosphatase and phosphate levels). Hypercalcemia occurs in about 50 percent of cases; increased urea nitrogen and hyperuricemia are sometimes observed.

These factors, along with the increased filtered load of free light chains, account for the frequency of renal insufficiency and amyloidosis. Other abnormalities, including reduced concentrations of normal immunoglobulins and reduced T-cell responses, may account for the increased tendency toward infectious disease in affected individuals. Neurologic complications, spinal root compression, and coagulation disorders may also be observed. Criteria for diagnosis include a marrow count with more than 20 percent plasma cells and a monoclonal serum spike of greater than 4 g/dl with Bence Jones proteins in excess of 0.5 g/24 hr, or a monoclonal serum spike of less than 4 g/dl with a concurrent reciprocal depression of all normal immunoglobins. Multiple myeloma disease is progressive: chemotherapy is available, but the mean survival time for those receiving treatment is about 30 mo.

Also called *Kahler's disease, myelomatosis,* and *plasma cell myeloma.* See also *gammopathy* and *plasmacytoma.*

multiple sclerosis see *multiple s.* under *sclerosis.*

multiple spike and slow-wave complex in electroencephalography, a sequence of two or more spikes (i.e., waves with pointed peaks that are 20–70 msec in duration) associated with one or more slow waves (i.e., waves longer than 125 msec in duration). The diagnostic value of this complex depends on the clinical circumstances in which it is found. Also called *polyspike and slow-wave complex.* See also *spike.*

multiple spike complex in electroencephalography, a sequence of two or more spikes (i.e., waves that are 20–70 msec in duration and characterized by pointed peaks). The diagnostic value of this complex depends on the clinical context in which it is found. Also called *polyspike complex.* See also *spike.*

multiple spike foci in electroencephalography, epileptiform discharges (spikes, sharp waves) that originate from at least one focus in each cerebral hemisphere and are recorded from at least three different areas of the scalp. This pattern is found most commonly in children under age 20 yr who experience seizures, whose neurologic examinations are abnormal, and who are intellectually impaired. The pattern is not characteristic of a particular pathologic process, but rather is caused by a variety of neurologic disorders. See also *epileptiform pattern.*

multiplex (mul′tĭ-pleks) [*multi-* + L. *plex* fold] pertaining to the simultaneous transmission of two or more signals over a single channel. There are two types of multiplexing: in time division multiplexing, the channel is time shared, and the different signals are interleaved bit by bit or character by character; in frequency division multiplexing, the bandwidth is shared; each signal modulates a different carrier frequency. In the laboratory, analog multiplexers are used to allow a single analog-to-digital converter to digitize signals from several sources.

multiplexer (mul″tĭ-plek′ser) a device that combines several signals in coded form for simultaneous transmission over a single communications channel. Multiplexers are available for either analog or digital signals and allow one analog-to-digital converter or one digital processor to service multiple inputs or outputs. The logic for scanning the inputs and detecting service requests can be intrinsic to the multiplexer or can be supplied by the host device. Also called *scanner.*

multiplier (mul′tĭ-pli″er) 1. a resistor placed in series with a voltmeter to adjust the voltage range.

2. a digital or analog circuit that multiplies two inputs.

3. a number by which another number is multiplied.

multipolar (mul″tĭ-po′lar) [*multi-* + L. *polus* pole] having more than two poles or processes.

multiport (mul″tĭ-port′) a device that allows several input-output devices to be connected to a computer.

multiprogramming system (mul″tĭ-pro′gram-ing) a computer system in which several programs can be run concurrently. The central processing unit executes a few instructions in turn from each active program.

multitrichous (mul″tĭ-trĭ′kus) [*multi-* + Gr. *thrix* hair] a term used to describe a rod-shaped bacterial cell having a tuft of several flagella at one end. See also *flagellum.*

multivalent (mul″tĭ-va′lent) [*multi-* + L. *valere* to have value] 1. in chemistry, having a valence of greater than 1, or having more than one valence state.

2. in immunology, having more than one antigenic determinant. Also called *polyvalent.* Cf. *monovalent.*

3. in genetics, the object formed by synapsis of more than two partially homologous chromosomes during meiosis: a trivalent or quadrivalent. See also *reciprocal translocation.*

multivesicular body (mul″tĭ-vĕ-sik′u-lar) a membrane-bound sac found in various types of cells, such as those of the liver, in which there are numerous small vesicles. Its significance and its relationship to lysosomes are not known.

multivibrator (mul″tĭ-vi′bra-tor) an electronic circuit with two output voltage levels between which it switches back and forth.

astable m., a multivibrator that spends a set amount of time (controlled by circuit parameters) in each state. Its output is an equally spaced train of rectangular pulses. Also called free-running multivibrator.

bistable m., a multivibrator with two stable states. Each input pulse switches the state. The circuit thus serves as a binary counter or divide-by-two circuit. Also called *flip-flop.*

monostable m., a multivibrator that has one stable state and one state in which it spends a fixed time interval. When it is triggered by an input pulse, it produces a rectangular pulse output of fixed height (voltage) and width. Also called one-shot multivibrator.

multiwire proportional chamber (mul″tĭ-wir′) an experimental imaging radiation detector that uses the principle of the ionization chamber. It has good spatial and energy resolution but low detection efficiency. It has been used as a type of positron camera.

MUMPS (mumps) [acronym from *M*assachusetts General Hospital *U*tility *M*ulti-*P*rogramming *S*ystem] a high-level programming language suited for handling sparse, complex data sets, such as patient records.

mumps an acute, contagious viral disease characterized by swelling of the parotid glands and sometimes other salivary glands; the testes, ovaries, and pancreas may also be involved. The etiologic agent is the mumps virus, an RNA virus that is a member of the Paramyxoviridae family (related to the influenza virus). Mumps is found worldwide and has an increased incidence in the winter and spring seasons. Most cases involve children younger than 15 yr, although adults may also contract the disease. Humans are the only reservoir for the mumps virus; the disease is transmitted through droplet nuclei entering the upper respiratory tract of the new host. Subclinical infections with the mumps virus can occur. The incubation period is 14–24 da.

Once the virus attaches to respiratory epithelial cells, an immune response is provoked. Secretory IgA, lymphocytic infiltration, and increased vascular permeability cause symptoms in the upper and lower respiratory tracts. Eventually the virus invades the blood stream and reaches various glands, especially the salivary glands, as well as the central nervous system. The remarkable parotid swelling is due to interstitial edema caused by inflammation.

The clinical manifestations of mumps begin with a unilateral swelling of the parotid gland 2 da after the incubation period. Eventually the parotid swelling becomes bilateral. Fever, malaise, sore throat, headache, chills, and earache last 5–10 da. Certain cases of mumps may result in meningoencephalomyelitis, and in 15–35 percent of affected postpubescent males, orchitis may also occur.

The diagnosis of mumps is based on clinical symptoms and laboratory findings. A skin test (delayed hypersensitivity) can be used to determine if an individual was naturally infected or vaccinated; it is of limited diagnostic value, however, as it becomes positive only 3–4 wk after infection. The mumps virus may be isolated from saliva or urine and grown in a variety of tissue cultures, including chick embryo, in which the virus causes cytopathic effects. Antibodies to the mumps virus may be detected 1 wk after infection by a complement-fixation test, the hemagglutination inhibitor test, or indirect immunofluorescence.

Most individuals completely recover from the disease, although a small percentage of patients with involvement of CNS or orchitis may develop sequelae.

There is no effective antiviral chemotherapy at present for the mumps virus. However, a live attenuated vaccine is available for preventing mumps that is often combined with measles and rubella vaccines. It can be administered at any time after age 12 mo and should be given before puberty.

mumps antibody titer a value representing the relative amount of antibody to mumps virus present in an individual's serum. Hemagglutination inhibition is the assay used to determine the titer. The test is performed by incubating various dilutions of the individual's serum with mumps hemagglutinin and then adding erythrocytes. If the mumps antibody is present, the hemagglutinin is neutralized and no agglutination occurs. The titer is the inverse of the last dilution in which hemagglutination did not occur.

The mumps antibody titer test is not specific; a positive result is indicative of recent infection with mumps or any other member of the parainfluenza virus group. A negative test is more valuable than a positive one, as it suggests that the mumps virus is not involved.

Münchausen's syndrome (men-chow′zenz)

[named after Baron von *Münchhausen,* a famed teller of exaggerated tales] the repeated fabrication of acute, dramatic illness in order to obtain hospital treatment. The patient presents a convincing and accurate history of any of a variety of diseases. This syndrome is a complex psychiatric disorder and is associated with severe personality problems.

Munro microabscess a collection of pyknotic polymorphonuclear leukocytes located within the parakeratotic portion of the horny layer of the epidermis. The Munro abscess is one of the cardinal histologic features of active psoriasis and is found in greatest numbers in early lesions. It is also found occasionally in other dermatologic conditions.

MUP abbrev. See *motor unit potential.*

mural (mur'al) [L. *muralis,* from *murus* wall] pertaining to or occurring in the wall of a cavity.

muralium (mu-ral'e-um) a system of connecting sheets or walls.

muramic acid (mu-ram'ik) an amino sugar (a lactosyl ether of glucosamine) that occurs as the *N*-acetyl derivative uniquely in the peptidoglycan of bacterial cell walls.

muramidase (mu-ram'ĭ-dās) see *lysozyme.*

murein (mu're-in) see *peptidoglycan.*

mu rhythm in electroencephalography, a pattern of cerebral activity that has a frequency of 7–11 Hz and occurs during wakefulness. It has no diagnostic significance. In general, the mu rhythm is composed of waves having rounded electropositive and pointed electronegative components, and an amplitude of less than 50 μV. This pattern is best recorded over the centroparietal regions of the head. Mu rhythm is unaffected by eye opening but is attenuated by contralateral movement, intention and/or readiness to move, or tactile stimulation. Also called *arceau, comb rhythm,* and *wicket rhythm.*

muriform (mu'rĭ-form) having both transverse and longitudinal septa; wall-like, resembling a stone wall.

murine (mu'rin) [L. *mus, muris* mouse] pertaining to or affecting mice or rats.

murine typhus see *endemic murine t.* and under *typhus.*

murmur (mur'mur) [L.] a series of auditory vibrations, characterized as systolic, diastolic, or continuous, that are of a longer duration than normal heart sounds and originate within the heart or the great vessels. These vibrations may be described as blowing, high-pitched, rumbling, roaring, or musical. They may be classified as functional (physiologic) or organic (pathologic) and as ranging from grade I (least intense and barely audible) to grade VI (most intense and audible to the unassisted ear).

Murmurs are due to a number of physical mechanisms related to the flow of blood within the heart or vessels, including flow across a partial obstruction or an irregularity in the heart or its vessels, increased flow through normal structures, backward (regurgitant) flow across an incompetent heart valve, shunting of blood within the heart from areas of high to low pressures, or flow into a dilated chamber. Murmurs are principally analyzed according to their timing within the cardiac cycle, and also according to their location, intensity, frequency or pitch, quality, duration, and degree and direction of radiation.

The most common systolic murmur is the midsystolic murmur (beginning after S_1 and ending before S_2). It may be functional, innocent (occurring with no pathologic or physiologic disorders), or organic, and may be due to conditions such as aortic valve stenosis, pulmonic valve stenosis, and mitral regurgitation. Diastolic murmurs, which occupy part of the interval between S_2 and S_1, are primarily due to flow across the stenotic atrioventricular valves or across incompetent aortic and pulmonic valves; almost all indicate some form of heart disease. A third type of murmur, e.g., continuous murmur, occurs in both systolic and diastolic portions of the cardiac cycle. Examples are the murmur of a patent ductus arteriosus and a venous hum murmur.

Generally, murmurs are first detected on physical examination by auscultation with a stethoscope. Differentiation of timing and patterns may be assisted by phonocardiography (graphic representation of heart sounds picked up by chest wall microphones). The presence of a heart murmur may indicate some form of cardiac pathology and warrants further investigation by a variety of diagnostic cardiologic procedures, including electrocardiography, x-rays, and ultrasonography.

aortic m., a murmur heard at the aortic area and usually associated with aortic valve disease. Examples include the systolic murmur of aortic stenosis and the high-frequency, soft, blowing, diastolic murmur that occurs just after the second heart sound in aortic insufficiency.

apical m., a murmur that is best auscultated or recorded at the cardiac apex. Examples are the late systolic murmur of mitral valve prolapse, and the holosystolic murmur of rheumatic mitral insufficiency.

Austin Flint m., the rumbling, mid- to late diastolic murmur best heard or recorded from the cardiac apex in aortic regurgitation. Its onset is coincident with the third heart sound. The murmur results from turbulent flow across the mitral orifice when complete diastolic opening of the mitral valve leaflets is prevented by the hemodynamic consequences of a marked aortic reflux.

basal m., a murmur best heard or recorded from the base of the heart. The origin is usually in the outflow tract of the right or the left ventricle. Examples are the ejection murmur of aortic valve stenosis and the common innocent flow murmur that occurs in many children.

continuous m., a murmur initiated in the systolic portion of the cardiac cycle that continues without interruption beyond the second heart sound, usually ending in late diastole. The quality, duration, and intensity of the murmur varies with the pathologic hemodynamic condition underlying it. There are three general classes of abnormal states leading to continuous murmurs: (1) constriction in a peripheral vessel (artery or vein) that alters blood flow, (2) arteriovenous fistulas, or (3) communications between the aorta and pulmonary artery (as in patent ductus arteriosus). The venous hum murmur (due to altered venous flow) is the most frequently observed continuous murmur.

cooing m., a term descriptive of the "crying" or musical quality of a murmur that has a relatively narrow range of frequencies. The murmur is often the consequence of the vibration of valves or other cardiac structures. Also called seagull or musical murmur.

diastolic m., a murmur heard in the diastolic portion of the cardiac cycle. The exact timing, duration, and intensity of the murmur varies with the anatomic or pathologic derangement underlying it. For example, diastolic murmurs caused by blood flow across the atrioventricular (AV) valves (ventricular filling murmurs) are generally of a rumbling character and tend to be classified as middiastolic: i.e., there is a delay between the second heart sound and the onset of the murmur. Such murmurs occur when the size of the AV valve orifice is inadequate to handle the level of blood flow, which may be normal or increased (as in mitral and tricuspid regurgitation (left-to-right shunts). In contrast, diastolic murmurs that result from semilunar valve regurgitation begin with the aortic or pulmonic component of the second heart sound: i.e., they are early diastolic.

early systolic m., a murmur that originates coincident with the first heart sound and ends before the second sound, during mid- or midlate systole. It may occur with acute mitral regurgitation or with certain congenital heart diseases.

ejection m., the midsystolic murmur associated with ejection of blood into the root of one of the great vessels. Ejection murmurs begin in early systole (0.09–0.14 sec following the Q wave of the ECG), as the semilunar valves achieve their maximal opening. They can be heard in aortic and pulmonic valvular stenosis, and in pulmonary and systemic hypertension or other conditions causing dilation of the roots of the great vessels.

holosystolic m., a murmur with a duration that spans the entire time interval between the first and second heart sounds. It is associated with conditions that produce abnormal communication between the cardiac chambers, permitting a turbulent flow (ventricular septal defect) or retrograde flow (mitral or tricuspid regurgitation) that persists throughout the entire systole.

regurgitant m., a murmur due to regurgitation of blood through an incompetent valve.

venous hum m., a continuous murmur caused by rapid blood flow through the jugular vein as it is narrowed when an upright body posture is assumed. It is best auscultated over the great veins in the lower portion of the neck (i.e., from the right supraclavicular fossa); it is obliterated when recumbency is assumed, or with external compression of the vein. The venous hum murmur is an innocuous physical sign that is not uncommon in the normal child or in individuals in a state of circulatory hyperkinesia, such as that brought about by pregnancy, anemia, or thyrotoxicosis.

ventricular filling m., see under *diastolic m.*

Musca (mus′kah) [L. "fly"] a genus of sucking flies of the family Muscidae. The species *M. domestica,* the housefly, has a cosmopolitan distribution and is known to transmit pathogens such as *Salmonella typhosa, S. paratyphi, S. enteritidis, Shigella dysenteriae* complex, *Vibrio comma, Entamoeba histolytica,* and *Treponema pertenue* (yaws). Some cysts of protozoa and helminth ova are also carried by this species. *M. sorbens* has been incriminated in the transmission of conjunctivitis, trachoma, and other infections throughout the Orient, Indonesia, and Ethiopia. The larvae of the flies of this genus may cause human intestinal and urinary myiasis.

muscarine (mus′kah-rin) [L. *muscarius* pertaining to flies] a deadly toxin produced by the fly agaric mushroom, *Amanita muscaria,* and some other fungi.

muscarinic (mus″kah-rin′ik) producing effects similar to muscarine.

muscarinic receptor a receptor in the autonomic nervous system that can be stimulated by muscarine. See under *cholinergic receptors.*

Muscidae (mus′ĭ-de) a family of flies of the order Diptera. It includes the medically important genera *Fannia, Haematobia, Glossina, Musca, Muscina,* and *Stomoxys.*

muscle (mus″l) the contractile tissue of the body found in many tissues and organs, where it confers the capability of movement. Some muscles can be contracted at will and are termed voluntary muscles, whereas others are involuntary and under the control of the autonomic nervous system. The cells of muscle (muscle fibers) are elongated and contain contractile proteins in the form of small threads, the myofilaments (see the accompanying illustrations).

There are three basic histologic types of muscle tissue in the human body, each adapted for particular functional requirements. The most abundant is skeletal muscle, the flesh of the body. Cardiac muscle is confined to the walls of the chambers of the heart. Smooth muscle is ubiquitous within blood vessels other than the capillaries and sinusoids, and is present in the walls of tubular viscera such as the respiratory passages and alimentary canal.

See also *muscle fiber.*

cardiac m., the muscle of the heart. The cells of cardiac muscle are short, each containing a single, centrally located nucleus. The contractile proteins are the same in type and arrangement as those of skeletal muscle fibers; cardiac muscle is therefore seen as cross-striated by light microscopy. The heart muscle cells branch, and where they connect their neighbors the apposed cell membranes form an intercalated disk. At the disk, the cells are joined by desmosomes for adhesion, and by tight (nexus) junctions across which the impulse for contraction can be transmitted. Cardiac muscle cells can contract spontaneously, but their activity is coordinated by a network of specialized heart muscle cells, the neuromyocardium (see *heart*). The rate and force of contraction of the heart is adjusted through sympathetic and parasympathetic efferent nerves.

extrafusal fiber of m., the main contractile element of muscle.

fast twitch m., a muscle composed of anaerobically active fibers that can produce only rapid phasic contractions. Fast twitch fibers have few mitochondria and are poor in oxidative enzymes but rich in phosphorylases. They possess an extensive sarcoplasmic reticulum and fatigue quite rapidly. Also called type II or white muscle fiber.

intermediate fiber of striated m., a fiber that is structurally intermediate between slow twitch or red (type I) and fast twitch or white (type II) muscle fibers.

intrafusal fiber of m., a specialized fiber found only within muscle spindles. Intrafusal fibers are of two types: nuclear bag or nuclear chain. The nuclear bag fibers (one to three in number) are long, with nuclei that are grouped in the equatorial region of the cell. The nuclei of the three to seven chain fibers (shorter and smaller than the nuclear bag fibers) are found dispersed in a row along most of the cell length. See also *muscle spindle.*

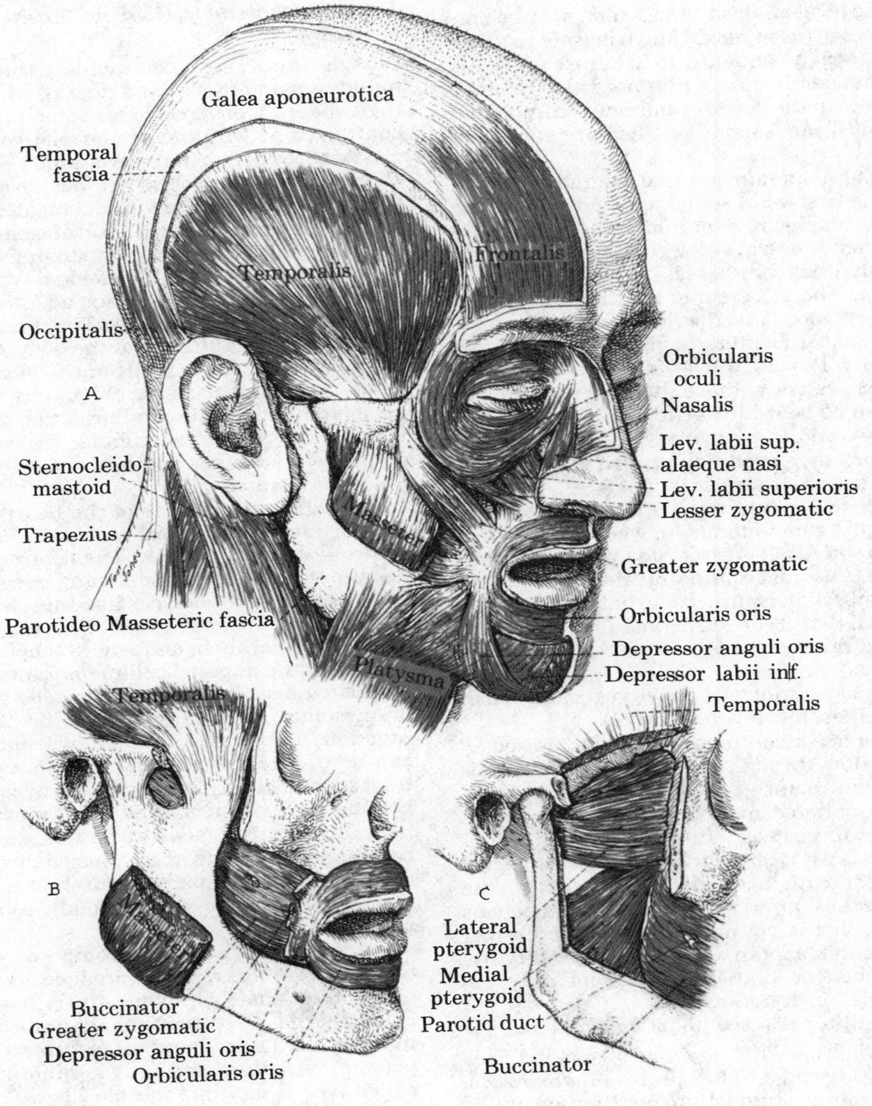

Muscle, Figure 1. Muscles of the head and face: *A,* muscles of face and scalp showing insertion of platysma; *B,* buccinator and orbicularis oris; and *C,* pterygoid muscles. (From Dorland's Illustrated Medical Dictionary. 26th ed. Philadelphia, W. B. Saunders Co., 1981.)

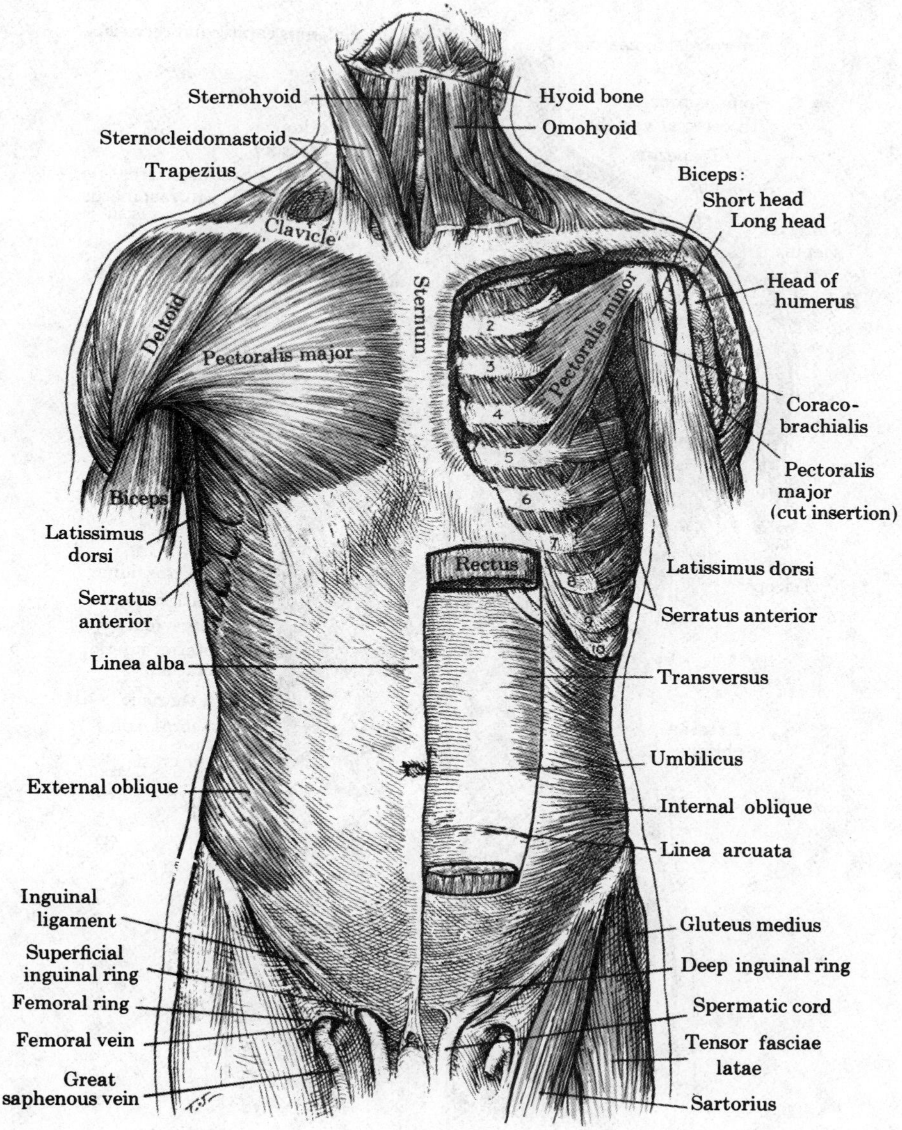

Muscle, Figure 2. Muscles of the trunk, anterior view. The left sternocleidomastoid, pectoralis major, external oblique, and a portion of the deltoid have been removed to show underlying muscles. A portion of the rectus abdominis has been cut away to expose the posterior part of its sheath. (From Dorland's Illustrated Medical Dictionary. 26th ed. Philadelphia, W. B. Saunders Co., 1981.)

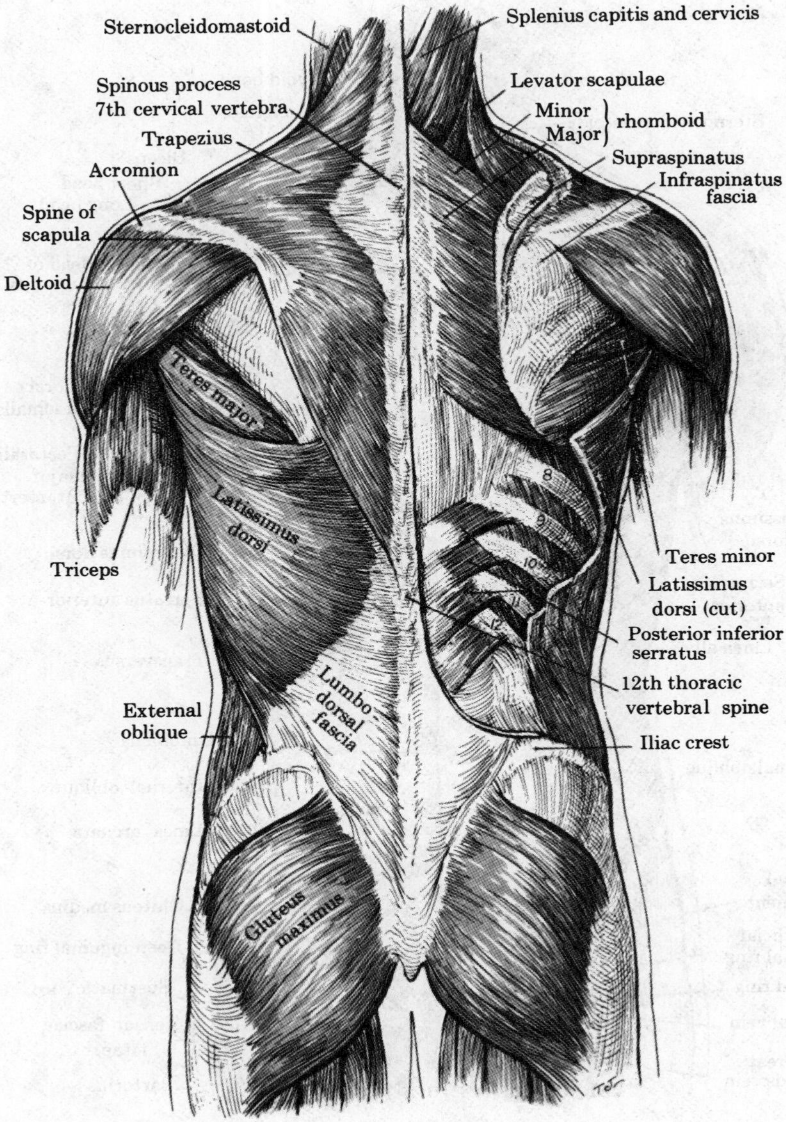

Muscle, Figure 3. Muscles of the trunk, posterior view. The latissimus dorsi and trapezius on the right side have been cut away to expose the underlying muscles. (From Dorland's Illustrated Medical Dictionary. 26th ed. Philadelphia, W. B. Saunders Co., 1981.)

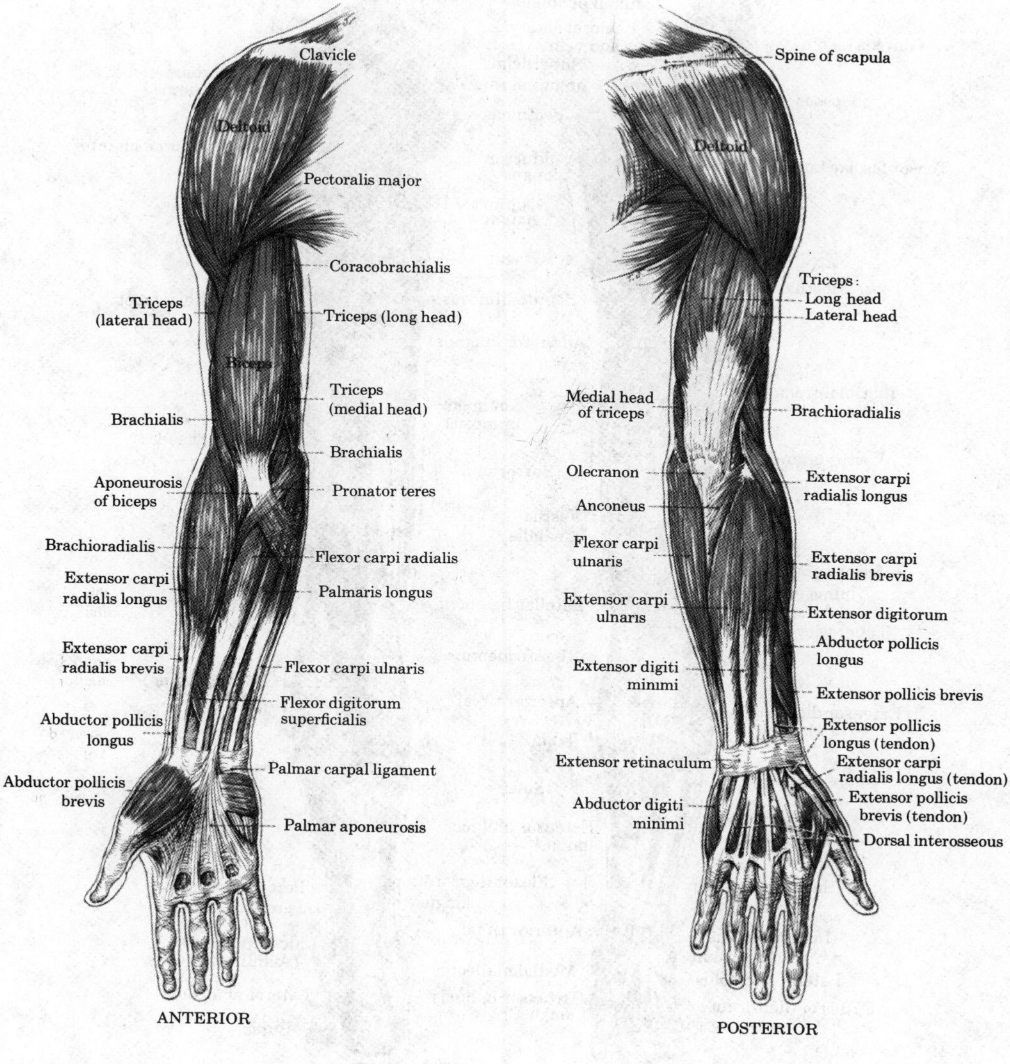

Muscle, Figure 4. Superficial muscles of the right upper extremity. (From Dorland's Illustrated Medical Dictionary. 26th ed. Philadelphia, W. B. Saunders Co., 1981.)

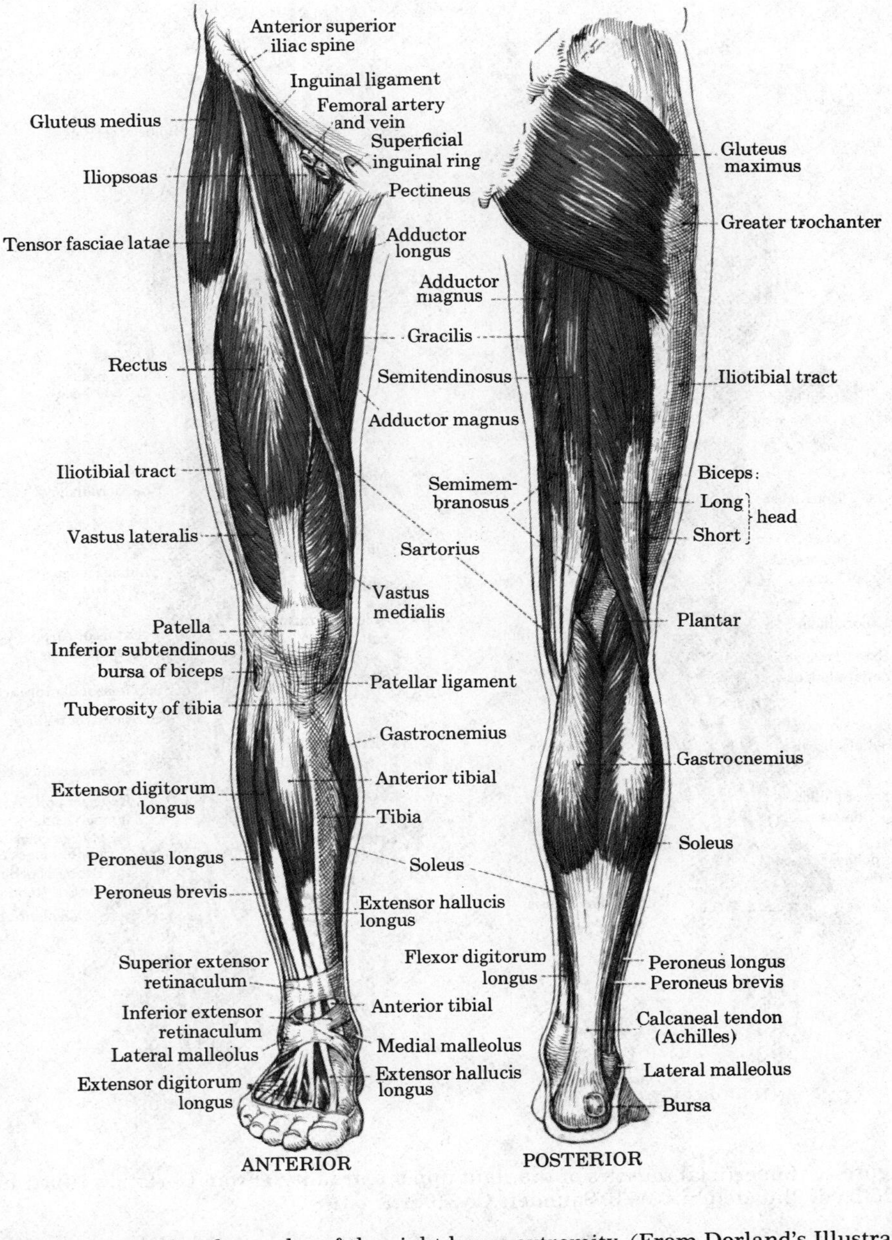

Muscle, Figure 5. Superficial muscles of the right lower extremity. (From Dorland's Illustrated Medical Dictionary. 26th ed. Philadelphia, W. B. Saunders Co., 1981.)

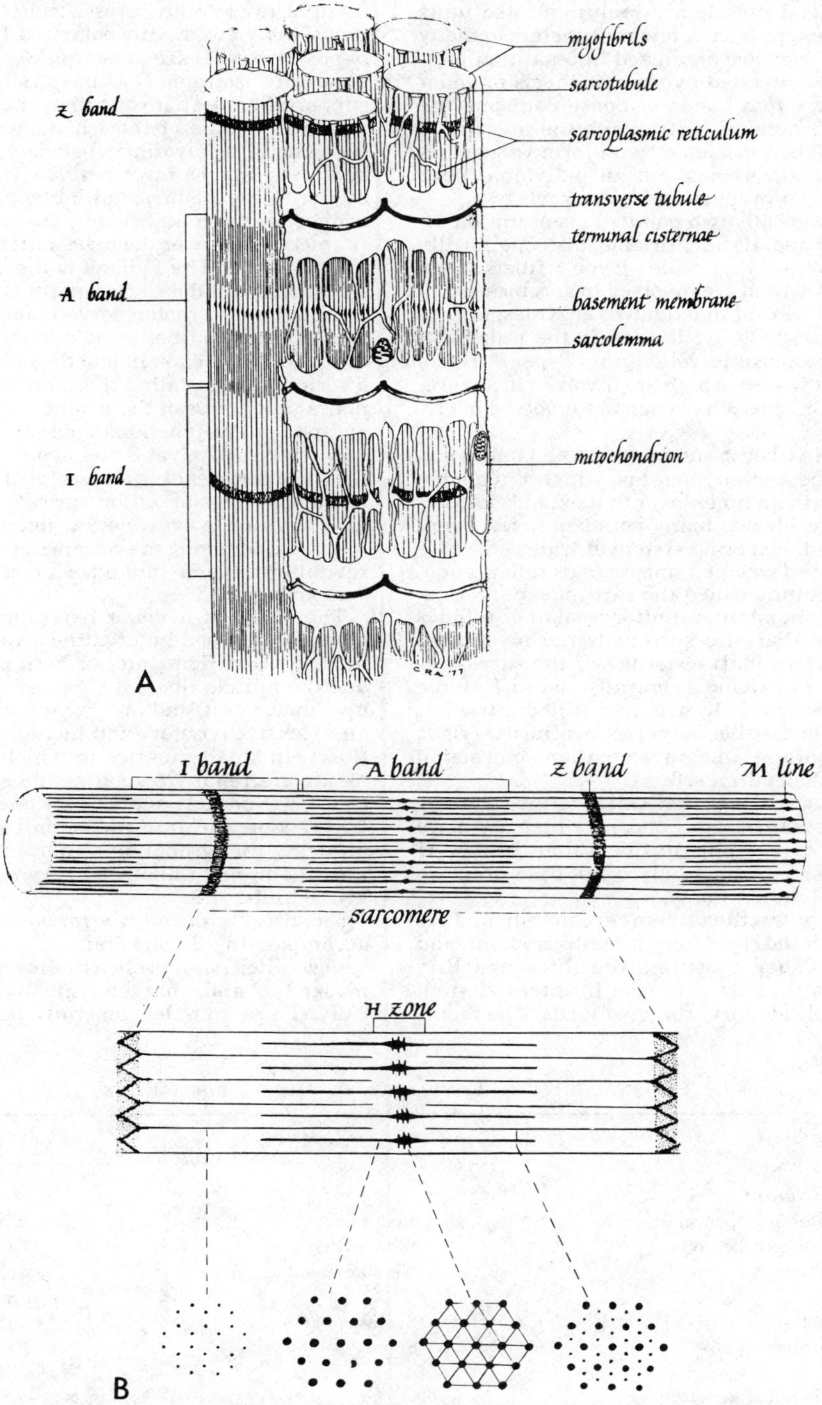

Muscle, Figure 6. *A,* Portion of a muscle fiber. The sarcomeres of the myofibrils are in register. Myofibrils are intimately surrounded by sarcoplasmic reticulum and mitochondria. It is these membranous organelles that are red with MGT stain and dark with NADH-TR reaction. The sarcoplasmic reticulum is closely related to the transverse tubules, which arise from the sarcolemma. A basement membrane covers the fiber. (AFIP 77-5174-7.) *B,* Arrangement of the myofilaments, resulting in the striated pattern. (AFIP 77-5174-10.) (From Armbrustmacher, V. W.: Skeletal muscle in denervation. In Sommers, S. C. (ed.) Pathology Annual, Pt 2. New York, Appleton-Century-Crofts, 1978.)

skeletal m., a striated muscle that is attached to bones and typically crosses at least one joint. The fibers of skeletal muscle are multinucleated units that vary in length from a few millimeters to many centimeters. They are organized into parallel bundles (fasciculi) invested by slender sheets of collagen, and insert into bands of dense collagen, the tendons and ligaments, that attach the muscles to the skeleton. The muscle fasciculi form various architectural arrangements, but an individual fiber can only shorten in length as it contracts.

There are basically two populations of muscle fibers (types I and II) identifiable histochemically (see the accompanying table). Type I fibers (slow twitch or red), which are involved in aerobic metabolism, tend to be rich in oxidative enzymes, the dehydrogenases, which are located in the mitochondria and sarcoplasmic reticulum. Type II fibers (fast twitch or white), which are involved in anaerobic metabolism, are rich in enzymes involved in glycogenolysis.

Each muscle fiber is surrounded by a continuous cell membrane, the sarcolemma, which is a double membrane with an inner layer that extends into the interior of the fiber at many points to invest every myofibril in an elaborate system of transverse or T tubules. A well-developed smooth (agranular) endoplasmic reticulum, called the sarcoplasmic reticulum, forms a membrane-limited system of tubules and cisternae that also surrounds the myofibrils. Two lateral (terminal) cisternae of the sarcoplasmic reticulum surround a centrally placed T tubule to form a characteristic structure called a triad at the A-I junction (see below) of the myofibrils. Triads play an important role in excitation-contraction coupling in skeletal muscle.

The cytoplasm of a muscle cell is termed the sarcoplasm. It contains mitochondria (which are more numerous in type I muscle fibers than in type II muscle fibers), ribosomes, glycogen, lipid droplets, and subsarcolemmal nuclei.

The main contractile proteins are myosin and actin, along with the regulatory proteins troponin and tropomyosin. They constitute the thick and thin myofilaments that are arranged in interdigitating parallel bundles to form the myofibrils. The recurring bands thus formed are in register across the fiber, so that a transverse periodicity is detectable by light microscopy (cross-striated muscle). When muscle is viewed with polarized light, the myosin bands (A bands) are anisotropic, whereas the actin bands are isotropic (I bands). Actin filaments are supported across a myofibril by the Z line that intersects the middle of the I band, and the recurring segment of a myofibril between two adjacent Z bands is termed a sarcomere. Actin filaments interdigitate with the myosin filaments and the two are connected by cross-bridges. On contraction, actin filaments slide over the myosin filaments to shorten the myofibril. The H band is the central zone of a sarcomere and does not contain actin filaments.

An axon of a motor nerve makes contact with a skeletal muscle fiber at its midpoint. The terminal branches of the axon indent the sarcolemma to form a series of folds called the junctional folds or subneural apparatus of the myoneural junction (motor end-plate). The junctional folds contain cholinesterase, which inactivates the acetylcholine liberated from the nerve ending on receipt of a nerve impulse. A wave of depolarization spreads along the sarcolemma from the myoneural junction and extends into the fiber along membranes of the sarcoplasmic reticulum to come into intimate contact with every sarcomere.

The axons of a motor nerve branch, with each anterior horn cell innervating a varying number of muscle fibers. The anterior horn cell, its branches, and the muscle fibers it supplies collectively make up a motor unit, and in large muscles it can occupy an extensive territory and include several hundred fibers. In small muscles in which intricate movements are required, such as the extraocular muscles, an axon may supply only one or a few fibers. Contraction within a motor unit is an all-or-none affair, so that gradation of movement in a muscle must be brought about by varying the number of active units.

See also *excitation-contraction coupling* and the accompanying illustration.

slow twitch m., muscle with fibers that are high in myoglobin and characteristically operate aerobically. These muscles generally possess narrow fi-

SKELETAL MUSCLE. COMPARISON OF MUSCLE FIBER TYPES

	TYPE I	TYPE II
Nomenclature		
Anatomic appearance	Red muscle	White muscle
Physiologic behavior	Slow twitch	Fast twitch
Biochemical property	Aerobic metabolism	Anaerobic metabolism
Function	Sustained action	Short bursts
Example	Soleus	Pectoralis
Histochemical Reactions		
Myofibrillar ATPase (pH 4.3)	High	Low
Phosphorylase	Low	High
Glycogen (PAS)	Low	High
Succinate dehydrogenase	High	Low
NADH-tetrazolium reductase	High	Low

Courtesy of Bruce Mackay, M.D., Ph.D.

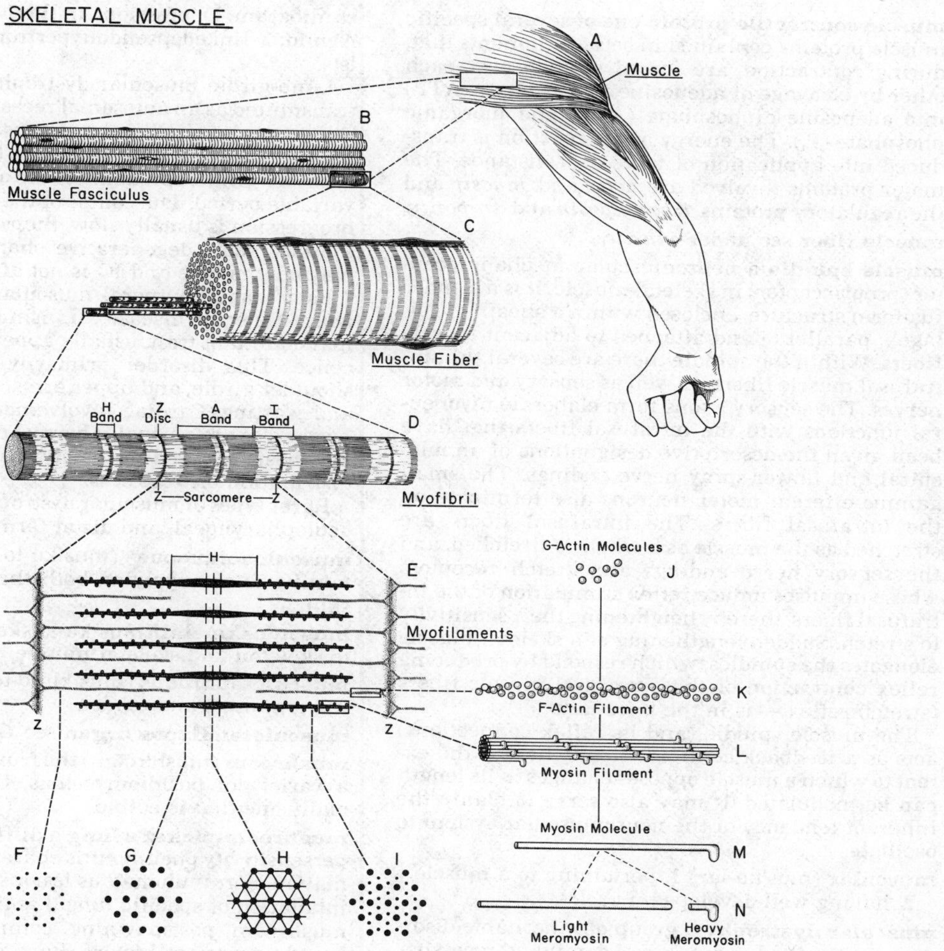

Skeletal muscle. Diagram of the organization of skeletal muscle from the gross to the molecular level. Diagram portions *F–I* are cross sections at the levels indicated. (Drawing by Sylvia Colard Keene.) (From Bloom, W., and Fawcett, D. W.: A Textbook of Histology. 10th ed. Philadelphia, W. B. Saunders Co., 1975.)

bers with poorly defined myofibrils. Slow twitch fibers are rich in mitochondria and oxidative enzymes but are poorly invested with phosphorylases. They are capable of slow, sustained contraction. Also called type I or red muscle fiber.

smooth m., nonstriated, involuntary muscle. The cells of smooth muscle are fusiform, and arranged in sheets so that by light microscopy the limits of individual cells may not be evident. Each cell has a single central nucleus. Some myosin is present, but the myofilaments are predominantly actin and are longitudinally aligned with the cell. The filaments are not arranged in myofibrils and do not form a banding pattern as in skeletal or cardiac muscle fibers. However, electron microscopy has revealed organized arrangements of myosin and actin, as well as lateral projections resembling cross-bridges, consistent with a sliding filament contractile mechanism, as seen in striated muscle.

Smooth muscle is generally classified into two types based on differing physiologic properties: single unit (visceral or unitary) and multiunit smooth muscle. Single unit smooth muscle cells are joined by oval plaques, and adjacent cells within a functional group are united by tight (nexus or gap) junctions; the impulse for contraction can be transmitted from one cell to the next across these low-resistance pathways. Thus, the spontaneous activity arising from pacemaker zones can excite adjacent cells and initiate contraction of large areas of the muscle at one time. Nervous mediation serves to coordinate and modulate the spontaneous, rhythmic contraction of this form of smooth muscle. Local factors (stretch, and humoral and hormonal factors) also influence its performance. Examples of single unit smooth muscle are those of the uterus, ureter, and gastrointestinal tract.

In contrast, contraction of multiunit, independently operative smooth muscle cells is almost entirely initiated by motor nerves of the autonomic nervous system that run close to the sarcolemma and release neurotransmitter substances. Examples of multiunit smooth muscle include those of the larger blood vessels and the iris, the ciliary muscles, and the pilomotor muscles.

muscle contractile protein one of several specific muscle proteins contained in sets of filaments that, during contraction, are forced to slide over each other by cleavage of adenosine triphosphate (ATP) into adenosine diphosphate (ADP) and inorganic phosphate (P_i). The energy of the reaction is transduced into application of force over distance. The major proteins involved are *actin* and *myosin* and the regulatory proteins *tropomyosin* and *troponin.*

muscle fiber see under *muscle.*

muscle spindle a neuromuscular mechanoreceptor (proprioceptor) in skeletal muscle. It is a slender fusiform structure, enclosed within a sheath of collagen, parallel to and attached to adjacent muscle fibers. Within the spindle there are several thin intrafusal muscle fibers, as well as sensory and motor nerves. The sensory axons form elaborate myoneural junctions with the intrafusal fibers that have been given the descriptive designations of annulospiral and flower-spray nerve endings. The small gamma-efferent motor neurons also terminate on the intrafusal fibers. The intrafusal fibers are stretched as the muscle as a whole is stretched, and the sensory nerve endings are stretch receptors whose impulses induce reflex stimulation of the intrafusal fibers, thereby heightening their sensitivity to stretch. Sudden lengthening of a skeletal muscle elongates the spindles, which respond by producing reflex contraction of the extrafusal muscle fibers (stretch reflex)—as in the knee jerk.

The muscle spindle (and its reflex connections) acts as a feedback control system whereby the extent to which a muscle opposes changes in its length can be modulated. It may also serve to clamp the inherent tendency of the neuromuscular system to oscillate.

muscular (mus′ku-lar) 1. pertaining to a muscle. 2. having well-developed muscles.

muscular dystrophy a group of inheritable disorders, transmitted as autosomal dominant, recessive, or X-linked recessive traits, that are characterized by progressive weakness and wasting of muscles and eventual degeneration of muscle fibers that is not due to any disturbance of the nerve supply to the muscles. The cause is unknown. Several types of muscular dystrophy are recognized and depend on age of onset, mode of inheritance, initial pattern of muscle involvement, and prognosis.

Pseudohypertrophic muscular dystrophy (Duchenne's disease), transmitted as a sex-linked recessive disorder in male children, may appear at any time from fetal life to age 7 yr. Initially, it affects the calves and thighs, with enlargement as a result of the infiltration of these muscles with fat and fibrous tissue. This results in progressive muscle weakness and contracture; pelvic and shoulder girdles are also affected, leading to a waddling gait and difficulty in climbing stairs. Those affected eventually become unable to walk at all, usually by about age 10 yr, and finally die from cardiac failure or respiratory infection at the end of their second decade. Diagnosis is based on the clinical picture; on biopsy of the affected muscles, which shows typical degenerative changes; and on the marked elevation (50–200 times normal) of the serum enzyme creatine kinase. Cardiac involvement is noted late in the disease and is characterized by tachycardia, prolongation of P-R intervals, slurring of the QRS complex, and elevation or depression of the ST segments in the electrocardiogram. Depressions in the IQ may also occur. A mild, X-linked, pseudohypertrophic form also exists.

Limb-girdle muscular dystrophy (Erb's disease), transmitted as an autosomal recessive trait in either sex, occurs later in life than the pseudohypertrophic type. Initially, it affects either the pelvic or the shoulder girdle, spreading to the other girdle after a variable period. The course of the illness varies, but progression is usually slow. Biopsies of the affected muscles show degenerative changes. Cardiac impairment is rare and IQ is not affected.

Facioscapulohumeral muscular dystrophy (Landouzy-Déjerine disease), transmitted as an autosomal dominant trait, usually appears during adolescence. This disorder primarily affects the face, shoulder girdle, and upper arms, causing weakness and wasting. Cardiac involvement is rare; life expectancies are normal. Abortive cases are common. Diagnosis is based primarily on the characteristic distribution of weakness.

Rarer types of muscular dystrophy include ocular, oculopharyngeal, and distal forms.

musculocutaneous (mus″ku-lo-ku-ta′ne-us) pertaining to or supplying both the muscles and the skin.

musculoskeletal (mus″ku-lo-skel′ĕ-tal) pertaining to skeleton and skeletal muscle.

musculotendinous (mus″ku-lo-ten′dĭ-nus) pertaining to muscle and tendon.

musculotendinous organ see *Golgi tendon organ.*

mushroom (mush′ro͞om) the fruiting body of any of a variety of basidiomycetous, fleshy fungi, especially one that is edible.

mushroom-picker's lung a diffuse, interstitial hypersensitivity pneumonitis characterized by the formation of granulomatous lesions in response to the inhalation of specific fungal antigens that occur in mushroom postspawning compost. Diagnosis is based on patient history, lung x-rays, and pulmonary function tests. See also *hypersensitivity p.* under *pneumonitis.*

mushroom poisoning poisoning due to the ingestion of mushrooms, most commonly *Amanita muscaria* and *A. phalloides. A. muscaria* contains muscarine, a parasympathomimetic, and various central nervous system toxins. Nausea, vomiting, diarrhea, and dyspnea occur within minutes after ingestion; death may occur within a few hours. *A. phalloides* contains heat-stable cytotoxins that may cause cell damage in the liver, kidneys, muscles, and brain. In about half of all poisonings caused by *A. phalloides,* death ensues in 5–8 da. See also *mycetismus.*

mustard gas (mus′tard) see *bis(2-chloroethyl)sulfide.*

mut/a (mu′tah) [L. *mutare* to change] a word element used in combining form to denote mutation or genetic change, e.g., mutant.

mutagen (mu′tah-jen) [acronym from *muta*tion + *gen*esis] an agent that induces a mutation in genetic material. Although several endogenous mutagens are known, the vast majority are exogenous. Included in this latter category are viruses, ionizing radiation, and chemicals. Viruses may act as mutagens by inserting their genetic material in host chromosomes and destroying their informational integrity. Ionizing radiation may alter individual bases in DNA or cause physical breaks in chromosomes. chemicals act as mutagens by attacking bases within the DNA and often combining with them, leading to altered structure and function.

Within the last 20 yr, there has been a growing realization that most cancer-causing agents are mutagens, and most carcinogens are mutagenic. As a result, many short-term screening tests to detect environmental carcinogens are now designed to detect the mutagenic potential of a compound. A large class consists of mutagens that are not direct-acting, requiring metabolic activation by the human body before they can exert their mutagenic potential. Many researchers believe it is necessary to remove mutagens from the environment in order to reduce the extent of human cancer.

See also *mutagenicity test* and *mutation.* Cf. *carcinogen* and *teratogen.*

mutagenesis (mu″tah-jen′ĕ-sis) 1. the production of change.

2. the process of inducing mutations in the genetic information of a cell, most often DNA. See also *mutagen* and *mutation.*

mutagenic (mu″tah-jen′ik) capable of inducing stable, heritable changes in the genetic information of a cell. See also *mutagen* and *mutation.*

mutagenicity (mu″tah-jĕ-nis′ĭ-te) the property of being able to induce genetic mutation.

mutagenicity test a test used to predict the carcinogenicity of a chemical based on the detection of its capacity for inducing damage to DNA in certain target cells. The rationale for using this test is based on the observation that there is a close correlation between mutagenicity, as assayed by mutagenicity testing, and carcinogenicity, as assayed by studies in laboratory animals.

Several forms of mutagenicity tests have been developed; most require the combination of the compound to be tested with tissue homogenates of mammalian cells, usually rat or human liver, to provide metabolism of the test chemical. After incubation of the test chemical and tissue homogenate, a genetic indicator is added and the degree of genetic damage assessed.

In the Ames test, initially used without mammalian activation systems, a special strain of *Salmonella* is used as the indicator, the end point being the number of revertant colonies growing out after plating compared with the number of spontaneous revertant colonies arising from untreated control specimens. Other methods of mutagenicity testing include the use of prophage λ in *Escherichia coli* K-12, *Drosophila* sperm, and human fibroblast cultures as genetic indicators. For these methods, the frequency of lysogenic induction, recessive lethal mutation rate, and DNA fragmentation and repair, respectively, are used as end points.

mutant (mu′tant) 1. an offspring that differs genetically from the parent and breeds true in respect to this difference. See also *mutation.*

2. a bacterial strain in which an inheritable change has occurred.

mutarotation (mu″tah-ro-ta′shun) the spontaneous change in the optical rotation of a freshly prepared solution of certain optically active compounds with time. The change in rotation is usually associated with the change of an optically pure single compound into a diastereoisomer of the original compound, often the result of the change in configuration of a single chiral center. Once equilibrium is established, a mixture of diastereoisomers is formed and the optical rotation of the product mixture is different from that of the pure material. The mutarotation of glucose is an important example of this phenomenon. Mutarotation is usually different from racemization, for in the latter process optical activity is always completely lost. See also *glucose.* Cf. *racemization.*

mutase (mu′tās) [*mut-* + *-ase*] one of a subclass of enzymes (intramolecular transferases, EC 5.4) of the isomerase class that catalyzes the transfer of an acyl-, phospho-, amino-, or other group from one position to another within one molecule. D-Phosphoglycerate 2,3-phosphomutase is an important enzyme in the Embden-Meyerhof pathway of carbohydrate metabolism.

mutation (mu-ta′shun) [L. *mutatio,* from *mutare* to change] 1. a change in form, quality, or some other characteristic.

2. in genetics, a term generally defined as a stable, heritable change in the genetic information of a cell, most often the DNA. The cause of many mutations in humans is unknown. Some arise spontaneously; others can be induced by a variety of exogenous agents including chemicals, viruses, and ionizing radiation.

The extent of the mutation to the genetic material may determine the phenotypic observable change. Some mutations are silent and do not produce an observable change; others may result in the production of biologic products with altered functional characteristics (e.g., alterations in hemoglobin leading to sickle cell anemia). Extensive mutations may be lethal and lead to cell death. Many theories propose that cancer is due to mutations in cellular genetic information.

Mutations may be as small as individual changes in the base composition of DNA. Deletion and insertion mutations may change the tripletic code reading of genetic information. Chromosomal mutations may occur through translocation or aberrant recombination during cell replication.

Mutations that occur in nongerm cell tissues may result in the production of a cellular population that differs from the nonmutated parent cell population. Such mutated populations may express biologic properties that differ dramatically from the cell population of their origin. The most common example of this is the creation of a neoplastic cell population. Mutations to germ cells may result in the propagation of the mutation to offspring.

See also *mutagen.*

amber m., a point mutation in a structural gene that changes a codon to the UAG termination codon, allowing the mutant gene to produce a shortened polypeptide. Cf. *ochre m.*

auxotrophic m., a mutation that results in the inability of bacteria to grow on minimal media. See also *auxotroph.*

clear plaque m., a mutation that results in clear plaque formation by a temperate phage that usually makes turbid plaques on bacterial lawns.

cold-sensitive m., a mutation that produces a gene that is functional at high temperatures and nonfunctional at low temperatures.

conditional lethal m., a mutation that results in death only under certain conditions, such as the absence of required growth factors.

constitutive m., a mutation that results in the formation of a product in the absence of the inducer, e.g., Lac I⁻ mutants synthesize all three genes: lac Z, lac Y, and lac A in the absence of lactose or other galactosides.

deletion m., a mutation that results from a deletion of one or more nucleotides from the DNA chain. Deletion mutations cannot revert to the wild-type state, because once lost the missing DNA cannot be restored.

feedback inhibition m., a forward mutation that results in a change of function—the loss of sensitivity to end-product feedback inhibition by enzymes in biosynthetic pathways. See also *forward m.*

forward m., a mutation that results in an abnormal phenotype. Cf. *reverse m.*

frameshift m., a mutation that results when one or two nucleotides are added or subtracted in a coding sequence. From the point of mutation, nucleotide triplets are read out of phase; a completely different set of amino acids is made into the protein.

host-range m., a phage mutation that overcomes the resistance of phage-resistant bacteria by alteration of their phage attachment sites. See also *phage-resistant m.*

insertion m., a mutation that results from an insertion of one or more nucleotides into the DNA chain. Insertion mutations can revert to the wild-type state by removal of the extra sequences.

lethal m., a mutation that prematurely kills every organism in which it is expressed. A recessive lethal kills only homozygotes; a dominant lethal also kills heterozygotes.

missense m., a genetic change that involves one codon of the DNA that codes for a protein. One amino acid is changed, usually causing the mutant protein to have a difference in stability or enzyme activity. Cf. *nonsense m.*

nonsense m., a genetic change involving one codon of the DNA that codes for a protein. The codon is changed to a stop codon, which causes the polypeptide chain to be prematurely terminated; the protein is almost always nonfunctional. Cf. *missense m.*

ochre m., a point mutation that changes a codon to the UGA termination codon. Cf. *amber m.*

phage-resistant m., a mutation that structurally modifies a bacterial cell wall to prevent attachment of a phage and to render the bacterium resistant to the injection of phage DNA into the cell.

pleiotropic m., a mutation that affects two or more phenotypic properties.

point m., a mutation that results from an alteration of a single nucleotide pair.

rapid-lysis m., a phage mutation resulting in the inheritable formation of a plaque different in appearance from that formed by normal phage. Normal plaques have a small, clear center surrounded by a turbid halo, whereas rapid-lysis plaques have a large, clear center and a sharp edge.

reverse m., a new mutation in the same structural gene, which restores the ability of the gene to produce a functional protein, the ability having been destroyed by a previous mutation. Cf. *forward m.*

semilethal m., a mutation that kills more than half (but not all) of the organisms in which it is expressed. Cf. *subvital m.*

sex-reversed m., a mutation found in mice that causes testicular development in the absence of any apparent Y chromosome. The individuals are karyotypically female (XX) but have small testes that do not contain germ cells. The male gonadal differentiation is probably mediated by the presence of the H-Y antigen. See also *H-Y antigen* and *sex differentiation.*

silent m., a point mutation that changes one codon to another codon that codes for the same amino acid. The mutation is detectable only by sequencing the DNA; it does not affect the protein encoded by the gene.

somatic m., a mutation occurring in a somatic cell. If the mutant cell can divide, the organism develops as a mosaic containing cell lines with two different genotypes. Somatic cell mutations have no genetic consequences but may have significance for the carrier. One proposed mechanism of aging is based on accumulation of somatic cell mutation of unspecified origin. See also *somatic cell genetics.*

spontaneous m., a mutation that occurs in the absence of known mutagenic treatment. The rate of spontaneous mutation is not constant, but rather is affected by environmental conditions. Known types include transition, transversion, mispairing, deletion, and insertion.

subvital m., a mutation that kills less than half (but a significant fraction) of the organisms in which it is expressed. Cf. *semilethal m.*

suppressor m., a mutation that totally or partially reverses the effect of another mutation although it occurs at a different site, usually owing to an altered anticodon in a tRNA gene.

temperature-sensitive (t-s) m., a conditional mutation that results in an abnormality at one temperature (s) and not at others. In lower organisms, cold-sensitive mutations tend to occur in genes coding for proteins with strict conformational requirements.

transition m., see *transition.*

transversion m., see *transversion.*

t-s m., see *temperature-sensitive m.*

ultraviolet light–induced m., a mutation caused by absorption of ultraviolet light by DNA, which most often results in the formation of pyrimidine dimers that distort the shape of the DNA molecule and interfere with normal base pairing.

mutation rate the rate at which mutations occur at a given gene locus, usually expressed as mutations per gamete per locus per generation in a given species.

mute (mūt) [L. *mutus* unable to speak, inarticulate] a person who is unable or unwilling to speak. Mutism may be due to anatomic abnormalities in the vocal organs, but most mutes are deaf (i.e., deaf mute). See also *mutism.*

mutism (mu'tizm) the inability or refusal to speak. The inability may result from structural impairment, as in anatomic abnormalities or damage (e.g., cancer of the throat), or from impairments in hearing and deafness, preventing the learning of speech. Mutism may also stem from psychologic or emotional disorders.

akinetic m., a state in which a patient lies silent and immobile, with an alteration of consciousness, and little if any evidence of mental activity. This can result from a number of lesions but especially from subacute communicating hydrocephalus, bilateral and extensive frontal lobe pathologic alteration, and pathologic alteration involving the reticular formation of the midbrain and diencephalon. Individuals may remain silent and immobile because of various psychologic disorders.

muton (mu′ton) [acronym from *mut*ation + Gr. *-on* quantum] in molecular genetics, the smallest element of DNA (a single base pair) whose alteration can cause mutation. Cf. *cistron, codon,* and *recon.*

mutualism (mu′tu-al-izm″) the symbiotic association between two organisms of different species in which the relationship is beneficial to both organisms and is occasionally essential for their existence.

mutualist (mu′tu-al-ist) one of the organisms existing in a beneficial relationship (mutualism).

MV abbrev. See *megavolt.*

mV abbrev. See *millivolt.*

μV abbrev. See *microvolt.*

MVV abbrev. See *maximal voluntary ventilation.*

M.W. abbrev. See *molecular weight.*

mW abbrev. See *milliwatt.*

μW abbrev. See *microwatt.*

M wave the response elicited from a muscle as a result of the application of an electrical stimulus to its motor nerve. It usually consists of a biphasic, compound action potential with a configuration that is relatively constant during repetitive stimulation.

By convention, the maximal-amplitude M wave (evoked by a stimulus of supramaximal intensity) is used in motor nerve conduction studies. In such studies, the duration of the M wave is generally measured solely as the duration of the first negative (upgoing) phase. The finding of decrementing or incrementing amplitudes of the M waves evoked by repetitive supramaximal stimuli is useful in characterizing abnormal neuromuscular transmission. Further, decreased amplitude of the M wave may have great clinical significance in peripheral neuropathy.

See also *motor n. c. s.* under *nerve conduction study.*

***m* wave** see under *electroretinogram.*

Mx abbrev. See *maxwell.*

my/o (mi′o) [Gr. *mys* muscle] a word element used in combining form to denote muscle, e.g., myocardial.

myalgia (mi-al′je-ah) [*my-* + G. *algos* pain + *-ia*] pain in a muscle or muscles. This condition may have a variety of causes, including overuse, systemic infections of viral or bacterial origin, trauma, and inflammation. Electromyography may be helpful in diagnosis, and serum concentrations of creatine kinase may be elevated.

myasis (mi-a′sis) see *myiasis.*

myasthenia gravis (mi″as-the′ne-ah grah′vis) [*my-* + Gr. *astheneia* weakness] a disease characterized by muscle weakness and fatigability, most commonly affecting the ocular, facial, bulbar, and limb muscles. It occurs at all ages and is twice as frequent in females as males. The onset is usually subacute; ptosis, diplopia, dysphagia, dysarthria, and limb fatigue are common early symptoms.

The disease has an autoimmune basis, resulting in abnormal neuromuscular transmission due to a reduction in the number of receptors for acetylcholine. Autoantibodies, present in the serum of 90 percent of all patients, are directed against acetylcholine receptors on the postsynaptic membranes of the neuromuscular junction. Many young females with this disease are positive for the HLA-B8 antigen. Thymic abnormalities are common in those affected, and 10 percent have a thymoma.

Diagnosis is based on the demonstration of abnormal muscle fatigue, which is reversed by anticholinesterase medication. Electrophysiologic studies (repetitive nerve stimulation) may confirm the diagnosis. Treatment modalities include anticholinesterase drugs, corticosteroids, thymectomy, and plasmapheresis in selected patients.

myatrophy (mi-at′ro-fe) [*my-* + Gr. *atrophia* atrophy] atrophy of a muscle, muscular atrophy.

myc/o (mi′ko) [Gr. *mykēs* fungus] a word element used in combining form to denote fungus or mold, e.g., mycosis.

mycelium (mi-se′le-um), pl. *mycelia* [*myc-* + Gr. *hēlos* nail] a mass of fungal hyphae. Filaments that grow into the medium are called basal or vegetative hyphae; those protruding into the air are aerial hyphae.

-myces (mi′sēz) [Gr. *mykēs* fungus] a suffix word element to denote a fungus, e.g., *Streptomyces.*

mycet/o (mi′set-o) [Gr. *mykēs* fungus] a word element used in combining form to denote relationship to fungi, e.g., mycetoma.

mycetismus (mi″sĕ-tiz′mus) a disease caused by the ingestion of fungi, often of poisonous mushrooms. There is no single test prior to ingestion to determine if a mushroom is poisonous. Expert fungal identification is necessary. Side-effects range from gastrointestinal disorders to hallucination, coma, and death. Children are more severely affected than adults. Mycetismus is categorized into five types, depending on the primary organ system involved.

m. cerebralis, poisoning resulting from the ingestion of mushrooms such as species of *Psilocybe, Panaeolus,* and a few other genera that contain two related hallucinogenic compounds, psilocin and psilocybin. Thirty minutes after ingestion, anxiety and confusion begin, followed by changes in sensory perception. Eventually, kaleidoscopic changes occur that resemble symptoms produced by lysergic acid diethylamide (LSD). See also *psilocin* and *psilocybin.*

m. choleriformis, a severe and often fatal mushroom poisoning following the ingestion of *Amanita phalloides* and a few other species. Two mycotoxins cause these symptoms, amaritine and muscarine. Characteristically, there is loss of large quantities of fluids (up to 3 l/da). A latent period follows ingestion, with lack of symptoms for up to 24 hr. This is followed by a quick onset of vomiting, diarrhea, fluid loss, dehydration, and muscle cramps. Affected individuals should be treated with atropine.

m. gastrointestinalis, a moderate reaction to the ingestion of poisonous mushrooms that occurs a few minutes after eating and may last up to 72 hr. Mushroom species that cause this illness include *Russula emetica, Boletus satanas, B. miniato-olivaceus, Lactarius torminosus,* and *Entoloma lividum.* The flavors produced by these mushrooms vary from pleasant to peppery. Symptoms include nausea, vomiting, diarrhea, cramps, and cerebral manifestations with dizziness.

m. nervosus, a common type of mushroom poisoning involving the parasympathetic nervous system and the GI tract. The symptoms begin early after ingestion of *Amanita muscaria, A. pantherina, Inocybe infelix, Clitocybe illudens,* and other species, and include profuse sweating, convulsions, delirium, coma, and cardiac and respiratory failure. Severe symptoms are due to large quantities of the mycotoxin muscarine.

m. sanguinarius, a mushroom poisoning due to the ingestion of *Helvella esculenta,* which causes hemoglobinuria and transient jaundice as the result of heat-labile hemolysins and one or more heat-stable toxins produced by this fungus. Mild symptoms may also result from the inhalation of fumes during the cooking of this mushroom.

mycetoma (mi″sĕ-to′mah) [*myceto-* + *-oma*] a chronic, localized abscess or granuloma caused by either true fungi or certain aerobic actinomycetes. Those due to true or filamentous fungi are known as eumycotic or maduromycotic mycetomas, the most common causative organisms being *Madurella mycetomi, Petriellidium boydii,* and *Acremonium* (*Cephalosporium*) species. The term actinomycotic mycetoma refers to those caused by actinomycetes belonging to the *Nocardia* and *Streptomyces* genera.

"Madura foot" was an early term used to describe a mycetoma because this disease was first described in the Madura area of India, and the foot is the part of the body most frequently affected; however, other parts of the body, such as the legs, hands, back, shoulders, and scalp, are also affected. Mycetoma is most frequently found in the tropics; the causal species varies with differences in its geographic occurrence. The mode of infection is by direct inoculation through minor trauma by such agents as thorns or wood splinters, as the causative organisms are saprobes; mycetomas are therefore most prevalent in jungle terrain.

Seventeen species of filamentous fungi are known to produce eumycotic mycetomas. *Nocardia*-induced actinomycotic mycetomas most often yield *N. asteroides* or *N. braziliensis* (especially in Mexico); both species are acid-fast. Also important are *Streptomyces madurae* and *S. pelletieri* (sometimes classified among the Nocardiae). The streptomyces of mycetomas respond poorly to the sulfonamide therapy used for *Nocardia* infections, so that surgery is more often needed.

A fully developed mycetoma appears as an abscess or granulomatous mass. Burrowing sinus tracts are common, and the lesions spread by extension, destroying soft tissue, fascia, and bone. Often the skin surface is broken and a chronic, suppurative ulcer develops that periodically becomes encrusted. The discharge contains colonies of mold or actinomycetes. It is necessary to determine which type is present as the causative agent (not contaminant), as the chemotherapeutic approach differs.

DIAGNOSIS: Exudate is examined grossly for granules and verified microscopically to distinguish between bacterial or eumycotic etiology. The actinomycetes in Gram-stained smears appear as thin, gram-positive interwoven filaments mixed with coccoid forms, whereas the true fungi in KOH preparations show broad, septate hyphae with large and bizarre swollen cells. Species identification requires much time and considerable skill.

Granules are cultivated on standard mycologic media, such as Sabouraud's glucose agar with chloramphenicol, both with and without cyclohexamide, with one set at 37°C and another at room temperature. Actinomycetes also grow on mycologic media; however, Löwenstein-Jensen media should be used for primary isolation. The histologic diagnosis of mycetoma has been brought to a high level of precision. The granules may be divided into three categories: (1) fungal, pigmented; (2) fungal, unpigmented; and (3) actinomycetes.

Diagnosis by skin and serum tests is not yet precise because of a lack of defined antigen. It is possible to distinguish between actinomycotic mycetoma and eumycotic mycetoma by skin tests and agar gel diffusion tests.

Also called *actinomycetoma* (bacterial form) and *maduromycetoma* (fungal form). For more information, see the accompanying table.

Mycobacteriaceae (mi″ko-bak-te″re-a′se-e) a family of bacteria of the order Actinomycetales. It consists of a single genus, *Mycobacterium,* which contains the organisms responsible for human tuberculosis and leprosy.

Mycobacterium (mi″ko-bak-te′re-um) [*myco-* + Gr. *bakterion* a small rod] a genus of bacteria of the family Mycobacteriaceae. It consists of slightly curved or straight rods that vary from coccoid to filamentous in appearance and are distinguished by acid-fast staining. Organisms of the genus are strictly aerobic and mostly slow-growing. The genus contains 30 species, including the highly pathogenic organisms that cause tuberculosis and leprosy. Brief descriptions of the clinically important species follow; for more information on the characteristics of the genus, as well as ecology and pathogenicity, see *mycobacterium.* See also *atypical mycobacterium.*

M. abscessus, an incorrect name for *M. chelonei.*

M. aquae, an incorrect name for *M. gordonae.*

M. avium, a species that causes tuberculosis in birds and swine but rarely in humans. It is slow-growing, growing optimally at 41°C. It forms smooth, buff- to yellow-colored, nonphotochromogenic colonies that do not hydrolyze Tween 80. *M. avium* and *M. intracellulare* are closely related species and are often referred to as *M. avium* complex or Battey-avium complex.

M. balnei, an incorrect name for *M. marinum.*

M. borstelense, an incorrect name for *M. chelonei.*

M. bovis, a virulent species that causes tuberculosis in cattle and, less frequently, in humans. It is closely related to *M. tuberculosis,* forming slow-growing, rough, nonpigmented colonies. It is differentiated from *M. tuberculosis* by being susceptible to inhibition by a 5-μg/ml concentration of T2H (thiophene 2-carboxylic acid hydrazide).

M. chelonei, an opportunist pathogenic species found in soil and water. It can produce soft tissue abscesses, from which it is readily recovered, and, less frequently, an osteomyelitis or disseminated infection. This rapidly growing species resembles *M. fortuitum,* forms buff-colored colonies, and produces arylsulfatase; it does not reduce nitrate. *M. abscessus* and *M. borstelense* are synonyms for the earlier recognized *M. chelonei.*

M. flavescens, a scotochromogen that is moderate- to slow-growing and forms smooth colonies. It is rarely pathogenic.

M. fortuitum, a potentially pathogenic opportunistic species found in soil and also in subcutaneous abscesses. It may produce lesions of lung, bone, or soft tissue following trauma, and expecially with prosthetic implants. It is rapid-growing, producing rough, buff-colored colonies and forming arylsulfatase. Also called *M. ranae.*

M. gastri, a nonpathogenic species that occurs as a contaminant in clinical specimens. It is slow-

MYCETOMA. COMMON CAUSATIVE ORGANISMS

ORGANISM	GEOGRAPHICAL LOCATION	CULTURE CHARACTERISTICS
Fungi		
Cephalosporium falciforme	South America, North Africa	White fluffy conidia produced singly on conidiophores; optimal growth temperature, 25-30°C
Exophiala jeanselmei (*Phialophora jeanselmei*)	America, India	Black, aerial mycelium; long, unbranched phialides
Leptosphaeria senegalensis	West Africa	Gray-brown colonies with a black reverse side
Madurella grisea	Western Hemisphere	Fast growing; no diffusible pigment
Madurella mycetoma	Africa, Asia, USA	Variable, gray-brown cylindric arthrospores and chlamydospores
Petriellidum boydii (*Allescheria boydii*)	Western Hemisphere	Rapid growth at 30-37°C; white velvety colony with single terminal spores
Pyrenochaeta romeroi	Venezuela, Africa	Rapid growing, dark aerial mycelium with pyonidia
Actinomycetes		
Actinomadura madurae (*Streptomyces madurae*)	Worldwide	Slow growing, waxy rugose colonies
Actinomadura pelletieri (*Streptomyces pelletieri*)	Africa, South America	Small red colonies
Nocardia asteroides	Worldwide	Orange colony with white fluffy surface
Nocardia caviae	America, Africa	Hard yellow colonies
Nocardia brasiliensis	Tropical America	Hard yellow colonies heaped, wrinkled, or folded
Streptomyces somaliensis	Africa, America	Rapid growing, spreading yellow colonies; optimal growth temperature, 30°C

growing, forming variable-surfaced, nonpigmented colonies. It hydrolyzes Tween 80 but does not produce catalase or arylsulfatase.

M. gordonae, a nonpathogenic species frequently found in sputum and gastric washings. It is slow-growing, producing rounded, smooth, yellow scotochromogenic colonies. It hydrolyzes Tween 80 in 5 da or less. Also called *M. aquae*.

M. haemophilum, a slow-growing species requiring hemin. It is a nonphotochromogen and forms rough colonies.

M. intracellulare, a species that occasionally causes chronic pulmonary disease in adults and lymph node infection in children. It is slow-growing, forms smooth, nonphotochromogenic colonies, and it does not hydrolyze Tween 80. *M. intracellulare* is a member of the *M. avium* complex, which consists of avian-like mycobacteria in Runyon Group III. Also called *Battey bacillus.*

M. kansasii, a species that causes a variety of human infections. It is slow-growing, forming mostly rough and smooth yellow photochromogenic colonies. It is usually niacin-negative and it reduces nitrate. Sometimes the bright orange crystals of β-carotene produced on the surface of colonies are useful in identification.

M. leprae, the causative agent of human leprosy. It cannot be cultured on an artificial medium; diagnosis depends on demonstration of acid-fast bacilli from suspect lesions. Typically, they occur in intracellular bundles called globi. They are abundant in lepromatous leprosy but are scarce in the tuberculoid variety. See also *leprosy*.

M. malmoense, a nonphotochromogen that grows slowly and forms smooth colonies. It is a pathogenic organism that may be associated with pulmonary infection.

M. marinum, a species that causes swimming pool granuloma and other superficial lesions. It is slow-growing, forming yellow photochromogenic colonies, with optimal growth at 24°–30°C and no growth or poor growth at 37°C. It does not reduce nitrate but hydrolyzes Tween 80 in 5 da. Also called *M. balnei*.

M. microti, a species that produces a tuberculosis-like disease in field mice but is not virulent for humans. It has been used as a live vaccine for human immunization. Also called *vole bacillus*.

M. nonchromogenicum, a nonpathogenic species that grows slowly, forms variably rough and smooth colonies, and does not produce pigment.

M. phlei, a nonpathogenic species in Runyon Group IV found in dust, plants, and soil. It is rapid-growing, producing rough, scotochromogenic, yellow-to-orange colonies. It grows at 45°C as well as at 30° and 37°C.

M. scrofulaceum, a potentially pathogenic species that causes lymph node infection in children; it is also found in the sputum and gastric washings from persons with no evidence of pulmonary disease. The species is slow-growing, forming small, yellow scotochromogenic, rounded and smooth colonies. The organisms do not hydrolyze Tween 80.

M. simiae, a rarely pathogenic, slow-growing photochromogen that forms smooth colonies.

M. smegmatis, a nonpathogenic, rapidly growing species, originally isolated from smegma, that forms variable-surfaced, nonphotochromogenic colonies. It grows at 45°C as well as at 30° and 37°C.

M. szulgai, a rarely pathogenic, slow-growing species with rough-to-smooth colonies that behaves either as a scotochromogen (37°C) or photochromogen (25°C). It is recovered from lung infections almost exclusively.

M. terrae, a nonpathogenic species in soil and water that forms slow-growing, smooth, nonpigmented colonies. It reduces nitrate, produces catalase, and hydrolyzes Tween 80 in 5 da.

M. triviale, a nonpathogenic species that contaminates sputum and gastric washings. It forms slow-growing, nonpigmented, rough colonies. Superficially, it resembles *M. tuberculosis,* but it produces catalase, not niacin.

M. tuberculosis, the causative agent of human tuberculosis. It is a pathogenic species that forms slow-growing, rough, nonpigmented colonies that become dry, wrinkled, and buff colored at 5 wk. It produces niacin but very little catalase and forms cords. Also called *tubercle bacillus.* See also *tuberculosis.*

M. ulcerans, a species that causes a chronic cutaneous lesions in humans. It is slow-growing, forming nonpigmented, rough colonies. It grows at 30°C but not at 37°C and does not hydrolyze Tween 80 in 5 da.

M. xenopi, a slow-growing opportunistic species, occasionally associated with chronic pulmonary disease. More frequently, it is isolated from tap water and human secretions without associated disease. It forms small, yellow, scotochromogenic smooth colonies and grows optimally at 42°–45°C.

mycobacterium (mi″ko-bak-te′re-um), pl. *mycobacteria.* a bacterium belonging to the genus *Mycobacterium.* These organisms are aerobic, nonsporulating, nonmotile rods that may form filaments as long as 10 μm. They stain poorly by the Gram method. The best known species are *M. tuberculosis* and *M. bovis,* which cause tuberculosis, and *M. leprae,* which causes leprosy. The 25 or more species are widely distributed in nature and often recovered from water, soil, domestic and wild animals, and birds. Some of these can produce human infections, usually as opportunistic pathogens.

STAINING AND CULTURE. Mycobacteria stain poorly with basic dyes, such as crystal violet, but staining methods are available that promote dye penetration. Once stained, mycobacteria are resistant to decolorization by acid-alcohol mixtures (e.g., 95 percent ethanol–3 percent HCl). This property is referred to as acid-fastness and is due to the high lipid content of mycobacterial cell walls. Methods used to stain mycobacteria include the Ziehl-Neelsen, in which smears are heated to steaming in the presence of carbolfuchsin in phenol; the Kinyoun, a carbolfuchsin staining procedure not requiring heat; and the Truant auramine-rhodamine, which requires a fluorescent microscope for examination. An advantage of the fluorescent procedure is that the smear may be scanned with a 25× microscope objective, allowing examination of a greater number of microscope fields in a shorter time. It is thought to be more sensitive but less specific than other techniques.

Acid-fast staining reveals slender, slightly curved or straight bacilli that may appear beaded. Some strains of *M. tuberculosis* grow as aggregated, thick strands of parallel cells or "cords." In Ziehl-Neelsen- or Kinyoun-stained smears, bacilli appear red against a blue or green background, depending on the counterstain used. If the fluorescent procedure is used, acid-fast bacilli appear bright yellow against a dark background.

STRUCTURE. The mycobacterial cell wall contains abundant lipid material, accounting for about 60 percent of the dry weight of the cell wall. The lipid-rich wall is responsible for both the relative impermeability of mycobacteria to stains and to their acid-fastness. Mycobacteria are also quite resistant to acid and alkali, and to cationic detergents such as quaternary ammonium compounds.

Among the cell wall lipids are true waxes and glycolipids. Mycolic acids are unique to cell walls of *Mycobacterium, Nocardia,* and *Corynebacterium* species. The presence of cord factor, a glycolipid, had been related to virulence and to the serpentine (cord) growth pattern seen with *M. tuberculosis.* Wax D cell wall glycolipid, present in *M. tuberculosis,* is used as an adjuvant to enhance the immunogenicity of various antigens with which it is mixed.

GROWTH. Mycobacteria are aerobic and can grow in simple synthetic media. Glycerol can be utilized as a sole carbon source and ammonium salts as a nitrogen source, but growth is stimulated by the addition of amino acids. Media containing egg yolk, such as Löwenstein-Jensen, produce better growth and are frequently used for primary isolation of mycobacteria from clinical specimens. *M. leprae,* the etiologic agent of leprosy, has not yet been cultivated in vitro.

The growth of mycobacteria is slow, except for certain rapidly growing species known as the rapid growers. The doubling time of *M. tuberculosis* in culture is 12–24 hr (for comparison, the doubling time of Enterobacteriaceae is about 20 min). Most of the pathogenic species require 2–6 wk for visible colonies to appear on solid media, but rapid growers, such as *M. fortuitum,* require less than 7 da.

Temperature requirements vary with the species. Some, including *M. tuberculosis* and *M. bovis,* grow only at restricted temperatures (approximately 37°C). *M ulcerans, M. haemophilum,* and *M. marinum,* all of which cause skin lesions, grow optimally at temperatures from 30°–32°C, whereas high temperatures (above 37°C) favor the growth of *M. xenopi* and *M. avium.*

The colony morphology of mycobacteria may be rough (e.g., *M. tuberculosis*) or smooth (as with *M. gordonae*).

Mycobacteria can be classified according to the production of carotenoid pigmentation. Photochromogens require light for pigment formation, whereas scotochromogens are pigmented in the presence or absence of light. Nonphotochromogens are not pigmented, even in the presence of light. Dark red β-carotene crystals may be observed on colonies of photochromogens when cultures are incubated continuously in the light.

ECOLOGY AND PATHOGENICITY. *M. tuberculosis,* the most commonly isolated species, causes pulmonary tuberculosis and extrapulmonary disease involving the lymph nodes, heart, kidneys, genitals, bones, joints, peritoneum, or central nervous system. Granulomatous lesions, called tubercles, are characteristic of the disease and consist of epithelioid cells (elongated macrophages) and giant cells (fused macrophages), often containing acid-fast bacilli.

Miliary tuberculosis is characterized by the presence of tubercles in many organs of the body. Tuberculosis is primarily transmitted by inhalation of airborne droplets containing mycobacteria. Other potential portals of the infection include the gastrointestinal tract, skin, and mucous membranes.

M. bovis causes tuberculosis in cattle and in humans who either consume unpasteurized milk from tuberculous cows or inhale the organism in aerosols. The pasteurization of milk and control of tuberculosis in cattle both have contributed to the virtual elimination of *M. bovis*–caused tuberculosis in the United States. An attenuated strain of *M. bovis,* bacille Calmette-Guérin (BCG) vaccine, has been used in the experimental immunotherapy of cancer patients and for the vaccination of populations at risk for tuberculosis.

Mycobacterial species other than *M. tuberculosis* or *M. bovis* were formerly called "atypical"; today, however, the terms "nontuberculous mycobacteria" or "mycobacteria, not *M. tuberculosis*" are preferable.

Runyon groups, as described by Runyon in 1959, divided mycobacterial species other than *M. tuberculosis* and *M. bovis* into four groups based on pigmentation and rate of growth, each group consisting of several species. Group I referred to slow-growing photochromogens; group II, to slow-growing scotochromogens; group III, to slow-growing nonphotochromogens; and group IV, to rapidly growing mycobacteria, maturing in less than 1 wk. There are limitations to the Runyon criteria. Furthermore, the current availability of species names and of tests for identification at the species level largely obviates the need for this classification. Thus, group designations are now descriptive terms, i.e., photochromogens, scotochromogens, nonphotochromogens, and rapidly growing mycobacteria. The nontuberculous mycobacteria can cause opportunistic infections, and also infections in otherwise normal humans.

M. ulcerans causes chronic, cutaneous ulcers in humans; it grows slowly, but optimally, at 31°C, and has been isolated mainly from individuals in Africa and Australia.

Slow-growing photochromogens include *M. kansasii, M. marinum,* and *M. simiae. M. simiae* has been isolated from water supplies but is rarely associated with human disease. *M. kansasii,* which has been isolated from water taps and water storage tanks, may cause lung disease, bone and joint infections, skin or soft tissue diseases, and, rarely, disseminated disease.

The slow-growing scotochromogens include the potential pathogens *M. scrofulaceum, M. szulgai, M. xenopi,* and species that are rarely human pathogens, *M. gordonae* and *M. flavescens. M. scrofulaceum* causes lymphadenitis in children and, rarely, pulmonary disease in adults. Some isolates from environmental or human clinical sources possess biochemical and pigment characteristics intermediate between those of *M. scrofulaceum* and the *M. avium* complex. Such isolates have been referred to as "MAIS intermediates" or "MAIS complex." *M. szulgai* may produce chronic lung disease or infections involving the lymph nodes or bursae. Strains of *M. szulgai* are generally scotochromogenic at 37°C but photochromogenic at 25°C.

M. xenopi, a thermophilic organism, may cause chronic pulmonary disease. Occasional nonpigmented strains may be observed. The organism has been isolated from hot-water tanks.

The nonphotochromogens include *M. avium, M. intracellulare* (Battey bacillus), *M. malmoense, M. haemophilum,* and the generally nonpathogenic species *M. gastri, M. terrae, M. triviale,* and *M. nonchromogenicum.*

Both *M. avium* and *M. intracellulare* are usually referred to together as the *M. avium* complex because these organisms are not readily distinguishable biochemically, although they can be distinguished serologically. Together with *M. kansasii,* the *M. avium* complex composes a large number of mycobacterial isolates in the clinical laboratory, ranking second to the isolation of *M. tuberculosis.* There appears to be geographic variation in the frequency of isolation of *M. kansasii* versus the *M. avium* complex.

Although generally nonphotochromogenic, pigmented strains of the *M. avium* complex may be isolated from environmental or clinical sources. Organisms having characteristics intermediate between those of *M. scrofulaceum* and the *M. avium* complex are known as the MAIS complex; they have been isolated from both environmental and clinical sources. The clinical significance of MAIS organisms is not yet known. The *M. avium* complex has been associated with human pulmonary disease, bone and joint infections, disseminated disease, and soft tissue infections. *M. avium* causes tuberculosis in birds and in swine. Human pulmonary disease caused by the *M. avium* complex is difficult to treat because of resistance to antituberculosis drugs.

M. malmoense has been associated with human pulmonary disease. *M. haemophilum* requires hemin for growth and has been isolated from a skin infection. Little is known about the distribution of these organisms.

The rapid-growing mycobacteria include the clinically significant species *M. fortuitum* and *M. chelonei,* together referred to as the *M. fortuitum* complex, and a variety of other mycobacterial species. The *M. fortuitum* complex has been isolated from soil and water. Human diseases associated with isolation of this complex are generally soft tissue abscesses, although osteomyelitis, infections of prosthetic heart valves, and disseminated disease have been reported.

Because nontuberculous mycobacteria can be isolated from a variety of environmental sources, as well as from occasional specimens from individuals free of disease, isolation from patient respiratory specimens or gastric aspirates may represent colonization. The possibility of contamination of laboratory reagents cannot be excluded. When isolated from sputum specimens or gastric aspirates, the significance of nontuberculous mycobacteria depends on: (1) evidence of a positive chest radiograph and elimination of other possible etiologies; and (2) either isolation of the same strain repeatedly from several specimens or isolation from a closed lesion, such as an abscess or biopsy tissue collected and transported under sterile conditions.

M. leprae (Hansen's bacillus) is the etiologic agent of leprosy, a disease involving the skin and the peripheral nerves. The organism has not been cultivated either on synthetic media or in tissue culture. Organisms may be observed in lesion biopsy specimens as acid-fast organisms, approximately 0.3 by 4–7 μm. The organisms are predominantly intracellular and can remain viable within macrophages.

LABORATORY DIAGNOSIS. Strict safety precautions must be followed when processing specimens or cultures containing mycobacteria. Production of infectious aerosols via Bunsen burners or centrifugation must be avoided. *M. tuberculosis, M. bovis,* and the *M. avium* complex are listed as class 3 agents by the U.S. Public Health Service Centers for Disease Control. Such agents, including specimens that may contain these agents, must be handled in a class 2 biologic safety cabinet equipped with a HEPA filter.

Specimens in which mycobacteria may be isolated are sputum; sputum induced by the aerosolization of warm saline; gastric washings; urine; pleural, spinal, joint, or other fluids; exudates; and biopsy specimens. Early morning sputum or urine specimens collected on three consecutive days are preferable to specimens collected later in the day. Gastric lavage specimens are useful for children or adults who swallow their sputum (saprophytic mycobacteria may be found in such specimens). Sterile containers should be used for specimen collection.

Specimens containing bacterial flora, such as sputum, bronchial and gastric washings, urine obtained by a nonsterile procedure, or autopsy specimens, must be processed as soon as possible after collection to remove bacterial contaminants. Processing methods not only serve to decontaminate specimens but also to digest or liquefy specimens. The centrifugation step serves to concentrate acid-fast bacilli.

Agents used for digestion and concentration of specimens include: sodium hydroxide alone; acetyl-cysteine, a mucolytic agent, and sodium hydroxide; or Zephiran–trisodium phosphate. The relative resistance of mycobacteria to alkali or to quaternary ammonium compounds (Zephiran) is utilized in these procedures. Strict adherence to alkali or detergent concentrations and times stated in these procedures is recommended. Specimens badly contaminated with gram-negative bacilli may be treated with oxalic acid or an increased alkali concentration, but the latter may kill mycobacteria. Aseptically collected urine; spinal, joint, or other body fluid; and surgically obtained biopsy specimens do not need to be processed.

Acid-fast staining procedures are performed on all specimens submitted for mycobacterial culture. Owing to the slow growth of most mycobacterial species, microscopy serves as an early detection mechanism for the presence of acid-fast bacilli. The numbers of bacilli observed may be used to determine the specimen dilution for direct susceptibility testing (see below) and to monitor the response to therapy. Smears are less sensitive than cultures. The absence of growth in spite of positive smears may be due to antimycobacterial drugs or to overly severe decontamination procedures. False-positive smears may result from contaminated stain solutions or tap water, and the carryover of material from a positive specimen or positive smear. The last can occur via contaminated immersion oil.

Culture media used for the isolation of mycobacteria include egg media, such as Löwenstein-Jensen, American Thoracic Society, or Petragnani media; and agar media, such as Middlebrook 7H10 or 7H11. The use of two types of media yields optimal results. Agents inhibiting the growth of bacterial contaminants may be added to either egg base or agar base media. Cultures are incubated at 37°C. Skin biopsy specimens or other specimens from external body areas should also be incubated at 30°C (or room temperature if a 30°C incubator is not available) to detect *M. marinum* or *M. ulcerans.* For growth on 7H10 or 7H11 media, 5–10 percent CO_2 is required and is stimulatory to growth on egg base media. Cultures are examined weekly for a minimum of 6–8 wk.

SPECIES IDENTIFICATION. Laboratories that do not process an adequate volume to maintain expertise should refer cultures to a reference laboratory for identification and sensitivity testing. *M. tuberculosis* may be identified easily by several criteria: the colonies grow slowly at 37°C and are characteristically rough and buff colored, and the niacin test is positive. Confirmatory tests include reduction of nitrate and loss of catalase activity after heating at 68°C.

Characteristics used for the identification of other mycobacterial species include the rate of growth, temperature necessary for growth, colony pigmentation in the presence and absence of light, morphology, and biochemical properties; see the accompanying table.

A number of biochemical tests are available as an aid to speciation of mycobacteria. Catalase is produced by all mycobacteria with the exception of some isoniazid-resistant strains of *M. tuberculosis, M. gastri,* and *M. kansasii.* A semiquantitative catalase test distinguishes mycobacterial species on the basis of high or low catalase production. Testing for the loss of catalase activity after heating at 68°C is useful for identification of *M. tuberculosis,* especially when used in conjunction with the niacin test.

A test of niacin production should be performed on acid-fast colonies that are suggestive of *M. tuber-*

culosis (nonpigmented, rough colonies). *M. simiae,* a photochromogen, and some strains of *M. bovis* are niacin-positive. Cyanogen bromide, a niacin test reagent, is hazardous. A safety paper strip method is available.

Several mycobacterial species, indluding *M. tuberculosis,* possess nitrate reductase. The nitrate reduction test is also available as a paper strip method.

The 3-da arylsulfatase test is useful for the differentiation of members of the potentially pathogenic *M. fortuitum* complex other rapidly growing mycobacteria. Other tests used for the identification of rapidly growing species of mycobacteria incude the iron uptake test, tests for growth in the presence of 5 percent NACl, and growth on MacConkey agar without crystal violet.

The 2-wk arylsulfatase test is useful for the identification of several species of slow-growing mycobacteria. Several species of the scotochromogen and nonphotochromogen groups hydrolyze Tween 80, releasing oleic acid. Generally, species that hydrolyze Tween 80 readily are seldom clinically significant. Reduction of a potassium salt of tellurite to black tellurium within several days is characteristic of *M. avium–intracellulare.*

Detection of the enzyme pyrazinamidase aids in the differentiation of *M. marinum* from *M. kansasii,* and *M. tuberculosis* from weakly niacin-positive *M. bovis.* Also used to differentiate *M. tuberculosis* (and other species) from *M. bovis* is a test for susceptibility to thiophene-2-carboxylic acid hydrazide (T2H). *M. bovis* is susceptible to concentrations of T2H as low as 5 μg/ml.

The urease test is useful for the differentiation of *M. scrofulaceum* from pigmented strains of *M. avium–intracellulare.*

SUSCEPTIBILITY TESTING. Newly diagnosed cases of tuberculosis are treated with two or more primary drugs: isoniazid, rifampin, ethambutol, or streptomycin. Isoniazid-resistant strains of *M. tuberculosis* have been isolated from individuals in the United States. If cultures continue to be positive for *M. tuberculosis* after a few months of therapy, the organism causing the infection may be resistant to one or more primary drugs. Susceptibility to secondary drugs, such as capreomycin, cycloserine, ethionamide, kanamycin, *p*-aminosalicylic acid, and pyrazinamide, may be tested for to select the appropriate drugs to be used in treating patients with multiple drug resistance. For slow-growing nontuberculosis mycobacteria, in vitro susceptibility test results may not correspond with treatment results.

Two methods for susceptibility testing of mycobacterial isolates are available: direct and indirect. In the direct testing method, the concentrated and decontaminated clinical specimen is utlized if acid-fast bacilli are observed in the smear of the concentrated specimen. The indirect method employs the organism that is isolated from the clinical specimen. It is used if the culture is to be referred for susceptibility testing or if the direct smear is negative but the culture is positive.

Disk diffusion tests such as those available for the rapidly growing Enterobacteriaceae are not applicable to the slow-growing mycobacteria, although a simple disk diffusion test procedure is available for testing the susceptibility of *M. fortuitum* and *M. chelonei* to amikacin, doxycyline, kanamycin, minocycline, sulfonamides, and trimethoprim. Testing of slow-growing mycobacterial isolates consists of inoculating a standardized suspension of microorganisms to a Middlebrook 7H10 or 7H11 agar medium containing standardized amounts of antibiotics. Several of the drugs are available in paper disk form. Strict attention must be paid to the time of incubation because of possible deterioration of the drug in the medium and subsequent growth of otherwise susceptible mycobacteria. Growth in the presence of antibiotics is compared with growth in the absence of antibiotics.

An automated, radiometric procedure (BACTEC) has been developed for detection of growth and for susceptibility testing of mycobacterial isolates.

mycobactin (mi″ko-bak′tin) a sideramine derivative of hydroxamic acid (*R*-$CONH_2OH$) required for growth by at least one species of the mycobacteria. It chelates ferric iron and facilitates its transfer into the cell. See also *sideramine.*

mycolic acid (mi-kol′ik) a large, saturated, branched-chain hydroxylated fatty acid of high molecular weight, which is characteristic of mycobacterial species; similar acids of lower molecular weight occur in the species of *Nocardia* and *Corynebacterium.* See also *antibacterial agents* and *mycoside.*

mycologist (mi-kol′o-jist) one who has a knowledge of fungi.

mycology (mi-kol′o-je) [*myco-* + *-logy*] the science and study of fungi. Microbiologically, fungi are a lower form of eukaryotes, and their analysis increases our knowledge of all eukaryotes. Medically, fungi cause morbidity and mortality in various cutaneous, subcutaneous, and systemic diseases. Moreover, certain fungi are a cause of toxic food poisoning. Fungi (particularly yeasts) are also important in industry where they are used for fermentation purposes and as a food (truffles and mushrooms).

mycomyringitis (mi″ko-mir″in-ji′tis) [*myco-* + L. *myringa* membrana tympani + *-itis*] a fungal infection of the eardrum, with a predominant inflammatory component.

Mycoplasma (mi″ko-plaz′mah) [*myco-* + Gr. *plasma* anything formed or molded] a genus of microorganisms of the family Mycoplasmataceae. It consists of highly pleomorphic, gram-negative cells that are spherical or slightly ovoid in shape and occur as animal parasites and pathogens. The organisms are bounded by a membrane but lack a true cell wall. The typical colony on agar has a central portion growing into the agar, surrounded by a light surface growth, giving it a “fried egg” appearance. Sterol is required for growth. The genus contains 36 recognized species widely distributed on the mucous membranes of humans and animals. They cause a wide variety of infections in animals, plants, and insects. A few species, notably *M. pneumoniae,* are primary human pathogens. See also *mycoplasma.*

M. fermentans, a relatively rare parasitic inhabitant of the mucosa of the genital tract. It ferments glucose, hydrolyzes arginine, and does not grow aerobically.

M. hominis, a common parasitic inhabitant of the lower genitourinary tract and the cervix. It is a potential pathogen of the female reproductive system, causing acute inflammation of the uterine tube; it is also a possible cause of pharyngitis and respiratory

MYCOBACTERIUM. SUMMARY OF CHARACTERISTICS OF MYCOBACTERIA[a]

Runyon Group	Species	Clinical Significance	Optimum Temperature	Colony Morphology[b]	Pigmentation[c]	Niacin	Nitrate	Catalase: Semiquantitative (> 45 mm)
	M. tuberculosis	+	37°	R	N	+	+	<
	M. bovis	+	37°	R	N	−	−	<
	M. ulcerans	+	31°	R	N	−	−	>
I	*M. kansasii*	+	37°	S, I	P	−	+	>
	M. marinum	+	31°, 24°	S, I	P	V	−	<
	M. simiae	+	37°	S	P	+	−	>
II	*M. scrofulaceum*	+	37°	S	S	−	−	>
	M. szulgai	+	37°	S, R	S, P	−	+	>
	M. xenopi	+	42°	S	S	−	−	<
	M. flavescens	−	37°	S	S	−	+	>
	M. gordonae	−	37°	S	S	−	−	>
III	*M. avium*	+	37°	S, R	N	−	−	<
	M. intracellulare	+	37°	S, R	N	−	−	<
	M. malmoense	+	37°	S	N	−	−	
	M. haemophilum[f]	+	31°, 24°	R	N	−	−	<
	M. gastri	−	37°	S, R, I	N	−	−	<
	M. nonchromogenicum	−	37°	I	N	−	+	>
	M. terrae	−	37°	I	N	−	+	>
	M. triviale	−	37°	R	N	−	+	>
IV	*M. fortuitum*[g]	+	37°	S, R	N	−	+	>
	M. chelonei[g]	+	37°	S, R	N	V	−	>
	M. phlei	−	37°	S, R	S	−	+	>
	M. smegmatis	−	37°	S, R	N	−	+	>
	M. vaccae	−	37°	S	S	−	+	>

[a] Plus = usually positive; minus = usually negative; V = variable; blank space = no data.
[b] S = smooth; R = rough; I = intermediate.
[c] N = nonphotochromogenic; P = photochromogenic; S = scotochromogenic. *M. szulgai* is scotochromogenic at 37°C and photochromogenic at 25°C. Pigmented *M. avium–M. intracellulare* stains may be isolated.
[d] Positive in 14 da.
[e] Thiophene-2-carboxylic acid hydrazide.

MYCOBACTERIUM. (*Continued*)

CATALASE: 68° pH 7.0	TWEEN HYDROLYSIS	TELLURITE REDUCTION	ARYLSULFATASE (3 da)[d]	UREASE	GROWTH ON 5% NaCl	PYRAZINAMIDASE	SUSCEPTIBILITY TO T2H (5 mg/ml)[e]	IRON UPTAKE
–	–	–	–	+	–	+	–	–
–	–	–	–	+	–	–	+	–
+	–	–	–	+	–	–	–	–
+	+	–	–	+	–	–	–	–
+	+	–	V[d]	+	–	+	–	–
+	–	–	–	+	–	–	–	–
+	–	–	–[d]	+	–	V	–	–
+	V	–	V[d]	+	–	–	–	–
+	–	–	–[d]	–	–	+	–	–
+	+	–	–	+	+	+	–	–
+	+	–	–	–	–	V	–	–
+	–	+	–	–	–	+	–	–
+	–	+	–	–	–	+	–	–
–	+	–	–	–		+		
–	–	–	–	–	–	+		–
–	+	–	–	+	–	–	–	–
+	+	–	–	–	–	+	–	–
+	+	–	–	–	–	V	–	–
+	+	–	V	–	+	+	–	–
+	V	V	+	+	+	+		+
+	–	V	+	+	V[h]	+		–
+	+	+	–	+	+	+		+
+	+	+	–	+	+	+		+
+	+	+	–	+	V	+		+

[f] Requires hemin for growth.
[g] *M. fortuitum* and *M. chelonei* grow on MacConkey agar.
[h] *M. chelonei* subspecies *abscessus*, +; *M. chelonei* subspecies *chelonei*, –.
Adapted from Lennette, E. H., et al.: Manual of Clinical Microbiology. 3rd ed. Washington, DC, American Society for Microbiology, pp. 152-153.

disease. *M. hominis* does not ferment glucose but hydrolyzes arginine, and it can be grown in both aerobic and anaerobic conditions.

M. orale, a normal inhabitant of the mouth and throat. The species consists of three strains (types 1, 2, 3), which can be differentiated by biochemical, cultural, and serologic characteristics. It does not ferment glucose but hydrolyzes arginine, and is predominantly anaerobic.

M. pneumoniae, the species that causes most cases of primary atypical pneumonia. The colonies are regular and spherical with a granular surface, although they do not have the typical "fried egg" appearance. The organism is presumptively identified by the nature of growth in highly selective culture media, and by hemadsorption to or beta hemolysis of guinea pig red cells. Conclusive identification depends on staining colonies with homologous fluorescein-labeled antibody or by inhibition of growth by the specific antibody. It ferments glucose, hydrolyzes arginine, and is facultative with respect to oxygen requirements. Also called *Eaton agent.* See also *pneumonia.*

M. salivarium, a common parasitic inhabitant of the oropharynx and gingival crevice. It does not ferment glucose but hydrolyzes arginine, and is microaerophilic.

mycoplasma (mi″ko-plaz′mah) a term for microorganisms belonging to the class Mollicutes, whose cells have a limiting membrane but no rigid wall. Although there is considerable taxonomic uncertainty about mycoplasmas, two families are currently accepted: Mycoplasmataceae, which contains two genera, and Acholeplasmataceae, which consists of a single genus. More than 70 different organisms have been recognized, 11 of which infect humans. Various species are common inhabitants of mucous membranes, and for most a pathogenic role, if any, is opportunistic.

Mycoplasmas constitute the smallest microorganisms capable of growth in a cell-free medium. They are extremely pleomorphic, ranging from small (0.3–0.5 μm) spheres to filaments as long as 150 μm. Because they lack the rigid peptoglycan cell wall of eubacteria, they stain poorly with conventional procedures such as the Gram stain. Mycoplasmas may be grown on artificial media, but their growth requirements are more exacting than those of most bacteria. Several characteristics that distinguish the mycoplasmas from some other prokaryotic organisms appear in Table 1. Classification of the mycoplasmas is based on morphologic, biochemical, nutritional, and serologic criteria, listed in Table 2. Mycoplasmas were for a long time confused with the L forms of various bacteria. However, in these L-phase variants, the loss of cell wall is generally reversible.

PATHOGENICITY. Mycoplasmas include important pathogens of animals, plants, and insects; they also constitute part of the normal flora of animals. In humans, a few species are often isolated from healthy respiratory tracts, especially *M. orale* and *M. salivarium. M. hominis* and *Ureaplasma urealyticum* are commonly found in the urogenital tract.

There is no doubt about the pathogenicity of *M. pneumoniae,* which is the etiologic agent of mycoplasmal pneumonia, first recognized in the 1930s and given the name primary atypical pneumonia. Unlike other mycoplasmas, *M. pneumoniae* can attach to the surface of respiratory epithelium by binding to neuraminic acid receptors. Cell damage may be the result of hydrogen peroxide release. Although respiratory infections with *M. pneumoniae* are generally mild, severe disease may result in some cases. In addition, a variety of extrapulmonary complications may occur as a consequence of respiratory infection (Table 3).

Two of the six species of mycoplasmas isolated from the urogenital tract have been associated with human disease. *U. urealyticum* (formerly designated as T-strain mycoplasmas) is capable of causing pelvic inflammatory disease; it is the probable agent in approximately 10 percent of cases of nongonococcal urethritis. A pathogenic role for *M. hominis* is much less certain, but it may act as an opportunist in infections of the female upper reproductive tract.

MYCOPLASMA, TABLE 1. CHARACTERISTICS OF MYCOPLASMAS AND SOME OTHER PROKARYOTIC ORGANISMS

PROPERTY	MYCOPLASMAS	SCHIZOMYCETES	CHLAMYDIAE	RICKETTSIAE	VIRUSES
Grows on cell-free medium	+	+*	−	−*	−
Cell wall or cell wall peptidoglycan absent	+	−	−	−	+
Generates metabolic energy	+	+	−	+	−
Depends on host cell nucleic acid for multiplication	−	−	−	−	+
Can synthesize proteins by own enzymes	+	+	+	+	−
Requires sterols	+†	−	−	−	−
Visible in optical microscope (× 1500)	+	+	+	+	−*
Filterable through 450-nm pore-size filters	+	−*	+	+	+
Contains both RNA and DNA	+	+	+	+	−
Growth inhibited by antibody alone	+	−	+	+	+
Growth inhibited by antibiotics acting on protein synthesis	+	+	+	+	−

* With few exceptions.
† Except *Acholeplasma* species.
From Tully, J. G., and Razin, S.: The Mollicutes "Mycoplasmas." Reprinted with permission from Handbook of Microbiology 2nd ed. Copyright The Chemical Rubber Co., CRC Press, Inc., 1977.

MYCOPLASMA, TABLE 2. TAXONOMY OF THE MYCOPLASMAS

CLASSIFICATION	
Class: Mollicutes	
Order: Mycoplasmatales	
Family I: Mycoplasmataceae	
	Sterol required for growth
	Genome size about 5 x 10^8 daltons
	NADH oxidase localized in cytoplasm
Genus I:	*Mycoplasma* (over 60 species)
	Do not hydrolyze urea
Genus II:	*Ureaplasma* (single species with serotypes)
	Hydrolyzes urea
Family II: Acholeplasmataceae	
	Sterol not required for growth
	Genome size about 10^9 daltons
	NADH oxidase localized in the membrane
Genus I:	*Acholeplasma* (8 species)

From Davis, B. D., et al. Microbiology. 3rd ed. Hagerstown, MD, Harper & Row, 1980, p. 787.

Recent reports of the direct isolation of mycoplasmas from the joints of individuals with acute arthritis, as well as studies in animal model systems, have restimulated interest in the arthritogenic potential of these agents.

LABORATORY DIAGNOSIS. Infection with *M. pneumoniae* is diagnosed by isolation of the organism and/or demonstration of a rise in the serum antibody titer. Isolation is accomplished by inoculating tubes of a selective broth medium or a selective di-

MYCOPLASMA, TABLE 3. CLINICAL SPECTRUM OF *Mycoplasma Pneumoniae* INFECTION

MANIFESTATION	FREQUENCY	PATHOPHYSIOLOGY
Pulmonary		
Upper respiratory illness	25%	Direct microbial injury to respiratory epithelium; indirect immunologic injury; autoimmunity reaction (?)
Pharyngitis	6-59%	
Otitis	12%	
Pneumonia	3-10%	
Reinfection	Occurs; frequency unknown	Host sensitization
Extrapulmonary complications	7% of patients hospitalized (21% no respiratory symptoms)	
Neurologic (meningoencephalitis, meningitis, ascending paralysis, transverse myelitis, cranial-nerve palsies)		Possibly microthrombo-embolism, direct microbial invasion, neurotoxin, or autoimmunity
Hematologic (hemolytic anemia, intravascular coagulation)	Clinically important >50 reported cases (subclinical form common)	Cold-agglutinin auto-immunity
Cardiovascular (myocarditis, pericarditis)	4.5%	Unknown but frequently associated with hemolytic anemia
Dermatologic (erythema multiforme, Stevens-Johnson syndrome and other rashes)	25%	Immune complex and/or direct microbial invasion
Musculoskeletal (myalgia, arthralgia, or arthritis)	14-45%*	Unknown
Gastrointestinal (anorexia, nausea, vomiting, transient diarrhea)	14-44%	Unknown
Acute glomerulonephritis	Unknown	Immune complex
Hepatitis, pancreatitis	Unknown	Possibly immune complex; autoimmunity

*Arthritis uncommon.
Modified from Cassal, G. H., and Cole, B.C.: Mycoplasmas as agents of human disease. Reprinted by permission of the New England Journal of Medicine *304*:80, 1981.

phasic (broth over agar) medium with a specimen such as sputum or nasopharyngeal or bronchial secretions. If growth occurs, as evidenced by the production of acid, the broth is subcultured to plates containing a medium enriched with horse serum and yeast extract. Following incubation, the plates are examined for very small (50–600 μm) colonies under 45× magnification. The central portion of the typical colony grows down into the agar medium, is opaque, and looks darker than the translucent peripheral zone, giving rise to the classic "fried egg" appearance. Group and genus identification is accomplished by placing filter paper disks containing a specific antiserum on the surface of an agar plate previously seeded with a pure culture of the isolate. A clear zone of inhibition around the disk identifies the species. *U. urealyticum* from the genitourinary tract can be isolated and identified on a selective urea medium by virtue of its unique property of hydrolyzing urea.

Serologic diagnosis involves demonstration of a fourfold rise in antibody titer between acute and convalescent phase specimens, generally using the complement-fixation test. Peak antibody titers are reached 3–4 wk after onset. A single complement-fixation titer greater than 1:64 is also suggestive of *M. pneumoniae* infection. About half of those with *M. pneumoniae* infection respond by producing an IgM autoantibody capable of agglutinating to a titer of greater than 1:64 their own erythrocytes at 4°C (cold agglutinins). Other less routine procedures for assessing antibody to *M. pneumoniae* include indirect hemagglutination, immunofluorescence, and growth-inhibition assays.

TREATMENT. Erythromycin and tetracycline reduce the duration of clinical symptoms of mycoplasmal pneumonia but fail to eliminate the organism. They are, however, the treatment of choice for *U. urealyticum* infections.

WALTER CEGLOWSKI, PH.D.

T-strain m., a strain that forms especially small (the T standing for tiny) colonies. It is a possible causative agent of nongonococcal urethritis and reproductive infertility in males. The organism hydrolyzes urea and is highly susceptible to erythromycin. The term T strain has no valid taxonomic standing and has been replaced by the species designation *Ureaplasma urealyticum.*

Mycoplasmataceae (mi″ko-plaz″mah-ta′se-e) a family of pleomorphic bacteria that requires sterol for growth. It contains two genera of medical interest, *Mycoplasma* and *Ureaplasma.*

mycoside (mi′ko-sid) a glycolipid that contains mycolic acid and a polysaccharide moiety. A distinctive mycoside found in the cell walls confers immunologic cross-reactivity on cells of *Corynebacterium, Mycobacteria,* and *Nocardia.*

mycosis (mi-ko′sis) [*myco-* + *-osis*] any disease caused by fungi. For more information, see the specific type of mycosis.

mycosis fungoides (MF) (mi-ko′sis fung-goid′ez) a cutaneous T-cell lymphoma with distinctive clinical and histologic features and a tendency for nodal and visceral involvement. Approximately 1 percent of deaths from lymphoma are attributable to mycosis fungoides. Most of those affected are in the fifth to seventh decades; it occurs in males almost twice as frequently as in females. MF lesions must be distinguished from those of other cutaneous lymphomas and from lymphomatoid papulosis.

The lesions may evolve over a period of 5 yr or longer, progressing from an initial erythematous stage through a plaque stage to a final tumor stage; often all three stages may coexist. In the d'emblee form of MF, the tumor stage develops rapidly. Lymphadenopathy is present in at least 50 percent of patients at the time of diagnosis, but more than half of biopsied lymph nodes show only dermatopathic lymphadenopathy. Nodal involvement by MF indicates an average survival time of under 18 mo. Visceral MF is seen in two-thirds of patients at some stage of their disease; the lung is the most common site of involvement. Survival time for this form is less than 1 yr. The Sézary syndrome is a part of the spectrum of MF. It is characterized by the presence of cells in the peripheral blood cytologically identical to those in the skin lesions of MF.

The features of the erythematous stage of MF are generally nonspecific. There are scattered reddish-brown, scaling patches resembling the cutaneous lesions seen in psoriasis and eczema. A bandlike infiltrate of mononuclear cells is seen in the superficial dermis. If the infiltrate includes the distinctive MF cells (T lymphocytes with markedly irregular—cerebriform—nuclear profiles), the diagnosis of MF may be suggested. The nuclear contour index of MF cells is greater than 6.5.

In indurated lesions of the plaque stage, the epidermotropic tendency of the MF cells may be evident in the form of Pautrier's microabscesses, in which groups of MF cells occupy sharply defined acantholytic spaces within the epidermis. The dermal infiltrate remains polymorphous but contains many MF cells.

In the tumor stage, raised reddish-brown and frequently ulcerated lesions are present. Much of the dermis becomes occupied by the infiltrate, which is dominated by MF cells. Those affected have low numbers of T cells and impaired cell-mediated immunity.

See also *nuclear contour index* and *Pautrier microabscess.*

mycotic (mi-kot′ik) pertaining to a mycosis.

mycotic keratitis (mi-kot′ik ker″ah-ti′tis) a fungal infection of the cornea. The infection is often initiated by trauma to the cornea by any object containing fungal spores. Moniliaceae, nonpigmented filamentary fungi, account for most corneal infections, *Fusarium solani* being the prime pathogen. Dematiaceae, pigmented filamentary fungi, are next in frequency, and yeasts are the least often involved. The resultant lesion is characterized by a raised epithelium with a white border and a circular margin of fungal elements. Unless treated, these lesions will invade the deep stroma of the cornea; there is often an acute inflammatory response. The treatment of choice is natamycin, a topical polyene antibiotic.

mycotoxicosis (mi″ko-tok-sĭ-ko′sis) a poisoning due to exposure, primarily through ingestion, to toxins of fungal or bacterial origin. The organisms responsible for the production need not be present to produce a mycotoxicosis. The term refers to an intoxication with or without a concomitant infection. See also *mycotoxin.*

mycotoxin (mi″ko-tok′sin) a toxic product of fungal

origin that includes numerous substances such as the toxins of mushroom poisoning, ergot alkaloids, and aflatoxins. Many mycotoxins are produced as secondary metabolites of fungi of the *Aspergillus, Penicillium, Fusarium,* and *Phoma* genera. Toxins are often elaborated on foodstuffs and consumed by humans, leading to a mycotoxicosis. Of the mycotoxins, the most well studied is aflatoxin, a toxic product of the fungus *Aspergillus flavus.* Aflatoxin ingestion has been linked to the high incidence of primary hepatocellular carcinoma in tropical Africa and Asia. See also *aflatoxin, ergot,* and *mushroom poisoning.*

mydriasis (mĭ-dri'ah-sis) [Gr.] dilation of the pupil.

myel/o (mi'ĕ-lo) [Gr. *myelos* marrow] a word element used in combining form to denote either spinal cord or bone marrow, e.g., myelocele or myeloblast.

myelapoplexy (mi"el-ap'o-plek"se) [*myel-* + *apoplexy*] a hemorrhage within the spinal cord.

myelencephalon (mi"ĕ-len-sef'ah-lon) [*myel-* + Gr. *enkephalos* brain] [NA], the part of the brain that includes the medulla oblongata and the posterior fourth ventricle, which develops from the posterior rhombencephalon.

myelin (mi'ĕ-lin) the substance of which the myelin sheath is composed, which includes phospholipids, proteins, glycoproteins, and lipoproteins.

myelinated (mi'ĕ-lĭ-nāt"ed) having a myelin sheath.

myelin basic protein (MBP) a protein (M.W. 18,000) released into the cerebrospinal fluid by the destruction of myelin, as in multiple sclerosis or other demyelinating diseases and acute infarction. MBP is determined by radioimmunoassay, and the amount correlates with the disease activity in multiple sclerosis. See also *myelin protein.*

myelin figures tightly packed membranous whorls observed within degenerating cells, reflecting lysosomal breakdown of endoplasmic reticulum.

myelinolysis (mi"ĕ-lin-ol'ĭ-sis) the destruction of myelin.

central pontine m., a rare disorder characterized by demyelination of the center of the base of the pons. This disease may result in quadriplegia but is often an incidental autopsy finding. It is most common in alcoholics and others who have suffered prolonged nutritional deprivation.

myelin protein peripheral and integral proteins of the myelin sheath of myelinated nerves. There are three fractions: myelin basic protein (M.W. 18,000), a single chain of 170 residues (see *myelin basic protein*); proteolipids (M.W. approximately 12,500–35,000), protein lipid combinations, which are insoluble in water but soluble in chloroform-methanol (the protein freed from lipid is soluble in both); and myelin acidic protein (M.W. over 50,000), a poorly characterized fraction. Several enzyme proteins are present in this fraction.

myelin sheath an insulating covering around the axon of a neuron, which increases the conduction velocity of the nerve impulse along the axon. It is formed from the cell membrane of a Schwann cell (in the peripheral nervous system) or of an oligodendrocyte (in the central nervous system). The cell is wrapped around the axon, forming several layers (lamellae). As all the cytoplasm is pushed to the body of the cell outside the sheath, each lamella consists of only two layers of cell membrane. When viewed in cross section, the line where the inside surfaces of the cell membrane contact, the major dense line, stains heavily. The line of contact of the outer surfaces, the interperiod line, is lighter staining (less electron-dense).

The length of an axon covered by a single Schwann cell is termed the internodal segment and is usually between 200 and 800 μm long. Between internodal segments, there is a brief unmyelinated gap, the node of Ranvier.

At some points in a myelin sheath, cytoplasm persists within the sheath, widening the major dense line in several consecutive lamellae: the area is called a cleft or incisure of Schmidt-Lanterman.

myelin staining methods 1. the Klüver-Barrera Luxol fast blue method. Formalin-fixed paraffin sections are stained in a 0.1 percent alcoholic solution of Luxol fast blue, then briefly placed in lithium carbonate solution and differentiated in 70 percent alcohol. Myelin sheaths and phospholipids stain deep blue. Oil red O, hematoxylin, periodic-acid–Schiff (PAS), and phosphotungstic acid–hematoxylin are commonly used counterstains.

2. methods based on chromate oxidation, which polymerizes lipids and binds them in an insoluble aggregate with chromium dioxide. The CrO_2 also serves as a mordant, binding hematoxylin and myelin phospholipids in an insoluble lake. Tissue blocks are fixed in formalin or Orth's fluid, then in 2.5 percent potassium dichromate solution for 2-8 da, processed in paraffin sections, and stained with hematoxylin. Myelin sheaths are stained blue-black.

3. osmic acid staining. Tissue blocks are stained in osmic acid and processed into paraffin or frozen sections. Myelin sheaths are black against a gray background.

See also *degenerating myelin methods.*

myelitis (mi"ĕ-li'tis) [*myel-* + *-itis*] an inflammation of the spinal cord. Three types of inflammatory processes have been distinguished. Viruses, mostly commonly the polio viruses and herpes zoster virus, primarily affect the gray matter. Subacute and chronic primary meningeal infections, including syphilis and tuberculosis, damage the spinal roots and outer surfaces of the spinal cord. A third variety of inflammation, which primarily affects the white matter, has no known cause, and leads to demyelination or necrosis. The cerebrospinal fluid may contain lymphocytes and mononuclear lymphocytes, and the protein may be increased.

acute transverse m., inflammation of both the gray and white matter in a discrete region of the spinal cord. It is characterized by sudden localized back pain and symptoms of spinal cord transection. Causes include bacterial and viral infections, multiple sclerosis and other demyelinative disorders, trauma, and ischemic necrosis. The CSF may contain mononuclear lymphocytes and a slightly increased protein level. Swelling of the cord may be seen on myelography. Subarachnoid blocks may occur at the level of the lesion.

myeloblast (mi'ĕ-lo-blast") [*myelo-* + Gr. *blastos* germ] the youngest identifiable cell of the granulocytic series, normally found only in the bone marrow; it is designated as M_1.

In Giemsa- or Wright-stained blood or bone marrow smears, these cells are 15–20 μm in diameter, with a large round or oval nucleus. The nucleus, which has a very fine chromatin pattern, contains between two and five round and pale blue nucleoli. The cytoplasm is blue and contains a few small azurophilic granules that are peroxidase-positive. See also *granulocytic series.*

myelocele (mi′ĕ-lo-sēl) [*myelo-* + Gr. *kēlē* hernia] the hernial protrusion of the spinal cord through a defect in the vertebral column.

myelocystocele (mi″ĕ-lo-sis′to-sēl) [*myelo-* + Gr. *kystis* sac + *kēlē* hernia] the cystic hernial protrusion of the spinal cord through a defect in the vertebral column.

myelocystomeningocele (mi″ĕ-lo-sis″to-mĕ-ning′-go-sēl) [*meylo-* + Gr. *kystis* sac + *mēninx* membrane + *kēlē* hernia] a cystic protrusion of the spinal cord and its meninges through a defect in the vertebral column.

myelocyte (mi′ĕ-lo-sīt) [*myelo-* + Gr. *kytos* hollow vessel] the stage of granulocytic maturation that follows the promyelocyte and precedes the metamyelocyte; it is designated as M_3 and M_4. The M_4 stage is more mature than the M_3 stage, having a more developed nucleus and a slightly condensed and smaller cell size (M_3, 16–20 μm in diameter; M_4, 10–16 μm). Myelocytes are normally found only in the bone marrow.

On bone marrow or peripheral blood smears, the nucleus of a myelocyte is smaller than that of a promyelocyte, and is round or oval and occasionally slightly indented. The chromatin pattern is coarse and sharply defined; the nucleolus is absent. In this stage, the cytoplasm becomes slightly acidophilic; specific granules (eosinophilic, basophilic, or neutrophilic) first appear and the production of azurophilic (primary) granules ceases.

Lysosomal hydrolases (acid phosphatase, arylsulfatase, β-glucuronidase, esterase, and 5-nucleotidase), cationic proteins, and lysozyme can be identified by special cytochemical stains, and the iron-binding protein lactoferrin and alkaline phosphatase appear.

See also *granulocytic series.*

myeloencephalitis (mi″ĕ-lo-en-sef″ah-li′tis) [*myelo-* + Gr. *enkephalos* brain + *-itis*] an inflammation of both the spinal cord and the brain.

myelofibrosis (mi″ĕ-lo-fi-bro′sis) [*myelo-* + L. *fibra* fiber + *-osis*] a myeloproliferative disorder characterized by the replacement of the marrow with varying amounts of fibrous tissue, abnormal growth of hematopoietic precursors (myeloid, erythroid, etc.), and myeloid metaplasia of the spleen and liver. The early features of the disease resemble chronic granulocytic leukemia. Myelofibrosis may occur without myeloid metaplasia. Clinically, splenomegaly and hepatomegaly with normochromic anemia are common. Anisocytosis and polychromasia with leukocytosis and nucleated red cells are seen in the peripheral blood.

Therapy with radiation or chemotherapeutic drugs has proved unsatisfactory. The course of the disease is variable with a median survival of 5 yr.

Also called *myelosclerosis* with myeloid metaplasia. See also *myeloproliferative syndrome.*

myelogenous (mi″ĕ-loj′ĕ-nus) [*myelo-* + Gr. *gennan* to produce] 1. produced in the bone marrow.

2. pertaining to cells of the granulocytic series.

myelogenous leukemia see *acute myelogenous l.* and *chronic myelogenous l.* under *leukemia.*

myelography (mi′ĕ-log′rah-fe) [*myelo-* + Gr. *graphein* to write] the radiographic examination of the spinal cord after the introduction of a contrast medium into the subarachnoid space by spinal puncture. The patient is then tilted until the medium flows into the region of interest.

gas m., myelography that employs air or oxygen as the contrast medium.

opaque m., myelography that employs iodophendylate or a water-soluble contrast medium.

radionuclide m., a procedure for imaging the subarachnoid space surrounding the spinal cord. It is rarely used, as the necessary information is better acquired by use of radiographic contrast media. The technique is the same as that of radionuclide cisternography.

myeloid (mi′ĕ-loid) [*myelo-* + Gr. *eidos* form] 1. pertaining to, derived from, or resembling bone marrow, particularly the myelocytic (granulocytic) series of cells.

2. pertaining to the spinal cord.

3. having the appearance of myelocytic cells but not derived from bone marrow.

myeloid depression see *bone marrow depression.*

myeloid/erythroid ratio the ratio of myeloid to erythroid cells, determined from an examination of bone marrow films. Approximately 300–500 nucleated cells are counted to determine the ratio, which in conjunction with a bone marrow differential and bone marrow biopsy, provides an accurate evaluation of the state of the bone marrow. Normal values have a range of 4:1–2:1; abnormal values are seen whenever a hematopoietic dyscrasia is present, including conditions of leukemias and anemias.

myeloid metaplasia in its primary form, a myeloproliferative disorder characterized by extramedullary hematopoiesis in the liver and spleen, with fibrosis of the marrow. The condition is self-perpetuating and thus resembles a neoplastic disease. Clinical manifestations include hepatosplenomegaly and anemia. The reticulocyte count is increased, with marked anisocytosis reflecting dyspoiesis or hemolysis, and white cell and platelet counts are commonly increased. In peripheral blood smears, a leukoerythroblastic blood picture may be seen, with immature forms of the granulocytic series, including myeloblasts and progranulocytes, as well as nucleated red blood cells. Myeloid metaplasia may be secondary to severe hemolytic anemias, leukemia, and metastatic neoplasms, infections, or poisonings involving the bone marrow.

Bone marrow aspirates are difficult to obtain, but closed needle or open surgical biopsy may demonstrate panhyperplasia with increased reticulin fibers, or severe myelofibrosis and osteosclerosis. Megakaryocytes are usually numerous. Other laboratory findings include increased serum alkaline phosphatase, normal or increased leukocyte alkaline phosphatase activity, and raised serum uric acid levels. The Philadelphia chromosome present in chronic granulocytic leukemia is absent.

The average survival is about 5 yr. In 20 percent of patients, this disorder progresses to an acute leukemic state. Therapy has thus far been ineffective.

See also *myelofibrosis.*

myeloid tissue the tissue (e.g., bone marrow) in

which hematopoiesis occurs; see under *bone marrow.*

myelolipoma (mi″ĕ-lo-lĭ-po′mah) a rare, benign neoplasm of the adrenal cortex composed of fat and bone marrow cells.

myelomalacia (mi″ĕ-lo-mah-la′she-ah) [*myelo-* + Gr. *malakia* softening] softening of the spinal cord secondary to spinal cord infarction.

myeloma protein the M component (monoclonal immunoglobulin) secreted by the neoplastic plasma cells of multiple myeloma; see *M component.*

myelomatosis (mi″ĕ-lo-mah-to′sis) see *multiple myeloma.*

myelomeningitis (mi″ĕ-lo-men″in-ji′tis) [*myelo-* + *meningitis*] inflammation of the spinal cord and its meninges. See also *meningitis* and *myelitis.*

myelomeningocele (mi″ĕ-lo-me-ning′go-sēl) [*myelo-* + *meningocele*] protrusion of the spinal cord and its meninges through a defect in the vertebral column. Neurologic deficits result from this condition, and hydrocephalus is commonly associated.

myelopathy (mi″ĕ-lop′ah-the) [*myelo-* + Gr. *pathos* disease] a general term for a functional disturbance and/or pathologic change in the spinal cord. Myelopathies can be caused by cervical spondylosis, infections, trauma, compression or infiltration by tumors, ischemia, metabolic disorders, and developmental anomalies.

myeloperoxidase (mi″ĕ-lo-per-ok′sĭ-dās) a hemoprotein having peroxidase activity that occurs in lysosomal granules.

myeloperoxidase deficiency a rare condition characterized by the lack of leukocyte myeloperoxidase, which is necessary for the normal intracellular killing of certain organisms, especially *Candida* species. The destruction of intracellular organisms is delayed but may reach normal levels with time. The leukocytes of affected individuals are normal in every other way. Such persons are highly susceptible to contracting candidal and staphylococcal infections.

Diagnosis can be established using a peroxidase stain of the peripheral blood cells. Chemiluminescence is abnormal. There is no specific treatment for myeloperoxidase deficiency other than antibiotic therapy for infections.

myeloperoxidase system a proposed mechanism by which polymorphonuclear leukocytes (PMNs) inactivate bacteria and viruses. The system involves the enzyme myeloperoxidase, which is present in the azurophilic granules of PMNs, hydrogen peroxide, and a halide (e.g., chloride). It has been demonstrated in vitro that the interaction of these components involves powerful antimicrobial activity. The mechanism of this activity has not been established but may involve the lethal halogenation of the microbe, generation of toxic oxygen intermediates (e.g., superoxide anion, hydroxyl radicals, or singlet oxygen), or the formation of aldehydes on the surface of bacterial membranes.

myelophthisic (mi″ĕ-lof-thiz′ik) characterized by myelopthisis.

myelophthisis (mi″ĕ-lof′thĭ-sis) [*myelo-* + Gr. *phthisis* wasting] infiltration of the bone marrow by abnormal cells, most often due to lymphoreticular malignancies, metastatic carcinoma, or myelofibrosis, which reduces effective hematopoiesis and disrupts the bone marrow–blood barrier, allowing the release of immature cells into the peripheral blood. Although myelophthisis is usually a feature of neoplastic disease, marrow replacement can be a manifestation of a variety of conditions, including granulomatous disorders and lipid storage diseases.

The signs and symptoms depend on the underlying disorder; however, lymph node enlargement, splenomegaly, hepatomegaly, neutropenia, bone pain, anemia (with marked anisocytosis and poikilocytosis), bleeding due to thrombocythemia, and hypercalcemia are common findings. Diagnosis is made by needle biopsy, which may reveal total or partial replacement of the marrow by neoplastic cells.

myelopoiesis (mi″ĕ-lo-poi-e′sis) [*myelo-* + Gr. *poiein* to arise] the formation of the bone marrow or blood cell precursors.

extramedullary m., formation of myeloid tissue outside the red marrow. Also called ectopic myelopoiesis. See also *myeloid metaplasia.*

myeloproliferative (mi″ĕ-lo-pro-lif″er-a′tiv) pertaining to or characterized by the medullary and/or extramedullary proliferation of bone marrow constituents.

myeloproliferative disorder a general term applied to a group of usually neoplastic diseases, which may be related histogenetically by a common multipotential stem cell, and which are characterized at varying times and in varying degrees by the medullary and extramedullary proliferation of one or more lines of bone marrow constituents, including erythroblasts, granulocytes, megakaryocytes, and fibroblasts. Examples include acute and chronic granulocytic leukemia, acute and chronic myelomonocytic leukemia, polycythemia vera, myelofibrosis, myeloid metaplasia, essential thrombocythemia, and erythroleukemia (Di Guglielmo syndrome).

There is a tendency for the slowly progressive, relatively benign form to evolve into a rapidly progressive form; e.g., chronic granulocytic leukemia may evolve to acute granulocytic leukemia. An interrelationship with the lymphoproliferative disorders does exist. Also called myeloproliferative syndrome. See also *lymphoproliferative disorders.*

myeloradiculitis (mi″ĕ-lo-rah-dik″u-li′tis) [*myelo-* + L. *radiculus* rootlet + *-itis*] an inflammation of both the spinal cord and the nerve roots.

myelorrhagia (mi″ĕ-lo-ra′je-ah) [*myelo-* + Gr. *rhēgnynai* to burst forth] a hemorrhage into the spinal cord.

myelosarcoma (mi″ĕ-lo-sar-ko′mah) a tumor of blood-forming cells, e.g., granulocytic leukemia, that presents in tissues and simulates a sarcoma. See also *chloroma.*

myeloschisis (mi″ĕ-los′kĭ-sis) [*myelo-* + Gr. *schisis* cleft] a developmental anomaly characterized by a cleft spinal cord, due to failure of the neural folds to close to form a complete neural tube; spina bifida inevitably ensues.

myelosclerosis (mi″ĕ-lo-sklĕ-ro′sis) see *myelofibrosis.*

myelosuppression (mi″ĕ-lo-soo-presh′un) the inhibition of hematopoiesis in the myeloid tissue.

myenteric (mi″en-ter′ik) pertaining to the myenteron.

myenteric plexus see *myenteric p.* under *plexus.*

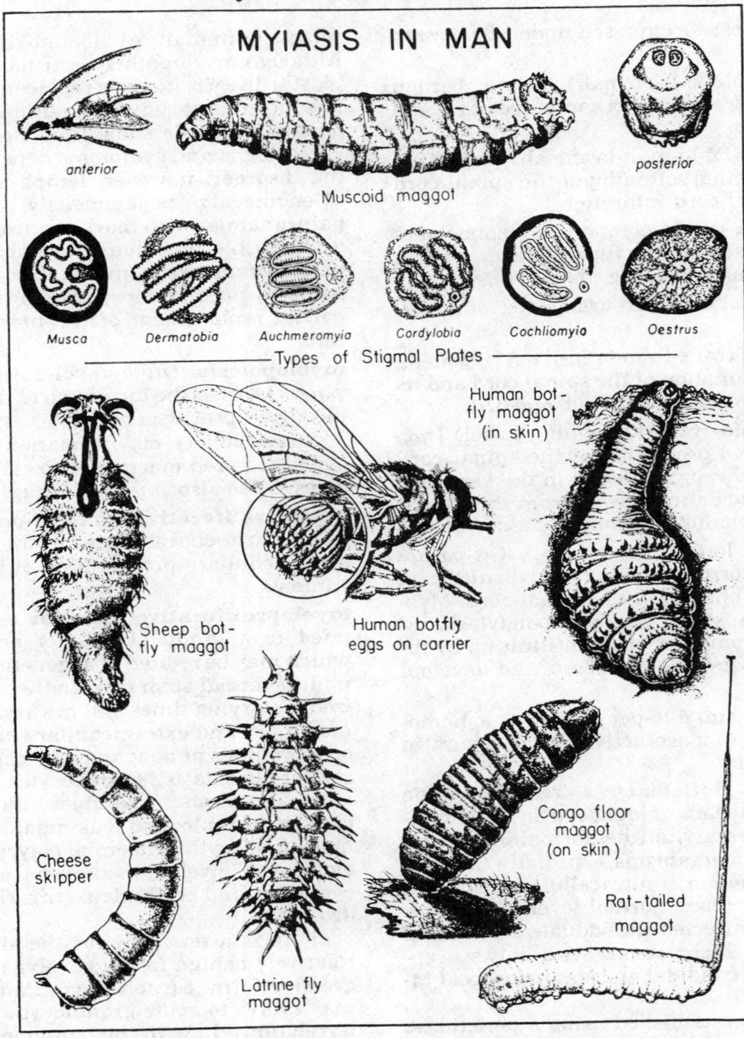

Myiasis, Figure 1. Dipterous larvae that cause myiasis in humans. (Courtesy of Centers for Disease Control, Public Health Service, U.S. Department of Health and Human Services, Atlanta, Georgia.)

myenteron (mi-en′ter-on) [*my-* + Gr. *enteron* intestine] the muscular coat of the intestine.

myiasis (mi′yah-sis) [Gr. *myia* fly + *-iasis*] a condition caused by infestation of the body by dipterous larvae (maggots). Several families of flies are involved and cause a variety of symptoms, depending on the type of larvae and the area affected. Infestation is generally classified according to the portion of the body affected, including cutaneous, facial, gastric, genitourinary, intestinal, and nasal myiasis. Also called *myasis* and *myiosis.* See also the accompanying illustrations.

cutaneous m., infestation of the skin by dipterous larvae, which invade unbroken skin or exposed areas of skin. Clinical symptoms include furuncular swelling, pruritus, and swollen skin lesions. When the larvae burrow in the skin in such a way that the progress may be followed as they advance, the term "creeping myiasis" is applied. Most larvae are removed surgically. The commonly found causative genera are *Auchmeromyia, Calliphora, Chrysomyia, Cordylobia, Dermatobia, Gasterophilus, Hypoderma,* and *Wohlfahrtia.*

facial m., the infestation of the face, most often the eyes, by dipterous larvae, resulting in inflammation of the conjunctiva or lacrimal duct. Clinical symptoms involve irritation, pain, congestion, and sometimes optic atrophy. Most larvae are removed aseptically. Flies of the genera *Hypoderma, Rhinoestrus, Oestrus,* and *Cuterebra* are most often incriminated.

genitourinary m., the accidental infestation of the urinary tract, including the bladder and genital passages of females, with dipterous larvae. Infestation is acquired by the larvae migrating from the intestinal tract or by flies depositing either eggs or larvae on the genital aperture, especially in females. Clinical symptoms may include obstruction, dysuria, hematuria, pyuria, or strangury. The larvae either pass spontaneously or are removed with the aid of a cystoscope. Some of the genera of flies thought to cause genitourinary myiasis include *Musca, Fannia, Psychoda, Muscina, Sarcophaga,* and *Calliphora.*

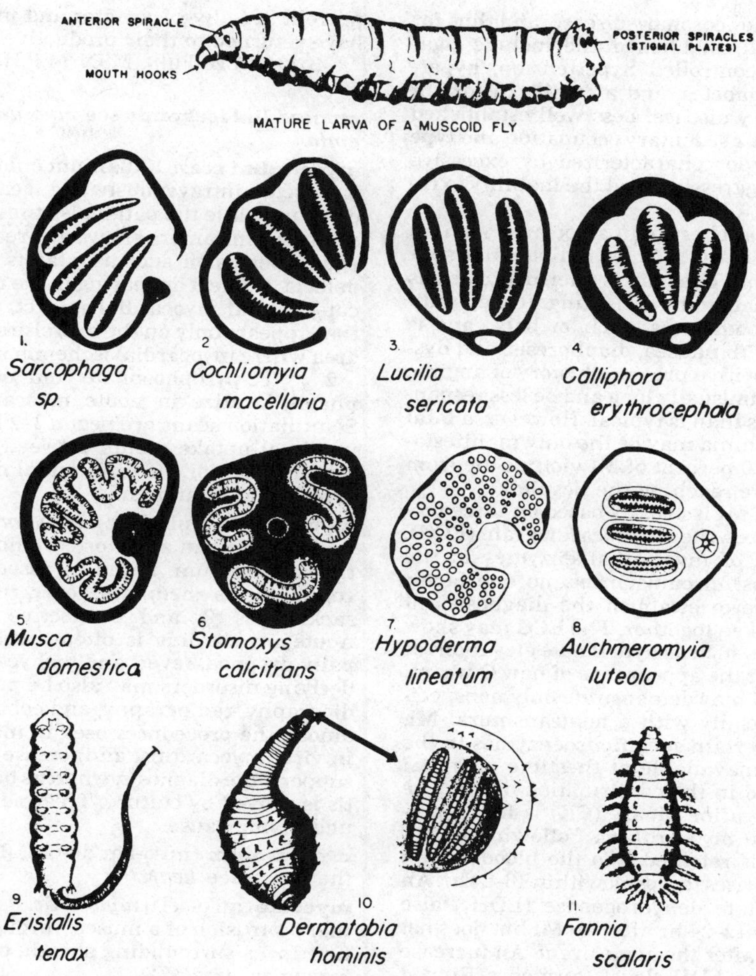

Myiasis, Figure 2. Key characters of myiasis-producing fly larvae. (Courtesy of Centers for Disease Control, Public Health Service, U.S. Department of Health and Human Services, Atlanta, Georgia.)

intestinal m., the presence of dipterous larvae in the stomach. The larvae enter the human host via ingestion of contaminated food. The presence of large numbers of larvae may provoke nausea, sharp pain, vertigo, and sometimes violent vomiting. When such vomiting results in expulsion of some of the larvae, a diagnosis can be made on the contents. Flies of the genera *Fannia, Musca, Calliphora,* and *Drosophila* are most often incriminated.

nasal m., the most common infection of dipterous larvae. The flies are attracted by an open wound or a discharge, and deposit their eggs on the skin nearby. The larvae enter the wound, causing local swelling. Most often the patient complains of intense pain and a "crawling" sensation. The larvae are removed by irrigation. Flies of the genera *Oestrus* and *Cochliomyia* are the most common cause of nasal myiasis.

myiosis (mi-yo′sis) see *myiasis.*

Mylar tradename for polyester plastic film.

myoblastoma (mi″o-blas-to′mah) [*myo-* + Gr. *blastos* germ + *-oma*] see *granular cell tumor.*

myocardi/o (mi″o-kar′de-o) [*myo-* + Gr. *kardia* heart] a word element used in combining form to denote heart muscle, e.g., myocarditis.

myocardial (mi″o-kar′de-al) pertaining to the muscular tissue of the heart.

myocardial infarction (MI) heart attack; the death of myocardial tissue that results from sudden, prolonged ischemia. At the present time, coronary heart disease is the most common cause of death in the United States. An estimated 1.25 million heart attacks occur annually, resulting in well over half a million deaths.

Nearly all MIs are a result of atherosclerosis of the coronary arteries (coronary artery disease). Far less common causes include coronary artery spasm (with or without accompanying atherosclerosis) or coronary embolism. Most MIs involve thrombosis at the site of an atheromatous plaque in a coronary artery, which cuts off an already diminished blood supply to the affected myocardium. Infarction usually results from simultaneous disease in two or more of the main coronary arteries or their major branches.

The risk factors for coronary disease, and thus for MI, have been well established and include cigarette smoking, uncontrolled hypertension, hypercholesterolemia, diabetes, and a family history of premature coronary disease. Less well established risk factors include a sedentary occupation and type A behavior (behavior characterized by excessive competitiveness, aggression, and the inability to relax).

Severe or unusual chest pain associated with an MI commonly causes the affected individual to seek emergency attention. The pain is often described as crushing, substernal, and unrelenting. It may radiate to the left or both arms, neck, or back, and is often associated with nausea, diaphoresis, and dyspnea. In someone with a previous history of angina, the pain may last unusually long and be less responsive to medications than is typical. However, a fatal ventricular arrhythmia may be the only manifestation. As many as 20 percent of MI victims die from arrhythmias before reaching the hospital.

The diagnosis of MI is usually based on three factors: clinical features, the electrocardiogram (ECG), and the presence of myocardial enzymes in the serum. Under most circumstances, no one factor can be used alone to establish the diagnosis; all three should be taken together. The ECG may show diagnostic changes such as hyperacute elevations of the ST segments or the appearance of new Q waves. However, the ECG may demonstrate only nonspecific changes, especially with a nontransmural MI. The presence of certain specific isoenzymes in the blood, although unavailable at the time of initial diagnosis, may aid in the confirmation of MI. The MB fraction of creatine kinase (CK) is found predominantly in the myocardium. Following an infarction, CK-MB is released into the blood within several hours and rises to a peak within 18–24 hr. An isoenzyme of lactate dehydrogenase (LDH_1) also rises in the serum 12–24 hr after an MI but does not peak for 48–72 hr after the acute event. An increase in LDH_1 above the LDH_2 level (termed a flipped LDH_1/LDH_2 ratio) is another diagnostic sign of an MI. Concentrations of the enzyme aspartate aminotransferase (AST) are also elevated 4–6 hr after an MI and peak in 24–36 hr. Rarely, additional diagnostic assistance such as radionuclide imaging is required.

Treatment is aimed at minimizing infarct size and preventing and treating complications. Pain is treated with nitrates and narcotics such as morphine. The patient is placed in a quiet environment and frequently sedated. The period of greatest danger is the first 24 hr following an MI, when ventricular arrhythmias are most common. These are usually treated successfully with antiarrhythmic drugs or electrocardioversion. Other complications include heart block, which may require a pacemaker, and heart failure, which signifies loss of a large portion of muscle. Newer therapies, such as administration of beta-adrenergic blockers, intracoronary infusions of streptokinase, and emergency coronary artery bypass grafting, are all being researched as ways to limit infarct size.

Arrhythmias were once the most common cause of death, but now result in a mortality rate of less than 10 percent of those admitted to a coronary care unit. Prognosis is clearly related to infarct size, but generally the early mortality is 15–30 percent in the first 4 wk. Of those who survive the first month, 88 percent are alive 1 yr later and many, if not most, have returned to their productive endeavors.

STEPHAN D. FIHN, M.D., M.P.H.

myocardial ischemia see *myocardial i.* under *ischemia.*

myocardial scan 1. thallium chloride tl 201 (^{201}Tl) is injected intravenously and localizes in the myocardium while the patient is at rest or exercising. A scintillation camera shows up areas that have inadequate perfusion, such as infarcts or lesions, as cold defects. A defect appearing in the resting study indicates an old myocardial infarct, whereas a defect that appears only on the exercise study indicates an area where myocardial ischemia is caused by stress.

2. ^{99m}Tc-pyrophosphate and other ^{99m}Tc phosphates localize in acute myocardial infarctions. Scintillation scans are begun 1–2 hr after injection; maximal uptake occurs between 2 and 6 da. This scan is used for the differential diagnosis of acute myocardial infarction.

myocarditis (mi″o-kar-di′tis) [*myo-* + Gr. *kardia* heart + *-itis*] an acute or chronic inflammation of the myocardium, found in association with such conditions as rheumatic fever, infection with coxsackievirus B, and connective tissue disorders. Acute myocarditis is often associated with chest pain, dyspnea, fever, and tachycardia; signs of underlying disorders may also be present. Electrocardiography, radiography, and echocardiography are among the procedures used in making a diagnosis; in viral myocarditis, an increase in antibody titers supports the diagnosis, whereas bacterial myocarditis is proved by culture. Treatment depends on the underlying cause.

myocardium (mi″o-kar′de-um) [NA], the muscle of the heart; see *heart.*

myocele (mi′o-sēl) [*myo-* + Gr. *kēlē* hernia] the hernial protrusion of a muscle through a defect or rupture in its surrounding sheath, often following injury or trauma.

myoclonic (mi″o-klon′ik) relating to or marked by myoclonus.

myoclonus (mi″o-klo′nus) [*myo-* + Gr. *klonos* turmoil] a sudden, involuntary, brief, nonrhythmic, shocklike contraction of a muscle or group of muscles. Myoclonus may be a normal reaction, as in the jerk of a limb as one falls asleep or in a startle reaction, or it may be a manifestation of convulsive disorder. It may occur in association with a progressive dementia, with certain inherited or acquired metabolic disorders, with severe anoxic encephalopathy, and in certain other neurologic disorders. If treatment is required, diazepam, clonazepam, or valproic acid may be helpful. See also *epilepsy.*

myocyte (mi′o-sīt) [*myo-* + Gr. *kytos* hollow vessel] 1. a muscle cell.

2. a type of cell found in the innermost layer of myonemes in the ectoplasm of certain protozoa of the order Gregarinida.

myoepithelial cell (mi″o-ep″ĭ-the′le-al) a modified smooth muscle cell located between the epithelial cells of exocrine acini and intercalated ducts and their basal lamina. The cell resembles a starfish in shape, with radiating arms of cytoplasm that encircle the acinus or duct and interweave to produce a meshwork—hence the synonym of basket cell. Slender bundles of smooth muscle myofilaments in the cell body and processes contract to express secretion from the acinus and duct. Contraction is stimulated by a transmitter substance that diffuses from axons adjacent to the basal lamina. See also *basket cell.*

myoepithelioma (mi″o-ep″ĭ-the″le-o′mah) a neoplasm composed of myoepithelial cells. These cells are a common component of tumors of the breast and salivary glands, but a pure myoepithelial neoplasm is rare.

myoepithelium (mi″o-ep″ĭ-the′le-um) tissue made up of myoepithelial cells.

myofibril (mi″o-fi′bril) a bundle of myofilaments within a muscle fiber; see under *muscle.*

myofibroblast (mi-o-fi′bro-blast) [*myo-* + L. *fibra* fiber + Gr. *blastos* germ] a fibroblast that contains smooth muscle myofilaments. The filaments generally are confined to slender bundles in the peripheral cytoplasm. Anchoring filaments connect the outer surface of the cell to surrounding collagen, providing a fulcrum for contraction. Myofibroblasts are responsible for the contraction of granulation and scar tissue, and are common in nonneoplastic fibroblastic proliferations such as nodular fasciitis and in the stromal proliferation associated with some infiltrating carcinomas. They may also be found in well-differentiated fibrosarcomas and in cells of the fibromatoses.

myofibrosis (mi″o-fi-bro′sis) [*myo-* + L. *fibra* fiber + *-osis*] the replacement of muscle tissue with fibrous tissue, often in response to trauma and injury.

myofibrositis (mi″o-fi″bro-si′tis) [*myo-* + L. *fibra* fiber + *-osis* + *-itis*] the inflammation of the perimysium, the sheath of collagen fibers that holds groups of muscle fibers together, often in response to infection or trauma.

myofilament (mi″o-fil′ah-ment) [*myo-* + L. *filamentum,* from *filum* thread] a threadlike aggregate of contractile protein. The myofibrils of striated muscle fibers are composed of oriented bundles of myofilaments of actin or myosin. See also *muscle.*

myoglobin (mi″o-glo′bin) a monomeric heme-containing protein that transports oxygen in mammalian muscles. Each molecule (M.W. 17,000) is composed of one heme group and one globin apoprotein structurally similar to the monomers of hemoglobin, and binds one molecule of oxygen. The oxygen dissociation curve exhibits no cooperativity; it is hyperbolic, not sigmoidal like that of hemoglobin. Myoglobin transports oxygen in the cytosol, bringing it from the cell membrane to the mitochondria. This transport by a carrier molecule is called facilitated diffusion.

Myoglobin is released into the blood and excreted in the urine when there is injury to skeletal muscle, as with a crushing injury or with extreme physical exercise. Differentiation of myoglobin from hemoglobin may be performed by electrophoresis, specific antisera, and by nature of differences in solubility, e.g., in ammonium sulfate solutions.

myoglobinemia (mi″o-glo″bin-e′me-ah) the presence of myoglobin in the blood.

myoglobin identification methods tests to distinguish myoglobin from hemoglobin in urine specimens after screening tests such as the *o*-toluidine test for occult blood have indicated the presence of a heme protein. Myoglobin and hemoglobin can be differentiated on the basis of their solubilities, absorption spectra, molecular size, or electrophoretic mobility. Adding 2.8 g of ammonium sulfate to 5 ml of urine produces an 80 percent saturated solution, which precipitates hemoglobin but no myoglobin. A positive *o*-toluidine test on the supernatant indicates myoglobin. The other tests use the clear supernatant from a centrifuged specimen. The absorbance of an alkalinized supernatant is measured at 600 and 580 nm. An A_{600}/A_{580} ratio greater than 0.8 indicates myoglobin. Hemoglobin will not pass through a Millipore filter with a pore diameter of 8–12 nm. A positive *o*-toluidine test on the ultrafiltrate indicates myoglobin. Myoglobin moves more rapidly in an electrophoretic field than does hemoglobin.

myoglobinuria (mi″o-glo″bin-ūr′e-ah) the presence of myoglobin in the urine, a condition that may occur when there is injury to skeletal or cardiac muscle. Myoglobinuria occurs with crush injuries and may occur with vigorous physical exercise.

***myo*-inositol** (mi″o-in-os′ĭ-tol) one of nine stereoisomeric forms of the carbocyclic hexitols (hexahydroxy-cyclohexanes) belonging to a class of compounds called cyclitols. *Myo*-inositol is the most important cyclitol and is widely distributed in microorganisms, higher plants, and animals. See also *cyclitol.*

myokinase (mi″o-ki′nās) [*myo-* + Gr. *kinein* to move + *-ase*] see *adenylate kinase.*

myokymia (mi″o-kim′e-ah) [*myo-* + Gr. *kyma* wave] the involuntary, repetitive contraction of muscle fibers that appears on the surface as a series of wormlike movements that ripple across the skin. This spontaneous quivering of muscle fibers can occur independently in different segments of the same muscle and may involve more than one muscle.

Electromyographic recordings reveal that the contractions are associated with individual potentials with the same parameters as those of normal motor units. These potentials may occur as a continuous, rhythmic discharge of single potentials or as iterative multiplets composed of 2–200 individual spikes.

myolipoma (mi″o-lĭ-po′mah) [*myo-* + Gr. *lipos* fat + *-oma*] a tumor composed of muscle and fat cells.

myolysis (mi-ol′ĭ-sis) [*myo-* + Gr. *lysis* dissolution] see *rhabdomyolysis.*

myoma (mi-o′mah), pl. *myomas, myomata* [*myo-* + *-oma*] a general term for a neoplasm composed of muscle cells. See also *leiomyoma* and *rhabdomyoma.*

myomalacia (mi″o-mah-la′she-ah) [*myo-* + Gr. *malakia* softening] a general term used to describe the pathologic softening of a muscle.

myometritis (mi″o-mĕ-tri′tis) [*myo-* + Gr. *mētra* uterus + *itis*] an inflammation of the myometrium, which may follow febrile amnionitis during labor. Fever, leukocytosis, and tachycardia may be present.

myometrium (mi-o-me′tre-um) [*myo-* + Gr. *mētra* uterus] the smooth muscle that forms the main mass of the uterus.

myonecrosis (mi″o-nĕ-kro′sis) [*myo-* + Gr. *nekrōsis* deadness] the necrosis or death of muscles or individual muscle fibers, often in response to trauma or to degenerative or infectious diseases such as clostridial gas gangrene. See also *clostridial m.* under *myositis* and *gas g.* under *gangrene.*

myoneme (mi'o-nēm) [*myo-* + Gr. *nēma* thread] a contractile fibril found in some protozoa.

myoneural junction (mi"o-nu'ral) see *neuromuscular junction.*

myopathy (mi-op'ah-the) [*myo-* muscle + Gr. *pathos* suffering, disease] a general term used to denote the primary and secondary disorders of muscles. A variety of external factors (e.g., metabolic or endocrine imbalances, vascular injury, or impairment in the trophic influences of nerves) may lead to the changes in the muscle fibers and surrounding connective tissue that are characteristic of a particular myopathy. Myopathies may also be inherited disorders.

The changes in muscle tissue that occur in specific myopathies either may take the form of degeneration, atrophy without accompanying degenerative changes, faulty maturation, or splitting and enlargement of the fibers, or may involve an impairment in excitability of the cell membrane.

Electromyographic examination of the recruitment pattern and configuration of motor unit potentials (MUPs) can be of use in determining whether a particular disorder is of myopathic origin. An increase in the incidence of polyphasic, short-duration, low-amplitude MUPs is commonly seen with myopathy but cannot be considered conclusive proof of the myopathic origin of a disorder.

Included under the classification of myopathy are the muscular dystrophies, congenital myopathies, and mitochondrial myopathies; glycogen and lipid storage diseases; periodic paralyses; myotonic disorders; polymyositis/dermatomyositis complex; and disorders associated with endocrine diseases. For more information, see under the individual diseases.

alcoholic m., a muscle weakness, particularly affecting the legs, that occurs in alcoholics. There is usually myoglobinuria and elevated serum concentrations of creatine kinase and aldolase. A cardiomyopathy and/or polyneuropathy may also occur in persons with chronic alcoholism. Muscle biopsies in those with alcoholic myopathy usually show only myofiber necrosis. See also *alcoholic c.* under *cardiomyopathy* and *alcoholic polyneuropathy* under *neuropathy.*

congenital m., a group of inherited genetic diseases of muscle that are often distinctive morphologically. They appear in infants, and lead to hypotonia and muscle weakness that generally are not progressive. The different types of congenital myopathy are classified morphologically on biopsy material and include central core disease; nemaline, centronuclear, and mitochondrial myopathies; and congenital fiber-type disproportion. There is no specific treatment.

corticosteroid m., a myopathy resulting from the administration of adrenal corticosteroids. There may be proximal muscle weakness and wasting. Muscle biopsy reveals selective type II fiber atrophy. At the ultrastructural level, large, abnormal mitochondria and subsarcolemmal accumulations of glycogen can be seen. Electromyograms show small but abundant action potentials. Serum creatine kinase and aldolase concentrations are elevated and there may be creatinuria. The condition is reversible when administration of the drug is tapered off or discontinued.

endocrine m., a group of neuromuscular disorders, usually characterized by proximal muscle weakness, associated with endocrine disease; they include thyrotoxicosis, hypothyroidism, hyperparathyroidism, acromegaly, Cushing's syndrome, Addison's disease, and hyperaldosteronism. Complete recovery from the myopathy frequently occurs following adequate treatment of the underlying endocrine disease. See also *corticosteroid m.*

nemaline m., a congenital, nonprogressive, myofibrillar abnormality in which small, threadlike rods of material are scattered throughout the muscle fiber. Infantile hypotonia and generalized muscle weakness are usually present.

myophosphorylase (mi"o-fos-fōr'ĭ-lās) muscle phosphorylase; see *glycogen phosphorylase.*

myopia (mi-o'pe-ah) [Gr. *myein* to shut + *ōps* eye + *-ia*] the decreased ability of the eyes to bring distant objects into focus. In this condition, the globe of the eye has an abnormally long anterior-posterior diameter; i.e., its focal length is too short. Whereas in a normally shaped eye images at a wide range of distances are brought into focus onto the retina, in myopic eyes distant images are brought into focus in front of the retina and thus appear blurred. On very rare occasions this condition may predispose to retinal detachment and blindness.

myorrhexis (mi"o-rek'sis) [*myo-* + Gr. *rhēxis* rupture] the rupture of a muscle. It may be caused by a violent strain leading to an abnormal bulge upon contraction, with loss of contractile power and pain. Most commonly, the biceps muscle is affected.

myos/o (mi'o-so) [Gr. *myos* of muscle] a word element used in combining form to denote muscle, e.g., myositis.

myosarcoma (mi"o-sar-ko'mah) a general term used to describe a malignant tumor arising from or differentiating toward muscle cells.

myosin (mi'o-sin) a large protein of which the thick myofilaments of striated muscle are composed; M.W. 470,000. Myosin has enzymatic properties (ATPase activity), the free form catalyzing the hydrolysis of ATP to ADP and P_i. See also *muscle.*

myositis (mi"o-si'tis) [*myos-* + *-itis* inflammation] inflammation in voluntary muscle, producing weakness and often pain in the proximal muscles. Known causes include bacteria, fungi, parasites, viruses, physical agents (heat and cold), and trauma. Repair of the damage caused in myositis depends on the extent of involvement; often, regeneration is incomplete and atrophy with fibrosis will remain. Electromyography may be helpful, and serum concentration of creatine kinase as well as the erythrocyte sedimentation rate are usually elevated. Muscle biopsy is useful in establishing the diagnosis.

clostridial m., an intense and rapidly progressing infection of muscle by bacteria of the genus *Clostridium.* Beginning in devitalized tissue, especially in anaerobic pockets of wounds, the infection spreads by extension. The high biochemical activity of these clostridia results in extensive tissue necrosis with the production of foul odors, serosanguineous exudate, and gas bubbles in the subcutaneous tissues and muscles (crepitation). Potent exotoxins may be produced that cause systemic involvement including toxemia, intravascular hemolysis, and irreversible shock. Without appropriate therapy, death is the likely consequence. Cf. *gas g.* under *gangrene* and *myonecrosis.*

m. ossificans, a condition characterized by the deposit of a bony substance in muscles following myo-

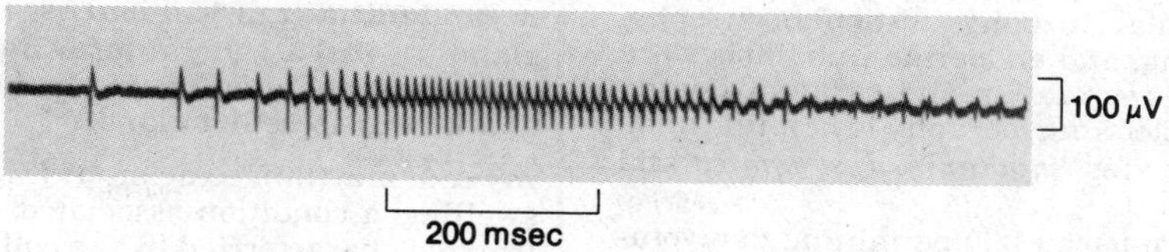

Myotonic discharge. A myotonic discharge evoked by electrode movement. (From Aminoff, M. J.: Electromyography in Clinical Practice. Menlo Park, CA, Addison-Wesley Publishing Co., 1978.)

sitis. Two types are recognized. One is a localized condition in a muscle that follows local trauma. A painful area develops, followed by fibrosis and deposition of bone. A visible bone mass appears on x-ray 4–7 wk after the initial damage. The other type is a progressive deposition of bone in muscles unrelated to trauma. It affects children and young adults, and is often accompanied by congenital anomalies. Initially, the radiographs are normal, but in 6–12 mo hard, calcific masses appear in a variety of muscles. Biochemical studies suggest that abnormal alkaline phosphatase activities may play an etiologic role in this disease.

proliferative m., a pseudosarcomatous lesion that forms a firm, scar-like nodule within skeletal muscle (a similar lesion in the subcutaneous tissue is termed proliferative fasciitis). The proliferating cells are plump with basophilic cytoplasm and prominent nucleoli; despite their resemblance to skeletal muscle, however, they are probably of myofibroblast origin. The lesion is benign and may represent a response to trauma. It is most common in adults, occurring in the shoulder region or thigh, and rarely is larger than 5 cm in diameter. Simple excision is the correct treatment.

myotome (mi′o-tōm) [*myo-* + Gr. *tomē* a cut] 1. in the developing embryo, the portion of a somite that is left after the emigration of the sclerotome mass to form a vertebra; the myotome thickens and differentiates into what will be muscle.

2. a group of muscles derived from a single embryonic myotome and innervated by a single segmental spinal nerve.

myotonia (mi″o-to′ne-ah) [*myo-* + Gr. *tonos* tension] a general term used to describe any disorder characterized by tonic muscle spasm provoked by percussion or voluntary muscle contraction, with delayed muscle relaxation.

m. congenita, an inherited disorder characterized by myotonia with difficulty in initiating movement and slowness of relaxation. The disorder typically presents at birth, and muscle spasm and hypertrophy are common. Myotonic discharges, which wax and wane in amplitude and frequency (and may be likened to a "dive bomber"), may be recorded on electromyography. Also called *Thomsen's disease.*

m. dystrophica, see *myotonic dystrophy.*

myotonic (mi″o-ton′ik) pertaining to or characterized by myotonia.

myotonic discharge the high-frequency (15–150 Hz) repetitive discharge of muscle action potentials that is evoked by insertion of a needle electrode, percussion, or voluntary contraction of a muscle. In order to be identified as myotonic discharge, the action potentials must both wax and wane in frequency and amplitude, and give rise to a characteristic "dive bomber" sound on the audio display of the electromyograph (see the accompanying illustration). This form of discharge is recorded from, but is not restricted to, muscle with the clinical signs of myotonia.

myotonic dystrophy a rare hereditary disease characterized by muscle weakness and myotonia. It may occur with variable severity at any age and often affects the face, jaw, foot, and hand muscles.

MYXOVIRUS. CHARACTERISTICS OF HUMAN MYXOVIRUSES

	Virion Diameter (nm)	Genome Size (daltons × 10^6)	Number of Gene Segments	Diameter of Ribonucleoprotein* (nm)	Nuclear Requirement for Replication
Orthomyxoviridae					
Influenza A & B	80–170	5	8	9	+
Influenza C	80–170	5	7 (?)	9	?
Paramyxoviridae					
Parainfluenza 1-4b	150–250	6	1	18	–
Mumps	150–250	6	1	18	–
Measles (Rubeola)	150–250	6	1	18	–
Respiratory syncytial virus	90–180	6	1	14	–

* Three size classes of ribonucleoprotein apparently exist, although their precise measurements vary with techniques of preparation.

From Braude, A. I.: Medical Microbiology and Infectious Disease. Philadelphia, W. B. Saunders Co., 1981, pp. 570–571.

Cataracts, muscular atrophy, testicular atrophy, premature balding, and endocrine imbalances are common. Mental retardation and cardiomyopathy may also occur. Electromyography is helpful in the diagnosis. Also called *myotonia dystrophica* and *Steinert's disease.*

myotubular (mi″o-too′bu-lar) pertaining to myotubules.

myriapod (mir′e-ah-pod) [Gr. *myrios* numberless + *podos* foot] a member of the superclass Myriapoda, which includes the centipedes and millipedes.

myring/o (mĭ-ring′go) [L. *myringa* drum membrane] a word element used in combining form to denote the eardrum, e.g., myringotomy.

myringitis (mir″in-ji′tis) [*myring-* + *-itis*] a general term used to describe an inflammation of the tympanic membrane, which is often due to viral, mycoplasmic, or bacterial infection.

bullous m., a form of middle ear inflammation due to viral, bacterial (particularly *Streptococcus pneumoniae*), or mycoplasmic infection. Serous or hemorrhagic blebs or bullae appear on the tympanic membrane and may spread to the adjacent wall of the acoustic meatus. Hearing loss and fever suggest bacterial infection.

myringomycosis (mĭ-ring″go-mi-ko′sis) [*myringo-* + Gr. *mykēs* fungus] fungal infection and disease of the tympanic membrane. See also *otomycosis.*

myristic acid (mĭ-ris′tik) *n*-tetradecanoic acid, $CH_3(CH_2)_{12}COOH$, a widely occurring saturated fatty acid, found in spermaceti, nutmeg butter, and other fats in the form of myristin.

myristica oil (mĭ-ris′tĭ-kah) [L.; Gr. *myrizein* to anoint] [NF], the volatile oil distilled with steam from the dried kernals of ripe seed of *Myristica fragrans,* used as a flavoring agent in pharmaceutic preparations. Also called *nutmeg oil.*

Myrmecia (mur-me′she-ah) [Gr. *myrmēx* ant] a genus of ants. *M. gulosa,* the bulldog ant, is found in tropical areas. It possesses a dangerous sting: the poisoning apparatus contains histamine, hyaluronidase, and a hemolytic factor.

myx/o (mik′so) [Gr. *myxa* mucus] a word element used in combining form to denote mucus, e.g., myxoma.

myxadenitis (mik″sad-ĕ-ni′tis) [*myx-* + Gr. *adēn* gland + *-itis*] a general term used to describe the inflammation, often caused by bacterial infection, of a mucus-secreting gland.

myxedema (mik″sĕ-de′mah) [*myx-* + Gr. *oidēma* swelling] a condition associated with hypothyroidism and characterized by the collection of hydrated mucopolysaccharides in the dermis and in other tissues of the body. Nonpitting peripheral edema, cardiomegaly, tongue and facial enlargement, and serous cavity effusions all result. Symptoms include lethargy, mental aberrations, dry skin, weak tendon reflexes, intestinal disorders, and menorrhagia.

Diagnosis is based on clinical signs and measurement of the serum levels of triiodothyronine (T_3) and thyroxine (T_4). Frequently, there also is hypercholesterolemia and increased serum levels of thyroid-stimulating hormone (TSH). Electrocardiographic alterations may be found. Treatment is accomplished by cautious restoration of thyroid hormone levels.

m. coma, a life-threatening, hypothermic, stuporous state accompanying advanced hypothyroidism.

m. heart, a cardiomyopathy associated with myxedema and hypothyroidism. This disorder is characterized grossly by a pale, flabby heart with marked right-side dilation. Microscopically, there is intercellular edema, degenerative alteration, and an increase in mucopolysaccharide ground substances between the myofibers.

m. madness, psychosis associated with advanced hypothyroidism.

pituitary m., myxedema and hypothyroidism due to the decreased secretion of thyroid-stimulating hormone (TSH) from the pituitary.

pretibial m., a symmetric, nonpitting, localized collection of hydrated mucopolysaccharides in the lower anterior legs. The skin over the deposits is edematous and shiny. It occurs most often with hyperthyroidism (Graves' disease).

myxochondroma (mik″so-kon-dro′mah) [*myxo-* + Gr. *chondros* cartiliage + *-oma*] a descriptive term for a chondroma that is at least partially composed of primitive mesenchymal tissue. See also *chondroma.*

MYXOVIRUS. (*Continued*)

Enzyme Activities					Cultivation of Primary Isolates		
RNA Polymerase	*Hemagglutinin*	*Neuraminidase*	*Hemolysin*	*Membrane Fusion*	*Embryonated Egg*	*Primary Human or Monkey Kidney*	*Continuous Cell Lines*
+	+	+	−	−	+	+	MDCK
+	+	−	−	−	+	−	MDCK
+	+	+	+	+	−	+	Some types only: MDCK, HeLa, HEp-2, WI-38
+	+	+	+	+	+	+	Vero, HeLa, LLC-MK2
+	+	+	+	+	+	+	HeLa, HEp-2, LLC-MK2
+	−	−	−	+	−	+	HEp-2, HeLa WI-38

myxofibroma (mik″so-fi-bro′mah) [*myxo-* + L. *fibra* fiber + *-oma*] see *m. of jaw* under *myxoma.*

myxofibrosarcoma (mik″so-fi″bro-sar-ko′mah) [*myxo-* + L. *fibra* fiber + Gr. *sarx* flesh + *-oma*] a malignant neoplasm of fibroblasts that has a predominant myxoid stroma.

myxoid (mik′soid) [*myxo-* + Gr. *eidos* form] a term applied to a tissue or neoplasm in which proteoglycans of the ground substance of connective tissue form a prominent component.

myxolipoma (mik″so-li-po′mah) [*myxo-* + Gr. *lipos* fat + *-oma*] a general term used to describe a neoplasm composed of cells of adipose origin that contain areas of myxomatous degeneration.

myxoma (mik-so′mah), pl. *myxomas, myxomata* [*myxo-* + *-oma*] an uncommon soft tissue neoplasm composed of mesenchyme-like cells loosely distributed in a myxoid stroma. Most myxomas occur in or near skeletal muscles; they are encapsulated and sometimes cystic. Myxomas are rarely malignant and thus must be distingushed from true myxoid sarcomas.

cardiac m., the most common type of primary heart tumor. It occurs most frequently in the left atrium and may contain calcium deposits that are visible on x-ray examination. Some lesions are merely organized thrombi. Diagnosis is based on the echocardiogram and selective angiocardiography. The lesion can obstruct blood flow.

m. of jaw, a myxoid neoplasm involving the jaw bones, composed of small stellate cells in an abundant myxoid stroma. On x-ray films it may form a distinctive "soap-bubble" appearance. It does not give rise to metastases but may infiltrate adjacent soft tissues, and recurrence is common. Most patients are young adults, and the maxilla is affected almost as frequently as the mandible. Odontogenic epithelial cells may be present, and the tumor is generally viewed as originating from the dental papilla. Some of the tumors are more fibrous (myxofibroma, odontogenic fibroma) then others.

myxosarcoma (mik″so-sar-ko′mah) [*myxo-* + Gr. *sarx* flesh + *-oma*] a sarcoma with myxoid stroma. The term is not a specific subclassification of a sarcoma and should be used only when more precise indication of the cell type is not possible. Also called myxoid sarcoma.

myxovirus (mik″so-vi′rus) a general name for a group of enveloped RNA viruses that contains two families: the orthomyxoviruses (influenza viruses) and the paramyxoviruses (the parainfluenza, measles, mumps, and respiratory syncytial virus). See also the accompanying table.

Myzomyia (mi″zo-mi′yah) [Gr. *myzan* to suck + *myia* fly] a subgenus of mosquitoes of the tribe Anophelini, several species of which are carriers of the malarial parasites.

Myzorhynchus (mi″zo-ring′kus) [Gr. *myzan* to suck + *rhynchos* snout] a subgenus of mosquitoes of the tribe Anophelini, many species of which are vectors of malaria.

N

N symbol for *asparagine;* neutron number; *newton;* the chemical element *nitrogen;* normal solution, the concentration of a solution expressed in equivalents/liter (use of this symbol is discouraged in the SI system); number of molecules; population size.

NR abbrev. See *Reynold's number.*

n symbol for index of refraction, *nano-, neutron,* number density of molecule (see under *mole fraction*), sample size.

ν the lower case form of the Greek letter *nu;* symbol for frequency, neutrino, number of degrees of freedom.

NA abbrev. See *Nomina Anatomica, numerical aperture.*

Na [L. *natrium*] symbol for the chemical element *sodium.*

NAACLS abbrev. See *National Accrediting Agency for Clinical Laboratory Sciences.*

nabothian cyst (nah-bo'the-an) [Martin *Naboth,* Leipzig anatomist, 1675–1721] see *nabothian c.* under *cyst.*

NAD⁺ abbrev. for the oxidized form of the redox coenzyme *nicotinamide adenine dinucleotide.*

NADH abbrev. for the reduced form of the redox coenzyme *nicotinamide adenine dinucleotide.*

NADH methemoglobin reductase see *cytochrome b_5 reductase.*

nadolol (na'do-lol) a beta-adrenergic blocking agent used for the treatment of hypertension. Like propranolol, it blocks both $beta_1$ and $beta_2$ receptors; it is not metabolized, however, and only one daily dose is required.

NADP⁺ abbrev. for the oxidized form of the redox coenzyme *nicotinamide adenine dinucleotide phosphate.*

NADPH abbrev. for the reduced form of the redox coenzyme *nicotinamide adenine dinucleotide phosphate.*

Naegeli leukemia (na'gĕ-lēz) [Otto *Naegeli,* Swiss hematologist, 1871–1937] an outmoded term infrequently used for an acute myelogenous leukemia. See *monomyelocytic l.* under *leukemia.*

Naegleria (na-gle'rĭ-ah) [F. P. O. *Nagler,* Australian bacteriologist, 20th century] a genus of ameboflagellates (amebas having both ameboid and flagellate phases in their life cycle) of the class Rhizopoda. The free-living soil ameba causes primary amebic meningitis. Infection is acquired by swimming in water contaminated with the amebas, which invade the nasopharynx and spread to the meninges.

Laboratory diagnosis requires identification of the organism (8–15 μ, possessing a blunt pseudopodia) in cerebrospinal fluid by light or phase microscopy, by tissue culture or culture on cell-free media, or by animal inoculation. See also *amebic n.* under *meningitis.*

nafcillin (naf-sil'in) a semisynthetic acid- and penicillinase-resistant penicillin, active as an antibiotic against gram-positive cocci and bacilli. Administered parenterally, it is used especially for severe infections by penicillin-resistant staphylococci. See also *antibacterial agents* and *penicillins.*

Nagler's reaction (nag'lerz) [F. P. O. *Nagler,* Australian bacteriologist, 20th century] an important test in the laboratory identification of *Clostridium perfringens.* The test culture is inoculated lightly to a plate of egg yolk agar, half of which has been spread with *C. perfringens* antitoxin. After overnight incubation, *C. perfringens* colonies on the control side are surrounded by precipitation due to the production of lecithinase; there is little or no precipitation on the antitoxin side. Three other species of *Clostridium* that are also Nagler-positive (*C. novi, C. septicum,* and *C. sordelli*) are rarely encountered in clinical specimens and are easily differentiated from *C. perfringens* by other means.

NaI(Tl) crystal abbrev. for thallium-activated sodium iodide crystal, used in gamma-ray detectors. See under *scintillation crystal.*

nail (nāl) [L. *unguis;* Gr. *onyx*] 1. the rectangular, horny, cutaneous plate attached proximally to the nail bed on the dorsal surface of the distal end of a finger or toe.

2. a rod of metal, bone, or other material used for fixation of the ends or fragments of fractured bones.

nail-patella syndrome (nāl pah-tel'ah) a hereditary disorder, transmitted as an autosomal dominant trait, that is characterized by multiple osseous abnormalities, flexion contractures of various joints, hypoplasia or absence of the nails, ocular abnormalities, and renal disease. X-ray examination may show absence or hypoplasia of the patella. Proteinuria is present in about half of those affected; microscopic hematuria and a defect in concentration of urine may also occur. About one-fifth of those with proteinuria slowly progress (over a period of 5–25 yr) to renal failure. No specific treatment is known. Also called hereditary onychoosteodysplasia.

nalbuphine hydrochloride (nal'bu-fēn) a synthetic narcotic agonist-antagonist chemically related to oxymorphone and naloxone. Used to treat severe pain, its analgesic effect is similar to that of morphine. Nalbuphine is less addictive than morphine, but physical and psychologic dependence can occur. Adverse effects include nausea, vomiting, sedation, and respiratory depression.

naled (na'led) a toxic organophosphate insecticide, dimethyl 1,2-dibromo-2,2-dichloroethyl phosphate. See also *organophosphate compounds.*

nalidixic acid (nal-ĭ-diks'ik) a synthetic chemotherapeutic agent, a synthetic derivative of 1,8-naphthyridine. It inhibits DNA synthesis, although the exact mechanism of inhibition has not been determined. Nalidixic acid has greater in vitro antibacterial activity against gram-negative rods than against gram-positive bacteria and is quite active against most Enterobacteriaceae. This drug concentrates primarily in the urinary tract and is therefore useful in the treatment of urinary tract infections. See also *antibacterial agents.*

nalorphine hydrochloride (nal'or-fēn, nal-or'fēn)

[USP], a narcotic agonist-antagonist used to treat respiratory depression due to narcotic overdosage; its action is by competitive inhibition of opiates. It may add to the respiratory depression produced by other drugs such as barbiturates. Nalorphine produces withdrawal symptoms when given to narcotic addicts. Adverse effects include anxiety and hallucinations.

naloxone hydrochloride (nal-oks'ōn) a pure narcotic antagonist derived from oxymorphone, lacking both agonist effects (respiratory depression, analgesia) and sympathomimetic effects (hallucinations). It is the drug of choice for treating respiratory depression produced by opiates, as well as synthetic narcotics such as propoxyphene or pentazocine. Naloxone produces withdrawal symptoms in narcotic addicts and also reverses narcotic analgesia. Abrupt reversal of narcotic effects may cause hypertension, tachycardia, or nausea. Naloxone is ineffective for treating overdoses of nonnarcotic drugs such as barbiturates.

NAME abbrev. See *National Association of Medical Examiners.*

NAND (from *NOT-AND*) the logical complement of the AND relations. The result is *false* only if all arguments are *true;* otherwise, the result is *true.* Cf. *AND.*

NAND gate an electronic circuit that produces the logical complement of the AND function: it is equivalent to an AND gate followed by an inverter. Its output is *false* only if all inputs are *true;* otherwise, the output is *true.* Also called NAND circuit.

nanism (na'nizm) [L. *nanus* dwarf] a general term used to describe a size that is markedly below normal; dwarfishness.

Nannizzia (nah-niz'ĭ-ah) a genus of fungi that represents the perfect (sexual) stage of *Microsporum.*

nano- (n) (nan'o) [Gr. *nanos* dwarf] a prefix attached to International System (S1) units of measurement to denote a unit that is one-billionth of the basic unit (10^{-9} unit).

nanocurie (nCi) (nan'o-ku″re) a unit of radioactivity equal to one-billionth of a curie (10^{-9} Ci).

nanofarad (nF) (nan'o-far″ad) a unit of electrical capacitance equal to one-billionth of a farad (10^{-9} F). Formerly called millimicrofarad (mμF).

nanogram (ng) (nan'o-gram) a unit of mass equal to one-billionth of a gram (10^{-9} g, 10^{-12} kg).

nanoliter (nl) (nan'o-le″ter) a unit of volume equal to one-billionth of a liter (10^{-9} l, 10^{-12} m^3, 10^{-3} mm^3).

nanometer (nm) (nan'o-me″ter) a unit of length equal to one-billionth of a meter (10^{-9} m), equivalent to 10 angstroms.

nanomole (nmol) (nan'o-mōl) a unit of amount of substance equal to one-billionth of a mole (10^{-9} mol).

nanosecond (ns, nsec) (na'no-sek″ond) a unit of time equal to one-billionth of a second (10^{-9} sec).

naphazoline hydrochloride (naf-az'o-lēn) [USP], an imidazoline derivative, a sympathomimetic drug, used to produce nasal decongestion due to vasoconstriction. Trademark, Privine.

naphtha (naf'thah) [L., from Gr., of Iranian origin] a term applied to distillation fractions from petroleum (petroleum naphtha) or from coal tar (coal-tar naphtha), which are used as solvents. Both are similar to petroleum ethers and ligroins.

naphthalene (naf'thah-lēn, nap'thah-lēn) [L. *naphthalinum*] a white crystalline solid, an aromatic hydrocarbon composed of two fused benzene rings, $C_{10}H_8$; M.W. 128.16. Naphthalene is a volatile, combustible substance with the odor of moth balls. It is used as a chemical intermediate in the dye and plastics industries and was formerly employed as a moth repellent and insecticide.

Ingestion, inhalation, or skin absorption of naphthalene can produce poisoning, with symptoms of eye irritation, headache, nausea, vomiting, hematuria, and fever. Severe poisoning can produce convulsions, coma, cataracts, hemolytic anemia, and liver damage.

naphthol (naf'thol) either of the two isomeric hydroxynaphthalenes, $C_{10}H_7OH$, 1-naphthol (α-naphthol) and 2-naphthol (β-naphthol); M.W. 144.16. Both are white crystalline solids, which darken slowly on exposure to air and light and which have a phenol-like odor. Both are weakly soluble in water but soluble in organic solvents and alkali hydroxides. They are used as intermediates in the synthesis of many important organic compounds, including pharmaceuticals. Both are toxic; ingestion of moderate amounts may lead to abdominal pain, nephritis, circulatory collapse, and convulsions. Skin contact causes skin peeling and pigmentation.

α-naphthol method see *Baker's hypochlorite α-naphthol method.*

α-naphthylthiourea (ANTU) (naf″thil-thi″o-u-re'ah) a gray, odorless powder, $C_{10}H_7NHCSNH_2$, used as a rat poison; M.W. 202.27. It produces massive pulmonary edema and pulmonary effusion in some species of rats, particularly *Rattus norvegicus,* and some other animals such as dogs, but is relatively nontoxic to humans.

Napier formol-gel test (na'pe-er) [Lionel Everard *Napier,* physician in India, b. 1888] a nonspecific precipitin test for detecting the increased serum globulin in kala-azar (visceral leishmaniasis). Formaldehyde is added to the patient's serum and mixed well. The test is positive if the serum turns white and opalescent.

napierian logarithm (nah-pir'e-an) [John *Napier,* Scottish mathematician, 1550–1617; inventor of logarithms] a logarithm to the base *e.* Also called *natural logarithm.*

Naprosyn (nah-pro'sin) trademark. See *naproxen.*

naproxen (nah-proks'en) an antiinflammatory, analgesic, and antipyretic nonsteroidal drug used for symptomatic relief in rheumatoid arthritis. It is an arylacetic acid derivative similar to ibuprofen, ketoprofen, and feneprofen. The most common side-effects are gastrointestinal intolerance (heartburn, nausea, dyspepsia), upper GI ulcer, bleeding, headache, drowsiness, itching, and skin eruptions. Trademark, *Naprosyn.*

narc/o (nar'ko) [Gr. *narkē* numbness] a word element used in combining form to denote numbness or stupor, e.g., narcotic.

narceine (nar'ce-ēn) an alkaloid that constitutes approximately 0.5 percent of raw opium.

narcolepsy (nar'ko-lep″se) [*narco-* + Gr. *lēpsis* a taking hold, a seizure] a syndrome characterized primarily by a sudden, almost irresistible urge to sleep for a brief period. Such attacks may occur during any activity or at any time of day. Cataplexy (temporary loss of muscle tone, often associated with sudden, intense emotion), sleep paralysis, and hypnagogic hallucinations are commonly experienced by narcolepsy patients. The cause of these disorders is unknown.

narcosis (nar-ko′sis) [Gr. *narkōsis* a benumbing] a reversible depression of neural activity accompanied by stupor.

narcotic (nar-kot′ik) [Gr. *narkōtikos* benumbing, deadening] 1. formerly, any substance that can produce narcosis.

2. legally, any opiate (drugs such as morphine and heroin isolated or synthesized from opium) or any extract of cocoa leaves containing cocaine or ecgonine. These drugs produce euphoria and analgesia; the opiates also produce physical dependence.

nares (na′rēz) [L. pl. of *naris*] [NA], the external orifices of the nose. Also called *nostrils*.

nas/o (na′zo) [L. *nasus* nose] a word element used in combining form to denote nose, e.g., nasosinusitis.

nasal (na′zal) [L. *nasalis*] pertaining to the nose.

nasal bone one of the paired skull bones that lie between the frontal processes of the maxillae in the bridge of the nose.

nasal cavity the proximal portion of the passages of the respiratory system; it extends from the nares to the nasopharynx.

nasal concha one of the shell-like bones of the nasal cavity. Only the inferior nasal conchae are separate bones, whereas the upper two pairs are processes of the ethmoid bone.

inferior n. c., one of the paired, scroll-like bones that lie horizontally in the lateral walls of the nasal cavity.

nasal myiasis see *nasal m.* under *myiasis*.

nascent (nas′ent, na′sent) [L. *nascens*] 1. just born; just coming into existence.

2. just liberated from a chemical combination, and hence more reactive because uncombined, e.g., nascent hydrogen, which is monatomic. This use of the term is now obsolete.

nasion (na′ze-on) [L. *nasus* nose] the point in the midsagittal plane at the root (top) of the nose where the frontonasal suture occurs, used as an anatomic landmark.

nasogastric (na″zo-gas′trik) [*naso-* + L. *gastricus*, from Gr. *gaster* stomach] pertaining to the nose and stomach.

nasolacrimal (na″zo-lak′rĭ-mal) [*naso-* + L. *lacrimalis*, from *lacrima* tear] pertaining to the nose and lacrimal apparatus.

nasolacrimal canal a canal in the medial wall of the orbit that communicates with the nasal passage and contains the nasolacrimal duct.

nasolacrimal duct see *nasolacrimal d.* under *duct*.

nasopharyngeal (na″zo-fa-rin′je-al) [*naso-* + L. *pharyngeus*] pertaining to the nasopharynx.

nasopharyngitis (na″zo-far″in-ji′tis) [*naso-* + *pharyngo-* + *-itis* inflammation] a general term to describe inflammation of the nasopharynx. See also *pharyngitis*.

nasopharyngography (na″zo-far-in-gog′rah-fe) [*naso-* + *pharyngo-* + *-graphy*] the radiographic examination of the nasopharynx.

nasopharynx (na″zo-far′inks) [*naso-* + Gr. *pharynx* pharynx] that part of the pharynx behind the nose and above the soft palate.

nasosinusitis (na″zo-si″nu-si′tis) [*naso-* + L. *sinus* a hollow + *-itis* inflammation] a general term to describe inflammation of the paranasal sinuses. See also *sinusitis*.

nasotracheal (na″zo-tra′ke-al) [*naso-* + L. *trachealis*] pertaining to the nose and trachea.

nat/i (na′te) [L. *natus* birth] a word element used in combining form to denote birth, e.g., neonate.

National Accrediting Agency for Clinical Laboratory Sciences (NAACLS) an organization responsible for accreditation of the clinical laboratory.

National Association of Medical Examiners (NAME) a professional organization of medical examiners.

National Bureau of Standards a department of the federal government that, in addition to other responsibilities, maintains primary reference standards and develops reference methods and reference materials.

National Certification Agency for Medical Laboratory Personnel (NCAMLP) a professional organization for the medical laboratory.

National Commission for Health Certifying Agencies (NCHCA) a professional health organization.

National Committee for Clinical Laboratory Standards (NCCLS) a voluntary organization involved in establishing clinical laboratory standards.

National Council of Health Laboratory Services (NCHLS) an intersociety of health care organizations in the United States that serves as a clearinghouse for those societies concerned with improving health-related laboratory services.

National Fire Protection Association (NFPA) an organization dedicated to promoting knowledge of methods of fire protection and to publication of standards relating to combustible and flammable materials, firefighting methods, safety of persons, and protection of property.

National Formulary (NF) a legally recognized book of standards and specifications for certain drugs that are not included in the United States Pharmacopeia. In 1974 the NF was acquired by the United States Pharmacopeial Convention, Inc. See also *United States Pharmacopeia*.

National Reference System in Clinical Chemistry (NRSCC) a concept proposed by the American Association for Clinical Chemistry to ensure the biologic relevance, chemical validity, and medical usefulness of clinical chemistry data. The system is based on the International System of units (SI) and has a hierarchical structure of interrelated methods (definitive, reference, and working methods) and materials (certified, matrixed, and control materials). It also envisions a defined relationship among professional, industrial, and govermental groups of scientific, medical, and technologic persons. See also the specific types of methods and materials.

National Registry in Clinical Chemistry (NRCC) a professional organization that certifies clinical chemists and clinical chemistry technologists.

National Registry of Microbiologists (NRM) a professional organization of microbiologists.

National Society for Histotechnology (NSH) a professional organization of histotechnicians.

native (na'tiv) [L. *nativus* born, native, natural] normal to a location; unaltered from its natural state.

native protein a protein in its normal conformation. It is said to be in the native state and has the conformation that endows the molecule with its specific biologic function.

natr/o (na'tro) [L. *natrium* sodium] a word element used in combining form to denote sodium, e.g., natremia.

natremia (na-tre'me-ah) [*natr-* + Gr. *haima* blood + *-ia*] see *hypernatremia.*

natrium (na'tre-um) gen. *natrii* [L.] modern Latin for *sodium.*

natriuresis (na"tre-u-re'sis) [*natr-* + Gr. *ourēsis* a making water] the excretion of abnormally large amounts of sodium in the urine. Polyuria, polydipsia, and large sodium requirements ensue. The condition is seen late in acute tubular necrosis, renal medullary cystic disease, and Bartter's syndrome.

natural (nat'u-ral) [L. *naturalis,* from *natura* nature] neither artificial nor pathologic.

natural gas an odorless mixture of combustible gases, found with petroleum below the surface of the earth, entrapped by rock structures. It contains methane (the principal component) plus ethane, propane, butane, carbon dioxide, nitrogen, and hydrogen sulfide. Natural gas is used primarily as a fuel. When supplied for household use, an odor is added to act as a warning of any asphyxiation hazard.

natural killer cell a member of a population of non-B, non-T lymphocytes having their own characteristic antigenic markers, which are completely marrow-dependent and found almost exclusively in the bone marrow and spleen. They are important in cytotoxicity directed against tumor cells, especially lymphoid tumors, and are the effector cells involved in the rejection of grafts of hematopoietic tissue. Also called *NK cell.*

natural logarithm a logarithm to the base *e.* Also called *napierian logarithm.*

nausea (naw'se-ah) [L.; Gr. *nausia* seasickness] a general symptom, usually described as an unpleasant sensation in the abdomen, which may culminate in vomiting. The condition may be due to systemic illness or pregnancy, or it may follow an upsetting visual experience or physical injury.

Navane (nav'ān) trademark. See *thiothixene.*

navicular (nah-vik'u-lar) [L. *navicula* boat] boat shaped, as in the navicular (one of the carpal) bone.

navicular cells boat-shaped, elongated cells of intermediate maturity seen in Papanicolaou smears of the squamous epithelium of the female genital tract. During pregnancy these cells are often predominant, and their cytoplasm accumulates yellow deposits of glycogen. A similar pattern may be seen in early menopause.

Nb symbol for the chemical element *niobium.*

NBS abbrev. See *National Bureau of Standards.*

NCAMLP abbrev. See *National Certification Agency for Medical Laboratory Personnel.*

NCCLS abbrev. See *National Committee for Clinical Laboratory Standards.*

NCF abbrev. for *neutrophil chemotactic factor.* See *polymorphonuclear neutrophil chemotactic factor.*

NCHCA abbrev. See *National Commission for Health Certifying Agencies.*

NCHLS abbrev. See *National Council of Health Laboratory Services.*

nCi abbrev. See *nanocurie.*

N:C ratio abbrev. See *nuclear-cytoplasmic ratio.*

Nd symbol for the chemical element *neodymium.*

Ne symbol for the chemical element *neon.*

nebulizer (neb'u-līz"er) an atomizer; a device for generating fine particles of a liquid suspended in a gas such as air. Nebulizers are used to administer medications to the airways or to stimulate a cough. They are also used as components on flame and atomic absorption photometers to produce a fine spray of the diluted sample for introduction into the flame. See also *atomizer.*

Necator (ne-ka'tor) [L. "murderer"] a genus of intestinal nematodes (hookworms).

N. americanus, the American or New World hookworm of worldwide distribution, parasitic in the small intestines of humans and causing hookworm disease. The adult worms are grayish-yellow (the males measuring 5–9 mm long; the females, 9–11 mm), with the head curving in opposition to the curvature of the body. It is characterized by a buccal cavity containing four plates, four pharyngeal lancets, and a dorsal conic tooth. Human infection is acquired by filariform larvae that penetrate the skin. The larvae migrate to the lungs, mature, and finally localize in the small intestines, where they attach and suck blood.

Laboratory diagnosis requires identification of the eggs (64–76 μm by 35–40 μm) in the feces by direct smears or by various concentrating methods, such as the formalin-ether sedimentation method or the AMS or zinc sulfate techniques. The worm burden can be determined by the Stoll dilution method, the Beaver direct smear method, the McMaster helminth techniques, and the Kato thick smear technique.

Also called *Uncinaria americana.* See also *hookworm.*

necatoriasis (ne-ka"to-ri'ah-sis) infection with hookworms of the genus *Necator.*

necessary and sufficient condition in logic, a proposition that is equivalent to another. That A is a necessary and sufficient condition for B means A and B are either both true or both false. Equivalent statements are "A implies B, and B implies A," and "B if and only if (iff) A." See also *necessary condition* and *sufficient condition.*

necessary condition in logic, a proposition that is required for another to hold. That A is a necessary condition for B means if A is false, then B is false; however, if A is true, then B may be either true or false. An equivalent statement is "B implies A." Cf. *sufficient condition.*

necr/o (nek'ro) [Gr. *nekros* dead] a word element used in combining form to denote death, e.g., necrosis.

necrobiosis (nek"ro-bi-o'sis) [*necro-* + Gr. *biōsis* life] 1. physiologic death, followed by normal replacement, of cells. Examples are the normal maintenance of cell populations of blood, endometrium, and skin.

2. a small region of tissue necrosis.

n. lipoidica diabeticorum, a disorder characterized by a plaquelike lesion that occurs predominantly on the legs, but also on the forearms, hands, neck, and face. The lesions have a yellow center and brown border. They show degeneration of collagen bundles, giant cells are often present, and ulceration of the lesion is common. More than half the cases of this skin disorder are associated with diabetes, and as many as 10 percent of cases precede overt diabetes.

necrophagocytosis (nek″ro-fag″o-si-to′sis) [*necro-* + Gr. *phagein* to eat + *kytos* hollow vessel + *-osis*] the ingestion of damaged or dying cells and cellular debris by monocytes and macrophages.

necrophilic (nek″ro-fil′ik) [*necro-* + Gr. *philein* to love] showing preference for dead tissue, as in necrophilic bacteria.

necropsy (nek′rop-se) [*necro-* + Gr. *opsis* view] the gross and microscopic examination of the body and viscera after death and the interpretation of these findings. Generally performed by a pathologist, this examination is a mechanism for instructing physicians on anatomy, disease processes, and effects of therapy; a means for correcting misdiagnosis; a source of material for investigation and epidemiologic studies; and an instrument for medico-legal examinations. Also called *autopsy* and *postmortem examination.*

necrosis (nĕ-kro′sis), pl. *necroses* [Gr. *nekrōsis* deadness] the death of an individual cell or groups of cells in living tissue. Cf. *apoptosis.*

acute tubular n., a renal disease that typically presents with clinical evidence of acute renal failure. The underlying injury to tubular epithelial cells can be produced either by ischemia secondary to hypotension, shock, or local renal vascular obstruction, or by toxic agents such as heavy metals (e.g., lead, cadmium, mercury, bismuth), mushroom poisoning, carbon tetrachloride, ethylene glycol, and miscellaneous chemicals and drugs.

The ischemia characteristically produces patchy or focal necrosis of the tubular epithelium, particularly in the proximal convoluted tubules, whereas toxins produce widespread uniform necrosis of the proximal convoluted tubular cells. The affected tubules, which contain interluminal casts of necrotic cells and debris, undergo sloughing of necrotic epithelial cells. Differentiation from acute tubular interstitial nephritis (tubulotubular interstitial nephropathy) is impossible when a prominent interstitial inflammatory reaction is present.

See also *tubulointerstitial nephropathy.*

aseptic n., necrosis that is due to interference with the vascular supply to the head of the femur, and that sometimes follows traumatic dislocation of the hip.

avascular n., necrosis due to deficient blood supply.

bridging hepatic n., confluent hepatic necrosis of sufficient severity to extend from centrilobular areas to portal tracts. Morphologically, it is characterized initially by parenchymal necrosis leading to condensation of the reticulin framework, and followed by the formation of fibrous septa. Bridging hepatic necrosis occurs in a minority of individuals with acute viral hepatitis. It signifies an increased risk of progression to cirrhosis and death.

caseous n., a form of necrosis in which the affected tissue changes into a dry, amorphous, semisolid mass resembling cheese. It is usually found in the central portion of soft granulomas, particularly in tuberculosis. The capsule of *Mycobacterium tuberculosis* contains materials that can denature protein and split lipids; these digest the dead cells to produce the cheesy necrosis.

central n., necrosis that affects the central portion of a bone or lobule of the liver.

coagulation n., necrosis of a portion of an organ or tissue resulting from the sudden interruption of the blood flow. Also called *ischemic n.*

cystic medial n., see *Erdheim's cystic medial n.*

Erdheim's cystic medial n., changes in the medial layer of the aorta, consisting of degeneration and necrosis of elastic and muscle fibers, mucoid infiltration, and cyst formation, often resulting in a dissecting aneurysm. Also called *medionecrosis of aorta.*

fat n., necrosis in which the neutral fats in the cells of adipose tissue are split into fatty acids and glycerol. It may affect subcutaneous fat depots, particularly in the female breast, as a result of trauma, forming a firm, circumscribed mass. Also called steatonecrosis.

focal n., the presence of a small area of necrosis.

gangrenous n., necrosis due to cell death caused by a combination of ischemia and superimposed bacterial infection.

hyaline n., see *Zenker's n.*

ischemic n., see *coagulation n.*

massive hepatic n., confluent necrosis of entire hepatic lobules that usually involves substantial portions of the liver. The causative agents include viruses, hepatotoxic chemicals (e.g., carbon tetrachloride, chloroform, cinchophen, mushroom poisons, and arsenicals), and certain drugs (e.g., iproniazid, *p*-aminosalicylic acid, tetracyclines, gold compounds, and halothane).

medial n., necrosis of the tunica media of a blood vessel, which may lead to its dissection or rupture.

peripheral n., necrosis of the peripheral portion of a liver lobule, as in puerperal eclampsia and phosphorous poisoning.

piecemeal n., hepatic cell necrosis at the junction of the hepatic parenchyma and portal tracts, which leads to replacement of necrotic hepatic cells by fibrous tissue. Morphologically, it is characterized by an irregular hepatic parenchyma–portal tract connective tissue boundary in involved portal tracts. It is one of the hallmarks of chronic aggressive hepatitis and is usually accompanied by a chronic inflammatory cell infiltrate, fibrosis, and small bile duct proliferation.

postpartum pituitary n., pituitary necrosis and panhypopituitarism resulting from circulatory collapse and thrombosis of the pituitary vasculature following delivery. Also called *Sheehan's syndrome.* See also *panhypopituitarism.*

pressure n., necrosis due to an insufficient local blood supply occasioned by occlusion of vessels from pressure, as in decubitus ulcers.

radiation n., death of tissue caused by radiation.

radium n., necrosis of the maxilla or mandible occurring in workers engaged in painting watch dials with radium-containing luminous paint. Also called osteoradionecrosis and radium jaw.

renal papillary n., an accompaniment of acute pyelonephritis, most often seen in diabetics, and characterized by necrosis of the renal papillae of one or both kidneys, with sharp demarcation between necrotic and living tissue. Also called necrotizing papillitis and necrotizing renal papillitis.

septic n., necrosis resulting from bacterial infection.

Zenker's n., the necrosis and hyaline degeneration of striated muscle. Also called *hyaline n.* and *Zenker's degeneration.*

necrotic (nĕ-krot′ik) pertaining to or characterized by necrosis.

needle (ne′d′l) [L. *acus*] 1. a sharp instrument for suturing or puncturing.

2. to puncture with a needle.

aspirating n., see *aspiration b.* under *biopsy.*

biopsy n., a large-bore carrier needle with an obturator and inner cutting needle. The needle is inserted into a tissue to remove a sample for pathologic examination. This biopsy technique has the advantage of allowing access to deeply situated tissues without requiring an open operation. See also the accompanying illustration and *aspiration b.* under *biopsy.*

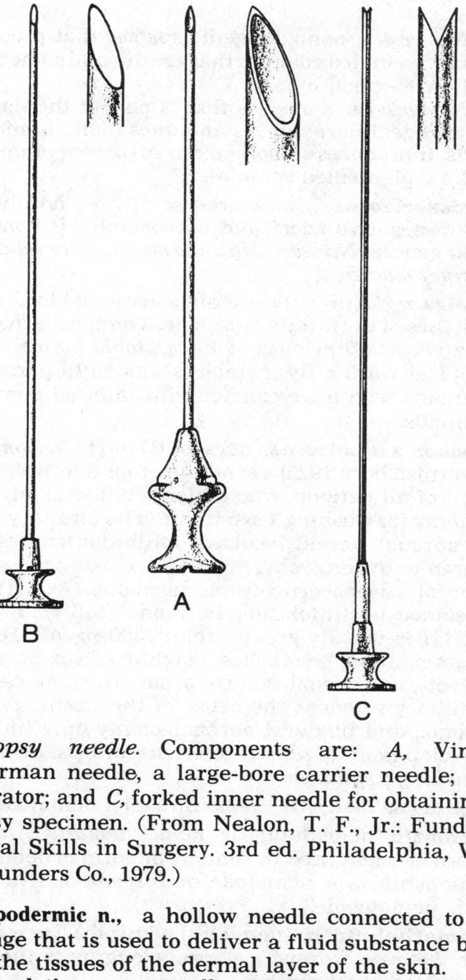

Biopsy needle. Components are: *A,* Vim-Silverman needle, a large-bore carrier needle; *B,* obturator; and *C,* forked inner needle for obtaining biopsy specimen. (From Nealon, T. F., Jr.: Fundamental Skills in Surgery. 3rd ed. Philadelphia, W. B. Saunders Co., 1979.)

hypodermic n., a hollow needle connected to a syringe that is used to deliver a fluid substance below the tissues of the dermal layer of the skin.

inoculating n., a needle consisting of a straight wire attached to a rod-shaped handle, which is used for inoculating a bacteriologic culture. Specifically, inoculating needles are employed in the preparation of stab cultures and for subculturing from single colonies on a culture plate.

spinal n., a long needle used to enter the spinal canal, either to withdraw cerebrospinal fluid for analysis or to inject anesthetic agents into the epidural space to effect regional anesthesia.

needle aspiration cytology a method of obtaining small amounts of cellular fragments for the diagnosis of palpable or radiologically or echographically detectable masses by the use of 21- to 25-gauge needles. The removal of tissue is accomplished with a syringe and negative pressure to draw biopsy material into the needle core.

The use of a needle to obtain diagnostic tissue had its origin in the nineteenth century, but it was not until 1904 that the first significant study, revealing trypanosomal organisms in lymph nodes by needle aspiration, was performed. In the United States, the rapid development and availability of surgical pathology hindered the development of this method. In Europe, however, where pathology was centralized and the transportation of large specimens was not practical, the use of small aspirate samples grew in popularity; in the last 35 yr the Europeans have developed needle aspiration cytology into a highly reliable technique. By the mid-1970s, needle aspiration cytology experienced a resurgence of interest in the United States that continues to this day.

Aspiration cytology has been shown to be useful in the diagnosis of primary tumors of all body sites and has been used extensively in the diagnosis of primary breast and thyroid masses. Aside from the detection of primary neoplastic diseases, metastatic deposits of a tumor may also be identified. Aspiration cytology has been shown to have high degrees of sensitivity and specificity: sensitivities and specificities of 90 and 97.1 percent have been reported for histologically proved breast malignancies; 92 and 95 percent, respectively, for thyroid neoplasms. Other body sites have yielded similar results.

The ability to obtain high-quality specimens and correct interpretation by this procedure is not difficult but does require training in histopathology, cytology, and biopsy technique. The aspiration of masses is performed by inserting a needle into a tumor mass and creating negative pressure in the attached syringe. While this vacuum is maintained, the needle is moved back and forth to sample various areas of the tumor. The vacuum is released and the needle and syringe are withdrawn. After the needle is detached, air is introduced into the syringe and the needle reattached. The needle is then positioned over a clean slide and the material forcibly expelled into it. The sample is smeared over the slide surface to form a monolayer sheet, and the material is wet fixed in 95 percent ethyl alcohol and stained by the Papanicolaou method. Air-dried material is treated with a Romanowsky stain.

Only two reported instances of tumor implantation along a fine-gauge (≤ 18) needle tract have been recorded. Mortality is extremely low, although death has been reported (e.g., exsanguination following liver and lung biopsies).

Also called *aspiration cytology, fine-needle biopsy, skinny-needle biopsy,* and *thin-needle biopsy.* See also *needle.*

THEODORE MILLER, M.D.

NEFA abbrev. for nonesterified fatty acids. See *nonesterified f. a.* under *fatty acids.*

negative (neg′ah-tiv) [L. *negativus*] 1. denying, opposing, or disparaging.

2. in mathematics, pertaining to a number having a value less than zero.

3. in laboratory medicine, pertaining to a test result and indicating a lack or absence, i.e., no pathogen, toxic substance, etc., is detected.

4. in physics and chemistry, pertaining to an electric charge that has the same sign as the charge on the electron, as a negative ion (anion) or negative electrode (cathode).

5. a photographic image in which dark areas of the object appear light on the film and light areas appear dark. Cf. *positive.*

negative interference in genetic mapping, the overabundant frequency of double cross-overs. Marker distances are not additive without correction of these double cross-overs. See also *genetic mapping.*

negative pressure a pressure that is less than atmospheric pressure.

negative pressure lavage see *Gravlee jet wash.*

negatron (neg′ah-tron) an electron. This term is used only to emphasize that the electron and positron are antiparticles, as in the contrast of negatron beta decay versus positron beta decay.

negatron beta decay see *beta decay.*

Negri body (na′gre) [Adelchi *Negri,* Italian physician, 1876–1912] a viral inclusion body seen in approximately 70 percent of brains affected with rabies, particularly in the cytoplasm of the pyramidal cells of the hippocampus or the Purkinje cells. Also called lyssa body. See also *rabies.*

Neisseria (nis-se′re-ah) [Albert Ludwig Siegmund *Neisser,* German physician, 1855–1916] a genus of bacteria, family Neisseriaceae, that consists of gram-negative, oxidase-positive cocci characteristically paired and shaped like coffee beans. These organisms are aerobic or facultatively anaerobic, and inhabit the mucous membranes of the oropharynx, nasopharynx, and genitourinary tract (see also *normal flora*). The genus includes two pyogenic species that are human pathogens, causing meningococcal meningitis and gonorrhea. Differentiation of species within the genus depends on carbohydrate fermentation reactions and cultural characteristics.

N. catarrhalis, see *B. catarrhalis* under *Branhamella.*

N. flavescens, a species occasionally recovered from the body fluids of individuals with meningitis and septicemia. It produces yellow pigmented colonies.

N. gonorrhoeae, a species that is an obligate human parasite; it can cause gonorrhea, urethritis, prostatitis, vulvovaginitis, epididymitis, cervicitis, salpingitis, proctitis, pharyngitis, perihepatitis, and ophthalmia in newborns.

N. gonorrhoeae is a fastidious microorganism, requiring 3–10 percent CO_2 and enriched media (chocolate agar) for growth. Morphologically, it is composed of small, translucent, raised, grayish-white colonies. Biochemically, they are oxidase-positive; that is, the bacterium produces the enzyme indophenol oxidase, which oxidizes the redox dye tetramethyl-*p*-phenylenediamine dihydrochloride from a red color to black. *N. gonorrhoeae* also ferments glucose when combined with a cystine trypticase agar base.

Microscopic examination of the infected exudate reveals gram-negative diplococci whose adjacent walls of paired cells are flattened; the diplococci are located intracellularly and extracellularly with respect to the leukocytes. Other laboratory methods for identification of the gonococci include a direct fluorescent antibody technique and the ability of gonococcal DNA to genetically transform an auxotrophic mutant of *N. gonorrhoeae* to prototrophy.

Also called *gonococcus.* See also *gonorrhea.*

N. lactamicus, a species that occurs frequently in throat and nasopharyngeal cultures and occasionally causes endocarditis and meningitis.

N. meningitidis, a species found frequently in the human nasopharyngeal area. Infection of susceptible persons leads to septicemia and epidemic meningococcal meningitis.

The species is divided serologically into four groups (A, B, C, D) and several provisional groups. Positive identification is based on fermentation tests and on agglutination techniques or fluorescence microscopy. Commonly called *meningococcus.*

N. sicca, a nonpathogenic species that produces small, wrinkled colonies that are dry and sometimes yellow-to-green in color.

N. subflava, a species that is part of the normal pharyngeal flora but is sometimes found in meningitis. It produces smooth and transparent or opaque yellow-pigmented colonies.

Neisseriaceae (nīs-se″re-a′se-e) a family of gram-negative cocci and coccobacilli. It contains four genera: *Neisseria, Branhamella, Moraxella,* and *Acinetobacter.*

Neivamyia (ni-vah′me-e″ah) a genus of blood-sucking flies of the family Muscidae. The species *N. lutzi* is a vector of the eggs of *Dermatobia hominis* (the tropical warble fly), which is known to parasitize humans who have contact with infested domestic animals.

Nelson's syndrome (nel′son) [Don H. *Nelson,* U.S. internist, born 1925] a syndrome found in 10–20 percent of all patients who undergo bilateral adrenalectomy for Cushing's syndrome. The pituitary's loss of adrenal steroid feedback inhibition causes this organ to hypertrophy, greatly increasing the secretion of adrenocorticotropic hormone (ACTH) and melanocyte-stimulating hormone (MSH). Plasma ACTH is usually greater than 2500 pg/ml. Hyperpigmentation, headaches, heightened sex hormone effects, and visual defects occur. In some cases a pituitary tumor is the cause of the Cushing's syndrome, and bilateral adrenalectomy only furthers development of the deleterious effects. See also *Cushing's syndrome.*

nema (ne′mah) [Gr. *nēma* thread] a nematode.

nemat/o (nem′ah-to) [Gr. *nēma, nēmatos* thread] a word element used in combining form to denote relationship to a nematode or threadlike structure, e.g., nematocide.

nemathelminth (nem″ah-thel′minth) [*nemat-* + Gr. *helmins* worms] a worm belonging to the phylum Nemathelminthes.

Nemathelminthes (nem″ah-thel-min′thēz) a phylum of worms in some systems of classification; it includes the Nematoda and sometimes the Acanthocephala.

nematocide (nem′ah-to-sīd″) [*nemato-* + L. *caedere*

to kill] any agent or preparation used to destroy nematodes.

Nematoda (nem″ah-to′dah) [*nemato-* + Gr. *eidos* form] roundworms, a class of tapered, cylindric helminths (phylum Aschelminthes) characterized by longitudinally oriented muscles and a triradiate esophagus. Many genera contain human parasites, including the intestinal roundworms *Ancylostoma, Ascaris, Enterobius, Necator, Strongyloides, Trichinella,* and *Trichuris,* and the filarial roundworms *Dipetalonema, Dracunculus, Loa, Mansonella, Onchocerca,* and *Wuchereria.*

nematode (nem′ah-tōd) any worm belonging to the phylum or class of Nematoda, depending on the system of classification. True roundworms, they are characterized by elongated, cylindric, and unsegmented bodies.

nematodiasis (nem″ah-to-di′ah-sis) being infected or having a disease caused by a nematode parasite.

nematologist (nem″ah-tol′o-jist) one who specializes in nematology.

nematology (nem″ah-tol′o-je) [*nemato-* + Gr. *logos* reasoned speech] the branch of zoology that deals with nematodes, or roundworms.

Nematomorpha (nem″ah-to-mor′fah) [*nemato-* + Gr. *morphē* form] a phylum of worms that includes the class Gordiacea (hairworms or hair snakes). The adult worms are elongated, cylindric, and unsegmented, measuring 10–15 cm long. In some systems of classification, they are a class of the phylum Aschelminthes. These worms are free-living in water; their larvae are parasitic in insects. Human infection is occasional and caused by accidental ingestion of insects contaminated with young worms or by ingestion of free-living adult worms.

nematosis (nem″ah-to′sis) [*nemat-* + *-osis*] infection with nematodes, or roundworms.

Nembutal (nem′bu-tal) trademark. See *pentobarbital.*

neo- (ne′o) [Gr. *neos* new] a prefix word element to denote new, e.g., neonate, neogenesis.

neodymium (Nd) (ne″o-dim′e-um) [*neo-* + *didymium* (a mixture of Nd and Pr, once reported as an element), from Gr. *didymos* twin] a soft, silvery-white metallic element that yellows on exposure to air; atomic number 60; atomic weight 144.24; a 4f transition element (lanthanide rare earth); oxidation state +3. See also *rare earth elements.*

neogenesis (ne″o-jen′ĕ-sis) [*neo-* + Gr. *genesis* production] 1. new growth of nonneoplastic tissue, e.g., angioneogenesis.

2. the formation of a new molecular structure, e.g., gluconeogenesis, the formation of glucose from molecules such as amino acids, lactate, and the glycerol portion of fats that are themselves not carbohydrate.

-neogenesis a suffix word element to denote the formation of a new substance or new tissue from a new source, e.g., angioneogenesis, gluconeogenesis.

neologism (ne-ol′o-jizm) [*neo-* + Gr. *logos* word] 1. a newly coined word.

2. the use of new words and phrases or of old words with new meanings.

neomycin (ne′o-mi″sin) an antibacterial aminoglycoside substance produced by the growth of *Streptomyces fradiae,* active against most gram-negative bacteria and against staphylococci. It is used for topical treatment of superficial lesions and to treat severe infections not responding to less toxic drugs. Systemic administration can cause irreversible deafness. See also *aminoglycosides* and *antibacterial agents.*

neon (Ne) (ne′on) [Gr. *neos* new] a colorless, odorless, inert, gaseous element; atomic number 10; atomic weight 20.179; Group 0 of the periodic table (the noble gases); only known oxidation state 0 (no compounds). It is used in electric discharge illuminating tubes and in lasers.

neopentyl- (ne″o-pen′til) a prefix word element used in organic chemistry to denote the 2,2-dimethylpropyl group, $—CH_2C(CH_3)_3$, e.g., neopentylamine, neopentyl alcohol. Cf. *isopentyl-* and *n-pentyl-.*

neoplasia (ne″o-pla′ze-ah) a disorder of cell proliferation and differentiation that results in the production of a new growth of tissue (neoplasm) commonly referred to as tumor.

neoplasm (ne′o-plazm) [*neo-* + Gr. *plasma* formation] an abnormal mass of cells typically exhibiting uncontrolled and progressive growth. Neoplasms are broadly classified into two categories: (1) according to the cell type from which they originate, major subdivisions being those derived from epithelial tissues and those from connective tissue; and (2) according to their biologic behavior, i.e., whether they are benign or malignant. (See *neoplastic growth.*)

Benign neoplasms are noninvasive, are frequently encapsulated, and do not metastasize. Typically, but not invariably, they are slow growing. Although they remain localized, benign neoplasms occasionally may cause death from complications such as compression of a critical structure, hemorrhage, or disseminated intravascular coagulation.

Malignant neoplasms generally grow more rapidly than benign neoplasms and can invade adjacent structures. A preinvasive stage of a malignant epithelial tumor is recognized and designated as in situ or intraepithelial carcinoma. When invasion does occur, the access of malignant cells to lymph and blood vascular channels provides the means for dissemination to distant sites in the body (metastasis). The newly established metastatic foci become centers for further growth as satellite tumors. Metastases are frequently the cause of death of the host, although either the primary tumor or a metastasis may interfere with the functions of vital organs. Other characteristic features of malignant tumors include the loss of normal architectural arrangements of cells; cellular aneuploidy (abnormal chromosome complement resulting in an abnormal nuclear DNA content and distribution), which cytologically is manifested by nuclear hyperchromasia; atypia and pleomorphism; altered regulation of cell proliferation; abnormal cell kinetics; misprogrammed gene function; nonspecific metabolic pathways; ectopic hormone production; and loss of isoantigens and transplant stability.

Neoplasms are classified according to their type as determined by histologic examination. Broad divisions include *adenoma* (a benign tumor of gland cells), *carcinoma* (a malignant tumor of epithelial cells), and *sarcoma* (a malignant mesenchymal tumor). The pathologist may attempt to indicate the degree of aggressiveness of a malignant tumor by assessing its histologic grade on the basis of criteria such as cellularity, degree of cellular pleomorphism, and mitotic activity (see *tumor grading*).

There are various methods available to treat patients with neoplasms; for more information, see, for example, *chemotherapy, hormonal therapy, immunotherapy,* and *radiation therapy.*
Also called *tumor.* See also *differentiation, metastasis,* and the accompanying table.

NEOPLASM. CLASSIFICATION OF TUMORS

TISSUE OF ORIGIN	BENIGN	MALIGNANT
I. Simple (composed of one single neoplastic cell type)		
A. Tumors of Mesenchymal Origin		*Sarcomas:*
(1) Connective Tissue and Derivatives		
Fibrous tissue	Fibroma	Fibrosarcoma
Myxomatous tissue	Myxoma	Myxosarcoma
Cartilage	Chondroma	Chondrosarcoma
Bone	Osteoma	Osteogenic sarcoma
Notochordal tissue	Chordoma	Chordoma (or better, chordosarcoma)
(2) Endothelial and Related Tissues		
Blood vessels	Hemangioma: Capillary Cavernous	Hemangiosarcoma (multiple sarcoma–Kaposi's sarcoma)
Lymph vessels	Lymphangioma	Lymphangiosarcoma
Synovia		Synovioma (synoviosarcoma)
Mesothelium (lining cells of body cavities)		Mesothelioma (mesothelio-sarcoma)
Brain coverings	Meningioma	
Glomus	Glomus tumor	
? Blood vessels of bone marrow		? Ewing's tumor (endotheliosarcoma)
(3) Blood Cells and Related Cells		
Hematopoietic cells		Granulocytic leukemia Monocytic leukemia
Lymphoid tissue		Malignant lymphomas Lymphocytic leukemia Plasmacytoma (multiple myeloma) ? Hodgkin's disease
(4) Muscle		
Smooth muscle	Leiomyoma	Leiomyosarcoma
Striated muscle	Rhabdomyoma	Rhabdomyosarcoma
B. Tumors of Epithelial Origin		*Carcinomas:*
Stratified squamous	Squamous cell papilloma	Squamous cell or epidermoid carcinoma
Skin adnexal glands:		
Hair follicles		Basal cell carcinoma
Sweat glands	Sweat gland adenoma	Sweat gland carcinoma
Sebaceous glands	Sebaceous gland adenoma	Sebaceous gland carcinoma
Epithelial lining:		
Glands or ducts—well-differentiated group	Adenoma Papilloma Papillary adenoma Cystadenoma	Adenocarcinoma Papillary carcinoma Papillary adenocarcinoma Cystadenocarcinoma
Poorly differentiated group		Medullary carcinoma Undifferentiated carcinoma (simplex)
Respiratory tract		Bronchogenic carcinoma Bronchial "adenoma"
Neuroectoderm	Nevus	Melanoma (melanocarcinoma)
Renal epithelium	Renal tubular adenoma	Renal cell carcinoma (hypernephroma)
Liver cells	Liver cell adenoma	Hepatoma or liver cell carcinoma
Bile duct	Bile duct adenoma	Bile duct carcinoma (cholangiocarcinoma)
Urinary tract epithelium (transitional)	Transitional cell papilloma	Papillary carcinoma Transitional cell carcinoma Squamous cell carcinoma
Placental epithelium	Hydatidiform mole	Choriocarcinoma
Testicular epithelium		Seminoma Embryonal carcinoma

NEOPLASM. (*Continued*)

TISSUE OF ORIGIN	BENIGN	MALIGNANT
II. Mixed (more than one neoplastic cell type, usually derived from one germ layer)		
Salivary glands	Mixed tumor of salivary gland origin (pleomorphic adenoma)	Malignant mixed tumor of salivary glandorigin
Renal anlage		Wilm's tumor
III. Compound (more than one neoplastic cell type, derived from more than one germ layer)		
Totipotential cells in gonads or in embryonic rests	Teratoma, Dermoid cyst	One or more elements become malignant

From Robbins, S. L., and Cotran, R. S.: Pathologic Basis of Disease. 2nd ed. Philadelphia, W. B. Saunders Co., 1979, pp. 144-145.

neoplastic (ne″o-plas′tik) pertaining to or like a neoplasm; pertaining to neoplasia.

neoplastic growth cell growth that is characteristically progressive and reflects defects in the normal regulatory controls of cell proliferation and differentiation.

Malignant neoplasms tend to invade surrounding tissues and may metastasize to distant organs; they grow more rapidly than do their benign neoplastic counterparts. Among malignant neoplasms, growth rates tend to increase with advancing degrees of malignancy, although there are many exceptions to this rule. Examples of the exceptions include certain benign neoplasms (e.g., leiomyomas) that may grow relatively fast, and certain malignant neoplasms that may grow quite slowly (e.g., adenoid cystic carcinoma of the salivary gland) and yet progress relentlessly to kill the host after many years. It should be noted that the growth rate of even the most malignant tumor is relatively slow when compared with that of the normal embryo or certain replicating adult tissues in humans and laboratory animals, such as bone marrow and gastrointestinal mucosal cells. Many tumors occurring in humans require years of growth to reach a size that is clinically detectable.

Specific factors relating to cell proliferation that contribute to the rate at which a given tumor grows include: (1) the length of the cell cycle of that tumor (generation time); (2) the proportion of tumor cells capable of entering and completing a cell cycle (growth fraction); and (3) the extent of tumor cell death, differentiation, and migration to distant sites (cell loss).

Studies of cell kinetics have modified many conventionally held ideas about tumor cell replication. These studies have shown that: (1) cells of solid malignant neoplasms usually replicate more slowly than do corresponding normal cells, (2) the growth fraction of a tumor is usually smaller than that of corresponding normal cells, (3) individual tumor cells replicate intermittently, and (4) replication of tumor cells is under regulatory controls similar to those of normal cells.

Our understanding of neoplastic growth in humans and laboratory animals has been obtained from in vivo and in vitro cell kinetic studies and from repeated measurements of growing tumors in situ. The growth rate of neoplasms is usually expressed in terms of the time required for a tumor to double its volume. Estimates of tumor volume doubling time in humans are based on serial measurements obtained directly by physical examination of superficial tumors, and indirectly from scans and radiographic studies of deep-seated tumors. From measurements of tumor diameter (D), assuming the tumor is spherical, the tumor volume can be approximated using the formula for a sphere ($\pi D^3/6$). Successive estimates of tumor volume calculated from serial measurements of tumor diameter provide a time/volume relationship from which the time required for a tumor to double its volume can be determined.

Because most tumors are not composed exclusively of neoplastic cells, and because factors such as hemorrhage, edema, and proliferation of fibrous tissue in the tumor can influence both tumor cells and gross rates of tumor growth. Estimates of tumor cell doubling time may vary greatly from those of tumor volume doubling time for the same tumor. Therefore, it is difficult to make direct comparisons between these two measurements. However, for purposes of the following hypothetical examples, a direct correlation between tumor cell and tumor volume doubling times is assumed.

Observations on the growth rate of carcinomas at various sites have revealed considerable heterogeneity in doubling times. For example, estimates of the volume doubling time of breast carcinomas from mammographic examinations in a number of studies have suggested mean doubling times of approximately 210 da with a range of approximately 40 to more than 400 da. Estimates of growth rates of metastatic breast carcinoma from chest wall recurrences and lung metastases have suggested shorter doubling times (faster growth) in these sites than in the primary tumor. These findings may be related to a late stage of the disease at the time metastases are present. In general, the mean volume doubling time for even the most rapidly growing tumors in metastatic sites is thought to be longer than 40 da, with the majority in the range of 100–500 da (see the accompanying illustration).

The observed growth rates for most malignant tumors are typically rapid and exponential while the tumor is still small, and become progressively slower as the tumor increases in size with time. Exponential growth in the initial stages of tumor development with progressive slowing is known as Gompertzian growth (a pattern of exponential growth with the growth rate decaying at an exponential rate over the duration of the life of the tumor).

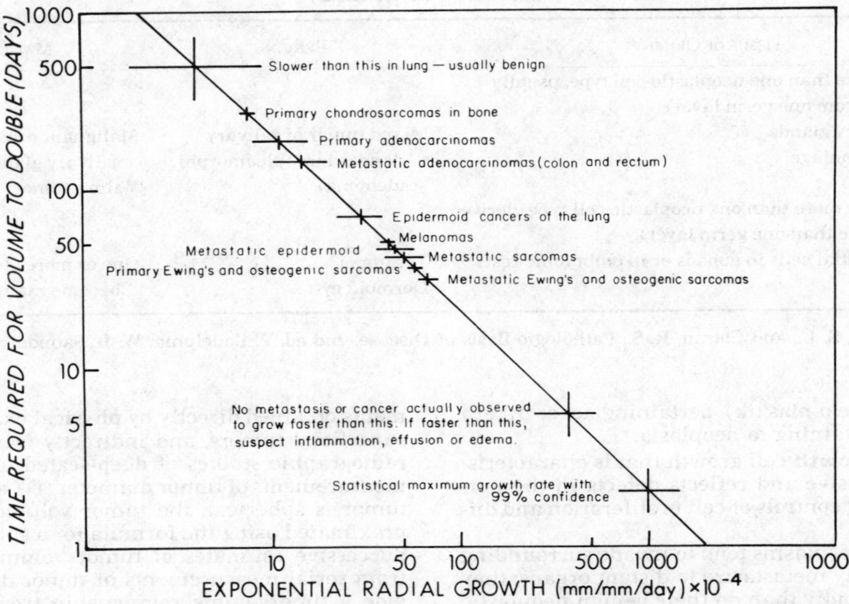

Neoplastic growth. This nomogram relates the time required in days for a growing spherical cancer to double its volume to the exponential radial growth rate in millimeters/millimeters/day. (From Spratt, J. S., and Spratt, J. A.: The prognostic value of measuring the gross linear radial growth of pulmonary metastases and primary pulmonary cancers. Journal of Thoracic and Cardiovascular Surgery *71*:274, 1976.)

It is often assumed that malignant neoplasms grow rapidly because they appear to reach substantial proportions in what seems to be a relatively short time. This perception arises largely because most tumors are difficult to detect when small, and grow silently for long periods until late in their development, when they become clinically evident. As the clinically detectable period of growth may be short until the patient dies, the impression is that of rapid growth.

A simplified illustration of the growth of a breast carcinoma provides a framework to better understand its mechanics. In the United States, the mean diameter of breast carcinomas detected by palpation is in the range of 3–4 cm in greatest diameter, and few tumors detected clinically are less than 1 cm in diameter. By the time a tumor does become clinically apparent, one or two doublings in cell volume are readily appreciated by the physician and patient, who tend to think of the inception of growth as being shortly before the tumor became detectable clinically. They therefore perceive the tumor as growing at an extremely rapid rate. In fact, a carcinoma of the breast enlarging from 1 cm (523 mm^3) to 4 cm (33500 mm^3) in diameter would involve slightly more than six doublings of the tumor cell volume and would require approximately 600 da if the tumor were 100 percent cellular, all cells were cycling, no cell loss occurred, and the tumor cell doubling time were 100 da. Using the same assumptions and beginning with one malignant cell 10 μ in diameter, it would take approximately 30 doublings or 3000 da for the tumor to reach 1 cm in diameter. In this example, growth from one cell to a tumor 4 cm in diameter requires 36 doublings and 3600 da, or nearly 10 yr. Such a tumor would be in the size range usually detectable clinically for less than 2 of the 10 yr of its growth. Another four doublings, or a total of 44 doublings (4400 da or 12 yr), would produce a tumor 26 cm in diameter (approx. 1 kg), which is thought to represent the maximal body burden of tumor consistent with life.

The potential clinical value derived from determinations of tumor growth rates includes their use in differential diagnosis and prognosis, the development of programs for early detection, and the planning and evaluation of therapy; correlation of growth rates with cell kinetic studies; and improved understanding of the natural history of neoplasms.

See also *cell cycle, chemotherapy,* and *radiation therapy.*

JACQUELINE HART, M.D.

neostigmine (ne″o-stig′min) a cholinesterase-inhibiting drug used to treat myasthenia gravis and as an antidote to the nondepolarizing neuromuscular blocking muscle relaxants tubocurarine, metocurine, and pancuronium. Adverse reactions are cholinergic effects of salivation, muscle fasciculations, and diarrhea. Overdosage may cause cholinergic crisis marked by muscle cramps, spasms and weakness, vomiting, bronchospasm, pulmonary edema, bradycardia, headache, coma, and convulsions. Weakness of respiratory muscles may be a cause of death in a cholinergic crisis.

n. bromide, [USP], a salt of neostigmine, used for oral administration.

n. methylsulfate, [USP], a salt of neostigmine, used for subcutaneous or intramuscular injection.

Neotestudina (ne″o-tes″tu′dīnah) a genus of loculoascomycete fungi that causes maduromycosis, found in individuals in Africa. The fungus is slow growing and produces grains that are brown in color. The medically important species is *N. rosatii.*

neotype (ne′o-tīp) [*neo-* + Gr. *typos* mark] a strain of bacteria that replaces a type strain which no longer exists, agrees with the original description of the strain, and is accepted by international agreement.

neper (Np) (ne′per) 1. a dimensionless unit of measurement used to express the ratio of two electrical voltages or currents. The number of nepers is the natural (napierian) logarithm of this ratio.

2. a unit used to express the ratio of two power levels. The number of nepers is the natural logarithm of the square root of this ratio. (This is equivalent to definition 1 when the power is proportional to the square of the voltage or current.) One neper equals. 8.686 dB.

nephel/o (nef′ĕ-lo) [Gr. *nephelē* cloud, mist] a word element used in combining form to denote relationship to cloudiness or mistiness, e.g., nephelometry.

nephelometer (nef″ĕ-lom′ĕ-ter) [*nephalo-* + Gr. *metron* measure] an optical device that measures the amount of light scattered by fine particles present in a suspension. The instrument measures the ratio of the intensity of light scattered by dispersion (and measured at an angle to the beam) to the intensity of the incident light; the intensities are compared with a standard of known concentration. A recent application of this technique is the immunochemical measurement of proteins.

nephelometric immunoassays (nef″ĕ-lo-met′rik) see *nonradioisotopic i.* under *immunoassays.*

nephelometric inhibition assay (NIA) see *nonradioisotopic i.* under *immunoassays.*

nephelometry (nef″ĕ-lom′ĕ-tre) a technique that uses a nephelometer to measure the number and size of particles in a suspension. The intensity of light, scattered by the particles, is measured with a detector at an angle to the incident light beam. One application of nephelometry is the quantitation of serum proteins (antigens). Varying amounts of antigen are added to constant amounts of specific antiserum, resulting in the formation of antigen-antibody complexes that are quantitated by nephelometry.

nephr/o (nef′ro) [Gr. *nephros* kidney] a word element used in combining form to denote kidney, e.g., nephritis, nephrology.

nephritis (nĕ-fri′tis), pl. *nephritides* [*nephr-* + *-itis* inflammation] an inflammation of the kidney; a focal or diffuse proliferative or destructive process that may involve the glomerulus, tubule, or interstitial renal tissue. See also *glomerulopathy* and *tubulointerstitial nephropathy.* Cf. *nephrosis.*

acute interstitial n., see *tubulointerstitial nephropathy.*

bacterial n., nephritis caused by microorganisms.

Balkan n., a very slowly progressive interstitial nephritis found geographically in several well-defined areas of Yugoslavia, Romania, Bulgaria, and Greece. The etiology is unknown. The disease is of particular interest because a relatively large percentage of affected individuals develop transitional cell carcinoma of the renal pelvis. Also called *Balkan nephropathy.*

chronic interstitial n., see under *tubulointerstitial nephropathy.*

interstitial n., see under *tubulointerstitial nephropathy.*

transfusion n., see *hemoglobinuric nephropathy.*

tubular n., see under *tubulointerstitial nephropathy.*

nephroblastoma (nef″ro-blas-to′mah) [*nephro-* + Gr. *blastos* germ + *-oma*] traditionally, a mixed renal tumor composed of metanephric blastema and its recognized stromal and epithelial derivatives at various stages of differentiation. The modern view expands the definition to include monoblastic neoplasms composed predominantly or exclusively of one of the histologic patterns common to the classical form of nephroblastoma. Also called *embryonal carcinosarcoma* (see *carcinosarcoma*), and *Wilms' tumor.* See also *renal tumors.*

nephrocalcinosis (nef″ro-kal″sĭ-no′sis) [*nephro-* + *calcium* + *-osis*] a condition characterized by the precipitation of calcium salts in the tubules and parenchyma of the kidneys. It most often follows chronic hypercalciuria and hyperphosphaturia, as seen in hyperparathyroidism, milk-alkali syndrome, hyperoxaluria, and excessive intake of vitamin D, calcium, or alkali. X-ray examination reveals minute calcific densities in the parenchyma of the kidneys near the papillae. Uremia may occur following impaired kidney function. Anemia is common, and blood chemistry tests reveal variable degrees of renal insufficiency.

nephrogenic (nef″ro-jen′ik) [*nephro-* + Gr. *gennan* to produce] forming kidney tissue.

nephrogenous (nĕ-froj′ĕ-nus) [*nephro* + Gr. *-genēs* born] originating in the kidney.

nephrolithiasis (nef″ro-lĭ-thi′ah-sis) [*nephro-* + Gr. *lithos* stone + *-iasis*] the condition of having renal calculi (kidney stones). See also *renal c.* under *calculus.*

nephrologist (nĕ-frol′o-jist) a specialist in nephrology.

nephrology (nĕ-frol′o-je) [*nephro-* + *-logy*] the scientific study of the kidney including its anatomy, histology, physiology, and pathology.

nephroma (nĕ-fro′mah) a general term used to denote a neoplasm that originates from renal parenchyma. See also *renal tumors.*

nephron (nef′ron) [*nephro-* + *on* neuter ending] the anatomic and functional unit of the kidney. By the three processes of filtration, secretion, and selective reabsorption, the nephron functions to determine the excretory and regulatory activity of the kidney. It consists of the renal corpuscle, proximal convoluted tubule, loop of Henle, distal convoluted tubule, and collecting duct. See also *kidney.*

nephropathy (nĕ-frop′ah-the) [*nephro-* + Gr. *pathos* disease] a general term for any disease of the kidneys. For more information see below and see the specific disease.

acute uric acid n., an acute condition characterized by the deposition of needlelike birefringent crystals of uric acid in the renal collection system, leading to urinary outflow obstruction and acute renal failure. This disorder is commonly seen in patients receiving cancer chemotherapy for leukemias and lymphomas. Peak serum uric acid concentrations are usually above 20 mg/100 ml. Careful monitoring of chemotherapeutic regimens will prevent this condition.

analgesic n., a condition characterized by tubulointerstitial inflammation and papillary necrosis. It is due to the excessive ingestion of analgesic preparations containing the combination of aspirin, phenacetin, and acetaminophen. Hematuria, renal colic, and secondary urinary infections are common. Urograms reveal ring shadows and cavities that are typical of papillary destruction. Elevated blood urea nitrogen, serum creatinine, and electrolytes (typical of renal failure) are often present. Individuals with this condition develop renal pelvic transitional cell carcinomas with a frequency greater than expected on the basis of chance.

Balkan n., see *Balkan n.* under *nephritis.*

diabetic n., a term for the kidney lesions observed in individuals with diabetes mellitus. These include glomerulosclerosis, arterionephrosclerosis, papillary necrosis, tubular lesions, and chronic interstitial nephritis. Renal dysfunction is the leading cause of death in diabetes. Glomerular lesions are most common and account for most of the clinical symptoms, including proteinuria, hypertension, and decreased glomerular filtration rate (GFR). For more information, see the specific disease.

gouty n., a chronic tubulointerstitial nephropathy seen in the prolonged hyperuricemia of gout. Crystalline deposits of uric acid and salts are seen in the parenchyma of the kidney, leading to urinary obstruction and inflammation. Infection, hypertension, and fibrosis may lead to renal failure. See also *gout.*

hemoglobinuric n., a form of acute tubulointerstitial nephropathy that results from acute renal damage secondary to the tubular infiltration of large amounts of soluble hemoglobin, usually following a transfusion reaction but occasionally occurring in other hemolytic processes. The disease presents with acute renal failure; renal damage is predominantly in the proximal convoluted tubular epithelium. Also called *transfusion nephritis.* See also *myoglobinuric n.* and *tubulointerstitial nephropathy.*

IgA n., see *Berger's disease.*

membranous n., see under *glomerulonephritis.*

myoglobinuric n., a form of acute tubulointerstitial nephropathy induced by a mechanism similar to that of hemoglobinuric nephropathy. This condition is usually secondary to crush injuries and burns that cause severe muscle damage. See also *hemoglobinuric n.* and *tubulointerstitial nephropathy.*

sickle cell n., a condition, seen in both heterozygous and homozygous forms of sickle cell disease, that is characterized by painless hematuria and failure of urinary concentration functions. Proteinuria is also common. Sickling leads to increased blood viscosity and microscopic infarcts in the renal cortex and adjacent structures and may progress to papillary necrosis. The condition may remit spontaneously.

tubulointerstitial n., see *tubulointerstitial nephropathy.*

nephroptosis (nef″-rop-to′sis) [*nephro-* + Gr. *ptōsis* falling] a downward displacement or other unusual mobility of the kidney due to congenital defects or trauma. This condition may predispose to infection in the upper urinary tract as a result of ureteral obstruction. The incidence of ureteral occlusion due to kidney movement is low.

nephropyelitis (nef″ro-pi″ĕ-li′tis) [*nephro-* + *pyelitis,* from Gr. *pylē* gate + *-itis* inflammation] an inflammation of the kidneys and the adjacent renal pelvis. See also *pyelonephritis.*

nephrosclerosis (nef″ro-sklĕ-ro′sis) [*nephro-* + Gr. *sklērōsis* hardening] a general term used to describe the vascular, renal tubular and glomerular changes caused by pre- or intrarenal vascular insufficiency in which the renal parenchyma undergoes atrophy and fibrosis and the glomeruli become scarred. Benign and malignant forms of nephrosclerosis are recognized.

benign n., a slowly evolving, diffuse, symmetric form of nephrosclerosis associated with benign hypertension and hyaline arteriolosclerosis (see also *arteriolosclerosis*). The morphologic changes seen in the kidneys include marked narrowing of the lumen of small intrarenal arteries and afferent arterioles caused by thickening and fibrosis of their walls, ischemic atrophy of the renal parenchyma including all portions of the nephron, and scarring, particularly of the glomeruli. Such changes are seen to varying degrees in the majority of kidneys examined at autopsy from individuals older than 60 yr. Benign nephrosclerosis rarely produces renal insufficiency; less than 5 percent of patients with well-developed benign nephrosclerosis die of renal failure.

malignant n., a form of nephrosclerosis that develops in individuals during the malignant phase of essential hypertension. It usually occurs in individuals younger than age 45 yr and is relatively uncommon, occurring in less than 5 percent of those with hypertension. The vascular lesions include fibrinoid necrosis of small arteries and afferent arterioles, and mucoid intimal hyperplasia of the interlobar arteries. Frequently there is concentric layering of collagen and fibroblasts, which imparts an onion-like appearance to the involved vessels. Vascular lumens are markedly narrowed and occasionally may be totally obliterated by proliferative endarteritis or may be occluded by fibrin thrombi. Cortical infarcts are common in those with severe vascular lesions.

Glomerular changes include fibrinoid necrosis of the capillary tufts, usually in continuity with similar changes in the corresponding afferent arteriole. Occasionally the entire glomerulus may be necrotic; more commonly, however, the necrosis affects only occasional glomerular lobules. In the most severe forms of malignant hypertension, glomerular proliferative changes with well-formed epithelial crescents may develop. Tubular atrophy and tubular loss, as well as progressive interstitial scarring and glomerular obsolescence, are common features of this condition.

In the absence of appropriate treatment, malignant hypertension is rapidly fatal with approximately 95 percent of individuals dying of renal failure and the remainder of either a cerebrovascular accident or cardiac disease within several months.

Also called hyperplastic arterionephrosclerosis. See also *hypertension.*

nephrosis (nĕ-fro′sis), pl. *nephroses* [*nephr-* + *-osis*] a syndrome characterized by proteinuria (in excess of 2 g/da, hypoalbuminuria, hyperlipidemia, and edema. The use of the term is frequently restricted to those who have the syndrome but who otherwise have normal renal function and normal urinary sediment. In such usage, the term is synonymous with primary or idiopathic nephrotic syndrome. The same constellation of findings can be found in individuals with renal insufficiency and abnormal urinary sediment, which signifies severe or advanced renal disease, usually of glomerular origin (secondary nephrotic syndrome).

amyloid n., see under *glomerulopathy.*

cholemic n., bile staining of the renal parenchyma in individuals with elevated bilirubin levels. It is not associated with intrinsic renal disease.

lipid n., see *lipoid n.*

lipoid n., a nonimmune complex renal disease characterized by alterations in basement membrane permeability to plasma proteins, and by reactive fusion of podocyte processes. It occurs predominantly in children younger than 8 yr, but may be associated with Hodgkin's disease and other neoplasms that alter T-cell function in older children and adults. The presenting features are usually those of the nephrotic syndrome, but the disease on occasion may present only with proteinuria. Also called epithelial cell disease, foot process fusion, *lipid nephrosis,* minimal change nephropathy, and minimal lesion. See also *glomerulopathy* and *nephrotic syndrome.*

toxic n., a form of nephrosis caused by toxic agents such as heavy metals (lead, cadmium, mercury, bismuth), mushroom poisoning, carbon tetrachloride, ethylene glycol, and miscellaneous chemicals and drugs. See also *acute tubular n.* and *tubulointerstitial nephropathy.*

nephrotic (nĕ-frot′ik) pertaining to, resembling, or caused by nephrosis.

nephrotic syndrome a clinical syndrome in which increased transglomerular passage of plasma proteins, primarily albumin, leads to heavy proteinuria, hypoalbuminemia, and edema. It may be associated with many different diseases. Diuretics and restriction of dietary sodium are used to control the edema; specific treatment depends on the underlying disorder.

Primary nephrotic syndrome due to lipoid nephrosis, focal glomerular sclerosis, membranous glomerulopathy, or proliferative or membranoproliferative glomerulonephritis accounts for about 90 percent of all cases in children and 75 percent in adults; the remaining cases are secondary conditions such as diabetes mellitus, amyloidosis, systemic lupus erythematosus, malignant neoplasms, infections, or nephrotoxic responses to drugs or poisons.

The characteristic clinical findings are proteinuria exceeding 3.0 g/da, plasma albumin below 3.0 g/dl, and hyperlipidemia with increased levels of cholesterol, phospholipids, triglycerides, and very-low-density lipoproteins.

See also *glomerulopathy.*

nephrotomography (nef″ro-to-mog′rah-fe) [*nephro-* + *tomography*] the tomographic demonstration of the kidneys. An opaque iodinated contrast medium is introduced intravenously by bolus injection or infusion or is injected directly into a cyst or tumor (percutaneous renal puncture).

nephrotoxin (nef″ro-tok′sin) an agent that causes toxic nephropathy. More specifically, the term connotes an exogenous chemical or abnormal endogenous substance that adversely affects the structure and/or function of the kidneys. Frequently, the damage is to the tubules, and, if severe, can lead to renal failure. Exogenous agents include heavy metals (gold, mercury, lead, bismuth), some antibiotics (amphotericin B, sulfonamides, polymyxins, aminoglycosides), analgesics (aspirin-phenacetin), radiographic contrast media, organic solvents (carbon tetrachloride), and pesticides.

nephrotuberculosis (nef″ro-tu-ber″ku-lo′sis) [*nephro-* + *tuberculosis*] tuberculosis involving the kidneys. Hematuria and "sterile" pyuria are the most common symptoms. Intravenous pyelography may reveal communication between the renal cortex and calyceal system due to cavity formation and erosion. The kidney is the second most frequent site of tuberculosis infection. See also *tuberculosis.*

nephrourography (nef″ro-u-rog′rah-fe) [*nephro-* + *urography*] the radiologic examination of the renal parenchyma, calices, and pelvis and the urinary tract following intravenous infusion of a water-soluble iodinated contrast medium such as diatrizoate or iothalmate. Nephrotomograms are made immediately and urograms at delayed intervals.

neptunium (Np) (nep-tu′ne-um) [from the planet *Neptune*] a silvery, metallic radioactive element; atomic number 93; most stable isotope, Np-237 (half-life, 2.14 million yr); a 5f transition element (actinide rare earth); oxidation states +3 through +7. It is used in neutron detectors.

Nernst equation (nernst) [Walther *Nernst,* German physicist, 1864-1941] an equation used to determine the electrode potential (voltage) of a half-cell or the membrane potential across a semipermeable membrane.

For a half-cell, $E = E^{\circ} - (RT/zF)\ln Q$, where E is the electrode potential, E° is the standard electrode potential (standard reduction potential), R is the gas constant (8.3143 J/mol·K), T is the absolute temperature, z is the number of electrons transferred in the redox reaction, F is the Faraday constant (96,487 C/mol), and Q is the reaction quotient of the half-reaction (in the simplest case, the concentration of the reduced species derived by that of the oxidized species). At 25°C this equation can be simplified to $E = E^{\circ} - (0.0592\ \text{V})(\log\ Q)/z$.

For a membrane, $E = (RT/zF)\ln Q$, where E is the membrane potential, Q is the ratio of the concentrations of any diffusible ion on the two sides of the membrane, and z is the ionic charge.

nerve (nerv) [L. *nervus;* Gr. *neuron*] a bundle of nerve cell processes with their investing connective tissue. The term gives no indication of the number of component processes and is loosely extended to include a single nerve cell or neuron. The terms nerve and nerve fiber are essentially synonymous. Nerves propagate electric impulses known as action potentials to their terminations (on structures such as muscles, glands, and other nerves), initiating specific responses in the structures that they innervate.

The structure of a nerve is a composite of its component parts, the cytoplasmic processes (axons) of neurons. Each axon is invested either by the cytoplasm of a series of Schwann cells, as in an unmyelinated nerve, or by multilayered wrappings of Schwann cell membranes (myelin sheath), as in a myelinated nerve. The myelin sheath is not continuous, but is interrupted periodically at the nodes of Ranvier. In the central nervous system, oligodendrocytes perform the same function as the Schwann cells of the peripheral nervous system. Unmyelinated and myelinated nerves supported by collagen are mingled in a peripheral nerve. Individual axons are invested by a connective tissue sheath (the endoneurium). Groups of axons are separated into bundles known as fascicles. Fascicles are delineated from one another by a connective tissue sheath (the perineurium) that is an extension of the epineurium, the outermost sheath of connective tissue that encases the entire nerve trunk.

An axon consists of its cytoplasm or axoplasm within which there are scattered mitochondria and longitudinally aligned fine filaments and microtubules. The neurofilaments provide some internal support and possibly play an orienting role in regeneration. The neurotubules are believed to facilitate passage of material down the axon from cell body to nerve ending. The axon is enclosed within a cell membrane across which there is a resting potential of approximately 90 mV. The diameter of an axon is proportional to its conduction velocity, and several classes of peripheral nerve fibers have been defined.

See also *action potential, myelin sheath, neuron,* and *Schwann cell.* For more information, see the accompanying illustrations and table.

fiber spectra of peripheral n., the range of fiber diameters in a nerve. The range of conduction velocities in a nerve is directly proportional to the range of fiber diameters.

nerve block regional anesthesia produced by the introduction of a local anesthetic near a nerve or nerves, thereby blocking conduction and producing anesthesia in the distribution of the nerve or nerves.

nerve cell a neuron, with its axon and dendritic processes, collaterals, and terminations; it is regarded as the structural unit of the nervous system. See also *neuron.*

nerve cell staining histologic techniques for staining nerve cells and their processes. Good general staining methods for nervous system tissues are hematoxylin and eosin, phosphotungstic acid–hematoxylin (PTAH), and periodic acid–Schiff (PAS); PTAH may be used after PAS. Some may also be combined with Luxol fast blue, used to stain myelin, or cresyl violet, used to stain Nissl granules.

There are several silver impregnation methods that are specific stains for nerve cell processes and neurofibrils; see *Bielschowsky's method, Bodian's method,* and *Holzer's method.*

The Golgi method is the classic one used for histologic study of the nervous system. Formalin-fixed tissue blocks are oxidized in potassium dichromate, impregnated with silver nitrate, dehydrated, embedded in paraffin, and cut in thick (100 μm) sections. Only about 1 percent of the neurons are stained, but these isolated cells are completely stained. All of their processes can be followed.

nerve conduction the self-propagation of an action potential along the nerve cell membrane. In an unmyelinated nerve, the action potential initiates a local, circular current flow that in turn causes the successive electrotonic depolarization to threshold level of that area of cell membrane immediately in front of the action potential. The cell membrane behind the moving impulse is refractory; thus, the wave of depolarization is spread only in the forward direction.

nerve conduction studies the noninvasive neurophysiologic methods used to evaluate the status of peripheral sensory and motor nerve function in patients with suspected peripheral neuropathy. These procedures may be employed to establish a diagno-

NERVE. TABLE OF VARIOUS FIBER TYPES

Fiber Type	Aα			Aδ	C
	Group I		*Group II*	*Group III*	*Group IV (Unmyelinated)*
Diameter (includes myelin sheath, where present)	5-20 μm			2-5 μm	0.1-1.5 μm
	12-20 μm		5-12 μm		
Conduction velocity	30-120 m/s			5-30 m/s	0.5-2 m/s
	70-120 m/s		30-70 m/s		
Receptor types	Primary endings in muscle spindles (IA) Golgi tendon organs (IB)		Secondary endings in muscle spindles Most other encapsulated endings Larger diameter mechanoreceptors and interoreceptors	Thermoceptors Nociceptors Smaller diameter mechanoreceptors and interoreceptors	
Other fiber types	α Motor fibers, 12-20 μm		γ Motor fibers, 2-8 μm	Autonomic preganglionic fibers 1.5-4 μm (B fibers)	Autonomic postganglionic fibers; olfactory nerve fibers, 0.1-1 μm

From Weiss L., and Greep, R. O.: Histology. 4th ed. New York, McGraw-Hill Book Co., 1977, p. 354.

sis, evaluate the extent of a peripheral nerve lesion, and determine the nature of the underlying pathology.

Nerve conduction studies examine evoked responses with respect to the various distances along the nerve at which the electric stimulus used to elicit them is applied. When the motor fibers of a peripheral nerve are stimulated (a procedure termed motor nerve conduction studies), the evoked compound muscle action potential is called the M response. In sensory nerve conduction studies, compound nerve action potentials are elicited.

The apparatus used in nerve conduction studies consists of a standard electromyograph system (see *electromyography*) into which a stimulator has been incorporated. The stimulator must be capable of delivering stimuli (repetitive or single) lasting approximately 0.05–0.2 msec, an amplitude of up to 300 V (i.e., of enough intensity to evoke maximal responses yet not so large as to spread to adjacent nerves), and a frequency of 0.5–50 Hz. The stimulus output is made to trigger the sweep of an oscilloscope and appear as a stimulus artifact on the cathode-ray screen.

Typically, surface (or less commonly, monopolar needle) electrodes are used for stimulation. When the stimulation is bipolar, the electrodes are placed as close as possible to the underlying nerve, with the cathode positioned nearest to the active recording electrode. Recording electrodes also are commonly of the surface type unless the evoked response is of low amplitude, in which case concentric needle electrodes are frequently used. In sensory conduction studies, the reference electrode is positioned over the nerve about 4 cm distal to the active recording electrode. In both types of studies, a ground electrode is placed between the stimulus and recording electrodes.

MOTOR NERVE CONDUCTION STUDIES. Such studies are an aid to distinguishing between peripheral nerve disorders and those disorders that involve anterior horn cells or the muscle itself. They can also help determine the site of a localized peripheral lesion, as the size and the shape of an M response evoked from above the lesion site often are different from those of a response evoked from more distal stimulation.

Another important measurement in studies of motor nerve conduction is the conduction velocity, which is the speed at which an impulse is propagated (in the largest fibers) between two points on a nerve; it can be calculated by dividing two easily measurable quantities. The difference between the conduction time or latency of the M responses evoked from two stimulation sites is divided into the distance along the nerve between the two sites, yielding a conduction velocity (meters per second). The two latencies are measured by evoking an M response from both distal and proximal nerve stimulation sites. In both instances, the time interval between the stimulus onset and the response (the latency) is determined from the distance between the stimulus artifact and the response on the oscilloscope screen. The length of the nerve segment between the two sites is measured on the skin surface. A reduced conduction velocity can be found in peripheral nerve disorders such as compression or entrapment neuropathies, diabetic neuropathy, Charcot-Marie-Tooth disease, and Guillain-Barré syndrome.

Other electric potentials can be evoked from a muscle when its motor nerve is stimulated. The H reflex is a monosynaptic reflex response to stimulation of Ia motor nerve fibers. Evoked by stimuli of a lower amplitude and frequency than those commonly used to elicit a maximal M response, it is most readily evoked from the soleus muscle innervated by the tibial nerve and the S1 root. Such a measurement is of use in the studies of unilateral S1 radiculopathy (the H reflex latency is absent or prolonged on the side affected) and of conduction velocity over long nerve segments; it may also be useful in the diagnosis of nerve dysfunction disorders such as Guillain-Barré syndrome. The F wave, most easily recorded from hand or foot small muscles, is thought to be the muscle response to antidromic activation. Its measurement is sometimes useful in the detection of lumbosacral root injury and of thoracic outlet syndrome, and in determining whether motor root avulsions are involved in injuries to the brachial plexus.

SENSORY NERVE CONDUCTION STUDIES. These studies record the compound nerve action potentials evoked by stimulation of the nerve at another point, and do not involve muscles or neuromuscular junctions, unlike motor nerve conduction studies. Clinical importance is given to the conduction velocity (in the fastest conducting fibers, the Ia fibers), the peak-to-peak amplitude, and the configuration of the evoked action potential. An approximation of conduction velocity is made by division of the latency (the time it takes an impulse to be propagated along the segment of nerve between the stimulating and recording electrodes) by the distance between the intervening nerve segment.

Sensory conduction studies that detect deviation in the shape, amplitude, and/or conduction velocity of sensory nerves can be useful in the diagnosis of peripheral neuropathies and also give objective data regarding its severity. Such studies are also helpful in distinguishing peripheral nerve disorders from those involving lesions proximal to the dorsal root ganglion.

In all studies of conduction in peripheral nerves, accurate interpretation of the results depends on use of the many standardized techniques developed for examination of each of the major nerves.

See also *conduction velocity, F wave, H reflex,* and *latency.*

nerve cord any trunk or bundle of nerve fibers.

nerve endings the peripheral terminations of an axon. Motor nerve endings are found in muscle and glands (see *motor end-plate*). The peripheral end of a sensory axon may display various types of structural specialization, which to some degree subserves the particular sensory function of the axon. Sensory nerve endings include Meissner's corpuscle, *Merkel cell,* and *pacinian corpuscle.*

annulospiral n. e., wide, ribbon-like sensory nerve endings that are wrapped around the intrafusal muscle fibers of a muscle spindle. See also *muscle spindle.*

flower-spray n. e., branched, slender sensory nerve endings on the sarcolemma of intrafusal muscle fibers of muscle spindles.

free n. e., the simplest type of sensory receptor, formed by the division of a peripheral nerve axon into fine arborizations devoid of specialized end-or-

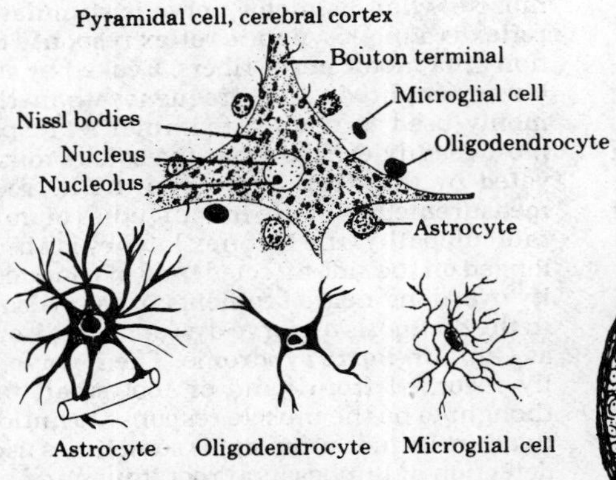

Three types of human neuroglial cell. (King and Showers.)

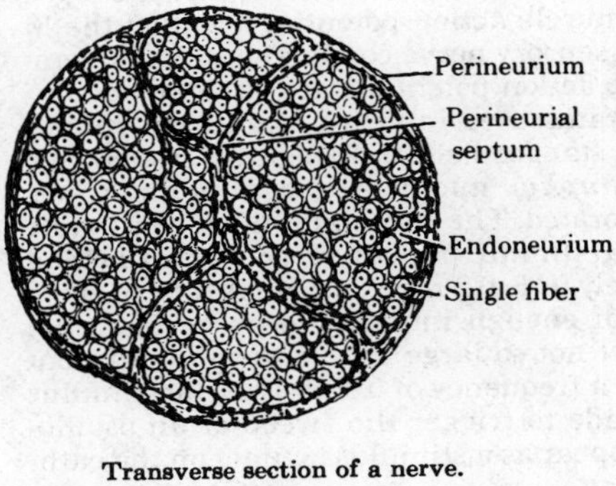

Transverse section of a nerve.

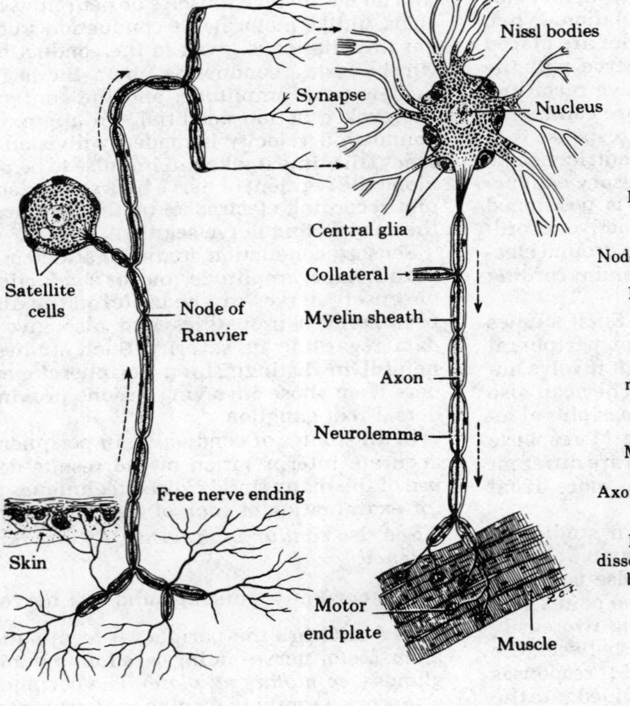

Diagrammatic representation of two types of neurons. (King and Showers.)

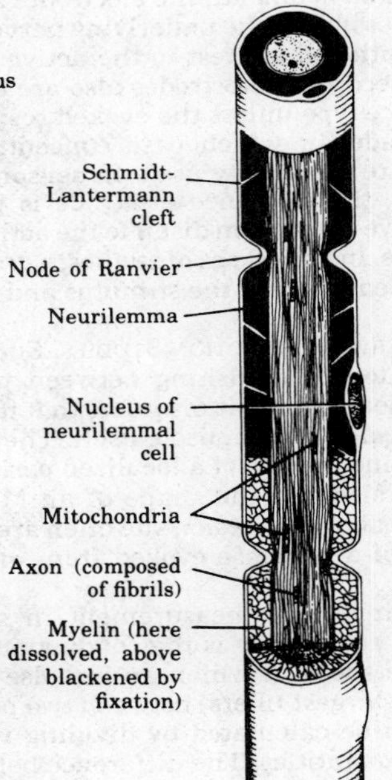

Longitudinal section of a nerve fiber (Leeson and Leeson).

Nerve, Figure 1. Details of the structure of components of nerve tissue. (From Dorland's Illustrated Medical Dictionary. 26th ed. Philadelphia, W. B. Saunders Co., 1981.)

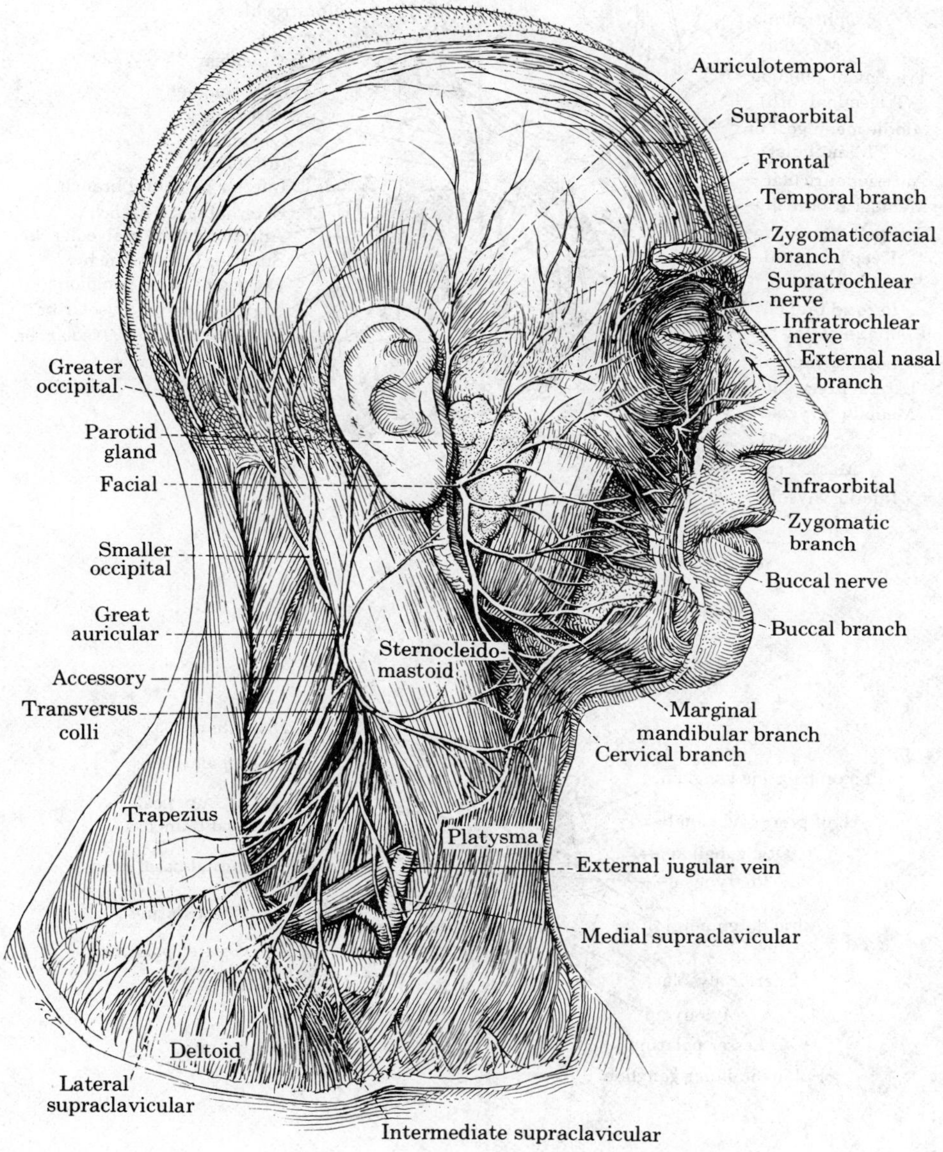

Nerve, Figure 2. Superficial nerves and muscles of the head and neck. (From Dorland's Illustrated Medical Dictionary. 26th ed. Philadelphia, W. B. Saunders Co., 1981.)

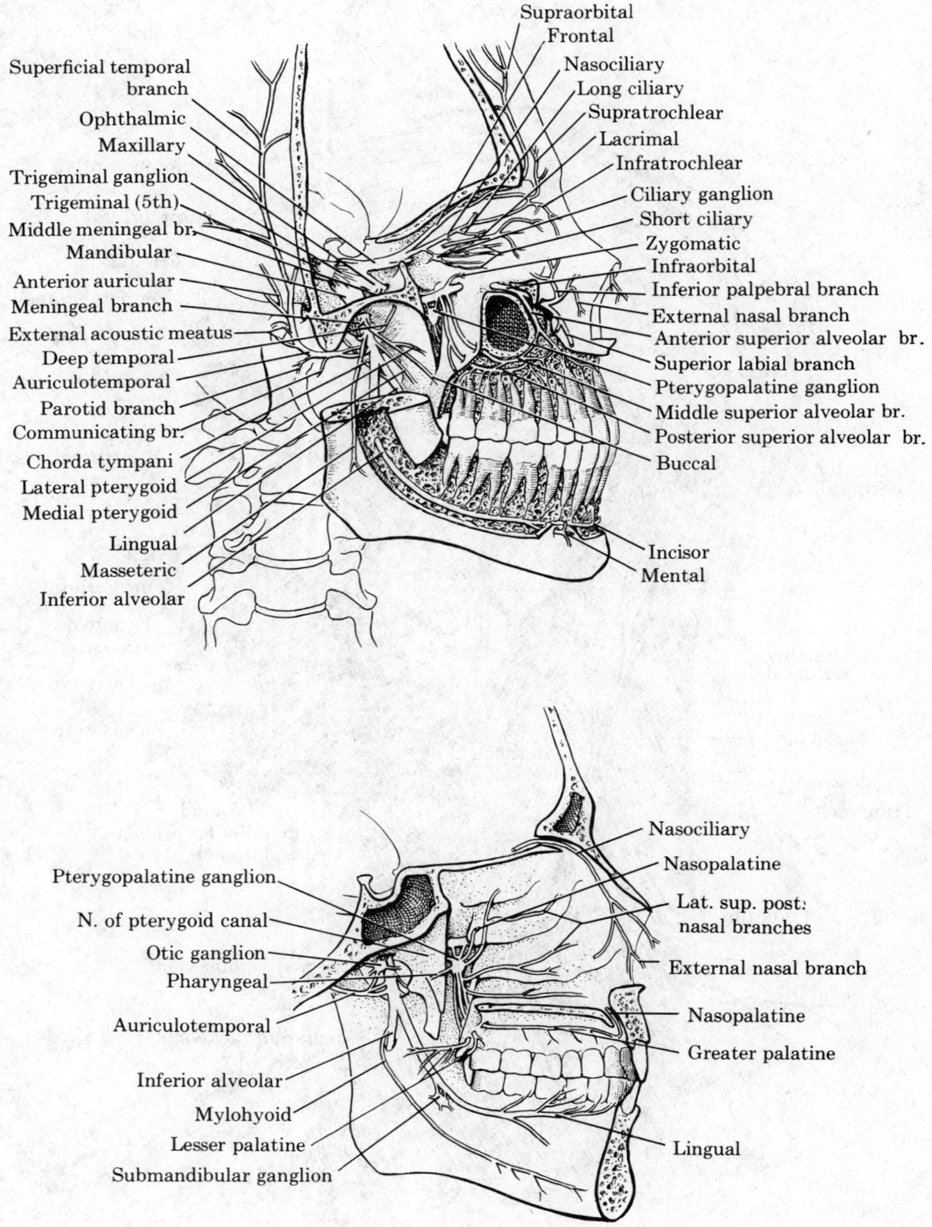

Nerve, Figure 3. Deep nerves shown in relation to the bones of the face. (From Dorland's Illustrated Medical Dictionary. 26th ed. Philadelphia, W. B. Saunders Co., 1981.)

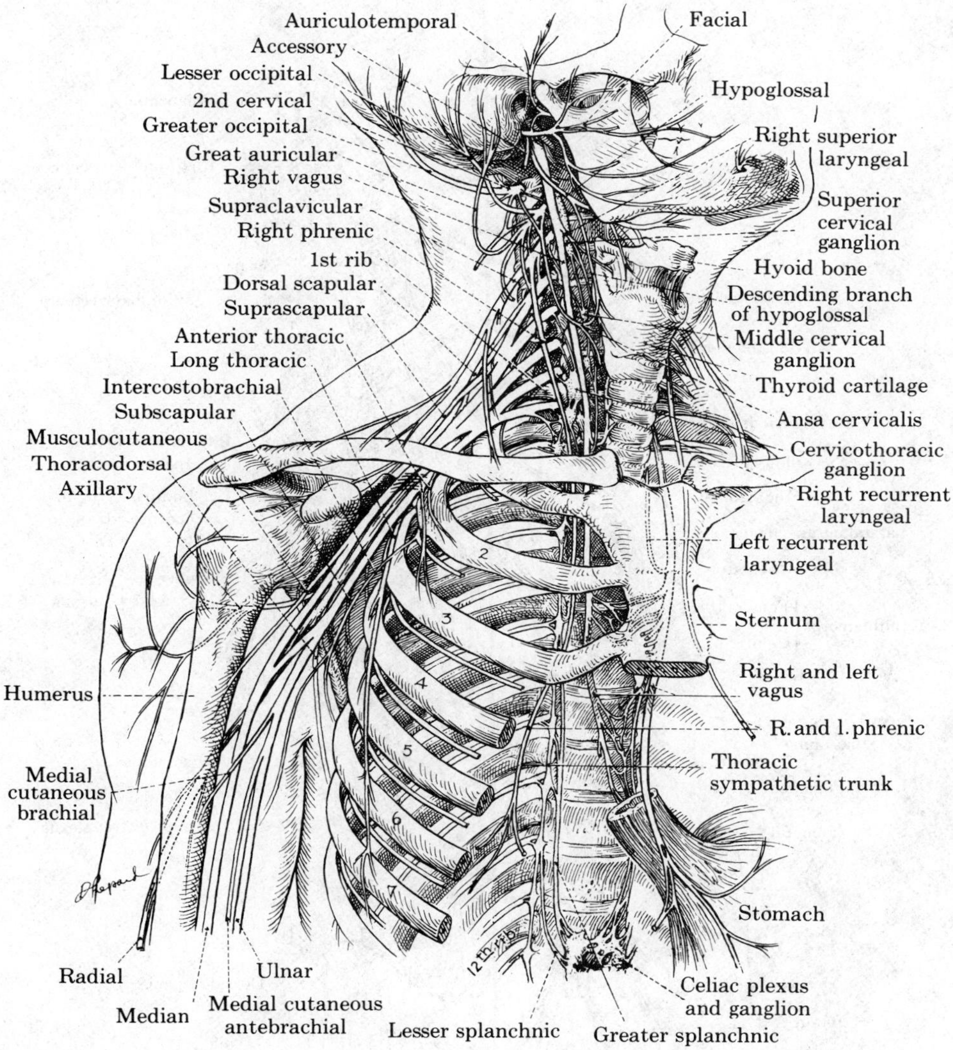

Nerve, Figure 4. Deep nerves of the neck, axilla, and upper thorax. (From Dorland's Illustrated Medical Dictionary. 26th ed. Philadelphia, W. B. Saunders Co., 1981.)

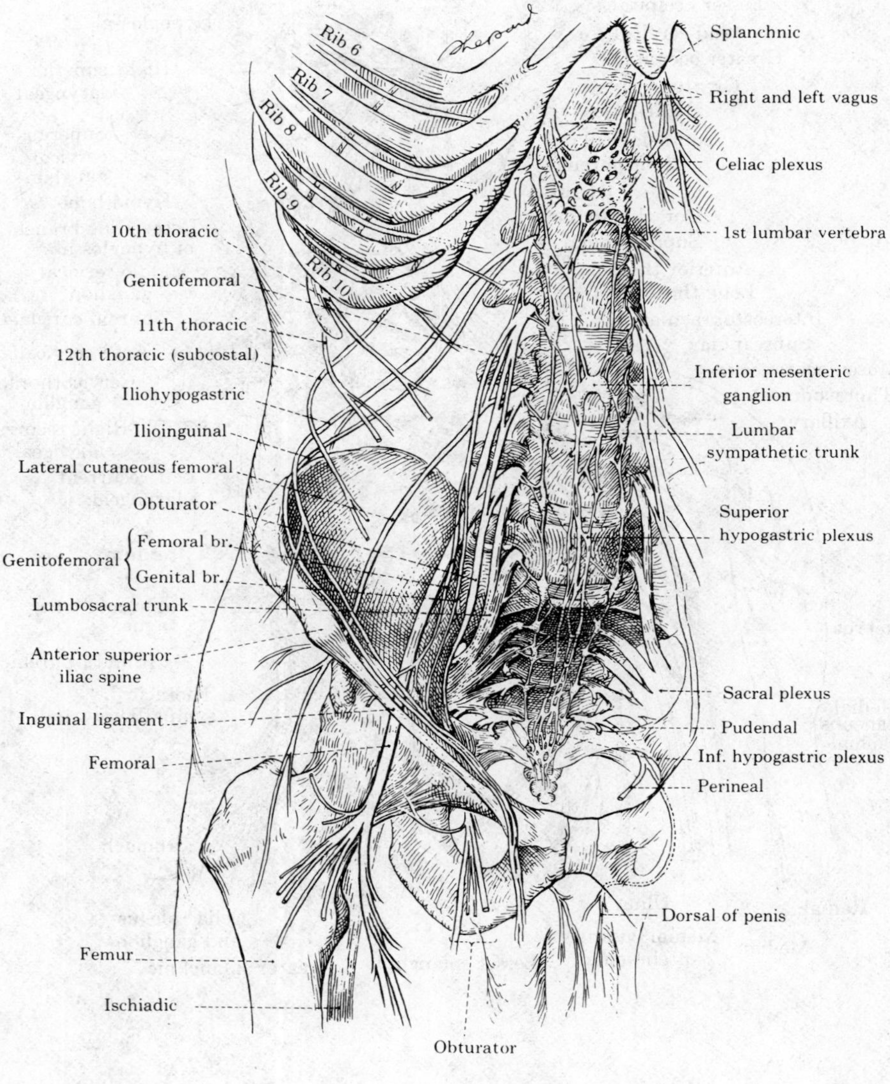

Nerve, Figure 5. Deep nerves of the lower trunk. (From Dorland's Illustrated Medical Dictionary. 26th ed. Philadelphia, W. B. Saunders Co., 1981.)

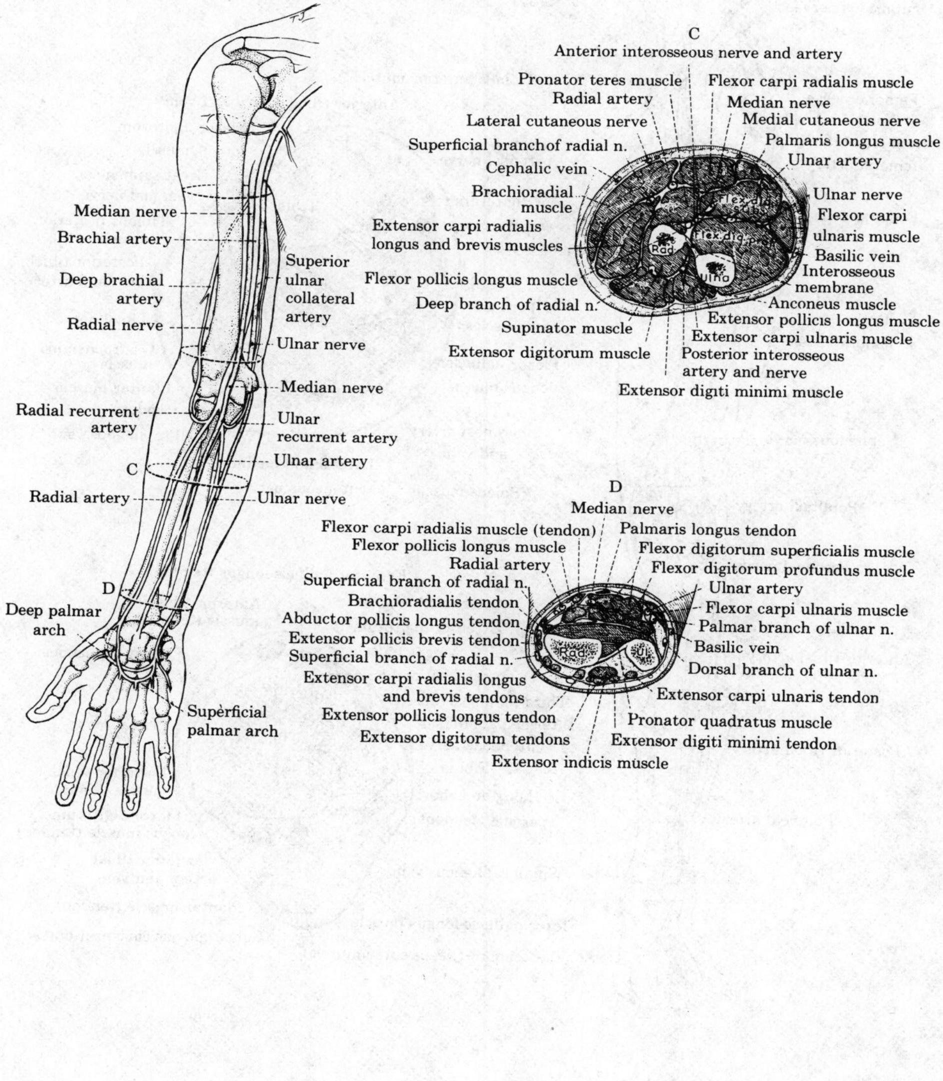
Median nerve
Brachial artery
Deep brachial artery
Radial nerve
Superior ulnar collateral artery
Ulnar nerve
Median nerve
Radial recurrent artery
Ulnar recurrent artery
C
Ulnar artery
Radial artery
Ulnar nerve
D
Deep palmar arch
Superficial palmar arch
C
Anterior interosseous nerve and artery
Pronator teres muscle
Flexor carpi radialis muscle
Radial artery
Median nerve
Lateral cutaneous nerve
Medial cutaneous nerve
Superficial branch of radial n.
Palmaris longus muscle
Ulnar artery
Cephalic vein
Brachioradial muscle
Ulnar nerve
Extensor carpi radialis longus and brevis muscles
Flexor carpi ulnaris muscle
Basilic vein
Flexor pollicis longus muscle
Interosseous membrane
Deep branch of radial n.
Anconeus muscle
Extensor pollicis longus muscle
Supinator muscle
Extensor carpi ulnaris muscle
Extensor digitorum muscle
Posterior interosseous artery and nerve
Extensor digiti minimi muscle
Rad
Ulna
D
Median nerve
Flexor carpi radialis muscle (tendon)
Palmaris longus tendon
Flexor pollicis longus muscle
Flexor digitorum superficialis muscle
Radial artery
Flexor digitorum profundus muscle
Superficial branch of radial n.
Ulnar artery
Brachioradialis tendon
Flexor carpi ulnaris muscle
Abductor pollicis longus tendon
Palmar branch of ulnar n.
Extensor pollicis brevis tendon
Basilic vein
Superficial branch of radial n.
Dorsal branch of ulnar n.
Extensor carpi radialis longus and brevis tendons
Extensor carpi ulnaris tendon
Extensor pollicis longus tendon
Pronator quadratus muscle
Extensor digitorum tendons
Extensor digiti minimi tendon
Extensor indicis muscle

Nerve, Figure 6. Nerves of the right upper extremity. (From Dorland's Illustrated Medical Dictionary. 26th ed. Philadelphia, W. B. Saunders Co., 1981.)

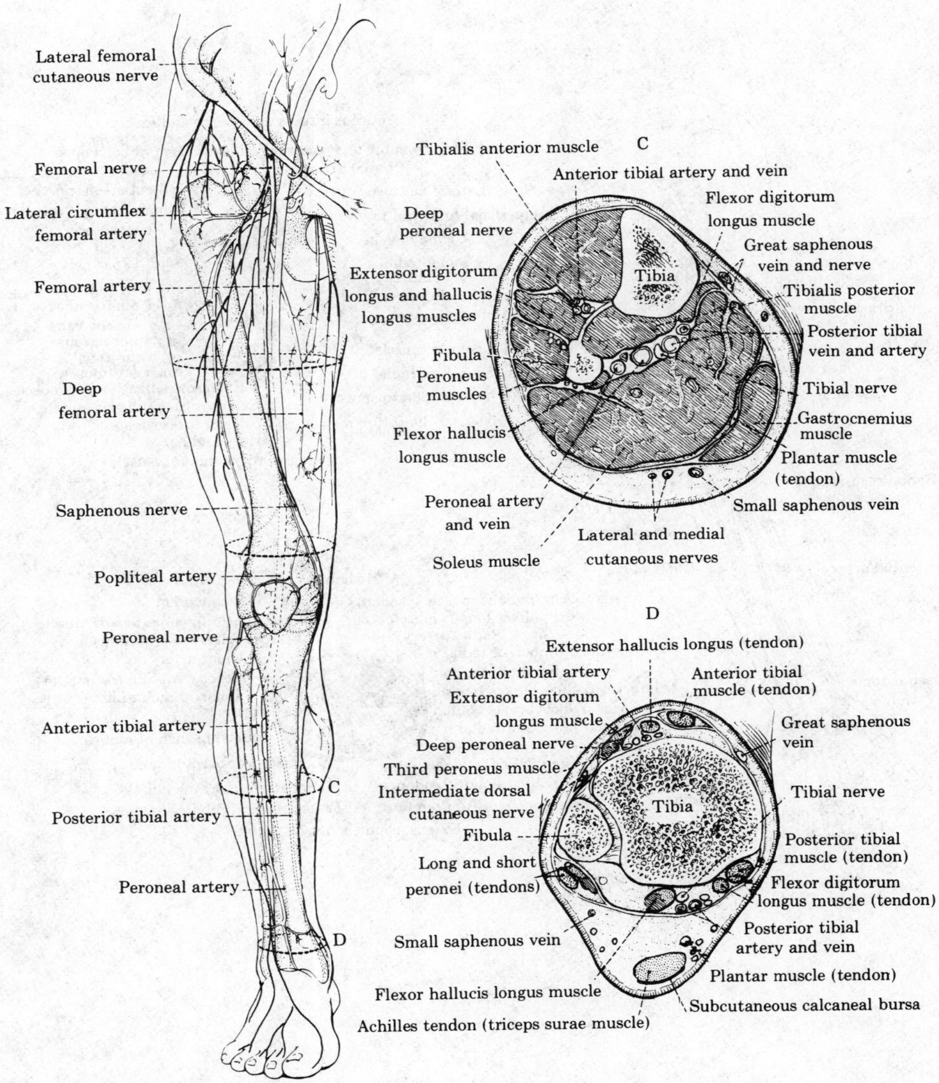

Nerve, Figure 7. Nerves of the right lower extremity. (From Dorland's Illustrated Medical Dictionary. 26th ed. Philadelphia, W. B. Saunders Co., 1981.)

gans. These nerve endings are found in the skin in contact with the outer root sheath epithelium of hair follicles, and some penetrate into the epidermis. The axons remain at least partially invested by Schwann cell cytoplasm up to the immediate vicinity of their termination. The function of free nerve endings in human skin and their relationship to specialized end-organs is uncertain, it is possible that the structural modifications of sensory axon terminals to some degree reflect their location, and the network of free endings may subserve all types of cutaneous sensory perception.

nerve fiber see *nerve.*

nervonic acid (ner-von′ik) an unsaturated fatty acid, *cis*-15-tetracosenoic acid, present as a constituent of brain sphingolipids, e.g., sphingomyelin.

nervous system the organ system composed of the brain, spinal cord, peripheral nerves, and receptor organs, which functions to enable the organism to respond appropriately to changes in its internal or external environment. The structural and functional cellular units of the nervous system are the neurons (or nerve cells) and glial cells. Changes in the membrane potential of the neurons (the action potential) in response to various stimuli are the signals transmitted by the nervous system.

Anatomically, the nervous system can be subdivided into the central nervous system (CNS), consisting of the brain and spinal cord, and the peripheral nervous system. The peripheral components can be subdivided physiologically into those elements or afferent fibers that convey action potentials from sensory receptors toward the CNS, and those efferent fibers that convey information from the CNS to the effector organs (skeletal, cardiac, or smooth muscle, and glandular tissue). Efferent fibers innervating skeletal muscles constitute the somatic nervous system, whereas those innervating cardiac or smooth muscle and glands constitute the autonomic nervous system.

See also *action potential, autonomic nervous system, brain, glial cell, nerve, neuron, nervous system, somatic nervous system,* and *spinal cord.*

nesidioblastosis (ne-sid″e-o-blas-to′sis) [Gr. *nēsdion* islet + *blastos* germ + *-osis*] islet cell hyperplasia and postnatal islet neogenesis evolving from pancreatic ductal cells. This condition has been observed in infants of diabetic mothers; in diabetic subjects receiving long-term sulfonylurea therapy; and experimentally with corticosteroids, glucagon-induced chronic hyperglycemia, and tolbutamide administration. Its finding in association with MEN (multiple endocrine neoplasia) syndrome has been explained by postulating that the stimulus for nesidioblastosis is inherited as an autosomal genetic defect with a high penetrance. The resulting chronic hypersecretion of one or more of the islet cell hormones may then trigger a neoplastic transformation of other endocrine glands in the body.

nesslerization (nes″ler-ĭ-za′shun) the formation of a colored product by adding Nessler's reagent to a solution containing ammonia.

Nessler reaction (nes′ler) [A. *Nessler,* German chemist, 1827–1905] the formation of a product (possibly $NH_2Hg_2I_3$), yellow to orange-brown in color, by reaction of Nessler's reagent, an alkaline solution of mercuric iodide and potassium iodide, with ammonia. It is a very sensitive and specific test for ammonia, which was previously used widely in the measurement of the concentration of urea and nonprotein nitrogen in body fluids.

nesting (nes′ting) 1. the inclusion of a block of data or a subroutine inside another block of data or subroutine.

2. in a computer program, the inclusion of a loop within the range of another loop so that the inner loop is executed several times during each execution of the outer loop.

nests of Brunn (Brōōn) [Albert von *Brunn,* German anatomist, 1849–1895] groups of transitional epithelial cells in the superficial lamina propria of the urinary bladder. They may be in contact with or detached from the overlying epithelium. Also called von Brunn's nests.

net (net) 1. a meshlike structure of fibers or strands. Also called *network* and *reticulum.*

2. a group of communications stations that are capable of direct intercommunication.

net protein ratio (NPR) see *dietary p.* see under *protein.*

net protein utilization (NPU) see *dietary p.* under *protein.*

network (net′werk) 1. an electrical circuit.

2. a graph consisting of a set of points linked by line segments. The points represent locations in a system, and the line segments represent flows of material or information between points. The line segments are assigned numbers indicating the capacity and direction of the flow. See also *flow chart* and *network analysis.*

3. see *net.*

network analysis 1. the derivation of the operating characteristics of an electrical circuit from its configuration and component values.

2. a management method used to analyze how to accomplish a specific objective on schedule. For each subtask of the objective, the time needed to accomplish it and the order in which it must be performed are determined. Paths are charted through the network of subtasks ordering them into that sequence in which each requires input from the preceding one. The critical path is the path that takes the most time and that determines the time required to complete the whole project. One form of this method is known as PERT, an acronym for program evaluation and review technique.

neur/o (nu′ro) [Gr. *neuron* nerve] a word element used in combining form to denote nerve, e.g., neuroblast.

neural (nu′ral) [L. *neuralis,* from Gr. *neuron*] pertaining to nerves.

neural crest a region of the early embryonic nervous system from which paraneuronal cells migrate to various peripheral locations.

Early in its third week, the embryo is a flattened oval disk formed by apposed ectoderm and endoderm. The two layers become separated by insinuating mesodermal cells but remain partially attached in the midline, where the ectoderm thickens (over the developing notochord). The lateral margins of this midline bar of ectoderm grow dorsally and then toward one another to fuse and create the neural tube. The column of cells lying in the line of fusion constitutes the neural crest.

Cells from the neural crest stream laterally and migrate to various parts of the body, where they form sensory neurons, Schwann cells, postganglionic autnomic neurons and the satellite cells of autonomic ganglia, some sensory receptor cells, a few of the APUD (amine precursor uptake and decarboxylation) series of cells, meningeal (pia-arachnoid) cells, odontoblasts, and melanocytes.

neuralgia (nu-ral'je-ah) [*neur-* + Gr. *algos* pain + *-ia* condition] a general term used to describe sudden and recurrent attacks of pain that occur along the distribution of the affected nerve. The pain is typically lancinating and severe, lasting only a few seconds.

glossopharyngeal n., a rare neurologic disorder characterized by paroxysmal attacks of sharp, stabbing pain in the distribution of the ninth cranial (glossopharyngeal) nerve. The attacks may occur spontaneously or be precipitated by movement (e.g., chewing, swallowing, sneezing, or talking), and the pain may last from seconds to minutes, affecting the base of the tongue and radiating to the ears or anterolateral neck. Generally, the cause of this condition is unknown and no pathologic lesions can be found. It usually occurs after age 40.

trigeminal n., a disorder, usually of uncertain etiology, characterized by episodes of severe facial pain, lasting typically for seconds or minutes, and often triggered by touching or moving the involved areas. The pain usually occurs in the distribution of the mandibular and maxillary branches of the trigeminal nerve (cranial nerve V). Similar symptoms may occasionally be a manifestation of multiple sclerosis or a posterior fossa space-occupying lesion.

neuralgic amyotrophy (nu-ral'jik ah"mi-ot'ro-fe) see *brachial neuritis.*

neural plate in the developing embryo, the thickened layer or plate of ectoderm that develops into the neural tube.

neural tube in the developing embryo, a tube formed during the fourth week by the development of the ectodermal neural plate, which forms the central nervous system.

neural tube defects two congenital malformations of the nervous system, anencephaly and spina bifida cystica, that are considered to be manifestations of a single entity because they occur together statistically more frequently than would be expected on the basis of chance. Neural tube defects are thought to involve multifactorial inheritance; the genetic component is small. There is a large geographic variation in the incidence (about 0.1–0.5 percent). The recurrence rate is 3–5 percent if there is one affected child and 5–10 percent if there are two or more. The sex ratio is two to three females to one male.

Amniocentesis is used for the prenatal diagnosis of neural tube defects. The amniotic fluid alpha-fetoprotein (AFP) concentration is elevated; the more open the defect, the more abnormal the AFP concentration. This test is 90 percent positive for anencephaly and 50 percent positive for spina bifida. AFP is also elevated in other anomalies, such as duodenal atresia, congenital nephrosis, omphalocele, and tetralogy of Fallot. Fetal bleeding produces false-positive results. Gross anomalies are confirmed by ultrasonography or amniography.

See also *anencephaly* and *spina bifida cystica.*

neuraminic acid (nur-ah-min'ik) 3,5-dideoxy-5-aminononulosonic acid, a nine-carbon pyranose keto-sugar molecule of D-configuration, created biosynthetically from derivatives of pyruvate and mannosamine. See also *N-acetylneuraminate.*

neuraminidase (nur-ah-min'i-dās) an enzyme of the hydrolase class (acylneuraminyl hydrolase, EC 3.2.1.18) that catalyzes the hydrolysis of glucosidic linkages between a sialic acid residue and a hexose or hexosamine at the nonreducing terminal of oligosaccharides present in glycoproteins, glycolipids, and proteoglycans. Neuraminidase, along with hemagglutinins, is located as spicules on the outer coat of the influenza virus. The virus attaches to the host cell by receptors for the hemagglutinins, causes its damage, and is then released from the host cell by neuraminidase, which digests the sialic acid in the glycoprotein receptor. A genetic deficiency of neuraminidase, transmitted as an autosomal recessive trait, leads to a condition known as mucolipidosis I. See also *influenza virus* and *sialidase digestion.*

neurapraxia (nu"rah-prak'se-ah) [*neur-* + Gr. *apraxia* absence of action] a partial or complete conduction block over a local segment of a nerve fiber that produces temporary paralysis. The pathologic basis for neurapraxia is segmental demyelination. Stimulation at a point distal to the block results in a normal conduction velocity and evoked muscle action potential.

neurasthenia (nu"ras-the'ne-ah) [*neur-* + Gr. *astheneia* debility] a syndrome characterized by abnormal fatigue, depression, physical and mental lethargy, and feelings of inadequacy. Originally regarded as an important neurosis, the diagnosis is now rarely made, as most patients with neurasthenia have either an anxiety neurosis or depression. Also called nervous prostration.

neurectoderm (nur"ek'to-derm) [*neur-* + Gr. *ektos* outside + *derma* skin] a slightly depressed region of thickened ectoderm dorsal to the notochord, which gives rise to the neural plate.

neurilemma (nu"rĭ-lem'mah) [*neur-* + Gr. *eilēma* a closely adhering sheath] a thin layer of loose connective tissue that surrounds a myelinated or unmyelinated nerve fiber.

neurilemmitis (neu"rĭ-le-mi'tis) inflammation of the neurilemma of a nerve. See also *neuritis.*

neurilemmoma (nu"rĭ-lem-mo'mah) See *schwannoma.*

neuroarthropathy (nu"ro-ar-throp'ah-the) [*neuro-* + Gr. *arthron* joint + *pathos* disease] central or peripheral nerve disease or damage that is associated with joint disease. The joint structure is often subject to cumulative damage and extensive degenerative changes, often with persistent effusion. Radiographic features include widespread destruction and hypertrophic changes.

neuroblast (nu'ro-blast) [*neuro-* + Gr. *blastos* germ] 1. in the embryo, primitive nerve cells, the precursors of the neurons of the central and peripheral nervous systems.

2. a cell of a neuroblastoma.

neuroblastoma (nu"ro-blas-to'mah) [*neuro-* + Gr. *blastos* germ + *-oma*] the malignant tumor of neuroblasts, precursor cells of elements of the nervous system. It is an aggressive neoplasm that occurs in early childhood—more than 80 percent of patients are under the age of 4 yr, but a few cases in adults have been reported. Most neuroblastomas arise within or near the adrenal glands, although some are located in the posterior mediastinum, head and neck region, and pelvis.

In localizing the primary tumor, x-ray studies including soft tissue radiographs, pyelograms, and CT scans are helpful. Neuroblastomas frequently have metastasized by the time the primary tumor is detected, and bone marrow spread is common.

In the diagnosis, measurements of the breakdown products of norepinephrine in the urine (vanillylmandelic acid, VMA, and homovanillic acid, HVA) may be useful, although their concentrations are not always elevated. The tumor must be biopsied for a precise diagnosis, and the light microscopic histology of sheets of small round cells (generally lacking cytoplasmic glycogen), with occasional rosettes, coupled with the clinical findings, may be sufficient to establish the diagnosis. Where other small round cell tumors such as Ewing's tumor, rhabdomyosarcoma, and leukemia/lymphoma cannot be excluded, electron microscopy should be employed: demonstration of the dendritic processes of the tumor cells containing microtubules and small, dense-core granules is diagnostic.

olfactory n., a neuroblastoma arising from, and showing differentiation toward, the olfactory epithelium. It arises in the nasal cavity above the middle turbinate, is initially unilateral but spreads to the other half of the nasal cavity, and may infiltrate the paranasal sinuses, retrobulbar orbit, or middle cranial fossa. True olfactory differentiation is relatively uncommon among nasal neuroblastomas: most tumors so diagnosed occur in older individuals and are better designated neuroendocrine carcinomas.

neurochoroiditis (nu″ro-ko″roi-di′tis) [*neuro-* + Gr. *choroid* + *-itis*] an inflammation of the optic nerve and choroid, often due to metabolic disorders such as the lipidoses and ataxias or infections with granulomatous inflammation. Frequently the retina is involved (neurochorioretinitis).

neurocutaneous (nu″ro-ku-ta′ne-us) [*neuro-* + *cutaneous*] relating to the nervous system and the skin.

neurocutaneous syndrome the association of a neurologic disorder with certain cutaneous abnormalities. The major disorders in this group include neurofibromatosis, tuberous sclerosis, von Hippel–Lindau syndrome, Sturge-Weber syndrome, and ataxia telangiectasia. For more information, see the individual diseases. Also called *phakomatosis.*

neurodermatitis (nu″ro-der″mah-ti′tis) [*neuro-* + Gr. *derma* skin + *-itis*] a general term for inflammations of the dermal layer of the skin that have a variety of causes, most commonly emotional factors. This condition is often classified as disseminated (atopic neurodermatitis) or localized (lichen simplex chronicus). See also *eczema* and *l. simplex chronicus* under *lichen.*

neuroencephalomyelopathy (nu″ro-en-sef″ah-lo-mi″ĕ-lop′ah-the) [*neuro-* + Gr. *enkephalos* brain + *myelos* marrow + *pathos* disease] a general term for any disease that affects the nerves, brain, and spinal cord.

neuroendocrine (nu″ro-en′do-krin) [*neuro-* + Gr. *endon* within + *krinein* to separate] pertaining to the nervous and endocrine systems, and especially to their interaction.

neuroendocrine carcinoma a general term for a small cell carcinoma of the dendritic, granule-containing cells of the diffuse neuroendocrine system. Histologically resembling a neuroblastoma, these neoplasms occur in adults in locations unusual for a primary neuroblastoma. Cutaneous neuroendocrine carcinomas are believed to be of Merkel cell origin. See also *Merkel cell tumor.*

neuroepithelioma (nu″ro-ep″ĭ-the″le-o′mah) [*neuro-* + *epithelium* + *-oma*] a term of imprecise connotation that has been used for certain primitive neoplasms of the central or peripheral nervous system. In the brain it may encompass medulloepitheliomas and primitive tumors of uncertain origin. In the peripheral nervous system, the term has been applied to tumors of probable Schwann cell derivation, in which epithelial elements are present or the cells have a pseudoepithelial appearance.

neuroepithelium (nu″ro-ep″ĭ-the′le-um) [*neuro-* + *epithelium*] 1. the simple columnar epithelium composed of specialized cells that serve as receptors of external stimuli and as the sensory cells of the cochlea, nasal mucosa, and tongue.

2. in the developing embryo, the epithelium of the ectoderm from which the cerebrospinal axis is formed.

neurofibril (nu″ro-fi′bril) [*neuro-* + L. *fibrilla* filament] see *neurofilament.*

neurofibroma (nu″ro-fi-bro′mah) [*neuro-* + L. *fibra* fiber + *-oma*] a neoplasm of Schwann cells that can arise adjacent to the spinal cord or anywhere in the peripheral nervous system. Neurofibromas involving the skin are common and often multiple. More collagen and fibroblasts are present than in schwannomas, but ultrastructurally the cells are similar. See also *neurofibromatosis.*

neurofibromatosis (nu″ro-fi″bro-mah-to′sis) a disorder characterized by the presence of multiple neurofibromas and numerous pigmented skin lesions commonly referred to as café au lait spots. Although this disease is transmitted as an autosomal dominant trait, many cases appear to arise as mutations. The neurofibromas may appear anywhere on the skin and internally. In a small percentage of patients, malignant transformation of a neurofibroma occurs. Other tumors of neural origin, including meningiomas, gliomas, and pheochromocytomas, also occur in association with this syndrome. Also called *von Recklinghausen's disease.*

neurofilament (nu″ro-fil′ah-ment) [*neuro-* + L. *filamentum*] a 10 nm–wide filament in the perikaryon of neurons. Also called *neurofibril.*

neurogenic (nu″ro-jen′ik) [*neuro-* + Gr. *gennan* to produce] 1. originating in the nervous system.

2. forming nervous tissue.

neurogenic bladder a condition characterized by impaired bladder control. Lesions in the spinal cord produce urgency and frequency of urination with small bladder capacity, strong reflex contractions, and poor voluntary control (spastic bladder). Lesions of the segmental innervation (S2, S3, S4) interfere with both voluntary and reflex control and produce impaired sensation of bladder fullness; incontinence may result (flaccid overflow bladder).

Neurogenic bladder almost always occurs in the setting of other neurologic dysfunction. Urinary tract infection is a common complication.

neuroglia (nu-rog′le-ah) [*neuro-* + Gr. *glia* glue] the supporting elements of the nervous system; nonexcitable cells that compose by weight more than 50 percent of the central nervous system. There are two basic classes of neuroglial cells: the macroglia, which includes the astrocytes and the oligodendrocytes, and the microglia.

neuroglia stains see *astrocyte staining, Holzer's method, Mallory's phosphotungstic acid–hematoxylin (PTAH) method,* and *Penfield's method.*

neurohypophysis (nu″ro-hi-pof′ĭ-sis) [*neuro-* + *hypophysis*] the part of the pituitary gland that is embryologically derived from a downgrowth (infundibulum) of the floor of the diencephalon. It includes the pars nervosa and the infundibular stalk. See also *hypophysis.*

neuroleptanalgesia (nu″ro-lep″tan-al-je′ze-ah) a state of dissociative anesthesia produced by the administration of a neuroleptic agent (such as droperidol) in combination with a narcotic analgesic (such as fentanyl).

neuroleptanesthesia (nu″ro-lep″tan-es-the′ze-ah) a state of neuroleptanalgesia and unconsciousness produced by the administration of nitrous oxide after neuroleptanalgesia has been established.

neuroleptic (neu″ro-lep′tik) [*neuro-* + Gr. *lēpsis* a taking hold] 1. pertaining to a drug that has antipsychotic activity without producing sedation.

2. a neuroleptic drug. Also called *antipsychotic drug* and *major tranquilizer.*

neurologic (nu-ro-loj′ik) pertaining to nerves or the nervous system.

neurologist (nu-rol′o-jist) a specialist in the nervous system or in the treatment of diseases of the nervous system.

neurology (nu-rol′o-je) [*neuro-* + *-logy*] the branch of medical science that deals with the nervous system, both normal and diseased.

neuroma (nu-ro′mah) [*neuro-* + *-oma*] a lesion formed by a tangle of regenerated nerve fibers, commonly following interruption of a peripheral nerve by trauma or amputation. The haphazardly grouped axons and Schwann cells are intermingled with collagen and fibroblasts.

acoustic n., see *schwannoma.*

amputation n., a traumatic neuroma occurring after amputation of an extremity or part.

Morton's n., a form of traumatic neuroma located in the interdigital space between the third and fourth toes. It is painful on weight bearing and tends to recur following excision. Also called *Morton's disease,* Morton's metatarsalgia toe or foot, and plantar neuroma.

mucosal n., a submucosal nodule, many of which involve the anterior tongue, lips, and tarsal plates of the eyes in MEN (multiple endocrine neoplasia) syndrome, type III (or IIb), in association with medullary carcinoma of the thyroid and pheochromocytoma. These structures have been called ganglioneuromas, as they contain ganglion cells in addition to haphazardly arranged axons intermingled with Schwann cells and collagenous tissue. The term mucosal neuroma, although not precise, avoids confusion with the neoplastic ganglioneuroma.

traumatic n., a neuroma arising after accidental or purposeful sectioning of the nerve.

neuromalacia (nu″ro-mah-la′she-ah) [*neuro-* + Gr. *malakia* softening] the abnormal softening of a nerve and, frequently, of its adjacent structures in response to disease.

neuromere (nu′ro-mēr) [*neuro-* + Gr. *meros* part] in the developing embryo, any of a series of masses of nerve tissue in the ventral lamina of the hindbrain that are separated by six transverse rhombic grooves. Neuromeres are closely associated with motor nuclei of some of the cranial nerves. Also called *rhombomere.*

neuromuscular (nu″ro-mus′ku-lar) pertaining to the nerves and muscles.

neuromuscular blockade a failure in neuromuscular transmission that can be induced by a variety of disturbances at the neuromuscular junction. In myasthenia gravis, neuromuscular blockade may be related to a reduction in the number of postsynaptic acetylcholine receptor sites. With botulism and myasthenic syndrome (Eaton-Lambert), release of acetylcholine from the presynaptic terminal is defective. Pharmacologic agents such as curare block neuromuscular transmission by competing with acetylcholine for available postsynaptic membrane receptor sites; others (physostigmine, neostigmine, edrophonium) may cause blockade through antagonism of the acetylcholinesterase system.

Abnormalities in neuromuscular transmission can be evaluated electrophysiologically by examination of the responses of the involved muscle to repetitive nerve stimuli action or through use of single-fiber electromyography.

neuromuscular blocker a drug that blocks the transmission of nerve impulses at the motor end-plate of skeletal muscles. See also *cholinergic receptors.*

neuromuscular junction the terminal of a motor neuron innervating a skeletal muscle fiber. Also called *myoneural junction.* See also *motor end-plate.*

neuromuscular transmission the chemically mediated transmission of an action potential from nerve to muscle across the neuromuscular junction. The arrival of a wave of depolarization at the presynaptic membrane brings about the liberation of 100–200 quanta of acetylcholine from the synaptic vesicles. The released acetylcholine diffuses across the synaptic cleft and, by reacting with receptor sites on the postsynaptic membrane, results in an increase in the permeability of the membrane to small cations. This increased permeability gives rise to a local depolarization of the postsynaptic membrane (the end-plate potential); when the depolarization reaches the threshold level, a propagated action potential is triggered and spreads from the muscle end-plate along the membrane of the fiber. Action of the acetylcholine ends when it is hydrolyzed by the enzyme acetylcholinesterase.

A disease (such as myasthenia gravis or botulism) that interferes with any of these physiologic events results in an impairment of neuromuscular transmission.

See also *neuromuscular blockade* and *neuromuscular junction.*

neuromyelitis (nu″ro-mi″ĕ-li′tis) [*neuro-* + Gr. *myelos* marrow + *itis*] a general term used to describe the inflammation of a nerve and its myelin sheaths.

n. optica, a condition characterized by bilateral inflammation of the optic nerves, with acute and selective demyelination. In many cases, there is subsequent spinal cord involvement. Blindness, pain, and loss of sphincter control may occur. This disorder is considered to be a variant form of multiple sclerosis. Also called Devic's syndrome.

neuromyositis (nu″ro-mi″o-si′tis) [*neuro-* + Gr. *myos* of muscle + *-itis*] a general term used to describe inflammation that affects a muscle and its nerves.

neuromyotonia (nu″ro-mi″o-to′ne-ah) [*neuro-* + Gr. *mys* muscle + *tonos* tension + *-ia*] a clinical syndrome that is associated with numerous types of electrical discharge. It is characterized by the continuous activity of skeletal muscle fibers, with associated stiffness and rippling of involved muscles.

neuron (nu′ron) [Gr. "nerve"] any of the excitable cells of the nervous system that are concerned with the reception, integration, transformation, and transmission of information. A neuron typically consists of a cell body, with its branching dendrites that conduct impulses toward the cell body, and axon, which conducts impulses away from the cell body.

afferent n., a neuron that conducts a nervous impulse from a peripheral sensory receptor toward the central nervous system.

efferent n., a neuron that conducts a nervous impulse from a center to an organ of response.

Golgi type I n.'s, pyramidal neurons with very long axons, that leave the gray matter of the central nervous system, traverse the white matter, and terminate in the periphery. Also called Golgi cells.

Golgi type II n.'s, stellate neurons with short axons that do not pass out of the gray matter in which the cell body lies; they are especially numerous in the cerebral and cerebellar cortices and in the retina. Also called Golgi cells and cells of van Gehuchten.

intercalated n., see *interneuron.*

motor n., see *motor neuron.*

multipolar n., a neuron with several to many processes; such neurons vary in shape, depending on the arrangement of the processes, with pyramidal and stellate (star) shapes being common. Also called polymorphic neuron.

postganglionic n.'s, neurons whose cell bodies are situated in the autonomic ganglia and whose purpose is to relay impulses beyond the ganglia.

preganglionic n.'s, neurons whose cell bodies lie in the CNS and whose efferent fibers terminate in the autonomic ganglia.

sensory n., any neuron possessing a sensory function; an afferent neuron conveying sensory impulses.

unipolar n., a neuron with a single process. True unipolar neurons are rare except in the early embryo, although they occasionally persist in the adult central nervous system.

neuronal (nu′ro-nal) pertaining to a neuron or neurons.

neuronophagia (nu″ron-o-fa′je-ah) [*neuro-* + *-phagia,* from Gr. *phagein* to eat] the process by which microglial cells surround and phagocytize degenerating nerve cells.

neuroparalysis (nu″ro-pah-ral′ĭ-sis) paralysis due to disease of a nerve or nerves.

neuropathic (nu″ro-path′ik) pertaining to, causing, or characterized by neuropathy.

neuropathology (nu″ro-path-ol′e-je) [*neuro-* + Gr. *pathos* disease + *-logy*] the study of diseases of the nervous system, as reflected in altered morphology.

neuropathy (nu-rop′ah-the) [*neuro-* + Gr. *pathos* disease] a general term used to describe a variety of diseases and disorders of the peripheral nervous system. These conditions may be acute, subacute, chronic, or chronic relapsing in nature; the causes may be known or unknown. The term applies to peripheral nerve lesions, whether inflammation is present or absent. Single or multiple (polyneuropathy) nerves may be involved. For more information, see below and see also the specific disease. Cf. *neuritis.*

alcoholic polyneuropathy, a form of neuropathy, which may be nutritional or due to the direct toxic effect of alcohol, that is characterized by paresthesias in the distal extremities. There is also distal symmetric muscle weakness and wasting that is greater in the legs than in the arms. The onset is usually insidious with slow progression, but it may be fulminant.

Diagnosis is aided by the finding of slowed nerve conduction velocity and axonal degeneration on electrophysiologic testing. Recovery, although often incomplete, usually occurs after treatment with thiamine and abstinence from alcohol.

Pathologically there is severe axonal degeneration of the peripheral nerves and, occasionally, the spinal roots. Degeneration is greater distally than proximally.

See also *alcoholic c.* under *cardiomyopathy* and *alcoholic m.* under *myopathy.*

amblyopia n., a disorder characterized by lesions of the papillomacular bundle of the optic nerve that result in a characteristic form of visual impairment. It is related to nutritional deficiencies and is thought to be influenced by alcohol and tobacco toxicities.

amyloid n., the neuropathy that results from accumulation of amyloid in the peripheral nervous tissue. When it occurs as an hereditary condition, transmitted as an autosomal dominant trait, it is characterized by paresthesias and pain in the extremities. The condition may also contribute to the development of an entrapment neuropathy such as carpal tunnel syndrome.

Studies of the conduction velocity of the affected nerves may reveal slowing. Electromyographic findings may reveal partial denervation consistent with peripheral neuropathy.

cis-platinum n., a distal sensory neuropathy that occasionally occurs after prolonged treatment with the cancer chemotherapeutic agent cis-platinum.

diabetic n., a disorder of nerves and nerve function that occurs in diabetes mellitus. It is characterized by segmental demyelination as well as axonal degeneration. It may involve single or multiple sensory and motor nerves as a mononeuropathy or polyneuropathy. The autonomic nervous system also is often affected. The pathogenesis is unknown, but both vascular and metabolic factors appear to be important.

entrapment n., a form of neuropathy that occurs when a nerve is subjected to compression, stretch, or angulation as it comes into contact with structures such as fibroosseous canals, space-occupying lesions, joints, or other anatomic passageways. Demyelination of the affected segment may occur, particularly in the largest fibers of the nerve. If the compression is severe, degeneration of axons may also be found.

Electromyographic and electroneurographic

techniques are of use in localizing the entrapment site, and generally reveal that conduction velocity is slowed or completely blocked across the affected site. Evoked responses are changed with respect to their size and shape and may be temporally dispersed, and electrical abnormalities may be present in muscles innervated by the affected nerve.

For more information about specific entrapment syndromes, see the individual entries (e.g., *carpal tunnel syndrome, injection palsy, sleep palsy,* and *thoracic outlet syndrome*).

hereditary sensory radicular n., a hereditary disorder, transmitted as an autosomal dominant trait, that is characterized by signs of radicular sensory deficit in the upper and lower extremities, shooting pains, marked loss of pain and temperature sensation, trophic ulceration of the feet, and sometimes deafness.

Electromyographic and electroneurographic examination can reveal evoked potentials that are abnormally low in amplitude, fibrillation potentials and indication of chronic denervation in the distal musculature, and motor nerve conduction velocities in the low range of normal. Conduction in sensory nerves is markedly abnormal. Degeneration of the dorsal root ganglia and (secondarily) of the olivary nuclei, optic nerves, and cerebellum can be revealed on pathologic examination.

hypertrophic interstitial n., a rare, progressive, usually hereditary disease, transmitted as a recessive or dominant trait, that is characterized by hyperplasia of the interstitial connective tissue of nerves and proliferation of the neurilemma cells (Schwann sheath). The peripheral nerves, ganglia, and roots become thickened, and axonal destruction occurs. Clinically, patients exhibit a motor and sensory polyneuropathy, with weakness, sensory loss, and depressed tendon reflexes. Nerve conduction velocities are markedly slowed. Diagnosis requires the histologic demonstration of hypertrophied nerves, with onion-bulb changes and hypomyelinated regions. No specific treatment is available.

peripheral n., a general term for any of the variety of disorders that involve degeneration and/or demyelination of a peripheral nerve or nerve root. The typical symptoms include paresthesias, pain and weakness. Hyporeflexia, impairment of sensation, and motor weakness tend to be most pronounced in the distal segments of the limbs. The cerebrospinal fluid protein concentration may or may not be elevated.

A peripheral neuropathy may occur as a consequence of trauma, infection, neoplasm, exposure to toxic compounds, or vascular and metabolic disorders. Electromyography, nerve conduction velocity testing, and muscle and nerve biopsies may help to distinguish the individual disorders.

See also *polyneuropathy.*

retrobulbar n., a condition characterized by impaired vision in one or both eyes, which may progress to blindness. In many cases the cause is unknown; however, demyelinating diseases, viral infections, vascular disorders, and tumors may be responsible. Demyelination in the optic nerve is commonly present. The CSF may contain increased numbers of lymphocytes and elevated protein. Visual evoked responses usually reveal slowed conduction in the optic nerve. Also called optic neuritis.

vincristine n., a peripheral neuropathy that results from the chemotherapeutic administration of *Vinca* alkaloids, especially vincristine. Neural involvement may be motor, sensory, or autonomic in nature. Weakness, pain, and sensory defects are common manifestations of this therapy; constipation and intestinal obstruction may also occur. These complications may require termination or interruption of vincristine chemotherapy.

neurophysiology (nu″ro-fiz″e-ol′o-je) [*neuro-* + *physiology*] the study of the physiology of the nervous system.

neuropil (nu′ro-pil) [*neuro-* + Gr. *pilos* felt] a dense, complex meshwork of interlacing axon terminals, dendrites, and neuroglial elements found in the central nervous system and in some parts of the peripheral nervous system.

neuroretinitis (nu″ro-ret″ĭ-ni′tis) [*neuro-* + *retina* + *-itis*] the inflammation of both the optic nerve and the retina, which may be due to trauma, infectious diseases, or metabolic disorders.

neuroretinopathy (nu″ro-ret″ĭ-nop′ah-the) [*neuro-* + *retina* + Gr. *pathos* disease] a general term used to describe diseases that affect the optic disk and the retina.

neurosarcoma (nu″ro-sar-ko′mah) one of several synonyms for a malignant tumor of Schwann cells. Others are neurofibrosarcoma, neurogenic sarcoma, and malignant schwannoma.

neurosclerosis (nu″ro-sklĕ-ro′sis) [*neuro-* + Gr. *sklēros* hard + *-osis* condition] the hardening of a nerve, nerve structure, or accessory nerve substance in response to a variety of pathologic conditions.

neurosecretory (nu″ro-se-kre′to-re) [*neuro-* + *secretory*] pertaining to the production of complex substances by neurons that are released from their terminals either onto effectors or into the blood stream.

neurosis (nu-ro′sis), pl. *neuroses* [*neur-* + *-osis* condition] a general term for psychologic disorders in which symptoms are due to emotional disorders. Most psychiatrists believe neurosis arises from a conflict between the instinctual drives (id) and conscious thought (ego). Behavior may be greatly affected although usually it remains within societal limits of acceptance. The principal manifestations of neurosis include excessive anxiety, hysterical symptoms, phobias, depression, and obsessive-compulsive behavior.

neuroskeletal (nu″ro-skel′ĕ-tal) pertaining to nervous and skeletal muscle tissue.

Neurospora (nu-ros′po-rah) a genus of fungi that belongs to the family Neurosporaceae, order Sphaeriales. It is commonly used by mycologists for genetic research and is utilized in the food industry of Indonesia.

neurosyphilis (nu″ro-sif′ĭ-lis) the central nervous system manifestations of syphilis, which can be divided into four groups; (1) asymptomatic neurosyphilis, diagnosed when there is a positive VDRL test in the cerebrospinal fluid; (2) meningovascular syphilis, which may result in cranial nerve palsies, meningitis, or cerebrovascular thrombosis and infarction; (3) tabes dorsalis, a progressive degenerative disease of the dorsal columns of the spinal cord with impairment of peripheral reflexes and proprioceptive sensation; and (4) general paresis, a chronic meningoencephalitis resulting in loss of cortical function and leading to personality changes, seizures, aphasia, and paralysis. See also *general p.* under *paresis, syphilis,* and *tabes dorsalis.*

neurotoxin (nu″ro-tok′sin) a substance that is poisonous or destructive to nerve tissue, especially the exotoxins secreted by *Corynebacterium diptheriae, Clostridium tetani* and *C. botulinum,* and *Shigella dysenteriae.* These organisms act by selectively blocking certain presynaptic terminals in the central nervous system. See also *exotoxins.*

neurotransmitter (nu″ro-trans′mit-er) a compound that serves to transmit a nervous impulse between cells, as at synapses and neuromuscular junctions. These compounds include acetylcholine, epinephrine, norepinephrine, dopamine, serotonin, γ-aminobutyrate, glycine, glutamate, and possibly some oligopeptides. Also called *synaptic transmitter.*

neurotubule (nu″ro-tu′būl) [*neuro-* + *tubule*] one of the long, straight microtubules, approximately 25 nm in diameter, longitudinally aligned within an axon or dendrite. See also *microtubule.*

neurovascular (nu″ro-vas′ku-lar) pertaining to the nerves that control the caliber of blood vessels.

neutr/o (nu′tro) [L. *neuter* neither] a word element used in combining form to denote neutral or neither acid nor base, e.g., neutrophil.

neutral (nu′tral) [L. *neutralis*] in chemistry, neither acidic nor basic; having neither a positive nor a negative charge.

neutral fats the most abundant group of lipids in nature, esters of fatty acids with glycerol. Mono-, di-, and triacylglyceryl esters occur, the triacylglycerols being the most abundant.

neutralization (nu″trah-lĭ-za′shun) the reaction of an acid with a base yielding a salt and water.

neutralization test see under *antistreptolysin O tests.*

neutralize (nu′tral-īz) to render neutral.

neutralizing antibody an antibody directed against a microorganism, in particular a virus, that prevents the microorganism from infecting the cells. The antibody may be titered by incubating serial dilutions of serum with fixed amounts of virus and cells in culture. The reciprocal of the highest dilution of serum that inhibits the virus's ability to infect the cells is the neutralizing antibody titer.

neutral red a basic aniline fluorochrome dye; C.I. 50040. It is used primarily in Schiff reagents, although it may be used as a pH-dependent indicator for potassium cyanide.

neutrino (nu-tre′no) [It. "little neutron"] an elementary particle that has zero rest mass and charge and spin 1/2. Neutrinos interact only by the weak force and thus have a negligible effect on matter. They are emitted by the beta-decay process.

neutron (n) (nu′tron) [*neutral* + *-on*] an elementary particle that has no charge, spin 1/2, and approximately the mass of a proton. A neutron has a half-life of 12 m but is stable when bound in an atomic nucleus. It is composed of three quarks.

neutron activation analysis an extremely sensitive, nondestructive technique for the quantitative determination of chemical elements. The sample is irradiated with neutrons, which interact with atoms in the sample and produce radioactive products.

These products can be identified by the characteristic energy spectrum of the emitted gamma rays. Arsenic-15, for example, absorbs neutrons to produce arsenic-76, which emits 559-keV gamma rays. Quantities of only a few nanograms—the amount found in about 50 hairs after a fatal poisoning—can be detected. This technique is too complicated for routine use but serves as a basis for reference procedures. It may be used to determine two-thirds of all the elements.

neutron capture a nuclear reaction in which a neutron is absorbed by a nuclide. Approximately 8 MeV of energy is immediately emitted, usually as gamma rays, an (n, γ) reaction. Protons, neutrons, and alpha particles can also be emitted, depending on the neutron speed and the target nuclide; these are (n, p), (n, 2n), and (n, α) reactions. Neutron capture reactions are the source of reactor-produced radioisotopes used in nuclear medicine.

neutropenia (noo″tro-pe′ne-ah) a reduction in the absolute neutrophil count below the lower reference limit, 2000 per mm^3 for white individuals and 1300 per mm^3 for blacks. It may be produced by several mechanisms including decreased or ineffective neutrophil production in the bone marrow, increased loss of neutrophils from the blood, and "pseudo" neutropenia in which there is a shift from the circulating granulocyte pool to the marginal granulocyte pool.

Neutropenia can be caused by the administration of drugs (particularly by cancer chemotherapy but also as an idiosyncratic response to many other drugs) and by exposure to radiation. It is associated with the acute leukemias, many infections, rheumatoid arthritis, congestive splenomegaly, and vitamin B_{12} deficiency. There are also several forms of congenital neutropenia.

neutrophil (nu′tro-fil) [*neutro-* + Gr. *philein* to love] a mature granulocytic leukocyte; also called *neutrophilic leukocyte.* See *polymorphonuclear neutrophil.*

neutrophilic granules (nu″tro-fil′ik) see *granules of developing neutrophils.*

neutrophilic leukemia see *chronic myelogenous l.* under *leukemia.*

neutrophilic leukocyte see *neutrophil.*

nevocarcinoma (ne″vo-kar″sĭ-no′mah) [*nevoid* + *carcinoma*] see *malignant m.* under *melanoma.*

nevoid (ne′void) [*nevus* + Gr. *eidos* form] associated with or resembling a nevus.

nevoxanthoendothelioma (ne″vo-zan″tho-en″do-the″le-o′mah) [*nevoid* + Gr. *xanthos* yellow + *epithelium* + *-oma*] see *xanthogranuloma, juvenile.*

nevus (ne′vus), pl. *nevi* [L. *naevus* birthmark, mole] any of a number of cutaneous hamartomas including melanocytic, epidermal, vascular, and connective tissue, most of which are apparent at birth.

blue n., a melanocytic nevus characterized by an aggregate of pigmented dendritic melanocytes within the dermis, forming a cutaneous nodule that is usually small and well circumscribed. Clinically, in natural light, this nevus has a bluish coloration.

cellular blue n., a blue nevus composed of nests of compact cells, ovoid to spindle-shaped, with associated dendritic pigmented melanocytes. See also *blue n.*

connective tissue n., a localized cutaneous lesion caused by either an increase or decrease of collagenous tissue, elastic tissue, or fat within the dermis or subcutaneous tissue.

epidermal n., a localized overgrowth of epidermis, which may involve the surface epidermis or epidermal appendages (see the accompanying table).

PRINCIPAL COMPONENTS OF EPIDERMAL NEVI (CUTANEOUS ORGANOID NEVI)

Surface Epidermis
Various forms of epidermal hyperplasia, hyperkeratosis, and dyskeratotic lesions
Inflammatory dermatosis-like nevi
Epidermal Appendages
Sebaceous glands
Sebaceous nevus of Jadassohn
Apocrine glands
Nevus syringocystadenoma papilliferum
Apocrine nevus
Eccrine glands
Eccrine nevus
Eccrine angiomatous hamartoma
Hair follicle
Nevus comedonicus
Trichofolliculoma

giant hairy n., a large, congenital melanocytic nevus, usually greater than 5–10 cm in greatest diameter, and generally associated with prominent hair formation in the distribution of the nevus.

halo n., a cutaneous melanocytic nevus surrounded by a depigmented zone indicating an early stage in the involution of the nevus.

n. of Ito, typically, a unilateral, patchy discoloration of the skin that is similar to the nevus of Ota but with a supraclavicular, scapular, and deltoid distribution. There may be an association with an ipsilateral or bilateral nevus of Ota.

malignant blue n., a blue nevus with cytologic evidence of malignant transformation and the capacity for metastasis. It is a rare condition. See also *blue n.*

melanocytic n., a localized collection of benign nevus cells (melanocytes). When the lesion is confined to the epidermal-dermal junction, it is designated a junctional nevus. If the nevus cells are only within the dermis, it is termed an intradermal (dermal) nevus. If the intradermal component is accompanied by junctional activity, it is called a compound nevus.

Such nevi may be acquired or congenital. The acquired melanocytic nevus makes its earliest appearance in childhood rather than at birth. Histologically, there are junctional (clinically flat), compound, and intradermal (clinically elevated) forms. The congenital melanocytic nevus is present at birth, and is found is sizes ranging from those several millimeters in diameter to those covering large portions of the body surface. Congenital nevi less than 5 mm are found in approximately 2 percent of newborns; those greater than 9 cm in maximal diameter occur in approximately 1 of every 20,000 live births.

n. of Ota, a unilateral pigmented lesion of the skin of the periorbital region; it appears in childhood and rarely becomes malignant.

spindle n., a dermal nevus composed of large spindle cells and round cells with plentiful cytoplasm, often with sparse junctional activity or pigmentation. It is more common in children and young adults. The appearance of the cells and the number of mitotic figures may occasion suspicion of melanoma. Also called *epithelioid nevus,* spindle and epithelioid cell nevus, and *Spitz nevus.* Formerly called *juvenile melanoma.*

vascular n., a localized overgrowth of blood vessels. Some, such as port wine stain (*stork bite, nuchal hemangioma*), are characterized by areas of flat or elevated erythema of various sizes resulting from an overgrowth of dilated but otherwise normal thin-walled vessels. Such lesions remain constant throughout the life of the affected individual. In contrast, the neonatal capillary hemangioma (*strawberry nevus*), which arises as a proliferation of small capillary-like vessels, usually goes through an evolution of growth and regression during the prepubertal years.

RICHARD W. SAGEBIEL, M.D.

nevus cell the dermal counterpart of the epidermal melanocyte; the cell that comprises melanocytic nevi.

newborn (nu'born) 1. a recently born infant. 2. newly born.

Newcastle disease (nu'kas-el) [from *Newcastle,* a seaport on the River Tyne in northeast England] a disease characterized by the transmission to humans of an avian virus that results in a viral conjunctivitis. Human exposure is most frequently from contaminated material; in 1–3 da it can result in a conjuntivitis, eyelid edema, and inflammation. Recovery is usually spontaneous in 10–14 da. Diagnosis may be accomplished by viral isolation in embryonated eggs.

Newman projection (nu'man) [Melvin Spencer *Newman,* U.S. organic chemist, born 1908] a particular convention used to represent a three-dimensional molecule in two dimensions; particularly valuable for showing conformation differences between structures. See also under *conformation.*

new methylene blue N a metachromatic thiazin basic dye used as a reticulocyte stain; C.I. 52030. Its orthochromatic color is blue and its metachromatic color is purple-red.

newton (N) (nu'ton) [Sir Isaac *Newton,* English mathematician, physicist, and astronomer, 1643–1727] the International System (SI) unit of force or weight equal to 1 kilogram-meter per second squared ($kg \cdot m/s^2$).

Newton's law of cooling stated as: the temperature change per unit time is proportional to the difference between the temperatures of an object and its surroundings.

newton-meter ($N \cdot m$) a unit of torque. It is dimensionally equivalent to the joule (J), which is used for energy, work, or heat.

New Zealand black (NZB) mouse an inbred strain of black mice that spontaneously develops autoimmune components and disorders, such as lupus erythematosus cells, antinuclear antibodies, hemolytic anemia, and immune complex glomerulonephritis. These mice are used as an animal model for human systemic lupus erythematosus. They are a useful research tool in that they have the following immunologic abnormalities: B lymphocytes that develop prematurely and produce excessive antibody responses, T lymphocytes that develop prematurely and are unable to maintain tolerance, loss of suppressor T-lymphocyte function, and loss of recirculating T lymphocytes. An F1 hybrid of a New Zealand black mouse and a New Zealand white mouse will develop an even more severe autoimmune disease.

New Zealand white (NZW) mouse an inbred strain of white mice that is often crossbred with New Zealand black mice to produce a hybrid useful in research on automimmune diseases. See also *New Zealand black mouse.*

nexus (nek'sus), pl. *nexus, nexuses*[L. "bond"] a type of cell junction adapted to provide a site of electrical coupling between cells. It is a disk-shaped structure in which adjacent cell membranes are separated by a narrow cleft approximately 3 nm wide, hence the synonym gap junction. The two membranes are in fact connected across the gap by a polygonal lattice of protein subunits, which facilitates the rapid passage of small molecules. Transmission of the contractile impulse between cells of cardiac muscle or smooth muscle is achieved by junctions of the nexus type. Also called gap junction.

Nezelof's syndrome (nez'e-lofz) [C. *Nezelof,* French pediatrician, 20th century] a condition characterized by marked T-cell immune deficiency and various degrees of B-cell deficiency. The cause is not known and there appears to be no genetic pattern; identified cases are sporadic. The primary defect may be within the thymus: the disorder may result from thymic hypoplasia with deficient interaction between B and T cells, and consequent formation of abnormal antibodies.

Affected individuals are susceptible to recurrent bacterial, fungal, viral, and protozoal infection; the spectrum of infections is similar to that occurring with other immunodeficiencies. However, patients frequently have marked lymphadenopathy and hepatosplenomegaly, in contrast to those with congenital hypogammaglobulinemia or severe combined immunodeficiency.

The principal immunologic findings associated with this condition are the reduction in total numbers of lymphocytes or T-cell rosettes and a decreased response of peripheral blood lymphocytes to T-cell mitogens, allogenic cells, and specific antigens. Delayed-type hypersensitivity responses are absent, and various degrees of B-cell deficiency are present. The number of circulating B cells is usually normal, and serum immunoglobulin levels may be decreased, normal, or high, with normal or abnormal distribution of the five immunoglobulin classes.

Biopsy of lymphoid tissues may reveal plasma cells, and the lymph nodes may be large and contain numerous histiocytes and macrophages with granuloma formation.

Because of the lack of uniformity of the clinical and laboratory characteristics, this disorder serves as a catch-all for poorly defined immunodeficiencies. Distinctions are possible, however. For example, persons with Wiskott-Aldrich syndrome have thrombocytopenia, whereas those with Nezelof's syndrome do not. Individuals with severe combined immunodeficiency have a complete absence of T- and B-cell immunity. Immunodeficiency disorders associated with enzyme deficiencies may have similar presentation but may be excluded on the basis of enzyme analysis of the red or white blood cells. Furthermore, the endocrine deficiencies associated with DiGeorge's syndrome are not present in Nezelof's syndrome.

Treatment includes aggressive therapy against infection; patients failing to respond to immunization should be given monthly immune globulin injections. Postural drainage may prevent chronic lung disease. Possibly owing to the unavailability of histocompatible donors, bone marrow transplants have not been very successful, although transfer factor therapy and thymus transplants have had some success. Graft-versus-host disease has not been shown to occur in this syndrome. Some patients may develop progressive encephalitis when given live attenuated viral vaccines. Long-term complications include the development of chronic lung disease, chronic fungal infection, and malignancy.

NF abbrev. See *National Formulary.*

nF abbrev. See *nanofarad.*

NFPA abbrev. See *National Fire Protection Association.*

ng abbrev. See *nanogram.*

NGU abbrev. See *nongonococcal urethritis.*

NHC protein abbrev. See *nonhistone chromosomal p.* under *protein.*

Ni symbol for the chemical element *nickel.*

NIA abbrev. for nephelometric inhibition assay. See *nonradioisotopic i.* under *immunoassays.*

niacin (ni'ah-sin) vitamin B_3, 3-pyridinecarboxylic acid; M.W. 123.11. Niacin is a water-soluble vitamin originally called the P-P factor, in reference to its pellagra-preventive ability. The amide form, niacinamide, is a constituent of the two coenzymes nicotinamide adenine dinucleotide (NAD) and nicotine adenine dinucleotide phosphate (NADP).

Niacin can be synthesized in the body from tryptophan. The average daily requirement for niacin in adults is 13–20 mg. Deficient intake may lead to pellagra.

Also called *nicotinic acid.* See also *pellagra.*

niacinamide (ni"ah-sin-am'id) the amide form of niacin.

niacin assays 1. microbiologic assay. The extent of the growth of *Lactobacillus plantarum,* upon the addition of graded amounts of niacin, is determined by measuring the turbidity of the cell suspension at 620 nm. A standard curve of niacin concentration against absorbance is plotted, from which the amount of niacin in the sample can be determined.

2. colorimetric assay. Niacin is treated first with cyanogen bromide to give a pyridinium compound, and then with an aromatic amine to yield a colored glutaconic dialdehyde derivative.

niacin test a test for the production of niacin used in the identification of *Mycobacterium* species. Niacin can be extracted from the mycobacteria by placing water or saline on colonies growing on egg medium for 15 min. On a porcelain spot plate, two drops of colony extract are mixed with two drops of aniline (4 percent in 95 percent ethanol) and two drops of 10 percent cyanogen bromide. If niacin is present, a complex yellow color compound is formed. A positive reaction is indicative of the human tubercle bacillus, *Mycobacterium tuberculosis.*

This procedure should be run under a chemical fume hood owing to tear gas production by cyanogen bromide. A positive control of niacin-producing mycobacteria should be run simultaneously.

See also *mycobacteria.*

nialamide (ni-al′ah-mīd) a monoamine oxidase (MAO) inhibitor formerly used therapeutically as an antidepressant.

niche (nich) [from Fr. *nicher* to nest] a recess in the wall of a hollow organ (such as an ulcerated area), which appears on a radiograph as a region filled with contrast medium. A niche has a wider neck than a diverticulum; it is more a pit than a sac.

nick (nik) a single-strand break in a double-stranded DNA molecule. A nick acts as a swivel, allowing the halves of the molecule on either side of the nick to rotate independently.

nickel (Ni) (nik′-el) [Swed. from Ger. *Kupfernickel* "copper demon" (its ores can be mistaken for copper ores)] a silvery-white metallic element; atomic number 28; atomic weight 58.71; a 3d transition element; oxidation states +1 through +4 (+2 is most common). It is used industrially as a catalyst, in batteries, and in copper, aluminum, and steel alloys. Contact with nickel or its alloys is a common cause of dermatitis (nickel itch).

nickel assays determination of the nickel concentration in biologic specimens by atomic absorption spectrometry. Acid digestion of urine, whole blood, or tissue or protein precipitation with trichloroacetic acid for serum is followed by complexing the nickel in the digest or protein-free supernatant with pyrrolidine dithiocarbamate. This is followed by extraction into methyl isobutyl ketone, followed by aspiration into an acetylene flame and reading at 232 nm. The coefficient of variation is about 10 percent. Gold and cadmium interfere slightly with this extraction procedure. Reference ranges for nickel in serum are: 1.1–4.6 $\mu g/l$, and for nickel in urine, 1.0–5.2.

nickel carbonyl a colorless, volatile liquid [tetracarbonylnickel(O), $Ni(CO)_4$] used in the industrial production of pure nickel. It has a sooty odor and is highly toxic. Acute poisoning causes nausea and dizziness, followed by cyanosis and dyspnea. Fatal lung and brain damage may occur. Chronic exposure is implicated in nasal and lung cancer.

nick translation a method of labeling DNA with ^{32}P-nucleotides used for preparing probes. DNA polymerase 1 acts as both a $5' \rightarrow 3'$ exonuclease and a $3' \rightarrow 5'$ polymerase. Starting at a nick, it removes bases from the free 5′ end and adds labeled nucleotides at the free 3′ end until the strand is completely replaced.

Nicollella (nĭ-ko-lel′ah) [Charles Jules Henri *Nicolle,* French physician, 1866–1936, noted for his discovery of the role of body lice in the transmission of typhus fever; winner of the Nobel Prize for Medicine in 1928] a genus of ciliate protozoa parasitic in the intestines of *Ctenodactylus gundi,* a northern African rodent.

Nicol prism (nik′ol) [William *Nicol,* Scottish physicist, 1768–1851] a polarizer composed of two prisms of calcite cemented together. Light entering the first prism is doubly refracted. The extraordinary ray (one plane polarization) passes through the interface and the other prism. The ordinary ray (the other polarization) is refracted more, striking the crystal-cement interface at an angle greater than the critical angle and undergoing total internal reflection. See also *birefringence.*

nicotinamide (nik″o-tin′ah-mīd) see *niacinamide.*

nicotinamide adenine dinucleotide (NAD, NAD^+) (nik″o-tin′ah-mīd ad′ĕ-nēn di-nu′kle-o-tīd″) a water-soluble, hygroscopic white powder, which yields on hydrolysis one molecule each of adenine and nicotinamide, and two each of D-ribose and phosphoric acid. In NAD^+, these parts are linked as follows: nicotinamide-ribose-phosphate-phosphate-ribose-adenine. It is a coenzyme in numerous dehydrogenase reactions, serving as a hydrogen transfer agent in the reversible reaction NAD $\rightleftarrows$ NADH. Formation or consumption of NADH is accompanied by a change in absorbance at 339 nm, which is frequently used as a measure of enzyme activity of dehydrogenases. In coupled enzyme reactions, the change in absorbance can be used to measure the activity of other enzymes (e.g., alanine aminotransferase, ALT, aspartate aminotransferase, AST) or the concentration of other compounds (e.g., glucose). Formerly called diphosphopyridine nucleotide (DPN), coenzyme I (Co I).

nicotinamide adenine dinucleotide phosphate (NADP, $NADP^+$) a grayish-white powder, soluble in water and methanol, that is a coenzyme in numerous dehydrogenase reactions (e.g., glucose-6-phosphate dehydrogenase, serum isocitrate dehydrogenase). NADP yields on complete hydrolysis one molecule each of adenine and nicotinamide, two of ribose, and three of phosphoric acid, linked in this manner: nicotinamide-ribose-phosphate-phosphate-ribose-phosphate-adenine. It is similar to nicotinamide adenine dinucleotide (NAD), differing only in an additional phosphate esterified at C-3 in the adenosine portion of the molecule.

As a coenzyme, NADP serves as a hydrogen transfer agent in the reversible reaction $NADP^+ + XH_2 \rightleftarrows NADPH_2 + X$ (where X is the donor compound). The formation or consumption of NADPH is accompanied by a change in absorbance at 340 nm, which is used as a measure of the activity of glucose-6-phosphate dehydrogenase. Generation of reduced NADP (NADPH) through the pentose phosphate pathway (glucose-6-phosphate dehydrogenase and 6-phosphogluconate dehydrogenase) is linked to glutathione reduction and is thus vital to the functions of enzymes that prevent the accumulation of methemoglobin in erythrocytes.

Formerly called *coenzyme II* and *triphosphopyridine nucleotide.*

nicotinamide mononucleotide (NMN) [nik″o-tin′ah-mīd mon″o-nu′kle-o-tid″] a nucleotide that can be formed from NAD during DNA synthesis or hydrolytically from NAD or NADP during their metabolism.

nicotine (nik′o-tēn, nik′o-tin) [L. *Nicotiana* a genus of plants that includes tobacco] a highly toxic liquid alkaloid (1-methyl-2-(3-pyridyl) pyrrolidine) with a pyridinelike odor and an acrid, burning taste. Extracted from leaves of the tobacco plant (*Nicotiana tabacum*) or obtained synthetically, nicotine is the primary active drug absorbed from tobacco smoking, producing vasoconstriction and slight central nervous system depression. It is habit forming. In addition to tobacco smoking, nicotine is used as a botanical insecticide.

Nicotine stimulates the nicotinic cholinergic receptors of the autonomic ganglia. Symptoms of acute poisoning include vomiting, muscular weakness and twitching, mental confusion, myocardial arrhythmias, convulsions, and respiratory paralysis. Death may occur rapidly.

Smokers have urine nicotine concentrations of 2–3 μg/ml. Blood concentrations above 10 μg/ml are toxic; concentrations above 20 μg/ml may be fatal.

nicotine assays 1. colorimetry. Steam distillation of the alkalinized sample is followed by formation of a white precipitate with silicotungstic acid. Other volatile alkaloids interfere.

2. ultraviolet spectrophotometry. Nicotine is extracted from the alkalinized sample into chloroform and reextracted into acid. The absorbance at 259 nm is compared with that of a reference solution. Other organic bases having similar absorbance spectra interfere.

3. gas chromatography. A flame ionization detector and a silicone column packing having intermediate polarity are used. Extraction is as in method two; methyprylon is used as the internal standard.

nicotinic (nik″o-tin′ik) producing effects similar to those of nicotine.

nicotinic acid see *niacin.*

nicotinic receptor a receptor in the autonomic nervous system that can be stimulated by nicotine; see under *cholinergic receptors.*

Niemann-Pick disease (ne′man pik) [Albert *Niemann,* German pediatrician, 1880–1921; Ludwig *Pick,* Berlin pediatrician, 1868–1935] a group of rare disorders transmitted as autosomal recessive traits, that are characterized by abnormal lipid metabolism and the excessive storage of phospholipids, especially sphingomyelin, in the reticuloendothelial system. Levels of sphingomyelinase, which hydrolyzes various phospholipids, may be severely reduced or absent. The infantile form is manifested in early life by central nervous system involvement, hepatosplenomegaly, xanthomas (rare), a cherry-red macular spot (in some cases), and vacuolated blood lymphocytes.

Diagnosis is based on biopsy and demonstration of sphingomyelinase deficiencies in white blood cells and cultured fibroblasts. No treatment is available. This disease is most common in families of Jewish descent.

Also called sphingomyelin lipidosis. See also *sphingolipidoses.*

adult N.-P. d., a group of disorders of sphingomyelin metabolism, which classically become manifest in the neonatal period with hepatosplenomegaly and severe mental retardation. Five varieties are currently recognized.

night blindness reduced or absent ability to see in dim light, as well as an abnormally slow visual adjustment from bright to dim light. Night blindness is considered to be an early manifestation of vitamin A deficiency, with a serum value below 20 μg/dl (normal, 20–50 μg/dl). The early rod dysfunction in night blindness may be diagnosed by dark adaptometry, rod scotometry, or electroretinography. Night blindness occasionally may have other causes, such as retinitis pigmentosa and glaucoma. Also called *nyctalopia.*

nightmare (nīt′mār) [M.E. *night* + *mare* spirit] a normal dream occurring during REM sleep causing anxiety. Cf. *pavor nocturnus.*

night terror see *parasomnias* and *p. nocturnus* under *pavor.*

nikethamide (nĭ-keth′an-mīd) a central nervous and respiratory system stimulant occasionally used to treat asphyxia in newborns and, formerly, to treat poisoning by CNS depressants. Overdosage may cause muscle spasms and convulsions. Trademark, Coramine.

Nikolsky's sign (nĭ-kol′skēz) [Petr Vasilyevich *Nikolsy,* Russian dermatologist, 1858–1940] the ready separation of the outer layer of the epidermis from the basal layer with skin sloughing by minor trauma. It may be present in pemphigus, scalded skin syndrome, exfoliative dermatitis, and a number of bullous disorders. Nikolsky's sign may be elicited on physical examination by exerting a sliding or rubbing pressure on the involved skin.

Nile blue sulfate a basic oxazine dye; C.I. 51180. It forms salts with free fatty acids and phospholipids, staining them blue. Commercial preparations contain a red oxazine derivative called Nile red; this neutral dye is soluble in neutral lipids (triglycerides and steroids) and stains them red. When acid (pH 1) Nile blue solutions are used, triglycerides are hydrolized and also stain blue.

ninhydrin (nin-hi′drin) triketohydrindene hydrate, a compound (oxidant) used for the detection and quantitation of alpha-amino acids. It reacts with the latter to form CO_2, NH_3, and an aldehyde with one less carbon. The CO_2 formed is a quantitative measure of alpha-amino acids. On heating, the NH_3 formed reacts with two reagent residues to form a blue-to-purple color with all alpha-amino acids except proline and hydroxyproline, which give a yellow color. This is the basis of the use of ninhydrin as a spray reagent in paper and thin-layer chromatography.

Under acid conditions, ninhydrin reacts with other primary and some secondary amines (e.g., ammonia, amphetamine, peptides, proteins, ephedrine) to also form a blue color, but with no CO_2 evolution.

ninhydrin-Schiff reaction (nin-hi′drin shif) a histochemical reaction used to demonstrate protein, which is stained magenta. Amino groups on protein undergo oxidative deamination to aldehyde by reaction with ninhydrin. These aldehyde groups react with Schiff reagent. See also *alloxan-Schiff reaction.*

niobium (Nb) (ni-o′be-um) [from *Niobe,* daughter of *Tantalus* in Greek mythology (niobium occurs in the ore tantalite)] a gray or silvery, ductile metallic element; atomic number 41; atomic weight 92.9064; a 4d transition element; oxidation states +2, +3, +4, +5 (the most common). It is used in metal alloys. Formerly called *columbium* (*Cb*).

nipple (nip″l) the pigmented projection at the tip of each breast, which gives outlet to milk in the breast. Each nipple is surrounded by the pigmented areola; its surface is dimpled with the openings of the lactiferous ducts.

niridazole (nĭ-rid′ah-zōl) a schistosomicidal and amebicidal drug. It should be used with caution because of its serious side-effects.

Nissl bodies (nis′l) [Franz *Nissl,* German neurologist, 1860–1919] clumps of basophilic material in the cytoplasm of nerve cells that are ribosomal in nature. They stain with basic aniline dyes such as toluidine blue, thionine, and cresyl violet. Also called Nissl granules and Nissl substance.

nit (nit) the egg of a louse, usually attached to hairs of infected individuals. Three types of lice are known to infest humans: *Pediculus humanus capitis,* head lice; *P. humanus corporis,* body lice; and *Phthirus pubis,* pubic or crab lice. Diagnosis is made by finding bites on the body, adult lice in hairy areas, or nits attached to hairs. The nits should be examined microscopically to ensure that they are really eggs.

nitrate (ni′trāt) 1. pertaining to the NO_3^- ion.

2. a compound that contains this ion.

3. an ester of an alcohol and nitric acid containing the —ONO_2 functional group. Several of these, particularly nitroglycerin (glyceryl trinitrate), are used as coronary vasodilators in the treatment of angina pectoris. Excessive intake of both inorganic and organic nitrates is hazardous.

The primary toxic effects of organic nitrates, usually occurring from industrial exposure, are hypotension, tachycardia, and severe headache. These disappear after tolerance develops. Ingestion of nitrate can cause methemoglobinemia. Nitrate is present in well waters, pickled meats, explosives, and some antiseptics.

nitrate reduction test a test for the reduction of nitrate to nitrite by a bacterial culture. A culture is examined for nitrites by combining a solution of sulfanilic acid and acetic acid (5 N) with alpha-naphthylamine and acetic acid (5 N) in the presence of the microorganisms in question. A red color develops if nitrites are present. The test is useful in identifying doubtful strains of Enterobacteriaceae, mycobacteria, and certain anaerobic bacteria.

nitrazepam (ni-trah′zĕ-pam) a benzodiazepine compound used as a hypnotic and anticonvulsant.

nitremia (ni-tre′me-ah) the presence of excess nitrogen in the blood. This excess may be due to increased blood protein; increased nonprotein nitrogen–containing compounds, such as creatinine and urea (azotemia); or increased nitrogen gas in the blood. Nitrogen inhalation under increased pressures (P_{N_2} of 6000 mmHg) may exert a narcoticlike effect, leading to nitrogen narcosis as seen in deep-sea divers. See also *azotemia.*

nitric (ni′trik) denoting a compound that contains nitrogen in a higher oxidation state than does the corresponding nitrous compound.

nitric acid a strong monobasic acid and oxidizing agent, HNO_3; M.W. 63.02. It is a colorless liquid with a choking odor. Nitric acid is highly toxic, caustic, and corrosive. Exposure to light causes slow decomposition to nitrogen dioxide, which gives the acid a yellow-red color.

nitric oxide a colorless gas, nitrogen monoxide, nitrogen(II) oxide, NO, used in the manufacture of nitric acid and in the preparation of nitro compounds; M.W. 30.01. It is a by-product of high-temperature combustion in air (such as occurs in internal combustion engines) and is an important air pollutant that contributes to the formation of photochemical smog. Upon exposure to air, it is oxidized to nitrogen dioxide, a highly toxic lung irritant.

nitrile (ni′tril) a compound that contains the nitrilo functional group, —CN, e.g., propanenitrile, C_2H_5CN.

nitrilo group (ni-tril′o) 1. the functional group ≡N occurring in nitriles; the prefix cyano- is usually used for this group.

2. the trivalent nitrogen atom in a tertiary amine; it is used in naming compounds of symmetric structure, e.g., nitrilotriacetic acid, $N(CH_2COOH)_3$.

nitrite (ni′trīt) 1. pertaining to the NO_2^- ion.

2. a compound that contains this ion.

3. an ester of an alcohol and nitrous acid that contains the —ONO functional group. Some of these, particularly amyl nitrite, have been used as coronary vasodilators in the treatment of angina pectoris.

nitro- (ni′tro) [L. *nitrum;* Gr. *nitron*] a prefix word element in organic chemistry used to denote the presence of the nitro functional group, —NO_2.

nitrobenzene (ni″tro-ben′zēn) a yellow, oily, combustible liquid with an almond odor, $C_6H_5NO_2$, used in industrial chemical synthesis; M.W. 123.11. It is highly toxic when ingested, absorbed, or inhaled, producing methemoglobinemia, cyanosis, headache, drowsiness, nausea, and vomiting.

nitroblue tetrazolium test (NBT) (ni″tro-blu′ tet″-ra-zo′le-um) an assay for the metabolism of phagocytosing neutrophils. Nitroblue tetrazolium is a clear yellow compound that upon reduction forms formazan, a blue dye. During phagocytosis there is an increase in hexose monophosphate shunt activity that generates reducing power. This reducing capability is indicated by a color change of nitroblue tetrazolium. Failure of dye reduction is indicative of disorders of neutrophil function, e.g., chronic granulomatous disease. False-positive and false-negative results may occur if a secondary disease is present.

nitrofurans (ni-tro-fu′ranz) a group of antimicrobial compounds containing a nitrofuran ring, NO_2—CH:CH—CH:C—. They are bacteriostatic for a variety of gram-positive and gram-negative bacteria, some fungi, and certain protozoa. The nitrofuran derivative, nitrofurantoin, is used principally for treatment of urinary tract infections because high urine concentrations can be achieved by oral administration. Other nitrofurans include *furazolidone* and *nitrofurazone.* See also *antibacterial agents.*

nitrofurantoin (ni″tro-fu-ran′to-in) a nitrofuran antibiotic that belongs to a class of organic substances characterized by a heterocyclic ring. It inhibits a variety of enzyme systems in bacteria, possibly by interfering with early stages of bacterial carbohydrate metabolism through the inhibition of acetyl coenzyme A.

Nitrofurantoin is active in vitro against a wide spectrum of gram-positive and gram-negative bacteria. Although most *Proteus* species and *Pseudomonas aeruginosa* are resistant, nitrofurantoin is, nevertheless, useful for the treatment of those urinary tract infections caused by susceptible organisms.

See also *antibacterial agents* and *nitrofurans.*

nitrofurazone (ni″tro-fu′rah-zōn) a synthetic nitrofuran with a broad antibacterial spectrum. Nitrofurazone is bactericidal against most bacteria that commonly cause skin and mucous membrane infections. It is used as a topical agent in the treatment of burns and skin grafts. See also *antibacterial agents* and *nitrofurans.*

nitrogen (N) (ni′tro-jen) [Fr. *nitrogène,* from Gr. *ni-*

tron niter (KNO_3) + *gennan* to produce] a colorless, odorless gaseous element; molecular form N_2; atomic number 7; atomic weight 14.007; Group V of the periodic table; common oxidation states −3 (in ammonia and nitrides) +3 (in nitrous acid and nitrites), +5 (in nitric acid and nitrates); all other oxidation states between −3 and +5 also occur.

Nitrogen is the major component of air, constituting 75.5 percent by weight and 78.06 percent by volume. It is used industrially as an inert atmosphere; as a cryogenic coolant (b. p. 77.36°K, −195.79°C); and in the production of nitrates, nitrites, and cyanides. Nitrogen is also used medicinally as a radiolucent contrast medium [USP], as a diluent for gases, and to displace air from pharmaceuticals.

In biologic systems, the element occurs primarily in amino acids; in the nitrogenous bases of nucleic acids; and in the waste products of their metabolism, ammonia and urea.

Although nitrogen gas (N_2) is metabolically inert, approximately 1 l is normally present in the body, about half of which is dissolved in body water, and the rest in fat.

An increase in the amount of dissolved nitrogen gas with pressure can produce serious problems for deep-sea divers. Nitrogen narcosis results from nitrogen dissolved in the lipid structures of the nervous system. It works like anethetics, producing first joviality, then drowsiness. Decompression sickness results from the formation of N_2 bubbles in the vascular system when decompression is too rapid for elimination of the nitrogen through the lungs. The formation of bubbles in blood vessels in the nervous system causes pain, dizziness, and, ultimately, paralysis, and in bones causes focal necrosis (see also *decompression sickness*).

nitrogen balance the relationship of the dietary intake of nitrogen to losses from the body. Nitrogen equilibrium is the characteristic condition in the adult, with losses just balanced by intake, so that the body composition remains relatively constant. To maintain nitrogen equilibrium, dietary proteins are needed to compensate for metabolic losses.

Negative nitrogen balance, or losses exceeding supply, is an obvious result of an inadequate intake. However, it is also characteristic of the ill and the injured, in whom cellular damage causes more nitrogen to be lost than is taken in. There is also a small negative nitrogen balance associated with aging.

Positive nitrogen balance occurs when tissues are growing. It is the characteristic state of pregnancy and the convalescent adult, as well as of growing young persons. Maintenance of positive nitrogen balance requires sufficient dietary protein from which to construct additional tissues being formed in addition to the amount required to replace metabolic losses.

nitrogen dietary requirement that amount of dietary protein nitrogen needed to maintain nitrogen equilibruim in a healthy adult of ideal body weight and in a state of basal (minimal) physical activity. For persons weighing 73 kg, this value is about 400 mmol of protein nitrogen (35 g of "protein") daily. The requirement must be met in terms not only of protein amount but also of protein quality, i.e., amino acid composition and digestibility. See also *nitrogen balance* and *dietary p.* under *protein.*

nitrogen dioxide a reddish-brown gas with an irritating odor, nitrogen(IV) oxide, NO_2, used in the production of nitric acid and as a nitrating and oxidizing agent; M.W. 46.01. It is highly toxic and causes delayed pulmonary inflammation and edema. A concentration of 100 ppm is dangerous; exposure to 200 ppm may be lethal.

Nitrogen dioxide is produced by the atmospheric oxidation of nitric oxide and is an important air pollutant. Commerical liquefied NO_2 is a mixture with its colorless dimer N_2O_4, dinitrogen tetroxide. Photodissociation of nitrogen dioxide is the first step in the production of photochemical smog.

See also *dinitrogen tetroxide.*

nitrogen fixation the reduction of molecular nitrogen (N_2) to ammonia, which in turn can proceed to the formation of an organic molecule. Nitrogen fixation is important because it is responsible for the regeneration of ammonia in the soil; most food sources for humans rely on ammonia as a nutritional requirement. Nitrogen fixation is an anaerobic process and is therefore inhibited by oxygen. It gives an organism the ability to use N_2 as a nitrogen source. Only certain bacteria are capable of employing this process, and some require a symbiotic relationship with specific plants. Overall nitrogen fixation involves the reduction of N_2 with six hydrogens to form two molecules of ammonia. This reaction is catalyzed by the enzyme nitrogenase, which has two components called ferredoxins, one part containing iron and molybdenum and the other containing iron.

nitrogen heterocycle a cyclic organic compound containing one or more nitrogen atoms in ring or rings. See also *heterocylic compound.*

nitrogen mustard any of a group of cytotoxic drugs including chlorambucil, cyclophosphamide, mechlorethamine, and melphalan, that act as biologic alkylating agents. They all contain the chemical group —$N(CH_2CH_2Cl)_2$. See also *cancer chemotherapy* and *Appendix A.*

nitrogen pentoxide a colorless, crystalline solid, dinitrogen pentoxide, nitrogen(V) oxide, N_2O_5, the anhydride of nitric acid; M.W. 108.02.

nitrogen-phosphorus (NP) detector see under *gas chromatography.*

nitrogen trioxide a blue liquid, dinitrogen trioxide, nitrogen(III) oxide, N_2O_3; M.W. 76.01. In the liquid phase and in solution it is partially dissociated: $N_2O_3 \rightleftarrows NO + NO_2$.

nitrogen washout curve the exponential curve that depicts the rate of elimination of nitrogen from the lungs (as measured by the nitrogen content of the expired alveolar air) during successive breaths of oxygen or other gases. Each inspiration dilutes the N_2 in the alveolar gas by an amount that reflects the size of the functional residual capacity (FRC); the rate of nitrogen washout increases at smaller FRC. The rates of washout are also less in poorly ventilated regions of the lung, a phonomenon that forms the basis for tests of the nonuniform distribution of ventilation such as the 7-min washout test and the single-breath N_2 test.

nitroglycerin (ni-tro-glis′er-in) a colorless liquid, 1,2,3-propanetriol trinitrate, the explosive in dynamite. It is also a coronary vasodilator; nonexplosive mixtures are used as sublingual tablets [USP] for the treatment of acute anginal pain. Slowly absorbed preparations are used for the prevention of angina attacks.

***p*-nitrophenol** (PNP) (ni″tro-fe′nol) 4-nitrophenol, used as a reagent and acid-base indicator; M.W. 139.11. Solutions are colorless at pH 5.6 and yellow above pH 7.6 (quinoid phenolate ion). PNP esters and glycosides are used as substrates for activity measurements of hydrolytic enzymes. The liberated PNP is measured at 402 (401–405) nm ($\epsilon = 18750$).

Some organophosphate insecticides, such as parathion, methyl parathion, EPN, and chlorothion, are PNP esters, and on hydrolytic detoxication liberate PNP, which is excreted in the urine.

***p*-nitrophenol assays** 1. spectrophotometry. The sample is extracted into an organic solvent and reextracted with an alkali; a colored product is then produced by reaction with *o*-cresol and titanium trichloride. The absorbance at 620 nm is compared with that of reference solutions.

2. gas chromatography. An electron capture detector and a nonpolar or slightly polar column packing are used. Extraction as in method 1 is followed by silation with hexamethyldisilazane. The specimen concentration is determined by comparing the specimen peak height with that of *p*-nitrophenol reference solutions.

nitroprusside (ni″tro-prus′id) see *sodium nitroprusside.*

nitroso- (ni-tro′so) a prefix word element in organic chemistry used to denote the presence of the nitrosyl functional group, —NO.

nitrous (ni′trus) denoting a compound that contains nitrogen in a lower oxidation state than does the corresponding nitric compound.

nitrous acid a weak acid, HNO_2, which decomposes in water to nitric oxide (NO) and nitric acid (HNO_3). It is formed by the action of acid on nitrite salts and is used to form organic diazonium salts from amines.

nitrous oxide a colorless gas, nitrogen(I) oxide, N_2O, having a sweet taste and pleasant odor; M.W. 44.02. Nitrous oxide is used as a general inhalation anesthetic, especially in dentistry. It does not produce full muscle relaxation but can be combined with other anesthetics for surgical anesthesia. Also called laughing gas.

NIXIE tube trademark for a digital readout device, which is a neon glow tube with 1 anode and 10 cathodes shaped like the decimal digits 0–9. When 55 V are applied between one of the cathodes and the anode, a glow discharge displays a digit. NIXIE tubes have been largely replaced by solid state readouts, which are more reliable and have a lower power consumption, as well as lower voltage requirements.

NK cell abbrev. See *natural killer cell.*

nl abbrev. See *nanoliter.*

N·m abbrev. see *newton-meter.*

nm abbrev. See *nanometer.*

NM(ASCP) a designation of certification for technologists in nuclear medicine. See under *nuclear medicine technologist.*

NMN abbrev. See *nicotinamide mononucleotide.*

nmol abbrev. See *nanomole.*

NMR abbrev. See *nuclear magnetic resonance.*

NNN medium See *Novy, MacNeal and Nicolle's medium.*

No symbol for the chemical element *nobelium.*

nobelium (No) (no-be′le-um) [Alfred Bernard *Nobel,* Swedish chemist and engineer, 1833–1896] a synthetic, metallic radioactive element; atomic number 102; most stable isotope, No-259 (half-life, 58 min); a 5f transition element (actinide element).

Nobel Prize (no-bel′) [Alfred Bernard *Nobel*] six awards, five of which were provided for in Alfred Nobel's will, that are given annually for outstanding achievement in chemistry, physics, medicine and physiology, literature, economics, and the promotion of world peace; first awarded in 1901.

Nocardia (no-kar′de-ah) [Edmond Isidore Étienne *Nocard,* French veterinarian, 1850–1903] a genus of bacteria of the family Nocardiaceae, order Actinomycetales, consisting of gram-positive aerobes with branching filaments that break into bacillary or coccal forms. The normal habitat is the soil. The two species that most often produce human infections are *N. asteroides* and *N. brasiliensis.*

N. asteroides, the etiologic bacterium of nocardiosis, an opportunistic pulmonary infection that has a predilection for spread to the central nervous system. The colonies appear folded, wrinkled, granular, and orange. A white overgrowth of aerial mycelia develops with time. Microscopically, gram-positive or partially acid-fast irregularly branching mycelia are found.

N. brasiliensis, a bacterium that causes a mycetoma characterized by a bumpy border around the lesions on the sinus tracts, as well as bone involvement. The grains on the lesion are small, are white to yellow in color, and may have clubs. The colonies appear heaped, wrinkled, and yellow to red with a white mycelial overgrowth. Microscopically, short partially acid-fast bacilli with some filamentation are seen. *N. brasiliensis* is partially acid-fast.

Nocardiaceae (no-kar″de-a′se-e) a family of bacteria, order Actinomycetales, that consists of three genera: *Nocardia, Nocardiopsis,* and *Actinomadura.*

Nocardiopsis (no-kar″de-op′sis) a genus of bacteria of the family Nocardiaceae, one of the actinomycetes. The organisms are gram-positive, aerobic, and nonacid-fast, forming dense, filamentous colonies with aerial mycelia and conidia in chains. These bacteria are similar to those of the genus *Nocardia,* but they differ in cell wall type and are not resistant to lysozyme. They can be pathogenic for humans, causing abscesses and granulomatous pulmonary lesions. The natural habitat apparently is soil.

nocardiosis (no-kar-de-o′sis) infection with *Nocardia,* whose habitat is the soil. It occurs either from inhalation of the organisms, causing primary pulmonary lesions resembling those of tuberculosis, or from contamination of skin wounds, causing abscesses (mycetoma) of the hands or feet. Pulmonary infection sometimes spreads to cause a brain abscess. See also *mycetoma.*

nociceptive (no″se-sep′tiv) [L. *nocere* to injure + *capere* to receive] painful; the term can be used to describe a sensory receptor that responds to noxious and damaging stimuli, which are perceived as painful sensations. It is also used to describe a reflex or response to such a noxious stimulus.

nociceptor (no″se-sep′tor) one of the nonadapting free nerve endings found in the skin (and in deeper tissues such as the arterial walls, periosteum, and surfaces of joints) that responds to one or more types of noxious or damaging stimuli. Such stimuli include extreme temperatures, mechanical trauma, and various chemical agents. Signals from these receptors are perceived centrally as pain.

noct/i (nok'te) [L. *nox* night] a word element used in combining form to denote night, e.g., nocturnal.

nocturia (nok-tu're-ah) [*noct-* + Gr. *ouron* urine + *-ia*] excessive urination during the night. It is an abnormal but nonspecific symptom of a variety of disease conditions, and often signifies renal disease with decreased concentrating capacity, as well as hepatic or cardiac disorders. Reduced bladder capacity due to prostatic enlargement, renal stones, infection, or tumors may led to nocturia. It may also be a normal consequence of excessive fluid intake in the evening.

nocturnal (nok-tur'nal) [L. *nocturnus,* from *nox* night] pertaining to or occurring at night.

nodal (no'dal) [L. *nodus* knot] pertaining to a node, particularly the atrioventricular node and lymph nodes.

nodal rhythm heart rhythm initiated in the specialized junctional tissue in or near the atrioventricular node.

node (nōd) [L. *nodus* knot] a small mass of tissue in the form of a swelling, knot, or protuberance.

atrioventricular n., an oval mass of specialized tissue located beneath the endocardium in the septal wall of the right atrium. It has pacemaker activity, which is normally superseded by the sinoatrial node. Also called *AV node.*

sinoatrial (SA) n., a flattened ellipsoid mass of specialized cardiac tissue located at the junction of the superior vena cava and the right atrium. Its cells exhibit a spontaneous discharge and normally initiate the cardiac cycle, so that the SA node is often called the pacemaker of the heart.

node of Ranvier the point on a myelinated axon where two adjacent Schwann cells meet. The nodes are separated by a short segment of naked axon, which is a region of high capacitance and low electric resistance; during passage of a nerve impulse, the wave of depolarization jumps from one node to the next, a manner of conduction termed "saltatory." Branching of axons occurs only at nodes.

nodular (nod'u-lar) resembling a node or nodule, used particularly to describe clearly demarcated, solid, or partially solid lesions of various tissues that are not linear, reticular, or diffuse. See also the illustration under *contour.*

nodular fasciitis see *nodular f.* under *fasciitis.*

nodule (nod'ūl) [L. *nodulus* little knot] a small, solid boss or node that can be detected by touch. The term is often used to designate a comparatively small aggregation of tissue. For more information, see the specific nodule.

noise (noiz) the random variations in a signal that do not carry any information about the source, caused by imperfections in the signal transmission.

pink n., the random noise that has equal energy in each octave band (doubling of frequency). The noise power P at frequency f is $P = P_0 2^{-f}$, where P_0 is the zero-frequency noise power. The noise level drops 3.1 dB/octave.

Poisson n., noise due to statistical fluctuations in the number of information carriers (e.g., electrons, photons) received by a detector, such as the "snow" on a television screen. In CT scans and scintillation photographs, Poisson noise is produced by two phenomena: (1) the statistical variation in the number of x-rays or gamma-rays received by the detector fom a given point in the subject, and (2) the statistical variation in the number of electrons produced by the detector (e.g., a photomultiplier and crystal) for each photon received.

Poisson noise can be reduced by increasing the counts that affect a picture element; this is accomplished by increasing the counting time, by increasing the radiation flux and the dose absorbed by the patient, or by reducing the resolution.

Also called counting noise, quantum noise, shot noise, and statistical noise.

thermal n., the noise produced by the thermal motion of electrons in electronic circuits. Semiconductor radiation detectors are cooled with liquid nitrogen to reduce thermal noise.

white n., random noise that has equal energy at every frequency.

nom/o (no'mo) [Gr. *nomos* law] a word element used in combining form to denote usage or law, e.g., nomotopic, nomogram.

noma (no'mah) [Gr. *nomai* eating sores] a rapidly progressive, ulcerative, gangrenous infection of the mucous membrane of the buccal area and mandible. A rare condition, it occurs in malnourished or debilitated small children in underdeveloped countries. The tissue destruction leads to severe disfigurement. Anaerobic bacteria are thought to play a role in its pathogenesis. Also called cancrum oris.

Nomarski optics see *Nomarski m.* under *microscope.*

nomenclature (no'men-kla"tūr, no-men'kla"tūr) [L. *nomen* name + *calare* to call] a classified system of names, as of anatomic structures, microorganisms, chemical compounds, or pathologic processes (e.g., tumors).

Nomina Anatomica (NA) (no'mĭ-nah an-ah-tom'ĭ-kah) [L. "anatomic names"] the official body of anatomic nomenclature; specifically, the revision by the International Anatomical Nomenclature Committee appointed by the Fifth International Congress of Anatomists held at Oxford in 1950.

nominal variable (nom'ĭ-nal) a variable that has nonnumerical values. See also *scale.*

nominal wavelength the wavelength at which a filter or other monochromator has the greatest transmittance.

nomogram (nom'o-gram) [*nomo-* + Gr. *gramma* mark] a chart that consists of three or more straight or curved graduated scales representing a mathematical or empirical relation between several variables. When a straight edge intersects two scales at specified values, the values of the other variables are then given by its intersections with the other scales; the *Siggaard-Andersen alignment nomogram* is one example. Also called *alignment chart* and *nomograph.*

nomograph (nom'o-graf) [*nomo-* + Gr. *graphein* to write] see *nomogram.*

non-A non-B hepatitis see under *hepatitis.*

noncombustible (non"kom-bus'tĭ-b'l) not combustible. Cf. *combustible, flammable,* and *nonflammable.*

nondisjunction (non"dis-junk'shun) the failure of homologous chromosomes or sister chromatids to separate during anaphase of a cell division, either mitosis, meiosis I, or meiosis II. If nondisjunction occurs during mitosis, one daughter cell receives both copies of a chromosome and is trisomic; the other has neither and is monosomic. The term can also refer to any failure of pairing that has the same result. Cf. *anaphase lag.*

primary n., nondisjunction that occurs during the division of a cell having the normal chromosome number and which, if it ocurs during metaphase, results in monosomic and trisomic cells.

secondary n., nondisjunction that results from the division of a trisomic cell. During meiosis, the extra chromosome segregates independently of its two homologues, producing monosomic and disomic gametes with equal frequency.

nonelectrolyte (non″e-lek′tro-līt) a solute that is not dissociated into ions in solution and cannot conduct electricity.

nonfermenting (non″fer-men′ting) not fermenting; said of bacteria that do not ferment sugars when cultured under specified conditions.

nonfilamented (non-fil′ah-men-ted) not having filamentous shape; said of bacterial colonies.

nonflammable (non-flam′ah-b′l) not flammable. Cf. *combustible, flammable,* and *noncombustible.*

nongonococcal urethritis (NGU) urethral inflammation not caused by gonococcal (e.g., *Neisseria gonorrhoeae*) bacterial pathogens; the causative organisms frequently are chlamydia.

nonheme iron protein (non′hēm) see *iron-sulfide protein.*

nonhemolytic (non″he-mo-lit′ik) not producing hemolysis.

non-Hodgkin's lymphoma see *malignant l.* under *lymphoma.*

nonidentity pattern (non″ī-den′tĭ-te) see under *Ouchterlony immunodiffusion.*

non-ionizing radiation (non-i′o-ni-zing) electromagnetic radiation (ultraviolet, visible, and infrared light, and radio waves) composed of photons with too little energy to ionize atoms.

nonlinear (non-lin′e-ar) pertaining to a mathematical function not described by a linear equation.

nonlinear circuit an electronic circuit in which a change in the input does not produce a proportional change in the output. The effect of the circuit cannot be described by a first-degree linear differential equation. Examples are circuits that provide exponential or logarithmic functions as outputs to a linear input.

nonmetal (non-met′al) any one of the group of chemical elements that form covalently bonded molecules or crystals or that form a monatomic gas at room temperature, e.g., carbon, chlorine, and neon. They have none of the properties of metals. Cf. *metal* and *semiconductor.*

nonmetallic (non″mĕ-tal′ik) 1. not containing metals.

2. pertaining to or composed of nonmetals.

nonmyelinated (non-mi′ĕ-lĭ-nāt″ed) not having a myelin sheath (also called *unmyelinated*); see under *nerve.*

nonnucleated (non-nu′kle-āt″ed) without a nucleus. Also called *anuclear.*

nonparalyzable detector (non″par-ah-līz′ah-b′l) a radiation detector, such as a proportional counter, that produces a characteristic maximal counting rate at very high radiation fluxes. After each particle that is counted there is a period known as the recovery time during which no particles can be counted. Cf. *paralyzable detector.*

nonparametric (non-par″ah-met′rik) pertaining to a statistic (such as a median or percentile) or a statistical test (such as a rank-sum test) that does not assume a specified mathematical form for the underlying distribution. Nonparametric tests are usually less powerful than parametric methods, which take advantage of a specified mathematical form for the underlying distribution, but they obviate the need for assuming or specifying the form.

nonpathogenic (non″path-o-jen′ik) not pathogenic.

nonpenetrance (non-pen′ĕ-trans) the lack of penetrance of a gene, i.e., the lack of phenotypic manifestation in certain individuals. Penetrance is an "all-or-none" quality but is dependent on the criteria used to define the phenotype. Cf. *expressivity.*

nonpenetrating radiation (non-pen′ĕ-trāt-ing) in dosimetry, radiation having a very short range in tissue so that most particles are absorbed in the organ where they are emitted. Cf. *penetrating radiation.*

nonpermissive (non″per-mis′iv) in microbial genetics, pertaining to the environmental conditions in which a conditional lethal mutant dies or cannot reproduce. Also called *restrictive.*

nonphotochromogen (non″fo-to-kro′mo-jen) [L. *non* not + Gr. *phōtos* light + *chrōma* color + *gennan* to produce] a microorganism that does not produce pigment in the presence of light. The term is specifically applied to mycobacteria that do not produce carotenoid pigmentation; included in this group are the common pathogens *Mycobacterium avium* and *M. intracellulare* (Battey bacillus).

nonproprietary (non″pro-pri′e-ter-e) not protected by copyright or patent. The nonproprietary name of a drug (also called the generic name) is chosen by an official organization such as the USAN Council to refer to a drug without specifying the manufacturer.

nonprotein nitrogen (NPN) (non″pro′tēn ni′tro-jen) the nitrogen of the nitrogenous constituents of blood exclusive of protein. It consists of nitrogen from urea (45–55 percent of total) and amino acids, peptides, uric acid, creatinine, creatine, and ammonia.

nonprotein nitrogen assays after removal of all proteins by precipitation, the organic nitrogen in the supernatant is converted to NH_4HSO_4 by means of a semimicro-Kjeldahl digestion with sulfuric acid in the presence of a catalyst. NH_3 is then released in the digestate and determined directly (or preferably after distillation) by the Berthelot procedure, by use of Nessler's reagent, or by microtitration.

Reference values for NPN are: for serum, 18–35 mg/dl; and for whole blood, 25–50. Serum NPN concentrations above 35 and whole blood concentrations above 50 suggest renal insufficiency. In terminal stages of renal failure, NPN levels may increase to more than 400. Other more sensitive and specific indices have largely replaced the NPN assay as the routine test for renal function.

nonREM sleep the deep, dreamless periods of

sleep that are interspersed between periods of REM (dreaming) sleep. See also *s. stages* under *sleep.*

nonrespiratory acidosis (non″re-spi′rah-to″re as″ĭ-do′sis) see *metabolic acidosis.*

nonrespiratory alkalosis (non″re-spi′rah-to″re al″-kah-lo′sis) see *metabolic alkalosis.*

nonsaponifiable fraction (non″sah-pon″ĭ-fi′ah-b′l) [L. *non* not + *sapo* soap + *facere* to make] the portion of total lipid that, after treatment with hot alkali, is insoluble in water and soluble in ether. Cf. *saponifiable fraction.*

nonsecretor (non″se-kre′tor) an individual who cannot secrete the ABH blood group antigen in saliva and other body fluids but who has the blood type (i.e., the antigen is present in red blood cells). See also *secretor factor.*

nonsense mutation see *nonsense m.* under *mutation.*

nonseptate (non-sep′tāt) without a septum or septa.

nonstress test (NST) a test performed to assess the respiratory function of the placenta and to determine whether the placenta and fetus can withstand the stress of labor. During spontaneous fetal activity or during activity induced by rubbing or gentle pressure on the mother's abdomen, the fetal heart rate can be monitored by ultrasound to determine the adequacy of respiratory reserve. See also *oxytocin challenge test.*

nonstriated muscle (non-stri′āt-ed) a muscle whose fibrils have no transverse striations and are not under direct voluntary control. Also called *involuntary muscle, plain muscle,* and *unstriated muscle.* See also *smooth m.* under *muscle.*

nontropical sprue (non-trop′ĭ-kal sproo) see *celiac s.* under *sprue.*

nonviable (non-vi′ah-b′l) not capable of surviving, dead.

Noonan's syndrome (noo′nanz) [Jacqueline Anne *Noonan,* U.S. cardiologist, 20th century] a dysmorphic syndrome having some phenotypic overlap with Turner's syndrome in which the affected individual possesses a normal chromosome complement. This syndrome is characterized by multiple abnormalities of the heart, skin, skeletal system, and gonads. There is a characteristic facial development, short stature, and retarded mental development. Valvular pulmonary stenosis is more common in Noonan's syndrome, whereas coarctation of the aorta is more common in Turner's syndrome. The syndrome affects both males and females and is sometimes dominantly inherited. See also *Turner's syndrome.*

NOR the complement of the logical OR function. The result is *false* if and only if any argument is *true.* See also *NOR gate.* Cf. *OR.*

nor- (nor) a prefix word element used in organic chemistry to denote (1) a compound (e.g., norleucine) having an unbranched chain isomeric with one (e.g., leucine) having a branched chain, or (2) a compound (e.g., norepinephrine) formed by the removal of one or more carbons and associated hydrogens from some parent compound (e.g., epinephrine).

noradrenalin (nor″ah-dren′ah-lin) see *norepinephrine.*

norbormide (nor-bor′mīd) a selective rat poison, 5-(α-hydroxy-α-2-pyridylbenzyl)-7-(α-2-pyridylbenzylidene)-5-norbornene-2,3-dicarboximide. It acts on receptors in the smooth muscle of peripheral vessels of the rat and causes irreversible vasoconstriction and death due to ischemia. Norbormide is essentially nontoxic to humans and to domestic animals, which apparently have receptors differing from those in the rat.

norbornane (nor-bor′nān) bicyclo [2.2.1] heptane, a compound that is the nucleus of terpene derivatives such as camphor and of the cyclodiene hydrocarbon pesticides.

norcodeine (nor-ko′dēn) *N*-desmethylcodeine, an opiate.

norepinephrine (nor″ep-ĭ-nef′rin) a hormone, α-(aminomethyl)-3,4-dihydroxybenzyl alcohol, secreted by certain neurons; M.W. 169.18. It is also secreted by the adrenal medulla in response to splanchnic stimulation. Norepinephrine is an excitatory neurotransmitter released at peripheral sympathetic postganglionic nerve terminals and at certain synapses in the central nervous system. It is synthesized from dopamine and stored in specialized granules or vesicles at the nerve endings. Its action on the target cells is mediated through alpha and beta receptors. Its effects include vasoconstriction of arterioles in the skin and splanchnic area (causing a rise in blood pressure), pupil dilation, and relaxation of the gut. Norepinephrine is inactivated via two major pathways, *O*-methylation and *N*-deamination. The main metabolites are normetanephrine and vanillylmandelic acid.

See also *adrenal m.* under *medulla* and *catecholamine.*

norepinephrine assays see *catecholamine assays.*

norepinephrine staining methods for demonstrating the presence of the catecholamine norepinephrine in tissue. Because fixation will destroy the reactivity of norepinephrine, fresh tissue must always be used.

In the iodate method for norepinephrine, fresh, thin slices of tissue are incubated in a potassium iodate solution. The slices are placed in formalin before cutting frozen sections. Cells containing norepinephrines will appear brown. Norepinephrine is rapidly oxidized by the iodate. In the case of epinephrine, this oxidation proceeds very slowly, taking up to 24 hr.

The fluorescent method for norepinephrine is relatively straightforward. Frozen sections of fresh tissue are cut and allowed to thaw in a calcium-formol solution. Once washed and mounted, the sections are examined with a fluorescent microscope. Cells containing norepinephrine exhibit a strong yellow-green fluorescence.

NOR gate an electronic circuit that produces the complement of the OR function. It is equivalent to an OR gate followed by an inverter. Its output is *false* if and only if at least one input is *true.* Cf. *OR gate.*

norm/o (nor′mo) [L. *norma* rule] a word element used in combining form to denote normal, rule, or order, e.g., normoblast.

norm (norm) a fixed or ideal standard.

normal (nor′mal) 1. agreeing with the regular and established type.

2. in chemistry, a former term for expressing concentration; the number of gram-equivalents of solute per liter of solution. A normal solution is the

Normal Flora. Microorganisms Commonly Colonizing Healthy Human Body Surfaces[1]

Organism	Skin	Conjunctivae	Outer Ear	Nose	Mouth and Pharynx	Esophagus and Stomach	Small Intestine	Large Intestine (Adult)	Anterior Urethra and External Genitalia	Vagina
Staphylococcus (coagulase-negative and micrococci)	++++	+++	++++	++++	++++		±	+	++++	+++
S. aureus	++	+		++	+			+	+	
Streptococcus sp.[2]	+	+		++	++++		+++	+++	+	++
Pneumococci		±	++	+	++					
Anaerobic cocci	+	+			++			++++	+	++
Neisseria and *Branhamella* sp.		±		+	+++					+
N. meningitidis					+					
Veillonella sp.					++++					
Bacillus sp.	+							+		+
Lactobacillus sp.		+			++	+	+++	+++		++++
Corynebacterium sp.	+++	+	++	++	++			++	+++	+++
Propionibacterium sp.	++++ (*P. acnes*)	+++						+	+	++
Bifidobacterium sp.								++++		
Enterobacteriaceae	+	±	+		++		++	++++	+	+
Pseudomonas sp.	+		++					+		
Moraxella sp.		±			+					
Acinetobacter sp.	++				+			+	±	+
Bacteroides sp.					++		+	++++	+	++
Fusobacterium sp.					++++			++++	+	
Clostridium sp.							+	++++		+
Hemophilus sp. (excepting *H. influenzae*)		+		+	+					+
H. influenzae		+		+	+					
Actinomyces sp.					+			+		
Mycobacterium sp. (excepting *M. tuberculosis*)	+					+	+	+	++	
Spirochetes					+++			+		
Mycoplasma sp.					+				+	+
Candida sp. (excepting *C. albicans*)	++				+			+	+	++
C. albicans	+				++			+	+	++
Pityrosporum sp.	+++									
Torulopsis glabrata					+				+	+
Trichomonas vaginalis									±	±

[1] Data are expressed as relative of isolation: ++++ = almost always present; +++ = usually present; ++ = frequently present; + = occasionally present; ± = rarely present. In the esophagus and stomach, bacteria exist in low numbers (<10/ml); surviving bacteria from food or upper respiratory tract are occasionally present.

[2] The streptococcal species in the skin, conjunctivae, and nose is *S. pyogenes*, ±; viridans streptococci (*S. pyogenes*, ±; other beta-hemolytic streptococci, ++) in the mouth and pharynx; enterococci, viridans streptococci in the small intestine; enterococci (other species, ±) in the large intestine and urethra and external genitalia; and enterococci (group B, ++; viridans streptococci, +) in the vagina.

Modified from Mandell, G. L.: Principles and Practice of Infectious Disease. New York, John Wiley & Sons, 1979.

same as a one-normal solution (1.0 N). A half-normal solution (0.5 N) has a concentration of 0.5 gram-equivalents per liter of solution (0.5 Eq/l). Because the definition of equivalent depends on the chemical reaction in which the compound is involved (e.g., acid-base, oxidation), a given solution can have more than one normality. Cf. *molal* and *molar.*

3. in names of chemical compounds, denoting a straight-chain hydrocarbon (abbrev. n), e.g., n-butane (butane) as opposed to isobutane (2-methylpropane).

normal distribution any member of the parametric family of probability distributions having symmetric, bell-shaped density functions:

$$f(x) = \frac{1}{\sigma\sqrt{2\pi}} \exp\left\{-\frac{(x-\mu)^2}{2\sigma^2}\right\},$$

where the parameters are μ as the mean and σ as the standard deviation. The random variable $Z = (X-\mu)/\sigma$ (called the standardized deviate, standard score, or Z score) has the standard normal distribution with mean 0 and standard deviation 1.

The sampling distribution of the mean of a sample of size n from a normal distribution has a normal distribution with mean μ and standard deviation $\sigma/\sqrt{n}$. The normal distribution is the only distribution with finite variance for which sampling distribution of the mean has the same shape as the parent distribution.

The sample mean and variance are independently distributed, and $(n-1)s^2/\sigma^2$ has the chi-squared distribution with $n-1$ degrees of freedom.

See also *central limit theorem, F distribution,* and *t distribution.*

normal flora in microbiology, the microorganisms that are more or less permanent residents of the superficial tissues. In any one body area the microbial population is invariably mixed but the composition is remarkably stable. Although there are constant fluctuations in the minor components, the same species remain numerically dominant in their own microenvironments. If the composition is altered by antibiotics or some other agent, the original composition is restored soon after the action of the drug or other agent is removed. Consequently, the types of microorganisms most likely to be cultured from any healthy body site can be predicted, allowing for some variation due to factors such as age, diet, and sanitation. However, there are significant and consistent differences in the major types present in the various regions of the body: *Staphylococcus epidermis* and *Propionibacterium acnes* predominate in the skin; lactobacilli, corynebacteria (diphtheroids), and staphylococci are most numerous in the vagina; and *Bacteroides* and bifidobacteria are found in the colon.

The accompanying table notes the relative frequencies with which the more important microorganisms (other than viruses) can be recovered from several body areas when appropriate culture methods are employed. This tabular summary, however, is not adequate for three of the body areas named—the skin, mouth and pharynx, and small intestine. Skin has both a transient and resident flora; the table includes both. Most of the organisms listed are transients, for the resident flora of dry skin is sparse with two exceptions: the two species named above are present in large numbers where sebaceous glands are located (e.g., the face), and *S. epidermidis* is found in all skin areas. Moist skin of the axillae and intertriginous areas harbors large numbers of gram-negative organisms, especially *Acinetobacter* species, instead of the gram-positive flora generally characteristic of skin.

The mouth and pharynx flora, although combined in the table, differ with respect to major types. Anaerobic cocci, bacilli, and spirochetes predominate on the teeth and gingiva, whereas viridans streptococci, *Neisseria,* and *Branhamella* species are the major types in the throat.

Except for the lower ileum, the microbial content of the small intestine is limited in both variety and number. Below the ileocecal valve, however, the flora increases enormously, reaching a level in the feces of about 3×10^{11}/g of dry weight. The numerical predominance of *Bacteroides* species is impressive, for they outnumber *Escherichia coli,* the traditional bacterium of the colon, by a ratio in the range of 1:1000–1:10,000.

Whether the body's commensals are beneficial or detrimental has been debated since Pasteur's time. The beneficial actions are better understood. Through the mechanism of bacterial antagonism, normal flora resists implantation and colonizaton of pathogenic species. The degree of protection provided by normal flora has become increasingly apparent since the advent of antibiotic therapy, especially through observation of the adverse effects of oral antibiotics on the gastrointestinal tract. Tetracycline or lincomycin, in doses that significantly alter the bowel flora, may give rise to severe enterocolitis due to the overgrowth of certain species, notably *Staphylococcus* or *Clostridium difficile.* In the laboratory it has been found that the number of *Salmonella enteritidis* needed to infect mice is reduced by a factor of 10^5 by a single oral dose of streptomycin, which drastically reduces the intestinal flora.

Humans develop maturation immunity between infancy and adulthood. This immunity results from repeated exposure to commensal antigens, originating in large part from enteric bacteria, and it accounts for the relative resistance of adults to many infectious agents that cause disease in infants and children. Its great importance became clear from observations of germ-free animals, which, by definition, have been deprived of this protective mechanism. Their lymphoid tissue is greatly undeveloped, their gamma-globulin (antibody) levels are exceedingly low, and their immunologic response to antigenic stimulation is slow and weak. Such animals are made sick by and sometimes die from oral introduction of a relatively few ordinarily innocuous bacteria, such as a *Lactobacillus* or *E. coli.*

Another benefit bestowed on the human host by the indigenous flora relates to nutrition. A significant proportion of the vitamin K absorbed by humans and animals from the digestive tracts is synthesized by bacteria, particularly *E. coli;* this is also the case with several B-complex vitamins.

Conversely, the normal intestinal flora may have harmful effects on the host. Incorporation of small quantities of antibiotic in animal feed (common practice in the livestock industry) significantly increases the growth rate of animals. The effect is clearly related to suppression of the normal gastrointestinal flora, although the mechanisms have not been fully explained.

Intestinal flora may harm the host in another way. It is widely held that gram-negative bacilli in the bowel are the source of antigenic endotoxins that are absorbed and that sensitize body tissues. Thus, constant absorption of endotoxin in small amounts is postulated to result in a mild but ever-present toxemia. In support of this belief is the severe reaction, such as hemorrhagic shock, that can occur during some gram-negative infections.

Also called autochthonous flora and indigenous flora. See also *opportunistic infection.*

KENNETH R. CUNDY, PH.D.

normality (nor-mal'ĭ-te) 1. the state of being normal.

2. the concentration of a solution expressed in gram-equivalents of solute per liter of solution (Eq/l). This expression of concentration is no longer recognized by the SI system. See also *normal.* Cf. *molality* and *molarity.*

normalize (nor'mah-līz) 1. in statistics, to convert a raw datum point to a standardized deviate.

2. see under *floating-point variable.*

normal probability paper graph paper used to plot the values of an experimental (random) variable against its cumulative frequency distribution (sample distribution function). Each observed value is plotted on one axis (a linear scale), and the percentage of trials having values less than or equal to that value is plotted on the other axis (a scale proportional to the error function of the scale length). If the sample has a distribution that is approximately normal, the plotted points will be close to a straight line (see the accompanying illustration).

normal sinus rhythm (NSR) the usual rhythm of the heart occurring when every impulse originating at a normal rate in the sinoatrial node is successfully propagated to the atria and ventricles. In the absence of physical exertion, emotion, neurohumoral factors, or fluctuation in body temperature, the normal sinus rhythm has a range of 60–100 beats/min in adults and about 130–160 beats/min in infants.

normal values in laboratory medicine, the range of values of some quantity within which values of a healthy individual are expected to fall. See also *reference values,* the preferred term, and *Appendix C.*

normetanephrine (nor-met"ah-nef-'rin) 1-(4-hydroxy-3-methoxyphenyl)-2-aminoethanol, a metabolite of norepinephrine that is excreted in the urine and is also found in certain tissues, such as those of the nervous system.

normoblast (nor'-mo-blast) [*normo-* + Gr. *blastos* germ] the immature nucleated cell in the erythrocyte series. Four developmental stages are recognized: in order of their development, they are pronormoblast, basophilic normoblast, polychromatophilic normoblast, and orthochromatic normoblast.

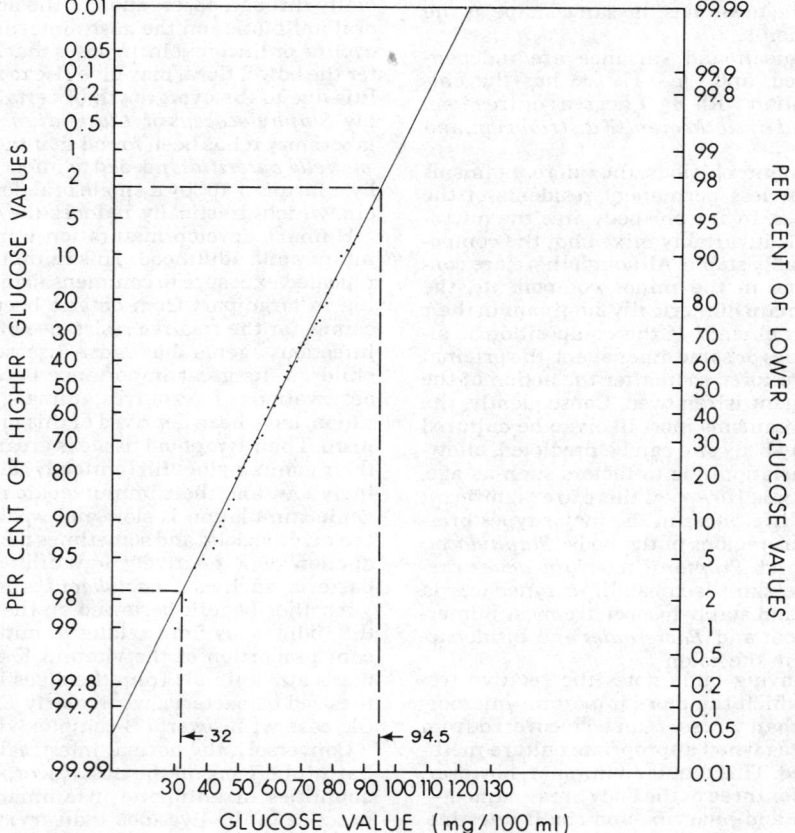

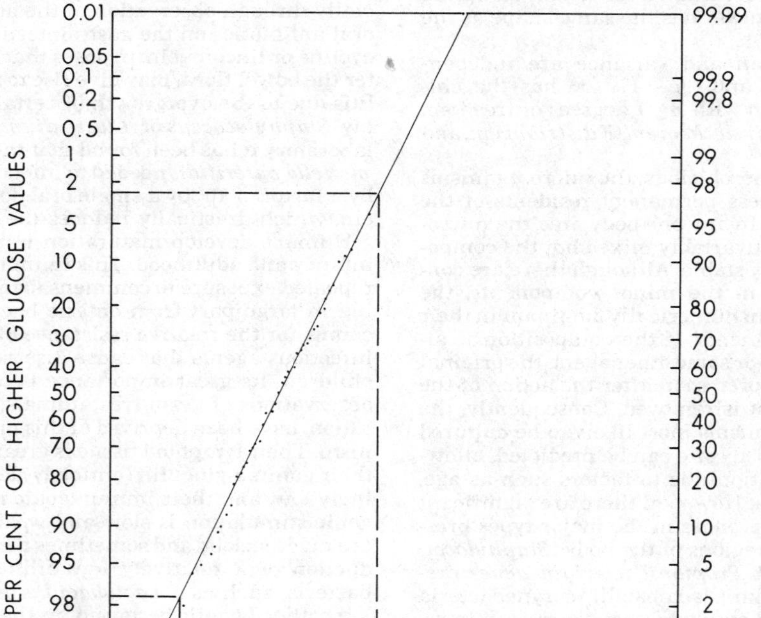

Normal probability paper. Cumulative frequency distribution of 105 glucose values plotted on normal probability paper. (From Tietz, N. W.: Fundamentals of Clinical Chemistry. 2nd ed. Philadelphia, W. B. Saunders Co., 1976.)

The term *megaloblast* refers to an immature, abnormal cell in certain disorders of erythropoiesis.

PRONORMOBLAST. The pronormoblast is the earliest recognizable precursor of the erythrocyte. The cell is 20–25 μm in diameter and has a nucleus that occupies eight-tenths of the cell diameter, with small clumps of chromatin and one or two small nucleoli often obscured by the perinuclear condensation of chromatin. The narrow band of nongranular cytoplasm stains dark blue (basophilic). The stage ends with mitosis. Also called *proerythroblast* (Ferrata) and *rubriblast* (an obsolete term).

BASOPHILIC NORMOBLAST. The basophilic normoblast represents the second stage in erythrocyte development, usually considered as two phases separated by a mitotic division: b. n. I (E_2) and b. n. II (E_3). The cell and nucleus are smaller, and the nuclear chromatin is more sharply defined than in the pronormoblast, appearing as coarse, granular material. The cytoplasm stains more deeply with basic dyes (basophilic) than that of the pronormoblast, the distinct nucleoli and cytoplasmic nucleotides have disappeared, and the protein production is reduced. Also called *basophilic erythroblast* (Ferrata), early erythroblast (Sabin), early normoblast (Custer), and *prorubricyte.*

POLYCHROMATOPHILIC NORMOBLAST. The polychromatophilic normoblast is the third stage in erythrocyte development, often considered in two phases separated by a mitotic division: p. n. I (E_4) and p. n. II (E_5). The stage is marked by the appearance of hemoglobin in the cytoplasm, which appears gray or grayish-pink, and it ends when the cytoplasm is no longer basophilic. As hemoglobin concentration increases, the nucleus becomes smaller (7–9 μm) and the nuclear chromatin becomes more condensed. The entire cell may be 12–15 μm in diameter. Also called intermediate normoblast (Custer), late erythroblast (Sabin), *polychromatic hormoblast,* and *polychromatophilic rubricyte.*

ORTHOCHROMATIC NORMOBLAST. The orthochromatic normoblast is the last stage in erythrocyte development before nuclear extrusion, in which cytoplasmic hemoglobin reaches its highest concentration (28×10^{-6} μg). The cytoplasm is said to be the color of a mature erythrocyte. The nuclear chromatin increasingly condenses as the nucleus disappears, and the cell volume decreases to 8–12 μm in diameter. Also called *acidophilic normoblast,* late normoblast (Custer), *metarubricyte,* and normoblast (Sabin). See also *erythrocyte* and *reticulocyte.*

normoblastic (nor″mo-blas′tik) relating to or having the characteristics of a normoblast.

normocalcemia (nor″mo-kal-se′me-ah) [*normo-* + *calcium* + Gr. *haima* blood + *-ia*] a condition characterized by a normal concentration of calcium in the blood. Reference ranges for calcium in serum are: 4.2–5.2 mEq/l, or 8.5–10.5 mg/dl; reference ranges for ionized serum calcium are: 2.1–2.6 mEq/l, or 4.2–5.2 mg/dl.

normochromic (nor″mo-kro′mik) [*normo-* + Gr. *chrōma* color] having a normal color; having a normal hemoglobin content.

normochromic anemia see *normochromic a.* under *anemia.*

normocrinic (nor″mo-krin′ik) [*normo-* + Gr. *krinein* to separate] pertaining to normal secretion or to the normal endocrine action of a gland.

normocyte (nor′mo-sit) [*normo-* + *-cyte*] an erythrocyte that is normal in size, shape, and color.

normocytic anemia (nor″mo-sit′ik) see *normocytic a.* under *anemia.*

normoglycemia (nor″mo-gli-se′me-ah) [*normo-* + Gr. *glykes* sweet + *haima* blood + *-ia*] a condition characterized by a normal concentration of glucose in the blood. Reference ranges for glucose in serum are 65–105 mg/dl in fasting individuals.

normokalemia (nor″mo-kah-le′me-ah) [*normo-* + L. *kalium* potassium + Gr. *haima* blood + *-ia*] a condition characterized by a normal concentration of potassium in the blood serum. Reference ranges for potassium in serum or plasma are 3.5–5.1 mmol/l.

normorphine (nor-mor′fēn) desmethylmorphine, an opiate that can produce physical dependence.

normotension (nor″mo-ten′shun) the state of normal tension, tone, or pressure, as in normal blood pressure.

normotensive (nor″mo-ten′siv) 1. characterized by normal tone, tension, or pressure.
2. an individual with normal blood pressure.

normothermia (nor″mo-ther′me-ah) [*normo-* + Gr. *thermē* heat + *-ia*] a normal body temperature. In humans it is 37°C or 98.6°F.

normovolemia (nor″mo-vo-le′me-ah) [*normo-* + *volume* + Gr. *haima* blood + *-ia*] the presence of a normal blood volume, which averages 60–70 ml/kg in males and 58–64 in females in different series. The range of total red cell volume or red cell mass is 26–32 for males and 23–29 for females and children. See also *blood volume measurements.*

Norpramin (nor′pram-in) trademark. See *desipramine.*

Norrie's disease (nor′ez) [Gordon *Norrie,* Danish ophthalmologist, 20th century] a genetic disorder, transmitted as an X-linked recessive trait, that is characterized by retinal malformations, abnormalities of mental development, and sensory disorders. Loss of both hearing and sight often occurs.

nortriptyline (nor-trip′tĭ-lēn) the generic name for a derivative of the tricyclic compound dibenzocycloheptadiene, which is used as an antidepressant. It is a metabolite of amitriptyline. For toxicity, see *tricyclic antidepressant.* Trademark for nortriptyline hydrochloride, *Aventyl.*

nortriptyline assays see *amitriptyline and nortriptyline assays.*

Norum's disease (nor′umz) see *lecithin–cholesterol acyltransferase deficiency.*

Norwegian itch (nor-we′ge-an) see *scabies.*

nos/o (nos′o) [Gr. *nosos* disease] a word element used in combining form to denote relationship to disease, e.g., nosocomial.

nose (nōz) [L. *nasus;* Gr. *rhis*] the specialized structure at the center of the face that serves both as an organ for the sense of smell and as part of the respiratory passages.

no-see-ums a common name for the adult fly of the genus *Culicoides,* family Heleidae (also called Ceratopogonidae). Several species are bloodsucking and serve as intermediate hosts for some filarial worms that are parasitic in humans.

nosocomial (nos″o-ko′me-al) [Gr. *nosokomeion,* from *nosos* disease + *komeion* to take care of] pertaining to or originating in a hospital or infirmary.

nosocomial anemia see *nosocomial a.* under *anemia.*

nosocomial infection hospital-acquired infection; infection that is not present or incubating when a patient enters the hospital, but generally occurs later than 72 hr after admission. Although the term is most often used to refer to patient disease, hospital personnel may also acquire nosocomial infection, and those involved in direct patient care are sometimes responsible for its transmission to patients.

There are several types of nosocomial infections: urinary tract infections (which account for 30–40 percent of all such infections), postoperative wound infections (20 percent), lung infections (15 percent), and blood stream infections (10–15 percent). The organisms most frequently involved in nosocomial infections are gram-negative rods (including the Enterobacteriaceae and *Pseudomonas aeruginosa*) and *Staphylococcus aureus,* which is the most common isolate from postoperative wound infections.

The organism most often isolated from nosocomial urinary tract infections is *Escherichia coli,* accounting for 30 percent of all isolates. *P. aeruginosa, Candida albicans,* and species of *Pseudomonas, Klebsiella, Enterobacter, Serratia, Proteus,* and *Providencia* are also isolated, and outbreaks caused by multiple resistant gram-negative bacilli can occur. The development of nosocomial urinary tract infection and bacteremia is associated with the use of indwelling Foley catheters. The risk of development of bacteriuria ($\geq 10^5$ colonies of bacteria per milliliter) is 5–10 percent for every day of catheterization. Bacteria may be introduced into the urinary tract at the time of catheter insertion in two ways: by ascent within the catheter lumen, and by ascent by way of the urethral mucus at the meatal-catheter interface.

Organisms commonly found in the sputum of patients with nosocomial pneumonia include *Pseudomonas* and *Klebsiella* species, *S. aureus,* anaerobes, viruses (including influenza A, respiratory syncytial virus, and hepatitis virus), and fungi (including species of *Candida*). Predisposing factors include old age, aspiration of gastric contents, anesthesia equipment, respiratory therapy, endotracheal or nasotracheal tubes, tracheostomies, bronchoscopy, cytotoxic drugs, steroids, and underlying disease such as leukemia, lymphoma, and diabetes mellitus.

Organisms that may be isolated from nosocomial bacteremia include Enterobacteriaceae, *S. aureus, P. aeruginosa,* and fungi. An important risk factor for bacteremia is a nosocomial infection at another site; for example, nosocomial bacteremia may result from the use of indwelling urinary tract catheters. Sepsis may also result from the use of contaminated intravascular solutions and devices.

Control of nosocomial infections involves the establishment of a hospital infection control program. Such programs include surveillance of infections occurring in the hospital; determination of endemic infection rates; review of data with hospital personnel; continuing education of hospital personnel; investigation of outbreaks; review of procedures for cleaning, sterilizing, and disinfecting the hospital environment and instruments used for invasive procedures; and establishment of isolation procedures. Such activities are usually overseen by an infection control committee.

Cf. *hospital-acquired penetration contact.*

nosologic (no″so-loj′ik) pertaining to nosology.

nosology (no-sol′o-je) [*noso-* + Gr. *logos* reasoned speech] the classification, description, and definition of diseases. Diagnosis is based on the nosologic picture, which comprises all the nosologic characters: symptoms, signs, and laboratory test results.

Nosopsyllus (nos″o-sil′us) [*noso-* + Gr. *psylla* flea] a genus of fleas.

N. fasciatus, the species commonly found on rats throughout North America and Europe. *N. fasciatus* is a known vector of murine typhus and possibly the plague. It is also an intermediate host of *Hymenolepis diminuta,* the rat tapeworm, which is occasionally parasitic in humans. Formerly called *Ceratophyllus fasciatus.*

nostrils (nos′trilz) see *nares.*

NOT ($\neg$ or $\sim$) a logical unary operation that is *true* if and only if its argument is *false.* See also *NAND.*

not/o (no′to) [Gr. *nōton* back] a word element used in combining form to denote relationship to the back, e.g., notochord.

NOT-AND gate see *NAND gate.*

notation (no-ta′shun) a particular symbolic method used in expressing a related group of mathematical concepts, quantities, and operations.

positional n., any method of expressing numbers, such as the familiar decimal system, in which the value of a digit depends on its place in the number, as opposed to a nonpositional notation, such as Roman numerals. See also *number system.*

notencephalocele (no″ten-sĕ-fal′-o-sēl″) [*noto-* + Gr. *enkephalos* brain + *kēlē* hernia] a hernial protrusion of the brain at the back of the head.

notencephalus (no″ten-sef′ah-lus) [*noto-* + Gr. *enkephalos* brain] a fetus affected with a developmental abnormality that leads to the formation of a hernial protrusion of cranial substance at the back of the head.

NOT gate see *inverter.*

notocord (no′to-kord) [*noto-* + Gr. *chordē* cord] in the developing embryo, the primitive backbone. An axial rod–shaped support that is characteristic of all species of Chordata, it is later replaced by the vertebral column.

Notoedres (no″to-ed′rēz) [N.L., from *noto-* + Gr. *hedra* abode] a genus of mites. The species *N. cati* (itch mite) is parasitic in cats and causes mange, and may temporarily infest humans.

novobiocin (no″vo-bi′o-sin) an antibiotic produced by *Streptomyces niveus.* It is a dibasic acid containing coumarin, a sugar, and a substituted phenol. Novobiocin is a narrow-spectrum drug; it was formerly used for penicillin-resistant staphylococcal infections but has been largely replaced by other drugs because of its toxicity. See also *antibacterial agents.*

Novocain (no′vo-kān) trademark. See *procaine hydrochloride.*

Novy, MacNeal and Nicolle's medium [Frederick George *Novy,* U.S. bacteriologist, 1864–1957; Ward J. *MacNeal,* U.S. bacteriologist, 1881–1946; Jules Henry *Nicolle,* Fr. bacteriologist, 1866–1936] a culture medium that consists of agar, salt, and rabbit or guinea pig blood. It is utilized in growing *Leishmania donovani* and *Trypanosoma cruzi.* Also called *NNN medium.*

noxious (nok′shus) [L. *noxius*] hurtful; unwholesome; pernicious.

NP abbrev. See *nurse practitioner.*

Np symbol for the chemical element *neptunium.*

NP detector abbrev. for nitrogen-phosphorus detector. See under *gas chromatography.*

NPN abbrev. See *nonprotein nitrogen.*

NRC abbrev. See *Nuclear Regulatory Commission.*

NRCC abbrev. See *National Registry in Clinical Chemistry.*

NREM sleep see *nonREM sleep.*

NRM abbrev. See *National Registry of Microbiologists.*

NRSCC abbrev. See *National Reference System in Clinical Chemistry.*

ns abbrev. See *nanosecond.*

NSAID abbrev. for nonsteroidal antiinflammatory drug. See under *prostaglandin.*

NSD abbrev. See *nominal single d.* under *dose.*

nsec abbrev. See *nanosecond.*

NSH abbrev. See *National Society for Histotechnology.*

NSILA-s abbrev. See *insulinlike activity, nonsuppressible.*

NSR abbrev. See *normal sinus rhythm.*

NST abbrev. See *nonstress test.*

5′NT abbrev. See *5′-nucleotidase.*

5′-NT abbrev. See *5′-nucleotidase.*

NTD abbrev. See *5′-nucleotidase.*

N-terminal referring to the amino acid residue with a free amino group at one end of a peptide chain. See *amino t.* under *terminal.* Cf. *C-terminal.*

NTP abbrev. See *5′-nucleotidase.*

nu N, ν (noo, nu) the thirteenth letter of the *Greek alphabet.*

nuchal (nu′kal) [L. *nucha* nape] pertaining to the back of the neck.

nuchal hemangioma see *vascular n.* under *nevus.*

nucle/o (nu′kle-o) [L. *nucleus* kernal, pit, stone] a word element used in combining form to denote nucleus, e.g., nucleoproteins.

nuclear (nu′kle-ar) pertaining to a nucleus.

nuclear contour index (NCI) a size-independent indicator of the shape of a nucleus, derived from its area and perimeter using the formula NCI = perimeter/area$^{1/2}$. It can be measured by tracing the nuclear membrane from an electron micrograph utilizing a graphic digitizer. The NCI gives a minimum value of 3.54 for a nucleus with a circular contour; the cerebriform nuclei of the cells in mycosis fungoides have an NCI of 6.5 or higher.

nuclear:cytoplasmic ratio (N:C ratio) the ratio of the volume (or diameter) of a cell nucleus to the volume of the cytoplasm (or the portion of the cell diameter occupied by the cytoplasm). In malignant cells, the N:C ratio is usually greater than normal.

nuclear envelope the structure that partitions the nucleus of a cell from its cytoplasm. It is composed of two unit membranes, separated by a space of about 15 nm, the perinuclear envelope or cisterna. The two membranes fuse at many places to form octagonal nuclear pores, about 70 nm in diameter, which allow the passage of molecules, e.g., mRNA. The outer membrane is continuous with the endoplasmic reticulum.

nuclear fast red the sodium salt of aminoanthraquinone sulfonic acid; C.I. 60760. It is used to demonstrate calcium deposits in tissues. Nuclear fast red forms a brillant red dye lake with calcium(II) ions, staining soluble and insoluble calcium salts with the exception of calcium oxalate. Laked with aluminum, it is used as a nuclear stain. It also forms lakes with Pb^{2+}, Fe^{3+}, Cu^{2+}, K^{+}, Sn^{4+}, and Sr^{2+}. Also called *calcium red* and *Kernechtrot.*

nuclear magnetic resonance (NMR) a phenomenon exhibited by all atomic nuclei having a magnetic moment: when placed in a constant magnetic field, the nuclei absorb electromagnetic radiation at a few characteristic frequencies. Nuclei with an even number of protons and neutrons, e.g., ^{12}C or ^{16}O, have zero spin and magnetic moment and do not exhibit NMR. Other nuclei have integral or half-integral spin quantum numbers (S) ranging from 1/2 to 9/2 for different nuclei. For a nucleus with spin S in a static magnetic field, there are 2S + 1 equally spaced energy levels representing different orientations of the spin (and magnetic moment) relative to the external field. The nucleus can absorb a photon in a transition to the next higher energy level or emit a photon in going to the next lower level.

Most NMR applications involve protons (^{1}H nuclei), which have spin 1/2 and thus two energy levels, with the spin parallel or antiparallel to the applied field. For an applied field of 1.4092 T, the NMR frequency for a free proton is 60 MHz, the radio frequency at which the photon energy is equal to the difference between the two spin energy levels. For a ^{1}H nucleus in a chemical compound, the NMR frequency is different because the magnetic field felt by the proton differs from the applied field as a result of additional magnetic effects due to other nearby electrons or nuclei. Each chemically different hydrogen in a compound thus absorbs at a slightly different frequency. Chemically identical hydrogens, those that can be superimposed by rotations about single bonds, such as the three hydrogens of a methyl group, or by reflections or rotations of the molecule, such as the six hydrogens of benzene, absorb at the same frequency. Each group of chemically identical hydrogens produces a single peak in the NMR spectrum, with a peak area proportional to the number of hydrogens in the group. The location of the peaks is given in terms of the chemical shift, which is the shift in frequency (in parts per million) from a reference peak, usually tetramethyl silane, $(CH_3)_4Si$, a compound with 12 identical hydrogens. The chemical shift is approximately proportional to the electron density near the carbon atom to which the hydrogen is attached; tables of approximate chemical shifts for particular groups in common molecular structures are available. It is usually possible to determine the structure of any unknown, relatively small compound from its molecular formula and NMR spectrum.

nuclear magnetic resonance (NMR) scanning an imaging technique that produces cross-sectional images superficially similar to x-ray computed tomography (CT). The technique is based on the fact that some atomic nuclei behave like tiny bar magnets; when a large external magnetic field is applied, these nuclei tend to align with the magnetic field. The alignment is not complete, and the nuclei precess like a top or gyroscope at a characteristic resonance frequency proportional to the magnetic field. To date, only hydrogen nuclei have been imaged, using a magnetic field of about 0.1^{T} and a resonance frequency of 4 MHz.

The images are produced by using a pulse of strong radio waves to selectively perturb the hydrogen nuclei in a cross-sectional slice and then monitoring the return of the nuclei to their equilibrium position. Several types of images can be produced: one is an anatomic map of the hydrogen distribution in the patient, which is analogous to the x-ray CT images; the more exciting possibilities are images that are maps of the nuclear spin relaxation times (T_1 and T_2), which represent the rates at which the nuclei recover from the perturbation. These response times are strongly dependent on the chemical environment of the hydrogen nuclei. The relaxation time images may provide completely new diagnostic information that will permit tissue identification. An additional important feature of NMR imaging is that, to the best of current knowledge, there is no risk to the patient, as no ionizing radiation is used.

ARTHUR E. BURGESS, PH.D.

nuclear magnetic resonance spectrometer an instrument for obtaining NMR spectra. The sample is placed between the poles of a powerful electromagnet having a spatially uniform, variable field and between the coils of a radio-frequency transmitter and receiver. One of two setups is used: the transmitter is maintained at a constant frequency and the magnetic field strength is varied, or the magnetic field is fixed and the microwave transmission is swept through the frequency range. The absorption peaks due to NMR are plotted on a chart recorder.

nuclear magneton (μ_N) a unit of magnetic moment defined as $eh/4\pi m_p c$ (where h is Planck's constant, c is the velocity of light, m_p is the proton mass, and e is the proton charge), which is equal to 5.051×10^{-27} J/T.

nuclear medicine the medical specialty concerned with the use of radioisotopes in the diagnosis and treatment of disease (except for the use of sealed sources in radiation therapy). Nuclear medicine is primarily concerned with the production and interpretation of diagnostic scintillation images and with in vivo tests that employ radioisotopes.

nuclear medicine quality control procedures to ensure maintenance of quality in nuclear medicine studies. Comprising three general categories, they include calibration and operational checks performed on scintillation cameras, rectilinear scanners, and scintillation counters; tests of the purity of radiopharmaceuticals prepared from manufacturers' kits; and strict adherence to established protocols for all clinical procedures.

The pulse-height analyzer (PHA) in a counter, camera, or scanner is calibrated daily. This involves setting the energy window controls for a standard-width window centered on the principal photopeak of a radionuclide, positioning a check source in the proper geometric relation to the detector, and adjusting the gain setting until the count rate is maximized. The maximal count is recorded as a check on PHA sensitivity. Because of the nonlinearity of PHA response, the PHA must be recalibrated using the radionuclide of interest whenever the nuclide being counted is changed. Long-lived substitutes with nearby photopeaks are often used, e.g., ^{57}Co for ^{99m}Tc, ^{129}I for ^{125}I, or ^{133}Ba for ^{131}I.

The energy resolution of the PHA is also checked regularly; this is performed by measuring the full width at half-maximum (FWHM) of the ^{137}Cs, ^{57}Co, or ^{99m}Tc photopeak either by using the multichannel analyzer if one is built into the instrument or by determining the count at 10-keV intervals and graphing the photopeak.

Additional checks for scanners include density and ratemeter calibration and contrast enhancement checks. A flood source in the focal plane is scanned and the scanner adjusted to produce the desired maximal film density, e.g., 1.6 at an information density of 800 counts/cm^2. By scanning a wedge transmission phantom, both the gray scale and the operation of the contrast enhancement controls can be checked. Dual-probe scanners must be adjusted so that both probes have the same response on all QC checks.

Additional checks for cameras are the imaging of a flood source and a bar phantom. The flood field image demonstrates field uniformity and camera sensitivity: the counting rate of the flood source should decline with the 271-da half-life of the ^{57}Co source. The bar phantom image demonstrates camera spatial resolution and linearity and also serves as a check for image size.

A nuclear medicine laboratory may also participate in an external quality control program, such as the proficiency survey of the College of American Pathologists (CAP). This type of evaluation involves sending phantoms with an unknown distribution of radioactivity to participating laboratories. After the external agency evaluates and compares the images, each laboratory is given an analysis of its results.

Imaging agents that have been prepared on-site from generator-produced nuclides and manufacturers' kits are checked for their specific activity and for some or all of the following properties: radionuclidic, radiochemical, and chemical purity; and pH, apyrogenicity, and sterility. Radionuclidic purity is demonstrated with a multichannel analyzer, radiochemical purity by thin-layer chromatography, and chemical purity by various chemical tests.

nuclear medicine technologist a health care professional whose duties include positioning and attending to patients undergoing nuclear medicine procedures, operating imaging devices (scintillation cameras and rectilinear scanners) under the direction of the nuclear medicine physician, preparing radiopharmaceuticals for administration to patients, making dose calculation for in vivo procedures, performing quality control procedures, and utilizing a knowledge of radiation physics and radiation safety to minimize radiation exposure. Educational preparation involves completion of an approved program; graduates are certified by one of three organizations: the American Registry of Radiologic Technologists (AART), the American Society of Clinical Pathologists (ASCP), and the Nuclear Medicine Technology Certification Board (NMTCB). Individuals certified by the AART are designated RT(N)(ARRT); those certified by ASCP are designated NM(ASCP); and those certified by the NMTCB are designated CNMT.

nuclear physician a specialist in nuclear medicine.

nuclear ploidy the number of sets of chromosomes or DNA content of a cell. See also *aneuploid, diploid, euploid, haploid,* and *polyploid.*

nuclear pore see under *nuclear envelope.*

nuclear reaction any process (fission, fusion, neutron capture, alpha decay, beta decay, or electron capture) that changes one or more nuclides into different nuclides.

nuclear reactor a device that produces energy by controlled fission of uranium or plutonium. It is a source of high-density neutron flux, which is used for neutron activation analysis and to produce many radioisotopes used in medicine.

Nuclear Regulatory Commission (NRC) an agency of the United States government that regulates the production, use, and disposal of radioactive materials; sets radiation exposure limits for both the public and for radiation workers; and licenses users of radioactive materials.

nuclear transplantation see *cellular c.* under *cloning.*

nuclease (nu′kle-ās) a general term for enzymes of the hydrolase class that split the phosphodiester linkages in nucleic acids to form nucleotides or oligonucleotides. The nucleases are classified in subgroups as exonucleases (EC 3.1.11–16) or endonucleases (EC 3.1.21–31). Important enzymes of the group are ribonucleases and deoxyribonuclease. In addition, there are also site-specific endodeoxyribonucleases that cleave both strands of DNA at specific sequences. They are usually isolated from bacteria. These enzymes are more commonly known as restriction endonucleases and have been widely used in recombinant DNA technology.

nucleated (nu′kle-āt″ed) [L. *nucleatus*] having a nucleus or nuclei.

nucleic acid a component of the utmost biologic importance in all organisms. It exists as either of the two macromolecules: deoxyribonucleic acid (DNA) or ribonucleic acid (RNA). Normally, all living organisms have both; some viruses, however, have just one or the other.

Nucleic acid is a polymer of nucleotides that consist of a pentose sugar with a phosphate group attached at the 5′ position of the sugar and nitrogen-containing portion (base) attached to the 1′ position. The combination of pentose and base without the phosphate constitutes a nucleoside. The pentose sugars are ribose or, lacking one oxygen atom at the 2′ position, deoxyribose. RNA contains ribose, DNA deoxyribose.

There are two types of bases: those that contain one carbon-nitrogen ring are the pyrimidines, whereas those that contain two fused rings are the purines. The two main pyrimidines found in DNA are cytosine (C) and thymine (T), whereas RNA contains cytosine and uracil (U). (See illustration under *base.*) Thymine is not ordinarily found in RNA nor uracil in DNA. The two main purines, adenine (A) and guanine (G), are found in both DNA and RNA.

Nucleic acids are linear polymers in which the nucleotides are linked together by means of phosphate-diester bridges with the pentose moiety. The bonds link the 3′ carbon of one nucleotide to the 5′ carbon in the pentose of the adjacent nucleotide. Thus, the backbone of nucleic acids consists of alternating phosphates and pentoses, with bases at the 1′ of the sugars of the backbone.

Although DNA base composition varies from species to species, striking regularities are found. In all cases the amount of thymine is equal to the amount of adenine found (i.e., A = T), and the number of cytosine and guanine bases is equal (i.e., G = C). Consequently, the total quantity of purines equals the total quantity of pyrimidines (i.e., A + G = C + T). Yet there exists considerable variation between species regarding the AT/GC ratio. Generally, in higher plants and animals AT exceeds GC, whereas in viruses, bacteria, and lower plants the reverse is more common.

The structure of DNA is composed of polynucleotide chains that form a right-handed double helix around the same central axis. The two strands are antiparallel: their 3′, 5′-phosphodiester links are in opposite directions, the two strands being held together by hydrogen bonds between pairs of bases. The only two possible pairings are AT and GC, with two hydrogen bonds between A and T and three bonds between G and C. In addition to the hydrogen bonds, hydrophobic interactions between stacked bases are important for stability of the helical structure. The axial sequence of bases along one polynucleotide chain may vary considerably, but the complementary pairing is exact. Most viruses have covalently closed circular DNA molecules that are supercoiled—this is associated with fewer turns in the DNA double helix.

The primary structure of RNA is similar to that of DNA, except for the presence of ribose and uracil in place of deoxyribose and thymine. The base composition does not follow as does DNA because RNA molecules form only one chain. RNA is synthesized within the nucleus, using only one strand of DNA as a template. There are three major classes of RNA: ribosomal RNA (rRNA), transfer RNA (tRNA), and messenger RNA (mRNA).

Although each RNA molecule is a single chain, it is not a simple, linear structure. RNA has extensive regions of complementarity in which hydrogen bonds between AU and GC pairs are formed between different regions of the same molecule. The result is that the molecule folds upon itself, forming hairpin loops. In this manner the RNA adopts a helical structure comparable with that of DNA.

The simplest infectious agents are viruses (viroids), consisting only of circular RNA molecules not covered by a protein coat. It is this naked molecule that is able to multiply in plant cells, disperse into the environment, and infect other plants.

DNA is primarily located in the nucleus, although it is also present in the mitochondria and chloroplasts. Its hydrolyzing enzyme is deoxyribonuclease (DNase). RNA is found in the cytoplasm, nucleolus, and chromosomes. Its hydrolyzing enzyme is ribonuclease (RNase). DNA acts as the genetic material of cells, carrying information in a coded form from cell to cell and from parent to offspring. When a gene is expressed, its information is copied into RNA, which in turn directs the synthesis of the ultimate gene products, the specific proteins. These concepts constitute the central dogma of molcular biology.

See also *deoxyribonucleic acid* and *ribonucleic acid.*

nucleography (nu″kle-og′rah-fe) [*nucleo-* + Gr. *graphein* to write] see *diskography.*

nucleohistone (nu″kle-o-his′tōn) the nucleoprotein that constitutes chromosomes, which is composed of DNA and histones. See *chromatin* and *nucleosome.*

nucleoid (nu′kle-oid) [*nucleo-* + Gr. *eidos* form] 1. resembling a nucleus.

2. the nuclear region of a bacterium, consisting of

a dense, centrally located, irregularly shaped region composed of DNA material that lacks a membrane. Also called nuclear body.

nucleolar (nu-kle′o-lar) pertaining to nucleolus.

nucleolar organizing site the region of certain chromosomes at which nucleoli form. In a condensed metaphase chromosome, it can be seen as the secondary constriction that separates a satellite from the rest of the chromosome. During telophase, as the chromatin uncoils, the nucleolus is synthesized. Also called nucleolus organizer.

nucleolar satellite see *Barr body.*

nucleolinus (nu″kle-o-li′nus), pl. *nucleolini* a spherical structure within the nucleolus composed of ribonucleoprotein. In electron micrographs, the nucleolini are electron-lucent and fibrillar; in light microscopy, they are deeply stained by toluidine blue molybdate. See also *anisonucleolinosis.*

nucleolonema (nu″kle-o″lo-ne′mah) [*nucleolus* + Gr. *nēma* thread] in light microscopy, a term used to describe the threadlike appearance of the fibers and granules of the nucleolus that wind through areas of lightly staining nucleoplasm.

nucleolus (nu-kle′o-lus), pl. *nucleoli* [L., dim. of *nucleus*] the region of the cell nucleus in which ribosomes are produced. It is absent in cells that are not synthesizing proteins and in all cells undergoing mitosis or meiosis. A nucleus may contain several nucleoli.

The nucleolus contains extended segments of DNA, which code for ribosomal RNA (rRNA); this is called nucleolar (or nucleolus-associated) chromatin. The rRNA is synthesized as long strands. These are cleaved into two pieces, which then combine with proteins to form the two ribosomal subunits. By electron microscopy the strands appear as fibrillar material (pars fibrosa) and the subunits as granular material (pars granulosa).

The nucleolus is stained by basophilic stains for DNA and is differentiated from the rest of the nucleus by stains that are specific for RNA, e.g., methyl green–pyronin.

nucleon (nu′kle-on) one of the particles composing an atomic nucleus—a proton or a neutron.

nucleophagocytosis (nu″kle-o-fag″o-si-to′sis) [*nucleo-* + Gr. *phagein* to eat + *kytos* hollow vessel + *-osis*] the ingestion of a nucleus by a phagocytic cell, e.g., as in a lupus erythematosus (LE) cell.

nucleophile (nu′kle-o-fīl″) [*nucleo-* + Gr. *philein* to love] a reagent that can donate an unshared electron pair; a reagent that is preferentially attracted to a site of low electron density in a substrate. The term is generally used to refer to a species with an unshared pair of electrons (*Lewis base*). Cf. *electrophile.*

nucleoprotein (nu″kle-o-pro′tēn) a complex formed from a nucleic acid combined with protein, particularly the coiled structure composed of acidic DNA and basic histones that make up the chromosome.

nucleoside (nu′kle-o-sīd″) a compound that contains a pentose (D-ribose or D-deoxyribose) linked to a purine or a pyrimidine base. The C-1 of the pentose is linked by a β-linkage to a nitrogen (N-1 of pyrimidine, N-9 of purine) of the base. Nucleosides may be obtained by the hydrolytic splitting of PO_4 from nucleotides. The major ribose and deoxyribose nucleosides are shown in the accompanying table.

nucleoside phosphorylase (nu′kle-o-sīd″ fos-for′ĭ-lās) see *purine nucleoside phosphorylase.*

nucleoside triphosphate (nu′kle-o-sīd″ tri-fos′fāt) a triphosphate ester of nucleosides. These triphosphates represent a reserve of stored energy as high-energy phosphate bonds for use in many reactions. Ribonucleoside triphosphates are involved in a number of the RNA chain elongation steps. See also *adenosine triphosphate, cytidine triphosphate, guanosine triphosphate, thymidine triphosphate,* and *uridine triphosphate.*

nucleosome (nu′kle-o-sōm) [*nucleus* + Gr. *sōma* body] a structure occurring in eukaryotic chromosomes that consists of a spherical particle containing two molecules each of the histones H2a, H2b, H3, and H4, plus a length of DNA of about 140 base pairs tightly coiled around the outside. The nucleosomes are separated by a 25–100 base pair length of DNA.

5′-nucleotidase (NTP, 5′NT) (nu″kle-ot′ĭ-dās) an enzyme of the hydrolase class (5′-ribonucleotide phosphohydrolase, EC 3.1.3.5) that catalyzes the reaction a 5′ribonucleotide + $H_2O \rightleftharpoons$ a ribonucleoside + orthophosphate. It is widely distributed throughout the body tissues. Serum NTP activity increases two to six times in obstructive jaundice, hepatobiliary disease, and intrahepatic cholestasis. The test is usually used to confirm that a high alkaline phosphatase activity is of hepatic origin. It is rarely used as a primary test.

5′-nucleotidase assays 1. methods based on liberation of phosphate. In these procedures, adenosine-5′-phosphate (5′-AMP) serves as substrate and is converted by the enzyme to adenosine and phosphate at pH 7.8. As this reaction is nonspecific, nickel ions are added to one set of reaction tubes to inhibit the enzyme. The difference in phosphate formed in the reaction with and without added Ni^{2+} is a measure of the enzyme activity. The test can also be performed by using both 5′-AMP and 2′-AMP as substrates. The former is acted on by both 5′-NT and alkaline phosphatase and the latter by alkaline phosphatase alone.

2. methods based on measurement of adenosine, a product of the reaction. Adenosine deaminase may be added to the reaction mixture to hydrolyze adenosine to ammonia, which may be measured by the Berthelot reaction. The NH_3 formed may also be measured by coupling the system to a third enzyme, glutamate dehydrogenase (with oxoglutarate and NADH) and measuring the decrease in NADH at

NUCLEOSIDE. TABLE OF THE MAJOR NUCLEOSIDES

BASE	NUCLEOSIDE
Adenine	Adenosine Deoxyadenosine
Guanine	Guanosine Deoxyguanosine
Cytosine	Cytidine Deoxycytidine
Uracil	Uridine
Thymine	Thymine ribonucleoside Thymidine

340 nm. Alternately, the decrease of adenosine may be measured by its absorbance at 265 nm.

The activity of ALP is suppressed by adding enough β-glycerophosphate, which saturates the ALP active center and thus prevents binding to 5′-AMP.

nucleotide (nu′kle-o-tīd) a phosphoric acid ester of nucleosides, one of the components into which nucleic acids are split by the action of nuclease. Nucleotides are composed of a nitrogen base (purine or pyrimidine), a sugar (ribose or deoxyribose), and a phosphate group. The last is linked to the sugar at either the 5′ position (most common) or at the 3′ or 2′ positions. The dinucleotides are composed of two nucleotides linked tail-to-tail via the phosphate groups (pyrophosphate). Both mono- and dinucleotides are known to occur free in biologic systems. Abbreviations for the major mononucleotides and two dinucleotides are listed in the accompanying table.

nucleotide cyclase (nu′kle-o-tīd″ si′klās) a subclass of the lyase class of enzymes (EC 4.6), consisting of those enzymes that eliminate pyrophosphate from a nucleoside triphosphate with the formation of a cyclic compound, such as adenylate cyclase.

nucleotide replacement site the locus on a DNA molecule at which a point mutation (the replacement of one base by another) has occurred.

nucleus (nu′kle-us) [L., dim. of *nux* nut] 1. the characteristic structure of the eukaryotic cell, a spheroidal body, usually 4–10 μm in diameter, separated from the cytoplasm by the nuclear envelope. It contains the chromosomes and nucleoli and is the site of DNA replication and transcription. The nucleus stains deeply with basic dyes such as hematoxylin because of its nucleic acid content. The chromosomal DNA is specifically stained by the Feulgen reaction.

2. in neuroanatomy, a group of cell bodies of neurons in the central nervous system.

3. the atomic nucleus, the small dense structure at the center of an atom. It is composed of protons and neutrons held together by strong forces and contains 99.9 percent of the mass of the atom in 1/10,000 of the atomic diameter. The rest of the atom consists of electrons orbiting the nucleus. The number of protons in the nucleus is the atomic number (A) and characterizes the chemical element of the atom; the number of protons plus neutrons is the mass number (Z), which characterizes the isotope.

4. in organic chemistry, a part of a compound, e.g., a benzene ring, that is characteristic of a group of compounds.

5. a minute particle that serves as the basis for the growth of a crystal in a saturated solution or a liquid droplet in a saturated vapor.

accessory n., see *Edinger-Westphal n.*

n. ambiguus, [NA], the cell bodies of a discrete group of motor neurons of the vagus, glossopharyngeal, and accessory nerves that innervate the striated muscles of the pharynx and larynx. Found deep in the reticular formation within the medulla oblongata, the nucleus ambiguus extends rostrally to the dorsal nucleus of the vagus, and caudally is continuous with the spinal nucleus of the accessory nerve.

n. amygdalae, see *amygdala.*

caudate n., an elongated, arched gray mass closely related to the lateral ventricle of the brain. It consists of a head, body, and tail. The caudate nucleus and putamen form a functional unit (neostriatum) of the corpus striatum.

Clarke's n., a well-defined column of cells in the

NUCLEOTIDE. TABLE OF ABBREVIATIONS FOR NUCLEOTIDES

NUCLEOTIDE	ABBREVIATION
Mononucleotides with Ribose as a Sugar	
Adenosine monophosphate (adenylic acid)	AMP
Adenosine diphosphate	ADP
Adenosine triphosphate	ATP
Cytidine monophosphate (cytidylic acid)	CMP
Cytidine diphosphate	CDP
Cytidine triphosphate	CTP
Guanosine monophosphate (guanylic acid)	GMP
Guanosine diphosphate	GDP
Guanosine triphosphate	GTP
Thymine ribonucleoside monophosphate (ribothymidylic acid)	TMP
Uridine monophosphate (uridylic acid)	UMP
Uridine diphosphate	UDP
Uridine triphosphate	UTP
Mononucleotides with Deoxyribose as Sugar	
Deoxyadenosine monophosphate (deoxyadenylic acid)	dAMP
Deoxycytidine monophosphate (deoxycytidylic acid)	dCMP
Deoxyguanosine monophosphate (deoxyguanylic acid)	dGMP
Thymidine monophosphate (thymidylic acid)	dTMP
Dinucleotides	
Flavin adenine dinucleotide	FAD
Nicotinamide adenine dinucleotide	NAD

medial part of the base of the posterior gray column of the spinal cord, extending from the seventh or eighth cervical segments to the second or third lumbar level. The cells give rise to the posterior spinocerebellar tract. Also called *n. thoracicus.*

cuneate n., a nucleus in the medulla oblongata at the rostral end of the fasciculus cuneatus, in which the fibers of this fasciculus synapse. The cells project to the thalamus via the medial lemniscus.

Deiters' n., the lateral vestibular nucleus.

dentate n., the largest of the deep cerebellar nuclei. It lies in the white matter of the cerebellum just lateral to the emboliform nucleus, and receives Purkinje cell fibers from the neocerebellum. Its axons form most of the superior cerebellar peduncle and project chiefly to the contralateral red nucleus and thalamus.

diploid n., a cell nucleus containing the number of chromosomes typical of the somatic cells of the particular species.

Edinger-Westphal n., a group of multipolar neurons located dorsal to the oculomotor nucleus that supply parasympathetic efferents via the ciliary ganglion to the ciliary muscle and the pupillary sphincter muscle. Also called *accessory n.*

n. gracilis, a nucleus in the medulla oblongata at the rostral end of the fasciculus gracilis of the spinal cord, in which the fibers of the fasciculus gracilis synapse; the cells project to the thalamus via the medial lemniscus. Also called Goll's nucleus.

hypothalamic n., a biconvex mass of gray matter on the medial side of the junction of the internal capsule and the crus cerebri; its chief connections are with the globus pallidus.

motor n., any collection of cells of the central nervous system that gives origin to the motor fibers of a nerve.

olivary n., a folded band of gray substance enclosing a white core that produces the elevation on the medulla oblongata known as the olive. It is a nuclear complex that receives projections from the spinal cord, mesencephalon, and cerebral cortex; it projects fibers, via the opposite inferior cerebellar peduncle, partly to the vermis, but principally to the neocerebellum.

pontine n., groups of nerve cell bodies in the portion of the pyramidal tract within the pars ventralis of the pons on which the fibers of the corticopontine tract synapse, and whose axons in turn cross to the opposite side and form the middle cerebellar peduncle, which projects fibers to the neocerebellum.

n. pulposus, see *intervertebral d.* under *disk.*

red n., a distinctive oval nucleus (having a pink appearance in fresh specimens owing to its relatively high vascularity) centrally placed in the upper mesencephalic reticular formation. It receives fibers from the deep cerebellar nuclei and cerebral cortex, and projects fibers to the cerebellum, brain stem, and spinal cord, and probably to the thalamus.

sensory n., the nucleus of termination of the afferent fibers of a peripheral nerve.

n. thoracicus, see *Clarke's n.*

vesicular n., a form of cell nucleus, the periphery of which stains deeply, whereas the central part is rather pale.

vestibular nuclei, four cellular masses in the floor of the fourth ventricle: the superior, lateral, medial, and inferior vestibular nuclei. The nuclei give rise to a widely dispersed special sensory system through projections to motor nuclei in the brain stem and cervical cord via the medial longitudinal fasciculi, to the cerebellum, and to motor cells throughout the spinal cord. Additional connections of the nuclei provide for conscious perception of, and autonomic reactions to, labyrinthine stimulation.

nuclide (nu'klīd) a species of atom characterized by the number of protons and neutrons in its nucleus, or equivalently by the atomic (or the element it specifies) and the mass number. Isomers are not separate nuclides; Tc-99m is the metastable excited state of the Tc-99 nuclide.

null balance in potentiometry, the condition in which the unknown voltage being measured is exactly opposed by the voltage produced by the potentiometer circuit and no current flows between them, as indicated by the galvanometer.

null cell 1. a lymphocyte that lacks the surface antigens characteristic of T and B lymphocytes and that can kill cultured tumor cells in vitro. These cells are seen in, for example, systemic lupus erythematosus. 2. a leukemic cell that lacks T- or B-lymphocyte characteristics.

null hypothesis (H_0) [L. *nullus* none] an assumption made about the parent population of a statistical sample that determines the sampling distribution of a specified test statistic. See also *hypothesis testing.*

nullipara (nu-lip'ah-rah) [L. *nullus* none + *parere* to bring forth] the term used to designate a woman who has not produced a viable offsping. Also called para 0.

nullisomatic (nul"ĭ-so-mat'ik) [L. *nullus* none + Gr. *sōma* body] lacking a pair of chromosomes.

number system a positional notation for the representation of numbers, such as the familiar decimal (base 10) system. Because computer logic circuits have only two states (on and off), computers use the binary (base 2) system for internal calculations. The octal (base 8) and hexadecimal (base 16) systems, in which each digit corresponds to three or four bits, are used to represent binary numbers in output.

The binary system uses only the digits 0 and 1; the octal system, 0–7; and the hexadecimal system, 0–9 and A–F (the letters represent the decimal numbers 10–15).

In the decimal system, the places to the left of the decimal point count ones (10^0), tens (10^1), hundreds (10^2), whereas the places to the right count tenths (10^{-1}), hundredths (10^{-2}), etc. Similarly, in the binary system, places to the left of the radix, or base, point count ones (2^0), twos (2^1), fours (2^2), etc., and places to the right count halves (2^{-1}), quarters (2^{-2}), etc. The accompanying table gives the first 16 numbers in all four systems.

numbness (num'nes) abnormal decrease or absence of sensation. The causes are varied and include lesions in the peripheral or central nervous system.

numeric (noo-mer'ik) in automatic data processing, pertaining to data consisting of numbers or character-string data composed of the decimal digits 0–9 or the hexadecimal digits 0–9, A–F.

numerical aperture (NA) (noo-mer'ĭ-kal) a number that measures the resolving power of a microscope objective lens. The smallest distance that can

NUMBER SYSTEM

DECIMAL	BINARY	OCTAL	HEXADECIMAL
1	1	1	1
2	10	2	2
3	11	3	3
4	100	4	4
5	101	5	5
6	110	6	6
7	111	7	7
8	1000	10	8
9	1001	11	9
10	1010	12	A
11	1011	13	B
12	1100	14	C
13	1101	15	D
14	1110	16	E
15	1111	17	F
16	10000	20	10

be resolved is the wavelength of light divided by twice the NA. The formula is NA = $n \sin u$, where n is the refractive index of the optical medium (1 for air and up to 1.5 for immersion oil), and u is half the angle made at the front lens by rays from the edge of the field of view.

numerical taxonomy the classification of organisms using as criteria only their observable characters, that is, their phenotypes, as opposed to classical taxonomy in which organisms are classified in groups (taxa) known or believed to be descended from a common evolutionary ancestor. This system has been used primarily in the classification of bacteria.

By comparing the organisms (practically accomplished by means of a computer program), a similarity coefficient for each pair or organisms can be computed. When binary (two-state) characters are used, the similarity coefficient can be defined as the number of character matches (as a percentage of the total number of characters). More complicated measures of similarity (or taxonomic distance) use quantitative characters and weighting of the characters. The computer then divides the organisms into taxonomic groups that are similarity clusters or phenons (organisms that have some specified mutual similarity). As the specified similarity decreases, the groups coalesce to form larger groups.

nurse (nurs) 1. a health care professional responsible for the observation, care, and counsel of the ill, injured, or infirm; for the administration of medications or treatments prescribed by a physician; and for the maintenance of health or prevention of illness in clients or patients.

2. to perform the duties of a professional nurse.
3. to breastfeed an infant.

n. clinician, a registered nurse who has well-developed competencies in utilizing a broad range of cues. These cues are used for prescribing and implementing both direct and indirect nursing care and for articulating nursing therapies with other planned therapies. Nurse clinicians demonstrate expertise in nursing practice and ensure ongoing development of expertise through clinical experience and continuing education. Generally, minimal preparation for this role is the baccalaureate degree.

n. practitioner, a registered nurse with advanced skills in the assessment of the physical and psychosocial health-illness status of individuals, families, or groups in a variety of settings through health and development history taking and physical examination.

registered n., a graduate nurse registered and licensed to practice by a State Board of Nurse Examiners or other state authority.

nutmeg liver a term used to describe the appearance of the liver in chronic passive congestion. The central regions of lobules appear dark red. Because these hyperemic zones are surrounded by yellow-brown normal hepatic parenchyma, the pattern of the cut surface of the liver resembles that of the cut surface of a nutmeg.

nutmeg oil see *myristica oil.*

nutrient (nu'tre-ent) [L. *nutriens*] 1. nourishing; aiding nutrition.

2. a nourishing substance or food.

nutrition (nu-trish'un) [L. *nutritio*] 1. the process involved in taking in nutrients, assimilating them, and utilizing them to satisfy body needs.

2. the scientific study of dietary requirements for nutrients, their use by the body, and the effects produced by the lack of specific nutrients.

nutritional cirrhosis a term that has been used in the etiologic classification of cirrhosis to describe a form of cirrhosis seen in alcoholic individuals, which corresponds approximately to micronodular cirrhosis. This concept is now known to be incorrect in that the etiology is alcohol abuse rather than a secondary nutritional deficiency. See also *cirrhosis.*

nyad (ni'ad) the nymph form in the life cycle of certain arthropods.

nyctalopia (nik"tah-lo'pe-ah) [Gr. *nyktalōps* night-blind, from *nyx, nyktos* night + *alaos* blind + *ōps* eye] see *night blindness.*

Nygmia a genus of moths. The species *N. phaeorrhoea,* the brown-tail moth of the order Lepidoptera, possesses poisonous hairs. It is found throughout Europe.

nylidrin hydrochloride (ni'lĭ-drin) [NF], a sympathomimetic amine, which acts primarily on the β-adrenergic receptors to produce peripheral vasodilation. It is used to increase the blood supply in treating peripheral vascular disease and circulatory disturbances of the inner ear. Adverse reactions include palpitations, trembling, and dizziness. Trademark, Arlidin.

nymph (nimf) [Gr. *nymphē* a bride] in the life cycle of certain arthropods, the late larval stage present before development into a true adult (as in mites or ticks).

Nyssorhynchus (nis"o-ring'kus) [Gr. *nyssa* prick + *rhynchos* snout] a subgenus of mosquitoes of the genus *Anopheles,* several species of which are known vectors of the malarial parasite in tropical areas of America.

nystagmus (nis-tag'mus) [Gr. *nystagmus* drowsiness, from *nystazein* to nod] the involuntary, rhythmic oscillation of the eyes in a vertical, horizontal, and/or rotary direction. It may be due to labyrinthine disorders, the ingestion of alcohol or other drugs such as barbiturates, or brain stem dysfunction. It may also occur on a congenital basis and in a variety of disorders in which central vision is lost early in life.

nystatin (nis'tah-tin) an antifungal agent, a polyene antibiotic, that is effective in vitro against a wide range of fungi including *Candida, Histoplasma, Paracoccidioides, Cryptococcus,* and *Blastomyces.* Nystatin works by disrupting the permeability of cell membranes that contain sterols. It is essentially insoluble in water, and is sensitive to heat, light, and oxygen. Some *Candida* species may be resistant to nystatin; these contain low amounts of ergosterol in their membranes. It is available in oral tablets or solutions and as a topical ointment.

NZB abbrev. See *New Zealand black mouse.*

NZW abbrev. See *New Zealand white mouse.*

O

O symbol for the observed number in a cell of a statistical table, the chemical element *oxygen.*

o- abbrev. See *ortho-.*

o the Greek lower case letter *omicron.*

Ω the Greek capital letter *omega;* symbol for ohm.

ω the Greek lower case letter *omega;* symbol for angular velocity.

OAF abbrev. See *osteoclast-activating factor.*

O antigen [Ger. *ohne* without] a bacterial antigen used in the serologic classification of enteric bacilli. The term was first applied by Weil and Felix in 1917 to nonswarming (nonflagellated) *Proteus* organisms because their discrete colonies were without the film of spreading growth surrounding the H (for *Hauch,* "film") colonies of motile organisms. Subsequently, the term was applied to the dominant agglutinating antigen of nonflagellated cells. It is a lipopolysaccharide-protein surface antigen. Agglutination of bacteria with O antiserum results in the formation of closely packed granular clumps. See also *H antigen.*

oasthouse urine disease (ōst′hows) [from the smell suggestive of an *oasthouse,* in which hops are dried] see *methionine malabsorption syndrome.*

oat cell carcinoma a type of carcinoma composed of small undifferentiated cells. The term is commonly associated with the bronchogenic carcinoma with this histology, although primary extrapulmonary small cell carcinomas have been described in various locations including the salivary glands, larynx, esophagus, colon, and other sites. For the bronchogenic oat cell carcinoma, the preferred term is small cell undifferentiated lung carcinoma.

Histologic subtypes have been described, but the criteria for their identification are imprecise and not consistently reproducible: the oat cell type is composed of small, round cells that resemble lymphocytes, whereas the intermediate variant has larger, often elongated cells. Confusion between the intermediate variant and a poorly differentiated adenocarcinoma of the lung can occur by light microscopy.

Small cell lung carcinomas are aggressive, spread rapidly, and are generally disseminated by the time they are diagnosed. The prognosis for affected individuals is poor, although occasional long-term survivors have been reported. Recent studies using combination forms of chemotherapy have produced some encouraging results:

See also *bronchogenic carcinoma, ectopic hormone production,* and *lung tumors.* Cf. *Merkel cell tumor* and *neuroendocrine carcinoma.*

object code the binary-coded machine language of a computer.

object-film distance (ofd, OFD) in radiology, the distance betweeen the x-ray film and the object making the image. This distance is always kept to a minimum (except in magnification) to ensure sharpness. Also called subject-film distance. See also *skin-film distance.*

objective (ob-jek′tiv) [L. *objectivus,* from *objectus* lying opposite or against] 1. perceptible to the external senses.

2. a result for whose achievement an effort is made.

3. a lens or system of lenses in a microscope that is nearest to the object under examination. Cf. *eyepiece.*

achromatic o., the standard type of microscope objective. Spherical aberration is corrected for one color, chromatic aberration for two. The correction is in the yellow-green part of the spectrum.

aplanatic o., a microscope objective that gives a flat field for use in photomicrography.

apochromatic o., the type of microscope objective that has the most correction. Spherical aberration is corrected for two colors, chromatic aberration for three. The objective is undercorrected and requires a special compensating eyepiece to bring all the colors of the image into focus.

dry o., any microscope objective designed to be used without an immersion medium.

flat-field o., a microscope objective that provides an image in which all parts of the field are simultaneously in focus.

fluorite o., a microscope objective containing one lens made of fluorite. It has a lower refractive index than glass, thus permitting more correction.

immersion o., an objective designed for use with an immersion medium (water or oil), which allows a greater resolving power than a dry objective.

semiapochromatic o., a type of microscope objective in which spherical aberration and chromatic aberration are both corrected for two colors.

object program the machine-language program that is produced by a compiler or assembler.

obligate (ob′lĭ-gāt) [L. *obligatus* bound, obliged] necessary; incapable of survival under different conditions. For example, an obligate aerobe such as *Mycobacterium tuberculosis* requires oxygen for growth. Cf. *facultative.*

oblique (ŏ-blēk, ŏ-blīk) [L. *obliquus*] slanting; inclined; between a horizontal and perpendicular direction. In radiology, the term pertains to a view or projection that is not directly anterior, posterior, or lateral.

obsessive-compulsive disorder (ob-ses′iv kom-pul′siv) a form of neurosis characterized by the intrusion of unwanted and disturbing thoughts, urges, or actions, such as the repeated and ritualistic performance of certain acts. Any departure from this behavior leads to intense anxiety. Symptoms may interfere with personal relationships, work, or the ability to enjoy life. If treatment is necessary, psychotherapy is the method of choice.

obstetrics (ob-stet′riks) [L. *obstetricia,* from *obstetrix* midwife] the branch of surgery that deals with the management of pregnancy, labor, and the puerperium.

obstruction (ob-struk′shun) [L. *obstructio,* from *obstruere* to obstruct] the act of blocking or clogging; the state of being blocked or clogged.

mesenteric vascular o., a disorder characterized by severe abdominal pain, bloody diarrhea, and protracted vomiting. The vascular obstruction is most commonly thrombotic, and may lead to bowel infarction and necrosis. Shock and severe prostration may intervene. Hemoconcentration and leukocytosis are common findings. Abdominal x-rays reveal gaseous distention and peritoneal fluid. The disease is often fatal.

urinary o., a blockage of the urinary tract that, if prolonged, may be characterized by atrophy of the renal parenchyma from back pressure; frequently there is urinary infection and stone formation. Causes of urinary blockage include congenital and neurologic defects, inflammation, prostatic hyperplasia, neoplasms, and urinary tract stones and strictures. Hematuria, crystalluria, and elevated blood urea nitrogen and serum creatinine are commonly seen.

obturator (ob″tu-ra′tor) [L. *obturare* to stop up] 1. that which closes or stops up an opening.

2. a structure associated with the obturator foramen.

obturator artery a branch of the internal iliac artery; it arises from the anterior division and leaves the pelvic cavity through the obturator canal, where it divides into anterior and posterior branches. An abnormal obturator artery (an enlarged pubic branch of the inferior epigastric artery, which replaces the normal obturator artery) is present in fewer than 30 percent of humans. Occasionally, this vessel follows the free margin of the lacunar part of the inguinal ligament; it may then be vulnerable during surgery on a femoral hernia.

obturator canal an opening in the obturator membrane for the passage of the obturator vessels and nerve. It is bounded by the free edge of the membrane and the border of the obturator groove of the pubic bone.

obturator membrane a fibrous membrane that closes the obturator foramen.

obturator nerve a nerve that arises from the lumbar plexus by the union of fibers from the second, third, and fourth lumbar nerves. It descends through psoas major and runs down the lateral wall of the pelvis to pass through the obturator foramen. It carries motor fibers for the adductor muscles.

occipital (ok-sip′ĭ-tal) [L. *occipitalis,* from *occiput* back of the head] pertaining to the back part of the head.

occipital artery a branch of the external carotid artery that runs to the posterior part of the scalp.

occipital bone the unpaired skull bone that surrounds the foramen magnum. It has an anterior basilar portion, two lateral condylar parts that articulate with the atlas vertebra, and an expanded squamous portion behind the foramen. The outer aspect of the squamous part of the occipital bone bears a median ridge, the external occipital crest, from which superior and inferior nuchal lines curve to the lateral edges of the bone.

occipitalization (ok-sip″ĭ-tal-ĭ-za′shun) a congenital malformation that results in the fusion of the first cervical vertebra to the skull. See also *Klippel-Feil syndrome.*

occipital lobe the posterior portion of the cerebral hemisphere, which extends from the posterior pole to the parietooccipital fissure on the medial surface and is continuous with the parietal lobe on the lateral surface.

occipitofrontal projection (ok-sip″ĭ-to-fron′tal) [L. *occiput* + *frontalis,* from *frons* forehead] a radiographic projection used to demonstrate the cranium, sella turcica, and ear. With the central ray perpendicular to the film, the patient is positioned in Valdini's position (the forehead resting against the grid and the infraorbitomeatal line making a 50° angle with the film). For demonstrating the external auditory canals, tympanic cavities, and eustachian tubes, a 50° angle with the orbitomeatal line is used.

occiput (ok′sĭ-put) [L.] [NA], the back part of the head.

occlusal (ŏ-kloo′zal) [L. *occlusus* shut, closed up] pertaining to closure, often used with regard to the teeth or the jaws.

occlusal plane the hypothetical horizontal plane formed by the contacting surfaces of the upper and lower teeth when the jaws are closed.

occlusion (ŏ-kloo′zhun) [L. *occlusio* closure] 1. the act of closure or state of being closed.

2. the trapping of a material, either liquid or gas, within cavities in a solid.

occult (ŏ-kult′) [L. *occultus* hidden] obscure or hidden from view.

occult blood blood present in such small amounts that it is detectable only by chemical analysis or by spectroscopic or microscopic examination, particularly the blood found in stools.

occult blood tests screening tests for hemoglobin in urine or feces to detect occult blood. These tests are based on the peroxidase activity of hemoglobin, myoglobin, and other heme proteins. Hemoglobin reduces hydrogen peroxide to water in the presence of a colorless chromogen, which acts as a hydrogen donor and is oxidized, forming a colored product. The most widely used chromogens are *o*-toluidine and guaiac. Commercially available reagent strips or tablet tests use a solid peroxide, such as strontium peroxide or cumene hydroperoxide.

These tests are very sensitive and have a high false-positive rate owing to peroxidases in foods, particularly meat, fish, poultry, celery, radishes, and horseradish. The sensitivity of chemical tests is about 100 mg of hemoglobin/100 g of feces (0.5–1.0 ml of blood/100 g of feces), and for reagent strips about 1–2 ml of blood/100 g of feces. The tests do not distinguish myoglobin from hemoglobin.

occupational lung disease a general term used to denote all damage and disease initiated by physical and chemical irritation of lungs as the result of occupational exposure to inhaled agents such as inorganic and organic dusts, chemical substances in the form of fumes or vapors, noxious gases, and airborne radioactive particles. These diseases or conditions include the various pneumoconioses (e.g., siderosis, silicosis, asbestosis, anthracosis, bagassosis, aluminosis, and farmer's lung), acute and chronic bronchitis, asthmatic reactions, airway obstruction, pneumonitis, interstitial pneumonia, diffuse interstitial pulmonary fibrosis, pulmonary edema, and neoplasia. For more information, see the specific diseases.

Occupational Safety and Health Administration (OSHA) an agency of the federal government, established by the Occupational Safety and Health Act of 1970, that is responsible for the establishment and enforcement of standards for the exposure of workers to harmful materials in the workplace and to other health hazards.

Although many laboratories are exempt from OSHA regulations and most are unlikely to be inspected for compliance with OSHA standards, the standards provide widely applicable useful guidelines; they may also supply the basis for civil suits following fires, explosions, personal injuries, or occupational illness that would not have occurred had there been compliance with the standards.

ochratoxin (ok″rah-tok′sin) a mycotoxin produced by *Aspergillus ochraceus* series or *Penicillium viridicatum* while growing in grain. This mycotoxin produces nephropathy and edema when ingested. There are three forms of ochratoxin: A, B, and C.

OCT 1. [acronym from *o*ptimal *c*utting *t*emperature], trademark for a synthetic water-soluble glycol and resin mounting medium. It is used to embed and mount tissue for cutting frozen sections.
2. abbrev. for *ornithine-carbamoyltransferase, oxytocin challenge test.*

octa- (ok′tah) [Gr. *oktō*, L. *octo* eight] a prefix word element to denote eight, e.g., octane, octigravida.

octal (ok′tal) pertaining to the base 8 number system or to the number 8. See also *number system.*

octane (ok′tān) a term used to refer to the normal alkane, $CH_3(CH_2)_6CH_3$, that occurs in petroleum. Branched-chain octanes, isomeric with normal octane, are also known.

octanoic acid (ok′tan-o″ik) see *caprylic acid.*

ocul/o (ok′u-lo) [L. *oculus* eye] a word element used in combining form to denote eye, e.g., oculopathy.

ocular (ok′u-lar) [L. *ocularis*, from *oculus* eye] 1. of, pertaining to, or affecting the eye.
2. see *eyepiece.*

oculocardiac reflex (ok″u-lo-kar′de-ak) the reflex bradycardia elicited by pressure on the eyeballs, a stimulus that increases cardiac vagal discharge. The reflex can be intentionally produced to convert atrial tachycardia or flutter to a normal sinus rhythm.

oculocerebrorenal syndrome (ok″u-lo-sĕ-re″bro-re′nal) an X-linked genetic disease affecting males that is characterized by congenital ocular defects (glaucoma and cataracts), hydrophthalmia, cerebral defects including mental retardation, and vitamin D–refractory rickets. An important aspect of this disorder is the associated renal pathology. Renal tubular dysfunction occurs in the processing of phosphate and neutral and dibasic amino acids, resulting in acidosis, aminoaciduria, and hypophosphatemia. Also called *Lowe's syndrome.*

oculomotor (ok″u-lo-mo′tor) pertaining to eye movements, or to the third cranial nerve.

oculomotor nerve cranial nerve III; a motor nerve whose fibers arise in the midbrain, run forward in the lateral wall of the cavernous sinus, and enter the orbit to supply most of the muscles of the orbit and eyeball. See also *cranial nerves.*

oculomycosis (ok″u-lo-mi-ko′sis) a general term used to describe any disease of the eye or its parts that is caused by a fungus. See also *ophthalmomycosis.*

OD abbrev. for *oculus dexter* (right eye), optical density (see *absorbance*), outside diameter, overdose.

Oddi's sphincter (od′ēz) [Ruggero *Oddi*, Italian physician of the 19th century] see *s. of Oddi* under *sphincter.*

odont/o (o-don′to) [Gr. *odous* tooth] a word element used in combining form to denote tooth, e.g., odontoid.

odontoameloblastoma (o-don″to-am″ĕ-lo-blas-to′-mah) [*odonto-* + Old Fr. *amel* enamel + Gr. *blastos* germ + *-oma*] an odontogenic neoplasm occurring in childhood that is characterized by the presence of enamel, dentin, and odontogenic epithelium. The overall appearance is similar to that of an ameloblastoma. On radiologic examination it appears as a well-defined area of mineralization.

odontoblast (o-don′to-blast) [*odonto-* + Gr. *blastos* germ] one of the tall, columnar cells of mesenchymal origin that secretes a collagenous matrix (which calcifies to beome dentin) and forms the outer layer of the dental pulp.

Odontobutis (o-don″to-bu′tis) a genus of freshwater fish. The species *O. obscurus* serves as a host for the encysted cercariae of the fluke *Metagonimus yokogawai.* These cercariae attach themselves under the scales in the skin or flesh of these fish, and then become encysted. Human infection is caused by ingestion of raw fish contaminated with the encysted cercariae.

odontogenic (o-don″to-jen′ik) [*odonto-* + Gr. *genesis* production] forming teeth; arising in tissues that form teeth.

odontogenic cyst an epithelium-lined cavity that arises in the jaws from tooth-forming tissues. Odontogenic cysts are classified according to the specific part of the tooth-forming apparatus from which they originate: primordial and dentigerous cysts develop from the enamel organ, gingival cysts from remnants of the dental lamina, and lateral and apical periodontal cysts from remnants of Hertwig's epithelial root sheath.

Primordial cysts develop from the enamel organ before the hard tissues of the tooth (enamel and dentin) are synthesized. Consequently, they are found in place of the tooth that would have differentiated from the enamel organ. The cells of the stellate reticulum of the enamel organ degenerate, leaving the enamel epithelium to form the primordial cyst lining. Primordial cysts are located most commonly in the posterior mandible and are lined by keratinized, stratified squamous epithelium.

The epithelial lining of the dentigerous cyst is derived from the reduced enamel epithelium that encircles the crown of a tooth after enamel and dentin formation, but before eruption of the tooth into the mouth. Dentigerous cysts are more common than primordial cysts and are usually associated with the crown of an unerupted mandibular third molar (wisdom tooth). The cyst wall consists of dense, fibrous connective tissue lined with stratified squamous epithelium.

During embryogenesis, the developing enamel organ is attached to the surface oral epithelium by a thin cord of cells called the dental lamina. As the calcified tissues of the tooth are deposited, the dental lamina degenerates, leaving behind in the connective tissue of the gingiva islands of odontogenic epithelium called rests of Serres. It is from these rests that gingival cysts arise. Gingival cysts differ from the other odontogenic cysts, being located in soft tissue rather than in bone.

The formation of the root portion of the tooth is initiated by an apical extension of the enamel organ called Hertwig's epithelial root sheath. Once root development is complete, this sheath degenerates. Epithelial remnants called rests of Malassez can be left behind in the periodontal ligament that attaches the teeth to alveolar bone of the jaws. These rests can proliferate to form lateral and apical periodontal cysts. Lateral periodontal cysts are found in the bone adjacent to the roots of the teeth. Mandibular cuspids are the teeth most frequently involved. Apical periodontal cysts arise from rests of Malassez in the periodontal ligament at the root apex of teeth with infected pulps. The rests proliferate in response to pulpal inflammation associated with dental caries.

See the accompanying illustrations.

J. ROBERT NEWLAND, D.D.S.

odontogenic tumor a neoplastic proliferation of tooth-forming tissues. Odontogenic tumors are divided according to their parent tissue into tumors of ectodermal origin, of mesodermal origin, and of mixed ectodermal and mesodermal origin (see the accompanying illustration).

Teeth develop from two types of embryonic tissue, ectoderm and mesoderm. The ectodermal component, called the enamel organ, forms from the surface epithelium that covers the alveolar bone of the jaws. The ameloblastic cells of the enamel organ synthesize the enamel layer of the tooth. The mesodermal component develops from the connective tissue beneath the enamel organ and is called the dental papilla. The cells of the dental papilla differentiate to form the dentin, cementum, and pulp tissue of the tooth.

The ameloblastoma is the most common odonto-

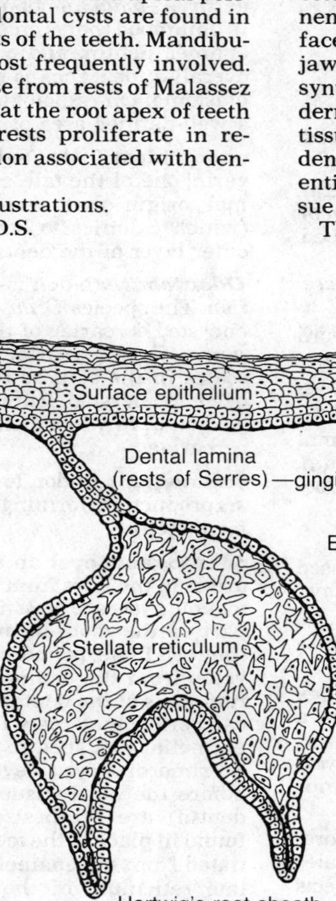

Odontogenic cyst, Figure 1. Histologic and morphologic features. (Courtesy of J. Robert Newland, D.D.S.)

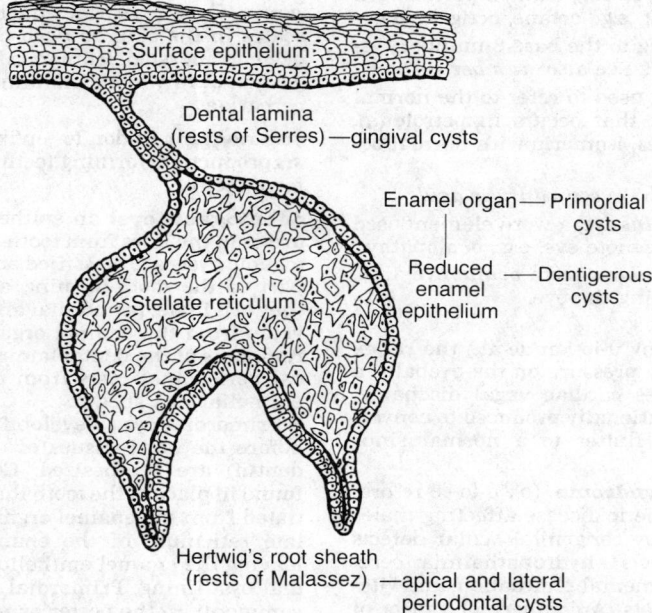

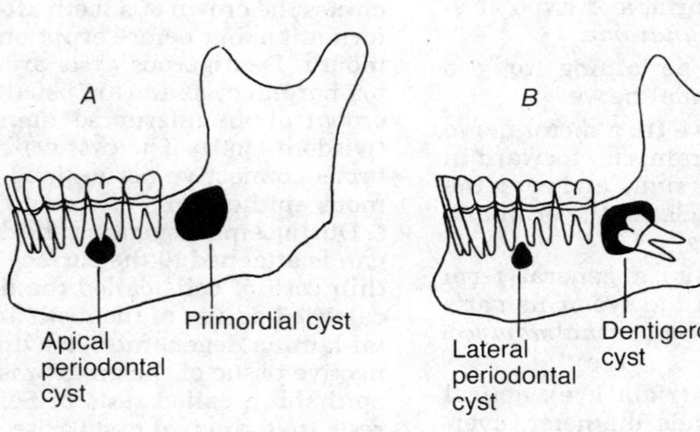

Odontogenic cyst, Figure 2. *A,* Location of apical periodontal and primordial cysts. *B,* Location of lateral periodontal and dentigerous cysts. (Courtesy of J. Robert Newland, D.D.S.)

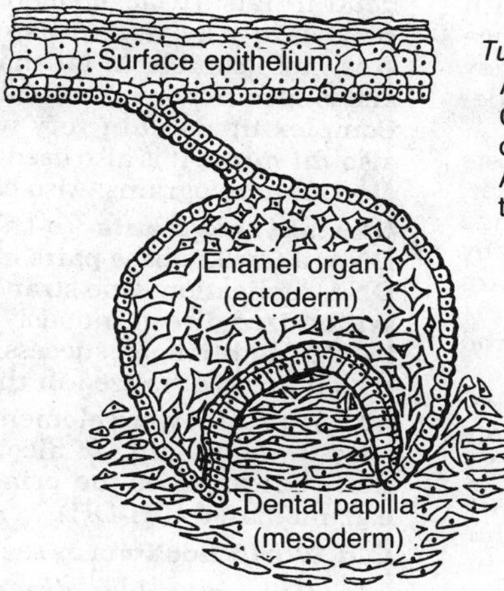

Odontogenic tumor. Histologic and morphologic features. (Courtesy of J. Robert Newland, D.D.S.)

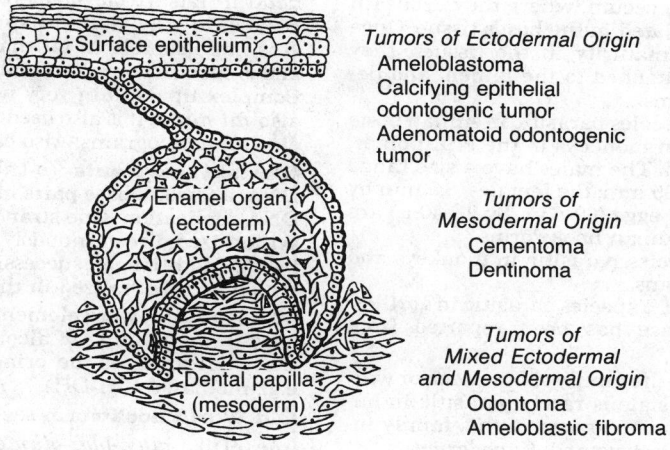

genic tumor of ectodermal origin. Histologically, it closely resembles the tissue of the enamel organ. Ameloblastomas are the most aggressive of the odontogenic tumors, tending to invade locally and to recur following removal. The posterior mandible is the usual site of occurrence. The calcifying epithelial odontogenic tumor and the odontogenic adenomatoid tumor (adenoameloblastoma) are odontogenic tumors of ectodermal origin that occur less frequently.

The most common odontogenic tumor of mesodermal origin is the cementoma. Cementum is the outermost layer of the tooth root, and thus tumors composed of cementum are usually either attached or in close proximity to the root of a tooth. Cementomas occur most often in the mandible. They are usually asymptomatic and are frequently discovered as incidental findings on routine dental x-ray examinations. A familial form of this tumor is the gigantiform cementoma, which involves all four quadrants of the jaw bones. The dentinoma is also of mesodermal origin. It develops from odontoblasts, the cells of the dental papilla that normally form the dentin layer of the tooth. Histologically, it consists of sheets of irregularly formed dentin and fibrous connective tissue. Dentinomas are usually found in the posterior mandible in association with an impacted molar tooth.

The odontoma is the most common of all odontogenic tumors and is of mixed ectodermal and mesodermal origin. Odontomas are composed of all the tissues normally found in teeth: enamel, dentin, cementum, and pulp tissue. These tissues are arranged in a haphazard fashion or in the shape of miniature teeth. Odontomas may arise in any part of the jaw bones. They are slow-growing and usually remain small; they can be easily removed and do not recur. The ameloblastic fibroma is a mixed odontogenic tumor composed of nests of odontogenic epithelium and proliferating fibrous connective tissue. This tumor is thought to represent a stage in the development of an odontoma before any calcified tissue has been synthesized.

J. Robert Newland, D.D.S.

odontology (o″don-tol′o-je) [*odonto-* + *-logy*] 1. the sum of knowledge regarding the teeth.
2. dentistry.

odontoma (o″don-to′mah) [*odonto-* + Gr. *ōma* tumor] an odontogenic lesion that is generally viewed as a hamartoma rather than a true neoplasm. It represents abnormal development of the tooth germ, and may contain all elements of tooth formation including enamel, dentin, cementum, and pulp. An odontoma is classified as complex if the components are randomly arranged and have not differentiated to the point of actual tooth formation; compound when a tooth regardless of form can be recognized; or ameloblastic if dental organ epithelium is present. The radiographic findings vary, depending on the components of the lesion. See also *odontogenic tumor.*

odyn/o (o-din′o) [Gr. *odynē* pain] a word element used in combining form to denote pain, e.g., odynophagia.

-odynia (o-din′e-ah) [Gr. *odynē* pain] a suffix word element to denote pain, e.g., pleurodynia.

odynophagia (od″ĭ-no-fa′je-ah) [*odyno-* + Gr. *phagein* to eat] the painful swallowing of food. This disorder may be associated with dysphagia. It is characterized by pain, burning sensations, and tightness on swallowing hot or cold food. It is commonly due to mucosal destruction in the esophagus following infection, gastroesophageal reflux, neoplastic invasion, or ingestion of harsh chemicals. Neurologic dysfunctions, such as achalasia or esophageal spasm, may also be involved in the etiology.

Oe abbrev See *oersted.*

oersted (Oe) (er′sted) [Hans Christian *Oersted,* Danish physicist, 1777–1851] the electromagnetic centimeter-gram-second (cgs) unit of magnetic field strength, defined as the intensity that produces a force of 1 dyne on a unit magnetic pole. It is equal in magnitude to the gauss, which is used for magnetic induction.

Oesophagostomum (e-sof″ah-gos′to-mum) [*oesophago-,* from Gr. *oisophagos* esophagus + *stoma* mouth] a genus of nematodes of the family Strongylidae that is occasionally parasitic in humans, although more commonly found in monkeys. Infection is caused by ingestion of ensheathed larvae, which localize in the cecum, where they exsheath and become encapsulated in the host's tissue. Once these worms reach maturity in the tissues, they break out, become attached to the lumen, and develop into adult worms.

O. apiostomum, a species parasitic in simian hosts in West Africa and in monkeys in the Philippines, Indonesia, and China. The males have a size range of 8–10 mm by 0.3–0.35 mm; the females, 8.5 mm by 0.295–0.325 mm. The eggs (60–63 μ by 27–40 μ) are similar to those of human hookworms.

O. bifurcum, a species parasitic in monkeys and occasionally in humans.

O. stephanostomum, a species parasitic in gorillas. A single human case has been reported from Mañaos, Brazil.

Oestridae (es′trĭ-de) the family of bot-, heel, or warble flies. The larval state is rarely parasitic in humans. The most common genera of this family include *Dermatobia, Oestrus,* and *Hypoderma.*

Oestrus (es′trus) [Gr. *oistros* gadfly] a genus of botflies. *O. ovis,* the common sheep botfly, has larvae that are parasitic in the nostrils and sinuses of sheep and goats; occasionally, the adult flies deposit larvae in human eyes, causing ophthalmomyiasis.

off-line pertaining to equipment that is not directly controlled by a computer or is temporarily disconnected. The off-line entry of data from analyzers is usually performed through manual entry or batch entry from punch cards, magnetic tape, etc. Cf. *on-line.*

Oguchi's disease (o-goo′chēz) [Chuta *Oguchi,* Japanese ophthalmologist, 1875–1945] a form of hereditary night blindness found in Japan. See also *night blindness.*

Ohara's disease (o-hah′rahz) [Hachiro *Ohara,* Japanese physician, born 1882] see *tularemia.*

ohm (Ω) (ōm) [Georg S. *Ohm,* German physicist, 1787–1854] the International System (SI) unit of electrical resistance equal to 1 volt per ampere.

Ohm's law (ōmz) [Georg S. *Ohm*] stated as: the potential difference (the voltage, V) across an electrical resistor is equal to the product of the resistance (R) and the current flowing through the resistor. The formula is $V = IR$. By analogy with this law, the resistance across a segment of the respiratory airways or of the vascular bed can be expressed as a ratio of the pressure drop across that segment to the rate of laminar flow (of air or blood) through it.

ohmmeter (ōm′me-ter) [*ohm* + *meter*] an instrument for measuring electrical resistance. See also *voltmeter.*

-oid (oyd) [Gr. *eidos* form, shape] a suffix word element to denote resembling, e.g., epidermoid.

oil (oyl) [L. *oleum*] 1. an unctuous, combustible substance, liquid or easily liquefiable on warming, that is soluble in ether but insoluble in water. Such substances, depending on their origin, are classified as animal, mineral, or vegetable oils; depending on their behavior upon heating, they are classified as volatile or fixed. For more information, see the specific oil.

2. a fat that is liquid at room temperature.

oil immersion lens a high-power microscopic objective lens used with a drop of immersion oil to form a liquid bridge between slide and lens. See also *microscope.*

oil red O the most commonly used dye for staining neutral fats (triacylglycerols), a red diazo dye, *p*-xylylazo-*p*-xylylazo-β-naphthol; C.I. 26125. Oil red O is more soluble in fat than in water or alcohols and is specific for neutral fats and some lipofuscins. Complex lipids stain very weakly or not at all; see also *fat stains.* It is also used for staining lipoprotein electrophoretograms. Also called *benzoyl oil red O.*

Okazaki segments (o-kah-zak′e) sequences of DNA, a few kilobase pairs in length, formed during DNA replication. One strand of the duplex DNA is synthesized discontinuously in the 3′ → 5′ direction by the addition of successive Okazaki segments, which are synthesized in the opposite direction.

-ol (ol) a suffix word element used in organic chemistry in the naming of alcohols and phenols when the —OH group is the principal functional group, e.g., methanol (CH_3OH).

Old World hookworm see under *hookworm.*

-ole (ōl) [L. *-olus, -ola, -olum* dim. suffix for little one] a suffix word element to denote little or small, e.g., nucleole.

oleandomycin (o″le-an″do-mi′sin) one of the macrolide group of antibiotics. See also *antibacterial agents* and *macrolide.*

oleate (o′le-āt) 1. any salt, ionic, or ester form of oleic acid, e.g., *cis*-9-octadecanoate, an 18-carbon, olefinic, fatty acid. The term is used alone or in combination with the name of the counterion, e.g., sodium oleate. When preceded by an organic substituent name, e.g., methyl oleate, it refers to an ester of oleic acid.

2. [L. *oleatum*], a solution of a chemical substance or drug in oleic acid, used as an ointment.

olecran/o (o-lek′ran-o) [Gr. *ōlekranon,* from *ōlenē* elbow + *kranion* head] a word element used in combining form to denote elbow, e.g., olecranarthropathy.

olecranarthropathy (o-lek″ran-ar-throp′ah-the) [*olecrano-* + Gr. *arthron* joint + *pathos* disease] a general term for any disease of the elbow joint. Two common conditions affecting this joint are olecranarthritis (inflammation of the joint due to infection or trauma) and olecranon bursitis (tenderness and inflammation of the bursa at the point of the elbow).

olecranon (o-lek′rah-non) [Gr. *ōlekranon*] [NA], the uppermost part of the ulna; a bony projection at the elbow that contributes to the trochlear notch.

olefin (o′le-fin) [Fr. *olefiant* ethylene] an unsaturated hydrocarbon, an alkene.

oleic acid (o-le′ik) *cis*-9-octadecenoic acid, a long-chain, unsaturated fatty acid found in animal and vegetable fats.

oleic acid I 125 a radioiodine-labeled fat; see under *fat absorption test.*

oleic acid uptake test see under *fat absorption test.*

oleo- (o′le-o) [L. *oleum* oil] a word element used in combining form to denote oil, e.g., oleoinfusion.

oleoresin (o″le-o-rez′in) [L. *oleoresina*] any natural combination of a resin and a volatile oil such as exudes from pines and other plants.

aspidium o., a thick, dark-green, liquid ether extract of male fern formerly used as a vermifuge or anthelmintic in the treatment of tapeworm infection. After its administration, the worms are evacuated. It is toxic and in large doses may cause vomiting, weakness, convulsions, coma, blindness, jaundice and kidney damage.

olfactory (ol-fak′to-re) [L. *olfacere* to smell] pertaining to the sense of smell.

olfactory glands small mucous glands in the olfactory submucosa. Also called *Bowman's glands.*

olfactory mucosa the specialized mucosa that lines the upper portion of the nasal cavity and subserves the sense of smell. It occupies an area approximately 5 cm^2 and extends onto the superior part of the nasal septum on each side. Three cell types have been identified: basal, sustentacular, and true sensory cells. The basal cells are small and located against the basal lamina. They probably function as reserve cells capable of replacing the sustentacular or supporting cells, tall columnar cells with apical microvilli that form a lipid secretion. The true sensory cells are neuroepithelial cells with a slender cell body that extends apically into a bulbous olfactory vesicle that bears specialized cilia and contains a few small dense-core granules. At the base of the cell, the cytoplasm continues through the basal lamina into a thin dendritic process that has longitudinally oriented microtubules, but few or no granules. This process unites with similar extensions from neighboring cells to form a nerve bundle that passes upward through the cribriform plate to the olfactory bulb.

olfactory nerve cranial nerve I; the sensory nerve for the sense of smell. Fibers originate as processes of the neuroepithelial cells of the olfactory mucosa in the upper part of the nasal cavity, and pass through the cribiform plate of the ethmoid to reach the olfactory bulb. See also *cranial nerves.*

olfactory neuroblastoma see under *neuroblastoma.*

olig/o (ol′ĭ-go) [Gr. *oligos* little] a word element used in combining form to denote scanty or little, e.g., oligospermia.

oligemia (ol″ĭ-ge′me-ah) [*oligo-* + Gr. *haima* blood + *-ia*] a reduction in blood volume. See also *hypovolemia.*

oligoclonal banding (ol″ĭ-go-klo′nal) [*oligo-* + Gr. *klōn* young shoot, twig] the occurrence of two or more discrete bands in the gamma-globulin region of protein electrophoretograms of spinal fluid. Positive findings have shown a good correlation with proved cases of multiple sclerosis and are also sometimes noted in neurosyphilis, sarcoidosis, chronic infection of the central nervous system, meningitis, and other inflammatory neurologic diseases. These bands belong to the IgG class of immunoglobulins; their origins and role in the course of multiple sclerosis have not been determined. See also *cerebrospinal fluid electrophoresis* and *protein electrophoresis.*

oligodendrocyte (ol″ĭ-go-den′dro-sīt) [*oligo* + Gr. *dendron* tree + *kytos* hollow vessel] one of the neuroglial cells of the central nervous system. These occur as intrafascicular cells between bundles of axons in myelinated tracts and as perineuronal cells that are intimately associated with the cell bodies in the gray matter. Connected with the myelin sheaths of their associated cells, they function to lay down myelin in the CNS. Also called *oligodendroglia.*

oligodendroglia (ol″ĭ-go-den-dro′gle-ah) [*oligo-* + Gr. *dendron* tree + *glia* glue] see *oligodendrocyte.*

oligodendroglia staining see under *Penfield's method.*

oligodendroglioma (ol″ĭ-go-den″dro-gli-o′mah) [*oligo-* + Gr. *dendron* tree + *glia* glue + *-ōma* tumor] a tumor of the central nervous system composed of oligodendrocytes in various stages of differentiation. Histologically, the cells are round, uniform, and compactly arranged in diffuse sheets. Admixture of other glial elements is found in roughly half the cases. The tumor can arise at any age, but is commonly found in the frontal lobes of adults. Approximately 6 percent of human brain tumors are oligodendrogliomas, but there is a much higher relative frequency in animals. The behavior of oligodendrogliomas cannot be predicted from their histology. Some tumors grow slowly over many years whereas others are aggressive, behaving like glioblastomas.

oligodynamic (ol″ĭ-go-di-nam′ik) [*oligo-* + Gr. *dynamis* power] active in very minute quantities, said especially of heavy metal ions, e.g., Hg^{2+}; some such substances can be used as antiseptics and disinfectants.

oligo-1,6-glucosidase (ol″ĭ-go-gloo-ko′sĭ-dās) an enzyme of the hydrolase class (dextrin-6-α-D-glucanohydrolase, EC 3.2.1.10) that catalyzes the hydrolysis of 1,6-α-D-glucosidic linkages in the isomaltose and dextrins produced from starch and glycogen by α-amylase. It is found in the intestinal mucosa. An inborn deficiency, disaccharidase deficiency, causes intolerance of ingested starches. It has not been possible to separate human sucrase and oligo-1,6-glucosidase into separate species. Also called *isomaltase.*

oligomenorrhea (ol″ĭ-go-men″o-re′ah) [*oligo-* + Gr. *mēn* month + *rhoia* flow] a reduced frequency of menstrual bleeding, periods having an interval range of 38–90 da. When the interval between menstruation periods is greater than 6 mo, the patient is considered to have amenorrhea. Causes of oligomenorrhea include emotional stress, marked weight loss, hormonal and endocrine dysfunctions, and systemic disorders. Ovulation rarely occurs.

oligomer (o-lig′o-mer) a polymer composed of only a few monomers (subunits), e.g., a dimer, trimer, or tetramer. The subunits may be all alike or different. The term is frequently applied to isoenzymes, proteins, and nucleic acids.

oligopeptide (ol″ĭ-go-pep′tid) see under *peptide.*

oligosaccharide (ol″ĭ-go-sak′ah-rīd) a carbohydrate that on hydrolysis yields 2–10 monosaccharides, as opposed to polysaccharides, that are composed of a large number of monosaccharide units.

oligospermia (ol″ĭ-go-sper′me-ah) [*oligo-* + Gr. *sperma* seed + *-ia*] a decreased density of spermatozoa in the semen. Clinically, this is defined as less than 20 million sperm per milliliter of semen, a value considered incompatible with fertility. The many causes of this condition include hormonal dysfunctions, neoplasms, trauma, drugs, and abnormal spermatozoa development.

oligotrophic (ol″ĭ-go-trof′ik) [*oligo-* + Gr. *trophē* nourishment] 1. pertaining to a state of poor (inadequate) nutrition.

2. poor in nutrients that support growth for specific organisms, as in lakes that do not support the growth of aerobic photosynthetic organisms. Cf. *eutrophic.*

oliguria (ol″ĭ-gu′re-ah) [*oligo-* + Gr. *ouron* urine + *-ia*] decreased urine volume in an average-sized adult down to levels of less than 400 ml/24 hr, a volume incompatible with the need to sustain life. The causes of acute oliguria may be extrinsic (fluid loss, hemorrhage, dehydration), postrenal extrinsic (prostatic hypertrophy, neoplasms, urinary tract stones), or intrinsic (the most common of which is acute renal tubular necrosis). Diagnostic tests to determine the specific cause include urinalysis and determinations of serum urea and creatinine, as well as determinations of urinary urea, creatinine, and sodium.

olive (ol′iv) [L. *oliva*] a smooth, rounded elevation between the anterolateral and posterolateral sulci and lateral to the upper part of the pyramids of the medulla oblongata. This swelling is caused by the underlying inferior olivary nucleus.

inferior o., a large, irregular, concave mass of gray matter with irregular scalloped walls that open medially. Intimately associated with the cerebellum, it receives input from the cerebral cortex, thalamus, basal nuclei, and midbrain, while projecting primarily to the cerebellum and the spinal cord.

superior o., a mass of gray matter lateral to the reticular formation at the pontomedullary junction. Concerned with auditory localization, it receives both ipsilateral and contralateral input from the cochlear nerves.

olivopontocerebellar degeneration (ol″ĭ-vo-pon″to-ser″ĕ-bel′ar) [L. *oliva* olive + *pons, pontis* bridge + *cerebellar,* from *cerebellum,* dim. of *cerebrum* brain] see under *spinocerebellar degeneration.*

Ollier's disease (ol″e-āz′) [Léopold Louis Xavier Edouard *Ollier,* French surgeon, 1830–1900] see *enchondroma.*

-ology (ol′o-je) [Gr. *logos* reasoned speech] a suffix word element to denote the study of, e.g., hematology.

olophonia (ol″o-fo′ne-ah) [Gr. *oloos* lost + *phōnē* voice + *-ia*] defective speech having organic causes, such as malformed vocal organs.

om/o (o′mo) [Gr. *ōmos* shoulder] a word element used in combining form to denote relationship to the shoulder, e.g., omarthritis.

-oma (o′mah) [Gr. *ōma,* perhaps adapted from *onkōma,* a swelling] a suffix word element to denote tumor, e.g., fibrosarcoma.

omalgia (o-mal′je-ah) [*om-* + Gr. *algos* pain + *-ia*] a general term used to describe any nonspecific pain in the shoulder. The causes include trauma, inflammation, and infection. Also called omodynia.

omega (o′me-ga, o-meg′ah) the twenty-fourth and last letter of the *Greek alphabet.*

omentitis (o″men-ti′tis) [*omentum* + *-itis* inflammation] an inflammation of the omentum; see also *peritonitis.*

omentum (o-men′tum), pl. *omenta* [L. "fat skin"] a fold of peritoneum that extends from the stomach to the liver (lesser omentum) or to the transverse colon (greater omentum). The lesser omentum forms the anterior wall of the lesser sac of peritoneum; the hepatic artery, portal vein, and common bile duct lie within its right margin in front of the opening into the lesser sac (foramen of Winslow). The greater omentum forms a large, apronlike structure filled with fat that hangs down in front of the intestines.

omicron (O, o) (om′ĭ-kron, o′mĭ-kron, o′mi-kron) the fifteenth letter of the *Greek alphabet.*

omitis (o-mi′tis) [*om-* + *-itis* inflammation] a general term used to describe inflammation of the shoulder. Also called omarthritis.

omnibus hypothesis (om′nĭ-bus″) [Fr., from L. *omnis* all] in analysis of variance, the null hypothesis (H_0) that there are no differences among the treatment groups.

omphal/o (om′fah-lo) [Gr. *omphalos* the navel] a word element used in combining form to denote relationship to the umbilicus, e.g., omphalomesenteric.

omphalelcosis (om″fal-el-ko′sis) [*omphal-* + Gr. *helkōsis* ulceration] an ulceration of the umbilicus, often due to infection with nosocomial staphylococci in the first days of life.

omphalitis (om″fah-li′tis) [*omphal-* + *-itis* inflammation] an inflammation of the umbilicus, most often occurring in the newborn. Common causes include infections, especially with the strains of staphylococci indigenous to hospitals.

omphalocele (om′fah-lo-sēl″) [*omphalo-* + Gr. *kēlē* hernia] a congenital umbilical hernia into which intestine, covered by amnion and peritoneum, protrudes through a widened umbilical opening. It results from the failure of the developing gut to return completely to the abdominal cavity from its embryonic location in the umbilical cord. See the accompanying illustration.

omphalomesenteric (om″fah-lo-mes″en-ter′ik) [*omphalo-* + Gr. *mesos* middle + *enteron* intestine] pertaining to the umbilicus and mesentery.

omphalomesenteric duct see *omphalomesenteric d.* under *duct.*

omphalomesenteric duct anomalies the failure of development that leads to the retention of remnants of the embryonic yolk sac. If the entire duct remains open, it is referred to as an omphalomesenteric or umbilical fistula; if the intestinal end is sealed and the umbilicus remains open, it is an umbilical sinus; if both ends are sealed and the middle remains patent, it is an enterocystoma. The most common remnant of the omphalomesenteric duct is Meckel's diverticulum. See also *Meckel's d.* under

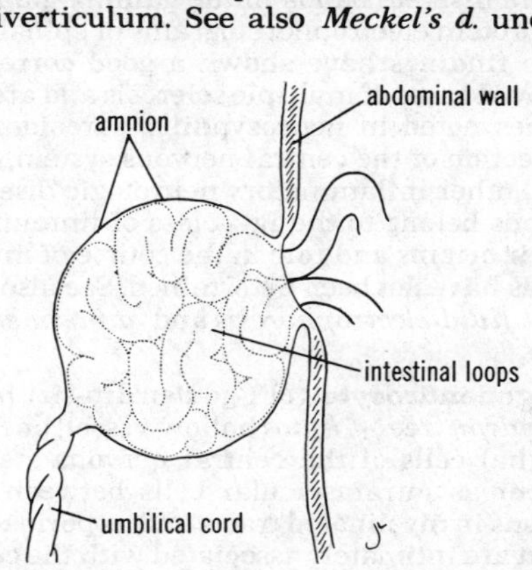

Omphalocele. Drawing showing herniated intestinal loops surrounded by a membranous sac formed by the amnion. (From Langman, J.: Medical Embryology. 4th ed. Baltimore, Williams & Wilkins Co., 1981.)

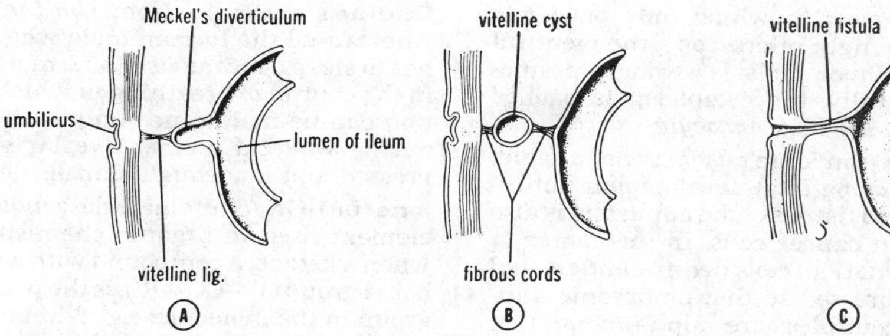

Omphalomesenteric duct anomalies. Remnants of the omphalomesenteric (vitelline) duct: *A,* Meckel's diverticulum combined with fibrous cord (vitelline ligament); *B,* vitelline cyst attached to the umbilicus and the wall of the ileum by vitelline ligaments; and *C,* vitelline fistula connecting the lumen of the ileum with the umbilicus. (From Langman, J.: Medical Embryology. 4th ed. Baltimore, Williams & Wilkins, 1981.)

diverticulum. See also the accompanying illustration.

Omsk hemorrhagic fever (omzk) [from *Omsk,* a city in the Asiatic region of the Soviet Union] an acute viral disease that originally occurred in the Omsk region of the Soviet Union; epidemics in Asia have also occurred. Appearing during the spring and summer, it is caused by a group B arbovirus and is transmitted to humans either by the bite of an infected *Dermacentor* tick or by the handling of infected muskrats. The disease is characterized by fever, headache, hemorrhage, and, rarely, neurologic disorders. Leukopenia is common.

-on (from *ion*) a suffix word element to denote a particle or quantum, e.g., electron or photon.

onc/o (ong′ko) [Gr. *onkos* mass, tumor, hook] 1. a word element used in combining form to denote a swelling or tumor, e.g., oncology, or barbed or hooked, e.g., onchium.

Onchocerca (ong″ko-ser′kah) [Gr. *onkos* hook + *kerkos* tail] a genus of nematodes of the superfamily Filarioidea. The adults live in the skin, subcutaneous connective tissue, and other tissues in humans, causing fibrous nodules. The microfilariae circulate in the lymph system and can be found in the eyes, subcutaneous connective tissue, and skin.

O. caecutiens, see *O. volvulus.*

O. cervicalis, a species parasitic in the cervical ligaments of horses and mules.

O. lienalis, a parasite found in cattle.

O. volvulus, a common parasite of humans, distributed through mountainous areas of the tropics and subtropics. The adult worms (the males measure 19–42 mm long; the females, 33–50 cm) live in coiled pairs in tumors (or nodules) in the subcutaneous connective tissues, especially around joints and in the back of the head. Black flies of the genus *Simulium* are the intermediate host: they become infected when feeding from infected hosts and transmit the filariae to humans.

Microfilariae are rarely found in the blood, but can be identified in aspiration of the nodules or in thin shavings of the skin. They have size ranges of 285–368 μm by 6–9 μm and 150–287 μm by 5–7 μm. They are unsheathed and the anterior end is blunt-rounded and enlarged, with no stylets. Also called *O. caecutiens.*

onchocerciasis (ong″ko-ser-ki′ah-sis) being infected with the filarial parasites of the genus *Onchocerca.* Black flies of the genus *Simulium* are the intermediate host and transmit the filariae to humans. This condition is found in persons living in hilly regions with swift-flowing streams, chiefly at altitudes of 1000–4000 ft in tropical Africa and parts of Mexico, Guatemala, and Venezuela. Early symptomatology includes a transient urticaria and eosinophilia, and sometimes insomnia and slight fever. The incubation period is usually 15–18 mo. The presence of the adult worm in nodules does not produce serious inflammation or illness.

The most serious manifestation of *Onchocerca* infection—involvement of the eyes—is believed to be caused by both living and dead microfilariae in the ocular tissue, and by toxic metabolic by-products of both microfilariae and adult worms acting locally and at a distance. As the ocular involvement progresses, there is development of more severe conjunctivitis; lesions of the iris, ciliary body, choroid, and retina; and corneal opacities. Eventually, involvement of the optic nerve and arterial blood supply may ensue, resulting in optic atrophy and blindness. This disease is known to present a variety of clinicopathologic features. Recent studies have revealed that some of these variations are caused by different strains of parasites and different species and strains of *Simulium.*

Intradermal tests have been used in diagnosis, but usually are not necessary, as skin biopsy for examination of microfilariae is an easier and more reliable method. The treatment of choice includes surgical excision of adult worms in nodules and combined chemotherapy with diethylcarbamazine and suramin.

Also called blinding filarial disease, mal morado, onchocercosis, river blindness, and vovulosis.

oncocyte [*onco-* + Gr. *kytos* hollow vessel] an epithelial cell characterized by abundant, granular, deeply eosinophilic cytoplasm, which at the ultrastructural level is seen to be due to the presence of numerous tightly packed mitochondria. Histochemically, oncocytes contain a high level of mitochondrial oxidative enzymes.

Oncocytes are found in a number of organs, particularly the parathyroid, thyroid, and salivary glands. They are also found in varying numbers as a component of both benign and malignant tumors of various organs.

oncocytoma (ong″ko-si-to′ma) [*oncocyte* + *-oma*] a tumor composed of mitochondrion-rich cells. As some are malignant, the term oncocytic tumor is preferable. Foci of oncocytic transformation may occur within salivary (oncocytic), thyroid (Hürthle cell), parathyroid (oxyphilic), bronchogenic, or renal tumors, but the term oncocytic tumor should be reserved for neoplasms in which only oncocytic cells are present. By light microscopy, the plentiful cytoplasm of the tumor cells is strongly eosinophilic; ultrastructurally, the cytoplasm is packed with mitochondria. See also *oncocyte.*

oncofetal antigen (on″ko-fe′tal) a gene product that is expressed during fetal development but repressed in specialized tissues of the adult, and is also produced by certain cancer cells. In the course of neoplastic transformation, cells dedifferentiate and genes can be derepressed so that embryonic antigens reappear. Examples are alpha-fetoprotein (AFP) and carcinoembryonic antigen (CEA).

oncogenesis (ong″ko-jen″ĕ-sis) [*onco-* + Gr. *genesis* production, generation] the process of forming and producing neoplasms or tumors. Although the causes of neoplasm formation are not entirely clear, factors such as chemicals, radiation, heredity, and viruses have been implicated for certain tumors. See also *cancer.*

oncogenic (ong″ko-jen′ik) a term used to indicate a process or agent that gives rise to tumor formation, e.g., the RNA-containing viruses that give rise to tumors in animals are called oncogenic viruses.

oncologist (ong″kol′o-jist) a physician whose primary interest is the practice of oncology. Physicians who specialize in the treatment of cancer by a particular technique and are trained in a particular branch of oncology have specific designations such as surgical, radiation, pediatric, and medical oncologists.

oncology (ong-kol′o-je) [*onco-* + *-logy*] the study of cancer and cancer-related diseases.

oncolysis (ong-kol′ĭ-sis) [*onco-* + Gr. *lysis* dissolution] the lysis or destruction of tumor cells.

oncolytic (ong″ko-lit′ik) pertaining to or causing oncolysis.

Oncomelania (ong″ko-mĕ-la′ne-ah) [*onco-* + Gr. *melas* black + *-ia*] a genus of snails; several species are the first intermediate host for the blood fluke, *Schistosoma japonicum.*

Oncorhynchus [*onco-* + Gr. *rhynchos* snout] a genus of trout and salmon naturally infected with the tapeworm *Diphyllobothrium latum.* Human infection is caused by the consumption of raw or undercooked flesh of infected fish.

oncosphere (ong′ko-sfēr) [*onco-* + Gr. *sphaira* sphere] the larva of tapeworm in the fully embryonated egg. In human tapeworms, the oncosphere usually has three pairs of hooklets and may be found in the feces.

oncotic (ong-kot′ik) pertaining to, caused by, or marked by swelling.

oncotic pressure the osmotic pressure exerted by colloidal particles suspended in a solvent. See also *osmotic pressure.*

Oncovirinae (on″ko-vi′rin-e) a subfamily of Retroviridae: the RNA tumor virus, which includes the mammary tumor virus of mice and the leukemia and sarcoma viruses of birds and mammals. Oncovirus DNA becomes integrated into host DNA during viral RNA replication. The host's new genetic information may or may not be expressed. See also *Retroviridae.*

on-demand system a data processing system in which information is retrieved or other services are performed at the time of the request.

Ondine's curse [F., from *Undine,* a water nymph who caused the human male who fell in love with her to sleep continuously] a term used for a disorder in the control of breathing in which normal ventilation can be maintained only with voluntary effort during wakeful hours. Alveolar ventilation is depressed and inadequate during sleep.

-one (ōn) [Gr. *-ōnē* female descendant] a suffix word element used in organic chemistry nomenclature when a ketone, a compound with a nonterminal carbonyl group (R—CO—R′), is the principal functional group in the molecule; e.g., 2-butanone, the systematic name for methyl ethyl ketone ($CH_3COC_2H_5$).

one-sided alternative an alternate hypothesis that a population parameter, such as the mean, is to one side of (i.e., greater than, less than) the value specified by the null hypothesis. The remaining alternatives (on the other side) are not tested because they are inconsequential. (For example, it may make no difference whether a new procedure is found to be identical in effect to the standard procedure or to be worse.) A one-tailed hypothesis test is used based on a test statistic estimating the parameter. See also *hypothesis testing* and *one-tailed test.* Cf. *two-sided alternative.*

one-tailed test a statistical hypothesis test in which the critical region consists either of all values of the test statistic below some specified critical value or of all values above some critical value. See also *hypothesis testing.* Cf. *two-tailed test.*

-onium (o′ne-um) a suffix word element used in chemistry to denote a cation in which the cationic atom has no hydrogens attached, e.g., $(CH_3)_4N^+$, tetramethylammonium; $(CH_3CH_2)_3O^+$, triethyloxonium. The term has also been used for cations with protons on that atom, e.g., ammonium, NH_4^+, and oxonium, H_3O^+, although this usage is no longer preferred. The term carbonium ion, referring to a trivalent, positively charged carbon atom has been replaced by the term carbenium ion.

on-line pertaining to equipment that is directly connected to a computer and interacting with it. Cf. *off-line.*

ONPG test a test for the production of beta-D-galactosidase. The reagent is *o*-nitrophenyl-beta-D-galactopyranoside. In bacteriology, this test serves to differentiate *Salmonella* from *Arizona,* and *Neisseria meningitidis* from *N. lactamicus.*

Onthophagus (on″thof′ah-gus) [N.L., from Gr. *onthos* dung + *phagein* to eat] a genus of dung beetles. Intestinal infestation with the species *O. unifasciatus* may cause enteritis.

ontogeny (on-toj′ĕ-ne) [Gr. *ōn* existing + *gennan* to produce] the origin and course of the development of the individual organism from fertilization through maturity to death, as distinguished from phylogeny, the evolutionary history of the race or species to which the individual belongs. Cf. *phylogeny.*

onych/o (on′ĭ-ko) [Gr. *onyx* nail] a word element used in combining form to denote a nail, e.g., onychomycosis.

onychatrophia (on″ik″ah-tro′fe-ah) [*onych-* + *a-* negative + Gr. *trophē* nutrition + *-ia*] atrophy of the nail(s). The condition may be congenital, or due to trauma or to vascular or neurologic disorders.

onycholysis (on″ĭ-kol′ĭ-sis) [*onycho-* + Gr. *lysis* destruction] the distal separation of the nails from the nail bed, which most commonly affects the fingers.

This disorder may be due to infection, most often fungal, and to excess exposure to harsh agents, such as detergents and alkali, as well as to water and soap. Keratolytic agents and nail hardeners may also be contributory. Systemic diseases such as hypothyroidism and hyperthyroidism (Plummer's disease) may play a role in this disorder. Also called onychoschizia.

onychomycosis (on″ĭ-ko-mi-ko′sis) [*onycho-* + Gr. *mykēs* fungus + *-osis*] any fungal infection of the nail. The organisms most commonly involved are *Candida albicans, Epidermophyton floccosum,* and *Trichophyton* species.

oo- (o′o) [Gr. *ōon* an egg] a word element used in combining form to denote an egg, e.g., oocyte.

oocyst (o′o-sist) [*oo-* + Gr. *kystis* sac, bladder] the encysted or encapsulated fertilized macrogamete in the life cycle of sporozoa; also, the encysted ookinete in the wall of a mosquito's stomach.

oocyte (o′o-sīt) [*oo-* + *-cyte*] the developing egg cell. A primary oocyte is one that has not completed the first meiotic division; a secondary oocyte is one that has not completed the second meiotic division. The primary oocyte is derived by differentiation of an oogonium; it divides, producing the secondary oocyte and first polar body. Division of the secondary oocyte produces the ootid and second polar body. See also *gametogenesis.*

oogenesis (o″o-jen′ĕ-sis) [*oo-* + Gr. *genesis* production] the process by which oocytes divide to produce ova. See under *gametogenesis.*

oogonium (o″o-go′ne-um) [*oo-* + Gr. *gonē* generation] an egg cell during fetal development; about the time of birth it becomes encapsulated in primordial follicle cells and enters prophase of meiosis I, thus becoming a primary oocyte.

oolemma (o″o-lem′ah) [*oo-* + Gr. *lemma* sheath] 1. the cell membrane of an oocyte.

2. the layer of the deep-staining substance that surrounds an oocyte; more commonly called *zona pellucida* or *zona radiata.*

oophor/o (o-of′o-ro) [Gr. *ōophoros* bearing eggs] a word element used in combining form to denote the ovary, e.g., oophoropathy.

oophoritis (o″of-o-ri′tis) [*oophor-* + *-itis* inflammation] a general term used to describe inflammation of the ovaries. See also *ovaritis.*

ootid (o′o-tid) one of the four haploid cells formed by the meiotic divisions of a primary oocyte; i.e., an ovum or a polar body.

O & P abbrev. for ova and parasites.

opac/o, opaq/o (o-pas′o, o-pak′o) [L. *opacus* shaded, dark] a word element used in combining form to denote dark or impervious to light rays, e.g., opacification, radiopaque.

opacity (o-pas′ĭ-te) [L. *opacitas*] 1. the condition of being opaque.

2. in photography, the light intensity incident on a developed film divided by the light transmitted. See also *density.*

opalescent (o″pal-es′ent) [L. *opalus,* from Sanskrit *upala* stone, jewel] showing a milky iridescence, such as that of an opal.

opaque (o′pāk) [L. *opacus* shaded, dark] not transmitting any light. Cf. *radiopaque, translucent,* and *transparent.*

OP code see *operation code.*

open-mouth position any radiographic position in which the parts of interest are projected through the open mouth, e.g., the anteroposterior transoral projection of the atlas and axis, the semiaxial transoral projection of the sphenoid sinuses, the lateral transoral projection of the temperomandibular articulations, or the transoral projection of the jugular foramina.

operand (op′er-and) [L. *operandum* something to be worked on] one of the quantities or variables on which a mathematical operation is performed.

operating cycle (op′er-āt″ing) the sequence of functions or steps performed repeatedly during the normal operation of a piece of equipment.

operating system a group of computer programs that control all the activities of a computing system, such as scheduling of user jobs; compiling, link-editing (adding subroutines from the system library), assigning memory, and loading user programs; controlling input and output; handling errors; and keeping accounting records.

operating time the total fraction of time that a piece of equipment is turned on and in use. Cf. *downtime.*

operation (op″er-a′shun) [L. *operatio,* from *operatus* (past part. of *operari* to work)] 1. a surgical procedure.

2. in mathematics and high-level computer languages, a function of one variable (a unary operation) or two variables (a binary operation) considered to be so basic that it deserves a special notation. The operation is indicated by a special symbol (operator), which is placed between the two operands of a binary operation or before the operand of a unary operation. In computer languages, the common operations (and symbolic operators) are the arithmetic operations: addition (+), subtraction (–), negation or unary minus (–), multiplication (*) division (/), and exponentiation (**); the comparison operations: less than (<, .LT.), equal to (=, .EQ.), greater than >, .GT.), less than or equal to (<=, .LE.), greater than or equal to (>=, .GE.), and not equal to (¬=, .NE.); the logical operators: AND (&, .AND.), OR (|, .OR.), and NOT (¬, .NOT.); and the string operator: concatenation (||).

3. in computer assembly languages, the action performed by the computer in the execution of a single instruction, e.g., load, shift, compare, branch or condition, add, AND, etc.

operation code the part of a computer instruction specifying the operation to be performed. Also called *OP code.*

operative (op′er-a″tiv) 1. pertaining to an operation.

2. effective; not inert.

operative angle in body-section radiography, the full angle through which the x-ray tube and film move during the process of making a tomogram. The part of this angle traversed during the actual exposure is the exposure angle. Also called tomographic angle.

operator (op′er-a-tor) [L. "worker"] 1. one who performs an operation or operates a mechanical device.

2. in prokaryotic genetics, a sequence of DNA that interacts with a repressor of operon to control the expression of adjacent structural genes. See also *operon.*

3. a symbol representing a mathematical operation.

operon (op′er-on) [L. *opera* exertion + Gr. *-on* neuter ending] a regulatory control model for gene expression, in which operator sites respond to external signals (proteins) and control the expression of adjacent structural genes. See also *genetic regulation.*

arabinose o., an operon that contains three enzymes whose synthesis is induced by arabinose, L-ribulose-5-phosphate-4-epimerase, L-arabinose isomerase, and L-ribulokinase. The three structural genes are linked and transcribed as a single polycistronic message.

A maximal rate of transcription is induced when the regulatory protein binds to arabinose. In the absence of arabinose, the regulatory protein functions as a repressor. The arabinose operon induction is an example of positive control enzyme induction. Cf. *lactose o.*

lactose o., an operon that contains three enzymes whose synthesis is induced by lactose, β-galactosidase, β-galactoside permease, and β-galactoside transacetylase. The three structural genes are linked and transcribed as a single polycistronic message.

The lactose regulatory molecule (repressor), which is coded for by a gene not linked to the operon, binds tightly to the operator site, and transcription is turned off. Transcription is delayed because the repressor alters the structure of a promoter region, which normally initiates transcription. Alternately, if allolactose (a lactose intermediate) binds to the repressor, the repressor cannot bind to the operator and transcription proceeds. The lactose operon model is an example of negative control enzyme induction. Cf. *arabinose o.*

transfer (tra) o., the genetic regulation mechanism of plasmid transfer that includes genes for conjugative plasmid transfer and pilus formation. Associated genes include those for DNA replication (rep) and incompatibility (inc). See also *p. transfer* under *plasmid.*

ophiasis (o-fi′ah-sis) [Gr., from *ophis* snake] a form of alopecia areata (patchy baldness) of unknown cause that occurs in a chronic pattern. It most often affects the temporal and occipital areas of the scalp. In severe cases, the baldness may form a continuous band. See also *a. areata* under *alopecia.*

ophidism (o′fĭ-dizm) [Gr. *ophidion* serpent] a general term used to describe poisoning by snake venom.

ophthalm/o (of-thal′mo) [Gr. *ophthalmos* eye] a word element used in combining form to denote the eye, e.g., ophthalmology.

ophthalmalgia (of″thal-mal′je-ah) [*ophthalm-* + Gr. *algos* pain + *-ia*] a general term used to describe a pain in the eye that has a variety of causes including trauma, infection, and inflammation.

ophthalmia (of-thal′me-ah) [*ophthalm-* + *-ia*] a severe inflammation of the eye, which may involve the conjunctiva or the deeper structures of the eyes.

adult gonococcal o., a rare disease characterized by a severe purulent conjunctivitis in adults following self-inoculation from a gonococcal genital lesion or acquired from a gonorrheal contact. Usually, one eye is affected, and symptoms appear 1–2 da after contact. Ulceration, abscess, and blindness may result.

gonorrheal o., see *b. adultorum* under *blennorrhea.*

o. neonatorum, a purulent conjunctivitis that occurs in newborn infants. The causative agents include *Neisseria gonorrhoeae,* herpes simplex virus type 2, *Chlamydia,* and, less commonly, staphylococci, streptococci, pneumonococci, and certain opportunistic baceteria. Infants' eyes become infected during passage through the birth canal; corneal ulceration and blindness may result.

The etiologic agent of the infection may be identified by culture and by Giemsa and Gram staining of scrapings of the conjunctiva and the exudates. Although a 1 percent solution of silver nitrate is inoculated routinely into the eyes of newborns to prevent this disease, this treatment does not prevent viral forms of the disease and has led to the emergence of *Chlamydia* inclusion conjunctivitis as a more common form of ophthalmia neonatorum.

Also called *blennorrhea neonatorum* and *conjunctivitis neonatorum.*

sympathetic o., a rare disorder of unknown cause characterized by severe, bilateral granulomatous uveitis, most frequently occuring 1 wk to many years following a penetrating injury near the ciliary body. The injured eye is first affected with inflammation, redness, photophobia, and blurred vision. These symptoms spread to the uninjured eye. Untreated, this disease progresses to atrophy and complete blindness. The only treatment is removal of the injured eye before the condition spreads to the uninjured eye. Also called *systemic uveitis.*

ophthalmic (of″thal′mik) [Gr. *ophthalmikos*] pertaining to the eye.

ophthalmitis (of″thal-mi′tis) [*ophthal-* + *-itis* inflammation] an inflammation of the eyeball from a variety of causes, including foreign body trauma and infection. Immediate medical attention should be sought for all such inflammations to minimize the risk of permanent damage.

ophthalmodynamometry (of-thal″mo-di″nah-mom′ĕ-tre) [*ophthalmo-* + Gr. *dynamis* power + *metron* measure] the measurement of the blood pressure of the retinal artery, usually accomplished with an ophthalmodynamometer. Increased pressure in the retinal artery is most frequently due to systemic disease and essential hypertension.

ophthalmology (of″thal-mol′o-je) [*ophthalmo-* + *-logy*] the branch of medicine that deals with the eye: its anatomy and physiology, and the treatment of eye disorders.

ophthalmomycosis (of-thal″mo-mi-ko′sis) [*ophthalmo-* + *mycosis*] a general term used to describe any disease of the eye caused by a fungus. The recent prolonged treatment of corneal ulcers with antibiotics and immunosuppressive drugs (i.e., corticosteroids) has increased the incidence of fungal infection of the eye. It has been suggested that sulfonamides be employed whenever feasible.

ophthalmopathy (of″thal-mop′ah-the) [*ophthalmo-* + Gr. *pathos* disease] a general term used to describe any disease of the eye.

infiltrative o., a disease condition associated with Graves' disease and marked by degeneration of the fibers of the eye muscles, retrobulbar tissue, and lacrimal glands, with infiltration of lymphocytes, mononuclear leukocytes, and lipoocytes. It is often associated with high levels of long-acting thyroid stimulator (LATS), but there is no evidence that LATS causes the condition. The condition may become self-limited, and therapy is difficult to evaluate.

ophthalmoplegia (of-thal"mo-ple'je-ah) [*ophthalmo-* + Gr. *plēgē* stroke + *-ia*] a paralysis of the eye muscles, most commonly due to neurologic (or) vascular disorders. Rare attacks may be associated with migraine headaches or direct trauma to the ocular muscles. Diplopia is the most common symptom, being most severe in the direction of the affected muscles. Pain and pupillary dilation may be observed. A full medical examination, in conjuction with extensive neurologic evaluation, may be necessary to determine the underlying causes. Treatment is based on removal or control of the underlying causes. Also called extraocular muscle palsy.

exophthalmic o., a weakness of the external ocular muscles associated with exophthalmos of Graves' disease. The exophthalmos is not invariably connected with muscle weakness, and both factors may precede the clinical signs of hyperthyroidism or follow its treatment. The weakness of the ocular muscles is occasionally unilateral, especially in the early stages of the disease. It may be seen with infiltrative ophthalmopathy.

intermittent o., a condition associated with ptosis, which occurs suddenly, lasts for a period of several weeks to months, and then recedes. This condition is unresponsive to neostigmine, and thyroid function tests appear normal. Electromyograms reveal decreased stimulation to the affected muscles through their nerve supply. An association with myasthenia gravis has been suggested.

ophthalmoscopy (of-thal-mos'ko-pe) [*ophthalmo-* + Gr. *skopein* to examine] the direct examination of the interior of the eye with an ophthalmoscope, an instrument that sends a bright, narrow beam of light through the lens, which is visualized by a series of perforated mirrors and lenses. Ophthalmoscopy may be used to disclose lesions of the cornea, lens, and retina. Abnormalities of the vitreous humors and optic nerve may also be detected.

Solutions of tropicamide (0.5 percent) or phenylephrine (2.5–5 percent) are often used to dilate the pupil to aid in the examination. Prolonged examination may require the administration of solutions of cyclopentolate or phenylephrine (10 percent) for prolonged pupil dilation.

ophthalmosteresis (of-thal"mo-stĕ-re'sis) [*ophthalmo-* + Gr. *steresis* loss] a general medical term used to describe the loss of an eye.

-opia (o'pe-ah) [Gr. *ōps* eye] a suffix word element to denote vision, e.g., diplopia.

opiate (o'pe-āt) [L. *opiatus* made with opium] a drug that contains opium or any extract or derivative; also, any drug that induces sleep.

opiate assays homogenous enzyme (EMIT) immunoassay, used for the detection of opiates in urine specimens of drug abusers. See also *morphine assays.*

opioid (o'pe-oid) [*opium* + Gr. *eidos* form] any substance that has properties similar to those of the opiates, but which is not derived from opium, e.g., synthetic narcotic analgesics and enkephalins and endorphins.

Opisthorchiidae (o-pis"thor-ki'ĭ-de) [N.L., from Gr. *opisthen* behind + *orchis* testicle] a family of digenetic trematodes or flukes of the superfamily Opisthorchioidea that are parasitic in humans and animals; infection is usually acquired through the ingestion of infested fish. An encysted late larval form of the parasite is freed in the digestive tract, and migrates to the liver. Opisthorchiidae are characterized by the absence of a cirrus pouch and the presence of the ovary anterior to the testes. Diagnosis depends on demonstration of the characteristic eggs in the feces, bile, or duodenal fluid, which can be obtained by intubation. The ovoidal eggs have a shell flair (shoulders) into which the operculum fits; some have a minute process, knob, or boss at the abopercular end.

Opisthorchioidea (o-pis"thor-ki-oi'de-ah) a superfamily of trematodes or flukes in the family Opisthorchiidae.

Opisthorchis (o"pis-thor'kis) [Gr. *opisthen* behind, at the back + *orchis* testicle] a genus of trematodes (flukes) parasitic in the liver and biliary tracts of birds and mammals, including humans. Two species, *O. felineus* and *O. sinensis* (*Clonorchis sinensis*), are common liver flukes that are parasitic in humans. Human infection is caused by ingestion of contaminated fish, which serve as intermediate hosts.

opisthorchosis (o"pis-thor-ko'sis) being infected with any species of the fluke *Opisthorchis.* Species of *Opisthorchis* are distributed throughout Europe and Asia. Most require an intermediate host (some even two) of freshwater fish or snails. Human infection is caused by ingestion of raw contaminated fish, and severe cases result in cirrhosis of the liver. Most are treated with oral dehydroemetine.

Laboratory diagnosis requires identification of eggs in the feces or by duodenal aspirtion. It is necessary to differentiate infections caused by liver flukes from other hepatic infections, such as amebic liver abscesses, cancer, and hydatid disease.

opisthotonos (o"pis-thot'o-nos) [*opistho-* + Gr. *tonos* tension] a form of spasm in which the head is retracted and the hips and knees are flexed. This condition is most often seen as an adverse effect of phenothiazine administration. Also called opisthotonos position.

opium (o'pe-um) [L.; Gr. *opion* poppy juice] [USP], the dried exudation from unripe opium poppies, which contains about 20 alkaloids, some of which are derivatives of phenathrene (e.g., morphine and codeine), and others of isoquinoline (e.g., papaverine). Opium and its extracts and derivatives are used as narcotics, analgesics, and antispasmodics. Because opiates produce physical dependence, their use is controlled by the U.S. Drug Enforcement Agency; certain opiates, e.g., heroin, are controlled substances.

Oppenheim's disease (op'en-hīmz) [Hermann *Oppenheim,* German neurologist 1858–1919] see *amyotonia congenita.*

opportunistic infection (op"or-tu-nis'tik) a disease produced by microorganisms of relatively low virulence, or by those ordinarily considered nonpathogenic, in individuals with impairment or defects in their host defense mechanisms. These may be impairments and defects of either natural resistance or specific immunity, and they can be grouped into four categories: (1) damage to, or penetration of, skin or mucosal barriers; (2) primary disease predisposing to secondary infection; (3) immunologic deficiencies; and (4) iatrogenic conditions.

Intact skin and mucous membranes constitute a physical barrier of primary importance in natural resistance to infection. Although a variety, and often enormous numbers, of microorganisms inhabit the

OPPORTUNISTIC INFECTION. PRINCIPAL PATHOGENS ASSOCIATED WITH IMPAIRED CELLULAR OR HUMORAL DEFENSES

BACTERIA	FUNGI	VIRUSES (DNA)	PARASITES
Gram-positive cocci	*Candida* spp.	Cytomegalovirus	*Toxoplasma gondii*
Pseudomonas	*Cryptococcus neoformans*	*Herpes simplex*	*Pneumocystis carinii*
Enterobacteriaceae	Phycomycetes	*Herpes zoster*	
Serratia marcescens	*Aspergillus*	Varicella	
Listeria monocytogenes			
Salmonella spp.			
Mycobacterium tuberculosis			
Nocardia asteroides			

Modified from LeFrock, J. L., and Klainer, A. S.: Nosocomial Infections. Kalamazoo, MI, Upjohn Company, 1976.

epithelial surfaces as normal flora, these commensals seldom enter deep tissues in any great number. This physical barrier is also effective in preventing entry of most low-grade pathogens. However, damage to tissue integrity by trauma, infections, catheterization, burns, and prostheses; by more subtle structural and biochemical changes; or by instrumental procedures diminishes the effectiveness of this barrier. It is bypassed entirely by deep wounds and many types of instrumentation.

Some primary diseases are associated with a high frequency of opportunistic infections, e.g., cystic fibrosis, diabetes mellitus, influenza, and some lymphomas. The primary disease may also be an infectious one, as in the case of pulmonary tuberculosis and secondary fungal disease. Although immunologic deficiencies overlap with the previous category to some degree, they are distinguishable as predominantly immunologic disorders. Some are related to humoral immunity and antibody, such as B-lymphocyte deficiency or dysfunction and acute leukemia. Others are due to disorders involving the thymic lymphocytes (T cells) of cellular immunity, e.g., Hodgkins's disease and chronic granulomata. Most frequently, the source of opportunistic infection in immunologically compromised individuals is endogenous.

As a consequence of therapeutic advances, opportunistic infections have increased considerably in recent years. X-irradiation and cytotoxic drugs depress the bone marrow and the process of lymphopoiesis; cortisone depresses the inflammatory response (a protective mechanism) and acts on some T-cell types. The antitumor immunosuppressive drugs produce severe side-effects such as leukopenia and hypogammaglobulinemia, which lower resistance to many bacterial, fungal, and parasitic diseases.

Superinfection with low-grade pathogens has been recognized since the early days of modern antimicrobial chemotherapy. Administration of penicillin, although effective in controlling the primary infection, often resulted in secondary infection with gram-negative bacteria or other types previously considered to be innocuous commensals. As the more susceptible species in the normal flora were replaced by these penicillin-resistant bacilli, their pathogenic potential, although low, became clinically apparent. Similarly, candidiasis of skin and mucous membranes often followed administration of tetracycline: a clear demonstration the the normal flora plays a role in defense against clinical infection by preventing the colonization of transient microorganisms.

Organisms with opportunistic capability are also frequently present, but only in small numbers; normally they have no deleterious effect on the host's tissues. In individuals with an impaired defense, however, even classic nonpathogenic commensals may become pathogenic. A slight shift of the host-parasite relationship in favor of the parasite is sufficient to permit overgrowth of low-grade pathogens. A greater shift toward lowered resistance has an even greater effect and allows commensals to produce harm, often because they escape into tissues ordinarily devoid of a normal flora, such as the urinary bladder and the alveoli of the lung.

Opportunistic microorganisms, such as *Pseudomonas aeruginosa*, various members of the Enterobacteriaceae, and certain fungi, are not usually pathogenic to individuals in good health. They are to be distinguished from primary pathogens such as group A streptococcus and *Salmonella typhi*, which are readily capable of causing disease in healthy persons.

The number of different organisms capable of becoming opportunists is increasing, as is recognition of their pathogenic potential. The source of such organisms may be exogenous or endogenous. In recent years, endogenous microbes have been most frequently incriminated. Many hospital-associated (nosocomial) infections caused by opportunistic organisms are often related to iatrogenic factors, e.g., the use of indwelling urinary or venous catheters.

See also *normal flora* and the accompanying table.

KENNETH R. CUNDY, PH.D.

opportunistic pathogen a microorganism that is usually of low virulence but is capable of establishing infections in individuals whose natural resistance has been reduced. These organisms may be part of the normal flora of the body or may be exogenous. The overzealous use of antibacterial antibiotics, immunosuppressive agents, cytotoxins, x-rays, and steroids can remove the normal floral defenses and allow opportunistic organisms to thrive. Two examples are the *Pseudomonas aeruginosa* organism, which may cause infections in burn patients and in cancer patients who have been treated with immunosuppressive drugs, and *Candida albicans*, which can cause vaginal infections in females taking tetracyclines for prolonged periods.

Cytomegaloviruses exhibit opportunistic behavior when the immune system is depressed. Multiple infections with opportunistic organisms are common. See also *opportunistic infection.*

opsin (op′sin) [Gr. *opsis* sight, vision] a protein of the retinal rods (scotopsin) and cones (photopsin) that combines with 11-*cis*-retinal to form the visual pigments. The opsins are named according to the color of the pigment, e.g., iodopsin (violet), porphyropsin (red), and rhodopsin (purple). The combination of retinal and opsin may involve Schiff's base formation with a lysine residue. See also *rhodopsin.*

opsoclonus (op″so-klo′nus) [Gr. *ōps* eye + *klonos* turmoil] a descriptive term used to indicate the constant, irregular movement of the eyes. These movements may be vertical, horizontal, or rotary. This movement is thought to be associated with cerebellar lesions, and is most commonly seen in viral encephalomyelitis such as poliomyelitis.

opsonin (op-so′nin) [Gr. *opsōnein* to buy provisions] a factor present in body fluids that can render microorganisms susceptible to phagocytosis. An opsonin may be an antibody capable of binding both a microorganism and a phagocyte; a product of the complement system; or any nonantibody, noncomplement material that aids in phagocytosis.

opsonization (op″so-nĭ-za′shun) the attachment of opsonins to microorganisms, or any other foreign particle, to aid phagocytosis.

opsy (op′se) [Gr. *opsis* vision] a word element used in combining form to denote view, e.g., autopsy.

optic (op′tik) [Gr. *optikos* of or for sight] pertaining to the eye, or to the second cranial nerve.

optical (op′tĭ-kal) pertaining to vision, the eye, or visible light.

optical activity the ability of chiral molecules to rotate the plane of polarization of plane-polarized light. If the plane of polarization is rotated clockwise (when the observer is looking at the light source), the compound is said to be dextrorotatory and is given the prefix (+) – (formerly *d*-). If the plane of polarization is rotated counterclockwise, the compound is said to be levorotatory and is identified by the prefix (–) – (formerly *l*-). The angle through which the plane of polarization is rotated is called the optical rotation. The optical rotation of a given compound varies with the wavelength of the light, path length, concentration, temperature, and solvent.

The variation with concentration and path length is removed from the specific rotation, which is the optical rotation divided by the product of the path length (decimeters) and the concentration (grams per 100 ml). For pure liquids, the concentration is replaced by density (grams per milliliter). Under identical conditions, the optical rotations of enantiomers are of equal magnitude but opposite sign. Thus a racemic (1:1) mixture has no optical activity; it is identified by the prefix (±) – (formerly *dl*-).

See also *isomerism.*

optical character reader a computer input device that reads special computer-readable characters, such as the numbers on credit cards.

optical character recognition (OCR) the technology involved in the automated reading of printed or handwritten characters.

optical density (OD) an obsolete term. See *absorbance.*

optical isomer one of a group of stereoisomers, most of which are optically active. This includes both enantiomorphs (true mirror image forms) and diastereomers. However, if there is more than one chiral center in the molecule, the optical centers may internally compensate for each other and thus be optically inactive. For example, *meso*-tartaric acid, an optical isomer of D(+)-tartaric acid and (L)(–)-tartaric acid. See also *isomerism.*

optical path 1. the integral of the refractive index of the material traversed by a light ray. It is proportional to the travel time and the phase shift of the light.

2. the path traversed by the source light in an instrument such as a spectrophotometer.

optical purity the specific rotation of a mixture of two enantiomers divided by the specific rotation of a pure enantiomer. A D-glucose mixture of 40 percent optical purity is 0.4 D-glucose and 0.6 DL-glucose, that is, 0.7 D-glucose and 0.3 L-glucose.

optical rotation see under *optical activity.*

optical rotatory dispersion (ORD) the variation of the optical rotation of a compound with the wavelength of light. The optical rotation in the neighborhood of an absorption peak can be either negative at wavelengths shorter than the peak wavelength and positive at longer wavelengths (the positive Cotton effect), or vice versa (the negative Cotton effect). Within a series of similar asymmetric compounds, the sign of the Cotton effect is correlated with the chirality of the molecules in the vicinity of the absorbing chromophore. See also *circular dichroism.*

optical scanner a computer input device that moves a spot of light over an image field and produces a signal corresponding to the reflected (or transmitted) light.

optic chiasma (ki-az′mah) a portion of the visual pathway located in front of the hypothalamus, in which the two optic nerves partially cross. The fibers from the nasal side of each retina (carrying sensations from the lateral field of view) cross to reach the opposite side of the brain, whereas the fibers from the lateral side of each retina go to the visual cortex on the same side. See also *hemianopia.*

optic disk the intraocular portion of the optic nerve, consisting of the converging fibers of retinal ganglion cell axons and the central retinal artery. No photoreceptors are present at this point on the retina. Also called the blind spot.

optic nerve cranial nerve II; the sensory nerve for sight. Fibers arise in the retina, converge, and run backward through the optic foramen to join the optic chiasma. In the chiasma, fibers from the nasal side of each retina decussate. The optic tract and radiation convey the fibers back to the visual center in the occipital pole of each cerebral hemisphere. See also *cranial nerves.*

optic nerve inflammation an inflammation of the optic nerve, usually in the area visible ophthalmoscopically. This lesion is often unilateral (depending on the etiology) and may lead to impairment or loss of vision. There are many causes of this condition, including chemical inflammations due to lead and methanol, infections (especially syphilis), and meningitis. Edema and hyperemia of the disk is often observable.

If this condition is treated early, vision is usually restored. Untreated cases may lead to optic nerve atrophy, with partial or complete vision loss. Treatment is aimed at the underlying cause, and corticosteroids may be of some value.

Also called optic neuritis.

optics (op'tiks) [Gr. *optikos* of or for sight] the branch of physics that deals with light and vision, the physics of the propagation of electromagnetic radiation.

geometric o., the description of light propagation in terms of rays of light that are reflected or refracted at the interfaces between different media.

physical o., the treatment of light as a wave phenomenon, which is necessary for the explanation of interference effects such as diffraction.

optimizing compiler a compiler that produces a more efficient machine-language program than the standard compiler for a computer language.

optochin susceptibility test a test for the identification of *Streptococcus pneumoniae.* See under *Streptococcus.*

OR (+, |, or V) a logical binary relation that is true if any argument is true, and false otherwise. For example, the result is true if A is true or B is true, etc. Also called *inclusive OR.* Cf. *exclusive OR* and *NOR.*

or/o (o'ro) [L. *os, oris* mouth] a word element used in combining form to denote mouth, e.g., oronasal.

-or (or) a suffix word element to denote one who, e.g., operator, or that which, e.g., repressor.

ora (o'rah) 1. pl. *orae.* [L.], an edge or margin.

2. [L.], plural of *os,* mouth.

o. serrata, the scalloped margin of the retina where it meets the posterior margin of the ciliary body on the internal surface of the eyeball.

Oragrafin (or-ah-graf'in) trademark for *ipodate calcium* and *ipodate sodium;* see under *ipodate.*

oral (o'ral) [L. *oralis*] pertaining to the mouth.

oral cavity the orifice shared by the gastrointestinal and respiratory systems, and through which food enters the alimentary canal and air can be drawn into the lungs. In the embryo, the oral cavity develops from a transverse cleft, the oral fossa, which is formed between the forebrain above and the heart below. The oral fossa is separated from the foregut by a thin partition called the buccopharyngeal membrane. During the third week of embryonic life the buccopharyngeal membrane ruptures, allowing direct communication between the oral cavity and the alimentary canal.

The oral cavity is lined by a mucous membrane of stratified squamous epithelium bound to a layer of fibrous connective tissue, the lamina propria. In the remainder of the alimentary canal, the lamina propria is separated from the submucosa by a thin band of muscle called the muscularis mucosae. The lamina propria is not present in the oral cavity, but instead merges imperceptibly with the underlying submucosa. The mucosa around the teeth and in the roof of the mouth is subjected to chewing forces and has a keratinized surface, whereas the rest of the oral mucosa is nonkeratinized.

The freely movable anterior and lateral walls of the oral cavity are formed by the lips and cheeks. The external surfaces of the lips are covered by the skin that blends with the oral mucous membrane. Beneath the mucous membrane is a band of striated muscle, the orbicularis oris, whose contractions open and close the lips. The roof of the oral cavity is divided into the hard palate, supported by the bone of the palatine processes, and the soft palate, which lacks bony support and is freely movable. The soft palate is elevated during speech and swallowing to close off the nasopharynx. The oral floor consists of the sublingual tissues and is the point of attachment for the tongue. The mucosa covering the oral floor is continuous with that of the ventral surface of the tongue. The dorsal surface of the tongue is covered with mucosa roughened by epithelial projections called papillae. Along the lateral walls and at the base of some of these papillae are specialized receptors called taste buds. Chemicals from food dissolved in saliva activate these receptors, stimulating the sense of taste. The tongue contains a complex system of striated muscles that function in speech, chewing, and swallowing.

The oral mucous membrane encircling the teeth and covering their supporting bone is called the gingiva (gums). The gingiva adjacent to the neck of the teeth is firmly attached to the periosteum of the alveolar process that anchors the teeth. The gingiva is separated from the mucosa of the lips and cheeks by the alveolar mucosa. A shallow trough called the mucobuccal fold is formed at the junction of the alveolar mucosa and the mucosa of the lips and cheeks.

In addition to the numerous accessory or minor salivary glands located in the submucosa of the lips, cheeks, and palate, there are three pairs of major salivary glands. The largest of these, the parotid salivary glands, are located in the retromolar fossa at the angle of the lower jaw. They discharge their secretions into the oral cavity through Stensen's duct, which opens on the mucosa of the cheek adjacent to the maxillary molar teeth. The submaxillary and sublingual salivary glands are buried in the soft tissues of the oral floor. They open into the oral cavity through ducts located on a crest of mucosa called the sublingual fold.

Salivary secretion is a reflex mediated by parasympathetic fibers of the autonomic nervous system. The reflex is stimulated by the sight, smell, and taste of food. Saliva, which contains enzymes initiating digestion, serves a variety of functions: it moistens food to facilitate swallowing, flushes food debris from around teeth, lubricates oral mucosa to aid speech, and contains secretory immunoglobulins that helps protect the oral mucosa from infection.

J. ROBERT NEWLAND, D.D.S.

oral pharynx (o'ral far'inks) the funnel-shaped extension of the oral cavity that directs food into the esophagus by the reflex action of swallowing and conducts air through the larynx into the lungs during respiration. The oral pharynx communicates with the oral cavity through the faucial isthmus, which consists of the soft palate above, the tonsillar pillars laterally, and the junction of the anterior two-thirds and posterior one-third of the tongue below.

Like the remainder of the alimentary canal, the oral pharynx is divided into three histologically distinct layers: a mucosa of nonkeratinizing squamous epithelium resting on a layer of fibrous connective tissue, the lamina propria; a submucosa containing blood vessels, lymphatic channels, and nerves; and a circular band of muscle whose contractions propel food into the esophagus during swallowing.

Nodules of lymphoid tissue called tonsils encircle the opening of the oral pharynx to form Waldeyer's ring. The largest of these, the palatine tonsils, are found in the lateral walls of the oral pharynx between the anterior and posterior tonsillar pillars. Their mucosal surface of stratified squamous epithelium is deeply furrowed by invaginations called tonsillar crypts. The pharyngeal tonsils or adenoids are located in the mucosa of the superior aspect of the posterior wall of the pharynx and are covered by respiratory epithelium without crypts. Multiple lymphoid nodules, called lingual tonsils, are present in the mucosa of the lateral borders of the posterior portion of the tongue.

Also called *oropharynx.*

J. ROBERT NEWLAND, D.D.S.

orange (or'anj) [Sanskrit *nāranga*] 1. any of several trees of the genus *Citrus* or its fruit.

2. a spectral color that corresponds to the perceived hue of monochromtic light having a wavelength between 597 and 662 nm (i.e., between red and yellow).

orange G an acid azo dye, $C_6H_5N{=}NC_{10}H_4(SO_3Na)_2OH$, used as a cytoplasmic stain; C.I. 16230.

orbiculus (or-bik'u-lus), pl. *orbiculi* [L., dim. of *orbis* orb, circle] [NA], a structure shaped like a small circle or disk, e.g., the orbicularis oris muscle.

orbiculus ciliaris (or-bik'u-lus sil"e-a'ris) [NA], the thin, smooth annular ring that comprises the major portion of the ciliary body. It is continuous posteriorly with the ora serrata.

orbit (or'bit) [L. *orbita* mark of a wheel] the bony cavity that contains the eyeball and its associated muscles, nerves, and vessels.

orbital (or'bĭ-tal) [L. *orbitalis*] 1. pertaining to the orbit.

2. a region in an atom that may contain either one or two opposite spin electrons; orbitals of various sizes and shapes may occur in a single atom.

orbital pneumotomography (or'bĭ-tal nu"mo-to-mog'rah-fe) tomography of the orbit after injection of oxygen into the muscle cone space, a procedure performed to outline tumors behind the eye.

orbitography (or"bĭ-tog'rah-fe) [*orbit* + Gr. *graphein* to record] the radiologic examination of the orbit after injection of a contrast medium into the muscle cone, the retrobulbar space. Both positive and negative contrast orbitography (called orbital pneumotomography) are used.

orbitomeatal line (or"bĭ-to-me-a'tal) [*orbit* + L. *meatus* passageway, path] the line passing through the outside corner of the eye (the outer canthus) and the center of the opening of the ear (the external auditory meatus); used in radiographic positioning. Also called *canthomeatal line.*

orbitoparietal projection (or'bĭ-to-pah-ri'ĕ-tal) [*orbit* + L. *parietalis*, from *paries* wall] a radiographic projection of the orbit, the exact opposite of the parietoorbital projection, used when a patient cannot be placed in the prone position.

Orbivirus (or'bĭ-vi"rus) a genus of RNA viruses belonging to the Reoviridae family. Orbiviruses are transmitted by arthropods and are the etiologic agents of Colorado tick fever, blue tongue, and African horse sickness. See also *Reovirus.*

orcein (or-se'in) a brown coloring matter produced by the oxidation of orcinol in ammonia water; C.I. 1242. It consists of 14 different compounds and is used in histology as a stain for elastic fibers, Australia antigen, or chromosomes. See also *acetic orcein* and *acid orcein.*

orch/o, orchi/o, orchid/o (or'ko, or'ke-o, or'kid-o) [Gr. *orchis* testis] a word element used in combining form to denote the testes, e.g., orchiectomy.

orchidoblastoma (or"kid-o-blas-to'mah) [*orchido-* + Gr. *blastos* germ + *-ōma* tumor] see *endodermal sinus tumor.*

orchiocele (or'ke-o-sēl) [*orchio-* + Gr. *kēlē* hernia] 1. the hernial protrusion of the testis beyond its tunica; a fairly uncommon disorder.

2. scrotal hernia.

3. tumor of the testis.

orchitis (or-ki'tis) [*orch-* + *-itis* inflammation] an inflammation of the testis. This condition may involve the epididymis as well, and may lead to testicular damage, scarring, and sterility. There is pain and swelling, and the testis may become hard. Orchitis has various causes. It often follows infection, e.g., gonorrhea, syphilis, tuberculosis, and mumps. Granulomatous orchitis may occur after trauma to the testis and is thought to have an autoimmune component. Less common causes include brucellosis, leprosy, typhoid, and meningococcal, rickettsial fungal, and parasitic infections.

orcin (or'sin) see *orcinol.*

orcinol (or'sĭ-nol) a white crystalline solid, 5-methylresorcinol, 1,3-dihydroxy,5-methyl benzene,5-methyl-1,3,-benzenediol, with a sweet but unpleasant taste; M.W. 124.14. It is a component of Bial's reagent for pentoses. Orcinol is corrosive and should be treated with the same care as phenols (carbolic acid). Also called *orcin.* See also *Bial's reagent* and *pentose assays.*

ORD abbrev. See *optical rotatory dispersion.*

order (or'der) [L. *ordo* a line, row, or series] a taxonomic group of organisms within a class; it may be further subdivided into families.

ordinal (or'dĭ-nal) [L. *ordino, ordinis* order] a specified postion in a numbered series or biologic order.

ordinal variable a variable that permits an ordering of observations. For any two values, it can be determined which is greater but not necessarily how much greater. See also *scale.*

ordinate (or'dĭ-nāt) the y-coordinate value of a point on a graph; the perpendicular distance from the x axis (horizontal axis); the value of the dependent variable. Cf. *abscissa.*

Oretic (o-ret'ik) trademark for hydrochlorothiazide; see under *thiazide diuretics.*

orexigenic (o-rek"sĭ-jen'ik) [Gr. *orexis* appetite + *gennan* to produce] a general term used to describe any compound or process that stimulates or increases the appetite.

organ (or'gan) [L. *organum;* Gr. *organnon*] any part of the body that performs a specific function or functions. See also the specific organ.

organ culture the growth and maintenance of small fragments of tissue in chemical media. Organ culture differs from tissue and cell culture in that tissue organization, i.e., relationships of cells to stroma and vessels, is maintained in the explanted fragment, whereas tissue culture refers to maintenance of a single cell type in a monolayer or suspension. Kidney, lungs, mammary gland, pancreas, and salivary gland have been successfully maintained in organ culture.

organelle (or″gan-el′) [N.L. *organella,* dim. of *organum* organ] a structure in the cytoplasm of a cell, specialized in its ultrastructure and biochemical composition to subserve a particular function. A limiting membrane selectively separates it from the surrounding cytoplasm. The common organelles in animal cells are the mitochondria (energy production), granular endoplasmic reticulum (protein formation), lysosomes (lytic enzymes), and Golgi complex (protein packaging and some synthetic activities). These organelles are found in most cells, but their relative numbers vary according to the functional requirements of the type of cell. In addition, chloroplasts, the photosynthetic organelles, are found in plant cells.

organic (or-gan′ik) [L. *organicus,* from Gr. *organikos* instrumental] 1. pertaining to an organ or organism.

2. derived or originating from living organisms.

3. pertaining to a class of chemical compounds characterized by carbon-carbon bonds, i.e., all compounds of carbon except carbides, carbonates, and oxides of carbon.

4. the branch of chemistry dealing with carbon compounds.

5. pertaining to food grown and processed using fertilizers, pesticides, and additives of animal or vegetable origin.

organic acid any organic compound capable of losing a proton to a base. Among the strongest types of organic acids are carboxylic acids (RCOOH) and sulfonic acids (RSO_3H). However, such compounds as ethanol (C_2H_5OH) and toluene ($C_6H_5CH_3$) function as weak organic acids in the presence of a strong base.

organic brain syndrome a complex syndrome of mental symptoms relating to impaired cerebral function. It includes defective perception and impairments of recall, logic, reasoning, and behavior; there may be disturbances of consciousness, and hallucinations and delusions may also be present. The syndrome may be acute and reversible, or irreversible and chronic. Various etiologies are known, including intoxication (alcohol, drugs, chemicals), drug withdrawal, postoperative states, fever, metabolic disturbances, endocrine disturbances, nutritional deficiencies, dementia, infections, trauma, cerebral neoplasms, cardiovascular disorders, epilepsy, sensory deprivation, and several systemic degenerative diseases. Often the etiology is multifactorial.

Electroencephalograms are often abnormal. This syndrome must be differentiated from nonorganic psychiatric syndromes.

organic phosphate any ester of phosphoric acid with an organic alcohol. Examples are sugar phosphates, phospholipids, phosphoproteins, nucleotides, coenzymes, nucleic acids, and other molecules. Some enzyme reactions proceed by forming an enzyme-phosphate intermediate (via serine), and other enzymes are regulated by the phosphorylation and dephosphorylation of the enzyme protein. Cell membranes are quite impervious to organic phosphates.

organism (or′gah-nizm) any individual living thing, whether animal or plant.

organization (or″gah-nĭ-za′shun) in electroencephalography, the degree to which the electrical activity of the brain, as recorded from an individual, conforms in character to that displayed by a large proportion of subjects of similar age who are free from neurologic, psychiatric, and other illnesses associated with brain dysfunction.

organo-chloro pesticides see *chlorinated hydrocarbon pesticides.*

organ of Chievitz (che′wits) [Johan Henrik *Chievitz,* Danish anatomist, 1850–1901] a small anatomic structure, located within the pterygoid fossa, that is composed of rests of epithelial cells with associated nerve fibers embedded in fibrous connective tissue. When it was noted that this body persists into adult life, it was named the juxtaoral organ of Chievitz. Possibly it is an embryologic remnant of an invagination of the stomodeal ectoderm, but a chemoreceptor function has also been proposed. Similar intraneural epithelial clusters have been reported within the bone of the maxilla. Also called paraparotid organ.

organometallic compound (or″gah-no-mĕ-tal′ik) a chemical compound in which a metal atom is bonded to a carbon atom, such as the gasoline additive tetraethyl lead, $Pb(C_2H_5)_4$.

organophosphate compounds (or″gah-no-fos′fāt) a large group of esters of phosphoric acid or thiophosphoric acid, used as insecticides and chemical warfare nerve gases. They are irreversible (noncompetitive) inhibitors of the enzymes acetylcholinesterase and pseudocholinesterase. The phosphate triesters, called direct inhibitors (e.g., Bidrin and DDVP), are covalently bonded to the enzyme active site by a phosphate ester bond. The phosphorothioate triesters (e.g., parathion and diazinon) and the phosphorodithioate triesters (e.g., malathion) are indirect inhibitors; they must undergo enzymatic oxidation to the corresponding oxo compound (for example, parathion is converted to paraoxon) before binding to cholinesterase. These esters thus are less toxic than their oxo analogs.

The primary effects of organophosphate poisoning are due to the accumulation of acetylcholine. Muscarinic effects include nausea, sweating, and heartburn; in severe poisioning there is excessive bronchial secretion, vomiting, involuntary defecation and urination, and bradycardia. Nicotinic effects include muscular weakness and twitching, difficulty in breathing, and tachycardia. Central nervous system effects include anxiety, headache, tremor, convulsions, and coma. The cause of death in fatal poisoning is usually asphyxiation due to respiratory failure and pulmonary edema.

Two antidotes are used in poisoning cases. Atropine reduces muscarinic effects by blocking the muscarinic receptors; pralidoxime reactivates cholinesterase by dephosphorylation and reduces both muscarinic and nicotinic effects.

organothiophosphate (or″gah-no-thi″o-fos′fāt) an organic ester of thiophosphoric acid (H_3PO_3S); see under *organophosphate compounds.*

organothiophosphate compound assays (or″gah-no-thi″o-fos′fāt) 1. thin-layer chromatography. Organic phosphate and thiophosphate esters are extracted from a specimen of blood, urine, tissue, or stomach content into pentane. The extracts are chromatographed on aluminum oxide G using two developing solvents that have different polarities. The plates may be sprayed with plasma (containing active cholinesterase) and acid-base indicator, and then with acetylcholine; the serum cholinesterase liberates acetic acid except at spots where it is inhibited by an organophosphate.

2. gas chromatography. Pentane extracts are chromatographed using a nonpolar silicone column packing and a halogen phosphorus (HP) or electron capture detector; methylstearate is used as the internal standard. The concentration is determined from the ratio of peak heights produced by the organophosphate and the internal standard. See also *cholinesterase assays.*

organotroph (or-gah'no-trōf) [Gr. *organnon* organ + *tropē* a turning] see *heterotroph.*

organotropism (or-gah-not'ro-pizm) a specific affinity manifested by chemical compounds or pathologic organisms for a particular tissue or organ of the body.

organ perfusion (or'gan per-fu'zhun) an in vitro technique used to obtain data concerning in vivo metabolic reactions. The perfusion of an isolate organ in vitro (or in situ in an anesthetized animal) makes possible the introduction of a substance; the fate of the perfused compound in that organ can be evaluated by analysis of the fluid emerging from the organ.

Organ perfusion is also used to maintain donor organs, e.g., the kidney, for short periods prior to transplantation.

OR gate (OR circuit) an electronic circuit that calculates the logical OR function. Its output is *true* if any input is *true,* and *false* otherwise. See also *NOR gate.*

Oriental blood fluke see *S. japonicum* under *Schistosoma.*

Oriental lung fluke see *P. westermani* under *Paragonimus.*

Oriental lung fluke disease see *paragonimiasis.*

orifice (or'ĭ-fis) [L. *orificium,* from *oris* mouth] 1. the entrance or outlet of any cavity in the body.

2. any foramen, meatus, or opening.

origanum oil (o-rig'ah-num) [L. wild marjoram] a substance composed of Spanish hop oil, thyme oil, or a mixture of the two, used as a clearing agent for stained tissue sections. It clears from 95 percent alcohol but tends to dissolve out aniline dyes.

Orinase (or'ĭ-nās) trademark. See *tolbutamide.*

Ormond's disease (or'mond) [John Kelso *Ormond,* U.S. urologist, born 1886] see *retroperitoneal f.* under *fibrosis.*

ornithine (or'nĭ-thin) [Gr. *ornithos* bird + *-ine*] a diaminomonocarboxylic acid. Ornithine is an intermediate in the synthesis of urea (urea cycle) and is not used for protein synthesis.

ornithine aminotransferase (or'nĭ-thin am"ĭ-no-trans'fer-as) see *ornithine–oxo-acid aminotransferase.*

ornithine carbamoyltransferase (OCT) (or'nĭ-thin kar'bah-moil-trans'fer-ās) an enzyme of the transferase class (carbamoylphosphate:L-ornithine carbamoyltransferase, EC 2.1.3.3) that catalyzes the reaction carbamoylphosphate + L-ornithine ⇄ orthophosphate + L-citrulline. The reaction is an important step in the Krebs-Henseleit cycle of urea synthesis. The enzyme occurs almost exclusively in the liver; elevated serum activity reflects liver injury or disease. Activities are markedly higher in individuals with hepatic necrosis and viral hepatitis. Also called *ornithine transcarbamoylase.*

ornithine carbamoyltransferase assays 1. enzyme assays using the forward reaction carbamoylphosphate + ornithine → citrulline + inorganic phosphate. The citrulline formed at pH 7.0 is reacted with diacetylmonoxime or dimethylglyoxime to produce a colored product, which is then quantitated photometrically. Interfering urea in the specimen is removed by urease.

2. enzyme assays using the reverse reaction citrulline + arsenate → ornithine + carbamoyl arsenate. The carbamoyl arsenate decomposes to ammonia plus CO_2. The ammonia formed can be measured using the Berthelot reaction or by using the glutamate dehydrogenase reaction involving oxoglutarate plus NADH and measuring the decrease in NADH. If ^{14}C-citrulline is used, the $^{14}CO_2$ formed can be isolated and measured radiometrically.

ornithine carbamoyltransferase deficiency a disorder of ornithine and glutamine metabolism, transmitted as an X-linked trait, that is due to a relative or absolute deficiency of the enzyme ornithine carbamyltransferase. It affects males most severely. This condition causes greatly increased levels of ammonia in the blood and glutamine in the blood and urine. Consequently, severely affected male infants have recurrent vomiting, irritability, lethargy, central nervous system dysfunctions, and protein intolerance, progressing to seizures, coma, or death; the clinical signs in females are more variable.

This disease may also lead to orotic aciduria without characteristic hematologic changes. Low-protein diets may yield some relief. Screening for detection of carriers is possible.

Also called *hyperammonemia I* and *ornithine transcarbamylase deficiency.* See also *aminoacidopathy.*

ornithine decarboxylase (or'nĭ-thin de"kar-bok'sĭ-lās) an enzyme of the lyase class (EC 4.1.1.17) that catalyzes the reaction L-ornithine ⇄ putrescine + CO_2. The reaction is important in the metabolism of arginine in the human body; it also occurs as a result of bacterial action in decaying meat. The presence of ornithine decarboxylase is used as a major differential criterion in the identification of closely related species among the Enterobacteriaceae and Vibrionaceae.

ornithinemia see *hyperornithinemia.*

ornithine–oxo-acid aminotransferase (or"nĭ-thin-ok"so-a'sĭd am"ĭ-no-trans'fer-ās) an enzyme of the transferase class (L-ornithine:2-oxo-acid aminotransferase, EC 2.6.1.13) that catalyzes the reaction L-ornithine + a 2-oxo acid ⇄ L-glutamate γ-semialdehyde + an L-amino acid. The reaction is important for the degradation of excess ornithine formed from excess arginine. A hereditary deficiency of the enzyme, causing excess ornithine accumulation, can cause atrophy of the retina and result in blindness. Also called *ornithine aminotransferase.*

ornithine transcarbamoylase (or'nĭ-thin trans-kar"bah-moi'lās) see *ornithine carbamoyltransferase.*

ornithine transcarbamylase deficiency (or'nĭ-thin trans-kor"bah-mil'ās) see *ornithine carbamoyltransferase deficiency.*

Ornithobilharzia (or″nĭ-tho-bil-har′ze-ah) [Gr. *ornithos* bird + *bilharzia,* from Theodor Maximilian *Bilharz,* German physician, 1825–1862] a genus of blood flukes parasitic in birds. The cercarial stage is known to cause dermatitis in humans exposed to the cercaria in infested waters.

Ornithodoros (or″nĭ-thod′o-ros) [Gr. *ornis, ornithos* bird + Gr. *doros* bag] a genus of soft-bodied ticks that transmits both spirochetes (of the genus *Borrelia,* which causes relapsing fevers) and *Trypanosoma cruzi* (causing Chagas' disease). See also the illustration under *tick.*

Ornithonyssus (or″nĭ-tho-nis′us) [Gr. *ornithos* bird + *nyssa* prick] a genus of mites. The species *O. bacoti* (the tropical rat mite) is known to feed on humans employed in granaries and food-supply houses where rats are common, causing dermatitis and occasionally a secondary infection when lesions are scratched. Other species, such as *O. bursa, O. nagayoi,* and *O. sylviarum,* also attack humans and cause dermatitis.

ornithosis (or″nĭ-tho′sis) [Gr. *ornis, ornithos* bird + *-osis*] primarily an infection of birds and originally thought to be limited to the psittacine or parrot family, hence the earlier name of psittacosis. However, a wide variety of birds harbor the causative agent, *Chlamydia psittaci,* with or without evidence of the disease. In humans, also, infection is often asymptomatic or produces only mild respiratory symptoms, although a severe and fatal pneumonia can develop.

Inhalation of the organism by contact with infected birds (including pets and poultry) is followed by an incubation period of 7–15 da. At onset there are fever, chills, coughing, headache, and prostration. The pneumonia most often is patchy but may change from day to day. The white blood cell count may be normal or shifted to the left, and proteinuria may be present.

Diagnosis is based on demonstration of a rise of complement-fixing and fluorescent antibodies against chlamydial group antigen. Isolation of the causative organism in eggs or cell culture is the best evidence. X-ray findings are not distinguishable from those in viral pneumonia or Q fever. This disease is effectively treated with tetracycline.

Also called *parrot fever* and *psittacosis.*

orofaciodigital syndrome (or″o-fa″she-o-dij′ĭ-tal) [*oro-* + L. *facies* face + *digitus* digit] a genetic syndrome, transmitted as an X-linked dominant trait, that is found only in females, probably because of male lethality. It is characterized by decreased mental abilities and severe developmental abnormalities of the tongue, mouth, fingers, and, frequently, the face.

orogenital syndrome (or″o-gen′ĭ-tal) [*oro-* + L. *genitalis* belonging to birth] mucocutaneous lesions similar to but distinct from those of pellagra that occur in Strachan's syndrome. These lesions consist of varying degrees of stomatoglossitis, genital dermatitis, and corneal degeneration. See also *Strachan's syndrome.*

oropharyngeal isthmus (or″o-fah-rin′je-al) [*oro-* + L. *pharyngeus*] see *i. of fauces* under *isthmus.*

oropharyngeal membrane in the developing embryo, a membrane that separates the primitive oral cavity from the developing pharynx. It ruptures in about the third week of development. Also called *buccopharyngeal membrane.*

oropharynx (o″ro-far′inks) [*oro-* + Gr. *pharynx* pharynx] see *oral pharynx.*

orosomucoid (or″ŏ-so-mu′koid) a plasma protein of the alpha$_1$-globulin group, an alpha$_1$-acid glycoprotein (42 percent carbohydrate). This is an acute-phase reactant and is increased along with other acute-phase reactants in any inflammatory condition. Elevations occur within a day of the injury, and decline after 4–5 da. Increased production of orosomucoid has been observed in disorders associated with enhanced cell proliferation (e.g., malignancies). Its exact function is not known, although it has been implicated in the regulation of spacing of collagen fibers. Also called *acid seromucoid* and *alpha$_1$-seromucoid.*

orotate phosphoribosyltransferase an enzyme of the transferase class (orotidine-5′-phosphate:pyrophosphate phosphoribosyltransferase, EC 2.4.2.10) that catalyzes the reaction orotidine-5′-phosphate + pyrophosphate ⇄ orotate + 5′-phospho-α-D-ribose-1-diphosphate. This enzyme and orotidylate decarboxylase are missing in type I orotic aciduria. Patients with this disorder are autotrophs for pyrimidine and therefore are treated with uridine.

orotic acid (o-rot″ik) uracil-6-carboxylic acid, a growth factor for certain microorganisms and an intermediate in the synthesis of pyrimidine nucleotides.

orotic aciduria (o-rot″ik as″ĭ-du′re-ah) a genetic condition, transmitted as an autosomal recessive trait, that involves the excretion of increased quantities of orotic acid (orange crystalluria) in the urine; it is characteristic of conditions presenting with some defects in pyrimidine metabolism.

In orotic aciduria type I, a deficiency is present in both orotate phosphoribosyltransferase and orotidine-5′-phosphate decarboxylase in all cells, whereas in type II, only the decarboxylase is deficient. Both conditions, in addition to presenting with orotic aciduria, are associated with megaloblastic anemia, and the former also with failure to thrive. Orotic aciduria type I responds to treatment with oral uridine; type II to uridine and orotidylic acid. Oral prednisone and pyrimidine (yeast extracts) may also be used. Orotic aciduria also accompanies a deficiency of ornithine transcarbamoylase, and the use of the drugs 6-azauridine and allopurinol is associated with high rates of orotic aciduria.

orotidine-5′-phosphate decarboxylase (o-rot′ĭ-dēn fos′fāt de″kar-bok′sĭ-lās) an enzyme of the lyase class (orotidine-5′-phosphate carboxy-lyase, EC 4.1.1.23) that catalyzes the reaction orotidine-5′-phosphate ⇄ uridine-5′-phosphate (UMP) + CO_2. The reaction occurs in the synthesis of pyrimidine nucleotides. A hereditary deficiency of the enzyme, known as orotic aciduria II, is characterized by the excretion of orotic acid. Also called *orotidylate decarboxylase.*

orotidylate decarboxylase (o-rot″ĭ-dĭ′lāt de″kar-bok′sĭ-lās) see *orotidine-5′-phosphate decarboxylase.*

Oroya fever (o-roi′yah) [La *Oroya,* a town in Peru] see *bartonellosis.*

orphenadrine (or-fen′ah-drēn) a derivative of diphenhydramine, having anticholinergic, analgesic, and weak antihistaminic activity. Adverse reactions include dryness of the mouth, blurring of vision, constipation, urinary retention, and mental confusion and hallucinations.

o. citrate, the salt of orphenadrine, used for relief of pain due to skeletal muscle tension. It has mild anticholinergic action.

o. hydrochloride, the salt of orphenadrine, used as an adjunct in the treatment of parkinsonism.

-orrhagia (or-a′je-ah) [Gr. *rhēgnynai* to burst forth] a suffix word element to denote a bursting forth of blood, e.g., menorrhagia.

-orrhaphy (or′ah-fe) [Gr. *rhaphē* a seam] a suffix word element to denote a suture, e.g., herniorrhaphy.

-orrhea (o-re′ah) [Gr. *rhoia* flow] a suffix word element to denote a flow or discharge, e.g., rhinorrhea.

-orrhexis (or-ek′sis) [Gr. *rhēxis* rupture] a suffix word element to denote a rupture, e.g., karyorrhexis.

Ortalidae (or-tal′ĭ-de) [N.L., from Gr. *ortalis* fowl] a family of flies whose larvae may cause intestinal myiasis in humans when food contaminated with their eggs is ingested.

Orth's fluid [Johannes J. *Orth,* German pathologist, 1847–1923] a dichromate-formalin fixative; see under *fixative.*

ortho- (or′tho) [Gr. *orthos* straight] 1. a prefix word element to denote straight, normal, correct, etc.

2. (abbrev. *o*-), a prefix word element in organic chemistry used to denote 1,2 substituted benzene (e.g., *ortho*-xylene, 1,2-dimethylbenzene), used only in trivial names. Cf. *meta*- and *para*-. See also the accompanying illustration.

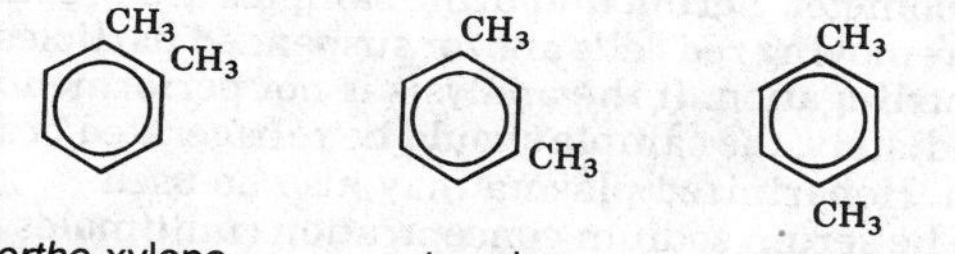

ortho-xylene *meta*-xylene *para*-xylene

ortho-. Structural formulas for *ortho*-, *meta*-, and *para*-isomers. (From Banks, J. E.: Naming Organic Compounds. 2nd ed. Philadelphia, W. B. Saunders Co., 1976.)

3. a prefix word element in inorganic chemistry used to denote the most hydrated acid or its salt, in contrast to the meta- or less hydrated acid or salt; e.g., orthoboric acid is H_3BO_3 and metaboric acid is HBO_2.

orthochromatic (or″tho-kro-mat′ik) [*ortho*- + Gr. *chrōma* color] in histochemistry, pertaining to the staining of a tissue with a dyestuff, resulting in a dye-tissue complex with the same color and absorption spectrum as the dye itself. Cf. *metachromatic.*

orthochromatic normoblast see under *normoblast.*

orthodiagraphy (or″tho-di-ag′rah-fe) [*ortho*- + Gr. *dia* through + *graphein* to record] the radiographic examination of the internal organs, particularly the long bones, to measure their exact size and shape. Image distortion is minimized by use of a long (6 ft or more) focal-film distance. Also called *orthoroentgenography.* See also *scanography.*

orthodromic conduction (or″tho-drom′ik) [Gr. *orthodromein* to run straight forward] the propagation of action potentials along an axon in the normal or physiologic direction, as in sensory nerve conduction from a peripheral receptor to the spinal cord. Cf. *antidromic conduction.*

orthoiodohippurate (or″tho-i-o″do-hip′u-rāt) see *iodohippurate.*

orthomyxovirus (or″tho-mik″so-vi′rus) [*ortho*- + *myxovirus,* from Gr. *myxa* mucus + *virus*] a family of myxoviruses that contains the influenza viruses types A, B, and C. These organisms are enveloped RNA viruses 80-120 nm in diameter that are pleomorphic, spherical, or filamentous. The genosome single-stranded RNA is transcribed to mRNA by a viral RNA transcriptase and exists as eight (types A and B) or fewer (type C) segments, one for each of the viral proteins. See also *influenza virus* and *myxovirus.*

orthophosphoric acid (or″tho-fos-for′ik) see under *phosphoric acid.*

orthophosphoric ester monohydrolase see *phosphoric monoester hydrolase.*

orthopnea (or″thop-ne′ah) [*ortho*- + Gr. *pnoia* breath] difficulty in breathing while lying down. It occurs in congestive heart failure, especially when associated with increased pulmonary venous and capillary pressure. The recumbent position further contributes to orthopnea by decreasing the vital capacity of the lungs and increasing pulmonary congestion. Orthopnea may be relieved by sitting erect or by standing. Cf. *platypnea.*

Orthopodomyia (or″tho-po″do-mi′e-ah) a genus of bloodsucking flies of the subfamily Culicinae that are transmitters of human diseases. It includes four species from North America.

Orthoptera (or-thop-ter-ah) [*ortho*- + Gr. *pteron* wing] an order of insects (grasshoppers, crickets, and cockroaches) of the class Insecta. Several species are intermediate hosts of incidental human helminths.

orthoroentgenography (or″tho-rent″gen-og′rah-fe) see *orthodiagraphy.*

Orthorrhapha (or-thor′rah-fah) [N.L., from *orth*- + Gr. *rhapē* a seam] a former suborder of flies of order Diptera, now divided into the suborders Nematocera and Brachycera.

orthostatic (or″tho-stat′ik) [*ortho*- + Gr. *statikos* causing to stand] pertaining to or caused by standing upright; standing erect.

orthostatic hypotension see *orthostatic h.* under *hypotension.*

orthotopic (or″tho-top′ik) [*ortho*- + Gr. *topos* place] occurring at the normal position of the body; in tissue transplantation, the term refers to a graft transferred to a position formerly occupied by tissue of the same kind.

orthotopic graft a tissue transplantation that places the graft in its proper location and orientation. Cf. *heterotopic graft.*

orthovoltage (or″tho-vol′tij) pertaining to x-ray radiation therapy using photon energies of about 200-500 keV, used for treatment of superficial neoplasms. See also *radiation therapy equipment.*

Os symbol for the clinical element *osmium.*

os (os), pl. *ora* [L. "an opening, or mouth"] [NA], the mouth; the opening of a structure, e.g., the external os of the endocervical canal.

oscillator (os′ĭ-la″tor) [L. *oscillare* to swing] an electronic circuit that produces an output with a definite periodic waveform (e.g., sine wave, square wave) and a definite frequency.

oscillopsia (os″ĭ-lop′se-ah) [L. *oscillare* to swing + Gr. *opsis* vision + *-ia* condition] a visual sensation in which stationary objects appear to move.

oscilloscope (ŏ-sil′o-skōp) [L. *oscillare* to swing + Gr. *skopein* to examine] an electronic device that uses a cathode-ray tube (CRT) to display an electrical waveform or other image on a screen. The image is produced by an electron beam of variable intensity striking the screen phosphors. The beam is produced, accelerated, focused, deflected, and controlled by the voltage on several electrodes or deflection plates, which determines the electrostatic attraction of the plate for the electrons (in some CRTs, magnetic coils are used for deflection). The X input controls the horizontal position of the dot produced on the oscilloscope face, the Y input controls the vertical position, and the Z input controls the intensity or brightness.

When the oscilloscope is used to display a waveform, the X input is swept (because the dot is moved across the screen at an even rate), while the waveform is applied to the Y input. This produces a graph of voltage versus time.

When an image is produced, the X and Y inputs control the beam position. In a scintillation camera, the Z input is unblanked (turned on) to record each count. In a CT scanner, the Z input is varied to produce a gray scale of pixel brightness.

storage o., an oscilloscope in which the image is held on the screen until it is erased. A storage mesh traps and stores the charge from the electron beam. An additional electron gun erases the image by flooding the screen with electrons.

Osgood-Schlatter disease (oz′good shlat′er) [Robert Bayley *Osgood,* Boston orthopedist, 1873–1956; Carl *Schlatter,* Zurich surgeon, 1864–1934] an inflammation of the apophysis of the tibial tuberosity that, when severe, may be accompanied by aseptic necrosis. It is most often seen in young, active individuals in their early or midteens; its cause is unknown. Swelling and tenderness are seen and tend to worsen with exercise. X-rays reveal irregular ossification of the tibial tubercle. Also called Schlatter-Osgood disease.

-osis (o′sis) [Gr.] a suffix word element to denote a condition or abnormal process, e.g., erythrocytosis.

Osler's nodes (ōs′lerz) [Sir William *Osler,* Canadian-born physician, 1849–1919] small (2–5 mm), tender, subcutaneous papules that develop on the pads or surfaces of fingers or toes and are associated with infectious endocarditis. Osler's nodes appear purple or erythematous and may persist for hours to days. Although they are found in about 10–25 percent of individuals with endocarditis, they also occur in those with collagen vascular disease and typhoid fever.

Osler-Vaquez disease (ōs′ler vak-āz′) [Sir William *Osler;* Louis Henri *Vaquez,* French physician, 1860–1936] see *p. vera* under *polycythemia.*

Osm abbrev. See *osmole.*

osm/o (oz′mo) 1. [Gr. *osmē* smell], a word element used in combining form to denote smells or odors, e.g., osmoscope.
2. [Gr. *ōsmos* impulse], a word element used in combining form to denote impulse or osmosis, e.g., osmophilic.

-osmia (oz′me-ăh) [Gr. *osmē* smell] a suffix word element to denote smell, e.g., anosmia.

osmic acid (oz′mik) 1. a dibasic acid, H_2OsO_4.
2. osmium tetroxide, OsO_4, the anhydride of true osmic acid.

osmiophilic (oz″me-o-fil′ik) [*osmic* acid + Gr. *philein* to love] staining easily with osmium tetroxide, usually said of lipids.

osmium (Os) (oz′me-um) [from Gr. *osmē,* odor because of the disagreeable odor of osmium tetroxide] a bluish-white, lustrous metallic element of the platinum group; atomic number 76; atomic weight 190.2; a 5d transition element; oxidation states +2 through +8 (+3, +4, and +6 are most common). Metallic osmium is not toxic. Osmium tetroxide, formed by burning osmium in air, is volatile and irritating to the eyes, skin, and respiratory tract.

osmium tetroxide (oz′me-um te-trox′id) an amorphous or crystalline solid, OsO_4, used as a secondary histologic fixative in electron microscopy and as a primary fixative when lipids are to be demonstrated in paraffin sections. Osmium tetroxide is also used in immunoperoxidase procedures to darken (enhance) the benzidine reaction product and to render it electron-dense. It is highly toxic when inhaled and is very irritating to the eyes and nose. See also *fixative* and *osmic acid.*

osmolality (os″mo-lal′ĭ-te) the concentration of a solution expressed in osmoles of solute particles per kilogram of solvent (Osm/kg). In clinical chemistry, osmolality of serum or urine is measured with an osmometer. Serum and urine samples are prepared by removing red cells and/or suspended particles by centrifugation. If the analysis is not performed immediately, the sample should be refrigerated or frozen. Heparinized plasma may also be used.

The serum sodium concentration (millimoles per liter) is normally 0.43–0.50 times the serum osmolality (milliosmoles per kilogram). A decrease in this ratio is caused by an increase in other osmolutes such as glucose or ketone bodies in diabetes mellitus, urea in uremia, or salicylate in salicylate poisoning.

Urine specimens are centrifuged to remove particles and analyzed immediately. If refrigeration is necessary, the specimens should be warmed before analysis to redissolve any precipitates.

Urine osmolality varies widely, depending on fluid intake (50–1400 mOsm/kg). A value of 900 mOsm/kg after a 12-hr fluid restriction shows normal ability of the renal tubules to concentrate urine. The osmolality of the urine is normally one to three times that of serum. Ratios below one are seen in cases of renal tubular deficiency and in diabetes insipidus.

See also *osmolarity* and *osmotic concentration.*

osmolarity (os″mo-lār′ĭ-te) the concentration of a solution expressed in osmoles of solute particles per liter of solution (Osm/l).

osmole (Osm) (os′mōl) the amount of substance that dissociates in solution to form one mole of particles. For a substance such as glucose, which does not dissociate, one mole equals one osmole. For a substance that completely dissociates into two ions per mole, there are two osmoles per mole.

osmolute a solute consisting of osmotically active

particles that are in solution (i.e., the concentration is measured in osmoles).

osmometer (oz-mom′ĕ-ter) a device that measures the osmolality of solutions. The most common type is the freezing point depression osmometer or cryoscope. In this device, the specimen is rapidly supercooled to below its freezing point. It is then removed from the cooling bath and stirred or vibrated to crystallize. The heat of fusion raises the temperature to the freezing point; then, while the specimen remains in equilibrium for several minutes, the temperature is measured by a thermistor. The osmolality is calculated from the molal freezing point depression of the solvent (for water, a 1-osmolal solution depresses the freezing point 1.86°C). A precision of $\pm$ 2 mOsm/kg can be obtained routinely.

Another type of osmometer measures the vapor pressure depression by measuring the dew point of the air in a closed chamber that contains a small (5 μl) sample. This measurement is automatically converted to osmolality.

osmometry (oz-mom′ĕ-tre) any technique for measuring the osmolality of a solution.

osmosis (oz-mo′sis, os-mo′sis) [Gr. *ōsmos* impulsion] the passage of solvent from a solution of lesser solvent concentration through a semipermeable membrane (one that does not permit passage of the solute particles) to a solution of greater solute concentration. Osmosis proceeds until the rates of diffusion in both directions are equal. This occurs when the mole fraction of the solvent (and thus the osmolality) is the same on both sides of the membrane, or when sufficient pressure is exerted on the side with the higher osmolality to force the solvent particles through the membrane at a matching rate.

osmotic (os-mot′ik) relating to osmosis.

osmotic coefficient (ϕ) the proportionality coefficient between the measured osmolality of a solution and the theoretic osmolality (the product of the molality and the number of particles into which each molecule can dissociate). It varies with the concentration.

osmotic fragility the susceptibility of erythrocytes to hemolyze when exposed to increasingly hypotonic saline solutions.

osmotic fragility test a test that reflects the surface/volume ratio of the erythrocyte, and hence its critical hemolytic volume. Red cells are suspended in a series of buffered saline solutions. The percentage of hemolysis is determined by comparing the supernatant of each dilution with a totally hemolyzed sample. Reference ranges for nonincubated samples are 0.3–0.5 percent NaCl.

Increased fragility (decreased resistance) is found in hereditary spherocytosis and in idiopathic and symptomatic acquired hemolytic anemia. Decreased hemolysis (increased resistance) is seen in obstructive jaundice, iron deficiency anemia, thalassemia, and sickle cell anemia; after splenectomy; and in other anemias exhibiting target cells.

The sensitivity of the test may be enhanced by incubating a sterile, defibrinated blood sample for 24 hr and again performing the procedure described above. Reference ranges after incubation are 0.465–0.590 percent NaCl. This additional procedure is useful in the diagnosis of mild hereditary spherocytosis.

osmotic hemolysis alteration in the permeability of the membrane of an erythrocyte, which allows the cell to gain water and lose hemoglobin and other macromolecules. Also called colloid-osmotic lysis and osmotic lysis.

osmotic pressure the force required to counterbalance the force of osmotic flow through a semipermeable membrane. This is directly related to the osmolality of a solution and also to the other three colligative properties of solutions: freezing point depression, vapor pressure depression, and boiling point elevation.

The colloidal osmotic pressure (or oncotic pressure) is the osmotic pressure due to colloidal particles. The oncotic pressure of blood is due to the plasma proteins, which cannot diffuse through the capillary walls. This attracts water from interstitial fluid into plasma but is counteracted by the hydrostatic blood pressure. When the protein concentration (particularly that of albumin, responsible for 80 percent of the normal oncotic pressure) falls, the plasma colloid osmotic pressure is reduced and water is forced into the tissues, producing edema. Very low plasma pressures are associated with death, usually from pulmonary edema.

osmotic shock any disruption in a cell that occurs when it is exposed to a markedly hypertonic or hypotonic medium.

osseous (os′e-us) [L. *osseus,* from *os* bone] composed of bone, bony.

osseous hydatid (os′e-us hi′dah-tid) [L. *osseus* + *hydatis* a drop of water] a type of unilocular cyst found in bone, caused by the hydatid worm *Echinococcus granulosus.* The parasite migrates along the bony canal as a naked protoplast, causing extensive erosion of the bone; the adjacent tissues are also frequently involved.

ossification (os″ĭ-fĭ-ka′shun) [L. *ossificatio*] the formation of bone. See also *bone.*

oste/o (os′te-o) [Gr. *osteon* bone] a word element used in combining form to denote bone, e.g., osteotomy.

ostealgia (os″te-al′je-ah) [*oste-* + Gr. *algos* pain + *-ia*] a general term used to describe bone pain. Also called osteodynia.

osteitis (os″te-i′tis) [*oste-* + *-itis* inflammation] a general term used to describe inflammation of bone. This inflammation may be localized, or it may encompass the haversian systems, canaliculi, and medullary cavities. Generally, there is bone tenderness, enlargement, and dull pain.

osteitis deformans a nonmetabolic disease of bone that is slowly progressive and of unknown cause. It is one of the most common skeletal diseases, and its frequency increases with age in people over 40 yr old. A familial incidence has been observed, but the mode of transmission is unknown. The disease is characterized by an osteolytic phase during which bone resorption occurs. V-shaped lesions, especially in the tibia, are observed. Following this, there is an osteoblastic phase characterized by the formation of new bone woven in a bizarre, patternless fashion, described as mosaic. The most commonly affected bones are the pelvis, femur, skull, tibia, clavicle, and humerus. Softening of bones leads to kyphosis and bowing, and frequent fractures are seen.

Laboratory findings include elevated alkaline phosphatase, urinary hydroxyproline, and urinary calcium levels. Blood phosphorus and calcium levels are normal. X-rays reveal increased bone density, cortical thickening, bowing, and bone overgrowth. Perpendicular lines of radiolucency and multiple-fissure fractures are evident in the long bones. Fluoride or technetium pyrophosphate bone scans may be helpful in assessing the activity of bone lesions. Complications of this disease include increased blood flow that, in rare instances when more than one-third of the skeleton is involved, may lead to high cardiac output, and osteosarcomatous changes that occur in less than 1 percent of those affected.

Also called *Paget's disease of bone.*

osteitis fibrosa cystica cystic lesions occurring in bone in hyperparathyroidism following excessive activation of osteoclasts. Histologically, the lesions resemble giant cell tumors. Hemosiderin deposition confers a brown color on the lesion, hence the synonym *brown tumor.* Also called *von Recklinghausen's disease of bone.*

osteoarthritis (os″te-o-ar-thri′tis) [*osteo-* + Gr. *arthron* joint + *-itis* inflammation] a progressive, degenerative joint disease characterized by the loss of articular cartilage, subchondral bone sclerosis, and hypertrophy of bone at articular surfaces. It commonly involves joints of the fingers, hips, and knees, the metatarsophalangeal joint of the big toes, and the cervical and lumbar portions of the spine. The cause is unknown; hereditary, mechanical, and metabolic factors have been implicated, and relationships to chronic trauma and to underlying joint disease have been established. There are no associated systemic manifestations, as in rheumatoid arthritis.

Osteoarthritis has a gradual onset. Those affected first experience joint stiffness and pain on motion that is localized to one or few joints. Symptoms most frequently occur after exercise and are relieved by rest. Joint deformity is usually minimal. The articular cartilage degenerates, and destruction and proliferation of chondrocytes occur simultaneously.

Laboratory tests are inconclusive and usually within normal limits. X-rays reveal narrowing of the joint spaces and the formation of osteophytes, cysts, and subchondral bony sclerosis.

Also called *degenerative joint disease.*

osteoarthropathy (os″te-o-ar-throp′ah-the) [*osteo-* + Gr. *arthron* joint + *pathos* disease] a disease of the joints and bones.

hypertrophic o., a condition characterized by the laying down of new bone matrix under the periosteum while endosteum is resorbed. Painful, enlarged distal extremities usually result, although other bones may be affected. Clubbing, periostitis, and arthritis are associated symptoms with a mononuclear infiltrate. The etiology is unknown, but cyanotic cardiovascular conditions and chronic lung disease—such as abscess, bronchiectasis, and most often carcinoma—are related. Thyroid and intestinal diseases have been implicated. The condition may be hereditary or idiopathic. Diagnosis is made on the basis of clinical signs and radiographic findings.

osteoblast (os′te-o-blast″) [*osteo-* + Gr. *blastos* germ] a cell associated with the production and calcification of bone. Cf. *osteoclast.*

osteoblastoma (os″te-o-blas-to′mah) [*osteo-* + Gr. *blastos* germ + *ōma* tumor] a solitary benign tumor of bone with some similarity to a large osteoid osteoma, but with more histologic variability and a tendency to affect the bones of the vertebral column. It can occur at any age, but most patients are adolescents or young adults. Histologically, areas of osteoid and primitive bone are present within a vascular connective tissue stroma that contains many osteoblasts. Confusion with osteosarcoma is possible on a small biopsy. The lesion is usually painful, and treatment is by curettage or, where feasible, conservative excision.

osteocartilaginous exostosis see *osteochondroma.*

multiple o. exostoses, see *multiple o.'s* under *osteochondroma.*

osteochondral (os″te-o-kon′dral) pertaining to bone and cartilage.

osteochrondritis (os″te-o-kon-dri′tis) [*osteo-* + Gr. *chondros* cartilage + *-itis* inflammation] inflammation of both bone and cartilage. The term is occasionally used incorrectly for noninflammatory conditions of bone; see *osteochondritis juvenilis* and *osteochondritis dissecans.*

osteochondritis dissecans a condition in which aseptic necrosis of bone leads to the formation of a small osteochondral body that is freed from an articular end of a bone and is usually extruded into the joint space.

osteochondritis juvenilis a condition characterized by avascular necrosis or infarction of all or part of an epiphysis, occurring in young persons during the growing phase of the epiphysis. Such infarcts frequently involve the subchondral bone and marrow as well as the epiphysis, and are thought to be related to traumatic interference with blood supply to the area. In spite of the name, inflammation is not a component of the disease process. Also called epiphyseal osteochondritis of growth centers, osteochondritis deformans, and *osteochondrosis.*

Eponymic terms for osteochondritis juvenilis of various sites include Legg-Calvé-Perthes disease (hip), Sever's disease (calcaneus), Kienböck's disease (lunate), Köhler's disease (navicular), and Preiser's disease (carpal scaphoid).

osteochondroma (os″te-o-kon-dro′mah) [*osteo-* + Gr. *chondros* cartilage + *ōma* tumor] a common, benign bone neoplasm that tends to occur in persons aged 10–20 yr. It presents as a slow-growing mass composed of cortical and medullary bone covered by a cartilaginous cap. Such tumors may occur in any bone that develops by enchondral ossification. Approximately 90 percent are solitary.

Also called *osteocartilaginous exostosis.*

multiple o.'s, a condition having a strong familial tendency in which tumors morphologically identical to solitary osteochondroma are found in multiple bones. A secondary chondrosarcoma is found in more than 10 percent of persons with this condition. Also called *multiple osteocartilaginous exostoses.*

osteochondrosis (os″te-o-kon-dro′sis) [*osteo-* + Gr. *chondros* cartilage + *-osis* condition] see *osteochondritis juvenilis.*

osteoclast (os′te-o-klast″) [*osteo-* + Gr. *-klastēs* breaker, destroyer] 1. a large, multinucleated cell associated with the absorption and removal of bone. These cells are important in the remodeling of bone and the maintenance of circulating calcium levels.

2. an instrument for use in the surgical fracture or refracture of bones. Cf. *osteoblast.*

osteoclast-activating factor (OAF) a product of activated T lymphocytes, which may have a role in the localized resorption of bone. It induces osteoclasts to resorb fetal bone matrix in organ cultures. This factor may also be involved in the localized destruction of bone. The production of OAF is macrophage dependent.

osteocyte (os′te-o-sīt″) [*osteo-* + Gr. *kytos* hollow vessel] the cell of mature bone. It is an osteoblast imprisoned within the bone matrix. It occupies a lacuna and maintains contact with other osteocytes and with osteoblasts via fine cytoplasmic processes that extend through channels called canaliculi.

osteogenesis (os″te-o-jen′ĕ-sis) [*osteo-* + Gr. *gennan* to produce] the formation of bone.

osteogenesis imperfecta a genetic disorder of mesenchymal tissue, transmitted as an autosomal dominant or autosomal recessive trait, of which there are two major recognized types: osteogenesis imperfecta congenita, which occurs in utero, is usually recessive, and is often fatal; and osteogenesis imperfecta tarda, which usually becomes apparent after birth as the infant becomes active. Both conditions are manifested by fragility of bones leading to pathologic fractures. Blue coloration of the sclerae and deafness are frequently associated with the dominant trait form. This condition is thought to be due to a disorder of connective tissue and may occur in more than 1 in every 20,000 births.

X-ray examinations reveal defects of the skull, vertebral column, and pelvis. In the usually recessively transmitted congenital form, "thick bones" with thin cortices and broad marrow cavities are seen. In the tarda form, "thin bones" with narrow shafts and reduced marrow cavities are observed. In general, severe expression of the congenital form results in death at or before birth. The tarda form is generally more benign, and the tendency to form fractures decreases after puberty, especially if the expression is less severe. No specific therapy is known.

Also called brittle bones, fragilitas ossium, and osteopsathyrosis.

osteogenic (os″te-o-jen′ik) derived from or composed of cells with osteoblastic potential.

osteogenic sarcoma see *osteosarcoma.*

osteoid (os′te-oid) [*osteo-* + Gr. *eidos* form] a thin layer of uncalcified preosseous tissue, no thicker than 1 μm, at the border of the matrix of a normal bone. It may be increased in quantity in conditions associated with abnormal osteogenesis such as rickets, or in osteosarcoma.

osteolysis (os″te-ol′ĭ-sis) [*osteo-* + Gr. *lysis* dissolution] the dissolution of bone, especially the loss of calcium from bone.

osteoma (os″te-o′mah) [*osteo-* + Gr. *ōma* tumor] a benign tumor of dense, bony tissue that involves the bones of the skull or face. Persons of almost any age may be affected. These tumors occur in association with intestinal polyposis in Gardner's syndrome. The dense bone is formed by broad trabeculae, and there may be an admixture of fat or hematopoietic tissue. Some of the neoplasms are highly vascular. Osteomas are of little clinical significance, but an enlarging lesion in a sinus may be resected if it produces symptoms. Neither recurrence nor malignant transformation is likely.

osteoid o., a small, benign lesion of bone, most common in the lower extremities of male children or young adults. It is typically painful and is usually excised for this reason. When located in the cortical region of the bone, it produces a surrounding zone of dense sclerosis, but the distinctive feature is the nidus of compactly grouped trabeculae with intervening connective tissue and vessels.

osteomalacia (os″te-o-mah-la′she-ah) [*osteo-* + Gr. *malakia* softness] a disorder of mineralization of the adult skeleton, which is considered to be the adult form of rickets. It results from a deficiency of calcium, phosphorus, or both, in bone. The causes include insufficient vitamin D, intestinal malabsorption syndromes, chronic acidosis, and renal tubular defects associated with hypophosphatemia (vitamin D–resistant rickets). Osteomalacia is most often associated with disorders of fat absorption, such as sprue, pancreatitis, and gastrectomy.

Serum calcium and phosphate levels are commonly low, whereas serum alkaline phosphatase is elevated. Intravenous calcium infusion tests result in 80–90 percent retention. Blood levels of 25-hydroxycholecalciferol are usually reduced. Primary steatorrhea or renal disease is commonly observed. On x-ray films, bone demineralization with subsequent bowing may be seen. Pseudofractures may be visible, and bone scintiscans may be useful in localizing these lesions. A definitive diagnosis may require bone biopsy.

Almost all forms of this disorder are associated with secondary hyperparathyroidism due to low calcium levels. Osteomalacia may also be associated with glycosuria and aminoaciduria (Fanconi's syndrome), chronic administration of anticonvulsants, and an inability to produce exogenous vitamin D owing to inadequate exposure to ultraviolet light.

See also *rickets.*

osteomyelitis (os″te-o-mi″ĕ-li′tis) [*osteo-* + Gr. *myelos* marrow + *-itis* inflammation] an infection of the bone and bone marrow, most commonly due to pyogenic microorganisms (such as *Staphylococcus aureus*), although a variety of gram-positive and gram-negative bacteria, fungi, rickettsiae, and viruses may be implicated. The route of infection may be hematogenous, direct (following fracture or other trauma), or through extension from adjacent infections. Fever, malaise, pain, swelling, and limitation of joint movement are symptoms. The disease appears in acute and chronic forms. *S. aureus* and β-hemolytic streptococci are most frequently the etiologic agents of the infection. Persons with sickle cell disease have a special susceptibility to *Salmonella* osteomyelitis.

Diagnosis is made by aspiration or biopsy culture. Repeated blood cultures (both aerobic and anaerobic) may be necessary. Leukocytosis is commonly absent, and anemia may also occur. The erythrocyte sedimentation rate is frequently elevated. X-ray examinations reveals extraosseous soft tissue swelling as the disease progresses, and xeroradiography may help to classify lesions. Radionuclide imaging may also be required, as changes in blood flow can be detected by technetium-99m scanning. Owing to the rapid systemic toxicity of this infection and its potential for bone destruction, antibiotic therapy should be instituted as early as possible.

osteomyelodysplasia (os″te-o-mi″ĕ-lo-dis-pla′se-ah) [*osteo-* + Gr. *myelos* marrow + *dys-* abnormal + *plassein* to form] a general term used to describe a condition in which there is thinning of the osseous tissue of bones, with concomitant thickening of the size of the marrow cavity. Such physiologic derangements often lead to decreases in the leukocyte population and to febrile episodes.

osteomyelosclerosis (os″te-o-mi″ĕ-lo-sklĕ-ro′sis) [*osteo-* + Gr. *myelos* marrow + *sklērōsis* hardening] a disorder characterized by fibrotic replacement of the marrow cells by a diffuse fibroplasia. There may be an accompanying thickening of bone due to osseous metaplasia. Areas of increased bone mass may be visible on radiographs. This disorder is often considered to be a phase of myeloproliferative syndromes and may be accompanied by extramedullary hematopoiesis.

osteon (os′te-on) [*osteo-* + Gr. *on* neuter ending] the basic structural unit of compact bone; it includes a haversian canal and its concentrically arranged lamellae, of which there may be 4–20 in each haversian system. Osteons are usually directed along the long axis of the bone.

osteonecrosis (os″te-o-ne-kro′sis) [*osteo-* + Gr. *nekrōsis* death] the death or necrosis of bone.

osteopathia (os″te-o-path′e-ah) [N.L.] see *osteopathy.*

osteopathy (os″te-op′ah-the) [*osteo-* + Gr. *pathos* disease] 1. a general term used to describe any disease involving bone. Also called *osteopathia.*

2. a branch of medicine that utilizes a system of therapy based on accepted medical practices and emphasizes the importance of normal body mechanisms and manipulations to detect and treat disease.

osteopenia (os″te-o-pe′nĭ-ah) [*osteo-* + Gr. *penia* poverty] a general term used to describe any condition that is characterized by a reduction in bone mass. It may occur in generalized conditions such as hyperparathyroidism or vitamin D deficiency, or in specific conditions such as osteoporosis. See also *osteoporosis.*

osteoperiostitis (os″te-o-per″e-os-ti′tis) [*osteo-* + *periostitis*] see *periostitis.*

osteopetrosis (os″te-o-pe-tro′sis) [*osteo-* + Gr. *petra* stone + *-osis* condition] a hereditary disease marked by the formation of abnormally dense bone, due presumably to defects in normal bone remodeling. Fractures are common, and bone encroachment on marrow cavities may lead to myelophthisic anemia. Radiographs reveal uniformly dense sclerotic bone. Bone deformities, neurologic abnormalities, and facial paralysis are not uncommon. Also called *Albers-Schönberg disease* and *marble bone disease.*

osteophyte (os′te-o-fit″) [*osteo-* + Gr. *phyton* plant] a bony outgrowth, a frequent feature of osteoarthritis.

osteopoikilosis (os″te-o-poi″kĭ-lo′sis) [*osteo-* + Gr. *poikilos* mottled] an abnormal condition of bone, transmitted as an autosomal dominant trait. It is characterized by the presence of dense spots of trabecular bone less than 1 cm in diameter, which are visible on radiographs and are located in and near the epiphyses. This condition is characteristically benign and without symptoms.

osteoporosis (os″te-o-po-ro′sis) [*osteo-* + Gr. *poros* passage + *-osis* condition] the most common metabolic disease of bone in the United States, characterized by an absolute decrease in the mass of bony tissue, especially trabecular bone. The primary features of this disorder are pain in the back and deformity of the spine due to collapse of the vertebrae. Fractures of the femur and distal end of the radius also are common. Osteoporosis most commonly affects females past middle age. Although the primary cause is unknown, suspected contributory factors include immobilization, lack of estrogens (postmenopausal osteoporosis), chronically low dietary levels of calcium, and malabsorption. The disease may also occur secondary to a number of systemic diseases such as hypercortisolism and multiple myeloma.

Serum calcium, phosphate, and alkaline phosphatase concentrations are normal; concentrations of urinary calcium may be elevated early in the course and normal later. X-rays reveal compression of the vertebrae and areas of demineralization of the spine and pelvis. Bone densitometry may help to confirm the diagnosis.

o. circumscripta, the lytic destruction and demineralization of bones, especially those of the skull (frontal, parietal, and occipital lobes). This condition is often observed in the early "lytic" phase of osteitis deformans. On x-ray examinations, the lesions of this disorder appear as areas of sharply demarcated radiolucency in the bones of the skull. See also *osteitis deformans.*

osteosarcoma (os″te-o-sar-ko′mah) [*osteo-* + Gr. *sarcoma*] a primary, highly malignant neoplasm of bone that arises from osteoblastic cells and is characterized by the formation of osteoid or bone. The peak age incidence is around 20 yr; it is infrequent over age 40. The knee region is most commonly affected and symptoms include pain, swelling, and tenderness.

X-ray findings include lytic and sclerotic patterns. Bone formation occurs in involved soft tissues. Elevated serum alkaline phosphatase is seen as the disease progresses. Where possible, the primary tumor is resected surgically.

Also called *osteogenic sarcoma.*

osteosclerosis (os″te-o-sklĕ-ro′sis) [*osteo-* + Gr. *sklērōsis* hardening] a general term used to describe the hardening and increased density of bone. This metabolic process may be seen in several conditions, most frequently in osteopetrosis. See also *osteopetrosis.*

Ostertagia (os″ter-ta′je-ah) [Robert von *Ostertag,* German veterinarian, 1864–1940] a genus of nematodes of the family Trichostrongylus, parasitic in cattle and other herbivorous mammals. The parasite is usually found in cysts on the wall of the abomasum (the fourth stomach) of cattle and other ruminants. Two species have been found in humans, *O. ostertagi* and *O. circumcincta.* Infections are thought to be caused by eating undercooked abomasum of cattle or sheep containing the nodular stage.

ostium (os′te-um) [L.] a door, or opening; in anatomy, a general term to designate an opening into a tubular organ, or between two distinct body cavities. Also called orifice and opening.

ostium primum (os′te-um pri′mum) [L.] see under *atrial septal defect.*

ostium secundum (os′te-um se-kun′dum) [L.] see under *atrial septal defect.*

-ostomy (os′to-me) [Gr. *stomoun* to provide with an opening, or mouth] a suffix word element to denote making a new opening, e.g., colostomy.

ot/o (o'to) [Gr. *ous, ōtos* ear] a word element used in combining form to denote the ear, e.g., otolaryngology.

otalgia (o-tal'je-ah) [Gr. *ōtalgia*] a general term used to describe a pain in the ear. Also called *earache* and *otodynia*.

otic (o'tik) [Gr. *ōtikos*] pertaining to the ear; aural.

otic vesicle (o'tik ves'i-k'l) in the developing embryo, a detached sac formed during the fifth week by the closure of the auditory pit, which develops into the inner ear. Also called *auditory vesicle*.

otitis (o-ti'tis) [*ot-* + *-itis* inflammation] a general term used to describe inflammation of the ear. It most commonly affects the outer or middle ear, and is generally marked by pain, fever, and disorders of hearing and balance.

chronic o. media, a chronic inflammation of the middle ear that is almost always associated with perforation of the tympanic membrane. The extent of the perforation varies and, depending on its severity, bone destruction, hearing loss, and cholesteatomas may result.

external o., an inflammation of the ear canal most commonly due to infection or allergies. It may be local or diffuse, and clinical manifestations may range from a diffuse, mild, eczematoid dermatitis to furunculosis. The most common etiologic agents are *Pseudomonas aeruginosa* and *Staphylococcus aureus*. Fungal organisms may be involved in secondary infections. Irritants and allergic agents may also be implicated. Predisposing factors include warm and moist climates, excessive bathing, trauma, and allergic dermatitis. Itching, pain, and scaling of the ear canal are symptoms. A purulent discharge and intermittent loss of hearing may also occur. Leukocyte counts may be elevated.

o. media, an acute bacterial or viral infection of the middle ear that is most commonly associated with an infection of the upper respiratory tract. The disease most often affects children (3 mo–3 yr), although it may occur at any age. There is pain, discharge, and variable hearing loss. Inflammation and suppuration may lead to perforation of the tympanic membrane and necrosis of the middle ear.

Laboratory studies usually reveal an elevation of white blood cells. The infectious agent isolated from culture of discharge from the ear or tympanocentesis most commonly proves to be pneumococcus; in infancy, *Hemophilus influenzae* is causative in more than one-third of cases. Hearing tests reveal conductive hearing loss.

serous o. media, an inflammation of the middle ear characterized by the accumulation of sterile fluid in the middle ear. This condition may result from obstruction of the eustachian tube or an unresolved acute infection. Obstruction may be due to inflammation, allergic reactions, or barotrauma such as from rapid descent in an aircraft. There is usually a feeling of fullness in the ear and slight hearing loss, but no pain or fever. Pneumatic otoscopic examination shows a ground-glass, amber discoloration and impaired mobility of the eardrum.

Otobius (o-to'be-us) [*oto* + Gr. *bios* manner of living] a genus of ticks (the spinous ear ticks) of the family Argosidae. The nymphs (a postembryonic stage) of two species, *O. lagophilus* (parasitic in rabbits) and *O. megnini* (found in cattle and other domestic animals), are ear-infesting parasites and may invade human ears. Also, the Colorado tick fever virus has been isolated from *O. megnini*, and *O. lagophilus* is naturally infected with *Rickettsia rickettsii* (causing Rocky Mountain spotted fever) in Mexico.

otoconia (o″to-ko'ne-ah) [*oto* + Gr. *konis* dust] see *otolith*.

otodynia (o″to-din'e-ah) [*oto-* + Gr. *odynē* pain] pain including the ears, nose, and throat; see *otalgia*.

otolaryngology (o″to-lar″in-gol'o-je) the medical specialty concerned with diseases of the ears and throat.

otolith (o'to-lith) [*oto-* + Gr. *lithos* stone] 1. one of the numerous calcium carbonate crystals within the gelatinous (otolithic) membrane covering the surfaces of the acoustic maculae. Also called *otoconia*.

2. a calciferous mass in the inner ear.

-otomy (ot'o-me) [Gr. *tomē* a cutting] a suffix word element to denote an incision or a cutting into, e.g., laparotomy.

otomycosis (o″to-mi-ko'sis) [*oto-* + Gr. *mykēs* fungus + *-osis* condition] any fungal infection of the pinna, external auditory meatus, or ear canal. In most cases the tympanic membrane is spared. The fungus that causes otomycosis of the external ear is usually one of the common contaminants, e.g., *Aspergillus niger*. Symptoms include scaling, pruritus, pain, and a feeling of fullness of the ear.

otorhinolaryngology (o″to-ri″no-lar″in-gol'o-je) [*oto-* + Gr. *rhis* nose + *larynx* + *-logy*] see *otolaryngology*.

otorrhagia (o″to-ra'je-ah) [*oto-* + Gr. *rhēgnynai* to burst forth] a hemorrhage from the ear, which may result from a fracture of the temporal bone, rupture of the tympanic membrane, or mucous membrane damage without perforation of the eardrum.

otorrhea (o″to-re'ah) [*oto-* + Gr. *rhoia* to flow] a general term used to describe a discharge from the ear. It is often used specifically to describe the leakage of cerebrospinal fluid from the ear, which is due to fracture of the base of the skull.

otosclerosis (o″to-skle-ro'sis) [*oto-* + Gr. *sklērōsis* hardening] a hereditary type of adult-onset hearing loss that is the most common form of both conductive deafness and of hearing loss in young adults who have a normal tympanic membrane. It is due to bony dysplasia, with the formation of spongy bone in the capsule of the labyrinth, causing ankylosis of the footplate of the stapes and conductive hearing loss. The disease process may accelerate during pregnancy.

otoscope (o'to-skōp) [*oto-* + Gr. *skopein* to examine] an instrument designed to inspect or auscultate the ear. It is designed primarily to examine the outer ear canal and tympanic membrane by means of light and air under moderate pressure, as with a pneumatic otoscope.

ototoxic (o″to-tok'sik) [*oto-* + L. *toxicum* poison] an agent or process that has a deleterious effect on either the ear (either in hearing or balance) or the eighth cranial nerve (the vestibulocochlear nerve).

ototoxic drugs a variety of therapeutic agents that exert a deleterious effect on the organ of hearing. These agents include aminoglycoside antibiotics, salicylates, antimalarials (quinine and derivatives), and diuretics (ethacrynic acid and furosemide). The auditory and vestibular portions of the inner ear and the organ of Corti are primarily affected. Hearing of highest frequencies is usually affected first, and tinnitus and vertigo may develop.

Inasmuch as most ototoxic drugs are eliminted by the kidneys, renal impairment may predispose to the accumulation of toxic levels of these agents in the blood, leading to ototoxicity. These agents should be avoided during pregnancy and in elderly patients. If possible, hearing levels should be monitored during treatment with these drugs.

ouabain (wah-ba'in) [USP], a cardiac glycoside similar to the digitalis glycosides. It is a white crystalline powder extracted from seeds of *Strophanthus gratus*, and consists of the aglycone ouabagenin and one rhamnose sugar residue.

Ouabain is administered intravenously to produce rapid digitalization in acute congestive heart failure, the full digitalis effect being obtained in 2 hr. It is more rapidly eliminated than the digitalis glycosides, having a half-life of about 21 hr, and is not suitable for maintenance of the digitalis effect. Ouabain is primarily excreted unchanged by the kidneys; there is also some gastrointestinal excretion.

Also called strophanthin G. See also *digitalis glycosides*.

Ouchterlony immunodiffusion [Orjan Thomas Gunnarsson *Ouchterlony*, Swedish bacteriologist, b. 1914] a method of antigen analysis: a double-diffusion–two-dimensional immunogel assay that compares two antigens; antigens and antibodies diffuse through agar, forming stable immune complexes. The antibodies (antiserum) and antigen are placed in separate wells cut out of agar; this procedure is often performed in a circular pattern. The antigen and antibody diffuse into the agar, forming precipitin bands that appear as arcs, at Ag/Ab equivalence. When the antigen is in excess, the precipitin bands are closer to the antibody well.

Four types of reactions, which can be visualized with indirect light, are commonly seen: identity, nonidentity, partial identity, and double partial identity (as in the accompanying illustration). In an identity reaction, both antigens are identical and fusion of precipitin lines occurs. In a nonidentity reaction, the antigens are totally unrelated, so the diffusion rates vary and the precipitin lines form a cross. A partial identity reaction involves the fusion of precipitin bands with a characteristic spur, the spur curving toward the unrelated antigen and antibody. Double partial identity is characterized by two spurs.

Ouchterlony immunodiffusion allows for the comparison of the serologic relationships among various antigens and antibodies, and demonstrates the presence of multiple antigenic determinants and the cross-reactivity of several antigens with an antibody.

Also called *double diffusion technique* and Ouchterlony analysis. Cf. *Oudin immunodiffusion*.

Oudin immunodiffusion (oo-da') [Paul *Oudin*, French physician, 1851–1923] a method for the detection of antigen-antibody reactions using single diffusion in agar. A small-bore tube is filled with agar containing antiserum, and is overlaid with an antigen onto the agar. After 2 da of diffusion, bands of precipitation form at the zone of equivalence (see *precipitin curve*). The number of bands formed indicates the minimal number of antigen-antibody systems present. Thus, the method demonstrates the heterogeneity of the antigens.

Single diffusion in agar shows that a band of precipitate migrates according to the equation $h = k\sqrt{t}$, where h is the distance migrated, k is a constant, and t is time. Antigen and antibody concentrations, viscosity of the gel, and the presence of contaminants determine the constant (k) value.

Also called *single diffusion technique*. Cf. *Ouchterlony immunodiffusion*.

-ous (us) [L. *-osus*] 1. a suffix word element to denote possessing, e.g., nitrogenous.

2. a suffix word element in inorganic chemistry, used to denote the lower of the two most common oxidation states of a metal cation, e.g., ferrous ion, the trivial name of the iron(II) ion, or of an oxo acid, e.g., sulfurous acid. Cf. *-ic*.

outflow tract the structures through which the blood flow leaves the ventricles. Left ventricular outflow tract obstruction refers to aortic, subaortic, or supravalvular aortic stenosis; corresponding obstructions also occur in the right ventricular outflow tract.

outlier (owt'li-er) a datum in a statistical sample far removed from the mass of data points found in a population. If there is no evidence of an experimental error, there is no generally accepted way to eliminate such data points from statistical analysis. One method is to eliminate all values beyond 3 SD (3 standard deviations), calculate a new mean and standard deviation, and again eliminate all values beyond 3 SD. This method is only appropriate for gaussian (normal) distributions. For small samples, a t-test should be used to set the rejection limit after

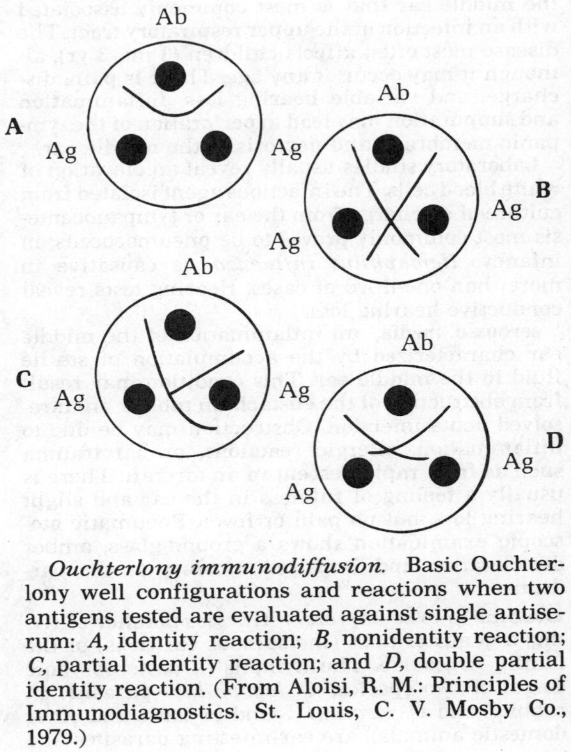

Ouchterlony immunodiffusion. Basic Ouchterlony well configurations and reactions when two antigens tested are evaluated against single antiserum: *A*, identity reaction; *B*, nonidentity reaction; *C*, partial identity reaction; and *D*, double partial identity reaction. (From Aloisi, R. M.: Principles of Immunodiagnostics. St. Louis, C. V. Mosby Co., 1979.)

having set the desired confidence level. Another method is to plot a histogram of the data and eliminate those values that appear to be far removed from the mass of data. Removal of selected discrepant values without knowledge of assignable cause is not usual statistical practice; trimming and windsorizing procedures are procedures that can be applied, when necessary, in order to avoid more ad hoc, post hoc editing. See under *mean.*

outpatient (owt-pa′shent) an individual who comes to a hospital or related medical facility for tests or treatment, but not as an admitted patient who occupies a bed overnight.

output (owt′poot) 1. in data processing, the result of a computational process, or the transfer of data from a computer (or other machine) to another computer, or to the user. Printed output is called "hard copy."

2. the yield or total amount of anything produced by any functional system of the body. Commonly described outputs include cardiac output (the volume of blood expelled by either heart ventricle per unit of time), energy output (the amount of energy expended in work or activity), and renal output (the amount of urine secreted by the kidneys).

output capacitor a coupling capacitor connected in series with the output of a circuit to remove the direct-current voltage level of the final amplifier stage output.

output impedance the impedance presented to a load by an electrical circuit defined as the change in the output signal voltage (produced by a change in the current drawn by the load) divided by the load current.

ov/i, ov/o (o′vĭ, o′vo) [L. *ovum* egg] a word element used in combining form to denote an egg, e.g., ovoid, ovary, oviduct.

ovalbumin (o″val-bu′min) [*ov-* + *albumin*] an albumin obtainable from the white of eggs.

ovale malaria (o-va′le) the least common of four types of malaria that infect humans. Caused by the parasite *Plasmodium ovale,* it is distributed throughout tropical Africa. See also *malaria.*

ovalocyte (o-val′o-sīt) [L. *ovalis,* from *ovum* egg + Gr. *kytos* hollow vessel] see *elliptocyte.*

ovalocytosis (o-val″o-si-to′sis) [L. *ovalis* + Gr. *kytos* hollow vessel + *-osis* condition] see *elliptocytosis.*

oval window an opening in the wall of the osseous labyrinth into which the footplate of the stapes fits, allowing for transmission of sound waves from the air-filled tympanic cavity to the fluid-filled vestibule of the inner ear. Also called *fenestra vestibuli.*

ovari/o (o-var′e-o) [L. *ovarium* ovary] a word element used in combining form to denote an ovary, e.g., ovarian.

ovarian (o-var′e-an) pertaining to the ovaries.

ovarian cycle see *menstrual cycle.*

ovarian cyst any of a wide variety of cysts that may occur in the ovary. Ovarian cysts may be classified as functional if they affect the elaboration or metabolism of sex steroids or hormones.

Follicular cysts are very common, occur primarily during the fertile years, and usually are multiple and bilateral. They most commonly are functional and lead to anovulation and endometrial hyperplasia.

Cysts of the corpus luteum classically arise in the first trimester of pregnancy in response to chorionic gonadotropin. They often are functional, most often are unilateral, and give rise to sudden amenorrhea. They may lead to intraperitoneal bleeding and are frequently mistaken for an ectopic pregnancy; they are considered not to undergo malignant transformation.

Theca lutein cysts occur in hydatidiform mole or choriocarcinoma. They often are multiple and bilateral, and are marked by amenorrhea and elevated levels of human chorionic gonadotropin. They may lead to hematoperitoneum or torsion of the ovaries but not to malignant transformation.

Inflammatory cysts, also called tubo-ovarian cysts, occur in association with acute salpingitis, are painful, and usually are multiple and bilateral. They are characterized by menometrorrhagia and anovulation. Although they do not become malignant, they may rupture and cause lethal peritonitis.

ovarian follicle a vesicular ovarian follicle; a maturing follicle with 6–12 layers of follicular cells. The eccentrically placed ovum is embedded in a stalk of these follicular cells, the cumulus oophorus, and extends into a fluid-filled cavity, the antrum. Also called *graafian follicle.* See also *meiosis* and *oogenesis.*

ovarian tumors neoplasms of the ovary. Constituting the fifth most common type of tumor in the female, roughly two-thirds occur during child-bearing years; however, only 5 percent in this age group are malignant, in contrast to 33 percent in postmenopausal females. Fewer than 2 percent of malignant ovarian tumors occur in children.

The broad range of histologic features encountered in ovarian tumors reflects the diversity of cell types present in the normal gonad. Most of the tumors may be categorized into one of three broad groups: tumors of the surface epithelium, germ cell tumors, and sex cord–stromal neoplasms. Soft tissue tumors of the ovary are infrequent. Metastatic involvement of the ovaries is relatively common. The term Krukenberg tumor is used to connote a signet-ring, mucin-forming adenocarcinoma in the ovary, metastatic from the stomach.

TUMORS OF THE SURFACE EPITHELIUM. More than 60 percent of all ovarian tumors and more than 85 percent of malignant tumors fall within this category. The clinical stage at the time of diagnosis is the most important prognostic factor: roughly two-thirds of those affected survive for at least 5 yr. Epithelial tumors derived from the mesothelium may show serous (tubal), endometrioid (endometrial), or mucinous (endocervical) differentiation, or a mixture of these types.

Serous tumors constitute approximately 30 percent of all ovarian tumors, and more than half are malignant. The lining cells are columnar, forming a single layer in the benign neoplasms, but becoming stratified in the more aggressive tumors, with solid areas developing. Psammoma bodies are common in serous tumors. Both ovaries are involved in more than half of those with serous carcinomas.

Mucinous tumors represent about 20 percent of all ovarian tumors; fewer than 15 percent are malignant. Both benign and malignant forms tend to be cystic and are composed of columnar, mucin-forming cells. The fluid within cystic spaces of these tumors contains a high content of mucopolysaccharides. Mucinous tumors are less likely to be bilateral than are serous carcinomas.

Endometrioid carcinomas represent approximately 10 percent of all ovarian tumors. A coexisting uterine adenocarcinoma is present in some individuals. Approximately 30 percent of endometrioid ovarian carcinomas are bilateral. Clear cell carcinomas arising in the ovary, formerly believed to be of mesonephric remnant origin, are probably derived from the surface epithelium and represent a variant of endometrioid carcinoma.

The Brenner tumor is a solid neoplasm composed of nests of urothelial-like cells in a dense, fibrous stroma. The great majority are benign, although a small number of malignant variants have been reported.

Germ Cell Tumors. Approximately 20 percent of ovarian tumors are of germ cell origin, of which 2 percent are malignant. However, in those under age 20 yr, 60 percent of ovarian tumors are of germ cell origin, of which more than 30 percent are malignant.

The dysgerminoma is the ovarian counterpart of the testicular seminoma. Most patients with dysgerminoma are between ages 10 and 30 yr. The tumor is highly sensitive to radiotherapy. The 5-yr survival rate of those treated by radiotherapy exceeds 90 percent.

Endodermal sinus (yolk sac) tumors are composed of distinctive papillary structures projecting into a network of anastomosing spaces that resemble those of the rodent placenta. Serum alpha-fetoprotein levels are usually elevated. The tumor is aggressive and tends to recur or metastasize.

Embryonal carcinomas are composed of primitive cells with the potential to mature into other germ cell tumor types. They may occur in pure form, be part of an immature teratoma, or be admixed with choriocarcinoma.

Choriocarcinoma is composed of an admixture of malignant cytoblastic and syncytiotrophoblastic cells. These tumors are particularly aggressive, and, in contrast to gestational choriocarcinomas, are resistant to chemotherapeutic agents.

Teratomas contain tissues that recapitulate the development of two or three of the embryonic layers; the components may be mature, immature, or mixtures of the two. Most of the immature tumors occur in children or adolescents. Benign cystic teratomas constitute 20 percent of ovarian tumors. Approximately 1 percent of teratomas are malignant. Malignant change (most frequently squamous carcinoma) in a benign teratoma occurs in fewer than 2 percent of such cysts.

Sex Cord–Stromal Tumors. Tumors of the ovary included in this group make up fewer than 10 percent of all ovarian neoplasms. The two most common forms are granulosa–theca cell and Sertoli–Leydig cell tumors, so designated because they resemble the sex cord and stromal components of the ovary. These tumors may be hormonally active. Their function cannot always be related to their histologic appearance. Some granulosa cell tumors are masculinizing, and occasional Sertoli cell tumors secrete estrogen.

The granulosa cell tumor can occur at any age, but is uncommon in children; it is usually seen during the reproductive years, and less frequently in older adults. The sheets or ribbons of tumor cells may contain microfollicular structures (Call-Exner bodies). Estrogen is secreted by more than 70 percent of the tumors that occur before puberty, causing sexual precocity. In older patients, menstrual disturbances or postmenopausal bleeding are usually present. Ten-year survival rates as high as 90 percent have been reported for patients with granulosa cell tumors. It is difficult to identify the aggressive tumors from their histology. Theca cell tumors, in contrast, are rarely malignant; they are derived from the ovarian stromal cell and may show varying degrees of luteinization.

Sertoli–Leydig cell tumors are composed of varying proportions of cells resembling Sertoli and Leydig cells. Most of these uncommon tumors have been reported in young females. A broad range of histologic appearances may be encountered within this group. Consequently, they may present problems in differential diagnosis. Generally, the tumors are not particularly aggressive; 5-yr survival rates as high as 90 percent have been reported. Also called *androblastoma* and *arrhenoblastoma.*

Gynandroblastoma is a rare tumor that shows histologic features of both granulosa–theca cell and Sertoli–Leydig cell neoplasms; when functional, it is usually masculinizing.

For more information, see the specific ovarian tumor.

ovaritis (o″vah-ri′tis) [*ovari-* + *-itis* inflammation] an inflammation of the ovaries. This condition is most often due to infection of the ovaries, often with *Neisseria gonorrhoeae,* gram-negative bacilli, gram-positive cocci, *Mycoplasma,* and viruses. Infections often begin intravaginally, usually following intercourse, insertion of an intrauterine device, recent childbirth, or abortion. Abscess formation may occur. Ovaritis may also be secondary to autoimmune disorders. Infertility may be a common complication following ovaritis. Also called *oophoritis.*

ovary (o′vah-re) [N.L. *ovarium*] the germinal reproductive organ of the female; each of the paired, almond-shaped structures is about 3 cm long by 1.5 cm wide and 1 cm thick. The ovaries are homologous to the male testes and, like the testes, develop within the abdominal cavity before descending into the pelvis prior to birth.

The position of the ovaries is somewhat variable, but in nulliparous women they are located in a small depression, the ovarian fossa, on the lateral wall of the pelvis. The ovaries are oriented with their broader tubal extremity pointed superiorly and are attached to the fimbria of the uterine tube and a fold of peritoneum, the suspensory ligament. The inferior end (uterine extremity) is more pointed and is attached to the lateral angle of the uterus by the cordlike ligament of the ovary, which courses through the broad ligament.

The ovaries have a thick cortex, which consists of a dense stroma of reticular fibers and fusiform cells with ovarian follicles and corpora lutea embedded within it. The medulla is composed of a loosely organized network of connective tissue with elastin fibers, smooth muscle cells, and numerous blood vessels.

At birth the ovaries contain many primary follicles. These consist of a large central cell, the oogonium, surrounded by a single layer of flattened follicular cells. Throughout prepubertal life, many of these follicles atrophy and disappear. From the onset of puberty until menopause, numbers of primary follicles develop into vesicular follicles, one of which ruptures to release an ovum approximately once each month. Those follicles that do not fully mature become atretic.

See also *ovulation.*

oven (uv′en) an enclosed space for heating objects used in the laboratory in procedures or experiments.

Relative to laboratory safety, laboratory ovens can overheat owing to failure of their temperature regulation devices; they can also ignite some materials because the surface temperature of the heat source is always much hotter than the oven. Placing paraffin solvent solutions or solvent-wet mixtures in a drying oven can be extremely hazardous, because the heating element for the oven is likely to be hotter than the ignition temperature of the solvents and other materials placed in the oven. For example, if the heating coils at the bottom of the drying oven are red hot, they will ignite any paraffin or combustible material that may reach the coils, including flammable vapors.

overdominance (o″ver-dom′ĭ-nans) a mode of inheritance in which the heterozygote has a more extreme phenotype than either homozygote, generally used in the sense that it is more fit. It is the opposite of intermediate inheritance, in which the heterozygote is intermediate in phenotype and fitness. Also called *superdominance.*

overflow (o′ver-flo) 1. the continuous escape of a fluid, as of tears or urine.

2. in a computer, an error condition caused by the execution of an arithmetic operation, which produces a result too large for the register or the memory location designated to hold it. Cf. *underflow.*

overlapping inversion (o″ver-lap′ing) a chromosomal inversion in which the inverted segment includes a section that was previously inverted.

oviduct (o′vĭ-dukt) [*ovi-* + L. *ductus* duct] see *fallopian tube.*

ovotestis (o″vo-tes′tis) [*ovo-* + L. *testis*] a gonad of a true hermaphrodite, which contains histologically identifiable ovarian and testicular tissue.

ovulation (o″vu-la′shun) the process of release of an ovum from a vesicular follicle of the ovary, occurring approximately once each month from puberty until menopause. During the maturation sequence of an ovum, the follicular cells multiply and form layers. A fluid-filled cavity forms and defines an inner layer (cumulus oophorus) surrounding the developing ovum and the outer layer (membrana granulosa) surrounding the entire follicle. The outer layer is ensheathed by cortical stromal cells that form the theca folliculi, which produces estrogens. The oogonium within the follicle develops into a primary oocyte, which during the first meiotic division divides into a secondary oocyte, releasing the first polar body.

At ovulation, the secondary oocyte (still surrounded by its cumulus oophorus) is extruded from the ovary and passes into the uterine tube. If fertilization does not take place the ovum soon disintegrates. If fertilization does occur, the second meiotic division ensues and the second polar body is then released.

After ovulation, the walls of the vesicular follicle collapse. The cells of the membrana granulosa swell appreciably and produce a yellow carotenoid pigment, lutein. These cells compose the bulk of the corpus luteum, which secretes progesterone. If fertilization does not occur, the corpus luteum atrophies, leaving a yellowish scar on the surface of the ovary.

See also *menstrual cycle.*

ovum (o′vum), pl. *ova* [L.] [NA], the mature female gamete. It is a round cell produced in the ovary, approximately 0.1 mm in diameter, with a large nucleus and a plentiful cytoplasm containing yolk granules. See also *gematogenesis* and *ovulation.*

oxa- (ok′sah) a prefix word element used in organic chemistry to denote the replacement of a methylene group (—CH_2—) by an oxygen atom (—O—), e.g., 2,4-dioxapentane-1,5,-diol ($HOCH_2OCH_2OCH_2OH$).

oxacillin sodium (oks″ah-sil′in) a semisynthetic isoxazolyl penicillin that is resistant to both penicillinase and gastric acidity. It can be administered orally and is most often used to treat staphylococci infections that are penicillin resistant. See also *antibacterial agents* and *penicillin.*

oxalate (ok′sah-lāt) a salt or ester of oxalic acid.

oxalic acid (ok-sal′ik) [L. *oxalis* wood sorrel, from *oxus* sour] a crystalline dicarboxylic acid, HOOCCOOH, occurring naturally in many plants including wood sorrel, spinach, rhubarb, and greasewood. Small amounts of oxalate are synthesized in humans by the metabolism of ascorbate and glyoxylate. The genetic disorder oxalosis or chronic ingestion of excessive amounts of oxalate may result in oxaluria and facilitate the formation of calcium oxalate kidney stones. Acute poisoning causes removal of calcium and magnesium from the blood and the deposition of oxalate kidney stones. The lethal dose is about 10 g.

oxalic acid assays 1. chemical methods. Oxalate can be isolated from urine by precipitation as calcium oxalate following the addition of calcium(II) ions at about pH 6.2. The precipitate is then analyzed by oxidation/reduction with permanganate or by complexometric titration of the unprecipitated calcium.

2. enzymatic methods. Oxalate may be analyzed by determining the amount of carbon dioxide liberated by the enzyme oxalate decarboxylase.

A newer enzymatic method employs the same enzyme but measures the amount of formate produced in this reaction. The indicator reaction in this assay involves formate dehydrogenase and the generation of NADH, which can be measured spectrophotometrically. In another procedure, oxalate oxidase is used, and the peroxide formed is measured using peroxidase and an appropriate oxygen acceptor.

3. gas chromatography. In another proposed method, oxalate is quantitated by GC of a methyl derivative.

oxalism (ok′sal-izm) poisoning by oxalic acid.

oxaloacetate (ok″sah-lo-as′ĕ-tāt) a salt of oxaloacetic acid.

oxaloacetate decarboxylase see *pyruvate carboxylase.*

oxaloacetic acid (ok-sah″lo-ah-se′tik) a dicarboxylic acid, $HOOC{\cdot}CH_2{\cdot}CO{\cdot}COOH$, an important intermediary metabolite. A major intermediate of the citric acid cycle, oxaloacetic acid functions in several major biochemical pathways.

oxalosis (ok″sah-lo′sis) a genetic disorder, transmitted as an autosomal recessive trait, that is characterized by the urinary excretion of large amounts of oxalic acid and by the formation of kidney stones and calcium deposits in the kidney, leading to early death from renal failure.

The disorder occurs in two forms, in both of which a defective enzyme causes the accumulation of excessive amounts of the oxalate precursor glyoxylate. In oxalosis I, glyoxylate is also excreted, and an enzyme catalyzing the synthesis of α-hydroxyl-β-ketoadipate from glyoxylate and α-ketoglutarate is defective. In oxalosis II, L-glycerate is also excreted, the reduction of glyoxalate to glycolate is decreased, and the reduction of hydroxypyruvate to D-glycerate is reduced. It is theorized that the same defective enzyme catalyzes both reactions or that the glycerate excess inhibits glyoxylate reductase.

oxaluria (ok″sah-lu′re-ah) see *hyperoxaluria* and *oxalosis.*

oxazepam (oks-az′ĕ-pam) [NF], a benzodiazepine minor tranquilizer and a metabolite of diazepam. See also *benzodiazepine.*

oxazine dyes (ok′sah-zēn) a group of dyes that are derivatives of phenoxazine. The category includes brilliant cresyl blue, cresyl violet, and Nile blue. Also called oxazin dye.

oxazolidinedione compounds (ok″sah-zol″ĭ-dēn-di′ōn) a group of anticonvulsant drugs (paramethadione, trimethadione) used to control absence (petit mal) seizures that do not respond to other drugs. In view of possible severe side-effects, a complete blood count, liver function tests, and urinalysis should be performed at monthly intervals during the first year of therapy. Adverse reactions include gastrointestinal intolerance, disturbance of vision, bone marrow depression, aplastic anemia, skin rash, dermatitis, systemic lupus erythematosus–like syndrome, and nephrotic syndrome. The drug is demethylated by liver microsomal enzymes. The metabolite is also active and is slowly excreted in the urine.

oxidant (ok′sĭ-dant) a compound that undergoes reduction or accepts electrons in an oxidation-reduction (redox) reaction. Also called *oxidizing agent.*

total o.'s, a measure of ambient oxidants in ambient air used as an index of the severity of photochemical smog. It includes ozone, peroxyacyl nitrates (PAN), and other unidentified components. Total oxidants are assayed by bubbling air through neutral buffered potassium iodide solution. The iodine (I_2) formed is measured by the absorption change at 352 nm.

oxidase (ok′sĭ-dās) any of the oxidoreductase class of enzymes (EC 1.9) that catalyze a reaction in which molecular oxygen acts as the direct acceptor of electrons from a substrate donor, resulting in the formation of water. Ascorbate oxidase is an example.

oxidase test a test of the ability of a microorganism to convert certain aromatic amines into colored products, determined usually by the presence of cytochrome *c* oxidase in the culture. In a positive test with the indophenol method, this enzyme acts as a catalyst to couple dimethyl-*p*-phenylenediamine or tetramethyl-*p*-phenylenediamine and α-naphthol, forming a bright blue product, indophenol blue. When performed by the Kovacs method using aqueous tetramethyl-*p*-phenylenediamine dihydrochloride, a pink color turning to black indicates a positive reaction.

This test is used to identify *Neisseria* and to differentiate the negative Enterobacteriaceae from oxidase-positive but similar organisms such as species of *Vibrio, Pasteurella,* most *Pseudomonas, Moraxella,* and *Alcaligenes.*

oxidation (ok″sĭ-da′shun) 1. a chemical reaction in which the oxidation number of an atom is increased; a loss of electrons. Oxidation occurs together with reduction. In an electrochemical cell, oxidation occurs at the anode.

2. originally, a chemical reaction in which oxygen combines with another compound; this meaning is now obsolete.

oxidation-fermentation test a test for glucose utilization by a bacterial culture. After duplicate tubes containing a medium with glucose as the sole carbon source are stab-inoculated, one tube is covered with sterile petrolatum or paraffin oil. Acid production is followed by a color change of the indicator. Acid only in the open tube indicates oxidative utilization, acid in both tubes indicates fermentation, and lack of acid in both tubes indicates the nonutilization of glucose.

oxidation number a number assigned to each atom in a molecule or ion, indicating the theoretical number of electrons gained (if the oxidation number is positive), or lost (if the oxidation number is negative), in converting the atom to the elemental form, which has an oxidation number of zero. Oxygen usually has the oxidation number −2, and hydrogen +1 (except in hydrides). The sum of the oxidation numbers for all the atoms in an ion equals the ionic charge, and for the atoms in a neutral compound equals zero. Oxidation numbers that satisfy these rules can be assigned to every atom in most compounds; e.g., in the sulfate ion SO_4^{2-}, sulfur has the oxidation number +6, oxygen −2, and the sum, $6 + 4 \times (-2) = -2$, the total charge.

To name a compound containing a positive ion of an element with several oxidation states, the oxidation number is written as a Roman numeral in parentheses after the name of the element, e.g., iron(II) chloride for $FeCl_2$.

Also called *oxidation state.*

oxidation-reducing potential see *redox potential.*

oxidation-reduction reaction a chemical reaction in which an oxidation and a reduction occur, e.g., $2H_2 + O_2 \rightarrow 2H_2O$. The oxidized substance (H_2) is called the reducing agent or reductant; the reduced substance (O_2) is called the oxidizing agent or oxidant. Also called *redox reaction.*

oxidation state see *oxidation number.*

oxidative (ok′sĭ-da-tiv) 1. having the power to oxidize.

2. an organism that has a respiratory metabolism, i.e., uses oxygen as the final hydrogen acceptor.

oxidative phosphorylation the final step in the aerobic catabolism of fuel molecules in which part of their energy content is captured and stored in the high-energy phosphate bond of ATP.

In eukaryotes, the reaction occurs in the inner mitochondrial membrane; in prokaryotes, in the cytoplasmic membrane. As an electron pair is transferred from the reduced coenzyme NADH to ubiquinone to cytochrome *c* to molecular oxygen, with each transfer one molecule of ATP is produced from ADP, making three molecules of ATP produced per atom of oxygen consumed (the P:O ratio). These transfers are catalyzed by organized enzyme complexes present in the mitochondrial membrane, which include NADH dehydrogenase, ubiquinol dehydrogenase, and cytochrome oxidase. The NADH is produced by the oxidation of a variety of alcohols by NAD-coupled substrate dehydrogenases in the mitochondrial matrix. Some substrates cannot be oxidized by NAD. For these, oxidative phosphorylation begins not with NADH but with the electron transfer to ubiquinone catalyzed by a flavoprotein dehydrogenase (such as succinate dehydrogenase) on the matrix surface of the inner mitochondrial membrane, and the P:O ratio is 2.

Three theories relate to the mechanism by which the electron transfers in the mitochondrial inner membrane are coupled to phosphorylation. In one, the formation of covalent high-energy intermediates is utilized to drive ATP synthesis; however, no such intermediates have been found. In the chemiosmotic or proton-motive hypothesis, the high-energy intermediate state is a proton concentration gradient, causing an electric potential across the inner membrane. This potential can drive ATP synthesis when protons flow back into the mitochondrion down the concentration gradient. In the conformation hypothesis, the high-energy state involves a conformational change and a release of protons into membrane-bound proteins, produced by the electron transfers. The proton gradient and the resultant electrical potential then move the protein back to its lower energy conformation, thus driving ATP synthesis. ATP is produced by an enzyme complex termed ATP synthase, which is embedded in the inner mitochondrial membrane and sticks out into the matrix.

oxidative phosphorylation inhibitors a variety of compounds that inhibit ATP synthesis by inhibiting transfer of high-energy phosphate to ADP. This also results in blocking electron transfer along the respiratory chain when coupled to oxidative phosphorylation.

Two antibiotics, oligomycin and rutamycin, block phosphorylation by combining with one of the proteins of the ATP synthase complex. Actractyloside (a plant compound) and bongkrekate (a bacterial toxin) block the operation of the ADP-ATP antiport on the inner membrane and block ATP synthesis by stopping the supply of substrate.

oxidative phosphorylation uncouplers a variety of compounds that block phosphorylation (ATP synthesis) while permitting continuance of electron transfer at the maximal rate, which causes oxygen consumption without ATP production. Some uncouplers act by affecting the distribution of monovalent cations across the mitochondrial inner membrane.

Ionophores are lipid-soluble compounds that can carry sodium and potassium across the membrane. Two of these, valinomycin and nonactin, form a complex with potassium ions and carry them into the mitochondrial matrix. Gramicidin forms a pore in the membrane, permitting the passive diffusion of ions across the membrane. 2,4-Dinitro-phenol is lipid soluble and transports hydrogen ions across the membrane. All of the compounds destroy the necessary electrochemical gradient and pH gradient across the membrane that drives ATP synthesis.

See also *chemiosmotic hypothesis.*

oxide (ok′sīd) [L. *oxidum*] 1. a binary compound of oxygen.

2. an epoxide, e.g., ethylene oxide. See *epoxide.*

oxidize (ok′sĭ-dīz) to cause a substance to undergo oxidation. In an oxidation-reduction (redox) reaction, the oxidizing agent is reduced. See also *oxidation-reduction reaction.*

oxidizer (ok″sĭ-di′zer) an agent that causes an element or radical to combine with oxygen or to lose electrons. Some oxidizers, such as some organic peroxides, are combustible and are either unstable or susceptible to spontaneous decomposition.

oxidizing agent (ok′si-diz″ing) see *oxidant.*

oxidizing gas a gas that supports combustion, such as oxygen or nitrous oxide.

oxidoreductase (ok″sĭ-do-re-duk′tās) any of a class of enzymes (EC 1) consisting of those that catalyze reactions in which one compound is oxidized and another compound is reduced. Clinically important enzymes of this class include alcohol dehydrogenase (AD), glucose-6-phosphate dehydrogenase (G-6-PD), isocitrate dehydrogenase (ICD), lactate dehydrogenase (LD), and 6-phosphogluconate dehydrogenase (6-P-GD). This class includes enzymes variously known as dehydrogenases, reductases, oxidases, peroxidases, hydroxylases, and oxygenases.

oximeter (ok-sim′e-ter) a photoelectric device that measures the oxygen saturation of blood by recording the amount of light transmitted by reduced versus oxygenated hemoglobin.

oxo- (ok′so) a prefix word element used in organic chemistry to denote the carbonyl group (C=O) when it is not the principal functional group in the molecule, e.g., 2-oxopentanedioic acid, the systematic name for α-ketoglutaric acid.

oxo acid an acid in which only oxygen is bound to the characteristic atom, e.g., sulfuric acid, periodic acid. It generally has a formula of the type H_xXO_m.

3-oxobutyric acid (ok″so-bu′tĭ-rik) see under *ketone bodies.*

oxoglutarate dehydrogenase (ok″so′gloo′tah-rāt de-hi′dro-jen″ās) a multienzyme complex (2-oxoglutarate:lipoamide oxidoreductase, EC 1.2.4.2), consisting of at least three distinct enzymes that catalyze the overall reaction 2-oxoglutarate + CoA-SH + $NAD^+ \rightarrow$ succinyl coenzyme A + NADH + H^+ + CO_2. This reaction is biologically irreversible. Thiamine diphosphate, lipoic acid, CoA, FAD, and NAD^+ are required as cofactors. The reaction is an essential part of the Krebs citric acid cycle. Also called *α-ketoglutarate dehydrogenase.*

2-oxoglutaric acid $COOH \cdot (CH_2) \cdot CO \cdot COOH$, an intermediate compound of the tricarboxylic acid cycle. Also called α-oxoglutaric acid.

2-oxoisovalerate dehydrogenase (ok″so-i″so-val′er-āt de-hi′dro-jen″ās) a multienzyme complex of the oxidoreductase class (2-oxoisovalerate:lipoamide oxidoreductase (decarboxylating), EC 1.2.4.4) that catalyzes the oxidative decarboxylation of the oxo-acids formed by transamination of valine, leucine, and isoleucine. A genetic absence of or defect in the enzyme causes elevation of serum levels of branched-chain amino acids and their excretion in the urine. The condition is associated with a characteristic odor (maple syrup urine disease). Also called *branched-chain α-keto acid dehydrogenase.* See also *aminoacidopathy* and *maple syrup urine disease.*

oxolinic acid (ok″so-lin′ik) a synthetic antibacterial agent that is very similar to nalidixic acid in its chemistry, properties, and antimicrobial spectrum. It is used chiefly as a urinary antiseptic.

oxonium ion (ok-so′ne-um) any ion containing a positive oxygen atom with bonds to three other atoms. Used alone it refers to H_3O^+, which is also called, less systematically, the hydronium ion. Atoms other than hydrogen may be attached as in the trimethyloxonium ion, $(CH_3)_3O^+$. See also *hydronium ion.*

5-oxoprolinase (ATP-hydrolyzing) (ok″so-pro′lĭ-nās) an enzyme of the hydrolase class (5-oxo-L-proline amidohydrolase (ATP-hydrolyzing), EC 3.5.2.9) that catalyzes the reaction ATP + 5-oxo-L-proline + $2H_2O$ ⇄ ADP + orthophosphate + L-glutamate. The enzyme catalyzes one step in the γ-glutamyl transfer cycle. Also called *pyroglutamase* and *pyroglutamate hydroxylase.* See also *γ-glutamyl transfer cycle.*

5-oxoproline (ok″so-pro′lēn) see *pyroglutamate.*

4-oxoproline reductase (ok″so-pro′lēn re-duk″tās) an enzyme of the oxidoreductase class (4-hydroxy-L-proline:NAD^+ oxidoreductase, EC 1.1.1.104) that catalyzes the reaction 4-hydroxyl-L-proline + NAD^+ ⇄ 4-oxoproline + NADH. A genetic deficiency of the enzyme results in hyperhydroxyprolinemia and excretion of large amounts of this amino acid in urine. There is a questionable association with mental retardation. The condition does not affect collagen metabolism and is probably inherited as an autosomal recessive trait. Also called *hydroxyproline oxidase.*

5-oxoprolinuria (ok″so-pro″lĭ-nu′re-ah) see *pyroglutamicaciduria.*

oxtriphylline (oks-trif′ĭ-lēn) [NF], choline theophyllinate, a bronchodilator used to treat bronchial asthma, chronic bronchitis, and emphysema. See also *theophylline.*

oxy- (ok′se) [Gr. *oxys* sharp, sour] 1. a prefix word element to denote the presence of oxygen (e.g., oxyhemoglobin), sharpness (e.g., oxyhydrocephalus), or acidity (e.g., oxyphil).

2. in organic chemistry; a prefix word element preceded by the name of an alkyl group, as in hexyloxy- and methoxy-, used as a prefix in naming ethers. It is also used as a prefix to name symmetric ethers; in this usage it is followed by the names of the groups attached, e.g., oxybismethane (methyl ether).

oxybiotin (ok″sĭ-bi′o-tin) a compound in which the sulfur of biotin is replaced by oxygen. It can substitute for biotin in the nutrition of most biotin-requiring species, and appears to be used unchanged, rather than being converted to biotin.

oxycodone hydrochloride (ok″se-ko′dōn) a semisynthetic narcotic analgesic, 14-hydroxydihydrocodeinone, with actions similar to morphine. It can produce physical dependence. Respiratory depression due to overdosage is reversed by the administration of naloxone, nalorphine, or levallorphan.

oxygen (O) (ok′sĭ-jen) [Gr. *oxy* sour, "acid" + *gennan* to produce] a nonmetallic element occurring as either a colorless, odorless gas (dioxygen, O_2) or a pungent bluish gas (ozone, O_3); atomic number 8; atomic weight 15.9994; Group VI of the periodic table; oxidation states −2, −1, +2. It occurs naturally as a component of air (20.95 percent), oxide rocks and ores, and water. Oxygen is present in many organic compounds, such as alcohols, aldehydes, ketones (e.g., as carbohydrates), and carboxylic acids (e.g., fatty acids).

In aerobic organisms (including humans), oxygen (O_2) is the ultimate electron acceptor in oxidative phosphorylation, the production of high-energy phosphate (adenosine triphosphate, ATP) from fuel molecules. When glucose is the fuel, three molecules of ATP are produced for each atom of oxygen that is reduced to water; when fat is the fuel, the phosphate:oxygen ratio is 2.8. Of all the energy used in the body, 85 percent is produced by reducing molecular oxygen.

Oxygen also is a substrate for certain catabolic enzymes, the oxidases; these include dioxygenases, which incorporate two atoms of oxygen into a substrate and reduce the other to water.

Oxygen is not very soluble in water. Only about 0.13 mmol/l is dissolved in blood plasma (0.9 mmol/l when breathing pure oxygen). A carrier protein is necessary for oxygen transport. In the blood this is hemoglobin (Hb), found in erythrocytes, which binds 4 mol of O_2/mol to Hb. In the muscles the transport protein is myoglobin (Mb), which binds 1 mol of O_2/mol to Mb and carries oxygen in the cytoplasm from the cell membrane to the mitochondria. Arterial blood normally contains 6.69–10.3 mmol/l; venous blood, 4.46–7.14 mmol/l.

The amount of oxygen bound to hemoglobin depends on the partial pressure of oxygen (Po_2) in the (imaginary) gas phase in equilibrium with the blood; it also depends on the acidity of the blood (pH) and the erythrocyte concentration of 2,3-diphosphoglycerate (2,3-DPG). The arterial Po_2 (83–108 mmHg) is lower than the atmospheric Po_2 (160 mmHg) and may be decreased (hypoxemia) owing to reduced atmospheric oxygen partial pressure, reduced pulmonary perfusion or ventilation, increased right-to-left shunting of blood in the heart, or reduced affinity of the hemoglobin for oxygen (as in methemoglobinemia or sulfhemoglobinemia). The lower limit for Po_2 in arterial blood is about 83 mmHg in younger subjects, decreasing to 70 mmHg in older subjects. A level of about 40 mmHg can be tolerated without producing cerebral hypoxia (marked by confusion or coma), but 50–55 mmHg is usually the minimal goal in treatment of respiratory failure.

The quantity of oxygen in the blood expressed as a percentage of the oxygen capacity of the blood hemoglobin (oxygen saturation, So_2) is a sigmoidal (S-shaped) function of the oxygen partial pressure (Po_2). The reference values for So_2 are 95–99 percent in arterial blood and 60–85 percent in venous blood.

The partial pressure of oxygen at half saturation (Po_2 [0.5] or P-50) is determined by calculation from the measured values of Po_2 and So_2; an increased value indicates a lowered affinity of hemoglobin for oxygen.

Oxygen [USP] is often administered to treat hypoxemia except when it is caused by cardiac shunting. The concentration usually is only moderately increased above normal (to 24–35 percent). There are two types of oxygen toxicity, chronic and acute. Chronic administration of high oxygen concentrations (above 50 percent) causes pulmonary edema and congestion due to a deficiency of pulmonary surfactant, which causes collapse of the alveoli. Acute oxygen toxicity is caused by breathing pure oxygen, especially at high pressure (as in deep-sea diving); symptoms include nausea, twitching, dizziness, convulsions, and coma. The toxic effect of pure oxygen is especially pronounced in newborns, in whom oxygen treatment may cause fibrosis in the eye with blindness (*retrolental fibroplasia*).

oxygen-15 (O 15, ^{15}O) a cyclotron-produced radionuclide, which decays with a 2.03-min half-life by positron beta decay, producing 511-keV annihilation radiation gamma rays. ^{15}O-oxygen is blood soluble and can be used to measure pulmonary perfusion and ventilation; the short half-life, however, makes this procedure generally impractical.

oxygen affinity the strength with which a hemoglobin binds oxygen; it is frequently measured as the partial pressure of oxygen at which the hemoglobin is half-saturated, and called the P-50 for that hemoglobin: P refers to the partial pressure of oxygen, 50 to the 50 percent saturation point on the O_2 dissociation curve.

Increased affinity shifts the dissociation curve to the right, increases the P-50, and impairs oxygen delivery to tissues. See also the illustration accompanying *oxygen-hemoglobin dissociation curve.*

oxygen analyzer an instrument used to measure continuously the concentration of oxygen (or partial pressure of O_2 in some models) in a stream (or static sample) of gas, particularly a continuous sample of respiratory gas.

Analysis in the paramagnetic models is based on measurement of the magnetic susceptibility of the analyzed gas. O_2 is unique in that it is strongly attracted into a magnetic field (i.e., it is paramagnetic), whereas most of the other common gases are weakly repelled from a magnetic field (i.e., they are diamagnetic). The magnetically susceptible gas O_2, then, has the ability to be temporarily magnetized when it is placed in a magnetic field. The paramagnetic O_2 analyzer cell contains a small, dumbbell-shaped test body that is suspended in a strong, nonuniform magnetic field by a quartz fiber. When a gas sample containing a magnetically susceptible gas such as O_2 is drawn into the cell, the quartz fiber (and thus the two spheres of the dumbbell) is rotated away from the region of maximal magnetic flux density by resulting changes in the magnetic field. The torque on the dumbbell caused by these magnetic forces can thus be used as a measure of the partial pressure of O_2 in the sample. The paramagnetic analyzer measures this partial pressure indirectly by supplying electrostatic forces that create a torque that balances those caused by the magnetic forces, bringing the test body to a null position. The voltage supplied to the test body, which becomes the output of the amplifier circuit of the analyzer, is thus equal to that needed to keep the test body in the null position against the forces exerted by the magnetic field.

In another type of analyzer, detection and measurement of O_2 is made through use of a polarographic sensor that is insensitive to other common gases. The sensor contains an anode, a cathode, a thin O_2-permeable membrane, and a thinly compressed layer of electrolyte gel. A small voltage is applied across the anode and cathode. O_2 is electrochemically reduced at the cathode when it diffuses through the membrane and passes through the electrolyte gel. This process produces an output current proportional to the partial pressure of O_2 in the sample.

The typical oxygen analyzer is used for pulmonary function tests, monitoring of patients in intensive care and on oxygen therapy, and animal research (particularly in studies of O_2 rate consumption when used as a measure of metabolic rate).

oxygenase (ok′sĭ-jĕ′nās) any of the enzymes of the oxidoreductase subclasses (EC 1.13 and 1.14) that catalyze the incorporation of oxygen from O_2 into one or two acceptor substrates. See also *dioxygenase* and *monooxygenase.*

oxygenation (ok″sĭ-jĕ-na′shun) the addition of oxygen; the term usually applies to molecular oxygen being dissolved in a liquid or being bound to hemoglobin in the blood.

oxygenator (ok″sĭ-jĕ-na′tor) a device used to oxygenate venous blood extracorporeally. See also under *heart-lung machine.*

oxygen capacity of blood the maximal quantity of oxygen that combines with the hemoglobin present in a specified volume of blood, usually measured in units of milliliters of oxygen (STPD) per 100 ml of blood (ml O_2/dl) or millimoles of oxygen per liter of blood (mmol/l). One gram of adult human hemoglobin in vitro will combine with about 1.34 ml of oxygen; human blood thus has an oxygen capacity of 21 ml/dl under conditions of 100 percent saturation of the 15.67 g of hemoglobin per 100 ml of whole blood found in an average healthy human.

oxygen consumption ($\dot{Q}_{O_2}$ or $\dot{V}_{O_2}$) 1. the rate of utilization of oxygen by tissue slices or cells respiring in vitro, measured as the $\dot{Q}_{O_2}$ in units of microliters of oxygen (STPD) per milligram of dry weight of tissue per hour (μl of O_2/mg/hr).

2. the total quantity of oxygen utilized by a whole organism, reflecting the sum of the amounts of oxygen utilized by all its metabolizing or active tissues. Oxygen consumption of the whole organism is generally expressed as a rate or volume utilized per unit of time ($\dot{V}_{O_2}$) in units of liters or milliliters of oxygen (STPD) per minute (l or ml of O_2/min). The oxygen consumption index is this quantity divided by the body surface area in square meters. The basal rate of oxygen consumption is most commonly measured clinically in units of milliliters of oxygen consumed per kilogram of body weight per minute (ml/kg/min). The basal rate so-measured is equal to about 3.5 ml/kg/min in healthy human adults, and can be used as an approximator of the basal metabolic rate.

Basal oxygen consumption of air-breathing animals (including humans) is commonly estimated by determining the amount of oxygen extracted by the lungs (oxygen intake) over a given period of time. The air expired from the lungs over this period is collected and its oxygen content analyzed. Oxygen consumption is then calculated as follows: $\dot{V}_{O_2}$ = (milliliters of oxygen consumed per liter of expired air) × (liters of air expired per minute of collection time). The milliliters of oxygen consumed per liter of expired air is equal to the difference between the oxygen content of the inspired room air and that of the expired air.

Cf. *oxygen uptake.*

oxygen content of blood the amount of oxygen in a given volume of blood, including both the physically dissolved oxygen and that bound to the hemoglobin molecule. It can be measured by the Van Slyke method or by gas chromatography of samples extracted in a Van Slyke apparatus. The oxygen content of blood exposed to a high oxygen tension is normally equal to the hemoglobin content, multiplied by 1.34 ml of oxygen per gram of hemoglobin, plus the dissolved oxygen that equals 0.003 ml/mmHg of oxygen tension.

oxygen cost of breathing the rate of oxygen consumption of the respiratory muscles during breathing. It is estimated by measuring the total oxygen intake ($\dot{V}_{O_2}$) at different ventilatory rates ($\dot{V}_E$), assuming that increases in $\dot{O}_2$ intake represent the cost of additional ventilation. A curve of $\dot{V}_{O_2}$ versus V_E is plotted, and the cost of breathing at rest is calculated by extrapolation of the curve to the $\dot{V}_{O_2}$ axis (resting ventilation). The O_2 cost of breathing in the healthy individual has a range of 0.5–1.0 ml of oxygen per liter of ventilation; this value is increased in obstructive lung disease.

oxygen debt the excess oxygen (over that required during resting metabolism) consumed during recovery from strenuous physical activity or a period of apnea. It is used to reconvert the accumulated lactic acid to glucose and the decomposed creatine phosphate and adenosine triphosphate (ATP) to their original higher-energy states; it is also used to restore alveolar and arterial P_{O_2} and the percentage of oxygen saturation of hemoglobin and myoglobin to normal levels. The oxygen debt compensates for or repays the oxygen and energy stores that were depleted during a period of anaerobic metabolism, in which tissue oxygen demand exceeded oxygen uptake or availability.

oxygen half-saturation pressure of hemoglobin (P-50) the partial pressure of oxygen required for the 50 percent saturation of hemoglobin under specific conditions of temperature, pH, and ionic strength. The oxygen half-saturation pressure of hemoglobin is a measure of (and varies inversely with) the affinity of hemoglobin for oxygen. An increase in P_{CO_2}, red blood cell 2,3-disphosphoglycerate concentration, or temperature, or a decrease in blood pH increases the P-50 (decreases the oxygen affinity), favoring the unloading of oxygen from the hemoglobin. At normal body temperature (37°C) and pH 7.4 (or P_{CO_2} of 40 mmHg), the oxygen half-saturation pressure for adult human hemoglobin is 27.0 mmHg.

oxygen-hemoglobin dissociation curve the graph of oxygen bound (percent) versus oxygen tension (mmHg) for hemoglobin under physiologic conditions (see the accompanying illustration). It is an S-shaped curve with the steepest slope near the half-saturation point (P-50).

The curve is shifted by changes in pH, P_{CO_2}, P_{O_2}, 2,3-diphosphoglycerate (2,3-DPG) concentration, and temperature. A decrease in pH or an increase in P_{CO_2} causes the dissociation curve to shift to the right (acid-Bohr effect), and an increase in blood pH or a decrease in blood P_{CO_2} causes the curve to shift to the left (alkaline-Bohr effect). Such changes occur, as blood bypasses the tissues, where metabolic

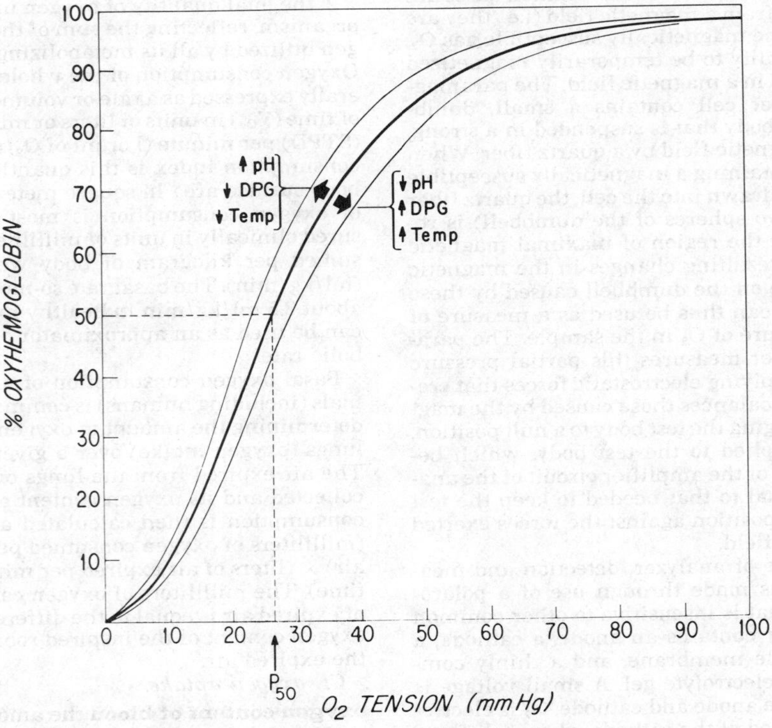

Oxygen-hemoglobin dissociation curve. The oxygen-binding curve for human hemoglobin A under physiologic conditions (dark curve). The affinity will be shifted by changes in pH, DPG concentration, and temperature as indicated. P_{50} represents the oxygen tension at half-saturation. (From Bunn, H. F., et al.: Human Hemoglobins. Philadelphia, W. B. Saunders Co., 1977.)

products decrease the pH and increase the P_{CO_2} of blood. As a result, the binding affinity of hemoglobin for O_2 decreases, and increased amounts of O_2 are released for use by the tissues.

An increase in 2,3-DPG also causes the dissociation curve to shift to the right, resulting in decreased affinity for O_2 and increased oxygen delivery to tissues. Such increase in 2,3-DPG and subsequent increase in O_2 delivery to tissues is an important compensatory mechanism in anemia and in conditions associated with the decreased functional capacity of hemoglobin, as in chronic carbon monoxide exposure.

oxygen pulse the quantity of oxygen consumed during a specified time interval, divided by the number of heartbeats occurring during that same interval, for any given level of physical activity. The oxygen pulse is commonly calculated as the oxygen uptake in millimeters per minute (ml/min) divided by the heart rate in beats per minute (beats/min). It is used as an index of an individual's cardiopulmonary physical fitness.

At rest, the oxygen pulse is approximately equal to 250 ml/min divided by 80 beats/min, or 3.1 ml/beat. With training and excellent cardiovascular fitness, the O_2 pulse ranges between 12 and 20 ml/beat, and during exercise efforts, between 20 and 40 ml/beat. In contrast, individuals with heart disease and an impaired cardiac output response to exercise often demonstrate a rapid increase in heart rate with increasing work and oxygen consumption; as a result, their oxygen pulse can be as low as 2–4 ml/beat during exercise efforts.

oxygen saturation (S_{O_2}) the ratio of the oxygen content of blood to its total oxygen-binding capacity. Specimens used consist of heparinized arterial blood or arterialized capillary blood. See also under *oxygen*.

oxygen saturation measurements 1. gasometric methods. Blood is treated with ferricyanide in a closed chamber (Van Slyke manometer, Natelson gasometer) to free the hemoglobin-bound oxygen. After absorbing any CO_2, the freed O_2 is measured directly, or indirectly, after absorption by cupric oxide (CuO) or dithionite. The oxygen measured in milliliters per liter (ml/l) or milliliters per deciliter (ml/dl) is compared with that obtained when the specimen is fully saturated with O_2 (as in a tonometer). Alternately, the percentage of O_2 saturation can be calculated by comparing the experimentally obtained O_2 value with a value obtained by multiplying the hemoglobin content (g/dl) by 1.34 (the amount of oxygen that can be bound by 1 g of hemoglobin).

2. spectrophotometric methods based on measuring the absorbance of a solution containing two forms of hemoglobin (oxyhemoglobin and deoxyhemoglobin) at two different wavelengths. The ratio of the two absorbances (e.g., 577/548 or 650/805 nm) is a function of the concentration of the two forms. An error in the measurement results if an appreciable concentration of a third hemoglobin form is present, but if readings at three wave lengths are made, all three forms may be measured and appropriate corrections made.

3. coulometric (polarographic) methods. The O_2 is measured using an oxygen electrode, obtaining the P_{O_2} of the solution. From this value and the pH, the percentage of saturation can be calculated.

4. gas chromatography. Special columns must be used to quantitate all dissolved gases in blood; this approach, however, has not been very successful for blood specimens.

oxygen tension see *p. p. of oxygen* under *partial pressure.*

oxygen therapy the administration of supplemental oxygen to alleviate the hypoxemia that accompanies many diverse disorders, including airway obstruction, pulmonary edema, adult respiratory distress syndrome (ARDS), chronic respiratory insufficiency, shock, and various cardiac disorders.

There are many modes of oxygen therapy; most commonly, oxygen is administered via a nasal cannula or Venturi mask. Oxygen is also administered in conjunction with mechanical ventilation and intermittent positive pressure breathing (IPPB) therapy. It is usually given in the lowest concentration that will achieve acceptable arterial Pa_{O_2} levels, generally 70–100 mmHg, although 50–60 mmHg is often considered satisfactory for patients with chronic respiratory insufficiency, particularly when carbon dioxide retention is present.

oxygen toxicity the pulmonary and neurologic manifestations that result from the prolonged inhalation of oxygen at high partial pressures at sea level (such as during controlled, mechanical ventilation or from breathing oxygen-enriched gases at high barometric pressures during diving). O_2 toxicity is concentration- and time-dependent. The pulmonary effects of inspiration of 100 percent O_2 at sea level (1 atmosphere absolute, ATA) become manifest after approximately 24 hr of continuous exposure. Pulmonary O_2 toxicity, however, may occur after continuous exposure to as little as 0.5 ATA of O_2. Prolonged exposure can lead to direct injury of the lung, with pathologic changes that resemble those found in acute respiratory failure: hemorrhage, edema, hyaline membrane formation in some alveoli, and morphologic changes in components of the alveolocapillary membrane. These changes can become lethal as a result of progressive impairment of gas exchange and resulting hypoxemia. The toxic effect of pure oxygen is especially pronounced in newborn infants, in whom oxygen treatment may cause retrolental fibroplasia.

Breathing pure O_2 at high barometric pressure (greater than 2.5 ATA) can produce a series of neurologic manifestations (twitching, nausea, dizziness, ringing in the ears) that may lead to convulsions even before any pulmonary problems have become apparent.

The cause of O_2 toxicity is still unknown, but it may involve the production of H_2O_2 and the superoxide anion (O_2^-). It is thought that these free radicals participate in chemical reactions that destroy cellular integrity because the defense mechanisms normally preventing these reactions have been upset by exposure to high O_2 levels.

oxygen uptake (V_{O_2}) the amount of O_2 removed from the environment by an organism, such as that removed by the lungs during inspiration. The O_2 uptake also includes the O_2 removed from alveolar gas by the pulmonary capillary blood and the removal of O_2 from the blood that perfuses an organ or tissue. It is commonly expressed as an uptake rate in units of liters or milliliters of O_2 per minute. The rate of O_2 uptake equals the rate of O_2 consumption under steady-state conditions in the respiratory and circulatory systems. Also called oxygen intake. Cf. *oxygen consumption.*

oxyhemoglobin (Hb O_2) fully oxygenated hemoglobin that contains four molecules of oxygen (O_2) per molecule of hemoglobin. See also *hemoglobin.*

oxymorphone hydrochloride (ok″se-mor′fōn) [NF], a narcotic analgesic, 14-hydroxydihydromorphinone, with an analgesic effect similar to that of morphine but producing less nausea, constipation, and respiratory depression. Its use can result in physical dependence.

oxyntic (ok-sin′tik) [Gr. *oxynō* to make acid] secreting acid, as the parietal (oxyntic) cells.

oxyntic cell see *parietal cell.*

oxyphenbutazone (ok″se-fen-bu′tah-zōn) [NF], an analgesic, antipyretic, antiinflammatory, and uricosuric nonsteroidal drug of the pyrazolone group. It is used for the treatment of gout, rheumatoid arthritis, osteoarthritis, and ankylosing spondylitis. It is a metabolite of phenylbutazone and is similar in its side-effects except that it causes less gastric irritation. See also *phenylbutazone* and *phenylbutazone assays.* Trademark, Tandearil.

oxyphil adenoma a parathyroid adenoma composed of mitochondrion-rich cells. Groups of oxyphilic cells are common within parathyroid adenomas but rarely compose the entire neoplasm. Some oxyphil adenomas are associated with hyperparathyroidism.

oxyphil cell (ok′se-fil) [*oxy-* + Gr. *philein* to love] a mitochondrion-rich cell of the parathyroid gland; a functioning cell that produces parathormone. Oxyphil cells are rare before puberty; they increase in number thereafter, and in older persons are quite numerous. They are also seen in adenomas and carcinomas of the parathyroid gland, kidneys, and other organs. See also *Hürthle cell* and *oncocyte.*

oxyphilic (ok″se-fil′ik) having an affinity for acid dyes. Also called *acidophilic.*

oxyphil inclusion bodies round or oval cytoplasmic inclusions, such as Negri bodies, Guarnieri bodies, or herpes bodies, which may be demonstrated with azure-eosin or other acid-base dye sequence methods such as the Stovall-Black method. Inclusion bodies stain dark red; nuclei, blue; and other structures, pink.

oxypurinol (ok″se-pūr′ĭ-nol) an isomer of xanthine useful for reducing blood uric acid concentration in hyperuricemic conditions such as gout. It is formed in vivo from administered allopurinol by an oxidation that introduces a second hydroxyl group. Oxypurinol acts as a noncompetitive inhibitor of xanthine oxidase, blocking formation of uric acid and resulting in excretion of the water-soluble hypoxanthine and xanthine.

oxyquinoline sulfate (ok″se-kwin′o-lēn) 8-hydroxyquinoline sulfate, used as a topical antiseptic.

oxytalan fiber (oks-it′ah-lan) a connective tissue fiber found in the periodontal tissues of humans and other primates. These fibers are extremely resistant to acid and can be stained only after oxidation with a strong acid such as performic or peracetic acid.

oxytetracycline (ok″se-tet″rah-si′klēn) a tetracycline antibiotic produced by *Streptomyces rimosus,* effective against a wide range of microorganisms. See also *antibacterial agents* and *tetracyclines.*

oxytocin (ok″se-to′sin) a cyclic peptide hormone consisting of eight amino acids, which acts on the female reproductive system; M.W. 1000. It is produced in the neurons of the supraoptic and paraventricular nuclei of the hypothalamus, along with vasopressin, and stored in the posterior lobe of the pituitary. The release of oxytocin is increased during labor. It stimulates the uterus, producing contraction of the myometrium and the mammary glands, resulting in lactation. Oxytocin is used clinically to hasten labor or to cause uterine contraction after delivery of the placenta.

oxytocin challenge test (OCT) a test performed to assess the respiratory function of the placenta and to determine whether the placenta and fetus can withstand the stress of labor. Oxytocin is administered to induce three or four uterine contractions, during which time the fetal heart rate is monitored by ultrasound to determine the adequacy of respiratory reserve. This test has now been largely replaced by the *nonstress test* (NST).

Oxytrema (ok″se-tre′mah) [*oxy-* + Gr. *trēma* hole] a genus of mollusks. The species *O. silicula* is the molluskan host of the fluke *Troglotrema salmincola,* which is associated with "salmon poisoning" in dogs and occasionally in humans.

Oxyurata (ok″se-ur′ah-tah) a suborder of nematodes that includes the superfamily Oxyuroidea.

oxyuriasis (ok″se-u-ri′ah-sis) infection with the nematode *Enterobius vermicularis* (the human pinworm or seatworm) or with other oxyurids. See also *E. vermicularis* under *Enterobius.*

Oxyuridae (ok″se-u′rĭ-de) a family of nematodes of the suborder Oxyurata and order Rhabditida.

Oxyuris (ok″se-u′ris) [*oxy-* + Gr. *oura* tail] a genus of intestinal nematodes of the superfamily Oxyuroidea.

O. vermicularis, see *E. vermicularis* under *Enterobius.*

Oxyuroidea (ok″se-u″roi-de′ah) a superfamily of nematodes (the oxyurids) that includes the pinworms and threadworms. These worms are parasitic in the intestines of humans and may infect invertebrates. They are small forms: the females are pin shaped, and the males resemble an inverted question mark, with phasmids and a bulbous esophagus. The most common species infecting humans is *Enterobius vermicularis.*

ozena (o-ze′nah) [Gr. *ozaina* a fetid polypus in the nose] a severe, chronic rhinitis characterized by a thick discharge with a foul odor, mucosal crusts, atrophy of turbinates, and sclerosis of mucous membranes, with abnormal patency of the nasal cavaties. Anosmia usually develops, and epistaxis (nosebleed) may be recurrent. The cause is unknown. Bacterial infections are thought to play a role, and cultures often reveal *Klebsiella ozaenae* and other gram-negative organisms.

ozone (o′zōn) [Gr. *ozē* stench] an allotropic form of oxygen, O_3; M.W. 48.00. Ozone, a common air pollutant, is a bluish gas with a distinctive odor that is produced by electrical discharges or ultraviolet light. It can be condensed to a blue liquid, with b.p. −112°C. Ozone is a stronger oxidizing agent than oxygen (O_2). Highly toxic by inhalation, it causes pulmonary edema with severe exposure and is irritating to the eyes and mucous membranes.

ozonization (o-zo-nĭ-zā′shun) see *ozonolysis.*

ozonolysis (o-zo-nol'ĭ-sis) the chemical reaction in which the carbon-carbon double bond of an alkene is cleaved by reaction with ozone. The reaction yields a cyclic peroxide, known as an ozonide, which is decomposed to a compound or compounds having carbonyl groups at the carbons that were initially connected by the double bond. Also called *ozonization*.

Ozzards's filaria (oz'zardz) [A.T. *Ozzard*, English zoologist, 19th century] a phasmid nematode (*Mansonella ozzardi*) that is parasitic in humans, causing filariasis. See also *M. ozzardi* under *Mansonella*.

P

P a phosphate group; *peta-;* the chemical element *phosphorus; poise; polarization; power; probability; proline.*

~P symbol for high-energy phosphate bond.

P-50 abbrev. See *oxygen half-saturation pressure of hemoglobin.*

P_L abbrev. See *transpulmonary pressure.*

p symbol for atomic orbital with angular momentum quantum number 1, *momentum, pico-, pressure, proton,* sample proportion (see under *binomial distribution*), the short arm of a chromosome.

p- abbrev. See *para-.*

Π the Greek capital letter *pi;* used in mathematics to indicate the product of a sequence: $\Pi_{i=1}^{n} X_i$ means $X_1 \times X_2 \times X_3 \times \ldots \times X_{n-1} \times X_n$; *i* is the product index, and 1 and *n* are the product limits.

π the Greek lower case letter *pi;* used in mathematics as a symbol for the ratio of circumference to diameter, approximately 3.1415926536.

PA abbrev. See *pernicious a.* under *anemia, phosphatidic acid, physician's assistant, posteroanterior.*

$P_{A_{CO_2}}$ abbrev. See *alveolar P_{CO_2}.*

$P_{A_{O_2}}$ abbrev. See *alveolar P_{O_2}.*

Pa symbol for *pascal,* the chemical element *protactinium.*

Pa_{CO_2} abbrev. See *arterial P_{CO_2}.*

Pa_{O_2} abbrev. See *arterial P_{O_2}.*

pA_2 see under *affinity constant.*

PAB abbrev. See *p-aminobenzoic acid.*

PABA abbrev. See *p-aminobenzoic acid.*

PAC abbrev. See *premature atrial contraction.*

pacemaker (pās′ma″ker) 1. in biochemistry, a substance that controls the rate at which a series of reactions occurs, i.e., one involved in the rate-determining step.

2. a region of tissue that controls the rate of rhythmic contraction of an organ. The term usually refers to the cardiac pacemaker, although contractions of the stomach and uterus are also controlled by pacemakers. The normal cardiac pacemaker is the sinoatrial (SA) node, a small, ellipsoidal mass of specialized muscle cells near the junction with the superior vena cava. At rest, the cell membranes of the SA fibers are slightly permeable to sodium ions. This phenomenon causes a gradual reduction in resting membrane potential until the threshold is reached, resulting in spontaneous SA node discharge. This phenomenon causes the fibers to fire rhythmically. Each of these pulses is carried by the conducting system of the heart to all of the muscle fibers. Other components of the conducting system can also spontaneously discharge at their own intrinsic rhythmic rates. However, they are suppressed from discharging by the more rapid rate of the SA node. In certain conditions a region can develop a discharge rate that is faster than that of the SA node and thus become an ectopic pacemaker.

3. an artificial cardiac pacemaker; an electronic device used to regulate the rhythm of the heart. Artificial cardiac pacing is most often used to treat atrioventricular (AV) block or sick sinus syndrome; it is also infrequently employed to treat some ventricular and supraventricular tachycardias. The pacing may be either temporary or permanent, and may use transvenous, endocardial, or direct myocardial electrode placement.

The pacing impulses are transmitted to the heart by one or more electrodes. For temporary pacing, the electrodes are placed by the transvenous route using the subclavian, internal jugular, femoral, or brachial vein. In addition, temporary leads may be loosely placed in the myocardium at the time of cardiac surgery. Transvenous electrode placement is used in 90 percent of those cases requiring permanent pacing. The major disadvantage of this is lead displacement, which occurs in about 5 percent of cases; however, the leads can usually be repositioned without thoracotomy. Although myocardial implantation necessitates thoracotomy with its accompanying perioperative mortality (2–5 percent), the leads are securely placed. This placement route is required for some modes of pacing.

The pulse generators of pacemakers now use lithium cells with an operating life of 5–10 yr. They are small (50–100 g) and usually implanted in a subcutaneous pocket beneath the clavicle.

The first pacemakers were fixed-rate devices, which now are rarely used; they have been replaced by various types of demand pacemakers. In this latter kind of pacemaker, the pacemaker output is inhibited when the patient's heart rate rises above the baseline rate of the pacemaker. This type of pacemaker is called an R wave–inhibited pacemaker. R wave–triggered pacemakers fire into the patient's QRS complex when the patient's rate rises above the base rate of the pacemaker. In the P wave–triggered mode, both atrial and ventricular electrodes are used. The pacemaker senses the patient's atrial contraction (P wave) and triggers ventricular contraction.

Pacemaker technology is changing rapidly; pacemakers currently are programmable and can be adjusted for pulse rate, current, voltage, duration, hysteresis, and sensitivity. They employ computer logic to identify the electrocardiographic waves and to respond to various conditions in a complex preprogrammed reaction.

pachy/o (pak′e-o) [Gr. *pachys* thick, clotted] a word element used in combining form to denote thick or heavy, e.g., pachymeningitis.

pachyacria (pak″e-a′kre-ah) [*pachy-* + Gr. *akron* end + *-ia*] a condition characterized by enlargement of the soft parts of the extremities.

pachycephaly (pak″e-sef′ah-le) [*pachy-* + Gr. *kephalē* head] a condition characterized by an abnormal thickening of the bones of the skull. Pachycephaly may be seen in a variety of disorders, such as acromegaly.

pachyderma (pak″e-der′mah) [*pachy-* + Gr. *derma* skin] a condition characterized by an abnormal thickening of the skin. It may be observed in a variety of conditions, such as osteomyelosclerosis.

p. laryngis, a condition characterized by the development of focal, wartlike, epithelial thickenings on the surface of the vocal cords. Also called pachyderma circumscripta.

p. oris, a condition that affects the mouth and is characterized by thickening of the oral epithelium, with raised white lesions and hyperkeratosis. It is thought to be due to chronic irritation of the oral epithelium. Upon removal of the irritant, the disorder heals within several weeks.

pachydermoperiostosis (pak″e-der″mo-per″e-os-to′sis) [*pachy-* + *derma* + N.L. *periosteum* periosteum + *-osis*] a condition characterized by a marked thickening of the skin of the face and hands, in addition to periosteal inflammation, new bone formation, arthritis, and clubbing of the fingers and toes. The exact cause of this disorder is unknown, but it is associated with diseases of the lungs, and as such is often called hereditary hypertrophic pulmonary osteoarthropathy. Also called Touraine-Salente-Golé syndrome.

pachygyria (pak″e-ji′re-ah) [*pachy-* + N.L. *gyrus* gyrus + *-ia*] the alteration of the cortex of the brain that results from arrested development. Mature gyral formation does not occur, so that there is a reduced number of gyri and a pattern characteristic of a fetal brain. This abnormality may be localized or diffuse.

pachynema (pak″e-ne′mah) [*pachy-* + Gr. *nēma* thread] see *pachytene.*

pachyonychia (pak″e-o-nik′e-ah) [*pachy-* + Gr. *onyx* nail + *-ia*] a general term used to describe an abnormal thickening of the nails.

p. congenita, a rare congenital abnormality, transmitted as an autosomal dominant trait, that is characterized by an excessive thickening of the nails, hyperkeratosis of the palms and soles, anomalies of hair, bullous lesions, and hyperkeratosis of the oral mucous membranes. Also called Jadassohn-Lewandowsky syndrome.

pachytene (pak′e-tēn) [Gr. *pachytēs* thickness] the third stage of prophase in meiosis I during which chromatids separate sufficiently for tetrads to be visible; crossover may occur. Also called *pachynema.* See also *meiosis.*

pacing (pa′sing) controlling a pace or rate, as by use of an artificial cardiac pacemaker.

pacinian corpuscle (pah-sin′e-an) [Filippo *Pacini,* Italian anatomist, 1812–1883] an encapsulated nerve ending, involved in the perception of pressure, that is found in the deeper layers of the dermis and throughout subcutaneous and some deeper tissues.

pack in computer programming, to convert data from a form in which each character or field is in a separate word or byte to a form in which two or more characters or fields are fitted into each word or byte. For example, decimal numbers can be represented in unpacked form (one binary coded–decimal [BCD] digit per byte) or in packed form (two digits per byte). The unpacked form is used for input and output, and the packed form is used for arithmetic. Cf. *unpack.*

packed cell volume see *hematocrit.*

packed red blood cells a concentrated unit of red blood cells with most of the plasma removed. The packed cells provide the same quantity of oxygen-carrying components as whole blood but in a smaller volume, thus helping to prevent circulatory overload. Additional components may also be prepared from the expressed plasma.

packet in bacteriology, a group of cells (usually eight in number) formed when parent cells divide progressively along three different axes and the cells remain together.

packing ratio the ratio of DNA length to chromatin fiber length. The DNA of each chromosome is packaged into chromatin fibers, which are shorter than the contained DNA. The packing ratio of interphase nuclei is about 50:1; the overpacking ratio of DNA in a metaphase chromosome is often greater than 10,000:1.

Paecilomyces (pe-sil″o-mi′sēz) a genus of fungi whose species resemble those of *Penicillium* except that phialides can be found singly along the hyphae as well as in a penicillate arrangement. Conidia are usually elliptic and in nonbranching chains.

paecilomycosis (pe-sil″o-mi-ko′sis) a fungal infection caused by the genus *Paecilomyces.* This organism has been isolated from the blood, thrombi, and emboli of patients who have undergone cardiac surgery. The resultant lesion of paecilomycosis is tuberculoma-like, with caseous necrosis and a cellular infiltrate of epithelioid and giant cells. *Paecilomyces lilacinus* has been reported as one of the causal agents of keratomycosis and endophthalmitis.

Paederus (pe′der-us) a genus of beetles of the family Staphylinidae (the rove beetles) that possess a dermal toxicant called pederin, which causes blistering of the skin in humans. These beetles are common in South America, Asia, and Africa.

PAF abbrev. See *platelet-activating factor.*

page (pāg) a division of the virtual memory of a computer.

Paget's disease (paj′ets) [Sir James *Paget,* English surgeon, 1814–1899] two separate disorders: Paget's disease of bone, also known as osteitis deformans; and Paget's disease of the skin, which affects the nipple and the vulvar or perianal region.

P. d. of bone, see *osteitis deformans.*

P. d. of the breast, a specialized form of ductal carcinoma that involves the skin of the nipple and areola. It often first appears as a unilateral dermatitis of the nipple with redness, crusting, and oozing. Sections show infiltration of the epidermis by malignant cells. An underlying duct cell carcinoma may be in continuity with the affected epidermis.

The disease is not common (approximately 3 percent of all breast cancers). If only the nipple is involved, metastases are infrequent (5 percent). If a breast mass is also present, the incidence of metastasis is higher and the prognosis is correspondingly poorer.

extramammary P. d., a condition, histologically similar to Paget's disease of the breast, that affects the skin of the vulva or perianal region. It appears as a plaquelike, crusted lesion, red to gray in color, with surrounding induration. In contrast to Paget's disease of the breast, approximately 70 percent of cases of extramammary Paget's disease are not associated with the presence of an underlying neoplasm.

paging system a computer memory that consists of a very large slow-access component divided into blocks, called pages, and a smaller fast-access component. The central processing unit communicates with the fast memory, which contains pages brought in from the slow memory as required.

pagophagia (pa″go-fa′je-ah) [Gr. *pagos* frost + *phagein* to eat] the abnormal desire to eat excessive amounts of ice, which may be related to iron deficiency or psychogenic factors. See also *pica.*

PAH abbrev. see *p-aminohippurate.*

pain (pān) [Old French *peine,* from L. *poena* punishment, pain] a feeling of distress, discomfort, or agony generated by specialized cells within the nervous system. It is considered to be a protective mechanism and is the most common symptom for which individuals seek treatment. Pain may be classified as physical (due to acute tissue injury), somatic (following dermatomal segments), and visceral (due to organ injury). Visceral pain often spreads along spinal afferent pathways and is classified as referred pain. Pain may also arise as a result of psychogenic factors, such as chronic tension, and may continue despite appropriate treatment.

Pain should always be treated with the mildest effective agent. Mild pain is often responsive to agents such as salicylates or propoxyphene. More severe pain may require narcotic agents such as codeine or morphine. Intractable pain may sometimes be relieved by surgical intervention to disrupt sensory pathways, but the results are unpredictable.

P-A interval the time required for a wave of depolarization to be conducted through the atria of the heart. It is measured from the onset of the P wave of the electrocardiogram to the onset of the A wave of the His bundle electrogram, and normally has a range of 5–40 msec.

pairing (pār′ing) 1. the act or process of joining into pairs.

2. in transplantation immunology, the process of selecting a compatible donor and host, usually by typing or matching.

3. in genetics, the synapsis of homologous chromosomes to form a bivalent during meiosis.

4. in molecular genetics, the hydrogen bonding of complementary base pairs in nucleic acids that form the double helix structure.

pairing segments the segments of the X and Y chromosomes that are homologous, synapse, and may cross over during meiosis. In humans, these are short segments at the tip of the short arm of each chromosome. The rest of the chromosomes are the differential segments.

pair production an interaction of high-energy gamma rays with a strong electric field, as in the vicinity of an atomic nucleus. A gamma-ray photon is converted into an electron and a positron. Because the positron is annihilated almost immediately, the overall result is the production of two 0.511-MeV photons from one photon having an energy in excess of 1.02 MeV. The excess energy is carried off as the kinetic energy of the electron.

Palaemonetes (pa-le-mo-ne′tēz) [N.L., from the Latin name of a sea god, from Gr. *palaimōn*] a genus of crayfish. The species *P. sinensis* serves as a second intermediate host for the liver fluke *Clonorchis sinensis. C. sinensis* has been found to infect humans in China who eat improperly cooked contaminated crayfish.

palat/o (pal′ah-to) [L. *palatum* palate] a word element used in combining form to denote palate, e.g., palatography.

palate (pal′at) [L. *palatum*] the partition that constitutes the roof of the mouth and the floor of the nasal cavity. The anterior two-thirds is bone (the hard palate), whereas the posterior one-third is a fleshy fold (the soft palate). The palate functions to secure food against the tongue during mastication and to close the pharyngeal isthmus during swallowing and speech.

The anterior hard palate is formed from the palatine processes of the maxillae and the horizontal plates of the palatine bones; it is covered on its upper surface by the mucous membrane of the nasal cavity and by squamous epithelium on its oral surface. A small conical process (the uvula) projects downward from the inferior surface of the soft palate.

cleft p., see *c. palate* under *cleft.*

palatine (pal′ah-tēn) [L. *palatinus*] pertaining to the palate.

palatine bone one of the paired skull bones that lie in the posterior part of the nasal cavity between the maxillae and the pterygoid processes of the sphenoid. They participate in the formation of the nasal cavity, orbital floors, palate, and pterygopalatine fossae. Each palatine bone is L shaped, with horizontal and perpendicular plates.

palatognathous (pal″ah-tog′nah-thus) [*palato-* + Gr. *gnathos* jaw] possessing a congenital cleft palate. See also *c. palate* under *cleft.*

palatography (pal″ah-tog′rah-fe) [*palato-* + Gr. *graphia,* writing, drawing, from *graphein* to write, draw] 1. the making of graphic records of the movements of the palate in speech.

2. the radiographic examination of the soft palate, usually employing barium sulfate as the contrast medium.

pali-, palin- (pal′e, pal′in) [Gr. *palin* backward, or again] a word element used in combining form to denote again, often used to indicate pathologic repetition, e.g., palindromic.

palindrome (pal′in-drōm) [Gr. *palindromos* running back, from *palin-* + *dromas* act of running] 1. a word or phrase that reads the same backward as forward.

2. in genetics, DNA that contains self-complementary sequences within each strand, which can fold back on itself to form double-stranded loops. In hybridization reactions, this DNA renatures even more rapidly than do highly repeated satellite sequences. Current data suggest that palindromes account for 5 percent or more of the total genomes of many eukaryotes.

A suggested role for palindromes is as recognition sites for regulatory proteins, as shown by the lactose operator in the bacterial lactose operon, which is an example of an imperfect palindrome. The operator binds to a regulatory molecule, the lactose repressor.

Restriction endonucleases, enzymes from bacterial cells that selectively hydrolyze double-stranded DNA at certain palindromic sequences, have become important research tools. These enzymes break both strands of DNA at special recognition sites, which may not be at the same point on both strands.

Also called *snapback DNA.* Cf. *hairpin loop.*

palisade (pal″ĭ-sād) [Fr. *palissade,* from L. *palus* stake] the arrangement of cells in stained smears of certain bacteria when two or more rods are arranged side by side like pales in a picket fence. The term is used to describe the arrangement of cells in regular rows in tissue sections, a characteristic of certain neoplasms, e.g., schwannoma.

palisading a histologic pattern seen particularly in some tumors of Schwann cells, less frequently in smooth muscle and other soft tissue neoplasms in which the nuclei form parallel rows. Also called Verocay body.

palladium (Pd) (pah-la′de-um) [N.L., from the asteroid *Pallas*] a ductile, silvery-white metallic element of the platinum group; atomic number 46; atomic weight 106.4; and 4d transition element; oxidation states +2, +4. It is used in alloys and as a catalyst. Palladium has low toxicity.

palladium chloride a dark brown crystalline solid, $PdCl_2$; used as a reagent to detect carbon monoxide, which reduces $PdCl_2$ to metallic platinum; M.W. 177.30. See also *carbon monoxide assays.*

palliate (pal′e-āt) [L. *palliatus* cloaked, covered, from *pallium* cloak] to relieve symptoms without necessarily evoking a cure. This term is often used to describe a drug (palliative drug) that can relieve the symptoms of a disorder without necessarily effecting a cure.

pallor (pal′or) [L.] paleness; absence of skin coloration.

palmar (pal′mar) [L. *palmaris,* from *palma* palm] pertaining to the palm.

palmitate (pal′mĭ-tāt) any salt, anion, or ester form of palmitic acid.

palmitic acid (pal-mit′ic) hexadecanoic acid, the most abundant fatty acid in humans.

palmitoleate (pal″mĭ-to′le-āt) any salt, anion, or ester form of palmitoleic acid.

palmitoleic acid (pal-mit′o-la-ik) *cis*-9-hexadecenoic acid, a naturally occurring monounsaturated fatty acid. It is found in the fat of marine animals, reptiles, avians, amphibians, and, to a lesser extent, mammals.

palpation (pal-pa′shun) [L. *palpatio,* from *palpare* to touch softly] an action of physical diagnosis in which the fingers are applied to the body surface to determine the condition of structures deeper within the body. It is useful for indicating organ enlargement, softening, and displacement, as well as the presence of tumors.

palpebra (pal′pĕ-brah), pl. *palpebrae* [L.] see *eyelid.*

palpitation (pal″pĭ-ta′shun) [L. *palpitatio,* from *palpitare* to throb] the conscious awareness of a forceful, rapid, or irregular heartbeat. It is not pathognomonic for any physical disease and may reflect a psychic rather than a physical disturbance. In many cases, the awareness of palpitation occurs during emotional or physical stress, for example, anxiety about heart disease or a long-standing emotional illness. Organic causes include anemias, thyroid disorders, fever, drugs, neoplasms of the adrenal medulla, and tachycardias.

palsy (pawl′ze) [Old English *palesie,* from Old French *paralysie,* from L. *paralysis*] a term used to connote paresis, or a condition of incomplete paralysis.

Bell's p., sudden paralysis of the muscles of one side of the face from unknown causes. It may occur at any age but is most common in patients aged 20–50 yr. The facial nerve (seventh cranial nerve), which innervates the muscles of facial expression, may possibly be affected by immune or viral agents. The affected muscles of the face become lax, so that the mouth may droop and drool and the patient may be unable to close one eye. The involved side of the face becomes flat, weak, and expressionless. Recovery usually occurs within 2–8 wk. Facial paralysis (prosopoplegia) may also have other causes, such as compression of the facial nerve by a neoplasm. Also called facial paralysis.

bulbar p., weakness or paralysis of the muscles supplied by the cranial nerves arising in the nuclei of the medulla oblongata, with nuclear involvement of the last four or five cranial nerves. The tongue, pharynx, larynx, and palate are affected, leading to difficulties in chewing, talking, and swallowing. Electromyography may be useful in diagnosis. True bulbar palsy may be associated with amyotrophic lateral sclerosis, with tumors, with congenital abnormalities, and with infections such as poliomyelitis. Treatment is directed at the underlying cause.

cerebral p. syndromes, nonprogressive, related motor disorders characterized by varying degrees of weakness and lack of muscle coordination. Cerebral palsy (CP) syndromes are due to gestational or perinatal central nervous system damage, and they affect 1–2 children per 1000. Although the causes are difficult to determine, lack of oxygen to the brain, infection, immune disorders, and injury have been implicated. These disorders may result in hemiplegia, paraplegia, or quadriplegia; spastic, dyskinetic, or ataxic syndromes; or combinations of these. Mental retardation, seizures, and visual disorders are also seen.

Early diagnosis is difficult and often may not be established until the second year of life. Tests to exclude metabolic, progressive, structural, or hereditary diseases are helpful. Treatment is designed to develop the patient's maximal capabilities within the limits imposed by the physical handicaps.

injection p., a peripheral neuropathy of the sciatic nerve, more frequent in infants, caused by the pressure or toxic effect exerted by a substance injected directly into or around the nerve. The symptoms, which may be immediate or delayed in onset, include pain, numbness, and weakness of the leg and thigh muscles supplied by the nerve.

sleep p., an entrapment syndrome of the radial nerve that occurs when the nerve is compressed as it exits the intermuscular septum distal to the axilla.

"Saturday night" palsy occurs in a patient, usually in an alcoholic stupor, whose arm has been draped over the back of a chair or bench for a prolonged period. The compression in "honeymoon" palsy is applied in the same location when a person's head has been resting in the crook of the patient's arm. The symptoms include paralysis or weakness of radial nerve–innervated muscles distal to the triceps. Hypesthesia and hypalgesia are generally slight.

Paludina (pal-u-de′nah) [L. *palud-,* from *palus* marsh + *-ina*] a genus of mollusks that serves as a first intermediate host for the fluke *Echinostoma revolutum,* which is parasitic in ducks, geese, and fowl, and occasionally in humans.

paludism (pal′u-dizm) see *malaria.*

pampiniform plexus (pam-pin′ĭ-form plek′sus) [L.] 1. in the male, a convoluted mass of veins arising from the testis and epididymis. It forms a major constituent of the spermatic cord.

2. in the female, a network of ovarian veins in the broad ligament.

PAN abbrev., used to refer either to the class of compounds, the peroxyacylnitrates (RCO_2ONO_2), or to the specific compound peroxyacetylnitrate, CH_3-CO_2ONO_2; see *peroxyacylnitrate.*

pan- (pan) [Gr. *pan* neuter form of *pas* "all"] a prefix word element to denote all, e.g., panagglutination.

panagglutination (pan″ah-gloo″tĭ-na′shun) [*pan-* + L. *agglutinare* to glue, from *gluten* glue] a condition in which a patient's serum agglutinates all the normal red blood cells owing to the presence of an antibody in the serum, such as anti-I against normal cells.

Pancoast's syndrome (pan′kōsts) [Henry Khunrath *Pancoast,* Philadelphia radiologist, 1875–1939] weakness and atrophy of the muscles of the arm and hand, often with pain and sensory loss, in association with a tumor (often bronchogenic carcinoma) in the apex of the lung. Horner's syndrome also may be present. These symptoms are due to neoplastic involvement of the brachial plexus and sympathetic ganglia at the base of the neck. Destruction of the ribs and vertebrae may also be seen. See also *Horner's syndrome.*

pancreas (pan′kre-as), pl. *pancreata* [*pan-* + Gr. *kreas* flesh] the mixed exocrine and endocrine gland that lies on the posterior wall of the abdomen, extending from the duodenum to the spleen. For descriptive purposes it is subdivided into a head, neck, body, and tail. The head is the expanded right end enclosed in the duodenal loop; its lower part forms a short uncinate process that curves to the left behind the superior mesenteric vessels. The neck is ill-defined but is considered to be about 1 in. long; it connects the head to the body, which constitutes the greatest part of the length of the pancreas. The body merges with the tail, which is the thickened left end that indents the spleen below its hilum.

Exocrine secretions are drained by the main pancreatic duct (duct of Wirsung), which begins at the tail and runs along the length of the body, receiving many tributaries. It curves downward in the head to reach the ampulla of Vater, where it enters the duodenum, generally in company with the common bile duct. Part of the head of the pancreas has a separate embryologic derivation from the rest of the organ, and its duct may persist instead of merging with the main duct, carrying secretions directly to the duodenum (duct of Santorini or accessory pancreatic duct).

The endocrine portion of the pancreas consists of a large number of clusters of cells distributed throughout the organ but more numerous in the body and tail. These are the islets of Langerhans, and they have a rich capillary network into which secretions of the cells are passed directly. The cells are of at least three types in the human pancreas: A or alpha cells, located at the periphery of the islets, forming glucagon; B or beta cells, the most numerous, occupying the central portion of the islet and forming proinsulin; and D or delta cells, mostly interposed between the A and B cells, forming somatostatin.

The cells of the exocrine pancreas are arranged in spherical clusters or acini, and pass their secretion into a small central cavity, the acinar lumen, which is continuous with an intercalated duct. Each acinar cell is a truncated pyramid, containing plentiful granular endoplasmic reticulum at its base and accumulated secretion in the form of zymogen granules in its more apical cytoplasm. The exocrine secretion is a clear alkaline fluid that contains electrolytes and enzymes. The electrolytes are formed by the intercalated duct cells and by similar-appearing cells within an acinus, the centroacinar cells. The pancreatic enzymes include proteolytic proenzymes (trypsinogen, chymotrypsinogen), lipase, and amylase. Exocrine secretion is induced by neural and hormonal stimuli. Parasympathetic (vagal) impulses cause the secretion of enzymes; and two hormones, secretin and cholecystokinin-pancreozymin (CK-PZ), formed by mucosal cells in the upper small bowel, promote the secretion of bicarbonate and enzymes, respectively. Gastrin has an effect on the pancreas similar to that of CK-PZ.

pancreas scan an imaging procedure in nuclear medicine that uses the imaging agent selenomethionine Se 75. This scan is most useful in cases of suspected pancreatic malignancy. The false-negative rate is less than 10 percent; however, there are a large number of false-positives. The scan also is sometimes used in the diagnosis of pancreatitis.

In the procedure, the agent is given intravenously and localizes in the pancreas and liver, sites of active protein synthesis. A scintillation camera is the preferred imaging system. Exposures are made at 10-min intervals; the concentration of radioactivity shifts throughout the course of the study, filling the head and the tail of the pancreas at different times. A technetium Tc 99m sulfur colloid liver scan is usually performed without moving the patient or the camera. If computerized digital image subtraction is available, the liver activity can be partially removed from the pancreas scan.

pancreat/o (pan″kre-at′o) [L. *pancreaticus*] a word element used in combining form to denote relationship to the pancreas, e.g., pancreatography.

pancreatic/o (pan″kre-at′ĭ-ko) [L. *pancreaticus*] a word element used in combining form to denote the pancreatic duct, e.g., pancreaticoduodenostomy.

pancreatic (pan″kre-at′ik) pertaining to the pancreas.

pancreatic colipase a small protein found in pancreatic juice that binds to lipase in a 2:1 molar complex; M.W. 10,000. It prevents surface denaturation of the lipase and in some way promotes the action of the lipase on a fat surface. Pancreatic colipase is noncatalytic by itself.

pancreatic islet cell antibody test an assay to detect antibodies against pancreatic islet cells. The test involves indirect immunofluorescence using the patient's serum with unfixed sections of human pancreas (from individuals with blood group O) or monkey pancreas as the substrate. A fluorescence microscope with epiillumination should be used to read the test.

Antibodies to pancreatic islet cells occur in 60–80 percent of those with insulin-dependent diabetes early after onset of the condition, and they decline as the disease progresses. The antibodies react with types A, B, and D islet cells. Their role in the pathogenesis of diabetes, and possibly of other diseases, is not well understood.

pancreatic islet stains differential stains that permit recognition of the three cell types in the pancreatic islets. Following fixation of fresh tissue in Bouin's fluid, sections are stained by the chrome alum hematoxylin-phloxine method or the aldehyde fuchsin method. Alpha cells and D cells are readily distinguished by the latter method, but not by the former. Islet cells can also be differentiated by immunohistochemical methods, which utilize specific antisera to the hormones produced by the cells, e.g., antiinsulin or antiglucagon.

pancreatic juice a bicarbonate-rich, alkaline, isotonic exocrine secretion of the pancreas that is transported to the intestine for use in digestion. Enzymes and zymogens present include trypsinogen, chymotrypsinogen, proelastase, procarboxypeptidases, prophospholipase, lipase, α-amylase, deoxyribonuclease, and ribonuclease. Daily volume in the human adult is 500–800 ml.

The HCO_3^- concentration increases with flow rate, from 25 mmol/l to as high as 130 mmol/l. The output of volume and HCO_3^- is stimulated by secretin; enzyme output, by cholecystokinin-pancreozymin.

See also *duodenal content examination.*

pancreatic lipase see *lipase.*

pancreatic tumors neoplasms of cells of the pancreas. Primary neoplasms can arise from the exocrine or endocrine cells. Tumors of the exocrine pancreas may be solid or cystic. The cystic lesions must be distinguished from nonneoplastic pancreatic cysts, the most common of which is the pancreatic pseudocyst that develops following damage to the exocrine pancreas through inflammation or trauma. Some pseudocysts are large and extend out of the organ into the peritoneal cavity. They contain clear or turbid fluid; although the fluid can be drained surgically, it tends to reaccumulate, and thus resection or marsupialization may be more effective. Retention cysts develop following obstruction of a portion of the pancreatic duct system. Developmental cysts of the pancreas are usually small and multiple and may form a component of von Hippel–Lindau disease.

Benign cystic neoplasms of the pancreas (cystadenomas) are uncommon. Typically, they contain many compartments into which protrude branching papillary projections covered by a single layer of columnar cells.

Most carcinomas of the exocrine pancreas develop from duct cells, whereas fewer than 5 percent are of acinar cell origin. Duct cell tumors form glandular aggregates and solid nests of cells within a fibrous stroma. The uncommon acinar cell carcinoma tends to form more organized microglandular or solid patterns and may be mistaken in sections for an islet cell tumor. Ultrastructurally, acinar cell tumors have abundant endoplasmic reticulum and large secretory granules. Rarely, a patient with a lipase-forming acinar cell tumor presents with polyarthropathy.

The incidence of pancreatic cancer in the United States is rising; smoking and dietary habits have been implicated. Most patients are older adults. The majority of the tumors occur in the head of the organ where they frequently occlude the common bile duct, producing obstructive jaundice. Tumors of the body and tail of the pancreas may be present for a long time before detection, and metastases, particularly to the liver, are frequent. Symptoms include gastrointestinal complaints, weight loss, back pain, and, occasionally, migratory venous thrombosis.

Radiologic procedures, including CT scans, are important in diagnosis, but tissue confirmation from a fine-needle aspiration or core needle biopsy, or an open biopsy at exploratory laparotomy, is necessary; good tissue preparations are important, as distinction from chronic pancreatitis can be difficult. The prognosis of pancreatic carcinoma is dismal. A few small lesions can be resected, but in most instances treatment is palliative, with 5-yr survival in only 2 percent of patients.

Tumors of the endocrine pancreas are collectively referred to as islet cell neoplasms. Usually occurring in adults, they may be benign (adenoma) or malignant (carcinoma). Hyperfunction is occasionally due to a diffuse hyperplasia of islet tissue. Most islet cell tumors can be shown by immunoperoxidase techniques to be forming one or several hormones; approximately 25 percent form multiple hormones, and some 10 percent do not give any positive staining reactions.

Histologically, the tumors commonly show a resemblance to normal islet cell tissue. Amyloid is often present in the stroma. Only 10 percent of insulin-forming islet cell tumors are malignant; in contrast, most gastrin- or glucagon-forming tumors give rise to metastases. Islet cell carcinomas can usually be identified only by the presence of invasion or metastases. Metastases usually involve regional nodes and the liver.

The more common clinical syndromes associated with pancreatic endocrine tumors are hypoglycemia with a beta-cell, insulin-forming neoplasm (insulinoma); anemia, diabetes, and necrolytic skin lesions with an alpha-cell, glucagon-forming tumor (glucagonoma); peptic ulceration from a gastrin-forming tumor, which in most instances is located in the pancreas (gastrinoma) and is less often found in the wall of the duodenum; and the watery diarrhea syndrome (WDHA), with hypokalemia and achlorhydria in which the islet cell tumor is forming vasoactive intestinal polypeptide (VIP) in about 50 percent of the cases. Islet cell tumors may coexist with other endocrine neoplasms in multiple endocrine neoplastic syndromes.

See also *gastrinoma, glucagonoma,* and *insulinoma.*

pancreatitis (pan″kre-ah-ti′tis) [*pancreat-* + *-itis*] an acute or chronic inflammation of the pancreas. In the acute form, pancreatic function and histology may return to normal following elimination of the cause. Chronic pancreatitis, however, persists even if the cause is removed, and may be associated with intermittent bouts of acute disease.

acute p., a severe inflammation of the pancreas associated with the escape of lytic pancreatic enzymes into the surrounding tissues. The exact pathogenesis of this disorder is unclear, and a number of clinical causes are known. Biliary tract disease is the most common underlying factor, followed by surgery, alcoholism, and infectious diseases. Frequently, the cause cannot be determined. Following the onset of acute pancreatitis, acute epigastric pain, nausea, vomiting, prostration, sweating, fever, hypotension, and mild jaundice are common. The abdomen is usually tender. A biopsy shows edema with acute inflammatory cells and varying degrees of necrosis of the acinar cells. Pseudocysts, abscess formation, and fat necrosis may occur.

Laboratory findings include leukocytosis, hypocalcemia, hypomagnesemia, hypokalemia, glycosuria, hyperglycemia, and elevated serum bilirubin. Serum amylase levels are elevated within 24 hr; serum lipase rises more slowly. An amylase/creatinine clearance ratio of greater than 5.5 percent usually indicates acute pancreatitis. X-rays may reveal calcification, gallstones, and a localized loop of gas-distended small bowel (sentinel loop). Ultrasonography and electrocardiography may provide information helpful in establishing the diagnosis. The prognosis in the severe form is poor; mortality rates may exceed 50 percent. In milder forms, the mortality rate is considerably lower.

chronic p., a long-term inflammation of the pancreas, resulting in progressive fibrosis and necrosis of the parenchyma. The causes include alcoholism, biliary tract disease, hypercalcemia, hyperlipoproteinemias, and hereditary pancreatitis. The affected individual experiences persistent or intermittent upper abdominal pain that may radiate to the back. Nausea, vomiting, constipation, gas, and anorexia are frequently observed. Steatorrhea, often in association with intestinal malabsorption, is seen. Attacks may last for hours or weeks.

Laboratory tests for the documentation of chronic pancreatitis include serum and urinary amylase, examination of the duodenal contents (volume, bicarbonate, amylase, etc., after intravenous administration of cholecystokinin-pancreozymin and secretin), chemical detection of fecal fat using triolein I 131, and glucose tolerance tests. Radiographs often reveal pancreatic calcification. Ultrasonography, endoscopic retrograde pancreatography, pancreatic nuclear scanning, and retrograde cholangiography may aid in establishing the diagnosis.

pancreatography (pan″kre-ah-tog′rah-fe) [*pancreato-* + Gr. *graphia* writing, drawing, from *graphein* to write or draw] a surgicoradiologic procedure in which a water-soluble iodinated contrast medium is injected into the main pancreatic duct and films are made while the abdomen is open. Also called direct pancreatography and operative pancreatography. See also *ERCP.*

reflux method of p., a type of operative pancreatography. In this procedure, following an injection of morphine to close the sphincter of Oddi, the contrast medium is injected into the cystic duct or the common bile duct and backs up into the main pancreatic duct. Several pancreaticograms are exposed during temporary respiratory arrest induced by the anesthetist. See also *ERCP.*

transduodenal p., a type of operative pancreatography in which the contrast medium is injected through a catheter passed through an incision in the duodenum.

pancreatolithiasis (pan″kre-ah-to-lĭ-thi′ah-sis) [*pancreato-* + Gr. *lithiasis* stone-disease, from *lithos* stone + *-iasis*] the presence of minute concretions or calculi in the ducts of the parenchyma of the pancreas. Such bodies may be seen in chronic pancreatitis when protein in the ducts precipitates and eventually becomes calcified. This may lead to ductal stenosis, fibrosis, and destruction of the substance of the pancreas.

pancreozymin (pan′kre-o-zi″min) see *cholecystokinin.*

pancuronium bromide (pan-ku-ro′ne-um bro′mīd) a nondepolarizing neuromuscular blocking drug used to induce skeletal muscle relaxation during surgery; it is five times as potent as tubocurarine. Adverse reactions, primarily respiratory depression, are due to excessive muscle relaxation; the intensity of the effect is increased by volatile inhalation anesthetics such as diethyl ether and halothane, and also by succinylcholine. A cholinesterase inhibitor, e.g., pyridostigmine or neostigmine, can be used to antagonize the relaxant action or to assist recovery.

pancytopenia (pan″si-to-pe′ne-ah) [*pan-* + *-cyte* cell, from Gr. *kytos* hollow container + *penia* poverty] the pathologic depression of all cellular elements of blood. Causes include aplastic anemia, hypersplenism, folate deficiency, hematologic malignancies, osteopetrosis, myelofibrosis, and several types of cancer chemotherapy and radiotherapy.

congenital p., see *aplastic a.* under *anemia.*

pandemic (pan-dem′ik) [*pan-* + Gr. *dēmos* people] an epidemic of a disease with unusually widespread distribution, often starting in one area and spreading from there throughout an entire country or continent, or the whole world. Examples of pandemic diseases include outbreaks of influenza A in 1918, 1957, and 1968; syphilis in the late fifteenth century; and plague during the sixth century, periodically throughout the Middle Ages, and in 1898.

panencephalitis (pan″en-sef″ah-li′tis) [*pan-* + Gr. *enkephaloc* brain + *-itis*] any disease characterized by inflammation of both gray and white matter.

subacute sclerosing p. (SSPE), a disease of the central nervous system that affects both gray and white matter and is characterized by the destruction of neurons and myelinated fibers, usually ending in death. Characteristic inclusion bodies are found in neurons and glial cells on pathologic examination. The disease rarely develops after age 18 yr; it is thought to be of viral origin and possibly associated with the measles virus. Thus, high levels of antibody to measles virus have been found in the serum and cerebrospinal fluid. Clinically, the disorder is characterized by personality changes, progressive intellectual deterioration, seizures, myoclonic jerking, visual loss, and various motor deficits, and usually follows a progressive course to a fatal outcome. The CSF contains an elevated gamma-globulin content.

The electroencephalogram shows a reduction in alpha rhythm and the appearance of recurrent generalized high-voltage, slow-wave complexes; these can last as long as 3 sec, are repeated regularly at 4- to 14-sec intervals, and may be temporally related to myoclonic jerking movements. There is no known treatment for the disorder.

panendoscopy (pan″en-dos′ko-pe) see *endoscopy.*

Paneth cell (pah′nāt) [Joseph *Paneth,* German physician, 1857–1890] one of the pyramidal epithelial cells that line the base of the small intestinal crypts; the large secretory granules in the apical cytoplasm may contain a peptidase or lysozyme.

Pangonia (pan-go′ne-ah) a genus of blood-sucking flies of the family Tabanidae. These flies (the zimbs) are common in Ethiopia and often attack humans.

panhypopituitarism (pan-hi″po-pĭ-tu′ĭ-tar-izm) [*pan-* + Gr. *hypo* under + *pituitary* + *-ism*] a generalized deficiency of all anterior pituitary hormones, including thyrotropin (TSH), corticotropin (ACTH), gonadotropins (LH and FH), growth hormone, and prolactin. Many symptoms may result, and dwarfism in children, sexual dysfunction, weight loss, easy fatigue, hypotension, and hypoglycemia may occur. Also called *Simmonds' disease.* See also *hypopituitarism.*

panmixis (pan-mik′sis) [*pan-* + Gr. *mixis* mixing, from *mignynai* to mix] see *random mating.*

panniculitis (pan-nik″u-li′tis) an inflammatory disorder of the subcutaneous fat. A number of forms occur, and in some there is an associated vasculitis. For certain types of panniculitis, an immunologic basis has been suggested, whereas others are associated with systemic conditions including infections and malignancy. In some instances the etiology is unknown.

In Weber-Christian disease, also known as systemic nodular panniculitis, extensive cutaneous involvement is accompanied by a broad spectrum of inflammation of deeper tissues, including joints and viscera. The disorder characteristically remits and recurs over a period of months, but eventual recovery is usual. Some individuals with pancreatic disease, including the rare lipase-producing acinar cell carcinoma, have focal inflammation of the subcutaneous fat lobules. The tender red lesions histologically show the changes of fat necrosis, and they heal leaving a small, depressed scar. In erythema induratum, painful nodules occur on the calves and may ulcerate. Histologic sections show an accompanying vasculitis. This form of panniculitis is seen in a number of systemic diseases, including tuberculosis and other infections. In erythema nodosum, the nodules usually occur in the pretibial region and remit spontaneously, and the histologic changes are nonspecific. A hypersensitivity type vasculitis is associated with a variety of infections and drug reactions. Adiposis dolorosa (Dercum's disease) is characterized by the occurrence of painful subcutaneous nodules in older obese females who have lost weight. A form of nodular panniculitis in children with rheumatic fever has been associated with the withdrawal of steroid therapy. The (inappropriate) term mesenteric panniculitis has been applied to an inflammatory disorder of undetermined etiology, occurring in older males, that is characterized clinically by intestinal obstruction, ascites, and steatorrhea. Histologic sections of the involved mesentery show fat necrosis.

See also *adiposis dolorosa, e. induratum* and *e. nodosum* under *erythema,* and *Weber-Christian disease.*

mesenteric p., an unusual lesion, occurring in the retroperitoneum and the mesentery, that is characterized by chronic fat necrosis. There is pain, fever, and a palpable mass. CT scans, arteriograms, and barium radiographic studies may help to localize the lesion. A biopsy may be required to confirm the diagnosis. There is no specific therapy and surgical removal is not recommended. Most frequently, the disorder regresses spontaneously.

metastatic p., an unusual form of chronic fat necrosis, characterized by inflammation and widespread adipose cell death. It is accompanied by fever, polyarthritis, malaise, and bone destruction. It is frequently associated with disorders of the pancreas. Although the precise cause is unknown, metastatic panniculitis is thought to be an immunologically mediated disease. The prognosis is poor, and death often follows within several months.

relapsing febrile nodular p., see *Weber-Christian disease.*

panniculus (pah-nik′u-lus), pl. *panniculi* [L., dim. of *pannus* cloth] a membranelike layer, e.g., panniculus carnosus.

p. adiposus, [NA], the subcutaneous fat.

pannus (pan′us) [L. "a piece of cloth"] 1. superficial vascularization of the cornea marked by ingrowth of blood vessels from the limbus in chronic corneal ulceration. Granulation tissue may form and cover the lesion.

2. folds of synovium that cover the surface of the articular cartilage and joint capsules, most commonly seen in rheumatoid arthritis. The pannus may destroy the articular cartilage and underlying subchondral bone, resulting in fibrous adhesions and bony ankylosis.

panography (pan-og′rah-fe) [*pan-* + Gr. *graphein* to write or draw] see *panoramic t.* under *tomography.*

panophthalmitis (pan-of″thal-mi′tis) [*pan-* + Gr. *ophthalmos* eye + *-itis*] a suppurative inflammation of the eye, usually extending to involve all three layers and leading to loss of vision. There is severe pain, swelling, rapid loss of vision, and extensive accumulation of pus. The eye quickly becomes shrunken and purulent; vomiting, fever, and systemic symptoms may occur. The pyogenic bacteria reach the eye through trauma, metastatic spread, corneal ulcers, or other routes.

pan-oral radiography (pan-or′al) see *panoramic t.* under *tomography.*

Panstrongylus (pan-stron′jĭ-lus) [*pan-* + Gr. *strongylos* round] a genus of triatomine bugs that are known to attack humans. Two species, *P. geniculatus* and *P. megistus,* are transmitters of *Trypanosoma cruzi* in Central and South America. Also called Mexican bedbug, cone-nosed bug, wild bedbug, assassin bug, or kissing bug.

pantetheine (pan″tĕ-the′in) a naturally occurring amide of pantothenic acid and β-mercaptoethylamine; an intermediate in the biosynthesis of CoA in mammalian liver and some microorganisms.

D-pantoic acid (pan″to-ik) a part of the molecule of the vitamin pantothenic acid, α,γ-dihydroxy-β,β-dimethylbutyric acid. It is combined in amide linkage with β-alanine to form pantothenic acid.

pantomography (pan″to-mog′rah-fe) [*pan-* + Gr. *tomos* slice + *graphein* to write or draw] see *panoramic t.* under *tomography.*

Pantopaque (pan-to-pāk′) trademark. See *iophendylate.*

pantothenic acid (pan″to-then′ik) [Gr. *pantothen* from all sides] a water-soluble vitamin, (*R*)-*N*-(2,4-dihydroxy-3,3-dimethyl-1-oxobutyl)-β-alanine; M.W. 219.23. It is an essential component of coenzyme A and acyl carrier protein, which function in the biosynthesis and degradation of fatty acids. Pantothenic acid is found in many foods, particularly eggs, kidney, liver, and yeast. As yet there is no well-established evidence for the existence of pantothenic acid deficiency in humans. See also *acyl carrier protein, coenzyme A,* and *pantetheine.*

pantothenic acid assays 1. microbiologic assay. On the addition of graded amounts of pantothenic acid, the extent of growth of *Lactobacillus plantarum* is determined by measuring the turbidity of the cell suspension at 620 nm. A standard curve of pantothenic acid concentration against increased absorbance is plotted, from which the amount of pantothenic acid in the sample can be determined.

pantoyl-β-alanine (pan′toil) pantothenic acid, a vitamin; pantoic acid combined in amide linkage with β-alanine.

panzootic (pan″zo-ot′ik) [*pan-* + Gr. *zōon* animal] a widespread occurrence of disease in an animal community.

PAO abbrev. for peak acid output; see under *gastric function tests.*

papain (pah-pa′in) [from Sp. *papaya*] an enzyme of the hydrolase class (EC 3.4.22.2) that catalyzes the hydrolysis of proteins and polypeptides to smaller polypeptides. It is derived from the papow plant, *Carica papaya.* Papain is used in medicine as a protein digestant in the topical treatment of insect stings and sloughing and infected wounds, and in immunology to split the immunoglobulin molecule into two Fab fragments and one Fc fragment. It is also used as a meat tenderizer. See also *immunoglobulin.*

Papanicolaou's stain (pap″ah-nik″o-la′o͞oz) [George Nicolas *Papanicolaou,* Greek physician, anatomist, and cytologist in the United States, 1883–1962] the most commonly used method of staining smears and millipore filtrates of cells from various body fluids and secretions from the respiratory, digestive, or genitourinary tracts. The smears are examined to detect malignancy as indicated by neoplastic changes in the exfoliated cells. Vaginal and cervical smears stained by this method are also suitable for assessing the individual's estrogen levels.

This technique produces a brilliant transparent stain, which reveals fine nuclear and cytoplasmic detail owing to the alcoholic phase staining. The nuclei stain blue; the cytoplasm stains various shades of pink, blue, green, yellow, and orange.

Smears are fixed in alcohol (95 percent ethyl alcohol) or in equal parts of alcohol and ether. The slides are then hydrated through graded alcohols, stained regressively in Harris' hematoxylin, and differentiated in hydrochloric acid or progressively in Mayer's hematoxylin (see hematoxylin). The slides are returned through graded alcohols to 95 percent alcohol, stained, cleared, and mounted.

See also *Pap test.*

papaverine hydrochloride (pah-pav′er-in) [L. *papaver* poppy] [USP], a benzylisoquinoline alkaloid extracted from opium, which produces vasodilation and smooth muscle relaxation but not analgesia. It is used to relieve smooth muscle spasms of bronchi, ureters, and the gastrointestinal tract, and to treat peripheral vascular disease and peripheral and pulmonary embolism.

paper chromatography a type of chromatography in which the stationary phase is a sheet of special-grade filter paper and the mobile phase is a solvent or solvent mixture. The sample, dissolved in a solvent, is applied to the paper as a spot and dried. The paper is then placed in a developing tank with the lower edge touching the solvent. As the solvent rises by capillary action through the pores in the paper, the sample separates into its components as a result of differences in solubility in the solvent components and differences in the affinity for the adsorbent. After this process (development), the paper is dried and the components are visualized by spraying with various reagents. Identification is by color reaction, or by R_f values, i.e., the ratio of the distance a spot moves to the distance the solvent front moves. In two-dimensional chromatography, the dried paper is rotated by 90° and rechromatographed in either the same or a different solvent mixture. See also *thin-layer chromatography.*

paper tape 1. a computer input-output medium; a continuous paper ribbon in which data are recorded by holes punched in the tape. Commonly, there are eight hole positions (channels) across the tape so that an eight-bit character can be recorded in each column. Also called *punched tape.*
2. the ASCII code in teletype applications.

paper tape punch a computer ouput device that writes data on paper tape.

paper tape reader a computer input device that senses data on paper tape.

papill/o (pap′ĭ-lo) [L. *papilla* a nipple] a word element used in combining form to denote nipplelike or fingerlike, e.g., papillary.

papilla (pah-pil′ah), pl. *papillae* [L. "a nipple"] any small cone- or nipple-shaped projection.

bile p., see *major duodenal p.*

circumvallate papillae, the largest papillae of the tongue; arranged in a V-shaped row in front of the terminal sulcus on the dorsal aspect of the tongue. Each of the papillae (8–12 in number) is surrounded by a circular depression.

dental p., the small mass of ectomesenchyme capped by the enamel organ that forms the tooth bud.

duodenal p., a small, rounded elevation on the interior of the posteromedial wall of the second part of the duodenum, 7–10 cm distal to the pylorus. The united common bile and main pancreatic ducts open into the duodenal lumen through its summit. An additional minor papilla is frequently found on the anteromedial aspect of the duodenum at the site of the opening of the accessory pancreatic duct.

filiform papillae, the smallest and most numerous papillae on the dorsal surface of the tongue. They are characteristically arranged in V-shaped rows from the foramen cecum forward.

foliate papillae, parallel mucosal folds on the margins of the tongue at the junction of its body and root.

fungiform papillae, the elevated, domelike papillae found mainly on the sides and apex of the tongue, but also scattered irregularly over its dorsal surface.

lingual papillae, the filiform, fungiform, vallate, foliate, and conical papillae of the tongue.

major duodenal p., a small elevation into the lumen of the duodenum at the site of the opening of the conjoined common bile duct and main pancreatic duct. Also called *bile p.*

minor duodenal p., a small elevation into the lumen of the duodenum at the site of the opening of the accessory pancreatic duct.

renal p., one of the rounded projections, the apices of the renal pyramids, that indent the walls of each minor calyx of the renal sinus; 10–40 collecting ducts perforate the summit of each papilla.

retinal p., the small raised disk on the retina corresponding to the blind spot, which is the point where the optic nerve penetrates the retina. The optic nerve, which consists of retinal ganglion cell axons, is pierced at its center by the central artery and vein of the retina. Also called nerve head, optic disk, and optic papilla.

urethral p., a slight elevation in the vestibule of the vagina on which is situated the external orifice of the urethra.

papillary (pap′ĭ-ler″e) 1. resembling a nipple.

2. having a structure characterized by the presence of one or more frond-like protrusions from a surface, e.g., papillary transitional cell carcinoma.

papillary carcinoma (pap′ĭ-ler″e kar″sĭ-no′mah) [*papill-* + *-ary*] a malignant neoplasm of epithelial origin that exhibits a microscopic pattern of finger-like projections.

papillary muscles conical muscular projections from the walls of the cardiac ventricles, attached to the cusps of the atrioventricular valves by the chordae tendinae. There is an anterior and a posterior papillary muscle in each ventricle, and a group of small papillary muscles on the septum of the right ventricle.

papillate (pap′il-āt) having or resembling papillae.

papilledema (pap″il-ĕ-de′mah) [*papill-* + Gr. *oidēma* swelling] the swelling of the head of the optic nerve, due to venous obstruction and congestion resulting from increased intracranial pressure. Causes include tumors and abscesses, edema, hemorrhage, and infections of the brain. It usually occurs bilaterally, with elevation of the optic disk, destruction of the physiologic cup, and blurring of the disk margins. Although vision is not initially affected except for enlargement of the blind spot, failure to relieve the increased intracranial pressure may lead to optic atrophy and loss of vision. Also called choked disk syndrome.

papillitis (pap″ĭ-li′tis) [*papill-* + *-itis*] a general term used to describe inflammation of the anal, lingual, or optic papillae.

anal p., an inflammation of the anal papillae, causing pain and burning on defecation and leading to papillary hypertrophy. This condition may be diagnosed on digital or anoscopic examination.

chronic lingual p., an inflammation of the lingual papillae, often with glossitis, that leads to pain and burning sensations. It may be associated with pernicious anemia, diuretics, nutritional deficiencies, infections, and diabetes mellitus. Often, no cause can be found. Treatment is symptomatic only. Also called glossodynia and glossopyrosis.

optic p., an inflammation of the optic nerve, resulting in reduced vision. The lesion is visible ophthalmoscopically and may follow viral illness, multiple sclerosis, or demyelinating diseases. Other causes include infiltrating tumor, chemical poisoning, immunologic reactions, and infectious diseases. Hyperemia and disk edema are present; complete blindness may occur within several days. The condition is most frequently unilateral and may last for months. Removal of the cause may lead to recovery of vision.

papilloma (pap″ĭ-lo′mah) [*papill-* + Gr. *oma* tumor] a benign neoplasm that protrudes as microscopic fingerlike projections from an epithelial surface.

inverted p., a squamous papilloma in which the projections and convolutions of stratified squamous epithelium with their supporting connective tissue cores do not form the typical exophytic lesion, but instead burrow into the underlying connective tissue. It is commonly encountered in the nasal cavity and nasopharynx.

papillomatosis (pap″ĭ-lo″mah-to′sis) [*papill-* + *-oma* + *-osis* condition] 1. hyperplasia and upward projection of the papillary layer of the dermis, producing an undulating surface of the overlying epithelium.

2. the development of multiple papillomas.

papillomatosis of breast the presence of multiple true intraductal papillomas. This term is frequently used incorrectly to describe nonpapillary forms of solid or fenestrated benign epithelial hyperplasia (epitheliosis). See also *epitheliosis* and *papilloma.*

papillomatous (pap″ĭ-lo′mah-tus) pertaining to or resembling a papilloma.

papova viruses (pap″o-vah) [acronym from *pap*illoma, *po*lyoma, and *va*cuolating agent] a group of DNA viruses, 45–55 nm in diameter, that includes the papilloma and polyoma viruses. These viruses form icosahedral capsids with 72 capsomeres.

pappataci fever [from *Phlebotomus papatasii*] see *phlebotomus fever.*

Pappenheimer body a phagosome (secondary lysosome) found in erythrocytes, that contains ferruginous granules. Because of their protein matrix, these granules stain positive with Perls' reaction and basophilically with Giemsa stain. They are rarely present in severe hemolytic anemia or sideroblastic anemia.

Pappenheim stain (pahp′en-hīm) [Artur *Pappenheim,* German physician, 1870–1916] the original methyl green–pyronine staining procedure, used for RNA and DNA.

PAPS abbrev. See *3′-phosphoadenosine-5′-phosphosulfate.*

PAP technique abbrev. for peroxidase-antiperoxidase technique. See under *immunoperoxidase technique.*

Pap test (pap) [from George Nicolas *Papanicolaou,* Greek physician, 1883–1962] a cytologic procedure for examining exfoliated cells from the female urogenital epithelium to detect dysplasias and carcinomas. It is less often utilized for an evaluation of endocrine function. Epithelial cells desquamated or scraped from the cervix and vagina are fixed, stained with Papanicolaou's stain, and then examined microscopically. See also *Papanicolaou's stain.*

papular (pap′u-lar) [L. *papularis*] pertaining to, resembling, or consisting of papules.

papule (pap′ūl) [L. *papula* pimple] an elevated lesion of the skin that is usually small (less than 5 mm across) and well circumscribed.

para (par′ah) [L. *parere* to bring forth, to bear] a female who has produced viable young, regardless of whether the child was living at birth. The term is used with Roman numerals to designate the number of pregnancies that have resulted in the birth of offspring.

para- (par′ah) [Gr. *para* beyond] 1. a prefix word element to denote beside, beyond, accessory to, apart from, against, e.g., paracardiac.

2. (abbrev. *p-*), a prefix word element in organic chemistry to denote a 1,4-substituted benzene used only in single-ring systems, e.g., *para*-xylene, 1,4-dimethylbenzene. Cf. *meta-* and *ortho-*. See also the illustration accompanying *ortho-*.

-para (pah′rah) [L. *parere* to bring forth, to bear] a suffix word element to denote births (viable offspring), e.g., multipara.

parabiosis (par″ah-bi-o′sis) [*para-* + Gr. *biōsis* way of life] 1. the fusion of two individuals as in conjoined twins.

2. the temporary suppression of nerve conduction.

3. the joining of the blood circulation of two individuals.

parabiotic (par″ah-bi-ot′ik) [*para-* + Gr. *biōtikos* pertaining to life] pertaining to or characterized by parabiosis.

parabola (pah-rab′o-la) [N.L., from Gr. *parabolē, from para-* + *bolē* a throw] a plane curve that is the locus of points equidistant from a fixed point (focus) and line (directrix). In rectangular coordinates the equation of a parabola with the focus at the point (c, 0) and the directrix at the line $x = -c$ is $y^2 = 4cx$. A parabolic reflector has the property that incident rays perpendicular to the directrix are reflected to the focus, and rays emitted by a source at the focus are reflected in a parallel beam.

Parabuthus (par-ah′bu-thus) a genus of scorpions that is extremely dangerous because of its neurotoxic venom.

paracasein (par″ah-ka′se-in) [*para-* + L. *caseus* cheese] a product of protease action on casein in the stomach of ruminants and humans. This action is the initial step in casein digestion in the infant stomach. Paracasein reacts with calcium to yield the insoluble curd.

paracentesis (par″ah-sen-te′sis) [*para-* + Gr. *kentēsis* puncture] the insertion of a needle (puncture) into a body cavity for the aspiration of fluid, e.g., the pleural space.

paracentric inversion (par″ah-sen′trik) [*para-* + Gr. *kentron* point, center of a circle] see under *inversion.*

Parachordodes (par″ah-kor-do′dēz) a genus of worms of the family Chordodidae, class Gordiacea. A few rare cases of human infection with members of this genus have been reported.

parachromatopsia (par″ah-kro″mah-top′se-ah) [*para-* + Gr. *chrōma* color + *opsis* vision + *-ia*] see *color blindness.*

paracoagulants (par″ah-co-ag′u-lants) [*para-* + L. *coagulans* present participle of *coagulare* coagulate] substances that induce paracoagulation. They include protamine sulfate, toluidine blue, ethanol, basic proteins from granulocytes, material from staphylococci, and platelet factor 4. See also *paracoagulation* and *paracoagulation test.*

paracoagulation (par″ah-co-ag″u-la′shun) [*para-* + L. *coagulatio* coagulation, from *coagulare* coagulate] the formation of soluble complexes of fibrin monomer produced when thrombin enzymatically splits fibrinogen. This results in the precipitation of fibrin, fibrin split products, or both. Clinical tests for the presence of fibrin monomer include the protamine sulfate precipitation test and the ethanol gelatin test.

paracoagulation test a test that demonstrates the presence of fibrin monomer in a plasma sample. The monomers, which are bound to fibrinogen or fibrin degradation products and which are present because fibrinolysis always accompanies intravascular coagulation, are dissociated by reagents such as protamine sulfate or ethanol. The monomer polymerizes and forms a precipitate, an indication that thrombin has acted on the fibrinogen. A positive test result is suggestive of disseminated intravascular coagulation. Agarose gel chromatography is the recommended research technique. See also *ethanol gelatin test* and *protamine sulfate test.*

Paracoccidioides (par″ah-kok-sid″e-oi′dēz) a genus of imperfect fungi that causes the systemic mycosis paracoccidioidomycosis. The genus has one medically important species, *P. brasiliensis.* See also *paracoccidioidomycosis.*

P. brasiliensis, a dimorphic fungus that grows as spherical or elliptic cells in tissue. These cells divide by budding and are connected to parent cells by a thin neck. The buds may be multiple, appearing as a circle of buds around one parent cell, giving this species its characteristic appearance. The mycelial form of *P. brasiliensis* grows slowly at room temperature or at 30°C, and microscopically appears as septated branching hyphae with chlamydospores. Also called *Blastomyces brasiliensis.*

paracoccidioidomycosis (par″ah-kok-sid″e-oi′do-mi-ko′sis) [*paracoccidioides* + Gr. *mykes* fungus + *-osis*] a systemic fungal infection caused by the dimorphic fungus *Paracoccidioides brasiliensis.* This disease is most often found geographically in Latin America; it usually affects individuals aged 15–19 and is more common in males than in females.

The fungus is inhaled and accumulates in the primary lymph nodes of the lungs, or enters by the gastrointestinal route and accumulates in the bowel. From the site of entry it may spread throughout the body hematogenously. In otherwise healthy individuals, the lesions heal, and the disease is self-limiting. In immunodeficient or debilitated persons, however, the primary lesion progresses, causing inflammation of the skeletal muscles, as well as mucocutaneous ulcers and granulomatous lesions.

The clinical manifestations of paracoccidioidomycosis may be grouped into four types: primary pulmonary, progressive pulmonary, disseminated, and acute juvenile. The primary pulmonary form is characterized by a mild, unrecognizable infection with lesions that heal without calcification. The progressive pulmonary form, which occurs in approximately 36 percent of cases, is a result of a reactivation of a primary lesion. Initially, there are nonspecific respiratory symptoms: cough, bloody sputum, fever, and thoracic pain, plus weight loss. Most cases of paracoccidioidomycosis are of the disseminated form, with lesions found in the mucous membranes, lymph nodes, skin, spleen, adrenal glands, intestine, and liver. Cervical lymph nodes are discrete, firm, and hard. The acute juvenile form is an infection of the reticuloendothelial system and causes malaise, fever, and lymphadenopathy; the liver and spleen become markedly enlarged.

The diagnosis of paracoccidioidomycosis is made with specimens taken from the lesion; the diagnosis is made serologically if the lesions are inaccessible for culture. Pus, exudate, or tissue from a lesion is cultured at both 25° and 35°C. Serologic diagnostic studies include immunodiffusion, immunoelectrophoresis, latex agglutination, and complement-fixation tests.

Also called *South American blastomycosis.*

paracolon bacillus (par″ah-ko′lun) [*para-* + Gr. *kōlon* member of the body] a name formerly used for certain enteric bacteria that did not readily ferment lactose. As these organisms can now be identified as to genus and species, the term is no longer useful.

paradoxical (par″ah-dok′sĭ-k′l) [Gr. *paradoxon* paradox, from *paradoxos* incredible] occurring at variance with the normal rule.

paradoxical respiration the movement of a part of the chest wall or diaphragm in an inappropriate direction for the time in the respiratory cycle at which the movement has occurred. Examples of paradoxical (and abnormal) motion during inspiration are an inward movement of the ribs over a portion of the chest wall and an upward movement of a hemidiaphragm.

Paradoxical respiration impairs ventilation in the underlying lung. Severe atelectasis and/or respiratory failure may ensue if the movement involves extensive areas of the thorax or diaphragm (such as an entire hemithorax or both hemidiaphragms). Also called paradoxical motion.

paradoxical sleep see *s. stages* under *sleep.*

paraffin (par'ah-fin) [L. *parum* little + *affinis* akin] 1. [NF], a purified mixture of solid hydrocarbons obtained from petroleum. It occurs as an odorless, tasteless, colorless or white, more or less translucent material. It has such uses as a stiffening agent, sealing compound, floor polish, and lubricant component.

2. a saturated hydrocarbon of the methane series, an alkane represented by the general formula C_nH_{2n+2}.

3. the embedding medium routinely used in histology; see also *embedding.*

paraffinoma (par"ah-fĭ-no'mah) [*paraffin* + *-oma* tumor] a chronic granuloma resulting from exposure of the lung parenchyma to paraffin, mineral oil, or other waxy substances. Lipoid pneumonitis is often present.

parafollicular cell (par"ah-fo-lik'u-lar) [*para-* + L. *folliculus* little bag, from *follis* bellows] see *C cell.*

paraformaldehyde (par"ah-for-mal'de-hīd) a polymer of formaldehyde, $H(CH_2O)_nOH$, used in histology; see under *fixative.*

Parafossarulus (par"ah-fos-sar'u-lus) [*para-* + L. *fossa* ditch + *arulus* diminutive ending] a genus of freshwater snails. The species *P. manchouricus* is an intermediate host of the flukes *Echinochasmus perfoliatus, Clonorchis sinensis,* and *Opisthorchis felineus,* and is geographically distributed throughout China and Japan.

paraganglioma (par"ah-gang"gle-o'mah) [*paraganglion* + *-oma* tumor] a neoplasm of paraganglion cells. These tumors are relatively uncommon and are often small and benign. They occur in the sites where paraganglia are found and may be classified according to the particular anatomic group from which they arise, e.g., branchiomeric, aorticosympathetic, intravagal; or to the specific location if known, e.g., carotid body paraganglioma. Histologically, they mimic the paraganglial structure, with nests of neoplastic paraganglionic cells (Zellballen) invested by supporting cells and separated by a connective tissue stroma. Ultrastructurally, the cells contain electron-dense granules. See also *carotid body tumor, chemodectoma,* and *paraganglion.*

paraganglion (par"ah-gang'gle-on), pl. *paraganglia* [*para-* + Gr. *ganglion* encysted tumor] an aggregate of cells of neural crest origin that forms a unit of the paraganglion system. The extraadrenal paraganglion system excludes the adrenal medulla and the chemoreceptor carotid and aortic bodies. It comprises small clusters of cells associated with the autonomic nervous system, which form catecholamines and store them as dense-core cytoplasmic granules. The paraganglia are principally distributed in the paraaxial regions of the trunk and in the neck; they include the branchiomeric, intravagal, aorticosympathetic and visceroautonomic paraganglia. See also *carotid body* and *chemoreceptor.*

intravagal p., an aggregation of chemoreceptors on the vagus nerve.

Paragon (par'ah-gon) trademark for a water-soluble mounting medium used in histology, primarily for fat stains. It has a refractive index of 1.4241 and a pH of 5.6.

paragonimiasis (par"ah-gon"ĭ-mi'ah-sis) [*paragonimus* + *-iasis*] an infection with the flukes of the genus *Paragonimus,* especially *P. westermani,* which are distributed throughout Africa, the Far East, Asia, Mexico, and Central and South America. It is caused by ingestion of uncooked crabs or crayfish infected with encysted larvae. These larvae are released in the stomach of the host and migrate to the lungs. Once the worms are established in the lungs and mature, they cause a pronounced tissue reaction, with the formation of pulmonic cysts; *Paragonimus* may rarely cause lesions in other sites such as the brain, peritoneum, and subcutaneous tissues. The disease is characterized by chills, fever, high eosinophilia, chronic cough, mucus production, and hemoptysis.

Laboratory diagnosis requires identification of the eggs in the feces or sputum. The eggs are operculate and unembryonated, and possess a moderately thick shell. For stool specimens, the AMS III technique (acid-sodium sulfate-triton-ether) is recommended. The eggs should be differentiated from fish tapeworm eggs, and the disease from other pulmonary infections. Examination of three stool and sputum specimens on successive days is recommended to increase the number of positive findings.

Also called *endemic hemoptysis, Oriental lung fluke disease,* and *pulmonary distomiasis.*

Paragonimus (par"ah-gon'ĭ-mus) [*para-* + Gr. *gonimos* productive; having generative power] a genus of trematodes (flukes) that is parasitic in humans and causes paragonimiasis. The parasite has two intermediate hosts: the snail or mollusk (such as *Melania* or *Semisulcospira*), followed by the crab or crayfish (such as *Potamon* or *Eriocheir*). The adult parasites are approximately 12 by 6 mm and are usually found encapsulated in the lungs.

P. africanus, a species occurring in Africa (in Zaire and the Cameroons) that is occasionally parasitic in humans. The eggs can be differentiated from those of *P. westermani:* they measure 67.9–113.2 μ long by 42.5–56.6 μ wide.

P. caliensis, a species occurring in Central and South America that is involved in human infections. The eggs have a thin, irregular shell and are 70–92 μ long by 38–54 μ wide.

P. heterotremus, a species responsible for one known human infection (in Thailand); it is ordinarily parasitic in rats, dogs, or cats. The eggs are usually symmetric and have a uniform eggshell.

P. kellicotti, a species occurring in the United States and Canada that is usually parasitic in dogs and minks. It has been incriminated in a human infection. *P. kellicotti* can be differentiated from *P. westermani* by the thickness of the metacercarial membrane.

P. mexicanus, a species occurring in Mexico that is parasitic in opossums and rarely in humans. The oval eggs are yellowish and measure 59.5–78.8 μ long by 38.5–49.0 μ wide.

P. westermani, the species of *Paragonimus* that is commonly parasitic in humans. It is geographically distributed throughout Japan, China, and southern Asia. The adult flukes measure 7.5–12 mm long by 4–6 mm wide, live encapsulated in the lungs, and have an oval- or pear-shaped body. The eggs are broadly ovoid with a flattened operculum, are golden-brown in color, and measure 80–118 μ long by 48–60 μ wide. Also called *Distoma pulmonum, D. ringeri, D. westermani,* and *Oriental lung fluke.*

Paragordius (par″ah-gor′de-us) a genus of worms of the family Chordodidae. Human infection with the species *P. cinctus, P. esvanianus, P. tricuspidatus,* and *P. varius* has been reported. Also called hairworm or hairsnake.

paragranuloma (par″ah-gran″u-lo′mah) [*para-* + L. *granulum* + *-oma*] a term from an early classification of Hodgkin's disease that described the most benign form. It is no longer used. See also *malignant l.* under *lymphoma.*

parahemophilia (par″ah-he″mo-fil′e-ah) a deficiency or absence of coagulation of Factor V, transmitted as an autosomal recessive trait, that is characterized by mild bleeding—usually nosebleeds and bruises on the skin. There may be severe menorrhagia. Clinical symptoms develop only when the gene is inherited from both parents. Parahemophilia may also occur as an acquired disorder due to the development of inhibitors (IgG or IgA) to Factor V; this has been associated with streptomycin therapy in some cases.

Laboratory studies show an abnormal prothrombin time and partial thromboplastin time. Diagnosis is confirmed by assay for Factor V. Replacement therapy is with fresh plasma.

Also called labile factor deficiency, Owren's disease, and proaccelerin deficiency.

parainfluenza antibody tests (par″ah-in″floo-en′zah) assays for detecting and quantitating antibody against the parainfluenza virus. The tests most routinely used are complement fixation and hemagglutination. In children younger than 6 mo and in the elderly, antibody levels may not be very high; these individuals may require more sensitive tests such as ELISA and virus neutralization. A fourfold rise in titer between acute and convalescent serum is required for diagnosis. Because the patient has usually recovered by the time the second serum sample is taken, serologic evidence of infection is more important as a retrospective confirmation than for primary diagnosis.

Mumps virus infection may cause a rise in parainfluenza antibody titer. Unchanging high levels of antibody in both acute and convalescent sera suggest recent virus infection. High levels may also indicate past infection with persistent high antibody levels or late collection of an acute serum.

parainfluenza virus one of a group of paramyxoviruses isolated from persons with upper respiratory tract disease of varying severity. Four distinct serologic types have been recovered from humans.

parakeratosis (par″ah-ker″ah-to′sis) [*para-* + Gr. *keras* horn + *-osis*] a pathologic skin condition characterized by abnormal keratinization, with the persistence of the nuclei of keratinocytes as they ascend into the stratum corneum. This condition often results in scaling of the skin.

paralbuminemia (par″al-bu″mĭ-ne′me-ah) [*para-* + *albumin* + Gr. *haima* blood + *-ia*] an asymptomatic genetic trait characterized by the presence of a variant serum albumin with abnormal electrophoretic mobility. See also *bisalbuminemia.*

paraldehyde (par-al′de-hīd) [USP], a colorless, volatile liquid, a cyclic polymer of acetaldehyde, $(CH_3CHO)_3$, used as a hypnotic and sedative. It has an unpleasant taste and is excreted in part by the lungs, giving odor to the breath. Adverse reactions include nausea, headache, dizziness, and coma. It may produce intoxication with excitement. Chronic use causes dependence; withdrawal may produce delirium tremens.

paraldehyde assays 1. ultraviolet spectrophotometry. Paraldehyde is hydrolyzed to acetaldehyde by heating with acid; acetaldehyde is separated from the sample by distillation and reacted with semicarbazide or Schiff reagent. The resulting semicarbazone is determined by its absorbance at 224 nm; the Schiff addition product by its absorbance at 560 nm.

2. gas chromatography. See *head space analysis.*

parallax (par′ah-laks) [Gr. "in turn"] a change in the relative position of two objects due to a change in the line of sight, as when looking first with one eye and then the other, or as in the left and right views made in stereoscopic radiography.

parallax method see under *foreign body localization.*

parallel (par′ah-lel) [Gr. *parallēlos* side by side] 1. in electronics, pertaining to processes carried out simultaneously or to components connected across the same two terminals.

2. in mathematics, referring to two coplanar lines or two planes that do not intersect.

parallel circuit an electric circuit in which the components are connected in parallel, i.e., in which the current is divided among the components. The voltage is the same across all the components, and the total current is the sum of the currents in the components. Capacitors connected in parallel are equivalent to one capacitor having the sum of their capacitances. Resistors connected in parallel combine differently; the reciprocal of the equivalent resistance is the sum of the reciprocals of the individual resistances ($1/R_{eq} = 1/R_1 + 1/R_2 + \ldots$). Inductances combine in the same way. Cf. *series circuit.*

parallel operation in digital logic circuitry, the processing of several related items of information, such as the bits of a word, at the same time.

paralysis (pah-ral′ĭ-sis), pl. *paralyses* [*para-* + Gr. *lyein* to loosen] weakness, which may result from an interruption in the motor pathway, located anywhere between the cerebral cortex and the contractile fibers of a muscle. A lesion in the corticospinal tracts produces an upper motor neuron lesion with spasticity, weakness, hyperreflexia, and a positive Babinski sign. A disturbance in the motor unit (anterior horn cell, peripheral nerve, neuromuscular junction, or muscle fiber) results in a lower motor neuron lesion with flaccid weakness, atrophy, and hyporeflexia.

Weakness may be caused by many different pathologic processes including cerebrovascular accidents (stroke), trauma, infection, inflammation, degenerative diseases, and neoplasm. The distribution of affected muscles depends on the location of the lesion.

Specialized tests such as nerve conduction tests and eletromyography may yield valuable diagnostic information when the weakness results from a lower motor neuron lesion.

Also called *palsy.*

p. agitans, see *parkinsonism.*

ascending p., a syndrome of progressive paralysis with an ascending pattern. Diseases that induce acute ascending paralysis include Guillain-Barré syndrome, porphyria, acute polyneuropathies associated with diphtheria, infectious mononucleosis, and hepatitis.

bulbar p., see *bulbar p.* under *palsy.*

familial periodic p., a rare group of diseases often transmitted as an autosomal dominant trait and characterized by episodes of severe weakness. Acquired forms of the disease also occur. Three types are known to exist: hypokalemic, hyperkalemic, and normokalemic. In the hypokalemic type, attacks may last for several hours to several days, during which time serum potassium concentrations are low. Attacks may be induced by the administration of glucose and insulin and may be relieved by the administration of potassium. The hyperkalemic type differs from the hypokalemic type in that the attacks are usually milder and of shorter duration and often occur during rest after physical exertion. Serum potassium is elevated during an attack. The hyperkalemic type of familial periodic paralysis is often associated with myotonia, usually occurs during infancy, and is also known as adynamia episodica hereditaria. The normokalemic form of this disorder is rare and has not been fully characterized.

ischemic p., see *Volkmann's p.*

Landry's p., see *Guillain-Barré syndrome.*

sleep p., a syndrome, usually associated with narcolepsy, characterized by brief attacks of paralysis upon falling asleep or on awakening. These episodes resemble the inhibition of motor function associated with REM (rapid eye movement) sleep.

Volkmann's p., ischemic paralysis associated with circulatory impairment. Most commonly, an occlusion of a major artery of an extremity results in ischemia of those muscles and nerves with a common blood supply. Also called *ischemic p.*

Werdnig-Hoffmann p., see *Werdnig-Hoffman paralysis.*

paralytic (par″ah-lit′ik) [Gr. *paralytikos*] affected with or pertaining to paralysis.

paralyzable detector (par″ah-līz′ah-b′l) a radiation detector, such as the typical Geiger-Müller counter, which cannot produce counts at very high radiation fluxes. It is unable to count any particles during a set period called the recovery time following the entrance of a particle into the detector, whether or not it is counted. Cf. *nonparalyzable detector.*

paramagnetic (par″ah-mag-net′ik) pertaining to materials in which some atoms or free radicals have intrinsic magnetic moments that tend to align with an external magnetic field. The alignment is opposed by the thermal motion of the atoms. Paramagnetic susceptibilities are typically about 10^{-4}–10^{-3} and are inversely proportional to the absolute temperature.

paramagnetic resonance of electrons see *electron spin resonance.*

Paramecium (par″ah-me′she-um, par″ah-me′se-um) [Gr. *paramēkēs* oblong] a genus of holotrichous ciliate protozoa.

P. coli, see *B. coli* under *Balantidium.*

paramedic (par″ah-med′ik) see under *emergency medical technician.*

paramesonephric duct (par″ah-mes″o-nef′rik) [*para-* + Gr. *mesos* middle + *nephros* kidney] see *müllerian d.* under *duct.*

parameter (pah-ram′ĕ-ter) [Gr. *parametrein* to measure one thing by another] 1. in statistics and mathematics, an arbitrary constant having a definite, fixed value in a particular problem (but different values in different problems), as opposed to a variable, which is varied in the context of the problem. For example, the mean and standard deviation of a normal distribution are the parameters that specify one particular distribution, whereas the mean and standard deviation of a sample are random variables.

2. a variable that is an indirect measurement of another quantity or function, which cannot be directly measured with precision. For example, blood pressure and pulse rate are parameters of cardiovascular function, and the level of glucose in blood and urine is a parameter of carbohydrate metabolism.

paramethadione (par″ah-meth″ah-di′ōn) [USP], an anticonvulsant drug similar to trimethadione but less toxic, used for the control of absence (petit mal) seizures that are not controlled by other drugs. Trademark, Paradione. See also *oxazolidinedione compounds.*

parametrium (par″ah-me′tre-um) [*para-* + Gr. *mētra* uterus] [NA], the loose connective tissue that lies between the two serous layers of the broad ligaments and separates the cervix from the urinary bladder.

Paramphistomatidae (par″am-fis″to-mah-ti′de) [N.L., from *para-* + Gr. *amphistomos* with a double mouth] a family of trematodes (flukes) that possesses a ventral sucker at the posterior extremity of the body. Two species that are parasitic in humans are *Watsonius watsoni* and *Gastrodiscoides hominis.*

paramyotonia (par″ah-mi″o-to′ne-ah) [*para-* + Gr. *mys* muscle + *tonos* tension + *-ia*] a general term used to describe a hereditary disease, characterized by weakness and myotonia, that typically is induced by cold. The weakness may be restricted or generalized, and often persists for several hours after cooling. The precise relationship of this disorder to the periodic paralysis syndromes is controversial.

p. congenita, a congenital disease, transmitted as an autosomal dominant trait, that is characterized by weakness, paralysis, and stiffness of the muscles of the throat, face, and mouth, as well as of the distal musculature, especially on exposure to cold. Prolonged exposure may lead to severe flaccid weakness and loss of deep reflexes. Muscle biopsies are normal. This disease may be closely related to hyerkalemic periodic paralysis; thus potassium therapy should not be used in these patients. Also called Eulenburg's disease. See also *m. congenita* under *myotonia.*

paramyxovirus (par″ah-mik″so-vi′rus) [*para-* + Gr. *myxa* mucus + *virus*] a family of myxoviruses that contains the parainfluenza, mumps, measles, and respiratory syncytial virus and related animal viruses. These organisms are spherical, enveloped RNA viruses 150–250 nm in diameter, containing an RNA transcriptase that transcribes the single-stranded RNA genome. See also *myxovirus*.

paranasal sinus (par″ah-na′sal) [*para-* + L. *nasus* nose] one of the cavities in the interior of certain of the skull bones that communicate with the cavity of the nose, and provide lightness for the skull and resonance for the voice. Each is lined with mucosa and is prone to extension of inflammatory processes from the nasal cavity (sinusitis). The named air sinuses are the frontal, ethmoid, sphenoid, maxillary, and palatine.

paraneoplastic syndrome (par″ah-ne″o-plas′tik) complexes of symptoms, seen in cancer patients, that are not directly attributable to local or distant metastatic spread of the neoplastic cells. Clinical findings may be very similar to those of unrelated primary endocrine, metabolic, hematologic, or neuromuscular disorders. The mechanism of generation of these symptoms is thought to involve the effects of tumor products, the effect of neoplastic destruction of normal tissue, or unknown factors. An example of the paraneoplastic syndrome is ectopic hormone production as, for example, in the production of adrenocorticotropic hormone (ACTH) or an ACTH-like factor by bronchogenic carcinomas.

The symptoms of the paraneoplastic syndrome can provide valuable clinical information that may lead to the early diagnosis of an occult neoplasm. The associated symptoms in some of the syndromes may prove more immediately life-threatening than the presence of the neoplasm, and therapy must be instituted to treat both the neoplasm and the accompanying paraneoplastic syndrome.

paraneuron (par″ah-nu′ron) [*para-* + Gr. *neuron* tendon, nerve] see under *diffuse neuroendocrine system*.

paranoia (par″ah-noi′ah) [*para-* + Gr. *nous* mind + *-ia* condition] a form of personality disorder characterized by a heightened sense of self-importance coupled with persistent persecutory delusions. The paranoid individual may suffer no impairment of intellectual, occupational, or normal daily functions but social functions may be inhibited. Paranoia tends to be a chronic disease developing over a long time, and there is usually no cure. Rapidly developing paranoid states may be attributable to systemic illness, organic brain disease, or drug toxicity.

paraparesis (par″ah-par′ĕ-sis) [*para-* + Gr. *paresis* paralysis] the gradual development of weakness and partial paralysis in the legs. It may occur in several diseases, including Friedreich's ataxia, multiple sclerosis, syphilitic infections, and spondylosis.

paraphimosis (par″ah-fi-mo′sis) [*para-* + Gr. *phimoun* to muzzle + *-osis* condition] a condition characterized by retraction of the foreskin of the penis, blocking replacement over the glans. The retraction may cause swelling, pain, and urethral constriction, leading to acute urinary retention. Prompt surgical treatment by circumcision may be required. This condition may be associated with phimosis. Cf. *phimosis*.

Paraplast (par″ah-plast′) trademark for a semisynthetic paraffin wax used in the embedding of tissue blocks.

paraplegia (par″ah-ple′je-ah) [*para-* + Gr. *plēgē* stroke + *-ia*] paralysis of the lower extremities. The condition is most frequently due to diseases of the spinal cord or spinal roots; the peripheral nerves may also be involved. Loss of voluntary control of the legs may be accompanied by sensory loss, and there is commonly associated alteration in the cerebrospinal fluid.

Paraplegia has many causes, including trauma, demyelinating diseases (multiple sclerosis), vascular disorders (hematomyelia, thrombosis), degenerative diseases (motor system diseases), neoplasms, and infections (bacterial, viral, tubercular, and fungal). Those affected may suffer from skin ulcers, bone deformities, and urinary, respiratory, or gastrointestinal dysfunctions.

Paraponera (par″ah-pōn′er-ah) a genus of ants. The species *P. clavata*, the large tucandeira ant, is found in central and northern South America. Its sting causes a painful, throbbing swelling (which produces a lesion about 18 cm in diameter). The swelling usually subsides in a few hours unless the victim has an allergic reaction to the venom, a mixture of histamine, 5-hydroxytryptamine, and acetylcholine.

parapraxia (par″ah-prak′se-ah) [*para-* + Gr. *praxis* doing + *-ia*] irrational behavior that may be coupled with a diminished ability to consciously perform purposeful movements.

paraprotein (par″ah-pro′tēn) [*para-* + *protein*, from Gr. *prōtos* first] a monoclonal immunoglobulin of blood plasma, observed electrophoretically as an intense extra band somewhere in the γ, β, or α_2 zones, that is due to an isolated increase in a single member of the immunoglobulins. Paraprotein is synthesized by a clone of many identical plasma cells, arising from abnormal rapid multiplication of a single cell. The cells comprising the clone all produce identical immunoglobulin molecules with the same mobility, giving an electrophoretically sharp monoclonal or M band (a paraprotein). The finding of a paraprotein in a patient's serum thus indicates the presence of a proliferating clone of immunoglobulin-producing cells.

paraproteinemia (par″ah-pro″tēn-e′me-ah) [*para-* + *protein* + Gr. *haima* blood + *-ia*] a condition characterized by the presence of excess homogeneous immunoglobulins or immunoglobulin fragments in the blood. The immunoglobulin may belong to any class (IgM, IgG, IgA, IgD, or IgE) and may be complete, single chains (heavy or light), or polypeptide fragments.

The disease is characterized by the uncontrolled proliferation of a plasma cell clone and may be associated with malignant, benign, or nonneoplastic diseases. The excess paraprotein may be detected as a homogeneous spike on serum electrophoresis. Despite an increase in the total immunoglobulin protein content of the serum, paraproteinemias may be associated with immune deficiency states.

See also *monoclonal gammopathy*.

parapsoriasis (par″ah-so-ri′ah-sis) [*para-* + Gr. *psōra* mange + *-iasis*] an uncommon group of disorders characterized by the formation of scaly, maculopapular plaques and papules on the skin. These conditions may occur in young and middle-aged adults, most often affecting the trunk and extremities. The histologic appearance of the lesions resembles that of a chronic dermatitis, but can be misdiagnosed as mycosis fungoides.

paraquat (par′a-kwat) a highly toxic bipyridyl herbicide. Heavy exposure to paraquat may cause fatal respiratory failure; lower doses produce pulmonary fibrosis and edema. Paraquat also causes skin irritation.

paraquat assays the determination of paraquat in the urine, stomach contents, or the supernatant remaining after tissue is macerated and the proteins are precipitated. Paraquat is detected by reducing it to the blue, free radical form with dithionite. This assay may be made quantitative by using ion-exchange chromatography to extract the paraquat, and spectrophotometry to measure the absorbance of the reduced free radical.

pararosaniline (par″ah-ro-zan′ĭ-lin) [*para-* + L. *rosa* rose + Arabic *al-nil* indigo plant] a red basic dye, $[C(C_6H_4NH_2)_3]^+$; C.I. 42500. See also *fuchsin* and *triphenylmethane dyes.*

Parasa (par′ah-sah) a genus of urticating caterpillars (saddle-back caterpillars) that possess spinous poisonous hairs. The species *P. chloris* and *P. indetermina* are distributed throughout the eastern United States, whereas *P. hilarata* is found in China and Korea. When the poison is introduced into the skin, a burning, stinging sensation is experienced and the site becomes erythematous.

parasite (par′ah-sīt) [Gr. *parasitos*] any organism (plant or animal) that lives on or in a host, usually a larger organism, that provides physical protection and nourishment. A parasite may be a single-celled or multicelled animal, bacterium, or fungus. Several types of relationships exist between a parasite and its host. See also *bacterial pathogenicity, host,* and *symbiosis.*

accidental p., an organism that parasitizes an animal other than the usual host. Also called incidental parasite.

ectozoic p., an animal ectoparasite (one that inhabits the outside of the body of the host).

entozoic p., any parasite that inhabits the lumen of the intestines.

extracellular p., a parasite that lives outside the cells of the host. Bacterial species that are extracellular parasites are usually destroyed rapidly when ingested by a phagocytic cell. Such organisms (e.g., streptococcus and pneumococcus) in general produce acute, short-term illnesses. Bacteriostatic and bactericidal drugs greatly increase the natural defenses of the host. Many fungi and most animal parasites also are extracellular.

facultative p., an organism that may be parasitic on another organism but is also capable of existing independently.

intermittent p., an organism that is parasitic in its natural host for certain periods and is free-living during the interval between host infections. Also called occasional parasite.

intracellular p., a parasite that can multiply or survive for a long time inside a cell. Bacterial species that are intracellular parasites (e.g., tubercle bacilli, brucellae, and typhoid organisms) ordinarily produce chronic and dormant diseases. They are less susceptible to the action of drugs than are extracellular parasites and are relatively resistant to the body's natural defense mechanisms. Viruses are obligatory intracellular parasites. Some fungi (e.g., *Histoplasma capsulatum*) and protozoa (*Plasmodium*) also exhibit intracellular parasitism, but the diseases they cause may be either chronic or acute.

malarial p., see *Plasmodium.*

obligate p., an organism that is totally dependent on a host for its survival.

periodic p., a parasite that inhabits its host for short periods.

permanent p., a parasite that completes its life cycle (early life to maturity or death) in its host.

spurious p., an organism that is parasitic to a host other than humans, but may pass through humans without causing damage.

temporary p., an organism that is free of its host during part of its life cycle.

parasitemia (par″ah-si-te′me-ah) [*parasitos* + Gr. *haima* blood + *-ia*] the presence of parasites, especially malarial forms or their products, in the blood. Identification of a parasite in the blood signifies the end of its biologic incubation period.

parasitic (par″ah-sit′ik) [Gr. *parasitikos*] pertaining to or caused by a parasite.

parasiticide (par″ah-sit′ĭ-sid) [*parasitos* + L. *caedere* to kill] any agent or chemical that is destructive to parasites.

parasitism (par′ah-si″tizm) 1. a symbiotic relationship of an individual (animal or organism) or a population that adversely affects another, but is totally dependent and cannot live without it.

2. an infection or infestation with parasites.

parasitize (par′ah-sĭ-tiz″) to inhabit within or on a host as a parasite.

Parasitoidea (par″ah-sit-oi′de-ah) a superfamily of mites of the order Acari. Two important species parasitic in humans are *Ornithonyssus bacoti* and *Dermanyssus gallinae.*

parasitologist (par″ah-sĭ-tol′o-jist) [*parasitos* + Gr. *logistēs* reasoner] a person knowledgeable in parasitology.

parasitology (par″ah-sĭ-tol′o-je) [*parasitos* + Gr. *logos* word, reason] the scientific study of parasites and parasitism.

parasomnias (par″ah-som′ne-ahz) [*para-* + L. *somnus* sleep] a class of sleep disorders in which complex behavior patterns occur during sleep or interrupt sleep. These disorders usually take place during sleep stages 3 or 4, involve partial arousal, and include sleepwalking (somnambulism), night terror (pavor nocturnus), and enuresis. They have a higher incidence in children than in adults, usually during the first few hours after falling asleep. The electroencephalogram during attacks is characterized by an intermixture of slow-wave, alpha, and beta activities, with movement artifacts often obscuring the recording. The disturbance of behavior usually is not remembered by the individual on the following morning. See also *p. diurnus* and *p. nocturnus* under *pavor,* and *somnambulism.*

paraspadias (par″ah-spa′de-ahz) [*para-* + Gr. *spadon* a rent] a congenital malformation of the urethral groove and canal that creates a urethral orifice on the side of the penis. This abnormality may be associated with aberrant testicular descent or bladder malformations. It may lead to urinary obstruction and bacterial infection. Proximal paraspadias may also interfere with normal ejaculation and cause sterility.

parasternal line (par″ah-ster′nal) [*para-* + Gr. *sternon* sternum] a vertical line midway between the mamillary line and the lateral sternal line (the edge of the sternum).

parasympathetic nervous system a division of the autonomic nervous system, with an outflow from the central nervous system in cranial nerves III, VII, IX, and X (the oculomotor, facial, glossopharyngeal, and vagal nerves, respectively) to supply visceral structures in the head, thorax, and upper abdomen, and the second, third, and fourth sacral spinal nerves to supply the pelvic viscera. The preganglionic fibers in both the cranial and sacral outflows synapse within ganglia on short postganglionic neurons that are in close proximity to, or distributed within, the visceral structures they supply. The neurotransmitter of both the pre- and postganglionic fibers is acetylcholine.

In general, the parasympathetic system influences the vegetative functions of the body. Specifically, stimulation of particular parasympathetic fibers effects the following: pupillary constriction and contraction of the ciliary muscle of the eye, resulting in increased curvature of the lens (accommodation); increased secretion from the lacrimal and salivary glands, and glands of the gastrointestinal and respiratory tracts; slowing of the heart (bradycardia), accompanied by decreased contraction of the atria, and slowing of impulse conduction over the bundle of His; constriction of the coronary vessels; increased mobility and decreased tone of the sphincters of the GI tract; contraction of the gallbladder; and erection of the penis and clitoris.

See also *autonomic nervous system* and its accompanying illustration.

parasympathomimetic (par″ah-sim″pah-tho-mĭ-met′ik) [*parasympathetic* + Gr. *mimētikos* imitative] producing effects resembling those involved in the stimulation of parasympathetic nerve fibers, as by the action of cholinergic agents such as acetylcholine, pilocarpine, or cholinesterase inhibitors. See also *cholinergic receptors.* Cf. *sympathomimetic.*

parathion (par″ah-thi′on) an agricultural insecticide (*O,O*-diethyl-*O*-[*p*-nitrophenyl]-phosphorothionate) that is highly toxic to humans and animals.

parathormone (par″ah-thor′mōn) see *parathyroid hormone.*

parathyrin (par″ah-thi′rin) see *parathyroid hormone.*

parathyroid/o (par″ah-thi′roid-o) [*para-* + *thyroid*] a word element used in combining form to denote the parathyroid glands, e.g., parathyroidism.

parathyroid (par″ah-thi′roid) 1. situated beside the thyroid gland.

2. pertaining to the parathyroid glands.

parathyroid glands small, yellowish-brown bodies in the region of the thyroid gland, ovoid or lentiform in shape, that are part of the endocrine system. Their secretion, parathyroid hormone, helps regulate the levels of calcium and phosphorus in the body. The glands usually are four in number: a right and left superior and a right and left inferior; occasionally, additional smaller glands are present. A normal parathyroid is usually not more than 4 mm in greatest dimension. The parathyroids develop from the third and fourth branchial pouches. The parathyroids from the third pouch become the inferior pair of glands and are occasionally drawn down by the descending thymus into the anterior mediastinum. They are more variable in their location and may be found within the thyroid gland or outside its fascia. The superior glands, which develop from the fourth branchial pouch, usually lie at the level of the middle of the thyroid lobes. The superior parathyroids usually lie dorsal to the recurrent laryngeal nerves, whereas the inferior pair of glands are commonly ventral.

The principal or chief cells of the parathyroid form irregular cords. They are polygonal cells with a rather small, round central nucleus and cytoplasm that appears clear by light microscopy. Sparse, small, dense-core granules are present in the vicinity of the Golgi complex. The chief cells may undergo transformation to mitochondrion-rich (oxyphil) cells, which become more numerous in older persons. In spite of the accumulation of mitochondria, the oxyphil cells retain their synthetic capability.

Parathyroid hormone influences calcium and phosphorus levels in conjunction with calcitonin and a derivative of vitamin D. Parathyroid hormone acts on osteoclasts, increasing the rate of release of calcium from bone into the blood. The rate of secretion of hormone from the parathyroids is determined by the concentration of serum calcium. Excess parathyroid secretion results in increased resorption of calcium from bones, producing osteitis fibrosa cystica. A deficiency of the hormone may result in tetanic muscle spasms due to a decreased ionized calcium concentration in serum.

See also *hyperparathyroidism, hypoparathyroidism,* and *parathyroid hormone.*

parathyroid hormone (PTH) a hormone secreted by the parathyroid gland, a single polypeptide; M.W. 9500. Its major function is to regulate calcium homeostasis in conjunction with calcitonin and vitamin D. When ionized calcium levels begin to drop in the plasma, PTH is secreted by the chief cells of the parathyroid gland; conversely, when ionized calcium reaches a certain level, PTH secretion ceases.

PTH directly mobilizes calcium from bone, decreases calcium clearance by increasing resorption in the kidney tubules, and increases the concentration of 1,25-dihydroxycholecalciferol, which in turn causes increased bone resorption and increased intestinal absorption of calcium. In addition, PTH acts to decrease plasma phosphate levels and increase phosphate excretion.

PTH consists of 84 amino acids; its intracellular biosynthesis is thought to occur by sequential cleavage of pre-pro-parathyroid hormone (115 amino acids) and pro-parathyroid hormone (90 amino acids). After PTH is bound to a high-affinity receptor in its target cell (e.g., bone, kidney), its activity is mediated by adenylate cyclase and cyclic AMP. In addition to intact and biologically active PTH being found in the serum, a biologically inactive C-terminal fragment and a biologically active N-terminal fragment are present. Amino acids 1–27 or possibly 1–34 are necessary for full biologic activity.

One of the major uses of PTH is in differentiating the hypercalcemia due to neoplasms from the hypercalcemia of primary hyperparathyroidism. If the calcium is increased because of a nonparathyroid malignancy, the PTH would normally be expected to be low or even undetectable. If a parathyroid adenoma is involved, the negative feedback mechanism is not functional, and PTH levels either are near the upper limit of normal or are elevated. PTH levels are sometimes used to localize parathyroid adenomas, a process accomplished by selective sampling of blood from the veins of the thyroid venous plexus.

Increased PTH levels in conjunction with elevated calcium (pseudohyperparathyroidism) can also be found in ectopic PTH-secreting tumors, the most common being renal cell and squamous cell carcinomas. PTH may be elevated, often significantly, in secondary hyperparathyroidism in response to hypocalcemia from hemodialysis, renal disease, malabsorption, and vitamin D deficiency. Pseudohypoparathyroidism, a rare genetic disease in which there is a failure of renal tubules to respond to PTH owing to lack of receptors, may also present with increased PTH levels. Decreased PTH values are seen in hypoparathyroidism and nonparathyroid hypercalcemia.

Owing to the fact that PTH results are expressed differently from laboratory to laboratory, reference values can be misleading. A variety of nomograms relating PTH and calcium have been constructed to aid in interpreting test results.

Also called *parathormone* and *parathyrin.* See also *calcitonin* and *vitamin D.*

parathyroid scan a procedure in nuclear medicine for the imaging of the parathyroid glands, which utilizes a rectilinear scanner (preferred) or a scintillation camera. It is useful in localizing parathyroid adenomas or carcinomas or hyperplastic thyroid tissue prior to surgery. This procedure is no longer widely used in clinical nuclear medicine.

Selenomethionine Se 75 is used as the imaging agent, being taken up by the parathyroid for incorporation into parathormone. Uptake by the thyroid is reduced by administration of the thyroid hormone triiodothyronine, and thyroid scans are made for comparison, to reduce the number of false-positive results. Although many scans are falsely negative (up to 40 percent), the parathyroids are well localized in many patients. Serial scans are begun 10 min after administration of the agent, using a medium-energy collimator, and are continued for 1–2 hr. The patient is immobilized in the supine position with the neck hyperextended.

parathyroid tumors neoplasms of the parathyroid glands. Benign tumors of the parathyroid glands (adenomas) are usually small and are more common in the lower glands. They may also occur in the mediastinum from ectopic parathyroid tissue drawn down to this location during descent of the thymus in the embryo. Most adenomas are composed of sheets or cords of chief cells, but areas of oxyphil cells can often be found; occasionally the entire lesion is composed of oxyphil cells. The location of the tumor may be determined preoperatively by selective venous catheterization of the neck and by assay for parathyroid hormone. Hyperfunction is seen mainly with adenomas containing chief cells, but immunoperoxidase staining for parathyroid hormone generally is also positive in the oxyphil cells. Malignant tumors of the parathyroid are uncommon; distinction from an adenoma in histologic sections may be difficult and may require evidence of invasive behavior or metastases. Spread may occur to the bones, lymph nodes, kidneys, and lungs. Some patients survive for many years.

paratyphoid fever (par″ah-ti′foid) [*para-* + *typhoid,* from Gr. *typhōdes* delirious] a prolonged febrile disease caused by *Salmonella* serotypes other than *Salmonella typhi,* clinically indistinguishable from typhoid fever. It is characterized by gastrointestinal symptoms, rose spots, splenomegaly, and decreased white blood cell counts. Positive blood and stool cultures most commonly reveal *S. enteritidis;* serotypes *paratyphi A* and *paratyphi B,* and *S. choleraesuis.* In general, paratyphoid is less severe and less likely to lead to a chronic carrier state than is typhoid fever. See also *typhoid fever.*

parenchyma (pah-reng′kĭ-mah) [Gr. "anything poured in beside"] the essential elements of an organ; the functional elements of an organ as distinguished from the supporting structures.

parenchymal (pah-reng′kĭ-mal) pertaining to or of the nature of parenchyma.

parent (par′ent) [L. *parens*] 1. a father or mother.

2. in nuclear medicine, a radionuclide that decays to produce another nuclide called the daughter or offspring. One example is the generator production of technetium-99m, the offspring of the parent molybdenum-99.

parenteral (pah-ren′ter-al) [*para-* + Gr. *enteron* intestine] administered not through the alimentary canal but by infusion or injection.

paresis (pah-re′sis, par′ĕ-sis) [Gr. "relaxation"] a general term for weakness.

general p., a late form of neurosyphilis, commonly affecting individuals aged 40–50 yr, that is characterized by brain atrophy and diffuse cortical neuron loss. The disorder was once a common cause of insanity, but is now rare. Symptoms usually develop about 10 or more yr after the original infection. Emotional disturbances, intellectual decline, tremors, dysarthria, delusions, psychosis, and dementia may progressively occur. Serologic tests for syphilis on blood and cerebrospinal fluid are positive. The CSF usually is characterized by increased numbers of lymphocytes, increased protein concentration, and an elevated gamma-globulin level; there is a first-zone colloidal gold reaction. Without treatment, death occurs in about 3 yr. Penicillin is the treatment of choice. Also called dementia paralytica.

-paresis a suffix word element to denote slight paralysis, e.g., hemiparesis.

pargyline hydrochloride (par′gĭ-lēn) [USP], an antihypertensive, a tertiary amine (hydrochloride), *N*-methyl-*N*-2-propynylbenzylamine hydrochloride; see under *monoamine oxidase inhibitors.*

parietal (pah-ri′ĕ-tal) [L. *parietalis,* from *paries* wall] 1. pertaining to the walls of a body cavity or hollow organ.

2. pertaining to or located near the parietal bones of the cranium, as the parietal lobe of the brain.

parietal bone one of the paired bones that form the upper and lateral parts of the vault of the skull.

parietal cell one of the large spheroidal or pyramidal cells interspersed among other epithelial cells of the gastric body and, less commonly, the pyloric glands. It secretes hydrochloric acid into the lumen of the glands from extensive invaginations of the apical cytoplasm, called the intracellular canaliculi. Also called *oxyntic cell.*

parietal lobe the upper central lobe of the cerebral hemisphere, which is separated from the temporal lobe below by the lateral fissure but is continuous at the posterior end of that sulcus, and is separated from the frontal lobe in front by the central sulcus. Posteriorly, it is continuous with the occipital lobe on the lateral surface, but separated from it by the parietooccipital sulcus on the medial surface.

parietoacanthal projection (pah-ri-ĕ-to-ah-kan′-thal) a radiographic projection of the maxillary sinuses. See under *Waters position.*

parietoorbital projection 1. a radiographic projection of the optic foramen in which the central ray passes along the optic canal inclined 37° laterally and 30° caudally (to the orbitomeatal line). See also *Camp-Gianturco method.*

2. any similar projection. Angulation of 20° laterally and 30° caudally is used to demonstrate the superior orbital fissure; angulation of 20° laterally and 20° caudally is used for the optic foramen and the anterior clinoid process (Lysholm positions); and angulation of 20° laterally and 7° caudally is used for the sphenoid strut (Hough position).

parietotemporal projections (pah-ri″ĕ-to-tem′-po-ral) two projections used for radiography of the petrous portions of the temporal bone. Both demonstrate the petrous apex, mastoid antrum, mastoid cells, internal acoustic canal, and labyrinth. The patient is placed in the semiprone position with the midpoint of the film directly beneath a localization point 1.5 in. anterior to the external auditory meatus. In the Löw-Beer position, the median sagittal plane is horizontal and the central ray is directed at angles of 33° toward the face and 10° toward the head. In the Lysholm position, the neck is flexed back to rotate the infraorbitomeatal line 5° past the transverse axis of the film, the median sagittal plane is tilted 15° toward the face, and the central ray is angled 30° toward the face. This position also demonstrates the carotid canal.

Parinaud's syndrome (pah-rĭ-nōz′) [Henri *Parinaud,* French ophthalmologist, 1844–1905] a syndrome characterized by paralysis of upward and sometimes downward gaze, fixed pupils, and divergence of the eyes. It is associated with tectal midbrain lesions, especially pinealomas.

Paris classification an identification of the human autosomes numbered 1–22 in order of decreasing size by means of their distinct banding patterns. See also *chromosome banding* and *chromosome nomenclature.*

Paris green trivial name for cupric acetoarsenite, $Cu(CH_3COO)_2 \cdot 3Cu(AsO_2)_2$, a larvacide used to destroy mosquitos in the larval stage of growth.

parity (par′ĭ-te) 1. [L. *parere* to bring forth, produce], the condition of a woman with respect to her having borne viable offspring. See also *nullipara* and *primipara.* Cf. *gravidity.*

2. [L. *paritas,* from *par* equal], equality; close correspondence or similarity.

3. in mathematics, a relation holding between two integers: if they are either both even or odd, they have the same parity; if one is odd and the other even, they have different parity.

4. in physics, a symmetry property of the quantum mechanical system: if the state function is unchanged by spatial inversion, the system has even parity; if the sign of the state function is reversed by inversion, the system has odd parity.

5. in computers, a method of checking the integrity of data in the presence of noise, where random bits may be set incorrectly. An extra "parity" bit is appended to a data word and is set so that the number of "1" bits, including the parity bit, is odd (if the convention in use is "odd parity") or even (if the convention is "even parity"). If the data are later found to have the wrong parity ("parity error"), the number is known to be incorrect. Parity checking can detect only single-bit errors; more complex techniques are used to detect and correct multiple-bit errors.

parity bit see under *parity.*

parity check a check for a read, write, or other data transmission error, which is based on the parity of the data groups or computer words. In an even parity check, all the words must have even parity; an odd parity word indicates machine or data transmission error.

Parkinson's disease (par′kin-sunz) [James *Parkinson,* English physician, 1755–1824] see *parkinsonism.*

parkinsonism (par′kin-sun-izm″) [James *Parkinson*] a chronic, progressive disorder of the central nervous system characterized by involuntary tremor, decreased motor power and control, postural instability, and muscular rigidity. The cause is unknown, and the disease most frequently affects individuals in their 50s and 60s. A similar syndrome may occur with phenothiazine administration, carbon monoxide poisoning, cerebral neoplasms, and head trauma.

The onset of the disease is insidious, with slowly progressing rigidity, tremor, and impairment (slowing) of voluntary activity. Ultimately, those affected may become incapable of looking after themselves. The most characteristic pathologic change is cell loss and depigmentation of the pigmented nuclei of the brain stem, especially the substantia nigra.

Diagnosis is based on the clinical picture. Although there is no cure, administration of levodopa (L-dopa) and of anticholinergic drugs may lead to a certain degree of symptomatic relief.

Also called *Parkinson's disease* and *paralysis agitans.*

paromomycin (par″o-mo-mi′sin) one of the aminoglycoside group of antibiotics isolated from various *Streptomyces* species; a bactericidal agent that inhibits protein synthesis. It is used as paromycin sulfate [USP] for the treatment of enteric bacterial and amebic infections and in the preoperative suppression of intestinal flora. Paromomycin is also an investigational drug for the treatment of tapeworm infestations. See also *aminoglycosides* and *antibacterial agents.*

paronychia (par″o-nik′e-ah) [*para-* + Gr. *onyx* nail + *-ia*] an inflammation and infection of the folds of tissue surrounding a fingernail. It is most frequently caused by staphylococci. A purulent lesion may occur and require surgical drainage. Chronic forms of this disorder may be resistant to topical treatment, necessitating the removal of the fingernail.

parotid (pah-rot′id) [*para-* + Gr. *ous* ear] 1. situated or occurring near the ear.

2. pertaining to the parotid gland.

parotid gland the largest of the salivary glands. Its regular shape allows it to fit into the hollow below the ear and behind the mandible. The gland envelops the external carotid artery, and branches of the facial nerve emerge from its upper, anterior, and lower borders. The parotid acini are composed of serous cells. Secretory nerve fibers from the ninth cranial nerve reach the gland via the lesser superficial petrosal nerve, otic ganglion, and auriculotemporal nerve. The parotid duct appears at the anterior border of the gland, and hooks around the masseter to pierce the buccal structures and open into the mouth opposite the second upper molar tooth.

parotiditis (pah-rot″ĭ-di′tis) see *parotitis.*

parotitis (par″o-ti′tis) [*para-* + Gr. *ous* ear + *-itis*] an inflammation of the parotid gland. It is frequently associated with obstruction of the parotid duct (Stensen's duct) by concretions or stones. These bodies may be detected by palpation or x-rays, occasionally with the injection of radiopaque material (sialography). Other causes of parotitis include viral infection leading to epidemic parotitis, or mumps, and bacterial infection, most commonly with *S. aureus,* leading to acute purulent parotitis. This is characterized by local pain, fever, and chills. Parotitis may also be associated with Mikulicz's disease, Sjögren's syndrome, and sarcoidosis. Also called *parotiditis.*

epidemic p., see *mumps.*

paroxysm (par′ok-sizm) [Gr. *paroxysmos*] 1. a sudden recurrence or intensification of symptoms.

2. a spasm, seizure, or burst of activity with sudden onset, rapid attainment of maximum intensity, and sudden termination.

paroxysmal (par″ok-siz′mal) occurring in paroxysms.

paroxysmal aciduria see under *aciduria.*

paroxysmal activity in electroencephalography, electrical activity of the brain that is characterized by an abrupt onset and termination and that clearly differs from the background activity. It can occur normally during hyperventilation in young adults or in response to sensory stimuli during sleep. In other circumstances, paroxysmal activity may relate to pathologic conditions, such as epilepsy; metabolic disorders (e.g., hyper- and hypoglycemia, hyper- and hypoparathyroidism); lesions of diencephalic or rostral midbrain structures; and traumatic, anoxic, or other severe encephalopathies. Such activity may occur with a regular periodicity in Creutzfeldt-Jakob disease, herpes simplex encephalitis, subacute sclerosing panencephalitis, and certain other disorders.

paroxysmal cold hemoglobinuria (PCH) an autoimmune or postviral disease in which IgG directed against the P blood group antigen is produced. It is marked by episodes of hemoglobinemia and hemoglobinuria after exposure to cold, and is diagnosed by the Donath-Landsteiner test. Treatment consists of protection from exposure to cold, and administration of prednisone; cyclophosphamide or similar drugs may be given if the condition is chronic.

paroxysmal depolarizing shift (PDS) large-amplitude depolarizations that can be recorded intracellularly from the soma of mammalian cerebral cortical cells in response to electrical stimulation, freeze lesions, or application of chemicals (strychnine, cobalt, alumina gel, penicillin) to the cortex. PDS with bursts of high-frequency discharges are the most characteristic feature of some "epileptic neurons." They are thought to be mediated by the synaptic activation of the cortical cells, but the nature and origination of the presynaptic influence is not yet known.

paroxysmal nocturnal cephalgia see *cluster h.* under *headache.*

paroxysmal nocturnal hemoglobinuria (PNH) an acquired anemia frequently accompanied by leukopenia and/or thrombocytopenia, which may be the presenting symptoms. Hemoglobinuria is episodic if present and is increased at night. Chronic hemolysis is the usual presentation. Complications include infection and thrombosis.

The disorder results from an abnormality of the red cell membrane, which renders the red cell unusually susceptible to lysis by complement. The PNH lesion is variable in distribution, with some red cell populations more affected than others. Predominantly a disease of young adults, PNH occurs in both sexes and in all races. It can accompany or follow aplastic or hypoplastic anemia and can lead to the development of acute or chronic leukemia.

Diagnosis of PNH depends on demonstration of complement-sensitive red cells. Laboratory findings include a positive acid serum lysis test (Ham test), a positive sucrose lysis test, an autohemolysis test that may demonstrate greater lysis than normal (which is not corrected by glucose and which is the same at 24 and 48 hr), and a normal osmotic fragility test (unless iron deficiency is present).

Also called *Marchiafava-Micheli syndrome.*

parrot fever see *ornithosis.*

Parrot's syndrome (par-ōz′) [Jules Marie *Parrot,* French physician, 1839–1883] a pseudoparalytic form of arthritis characterized by osteochondritis at the epiphyseal plate region, which leads to bone and articular cartilage destruction. It is seen in newborn infants and is the result of congenital syphilis. Diagnosis must be based on appropriate use of serologic tests for syphilis or darkfield examinations of scrapings from moist cutaneous or mucocutaneous lesions.

Parry's disease (par′ēz) [Caleb Hillier *Parry,* English physician, 1755–1822] see *Graves' disease.*

pars, pl. *partes* [L. "part"] [NA], a general term for a particular portion of a larger area, organ, or structure.

p. distalis, the anterior lobe of the hypophysis. See also *adenohypophysis* and *hypophysis.*

p. intermedia, the part of the adenohypophysis between the pars distalis and pars nervosa, which in adult humans consists of a band of follicles and chromophobic and basophilic cells.

p. nervosa, the posterior lobe of the pituitary gland. See also *neurohypophysis.*

p. tuberalis, the upward extension of the pars distalis (anterior lobe) of the pituitary gland over the anterior and lateral surfaces of the stalk of the infundibulum.

parthenogenesis (par″thĕ-no-jen′ĕ-sis) [Gr. *parthenos* virgin + *genesis* production] the development of an individual from an unfertilized egg, which can occur in some lower animals either naturally or by artificial induction. See also *fertilization.*

partial identity pattern see under *Ouchterlony immunodiffusion.*

partial pressure (P) the pressure that each component gas (in a mixture of gases) would exert if it were present alone. By Dalton's law of partial pressures, the sum of all the partial pressures equals the total pressure of an ideal gas mixture. The partial pressure of a component gas dissolved in a liquid refers to the partial pressure of that component gas in the gas phase that is in equilibrium with the liquid. The partial pressure of oxygen in blood, for example, is the pressure exerted by all the molecules of oxygen that are both dissolved in the plasma and combined with hemoglobin.

p. p. of carbon dioxide (P_{CO_2}), the portion of the pressure of a mixture of gases that is contributed by CO_2; for a fluid not directly in contact with a gas phase (e.g., blood), the P_{CO_2} refers to the pressure of CO_2 in an imaginary gas phase that would be in equilibrium with the fluid. The P_{CO_2} of dry atmospheric air at sea level and at 37°C is 0.3 torr (0.3 mmHg), or equal to the total barometric pressure (760 torr or mmHg) times the fraction of carbon dioxide in air (0.0004).

Reference ranges for P_{CO_2} in arterial blood are: for males, 35–45 mmHg; and for females, 32–43. Venous blood has a P_{CO_2} slightly higher than that of arterial blood. The highest P_{CO_2} observed in individuals breathing air is about 90 mmHg; the lowest is about 10 mmHg (with compensatory hyperventilation in metabolic acidosis).

An increased P_{CO_2} in blood (hypercapnia) is observed in respiratory acidosis, which may be caused by hypoventilation as a result of pulmonary disease, depressant drugs, or circulatory disorders. It may also be due to retention of CO_2 as a result of the compensatory respiratory mechanism in metabolic alkalosis. A decreased P_{CO_2} (hypocapnia) is observed in respiratory alkalosis, which is the result of increased alveolar ventilation. It may be caused by arterial respiratory stimuli, pharmaceuticals, anxiety, or hypoxia. A rapid lowering of P_{CO_2} from hypercapnic levels by controlled ventilation may cause convulsions and death. A decreased P_{CO_2} may also be the result of the respiratory compensatory mechanism in metabolic acidosis.

Also called *carbon dioxide tension.* See also *blood gas analysis.*

p. p. of nitrogen (P_{N_2}), the pressure exerted by nitrogen in a mixture of gases or its partial pressure in a liquid. The P_{N_2} of dry atmospheric air at sea level and at 37°C is equal to 600 torr or the total barometric pressure (760 torr) times the fraction of the air that is nitrogen (0.79).

p. p. of oxygen (P_{O_2}), the portion of the total pressure of a mixture of gases that is exerted by the O_2 in the mixture, or for a fluid (such as blood) that contains dissolved O_2, the pressure it exerts in an imaginary gas phase in equilibrium with the fluid. The P_{O_2} of dry atmospheric air at sea level and at 37°C is equal to 159 torr, or equal to the total barometric pressure (760 torr) times the fraction of O_2 in air (0.21).

Arterial blood has a P_{O_2} of 80–104 mmHg in healthy young males breathing room air. (Normal arterial oxygenation decreases steadily with age.) The reference for the P_{O_2} of venous blood under similar circumstances is 30–49 mmHg. The P_{O_2} of arterial blood (Pa_{O_2}) is considered to be a sensitive (although nonspecific) indicator of abnormal gas exchange. In other words, although a low Pa_{O_2}) (i.e., hypoxemia) indicates that abnormal gas exchange function of the lungs exists, it does not establish the underlying pathologic mechanism (i.e., $\dot{V}/\dot{Q}$ imbalance, alveolar hypoventilation, venous admixture, or diffusion defect) or disease. Although it is difficult to predict the exact level of hypoxemia that can threaten life, a Pa_{O_2} of about 50–55 mmHg is generally considered to be a minimal value to strive for in the therapeutic management of respiratory failure.

Also called *oxygen tension.* See also *blood gas analysis.*

p. p. of water vapor the partial pressure of water vapor in air. It varies directly with the ambient temperature and does not vary with changes in barometric pressure. Water vapor at sea level maintains a partial pressure in the inspired tracheal air (at a body temperature of 37°C) of 47 torr, leaving only 713 torr of the total barometric pressure (760 torr) for the sum of the partial pressures of CO_2, N_2, and O_2.

partial thromboplastin time test (PTT) a test that measures the coagulation factors of the intrinsic system present in plasma. Calcium chloride, a phospholipid substitute for platelets (partial thromboplastin), and an activator to ensure maximal activation of Factor XII (kaolin, celite, micronized silica, or ellagic acid) are added to plasma, and the time needed for fibrin formation is determined. The PTT is prolonged in the deficiency of Factors II, V, VIII, IX, X, XI, and XII (factor concentrations of 35 percent of normal, or less). The PTT can be used to screen for deficiency of Factors VIII, IX, XI, and XII when it is combined with a simultaneous PT that is not prolonged.

In addition, plasma may be screened for Fletcher factor deficiency by employing a partial thromboplastin reagent containing an activator other than ellagic acid. Low fibrinogen may also prolong the PTT and prothrombin time. The PTT may also be used to monitor heparin therapy.

Also called *activated partial thromboplastin time* (aPTT). See also *prothrombin time test.*

particle (par'tĭ-k'l) [L. *particula,* dim. of *pars* part] 1. any small mass of matter, such as a colloidal particle.

2. in physics, a body so small that it either has no internal structure or the internal structure is insignificant in most contexts. See also *alpha particle, beta particle, electron, elementary particle, gamma ray, neutron, nucleus, photon,* and *proton.*

particulate (par-tik'u-lāt) 1. composed of minute, solid particles.

2. having the form of minute particles.

settled p.'s, a component of air pollution measured by gravimetric analysis of the matter settling out of the air in an open-top cylinder.

suspended p.'s, a component of air pollution measured by high-volume filtration and gravimetric analysis.

partition coefficient (K_d) (par-tish'un) a measure of the relative solubility of a solute in two immiscible liquids defined as the equilibrium constant for the distribution of the solute between the two liquids, i.e., the constant ratio of the solute's concentration in the upper phase to its concentration in the lower phase. Also called *distribution coefficient.*

-partum (par'tum) [L. *partus,* past participle of *pario* to bear] a suffix word element to denote birth or labor, e.g., postpartum.

parturition (par"tu-rish'un) [L. *parturitio* the act or process of giving birth to a child] see *labor.*

Paryphostomum (par"e-fos'to-mum) a genus of flukes. The species *P. sufrartyfex* (also called *Artyfechinostomum sufrartyfex, Echinostoma sufrartyfex,* and *Euparyphium malayanum*), which is parasitic in humans in India, measures 9 mm long by 2.5 mm wide. The eggs are operculated and measure 90–125 μ by 60–75 μ. Infection resembles that of a fasciolopsiasis.

PAS abbrev. See *p-aminosalicylic acid, periodic acid–Schiff reaction.*

PASCAL (pas-kahl') [after Blaise *Pascal,* French scientist, 1623–1662, who designed the first calculating machine] one of the newer and more modern high-level computer programming languages. Its syntax and logic are designed to support the practice of structured programming, which is difficult and unnatural in most dialects of BASIC and FORTRAN, but is simple enough so that PASCAL (unlike PL/I) can be run on microcomputers; it is a good teaching language.

pascal (Pa) [Blaise *Pascal*] the International System (SI) unit of pressure defined as 1 newton per square meter (N/m^2). See also *atmosphere, millimeter of mercury,* and *torr.*

PAS reaction abbrev. *See periodic acid–Schiff reaction.*

Passavant's bar (pas'ah-vants) [Philip Gustav *Passavant,* German surgeon, 1815–1893] a rounded, horizontal bar that forms on the posterior wall of the pharynx below the level of the soft palate during swallowing, because of the contraction of the transverse fibers of the palatopharyngeal sphincter. It also appears during speech in persons with cleft palate. Also called Passavant's ridge and *pharyngeal ridge.*

passive agglutination (pas'iv) [L. *passivus,* from *pati* to suffer or undergo] see *indirect agglutination.*

passive cutaneous anaphylaxis (PCA) a reaction used in studies of antibodies causing immediate hypersensitivity. In the procedure an antibody or antiserum is injected intradermally into a laboratory animal and is followed about 24 hr later by intravenous injection of the specific antigen and a dye such as Evans blue, which labels albumin. Bluing of the skin at the intradermal injection site indicates altered vascular permeability by virtue of the pressure of the dye-labeled albumin.

passive immunity see under *immunity.*

passive transport (pas'iv) the inward translocation of ions or metabolites across a cell membrane with the concentration gradient. No energy (as adenosine triphosphate, ATP) is required, although specific mechanisms within the membrane may be present.

Passovoy factor a factor in the intrinsic pathway of blood coagulation, the deficiency of which leads to a hemorrhagic tendency resembling Factor XI deficiency. See also *coagulation factors* and *coagulation pathways.*

Pasteur effect (pas-ter') [Louis *Pasteur,* French chemist and bacteriologist, 1822–1895] a phenomenon in microorganisms, first observed by Pasteur, in which glycolysis can be diminished or abolished by limiting the availability of oxygen. The inhibitory effect of the large amounts of adenosine triphosphate (ATP) produced during aerobic metabolism on the regulatory properties of phosphofructokinase can account for most aspects of this phenomenon.

Pasteurella (pas'tĕ-rel'ah) [Louis *Pasteur*] a genus of gram-negative, nonmotile, facultatively anaerobic organisms of uncertain taxonomic status, which are ovoid to rodlike in shape. They are oxidase- and catalase-positive, are susceptible to penicillin, and show marked bipolar staining. *Pasteurella* organisms are primarily animal pathogens, causing fowl cholera, cattle "shipping fever," and hemorrhagic septicemia in many animals and birds. They are also known to be the cause of a variety of human diseases, ranging from local abscesses to fatal septicemias.

P. haemolytica, the cause of disease in fowl, sheep, and cattle, and a potential human pathogen.

P. multocida, a pathogenic species causing disease in animals and humans, such as local infections following a cat scratch or animal bite, chronic pulmonary infections, or systemic infections with meningitis or bacteremia. The organism is very sensitive to penicillin; several biotypes and serologic types are recognized. Formerly called *P. septica.*

P. pestis, see *Y. pestis* under *Yersinia.*

P. pneumotropica, a species occasionally isolated from human sources but of no known pathogenicity in humans.

P. pseudotuberculosis, see *Y. pseudotuberculosis* under *Yersinia.*

P. septica, the obsolete name for *P. multocida.*

P. tularensis, see *F. tularensis* under *Francisella.*

P. ureae, the only species of the genus with no known animal host. It has been isolated from human infections of the upper respiratory tract.

pasteurellosis (pas"ter-ĕ-lo'sis) [*Pasteurella* + *-osis*] infection by microorganisms of the genus *Pasteurella,* especially *P. multocida.*

pasteurization (pas"ter-ĭ-za'shun) [Louis *Pasteur*] the process of heat treatment devised by Pasteur to destroy microorganisms in wine and beer that would otherwise cause spoilage. It is now used widely to make beverages (especially milk) and foods safe for consumption by killing any pathogenic microorganisms, such as tubercle bacilli, that might be present. Milk is heated gradually to 62°C for 30 min, or rapidly to 80°C for 15–30 sec (flash pasteurization). Many harmless bacteria survive and the desirable properties are in large part retained.

Pasteur pipet [Louis *Pasteur*] a pipet fitted with a rubber bulb for suction, used to avoid oral contact when transferring cultures of pathogenic microorganisms or toxic solutions.

patch test (pach) [L. *pittacium,* Gr. *pittakion*] an immunologic skin test that detects hypersensitivity to a specific antigen. The antigen in question is applied to the skin and then covered with an impervious dressing for 48 hr. Positive hypersensitivity is shown by an eczematous skin eruption. The skin test for allergy to poison ivy or oak extract is one example of a patch test.

patell/o (pah-tel'o) [L. *patella* patella] a word element used in combining form to denote patella, e.g., patelliform.

patella (pah-tel'ah) [L., dim. of *patera* a shallow dish] the largest of the sesamoid bones, which is embedded in the quadriceps tendon in front of the knee joint. Its posterior aspect is largely occupied by an articular surface for the femur.

patency (pa'ten-se) [L. *patens* open] the condition of being open.

patent (pa'tent) 1. open, unobstructed, exposed.
2. apparent, evident.

patent blue V a triphenylmethane acid dye; C.I. 42051. it is used in the leuko patent blue stain for hemoglobin peroxidase. Also called *alphazurine 2G.*

patent ductus arteriosus (pa'tent duk'tus arte're-o-sus) a ductus arteriosus that remains open after birth. The normal ductus arteriosus closes at birth and becomes occluded permanently through intimal proliferation and fibrosis in the early postnatal months. Persistent patency is relatively common and may coexist with other cardiovascular malformations. The clinical effects of a patent ductus depend on the relative pressures in the systemic and pulmonary circulations and the caliber and length of the connecting channel. Usually there is a shunt from aorta to pulmonary artery throughout the cardiac cycle, and a "machinery" murmur is produced. Venous return from the lungs is increased, resulting in dilation of the left atrium and ventricle. In the absence of contraindications such as associated anomalies of the heart, or lung disease, surgical correction by ligation or division is commonly performed.

paternity [L. *paternus* fatherly, from *pater* father] the state of fatherhood, or descent on a father's side.

paternity testing any laboratory procedure performed to aid in the evaluation of disputed parentage, primarily paternity. Tests performed on blood samples of the offspring and its alleged parents include examination of red blood cell antigens, serum proteins, red blood cell enzymes, and HLA antigens. By employing all these procedures, various genetic markers may be determined, and an exclusion rate greater than 98 percent is possible. Care must be taken during laboratory procedures regarding patient identification and confidential information to avoid compromising test results.

Paterson-Kelly syndrome [Donald Rose *Paterson*, Welsh laryngologist, 1863–1939; Adam Brown *Kelly*, 1865–1941] see *Plummer-Vinson syndrome.*

path/o (path′o) [Gr. *pathos* disease] a word element used in combining form to denote disease, e.g., pathology.

pathogen (path′o-jen) [*patho-* + Gr. *gennan* to produce] any microorganism or agent that is capable of producing disease. The term is usually restricted to living agents. See also *bacterial pathogenicity.*

pathogenesis (path″o-jen′ĕ-sis) [*patho-* + Gr. *genesis* origin] the development of morbid conditions or disease, more specifically the biochemical and physiologic mechanisms by which the disease progresses. Cf. *etiology.*

pathogenic (path-o-jen′ik) able to cause disease.

pathognomonic (path″og-no-mon′ik) [*patho-* + Gr. *gnōmonikos* fit to give judgment] specifically distinctive or characteristic of a disease; said of a sign, symptom, or test result on which a diagnosis can be made because the range of values or findings observed in diseased individuals does not overlap the range of values observed in healthy persons.

pathologic (path″o-log′ik) 1. diseased; exhibiting abnormal function, structure, or appearance.
2. pertaining to pathology.

pathologic fracture a fracture due to weakening of the bone structure from a pathologic process such as a neoplasm or osteomyelitis.

pathologist (pah-thol′o-jist) a specialist in the structural and functional changes caused by the disease process.

pathology (pah-thol′o-je) [*patho-* + Gr. *logos* word or reason] the branch of medicine that deals with the basis of disease, especially those structural and functional changes in organs and tissues causing or caused by disease.

anatomic p., the subspecialty of pathology that deals with the diagnosis of disease from the gross and microscopic examination of tissues and cells removed from patients during surgery, by biopsy, or during postmortem examination.

clinical p., the subspecialty of pathology that deals with the use of laboratory methods (clinical chemistry, microbiology, hematology, immunology, cytogenetics, etc.) in the diagnosis and treatment of disease.

experimental p., the study of artificially induced disease processes and animal models of disease.

geographic p., the study of the relationship of geography and climate to disease.

surgical p., the subspecialty of pathology that deals with the diagnosis of disease from the examination of tissue removed from patients during surgery or by biopsy.

-pathy (path′e) [Gr. *pathos* disease] a suffix word element to denote a disease process, e.g., endocrinopathy.

patient (pa′shent) [L. *patiens*] a person who is undergoing medical treatment.

Paul-Bunnell test [John Rodman *Paul*, U.S. physician, 1893–1971; Wallis Willard *Bunnell*, U.S. physician, born 1902] a hemagglutination test for the presence of heterophil antibodies in blood, which is suggestive of infectious mononucleosis. The serum from an individual with infectious mononucleosis can agglutinate sheep red blood cells. The level of heterophil antibodies in the blood can be expressed as agglutination titer. The antibody responsible for the sheep cell agglutination in this test is called the heterophil antibody. The determination of heterophil antibody specific for infectious mononucleosis is made by the Davidson differential test. See also *infectious mononucleosis.*

paurometabolous [Gr. *pauros* little + *metabolē* change] a gradual metamorphosis characteristic of some insects of the class Insecta.

Pautrier microabscess (po′tre-a) [Lucien Marius Adolphe *Pautrier*, French dermatologist, 1876–1959] a collection of mycosis cells (malignant lymphoid cells of T-cell origin) and nonspecific inflammatory cells, usually located in the lower epidermis but occasionally present in the upper portions of hair follicles. When present, this finding is almost pathognomonic of mycosis fungoides.

pavor (pa′vor) [L.] terror.

p. diurnus, attacks of fear in children during the afternoon nap.

p. nocturnus, "night terror," a sleep disorder that occurs most frequently in children during the first hours after falling asleep. It occurs in association with sleep stages 3 and 4, and is characterized by anxiety, increased heart rate and respiration, vocalizations (such as screaming or crying), and motor activity for a few minutes, after which the individual quiets down again. Rarely are more than fragments of content remembered. The electroencephalogram during the attacks displays a mixture of slow-wave, alpha, and beta activities. Pharmacologic agents that interfere with the metabolism of norepinephrine or serotonin have been used to treat this disorder. Also called *sleep terror disorder.*

Pb [L. *plumbum*] symbol for the chemical element *lead.*

PBG abbrev. See *porphobilinogen.*

PBI abbrev. for protein-bound iodine. See under *thyroxine assays.*

P blood group see under *blood groups.*

π bond see *pi b.* under *bond.*

PBS abbrev. for phosphate-buffered saline.

PC abbrev. See *phosphatidylcholine, printed circuit.*

PCA abbrev. See *passive cutaneous anaphylaxis.*

PCB abbrev. See *polychlorinated biphenyl.*

PCH abbrev. See *paroxysmal cold hemoglobinuria.*

pCi abbrev. See *picocurie.*

PCO_2 abbrev. See *p. p. of carbon dioxide* under *partial pressure.*

Π-complex an adduct formed between two molecules or two parts of one molecule in which the bond between them involves electron-pair donation from a Π-orbital in the donor to a σ-orbital in the acceptor, from a σ- to a Π-orbital, or from a Π- to a Π-orbital. See also *charge-transfer complex.*

PCP abbrev. See *pentachlorophenol.*

PCV abbrev. for packed cell volume. See *hematocrit.*

Pd symbol for the chemical element *palladium.*

PDS abbrev. See *paroxysmal depolarizing shift.*

PE abbrev. for paper electrophoresis (see under *electrophoresis*), *phosphatidylethanolamine, photographic effect.*

peak (pēk) 1. the maximal value of a physical quantity, such as electrical current or voltage.

2. on a graph or chart, such as the output of a gas chromatograph or recording spectrophotometer, the portion of the curve rising from one minimum to a maximum and falling to a minimum.

peak acid output (PAO) the rate of acid secretion (millimoles of titratable acidity per hour) by the stomach after maximal stimulation by pentagastrin or betazole (Histalog). Generally, six 15-min specimens are collected, and the PAO is calculated on the basis of the two 15-min specimens with the highest acid output. See also *gastric function tests.*

peak amplitude the maximal deviation from zero in a positive or negative direction of an alternating-current waveform.

peak area on a gas chromatogram, the area (above the baseline) under a peak. The peak area can be measured manually (using a planimeter), mechanically (using a disk integrator), or electronically (using digital logic circuitry). For some analyses, it is a better measure of the amount of sample component present than is peak height.

peak broadening in gas chromatography, the phenomenon that the peak width of the various components increases with their retention time.

peak expiratory flow rate (PEFR) a clinical test of pulmonary function involving measurement of a single expiration, commonly used to detect obstructive pulmonary disease. The subject inhales maximally, then expires rapidly, with maximal expiratory force. The highest instantaneous flow velocity (in liters per minute) achieved during the maximal forced expiration is recorded, usually with a Wright peak-flow meter. Dynamic compression of the airways with the progressively increasing expiratory force limits the expiratory air flow to a maximum of 6–12 l/min (0.1–0.2 l/sec) in a healthy subject; this amount decreases markedly in a patient with emphysema or asthma.

peak height on a gas chromatogram, the maximal height (above the baseline) of a peak, commonly used as a measure of the amount of the sample component represented by the peak.

peak kilovoltage (pkV, kVp) the highest voltage applied to an x-ray tube. The power supply produces a pulsed DC output; pkV is the maximal voltage produced, not the average. Also called kilovolts peak.

peak-to-peak amplitude the sum of the positive and negative peak amplitudes; for a symmetric alternating-current waveform, it is double the peak amplitude.

peanut oil the refined fixed oil (triglycerides) obtained from the seed kernels of one or more of the cultivated varieties of *Arachis hypogaea;* used, [USP grade], as a solvent for drugs and in veterinary medicine as a laxative. Peanut oil is an important food oil. Also called *groundnut oil.*

pearl (perl) a compact whorl to crescentic, concentrically grouped, keratinized squamous cells found in stratified squamous epithelium and disorders such as keratoacanthoma and squamous carcinoma.

pectenosis (pek″tĕ-no′sis) [L. *pecten* comb + *-osis*] stenosis of the anal canal, causing pain on defecation and bleeding; when severe, the condition may be associated with intestinal obstruction. It is caused by constriction about the pectineal line, the area between the anal groove and the anal crypts.

pectin (pek′tin) [Gr. *pēktos* congealed] [NF], a homosaccharidic polymer of galacturonic acid, with the carboxyls partly or fully methylated, that is present in plant cell walls. Pectin is generally used in conjunction with opiates and, with an adsorbant such as kaolin, to control diarrhea. At the proper pH, it forms gels with sugar, and is used in cooking and as a surface protectant.

pectinate (pek′tĭ-nāt) [L. *pecten* comb] shaped like a comb.

pectinate body a descriptive term for certain fungal hyphae that project outward, like the teeth of a comb. This type of structure is sometimes found in dermatophytes, especially *Microsporum audouinii.*

Pectinibranchiata an order of operculate snails of the class Gastropoda.

Pectobacterium (pek″to-bak-te′re-um) a genus of bacteria of the family Enterobacteriaceae. These organisms are of unknown clinical significance but may be confused with species of *Enterobacter, Hafnia,* and *Serratia.* They are also plant pathogens. See also *Enterobacteriaceae.*

pector/o (pek′tor-o) [L. *pectus* breast] a word element used in combining form to denote the chest, e.g., pectoral.

pectoral (pek′to-ral) [L. *pectoralis,* from *pectus* breast] of or pertaining to the breast or chest.

pectus (pek′tus) [L.] the breast, chest, or thorax.

p. excavatum, see *funnel chest.*

ped/o (pe′do) 1. [Gr. *pais, paidos* child], a word element used in combining form to denote child, e.g., pedology, pediatric.

2. [L. *pes, pedis* foot], word element used in combining form to denote relationship to a foot, e.g., pedopathy.

pederin (ped′er-in) [N.L. *Paederus* genus of beetles] a compound in the body fluids of rove beetles of the genus *Paederus,* family Staphylinidae. Contact with the skin causes a necrotizing lesion with desquamation (shedding of epithelial cells in scales or sheets), which heals very slowly. The fluid is discharged when the beetle is crushed. Rove beetles are common in early spring and summer.

pedia- (pe′de-ah) [Gr. *pais, paidos* child] a word element used in combining form to denote relationship to a child, e.g., pediatrics. See also *ped/o.*

pediatrician a physician who specializes in pediatrics.

pediatrics (pe″de-at′riks) [*ped-* Gr. *iatrikē* surgery, medicine] the branch of medicine that deals with the development, problems, and diseases of infants, children, and adolescents.

pedicel (ped′ĭ-sel) [N.L. *pedicellus,* dim. of L. *pediculus,* dim. of *pes* foot] one of the footlike terminal processes of the podocytes of the renal glomeruli. Each interdigitates with those of neighboring podocytes, forming a complex system of narrow intercellular clefts (slit pores). See also *podocyte.*

pedicle (ped′ĭ-k′l) [L. *pediculus,* dim. of *pes* foot] a footlike or stalklike portion of structure, as the footlike synaptic terminals of cone cells in the retina or the narrow anterior region of the vertebral arch. See also *cone cells.*

graft p., a narrow strip of tissue that connects a graft with the original donor site. Pedicle flaps orginate from donor areas such as the neck, the thoracoabdominal region of the trunk, and the anteromedial aspect of the thighs. They have largely been replaced by free flap procedures.

pediculosis (pe-dik″u-lo′sis) [L. *pediculus,* dim. of *pedis* louse + *-osis* condition] infestation with lice. Infestation is commonly found among prisoners, soldiers during wartime, and in general among those living in crowded, unhygienic conditions.

Humans are infested by three types of lice, which are obligate bloodsuckers (1) the head louse, *Pediculus humanus capitis,* usually found on the back of the neck, which occurs more often in children than in adults; (2) the body louse, *P. humanus corporis,* found on any part of the body where nymphs or adults feed, which produces cutaneous lesions and which can transmit typhus, relapsing fever, and trench fever; and (3) the pubic or "crab" louse, *Phthirus pubis,* which inhabits the pubic region. It transmits no disease.

Active forms and nits can usually be recognized with the naked eye, but a hand lens and flashlight may be helpful in searching for *P. humanus capitis.* The examiner should take care to avoid infestation. Microscopic examination of hair casts and globules will differentiate the pseudonits from eggs of lice.

See also *louse, P. humanus capitis* and *P. humanus corporis* under *Pediculus,* and *P. pubis* under *Phthirus.*

Pediculus (pe-dik′-u-lus) [L., dim of *pedis* louse] a genus of wingless sucking lice of the family Pediculidae, two species of which infest humans.

P. humanus capitis, the head louse, measuring 2–3 mm long, which inhabits the head, neck, and ears of its host. It obtains nourishment by biting and sucking on the human host. These insects have a cosmopolitan distribution.

Diagnosis requires the finding of adults in hairy areas and the microscopic examination of suspected nits to determine that they are truly eggs.

See also *vagabond's disease.*

P. humanus corporis, the body louse, measuring 2–3 mm in size, which is longer and less crablike than the pubic louse. These lice are found around the armpits, waist, neck, shoulders, and crotch—wherever the body and clothing are in close contact. The female louse deposits her eggs in the seams of clothing, and subsequent infection is acquired from contact with the clothing or from infested people. When the bites caused by lice are scratched, feces are introduced into the abrasions, thus transmitting any diseases present. The body louse is the vector of typhus, trench fever, and relapsing fever. Microscopic examination of eggs in clothing confirms the diagnosis. See also *vagabond's disease.*

pedigree chart in genetics, a diagram used to summarize the family history of a genetic defect for the purpose of determining the mode of inheritance or assessing the risk of genetic defects. An example is shown in the accompanying illustration.

pedogenesis (pe″do-jen′ĕ-sis) [*pedo-*(1) + Gr. *genesis* reproduction] the process by which the larval stages of insects, especially flies, produce parthenogenetic eggs that give rise to more larvae. Some of these larvae undergo metamorphosis into adults, both male and female, which mate and produce fertilized eggs.

peduncle (pe-dung′k′l) [N.L. *pedunculus,* dim. of L. *pes* foot] a stemlike connecting part; a general term for collections of nerve fibers coursing between different areas in the central nervous system.

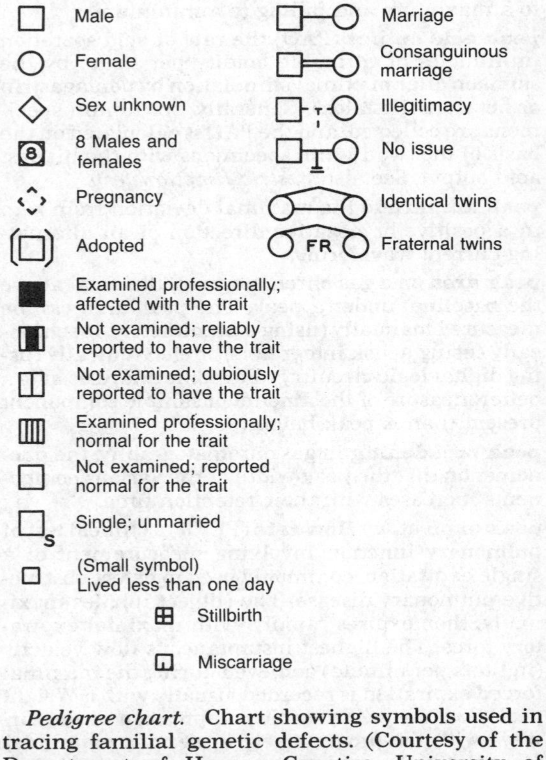

Pedigree chart. Chart showing symbols used in tracing familial genetic defects. (Courtesy of the Department of Human Genetics, University of Michigan, Robert P. Erickson, M.D.)

cerebellar p., one of the thick trunks of fibers that connect the cerebellum with the brain stem and higher areas of the brain. These fibers are divided into three paired branches; the inferior branches, which connect the cerebellum with the medulla oblongata and the spinal cord; the middle branches, which transmit information from the cerebral cortex to the cerebellum by way of the pontine nuclei; and the superior trunks, which carry fibers from the cerebellum to the midbrain, primarily the red nuclei, and to the thalamus.

pedunculated (pĕ-dung′ku-lāt-ed) stalked, having a peduncle. Cf. *sessile.*

PEEP abbrev. See *positive end-expiratory pressure.*

PEFR abbrev. See *peak expiratory flow rate.*

PEG abbrev. See *pneumoencephalography, polyethylene glycol.*

Pel-Ebstein fever (pel eb′stīn) [Pieter Klaases *Pel,* Dutch physician, 1852–1919; Wilhelm *Ebstein,* German physician, 1836–1912] a cyclic fever pattern characterized by several days or weeks of fever alternating with afebrile periods. This symptom has been observed in Hodgkin's disease.

Pelger-Huët anomaly (pel′ger hyoo′et) [Karel *Pelger,* Dutch physician, 1885–1931; G.J. *Huët,* Dutch physician, born 1879] a familial condition, transmitted as a mendelian dominant trait, that is characterized by polymorphonuclear leukocytes that are pedominantly unsegmented, with only occasional cells having bilobed nuclei. This condition has no known clinical significance in humans.

pellagra (pĕ-la′grah, pĕ-lag′rah) [It. *pelle* skin + *agra* rough] a deficiency disorder due to a diet insufficient in niacin or tryptophan. It is characterized by weakness, chronic dermatitis, diarrhea, and central nervous system disorders that resemble dementia (the "three D's" of pellagra are a mnemonic for dermatitis, diarrhea, and dementia). The mucous membrane of the mouth and tongue may also be affected. There is no definitive diagnostic biochemical test for pellagra. Treatment is centered on niacin replacement.

Pellegrini's disease (pel″ĕ-gre′nēz) [Augusto *Pellegrini,* Italian surgeon, 20th century] calcification of the medial collateral ligament of the knee due to trauma, often repeated, to the area.

pellicle (pel′ĭ-k′l) [L. *pellicula,* dim. of *pellis* skin] a continuous or fragmentary skin or film that may form on the surface of a liquid culture of bacteria or fungi.

pellucid (pĕ-lu′sid) [L. *pellucidus,* from *per* through + *lucere* to shine] translucent.

pelv/i, pelv/o, pelvi/o (pel′vĭ, pel′vo, pel′ve-o) [L. *pelvis* basin] a word element used in combining form to denote the pelvic bone or hip, e.g., pelvimetry.

pelvic (pel′vik) pertaining to the pelvis.

pelvicephalography (pel″vĭ-sef″ah-log′rah-fe) [*pelvi-* + Gr. *kephalē* head + *graphein* to write] see *roentgen p.* under *pelvimetry.*

pelvicephalometry (pel″vĭ-sef″ah-lom′ĕ-tre) [*pelvi-* + Gr. *kephalē* head + *metron* measure] see *roentgen p.* under *pelvimetry.*

pelvic inflammatory disease (PID) see *salpingitis.*

pelvimetry (pel-vim′ĕ-tre) [*pelvi-* + Gr. *metron* measure] any method of measurement of the pelvic outlet, or other pelvic diameters.

Caldwell-Moloy method, a method of radiographic pelvimetry in which three views of the pelvis are obtained. The first is a stereoscopic anteroposterior projection with the patient supine; the fetal head and pelvic diameters are determined by measuring the three-dimensional phantom image produced by the precision stereoscope. The second is a lateral projection with the patient erect; it demonstrates the sacrum and sciatic notches in which true distances are indicated by a metal rule placed in the midgluteal fold. The third is an inferosuperior anteroposterior projection (45° angulation) with the patient supine, which demonstrates the lower pelvis and semipubic arch.

Colcher-Sussman method, a method of roentgen pelvimetry using an anterior projection (supine position) and a lateral projection (lateral position). A Colcher-Sussman pelvimeter (a perforated metal ruler and adjustable holder) is used to correct for magnification by placement in the posterior view at the level of the ischial tuberosities and in the lateral view at the level of the gluteal fold.

roentgen p., a radiologic measurement, performed to determine whether delivery by cesarean section is necessary, which assesses the diameters of the head of the unborn fetus and the maternal pelvic outlet. Among the methods devised for correcting for magnification and distortion in the radiographs of these structures are: (1) the use of rulers or grids (pelvimeters), which are placed at the same object film distance as the diameters to be measured so that they are subject to the same magnification; (2) the use of tables or nomograms that allow correction factors for a view to be determined from measurements made on a perpendicular view; and (3) the use of teleradiography to minimize magnification. Also called *pelvicephalography, pelvicephalometry, pelvioradiograhy,* and *pelviradiography.*

Thoms method, a method of roentgen pelvimetry that uses a lateral view, in which true distances are indicated by a metal rule held in the midgluteal fold, and an inlet view, in which true distances are indicated by a perforated metal grid placed in the plane of the pelvic inlet for a second exposure after the patient has been removed.

pelvioradiography (pel″ve-o-ra″de-og′rah-fe) [*pelvio-* + *radiography*] see *roentgen p.* under *pelvimetry.*

pelviradiography (pel″vĭ-ra″de-og′rah-fe) [*pelvi-* + *radiography*] see *roentgen p.* under *pelvimetry.*

pelvis (pel′vis), pl. *pelves* [L. "basin"; Gr. *pyelos* an oblong trough] 1. [NA], the lower (caudal) portion of the trunk. It forms a basin bounded anteriorly and laterally by the two innominate bones and posteriorly by the sacrum and coccyx.

2. any basinlike structure, e.g., the renal pelvis.

pemphigoid (pem′fĭ-goid) [Gr. *pemphix* blister + *eidos* form] a group of skin diseases that resembles, but is less severe than, pemphigus. Differentiation from pemphigus is aided by histologic and immunofluorescent examination of a biopsy specimen of a lesion. Cf. *pemphigus.*

bullous p., a chronic and relatively self-limited form of blistering disease, seen primarily in older individuals (above age 60); its cause is unknown. The disease is characterized by subepidermal bullae occuring anywhere on the skin. Immunofluorescent studies reveal antibodies of the IgG class, which react specifically against antigens in the basement membrane of the subepidermal lesions. It should be distinguished from pemphigus, a much more serious disorder.

pemphigus (pem′fĭ-gus) [N.L., from Gr. *pemphix* blister] a rare group of cutaneous disorders of unknown etiologies, occuring primarily in adults and characterized by the formation of vesicles and bullae. This disease may appear in several forms, of which pemphigus vulgaris is the most important clinical entity. It is a chronic disease characterized by the appearance of bullae of the skin near the mouth, nose, and scalp, and often the axilla and groin. These blisters break, leaving eroded patches of raw and tender skin where secondary bacterial infections may occur.

The disease eventually becomes generalized, leading to weakness, electrolytic imbalances, and, frequently, death.

Diagnosis is based on histologic examination of a biopsy of a lesion. Characteristic features include intercellular edema and loss of intercellular bridge attachments in the lower epidermis, leading to a loss of cohesion between epidermal cells (acantholysis). Immunofluorescent studies reveal serum antibodies of the IgG class to intercellular substances in the skin and mucous membrane. Treatment is with corticosteroids and immunosuppressive agents.

Cf. *pemphigoid.*

benign familial p., a recurrent hereditary form of pemphigus, characterized by vesicles and blisters involving the neck, groin, and axilla. These eruptions often give off a foul odor and can persist for long periods. Also called *Hailey-Hailey disease.*

p. neonatorum, bullous impetigo. See under *scalded skin syndrome.*

p. vulgaris, the most severe of the various forms of pemphigus.

penetrability (pen″ĕ-trah-bil′ĭ-te) the intensity of an x-ray beam, based on the thickness of aluminum or other material penetrated by the beam as measured with a penetrometer.

penetrance (pen′ĕ-trans) [L. *penetrare* to enter into] 1. the extent to which a substance is entered or infiltrated by another substance or object.

2. in genetics, the fraction of individuals having a particular genotyope that exhibit the corresponding mutant phenotype. Individuals not showing the trait are said to be nonpenetrant. Cf. *expressivity.*

complete p., the appearance in all individuals of the phenotype of a single dominant gene or of homozygous recessive genes.

incomplete p., the appearance in only some individuals of the phenotype of a single dominant gene or of homozygous recessive genes.

penetrating radiation (pen′ĕ-trāt-ing) in dosimetry, radiation having a long range in tissue so that particles emitted in one organ produce a significant absorbed dose in another. Cf. *nonpenetrating radiation.*

penetrometer (pen″ĕ-trom′ĕ-ter) a device used to measure the penetrability of x-rays or other penetrating radiation. In radiology, the device employed is an aluminum step wedge. The penetrability is determined as the thickness of aluminum that can be penetrated.

Penfield's method a histologic staining method for oligodendrocytes and microglia. In this procedure, tissue is fixed in Cajal's formalin ammonium bromide or in buffered neutral formalin, frozen sections 15–20 μm thick are cut, and the sections are washed overnight in dilute ammonia water. They are then serially placed in solutions of hydrobromic acid, sodium carbonate, and Hortega's ammoniacal silver solution. Following this, the sections are developed in a dilute formalin solution, toned with gold chloride, and fixed with sodium thiosulfate. Oligodendrocytes and microglia stain black and the background yellow-brown.

-penia (pe′ne-ah) [Gr. *penia* poverty, need] a suffix word element to denote decreased number, e.g., lymphopenia.

penicillamine (pen″ĭ-sil′am-ēn) [USP], D-3-mercaptovaline, a chelating agent used in the treatment of Wilson's disease, lead poisoning, cystinuria, and rheumatoid arthritis. It forms a tightly bound complex with copper or lead and a mixed disulfide with cystine. Penicillamine is the treatment of choice for Wilson's disease, because it removes excess copper from the blood; it also prevents the formation of renal calculi from cystine. Its mechanism of action in rheumatoid arthritis is unknown, but the chemical does reduce the serum concentration of IgM rheumatoid factor and depresses T-cell activity.

D-Penicillamine is relatively nontoxic. Many reports on its toxicity relate to the L- or DL- forms. Some adverse reactions include aplastic anemia, thrombocytopenia, agranulocytosis, drug fever and other allergic reactions, and toxic glomerulonephritis. When penicillamine is used, laboratory measurements of white blood cell count, platelet count, and urine protein should be made periodically to detect bone marrow depression or kidney damage.

penicillinase (pen″ĭ-sil′ĭ-nās) an enzyme of the hydrolase class (EC 3.5.2.6) that catalyzes the hydrolysis of the beta-lactam ring of penicillin, forming penicilloic acid, which is inactive as an antibiotic. The enzyme is produced by certain bacteria such as staphylococci, making them resistant to penicillin. Also called *β-lactamase.* See also *antibacterial agents.*

penicillin-fast resistant to the action of penicillin; said of certain strains of bacteria.

penicillinosis (pen′ĭ-sil″lin-o′sis) [*Penicillium* + *-osis*] a fungal infection caused by the common blue-green mold *Penicillium.* Although *Penicillium* is ubiquitous in nature, it has been known to cause several diseases in humans: some species produce toxins that can result in gastrointestinal disturbances, whereas others are capable of causing external ear, systemic, and urinary tract infections, and bronchopulmonary disease. For those individuals with allergies to penicillin, penicillinosis can result in an allergic disease. Persons affected by penicillinosis usually have a second predisposing debilitating disease.

penicillins (pen″ĭ-sil′ins) [*Penicillium* + *-in*] a group of antibiotics that contain the active principal 6-aminopenicillanic acid (a binuclear compound containing beta-lactam and thiazolidine rings). Penicillin, discovered in 1929 in London by Sir Alexander Fleming, was the first of the modern "wonder drugs." Flemming thought it too unstable to be useful. It was 10 yr later that Florey and Chain at Oxford found that it was a stable substance when purified.

STRUCTURE. The term penicillin includes both natural and semisynthetic penicillins. The basic structure is a thiazolidine ring, a beta-lactam ring, and a side-chain that helps to determine the antibacterial spectrum and pharmacologic properties of a particular penicillin. The penicillin nucleus 6-aminopenicillanic acid, derived from the mold *Penicillium notatum,* is required for biologic activity. The side-chain may be modified to produce penicillins with specific desirable properties, such as resistance to hydrolysis by beta-lactamases, resistance to gastric acid, and increased activity against gram-negative species.

MECHANISM OF ACTION. The target of penicillin is cell wall peptidoglycan synthesis, but the precise mechanism of action on growing cells is not well defined. A number of cell membrane–associated beta-lactam binding proteins have been isolated from bacterial cells. Some of these binding sites represent enzymes involved in cell wall synthesis. It is thought that the action of autolytic enzymes results in lysis and ultimate death of penicillin-treated bacteria.

RESISTANCE. An important mechanism of bacterial resistance to penicillin is the production by a variety of gram-positive and gram-negative bacteria of beta-lactamases. Enzymatic hydrolysis of the beta-lactam bond by beta-lactamases leads to loss of activity of the penicillin molecule. Other mechanisms of resistance include lack of permeability to penicillin molecules and alterations of the peptidoglycan target so that it is no longer susceptible to inhibition by penicillins. Tolerance refers to inhibition of bacterial growth but lack of killing. A defect in bacterial autolytic enzymes has been implicated in tolerance to penicillins.

CLINICAL USE. Pencillins are drugs of choice when treating infections caused by susceptible organisms. Penicillin G (benzylpenicillin) is the primary agent for treatment of *Streptococcus pyogenes* respiratory tract infections, as well as infections caused by *S. pneumoniae.* Resistant isolates of *S. pneumoniae* have been reported but are rare in the United States. *Neisseria meningitidis* is susceptible to penicillin G, and the drug is also used to treat infections caused by *N. gonorrhoeae;* however, resistant beta-lactamase–producing *N. gonorrhoeae* have been reported. Penicillin G is also effective in the treatment of treponemal infections and puerperal infections due to anaerobic streptococci or group B streptococci.

Extended-spectrum penicillins include mezlocillin and piperacillin. Piperacillin is similar in activity to ampicillin against gram-positive species and to carbenicillin against *Pseudomonas aeruginosa.* Another penicillin-related compound under investigation is mecillinam, a 6-β-acylaminopenicillanic acid. Although the drug has poor antigram-positive activity, it is extremely active against *Escherichia coli,* and species of *Shigella, Salmonella, Klebsiella, Enterobacter,* and *Citrobacter.* Its activity is not inhibited by beta-lactamases.

Semisynthetic, penicillinase-resistant penicillins (methicillin, nafcillin, cloxacillin, dicloxacillin, oxacillin) are drugs of choice for penicillin-resistant *Staphylococcus aureus* and other *Staphylococcus* species. Ampicillin and amoxicillin (aminopenicillins) are useful against gram-negative bacilli and enterococci. Most *Escherichia coli* isolates are susceptible, although plasmid-mediated resistance is common in hospital isolates. Most *Enterobacter, Klebsiella, Serratia, Acinetobacter,* indole-positive *Proteus, Pseudomonas,* and *Bacteroides fragilis* strains are resistant to aminopenicillins.

Among the anti-*Pseudomonas* penicillins are carbenicillin and ticarcillin. Aside from their activity against *P. aeruginosa,* these penicillins are also active against *E. coli, Proteus mirabilis, Salmonella,* and *Shigella* species.

For more information, see also *6-aminopenicillanic acid, amoxicillin, ampicillin, antibacterial agents, benzylpenicillin, methicillin,* and *phenoxycillin.*

p. G, benzylpenicillin, the most potent of the original natural penicillins and still the most commonly used and inexpensive form. Benzathine, potassium, and procaine salts are the most widely used clinically.

p. V, phenoxymethyl penicillin, a natural penicillin that is acid-stable and more suitable for oral administration. Also called *phenoxypenicillin.* Trademark, *V-Cillin.*

Penicillium (pen″ĭ-sil′e-um) [N.L., from L. *penicillus* brush, roll] a genus of fungi that belongs to the class Fungi Imperfecti. Some have perfect states and are affiliated with the Ascomycetes. Microscopically, *Penicillium* resembles a broom or the bones of a hand and fingers (see accompanying illustration). This mold is ubiquitous in nature, and certain species can produce an antibiotic. Although usually nonpathogenic, the following species have been implicated in diseases occurring in humans: *P. barbae, P. bouffardi, P. crustaceum, P. glaucum, P. minimum,* and *P. montoyai.*

penicillus (pen″ĭ-sil′us), pl. *penicilli* [L. "a brush"] one of the brushlike groups of straight, slender branches of a central artery, two to six in number, that are located in the red pulp of the spleen.

penile (pe′nīl) pertaining to or affecting the penis.

penis (pe′nis) [L.] [NA] the male organ of copulation and urination. It consists of three cylindric masses of cavernous tissue: two, the corpora cavernosa, lie side by side on the dorsum, and one, the corpus spongiosum, lies ventrally in the medial plane. The corpora are bound by fibrous tissue and covered by skin. The conical glans penis is at the distal end, with the external urethral orifice at its summit. The skin forms a fold, the prepuce, at the base of the glans.

penta- (pen′tah) [Gr. *pente* five] a word element used in combining form to denote five, e.g., *pentamer.*

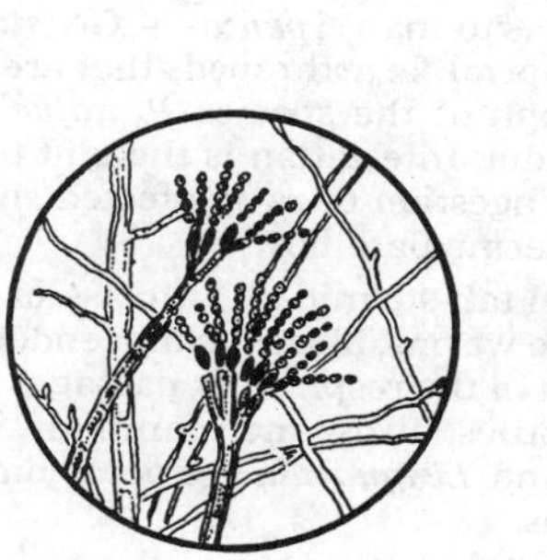

Penicillium (de Rivas).

Penicillium. Drawing of the microorganism *Penicillium* (de Rivas). (From Dorland's Illustrated Medical Dictionary, 26th ed. Philadelphia, W. B. Saunders Co., 1981.)

pentachlorophenol (PCP) (pen″tah-klor″o-fe′nol) a white crystalline solid, C_6Cl_5OH, used as a fungicide, insecticide, herbicide, bactericide, algicide, and wood preservative; M.W. 266.35. It is toxic when ingested, inhaled, or absorbed through the skin. By increasing the metabolic rate as a result of the uncoupling of oxidative phosphorylation, pentachlorophenol causes gastric upset, fever, rapid respiration, tachycardia, collapse, convulsions, and coma. It also produces contact dermatitis and damage to the lungs, liver, and kidneys.

pentaene (pen″tah-ēn) [Gr. *pente* five] 1. having five conjugated double bonds.

2. a group of antifungal antibiotics (e.g., filipin and chainin). See also *polyene antibiotics.*

pentaerythritol tetranitrate (PETN) (pen″tah-e-rith′rĭ-tol tet″rah-ni′trāt) an organic nitrate, $C(CH_2ONO_2)_4$, which is highly explosive.

p. t., diluted, a nonexplosive mixture that contains pentaerythritol tetranitrate, used as a coronary vasodilator in the treatment of angina pectoris.

pentagastrin (pen″tah-gas′trin) a pentapeptide, which includes the C-terminal tetrapeptide sequence of gastrin, responsible for its biologic activity. It is used as an HCl stimulant in tests of gastric secretion. See also *gastrin.*

pentamer (pen′tah-mer) [*penta-* + Gr. *meros* part] 1. a polymer composed of five monomers; the IgM immunoglobulins are examples.

2. a viral capsomer composed of five polypeptide units; see under *capsid.*

pentamidine (pen-tam′ĭ-dēn) 4,4′-diamidinodiphenoxy-15-*n*-pentane, used to treat early cases of *Trypanosoma gambiense* and *T. rhodesiense;* it is also used to treat *Pneumocystis carinii* infections. Pentamidine is administered intramuscularly and does not penetrate the blood-brain barrier (and thus is ineffective in latter stages of the disease with central nervous system involvement). Herxheimer reactions can occur and may be prevented by pretreatment with corticosteroids. Side-effects include hypotension, vomiting, blood dyscrasias, renal damage, and pain at the injection site.

pentane (pen′tān) *n*-pentane; an aliphatic hydrocarbon, C_5H_{12}, obtained by distillation of petroleum. It occurs as a clear, colorless, flammable liquid. When pentane is inhaled, ingested, or injected, it produces anesthesia. The branched-chain isomers of normal pentane may also be referred to as pentanes.

Pentastoma (pen-tas′to-mah) [*penta-* + Gr. *stoma* mouth] a genus of wormlike arthropods that are endoparasites. A nymph of the species *P. najae* has been reported in India. Infestation is thought to be acquired from the ingestion of raw infected snake meat (the usual intermediate host).

Pentastomida (pen″tah-sto′mid-ah) a class of Arthropoda, the tongue worms, bloodsucking endoparasites usually found in the respiratory passages and body cavities of reptiles, birds, and mammals. The genera *Armillifer* and *Linguatula* are occasionally parasitic in humans.

Pentatrichomonas (pen″tah-trik″o-mo′nas) [*penta-* + *Trichomonas*] see *Trichomonas.*

P. ardin delteili, see *T. hominis* under *Trichomonas.*

pentavalent (pen″tah-va′lent) [*penta-* + *valent*] in chemistry, having a valence of five. Also called *quinquevalent.*

pentazocine (pen-taz′o-sēn) [USP], a synthetic narcotic, a derivative of benzmorphan. It is used to treat severe pain; its analgesic effect is similar to that of codeine and about one-third that of morphine. Pentazocine is less addicting than morphine, but physical and psychologic dependence can occur. Adverse reactions include gastrointestinal upset, euphoria, sedation, and tissue damage at the site of multiple injections. Overdose effects can be reversed by naloxone.

p. hydrochloride, [USP], the form of pentazocine used for oral administration.

p. lactate, [USP], the form of pentazocine used for parenteral injection.

pentene (pen′tēn) one of the isomeric alkenes: 1-pentene, *cis*-2-pentene, or *trans*-2-pentene. The branched-chain isomers may also be referred to as pentenes. All these compounds may be called by the older name, amylene. See also *alkene.*

pentobarbital (pen″to-bar′bĭ-tal) a short-acting barbiturate used as a sedative and to control convulsions due to poisoning. See also *barbiturate.* Trademark, *Nembutal.*

p. sodium, [USP], the salt of pentobarbital, given by injection or capsule.

pentose (pen′tōs) a generic name for 5-carbon monosaccharides, encountered in aldose and ketose forms. Xylose and ribose occur in food and thus may be found in urine. As they are reducing sugars, they must be distinguished from glucose in the detection of glycosuria in diabetes. See also *pentosuria.* Cf. *ribanose* and *xylose.*

pentose assays Bial's test for pentoses in urine, using Bial's reagent (orcinol, hydrochloric acid, and ferric chloride). When urine is heated with hydrochloric acid, pentoses are converted to furfural, which reacts with orcinol to form green-colored compounds. All pentoses react, as do heptuloses and, occasionally, uronic acids. Pentoses may also be isolated and detected by thin-layer chromatography.

pentose phosphate pathway a major branch of the Embden-Meyerhof pathway (glycolysis) of carbohydrate metabolism that occurs in the cytoplasm of cells. Glucose-6-phosphate undergoes two successive oxidations by NADP, the final one being an oxidative decarboxylation to form ribose-5-phosphate. These oxidations are sufficiently exergonic to create a high [NADPH]/[NADP] ratio. They provide NADPH for reductive synthesis reactions, e.g., fatty acid synthesis, cholesterol synthesis, and the conversion of oxidized glutathione to reduced glutathione, and they provide pentose phosphates for the synthesis of nucleotides.

The handling of the excess pentose phosphates involves a redistribution of carbons by a transketolase and a transaldolase. Pentose phosphates can be stoichiometrically converted to fructose-6-phosphate and glyceraldehyde-3-phosphate, which can be returned to the Embden-Meyerhof pathway. The redistribution reactions also serve as a means for the metabolism of dietary or other excess pentoses.

Also called *hexose monophosphate shunt* and *pentose shunt.*

pentose shunt see *pentose phosphate pathway.*

pentoside (pen′to-sīd) a combination of a pentose

(ribose or deoxyribose) with a purine or pyrimidine base. See also *mononucleotide.*

pentosuria (pen″to-su′re-ah) [*pentose* + Gr. *ouron* urine + *-ia*] the urinary excretion of one or more of the pentose sugars. Pentosuria may be benign (alimentary) or may be the result of a genetic defect (essential pentosuria) that gives rise to the excretion of excessive amounts of L-xylulose.

alimentary p., the presence of pentose sugars, e.g., xylose and arabinose, in the urine, which occurs after the ingestion of large quantities of fruit or fruit juices, especially plums, prunes, and cherries. Normally, pentoses cannot be detected in urine.

essential p., see *idiopathic p.*

idiopathic p., a benign hereditary disorder, transmitted as an autosomal recessive trait, that occurs extremely rarely but almost exclusively in Ashkenazi Jews. Those affected excrete 1–4 g of the pentose L-xylulose in their urine each day.

The disease is caused by an error of metabolism of glucuronic acid due to a deficiency in the activity of the enzyme xylitol dehydrogenase; normally, glucuronic acid is reduced to L-gulonic acid, which is oxidized to L-xylulose. This is reduced by NADPH to xylitol, which is oxidized by NAD to D-xylulose. The enzyme catalyzing the reduction of L-xylulose to xylitol (xylitol dehydrogenase) is deficient in hereditary pentosuria. Also called *essential p.* and *L-xylulosuria.*

Pentothal (pen′to-thal) trademark. See *thiopental sodium.*

pentyl- (pen′til) a prefix word element in systematic organic chemical nomenclature to denote the *n*-pentyl group, $CH_3CH_2CH_2CH_2CH_2$—, e.g., 6-pentylundecane, $(C_5H_{11})_3CH$.

***n*-pentyl-** a prefix word element (meaning normal pentyl-) used in organic chemistry to denote the pentyl group, —$CH_2CH_2CH_2CH_2CH_3$, e.g., *n*-pentylamine, *n*-pentyl alcohol. Cf. *isopentyl-* and *neopentyl-.*

pentylenetetrazol (pen″ti-lēn-tet′rah-zol) an analeptic central nervous system stimulant drug that may be of value in treating elderly persons with mental confusion and memory defects. Overdoses may cause clonic convulsions followed by medullary depression and respiratory paralysis.

penumbra (pĕ-num′brah) [L. *paene* almost + *umbra* shadow] 1. the region of partial shadow at the edge of a full shadow (umbra) where only part of the radiation source is seen by the detector. In radiology, the penumbra is the blurred edge of the radiographic image where x-rays from one side of the focal spot reach the film, and x-rays from the other side are absorbed by a dense object. The unsharpness is increased when either the size of the focal spot or the object-film distance is increased.

2. the region where a point radiation source is seen by only part of a collimated radiation detector.

PEP abbrev. See *phosphoenolpyruvate.*

-pepsia (pep′se-ah) [Gr. *pepsis* digestion, from *peptein* to digest] a suffix word element to denote digestion, e.g., dyspepsia.

pepsin (pep′sin) [L. *pepsinum,* from Gr. *pepsis* digestion] a general name for several hydrolase enzymes (pepsin A, B, C; EC 3.4.23.1–3) secreted by the gastric mucosa of many species that catalyze the hydrolysis of proteins to a mixture of polypeptides. Commercial preparations have been used to split the immunoglobulin molecule into a large F(ab′)$_2$ fragment and an extensively degraded Fc fragment. For the human gastric enzyme, see *pepsin A.* See also *F(ab′)$_2$.*

pepsin A (PPS) an enzyme of the hydrolase class (EC 3.4.23.1), an endopeptidase that preferentially splits peptide bonds adjacent to phenylalanine or leucine to form polypeptide molecules. Pepsin is produced in and secreted by the stomach; a small amount enters the blood stream and is excreted in the urine (referred to as uropepsin). The precursor of this enzyme, pepsinogen, may also be excreted.

A decreased level of activity usually is seen in individuals with gastritis and gastric carcinoma, and also in those with myxedema, Addison's disease, and hypopituitarism. Absence of pepsin secretion is observed in persons with achlorhydria, and may suggest pernicious anemia. Increased activity is seen in patients with duodenal ulcer and Zollinger-Ellison syndrome.

See also *pepsinogen.*

pepsinogen (pep-sin′o-jen) [*pepsin* + Gr. *gennan* to produce] the precursor of pepsin, synthesized and excreted by the chief cells of the stomach. It is inactive, but at acid pH it is autocatalytically converted to the active enzyme pepsin. Also called propepsin. See also *pepsin A.*

pepsinogen assays determination of the amount of pepsinogen in serum or urine (in the urine, called uropepsinogen). The proenzyme is converted to the active enzyme (pepsin or uropepsin) by incubating the specimen with HCl at pH 1.5–1.8. The pepsin activity can then be measured by a variety of procedures: (1) as rennin activity, measuring the time required to clot a standard milk preparation; (2) using hemoglobin as substrate and measuring tyrosine formed with the Folin-Ciocalteau reagent; (3) by the measurement of heme pigment formed from hemoglobin, after protein precipitation with trichloroacetic acid; and (4) colorimetrically, using pepsin-specific synthetic substrates.

peptic (pep′tik) [Gr. *peptikos,* from *peptein* to digest] pertaining to pepsin or to digestion; related to the action of gastric juices.

peptic cell see *chief cell.*

peptic ulcer see *peptic u.* under *ulcer.*

peptidase (pep′tĭ-dās) any one of seven sub-subgroups of enzymes (EC 3.4.11–17) in the hydrolase class. These groups consist of enzymes that hydrolyze carboxy or amino terminal peptide bonds in a small polypeptide to produce smaller peptides and free amino acids or dipeptides. Also called exopeptidase and peptide hydrolase.

peptide (pep′tīd) any compound formed by the linkage of two or more amino acids by amide bonds (peptide bonds), usually referring to a polymer of α-amino acids formed by mRNA-directed synthesis by ribosomes in which the α-amino group of each amino acid residue (except the NH_2-terminal) is linked to the α-carboxy group of the next residue in a linear chain. The terms di-, tri-, tetrapeptide, etc., are used to specify the number of amino acid residues in the chain.

The terms peptide and polypeptide are used synonymously to refer to this class of compounds. In some contexts, however, the terms are restricted in order to indicate sizes. Then, the term peptide or oligopeptide is used to refer to those with few amino acid residues, whereas polypeptide is used to refer to those with many. The largest members of this class are referred to as proteins. The dividing line between polypeptides and proteins is arbitrary, but may be taken to be about 50–100 amino acid residues or a molecular weight of 5,000–15,000. Some proteins consist of several polypeptide chains linked by disulfide bridges and noncovalent bonds; in this case the term protein refers to the molecule with biologic function, and the term polypeptide to its component chains.

peptide bond see *peptide b.* under *bond.*

peptidoglycan (pep″tĭ-do-gli′kan) a high-molecular-weight polymer that forms the tough, rigid structure of bacterial cell walls. It is made up of three parts: (1) a backbone, composed of alternating *N*-acetylglucosamine and *N*-acetylmuramic acid; (2) a set of identical tetrapeptide side-chains attached to *N*-acetylmuramic acid; and (3) a set of identical peptide cross-bridges. The backbone is the same in all bacterial species; however, the tetrapeptide side-chains and the peptide cross-bridges vary from species to species. Also called *mucopeptide* and *murein.* See also *antibacterial agents.*

pepto- (pep′to) [Gr. *peptein* to digest] a word element used in combining form to denote digestion, e.g., peptone.

Peptococcaceae (pep″to-kok-a′se-e) a family of bacteria consisting of gram-positive, anaerobic cocci. It contains two medically important genera: *Peptococcus* and *Peptostreptoccus.*

Peptococcus (pep″to-kok′us) [*pepto-* + Gr. *kokkos* berry] a genus of gram-positive, obligately anaerobic, coccoid bacteria of the family Peptococcaceae. The colonies are small, convex, opaque, and grayish-white in color. The organisms are generally nonfermentative and negative for catalase, nitrate, and esculin. Part of the normal human flora of the mouth, upper respiratory tract, and large intestine, they are also important pathogens, causing infections of soft tissues and bacteremias. Species identification depends on biochemical reactions and identification of the products by gas-liquid chromatography.

P. asaccharolyticus, an indole-positive species commonly recovered from clinical specimens.

P. magnus, a species with large (1–2 μm in diameter) cells that is the species most frequently recovered from clinical specimens. It is a significant cause of septic arthritis and soft tissue infections.

P. prevotii, a species commonly recovered from clinical specimens, which is indole-negative and nonfermentative. Definitive identification is made by a combination of gas-liquid chromatography and biochemical tests.

peptone (pep′tōn) [Gr. *peptōn* digesting] a hydrolytic product of protein having less than 40 amino acid residues. It is not coagulable by heat and is not precipitated by saturating solutions of ammonium sulfate or by trichloroacetic acid + K_2HgI_4; however, it is precipitated by tannic acid and phosphotungstic acid. Peptones are widely used as a component of bacteriologic culture media. See also *culture media* and *proteose.*

Peptostreptococcus (pep″to-strep″to-kok′us) [*pepto-* + *streptococcus*] a genus of gram-positive, obligately anaerobic, coccoid bacteria of the family Peptococcaceae. The colonies are small, convex, opaque, and grayish-white in color. The organisms are catalase- and indole-negative. Part of the normal human flora of the mouth, upper respiratory tract, and large intestine, they are also opportunistic pathogens, causing infections of soft tissues and bacteremias. Species identification depends on biochemical reactions and identification of the products by gas-liquid chromatography.

P. anaerobius, a species that ferments glucose only.

P. micros, a nonfermentative species that is distinguished by its small cell size.

per- (per) [L. *per* through] 1. a prefix word element to denote throughout, completely, or extremely, e.g., peracidity.

2. a prefix word element in chemistry used to denote a compound containing an element in its high-oxidation state, as in perchlorate, pertechnetate, or periodic acid; one containing the peroxy (—O—O—) group, as in peracetic or perchromic acid; or one that has undergone complete addition or substitution by another reagent, often a halogen, as in perchloroethylene, $Cl_2C{=}CCl_2$, and perfluorokerosene (kerosene in which all hydrogen atoms have been replaced by fluorine atoms). See also *peracid.*

peracetic acid (per″ah-se′tik) a colorless liquid with an acrid odor, CH_3COOOH; M.W. 76.05. Peracetic acid is a strong irritant and oxidizing agent, prepared by reacting acetic acid with hydrogen peroxide, using sulfuric acid as a catalyst. It explodes at 115°C. Systematic names are ethaneperoxic acid and peroxyacetic acid.

peracetic acid–Schiff reaction see the similar *performic acid–Schiff reaction.*

peracid (per-as′id) a member of a class of compounds related to the carboxylic acids and having an oxygen-oxygen single bond: RCO_3H. Examples include peracetic, perbenzoic, and peroxytrifluoroacetic acids.

percent (per-sent′) (p. c., pct, %) [L. *per centum* by the hundred] a term that indicates that the preceding number is a percentage.

percentage (per-sen′tij) a ratio that has been multiplied by 100 is thus expressed as a comparison to 100; e.g., 0.3 is equivalent to 30 per cent.

percentile (per-sen′tīl) any value that divides the range of a probability distribution or sample distribution into two groups so that a specified percentage of the distribution lies below this value, e.g., 45 percent of the population scores below the forty-fifth percentile. Cf. *decile, median, quantile,* and *quartile.*

perchlorate (per-klo′rāt) a salt, ester, or dissociated form of perchloric acid.

perchlorate discharge test see under *thyroid uptake tests.*

perchloric acid (per-klor′ik) $ClHO_4$, used in analytical chemistry as an oxidant; M.W. 100.47. Perchloric acid decomposes when distilled at atmospheric pressure, sometimes with explosive violence. The aqueous acid is very caustic and may deflagrate in contact with oxidizable substances; it is corrosive to the skin and mucous membranes.

perchloroethylene (per-klor″o-eth′ĭ-lēn) see *tetrachloroethylene.*

percolate (per′ko-lāt) [L. *percolare* to strain through] 1. to strain; to submit to percolation; to pass a liquid gradually through small spaces or a porous substance.

2. to trickle slowly through a substance; to pass or ooze through small interstices or pores.

3. a liquid that has been subjected to percolation; a product of percolation.

percolation (per″ko-la′shun) [L. *percolatio,* from *percolare* to strain through] the extraction of the soluble parts of a solid mixture by means of a liquid solvent flowing slowly through interstices in the mixture.

percussion wave (per-kush′un) [L. *percussio,* from *percutere* to strike] a early systolic peak in the recorded or palpated pulse of the central arteries, attributable to the transmission of the abrupt shock caused by left ventricular ejection. It is the most positive wave of the pulse in normal individuals.

percutaneous (per″ku-ta′ne-us) [*per-* + L. *cutis* skin] performed through the skin, as in the injection of a radiopaque contrast medium in a radiologic examination, or the removal of tissue for a biopsy accomplished with a needle or catheter inserted through the skin.

percutaneous renal puncture 1. a radiologic procedure used to examine renal cysts and tumors after the injection of a radiopaque contrast medium through a needle inserted under radioscopic control directly into the cyst.

2. a cytologic procedure used to obtain fluid from a renal cyst for examination.

perester (per-es′ter) the ester of an alcohol and a peroxyacid. See also *functional group.*

perforating (per′fo-rāt″ing) [L. *perforare* to pierce through] piercing with holes, or passing through a part.

perforating fibers of Sharpey slender bundles of calcified connective tissue that penetrate the periosteum and outer cortex of a bone and aid in holding the lamellae together.

perforation (per″for-a′shun) 1. a hole or series of holes punched or drilled into or through an object.

2. the act of perforating.

performic acid (per-for′mik) a colorless liquid, HCOOOH; M.W. 62.03. It is a strong irritant and oxidizing agent prepared by reacting formic acid with hydrogen peroxide, using sulfuric acid as a catalyst. It explodes on contact with metals or metal oxides, or when shocked or heated. Performic acid solutions deteriorate after about 2 hr and must be prepared daily. Systematic names are methaneperoxic acid and peroxyformic acid.

performic acid–Schiff reaction (PFAS) a specific histochemical reaction for unsaturated lipids (e.g., phospholipids or cerebrosides). Performic (or peracetic) acid oxidizes the carbon-carbon double bond to two aldehyde groups, which react with Schiff reagent.

The mercapto group in cystine also reacts; it is oxidized to sulfonate, which reacts with Schiff reagent; however, only proteins rich in cystine; e.g., keratin, react noticeably. Unsaturated lipids and keratin are stained red-purple; chromatin may also be stained (by the Feulgen reaction).

perfusate (per-fu′zāt) [L. *perfusus,* past participle of *perfundere* to pour over] a liquid that has been passed over or through the vessels of an organ or tissue.

perfuse (per-fūz′) [L. *perfundere* to pour over] to pour over or through.

perfusion (per-fu′zhun) 1. the act of pouring over or through, especially the artificially enforced passage of fluid through the vessels of a specific tissue or of an entire organism.

2. the circulation of blood through a vascular bed.

p. pressure, the difference between the mean pressures at the arterial and venous ends of the circulation at the organ or tissue level. The blood flow of a particular organ or tissue is equal to the effective perfusion pressure divided by the vascular resistance to the flow.

pulmonary p., blood flow through the pulmonary capillaries. Perfusion is not evenly distributed throughout normal human lungs. Radioactive gas methods for studying the regional distribution of blood flow have identified four horizontal zones, differentiated on the basis of the relative magnitude of the pressures determining capillary blood flow. In Zone 1, extending from the apex to about 4 cm below the apex of the lung, alveolar pressure (PA) exceeds pulmonary arterial pressure (Pa), and flow per alveolus is nearly zero. The flow increases linearly throughout Zone 2, owing to a linear increase in the driving pressure (Pa-PA). The flow also increases somewhat in Zone 3 despite a constant perfusion pressure (Pa-Pv, where Pv equals pulmonary venous pressure), perhaps because of greater distention of the vessels with downward progression through the zone. There is an area of reduced flow at the base of the lungs (Zone 4), possibly owing to a greater interstitial pressure surrounding the capillaries in this region.

Blood flow per alveolus is more uniform when measured at a smaller lung volume (i.e., at residual volume rather than at total lung capacity).

Also called *pulmonary blood flow.* See also *ventilation/perfusion ratio.*

perfusion lung scan see *pulmonary perfusion scan.*

peri- (per′e, per′ĭ) [Gr. *peri* around] a prefix word element to denote around, near, or surrounding, e.g., perihepatic.

perianal (per″e-a′nal) [*peri-* + L. *anus* anus] located around the anus.

periapical (per″e-a′pĭ-kal) [*peri-* + L. *apex* tip] referring to the area surrounding the apex of the root of the tooth.

periapical abscess acute or chronic purulent inflammation of the area surrounding the root apex of a tooth. It is frequently a cariogenic infection of dental pulp, but may also follow trauma. The most common etiologic agents are alpha-hemolytic streptococci or staphylococci. Percussion, pulp testing, and X-ray examination may confirm the diagnosis. Also called apical abscess.

periapical projection a radiographic projection used to demonstrate the roots of the teeth; see under *dental radiography.*

periarteritis (per″e-ar″tē-ri′tis) [*peri-* + Gr. *artēria* artery + *-itis*] a general term used to describe inflammation of the coats of an artery that may extend to involve surrounding tissues. Also called *polyarteritis.*

p. nodosa, an inflammatory disease characterized by the segmental necrosis of small- and medium-sized arteries and adjacent veins, but not capillaries. These lesions may be widespread throughout the body and lead to secondary ischemia of tissues supplied by the involved vessels. Young adult males are most commonly affected. The prognosis for recovery is always guarded. The cause is unknown but may be associated with the use of certain drugs (allopurinol, sulfonamides), allergies, immune complex disorders, and hepatitis B antigen.

Laboratory findings include elevated leukocyte counts (20,000–40,000/μl), proteinuria, and hematuria. The erythrocyte sedimentation rate is frequently elevated. Although there is no specific biochemical or serologic test for this disease, angiography has been increasingly important in supporting other clinical information to establish the diagnosis. Histologic examination of biopsies of the affected vessels is essential for establishing the diagnosis. Involvement of vessels in testicular tissue is frequent and is often a preferred biopsy site in males.

Also called *periarteritis nodosa.*

pericardial (per″ĭ-kar′de-al) [*peri-* + Gr. *kardia* heart] pertaining to the fibroserous sac enclosing the heart and the roots of the great vessels (pericardium).

pericardial effusion the increased formation of fluid in the pericardial sac, usually associated with inflammation of the pericardium; it may occur as either an acute or a chronic process. The causes are many and include viral and bacterial infection, connective tissue disorders, trauma, uremia, and the pericarditis with effusion that follows myocardial infarction. Pericardial effusion and pericarditis are manifested by a nagging anterior chest pain, which is usually aggravated by inspiration and partially relieved by sitting forward.

On physical examination, a friction rub may be heard. Diagnosis is aided by ultrasound studies of the heart. The electrocardiogram may show a characteristic diffuse ST segment elevation. Occasionally, serum glutamic oxaloacetic transaminase (SGOT) concentration is elevated (normal range, 6–18 IU/l). In some cases, contrast radiography of the heart and/or pericardiocentesis is necessary to establish the diagnosis.

When of rapid onset, a pericardial effusion may cause life-threatening compromise of cardiac function, and result in symptoms of right- and left-sided cardiac failure, with diminished cardiac output, hypotension, and shock.

pericardial fluid the small quantity of slightly viscous serous fluid that occupies the pericardial cavity.

pericardial fluid examination the study of pericardial fluid by routine and special procedures to determine the etiology of an effusion, which can demonstrate the presence of a disease process involving the pericardium. Normal fluid is pale yellow and clear; specific gravity, 1.010–1.026; total protein, 0.3–4.1 g/100 ml (albumin, 50–70 percent; globulin, 30–45 percent; fibrinogen, 0.3–4.5 percent); and pH, 6.8–7.6. The normal total amount of fluid is 10–50 ml. See also *pericardial effusion.*

pericardial rub an abnormal scratching or leathery grating noise heard as the heart beats. It may be systolic or systolic and early diastolic; when atrial contraction adds a presystolic noise, as many as three sounds may be heard. Pericardial rub is most frequently associated with pericarditis. Also called pericardial friction rub. See also *acute p.* under *pericarditis.*

pericardial tamponade see *cardiac tamponade.*

pericardiocentesis (per″ĭ-kar″de-o-sen-te′sis) [*pericardium* + Gr. *kentēsis* puncture] the surgical puncture of the pericardial cavity. This procedure may be employed to relieve tamponade and/or to obtain pericardial fluid for diagnosis.

pericarditis (per″ĭ-kar-di′tis) [*pericardium* + *-itis*] inflammation of the pericardium. It can result from a wide variety of causes; the three principal syndromes are acute pericarditis, pericardial effusion, and constrictive pericarditis. The major clinical consequences are pain, pericardial friction rub, and compromised cardiac function.

acute p., active inflammation of the pericardium, of recent onset. Etiologic factors include infections, acute myocardial infarction, connective tissue disorders, and trauma. Some cases are idiopathic. The causative factors may persist and produce subacute and chronic pericarditis, or recurrent episodes of acute inflammation may occur.

acute benign p., see *idiopathic p.*

adhesive p., a complication of pericardial inflammation in which adhesions are present between the two pericardial layers or between the parietal pericardium and the surrounding mediastinal structures. It does not interfere with cardiac filling and is of little clinical or hemodynamic significance, in contrast to constrictive pericarditis.

bacterial p., inflammation of the pericardium due to bacterial infection that may reach the pericardium by extension from intrathoracic infection, from blood-borne bacteria, or from penetrating trauma. Staphylococci are frequently the causative organisms, but many other types are also implicated.

benign p., a misnomer for nonspecific or idiopathic pericarditis; see *idiopathic p.*

bile p., see *choleperitoneum.*

cholesterol p., a condition in which an elevated level of cholesterol occurs within a pericardial effusion. Hypothyroidism is the most common cause. The pericardial surfaces have a smooth, shiny appearance. The effusion develops slowly and is nonconstrictive, but may be large and cause cardiac compression.

chronic p., a persistent or long-standing inflammation of the pericardium, often following repeated exacerbations of acute pericarditis. It is associated with varying degrees of fibrosis and adhesion formation, and may lead to the development of constrictive pericarditis.

chronic constrictive p., a disorder, severe enough to compress the heart and interfere with cardiac filling, that results from scarring of the parietal and/or visceral pericardium. Pericardial calcification may aggravate these pathologic processes.

The common signs and symptoms include dyspnea, peripheral edema, abdominal swelling, hepatomegaly, and distention of the neck veins. Causes include infections (especially tuberculosis), invasion by malignant neoplasm, trauma, and radiation therapy.

Important diagnostic findings include a prolonged arm-to-tongue circulation time, flat T waves, and atrial fibrillation. Radiographs reveal cardiac enlargement. Ultrasonic and echocardiographic examinations may provide important diagnostic information.

chylous p., a condition in which a pericardial effusion contains a milky, chylous fluid. It develops following traumatic rupture or obstruction of the thoracic duct, the latter usually by a neoplastic process. In the majority of cases, however, a specific etiology cannot be determined.

constrictive p., a complication of acute or chronic pericarditis in which fibrous thickening of the pericardial membranes creates a rigid sac that restricts movement of the heart. The clinical effects depend on whether the process is focal or diffuse, and on its severity. The basic consequence is a progressive decrease in cardiac filling with resultant fall in cardiac output and peripheral venous pooling. The effects may be made more severe by the coexistence of a pericardial effusion. Thoracotomy with pericardial stripping may be necessary.

drug-induced p., inflammation of the pericardium that develops as a response to a particular drug. It has been observed as an allergic response to penicillin, and following prolonged use of procainamide, hydralazine, and isoniazid for the prevention of cardiac arrhythmias.

fibrinous p., an acute or chronic form of pericarditis characterized by the development of a fibrinous exudate on the pericardial surface, which can lead to adhesions between the peripheral and parietal layers of the serous pericardium.

fungal p., an uncommon form of pericardial inflammation induced by a fungal infection, usually seen in immunosuppressed patients. The most frequent causative agents are opportunistic species of *Candida* and *Aspergillus.*

hemorrhagic p., pericardial inflammation associated with the development of a bloody pericardial effusion. It is seen particularly in malignant involvement of the pericardial membranes.

idiopathic p., the most common type of acute pericarditis in adults. Although a viral infection and hypersensitivity reaction have been postulated, there is no proof that either is the cause. Affected individuals are usually adolescents or young adults. The condition lasts for one to a few weeks and usually subsides without the development of sequelae. However, recurrent attacks and serious complications may develop. Also called (inappropriately) *benign p.*

infectious p., inflammation of the pericardium due to viral, bacterial, fungal, or parasitic infection.

metabolic p., pericardial inflammation occurring in the course of uremia, myxedema, and, infrequently, other metabolic disorders.

neoplastic p., inflammation of the pericardium due to involvement of malignant neoplasms, either from direct extension or metastasis. The tumors most often responsible are bronchogenic carcinomas in males and breast carcinomas in females. Other forms of neoplasia include melanoma, leukemia, and lymphomas; primary tumors of the pericardium are uncommon. When the pericardium is involved by a malignant infiltrate, the effusion is usually bloody, and may contain cells that can be recovered for cytologic examination by pericardiocentesis.

obliterative p., an extensive adhesive pericarditis that totally obliterates the pericardial cavity.

parasitic p., an infrequent cause of pericardial inflammation. Causative organisms include *Entamoeba histolytica, Echinococcus, Toxoplasma,* and *Cysticercus.*

postmyocardial infarction p., a syndrome that develops weeks or months following an acute myocardial infarction. It is characterized by pericardial pain that tends to occur with position changes, respiration, or coughing. A friction rub may be audible and an effusion may accumulate, but the need for pericardiocentesis is rare. The condition must be distinguished from recurrent infarction by clinical findings, electrocardiography, echocardiography, x-rays, and cardiac enzyme levels. Also called Dressler's syndrome.

postpericardiotomy p., a syndrome characterized by fever, substernal chest pain, and pericardial rub. It is seen in 10–30 percent of patients undergoing cardiac surgery. The condition may be manifested 2–4 wk after the surgery. The etiology is thought to involve both autoimmune responses and viral agents.

posttraumatic p., pericardial inflammation developing following injury to the chest. It may be produced by blunt trauma such as steering wheel injury, or by a penetrating wound, in which case bacterial infection is sometimes the cause.

purulent p., acute pericarditis accompanied by the accumulation of pus within the pericardial sac. Resolution is usually accompanied by the development of adhesions.

radiation-induced p., inflammation of the pericardium following therapeutic radiation to a field that includes the heart.

rheumatic p., a form of pericardial inflammation, seen particularly in some children and young adults with acute rheumatic fever. Other connective tissue disorders are also responsible for its development. A similar pericarditis in individuals with systemic lupus erythematosus, rheumatoid arthritis, and scleroderma may produce an identical form of inflammation.

serous p., pericardial inflammation associated with the accumulation of a clear serous fluid with a relatively low protein content. This type of exudate is seen early in the development of most forms of acute pericarditis. See also *pericardial fluid examination.*

suppurative p., severe purulent pericarditis; see *purulent p.*

tuberculous p., at one time a relatively common form of pericarditis associated with a high incidence of development of constrictive pericarditis. It is usually secondary to pulmonary tuberculosis. Confirmation of the diagnosis requires histologic examination and positive staining for acid-fast bacteria and/or growth of mycobacteria in cultures of the pericardium obtained at thoracotomy.

uremic p., pericardial inflammation, often associated with the development of a fibrinous or hemorrhagic pericardial effusion, occurring in the late stages of uremia. It is seen more frequently with the extended use of renal dialysis in patients with renal failure. In patients receiving dialysis, the procedure causes a resolution of the symptoms in some, but not in others.

viral p., viral inflammation of the pericardium. The most frequent causative agents are the enteroviruses, especially the group B coxsackieviruses. A viral etiology for idiopathic pericarditis has been postulated but not proven.

pericardium (per″ĭ-kar′de-um) [*peri-* + Gr. *kardia* heart] [NA], the sac that encloses the heart and roots of the great vessels, located in the mediastinum posterior to the body of the sternum. It consists of a tough external sac of fibrous tissue (fibrous pericardium), lined by an inner sac of two apposed layers of serous membrane (serous pericardium). The pericardium resists overdistention of the heart, holds it in position, and reduces friction on its moving surfaces during contraction.

fibrous p., the cone-shaped outer sac of the pericardium, into which the heart is invaginated; it is composed of a dense network of collagenous and elastic fibers. The fibrous pericardium is continuous at its apex with the tunica adventitia of the great vessels and is attached at its base to the central tendon of the diaphragm.

parietal p., the outer layer of the serous pericardium; its subserosal areolar connective tissue blends with that of the fibrous pericardium.

serous p., the inner layers of the pericardium. They form a closed membranous sac, the inner visceral layer of which covers the heart and, at the roots of the great vessels, is reflected back to form an outer parietal layer that is apposed to the inner surface of the fibrous pericardium. The opposing surfaces of the two serous layers are lined by mesothelial cells resting on areolar connective tissue, and are separated by a film of fluid.

visceral p., see *epicardium.*

pericentric inversion (per″ĭ-sen′trik) [*peri-* + Gr. *kentron* center of a circle] see under *inversion.*

pericholangitis (per″ĭ-ko″lan-ji′tis) [*peri-* + Gr. *cholē* bile + *angeion* vessel + *-itis*] inflammation of tissues that surround the bile ducts. Bile ductules and portal triads show mixed inflammatory reactions, and Kupffer cells are swollen. Affected individuals may experience fever, jaundice, and hepatic fibrosis, but cirrhosis is uncommon. Laboratory tests for hepatic function are usually only mildly abnormal.

perichondrium (per″ĭ-kon′dre-um) [*peri-* + *chondros* cartilage] [NA], the dense, fibrous connective tissue that ensheathes all cartilage except the articular cartilage of synovial joints. The innermost cells possess chondrogenic properties.

pericyte (per′ĭ-sīt) [*peri-* + Gr. *kytos* hollow vessel] a flattened satellite cell with cytoplasmic extensions, which wraps around an arteriole, capillary, or sinusoid, and is attached to the outer aspect of the endothelial cell of capillaries. It contains actin filaments and may have a contractile function, but its precise nature and significance are not known. See also *hemangiopericytoma* and *Rouget cell.*

periductal mastitis (per″ĭ-duk′tal mas-ti′tis) [*peri-* + L. *ductus* duct; Gr. *mastos* breast + *-itis*] see *mammary duct ectasia.*

perikaryon (per″ĭ-kar′e-on) [*peri-* + Gr. *karyon* nut] the cell body of a neuron.

perilymph (per′ĭ-limf) [*peri-* + L. *lympha* water, lymph] the viscous fluid that occupies the spaces between the membranous and osseous labyrinths of the inner ear. It is similar in composition to the extracellular or cerebrospinal fluids. Cf. *endolymph.*

perimysium (per″ĭ-mi′se-um), pl. *perimysia* [*peri-* + Gr. *mys* muscle] [NA], the connective tissue sheath that envelops each fascicle of fibers within a skeletal muscle.

perinatal (per″e-na′tal) [*peri-* + L. *natus* born] pertaining to or occurring shortly before or after birth.

perine/o (per″ĭ-ne′o) a word element used in combining form to denote the perineum, e.g., perineotomy.

perineal (per″ĭ-ne′al) pertaining to the perineum.

perineal body a fibromuscular nodule located between the anal canal and the perineal membrane, into which surrounding muscles insert.

perinephric (per″ĭ-nef′rik) [*peri-* + Gr. *nephros* kidney] a general term used to designate the area around the kidney.

perinephric abscess a pyogenic inflammation of the area surrounding the kidney, usually due to the rupture of a kidney abscess as a complication of pyelonephritis. It is most frequently caused by those organisms causing pyelonephritis (e.g., *Escherichia coli, Proteus,* and *Klebsiella*). Affected individuals experience fever, pain, weakness, and dysuria. Leukocytosis, pyuria, positive urine cultures, and bacteremia are present. Excretory urograms and ultrasonic examination may aid in the diagnosis.

perineum (per″ĭ-ne′um) [Gr. *perineos* the space between the anus and scrotum] [NA], the roughly diamond-shaped area and associated structures overlying the pelvic outlet, delimited on the surface of the body by the anus, external urogenital organs, and medial sides of the thighs. Its deeper boundaries are formed anteriorly by the pubic arch, posteriorly by the coccyx, and on each side by the ischial tuberosity.

perineural (per″ĭ-nu′ral) [*peri-* + Gr. *neuron* nerve] surrounding a nerve or nerves.

perineurium (per″ĭ-nu′re-um) [*peri-* + Gr. *neuron* nerve] a connective tissue sheath that envelops fascicles of nerve fibers within a peripheral nerve. Its cells are flattened and the attenuated cytoplasm contains many pinocytotic vesicles. The perineurium is continuous with the meninges at the origin of spinal nerves and is believed to function as a selective diffusion barrier around the nerve.

perinuclear (per″ĭ-nu′kle-ar) [*peri-* + *nuclear*] situated on or occurring around a cell nucleus.

perinuclear cisterna see under *nuclear envelope.*

perinuclear space see under *nuclear envelope.*

period (pe′re-od) [Gr. *periodos,* from *peri-* + *hodos* way] 1. an interval or division of time; the time for the regular recurrence of a phenomenon.

2. in electrophysiology, the duration of an individual component of a sequence of electroencephalogram waves, which is the reciprocal of the frequency ($1/f$).

periodic (pe″re-od′ik) [Gr. *periodikos,* from *periodos* period] recurring at regular intervals, e.g., intervals of time or space.

periodic acid one of the series of acids derived from I_2O_7: HIO_4, H_5IO_6 (or $HIO_4 \cdot 2H_2O$), etc. The term usually refers to $HIO_4 \cdot 2H_2O$, a white crystalline solid, which is a weak acid in aqueous solution but a strong oxidizing agent.

periodic acid–Schiff (PAS) reaction oxidation by periodic acid followed by staining with Schiff reagent. Hydroxy groups on adjacent carbons (a 1,2-glycol) are oxidized to aldehyde groups by periodic acid. This reaction breaks the pyranose ring of many sugars, producing a dialdehyde that reacts with Schiff reagent.

Most substances that contain hexoses or hexosamines are PAS-positive. These include polysaccharides, glycoproteins, and glycolipids. Some unsaturated lipids and phospholipids are also PAS-positive. Acid mucopolysaccharides (glycosaminoglycans) are PAS-negative; acetylation of the 1,2-glycol group by acetic anhydride blocks the PAS reaction. PAS-positive material that is negative after acetylation and does not stain with Schiff reagent alone is considered to be polysaccharide.

periodic complexes in electroencephalography, a pattern of cerebral electrical activity characterized by paroxysmal high-voltage slow activity and/or sharp waves recurring at regular intervals. Periodic complexes have been associated particularly with subacute sclerosing panencephalitis, Creutzfeldt-Jakob disease, and herpes encephalitis. Repetitive bursts of activity, with less regular rhythmicity, may also be found with deep anesthesia, cardiac arrest, head injury, anoxic states, and cerebral lipidoses, and occasionally after tonic-clonic (grand mal) attacks. The diagnostic value of these complexes depends on the clinical circumstances in which they are found.

Also called *periodic patterns.* See also *burst suppression, paroxysmal activity,* and *periodic lateralized epileptiform discharges.*

periodicity (pe″re-o-dis′ĭ-te) 1. recurrence at regular intervals of time.

2. in parasitology, the periodic increase of microfilaria in the peripheral blood (*Wuchereria bancrofti* and *Brugia malayi* exhibit a nocturnal periodicity, whereas *Loa loa* is diurnal), and the somewhat regular recurrence of symptoms in individuals with malaria is due to the development of a new generation of parasites in the body.

3. in anatomy, a regularly repeating feature, such as the banding pattern of a myofibril or collagen fibril.

periodic lateralized epileptiform discharge (PLED) in electroencephalography, repetitive, paroxysmal, slow- and/or sharp-wave activity that occurs with a regular periodicity on either the right or left side of the head, or independently on both sides. Such activity is frequently found in individuals with an acute hemispheric lesion due to cerebral infarction or tumor.

periodic paralysis see *familial periodic p.* under *paralysis.*

periodic patterns see *periodic complexes.*

periodontal (per″e-o-don′tal) [*peri-* + Gr. *odous* tooth] a general term used to describe the area around a tooth, including the tissues that support and invest the tooth, i.e., cementum, periodontal ligament, alveolar bone, and gingiva.

periodontal disease inflammation and degeneration of the tissues that surround and support the teeth; its prevalence is almost universal. The major etiologic factor in periodontal disease is the microflora that colonize the surface of teeth (plaque); the specific microorganisms have not yet been isolated. Periodontal disease is the major cause of tooth loss after age 20 yr. It begins most commonly as gingivitis and may progress to periodontitis. Diagnosis is based on the findings of erythema, bleeding, gingival swelling, pocket formation, suppuration, osseous destruction, and loosening of the teeth. Treatment involves the elimination or control of the microorganisms. See also *gingivitis* and *periodontitis.*

periodontal ligament the connective tissue that attaches the cementum of the root of a tooth to its bony socket; it suspends the tooth and allows for some degree of movement. The orientation of its collagen fiber bundles varies over different parts of the tooth.

periodontitis (per″e-o-don-ti′tis) [*peri-* + Gr. *odous* tooth + *-itis*] the extension of gingivitis to underlying periodontal tissue (periodontal membrane, cementum of the teeth, and alveolar bone). Inflammation spreads from the gingivae to the underlying alveolar bones and periodontal ligaments, resulting in bone resorption, pocket formation, and loosening of teeth. Destruction of osseous tissue is the earliest observation on x-ray examination. Bacterial infection of diseased tissue is common. Treatment involves the elimination or control of bacterial plaque. Formerly called *pyorrhea.*

periodontium (per″e-o-don′she-um) [N.L., from *peri-* + Gr. *odous* tooth] a term used to describe the investing and supporting tissues of the teeth including the gingiva, periodontal ligament, cementum, and alveolar bone.

periodontology (per″e-o-don-tol′o-je) [*peri-* + Gr. *odous* tooth + *-logy*] the science and study of the periodontium.

perionychium (per″e-o-nik′e-um) [N.L., from *peri-* + Gr. *onyx* nail] the epidermis bordering a nail.

periosteum (per″e-os′te-um) [N.L., from *peri-* + Gr. *osteon* bone] [NA], the tissue membrane that covers the free surface of bone. It consists of a dense, fibrous outer layer and a deeper layer of thin elastic fibers in a loosely arranged network of collagen fiber bundles. With age, the periosteum of bone becomes progressively less vascular, and periosteal cells become flattened and quiescent but retain potential to form bone.

periostitis (per″e-os-ti′tis) [*periosteum* + *-itis*] inflammation of the periosteum. It may occur in congenital or acquired syphilis. Bone involvement is commonly symmetric, and proliferation is more frequent than resorption. Radiographs reveal proliferation along bone crests, such as the tibia, leading to "saber shin." In adults, radiographic examination is not diagnostic. Also called *osteoperiostitis.*

peripheral (pĕ-rif′er-al) [Gr. *periphereia,* from *peri-* + *pherein* to carry] 1. pertaining to or situated near the periphery; situated away from a center or central structure.

2. a separate device that works with a computer, usually an input-output device or a bulk memory device.

peripheral blood see *peripheral b.* under *blood.*

peripheral blood smear see *peripheral blood s.* under *smear.*

peripheral nervous system the division of the nervous system composed of the nerves and ganglia outside the brain and spinal cord. It is subdivided into the somatic and autonomic systems. See also *autonomic nervous system* and *peripheral nerve.*

peripheral neuropathy see *peripheral n.* under *neuropathy.*

peripheral perfusion scan a procedure used in nuclear medicine, similar to the pulmonary perfusion scan except that the technetium (Tc 99m) albumin microspheres are injected into an artery rather than a vein, and are trapped in the capillary beds supplied by the artery rather than in the lungs. It is now rarely used to evaluate arterial occlusion. The percentage of peripheral arteriovenous shunting may be determined with this study (the fraction of the administered radioactive material that lodges in the lungs, expressed as a percentage of the fraction that lodges there when the agent is injected into a vein in the same extremity).

peripheral proteins see under *cell membrane.*

peripheral resistance unit (PRU) a unit of vascular resistance equal to a pressure of 1 mm of mercury divided by a flow rate of 1 ml/sec (1 mmHg·s/ml).

Periplaneta (per″ĭ-plah-ne′tah) [*peri-* + Gr. *planētēs* wanderer] a genus of roaches. The American cockroach, *P. americana,* has been incriminated as intermediate host of *Hymenolepis diminuta, Raillietina* species, *Gongylonema pulchrum,* and *Moniliformis moniliformis.*

periplasm (per′ĭ-plazm) [*peri-* + Gr. *plasma* something molded] the space between the inner and outer membranes of a bacterial cell. In the periplasmic space, much excreted protein, including potentially destructive enzymes, is retained in a manner analogous to that of liposomes in animal cells.

periplast (per′ĭ-plast) [*peri-* + Gr. *plassein* to mold] the peripheral protoplasm of a cell; cytoplasm.

periportal (per″ĭ-por′tal) [*peri-* + *portal*] referring to the region around a portal tract.

peristalsis (per″ĭ-stal′sis) [*peri-* + Gr. *stalsis* contraction] the rhythmic muscular contractions that propel forward the contents of the gastrointestinal tract, bile ducts, ureters, or other tubular structures with longitudinal and circular layers of smooth muscle fibers. Distention of a segment of the tube by an increase in its contents stimulates contraction of the smooth muscle. The contractile ring thus formed is transmitted in waves along the tube, propelling forward any material in front of the ring. In the case of the GI tract, peristaltic movements cause food to progress along the tract at a rate suitable for digestion and absorption.

peristaltic (per″ĭ-stal′tik) of the nature of peristalsis.

perithecium (per″ĭ-the′se-um) [*peri-* + Gr. *thēkē* case] a globular or flask-shaped ascocarp that contains asci and ascospores for the fruitification of certain fungi.

peritone/o (per″ĭ-to-ne′o) [L.; Gr. *peritonaion,* from *peri-* + *teinein* to stretch] a word element used in combining form to denote the peritoneum, e.g., peritoneocentesis.

peritoneal (per″ĭ-to-ne′al) pertaining to the peritoneum.

peritoneal cancer a mesothelioma derived from the lining cells of the peritoneal cavity, or a tumor secondarily involving the peritoneum. The latter may be metastatic from intraabdominal or pelvic locations, particularly the gastrointestinal tract or ovary. Cells from a peritoneal tumor can usually be obtained by paracentesis for cytologic examination. See also *mesothelioma.*

peritoneal cavity see *visceral p.* under *peritoneum.*

peritoneal fluid the thin layer of liquid, composed of water, electrolytes, and proteins, that covers the visceral and parietal peritoneum. Normally, the cellular constituents include desquamated mesothelial cells, macrophages, mast cells, lymphocytes, and other leukocytes. Substances introduced into the peritoneum are readily absorbed across this fluid layer and the mesothelium into the general circulation.

peritoneal fluid examination the study of peritoneal fluid by routine and special procedures to determine its etiology or the presence of a disease process involving the peritoneum. It is pale yellow and clear; specific gravity, 1.010–1.026; total protein, 0.3–4.1 g/100 ml (albumin, 50–70 percent; globulin, 30–45 percent; fibrinogen, 0.3–4.5 percent); and pH, 6.8–7.6. The normal total amount of fluid is 30–50 ml. See also *ascites.*

peritoneal hemodialysis see under *hemodialysis.*

peritoneal lavage see *peritoneal l.* under *lavage.*

peritoneography (per″ĭ-to-ne-og′rah-fe) [*peritoneo* + Gr. *graphein* to write or draw] the radiologic examination of the peritoneum.

positive contrast p., a procedure used to evaluate abnormalities such as hernias, in which a water-soluble iodinated contrast medium is introduced into the peritoneal cavity. Also called herniography.

peritoneum (per″ĭ-to-ne′um) [L.; Gr. *peritonaion*] [NA], the serous membrane with a smooth, glistening surface that lines the abdominal cavity (parietal peritoneum) and covers the viscera (visceral peritoneum) contained within the cavity. In the male it forms a closed sac; in the female it is perforated by the lateral ends of the oviducts.

lesser sac of p., a large, irregularly shaped potential space situated between the stomach and the posterior abdominal wall. It is formed by the peritoneum that lines the abdominal wall and stomach, as well as by a fold of the greater omentum, and is thought to facilitate movement of the stomach against the posterior abdominal wall. The lesser sac communicates with the greater sac via the epiploic foramen. Also called *omental bursa.*

parietal p., the peritoneum that lines the abdominal and pelvic walls and the undersurface of the diaphragm.

visceral p., a continuation of the parietal peritoneum reflected at various places over the viscera, forming a complete covering for the stomach, spleen, liver, ascending portion of the duodenum, jejunum, ileum, transverse colon, sigmoid flexure, upper end of the rectum, uterus, and ovaries. It also partially covers the descending and transverse portions of the duodenum, cecum, ascending and descending colon, middle part of the rectum, posterior wall of the bladder, and upper portion of the vagina. The peritoneum serves to hold the viscera in position by its folds, some of which form the mesenteries, connecting portions of the intestine with the posterior abdominal wall. Other folds, the omenta, are attached to the stomach, and still others form the ligaments of the liver, spleen, stomach, kidneys, bladder, and uterus. The space between the visceral and the parietal peritoneum is the peritoneal cavity, which includes the pelvic peritoneal cavity below and the general peritoneal cavity above. The general peritoneal cavity communicates by the epiploic foramen with the cavity of the greater omentum, which is also known as the lesser peritoneal cavity or lesser sac.

peritonitis (per″ĭ-to-ni′tis) [*peritoneum* + *-itis*] a generalized or localized inflammation of the visceral or parietal peritoneum that may occur in acute or chronic forms. It is most commonly due to perforation of the intestinal tract (appendicitis, peptic ulcer, and perforations associated with diverticulitis and gangrenous gallbladder). Other causes include the spread of pelvic infections, trauma, carcinoma, and leakage of pancreatic enzymes.

Peritonitis is an important complication of a wide variety of acute abdominal disorders. Systemic symptoms include nausea, malaise, fever, leukocytosis, and electrolyte imbalances. The primary symptomatology is centered in the abdomen. Pain, tenderness, and muscle rigidity are common. Intestinal motility is severely diminished. Hypotension and leukocytosis (more than 20,000 cells/mm^3) are seen. Radiographs reveal fluid collection and generalized dilation. Diagnostic paracentesis and barium enemas may be helpful. Cultures reveal *Escherichia coli* and *Streptococcus faecalis* to be the most common infecting organisms.

bile p., peritonitis resulting from the presence of bile in the peritoneum. Also called *choleperitoneum.*

chemical p., peritonitis due to chemical irritation.

diffuse p., peritonitis that is not limited to a portion of the peritoneum.

gonococcal p., generalized peritonitis due to the spread of a gonococcal infection, usually from a primary focus in the female reproductive tract. The inflammation may be limited to the pelvis or may spread to involve the capsule of the liver.

localized p., peritonitis that is limited to a portion of the peritoneum.

meconium p., peritonitis arising from perforation of the bowel and escape of meconium shortly after birth. It occurs most often as a complication of meconium ileus in infants with fibrocystic disease of the pancreas.

septic p., peritonitis due to a pyogenic microorganism.

starch p., an acute granulomatous inflammation of the peritoneum caused by starch. In the past, it was frequently secondary to surgery, caused by the starch on surgeons' gloves. The condition is rarely seen as a result of glove powders currently being used.

peritonsillar (per″ĭ-ton′sĭ-lar) [*peri-* + L. *tonsillae* tonsils] a general term used to describe the area around a tonsil.

peritonsillar abscess an acute infection, often following acute tonsillitis, that occurs between the tonsil and the superior constrictor muscle of the pharynx. The etiologic agent is almost always group A β-hemolytic streptococci, which is readily recovered on culture. The abscess usually drains but the pus does not regularly contain the causative organism. Fever, cervical lymphadenopathy, dysphagia, and soft palate swelling are frequently present. Also called *quinsy.*

peritrichous (pĕ-rit′rĭ-kus) [*peri-* + Gr. *thrix, trichos* hair] referring to a bacterial cell or other unicellular organism that has flagella distributed randomly over the entire surface. See also *flagellum.*

Perls' reaction (perlz) [Max *Perls,* German pathologist, 1843–1881] the Prussian blue test for ferric iron; see under *iron-positive pigment demonstration.*

permanganate (per-man′gah-nāt) the MnO_4^- ion or a salt of this ion. Permanganate is a strong oxidizing agent. Aqueous solutions and salts are dark purple.

permeability (per″me-ah-bil′ĭ-te) [L. *permeabilis,* from *permeare* to pass through] 1. the property or state of being permeable. See also *osmosis.*

2. (symbol μ), in paramagnetic and diamagnetic materials, the ratio of the magnetic induction (**B**) to the magnetic field strength (**H**):**B** = μ**H.** See also *magnetic susceptibility.*

permeability of vacuum (μ_0) the ratio of the magnetic induction to the magnetic field strength when no magnetization is present. When International System (SI) units are used, $\mu_0 = 4\pi \times 10^{-7}$ Hz/m.

permeable (per′me-ah-b′l) not impassable; pervious; permitting substances to pass through.

permease (per′me-ās) originally, the specific inducible binding protein in a bacterial membrane transport system, e.g., in β-galactoside transport in *Escherichia coli.* The term is also used to designate the entire inducible transport system.

permissible exposure limits (per-mis′ĭ-b′l) the limits adopted by the Occupational Safety and Health Administration (OSHA) for permissible exposures to airborne concentrations of chemicals. These limits are based on recommended threshold limit values of the American Conference of Government and Industrial Hygienists (ACGIH); OSHA uses the limits as enforceable regulatory standards. For limits that are not ceiling values or that are based on effects other than toxicity, OSHA enforcement guidelines allow some higher exposures without citation for a serious violation. See also *threshold limit values.*

permissive (per-mis′iv) in microbial genetics, pertaining to the environmental conditions in which a conditional lethal mutant grows and reproduces normally.

Permitil (per′mĭ-til) trademark. See *fluphenazine.*

permittivity (ϵ) [L. *permittere* permit] the product of the dielectric constant and the permittivity of vacuum.

permittivity of vacuum (ϵ_0) the ratio of the electric displacement to the electric field strength when no polarization is present. When International System (SI) units are used, $\epsilon_0 = 8.854 \times 10^{-12}$ F/m, which is $1/\mu_0 c^2$, where μ_0 is the permeability of vacuum and c is the velocity of light.

Permount (per′mount) trademark for a synthetic resin mounting medium used in histology, a polymer of β-pinene. Permount has an index of refraction ranging from 1.5144 (60 percent toluene solution) to 1.5286 (the solid).

permutation (per″mu-ta′shun) [L. *permutatio,* from *per-* (1) + *mutare* to change] 1. an arrangement of an ordered set of objects. There are $n!$ (n factorial) permutations of n objects.

2. the number of different arrangements of r objects selected from a set of n objects: ${}_nP_r = n!/(n-r)!$.

Permutit (per′mu-tit) trademark for ion-exchange resins made from a variety of synthetic polymers. Permutit-Folin, used in clinical chemistry as an ammonia adsorbent, is a gel-like precipitated form of sodium aluminosilicate.

pernicious (per′nish′us) [L. *perniciosus,* from *pernicies* destruction, ruin] fatal, very destructive, severe; that which is noxious or deleterious to physical or mental health.

pernicious anemia see *pernicious a.* under *anemia.*

perone/o (per-o-ne′o) [Gr. *peronē* fibula] a word element used in combining form to denote the fibula, e.g., peroneal.

peroneal muscular atrophy an inherited, gradually progressive peripheral neuropathy, transmitted as an autosomal dominant trait in some families, an autosomal recessive trait in others, and an X-linked recessive trait in still others. It produces atrophy of the muscles of the legs and forearms. Contractures and deformity of the limbs occur, most notably an arched equinovarus deformity of the feet, and there is concomitant sensory impairment with paresthesias, pain, and distal sensory loss. Although the disease is inherited, no enzymatic abnormality has yet been found. Also called *Charcot-Marie-Tooth disease* (the autosomal dominant form), and hereditary motor and sensory neuropathy.

peroneal nerve, common a terminal branch of the sciatic nerve. It arises above the knee joint, and descends obliquely through the popliteal fossa to wind around the neck of the fibula and divide into superficial and deep peroneal nerves.

peroxidase (per-ok′sĭ-dās) an enzyme of the oxidoreductase class (EC 1.11.1) that acts on a substrate (electron donor) with hydrogen peroxide as the electron (or hydrogen) acceptor. The enzyme serves to remove toxic peroxides within the cell, e.g., glutathione reductase, and catalase. In clinical chemistry, it is widely used in conjuction with specific enzymes for the measurement of glucose, uric acid, and other analytes.

peroxidase-antiperoxidase (PAP) complex a soluble antigen-antibody complex of horseradish peroxidase (antigen) and antihorseradish peroxidase (antibody), which is used in the immunoperoxidase technique. The complex is stored frozen and is diluted with buffer-saline before use. See also *immunoperoxidase technique.*

peroxidase-antiperoxidase (PAP) technique see *immunoperoxidase technique* and *peroxidase staining methods.*

peroxidase staining methods any of several histochemical procedures for the demonstration of peroxidases in frozen or freeze-dried tissue sections or alcohol-fixed smears (for leukocytes). The specimens are incubated in a solution containing hydrogen peroxide and a substance that serves as a hydrogen donor; as peroxide is reduced to water, the hydrogen donor is oxidized from a colorless form to a colored form. Commonly used reagents are benzidine (*p*-diaminodiphenyl, which is oxidized to a brown diimino compound), α-napthol (which is oxidized to red or purple-red naphthoquinones), and leuko-dyes. The latter are reduced forms of common dyes such as patent blue or acid fuchsin, made by reaction with metallic zinc in acetic acid or with nascent hydrogen. They are oxidized by the peroxidase back to the original dye.

Another reagent is 3,3′-diaminobenzidine (DAB), which is oxidized to an insoluble yellowish-brown polymer in immunocytochemistry methods. DAB is used to react with the PAP (peroxidase-antiperoxidase) complex to form a stable colored product at the antigen site. For electron microscopy this polymer can be reacted with osmium tetroxide to produce electron-dense, insoluble osmium black.

peroxide (per-ok′sīd) 1. any compound containing the functional group —O—O—. Organic peroxides such as lauroyl peroxide are highly reactive oxidizing agents, used industrially as bleaching agents and polymerization catalysts. They are strong skin irritants capable of producing burns and damage to the eyes; some are so unstable as to be explosive.

2. hydrogen peroxide, HOOH.

peroxisome (per-oks′ĭ-sōm) a small, electron-dense, membrane-bound, cytoplasmic vacuole found in most cells. Peroxisomes are numerous in hepatocytes. They contain peroxidase, catalase, and oxidases and are involved in catabolic reactions that release hydrogen peroxides. Also called *microbody.*

peroxyacylnitrate (PAN) (per-ok″se-a″sil-ni′trāt) a type of compound occurring in photochemical smog, $RCOOONO_2$. The simplest PAN is peroxyacetylnitrate, $CH_3COOONO_2$. All PANs are highly irritating to the eyes and respiratory tract and are destructive to vegetation, fabrics, and rubber.

perphenazine (per-fen′ah-zēn) [*per-* + *phenazine*] [USP], a piperazine-type phenothiazine major tranquilizer used in the management of psychotic disorders and for control of nausea and vomiting. See also *phenothiazine tranquilizers.* Trademark, *Trilafon.*

Persantine (per-san′tēn) trademark. See *dipyridamole.*

persistent filaria see *Dipetalonema perstans.*

persistent vegetative state a condition resulting from extreme damage to the brain from such causes as head injury or cardiopulmonary arrest. Patients may survive in this state for months or years. They lie quietly with their eyes open and roving, or closed. Externally applied stimuli produce such responses as eye movements, grimacing, and postural reflexes, but patients otherwise seem unaware of their environment and cannot communicate with others. Such individuals have been described as being capable of "wakefulness without awareness." The electroencephalogram can vary from low-voltage activity to highly organized patterns. Also called anoetic symptom complex, *apallic syndrome,* and *vegetative survival.* See also *akinetic m.* under *mutism.*

persister (per-sĭs′ter) [L. *persistere* persist, from *per-* through + *sistere* to stand still] in bacteriology, a microorganism that resists a generally toxic level of a drug but that is not genetically resistant. It is often seen in laboratory studies with chemotherapeutic agents.

perspiration (per″spĭ-ra′shun) [L. *perspirare* to breathe through] 1. sweat.

2. sweating; the functional secretion of sweat. Insensible perspiration refers to those evaporative losses of water from the moist surfaces of the body (such as the skin and the respiratory tree) that are not due to the secretory activity of glands. This perspiration results in the loss of essentially pure water, and may amount to 600–700 ml/da for an adult.

Sensible perspiration (visible sweat) is that due to the secretory activity of the sweat glands. When visible sweat is produced, its volume and composition are determined by rate of evaporation, the previous fluid intake of the individual, the external temperature and humidity, and hormonal factors. Volumes as large as 14 l/da have been recorded. Both volume and salt content of sensible perspiration are influenced by the acclimatization of the individual.

PERT (acronym from *p*rogram *e*valuation and

review technique) a form of network analysis. See also *network analysis.*

pertechnetate (per-tek′nĕ-tāt) see under *technetium-99m.*

Pertofrane (per′to-frān) trademark. See *desipramine.*

pertussis (per-tus′is) [*per-* + L. *tussis* cough] see *whooping cough.*

Peruvian balsam a dark brown viscous liquid, obtained from *Myroxylon pereirae.* It is used in ointments or alcohol solutions as a topical protectant and is also an ingredient in many cough syrups.

pes (pās), pl. *pedes* [L. "foot"] [NA], a foot or a footlike structure.

p. cavus, exaggerated height of the longitudinal arch of the foot, present from birth or appearing later because of contractures or disturbed balance of the muscles controlling the arch of the foot.

p. valgus, flatfoot, a condition in which one or more of the arches of the foot have flattened out.

pesticide (pes′tĭ-sīd) [L. *pestis* pest + *caedere* to kill] a substance used to kill or inhibit the growth of plant or animal pests. Pesticides are categorized into three main classes: compounds of toxic heavy metals, such as arsenic and lead; natural organic compounds, such as rotenone, pyrethrins, and nicotine; and synthetic organic compounds. The synthetic pesticides are further differentiated into chlorinated hydrocarbons, such as DDT and dieldrin; organophosphate esters, such as malathion and parathion; bipyridyl compounds, such as paraquat and diquat; chlorphenoxy herbicides, such as 2,4-D and 2,4,5-T; carbamates, such as Temik; and dinitrophenols, such as DNOC.

PET abbrev. See *positron-emission tomography.*

peta (P) a prefix attached to International System (SI) units of measurement to denote a unit equal to 1 quadrillion of the basic unit (10^{15} unit).

-petal (pĕ-t″l) [L. *petere* to seek] a suffix word element to denote directed or moving toward, e.g., centripetal.

petechia (pe-te′ke-ah), pl. *petechiae* [L.] a hemorrhage into the skin less than 3 mm in diameter. Cf. *ecchymosis.*

petit mal attack (pĕ-te′ mahl′) [Fr. "little illness"] former name for *absence attack.*

PETN see *pentaerythritol tetranitrate.*

Petri dish (pe′tre) [Julius Richard *Petri,* German bacteriologist, 1852–1921] a round, shallow, flat-bottomed, transparent glass or plastic dish with a slightly larger, similarly shaped dish that forms a cover. It is used in bacteriology to hold a layer of solid medium for growing cultures.

petriellidiosis pulmonary infection caused by the fungus *Petriellidium boydii,* which occurs rarely in humans. It may be associated with a number of other respiratory conditions. Sometimes incorrectly called *allescheriosis.*

Petriellidium (pe″tre-el-id′e-um) a genus of perfect fungi of the class Ascomycetes. The species *P. boydii* (also called *Allescheria boydii*), which is the causative agent of necrotizing pneumonia, mycetoma, and generalized infections in immunosuppressed patients, has been isolated from sputum samples. It produces ascocarps that are spherical, submerged, and often covered with septate hyphae that are brown, thick-walled, and 2–3 μm wide. At maturity the ascocarps produce eight-spored asci; the spores are straw colored and measure 6–7 μm long by 3.5–4.0 μm wide. Also called *Pseudoallescheria.*

petrolatum (pet″ro-la′tum) [L.] [USP], a purified mixture, colorless to yellow, of semisolid hydrocarbons obtained from petroleum, used as an ointment base. It is also used as a protective dressing and soothing application to the skin. Also called mineral jelly, paraffin jelly, and *petroleum jelly.*

hydrophilic p., [USP], a mixture of cholesterol, stearyl alcohol, white wax, and white petrolatum; used as an ointment base and protective dressing.

liquid p., see *mineral oil.*

red p., a topical sunscreen that absorbs ultraviolet and visible light with a wavelength above 340 nm, but that passes the ultraviolet wavelengths of light that causes tanning and sunburn. Trademark, RVP.

white p., [USP], similar to petrolatum except that it is colorless and never yellow.

petroleum (pĕ-tro′le-um) [L., from *petra* stone + *oleum* oil] a thick natural oil obtained from beneath the earth. It consists of a mixture of various hydrocarbons, chiefly of the paraffin and olefin series. Petroleum has many uses, not only as a source of gasoline, kerosene, and other petroleum fractions, but also as a lubricant and as a source of chemicals for commercial use in the synthesis of a great number of compounds.

petroleum ether one of several commercial mixtures of low-boiling hydrocarbons (not ethers in the modern sense of the word), obtained as distillation fractions from petroleum and used as organic solvents. Low-boiling petroleum ether (boiling range, approximately 30°–60°C) is a mixture principally of pentanes and hexanes; it is usually called petroleum ether without a modifier. Higher-boiling petroleum ether (e.g., 60°–80°C) sometimes is also called ligroin.

petroleum jelly see *petrolatum.*

petrositis (pet″ro-si′tis) [*petrosa,* from L. *petrosus* rocky + *-itis*] a general term used to describe an inflammation of the petrous portion of the temporal bone of the skull.

petrous (pet′rus) [L. *petrosus* rocky, from *petra* rock] resembling a rock, hard, stony.

PETT abbrev. for positron-emission transverse tomography. See *positron-emission tomography.*

Peutz-Jeghers syndrome [J. L. A. *Peutz,* Dutch physician, 20th century; Harold *Jeghers,* U.S. physician, 20th century] an uncommon condition, transmitted as an autosomal dominant trait, that is characterized by multiple polyps of the stomach, small bowel, and colon. The polyps resemble hamartomas rather than true neoplasms. Persons affected have melanin spots of the skin, lips, buccal and mucous membranes, and fingers. The malignant potential of these polyps is small. Laboratory studies may reveal anemia and occult fecal blood; barium radiographs of the bowel reveal multiple polyps. See also *familial p.* under *polyposis.*

-pexy (pek′se) [Gr. *pēxis* a fixing, putting together] a suffix word element to denote fixation, e.g., nephropexy.

Peyer's patches (pi′erz) [Johann Conrad *Peyer,* Swiss anatomist, 1653–1712] the oval-shaped groupings of lymphoid tissue located on the antimesenteric aspect of the mucosa of the ileum. Peyer's patches constitute a major component of the gut-associated lymphoid tissue.

peyote (pa-o′te) [Sp.] 1. the cactus *Lophophora williamsii,* native to the southwestern United States and Mexico. Also called *mescal.*

2. the dried tubercles (flowering heads) of this cactus, which contain the hallucinogen mescaline. Peyote is used ritualistically by certain Indian tribes of the region. Also called *mescal* and mescal buttons. See also *mescaline.*

Peyronie's disease (pa-ron-ēz′) [François de la *Peyronie,* French surgeon, 1678–1747] the sclerotic induration of the corpora cavernosa of the penis, resulting in a fibrous thickening of the covering fascia. This condition occurs in adult males; the cause is unknown, but it may be associated with sclerosing processes elsewhere. It causes painful erection and may prevent sexual intercourse.

pF abbrev. See *picofarad.*

PFAS abbrev. See *performic acid–Schiff reaction.*

Pfeiffer-Comberg method a radiographic method of localizing foreign bodies in the eye that uses lateral and anterior views and a contact lens with four lead markers in a square pattern. The eye is anesthetized, and the contact lens inserted and aligned so that the markers are directly above, below, and to the sides of the center of the cornea. With the patient gazing directly ahead, the posteroanterior projection (Waters position) and lateral projection (central ray through the outer canthi) are obtained without moving the patient. The positions of the object on a front view and horizontal section are taken directly from the anterior and lateral views, using the known spacing of the lead markers. See also *foreign body localization.* Cf. *Sweet method.*

Pfeiffer's disease (pfi′ferz) [Emil *Pfeiffer,* German physician, 1846–1921] see *infectious mononucleosis.*

Pfeiffer phenomenon (pfi′fer) [Richard Friedrich Johann *Pfeiffer,* bacteriologist in Breslau, 1858–1945] a reaction in which *Vibrio cholerae* is lysed by antibody in the presence of complement in the absence of cells. This phenomenon was first demonstrated in 1894, when *V. cholerae* was injected into the peritoneum of previously immunized guinea pigs; the bacteria lost motility, clumped together, and lysed. This was one of the initial descriptions of humoral immunity.

PFP abbrev. See *platelet-free plasma.*

PG abbrev. See *phosphatidylglycerol, pituitary gonadotropin, prostaglandin.*

pg abbrev. See *picogram.*

PGA abbrev. See *p. A* under *prostaglandin.*

PGA_1 abbrev. for prostaglandin A_1. See *p. A* under *prostaglandin.*

PGA_2 abbrev. for prostaglandin A_2. See *p. A* under *prostaglandin.*

PGA_3 abbrev. for prostaglandin A_3. See *p. A* under *prostaglandin.*

PGB abbrev. See *p. B* under *prostaglandin.*

PGD abbrev. See *phosphogluconate dehydrogenase.*

PGD_2 abbrev. See *p.* D_2 under *prostaglandin.*

PGE_1 abbrev. See *p.* E_1 under *prostaglandin.*

PGE_2 abbrev. See *p.* E_2 under *prostaglandin.*

$PGF_{1\alpha}$ abbrev. See *p.* $F_{1\alpha}$ under *prostaglandin.*

$PGF_{2\alpha}$ abbrev. See *p.* $F_{2\alpha}$ under *prostaglandin.*

PGG_2 abbrev. See p. G_2 under *prostaglandin.*

PGH_2 abbrev. See p. H_2 under *prostaglandin.*

PGI_2 abbrev. See prostaglandin I_2. See *prostacyclin.*

PGK abbrev. See *phosphoglycerate kinase.*

PGO spike abbrev. for ponto-geniculo-occipital spike. See under *rapid eye movement.*

PgR abbrev. See *progesterone receptor.*

Ph^1 abbrev. See *Philadelphia c.* under *chromosome.*

pH a measure of the effective acidity or alkalinity of a solution, defined as the negative logarithm of the hydrogen ion activity; $pH = -\log_{10} a_{H^+}$. In dilute solutions, this is approximately equal to the negative of the logarithm of the hydrogen ion concentration: $pH = -\log_{10}[H^+]$, because the activity coefficient $f_{H^+} = a_{H^+}/[H^+]$ approaches 1 as the concentration approaches zero. Because the ionization equilibrium varies with temperature, the pH is slightly temperature dependent.

The pH of a solution may be accurately measured by using a pH meter (potentiometer); semiquantitative determinations, as in urinalysis, can be made by using acid-base indicator papers, paper strips treated with dyes that change color when protonated. As a result, the color of these papers changes with the pH of the solution.

The pH of the blood and of the intracellular fluid is maintained within a narrow range by the blood buffer system, by the renal mechanism (which eliminates excess acid or retains acid as needed), and by the respiratory system. The combined efforts of these three systems control the pH of blood very rigidly.

The reference range for pH in venous blood is: 7.35–7.45 (average, 7.40); the difference between arterial and venous blood ranges between 0.01 and 0.3. Acidemia and alkalemia refer to blood pH values below and above the normal range, respectively. The terms acidosis and alkalosis refer to a physiologic condition with abnormal amounts of acid or base in the body as a whole.

The average pH of adult urine is about 6, varying from 4.6 to about 8.0. After a meal, urine (just as blood) becomes more basic (alkaline tide) as acid is secreted into the stomach.

pH_I abbrev. See *isoelectric point.*

Φ the Greek capital letter *phi;* symbol for magnetic flux.

ϕ the Greek lower case letter *phi;* used in mathematics as an angular coordinate variable.

PHA abbrev. See *phytohemagglutinin, pulse height analyzer.*

phac/o (fak′o) [Gr. *phakos* lentil or a lentil-shaped object] a word element used in combining form to denote relationship to a lens, e.g., phacosclerosis.

phacomalacia (fak″o-mah-la′she-ah) [*phaco-* + Gr. *malakia* softness] a condition characterized by the softening of the lens of the eye. The term is also used to describe soft cataracts (without a hard nucleus). Cf. *phacosclerosis.*

phacosclerosis (fak″o-skle-ro′sis) [*phaco-* + Gr. *sklērōsis* hardening] a condition characterized by the hardening of the lens of the eye. The term is also used to describe hard cataracts (with a hard nucleus). Cf. *phacomalacia.*

Phaenicia (fe-nĭ′she-ah) a genus of greenbottle flies, also referred to as *Lucilia.*

P. sericata, see under *Lucilia.*

phag/o (fag′o) [Gr. *phagein* to eat] a word element

used in combining form to denote eating or engulfing, e.g., phagocyte.

phage (fāj) [Gr. *phagein* to eat] see *bacteriophage.*

phage genetics see *bacteriophage g.* under *genetics.*

-phagia (fa′je-ah) [Gr. *phagein* to eat] a suffix word element to denote eating or swallowing, e.g., dysphagia.

phagocyte (fag′o-sīt) [*phago-* + *-cyte* from Gr. *kytos* hollow vessel] any cell that ingests bacteria or other particles by the process of phagocytosis. In humans, there are three types of phagocytes: macrophages, granulocytes, and monocytes. All three types are attracted to bacteria and certain other particles by substances released by the particles (the process of chemotaxis). They then pin the particle against a surface and engulf it.

The coating of particles by certain antibodies, lysins, or opsonins, or by complement fractions, enhances phagocytosis. Some macrophages, particularly the alveolar macrophages of the lungs, can ingest particles such as dust and pollutants without this immunologic phagocytic recognition.

See also *chemotaxis.*

phagocytic (fag″o-sit′ik) pertaining to or produced by phagocytes.

phagocytosis (fag″o-si-to′sis) the engulfment of microorganisms or particles, the process by which specialized cells engulf and process extracellular material. The steps in this process involve: recognition, ingestion, phagolysosome formation, killing, and digestion.

RECOGNITION. Phagocytes (granulocytes, monocytes, and macrophages) need to recognize that the particle is a candidate for phagocytosis. Opsonization prepares the particle for phagocytosis by adding opsonins (for which phagocytes have receptors) to the particle's surface. The Fc portion of immunoglobulin acts as a nonheat-labile opsonin for phagocytes after binding by its antigen-binding segment (Fab) to the foreign antigen's surface. Phagocytes have receptors for the Fc portion of various immunoglobulins, as well as a receptor for some complement fragments, the most important of which is C3b. The C3b fragment is formed by activation of either the classical or the alternative complement pathway. Classical pathway activation requires antigen-antibody complex interaction with C1q and then subsequent C4, C2, and C3 activation. The alternative pathway does not require antigen-antibody complexes and thus is not specific.

The heat lability of both the classical and alternative complement pathways allows one to distinguish between antibody and complement as opsonins, because antibodies are heat-stable. Immunoglobulins of the IgG subclasses 1 and 3 are the most effective immunoglobulins for opsonization. The receptor recognition of C3b and the Fc portion of immunoglobulin with phagocytes promotes their uptake into phagocytic vacuoles called phagosomes.

INGESTION. Without opsonization, phagocytes may ingest inert particles, such as latex beads, iron filings, or carbon particles, but the rate of ingestion is slow and does not show a significant energy dependence. In the ingestion of opsonized particles there is a significant increase in intracellular metabolic activity. The process is energy-dependent and appears to require the divalent cations Ca^{2+} and Mg^{2+}. Cytochalasin B, a fungal metabolite that disrupts microfilaments, has been shown to reversibly impair ingestion. Metabolic inhibitors of glycolysis and low temperatures also impair ingestion of opsonized particles.

PHAGOLYSOSOME FORMATION. The vacuole with the ingested particle fuses with a preformed granule, the lysosome, forming a phagolysosome. The lysosome releases its contents into the phagosome in a process called degranulation. The granule contents vary among macrophages, polymorphonuclear leukocytes, and eosinophils, but they all contain various enzymes such as hydrolases, lipases, etc., that can act on the ingested particle.

KILLING. After formation of a phagolysosome, the phagocyte proceeds with the respiratory burst, which involves increased glycolysis, increased hexose monophosphate shunt activity, utilization of the tricarboxylic acid pathway in certain macrophages, increased O_2 consumption, and production of hydrogen peroxide and lactic acid. The phagocytic mechanisms that kill microorganisms may be divided into oxygen-dependent and oxyen-independent systems. The combination of hydrogen peroxide, halides, and myeloperoxidase is one type of oxygen-dependent antimicrobial system, which results in the halogenation of bacterial proteins, eventually leading to cell death. Another type of oxygen-dependent antimicrobial system involves hydrogen peroxide alone or in the superoxide anion (O_2^-). The superoxide anion is a product of the univalent reduction of molecular oxygen and is a toxic high-energy free radical effective in killing bacteria. In the granules of some polymorphonuclear leukocytes, superoxide anions may be further reduced by the enzyme superoxide dismutase producing hydrogen peroxide, which is also bacteriostatic. Granular cationic proteins and lactic acid are factors involved in oxygen-dependent bactericidal activity.

DIGESTION. The process of degradation of the ingested material is accomplished by the various hydrolases in the granules (proteinases, lipases, and saccharidases).

LABORATORY METHODS FOR THE EVALUATION OF PHAGOCYTOSIS. Phagocytic activity may be analyzed by three general approaches: ingestion, degranulation, and oxygen metabolism. The evaluation of ingestion by blood phagocytes is made by making available to the phagocytes *Escherichia coli* lipopolysaccharide-coated oil droplets containing oil red O. These particles are pretreated with fresh human serum for opsonization. Ingestion proceeds for 5 min, after which the uningested oil droplets are separated from the phagocytes. The phagocytes are pelleted and washed, and the concentration of oil red O is measured spectrophotometrically.

Ingestion may also be measured indirectly using nitroblue tetrazolium, a redox dye that measures the production of superoxide anion (O_2^-) or other oxidizing agents. When nitroblue tetrazolium is reduced by superoxide anion, it turns from yellow to purple (formazan). Formazan production may be quantitated spectrophotometrically.

Phagocytic degranulation may be evaluated by the measurement of β-glucuronidase activity. During phagocytosis, granule-associated enzymes are released into the extracellular environment. After ingestion is completed, β-glucuronidase is detected using the substrate *p*-nitrophenyl-β-glucuronide in Triton X-100. Sodium hydroxide is added to this mixture, and the product is measured spectrophotometrically at 410 nm.

The bactericidal activity of a phagocyte may be determined by lysing the phagocyte after ingestion and measuring the survival of phagocytosed bacteria. Adherent bacteria must be eliminated by vigorous washing or, in the case of staphylococci, by use of lysostaphin, an agent that selectively lyses staphylococci.

Cf. *pinocytosis.*

GERALD B. KOLSKI, M.D., PH.D.

phagolysosome (fag″o-li′so-sōm) [*phago-* + Gr. *lyein* to loose + *sōma* body] a digestive vacuole formed by the aggregation of lysosomes around a phagosome; the lysosomal membranes fuse with the phagosome, and their hydrolytic enzymes digest the phagocytosed material. See also *heterophagic vacuole.*

phagosome (fag′o-sōm) [*phago-* + Gr. *sōma* body] see under *phagocytosis.*

phakomatosis (fak″o-mah-to′sis), pl. *phakomatoses* [Gr. *phako* lentil + *-oma* swelling + *-osis*] an unusual group of diseases in which neurologic abnormalities are combined with congenital defects of the retina, brain, skin, and other organs. The diseases include neurofibromatosis (von Recklinghausen's disease), tuberous sclerosis (Bourneville's disease), cerebelloretinal hemangioblastomatosis (von Hippel-Lindau disease), and encephalotrigeminal syndrome (Sturge-Weber syndrome). It has been suggested that ataxia telangiectasia be included in this group. For further information, see under the individual diseases.

phalang/o (fah-lan′jo) [Gr. *phalanges,* pl. of *phalanx* a line or array of soldiers] a word element used in combining form to denote the phalanges (finger or toe bones), e.g., phalangitis.

phalangeal (fah-lan′je-al) pertaining to a phalanx.

phalanx (fa′lanks), pl. *phalanges* [Gr.] one of the miniature long bones that form the skeleton of the fingers and toes. The thumb or big toe contains two; there are three in each of the other digits.

phalloidin (fah-loid′in) one of the heat-stable, bicyclo hexapeptide poisons from the mushroom *Amanita phalloides.* Also called phalloidine. See also *amanitin.*

phantom (fan′tom) [Old French *fantome,* from L. *phantasma* an appearance] 1. a model of the body or a specific part thereof.

2. in radiology and nuclear medicine, an object used to simulate the body in tests of imaging systems or to estimate radiation dose effects. Two types of phantoms are used in nuclear medicine quality control: imaging phantoms and transmission phantoms.

An imaging phantom or organ phantom is a plastic dummy of the organ or body part, which has compartments filled with radioactive solutions to simulate lesions. These are used to check the general performance of a scintillation camera or rectilinear scanner. The College of American Pathologists (CAP) provides organ phantoms with unknown distributions of radioactivity. Images of CAP phantoms are used in outside evaluation of laboratory performance.

Transmission phantoms are used to test the spatial resolution and the lack of distortion of scintillation cameras. These are usually bar phantoms, which are parallel bars of lead set in plastic and separated by equal spacing. They are usually attached to the collimator face with a flood source attached behind. The camera system's ability to resolve the bar is a check of its total spatial resolution. The same test with the collimator removed checks intrinsic spatial resolution. A parallel-line equal-space (PLES) phantom is a repeating pattern of bars and spaces of equal width that tests the lower limit of camera resolving power (about 1/4–1/8 in). Two images with the phantom rotated 90° test resolution, linearity, and distortion. A four-quadrant bar phantom (standard bar phantom) is like four small PLES phantoms with four different separations arranged in a square: which set of bars is resolved provides a measure of the variation in resolving power under varying conditions.

bar p., a square sheet of plastic with four sets of uniformly spaced flat lead bars used for evaluating scintillation camera resolution. If used with a collimator, the bar phantom indicates extrinsic characteristics; if used without, intrinsic characteristics.

flood p., a large plastic container having a disk-shaped cavity filled with liquid radioactive material. It is used as a flood source.

four-quadrant bar p., a transmission phantom used to check the spatial resolution of a scintillation camera. Each quadrant consists of a series of bars having equal width and spacing.

Hine-Duley p., in scintillation cameras, a transmission bar phantom used in quality control to check linearity, distortion, and resolution. It has five groups of bars that have three different spacings: 3/16, 1/4, and 1/2 in.

phantom spike and wave see *six-Hertz spike and slow waves.*

pharmac/o (fahr′mah-ko) [Gr. *pharmakon* medicine] a word element used in combining form to denote a drug or chemical, e.g., pharmacologic.

pharmaceutic, pharmaceutical (fahr-mah-su′tik, fahr-mah-su′tĭ-kal) pertaining to pharmacy or drugs.

pharmacist (fahr′mah-sist) an individual licensed to prepare and sell or dispense drugs and compounds, and to make up prescriptions.

pharmacodynamics (far″mah-ko-di-nam′iks) [*pharmaco-* + Gr. *dynamis* power] the body of knowledge concerning the biochemical and physiologic effects of drugs and their mechanisms of action and structure-activity relationships.

pharmacogenetics (fahr″mah-ko-jĕ-net′iks) the study of the genetically determined variation in response to drugs. Examples of such genetic variations are (1) pseudocholintesterase deficiency, which produces a sensitivity to the muscle relaxant succinylcholine; (2) slow inactivation of the antituberculosis drug isoniazid, which causes an increase in toxic reactions; and (3) glucose-6-phosphate dehydrogenase deficiency, which is the basis of hemolytic anemia induced by the antimalarial drug primaquine, by sulfonamides, and by aspirin (in very large doses).

pharmacokinetics (fahr″mah-ko-kĭ-net′iks) [*pharmaco-* + Gr. *kinētikos* of or for putting into motion] referring to the rate of absorption, systemic distribution, and clearance of a drug in the body over a period of time.

pharmacologic (fahr″mah-ko-loj′ik) pertaining to pharmacology or to the properties and reactions of drugs.

pharmacology (fahr″mah-kol′o-je) [*pharmaco-* + *-logy*] the science that deals with the chemistry, effects, and therapeutic uses of drugs.

pharmacopeia (far″mah-ko-pe′ah) [*pharmaco-* + Gr. *poiein* to make] an authoritative treatise on drugs and their preparation, which contains descriptions and formulations of the drugs plus standards, tests, and assays for their strength, quality, and purity. See also *United States Pharmacopeia.*

pharyng/o (fah-ring′go) [Gr. *pharynx* throat] a word element used in combining form to denote the pharynx, e.g., pharyngopathy.

pharyngeal (fah-rin′je-al) [L. *pharyngeus*] pertaining to the pharynx.

pharyngeal ridge see *Passavant's bar.*

pharyngitis (far″in-ji′tis) [*pharyng-* + *-itis* inflammation] acute or chronic inflammation of the pharynx. Acute inflammations of the pharynx most frequently are viral in origin but may also be due to a group A β-hemolytic streptococcus, pneumococcus, gonococcus, a coagulase-positive staphylococcus, or *Mycoplasma hominis.* The throat is sore and dry, there is pain on swallowing, and usually fever or malaise. The inflammation involves the mucosa of the pharynx and may spread to involve the nose (nasopharyngitis), larynx (pharyngolaryngitis), sinuses (sinusitis), or surrounding lymphatic structures. Pharyngitis may also be observed as part of systemic diseases (e.g., measles and whooping cough). Specific antibiotic therapy is indicated in bacterial infections; in others, treatment is symptomatic. In viral pharyngitis, the disease is usually self-limiting within several days.

Chronic inflammations may produce a dry throat, thick secretions of mucus, and swelling of the mucosa. Treatment is based on removing the underlying causes, such as chronic nasal or sinus infections, and restricting exposure to irritants.

Pharyngobdellida (fah-ring″gob-del′e-ah) [*pharyngo-* + Gr. *bdella* leech] an order of leeches.

pharyngoconjunctival fever (fah-ring″go-kon″-junk-ti′val) [*pharyngo-* + N.L. *conjunctiva* conjunctiva] a communicable disease that may be water-borne. It is thought to be due to adenovirus types 3 and 7, and occurs after an incubation of 5–8 da. It primarily affects school children and is characterized by fever, pharyngitis, and conjunctivitis. The conjunctivitis usually is unilateral, is follicular, and may be severe. The pharyngitis may extend to involve the lower respiratory tract. The disease is usually self-limiting within 7 da.

pharyngolaryngitis (fah-ring″go-lar″in-ji′tis) [*pharyngo-* + Gr. *larynx* larynx + *-itis*] the inflammation of both the pharynx and the larynx. It can be either bacterial or viral in origin, and may result from the extension of a pharyngeal or laryngeal inflammation. See also *laryngitis* and *pharyngitis.*

pharyngotympanic tube (fah-ring″go-tim-pan′ik) [*pharyngo-* + L. *tympanum* drum] see *auditory tube.*

pharynx (far′inks) [Gr. "throat"] [NA], a musculomembranous pouch between the nasal cavity, mouth, and larynx. A part of the alimentary canal, the pharynx is continuous with the esophagus and the nasopharynx, and communicates with the tympanic cavities through the auditory tubes.

phas/o (fa′zo) [Gr. *phasis* speech, from *phanai* to speak] a word element used in combining form to denote speech, e.g., dysphasia.

phase (fāz) [Gr. *phasis* an appearance, from *phainen* to make appear] 1. any one of the varying aspects or stages through which a disease or biologic process may pass.

2. any distinct or separable portion of a physical system or chemical process.

continuous p., a phase that is physically continuous; the continuous portion of a colloid system.

disperse p., the internal or discontinuous portion of a colloid system; it is analogous to the solute in a solution. Also called internal phase.

exponential p., see *logarithmic p.*

inductive p., the time elapsed between the administration of antigen and the development of a detectable immune response.

lag p., in microbiology, the time between the initial planting of an inoculum into the new medium and the beginning of cell multiplication; a period of stationary population during which the cells readjust to the new environment and begin to synthesize and accumulate the enzymes and intermediates for the next phase. Also called *lag.*

p. lag, see *lag.*

logarithmic p., the stage in the growth of a bacterial culture when a plot of the logarithm of the number of cells against time gives a straight-upward line. Also called *exponential p.*

meiotic p., that stage in meiosis in which the reduction of the chromosomes occurs. Also called reduction phase. See also *meions.*

mobile p., see *moving p.*

moving p., in chromatography, the fluid medium that carries the sample. Also called *mobile p.* See also *chromatography.*

stationary p., 1. the stage in the growth of a bacterial culture when the bacteria undergoing division are in equilibrium with those dying, and the number of bacterial cells remains nearly constant.

2. in chromatography, the sorbent that separates the sample into components by differences in their affinity for the sorbent. See also *chromatography.*

phasmid (faz′mid) 1. a type of caudal sensory organ thought to be an olfactory receptor (or chemoreceptor); usually found in pairs and associated with glands. It occurs in nematodes of the class Phasmidia.

2. any nematode that has phasmids. Cf. *aphasmid.*

Phasmidia (faz-mid′e-ah) a class of nematodes (roundworms), which includes the orders Rhabditida and Spirurida, whose members possess phasmids (olfactory receptors).

Ph.D. abbrev. for Doctor of Philosophy (L. *Philosophiae Doctor*), generally the highest postbaccalaureate academic degree granted by arts and sciences institutions.

Phe abbrev. See *phenylalanine.*

phe/o (fe′o) [Gr. *phaios* dusky, darkish] a word element used in combining form to denote dusky, e.g., pheochromocytoma.

phen/o (fe′no) [Gr. *phainein* to show] 1. a word element used in combining form to denote a show or display, e.g., phenotype.

2. a word element in combining form in organic

chemistry, to denote derived from or related to benzene, or containing phenyl, e.g., phenolsulfonphthalein.

phenacemide (fe-nas′ĕ-mīd) [USP], an anticonvulsant drug, phenylacetylurea, used in the control of severe psychomotor seizures that are unresponsive to other drugs. Adverse reactions include personality change, liver damage, and bone marrow depression (particularly aplastic anemia or leukopenia). Liver function tests and complete blood counts should be performed at regular intervals to detect toxic reactions. Trademark, Phenurone.

phenacetin (fe-nas′ĕ-tin) [USP], an analgesic and antipyretic drug, related to acetaminophen, that is often used in combination with aspirin and caffeine (APC, or acetylsalicylic acid, phenacetin, and caffeine) or with aspirin and codeine. Adverse reactions include cyanosis due to methemoglobinemia, dyspnea, and convulsions; long-term use may cause kidney damage, and chronic use in high doses has been associated with papillary necrosis and transitional carcinoma of the renal pelvis.

phenaceturic acid (fen″ah-se-tu′rik) the glycine conjugate of phenylacetic acid, $C_6H_5CH_2 \cdot CO \cdot NH \cdot CH_2 \cdot COOH$. It is formed from phenylacetic acid, which either is administered or arises metabolically.

phenanthrene (fe-nan′thrēn) a colorless, carcinogenic, crystalline hydrocarbon that comprises three fused rings. These rings have the same structural relationship to each other as do the A, B, and C rings of the steroid ring system. See also *steroids*.

phenazopyridine hydrochloride (fen′ah-zo-pēr′ĭ-dēn) [USP], an azo dye used for symptomatic relief of pain due to irritation of lower urinary tract mucosa. Overdosage may cause methemoglobinemia or hemolytic anemia. Poor kidney or liver function is a contraindication for its use.

phencyclidine (PCP) [fen-si′klĭ-dēn] 1-(1-phenylcyclohexyl)piperdine, one of the most dangerous hallucinogenic illicit drugs, most often referred to by its abbreviation, PCP. Psychotic reactions such as extreme anxiety or panic and hypertensive crisis and seizures are common; many fatalities have occurred through its abuse.

phencyclidine assays 1. gas chromatography. A flame ionization detector and silicone column packing of intermediate polarity are used. PCP is extracted from alkalinized samples into an organic solvent and silanized using dimethyldichlorosilane. The amount of PCP is determined by comparing the ratio of the peak heights of PCP and the internal standard ketamine with a previously prepared standard curve.

2. Emit homogeneous enzyme immunoassay for phencyclidine in urine specimens of suspected drug abusers.

phene (fēn) [Gr. *phainein* to make appear] a phenotypic character controlled by one or more genes.

phenelzine sulfate (fen′el-zēn) [USP], 2-phenylethylhydrazine, an antidepressant; see under *monoamine oxidase inhibitors*.

phenformin hydrochloride (fen-for′min) a biguanide oral hypoglycemic drug, now banned in the United States because of the unacceptably high risk of fatal lactic acidosis associated with its use.

phenindamine tartrate (fē-nin′dah-mēn) an antihistaminic and anticholinergic agent. Used in decongestant preparations, it has mild stimulant activity but rarely any sedative action.

pheniramine maleate (fen-ir′ah-mēn) an antihistamine that is used as a decongestant.

phenmetrazine hydrochloride (feh-met′rah-zēn) [USP], a sympathomimetic amine, similar to amphetamine, used as an anorectic (diet pill). Adverse reactions are similar to those of amphetamines and include the possibility of physical dependence or fatal overdosage. Trademark, *Preludin*.

phenobarbital (fe″no-bar′bĭ-tal) [USP], a long-acting barbiturate used to control convulsions caused by poisoning or fever and to control tonic-clonic (grand mal), focal, or psychomotor epileptic seizures. It also has use as a sedative or sleeping aid. See also *barbiturate*.

phenobarbital assays see *babiturate assays*.

phenocopy (fe′no-kop″e) 1. a phenotypic variation produced by environmental factors, which imitates one determined by a specific genotype. Rickets, produced by vitamin D deficiency, is an example of a phenocopy of the X-linked trait hypophosphatemia (vitamin D–resistant rickets).

2. an organism having this kind of phenotype.

phenodeviant (fe″no-de′ve-ant) [*pheno-* + L. *de* away from + *via* way] an extreme phenotype, representing a great variation from the norm for quantitative inherited traits.

phenogenetics (fe″no-jĕ-net′iks) see *developmental genetics*.

phenol (fe′nol) 1. [USP], the systematic name for hydroxybenzene, a weak organic acid (pK_a 10, pH about 6); M.W. 94.11. It forms crystals that are colorless, white, or red (if impure), and has a characteristic odor and a sharp burning taste. Phenol is used as a topical antiseptic and as an antimicrobial agent in solutions of 1–2 percent in lotions and mouthwashes.

Phenol and its derivatives are widely used in industry, especially in the manufacture of plastics. It is highly toxic and caustic when ingested; amounts as small as 1 g can be fatal, but 15 g is the average fatal dose. Symptoms of acute poisoning include nausea, vomiting, dark-colored urine, necrosis of the mouth and gastrointestinal tract, paralysis, convulsions, coma, respiratory depression, and cardiac arrest. Fatal poisoning can also occur by skin absorption when phenol is applied to large portions of body surfaces. Chronic poisoning can cause kidney and liver damage. Also called *carbolism*.

Phenol is a metabolite of benzene and some drugs; it is excreted in the urine in conjugated form as the sulfate or glucuronide. Also call *carbolic acid*.

2. the generic name for any compound that has a hydroxy group directly attached to an aromatic ring, e.g., naphthol, catechol, cresol, or resorcinol. All are weak acids (pK_a 10), yet are much more strongly acidic than aliphatic alcohols. The generic formula is ArOH.

phenol assays 1. colorimetric test. Phenols may be separated from an acidified sample by steam distillation. Million's reagent is added to the distillate, which is then boiled; a red color indicates a phenolic compound. Alternate color reagents are ammonium hydroxide and bromine, which give a yellow precipitate; ammonium hydroxide and sodium hypochlorite, which give a green to blue-green color; or ferric chloride, which gives a violet color. None are specific for phenol.

2. titration. Phenol in the steam distillate (method 1) is brominated. Iodide is reduced to iodine by the tribromophenol. The iodine is titrated with sodium thiosulfate solution, using starch as the indicator.

3. ultraviolet spectrophotometry. Phenolic compounds, separated by steam distillation (method 1) or extracted by organic solvents from acidified specimens, are identified by their characteristic ultraviolet absorption spectra.

phenol coefficient a measure of the bactericidal activity of a chemical compound in relation to that of phenol as determined under a standard test condition.

phenolphthalein (fe″nol-thal′e-in) [USP], a drug used as a laxative and purgative that has continuous action for 3–4 da. Adverse reactions include skin rash and renal irritation. Phenolphthalein is also used as an acid-base indicator dye; it is colorless below pH 8.5 and deep red above pH 9.0.

phenol sulfatase See *arylsulfatase.*

phenolsulfonphthalein (PSP) (fe″nol-sul″fōn-thal′e-in) an acid-base indicator with a pH range of 6.8 (yellow)–8.4 (red). In diagnostic medicine, the excretion rate of PSP dye was once used as a test for measuring renal tubular secretory function. Also called phenol red.

phenolsulfonphthalein test a renal function test that is primarily a measure of renal secretory function. It is rarely used today. A standard dose (usually 6 mg) of PSP dye is injected, and the fraction cleared by the kidneys in specified time intervals is determined. Eighty percent of PSP is excreted by the kidneys (94 percent of which is by tubular excretion and 6 percent by glomerular filtration) and 20 percent by the liver.

The individual is hydrated and 1 ml of sterile PSP solution injected intramuscularly. Urine specimens are collected at 15-, 30-, 60-, and 120-min intervals (some hospitals use only a 15-min specimen). The PSP concentration (used to calculate the fraction excreted) is then determined spectrophotometrically at 540 nm after alkalinizing the urine. The reference range is 25–35 percent dye excretion in the first 15 min.

phenom (fe′nom) see *phenon.*

phenomenon (fĕ-nom′ĕ-non), pl. *phenomena* [Gr. neuter present participle of *phainesthal* to appear] any sign or objective symptom; any observable occurrence or fact.

phenon (fe′non), pl. *phena, phenons* using numerical taxonomy, a group of organisms classified together on the basis of their phenotypes. Also called *phenom.*

phenothiazine (fe″no-thi′ah-zēn) a compound used as a veterinary anthelmintic, as an insecticide, and in industrial synthesis. Also called dibenzothiazine and thiodiphenylamine.

phenothiazine tranquilizers a large group of major tranquilizers that are derivatives of phenothiazine, and are chemically and pharmacologically similar to the thioxanthenes. They are used in the management of psychotic disorders (e.g., schizophrenias) and other psychiatric conditions. Adverse reactions include drowsiness, orthostatic hypotension, and extrapyramidal effects such as restlessness, tremor, muscular rigidity, slowness of movements, and other parkinsonian symptoms. Persistent tardive dyskinesia may appear during or after long-term therapy on phenothiazines; this syndrome is characterized by involuntary movements of the face, mouth, tongue, and (in some cases) the extremities. Phenothiazines have a high therapeutic index; very large doses are rarely fatal.

There is no known correlation between the blood levels of phenothiazines and the therapeutic response; screening assays are performed primarily to show whether the patient is taking the medication. Some of the phenothiazines have hundreds of metabolites, many of which may be active. Some of the metabolites continue to be excreted in the urine for months after treatment is stopped.

Phenothiazines are divided into three derivative types based on the chemical group in the side-chain. Alkyl derivatives produce more sedation and hypotension; piperazine derivatives are more potent, less sedating, and more likely to produce dyskinesia; and piperidine derivatives produce extrapyramidal symptoms less frequently but can produce hypotension and (rarely) toxic retinitis.

phenothiazine tranquilizers assays 1. urine ferric chloride screening test. FPN reagent (ferric chloride, perchloric acid, and nitric acid solution) is added to a urine specimen; a blue, purple, or red color may indicate the presence of a phenothiazine or derivative. False-negatives may occur, particularly with therapeutic doses of the most potent phenothiazines, e.g., fluphenazine; large overdoses should give a positive indication. False-positives may also occur.

2. thin-layer chromatography. Silica gel plates and a polar developing solvent are used. Phenothiazines are detected by converting them to sulfoxides by oxidation with hydrogen peroxide. Positive identification can be made by eluting the sulfoxide and determining the ultraviolet absorption maxima.

3. gas chromatography. The drug and its metabolites are extracted from alkalinized plasma by a mixed organic solvent, purified by differential extractions, and injected onto a column of intermediate polarity using an electron capture detector. Sensitivity is 0.01 μg/ml.

See also *chlorpromazine assays* and *thioridazine assays.*

phenotype (fe′no-tīp) [*pheno-* + Gr. *typos* type] 1. all the characteristics of an organism that result from the interaction of its genetic make-up with the environment; also one such characteristic.

2. an organism or group of organisms having a particular phenotype.

phenotypic variance (fe′no-tip′ik) the total range of variation observed in one character.

phenoxybenzamine hydrochloride (fĕnok″se-ben′zah-mēn) [USP], a long-acting alpha-adrenergic receptor blocking drug used in the treatment of pheochromocytoma. It produces a stable alpha-adrenergic blockade that controls the hypotension produced by the catecholamines secreted from the tumor. The drug is also used to reduce peripheral vasospasm, as occurs in Raynaud's syndrome. Adverse reactions include postural hypotension and tachycardia. Trademark, *Dibenzyline.*

phenoxypenicillin (fe-nox″e-pen″ĭ-sil′in) see *p. V* under *penicillins.*

phensuximide (fen-suk′sĭ-mīd) [USP], an anticonvulsant drug similar to ethosuximide but sometimes less effective, used to treat absence (petit mal) epilepsy. Trademark, Milontin.

phentermine hydrochloride (fen′ter-mēn) a sympathomimetic amine, similar to the amphetamines, used as an anorectic (diet pill). Adverse reactions are similar to those of amphetamines and include the possibility of physical dependence and fatal overdosage. It is also available as a cationic exchange resin complex (phentermine resin).

phentolamine (fen-tol′ah-mēn) a short-acting alpha-adrenergic receptor blocking drug used in the diagnosis of pheochromocytoma and in the control of hypertensive crises produced by the catecholamines secreted by the tumor. Intravenous administration produces an immediate fall in blood pressure in individuals having an elevated blood level of norepinephrine; the drug does not, however, reduce hypertension due to other causes. Overdosage may produce a hypotensive reaction, which is reversed by administration of norepinephrine. Trademark, *Regitine.*

p. hydrochloride, [USP], the salt of phentolamine used for oral administration.

p. mesylate, [USP], the salt of phentolamine used for parenteral administraton.

phenyl- (fen′il) a prefix word element used in organic chemistry to denote the benzene ring when it is treated as a substituent (—C_6H_5, sometimes symbolized by the Greek letter phi, ϕ, or by Ph) attached to some parent compound, e.g., phenylalanine (2-amino-3-phenylpropanoic acid, $C_6H_5CH_2$-$CH(NH_2)COOH$).

phenylacetic acid (fen″il-ah-se′tik) a decarboxylation product of phenylpyruvic acid, $C_6H_5 \cdot CH_2 \cdot$ COOH, formed in the metabolism of phenylalanine in the body, especially in phenylketonuria. It is conjugated with glutamine, forming phenylacetylglutamine, and is excreted in the urine.

phenylacetylglutamine (fen″il-as″e-til-gloo′tah-mēn) an excretory product of phenylacetic acid that is found in the urine, $C_6H_5 \cdot CH \cdot CO \cdot NH \cdot CH$-$(COOH) \cdot (CH_2)_2 \cdot CO \cdot NH_2$, especially in phenylketonuria.

phenylalanine (Phe, F) (fen″il-al′ah-nēn) 2-amino-3-phenylpropanoic acid, $C_6H_5CH_2CH(NH_2)$-COOH, a naturally occurring essential amino acid; M.W. 165.19. It serves as a constituent of proteins and as a precursor for a number of important biologic molecules, e.g., tyrosine, epinephrine, norepinephrine, 3,4-dihydroxyphenylalanine (DOPA), 3,4-dihydroxyphenylethylamine (dopamine), and melanin. The source of phenylalanine is protein in the diet. Special diets low in phenylalanine are utilized in treating patients with phenylketonuria. See also under *amino acids.*

phenylalanine agar see *phenylalanine a.* under *agar.*

phenylalanine assays 1. Guthrie screening test. A microbiologic procedure primarily used to detect the presence of elevated levels of phenylalanine (Phe) in blood or serum. A strain of *Bacillus subtilis* requiring phenylalanine as a growth factor is cultivated on a medium containing essential nutrients plus the phenylalanine antagonist β-2-thienylalanine. The level of antagonist is such that no growth occurs with Phe present at concentrations normally present in blood. Elevated levels of the Phe overcome the antagonism and thus permit growth, the extent dependent on the concentration of Phe. The specimen is added to the culture plate in the form of a paper disk saturated with dried blood. The size of the bacterial growth rings depends on the Phe level. A series of Phe standards permits semiquantitation.

2. quantitative fluorometric procedure. A trichloroacetic acid filtrate is heated with Ninhydrin in the presence of a dipeptide to form a fluorophor; fluorescence is measured at 515 nm (activation at 365 nm) in the presence of alkaline copper and is proportional to the Phe concentration.

3. extraction of Phe from blood and measurement by thin-layer chromatography, a less accurate procedure than methods 1 and 2.

phenylalanine hydroxylase see *phenylalanine-4-monooxygenase.*

phenylalanine-4-monooxygenase an enzyme of the oxidoreductase class (EC 1.14.16.1) that catalyzes the reaction L-phenylalanine + tetrahydropteridine + $O_2 \rightleftarrows$ L-tyrosine + dihydropteridine + H_2O. This enzyme occurs primarily in the liver. The reaction is the first step in the metabolism of dietary phenylalanine. A genetic deficiency of the enzyme, known as phenylketonuria, leads to the accumulation of phenylalanine and its metabolites in the tissues and phenylpyruvate excretion in the urine. Also called *phenylalanine hydroxylase.* See also *aminoacidopathy.*

phenylalanine tolerance index a diagnostic tool proposed to aid the identification of carriers (heterozygotes) of the phenylketonuria gene. Serum phenylalanine levels are determined 1, 2, and 4 hr after administration of a 100-mg/kg oral dose of phenylalanine. The index is the sum of the three measurements. Another method used to detect carriers for phenylketonuria involves determination of the ratio of phenylalanine to tyrosine in serum.

phenylalanyl (fen″il-al′ah-nil) the acyl radical derived from or relating to phenylalanine.

phenylbutazone (fen″il-bu′tah-zōn) [USP], an analgesic, antipyretic, antiinflammatory, and uricosuric nonsteroidal drug of the pyrazolone group. It is used for the treatment of gout, rheumatoid arthritis, osteoarthritis, and ankylosing spondylitis. Phenylbutazone has many serious side-effects, including gastric irritation, peptic ulcers, fluid retention, allergic skin rashes, and bone marrow suppression that causes aplastic anemia or agranulocytosis. Patients taking phenylbutazone must be regularly examined for edema and other signs of toxicity; blood counts should also be performed.

Overdosage may cause acidosis, impaired kidney and liver function, and respiratory depression.

Trademarks, Azolid and Butazolidin.

phenylbutazone assays 1. ultraviolet (UV), spectrophotometry. Phenylbutazone and its two major metabolites—oxyphenbutazone, which also has antiinflammatory activity, and γ-hydroxyphenylbutazone—are extracted from acidified biologic specimens into organic solvents, and then back into water at alkaline pH. Oxyphenbutazone can be separated from phenylbutazone by extraction into alkaline solution from ethylene dichloride; the phenylbutazone remains in the ethylene dichloride. The absorbance at 265 nm for phenylbutazone and 253 nm for oxyphenbutazone is determined in both acidic and basic solution. The phenylbutazone concentration is proportional to the difference between the absorbance in base and in acid.

2. thin-layer chromatography (TLC). After extraction as in method 1, phenylbutazone and its metabolites are separated by TLC on silica gel plates using a polar developing solvent (chloroform-methanol or ethyl acetate-methanol-ammonium hydroxide). Potassium permanganate or ammonium vanadate with sulfuric acid overspray can be used as the spray reagent.

3. gas chromatography (GLC). After extraction, the compounds with appropriate internal standards are derivatized by methylation and chromatographed using a slightly polar silicone stationary phase and a flame ionization detector. The peak ratios of the drugs to their internal standards are compared to those for reference standards.

phenylcarbinol (fen″il-kar′bĭ-nol) see *benzyl alcohol.*

phenylephrine (fen″il-ef′rin) a sympathomimetic amine that is a strong α-adrenergic stimulating agent. It is used as a vasoconstrictor and pressor in the emergency treatment of shock or hypotension, in the treatment of paroxysmal supraventricular tachycardia, as a decongestant for rhinitis, and in ophthalmology as a mydriatic.

p. bitartrate, a salt of phenylephrine used in aerosol inhalers.

p. hydrobromide, a salt of phenylephrine used in liquid oral preparations.

p. hydrochloride, [USP], a salt of phenylephrine administered orally, by injection, topically, and in nasal sprays or inhalants.

p. tannate, a salt of phenylephrine administered orally in tablets and suspensions.

phenylhydrazine (fen″il-hi′drah-zēn) an oily, colorless liquid, $C_6H_5NH \cdot NH_2$, used as a reagent for carbonyl compounds (ketones and aldehydes) and for reducing sugars in particular.

phenylketonuria (PKU) (fen″il-ke″to-nu′re-ah) a genetic condition, transmitted as an autosomal recessive trait with a frequency of 1 in every 10,000–15,000 births, that is characterized by the accumulation of plasma phenylalanine. The disease results from an inborn error of metabolism in which the enzyme activity of phenylalanine hydroxylase is almost or completely absent. This enzyme deficiency prevents the normal degradation of phenylalanine to tyrosine. As a result, phenylalanine accumulates in the blood and is eventually degraded in secondary metabolic pathways to phenylpyruvic acid, phenyllactic acid, and phenylacetic acid, which are execreted in the urine. In the fully expressed state, there is a persistent hyperphenylalaninemia greater than 1 mmol (16.5 mg/100 ml). Clinical symptoms are virtually absent in the newborn period. Untreated, the disease progresses, causing mental retardation. A "mousy" odor is frequently present in the urine.

The exact mechanism by which the accumulation of phenylalanine leads to mental retardation is unknown. Although phenylketonuria cannot be cured, its severity may be lessened by proper dietary management. Affected infants are fed a diet that contains enough phenylalanine to meet the body's needs in growth and development. Because phenylalanine is an essential amino acid and approximately 4 percent of all protein is phenylalanine, it is impossible to satisfy the body's protein demand with normal foods without exceeding the phenylalanine tolerance levels. Therefore, casein hydrolysates treated to remove phenylalanine, or mixtures of amino acids deficient in phenylalanine, are prescribed. Assays of plasma phenylalanine levels should be routinely performed to test the effectiveness of the diet.

PKU is the first disease in which a biochemical mechanism for mental retardation was elucidated. On the basis of this information, a logical dietary approach to control the disease was predicted, and early identification of affected infants with a more favorable outcome was made possible. Screening programs have revealed several variants, including dihydropteridine reductase deficiency.

Also called classic phenylketonuria, phenylalaninemia, and *phenylpyruvic oligophrenia.* For more information on the diagnostic procedure for PKU, see under *genetic screening, phenylalanine assays, phenylalanine tolerance index,* and *phenylpyruvic acid tests.* See also *aminoacidopathy* and *hyperphenylalaninemia.*

phenyllactic acid (fen″il-lak′tik) an acid, $C_6H_5CH_2$-CHOHCOOH, formed reductively from phenylpyruvic acid. It appears in the urine in phenylketonuria.

phenylpropanolamine hydrochloride (fen″il-pro″pah-nol′am-ēn) [USP], a sympathomimetic amine used in over-the-counter preparations as a vasoconstrictor and bronchodilator, usually in combination with an antihistamine drug. Use with other sympathomimetic amines or monoamine oxidase inhibitors should be avoided.

phenylpyruvic acid (fen″il-pi-roo′vik) a deamination product in the metabolism of phenylalanine, $C_6H_5 \cdot CH_2 \cdot CO \cdot COOH$. Ordinarily, this pathway is minor compared with the conversion phenylalanine to tyrosine, but it becomes the main pathway in phenylketonuria, where this conversion is decreased or blocked owing to a genetic deficiency of the enzyme phenylalanine-4-monooxygenase.

phenylpyruvic acid tests a urine screening test. Ferric chloride reagent reacts with phenylpyruvic acid to produce a transient green to blue-green color. Imidazolepyruvic acid and bilirubin, if present, can yield false-positive reactions. A commercial product, an impregnated reagent strip Phenistix, is also based on the $FeCl_3$ reaction.

phenylpyruvic oligophrenia see *phenylketonuria.*

phenylthiocarbamide (PTC) (fen″il-thi″o-kar-bam′īd) see *phenylthiourea.*

phenylthiocarbamoyl (PTC) peptide (fen″il-thi-o-kar′bah-moil) a derivative of a peptide or protein made by reaction of the amino-terminal residue with Edman's reagent, phenyl isothiocyanate. On treating with weak acid, this derivative liberates the phenylthiohydantoin of the *N*-terminal amino acid, which can then be identified. The procedure can then be repeated with each amino acid in turn. This permits sequencing of a peptide or protein; the procedure can be performed with automated equipment. See also *Edman reaction.*

phenylthiourea (fen″il-thi″o-u-re′ah) a compound, $C_6H_5NHCSNH_2$, used in genetic research. The ability to taste it is inherited as a dominant trait, the compound being intensely bitter to approximately 70 percent of the population, and nearly tasteless to the remainder. Also called *phenylthiocarbamide* or PTC.

phenyltoloxamine (fen″il-tol-ok′sah-mēn) a mild

antihistamine used in analgesic and decongestant preparations.

phenytoin (fen'ĭ-to-in) [USP], generic name for 5,5-diphenyl-2,4-imidazolidinedione, an anticonvulsant used to treat epilepsy. Toxic effects, which occur at blood concentrations only slightly higher than therapeutic levels, include dizziness, headache, vomiting, and constipation. Severe complications, some fatal, include cardiac irregularities and irregularities in blood cell production. Phenytoin interferes with several clinical laboratory tests, including the metyrapone and dexamethasone tests for adrenocorticotropin hormone (ACTH) and the protein-bound iodine tests. Also called *diphenylhydantoin.* Trademark (for phenytoin sodium), *Dilantin.*

phenytoin assays 1. extraction from serum and conversion to benzophenone, which is detected by ultraviolet absorption at 247 nm.

2. extraction from blood or urine into toluene, followed by derivatization by trimethylanilinium hydroxide and detection by gas chromatography.

3. EMIT or RIA immunoassays, using commercial kits.

pheochrome body (fe'o-krōm) [*pheo-* + Gr. *chrōma* color] see *paraganglion.*

pheochromocytoma (fe-o-kro″mo-si-to'mah) [*pheo-* + Gr. *chroma* color + *kytos* hollow vessel + ōma swelling] a chromaffin-positive tumor composed of neuroepithelial cells arising from the paraganglion system. In the adrenal, pheochromocytomas may secrete epinephrine, norepinephrine, or both; in extraadrenal sites, they usually secrete only norepinephrine.

Pheochromocytomas occur most commonly in the adrenal (90 percent of cases), where they arise from the adrenal medulla; approximately 10 percent are bilateral. Extraadrenal pheochromocytomas may arise from paraganglionic tissue located in the retroperitoneum, organ of Zuckerkandl, urinary bladder, mediastinum, and, occasionally, carotid body or glomus jugulare.

In both adrenal and extraadrenal sites, approximately 90 percent of pheochromocytomas occur in adults, and both sexes are affected with equal frequency. Approximately 10 percent of the tumors are malignant.

Familial cases of pheochromocytoma have been reported in association with hyperparathyroidism and medullary carcinoma of the thyroid (the constellation known as MEN II [multiple endocrine neoplasia] or Sipple syndrome). Instances of pheochromocytoma associated with neurofibromatosis, cerebellar hemangioblastoma, or renal artery stenosis have also been reported.

Less than 25 percent of pheochromocytomas are hormonally active. Symptoms produced by hormonally active tumors are the same as those produced by the injection of large amounts of epinephrine, e.g., headache, excessive sweating, palpitations, anxiety, and pallor with subsequent flushing. Hypertensive attacks are usually intermittent. They may be precipitated by palpation of the tumor, abdominal compression or massage, emotional trauma, or physical exertion.

Diagnosis of pheochromocytoma is directed at demonstrating hypermetabolism and/or diabetes mellitus, which may be associated with this tumor, and the measurement of plasma or urinary levels of catecholamines, primarily epinephrine and norepinephrine or their breakdown products. Radiologic techniques to demonstrate the presence of a lesion include radiographs of the chest, abdomen, and retroperitoneum; nephrotomography; retroperitoneal pneumography; and angiography. Recently, computerized tomography has supplanted these techniques and offers the most accurate, noninvasive preoperative diagnostic evaluation for suspected pheochromocytoma. Because malignant pheochromocytomas have a propensity for metastasizing to the skeletal system, particularly the spine and ribs, a preoperative bone scan is recommended for all patients suspected of having this tumor.

The treatment of pheochromocytoma is surgical removal in conjunction with alpha- and beta-adrenergic blocking agents.

pheomelanin (fe-o-mel'ah-nin) [*pheo-* + Gr. *melas* black] a yellowish-red melanin pigment in which some sulfur-containing compounds are also polymerized. It is a pigment of red hair. See also *melanin.*

pheresis (fĕ-re'sis) [Gr. *aphairesis* removal] a procedure in which whole blood is withdrawn from the patient, a portion of the blood separated and retained (e.g., plasma, platelets, leukocytes), and the remainer retransfused into the patient. Also called *hemapheresis.*

-pheresis a suffix word element to denote removal, e.g., plasmapheresis.

phi (Φ, ϕ) (fi) the twenty-first letter of the *Greek alphabet.*

phialide (fi'ah-lid) [Gr. *phialis,* dim. of *phialē* a broad, flat vessel] a tubular or flasklike conidiophore from which arise the conidia (phialospores). The phialide is well developed in the *Phialophora* species. Cf. *annellophore* and *sterigma.*

Phialophora (fi″ah-lof'o-rah) [Gr. *phialis* + *phoros* bearing, from *pherein* to bear] a genus of fungi that causes chromomycosis.

P. compactum, see *F. compactum* under *Fonsecaea.*

p. dermatitidis, see *F. dermatitidis* under *Fonsecaea.*

P. gougerotii, a fungus that is the most common cause of cystic chromomycosis, which usually results from infection of cysts in a puncture wound. The colony morphology is moist, glistening, and olive to black in color—similar in morphology to *Fonsecaea dermatitidis* and *P. jeanselmei.* Microscopically, pleomorphic, budding, yeastlike cells are seen and, in the mycelial stage, hyphae form branches of phialophores with elongated conidia.

P. jeanselmei, former name for the fungus *Exophiala jeanselmei.*

phialophore (fi'ah-lo-fōr) the branch of the mycelium of certain fungi that bears the phialospore at its tip.

phialospore (fi'ah-lo-spōr) [Gr. *phialis* + *sporos* seed] a spore borne at the end of a phialide or phialophore in some fungi.

Philadelphia chromosome [*Philadelphia,* a city in Pennsylvania] see *Philadelphia c.* under *chromosome.*

-philia (fil'e-ah) [Gr. *philein* to regard with affection, to love] a suffix word element to denote attraction for, e.g., eosinophilia.

phimosis (fi-mo'sis) [Gr. *phimōsis* a muzzling or

closure] a condition characterized by the presence of an unretractable foreskin on the penis. This disorder may have congenital or developmental causes (a foreskin with an abnormal opening) or may be due to inflammation, leading to scarring constriction of the prepuce. Phimosis favors the accumulation of debris under the foreskin, encouraging secondary bacterial infections. Surgical enlargement or removal (circumcision) of the prepuce may be necessary. Cf. *paraphimosis.*

pH indicator an organic compound that changes color to indicate when the acid form changes into the ionic (or salt) form. In bacteriology, pH indicators are incorporated in culture media to indicate an increase or decrease in the acidity, which is due to the accumulation of metabolic products during bacterial growth. The accompanying table lists the principal pH indicators. For more information, see the individual indicators.

pHisoHex (fi'so-heks) see under *hexachlorophene.*

PHLA abbrev. See *postheparin lipolytic activity.*

phleb/o (fleb'o) [Gr. *phleps, phlebos* vein] a word element used in combining form to denote the vein, e.g., phlebitis.

phlebectasia (fleb"ek-ta'ze-ah) [*phleb-* + Gr. *ektasis* dilation + *-ia*] a condition characterized by the dilation of a vein, or a plexus of veins, leading to a varicose lesion. It may occur in the jejunum, buccal mucosa, lips, or scrotum. When it occurs in the esophagus or GI tract, it is often in association with gastrointestinal bleeding.

phlebitis (flĕ-bi'tis) [*phleb-* + *-itis* inflammation] see *thrombophlebitis.*

phlebogram (fleb'o-gram) [*phlebo-* + Gr. *gramma* a mark] a radiograph of an opacified vein demonstrating the venous circulation Also called *venogram.*

phlebography (flĕ-bog'rah-fe) [*phlebo-* + Gr. *graphein* to write or draw] the radiologic examination of a vein after the injection of a radiopaque contrast medium. In common usage, phlebography refers to the radiologic examination of the leg veins to demonstrate the location, extent, and degree of attachment of a thrombosis. Phlebography is the most accurate and complete way to demonstrate this lesion. Venous blockage, filling defects, and flow diversions may be visualized. Even though not all leg veins may be demonstrable by this procedure (such as profunda femoris and internal iliac), it accurately detects more than 90 percent of thrombi. Because of the time, expense, and discomfort of this procedure, it is not used in screening; repeated use may lead to leg vein thrombosis. Also called ascending contrast phlebography and peripheral venography. See also *venography* and *venous thrombosis scanning.*

phleborheography (fleb"o-re-og'rah-fe) [*plebo-* + Gr. *rheos* stream, from L. *rhein* to flow + *graphein* to write or draw] a newly developed technique that measures the changes of volume of an extremity as a result of the obstruction of venous outflow. The instrument employed, a phleborheograph, uses multiple strain-gauge plethysmographs. This technique is proving to be a very accurate means of detecting venous obstruction and thrombosis in the pelvis, thighs, and calves.

phlebosclerosis (fleb"o-sklĕ-ro'sis) [*phlebo-* + Gr. *sklērōsis* hardening] thickening and hardening of the walls of veins due to fibrous intimal proliferation and medial muscular hypertrophy, frequently associated with degeneration of elastic tissue and calcification in the media. Common sites of occurence are the inferior vena cava and the iliac, popliteal, and portal veins.

phlebothrombosis (fleb"o-throm-bo'sis) [*phlebo-* + Gr. *thrombos* clot] the development of a venous thrombus. This term was once used to describe the formation of a thrombus without venous inflammation; however, it is now considered to be a part of the overall pathologic process of thrombophlebitis, as the development of a thrombus inevitably leads to inflammatory changes within the wall of the vein. See also *thrombophlebitis.*

Phlebotominae (flĕ-bot-om-in'e-e) [N.L. from *phlebo-* + Gr. *tomos* a cutting + L. *-inus* of the nature of] a subfamily of bloodsucking flies of which the genus *Phlebotomus* is a member.

Phlebotomus (flĕ-bot'o-mus) [*phlebo-* + Gr. *tomos*

pH INDICATOR. TABLE OF THE PRINCIPAL pH INDICATORS

NAME	pH RANGE	COLOR IN ACID	COLOR IN BASE
Bromocresol green	3.8–5.4	Yellow	Green
Bromocresol purple	5.2–6.8	Yellow	Purple
Bromophenol blue	3.0–4.6	Yellow	Blue
Bromothymol blue	6.0–7.6	Yellow	Blue
Chlorophenol red	5.2–6.8	Yellow	Red
Congo red	3.0–4.5	Blue	Red
Cresol red	7.2–8.8	Yellow	Red
Litmus	4.5–8.3	Red	Blue
Methyl orange	3.0–4.4	Red	Orange-yellow
Methyl red	4.4–6.2	Red	Yellow
Neutral red	6.8–8.0	Red	Yellow
Phenol red	6.8–8.4	Yellow	Red
Phenolphthalein	8.3–10.0	Colorless	Red
Thymol blue (acid range)	1.2–2.8	Red	Yellow
Thymol blue (alkaline range)	8.0–9.6	Yellow	Blue
Thymolphthalein	9.3–10.5	Colorless	Blue

a cutting] a genus of biting flies (the sandflies) of the family Psychodidae. These are small, hump-backed flies that usually inhabit warm climates. The females are bloodsucking. Some species of *Phlebotomus* are transmitters of various diseases such as kala-azar (via *P. argentipes, P. chinensis, P. martini, P. orientalis, P. perniciosus*), Carrión's disease or bartonellosis (via *P. noguchi, P. verrucarum*), cutaneous leishmaniasis (via *P. sergenti*), and phlebotomus fever (via *P. papatasii*).

phlebotomus fever an acute infectious disease caused by an arbovirus (25–60 μμ), transmitted by the sandfly *Phlebotomus papatasii.* The disease is characterized by fever, malaise, severe headache, orbital pain, and leukopenia. It is found geographically in Mediterranean and Middle Eastern countries.

Phlebotomus fever should be distinguished from acute rhinopharyngitis, gastroenteritis, malaria, and other acute febrile diseases. The disease occurs only during the breeding season of *P. papatasii,* and can be transmitted only by females.

In laboratory diagnosis, urine and spinal fluid samples are negative for abnormalities and for the virus. Red blood cells are normal. There is a reduction in the number of mature neutrophils and an increase in immature neutrophils; the monocytes are usually normal in appearance and number.

Also called *pappataci fever* and *sandfly fever.*

phlebotomy (flĕ-bot′o-me) [*phlebo-* + Gr. *tomē* a cutting] the withdrawing of blood. This procedure may be used diagnostically to obtain blood or serum specimens for laboratory analysis, and therapeutically to reduce blood volume in cor pulmonale, to reduce the number of erythrocytes in polycythemia vera, or to mobilize and deplete excessive body iron stores in hemochromatosis.

phlegm (flem) [Gr. *phlegma*] the common name for secretions of thick and viscid mucus from the respiratory tract. Abnormally large amounts of phlegm may be produced and excreted in respiratory tract infections and inflammations.

phlegmasia (fleg-ma′ze-ah) [Gr. "heat, inflammation"] inflammation.

p. alba dolens, an iliofemoral venous thrombosis that occurs most frequently in the third trimester of pregnancy, following delivery, or after acute febrile illness. It is characterized by painful swelling of the extremities, with tenderness over the involved veins. Arterial spasm, diminished pulse, and a cool, pale leg are also symptomatic. In pregnancy this condition may be associated with changes in platelets and clotting factors. Also called milk leg.

p. cerulea dolens, a severe form of iliofemoral or deep vein thrombosis that is characterized by marked obstruction of venous outflow, leading to cyanosis. The affected extremity displays a diminished arterial pulse and becomes swollen and cool. If obstruction in the venous outflow in a given area becomes massive and nearly complete, there may be a rapid rise in tissue pressure, compromising arterial inflow. Also called *blue phlebitis.*

phlegmon (fleg′mon) [Gr. *phlegmonē* inflammation, boil] 1. a spreading, diffuse inflammatory reaction that forms a long, flat abscess, often caused by streptococci. It may extend into the deep subcutaneous areas and muscles and produce edema, suppuration, and occasional pockets of gas. See also *cellulitis.*

2. an abdominal mass that results from a swollen and inflamed pancreas. It may last for several weeks and require draining. There are patchy areas of necrosis that are prone to secondary infections. Differentiation from a pancreatic pseudocyst may be accomplished by sonography.

phloroglucin (flo″ro-gloo′sin) [*phlorizin* + Gr. *glykys* sweet] 1,3,5-trihydroxybenzene, the aglycone of many glycosides. Obtained from the bark of apple and other trees, it is used as a reagent for some carbohydrates and for hydrochloric acid in gastric juice. Phloroglucin is an excellent decalcifier of bone specimens. Also called *phloroglucinol.*

phloroglucinol (flo″ro-gloo′sĭ-nol) see *phloroglucin.*

phloxine B (flok′sin) [Gr. *phlox* flame] a red acid dye used in histology as a plasma stain; C.I. 45410.

phlyctenule (flik-te′nūl) [L. *phlyctaenula,* from Gr. *phlyktaina* blister] a discrete, ulcerated nodule of inflammation that appears at the junction of the conjunctiva and the cornea. The nodules may last for several days to several weeks and disappear without scarring. If the cornea is affected, there may be corneal tearing, photophobia, and pain. Repeated episodes of this disease can lead to corneal opacity.

pH meter an instrument that measures pH electrochemically (potentiometrically). It consists of two electrodes, a hydrogen ion–sensitive glass electrode and a calomel reference electrode, as well as a high-impedance potentiometer (drawing less than 10^{-10} A of current) for measuring the voltage difference that exists when the electrodes are immersed in the solution whose pH is being sought. The pH is a linear function of the voltage measured.

The instrument is calibrated by setting the meter to indicate the correct pH of two standard buffer solutions having defined pH values, as certified by some appropriate body, such as the National Bureau of Standards. Usually the meter has a means of compensating for change in the standard potential of the reference electrode with change in temperature if readings are made at other than 25°C.

See also *pH.*

PH_2O abbrev. See *p. p. of water vapor* under *partial pressure.*

Phobetron (fo-be′tron) [Gr. *phobē* lock of hair] a genus of urticating caterpillars (the hag moth). The species *P. pithecium,* found in the eastern United States, possesses spine-type poisonous hairs. When the poisonous substance is introduced into the skin, a burning, stinging sensation is experienced and the site usually becomes erythematous.

phobia (fo′be-ah) [Gr. *phobos* fear + *-ia*] a persistent, abnormal dread or fear characterized as a form of "displacement" in which the individual transfers feelings of anxiety and fear from their true source to some other object or situation. Those affected usually recognize that there is no realistic basis for their fear but they are unable to master their reaction to it. Phobias represent ineffective defense mechanisms and tend to increase in scope, frequency, and intensity. Individuals act unreasonably and uncontrollably when confronted by objects or situations they fear. Opinions are divided as to the effectiveness of therapies such as psychotherapy, psychoanalysis, and behavioral therapy; some believe phobias may be due to unknown biochemical or neurophysiologic disorders. Examples of more common phobias include acrophobia (fear of heights), agoraphobia (fear of open or public places), claustrophobia (fear of closed places), and xenophobia (fear of strangers).

-phobia (fo′be-ah) a suffix word element to denote fear, e.g., hydrophobia.

phocomelia (fo″ko-me′le-ah) [Gr. *phōkē* seal + *melos* limb + *-ia*] a congenital malformation that results in the absence of a limb or limbs and the direct attachment of a hand or foot to the trunk ("seal extremity"). Such birth defects have been linked to certain drugs (e.g., thalidomide) taken during pregnancy. See also *meromelia* and *micromelia.* Cf. *amelia.*

phon/o (fo′no) [Gr. *phōnē* voice] a word element used in combining form to denote sound or voice, e.g., phonoreception, phonocardiogram.

phonation (fo-na′shun) the utterance of vocal sounds. In radiology, laryngograms are often obtained with phonation to demonstrate the function of the soft palate, larynx, and pharynx.

inspiratory p., the production of sounds during inhalation, which demonstrates the laryngeal ventricle. Also called aspirant maneuver and reverse phonation.

normal p., the production of sounds during exhalation, which tests the adduction of the vocal cords. Also called expiratory phonation.

phonendoscope (fōn-en′do-skōp) [*phon-* + Gr. *endon* within + *skopein* to examine] an instrument that functions like a stethoscope to magnify and intensify auscultatory sounds. It may be used to detect normal heart sounds that are the lower limit of unassisted human hearing (S_3 and S_4) or to detect faint abnormal sounds such as murmurs.

-phonia (fo′ne-ah) [Gr. *phōnē* voice + *-ia*] a suffix word element to denote voice or sound, e.g., dysphonia.

phonoangiography (fo″nō-an″je-og′rah-fe) [*phono-* + Gr. *angeion* vessel + *graphein* to write or draw] the recording and analysis of arterial bruits to estimate the extent of arterial stenosis.

phonoauscultation (fo″no-aws″kul-ta′shun) [*phono-* + L. *auscultare* to listen] auscultation in which a tuning fork is placed over the organ to be examined and its vibrations are listened to through a stethoscope placed over the same organ.

phonocardiogram (fo″no-kar′de-o-gram) [*phono-* + Gr. *kardia* heart + *gramma* a mark] the graphic record produced by phonocardiography.

phonocardiograph (fo″no-kar′de-o-graf) [*phono-* + Gr. *kardia* heart + Gr. *graphein* to write or draw] the instrument used in phonocardiography.

phonocardiography (fo″no-kar″de-og′rah-fe) the recording of heart sounds and murmurs using a piezoelectric microphone. The microphone, applied directly to the skin or air-coupled by means of a rubber suction bell, has two advantages over auscultation: it is more sensitive to low-frequency sounds than is the human ear, and the graphic recording produced (phonocardiogram) is useful in the precise timing of cardiac sounds and murmurs, providing a permanent record for comparison with later measurements. The phonocardiogram is normally recorded in conjunction with a carotid pulse tracing and electrocardiogram, and is sometimes also recorded in conjunction with a jugular venous pulse tracing echocardiogram and apexcardiogram. Such a record permits a visualization of the sequence of abnormal events during the cardiac cycle. See also *echophonocardiography.*

phonocatheterization (fo″no-kath″e-ter-ĭ-za′shun) [*phono-* + *catheter* from Gr. *kathetēr,* from *kathienai* to send down] the use of a phonocatheter for the detection of sounds produced by the circulatory system.

phonogram (fo′no-gram) [*phono-* + Gr. *gramma* mark] a graphic record of a sound, as of a heart sound.

phonorenogram (fo″no-re′no-gram) [*phono-* + L. *renes* kidneys + Gr. *gramma* a mark] a graphic representation of the flow of blood through a renal artery. It is produced by recording the sounds of blood pulsation as measured by a phonocatheter introduced into the ureter and passed into the renal pelvis. A phonorenogram may be used to differentiate abnormal kidney function due to occlusion from that caused by narrowing of the renal artery.

-phor, -phore (fōr) [Gr. *phoros* bearing] a suffix word element to denote a carrier of the element designated by the stem to which it is affixed, e.g., melanophore.

phorate (for′āt) a highly toxic, organothiophosphate insecticide, *O,O*-diethyl S-(ethylthio)methyl phosphorodithioate. See also *organophosphate compounds.*

-phoresis (fo-re′sis) [Gr. *phorēsis* transport, a being borne] a suffix word element to denote carrying or transmission, e.g., electrophoresis.

phoria (fo′re-ah) [Gr. *phoros* bearing + *-ia*] a visual disorder characterized by a tendency of the affected eye to deviate from parallel vision with the unaffected eye. It is due to a muscle imbalance and often is apparent only when fusional stimuli are removed. Phoria is considered a form of latent strabismus that is overridden by cortical centers. The disorder, unless extreme, rarely produces symptoms.

-phoria a suffix word element to denote feeling, e.g., euphoria.

Phoridae (for′ĭ-de) a family of flies. Gravid female flies may cause human intestinal myiasis when they deposit their eggs on food.

Phormia (for′me-ah) a genus of blue, black, or green flies (the blackbottle flies) of the family Calliphoridae. *P. regina* (the black blowfly) may cause myiasis in humans.

phosgene (fos′jēn) [Gr. *phos* light + *-genēs* born] carbonyl chloride, $COCl_2$, a highly toxic, colorless or pale yellow gas (b. p., 8.2°C) with a stifling odor; M.W. 98.92. It is used in industrial organic synthesis and has been employed as a war gas. When inhaled, phosgene hydrolyzes and produces hydrochloric acid, which causes pulmonary congestion, edema, and pneumonia.

phosph/o (fos′fo) [N.L., from Gr. *phōsphoros* light-bearing] 1. a word element used in combining form to denote relationship to phosphorus or compounds that contain phosphorus, e.g., phosphine.

2. a word element in organic chemistry used to denote the presence of a phosphate group, e.g., phosphoglyceraldehyde.

phosphagen (fos′fah-jen) see *phosphocreatine.*

phosphatase (fos′fah-tās″) [*phosphate* + *-ase*] any of the phosphoric monoester hydrolases (EC 3.1.3) with broad specificity that catalyze the reaction: organic phosphate + $H_2O \rightleftharpoons$ an alcohol + inorganic phosphate, or the phosphate transfer reaction: organic phosphate + phosphate acceptor $\rightleftharpoons$ alcohol + inorganic phosphate–phosphate acceptor (e.g., AMP buffer). The phosphatases are found in practically all tissues, body fluids, and cells. See also *acid phosphatase* and *alkaline phosphatase.*

phosphate (fos′fāt) any salt or ester of one of three phosphoric acids (ortho-, meta-, and pyro-). Phosphates are distributed throughout the body. Inorganic phosphates occur chiefly in the skeleton, in association with calcium as the orthophosphate and as hydroxyapatite in a crystal structure. They also occur in body fluids, where they play a role as a component of the buffer base, and in cells as metabolic and enzyme substrates. Organic phosphates occur as sugar phosphates, phospholipids, phosphoproteins, nucleotides, and nucleic acids (see *organic phosphate.*)

The inorganic phosphate (P_i) in plasma is largely orthophosphate, with HPO_4^{2-} and $H_2PO_4^-$ present in a ratio of approximately 4:1. All the plasma P_i is diffusible and filterable through the glomerulus. Small quantities of several sugar phosphates are also present in plasma. Reference ranges of P_i in plasma are: for children, 4–7 mg/dl; and for adults, 2.5–4.5 mg/dl; this concentration is regulated homeostatically.

In urine, HPO_4^{2-} can contribute to the excretion of H^+ through the formation of $H_2PO_4^-$. At a urine pH of approximately 4.5, nearly all HPO_4^{2-} is converted to $H_2PO_4^-$.

See also *inorganic phosphate* and *inorganic pyrophosphate.*

acid p., any orthophosphate salt in which only one or two of the three replaceable hydrogen atoms are substituted by a metal ion, e.g., KH_2PO_4, potassium dihydrogen phosphate, and $CaHPO_4$, calcium monohydrogen phosphate.

ammonium magnesium p., a double salt of ammonium and magnesium with orthophosphoric acid, $Mg(NH_4)PO_4 \cdot 6H_2O$. It is encountered as a bladder stone and occasionally as a kidney stone.

calcium p., a compound that contains calcium and the phosphate radical; the fully neutralized salt of calcium and orthophosphoric acid, $Ca_3(PO_4)_2$. It is found as a common component of kidney stones.

carbamyl p., an important intermediate compound in the formation of pyrimidine and citrulline, the latter being a step in the formation of arginine and urea. Also called carbamoyl phosphate.

triple p., a mixed salt of ammonium, calcium, and magnesium with orthophosphoric acid. It occasionally forms renal calculi and is found in the urine.

phosphate group transfer potential a measure of the tendency to transfer a phosphate group from one compound to another. Adenosine triphosphate (ATP) has an intermediate group transfer potential value when compared with other biologically important phosphorylated molecules. Compounds with a higher phosphate transfer potential, e.g., phosphoenolpyruvate, can transfer their phosphate groups to adenosine diphosphate (ADP), converting it to ATP. Similarly, ATP can transfer its phosphate group to compounds such as glucose, converting it to glucose-6-phosphate, which has a lower phosphate transfer potential than ATP. Thus, ATP functions as an efficient carrier of phosphate groups and has a central role in metabolism. The phosphate group transfer potential is measured as $\Delta G^{o\prime}$ values. Compounds with greater negative values transfer their phosphate groups to compounds with less negative values.

phosphate (inorganic) assays see *phosphorus assays.*

phosphatemia (fos″fah-te′me-ah) [*phosphate* + Gr. *haima* blood + *-ia*] an excess of phosphates in the blood. See also *hyperphosphatemia.*

phosphatidalcholine (fas″fah-ti″dal-ko′lēn) a plasmalogen as well as a compound homologous to phosphatidylcholine in which position one of glycerol is linked to an aldehyde moiety in a vinyl ether linkage. Upon complete hydrolysis, higher fatty aldehydes as well as fatty acids are released. This phospholipid is present in blood platelets.

phosphatidalethanolamine (fos″fah-ti″dal-eth″-ah-nol-am′ēn) a plasmalogen with structural similarity to phosphatidylethanolamine, in which position one of glycerol is linked to a fatty aldehyde moiety in a vinyl ether linkage. Upon complete hydrolysis, equimolar amounts of higher fatty aldehydes, higher fatty acids, glycerol, phosphoric acid, and ethanolamine are released. This phospholipid is present in blood platelets.

phosphatidate (fos″fah-ti′dāt) a salt or anion form of 1,2-difatty acyl-glycerol-3-phosphoric acid. See also *phosphatidic acid.*

phosphatidic acid (fos″fah-tid′ik) a glycerophosphatide; a 1,2-difatty acyl-glycerol-3-phosphoric acid.

phosphatidylcholine (PC) (fos″fah-ti″dil-ko′lēn) any of a group of phospholipids consisting of esters of glycerol with two molecules of long-chain aliphatic acids on carbons 1 and 2, phosphoric acid ion carbon 3, the latter being esterified with the alcohol group of choline. Phosphatidylcholines are found in animal tissues, especially in nerve tissue, the liver, semen, and egg yolk, and in smaller amounts in bile and blood. They differ from each other in the nature of their long-chain acyl groups. Also called *lecithin.*

phosphatidylcholine-cholesterol acyltransferase (fos″fah-ti″dil-ko′lēn ko-les′ter-ol as″il-trans′-fer-ās) see *lecithin-cholesterol acyltransferase.*

phosphatidylethanolamine (PE) (fos″fah-ti″dil-eth″ah-nol-am′ēn) 1. a monoamino-monophosphatide, a glycerophosphatide composed of 1,2-difatty acyl-glycerol-3-phosphate esterified to ethanolamine, that exists in brain, nerve, and other tissues, and in egg yolk.

2. one of the prothromboplastic phosphatides contained in blood platelets. See also *cephalin.*

phosphatidylglycerol (PG) (fos″fah-ti″dil-glis′er-ol) a phospholipid whose presence in amniotic fluid appears to correlate well with fetal lung maturity. PG is the second most abundant pulmonary surfactant, and its measurement enhances the reliability of the lecithin-sphingomyelin (L/S) ratio in predicting hyaline membrane disease, especially in complicated pregnancies and in amniotic fluid contaminated with blood. See also *lecithin-sphingomyelin ratio.*

phosphatidylinositide (fos″fah-ti″dil-in-o′sĭ-tīd) any of a group of compounds containing phosphatidylinositol, as well as its derivatives, which have either one or two additional phosphate residues esterified to the inositol. Also called phosphoinositide.

phosphatidylinositol (PI) (fos″fah-ti″dil-in-o′sĭ-tol) a phosphatidic acid esterified at the phosphate residue with inositol.

phosphatidylserine (PS) (fos″fah-ti″dil-se′rīn) a glycerophosphatide homologous in structure to phosphatidylethanolamine, one of the components of the prothromboplastic phosphatides in blood platelets. It is one of the components of the crude phospholipid fraction cephalin, and can be converted directly to phosphatidylethanolamine by the enzyme phosphatidylserine decarboxylase. See also *cephalin.*

phosphaturia (fos″fah-tu′re-ah) [*phosphate* + Gr. *ouron* urine + *-ia*] an excess of phosphates in the urine. See also *hyperphosphaturia.*

phosphine (fos′fēn) 1. hydrogen phosphide, PH_3, a highly toxic and flammable gas with the odor of decaying fish; M.W. 34.00. It is produced by the reaction of water with metallic phosphides such as zinc phosphide, a rat poison. Inhalation of phosphine or ingestion of phosphides causes severe gastrointestinal irritation and can result in severe bronchitis and fatal pulmonary edema.

2. an alternate name for chrysaniline yellow, a fat-soluble dye used as a fluorescent stain and in fluorochrome Schiff reagent.

phosphoadenosine diphosphosulfate (PAPS) (fos″fo-ah-den′o-sēn di-fos″fo-sul′fāt) see *3′-phosphoadenosine-5′-phosphosulfate.*

3′-phosphoadenosine-5′-phosphosulfate (PAPS) (fos″fo-ah-den′o-sēn fos″fo-sul′fāt) an important activated sulfate molecule used for formation of sulfate esters of alcohols, phenols, polysaccharides, and some lipids in most living forms, including mammals. It is a high-energy sulfate compound having a mixed anhydride of sulfuric and phosphoric acids esterified with a phosphoadenosine group. Also called *phosphoadenosine diphosphosulfate.*

phosphocholine (fos″fo-ko′lin) an ester of phosphoric acid with choline, $(CH_3)_3N^+(CH_2)_2OPO_3^{2-}$, which serves as an intermediate in the synthesis of phosphatidylcholine and sphingomyelin.

phosphocreatine (fos″fo-kre′ah-tēn) a creatine phosphamic acid compound, $(OH)_2PO{\cdot}NH{\cdot}C(:NH){\cdot}N{-}(CH_3){\cdot}CH_2{\cdot}COOH$, which can provide energy in muscles and nerves, liberating creatine and inorganic phosphate in the process. It can react reversibly with adenosine diphosphate (ADP) to form adenosine triphosphate (ATP) and creatine catalyzed by creatine kinase. Phosphocreatine degrades slowly in vivo to produce an excreted metabolite (creatinine) and inorganic phosphate. It serves as a store of available high-energy phosphate in muscle. Also called *phosphagen.* See also *creatine kinase.*

phosphodiesterase (fos″fo-di-es′ter-ās) any enzyme of the sub-subclass of hydrolases (EC 3.1.4) that catalyzes the hydrolysis of one of the two ester linkages of a phosphodiester, a compound ($R{-}O{-}PO_2^-{-}O{-}R'$) in which the phosphate group is joined to two alkyl residues.

phosphoenolpyruvate (PEP) (fos″fo-e″nol-pi′roo-vāt) an intermediary metabolite, $CH_2{=}C(OPO_3^{2-})COO^-$, important in the reactions of glycolysis, gluconeogenesis, and the glyoxylate pathway.

phosphoethanolamine (fos″fo-eth″ah-nol-ah′mēn) an ester of phosphoric acid with ethanolamine, $^{2-}O_3PO{\cdot}(CH_2)_2{\cdot}NH_2$, which serves as an intermediate in the synthesis of phosphatidylethanolamine.

6-phosphofructokinase (fos″fo-fruk″to-ki′nās) an enzyme of the transferase class (ATP:D-fructose-6-phosphate-1-phosphotransferase, EC 2.7.1.11) that catalyzes the reaction D-fructose-6-phosphate + ATP → D-fructose-1,6-bisphosphate + ADP. The reaction is essentially irreversible. The enzyme is a key step in the Embden-Meyerhof pathway of glucose metabolism and in the regulation of carbohydrate metabolism. A genetic deficiency of the muscle enzyme, transmitted as an autosomal recessive trait, is found in glycogen storage disease type VII. Also called *phosphohexokinase.*

phosphofructokinase deficiency a hereditary disorder, transmitted as an autosomal recessive trait, that is characterized by abnormal glycogen metabolism and deposition in the skeletal muscle. The disease is due to an absolute or relative deficiency of the enzyme phosphofructokinase. Symptoms, which include muscle pain, contracture, weakness after exercise without a rise in blood lactate, and myoglobinuria, result from a block of glycolysis in muscle due to the enzyme deficiency; they first appear in early childhood and become slowly progressive. Diagnosis is based on the determination of specific enzyme activity in a sample of striated muscle obtained by biopsy. Also called glycogen storage disease type VII (Cori type VII). See also *6-phosphofructokinase.*

phosphoglucomutase (fos″fo-gloo″ko-mu′tās) an enzyme of the transferase class (α-Dglucose-1,6-bisphosphate:α-D-glucose-1-phosphate phosphotransferase, EC 2.7.5.1) that catalyzes the apparent intramolecular reversible transfer of a phosphate group from carbon 1 to carbon 6 of glucose; the actual reaction is α-D-glucose-1,6-bisphosphate + α-D-glucose-1-phosphate ⇄ α-D-glucose-6-phosphate + α-D-glucose-1,6-bisphosphate.

6-phospho-D-gluconate (fos″fo gloo′ko-nāt) a phosphate ester of a sugar acid, $^{2-}O_3PO{\cdot}CH_2{\cdot}(CHOH)_4COO^-$, which is an intermediate of the pentose phosphate pathway of the metabolism of glucose.

phosphogluconate dehydrogenase (decarboxylating) (PGD, 6-PGD) an enzyme of the oxidoreductase class (6-phospho-D-gluconate:$NADP^+$ 2-oxidoreductase [decarboxylating], EC 1.1.1.44). It catalyzes the reaction 6-phospho-D-gluconate + $NADP^+$ ⇄ D-ribulose-5-phosphate + CO_2 + NADPH, a step in the pentose phosphate shunt of glucose metabolism. Elevated serum levels have been reported in individuals with hepatic disease.

6-phosphogluconate dehydrogenase assays see under *glucose-6-phosphate dehydrogenase assays.*

phosphogluconate oxidative pathway see *pentose phosphate pathway.*

6-phosphogluconic acid (fos″fo-gloo-con′ik) the phosphate ester, $HOOC{\cdot}(CHOH)_4{\cdot}CH_2{\cdot}O{\cdot}PO_3^{2-}$, of a sugar acid; an intermediate in the pentose phosphate pathway of the metabolism of glucose.

6-phospho-D-gluconolactone (fos″fo-gloo″ko′no-lak″tōn) an intermediate formed by oxidation of carbon 1 of glucose-6-phosphate to a carbonyl group, which occurs in the pentose phosphate pathway of the metabolism of glucose.

3-phosphoglyceraldehyde (fos″fo-glis″er-al′dĕ-hīd) see *glyceraldehyde-3-phosphate.*

2-phospho-D-glycerate (fos″fo-glis′er-āt) a phosphorylated intermediate, $CH_2OH \cdot CHOPO_3^{2-} \cdot COO^-$. It exists in the glycolytic pathway of the metabolism of glucose and in the gluconeogenic pathway.

3-phospho-D-glycerate a phosphorylated intermediate, $CH_2OPO_3^{2-} \cdot CHOH \cdot COO^-$. It exists in glycolytic and gluconeogenic pathways of glucose and in the pathway of synthesis of serine from glucose.

phosphoglycerate kinase (PGK) (fos″fo-glis′er-āt ki′nās) an enzyme of the transferase class (EC 2.7.2.3) that catalyzes the reaction ATP + 3-phospho-D-glycerate ⇄ ADP + 3-phospho-D-glyceroyl phosphate. The reaction is an important energy-yielding step in the Embden-Meyerhof scheme of carbohydrate metabolism. A genetic deficiency of the enzyme in erythrocytes, transmitted as an X-linked trait, is associated with some types of hemolytic anemia.

phosphoglycerides (fos″fo-glis′er-īdz) a group of glycerol-containing lipids, including all the phosphatidyl- compounds, that are derivatives of L-glycerol-3-phosphate.

phosphoglyceromutase (fos″fo-glis″er-o-mu′tās) an enzyme of the transferase class (2,3-bisphospho-D-glycerate: 2-phospho-D-glycerate phosphotransferase, EC 2.7.5.3) that catalyzes the reaction 2-phospho-D-glycerate + 2,3-bisphospho-D-glycerate ⇄ 3-phospho-D-glycerate + 2,3-bisphospho-D-glycerate. The reaction is an important step in the Embden-Meyerhof scheme of glycolysis.

phosphoguanidine (fos″fo-gwan′ĭ-dēn) any of a group of phosphorylated derivatives of guanidine compounds that occur in tissue and serve as a store of high-energy phosphate. Compounds found in various phyla are phosphocreatine (in vertebrates), phosphoarginine (in invertebrates), and the less common forms of phosphotaurocyamine and phospholombricine (found in annelids).

phosphohexoisomerase (fos″fo-hek″so-i-som′er-ās) see *glucosephosphate isomerase.*

phosphohexokinase (fos″fo-hek″so-ki′nās) see *6-phosphofructokinase.*

phospholipase (fos″fo-lip′ās) any one of several enzymes that catalyzes the hydrolysis of a specific bond of a phospholipid, such as lecithin or lysolecithin, with the release of a free fatty acid anion and glycerophosphocholine, diacylglycerol, or phosphorylcholine.

p. A_2, an enzyme of the hydrolase class phosphatide 2-acylhydrolase (EC 3.1.1.4) that catalyzes the reaction lecithin + H_2O ⇄ 1-acylglycerophosphocholine + an unsaturated fatty acid anion. It is secreted by the pancreas as a proenzyme. After activation it acts to release free fatty acids from dietary phospholipids. Also called *lecithinase A.*

p. B, see *lysophospholipase.*

p. C, an enzyme of the hydrolase class (EC 3.1.4.3) that catalyzes the reaction phosphatidylcholine + H_2O ⇄ 1,2-diacylglycerol + choline phosphate. The enzyme, found in the bacterial species *Clostridium perfringens,* is known as alpha-toxin; the same or similar exotoxins are found in other strains of *Clostridium.* Also called *lecithinase C.*

phospholipid (fos″fo-lip′id) [*phospho-* + Gr. *lipos* fat] a lipid that contains phosphorus; one of a group of compounds that includes phosphatidates, phosphatidyl compounds (lecithin), phosphatidyl glycerol, cardiolipins, phosphatidal compounds (plasmalogens), and sphingomyelins.

Reference ranges for phospholipid in serum are: for newborns, 30–90 mg/dl; for males <60 yr, 175–275; for nonpregnant females, 160–230; for females in early pregnancy, 205–290; and for males and females aged 60–88 yr. 195–365.

phospholipid assays the determination of phospholipids in serum. The oxidative digestion of the purified lipid extract is followed by measurement of the inorganic phosphorus liberated. Oxidizing agents used include hot concentrated sulfuric acid in conjunction with hydrogen peroxide, nitric acid, or perchloric acid. Virtually all procedures depend on the formation of the phosphomolybdate ion, which is then reduced by a suitable reagent to the complex "heteropoly blue," a colloidal dispersion of unknown composition.

phospholipid staining a staining technique to localize phospholipids in tissue. The McManus method involves staining sections in a saturated solution of Sudan black B in 70 percent ethanol followed by counterstaining in 1 percent aqueous neutral red. Phospholipids stain blue-black to brownish-black; nuclei stain red. The Baker acid hematein method requires fixation in calcium-formalin and chromation with potassium dichromate. Sections are stained with acid hematein and differentiated with borax-ferricyanide solution.

Phospholipids stain dark blue to blue-black; their presence cannot be confirmed by this technique unless paired sections are negative following extraction of the phospholipids with pyridine. Tissue must be fixed in a solution that prevents extraction of the lipid during subsequent processing; acrolein and osmium tetroxide preserve phospholipids, as does fixation in calcium-formalin or chromation with potassium dichromate during or after fixation.

phospholipid vesicle a type of liposome.

5-phosphomevalonic acid (fos″fo-mev″a-lon′ik) an intermediate in the biosynthesis of cholesterol from acetyl CoA, $HOOC \cdot CH_2 \cdot C(CH_3)OH \cdot (CH_2)_2OPO_3^{2-}$.

phosphomolybdic acid (fos″fo-mo-lib′dik) a bright yellow crystalline solid, with suggested formula $24 MoO_3 \cdot 2H_3PO_4 \cdot xH_2O$, which behaves as a strong oxidizing agent in aqueous solution. Phosphomolybdic acid is used as a protein precipitant and color reagent. Many substances (e.g., alkaloids, xanthine, and uric acid) reduce phosphomolybdic acid to molybdenum blue, a phospho-12-molybdate complex, which is measured by its absorbance in the red or infrared wavelengths (670–850 nm).

In histology, it is used as a mordant, forming lakes with several basic dyes, e.g., hematoxylin, and reacting with any amino groups in acid dyes, such as aniline blue and light green SF.

phosphomonoesterase (fos″fo-mon″o-es′ter-ās) see *phosphoric monoester hydrolase.*

phosphonoacetic acid (fos″fo-no-ah-se′tik) an antiviral agent that affects the replication of viral nucleic acids as an inhibitor of viral coded DNA polymerase. See also *antiviral agent.*

4′-phosphopantetheine (fos″fo-pan-tě-the′in) 1. that portion of the coenzyme A (CoA) molecule linked through its phosphate to a serine residue of protein in the fatty acid synthase complex or to an acyl carrier protein. It is composed of residues of (β-mercaptoethylamine)-(β-alanine)-(D-pantoic acid)-(phosphoric acid).

2. an intermediate in the biosynthesis of CoA from pantothenic acid.

phosphoprotein (fos″fo-pro′tēn) [*phospho-* + *protein*] a protein that has been modified by the conversion of at least one hydroxyl group (e.g., in a serine or threonine residue) to a phosphate ester or of an amino group (e.g., in an arginine, lysine, or histidine residue) to a phosphate amide. This mechanism is involved in activating or deactivating some enzymes. See also *sulfoprotein.*

phosphopyridoxal (fos″fo-pi″rĭ-dok′s'l) see *pyridoxal-5′-phosphate.*

phosphor (fos′for) [Gr *phōs* light + *phoros* bearing, from *pherein* to bear] a material that emits light after absorbing radiant energy, particularly one that emits the light after a short delay (a microsecond or longer), e.g., the material on the screen of a cathode-ray tube that emits light when struck by the electron beam.

phosphorescence (for″fo-res′ens) the emission of light without appreciable heat; the property of continuing to be luminous in the dark after exposure to light or other radiation.

phosphorescent (fos″fo-res′ent) pertaining to or exhibiting phosphorescence.

5-phosphoribosyl-1-amine (fos″fo-ri′bo-sil ah-mēn′) a derivative of ribose, with the carbon 1 hydroxyl replaced with an amino group and the phosphate esterified to the carbon 5 hydroxyl. Formation of this compound is the committed metabolic step in purine biosynthesis and is subject to feedback inhibition by purine nucleotides.

α-5-phosphoribosyl-1-pyrophosphate (fos″fo-ri′bo-sil pi″ro-fos′fāt) a biosynthetic intermediate formed from ribose-5-phosphate by having a pyrophosphate group esterified to the carbon 1 hydroxyl group. This compound is essential to the biosynthesis of both purine and pyrimidine nucleotides and in salvaging the preformed purines and pyrimidines.

phosphoric acid (fos-for′ik) a strong, corrosive, tribasic inorganic acid, H_3PO_4; M.W. 98.00. The pure acid is a crystalline solid (m. p., 42°C). Commercial phosphoric acid is usually prepared as a syrupy solution, 85 percent in water. When it is heated, a polymer (polyphosphoric acid, $H(HPO_3)_nOH$) forms. The dimer, $H_4P_2O_7$, is called pyrophosphoric acid; the longer polymers, metaphosphoric acid. The monomer is sometimes called orthophosphoric acid.

phosphoric monoester hydrolase one of a sub-subgroup (EC 3.1.3) of enzymes of the hydrolase class, composed of those that catalyze the hydrolysis of orthophosphoryl esters of alcohol (R—O—P). Examples are the clinically important acid and alkaline phosphatases. Also called *orthophosphoric ester monohydrolase* and *phosphomonoesterase.*

phosphorus (P) (fos′fŏ-rus) [L., from Gr. *Phosphoros* the morning star, from *phōs* light + *phoros* bearing] a nonmetallic element; atomic number 15; atomic weight 30.9738; Group V of the periodic table; oxidation states –3, +3, +5. It has three allotropic forms; white (also called yellow), red, and black phosphorus.

Phosphorus is an essential mineral nutrient; the recommended daily allowance is 1200 mg/da for adolescents and pregnant and lactating females, and 800 mg/da for most other individuals. It occurs as inorganic phosphate, primarily in bones and teeth. It also occurs as organic phosphate, primarily as the high-energy phosphates adenosine tri- and diphosphate (ATP and ADP) in muscle and neural tissue, and in many other high-energy compounds and in nucleic acids. Reference ranges for inorganic phosphate–phosphorus (P_i) in serum are: for adults, 2.9–4.6 mg/dl (1.0–1.5 mmol/l); and for children, 4.0–7.2 (1.3.–2.3), although the values vary somewhat, depending on the growth phase.

White phosphorus is a waxy, crystalline solid that ignites spontaneously in air at 86°F. It slowly oxidizes, accompanied by phosphorescence at lower temperatures or when moist. It is extremely toxic. Chronic poisoning of industrial workers due to inhalation of white phosphorus causes "phossy jaw," a painful and disfiguring necrosis of the jawbone. Acute poisoning (as from ingesting phosphorus rat poison) causes severe gastrointestinal irritation and hemorrhage, and may cause death from cardiovascular collapse or fatty necrosis of the liver. An ingested dose of 50 mg is usually fatal. Skin contact can cause severe chemical burns.

Phosphorus is used in the manufacture of phosphoric acid, bronze alloys, semiconductors, and incendiary materials. Red phosphorus is a red-violet amorphous or crystalline solid that is more stable than white phosphorus and much less toxic, ignitable only by high temperature or strong oxidizing agents; it is used in safety matches. Black phosphorus is a crystalline or amorphous solid similar to graphite.

phosphorus-32 (^{32}P, P 32) a reactor-produced radionuclide with a half-life of 14.3 da. It is a pure beta emitter of particles with a maximal energy of 1.7 MeV, which corresponds to a range in tissue of about 7 mm. See also *sodium phosphate P 32.*

phosphorus assays 1. the determination of inorganic phosphate (P_i, orthophosphate) in serum or urine. Most of the methods are based on the formation of the yellow-green heteropoly compound, ammonium phosphomolybdate (ammonium 12-molybdophosphate; $(NH_4)_3[PO_4(MoO_3)_{12}]$) by reaction with ammonium molybdate under suitable conditions. This compound is reduced to molybdenum blue (structure and Mo valence not yet elucidated) by any one of a variety of reducing agents; stannous chloride, ferrous sulfate, hydroquinone, ascorbic acid, *p*-methylaminophenol, *N*-phenyl-*p*-phenylenediamine, *p*-aminonaphtholsulfonic acid. The resulting blue color is measured at some red (or preferably infrared) wavelength. Extraction of the blue color into an organic solvent can increase the sensitivity (usual is 0.5 μg/cuvet). Alternate procedures use vanadate (yellow color) in place of the molybdate and read the unreduced 12-molybdophosphate at 310 nm.

Decreased concentrations of P_i in serum are seen in primary hyperparathyroidism, in vitamin D deficiency, and in severe intestinal malabsorption and steatorrhea. Increased concentrations in serum are encountered in renal disease (especially renal failure), in hypervitaminosis D, and often in hypoparathyroidism. An increased urinary output of phosphorus is observed in hyperparathyroidism.

2. measurement of phosphorus in suspected phosphorus poisoning by yellow phosphorus or phosphide. A specimen of tissue or organ contents is acidified, distilled under nitrogen gas, and the phos-

phorus or phosphine (PH_3) is trapped on filter paper impregnated with silver nitrate, giving a brownish-gray stain. The latter is then oxidized to phosphate by chlorine. The phosphate is determined colorimetrically as in the first method by reaction with ammonium molybdate and a reducing agent.

phosphorylase (fos-fŏr′ĭ-lās) an enzyme of the transferase class (1,4-α-D-glucan:orthophosphate α-D-glucosyltransferase, EC 2.4.1.1) that catalyzes the reaction (1,4-α-D-glucosyl)$_n$ + orthophosphate ⇄ 1,4-α-D-glucosyl)$_{n-1}$ + α-D-glucose 1-phosphate. The reaction degrades various glucose polymers by phosphorylation of the terminal unit. The name is qualified in each instance by adding the name of the natural substrate (e.g., maltodextrin phosphorylase, starch phosphorylase, glycogen phosphorylase). See also *glycogen phosphorylase.*

phosphorylase deficiency a term referring either to glycogen storage disease type V (see *McArdle's disease*) or to glycogen storage disease type VI (see *Hers' disease*).

phosphorylase kinase (fos-for′ĭ-lās ki′nās) an enzyme of the transferase class (EC 2.7.1.38) that catalyzes the reaction ATP + phosphorylase b (inactive) ⇄ ADP + phosphorylase a (active). The enzyme catalyzes the activation of glycogen phosphorylase, which then catalyzes the mobilization of glycogen, and is important in the regulation of glycogen metabolism. A genetic defect, transmitted as an X-linked recessive trait, is probably present in glycogen storage disease type VIII.

phosphorylation (fos″for-ĭ-la′shun) the introduction of a phosphate group into a molecule, e.g., the phosphorylation of adenosine diphosphate (ADP) to form adenosine triphosphate (ATP). See also *oxidative phosphorylation.*

3-phosphoserine (fos″fo-ser′ēn) a serine molecule with phosphate esterified to the hydroxyl group at carbon 3; it is an intermediate in the synthesis of serine from glucose. These residues are found in histones, caseins, and other proteins. The activity of some enzymes is regulated by phosphorylations or dephosphorylations (e.g., enzymes of glycogen synthesis and breakdown of these residues).

phosphotransferase (fos″fo-trans′fer-ās) any one of a large subclass of enzymes of the transferase class (EC 2.7.1–5) consisting of those that catalyze the transfer of a phosphate group. Adenosine triphosphate is the most common donor of the phosphate group, but other donors exist. Examples of phosphotransferases are hexokinase, myokinase, and phosphoglyceromutase.

phosphotungstic acid (fos″fo-tung′stik) a yellowish-white solid, $24WO_3 \cdot 2H_3PO_4 \cdot 48H_2O$ (the water content varies), which is a strong oxidizing agent in aqueous solution. It is used as a protein precipitant and color reagent. Many substances, e.g., uric acid, alkaloids, nitrogen bases, and amino acids, reduce phosphotungstic acid to tungsten blue, a phosphotungstite complex, which is measured by its absorbance at 710 nm.

In histology, it is used as a mordant; forming lakes with several basic dyes such as hematoxylin.

phosphotungstic acid hematoxylin (PTAH) a stain used particularly for the nervous system and to demonstrate mitochondria and muscle striations. Nuclei, centrioles, mitotic spindles, mitochondria, neuroglial fibrils, and myofibrils in striated muscle stain blue with PTAH; bone, cartilage, collagen, and elastin stain yellow-orange to brownish red.

Sections are fixed or postmordanted in Zenker's fluid, the mercury deposits are removed with alcoholic iodine, and Mallory bleach is added; the sections are oxidized in a solution of potassium permanganate and bleached with a solution of oxalic acid. They are then stained overnight in PTAH (1 g of hematoxylin and 20 g of phosphotungstic acid per liter of distilled water).

phot/o- (fo′to) [Gr. *phōs, phōtos* light] a word element used in combining form to denote light, e.g., photosynthesis.

phot (fōt, fot) a unit of illuminance (luminous flux density) equal to 1 lumen per square centimeter or 10,000 lux (10^4 lx).

photalgia (fo-tal′je-ah) [*phot-* + Gr. *algos* pain + *-ia*] a general term used to describe a painful sensation in the eye following exposure to light. See also *photophobia.*

photic (fo′tik) pertaining to light.

photic driving in electroencephalography, the rhythmic electrical activity recorded from the occipital region of the head in response to repetitive photic stimulation at up to about 30 Hz when this activity is time-locked to the stimulus and is of an identical or harmonically related frequency. Also called *driving response.* Cf. *visual e. p.* under *evoked potential.*

photic stimulation in electroencephalography, the delivery of flashes of light to the eyes. A stroboscope is used to produce intermittent flashes at rates of up to 30 flashes/sec while the electroencephalogram (EEG) is recorded for 5 sec over the occipital and parietal regions of the head. The procedure is undertaken while the patient lies quietly with the eyes closed and is then repeated with the eyes open.

In normal subjects, EEG activity of identical or harmonically related frequency to that of the light flashes is produced. The amplitude of the activity may be greater over the nondominant hemisphere. In normal children, paroxysmal activity can sometimes be provoked. Spike discharges originating in muscles and associated with fluttering of the eyelids can sometimes be recorded over the scalp following the light flashes in normal subjects.

Photic stimulation is one of the activation procedures used in patients with suspected epilepsy, as it may provoke epileptiform activity characterized by slow-wave and spike or polyspike activity having a frequency unrelated to that of the light flashes. Such activity is usually generalized, is bilaterally symmetric and bisynchronous, outlasts the stimulus, and is potentiated by hypoglycemia. Red light has been found to be more effective than blue-white light in inducing such abnormal responses. Speech arrest, transient absence, or deviation of the eyes may accompanay the EEG changes, and if photic stimulation is continued, a convulsion may eventually occur.

See also *photomyogenic response* and *photoparoxysmal response.*

photoallergic (fo″to-al-ler′jik) pertaining to or characterized by heightened delayed sensitivity to contact with light.

photoallergy (fo″to-al′er-je) [*photo-* + allergy] an acquired immune response that occurs following drug treatment and exposure to light. The absorbed light catalyzes a biochemical reaction that results in the binding of the drug (hapten) to body proteins and produces a conjugate with antigenic properties capable of eliciting an immune response. Long-wavelength light (320–400 nm) of low intensity is implicated in association with a variety of drugs, including sulfonamides, quinethazone, griseofulvin, and triacetyldiphenolisatin. Photoallergic reactions may lead to urticarial, eczematous, or papular lesions in the presence of edema or vasodilation. Cf. *phototoxicity.*

photoautotroph (fo″to-aw′to-trōf) [*photo-* + Gr. *autos* self + *trophos* feeder, from *trephein* to nourish] an autotrophic organism that can derive the energy it needs from the absorption of visible light. Such organisms include plants, algae, and a few bacteria. Also called *photolithotroph.* See also *autotroph* and *chemoautotroph.*

photoautotrophic (fo″to-aw″to-trōf′ik) pertaining to photoautotrophs.

photocatalysis (fo″to-kah-tal′ĭ-sis) an increase in the rate of a chemical reaction produced by irradiating the reactants with light (electromagnetic radiation).

photocatalyst (fo″to-kat′ah-list) a substance, e.g., chlorophyll, necessary for the occurrence of a photocatalytic process.

photocell (fo″to-sel′) any solid-state device used for measuring light or for producing electricity from light.

A photovoltaic cell produces a current in response to light. It consists of a layer of a semiconductor (such as silicon) backed by a layer of metal. Light falling on the semiconductor causes electrons to flow to the metal. This type of photocell is used in some photometers and colorimeters. Because their response is slow, photocells are not used in instruments that use chopped light beams. The output is very temperature-dependent, so photocells must be insulated from the heat produced by the lamp or burner. Also called *barrier layer cell* and solar cell.

A photoconductive cell changes its resistance in response to light. Some photovoltaic cells also exhibit this resistance change. Both photovoltaic cells and photoresistors are normally used in double-beam configurations to compensate for drift due to temperature change and for fluctuations in the light source. Also called *photoresistor.* See also *photodiode* and phototransistor.

photochemical (fo″to-kem′ĭ-kal) pertaining to the chemical properties of light; chemically reactive in the presence of light or other radiation.

photochemical reaction a chemical reaction in which energy is supplied by light (electromagnetic radiation), as in photography, photosynthesis, and vision. Also called *photoreaction.*

photochemical smog a type of air pollution produced by the effect of sunlight on hydrocarbons, oxides of nitrogen, and atmospheric oxygen. It appears as a brown haze and is highly irritating to the eyes and respiratory tract; it also damages rubber, fabrics, and vegetation.

Nitric oxide (NO) is produced from atmospheric oxygen and nitrogen by high-temperature combustion in air, as occurs in automobiles and power plants. NO reacts with oxygen (O_2) to form nitrogen dioxide (NO_2). NO_2 is broken down by sunlight to NO and atomic oxygen (O), which then combines with molecular oxygen (O_2) to form ozone (O_3). The reaction $O_3 + NO \rightarrow NO_2 + O_2$ closes the cycle. Ozone and oxygen atoms react with hydrocarbons produced by incomplete combustion to form radicals and aldehydes. These products react further to produce a complex mixture that includes some of the major irritants in smog, aldehydes, ozone, and peroxyacylnitrates (PAN).

See also *peroxyacylnitrate.*

photochemistry (fo″to-kem′is-tre) the study of the chemical and physical changes produced by the absorption or emission of light.

photochemotherapy (fo″to-ke″mo-ther′ah-pe) the treatment of disease by exposure to non-ionizing electromagnetic radiation (ultraviolet or visible light) in combination with the administration of a systemic, photoreactive agent. UV-A radiation (320–400 nm) is used in combination with oral psoralen in the treatment of psoriasis, vitiligo, eczema, and mycosis fungoides. On photoactivation, psoralen forms cross-links with the strands of DNA, leading to the inhibition of DNA synthesis and cell death. Methoxsalen also is now used as a photoactive agent.

Photochemotherapy usually requires numerous treatments over long periods and has been linked to the formation of skin cancer; cataracts; and premature, irreversible aging of blood vessels, connective tissue, and keratinocytes. However, when this form of therapy for psoriasis and vitiligo is compared with alternate forms of therapy, there appears to be an acceptable risk-to-benefit ratio. Cf. *phototherapy.*

photochromogen (fo″to-kro′mo-jen) [*photo-* + Gr. *chrōma* color + *gennan* to produce] a microorganism producing colonies that develop color when exposed to light. See also *Mycobacterium.*

photochromogenicity (fo″to-kro″mo-je-nis′ĭ-te) the propensity of microorganisms to form pigment consequent to light exposure; induction occurs within a few minutes in the shorter wavelengths of visible light, pigmentation takes place within 24 hr if conditions permit continued growth. For example, *Mycobacterium kansasii* becomes yellow 6–12 hr after an hour of exposure to bright light.

photocoagulation (fo″to-ko-ag″u-la′shun) the use of high-intensity light sources to condense proteins or to coagulate moving columns of blood. This technique is most frequently employed in the treatment of diabetic retinopathy. Three types of light sources are widely used. The xenon arc uses a white light that preferentially affects the pigmented epithelium. It is effective in destroying new blood vessels that appear at the surface and within the retina, but tends to produce large lesions (>500 μm in diameter). The ruby laser uses a monochromatic red light and produces smaller lesions than the xenon arc. Argon lasers use a green light that specifically affects hemoglobin, leading to coagulation. Argon laser photocoagulation produces small lesions of about 50 μm and is especially valuable in destroying new vessels that extend into the retrovitreal space.

These therapeutic techniques are particularly valuable in reducing the progressive loss of vision due to retinopathy. Indications for their use include moderate or severe growth of new vessels in the region of the optic disk, mild growth of new vessels in the area of the optic disk if fresh bleeding is present, or moderate to severe growth of new vessels elsewhere in the eye if fresh bleeding is present. Photocoagulation should be considered in all patients with early signs of proliferative disease and ocular complications due to diabetes. This form of therapy also may be of value in certain cases of minimal retinal detachment, by sealing small retinal tears before widespread detachment occurs.

Deleterious side-effects include vitreal bleeding and contraction, macular edema, retinal detachment, and visual field losses. In rare cases, there may be inflammation of the iris.

photoconductive cell (fo″to-kon-duk′tiv) see under *photocell.*

photoconvulsive response (fo″to-kon-vul′siv) see *photoparoxysmal response.*

photodecomposition (fo″to-de″kom-po-zish′un) the breakdown of a chemical compound induced by absorption of light. See also *phototherapy.*

photodermatitis (fo″to-der″mah-ti′tis) [*photo-* + Gr. *derma* skin + *-itis* inflammation] an acute or chronic inflammation of the skin in which light, especially sunlight, plays a causative role. Such skin reaction may be due to overexposure to sunlight, drug-induced photosensitization of the skin, or hypersensitivity to sunlight because of genetic or metabolic abnormalities (such as porphyria, phenylketonuria, and xeroderma pigmentosum). The cutaneous inflammation may be accompanied by pain, fever, and gastrointestinal disorders. Redness, swelling, vesicle formation, exfoliation, and pigmentary changes in the skin are also seen. Also called actinic dermatitis, erythema solare, polymorphous light sensitivity, and *sunburn.*

photodetector (fo″to-de-tek′tor) any device used to measure or indicate the presence of light, e.g., a photocell.

photodiode (fo″to-di′ōd) a semiconductor diode in which light focused on the *p-n* junction causes a reverse current. Photodiodes are used as detectors in some flame photometers and in computer card readers.

photodissociation (fo″to-dis-so″she-a′shun) [*photo-* + L. *dissociare* to separate] the separation of a molecule into mono- or polyatomic fragment(s) following the absorption of a photon.

photodynamic (fo″to-di-nam′ik) [*photo-* + Gr. *dynamis* power] pertaining to a fluorescent dye (e.g., methylene blue, rose bengal, eosin) that, when activated by visible light, can oxidize proteins, lyse red blood cells, kill bacteria, and inactivate viruses.

photoelectric (fo″to-e-lek′trik) pertaining to the electric effects of light or other radiation.

photoelectric effect the ejection of electrons from a surface by incident light. The number of photoelectrons emitted is proportional to the number of incident photons. The energy of the photoelectron is the difference between the photon energy and the work function of the material (the bonding energy of the electron). Photons with less energy (having longer wavelengths) than the work function cannot produce photoelectrons.

photoelectron (fo″to-e-lek′tron) an electron produced by the photoelectric effect.

photofluorography (fo″to-floo″or-og′rah-fe) a technique that utilizes the recording of fluoroscopic images on photographic film. Also called abreuography, fluorography, fluoroentgenography.

photographic effect (PE) (fo″to-graf′ik) the response of photographic film to light or x-rays. In radiography, film blackening (radiographic density) is proportional to the product of the millamperage, exposure time, and square of the kilovoltage, divided by the square of the focal-film distance.

photography (fo-tog′rah-fe) [*photo-* + Gr. *graphein* to record] the process of making images on a film coated with an emulsion of silver halide crystals, which are activated on exposure to light. The film is then developed, a process in which the film is placed in a weak reducing agent, which reduces activated crystals to black metallic silver and leaves the unactivated crystals unaffected. See also *film processing.*

photoheterotroph (fo″to-het′er-o-trōf) [*photo-* + Gr. *heteros* other + *trophos* feeder, from *trephein* to nourish] a photosynthetic bacterium that uses organic compounds, rather than CO_2, as its principal carbon source. Also called *photoorganotroph.* See also *heterotroph.*

photoheterotrophic (fo″to-het″er-o-trōf′ik) pertaining to photoheterotrophs.

photolithotroph (fo″to-lith′o-trōf) [*photo-* + Gr. *lithos* stone + *trophos* feeder, from *trephein* to nourish] see *photoautotroph.*

photoluminescence (fo″to-lu″mĭ-nes′ens) [*photo-* + L. *lumen* light] the quality of being luminescent after exposure to light.

photolysis (fo-tol′ĭ-sis) [*photo-* + Gr. *lysis* dissolution, from *lyein* to lose] chemical decomposition induced by the action of light.

photolytic (fo″to-lit′ik) decomposed by the action of light or radiant energy.

photometer (fo-tom′ĕ-ter) [*photo-* + Gr. *metron* measure] a device for measuring light intensity. For more information, see the specific type, e.g., *colorimeter* and *spectrophotometer.*

photometrazol threshold the total quantity of leptazol needed to produce clinical myoclonus and electroencephalographic polyspike or wave and spike discharges in response to photic stimulation. it is measured in milligrams per kilogram of body weight, with leptazol injected intravenously at a rate of 50 mg per 30 sec. A zero photometrazol threshold is taken as spontaneous or photic-initiated paroxysmal activity. The threshold is unaffected by anxiety states and may vary during the course of an illness; it is low (<5 mg/kg) in those with centrencephalic epilepsy, and certain other disorders including schizophrenia and hysteria. Although the threshold is a useful diagnostic (activation) tool, it is of no value in predicting the occurrence of spontaneous epileptic seizures. See also *photometrazol a.* under *activation.*

photometric (fo-to-met′rik) pertaining to the measurement of light intensity.

photometric accuracy a measure of how accurately a photometer indicates the amount of light falling on the detector. It measures both meter accuracy and detector linearity.

photometric linearity the ability of a photometer to indicate accurately the linear change of absorbance with concentration for solutions known to obey Beer's law. It is usually expressed as the absorbance range at a given wavelength or range of wavelengths.

photometric reproducibility the ability of a photometer to produce identical readings in repeated measurements.

photomicrograph (fo″to-mi′kro-graf) [*photo-* + Gr. *mikros* small + *graphein* to record] a photograph of an object taken through a light microscope.

photomicrography (fo″to-mi-krog′rah-fe) the technique in which photographs are taken of objects through a light microscope.

photomicroscope (fo″to-mi′kro-skōp) [*photo-* + Gr. *mikros* small + *skopein* to examine] a microscope with camera attached for making photomicrographs.

photomultiplier tube (PM) (fo″to-mul′tĭ-pli-er) an electronic device (a vacuum tube), used in most scintillation detectors and in some spectrophotometers. PM tubes detect faint light pulses containing only one or a few photons. The output, a voltage pulse, is proportional to the number and energy of the photons in the light pulse.

In this process, photons strike a thin metal plate, the photocathode, producing photoelectrons. Behind the photocathode are a series of 10–12 plates, called dynodes, with successively higher voltages. When a photoelectron is accelerated toward the first dynode, it strikes it, knocking loose several more electrons, which are accelerated toward the next. The process continues, producing a cascade of 10^5–10^8 electrons (depending on the applied voltage), which are collected by the anode. The efficiency depends on the probability that a photon will produce a photoelectron. Some tubes have an efficiency of 30 percent.

photomyoclonic response (fo″to-mi″o-klon′ik) [*photo-* + Gr. *myos* muscle + *klonos* turmoil] see *photomyogenic response.*

photomyogenic response (fo″to-mi″o-jen′ik) [*photo-* + Gr. *myos* muscle + *gennan* to produce] in electroencephalography, a response to high-intensity, rhythmic photic stimulation, consisting of frontally predominant repetitive spikes that follow each flash of light, increase in amplitude as the stimulus continues, cease when the stimulus is withdrawn, and are muscular in origin. The photomyogenic response may be accompanied by eyelid flutter and by jerking of the facial and scalp muscles; it is found in some normal individuals. Also called *photomyoclonic response.*

photon (foton) [*photo-* + *-on*] a particle that has zero mass or charge and unit spin, the quantum of the electromagnetic field and carrier of the electromagnetic force. The energy (E) and frequency (ν) of a photon are related by the equation $E = h\nu$, where h is Planck's constant.

photon counting the measurement of the intensity of light or other electromagnetic radiation by a device with enough sensitivity and a response time fast enough to record the arrival of different photons as discrete events. Most photon-counting systems use a photomultiplier tube detector, the output of which is fed to a discriminator circuit, which separates pulses that correspond to photons from lower-level noise pulses.

photoophthalmia (fo″to-of-thal′me-ah) [*photo-* + Gr. *ophthalmos* eye + *-ia*] ophthalmia caused by intense lights, such as electric light, rays of a welding arc, or reflection from snow (snow blindness). Also called *photoretinitis.*

photoorganotroph (fo″to-or-gah′no-trōf) [*photo-* + Gr. *organon* organ + *trophos* feeder, from *trephein* to nourish] see *photoheterotroph.*

photoparoxysmal response (fo″to-par″ok-siz′mal) in electroencephalography, a response to intermittent photic stimuli consisting of generalized, bilaterally symmetric, synchronous, slow-wave and spike or polyspike complexes. The discharge may outlast the stimulus by a few seconds and is sometimes associated with an impairment of consciousness. It may be found in patients with generalized seizures or certain metabolic disorders and sometimes in normal subjects, and it may have a familial basis. If photic stimulation is prolonged after the appearance of this response, it can lead to a major convulsion. Also called *photoconvulsive response.*

photopeak (fo′to-pēk) a peak corresponding to the energy of detected photons in the graph of a gamma-ray spectrum recorded with a scintillation detector, as opposed to a peak due to a process occurring in a crystal. The energy resolution of the detector measuring a photopeak is calculated as the full width of the photopeak measured at half the maximal count (FWHM), expressed as a percentage of the energy of the peak maximum. See also the accompanying illustration.

photopeak detection efficiency the fraction of the gamma rays entering a scintillation crystal that produce an output pulse in the photopeak energy window. Only these photons contribute to the image in a scintillation camera. The efficiency increases with increasing crystal thickness and decreases with increasing photon energy. A scintillation camera is about 3.7 times as efficient at detecting the 140-keV photons of Tc-99m as it is at detecting the 360-keV photons of I-131. Also called photopeak detection sensitivity.

photophobia (fo″to-fo′be-ah) [*photo-* + Gr. *phobein* to be frightened by] an abnormal visual intolerance to light. It is more common in light-skinned people and may often be relieved by wearing dark glasses. This condition occurs in association with a variety of disorders, including corneal inflammation, iritis, ocular albinism, aphakia, keratoconjunctivitis, acute glaucoma, and corneal abrasions. It may also appear as a complication of several febrile viral diseases, especially measles.

photopic (fo-top′ik) [*phot-* + Gr. *ōps* eye] pertaining to vision at high levels of illumination, i.e., in the light.

photopic vision vision under daylight conditions, characterized by predominantly cone receptor functioning, high visual acuity at the center of the fovea, and rapid temporal resolution of changing visual patterns.

photoptometer (fo″top-tom′ĕ-ter) [*phot-* + Gr. *optos* seen + *metron* measure] an instrument used to measure visual acuity in dim light. An examination with this instrument determines the least amount of light that renders an object just visible.

photoreaction (fo″to-re-ak′shun) see *photochemical reaction.*

photoreactivation (fo″to-re-ak″tĭ-va′shun) a process of DNA repair that occurs in bacteria and other species but not in mammals, and reverses the lethal biologic effects of thymine dimers induced by ultraviolet radiation. Visible light in the blue range activates an exonuclease that excises thymine dimers.

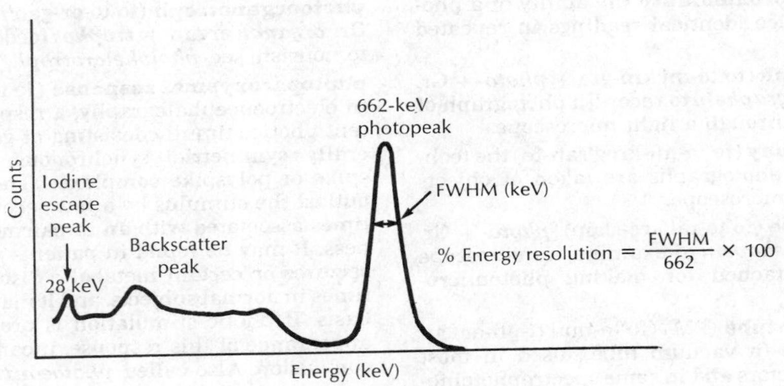

Photopeak. Cesium-137 spectrum illustrating iodine escape peak and concept of energy resolution as measured by FWHM (full-width half-maximum). (From Rollo, F.D.: Detection and measurement of nuclear radiations. In Rollo, F. D. (ed.) Nuclear Medicine Physics, Instrumentation, and Agents. St. Louis, C. V. Mosby Co., 1977.)

The strand is then repaired using the complementary strand as a template. See also *DNA repair.* Cf. *dark reactivation.*

photoreceptor (fo″to-re-sep′tor) one of the cell types in the retina that sense light. There are two types, rods and cones. Both are long, thin cells (1–8 μm in diameter and 40–60 μm long) that extend vertically from the middle layer of the retina to its outer surface.

Humans have 115–130 million photoreceptors (about four rods to a cone). The cones, which distinguish colors, are concentrated in the area of high visual acuity, the fovea, where rods are absent. The rods are light, but not color, sensitive.

The light-sensitive part of a rod or cone is the outer segment composed of disks that are approximately 14 nm thick, contain pigment (rhodopsin in rods, iodopsin in cones), and are enveloped by infoldings of the cell membrane. (In the cones the stack of disks tapers to a point.) Except in the fovea, light passes through the cell bodies of the interneurons and rods and cones before reaching the outer segments. A single photon entering an outer segment changes the prosthetic group of rhodopsin (or iodopsin) from 11-*cis*-retinene to its isomer all-*trans*-retinene, which is released from the apoprotein opsin. In the process, the cell membrane is made less permeable to sodium ions and the membrane potential increases, possibly owing to a release of calcium ions when the pigment decomposes. Thus, unlike other sensory receptors and neurons, photoreceptors (and the bipolar cells and horizontal cells with which they synapse) respond to a stimulus by hyperpolarizing rather than by depolarizing. The total response of a photoreceptor is approximately proportional to the logarithm of the light intensity.

See also *color vision, iodopsin,* and *rhodopsin.*

photorecorder (fo″to-re-kor′der) the primary display device of many rectilinear scanners. It consists of a light source that is moved back and forth over an x-ray film, matching the motion of the detector. In some cases, the travel is reduced by one-half or one-fifth, producing a minified image. The light source flashes once for each count or once each time that a preset number of counts (the regularization ratio) have been detected. The intensity and the duration of each flash are adjusted so that the maximal film density is produced in the region with the highest count density. Also called *photoscanner.*

photoresistor (fo″to-re-zis′ter) see under *photocell.*

photoretinitis (fo″to-ret″ĭ-ni′tis) [*photo* + *retina* + *-itis* inflammation] see *photoophthalmia.*

photoscan (fo′to-skan) the image produced by a rectilinear scanner that uses a photorecorder. It shows the distribution of a gamma-ray–emitting isotope in the subject.

photoscanner (fo″to-skan′ner) see *photorecorder.*

photosensitive (fo″to-sen′sĭ-tiv) [*photo-* + L. *sentire* to feel] 1. an abnormally heightened reactivity of the skin to sunlight.

2. responding to light, e.g., as by a photocell or photographic film.

photosensitivity (fo″to-sen″sĭ-tiv′ĭ-te) abnormally severe reactions of the skin on exposure to sunlight. Although acute sunburn and chronic actinic keratoses may be considered "normal" reactions to the overexposure of the skin to sunlight, photosensitivity reactions are classified as those occurring only after a few minutes of exposure to sunlight. Erythema, dermatitis, urticarial and erythematous lesions, and thick, scaling patches may result.

This condition may be associated with systemic disease (systemic lupus erythematosus, herpes simplex, or xeroderma pigmentosum), ingestion of various photosensitizing drugs (sulfonamides, griseofulvin, tetracyclines), or application of certain topical agents (toilet waters, perfumes, coal tars). Idiopathic photosensitivity reactions may also occur.

photosensitization (fo″to-sen″sĭ-tĭ-za′shun) the development of abnormally heightened skin reactivity to sunlight.

photostable (fo′to-sta″b′l) unchanged by exposure to light.

photosynthesis (fo″to-sin′thĕ-sis) [*photo-* + Gr. *synthesis* putting together; from *syn-* together + *thesis* setting, placing] a chemical combination caused by the action of light. Specifically, the term refers to the series of complex reactions leading to the formation of carbohydrates from carbon dioxide and water in the chlorophyll-containing organelles of plants with energy provided by visible light.

photosynthetic organism (fo″to-sin-thet′ik) one of a group of organisms that can use radiant solar energy to support biosynthesis and growth, a unique property of this major group. See also *photoautotroph* and *photoheterotroph.*

phototaxis (fo″to-tak′sis) [*photo-* + Gr. *taxis* arrangement] an orientation movement of a motile organism toward (positive phototaxis) or away from (negative phototaxis) light.

phototherapy (fo″to-ther′ah-pe) the treatment of disease by exposure to ultraviolet (290–320 nm) or visible light, without the concomitant use of systemic drug therapy. Therapy with blue light (wavelength, 430–500 nm) enhances the breakdown and excretion of bilirubin in jaundiced newborn infants. As bilirubin absorbs light, it produces an excited state that causes the bilirubin to combine with oxygen to form biliverdin and other oxidation products. Exposure to ultraviolet radiation (290–320 nm) has also been used in the treatment of skin disorders such as psoriasis and pityriasis rosea. Cf. *photochemotherapy.*

phototimer (fo″to-tīm′er) a device used in photography and radiography to control the exposure interval. In radiography, it is used to produce repeated exposures with the same radiographic density. A cassette without lead backing is used: the remnant x-rays pass through the cassette and strike a fluorescent screen, emitting light that is measured by a photocell. The exposure is terminated when the total amount of light energy (intensity times time) measured reaches a preset quantity.

phototoxic (fo″to-tok′sik) [*photo-* + L. *toxicum* poison] pertaining to or characterized by heightening of the sunburn response to ultraviolet light, without any allergic effect (immune response) being involved.

phototoxicity (fo″to-tok-sis′ĭ-te) a reaction of the skin seen in association with the ingestion or application of certain drugs and exposure to sunlight. It is characterized by an exaggerated sunburn often accompanied by edema. Hyperpigmentation and desquamation may also occur. These reactions are usually confined to the site of exposure and reach maximal intensity within 12–24 hr. This reaction is not thought to be mediated by the immune system. Drugs implicated in phototoxicity reactions include sulfonamides, acridine dyes, griseofulvin, phenothiazine, and sulfonylurea hypoglycemic agents. Cf. *photoallergy.*

phototransistor (fo″to-tran-zis′tor) a transistor in which light focused on the base controls the current flow. Its uses are similar to those of the photodiode.

phototrophic (fo″to-trōf′ik) [*photo-* + Gr. *trophē* nourishment] utilizing light as a source of energy, as in photosynthesis, which occurs in plants, certain bacteria, and algae.

phototropism (fo″to-tro′pizm) [*photo-* + Gr. *tropos* a turning] the tendency of an organism to turn or move toward (positive phototropism) or away from (negative phototropism) light.

phototube (fo″to-tūb′) a diode vacuum tube that detects light. Photoelectrons produced by light falling on the photocathode are attracted to the anode. This produces a current proportional to the amount of incident light. Some phototubes are gas-filled; the avalanche effect amplifies the photocurrent in the photomultiplier type of phototube.

photovoltaic cell (fo″to-vol-ta′ik) see under *photocell.*

phren/o (fren′o) [Gr. *phrēn* diaphragm, mind] a word element used in combining form to denote diaphragm or mind, e.g., phrenodynia, schizophrenia.

phrenic (fren′ik) pertaining to the diaphragm or the mind.

phrenic nerve the motor nerve to the diaphragm. It arises from the cervical plexus, mainly from fibers of the fourth cervical nerve, and descends through the neck and thorax to reach the diaphragm.

phrenosin (fren′o-sēn) a galactocerebroside that contains a 24-carbon fatty acid with a 2-hydroxyl group, cerebronic acid. See also *cerebroside.*

phthalic acid (thal′ik) a colorless, crystalline solid, 1,2-benzenedicarboxylic acid; M.W. 166.13. The monopotassium salt is used as a primary acid-base standard. The combination of free acid and monovalent ion gives buffers, effective in the pH range of 2.2–3.8, and the combination of mono- and divalent ions gives buffers effective in the range of 4.2–6.0.

phthalylsulfathiazole (thal″il-sul″fah-thi′ah-zōl) see *sulfonamide.*

phthiriasis (thir-i′ah-sis) [Gr. *phtheiriasis,* from *phtheir* louse] being infested with lice of the species *Phthirus pubis.*

Phthirus (thir′us) [Gr. *phtheir* louse] a genus of sucking lice of the order Anoplura.

P. pubis, the pubic or crab louse. These crablike insects, measuring 1.5-2 mm, infest the hair of the pubic region (and occasionally in heavy infestations, the eyebrows and eyelashes). They are most frequently transmitted through sexual contact.

Microscopic examination of the eggs (nits) attached to the hair confirms the diagnosis.

phyc/o (fi′ko) [Gr. *phykos* seaweed] a word element used in combining form to denote relationship to seaweed or algae, e.g., Phycomycetes.

Phycomycetes (fi″ko-mi-se′tēz) [*phyco-* + Gr. *mykēs* fungus] a group of lower fungi that previously included Mastigomycotina (Chytridiomycetes, Oomycetes, Hyphochytridiomycetes) and Zygomycetina. Taxonomically, true fungi (Eumycota) are often divided into five subphyla: Mastigomycotina, Zygomycotina, Phycomycetes, Ascomycotina, Basidiomycotina, and Deuteromycotina. The term Phycomycetes is obsolete and has no taxonomic status.

phycomycosis (fi″ko-mi-ko′sis) [*phyco-* + Gr. *mykēs* fungus + *-osis* condition] a general term frequently used for mucormycosis. Phycomycosis is a general term for all the non-septate fungi that cause mucormycosis plus some additional mycoses. See also *mucormycosis.*

phylactic (fi-lak′tik) [Gr. *phylaktikos* preservative] serving to protect; producing phylaxis.

-phylaxis (fi-lak′sis) [Gr. "a guarding," from *phylax* a guard] a suffix word element to denote protection, e.g., prophylaxis.

phyllode (fil′ōd) [Gr. *phyllon* leaf + *eidos* form] resembling a leaf; a term applied to tumors that on section show a lobulated, leaflike appearance. See also pseudosarcoma phyllodes.

phylloquinone (fil″o-kwin′ōn) see *vitamin K_1.*

phylogeny (fi-loj′e-ne) [Gr. *phylon* tribe + *genesis* generation] 1. the evolutionary development of a genetically related group of organisms or of a race or species of animals or plants from the simplest form.

2. the evolution of the species as distinguished from ontogenesis, the evolution of the individual. Cf. *ontogeny.*

phylum (fi′lum), pl. *phyla* [N.L., from Gr. *phylon* tribe] a taxonomic division that groups together several classes within a kingdom. The term is now used only for animals; plants and prokaryotes are classified in divisions.

Physa (fi′sah) a genus of snails. The species *P. parkeri* is a host for the fluke *Schistosoma,* which can cause schistosomal cercarial dermatitis, or swimmer's itch.

physaliferous (fis″ah-lif′er-us) [Gr. *physallis* bubble + L. *ferre* to bear] see *physaliphorous.*

physaliphorous (fis″ah-lif′o-rus) [Gr. *physallis* bubble + *phoros* bearing] a term applied to cells with a frothy or vacuolated cytoplasm, as in the jellyfish, which are characteristic of chordoma.

Physaloptera (fis″ah-lop′ter-ah) [Gr. *physallis* bubble + *pteron* wing] a genus of nematodes of the family Spiruroidea, which is parasitic in the stomachs of humans.

P. caucasica, a species of large worms found in South America and Africa; the males measure 14–50 mm long; the females, 24–100 mm. Several cases of infection with this organism in humans have been reported. The eggs are smooth, thick-shelled, and ovoid, measuring 44–65 μ by 32–45 μ. Human infection is thought to be caused by the accidental ingestion of intermediate hosts such as beetles and cockroaches.

Laboratory diagnosis requires identification by the formalin-ether sedimentation technique of eggs in feces. Also called *P. mordens.*

P. mordens, see *P. caucasica.*

physalopteriasis (fis″ah-lop″ter-i′ah-sis) infection with worms of the genus *Physaloptera.*

Physalopteridae (fis″ah-lop-ter′ĭ-de) a family of nematodes that includes the genus *Physaloptera.*

physi/o (fiz′e-o) [Gr. *physis* nature] a word element used in combining form to denote nature or physiology, e.g., physiologic, physiotherapy.

physiatrics (fiz″e-at′triks) [*physi-* + Gr. *iatrikē* medicine, surgery] the branch of medicine that deals with physical therapy and physical agents (water, heat, light, electricity, and mechanical manipulations) in the diagnosis, treatment, and prevention of disease and body disorders.

physician (fĭ-zish′un) [Old French *fisicien,* from *fisique* medicine] an authorized practitioner of medicine, e.g., one graduated from a college of medicine or osteopathy and licensed by state certification. For more information, see the specific physician specialty.

physician's assistant (PA) a health care professional who carries out certain duties usually performed by physicians. Such personnel may serve as assistants to the primary care physician or as surgeon's assistants. Among a PA's responsibilities, carried out under physician supervision, are the taking of patient histories, performing physical examinations, drawing blood samples, performing electrocardiographic examinations, and routine therapeutic procedures such as injections, immunizations, and wound suturing. Educational preparation involves completion of an approved program; graduates are certified by the American Academy of Physician's Assistants and are designated PA–C, Physician's Assistant–Certified. See also *nurse practitioner.*

physicochemical (fiz″ĭ-ko-kem′ĭ-kal) 1. of or pertaining to both physical and chemical properties, changes, and reactions.

2. of or according to physical chemistry.

physics (fiz′iks) [Gr. *physis* nature] the science that studies the various types of matter and energy, and accounts for natural phenomena by laws that describe the motion and interaction of the two.

physiognomy (fiz″e-og′no-me) [*physio-* + Gr. *gnōmōn* a judge] a technique that utilizes facial expression and appearance as an aid in the diagnosis of disease processes.

physiologic (fiz″e-o-loj′ik) [Gr. *physiologikos* pertaining to natural science] 1. normal, not pathologic.

2. pertaining to physiology.

physiologic chemistry a branch of biochemistry concerned with the chemical processes and reactions associated with the functioning of animals (and in particular, the human) in both health and disease.

physiologic dead space the total portion of each tidal volume that does not participate in gaseous exchange in alveoli; the functional sum of the alveolar and anatomic dead spaces. The increase in the ratio of this quantity to the total tidal volume (estimated by the Bohr equation), which occurs with age and in certain pulmonary disorders, indicates a loss of efficiency in oxygenation and elimination of carbon dioxide with each unit of ventilation.

physiologic hypogammaglobulinemia a temporary form of hypogammaglobulinemia, which is a normal occurrence in infants at about age 3–6 mo when maternal IgG levels wane, and before the onset of the normal snythesis of IgG by the infant.

physiologist (fiz″e-ol′o-jist) [*physio-* + Gr. *logistēs* reasons] a specialist in the science of physiology.

physiology (fiz″e-ol′o-je) [*physio-* + Gr. *logos* word, reason] 1. the science that deals with the functioning of living organisms and of the physical and chemical factors and processes involved.

2. the vital processes of a living organism.

physis (fi′sis) [Gr. *physis* origin, nature, from *phyein* to produce] a suffix word element to denote growth, e.g., epiphysis.

physisorption (fiz″ĭ-sorp′shun) see *physical a.* under *adsorption.*

Physopsis (fī-sop′sis) a subgenus of snails (genus *Bulinus*) that serves as host for the blood fluke, *Schistosoma haematobium.*

physostigmine salicylate (fi″so-stig′mēn) an anticholinesterase, the salicylate salt of physostigmine, an alkaloid extracted from the calabar bean, *Physostigma venenosum.* It is used as an antidote to overdoses of anticholinergic drugs, e.g., atropine, and in the treatment of glaucoma. Physostigmine poisoning can cause cholinergic crises with life-threatening convulsions, arrhythmias, and coma.

phyt/o (fi′to) [Gr. *phyton* plant] a word element used in combining form to denote relationship to plants, e.g., phytol, phytomitogen.

phytanic acid (fi-tan′ik) 3,7,11,15-tetramethylhexadecanoic acid; a 20-carbon atom, branched-chain fatty acid that accumulates in large amounts in the tissues and serum of individuals with Refsum's disease. Phytanic acid is derived metabolically from the phytol, which is a substituent of chlorophyll in plants. Serum phytanic acid concentrations can be determined by gas chromatography of fatty acid methyl esters. See also *Refsum's disease.*

phytic acid (fi'tik) the hexaphosphate of *myo*-inositol found in plant tissues, especially cereals. High concentrations of phytates in the diet not hydrolyzed in the intestine can chelate Ca^{++}, Fe^{++}, and Zn^{++}, and prevent their absorption from the intestine.

phytin (fi'tin) the mixed calcium-magnesium salt of phytic acid present in plant tissues such as cereal grains. See also *phytic acid.*

Phytobdella (fi"tōb-del'ah) [*phyto-* + Gr. *bdella* leech] a genus of terrestrial leeches, of which the species *P. catenifera* is known to attack humans in Malaysia.

phytobezoar (fi"to-be'zōr) [*phyto-* + Persian *bezoar* protecting against poison] a gastric concretion composed primarily of vegetable matter. See also *bezoar.*

phytohemagglutinin (PHA) (fi"to-hem"ah-gloo'tĭ-nin) [*phyto-* + Gr. *haima* blood + L. *agglutinare* to glue to + *-in*] a plant lectin extracted from the red kidney bean, *Phaseolus vulgaris.* It is a glycoprotein that causes the agglutination of red blood cells by binding to *N*-acetyl-β-galactosamine. It is also a mitogen and inducer of lymphocyte proliferation. PHA generally stimulates T cells, and is used to evaluate T-cell function and to induce mitosis in peripheral leukocyte cultures for cytogenetic tests. See also *concanavalin A* and *pokeweed mitogen.*

phytol (fi'tol) 3,7,11,15-tetramethylhexadecen-2-ol, a terpene (isoprenoid) alcohol that exists as an ester in chlorophyll. It is used in the preparation of vitamin E and phytonadione, a prothrombogenic agent. A hereditary disturbance in its ultimate metabolism results in Refsum's disease.

Phytomastigophora (fi"to-mas"tĭ-gof'o-rah) [*phyto-* + Gr. *mastix, mastigos* whip + *phoros* bearer, from *pherein* to bear] a class of small, plant-like, flagellate protozoa of the superclass Mastigophora.

phytomitogen (fi"to-mi'to-jen) [*phyto-* + Gr. *mitos* thread + *gennan* to produce] a substance of plant origin that stimulates DNA synthesis and blast formation in lymphocytes. See also *lectin, mitogen,* and *phytohemagglutinin.*

phytophotodermatitis (fi"to-fo"to-der"mah-ti'tis) [*phyto-* + Gr. *phōs* light + *derma* skin + *-itis* inflammation] an inflammation of discrete skin areas, which results from the combination of applying certain plant products to the skin and subsequently exposing that skin to the sunlight. A mild-to-severe erythema may result, often in association with vesicles and bullae. Dense hyperpigmentation may follow 3–5 da later. Implicated products belong to the plant families Rutaceae and Umbelliferae (e.g., celery, parsley, certain limes, and figs). Plant oils contained in certain perfumes may also be involved.

PI abbrev. See *phosphatidylinositol.*

Pi, P_i symbol for *inorganic phosphate.*

pi (Π, π) (pi) the sixteenth letter of the *Greek alphabet.*

pI abbrev. See *isoelectric point.*

pia-arachnitis (pi'ah ar"ak-ni'tis) an inflammation of the pia mater and the arachnoid (known together as the leptomeninges). Also called piarachnitis. See also *leptomeningitis.*

pia-arachnoid (pi"ah ah-rak'noid) [*pia* + *arachnoid*] the pia mater and arachnoid mater considered together as one functional unit. See also *pia mater.*

pia mater (pi'ah ma'ter) [L. "tender mother"] a loose connective tissue sheath, containing elastin, collagen, and reticular fibers, that forms the innermost meningeal covering of the brain and spinal cord. It also forms the choroid plexuses of the lateral, third, and fourth cerebral ventricles, as well as the sheaths for the cranial and spinal nerve roots. The pia mater closely covers the neural tissue, penetrating the cerebral gyri and cerebellar lamina; it functions as a mechanical barrier against infection for the neural tissue, and also as a support structure that covers the precapillary blood vessels that penetrate the cerebral hemispheres.

The pia mater has its embryologic origin in the mesenchyme and cells of the neural crests. Because it develops simultaneously with the arachnoid mater, the two meningeal coverings are often referred to as the pia-arachnoid.

p. m. encephali, [NA], the pial membrane associated with the brain.

p. m. spinalis, [NA], the pial covering of the spinal cord.

pian (pe-ahn') [Fr.] see *yaws.*

pica (pi'kah) [L. "magpie"] a craving to eat objects that are inedible or not normally considered to be food. Pica may be seen in adults who have iron deficiency anemia: starch, ice cubes, and ice chips are commonly eaten (see *pagophagia*). In infants, pica may involve the eating of lead-based paint chips and plaster, which leads to acute or chronic lead poisoning.

Pichia a genus of fungi; the asexual stages (anamorphs) are species of *Candida.*

Pick's bodies (piks) [Arnold *Pick,* Czechoslovakian neurologist and psychiatrist, 1851–1924] spherical, argyrophilic masses found close to the nucleus of degenerating neurons in Pick's disease. The accumulated material distends the cell body, giving it a ballooned appearance. This distinctive microscopic pathology is not found in similar degenerative neurologic disorders and, together with the focal nature of the cerebral degeneration, serves to distinguish Pick's disease from conditions such as Alzheimer's disease.

Pick's cells [Ludwig *Pick,* German pathologist, 1868–1935] round, oval, or polyhedral cells with foamy, lipid-containing cytoplasm found in the bone marrow and spleen in Niemann-Pick disease.

Pick's disease 1. [Arnold *Pick*], a degenerative disease that affects the frontal and temporal lobes of the brain in middle and later life (presenile period). It cannot be distinguished from Alzheimer's disease except at autopsy, when a distinct line of demarcation is found between the atrophy of the affected lobes and the normal brain, and a number of histologic changes are seen. The cause of this rare disease is unknown, but familial cases have occasionally been described. The course of the atrophy is slow and progressive, leading to intellectual and behavioral deterioration, and ultimately death, usually within 7 yr of onset of the disorder.

2. [Friedel *Pick,* Prague physician, 1867–1926], ascites and fibrotic liver disease that is associated with constrictive pericarditis. Also called pericardial pseudocirrhosis of the liver.

3. [Ludwig *Pick*], see *Niemann-Pick disease.*

picket cell a term sometimes used for the tall, mucus-producing cell that makes up the endocervical columnar epithelium. These cells have a clear apical cytoplasm with oval nuclei that usually have a basal location but this may vary with hormonal effects.

pickwickian syndrome (pik-wik′e-an) [from the description of the fat boy in Dickens' *Pickwick Papers*] the occurrence of chronic alveolar hypoventilation, somnolence, and polycythemia in the obese individual. See also *alveolar hypoventilation.*

picloram (pi-klor′am) a toxic herbicide, 4-amino-3,5,6-trichloropicolinic acid, used as a chemical warfare agent (defoliant).

pico- (p) (pi′ko, pe′ko) [Sp. *pico* small amount; It. *piccolo* small] a prefix word element attached to International System (SI) units to denote a unit that is one-trillionth of the basic unit (10^{-12} unit).

picocurie (pCi) (pi″ko-ku′re, pe″ko-ku′re) a unit of radioactivity equal to one-trillionth of a curie (10^{-12} Ci).

picofarad (pF) (pi″ko-far′ad, pe″ko-far′ad) a unit of electrical capacitance equal to one-trillionth of a farad (10^{-12} F). Formerly called micromicrofarad ($\mu\mu$F).

picogram (pg) (pi′ko-gram, pe′ko-gram) a unit of mass equal to one-trillionth of a gram (10^{-12} g, 10^{-15} kg).

picometer (pm) (pi′ko-me″ter, pe′ko-me″ter) a unit of length equal to one-trillionth of a meter (10^{-12} m).

picornavirus (pi-kor″nah-vi′rus) [acronym from *pico-* + *r*ibo*n*ucleic *a*cid + *virus*] one of a group of small RNA animal viruses that belong to the Picornaviridae family. The virion is 20–30 nm in size, has an icosahedral symmetry with 60 capsomers, and is not enveloped with a lipid coat. The RNA is single stranded, linear, and nonsegmented, and serves as a template for RNA synthesis and protein translation in the cytoplasm of the host cell. There are four genera of picornaviruses, *Enterovirus, Cardiovirus, Rhinovirus,* and *Aphthovirus.* Within the *Enterovirus* genus, there are five subgenera, *Poliovirus, Coxsackie A virus, Coxsackie B virus, Echovirus,* and *Enterovirus.*

Picornaviruses play a significant role in human infection, with the exception of the aphthoviruses, which infect only cloven-footed animals, and the cardioviruses, which cause a rare cephalomyocarditis in humans.

For more information, see the individual genus and the accompanying table.

picosecond (ps, psec) (pi′ko-sek″ond, pe′ko-sek″-ond,) a unit of time equal to one-trillionth of a second (10^{-12} sec).

picr/o [Gr. *pikros* bitter] 1. a word element used in combining form to denote bitter, e.g., picronigeusia, picrotoxin.

2. in histology, a word element used in combining form to denote the presence of picric acid in a formulation, e.g., picrofuchsin.

picrate (pik′rāt) any salt of picric acid.

picric acid (pik′rik) [Gr. *pikros* bitter] the trivial name for 2,4,6-trinitrophenol; pale yellow, odorless crystals; M.W. 229.11. Picric acid is a component of some histologic fixatives and is used as a yellow acid dye, primarily as a counterstain in combination with other dyes, e.g., in van Gieson's stain. In clinical chemistry it is widely used in the Jaffe procedure for the measurement of creatinine. This acid explodes on rapid heating or by percussion, and should be stored in a cool place.

PICORNAVIRUS. A CLASSIFICATION OF THE FAMILY PICORNAVIRIDAE

			Distinctive Properties			
Genus	Subgenus[a]	Number of Immunotypes (Species)	*Infectivity at pH 3*	*Infectivity at pH 6*	*Density in CsCl (g/cm³)*	*Optimal Growth Temperature*
Enterovirus	Poliovirus	3				
	Coxsackievirus A	23[b]				
	Coxsackievirus B	6	+	+	1.33–1.35	37°C
	Echovirus	30[c]				
	Enterovirus	4				
Cardiovirus	–	2	+	–[d]	1.34	37°C
Rhinovirus	–	>115	–	±[e]	1.38–1.41	33°C
Aphthovirus	–	7	–	±[f]	1.43–1.45	37°C

[a] The designation subgenus has not been proposed by the International Committee on Taxonomy of Viruses but is used here for convenience simply to indicate a taxon smaller than a genus but larger than a species.
[b] Coxsackieviruses A1–A24; coxsackievirus A23 has been reclassified as echovirus 9.
[c] Echoviruses 1–34; echoviruses 1 and 8 are identical; echovirus 10 has been reclassified as reovirus 1, and echovirus 28 as rhinovirus 1A; echovirus 34 is a variant of coxsackievirus A24.
[d] Cardioviruses are stable at pH 4–10, but in the presence of chloride ions they are unstable in the region of pH 6.
[e] Rhinoviruses are borderline stable at pH 6 and unstable at lower pH.
[f] Aphthoviruses are unstable below pH 7 at low ionic strength but stable at pH 5–6 in high ionic strength.
Modified from Braude, A. I.: Medical Microbiology and Infectious Disease. Philadelphia, W. B. Saunders Co., 1981, p. 586.

picrotoxin (pik″ro-tok′sin) [*picro-* + *toxin*] an analeptic drug extracted from the fishberry plant, *Cocculus indicus.* Picrotoxin was formerly used as a stimulant in the treatment of barbiturate poisonings; although no longer considered a useful therapeutic agent, it is an important means of studying inhibition of the central nervous system.

PID abbrev. for pelvic inflammatory disease. See *salpingitis.*

piedra (pe-ĕ′drah) [Sp. stone] a fungal infection of the hair shaft characterized by irregular nodules composed of aggregated fungal elements. There are two types: white piedra, caused by *Trichosporon cutaneum,* and black piedra, caused by *Piedraia hortae.* The disease is cosmetic in nature, causing no pain or physical reaction. See also *Piedraia.*

Piedraia (pi″ĕ-dri′ah) a genus of fungi that belongs to the family Piedraiaceae, order Myriangiales; the etiologic agent of black piedra. There is only one medically important species, *P. hortae. Piedraia* grows slowly at 25°C as a dark brown conical colony, often with a raised center. Microscopically, there are thick-walled septate hyphae; chlamydospores; and swollen, irregular cells.

Pierre Robin developmental field complex (pe-yair′ ro-ba′) [*Pierre Robin,* French dentist, 1867–1950] a congenital defect characterized by micrognathia and glossoptosis, frequently with cleft palate. Affected infants have difficulty with feeding, and the tongue may be sucked backward, obstructing the laryngeal airway. If respiratory problems develop, a tracheostomy may be necessary. This congenital malformation occurs in a number of syndromes and as an isolated hypoplasia.

PIE syndrome [acronym from *p*ulmonary *i*nfiltrate with *e*osinophilia] a general term that includes a variety of disease entities in which pulmonary infiltration occurs in conjunction with local or systemic eosinophilia.

piezoelectric effect (pi-e″zo-ĕ-lek′trik, pe-a″zo-ĕ-lek′trik) [Gr. *piezein* to compress + *electric*] a phenomenon exhibited by certain crystals, in which an applied mechanical stress produces a proportional electric polarization in the crystal, and an applied voltage produces a proportional mechanical force exerted by the crystal.

PIF abbrev. See *prolactin inhibiting factor, proliferation inhibitory factor.*

pigment (pig′ment) [L. *pigmentum* paint] 1. any normal or abnormal coloring matter of the body. See also *endogenous p.'s and deposits, exogenous p.'s and deposits,* and the specific pigment.

2. in chemistry, any material used as a coloring agent (those that chemically bind to other materials are more commonly called dyes).

3. a paintlike medicinal preparation applied to the skin.

endogenous p.'s and deposits, pigments and deposits derived from material normally present in the body. These may be divided into hemoglobin-derived pigments, lipid pigments, melanins, and endogenous deposits.

Hemoglobin and its breakdown products occur as pigments. Hemosiderin is a yellow-brown pigment that contains ferric hydroxide bound to the protein apoferritin, forming ferritin. It is the storage form of iron normally found in reticuloendothelial cells that break down red cells. It is also found at sites of hemorrhage and in many tissues in cases of systemic iron overload. The porphyrin portion of heme is metabolized to bilirubin and other bile pigments. These are termed hematoidin when they appear as yellow-brown deposits at the sites of old hemorrhages. Hematin is a dark brown pigment produced from hemoglobin by the action of malarial or schistosomal parasites (the similar appearing formalin pigment is a fixation artifact).

The endogenous lipid pigments include lipofuscin, a yellow-brown pigment found in atrophic tissue, where it is produced by the lysosomal oxidation of lipids. Ceroid found in cirrhotic livers and hemofuscin produced in hemochromatosis are also lipofuscin material.

Melanins are granular yellow, brown, or black pigments formed by the polymerization of tyrosine catalyzed by the enzyme tyrosinase. They occur normally in the skin and hair, in the iris and choroid of the eye, and in the meninges and substantia nigra of the brain. They also occur in malignant melanomas. (Chromaffin and enterochromaffin are similar pigments produced from the hormones epinephrine, norepinephrine, and serotonin by chromate fixation).

Common endogenous deposits include calcium, urates, oxalates, alcoholic hyaline and amyloid, and various materials produced by inborn errors of metabolism.

exogenous p.'s and deposits, pigments and deposits inhaled or ingested and found in the lungs or other tissues. These include carbon, silica, and beryllium dusts; asbestos and sugar cane fibers; aspirated oils and oily radiographic contrast media; and heavy metals. Carotenes ingested in excess stain adipose tissue and are termed lipochromes.

pigmentation (pig″men-ta′shun) 1. the deposition of coloring matter.

2. coloration, especially abnormally increased coloration of a part by the deposition or formation of a pigment.

pigment granules small masses of dense, colored material in the cytoplasm of cells, e.g., melanosomes.

pil/o (pi′lo) [L. *pilus* hair] a word element used in combining form to denote hair, e.g., pilocytic, pilomatrixoma.

Pila (pi′lah) a genus of freshwater snails. In the Philippines, the species *P. conica* is the second intermediate host of *Echinostoma ilocanum.*

pili (pi′li) [L.] plural of *pilus.*

Pilidae (pil′ĭ-de) a family of freshwater snails that includes the species *Pila conica,* the second intermediate host of *Echinostoma ilocanum.*

pilin (pi′lin) the phosphoprotein that composes the F pilus; M.W. 11,800. It forms a hollow tube when viewed under the electron microscope.

pill (pil) [L. *pila* ball] 1. a small oval or globular medicated mass to be swallowed. Cf. *tablet.*

2. a colloquial term for oral contraceptive; when so used, it generally is capitalized and has the definite article, i.e., the Pill.

pilocarpine (pi″lo-kar′pin) a cholinergic drug extracted from shrubs of the genus *Pilocarpus.* It stimulates the postganglionic parasympathetic (muscarinic) receptors, producing contraction of the pupil (miosis), sweating, and increased peristalsis and salivary and bronchial secretion.

Pilocarpine is applied topically to the eyes for the treatment of chronic open angle glaucoma and acute angle closure glaucoma; it improves drainage from the interior chamber, reducing interocular pressure. When taken internally, it produces adverse reactions including bradycardia, hypotension, nausea, and vomiting.

In clinical chemistry, pilocarpine is introduced into the skin by iontophoresis to produce sweating; see also *sweat test.*

pilomatrixoma (pi″lo-ma-trik-so′mah) [*pilo-* + L. *matrix* womb + Gr. *ōma* swelling] a benign neoplasm that differentiates toward hair cells. It forms a well-circumscribed, deep dermal nodule (1 mm to several cm in diameter) on the face, neck, or arms. Most of those affected are young individuals. The tumor contains islands of basophilic and "shadow" cells, and keratin, which is focally calcified.

pilonidal (pi″lo-ni′dal) [*pilo-* + L. *nidus* nest] characterized by a nidus or tuft of hair.

pilonidal sinus an acute abscess or chronic draining sinus in the sacrococcygeal area, associated with an underlying cyst that contains granulation tissue, fibrosis, and hair shafts. Infection, irritation, and acute suppuration are common. Treatment usually involves surgical incision and drainage, as well as removal of the hair, which acts as a foreign body and perpetuates the infection.

pilus (pi′lus), pl. *pili* [L. hair] 1. a filamentous appendage possessed by many gram-negative bacilli. Shorter and thinner than flagella, pili arise from the cytoplasmic membrane and contain the protein pilin. Their function is not known. Also called fimbria (L. "a fringe"). See also the accompanying illustration.

2. see *hair.*

F p., a hollow, tubular pilus on a male bacterial cell that forms a bridge with a female cell in bacterial conjugation to allow the transfer of genetic material. The letter F denotes fertility. See also the accompanying illustration.

sex p., see *F p.*

pimple (pim′p′l) a papule or pustule that may occur in any area of skin but most frequently appears on the face, neck, or upper back.

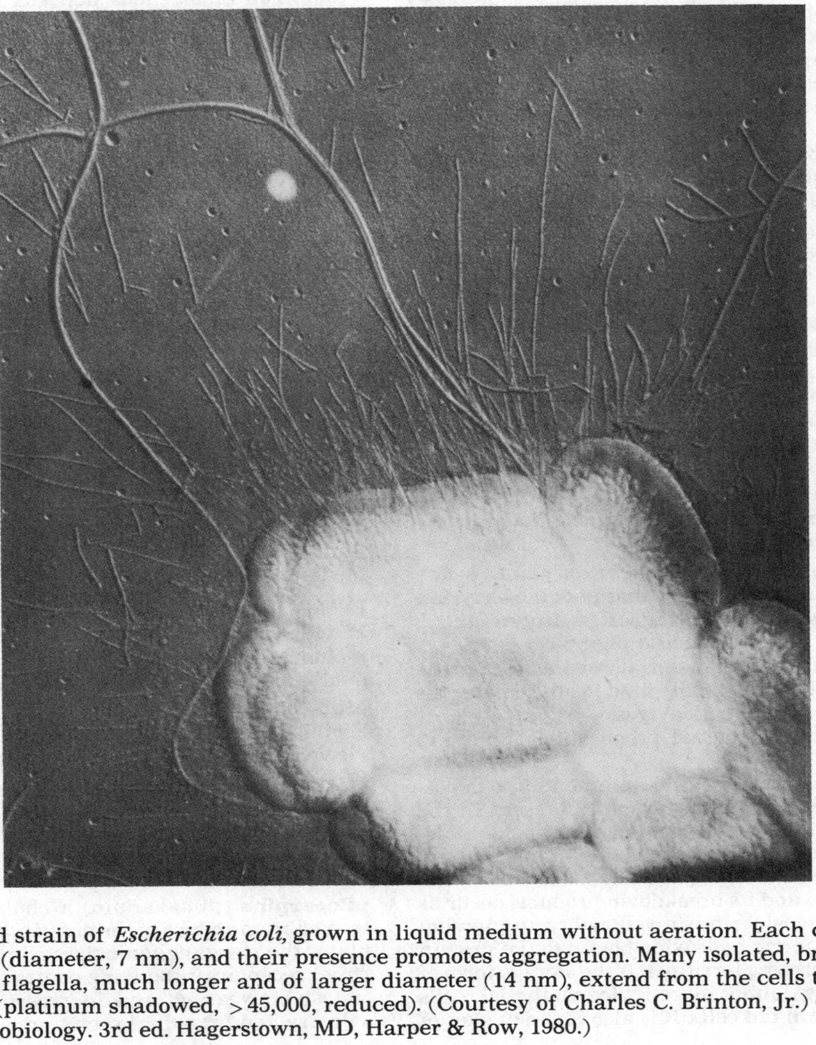

Pilus. Piliated strain of *Escherichia coli,* grown in liquid medium without aeration. Each cell possesses hundreds of pili (diameter, 7 nm), and their presence promotes aggregation. Many isolated, broken pili are also seen. A few flagella, much longer and of larger diameter (14 nm), extend from the cells to the edge of the photograph (platinum shadowed, >45,000, reduced). (Courtesy of Charles C. Brinton, Jr.) (From Davis, B. D., et al.: Microbiology. 3rd ed. Hagerstown, MD, Harper & Row, 1980.)

pine/o [L. *pinea* pine cone] a word element used in combining form to denote relationship to the pineal gland, e.g., pineoblastoma.

pineal (pin′e-al, pi-ne′al) [L. *pinealis*, from *pinea* pine cone] pertaining to the pineal gland.

pineal gland a small, cone-shaped body, weighing less than 200 mg, that lies between the superior colliculi on the dorsal surface of the upper midbrain; it is attached by a short stalk to the caudal end of the roof of the diencephalon.

The pineal gland is composed of two cell types, pinealocytes or parenchymal cells, and interstitial cells, which resemble glial cells and probably have a supporting function. The pinealocytes, which are grouped in cords and clusters, are stellate cells with cytoplasmic extensions that terminate in bulbous expansions on capillaries. They contain relatively large mitochondria, considerable amounts of smooth endoplasmic reticulum, and numerous microtubules.

A number of neurotransmitter substances have been located in the pineal gland, including melatonin, a 5-hydroxyindole, which the pinealocytes synthesize from tryptophan. In amphibians, this hormone inhibits the melanocyte-stimulating hormone; in humans, it is postulated that it may regulate some of the activities of the endocrine system. The pineal gland is innervated by sympathetic nerve fibers and is inhibited by light. As its activity increases with darkness, it may be responsible for inducing drowsiness.

Tumors of the pineal gland are uncommon. They may affect the hypothalamus, or compress the aqueduct and produce hydrocephalus. In young males, they have been associated with precocious puberty. Surgical removal of the pineal tumor is usually difficult; some are radiosensitive.

Also called pineal body.

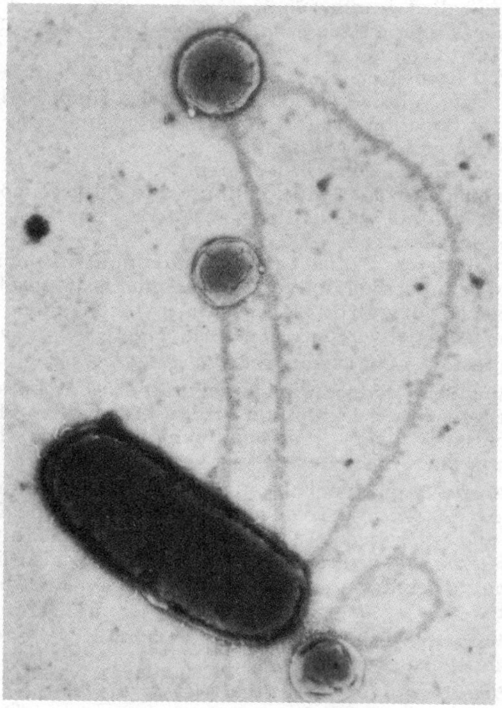

F pilus. Attachment of an F^+ *Escherichia coli* cell, by means of F pili, to three F^- minicells (products of mutants that occasionally separate a small cell without a nucleus.) The few long F pili are covered with F-specific MS2 phage particles. These phages are icosahedral; other filamentous, male-specific phages have been found to adsorb only to the tips of F pili. (From Davis, B. D., et al.: Microbiology. 3rd ed. Hagerstown, MD, Harper & Row, 1980; after Curtiss, R., III, et al.: Early stages of conjugation in *Escherichia coli.* Journal of Bacteriology *100*:1091, 1969.)

pinealocyte (pin′e-ah-lo-sit″) [L. *pinealis* pineal + Gr. *kytos* hollow vessel] one of the large, melatonin-secreting cells that comprise the bulk of the pineal gland. Its large, dark-staining nucleus has one or more prominent nucleoli, and processes of the pale-staining cytoplasm may terminate as bulbous swellings near or within the perivascular space. Also called *chief cell.*

pinealoma (pin″e-ah-lo′mah) [L. *pinealis* pineal + Gr. *ōma* swelling] the term proposed for a neoplasm that originates in the vicinity of the pineal gland, now believed to arise from ectopic germ cells and more appropriately designated as germinoma. See also *pineoblastoma* and *pineocytoma.*

pineoblastoma (pin″e-o-blas-to′mah) [*pineo-* + Gr. *blastos* bud + *ōma* swelling, tumor] a tumor of pineal cells, arising in the young, that resembles medulloblastoma and neuroblastoma in its histology and behavior. The tumor cells infiltrate and spread through the cerebrospinal fluid. Histologically, cytoplasmic processes are sparse (in contrast to pineocytoma), and Homer-Wright rosettes are seen. The tumor grows rapidly but is radiosensitive.

pineocytoma (pin″e-o-si-to′mah) [*pineo-* + Gr. *kytos* hollow vessel + *ōma* swelling, tumor] a tumor of pineal cells, occurring in adults, that is characterized by numerous cytoplasmic processes, rosette formation, and giant cells. It grows more slowly than a pineoblastoma, forming a circumscribed mass that projects into the third ventricle.

pine oil [NF], the volatile oil obtained by steam distillation of the wood of *Pinus palustris* and other species of *Pinus.* It is used as a deodorant and disinfectant.

ping-pong mechanism a double displacement reaction mechanism for a bisubstrate enzymatic reaction such as $A + B \rightleftarrows C + D$. Substrate A adds to the enzyme to give an EA complex, after which product C is released to give the stable enzyme intermediate E^* that differs from E. Intermediate E^* then reacts with (the second) substrate B to give the enzyme substrate complex EB, which yields (the second) product D, thus freeing enzyme E for another cycle.

pinguecula (ping-gwek′u-lah) [L. *pinguis* fat] a common degenerative condition that affects the cornea, particularly in the interpalpebral region where it produces a thickened yellowish area. It may be induced by actinic damage to the subepithelial collagen; histologic sections show an appearance similar to that of cutaneous actinic keratosis, often with some degree of epithelial atrophy, but occasionally, in the case of a large inflamed lesion, accompanied by pseudoepitheliomatous hyperplasia.

pinkeye (pink′i) a popular term for a highly contagious form of conjunctivitis caused by the Koch-Weeks bacillus (*Hemophilus aegyptius*). See also *conjunctivitis.*

pinocytosis (pi″no-si-to′sis) [Gr. *pinein* to drink + *kytos* cell + *-osis* condition] the process in which a cell imbibes fluids, seen to good advantage in endothelial and smooth muscle cells. A pocket forms in the cell membrane, which then closes over to engulf the particle and enclose it in a membrane-bound vesicle (pinosome) detached from the cell membrane. Cf. *phagocytosis.*

pinocytotic (pi″no-si-tot′ik) pertaining to or characterized by pinocytosis.

pinosome (pin′o-sōm, pi′no-sōm) [Gr. *pinein* to drink + *sōma* body] see under *pinocytosis.*

pinta (pēn′tah) [Spanish "painted"] a nonvenereal spirochetal infection caused by *Treponema carateum.* It occurs endemically in individuals living in areas of Central and South America and the Pacific. As pinta primarily affects the cutaneous areas, resulting in marked changes in skin color without affecting the viscera, the main problem is cosmetic disfigurement.

The primary stage is characterized by a nonulcerative, erythematous primary papule that progresses in a few months to an erythematous plaque. Secondary papulosquamous plaques with a variety of color changes (slate, lilac, black) develop on the face and extremities within a year. The final stage of the disease is marked by depigmentation of the lesions, which becomes mottled and porcelain-white. Hyperkeratosis of the soles and palms may occur.

Diagnosis of the disease is based on the appearance of typical signs in a patient living in endemic areas. The VDRL and FTA-ABS tests are positive but do not distinguish this condition from venereal syphilis. Darkfield examination is positive for spirochetes, which are indistinguishable from *Treponema pallidum.* Treatment with penicillin is effective.

Also called azul, carate, mal del pinto, and purupuru. See also *spirochete.*

pinworm (pin′werm) any oxyurid of the genus *Enterobius,* especially *E. vermicularis.* See also *E. vermicularis* under *Enterobius.*

pion (pi′on) [acronym from Gr. letter *pi* + *-on*] one of the three particles (π^-, π^0, π^+) that carry the strong force, i.e., the attraction between nucleons (protons or neutrons). The nuclei of atoms are held together by this force. Each pion is composed of a quark and an antiquark. Formerly called pi meson.

piperacetazine (pip″er-ah-set′ah-zēn) [USP], a piperidine-type phenothiazine major tranquilizer used in the management of psychotic disorders. See also *phenothiazine tranquilizers.* Trademark, *Quide.*

piperacillin (pip″er-ah-cil′in) see *penicillins.*

piperazine (pi-per′ah-zēn) [USP], a compound, diethylenediamine, used as an anthelminthic against *Ascaris lumbricoides* and *Enterobius vermicularis.* It blocks the effect of acetylcholine on worm muscle, resulting in a flaccid paralysis and expulsion of the worm by peristalsis.

piperidolate hydrochloride (pi″per-id′o-lāt) [USP], a synthetic parasympatholytic drug used as an antispasmodic for the gastrointestinal tract.

piperocaine hydrochloride (pi′per-o-kān″) a local anesthetic drug used primarily for surface anesthesia and also for infiltration and regional nerve block. Its toxicity and mechanism of action are similar to those of procaine.

pipet (pi-pet′) [Fr. *pipette* little tube, dim. of *pipe* tube] 1. a glass or transparent plastic tube used to measure or transfer small quantities of liquid. A pipet calibrated to contain less than 1 ml is often called a micropipet.

2. to use a pipet.

blowout p., a pipet calibrated to deliver its nominal volume, contained between the tip and a calibration mark, by permitting it first to drain and then by blowing out the last drop held in the tip. Blowout pipets are identified by the presence of an etched ring (or a pair of lines) at the mouth end of the pipet. Long, tube-type pipets are referred to as "serologic" pipets; those having their bulb close to the tip (to reduce the surface area) are called Ostwald pipets and are used for viscous fluids such as blood. This is one type of TD (to deliver) pipet.

graduated p., a pipet with a plain, narrow tube drawn out to a tip and graduated uniformly along its length. There are two types: Mohr, which is calibrated between two marks on the stem, and serologic, which has graduation marks down to the tip. Also called *measuring p.*

measuring p., see *graduated p.*

TC (to contain) p., see *washout p.*

TD (to deliver) p., a pipet calibrated to deliver a specific volume without rinsing with fluid. If the pipet is calibrated for blowout, an opaque ring is etched near the mouthpiece.

transfer p., see *volumetric p.*

volumetric p., a pipet calibrated to deliver a specific volume when filled to an etched mark. Also called *transfer p.*

washout p., a pipet calibrated to contain its nominal volume; after delivery of the contents, it must be washed out with diluting solution, which is added to the fluid delivered. Also called *TC p.*

pipette (pi-pet′) see *pipet.*

pipradrol hydrochloride (pi′prah-drol) a central nervous system stimulant drug used as an antidepressant. Adverse reactions include insomnia and anorexia.

Pirenella (pi″rĕ-nel′ah) a genus of snails. The species *P. conica,* a freshwater snail geographically found in Egypt, is the host of the intestinal fluke *Heterophyes heterophyes.* These snails may also discharge cercariae, which cause schistosome dermatitis.

piriform (pir′ĭ-form) [L. *pirum* a pear + *forma* shape] pear shaped.

Piroplasma (pi″ro-plaz′mah) [L. *pirum* pear + Gr. *plasma* something formed] the former name given to the genus *Babesia,* a protozoan parasitic in the red blood cells of animals. The species *P. donovani* is synonymous with *Leishmania donovani.*

Pirquet's reaction (per-kāz′) [Clemens Freiherr von *Pirquet,* Austrian pediatrician, 1874–1929] a tuberculin skin test used to determine previous infection with the tubercle bacilli. A positive reaction is determined by the presence of a raised red papule 24–48 hr after introduction of several drops of Old tuberculin into the cutaneous area. See also *Mantoux test.*

Pisces (pi′sēz) [L. *piscis* fish] a superclass of fishes, several species of which serve as secondary intermediate hosts of trematodes and tapeworms parasitic in humans. Others have poisonous spines and flesh that produce systemic intoxication.

pit (pit) 1. a hollow fovea or indentation.
2. to indent or become indented.

PITR abbrev. for plasma iron turnover rate. See under *ferrokinetics study.*

pitting function see under *spleen.*

pituitary (pĭ-tu′ĭ-tār″e) [L. *pituita* phlegm] 1. pertaining to the pituitary gland or its hormones.
2. the pituitary gland; see *hypophysis.*

anterior p., the anterior lobe of the pituitary gland (hypophysis). Also called *adenohypophysis.* See under *hypophysis.*

posterior p., the posterior lobe of the pituitary gland (*neurohypophysis*). Extracts of the posterior lobe of the pituitary gland of domestic animals contain oxytocin and antidiuretic hormone (ADH) which are used in the treatment of diabetes insipidus. See under *hypophysis.*

pituitary function test any test of pituitary function; see *adrenocorticotropic hormone stimulation test* and *metyrapone stimulation test.*

combined p. f. t., the simultaneous administration of thyrotropin-releasing hormone (TRH), luteinizing hormone–releasing hormone (LHRH), and insulin-induced hypoglycemia. The releasing hormones are used for the evaluation of gonadotropin and thyroid-stimulating hormone secretion, whereas insulin-induced hypoglycemia is used for investigating somatotropin, prolactin, and corticotropin secretion.

pituitary gonadotropin (PG, hPG) one of a group of hormones secreted by the pituitary, which enhances maturation of the testes and the ovaries. PG hormones include follicle-stimulating hormone and luteinizing hormone. For more information, see the specific hormones.

pityriasis (pit″ĭ-ri′ah-sis) [Gr. *pityron* bran + *-iasis* condition] a name originally applied to a group of skin diseases characterized by the formation of fine, branny scales. The term is now used only with a modifier.

p. alba, a chronic condition with patchy scaling and hypopigmentation of the facial skin.

p. rosea, a common mild, noncontagious, acute inflammatory skin disease of unknown etiology. It is characterized by the production of oval, fawn-colored eruptions of scales that follow skin cleavage lines, primarily on the trunk. These patches usually resolve spontaneously within 6 wk and confer a long-lasting immunity; the chronic form is rare. The lesions may be confused with those of mycotic infections (from which it should be differentiated by a potassium hydroxide test) or secondary syphilis (from which it should be differentiated by serologic tests).

p. rubra pilaris, a chronic inflammatory skin disease characterized by pink scales, macules, and follicular papules. It is associated with severe cases of seborrhea, especially of the face and head, and keratoderma of the palms and soles.

p. versicolor, see *tinea versicolor.*

Pityrosporum (pit″ĭ-ros′po-rum) [Gr. *pityron* bran + *sporos* seed] a genus of imperfect fungi of the family Cryptococcaceae. It is part of the normal endogenous flora of the skin and is an opportunistic pathogen, causing disease only under certain conditions. For example, a decreased rate of epithelial cell turnover enables *Pityrosporum* to cause tinea versicolor. There are two medically important species, *P. orbiculare* and *P. pachydermatis.* Also called *Malassezia.* See also *tinea versicolor.*

P. furfur, see *P. orbiculare.*

P. orbiculare, an opportunistically pathogenic fungus that causes tinea versicolor. It is part of the normal microbial flora of the skin. Microscopic examination shows a cluster of round, budding yeast cells mixed with short, septate hyphae. This appearance is sometimes described as "spaghetti and meatballs." *P. orbiculare* grows well at 37°C on malt agar or Sabouraud agar containing streptomycin, penicillin, and cycloheximide. Also called *Malassezia furfur, P. furfur,* and *P. ovale.*

P. ovale, see *P. orbiculare.*

pixel (pik′sel) [loosely, acronym from *pic*ture *el*ement] an element of a picture that has been divided into an array of small squares. The density of each pixel is represented by a number for computer processing. See also *computed tomography.*

Pizzolato's peroxide-silver method a staining method used to detect the presence of calcium oxalate in tissue sections. Slides are flooded with a solution of hydrogen peroxide and silver nitrate. The slides are briefly exposed to a bright white light to reduce the silver and then counterstained with safranin in acetic acid. The stain, which is specific for calcium oxalate, renders nuclei red and calcium oxalate deposits black.

PK abbrev. See *pyruvate kinase.*

p*K* the negative logarithm of the dissociation constant.

p*K′* the negative logarithm of the dissociation constant of an acid ($-\log K_a'$), where K_a' is expressed in terms of concentration (not activity), and concentration of water is included in the value of K_a'. The deviation from activity values is largely due to matrix effects such as ionic strength and viscosity, which can be observed in biologic fluids such as serum. For carbonic acid in serum, the pK' is 6.10. See also *pK.*

pK_a a measure of the strength of an acid defined as the negative of the logarithm of the acid ionization constant (K_a); $pK_a = -\log_{10} K_a = -\log_{10}([A^-][H^+]/[HA])$, where [HA], [A$^-$], and [H$^+$] are the undissociated acid, conjugate base, and hydrogen ion concentrations (taken to be equal to the activities) measured in moles per liter. In a solution having a pH equal to pK_a, the concentrations of the acid (HA) and its conjugate base (ionized form, A$^-$) are equal. The lower the value of pK_a, the stronger is the acid.

PK reaction abbrev. See *Prausnitz-Küstner reaction.*

PKU abbrev. See *phenylketonuria.*

pkV abbrev. See *peak kilovoltage.*

PL/I [acronym from *p*rogramming *l*anguage *one*] a high-level computer language developed by IBM for its Model 360 and 370 computers. It is flexible but complex and intended for both business and scientific applications.

placebo (plah-se′bo) [L. *placebo* "I will please"] an inactive substance, procedure, or preparation with no intrinsic therapeutic value, given to patients for various reasons. A placebo may be prescribed to satisfy the patient's symbolic need for drug therapy.

The "placebo effect" of influencing a person's threshold of pain through psychic or emotional factors is well documented.

Placebos are also used in controlled therapeutic trials to provide a basis of comparison for evaluating the efficacy of a medicinal preparation. With this procedure, the placebo is given to some individuals, whereas others receive the active drug. This method distinguishes between actual effects due to the drug and placebo effects due only to suggestion.

placenta (plah-sen′tah), pl. *placentas* or *placentae* [L. "a flat cake"] a transient, highly vascular structure connecting mother and fetus that functions as both an organ of exchange and an endocrine organ during gestation. At term, the placenta is a flattened, disk-shaped structure weighing approximately 500 g and possessing a smooth fetal surface and a roughened maternal surface. The maternal surface attaches to the uterine fundus and is separated from the muscular uterine wall by a layer of endometrial decidua. The fetal surface is in continuity with the fetal membranes (gestational sac). The fetal membranes consist of the inner smooth amnion and an outer roughened chorion. The former is lined by a simple squamous epithelium, whereas the latter is composed of an attenuated layer of chorionic villi (see below). The umbilical cord normally inserts near the center of the fetal surface, and supports two arteries and one vein embedded in a jelly-like matrix. The centrifugal branches of these vessels are visible under the amnion. These vessels connect the fetal circulation with the placental villous capillary network distributed throughout the chorionic villi. These in turn are exposed to the maternal blood that percolates through the placental sinuses. The maternal surface is roughened and fissured. The fissures are produced by placental septae, which delimit lobular units (lobules), sometimes incorrectly referred to as cotyledons.

The placenta develops from the outer layers of the implanting blastocyst (the trophoblastic cell mass). Early in development, this trophoblastic shell completely surrounds the amnionic sac and its enclosed developing embryo, but later there is accentuated growth of the trophoblastic layer at the implantation site to form the definitive placenta. The other portions of the trophoblastic shell disintegrate to form the attenuated chorionic membrane (chorion laeve).

Microscopically, the fully developed placenta consists of numerous branching chorionic villi immersed in pools of maternal blood. Chorionic villi have an inner core of stroma, which contains fetal capillaries, and an outer bilaminar layer of trophoblastic cells. The inner layer of cells—the cytotrophoblastic layer—is composed of cells possessing a single nucleus and clear cytoplasm. The outer syncytiotrophoblastic layer develops from the cytotrophoblast and is composed of cells with multiple nuclei and abundant eosinophilic cytoplasm. These cells possess a prominent microvillous border, visible ultrastructurally, that greatly increases their exchange surface. Early in gestation, both of these trophoblastic layers are prominent; in the last trimester, however, the cytotrophoblastic layer diminishes.

The placenta is the sole source of oxygen and nutrients for the embryo and its only means of excreting carbon dioxide and metabolites. In addition, large numbers of important small molecules (such as antibodies and hormones) are transmitted by the placenta from mother to conceptus. The placenta produces a wide variety of steroidal hormones and polypeptides. In particular, human chorionic gonadotropin (hCG) is produced by the syncytiotrophoblast. Its detection by assays of maternal blood or urine is the basis of pregnancy tests.

See also the accompanying illustration.

MICHAEL R. HENDRICKSON, M.D.

abruptio placentae, see *abruptio placentae.*

p. previa, the implantation and development of the placenta near the internal os of the cervix. The degree of resulting cervical occlusion may be partial or complete. This condition occurs approximately once in every 200 deliveries, and is more common in females experiencing their first delivery or who have abnormalities of the uterus. The primary symptom is acute, but painless, vaginal bleeding late in the third trimester. Extensive bleeding may necessitate cesarean section and blood transfusions. Diagnosis of this condition may require isotopic localization, soft tissue density radiographs or ultrasonic examination and localization of the placenta.

placental (plah-sen′tal) pertaining to the placenta.

placental and fetoplacental function tests the determination of human placental lactogen (hPL) and estriol in maternal serum during the third trimester. The synthesis of estriol involves both the placenta and the fetal adrenal glands; thus, the level of unconjugated estriol in serum is considered the best indicator of fetoplacental well-being. Serial determinations should be performed; a 50 percent decrease from one sample to the next is considered and indicative of fetal distress. hPL measurement is primarily a measurement of placental function.

placental lactogen, human (hPL) a single-chain polypeptide hormone formed by the trophoblast; M.W. 38,000. The placenta begins secreting this hormone in the fifth week of pregnancy. hPL has great structural similarity to growth hormone and possesses lactogenic and somatotropic activity. It promotes growth of the breasts and enhances milk production; it also has metabolic effects similar to those of growth hormone, e.g., inhibition of glucose uptake, stimulation of lipolysis, and enhancement of nitrogen and calcium retention.

hPL has clinical significance as a diagnostic and prognostic index of the functional status of the placenta. It is determined in maternal plasma by radioimmunoassay; the normal cencentration of plasma increases from 1 μg/ml at the twenty-second week of pregnancy to 8 μg/ml by end of term. Maternal serum hPL reflects the function of the placenta and in turn relates to the health of the fetus. hPL concentration usually exceeds 4 μg/ml after the thirtieth week of gestation; values that fall below this level are termed abnormal and in the fetal danger (FD) zone.

Also called *chorionic somatomammotropin* (CS).

placental villi see *chorionic villi.*

placentography (plas″en-tog′rah-fe) [L. *placenta* + Gr. *graphein* to write or draw] the radiologic imaging of the placenta after the injection of a contrast medium. The procedure is now usually replaced by ultrasonographic imaging.

Placidyl (plas′ĭ-dil) trademark. See *ethchlorvynol.*

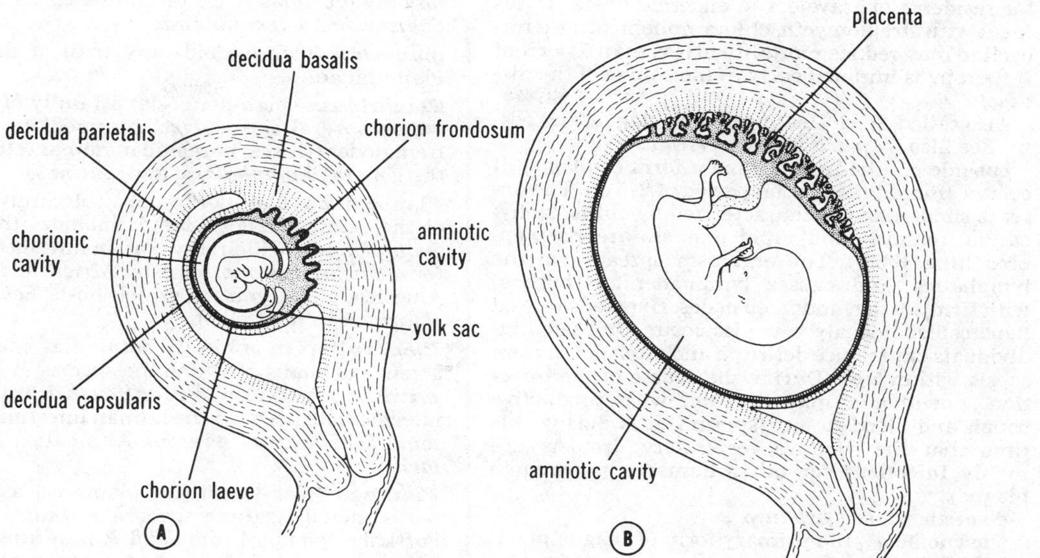

Placenta. Schematic drawing showing the relation of the fetal membranes and the wall of the uterus. *A*, End of the second month: note the yolk sac in the chorionic cavity between the amnion and chorion; at the abembryonic pole the villi have disappeared (chorion laeve). *B*, End of the third month: the amnion and chorion have fused, and the uterine cavity is obliterated by fusion of the chorion laeve and decidua parietalis. From Langman, J.: Medical Embryology. 4th ed. Baltimore, Williams & Wilkins Co., 1981.)

placode (plak′ōd) [Gr. *plax* plate + *eidos* form] a specialized patch or plate of embryonic ectoderm that, when in association with cells from other sources, develops into various sensory receptors and their accessory structures. Possessing a number of characteristics in common with neural crest cells, placodes develop into olfactory receptors of the nasal mucosa; epithelial walls of the membranous labyrinth and receptors in the semicircular canals; various primary sensory neurons associated with cranial nerves V, VII, VIII, IX, and X; the crystalline lens of the eyes; and some cells of the APUD system.

plagiocephaly (pla″je-o-sef′ah-le) [Gr. *plagios* oblique + *kephalē* head] a congenital malformation of the skull that results from the premature closure of the coronal and lambdoid sutures on one side. See also *craniostenosis.*

Plagiorchiidae (pla″je-or-ki′ĭ-de) a family of trematodes (flukes) of which the species *Plagiorchis javensis* is a member.

Plagiorchioidea (pla″je-or″ke-oi′de-ah) a superfamily of trematodes (flukes) parasitic in the intestines or lungs of vertebrates.

Plagiorchis (pla″je-or′kis) a genus of trematodes (flukes) of which the species *P. javensis, P. muris,* and *P. philippinensis* are rarely parasitic in humans.

plague (plāg) [L. *plaga,* probably from Gr. *plēgē* stroke] a severe, acute, febrile infection, which may occur in bubonic or pneumonic forms; it is caused by the gram-negative facultative or aerobic rod *Yersinia pestis.* This disease has a long history of precipitating massive human pandemics (e.g., the Black Death of the Middle Ages) and is still responsible for outbreaks of human disease in endemic areas of Asia and Africa.

Y. pestis frequently is endemic in rodents (rats, mice, squirrels, or prairie dogs) found in urban or wooded environments. This organism is usually transmitted from the infected rodent by a blood-sucking flea (often *Xenopsylla cheopis*), which acts as a transmission vector for humans. The flea inoculates the organism by regurgitation or defecation into a bite wound, establishing the primary site of infection. Local lymph nodes enlarge and become necrotic buboes—hence the name bubonic plague. When untreated, septicemia and secondary pneumonic plague ensue; terminally, petechiae and massive ecchymoses appear—hence the name Black Death.

Diagnosis is based on the isolation and culture of *Y. pestis* from needle aspirates of infected lymph nodes, blood, or sputum. *Y. pestis* is nonmotile, and stains in a bipolar "safety pin" pattern with Wayson or Giemsa stain. Smears stained with Wayson stain usually provide rapid presumptive diagnosis. Peripheral white blood cell counts in affected individuals usually are in the range of 12,000–20,000/μl, with a marked neutrophilia. There is disseminated intravascular coagulation, which may lead to purpuric spots on the skin. Electrocardiograms and liver function tests are usually normal. Serologic tests, including complement fixation, passive hemagglutination, and immunofluorescent staining, may also be required for diagnosis. Radiographic findings of pulmonary infiltration are suggestive of pulmonic involvement and require rapid and strict patient isolation.

Prevention of plague is based on rodent control and the use of repellents to reduce flea attacks. Immunization with killed plague vaccine is beneficial for residents or travelers in endemic areas. Treatment with streptomycin, chloramphenicol, or tetracycline may reduce mortality to less than 5 percent if therapy is initiated early in the course of the disease.

Also called Black Death, bubonic plague, and pestis. See also *Y. pestis* under *Yersinia.*

bubonic p., the most common form of plague. It occurs after an incubation period of 2–5 da. The onset is sudden and is characterized by chills, tachycardia, malaise, and rapid temperature rise (approaching 106°F). The organism spreads via the lymphatics, and causes lymphadenitis (buboes) with firm, tender, and fixed nodes. Hypotension and hepatosplenomegaly may also occur. Untreated individuals experience delirium and often death from sepsis within 5 da. During the course of the infection, pneumonia may develop, with productive cough and blood-stained sputum. It is during this time that the victim's respiratory droplets are highly infectious for other humans (pneumonic plague).

domestic p., see *urban p.*

pneumonic p., the primary form of plague pneumonia. It is transmitted among humans via inhalation of infectious droplets. After an incubation period of 2–3 da, there is high fever, tachycardia, severe headache, frothy and bloody sputum, and sepsis; death usually ensues unless treatment is rapidly initiated.

sylvatic p., a plague that occurs as an epizootic among wild forest rodents (e.g., squirrels, rabbits, pack rats, and prairie dogs). This reservoir represents a potential source for sporadic human infections. In the United States, sylvatic plague occurs in approximately 15 western states. Also called *wild p.*

urban p., a plague that has a primary animal reservoir consisting of wild urban rodents. Also called *domestic p.*

wild p., see *sylvatic p.*

plague bacillus see *Y. pestis* under *Yersinia.*

plain muscle see *nonstriated muscle.*

Planck's constant (*h*) (planks) [Max Karl Ernst Ludwig *Planck,* German physicist, 1858–1947] a fundamental physical constant; the quantum of action, 6.625×10^{-35} joule-second (J·S). See also *quantum mechanics.*

Planck radiation law [Max Karl Ernst Ludwig *Planck*] see under *blackbody radiation.*

plane (plān) [L. *planus*] 1. a flat surface that contains any straight line connecting two points lying in it. For more information, see the particular plane.
2. a specified level, e.g., a plane of anesthesia.
3. to rub away or abrade.

plan/i, plan/o (pla'nĭ, plan'o) [L. *planus*] a word element used in combining form to denote a plane or level, flat, e.g., planigraphy.

planigraphy (plah-nig'rah-fe) [*plani-* + Gr. *graphein* to write or draw] a type of body-section radiography. See under *tomography.*

planimeter (plah-nim'ĕ-ter) [*plani* + Gr. *metron* measure] an instrument used in measuring the area and perimeter of surfaces.

planimetry (plah-nim'ĕ-tre) the measurement of surface areas and perimeters by tracing the boundaries. Planimetry on photomicrographs or projected images is often used to evaluate the size of cells.

Planorbarius (pla"nor-bār'e-us) a genus of mollusks, which has been incriminated as a host of *Schistosoma haematobium.*

planorbid (plah-nor'bid) any snail of the family Planorbidae.

Planorbidae (plah-nor'bĭ-de) a family of snails of which several species are intermediate hosts for trematodes (flukes) parasitic in humans. It includes the genera *Biomphalaria* and *Bulinus.*

Planorbinae (plah-nor'bĭ-ne) a subfamily of snails of the family Planorbidae. It includes the genera *Biomphalaria,* which serves as an intermediate host for *Schistosoma mansoni* in Africa and tropical America, and *Gyraulus,* which hosts *Echinostoma ilocanum* in the Orient.

Planorbis (plan-or'bis) [L. *planus* flat + *orbis* ring] a genus of snails of which the species *P. guadaloupensis, P. olivaceus,* and *P. antiguensis* are the main intermediate hosts for the human intestinal schistosome *Schistosoma mansoni.* Also called *Biomphalaria.*

Plantago (plan-ta'go) [L. "plantain"] a genus of herbs including three species, *P. indica, P. ovata* Forskal (blond psyllium), and *P. psyllium* L. (Spanish *psyllium*), whose seeds (plantago, or psyllum seeds) are used as a cathartic. A preparation of the separated mucilaginous outer layers of the seeds of *P. ovata* is used as a bulk laxative.

plantar (plan'tar) [L. *planta* sole] pertaining to the sole of the foot. Cf. *dorsal.*

plantar wart a wart that grows on the plantar surface of the foot (sole); it usually becomes flattened, is covered by cornified epithelium, and may be exquisitely painful. These lesions represent benign epidermal proliferations due to infection with a human wart virus. If they occur in small, tight clusters, they may be referred to as mosaic warts. Also called *verruca plantaris.*

plantodorsal (plan"to-dor'sal) pertaining to a radiographic projection of the foot, in which the central ray passes from the plantar surface to the dorsal surface or to the calf.

plaque (plak) [Fr.] a general term used to describe any patch or flat area.

atheromatous p., a lesion of a large or medium-sized artery (especially the aorta and the iliac, femoral, coronary, and cerebral arteries), associated with atherosclerosis. Clinically significant plaque usually contains smooth muscle cells, connective tissue, and a mixture of intracellular and extracellular lipids and lipid complexes. Cell necrosis and calcification are also prominent. Atheromatous plaques may be associated with thrombotic occlusion of the lumen of an artery, rupture and release of plaque components, hemorrhage into the plaque, and dissection of the arterial wall. The pathogenesis of this lesion is unclear, but it appears to progress through three stages: fatty streaks of raised, soft, yellow accumulations of lipid within the arterial wall; fibrous plaque of raised, grayish-white, focal accumulations that contain both lipid and connective tissue cells; and complicated lesions, which contain all components of the atheromatous plaque.

See also *atherosclerosis.*

dental p., an accumulation of extracellular polysaccharides, bacteria (especially *Lactobacillus acidophilus, Streptococcus mutans,* and *Actinomyces viscosus*), and salivary glycoproteins on the surface of the teeth. It provides a suitable substrate and environment for bacterial adherence and multiplication and acid production. Accumulations of plaque are responsible for dental caries (tooth decay) and periodontal disease. See also *caries.*

Hollenhorst p., an atheromatous embolus seen in the retinal arteries, which frequently contains cholesterol crystals. These structures are seen on funduscopic examination as shiny, irregular, yellow patches.

skin p., a cutaneous lesion characterized by a group of papules that become confluent and create a raised, large, and well-circumscribed patch. Skin plaques may be associated with many cutaneous diseases, including psoriasis, syphilis, lichen planus, seborrheic and actinic keratosis, and epitheliomas.

-plasia (pla'ze-ah) [Gr. *plassein* to form] a suffix word element to denote formation, development, or growth, e.g., hyperplasia, aplasia.

plasm/o (plaz'mo) [Gr. *plasma* anything formed or molded] a word element used in combining form to denote plasma or the substance of a cell, e.g., plasmocyte, plasmapheresis.

-plasm (plazm) [Gr. *plasma*] a suffix word element to denote growth or formation, e.g., neoplasm.

plasma (plaz'mah) [Gr.] 1. a clear, yellowish fluid that accounts for about 55 percent of the total volume of the blood. It consists of 92 percent water, 7 percent proteins, and less than 1 percent of inorganic salts, and organic substances other than proteins, dissolved gases, and hormones. Plasma from which fibrinogen has been removed is called serum.

High-molecular-weight proteins dissolved in plasma include enzymes, as well as prothrombin and fibrinogen, which are associated with the clotting mechanism; immunoglobulins and complement proteins, all of which are involved in the immune response; and lipoproteins and glycoproteins. Small-molecular-weight organic substances include polypeptides, which function as hormones.

The plasma contains relatively high concentrations of sodium and chloride ions; other physiologically important ions found in the plasma include potassium, calcium, phosphate, magnesium, and bicarbonate. Glucose, amino acids, fats in the form of chylomicrons, VLDL, LDL, and HDL, and free fatty acids circulate in the plasma.

The analysis of the changes in the composition of blood plasma is a powerful diagnostic tool for indicating those metabolic activities that are not normal. Plasma volume is sometimes measured in order to calculate the total blood volume.

2. cytoplasm or protoplasm.

3. a highly ionized gas that contains an approximately electrically neutral mixture of free electrons and positive ions.

plasmablast (plaz'mah-blast) [Gr. *plasma* + *blastos* germ] a former term for an immature plasma cell. It is now recognized that plasma cells develop from transformed B lymphocytes. Immature forms seen in myeloma may display an abnormal nuclear-cytoplasmic ratio.

plasma cell a cell differentiated from the B lymphocyte and found in the lymph nodes, spleen, and connective tissue (particularly the intestinal mucosa); it participates in the body's humoral immune response through the production of antibody. The plasma cell has an abundant, basophilic cytoplasm, and a nucleus, which tends to be positioned asymmetrically. It can be recognized by the characteristic clumping of its nuclear chromatin around the periphery of the nucleus, giving it the appearance of the spokes of a wheel. Electron microscopy reveals a network of cisternae of rough endoplasmic reticulum, numerous attached ribosomes, and a prominent paranuclear Golgi complex. The cells sometimes contain eosinophilic granules or Russell bodies.

During an acute humoral immune response, greatly increased numbers of plasma cells can be seen in the lymph nodes and spleen. Immature forms enter the lymph and (in small numbers) the blood in response to the presence of a foreign antigen.

plasma cell dyscrasias a group of diseases characterized by an apparently uncontrolled proliferation of cells normally involved in antibody production, along with the production of a homogenous gamma globulin or its subunits. These diseases include multiple myeloma, Waldenström's macroglobulinemia, heavy-chain disease, amyloidosis, and "benign" monoclonal hypergammaglobulinemia. See also *lymphoproliferative disorder* and *monoclonal g.* under *gammopathy.*

plasmacytoma (plaz"mah-si-to'mah) [Gr. *plasma* + Gr. *kytos* hollow vessel + *ōma* swelling] a solitary neoplasm of plasma cells forming a discrete nodule that may be accompanied by sufficient immunoglobulin formation to be detectable by electrophoresis. Plasmacytomas may not be distinguishable histologically from foci of multiple myeloma, and they may be malignant (e.g., Waldenström's macroglobulinemia and multiple myeloma). See also *multiple m.* under *myeloma.*

plasmacytosis (plaz"mah-sĭ-to'sis) [Gr. *plasma* + *kytos* hollow vessel + *-osis* condition] the presence of excess plasma cells. Such a finding in the bone marrow or a soft tissue lesion is required for a definitive diagnosis of multiple myeloma; however, the condition can also occur in other diseases including collagen, vascular, and immune disorders, and in damaged marrow. A relative plasmacytosis may be seen in a depleted or hypoplastic bone marrow.

plasma exchange the removal of plasma from withdrawn blood, usually to a greater extent than in plasmapheresis, transfusion of the formed elements back into the donor; performed for removal of circulating antibodies or abnormal plasma constituents. The plasma removed is replaced by type-specific frozen plasma or albumin.

plasma iron turnover rate (PITR) see under *ferrokinetics study.*

plasmalemma (plaz"mah-lem'ah) [Gr. *plasma* + *lemma* husk] see *cell membrane.*

plasmalogen (plaz-mal'o-jen) see *phosphatidylcholine* and *phosphatidylethanolamine.*

plasma membrane see *cell membrane.*

plasmapheresis (plaz"mah-fĕ-re'sis) [Gr. *plasma* + *aphairesis* removal] the removal of blood, separation of plasma by centrifugation, and transfusion of packed cells suspended in a suitable anticoagulant medium back into an individual. Plasmapheresis is used to obtain plasma without wasting RBC and other blood cells in the treatment of certain diseases, such as macroglobulinemia syndromes. It is the treatment of choice for removal of excess IgM from the blood of individuals with Waldenström's macroglobulinemia.

plasma protein fraction (PPF) a heat-treated protein preparation derived from pooled human plasma. It contains albumin, alpha and beta globulins, and electrolytes, and is isotonic and isooncotic with normal plasma. PPF can be used for replacing intravascular volume and colloid without the risk of hepatitis. Care must be taken to avoid hypovolemic shock when infusing it, as vasoactive kinins may be present in the PPF and can precipitate a hypotensive episode.

plasma-thrombin clot method see under *cell block preparation.*

plasma thromboplastin antecedent (PTA) see *Factor XI.*

plasma thromboplastin antecedent (PTA) deficiency see *h. C* under *hemophilia.*

plasma thromboplastin component (PTC) see *Factor IX.*

plasma volume (PV) see under *blood volume measurements.*

plasma volume expander a preparation used to maintain blood volume until it can be replaced by physiologic processes, as in the treatment of shock or postoperative hypovolemia; as a primer fluid for heart-lung machines; and for volume replacement during leukapheresis. Examples are albumin, dextran, and hetastarch.

plasmid (plaz′mid) [*plasm-* + *-id*] an extrachromosomal genetic element that contains autonomously replicating, cyclic double-stranded DNA distinct from the bacterial chromosome. Plasmids contain genes that are not essential for bacterial growth. They are classified into incompatibility and compatibility groups. The number of plasmids within a cell is regulated by a replication repressor. If the plasmids within a cell line have the same repressor (incompatible), most cells end up with the same kind of plasmid. Incompatible plasmids cannot coexist within the same cell in the absence of strong selection for each type of plasmid. If plasmids are regulated by different repressors (compatible), each different type of plasmid can be maintained for generations within a cell line.

Classification of plasmids on the basis of phenotypic effects has decreased in importance since the finding that plasmids carry genes other than those for antibiotic resistance. Observed phenotypic effects include resistance to serum bactericidal activity; production of proteases, exotoxins, enterotoxins, surface antigens, H_2S, and chloramphenicol; and metabolism of various sugars and hydrocarbons. Some plasmids are cryptic, i.e., they have no phenotypic effect.

Replication of large plasmids is symmetric and bidirectional and is generally synchronous with host chromosome replication. Large plasmids use the cellular machinery for replication, but initiation is controlled by plasmid gene products. Small plasmids replicate usually in one direction and asynchronously with the host chromosome; they may not require any plasmid gene products. Plasmids are transferred during conjugation between sex pili and receptor sites of bacterial cells (see *conjugative p.*).

Theories on plasmid origin suggest that they were derived from cell chromosomes as small excisions of DNA that included the controls for autonomous replication. Plasmids developed a symbiotic relationship by assimilating genes useful to the bacterial host.

Plasmids are best known for the spread of microbial resistance to antibiotics (R plasmids). They also allow certain strains of bacteria to inhibit other strains (bacteriocinogens) and are fertility factors of bacterial conjugation (F plasmid). Plasmids are used in gene cloning and splicing. See also *cloning* and *gene splicing.*

conjugative p., a plasmid that is transferred from one bacterial cell to another during conjugation. See also *p. transfer.*

F p., a conjugative plasmid found in F^+ bacterial cells that leads with high frequency to its transfer and much less frequently to transfer of the bacterial chromosome. The F^+ cell (male donor) transfers the F plasmid across a conjugation bridge (F pilus) of pilin to the F^- cell (female recipient). Genetic material can be transferred in $F^+ \times F^+$ crosses, although $F^- \times F^-$ crosses are sterile.

An F plasmid can become integrated into the host chromosome of the F^+ cell, resulting in a 1000-fold increase in recombination. The F^+ cell is then an Hfr mutant and the integration is reversible at low frequency, usually restoring the original F^+. However, if the integrated F plasmid is excised imprecisely so that it carries part of the host chromosome, the resulting hybrid is called F′.

Also called *fertility factor.* See also *conjugation, F^+ cell, F^- cell, high-frequency recombination* (*Hfr*) *mutant,* and *integration.*

F′ p., a hybrid F plasmid that contains a segment of the host chromosome. These hybrids are transmitted to F^- cells with high efficiency, are easily separated from the chromosome in lysates, and are very useful for the transfer and isolation of selected genes. See also *F-duction.*

p. integration, the insertion of a plasmid into a bacterial host chromosome, which is achieved by a single cross-over between the two; in detachment, the cross-over is reversed. Most crossover sites are between insertion sequences in the plasmid and specific regions in the chromosome.

oligomeric p., a plasmid that contains tandem repeated segments of the R determinant or of an R gene within it formed by recombination between strands during replication; i.e., gene amplification has occurred. In cells resistant to a certain drug owing to the presence of an R plasmid, the addition of a subinhibitory concentration of the drug causes the cells to exhibit high resistance as a result of the selection of oligomeric plasmids.

R p., a conjugative plasmid that is responsible for resistance to various elements in bacterial cells, including antibiotics, metal ions, ultraviolet radiation, bacteriophage, and ethidium bromide. R plasmids are large, with two functionally distinct parts: a resistance transfer factor (RTF) consisting of genes for autonomous replication and conjugation, and a resistance determinant (R determinant) containing genes for drug resistance (R genes).

The selection for R plasmids by antibiotic therapy and the transfer of plasmids between bacterial species threatens the use of antibiotics as treatment for bacterial diseases. Plasmids have been found in Enterobacteriaceae and in the most prevalent anaerobic enteric organism, *Bacteroides.* Penicillinase-producing R plasmids were found in *Neisseria gon-*

orrhoeae after two decades of spread in enteric bacteria. Nonconjugative penicillinase-producing plasmids have been isolated from *Staphylococcus.*

Also called *R factor* and *resistance plasmid.* See also *antibacterial agents.*

p. transfer, the process by which a plasmid is passed from a bacterial donor cell to a recipient cell. For instance, during conjugation the F pilus of the F^+ cell attaches to an F^- cell receptor site. This process is associated with asymmetric DNA replication: one strand is nicked, transferred, and released; the cells then separate. The recipient cell synthesizes a complementary strand to the transferred strand and forms a circle.

Transfer is initiated at the origin (oriT) of the plasmid by a nick of the DNA sequence by a plasmid endonuclease. The mechanism of transfer is mediated by a transfer (tra) operon of localized genes for transfer and at least eight genes for the formation of the F pilus. Many other genes are associated with operon, such as those for DNA replication (rep) and incompatibility (inc). The transfer operon is repressed by fertility-inhibition (fin) genes, but derepressed by fin^- genes that form F pili. Most conjugative plasmids (such as R) do not form pili without this mutation. Other controls of the transfer operon include entry exclusion (cells that form the same type of pilus rarely mate), so that identical donors do not make useless exchanges, and the phenomenon of transient derepression, which ultimately results in low-frequency transfer.

The F plasmid can be transferred across species, e.g., *Escherichia* to *Salmonella* or *Shigella;* the efficiency of such transfers varies greatly.

See also *conjugation, integration,* and *transient derepression.*

plasmin (plaz′min) [*plasm-* + *-in*] an enzyme of the hydrolase class (EC 3.4.21.7), an endopeptidase formed from plasminogen by proteolysis, which results in multiple forms of the active plasmin. It hydrolyzes certain arginine and lysine peptide bonds, and catalyzes the hydrolysis of the insoluble fibrin of a blood clot into soluble components. Fibrin (fibrinogen) degradation products are produced when fibrin and fibrinogen are digested by plasmin. Normally, plasmin is neutralized by $alpha_2$-antiplasmin.

Activation of plasminogen can occur by an intrinsic pathway, partly dependent on activation of Factor XII to Factor XIIa, so that an event triggering clot formation may also trigger fibrinolysis. An extrinsic pathway is mediated by poorly characterized serine proteases, whose release from endothelial cells is induced by exercise, bradykinin, and a variety of drugs.

Also called *fibrinolysin.* See also *fibrin (fibrinogen) degradation products* and *fibrinolysis.*

plasminogen (plaz-min′o-jen) [*plasmin* + *-gen,* from Gr. *gennan* to produce] a beta globulin, zymogen (proenzyme); the inactive precursor of the fibrinolytic enzyme plasmin, found most abundantly in plasma but present in all body fluids. It can be activated by streptokinase, urokinase, and a proteolytic vascular tissue factor, and it coprecipitates with fibrin at the site of fibrin deposition. Also called *profibrinolysin.*

plasminogen activator a proteolytic enzyme that is capable of hydrolyzing arginine and/or lysine bonds and is highly specific for activating plasminogen. Only the activators in blood vessels (both veins and capillaries) are readily released by physiologic stimuli such as exercise, epinephrine, bradykinin, and many pharmacologic agents. Urokinase may be released during urologic surgery or in prostatic neoplasm. Streptokinase is used therapeutically for the dissolution of thrombi.

Plasmodiidae (plaz″mo-di′ĭ-de) a family of protozoa of the order Haemosporidia; it has a single genus, *Plasmodium,* which causes malaria in humans.

Plasmodium (plaz-mo′de-um) [*plasmo-* + Gr. *-odēs* like] a genus of sporozoa of the family Plasmodiidae, order Haemosporidia, that causes malaria in humans throughout the tropics in South America, Africa, India, and South Asia. The disease is parasitic in the red blood corpuscles of humans. Mosquitoes of the genus *Anopheles* are the host of the exogenous or anopheline phase of the parasites's life cycle. Four species occur naturally in humans: *P. falciparum, P. malariae, P. ovale,* and *P. vivax.* See also *malaria.*

P. vivax, the most common malarial parasite, which causes benign tertiary malaria. Vivax infections, transmitted by infected mosquitoes of the genus *Anopheles,* are found in areas in which malaria is endemic. Most infections are common in temperate zones as well as in tropical regions.

Clinical manifestations following an incubation period of approximately 10–17 da after infection include headache, muscular aches and pains, anorexia, nausea, occasional vomiting, and irregular remittent fever. Anemia and jaundice may occur. After a few days, the typical paroxysm is experienced: a sudden, shaking chill with an elevated temperature, followed by hot and then sweating stages. Initially, the periodicity of the paroxysms is usually irregular but is followed by establishment of a regular 48-hr cycle. A delayed attack of this relapsing species of malaria may occur within a few months and occasionally even up to a year or more after the patient's return from the malarious area.

Identification of the parasite in the peripheral blood with Giemsa- or Romanowsky-stained smears or thick films substantiates the clinical diagnosis. The trophozoites are ameboid, occupying one-third the diameter of the red blood cell, with a single chromatin dot. Schüffner's dots are present in the cytoplasm; the erythrocytes appear pale (hypochromic). Hemoglobin and red blood cell counts are usually reduced. Macrocytosis may be present owing to the increased number of reticulocytes and the enlargement of parasitized red blood cells.

Malaria caused by *P. vivax* is also called benign tertian malaria and *vivax malaria.* See also *malaria.*

plasmodium (plaz-mo′de-um), pl. *plasmodia* 1. a parasite of the genus *Plasmodium.*

2. a multinucleated cell or cell mass formed by repeated nuclear division without corresponding cytoplasmic fission.

plasmolysis (plaz-mol′ĭ-sis) [*plasmo-* + Gr. *lysis* dissolution, from *lyein* to loose] the contraction or shrinking of the protoplast away from the wall of a bacterial cell, due to exposure to a hypertonic solution.

plasmon (plaz′mon) the total extrachromosomal genetic material of an organism, which in humans consists primarily of the mitochondrial genes. Also called *plasmotype.*

plasmoptysis (plaz-mop′tĭ-sis) [*plasmo-* + Gr.

ptyein to split] escape of protoplasm from a cell through a ruptured cell wall.

plasmotype (plaz'mo-tip) [*plasmo-* + Gr. *typos* type] see *plasmon.*

plastic (plas'tik) [L. *plasticus;* Gr. *plastikos* from *plassein* to form] 1. tending to build up tissues or to restore a lost part.

2. conformable; capable of being molded.

3. a high-molecular-weight polymer containing additives such as plasticizers, filler, and dyes. It can be thermosetting or thermoplastic; thermosetting refers to formation by heating with the production of cross-linked hard, infusible products, whereas themoplastic refers to noncross-linked products that merely soften, without chemical change, on heating.

4. material that can be molded.

plasticizer (plas'tĭ-si″zer) any of a group of agents added to other organic or synthetic polymers to make them soft and flexible. Nonvolatile liquids and low melting point solids are common plasticizers. Copolymerization (such as that between ethyl acrylate and methacrylate to form Plexiglas) can also produce the desired flexibility; the result is "internally plasticized" polymers.

-plasty (plas'te) [Gr. *plassein* to form, mold, shape] a suffix word element to denote surgical repair, e.g., pyloroplasty.

plate (plāt) [Gr. *platys* broad, flat] 1. a flat structure or layer, chiefly of bone; see also *lamina* and *layer.*

2. in bacteriology, a flat vessel containing sterile solid medium for the culture of microorganisms, e.g., a Petri dish.

3. to inoculate a culture plate.

4. see *counting plate.*

limiting p., the layer of hepatic cells abutting the periphery of a portal tract.

liver cell p., the radially arranged lamina of hepatic epithelial cells. The normal adult liver plate is one cell thick and bounded on either side by vascular channels (hepatic sinusoids).

pour p., a bacterial culture poured into a sterile Petri dish from a test tube of melted and semicooled medium that has just been inoculated. This step is performed to obtain a pure culture or to count bacteria in a liquid by preparing dilution pour plates.

streak p., a plate of solid culture medium that has been inoculated by streaking an inoculum across the surface to obtain isolated bacterial colonies.

platelet (plāt'let) [*plate* + *-let* diminutive suffix] a disk-shaped nonnucleated cell structure, 2 μ in diameter, which is formed in the bone marrow from giant polyploid megakaryocytes. Platelets normally found in peripheral blood number 150,000–450,000 mm^3; in Wright-stained blood smears they appear as small, blue-gray disks containing red granules.

Platelets help to form the hemostatic plug by adhering to subendothelial connective tissue and aggregating with other platelets. When stimulated by very small amounts of thrombin formed very early in the process of coagulation or by connective tissue, platelets undergo "activation" and the "release reaction," releasing from their intracellular granules such potent substances as adenosine diphosphate (ADP), thromboxane A_2, prostaglandin endoperoxide PGG_2, and lysosomal enzymes. Additionally, platelets provide the surface for the activation of soluble coagulation factors and platelet factor 3, and are responsible for clot retraction.

Also called *thrombocyte.*

platelet-activating factor (PAF) a mediator of immediate hypersensitivity that is a poorly characterized lipid released from basophils during IgE-induced mediator release. It induces platelet aggregation and release of vasoactive amines, lysosomal enzymes, and prostaglandins from platelets.

platelet adhesiveness test a test that measures the adhesiveness of platelets to a foreign surface. A platelet count is performed before and after whole blood is exposed to a foreign surface for a standardized period of time. Diminished adhesion is seen in von Willebrand's disease and in some qualitative platelet disorders. Increased adhesiveness has been reported in individuals predisposed to thrombosis, but this is controversial.

Platelet adhesiveness methods include: (1) the Salzman method, which measures platelet adhesion (retention) when whole blood is exposed to a glass-bead column; (2) the Borchgrevink method, which measures platelet adhesion at the site of a small incision; (3) the Baumgartner method, which measures the adhesion and aggregration of platelets to the subendothelium of rabbit aorta; and (4) the H. P. Wright method, which measures platelet adhesion to the wall of a slowly rotating glass flask.

See also *Salzman method.*

platelet aggegation test a test that determines the response of platelets to a variety of aggregating agents including adenosine diphosphate (ADP), epinephrine, collagen, ristocetin, and arachidonic acid. Platelet aggregation is determined by measuring change in the optical density of stirred, platelet-rich plasma after the addition of an aggregating agent. The normal concentration of aggregating agents required to produce the characteristic response varies with the technique used.

In all methods, normal platelets reacted with ADP and epinephrine exhibit a primary- and secondary-phase reaction, and those with collagen, a single-phase reaction. Ristocetin is used to help rule out von Willebrand's disease, demonstrating a severely decreased or absent aggregating response. Arachidonic acid is used to eliminate aspirin as a possible cause of abnormal platelet aggregation; arachidonic acid does not overcome an aspirin-induced defect, and in that case will not produce normal platelet aggregation.

Defective aggregation is seen in a number of inherited and acquired thrombocytopathies such as thrombasthenia, von Willebrand's disease, and Bernard-Soulier syndrome.

platelet autoantibodies see under *antiplatelet antibodies.*

platelet concentrate a concentrated suspension of platelets harvested by centrifugation from freshly drawn whole blood. Platelet concentrate transfusion is indicated in the prevention of bleeding in patients with thrombocytopenia subsequent either to hypoplastic anemia, or to marrow failure due to chemotherapy or malignancy.

The platelets should be ABO-compatible with the recipient to maximize the therapeutic response, although ABO-incompatible platelets may be used if ABO-compatible platelets are not available. A single unit contains 5.5×10^{10} platelets, which should raise the platelet count of an average adult by $5–6 \times 10^3$

mm³. The platelets may be stored at room temperature (20–24°C) for up to 72 hr with gentle agitation.

platelet count the number of platelets in a representative blood sample, usually of venous blood using EDTA as an anticoagulant. Platelet counts can be performed by manual or automated techniques. Frequently used manual methods include the Brecher-Cronkite and Reese-Ecker methods. In the Brecher-Cronkite method (the reference method), the platelets are counted in a counting chamber using a phase microscope after the dilution of whole blood or plasma with 1 percent ammonium oxalate, which hemolyzes the red cells. In the Reese-Ecker method, whole blood is diluted in a solution containing brilliant cresyl blue, which stains the platelets a light blue. They are then counted in a counting chamber. Normal platelet counts have a range of 150,000–450,000/mm³, with a mean of approximately 250,000.

See also *blood cell count.* For information on automated methods, see *blood cell count automation.*

platelet-derived growth factor a protein contained in the alpha-granules of platelets (together with platelet factor 4 and beta-thromboglobulin), which stimulates the growth of human arterial smooth muscle cells and mouse fibroblasts in culture.

platelet factor 1 historically, absorbed Factor V from plasma. However, as platelets are now known to contain Factor V, the term is no longer in use.

platelet factor 2 historically, a platelet protein that accelerates the thrombin-activated conversion of fibrinogen to fibrin by increasing the peptide release from fibrinogen. The term is no longer in use.

platelet factor 3 a lipoprotein (phospholipid) component of the platelet membrane. Although the platelet membrane, including its lipoprotein content, continues to be a subject of intense interest and research in blood coagulation, this term is now seldom used.

platelet factor 4 antiheparin factor, a protein contained in the alpha-granules of platelets (together with beta-thromboglobolin and platelet-derived growth factor) and released following ADP-, thrombin-, or epinephrine-induced aggregation. It is capable of neutralizing the antithrombotic activity of heparin.

platelet-free plasma (PFP) a plasma preparation required for some coagulation studies obtained by prolonged centrifugation (30 min or more at high speeds, 8000 *g*).

platelet isoantibodies see under *antiplatelet antibodies.*

plateletpheresis (plāt″let-fĕ-re′sis) [*platelet* + Gr. *aphairesis* removal] the separation of platelets from donor whole blood by centrifugation and the return of the platelet-poor red blood cells and plasma to donor. This procedure can be performed in multiple-bag systems or in equipment especially designed for plateletpheresis. Common devices now available use continuous-flow or intermittent-flow centrifugation systems.

platelet-poor plasma (PPP) the plasma preparation used for most coagulation studies obtained by fast centrifugation (1600–2000 *g* for 5–10 min).

platelet retention test see *Salzman method.*

platelet-rich plasma (PRP) the platelet preparation required in some coagulation studies, as plasma obtained by slow centrifugation (at 75–100 *g* for 5–10 min or 300 *g* for 2 min) of whole blood.

platelet survival test a technique that measures the survival of platelets in the circulation. The patient's own or donor platelets labeled with ^{51}Cr sodium chromate or indium 111 in vitro are injected intravenously into the patient, and their survival studied. The normal survival time is 7–10 da. Shorter survival times are found in disorders that cause shortened platelet survival. Intravenously injected isotopes that are incorporated into the megakaryocyte—^{32}P sodium phosphate, ^{75}Se selenomethionine, and ^{32}P diisopropylfluorophosphate—have also been used to measure platelet survival.

platelike shaped like a plate, i.e., a cylinder with no appreciable thickness. See also the illustration under *contour.*

plating (plāt′ing) in microbiology, the act of applying an inoculum to the surface of a sterile solid medium in a Petri dish; the cultivation of bacteria, or preparing pour plate cultures. See also *pour p.* under *plate.*

platinosis (plat″ĭ-no′sis) [*platinum* + *-osis*] a form of occupational asthma that results from an individual's exposure, usually in refineries, to soluble, complex platinum salts. It is most commonly characterized by upper respiratory tract symptoms, including rhinorrhea, bronchospasm, and allergic skin reactions, including urticaria. Diagnosis is based on a history of occupational exposure, the presence of respiratory symptoms, documentation of immunologic sensitization to platinum, and abnormal pulmonary function studies.

platinum (Pt) (plat′ĭ-num) [Sp. *platina,* dim. of *plata* silver, metal plate] a malleable, ductile, silvery-white metallic element; atomic number 78; atomic weight 195.09; a 5d transition element; oxidation states +2, +4, and rarely, +1, +5, +6.

Platinum is employed (usually alloyed with other platinum group metals) in jewelry, electrical components, platinum resistance thermometers, thermocouples, and electrochemical electrodes; in the forms of platinum black (a powder) and platinum sponge (a gray, porous mass); it is used as a catalyst in the manufacture of acids and automobile catalytic converters. Platinum has low toxicity for most indivduals, although with chronic exposure, it may cause platinosis.

platinum group six metallic elements very similar in physical and chemical properties that are used together in corrosion-resistant alloys and as catalysts. They are the 4d transition elements—ruthenium (atomic number 44), rhodium (45), and palladium (46), and the corresponding 5d transition elements—osmium (76), iridium (77), and platinum (78).

platy- (plat′e) [Gr. *platys* broad] a word element used in combining form to denote broad or flat, e.g., platypodia.

platybasia (plat″ĕ-ba′se-ah) [*platy-* + Gr. *basis* base (of the skull) + *-ia*] a congenital or acquired malformation, which may be genetic or metabolic in origin; it is characterized by a flattening of the base of the skull, resulting in an increase in the angle between the orbital plates of the anterior fossa and the clivus of the posterior fossa of the skull. The normal angle, which is 135°, may be increased to 145° or more, as demonstrated by lateral radiographs of the skull.

Congenital platybasia is associated with Klippel-Feil syndrome, Arnold-Chiari malformation, and other congenital abnormalities. The acquired form is associated with metabolic bone diseases, such as rickets, osteitis deformans, osteomalacia, and osteogenesis imperfecta. If mild, this condition may be asymptomatic. Severe platybasia may cause neurologic signs, especially when the medulla, cervical spinal cord, and cranial nerves are displaced.

platyhelminth (plat″e-hel′minth) any member of the phylum Platyhelminthes.

Platyhelminthes (plat″e-hel-min′thēz) [*platy-* + Gr. *helmins* worm] a phylum of flatworms that is leaflike or tapelike and bilaterally symmetric, with three body layers; members of this phylum lack a body cavity and a circulatory system. The phylum consists of three classes: Trematoda (flukes), Cestoidea (tapeworms), and the free-living Turbellaria.

platykurtic (plat″e-kur′tik) pertaining to a probability distribution curve with a broad, flat peak. See also *kurtosis.*

platypellic (plat″e-pel′ik) [*platy-* + Gr. *pella* bowl] having a wide, broad pelvis with a pelvic index below 90.

platypelloid (plat″e-pel′oid) [*platy-* + Gr. *pella* bowl + *eidos* form] a term used to describe a pelvis that is flattened at the brim and has a shortened anteroposterior dimension. The promontory of the sacrum is usually pushed forward, but the transverse diameter is often normal. This type of pelvis is found in fewer than 5 percent of Caucasian females and even less frequently in persons of other races.

platypnea (plah-tip′ne-ah) [*platy-* + Gr. *pnoia* breath] dyspnea induced by an upright position and relieved by a recumbent position. Cf. *orthopnea.*

ple/o (ple′o) [Gr. *pleōn* more] a word element used in combining form to denote more, e.g., pleomorphic.

pleated sheet a type of secondary structure in protein molecules in which portions of extended polypeptide chains are arranged linearly and side by side. The direction of the side-by-side chains may be either parallel (i.e., NH_2^- terminal to $COOH^-$ terminal residues running in the same direction) or antiparallel (i.e., chains running in opposite directions). Also called *β-stucture.* See also under *protein.*

PLED abbrev. See *periodic lateralized epileptiform discharge.*

-plegia (ple′je-ah) [Gr. *plēgē* a blow, stroke] a suffix word element to denote paralysis and palsy, e.g., paraplegia.

pleiotropy (pli-ot′ro-pe) [Gr. *pleiōn* more + *tropē* a turning] the production of diverse phenotypic effects produced by a mutation in a single gene. Also called *polypheny.*

pleocytosis (ple″o-si-to′sis) [*pleo-* + Gr. *kytos* hollow vessel + *-osis*] a general term used to refer to a greater-than-normal number of cells in a given area.

pleomorphic (ple″o-mor′fik) [*pleo-* + Gr. *morphē* form] occuring in various distinct forms; exhibiting pleomorphism; a common property of certain types of microorganisms and neoplastic cells.

pleomorphic lipoma a rare benign neoplasm of fat cells, characterized by an admixture of lipocytes, spindle cells, and bizarre giant cells. Pleomorphic lipoma must be distinguished histologically from liposarcoma or myxoid malignant, fibrous histiocytoma.

pleomorphism (ple″o-mor′fism) [*pleo-* + Gr. *morphē* form] 1. the ability of an organism or species to exist in several sizes or forms.

2. in cytology, the abnormal, irregular, and bizarre cell and nuclear shapes that characterize neoplastic cells in contrast to the regularity and uniformity of normal cells.

3. variation in the size and shape of cells or nuclei.

pleonosteosis (ple″on-os″te-o′sis) [*pleo* + Gr. *osteon* bone + *-osis*] a general term that refers to abnormally increased ossification of bones.

Léri's p., a hereditary congenital condition, transmitted as an autosomal dominant trait, that is characterized by abnormally increased ossification of the epiphyses of long bones; shortening of the extremities; limitation of movement; and swollen, deformed joints.

plerocercoid (ple″ro-ser′koid) [Gr. *plēroun* to complete + *kerkos* tail + *eidos* form] one of the four main types of larval stages of certain cestode tapeworms parasitic in the tissues of vertebrates and invertebrates. These larvae are solid and elongated, with the head invaginated only into the neck.

plerocercus (ple″ro-ser′kus) [Gr. *plēroun* to complete + *kerkos* tail] a type of larval stage of certain cestode tapeworms found in the tissues of vertebrates and invertebrates. The larvae are solid and relatively globular, with the head of the worm invaginated into the body.

plesiocassette (ple″se-o-kah-set′) a type of multiscreen cassette. See also *simultaneous multifilm t.* under *tomography.*

Plesiomonas (ple″se-o-mo′nas) [Gr. *plesios* near + *monas* monad, e.g., near to *Aeromonas*] a genus of bacteria of the family Vibrionaceae, which are of gram-negative, facultatively anaerobic rods with polar flagella. It occurs primarily in water and may infect humans, causing diarrhea, especially in tropical and subtropical areas. The organisms are catalase- and oxidase-positive, and ferment glucose, lactose, and inositol. There is a single species, *P. shigelloides.*

plethysmogram (ple-thiz′mo-gram) [Gr. *plēthysmos* increase + *gramma* a mark] the graphic record of volume changes made by a plethysmograph.

plethysmograph (ple-thiz′mo-graf) [Gr. *plēthysmos* increase + *graphein* to write] an instrument used to determine and record changes in the volume of an organ, limb, or part, or in the amount of blood flow through these structures.

finger p., a device to record rapid changes in the volume of a finger reflecting variation in the quantity of the blood flowing through it.

whole body p., an airtight body box (large enough to accommodate a seated individual) connected to a sensitive pressure transducer that allows for the recording of alveolar pressure (and thoracic volume) changes during the respiratory cycle.

plethysmography (pleth″iz-mog′rah-fe) a technique designed to record small variations in the volume of an organ, limb, or whole body. Limb impedance plethysmography is a sensitive and specific means of diagnosing and following acute venous obstruction and arterial insufficiency. It measures the change in the volume of the limb with each arterial pulsation and during cuff occlusion of the venous flow from the limb. Careful manipulation of the occluding cuff allows an observer to evaluate either arterial or venous flow in the limb. Whole body plethysmography can be used to measure the total volume of gas in the lungs, including air that may be trapped behind poorly communicating air spaces. This type of measurement is important to the diagnosis of chronic obstructive pulmonary disease (COPD).

venous occlusion p., a technique used to measure the blood flow into a limb. The limb is placed in a watertight chamber (plethysmograph) connected to a volume recorder. Any changes in the volume of the limb are recorded as displacements in the volume of water in the chamber.

Venous flow from the limb is briefly occluded by a pressure cuff. During the first few seconds after occlusion, the limb volume increases at a rate that is a function of the arterial blood flow. The rate of arterial flow (measured in milliliters per minute) equals the slope of the volume record.

whole body p., a technique that can be used to record thoracic gas volume (TGV), airway resistance, and pulmonary capillary blood flow by means of an airtight chamber (plethysmograph) connected to a volume recorder. The pressure in the chamber is recorded with a sensitive transducer, and is found to increase and decrease as the subject's chest expands and contracts with inspiration and expiration, respectively (owing to alternate expansion and compression of the alveolar gas).

In the measurement of TGV, the subject breathes the surrounding air while pressures in the plethysmograph and airway pressure are simultaneously recorded. It is assumed that alveolar pressure is equal to the airway pressure when airflow stops, or to atmospheric pressure at end-expiration; the TGV is unknown at this point. When the subject is made to inspire against an occluded airway, a new gas volume and pressure are measured, providing the data needed to calculate the original, unknown TGV through application of Boyle's law.

In the measurement of airway resistance, pressure in the plethysmograph and airflow (using a pneumotachograph) are simultaneously measured while the subject pants. The product of airway resistance and lung volume can be found as the slope of the sigmoidal X-Y plot relating the flow and pressure changes. The airway is then occluded while the subject again pants. The slope of the linear X-Y plot of the resulting pressure changes at the mouth and chest is equal to the lung volume. Airway resistance can then be calculated as the product of resistance and lung volume divided by the lung volume.

Pulmonary capillary blood flow can be measured when a subject in a plethysmograph inhales a mixture of 80 percent nitrous oxide and 20 percent oxygen from a bag. As this mixture gradually dissolves in the pulmonary capillary blood, pressure in the plethysmograph gradually decreases. The pulsatile flow of the pulmonary capillary blood can thus be traced. Instantaneous flow can be calculated through the use of alveolar volume (plethysmographic) measurements and knowledge of the alveolar N_2O pressure and solubility of the gas in the blood.

pleur/o (ploor′o) [Gr. *pleura* rib, side] a word element used in combining form to denote the pleura, e.g., pleuritis.

pleura (ploor′ah), pl. *pleurae* [Gr. "rib, side"] [NA], the thin, serous membrane that lines the thoracic cavity and invests the lungs. The pleurae form two distinct sacs, right and left, within which the visceral pleura covers the surface of the lungs and the parietal pleura lines the chest cavity and diaphragm and covers the mediastinum. The pleura is well invested with capillaries and lymphatic vessels, which aid in producing a serous secretion that moistens the mesothelial surfaces, thereby facilitating movements of the lungs.

localized fibrous tumor of p., a lesion of the pleura that commonly has a plaquelike appearance. It is composed of fibroblasts in a collagenous stroma. These lesions may represent focal areas of reactive fibrosis rather than true neoplasms.

pleural (ploor′al) pertaining to the pleura.

pleural effusion the accumulation of fluid within the pleural spaces that occurs either as a result of disease involving the pleurae or as a result of diseases of other organs that affect the dynamics of pleural fluid production. Many diseases of the lungs and pleurae, including pleural or malignant pulmonary neoplasms (primary or metastatic), tuberculosis, connective tissue diseases, pneumonia, and lung trauma, may produce pleural effusions. In addition, diseases affecting other organs (e.g., congestive heart failure, pancreatitis, subdiaphragmatic abscess, certain ovarian tumors) are often the cause. Pleural effusions, especially those associated with inflammation of the pleurae (pleurisy), are frequently accompanied by pain (pleuritic pain), often at or near the site of involvement, that characteristically increases with deep inspiration.

Radiographs of the chest show a characteristic upwardly convex fluid level at the costophrenic angles or even across one or both diaphragms. Collections of pleural fluid within the major and minor fissures of the lungs produce rounded densities on the radiographs, which have the appearance of tumors within the lung—so called "pseudotumors." Diagnosis of the underlying process often depends on analysis of the pleural fluid. Fluids that are primarily transudates (containing electrolytes, a small amount of protein, and few cellular elements) are formed by processes resulting in increased hydrostatic pressure or capillary permeability, and are often associated with diseases not directly involving the pleurae. Exudative fluid, containing large amounts of protein and cellular elements, including inflammatory cells, is characteristic of diseases that cause damage to the pleura themselves, local inflammation, or failure of lymphatic protein removal.

See also *pleural fluid examination.*

pleural fibroma a benign, spindle cell neoplasm arising from the pleural surface, which is composed of fibroblasts or myofibroblasts within a collagenous stroma.

pleural fluid the thin, serous fluid that covers the pulmonary and parietal pleura, and provides lubrication for the lungs and thoracic wall during ventilation. A rise in intrapleural pressure during expiration forces excess fluid into the lymphatic channels of the mediastinum and parietal pleura.

pleural fluid examination the study of pleural fluid by routine and special procedures to determine its etiology or the presence of a disease process. The color is pale yellow and clear; specific gravity, 1.010–1.026; total protein, 0.3–4.1 g/100 ml (albumin, 50–70 percent; globulin, 30–45 percent; fibrinogen, 0.3–4.5 percent); and pH, 6.8–7.6. Glucose is less than 60 mg/dl. The normal total amount of fluid is less than 20–30 ml.

Pleural transudates generally have specific gravity values of less than 1.015, total protein contents of less than 2.5 g/100 ml, low cell counts, ratios of pleural fluid to serum lactic dehydrogenase (LDH) that are less than 0.6, and pleural fluid LDH concentrations of less than 200 IU. Pleural exudates generally have specific gravity values of greater than 1.018, total protein contents of greater than 3 g/100 ml and ratios of pleural fluid to serum LDH that are greater than 0.6.

See also *pleural effusion.*

pleuralgia (ploor-al′je-ah) [*pleur-* + Gr. *algos* pain + *-ia*] a general term used to describe pain in the pleura. It is the most common symptom of pleural disease originating in the parietal pleura. The pain tends to be sharp, is aggravated by respiration and coughing, and is referred to different locations in the body. Respiratory movements may be affected by pleuralgia. Common causes of this symptom include pericarditis, pneumonia, pleurisy, pneumothorax, neoplasms, and fibromyositis. See also *pleurisy.*

pleurisy (ploor′ĭ-se) [*pleur-* + Gr. *-itis* inflammation] an inflammation of the pleura occurring as a result of injury (such as pneumonia or pulmonary infarct), infection, irritation, or invasion by neoplastic cells. The pleura becomes swollen and congested, and inflammatory cell infiltration, fluid exudation, and fibrosis may occur. Healing frequently results in fibrous adhesions.

Onset of pleurisy is often sudden. Pain, aggravated by coughing or breathing, is the most frequent symptom. As a result, respiration is often rapid and shallow, and dyspnea is common. If pleural effusion develops, the pain subsides and decreased breath sounds, percussion dullness, and egophony may be heard.

Diagnosis is based primarily on the association of pleuritic pain with pleural friction rubs and/or effusion. Rubs may present as fine crackles, harsh grating, or creaking sounds on inspiration and expiration. Chest radiographs may demonstrate the presence of pleural effusion or pleural thickening. Thoracentesis is used to obtain fluid for chemical, bacteriologic, and cytologic examinations.

Also called *pleuritis. See also pleural fluid examination.*

pleuritis (ploo-ri′tis) see *pleurisy.*

Pleuroceridae (ploor″o-ser′ĭ-de) a family of mollusks of which several species are intermediate hosts of *Paragonimus westermani, Clonorchis sinensis,* and *Troglotrema salmincola.*

pleurodynia (ploor″o-din′e-ah) [*pleuro-* + Gr. *odynē* pain] a paroxysmal and spasmodic pain in the intercostal muscles, most commonly due to infection with group B coxsackieviruses.

epidemic p., an acute, febrile infectious disease, due to infection with group B coxsackieviruses or other enteroviruses, that is characterized by sudden, sharp, and spasmodic pain in the intercostal region of the chest or abdomen. It is most common in children; those affected may experience prodromal symptoms (headache, anorexia, and myalgia) followed by spasmodic pain in the lower rib cage or upper abdomen. This pain is aggravated by respiration, moving about, coughing, and sneezing. Fever, tenderness, sore throat, and muscle swelling may be present. The disease usually appears in epidemics, lasts for 3–7 da, and tends to recur.

Diagnosis is based on recovery, and identification of the virus from throat washings or feces and demonstration of a rise in specific antivirus antibodies. Complication include orchitis, pleurisy, aseptic meningitis, and hepatitis. Involvement of the lower abdomen may simulate acute surgical conditions. Treatment is symptomatic.

Also called *Bornholm disease,* devil's grip, epidermic myalgia, and *Sylvest's disease.*

pleurography (ploo-rog′rah-fe) [*pleuro-* + Gr. *graphein* to write] the radiographic examination of the pleural cavity and the pleura. The normal quantity (20–30 ml) of pleural fluid usually is not visible in radiographs of the chest in upright patient and is only slightly visible in decubitus films. However, fluid accumulations, as well as other forms of pleural disease, may be diagnosed with this procedure; it may also serve as a guide for the selection or appropriate therapy.

pleurohepatitis (ploor″o-hep″ah-ti′tis) [*pleuro-* + Gr. *hēpar* liver + *-itis*] the inflammation of both the liver and the portion of the pleura near the liver. This condition may occur in association with hepatic abscesses or hepatitis, and commonly ascends by continuity through the diaphragm to involve the pleural spaces, usually on the right side.

pleuropneumonia (ploor″o-nu-mo′ne-ah) [pleuro- + Gr. *pneumonia* pneumonia, from *pneumōn* lung] 1. a pneumonia that also involves the pleural surfaces (pleurisy).

2. a disease attributable to infection with pleuropneumonia-like organisms (i.e., *Mycoplasma*). See also *primary atypical p.* under *pneumonia.*

pleuropneumonia-like organisms (PPLO) see under *mycoplasma.*

pleuroscopy (ploor-os′ko-pe) [*pleuro-* + Gr. *skopein* to examine] a procedure used to visually assess the pleura; it may be performed in association with mediastinoscopy. Pleuroscopy is primarily indicated to obtain diagnostic information about thoracic disease and to assess the extent and involvement of inflammatory disease or metastatic malignancies affecting the pleura.

plex/o (plek′so) [L. *plexus* a plait] a word element used in combining form to denote plexus or nerve network, e.g., plexitis.

plexiform (plek′sĭ-form) [L. *plexus* plait + *forma* form] resembling a plexus or network.

Plexiglas (pleks′ĭ-glas) trademark for transparent, thermoplastic polymers of the methyl methacrylate type, made by the copolymerization of methyl methacrylate with a small amount of ethyl acrylate. Plexiglas is available in beads, granules, and sheets for such diverse uses as in the manufacture of lenses, ornaments, light diffusers, glazing, chalkboards, windshields, and letters for signs, canopies, and windows.

plexitis (plek-si′tis) [*plex-* + *-itis* inflammation] a general term used to describe the inflammation of a plexus of nerves, usually the brachial plexus. It has a variety of causes including infection, trauma, and allergic reactions. Also called brachial plexus neuritis and Parsonage-Turner syndrome. See also *plexus neuropathies.*

plexus (plek′sus), pl. *plexus* or *plexuses* [L. "plait"] a general term for a network of interconnected, linear structures, such as lymphatic vessels, nerves, or veins.

Auerbach's p., see *myenteric p.*

brachial p., a neural plexus originating from the ventral branches of the last four cervical and first thoracic spinal nerves. Situated in the neck and axilla, one part is situated next to the subclavian artery and gives off the dorsal scapular, long thoracic, subclavian, and suprascapular nerves. Another part is situated along the axillary artery and gives off branches to the medial and lateral pectoral, median brachial cutaneous, median antebrachial cutaneous, median, ulnar, radial, subscapular, thoracodorsal, and axillary nerves.

cervical p., a plexus formed by the ventral rami of the upper four cervical nerves. Its branches are distributed to parts of the head, neck, chest, and diaphragm.

enteric p., a network of autonomic nerve fibers within the wall of the digestive tract, composed of the myenteric, submucosal, and subserosal plexuses. Its components are visceral afferent fibers; sympathetic postganglionic fibers; parasympathetic preganglionic and postganglionic fibers; and parasympathetic postganglionic cell bodies. The enteric plexus regulates the tone and coordinates the movement of the gastrointestinal smooth muscle.

lumbar p., a nerve plexus in the posterior part of the psoas major, formed by the ventral branches of the first three lumbar nerves and part of the fourth.

Meissner's p., *see submucosal p.*

myenteric p., part of the enteric plexus. It lies between the circular and longitudinal layers of the external muscle of the GI tract. Also called *Auerbach's plexus.* See also *enteric p.*

submucosal p., the portion of the enteric plexus located on the submucosal surface of the external smooth muscle layer of the GI tract. Also called *Meissner's plexus.* See also *enteric p.*

subserosal p., the portion of the enteric plexus deep to the serosal layer of the digestive tube.

plexus block the administration of an analgesic to a nerve plexus to block pain and temperature sensations from the peripheral nerves, a procedure that requires a detailed knowledge of nerve distribution, fascial planes, and anatomic structures.

plexus neuropathies disease processes that involve major nerve plexuses, primarily the brachial and lumbosacral plexuses. Injury to the brachial plexus may be idiopathic or due to traction, wounds, compression, infection, or allergic reactions. Onset is associated with paresthesia, and muscle weakness. Recovery is usually complete but may require months or years.

Neurologic examination and electromyography may help to establish the degree of extremity involvement. Myelography may be required to rule out a spinal cord lesion.

See also *plexitis.*

plica (pli′kah), pl. *plicae* [L.] a general term for a ridge or fold, as of peritoneum or other membrane. See also *fold.*

plicate (pli′kāt) [L. *plicatus,* past participle of *plicare* to fold] plaited or folded.

ploidy (ploi′de) [Gr. *-ploos* -fold, as in *diploos* twofold + *-oeidēs* having the form of, from *eidos* form] the status of a chromosome set in the karyotype.

-ploidy a suffix word element to denote the degree of multiplication of chromosome sets, as in aneuploidy, diploidy, haploidy, etc.

plotter (plot′er) 1. a computer output device that produces charts and graphs by making a pen-and-ink drawing under program control. Also called XY plotter.

2. an electromechanical device that produces a graph, such as a chart recorder.

plug (plug) an obstructing mass that closes or blocks an opening or lumen of a tube. Plugs may be epithelial, such as those found in the external nares of the fetus at birth, or mucous, such as that closing the cervical canal during pregnancy.

plumbism (plum′bizm) [L. *plumbum* lead] a chronic form of lead poisoning due to the inhalation, absorption, or ingestion of lead or lead salts. For the symptoms of lead poisoning, see under *lead.*

Plummer's disease (plum′erz) [Henry Stanley *Plummer,* American physician, 1874–1937] a disorder characterized by the overproduction of thyroid hormone by one or more hypersecreting, autonomous, adenomatous nodules or a multinodular toxic goiter. The disease tends to occur in older people and may not always present with thyrotoxicosis.

Serum T_3 concentration is always elevated; serum T_4, T_3,-resin uptake, and radioiodine uptake may be elevated. The nodules of Plummer's disease are autonomous and not under the control of the normal hypothalamic-pituitary axis. Suppression of TSH secretion does not inhibit ^{131}I uptake in these nodules. Also called *nodular toxic goiter.* See also *hyperthyroidism.*

Plummer's nails [Henry Stanley *Plummer*] fingernail changes that are characteristic of Plummer's disease: the nails are thin and the nail beds receded. Concave erosions may be visible under the distal end of the nails, especially those of the fourth digits. Similar changes are also due to onycholysis. See also *hyperthroidism, oncholysis,* and *Plummer's disease.*

Plummer-Vinson syndrome (plum′er vin′son) [Henry Stanley *Plummer*; Porter Paisley *Vinson,* American surgeon, born 1890] a syndrome with signs and symptoms of cutaneous, gastrointestinal, and hematologic disease; it is characterized by angular stomatitis, oral mucosal hyperkeratosis, brittle nails, atrophic glossitis, esophageal webs, and microcytic hypochromic (iron deficiency) anemia. This disease occurs most frequently in premenopausal females, and presents initially with dysphagia. Crescent-shaped diaphanous fibrous webs in the anterior portion of the cricopharyngeal area may be associated with mucosal atrophy and inflammation of the hypopharynx. Achlorhydria may also be present.

Techniques for the diagnosis of this syndrome include barium swallow, esophagoscopy, endoscopy, and fluoroscopy with a radiopaque bolus. Most symptoms disappear following treatment of the underlying anemia. Individuals with Plummer-Vinson syndrome have an increased risk of developing pharyngeal carcinoma.

Also called *Paterson-Kelly syndrome* and *sideropenic dysphagia.*

pluripotent myeloid stem cell (ploor″ĭ-po′tent) a

hematopoietic stem cell that gives rise to the myeloid stem cell lines. See under *stem cell.*

plutonium (Pu) (ploo-to′ne-um) [from the planet *Pluto*] a silvery-white, metallic radioactive element; atomic number 94; most stable isotope, Pu-244 (half-life 8.1×10^7 yr); a 5f transition element (an actinide element); oxidation states +3 through +7 (+4 is most common).

Produced in reactors from U-238 by neutron capture followed by beta decay; Pu-239 is fissionable, and is used as reactor fuel and to make the trigger mechanism for hydrogen bombs.

Plutonium is one of the most toxic of all substances. It is carcinogenic when ingested or inhaled, causing bone, lung, and other cancers.

Pm symbol for the chemical element *promethium.*

pm abbrev. See *picometer.*

PMA abbrev. See *p-methoxyamphetamine.*

PML abbrev. See *progressive multifocal leukoencephalopathy.*

PMN abbrev. See *polymorphonuclear neutrophil.*

PMR abbrev. See *proportionate mortality r.* under *ratio.*

P_{N_2} abbrev. See *p. p. of nitrogen* under *partial pressure.*

pne/o (ne′o) [Gr. *pnein* to breathe] a word element used in combining form to denote breathing, e.g., pneograph.

-pnea (ne′ah) [Gr. *pnoia* breath] a suffix word element to denote breathing, e.g., dyspnea.

pneum/o (nu′mo) [Gr. *pneumōn* lung] a word element used in combining form to denote the lung or air, e.g., pneumomycosis.

pneumarthrosis (nu″mar-thro′sis) [*pneum-* + Gr. *arthron* joint + *-osis*] the presence of gas or air in a joint. This condition may be induced clinically to enhance x-ray contrast, or it may occur pathologically, as in trauma or in the "bends" of decompression sickness.

pneumat/o (nu-mat′o) [Gr. *pneuma,* genitive *pneumatos* air] a word element used in combining form to denote relationship to air or gas, or to respiration, e.g., pneumatosis.

pneumatic (nu-mat′ik) pertaining to air or respiration.

pneumatic bone bone that contains air-filled cavities or sinuses.

pneumatization (nu″mah-tĭ-za′shun) the formation of air cells or cavities in tissue, especially those in the mastoid process of the temporal bone.

pneumatocele (nu-mat′o-sēl) [*pneumato-* + Gr. *kēlē* hernia] 1. herniation of the lung due to a defect in the chest wall. Such defects may be the result of surgery, trauma, or abnormal development. Most pneumatoceles occur in a thoracic location, although cervical and diaphragmatic types are also seen. The lesion may cause pain and dyspnea but more commonly is asymptomatic. Diagnosis is normally accomplished by physical examination. Treatment may require surgery.

2. a thin-walled, air-containing cyst in the lung, often seen in staphylococcal pneumonia.

pneumatosis (nu″mah-to′sis) [*pneumat-* + *-osis,* condition] a general term used to describe air or gas in an abnormal location in the body.

p. cystoides intestinalis, a condition characterized by thin-walled gas cysts in the wall of the intestines. Usually it involves the ileum and jejunum, and less often, the stomach and large intestine and duodenum. There is usually an associated peptic ulcer in adults and severe gastroenteritis or necrotizing enterocolitis in children; the cysts may be submucosal or subserosal and in extreme cases may extend into the mesentery. Radiography can be used for diagnosis. Also called gas cyst.

pneumatotherapy (nu″mah-to-ther′ah-pe) the treatment of disease by rarefied or compressed air. See also *hyperbaric oxygenation.*

pneumaturia (nu″mah-tu′re-ah) [*pneumat-* + Gr. *ouron* urine + *-ia*] the presence of air or gas in the urine, usually appearing as small gas bubbles or froth during micturition. Its causes include fistulas between the urinary tract and either the intestinal tract or the vagina, which may be due to diverticulitis with abscess formation, trauma, surgery, neoplasms, or enterocolitis. Rarely, gas-forming bacteria (*Escherichia coli* or *Enterobacter aerogenes* organisms) may initiate pneumaturia, especially in elderly females. X-rays of the bladder may reveal a gas outline in severe cases.

pneumoarthrography (nu″mo-ar-throg′rah-fe) [*pneumo-* + Gr. *arthron* joint + *graphein* to write or draw] the radiographic examination of a joint after injection of air into the capsular space. See also *arthrography.*

pneumococcus (nu″mo-kok′us), pl. *pneumococci* [*pneumo-* + Gr. *kokkos* berry] the *Streptococcus pneumoniae* organism; see under *Streptococcus.*

pneumoconiosis (nu″mo-ko″ne-o′sis) [*pneumo-* + Gr. *konis* dust + *-osis* condition] any of a group of chronic lung disorders caused by the inhalation of inorganic (mineral) dust and deposition of these particles in the lungs. These conditions primarily result from occupational or environmental exposure to inorganic dusts, and vary in severity directly with the duration of exposure.

Generally, the initial symptoms of these disorders that are similar include dyspnea and chronic productive cough. The pathologic reactions of the lungs vary markedly and depend on the chemical and physical properties of the particulate matter. Silica inhalation (silicosis) results in a discrete nodular pulmonary fibrosis that progresses well after exposure, and renders the lungs susceptible to tuberculosis and emphysema. Inhalation of asbestos leads to a diffuse interstitial fibrosis (asbestosis), alveolar thickening, pleural mesothelial cell proliferation, and calcification. The incidence of both bronchogenic carcinoma and mesothelioma is increased following exposure to asbestos. Exposure to beryllium (berylliosis) may initiate an acute disorder, characterized by patchy pulmonary infiltration resembling pneumonia, or a chronic disorder (after 6–18 mo), characterized by fine nodular septal fibrosis, granulomas and elastic tissue damage (leading to emphysema) without fibrosis. Inhalation of bauxite (aluminosis) results in pulmonary fibrosis, hilar lymph adenopathy, and pulmonary atelectasis after an exposure time of several months to 2 yr. Anthracosis and siderosis, arising from inhalation of coal dust or iron and iron ore particles, respectively, result in "fibrosis" and emphysema after years of exposure. Radioactive dust inhalation (e.g., by uranium miners) may increase the incidence of pulmonary neoplasia. All types of inorganic dusts may lead to chronic bronchitis, if inhaled in sufficient amounts. Other compounds implicated in the pneumoconioses include mica, talc, graphite, diatomaceous earth, tin, barium, and other forms of carbon.

There is no specific treatment for these pneumoconioses other than symptomatic relief. It is essential to obtain a history of the patient's occupational or environmental exposure in order to make a differential diagnosis.

For more information, see the specific disorder.

Pneumocystis (nu″mo-sis′tis) [*pneumo-* + Gr. *kystis* bladder] a genus of parasites of uncertain status, probably a coccidian, of worldwide distribution. The species *P. carinii* causes interstitial pneumonia in infants, children, and individuals with congenital or acquired immunodeficiency diseases. The organism is spread by the respiratory route from carriers or individuals with asymptomatic infections. It is thought that the organism colonizes a high proportion of healthy persons early in life but does not disclose its presence until an individual is immunosuppressed.

Laboratory diagnosis requires identification of the organism in pulmonary material obtained by lung biopsy, bronchial washings, or transthoracic needle aspirates. The cysts, measuring 4–6μ in diameter, contain eight nucleated bodies. They are seen best in Giemsa, Grocott, or Gomori silver stains.

pneumocystosis (nu″mo-sis-to′sis) an acute pulmonary infection due to the organism *Pneumocystis carinii.* Pneumocystosis is characterized by a pneumonia with diffuse involvement, tachypnea, dyspnea, a nonproductive cough, respiratory insufficiency, and cyanosis. Diagnosis is based on cytologic demonstration of the organism obtained by bronchial secretions, tracheal lavage, endobronchial brush biopsy, or percutaneous needle aspiration of the lung, and staining of the removed materials with methenamine silver, Gram-Weigert, or Giemsa stains. Mortality rates are uncertain; untreated cases may be fatal.

Also called *interstitial plasma cell pneumonia.* See also *Pneumocystis.*

pneumocystography (nu″mo-sis-tog′rah-fe) [*pneumo-* + Gr. *kystis* bladder + *graphein* to write or draw] the radiographic demonstration of the bladder after filling it with air, usually a double-contrast study. After the bladder lining is coated with an opaque contrast medium (introduced by urinary catheter), the lumen is filled with air. Also called air cystography.

pneumocyte (nu-mo-sit′) [*pneumo-* + Gr. *kytos* hollow vessel] see *type I pneumocyte* and *type II pneumocyte* under *alveolar cell.*

pneumoencephalography (PEG) (nu″mo-en-sef″-ah-log′rah-fe) [*pneumo-* + Gr. *enkephalos* brain + *graphein* to write or draw] the radiographic imaging of the ventricles and cisterns of the brain. See also *cerebral p.* under *pneumoradiography.*

pneumogram (nu′mo-gram) [*pneumo-* + Gr. *gramma* a mark] the tracing of graphic record of the movements of the chest during respiration.

pneumograph (nu′mo-graf) [*pneumo-* + Gr. *graphein* to write] an instrument (such as an inflated coil that is placed around the chest) used to detect the movements of the chest with each respiratory cycle. When used in conjunction with an appropriate amplification and recording system, the pneumograph can measure the rate and, less accurately, the depth of breathing.

pneumography (nu-mog′rah-fe) see *pneumoradiography.*

pneumomediastinum (nu″mo-me″de-as-ti′num) [*pneumo-* + *mediastinum*] the presence of air or gas in the mediastinum, which may interfere with respiration and circulation and may lead to conditions such as pneumothorax or pneumoperitoneum. It is usually due to trauma, although air is sometimes deliberately introduced into the mediastinum as a diagnostic procedure.

pneumon/o (nu-mon′o) [Gr. *pneumōn* lung] a word element used in combining form to denote the lungs, e.g., pneumonitis.

pneumonia (nu-mo′ne-ah) [Gr. "lung disease," from *pneumōn* lung] an acute infection and inflammation of the pulmonary parenchyma that occurs in areas distal to the terminal bronchioles (respiratory bronchioles, alveolar ducts and sacs, and alveoli). A variety of microorganisms may cause bacterial pneumonia, including pneumococci, staphylococci, group A streptococci, *Klebsiella pneumoniae, Hemophilus influenzae, Neisseria meningitidis,* and several gram-negative anaerobes and enteric bacteria. Other agents causing include viruses, rickettsia, chlamydia, fungi, tubercle bacilli, or mycoplasmas.

The types of pneumonia are classified according to their pattern of parenchymal involvement, i.e., lobar (involving an entire lobe), segmental or lobular (involving parts of a lobe), or bronchial (involving alveoli contiguous to a bronchus).

Pneumonia once represented a leading cause of death in the United States. Though its control and cure have improved with the advent of antibiotic therapy, pneumonia is still a leading cause of death in the very young, the elderly, and debilitated individuals. Predisposing factors include upper respiratory tract infections, alcoholism, malnutrition, coma, bronchial neoplasms, aspiration of foreign substances (such as vomitus), and immunosuppressive therapy. In those affected, there is typically fever, cough, dyspnea, chest pain, and sputum production. Tachycardia and tachypnea in the presence of hypoxia and cyanosis are common. Findings on physical examination include dullness on percussion, decreased respiratory excursion, end-inspiratory crackles, and bronchial breath sounds.

Diagnostic studies include radiologic examination of the lungs and Gram staining or acid-fast staining and culturing of sputum samples. If sputum samples are unobtainable, transtracheal aspiration may be required. Blood cultures should also be examined. Nonbacterial pneumonias are often diagnosed by serologic comparison of acute and convalescent samples for changes in viral antibody titers.

alcoholic p., a pneumonia that is associated with alcoholism. Pneumonia is a common accompaniment to alcoholism, when infection with *Klebsiella pneumoniae* is often seen.

aspiration p., a severe type of pulmonary damage due to the inhalation of gastric contents and often of microorganisms in the upper respiratory tract. It may follow anesthesia, alcohol intoxication, drug abuse, convulsive disorders, or disturbances of consciousness associated with vomiting. There is patchy pulmonary edema, necrosis, and bronchospasm due to the acidic content of the gastric aspiration. The resultant pneumonias may or may not have a bacterial component.

Friedländer's p., see *Klebsiella p.*

fungal p., a primary lung infection by such fungal organisms as *Histoplasma capsulatum, Coccidioides immitis,* and (less commonly) *Candida, Cryptococcus,* and *Blastomyces.* Fungal pneumonias are most frequently seen in debilitated individuals and in patients with impaired immune systems on antimicrobial therapy or cancer chemotherapy. Signs and symptoms range from those of an acute, mild viral illness to those of chronic pulmonary disease.

Some fungal pneumonias are endemic in certain geographic areas, which, combined with clinical symptoms, should suggest a diagnosis. Serologic studies and skin tests may assist in establishing the diagnosis. Regardless of the etiologic agent, treatment is limited to a small number of available antifungal agents, including amphotericin B, miconazole, ketoconazole, and flucytosine.

For more information, see the specific fungal organism (e.g., *Histoplasma capsulatum*) and the resultant disease (e.g., *histoplasmosis*).

***Hemophilus influenzae* p.,** an infection of the lung parenchyma due to *Hemophilus influenzae,* most frequently type b. It primarily affects infants, young children, and adults over age 50 who have chronic obstructive pulmonary disease, immune deficiency, cardiac disease, or alcoholism. Major complaints are chills, fever, cough, dyspnea, and chest pain.

Radiographs of the lungs typically reveal a bronchopneumonia. The white blood count is elevated with a shift to the left. The diagnosis is based on demonstration of many small, pleomorphic, gram-negative coccobacilli, especially in and around abundant neutrophils, on Gram-stained sputum, and identification of *H. influenzae* in cultures of sputum and blood. Organism typing by capsular swelling reaction should be performed.

See also *H. influenzae* under *Hemophilus.*

interstitial plasma cell p., see *pneumocystosis.*

***Klebsiella* p.,** a rare infection of the pulmonary parenchyma due to *Klebsiella pneumoniae.* It accounts for less than 1 percent of all bacterial pneumonias, occurring most frequently in persons over age 40 who are alcoholics, malnourished, or debilitated. The signs and symptoms of *Klebsiella* pneumonia are similar to those of other pneumonias caused by gram-negative enteric bacteria, i.e., acute onset of chills, fever, dyspnea, and cyanosis. The characteristic finding is dark brown or red, sticky, and extremely mucoid sputum that is difficult to expectorate. The disease may be fulminant and rapidly progressive, leading to lung necrosis, abscess formation, and death.

Diagnosis of pneumonia due to *Klebsiella pneumoniae* or other gram-negative enteric bacilli is established by demonstration of gram-negative rods in the sputum and identification of *K. pneumoniae* in cultures of sputum and blood. Radiographs of the lungs reveal lobar or multilobar consolidation. *K. pneumoniae* is associated with the aspiration of oropharyngeal secretions and is frequently nosocomial. Mixed infection, particularly with anaerobes, is also common. Recovery is usually slow, and residual fibrosis, abscesses, and necrosis are frequent sequelae. Despite therapy, mortality remains about 30 percent.

Also called *Friedländer's penumonia.* See also *K. pneumoniae* under *Klebsiella.*

lipid p., the patchy or diffuse pulmonary damage resulting from the aspiration of a variety of oils or oily medications. It may be seen in infants who are forced to swallow lipid medications, or in adults who use oily nosedrops or who use mineral oil as a laxative. Radiographs of the lungs may reveal scattered lobar densities and central cavitation. Histologically, consolidation fibrosis, and, occasionally, macrophages containing oil droplets are seen. Lipid pneumonia is rarely a cause of primary clinical disease. Treatment is nonspecific and symptomatic, including the patient's avoidance of the offending lipid agent.

mycoplasmal p., an infection of the lung parenchyma due to the organism *Mycoplasma pneumoniae* (which is also called the *pleuropneumonia-like organism* (PPLO) and *Eaton agent*). It is the most common cause of nonbacterial pneumonia and primarily affects children, young adults, and military recruits. This form commonly spreads through family members and may also cause community epidemics. After an incubation period of 2–3 wk, there is a gradual onset of headache, myalgia, slow-rising fever, and increasing cough with scanty sputum. The course of the disease is variable and may persist for from 3 da to 4–6 wk. Recovery is generally slow. Relapse may occur, but death is rare.

Physical examination reveals minimal rales and consolidation, and frequently x-ray findings that seem out of proportion to the physical findings. White blood cell counts are usually normal. Diagnosis may be made by serologic studies (especially the complement-fixation test), or by culturing the organism on special media for several weeks. About half of those affected develop nonspecific cold hemagglutins ($>$1:64) to human type O red cells at 4°C by the end of the first week.

See also *M. pneumoniae* under *Mycoplasma.*

pneumococcal p., an acute febrile infection of the pulmonary parenchyma due to *Streptococcus pneumoniae* (pneumococcus). This is the most common form of pneumonia, accounting for up to 40 percent of all cases. It occurs at any age and is more severe in the very young and very old, in immunosuppressed patients, and in those with impaired respiratory defenses. The pneumococci (types 1–9 and 12 in adults; types 6, 14, 19, and 23 in children) reach the lungs through the respiratory passages. In the early stages (12–48 hr), there is consolidation, pulmonary edema, and extravasation of red blood cells into the alveoli (red hepatization). Large numbers of neutrophils and macrophages are mobilized to the lungs, and the individual experiences sudden chills, chest pains, high fever, cough, and blood-streaked sputum. Acute illness is the rule. Resolution of consolidation may require 8–10 wk.

Physical examination reveals absent breath sounds, dullness on percussion, and decreased respiratory excursion. Leukocytosis is frequently present. Chest radiographs reveal pulmonary consolidation in a lobar or segmental pattern. Diagnosis is based on the demonstration of single or paired gram-positive cocci with many red and white blood cells in the sputum and identification of pneumococci in the sputum and blood cultures. Identification of pneumococci in fresh sputum is aided by the Quellung reaction with pooled antiserum.

About 90–95 percent of treated patients survive. The prognosis is poorer if there is bacteremia, leukopenia, or an underlying chronic illness. Complications of pneumococcal pneumonia include pleural effusion, lung abscess, empyema, endocarditis, pericarditis, and meningitis. Rarely, resolution of the pneumonia may lead to fibrous organization. Although any cultured organism should be tested for antibiotic sensitivity, the pneumococci are generally sensitive to penicillin. A polyvalent vaccine is commercially available that offers prophylactic protection to those at high risk.

See also *S. pneumoniae* under *Streptococcus.*

primary atypical p., the former designation of pulmonary infections that developed in a pattern different from that seen in classic lobar pneumococcal pneumonia. Frequently, it referred to the pneumonia caused by *Mycoplasma pneumoniae.* See also *mycoplasmal p.*

primary influenza virus p., a severe and usually fatal pneumonia caused by the influenza virus. There is a sudden onset of high fever (40°C, 104°F), a productive cough with bloody sputum, poor air exchange, cyanosis, but no pulmonary parenchymal consolidation. Primary influenza virus pneumonia is generally limited to individuals with preexisting cardiac disease, especially mitral stenosis, or pulmonary disease or it is a complication of pregnancy. Secondary bacterial pneumonia is often a complicating factor.

staphylococcal p., an infection of the lung parenchyma due to coagulase-positive *Staphylococcus aureus.* This disease is a frequent complication of influenza; it may occur in a primary form in the very young and very old. It accounts for 5 percent of all bacterial pneumonias. Staphylococcal pneumonia is also common in hospitalized newborn infants and in older hospitalized patients, especially following surgery, tracheostomy, immunosuppressive drug therapy, and generalized debility. Pulmonary infection with staphylococci may also follow hematogenous spread.

Those affected display symptoms that include high fever and chills; they have a severe cough with blood-streaked sputum, which may be copious and salmon-colored. Infants tend to develop a bronchogenic form of pneumonia, with pneumatoceles and pyopneumothorax. Older and debilitated patients tend to develop tracheobronchitis, lobar or diffuse pneumonia. In both cases, pleural effusion, empyema, and tension pneumothorax may occur. Leukocytosis and abscesses are common, and peripheral vascular collapse may occur.

Diagnosis is made by demonstration of gram-positive cocci, both intra- and extracellular, in the sputum or tracheobronchial secretions, and by identification of *Staphylococcus aureus* in the sputum, pleural fluid, or blood. Blood cultures are rarely positive unless the pneumonia has developed secondarily to a staphylococcal bacteremia. Radiographic evidence of multiple cavities within the lung is also suggestive of the disease. Sensitivity tests must be performed to select appropriate antibiotic therapy; even with treatment, however, the mortality rate is high (15–20 percent). Bronchiectasis can be a consequence of this form of pneumonia.

See also *S. aureus* under *Staphylococcus.*

streptococcal p., an infection of the lung parenchyma due to group A hemolytic streptococci. Once common but now rare, streptococcal pneumonia usually follows a viral infection, most commonly influenza, but it may also occur in individuals following streptococcal sore throat or scarlet fever or in those with underlying pulmonary disease. Those affected have an abrupt onset of fever, chills, dyspnea, pleuritic chest pain, and pink, thin sputum. The pneumonia is lobular in distribution, and there is a high incidence of copious pleural effusion with rapid accumulation of thin, serosanguineous, empyemic fluid. Bacteremia is rare but purulent pericarditis, mediastinitis, pneumothorax, and bronchiectasis are recognized complications.

Diagnosis is established by isolation of group A hemolytic streptococci from cultures of sputum, pleural fluid, or blood, and demonstration of chains of gram-positive cocci with Gram stains of sputum or pleural fluid. Recovery is generally slow; abscesses and fibrosis may be sequelae.

See also *S. group A* under *Streptococcus.*

viral p., an infection of the pulmonary parenchyma due to a number of viral agents, e.g., influenza and parainfluenza viruses; adenovirus; respiratory syncytial virus; cytomegalovirus (CMV); coxsackie-, echo-, and reovirus; and viruses of the childhood exanthems (e.g., varicella and measles).

Headache, anorexia, fever, myalgia, and cough are common symptoms. Most viral infections of the lungs involve more than one pulmonary segment, and entire lobes occasionally become consolidated.

pneumonic plague (nu-mon′ik) see *pneumonic p.* under *plague.*

pneumonitis (nu″mo-ni′tis) [*pneumon-* + *-itis* inflammation] a general term used to describe an inflammation of the lung that is not necessarily associated with lung infection.

Although many types of pneumonitis are described, there are three main categories: hypersensitivity, an immunologically mediated allergic response to a variety of inhaled organic dusts; chemical, an inflammatory reaction to inhaled noxious chemical agents and gases; and desquamative interstitial, an interstitial fibrosis of unknown causes with aggregations of mononuclear cells.

See also *delayed hypersensitivity* and *immediate hypersensitivity.* Cf. *pneumonia.*

aspiration p., see *aspiration p.* under *pneumonia.*

chemical p., an inflammation of the lungs caused by the inhalation of chemical irritants, such as sulfur dioxide (SO_2), ammonia (NH_3), chlorine (Cl_2), phosgene (Cl_2CO), hydrogen fluoride (HF), osmium tetroxide (OsO_4), vanadium pentoxide (V_2O_5), and zinc chloride ($ZnCl_2$). Most often these chemicals are inhaled as vapors; they are soluble in biologic fluids in the upper airways and deep in the bronchial tree and the alveoli; the chemical irritation causes inflammation, mucosal edema, and hypersecretion. Occasionally, extensive tissue damage leads to necrosis. Clinically, there is burning of the throat, laryngitis, airway obstruction, cough, and severe hypoxemia. Severe alveolitis can result in pulmonary edema. Diagnosis is made on the basis of clinical symptoms, a history of exposure to chemical vapors, and evidence of damage to the respiratory mucosa.

desquamative interstitial p. (DIP), an interstitial, fibrosing pneumonitis characterized by the aggregation of desquamated histiocytes (mononuclear) within the alveolar spaces and the presence of an interstitial inflammatory cell reaction. Those affected usually display a persistent cough, dypsnea, clubbing of the fingers, and cyanosis. DIP and alveolitis may be the initial phase of a diffuse process that ultimately leads to pulmonary fibrosis. Although the exact cause of the disorder is unknown, it may represent an abnormal pulmonary parenchymal reaction to viral, toxic, or immunologic injury.

Pulmonary function tests characteristically reveal a reduction in lung volume, diffusing capacity, and arterial oxygenation. The radiographic picture is variable but usually is characterized by an increase in interstitial lung markings.

See also *pulmonary f.* under *fibrosis.*

hypersensitivity p., an immunologically induced inflammation of the lungs due to antigenic stimulation by inhaled organic dust, which can cause this allergic response. It is most often caused by fungal, animal, or vegetable proteins. Type III (antigen-antibody complex–mediated) and type IV (cell-mediated) hypersensitivity reactions are probably the important immunologic mechanisms involved in hypersensitivity pneumonitis, but complement-mediated reactions may also play a role. The acute phase is characterized by fever, cough, chills, and dyspnea, which develop 4–8 hr after reexposure to the antigen.

Diagnosis is based on a meticulous history of exposure to specific antigens, serologic demonstration of precipitins to the suspected antigen (positive in > 90 percent of patients with clinical disease), a polyclonal elevation of serum IgG, and a positive Arthus skin reaction to intradermal testing with the suspected antigen.

usual interstitial p., see *pulmonary f.* under *fibrosis.*

pneumonocyte (nu-mon′o-sit) [*pneumono-* + Gr. *kytos* hollow vessel] see *alveolar cell.*

pneumoperitoneum (nu″mo-per″ĭ-to-ne′um) [*pneumo-* + L. *peritoneum*] the presence of air or gas in the peritoneal cavity. It may occur spontaneously, e.g., peptic ulcer perforation, or it may be induced as a radiolucent contrast medium in abdominal pneumoradiography.

pneumopyelography (nu″mo-pi″ĕ-log′rah-fe) [*pneumo-* + Gr. *pyelos* pelvis + *graphein* to write] a negative contrast radiologic examination of the ureters and the renal pelvis and calyces, using air injected through a catheter. See also *pneumocystography.*

pneumoradiography (nu″mo-ra″de-og′rah-fe) [*pneumo-* + *radiography*] the radiologic examination of a part after introduction of a gaseous medium into an internal space of the part or into a space surrounding the part. Also called *pneumography.* See also *pneumoencephalography* and *ventriculography.*

abdominal p., the radiologic examination of the abdominal viscera after the introduction of a gaseous contrast medium (usually air, oxygen, or nitrous oxide) through a hollow needle passed percutaneously into one of the spaces surrounding the organ of interest. The position, contour, and mobility of the organs and the presence of space-occupying lesions may be demonstrated by this technique. The intestinal tract must first be cleared of gas and feces by administration of a cathartic and a cleansing enema before the examination is performed.

perirenal p., retroperitoneal pneumoradiography in which gas is introduced into the perirenal space for demonstration of the kidneys. Also called perirenal gas insufflation.

presacral p., abdominal pneumoradiography in which gas is introduced into the presacral retroperitoneal space and rises into the upper retroperitoneal space for demonstration of the kidneys and adrenal glands. This technique is now replaced by computed tomography.

retroperitoneal p., see *presacral p.*

pneumoretroperitoneum (nu″mo-re″tro-per″ĭ-to-ne′um) [*pneumo-* + L. *retro* behind *peritoneum*] the presence of air or gas in the retroperitoneal space, as in presacral pneumoradiography.

pneumotachogram (nu″mo-tak′o-gram) [*pneumo-* + Gr. *tachys* swift + *gramma* writing, a record] the record produced by a pneumotachograph of changes in respired air flow as a function of time.

pneumotachograph (nu″mo-tak′o-graf) [*pneumo-* + Gr. *tachys* swift + *graphein* to write] an instrument used to record the instantaneous flow of respired air at the mouth or, when the pneumotachograph signal is integrated, the volume of air that enters the lungs. In tests of pulmonary function, it can be used (in conjunction with an esophageal balloon) to measure static lung compliance or airway resistance (in conjunction with a whole body plethysmograph).

pneumothorax (nu″mo-tho′raks) [*pneumo-* + Gr. *thōrax* thorax] an accumulation of air or gas in the pleural space. It may occur spontaneously or as a result of trauma or other pathologic processes. Air may be introduced into the pleural space deliberately for collapse of the lung (therapeutic pneumothorax) or for radiologic demonstration of the pleurae (diagnostic pneumothorax).

pneumoventriculography (nu″mo-ven-trik″u-log′rah-fe) [*pneumo-* + L. *ventriculus* ventricle + Gr. *graphein* to write or draw] the radiographic imaging of the ventricles of the brain. See also *cerebral p.* under *pneumography.*

PNH abbrev. See *paroxysmal nocturnal hemoglobinuria.*

Po_2 abbrev. See *p. p. of oxygen* under *partial pressure.*

Po symbol for the chemical element *polonium.*

pod/o (pod′o) [Gr. *pous, podos* foot] a word element used in combining form to denote the foot, e.g., podiatry.

podocyte (pod′o-sit) [*podo-* + Gr. *kytos* hollow vessel] [NA], a flattened, stellate, epithelial cell of the visceral layer of the renal corpuscle. Podocytes have cytoplasmic extensions with end processes called pedicels, which interdigitate to produce the slit pores of the glomerular filtration barrier.

podophyllin (pod″o-fil′in) [*podo-* + Gr. *phyllon* plant + *-in*] a mixture of resins, prepared from the plant *Podophyllum peltatum,* that is a potent inhibitor of mitosis. It is sometimes used in the treatment of certain mucosal lesions, e.g., condyloma acuminatum. Also called podophyllum resin.

pogonion (po-go′ne-on) [Gr., dim. of *pōgōn* beard] the most anterior point of the chin lying in the midsagittal plane. Also called *mental point.*

pOH a measure of the acidity or alkalinity of a solution. It is related to pH as $pH + pOH = 14.0$, and is defined as the negative logarithm of hydroxide ion activity ($-\log a_{OH^-}$). In dilute solutions, activity becomes identical with concentration [OH^-]. See also *pH.*

-poiesis (poi-e′sis) [Gr. *poiein* to make] a suffix word element to denote formation, e.g., hematopoiesis.

poikil/o (poi′kĭ-lo) [Gr. *poikilos* spotted, mottled; varied] a word element used in combining form to denote varied or irregular, e.g., poikilocytosis.

poikilocyte (poi′kĭ-lo-sīt) [*poikilō* + Gr. *kytos* hollow vessel] an abnormally shaped red cell.

poikilocytosis (poi″kĭ-lo-si-to′sis) [*poikilo-* + Gr. *kytos* hollow vessel + *-osis* condition] the presence of erythrocytes in the blood with abnormal variations in shape.

pointer variable a computer language variable that can have a value representing an address; it points to another variable. Also called indirect addressing.

point mutation see *point m.* under *mutation.*

point of inflection the point on a graph of a function at which the curvature changes from concave to convex and the second derivative is zero.

poise (P) (poiz; Fr. pwahz) [Jean Leonard Marie *Poiseuille,* French physiologist, 1799–1869] the CGS unit of viscosity, 1 dyn·sec/cm^2. The convenient unit is the centipoise (cP), equal to 0.01 poise.

Poiseuille's law (pwah-zuh′yez) [Jean Leonard Marie *Poiseuille*] stated as: the rate of laminar flow (Q) of a newtonian fluid through a segment of a rigid tube is directly proportional to the pressure drop ($P_{-1} - P_{-2}$) along the length of the segment and to the fourth power of its radius (r), and inversely proportional to the length of the segment (L) and to the viscosity of the fluid (η). The mathematical relationship is: $Q = \pi(P_{-1} - P_{-2})\ r^4/8L\eta$. It is commonly used to approximate the rate of flow of blood in vessels or of air in the respiratory passages.

poison (poi′zun) [L. *potio* a drink] 1. a substance that can cause injury, disease, or death to living tissues. Because most chemical substances can be hazardous to health, depending on the circumstances, whether a substance is considered a poison depends on the characteristics of exposure and the dose. See also *toxin* and *toxicity.*

2. in the labeling of hazardous materials, a substance that is extremely toxic.

3. in chemistry, a substance that inhibits the activity of a catalyst.

4. in nuclear technology, a substance that absorbs neutrons and that can inhibit a fission chain reaction.

industrial p., toxic materials used in commerce, such as pesticides and toxic industrial wastes. See also *pesticide.*

Poison Control Center a source from which information helpful in dealing with poisonings can be obtained by telephone. Information on the toxic constituents of common household products and on antidotes, first aid, and treatment is available from more than 500 Poison Control Centers throughout the United States. Recently, consolidation of individual centers into Regional Centers has provided improved informational resources as well as effective centers for treatment of poisoning.

poisoning (poi′zun-ing) the morbid condition produced by a poison; see also *intoxication.*

Poisson distribution (pwah-sawn′) [Siméon Denis *Poisson,* French mathematician, 1781–1840] the probability distribution of a random variable X, the number of events observed in a specified time interval, when events occur independently and at a constant rate. (The number of events occurring in different intervals is unrelated.) The events are randomly distributed in time; the Poisson distribution also describes events randomly distributed over a spatial interval, area, or volume. Examples of Poisson processes are the number of radioactive decays counted in a time interval that is short compared with the half-life of the radioactive isotope, the number of blood cells counted in a specified volume (if the dilution is enough so that the cells are not crowded together), and the number of x-ray photons absorbed in a particular volume element of a CT scan.

The probability of observing n counts is $P(X = n) = \lambda^n e^{-\lambda}/n!$, where $n!$ is n factorial and λ is the mean of the distribution rate (or average density) of events multiplied by the length of the time interval (or spatial length, area, or volume). The variance of the distribution is λ; thus, the coefficient of variation (CV) is $1/\sqrt{\lambda}$. If 100 events are counted, the CV is 10 percent; if 10,000 events are counted, the CF is 1 percent.

pokeweed mitogen (PWM) (pōk′wēd mi′to-jen) a plant lectin extracted from the roots, stems, and berries of the pokeweed, *Phytolacca americana.* It is a glycoprotein that causes the agglutination of red blood cells; it is also a mitogen, an inducer of lymphocyte proliferation. PWM stimulates B cells more than T cells, and is used to induce mitosis in peripheral leukocyte cultures for cytogenetic tests. See also *concanavalin A* and *phytohemagglutinin.*

polar (po′lar) [L. *polaris,* from *polus* pole] 1. of or relating to a pole.

2. in bacteriology, a term used to describe a rod-shaped bacterial cell having flagella or endospores only at the ends of the cell; see *flagellum.*

3. in physics and chemistry, having an electric or magnetic dipole moment. In covalent chemical compounds, a polar covalent bond exists when the electron pair of a bond between atoms of two different elements is shared unequally, and the electron charge density is greater near the more electronegative atom. If the electric dipoles of the polar bonds do not cancel (as in a symmetric molecule), the molecules have an overall dipole moment and are electrostatically attracted to other dipoles. In general, polar molecules or compounds are those with a permanent dipole moment. Polar and ionic compounds (such as salts and proteins) are generally more soluble in polar solvents (e.g., water, alcohols, and ketones) than in nonpolar solvents (e.g., hydrocarbons).

polar body an incomplete cell produced during cogenesis by the unequal division of cytoplasm. In the first meiotic division, the first polar body is expelled and rapidly fragments. The secondary oocyte retains most of the cytoplasm and divides to form the ovum and a small second polar body, which disappears soon after fertilization.

polar compound see *polar.*

polarimeter (po″lah-rim′ĕ-ter) [*polar* + Gr. *metron* measure] an instrument for measuring optical activity. It consists of a monochromatic light source, polarizer, sample holder, and analyzer. The polarizer and analyzer are devices, such as Nicol prisms, that transmit light polarized in one plane but not in the perpendicular plane. The light beam passes from the source through the polarizer, sample, and analyzer. The analyzer is rotated until the intensity of the transmitted beam is brightest, when the angle between the polarization planes of the polarizer and analyzer equals the optical rotation produced by the sample.

polarimetry (po″lah-rim′ĕ-tre) the measurement of optical rotation, the amount by which the plane of polarization of a light beam is rotated by an optically active material. See also *optical activity* and *polarimeter.*

polarity (po-lar′ĭ-te) 1. the physical property of having two opposite poles like a magnetic or electric dipole.

2. the sign (positive or negative) of a physical property at a pole or electrical terminal.

3. in chemistry, a property of molecules or solvents relating to the extent of the presence in the molecules of ionic functional groups or strong, permanent, electric dipoles. Polar solvents readily dissolve polar molecules, and nonpolar solvents readily dissolve nonpolar molecules.

4. the exhibition of opposite effects at the two extremities.

5. the presence of an axial gradient and exhibition by a nerve of both anelectrotonus and catelectrotonus.

6. the orientation of intracellular structures to the tissue as a whole.

polarizability (po″lah-rīz″ah-bil′ĭ-te) the induced electric dipole moment divided by the applied electric field strength. The polarizability of molecules of a substance is directly related to its refractive index, dielectric constant, and solubility in polar solvents.

polarization (po″lar-ĭ-za′shun) 1. the orientation of the plane of vibration of a light wave, which can be vertical or horizontal. In circularly polarized light, the plane of polarization rotates to the right or left, along the direction of propagation. Unpolarized or partially polarized light is a mixture of polarizations.

2. the separation of electric charge in an object, such as a molecule or an electrochemical cell, in response to an applied electric field.

3. (symbol *P*), the electric dipole moment per unit volume of a material. See also *dielectric.*

4. in neurophysiology, the existence of a potential difference across the membrane of an excitable cell; the process of transmembrane charge separation.

polarize (po′lar-īz) to induce a specific polarization.

polarized light light in which the polarization is nonrandom. The oscillating electric field vector is perpendicular to the direction of propagation. In plane-polarized light the electric field vector remains in one plane, whereas in circular-polarized light its direction rotates around the direction of propagation. Elliptic-polarized light is a combination of the first two types of polarized light.

polarizer (po′lah-rīz″er) a device that polarizes light. See also *birefringence* and *polarization.*

polarogram (po-lar′o-gram) [*polar* + Gr. *gramma* a mark] in polarography, a graph of current as a function of voltage across the electrochemical cell.

polarography (po″lar-og′rah-fe) [*polar* + Gr. *graphein* to write or draw] an electrochemical method in which the voltage across the cell is increased until a current flows. If the electrolyte is pure water, hydrogen will be reduced at the cathode, liberating gas bubbles. If other, more easily reduced substances are present, they will be reduced at a lower voltage: e.g., oxygen will be reduced to hydroxide. The current that flows (the diffusion current) is proportional to the concentration of the substance being reduced. The voltage at which the diffusion current begins to flow (measured at half the maximal current), the half-wave potential, identifies the substance being reduced. This is the method used to measure the partial pressure of oxygen in blood (Po_2) by automatic blood gas analyzers.

Polaroid (po′lar-oid) trademark for a type of instant photography. It is used in medicine particularly for making prints of images on a cathode-ray tube (CRT), e.g., the readout produced by a scintillation camera or CT scanner.

poli/o (po′le-o) [Gr. *polios* gray] a word element used in combining form to denote the gray matter of brain and spinal cord, e.g., poliomyelitis.

polio see *poliomyelitis.*

poliomyelitis (po″le-o-mi″ĕ-li′tis) [*polio-* + Gr. *myelos* marrow + *-itis*] an acute, highly contagious viral disease caused by a poliovirus infection, which exists in three forms: abortive, nonparalytic, and paralytic. Poliomyelitis is characterized by fever, headache, muscle pain, nausea, and sometimes a flaccid paralysis, and it ranges greatly in severity. Before the use of polio vaccine (in use since the 1950s), this disease caused epidemics in developed areas of Western Europe and North America. The poliovirus infects certain primates (particularly humans) and has no other known reservoir. It is transmitted in humans by the fecal-oral route. Unfortunately, public apathy and individual avoidance of vaccination have prevented complete eradication of the poliovirus infection.

The poliovirus is a small RNA enterovirus. There are three immunologic types (1, 2, and 3), which confer no cross-immunity; survival of an infection by one type of poliovirus provides the individual with lifelong immunity only to that particular serotype. Most poliovirus infections are asymptomatic, and thus many people have antibodies to the virus at an early age.

The infectious process begins with poliovirus multiplication in the oropharynx without clinical symptoms. The virus then spreads to the lymph nodes, blood, and central nervous system, causing neuronal damage due to viral multiplication.

Abortive poliomyelitis is a transient infection with only minor symptoms of disease and no CNS involvement. The clinical manifestations of nonparalytic and paralytic poliomyelitis are biphasic. Initially, there is a viremia with dissemination, during which time CNS involvement may occur. Nonparalytic poliomyelitis, the least acute of the CNS forms, begins with a general malaise, sore throat, muscle pain, headache, chills, fever (38.5°–40°C), flushed skin, sweating, stiff neck, and nausea. Paralytic poliomyelitis combines the nonparalytic symptoms with the development of a flaccid paralysis. Onset of the paralysis may be indolent or rapid, progressing from weakness to total tetraplegia within a few hours. (This form of poliomyelitis is also called *infantile paralysis.*) Bulbar palsy is a life-threatening type of paralytic poliomyelitis with a poor prognosis. It may rapidly progress to delirium, with stupor, myoclonic twitches, and various abnormalities in the motor cranial nerves. The most serious complications include impaired swallowing and respiratory failure.

Diagnosis is difficult if there is no CNS involvement. The most helpful indications are persistent fever with other clinical symptoms and analysis of the cerebrospinal fluid. It shows pleocytosis with a white blood cell count up to 3000 cells/ml. Initially, polymorphonuclear leukocytes predominate, followed by lymphocytes. Concentration of the CSF protein is increased, but pressure, glucose, and electrolytes are normal. The virus may be recovered from the pharynx, nasopharyngeal secretions, or feces.

The long-term prognosis of poliomyelitis is quite varied and often unpredictable, although the absence of voluntary movement of specific muscles for 3 mo usually indicates a permanent loss of function.

The key to the reduction of poliomyelitis is prevention by vaccination. Two types of polio vaccines exist: an inactive one and an attenuated oral one. The inactive vaccine should be administered to first-exposure adults. In children and young adults, the oral vaccine is more effective, in that it also elicits a secretory antibody response in the gastrointestinal tract, reducing transmission. The vaccine should be given in three doses beginning at age 2 mo, with the second and third doses at 8-wk intervals. Additional doses during grade school, up to seventh grade, ensure lifelong immunity.

Also called *polio.*

poliovirus (po″le-o-vi′rus) [*polio-* + *virus*] a picornavirus that is the etiologic agent of poliomyelitis. There are three immunotypes, designated 1, 2, and 3. See also *picornavirus* and *poliomyelitis.*

Polistes (po-lis′tēz) a genus of wasps, of which the species *P. gallicus* is a known disseminator of the eggs of *Ascaris* (an intestinal roundworm), the hookworm, the whipworm, and the rhabditoid larvae of the hookworm. They transport the eggs on their wings, legs, body, and mouth parts, but not in the digestive tract.

Pollenia (pol-e′ne-ah) a genus of flies, of which the species *P. rudis* (the cluster fly) may transmit pathogens to humans. It does so by carrying the microorganisms on its external hairs, bristles, foot pads, or mouth parts, or in its digestive tract.

pollex (pol′eks), pl. *pollicies* [L.] [NA], the thumb, the first digit of the hand. See also *thumb.*

polonium (Po) (po-lo′ne-um) [M.L. *Polonia* Poland, where it was discovered by M. Curie] a radioactive metallic element; atomic number 84; most stable isotope, ^{209}Po (half-life, 102 yr); Group VI of the periodic table; oxidation states +2, +4 (the most common), +6. ^{210}Po, a decay product of radium, and ^{214}Po and ^{218}Po, decay products of radon, are all alpha emitters and are highly carcinogenic when ingested or inhaled.

poly- (pol′e) [Gr. *polys* many] a prefix word element to denote many, e.g., polychromatophil.

poly(A) abbrev. See *polyadenylic acid.*

polyacrylamide (pol″e-ah-kril′ah-mīd) a polymer of acrylamide, which may be soluble or insoluble in water. It can be prepared by heating acrylamide with a variety of catalysts, with and without cross-linking agents. Polyacrylamide gels are used in clinical laboratories as media for zone electrophoresis.

polyadenylate (polyA) tail a structure that terminates the 3′ end of most eukaryotic messenger RNA (mRNA), which consists of about 100 adenylate residues; it may have a function in the transport of mRNA from the nucleus to the cytoplasm and in slowing the cytoplasmic degradation of mRNA. The polyA tail is used for the in vitro separation of mRNA from other RNA, using complementary polyU chains covalently bound to Sepharose or oligo-dT-cellulose.

polyadenylation (pol″e-ah-den″ĭ-la′shun) a step in the posttranscription processing of mRNA, in which the polyA tail is added by the enzyme polyadenylate polymerase.

polyadenylic acid (pol″e-ah-den′e-lik) a synthetic polynucleotide containing a single nucleotide base, adenine. Also called *poly(A).* See also *poly A·U.*

polyagglutination (pol″e-ah-gloo″tĭ-na′shun) [*poly-* + L. *agglutinare* to glue to] the condition in which a patient's red blood cells are agglutinated by most human sera. An abnormal state for the red cells, it can develop in vivo or in vitro and occurs when abnormal red cell membrane receptors become available to antibodies that are present in normal serum.

polyamide (pol″e-am′īd) a condensation polymer formed by the linking together of relatively small molecules by amide bonds, e.g., nylon.

polyamine (pol″e-ah-mēn′) one of a group of aliphatic amines derived biosynthetically from ornithine, including putrescine, spermidine, and spermine. Putrescine and spermidine, present in increased amounts in the S phase of the cell cycle, may in some way be involved in the functioning of DNA or RNA; putrescine also occurs through the action of bacteria on decaying meat. Spermidine and spermine are known to be present in human semen. Examination of stains for crystals of spermine phosphate is a technique used in forensic medicine for identification of semen. See also *cadaverine.*

polyarteritis (pol″e-ar″tĕ-ri′tis) [*poly-* + Gr. *artēria* artery + *itis* inflammation] see *periarteritis.*

p. nodosa, see *p. nodosa* under *periarteritis.*

poly A·U a synthetic polynucleotide consisting of one strand of polyadenylate (polyA) and one strand of polyuridylate (polyU), which has been used in the laboratory to enhance general immune response. Its target is probably the T-lymphocyte cell membrane; addition of poly A·U and antigen stimulate helper T cells, delayed sensitivity, and cell-mediated cytotoxicity. Some evidence exists that poly A·U also acts on B lymphocytes to increase antibody production. Its clinical uses are still under study.

polybasic acid an acid that contains two or more replaceable hydrogen atoms, e.g., H_3PO_4. See also *dibasic acid* and *tribasic acid.*

polychlorinated biphenyl (PCB) any of the chlorine-substituted derivatives of biphenyl, used industrially as insulating fluids or heat-exchange fluids. PCBs are no longer manufactured because they are highly toxic and persist in the environment.

polychlorinated biphenyl assays gas chromatography using an electron capture detector and a column packed with a mixture of nonpolar silicone and polar fluorinated silicone. The PCB is extracted from the specimen into hexane, and the concentration is then determined by comparing the peak heights produced by the specimen and a reference solution.

polychromasia (pol″e-kro-ma′ze-ah) [Gr. *polychrōmos* many-colored, from *poly-* + *chrōma* color] 1. a variation in the hemoglobin content of the erythrocyte.

2. see *polychromatophilia.*

polychromatia (pol″e-kro-ma′she-ah) see *polychromatophilia.*

polychromatic (pol″e-kro-mat′ik) multicolored; exhibiting many colors.

polychromatic normoblast see polychromatophilic normoblast under *normoblast.*

polychromatocyte (pol″e-kro-mat′o-sīt) [*poly-* + Gr. *chroma* color + *kytos* hollow vessel] a cell stainable with various stains or colors.

polychromatocytosis (pol″e-kro″mah-to-si-to′sis) [*poly-* + Gr. *chrōma* color + *kytos* hollow vessel + *-osis* condition] see *polychromatophilia.*

polychromatophil (pol″e-kro-mat′o-fil) [*poly-* + Gr. *chrōma* color + *philein* to love] a polychromatophilic cell or tissue element.

polychromatophilia (pol″e-kro″mah-to-fil′e-ah) 1. the quality of being stainable with various stains or tints; an affinity for all sorts of stains.

2. the bluish-gray tint characteristic of young erythrocytes stained with Romanowsky-type stains, e.g., Wright stain; hemoglobin has an affinity for the acidic component and RNA for the basic component of the stain. Polychromatic red cells are paler and larger than mature red cells and may also lack the central pallor. These cells are shown to be reticulocytes when stained supravitally with brilliant cresyl blue. Thus, increased polychromasia implies reticulocytosis. It is most evident in conditions of hemolysis or acute blood loss. Also called *polychromasia, polychromatia,* and *polychromatocytosis.*

polychromatophilic (pol″e-kro″mah-to-fil′ik) pertaining to or characterized by polychromatophilia.

polychromatophilic normoblast see under *normoblast.*

polychromatophilic rubricyte see polychromatophilic normoblast under *normoblast.*

polychromatosis (pol″e-kro″mah-to′sis) [*poly-* + Gr. *chrōma* color + *-osis*] an excess of polychromatophilic erythrocytes in the blood, reticulocytosis.

polyclave (pol′e-klāv″) [*poly-* + L. *clavis* key] a multiple-entry key. See under *key.*

polyclonal (pol″e-klōn′al) [*poly-* + *clone*] derived from different cells; of or pertaining to several clones. The term is most frequently used in the description of an antibody response.

poly C·poly I see *antiviral agent.*

polycystic kidney disease (pol″e-sis′tik) [*poly-* + Gr. *kystis* cyst] a term used to describe two different and genetically distinct disorders, an infantile and an adult form, each characterized by bilateral renal cysts that increase total kidney size while reducing by compression the amount of functional kidney tissue.

The infantile form, transmitted as an autosomal recessive trait, may represent a heterogenous group with as many as four overlapping conditions. The earlier the onset, the more severe it is: perinatal onset is associated with a very early death, whereas juvenile onset may result in survival into the third decade with surgical treatment (portacaval shunting).

The adult form of the disease affects roughly 1 in 500 persons. It is transmitted as an autosomal dominant trait, with a penetrance that approaches 100 percent. Not all individuals with morphologic manifestations of the disease are symptomatic. Symptoms, when present, include flank pain, hematuria, infection, and (eventually) uremia. Hypertension and renal failure develop as the condition progresses. Pancreatic and hepatic cysts may also occur.

Laboratory results reflect the degree of renal involvement and may include proteinuria, hematuria, and pyuria. Diagnosis is accomplished by excretory urograms and radionuclide scanning.

polycythemia (pol″e-si-the′me-ah) [*poly-* + Gr. *kytos* hollow vessel + *haima* blood + *-ia*] a general term used to describe a condition in which the red blood cell (RBC) count (and usually hemoglobin concentration and hematocrit) is increased above normal. It takes two forms, relative and absolute.

Relative polycythemia is characterized by an increase in RBC concentration due to a reduction in plasma volume. This may occur in conditions of dehydration or stress, in which case it is not considered a true hematologic disorder.

Absolute polycythemia is characterized by an increase in RBC concentration due to an increase in RBC numbers, and is a true hematologic disorder. It is characterized by marrow hyperactivity and increased reticulocyte counts, serum iron turnover, blood volume, and blood viscosity. As a consequence, there is venous engorgement, cardiovascular stress, and nasal and gastric bleeding. This form may be further classified as primary (polycythemia vera) or secondary.

The secondary form is characterized by increased erythropoietin due to either appropriate or inappropriate stimuli. Examples of appropriate stimuli, viewed as an adaptive response, include living at high altitudes ($>$ 7000 ft), pulmonary disease (fibrosis and chronic obstructive diseases), alveolar hypoventilation, cardiac disease (especially with right-to-left shunts), defective hemoglobin (genetic or carbon monoxide exposure), and certain drugs (cobalt, testosterone, and exogenous erythropoietin). Inappropriate stimuli, which do not constitute an adaptive response, include renal disease, hepatic erythropoietin production, Cushing's syndrome, and cerebellar hemangioblastoma.

The differential diagnosis of the various forms of polycythemia is considered difficult and may require ^{51}Cr determination of RBC volume, ^{131}I-labeled albumin determination of plasma volume, determinations of blood cell morphology, absolute basophil counts, leukocyte alkaline phosphatase measurements, and bioassay of urinary erythropoietin excretion. Therapy is directed at reducing the number of red blood cells, often through phlebotomy.

Also called *erythremia* and *erythrocytosis.* For the classification of polycythemias, see the accompanying illustration.

p. vera, a form of primary absolute polycythemia, classified as a myeloproliferative disorder, that is characterized by an increase in the number of circulating red blood cells (RBC), white blood cells (WBCs), and platelets. The bone marrow is hyperactive, and erythroprotein concentration is depressed. RBC mass, hemoglobin concentration, and hemato-

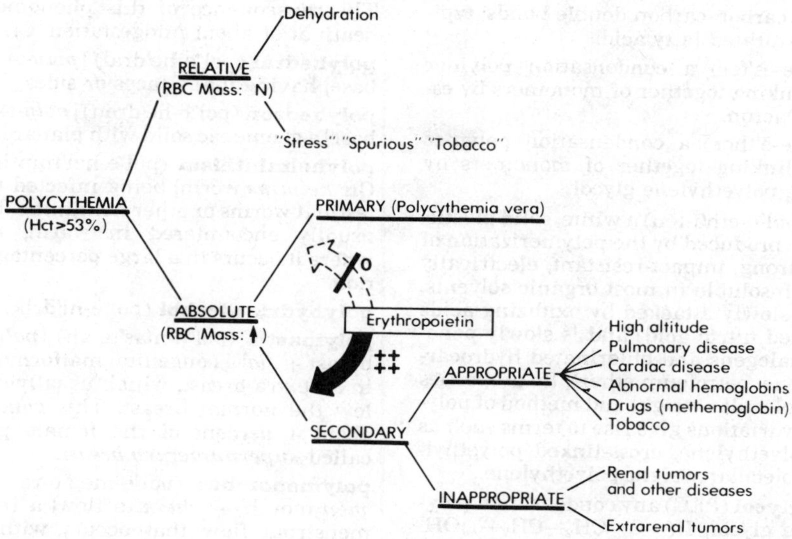

Polycythemia. Classification of the polycythemias. (From Wyngaarden, J. B., and Smith, L. H., Jr., eds.: Cecil Textbook of Medicine. 16th ed. Philadelphia, W. B. Saunders Co., 1979.)

crit counts are elevated. This disease is most common in middle age, occurring more frequently in males than in females.

Symptoms arise as a result of the increased blood viscosity and hypermetabolism. Splenomegaly and dusky redness of the skin, mucous membranes, and conjunctiva are commonly seen. Headache, weakness, hearing loss, and pruritus are frequent complaints.

Laboratory tests reveal RBC counts in the range of 6–10 million cells/μl. Hemoglobin concentration is elevated ($>$ 18 gm/100 ml in males, $>$ 16 gm/100 ml in females), as are the hematocrit ($>$ 54 percent in males, $>$ 49 percent in females), and RBC volume ($>$ 36 ml/kg in males, $>$ 32 ml/kg in females). Increases may also be seen in the WBC counts ($>$ 20,000/μl) and platelet counts ($>$ 400,000/μl). Other parameters that may be elevated include leukocyte alkaline phosphatase (score $>$ 100), serum B_{12} ($>$900 pg/ml), serum uric acid ($>$ 10–30 mg/100 ml), and blood and urine histamine. The bone marrow shows a hyperactivity of all elements with a decrease in fat, and the arterial oxygen saturation is normal or slightly depressed (although always above 91 percent).

The diagnosis of polycythemia vera should be suspected in any individual with an elevated hematocrit who is not on testosterone or diuretic therapy, who does not have congestive heart failure, or who does not live above 7000 ft; minimal criteria necessary for diagnosis include an increased RBC mass, an arterial oxygen saturation of $>$ 92 percent, and enlarged spleen. Complications of this disease include hemorrhage, thrombosis, and secondary gout. A few of those affected develop myelofibrosis and acute leukemia. Treatment may require phlebotomy, radiophosphorus (^{32}P), and chemotherapy; the average survival time following diagnosis and treatment is approximately 13 yr.

Also called *Osler-Vaquez disease* and polycythemia rubra vera.

polydactyly (pol″e-dak′tĭ-le) [*poly-* + Gr. *daktylos* finger + *-ia*] a congenital malformation of limbs that consists of the presence of extra fingers or toes. The extra digit generally lacks full muscular connections. If the hand is affected, the extra finger is most commonly on the ulnar side; if the foot is affected, the extra toe is most commonly on the fibular side.

polydeoxyribonucleotide synthetase (ATP) (po″lĭ-de-ok″se-ri″bo-nu′kle-o-tid sin′the-tās) an enzyme of the ligase class (poly (deoxyribonucleotide): poly (deoxyribonucleotide) ligase (AMP-forming), EC 6.5.1.1) that catalyzes the reaction ATP + (deoxyribonucleotide)$_n$ + (deoxyribonucleotide)$_m$ ⇄ AMP + pyrophosphate + (deoxyribonucleotide)$_{n+m}$. The reaction is important in the repair and synthesis of DNA. Also called *DNA ligase.*

Polydesmus (pol″e-dez′mus) a genus of millipedes of which the species *Polydesmus* has been reported in the digestive and urinary tracts of humans.

polydipsia (pol″e-dip′se-ah) [*poly-* + Gr. *dipsa* thirst + *-ia*] excessive thirst that persists for long periods, as in diabetes mellitus.

polyelectrolyte (pol″e-e-lek′tro-lĭt) in organic chemistry, a natural or synthetic high-molecular-weight polymer having ionizable side-chains, such as a protein or an ion-exchange resin.

polyene (pol′e-ēn) a chemical compound containing several double bonds, conjugated or nonconjugated.

polyene antibiotics a group of antibiotics, consisting of a macrocyclic lactone molecule containing several conjugated double bonds, that are synthesized by various species of *Streptomyces.* These compounds form complexes with sterols in the cell membranes of fungi, causing leakage of intracellular compounds; they are not active against most bacteria. See also *amphotericin B, antibacterial agents, candicidin,* and *nystatin.*

polyenoic acid (pol-e-e″no′ik) an organic acid having two or more carbon-carbon double bonds; typically, a polyunsaturated fatty acid.

polyester (pol″e-es′ter) a condensation polymer formed by the linking together of monomers by ester bonds, e.g., Dacron.

polyether (pol″e-ē′ther) a condensation polymer formed by the linking together of monomers by ether bonds, e.g., polyethylene glycol.

polyethylene (pol″e-eth′ĭ-lēn) a white, solid plastic, $[-CH_2-CH_2-]_x$, produced by the polymerization of ethylene. It is strong, impact-resistant, electrically insulating, and insoluble in most organic solvents. Polyethylene is slowly attacked by oxidizing acids (e.g., concentrated nitric acid) and is slowly penetrated by free halogens and chlorinated hydrocarbons (e.g., benzene, petroleum ether). Its properties vary with the molecular weight and method of polymerization; the variations give rise to terms such as high-density polyethylene, cross-linked polyethylene, and low-molecular-weight polyethylene.

polyethylene glycol (PEG) any condensation polymer of ethylene glycol, $H(-O-CH_2-CH_2-)_nOH$. The different preparations or formulations vary in average molecular weight of the product and in viscosity. The melting point increases with the molecular weight; the density and refractive index also vary with the molecular weight, but less consistently. PEGs are soluble in water, alcohol, and aromatic hydrocarbon solvents, forming sols/gels of varying viscosity. Those PEG preparations of relatively low molecular weight, PEG 200 to PEG 600, are liquids that are clear and essentially colorless, with the viscosity increasing from 4.3 to 10.5 cP, and the melting point increasing from –65° to 22°C. PEG 1000 to PEG 20,000 are white, waxy, and powdery or flaky solids, with viscosity values increasing from 17.4 to over 3200 (measured at 99°C), and melting points increasing from 28°C to 65°C. The industrial products are referred to by the trademark Carbowax. The designated molecular weights vary by about ±5 percent for preparations up to PEG 1000, and by roughly ±10 percent for the larger molecular forms.

In pharmaceutical work, the various PEGs are used as water-soluble ointment bases and solvents, suppository bases and vehicles, and tablet excipients. In the laboratory, PEG 400 and 600 are used as safe, inert, heat-stable, nonodorous heating bath fluids. PEG 4000 and 6000 may be used as osmotic agents to concentrate protein solutions. PEG is also used as histologic embedding medium.

polygenic (pol″ĕ-jen′ik) [*poly-* + Gr. *gennan* to produce] pertaining to or determined by the action of several different genes. See also *polygenic i.* under *inheritance.*

polygon (pol′e-gon) [*poly-* + Gr. *gōnia* angle] a plane geometric figure with straight sides.

polygraphic record (pol″e-graf′ik) [*poly-* + Gr. *graphein* to write] the record obtained from the simultaneous measurement of a number of physiologic parameters, such as the electroencephalogram, electrocardiogram, blood pressure, temperature, skin resistance, respiration, eye movement, electromyogram, and oxygen consumption.

polygyny (po-lij′ĭ-ne) [*poly-* + Gr. *gynē* woman] the failure of an oocyte to release the second polar body. The fertilized egg therefore contains one male pronucleus and two female pronuclei and is triploid. The consequence of this phenomenon is usually death at or about midgestation. Cf. *polyspermy.*

polyhedral (pol″e-he′dral) [*poly-* + Gr. *hedra* seat, base] having many faces or sides.

polyhedron (pol″e-he′dron) [*poly-* + Gr. *hedra* seat, base] a geometric solid with planar faces (polygons).

polyhelminthism (pol″e-hel′minth-iz′m) [*poly-* + Gr. *helmins* worm] being infected with several intestinal worms or other helminths. This condition is usually encountered in warm, moist climates, where it occurs in a large percentage of the population.

polyhydric alcohol (pol″e-hi′drik) see *polyol.*

polymastia (pol″e-mas′te-ah) [*poly-* + Gr. *mastos* breast + *-ia*] a congenital malformation that results in an extra breast, which usually develops just below the normal breast. This condition occurs in about 1 percent of the female population. Also called *supernumerary breast.*

polymenorrhea (pol″e-men″o-re′ah) [*poly-* + Gr. *mēn* month + *rhein* to flow] a relatively normal menstrual flow that occurs with abnormal frequency, i.e., in cycles less than 21 da apart.

polymer (pol′ĭ-mer) [*poly-* + Gr. *meros* part] a molecule formed by the binding together of many identical or similar subunits called monomers. A polymer may be a linear chain of monomers linked by the same type of bond (e.g., the peptide bond in proteins), or it may have a branched chain; synthetic polymers may have many cross-links between chains. If it consists of fewer than five monomers, it is called an oligomer.

addition p., a polymer formed by an addition reaction in which one unsaturated monomer unit is added to another so that no by-products are formed, e.g., polystyrene.

condensation p., a polymer formed by a condensation reaction in which monomers are joined into chains by the removal of water or some other small by-product. Biologic polymers are often of this type, e.g., proteins, polysaccharides, and nucleic acids.

polymerase (pol-im′er-ās, pol″ĭ-mer′ās) any enzyme that catalyzes polymerization, e.g., DNA polymerase.

polymerization (pol″ĭ-mer″ĭ-za′shun) the chemical reaction that forms a polymer.

polymerize (pol′ĭ-mer-īz) to subject to or to undergo polymerization.

polymetaphosphate (pol″e-met″ah-fos′fāt) a polymer of phosphate that occurs as a metachromatic granule in microorganisms and serves as a reserve of phosphate. Such granules are metachromatic, meaning that there is a change in color when they are stained by dyes such as methylene blue and toluidine blue.

poly-(methyl methacrylate) polymer (pol″e-meth″il-meth-ak′kril-āt) see *Plexiglas.*

polymicrobial (pol″e-mi-kro′be-al) [*poly-* + *microbe*] characterized by the presence of several species of microorganisms.

polymorphism (pol″e-mor′fizm) [*poly-* + Gr. *morphē* form] 1. the quality or character of occurring in several different forms.

2. in genetics, the occurrence in the same population of two or more alleles at a genetic locus, with at least one minor allele having a frequency greater than 1 percent. Thus, there are several normal

forms of the protein controlled by a polymorphic locus. Blood group (erythrocyte) and HLA (leukocyte) antigens are polymorphic and are detected using specific antisera. Many enzymes are polymorphic and the variants can be separated by electrophoresis (e.g., α-antitrypsin).

3. see *allotropy.*

balanced p., a genetic polymorphism that is maintained in a population, probably because heterozygotes have a selective advantage over both types of homozygote.

polymorphonuclear (pol″e-mor″fo-nu′kle-ar) [*poly-* + Gr. *morphē* form + *nucleus*] having a nucleus deeply lobed or so divided that it appears to be multiple.

polymorphonuclear leukocyte a mature form of one of the granulocytic series of blood cells (neutrophil, eosinophil, basophil). The term is sometimes used imprecisely to designate a neutrophil, and is often abbreviated as polymorph or poly.

polymorphonuclear neutrophil (PMN) an intensely phagocytic granular leukocyte formed in the bone marrow, which has a multilobed nucleus connected by slender threads of chromatin. The PMN is the mature cell of the granulocytic series and is designated M_6 and M_7. Of these two forms, the nonsegmented, less mature neutrophil (M_6), also known as the band form or stab cell, has a sausage-shaped nucleus (sometimes with indentations indicating future segmentation). The segmented neutrophil (M_7) is characterized by segmentation of the nucleus into separate lobes. Normally there are two to five lobes, with at most 5 percent of the cells containing five lobes; the majority contain three lobes. Under pathologic conditions there may be hypersegmentation into 6–10 lobes, which is referred to as a shift to the right; an increase in the number of band cells is referred to as a shift to the left (see *Arneth count*). Congenital hereditary hypersegmentation and hyposegmentation (Pelger-Huët anomaly, with unsegmented or bilobed nuclei) exist and are not associated with any functional cellular abnormality.

The cytoplasm of the PMN is slightly acidophilic and contains specific reddish-purple azurophilic granules. Because azurophilic granules are not produced after the myelocyte stage and decrease in number as a result of cellular division, they are greatly outnumbered by specific granules in the mature PMN. Although no longer produced in the mature PMN, the proteins and enzymes contained in these granules (myeloperoxidase, acid phosphatase, and β-glucuronidase in the azurophilic granules and acid phosphatase and proteins called phagocytins in the specific granules) play an important role in phagocytosis and cellular metabolism.

Highly phagocytic, PMNs are part of the body's first-line immune response. Being very adhesive and motile, they can ingest and digest microorganisms, other cells (erythrocytes and leukocytes), and inorganic material (crystals and other particulate matter). PMNs leave the bone marrow where they are formed from metamyelocytes and enter the circulation by active diapedesis; they can also migrate to the tissues by active diapedesis in response to an antigenic challenge.

Three pools of PMN exist in the body: the bone marrow pool, in which the mature cells remain in the bone marrow as a reserve; the marginal pool, which consists of cells that adhere for a time to vessel walls but continuously exchange with circulating PMNs; the tissue pool, which consists of PMNs that leave the peripheral blood and enter the tissues or body cavity. (These cells cannot reenter the circulation.)

Nuclear appendages are useful markers for making sex determination on blood specimens. A drumstick-shaped appendage, resulting from condensation of the inactive X chromosome, is present in 1–5 percent of the circulating granulocytes in females. The Y chromosome, which forms small clubs rather than drumsticks, is found in 3.5 percent of the PMNs circulating in males. They can be seen by their fluorescence after quinacrine staining.

Also called *neutrophil* and segmented leukocyte. See also *Barr body, Döhle bodies, erythrophagocytosis, LE cell, May-Hegglin bodies, tart cell,* and *toxic granulation.*

polymorphonuclear neutrophil chemotactic factor (NCF) a high-molecular-weight protein (M.W. 750,000) produced by activated mast cells, which is responsible for the chemotactic attraction of neutrophils and for neutrophil deactivation. Eosinophil chemotactic factor (ECF) may also be an attractant for neutrophils.

polymyalgia rheumatica (pol″e-mi-al′je-ah roomat′ik-ah) [*poly-* + Gr. *mys* muscle + *algos* pain; L. *rheumaticus* rheumatic] a rare disorder characterized by pain and stiffness in the proximal muscles, fever, malaise, weight loss, and a markedly elevated erythrocyte sedimentation rate (ESR). The onset can be either acute or gradual and usually does not appear before age 50 yr. The etiology is unknown. Many affected individuals develop temporal arteritis with associated pain and vision loss. Laboratory studies show an elevated ESR (often 100 mm/hr by the Westergren method). There may also be nonhemolytic anemia, and elevated alpha$_2$-globulins and fibrinogen. Corticosteroids are used in therapy; response is rapid and complete. Even without treatment, the disorder is usually self-limited.

polymyositis (pol″e-mi″o-si′tis) [*poly-* + Gr. *mys* muscle + *-itis* inflammation] a condition that produces weakness of the muscles of the shoulders, hips, and neck, usually associated with muscle pain and tenderness. Dysphagia, Raynaud's phenomenon, and arthritis are common associated findings. Polymyositis primarily affects females, its peak incidence occurring in the young and in those of late middle age. Histologically, it is characterized by myofiber necrosis, phagocytosis of degenerating muscle cells and infiltration by chronic inflammatory cells. Some individuals have an associated connective tissue disease (e.g., systemic lupus erythematosus, rheumatoid arthritis).

Diagnosis is aided by the finding of elevated serum creatine kinase levels and erythrocyte sedimentation rate, by electromyography, and by muscle biopsy.

polymyxins (pol″e-mik′sins) an antibiotic complex, produced by *Bacillus polymyxa,* that consists of cyclic polypeptides containing α, γ-diaminobutyrate and fatty acid side-chains. Polymyxins bind to cell membranes and alter the structure so that there is leakage of metabolites; thus, they act like cationic detergents and are bactericidal.

Resistance to polymyxins may result from an alteration in the cell envelope so that polymyxins cannot act at the target site. Polymyxin B and polymyxin E (colistin) are useful clinically. They are active against gram-negative bacilli, including *Pseudomonas aeruginosa* and coliform bacilli. *Proteus, Providencia, Serratia,* and *Neisseria* species are usually resistant. Polymyxins are used parenterally for serious life-threatening *Pseudomonas* infections or infections with gram-negative bacilli that are resistant to other drugs. Because they are toxic for human cell membranes as well as those of the target bacteria, use is indicated only for treatment of serious systemic infections by susceptible organisms and topical application for skin infections by susceptible organisms.

See also *antibacterial agents.*

p. B sulfate, the sulfate salt of polymyxin, used in the treatment of systemic *Pseudomonas* infections and, in combination with other antibiotics, for topical use.

p. E, see *colistin sulfate.*

polyneuritis (pol″e-nu-ri′tis) [*poly-* + Gr. *neuron* nerve + *-itis* inflammation] a condition that produces a weakness and sensory loss in the limbs as a result of inflammation in peripheral nerves. More recently, this term has been used to refer specifically to an autoimmune process that produces multifocal demyelination in the peripheral nerves in a patchy distribution. The prototype of this disorder is acute idiopathic polyneuritis, or Guillain-Barré syndrome. Profound slowing is evident on nerve conduction studies.

acute idiopathic p., see *Guillain-Barré syndrome.*

polyneuropathy (pol″e-nu-rop′ah-the) [*poly-* + Gr. *neuron* nerve + *pathos* disease] a degenerative or demyelinating dysfunction of the peripheral nervous system that affects more than one nerve.

polynuclear (pol″e-nu′kle-ar) [*poly-* + *nuclear*] 1. pertaining to or having several nuclei; polynucleate. 2. polymorphonuclear.

polynucleate (pol″e-nu′kle-āt) [*poly-* + *nucleate*] having several nuclei. Also called multinucleate.

polynucleolar (pol″e-nu-kle′o-lar) [*poly-* + *nucleolar*] having several nucleoli.

polynucleotide (pol″e-nu′kle-o-tīd) [*poly-* + *nucleotide*] any polymer of mononucleotides; nucleic acid. Some of these, such as polyadenylic acid, poly(A), or polyuridylic acid, poly(U), are synthetic.

polynucleotide ligase see *polydeoxyribonucleotide synthetase.*

polyol (pol″e-ol′) an alcohol with three or more hydroxy groups, e.g., a sugar alcohol or an inositol. Also called *polyhydric alcohol.*

polyol dehydrogenase see *iditol dehydrogenase.*

polyolefin (pol″e-o′le-fin) a thermoplastic polymer formed by the polymerization of simple olefins (alkenes); see *polyethylene* and *polypropylene.*

polyostotic (pol″e-os-tot′ik) [*poly-* + L. *os* bone] pertaining to or affecting several bones.

polyostotic fibrous dysplasia a congenital dysplasia of bone in which normal bone is replaced by fibrous tissue and poorly formed, woven bony trabeculae. Symptoms include segmental, painless swelling of the involved bones and brown pigmentation of the overlying skin. When associated with true precocious puberty in females, the condition is known as Albright's syndrome.

Radiographs characteristically reveal bone cysts and hypertrophy of bone; fractures and other deformities may also be evident. Serum concentrations of calcium and phosphorus are usually normal; alkaline phosphatase and urinary hydroxyproline concentration may be elevated.

See also *Albright's syndrome.*

polyp/o (pol′e-po) [Gr. *polypous* octopus, many-footed, from *poly-* + *pous* foot] a word element used in combining form to denote polyps or growths, e.g., polyposis.

polyp (pol′ip) a clinical or macroscopic term used to describe a circumscribed tumor that projects above the normal flat surface of the skin or a mucous membrane. Polyps may be sessile with a broad base or pedunculated with a stalk of variable length and diameter. See also *colon tumors* and the accompanying table.

adenomatous p., a neoplastic polyp, adenoma, composed of proliferating epithelial tubules that form caricatures of normal glands. Adenomatous polyps can arise on any mucous membrane, but are most common in the gastrointestinal tract, particularly in the colon. The spectrum of histologic patterns of adenomas in the colon ranges from that of tubular adenoma through tubulovillous adenoma to villous adenoma (see *colon tumors*).

aural p., a projection of granulation tissue from the middle ear into the external ear canal. In

POLYP. HISTOLOGIC CLASSIFICATION OF POLYPS OF THE LARGE INTESTINE

TYPE	SINGLE OR ISOLATED MULTIPLE POLYPS	POLYPOSIS
Neoplastic	Adenoma	Adenomatosis (familial polyposis)
Hamartomatous	Juvenile polyp	Juvenile polyposis
	Peutz-Jeghers polyp	Peutz-Jeghers syndrome
Inflammatory	Benign lymphoid polyp	Benign lymphoid polyposis
		Inflammatory polyposis, e.g., in inflammatory bowel disease
Unclassified	Hyperplastic (metaplastic) polyp	Hyperplastic polyposis

Modified from Morson, B.: Introduction. *In* Bennington, J. L. (ed.). The Pathogenesis of Colorectal Cancer. Major Problems in Pathology, Vol.10. Philadelphia, W. B. Saunders Co., 1978, p. 3.

chronic otitis media the tissue protrudes through a perforation in the tympanic membrane.

cervical p., a common benign polyp, usually pedunculated, that occurs after menarche but rarely after menopause. It may cause irregular vaginal bleeding, especially after trauma from intercourse or douching. The cause is not known, but irritation and inflammation may play a role in the etiology. These lesions may occur singly or multiply. If they are not visible on pelvic examination—occurring high within the cervical canal—hysterosalpingography or dilation of the cervix may be required for detection.

cholesterol p., a nonneoplastic lesion of the gallbladder, attached to the mucosa by a fragile, easily broken stalk; it is characterized by a focal accumulation of cholesterol-filled histiocytes in the submucosa. It may play a role in the genesis of gallstones.

colorectal p., a mass of tissue that projects from the colonic or rectal mucosa and protrudes into the lumen. There are a variety of types of colorectal polyps: sessile, pedunculated, or hyperplastic, and benign or malignant. The incidence increases with age.

The most common form of colorectal polyp is the adenomatous polyp. These benign neoplasms may be single or multiple, and sessile or pedunculated. They are more common in the rectum and sigmoid than elsewhere in the colon and are usually asymptomatic. They are important because of their propensity for malignant transformation.

Hyperplastic and lymphoid polyps are small, hyperplastic reactions of normal mucosa to initiation or inflammation. They are considered to hold no greater potential for malignant transformation than normal colonic mucosa.

Most polyps are asymptomatic, especially when small. Larger polyps may cause painless rectal bleeding. Copious mucus production is common with villous adenomas and may produce watery diarrhea, potassium loss, and dehydration. Multiple colonic polyps of various type, distribution, and malignant potential are associated with a number of syndromes, including familial colonic polyposis, Gardner's syndrome, multiple polyps, Peutz-Jeghers syndrome, and juvenile polyposis.

See also *polyposis* and the specific syndrome.

endometrial p., a small sessile or pedunculated projection of the endometrial mucosa. Endometrial polyps are usually single but may be multiple. They are most common at or near the time of menopause. Most are benign, but some show malignant transformation. Histologically, they are characterized by a polypoid configuration, stromal fibrosis, arterial sclerosis, chronic inflammation, and mucosal glands in various stages of cystic dilation.

gastric p., a relatively rare lesion of the stomach that may take the form of a small mucosal protrusion, pedunculated lesion, or large mass on the mucosal surface. Such lesions may be hyperplastic or adenomatous.

Hyperplastic polyps in the stomach are usually small (1–2 cm in diameter) and multiple; they rarely have stalks. Adenomatous polyps are single or multiple and pedunculated or sessile. As with colonic polyps, the adenomatous polyp may undergo malignant transformation.

hyperplastic p., a common benign polyp of the colon that is usually multiple and increases in frequency with advancing age. Usually sessile, the lesions rarely grow larger than 0.5 cm and may regress spontaneously. The pathogenesis is an alteration of the maturation of the normal mucosal epithelium, but the etiology is not known. Histologically, the polyp is characterized by elongated, cystically dilated tubular glands lined by an epithelium with patchy flattening of the cells, which produces a scalloped appearance; goblet cells are reduced in number. Also called metaplastic polyp.

inflammatory p., a polyp formed by mucosal tags of various sizes and shapes, which arises by the ulceration and undermining of adjacent mucosa. A variety of inflammatory diseases, including ulcerative colitis, Crohn's disease, and colitis of infectious origin, may give rise to this polyp form. Also called pseudopolyp.

juvenile p., a polyp most often found in the rectum, usually within 5 cm of the anus, of individuals generally younger than age 20 yr. It is less frequently found in the proximal large intestine, and in the stomach, small intestine, and appendix. The typical juvenile polyp exhibits cystic dilation of glands separated by an excess of lamina propria. Because most are associated with inflammation, an inflammatory basis for the origin of juvenile polyps has been postulated; currently, however, such polyps are generally regarded as hamartomas. Such polyps are generally symptomless and frequently undergo torsion with autoamputation, producing painless rectal bleeding.

laryngeal p., a smooth, small, rounded sessile or pedunculated nodule, most common in adult males, that occurs on the true vocal cords in response to voice abuse, chronic allergic reactions of the larynx, or chronic irritation from industrial fumes or cigarette smoke. It is unclear whether these nodules are inflammatory overgrowths of normal tissue or true benign neoplasms. Laryngeal polyps may produce changes in voice quality (e.g., hoarseness). Biopsy should be performed to exclude carcinoma, and surgical removal may be required.

lymphoid p., a polyp of the colon that usually occurs in the lower one-third of the rectum; it is generally solitary and typically is found in middle-aged individuals. Approximately 25 percent are pedunculated; the remainder are sessile. The lesion represents the extranodal equivalent of reactive follicular lymphoid hyperplasia.

Histologically, the lymphoid proliferation is centered in the submucosa. It includes lymphocytes in all stages of normal maturation and exhibits a distinct follicular pattern. This lesion must be differentiated from malignant lymphoid lesions of the intestine.

multiple p., a condition in which an individual has more than five adenomatous polyps of the colon but usually no more than 100 and does not derive the propensity for these polyps from the inheritance of an autosomal dominant character. Also called *multiple adenoma.* See also *colorectal p.* Cf. *familial colonic p.* under *polyposis.*

nasal p., a teardrop-shaped lesion that results from edema and hyperplasia of the submucosal connective tissue; it occurs most frequently around the ostia of the maxillary sinuses. These lesions are usually due to allergic rhinitis or to acute or chronic infections, and are frequently inflamed (inflammatory polyps). In addition to inflammatory polyps of the nasal cavity, dysplastic lesions and carcinomas may present as polyps.

Peutz-Jeghers p., a polyp derived from intestinal glandular epithelium, which may occur anywhere in the gastrointestinal tract. These polyps may be found singly without association with the Peutz-Jeghers syndrome, or as multiple polyps in association with the syndrome. In either case, the histologic appearance is identical. The lesions are characterized by a prominent branching fibromuscular scaffolding covered by a mucosecretory epithelium that forms elongated convoluted glands. Dysplastic changes are uncommon and malignant change is exceptionally rare. See also *Peutz-Jeghers syndrome.*

small intestine p., a lesion of the small intestine that protrudes above the mucosa that occurs in the various morphologic forms seen in mucosal polyps of the stomach and colon. They may be single or multiple. They are usually asymptomatic but may lead to partial obstruction, bleeding, volvulus, or intussusception. Multiple pedunculated polyps occur in the small intestine in association with familial colonic polyposis (see under *polyposis*) or *Peutz-Jeghers syndrome.*

villous p., a polyp that is usually large, sessile, and grossly covered by thin delicate fronds formed by markedly elongated tubular glands. It represents the extreme in the histologic spectrum, from tubular to villous. Also called *villous adenoma* and villous papilloma. See also *colorectal p.*

polyparasitism (pol″e-par′ah-si-tizm) infection or infestation by more than one variety of parasite.

polypeptide (pol″e-pep′tīd) [*poly-* + *peptide*] a peptide that on hydrolysis yields more than approximately 20 amino acids, according to the number of amino acids contained. See also *peptide.*

vasoactive intestinal p. (VIP), a putative gastrointestinal polypeptide hormone consisting of 28 amino acids, which is a member of the glucagon-secretin family of hormones; M.W. 3100. VIP is found not only in the GI tract (small intestine and colon) but also in other tissues, namely, the pancreas, peripheral nervous system, and brain. Its physiologic actions include stimulation of watery pancreatic bicarbonate juice, hyperglycemia due to hepatic glycogenolysis, inhibition of gastric secretion, stimulation of insulin and glucagon release, lowering of blood pressure by peripheral vasodilation (although it is an inotrophic agent), stimulation of small intestinal juice production, activation of mucosal adenylate cyclase, and inhibition of gastric motility. High plasma levels of VIP have been observed in the Verner-Morrison syndrome, which is caused by an APUD tumor of the endocrine pancreas. See also *Verner-Morrison syndrome.*

polyphase (pol′e-fāz) [*poly-* + *phase,* from Gr. *phasis* appearance] 1. having several phases.
2. containing colloid of several types.
3. pertaining to a three-phase, alternating-current power source or to equipment that requires a three-phase source.

polyphenism (pol″e-phēn′is′m) [*poly-* + Gr. *phainein* to show] the occurrence of different phenotypes that correspond to the same genotype.

polypheny (pol″e-fēn′e) see *pleiotropy.*

polyphosphoric acid (pol″e-fos-for′ik) see under *phosphoric acid.*

Polyplis (pol′e-plis) a genus of mollusks that serves as host of dermatitis-producing schistosome cercariae.

polyploid (pol′e-ploid) [*poly-* + Gr. *ploos* fold + *eidos* form] referring to an increase in the chromosome number (and, by extension, to nuclear DNA content) by multiples of the value in postmitotic diploid cells.

polyploidy (pol′e-ploi″de) the condition of having more than two full sets of homologous chromosomes. Cf. *polyteny.*

polypnea (pol″ip-ne′ah) [*poly-* + Gr. *pnoia* respiration] see *tachypnea.*

polyposis (pol″ip-o′sis) [*polyp* + *-osis* condition] the formation of numerous mucosal polyps. See also *polyp.*

familial colonic p., a rare hereditary condition, transmitted as a heterozygous and autosomal dominant trait, that is characterized by the formation of numerous (more than 100, and usually between 500 and 2500) adenomatous polyps that involve the entire colon and rectum, and occasionally extend to the stomach. The lesions most commonly appear in childhood and adolescence, and may cause rectal bleeding and diarrhea. Untreated individuals eventually develop malignant transformation of a polyp or polyps.

Diagnosis is based on family history, sigmoidoscopy, and barium enema. Cf. *multiple p.* under *polyp.*

juvenile p., a condition characterized by the appearance of multiple hamartomas or inflammatory polyps in the colon or small intestine of children; it may have a familial basis. The lesions may be true benign neoplasms or may represent congenitally malformed glands that give rise to mucous retention cysts. These polyps rarely, if ever, undergo malignant transformation.

multiple p., a group of conditions characterized by multiple polyps of the intestine, particularly the colon. In Gardner's syndrome, colonic polyposis is associated with epidermoid cysts, fibromas, osteomas of the skull, and supernumerary teeth. In Peutz-Jeghers syndrome, mucocutaneous pigmentation (particularly of the lips) is associated with hamartomatous polyps of the intestine, particularly the small bowel. In Canada-Cronkhite syndrome, multiple polyposis is associated with ectodermal abnormalities. In Turcot syndrome, colonic polyposis is associated with gliomas of the central nervous system. In familial multiple polyposis, which is transmitted as an autosomal dominant trait, the polyps are detected in children or adolescents, and the incidence of malignant transformation is high.

polypropylene (pol″e-pro′pĭ-lēn) a polyolefin plastic, $H[CH(CH_3)CH_2]_xH$, similar in properties and uses to polyethylene, although harder and more rigid.

polypyrrylmethane (pol″e-pir″il-meth′ān) an intermediate in the biosynthesis of heme from porphobilinogen. Chemically, it is a polymer of substituted pyrrole rings linked alternately with methene ($—CH_2—$) bridges.

polyribosome (pol″e-ri′bo-sōm) [*poly-* + *ribosome*] see *polysome.*

polysaccharide (pol″e-sak′ah-rīd) [*poly-* + *saccharide*] a carbohydrate (e.g., starch, inulin, cellulose) that contains a relatively large number of monosaccharide units per molecule. Polysaccharides may be hydrolyzed by acids or enzymes into their component monosaccharides.

polysome (pol′e-sōm) [*poly-* + Gr. *soma* body] a subcellular structure involved in protein synthesis. A strand of messenger RNA (mRNA), which carries the coding for one or more polypeptides, is transcribed from DNA in the nucleus and then moves into the cytoplasm. Ribosomes then attach the mRNA strand and travel along it, reading the code and producing a polypeptide chain (adding amino acids at a rate of 100–150 per min). With use of the electron microscope, the polysome appears as a string of beads (ribosomes about 20 nm in diameter) separated by about 34 nm and strung on an mRNA strand 300–600 nm long. Also called *polyribosome.*

polysomic (pol″e-so′mik) 1. pertaining to or exhibiting polysomy.
2. an individual exhibiting polysomy.

polysomnogram (PSG) (pol″e-som′no-gram) [*poly-* + L. *somnus* sleep + Gr. *gramma* a record] the record obtained from polysomnography.

polysomnography (pol″e-som-nog′rah-fe) [*poly-* + L. *somnus* sleep + Gr. *graphein* to write or draw] the continuous polygraphic recording of various physiologic parameters during sleep. The record obtained, the polysomnogram (PSG), is used in the diagnosis of various sleep and neurologic disorders. Parameters commonly recorded are the electroencephalogram, respiratory air flow, breath sounds, heart rate, diaphragmatic and leg movements, oxyhemoglobin content of the blood, and the occurrence of enuresis.

polysomy (pol″e-so′me) [*poly-* + chromo*some*] the presence of extra chromosomes in excess of the normal diploid number. Trisomy is the presence of one excess chromosome; tetrasomy, the presence of two excess homologous chromosomes (four homologues in all); and double trisomy, the presence of two excess nonhomologous chromosomes.

polysorbate (pol″e-sor′bāt) [USAN], the generic name for a group of non-ionic surfactants (detergents). They are used as pharmaceutical aids (emulsifiers), as dispersing agents, and as substrates in histochemical staining methods for esterases. The esters are copolymers of 1 mol of sorbitan (sorbitol anhydride) with 20 mol of ethylene oxide esterified to 1 or 3 mol of a fatty acid. The fatty acid groups are indicated by numbers: 20 for monolaurate, 40 for monopalmitate, 60 for monostearate, 65 for tristearate, 80 for monooleate, and 85 for trioleate; e.g., polysorbate 80 [USP], which is polyoxyethylene 20 sorbitan monooleate. Trademark, *Tween.*

polyspermy (pol″e-sper′me) [*poly-* + Gr. *sperma* seed] the penetration of the ovum by more than one spermatozoon during fertilization. Cf. *polygyny.*

polyspike and slow-wave complex (pol′e-spīk) see *multiple spike and slow-wave complex.*

polyspike complex see *multiple spike complex.*

polystyrene (pol″e-sti′rēn) a polymer formed from styrene (vinyl benzene), a common plastic.

polytene chromosome (pol′e-tēn) [*poly-* + L. *taenia* band, from Gr. *tainia*] giant chromosomes that consist of many chromatids (perhaps thousands, in some cases) associated along their length. These are found in some species of flies and are used in genetic research, as the chromosome banding pattern is easily mapped. See also *gene a.* under *amplification.* Also called *Balbiani chromosome.*

polyteny (pol″e-te′ne) the reduplication of chromosomes not followed by the separation of the sister chromatids, forming a multistranded chromosome. Cf. *polyploidy.*

polytetrafluoroethylene (TFE) (pol″e-tet″rah-floor″o-eth′ĭ-lēn) see *Teflon.*

polythiazide (pol″e-thi′ah-zīd) [NF], see under *thiazide diuretics.*

poly(U) abbrev. See *polyuridylic acid.*

polyunsaturated (pol″e-un-sach′ĕ-ra″ted) having many unsaturated bonds and tending to be liquid at room temperature; said of fats and oils.

polunsaturated fatty acid a fatty acid that contains more than two unsaturated carbon-carbon bonds in the molecule.

polyuria (pol″e-u′re-ah) [*poly-* + Gr. *ouron* urine + *-ia*] the passage of a large volume of urine in a given period, characteristic of diabetes.

polyuridylic acid (pol″e-ūr″ĭ-dil′ik) a synthetic polynucleotide containing a single nucleotide base, uracil. Also called *poly(U).* See also *poly A · U.*

polyvalent (pol″e-va′lent) 1. in chemistry, having two or more different valences or having a valence greater than 2.
2. see *multivalent.*

polyvinyl alcohol fixative method (pol″e-vi′nil) see *PVA fixative method.*

polyvinyl chloride (PVC) a white or colorless synthetic thermoplastic, $(\text{—}CH_2CHCl\text{—})_x$. Because there is a possibility of migration of the carcinogenic vinyl chloride, the use of PVC in some types of food packaging has been restricted by the U.S. Food and Drug Administration (FDA).

polyvinylpyrrolidone (PVP) (pol″e-vi″nil-pir-rol′ĭ-dōn) see *povidone.*

Pomatiopsis (po-mat″e-op′sis) a genus of freshwater snails, found in the United States, of which the species *P. lapidaria* is the first intermediate host of *Paragonimus kellicotti.*

Pompe's disease (pomps) [J. C. *Pompe,* Dutch physician, 20th century] a hereditary disorder, transmitted as an autosomal recessive trait, that is characterized by the abnormal metabolism and deposition of glycogen in all tissues. It is uniformly fatal by age 1 yr in the severe form (IIa), although in another form it may not appear until later in life (IIb). The disease is due to a relative or absolute deficiency of the enzyme α-1,4-glucosidase (acid maltase) in lysosomes. This defect leads to a cretinoid appearance, macroglossia, muscular hypotonicity, and cardiomegaly.

Electromyograms demonstrate myotonic discharges. Electrocardiograms show left ventricular hypertrophy with interventricular involvement. Histologic examination reveals vacuolar myopathy, thought to be associated with glycogen-filled lysosomes. Diagnosis is based on demonstration of the enzyme deficiency in muscle homogenates or the urine. Skin fibroblast cultures may also be useful. Prenatal diagnosis using cultured amniotic cells is possible.

Also called glycogenosis type II (Cori type II). See also *glycogenoses.*

ponceau 2R (pon′so) a red monoazo acid dye; C.I. 16150. It is used in histology as a plasma stain.

ponceau S a red acid dye; C.I. 27195. It is used primarily as a protein stain, particularly for staining the protein bands in serum protein electrophoretograms on cellulose acetate strips.

ponos (po′nos) [Gr. "suffering, pain"] see *kala-azar.*

pons (ponz), pl. *pontes,* gen. *pontis* [L. "bridge"] [NA], the part of the brain stem between the midbrain and the medulla oblongata, ventral to the cerebellum.

pont/o (pon′to) [L. *pons, pontis* bridge] a word element used in combining form to denote the pons, e.g., pontocerebellar.

Pontiac fever (pon′te-ak) [*Pontiac,* a city in SE Michigan] a nonpneumonic, self-limited, acute febrile illness without associated deaths. First noted in an outbreak in 1968 in Michigan, it is now known to be caused by a strain of *Legionella pneumophila.*

pontine (pon′tēn, pon′tin) pertaining to the pons.

ponto-geniculo-occipital (PGO) spike (pon″to-je-nik″u-lo-ok-sip′ĭ-tal) see under *rapid eye movement.*

pool (pōōl) 1. a common reservoir on which to draw.
2. to mix plasma from several donors.
3. an accumulation, as of blood in any part of the body, due to retardation of the venous circulation. See also *gene pool* and *metabolic pool.*

pooled estimate an estimate of the common variance of two populations given by the formula: $[(n_1-1)s_1^2+(n_2-1)s_2^2]/(n_1+n_2-2)$, where n_1 and n_2 are the population sizes and s_1^2 and s_2^2 the population variances.

POP a scintillator, 2,5-diphenyloxazole. POP and POPOP dissolved in toluene are used in most scintillation counters. Beta particles interact with POP (the primary scintillator), which emits a photon absorbed by POPOP (the secondary scintillator). POPOP then emits a photon at a wavelength good for detection by a photomultiplier tube.

popliteal (pop-lit′e-al, pop″lĭ-te′al) [L. *poples* ham] pertaining to the area behind the knee.

popliteal artery the continuation of the femoral artery. It begins at the opening in adductor magnus and runs down through the popliteal fossa to divide at the lower border of the popliteus muscle into anterior and posterior tibial arteries.

popliteal vein the vein formed by the junction of the anterior and posterior tibial veins. It ascends through the popliteal fossa to end at the opening in the adductor magnus, where it becomes the femoral vein.

POPOP a scintillator, 1,4-bis-(5-phenoxazole)benzene. See under *POP.*

population (pop″u-la′shun) [L. *populatio*] 1. the individuals collectively constituting a certain category or inhabiting a specified geographic area.
2. in statistics, the totality of possible individuals or observations from which a sample is selected. If the sample is random, the procedures of statistical influence can be applied validly.

P:O ratio the number of molecules of high-energy ATP produced from ADP per atom of oxygen gas consumed by an actively respiring mitochondrial system. It is a commonly used index of energy conversion in oxidative metabolism.

pore (pōr) [L. *porus,* from Gr. *poros* passage, from *peran* to pass through] a small opening or empty space.

alveolar p., any of the small openings in the alveolar wall that allow for the flow of air between adjacent alveoli of the lung (collateral airdrift); by providing an alternate avenue of escape for air otherwise trapped in isolated parts of the lung, they may help prevent alveolar collapse (atelectasis). Also called *pore of Kohn* and interalveolar pore.

gustatory p., the small opening of a taste bud onto the surface of the tongue.

p. of Kohn, see *alveolar p.*

nuclear p.'s, small openings in the nuclear envelope formed by fusion of the two layers of the envelope around a circular orifice that appears to contain a thin diaphragm.

slit p.'s, small, slitlike spaces between the pedicels of the podocytes of the renal glomerulus. Also called filtration slits. See also *glomerulus.*

sweat p., the opening of a duct of a sweat gland on the surface of the skin.

pork tapeworm see *T. solium* under *Taenia.*

Porocephalus (po″ro-sef′ah-lus) [Gr. *poros* passage + *kephalē* head] a genus of wormlike arthropods. The species that are parasitic in humans are now assigned to other genera; these include *P. armillatus* (*Armillifer armillatus*), *P. constrictus* (*A. armillatus*), and *P. denticulatus* (*Pentastoma denticulatum*).

-porosis (po-ro′sis) [Gr. *poros* passage] a suffix word element to denote passage, e.g., osteoporosis.

porosity (po-ros′ĭ-te) 1. the condition of being porous.
2. a pore.

porous (po′rus) characterized by numerous pores.

porphin (por′fin) the fundamental ring structure of four pyrrole nuclei linked by methyne bridges (—CH=) in an alternating double-bond super ring system. The porphyrins, hemin, the cytochromes, and chlorophyll are derivatives of porphin that contain various substituents on the β-carbons of the pyrroles and various metal ions chelated to the pyrrole-nitrogens.

porphobilinogen (PBG) (por″fo-bi-lin′o-jen) an unstable intermediary product in the biosynthesis of heme. It is a pyrrole derivative formed by the condensation of two molecules of δ-aminolevulinic acid (DALA) by cytoplasmic DALA-dehydratase; four molecules condense to form the PBG ring structure. It is rapidly converted to uroporphyrinogen, and steady-state plasma levels are low under normal circumstances; the urinary output is less than 2.5 mg/da. A significant increase in urinary output is characteristic of the acute intermittent form of hepatic porphyria. PBG gives a characteristic red color with Ehrlich's reagent, consisting of acid *p*-dimethylaminobenzaldehyde.

porphobilinogen assays and tests 1. the Watson-Schwartz test for urobilinogen and porphobilinogen in urine. See under *urobilinogen assays.*
2. quantitative assay. Porphobilinogen is adsorbed onto styrene-divinyl benzene copolymer anion exchange resin (Dowex 2) and eluted with acetic acid after the resin is washed to remove interfering substances. A red product is formed by adding Ehrlich's reagent (*p*-dimethylaminobenzaldehyde in hydrochloric acid) and quantitated spectrophotometrically at 555 nm.

porphobilinogen deaminase see *uroporphyrinogen I synthase.*

porphobilinogen synthase an enzyme of the lyase class (5-aminolaevulinate hydro-lyase, EC 4.2.1.24) that catalyzes the reaction 2,5-aminolevulinate ⇄ porphobilinogen + 2 H_2O. The reaction is an important step in heme biosynthesis. It is inhibited by lead in minute quantities, and a decreased level of the enzyme in erythrocytes is an indication of lead poisoning. Also called *δ-aminolevulinate dehydratase.*

porphobilinogen synthase assays a test for lead intoxication, based on determination of the porphobilinogen synthase [aminolevulinate (ALA) dehydratase] activity in erythrocytes, which may be depressed in the presence of lead even in concentrations that may not produce clinical symptoms. A buffered hemolysate of suspected red cells is permitted to act on a preparation of 5-aminolevulinate, and the free amount of porphobilinogen (PBG) formed in a fixed time period, compared with an appropriate control, is calculated. The PBG is measured using Ehrlich's reagent.

The test should be performed on fresh blood whenever possible. The pH must be rigidly controlled, and chelating anticoagulants such as EDTA must not be used; heparin is preferred.

Also called *δ-aminolevulinate dehydratase assay.*

porphyria (por-fe′re-ah, por-fi′re-ah) [Gr. *porphyra* purple] a heterogeneous group of hereditary or acquired disorders of heme biosynthesis, resulting in the overproduction and excretion of precursors in the heme biosynthetic pathway. The individual hereditary disorders are thought to result from specific enzymatic deficiencies. The principal pathologic abnormalities in the porphyrias are neurologic dysfunctions and/or skin photosensitivity. The neurologic manifestations are usually linked to the ingestion of certain drugs, such as barbiturates, and are characterized by abdominal pain, neuropathies of the peripheral nerves, and mental dysfunctions. Skin sensitivities result from the accumulation of porphyrin, and are expressed as scarring and mutilation. Clinical expression in the porphyrias may be extremely variable. These syndromes are classified as either erythropoietic or hepatic porphyrias, depending on the site of heme synthesis where the metabolic errors occur.

acute intermittent p., a genetic disease, transmitted as an autosomal dominant trait, that is characterized by repeated attacks of neurologic dysfunction and psychiatric disorders. (The skin photosensitivity exhibited in erythropoietic porphyria is not observed in this disorder). This form is a hepatic porphyria, with the abnormal enzyme uroporphyrinogen-1-synthetase involved in heme biosynthesis in the liver. Characteristic symptoms are rarely expressed before puberty. Abdominal pain, vomiting, and nausea are commonly the first complaints. Neurologic impairment occurs, including paresthesia, neuritic pain, psychoses, convulsions, and quadriplegia. Acute attacks are considered to be provoked by four factors: drugs (barbiturates, sulfonamides, and griseofulvin), steroids (estrogens and contraceptive steroids), starvation, and infection.

Laboratory diagnosis is accomplished by the demonstration of increased urinary levels of only the porphyrin precursors, aminolevulinic acid and porphobilinogens, particulary in the latent carrier. Lack of accumulation of preformed porphyrins explains the absence of skin photosensitivity. Freshly passed urine is colorless and turns dark when left standing in light and air. Values for conventional liver function tests are, for the most part, within normal limits, except for the bromsulphalein (BSP) retention test. Acute attacks, often aggravated by fluid imbalance, frequently used to be fatal, but with modern treatment the mortality rate has dropped to 5 percent or less.

Also called pyrroloporphyria.

congenital erythropoietic p., a rare genetic disorder, transmitted as an autosomal recessive trait, that is characterized by chronic sensitivity to light and by hemolytic anemia; heterozygous individuals are not clinically affected. This disorder is due to a defective enzyme in the erythroid developmental series in the bone marrow. As a result, there is massive overproduction of uroporphyrinogen I, which cannot be used for heme synthesis but is converted to coproporphyrinogen I. This latter compound cannot be metabolized further; along with its precursor, it accumulates in the body tissues and is excreted in the urine and feces. Porphyrin accumulation leads to skin photosensitivity and the progressive formation of skin vesicles and bullae, which degenerate to produce scarring and mutilation. Red cells are short-lived, resulting in hemolytic anemia. A red discoloration of the teeth and bones is also common.

Diagnosis is based on demonstration of high concentrations of uroporphyrin I and coproporphyrin in the urine, which color it red. The normoblasts and reticulocytes contain large quantities of uroporphyrin I, a condition that leads to an intense red fluorescence on examination. Those affected often die during childhood, and few survive past age 40.

Also called congenital photosensitive porphyria, erythropoietic uroporphyria, and Günther's disease. See also *uroporphyrinogen III cosynthase.*

p. cutanea tarda, the most common form of hepatic porphyria, transmitted as an autosomal dominant trait, that is characterized by chronic skin lesions without any neuropsychiatric dysfunction. The inherited trait responsible for this disorder seems to be a partial deficiency of the enzyme uroporphyrinogen decarboxylase. The disease may present in an overt, subclinical, or latent form. It is seen most frequently in individuals of middle age and is invariably associated with a form of liver dysfunction, such as alcoholic liver disease or hepatic siderosis. Skin lesions include hyperpigmentation, erythema, and ulcerative vesicles. Sclerodermatous changes and increased skin sensitivity to trauma are also observed. The urine may be pink or brown because of the increased urinary excretion of uroporphyrin and coproporphyrin.

Diagnosis is established by noting the skin sensitivity, liver disease, increased urinary levels of uroporphyrin, and a lack of either porphyrin precursor accumulation or neurologic dysfunction.

Also called symptomatic cutaneous hepatic porphyria and symptomatic porphyria.

hereditary coproporphyria, a genetic disorder, transmitted as an autosomal dominant trait, that is characterized by neurologic dysfunctions, psychiatric disorders, and, infrequently, skin photosensitivity, which resemble the symptoms observed in acute intermittent porphyria. However, in contrast to that disorder, this disease process is much milder; more than half of those affected are asymptomatic. The primary genetic defect is thought to be a deficiency of coproporphyrinogen oxidase, which leads to massive excretion of coproporphyrin III in the feces and, to a lesser extent, in the urine. The enzyme deficiency can be demonstrated in the leukocytes, erythrocytes, and cultured skin fibroblasts. Acute attacks may be precipitated by the same factors precipitating attacks of intermittent acute porphyria and variegate porphyria: drugs, steroids, starvation, and infection. The onset of the disorder's acute phase is often associated with concurrent liver disease.

protoporphyria, a genetic disease, transmitted as an autosomal dominant trait, that is characterized by mild skin photosensitivity and increased concentrations of protoporphyrin in erythrocytes, and occasionally in the liver. This metabolic disorder is due to a deficiency of ferrochelatase, which can be demonstrated in the liver, peripheral blood, bone marrow, and cultured skin fibroblasts of those affected. The photosensitivity, which is due to increased levels of protoporphyrin, is manifested by pruritus, erythema, edema, and solar eczema following exposure to sunlight. The extent of expression of these cutaneous symptoms is variable, and the hyperpigmentation, hypertrichosis, and neuropsychiatric dysfunctions of other porphyrias are not seen. Although this disease is generally mild, liver and biliary disease leading to massive cirrhosis and cholelithiasis, presumably due to deposition of protoporphyrin, has been reported.

Diagnosis is based on erythrocyte examination with fluorescent microscopy. Increased concentrations of protoporphyrins in these cells impart a characteristic red fluorescence pattern. Concentrations of protoporphyrin may also be increased in the plasma and feces.

Also called erythrohepatic protoporphyria and erythropoietic protoporphyria.

variegate p., a genetic disease, transmitted as an autosomal dominant trait, that is characterized by acute attacks of neurologic dysfunction and psychoses and skin sensitivity to sunlight and mechanical trauma. It was first recognized in the Afrikaaners of South Africa and is now known to occur worldwide. The enzymatic abnormality responsible for this disorder has not been conclusively identified, but a deficiency in either protoporphyrinogen oxidase or ferrochelatase has been suggested as a possible mechanism. Overt disease does not appear until the second or third decade of life. Abdominal pain, neurologic and psychiatric abnormalities, and skin lesions may occur during an acute attack. Mechanical fragility, especially of sun-exposed skin, leads to pigmented scars, hyperpigmentation, and delayed healing after trivial injury. As in acute intermittent porphyria, drugs and steroids may precipitate acute attacks. Large amounts of protoporphyrin are excreted in the bile and feces. The chronic excessive excretion of protoporphyrin and, to a lesser extent, coproporphyrin, is observed in the urine. During an acute attack, there is increased urinary excretion of aminolevulinic acid and porphobilinogens. Erythrocyte porphyrin levels are normal, however, distinguishing this condition from protoporphyria. Also called South African genetic porphyria.

porphyrin (por′fĭ-rin) any one of a group of iron-free or magnesium-free porphyrin derivatives that occur universally in protoplasm and differ in substituents on the β-positions in the pyrrole ring. These include chlorophyll and a number of intermediates leading to the biosynthesis of heme.

porphyrin assays 1. spectrophotometry or fluorometry. Porphyrins have characteristic absorbance peaks in the wavelength range of 400–410 nm. On excitation at this wavelength, they exhibit an intense pink-orange fluorescence in the range of 590–620 nm. In screening tests, specimens are acidified with acetic acid and then extracted into ethyl acetate (total porphyrins) or diethyl ether (coproporphyrins). The porphyrins are then reextracted into dilute HCl. The latter is examined for pink-orange fluorescence using a long-range ultraviolet (black light) lamp.

For quantitative determination, coproporphyrin is extracted from urine at pH 4.8 into ethyl acetate and then back into 0.1 mol/l of HCl. The absorbance of the solution is read at 401 nm using the Allen correction technique, or the coproporphyrin is measured fluorometrically. Uroporphyrin is extracted into *n*-butanol and reextracted into 0.5 mol/l of HCl and the absorbance read at 405 nm. Protoporphyrin in erythrocytes and stool is reextracted into 3.0 mol/l of HCl.

2. separation by thin-layer chromatography. For qualitative analysis, the plates can be inspected directly under UV light; for quantitative analysis, the individual spots are scraped off, eluted with appropriate HCl solutions, and measured fluorometrically.

porphyrinuria (por″fĭ-rĭ-nu′re-ah) [*porphyrin* + Gr. *ouron* urine + *-ia*] the presence of porphyrin and/or porphyrinogens in the urine in excess of the normal amount. Abnormal excretion of porphyrins is seen in diverse disorders, such as alcoholism, lead poisoning, and hemolytic disease, as well as in some of the true porphyrias. The porphyrins may be of the uro- or copro- forms, and of either type III or type I.

porphyropsin (por″fĭ-rop′sin) [Gr. *porphyra* purple + *ōps* eye + *-in*] a purple photosensitive pigment in the retinal rods of all true freshwater fish; its absorption maximum is near 522 nm. Like rhodopsin contained in the retinas of mammals, birds, amphibia, marine fish, and invertebrates, the porphyropsin system undergoes cyclic changes of bleaching and regeneration in which the vitamin A_2 derivatives retinol$_2$ and retinal$_2$ replace their vitamin A_1 analogs of the rhodopsin system. Vitamin A_2 differs from A_1 by having one additional double bond in the ring. See also *rhodopsin.*

port (port) [L. *portus* port] an access to a system or circuit; a connection to a computer by an input-output device.

porta (por′tah) [L. "bridge, entrance"] an entrance or gateway, especially the point at which blood vessels and other supplying or draining structures enter an organ, e.g., the porta hepatis.

p. hepatis, a deep fissure on the inferior surface of the liver between the quadrate lobe and the caudate process where the hepatic artery, portal vein, and hepatic nerves enter and the hepatic ducts and lymph vessels emerge. Also called hepatic portal.

portal (por′tal) [L. *porta* entrance] 1. an avenue of entrance.

2. pertaining to an entrance, especially the porta hepatis.

portal canal the connective tissue sheath that encloses small branches of the portal vein, hepatic artery, and bile duct. It lies at the center of a portal lobule of the liver, i.e., at the periphery of a classical lobule.

portal cirrhosis a term that has been used in the anatomic classification of cirrhosis to describe a form of cirrhosis that corresponds approximately to micronodular cirrhosis. See also *cirrhosis.*

portal hypertension see *portal h.* under *hypertension.*

portal lobule a functional unit of the liver; a roughly triangular area of hepatic tissue whose axis is the interlobular bile duct of the portal canal.

portal system an arrangement of vessels in which blood collected from one set of capillaries passes through a large vessel or vessels and then through a second set of capillaries before passing back into the systemic circulation.

hepatic p. s., a system of blood vessels that carries venous blood from the intraabdominal digestive tract, pancreas, gallbladder, and spleen to the liver. Blood from the capillary network of these organs is transported via the portal vein to the liver where it enters a second network of capillaries, the liver sinusoids.

hypothalamic-hypophyseal p. s., a system of long and short portal vessels that extends from the capillary plexuses of the median eminence, infundibulum, and neurohypophysis to the capillary network in the anterior pituitary. Releasing and inhibitory factors from the hypothalamus are conveyed by these vessels to the anterior pituitary to modulate its secretory activities.

portal triad a group of three structures: the small branches of the hepatic artery, the portal vein, and the bile duct, which are ensheathed by connective tissue between liver lobules.

portal vein the vein formed by the junction of the superior mesenteric and splenic veins behind the neck of the pancreas. It passes upward in the free edge of the lesser omentum in company with the hepatic artery and common bile duct, and enters the liver through the porta hepatis.

Porter-Silber reaction [Curt C. *Porter,* U.S. biochemist, born 1914; Robert H. *Silber,* U.S. biochemist, born 1915] a color reaction used in the determination of 17,21-dihydroxy-20-ketocorticosteroids, including cortisol, cortisone, 11-deoxycortisol (compound S), and their tetrahydro derivatives. In acid solution, these compounds rearrange to form a 21-aldehyde, which reacts with phenylhydrazine to form a yellow hydrazone having an absorbance maximum at 410 nm. The reaction is nonspecific; other aldehydes and ketones also form hydrazones. Compounds undergoing this reaction are called Porter-Silber chromogens. In assays of urinary corticosteroids, conjugates are hydrolyzed by β-glucuronidase and extracted into organic solvents such as chloroform before the formation of the hydrazone.

Porthetria (por-thet′re-ah) a genus of caterpillars; the species *P. dispar* (the gypsy moth), which possesses poisonous hairs, is found throughout Europe.

position (po-zish′un) [L. *positio,* from *ponere* to place] 1. a body posture or attitude assumed by the patient to achieve comfort in certain conditions, or the particular placement of the body and extremities to facilitate the performance of certain diagnostic or therapeutic procedures.

2. in obstetrics, the situation of the fetus in the pelvis, determined and described by the relation of a given arbitrary point (point of direction or reference point) in the presenting part to a given arbitrary point in the coronal plan of the maternal pelvis. Cf. *presentation.*

anatomic p., the position of the human body standing erect, with the palms of the hands turned forward; it is used as the position of reference in describing the site or direction of various structures or parts as established in official anatomic nomenclature.

decubitus p., the position of an individual lying on a horizontal surface; it is designated according to the portion of the body resting on the surface as dorsal decubitus (lying on the back); left lateral decubitus (on the left side); right lateral decubitus (on the right side); or ventral decubitus (on the abdomen).

lithotomy p., a position in which the patient lies in dorsal decubitus with hips and knees flexed and the thighs abducted and externally rotated.

obstetric p., a position in which the patient lies on the left side, the right thigh and knee drawn up. Also called English position and lateral recumbent position.

occipitoanterior p., a position of the fetus in cephalic presentation in labor, with the occiput directed toward the right (ROA) or left (LOA) anterior quadrant of the maternal pelvis.

occipitoposterior p., a position of the fetus in cephalic presentation in labor, with the occiput directed toward the right (ROP) or left (LOP) posterior quadrant of the maternal pelvis.

occipitotransverse p., a position of the fetus in cephalic presentation in labor, with the occiput directed toward the right (ROT) or left (LOT) iliac fossa of the maternal pelvis.

opisthotonos p., see *opisthotonos.*

prone p., a position in which the patient lies face down.

radiographic p., the specific body position of the patient during the exposure of a radiograph, e.g., prone, right lateral decubitus. Certain positions, especially those named after their originators, also imply a particular projection (path of the central ray) and part-film relationship. For this reason, the term position is sometimes used as a synonym for projection.

positioning (po-zish′un-ing) the relative placement of patient, film, or x-ray tube in the exact alignment necessary for making a diagnostic radiograph of a particular part.

positive (poz′ĭ-tiv) [L. *positivus,* from *ponere* to place or assert] 1. affirming or cooperating.

2. having a numerical value greater than zero.

3. the presence of a condition or substance in a test or assay.

4. referring to an electric charge having the same sign as the charge on the proton, as a positive ion (cation) or positive electrode (anode).

5. a photographic image in which the light and dark areas are like the original object; usually a print made from a developed negative. Cf. *negative.*

positive end-expiratory pressure (PEEP) a form of positive pressure breathing used during continuous mechanical ventilation in which airway pressure is increased at the end of the expiratory phase. The desired level of positive end-expiratory pressure (usually 5–15 cm of H_2O) is set by adjustment of the expiratory valve of the ventilator so that expiratory flow is impeded by the necessary amount.

Application of positive end-expiratory pressure acts to increase the number of alveoli that remain open at end-expiration, serving to increase the functional residual capacity and reduce any shunt or alveolar-arterial Po_2 difference. Its use is therefore indicated in forms of adult respiratory distress syndrome that lead to airway closure or alveolar collapse at end-expiration. As in other forms of positive pressure breathing, monitoring of blood pressure and cardiac output and blood gas analysis (mixed venous O_2 content and arteriovenous difference in O_2 content) are utilized to ensure that venous return is not restricted during inspiration and expiration.

positive occipital sharp transient of sleep in electroencephalography, a sharp wave that is maximal over occipital regions, where it is positive in relation to other brain areas. Its amplitude varies but is usually less than 50 μV. Such waves occur spontaneously, either singly or repetitively, during light sleep (Stage 2). Also called *lambdoid wave.*

positive pressure a pressure greater than atmospheric pressure.

positive pressure breathing (PPB) a method used to assist alveolar ventilation. In this procedure, the lungs are inflated and the thorax expanded by the breathing of gas at a pressure above atmospheric (usually 20–30 torr) through a mask, mouthpiece, or endotracheal or tracheostomy tube. Room air, 100 percent O_2, or a gaseous mixture at a positive pressure can be supplied continuously (continuous positive pressure breathing) when respiration is spontaneous, or in bursts (intermittent positive pressure breathing.

Intrapleural pressure is negative in both the inspiratory and expiratory phases of a normal, spontaneous respiration. Inspiration accentuates the negative intrapleural pressure, facilitating venous return from the peripheral veins to the heart. In contrast, intrapleural pressure is positive during inspiration in positive pressure breathing; venous return may be impeded during this phase of the respiratory cycle, resulting in a decreased cardiac output.

These hemodynamic consequences are aggravated in individuals with hypovolemia or inadequate left ventricular function. An adequate expiratory time (during which time intrapleural pressure may again approach subatmospheric values) is thus a necessary part of positive pressure breathing.

continuous p. p. b. (CPPB), the continuous application of gas at a positive pressure to the airways during spontaneous breathing. The pattern of breathing during CPPB consists of intermittent forced (active) expirations interspersed with passive inspirations from the source of positive pressure, usually an air compressor or compressed gas cylinder. One consequence of CPPB is that unless the subject forcibly inhales in order to reduce intrathoracic pressure, the pressure may be sustained at values greater than atmospheric, thus impeding venous return.

This form of assisted ventilation is most useful clinically in the prevention of airway collapse during expiration or in the treatment of infant respiratory distress syndrome.

Also called *continuous positive airway pressure.*

intermittent p. p. b. (IPPB), a form of assisted ventilation in which the lungs are inflated by bursts of room air, pure O_2, or a gaseous mixture under positive pressure. As pressure in the mouthpiece or mask used to deliver the gas decreases between bursts, passive exhalations can occur.

IPPB systems can be adjusted so that the inspiratory phase is triggered by a desired level of inspiratory effort (level of subatmospheric pressure) and is halted by any desired cut-off value of peak inspiratory pressure. Inspiratory and expiratory flow rates can also be set to optimal levels.

Use of IPPB is indicated in conditions such as pulmonary edema, respiratory arrest, and atelectasis, and in conditions in which the work of breathing has greatly increased.

positive sharp wave the brief burst, usually 10–100 msec in duration, of biphasic electrical activity recorded from muscle fibers mechanically stimulated or injured by electrode insertion or other electrode movement. After the rapid onset of an initial positive deflection of less than 5-msec duration and 1-mV amplitude, a smaller-amplitude negative phase occurs. These positive-negative potential changes are repeated with a generally regular rhythm at a rate of 2–10 Hz in a sequence known as a train of positive sharp waves. These characteristic waves may also occur spontaneously in certain myopathic disorders and in denervated muscle. See also the accompanying illustration.

positron (e^+) (poz′ĭ-tron) [*posi*tive + elec*tron*] the antiparticle of the electron. Positrons are emitted by some radionuclides; they immediately collide with electrons in the surrounding matter and are annihilated. The resulting 511-keV gamma rays can be used for scintillation imaging or computed tomography.

positron annihilation the conversion of a positron and an electron to energy in the form of two 511-keV gamma-ray photons, which travel in opposite directions.

positron beta decay see *beta decay.*

positron-emission tomography (PET) an imaging device used in nuclear medicine to produce an image of the distribution of a positron-emitting radioisotope through the body in a transverse plane.

Except for the detector, PET is the same as computed tomography (CT): the image is produced by a computer program (reconstruction algorithm) from data giving the distribution of the isotope along lines lying in the imaging plane. These lines correspond to the path of the two gamma rays emitted almost exactly in opposite directions during a positron annihilation. When two rays are received si-

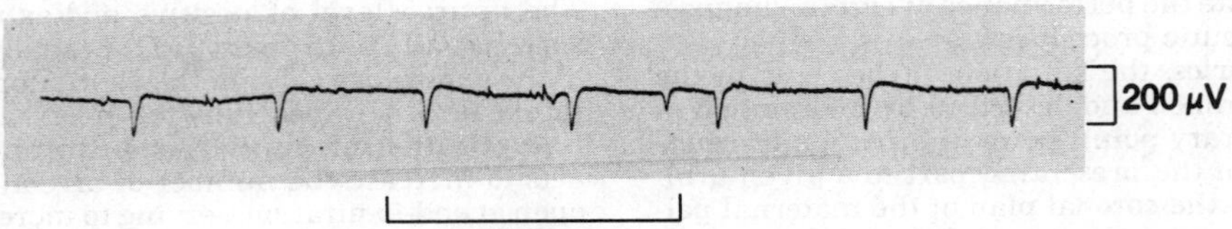

Positive sharp wave. Positive sharp waves recorded in partially denervated muscle. From Aminoff, M. J.: Electromyography in Clinical Practice. Menlo Park, CA, Addison-Wesley Publishing Co., 1978.

multaneously, a positron emission is assumed to have occured on the line connecting the two detectors.

This assumption is not precisely correct because when a positron emission occurs, the positron travels approximately 2 mm while it is being stopped by electrostatic interactions with electrons. It then annihilates an electron with the emission of two 511-keV gamma rays. Owing to the thermal motion of the electron and positron, the angle between the emitted photons is not exactly 180°.

The detector array is a ring of thallium-activated sodium iodide [NaI (Tl)] scintillation crystals and photomultiplier tubes; a typical array has 64 crystals, each 2 cm in diameter. Positron decays are recorded by coincidence-counting circuitry when gamma rays arrive at two detectors at the same time. The computer stores the number of decays that occur on each projection (the line between two detectors) and reconstructs the image. Spatial resolution of the image depends on the detector size, pixel area, counting statistics (noise), and uncertainty of the decay position due to motion of the positron, but is typically a few millimeters.

PET is an expensive procedure because the most useful radioisotopes—^{15}O, ^{13}N, ^{11}C, and ^{18}F—have very short half-lives. They must be produced in an on-site cyclotron and chemically attached to a tracer substance within a period of minutes. However, PET is important because it provides information that cannot be obtained by other means. For example, by labeling blood with ^{11}C–carbon monoxide, which binds to hemoglobin, tomographic blood pool images can be obtained to show the regional perfusion of an organ in multiple planes. Images of the distribution of metabolic activity throughout an organ can be obtained by using labeled metabolites. ^{15}O-oxygen and ^{11}C-glucose have been used for brain imaging and ^{11}C-palmitate for heart imaging. Rubidium-81, which is distributed like potassium, is also used for heart imaging. Use of labeled neurotransmitters, hormones, and drugs makes PET an important research tool; by mapping the distribution of receptors for these substances in the central nervous system, scientists expect to make important advances in the fields of neurophysiology and neuropharmacology.

Also called positron-emission transverse tomography. See also *computed tomography.*

post- (pōst) [L. *post* after] a prefix word element to denote after or behind, e.g., postnatal.

postabsorptive state (pōst″-ab-sorp′tiv) the metabolic state of the body after the digestion and absorption of a meal is completed; it is characterized by decreased concentrations of glucose, insulin, and lipids in the blood, and also by glycolysis and lipolysis. The body returns to the postabsorptive state within 6 hr after the meal. In many cases blood samples for chemical analysis are drawn during this period. Cf. *absorptive state.*

postactivation exhaustion (pōst″ak-tĭ-va′shun) a decrease in the amplitude of the initial M wave and/or the appearance of or increase in a decrementing response that occurs immediately following a brief period (10–30 sec) of muscle exercise (strong, voluntary isometric contractions). It also occurs after an interval of repetitive stimulation that has resulted in tetanic contraction. Cf. *postactivation facilitation.*

postactivation facilitation an increase in the amplitude of the initial M wave and/or the disappearance of or decrease in a decrementing response that appears immediately after a period of muscle exercise. It also occurs after a brief period of repetitive nerve stimulation following a tetanic contraction. Also called postactivation potentiation. Cf. *postactivation exhaustion.*

postauricular (pōst″aw-rik′u-lar) [*post-* + L. *auriculus,* dim. of *auris* ear] located behind the ear.

postauricular region the region of the upper neck posterior to the ear.

postchromation (pōst″kro-ma′shun) [*post-* + Gr. *chroma* color] the use of dichromate fixatives after primary fixation in formalin to render certain lipids (especially phospholipids) insoluble in the usual lipid solvents; it enhances the demonstration of myelin in paraffin sections.

postdiction (pōst-dik′shun) a statement about the probability of an event after the random experiment has been performed and thus the probability no longer technically exists (the known outcome of the experiment is a certainty).

poster/o (pos′ter-o) [L. *posterus* behind] a word element used in combining form to denote the back of the body or a structure, e.g., posteromedial.

posterior (pos-tēr′e-or) [L.] situated in back of, or in the back part of, a structure; [NA], a term used in reference to the back or dorsal surface of the body. In radiology, a posterior view is one made with the posterior side of the subject closest to the film.

posterior axillary line the vertical line that passes through the posterior axillary fold.

posterior chamber of the eye the chamber in front of the lens and suspensory ligament and behind the iris. This chamber is bathed in aqueous humor and communicates with the anterior chamber by way of the pupil.

posterior oblique see *left posterior oblique* or *right posterior oblique.*

posterior perforated substance a small, gray, depressed area that occupies the caudal portion of the floor of the interpeduncular fossa at the divergence of the cerebral peduncles. The substance is pierced by numerous small branches of the posterior cerebral artery that supplies the anterior thalamus, the lateral wall of the third ventricle, and the globus pallidus. See also *anterior perforated substance.*

posterior pituitary [USP], an extract of the posterior lobe of the pituitary gland of domestic food animals, which containes the hormones oxytocin and vasopressin used in the treatment of diabetes insipidus.

posteroanterior (PA) (pos″ter-o-an-tēr′e-or) [*postero-* + L. *anterior* in front] in radiology, pertaining to a projection made by passing the x-ray beam from back to front through the subject. Cf. *anteroposterior.*

posterolateral (pos″ter-o-lat′er-al) [*postero-* + L. *latus,* genitive of *lateris* side] pertaining to an oblique radiographic projection, in which the central ray passes through a part (e.g., a knee) from the posterior medial surface to the anterior lateral surface.

posteromedial (post″ter-o-me′de-al) [*postero* + L. *medius* middle] pertaining to an oblique radiographic projection, in which the central ray passes through a part (e.g., a knee) from the posterior lateral surface to the anterior medial surface.

postheparin lipolytic activity (PHLA) (pōst″-hep′ah-rin) a measure of the level of plasma lipoprotein lipase activity after an intravenous administration of heparin, which releases the enzyme from capillary endothelial cells. In normal individuals, such activity is indicated by the disappearance of plasma chylomicrons or by the increased mobility of the lipoprotein bands (especially the beta and pre-beta bands) in lipoprotein electrophoresis. A very low PHLA results in primary exogenous hypertriglyceridemia.

posthepatic cirrhosis a term used in the etiologic classification of cirrhosis to describe a form of cirrhosis seen following viral hepatitis. It is characterized by preservation of portal tracts and central veins, and by fine, frequently incomplete fibrous septa that separate macronodules of regenerated hepatic parenchyma. The term corresponds approximately to macronodular cirrhosis. See also *cirrhosis.* Cf. *postnecrotic cirrhosis.*

postmenopausal (pōst″men-o-paw′zal) [*post-* + Gr. *mēn* month + *pauein* to cause to stop] a general term used to describe any event that happens after cessation of the female menstrual cycle.

postmenopausal vaginal bleeding any bleeding from the vagina 6 mo or more following cessation of menses; it may originate anywhere along the reproductive tract. Important causes include cancer of the cervix or endometrium, and the noncyclic or excessive administration of estrogens.

Vaginal and cervical smears for cytologic examination, dilation and curettage (D&C) of the endometrium, cervical biopsy, and laparoscopic examination are diagnostic tools employed in the evaluation of the patient with postmenopausal bleeding.

postmordanting (pōst-mor′dant-ing) [*post-* + Fr. *mordant,* present participle of *mordre* to bite, from L. *mordere* to bite] the use of a second type of fixative after sectioning but before staining in order to improve the staining.

postmortem (pōst-mor′tem) [L. "after death"] occurring after death.

postmortem examination see *autopsy* and *necropsy.*

postnecrotic cirrhosis a term used in the etiologic classification of cirrhosis to describe the form of cirrhosis seen following viral hepatitis. It is characterized by massive collapse of the hepatic parenchyma; formation of broad, fibrous septae; and loss of identifiable portal tracts and central veins. The term corresponds approximately to macronodular cirrhosis. Also called postcollapse cirrhosis. See also *cirrhosis.* Cf. *posthepatic cirrhosis.*

postpartum (pōst″par′tum) [L. "after birth"] the period occurring after childbirth. The term is frequently used to imply that an occurrence is directly or indirectly related to that childbirth.

postpartum hemorrhage a condition characterized by the loss of more than 500 ml of blood during or following the third stage of labor; the major cause of maternal death in the United States. The most common causes include blood coagulation defects, uterine lacerations, and uterine atony. Prolonged labor, placenta previa, uterine infection, polyhydramnios, and abruptio placentae all predispose to postpartum hemorrhage. Laboratory studies should include a coagulation screen to detect any blood coagulation defects.

postpericardiectomy syndrome (post-per″e-kar″-de-ek′to-me) [*post-* + *pericardium* + Gr. *ektomē* excision] a condition characterized by the appearance of fever, chest pains, and pericardial friction rub following opening of the pericardium. It occurs in approximately 10 percent of patients undergoing cardiac surgery. Although the syndrome may occur as soon as 1 wk after surgery, it usually does not appear until several weeks or months later. Fever, electrocardiogram changes, and an elevation of the erythrocyte sedimentation rate may accompany the syndrome, which is treated with antiinflammatory agents.

posttransfusion hepatitis (post″trans-fu′shun) see under *hepatitis.*

postulate (pos′tu-lāt) [L. *postulatum* demanded, past participle of *postulare* to demand] a statement asserted without proof from which certain inferences are deduced.

postural (pos′chur-al) [L. *positura* position] a general term used to describe posture or position.

postural drainage a procedure performed to facilitate the flow of pulmonary secretions from the distal bronchi to the main bronchi and trachea. The patient is placed in a position that allows gravity to help the movement of secretions from alveoli and small airways into major airways where the cough mechanisms are more effective. It may be performed in those who are acutely ill and hospitalized, as well as in those who are chronically ill but ambulatory. The technique is most useful in the supportive treatment of patients with severe bronchiectasis, especially when profuse secretions are present. It may include turning the patient side to back to side every 2 hr so that pooling of secretions does not occur in one segment of the bronchial tree. Chest wall percussion and vibration are also frequently employed during postural drainage to create shock waves to dislodge secretions and move them to large airways where they can be coughed up.

potable (po′tah-b′l) [L. *potabilis,* from *potare* to drink] fit to drink; having acceptable physical qualities, although not necessarily free of pathogenic microorganisms or their noxious products.

Potamidae (pot-am′ĭ-de) [Gr. *potamos* river + *-ides* son of] a family of snails found in marine and brackish waters. Several genera serve as intermediate hosts of parasites that cause dermatitis and heterophyiasis in humans.

Potamon (pot′ah-mon) [Gr. *potamos* river] a genus of freshwater crabs, of which the species *P. denticularis, P. dehaani,* and *P. rathbuni* are the secondary hosts of the metacercariae of *Paragonimus westermani.*

potassium (K) (po-tas′e-um) [from potash (K_2CO_3 or KOH), from pot ashes; L. *kalium*] a soft, silvery metallic element; atomic number 19; atomic weight 39.102; Group I of the periodic table (the alkali metals); oxidation state +1. It oxidizes spontaneously and reacts with water to produce hydrogen, evolving enough heat to ignite the hydrogen. Metallic potassium is extremely caustic. Ionic potassium (K^+) is an essential bulk mineral and is contained in many foods; a normal diet (containing 80–200 mmol/da) satisfies the body's requirements.

Potassium is the major intracellular cation. Tissue cells contain 150 mmol/l and red blood cells contain 105 mmol/l, whereas blood plasma normally contains only about 3.5–5.3 mmol/l. This concentration gradient is accomplished by coupled active transport of potassium and sodium ions. The urinary excretion varies with the diet; it is normally 25–120 mmol/da.

Potassium is involved in the transmission of nerve and muscle impulses, and abnormal concentrations of potassium adversely affect these tissues. It is an obligate activator of many enzymes, e.g. pyruvate kinase and acetyl CoA synthetase.

A low serum potassium concentration, hypokalemia, can be produced by gastrointestinal fluid loss (vomiting or diarrhea), renal diseases, increased levels of mineralocorticosteroids (especially aldosterone), or the administration of diuretic drugs. It can also be produced by alkalosis, because $K^+$is excreted in exchange for $H^+$by the distal tubules, and K^+moves into cells in exchange for H^+. An elevated serum potassium concentration, hyperkalemia, can be produced by acute or chronic renal disease or by renal tubular acidosis.

See also *active transport, hyperkalemia, hypokalemia,* and *sodium.*

total exchangeable p. measurement, in nuclear medicine, a procedure that determines the body exchangeable potassium (K_{ex}) by the isotope dilution technique. A known activity of potassium-42 is administered intravenously (or orally to a fasting patient) and allowed to equilibrate for 24–72 hr, during which time all urine is collected, and after which several spot samples are collected. The activity of the urine is determined by liquid scintillation counting, and the potassium concentration (^{42}K plus nonradioactive ^{39}K) is determined by flame photometry or atomic absorption spectrophotometry.

The K_{ex} is the spot sample potassium concentration ($[^{39}K]$) multiplied by the ratio of the activity remaining in the body ($^{42}K_{body}$, which is the activity administered minus the activity excreted) to the activity of the urine spot sample ($^{42}K_{urine}$): $K_{ex} = [^{39}K](^{42}K_{body}/^{42}K_{urine})$.

Because potassium is the major intracellular cation, K_{ex} is related to total body water and lean body mass; normal values are 37.3–48.1 mmol/kg of body weight for males and 29.7–38.3 mmol/kg for females.

potassium-42 (^{42}K, K 42) a reactor-produced radionuclide with a half-life of 12.36 hr. It undergoes beta decay, emitting 3.52-MeV beta particles and 31-keV and 1.52-MeV gamma rays. Potassium-42 is used as a tracer of naturally occurring stable potassium-39.

potassium acidosis the metabolic acidosis promoted by an excess serum K^+ concentration (hyperkalemia), which increases the renal tubular secretion of K^+. Because K^+ and H^+ compete for the sodium ions that are available in the tubular fluid and are both excreted in exchange for Na^+, the excess K^+ secretion inhibits H^+ secretion, and acidosis is thus promoted. See also *electrolyte balance and homeostasis.*

potassium arsenite solution (po-tas′e-um ar′sĕ-nīt) an aqueous solution of arsenic trioxide, potassium bicarbonate, and alcohol, formerly used in the treatment of leukemia and dermatitis. Also called *Fowler's solution.*

potassium assays see *sodium and potassium assays.*

potassium chlorate (po-tas′e-um klor′āt) a salt, $KClO_3$; M.W. 122.55. It is a strong oxidizing agent that is explosive when mixed with combustible materials.

potassium chloride (po-tas′e-um klor′īd) a salt, KCl; M.W. 74.56. It is used as a potassium supplement in cases of hypokalemia and as a salt substitute in low-sodium diets.

potassium cyanide (po-tas′e-um si′ah-nīd) a highly poisonous salt, KCN; M.W. 65.11. See also *cyanide.*

potassium dichromate (po-tas′e-um di-kro′māt) an orange-red crystalline salt, $K_2Cr_2O_7$; M.W. 294.11. Highly corrosive, it is used as a cleaning agent and as an oxidizer in histologic techniques, as in eliciting the chromaffin reaction.

potassium ferrocyanide (po-tas′e-um fer″o-si′ah-nīd) a salt, $K_4Fe(CN)_6$, used as a dye; M.W. 386.34. See also *ferrocyanide.*

potassium hydroxide (po-tas′e-um hi-drok′sīd) a strong base, KOH; M.W. 56.10. Solid KOH or concentrated solutions are caustic and extremely corrosive to tissue.

potassium hydroxide (KOH) test a simple examination to detect the presence of fungus in a skin infection. A sample of skin scraping is heated with 10 percent KOH and methylene blue. The clearing action of KOH reveals any fungal elements present under microscopic examination. The slide mounts can be preserved for a few days by adding a small amount of glycerol to the KOH solution. Dimethyl sulfoxide (DMSO) can be added to clear nail materials.

potassium iodide (po-tas′e-um i′o-dīd) a salt, KI, administered as a source of iodine in iodine deficiency; M.W. 166.02. It is a component of iodine solutions (Gram's iodine, Lugol's solution).

potassium perchlorate (po-tas′e-um per-klor′āt) a white crystalline solid, $KClO_4$, a strong oxidizing agent; M.W. 138.55. It is administered orally 30–60 min before nuclear medicine procedures that involve injection of ^{99m}Tc-pertechnetate ($^{99m}TcO_4^-$). Perchlorate (ClO_4^-) is taken up by the thyroid and salivary glands and by the choroid plexus. It blocks the subsequent concentration of pertechnetate in these organs, thereby reducing both undesirable choroid plexus activity in brain scanning and the organ radiation dose received during brain scans and blood-pool imaging.

potassium permanganate (po-tas′e-um per-man′-gah-nāt) odorless crystals that are dark purple–bronze in color, $KMnO_4$; M.W. 158.03. The chemical has a sweet astringent taste, is a strong oxidizing agent, and is a fire and explosion hazard when in contact with organic materials. Its aqueous solutions are irritating or corrosive when ingested.

[USP], used as a topical antiseptic for skin (1:2000–1:1000 solution), used as a topical antiseptic (1:10,000–1:5000 solution) for mucous membranes. A former use—administration by gastric lavage of a 1:5000 solution as an antidote (oxidizing agent) for alkaloids such as nicotine, physostigmine, quinine, or strychnine—has generally been replaced by other measures.

potassium phosphate (po-tas′e-um fos′fāt) a salt of potassium and phosphate.

dibasic p. p., dipotassium hydrogen phosphate, K_2HPO_4; M.W. 174.18.

monobasic p. p. (MKP), potassium dihydrogen phosphate. KH_2PO_4; M.W. 136.09.

tribasic p. p., tripotassium phosphate, K_3PO_4; M.W. 212.27.

potassium thiocyanate (po-tas′e-um thi″o-si′ah-nāt) a salt, KSCN; M.W. 97.18. It is used as a reagent in chemistry and film developing.

potency (po′ten-se) [L. *potentia* power] 1. the ability of a male to perform sexual intercourse.

2. the relative effectiveness of a drug compared with equal weights of similar drugs.

potential (po-ten′shal) [L. *potentia* power] 1. that which is possible that has not yet occurred.

2. in physics, a field that determines a physical vector quantity, such as a force or the electric or magnetic field strength. The components of the force are determined by the first partial derivatives of the field.

3. a voltage (electric potential); in neurophysiology, the term is loosely used to refer to an action potential or a wave.

corneoretinal p., the electric potential difference across the eye between the cornea (positive) and retina (negative), about 1 mV in the adult human. This potential creates an electric field in the front of the head that can be detected by electrodes placed on the skin around the eyes. Movements of the eyeballs (nystagmus, saccades, and tracking) can therefore be recorded as changes in this electric field. See also *electrooculogram.*

resting membrane p., the difference in electric potential that exists across the membrane of a cell under steady-state conditions. At equilibrium, the cell interior reaches a negative potential of approximately –70 to –90 mV relative to the exterior. The resting potential is the result of transmembrane differences in the concentrations of various species of ions. Cf. *action potential.*

potentiometer (po-ten″she-om′e-ter) [L. *potentia* power + Gr. *metron* measure] 1. an instrument that measures a voltage by comparing it with a known reference voltage.

2. a variable resistor, particularly one adjusted by rotating a shaft. For instruments that use analog electronics, setting of the slope and offset (zero point) is accomplished with manually set potentiometers. Also called pot (slang).

direct-reading p., a voltmeter that has a very high resistance so that almost no current flows through the electrochemical cell when the potential is measured. Cf. *null-point p.*

null-point p., an instrument that measures a voltage by adjusting an opposing voltage until no current flows in the circuit. Also called balancing potentiometer and compensation potentiometer.

slide-wire p., a variable resistor with a contact that slides along a straight resistance wire. A common example is the potentiometer used in a servo-driven strip chart recorder: the potentiometer acts as a voltage divider, which is driven by the servomotor until the voltage output equals the signal voltage input to the servoamplifier.

potentiometric titration (po-ten″she-o-met′rik ti-tra′shun) a titration in which the end point is determined by potentiometry.

potentiometry (po-ten″she-om′e-tre) the measurement of the electric potential difference (voltage) between the two electrodes of an electrochemical cell, which indicates the concentration of the substance that undergoes an electrochemical reaction at the indicator electrode. See also *electrochemical cell.*

Pott's disease (pots) [Sir Percival *Pott,* English surgeon, 1714–1788] a serious form of skeletal tuberculosis in which the infection involves the vertebral body near an intervertebral disk, which can lead to destruction of that disk. As a result, shortening and angulation of the spine may occur as well as abscess formation. Clinical manifestations include weight loss, lower back pain, abdominal disorders, weakness, or paralysis of the legs. Antimicrobial therapy for more than 2 yr is essential to eliminate infection. Spinal cord compression may necessitate surgery. Also called *tuberculous spondylitis.*

Potter-Bucky diaphragm (pot′er buk′e) [Hollis Elmer *Potter,* U.S. radiologist, born 1880; Gustav *Bucky,* U.S. radiologist, 1880–1963] see *Bucky-Potter g.* under *grid.*

pouch (powch) [Old French *pouche* small bag] a pocketlike space or sac.

branchial p., see *pharyngeal p.*

p. of Douglas, a sac or recess formed by a fold of the peritoneum that dips down between the rectum and the uterus. Also called *rectouterine p.* and *rectovaginal p.*

Pavlov's p., a pocket of stomach that has been surgically separated from the body of the stomach by a mucosal septum, but which retains vagal innervation and muscular connection, and which drains to the exterior; used in the experimental study of gastric physiology.

pharyngeal p., one of a series of lateral diverticula of the pharynx that approximate to corresponding grooves in the ectoderm. It forms a closing plate that may rupture and complete the gill slit condition observed in lower vertebrates. Also called *branchial p.* See also *branchial region.*

Rathke's p., see *Rathke's pouch.*

rectouterine p., see *p. of Douglas.*

rectovaginal p., see *p. of Douglas.*

rectovesical p., in the male, the space in the peritoneal cavity between the rectum and the bladder.

uterovesical p., in the female, the space in the peritoneal cavity between the bladder and the uterus.

povidone (po′vĭ-dōn) [USP], a linear polymer of 1-ethenyl-2-pyrrolidinone; M.W. 10,000–700,000. It is a white- to cream-colored powder, which disperses in water to form colloidal solutions, and is used as a pharmaceutical aid and as a dispersing and suspending agent; it has also been used as a plasma volume expander. As dry powder or as concentrated solutions, povidone has been used as a dehydrating material to concentrate solutions of proteins or other macromolecules. Former generic drug name, polyvinylpyrrolidone (PVP).

povidone-iodine (po′vĭ-dōn i′o-dīn) [USP], a complex of the polymer povidone and iodine, which occurs as a yellowish-brown amorphous powder or liquid. It is used as an antiseptic and germicide applied to the skin or mucosa. Povidone-iodine has the same effectiveness as iodine, killing many bacteria, fungi, viruses, protozoa, and yeasts. Trademark, *Betadine.*

power (pow′er) [L. *posse* to have power] 1. capability; potency; the ability to act.

2. a physical quantity, the rate at which work is

done or energy consumed. The International System (SI) unit of power is the watt (W).

3. in mathematics, the exponent of a number (indicated by a superscript) or the value of the number raised to that exponent; i.e., x^3 *is x* raised to the third power and is also the third power of *x*.

4. in statistical hypothesis testing, the probability that the alternate hypothesis is accepted when it is in fact true. One minus the power $(1 - \beta)$ is the probability of a Type II error.

power supply 1. any source of electric power, such as a battery or power line.

2. the circuit in an electronic device that has AC line current as input and the various DC voltages required by the tubes and semiconductor devices as output. It consists of four sections: a transformer, which steps the alternating current up or down to the required voltage; a rectifier, which changes the alternating current to pulsed direct current; a filter, a bank of capacitors that smooths the direct current; and a regulator, an electronic circuit that maintains the output voltage under changing load conditions by comparing it with a reference voltage and correcting any error. The voltage output of an unregulated power supply changes with changes in load or input voltage; that of a regulated power supply is stable over a broad range of loads and input voltages.

The power supply of an x-ray generator consists only of a transformer and rectifiers, because some ripple voltage in the x-ray tube supply is acceptable. Fluctuation in the x-ray dose rate is reduced by use of a polyphase generator.

poxvirus (poks-vi′rus) [*pox,* plural of *pock* pustule + *virus*] any of a group of double-stranded DNA viruses, which are characterized as the largest animal viruses known. The poxviruses are the etiologic agents of smallpox or vaccinia. This virus is enveloped with a double membrane, which is synthesized by the virus itself. Although there are six genera of poxviruses, only *Orthopoxvirus* affects humans. The poxviruses are phagocytosed by host cells, the envelope is degraded, and they multiply in the cytoplasm while preventing host cell protein synthesis. At the World Health Assembly in May 1980, the World Health Organization (WHO) declared the world free of smallpox as a result of the successful vaccination programs against the disease.

PP abbrev. for *postprandial* (after meals).

PP_i abbrev. See *inorganic pyrophosphate.*

P-5′-P abbrev. See *pyridoxal-5′-phosphate.*

PPB abbrev. See *positive pressure breathing.*

ppb abbrev. for *p*arts *p*er *b*illion, a weight per weight (w/w) concentration of 1 μg/kg.

PPD abbrev. See *purified protein derivative.*

PPF abbrev. See *plasma protein fraction.*

Ppl abbrev. See *intrapleural pressure.*

PPLO abbrev. for *pleuropneumonia-like organisms.* See under *Mycoplasma.*

ppm abbrev. for parts per million, a weight per weight (w/w) concentration of 1 mg/kg.

PPP abbrev. See *platelet-poor plasma.*

PPS abbrev. See *pepsin A.*

Pr symbol for the chemical element *praseodymium.*

PRA abbrev. See *plasma r. activity* under *renin assays.*

pralidoxime chloride (PAM, 2-PAM) (pral″ĭ-doks′ēm klor′īd) an antidote to poisoning by organophosphate compounds, 2-pyridine aldoxime methylchloride. It reactivates cholinesterase by removing the organophosphate group causing the enzyme inhibition. Pralidoxime cannot cross the blood-brain barrier and does not reverse the effects of the poison on the central nervous system. It is used in combination with atropine. See also *organophosphate compounds.*

pramoxine hydrochloride (pram-ok′sēn hi″dro-klor′īd) [USP], a surface analgesic used for relief of pain and itching; it is chemically unrelated to procaine and similar benzoate esters.

-prandial (pran′de-al) [L. *prandium* breakfast] a suffix word element to denote a meal, e.g., postprandial.

praseodymium (Pr) (pra″ze-o-dim′e-um, pra″se-o-dim′e-um) [Gr. *prasios* leek-green + *didymium* (a mixture of Pr and Nd, once reported as an element), from Gr. *didymos* twin] a soft, silvery metallic element that forms green salts; atomic number 59; atomic weight 140.9077; a 4f transition element (lanthanide rare earth); oxidation states +3, +4. See also *rare earth elements.*

Prausnitz-Küstner reaction (PK reaction) (prows′nits kist′ner) [Carl Willy *Prausnitz,* German hygienist, b. 1876; Heinz *Küstner,* German gynecologist, b. 1897] a skin reaction formerly used to measure and detect IgE. When the serum from a sensitized individual is injected into the skin of a nonsensitive recipient, IgE attaches to the mast cells in the skin, whereas most other immunoglobulins do not. After 12 hr, the recipient is challenged with antigen; a wheal-and-erythema reaction results. This test is no longer used in humans owing to the high risk of the transfer of serum hepatitis and other blood-borne diseases.

prazepam (prāz′ĕ-pam) a long-acting benzodiazepine used as an antianxiety medication. Trademark, Centrax.

prazosin hydrochloride (prah′zo-sin hi″dro-klor′-īd) a quinazoline derivative used in the treatment of hypertension. It acts by blocking the postsynaptic alpha-adrenergic receptors on vascular smooth muscle. Unlike nonselective alpha-blockers, it does not produce reflex tachycardia. Common adverse reactions include syncope due to postural hypotension, dizziness, headache, drowsiness, weakness, palpitations, and nausea. Trademark, *Minipress.*

PRC abbrev. See *plasma r. concentration* under *renin assays.*

pre- (pre) [L. *prae* before] a prefix word element to denote before or in front of, e.g., precancerous.

preadaptation (pre-ad″ap-ta′shun) referring to a characteristic or trait of a species, which develops to perform one function, but later in its evolutionary history is also able to perform a different function, to which it is said to be preadapted.

prealbumin (pre″al-bu′min) a blood serum protein that migrates ahead of albumin on paper electrophoresis; M.W. 55,000. It binds and transports thyroxine and binds retinol in blood. Its concentration in plasma is 10–40 mg/100 ml.

preamplifier (pre-am′plĕ-fi″er) an amplifier used to boost a weak signal from a detector or transducer to avoid signal degradation by system noise.

preauricular (pre″aw-rik′u-lar) in front of the auricle of the ear.

preauricular point in electroencephalography, one of the reference points used to determine the placement of electrodes on the scalp.

preauricular region the region of the face anterior to the ear.

pre–B cell an immature lymphoid cell containing cytoplasmic IgM. A pre–B cell differentiates into a mature B lymphocyte. See also *B l.* under *lymphocyte.*

pre-beta-lipoprotein a lipoprotein that consists mainly of very-low-density lipoproteins. Increases are characteristically seen in types IV and V hyperlipidemias. See also *very-low-density l.* under *lipoprotein* and *lipoprotein assays.*

precancerous (pre-kan′ser-us) pertaining to a pathologic process that tends to become malignant.

precipitant (pre-sip′ĭ-tant) [L. *praeciptans,* present participle of *praecipitare* to cast down] a substance that causes precipitation. Cf. *precipitate.*

precipitate (pre-sip′ĭ-tāt) 1. [L. *praecipitatum*], a deposit formed of small particles that have settled out of a solution or a gas. The particles may be formed by a chemical reaction that yields the substance in excess of its solubility, by a lowering of temperature so that the solubility is lowered, by the crystallization of a supersaturated solution, or by the agglomeration of colloidal particles as the result of an application of an electric charge.

2. [L. *praecipitare* to cast down], to cause precipitation.

3. to separate from a medium (a solution or a gas) as a precipitate.

4. in immunology, a large insoluble complex of antigen and antibody; see also *precipitin curve.*

precipitation (pre-sip″ĭ-ta′shun) [L. *praecipitatio,* from *praecipitare* to cast down] the settling out of a precipitate; the state of being precipitated (as from a solution). See also *precipitate.*

precipitin (pre-sip′ĭ-tin) [*precipi*tate + *-in*] an antibody to soluble antigen that reacts with the antigen in vivo or in vitro to give a visible precipitate.

precipitin curve the curve that results from the plotting of increasing antigen concentrations on the abscissa and increasing amounts of immune precipitate formed on the ordinate. The optimal antigen-antibody ratio, called the zone of equivalence, gives the greatest amount of precipitate. See also the accompanying illustration.

precision (pre-sizh′un) 1. in statistics, a measurement of the agreement between repeated measurements; an indication of the random error. The standard deviation, variance, or coefficient of variation may be used as a measure of the precision; the smaller the variance, the greater the precision. Cf. *imprecision.*

2. in computer terminology, the number of digits or bytes reserved for the fractional part of a real (floating-point) number. Available sizes depend on the computer hardware; these are usually called single precision, double precision, and (if available) extended precision.

precocious (pre-ko′shus) [L. *praecox* ripe before its time] more developed than is usual at a given age.

precursor (pre′kur-sor) [L. *praecursor* a forerunner] 1. something that precedes.

2. in the chain of metabolic reactions necessary to produce some end product (e.g., enzyme, hormone, vitamin), any of the compounds produced by and consumed in some of the intermediate reaction steps.

3. the inactive form of an important metabolite, which is converted into the active form by a converting enzyme or other process; e.g., trypsinogen is the precursor of trypsin, and β-carotene is a precursor of retinol.

precursor lesion an abnormality of epithelium that may develop into a carcinoma. See also *atypical hyperplasia* and *carcinoma in situ.*

predaceous mite (pre-da′shus) [L. *praeda* prey] one of the species of mites of the genus *Pyemotes,* especially *P. ventricosus,* that causes grain itch or straw itch. See also *Pyemotes.*

predator (pred′ah-tor) [L. *praedator* a plunderer, pillager, from *praeda* plunder] an organism that attacks and destroys another organism or another species to obtain elements essential for its existence. A predator usually feeds on smaller or weaker organisms.

prediabetes (pre-di″ah-be′tēz) a retrospective state of known diabetics at which time these individuals had normal glucose concentrations and were asymptomatic. See also *diabetes.*

predictive value of a negative test the conditional probability of a person not having a specific disease, given that a certain test result is negative. If $P(A \mid B)$ is the predictive value of a positive test, where A denotes the presence of disease, and B denotes a positive test result, then $P(\text{not } A \mid \text{not } B)$ is the predictive value of a negative test. See also *Bayes's theorem, sensitivity,* and *specificity.*

predictive value of a positive test the conditional probability of a person having a specific disease,

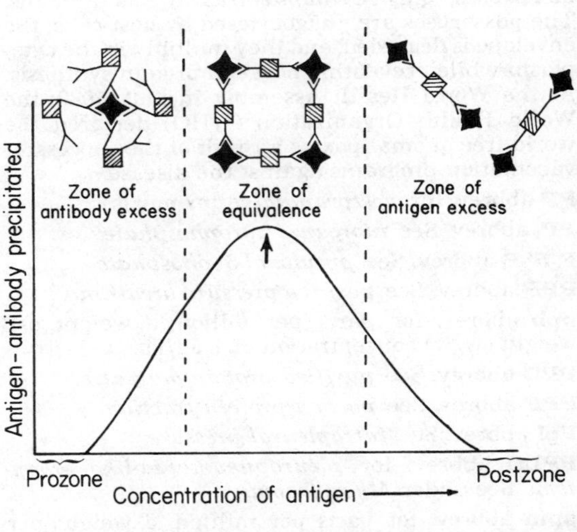

Precipitin curve. The plot is obtained by adding increasing amounts of a soluble antigen to fixed volumes of monospecific antiserum. Maximum precipitate (↑) is formed at an optimal ratio of antigen to antibody called the equivalence point. (From Henry, J. B.: Clinical Diagnosis and Management. 16th ed. Philadelphia, W. B. Saunders Co., 1979.)

given that a certain test result is positive; see also *Bayes's theorem, sensitivity,* and *specificity.*

prednisolone (pred-nis′o-lōn) [USP], a synthetic corticosteroid (Δ^1-cortisol) with glucocorticoid activity; used in the treatment of various conditions, such as rheumatoid arthritis, collagen diseases, allergic diseases, bronchial asthma, and skin diseases, and for substitution therapy in adrenal insufficiency. See also *corticosteroids.*

prednisone (pred′nĭ-sōn) [USP], a synthetic corticosteroid (Δ^1-cortisone) with glucocorticoid activity; used as an antiinflammatory agent in the treatment of various conditions, such as rheumatoid arthritis, collagen diseases, allergic diseases, bronchial asthma, and skin diseases. It may also be used for substitution therapy in adrenal insufficiency, and to inhibit poorly differentiated lymphoid cells in the treatment of Hodgkin's disease, usually in a treatment regimen in combination with an alkylating agent and a vinca alkaloid. See also *corticosteroids.*

preeclampsia (pre″e-klamp′se-ah) [*pre-* + Gr. *eklampsis* a shining out] a syndrome occurring in the third trimester of pregnancy, characterized by hypertension, proteinuria, and sometimes edema. It may progress to decreased renal function or convulsions (eclampsia). Rarely a similar condition associated with hydatidiform mole is seen in the first trimester. Preeclampsia occurs in 5–10 percent of pregnancies, depending on socioeconomic and geographic factors. The etiologic factors responsible for its development are not understood, but toxemia is more common when there is preexisting hypertension, renal disease, or diabetes. The common factor is probably impaired maternal utero-placental blood flow, which somehow leads to the generation of the syndrome. An important aspect of prenatal care is monitoring for the possible development of hypertension and proteinuria.

Preeclampsia may be associated with a consumptive coagulopathy and thrombocytopenia, and fibrin degradation products may be elevated in the serum and urine. Thrombotic changes occur in the vessels of the uterus, and placental infection is common. Glomerular changes include deposition of fibrin in the endothelium and the mesangium.

Mild degrees of preeclampsia may be managed by bed rest and monitoring in the hospital, but antihypertensive drugs are necessary in more severe cases, and the pregnancy may have to be terminated. Magnesium sulfate infusion is used to prevent convulsions. Blood pressure returns to normal some weeks after delivery, unless the preeclamptic syndrome was associated with underlying renal or vascular disease.

Also called *toxemia of pregnancy.*

preejection period (PEP) (pre″e-jek′shun) see under *systolic time interval.*

preexcitation syndrome (pre-ek″si-ta′shun) see *Wolff-Parkinson-White syndrome.*

prefibrinolysin (pre-fi″brĭ-nol′ĭ-sin) see *plasminogen.*

pregnancy (preg′nan-se) [L. *praegnans* pregnant] the condition of having a developing embryo or fetus in the body. Human pregnancy lasts about 9 mo (266 da).

pregnancy tests methods that detect the presence of human chorionic gonadotropin (hCG) produced by trophoblastic tissue in the placenta, used not only to confirm pregnancy but also to diagnose ectopic pregnancy and trophoblastic tumors.

General methods used to measure hCG levels are: (1) immunoassay (hemagglutination inhibition [HAI]), (2) latex particle agglutination inhibition (LAI), (3) direct agglutination of latex particles, (4) radioimmunoassay (RIA), and (5) radioreceptor assay (RRA). HAI involves the incubation of anti-hCG serum and hCG-coated erythrocytes with the urine specimen of the patient. The presence of hCG neutralizes the antiserum; the erythrocytes do not agglutinate, but settle on the round bottom of the test tube in a characteristic ring or "doughnut" pattern. Absence of hCG results in agglutination due to reaction between the anti-hCG and the hCG coated on the erythrocytes, which produces a diffuse mat. LAI is similar to HAI, except that latex particles coated with hCG are substituted for hCG-coated erythrocytes. LAI procedures are usually slide tests requiring only a few minutes. Direct latex particle agglutination tests utilize anti-hCG directly adsorbed on latex particles. If hCG is present, agglutination occurs.

Most RIA techniques for hCG use antiserum specific for the beta subunit of hCG. This avoids cross reactions with luteinizing hormone. RRA for hCG utilizes receptors isolated from the corpora lutea of pregnant cows. The assay is more rapid but less specific than the beta subunit RIA.

pregnanediol (preg″nān-di′ol) 5β-pregnane-3α, 20α-diol, the major metabolite of progesterone in the urine; M.W. 320.50. Pregnanediol is formed by the reduction of progesterone to a dihydroxy derivative. Following enzyme or acid hydrolysis of urinary pregnanediol glucuronide and extraction with a suitable solvent, it is quantitated either by colorimetry or gas chromatography. The determination of urinary pregnanediol has clinical significance, as it indicates ovulation and the normal function of the corpus luteum in nonpregnant women. Reference ranges for pregnanediol are: for males, < 1.2 mg/da; for females, 0.2–7.0; and for females during pregnancy, 5.0–63.0.

pregnanediol assays 1. colorimetric assay. The sample is subjected to acid hydrolysis to release pregnanediol from its conjugates. Pregnanediol is then extracted with toluene and oxidized with permanganate solution. The residue is purified with column chromatography and treated with sulfuric acid to produce a chromogen that absorbs at 430 nm and can be determined spectrophotometrically.

2. gas chromatography. The sample is subjected to acid hydrolysis, extracted with toluene or benzene and washed with alkali, then water. The sample is acetylated with a mixture of acetic anhydride and pyridine or by reacting pregnanediol in tetrahydrofuran with hexamethyldisilazane and trimethylchlorosilane. Then it is injected into the gas chromatograph. Quantitation is accomplished by comparing the peak area of the pregnanediol to that of an internal standard such as cholesterol propionate. This procedure is generally more specific than the colorimetric assay.

pregnanetriol (preg″nān-tri′ol) 5β-pregnane-3α, 17α, 20α-triol, a reduced metabolite of 17-hyydroxyprogesterone; M.W. 336.50. It normally occurs in body fluids and urine in small amounts, but increases greatly in disorders of the adrenal cortex in which 21-hydroxylation or 11β-hydroxylation of the steroid nucleus is impaired. After enzymatic hydrolysis of the conjugates in the urine, pregnanetriol is extracted with an organic solvent such as dichloromethane and quantitated by gas chromatography. Reference values for pregnanetriol in 24-hr urine specimens are: for children, <0.5 mg/da; and for adults, up to 2.0.

pregnenolone (preg-nen′o-lōn) 3-β-hydroxypregn-5-en-20-one, an important precursor in the biosynthesis of steroid hormones; M.W. 316.47. Pregnenolone is formed from cholesterol by two successive hydroxylations and a side-chain cleavage. Because its formation involves the initial rate-limiting side-chain hydroxylation of cholesterol, pregnenolone exerts a regulatory influence on steroidogenesis.

preictal (pre-ik′tal) [*pre-* + L. *ictus* stroke] occurring before an ictus.

preinvasive (pre″in-va′siv) not yet invading other tissues. See also *carcinoma in situ.*

Preiser's disease (pri′zerz) [Georg Karl Felix *Preiser,* German orthopedic surgeon, 1879–1913] see under *osteochondritis juvenilis.*

preleukemia (pre-lu-ke′me-ah) a syndrome that in time (sometimes years) may develop into overt monocytic, or stem cell leukemia; it is characterized by bone marrow dysfunction manifested by anemia, neutropenia, thrombocytopenia, and a combination of physical findings, i.e., splenomegaly, hepatomegaly, or lymphadenopathy. Conversion to acute leukemia is often abrupt, and there is usually a poorer response to therapy than in cases of acute leukemia that have no preleukemic phase. See also *refractory a.* under *anemia.*

preload (pre′lōd) the load on a muscle prior to contraction. The preload on the heart is estimated by the end-diastolic volume, end-diastolic pressure, or left ventricular filling pressure. Within limits, the cardiac performance increases with preload. Cf. *afterload.*

Preludin (pre-loo′din) trademark. See *phenmetrazine hydrochloride.*

prelytic sphere (pre-lit′ik) see *spherocyte.*

premature (pre-mah-tūr′) [L. *praematurus* ripe early] 1. occurring before the proper time.
2. referring to an infant born before full term.

premature atrial contraction (PAC) an early electrical impulse that arises within the atria from a reentry or automatic site other than the sinoatrial node, which activates an atrial contraction occurring prior to the normal expected one. The electrocardiographic features of a PAC include a prematurely occurring P wave often with an abnormal shape, which is usually followed by a QRS complex and T wave of normal configuration and polarity; other features depend on the degree of prematurity and the location of the ectopic site with respect to the sinoatrial and atrioventricular nodes. Occasionally, conduction to the ventricles is aberrant, and the resulting abnormal QRS may be mistaken for premature ventricular contraction (PVC). Fully compensatory pauses usually do not occur with PACs in contrast to PVCs.

PACs may occur frequently in individuals with normal hearts, or may be initiated by conditions such as excitement or excessive use of cigarettes, coffee, or alcohol. PACs that occur in diseased hearts may required management with antiarrhythmic drugs.

Also called *atrial premature beat, atrial premature contraction,* and *atrial premature depolarization.*

premature contraction a heartbeat occurring prior to the time normally expected in the cardiac cycle. It is initiated as the result of an impulse that has arisen in some portion of the heart other than the functioning pacemaker of the heart. Premature contractions may alternate in a regular or sporadic fashion with the normal contractions. Also called ectopic contraction, *extrasystole,* and premature beat. See also *premature atrial contraction* and *premature ventricular contraction.*

premature infant an infant born before the thirty-seventh week of gestation. Such newborn infants usually have a low birth weight and little subcutaneous fat, and in general suffer from underdevelopment of their organ systems. No definitive cause for premature delivery has been established, but many premature infants are born to mothers who have had poor prenatal care and nutrition. Problems associated with such infants include hyperbilirubinemia and kernicterus, plus a greater risk of developing neonatal sepsis or meningitis, metabolic acidosis due to undeveloped kidney function, and respiratory distress syndrome due to lack of pulmonary surfactant. Retrolental fibroplasia also has been known to develop in individuals who, as premature infants, were treated with excess oxygen to the point of toxicity.

premature separation of the placenta see *abruptio p.* under *placenta.*

premature ventricular contraction (PVC) an early abnormal activation sequence arising from an impulse that originates in a ventricle. Electrocardiographic features of a PVC commonly include a premature, prolonged, high-voltage, and bizarrely shaped QRS complex, followed by a T wave that is commonly opposite in direction. The discharge of the sinoatrial node is rarely disrupted. Other features vary, depending on the degree of prematurity and the location of the ectopic focus; for example, a PVC may occur so early that the resulting R wave is superimposed on the T wave of the preceding complex (R-on-T phenomenon). A PVC is usually conducted over a relatively stable reentry pathway; thus, the QRS complex resulting from a single focus has a fixed configuration and relation to the normal complexes.

The necessity for treatment generally depends on the site and mechanism of origin, degree of prematurity, form and frequency of repetition, and presence of adverse symptoms. Infrequent PVCs commonly occur in normal hearts without adverse consequences and do not require therapy. PVCs occurring in individuals with ischemic heart disease, idiopathic subaortic stenosis, mitral valve prolapse syndrome, or other conditions may increase the likelihood of more serious arrhythmias or cardiac arrest; antiarrhythmic drugs (lidocaine, procainamide, quinidine, disopyramide, propranolol) may be used to reduce the frequency of PVCs in these instances.

Also called *ventricular premature beat, ventricular premature contraction,* and *ventricular premature depolarization.* See also the accompanying illustration.

premenopausal (pre″men-o-paw′zal) [*pre-* + Gr. *mēn* month + *pauein* to cause to stop] a general

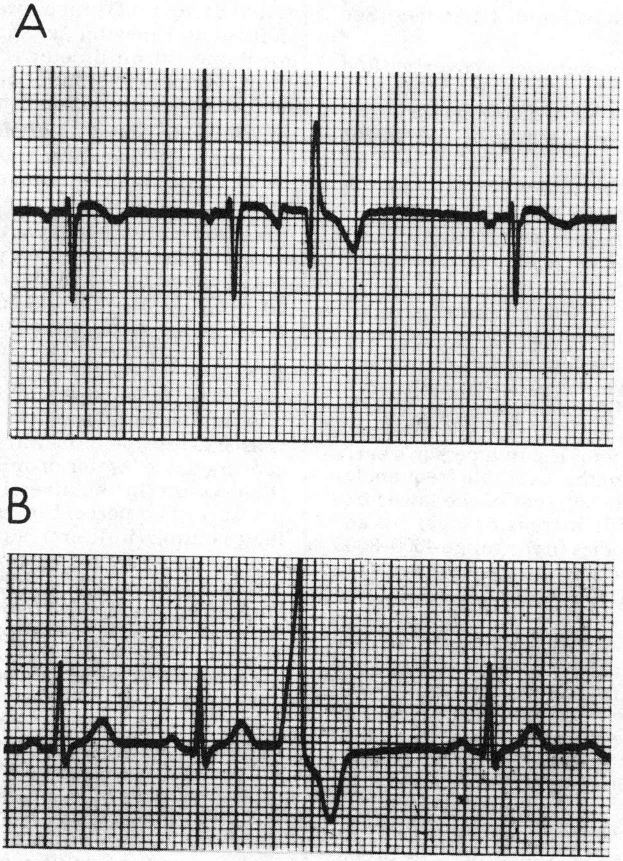

Premature ventricular contraction. Comparison of *A*, premature atrial beat (PAB), and *B*, premature ventricular beat (PVB). In both A and B, a wide QRS premature beat follows two sinus beats. In A, this extrasytole is due to an atrial premature beat, which causes a deformity of the T wave of the preceding sinus beat. In *B*, however, the premature ventricular beat shown is not preceded by any evidence of atrial activity. (From Wyngaarden, J. B., and Smith, H. L., Jr.: Cecil Textbook of Medicine. 16th ed. Philadelphia, W. B. Saunders Co., 1982.)

term used to describe any event that happens before cessation of the menstrual cycles.

premenstrual tension (pre-men′stroo-al) [*pre-* + L. *menstrualis* menstrual, from *menstruus* monthly] a recurrent, periodic condition characterized by generalized edema, pain in the breasts, headache, and emotional irritability; it occurs 5–10 da before menstruation, disappearing at its onset. Approximately 50 percent of all females may be affected to some degree. The cause of the symptoms is not well understood, although it is thought to be related to the fluid-retaining effects of estrogen. Laboratory findings may show slight functional hypoglycemia and elevated serum prolactin concentrations during this time.

premorbid (pre-mor′bid) [*pre-* + L. *morbidus* diseased, from *morbus* disease] occurring before the onset of a disease.

prenatal (pre-na′tal) [*pre-* + L. *natalis* natal] existing or occurring before birth.

prenatal diagnosis see *antenatal diagnosis.*

prenyl groups (pre′nil) isoprene groups with the formula —CH_2—$C(CH_3)$=CH—CH_2—. They are basic building block units of polyprenyl compounds in steroids, ubiquinone side-chains, carotenes, rubber, and cyclic terpenoid compounds (camphor, pinene, limonene, and many others).

preparation (prep″ah-ra′shun) [L. *praeparatio,* from *praeparare* to prepare] 1. anything prepared for use or examination, such as a medicine or a histologic specimen.

2. that which is prepared.

preproprotein (pre″pro-pro′tēn) a precursor of a protein molecule that lacks biologic activity. It is initially translated and transported into the endoplasmic reticulum and, by proteolysis, converted into a proprotein. The second stage of proteolysis, which occurs either in the intracellular granules or outside the cell, converts the proprotein to the active protein molecule by proteolytic removal of a polypeptide fragment from the preprotein. Examples of extracellular activation are digestive enzymes, which are activated after entry into the intestines, and tissue blood-clotting enzymes, which are activated when tissues are damaged. Examples of intracellular activation are the protein hormones. See also *proprotein.*

prepuce (pre′pūs) [L. *praeputium*] a covering fold of skin.

p. of clitoris, the fold of tissue formed by the union of the anterior labia minora that covers over the clitoris.

p. of penis, the fold of skin that covers the glans penis. Also called the *foreskin.*

presby/o (pres′be-o) [Gr. *presbys* old] a word element used in combining form to denote old age, e.g., presbyopia.

presbycardia (pres″be-kar′de-ah) [*presby-* + Gr. *kardia* heart] aging changes of the myocardium.

presbycusis (pres″be-ku′sis) [*presby-* + Gr. *akousis* hearing] a bilaterally symmetric, progressive sensorineural hearing loss that develops as a part of the aging process. Males are usually affected more often and more severely than females. In a person's early twenties, hearing of the highest audible frequencies (18,000–20,000 Hz) is affected; that of the lower frequencies is affected with increasing age. By age 55–65, hearing of frequencies in the range 4000–8000 Hz is often affected. There is, however, great variability in the degree of impairment among individuals.

presbyopia (pres″be-o′pe-ah) [*presby-* + Gr. *ōps* eye + *-ia*] a decrease in the ability of the lens of the eye to accommodate, which develops with advancing age. Beginning in adolescence, the lens gradually loses its elasticity and eventually cannot be made convex enough to focus on nearby objects. In most cases, corrective lenses are not necessary until after age 40.

prescription (pre-skrip′shun) [L. *praescriptio*] a directive written by a physician that orders the preparation and administration of a drug or other treatment. By federal law, certain types of drugs are dispensed only by prescription.

Traditionally, a prescription consists of four parts: superscription, inscription, subscription, and signature. The superscription is the symbol ℞, which stands for the Latin *recipe,* "take thou"; the inscription consists of the names and amounts of the ingredients; the subscription consists of directions to the pharmacist; and the signature (from the Latin *signa,* "mark or label") consists of the directions to the patient.

Prescription orders for prescription drugs must also indicate how many times (if any) the prescription may be refilled. Orders for drugs listed in the Controlled Substances Act must also contain the date; patient's name and address; and physician's name, address, and DEA (Drug Enforcement Administration) number.

presenile dementia (pre-se′nīl) [*pre-* + L. *senilis* senile, from *senex* old] see *Alzheimer's disease.*

preservative (pre-zer′vah-tiv) in biologic specimens, a chemical added to a product, liquid or solid, to inhibit the multiplication rate of microorganisms that may be present and would otherwise cause undesirable changes or even spoilage.

pressor (pres′or) [L. "that which presses," from *premere* to press] that which increases the blood pressure.

pressure (p) (presh′ur) [L. *pressura*] the force per unit area exerted on a surface. A static fluid exerts a uniform pressure in all directions. The International System (SI) unit of pressure is the pascal (Pa), defined as 1 newton per square meter (1 N/m^2). In medicine, the millimeter of mercury (mmHg) is the most commonly used unit of pressure because of the continued use of mercury manometers.

pressure crescent an artifact on a radiograph, appearing as a black, crescent-shaped mark, that is caused by rough handling of the film either before or after exposure.

pressure-volume curve the graphic representation of the intrapulmonary pressure that can be passively or actively developed at specific lung volumes. The pressure-volume relationship is measured under conditions of zero airflow following inflation or deflation of the lungs to various volumes. The curve is used to characterize the elastic properties of the lung-chest wall system.

When the curve is plotted, the X axis of the graph is used to represent the intrapulmonary pressure (in centimeters of water or millimeters of mercury) or the pressure in the alveoli relative to atmospheric pressure. The percent of vital capacity or absolute lung volume (in liters) is plotted on the Y axis.

A passive (relaxation) pressure curve can be generated as follows: the subject inhales from residual volume or functional residual capacity to a certain lung volume. After inhaling, the subject relaxes the respiratory muscles with the glottis open against a pressure-measuring device within the breathing apparatus. As the subject relaxes, alveolar pressure reaches the level required to maintain the lung and chest wall at that particular volume. This maneuver is repeated for other inhaled volumes within the vital capacity range. A passive deflation curve can be similarly generated by having the subject expire to various volumes from total lung capacity. During both maneuvers, volume can be measured plethysmographically, or by spirometry, bag-box circuit, or integration of the pneumotachograph signal.

The relaxation pressure curve has the following features: the total pressure in the respiratory system is zero (atmospheric) at the relaxation volume, the point at which the elastic recoil pressures of the lung and chest wall are exactly balanced (opposite and equal). The relaxation volume of the normal lung defines the functional residual capacity (FRC), the volume of air remaining in the lungs following a quiet expiration. At volumes above the relaxation volume, the pressure is above atmospheric pressure because the forces that tend to collapse the lungs exceed the opposing forces that tend to expand the chest wall. At volumes below the FRC, relaxation pressures are subatmospheric. The relaxation curves developed during inflation and deflation of the lungs form a hysteresis loop: the prior inflation history of the lungs influences the pressure that is developed at a specific volume. The slope of the relaxation curve (inflation or deflation) in the tidal volume range is equal to the static compliance, a measure of the elastic properties of the lungs.

Maximal (active) inspiratory and expiratory curves can be developed by having the subject inhale or exhale to a certain volume. After relaxation to the intrapulmonary pressure at which the chest wall and lungs are maintained at that volume, the subject forcibly inhales or exhales against the pressure-sensing device. The distance on the X axis between these maximal pressure curves and the relaxation curve represents the net pressure actively developed by the respiratory muscles. It can be used as a measure of the strength of these muscles.

Emphysematous lungs exhibit relaxation pressure-volume curves that are displaced upward and to the left of the curve for the normal lung, whereas conditions such as interstitial pulmonary fibrosis displace the normal curve in the opposite direction (see the accompanying illustration).

See also *elastic recoil* and *static c.* under *compliance.*

presumptive heterophile test (pre-sump'tiv het'er-o-fil) see under *infectious mononucleosis.*

prevalence (prev'ah-lens) [L. *praevalere* to have more power] the total number of cases of a disease in existence at a certain time in a designated area. See also *prevalence r.* under *rate.* Cf. *incidence.*

preventive medicine (pre-ven'tiv) the branch of medicine that deals with the prevention of disease.

previous value check see *delta check.*

PRH abbrev. See *prolactin releasing hormone.*

priapism (pri'ah-pizm) [L. *priapismus;* Gr. *priapismos,* from *Priapus,* Greco-Roman god of procreation] a persistent, painful, abnormal erection of the penis without sexual desire. Causes of the disorder include sickle cell anemia, leukemia, other blood disorders, spinal cord injuries, and other neurologic abnormalities. The condition is probably secondary to stasis within the penile vascular network. Treatment is difficult and often unsuccessful; the underlying disorders must also be treated. Unrelieved, the persistent erection can lead to fibrosis of the corpora and permanent loss of sexual function.

Price-Jones curve (Cecil *Price-Jones,* English physician, 1863–1943) a frequency distribution curve of the diameters of individual red cells in a peripheral blood smear, estimated visually with the aid of an ocular micrometer. This curve has been replaced by the frequency distribution curve of red cell volumes obtained by electronic cell counter.

prilocaine hydrochloride (pril'o-kān) [USP], a water-soluble local analgesic of the amide type, similar to lidocaine but having a longer action. It is used for infiltration and nerve block. Adverse reactions due to overdosage or rapid absorption include excitation (possibly followed by convulsions), unconsciousness, and respiratory arrest. A metabolite, *o*-toluidine, causes methemoglobinemia; overdosage may cause cyanosis, which is treated with methylene blue.

primaquine phosphate (prim'ah-kwin) [USP], one of the 8-aminoquinoline antimalarial drugs; it kills the exoerythrocytic schizonts and gametes, and is the drug of choice when used with one of the 4-aminoquinolines that kill the erythrocytic forms of the parasite. Adverse effects include methemoglobinemia and hemolytic anemia. There is a genetic X-linked sensitivity to primaquine.

primaquine sensitivity a widespread (inherited) disorder in which the administration of a variety of agents, including the antimalarial drug primaquine, causes hemolysis of erythrocytes. Primaquine-sensitive erythrocytes are present in individuals with glutathione reductase deficiency or, more frequently, with glucose-6-phosphate dehydrogenase deficiency. Hemolysis is thought to be related to a hypersensitivity to peroxides as a consequence of a low concentration of reduced glutathione (GSH). Both enzymes are involved in maintaining the GSH concentrations needed to remove peroxides. See also *glutathione reductase deficiency* and *glucose-6-phosphate dehydrogenase deficiency.*

primary (pri'mar-e) [L. *primarius* principal, from *primus* first] 1. first in order or in time of development; principal.

2. in organic chemistry, principal, with use in several contexts: a primary carbon is bonded either to one other carbon or to none (e.g., all the carbons in ethyl bromide, CH_3CH_2Br, can be designated as primary carbons); a primary substituent is one in which the point of attachment to the parent compound is a primary carbon; a primary amine is one having a nitrogen atom with one carbon atom and two hydrogen atoms attached; and a primary alcohol is one in which the hydroxy group is attached to a primary carbon. See also *primary structure.*

primary active transport see under *active transport.*

primary beam the beam emerging from the port of an x-ray tube before the softer x-rays have been removed by a filter.

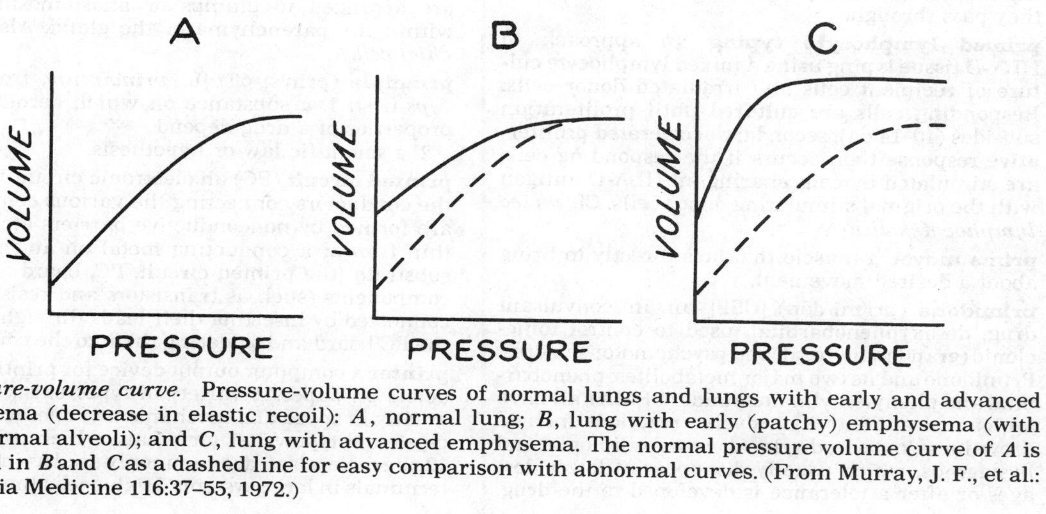

Pressure-volume curve. Pressure-volume curves of normal lungs and lungs with early and advanced emphysema (decrease in elastic recoil): *A*, normal lung; *B*, lung with early (patchy) emphysema (with some normal alveoli); and *C*, lung with advanced emphysema. The normal pressure volume curve of *A* is repeated in *B* and *C* as a dashed line for easy comparison with abnormal curves. (From Murray, J. F., et al.: California Medicine 116:37–55, 1972.)

primary coil the input coil of a transformer.

primary constriction see *centromere.*

primary culture see *primary c.* under *culture.*

primary fibrinolysis a rare disorder, occurring when the fibrinolytic system is activated, that results in the proteolytic action of plasmin on fibrin and other plasma proteins. Sometimes it arises as a complication of severe liver disease, but it can also occur spontaneously. It is difficult to differentiate primary fibrinolysis from disseminated intravascular coagulation because secondary fibrinolysis is activated by the intravenous fibrin deposition.

Laboratory findings include rapid lysis of clotted whole blood, rapid euglobulin lysis time, abnormal prothrombin time and activated partial thromboplastin time, hypofibrinogenemia, significantly elevated levels of fibrin and fibrinogen degradation products, and a normal platelet count.

primary granule see *azurophilic granule.*

primary reference materials see *reference materials.*

primary sex character see under *character.*

primary standard a highly purified chemical of well-defined composition that meets specifications prepared by the Committee on Analytical Reagents of the American Chemical Society or by other qualified certifying agencies, such as the National Bureau of Standards. A variety of materials are now made available by the latter as standard reference materials (SRM). Such materials should not be hygroscopic, and can be dried without change and handled easily when weighed in the preparation of standard solutions. These compounds generally have a high equivalent weight in order to minimize weighing errors. The analysis for contaminating materials (as to kind and quantity) is usually supplied with the material. See also *reference materials.*

primary structure the sequence of amino acid residues along a polypeptide chain in a protein or the sequence of nucleotide residues along a polynucleotide chain in a nucleic acid. The primary structure completely determines the secondary, tertiary, and quaternary structures.

primary x-rays the x-rays in the collimated x-ray beam, as opposed to secondary x-rays produced by the scattering of the primary x-rays in the objects they pass through.

primed lymphocyte typing an approach to HLA-D tissue typing using a mixed lymphocyte culture of recipient cells and irradiated donor cells. Responding cells are cultured until proliferation subsides (10–14 da); secondary accelerated proliferative response then occurs if the responding cells are stimulated by cells sharing an HLA-D antigen with the original stimulating donor cells. Cf. *mixed lymphocyte culture.*

prime mover a muscle that acts directly to bring about a desired movement.

primidone (pri′mĭ-dōn) [USP], an anticonvulsant drug, desoxyphenobarbital, used to control tonic-clonic (grand mal), focal, and psychomotor seizures. Primidone and its two major metabolites, phenobarbital and phenylethylmalonamide (PEMA), all have anticonvulsant activity. Adverse reactions include drowsiness, nausea, dizziness, vertigo, diplopia, and nystagmus, which usually disappear at lower dosages or after a tolerance is developed to the drug. Acute poisoning causes coma and respiratory depression. Therapeutic serum concentrations of primidone are usually in the range of 5–12 μg/ml. Trademark, Mysoline.

primidone assays 1. gas chromatography using a moderately polar column packing and a flame ionization detector. Primidone, phenobarbital, and phenytoin are extracted from a sample of blood, plasma, urine, or reference solution to which the internal standard *p*-methylphenobarbital has been added to an organic solvent. After evaporation, the residue is dissolved in methanol. The drugs are then methylated by reaction with trimethylanilinium hydroxide (TMAH), and the concentration of each is calculated from either the peak height ratio or peak area ratio.

2. EMIT homogeneous enzyme immunoassay used for the therapeutic drug monitoring of serum primidone levels.

primigravida (pri″mĭ-grav′ĭ-dah) [L. *prima* first + *gravida* pregnant] a female who is pregnant for the first time. Also called gravida I and *unigravida.*

primipara (pri-mip′ah-rah) [L. *prima* first + *parere* to bring forth] a female who has had one pregnancy resulting in a viable child. Also called para I and *unipara.*

primitive (prim′ĭ-tiv) [L. *primitivus,* from *primus* first] existing in a simple or early form; showing little evolution.

primitive erythroblasts the cells that arise in the blood islands during the first month of prenatal life. They are large and megaloblastic, are formed intravascularly, and retain their nuclei. See also *blood island.*

primitive streak in the early embryo, a narrow groove that forms on the surface of the ectoderm of the germ disk, into which ectodermal cells migrate and then extend laterally between ectoderm and endoderm as the developing mesoderm.

primordium (pri-mor′de-um), pl. *primordia* [L. "the beginning"] in the developing embryo, a grouping of cells that shows the first signs of the organ or part into which they will develop. Also called *anlage.*

principal cell (prin′sĭ-pal) a polygonal parathyroid cell that secretes parathyroid hormone. It has a round, centrally placed vesicular nucleus. The cells are arranged in clumps or anastomosing cords within the parenchyma of the gland. Also called *chief cell.*

principle (prin′sĭ-p′l) [L. *principium,* from *princeps* first] 1. a substance on which certain of the properties of a drug depend.

2. a scientific law or hypothesis.

printed circuit (PC) an electronic circuit in which the conductors connecting the various components are formed by nonconductive barriers etched in a thin film of a conducting metal on an insulating substrate (the printed circuit, PC, board). Discrete components (such as transistors and resistors) are connected by inserting their leads through holes in the PC board and soldering them to the conductors.

printer a computer output device for printing characters on paper. A variety of types exist, differing greatly in speed and mechanism of operation. Teletypes and typewriter terminals, which print about 12 characters/sec, are commonly used as interactive terminals in large systems. High-speed line printers are used for batch output. Impact printers that use drums or chains for printing have speeds of 200–3000 lines/min. Electrostatic printers (dot matrix printers), which generate characters or graphs from a pattern of small dots, can print 5000 lines/min. Ink-jet printers form dot matrix characters from drops of ink that are squirted from a nozzle and directed to the proper spot on the paper by electrostatic deflection. Microcomputer systems often use a low-speed dot matrix printer or a daisy wheel printer, which is a medium-speed character printer.

P-R interval the duration of time between the onset of atrial depolarization (beginning of the P wave) and the onset of ventricular depolarization (beginning of the QRS complex), including the AV node conduction time, as measured from the electrocardiogram. The average P-R interval of 0.16 sec may be shortened or prolonged in various abnormalities of cardiac function or during treatment with antiarrhythmic drugs.

printout the output of a computer printer.

Prinzmetal's angina (prins′met-als) [Myron *Prinzmetal,* U.S. internist, born 1908] see *Prinzmetal's a.* under *angina.*

Prionurus (pri″o-noo′rus) a genus of scorpions found throughout the Mediterranean whose sting produces a local reaction in humans.

prism (prizm) [Gr. *prisma*] 1. a geometric solid produced by the parallel translation of a polygon, i.e., a polyhedron having two congruent polygonal faces and parallelograms for the rest of the faces (sides).
2. a glass prism with a triangular base and rectangular sides, used to disperse a beam of white light into a spectrum or to reflect a beam of light.
3. see *Nicol prism.*

prismatic (priz-mat′ik) shaped like a prism; produced by a prism.

pristanic acid (pris″tan′ik) a tetramethylpentadecanoic acid, which is an enzymic oxidation product of phytanic acid. After conversion to its CoA thioester, it undergoes beta oxidation.

private antigen an antigen of a low-frequency blood group, so-called because many are found only in members of a single kindred. Cf. *public antigen.*

PRM abbrev. for Primary Reference Material. See under *reference materials.*

prn abbrev. for *pro re nata* (as required).

Pro abbrev. See *proline.*

pro- (pro) [L., Gr. *pro* before] a prefix word element to denote before, e.g., proactivator.

proaccelerin (pro″ak-sel′er-in) [*pro-* + L. *accelerare* to hasten + *-in*] see *Factor V.*

probabilistic (prob″ah-bĭ-lis′tik) pertaining to a process described by a specified probability distribution, possibly a conditional distribution that depends on the values of a number of parameters. Cf. *deterministic* and *stochastic.*

probability (P) (prob″ah-bil′ĭ-te) [L. *probabilitas,* from *probabilis* probable, from *probare* to examine, prove] the likelihood of the occurrence of an event (A) denoted $P(A)$ or $Pr(A)$. It is a number between zero and one and corresponds to the long-run frequency at which A occurs in a sequence of independent trials under identical conditions.
If A always occurs, $P(A) = 1$; if A never occurs, $P(A) = 0$. The probability that A does not occur is given by $P(\text{not } A) = 1 - P(A)$.
The addition rule relates the probabilities of two events A and B: $P(A \text{ or } B) = P(A) + P(B) - P(A \text{ and } B)$. If A and B are mutually exclusive events, $P(A \text{ and } B) = 0$, and the addition rule reduces to $P(A \text{ or } B) = P(A) + P(B)$.
The multiplication rule governs conditional probabilities: $P(B \mid A)$ denotes the probability of the event B, given that A has occurred. The rule is $P(A \text{ and } B) = P(B \mid A) \cdot P(A)$.
Two events are said to be independent if $P(B \mid A) = P(B)$ and therefore $P(A \text{ and } B) = P(A) \cdot P(B)$.

probability distribution a mathematical function that assigns to each measurable event A in the sample space the probability $P(A)$ that the event will occur. For a univariate (one-dimensional) distribution, the probabilities are determined by the distribution function (also called the cumulative distribution function, abbrev. cdf) $F(x) = P(X = x)$ which is the probability that the observed value X will be less than or equal to x. It is a nondecreasing function of x with $F(-\infty) = 0$ and $F(\infty) = 1$.
The distribution function of a discrete distribution is a step function that assigns a nonzero probability to each point of a finite or countable sequence of points, which constitutes the sample space. In practice, discrete random variables are usually integer-valued. The probability that the value k is observed is written $p_k = P(X = k)$, then $F(x) = \Sigma_{k \leq x} P_k$, and $\Sigma P_k = F(\infty) = 1$.
The distribution function of a continuous distribution is continuous, so that the probability assigned to each point is zero. The probability of the interval $a \leq X \leq b$ is $F(b) - F(a)$.
A function $Y = g(X)$ defined on the sample space is called a random variable; the average value of Y is called its expectation $E(Y)$. When X is discrete, the expectation is defined by the formula $E(Y) = \Sigma_x g(x) P_x$, if the sum is finite. When X is continuous, the expectation is defined (if it exists) by the integral $\int g(x) f(x) dx$, where $f(x)$, the density function, is the derivative of the distribution function. The average values $Y_n = \Sigma_{k=1}^{n} Y_n/n$ of a sequence of experimental observations Y_k converge to $E(Y)$ as the number of observations increases.
See also *mean* and *variance.* For specific examples, see *binomial distribution* and *normal distribution.*

probability paper graph paper especially designed for plotting the cumulative frequency of a sample against the measurement scale to check the form of the observed distribution against a theoretic distribution, such as a normal or logistic distribution. The paper is designed to yield a straight line if the observed distribution is well approximated by the theoretic distribution. See also *normal probability paper.*

probable error in statistics, the absolute deviation from the mean that is exceeded with probability one-half. For the normal distribution, the probable error is 0.6745 times the standard deviation.

proband (pro′band) [Ger., from L. *probare* to test] see *propositus.*

probe (prōb) [L. *proba,* from *probare* to test] 1. a slender, flexible instrument designed for introduction into a wound, cavity, or sinus tract for purposes of exploration.
2. the detector of a radiation-measuring device,

particularly a movable one, such as the detector of a rectilinear scanner or a scintillation counter.

3. in recombinant DNA technology, a labeled (usually 32p) sequence of DNA or RNA used to visualize a specific DNA sequence. After a mixture of DNA fragments is separated electrophoretically and transferred to a nitrocellulose sheet, the probe is added. It hybridizes with any fragments containing its complementary sequence, allowing them to be visualized by autoradiography.

probenecid (pro-ben'ĕ-sid) [USP], a uricosuric drug used to treat the hyperuricemia of gout and gouty arthritis, although not crisis attacks. It promotes the excretion of uric acid by blocking its reabsorption in the proximal tubules of the kidney. Major side-effects include headache, gastrointestinal intolerance, and hypersensitivity. Probenecid is also administered with certain antibiotics, such as ampicillin and penicillin G, to delay their excretion. Trademark, Benemid.

probit transformation (pro'bit) the transformation of an observed cumulative distribution using an inverse normal distribution with mean five and unit standard deviation. It is used in quantal biologic assay to fit a dose-response curve to the observed proportion responding to assigned dose levels, assuming an underlying normal distribution of tolerance or thresholds.

proboscis (pro-bos'is) [*pro-* + Gr. *boskein* to feed, graze] an abnormal, tubular nose associated with cyclopia.

probucol (pro'bu-kōl) an antilipidemic drug used in the treatment of hyperlipoproteinemia to reduce serum cholesterol levels. The most common adverse effects are diarrhea and other gastrointestinal reactions. Trademark, Lorelco.

procainamide (pro-kān'ah-mid) an analog of procaine having an amide bond replacing an ester bond, used as procainamide hydrochloride [USP] for the treatment of various cardiac arrhythmias, particularly premature beats, and for the treatment of atrial fibrillation or tachycardias after direct-current electrical cardioversion. It acts by prolonging the refractory period of repolarization that is necessary between successive depolarizations (beats), and slows the conduction velocity of the excitation wave. Adverse reactions include hypotension, ventricular asystole or fibrillation, hypersensitivity, and agranulocytosis; a syndrome similar to lupus erythematosus accompanied by a positive antinuclear antibody titer may develop with long-term use.

Therapeutic serum concentrations are 3–10 μg/ml, usually 4–8 μg/ml; toxic effects most often occur above 16 μg/ml.

Procainamide is primarily excreted in the urine. About 60 percent is unchanged; some of the remainder is hydrolyzed to *p*-aminobenzoic acid (PABA). The major metabolite, *N*-acetylprocainamide (NAPA), is also antiarrhythmic. Trademark, *Pronestyl.*

procainamide assays 1. colorimetry. Procainamide is extracted from an alkalinized serum or reference solution sample into an organic solvent. The solvent is evaporated, and the drug is diazotized with sodium nitrite and coupled with *N*-(1-naphthyl)ethylenediamine. The resulting chromophore is read at 550 nm and compared with standards. The sensitivity of the assay is 0.5 μg/ml; the metabolite *N*-acetylprocainamide (NAPA) is not measured.

2. gas chromatography. Procainamide, NAPA, and the internal standard *p*-amino-*N*-(2-dipropylaminoethyl)benzamide are extracted from alkalinized serum or reference solution samples into an organic solvent, and are chromatographed using a nonpolar column packing and a flame ionization detector. The specimen concentration is determined by comparing the ratio of the procainamide or NAPA and internal standard peak heights with a standard curve.

The sensitivity of the method for the parent drug and its metabolite is less than 1 μg/ml.

3. high-performance liquid chromatography. An extraction is carried out as for gas chromatography, and a portion of the concentrated extract is injected onto a silica gel column using buffered acetonitrile as mobile phase and a detector set at 254 nm. Sensitivity for procainamide and its metabolite is 0.1 μg/ml.

4. EMIT homogeneous enzyme immunoassay for procainamide. Its major metabolite, NAPA, can also be determined in serum with this technique.

procaine hydrochloride (pro'kān) [*pro-* + *cocaine*] [USP], a water-soluble salt of a local analgesic drug used for infiltration, nerve and spinal block. It acts to prevent the transmission of nerve impulses by blocking the entry of sodium ions, a necessary condition for propagation of the action potential. It is the ester of *p*-aminobenzoic acid and diethylaminoethanol and is rapidly metabolized to these inactive compounds. Adverse reactions due to overly rapid absorption include excitation of the central nervous system, which may be followed by convulsions, and respiratory depression. Trademark, *Novocain.*

procaryote (pro-kar'e-ōt) [*pro-* + Gr. *karyon* nut] see *prokaryote.*

procedure (pro-se'jur) [L. *procedure,* from *pro-* + *cedere* to move] 1. a series of steps by which a desired result is accomplished.

2. an act or process, such as a surgical or diagnostic procedure.

3. a computer subprogram or subroutine used with various programming languages.

procentriole (pro-sen'tre-ol) the precursor of a centriole. See also *centriole.*

procentriole organizer a dense amorphous mass around which a procentriole forms. Also called *deuterosome.*

process (pros'es) [L. *processus,* from *procedere* to go forward] 1. a prominence or projection, as of bone. For more information, see also the specific process.

2. a series of operations, events, or steps leading to the achievement of a specific result.

acromion p., see *acromion.*

alveolar p., that portion of the mandible or maxilla that surrounds and supports the teeth.

articular p., one of the paired superior and inferior projections of a vertebra. They serve as points of articulation between adjacent vertebrae.

caudate p., a narrow projection of liver tissue that connects the caudate lobe with the right lobe of the liver.

ciliary p., one of the 70–80 ridges or folds that radiate from the base of the iris to the orbiculus ciliaris.

clinoid p., one of the bony projections of the sphenoid bone arranged around the hypophyseal fossa. The two anterior processes are on the lesser wing of the sphenoid; two middle processes may be present and can be continuous with each anterior process; and the posterior processes are the upper corners of the dorsum sellae.

coracoid p., see *coracoid.*

coronoid p., a prominence on the front of the upper ulna that forms the lower part of the trochlear notch. The head of the radius articulates with its lateral surface.

costal p., a prominence of the primitive vertebral arches. In the thoracic region, these structures develop into precartilaginous ribs and finally into true ribs. In other regions, they are incorporated into the transverse processes.

dendritic p., the fine, usually branched extensions of a neuron that serve as a receptive surface for the neuron.

falciform p., an extension of the sacrotuberous ligament running along the inner border of the ramus of the ischium.

mastoid p., a conical projection from the petrosal part of the temporal bone. Angled forward and downward, it serves as a point of attachment for muscles.

odontoid p., a rigid, toothlike process that projects vertically upward from the body of the axis. Also called *dens.*

olecranon p., see *olecranon.*

pterygoid p., one of a pair of bony projections of the sphenoid bone, consisting of lateral and medial plates, that extend downward from the junction of the greater wings and body, behind the maxilla.

spinous p., a bony process that projects dorsally and downward from the dorsomedial surface of a vertebra. It serves as a point of attachment for the muscles of the back. Also called spine of vertebra.

styloid p., a long, slender, bony projection from the inferior surface of the temporal bone. Situated in front of the mastoid process, it is directed forward and downward.

Tomes' p., see *Tomes' fiber.*

transverse p., one of the lateral projections from the body of a vertebra, which serves as a point of attachment for muscles and articulates with the tubercle of a rib.

uncinate p. of pancreas, an extension of pancreatic tissue that projects from the lower left border of the head of the pancreas and hooks around behind the superior mesenteric vessels.

xiphoid p., a pointed process of cartilage and bone that projects downward from the lower end of the sternum.

process control the automatic control of a continuous mechanical process by a computer.

processor (pros′es-or) 1. the central processing unit (CPU), the part of a computer that carries out the arithmetic and logical operations.

2. the entire collection of computer hardware and software that supports some function, such as the CPU, input-output devices, compiler, and subroutine library necessary for running a program written in a high-level language.

processus (pro-ses′us) [L., from *procedere* to go forward] a process or projection; a general term for a mass projecting from a larger anatomic structure, especially the processus vaginalis testis.

p. vaginalis testis, a tubular diverticulum of the peritoneum that protrudes through the inguinal canal along the gubernaculum. After descent of the testes, it becomes the tunica vaginalis testis; vestiges of the processus may occasionally be seen in the spermatic cord.

prochlorperazine (pro″klōr-per′ah-zēn) [USP], a piperazine-type phenothiazine major tranquilizer used in the management of psychotic disorders and the control of nausea and vomiting. The free base is used in suppositories. See also *phenothiazine tranquilizers.* Trademark, *Compazine.*

p. edisylate, [USP], the salt of prochlorperazine, administered orally or intramuscularly.

p. maleate, [USP], the salt of prochlorperazine, administrated orally.

procidentia (pro″si-den′she-ah) [L., from *procidere* to fall forward] see under *prolapse.*

procoagulant (pro″ko-ag′u-lant) 1. tending to favor the occurrence of coagulation.

2. a precursor of a natural substance necessary for coagulation of the blood.

procollagen (pro-kol′ah-jen) [*pro-* + Gr. *kolla* glue + *gennan* to produce] a precursor polypeptide used in the synthesis of collagen. Hydroxylation of prolyl and lysyl residues on the polypeptide begins before ribosomal translation is completed. The procollagen chains combine into a triple helix in the next step of collagen formation.

proconvertin (pro″kon-ver′tin) see *Factor VII.*

proct/o (prok′to) [Gr. *prōktos* anus] a word element used in combining form to denote the anus or rectum, e.g., proctitis, proctoscopy.

proctatresia (prok″tah-tre′ze-ah) [*proct-* + Gr. *trēsis* perforation] see *imperforate anus.*

proctectasia (prok″tek-ta′ze-ah) [*proct-* + Gr. *ektasis* dilation + *-ia*] the dilation of the anus or rectum.

proctitis (prok-ti′tis) [*proct-* + *-itis* inflammation] an inflammation of the rectal mucosa. Symptoms include painful diarrhea with the passage of blood, mucus, and pus, and general rectal discomfort. Ulcerative colitis and regional enteritis are associated with proctitis in the United States.

Diagnosis is confirmed by histologic examination of a rectal biopsy. Proctitis due to specific infectious agents can be diagnosed by stool culture, examination of swabs or scrapings from the rectal mucosa, and by histologic examination of rectal biopsy.

See also *Crohn's disease* and *ulcerative c.* under *colitis.*

proctocele (prok′to-sēl) [*procto-* + Gr. *kēlē* hernia] see *rectocele.*

proctoptosis (prok″top-to′sis) [*procto-* + Gr. *ptōsis* fall] prolapse of the rectum and anus. See also *rectal p.* under *prolapse.*

proctoscopy (prok-tos′ko-pe) [*procto-* + Gr. *skopein* to examine] a diagnostic procedure performed to examine the lower part of the intestine (14–18 cm from the anus) by means of a rigid speculum or tubular instrument (proctoscope) containing a light source. This technique may reveal approximately 70 percent of all rectal lesions below the pelvic peritoneal reflection and provides a means for obtaining rectal biopsies for histologic examination.

proctosigmoidoscopy (prok″to-sig″moi-dos′ko-pe) [*procto-* + *sigmoid* (colon), from Gr. *sigmoeidēs* shaped like the letter sigma + *skopein* to examine] see *sigmoidoscopy.*

procyclidine hydrochloride (pro-si′klĭ-dēn) [USP], an anticholinergic drug used in the palliative treatment of Parkinson's disease and of parkinsonian adverse reactions to antipsychotic drugs. It relieves muscle rigidity and, to a lesser extent, tremor. Adverse side-effects include dryness of the mouth, blurring of vision, dizziness, gastrointestinal intolerance, and constipation; confusion, disorientation, and hallucinations, especially in older persons. Trademark, *Kemadrin.*

prodigiosin (pro-dij″e-o′sin) a tri-pyrrole compound; a red, nondiffusible pigment produced especially at room temperature by certain strains of *Serratia marcescens.*

prodromal (pro-dro′mal) [Gr. *prodromos* going before] premonitory; indicating the onset of a disease.

product (prod′ukt) [L. *producere* to bring forth] 1. anything that is produced.

2. in chemistry, one of the substances produced by a chemical reaction. Because most chemical reactions are reversible, the products become reactants (and vice versa) when the reaction is considered as going in the opposite direction. Cf. *reactant.*

3. in mathematics, the result of a multiplication.

production-defect anemia see *production-defect a.* under *anemia.*

proenzyme (pro-en′zīm) an inactive precursor of an enzyme converted to the active enzyme by being partially hydrolyzed to remove an inhibiting polypeptide section. This process may be catalyzed by acids, alkalis, another enzyme, or the enzyme itself. Also called *zymogen.*

proerythroblast (pro-ĕ-rith′ro-blast″) the earliest recognizable precursor of the erythrocyte; see under *normoblast* and the illustration under *stem cell.*

professional (pro-fesh′un-al) [L. *professio* profession, from *profiteor* to acknowledge] 1. pertaining to a profession.

2. one who is a specialist in a particular profession or occupation.

Professional Standards Review Organization (PSRO) a federally mandated professional health care organization established to ensure ongoing physician review of standards of health care.

profibrinolysin (pro-fi″brĭ-no-li′sin) see *plasminogen.*

proficiency survey an external quality control program in which test materials are prepared by a recognized public or private agency such as the College of American Pathologists (CAP) or the Center for Disease Control (CDC). These are sent to participating clinical laboratories for analysis according to regular, routine procedures, and the results returned to the agency. After the results from all participating laboratories are analyzed and compared, a report indicating the relative level of performance of each laboratory is written and distributed. Also called *survey program.* See also *quality control.*

profile (pro′fīl) [Italian *profilare* to draw in profile, from L. *pro* for + *filum* thread] 1. the outline of an object, such as the head, when viewed from the side.

2. a graph that represents quantitatively a set of tested characteristics.

3. a panel of tests providing related or complementary information.

progenitor (pro-jen′ĭ-tor) [L.] a parent or ancestor.

progeny (proj′ĕ-ne) [L. *progignere* to bring forth] offspring or descendants.

progeria (pro-je′re-ah) [*pro-* + Gr. *gēras* old age + *-ia*] premature old age; a condition occurring in childhood that is marked by the general appearance of old age and is characterized by short stature, gray hair, wrinkled skin, and lack of facial and pubic hair. The manner of inheritance is unclear and there are no detectable abnormalities in pituitary, adrenal, thyroid, or parathyroid function or in response to growth hormone. Affected children show insulin resistance, abnormal collagen, an increased metabolic rate, and various abnormalities in serum lipids. Such children are usually considered normal at birth, but exhibit profound growth failure and an aged appearance in the first 2 yr of life. Those affected develop atherosclerosis and die of cardiac or cerebrovascular disease between 7 and 27 yr of age.

progestational (pro″jes-ta′shun-al) [*pro-* + L. *gestatio* a bearing, from *gestare* to bear] 1. a term applied to that phase of the menstrual cycle, just before menstruation, when the corpus luteum is active and the endometrium is secretory.

2. denoting a class of agents having effects similar to those of progesterone, used in the treatment of endometrial cancer and such disorders as dysfunctional uterine bleeding and recurrent abortion. Synthetic progestational hormones form part of most oral contraceptives.

progestational hormones a group of hormones secreted by the corpus luteum and the placenta, including progesterone, Δ^4-3-ketopregnene-20(α)-ol and Δ^4-3-ketopregnene-20(β)-ol.

progesteroid (pro jes′tĕ-roid) a progesterone-like compound. The term is sometimes used to describe progesterone and all other compounds that have progestational effects.

progesterone (pro-jes′tĕ-rōn) pregn-4-ene-3,20-dione, a major female sex hormone; M.W. 314.45. This steroid is primarily involved in the preparation of the uterus for pregnancy, in its maintenance during pregnancy, and in the preparation of the breasts for lactation. In nonpregnant females, progesterone is synthesized almost entirely by the corpus luteum, whereas during pregnancy this role is taken over by the placenta. Because progesterone is a precursor for androgens and corticosteroids in males, it is also produced in small amounts by the testes and adrenals.

Acetone, cholesterol, and pregnenolone are all precursors of progesterone, and its metabolities are formed by successive reductions, yielding pregnanediones, pregnanolones, and pregnanediols. These substances are subsequently conjugated with glucuronic acid in the liver and excreted as water-soluble glucuronides in the urine. The major end product is pregnanediol, which accounts for 10 percent of the progesterone when measured in the urine.

Progesterone concentrations in the serum are low during the follicular stage of the menstrual cycle, increase soon after ovulation to a maximum in 3–5 da, and return to baseline levels 24 hr before menstruation. When administered between the fifth and twenty-fifth days of the menstrual cycle, progesterone has an antiovulatory effect. This characteristic is also possessed by progestins, synthetic steroids with progesterone-like activity, which are used as oral contraceptives.

Progesterone is transported in the blood bound to transcortin and can be measured in the plasma or serum as progesterone or in the urine as pregnanediol, its major metabolite. Progesterone measurements are used to evaluate the menstrual cycle, the corpus luteum, and the placenta during pregnancy. Sequential concentrations are usually determined to detect luteal insufficiency, defective ovulation, or malfunctioning placentas.

Reference values for progesterone in females are: in the follicular stage of the menstrual cycle, less than 1.5 ng/ml; in the midluteal stage of the menstrual cycle, up to 20; in the first trimester of pregnancy, 15–50; and in the third trimester of pregnancy, 80–200. Reference values for progesterone in males are less than 1 ng/ml.

See also *pregnanediol.*

progesterone assays determination of the progesterone concentration of serum or plasma by radioimmunoassay using rabbit antibodies to progesterone conjugated to a protein, such as bovine serum albumin. Depending on the specificity of antisera, the assay may be performed directly on the specimen, or the specimen may be extracted with an organic solvent (e.g., petroleum ether or hexane), the solvent evaporated, and the residue redissolved in an appropriate buffer. Progesterone assays are generally performed to assess the functional status of the corpus luteum and the placenta. Because progesterone concentration can have a range of < 1–200 ng/ml, it is helpful to know when the specimen was taken relative to the menstrual cycle or duration of pregnancy, to avoid assaying the specimen at several different dilutions.

It should be noted that some antibody preparations to progesterone cross react with other steroids, especially pregnenolone and the corticosteroids.

progesterone receptor (PgR) a specific protein, found in the cytoplasm of a target cell, that has a high affinity for progesterone. Although such receptors are present in various tissues, those in cells of breast cancer are receiving the greatest attention, as the presence of progesterone and estrogen receptors suggest that estrogen therapy may be indicated.

As PgR synthesis appears to be estrogen-dependent, measurement of PgR activity would seem to be a useful indicator of estrogen receptor (ER) concentration. Patients with tumors that are ER^+ and PgR^+ have a response rate to endocrine therapy of greater than 75 percent, whereas those with tumors that are ER^+ and PgR^- have only a 30 percent response rate.

See also *estrogen receptor* and *hormonal therapy.*

progestin (pro-jes′tin) the name originally given to the crude hormone of the corpus luteum. Progestin has since been isolated in pure form, as a substance known as progesterone. The name progestin is used for certain synthetic or natural progestational agents. See also *progesterone.*

progestogen (pro-jes′to-jen) a term used to describe any substance possessing progestational activity. Progestogens have been used in the treatment of uterine cancer and menstrual disorders and form part of most oral contraceptives.

proglottid (pro-glot′id) [*pro-* + Gr. *glōttis* glottis] any one of the chain of egg-producing segments making up the body of a tapeworm (Fig. 1). The proglottid develops from the distal end of a scolex (the attachment organ that anchors the tapeworm to the host's intestinal wall). Three stages of proglottids may be seen in a tapeworm: immature, mature, and gravid. The entire chain of proglottids is called the strobila. The shape and pattern of the gravid uterus are usually diagnostic of the species (Fig. 2).

prognathism (prog′nah-thizm) [*pro-* + Gr. *gnathos* jaw] the abnormal protrusion of the jaw, especially the lower jaw.

prognosis (prog-no′sis) [Gr. *prognōsis* foreknowledge] the expected outcome or course of a pathologic process; the prospects of recovery from a disease.

program (pro′gram) [Gr. *programma* agenda, from *prographein* to write beforehand] a procedure for performing a specific task. In computer science, a program is a set of instructions to a computer. Some

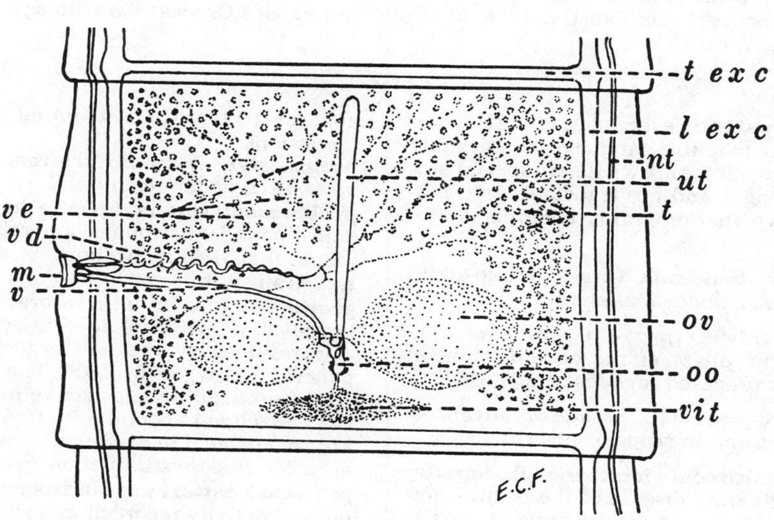

Proglottid, Figure 1. Proglottid of *Taenia saginata*, showing important organs: *l exc*, lateral excretory trunk; *m*, ⚥ pore or genital atrium; *nt*, lateral nerve trunk; *oo*, ootype; *ov*, ovary; *t*, testes; *t exc,* transverse excretory canal; *ut*, uterus; *v*, vagina; *vd*, vas deferens; *ve*, vasa efferentia; and *vit*, "vitellaria," ×10. (Original, from Faust's *Human Helminthology,* Lea & Febiger.) (From Faust, E. C., et al.: Craig and Faust's Clinical Parasitology. 8th ed. Philadelphia, Lea & Febiger, 1970.)

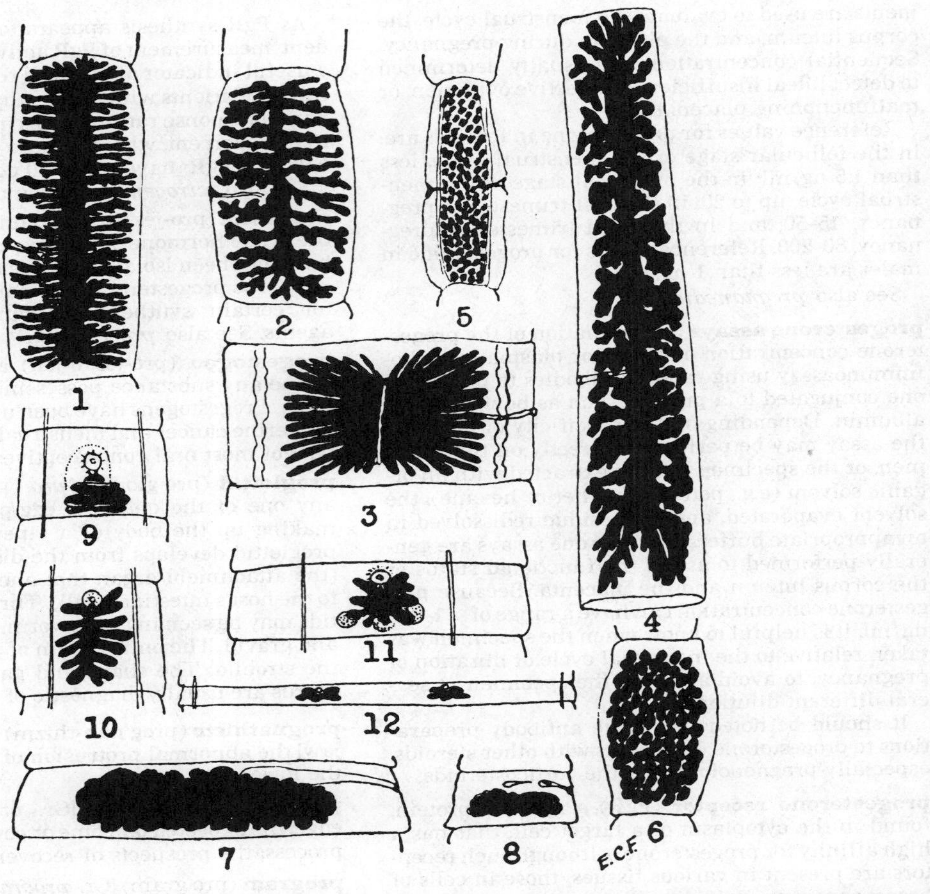

Proglottid, Figure 2. Gravid proglottids of human tapeworms, showing characteristic uterine patterns: 1, *Taenia saginata;* 2, *T. solium;* 3, *T. africana;* 4, *T. confusa;* 5, *Dipylidium caninum;* 6, *Inermicapsifer madagascariensis;* 7, *Hymenolepis diminuta;* 8, *H. nana;* 9, *Spirometra mansoni;* 10, *Diphyllobothrium cordatum;* 11, *D. latum;* and 12, *Diplogonoporus grandis.* (Original, from Faust, compiled and adapted from various authors.) (From Faust, E. C., et al.: Craig and Faust's Clinical Parasitology. 8th ed. Philadelphia, Lea & Febiger, 1970.)

programs directly specify every operation the computer executes (a machine language or assembly language program). Some are written in special programming languages and are translated into machine language by other programs (compilers or interpreters).

progranulocytic leukemia (pro-gran″u-lo-sĭ′tik) see *promyelocytic l.* under *leukemia.*

progravid (pro-grav′id) [*pro-* + L. *gravidus* pregnant] denoting the phase of the endometrium at which point it is prepared for pregnancy.

progressive (pro-gres′iv) [L. *progressus* advanced] advancing; increasing in scope of severity.

progressive multifocal leukoencephalopathy (PML) a demyelinating disease of the central nervous system probably caused by a virus. It usually occurs in the immunosuppressed patient or in the context of chronic neoplastic disease. PML is characterized by a sudden onset of impaired motor function, vision, sensation, and speech. Although no specific microbiologic laboratory procedures are available for diagnosis, CT scanning may help localize the lesions.

progressive systemic sclerosis see *progressive systemic s.* under *sclerosis.*

prohormone (pro-hor′mōn) a hormone precursor. Some peptide hormones are released as prohormones that yield active hormones after proteolysis, e.g., proinsulin.

proinsulin (pro-in′su-lin) a precursor of insulin; a single-chain polypeptide consisting of 86 amino-acid residues, synthesized in the beta cells of the pancreas; M.W. 8000-10,000. The proteolytic cleavage of proinsulin yields active insulin and biologically inactive C peptide. Plasma proinsulin levels are not elevated in diabetics or in normal individuals after glucose stimulation. See also *C peptide.*

projected patterns in electroencephalography, abnormal activity recorded at a site remote from the location of the cerebral disturbance that has given rise to it.

projection (pro-jek′shun) [*pro-* + L. *jacere* to throw] 1. a throwing forward, especially the act of referring impressions made on sense organs to their source.

2. a connection between the cerebral cortex and other parts of the nervous system or organs of special sense.

3. a part that juts out.

4. in radiology, the passage of the central ray of an x-ray beam through the part being radiographed; e.g., in an anteroposterior projection, the beam passes from the front of the subject to the back.

Prokaryotae (pro″kar-e-o′te) [*pro-* + Gr. *karyon* nut] a kingdom of microorganisms of prokaryotic cell structure, which contains two divisions: (1) the cyanobacteria (the blue-green photobacteria, formerly called blue-green algae) and (2) prokaryotic cells that are not cyanobacteria (including the nonphotosynthetic bacteria and the red and green photobacteria). The latter group contains the bacteria commonly encountered in human and veterinary biology and medicine.

prokaryote (pro-kar′e-ōt) an organism whose nuclear material is not bounded by a membrane and consists of a single chromosome formed by a circular DNA molecule. Prokaryotes usually have a rigid cell wall; they lack internal cellular structures such as mitochondria. Cf. *eukaryote.*

prokaryotic (pro″kar-e-ot′ik) having the characteristics of a prokaryote.

prolactin (pro-lak′tin) [*pro-* + L. *lac* milk] a protein hormone produced by lactotrophic cells in the pituitary gland; M.W. 22,500. It is mammotropic and lactogenic in the breast that has been primed by estrogens, progestins, corticosteroids, and insulin. Prolactin induces ductal growth and development of the lobule alveolar system. Lactogenesis cannot occur without prolactin. Specific milk proteins, including casein and alpha lactalbumin, are induced by prolactin. The hormone is under hypothalamic control, primarily through a tonic inhibition of release by prolactin-inhibiting factor (PIF), which in turn is regulated by dopaminergic mechanisms. A physiologic elevation of prolactin levels occurs in the fetus and newborn infant, in adults during sleep and stress, and in females during pregnancy and while nursing. In addition, exercise, surgical trauma, pain, insulin-induced hypoglycemia, and other such stresses usually result in physiologic hyperprolactinemia. The pathologic causes of hyperprolactinemia include functional hypothalamic disorders (e.g., Chiari-Frommel syndrome), autonomous prolactin production (e.g., pituitary chromophobe adenoma), and endocrine metabolic disorders such as acromegaly, hypothyroidism, and chronic renal failure. Prolactin in certain mammals such as the rat shows luteotropic activity.

Prolactin concentrations in blood are measured by radioimmunoassay techniques utilizing highly purified human pituitary prolactin as standard and labeled antigen and anti-human pituitary prolactin antibody. Values of prolactin in serum are: for males, 5–18 ng/ml; and for females, 6–22.

Also called lactogenic hormone, *luteotropic hormone* (LTH), *luteotropin,* and *mammotropin.*

prolactin-inhibiting factor (PIF) a hypothalamic factor that inhibits the release of the hormone prolactin. Also called *prolactin release-inhibiting hormone.*

prolactin release-inhibiting hormone (PRIH) see *prolactin-inhibiting factor.*

prolactin-releasing hormone (PRH) a hypothalamic factor that stimulates the release of the hormone prolactin.

prolapse (pro-laps′) [L. *prolapsus,* from *prō* + *labi* to fall] the falling down or sinking of an organ or other part; procidentia, ptosis.

rectal p., a condition, in which the rectal mucosa or a portion of the rectum protrudes through the anus (proctoptosis). In adults the condition is acquired and generally appears after pelvic surgery, after childbirth, or with increasing age; in children it is common in those with cystic fibrosis of the pancreas, or it may be a congenital condition related to a lack of skeletal support and fixation. Initially, the prolapse is small and appears only with straining; however, further progression leads to an irritated, bloody mucosa, a dilated anal sphincter, and incontinence.

Sigmoidoscopy and barium enema examination should be performed to rule out other disorders. Endoscopy shows an engorged and thickened mucosa in the prolapsed area. Treatment involves stool softeners and surgery.

uterine p., a downward displacement of the uterus that usually occurs in multiparous females. The condition is caused by laxity of the muscular and fascial structures of the pelvic floor due to the stress of childbirth, the effects of gravity in the standing position, and the loss of tone associated with the hormonal withdrawal of menopause.

proliferation (pro-lif″ĕ-ra′shun) [L. *proles* offspring + *ferre* to bear] to increase in number, the reproduction or multiplication of similar forms, especially referring to cells in normal and neoplastic tissues.

proliferation inhibitory factor (PIF) a lymphocyte effector that causes reversible and irreversible growth inhibition, as does a similar lymphocyte effector, cloning inhibitory factor (CIF). There is evidence that PIF and CIF are the same substance as lymphotoxin (LT). The activities are concentration-dependent: high concentrations of stimulated lymphocyte culture supernatants have LT activity, whereas lower concentrations show reversible growth inhibition. Also, both activities parallel each other during purification steps. See also *lymphotoxin.*

proliferative (pro-lif′er-a-tiv) characterized by proliferation.

proliferative glomerulopathy see under *glomerulopathy.*

proliferative myositis a lesion of skeletal muscle, probably formed in response to injury, which, because of its clinical presentation and histologic features, may be mistaken for a neoplasm. It commonly occurs in the muscles of the shoulder region or thigh of adults, and forms a firm mass several centimeters in diameter, with a scarlike appearance on the cut surface. Histologically, loosely arranged round cells with eosinophilic cytoplasm and prominent nucleoli within round nuclei are typical, but a spindle cell component may also be present. Degeneration, regeneration, and phagocytosis of myofibers is common and may be associated with chronic inflammation. The surrounding skeletal muscle is normal. Treatment consists of simple excision.

proline (Pro, P) (pro′lēn) [Ger. *prolin,* from *pyr rol*-*id in* pyrrolidine] a heterocyclic compound, 2-pyrrolidinecarboxylic acid, $(C_4H_8N)COOH$, a naturally occurring nonessential amino acid; M.W. 115.13. It is a major amino acid of connective tissue proteins, e.g., collagen, elastin, and tooth enamel protein. Proline can give rise to glutamic acid metabolically. Because of its structure, it can destabilize both the beta-structure and alpha-helix of polypeptides. It is present in many dietary proteins and can be formed from glutamic acid. See also under *amino acids.*

proline dehydrogenase see *pyrroline-5-carboxylate reductase.*

proline hydroxylase see *proline,2-oxoglutarate dioxygenase.*

prolinemia (pro″lĭ-ne′me-ah) [*proline* + Gr. *haima* blood + *-ia*] see *hyperprolinemia.*

proline oxidase see *pyrroline-5-carboxylate reductase.*

proline,2-oxoglutarate dioxygenase an enzyme of the oxidoreductase class (EC 1.14.11.2) that catalyzes the reaction prolyl-glycyl-containing–peptide + 2-oxoglutarate + O_2 ⇄ hydroxyprolyl-glycyl-containing–peptide + succinate + CO_2. The presence of ferrous iron and ascorbate is required. It is important in the conversion of prolyl to hydroxyprolyl residues to form collagen. Also called *proline hydroxylase.*

prolinuria (pro″lĭ-nu′re-ah) [*proline* + Gr. *ouron* urine + *-ia*] iminoglycinuria. See under *hyperglycinuria.*

Prolixin (pro-lik′sin) trademark. See *fluphenazine.*

prolyl (pro′lyl) the acyl radical of proline.

PROM abbrev. See *programmable r. o. m.* under *read only memory.*

promastigote (pro-mas′tĭ-gōt) [*pro-* + Gr. *mastix* whip] a morphologic stage in the development of protozoa of the family Trypanosomatidae, characterized by a free anterior flagellum and resembling the typical adult form of *Leptomonas.*

promegakaryoblast (pro-meg″ah-kar′e-o-blast″) the earliest recognizable precursor of the bone marrow cell that forms platelets; see under *stem cell* and *thrombocytopoiesis.*

prometaphase (pro-met′ah-fāz) [*prophase* + *metaphase*] the stage of cell division, covering late prophase and early metaphase, during which the nuclear membrane disappears and the centrioles move to the poles of the spindle. See also *meiosis* and *mitosis.*

promethazine hydrochloride (pro-meth′ah-sēn) [USP], an anticholinergic and antihistaminic phenothiazine derivative used as a sedative and antiemetic and in the treatment of allergic reactions. Adverse reactions include dryness of the mouth, blurring of vision, dizziness, and drowsiness. Overdosage may cause respiratory depression and coma. Trademark, Phenergan.

promethium (Pm) (pro-me′the-um) [from the Titan god Prometheus in Greek mythology, who gave fire to humans] a reactor-produced radioactive element, atomic number 61; most stable isotope, Pm-145 (half-life, 17.7 yr); a 4f transition element (lanthanide or rare earth); oxidation state +3. See also *rare earth elements.*

promonocyte (pro-mon′o-sīt) one of the recognizable precursors of the monocyte; see *monohistiocytic series* and the illustration under *stem cell.*

promoter (pro-mo′ter) [*pro-* + L. *moveo,* past participle *motus* to move] 1. in molecular genetics, a DNA segment to which RNA polymerase binds and initiates the transcription of genetic information from DNA to messenger RNA. This binding is the beginning of protein synthesis. See also *bacterial g.* under *genetics* and *genetic regulation.*

2. in chemistry, a substance that increases the effect of a catalyst.

3. see *tumor p.*

tumor p., a chemical substance, possessing little or no carcinogenic potential itself, that can increase the incidence of neoplasms in tissue previously exposed to an initiating carcinogenic chemical. Classical evidence for tumor promoters comes from experiments with mice, in which a small amount of a chemical carcinogen (the initiator) is painted on the skin in a dose insufficient to cause the formation of neoplasms. Weeks to months later, however, an irritating substance such as croton oil (the promoter) is repeatedly applied to the same skin site, which was originally treated with the initiator; this results in the formation of a neoplasm. If the promoting substance alone is applied (before the initiator), or if it is applied in a single dose, no neoplasm develops. This sequence of events has led to the hypothesis of a two-stage mechanism of carcinogenesis. It is suggested that the initiator produces some form of cellular alteration that primes the cell for neoplastic transformation. A promoter is necessary to induce these cells to divide and express their acquired carcinogenic potential.

Early studies on tumor promoters used crude irritants such as croton oil. The active ingredients have since been determined to be the phorbol esters, of which 12-O-tetradecanoylphorbol-13-acetate (TPA) is the best characterized. The role of tumor promoters in humans is not well known. Some studies have suggested that cigarette smoke and saccharine may act as promoters in bronchogenic carcinoma and bladder cancer, respectively.

See also *cancer.*

promyelocyte (pro-mi′ĕ-lo-sīt″) the second stage in granulocytic maturation, designated M_2, which follows the myeloblast and precedes the myelocyte. A promyelocyte is the largest cell of the granulocytic series (15–20 μm in diameter) and is normally found only in the bone marrow.

On a blood or bone marrow smear stained with Giemsa or Wright stain, the nucleus is oval with a slightly condensed chromatin pattern; occasionally it has small nucleoli hidden behind perinuclear chromatin. The cytoplasm is slightly blue and contains azurophilic granules. It also contains a large centrosome, detectable as a light juxtanuclear zone adjacent to a slight depression in the nucleus; this clear zone does not contain granules. The presence of azurophilic granules (primary granules), which vary in shape and size, allows the persistence of the peroxidase-positive cytochemical reaction.

See also *granulocytic series.*

pronation (pro-na′shun) [L. *pronatio,* from *pronare* to bend forward] 1. the act of assuming the prone position, or the state of being prone.

2. the act of turning the forearm so that the palm faces backward (posteriorly).

3. the combination of eversion and abduction of the foot, resulting in the lowering of the medial margin of the foot and of the longitudinal arch. Cf. *supination.*

prone (prōn) [L. *pronus* inclined forward] lying face down, on the anterior or ventral surface.

Pronestyl (pro-nes′til) trademark. See *procainamide hydrochloride.*

pronormoblast (pro-nor′mo-blast) see under *normoblast.*

pronucleus (pro-nu′kle-us) the haploid nucleus of an ovum (the female pronucleus) or sperm (the male pronucleus) after fertilization but before the two pronuclei are combined to form the nucleus of the zygote.

propanenitrile (pro″pān-ni′tril) a liquid, C_2H_5CN, that is highly toxic, flammable, colorless, and volatile; M.W. 55.08. It is used as a solvent, dielectric, and reagent. Also called *ethyl cyanide* and *propionitrile.*

propanoic acid (pro″pah-no′ik) see *propionic acid.*

1-propanol (pro′pah-nol) a colorless, flammable liquid, C_3H_8OH, used as solvent and chemical intermediate; M.W. 60.09. In toxicity it is similar to ethanol. Also called *propyl alcohol.*

2-propanol isopropyl alcohol, $CH_3CHOHCH_3$, a volatile, colorless liquid used as a rubbing compound, antiseptic, and denaturing agent for ethyl alcohol; M.W. 60.09. Ingestion or inhalation of the vapors causes nausea, vomiting, and dizziness; larger quantities produce mental depression, narcosis, anesthesia, and coma. 2-Propanol is metabolized to acetone.

propantheline bromide (pro-pan′thĕ-lēn) [USP], an anticholinergic sympatholytic drug that reduces gastric secretion and motility. It is used in the management of peptic ulcer and to reduce duodenal motility during hypotonic duodenography. Adverse reactions are similar to those of atropine and include drying of salivary and other secretions, decreased sweating, rapid heartbeat, blurred vision, and inability to urinate. Conditions in which it is contraindicated include glaucoma, prostatic hypertrophy, and cardiovascular disease.

propenal (pro′pen-al) see *acrolein.*

propepsin (pro-pep′sin) see *pepsinogen.*

properdin (pro′per-din) a heat-labile glycoprotein; M.W. 185,000. With several other factors, properdin can activate the alternative complement pathway and result in the destruction of gram-negative bacteria and viruses; it also plays a role in the lysis of erythrocytes. In examination of serum proteins by electrophoresis, properdin can be seen to migrate as a $gamma_2$-globulin. Reference ranges for properdin in serum are 17.2–29.4 μg/ml (mean, 24.7 $\pm$ 3.9). See also *alternative complement pathway.*

properdin assays a test for quantitating the amount of properdin in serum. The most commonly used assay is radial immunodiffusion. It is still used primarily as a research tool.

properdin system see *alternative complement pathway.*

prophage (pro′fāj) [*pro-* + *phage*] the stage of a bacterial virus in which the genome is integrated into the bacterial chromosome. It is a stable, inherited, noninfectious form of the virus. Also called probacteriophage.

prophase (pro′fāz) a stage of cell division during which the chromosomes become visible and the centrioles separate. In meiosis I, prophase is further divided into five stages (leptotene, zygotene, pachytene, diplotene, and diakinesis) during which cross-over occurs. See also *meiosis* and *mitosis.*

prophylactic (pro″fĭ-lak′tik) [Gr. *prophylaktikos,* from *prophylax* advance guard, from *phylax* guard] 1. tending to ward off disease; pertaining to prophylaxis.

2. an agent that tends to ward off disease.

prophylaxis (pro″fĭ-lak′sis) [Gr. *prophylassein* to keep guard before] the prevention of disease; preventive treatment.

β-propiolactone (BPL) (pro″pe-o-lak′tōn) hydroacrylic acid β-lactone; a water-miscible, nonflammable liquid used as a disinfectant and sterilizing agent. It is a powerful bactericide, viricide, and fungicide, and kills bacterial endospores more rapidly than do most sporicidal chemicals. The greatest use of BPL is in decontamination of closed spaces. BPL is a toxic chemical; it is a respiratory irritant, strong lacrimator, and vesicant. Carcinogenic properties have been demonstrated in animals; however, the half-life of a 1 percent solution is only 3–4 hr, and the hydrolysis product is a nontoxic isomer of lactic acid.

propiomazine hydrochloride (pro″pe-o-ma′zēn) [USP], a phenothiazine derivative having sedative and antihistamine activity, used as an adjunct to anesthesia.

propionate carboxylase (pro′pe-o-nāt) see *propionyl-CoA carboxylase.*

propionate metabolism a process involving conversion in several steps to succinyl coenzyme A, requiring biotin and vitamin B_{12}, which then enters the tricarboxylic acid cycle. Propionate is formed from oxidation of odd-numbered C-chain fatty acids and from branched-chain aliphatic amino acids in animal tissues.

Propionibacteriaceae (pro″pe-on″e-bak-te″re-a′se-e) a family of gram-positive, nonspore-forming, anaerobic, rod-shaped bacteria closely related to the actinomycetes. The family includes two genera, *Propionibacterium* and *Eubacterium.*

Propionibacterium (pro″pe-on″e-bak-te′re-um) [*pro-* + Gr. *piōn* fat + *baktērion* little rod] a genus of bacteria of the family Propionibacteriaceae, composed of gram-positive, anaerobic or facultatively anaerobic, nonsporulating rods. These organisms are normal inhabitants of mammalian and human cavities and skin, occasionally causing infections of soft tissue. They are small, club-shaped rods that frequently form configurations resembling Chinese letters. Catalase is usually produced.

propionic acid (pro″pĭ-on′ik) systematic name, propanoic acid, CH_3CH_2COOH, an oily liquid with a pungent odor; M.W. 74.08. It is produced by some bacteria and occurs in animals as propionyl coenzyme A, an intermediate in the oxidation of odd-chain or branched-chain fatty acids and the metabolism of some amino acids (e.g., valine). It is used medicinally as a topical antifungal agent.

propionic acidemia a rare genetic defect, transmitted as an autosomal recessive trait, of branched-chain amino acid metabolism. Impairment of propionyl CoA carboxylase is the defect. Symptoms include repeated bouts of vomiting, metabolic acidosis, neutropenia, high serum glycine, developmental retardation, high serum and urine propionic acid, and intolerance to protein. Large doses of biotin may be helpful in selected cases.

Propionyl CoA is derived primarily from branched-chain amino acids and, in small part, from odd-numbered carbon-chain fatty acids. The accumulation of glycine is not well understood.

See also *aminoacidopathy* and *ketotic h.* under *hyperglycinemia.*

propionic aciduria the excretion of excess amounts of propionic acid in urine. It can occur as a consequence of biotin deficiency or as a genetic defect with impairment of propionyl CoA carboxylase. See also *propionic acidemia.*

propionitrile (pro″pe-o-ni′tril) see *propanenitrile.*

propionyl CoA (pro′pe-o-nil) the coenzyme A thioester of propionic acid formed during the oxidative metabolism of odd-number carbon atom fatty acids and branched-chain amino acids.

propionyl-CoA carboxylase an enzyme of the lyase class (EC 4.1.1.41) that catalyzes the reaction (R)-methylmalonyl-CoA ⇄ propionyl-CoA + CO_2, a reaction important in the metabolism of amino acids and fatty acids. A genetic defect, transmitted as an autosomal recessive trait, is characterized by the absence or deficiency of this enzyme. This condition may lead to neonatal ketotic hyperglycinemia and propionic acidemia, as well as failure to thrive and other nonspecific symptoms. Measurement of the enzyme activity in cells of the amniotic fluid can be used in prenatal screening. Also called *methylmalonyl-CoA decarboxylase* and *propionate carboxylase.*

proportional counter a radiation detector used primarily for counting alpha and beta particles; it is a gas-filled chamber (usually a mixture of argon and methane). Particles entering the chamber produce ions that are accelerated toward two electrodes, producing more ions (a process called gas amplification). The voltage is set so that the amplification factor is about 1000, and the output pulse is proportional to the number of ions produced directly by the particle.

propositus (por-poz′ĭ-tus), pl. *propositi* [L. *proponere* to put on view] in a genetic diagram, or pedigree, the index individual; i.e., the original person presenting with a clinical disorder whose case initiates a genealogic study of the family. In pedigree analysis, the propositus is usually omitted from calculations of the proportion of the family affected. Also called *index case* and *proband.*

propoxur (pro-poks′oor) a toxic carbamate insecticide, *O*-isopropoxyphenyl-*N*-methylcarbamate. It can be ingested, inhaled, or absorbed through the skin, and produces cholinesterase inhibition with symptoms resembling poisoning by organophosphate compounds. Atropine (but not pralidoxime) is used to treat carbamate poisoning. Trademark, Baygon.

propoxyphene (pro-pok′se-fēn) a mild analgesic, chemically similar to methadone, that is often used in combination with aspirin or acetaminophen for relief of mild-to-moderate pain. The potential for abuse of propoxyphene is similar to that of codeine; it can produce psychic and physical dependence and tolerance. The effects of propoxyphene and other central nervous system depressants (e.g., tranquilizers, alcohol, and sedatives) are additive. Adverse reactions include dizziness, sedation, and gastrointestinal disturbances. Acute toxicity is similar to narcotic overdose and can produce respiratory depression, coma, and death. The narcotic antagonist naloxone is used to reverse respiratory depression.

Propoxyphene is rapidly bound to tissue; concentrations in the brain, lungs, liver, and kidneys are much higher than in blood. The serum concentration in fatal poisonings is more than 1 μg/ml (usually more than 5 μg/ml), and liver concentrations are more than 15 mg/kg (usually more than 50 mg/kg).

propoxyphene assays 1. ultraviolet (UV) spectrophotometry. The product of acid hydrolysis of the sample is extracted into ether. The absorbance at 254 nm is proportional to the concentration. This procedure can be made more specific for propoxyphene by irradiating the extract with UV light at 257.3 nm, which produces a large increase in the absorbance of the product at 254 nm; the concentration is proportional to the absorbance increase.

2. gas chromatography. A flame ionization detector and a nonpolar silicone column packing are used. An alkalinized sample is extracted with an organic solvent and reextracted into acid. Pyrroliphene is used as the internal standard. This procedure separates propoxyphene from its major metabolite norpropoxyphene (which spectrophotometry does not); however, several basic drugs, including doxepin, atropine, and cocaine, are not completely separated.

3. EMIT homogenous enzyme immunoassay for propoxyphene in urine specimens.

propranolol (pro-pran′o-lōl) a beta-adrenergic blocking drug used as propranolol hydrochloride [USP] in the treatment of hypertension, cardiac arrhythmias, and angina pectoris. Beta blockade reduces blood pressure, heart rate, and cardiac output (β_1-effects) and also produces bronchial constriction (a β_2-effect). Cardiac depressant effects similar to those of quinidine are produced at higher dosages. Adverse reactions include precipitation of heart failure, bradycardia, hypotension, bronchospasm, and hypoglycemia.

Serum concentrations do not correlate well with either the oral dosage or the drug effects; however, a level of 50–100 ng/ml produces beta blockade in most individuals. The metabolite 4-hydroxypropranolol also contributes to the beta blockade. Trademark, *Inderal.*

propranolol assays 1. fluorescence spectrophotometry. Propranolol is extracted from samples of alkalinized blood, tissue, stomach content, or reference solution into toluene and reextracted into dilute acid. The acidic extract is read at an excitation wavelength of 290 nm for propranolol (emitting at 358 nm) and 320 nm for the metabolite 4-hydroxpropranolol (emitting at 510 nm). The sensitivity of the assay is 0.015 μg/ml.

2. gas chromatography. Propranolol and the internal standard oxprenolol are extracted from alkalinized plasma with an organic solvent. After forming the trifluoroacetylated derivatives, they are injected into a moderately polar column utilizing an electron capture detector. The sensitivity of the assay is 0.001 μg/ml. Effective plasma concentrations are 0.05–0.1 μg/ml for propranolol and 0.02–0.16 for the 4-hydroxypropranolol metabolite.

proprioceptive (pro′pre-o-sep′tiv) receiving stimuli within the tissues of the body, as within muscles and tendons, a function that may be temporarily diminished by prolonged immobilization of a part, such as in a cast, or by prolonged bed rest. Diminished proprioceptive sensation is seen in such conditions as tabes dorsalis, hereditary sensory neuropathy, Friedreich's ataxia, and subacute combined degeneration (secondary to vitamin B_{12} deficiency). See also *proprioceptor.*

proprioceptive receptor a sensory nerve ending, which is located in muscles, tendons, and the inner ear, that receives information concerning the position and movements of the body. Cf. *exteroceptor, Golgi tendon organ, interoceptor, muscle spindle,* and *receptor.*

proprotein (pro-pro'tēn) a masked form of an active protein molecule formed by proteolytic removal of a polypeptide fragment from a preproprotein. By proteolysis, intra- or extracellularly, it is converted to the active protein molecule. See also *preproprotein.*

proptometer (pro-tom'ĕ-ter) [Gr. *proptōsis* a fall forward + *metron* measure] an instrument used to measure the degree of protrusion; for example, in exophthalmos, an instrument to measure the degree of protrusion of the eyeball.

proptosis (prop-to'sis) [Gr. *proptōsis* a fall forward] see *exophthalmos.*

propyl- (pro'pil) a prefix word element used in systematic organic chemical nomenclature to denote the *n*-propyl group, $CH_3CH_2CH_2$—, e.g., 4-propylheptane, $(C_3H_7)_3CH$.

***n*-propyl-** a prefix word element (meaning normal propyl) used in organic chemistry to denote the propyl group, —$CH_2CH_2CH_3$, e.g., *n*-propylamine and *n*-propyl alcohol. Cf. *isopropyl-.*

propyl alcohol see *1-propanol.*

propylene (pro'pĭ-lēn) a gaseous unsaturated hydrocarbon, propene, $CH_3CH{=}CH_2$.

p. glycol, [USP], a clear, colorless, nearly odorless, viscous liquid, 1,2-propanediol, $CH_3CHOHCH_2OH$. Propylene glycol has a slight, characteristic taste and absorbs moisture on exposure to air; it is used as a humectant and solvent.

propylhexadrine (pro"pil-hek'sĕ-drēn) [USP], a volatile sympathomimetic amine with only slight stimulant effect, inhaled as a nasal decongestant. Trademark, *Benzedrex.*

propyliodone (pro"pil-i'o-dōn) [USP], a radiopaque contrast medium used in bronchography. Trademark for a suspension of propyliodone in peanut oil, *Dionosil.*

propylthiouracil (pro"pil-thi"o-u'rah-sil) [USP], a thioamide drug that inhibits the synthesis of thyroid hormones; used for the treatment of hyperthyroidism. A rare adverse reaction is its interference with the formation of blood cells, causing agranulocytosis. If this occurs, drug therapy is stopped and alternate modalities (surgery, radioactive iodine) are used. Thioamides interfere with thyroid function tests.

prorubricyte (pro-roo'brĭ-sīt) see basophilic normoblast under *normoblast.*

pros/o (pros'o) [Gr. *prosō* forward] a word element used in combining form to denote forward or anterior, e.g., prosocoele.

prosection (pro-sek'shun) [Late latin *prosecare* to cut up, from *pro-* + *secare* to cut] careful dissection of a cadaver for the demonstration of anatomic structures.

prosencephalon (pros"en-sef'ah-lon) [*prosō-* + Gr. *enkephalos* brain] 1. [NA], the part of the brain comprising the diencephalon and telencephalon with the third ventricle.

2. in the developing embryo, the most anterior of the developing brain vesicles, which later divides into the telencephalon and diencephalon.

prosodemic (pros"o-dem'ik) [*proso-* + Gr. *dēmos* people] passing directly from one person to another, rather than to a large number of people at once; said of a disease (e.g., syphilis) transmitted in such a manner.

prosop/o (pros'o-po) [Gr. *prosōpon* face] a word element used in combining form to denote relationship to the face, e.g., prosopoplegia.

prosopagnosia (pros"o-pag-no'se-ah) [*prosopo-* + *a* neg. + Gr. *gnōsis* perception + *-ia*] a type of visual agnosia characterized by the inability to recognize the faces of other individuals, or even one's own face. The severely prosopagnosic patient, for example, may be unable to recognize members of his or her own family unless they speak. Usually this disorder is associated with agnosias for color, places, and objects. At autopsy, there are lesions in the right anterior-inferior occipital region and usually an additional lesion in the left hemisphere that is often, but not always, symmetric with that on the right.

prosopoplegia (pros"o-po-ple'je-ah) [*prosopo-* + Gr. *plēgē* stroke + *-ia*] facial paralysis. See also *Bell's p.* under *palsy.*

prosostomate trematodes (pros-os'to-māt) [*proso-* + Gr. *stoma* mouth] a descriptive term used to denote those trematodes having a mouth at the anterior end of the body, which is surrounded by a sucker. The trematodes that are parasitic in humans are of this type.

prospective study a study in which the event of interest is expected to occur in the future relative to the investigator's place in time. For example, a study to ascertain the effect of decreasing dietary fat on heart disease is a prospective study. Individuals may be exhorted in the present by a physician to reduce their fat intake, but the effect (and measurement of that effect) takes place in the future. All experimental studies are prospective. The term cohort study is frequently used synonymously with prospective study, a usage that should be avoided as the former refers to the selection of the group to be studied, whereas the latter refers to the chronology of event occurrence relative to the investigator.

prostacyclin (PGI_2) (pros"tah-si'klin) 9-deoxy-6,9α-epoxy-Δ^5-$PGF_{1\alpha}$, a prostaglandin derived from arachidonic acid (20:4) and produced mainly by the blood vessels, heart, kidneys, and lungs; M.W. 352.48. Prostacyclin is a potent vasodilator and is among the most potent naturally occuring inhibitors of platelet aggregation. This inhibition is mediated by elevation of platelet cAMP. At physiologic pH, prostacyclin is unstable ($t_{1/2}$ = 10.4 min at 22°C) and it decomposes to a biologically inactive metabolite, 6-keto-prostaglandin $F_{1\alpha}$, which is further metabolized in the body. Stable prostacyclin analogs may have potential clinical use as antihypertensive or antiplatelet drugs. Also called *prostaglandin I_2.*

prostaglandin (PG) (pros"tah-glan'din) one of a group of naturally occurring, cyclic, 20-carbon, hydroxy fatty acids that have numerous and diverse biologic actions, exerting their effects in nanogram concentrations; M.W. about 360. Among other effects, prostaglandins may increase or decrease cAMP production, constrict or dilate blood vessels, induce or inhibit platelet aggregation, inhibit gastric acid secretion, change renal electrolyte balance, induce labor at term, and terminate pregnancy. The effects of prostaglandins are diverse and sometimes contradictory to each other, depending on the type of prostaglandin or the target tissue involved.

First discovered in seminal fluid and extracts of the accessory genital glands of humans and sheep, prostaglandins have been found to be produced by most mammalian tissues except red blood cells. Prostaglandins can be regarded as derivatives of a hypothetical 20-carbon compound, prostanoic acid, that contains a cyclopentane ring. Some related compounds, namely thromboxanes, have a six-member oxane ring instead. Prostaglandins are divided into types A through I, on the basis of their functions in the cyclopentane ring. Their numerical subscripts (1, 2, and 3) refer to the number of double bonds in the side-chains, whereas α and β subscripts refer to the configuration of the substituents in the ring.

Three 20-carbon fatty acids have been found to be precursors for prostaglandin biosynthesis: dihomo-gammalinoleic acid (DLL), arachidonic acid (AA), and eicosapentaenoic acid (EPA), AA being quantitatively by far the most significant. The initial step of the synthesis involves oxygenation by cyclooxygenase, a unique enzyme that yields a cyclic endoperoxide, prostaglandin G (PGG), which is subsequently reduced to PGH, a chemically unstable and very potent compound. These two prostaglandins are obligatory intermediates for the synthesis of all other prostaglandins or thromboxanes. Prostaglandin biosynthesis is selectively inhibited by nonsteroidal antiinflammatory drugs (NSAID) such as aspirin and indomethacin.

Some prostaglandins are in the clinical trial stage, but so far only one stable derivative ($PGF_{2\alpha}$) has gained use as an abortive drug. Prostaglandins are assayed by gas chromatography–mass spectrophotometry, radioimmunoassay, and spectroscopic methods, primarily in research laboratories. No diagnostic value has yet been found.

See also *aspirin* and *naproxen.*

p. A (PGA), 15-hydroxy-9-oxoprostanoic acid, a prostaglandin formed by acid-catalyzed dehydration of prostaglandin of the E series; M.W. about 338. PGA, A_2, or A_3 can be formed from the corresponding parent fatty acids. PGA_2 is found mainly in the mammalian kidneys; interestingly, it is also formed in relatively large quantities in a marine coelenterate, the gorgonian *Plexaura homomalla,* a species of Caribbean coral. PGAs can also be formed by acid-catalyzed reduction of PGEs. PGA_2 acts as a weak vasodilator, and can increase renal blood flow and induce natriuresis.

p. B (PGB), 15-hydroxy-prostanoic acid, a prostaglandin formed by isomerization of PGA in basic conditions; M.W. about 324. Prostaglandins of the B series have an absorption maximum at 237 nm, a fact used in the quantitative determination of prostaglandins from the E series, which are converted to PGFs and subsequently to PGBs.

p. D_2 (PGD_2), 9,15-dihydroxy-11-oxoprost-5,13-dienoic acid, a prostaglandin derived from arachidonic acid (20:4) and formed in platelets and several rat tissues and sheep lung; M.W. 352.48. PGD_2 is a potent inhibitor of human platelet aggregation via an elevation of cAMP, and also increases vascular permeability. PGD_2 can also be formed by nonenzymatic decomposition of PGH_2.

p. E_1 (PGE_1), 11,15-dihydroxy-9-oxoprost-13-enoic acid, a prostaglandin found mainly in seminal vesicles and formed from eicosa-8,11,14-trienoic acid (20:3) through the actions of cyclooxygenase and PGE isomerase; M.W. 354.49. PGE_1 stimulates adenylate cyclase, inhibits lipolysis, inhibits platelet aggregation, dilates blood vessels, and modulates some immunologic responses.

p. E_2 (PGE_2), 11,15-dihydroxy-9-oxoprost-5,13-dienoic acid, a prostaglandin derived from arachidonic acid (20:4) and found in most mammalian tissues; M.W. 352.48. PGE_2 dilates certain vascular smooth muscles, constricts uterine and gastrointestinal smooth muscle, enhances platelet aggregation, stimulates Ca^{++} mobilization from bone, and inhibits Na^+ excretion in the kidneys.

p. $F_{1\alpha}$ ($PGF_{1\alpha}$), 9,11,15-trihydroxy-prost-13-enoic acid, a prostaglandin derived from eicosa-8,11,14-trienoic acid and found mainly in sheep seminal vesicles; M.W. 356.49. It has similar properties to $PGF_{2\alpha}$, with less potency.

p. $F_{2\alpha}$ ($PGF_{2\alpha}$), 9,11,15-trihydroxy-5,13-dienoic acid, a prostaglandin derived from arachidonic acid (20:4) and found in most mammalian tissues; M.W. 354.49. $PGF_{2\alpha}$ can also be formed by chemical decomposition of PGH_2 or by enzymatic reduction of PGE_2. $PGF_{2\alpha}$ constricts blood vessels and bronchial smooth muscles. It also stimulates uterine activity during labor, causing expulsion of the fetus and placenta. Thus, $PGF_{2\alpha}$ and its synthetic analogs are used to induce abortion. In addition, $PGF_{2\alpha}$ produces luteolysis of a functional corpus luteum and can thus facilitate interruption of pregnancy by the reduction of progesterone in blood levels.

p. G_2 (PGG_2), 15-hydroperoxy-9α-11α-peroxidoprosta-5,13-dienoic acid, an unstable prostaglandin derived from arachidonic acid (20:4) by the action of cyclooxygenase and formed in almost every tissue; M.W. 368.48. PGG_2 is an obligatory intermediate in the formation of all prostaglandins, is a very potent vasoconstrictor, and induces platelet aggregation. See also *prostaglandin endoperoxide.*

p. H_2 (PGH_2), 15-hydroxy-9,11-peroxidoprosta-5,13-dienoic acid, an unstable prostaglandin derived from arachidonic acid (20:4) and formed in almost every tissue by peroxidase-mediated reduction of PGG_2; M.W. 352.48. PGH_2 is an obligatory intermediate in the formation of all prostaglandins, is a very potent vasoconstrictor, and induces platelet aggregation. See also *prostaglandin endoperoxide.*

p. I_2 (PGI_2), see *prostacyclin.*

prostaglandin endoperoxide a group of unstable and biologically potent prostaglandins, containing a cyclic peroxide bridge between carbon 9 and 11 on the cyclopentane ring. These prostaglandins, i.e., PGG and PGH, are produced by the action of cyclooxygenase on the parent fatty acids, and are obligatory intermediates in the synthesis of all other prostanoids. Prostaglandin endoperoxides are potent vasoconstrictors and induce platelet aggregation. PGG and PGH are unstable compounds that decompose in aqueous solution to hydroxy-hepta-decatrienoic acid (HHT), malondialdehyde (MDA), PGE, PGD, and PGF. Prostaglandin endoperoxides were once called *rabbit aorta contract-*

ing substance (*RCS*). See also *p.* G_2 and *p.* H_2 under *prostaglandin.*

prostanoic acid (pros″tă-no′ik) a cyclic, 20-carbon fatty acid of which prostaglandins can be considered derivatives. See also *prostaglandin* and the accompanying illustration.

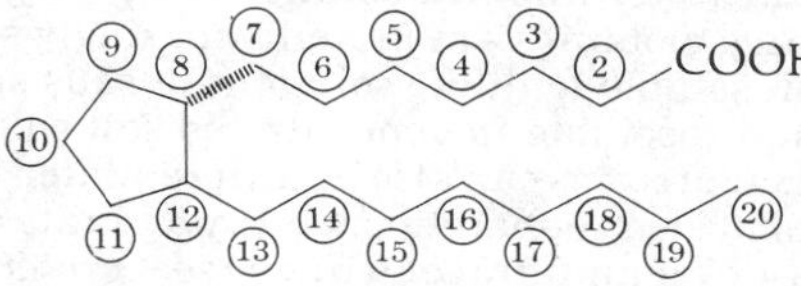

Prostanoic acid. Carbon skeleton of prostanoic acid. (From White, A., et al.: Principles of Biochemistry. 6th ed. New York, McGraw-Hill Book Co., 1978.)

prostat/o (pros′tah-to) [Gr. *prostatēs* standing before] a word element used in combining form to denote the prostate gland, e.g., prostatitis.

prostate (pros′tāt) [Gr. *prostatēs*] a gland, partly glandular and partly fibromuscular, that encircles the urethra of the male at its juncture with the bladder. It is composed of a single median and two lateral lobes with ducts emptying into the prostatic urethra. The prostate produces a slightly acid secretion containing acid phosphatase and citric acid, as well as a number of proteolytic enzymes that contribute to the seminal fluid.

prostatic tumors neoplasms of the prostate gland. Carcinoma of the prostate occurs almost exclusively in older adults (prostatic neoplasms in childhood or adolescence are rare—usually rhabdomyosarcomas). The cause of adenocarcinoma of the prostate is not known, although hormonal factors have been suggested, as these carcinomas are endocrine-dependent prostatic carcinomas that usually arise near the capsule of the gland in the posterior lobe. The extent of gland formation and anaplasia is taken into account in determining histologic grade.

Diagnosis is often made on specimens obtained by needle biopsy. Occult foci of prostatic adenocarcinoma are often an incidental finding at autopsy of individuals who have died from other causes. Spread of carcinomas is commonly to bone, most commonly to the axial skeleton. Osteoblastic metastases are typical. Serum prostatic acid phosphatase concentrations are usually elevated by the time the prostatic capsule becomes involved. Alkaline phosphatase levels are associated with osteoblastic metastases.

prostatitis (pros″tah-ti′tis) [*prostat-* + *-itis* inflammation] an acute or chronic inflammation of the prostate gland that is usually associated with urethritis, cystitis, or inflammation elsewhere in the urinary tract. Symptoms may include low back and perineal pain, fever, urinary frequency, dysuria, and even hematuria. Leukocytosis is usually present. *Escherichia coli* and *Klebsiella* are the bacteria most commonly responsible for bacterial prostatitis. A urine culture or culture of expressed prostatic secretion is used to identify the causative organism.

prostatocystitis (pros-ta″to-sis-ti′tis) [*prostato-* + Gr. *kystis* bladder + *-itis*] an inflammation of the bladder and prostate gland. See also *cystitis* and *prostatitis.*

prostatography (pros″tah-tog′rah-fe) [*prostato-* + Gr. *graphein* to write or draw] the radiologic examination of the prostate gland to detect calcifications or enlargement. The term is applied both to plain film studies and to cystography or vesiculography performed for the detection of prostate abnormalities.

prostatolith (pros-tat′o-lith) [*prostato-* + Gr. *lithos* stone] a concretion composed of calcium carbonate and phosphate, which is formed in the normal prostate.

prosthetic (pros-thet′ik) [Gr. *prosthetikos* adding] serving as a substitute; pertaining to the use or application of prostheses.

prosthetic group a component nonprotein or non-amino acid, added to a polypeptide (apoprotein) to form a complete, functional protein. An example is hemoglobin, which involves the action of two components—the prosthetic group heme (iron(II)-porphyrin) and the polypeptide (apoprotein) globin.

prosthetic valve an artificial device used to replace a heart valve. There are two types: one (synthetic) composed of a moving plastic obturator in a metal cage, and the other (principally organic) composed of animal heart valve (usually porcine) treated with glutaraldehyde and mounted in a stent (a device that supports the valve).

prosthion (pros′the-on) [Gr. *prosthion,* neuter of *prosthios* the foremost] the most anterior point on the upper jaw; the point of the alveolar process in the midsagittal plane. Also called *alveolar point.*

prot/o (pro′to) [Gr. *prōtos* first] a word element used in combining form to denote first, e.g., protoporphyrin.

protactinium (Pa) (pro″tak-tin′e-um) [*prot-* + L. *actinium*] a shiny, malleable, metallic radioactive element; atomic number 91; atomic weight 231.0359; a 5f transition element (actinide element); oxidation states +4, +5; most stable isotope, Pa-231 (half-life, 3.28×10^4 yr).

Protactinium occurs naturally as a decay product of thorium and is a highly toxic radiation hazard when ingested or inhaled.

protamine (pro′tah-mēn) [*prot-* + *amine*] one of a class of basic proteins of low molecular weight, occurring in the spermatozoa of fish. These proteins do not coagulate by heat and yield large amounts of diamino acids on hydrolysis.

p. sulfate, [USP], an antidote to heparin overdosage, which forms a stable, inactive salt with heparin (which is strongly acidic). Because protamine by itself is an anticoagulant, only the amount required to neutralize the heparin is administered. Coagulation tests, e.g., the plasma thrombin time or the heparin titration test with protamine, are used to determine the correct dosage. Adverse reactions include flushing, a fall in blood pressure, bradycardia, and difficulty in breathing.

protamine sulfate test a simple screening test to detect the presence of intravascular fibrin formation. Fibrin monomers created by the enzymatic action of thrombin on fibrinogen form a soluble complex with the early fibrin degradation products X and Y. Protamine sulfate dissociates these complexes, whereupon the fibrin monomer polymerizes and precipitates with the large fibrin (fibrinogen) degradation products. Although the test is relatively insensitive, it suggests intravascular coagulation when positive.

protamine titration test a test used to estimate the minimal dose of protamine needed to neutralize the heparin used in open heart surgery. At the end of 15 min, tubes containing whole blood and varying dilutions of protamine are titered to determine the lowest concentration of protamine sulfate needed to clot the blood.

protan (pro′tan) an individual who has protanomaly or protanopia.

protanomaly (pro″tah-nom′ah-le) [*prot-* + *Gr. anōmalia* irregularity] defective color vision of the trichromatic type in which red vision is anomalous (weak).

protanopia (pro″tah-no′pe-ah) [*prot-* + *an-* neg. + Gr. *ōpē* sight + *ia*] defective color vision of the dichromatic type in which red cones are lacking and the color red cannot be perceived.

Protargol (pro-tar′gōl) trademark for strong silver protein, which is used as an antibacterial and in histology in Bodian's staining method for nerve cells.

prote/o (pro′te-o) [Gr. *proteios* primary] a word element used in combining form to denote protein, e.g., proteolysis.

protease (pro′te-ās) a general term for a proteolytic enzyme. See also *peptidase* and *proteinases.*

protein (pro′tēn) [Fr. *protéine,* from Gr. *proteios* primary, from *protos* first] the major functional entity of all living things. Proteins are the many complex nitrogenous substances found in the cells of all animals, plants, and microorganisms; they are macromolecules with a molecular weight of 5000 to many millions.

Proteins are chains of α-amino acids. The polymerization is accomplished by the elimination of a water molecule between the amino group of one amino acid and the carboxyl group of the next amino acid. The repetition of this process with many amino acids yields a polymer referred to as a polypeptide. The bond formed between two amino acid residues is known as a peptide bond. The end of the peptide chain that contains the free amino group is called the amino terminus, and that bearing the carboxyl group is called the carboxyl terminus. One or more polypeptides may form a protein. Proteins may be conjugated with other molecules, such as carbohydrates or fats.

CLASSIFICATION. Two broad classes of proteins are generally acknowledged: globular and fibrous. Globular proteins are spherical or ellipsoidal, and have a general structural design as seen for cytochrome C and hemoglobin. Fibrous proteins are a heterogeneous group of proteins that contain one or more polypeptide chains; they are elongated, very asymmetric molecules whose length may be many times their diameter, and are often laterally cross-linked by a variety of types of chemical bonding to confer mechanical strength and water insolubility to these proteins. Thus, fibrous proteins are found primarily as structural proteins of connective, elastic, and contractile tissue, and the insoluble substance of hair and skin.

Proteins are often described in terms of their prosthetic group; thus, hemoglobin is a hemeprotein, and proteins that contain lipids, carbohydrates, or metals are called lipoproteins, glycoproteins, and metalloproteins, respectively. The great majority of known proteins are globular proteins.

Older attempts to classify globular proteins on the basis of their solubility in aqueous media are less meaningful today than formerly. For example, albumin is the name used to describe proteins readily soluble in water and salt solutions and coagulable by heating; globulins are proteins sparingly soluble in water, soluble in dilute solutions of salts such as NaCl, and insoluble in concentrated salt solutions. Individual proteins can also be differentiated by differences in electrophoretic mobility and rate of sedimentation in an ultracentrifuge (see *protein electrophoresis* and *sedimentation velocity-diffusion*).

STRUCTURE. The structure of protein is considered at four levels—primary, secondary, tertiary, and quaternary—for proteins containing two or more separate polypeptide chains or subunits.

The primary structure describes the number and sequence of amino acids in a polypeptide.

The secondary structure is determined by interactions between amino acids close to each other in the primary segments. It includes the α-helical conformation produced by intrachain hydrogen bonding, β-pleated sheet structure formed by intramolecular hydrogen bonding between the stretched out neighboring polypeptide chains, random coil (a sequence without secondary structure stabilized by hydrogen bonding), and chain reversal formed by a polypeptide chain folding back on itself (β-turns).

The tertiary structure refers to interactions among amino acids far apart in the primary sequence. It is achieved by coiling and folding of the polypeptide chain in attaining a final molecular shape (e.g., globular). The tertiary structure is largely determined by the nature of noncovalent interactions between the side-chains (commonly called R- groups) of the amino acid residues, e.g., hydrophobic interactions and electrostatic attraction or repulsion. However, if a polypeptide contains cysteine residues appropriately positioned, the formation of disulfide bonds (—S—S—) can also contribute to tertiary structure. Most proteins are highly compact and convoluted molecules. The position of each amino acid residue in relation to others is precisely established and is important in terms of its function.

The quaternary structure deals with proteins that contain two or more polypeptides, which form oligomeric forms with varying biologic activity. The quaternary structure is stabilized by noncovalent forces. The description of the folding nature of a polypeptide into its three-dimensional structure or a particular association of subunits is known as conformation. Conformational changes can bring about alterations in biologic properties (conversion from a less active state to a more active state or vice versa).

PRINCIPLES. Three major principles pertaining to protein structure, function, and assembly may be recognized. (1) The amino acid sequence in a polypeptide chain is determined by the DNA template that directs its synthesis via a messenger RNA intermediate (see *protein synthesis*). Side-chains of some of the amino acid residues, however, may be modified (e.g., hydroxylation, phosphorylation, acetylation) in some proteins. These modifications occur after the amino acid is incorporated into the polypeptide structure (posttranslational alteration). (2) The three-dimensional conformation of a polypeptide chain is determined entirely by the amino acid sequence. Changes in sequence resulting from genetic mutations usually yield conformationally altered (and often less stable, less active, or inactive) proteins. (3) The specific activity of a protein as an enzyme, hormone, oxygen carrier, etc., depends on its specific conformation, changes of which can lead to loss of biologic activity.

SIDE-CHAINS. The amino acid side-chains extending outward from a polypeptide chain structure may be either hydrophilic or hydrophobic. The most hydrophilic, or water loving, are those with net ionic charges. Nonpolar side-chains tend to cluster together in the interior of protein molecules to avoid exposure to water. The force causing this comes only from the propensity of the surrounding water to resist being forced into ordered structures by the presence of nonpolar groups. The so-called hydrophobic bond is actually an association created by spurned water.

FUNCTIONS. Proteins with specific biologic functions (e.g., enzymes, hormones and proteins involved in the transport and storage of small molecules and membranes) depend on their conformation for such functions; disturbances in the conformation may lead to a loss of activity. A protein in its normal conformation is said to be in the native state. Rather mild changes in physical conditions can disrupt conformation, causing the protein to undergo biologic activity and structure denaturation.

dietary p., protein derived from food; for humans, the major sources are animal proteins such as those present in meat, fish, eggs, milk, and vegetable proteins. Dietary protein is digested in the stomach, duodenum, and remainder of the small intestine by proteolytic enzymes that are specific for individual peptide linkages. Proteins first undergo hydrolysis in the stomach by pepsin, which breaks them down into polypeptides of various sizes (and some amino acids). In the small intestine, the pancreatic enzymes trypsin, chymotrypsin, and carboxypolypeptidase hydrolyze these products into shorter peptides, which are finally broken down to individual amino acids by enzymes secreted by intestinal epithelial cells, polypeptidase, aminopeptidases, and dipeptidases. These amino acids are actively absorbed into the blood, where they are transported to other organs to be used for the building and repair of body tissue (muscle, heart, etc.), for the synthesis of enzymes and some hormones, or as a reserve (liver, plasma).

Dietary proteins also play a crucial role in protein synthesis. All 20 amino acids must be present for protein synthesis to occur; however, only 10 can be made in the body from glucose and amino acid nitrogen (nonessential amino acids). These amino acids are either synthesized in the cells where they are utilized or are supplied through the blood from the liver, the main site of amino acid synthesis and metabolism. The other 10 (designated essential amino acids: valine, leucine, isoleucine, methionine, lysine, threonine, tryptophan, phenylalanine, histidine, and arginine) cannot be synthesized in the body and must be supplied by the diet. Arginine and histidine are required by growing children because they cannot synthesize sufficient amounts, but are not required by adults. Thus, ingestion of sufficient high-quality protein (i.e., protein that provides a relatively high proportion of all the essential amino acids in the correct proportions) and the ability to successfully absorb these amino acids are both necessary to maintain life.

The ability of foods to satisfy dietary protein requirements depends on their total protein content, on the amino acid composition of the proteins, and on the digestibility of the food. Protein quality may be stated in terms of nitrogen utilization or weight gain, or in terms of the amino acid pattern.

In the first method, test subjects are placed on a protein-free diet for a week or more to deplete labile protein; nitrogen loss through the feces, urine, and skin is then estimated. The subjects are then fed measured quantities of a particular food, and the nitrogen loss is estimated again. The retained nitrogen is the dietary nitrogen consumed minus the difference between the nitrogen loss after feeding and the basal nitrogen loss. The retained nitrogen, expressed as a percentage of the dietary nitrogen consumed, is termed the net protein utilization (NPU). Retained nitrogen expressed as a percentage of absorbed dietary nitrogen (nitrogen consumed minus fecal nitrogen of food origin lost) is termed the biologic value of the protein.

A similar measure, the net protein ratio (NPR), is defined as the sum of the weight gain of a test group fed a particular food plus the weight loss of a control protein consumed.

The amino acid composition of a food is compared with the reference pattern, the composition of an effectively used protein, such as human milk protein. The chemical score is the mole fraction of the most limiting amino acid expressed as a percentage of its mole fraction in the reference pattern, the most limiting amino acid being the essential amino acid with the lowest relative mole fraction.

nonhistone chromosomal (NHC) p., a diverse group of proteins found in chromatin not removed by acid extraction. Several enzymes are included: DNA and RNA polymerases, nucleases, and protein phosphokinases. A regulatory role for NHC proteins is indicated from DNA reconstitution experiments. From chromatin separation experiments, it is inferred that NHC proteins regulate transcription by reversing some of the repression of template activity caused by histone proteins. Various information suggests that NHC molecules may also act as negative regulators that suppress specific genes. Cf. *histone.*

proteinases (pro′tēn-ās″es) enzymes belonging to one of the four sub-subclasses of the hydrolases (EC 3.4.21–24), consisting of enzymes that hydrolyze the interior peptide bonds in a protein to produce polypeptides. Also called endopeptidases, peptidyl-peptide hydrolases, and proteolytic enzymes.

protein assays 1. Kjeldahl digestion plus titration. Proteins in biologic specimens are precipitated with trichloroacetic acid and the nonprotein nitrogen removed by washing and decantation. The precipitate is digested with boiling sulfuric acid (plus catalysts), which converts all organic nitrogen to ammonium ions. The digestate is made alkaline with NaOH, and the ammonia is distilled into standard acid and quantitated by back titration with standard base. By common practice, this value of protein-nitrogen is converted to protein by multiplying by the factor 6.25, based on the assumption that the protein had a nitrogen content of 16.0 percent. This value is valid only for serum albumin; the actual nitrogen content of a normal mixture of serum proteins is probably closer to 15.7 percent (factor, 6.40). Proteins in other body fluids and biologic materials may have a range of 12–18 percent. This procedure gives accurate results if the nitrogen content of the protein being measured is known. For a number of years, it served as a reference method, crystalline bovine serum albumin of known nitrogen content being the usual standard.

2. Kjeldahl digestion with colorimetric ammonia determination. The ammonia in the digestate or distillate (see above) is measured spectrophotometrically, using either the Nessler or Berthelot reagents and methods (see *Nessler* and *Berthelot reaction*).

3. biuret reaction. This is a direct method for protein, the reagent measuring the number of peptide bonds in the specimen. Cupric ions, in an alkaline medium, chelate with the peptide nitrogen and carbonyl oxygen, about two each per Cu^{2+}, to form a violet-colored soluble complex, which is measured at 540–550 nm against a reagent blank. The procedure is standardized against a pure protein standard (bovine serum albumin), or indirectly against a serum of known protein content. The sensitivity is 1–6 mg/ml of reaction volume.

4. use of the Folin phenol reagent. This procedure measures proteins by virtue of their content of tyrosine. The specimen, free of all free amino acids, is dissolved in weak alkali and treated with the Folin-Ciocalteau reagent to form a bluish-black color, which is measured at 680–750 nm. This procedure is applicable to measuring relatively pure or isolated proteins of known tyrosine content, such as fibrinogen, or to compare the protein content in similar materials. The method is nearly one hundred-fold more sensitive than the biuret procedure.

5. refractometry. This is a semiquantitative method. The increment in refractive index value of a protein solution is proportional to its protein content, provided the concentration of salt ions and other solutes is essentially the same in the protein specimens. Gross errors are introduced if the specimen is lipemic.

6. absorbance at specific ultraviolet wavelengths. Absorbance at 210–215 nm reflects the presence of the peptide bond and is thus a good measure of the total amount of mixed proteins. This approach is very sensitive but technically difficult because of contamination problems.

The absorbance at 270–280 nm reflects the presence of aromatic amino acids (tyrosine, tryptophan, phenylalanine). Inasmuch as proteins vary widely in composition in regard to aromatic amino acids, this method is useful only to compare specimens of similar origin or source, as in following the purification of an enzyme or protein.

7. Lowry procedure. The reagent consists of a combination of the biuret and Folin-Ciocalteau reagents. This method, once widely used, is somewhat more sensitive than the Folin procedure, but as the values obtained are independent of tyrosine content, this method can be used for measuring all proteins.

8. turbidimetric methods. Dilute solutions of proteins in saline are treated with protein-precipitating reagents under conditions permitting the formation of fine, uniform, nonsettling precipitates that can be measured spectrophotometrically at wavelengths such as 620 or 480 nm. Trichloroacetic acid and sulfosalicylic acid at concentrations of 30 g/l are the most commonly used reagents. However, not all proteins produce equivalent degrees of turbidity at any given concentration. The sensitivity is 20–200 μg/ml of reaction volume.

9. dye-binding methods. These are special methods with limited applicability. A variety of acid-base dyes bind to albumin (and also to other proteins). Most interest has centered around methods for serum albumin; the most widely used dye is bromocresol green (BCG), but bromocresol purple, methyl orange, *p*-hydroxyazobenzene-benzoic acid (HABA), and bromphenol blue (urine protein) are also used. When protein is added to a buffered solution of the dye, a dye-protein complex is formed with a shift in absorbance pattern. For BCG, the absorbance peak of the dye at 615 nm is shifted, and the decrease of absorbance at 615 nm is proportional to the albumin concentration.

10. nephelometry. Proteins may be measured nephelometrically by use of antihuman serum protein as antibody.

protein-bound iodine-131 test ($PB^{131}I$) the determination of the fraction of an administered dose of radioactive iodine present as protein-bound iodine 72 hr later. If more than 0.27 percent has been incorporated into hormones and released into the blood by the thyroid, hyperthyroidism may be present. The conversion ratio is the activity of protein-bound ^{131}I divided by the activity of the total plasma ^{131}I. A conversion ratio greater than 50 percent may indicate hypothyroidism. These tests now are rarely used as clinical tests of thyroid function, having been superseded by measurements of the concentrations of serum thyroxine (T_4) and triiodothyronine (T_3).

protein breakdown 1. the enzymatic degradation of proteins through the processes of food digestion, by which amino acids and short polypeptides are formed.

2. the catabolism of proteins in the body as a result of metabolic processes.

3. the degradation of proteins (enzymatic or by acid or base hydrolysis) with the object of ascertaining the chemical structure of the given protein molecule or preparational polypeptide chain structure or amino acid composition.

starvation-induced p. b., the degradation of protein under conditions of negative carbon, nitrogen, and essential amino acid balance. The breakdown of storage, plasma, and some structural proteins provides amino acids for the synthesis of more vital (essential) enzymes and other proteins needed to maintain life.

protein denaturation any nonproteolytic change in the native structure of a protein that causes it to lose some or all of its specific biochemical and physical characteristics, such as solubility, enzymatic activity, and physiologic activity. During denaturation the original ordered conformation is unfolded to a more or less random coil. Early phases of denaturation are wholly or partially reversible; later stages are irreversible. Mechanical, surface heat, and light energy as well as organic solvents and salt solutions are agents that cause denaturation.

protein electrophoresis 1. routine serum protein electrophoresis. This process separates the plasma proteins into seven bands (prealbumin, albumin, $alpha_1$, $alpha_2$, $beta_1$, $beta_2$, and gamma globulin). The main protein and lipoprotein constituents of the bands and the changes in their levels that occur in various diseases are summarized in the accompanying table.

The most popular methods use cellulose acetate or agar gels as support media and pH 8.6 barbital buffer with an ionic strength of 0.025–0.075. A higher ionic strength gives a sharper resolution of the zones but decreased migration rates. The voltage or current setting used to form the electric field varies with the equipment and support used; typical electrophoresis runs take 20–30 min. The protein bands are visualized by fixing onto the medium and staining with a protein-binding dye such as Ponceau S.

Abnormalities of the electrophoretic pattern are evident on visual examination of the strip. Quantitation is performed by measuring the amount of bound dye with a densitometer using light absorbance or reflectance.

2. routine protein electrophoresis of specimens of urine or cerebrospinal fluid. The protein in the specimen must initially be concentrated twenty- to fifty-fold by using centrifugal membrane ultrafiltration, negative pressure ultrafiltration, or other concentrating techniques. The separation techniques are the same as for serum.

proteinemia (pro″tēn-e′me-ah) [*protein* + Gr. *haima* blood + *ia*] an excess of protein in the blood.

protein hydrolysate (pro′tēn hi-drol′ĭ-zāt) [USP], a mixture of amino acids produced by the hydrolysis of protein. It is used in special diets for those patients unable to ingest, digest, or absorb proteins in their food (e.g., after an operation or severe illness).

proteinosis (pro″te-in-o′sis) [*protein* + *-osis* condition] the accumulation of excess protein in the tissues.

alveolar p., an infiltrative disease of the lungs characterized by a gradual filling of the alveoli with a granular, proteinaceous, lipid-rich precipitate that prevents adequate ventilation of the affected areas. Persons affected may exhibit weakness, cough with slight mucus expectoration, and progressive hypoxemia and dyspnea.

The cause and pathogenesis of alveolar proteinosis is still uncertain, but it may involve an accumulation of surfactant material resulting either from an excessive production by hyperplastic type II pneumocytes, or from a decreased degradation by defective alveolar macrophages.

Pulmonary function tests reveal varying degrees of reduction in the diffusing capacity of the lungs but are generally otherwise normal. X-rays examination shows a focal-to-confluent airspace consolidation over large areas of the central and middle zones of both lungs; the pattern of distribution has a characteristic butterfly shape. Histologic examination of the lungs reveals a normal septal structure, with filling of the alveoli and bronchioles with a granular, eosinophilic, PAS-positive material rich in proteins and lipids. The condition frequently resolves spontaneously, or may be treated with steroids or repeated whole-lung, volume-controlled lavage.

lipid p., a rare hereditary disorder, transmitted as an autosomal recessive trait, that is characterized by the deposition of a hyalinlike material in the mucous membranes of the mouth, tongue, and larynx; yellowish-white papules on the face, arms, and trunk, which may coalesce into plaques or nodules; and hoarseness due to infiltration of the vocal cords. No consistent biochemical abnormalities have been identified. The disorder is usually benign and compatible with a long life but tracheotomy may be necessary owing to infiltration of the vocal cords.

protein separation methods 1. salt or solvent fractionation, based on the different solubilities of proteins in solutions that contain dehydrating solvents or ionic solutes. In water solution, protein molecules are surrounded by a layer of water molecules attracted by the interaction between the dipolar water molecule and charged groups on the protein. At low concentrations, inorganic ions also interact with charged groups on the protein and increase solubility, a process known as the salting-in effect. At high concentrations, the ions interact more with the water molecules and decrease solubility—the salting-out effect.

Organic solvents miscible in water, such as methanol or acetone, also reduce solubility because they are less polar than water. A protein is least soluble at its isoelectric point (pI). Many proteins can be selectively precipitated by using the appropriate pH and type and concentration of salt or solvent. Plasma protein fractions are commercially prepared using these methods.

2. ultracentrifugation, based on differences in densities of protein molecules. This method is used in research to characterize proteins by virtue of their sedimentation velocities or coefficients. Its clinical use is limited to the separation of lipoprotein fractions (see *lipoprotein assays*).

3. ion-exchange chromatography, using the ionic interaction between charged groups on the proteins and the ion-exchange medium. Proteins are adsorbed on the medium and then selectively eluted. Each protein washes out with a buffer with a pH near the pI of the protein.

4. gel-filtration chromatography, based on the difference in size and shape of the protein molecules.

5. affinity chromatography, in which the stationary phase consists of a binding protein covalently bonded to a solid matrix. The binding protein has a high affinity for specific ligands, which are separated from mixtures passing through the column. The binding protein may be: (1) an antibody directed against a specific protein; (2) an enzyme with a high affinity for its substrates or for other compounds of similar structure that fit the active site; or (3) a receptor protein with a high affinity for its specific hormone, for a neurotransmitter, or for a drug that is its agonist or antagonist.

6. electrophoresis using a variety of different media that utilize the different charges of the molecules to effect the separation of different proteins when an electrical current is applied across the medium. Separation is influenced by the net electrical charge of the molecules, size and shape of the molecules, electrical field strength, nature of the supporting medium, and temperature of the operation.

protein synthesis see *translation.*

proteinuria (pro″tēn-u′re-ah) [*protein* + Gr. *ouron* urine + *-ia*] the presence of proteins in the urine, at concentrations in excess of normal. The type and quantity of proteins excreted in the urine in various diseases depends on five processes: (1) The most frequently observed process is glomerular leakage of plasma proteins, which may be selective, allowing smaller proteins such as albumin to pass through while larger proteins such as macroglobulins are excluded, or nonselective, allowing proteins of any size to pass through, which indicates a greater de-

PROTEIN ELECTROPHORESIS. ELECTROPHORETIC FRACTIONS AND THEIR MAIN CONSTITUENTS

Electrophoretic Bands	*Normal Range—Depth of Staining of Electrophoretic Fractions (g/100 ml)*	*Main Constituents and Their Relative Molecular Weight*	
Albumin	3.5–5.0	*Albumin* (Alb)	65,000
α_1	0.17–0.33	*α_1-Anti-trypsin* (α_1ATr). Cause of band on protein staining	45,000
		α_1-Lipoprotein (α_1Lp) (apoprotein A). Cause of band on fat staining	200,000
		Orosomucoid (α_1AGp) (α_1-acid-glycoprotein, seromucoid). Stains only faintly with protein stain	44,000
α_2	0.42–0.90	*α_2-Macroglobulin* (α_2M)	820,000
		Haptoglobin (Hpt)	From 85,000 up to more than 1,000,000 in higher polymers
		Pre-β-lipoprotein (VLDL) (apoprotein A, B, and C). Seen only on fat staining	Very large
β_1	0.52–1.05	*Transferrin* (Tr) (siderophilin)	80,000–90,000
		Hemopexin (Hpx). Stains poorly	80,000
		β-Lipoprotein (βLp) (apoprotein B). Requires fat stain	About 3,000,000
β_2	0.08–0.14 (only present in fresh serum)	β_1c	
	0.71–1.65	Immunoglobulin G (IgG)	150,000
		Immunoglobulin A (IgA)	180,000 (higher when polymerized)
		Immunoglobulin M (IgM)	900,000 (higher when polymerized)

*Some levels vary with season, age, or sex. Values may also differ in accordance with the method employed (e.g., electrophoresis vs. immunochemical techniques).

Modified from Tietz, N. W.: Fundamentals of Clinical Chemistry. 2nd ed. Philadelphia, W. B. Saunders Co., 1976, pp. 306-307.

PROTEIN ELECTROPHORESIS. (*Continued*)

Average Values and Approximate Reference Ranges of Individual Proteins (g/100 ml)*	*Biologic Function*	*Main Pathologic Abnormalities*
4.4 (3.5–5.0)	Transport of fatty acids, etc. Regulation of plasma volume by colloid osmotic pressure. Provides main protein reserve	Reduced in cirrhosis and nephrotic syndrome, malnutrition, protein losing enteropathy and hemodilution
0.25 (0.2–0.4)	Proteinase inhibitor	Increased in acute phase reaction. Its congenital deficiency leads to emphysema and neonatal liver necrosis
0.36 (0.29–0.77)	Transport of lipids, fat-soluble vitamins, and hormones	Reduced in liver disease
0.09 (0.05–0.14)	Not established	Increased in acute phase reaction, chronic inflammation, rheumatoid arthritis, and malignancy
Males: 0.24 (0.15–0.35) Females: 0.29 (0.17–0.42)	Plasmin inhibitor	Increased in nephrosis, liver disease, and diabetes
0.1–0.3 (depending on type)	Binds hemoglobin, preventing loss of iron	Reduced in hemolysis and liver failure. Increased in acute phase reaction
	Transports lipids, especially triglycerides	Increased in primary and secondary hyperlipidemias Fredrickson Type IV
0.29 (0.2–0.4)	Iron transport	Increased in iron deficiency. Reduced in nephrotic syndrome.
0.10 (0.07–0.13)	Heme binding	Reduced in hemolytic anemia
0.53 (0.29–0.95) (depending on age and sex)	Lipid transport, especially cholesterol, fat-soluble vitamins, and hormones.	Increased in primary and secondary hyperlipoproteinemia Fredrickson Type II
0.11 (0.08–0.14)	Complement factor C3. On standing converted to β_{1A}.	Reduced in autoimmune diseases, e.g., glomerulonephritis, and SLE
1.16 (0.8–1.4) (125 IU/ml)	Antibodies	Polyclonal increase in liver disease and chronic infections. Monoclonal increase in myeloma. Reduced in immune paresis
0.21 (0.09–0.45) (116 IU/ml)	Antibodies, especially in secretions	Increased in portal cirrhosis. Otherwise similar to IgG
0.1 (0.06–0.25) (140 IU/ml)	Antibodies formed first; confined to blood	Monoclonal increase in Waldenström's macroglobulinemia. Otherwise similar to IgG

gree of damage to the glomeruli. (2) There may be an overflow of filtered (low-molecular-mass) proteins due to elevations of the serum concentrations of these proteins, e.g., Bence Jones proteins and lysozymes. (3) Failure of tubular reabsorption of filtered protein may occur because the tubules are damaged and cannot reabsorb low-molecular-weight proteins such as α_2- and β_2-microglobulins. (4) Another process is the secretion of proteins, e.g., Tamm-Horsfall mucoprotein and IgA by the kidney. (5) The breakdown of kidney tissue releases products such as basement membrane fragments.

proteoglycan (pro″te-o-gli′kan) a substance occurring primarily in the ground substance of connective tissue, consisting of about 95 percent polysaccharides and 5 percent protein. Proteoglycan aggregates consist of a long backbone of hyaluronic acid to which proteoglycan subunits are attached every 20–30 nm by a noncovalent linkage involving a link protein. The subunits have a polypeptide backbone (core protein) to which heteropolysaccharide (glycosaminoglycan) chains are attached at regular intervals by covalent linkages like those of glycoproteins. The protein subunits may contain several different types of glycosaminoglycans.

Because glycosaminoglycans have many anionic charged groups, the chains repel each other. These large polyanions bind cations and water, thus forming the ground substance. In water they stand out straight from the backbone, giving both the subunits and the aggregates the shape of a bottle brush. The volume occupied by a proteoglycan molecule (its domain) is filled mostly with water and is thousands of times the volume of a densely packed molecule of the same mass. The proteoglycans act as molecular sieves by excluding large molecules from their domains. They also have high viscosity, elasticity, and resistance to compression.

See also *glycosaminoglycan, mucopolysaccharide,* and *mucoprotein.*

proteolipid (pro″te-o-lip′id) [*proteo-* + *lipid*] a protein-lipid combination extractable from brain tissue. It differs from water-soluble lipoprotein in that it is insoluble in water but soluble in chloroform-methanol mixtures. A major protein of myelin sheath is an acidic proteolipid. Cf. *lipoprotein.*

proteolysis (pro″te-ol′ĭ-sis) [*proteo-* + Gr. *lysis* dissolution] the splitting of proteins by hydrolysis of the peptide bonds with the formation of smaller polypeptides and amino acid fragments; the process may be catalyzed by proteolytic enzymes, or by hydrolysis with acids or bases.

proteolytic (pro′te-o-lit′ik) pertaining to or promoting proteolysis, the hydrolysis of proteins into smaller chemical entities.

proteose (pro′te-ōs) [*prote-* + *-ose*] a large polypeptide hydrolytic product of protein having less than some 40 amino acid residues. It is not coagulable by heat and is precipitable with ammonium sulfate, in some cases by half-saturation and in others by saturation. See also *peptone.*

Proteus (pro′te-us) [Gr. *Prōteus,* a sea god who could assume many shapes] a genus of microorganisms of the tribe Proteeae, family Enterobacteriaceae, that consists of gram-negative, pleomorphic, motile, rod-shaped bacilli. These organisms are facultative anaerobes, being lactose-negative and urease-positive. They are found in normal human feces, especially in patients being treated with oral antibiotics. Potential pathogens, they are frequently associated with urinary tract infections, and are also seen in bacteremia and in abdominal and wound infections. See also *Enterobacteriaceae.*

P. inconstans, see *Providencia.*

P. mirabilis, the *Proteus* species most frequently isolated from human clinical material, and a leading cause of urinary tract infections. The swarming phenomenon of moist agar is pronounced; however, unlike other species, most strains are indole-negative and susceptible to penicillin.

P. morganii, See *M. morganii* under *Morganella.*

P. rettgeri, a species that does not swarm spontaneously; unlike other *Proteus* species, it ferments inositol and mannitol. *P. rettgeri* is both biochemically and genetically more closely related to *Providencia* than to *Proteus,* although it does produce urease, a prime characteristic of the *Proteus* genus. It has been proposed that this species be named *Providencia rettgeri.*

P. vulgaris, a species that forms a thin, spreading swarm on moist agar; it is urease-and indole-positive, and is widely distributed in nature. See also *Weil-Felix reaction.*

prothrombin (pro-throm′bin) [*pro-* + Gr. *thrombos* clot + *in* chemical suffix] see *Factor II.*

prothrombinase (pro-throm′bin-ās) a complex composed of Factor Xa, Factor V, phospholipid, and calcium, which acts as an enzyme, catalyzing the conversion of prothrombin to thrombin.

prothrombin complex a concentrate of the vitamin K–dependent coagulation factors (Factors II, IX, and X; most contain Factor VII and some both Factor VII and Factor XI). From large quantities of pooled plasma, it is prepared, lyophilized, and packaged.

The prothrombin concentrates are used in severe congenital Factor IX deficiency (hemophilia B), as well as in the other rare vitamin K–factor deficiencies. Prothrombin complex has also been used to promote hemostasis in hemophiliacs (Factor VIII deficiency) who have developed high titer inhibitors to Factor VIII. The hemostatic promoting mechanism of the prothrombin complex (activated prothrombin complex) in this instance is not clear.

Complications include hepatitis, and accelerated blood clotting with localized or generalized thrombosis.

prothrombin consumption test a technique for measuring the residual procoagulant activity of serum after clotting is completed. It is determined by performing a prothrombin time on serum.

The concentration of prothrombin in serum will be high and the serum prothrombin time short when any one of the following conditions exists: (1) when clotting factors active in the intrinsic pathway other than prothrombin are sufficiently deficient, (2) when platelets are inadequate in number or are qualitatively abnormal, or (3) when an anticoagulant retards the generation of prothrombin-converting activity.

The test is not sensitive enough to exclude minor defects in the intrinsic pathway. The reference value is greater than 20 sec. Since the advent of the activated partial thromboplastin time and better individual coagulation factor assays, this test is seldom used.

Also called *serum prothrombin activity* and *serum prothrombin time.*

prothrombin deficiency see under *Factor II.*

prothrombin time test (pro-time, PT) a test to determine the activity of Factors I, II, V, VII, and X, which participate in the extrinsic pathway of coagulation. It is performed by measuring the time needed for clot formation of citrated plasma after the addition of tissue extract (brain) and calcium. A PT test is used to monitor individuals undergoing anticoagulant therapy with coumarin drugs, and in the study of acquired or congenital coagulation disorders. Also called one-stage prothrombin time and Quick's test.

two-stage PT t., a test for determining the concentration of prothrombin in plasma. The amount of thrombin formed from converted prothrombin is assumed to reflect the concentration of prothrombin in the original plasma; it is calculated by determining the dilution of plasma that will clot a standard fibrinogen reagent in a specific period of time. One unit of prothrombin will generate one unit of thrombin, and one unit of thrombin will clot 1 ml of standardized fibrinogen solution in 15 sec. Sufficient amounts of Factors V, VII, and X must be present for the test to be valid. Also called *Warner-Brinkhous-Smith method.*

proticity (pro'tis-ĭ-te) the flow of protons from high to low protic potential, which is analogous to an electric circuit.

protic solvent (pro'tik) a solvent that is a hydrogen-bonding solvent, e.g., H_2O, HCOOH, and CH_3-OH. Cf. *aprotic solvent.*

pro-time abbrev. for *pro*thrombin *time.* See *prothrombin time test.*

protirelin (pro-ti'rĕ-lin) generic drug name (USAN) for thyrotropin-releasing hormone (TRH), which is used as a diagnostic aid.

protist (pro'tist) [Gr. *prōtistos* the very first] a collective name for unicellular eukaryotic organisms, including the protozoa, fungi, algae, and bacteria.

Protista (pro-tis'tah) [Gr. "the very first," from *prōtos* first] formerly, a kingdom composed of all unicellular organisms, now classified as either eukaryotes or prokaryotes. See also *protist.*

protium (pro'te-um) [Gr. *prōtos* first] hydrogen 1 (^1H), the abundant isotope of hydrogen. Also called light hydrogen. Cf. *deuterium* and *tritium.*

protocol (pro'to-kol) [Gr. *prōtokollon* first sheet of a papyrus roll, bearing official authentication and date of manufacture] an explicit, detailed statement of all the steps involved in an experimental procedure. The protocol has two functions: in a large study with many investigators, rigid adherence to the protocol ensures that all investigators follow the same procedures; also, after an experiment is completed, the protocol tells other investigators exactly what was done and enables them to reproduce the results.

protodiastole (pro"to-di-as'to-le) [*proto-* + Gr. *diastolē* dilation, from *diastellein* to dilate] the early part of ventricular diastole, that is, immediately following the second heart sound.

protohemin IX (pro"to-he'min) see *metheme.*

proton (p) (pro'ton) [Gr., neuter of *prōtos* first] an elementary particle that has the same charge as an electron, spin 1/2, and approximately the mass of a neutron. It is composed of three quarks, and is stable or has a lifetime too long to measure. Protons and neutrons are the building blocks of atomic nuclei.

proton acceptor a molecule with an unshared pair of electrons, a base.

proton acid see *proton donor.*

proton donor a molecule that can donate a proton, as to a base; a Bronsted-Lowry acid. Also called *proton acid.*

protonephridium (pro"to-nef-rid'e-um) [*proto-* + Gr. *nephros* kidney + L. *-idium,* from Gr. *-idium* lesser] see *flame cell.*

proton irradiation therapy see *heavy particle therapy.*

proton-motive hypothesis see *chemiosmotic hypothesis.*

protoplasm (pro'to-plazm) [*proto-* + Gr. *plasma* anything formed] a general term for the substance of a living cell.

protoplast (pro'to-plast) [*proto-* + Gr. *plastos* formed] a membrane-bound spherical form that results from the enzymatic removal of cell wall constituents from a bacterial, yeast, or fungal cell in a hypertonic medium. Cf. *spheroplast.*

protoplast fusion a technique for producing genetic recombination of bacteria. The cell walls are removed with enzymes, leaving protoplasts with intact cell membranes and contents. Protoplasts are fused by exposure to isotonic polyethylene glycol solution. After new cell walls are snythesized, about 1 in 10,000 cells is a stable haploid recombinant.

protoporphyria (pro"to-por-fĭr'e-ah) [*proto-* + Gr. *porphyra* purple + *-ia*] an erythropoietic porphyria, a genetic disorder transmitted as an autosomal dominant trait, that is characterized by skin photosensitivity and increased levels of protoporphyrin in the erythrocytes, plasma, and feces. See also *porphyria.*

protoporphyrin (pro"to-por'fĭ-rin) see *protoporphyrin IX.*

protoporphyrin IX 1,3,5,8-tetramethyl-2,4,-divinylporphin-6,7-dipropionic acid; the substituted porphin that, with iron, forms the heme of hemoglobin and other heme proteins. The presence of four methyl groups, two vinyl groups, and two propionic side-chains permits the formation of 15 isomers; that isomer, with substituents in the order given in the systematic name, is referred to as protoporphyrin IX. This compound is identical to protoporphyrin III, which is derived from coproporphyrin III.

protoporphyrin assays see under *porphyrin assays.*

protoporphyrinogen oxidase (pro"to-por"fĭ-rin'o-jen ok'si-dās) an enzyme of the oxidoreductase class (EC 1.3.3.4) that catalyzes the reaction protoporphyrinogen-IX + O_2 ⇄ protoporphyrin-IX + H_2O. The reaction is one of the terminal reactions in the sequence of heme synthesis.

Prototheca (pro"to-the'kah) a genus of achloric algae organisms with yeastlike characteristics that cause protothecosis. *Prototheca* organisms are ubiquitous in nature; cells stain well with Gomori methenamine silver or PAS, and often contain two to eight endospores in each cell or sporangium. The species *P. wickerhamii* has been the agent in most human cases except for an occasional case due to *P. zopfii* (also called *P. segbwema*).

protothecosis (pro"to-the-ko'sis) [*Prototheca* + *-osis* condition] an infection caused by the yeastlike algae *Prototheca.* The resultant disease varies from cutaneous papular lesions to a spreading disease, with this opportunistic pathogen, producing a systemic infection. Individuals with protothecosis most often have a second debilitating disease. Surgical excision of the lesions and intravenous treatment with amphotericin B have both been successful. *Prototheca* species are resistant to 5-fluorocytosine.

prototype (pro'to-tīp) [*proto-* + Gr. *typos* type] 1. the original type or form after which other types or forms are developed.

2. in microbiology, the standard reference strain with which other strains are compared.

Protozoa (pro"to-zo'ah) [*proto-* + Gr. *zōa,* plural of *zōon* animal] a phylum composed of simple unicellular organisms of the animal kingdom, ranging in size from microscopic to macroscopic. The majority are free-living, but they may also live a commensalistic, mutualistic, or parasitic existence. The phylum is divided into four subphyla: Sarcodina (amebae), Mastigophora (flagellates), Ciliophora (ciliates), and Sporozoa.

protraction (pro-trak'shun) [L. *protrahere* to drag out] in radiation therapy, the extension of the time required to deliver a specific total radiation dose by administering radiation at a lower dose rate.

protransglutaminase (pro-tranz"gloo-tam'in-ās) the inactive form (zymogen) of transglutaminase (glutaminyl-peptide γ-glutamyltransferase), which circulates in the blood. This form, blood-clotting Factor XIII, is converted by thrombin to the active enzyme.

protriptyline (pro-trip'tĭ-lēn) generic name for a derivative of the tricyclic compound dibenzocycloheptadiene, used as an antidepressant. For toxicity, see *tricyclic antidepressant.* Trademark for protriptyline HCl, *Vivactil.*

protriptyline assays protriptyline concentrations may be determined by fluorometry using an excitation wavelength of 300 nm and an emission wavelength of 375 nm. Newer methods employ either gas chromatography using nitrogen, electron capture, or mass fragmentography detection; or high-pressure liquid chromatography.

protuberance (pro-tu'ber-ans) [*pro-* + L. *tuber* bulge] a projecting part or prominence.

external occipital p., a prominence on the external surface of the occipital bone in the midline above the foramen magnum, which serves as a point of attachment for the nuchal ligament.

internal occipital p., an irregular midline prominence on the internal surface of the occipital bone.

mental p., a triangular raised area on the midline of the anterior surface of the mandible.

Providencia (prov"ĭ-den'se-ah) a genus of microorganisms of the tribe Proteeae, family Enterobacteriaceae, that consists of gram-negative motile rods. These organisms are facultative anaerobes, being lactose-negative and urease-negative, but positive in phenylalanine deaminase. They occur in human feces normally, but are potential pathogens, being recovered frequently from urinary tract infections, and secondary tissue infections. This genus and its species were formerly called *Proteus inconstans.* See also *Enterobacteriaceae.*

P. alcalifaciens, a species that ferments adonitol. Formerly called *Proteus inconstans.*

P. stuartii, a species that does not ferment adonitol. Formerly called *Proteus inconstans.*

provitamin (pro-vi'tah-min) a precursor of a vitamin; a substance from which the animal organism can form vitamins. For example, carotene is provitamin A and ergosterol is provitamin D.

provocation (prov"o-ka'shun) see *activation.*

provocative chelation test (pro-vok'ah-tiv ke-la'-shun) see under *lead assays.*

Prower factor [*Prower,* the patient in whom Factor X deficiency was first described] see *Factor X.*

proxim/o (prok'sĭ-mo) [L. *proximus* next] a word element used in combining form to denote near, e.g., proximolingual.

proximal (prok'sĭ-mal) [L. *proximus*] nearest; closer to any point of reference or place of attachment. Cf. *distal.*

proximal convoluted tubule the first segment of a renal tubule. It is continuous with the glomerular capsular space proximally and with the distal convoluted tubule distally. It lies in the renal cortex. It is the site of active resorption of many substances in the glomerular filtrate, including glucose, amino acids, phosphates, and sodium.

proximal latency see *proximal l.* under *latency.*

prozone phenomenon (pro'zōn) [*pro-* + *zone*] the phenomenon exhibited by some sera, which give effective agglutination reactions when diluted several hundred- or thousand-fold but do not visibly react with the antigen when undiluted or only slightly diluted. The phenomenon is not simply due to antibody excess, but often involves a special class of antibodies (blocking or incomplete), which react with the corresponding antigen in an anomalous manner. The bound antibody not only fails to elicit agglutination, but actively inhibits it. The phenomenon may also occur with precipitation or other immunologic reactions.

PRP abbrev. See *platelet-rich plasma.*

P-R segment the portion of the electrocardiogram between the end of the P and the beginning of the QRS complex. Depression of the P-R segment may occur with cardiac abnormalities, such as tricuspid stenosis.

PRU abbrev. See *peripheral resistance unit.*

prurigo (proo-ri'go) [L. "the itch"] a general classification for a variety of skin diseases characterized by the presence of several itchy, dome-shaped skin lesions topped with a small transient vesicle. The lesions resolve by crusting over and lichenification. The cause is unknown, but certain types appear to be associated with pregnancy.

pruritus (proo-ri'tus) [L., from *prurire* to itch] itching; an unpleasant sensation that makes one want to scratch the skin to obtain relief. It may be present with a primary skin disease or with systemic illness, such as uremia, diabetes, lymphoma, leukemia, obstructive biliary disease, or polycythemia vera. Some drugs and the later months of pregnancy may also cause itching. Prolonged scratching can lead to pigmented, lichenified patches on the skin.

p. ani, itching in the anal and perianal area. The causes include infectious or parasitic agents, anorectal disease, irritating soaps and clothing, allergic conditions, and systemic illness. Stool examination may show parasites, e.g., the eggs of *Enterobius vermicularis.* Culture and microscopic examination of tissue scrapings may reveal *Sarcoptes scabiei,* yeasts, or fungi. Urinalysis and blood tests may reveal systemic disorders.

essential p., itching of unknown cause on any part of the body.

p. vulvae, itching of the vulva. A common gynecologic complaint, this form of pruritus may be caused by vulvovaginitis, dermatologic disorders, estrogen deficiency, systemic disorders, or rectal disease. It may be the initial symptom of vulvar carcinoma. *Candida albicans, Trichomonas vaginalis, Pediculosis pubis,* and *Sarcoptes scabiei* may also be associated with the condition.

Culture and Gram stain of vaginal discharge may reveal a causative organism, and cytologic examination may show estrogen deficiency.

Prussian blue (prush′an) a dark blue dye, ferric ferrocyanide, $Fe_4(Fe(CN)_6)_3$; M.W. 859.28. In histology, Prussian blue is the colored end product formed in the reaction to demonstrate ferric ion. See under *iron-positive pigment demonstration.*

PS abbrev. See *phosphatidylserine.*

ps abbrev. See *picosecond.*

Ψ the Greek capital letter *psi.*

ψ the Greek lower case letter *psi;* symbol for wave-function.

psamm/o (sam′o) [Gr. *psammos* sand] a word element used in combining form to denote sand or sandlike material, e.g., psammoma bodies.

Psammolestes (sam″ol′es-tēs) a genus of bugs of the family Triatomidae. The species *P. coreodes,* found in northern Argentina, and *P. arthuri* and *P. rubrotuberculatus,* found in Venezuela, are naturally infected with *Trypanosoma cruzi.*

psammoma body (sam-o′mah) [Gr. *psammos* sand + *-oma*] a discrete, concentrically laminated, mineralized body that is seen histologically in the stroma of certain tumors, particularly meningiomas, papillary carcinoma of the thyroid, and papillary serous tumors of the ovary. The exact significance of these bodies is unknown; however, their presence may be helpful in the histologic identification and classification of some tumors.

psec abbrev. See *picosecond.*

Pselaphephilia (sel″ah-fĕ-fil′ĭ-ah) a genus of non-bloodsucking muscoids that are vectors of *Dermatobia hominis.*

pseud/o (su′do) [Gr. *pseudēs* false] a word element used in combining form to denote false, e.g., pseudopodia.

pseudarthrosis (soo″dar-thro′sis) [*pseud-* + Gr. *arthrōsis* joint] a false joint caused by the inadequate immobilization of a fractured bone. The continuation of abnormal mobility can slow or even stop the laying down of an osseous callus, and the callus will instead be composed of fibrous tissue that has no structural strength, thus forming a false joint. With adequate immobilization and removal of any interposing soft tissues in the false joint, a normal osseous callus may be formed.

pseudesthesia (soo″des-the′ze-ah) [*pseud-* + Gr. *aisthēsis* perception] a sensation felt without any external stimulus or one that is referred to an absent limb.

pseudoacini (soo″do-as′ĭ-ni) [*pseudo-* + L. *acinus* grape, grape seed] glandlike structures (rosettes) formed by liver cell plates two cells thick seen on cross section of the liver. Their presence is a manifestation of regenerative hyperplasia.

pseudoalleles (soo″do-ah-lēlz′) [*pseudo-* + Gr. *allēlōn* of one another] genes that are involved in the same function and are so closely linked that cross-over rarely occurs between them; thus, they appear to be alleles but are actually at separate loci. See also *cis-trans test.*

pseudoaneurysm (soo″do-an′u-rizm) [*pseudo-* + Gr. *aneurysma* a widening] false-positive evidence of an aneurysm, based on physical or x-ray findings. An enlarged and tortuous vessel, or a contained rupture of the left ventricle or of a large blood vessel, all of which can give the appearance of an aneurysm.

pseudocholesteatoma (soo″do-ko″les-te-ah-to′-mah) [*pseudo-* + Gr. *chōle* bile + *steatos* fat + *ōma* tumor] a mass of cornified epithelial cells found in the middle ear in chronic middle ear inflammation and resembling cholesteatoma. See also *cholesteatoma.*

pseudocholinesterase (soo″do-ko″lin-es′ter-ās) see *cholinesterase.*

pseudocholinesterase deficiency a condition, transmitted as an autosomal recessive trait, that reflects the presence of variant enzyme; it is found in 0.3–0.5 percent of the population. Two variant loci (E_1 and E_2) are found, both probably on chromosome 1. The E_1 locus has four alleles: normal ($E_1{}^u$); atypical ($E_1{}^a$), which produces enzyme having weak activity and less inhibition by dibucaine than normal; $E_1{}^f$, which produces enzyme having diminished activity and less inhibition by fluoride ions than normal; and silent ($E_1{}^s$), which produces an inactive enzyme. Persons of a phenotype containing no normal gene, $E_1{}^u$, are sensitive to the muscle relaxant drug succinylcholine, which is normally inactivated by pseudocholinesterase; administration of this drug to such patients may cause prolonged paralysis and respiratory failure. Also called succinylcholine sensitivity.

pseudocirrhosis (soo″do-sĭ-ro′sis) [*pseudo-* + *cirrhosis,* from Gr. *kirrhos* orange yellow + *-osis* condition] a clinical condition mimicking, but not due to, cirrhosis of the liver. It is caused by severe hepatic congestion, such as that found in chronic heart failure.

pseudocyesis (soo″do-si-e′sis) [*pseudo-* + Gr. *kyēsis* pregnancy] false pregnancy.

pseudocylindroid (soo″do-sĭ-lin′droid) [*pseudo-* + Gr. *kylindros* cylinder + *eidos* form] a piece of mucin found in the urine. It is shaped like a fusiform cylinder, tapering to a tail that often has a twist.

pseudocyst (soo′do-sist) [*pseudo-* + Gr. *kystis* sac, bladder] an abnormal or dilated cavity resembling a cyst but not lined by epithelium.

pseudodiploid (soo″do-dip′loid) [*pseudo-* + Gr. *diploos* twofold] pertaining to a chromosomal complement that has the normal diploid number (46 in humans) but in which the normal diploid complement is not present owing to chromosomal aberrations.

pseudoephedrine hydrochloride (soo″do-ĕ-fed′-rin) [USP], a sympathomimetic amine used as a nasal decongestant (vasoconstrictor) and bronchodilator. Unlike its stereoisomer ephedrine, it has almost no pressor activity. Mild stimulation is produced in some individuals. Trademark, *Sudafed.*

pseudoepitheliomatous hyperplasia (soo″do-ep-ĭ-the″le-o′mah-tus) [*pseudo-* + Gr. *epi* on + *thēlē* nipple + *-oma* tumor] a term applied to a hyperplastic proliferation of stratified squamous epithelium to the degree that epidermoid carcinoma is simulated. It may occur over an underlying dermal or subcutaneous lesion, e.g., granular cell myoblastoma, or it may reflect response to an epithelial irritant, e.g., inflammation or ulcer.

Pseudogordius (soo″do-gor′de-us) a genus of worms of the family Chordodidae, of which the species *P. tanganyikae* has been recovered from a human in East Africa.

pseudogout (soo″do-gowt) a form of chondrocalcinosis, usually occurring in older individuals in which the predominant calcium salt found in the synovial fluid is calcium pyrophosphate dihydrate (CPPD). The disease may progress to calcification of articular cartilage and degenerative joint disease. See also *chondrocalcinosis.*

Pseudohazis a genus of caterpillars. The species *P. hera* and *P. eglanterina,* which possess poisonous hairs, are found geographically throughout the western United States.

pseudohermaphroditism (soo″do-her-maf′-ro-di-tizm″) a genetic malformation that results in individuals with well-defined male or female gonads but with other reproductive organs that are either ambiguous or of the opposite sex. Pseudohermaphrodites are designated male or female on the basis of their karyotype, not their external sexual phenotype. See also *sex determination.*

pseudohyperkalemia (soo″do-hi″per-kal-e′me-ah) [*pseudo-* + Gr. *hyper* above + L. *kalium* potassium + Gr. *haima* blood + *-ia*] a spurious elevation of the serum concentration of potassium while the plasma concentration remains normal. It occurs most commonly in myeloproliferative disorders due to leukocytosis or marked thrombocytosis, which promote the release of potassium from the cells.

pseudohypoparathyroidism (soo″do-hi″po-par″-ah-thi′roi-dizm) [*pseudo-* + Gr. *hypo* under, below + *parathyroid* + *-ism* condition] a condition clinically resembling hypoparathyroidism, transmitted as an X-linked dominant trait, that is caused by end-organ unresponsiveness to parathyroid hormone. Hypocalcemia, hyperphosphatemia, short stature, obesity, round face, short metacarpals and metatarsals, and ectopic calcifications are present; mental deficits may also be evident. Increased neuromuscular excitability and tetany may be caused by the hypocalcemia.

Low serum calcium, high serum PO_4, normal alkaline phosphatase, low urinary PO_4, and low or absent concentrations of urinary calcium are characteristic. Skull radiographs may show calcification of the basal ganglia, and slit-lamp examination of the eye may reveal early cataracts. The condition may be distinguished from true hypoparathyroidism by the absence of phosphaturia after administration of parathyroid hormone, the presence of normal or increased concentrations of circulating parathyroid hormone, and the associated skeletal abnormalities.

pseudoisochromatic (soo″do-i″so-kro-mat′ik) [*pseudo-* + Gr. *isos* equal + *chrōma* color] seemingly of the same color throughout; applied to charts containing two pigments or colors that can be detected with normal eyesight but cannot be differentiated by colorblind persons.

pseudolymphoma (soo″do-lim-fo′mah) [*pseudo-* + *lymphoma,* from L. *lympha* water + *ōma* swelling] a diffuse proliferation of lymphocytes that occasions suspicion of a lymphoma on histologic examination.

pseudolymphoma of Spiegler-Fendt [Eduard *Spiegler,* Austrian dermatologist, 1860–1908; Heinrich *Fendt,* German physician, 19th century] a nonmalignant lymphoid infiltrate of the skin, usually occurring as a solitary nodule and most frequently presenting on the face. The lesions heal spontaneously but may recur. The etiology and pathogenesis are not known. Histologically, the lesions are characterized by nodular dermal infiltrates of large and small lymphocytes that are admixed or that form structures resembling lymphoid follicles. Plasma cells and occasionally eosinophils are present in the infiltrates. The principal differential diagnostic consideration is malignant lymphoma, and the distinction may be difficult. Also called cutaneous lymphoid hyperplasia, *lymphocytoma cutis,* and *Spiegler-Fendt sarcoid.*

pseudomelanosis pigment (soo″do-mel″ah-no′sis) [*pseudo-* + Gr. *melas* black + *-osis*] a dark brown granular pigment deposited in phagocytic mononuclear cells of the mucosae of the large bowel and appendix in an asymptomatic condition called melanosis coli. The pigment is thought to be formed from absorbed aromatic protein degradation products converted by tyrosinase into a melanin-like pigment. It is PAS-positive and gives a positive result in the ferric ferricyanide reduction test.

pseudomembranous colitis (soo″do-mem′brah-nus) [*pseudo-* + L. *membranosus*] see *pseudomembranous c.* under *colitis.*

pseudomonad (su′do-mo″nad) any member of the genus *Pseudomonas.*

Pseudomonadaceae (soo″do-mo″nah-da′se-e) a family of gram-negative strict aerobic bacteria. The Pseudomonadaceae are straight or curved rods that are catalase- and oxidase-positive; they oxidize organic compounds and are motile with polar flagella. The family includes four genera, *Pseudomonas, Xanthomonas, Zoogloea,* and *Gluconobacter,* but only the first-named is of medical importance.

Pseudomonadales (soo″do-mo″nah-da′lēz) one of the orders formerly in the class Schizomycetes, the true bacteria, consisting of those that have polar flagella. This order is now obsolete according to modern classification.

Pseudomonas (soo″do-mo′nas) [*pseudo-* + Gr. *monas* unit] a genus of the family Pseudomonadaceae, consisting of gram-negative, straight or curved, rod-shaped organisms. They are motile with polar flagella and have respiratory rather than fermentative, energy-yielding metabolism. Most species are strict aerobes. Some produce yellow, green, or blue pigments. They are widely distributed in soil and water, and some are opportunistic human pathogens, causing many hospital-acquired infections in debilitated patients.

P. acidovorans, a rarely opportunistic pathogen of widespread occurrence. It is nonoxidative in glucose oxidative-fermentative (O-F) medium, does not grow at 42°C, and has a polar tuft of three or more flagella. Also call *Comamonas terrigena.*

P. aeruginosa, a species that is a major agent of hospital-acquired infections, especially in patients debilitated by burns, cystic fibrosis, various chronic illnesses, or surgery, or those who are on antibiotics, immunosuppressive drugs, or inhalation therapy. It causes severe and often fatal infections, most commonly involving the urinary tract, wounds, abscesses, or the blood stream. It is also responsible for eye infections in those who wear contact lenses. Its resistance to most antibiotics makes treatment difficult.

The organism is oxidase-positive and is oxidative in glucose O-F medium. Most stains produce pyocyanin and fluorescein, giving the medium a characteristic blue-green color. The organism also produces endo- and extracellular toxic products (see *endotoxin* and *exotoxins*). Three methods have been used to differentiate among its many strains for epidemiologic study: bacteriophage, pyocin, and serologic typings.

Formerly called *Bacillus pyocyaneus.*

P. alcaligenes, a rarely infectious species found in water reservoirs and occasionally isolated from an individual's blood. It grows at 42°C and produces alkali in open tubes of glucose O-F medium.

P. cepacia, an opportunistic pathogen, with widespread geographic distribution, that is isolated from a wide variety of clinical material, hospital equipment, and supplies. It has been identified as the cause of outbreaks of hospital-acquired infections. The organism has a polar tuft of three or more flagella, is lysine-decarboxylase–positive, produces yellow pigment on iron-containing media, and is oxidative in glucose O-F medium. Formerly called *P. multivorans* and *P. kingii.*

P. fluorescens, a species that is an environmental contaminant and occasionally an opportunistic pathogen for humans. It also occurs as a contaminant of the blood and blood products used for transfusions. The species produces the yellow fluorescent pigment pyoverdin; it does not grow at 42°C but does grow at 4°C. It is oxidative in glucose O-F medium.

P. mallei, a nonmotile species that causes disease (glanders) in horses and occasionally in humans. It is oxidative in glucose O-F medium and does not produce pigment. See also *glanders.*

P. maltophilia, a widespread species; an occasionally opportunistic pathogen that causes infections in the upper respiratory tract and in wounds, blood, and urine. The organism has a polar tuft of three or more flagella, produces acid oxidatively from glucose and maltose, and is oxidase-negative.

P. pseudomallei, the species that causes melioidosis in humans, especially in Southeast Asia. It is oxidative in glucose, lactose, and maltose O-F media and does not produce pigment. Other distinguishing characteristics are bipolar tufts of flagella and the production of arginine dehydrolase. See also *melioidosis.*

P. stutzeri, a widespread species often recovered from clinical specimens although not usually considered etiologically significant. It is a polar-monotrichous, nonfluorescent organism that is oxidative in glucose O-F medium. Dry, wrinkled, yellowish colonies are characteristic.

pseudomyiasis (soo″do-mi-i′ah-sis) [*pseudo-* + Gr. *myia* fly + *-iasis*] the accidental ingestion of dead or living fly larvae, which may cause diarrhea and other symptoms if present in large quantities.

pseudomyxoma peritonei (soo″do-mik-so′mah per″i-to-ne′i) [N.L.; *pseudo-* + Gr. *myxa* mucus + *-oma* tumor; L. *peritonei* genitive case of *peritoneum*] a condition characterized by abdominal distention, resulting from extensive seeding of the peritoneum by mucus-secreting tumor cells. The cause is commonly rupture of a mucinous adenocarcinoma of the ovary or appendix. Gelatinous material containing nests of tumor cells coat the peritoneal surface. Surgical removal of the primary tumor and as much mucin as possible, along with intraperitoneal instillation of an alkylating agent, is the present mode of treatment. Because tumors producing pseudomyxoma peritonei rarely metastasize widely, the disease is usually chronic, characterized by malnutrition and recurrent bouts of intestinal obstruction.

pseudoparakeratosis (soo″do-par″ah-ker″ah-to′sis) [*pseudo-* + Gr. *para* resembling + *keras* horn + *-osis* condition] a condition of the epithelium of the uterine cervix that resembles parakeratosis of the skin. It is characterized by several layers of small, keratinized squamous cells at the surface of the squamous mucosa.

pseudopelade (soo″do-pe′lād) [*pseudo-* + Fr. *pelade,* from *peler* to remove or loosen hair, to peel] a patchy, scarring alopecia of the scalp, similar in appearance to alopecia areata. In the early stages, little fibrosis is apparent, and hairs can be easily removed. Later, extensive fibrosis may be seen.

pseudoperiodic (soo″do-pe″re-od′ik) see *quasiperiodic.*

Pseudophyllidea (soo″do-fĭ-lid′e-ah) [*pseudo-* + Gr. *phyllon* leaf] an order of cestodes in which the scolex has two opposite sucking organs. It includes the family Diphyllobothriidae.

pseudophyllidean (soo″do-fĭ-lid′-e-an) pertaining to or caused by cestodes (tapeworms) of the family Pseudophyllidea.

pseudopodium (soo″do-po′de-um), pl. *pseudopodia* [L., from *pseudo-* + Gr. *podion,* diminutive of *pous* foot] a temporary protrusion of cytoplasm from an ameboid cell, serving the functions of locomotion or the engulfing of food.

pseudopolyposis (soo″do-pol″ĭ-po′sis) [*pseudo-* + *polyp,* from Gr. *polypous* many-footed + *-osis* condition] the occurrence of a large number of inflammatory polyps in the colon, most frequent in association with ulcerative colitis. Ulceration of large areas of colonic mucosa leaves scattered islands of hyperemic, edematous mucosa with undermined edges. Free ends of the ulcerated mucosa form the pseudopolyps. In moderately severe cases, the pseudopolyps can be visualized radiographically.

pseudo-pseudohypoparathyroidism (soo″do-soo″do-hi″po-par″ah-thi′roid-izm) a hereditary condition, with physical features resembling pseudohypoparathyroidism, that lacks the associated end-organ unresponsiveness to parathyroid hormone. Affected individuals demonstrate short stature, obesity, round face, and shortened metacarpals and metatarsals; however, all serum concentrations of calcium, phosphate, and parathyroid hormone are normal. An individual may have pseudohypoparathyroidism at one time and pseudo-pseudohypoparathyroidism at different times; the two disorders are thought to be different manifestations of the same gene.

pseudorosette (soo″do-ro-zet′) a histologic grouping of neoplastic cells characterized by a circle of cells that form a structure resembling a true rosette, but with the central zone occupied by a small vessel. Cf. *rosette.*

pseudosarcoma (soo″do-sar-ko′mah) [*pseudo-* + *sarcoma,* from Gr. *sarkos* flesh + *-oma* swelling] sarcomatoid transformation of a carcinoma histologically simulating a sarcoma. The most common form of pseudosarcoma is the spindle cell variant of squamous carcinoma, which may arise on the skin or mucosa, particularly in the head and neck region.

pseudostratified (soo″do-strat′ĭ-fīd) seemingly composed of layers. Cf. *stratified.*

pseudostratified epithelium a simple columnar epithelium in which the nuclei lie at different levels, creating the impression of stratification. The epithelium that lines most of the respiratory passages is pseudostratified ciliated columnar epithelium. Also called *respiratory epithelium.*

Pseudothelphusa (soo″do-thel-fu′sah) a genus of crabs, of which the species *P. iturbei,* found in Venezuela, is the secondary host of the metacercariae of *Paragonimus westermani.*

pseudotumor (soo″do-too′mor) [*pseudo-* + *tumor,* from L. *tumere* to swell] a firm nodule of inflammatory tissue, often with a component of plump reactive fibroblasts, that simulates a true neoplasm.

pseudotumor cerebri see *benign intracranial hypertension.*

pseudouridine (Ψ) (soo″do-ur′ĭ-dēn) a nucleoside in which the ribose moiety is attached to uracil at the 5 position rather than at the 1 position as in uridine; formed from uridine by posttranscriptional enzymatic modification in rRNAs and tRNAs. Catabolism of RNAs results in free nucleosides that are excreted in urine. Elevated concentrations of both pseudouridine and methylated nucleosides in blood and urine have been demonstrated in many types of cancer.

pseudoxanthoma elasticum (soo″do-zan-tho′mah e-las′tĭ-kum) [*pseudo-* + Gr. *xanthos* yellow + *ōma* swelling; Gr. *elastikos* elastic] a rare, inherited, generalized disorder of the connective tissue. It is characterized by small yellow macules and papules, and thickened, inelastic, redundant skin, most notably present in the neck, axillae, and inguinal and periumbilical areas. Angioid streaks of the retina, gastrointestinal bleeding, and cardiovascular abnormalities—including weak or absent pulses, intermittent claudication, and coronary artery disease—are also present. The basic abnormality is unknown but probably involves a defect in elastic fibers.

Radiographs may show arterial calcification, and brachial arteriography may reveal radial and ulnar artery occlusion, along with dilated interosseous arteries. Deaths from cerebrovascular accidents, cardiac disease, or hemorrhage related to the disorder have been reported in individuals whose ages ranged from 30 to 70 yr. No specific treatment is known.

PSG abbrev. See *polysomnogram.*

psi (Ψ,ψ) (si, psi) the twenty-third letter of the *Greek alphabet.*

psilocin (si′lo-sin) a hallucinogenic toxin, 4-hydroxy-*N,N*-dimethyltryptamine, produced by various mushrooms and related to psilocybin. Psilocin is formed in the body by the dephosphorylation of psilocybin. See also *m. cerebralis* under *mycetismus.*

psilocybin (si″lo-si′bin) a hallucinogen, the phosphate ester of psilocin, found in several genera of mushrooms, such as species of *Psilocybe* and a few other genera. It is somewhat less toxic than mescaline but in children can cause fatalities from fever and convulsions. As with other hallucinogens, it may produce anxiety attacks or panic states. See also *m. cerebralis* under *mycetismus.*

psittacosis (sit″ah-ko′sis) [Gr. *psittakos* parrot + *-osis*] see *ornithosis.*

psoriasis (so-ri′ah-sis) [Gr. *psōriasis,* from *psōra* itch] a common, benign inflammatory disease of the skin characterized by dry, well-circumscribed, silvery scales on bright red plaques; it may be acute or chronic. This disease is commonly found among those aged 10–40 yr, but it may occur at any age. The cause is unknown, although familial transmission (through specific human leukocyte antigen, HLA, loci), immune phenomena, and biochemical abnormalities (decreased cyclic adenosine monophosphate, cAMP, and prostaglandin E_1 insensitivity) have been suggested.

Onset is gradual. Lesions often appear on the scalp, extensor surfaces, back, and buttocks. Sterile pustules (pustular psoriasis) may occur on the palms and soles, and psoriatic lesions of the nails are also common. Occasionally, eruptive episodes of focal or generalized psoriasis may occur, especially after trauma, infection, or stress. Severe cases are characterized by exfoliative dermatitis and/or arthritis.

Diagnosis is based on visual inspection and histologic examination of a biopsy of affected skin.

Also called psoriasis vulgaris. See also *Munro microabscess.*

Psorophora (so-rof′o-rah) [Gr. *psōra* itch + *phoros* bearing, from *pherein* to bear] a genus of large mosquitos. The species *P. ferox, P. lutzi,* and *P. cyanescens* are carrier hosts of the eggs of the tropical bot fly, *Dermatobia hominis.*

PSP abbrev. See *phenolsulfonphthalein.*

PSRO abbrev. See *Professional Standards Review Organization.*

psych/o (si′ko) [Gr. *psychē* soul] a word element used in combining form to denote the mind, e.g., psychogenesis.

psychalgia (si-kal′je-ah) [*psych-* + Gr. *algos* pain + *-ia*] a pain of mental or nonorganic origin; pain resulting from mental efforts.

psychataxia (si″kah-tak′se-ah) [*psych-* + Gr. *ataxia* disorder] a mental condition characterized by inability to maintain fixed attention or to maintain any sort of continuous mental effort.

psychiatry (si-ki′ah-tre) [*psych-* + Gr. *iatreia* healing] the branch of medicine that deals with the study, treatment, and prevention of mental illness.

psychology (si-kol′o-je) [*psycho-* + *-logy*] the branch of science that deals with the mind and mental processes, especially in relation to behavior.

psychomotor variant (si″ko-mo′tor) see *rhythmic temporal theta burst of drowsiness.*

psychosine (si-ko′sēn) a glycoside, β-galactosylsphingenine, which can be obtained by the partial hydrolysis of cerebrosides or by direct glycosylation of sphingenine using UDP-galactose, which is catalyzed by the glycosyl transferase of brain cell microsomes. It can serve as an intermediate of cerebroside synthesis.

psychosis (si-ko′sis), pl. *psychoses* [*psych-* + *-osis* condition] a disorder of major mental processes, which may have organic or emotional (functional) causes, and is characterized by severe personality changes and loss of contact with reality. Often the affected individual may experience illusions, delusions, or hallucinations. Common forms include schizophrenia, paranoia, manic-depressive psychosis, and involutional reactions. Cf. *neurosis.*

affective p., a severely disabling disorder of mood or emotional feeling, with profound effect on thought and behavior, that occurs as the predominant feature of a psychotic reaction.

Korsakoff's p., see under *Wernicke-Korsakoff syndrome.*

psychrophile (si′kro-fil) [Gr. *psychros* cold + *philein* to love] a microorganism, usually one of the pseudomonads, that can multiply at low temperatures such as 4°C. Cf. *mesophile* and *thermophile.*

psyllium hydrophilic mucilloid (sil′e-um) a mucilaginous paste made from seeds of the herb *Plantago ovata* (blond psyllium), which is used as a bulk laxative. Also called psyllium hydrocolloid.

Pt symbol for the chemical element *platinum.*

PTA abbrev. for plasma thromboplastin antecedent. See *Factor XI.*

PTAH abbrev. See *phosphotungstic acid hematoxylin.*

PTC abbrev. for plasma thromboplastin component. See *Factor IX.*

PTC peptide abbrev. See *phenylthiocarbamoyl peptide.*

pteridine (ter-ĭ-dēn) a nitrogenous base that characterizes the pterins.

pterin (ter′in) [Gr. *pteron* wing] any one of a class of nitrogenous compounds first observed in the wings of butterflies. Basically they are the pteridine base with various substitutions. Examples include aminopterin, leucopterin, uropterin, and xanthopterin.

pterion (te′re-on) [Gr., diminutive of *pteron* wing] a small, circular area at the junction of the frontal, sphenoid, parietal, and squamous portions of the temporal bone.

pteroic acid (ter′o-ik) a compound containing a pterin linked to the nitrogen of *p*-aminobenzoic acid. It in turn is a part of the folic acid (pteroylglutamic acid) molecule.

pteroylglutamic acid (ter″o-il-gloo-tam′ik) see *folic acid.*

pteroylpolyglutamate (ter″o-il-pol″ē-gloo′tah-māt) a folic acid (folate) precursor for humans, present in plant food stuffs; pteroic acid linked to an oligopeptide of glutamic acid. The intestinal mucosa enzymatically removes all but one of the glutamyl residues, and ultimately the monopteroylglutamate (H_4 folate) is absorbed.

pterygium (tĕ-rij′e-um) [L., from Gr. *pterygion,* diminutive of *pteryx* wing] a lesion of the conjunctiva that arises at the limbus and progresses into the cornea, producing a yellow elevation covered by atrophic epithelium. It is similar to a pinguecula but more serious because of its location.

pterygium colli (tĕ-rij′e-um col′i) [L. *pterygium;* L. *collum* neck] a thick fold of skin, usually occurring congenitally, that extends from the mastoid region to the acromion on the lateral aspect of the neck. It is generally found in association with Turner's syndrome and Noonan's syndrome.

Pterygota (ter″ĭ-go′tah) [Gr. *pteryx* wing] a subclass of winged and wingless insects, including lice, cockroaches, bugs, beetles, wasps, ants, moths, flies, and fleas.

PTH abbrev. See *parathyroid hormone.*

ptilosis (ti-lo′sis) [Gr. *ptilōsis,* from *ptilon* down, feathers] a general term used to describe a loss of the eyelashes.

ptosis (to′sis) [Gr. *ptōsis* fall] a congenital or acquired drooping of the upper eyelid. It can be caused by paralysis of the oculomotor nerve, or by paralysis of the superior cervical sympathetic nerve on the affected side, which is usually accompanied by miosis and anhidrosis. See also *Horner's syndrome.*

-ptosis (to′sis) a suffix word element to denote drooping, sagging, or prolapse, e.g., visceroptosis.

PTT abbrev. See *partial thromboplastin time test.*

-ptysis (ti′sis) [Gr. *ptysis* spitting] a suffix word element to denote spitting, e.g., hemoptysis.

Pu symbol for the chemical element *plutonium.*

pub/o (pu′bo) [L. *pubes* adulthood, the signs of puberty] a word element used in combining form to denote pubis, e.g., pubofemeral.

pubarche (pu-bar′ke) [*pub-* + Gr. *arche* beginning] a condition characterized by the premature development of pubic and/or axillary hair unaccompanied by the development of other sexual characteristics. Cf. *precocious p.* under *puberty* and *thelarche.*

puberty (pu′ber-te) [L. *pubertas,* from *puber* young adult] the period in life during which the secondary sex characteristics appear and the reproductive organs become capable of functioning. Although onset varies greatly, females usually reach puberty by age 11–13 yr, males by age 13–15. Females show broadening of the hips, development of the breasts, onset of menstruation, and the appearance of pubic hair. Males show broadening of the shoulders, genital enlargement, deepening of the voice, and the appearance of facial and pubic hair.

precocious p., a condition characterized by the onset of sexual maturation before age 8 yr in females and 10 yr in males. It may be accompanied by either ovulation or spermatogenesis (true precocious puberty) or immature gonads and lack of ovulation or spermatogenesis (false precocious puberty). Causes of true precocious puberty include hypothalamic lesions, encephalitis, tumors, juvenile hypothyroidism, and (in girls) Albright's syndrome. In 90 percent of all girls and 40 percent of all boys, however, there is no underlying abnormality. Causes of false precocious puberty include adrenal hyperplasia or tumor, gonadal tumors, and (in girls) ingestion of estrogen-containing pills.

Diagnostic studies should include skull x-rays, 24-hr urinary 17-hydroxycorticosteroid and 17-ketosteroid determinations, and serum luteinizing hormone, follicle-stimulating hormone, and serum thyroxine measurements. In true precocious puberty, in which no identifiable cause is found, CT scans of the brain should be made.

Treatment is directed at the underlying abnormality. If untreated, growth will be affected as a result of the premature closure of the epiphyses.

pubic (pu′bik) pertaining to the pubes.

pubic region the lower central region of the abdomen below the umbilical region and between the inguinal regions. Also called *hypogastric region.* See illustration under *abdominal regions.*

pubic symphysis the union of the pubic bones in the median plane by a plate of fibrocartilage; the center of the front of the pelvis. Also called symphysis pubis.

public antigen an antigen of a high-frequency blood group, so-called because it is found in an appreciable fraction of the population. Cf. *private antigen.*

Puchtler's alkaline Congo red method a method for demonstrating amyloid. After staining with Congo red dye, examination with polarized light produces a green birefringence dichroism. The alkaline medium of the Congo red dye prevents nonspecific staining.

Sections are first stained in Mayer's acid hemalum and then placed in a saturated sodium chloride solution in basic ethanol before staining in alkaline Congo red. Amyloid stains deep pink to red and fluoresces brightly in ultraviolet light from a BG 12/3-mm exciter filter.

Puchtler Sirius red method a method for selectively staining amyloid. Sections are stained in hot (60°C) Sirius red 4B in 1 percent sodium chloride and counterstained with alum hematoxylin. Amyloid stains red, whereas other tissue components remain unstained except for elastin fibers and red blood cells.

pudendal (pu-den′dal) pertaining to the pudenda, the external genitalia.

pudendal nerve a branch of the sacral plexus, which receives fibers from the second, third, and fourth spinal nerves. It leaves the pelvis through the greater sciatic foramen, then passes with the internal pudendal artery through the lesser sciatic foramen into the pudendal canal.

pudendum (pu-den′dum), pl. *pudenda* [N.L., from L. *pudendus,* from *pudere* to be ashamed] the external genitalia of humans, especially of females.

p. femininum, see *vulva.*

p. muliebre, see *vulva.*

puerpera (pu-er′per-ah) [L., from *puer* child + *parere* to bring forth, to bear] a female who has just given birth to a child.

puerperal (pu-er′per-al) [L. *puerperalis*] pertaining to the puerpera or the puerperium. The term usually refers to conditions that arise in females 48–72 hr after giving birth.

puerperal infection an infection in the mother, occurring within 1–3 da of childbirth, that is characterized by an elevated temperature (100.4°F, 38°C) for two successive days. These infections are commonly due to *Escherichia coli,* β-hemolytic streptococci, *Streptococcus faecalis,* or anaerobes such as *Clostridium perfringens.* The source of the organisms may be exogenous (unsterile procedures) or endogenous (normal vaginal flora).

Those affected experience chills, malaise, anorexia, headache, pallor, and tachycardia. Excessive bleeding and pain originating in the abdomen and spreading to the pelvic, chest, and leg areas are common.

Examination reveals a large, tender uterus and foul-smelling discharge. Leukocytosis is often seen. Blood and urine cultures, along with chest and uterine examination, should be performed. Complications include peritonitis, thrombophlebitis, and septicemia. If gram-negative organisms are involved, endotoxic shock frequently associated with acute tubular necrosis may result.

puerperium (pu″er-pe′re-um) [L. "childbirth"] the period or state of confinement after childbirth.

Pulex (pu′leks) [L. "flea"] a genus of fleas that are parasitic on the skin of humans, dogs, and cats. The bite of the species *P. irritans* (the common flea or human flea) produces itching. This species is also known to host *Dipylidium caninum, Hymenolepis diminuta,* and *H. nana.* See also the illustration accompanying *flea.*

Pulicidae (pu-lis′ĭ-de) a family of fleas that includes the species *Pulex irritans* (the human flea) and several species of *Xenopsylla,* which are thought to transmit the plague.

pulmon/o (pul′mo-no) [L. *pulmo* lung] a word element used in combining form to denote the lungs, e.g., pulmonic.

pulmonary (pul′mo-ner″e) [L. *pulmonarius,* from *pulmo* lung] pertaining to the lungs.

pulmonary blastoma a rare, malignant tumor of the lung composed of epithelial and mesenchymal elements, reminiscent of fetal pulmonary tissue. Initially called embryoma, the term blastoma was introduced because the tumor was viewed as the pulmonary counterpart of nephroblastoma. Others consider it to be a distinctive form of carcinosarcoma. Most of those affected are male, and the average age is younger than that for individuals with carcinoma of the lung. Typically, the tumor is large, peripheral, and unilateral. About half of those affected rapidly develop metastases; the remainder have a protracted course.

pulmonary blood flow see *pulmonary p.* under *perfusion.*

pulmonary capillary blood volume (V_C) the total volume of blood in the pulmonay capillaries at any one time in the healthy adult, normally amounting to 60 ml at rest and 95-120 ml during hard physical work or exercise. It is one of the factors that determines the total diffusion capacity of the lung.

pulmonary circulation the segment of the circulation that functions in external respiration by exposing the blood to alveolar air, enabling gas exchange to take place. The pulmonary circuit is arranged so that the right ventricular output (deoxygenated blood) is pumped into the pulmonary artery. The pulmonary artery branches into many smaller arteries following the course of the segmental and subsegmental bronchi. At the level of the alveolar ducts, these smaller branches become terminal arterioles, with a diameter close to 50 μ; the terminal arterioles further subdivide into pulmonary capillaries (7–9 μ in diameter), which form a dense, anastomosing network juxtaposed between the alveolar walls. The blood is oxygenated by gaseous diffusion across the alveolo-capillary wall. The pulmonary capillaries join to form venules that eventually coalesce to form the pulmonary veins (two veins from each lung). The pulmonary veins empty into the left atrium, conveying oxygenated blood for distribution to the systemic circulation by the pumping action of the left ventricle.

In general, the vessels of the pulmonary circulation differ anatomically from their systemic counterparts in that they have less smooth muscle and elastin content in their thinner, more compliant walls. The pulmonary circuit also differs hemodynamically from the systemic circuit with which it is in series. It is a low-resistance, low-pressure system that receives a higher blood flow (the entire cardiac output) than any other organ. Pulmonary vascular resistances and thus the regional distribution of pulmonary blood flow is greatly influenced by hydrostatic pressure (both intravascular and vascular components), a factor that varies widely between the apex and base of the lung during each respiratory cycle.

Because of its high distensibility, the pulmonary vasculature can also function as a blood reservoir; the pulmonary blood volume can increase significantly during exercise, with assumption of a supine body position, and in pathologic conditions such as left heart failure.

pulmonary distomiasis see *paragonimiasis.*

pulmonary edema see *pulmonary e.* under *edema.*

pulmonary embolism see *pulmonary e.* under *embolism.*

pulmonary fibrosis see *pulmonary f.* under *fibrosis.*

pulmonary hypertension see *pulmonary h.* under *hypertension.*

pulmonary infarction see *pulmonary i.* under *infarction.*

pulmonary mechanics the study of the behavior of the lung–chest wall unit under the influence of the forces that determine its movement with each breathing cycle. See also *compliance, elastic recoil,* and *pressure-volume curve.*

pulmonary perfusion see *pulmonary p.* under *perfusion.*

pulmonary perfusion scan a scintillation camera scan or rectilinear scan of the lungs. This technique uses radioactive particles (technetium-99m albumin microspheres or Tc 99m macroaggregated albumin are the usual radioactive agents) injected intravenously that become trapped in those areas of the pulmonary capillary bed that are adequately perfused. Regions of obstructed blood flow due to embolism, carcinoma, edema, bronchitis, emphysema, etc., are seen as nonradioactive defects. Chest radiographs and ventilation scans aid in the diagnosis.

pulmonary pressure the blood pressure exerted against the walls of the pulmonary artery, approximately equal to the maximal right ventricular pressure of 22 mmHg during systole, and 8 mmHg during diastole after the pulmonary valve has closed.

pulmonary tissue resistance the frictional resistance to the deformation of tissue that opposes the movement of the lungs, diaphragm, thoracic cage, and abdomen during inspiration and expiration. It constitutes 20 percent of the pulmonary resistance in the normal young male (the remaining 80 percent is the airway resistance). Tissue resistance may increase in conditions such as pulmonary fibrosis, sarcoidosis, kyphoscoliosis, and asthma.

pulmonary trunk the artery that arises from the right ventricle and extends backward and upward for approximately 2 in. to end below the aortic arch by dividing into the right and left pulmonary arteries.

pulmonary vein one of the veins that return oxygenated blood from the lungs to the left atrium. There usually are two right and two left pulmonary veins, which open separately into the atrium.

pulmonary ventilation scan a scintillation camera scan of the lungs, most commonly using xenon-133 gas as the imaging agent. The gas is inhaled with a deep breath and the single breath image is taken; then, the Xe 133 is rebreathed for several minutes and the equilibration image is taken. The breath is held, if possible, during imaging. Finally, room air is inhaled and the Xe 133 exhaled while a washout series of images is taken. This scan is used in the diagnosis of various obstructive lung diseases and in the evaluation of pulmonary function prior to surgery.

pulmonary wedge pressure the pressure measured through a catheter advanced through the right heart and tightly lodged in a small branch of the pulmonary artery, approximately equal to 10 mmHg. It is used to estimate left atrial pressure, particularly during studies of the dynamics of the left heart during congestive heart failure.

pulmonology (pul″mo-nol′o-je) [*pulmono-* + *logy*] the science concerned with the anatomy, physiology, and pathology of the lungs.

pulp (pulp) [L. *pulpa* flesh] any soft, juicy animal or vegetable tissue.

dental p., the connective tissue filling the pulp chamber of a tooth. It is surrounded by dentine and has a rich blood and nerve supply. The pulp serves a nutritive and sensory function for the dentine.

pulse (puls) [L. *pulsus* a beat, pulse] the palpable expansion of a blood vessel wall as the pressure wave travels through it. The arterial pulse, commonly felt from the radial artery at the wrist, can be used to determine the heart rate. In adults, resting heart rate is normally between 60 and 100 beats/min, although in some well-trained athletes it may consistently be below 60. In infants, resting heart rate may be normally as high as 170 beats/min. Evaluation of the strength of the arterial pulse, which is related to the magnitude of pulse pressure, can be used in the diagnosis of circulatory disorders. Pulse pressure is determined by subtracting diastolic from systolic pressure; normally, it averages about 40 mmHg. Decreasing peripheral resistance or decreasing heart rate tend to increase pulse pressure. Pathologic conditions that increase pulse pressure include arteriosclerosis, aortic valvular insufficiency, patent ductus arteriosus, and arteriovenous malformations.

As felt in clinical examination, the pulse wave has a characteristic shape or contour, normally with a smooth upward rise and a somewhat less rapid fall; this arterial pressure wave can also be measured directly by an arterial catheter. Changes in pulse contour can often aid in the diagnosis of cardiac disease.

See also *pulsus.*

alternating p., a pulse that occurs with a regular rhythm, but with consistent alterations in strength. Pulse pressure alternately decreases or increases by at least 20 mmHg on successive beats. This condition is indicative of a serious depression of myocardial function.

anacrotic p., a pulse in which a small, transient drop or pause in the upstroke of the beat (anacrotic notch), normally recorded but not palpated, becomes perceptible. The two separate systolic waves may be palpated during conditions such as aortic stenosis.

bigeminal p., a coupled pulse in which each pair of beats is separated from the following pair by a longer interval. It may result from the regular occurrence of premature ventricular contractions (ventricular bigeminy) or premature atrial contractions (atrial bigeminy). Other mechanisms such as 3:2 atrioventricular block can also produce a bigeminal pulse.

bisferiens p., the occurrence of two systolic peaks (attributable to the percussion and tidal waves) within a single beat, most readily palpable from the carotid artery. It is rarely seen in normal individuals but is commonly detected in those with aortic regurgitation or hypertrophic subaortic stenosis.

carotid p., the wave of pulsation in the carotid arteries or the pulse over the carotid arteries. It may be recorded by placing a transducer on the skin over the point of arterial pulsation in the midneck region. The carotid pulse has a rapid rise, beginning about 0.15 sec after initiation of the QRS complex. Following the rapid ejection of blood from the left ventricle, it declines to a dip, the dicrotic notch, which is caused by aortic valve closure. After a slight rise, it again declines until the start of the next cycle.

p. deficit, the failure to palpate a beat in the radial artery, which can be heard with the aid of a stethoscope placed over the heart. It is noted in conditions such as atrial fibrillation, or with ectopic beats, when two beats occur so closely together that there is inadequate ventricular filling time between them; the second systole therefore results in little or no ejection of blood into the systemic circulation.

dicrotic p., a pulse characterized by two marked expansions in each single beat of the artery, which is caused by an exaggeration of the normally small wave that follows the dicrotic notch. It usually accompanies conditions in which the normal elasticity of the aorta is maintained, yet the stroke volume is abnormally low: for example, hypovolemic shock, severe heart failure, and cardiac tamponade.

jugular venous p., the pulsations of the jugular vein caused by backward transmission of the changes in right atrial pressure during each cardiac cycle. The pressure changes can be recorded without catheterization by placing a transducer on the skin of the neck (just above the medial clavicle), where the jugular venous pulsations are visible.

Three characteristic waves can be seen with each cycle: an a wave, which is caused by atrial systole; followed by a small c wave, which reflects the rise in atrial pressure that occurs when the tricuspid valve bulges upward during isometric ventricular contraction; and finally a v wave, which is due to filling of the atria against a closed tricuspid valve during diastole.

Although recordings of jugular venous pulse now are seldom made except for educational purposes, observation of the pulse can be useful in the diagnosis of conditions such as pericardial tamponade and constriction, tricuspid insufficiency or stenosis, and certain arrhythmias.

paradoxical p., an accentuation of the normal weakening and strengthening of the arterial pulse (due to an alternate decrease and increase in cardiac output) that occurs with the inspiratory and expiratory phases of respiration. Conditions such as pericardial tamponade, constrictive pericarditis, and deep breathing can exaggerate these normal changes in pulse strength.

Quincke's p., the finding of visible pulsation in the color of the nail bed, indicative of aortic regurgitation and other conditions with a greatly widened pulse pressure. The nail bed is seen to flush with each heart beat, which can be readily detected by pressing a flashlight against the terminal digits.

water-hammer p., the pulse characteristic of aortic regurgitation, consisting of an abrupt, forceful expansion followed by a sudden collapse later in systole. Also called collapsing pulse and *Corrigan's pulse.*

pulse height analyzer (PHA) 1. an electronic circuit that accepts pulses only in a certain range of amplitudes. PHAs are used in scintillation cameras, scintillation counters, and rectilinear scanners to reject unwanted pulses. They consist of two discriminators and an anticoincidence circuit. The discriminators produce an output pulse only when the input pulse exceeds a preset amplitude level, whereas the anticoincidence circuit produces an output pulse only when one (but not both) discriminators produces an output pulse. The controls usually set the lower discriminator level (called the baseline, threshold, or E setting) and difference between the upper and lower levels (called the window, or ΔE setting). The gamma photons with the photopeak energy produce pulses in the window. Background radiation, scattered photons, and photons emitted by other isotopes are largely rejected. Also called *gamma spectrometer.*

2. see *multichannel analyzer.*

pulse pressure see under *arterial pressure.*

pulsus (pul'sus), pl. *pulsus* [L.] pulse.

p. parvus, a pulse with a small amplitude, usually attributable to a reduced stroke volume.

p. tardus, a pulse with a slow rate of systolic rise, suggesting the presence of an obstruction to outflow from the left ventricle.

pulvinar (pul-vi'nar) [L. "cushioned couch"] [NA], the expanded posterior end of the thalamus that lies superior to and slightly overhangs the superior colliculus. It is the most caudal of the thalamic nuclei and receives fibers from the lateral geniculate, medial geniculate, and amygdaloid complex. The pulvinar projects to most areas of the cortex, with particularly profuse connections to the speech area.

punched card a stiff paper card used to code data for computer input. The standard card (a Hollerith punched card) measures 3-1/4 in. by 7-3/8 in. and has 80 columns and 12 rows of hole positions. There is also a smaller 96-column punched card (the IBM System/3 card). The punches in each column represent one character. See also *card punch, card reader,* and *Hollerith code.*

punched tape see *paper tape.*

punctate (punk'tāt) [L. *punctum* point] marked with points or dots.

punkies (pun'kēs) see *Heleidae.*

Puntius (pun'te-us) a genus of freshwater fish, of which the species *P. orphoides* serves as a second host for the trematode *Opisthorchis felineus.*

pupil (pu'pil) [L. *pupilla* girl] the central orifice in the iris through which light must pass before entering the vitreous chamber of the eye.

pupill/o (pu'pĭ-lo) [L. *pupilla* girl] a word element

used in combining form to denote the pupil, e.g., pupillatonia.

pure red cell aplasia see *pure red cell aplasia* under *anemia.*

purified protein derivative (PPD) a partially purified antigenic preparation from a culture of *Mycobacterium tuberculosis* that is used in the tuberculin skin test. The culture filtrate of *M. tuberculosis* is partially purified by ammonium sulfate precipitation and then standardized for biologic activity (expressed in tuberculin units). For the skin test, five tuberculin units are administered intradermally. After 48–72 hr, 10 mm or more of erythema and induration constitutes a positive response. See also *Mantoux test.*

purine (pu′rēn) [L. *purum* pure + N.L. *uricum* uric acid + *-ine*] a heterocyclic organic compound, $C_5H_4N_4$, which is the fundamental form of a group of compounds known as purines or purine bases. Some of these bases are constituents of nucleic acid. In humans, uric acid is the metabolic end product of these bases. See also *purine and pyrimidine b.'s* under *base.*

purine nucleoside phosphorylase (pu′rēn nu′kle-o-sīd fos-for′ĭ-lās) an enzyme of the transferase class (EC 2.4.2.1) that catalyzes the reaction purine nucleoside + orthophosphate ⇄ purine + α-D-ribose 1-phosphate. It also catalyzes the analogous phosphorolytic cleavage of inosine to hypoxanthine. The reaction is a step in the degradation of nucleotides, nucleic acids, and purine residues, as well as in the pathway of purine salvage (reverse reaction). A genetic deficiency of this enzyme, transmitted as an autosomal dominant trait, results in defective T-cell immunity. Also called inosine phosphorylase (IP) and nucleoside phosphorylase.

purity (pūr′ĭ-te) [L. *puritas,* from *purus* pure] 1. the state of being a pure chemical compound.

2. the degree to which a substance is pure, e.g., 99.99 percent pure.

Purkinje cells (pur-kin′je) [Johannes Evangelista von *Purkinje,* Bohemian anatomist, physiologist, and microscopist, 1787–1869] large, branching neurons in the deepest region of the molecular layer of the cerebellar cortex.

Purkinje fibers [Johannes Evangelista von *Purkinje*] a subendocardial network of modified cardiac muscle cells that constitute the terminal ramifications of the neuromyocardium. The cells of Purkinje fibers may be wider and shorter than the typical myocardial fibers; they contain many mitochondria, sparse myofibrils, plentiful glycogen, and many tubules of sarcoplasmic reticulum. Impulses are conducted along Purkinje fibers at 2–3 m/sec, which is four or five times faster than the conduction velocities in the surrounding myocardium.

Purkinje network [Johannes Evangelista von *Purkinje*] see *Purkinje fibers.*

purpura (pur′pu-rah) [L. "purple"] 1. a small hemorrhage (up to about 1 cm in diameter) occurring on the skin, mucous membranes, and serosal surfaces. It has a variety of causes, including blood disorders, vascular abnormalities, and trauma. Cf. *ecchymosis* and *petechia.*

2. a group of vascular or hemorrhagic diseases characterized by hemorrhage into skin, mucous membranes, or serosal surfaces, resulting in purpuric hemorrhages, ecchymoses, and the tendency to bruise easily. These diseases may be due to decreased platelet counts, the presence of abnormal platelets (in uremia, gammaglobulinopathies, and reactions to drugs, especially aspirin), and vascular defects (hereditary disorders, autoimmune diseases, or infection).

allergic p., a nonthrombocytopenic purpura characterized by the formation of an urticarial rash, petechiae, and ecchymoses. These lesions primarily affect children, and occur on the skin and mucous membranes, particularly of the gastrointestinal tract. Colicky pains, melena, vomiting, and intussception may occur, and hematuria and renal dysfunction are commonly associated findings. This disorder may result from a hypersensitivity reaction to streptococcal upper respiratory tract infections, but other allergens may also be causative. In the absence of complications, the disorder is self-limiting. Also called *Henoch-Schönlein syndrome.*

anaphylactoid p., see *Henoch-Schönlein syndrome.*

p. annularis telangiectodes, see *Majocchi's disease.*

Henoch-Schönlein p., see *Henoch-Schönlein syndrome.*

thrombotic thrombocytopenic p., a rare, severe, acute, multisystem illness of unknown origin characterized by fever, hemolytic anemia, jaundice, thrombocytopenic purpura, changing neurologic signs, and nephropathy. Laboratory findings include a negative Coombs' test, leukocytosis, normal red cell enzymes, proteinuria, and hematuria. Pathologically, the condition is characterized by hyaline thrombi in the small blood vessels. Plasmapheresis, fresh frozen plasma transfusions, and antiplatelet drugs have been successful in treating what has often been a fatal illness.

purulent (pu′roo-lent) [L. *purulentus,* from *pus, puris* pus] consisting of, containing, or forming pus.

pus (pus) [L.] a protein-rich product of liquefaction necrosis that is pale yellow to yellow-green in color and contains leukocytes and cellular debris.

pustule (pus′tūl) [L. *pustula,* from *pus*] an elevation of the skin that contains a purulent exudate filled with neutrophils. Bacteria may or may not be present. Pustules develop from vesicular lesions of any cause that become infected with bacteria.

putrefaction (pu″tre-fak′shun) [L. *putrefactio,* from *putrefacere* to make rotten, from *puter* rotten + *facere* to make] the anaerobic decomposition of proteins with the production of foul-smelling compounds, such as hydrogen sulfide, ammonia, cadaverine, and putrescine; especially decomposition by proteolytic bacteria, such as species of *Clostridium.*

putrescine (pu-tres′in) $NH_3^+(CH_2)_4NH_3^+$, a polyamine present in cells. It is formed by the decarboxylation of ornithine, and has growth-promoting action both in mammalian and bacterial cells. This property is presumably related to putrescine's ability to stimulate RNA synthesis. See also *polyamine.*

PV abbrev. for plasma volume. See under *blood volume measurements.*

$P\bar{v}_{CO_2}$ abbrev. See *mixed venous P_{CO_2}.*

$P\bar{v}_{O_2}$ abbrev. See *mixed venous P_{O_2}.*

PVA fixative method a method for preserving trophozoites of amebae and a fairly adequate method for detecting protozoan cysts. The fixative consists of polyvinyl alcohol mixed with glycerol, glacial acetic acid, and Schaudinn's solution, which is heated until dissolved. The specimen may be fixed in a vial, and films for staining prepared on microscope slides later, or a film made from a fresh specimen may be fixed on microscope slides and stained when dry. Heidenhain's iron-hematoxylin and trichrome stains are recommended for PVA film staining.

PVA-lacto-phenol medium a mounting medium that combines the clearing and mounting processes for small nematodes. It consists of polyvinyl alcohol, phenol, and lactic acid.

P value see *significance probability.*

PVC abbrev. See *polyvinyl chloride, premature ventricular contraction.*

P wave the deflection in the electrocardiogram that is the result of electric currents generated during the excitation (depolarization) of the atria that precedes atrial contraction. It has an average duration of 90 msec and an amplitude of less than 0.3 MV.

PWM abbrev. See *pokeweed mitogen.*

py/o (pi′o) [Gr. *pyon* pus] a word element used in combining form to denote pus, e.g., pyogenic, pyoderma.

pyel/o (pi′ĕ-lo) [Gr. *pyelos* basin] a word element used in combining form to denote the renal pelvis, e.g., pyelonephritis.

pyelitis (pi″ĕ-li′tis) [*pyel-* + *-itis*] inflammation of the renal pelvis. See also *pyelonephritis.*

pyelogram (pi′ĕ-lo-gram″) [*pyelo-* + Gr. *gramma* mark] the radiologic visualization of the urinary tract following direct injection into it of a radiopaque contrast agent. See also *pyelography.*

pyelography (pi″ĕ-log′rah-fe) [*pyelo-* + Gr. *graphein* to draw] radiography of the renal pelvis or other parts of the urinary tract. See also *urography.*

pyelonephritis (pi″ĕ-lo-nĕ-fri′tis) [*pyelo-* + Gr. *nephros* kidney + *-itis*] the inflammation of the renal pelvis and interstitium, most commonly due to infection. See also *tubulointerstitial nephropathy.*

acute p., an acute, suppurative bacterial infection of the renal pelvis and renal parenchyma that is diffuse and often bilateral. It most frequently follows an ascending urinary tract infection. Acute pyelonephritis may occur with or without an associated cystitis. Gram-negative bacilli, most commonly *Escherichia coli,* are the usual etiologic agents. Others include species of *Proteus, Klebsiella, Enterobacter, Pseudomonas, Staphylococcus,* and *Streptococcus.* Poor perineal hygiene, pregnancy, urinary tract obstruction or trauma, vesicoureteral reflex, renal disease, malnutrition, and diabetes are factors that predispose to the disease. Those affected experience rapidly progressive fever, chills, vomiting, nausea, diarrhea, deep abdominal pain, and leukocytosis.

Laboratory tests reveal blood, leukocytes, and bacteria in the urine. Urine cultures grow more than 100,000 organisms/ml, and urinalysis may reveal an alkaline pH, minimal proteinuria, and white blood cell casts. Dangerous complications include necrotizing papillitis in patients with diabetes and those with urinary tract obstruction, pyonephrosis in patients with complete obstruction near the pelves, and perinephric abscess. Acute pyelonephritis is seen frequently in hospitalized patients with long-term indwelling urinary catheters.

chronic p., a chronic inflammation of both the renal pelvis and the renal parenchyma, resulting in irregular scarring, fibrosis, and deformity of these structures. The disease is thought to follow acute pyelonephritis, but only in those with underlying urologic abnormalities such as obstruction, vesicoureteral reflux, or neurogenic bladder. Chronic pyelonephritis accounts for 10–15 percent of patients requiring renal dialysis owing to end-stage renal failure.

The early signs of this disease include pyuria, bacteriuria, white blood cell casts, and evidence of stasis; urography shows diffuse renal, pelvic, and caliceal scarring. The signs vary in severity and may be associated with hypertension and elevated blood urea nitrogen. As the disease progresses, the glomerular filtration rate and renal blood flow decline, leading to decreased renal function. Proteinuria is usually minimal.

Pyemotes (pi″ĕ-mo′tēz) a genus of parasitic mites. The species *P. ventricosus* (the grain itch mite) is a predaceous mite that attacks the larvae of numerous insects infesting seeds and grain. These mites develop in the insects and are discharged when mature. They cause a vesiculopapular dermatitis on individuals who come into contact with grain, straw, or hay harboring the mites. The lesions produce a burning pruritus with fever and sweating. The dermatitis is often confused with pediculosis, scabies, and allergy. See also the illustration under *mite.*

Pyemotidae (pi″ĕ-mo′tĭ-de) a family of mites. It includes the genus *Pyemotes,* which causes grain or straw itch.

pyknosis (pik-no′sis) [Gr. *pyknōsis* condensation, from *pyknoun* to condense] a degenerative change in the nucleus of a cell, in which the chromatin becomes condensed and its pattern obliterated; these changes are accompanied by shrinking of the nucleus.

pyknotic (pik-not′ik) [Gr. *pyknōtikos*] pertaining to pyknosis.

pylor/o (pi-lo′ro) [Gr. *pylōros,* from *pylē* gate + *ouros* guard] a word element used in combining form to denote the pylorus, e.g., pylorospasm.

pyloric (pi-lor′ik) pertaining to the pylorus.

pyloric canal the short, narrow part of the stomach that extends from the pyloric antrum to the gastroduodenal junction.

pyloric stenosis obstruction of the pyloric orifice of the stomach. It may be congenital, or acquired as the result of peptic ulceration or prepyloric carcinoma.

pylorus (pi-lo′rus) [L., from Gr. *pylōros,* from *pylē* gate + *ouros* guard] [NA], the distal portion of the stomach, terminating as a thickened band of circular muscle, the pyloric sphincter, which controls passage of the gastric contents into the duodenum. The term is variously used to describe the pyloric region of the stomach, pyloric antrum, pyloric canal, and pyloric sphincter.

pyocin (pi′o-sin) [*pyo-* + *-cin* from L. caedere to kill] a protein substance, produced by some strains of *Pseudomonas,* that inhibits the growth of other pseudomonads. See also *bacteriocin.*

pyocyanin (pi″o-si′ah-nin) [*pyo-* + Gr. *kyanos* blue + *-in* a chemical suffix] a blue phenazine pigment produced by one *Pseudomonas* species, *P. aeruginosa.* It is the cause of "blue pus" in pseudomonal infections.

pyogenic (pi″-o-jen′ik) [*pyo-* + Gr. *gennan* to produce] producing pus.

pyorrhea (pi″o-re′ah) [*pyo-* + Gr. *rhoia* flow] the former name for periodontal disease, especially periodontitis. See also *periodontal disease* and *periodontitis.*

pyoverdin (pi″o-ver′din) [*pyo-* + Fr. *vert* green + *in* a chemical suffix] a yellow-green fluorescent pigment produced by the fluorescent pseudomonads. Also called *fluorescein.*

pyr/o (pi′ro) [Gr. *pyr* fire] a word element used in combining form to denote fever, e.g., pyrogenic.

pyramidal (pĭ-ram′ĭ-dal) [L. *pyramidalis,* from Gr. *pyramis* pyramid] shaped like a pyramid.

pyramidal cells large multipolar neurons of the cerebral cortex that are shaped like cones or pyramids.

pyramidal tracts a term used to describe the corticospinal and corticobulbar tracts of the central nervous system. Originally so-named because the corticospinal tracts pass through the pyramids of the medulla oblongata, the term also generally includes the corticobulbar tracts, which terminate above this level onto the motor nuclei of the cranial nerves. See also *corticobulbar tract* and *corticospinal tract.*

pyran (pi′ran) a member of a class of compounds having a pyran ring, which is a six-membered ring containing one oxygen atom, five carbon atoms, and two carbon-carbon double bonds.

pyranose (pi′rah-nōs) a sugar in which the hemiacetal or hemiketal ring contains six atoms; glucose and galactose in their cyclic forms are pyranoses. The name is derived from the relationship to pyran, C_5H_6O, which has a six-membered ring composed of five carbon atoms and an oxygen atom. Cf. *furanose.*

pyranoside (pi-ran′ō-sīd) a glycoside of a pyranose sugar.

pyrazinamide (pi″rah-zin′ah-mīd) [USP], pyrazinecarboxamide, an antibacterial derivative of nicotinamide; M.W. 123.11. Used in the treatment of tuberculosis, it is relatively toxic and is generally employed only in the presence of allergy or resistance to other drugs.

Pyrazus (pi-ra′zus) a genus of mollusks found geographically in Australia, of which the species *P. ebeninus* is the host of dermatitis-producing schistosome cercariae.

Pyrenochaeta (pi″rĕ-no-ke′tah) a genus of fungi, closely related or identical to *Madurella grisea,* that can cause black-grained maduromycosis. The genus produces black pycnidia of various shapes and sizes. On agar, the colony is floccose and gray to black in color, with an optimal growing temperature of 30°C. The only medically important species is *P. romeroi.*

pyrethrins (pi-re′thrinz) [from *pyrethrum*] pyrethrin I and II, active principals of pyrethrum flowers, which also contain two other toxic constituents, cinerin I and II. Pyrethrins are used in combination with a synergist, piperonyl butoxide, in common household rapid knock-down spray insecticides, and medicinally in topically applied liquids or gels to kill head, body, and pubic lice. Pyrethrins are potent skin sensitizers and can cause an allergic reaction; they cross react with ragweed. Poisoning by ingestion of large amounts can cause central nervous system disturbances and respiratory failure.

pyrethrum (pi-re′thrum) [Gr. *pyrethron* the feverfew (*Chrysanthemum parthenium*)] an extract of dried flowers of the genus *Chrysanthemum,* used as an insecticide. Also called pyrethrum extract and pyrethrum flowers. See also *pyrethrins.*

Pyrex trademark. See *heat-resistant g.* under *glass.*

pyridine (pēr′ĭ-dēn) a colorless, weakly basic liquid, C_5H_5N, with a disagreeable odor. Pyridine is a nitrogen analog of benzene and is considered to have an aromatic ring. It is a constituent of coal tar and can also be derived from tobacco and various organic matters. Many pyridine derivatives occur in nature.

In histology, it is used as a solvent and to extract lipids from tissues.

pyridine nucleotide a term used to refer to the diphosphopyridine (DPN) or triphosphopyridine (TPN) nucleotides. These nucleotides contain a pyridine moiety as part of their molecular structures. They are important enzyme cofactors and participate in oxidation-reduction reactions. Also called *nicotinamide adenine dinucleotide* (*NAD*) and *nicotinamide adenine dinucleotide phosphate* (*NADP*).

pyridostigmine bromide (pēr″ĭ-do-stig′mēn) [USP], a cholinesterase-inhibiting drug, used to treat myasthenia gravis and also as an antidote to the curariform muscle relaxants. For adverse reactions, see the similar drug *neostigmine.*

pyridoxal-5′-phosphate (pēr″ĭ-dok′sal fos′fāt) the anion form of the phosphoric acid ester of pyridoxal, one of the forms of vitamin B_6; M.W. 247.15. It is a coenzyme in many reactions involving free amino acids, e.g., amino transferase, amino acid decarboxylase, and glycine dehydrogenase, in which it is transformed into and from pyridoxamine-5′-phosphate. Also called *phosphopyridoxal.*

pyridoxamine (pēr″i-dox′ah-mēn) one of the three active forms of vitamin B_6. See also *vitamin B_6.*

4-pyridoxic acid (pēr″ĭ-dok′sik) the predominant urinary metabolite of vitamin B_6, 3-hydroxy-5-(hydroxymethyl)-2-methyl-4-pyridinecarboxalic acid; M.W. 183.16.

pyridoxine (pēr″ĭ-dok′sēn) a form of vitamin B_6, 5-hydroxy-6-methyl-3,4-pyridinedimethanol; M.W. 169.18. Pyridoxine is converted to the more active forms of vitamin B_6, namely, pyridoxal and pyridoxamine phosphates. See also *vitamin B_6.*

pyriform (pēr′ĭ-form) see *piriform.*

pyrilamine maleate (pēr-il′ah-mēn) [NF], an antihistamine used in many analgesic, decongestant, cold, and allergy preparations. It has the side-effect of mild drowsiness.

pyrimethamine (pēr″ĭ-meth′ah-mēn) [USP], an antimalarial drug that inhibits folic acid synthesis in microorganisms. It is used against chloroquine-resistant strains of malaria and severe infections caused by the *Toxoplasma* parasite.

pyrimethamine assays gas chromatography. Pyrimethamine is extracted from samples of alkalinized plasma, urine, or reference solution into chloroform, and chromatographed using a moderately polar column packing and a flame ionization detector. It is determined qualitatively by its retention index and quantitatively by the ratio of its peak area to that of *n*-octacosane.

pyrimidine (pi-rim′ĭ-dēn) a heterocyclic organic compound, $C_4H_4N_2$, the fundamental form of pyrimidine bases. Some of these bases are constituents of nucleic acid. Metabolic products of pyrimidines are urea and ammonia. See also under *purine and pyrimidine b.'s* under *base.*

pyrithione zinc (pēr″ĭ-thi′ōn) an antifungal, antibacterial, and antiseborrheic compound used in dandruff shampoos.

pyrogallol (pi″ro-gal′ol) a white crystalline solid, 1,2,3-trihydroxybenzene, $C_6H_3(OH)_3$. It is used in histology as a reducing agent and in medicine as a topically applied treatment for skin disorders.

pyrogen (pi′ro-jen) [*pyr-* + Gr. *gennan* to produce] a fever-producing substance. Fever results when an activating agent induces the production of pyrogenic proteins (endogenous pyrogens) by immunologically active phagocytic cells. Endogenous pyrogens are heat-labile (50°) proteins produced by neutrophils, eosinophils, monocytes, Kupffer cells, and macrophages. These proteins circulate to the central nervous system, altering the thermoregulatory set point. The exact mechanism by which the set point is elevated is still unclear. Several experimental studies suggest that pyrogens exert a direct or indirect effect on the cells of the preoptic area, hypothalamus, and midbrain by altering prostaglandin and/or cyclic 3′,5′-adenosine monophosphate (cyclic AMP) synthesis or the ratio of cellular or intracellular sodium to calcium.

The official pyrogen test for pharmaceuticals is to inject rabbits with the agent; a febrile response indicates pyrogenicity. A more sensitive test uses a lysate of blood cells from the horseshoe crab, *Limulus polyphemus;* endotoxins cause coagulation of the lysate to a gel. The specificity of this latter test, however, is not established.

pyrogenic (pi″ro-jen′ik) inducing fever.

pyroglobulin (pi″ro-glob′u-lin) [*pyro-* + *globulin*] a plasma globulin that irreversibly precipitates from serum heated to 56°C. Pyroglobulins are often monoclonal immunoglobulins found in individuals with multiple myeloma.

pyroglobulinemia (pi″ro-glob″u-li-ne′me-ah) the presence of pyroglobulins in the blood. Pyroglobulinemia is often discovered when serum is heated to inactivate complement before a routine serologic test. The condition is found in those with myeloma or lymphosarcoma.

pyroglutamase see *5-oxoprolinase (ATP-hydrolyzing).*

pyroglutamate (pi″ro-gloo′tah-māt) a heterocyclic amino acid residue formed by amide bond linkage between the 5-carboxyl group of glutamine with the α-amino group of the same molecule, with liberation of ammonia. This residue can occur as the *N*-terminal residue in some proteins. It is also an intermediate in the γ-glutamyl transfer cycle. Also called *5-oxoproline* and *pyrrolidone carboxylate.*

pyroglutamate hydroxylase see *5-oxoprolinase (ATP-hydrolyzing).*

pyroglutamicaciduria (pi″ro-gloo″tah-mik-as″ĭ-du′re-ah) a hereditary disorder, transmitted as an autosomal recessive trait, in which large amounts of pyroglutamate (5-oxoproline) are present in the urine and plasma. It is characterized by hemolytic anemia, mental retardation, chronic metabolic acidosis, and a cerebellar disorder with ataxia, spastic quadraparesis, intention tremor, and dysarthria. Enzyme studies of red blood cells of patients with pyroglutamic aciduria (or acidemia) show a deficiency not of 5-oxoprolinase but of glutathione synthetase. γ-Glutamylcysteine appears to be an alternate substrate for the transferase and the cyclotransferase, so that pyroglutamate accumulates beyond the capacity of 5-oxoprolinase to catabolize it. Also called *5-oxoprolinuria.* See also *γ-glutamyl transfer cycle.*

pyrolysis (pi-rol′ĭ-sis) [*pyro-* + Gr. *lysis* dissolution] the decomposition of organic substances by heat.

pyronin (pi′ro-nin) any of several basic dyes that produce stains pink-red to purple-red in color, used as specific stains for RNA. Also called pyronine.

p. B, bis(diethylamino)xanthene; C.I. 45010.

p. Y, bis(dimethylamino)xanthene; C.I. 45005. Also called pyronin G.

pyrophosphate (pi″ro-fos′fāt) the $P_2O_7^{4-}$ ion. In living organisms, this ion is formed by the cleavage of nucleoside triphosphates (e.g., adenosine triphosphate, ATP). It is broken down to phosphate by the enzyme inorganic pyrophosphatase. See also *inorganic pyrophosphate.*

pyrophosphoric acid (pi″ro-fos-for′ik) see under *phosphoric acid.*

pyroracemic acid (pi″ro-ra-se′mik) see *pyruvic acid.*

pyrrobutamine phosphate (pēr″ro-bu′tah-mēn) [USP], an antihistamine used to treat rhinitis. Adverse reactions include sedation and dryness of the mouth.

pyrrole (pēr′ōl) a five-member heterocyclic ring compound constituted of four carbons and one nitrogen (C_4H_4NH), the basic unit of porphyrins and heme derivatives. Porphyrins contain four pyrrole-like rings linked by four methene bridges in an alternating double-bond system.

pyrrolidone carboxylate (pēr-ōl′ĭ-dōn kar-bok′sĭ-lāt) see *pyroglutamate.*

1-pyrroline-5-carboxylate dehydrogenase (pēr′-o-lin) an enzyme of the oxidoreductase class (EC 1.5.1.12) that catalyzes the reaction 1-pyrroline-5-carboxylate + NAD^+ H_2O ⇄ L-glutamate + NADH + H^+. The reaction is a step in the metabolism of dietary proline. A genetic defect, transmitted as an autosomal recessive trait, is found in type II hyperprolinemia.

pyrroline-5-carboxylate reductase an enzyme of the oxidoreductase class (EC 1.5.1.2) that catalyzes the reaction L-proline + $NAD(P)^+$ ⇄ 1-pyrroline-5-carboxylate + NAD(P)H. The reaction is the first step in the metabolism of dietary proline. A congenital defect, transmitted as an autosomal recessive trait, is characterized by the absence of the liver enzyme; it is found in type I hyperprolinemia. Also called *proline dehydrogenase* and *proline oxidase.*

pyruvate (pi′roo-vāt) a salt, ester, or dissociated form of pyruvic acid.

pyruvate carboxylase (pi′roo-vāt kar-bok′sĭ-lās) an enzyme of the ligase class (pyruvate:carbon-dioxide ligase (ADP-forming), EC 6.4.1.1) that catalyzes the reaction ATP + pyruvate + CO_2 + H_2O ⇄ ADP + orthophosphate + oxaloacetate. An error of metabolism (Leigh's necrotizing encephalomyelopathy), transmitted as an autosomal recessive trait, is due to a genetic deficiency of the enzyme and leads to infantile degeneration of the brain, with physical and mental retardation. Also called *oxaloacetic decarboxylase.*

pyruvate kinase (PK) (kī′nās) an enzyme of the transferase class (ATP:pyruvate 2-*O*-phosphotransferase, EC 2.7.1.40) that catalyzes the reaction phosphoenolypyruvate + ADP ⇄ pyruvate + ATP. This is the final reaction in the Embden-Meyerhof scheme of glycolysis, one of the two reactions resulting in production of adenosine triphosphate. A genetic deficiency of the enzyme in red blood cells causes both a lowered ATP and defective cell membranes, leading to nonspherocytic hemolytic anemia. Screening tests may be conducted to detect PK deficiency in infants.

pyruvate kinase assays 1. screening test to detect PK deficiency in red cells. Leukocytes, which contain ≈300 times the amount of PK in erythrocytes, are first removed by centrifugation of the specimen and complete aspiration of the buffy coat. The red cells are lysed by suspension in a hypotonic solution, and the lysate is incubated with buffered phosphoenolypyruvate, ADP, and NADH. The pyruvate formed in this reaction oxidizes NADH to NAD^+, which can be followed by the decrease in ultraviolet fluorescence. The reaction can be carried out by placing one spot of reaction mixture on nonfluorescing filter paper at the beginning of the reaction and a second spot after a 30-min incubation at 37°C. The dried spots are examined under long-wave UV light. Fluorescence on the second spot indicates PK deficiency.

2. quantitative method. The same principle is applied as in the screening test, except that decrease of NADH is measured by the decrease in the absorbance at 340 nm. The assay is performed at different substrate concentrations to detect mutant kinase enzymes that show normal activity at artificially high substrate concentrations but decreased activity at the lower, physiologic concentration of phosphoenolypyruvate.

pyruvic acid (pi-roo′vik as′id) a colorless liquid, $CH_3CO \cdot CO_2H$, with an odor similar to acetic acid, which can be formed by the dry distillation of racemic or tartaric acid. It is unstable and easily polymerizes. Pyruvic acid is an important intermediate in the metabolism of carbohydrates and some amino acids. Metabolically, it can be oxidized to acetyl CoA, which then enters the tricarboxylic acid cycle. In fermentation (yeasts), it is decarboxylated to acetaldehyde and then reduced to alcohol. Also called *pyroracemic acid.*

pyruvic acid assays 1. enzymatic method. Heparinized blood is immediately deproteinized with metaphosphoric acid. Pyruvate is stable for days in metaphosphoric acid filtrates. The filtrate is reacted with NADH and lactate dehydrogenase at pH 7.5, and the change in NADH absorbance at 340 nm is used to determine the pyruvate concentration. Reference ranges for fasting venous blood withdrawn with the patient at rest are 0.034–0.102 mmol/l.

2. chemical method. Pyruvic acid is reacted with 2,4-dinitrophenylhydrazine to form a hydrazone, which is extracted into ethyl acetate and then into aqueous sodium bicarbonate. Alkali is added and the brown hydrazone product is quantitated photometrically. This reaction is not specific for pyruvate; it measures total keto acids in serum.

pyuria (pi-u′re-ah) [*py-* + Gr. *ouron* urine + *-ia*] the presence of pus in the urine.

Q

Q symbol for *glutamine,* quantity of electric charge, quantity of heat.

Q_{O_2} abbrev. See *oxygen consumption.*

q symbol for electric charge, the long arm of a chromosome.

Q banding (quinacrine banding) see under *chromosome banding.*

QC abbrev. See *quality control.*

qd abbrev. for *quaque die* (every day).

Q-enzyme see *1,4-α-glucan branching enzyme.*

QF abbrev. for *quality factor.* See *relative biological effectiveness.*

Q fever [*q* from query] an acute, self-limiting rickettsial disease caused by inhalation of *Coxiella burnetii* and characterized by headache, fever, and abdominal pain; in about 50 percent of those affected, there is also interstitial pneumonitis. This disease is considered an unusual infection because the agent is most commonly inhaled. In contrast to other rickettsial infections, no agglutinins develop against *Proteus* strains and no rash is present. After inhalation and an incubation period of approximately 20 da, severe fever, headache, myalgia, malaise, and nonproductive cough, with marked pulmonary infiltration seen on chest radiographs. The mortality is very low; most cases resolve, although chronic and relapsing forms of the disease do occur and may lead to endocarditis or severe hepatitis.

Q fever occurs in a worldwide distribution with endemic foci. It represents an occupational hazard for those exposed to domestic animals or their by-products. *C. burnetii* is maintained in wild animal populations and may be transmitted from animal to animal by tick bite (*Dermacentor andersoni*). Ticks may also transmit the organism to domestic animals, especially cattle, sheep, and goats, producing a mild infection. The organism is excreted through milk, placenta, and feces, and dusts or droplets containing viable organisms represent the primary transmission route to humans. Human infection occurs through inhalation of infected dust, or from infected milk, tick bites, or contact between individuals. A sporogenic cycle discovered in *C. burnetii* could be responsible for its high stability in the environment.

C. burnetii may also be isolated from blood in acutely infected individuals. Leukopenia, specific complement-fixing (CF) antibodies, and specific agglutinins may be found. The Weil-Felix test is negative. Specific fluorescent antibody tests are available. Liver function tests may reveal subclinical hepatitis.

Prevention is based on interruption of animal-to-human transmission, including proper disposal of animal products. Affected individuals should be isolated.

Also called Australian Q fever, hibernoverna1 bronchopneumonia, and nine-mile fever. See also *Rickettsiaceae.*

qh abbrev. for *quaque hora* (every hour).

qid abbrev. for *quater in die* (four times daily).

qn abbrev. for *quaque nocte* (every night).

qns abbrev. for *q*uantity *n*ot *s*ufficient.

QRS complex the deflection in the electrocardiogram, consisting of the Q, R, and S waves, that is the result of electric currents generated during the excitation (depolarization) of the ventricles preceding ventricular contraction. It has an average duration of 80 msec and an amplitude of 1.0 MV. The QRS complex pattern may be prolonged or bizarre in conditions such as cardiac hypertrophy, premature ventricular contraction, bundle branch block, myocardial infarction, or ventricular fibrillation.

QRS interval the duration of the QRS complex measured from the beginning of the initial wave to the end of the final wave in an electrocardiogram, which represents the duration of ventricular depolarization.

QRS loop the loop, traced by the QRS vectors in vectorcardiography, that represents ventricular depolarization.

QRS-ST junction in the electrocardiogram, the junction between the QRS complex and the ST segment.

QRS-T angle the angle between the mean QRS and T vectors in vectocardiography. See also *vectorcardiography.*

Q-T interval the time from the beginning of the QRS complex to the end of the T wave, which represents the duration of ventricular depolarization and repolarization as measured from the electrocardiogram.

Quaalude (kwa′lo͞od) trademark. See *methaqualone.*

quadrant (kwod′rant) [L. *quadrans* quarter] 1. one quarter of a circle; a sector subtending an angle of 90°.

2. one of the four quarters into which the *xy* plane is divided by the *x* and *y* axes of a cartesian coordinate system.

3. one of the four quarters into which a body part is divided by bisecting transverse and axial planes; e.g., the abdomen is divided into right and left upper and lower quadrants.

quadri- (kwod′rĭ) [L., from *quattuor* four] a prefix word element to denote four or fourfold, e.g., quadriceps.

quadriplegia (kwod″rĭ-ple′je-ah) [*quadri-* + Gr. *plēgē* a blow, stroke + *-ia*] paralysis of all four limbs. This condition may be caused by any lesion that affects the cervical segments of the spinal cord. Acute quadriplegia may thus follow trauma, vascular lesions of the cord, demyelinating diseases, neoplasms, infections, and spondylosis. Quadriplegia may also arise from diseases or damage involving the spinal cord diffusely or both the cervical and lumbar enlargements, or the pyramidal tract (bilaterally) anywhere in the brain. A severe peripheral neuropathy or disordered neuromuscular transmission may also cause weakness or paralysis of all four extremities. In all such cases, secondary effects such as skin erosion (as decubitis ulcers), fecal impaction, and urinary tract infections represent serious health threats. Also called *tetraplegia.*

quadriradial (kwod″rĭ-ra′de-al) [*quadri-* + L. *radialis,* from *radius* spoke of a wheel] a four-armed structure formed by the synapsis of partially homologous (especially translocated) chromosomes.

quadrivalent (kwod″rĭ-va′lent) [*quadri-* + L. *valens* powerful] 1. in chemistry, having a valence of 4. Also called *tetravalent.*

2. in genetics, the object formed by the synapsis of four partially homologous chromosomes during meiosis. See also *reciprocal translocation.*

qualitative (kwol′ĭ-ta″tiv) [L. *qualitativus*] 1. pertaining to quality.

2. pertaining to a test or measurement that determines the presence or absence of a particular property or condition. Cf. *quantitative* and *semiquantitative.*

qualitative analysis see *qualitative a.* under *analysis.*

quality (kwol′i-te) [L. *qualitas*] 1. a distinguishing or identifying characteristic.

2. the degree of excellence, or the degree of conformance to a predetermined standard.

3. in radiology, pertaining to those properties of x-rays controlled by the kilovoltage: wavelength and energy of the x-ray photons and hardness and penetrability of the beam. Cf. *quantity.*

quality control (QC) a system instituted to maintain either the quality of performance or the output of a technical operation at a level that has been established as acceptable to the user. It involves the setting of quality standards, continual appraisal of conformance to these standards, and (in the absence of conformance) taking corrective action to establish or maintain the predetermined levels of performance. Both intra- and interlaboratory QC are utilized in the clinical laboratory.

Intralaboratory QC extends to all facets of the testing process. It involves the selection and use of laboratory methods, performances of tests, and reporting of test results; the collection and handling of specimens; the selection, calibration, and maintenance of equipment; the selection and use of reagents, controls, standards, and supplies; the selection, monitoring, and education of personnel; and the development, documentation, use, and review of all testing processes.

Interlaboratory QC has two principal forms: survey programs (proficiency surveys), in which large numbers of laboratories analyze the same unknown specimen, and regional QC programs, in which laboratories in a geographic area use the same lots of QC specimens on a daily basis. In both forms, the results obtained by an individual laboratory are compared with those of the group as an indicator of the current level of performance.

Also called quality assurance. For more information, see the related information under blood banking, clinical chemistry, clinical microbiology, hematology, and nuclear medicine. See also *calibration, proficiency survey,* and *quality control chart.*

quality control chart a plot of the results of analysis for some component of a control specimen or material as a function of time (daily, twice daily, etc). Generally, it is a part of a formal QC program (e.g., Shewhart or Levy-Jennings charts). The value of the mean (or expected value) is shown by a line, as are the established limits of permissible deviation from this expected value (warning and action limits). The chart is examined not only for analytic values falling outside the established acceptable limits of variation, but also for shifts and trends that suggest the presence of nonrandom variations, reflecting systematic changes in the analytic procedure.

quality factor (QF) see *relative biological effectiveness.*

quantile (kwan′tīl) [L. *quantus* how much] in statistics, any value that divides the range of a probability distribution into two groups so that a specified fraction of the distribution lies below this value. If x_p denotes the quantile that gives an individual the probability p of having a value less than x_p and the probability $1 - p$ of having a value greater than x_p, then x_p is often called the 100pth percentile; $x_{1/2}$ the median; and $x_{1/4}$ and $x_{3/4}$ the first and third quantiles.

quantitative (kwon′tĭ-ta″tiv) [L. *quantitativus*] 1. pertaining to quantity.

2. pertaining to a precise numerical measurement. Cf. *qualitative* and *semiquantitative.*

quantitative analysis see *quantitative a.* under *analysis.*

quantity (kwon′tĭ-te) [L. *quantitas*] 1. any number or amount, any measurable property of an object or physical process.

2. in mathematics, any expression that can be evaluated to produce a numerical value.

3. in radiology, the exposure produced by an x-ray beam; the product of beam intensity and exposure time. At fixed kilovoltage, quantity is proportional to the product of time and milliamperage. Cf. *quality.*

quantum (kwon′tum), pl. *quanta* [L. "as much as"] 1. a unit of some physical quantity, such as energy, mass, momentum, or angular momentum. The possible states of a physical system, such as an atom or the electromagnetic field, are restricted to a discrete set of quantum states. As the system changes from one state to another, a whole quantum must be added or subtracted; an infinitesimal change is not possible. This is called a quantum jump or transition.

The quanta of the electromagnetic field are called photons; each has an energy equal to the product of Planck's constant and its frequency. The electrons in an atom are in quantum states (often called orbitals), each characterized by definite states of the quantized variables, energy and angular momentum. An electron can jump from one state to another by emitting or absorbing a photon, which supplies the energy and angular momentum difference between the states. All the possible states can usually be tagged with one or more numbers, called quantum numbers, which order the states by increasing values of quantized variables starting with the lowest or ground state. The branch of physics and chemistry that describes the possible states and interactions of quantized systems is called quantum mechanics.

2. in neurophysiology, a small, discrete packet of a neurotransmitter substance that is released from a single synaptic vesicle.

quantum yield the number of molecules of a specified reactant consumed (or molecules of product produced) in a photochemical reaction or in a photophysical process (such as fluorescence) for each quantum of light absorbed. It is equivalent to moles of reactant per einstein of absorbed light.

quarantine (kwor′an-tēn) [Ital. *quarantina*] one of the earliest methods employed to stop the spread of disease, involving restriction of physical contact between individuals or of entrance to or exit from a place where communicable disease is present. In most cases quarantine is ineffective owing to the occurrence of human reservoirs of infection in symptomless carriers in prodromal, casual, or chronic states. Today the efficiency of this method is further compromised because of extensive air travel. Quarantine is still encouraged by the World Health Organization, however, to protect susceptible populations from plague, cholera, and yellow fever.

quark (quawrk) [from a line in Joyce's *Finnegan's Wake,* "three quarks for Mr. Marks"] any of a group of particles having spin 1/2 and charge either 1/3 or 2/3 of the electron charge. Quarks constitute all particles except leptons; there are three in baryons and two in mesons. There are six known quarks, which have been given the whimsical names of up, down, strange, charmed, bottom, and top. They interact by the so-called color force, which increases with distance, making it impossible to produce an isolated quark.

quartile (kwar′til) [L. *quartas* one-fourth] in statistics, one of the values that divides a population or sample into four equal parts with regard to frequency; e.g., in the frequency distribution, one-fourth score below the first quartile, one-half below the second quartile (median), and three-fourths below the third quartile. See also *percentile* and *quantile.*

quartz (kworts) [Ger. *Quarz*] crystalline silicon dioxide (silica), SiO_2. Quartz glass cuvets are used for ultraviolet spectrometry (wavelengths below 340 nm) because they are transparent in this region of the spectrum and ordinary glass is not.

quasi- (kwa′zi) [L. "as if, as though"] a prefix word element to denote seemingly, or resembling, e.g., quasidiploid.

quasidiploid (kwa″zi-dip′loid) [*quasi-* + *diploid,* from Gr. *diploos* twofold] 1. having two sets of chromosomes but with an abnormal distribution; e.g., a chromosome of one pair may be missing and may be replaced by an extra chromosome from another pair. Discovered during the analysis of the chromosomal constitution of cultured tissue cells, this phenomenon is important in genetic studies.

2. an organism or cell that is quasidiploid. Cf. *diploid.*

quasiperiodic (kwa″zi-pe″re-od′ik) [*quasi-* + *periodic*] in electroencephalography, a term used to describe any pattern of electric activity occurring at intervals that approach regularity but in fact are not regular. Also called *pseudoperiodic.*

quaternary (kwah′ter-ner″e, kwah-ter′nah-re) [L. *quaternarius,* from *quattuor* four] fourth in order or containing four elements or groups. In organic chemistry, quaternary refers to a carbon or nitrogen atom that is bonded to four carbon atoms, i.e., CR_4, or R_4N^+ (a quaternary ammonium ion). Quaternary ammonium compounds are widely used for antisepsis and for disinfecting food utensils and medical instruments. They act by disrupting cell membranes and, through their detergent action, dissolving lipid films that may protect bacteria.

quaternary structure the association of several protein monomers into a larger unit. The monomers are held together by the same forces that create secondary and tertiary structure, hydrophobic bonding being the most important. For example, hemoglobin, A, $\alpha_2\beta_2$, is composed of two alpha monomers and two beta monomers.

Queckenstedt's test (kwek′en-stets″) [Hans Heinrich Georg *Queckenstedt,* German physician, 1876–1918] a maneuver performed in conjunction with a lumbar puncture to determine whether there is a block in the cerebrospinal fluid pathway in the spinal subarachnoid space. Following lumbar puncture, CSF pressure is recorded using a manometer. Bilateral manual pressure is exerted on the jugular veins, hindering blood flow from the cranium and thus raising the intracranial pressure. If no CSF pathway block is present, the CSF pressure will increase. If a block is present, however, this manipulation will have little or no effect on CSF pressure in the lumbar sac.

Contrast-medium myelography may be required for determination of the cause of any obstruction that is present. This test should not be performed if intracranial disease is suspected, particularly when there is increased intracranial pressure, as further pressure increases may force the medulla and cerebellum through the foramen magnum, with potentially fatal consequences.

Quellung test (kwel′lung) [Ger. "swelling"] a serologic test for the identification of the pneumococcus. A suspension of bacteria from a colony suspected of being pneumococci is mixed with specific antiserum and a dye, and examined microscopically. A positive reaction (a greatly swollen capsule surrounding each bacterium, called Quellung) identifies the organism as *Streptococcus pneumoniae.* The reaction is type-specific for the capsular antigen. Both polyvalent combined antisera and monotypic antisera are employed in practical laboratory identification. Before the advent of antibiotics, pneumococcus typing was a necessary diagnostic tool for determining the proper antiserum to use for therapy.

quenching (kwench′ing) any type of interference that reduces the intensity of fluorescence, such as the transfer of excitation energy from a fluorescent molecule to a nonfluorescent molecule, the absorption of fluorescent energy by colored compounds in the sample or by the cuvet surface, or the binding of the fluorescent molecule by chemical agents so that fluorescence is either shifted in wavelength or eliminated. See also *fluorometry* and *liquid scintillation counter.*

queue (kew) a computer data structure that provides first in, first out (FIFO) access to the data. Only the first item placed in the queue is available for use until it is removed. When an item is removed, the next item becomes available. Cf. *stack.*

queuing theory a branch of probability theory that deals with the behavior of queues (waiting lines). The theory is used to determine parameters of interest, such as the average waiting time for a customer and the average amount of time each server is busy.

Customers arrive at various times (arrival times) and either are waited on by a free server or join a queue if all servers are busy. If either the service times, the arrival times, or both are random processes, the customer waiting times, the number of customers in line, and the number of busy servers are all random variables.

In industrial engineering, queuing theory is used to determine the relation between the number of items being processed by a system, the number of items in the queue, and the percentage of time that the system is productive (the load factor).

Quide (kwīd) trademark. See *piperacetazine.*

quiet wakefulness see *s. stages* under *sleep.*

quinacrine hydrochloride (kwin′ah-krin) [USP], a synthetic drug similar to quinine and formerly used to treat malaria. In cytogenetics, it is used as a fluorescent stain. Trademark, *Atabrine.* See under *chromosome banding.*

quinethazone (kwin-eth′ah-zōn) [USP], a thiazide-like diuretic; see under *thiazide diuretics.*

quinhydrone electrode (kwin″hi-drōn′) a reference electrode consisting of a gold or platinum electrode in a suspension of quinhydrone in an electrolyte. Quinhydrone is an equimolar compound of quinone and hydroquinone. This electrode can be used in conjunction with the calomel electrode for measurement of the hydrogen-ion activities of water solutions.

quinidine (kwin′ĭ-din) a dextrorotatory isomer of quinine, used for the treatment of various cardiac arrhythmias, particularly premature beats, and for the maintenance of normal heart rhythm after direct current electrical cardioversion of atrial fibrillation of tachycardia. It acts by lengthening the refractory period of repolarization necessary between successive depolarizations (beats), slows the conduction velocity of the excitation wave, and also produces the anticholinergic effects of vasodilation and hypotension, particularly in large doses. Adverse reactions include gastrointestinal intolerance, hypersensitivity, cinchonism (ringing in the ears, headache, and visual disturbances), and cardiac arrhythmias.

Therapeutic quinidine concentrations in plasma are 2.3–5 μg/ml; toxic concentrations are above 10 μg/ml.

q. gluconate, [USP], a salt of quinidine used for oral intramuscular, and intravenous administration.

q. polygalacturonate, a salt of quinidine used for oral administration.

q. sulfate, [USP], a salt of quinidine used for oral administration.

quinidine assays 1. fluorometric assay based on the fluorescence of quinidine and several metabolites in acid. See under *quinine assays.*

2. EMIT homogeneous enzyme immunoassay for quinidine in serum.

3. high-pressure liquid chromatography (HPLC). After extraction of alkalinized plasma with toluene, the extract is chromatographed on a reverse-phase column using an ultraviolet detector.

quinine (kwin′in, kwin-ēn′, kwi′nīn) [Sp. *quina* cinchona bark, from Quechuan (Inca) *kina* bark] a bitter alkaloid extracted from the bark of the cinchona plant, first found to cure malaria in the fifteenth century. Quinine is still used, often with pyrimethamine and a sulfonamide, to treat strains of malarial parasites that are resistant to less toxic drugs such as chloroquine. To treat severe cases and complications such as cerebral malaria, quinine is administered intravenously. Adverse effects include upset stomach, mental dullness, and headache; mild overdoses cause visual and hearing disturbances (cinchonism); large overdoses can cause hypotension and heart failure.

q. dihydrochloride, the form of quinine used for intravenous administration.

q. sulfate, [USP], the form of quinine used for oral administration.

quinine assays 1. fluorometric determination. Quinine and its isomer quinidine are extracted from samples of alkalinized plasma, urine, or reference solution into an organic solvent and reextracted into dilute acid. Quinine and quinidine fluoresce at 445–450 nm when excited at 250 nm.

2. thin-layer chromatography. Quinidine and quinine can be separated by extraction as in method 1 and by chromatography, using silica gel G plates and cyclohexane-chloroform-diethylamine (5:4:1) developing solvent. Quinine has an R_f value of approximately 0.07 and quinidine 0.15. The spots are detected by spraying with dilute acid and irradiation with 255-nm ultraviolet light.

3. ultraviolet spectrophotometry. Extraction is as in method 1; the concentration of quinine or quinidine at 250 nm is proportional to the sample concentration. Papaverine, primaquine, and chloroquine have similar spectra.

4. gas chromatography. A moderately polar column packing and a flame ionization detector are used. Quinine and quinidine are extracted into organic solvent, methylated using trimethylanilinium hydroxide (TMAH), and chromatographed; their retention times are the same. The sample concentration is proportional to the ratio of the quinine peak height compared with that of the internal standard, cinchonidine. The sensitivity of the assay is 0.2 μg/ml.

quinolinic acid (kwin″o-lin′ic) a dicarboxylic acid formed from the metabolism of tryptophan. It is an intermediate in the biosynthesis of NAD^+.

quinone (kwi-nōn′, kwin′ōn) 1. a yellow crystalline solid with an irritating odor, 2,5-cyclohexadiene-1,4-dione, the oxidized form of hydroquinone. It is a strong irritant to the skin and respiratory tract. Also called benzoquinone.

2. any compound formed by the oxidation of an aromatic diol, producing two carbonyl groups conjugated with the double bonds in a fully unsaturated ring. Cf. *hydroquinone.*

quinovose (kwin′o-vōs) 6-deoxy-D-glucose, occurring in some plant glycolipids. Also called epifucose, D-epirhamnose, D-isorhamnose, and isorhodeose.

quinquevalent (kwing″kwĕ-va′lent) [L. *quinque* five + *valens* powerful] see *pentavalent.*

quinsy (kwin′ze) [L. *quinancia,* from Gr. *kynanchē* sore throat] see *peritonsillar abscess.*

quotient (kwo′shent) the result of the division of one number by another.

Q wave any initial negative deflection that occurs at the onset of the QRS complex of the electrocardiogram and is followed by a positive deflection (R wave). The term Q wave is part of a terminology representative of the order and polarity of the deflections constituting the QRS complex.

R

R symbol for *arginine,* the *gas constant, resistance, roentgen.*

R- (L. *rectus* right) a stereodescriptor used to indicate the configuration at an asymmetric carbon atom, e.g., (*R*)-2,3,dihydroxypropanal (D-glyceraldehyde); see also *isomerism.*

R_E abbrev. See *respiratory exchange ratio.*

R_e abbrev. See *Reynold's number.*

R_f in paper or thin-layer chromatography, the distance that a spot of a substance has moved from the point of application, expressed as a fraction of the distance that the solvent front has moved. The R_f value of a substance depends on the adsorbent and solvent system being used, but substances can be identified by their R_f values in one or more developing systems. R_f values also vary somewhat with temperature and developing time. Cf. R_{st}.

R_{st} in paper or thin-layer chromatography, the distance that a spot of a substance has moved, relative to the distance that a reference standard spot has moved, expressed as a ratio. Cf. R_f.

r symbol for the radius (of a circle), *ribose,* ring chromosome, sample correlation coefficient.

ρ the Greek lower case letter *rho;* symbol for: (1) correlation coefficient, (2) mass density, (3) electric charge density.

RA abbrev. See *rheumatoid arthritis.*

Ra symbol for the chemical element *radium.*

rabbit aorta–contracting substance (RCS) a mixture of prostaglandins, i.e., PGG_2, PGH_2, and TXA_2, released during anaphylaxis in the lungs of sensitized rabbits; it causes strong bronchoconstriction. See also *prostaglandin endoperoxide.*

rabbit papilloma a viral disease of rabbits marked by the formation of horny warts. These papillomas were the first mammalian tumors shown to be induced by a virus and the first to be transmitted by purified viral DNA. Also called *Shope papilloma.*

rabies (ra′bēz, ra′be-ēz) [L. "madness," from *rabere* to rage] an acute, infectious viral disease of the central nervous system that affects all mammals including humans. This disease is transmitted from the saliva of an infected animal to a new host through bites or the licking of open wounds. The etiologic agent of rabies is the rabies virus, a bullet-shaped, double-stranded RNA virus belonging to the rhabdovirus group. The most common source of infection worldwide is the dog, with cats as the second most common source; in the United States, skunks and bats are currently the most common reservoir. Rats, squirrels, and foxes also are sources of infection.

The incubation period of the rabies virus in humans varies from 10 da to 1 yr, depending on the size of the inoculum and the site of infection. Initially there is fever, anorexia, headache, malaise, sore throat, and abnormal sensation around the site of infection. If the disease progresses, there are spasmodic contractions of the throat, hydrophobia, convulsive seizures, paralysis, and eventually death.

The virus may be isolated from the saliva or infected tissue by intracerebral inoculation into suckling mice. Rabies viral antigens may be demonstrated in tissue by using the fluorescent antibody staining technique. Neutralizing antibodies to rabies virus in serum increase at least fourfold during acute infection. Histologically, neurons show intracytoplasmic inclusion bodies known as Negri bodies.

If the biting animal can be captured, it should be observed for signs of illness for at least 10 da. The bite wound should be cleaned with a soap solution, then with solutions of alcohol, iodine, or quaternary ammonium compounds, to reduce the number of virus particles. Rabies vaccine is sufficient for minor exposures, if postexposure treatment is necessary. Today, human diploid cell vaccine is preferred to duck embryo vaccine, as the former has lower rates of all serious adverse reactions than the latter.

In the past, rabies has been 100 percent fatal in injected humans; in recent years, however, instances of recovery have been seen following vigorous supportive therapy.

See also *rhabdovirus.*

rabies virus a bullet-shaped virus that is the etiologic agent of rabies and belongs to the rhabdovirus group. The envelope of the rabies virus causes the production of neutralizing and hemagglutination-inhibition antibodies; the nucleocapsid elicits a complement-fixing antibody response. See also *rabies.*

race (rās) a subspecies, i.e., an interbreeding population distiguishable from the rest of the species by a difference in several characteristic gene frequencies. The term is usually applied to geographically isolated groups. Also called *subspecies.*

RA cell abbrev. See *ragocyte.*

racemase (ra′sĕ-mās) a subclass of enzymes in the isomerase class (EC 5.1) that catalyzes the racemization of a center of chirality in a substrate.

racemate (ra′sĕ-māt) a crystalline compound formed when many racemic modifications crystallize. Racemates are 1:1 association compounds that melt above, below, or at the same temperature as the separate enantiomers. In the solid state, a racemic modification may also exist as a conglomerate or racemic mixture (eutectic mixtures), with the melting point always below that of the separate enantiomers.

racemic (ra-se′mik) being composed of two enantiomorphic isomers and therefore optically inactive.

racemic mixture one of the crystalline forms of a racemic form. It is a simple 1:1 eutectic mixture of the two enantiomers in which each crystal is a single enantiomer. The racemic mixture has a lower melting point than that of the separate enantiomers. Also called *conglomerate.* See also *racemate.*

racemic modification an equimolar (1:1) mixture of enantiomers. Because the optical rotations of the two enantiomers cancel, the racemic modification has no optical activity. A racemic modification is indicated by the prefix (±)- (formerly *dl-*) for example, (±)-tartaric acid.

racemization (ra″sĕ-mĭ-za′shun) the process by

which a single enantiomer is reversibly converted into a racemic modification. In this process the optical rotation proceeds from some finite value (+ or –) toward zero when equilibration is complete. See also *isomerism*. Cf. *mutarotation*.

rachi/o (ra′ke-o) [Gr. *rhachis* spine] a word element used in combining form to denote the spinal column, e.g., rachischisis.

rachischisis (ra-kis′kĭ-sis) [*rachi-* + Gr. *schisis* cleft] a congenital condition characterized by fissure, incomplete closure, or absence of vertebrae of the spinal column. Cord aplasia is seen, and neural covering elements are frequently absent. This condition may be minor and asymptomatic or incompatible with life, depending on the severity of the defect. Diagnosis is based on clinical appearance and radiographic profiles. See also *s. b. cystica* under *spina bifida*.

r. posterior, see *s. b. cystica* under *spina bifida*.

racial (ra′shul) pertaining to a particular race.

racquet hypha (rak′et hi′fah) a type of hypha in which one end of each segment is larger than the other end, the overall appearance being similar to a chain of tennis racquets. Also called racquet mycelium.

rad (rad) [acronym from *r*adiation *a*bsorbed *d*ose] 1. a unit of absorbed dose of ionizing radiation defined as the transfer of 100 ergs of energy per gram of absorber (0.01 J/kg). Cf. *rem*.
2. abbrev. See *radian*.

Radford nomogram a nomogram used to predict the minimal (basal) tidal volume necessary for adequate alveolar ventilation in individuals with various body weights and breathing frequencies (or rates of mechanical ventilation). The minimal tidal volume is the point on the nomogram where the straight line that connects the body weight (in kilograms or pounds) and breathing frequency (in cycles per minute) intersects the predicted basal tidal volume line. Corrections must be made for the presence of physical activity, fever, apparatus used to assist breathing, and tracheostomy, and for the dead space volume of masks or other apparatus. A larger tidal volume than that predicted is needed to adequately oxygenate the blood of individuals with abnormal lungs.

radi/o (ra′de-o) a word element used in combining form to denote radius, rays, or radiation, e.g., radiocarpal, radioactivity.

radial (ra′de-al) [L. *radialis*] pertaining to a radius, directed parallel to a radius.

radial artery one of the two terminal branches of the brachial artery. It begins just below the elbow joint, runs around the radial side of the forearm to the wrist, then between the first and second metacarpal bones into the palm, where it meets the deep branch of the ulnar artery in the deep palmar arch.

radial immunodiffusion a method for determining the concentration of antigen or antibody. Either the antigen or (more commonly) the antibody is uniformly contained in agar. The remaining reactant, antigen or antibody, is placed into a well cut into the agar. A series of wells are formed to allow a range of reactant concentrations. With time, the antigen (or antibody) diffuses radially into the agar, forming a precipitin ring at the zone of equivalence (see *precipitin curve*).

The diameter of the ring is quantitatively related to the concentration of the reactant. If the reaction is allowed to proceed until the ring stops enlarging, the method is known as limit diffusion. In this procedure, the diameter of the ring squared is linearly proportional to the concentration of the reactant. If the method is timed with respect to ring enlargement, the logarithm of the reactant concentration will be linearly proportional to the ring diameter. Therefore, known standards are run at the same time as the unknown antigen or antibody, and a standard curve is generated on which unknown concentrations are determined.

Mancini radial immunodiffusion is most often used to detect certain antigens related to specific infectious disease, e.g., the concentrations of immunoglobulins IgG, IgM, or IgA, or certain complement proteins, especially C3 and C5, in a patient's serum.

radial nerve a nerve that arises from the posterior cord of the brachial plexus. It descends behind the axillary and brachial arteries and runs around the back of the humerus to pierce the lateral intermuscular septum and enter the anterior compartment of the arm. On the front of the lateral epicondyle, it divides into superficial and deep branches. The superficial branch continues down the lateral side of the forearm to form four or five dorsal digital nerves. The deep branch (posterior interosseous nerve) curves backward around the radius to the back of the forearm to supply extensor muscles and the wrist joint.

radian (ra′de-an) a measure of angle defined as $1/2\pi$ of a full circle. It is approximately equal to 57.295°.

radiant (ra′de-ant) [L. *radians*, present participle of *radiare* to emit rays] 1. diverging from a center.
2. emitting rays of light.

radiant energy energy propagated through space. Usually, the energy carried by photons (light, x-rays, or gamma rays) is the intended reference, but the term may also refer to energy carried by other particles.

radiation (ra″de-a′shun) [L. *radiatio*] 1. divergence from a common center or a common origin.
2. a structure composed of divergent elements, as one of the fiber tracts in the brain.
3. the propagation of waves through space or through a material medium, e.g., electromagnetic waves or sound waves.
4. a stream of particles emitted by a radioactive material.

radiation dose see *radiation d.* under *dose*.

radiation effects the biologic effects of ionizing radiation, which may be classified as short-term somatic, long-term somatic, and genetic effects.

Short-term somatic effects, ranging from erythema (skin reddening) to death, are usually due to rather large doses received within a short period. The interval between dose and effect is generally hours to weeks. These effects have thresholds in the sense that the probability of the effect changes rapidly from nearly zero percent to nearly 100 percent over a relatively narrow range (e.g., 200–600 rads for death).

Long-term somatic effects include induction of leukemia and other malignant neoplasms. These radiation-induced effects are indistinguishable from those occurring naturally. There can be a latency period of years or decades between receipt of radiation and clinical onset of disease. The relationship between dose and effect at high-radiation doses has been established by the statistical study of disease incidence in irradiated populations, such as the survivors of the Hiroshima and Nagasaki atomic blasts. It has been very difficult, however, to establish reliable estimates of the dose-response relationship at low doses because of the low probability of effect. The topic is highly controversial, but there seems to be a consensus that there is no threshold dose or dose rate below which somatic effects are nonexistent. A linear relationship between dose and effect is often assumed.

Cellular growth and development can be affected by radiation. This is of particular concern for fetuses and infants, as rapidly growing and dividing cells are particularly sensitive to radiation damage, and it has led to a careful assessment of the necessity of medical irradiation of females who are or may be in the earliest stages of pregnancy.

Genetic effects are radiation-induced mutations or abnormalities in subsequent generations. These effects are assumed to have no threshold and a linear dose-response relationship. Radiation-induced genetic effects are indistinguishable from those occurring naturally. It has been estimated that natural genetic defects cause approximately 10 percent of all humans to fail to reproduce, or to die before maturity. The best estimate of genetically permissible doses is provided by naturally occurring radioactivity (about 0.1 rad/yr at sea level).

ARTHUR E. BURGESS, PH.D.

radiation hazard a danger to health due to exposure to ionizing radiation.

radiation measuring units units of activity and radiation dose. The activity of a radioactive source is measured in terms of the curie (Ci), defined as 3.7×10^{10} disintegrations/sec. A new coherent International System (SI) unit, the bequerel (Bq), has been proposed; it is defined as 1 disintegration/sec ($1\ s^{-1}$). Thus, 1 Ci = 37 GBq, and 1 μCi = 37 kBq. Radiation dose is the energy deposited in an absorber by radiation and is measured in three different kinds of units: the roentgen; the rad and its SI equivalent, the gray; and the rem.

The roentgen (R) is used only for x-rays and gamma rays. It is defined in terms of the ionization produced in a sample of air at standard temperature and pressure (STP): 2.58×10^{-4} coulombs of ions of each polarity are released per kilogram of air.

The rad applies to all types of radiation. It is defined as a depression of 100 ergs of energy per gram of absorber. The new SI unit, the gray (Gy), is defined in terms of joules per kilogram—1 J/kg; therefore, 1 Gy = 100 rads.

The rem measures the biologic effect of radiation. It is defined as the amount of radiation that produces the same biologic effect on living tissue as a standard dose of gamma rays. For beta, gamma, and x-radiation, the rem is approximately equal to the rad. For alpha radiation, 1 rad = approximately 20 rem.

Radiation detection devices are usually calibrated in millirems per hour (mrem/hr) or counts per minute (cpm) for survey meters, and in roentgens or rems for personnel monitoring devices.

radiation oncology see *radiation therapy.*

radiation physicist a physicist who is responsible for certain technical aspects of radiation therapy, such as preparation of isodose curves, preparation of wedge and compensating filters, calibration of teletherapy equipment, and supervision of radiation safety procedures.

radiation protection the establishment and implementation of safety standards with regard to ionizing radiation for the protection of users and the public. Radiation protection is achieved by five main methods: (1) surrounding the radiation sources with highly attenuating materials such as lead; (2) ensuring the physical containment of sources (radioisotopes) that are continually emitting radiation; (3) taking advantage of the reduction of radiation intensity as the inverse square of the distance from the source; (4) carefully limiting exposure time to avoid exceeding the maximal permissible dose; and (5) providing personal radiation monitoring devices to radiation workers to measure the amount of radiation dose received.

International safety standards were first established in 1928. This led to the introduction of a maximal permissible annual dose (MPD) for radiation workers. The value of the MPD was considered to be "safe," given the state of knowledge of the biologic effects on radiation; significantly, it has been reduced a number of times in the light of new knowledge.

Establishing dose limits is difficult because there appears to be no threshold radiation dose or dose rate below which radiation is completely safe. Additionally, radiation effects are very infrequent at low doses; hence, it is an enormous undertaking to measure reliably the relationship between radiation dose and biologic effects when the probability of an effect is in the range of one in one million. The standards are based on a careful subjective assessment of both the benefits and risks of ionizing radiation. The MPD for adults exposed in the course of their work is 5 rem/yr. The limit for members of the public is 0.5 rem/yr. This does not include doses received in the course of medical diagnostic or therapy procedures.

The principal authority is the International Commission on Radiological Protection; a number of countries also have national commissions—the National Council on Radiation Protection and Measurements (NCRP) of the United States, for example. These bodies occasionally publish recommendations on the control and disposal of radioisotopes, radiation measurement methods and instruments, and methods of protection against various types of radiation (e.g., x-rays, high-energy electrons, and neutrons).

ARTHUR E. BURGESS, PH.D.

radiation therapist a physician who specializes in the treatment of disease by means of ionizing radiation. Also called radiation oncologist. Cf. *radiologist.*

radiation therapy the use of high-energy radiations (ionizing radiations) in the treatment of malignant neoplasms and occasionally in the treatment of certain benign conditions. Depending on the type of cancer, its stage of development or spread, and its location within the body, radiation therapy may be used as the primary curative treatment for cancer, as adjunctive treatment to surgery and/or chemotherapy, or for palliation of symptoms in patients who have incurable disease. Some types of cancer are more sensitive to radiation therapy than others. For example, lymphomas are generally very radiosensitive, whereas sarcomas are generally very radioresistant.

Ionizing radiations include high-energy photon radiations (x-rays and gamma rays) as well as high-energy particle radiations (beta rays, electrons, neutrons, or heavy-charge particles). Most commonly, x-rays, gamma rays, and electrons are used in the treatment of cancer.

External radiation therapy (teletherapy) is administered using x-ray, gamma-ray, or electron-producing machines. The more superficial x-ray machines are known as orthovoltage machines and are used in treatment of very superficial cancers, e.g., skin cancer. Higher-energy x-ray (supervoltage or megavoltage) machines (linear accelerators, betatrons, Van de Graaff generators) are used to treat deep-seated tumors. Gamma-ray machines employing cesium-137 are used to treat moderately deep-seated tumors, whereas cobalt-60 is comparable with high-energy x-ray machines for the treatment of deep-seated tumors.

Internal radiation therapy (brachytherapy) is the insertion of radioactive isotopes directly into tumors or tissues surrounding tumors to produce a local concentration of radiations. These implants may be either permanent or removable, depending on the type, location, and condition. The types of radiations used are usually radium-226, cesium-137, cobalt-60, iridium-192, iodine-125, and gold-198.

The selection of which type of teletherapy machine or brachytherapy isotopic source to use depends on the type of cancer being treated, its location, and its responsiveness to radiation. These judgments require the experience of a radiation therapist, a physician trained and specializing in this specialty.

Radiation sensitivity is highly dependent on the oxygen tension within a tissue or tumor. Tumors, particularly in their centers, tend to have less oxygen tension than the normal tissue around them. As the tumors regress under radiation treatments, they become progressively more oxygenated and therefore more sensitive to the radiation. The standard practice of radiation therapy is to fractionate it into many daily treatments, allowing for the recovery of injury to normal tissues and for the reoxygenation of tumor tissues.

Radiation therapy is most useful in treating regional and local disease; only occasionally is it used to treat widespread disease (whole body irradiation). In the treatment of regional and local disease, a "volume of interest" is identified by radiation therapists on the basis of their knowledge of the patterns of spread and involvement of the cancer. Having selected the volume of interest, a prescription is based on a treatment plan that takes into account the location of the tumor and the patterns of potential spread, as well as the normal tissue and organ structures that will be involved within that volume. Doses of radiations delivered are measured in rads, and the distribution of those doses within tissue determines the amount of radiation to be delivered each day, and the length of time involved. Tolerance of normal tissues is determined by these three factors—time, dose, and volume relationship.

Combining radiation treatments with surgery and/or chemotherapy may result in more effective cancer treatment, but the interactions of radiation therapy with normal tissues also may be altered by surgery and/or chemotherapy. These considerations must be included in the treatment plan.

In general, ionizing radiations damage cells by injuring the genetic material (DNA) of the cell. The radiation sensitivity of a tissue or tumor is dependent on how well it is oxygenated, how rapidly it is growing, and its ability to repair injury. More rapidly dividing cells are more easily injured by the radiation therapy. Radiosensitivity is defined as the ability of radiations to change cells within a tumor or a tissue. Radioresponsiveness can be measured in terms of the rate at which these changes take place. Radiocurability is the ability of ionizing radiations to cure malignant tumors for the lifetime of the person being treated, regardless of radiosensitivity or radioresponsiveness. Factors that reduce radiosensitivity, radioresponsiveness, and radiocurability are those factors that reduce the oxygenation of tissues (such as trauma, infection, and necrosis) or in some other way interfere with direct cell injury or cell repair.

In general, patients who are otherwise well and who have good nutrition tolerate radiation therapy best, and very young or old people may tolerate such therapy poorly. In the growing child, radiation therapy may interfere with skeletal and other organ development, and this must be given special consideration when patients in this age group are being treated.

Radiation side-effects are both acute and chronic. Acute side-effects are generally related to the organs being treated and are temporary (diarrhea, soreness of the mouth, redness of the skin). Long-term side-effects, which are the most important, are confined to those organs directly within the path of the radiation and are the limiting factors in determining the total dose of radiations that can be given to a cancer patient.

Also called *radiation oncology, radiotherapy,* and *x-ray therapy.*

SIMEON T. CANTRIL, M.D.

radiation therapy equipment machines using beams of particle energy such as x-rays, gamma rays, or electrons to treat individuals with various types of cancers. The development of radiation therapy (radiotherapy) equipment has progressed from the early x-ray equipment of the first two decades of the twentieth century to the sophisticated high-energy x-ray and particle beam equipment now in daily use. The energy of a beam of radiation, expressed in kilovolts or megavolts, determines both the depth of penetration into the body tissues and the energy of the electrons produced by secondary ionization within the tissues. It is these electrons that cause the desired clinical effect. Beam therapy equipment can be classified into three types:

SUPERFICIAL THERAPY. This utilizes x-ray energies in the range of 10–120 kV. Generally, in the treatment of malignant neoplasms, energies above 45 kV are preferred. Superficial x-ray beams do not penetrate far into the tissues. Almost all the energy is dissipated in the superficial tissues: 80 percent of the beam penetrates just 0.5 cm and 50 percent reaches 2 cm; only 10 percent reaches a depth of 5 cm. Because the energy of the beam is released in the superficial tissue, this type of radiation treatment is used almost exclusively in the treatment of skin cancers.

ORTHOVOLTAGE THERAPY. This utilizes x-ray beams produced by electric energies in the range of

200–500 kV. Such standard x-ray energies were the mainstay of radiotherapy until the development of megavoltage equipment in the 1950s. These beams are more penetrating than superficial x-rays: approximately 50 percent of the beam reaches 10 cm. With several beams approaching a deep-seated tumor from different directions, the amount of radiation delivered to the tumor can be increased to more than that received by the surrounding normal tissues; in this way the normal tissues are protected from excessive radiation. Such orthovoltage beams suffered from a number of drawbacks, which were overcome by the advent of megavoltage therapy.

MEGAVOLTAGE THERAPY. This utilizes beams of radiation with energy in excess of 1 MV. The gamma radiation emitted by cobalt-60 and developed into beam therapy equipment in the early 1950s has a spectrum of energy equivalent to 1.1 MeV and is therefore classified as megavoltage. High-energy x-rays, neutrons, electrons, and other forms of particle therapy fall into the megavoltage classification. Megavoltage beam therapy has three principal advantages over orthovoltage treatment: the depth of penetration is superior, with 70–80 percent of the beam penetrating 10 cm; the maximal energy of the beam is below the surface, resulting in a sparing of radiation to the skin and superficial tissues; and there is less differential absorption of the beam in high-density tissues such as bone, which has resulted in a major reduction in the incidence of bone and cartilage damage from radiation treatment. With the introduction of sophisticated electronics and mechanical systems, these modern beam therapy units are able to deliver radiation treatment in an extremely accurate physical manner and in a short period of time.

S. M. JACKSON, M.D.

radiation therapy technologist a health care professional who delivers courses of radiation therapy under the supervision of a radiation therapist. Duties include positioning and caring for patients; calibrating teletherapy equipment; preparing brachytherapy equipment and handling radioactive materials; assisting the radiation physicist in the preparation of isodose curves, performance of computer estimations, and preparation of wedge and compensating filters; observing the patient for signs of clinical progress or complications that require consultation with the physician; and observing radiation safety measures. Educational preparation involves completion of an accredited program; graduates are certified by the American Registry of Radiologic Technologists and are designated RT(T)(ARRT), Registered Technologist. See also *radiologic technologist.*

radiative capture the capture of a particle (such as a thermal neutron) by a nucleus, in which the gain in binding energy (8 MeV for a neutron) is emitted in the form of gamma rays instead of particles.

radical (rad′ĭ-kal) [L. *radicalis* "having roots," from *radix* root] 1. directed to the cause; directed to the root or source of a pathologic process, e.g., radical surgery.

2. a part of a molecule (often a hydrocarbon portion) in which a group of atoms is considered together as a unit; often called a substituent group.

3. a species that has an unpaired electron. Paramagnetic metal ions are not usually called radicals. This term is preferred by some (e.g., IUPAC) to the equivalent term free radical.

radical scavenger a substance, e.g., diphenylpicrylhydrazyl, that reacts with and removes free radicals formed during a chemical reaction.

radiculitis (rah-dik″u-li′tis) [L. *radicula* radicle, diminutive of *radix* root + *-itis*] a nerve root disorder characterized by inflammation of a spinal nerve, most frequently in the area between the spinal cord and intervertebral canal. This condition may be due to compression, metastatic tumor, infection, or systemic disorders. Ventral root involvement leads to a flaccid muscle weakness, and to atrophy if the condition is chronic. Dorsal root involvement results in sensory loss or pain in the dermatome of that root. Tendon reflexes also are commonly diminished. Radiography, electromyography, computerized tomographic scanning, and myelography may be useful in the diagnosis.

radiculoganglionitis (rah-dik″u-lo-gang″gle-o-ni′tis) [L. *radicula,* dim. of *radix* root + *ganglion* + *-itis*] inflammation of the posterior spinal nerve roots and their ganglions.

radiculomeningomyelitis (rah-dik″u-lo-mĕ-ning″go-mi″ĕ-li′tis) [L. *radicula* + Gr. *meninx* membrane + *myelos* spinal cord + *-itis*] inflammation of the nerve roots, meninges, and spinal cord.

radiculomyelopathy (rah-dik″u-lo-mi″ĕ-lop′ah-the) [L. *radicula* + Gr. *myelos* spinal cord + *pathos* suffering] disease of the nerve roots and spinal cord.

radiculoneuropathy (rah-dik″u-lo-nu-rop′ah-the) [radicula + Gr. *neuron* nerve + *pathos* suffering] a general term for any disease of the nerve roots and spinal nerves.

radiculopathy (rah-dik″u-lop′ah-the) [*radicula* + Gr. *pathos* suffering] a clinical condition associated with a lesion of a spinal nerve or nerve root that may be accompanied by a severe weakness and atrophy of the segmentally innervated muscles. The most common abnormal associated diagnostic finding is the appearance of positive waves in the electromyogram; fibrillation potentials and an increased incidence of polyphasic potentials may also occur.

The positive waves or other abnormal electrical activity found in a particular nerve root distribution generally appear first in the paraspinous muscles.

radio- (ra′de-o) [L. *radius* ray] a word element used in combining form to denote relationship to a ray or radiation. The term is sometimes employed with specific reference to the emission of radiant energy (e.g., radioactive), to radium, or to the radial bone of the forearm (e.g., radiocarpal); it may also be affixed to the name of a chemical element to designate a radioactive isotope of that particular element, e.g., radiocarbon, radioiodine.

radioactive (ra″de-o-ak′tiv) having the property of radioactivity.

radioactive concentration the activity of a designated radionuclide divided by the volume in which it is dissolved, usually expressed in curies per milliliter (Ci/ml).

radioactive constant see *decay constant.*

radioactive decay the spontaneous transformation of one nuclide into another nuclide by the emission of particles, or the spontaneous fission of a nuclide into several nuclides and particles.

radioactive drug any therapeutic or diagnostic

agent, in the usage of the Food and Drug Administration, that contains a radionuclide that emits nuclear particles or photons; the term also refers to nonradioactive reagent kits or radionuclide generators used in the preparation of such agents. The term does not refer to drugs containing traces of naturally occurring radionuclides, such as carbon-14.

radioactive iodine uptake test (RAIU) see under *thyroid uptake tests.*

radioactive waste radiochemicals and any material that has become contaminated with radioactivity and that has no further use. Such materials must be handled, stored, and disposed of in accordance with government regulations.

radioactivity (ra″de-o-ak-tiv′ĭ-te) 1. a phenomenon exhibited by unstable isotopes of chemical elements (radioisotopes) that undergo radioactive decay by various modes (alpha decay, beta decay, positron emission, electron capture, isomeric transition, or spontaneous fission) emitting various high-energy particles: alpha particles (helium nuclei), beta particles (electrons), positrons, gamma rays (photons), and neutrons. A constant fraction of the remaining (undecayed) atoms decay in every unit time period; this fraction is λ, the decay constant.

The number of remaining atoms constantly decreases; as does the number of decaying atoms. The amount of radioisotope remaining at time t is given by the equation $A = A_0e^{-\lambda t}$, where A_0 is the amount at $t = 0$. The time required for the amount to decrease by half is called the half-life ($T_{1/2}$).

2. the particles emitted by a radioactive substance.

3. the rate at which a radioactive substance decays, usually termed its activity (A); it is expressed in terms of the curie (Ci), 3.7×10^{10} decays/sec, or the new SI unit of activity, the bequerel (Bq), 1 decay/sec.

radioallergosorbent test (RAST) (ra″de-o-al″ergo-sor′bent) a radioimmunoassay test for detecting specific IgE antibody, which involves coating a sorbent matrix with allergen. The most commonly used sorbents are complex carbohydrates such as Sephadex, microcrystalline cellulose particles, or agarose beads. Paper disks or polystyrene tubes, which are most convenient but do not have the sensitivity of the carbohydrates, may also be used.

In this procedure, the test serum is added to the allergen-coated particles and incubated. Excess serum is then washed away and radiolabeled anti-IgE is added. The excess is washed away, and the radioactivity bound to the antibody on the allergen-sorbent complex is then measured. The amount of antibody present is quantitated by comparing it with a standard reference serum.

RAST generally provides no more information than direct skin testing, which is less expensive and provides immediate results. Thus, skin testing is currently the preferred means for diagnosing IgE-mediated disorders. There are clinical situations, however, in which RAST may be useful: e.g., in severe dermatitis, which makes skin tests difficult to interpret, or in patients taking antihistamines that cannot be withdrawn. RAST may also be useful for those with highly suggestive clinical histories but negative skin tests.

The principal problem with RAST at this time is the difficulty of transforming the results into clinically significant data. Correlation between RAST and skin testing is good if the same allergen is used for both. Unfortunately, the availability of the same allergen for both tests is rare; none of the commercially available RAST kits is standardized with respect to skin testing. Two additional problems frequently occur with commercially available RAST kits: (1) many kits are provided for allergies that have never been proved to be IgE-mediated, including many foods and drugs such as codeine and local anesthetics; and (2) a number of scoring schemes have been promoted that supposedly increase the sensitivity of the assay, when actually they result in false-positive reactions.

radioassay (ra″de-o-as′a) any assay in which a radioactively labeled material is used directly or indirectly in carrying out the analysis; for example, (1) the quantitation of some analyte by dilution of a known volume of specimen with a known quantity of radio-tagged analyte and measurement of the degree of dilution of the labeled analyte (e.g., serum calcium with ^{45}Ca); (2) a term used to designate a form of ligand assay in which the compound to be measured and a radioactively tagged form of the same compound compete for the same binding sites on some specific binding protein (e.g., thyroxine competing with labeled T_4 for thyroxine antibody binding sites); (3) the assay of some protein or other compound with specific binding properties, which is carried out by adding an excess of radioactively labeled ligand and measuring the quantity of ligand bound by the compound (e.g., transferrin with ^{59}Fe); and (4) the quantitation of enzyme activity by measuring the rate of incorporation of a radioactively labeled substrate into a product (e.g., TdT activity).

radioautography (ra″de-o-aw-tog′rah-fe) see *autoradiography.*

radiobiology (ra″de-o-bi-ol′o-je) [*radio-* + Gr. *bios* life + *logos* reason, discourse] the branch of science concerned with effects of light and of ultraviolet and ionizing radiations on living tissue or organisms.

radiocarpal (ra″de-o-kar′pal) [*radio-* + L. *carpus,* from Gr. *karpos* wrist] pertaining to the region of articulation between the radius and carpus.

radiocarpal joint see *wrist joint.*

radiochemical purity in a radiopharmaceutical, the percentage of total activity of the designated radionuclide emitted by the desired chemical form of the nuclide.

radiochromatogram (ra″de-o-kro-mat′o-gram) [*radio-* + Gr. *chrōma* color + *gramma* mark, drawing] a graphic record of the separation of radioactive substances by paper or thin-layer chromatography. The radioactivity along the chromatogram can be measured by passing it through appropriate counters. The measured radioactivity is plotted as a function of the R_f value; each separated radioactive substance produces a distinct peak. Autoradiography with an emulsion applied directly to a thin-layer chromatography (TLC) plate or paper chromatogram is also used.

radiocurability (ra″de-o-kūr″ah-bil′ĭ-te) the degree to which a type of tumor can be cured by radiation therapy. See also *radiation therapy.*

radiodense (ra″de-o-dens′) [*radio-* + L. *densus* thick, dense] absorbing x-rays; radiopaque.

radiodensity (ra″de-o-den′sĭ-te) the resistance of a material to the passage of radiation; radiopacity.

radiodermatitis (ra″de-o-der-mah-ti′tis) [*radio-* + Gr. *derma* skin + *-itis*] a cutaneous inflammatory reaction to exposure to biologically effective levels of ionizing radiation; x-ray dermatitis.

radioencephalography (ra″de-o-en-sef″ah-log′-rah-fe) the recording of changes in the electric potential of the brain without direct attachment between the recording apparatus and the subject, the impulses being beamed by radio waves from the subject to the receiver. See also *electroencephalography.*

radiograph (ra′de-o-graf″) [*radio-* + Gr. *graphein* to write or draw] the permanent record on photographic film of a radiologic examination. The film shows the radiographic shadows produced by differences in radiodensity among the various structures or introduced contrast media through which the beam has passed. It demonstrates the presence or absence of certain pathologic or traumatic changes in these structures. Also called *roentgenogram.* Formerly called skiagram.

radiographer (ra″de-og′rah-fer) a radiologic technologist whose work is the making of diagnostic radiographs. Duties include positioning patients for radiologic examinations; determining the proper voltage, current, and exposure time for each radiograph and adjusting the x-ray equipment; producing those radiographs requested by the physician; developing the x-ray film; and assisting the radiologist in special procedures. Educational preparation involves completion of an approved program; graduates are certified by the American Registry of Radiologic Technologists and are designated RT(ARRT), Registered Technologist. See also *radiologic technologist.*

radiographic (ra″de-o-graf′ik) pertaining to the making of radiographs.

radiographic effect the image density produced by x-rays falling on a film. The radiographic effect (re) is proportional to the milliamperage (mA) and the exposure time (s), is inversely proportional to the focal-film distance (d), and is approximately proportional to the square of the kilovoltage (kVP): re = (mA) (s) $(\text{kVp})^2/d^2$.

radiography (ra″de-og′rah-fe) [*radio-* + Gr. *graphein* to write] the making of diagnostic radiographs.

radioimmunoassay (RIA) (ra″de-o-im″u-no-as′a) a laboratory procedure that measures minute quantities of a variety of substances by combining the sensitivity of a radioisotope measurement with the specificity of an antibody. A number of other techniques such as radioligand assay, competitive protein binding, saturation analysis, and displacement analysis use the same basic principle. When a receptor or high-affinity protein rather than an antibody is employed as the binder, these assays are named radioassays, radioreceptor assays, competitive protein binding assays, or radioligand assays. RIAs should not be confused with immunoradiometric assays, in which an antibody instead of an antigen is labeled and no competition or displacement occurs.

Since the pioneering work of Berson and Yalow with insulin in the 1950s, RIA has been used to detect a variety of compounds. Substances now routinely measured by this technique include hormones, vitamins, drugs, cancer antigens, enzymes, receptors, viruses, antibodies, polypeptides, and other proteins. Before the use of RIA, many of these compounds either could not be quantitated or were measured by time-consuming and laborious procedures (e.g., bioassays) not readily adaptable to the clinical laboratory on a routine basis. RIA has advanced over a 10-yr period from manual to semiautomated, and finally to totally automated methodology. RIA has had far-reaching effects on a variety of disciplines, including endocrinology, pharmacology, immunology, microbiology, oncology, and hematology.

A requirement for RIA is the availability of substance to be measured in a pure form. Once obtained, this substance is utilized to produce antibodies for the preparation of a tracer by attaching a radioactive isotope to it and for the preparation of standards. In the case of proteins, obtaining the antigen in an uncontaminated form is often a problem and usually involves exhaustive purification procedures that usually provide low yields of the material of interest. This has made it difficult, if not impossible, to standardize some assays adequately. Recombinant DNA methodology offers a means by which purified human proteins can be synthesized, and potentially could solve some existing standardization problems. Many of the polypeptide hormone assays are currently being standardized against World Health Organization (WHO) preparations of highly purified substances.

The clinical utility of a radioimmunoassay is heavily dependent on the production of a suitable antibody. For the higher-molecular-weight substances (usually proteins or glycoproteins with M.W. $>10{,}000$), this involves injecting animals (most commonly rabbits, goats, and sheep) with the purified substance to be measured on a regular schedule, and bleeding them periodically until the appropriate titer of antibody is obtained. Not all animals respond, and those that do often produce different families of antibodies with different titers. The relatively new hybridoma technique to produce monoclonal antibodies is becoming popular and may eventually replace the older methods of producing antibodies. Substances of low molecular weight (<3000) that cannot directly elicit antibody production are called haptens and require a different approach for assay. By one of a variety of methods, haptens are covalently linked to substances of higher molecular weight, such as bovine serum albumin, so that the antigenic response can be elicited against the attached hapten. The site of the covalent bond is important so that the antibody will recognize the functional group of the hapten.

Some common techniques for radioactive labeling of the antigen are the use of chloramine-T lactoperoxidase iodination, Bolten-Hunter iodination, and tritiation. Following the radiolabeling procedure, it is necessary to purify the labeled substance, usually by chromatography, to ensure that the only labeled compound in the assay is the particular antigen of interest. The radioactive half-life of a particular isotope is predictable and important in establishing how long a tracer can be used before the count rate is no longer acceptable. The chemical stability of the compound is equally important, and care must be exercised in the radiolabeling process to ensure a stable and immunoreactive product.

The purified unlabeled antigen is aliquoted into a set of standards, the values of which are determined by the reference ranges in a normal population, and in which maximal sensitivity is required to differentiate normal from abnormal results. It is necessary to add protein (for example, albumin) for stability and also to ensure that the standards and the patient samples being tested react in a similar manner with the antibody. The stability of the antigen often dictates how frequently standards have to be prepared, stored, aliquoted, reconstituted, and so forth.

Owing to the heterogeneity of hormones (for example, parathormone) in particular, and proteins in general, it is often difficult to determine which particular form of the hormone or protein to purify and use as the standard. Indeed, it may not even be possible to utilize a human standard because of the lack of an appropriate source, although recombinant DNA research may overcome this problem. The choice of standard is also determined by the clinical utility of the procedure and the various disease processes that are being diagnosed. The immunologic activity of a protein as measured by RIA may not necessarily correlate with its biologic activity; thus, it is critical to understand the metabolism of the compound in order to better interpret the results.

The basic theory of an RIA is illustrated by the formula $Ag + Ag^* + Ab \rightleftarrows AgAb + Ag^*Ab$, where Ag is unlabeled antigen, either in the form of a standard or unknown (specimen, control); Ag* is radioactive antigen; Ab is antibody; AgAb is unlabeled antigen bound in antigen-antibody complex; and Ag*Ab is radioactive antigen bound in antigen-antibody complex. Once the buffer system has been chosen, a variety of combinations of differing concentrations of antibody, unlabeled antigen, and labeled antigen are tried until the resulting standard curve has been maximized for precision, sensitivity, and clinical utility. The final standard curve is then set up with a fixed amount of radioactive antigen (Ag*) and antibody (Ab) and varying concentrations of standards. Certain antigens require a pretreatment of the sample before the RIA is performed, to remove interfering substances or to release the compound being measured. Folic acid and vitamin B_{12} are released from their protein binder; carcinoembryonic antigen is precipitated and dialyzed; estrogen receptors are separated in the cytosol and ultracentrifuged; and steroids are often extracted into an organic phase, dried down, and redissolved in buffer.

Depending on any structural differences between the antigen and antibody, the assay is set up either as a true equilibrium, where the antibody is added to a premixed solution of Ag and Ag*, or as a "sequential saturation," where the addition of the Ag and Ab is followed by an incubation and subsequent addition of Ag*. Once equilibrium has been reached, one of the most critical steps in the procedure is the separation of bound from free Ag* without disturbing this equilibrium. This is made easier because of the high affinity constant of the Ab and thus the minimal dissociation of the complex. The actual separation is accomplished by a variety of techniques, involving charcoal, dextran-coated charcoal, double antibody, ammonium sulfate, polyethylene glycol, antibody polymers, antibody-coated tubes, antibody covalently linked to resins and glass beads, chromatography, and antibodies attached to magnetic particles. Once separated, either the bound or free fractions are counted in a suitable beta or gamma counter and the standard curve is plotted. If the bound (Ag*Ab) portion is counted, there is an inverse relationship between the count rate and the amount of unlabeled antigen (Ag) present. This is because, as the latter increases, with a constant amount of Ag* and Ab less Ag* will be bound. If the free portion is counted, there is a direct relationship between count rate and amount of Ag. The counts for the unknown (control or patient) samples are then compared with the standard curve, and the results calculated accordingly. The reduction of RIA data has received considerable attention; some of the commonly used methods include Scatchard plot, logit-log, probit, arc sine, hyperbolic, point to point, B/B_0, B/F, quadratic logit, and spline. Not all curve fitting or linearization methods are applicable to a particular assay, and care must be exercised in choosing the appropriate calculation method.

A number of evaluation studies should be performed before an assay is ready to be used clinically, such as parallelism analysis, to detect interfering factors; cross-reactivity, to determine to what degree structurally related compounds will react with the antibody; recovery, to see if known amounts of the substance to be tested can be accurately detected; precision, to assess the reproducibility of the results; sensitivity, to determine the least amount of the substance that can be detected with acceptable precision; and nonspecific binding, to correct for the binding or trapping of radioactivity in the absence of the antibody. The accuracy factor is often difficult to assess, owing to the previously mentioned problems of obtaining homogeneous, pure substances to be used as standards. Probably the most important factor in assessing the utility of a particular radioimmunoassay is the degree of correlation of the result with the clinical status of the patient. Although this is certainly true for any test result, it is especially so for RIA procedures.

Cf. *nonradioisotopic i.* under *immunoassay.*

radioimmunoassay automation partially or fully automated instrumentation for the performance of radioimmunoassays (RIAs) and other radioligand assays. The primary purposes of these systems are to reduce time-consuming manual manipulations in these tests and to reduce interassay coefficients of variation (typically around 10 percent for manual methods and near 5 percent for completely automated methods).

Partially automated systems involve the automation of discrete steps in the test procedure. For example, an automated pipetting station can be used for rapid and consistent pipetting of patient samples and test reagents or after manual incubation and separation of bound and free ligand, radioactivity in all samples can be counted automatically and the data computer reduced to generate test results.

Owing to the heterogeneity of RIA reagents and assay techniques, these procedures are very difficult to automate fully. Completely automated systems eliminate all manual steps in the assay and have automated sample and reagent pipetting, mixing, incubation, separation of bound and free ligand, counting, and data reduction. However, to apply one type of instrument to a variety of RIA procedures, some assay steps, such as incubation time and separation technique, must be uniform for all procedures run on that instrument. The final set of test conditions may not be optimal for or applicable to the procedures being run in a given RIA laboratory. Such systems are used for high-volume assays with capabilities of performing 30–240 tests/hr. Assays currently available on most fully automated systems are digoxin, T_4, T_3-resin uptake, and cortisol, with others under development. Reagents from the manufacturer of the system must be used on their own equipment.

Complete systems can be classified as discrete, in which the tests are performed in separate tubes, or as continuous flow, in which samples pass through the system as a continuous stream of fluid separated by air bubbles. A major difference between automated systems is the type of method for separating bound from free ligand. Examples are the use of resin/charcoal columns, immobilized antibody chambers, antibody-coated tubes, and filtration.

radioimmunoelectrophoresis (ra″de-o-im″u-no-e-lek″tro-fo-re′sis) see *radio-i.* under *immunoelectrophoresis.*

radioisotope (ra″de-o-i′so-tōp) [*radio-* + Gr. *isos* equal + *topos* place] an unstable isotope of a chemical element, i.e., one that is radioactive.

radioligand assay (ra″de-o-li′gand) [*radio-* + L. *ligare* to bind] a technique in which unlabeled and radioactively labeled molecules of the same species compete for a limited number of binding sites on a specific binding protein. The binding protein may be an antibody, transport protein, hormone receptor, or any other cell-associated receptor or tissue component. The unlabeled ligand is the substance being assayed. In the procedure, after a suitable reaction period, the bound ligand (both labeled and unlabeled) is separated from the free ligand, and the radioactivity of either fraction is measured. Standards are included in the assay, and the concentration of unlabeled ligand can be determined from a standard curve. Also called displacement analysis, and saturation analysis (the term competitive protein binding assay is used for ligand assays in which the binding protein is a transport protein or enzyme; radioreceptor assay is used when it is a receptor; and radioimmunoassay is used when it is an antibody). See also *radioimmunoassay* and *radioreceptor assay.*

radiologic (ra″de-o-loj′ik) pertaining to radiology.

Radiological Society of North America (RSNA) a professional organization of radiologists.

radiologic technologist a health care professional skilled in the theory and practice of the technical aspects of the x-rays and radioisotopes used in the diagnosis and treatment of disease. Radiologic technologists can specialize in radiography, radiation therapy, or nuclear medicine. See also *nuclear medicine technologist, radiation therapy technologist,* and *radiographer.*

radiologic technology the allied health profession that deals with the use of ionizing radiation, as in the making of diagnostic radiographs, radiation therapy, and nuclear medicine technology.

radiologist (ra″de-ol′o-jist) a physician who specializes in the diagnostic and therapeutic use of x-rays and other forms of radiation. Also called *roentgenologist.* Cf. *radiation therapist.*

radiology (ra″de-ol′o-je) [*radio-* + Gr. *logos* reason, discourse] the branch of medicine that deals with the diagnosis and treatment of disease by means of ionizing and nonionizing radiation (e.g., ultrasound and nuclear magnetic resonance). Formerly called *roentgenology.*

radiolucency (ra″de-o-lu′sen-se) [*radio-* + L. *lucere* to shine] the degree to which a tissue is penetrable by x-rays. Increased radiolucency (also called hyperlucency) corresponds to a decreased density of tissue.

radiolucent (ra″de-o-lu′sent) permitting the passage of x-rays, although with some absorption. Adipose tissue is moderately radiolucent and is the most penetrable type of tissue. Air and other gases are very radiolucent. Water and most soft tissue (such as muscle, epithelium, and connective tissue) have intermediate penetrability and are neither radiopaque nor radiolucent. Cf. *radiopaque.*

radiolysis (ra″de-ol′ĭ-sis) [*radio-* + Gr. *lysis* a loosening] the chemical decomposition of a substance due to the action of ionizing radiation. See also *autoradiolysis.*

radiometer (ra″de-om′ĕ-ter) [*radio-* + Gr. *metron* measure] an instrument that measures radiant energy, e.g., a bolometer.

radionecrosis (ra″de-o-nĕ-kro′sis) [*radio-* + Gr. *nekrōsis* necrosis, from *nekroun* to cause to die] tissue destruction due to radiant energy.

radionuclide (ra″de-o-nu′klīd) an unstable (radioactive) nuclide; see the accompanying table.

radionuclidic purity the percentage of the total activity of a radiopharmaceutical emitted by the designated radionuclide.

radiopacity (ra″de-o-pas′ĭ-te) [*radio-* + L. *opacus* dark] the degree to which a tissue absorbs x-rays. Increased radiopacity corresponds to an increased density of tissue.

radiopaque (ra″de-o-pāk′) not permitting the passage of x-rays. Bone and other tissues that contain calcium salts are moderately radiopaque and are the least penetrable tissues. Barium sulfate and iodinated contrast media are very radiopaque. Cf. *radiolucent.*

radiopharmaceutical (ra″de-o-far″mah-su′tĭ-kal) a sterile, apyrogenic diagnostic or therapeutic agent containing a radionuclide. Radiopharmaceuticals containing generator-produced nuclides, such as technetium-99m, are formulated using prefabricated sterile kits.

radiopulmonography (ra″de-o-pul″mo-nog′rah-fe) [*radio-* + L. *pulmo* lung + Gr. *graphein* to write or draw] a rapid method for estimating the ventilation of localized lung areas. It is based on the measurement of variation in intensity of low-voltage x-rays passed through the lungs during breathing.

radioreceptor (ra″de-o-re-sep′tor) 1. a receptor for the stimuli that are excited by radiant energy, such as light and heat.

2. see *radioreceptor assay.*

radioreceptor assay a type of radioligand assay in which the binding protein is a hormone receptor. Target tissues containing specific receptors are used for the source, e.g., uterus (for estrogens), prostate and seminal vesicles (for dihydrotestosterone), thymus (for glucocorticoids), and kidney and toad bladder (for mineralocorticoids). See also *competitive protein binding assays, radioimmunoassay,* and *radioligand assay.*

radiorenography (ra″de-o-re-nog′rah-fe) [*radio-* + L. *renes* kidneys + Gr. *graphein* to write or draw] a

RADIONUCLIDE. PHYSICAL CONSTANTS FOR SOME IMPORTANT RADIONUCLIDES

Nuclide	Half-life	Decay Mode*	Major Photons †
Carbon-11	20.3 min	$\beta+$	511
Cesium-137	30.0 yr	β^-	662
Chromium-51	27.8 da	E.C.	320
Cobalt-57	270 da	E.C.	122
Cobalt-60	5.26 yr	β^-	1173
Gallium-67	78 hr	E.C.	93, 184, 296
Gold-198	2.7 da	β^-	412
Indium-111	2.8 da	E.C.	173, 247
Indium-113m	100 min	I.T.	393
Iodine-123	13.3 hr	E.C.	159
Iodine-125	60 da	E.C.	28
Iodine-131	8.05 da	β^-	364
Iron-59	45 da	β^-	1095, 1292
Mercury-197	65 hr	E.C.	77
Nitrogen-13	10.0 min	$\beta+$	511
Oxygen-15	124 sec	$\beta+$	511
Phosphorus-32	14.3 da	β^-	None
Selenium-75	120 da	E.C.	121, 136, 265, 280, 400
Technetium-99m	6.0 hr	I.T.	140
Thallium-201	73 hr	E.C.	71, 135
Xenon-133	5.3 da	β^-	81
Ytterbium-169	31.8 da	E.C.	117, 198

* Decay modes include: β^-, beta decay; $\beta+$, positron emission; E.C., electron capture; I.T., isomeric transition.
† Major photons are energies in kiloelectron volts of gamma rays or x-rays emitted by the radionuclide or short-lived daughters.
Courtesy of Jerold M. Lowenstein, M.D.

nuclear medicine study of kidney function. See also *renogram.*

radioresistant (ra″de-o-re-sis′tant) resistant to the effects of ionizing radiation, e.g., radioresistant tumors.

radioresponsiveness (ra″de-o-re-spon′siv-ness) the rate at which changes occur in a tumor or other tissue in response to radiation treatment. See also *radiation therapy.*

radioscopic (ra″de-o-skop′ik) pertaining to the equipment or procedures used in radioscopy.

radioscopy (ra″de-os′ko-pe) [*radio-* + Gr. *skopein* to examine] x-ray examination using a fluoroscope or image intensifier, which produces a realtime image of the structures being examined. Also called *fluoroscopy.*

radiosensitivity (ra″de-o-sen″sĭ-tiv′ĭ-te) sensitivity of tissue (e.g., skin or tumors) to the effects of ionizing radiation. See also *radiation therapy.*

radiotherapeutics (ra″de-o-ther″ah-pu′tiks) the art and science of radiation therapy.

radiotherapy (ra″de-o-ther′ah-pe) [*radio-* + Gr. *therapeia* cure] see *radiation therapy.*

radium (Ra) (ra′de-um) [L. *radius* ray, from its radioactivity] a radioactive, white, metallic element; atomic number 88; atomic weight 226.0254; Group II of the periodic table (the alkaline earths), oxidation state +2, most stable isotope, Ra-226 (1.62×10^3 yr).

Radium turns black in air; it also reacts in water, releasing hydrogen. Four isotopes of radium, decay products of uranium and thorium, occur naturally; when ingested or inhaled, they localize in bone and can cause bone and lung cancer.

radium-226 (^{226}Ra, Ra 226) an isotope used as an implanted radiation source in cancer radiation therapy. It is the longest lived isotope of radium (half-life, 1620 yr). Radium-226 disintegrates by alpha decay (also emitting 187-keV gamma rays) to radon-222, another alpha emitter.

radius (ra′de-us), pl. *radii* [L. "spoke of a wheel"] [NA], the more lateral of the two bones of the forearm. The upper end forms a circular flattened head that articulates with the capitulum of the humerus and is held against the radial notch of the ulna by its encircling annular ligament. A tuberosity below the head provides attachment for the biceps tendon. The lower end of the radius participates in the wrist joint and has a short, thick styloid process.

radius of resolution a measure of the spatial resolution of a focusing collimator; the radius of view in the focal plane of the collimator.

radius of view (R_v) a measure of the spatial resolution of a collimator; the radius of the circle in a plane parallel to the collimator face that is seen by the detector through a single-hole collimator or through one hole of a multihole collimator.

It increases with the distance of the plane from the collimator face. The true R_v is the R_v when air is the scattering medium; the apparent R_v is the R_v from which photons can be emitted, be scattered by the intervening medium, and then pass through the collimator hole.

radix (ra′diks), pl. *radices* [L.] 1. [NA], a general term for the lowermost part, or a part by which a structure is anchored; e.g., the portion of the hair, nail, or tooth that is buried in the tissues, or the part of a nerve adjacent to its origin in the brain or spinal cord. Also called *root.*

2. the base of a number system.

radix point the analog of the decimal point in a number system with a different base. See also *number system.*

radon (Rn) (ra′don) [from radium] a colorless, odorless, inert, gaseous, radioactive element; atomic number 86; most stable isotope, radon-222 (half-life, 3.8235 da); Group O of the periodic table (the noble gases; oxidation states +2, +4. ^{222}Rn, a decay product of radium, ^{220}Rn, a decay product of thorium, and ^{219}Rn, a decay product of actinium, occur naturally as radioactive gaseous emanations from these elements and their ores. Their decay products (^{218}Po, ^{214}Pb, ^{214}Bi, and ^{214}Po) become attached to dust particles and are also inhaled. All these isotopes are alpha emitters and can cause cancer when inhaled or ingested.

raffinose (raf′ĭ-nōs) a trisaccharide occurring in the seeds of some lentils, such as peas and soybeans. Raffinose may be regarded as sucrose with D-galactose linked (1,6) to the glucose residue of the sucrose. Because of the galactose (1,6)-glucose link, it cannot be hydrolyzed by digestive glycosidases and thus cannot be absorbed. Also called *melitose.*

ragocyte (RA cell) (rag′o-sīt) a type of polymorphonuclear cell that contains dense cytoplasmic inclusion bodies consisting of IgG aggregates, rheumatoid factor, complement, and fibrin. It can be found in the synovial fluid of persons with rheumatic disease.

RAI abbrev. for radioactive iodine.

Raillietina (ri″le-ĕ-ti′nah) [N.L., from A. *Railliet,* French biologist, 19th century] a genus of tapeworms of the family Davaineidae that is parasitic in birds, domestic fowls, and mammals. A few species, including *R. demerariensis, R. celebensis, R. asiatica, R. garrisoni,* and *R. siriraji,* have been reported to parasitize humans.

RAIU abbrev. for radioactive iodine uptake.

rale (rahl) [Fr. *râle* rattle] an abnormal respiratory sound heard in auscultation of the chest.

RAM see *random-access memory.*

Raman spectroscopy (ram′an) [Sir Chandrasekhara Venkata *Raman,* Indian physicist, 1888–1970, winner of the Nobel Prize for physics in 1930] the recording of the spectrum of light scattered by a transparent medium at right angles in the incident beam of monochromatic light. A peak in the Raman spectrum (a frequency shift in the scattered light) corresponds to a vibrational or rotational mode of the scattering molecules. This is the same kind of information as that provided by infrared spectrophotometry; the two processes are complementary rather than similar, however, because they excite different modes.

ramus (ra′mus), pl. *rami* [L.] [NA], a branch; a smaller structure given off by a larger one, or into which the larger structure divides, as with a blood vessel or nerve.

r. communicans, a general term for a small branch to and from a ganglion of the sympathetic chain, which connects the ganglion with a ventral branch of a spinal nerve. A white ramus of myelinated axons provides a pathway for a preganglionic sympathetic fiber of a spinal nerve to reach the sympathetic ganglia. The unmyelinated fibers of gray rami connect postganglionic neurons in the sympathetic chain to spinal nerves at all levels of the cord.

dorsal r., the posterior branch of a spinal nerve that passes backward to supply the muscles and skin of the back and neck. Cf. *ventral r.*

ventral r., the anterior branch of a spinal nerve. It is longer than the dorsal ramus and supplies the limbs and the anterior aspects of the trunk. Cf. *dorsal r.*

rancid (ran′sid) [L. *rancidus*] having a musty, rank taste or smell. The term is applied to fats that have decomposed by reaction with oxygen from air, producing fatty acids.

rancidification (ran-sid″ĭ-fĭ-ka′shun) the decomposition of a substance by reaction with oxygen from air to produce fatty acids. The term is especially applied to the decomposition of fats.

rancidity (ran-sid′ĭ-te) the quality of being rancid.

random (ran′dom) [Old French *randon* violence] pertaining to a chance-dependent process, particularly one that occurs according to a known probability distribution.

random access pertaining to a computer memory or other storage device that has approximately the same access time for every stored datum. Also called *direct access,* particularly when referring to disk or drum.

random-access memory (RAM) a read/write computer memory, i.e., one in which data can be stored and then recalled; the main memory of a computer, in which user programs and data are stored. Cf. *read-only memory.*

random coil one type of secondary structure of protein molecules, being random in the sense that there is no repeating pattern in which each residue interacts with other residues (as in an alpha helix).

random error an error in a measurement process that has a specific probability distribution (usually, a normal distribution with zero mean and when unknown variance is assumed). The effects of random errors on data can be measured by statistical techniques. Cf. *systematic error.*

randomization (ran′dom-ĭ-za′shun) the random assignment of individual units (e.g., patients, animals, test tubes) to the different treatment and control groups in a planned experiment, usually carried out by using a table of random numbers or a computer algorithm.

random mating an assortment of gametes with one genotype at a locus having a purely random probability of combining with any other genotype at that locus. The frequencies of different kinds of mating are dependent only on the frequencies of the genotypes in the population. Random mating is rare in natural populations. The Hardy-Weinberg equilibrium of genotype frequencies is maintained only if there is random mating. Also called *panmixis.* Cf. *assortative mating.*

random number 1. a number produced by a process that generates numbers with a specified probability distribution. Random digits (0, 1, . . . 9) are produced by a process that has equal and independent probabilities of producing each of the 10 decimal (or 2 binary) digits. *n*-Digit random numbers are produced by taking the digits in a table or random digits in groups of *n* digits.

A random sample (without replacement) from a

numbered population is chosen by selecting the members corresponding to a sequence of random numbers. Random numbers that are larger than the population size or that are repeats of previously selected members are ignored.

Uniform random numbers, a random sample of points in the interval between zero and one, are produced by considering the random numbers with a decimal point at the right. If $F^{-1}(x)$ is the inverse function of a probability distribution function $F(x)$ of a continuous distribution, then the sequence of numbers $F^{-1}(x)$, where x is a sequence of uniform random numbers, is a random sample from the distribution F.

2. a pseudorandom number. See under *random number generator.*

random number generator a method, machine, or mathematical algorithm (often run on a computer) that produces a sequence of numbers that behave like true random numbers for certain practical purposes. Each number occurs in a produced sequence with the specified frequency, consecutive numbers are almost uncorrelated, and the sequence passes other statistical tests for randomness.

random sample a sample chosen from a population in such a way that every member of the specified population has a well-defined probability of being chosen as a member of the sample.

multiple stage r. s., a sample obtained by sequential steps, each involving a random sampling procedure. For example, the population might be divided into mutually exclusive groups, and a simple random sample of the groups might be selected, followed by a simple random sampling of the individuals in each of these groups.

simple r. s., 1. a random sample chosen so that every member of the population has an equal and independent probability of being chosen for the sample.

2. observations in a set of independent and identically distributed random variables.

stratified r. s., a sample obtained by dividing the population into mutually exclusive groups called strata and taking a simple random sample from each stratum.

random urine specimen a specimen not obtained at a specified time or over a specified collection period.

random variable see under *probability distribution.*

Raney nickel (ra'ne) [Murray *Raney,* U.S. engineer and manufacturer, 1885–1966] a catalyst used in hydrogenation; a finely divided nickel already saturated with hydrogen. It is prepared by dissolving a nickel-aluminum alloy with aqueous sodium hydroxide. The hydrogen, which is a product of the reaction, is adsorbed on the nickel surface. This catalyst is used to add hydrogen to unsaturated functional groups and to cause hydrogenolysis of the carbon-sulfur and carbon-oxygen single bonds.

range (rānj) the difference between the upper and lower limits of a variable or of a series of values; in statistics, the term refers to the difference between the highest and lowest values in a random sample.

rank (rank) in statistics, the position of a sample observation in the ordering of the observations according to their values. In a sample size n, there are $k - 1$ observations less than the observation with rank k, and $n - k$ greater than it. When some of the observations are tied (having the same value), they are usually assigned an average rank, i.e., the average of the ranks that would have been assigned if the values had been slightly different. If an observation is just greater than the kth observation and tied in a group of d observations, it is assigned the rank $k + (d + 1)/2$.

rank correlation coefficient (r_S) a nonparametric statistic that measures the association between two variables X and Y. It is the correlation coefficient that is produced when the ranks of the X and Y values are substituted for the actual values. It is calculated using the formula $r_S = 1 - 6\Sigma_i d_i^2 / n(n^2 - 1)$, where n is the number of data points (X_i, Y_i) and d_i is the difference between the rank of X_i among the X values and the rank of Y_i among the Y values.

In the exact sampling distribution of r_S under the null hypothesis that X and Y are independent, continuous random variables has been tabulated for small sample sizes. The normal approximation, treating $r_S \sqrt{n-1}$ as a standard normal variable, is used for larger sample sizes.

Also called *Spearman's rank correlation coefficient.*

ranked data data composed of data points or observations that can be arranged in order and ranked according to their place. See also *scale.*

Rankine temperature scale (rang'kin) [William J. M. *Rankine,* Scottish physicist, 1820–1872] a scale of absolute temperature with degrees of the same size as the degree Fahrenheit. See also *temperature.*

rank sum test a nonparametric statistical test for the difference between the medians of two random variables X and Y that are assumed to have continuous distributions differing only in location; that is to say, X and $Y - \Delta$ have the same distribution, where Δ, the shift parameter, is the difference of the medians. The test statistic is the Wilcoxson rank sum statistic W, which is the sum of the ranks of the X observations in the joint ranking of the two samples.

Under the null hypothesis ($\Delta = 0$), W has a symmetric distribution with mean $\mu = n(N + 1)/2$ and variance $\sigma^2 = mn(N + 1)/12$, where n and m are the sizes of the X and Y samples and $N = n + m$.

The exact null sampling distribution of W is tabulated for small sample sizes. For larger samples, the normal approximation is used: the upper tail probabilities are approximated by the area under the normal curve to the right of $(W - \frac{1}{2} - \mu)/\sigma$.

The null hypothesis is rejected, and the alternative that the median of X is greater than the median of Y is accepted if W exceeds the upper α percentile point of the null distribution. The alternative that the medians are different is accepted if W or $n(N + m + 1)/2 + 1 - W$ exceeds the upper $\alpha/2$ percent point.

If X and Y have discrete distributions, average ranks are used in case of ties. The test is overly conservative when ties occur. The conditional variance of W is $\sigma_T^2 = \sigma^2 - mn\Sigma_i (f_i^3 - f_i)/12N(N-1)$, where for each distinct average rank, f_i is the number of observations tied at that rank ($f_i = 1$ if there is no tie); σ_T is substituted for σ in the normal approximation.

The interval and point estimates for Δ associated with the rank sum test are based on the ordered X, Y differences D_k. (The mn differences $D = X - Y$ are arranged in order, and D_k is the difference larger than exactly $k - 1$ other differences.) The median difference ($D_{(mn+1)/2}$ for odd mn, $\frac{1}{2}(D_{mn/2} + D_{mn/(2+1)}$ for even mn) is an unbiased estimator for Δ.

The confidence interval uses the Mann-Whitney form of the rank sum statistic, $U = W - n(n+1)/2$, which is the number of positive X, Y differences. If u is the upper $\alpha/2$ percentile point of the null distribution of U, then $D_{mn+1-u} \leq \Delta < D_u$ is a $100(1-\alpha)$ percent confidence interval for Δ. Inclusion of the lower limit in the interval provides a conservative estimate that remains valid when the parent population is discrete.

ranula (ran′u-lah) [L., dim. of *rana* frog] a mucin-filled cystic lesion in the floor of the mouth thought to arise from blockage of the submandibular or sublingual salivary gland ducts. It is usually slow-growing and asymptomatic. Treatment is by simple excision or marsupialization (unroofing).

Ranvier node (rahn-ve-a′) [Louis Antoine *Ranvier*, French pathologist, 1835–1922] see *node of Ranvier*.

RAO abbrev. See *right anterior oblique*.

Raoult's law (rah′ōlz) [François Marie *Raoult*, French physicist, 1830–1901] stated as: the vapor pressure of a liquid in solution (a solvent or solute) is proportional to the mole fraction of that liquid. The other colligative properties of the solution (freezing point depression, boiling point elevation, and osmotic pressure) are proportional to the (solvent) vapor pressure depression. The law holds exactly only for ideal solutions; the behavior of some nonideal solutions (e.g., azeotropes) deviates significantly.

rape (rāp) [L. *rapere* to take by force] an act of violence that involves involuntary sexual intercourse; 95 percent of the victims are females. Approximately 50,000 rapes are reported annually in the United States; 40 percent have previous knowledge of their attackers. The level of force varies; 5–10 percent of rape victims require serious medical attention.

Medical examination of the rape victim is very important and serves several purposes: to collect forensic evidence, to check the victim's physical condition, to treat injuries, and to prevent sexually transmitted disease. Included in the laboratory testing should be cultures to test for *Neisseria gonorrhoeae* organisms, wet mount preparations to detect the morphology and motility of any sperm present, an acid phosphatase test, and a blood group antigen test. The victim should have follow-up testing 6 wk later, at which time a VDRL (Venereal Disease Research Laboratory) test should be performed to detect syphilis, cultures taken again to detect gonorrhea, and pregnancy testing done if the victim is of child-bearing age.

raphe (ra′fe) [Gr. *rhaphē* seam, suture] [NA], a general term for the line of union of halves of various symmetric parts.

rapid eye movement (REM) in sleep, the phasic, rapid conjugate eye movements occurring during the stage characterized by low-voltage, fast activity on the electroencephalogram in humans and experimental aminals. These eye movements are preceded and accompanied by neural activity arising from the pontine reticular formation. This activity is projected to the lateral geniculate nuclei, and from there relayed to the visual cortex. High-voltage waves called ponto-geniculo-occipital (PGO) spikes accompany the REM and can be recorded in the electrocorticogram of certain laboratory animals such as the cat. See also *s. stages* under *sleep*.

rapid grower a mycobacterium that grows completely to maturity within 1 wk at optimal temperature. See *mycobacterium*.

rapidly progressive glomerulonephritis see crescentic glomerulopathy under *glomerulopathy*.

rapid plasma reagin (RPR) test a test for antibodies against *Treponema pallidum*, the organism that causes syphilis. The test is very similar to the VDRL (Venereal Disease Research Laboratory) test in that it applies unheated serum or plasma to cardiolipin antigen bound to charcoal particles. This test offers several advantages: (1) it is provided commercially as a test kit, which contains all necessary reagents; (2) unheated serum is used; (3) the reaction can be read macroscopically; and (4) the materials are disposable. A disadvantage is that it cannot be used as a test for cerebrospinal fluid. See also *VDRL test*.

rapid-sequence film changer a device that unrolls x-ray film and passes it between two intensifying screens for exposure (as many as 12 exposures/sec) or one that changes loaded cassettes (as many as 2 exposures/sec). It is used, for example, in angiocardiography, where serial films are commonly made simultaneously in two different planes (e.g., frontal and lateral).

Rare Donor File a listing of potential blood donors with rare phenotypes, representing less than 2 percent of random donors. It was established by and is available from the American Association of Blood Banks.

rare earth elements a group of lustrous, silvery-white metallic elements, most of which readily oxidize in air. They occur naturally as oxides (earths), but in fact are not rare elements. Their natural occurrences are relatively high. They are used in alloys, as catalysts, and as color television tube phosphors. Poorly absorbed from the gastrointestinal tract, rare earth elements have low toxicity, although many act as anticoagulants.

The rare earths include the 4f transition elements (atomic numbers 57–71; the lanthanide series). Because of their similar chemistry, scandium and yttrium sometimes are also included. All these elements are very similar in their physical and chemical properties. See also *lanthanide* and *periodic table of the elements*.

rash (rash) [Old French *rache*] a temporary eruption on the skin, as in urticaria; a drug eruption or viral exanthem.

RAST abbrev. See *radioallergosorbent test*.

rat (rat) [Anglo-Saxon *raet*] a small, aggressive, and omnivorous rodent of the genus *Rattus* and related genera of the family Muridae, commonly found around human habitations. Rats cause great economic loss and are vectors of human disease; they harbor intestinal parasites that can be transmitted to humans, such as tapeworms, roundworms, and trichinae, and they are reservoirs for the infectous agents of plague, typhus, Weil's disease, and rat-bite fever. Albino mutants of both *R. rattus* and *R. norvegicus* are widely used as laboratory animals.

rat-bite fever an infection transmitted to humans by the bite of a rat or other rodent; it occurs as two clinically similar but etiologically distinct diseases. The streptobacillary form is caused by the gram-negative pleomorphic bacillus *Streptobacillus moniliformis,* whereas the spirillary form (also called sodoku) is caused by infection with *Spirillum minor.*

Streptobacillary rat-bite fever is more common in the United States and is seen most frequently in crowded areas having substandard housing conditions, in other types of economically deprived areas, and among laboratory animal handlers. The disease occurs in approximately 10 percent of those who are bitten. Although the primary wound heals promptly, a viral-like disease develops within 10 da. Chills, fever, vomiting, and headache, with polyarthralgia and a petechial rash, are common. Rarely, subacute bacterial endocarditis and brain abscesses develop. White blood cell counts are 6000–30,000/mm³.

Diagnosis is established by culturing the organism (in ordinary media, 20 percent horse serum, and 5–10 percent CO_2). Agglutinins usually develop within 2–3 wk, and there are false-positive serologic test results for syphilis. If untreated, streptobacillary rat-bite fever may mimic the clinical features of relapsing fever.

Spirillary rat-bite fever leads to inflammation at the primary wound site, with fever and lymphadenitis developing 10 da after the bite. A relapsing fever may also occur in this form of the disease; arthritis and rashes are rare. Subacute bacterial endocarditis is seen very infrequently. Most infections subside within weeks. During the acute phase, white blood cell counts are elevated (as high as 30,000/mm³) and false-positive syphilis test results are common.

S. minor may be identified microscopically in darkfield preparations of blood and tissue smears from infected wounds and lymph nodes; the organism has not been cultured on laboratory media. Intraperitoneal injection of infected material into mice produces growth of organisms within 5–15 da, which can be demonstrated with Giemsa stain or darkfield microscopy.

Rat-bite fever may be confused with tularemia, malaria, meningococcemia, or *Borrelia recurrentis* infections, all of which are characterized by relapsing fever.

rate (rāt) [L. *rata,* from *ratus,* past participle of *reri* to calculate] 1. the time rate of change of a quantity. 2. the frequency of an event in a specified population. In epidemiology, demography, and actuarial science, rate refers to a fraction in which the numerator is the number of cases of a disease, or the number of deaths, in a population in a specified time period, and the denominator is the population size during that period. Rates are often multiplied by a power of 10 to yield values in a convenient numerical range, e.g., the annual death rate is usually expressed as cases per 1000 population.

adjusted r., a fictional summary rate that has been statistically adjusted to remove the effect of the demographic structure of the population by estimating the rate that would be observed in a population with an arbitrarily chosen standard population structure. The demographic variable most commonly adjusted for is age, but the method can also be used to adjust for other variables, such as sex or race. There are two common methods of adjustment: the direct and the indirect.

The direct method uses the specific rates for the study population and the demographic structure of a real or hypothetical standard population. To determine an age-adjusted rate, the number of expected events (cases of disease or deaths) is calculated. The age-specific rate for each age group in the study population multiplied by the size of that age group in the standard population gives the expected number of events in that age group. The numerator is then the expected number of events for all age groups, and the denominator is the size of the standard population.

The indirect method is especially useful when the specific rates for the study population are unavailable or are unstable because of small sample size. It uses the specific rates for a real standard population, e.g., age-specific death rates for the United States population and the demographic structure of the study population. Multiplying the number of individuals in each age group by the age-specific death rate for the standard population yields the expected deaths in that group. The sum over all groups is the total of expected deaths. The standard mortality ratio (SMR) is defined as the ratio having observed deaths in the study group as the numerator and expected deaths as the denominator. If the specific morbidity rates are used, the ratio of observed cases to expected cases is called the standard morbidity ratio (the word "rate" is not appropriate because the denominators are not population sizes). The SMR multiplied by the crude standard population mortality (or morbidity) rate gives the adjusted rate.

Also called *standardized r.* Cf. *crude r.* and *specific r.*

age-specific r., a rate computed for a specified age group.

attack r., an incidence rate, particularly one that varies with time, e.g., the incidence rate during an epidemic. See also *incidence r.* and *secondary attack r.*

case fatality r., a rate in which the numerator is the number of deaths from a disease and the denominator is the number of diagnosed cases of the disease. It is a commonly used measure of the severity of a disease; for most diseases, however, it overstates the severity of the disease because the denominator is too small, as unapparent or mild cases do not come to medical attention.

cause-specific death r., a mortality rate in which the numerator is the number of deaths due to a particular cause. Cf. *proportionate mortality r.* under *ratio.*

crude r., an actuarial summary rate in which the numerator is the actual number of events in a total population and the denominator is the total population. Cf. *adjusted r.* and *specific r.*

dose r., the amount of any therapeutic agent administered per unit of time, and often standardized to some measure of body size, usually per kilogram of body weight or per square meter of body surface.

incidence r., a rate in which the numerator is the number of new cases of a disease in a population during a specified time and the denominator is the numbers in the population at risk. Persons who already have the disease or who are not susceptible to it (e.g., because of immunization) may be excluded from the denominator. In the latter situation, the incidence rate is meant to measure the true risk of disease. See also *attack r.* Cf. *prevalence r.*

morbidity r., a rate in which the numerator is the

number of cases of disease. See also *incidence r.* and *prevalence r.*

mortality r., a rate in which the numerator is the number of deaths in a population in a specified time (usually 1 yr) and the denominator is the population size.

prevalence r., a rate in which the numerator is the number of existing cases of a disease in a population at a point in time and the denominator is the total population, also called the point prevalence rate. In a period prevalence rate, the numerator is the number of existing cases during a period of time, and the denominator is the average population or the population at the midpoint of the time period. Prevalence rate is useful in estimating the workload of health care personnel. If the incidence is stable over time, the prevalence is the product of the incidence and the average duration of the disease. Cf. *incidence r.*

secondary attack r., the attack rate among a closed group, such as a household. The numerator is the number of new cases of the disease in the group and the denominator is the number of susceptible persons in the group. Both the numerator and denominator exclude the index case, which brings the group to the attention of the investigator, and also other initial cases that are considered to have occurred too early to be related to the index case.

specific r., a rate that applies to a specific demograhic group, e.g., individuals of a specific age, sex, and/or race. Cf. *adjusted r.* and *crude r.*

standardized r., see *adjusted r.*

rate constant the temperature-dependent magnitude that characterizes the velocity of a chemical reaction, as a function of the concentration of one of the reactants. It has the unit: (concentration)$^{1-n}$ × (time)$^{-1}$, where n is the order of the reaction. See also *kinetics.*

rate-controlling step the single reaction in a reaction sequence that proceeds at the slowest rate and thereby controls the overall rate of the sequence of reactions.

rate meter an electronic device that indicates the rate at which counts are detected by a radiation detector. The counts are averaged by a resistance-capacitance circuit, and the output is indicated by a meter or chart recorder. Rate meters are widely used to measure radioactivity in organs, samples, contamination, and the like, in which the count rate recorded can be related to the amount of radioactivity present. They are also used to indicate the count rate received in some rectilinear scanners or scintillation camera systems, and to average the output of the scintillation probes used in making renograms. Also called *count rate meter.*

Rathke's pouch (rahth'kez) [Martin Heinrich *Rathke,* German anatomist, 1793–1860] in the embryo, an outpouching of the floor of the primitive oral cavity that grows dorsally to meet the developing infundibulum of the diencephalon. Rathke's pouch loses its connection with the oral cavity and forms the adenohypophysis. Rarely, a group of anterior pituitary cells persists at its site of origin to form a pharyngeal pituitary. Also called craniopharyngeal diverticulum.

ratio (ra'she-o) [L. "calculation," from *ratus,* past participle of *reri* to calculate] the relative magnitude of two quantities, usually given as a reduced fraction; e.g., the ratio of 10 to 5 is usually written 2:1 or 2/1.

proportionate mortality r. (PMR), the ratio of the number of deaths from a particular cause to the total number of deaths in the same period of time; it equals the cause-specific death rate divided by the crude death rate. Usually expressed as a percentage, the PMR indicates the relative importance of a disease as a cause of death, whereas the cause-specific rate indicates the risk of death from the cause. The PMR is not a rate because the denominator is not a population size. Cf. *cause-specific death r.* under *rate.*

standard morbidity r., see *adjusted r.* under *rate.*

standard mortality r., see *adjusted r.* under *rate.*

rational (rash'un-al) [L. *rationalis,* from *ratio*] based on reason; having possession of reason.

rationale (rash"un-al') [L., neuter of *rationalis*] a logical or rational basis or explanation for something.

ratio scale a numerical scale that has the property that observation or measurement is proportional to the quantity measured. See also *scale.*

rat tapeworm se *H. diminuta* under *Hymenolepsis.*

Rattus (rat'us) a genus of rats, of which the species *R. brevicaudatus,* found in Java and Japan, is a common reservoir host of *Gastrodiscoides hominis.*

Rauwolfia (rah-wul'fe-ah, rou-wul'fe-ah) [Leonhard *Rauwolf,* German botanist, died 1596] a genus of tropical trees and shrubs native to Asia, many of which, particularly *R. serpentina,* have been used as a source of medicinal alkaloids.

rauwolfia serpentina (ser"pen-te'nah) [NF], an extract of the root of *R. serpentina* containing many indole alkaloids, e.g., reserpine, rescinnamine; used as an antihypertensive, sedative, and tranquilizer. See also *reserpine.*

RAW abbrev. See *airway resistance.*

ray (ra) [L. *radius* spoke of a wheel, ray] 1. a photon or other particle of ionizing radiation. See also *alpha ray, beta ray, delta ray, gamma ray,* and *x-ray.*

2. a line followed by a beam of light. It is straight in homogeneous media and forms angles where light is reflected by mirrors or refracted at lens surfaces.

3. in computed tomography, a line that connects the x-ray source and detector. The attenuation by the tissues of x-ray beams traversing many rays is used to reconstruct the image.

4. in mathematics, a half-line projecting from a point.

Raynaud's disease (ra-nōz') [A. G. Maurice *Raynaud,* French physician, 1834–1881] a vasospastic disease of the small arteries and arterioles, primarily affecting the extremities (the fingers more than the toes), that is characterized by paroxysmal pallor and cyanosis, especially following exposure to cold or after emotional stress.

Raynaud's disease occurs in a bilateral symmetric pattern and primarily affects females under age 40. The vascular spasms may last from minutes to hours, and are usually accompanied by numbness and tingling or burning sensations. The fingers turn white, then blue; on rewarming, they turn red. Attacks remit spontaneously. The disease usually follows a benign course but very rarely is progressive. Trophic changes, skin and muscle atrophy, and small areas of ischemic necrosis may (rarely) develop. The causes of Raynaud's disease are unknown, but a defect leading to hyperlability of the autonomic nervous system's input to the affected vessels has been implicated in the etiology. A variety of experimental drugs and treatments, including local injection of prostaglandin E_1 (PGE_1), are under evaluation.

Cf. *Raynaud's phenomenon.*

Raynaud's phenomenon [A. G. Maurice *Raynaud*] a vasospastic condition that affects the small arteries and arterioles and is secondary to some form of systemic disease. Among the systemic diseases implicated are collagen vascular disease, progressive systemic sclerosis, systemic lupus erythematosus, thromboangiitis obliterans, drug and metal toxicities, pulmonary hypertension, and myxedema.

The condition is often unilateral and may involve only one or two fingers. The pattern of extremity involvement is very similar to that seen in Raynaud's disease; it may also precede scleroderma and frank necrosis. Serum protein and serologic abnormalities, including the presence of autoantibodies and depression of levels of the third component of complement, are more marked than those of Raynaud's disease.

Cf. *Raynaud's disease.*

razoxane (rah-zok'sān) a cancer chemotherapeutic drug. For more information, see *Appendix A.*

Rb symbol for the chemical element *rubidium.*

R banding (reverse banding) see under *chromosome banding.*

RBC abbrev. for *r*ed *b*lood *c*ell. See *erythrocyte.*

RBE abbrev. See *relative biological effectiveness.*

RBP abbrev. See *retinol-binding protein.*

RC circuit an electronic circuit containing a resistor and capacitor in series. When a voltage (V) is placed across the circuit, the capacitor will charge. The current in the circuit (i) is given by the formula $i = (V/R)e^{-t/RC}$, where R is resistance, C is capacitance, and t is time. The voltage across the capacitor (V) is given by the formula $e = V(1 - e^{t/RC})$. RC, the time it takes the capacitor to charge to 63.2 percent of the applied voltage, is called the time constant of the circuit. RC circuits are extensively used in designing filters to block selected frequencies.

RCF abbrev. *See relative centrifugal force.*

RCITR abbrev. for *r*ed *c*ell *i*ron *t*urnover *r*ate. See under *ferrokinetics study.*

R colony abbrev. See *rough c.* under *colony.*

RCRA abbrev. See *Resource Conservation and Recovery Act.*

RCS abbrev. See *rabbit aorta–contracting substance.*

RCV abbrev. for red cell volume. See under *blood volume measurements.*

R determinant abbrev. for resistance *determinant.* See *R p.* under *plasmid.*

rDNA abbrev. See *ribosomal DNA.*

RDW abbrev. See *red cell distribution width.*

Re symbol for the chemical element *rhenium.*

re- (re) [L.] a prefix word element to denote back, e.g., reflux.

reabsorb (re″ab-sorb′) to absorb again.

reabsorption (re″ab-sorp′shun) the process of absorption again, such as the selective absorption in the renal tubules and return to the blood of substances (e.g., glucose, amino acids, electrolytes) filtered by the glomeruli.

react (re-akt′) [*re-* + L. *agere* to do] 1. to respond to a stimulus.

2. to enter into a chemical reaction.

reactance (re-ak′tans) (X) the ratio of the peak voltage (V_p) to the peak alternating current (I_p) in a capacitor or inductor; $V_p = I_pX$. Because the current and voltage are 90° out of phase, this relation does not hold between the instantaneous voltage and current. The International System (SI) unit of reactance is the ohm (Ω).

capacitive r. (X_C), the reactance of a capacitor equal to $1/\omega C$ or $1/2\pi fC$, where C is capacitance, ω is angular frequency, and f is frequency. It becomes infinite at zero frequency, because a capacitor does not conduct direct current.

inductive r. (X_L), the reactance of an inductor equal to ωL or $2\pi fL$, where L is inductance, ω is angular frequency, and f is frequency.

reactant (re-ak′tant) any of the substances that enter into and undergo a change in a chemical reaction. Because most chemical reactions are reversible, the reactants become products (and vice versa) when the reaction is considered as going in the opposite direction. In an enzyme-catalyzed reaction, the reactants are usually referred to as substrate(s) of the enzyme. Cf. *product.*

limiting r., the reactant that determines the maximal amount of product that can be formed in a chemical reaction. If the reaction goes to completion, the reactant is totally incorporated into the products. Other reactants are said to be present in excess.

reaction (re-ak′shun) [*re-* + L. *agere* to act] 1. the reciprocal action of chemical agents on each other.

2. the physiologic response to stimulation, as for example, of a muscle or nerve.

3. in physics, the equal and opposite force opposed to a specified force (the action).

4. the specific cellular effect produced by foreign matter, as in testing for allergies. For more information, see the specific reaction.

chemical r., any single process or operation involving the interconversion of chemical species; i.e., the conversion of one or more chemical species (reactants) to other chemical species (products).

A chemical reaction that evolves heat is called an exothermic reaction; when heat is absorbed it is called an endothermic reaction. If the reaction also proceeds backward from products to reactants at an appreciable rate, the system eventually reaches chemical equilibrium in which the reaction rate is the same in both directions: a reversible reaction. Otherwise, the reaction goes to completion, the maximal amount of product is formed, and the limiting reactant is completely consumed.

See also *chemical e.* under *equation.*

false-negative r., an erroneously negative reaction to a test.

false-positive r., an erroneously positive reaction to a test.

reaction intermediate a short-lived chemical species that is formed from the reactants and that reacts further to give the products of a chemical reaction.

reaction order see under *kinetics.*

reaction quotient the equivalent of an equilibrium constant for a chemical reaction that has not reached equilibrium: the product of the activities (concentrations or partial pressures) of the reaction products, each raised to a power equal to its coefficient in the equation for the reaction, divided by the product of the reactant activities raised to their coefficients. See also *equilibrium constant.*

reaction rate the speed (in moles per second) at which products are produced and reactants consumed in a chemical reaction. It is a product of three factors: the frequency of molecular collisions, the fraction of collisions in which the molecules have energy in excess of the activation energy, and the probability that the molecules have the necessary spatial orientation. The first factor is proportional to the concentrations of the reactants. Thus, for a bimolecular reaction, rate = k[A] [B], where k is the rate constant at a specific temperature, and [A] and [B] are the concentrations of the two species that combine to form the transition state (activated complex). See also *kinetics.*

reactive material a material that is unstable and likely to decompose vigorously or violently if exposed to friction, pressure, impact, or heat; or is vigorously reactive with air or water; or exhibits other properties of reactivity.

reactivity 1. a property exhibited by a chemical waste if a representative sample of the waste has any of the following properties: (1) it is normally unstable and readily undergoes violent change without detonating; (2) it reacts violently with water; (3) it forms potentially explosive mixtures with water; (4) it generates toxic gases, vapors, or fumes when mixed with water in a quantity sufficient to present a danger to human health or the environment; (5) it is a cyanide- or sulfide-bearing waste that, when exposed to pH conditions between 2 and 12.5, can generate toxic gases, vapors, or fumes in a quantity sufficient to endanger humans or the environment; (6) it is capable of detonation or explosive reaction if subjected to a strong initiating source or if heated under confinement; and (7) it is a forbidden explosive, or a Class A or B explosive, as defined in DOT (Department of Transportation) regulations.

Such wastes are classified as hazardous and are regulated by standards established by the Environmental Protection Agency (EPA) and the Resources Conservation and Recovery Act (RCRA).

2. in electroencephalography, the ease with which a particular pattern of electric activity is altered by means of sensory stimulation of the patient or other physiologic actions.

reactivity hazard ratings a system for rating degrees of reactivity or instability of the several hundred common chemicals identified by the National Fire Protection Association (NFPA 704-1980 and NFPA 49-1975).

read (rēd) 1. to transfer data from a computer input device to memory, or the operation or statement of a program that accomplishes this transfer.

2. to recall data from computer memory to a register for processing; an operation usually called a *load.*

readability (re″dah-bil′ĭ-te) the smallest fraction of a scale division that can be accurately determined on a measuring device.

readiness potential in electroencephalography, a slowly increasing negative potential that is recorded maximally from the central regions of the brain just prior to limb movements. This potential contributes to the contingent negative variation. Also called *Bereitshaftspotential.*

reading (rēd′ing) the process by which the nucleotide sequence of a messenger RNA is decoded by the translation mechanism, every three nucleotides (a codon) specifying one amino acid of a polypeptide sequence. See also *translation.*

reading frame the division of the nucleotide sequence of a nucleic acid into consecutive three-nucleotide codons. There are three different reading frames (starting a codon with the first, second, or third nucleotide). Generally, only one reading frame encodes a polypeptide; this frame is specified by the location of the initiation codon of the polypeptide.

The deletion or addition of a nucleotide throws off the reading frame after that point, making nonsense of the remaining code; this is called a frameshift mutation.

read-only memory (ROM) a computer memory from which data can only be recalled; the contents cannot be changed by the user. It is used in microcomputers to store permanent programs and data, and also in larger computers to store microprograms. Cf. *random-access memory.*

erasable programmable r.-o. m. (EPROM), a ROM that can be erased (all bits reset to zero) and reprogrammed several times. Special equipment is required for reprogramming, and the memory contents cannot be changed while the EPROM is in use.

programmable r.-o. m (PROM), a read-only memory for which the stored data are specified by the user. Some PROMs are programmed by the user; others must be programmed by the manufacturer. Once programmed, a PROM cannot be erased and reprogrammed, nor can the data be lost.

readout (rēd′out) a device that displays information, such as a meter, chart recorder, digital readout, or computer output device.

readthrough (rēd′throo) transcription of DNA into mRNA that goes beyond the end of a transcription unit because of a failure of recognition of the termination sequence by RNA polymerase.

read-write head a wire coil used to record or sense signals on a magnetic tape or disk.

read-write memory see *random-access memory.*

reagent (re-a′jent) [*re-* + L. *agere* to act] 1. any chemical compound used as a reactant in a chemical reaction. A distinction is made between the various reactants (which lead to products), e.g., the one on which attention is arbitrarily focused, the substrate, and the other, commonly an inorganic or simple organic substance, the reagent; such a distinction, however, is often meaningless. Analytic reagents are those used in detecting, measuring, or analyzing other substances.

2. an indication of the purity of some commercially available chemical compounds, as in reagent grade or reagent chemicals.

reagent grade a degree of purity of chemicals that is sufficient for their use in sensitive qualitative analyses and in precision quantitative measurements. The term purity is a relative one; the degree of purity varies with the specific analytic problem, the state of the chemical industrial art, and the sophistication of available measuring devices. In the United States, the specifications prepared by the Committee on Analytical Reagents of the American

Chemical Society are those generally recognized and accepted.

Two forms of reporting grade are used in practice: lot-analyzed reagents, for which the manufacturer analyzes each individual lot and reports the quantity of all significant impurities, and maximum impurities reagents, for which the report lists only the maximal allowable level of significant impurities.

Also called ACS grade and analytical reagent grade.

reagent strip a paper strip with one or more areas impregnated with reagents that undergo a color change when reacted with specific substances in aqueous solution, e.g., glucose, ketones, protein, and certain amino acids. Substance concentrations in the specimen (usually urine) are indicated by changes in color, which are compared with a color chart prepared by the manufacturer. Semiquantitative results are usually reported on a scale that has a range of 0–4: 0, trace, +, ++, +++, ++++; the last three steps are also written 2+, 3+, and 4+.

reagin (re′ah-jin) an IgE antibody or a substance that behaves like an antibody in complement fixation. Reagin reacts in the Wassermann reaction with cardiolipin as a diagnostic test for syphilis.

reaginic antibody an antibody produced in individuals affected with syphilis, which reacts with a component of mitochondrial membranes known as cardiolipin. Many serologic tests for syphilis, such as the VDRL and Wassermann tests, function by detecting reaginic antibody.

real (rēl) [L. *realis* real, from *res* thing] 1. having an actual existence.

2. pertaining to the real numbers.

3. in computer languages, a data type referring to floating-point numbers expressed using a fixed number of digits. The most common precision is 32 bits or 6 hexadecimal digits.

real number the limit of a sequence of rational numbers. The real numbers can be identified with the continuum of points on a line or with all of the numbers that can be expressed using an infinite number of decimal places.

real-time pertaining to a computer application in which data are processed at a rate necessary to keep pace with external events, as in a real-time ultrasound scanner, or fast enough to provide the information necessary for an imminent decision.

real-time clock a circuit in the central processing unit of a computer containing a register that is incremented at regular intervals and can be read by programs for timing purposes. It also interrupts user programs after a preset interval, which allows the operating system to schedule time-shared user programming or to synchronize control of input-output devices.

recalcification time (re-kal″sĭ-fi-ka′shun) the interval required for clot formation when calcium ions are replaced in anticoagulated platelet-rich plasma. It is an insensitive measure of hemostasis.

receiver operating characteristic (ROC) a plot of the sensitivity of a diagnostic test as a function of nonspecificity. The sensitivity is the probability that the test positively identifies a disease (later established by reference test results or pathologic findings). The nonspecificity (one minus the specificity) is the probability that the test incorrectly indicates the presence of a disease. Requiring stricter, more decisive evidence for a positive test result increases both the sensitivity and the nonspecificity. Less strict criteria lower both.

The ROC curve indicates the intrinsic properties of the test technology and is applied in comparing the relative merits of competing procedures (e.g., computed tomography versus radionuclide scintiphotography). If the ROC curves intersect, a preference for one of the tests depends on the relative costs of false-negative and false-positive diagnosis; otherwise, the more sensitive test is better.

receptor (re-sep′tor) [L., from *recipere* to receive] 1. a sensory nerve terminal; see under the specific type, e.g., photoreceptor.

2. a specific molecule on the surface of an immunocompetent cell that binds with antigen complement components, or lymphokines.

3. a specific molecule on the surface of a neuron or target cell that binds to a neurotransmitter or hormone. See also *adrenergic receptors, cholinergic receptors,* and H_1-receptors and H_2-receptors under *histamine.*

recessive (re-ses′iv) [L. *recessus,* past participle of *recedere* to go back] in genetics, pertaining to a trait that is expressed only in homozygous individuals, i.e., only when both homologous alleles of a gene code for the trait.

The term is also applied to the allele or gene for a recessive trait. Usually, a recessive allele codes for a nonfunctional protein. In the homozygous individual, the lack of the protein produces a genetic defect, whereas in the heterozygous individual the single copy of the normal allele produces enough normal protein to permit normal function.

For some recessive traits, such as Tay-Sachs disease, sickle cell anemia, and thalassemia, heterozygotes (carriers) can be identified by biochemical tests for the abnormal protein produced by the recessive allele even though there are no phenotypic effects that identify a carrier.

See also *autosomal recessive i.* and *X-linked recessive i.* under *inheritance,* and *codominance.* Cf. *dominant.*

recessive gene see *recessive c.* under *character.*

recessus (re-ses′sus), pl. *recessus* [L., from *recedere* to go back, withdraw] [NA], a general term for a small empty space, hollow, or cavity.

recipient (re-sip′e-ent) [L. *recipiens* present participle of *recipere* to receive] one who receives, as in blood transfusion or a tissue or organ graft. In bacteriology, a recipient is a cell that receives genetic material from another (donor) cell. See also *bacterial g.* under *genetics* and *conjugation.*

reciprocal (re-sip′ro-kal) [L. *reciprocus* alternating] 1. pertaining to each of two or more separate entities; complementary.

2. in mathematics, the reciprocal of a number is that number divided into 1. Thus, the reciprocal of 3 is 1/3; the reciprocal of 2/3 is 3/2.

reciprocal translocation a chromosomal aberration in which two nonhomologous chromosomes are broken and repaired so that two monocentric chromosomes, composed of a piece from each of the originals, are formed. Because no genetic material is lost, there is no phenotypic effect. Abnormal gametes are formed, however. During meiosis, each aberrant chromosome synapses with the two normal chromosomes that are their partial homologues, thus forming a quadrivalent.

Three possible types of gametes can be formed: a normal gamete with the two untranslocated chromosomes, a gamete with both translocated chromosomes (which will produce an offspring who is a translocation heterozygote or balanced carrier like the parent), and a gamete with one untranslocated and one translocated chromosome (which will produce a child with a partial duplication deficiency: one end of the translocated chromosome is duplicated on the untranslocated chromosome, and the material that this end replaces is deleted). When one of the chromosome breaks occurs near the end of an arm, an almost pure partial trisomy or monosomy may be formed.

Cf. *robertsonian translocation.*

recombinant (re-kom′bĭ-nant) a genome or organism produced by genetic recombination.

recombinant DNA see *molecular c.* under *cloning.*

recombination (re″kom-bĭ-na′shun) in genetics, the occurrence of new genetic combinations in which alleles that were on different homologous chromosomes in a parent are located on the same chromosome in an offspring. This is because of a cross-over that occurred between the loci during meiosis.

recombination frequency the frequency with which two genetic loci are recombined, i.e., the number of recombinants divided by the total number of progeny. The term is used in gene mapping. See also *centimorgan.*

recon (re′kon) [acronym from *rec*ombination + Gr. *-on* quantum] in molecular genetics, the smallest unit of DNA capable of recombination, i.e., the distance between two base pairs. Cf. *cistron, codon,* and *muton.*

record (rek′ord) [L. *recordari* to recollect, from *re-* + *cor* heart, mind] 1. a permanent or long-lasting account of something, as preserved in writing or on film.

2. in data processing, a unit of data. A record may be several characters or several hundred characters long; conceptually, a record is "one line of data."

logical r., a set of logically related data items processed together by the system input-output programs.

medical r., the official written record of data kept by a health care facility pertaining to a single patient. Two different systems are used: the source record (the traditional "chart") and the problem-oriented record (POR). In the first, each discipline or department records separate notes, e.g., the physician's orders, physician's progress notes, nurse's notes, laboratory data, and radiologic findings. The POR is divided into four sections: the database, which contains information from the history, physical examination, laboratory reports, and other assessment methods; the problem list, which contains the major problems currently needing medical attention; the plan, which contains the diagnosis and treatment plan for each problem; and the progress notes (or narrative notes), which are presented in the SOAP format (an acronym from *s*ubjective data obtained from the patient or family, *o*bjective data obtained by physical examination or diagnostic studies, *a*ssessment of the patient status, and *p*lan of treatment).

physical r., a set of data characters processed together by an input-output device, such as the 80 columns of a punched card or a print line of a high-speed printer.

recorder (re-kor′der) a device that produces a permanent record of an electronic signal, such as a chart recorder or a tape drive.

recovery time in the operation of a Geiger-Müller counter, the time interval that elapses after a count has been recorded before the tube can again produce a maximal pulse. See also *dead time* and *resolving time.*

recruitment (re-kroo͞t′ment) the orderly, programmed increase in the number of active motor units with increasing strength of voluntary muscle contraction. This stepwise activation of motor units with successively higher thresholds is in part responsible for the smooth, graded nature of normal skeletal muscle activity.

rect/o (rek′to) [L. *rectum*] a word element used in combining form to denote relationship to the rectum, e.g., rectosigmoid. See also words beginning *procto-.*

rectal (rek′tal) pertaining to the rectum.

rectification (rek″tĭ-fĭ-ka′shun) [L. *rectificatio*] the conversion of alternating current to unidirectional (pulsating direct) current.

rectifier (rek′tĭ-fi″er) an electric component, such as a semiconductor diode, that permits current flow only in one direction, or a circuit using such components that produces unidirectional (pulsating direct) current from alternating current.

bridge r., a type of full-wave rectifier that uses four diodes to direct the current through the load (see the accompanying illustration).

full-wave r., a rectifier circuit, such as a bridge rectifier, that passes both the positive and negative halves of each alternating current cycle through the load. The half cycles go along different paths so that they pass through the load in the same directions. The full-wave rectifier passes all the available power and produces a much smaller ripple voltage (48 percent of the DC voltage) than does the half-wave rectifier.

half-wave r., a rectifier circuit that passes the positive half of each alternating current cycle through the load and blocks the other half, thus wasting half of the available power and producing a very large ripple voltage (121 percent of the DC voltage).

rectilinear (rek″tĭ-lin′e-ar) [L. *rectilineus* straight] characterized by a straight line or lines.

rectilinear scanner a moving detector imaging device used in nuclear medicine to produce two-dimensional images of the three-dimensional distribution of radioactivity in an object. It consists of one or two detector probes; a pulse-height analyzer (PHA), ratemeter, and associated electronics; and a photorecorder (as shown in the accompanying illustration). The probe moves back and forth, above or below the object, in an equally spaced pattern of parallel scan lines. A light source in the photorecorder moves in synchronization with the probe in an identical or minified pattern over an x-ray film. Counts received by the detector and accepted by the electronic processor are recorded by a light flash, making a mark on the film. Dual-probe scanners simultaneously produce anterior and posterior views.

The probe consists of a multiholed focused collimator, scintillation crystal, photomultiplier tube,

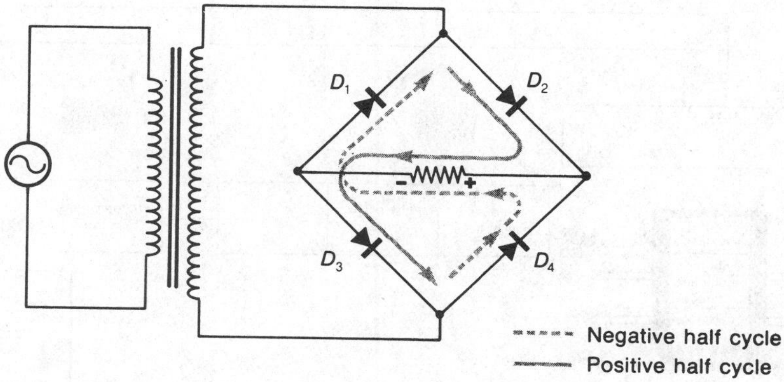

Bridge rectifier. Schematic drawing of a bridge rectifier circuit. (From Diefenderfer, A. J.: Principles of Electronic Instrumentation. 2nd ed. Philadelphia, W. B. Saunders Co., 1979.)

and preamplifier. Owing to the focusing effect of the collimator, images of objects situated above or below the focal plane are blurred, which produces a tomographic effect. The same number of counts is received, but the image of a point is spread out over a circle with a radius proportional to the distance of the point from the focal plane.

The PHA removes counts produced by scattered radiation, accepting those produced by photons within a range (the "energy window") around the principal photopeak of the radionuclide. Photons that lose energy being scattered in the object or collimator do not contribute to the image. The ratemeter measures the counting rate averaged over a period of time controlled by setting the time constant of the meter. Before a scan, the count rate over the region of greatest activity is used to set the maximal count information density (counts per square centimeter) by setting the scan speed, line spacing, and scaling factor (accepted counts per light flash).

Several methods of image modification are used. Background erase inhibits the photorecorder when the count rate is below a preset level. Contrast enhancement produces a scan in which the film blackening is not proportional to the activity in the object. In linear contrast enhancement there is a linear variation of optical density with count rate, but zero density corresponds to the background threshold, whereas in nonlinear contrast enhancement the change in density with count rate increases at higher count rates, thereby reducing the statistical noise in the image. Because any of these modification techniques can remove clinically significant information from the image, there is growing use of digital image processing in which all the accepted counts are stored in a computer; different levels of background erase and contrast enhancement can be experimented with until the optimal image is produced.

See also *multiplane tomographic scanner.*

rectocele (rek′to-sēl) [*recto-* + Gr. *kēlē* hernia] the hernial protrusion of part of the rectum into the vagina caused by rupture of the fibrous connective tissue layer that separates the rectum and the vagina. The condition usually becomes apparent in women above the 35–40 age group. Often, there is a frequent urge to defecate and a sense of rectal and vaginal fullness. The condition is diagnosed clinically but x-ray examination with a barium enema can demonstrate the abnormality. Also called *proctocele.* Cf. *enterocele.*

rectum (rek′tum) [L. "straight"] [NA], the portion of the large intestine that connects the sigmoid colon with the anal canal. It is about 12.5 cm long and begins in front of the middle of the sacrum, following the curve of the sacrum and coccyx. Below the tip of the coccyx, it curves posteriorly to become the anal canal. The lower rectum is expanded as an ampulla. Peritoneum clothes the front and sides of the upper third of the rectum, but is then reflected onto the bladder or vagina to form the rectovesical or rectovaginal pouch.

The wall of the rectum is histologically similar to that of the colon, and most of the epithelial cells form mucin. The taeniae coli of the descending colon spread to form a continuous layer of longitudinal smooth muscle. Functionally, the rectum is essentially a conduit between the colon and exterior via the anal canal; it is usually empty, as fecal material is commonly stored in the sigmoid colon. Entry of fecal material into the rectum triggers a defecation reflex, probably through pressure on the rectal wall.

recumbent (re-kum′bent) lying down. In radiography, this term is applied only to vertical ray projections. Cf. *decubitus.*

dorsal r., lying on one's back. Also called *supine.*

lateral r., lying on one's side.

ventral r., lying face down. Also called *prone.*

recurrence (re-kur′ens) [*re-* + L. *currere* to run] the return of a disease or its symptoms after a remission.

recurrence risk the probability that a genetic defect affecting one or more individuals in a family will also affect future children; the degree of risk varies, depending on the relationship of the potential offspring to the affected individuals.

recursion (re-kur′zhun) 1. a recursive definition. 2. a computation that used a recursive subroutine or algorithm.

recursive definition (re-kur′siv) a definition of a mathematical function in terms of the function itself. The definition is not circular because it allows complex cases to be reduced to simpler ones, and repeated application of the recursive definition pro-

A

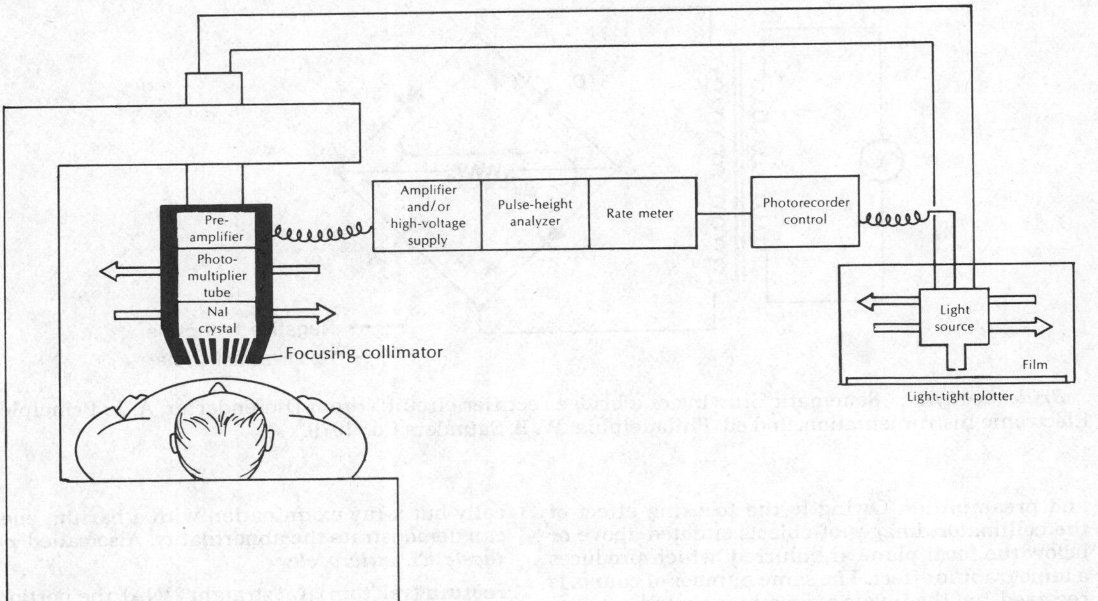

Rectilinear scanner. Block diagram of scanner components. (From Johnson, R. F., Jr.: Operation and quality control of the rectilinear scanner. *In* Rollo, F. D. (ed.): Nuclear Medicine Physics, Instrumentation, and Agents. St. Louis, C. V. Mosby Co., 1977.)

duces a basic, independently defined case. For example, the definition of the factorial function ($n!$) as $n! = n(n-1)!$ is recursive, requiring separate definition of the special case $0! = 1$.

recursive subroutine a computer subroutine that calculates a recursively defined function by calling itself. This requires the subroutine to keep a list of all the values of its variables and of the return addresses for each time it has been entered and reentered without returning to the calling program. Recursive subroutines are a feature supported by only a few high-level languages, such as ALGOL and PL/I.

red (red) [A.S. *rēad*] a spectral color that corresponds to the perceived hue of monochromatic light, having a wavelength between 622 and 770 nm (i.e., between orange and near-infrared).

red blood cell (RBC) see *erythrocyte.*

red blood cell count the number of red blood cells in a representative blood sample; see also *blood cell count.*

red cell a red blood cell. See also *erythrocyte.*

red cell distribution width (RDW) an erythrocyte parameter that reflects dispersion of red cell size (degree of anisocytosis). It is performed by measuring the width of the size distribution curve obtained in automated electronic instruments in which red cells produce pulses, the height of which is proportional to their size.

red cell indices quantitative parameters used as the basis for the morphologic classification of anemias, including mean corpuscular volume (MCV), mean corpuscular hemoglobin (MCH), and mean corpuscular hemoglobin concentration (MCHC). In electronic counters, the MCV is measured directly as the mean of appropriately calibrated pulse heights, which are proportional to the size of individual red cells passing through the counter. In manual methods, the MCV is computed as the hematocrit divided by the red cell count, the MCH is computed as hemoglobin concentration divided by red cell count, and the MCHC is computed as hemoglobin concentration divided by packed cell volume. In automated counters, the MCHC is computed as hemoglobin concentration divided by the red blood cell count times MCV. These indices detect deviations of red cell populations from the normal but give only an average value, sometimes missing abnormalities in blood having mixed red cell populations and particularly a minor, but pathologically significant, second red cell population. Because of this, a peripheral smear should be examined and compared with the values of the red cell indices. See also *blood cell count automation* and the specific indices.

red cell iron turnover rate (RCITR) see under *ferrokinetics study.*

red cell survival test a procedure in nuclear medicine that measures the fraction of the red blood cells in circulation at one time that are still in circulation at later times. An individual's red blood cells are labeled with ^{51}Cr sodium chromate (the chromium(VI) ion binding to hemoglobin) and reinjected; the samples are taken every 2 da to measure the surviving fraction. In normal persons, half the cells will survive for 26–30 da; this is shorter than the normal 120-da life span of red cells because old and young cells are both labeled and because there is some elution of the label, although it is reproducible.

The radioactivity over the heart, liver, and spleen is also measured. A high ratio of spleen to liver or a high ratio of spleen to precordium indicates splenic sequestration of red cells. A survival half-time of less than 20 da shows significant blood loss or hemolysis

See also *ferrokinetics study.* Cf. *cohort labeling.*

red cell volume (RCV) see under *blood volume measurements.*

red mite see *Trombicula.*

red muscle the darker colored muscle of some higher mammals that contains large amounts of myoglobin. These muscles are rich in mitochondria and oxidative enzymes but are deficient in phosphorylases. They react slowly and are used for sustained action. They are generally referred to as slow twitch muscles. See also *muscle.* Cf. *white muscle.*

redox couple (re′doks) a substance that can undergo oxidation-reduction reactions and therefore can exist as an oxidized form (A) and a reduced form (A^-). The redox electrochemical potential generated by this couple can be established by measuring the electromotive force generated when compared with a standard reference redox couple. Also called *conjugate redox pair.*

redox potential (E, E_h) the emf of an oxidation-reduction half-reaction, written as a reduction; it is equal to the electrode potential of an electrochemical half-cell that involves the redox couple. If the reaction is written as an oxidation, the redox potential has the same value but the opposite sign.

The redox potential of a solution containing several redox couples refers to the potential of an inert electrode placed in the solution relative to the standard hydrogen electrode; it does not indicate the state of any particular redox couple in the system.

In bacteriology, E_h is used to characterize the reducing capacity of certain bacterial culture media; it becomes more negative as the hydrogen ion concentration decreases. E_h is usually measured electrically, but it can also be estimated by the reduction of certain dyes to a colorless (leuko) form. At pH 7.0, this occurs with methylene blue at −11 mV and with resazurin at 42 mV.

Also called *oxidation-reduction potential.*

redox reaction see *oxidation-reduction reaction.*

reduce (re-dūs′) [*re-* + L. *ducere* to lead] 1. to cause a substance to undergo reduction.

2. in organic chemistry, to add hydrogen to a double or triple bond.

3. to restore to the normal place or relation of parts, as to reduce a fracture. See also *reduction.*

reducing agent see *reductant.*

reducing substances in urine a heterogeneous group of substances characterized by their ability to reduce cupric ions in hot alkaline solution (Benedict's test, Clinitest). Among the reducing substances that may occur in urine are the sugars glucose, fructose, galactose, lactose, maltose, arabinose, xylose, and ribose, as well as other substances such as amino acids, cysteine, tyrosine, homogentisic acid, ascorbic acid, uric acid, creatinine, ketone bodies, and many drugs and some x-ray contrast media. See also *glucose assays.*

reductant (re-duk′tant) a compound that undergoes oxidation or donates electrons in an oxidation-reduction (redox) reaction. Also called *reducing agent.* Cf. *oxidant.*

reductase (re-duk′tās) an enzyme of the oxidoreductase class (EC 1) that catalyzes the reduction of an organic compound. Clinically important examples are *acetoacetyl-CoA reductase, cytochrome b_5 reductase,* and *4-oxoproline reductase.*

reduction (re-duk′shun) [L. *reductio*] 1. a chemical reaction in which the oxidation number of an atom is decreased; it always occurs together with oxidation. In an electrochemical cell, reduction occurs at the cathode.

2. in organic chemistry, the addition of hydrogen to a double or triple bond is commonly called reduction. This reaction does involve a decrease in the oxidation number of the carbons affected.

3. the correction of a bone fracture, joint dislocation, or hernia.

closed r., the manipulative reduction of a fracture without incision.

open r., the reduction of a fracture after incision into the fracture site.

reduction potential see *electrode potential.*

reduviid (re-du′vĭ-id) belonging to the family Reduviidae.

Reduviidae (re″du-vi′ĭ-de) a family of winged hemipterous insects, the kissing or cone-nose bugs, of which many species (called assassin bugs) feed on insects and humans. Some species are vectors for *Trypanosoma cruzi,* which causes Chagas' disease. This family includes the genera *Eratyrus, Eutriatoma, Panstrongylus, Reduvius, Rhodnius,* and *Triatoma.*

Reduvius (re-du′ve-us) a genus of blood-sucking insects of the family Reduviidae. The species *R. personatus* has a painful bite, which is caused by a potent salivary toxin.

Reed-Sternberg cell [Dorothy *Reed,* American pathologist; Carl *Sternberg,* Austrian pathologist, 1872–1935] an enlarged cell of disputed (lymphocyte or macrophage) lineage, which is characterized by two or more nuclei, each containing a large nucleolus. It is a diagnostic histologic feature in Hodgkin's disease, but similar cells are occasionally seen in other disorders. Also called *Sternberg-Reed cell.*

reentry (re-en′tre) in cardiology, one of the major mechanisms postulated to explain the observation of premature heart beats and their coupling to the normal cardiac rhythm. The premature beats may be atrial, A-V nodal, or ventricular in origin. Reentry requires the pathologic slowing of impulse conduction through the heart. Local ischemia or mechanical stress may be responsible for the decreased responsiveness of an area of the myocardium so that the normal sinus impulse cannot activate the injured area at the normal rate. When the impulse eventually exits the area of decreased conduction velocity, it encounters the adjacent normal myocardium that has already conducted the impulse and recovered electrically. The impulse then "reenters" the normal myocardium from the injured area and elicits a premature contraction. Conduction may be slowed in a diseased area of the heart so that a unidirectional block of impulse conduction occurs. Reexcitation of normal myocardium may then produce retrograde repetitive stimulation of the injured area, resulting in a sustained tachyarrhythmia.

Rees's culture medium (rēs′ez) a culture medium for the cultivation of hemoflagellates, such as *Leishmania donovani, L. braziliensis, L. tropica, Trypanosoma gambiense, T. cruzi,* and the intestinal flagellate *Balantidium coli.* The medium consists of a modified Ringer's solution, with human or horse serum and rice powder. Blood or biopsies of lymph nodes, spleen, liver, or bone marrow are inoculated on the culture and incubated at 36°C.

Reese-Ecker method a method of enumerating blood platelets; see under *platelet count.*

reference materials three distinct classes of reference materials can be identified: primary, secondary, and control materials. Reference materials have been tentatively defined by the International Standards Organization (ISO) to be "a material or substance, one or more physical or chemical properties of which are sufficiently well established to be used for the calibration of an apparatus or the verification of a measurement method."

PRIMARY REFERENCE MATERIALS

Primary Reference Material. This is a term reserved for well-characterized, stable, homogeneous materials of which one or more physical or chemical properties have been experimentally determined within stated measurement uncertainties. When available, values should be assigned by analysis with a Definitive Method or a number of independent methods of established high accuracy. Impurities should be identified and quantitatively evaluated. Homogeneity of the material should be determined and stability established.

Primary Reference Materials are used in calibrating Definitive Methods, in the development, evaluation, and calibration of Reference Methods, and for assigning values to Secondary Reference Material.

Certified Reference Material (CRM). [This] is a term used for reference materials that are accompanied by a certificate stating the property values concerned and issued by an organization which is generally accepted as technically competent, such as the National Bureau of Standards, which is now the world's chief source. Other CRMs are being prepared by the European Community Bureau of Reference, National Physical Laboratory (United Kingdom), and the Bureau National de Metrologie (France).

Biological Matrix Reference Materials. The exact composition of biological matrix reference materials will depend on the intended use. In general, such materials are essentially identical to the actual samples being measured, e.g., pooled serum in which the quantity of one or more analytes has been determined by a Definitive Method. Pooled sera, however, will differ from a patient's sample in regard to the exact concentration of the individual components and possibly of exogenous substances (e.g., drugs that may be present).

Simulated Matrix Reference Materials. These materials have a matrix with properties closely resembling those of the test specimens.

Both Biological Matrix and Simulated Matrix Reference Materials are well-characterized in regard to one or more of the analytes. The assigned values for analytes must be determined by either a Definitive Method or a number of independent methods of high accuracy. Known or potential interfering substances must be specified qualitatively and quantitatively.

Matrix Reference Materials are useful for assessing the reliability and performance of an analytical procedure; for the understanding and elimination of the bias (matrix effects) in Reference or Field Methods under development; and for interrelating results of Definitive, Reference, and Field Methods.

SECONDARY REFERENCE MATERIALS (CALIBRATION AND TEST MATERIALS)

This group of reference materials includes pure substances (usually in solution in aqueous and/or organic solvents) and materials in a matrix that reproduces or simulates the expected matrix. These materials are frequently prepared commercially or in the user's laboratory and are utilized for the calibration of a Field Method. The pure, simple substances could be Primary Reference Materials or they should be materials that have assigned values relative to the Primary Reference Material. Values for analytes in matrix material should be established by analysis with the Reference Method, when available, or values should be traceable to those for a Primary Reference Material. These materials are mainly used to standardize Field Methods and, in conjunction with Reference or Field Methods, to assign values to Control Material.

CONTROL MATERIALS

These materials are primarily used in routine internal and external quality-assurance programs. They are not intended for use as a calibrator and are available assayed or unassayed. Values may be assigned by using a Reference Method or a Field Method together with the appropriate Reference Material (Primary or Secondary, respectively).

(*Reprinted with permission from Tietz, N. W.: A model for a comprehensive measurement system in clinical chemistry. Clinical Chemistry 25: 837-838, 1979.*)

reference strain a strain of bacteria or other microorganisms used as a standard of reference, which appears to meet the criteria of the type strain but is not officially accepted as a neotype.

reference values a range of values of some quantity (physiologic parameter) within which the measurements of most healthy individuals fall. This range, or reference interval, is determined by testing a sample of a well-characterized population of healthy individuals (usually 100–300 people) and calculating an interval that contains 95 percent of the values found in the healthy general population. On the average, values for 1 in 20 healthy persons fall outside the reference interval. Values outside this interval may not necessarily indicate the presence of a pathologic process, but may be caused by special circumstances, e.g., the high protein content of urine in an athlete engaged in rigorous exercise.

The reference interval depends on the choice of the measurement method and on the definition of the health state, and is possibly interrelated to details of the sampling technique and the exact composition of the population studied. Thus, except for commonly used methods, each laboratory may have to establish its own reference values. In addition, subpopulations of infants, children, adults, and older adults may have values that differ widely and thus need separate reference intervals. Even factors such as body build, body position (whether values obtained with patient in upright or recumbent position), and smoking habits of the population may influence the reference interval.

If data from the sample appear to fit a (normal) gaussian distribution, the reference interval may be calculated as the mean plus or minus 2 standard deviations (SD). This reference interval was formerly called the normal range (and the values called normal values), but this terminology is now discouraged because of confusion regarding the meaning of "normal" versus "healthy." If the data do not seem to fit a gaussian distribution, the logarithms of the values may be substituted. If this leads to a gaussian distribution (in this case called "lognormal distribution"), ± 2 SD may be calculated as above. For the nongaussian distribution of values, the use of ± 2 SD gives invalid data; in this case, nonparametric procedures may be used or the central 95th percentile (values between the 2.5th and 97.5th percentile) of the sample may be calculated and used as the reference interval.

If healthy individuals are not available, the interval may be based on a sample of a hospital population, although this is less satisfactory. Statistical techniques are used to identify the data from sick individuals, which are eliminated from the sample.

Previously obtained values for a given individual in a healthy condition may also be used as reference values for comparison with present values that may be indicative of illness. This is the concept of the individual reference values.

For more information on reference ranges and laboratory values of clinical importance, see *Appendix C.*

reflection (re-flek′shun) [L. *reflexio*] 1. the turning back of waves or particles from a surface.

2. the symmetry operation that superimposes an object on its mirror image. The mirror plane is called a reflection plane or symmetry plane.

diffuse r., reflection, as from a matte surface, in which the incident rays are scattered in all directions.

specular r., reflection, as from a mirror, in which the incident and reflected rays make equal angles with a perpendicular to the surface.

total internal r., the reflection of light traveling in a dense medium (e.g., glass) from the interface with a less dense medium (e.g., air) when the angle of incidence is greater than the critical angle (approximately 42° for a glass-air interface). The light is reflected from the surface without any loss.

In binocular microscopes, prisms are used to reflect light beams; the beam enters perpendicularly at one face, is totally internally reflected from a second (the hypotenuse), and exits perpendicularly through the third. In fiberoptic equipment, light is transmitted through a light pipe of flexible glass fibers. As long as the curvature of the light pipe is not too great, the light always strikes the walls at glancing angles and is totally internally reflected with no light loss.

reflex (re′fleks) [L. *reflexus*] a sequence of events initiated in response to an environmental or internal stimulus. The sequence culminates in a response that consists of a stereotypical involuntary activity or movement, or an onset of function in an organ or part.

accommodation r., one of the pupillary reflexes: the coordinated changes that occur when the eye adapts itself for near vision; they are constriction of the pupil, convergence of the eyes, and increased convexity of the lens.

audiocular r., the slight reflex contraction of the orbicularis oculi muscles causing momentary closure of the eyes, or the reaction of the iris, to a sudden loud sound. The absence of this reflex is one of the necessary criteria for establishing brain death. See also *cochleopupillary r.*

autonomic r., a variety of autonomic responses, including changes in the tone of the bladder, gastrointestinal tract, and vascular smooth muscle; in the secretion of the glands; and in the rate and force of contraction of cardiac muscle. These responses are elicited by a number of different stimuli and integrated at various levels of the central nervous system.

axon r., a reflex in which afferent impulses initiated in the terminal branches of sensory nerves from the skin are conducted antidromically down other branches of the same nerves. This is held to account for the flare component of the triple response to local injury, nerve impulses being conducted antidromically to cutaneous arterioles, causing localized vasodilation. Chemical or mechanical irritation of the skin elicits the response.

Bainbridge r., the compensatory increase in heart rate and force of contraction produced when central venous pressure and/or venous return are suddenly increased. The receptors involved may be type A atrial stretch receptors with vagal afferents.

baroreceptor r., a reflex initiated by stretch receptors, primarily distributed in the walls of the carotid sinus and aortic arch, that acts to stabilize arterial blood pressure. When blood pressure increases, the arterial walls are stretched and the baroreceptor afferent nerves increase their firing rate. Incoming baroreceptor impulses exert an inhibitory effect on the medullary vasomotor center and an excitatory effect on the vagal center. Peripheral vasodilation and decrease in cardiac output occur; the net effect is a compensatory decrease in arterial blood pressure. The reverse occurs in response to an initial decrease in blood pressure. Also called *baroreflex.*

Bezold-Jarisch r., the bradycardia and hypotension from enhanced vagal activity that follow chemical stimulation (by veratroidine, for example) of left ventricular myocardial chemoreceptors. This reflex (induced by substances released from the damaged tissue) may account for some of the hypotension that is a frequent complication of myocardial infarction.

carotid sinus r., a baroreceptor reflex initiated by stretch receptors (located in the wall of the carotid sinus) in response to changes in the arterial blood pressure. Impulses from the receptors are transmitted to the central nervous system via the sinus or Hering nerve, a branch of the glossopharyngeal nerve. External application of pressure to the neck at the level of the carotid bifurcation can also elicit a baroreceptor-mediated reflex decrease in blood pressure and heart rate. See also *carotid sinus syndrome.*

ciliospinal r., one of the pupillary reflexes: the dilation of both pupils in response to painful stimulation of the skin; it is effected through the efferent sympathetic pathways. The reflex is elicited most easily by pinching the neck, face, or upper trunk.

cochleopupillary r., a dilation, or constriction followed by a dilation, of the pupils in response to a sudden loud sound. See also *audioocular r.*

conditioned r., a reflex response to a stimulus (the conditioned stimulus) that normally would not be expected to elicit this response. The response becomes associated with the conditioned stimulus as the result of repeated pairing of the stimulus with another stimulus (the unconditioned stimulus), that normally elicits the response. In Pavlov's experiments with dogs, the onset of salivation (conditioned reflex), usually elicited by the placing of food in an animal's mouth (unconditioned stimulus), was eventually elicited by the ringing of a bell (conditioned stimulus) after the conditioned and unconditioned stimuli had been paired a number of times.

corneal r., the reflex closure of both eyes and tearing when the cornea of one eye is stimulated. This reflex, tested by touching the cornea with a wisp of cotton, is used to assess the integrity of the fifth and seventh cranial nerves. The absence of the reflex can be used to ascertain the plane of surgical anesthesia and is one of the necessary criteria for establishing brain death. Also called blink reflex.

cough r., the coordinated sequence of events that is initiated by chemical or mechanical irritation of the nerve endings in the walls of the respiratory passages. When these endings are stimulated by such foreign matter as smoke or noxious gases, afferent impulses to the CNS (mainly via the vagus nerve) result in the following actions, triggered by the neuronal circuitry of the medulla: the inspiration of about 2.5 l of air, and an increase in intrapleural pressure to as much as 100 mmHg (caused by closure of the glottis, then forceful contraction of the expiratory muscles against the closed glottis), followed by a sudden opening of the glottis so that the air under pressure within the lungs flows rapidly down a steep pressure gradient and is explosively expelled. In addition, dynamic compression of the noncartilaginous portion of the trachea acts to increase the velocity of expulsion. The foreign matter is dislodged and swept out with the exhaled air. See also *cough*.

Cushing r., the compensatory increase in arterial pressure and the decrease in heart rate that occur when intracranial pressure (cerebrospinal fluid pressure) becomes great enough to compress the arteries in the brain. The decrease in blood supply (and resulting hypoxia and hypercapnia) stimulates a CNS ischemic response; the arterial pressure is thus brought to a value exceeding the CSF pressure, and blood flow is restored. The bradycardia is a secondary reflex response caused by stimulation of the arterial baroreceptors by the increase in arterial pressure.

enterogastric r., a neurally mediated slowing of gastric motility and inhibition of gastric emptying that is elicited by duodenal distention, irritants (especially excess hydrogen ions), the presence of products of protein digestion in the duodenal chyme, or a hypo- or hypertonic duodenal chyme.

Hering-Breuer r., the reflex responses to the inflation and deflation of the lungs. Inflation during inspiration activates pulmonary stretch receptors; signals from the receptors are transmitted through vagal afferent fibers to the inspiratory center in the medulla, causing the duration of the inspiration to be limited. The reverse happens when the lungs are deflated: the reflex serves to limit the extent of the respiratory excursions of the lungs.

ischemic r., the compensatory rise in arterial blood pressure, sometimes to maximal levels, that occurs in response to cerebral ischemia. The decreased blood flow to the medullary vasomotor center directly excites a massive sympathetic vasoconstriction of the peripheral vasculature, which acts to restore the blood supply. Also called CNS ischemic response.

light r., one of the pupillary reflexes: the constriction of the pupil in response to exposure of the same eye (direct light reflex) or opposite eye (consensual light reflex) to a bright light.

mass r., the simultaneous initiation of many segmental autonomic and somatic spinal reflexes in an animal with high transection of the spinal cord. A noxious stimulus (to the skin, for example) excites a massive discharge of large areas of the spinal cord. As a result, there may be a marked increase in arterial blood pressure, and involuntary defecation, urination, sweating, and intensive flexor spasm of the limbs. A mild mass reflex can be intentionally evoked to give paraplegics some degree of control over their bowel and bladder function.

milk let-down r., the neuroendocrine reflex elicited when nipple mechanoreceptors are stimulated by the suckling of an infant. Stimulation of the receptors causes release from the posterior pituitary of oxytocin, which acts on the myoepithelial cells that surround the alveoli of the lactating breast to stimulate their contraction. Milk is ejected out of the alveoli into the ducts, and begins to flow.

monosynaptic r., the most simple reflex arc, one in which there is only one synapse between the afferent (sensory) and efferent (motor) neurons. Stretch reflexes are the only monosynaptic reflexes known to occur normally in humans.

oculocephalic r., the reflex, conjugate movement of the eyes in response to turning or tilting of the head quickly. In a conscious individual, the eyes move unpredictably in such circumstances. In a comatose patient, however, the eyes may move in a direction opposite to that of the turn (preserved oculocephalic reflex); this indicates the functional integrity of certain brain stem structures. The absence of this reflex response suggests a lesion of the midbrain or pons and is one of the necessary criteria for establishing brain death. Also called *doll's eye movements.*

oculovestibular r., a reflex elicited by briskly turning or tilting the head, when movement of the eyes occurs conjugately in the opposite direction. Such a response is not present in healthy individuals. If present in a comatose person, it indicates that the tegmental structures of the upper brain stem are intact.

orienting r., the behavioral response to the presentation of a novel stimulus, consisting of an increase in attentiveness and alertness.

patellar tendon r., see *knee jerk.*

polysynaptic r., a reflex arc in which at least one interneuron separates the afferent and efferent neural pathways.

postural r., any one of the series of reflexes that act to keep the body upright and provide the continual adjustments needed for the maintenance of a stable postural framework for voluntary motor activity. The principal postural reflexes are positive and negative supporting reactions; stretch, righting, and tonic labyrinthine and neck reflexes; and the hopping and placing reactions.

pupillary r.'s, see *accommodation r., ciliospinal r.,* and *light r.*

righting r.'s, the series of dynamic reactions (largely integrated in midbrain nuclei) by which higher animals operate to return to a standing position (with the head upright) after changes in position have occurred. They include the labyrinthine, body on head, body on body, neck, and optical righting reflexes.

spinal r., any reflex that is integrated at the level of the spinal cord.

stretch r., a contraction of a skeletal muscle in response to passive changes in its length. Passive stretch of the muscle fibers stimulates the muscle spindle stretch receptors to increase their firing rate. The impulses from the receptors are transmitted from the periphery via fast sensory afferent fibers, which form excitatory synapses directly on the alpha–motor neurons in the spinal cord that innervate the muscle that was stretched. The corresponding motor units are excited, causing contraction of the muscle.

tonic r., a reflex response that persists for an appreciable time, especially the contraction of muscles in certain postural reflexes.

withdrawal r., a polysynaptic reflex that is elicited when a noxious sensory stimulus is applied to the skin or subcutaneous tissue. The response is a strong contraction of the flexor muscles and an inhibition of the antagonist muscles (reciprocal inhibition), so that the stimulated portion of the body is withdrawn from the stimulus. When the stimulus is applied to a limb, the opposite limb is in addition reflexly extended (crossed extensor reflex). Also called flexor reflex.

reflex arc the sequence of events and structural pathways through which a change in the internal or external environment (a stimulus) is perceived, integrated, and directed into a compensatory change in activity known as the response. This information transfer system has the following components: a receptor (the stimulus acts on the receptor to change its firing rate), an afferent pathway to a control or integrating center, and an efferent pathway to an effector that brings about the response.

reflux (re′fluks) [*re-* + *fluxus* flow] 1. in a fractional distillation process, liquid that condenses from the vapor rising in the fractionating column and trickles back down the column to the distillation flask.

Refluxing improves separation because of the heat exchange between the reflux and rising vapor, in which the more volatile components are transferred from the reflux to the vapor and the less volatile components from the vapor to the reflux.

2. a backward or return flow. See also *vesicoureteral r.*

hepatojugular r., distention of the jugular veins, induced by applying manual pressure over the liver, which suggests failure of the right heart.

vesicoureteral r., the flow of urine from the bladder back up into the ureter. Also called vesicoureteral regurgitation.

refract (re-frakt′) [L. *refringere* to break apart] 1. to cause to deviate.

2. to ascertain errors of ocular refraction.

refraction (re-frak′shun) the bending of light rays at the interface between two different media. This principle is used in the refractometer, which measures the refraction caused by the solution being measured. The amount of bending depends on the index of refraction (n) in each medium, which is the ratio (always greater than one) of the velocity of light in a vacuum (c) to the velocity of light in the medium (v): $n = c/v$. Snell's law gives the relation between the angle of incidence (i, the angle between the incident light ray and the normal [perpendicular line] to the surface) and the angle of refraction (r, the angle between the refracted ray and the normal); the formula is $n_i \cdot \sin i = n_r \cdot \sin r$, where n_i and n_r are the indexes of refraction of the first and second media.

The angle (of incidence or refraction) is always greater in the less dense medium. For light traveling from the denser medium with an angle greater than the critical angle (θ, where $\sin \theta = n_r/n_i$); Snell's law gives a sin r greater than one, which is impossible. In this case, the light is reflected back into the denser medium, a phenomenon called total internal reflection.

See also *index of refraction* and *refractometer.*

double r., see *birefringence.*

refractive (re-frak′tiv) pertaining to refraction; having the power to refract.

refractive index see *index of refraction.*

refractometer (re″frak-tom′ĕ-ter) [*refraction* + Gr. *metron* measure] 1. an instrument for measuring the refractive power of the eye.

2. an instrument for determining the refractive index of various substances. In clinical chemistry, refractometers are used as tools for the indirect measurement of total dissolved solids in urine (usually estimated by specific gravity) and of total protein in serum.

refractory (re-frak′to-re) [L. *refractarius*] 1. not readily yielding to treatment.

2. capable of enduring high temperatures.

refractory anemia see *aplastic a.* and *refractory a.* under *anemia.*

refractory sideroblastic anemia see *sideroblastic a.* under *anemia.*

Refsum's disease (ref′soomz) [Sigvald *Refsum,* Norwegian physician] a rare inherited disorder of lipid metabolism, transmitted as an autosomal recessive trait, that results in the marked accumulation of phytanic acid in the blood and tissues. The disorder is considered to result from a deficiency of phytanic acid hydroxylase, an enzyme required to clear and metabolize phytanic acid. It is characterized by neuropathies of the peripheral nerves, retinitis pigmentosa, cerebellar motor disturbances, various sensory defects including impaired hearing, and abnormal electrocardiographic measurements. Ichthyosis and bone abnormalities are observed. Elevated cerebrospinal fluid protein levels are also found. Antenatal diagnosis of Refsum's disease is now considered feasible. Also called phytanic acid storage disease.

Regan isoenzyme an isoenzyme of alkaline phosphatase (ALP) found in the serum of about 5 percent of individuals with a variety of carcinomas. It resembles placental ALP in its electrophoretic mobility and in its degree of inhibition by phenylalanine, heat, or urea.

regeneration (re-jen″er-a′shun) [*re-* + L. *generare* to produce, bring to life] 1. the natural renewal of a structure, as of a lost tissue or part.

2. the restoration of function to a system that has undergone chemical modification, e.g., the renewal or reactivation of a desiccant, catalyst, or ion-exchange resin.

3. renewal of information that is subject to decay, such as the image on a storage oscilloscope or a cathode ray tube display terminal.

4. see *positive feedback.*

regimen (rej′ĭ-men) [L. "guidance"] a strictly regulated scheme of diet, exercise, or therapeutics.

region (re'jun) a plane with more or less definite boundaries. For more information, see the specific region.

regional enteritis (re'jun-al) see *Crohn's disease.*

region of interest (ROI) a region of a scintiphotograph obtained using computerized data acquisition that is marked for further computer processing. The region is drawn on the display screen with a light pen or cursor. The computer can then construct an activity-time curve, a plot of the total activity in the ROI recorded in successive intervals.

register (rej'is-ter) a computer hardware circuit that holds one word of data on which operations are performed or which is used in controlling the program. Registers are used to hold the instruction being processed and its address and operation code; the data are transferred to and from memory and the memory address for the transfer, the indexes are used to calculate the addresses of operands, and the data are manipulated by arithmetic or logical operations. A single arithmetic/logical register is usually called the accumulator. Large computers usually have several registers used for both arithmetic and indexing, as well as special registers for floating-point arithmetic.

registry (rej'is-tre) 1. an organization that lists available professionals in certain fields or those meeting certain qualifications.

2. a central agency for the collection of pathologic material (tissue and slides), related clinical laboratory data, and radiographs, and the organization of these materials for the purpose of making them available for study.

3. a central agency for the collection of clinical information; laboratory, radiologic, and pathologic data; methods of treatment; and follow-up on patient response to therapy for neoplastic diseases. Also called *tumor registry.*

Regitine (rej'ĭ-tēn) trademark. See *phentolamine.*

regression (re-gresh'un) [L. *regressio* a return] 1. a return to a former or earlier state.

2. a subsidence of symptoms or of a disease process.

3. in statistics, a relationship between a dependent random variable and one or more independent variables. See also *least-squares regression* and *linear regression.*

regression curve a function that represents the dependence of one random variable, *Y*, on another, *X*. For each value of *X*, it gives the conditional mean (or median) of *Y*, i.e., the average (or middle) value of *Y* observed when *X* is fixed. The regression curve minimizes the conditional average squared deviation (or absolute deviation) of *Y* from the curve. This makes it the best predictor (in the sense of least squares, for example) of which *Y* will occur with a given *X*. Also called the regression curve of *Y* on *X* to emphasize that *Y* is the dependent variable; the regression curve of *X* on *Y* is different, except in the case of perfect correlation. See also *linear regression.*

regulated area an area defined in OSHA (Occupational Safety and Health Administration) standards as one "in which entry and exit is restricted and controlled." The standards for some specific chemicals known or suspected to be carcinogens include a number of requirements for use of the chemicals, including establishment by an employer of a regulated area where the chemicals are processed, used, repackaged, released, handled, or stored.

regulation (reg"u-la'shun) [L. *regula* rule] 1. the control of the form or behavior of an organism that is mediated by the nervous and endocrine systems or other homeostatic mechanisms.

2. a governmental order issued by an executive agency, which has the force of law.

regulator 1. a device that maintains a quantity at some present level despite variations in external conditions. See also *current regulator* and *voltage regulator.*

2. a biologic entity, such as an enzyme or hormone, that functions to maintain a biologic equilibrium.

regulatory gene a gene that contains information that controls gene function in various ways, such as by enzyme induction, repression, metabolic regulation, controlling transcription and translation, and RNA processing. See also *gene.*

regulatory sequence a DNA sequence involved in regulating gene expression, e.g., a promoter or operator, rather than encoding a polypeptide.

regurgitation (re-ger"jĭ-ta'shun) [*re-* + L. *gurgitare* to flood] a backward flowing, as in the casting up of undigested food or the backflow of blood through a defective heart valve. See also *aortic regurgitation, mitral regurgitation,* and *tricuspid regurgitation.*

rehydration (re"hi-dra'shun) 1. physiologically, the correction of a fluid volume deficit.

2. in histology, to reverse the process of dehydration.

Reid's base line (rēdz) [Robert William *Reid,* Scottish anatomist, 1851–1939] an imaginary reference line used in radiography, which passes through the infraorbital ridge of the orbit and the middle of the external auditory meatus.

Reid index (rēd) the ratio of bronchial mucous glands to bronchial wall thickness, which is used to quantitate the degree of mucous gland hyperplasia in conditions such as chronic bronchitis. Most individuals with chronic bronchitis have a Reid index above 0.55.

reinfection (re"in-fek'shun) a second infection with the same pathogenic agent.

reinnervation (re"in-er-va'shun) 1. the operative procedure by which a live nerve is grafted into a paralyzed muscle to restore its function.

2. the process by which denervated muscle fibers are rescued by neighboring functional motor units. Motor units sprout axonal twigs that grow toward and eventually contact the denervated fibers. At the points of contact, new myoneural junctions are formed. A muscle cell thus reinnervated will adapt its fiber type to match that of the rescuing motor unit.

Reinsch test see under *arsenic assays.*

Reissner's membrane (rīs'nerz) [Ernst *Reissner,* German anatomist, 1824–1878] the thin bilaminar wall that forms the roof of the scala media (cochlear duct), partitioning it from the scala vestibuli. Also called *vestibular membrane.*

Reiter's syndrome (ri'terz) [Hans *Reiter,* German hygienist, born 1881] a disorder occurring in young adult males that is characterized by arthritis, conjunctivitis, urethritis, and frequent cutaneous lesions. The etiology is unknown, but in some cases venereal transmission is evident, with mycoplasma and chlamydia suspected as causative organisms. The arthritis is usually asymmetric and involves multiple, large weight-bearing joints, primarily in the lower extremities. Laboratory findings are non-specific, except for a high incidence of HLA-B27. Most signs of the disease disappear within weeks, but the arthritis may persist for months or even years. Treatment is symptomatic.

relapse (re-laps') [L. *relapsus*] the return of a disease weeks or months after its apparent cessation.

relapsing fever (re-laps'ing fe'ver) an acute infectious disease due to several species of spirochetes of the *Borrelia* genus. It is characterized by recurrent paroxysmal fever and lasts for 3–10 da, followed by periods of apparent recovery. The main reservoirs for the spirochetes are rodents and humans, with the infection transmitted by the bite of a soft-backed tick (*Ornithodoros*) or by the bite of the body louse (*Pediculus humanus*). The tick-borne form is more common in the United States, especially in the West where *O. hermsi* is the principal vector.

About 2–15 da after an individual is bitten by either vector, there is onset of fever, chills, nausea, arthralgia, and severe headaches. Splenic and hepatic enlargement is common. Rashes, delirium, neurologic and psychic disturbances, and tachycardia are common during the acute phase. Casts, albumin, and polymorphonuclear leukocytosis in the urine may also be seen. The acute attack ends suddenly within 3–10 da, to be followed 10–20 da later by a relapse. Most relapse phases are milder than the acute phase, and after 2–10 similar episodes recovery occurs and immunity develops. Clinical forms of recurrent paroxysmal fever may be seen in tularemia, meningococcemia, malaria, and rat-bite fever.

Laboratory diagnosis requires demonstration of large spirochetes (usually *B. recurrentis*) in blood smears stained with Wright or Giemsa stain. The organisms grow in mouse blood and are recoverable 3–5 da after inoculation. Anti-*Borrelia* antibodies develop and false-positive syphilis test results are seen. Meningeal involvement may lead to altered cerebrospinal fluid. Anemia and thrombocytopenia with normal white blood cell counts also occur. Mortality rates are approximately 5 percent but are higher in very young or very old individuals. Tetracycline or penicillin therapy usually reduces the severity and shortens the course of the disease; however, a Jarisch-Herxheimer reaction may develop and complicate the disease process following initial treatment.

Also called yellow famine fever and yellow plague. See also *spirochete*.

relation (re-la'shun) 1. a mathematical or logical association or function holding between variables. 2. a person connected to another by kinship.

relative biological effectiveness (RBE) a measure of the amount of specific radiation damage produced by exposure to ionizing radiation, as compared with the damage produced by the same absorbed dose (in rads) of high-energy x-rays. The RBE is 1 for x-rays, gamma rays, and beta particles; 20 for fast alpha particles; and 10 for fast neutrons and protons (30 for exposure to the eye). Also called *quality factor*. See also *rem*.

relative cardiac volume an estimate of the size of the heart, calculated from direct measurements of three standard dimensions of the cardiac silhouette on chest x-rays. Relative cardiac volume is calculated as: $L \times S \times D \times K$/body surface area, where L represents the long axis of the heart, S is the short axis, D is the largest anteroposterior diameter, and K is a constant used to adjust for the distance between the film and the x-ray tube. A value greater than 490 cc/m² for females or 540 cc/m² for males indicates an enlargement of the heart and is a sign of cardiac disease.

relative centrifugal force (RCF) the weight of a particle in a centrifuge relative to its normal weight, the centrifugal force per unit mass in gravities: $RCF = 11.18 \times 10^{-6} \times r \times N^2$, where r is the radius of the centrifuge (from the shaft center to the bottom of the tube), and N is the number of revolutions per minute. Also called relative centrifugal field.

relative standard deviation (RSD) the standard deviation divided by the mean, i.e., expressed as a fraction of the mean. Also called *coefficient of variation*.

relaxation volume (Vr) (re"lak-sa'shun) the point on the pressure-volume curve of the relaxed lung at which the opposing elastic recoil pressures of the chest wall are in balance, and total pressure in the respiratory system is atmospheric (zero). The relaxation volume is normally equivalent to the functional residual capacity.

relaxin (re-lak'sin) a polypeptide secreted by the corpus luteum during pregnancy; M.W. about 6000. This polypeptide has a structural similarity to insulin and is thought to be synthesized in the ovaries as a prohormone. Relaxin causes dilation and softening of the cervix, inhibition of uterine contractions, and relaxation of the pubic symphysis and other pelvic joints. It has been used in treatment of dysmenorrhea and premature labor, and to facilitate labor at term. Administration of relaxin early in a pregnancy will promote resorption of the fetus.

relay (re'lay) an electromechanical switching device in which the contacts are closed by the movement of an armature in response to the current passing through a magnetic coil. Because relays are slow and unreliable, newer equipment usually has semiconductor switching devices. See also *solenoid*.

mercury-wetted r., a reed relay in which the reed and contacts are covered by a film of mercury, which extends the operating life of the relay and prevents bouncing of the contacts on closure.

reed r., a relay having the contacts mounted on magnetic reeds sealed in a glass tube. Some can be directly activated by transistor-transistor logic (TTL) and are used for switching instrumentation output signals. In general, they can be activated by low-voltage and current levels and have current ratings in the milliampere range.

releasing hormone (RH) any of a class of hypothalamic, low-molecular-weight polypeptides that arrive at the pituitary through the portal veins and influence the release of the pituitary hormones.

relief (re-lēf) [L. *relevatio*] the mitigation or removal of pain or signs and symptoms of a disease.

relieve (re-lēv) [L. *relevare* to lighten] to provide relief.

REM abbrev. See *rapid eye movement*.

rem (rem) [acronym from *r*oentgen *e*quivalent *m*an] a unit of ionizing radiation exposure equal to the exposure that produces the same damage to humans as 1 rad of high-energy x-rays. The rem/rad ratio is called the relative biological effectiveness (RBE). The RBE has been legally established by federal regulations as 1 for beta, gamma, and x-radiation, and 20 for alpha radiation; that is, the rad and rem are equivalent quantities of beta-, gamma-, and x-radiation exposure, but for alpha radiation, 20 rads equals 1 rem.

remission (re-mish′un) [L. *remissio*] 1. a diminution or abatement of the symptoms of a disease.

2. the period during which such abatement occurs.

remnant (rem′nant) something remaining; a residue or vestige.

remnant rays in radiology, the x-rays that emerge from the object and produce the radiographic image. They consist of primary rays not absorbed in the object and secondary rays produced in the object.

ren (ren), pl. *renes,* gen. *renis* [L.] [NA], either of the two renal organs (i.e., the kidneys) in the lumbar region that excrete urine.

ren/o (re′no) a word element used in combining form to denote the kidney, e.g., renotrophic.

renal (re′nal) [L. *renalis*] pertaining to the kidney.

renal adenocarcinoma see under *renal tumors.*

renal artery one of the paired branches that arise from the sides of the abdominal aorta and run directly to the corresponding renal hilum.

renal calyx one of a system of collecting sacs into which urine passes after it leaves the renal parenchyma through the apices of the medullary pyramids. The calyceal system is made up of a series of 12–16 minor calyces, each a funnel-shaped structure that caps one of the pyramids, and a smaller number of major calyces into which the minor calyces empty. The major calyces are in continuity with the renal pelvis. The calyces are lined by transitional epithelium, and their walls contain two layers of smooth muscle with a complex orientation that facilitates movement of urine into the pelvis and ureter. See also *kidney.*

renal corpuscle the commencement of a nephron, formed by the capillaries of the glomerulus and the double-walled expanded portion of the renal tubule.

renal cortex the outer zone of the kidney, which surrounds the medulla and is covered by the renal capsule. The glomeruli and proximal and distal convoluted tubules are located within the cortex. See also *kidney.*

renal failure a loss of normal function of the kidneys.

acute r. f. (ARF), kidney dysfunction involving a sudden fall in the glomerular filtration rate (GFR); the normal GFR is approximately 70 ml/min/m^2 of body surface area. At the glomerulus of the kidney, whole blood is filtered, producing a cell-free, protein-free filtrate. This failure is preceded by azotemia, i.e., a buildup of nitrogenous wastes, especially blood urea nitrogen and creatinine. An acute decrease in the amount of the glomerular filtrate produced can be caused by three basic mechanisms: prerenal, postrenal, and intrarenal failure.

Prerenal failure, accounting for 25 percent of all ARF, arises as a consequence of a decreased volume of blood reaching the kidneys. This decreased perfusion may be secondary to actual loss of blood volume, or to an effective decrease of blood volume at the level of the kidneys due to poor cardiac pumping function, increased systemic vasodilation, increased renal arterial resistance, or renal artery occlusion. Postrenal failure (10 percent of all cases) is a result of mechanical obstruction to urine flow at the level of the ureters, bladder, or urethra. The remaining 65 percent of episodes of ARF are intrarenal in origin, and their causes include renal ischemia or nephrotoxicity (often referred to as acute tubular necrosis, ATN, and accounting for 99 percent of all cases of intrarenal failure), substances that are specifically toxic to the kidneys (e.g., aminoglycoside antibiotics, mercury, lead, ethylene glycol, carbon tetrachloride, x-ray contrast material), acute glomerulonephritis, vasculitis, malignant hypertension, infection, tubular obstruction (often with myeloma protein, uric acid, myoglobin, or hemoglobin), renal vein thrombosis, and necrosis of portions of the kidney itself.

Many laboratory tests and other diagnostic studies help to determine the cause of ARF. Postrenal failure is suggested by the complete absence of urine (anuria) and is best diagnosed by ultrasound, computed tomography, intravenous pyelography, or retrograde pyelography. Prerenal and intrarenal failure generally produce oliguria (decreased urine volume), although nearly half of all patients with acute tubular necrosis may, in fact, by nonoliguric. (Azotemia still ensues despite good urine volume.) Laboratory studies are most helpful in distinguishing prerenal from intrarenal failure. These differences are outlined in the accompanying table.

The clinical course varies, depending on the patient's state of health and the underlying cause of the renal failure. In general, those patients who do survive regain complete renal function. Prior to recovery, one must monitor fluid and electrolyte balance. In particular, potassium levels can become dangerously high, leading to muscular paralysis and cardiac failure. Management generally includes dialysis to control the azotemia, fluid volume, and electrolyte levels. The major causes of mortality are infection and gastrointestinal hemorrhage.

chronic r. f. (CRF), the progressive loss of renal function, and therefore GFR, due to an irreversible process whereby individual nephrons are destroyed by some intrinsic renal disease. CRF may take years to become clinically apparent because, as individual nephrons are destroyed, the remaining nephrons hypertrophy and may almost compensate for the loss of function. Major causes of CRF include the glomerulonephropathies (50–60 percent), diabetic nephropathy, hypertension, polycystic kidney disease, vesicoureteral reflux, drugs (especially phenacetin), chronic pyelonephritis and tuberculosis, collagen vascular disease (e.g., systemic lupus erythematosus), and congenital anomalies.

During the early stages of CRF the individual often remains asymptomatic. However, the severity of the disease may be judged by a laboratory measurement of creatinine clearance or inulin clearance, which roughly approximates to the GFR. Symptoms may not appear until the kidneys have lost 80–85 percent of their normal functioning ability, at which point the syndrome of uremia becomes apparent. It is not currently known whether the toxic effects of uremia are caused by urea and creatinine or by some other metabolic intermediate or product.

RENAL FAILURE. COMPARISON OF VALUES FOUND IN PRERENAL AND INTRARENAL FAILURE*

VALUE	PRERENAL FAILURE	INTRARENAL FAILURE
BUN/creatinine	> 10:1	< 10:1
Urine sediment	Hyaline casts	Granular casts, epithelial cells
Creatinine	< 5 mg/dl	> 5 mg/dl
Urine osmolarity	> 500 mOsm/kg	< 350 mOsm/kg
Urine Na	< 20 mmol/l	> 40 mmol/l
Urine/plasma BUN	> 8	< 3
Urine/plasma creatinine	> 40	< 20
Fractional excretion of Na $\left(\frac{U/P\ Na}{U/P\ Cr} \times 100\right)$	< 1.0	> 1.0

Note: Chronic postrenal failure values tend to be similar to ATN except FeNa, which is usually < 1.0.

Manifestations of uremia include peripheral neuropathy, encephalopathy, anemia, bleeding, pericarditis, hypertension, anorexia, nausea and vomiting, glucose intolerance, infertility, bone disease, hyperparathyroidism, pruritus, psychologic disorders, edema, hyponatremia, hyperkalemia, acidosis, and fluid disturbance. In children, CRF has the additional effect of interfering with normal growth and development.

Management includes compensation for or correction of the various malfunctions present in uremia. Laboratory tests are most useful in measuring the particular electrolytes, hematologic variables, hormones, etc., that are altered by CRF, as well as in determining the GFR.

Advanced, end-stage renal disease poses difficult clinical decisions regarding the use of transplantation or chronic dialysis in order to maintain life. The stage at which these decisions must be made is highly variable, but is generally the serum creatinine exceeds 15 mg/dl, BUN is >100 mg/dl, and GFR falls below 5 ml/min.

Also called *uremia.*

SANDRA L. WATKINS, M.D.

renal medulla the inner part of the kidney, surrounded by the renal cortex. It is composed of a series of 12–16 conical projections, the pyramids; the base of a pyramid lies next to the cortex, and its apex projects into the hilus and is covered by a minor calyx. The medulla contains the thin segments of the nephrons and the collecting ducts. See also *kidney.*

renal pelvic carcinoma see under *renal tumors.*

renal pelvis a pouch shaped like a curved funnel that connects the renal calyces with the ureter. Like the calyces, it is lined by transitional epithelium and contains two layers of smooth muscle within its wall. The pelvis and calyces can be demonstrated radiologically by intravenous or retrograde pyelography. See also *kidney.*

renal pyramid a conical mass of tissue in the renal medulla. The apices of the pyramids project into the renal pelvis. Within the pyramids are the loops of Henle, the collecting ducts, and the vasa recta.

renal threshold the blood concentration of a substance (e.g., glucose) above which the substance cannot be reabsorbed by the renal tubules and thus is excreted into the urine.

renal tumors in the strict sense, a term to denote neoplasms derived from cells of the renal parenchyma; in common usage, however, it also includes neoplasms derived from cells of the renal pelvis.

Those tumors with an origin in the renal parenchyma are of diverse histogenesis and may be composed of metanephric blastema, differentiated proximal convoluted tubular epithelium, and mesenchyme (see the accompanying table). Major categories of renal parenchymal tumors are unrelated epidemiologically; however, renal adenocarcinoma and renal pelvic carcinoma, which are embryologically and morphologically dissimilar, may share certain etiologic factors.

Benign renal tumors are principally of stromal origin, and for the most part are asymptomatic and found incidentally at autopsy. Primary malignant neoplasms of the kidney are relatively uncommon, ranking thirteenth among human cancers. Approximately 1.5 percent of all human cancers arise in the kidney (1.2 percent of renal parenchymal and 0.3 percent of renal pelvic origin). Most of those arising in the renal parenchyma are renal adenocarcinomas (85.7 percent); the remainder are nephroblastomas (11.6 percent) and sarcomas (2.7 percent).

Renal adenocarcinomas occur almost exclusively in adults, an age group in which nephroblastomas are rare. As such, in adults, this neoplasm represents approximately 97 percent of all malignant tumors of the renal parenchyma. Malignant tumors of the renal pelvis are almost exclusively transitional carcinomas.

RENAL ADENOCARCINOMA. This type of renal neoplasm shows differentiation toward cells of the proximal convoluted tubule. It is rare in children, is uncommon in persons under age 30 yr, and thereafter shows an increase in frequency with advancing age. Males are affected three times as often as females. An increased frequency is noted among tobacco users. An association with von Hippel–Lindau disease is also recognized, with approximately two-thirds of such patients developing renal adenocarcinomas at some stage of their illness. In 70–75 percent of those with renal adenocarcinoma, the tumor is discovered because of urologic symptoms; the remaining tumors are diagnosed because of other manifestations of this disease, approximately 10 percent because of symptoms of metastasis.

CONGENITAL MESOBLASTIC NEPHROMA. Most mesoblastic nephromas are present at birth and diag-

Renal Tumors. Classification of Renal Tumors

Classification/Derivation
I. *Renal Parenchyma*
A. Derived from Proximal Convoluted Tubule
1. "Renal Adenoma"
2. Renal Adenocarcinoma
B. Derived from Metanephric Blastema
1. Congenital Mesoblastic Nephroma
2. Nephroblastomatosis
3. Nephroblastoma
4. Multilocular Cystic Kidney?
C. Derived from Mesenchymal Structures
Benign
1. Lipoma
2. Leiomyoma
3. Angiomyolipoma
4. Hemangioma
5. Juxtaglomerular Tumor
6. Lymphangioma
7. Renomedullary Interstitial Cell Tumor (Medullary Fibroma)
Malignant
1. Leiomyosarcoma
2. Liposarcoma
3. Fibrosarcoma
4. Fibroxanthosarcoma
II. *Renal Pelvis*
A. Derived from Epithelium
Benign
1. Papilloma
2. Fibroepithelial Polyp
Malignant
1. Transitional Carcinoma
2. Squamous Carcinoma
3. Adenocarcinoma
B. Derived from Mesenchymal Structures
Benign
1. Leiomyoma
2. Angioma
Malignant
1. Miscellaneous Sarcomas

Courtesy of James L. Bennington, M.D.

nosed within the early months of life. The presenting feature is usually an abdominal mass, occasionally with a history of recent rapid growth. Association with other syndromes such as hemihypertrophy and aniridia, as occurs with nephroblastoma, has not been reported. Nephrectomy has effected a cure in virtually all patients with mesoblastoma, although there are a few reports of recurrence.

Nephroblastoma. Classically, nephroblastomas are tumors composed of an admixture of epithelial stromal and blastemal components, although either one component may predominate. Although nephroblastomas are found in all age groups, the vast majority occur in children under the age of 10 yr, with the peak occurrence at 1–2 yr; the childhood incidence is approximately 1 per 100,000 live births. The rate is the same for males and females. In some cases, hereditary factors are thought to influence occurrence. Both tumor stage and histologic classification of nephroblastoma correlate with prognosis. Chemotherapy and radiation therapy are highly effective, contributing to an overall cure rate in excess of 80 percent.

Multilocular Cystic Kidney. This type of tumor is of uncertain pathogenesis; it has been postulated to represent either a benign neoplasm arising from metanephric blastema (perhaps analogous to the mesoblastic nephroma it resembles), a nephroblastoma that has undergone benign differentiation, or a developmental abnormality. It has been noted at all ages, but the number reported is relatively small. About half of all cases occur in young children (approximately 8 per 100,000 live births), and the remainder in adults. In some cases, particularly those in children, tumors described as multicystic kidney may represent other entities such as cystic mesoblastic nephroma and cystic partially differentiated nephroblastoma.

The lesion presents most commonly as an abdominal mass; less frequently reported symptoms are hematuria and hypertension. Multicystic kidney appears to be a benign lesion adequately treated with nephrectomy.

Angiomyolipoma. This type of renal tumor is generally unilateral and solitary. It is multiple in 13–30 percent of cases, and when multiple may involve one or both kidneys. The tumor is relatively uncommon, with a mean age of occurrence of 41 yr. There is a predominance of females over males (a ratio of 2.6:1). Among patients who are symptomatic, the usual presenting symptom is flank pain, which may be sudden and severe, and is usually due to intra- or perirenal hemorrhage into the tumor. Occasionally, hematuria or hypertension is the presenting symptom. An association with tuberous sclerosis is well established. Approximately 40 percent of persons with renal angiomyolipoma have tuberous sclerosis, and about 80 percent of those with tuberous sclerosis have symptomatic or asymptomatic angiomyolipomas. Angiomyolipomas may occasionally invade adjacent organs. However, it is doubtful that distant metastasis ever occurs.

Renal Pelvic Carcinoma. Carcinomas of the renal pelvis rarely arise under age 30 yr, but thereafter increase in frequency with advancing age. The ratio of males to females is 3:1. Geographic factors may influence the frequency of occurrence, but no hereditary influence has been identified. Certain chemical agents are associated with increased frequency of carcinomas of the renal pelvis, e.g., industrial chemicals such as dye stuffs, rubber, plastic, and gas. In addition, certain habits such as smoking and the taking of large amounts of phenacetin predispose to carcinomas of the renal pelvis at rates substantially higher than those expected of the normal population. Presenting features are predominantly those of hematuria (80 percent), pain (24 percent), and dysuria; frequency, abdominal mass, and pyuria each present with an occurrence of 10 percent.

Because carcinomas of the renal pelvis are often

multicentric, recurrences are likely in patients treated with less than total nephrectomy. The prognosis appears to be directly related to tumor grade and extent of invasion. Reports of the relative frequency of the various histologic types of carcinoma found in the renal pelvis are usually in the range of 90–92 percent (transitional carcinoma), 8 percent (squamous cell carcinoma), and less than 1 percent (adenocarcinoma). In general, squamous cell carcinoma and adenocarcinomas appear to have a shorter natural history than does transitional carcinoma of the renal pelvis.

renal vein the vein that drains blood from the corresponding kidney to the inferior vena cava.

Rendu-Weber-Osler disease (ron-du′ web′er ōs′ler) [Henri Jules Louis Marie *Rendu,* French physician, 1844–1902; Frederick Parkes *Weber,* British physician, 1863–1962; Sir William *Osler,* Canadian-born physician, 1849–1919] see *hereditary hemorrhagic t.* under *telangiectasia.*

reniform (ren′ĭ-form) [*ren* + L. *forma* form] shaped like a kidney.

renin (re′nin) a proteolytic enzyme of the hydrolase class (EC 3.4.99.19) that catalyzes the conversion of angiotensinogen to angiotensin I in the plasma; it is produced and stored in the juxtaglomerular cells of the kidneys. Renin is synthesized in a larger form (prorenin or big renin) and converted to its enzymatically active form, being released into the blood in response to decreased plasma volumes, sodium depletion, fluid transudation, decreased arterial pressure, hemorrhage, and increased potassium. Increased blood volumes, acute increases in blood pressure, and potassium loss suppress renin release.

Renin activity is increased in some types of hypertension, adrenocortical insufficiency, renin-secreting tumors, and salt-losing nephropathies. Decreased values are observed in some types of hypertension, primary aldosteronism, and adrenal carcinomas. Antidiuretic hormone therapy and salt-retaining steroids tend to decrease renin values, whereas specimens drawn in the morning and in upright position and low salt diets yield higher values.

Reference values for renin in plasma are: for adults in an upright position and with normal salt intake, 0.4–4.5 ng/ml/hr.

See also *hypertension, plasma renin activity, plasma renin concentration,* and *renin-aldosterone axis.*

renin-aldosterone axis see *renin-angiotensin-aldosterone system.*

renin-angiotensin-aldosterone system a related group of physiologically active compounds involved in the regulation of plasma sodium and potassium balance, arterial fluid volume, and blood pressure.

Renin is released from the cortex of the kidney into the circulatory system when the blood volume decreases and the arterial pressure falls following a reduction in kidney perfusion.

This condition may occur as a result of hemorrhage, sodium depletion, fluid transudation, or alimentary loss. The renin then converts a plasma globulin (angiotensinogen) to angiotensin I, which is converted to angiotensin II by an enzyme originating from the lung capillaries. Angiotensin II possesses pressor activity and also stimulates aldosterone secretion, which in turn causes the kidneys to retain sodium. This process results in retention of water, expansion of extracellular fluid, increase in blood pressure, restoration of normal potassium levels, and restoration of renal perfusion. Conversely, when the blood volume expands or blood pressure increases, there is cessation of renin secretion and loss of sodium.

Also called *renin-aldosterone axis.* See also *aldosterone* and *renin.*

renin assays 1. plasma renin activity (PRA), a measure of the activity of the enzyme renin. This is usually accomplished by a radioimmunoassay of angiotensin I, formed as a result of incubation of plasma at 37°C in the presence of inhibitors that prevent the enzymatic conversion of angiotensin I to angiotensin II. Endogenous substrate concentration, and hence the PRA, are increased in the presence of Addison's disease, primary salt-losing nephropathy, diuretic therapy, hemorrhage, pregnancy, and oral contraceptives.

2. plasma renin concentration (PRC), a measure of the concentration of renin in terms of its activity. This is accomplished by inactivating the endogenous substrate, adding an excess of exogenous substrate, and measuring the generation of the product angiotensin I by radioimmunoassay. As zero-order kinetics is followed, the PRC is independent of substrate concentration and is proportional to the renin concentration. Owing to the difficulty of performing the plasma renin concentration assay, most laboratories utilize some form of the plasma renin activity assay.

rennin (ren′in) see *chymosin.*

Renografin (re″no-graf′in) trademark. See under *diatrizoate.*

renogram (re′no-gram) a graph that indicates kidney function. A radiopharmaceutical capable of being filtered only by the kidney is injected; ^{131}I orthoiodohippurate (sodium hippurate I 131) is preferred. The radioactivity of each kidney is separately measured during the 30 min it takes to filter the agent, and the variation over time is charted. An abnormal difference in the function of the two kidneys or a significant obstruction or loss of function in a kidney can be detected.

This procedure may be performed using two scintillation probes placed over the kidneys, although better results can be obtained with a scintillation camera having computer data analysis. Regions of interest are specified using the images of the kidneys.

For radiography of the kidney, see *pyelography* or *urography.*

Reno-M-DIP trademark for a preparation of diatrizoate meglumine administered by drip infusion in pyelography and computed tomography.

Renovue trademark. See *iodamide meglumine.*

Renshaw cell an interneuron in lamina IX of the ventral horn of the spinal cord that makes inhibitory contact with motor neurons.

Reovirus (re″o-vi′rus) [acronym from *r*espiratory and *e*nteric *o*rphan + *virus*] a genus of double-stranded RNA viruses that can cause respiratory and gastrointestinal diseases in children. The nucleic acid is divided into 10–12 molecules of RNA and the virion contains its own transcriptase. This virus is a common inhabitant of sewage and is stable at pH 3.

Three immunotypes of *Reovirus* are distinguishable by hemagglutination-inhibition or neutralization tests. Reoviruses can be grown on primate kidney, HeLa, and mouse L cell lines. This results in cytoplasmic inclusions and cytopathic effects such as the inhibition of DNA and protein synthesis and the inhibition of interferon induction. There are no known sequelae after a *Reovirus* infection. Laboratory identification is made either by growth and isolation in specific cell lines or by the detection of *Reovirus* antigens by immunofluorescence or immunoperoxidase techniques.

repair (re-pār) 1. the restoration of damaged tissues, especially the replacement of dead or damaged cells in a body tissue or organ by healthy new cells or by fibrous tissue (scar tissue).

2. a surgical procedure to correct a defect.

reparative granuloma see *giant cell reparative g.* under *granuloma.*

repeated DNA sequences nucleotide sequences present in multiple copies per haploid genome in all cells of an organism, including haploid gametes. Repetition is measured by renaturation reactions in which double-stranded DNA is fragmented into standard-size pieces, usually 400–500 nucleotide pairs in length. These are then separated by heating and/or denaturing agents into single strands and cooled or removed from denaturing agents. Complementary strands renature into double helices.

Renaturation of repeated sequences proceeds more rapidly than that of unique DNA. Renaturation rates are related to gene complexity (complexity being the number of nucleotide pairs required to make one single copy of every coding sequence in the DNA) by initial DNA concentration (C_0) and the amount of time the reaction is in progress (t). The relationship is the cot value expressed in moles times seconds per liter (mol·sec/l). The half reaction, $cot_{1/2}$, is equal to the reciprocal of the reaction rate (k). See also *cot value.*

Separation of DNA by renaturation reactions yields three fractions: highly repeated sequences present as about 10^6 copies or more per haploid genome, moderately repeated sequences present as about 10^2–10^5 copies, and unique sequences present as only one or a few copies.

Highly repeated sequences are usually termed satellite DNA. One of the most studied satellites is mouse satellite DNA, which is 110–140 nucleotides repeated over 10^6 times per haploid genome. It has been suggested that highly repeated sequences play a role in chromosome structure. The human Y chromosome contains a highly repeated sequence of DNA that constitutes more than 50 percent of the DNA of that chromosome. See also *satellite DNA.*

Moderately repeated sequences of 10^2–10^5 copies are considered as potential sites for the regulation of gene expression. More than half the human genome consists of unique sequences, interspersed with moderately repeated sequences, which could serve as binding sites for molecules that regulate transcription of adjacent unique sequences. The genes for the histones, rRNA, and tRNA are moderately repeated sequences.

Unique DNA represents as much as 70 percent of the total mammalian genome. Most of the mRNA in eukaryotic cells is unique sequence.

Cf. *gene a.* under *amplification.*

repetitive stimulation the application of a train of supramaximal electric stimuli to a motor nerve to evoke M waves from the muscles it innervates. Descriptions of the types of responses that may be seen with repetitive stimulation can be found under specific entries such as *decrementing response, postactivation exhaustion,* and *postactivation facilitation.*

replenisher (re-plen′ish-er) in film processing, a solution that is added periodically to the developer to replace chemicals used up in the development process; it also refers to a solution added to the fixer for the same purpose.

replication (rep″lĭ-ka′shun) 1. a turning back of a part so as to form a duplication.

2. the repetition of an experiment to ensure accuracy.

3. the process by which double-stranded DNA is unwound and two new daughter strands are synthesized using the parent strands as templates. See also *DNA synthesis.*

replication cycle see *cell cycle.*

replication fork a point at which the two strands of a DNA double helix are unwound and separated during replication.

replicon (rep′lĭ-kon) 1. in genetics, the unit of DNA replication. Each replicon has an initiation site, recognized perhaps by a specific initiating protein. Some bacteria (e.g., *Escherichia coli*) have only one replicon; mammalian cells have 30,000–40,000. See also *bacterial g.* under *genetics.*

2. in gene cloning, a segment of DNA capable of independent reproduction in a bacterial cell, e.g., plasmid or phage DNA, used for cloning foreign genes spliced into the replicon.

repolarization (re-po″lar-ĭ-za′shun) a return in the polarity of an excitable cell in the direction of the resting membrane potential after depolarization.

repression (re-presh′un) [L. *reprimare, repressus* to hold back, from *premere* to press] the act of inhibiting.

catabolite r., repression based on the availability and preferential use of glucose. First discovered in mammalian cells, it was later shown to be present in bacteria also. The repressor, originally thought to be a catabolite, is now known to be cyclic adenosine monophosphate (cAMP). This action represses the synthesis of enzymes that would not be useful when glucose alone can supply the cell's carbon and energy needs. See also *genetic regulation* and *positive control e. i.* under *enzyme induction.*

end-product r., repression resulting from the preferential use of exogenous nutrients when available, rather than endogenous nutrients. The operons coding for the enzymes needed for endogenous synthesis of nutrients are repressed by the presence of the exogenous substrates. Also called *enzyme repression.* See also *genetic regulation.*

negative control r., a transcriptional control mechanism in which an activated repressor binds to an operator site and reduces the initiation of transcription of the operon in the presence of excess substrate. An example is the tryptophan operon.

positive control r., a transcriptional control mechanism in which a corepressor binds a regulatory molecule, rendering it incapable of starting transcription. An example is the repression of histidine synthesis by histidyl tRNA.

repressor (re-pres′or) [L. "a restrainer"] 1. a molecule, usually a protein, that regulates the transcription of bacteria operon genes by binding to the operator site. Transcription is turned off when the repressor is present. See also *bacterial g.* under *genetics* and *lactose o.* under *operon.*

2. a cytoplasmic factor carried by a prophage that prevents multiplication of an exogenous phage genome introduced into a lysogenic cell and holds in check the endogenous prophage to maintain the lysogenic condition. Also called *immunity substance.*

reproduction (re″pro-duk′shun) [*re-* + L. *productio* production] procreation, the process by which living organisms produce new organisms of the same species.

asexual r., reproduction without the recombination of genetic material; the division of unicellular organisms by mitosis and the propagation of plants and primitive animals by budding or division. Except for new mutations, the offspring are genetically identical to (i.e., are clones of) the parent.

sexual r., reproduction with recombination of genetic material. In diploid eukaryotic organisms, the offspring are formed by the fusion of two haploid sex cells (gametes). A diploid cell zygote is formed, which then develops into a new organism by mitotic cell division. The adult organism then produces haploid gametes by meiotic cell division in which the chromosomes cross over to produce new genetic combinations.

In bacterial conjugation, part of the DNA of one bacterium is transferred to another, producing a partially diploid organism (a merozygote). Crossing over occurs between the donor fragment and the recipient chromosome, producing (as in eukaryotes) new genetic combinations.

reproductive (re″pro-duk′tiv) serving purposes of reproduction.

reproductive system the organs of reproduction.

female r. s., those organs in the female, situated in the pelvis, that include the ovaries, uterine tubes, uterus, vagina, and external genitalia.

male r. s., those organs in the male consisting of the primary sex organs (testes, epididymis, vas deferens, ejaculatory duct, and penis), as well as the accessory glands (seminal vesicles, prostate, and bulbourethral glands).

reptilase (rep′til-ās) an enzyme of the hydrolase class (*Bothrops atrox* serine proteinase, EC 3.4.21.29) that hydrolyzes predominantly fibrinopeptide A from intact fibrinogen and can release fibrinopeptide B from the *N*-terminal fragments of fibrinogen.

reptilase fibrin fibrinopeptide A. See under *fibrinopeptide.*

Reptilia (rep-til′e-ah) a class of amniotic vertebrates, of which many species may be second intermediate hosts of trematodes and tapeworms parasitic in humans.

repulsion (re-pul′shun) [*re-* + L. *pellere* to drive] 1. the act of driving apart or away.

2. in physics, a force that tends to drive two bodies apart, such as the electric force between like charges; the opposite of attraction.

3. in genetics, the occurrence on opposite chromosomes (homologues) in a double heterozygote of the two mutant alleles of interest. The genes are said to be linked in repulsion. Cf. *coupling.*

resazurin (re-sa′zu-rin) 7-hydroxy-3H-phenoxazin-3-one 10-oxide; a quinone-imine compound used as a pH indicator with a pH range of 3.8 (orange)–6.5 (violet). It is also used as an indicator of oxidation-reduction potential (E_h). At pH 7.0, fully oxidized resazurin is blue, becoming pink when reduced and colorless when fully reduced. See also *redox potential.*

rescinnamine (re-sin′ah-min) a rauwolfia alkaloid whose action and effects are similar to those of reserpine. It is used for the treatment of hypertension.

resection (re-sek′shun) [L. *resectio*] the excision of a portion of an organ or other structure.

wedge r., the removal of a triangular mass of tissue, as from an ovary.

reserpine (res′er-pēn, rĕ-ser′pēn) [USP], an alkaloid, extracted from roots of *Rauwolfia serpentina,* that acts by depleting the body's stores of catecholamines. It is used in the treatment of hypertension and as an antipsychotic medication. The antihypertensive effect is due to a lack of norepinephrine, which produces alpha-adrenergic blockade. Its effects on the central nervous system are caused by depletion of dopamine and serotonin (5-HT). Adverse reactions include depressed respiration, drowsiness, nightmares, nasal congestion, gastrointestinal intolerance, and severe mental depression. The drug must be stopped at the first sign of depression.

reserve (re-zerv′) 1. to hold back for future use.

2. a supply, beyond that ordinarily used, that may be utilized in an emergency.

reserve cell a small cell lying at the base of an epithelium, that has the capability of differentiating into a mature epithelial cell.

reservoir (rez′er-vwar) 1. a place or cavity for storage.

2. an alternate host or passive carrier harboring pathogenic microorganisms, without injury to itself, which may be transmitted at any time to humans, producing disease.

reset (re′set) 1. to set a binary logic circuit to the 0 state. Cf. *set.*

2. the input line of a flip-flop to which a reset signal is applied.

residual (re-zid′u-al) [L. *residuus*] remaining or left behind.

residual body material remaining in the cytoplasm after digestion has ceased within an autophagic or heterophagic vacuole.

residual latency see *residual l.* under *latency.*

residual urine volume measurement a procedure in nuclear medicine that detects an abnormally large volume of urine in the bladder after voiding has occurred. In the procedure, ^{99m}Tc-Sn-DPTA (technetium Tc 99m stannous pentatate sodium) is injected and filtered into the urine by the kidneys. The radioactivity of the bladder is counted before and after voiding, using a scintillation probe or scintillation camera. Residual urine volume is the voided volume multiplied by the postvoiding activity divided by the difference of the prevoiding and postvoiding activities. This test may also be performed after a renogram, using ^{131}I orthoiodohippurate. See also *retrograde c.* under *cystography.*

residual volume (RV) the volume of air that cannot be emptied from the lungs despite a maximal voluntary expiratory effort; it remains in the alveoli to aerate the blood between breaths. This quantity, normally equal to 1000–1200 ml in the young adult male, cannot be measured directly, and is usually determined by measuring the functional residual capacity by a gas dilution technique and then subtracting the expiratory reserve volume.

residue (rez′i-du) [L. *residuum,* from *re-* + *sidere* to sit] 1. a remainder; that which remains after the removal of a part.

2. the material remaining after an abstractive chemical or physical process, e.g., evaporation, filtration, or combustion.

3. in biochemistry, a part of a molecule that has been incorporated into another molecule, e.g., an amino acid residue in a polypeptide. Cf. *moiety.*

resin (rez′in) [L. *resina*] 1. a solid or semisolid, amorphous, organic substance, of vegetable origin or produced synthetically. Natural resins are insoluble in water but are readily dissolved in alcohol, ether, and volatile oils. Synthetic resins are the polymers from which plastics are made; some are soluble in water.

2. see *rosin.*

resistance (re-zis′tans) [L. *resistentia*] 1. (symbol *R*), electric resistance, the opposition of a resistor to the flow of current equal to the voltage drop across the resistor divided by the current. The International System (SI) unit of resistance is the ohm (Ω), 1 V/A. The reciprocal of resistance (1/R) is called the conductance. See also *parallel circuit* and *series circuit.*

2. (symbol *R*), vascular resistance, the opposition to blood flow in a vessel equal to the pressure drop between the ends divided by the flow rate. The commonly used unit of resistance is the peripheral resistance unit (PRU), 1 mmHg · sec/ml. The reciprocal of vascular resistance is also called the conductance, and the formulas for resistances connected in series and in parallel are the same as those for electric resistance. The conductance of a vessel is proportional to the fourth power of the vessel radius and inversely proportional to the blood viscosity (η) and vessel length.

3. the ability of a human being, lower animal, or plant to withstand a noxious influence in its environment, e.g., a resistance to a poison, toxin, irritant, or pathogenic microorganism.

4. in microbiology, a species that may be relatively unaffected by a chemical or physical agent (natural resistance). After exposure, usually repeated, a species normally inhibited by certain antimicrobial agents such as antibiotics may give rise by selective mutation to a strain that is no longer affected (acquired resistance).

electrode r., the resistance to the flow of a direct current across the interface between an electrode and the part of the body with which it is in contact. It is measured in ohms. Cf. *electrode i.* under *impedance.*

total peripheral r., the vascular resistance of the systemic circulation, normally approximately 1 PRU. (The difference between the mean arterial pressure and the right atrial pressure is about 100 mmHg; the venous return is about 100 ml/sec and varies in the range of 0.25–4 PRU.)

total pulmonary r., the vascular resistance of the pulmonary circulation, normally approximately 0.09 PRU at rest.

resistance determinant see *R p.* under *plasmid.*

resistance plasmid see *R p.* under *plasmid.*

resistance transfer factor see *R p.* under *plasmid.*

resistivity (re″zis-tiv′i-te) the electric resistance of a resistor multiplied by its cross-sectional area divided by its length, measured in ohm-meters (Ω · m). Resistivity is the reciprocal of conductivity and is a physical property of the resistor material. Also called specific resistance.

resistor (re-zis′tor) an electric component used to provide a fixed resistance in a circuit.

carbon r., a resistor made from powdered graphite and a ceramic binder, and usually consisting of a cylinder with leads attached at the ends. Carbon resistors are manufactured with various tolerances (the agreement between the nominal value and the actual resistance, usually to within 5 or 10 percent) and wattage ratings (the amount of power that can be dissipated as heat). They are generally marked using the resistor color code. Also called *composition r.*

carbon-film r., a resistor made by depositing a thin carbon film on a ceramic base.

composition r., see *carbon r.*

power r., a resistor that has a large heat-dissipating capacity. Wire-wound power resistors are available with capacities up to 50 W.

precision r., a resistor that has a tolerance of less than 5 percent. The exact tolerance (e.g., 1 percent, 0.1 percent) is marked on the body of the resistor. Precision resistors are usually either carbon-film or wire-wound resistors.

trimming r., see *variable r.*

variable r., a component that provides a continuously variable resistance. Also called *potentiometer* (when its function is to regulate voltage), *rheostat* (particularly when its function is to regulate current), or *trimming r.* (when its function is to set specified parameters in a circuit before the circuit is put into operation).

wire-wound r., a resistor made by winding high-resistance wire around an insulating form. It is usually embedded in ceramic, which increases its capacity to dissipate heat.

resistor color code a method of designating the resistance and tolerance values on resistors with colored bands according to the established code of black = 0, brown = 1, red = 2, orange = 3, yellow = 4, green = 5, blue = 6, violet (purple) = 7, gray = 8, and white = 9.

The resistance is obtained by the digits represented by the first two bands, followed by the number of zeros indicated by the third band. When the third band is a gold color, it indicates the decimal point goes between the two digits, whereas silver indicates the decimal point precedes the first digit. The fourth band indicates the tolerance: silver = 10 percent, gold = 5 percent, and no band = 20 percent. For example, a resistor with a code of orange, white, red, and silver means 3900 ohms (3.9 KΩ) ± 10 percent. A wire-wound resistor is indicated by a double-width first band.

resolution (rez″o-lu′shun) [L. *resolatum,* from *resolvere* to unbind] 1. the subsidence of a pathologic state, as of an inflammation or swelling.

2. the ability of an instrument to distinguish separate objects. See also *energy resolution, resolving power,* and *spatial resolution.*

3. the separation of the enantiomers of a racemic mixture.

resolve (re-zolv′) [L. *resolvere*] 1. to restore to the normal state after some pathologic process.

2. to separate a thing into its component parts.

resolving power 1. the ability of a microscope to separate the diffraction disks produced by two point sources and thus distinguish them as separate points; usually defined as the smallest linear or angular separation that can be resolved according to the Rayleigh criterion (each disk falls off to half its maximal intensity at the midpoint). The resolving power is directly proportional to the wavelength of the illumination being used. Also called *resolution.*

2. the ability of a spectrophotometer or monochrometer to separate spectral lines, usually defined as the average wavelength of two equally strong absorption peaks divided by the difference in their wavelengths, when the lines are resolved according to the Rayleigh criterion. Also called *spectral resolution.*

resolving time the minimal time interval that must elapse after a device (such as a radiation detector or electronic counter) registers an event before it can respond to another event. All events occurring within one resolving time constitute only one count. See also *dead time* and *recovery time.*

resonance (rez′o-nans) [L. *resonantia*] 1. the phenomenon associated with molecules, radicals, or ions that cannot be represented adequately by a single Lewis structure. The true structure of such a species, in which some of the electrons (some π electrons) are said to be delocalized (not localized on individual atoms), can be taken as a weighted average of several Lewis structures (resonance forms), none of which alone has any real existence.

Benzene is a classic example of a molecule that is a resonance hybrid. At least two resonance forms are used to represent its true structure. The bond lengths in benzene are not alternately long (single) and short (double) but are all equal with a length between those two extremes. Resonance is conventionally indicated by a double-headed arrow; equilibrium, in contrast, is indicated by opposed double arrows (see below). The term resonance is often used as an adjective, as in resonance energy and resonance forms.

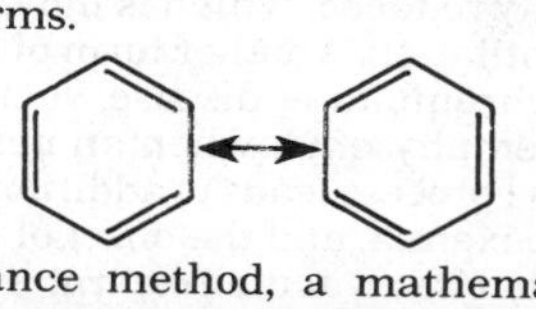

The resonance method, a mathematical treatment based on quantum mechanics, is only one of the methods that can be used to describe delocalized molecules or ions.

2. in physics, a harmonic oscillator is said to be in resonance with a driving agent when the natural frequency of the oscillator equals the frequency of the driving force. This principle is the basis for the resonance absorption of electromagnetic radiation by atoms, ions, and molecules in many spectroscopic methods; e.g., nuclear magnetic resonance.

resonance fluorescence the absorption of a photon by an atom followed by the emission of a photon of the same energy.

resonance line a wavelength at which an element exhibits resonance fluorescence.

resorcin (rĕ-zor′sin) see *resorcinol.*

resorcin-fuchsin (rĕ-zor′sin fook′sin) a stain for elastic fibers that contains basic fuchsin and an oxidizer (ferric chloride). Elastic fibers are stained blue-black to black. Overstained sections may be differentiated in acid alcohol.

Resorcin-fuchsin may be obtained commercially, or prepared by boiling a solution of basic fuchsin and resorcinol in water and adding a solution of 29 percent aqueous ferric chloride. When the filtered and dried precipitate is dissolved in a solution of alcohol, concentrated hydrochloric acid is added. Crystal violet or other basic dyes may be substituted for the fuchsin.

Also called Weigert's resorcin-fuchsin.

resorcinol (rĕ-zor′sĭ-nol) 1. a white crystalline solid with a sweet taste, 1,3-benzenediol, used in the manufacture of resins, dyes, and drugs; M.W. 110.11. It is irritating to the skin and mucous membranes and is toxic when ingested. Also called *resorcin.* See also *phenol.*

2. [USP], a preparation of resorcinol used for the treatment of acne vulgaris. It causes drying and peeling of the skin.

r. monoacetate, [USP], an ester that has the same uses as resorcinol.

resorption (re-sorp′shun) [L. *resorbere* to swallow again] the removal by absorption of something already secreted or formed in the body, such as reabsorption in the renal tubules of materials filtered by the glomeruli into the urine, or the process of reabsorption of minerals from bone or from teeth.

resorption lacunae see *Howship's lacuna.*

Resource Conservation and Recovery Act (RCRA) a federal law empowering the EPA (Environmental Protection Agency) to adopt regulations that define hazardous wastes and that establish requirements for generators of hazardous wastes, including quantities for which reporting and compliance are required.

respiration (res″pĭ-ra′shun) [L. *respiratio*] 1. the exchange of oxygen and carbon dioxide between the atmosphere and the cells of the body. This includes the absorption of oxygen and the release of carbon dioxide at the lungs by the process of ventilation (inspiration and expiration), diffusion of these respiratory gases between the alveoli and capillary red blood cells, and transport of gas between the lungs and tissues.

2. the aerobic metabolism of living cells, consisting of the oxidation of substrates with molecular oxygen as the terminal electron acceptor, which provides energy for the cell.

3. anaerobic respiration, which is unique to bacteria that can carry on respiratory metabolism under anaerobic conditions by using inorganic compounds such as nitrate, sulfate, and carbonate as the terminal electron acceptor.

aerobic r., the series of mitochondrial, enzyme-catalyzed oxidation-reduction reactions in which electrons are transferred from organic fuel molecules to the final electron acceptor, molecular oxygen, and in the process of which CO_2 and H_2O are released.

Because the transport of electrons to oxygen is coupled to the oxidative phosphorylation of ATP, 38 percent of the free energy otherwise released in the electron transport process is conserved as chemical energy that can be utilized for cellular endergonic processes.

See also *electron transport chain, oxidative phosphorylation,* and *tricarboxylic acid cycle.*

anaerobic r., an ATP-generating metabolic process in which inorganic compounds other than oxygen serve as the ultimate electron acceptor and therefore become reduced. Such inorganic compounds, including nitrates, sulfates, and carbonates, are used by various bacteria. Examples of bacteria capable of anaerobic respiration include denitrifiers: $H_2 + NO_3^- \rightarrow N_2O, N_2, NH_3$, *Desulfovibrio*: $H_2 + SO_4^{-2} \rightarrow S$ or H_2S, methane bacteria: $4\ H_2 + CO_2 \rightarrow CH_4 + 2\ CH_2O$, and *Clostridium aceticum*: $4\ H_2 + 2\ CO_2 \rightarrow CH_3COOH + 2\ H_2O$.

respirator (res′pĭ-ra″tor) a mechanical device used to substitute for or assist with the respirations of a patient who has pulmonary insufficiency. The preferred terminology is *ventilator.*

body r., a machine that inflates the lungs by surrounding the thorax with a subatmospheric (negative) pressure. It is used to maintain adequate alveolar ventilation when spontaneous breathing is lacking in patients under the influence of deep anesthesia or neuromuscular blocking agents, or in patients with pathologic conditions such as poliomyelitis. The airway must be patent for the body respirator to provide adequate ventilation.

In the Drinker type of body respirator ("iron lung"), the entire body below the neck is encased in a plastic or metal tank. A pump decreases the pressure in the tank to subatmospheric values, thus expanding the chest and lowering intraalveolar pressure; this causes ambient air at atmospheric pressures to flow into the lung. After this inspiration, the pressure in the tank is allowed to return to atmospheric, allowing for expiration through passive elastic recoil of the lungs and thorax. The respirator can be adjusted to repeat this inspiratory-expiratory cycle at a desired frequency and amplitude.

More recently developed portable body respirators operate on the same principle as the Drinker respirator but enclose only the anterior chest.

Also called tank respirator.

Drinker r., a type of body respirator that controls alveolar ventilation in apneic patients by cycling the pressure within an airtight tank that encases the body (except for the head). Also called *iron lung.* See also *body r.*

respiratory (re-spi′rah-to″re) [*re-* + L. *spirare* to breathe] pertaining to respiration.

respiratory acidosis a shift in the body acid-base balance so that one becomes acidotic. It is caused by the failure of the lungs to eliminate CO_2 from the body as rapidly as it is formed metabolically. This leads to hypercapnia and a lowering of blood pH before compensation occurs. Also called *hypercapnic acidosis.* See also *acid-base balance.* Cf. *metabolic acidosis.*

respiratory alkalosis a shift in the body's acid-base balance, so that one becomes alkalotic owing to hyperventilation (when the level of alveolar ventilation exceeds that necessary to eliminate the CO_2 formed metabolically). Arterial P_{CO_2} is lowered and blood pH is elevated before compensation occurs. See also *acid-base balance.* Cf. *metabolic alkalosis.*

respiratory chain see *electron transport chain.*

respiratory epithelium see *pseudostratified epithelium.*

respiratory exchange ratio (R_E) the ratio of carbon dioxide output to the rate of oxygen uptake in the lungs, used when these quantities are determined by analysis of mixed expired gas. During steady-state conditions, it is equal to the respiratory quotient.

respiratory failure hypoxemia (reduction in arterial P_{O_2} below 60 mmHg) and/or hypercapnia (elevation of P_{CO_2} above 49 mmHg) subsequent to the temporary or prolonged impairment of respiratory function (ventilation, diffusion, perfusion, or control of breathing). Respiratory failure may be classified as acute or chronic, depending on the time course of development of the underlying disturbance to normal gaseous exchange. Included among the many disease factors or traumatic events that may precipitate the condition are diseases that cause acute and chronic airway obstruction and parenchymal infiltration, pulmonary edema and embolism, hyaline membrane diseases, neuromuscular disorders, pulmonary vascular diseases, shock, burns, acute thoracic injury, carbon monoxide poisoning, and administration of respiratory depressants.

The diagnosis of respiratory failure is primarily based on arterial blood gas analysis (to determine whether hypoxemia, hypercapnia, or both are present). Clinical manifestations of the condition are diverse, varying with the underlying causative condition, and may represent unreliable diagnostic criteria.

acute r. f. (ARF), a syndrome of acute hypoxemia that is the consequence of numerous and disparate factors and diseases that lead to an impairment of the normal exchange of oxygen and carbon dioxide (CO_2). Patients recovering from shock, hemorrhage, sepsis, or severe trauma are at an especially high risk for developing this syndrome. As a medical term, ARF has been used in recent years to denote severe hypoxemia secondary to a diffuse pulmonary disease of rapid onset in an individual with little or no previous pulmonary disease. Used in this way, the term is synonymous with "adult respiratory distress syndrome." The characteristic presentation of this particular form of respiratory failure is one of severe abnormality in arterial blood oxygenation without CO_2 retention. In fact, the arterial CO_2 tension is usually reduced, which is indicative of alveolar hyperventilation. Another form of ARF occurs in those with chronic lung disease, such as advanced obstructive emphysema, when an acute worsening in the disease process leads to additional respiratory distress, hypoxemia, and the onset of CO_2 retention; the last gives rise to acute respiratory acidosis.

Four phases can be characterized in the progression of ARF. In the initial stage of resuscitation that follows hemorrhage, infection, or injury, no evidence of respiratory stress may be present. Hyperventilation, generally the earliest and most significant sign of incipient ARF, does not usually appear until after a second phase (usually 5–7 da) during which the circulation has stabilized and tissue perfusion has returned to normal. In this phase, although Pa_{O2} may be only slightly decreased, the measurement of Pa_{O2} following 20 min of inhalation of 100 percent O_2 reveals a large $(A\text{-}a)D_{O2}$, indicative of extensive intrapulmonic shunt. Progressive respiratory distress, characterized by increasingly severe hypoxemia, tachypnea, and hypocapnia, is present in the third phase. Diffuse, patchy infiltrates (consistent with bronchopneumonia), which eventually show as large areas of consolidation, are first apparent on radiographs of the chest. *Klebsiella, Serratia,* and *Pseudomonas* species may be isolated from sputum cultures. Hypocapnia gradually gives way to progressive hypercapnia. The respiratory drive gradually weakens, mixed venous oxygen tension drops, and the patient enters a comatose state. In a brief terminal phase, the degree of hypercapnia (and accompanying metabolic acidosis), intrapulmonic shunt, and coma progressively worsen. Tissue perfusion becomes inadequate as cardiac output begins to drop. Ventricular and atrial arrhythmias may appear. The death of the patient is frequently preceded by a bradycardia and terminal asystole.

Pathologic features of the lungs following ARF commonly include the formation of a hyaline membrane, atelectasis, bronchopneumonia, the presence of pulmonary capillary microaggregates composed of leukocytes and platelets, marked proliferation of type II alveolar cells, hemorrhage and edema, and the destruction and swelling of the capillary endothelium.

chronic r. f. (CRF), a condition in which Pa_{O_2} is consistently subnormal and Pa_{CO_2} consistently elevated as the result of an underlying chronic disorder that impairs respiratory function. CRF is accompanied by arterial blood acid-base findings that are indicative of chronic respiratory acidosis, such as elevated P_{CO_2}, elevated bicarbonate (compensatory), and an acid pH. Whenever CO_2 retention is present, hypoxemia must also be present if the individual is breathing room air. In general, the arterial oxygen tension values in CRF are less than 60 torr. Periodic, life-threatening, acute worsenings of the hypoxemia and hypercapnia are superimposed on the chronic syndrome.

respiratory minute volume ($\dot{V}_E$) the amount of air ventilated each minute, normally equal to about 6 l. It is measured by recording spirometry, by use of a flowmeter (pneumotachograph), or by collection of the expired gas into a tank or Neoprene bag. The volume collected is measured with a volume meter or in a Tissot spirometer. If an assumed value for the total volume of the dead space is used, resting minute volume can be used to estimate the alveolar ventilation.

The determination of minute volume is usually of little value in routine assessment of pulmonary function, because it is almost always normal, even in those with advanced states of lung disease. In individuals in danger of respiratory failure due to hypoventilation, as can occur in barbiturate intoxication, in neuromuscular disorders, or in postoperative states, minute volume becomes an important vital sign. Also called minute ventilation and pulmonary ventilation.

respiratory protein any of the various O_2-transport proteins present in animals. The respiratory proteins in vertebrates are myoglobin and hemoglobin (M.W. 17,000 and 64,500, respectively).

respiratory quotient (RQ) the ratio of the volume of carbon dioxide (CO_2) produced to the volume of oxygen (O_2) consumed during the metabolism of food in the body. RQ can be used to estimate the relative rates of carbohydrate and fat metabolism in the body. The RQ values for the metabolism of different fuels are 1 for glucose, 0.7 for fatty acids, $\approx$ 0.85 for a mixed diet, and $\approx$ 0.8 for protein (the last RQ is difficult to measure).

respiratory rate see *breathing frequency.*

respiratory syncytial virus (RSV) a single-stranded RNA virus that belongs to the paramyxovirus family, genus *Pneumovirus.* This virus infects the respiratory mucosa after an incubation period of 4–5 da, and can result in bronchiolitis, pneumonitis, and croup. Children over 6 mo of age are most commonly infected. RSV may be isolated from the respiratory secretions of infected individuals or detected in the serum by the complement-fixation serologic technique. In addition, direct examination of RSV in nasopharyngeal secretions by fluorescent-antibody techniques can be useful. Infections with this virus are most common in the winter months of January, February, and March.

respiratory syncytial virus antibody tests assays for detecting antibody against respiratory syncytial virus. These include complement fixation, neutralization, and ELISA. The complement-fixation test is used usually routinely in diagnostic laboratories, and is performed by reacting serial dilutions of the test serum with a constant amount of viral antigen and then adding guinea pig complement. A serologic diagnosis requires a fourfold rise in titer between acute and convalescent sera. Unchanging high titers suggest recent viral infection or persistent antibody levels from a past infection.

Often, children younger than 6 mo do not develop enough antibody to be detected by complement fixation; the ELISA can be useful in these cases as it is more sensitive. Virus neutralization is not practical for routine use and is employed only in special cases. Because the individual has usually recovered from the virus infection by the time the convalescent serum is collected, serologic tests are used for retrospective diagnosis or epidemiologic information.

Rapid diagnosis may be accomplished by the use of indirect immunofluorescence to detect viral antigens in respiratory tract tissues or secretions.

See also *respiratory syncytial virus antigen test.*

respiratory syncytial virus antigen test an indirect immunofluorescence test for detecting respiratory syncytial virus antigen in respiratory tract mucosal cells and nasal secretions. The test is performed by obtaining nasal mucosal cells, using a saline wash or rhinorrhea fluid. The cells are washed in phosphate buffered saline (PBS), smeared on a slide, and fixed in acetone. Bovine antibody to respiratory syncytial virus is then added to the cells. Finally, fluorescein-labeled antibovine immunoglobulin antibody is added.

respiratory therapist a health care professional skilled in the treatment, management, and care of patients with respiratory problems. Clinical tasks include administration of medical gases (oxygen, helium, and carbon dioxide), aerosol and humidity therapy, intermittent positive pressure breathing (IPPB) therapy, incentive spirometry, artificial mechanical ventilation, arterial blood gas analysis, and pulmonary function testing. The respiratory therapist also has a knowledge of cardiopulmonary anatomy, physiology, and pharmacology, and often a good working knowledge of many aspects of chest medicine. Educational preparation involves completion of an associate degree program; graduates are certified by the National Board for Respiratory Therapy and are designated RRT, Registered Respiratory Therapist.

respiratory therapy an area of clinical specialization dealing with the treatment, management, and care of those with respiratory problems including the administration of medical gases (oxygen therapy, carbon dioxide–oxygen therapy, and helium-oxygen therapy), aerosol therapy, humidity therapy, mechanical ventilation, intermittent positive pressure breathing (IPPB) therapy, incentive spirometry, pulmonary function testing, and arterial blood gas analysis. Practitioners are called respiratory therapists and respiratory therapy technicians.

respiratory therapy technician a health care professional who, under the supervision of a respiratory therapist, performs routine care, management, and treatment of patients with respiratory problems. Educational preparation involves completion of a 1-yr approved program; graduates are certified by the National Board for Respiratory Therapy and are designated CRTT, Certified Respiratory Therapy Technician.

respirometer (res″pĭ-rom′ĕ-ter) 1. an instrument used to measure the volume of expired air or to analyze its contents.

2. an instrument used to measure the tissue O_2 consumption or CO_2 production, or the oxygen uptake of an entire organism.

Wright r., a portable instrument used to measure resting minute ventilation. As expired air enters the respirometer, it passes through tangential slots to turn a two-bladed rotor at a number of revolutions per second proportional to the respiratory minute volume.

resting cell a cell that is not dividing (i.e., which is in the interphase period).

restriction endonuclease an enzyme from bacterial cells that selectively hydrolyzes double-stranded DNA at the ends of certain palindromic sequences. Such enzymes are important tools in molecular genetics research.

Restriction endonucleases break both strands of native double-stranded helical DNA at specific recognition sites that have twofold symmetry and a particular base sequence. Two examples are Eco RI (from *Escherichia coli*) and HIND III (from *Hemophilus influenzae*). Such enzymes permit large genomes to be cut into a number of pieces for detailed analysis and sequencing. Many restriction endonucleases do not cleave both DNA strands at the same point, leaving staggered ends that permit the joining of pieces from two dissimilar DNAs that have both been cleaved with the same enzyme (DNA recombination).

restrictive (re-strik′tiv) see *nonpermissive.*

restrictive lung disease a pattern of pathologic changes in ventilatory function that results in a limitation in the amount of air moved into the lungs with each breath. The hallmarks of the restrictive pattern of ventilatory disorder are a reduction in vital capacity (and in other lung volumes such as the total lung capacity) and in the FEV (the forced expiratory volume over the first second of a maximally fast expiration). The residual volume, functional residual capacity, and maximal voluntary ventilation can be normal early in the process, eventually becoming decreased, whereas the RV/TLC, maximal midexpiratory flow rate, and FEV/FVC are normal or increased.

Among the many diseases that can lead to the development of restrictive lung disorders are those that limit the expansion of the chest wall (pectus excavatum, myasthenia gravis), those that result in a loss of lung tissue or in a reduction in lung volume by occupying space in the thorax (pneumonectomy, tumors, cardiac enlargement, effusions), those that cause infiltrations in the air spaces and/or alveolar walls (pulmonary edema, diffuse interstital fibrosis), and those that cause changes in the pleura (pleural thickening).

Cf. *chronic obstructive lung disease.*

resuscitation (re-sus″ĭ-ta′shun) [L. *resuscitare* to revive] the restoration to life or consciousness of one apparently dead or whose respirations have ceased. See also *artificial respiration, cardiac massage, cardiopulmonary resuscitation, cardioversion,* and *defibrillation.*

rete (re′te), pl. *retia* [L. "net"] a net or meshwork; used as a general term to designate a network, especially of arteries or veins.

r. pegs, inward projections of epidermis into the dermis at the dermoepidermal junction.

r. testis, [NA], a network of channels or canals in the posterior portion of the testes, which traverses the mediastinum testis. Their lumen is lined with low columnar or cuboidal epithelial cells, many of which possess short microvilli. The contents of the seminiferous tubules pass through the rete testis to the epididymis.

retention (re-ten′shun) [L. *retentio*, from *retentare* to hold firmly back] the process of holding in the body as opposed to normal or abnormal expulsion, as in the retention of food, fluids, urine, or feces.

retention index a standard measure of retention time, used in gas chromatography, that compares the retention time of a compound with those of the straight-chain saturated hydrocarbons (*n*-alkanes). It is independent of operating parameters and is primarily a function of the polarities and chemical similarity of the compound and the stationary phase. The logarithm of the corrected retention time (CRT) of *n*-alkanes is approximately proportional to chain length. The retention index is the logarithm of the CRT of a compound multiplied by a factor chosen to give each *n*-alkane a retention index of 100 times its chain length (e.g., *n*-heptane is 700) for every temperature and for every liquid phase. Also called *Kovats index.*

retention time in column chromatography, the time interval during which a particular substance remains in the column. Retention time varies with the column size, stationary phase, column loading, carrier gas flow rate, and temperatures of the injection port and column.

absolute r. t. (ART), the total time interval between injection of the specimen and arrival of a particular specimen component or reference standard at the detector.

corrected r. t. (CRT), the difference between absolute retention time and dead time, which is the absolute retention time either of air injected with the sample or of the sample solvent; i.e., the CRT is the time interval between the air peak or solvent peak and a sample component peak.

relative r. t. (RRT), the ratio of the corrected retention times of a sample component and of some arbitrary substance chosen as a standard. The RRT is relatively independent of the operating parameters of the chromatograph, and is primarily a function of the polarities and chemical similarities of the stationary phase, sample component, and standard substance.

retention volume in gas chromatography, the product of the retention time and flow rate.

reticul/o (re-tik′u-lo) a word element used in combining form to denote a network, e.g., reticulum.

reticular (rĕ-tik′u-lar) [L. *reticularis*] resembling a net, used in describing the internal appearance of an organ or part. See also the illustration under *contour.*

reticular cell a branched fibroblastic cell forming the reticular fibers that are characteristic of reticular connective tissue. These cells are found in the spongy framework of the bone marrow, spleen, and lymph nodes. See also *reticular fibers.*

reticular fibers slender bundles of collagen fibrils that form the delicate sheets of the connective tissue framework of hematopoietic organs. The term is also applied to the irregularly arranged collagen fibrils subjacent to a basal lamina. Also called *reticulin.*

reticular lamina the tissue layer composed of reticular fibers and ground substance that lies beneath the basal lamina of epithelial tissue.

reticulin (rĕ-tik′u-lin) the material of which reticular fibers are composed, now known to be collagen assembled in a loose network of fibrils. The difference between the argyrophilia of reticular fibers and that of collagenous fibers is thought to be due to associated proteoglycans and glycoproteins. Also called *reticular fibers.*

reticulin staining any of a large variety of similar methods of silver impregnation of reticular fibers. Reticulin stains are useful in identifying tumors of mesodermal origin (which produce abundant reticulin), cirrhosis of the liver, fibrosis of bone marrow, and certain lesions of the kidney. These methods use ammoniacal solutions of silver carbonate or silver oxide, which contain the diammine silver ion, $[Ag(NH_3)_2]^+$. Aldehyde groups of reticulin react with this ion to form a precipitate of silver oxide, which is then reduced to metallic silver by formalin.

Formalin-fixed paraffin sections are most commonly used. They are first oxidized in dilute potassium permanganate solution for a few minutes (some methods use periodic acid or chromic acid), and then bleached in oxalic acid. This is sometimes followed by treatment with a so-called sensitizer such as silver nitrate, uranyl nitrate, ferric chloride, or iron alum. The sections are next placed first into the ammoniacal silver solution and then into the formalin solution. This is followed by gold toning, replacement by immersion in gold chloride of the yellow colloidal silver background by grayish metallic gold. The last step, fixing the sodium thiosulfate, removes unreduced silver and gold.

Reticular fibers stain purplish to black; collagenous fibers stain gray to lavender. Note the warning under *ammoniacal silver solutions.*

reticulocyte (rĕ-tik′u-lo-sit″) the stage of red cell development immediately following extrusion of the normoblast nucleus in the bone marrow, characterized by the presence of RNA. Reticulocytes normally mature (progressively lose their residual RNA) in 3–4 da in the marrow and an additional day in the peripheral blood. They become mature cells when all the RNA has been lost. Normally, the reticulocyte count in the peripheral blood is 1 percent, or $50{,}000/mm^3$. See also *reticulocyte count, reticulocyte production index,* and *reticulocytopenia.*

shift r., a reticulocyte, either normal or large (macro-stress) in size, that is released (shifted) from the bone marrow under moderate or severe erythropoietic stress to compensate for anemia. The fraction of reticulocytes shifted into the periphery increases progressively with decreasing hemoglobin levels. See also *reticulocyte production index.*

stress r., a reticulocyte up to twice the normal size, which has a corresponding increase in hemoglobin content. It is produced in the bone marrow from macronormoblasts in response to a severe stress on the erythropoietic system, i.e., severe anemia with elevated erythropoietin levels. This response is mediated by erythropoietin. Also called *macroreticulocyte.*

reticulocyte count a method for enumerating reticulocytes in the peripheral blood. One or more drops of fresh blood are mixed with an equal quantity of a supravital dye, such as new methylene blue or brilliant cresyl blue, which precipitates residual RNA in immature red cells. The precipitate appears as granules or a fibrillar network, originally called substantia reticulofilamentosa, which accounts for the designation of reticulocyte. Results are reported as a percentage or in absolute numbers per cubic millimeter (normal being 1.0 ± 0.5 percent, or $50{,}000/mm^3$).

reticulocyte production index a more useful measure of red cell production than the uncorrected reticulocyte count.

In anemia, the reticulocyte count may appear to be falsely elevated for two reasons: (1) At normal red blood cell (RBC) counts of 5 million, the 1 percent reticulocyte level obtained from a reticulocyte count indicates the production of 50,000 RBC per day. In anemia, if the total RBC count has dropped to 3.5 or 2.5 million, a 1 percent reticulocyte count may indicate only 35,000 or 25,000 RBC per day. Consequently, it is necessary to normalize the reticulocyte count by multiplying it by the actual hematocrit divided by 45, or by the actual RBC count divided by 5 million. (2) The early release of reticulocytes (shift reticulocytes) in anemia results in their maturing in the peripheral blood for 1.5, 2.0, or 2.5 da at hematocrits of 35, 25, and 15, respectively, rather than 1 da at a hematocrit of 45. Thus, the reticulocyte count must be further corrected by dividing by 1.5, 2.0, or 2.5, depending on the level of anemia. When both corrections are used, raw reticulocyte counts of 2, 3, and 4 percent often give corrected values of 1 percent or less, indicating that production rates are not increased. Raw reticulocyte counts of 5 percent or higher usually indicate increased production rates even after correction.

If reticulocyte counts are given in absolute numbers per cubic millimeter, only the correction for shift reticulocytes needs to be made to make counts directly comparable with the normal value of 50,000; see also *shift reticulocyte.*

reticulocyte response a temporary marked increase in reticulocytes in response to "specific" therapy in anemia, such as iron therapy in iron deficiency anemia, vitamin B_{12} in pernicious anemia, or folic acid in folic acid deficiency. The increase usually occurs 4–10 da after the start of adequate therapy, and returns to levels only slightly higher than normal during continued therapy and improvement. The height of the response depends on the severity of the anemia.

reticulocytopenia (rĕ-tik″u-lo-si″to-pe′ne-ah) [*reticulocyte* + Gr. *penia* poverty] a decrease in the number of reticulocytes in the blood.

reticulocytosis (rĕ-tik″u-lo-si-to′sis) an increase in the number of reticulocytes in the peripheral blood.

reticuloendothelial system (rĕ-tik″u-lo-en″do-the′le-al) pertaining to tissues having both endothelial and phagocytic properties, such as fixed macrophages in the walls of sinusoids. The concept of a reticuloendothelial system of cells was developed by Aschoff (1924) as an extension and revision of the phagocytic series of cells described by Metchnikoff (1892). Endothelial cells and fibroblasts were omitted from the revision because of their low phagocytic capability. The concept has been frequently reviewed and criticized, and alternative terms such as mononuclear phagocyte system have been proposed. See also *mononuclear phagocyte system.*

reticulohistiocytoma (rĕ-tik″u-lo-his″te-o-si-to′-mah) a lesion of large, lipid-laden histiocytes involving the skin and mucosal surfaces, which may occur as single or multiple nodules. One-third of those affected also have a destructive arthritis (lipid dermatoarthritis). Also called giant cell reticulohistiocytoma and multicentric reticulohistiocytosis.

reticulum (rĕ-tik′u-lum), pl. *reticula* [L. dim. of *rete* net] a network, such as one formed of collagen fibrils. See also *endoplasmic reticulum* and *sarcoplasmic reticulum.*

retin/o (ret′ĭ-no) a word element used in combining form to denote the retina, e.g., retinoblastoma.

retina (ret′ĭ-nah) [L.] [NA], the innermost of three coats of the eyeball that lines the posterior segment of the eye from the ora serrata to the optic nerve, and is the site of photoreception. It is transparent except for the most peripheral layer, the pigmented epithelium. The retina is laminated into 10 parallel layers. Along the visual axis of the eye lie the fovea, a depression or thin area of the retina that corresponds to the area of greatest sensitivity and the highest density of cone photoreceptors. In addition to seven types of neurons contained in the retina, there are supporting neuroglial elements, the Müller cells. Offset from the visual axis in each eye is the site of exit of the ganglion cell axons; this is the point of formation of the optic nerve and is known as the blind spot because of the absence of receptors.

retinaculum (ret″ĭ-nak′u-lum), pl. *retinacula* [L. "a rope, cable"] [NA], a general term for a structure that retains an organ or tissues in place.

retinal (ret′ĭ-nal, ret-in-el′) 1. pertaining to the retina.

2. the aldehyde of retinol, formed by the oxidative enzymatic splitting of absorbed dietary carotene, and having vitamin A activity. In the retina, retinal combines with opsins to form visual pigments. One isomer, 11-*cis*-retinal, combines with opsin in the rods to form rhodopsin or visual purple. Another, all-*trans* retinal, present in visual yellow, results from the bleaching of rhodopsin by light, during which the 11-*cis* form is converted to the all-*trans* form. Retinal also combines with opsins in the cones to form the three pigments responsible for color vision. Retinal and retinol equilibrate through the action of retinal reductase, an alcohol dehydrogenase. It is thought that the *trans*-retinal is converted to the 11-*cis* form by a retinal isomerase, but nothing is known of this enzyme.

retinal detachment a condition in which the inner layers of the retina (neural retina) are separated from the pigment epithelium. It can result from accumulation of fluids or blood, from the presence of a tumor, or through traction from fibrous tissue in the vitreous, as, for example, following cataract surgery. Focal distortion of the visual image is produced, the affected eye seeing sudden curvature or angulation of a normally straight line. If not promptly corrected, the detached layer may shrink, producing a permanent fold, or it may atrophy.

retinitis (ret″ĭ-ni′tis) a general term used to describe an inflammation of the retina.

retinitis pigmentosa a noninflammatory, slowly progressive bilateral degeneration of the retina. It is a genetic defect, most often transmitted as an autosomal recessive trait, although autosomal dominant and X-linked transmission patterns have been described. This disease is characterized by degeneration of rod and cone cells, with displacement of cells of the pigmented epithelium. Rod-mediated night vision is first affected, often in childhood. A midperipheral ring scotoma gradually widens, leading to a reduction of central vision and possibly blindness by middle age.

Ophthalmoscopic examination most frequently reveals dark peripheral pigmentation of the retina and pale optic disks. Diagnosis may require specialized testing, including dark adaptation, electroretinography, and fluorescein angiography. This condition is often associated with deaf-mutism, hereditary ataxias, familial neuropathies, and, occasionally, certain neuronal lipidoses. As therapy is not available, genetic counseling and screening of family members may be advisable.

retinoblastoma (ret″ĭ-no-blas-to′mah) a tumor of the retinal cells. It is the most common intraocular tumor of childhood. It may be present at birth, but is usually diagnosed between the ages of 1 and 2 yr. The tumor is bilateral in about 30 percent of cases, but a familial form also occurs and in almost all such cases the tumor is bilateral; it is transmitted as an autosomal dominant trait with incomplete penetrance. Retinoblastoma forms an elevation growing out from the retina. Histologically, it is composed of small, densely packed cells with frequent rosettes. The ultrastructural features are not specific, but short dendritic processes and small neurosecretory granules have been described in some cases.

If the tumor is large, or has extended deeply into the optic nerve or reached the meninges, it may recur following enucleation; postoperative radiotherapy is usually given. Examination of family members, particularly newborns, should be performed, and genetic counseling is advisable for other family members of reproductive years.

retinoic acid (ret′ĭ-no-ik) a compound in which the alcohol function of retinol (vitamin A) has been oxidized to a carboxyl.

retinol (ret′ĭ-nol) vitamin A_1, the form of vitamin A found in mammals; a 20-carbon alcohol that is reversibly dehydrogenated by enzymatic action into its aldehyde, retinal. Also called retinol$_1$ and vitamin A_1.

retinol-binding protein (RBP) a transport protein of retinol in blood plasma. It is an α_1-globulin; M.W.

21,000. It forms an equimolar complex with prealbumin, which functions as a thyroxine-binding protein.

retinopathy (ret″ĭ-nop′ah-the) [*retino-* + Gr. *pathos* disease] a general term for any noninflammatory disease of the retina.

diabetic r., the pathologic retinal changes that are associated with diabetes mellitus. Diabetic retinopathy represents a leading cause of blindness, occurring more frequently in juvenile (insulin-dependent) diabetes than in other forms. Its occurrence and severity are thought to be related to the length of the disease and the effectiveness of control of hypoglycemia. Two categories of changes are seen: background lesions, which include microaneurysms, dot and blot hemorrhages, cotton wool spots, and hard exudates; and proliferative lesions, which include new vessel formation, vitreous hemorrhage, scars (retinitis proliferans), and retinal detachment.

The oscillatory potentials of the electroretinogram (ERG) are reduced in individuals with diabetic retinopathy, even when no ophthalmoscopic changes in the retina can be detected. In the later stages of the disease, the *b* wave of the ERG is also reduced.

The treatment of choice is photocoagulation.

See also *d. mellitus* under *diabetes.*

retinoscopy (ret″ĭ-nos′ko-pe) [*retino-* + Gr. *skopein* to examine] the observation of the pupil and retina under a beam of light projected into the eye as a means of determining refractive errors of the eye. Also called *skiametry.*

retinotopic (ret″ĭ-no-top′ik) referring to the phenomenon in which a specific receptor or group of receptors in the retina project to a specific point in the central nervous system; related to a particular point on the retina.

Retortamonas (re″tor-tam′o-nas) [L. *retortus* bent back + Gr. *monas* unit] a genus of biflagellate protozoa.

R. intestinalis, a nonpathogenic intestinal flagellate of cosmopolitan distribution. The trophozoite is small and ovoid, measuring 4–9 μm long. The cyst is oval or pear-shaped, and 4–7 μm long. Transmission is thought to occur by the ingestion of cysts. Laboratory diagnosis requires identification of the cysts or trophozoites in the feces.

retraction (re-trak′shun) [L. *retractio,* from *re-* + *trahere* to draw] the act of drawing back, or condition of being drawn back.

clot r., see *clot retraction.*

retro- (ret′ro) [L. "backward"] a prefix word element to denote behind, e.g., retroperitoneal.

retrograde (ret′ro-grād) [*retro-* + L. *gradi* to step] degenerating, deteriorating, or catabolic; moving backward or against the usual direction of flow, as retrograde urography or aortography. Cf. *anterograde.*

retrolental (ret″ro-len′tal) behind the lens of the eye.

retrolental fibroplasia bilateral abnormality of the retinal vessels, with dilation, increased permeability, fibrovascular proliferation, retinal detachment, and blindness. It is seen in infants, especially premature infants weighing less than 1500 g, and is related to postnatal incubator exposure to high oxygen concentrations (greater than ambient air levels). Changes may appear months to a year or more after exposure and may contribute to glaucoma, retinal detachment in adulthood, and mental retardation. The lowest concentration of oxygen required for maintenance of the infant should be used. If higher concentrations are required (above 40 percent), the radial or temporal arterial oxygen tensions should be checked to maintain a level of 50–80 mmHg.

retroperitoneum (re″tro-per″ĭ-to-ne′um) the area between the posterior abdominal wall and the posterior parietal peritoneum. It contains the kidneys, adrenal glands, ureters, duodenum, ascending and descending colon, pancreas, abdominal aorta, inferior vena cava, and other large vessels and nerves.

retrospective study a study in which the event of interest has occurred in the past relative to the investigator's place in time. For example, a study seeking to ascertain the association between exposure to a certain agent and subsequent development of a disease may compare the exposure rate in individuals with, to those without, the disease. In this case, the disease is already present or absent, and the investigator must look backward in time to establish the presence or absence of a possibly causative antecedent factor. The term case-control study is frequently used synonymously with retrospective study, a usage that should be avoided as it is possible to do a retrospective cohort study, i.e., to study a cohort that existed in the past. For example, a study to show the association between radiation exposure and hematologic neoplasms may follow the inhabitants of Hiroshima who survived the 1945 atom bomb. In this instance, the group under study, i.e., the cohort, existed in the past relative to the investigator's frame of time, and this is thus a retrospective cohort study.

Retroviridae a family of RNA viruses characterized by the possession of reverse transcriptase (RNA-dependent DNA polymerase) in the virion. During viral replication, viral DNA becomes integrated into host cell DNA, thus donating new properties to the host cell. Retroviridae is divided into three subfamilies; Oncovirinae, Spumavirinae, and Lentivirinae. All retroviruses are enveloped, are sensitive to ether, and assemble their capsids in the host cytoplasm.

return (rĕ-turn′) in computer programming, to transfer control from a subroutine back to the calling program, usually to the instruction immediately following the calling instruction.

return address in computer programming, the address of the first statement in the calling program executed after the return from a subroutine. The return address is supplied by the calling program with each subroutine call.

reversal (re-ver′sal) a turning or change in the opposite direction.

reverse (re-vers′) turned backward; opposite.

reverse agglutination the process of detecting the presence of an antigen by mixing the sample fluid with antibody-coated latex particles or red blood cells. If a specific antigen is present, it clumps in the presence of the antibody.

reverse bias a voltage across a diode or *p-n* junction that does not cause conduction. The *n*-terminal is positive with respect to the *p*-terminal. Cf. *forward bias.*

reverse grouping a confirmatory technique for determining an ABO blood group. Serum is mixed with known A and B cells, centrifuged, and examined for agglutination. Group A individuals have naturally occurring anti-B; group B, anti-A; group O, both anti-A and anti-B; and group AB, neither. Also called back testing.

reverse T_3 abbrev. See *reverse triiodothyronine.*

reverse transcriptase RNA-dependent DNA polymerase. This enzyme is able to use RNA as a template for the synthesis of single-stranded DNA, whose sequences are complementary to the RNA. Such DNA is referred to as complementary DNA (cDNA). The enzyme adds nucleotides to the 3′-OH end of short RNA primers in much the same way as bacterial DNA polymerases.

Necessary for viral replication, reverse transcriptase is found in the leukoviruses and RNA tumor viruses of eukaryotic cells. Its activity can be inhibited by certain rifamycins.

See also *viral carcinogenesis in c. e.* under *cancer etiology.*

reverse triiodothyronine (reverse T_3; rT_3) (tri″-i-o″do-thi′ro-nēn) 3′,5′,3-triiodothyronine, a major metabolite of thyroxine having little or no calorigenic activity; M.W. 651.01. It is produced almost exclusively by extrathyroidal monodeiodination at the 5 position, and represents less than 1 percent of total iodine in the body. The metabolism of thyroxine to reverse T_3 or to T_3 represents a mechanism that potentially can respond to the energy needs of the body in a variety of different physiologic states.

Reverse T_3 is often elevated in hyperthyroidism, hepatic disease, renal disease, malnutrition, starvation, fasting, and acute heat load, and in newborn infants. Reference values for reverse T_3 in serum are 18–60 ng/dl.

See also *thyroxine* and *triiodothyronine.*

reversible (re-ver′si-b′l) capable of going through a series of changes in either direction, forward or backward, as a reversible chemical reaction.

Reye's syndrome an acute disease in children and young adults (aged 6 mo–18 yr) that is characterized by acute encephalopathy and fatty degeneration of the liver and renal tubules; its cause is unknown. It is thought to be a rare and severe complication of certain viral infections, especially those caused by influenza, parainfluenza, varicella, and coxsackie- and echoviruses. A similar syndrome has been associated with the ingestion of aflatoxin, a fungal toxin. There may be an increased incidence of the syndrome following nonspecific febrile illnesses in children who have received aspirin. Hours to several days after apparent resolution of the preceding viral infection, there is vomiting, headache, and prominent mental changes that rapidly progress to stupor and coma, followed in severe cases by death.

Pathologic findings include acute cerebral swelling and organomegaly with fatty infiltration. Cerebral edema and astrocytic swelling lead to severe intracranial hypertension. Visceral changes include fatty changes in the liver, pancreas, heart, kidneys, spleen, and lymph nodes.

Liver function tests reveal increased transaminases, increased blood ammonia, and bilirubin levels of less than 2.5 mg/100 ml. Prothrombin time is less than 60 percent of normal. Cerebrospinal fluid changes include increased pressure, fewer than 8–10 white blood cells per cubic millimeter, and increased glutamine. Glucose concentration in both the blood and CSF may be reduced. Serum levels of amino acid, medium-chain fatty acids, amylase, and creatine kinase (CK) are elevated. Neurogenic hyperventilation leads to respiratory alkalosis, but metabolic acidosis and electrolyte imbalances are also common. Abnormalities in the electroencephalogram are usually nonspecific and diffuse. A biopsy of the liver for histologic examination is important in establishing the diagnosis.

The prognosis is dependent on the severity of the condition: survivors may make a complete recovery, and recurrence is uncommon. Neurologic sequelae, if present, are usually related to the severity of the coma. Currently, there is no specific treatment available for Reye's syndrome except supportive therapy aimed at reducing intracranial pressure and correcting the metabolic disturbances.

Reynold's number (R_e or N_R) (ren′oldz) a dimensionless number used to predict the tendency toward the turbulent flow of gas or fluid molecules through a tube, particularly the flow of air through the respiratory tract or of blood in the vascular system.

The R_e is related to the density (ρ) and viscosity (η) of the fluid or gas, the diameter of the tube (D), and the average linear velocity of flow (V) in the following equation: $R_e = \rho DV/\eta$. As predicted by the equation, turbulent flow occurs at lower velocities in tubes with larger diameters. Flow becomes turbulent when a critical linear velocity or value for the R_e (2000 for the vascular system and respiratory airways) is exceeded, as may occur in the presence of stenotic valves; narrowing of the arterial lumen; or reduction in caliber, obstruction, or irregularity in the respiratory tract.

R factor see *R p.* under *plasmid.*

RH abbrev. See *releasing hormone.*

Rh symbol for the chemical element *rhodium.*

rhabd/o (rab′do) [Gr. *rhabdos* rod] a word element used in combining form to denote rod-shaped, e.g., rhabdoid.

Rhabdiasoidea (rab″dĭ-ah-soi′de-ah) a superfamily of phasmids in some classifications, including the genera *Strongyloides* and *Rhabditis.*

Rhabditata a suborder of phasmids of the class Phasmidia, including the superfamily Rhabdiasoidea.

Rhabditida an order phasmids of the class Phasmidia, including the superfamily Rhabdiasoidea.

Rhabditis (rab-di′tis) [Gr. *rhabdos* rod] a genus of free-living, minute phasmid nematodes, which are accidental parasites of humans. These nematodes live in damp earth. The early rhabditoid stage is almost identical to that of *Strongyloides.* The species *R. hominis* and *R. intestinalis* have been found in human stools.

rhabdomy/o (rab-do-mi′o) [*rhabdo-* + Gr. *mys* muscle] a word element used in combining form to denote striated muscle, e.g., rhabdomyoblastoma.

rhabdomyolysis (rab″do-mi-ol′ĭ-sis) [*rhabdomyo-* + Gr. *lysis* dissolution] the destruction or degeneration of muscle tissue due to a variety of causes, especially trauma.

rhabdomyoma (rab″do-mi-o′mah) a benign proliferation of skeletal muscle cells. Tumors occurring in the heart with this appearance are often associated with the tuberous sclerosis complex and are probably hamartomas. Extracardiac rhabdomyomas are, in contrast, true benign neoplasms. They are most commonly found in the head and neck region, including the larynx and pharynx, forming circumscribed lesions. Individual cells resemble normal skeletal muscle cells in their eosinophilic cytoplasm, but they are typically round and a banding pattern may not be evident by light microscopy. Ultrastructurally, the cells contain many short segments of myofibrils, often with hypertrophied Z disks, numerous mitochondria, and plentiful glycogen. The tumor cells may resemble those of the granular cell tumor although the two are not related. An uncommon form of rhabdomyoma that occurs in the head and neck region of infants is composed of immature skeletal muscle cells and undifferentiated mesenchymal cells within an edematous stroma, and has been termed a fetal rhabdomyoma.

rhabdomyosarcoma (rab″do-mi″o-sar-ko′mah) a malignant tumor of cells with the potential for skeletal muscle differentiation. It represents up to 8 percent of malignant tumors in children under the age of 15 yr, and occurs in older patients with a frequency that diminishes with age. It is an aggressive tumor, but combination forms of therapy are improving the outlook, and survival figures above 50 percent at 3 yr are being reported.

The tumor cells display a range of differentiation, from small and round or oval cells with scanty cytoplasm, to plump eosinophilic cells containing many myofilaments, or elongated multinucleated units in which cross striations are visible by light microscopy. Subtypes have been defined on the basis of histologic patterns, but there is considerable overlap among them. Embryonal rhabdomyosarcomas are composed of cells similar to those seen in an early stage of development of skeletal muscle in the embryo; they are most commonly found in the head and neck in children, but also occur in the urogenital tract, retroperitoneum, and extremities. When the tumor is located in submucosal connective tissue, the edematous stroma contributes to the formation of spherical grapelike protrusions characteristic of the so-called botryoid sarcoma. Alveolar rhabdomyosarcomas occur predominantly in adolescents and are seen most commonly in the upper limbs and pelvic region; the tumor cells adhere to a branching framework of fibrous connective tissue, but many cells lie free within the alveolar spaces and are individually similar to those seen in embryonal tumors. Mixtures of the two types occur. Pleomorphic rhabdomyosarcoma occurs in older individuals. Many tumors formerly designated as rhabdomyosarcomas are now recognized as malignant fibrous histiocytomas.

rhabdovirus (rab″do-vi′rus) [*rhabdo-* + *virus*] a group of viruses that contain the rabies virus and the Marburg agent. These viruses are bullet-shaped (75 by 175 nm) and enveloped. They contain a single-stranded RNA genome. The nucleocapsid shows a helical arrangement. The envelope of the rhabdovirus is partially composed of hemagglutinin and lipoprotein. The virion has the enzyme transcriptase. This group of viruses comprises a large variety of agents that parasitize hosts across both animal and plant kingdoms.

rhagades (rag′ah-dēz) [pl. of Gr. *rhagas* rent] fissures, cracks, or fine scars in the skin, especially around the mouth or other regions subjected to frequent movement.

-rhage [Gr. *rhēgnynai* to burst forth] a suffix word element to denote breaking or bursting forth; a profuse flow, e.g., hemorrhage.

β-L-rhamnose (ram′nōs) 6-deoxy-β-L-mannose, a 6-deoxy-hexose monosaccharide, one of the few monosaccharides of the L-configuration that occur in plants and animals.

Rh blood group see under *blood groups.*

Rh_0(D) immune globulin a concentrated preparation of specific immunoglobulin (IgG), derived from human plasma and administered intramuscularly for passive immunization in order to prevent the active immunization of Rh_O(D)–negative individuals exposed to Rh_O-positive red cells. Trademark, *RhoGAM.* See also *Rh isoimmunization syndrome.*

rhe/o (re′o) [Gr. *rheos* current] a word element used in combining form to denote an electric current or flow, e.g., rheostat, rheology.

rhenium (Re) (re′ne-um) [L. *Rhēnus* the Rhine river] a metallic element occurring as a silvery-white solid or gray powder; atomic number 75; atomic weight 186.207; a 5d transition element; oxidation states –1, +1 through +7. Rhenium has low toxicity and is used in corrosion-resistant alloys.

rheobase (re′o-bās) [*rheo-* + Gr. *basis* step] the intensity of electric current just sufficient (when acting over an infinite period of time) to stimulate a muscle contraction.

rheostat (re′o-stat) [*rheo-* + Gr. *histanai* to place] a continuously variable electric resistor. Also called *potentiometer.*

rheumatic (roo-mat′ik) [Gr. *rheumatikos*] pertaining to or affected with rheumatism.

rheumatic fever an acute, subacute, or chronic nonsuppurative inflammatory disease that is a sequela to a group A hemolytic streptococcal infection, which may be inapparent. Rheumatic fever is a reaction (probably immunologic) occurring after the infection, rather than an infection itself. It is noted about 3 wk after a streptococcal pharyngitis, most commonly among children aged 4–18 yr. In past epidemics, up to 3 percent of those affected with group A streptococcal pharyngitis subsequently developed rheumatic fever. Antimicrobial therapy for streptococcal infections that eradicates the organisms can prevent the subsequent development of this disease.

The cardinal clinical manifestations of rheumatic fever are called the Jones diagnostic criteria, which are divided into major and minor symptoms. An individual may have one or more of the five major symptoms: carditis, arthritis, chorea, subcutaneous nodules, and erythema marginatum. Minor criteria include arthralgia, fever, elevated erythrocyte sedimentation rate (ESR), elevated C-reactive protein, leukocytosis, and a prolonged P-R interval on electrocardiogram.

When arthritis occurs in rheumatic fever, it is usually a migratory polyarthritis, i.e., it affects multiple joints at different times. The carditis is often associated with palpitations and chest pain, and may lead to cardiac failure and later to valve deformity. Erythema marginatum is seen only in approximately 20 percent of affected individuals, appearing as a roughly circular macular lesion on the trunk or extremities, which leaves a clear center as it grows. Subcutaneous nodules strongly support the diagnosis of rheumatic fever, but they are not usually present. Sydenham's chorea may be the sole symptom; onset begins slowly with involuntary movements and a loss in coordination, as evidenced by the individual's dropping or spilling things.

Laboratory diagnosis of rheumatic fever involves hematology, chemistry, microbiology, and serology. Leukocytosis (up to 24,000 cells/mm^3), anemia, and an increased ESR are common. Evidence of a previous group A streptococcal throat infection is important, although the organisms may not still be present. To determine a recent history of streptococcal pharyngitis, serologic analysis of antistreptococcal antibodies (antistreptolysin O or others) is helpful.

See also *streptococci.*

rheumatic nodules subcutaneous nodules seen in rheumatic fever, usually in association with rheumatic carditis. They have a concentric zoned composition with a central focus of necrosis surrounded by a radial array of histiocytes and fibroblasts.

rheumatid (roo′mah-tid) any skin lesion that is etiologically associated with rheumatism.

rheumatism (roo′mah-tizm) [L. *rheumatismus;* Gr. *rheumatismos*] 1. any of a variety of disorders marked by inflammation, degeneration, or metabolic derangement of the connective tissue structures, especially the joints and related structures, and attended by pain, stiffness, or limitation of motion.

2. a term applied by laymen to such disorders as arthritis, osteoarthritis, and bursitis.

rheumatoid (roo′mah-toid) [Gr. *rheuma* flux + *eidos* form] resembling rheumatism.

rheumatoid agglutinator an immunoglobulin for a specific immunoglobulin allotypic marker, normally present in serum of individuals with rheumatoid arthritis.

rheumatoid arthritis a chronic, systemic inflammatory disease of unknown cause. The characteristic lesion is a diffuse progressive synovitis, in which the synovial lining becomes a highly vascularized mass of inflammatory tissue (the pannus). Lymphocytes, macrophages, plasma cells, and leukocytes (primarily neutrophils) are found in the synovial fluid. The pannus and products of the inflammatory reaction are capable of eroding the underlying articular cartilage, subchondral bone, ligaments, and tendons. Extraarticular manifestations, as well as pulmonary involvement, may occur.

There is great variation among patients in the mode of onset of rheumatoid arthritis, in the pattern of joint involvement, and in the frequency of extraarticular manifestations. The clinical course is also highly variable: 10 percent of those affected experience crippling disease, 10–20 percent have complete remissions, and the remainder have sustained but fluctuating disease activity.

Criteria diagnostic of rheumatoid arthritis include radiographic changes indicative of demineralization in periarticular bone; a positive test for rheumatoid factor in serum (a group of IgM, IgG, and IgA autoantibodies that react with the Fc regions of IgG molecules forming soluble complexes); poor mucin clot formation in the mucin clot test on synovial fluid; characteristic synovial histopathology, and histopathology characteristic of biopsied rheumatoid nodules.

The presence of rheumatoid factors in the serum of about 80 percent of RA patients and in the synovial fluid of about 60 percent of those affected with RA has led to the classification of rheumatoid arthritis as an autoimmune disease although there is no conclusive evidence that autoimmune processes are either the initial event in the disease process or the direct cause of pathology.

See also *autoimmune disease* and *rheumatoid factor.*

rheumatoid factor an immunoglobulin specific for denatured IgG, found in individuals with rheumatoid diseases such as rheumatoid arthritis. This factor is associated with such diseases as idiopathic interstitial pulmonary fibrosis, immune complex glomerulonephritis, some rheumatoid afflictions of the eye, and systemic lupus erythematosus. More specifically, classical rheumatoid factor is a 19S IgM antibody directed against 7S IgG, but it may also be an IgG or IgA protein.

rheumatoid factor tests assays for the detection of rheumatoid factor. The most commonly used tests are latex fixation and sheep red blood cell agglutinations.

The latex-fixation tests can be performed in two ways. In the slide test, human IgG-coated latex beads are added to a 1:20 dilution of heat-inactivated test serum and allowed to react. The serum must be heat-inactivated to destroy C1q, which could give a false-positive result. If rheumatoid factor is present, it causes the formation of visible clumps of the latex particles. In the tube dilution method, the IgG-coated latex beads are added to serial dilutions of the test serum in test tubes and centrifuged after incubation. The flocculation reaction is read by gently tapping the tube to dislodge the pellet. If the precipitate breaks into small particles and the supernatant remains clear, the reaction is positive; if the precipitate breaks up in a hazy pattern, it is negative. The highest tube dilution showing flocculation is the rheumatoid factor titer. A titer greater than 1:160 is considered significant.

The other commonly used test, the sheep cell agglutination test, is performed using sheep red blood cells coated with rabbit IgG antibodies specific for sheep red blood cells. The test serum is incubated with sheep red blood cells to absorb out heterophil antibody. After centrifugation, the antibody is serially diluted and antibody-coated cells are added. An agglutination titer of greater than 1:16 is considered significant.

These tests primarily detect IgM. Rheumatoid factors may also be IgG or IgA, but detection of these isotypes requires more sophisticated techniques and is not necessary for routine clinical purposes. Rheumatoid factor is used to differentiate rheumatoid arthritis from other chronic inflammatory arthritides. It may also aid in the diagnosis of immunologically mediated diseases in individuals with an autoimmune disorder or chronic inflammation, e.g., systemic lupus erythematosus or subacute bacterial endocarditis.

Sheep red blood cell agglutination is more specific for rheumatoid factor, as it uses rabbit immunoglobulin, whereas latex fixation detects any antibodies to human immunoglobulin. The latex test is easier to perform and therefore is used at least for preliminary screenings. All tests for rheumatoid factor are inhibited by serum IgG. In extreme cases, it may be necessary to dilute IgG from the serum.

The latex-fixation test detects rheumatoid factor

in 1–4 percent of the general population. The highest incidence of rheumatoid factor is in persons older than 65, reaching 20 percent with the latex-fixation test.

The clinical significance of elevated rheumatoid factor should be interpreted cautiously. Increased titers may occur during acute immune responses, especially viral infections, and in normal elderly persons. High titers (> 1:160) are highly suggestive. Titers with a range of 1:20–1:80 are more difficult to interpret; they can indicate early rheumatoid arthritis or be a nonspecific finding.

Another type of rheumatoid factor, termed cold-reacting rheumatoid factor, may be present in immunologically mediated diseases or chronic infections. Unlike common rheumatoid factor, it tends to be monoclonal and reacts with IgG at 4°C. This type of factor is detected by measuring circulatory cryoglobulins, solubilizing the cryoprecipitate at 37°C, and subsequently determining the concentration of rheumatoid factor.

rhin/o (ri′no) [Gr. *rhis* nose] a word element used in combining form to denote the nose, e.g., rhinoplasty.

rhinal (ri′nal) [Gr. *rhis* nose] pertaining to the nose.

rhinitis (ri-ni′tis) [*rhin-* + *-itis*] a common upper respiratory tract infection characterized by inflammation of the nasal mucosal membranes, airway obstruction, and nasal discharge. Acute forms occur in viral respiratory infections (e.g., the common cold) and nasal infections by gram-positive cocci. Chronic forms are due to granulomatous infections (e.g., tuberculosis, fungi, etc.) and are characterized by tissue destruction. Diagnosis is based on the clinical picture and, when appropriate, identification of the infectious organism. Nonviral rhinitis may be treated by antibiotic therapy.

allergic r., a seasonal (hay fever) or nonseasonal (perennial) form of upper respiratory tract infection that results from the contact of a sensitized individual with a particular antigen. This allergic reaction is considered to be a type IV (IgE-mediated) response. Offending allergens are varied and include pollen and fungi. Following contact with the allergen, histamine and other mediators are released, leading to nasal congestion, watery rhinorrhea, sneezing, lacrimation, and itching of the nose, pharynx, and eyes. The conjunctiva is infected, and the nasal mucosa is pale and boggy. Inflammatory nasal polyps may be found in association with allergic rhinitis.

Laboratory tests reveal the presence of increased numbers of eosinophils in nasal secretions. Diagnosis is based on the clinical findings. Skin tests may help to determine the specific allergen.

atrophic r., a chronic form of nasal inflammation characterized by atrophy and sclerosis of the nasal mucosal membranes, leading to obstruction of the nasal airways. The etiology is unknown. Characteristically, the mucosal membranes become encrusted and covered with stratified squamous epithelium. Insomnia, frequent epistaxis, and a foul breath result. Also called ozena.

vasomotor r., a chronic form of rhinitis characterized by engorgement of the nasal mucosal membranes, leading to obstruction, sneezing, and watery nasal discharge. Although this condition resembles allergic rhinitis in its signs and symptoms, it does not have an allergic etiology. The cause of vasomotor rhinitis is uncertain.

Rhinoestrus (rīn-es′trus) a genus of flies of the family Oestridae. The species *R. nasalis,* the Russian gadfly, may parasitize humans, as may *R. purpureus,* which has caused ophthalmomyiasis.

rhinopharyngitis (ri″no-far″in-ji′tis) an inflammation of the nasopharynx.

rhinorrhea (ri″no-re′ah) [*rhino-* + Gr. *rhoia* flow] the discharge of a thin nasal mucus.

cerebrospinal r., the discharge of cerebrospinal fluid through the nose, usually due to a fracture of the anterior cranial fossa.

rhinoscleroma (ri″no-sklĕ-ro′mah) [*rhino-* + Gr. *sklērōma* a hard swelling] a disease of the nose and nasopharynx due to infection with the organism *Klebsiella rhinoscleromatis,* primarily found in persons living in the Middle East, Eastern Europe, and Central and South America. The disease develops slowly and insidiously over many years. It is characterized by granulomatous inflammation with the formation of hard, patchy, painful nodules that tend to enlarge. The characteristic nasal configuration is called the Hebra nose.

rhinovirus (ri″no-vi′rus) a virus that is the most frequent etiologic agent of the common cold. In the very young and very old, rhinovirus may cause chronic pneumonia and bronchitis and, rarely, viremia. *Rhinovirus* is a genus in the family Picornaviridae, which are small, nonenveloped RNA viruses. Clinical symptoms of the common cold include a prodromal irritation and congestion of the nose, headache, dry cough, sore throat, and little or no fever. The incubation period is 1–5 da with a mean of 2 da. The period of clinical symptoms is 4–24 da with a mean of 7 da. The shedding of virus begins with the onset of symptoms and may continue for 1 wk.

Rhinovirus is most efficiently transmitted from person to person, although particle aerosols are also responsible. Rhinovirus infections occur the year round, with peaks in the fall and spring. Common colds during the winter season are more frequently due to coronavirus and paramyxovirus. The common cold is often incorrectly associated with winter, cold, and wetness. A high incidence of colds is more correctly associated with many people interacting within closed environments.

There are more than 110 immunotypes of rhinovirus, which explains, in part, why contracting a cold does not confer immunity to subsequent colds. The average person gets two to six colds per year, each with a separate immunotype. In addition, there are several immunotypes of rhinovirus present in the environment at any given time, unlike influenza, which is present as only one immunotype at a given time. Rhinoviruses do undergo antigenic shifts.

Host immunity is type-specific and consists of local IgA production in nasal secretions and circulating IgG. Type-specific immunity remains for a few years. The rhinovirus grows best in tissue culture at 37°C, and at a neutral or slightly alkaline pH. Incubation of rhinovirus at 33°C at pH 3.0 for 3 hr causes a loss of infectivity. This is probably why this virus causes only a local infection, unlike its relative the enterovirus, which is pH-resistant and can survive at the low pH of the stomach.

Laboratory identification of rhinovirus is usually performed for epidemiologic purposes. The rhinovirus can be isolated from nasal or pharyngeal washings collected 3 da after the onset of symptoms. If the specimen is not inoculated within 3 hr, it may be stored for a short time at 4°C and a longer time at –70°C. The tissue cultures of choice for the growth of rhinovirus are human fetal kidney cells and diploid strains of human embryonic lung. Incubation should be achieved by rotating the cultures on a roller drum at 33°C and at neutral pH.

Serologic diagnosis is not simple, owing to the large number of immunotypes. The neutralization test is the optimal assay for the detection of rhinovirus antibody, and is used for numbering immunotypes. The acute-phase serum should be collected at the onset of symptoms. The convalescent-phase serum should be collected after 3 wk. The viral neutralization test result is considered positive if there is a fourfold increase in antibody titer between acute and convalescent sera.

Treatment of the common cold due to rhinovirus is symptomatic, as there is no effective antiviral chemotherapy. Vaccines are of little use owing to the large number of immunotypes.

Formerly called *coryzavirus.*

Rhipicentor (ri″pĭ-sen′tor) [Gr. *rhipis* fan + *kentein* to prick or stab] a genus of ticks. Several species are transmitters of diseases such as Rocky Mountain spotted fever, tick-borne relapsing fever, and Colorado tick fever. The species *R. bicornis* is known to cause a high fever in human adults, and even death in children.

Rhipicephalus (ri″pĭ-sef′ah-lus) [Gr. *rhipis* fan + *kephalē* head] a genus of ticks that are parasitic in cattle and dogs. Several species are transmitters of the spotted fever group rickettsiae (causing Rocky Mountain spotted fever), and others are unpleasant pests to humans.

Rh isoimmunization syndrome a condition involving the immunization of a mother with Rh-negative blood against the red cell antigens (D factor or Rh_o) of her Rh-positive fetus, which produces hemolytic disease of the fetus or newborn infant. Red cell hemolysis is caused by maternal antibodies crossing the placenta during pregnancy. Sensitization of the mother is due to previous transfusion of Rh-incompatible blood or to transplacental hemorrhage during a previous pregnancy. Such sensitization can be prevented by passive immunization with Rh_o(D) immune globulin immediately after the birth of an Rh-positive infant, which prevents active immunization.

Rh isoimmunizaton is assessed by monitoring maternal antibody titers, and, when the titer reaches critical levels, by amniocentesis. Bilirubin and other pigment breakdown products of hemoglobin are detected in amniotic fluid by spectrophotometry. A scan of the absorbance between 350 and 700 nm shows a peak at 450 nm. The net absorbance at 450 nm (measured baseline to peak) is proportional to the bilirubin concentration; it measures the severity of the disease and is helpful in predicting fetal survival.

When the fetus is not likely to survive to term without intervention, an intrauterine transfusion is performed. Rh-compatible blood is transfused into the fetal peritoneal cavity.

rhiz/o (ri′zo) [Gr. *rhiza* root] a word element used in combining form to denote relationship to a root, e.g., rhizopodium, rhizotomy.

Rhizobiaceae (ri-zo″bi-a′se-e) [*rhizo-* + Gr. *bios* life + *aceae*] a family of aerobic, gram-negative bacteria that inhabits the soil. There are two genera, *Rhizobium* and *Agrobacterium. Rhizobium* species produce nodules on the roots of leguminous plants and fix nitrogen within these nodules. Three of the four species of *Agrobacterium* are phytopathogens, causing crown-gall in many kinds of plants. The fourth species, *A. radiobacter,* is not known to cause plant disease and is occasionally recovered from clinical species; although not considered pathogenic, this species does need to be differentiated from other oxidase- and nitrate-positive, motile, glucose oxidizers.

rhizoid (ri′zoid) [*rhizo-* + Gr. *eidos* form] rootlike; a descriptive term for hyphae with rootlike structures found in the fungi *Rhizopus* and *Absidia.* The location of a rhizoid on the mycelium is a distinguishing characteristic of these fungi and is useful in microscopic identification.

Rhizopodea (ri-zop′o-de-ah) [*rhizo-* + Gr. *pous* foot] a class of protozoa that includes the order Amoebida (the amebae).

Rhizopus (ri-zo′pus) a genus of fungi that are zygomycetes and belong to the family Mucoraceae, order Mucorales; it can be an etiologic agent of mucormycosis. The *Rhizopus* fungus is characterized by simple sporangiophores that arise from nodes (swollen areas) along a stolon. Rhizoids are present, also attached to the nodes. This sporangiophore-rhizoid relationship to the node differs from *Absidia,* whose sporangiophores arise between the nodes. Medically important species include *R. oryzae, R. arrhizus,* and *R. rhizopodoformis.* See also *Absidia, Mucor,* and *mucormycosis.*

Rh negative lacking the Rh_0(D) antigen; the notation Rh_0-negative or D- should be used to avoid ambiguity, as there are other Rh antigens in use.

rho (Ρ, ρ) (ro) the seventeenth letter of the *Greek alphabet.*

rhodamine (ro-dah′min) [Gr. *rhodon* rose + *amine*] any of several related fluorochrome dyes. The two most commonly used are rhodamine B C.I. 45170, a carboxyphenyl derivative of pyronine B, and sulforhodamine B C.I. 45100, a disulfophenyl derivative.

Rhodesian trypanosomiasis see *African t.* under *trypanosomiasis.*

rhodium (Rh) (ro′de-um) [Gr. *rhodon* rose, from the color of its compounds] a ductile metallic element of the platinum group; atomic number 45; atomic weight 102.9055; oxidation states +1 through +6 (+1 and +3 are common). It is used in alloys and as a catalyst. Rhodium has low toxicity.

Rhodnius (rod′ne-us) a genus of insects of the family Reduviidae. Several species are known vectors of *Trypanosoma rangeli* and *T. cruzi.*

rhodo- (ro′do) [Gr. *rhodon* rose] a word element used in combining form to denote red, e.g., rhodopsin.

rhodopsin (ro-dop′sin) [*rhodo-* + Gr. *opsis* vision] visual purple; a photosensitive, purple-red chromoprotein in the retinal rods that is bleached to visual yellow (all-*trans* retinal) by light, thereby producing stimulation of the retinal sensory endings. Rhodopsin is a thermolabile conjugated glycoprotein (M.W. about 35,000), the prosthetic group of which is 11-*cis*-retinal.

When bleached by light, and studied at low temperature, a series of some half-dozen or more intermediate pigments, with characteristic spectral absorption maxima, are formed before 11-*trans*-retinal and opsin are released by the photochemical event. Transformation of rhodopsin to retinal and opsin is endergonic, the energy for which is supplied by an absorbed photon. Regeneration of rhodopsin is an exergonic process, occurring spontaneously by reaction of opsin with 11-*cis*-retinal.

Rhodotorula (ro″do-tor′u-lah) a genus of yeasts. It resembles *Cryptococcus* in rate of growth, colony morphology, cell size and shape, occasional rudimentary pseudomycelium, presence of a capsule, ability to split urea, and lack of fermentative ability. Its lack of pathogenicity and presence of conspicuous carotenoid pigment have maintained *Rhodotorula* as a distinct genus. *Rhodotorula* species is commonly found airborne or as a contaminant. Often this genus is isolated from sputum or moist skin as a commensal. When *Rhodotorula* species is repeatedly isolated from blood with contamination ruled out, it may be considered pathogenic.

R. rubra, a species that is coral red when grown on culture media, owing to carotenoid pigments. It has caused transient blood-stream fungemia but not actual infection of host tissues.

rhodotorulosis a rare yeast infection caused by *Rhodotorula* species. Individuals with this infection usually have an underlying debilitating disease.

rho factor (ro fak′tor) [L. "maker"] an oligomeric protein that has the ability to depress in vitro the amount of RNA formed by the RNA polymerase holoenzyme by causing chain termination; M.W. 50,000.

RhoGAM (ro′gam) trademark for a preparation of Rh_0(D) immune globulin; see *Rh_0 (D) immune globulin.*

rhombencephalon (rom″ben-sef′ah-lon) [Gr. *rhombos* rhomb + *enkephalos* brain] 1. [NA], the part of the brain composed of the pons, medulla oblongata, and cerebellum.

2. in the developing embryo, the most caudal of the three primary brain vesicles. Also called *hindbrain.*

rhombomere (rom′bo-mēr) see *neuromere.*

Rhombomys a genus of rodents. The species *R. opimus* is a common reservoir of *Leishmania tropica* and is found in Iran.

rhonchus (rong′kus), pl. *rhonchi* [L.; Gr. *rhonchos* a snoring sound] a rattling in the throat; also, a dry, coarse rale in the bronchial tubes due to partial obstruction.

rhopheocytosis the microphagocytic incorporation of particles (carbon, silica, gamma globulin) into a cell. The process is initiated by adherence of the particles to the cell surface, invagination of that portion of the cell surface, formation of an intracytoplasmic vacuole containing the particles, and eventual liberation of the particles into the cytoplasm. The best known and studied example is the incorporation of ferritin into erythroblasts. The process differs from micropinocytosis, in which the cell surface throws out veils that then surround part of the adjacent medium, eventually incorporating (phagocytosing) it into the cell cytoplasm.

Rh positive having the Rh_0(D) antigen; the notation Rh_0-positive or D+ should be used to avoid ambiguity, as there are other Rh antigens in use.

Rh typing see *blood typing.*

rhythm (rith′m) [L. *rhythmus;* Gr. *rhythmos*] 1. a measured movement; the recurrence of an action or function at regular intervals.

2. in electroencephalography, a pattern of waves of approximately constant period.

3. in cardiology, referring to the particular site of initiation of the heart rhythm, e.g., *idioventricular rhythm, nodal rhythm, normal sinus rhythm.*

rhythmic temporal theta burst of drowsiness in electroencephalography, a burst of 4- to 7-Hz electric activity (theta frequency) usually notched by faster waves, recorded from the temporal region of the scalp during drowsiness. The occurrence of this pattern is rare and its pathologic significance is controversial. Also called *psychomotor variant.*

rhythm of alpha frequency in electroencephalography, any activity with a frequency of 8–13 Hz (alpha band) that differs from alpha rhythm in its reactivity to various stimuli and/or its distribution over the scalp. See also *alpha rhythm.*

RIA abbrev. See *radioimmunoassay.*

rib/o (ri′bo) a word element used in combining form to denote sugar, e.g., ribosome.

rib (rib) a slender, flattened, curved strip of bone attached posteriorly to the thoracic vertebrae and connected anteriorly to the sternum by strips of costal cartilage. There are 12 pairs of ribs, which enclose and protect the thoracic cavity. The lower five pairs of ribs are called false ribs because they lack a direct articulation with the sternum. The anterior ends of the eighth, ninth, and tenth ribs are joined to the rib above by cartilage. The eleventh and twelfth ribs are not attached anteriorly and are therefore called floating ribs.

Each rib has a head, neck tubercle, shaft, and costal cartilage. The ribs become longer down to the seventh or eighth, after which their size diminishes down to the twelfth rib. The first rib is sharply curved and has upper and lower surfaces; the other ribs have outer and inner surfaces.

ribavirin (ri″bah-vi′rin) an antiviral agent that is an analog of purine (guanosine) nucleoside. It is effective against herpesvirus and influenza virus. Its mode of action involves the inhibition of synthesis of guanylic acid nucleotides. Ribavirin is teratogenic and should not be used during pregnancy. See also *antiviral agent.*

riboflavin vitamin B_2, 6,7-dimethyl-9-[1′-D-ribityl]-isoalloxazin; M.W. 376.36. This is a fat-soluble vitamin found in the body in the liver, muscle, and kidneys; it also occurs in eggs, malt, and leafy vegetables, See also *flavin.*

riboflavin assays 1. fluorometric spectroscopy. The urine sample is treated with permanganate, which oxidizes and destroys interfering substances. Riboflavin is then extracted into a butanol-pyridine solution, and its fluorescence is determined at 530 nm. A urine blank, in which riboflavin has been destroyed by radiation, is prepared. The concentration of the sample is calculated after subtracting the blank fluorescence from the fluorescence obtained from the sample.

2. microbiologic assay. The rate of growth of *Lactobacillus casei,* a riboflavin-dependent microorganism, is measured photometrically at 620 nm. The amount of riboflavin in the sample is calculated from a standard curve, where the amount of riboflavin per tube is plotted against the absorbance.

3. enzymatic assays for flavin mononucleotide (FMN) and flavin adenine dinucleotide (FAD). For spectrophotometric assay of FAD based on the oxidation of D-alanine by D-amino oxidase, when coupled to the lactic acid dehydrogenase system; when all substrates except FAD are in excess, the decrease in absorbance at 340 nm due to NADH consumption is directly proportional to the amount of FAD in the reaction mixture. For FAD spectrophotometric assay based on the reduction of reduced glutathione by the enzyme glutathione reductase: NADH is oxidized to NAD^+ in this reaction and the decrease in absorbance at 340 nm is measured. The degree of stimulation by added FAD is measured, and the amount of FAD in the sample is determined by comparison with the standard FAD.

riboflavin-5′-phosphate (ri″bo-fla′vin fos′fāt) a phosphate ester derivative of riboflavin, which consists of a three-ring system (dimethylisoalloxazine) attached to an alcohol (ribitol). See also *f. mononucleotide* under *flavin.*

ribonuclease (RNase, RNAase) (ri″bo-nu′kle-ās) enzymes of the hydrolase subclass (EC 3.1.13,14,26,27,30,31) that catalyze the hydrolysis (depolymerization) of a ribonucleic acid by hydrolysis of a phosphate ester linkage. These enzymes, found in various bacterial, plant, and animal sources, are important in the degradation of ribonucleic acids.

ribonucleic acid (RNA) (ri″bo-nu′kle-ik) a polymer of ribonucleotides that consists of three components: a nitrogenous base, D-ribose, and a phosphate residue derived from phosphoric acid. The bases occurring in all RNAs are the purines adenine (A) and guanine (G) and the pyrimidines cytosine (C) and uracil (U), an analog of thymine (T), which occurs in DNA. The furanose form of ribose is bonded by a β-glycosidic linkage to the 1′ position of the pyrimidine or to the 9′ position of the purine residue. The sugar and base together are referred to as a nucleoside. Mononucleotides of RNA have the phosphoric acid group esterified to one of the free hydroxyls occurring at the 2′, 3′, and 5′ of ribose, with 5′-ribonucleotides the most common. Generally, the nucleoside 5′-diphosphates occur as complexes with Ca^{2+}, or with Mg^{2+} (more prevalent). Polynucleotide backbones of the common kinds of RNA are built from mononucleotides linked covalently via phosphodiester bridges between the 3′ position of one unit and the 5′ position of the next. Other polymers are also found in biologic systems.

Almost all RNA molecules are synthesized from a DNA template by one of the RNA polymerases, a process called transcription (a few viruses produce enzymes that can replicate RNA). The base sequence of the RNA is complementary to its DNA template. The pairing rules are A to U, T to A, C to G, and G to C. After transcription, RNAs are modified by enzymes that add cap and tail pieces or that modify some of the bases.

All cells contain three kinds of RNAs: messenger RNA (mRNA), transfer RNA (tRNA), and ribosomal RNA (rRNA). In eukaryotes there is another class, heterogeneous nuclear RNA (hnRNA).

MESSENGER RNA. This is a transcript of a structural gene from which a polypeptide chain is synthesized, a process called translation. In eukaryotic cells, the primary transcript is modified by several processes before translation. A cap and tail are added and, for most genes, several intervening sequences (introns) must be cut out, and the coding sequences (exons) must be spliced together to form an mRNA, which then moves to the cytosol. Heterogeneous nuclear RNA refers to the primary transcripts, which include introns that will be removed from transcripts and other RNAs having a regulatory function that are found in the nucleus.

The structure of eukaryotic mRNA is complex. There is a 5′ cap (Cap I or Cap II); Cap I consists of 7-methylguanosine, which is connected in 5′-5′-triphosphate linkage to the 5′ end of the mRNA molecule, plus a 2′-O-methyl substitution on the first nucleotide in the regular portion of the RNA. Cap II is of the same structure, except that the second nucleotide is also methylated. Recent data suggest that the 5′ caps play important roles in protein synthesis because removal of the caps greatly reduces initiation. After the cap, there is a leader sequence (5′ untranslated segment) before the actual structural gene begins and an untranslated trailer sequence at the 3′ end of the message. Many (but not all) types of eukaryotic mRNA contain a poly A sequence at the 3′ end varying in length from 30 to 200 nucleotides. See also the accompanying illustration.

Messenger RNA exhibits a broad range of molecular weights. In general, the distribution of the bulk cellular RNA is found to be between 8 and 30S or 1–15 daltons. A short lifetime is often cited as a characteristic property of mRNA. Long-lived mRNA may be produced when a cell becomes committed to synthesizing one or a few kinds of proteins. Under conditions of mRNA excess, in which the rate of translation is limited by components of the translational machinery, some types of message are used more effectively than others.

TRANSFER RNA. The secondary structure of tRNA is a cloverleaf. Complementary sequences in different parts of the molecule pair up, forming three loops. The function of tRNA is to translate the genetic code, i.e., to match codons on mRNA to amino acids. There are four significant regions on tRNA molecules: the anticodon that binds to the codon, the CCA acceptor stem where the amino acid is attached, the region that is recognized by a specific aminoacyl tRNA synthetase, and the site that binds to a complementary sequence on 55 rRNA.

One of the functions of tRNA is to carry the anticodon in a prominent position so that it can base-pair with its complementary codon in mRNA. A second function of tRNA is to bind to amino acids. The actual bond forms between the 3′ terminal adenine of the tRNA and the carboxyl group of the amino acid. All known tRNAs end with the CCA sequence, and this sequence is added enzymatically to each molecule during maturation. Specificity of tRNA is provided by the aminoacyl-tRNA synthetases. There are at least 20 different kinds of such synthetases in a cell for each amino acid. They mediate the joining of an amino acid to its tRNA molecule.

There are probably about 60 different forms of tRNA molecules; it follows that several tRNAs are carriers for the same amino acid. A particular tRNA is identified according to the amino acids it can carry; $tRNA^{Met}$ is a methionine-carrying tRNA.

Transfer RNA is relatively stable compared with mRNA. The molecules are small, containing only 70–80 nucleotides; each has a molecular weight of approximately 30,000 and a sedimentation coefficient of 4S.

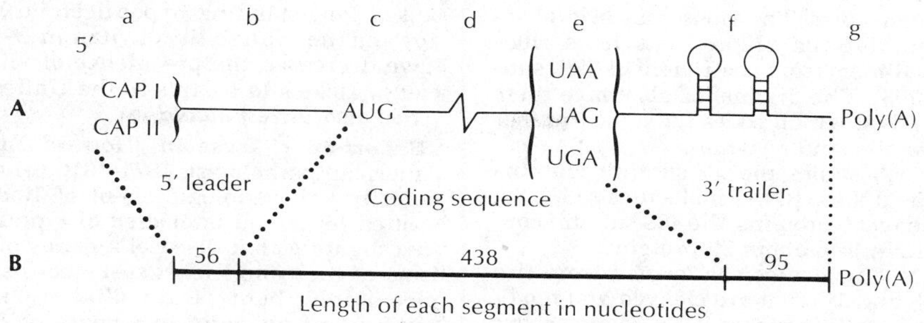

Ribonucleic acid. Schematic representation of eukaryotic mRNA. *A*, Expanded view of noncoding sections of a typical mRNA. *a* = CAP I ($m^7G(5')pppX^mpYpZp$ . . .) or CAP II ($m^7G(5')pppX^mpY^mpZp$ . . .); *b* = untranslated region at 5′ end; *c* = initiation codon; *d* = translated sequence; *e* = termination codon; *f* = untranslated sequence at 3′ end, including possible self-complementary loop forming sequences; and *g* = poly(A) (not present in all mRNAs). *B*, Scale drawing of rabbit beta globulin mRNA with loops straightened out. (From Ham, R. G., and Veomett, M. J.: Mechanisms of Development. St. Louis, C. V. Mosby Co., 1980.)

RIBOSOMAL RNA. The rRNAs are an integral, permanent part of the ribosome structure, yet do not code for protein amino acid sequences. All cytoplasmic ribosomes in a given species have identical rRNA sizes identified by sedimentation coefficients. Prokaryotic rRNA consists of 23S RNA (M.W. 1.2×10^6), 16S RNA (M.W. 6×10^5), and 5S RNA (M.W. 4×10^4). Eukaryotic rRNA consists of 28S RNA (M.W. 1.7×10^6), 18S RNA (M.W. 7×10^5), 5.8S RNA (M.W. 5×10^4), and 5S RNA (M.W. 4×10^4). In both prokaryotic and eukaryotic organisms, the largest of the rRNA species is associated with the larger of the two ribosomal subunits, whereas the rRNA next in size is associated with the small ribosomal subunit. These two species of rRNA contain 1–2 percent nucleotides that are methylated either on the 2′ hydroxyl of ribose or on the base. Ribosomal RNA is the most abundant of RNAs in the cell, comprising 60–80 percent of the total cellular RNA.

See also *nucleic acid, protein synthesis, RNA processing, transcription,* and *translation.* Cf. *deoxyribonucleic acid.*

ribonucleoprotein (RNP) complex (ri″bo-nu″-kle-o-pro′tēn) a ribonucleic acid (RNA) protein particle. Both heterogeneous nuclear RNP (hnRNP) and messenger RNP (mRNP) complexes exist. It is considered likely that the proteins that bind to RNA play significant roles in RNA processing, the transport of RNA across the nuclear membrane to the cytoplasm, or the translation of the RNA to which they attach. The binding of mRNP to the ribosome has been found to be more efficient in some cases than that of free mRNA.

Association of hnRNA with protein complexes has been shown both biochemically and by cytologic observation. The protein composition of hnRNP is unclear. Some researchers claim hnRNP particles to be hnRNA molecules associated with a single protein species. Others find a more heterogeneous population of protein complexed to the hnRNA. Reports that different cells contain different RNA-bound populations have led to speculation that there may be specific interactions between certain proteins and certain message sequences. It is suggested that mRNP particles contain proteins that are distinct from those in hnRNP particles.

ribonucleoside (ri″bo-nu′kle-o-sīd) the glycosidic combination of ribose with either a purine or a pyrimidine.

ribonucleotide (ri″bo-nu′kle-o-tid) a nucleotide containing ribose; the 5′-phosphate, pyrophosphate, or triphosphate of a ribonucleoside.

ribose (r) (ri′bōs) an aldopentose, a 5-carbon sugar that forms a part of the structure of ribonucleic acids.

ribose-1-phosphate (ri′bos fos′fāt) [L. *phosphos*] a phosphate ester of ribose. It is interconvertible with ribose-5-phosphate through the action of phosphoglucomutase.

ribose-5-phosphate the 5-phosphate derivative of ribose, an important intermediate in the pentose shunt of glucose metabolism and a constituent of ribonucleic acid. See also *ribose.*

ribosomal (ri″bo-so′mal) pertaining to ribosomes.

ribosomal DNA (rDNA) the genes that code for the 18S and 28S rRNAs. The genes for these RNA end products are arranged in tandem along the DNA molecules in transcription units containing a spacer region, the 18S-rRNA gene, a second spacer region (a portion of which later becomes the 5.8S rRNA), and the 28S-rRNA gene. Between each transcription unit there is a longer, nontranscribed spacer sequence.

Ribosomal DNA can be separated from the rest of the cell DNA by cesium chloride density gradient centrifugation. Its high content of guanine and cytosine makes it more dense than other DNA.

ribosomal RNA (rRNA) see under *ribonucleic acid.*

ribosome (ri′bo-sōm) an intracellular ribonucleoprotein particle involved in protein synthesis. Ribosomes consist of reversibly dissociable units, and occur either bound to membranes or free in the cytoplasm. Ribosomes within cellular organelles and in prokaryotic cells generally are smaller than the cytoplasmic ribosomes of eukaryotic cells.

Cytoplasmic ribosomes have a diameter of 30 nm and a sedimentation coefficient of 80S. They have two subunits (sedimentation coefficients 60S and 40S) that associate and dissociate during protein synthesis. Each is constructed from proteins and specific RNA molecules. The ribosomes of prokaryotes, mitochondria, and chloroplasts have ribosomes with a sedimentation coefficient of 70S (subunits 50S and 30S). The organelles also have their own supply of DNA, which codes for some (but not all) of their proteins and enzymes.

In eukaryotic ribosomes, the 60S subunit contains three ribosomal RNA (rRNA) molecules (5S, 5.8S, and 28S) and about 50 proteins; the 40S subunit contains an 18S rRNA and about 30 proteins.

The four rRNA molecules are formed from two precursors (45S and 5S) that are cleaved and modified to yield the four RNA pieces. The precursors are transcribed from DNA. The modifications of the precursors include cleavage, hydrolysis, removal of some nucleotide sequences, methylation of some ribosyl moieties and bases, and formation of pseudouridine from uridine.

The function of a ribosome is to synthesize polypeptide chains having amino acid sequences specified by the genetic code of messenger RNA (mRNA) molecules. Many ribosomes can be translating a single mRNA at the same time; the resulting structure is called a polysome.

See also *translation.*

ribosuria (ri″bo-su′re-ah) elevation of urinary levels of D-ribose; associated with muscular dystrophy.

ribothymidylic acid (ri″bo-thi′mi-dĭ″lic) see *thymine ribonucleoside-5-phosphate.*

ribulose (ri′bu-lōs) the 2-ketose isomer of ribose.

ribulose-5-phosphate (ri′bu-lōs fos′fāt) [L. *phosphos*] the 2-ketose isomer of ribose-5-phosphate. It is an important intermediate of the pentose shunt, the hexosemonophosphate pathway of the metabolism of glucose.

rice water stool stool that is watery, contains mucus, and is flecked with fragments of necrotic mucosal epithelium; the term is used to describe the feces of a person with an acute cholera infection. See also *cholera.*

Richter's syndrome a complication of chronic lymphocytic leukemia in which transformation to large cell lymphoma occurs. The subsequent course is aggressive, and most individuals so affected survive for less than 15 mo.

ricin (ri′sin) a poisonous substance (phytotoxin, a plant protein) found in the seeds of the castor oil plant (*Ricinus communis*). It is an inhibitor of protein synthesis, interfering with elongation of eukaryotic ribosomes by binding to the 60S subunit. Ricin agglutinates red blood cells.

ricinoleic acid (ri-sin-o″le′ic) 12-hydroxyoleic acid, an unsaturated hydroxy acid, found as a glyceride in castor oil.

rickets (rik′ets) a metabolic bone disease, most often seen in children, that is due to a deficiency of vitamin D. Certain forms of rickets occur as a familial disorder, genetically transmitted. The disease is caused by inadequate dietary intake of vitamin D, inadequate exposure to sunlight, malabsorption syndromes, and renal tubular defects.

Characteristic radiographic findings in the growing child include the appearance of wide, "motheaten" epiphyses. Serum calcium and phosphate levels are usually low. Serum alkaline phosphatase levels are frequently elevated. Bone scintiscans and biopsies may be used in establishing the diagnosis. Chronic rickets may lead to rachitic tetany as a result of long-standing hypocalcemia. Vitamin therapy and the availability of vitamin D–fortified milk have decreased the prevalence of vitamin D deficiency rickets in infants in the United States.

See also *osteomalacia.*

Rickettsia (rĭ-ket′se-ah) [Howard Taylor *Ricketts,* American pathologist, 1871–1910, who in 1909 first described the etiologic agent of Rocky Mountain spotted fever and later died of typhus fever while investigating that disease] a genus of microorganisms of the tribe Rickettsieae, consisting of small, pleomorphic but typical rodlike organisms that are often found in pairs in smears of infected cells. These organisms have bacterial cell walls, possess no flagella, are gram-negative, and multiply only inside host cells. They grow in one or more arthropods and have natural reservoirs in one or more vertebrate hosts. Highly pathogenic species cause spotted fever and typhus.

The laboratory diagnosis of rickettsial disease is usually by analysis of specific serum antibodies with the Weil-Felix test. Smears of infected tissue may be examined using the Giménez or Giemsa stain, or by fluorescent microscopy. Cultural isolation (in laboratory animals) and identification are precluded in most clinical laboratories because of the pathogenicity of the organism.

See also *Rickettsiaceae.*

R. akari, a species that causes rickettsialpox in rodent- and mite-infested urban areas. Infection is transmitted to humans by the bite of a mite that has fed on an infected mouse or other rodent.

R. australis, a species, found in Australia, that causes tick typhus. Infection is transmitted to humans by the bite of a tick that has fed on infected marsupials, particularly during the rainy season.

R. conorii, a species that causes boutonneuse fever in Mediterranean countries, the Middle East, and India. It is transmitted to humans by the bite of a tick that has fed on infected dogs or rodents.

R. prowazekii, a species that causes worldwide epidemic typhus and Brill-Zinsser disease in North America and Europe. It is transmitted to humans by cutaneous penetration of deposited feces by the infected human body louse from a human reservoir.

R. rickettsii, a species that causes Rocky Mountain spotted fever in the Western hemisphere. It is transmitted to humans by the bite of a tick that has fed on infected rodents, dogs, or foxes. See also *Rickettsiaceae.*

R. sibirica, a species that causes Siberian tick typhus in Siberia, Central Asia, and Mongolia. It is transmitted to humans by the bite of a tick that has fed on infected rodents.

R. tsutsugamushi, a species that causes scrub typhus in Asia, Australia, the Pacific islands, and the Indian subcontinent. It is transmitted to humans by the bite of a mite that has fed on infected rodents.

R. typhi (mooseri), a species that causes worldwide murine typhus. It is transmitted to humans by cutaneous penetration of the deposited feces of infected rat fleas.

Rickettsiaceae (rĭ-ket″se-a′se-e) [Howard Taylor *Ricketts*] a family of microorganisms consisting of three genera: *Rickettsia,* composed of 10 species; *Rochalimaea,* with only one species, *R. quintana;* and Coxiella, with a single species, *C. burnetii.* Generally referred to collectively as the rickettsiae, they are obligate, intracellular parasites with the microscopic appearance of small (0.3–0.5 μm) coccobacillary bodies. They occur singly, in pairs or in filaments that can be visualized with Giemsa or Macchiavello stain. Rickettsiae proliferate by transverse binary fission in the manner of bacteria, and have cell walls resembling those of the gram-negative bacteria in that they contain peptidoglycan and lipopolysaccharide. In addition, rickettsiae contain RNA and DNA in a ratio of 3.5:1, which is similar to that of many bacteria. They also possess the complement of enzymes required for the oxidation of pyruvic, succinic, and glutamic acids.

Studies of rickettsial physiology have been complicated by the observation that purified rickettsiae rapidly lose biologic activity even when stored at 0°C. This loss can be prevented or reversed in large part by the addition of glutamate, potassium, glucose, and/or nicotinamide adenine dinucleotide (NAD) to the medium. Growth studies of rickettsiae in tissue culture systems have revealed generation times in the range of 8–10 hr. To date, with the exception of *Rochalimaea quintana,* none of the rickettsiae has been propagated in a cell-free medium. *R. quintana* may be cultivated on blood agar when incubated in a 10 percent CO_2 atmosphere. The properties of the rickettsiae, as compared with those of other pathogenic agents, are listed in Table 1.

The rickettsiae capable of inducing disease in humans are divided on the basis of antigenic relationships into the typhus group; spotted fever group; and the causative agents of scrub typhus, trench fever, and Q fever, respectively. See also Table 2.

CLINICAL CHARACTERISTICS. The prototype disease of the typhus group is epidemic typhus fever, an acute infection characterized by a sustained high fever, severe headache, and generalized macular or maculopapular rash that usually terminates in 14–18 da. The fatality rate in epidemics is around 20 percent. Brill-Zinsser disease represents a recrudescence of epidemic typhus fever in a relatively mild form, usually years after the primary infection. Murine or endemic typhus closely resembles louse-borne typhus, but is a milder acute febrile disease approximately 2 wk in duration and characterized by a headache and macular rash.

The spotted fever group consists of several very similar diseases widely distributed geographically but caused by *R. rickettsii* and closely related organisms that are probably antigenic variants. Rocky Mountain spotted fever is characterized by chills; pronounced headache; extreme pain in the muscles, joints, and bones; and a rapidly rising fever. A distinctive rash first appears on the ankles and wrists on the second to fourth day of the disease. The rash subsequently spreads over the entire body with the development of a maculopapular rash. Boutonneuse fever (tick-borne typhus) is a generally mild, febrile disease with a maculopapular rash that covers the entire body, including the palms and soles. Rickettsialpox differs from the others in that it is transmitted by a blood-sucking mite, whose mammalian reservoir is the house mouse, and its rash is vesicular like that of chickenpox. Scrub typhus, also known as tsutsugamushi disease, is characterized by a sudden onset, with fever, chills, and severe headache. Unlike other rickettsial infections, it is followed by generalized moderate lymphadenopathy. A macular rash appears on the trunk in 5–8 da and may extend to the arms and legs.

Trench fever, an infection of humans only, shows the typical rickettsial manifestations of headache, fever, exhaustion, and roseolar rash.

Q fever is an acute systemic disease usually acquired by inhalation of contaminated dust. A sudden febrile onset is accompanied by severe headache. Interstitial pneumonia often develops subsequently. No skin rash is observed, in contrast to other rickettsial diseases.

In the continental United States, Rocky Mountain spotted fever is currently the predominant human rickettsial disease. In 1979, 1070 cases were reported, 57 percent of them in the Southeast. The next most prevalent rickettsial disease in 1979 was murine typhus; 85 percent of these cases were reported from Texas. The reporting of Q fever is not mandatory in the United States, so that information

RICKETTSIACEAE, TABLE 1. COMPARISON OF RICKETTSIAE WITH OTHER PATHOGENIC AGENTS

	CHLAMYDIAE	BACTERIA	RICKETTSIAE	MYCOPLASMAS	VIRUSES
Growth outside host cell	0	+	0*	+	0
Independent protein synthesis	+	+	+	+	0
Generation of metabolic energy	0	+	+	+	0
Rigid cell envelope	Variable	+	+	0	Variable
Antibiotic susceptibility	+	+	+	+	0
Mode of reproduction	Fission	Fission	Fission	Fission	Host cell synthesis of subunits; then assembly of virion
Nucleic acids	DNA & RNA	DNA & RNA	DNA & RNA	DNA & RNA	DNA or RNA, not both

* Except *Rochalimaea quintana.*
From Davis, B. D., et al.: Microbiology. 3rd ed. Hagerstown, MD, Harper & Row, 1980, p. 777.

RICKETTSIACEAE, TABLE 2. RICKETTSIAL DISEASES OF HUMANS

Antigenic Category	Etiologic Agent	Diseases and Synonyms	Transmission to Humans	Incubation (Days)	Geographic Distribution	Natural Infection Cycle: *Arthropod Vector*	Natural Infection Cycle: *Vertebrate Host*
TYPHUS GROUP	*R. prowazekii*	Epidemic typhus, louse-borne typhus, exanthematous typhus	Infected louse feces into broken skin or inhaled	6–15	World-wide	Body louse	Human
	R. prowazekii	Brill-Zinsser disease, sporadic typhus, recrudescent typhus	Reactivation of latent infection years after primary epidemic typhus		World-wide	—	—
	R. typhi	Murine typhus, endemic typhus, urban typhus, shop typhus, flea-borne typhus	Infected flea feces into broken skin	6–14	World-wide	Rat flea	Commensal rats
SPOTTED FEVER GROUP	*R. rickettsii*	Rocky Mountain spotted fever, fiebre manchada, São Paulo typhus, tobia fever	Tick bite	3–12	Western Hemisphere	Tick	Small and medium-sized wild mammals, birds, dogs
	R. conorii	Boutonneuse fever, Marseilles fever, South African tick-bite fever, Kenya tick typhus, Indian tick typhus	Tick bite	5–7	Mediterranean countries, Africa, India	Tick	Small wild animals, dogs
	R. australis	Queensland tick typhus	Tick bite	7–10	Australia	Tick	Small wild rodents, marsupials
	R. siberica	Siberian tick typhus, North Asian tick-borne rickettsiosis	Tick bite	2–7	Siberia, Mongolia	Tick	Wild and domestic animals, birds
	R. akari	Rickettsialpox, vesicular rickettsiosis	Mite bite	7–10	Northeast U.S.A., U.S.S.R.	Gamasid mite	House mouse
SCRUB TYPHUS	*R. tsutsugamushi*	Scrub typhus, tsutsugamushi disease, mite-borne typhus, tropical typhus, rural typhus	Chigger bite	6–21	Asia, Australia, Pacific Islands	Trombiculid mite	Small wild rodents, birds
TRENCH FEVER	*R. quintana*	Trench fever, Wolhynian fever, five-day fever	Infected louse feces into broken skin	9–17	Europe, Middle East, North Africa, Mexico	Body louse	Humans
Q FEVER	*C. burnetii*	Q fever, Balkan grippe	Inhalation of infected aerosol	7–17	World-wide	Tick	Small wild mammals
						Cattle, sheep, goats without arthropod vector	

*Modified from Lennette, E. H., and Schmidt, N. J.: Diagnostic Procedures for Viral and Rickettsial Infections. 4th ed. New York, American Public Health Association, 1969, p. 829.

regarding the incidence of this disease is incomplete, but there were reports from 11 states, with California accounting for 34 of the 57 cases.

LABORATORY DIAGNOSIS. The isolation and subsequent identification of the rickettsiae is technically demanding and hazardous. Consequently, it should be attempted only in laboratories (most frequently state, national, or military) that have the proper containment facilities and technical expertise. Even in these circumstances, a number of laboratory-acquired infections have been documented.

For isolation, whole blood from individuals is inoculated into guinea pigs and mice. Rickettsiae can induce fever, necrosis, and, in rare cases, death of laboratory animals.

When fever or lesions develop in the inoculated animals, representative tissues may be obtained and smears prepared and examined microscopically for the presence of rickettsiae. In addition, immunofluorescent assays utilizing group-specific antisera may be performed to identify the appropriate antigenic group to which an isolate may be assigned. Further studies, including complement-fixation tests, agglutination tests, toxin neutralization assays, and/or immunity and vacination challenge tests, are required to identify the species or strain. Additional studies involve serologic testing of the serum obtained from animals inoculated with human blood for evidence of infection.

Serologic studies to assist the diagnosis of rickettsial infections involve the demonstration of a rise in the titer of specific antibodies during the course of illness and convalescence. It is important that the first blood be drawn early in the disease, with subsequent specimens collected 10–14 and 21–28 da later. Levels of specific antibody in the serum may be detected by means of complement-fixation, indirect immunofluorescence, and agglutination tests.

For routine diagnostic laboratories, the most feasible serologic aid in the diagnosis of rickettsial infections is the Weil-Felix test. A positive reaction is agglutination by the patient's serum of certain strains of *Proteus,* particularly the OX19 and OX2 strains of *P. vulgaris* and the OXK strain of *P. mirabilis.* These agglutinins usually appear by the twelfth day of the disease, reach peak titers early in the convalescent phase, and subsequently decline over a period of months. The expected Weil-Felix reactions are listed in Table 3. Urinary tract infections with *Proteus* species may give rise to a false-positive reaction.

See also *B. bacilliformis* under *Bartonella.*

WALTER S. CEGLOWSKI, PH.D.

rickettsia (ri-ket′se-ah), pl. *rickettsiae.* an individual organism of the family Rickettsiaceae.

rickettsiae (rĭ-ket′se-e) 1. plural of rickettsia.
2. a group of microorganisms that includes the clinically important Rickettsiaceae, Bartonellaceae, and Chlamydiaceae.

rickettsial (rĭ-ket′se-al) caused by rickettsiae.

rickettsialpox (rĭ-ket′se-al-poks″) a mild febrile disease caused by infection with *Rickettsia akari,* which is transmitted to humans by the bite of a mite infected by a house-mouse host. The initial lesion forms a red papule that becomes covered by a black scar (eschar) and is followed by sudden onset of fever, chills, photophobia, headache, and myalgia. A maculopapular rash with intraepidermal vesicles may appear on the body, except on the palms and soles, leading to confusion with chickenpox and smallpox.

Diagnosis may be established by complement-fixation, microscopic agglutination, and immunofluorescent antibody tests. The Weil-Felix test is generally negative.

Also called vesicular rickettsiosis.

ridge (rij) a long, narrow projection or projecting structure. See also *crest.*

Riedel's lobe (re′delz) [Bernhard Moritz Carl Ludwig *Riedel,* surgeon in Jena, 1846–1916] an anomalous, broad, tonguelike mass of tissue projecting downward from the right lobe of the liver.

Riedel's thyroiditis [Bernhard M. C. L. *Riedel*] see *invasive fibrous t.* under *thyroiditis.*

rifamide (rif′ah-mid) see *rifamycins.*

rifampicin (rif″am′pi-sin) see *rifampin.*

RICKETTSIACEAE, TABLE 3. WEIL-FELIX REACTION

RICKETTSIAL DISEASES	MAGNITUDE OF ANTIBODY RESPONSE		
	Proteus Antigens		
	OX19	*OX2*	*OXK*
Epidemic typhus (primary)	++++	+	0
Murine typhus	++++	+	0
Rocky Mountain spotted fever	++++	+	0
and other tick-borne Spotted Fever Group infections	+	++++	0
Rickettsialpox	0	0	0
Scrub typhus	0	0	++++
Q fever	0	0	0
Trench fever	0	0	0

Modified from Lennette, E. H., and Schmidt, N. J.: Diagnostic Procedures for Viral and Rickettsial Infections. 4th ed. New York, American Public Health Association, 1969, p. 855.

rifampin (rif″am′pin) [USP], a member of a group of complex macrocyclic antibiotics. It inhibits initiation of bacterial RNA synthesis by inhibiting DNA-dependent RNA polymerase activity. Rifampin has a wide antibacterial spectrum of activity and is especially effective against many gram-positive organisms, *Neisseria meningitidis,* and *Mycobacterium tuberculosis.* See also *antibacterial agents.*

rifamycins (rif″ah-mi′sins) a group of antibiotics produced by certain strains of *Streptomyces mediterranei* with a highly substituted macrocyclic ring structure. Rifamycins inhibit bacterial protein synthesis by binding to DNA-dependent RNA polymerase and blocking the initiation of transcription. These agents are active against gram-positive and some gram-negative bacteria, and also have antiviral activity. They are also important oral drugs in the treatment of tuberculosis and leprosy. Rifampin, rifambin, and rifamide are semisynthetic derivatives of the naturally occurring rifamycin. See also *antibacterial agents.*

rifomycin see *rifamycins.*

Rift Valley fever a viral disease of animals that is transmissible to humans, resulting in an acute febrile illness of short duration; it has widespread occurrence in areas of Africa. The causative agent is an RNA-containing arbovirus that affects wild game animals and domestic livestock. Rift Valley fever is transmitted to humans by the bite of a mosquito (*Aedes* and *Culex* species) or by the handling of the tissue of infected animals. Following an incubation period of 3–6 da, there is headache, myalgia, malaise, anorexia, saddleback fever, photophobia, and leukopenia. Most cases spontaneously resolve, although hemorrhagic, hepatic, and retinal complications have been noted.

Diagnosis is based on isolation of the virus from the blood and on serologic examination of paired sera. Leukopenia is present and may be severe. There is no treatment; complete recovery is the rule. Because of the serious potential for infection of both humans and domestic livestock in nonendemic areas, importation of the virus into the United States, even for experimental purposes, is prohibited.

right anterior oblique (RAO) in radiology, pertaining to a view with the right anterior aspect of the patient closest to the film and an obliquity of 45° unless otherwise stated.

right axis deviation in electrocardiography, deviation of the mean QRS vector in the frontal plane to a direction more positive than +200°; seen in right ventricular hypertrophy and left posterior hemiblock. Reference values differ in various age groups and may be as positive as +175° in normal infants.

right-handed α-helix a rodlike helical structure that is one of the most common secondary structures found in proteins. It is stabilized by hydrogen bonds that are formed between the CO group of each amino acid residue and the NH group of the amino acid that is present four residues ahead in the linear sequence. The helix makes a complete turn for each 3.6 residues.

right posterior oblique (RPO) in radiology, pertaining to a view with the right posterior aspect of the patient closest to the film and an obliquity of 45° unless otherwise stated.

right-to-know laws laws or ordinances that require dissemination of information about hazardous substances. They have been adopted in several governmental jurisdictions: employers must provide employees with precautionary labels noting safety and health hazards on all hazardous substances used in the workplace. Employers must also provide training programs to explain the information on the labels and on material safety data sheets, and other supplemental information.

rigidity (rĭ-jid′ĭ-te) [L. *rigiditas; rigidus* stiff] increased muscle tone in response to passive stretch. Unlike spasticity, the increased tone is uniform throughout the range of motion of the joint, as in bending a lead pipe.

cogwheel r., a special type of increased muscle tone that gives way in little jerks when the muscle is passively stretched; it is seen in paralysis agitans and represents an associated tremor superimposed on rigidity.

decerebrate r., the rigid extension and internal rotation of the limbs in a comatose patient, which occurs either spontaneously or following a noxious stimulus. Usually, this posture is produced by lesions in the upper brain stem.

rigor (rig′or, ri′gor) [L.] a chill; rigidity.

r. mortis, the stiffening of a dead body that accompanies depletion of adenosine triphosphate in the muscle fibers.

rigorous (rig′or-us) 1. severe, trying, or strenuous. 2. strict or precise. In logic, a rigorous proof is one conforming exactly to the rules of argument, a complete argument from stated premises. Cf. *heuristic.*

Riley-Day syndrome see *familial d.* under *dysautonomia.*

ring (ring) [L. *annulus, circulus, orbiculus*] a circular or continuous structure, as one surrounding an opening in an organ or body wall; in chemistry, the term is used to refer to a collection of atoms united in a continuous or closed chain.

Kayser-Fleischer r., a pigmented ring, green to brown in color, located at the limbus of the cornea. It is caused by an accumulation of copper in Descemet's membrane and is indicative of Wilson's disease and pseudosclerosis.

Ringer's solution (ring′erz) [Sydney *Ringer,* English physiologist, 1835–1910] a sterile solution containing sodium chloride, potassium chloride, and calcium chloride in purified water, that is used for topical application.

ringworm (ring′wurm) see *tinea corporis* and *tinea cruris.*

ringworm of the foot see *tinea pedis.*

Rinne's test (rin′nĕz) [Heinrich Adolf *Rinne,* German otologist, 1819–1868] a simple hearing test designed to differentiate conductive hearing loss and sensorineural hearing loss. A tuning fork (preferably at 512 cps) is struck and the stem placed against the mastoid process. The patient is asked to indicate when the fork can no longer be heard, at which time the fork is moved to within an inch of the pinna. In the normal ear, the stimulus is heard louder and longer by air conduction (AC) than by bone conduction (BC), so the fork is still audible when held near the ear (AC > BC). In conductive hearing loss, however, the bone conduction stimulus is heard longer and louder (BC > AC), and in sensorineural hearing loss, both air and bone conduction are reduced, although air conduction stimuli are still louder and longer (AC > BC). Because of the ease with which bone-conducted stimuli pass through the skull, the untested ear should be masked by rattling paper or a ticking clock whenever this test is performed. Cf. *Weber's test.*

ripple factor the root-mean-square ripple voltage divided by the DC voltage level.

ripple voltage a small alternating current (AC) voltage superimposed on the direct current (DC) voltage output of a power supply, i.e., the fluctuation in the output voltage.

rise time 1. by convention, the time required for a waveform to rise from 10 percent to 90 percent of the peak amplitude, as measured from the baseline.

2. in neurophysiology, the minimal elapsed time interval between the peak of the positive phase of a wave to that of the negative phase.

risk factor a clearly defined occurrence or characteristic that has been associated with the increased rate of a disease.

ristocetin cofactor (ris″to-se′tin) see *von Willebrand factor.*

Ritter's disease (rit′erz) [Gottfried *Ritter* von Rittershain, German physician, 1820–1883] see under *scalded skin syndrome.*

RM abbrev. See *reference materials.*

R-meter a radiation-detecting device used to measure the radiation intensity produced by x-ray therapy machines. It contains an electroscope (like a pocket dosimeter); the device is charged (set to zero), and the ionization produced in a specific time period is indicated in roentgens (R). Also called *roentgen-meter.*

RMS abbrev. See *root-mean-square.*

Rn symbol for the chemical element *radon.*

RNA abbrev. See *ribonucleic acid.*

RNAase see *ribonuclease.*

RNA nucleotidyltransferase (nu″kle-o-tid′il-trans′fer-ās) an enzyme of the transferase class (EC 2.7.7.6) that catalyzes the reaction *n*-nucleoside triphosphate ⇄ *n*-pyrophosphate + RNA_n. It requires DNA as a template and is important in the synthesis and repair of RNA. Also called *RNA polymerase.*

RNA polymerase see *RNA nucleotidyltransferase.*

RNA processing the operations required to convert newly synthesized RNA sequences into functional RNA. Most if not all classes of mature RNA in eukaryotic cells are different from the initial product of transcription.

The first types of RNA processing involve mRNA. They include removal of excess nucleotides, modification of both ends of the remaining message-containing sequence, and transport across the nuclear membrane to the cytoplasm, probably as a ribonucleoprotein (RNP) complex. Genes for certain eukaryotic proteins contain noncoding sequences (introns) interspersed with coding sequences (exons); this has important implications for processing transcribed nuclear RNA (hnRNA) into cytoplasmic mRNA.

There are two possible mechanisms whereby mRNA transcripts that lack intervening sequences could be produced from insertion-containing genes: either the gene is transcribed in pieces that are joined together later, or the entire gene (including introns) is transcribed and the noncoding sequences later removed and the exons spliced. Recent data favor the latter mechanism.

The type of RNA processing currently best understood is the series of reactions leading to formation of 18S, 28S, and 5.8S rRNA from a single large transcript. All three tRNA sequences are closely linked within a single large molecule of 40S in amphibians and 45S in mammals. This large transcription unit includes three transcribed spacer sequences that are subsequently degraded. The transcription units alternate with nontranscribed spacers in a repeated, tandem pattern.

The processing consists of selective methylation in those sections destined to become rRNA, followed by nuclease cleavage to yield the 5.8S, 18S, and 28S sequences. Methylation appears to protect the sequences from degradation.

Similar processing steps are involved in the maturation of tRNA. Processing includes removal of 15–35 nucleotides from a large precursor transcript and extensive modification of specific bases to yield the unusual bases found in the tRNA cloverleaf. Processing of 5S rRNA has been difficult to demonstrate.

See also *heterogeneous nuclear RNA.*

RNase see *ribonuclease.*

RNP complex abbrev. See *ribonucleoprotein* (RNP) *complex.*

robertsonian translocation a particular type of reciprocal translocation that involves acrocentric chromosomes. Breaks occur near the centromere; one new chromosome gets most of both long arms. The other new chromosome is formed from the small satellite regions and is normally lost.

There is no phenotypic effect, but abnormal gametes are formed. During meiosis, the aberrant chromosome synapses with its two partial homologues, forming a trivalent.

Four possible types of gametes can be formed: a normal gamete with the two untranslocated chromosomes, a gamete with the translocated chromosome (which will produce a child who is a translocation heterozygote or balanced carrier like the parent), a gamete with the translocated chromosome and one of its partial homologues (which will produce a defective child with a trisomy for the translocated material), and a gamete with only one of the normal chromosomes (which will produce a lethal monosomy).

Also called *centric fusion* and *whole arm fusion.* See also the accompanying illustration.
Cf. *reciprocal translocation.*

Robin's syndrome (ro-baz′) [Pierre *Robin,* French dentist, 1867–1950] see *Pierre Robin syndrome.*

robust in statistics, a general term used to describe a test or estimate that is relatively insensitive to failure to satisfy all the assumptions of its statistical model, or a test that makes few assumptions.

ROC abbrev. See *receiver operating characteristic.*

Rochalimaea (ro″kah-li-me′ah) a genus of microorganisms of the tribe Rickettsieae, which closely resemble *Rickettsia* but which reside extracellularly in the arthropod host. These organisms are capable of cultivation in cell-free media. See also *Rickettsiaceae.*

R. quintana, the species that causes trench fever in Europe, Africa, and North America. It is transmitted to humans from a human reservoir by the bite of an infective body louse, or the infectious

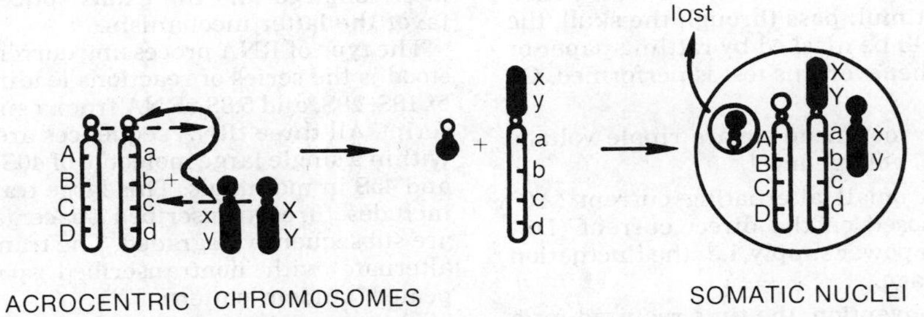

Robertsonian translation. (Modified from Raphael, S. S.: Lynch's Medical Laboratory Technology. 3rd ed. Philadelphia, W. B. Saunders Co., 1976.)

agent may enter the body through skin lesions in the deposited feces of an infective louse.

rocket immunoelectrophoresis see *rocket i.* under *immunoelectrophoresis.*

Rocky Mountain spotted fever an acute illness caused by infection with the organism *Rickettsia rickettsii,* which is harbored by ticks. Infections in humans are almost always the consequences of a tick bite, primarily by *Dermacentor andersoni* (the wood tick) and *Dermacentor variabilis* (the dog tick). Once a human is infected there is usually an incubation period of 3–12 da, which is followed by the rapid onset of headache, myalgia, nausea, vomiting, fever, and rigor. A rash, first erythematous and macular, appears 2–6 da after the initial onset of symptoms. It occurs primarily on the palms, soles, wrists, ankles, and forearms. The rash gradually becomes petechial and confluent, occasionally resulting in sloughing and necrosis of some overlying skin.

Those affected become hypotensive and dehydrated; shock, coma, or anuric renal failure are frequent complications. Additional complications include bronchopneumonia, parotitis, otitis media, and gangrene of distal extremities as a result of arterial thrombosis. Abnormal results of liver function tests as well as hypoproteinemia are common.

An aid to diagnosis is the finding of serum agglutinins directed against *Proteus* OX-2 and OX-19 in the Weil-Felix reaction.

Rocky Mountain spotted fever antibody tests assays for the detection of antibodies to *Rickettsia rickettsii,* the organism that causes Rocky Mountain spotted fever. The tests include indirect immunofluorescence, indirect hemagglutination, complement fixation, and the Weil-Felix test. The indirect immunofluorescence and indirect hemagglutination tests are highly specific, whereas complement fixation is less specific, and the Weil-Felix test is not specific, showing only a 4–18 percent correlation with indirect fluorescence.

The indirect immunofluorescence test is performed using rickettsiae that have been grown with chicken yolk sacs or cell culture as the substrate, or using skin biopsy of a rickettsial lesion. Dilutions of the patient's serum are added, as is fluorescein-conjugated antihuman immunoglobulin. A fourfold rise in titer, a titer of 1:128 or greater, or any IgM titer (suggestive of recent infection) is significant.

The indirect hemagglutination test is performed with sheep erythrocytes coated with erythrocyte-sensitizing substance (ESS). ESS is prepared by treating the complement-fixing antigens from diethyl ether–treated rickettsiae with hot alkali. The sensitized erythrocytes are added to serial dilutions of the test serum. A fourfold rise in titer is diagnostic.

The complement-fixation test uses dilutions of the test serum, complement-fixing antigen, and bovine complement. A fourfold rise in titer or a single titer of 1:16 or greater is considered diagnostic.

The Weil-Felix test takes advantage of the fact that rickettsial and *Proteus* antigens cross react. Dilutions of the test serum are tested for their ability to agglutinate unflagellated *Proteus vulgaris* strains OX-19 and OX-2. A fourfold rise in titer or a single titer of 1:160 or greater is considered diagnostic. Because of the cross-reactivity, results must be interpreted with caution.

See also *Rickettsiaceae.*

rod (rod) 1. a straight, slim mass of substance.
2. one of the retinal photoreceptors. See under *photoreceptor.*

rodent (ro′dent) a member of the order Rodentia, consisting of mammals such as the mouse, rat, and squirrel, which are characterized by large incisors used for gnawing and nibbling.

rodenticide (ro-den′tĭ-sid) a pesticide, such as warfarin, squill, norbornide, and sodium fluoroacetate, used to kill rats and other rodents.

rodent ulcer see *basal cell carcinoma.*

roentgen/o (rent′gen-o) a word element used in combining form to denote x-rays, e.g., roentgenograph.

roentgen (R) (rent′gen) [Wilhelm Konrad *Roentgen,* German physicist, 1845–1923, the discoverer of x-rays, winner of the Nobel Prize for physics in 1901] a unit of exposure dose of x-rays or gamma rays defined as the amount of radiation that will produce 1 electrostatic unit (esu) of ions of each sign in passing through 1 cubic centimeter of dry air at standard temperature and pressure (i.e., 2.58×10^{-4} coulombs of ions per kilogram of air).

roentgenkymography (rent″gen-ki-mog′rah-fe) a technique of graphically recording the movements of an organ on a single x-ray film.

roentgen-meter see *R-meter.*

roentgenogram (rent-gen′o-gram) see *radiograph.*

roentgenologist (rent″gĕ-nol′o-jist) see *radiologist.*

roentgenology (rent″gĕ-nol′o-je) [*roentgeno-* + *-logy*] see *radiology.*

roentgen rays see *x-rays.*

Roger's disease (ro-zhāz′) [Henri Louis *Roger*, French physician, 1809–1891] a congenital anomaly characterized by a small defect in the membranous portion of the ventricular septum. The resulting small left-to-right shunt causes increased pulmonary blood flow and a holosystolic murmur along the left border of the sternum. Cyanosis is not present and the condition is usually asymptomatic. Diagnosis is frequently made by auscultation at an infant's first examination. Also called *maladie de Roger.*

ROI abbrev. See *region of interest.*

Rokitansky-Aschoff sinus (ro″kĭ-tan′skee ash′of) [Karl Freiherr von *Rokitansky*, pathologist in Vienna, 1804–1878; Karl Albert Ludwig *Aschoff*, German pathologist, 1866–1942] an invagination of the surface epithelium of the gallbladder into its wall, generally thought to indicate pathologic change. These crypts may extend through the lamina propria and the muscular layers.

rolandic epilepsy (ro-lan′dik) [Luigi *Rolando*, Italian anatomist, 1773–1831] see *benign focal e.* under *epilepsy.*

roll tube a test tube utilized in anaerobic bacteriology. After liquid agar culture medium is instilled into the tube, the tube is chilled and rotated so that its inside surface becomes coated with the culture medium.

roll-tube technique a technique used for counting viable bacteria in a sample. The melted agar medium is inoculated with a measured volume of the specimen, and then rotated in the culture tube while immersed in an ice bath to form a thin layer on the inner surface. In culturing anaerobes the tubes are kept tightly closed, and are opened only in the presence of oxygen-free gas.

ROM see *read-only memory.*

Romaña's sign (ro-mahn′yahz) [Cecilio *Romaña*, Brazilian physician] the characteristic swelling of one or both eyelids in Chagas' disease.

Romanowsky's stains (ro″man-of′skēz) [Dimitri Leonidovich *Romanowsky*, Russian physician, 1861–1921] a group of eosin-methylene blue stains for blood smears, including Wright, Leishman, and Giemsa stains. These are generally used to stain blood or marrow cells, protozoa, and bacteria. Cytoplasm usually stains medium blue with deep-purple nuclei in blood cells, whereas malarial parasites and trypanosomes have red-purple nuclei.

ronnel (ron′el) a moderately toxic organothiophosphate insecticide, *O,O*-dimethyl *O*-(2,4,5-trichlorophenyl) phosphorothioate. See also *organophosphate compounds.*

root (root) 1. the lowermost part, or a structure by which something is firmly attached, e.g., root of a tooth or a spinal nerve. Also called *radix.*

2. a number that is multiplied by itself *n* times (i.e., raised to the *n*th power) to produce a specified number, indicated $\sqrt[n]{x}$.

3. a solution of the equation $f(x) = 0$, particularly used when f is a polynominal function. Also called zero.

4. see *teeth.*

r. of lung, the structures entering and emerging at the hilus of the lung, which attach the lung to the heart and trachea.

root canal the narrowed portion of the pulp cavity in the root of a tooth that extends from the pulp chamber to the apical foramen.

root-mean-square (RMS) a term denoting the square root of the average of the squared values of some quantity. The standard deviation used in statistics is the RMS deviation; the effective current (or voltage) of alternating current is the RMS current (or voltage). The average is taken over a complete cycle of the waveform.

Ropes test see *mucin clot test.*

rosacea (ro-za′she-ah) a chronic disease that affects the skin of the nose, forehead, and cheeks; it is marked by flushing and followed by red coloration due to capillary dilation, with the appearance of papules and acne-like pustules. Also called acne rosacea and brandy face.

Rosai-Dorfman disease see *sinus histicytosis with massive l.* under *lymphadenopathy.*

rosaniline (ro-zan′ĭ-lin) a reddish-brown basic dye, methylpararosaniline; C.I. 42510. See also *triphenylmethane dyes.*

rose bengal sodium I 131 [USP], a labeled dye that is cleared from the blood by hepatocytes and excreted in bile.

Rosenmüller's organ (ro′zen-mil″erz) [Johann Christian *Rosenmüller*, German anatomist, 1771–1820] see *epoöphoron.*

Rosenthal's syndrome see *h. C* under *hemophilia.*

roseola (ro-ze′o-lah, ro″ze-o′lah) [L.] a rose-colored rash, as in measles and syphilis; sometimes used alone to mean roseola infantum.

rosette (ro-zet′) [Fr.] a histologic grouping of cells in which a central fibrillary space is surrounded by a circle of cells. They are characteristic of some examples of certain tumors of the nervous system, notably neuroblastoma, in which the central zone is formed by a tangle of dendritic cell processes. Cf. *pseudorosette.*

Rose-Waaler test a passive hemagglutination test for detecting the presence of rheumatoid factors in serum. The basis of the test is the immunologic cross-reactivity of rabbit IgG and human S IgG. When tanned sheep red blood cells are coated with small amounts of rabbit IgG and mixed with the serum in question, the red blood cells will agglutinate if rheumatoid factor is present. Also called *sheep cell agglutination test.* See also *rheumatoid factor tests.*

rosin (roz′in) [L. *resina*] [USP], chiefly abietic acid anhydride, the solid resin obtained from the distillation of the turpentine from *Pinus palustris* and other species. Rosin occurs as sharply angular, translucent, amber-colored fragments, frequently covered with yellow dust. It is used as a stiffening agent in the preparation of plasters and ointments, and as an ingredient in paints and varnishes. Formerly called colophony.

rotamer (ro′ta-mer) one of a group of isomers that can be interconverted by rotation about a single bond. Also called conformational isomers, conformers, rotomers, and torsional single bond isomers. See also *conformation.*

rotation (ro-ta′shun) [L. *rotatio*, *rotare* to turn] a rigid motion of an object in which all the points along a line, the axis of rotation, remain fixed.

rotavirus (ro′tah-vi″rus) a group of double-stranded RNA viruses having diameters of 70–75 nm that cause 60–80 percent of cases of viral gastroenteritis in infants. Rotavirus often exhibits a seasonal prevalence in temperate climates; infection occurs almost exclusively in the cold winter months.

rotenone (ro′tĕ-nōn) [Jap. *rōten* derris plant] a moderately toxic insecticide extracted from roots of the derris and cube plants. The substance is practically insoluble in water but is soluble in most organic solvents. Inhalation or ingestion may cause numbness of mouth, nausea, or tremors. Lethal doses produce respiratory paralysis. Chronic poisoning may cause fatty changes in the liver and kidney. Rotenone is more toxic when inhaled than when ingested.

Roth's spot (rōts) [Moritz *Roth,* Swiss physician, 1839–1915] round or oval white spots, with or without surrounding hemorrhage, sometimes seen in the retina in the course of subacute bacterial endocarditis.

Rotor's syndrome a rare genetic disorder, transmitted as an autosomal recessive trait, that is characterized by a faulty excretory function of hepatocytes, leading to a mild conjugated hyperbilirubinemia. This syndrome is similar to Dubin-Johnson syndrome, but the liver is not pigmented and there is normal gallbladder filling on oral cholecystography. There is delayed excretion of sulfobromophthalein (BSP), with plasma concentrations of BSP greater at 120 min than at 45 min in the standard retention test. Urinary coproporphyrin excretion is abnormal. See also *hyperbilirubinemia.*

rot value see under *cot value.*

Rouget cell (roo-zhāz′) [Charles Marie Benjamin *Rouget,* French physiologist and anatomist, 1824–1904] see *pericyte.*

rough (ruf) not smooth; having an irregular, uneven surface.

rough endoplasmic reticulum see under *endoplasmic reticulum.*

rough-smooth variation see *smooth-rough* (*S–R*) *variation.*

rouleau (roo-lo′), pl. *rouleaux* [Fr. "roll"] an aggregate of erythrocytes stacked like a pile of coins. The speed of the erythrocyte sedimentation rate (ESR) corresponds to the length of the rouleaux formation. Increases in fibrinogen (from infections) or globulins (from infections or multiple myeloma) will produce long rouleaux that are difficult to disperse, whereas red cell shape changes that prevent the cells from adhering to each other (as in hereditary spherocytosis) produce decreased rouleaux formation.

rounding (roun′ding) in numerical analysis and computing, dropping low-order digits and retaining a resultant number that is the closest possible in precision to the original number. See also *truncation.*

round window a round opening, covered by the secondary tympanic membrane, that connects the tympanic cavity (middle ear) to the scala tympani of the cochlea. Also called *fenestra cochleae.*

roundworm (rownd′worm) any worm or nematode of the class Nematoda.

Roux bottle (rōō) [Pierre Paul Emile *Roux,* French bacteriologist, 1853–1933] a flat-bottomed rectangular glass container with a short straight neck on the side, used in bacteriology.

RP film abbrev. See *rapid processing f.* under *film.*

R plasmid see *R p.* under *plasmid.*

rpm abbrev. for revolutions per minute, used as a unit of angular velocity, e.g., for centrifuge speed.

RPO abbrev. See *right posterior oblique.*

RPR abbrev. See *rapid plasma reagin test.*

RQ abbrev. See *respiratory quotient.*

rRNA abbrev. for ribosomal ribonucleic acid. See under *ribonucleic acid.*

RRT abbrev. See *relative r.t.* under *retention time.*

RSD abbrev. See *relative standard deviation.*

RSNA abbrev. See *Radiological Society of North America.*

RSV abbrev. See *respiratory syncytial virus.*

R-S variation see *smooth-rough* (*S-R*) *variation.*

rT_3 abbrev. See *reverse triiodothyronine.*

RTF abbrev. for resistance transfer factor. See *R p.* under *plasmid.*

RT N(ARRT) the designation for a Registered Technologist specializing in Nuclear Medicine Technology. See under *American Registry of Radiologic Technologists* and *nuclear medicine technologist.*

RT R(ARRT) the designation for a Registered Technologist specializing in Radiography. See under *American Registry of Radiologic Technologists.*

RT T(ARRT) the designation for a Registered Technologist specializing in Radiation Therapy Technology. See under *American Registry of Radiologic Technologists.*

Ru symbol for the chemical element *ruthenium.*

rub (rub) an auscultatory sound caused by the rubbing together of two dry or roughened surfaces, such as inflamed serous surfaces.

pericardial friction r., the sound produced when two inflamed layers of the pericardium, roughened by a fibrous exudate, slide over one another during those portions of the cardiac cycle in which movements of the heart are maximal. When auscultated, the sound seems to be close to the ear and is variously described as scratchy, grating, scraping, or leathery. The rub is usually most readily auscultated just to the left of the sternum or in the midclavicular line in the second, third, or fourth intercostal spaces. Atrial systolic, ventricular systolic, and early ventricular diastolic components may be heard producing one, two, or three component rubs.

Pericardial friction rubs may be audible in disorders such as acute pericarditis, acute myocardial infarction, and uremia.

pleural-pericardial friction r., a sound produced when inflamed pleura rubs against parietal pericardium on inspiration.

rubber (rub′er) 1. natural rubber, a mixture of hydrocarbons that are linear polymers of isoprene, *cis*-1,4-polyisoprene.

2. synthetic rubber, any of a group of elastomers with properties similar to those of natural rubber.

rubella (roo-bel′ah) an acute, contagious, systemic viral infection affecting children and young adults; it is characterized by a pink, confluent, macular exanthem and cervical lymphadenitis. Most often rubella is trivial; however, if a woman contracts this disease in the first trimester of pregnancy, there is a good probability that the fetus may also be infected (congenital rubella syndrome). The etiologic agent of rubella is a togavirus, which is not arthropod-borne. Rubella virus is not serologically related to other viruses and is not similar to measles virus (paramyxovirus). There is only one serotype.

Rubella virus enters the respiratory tract in droplets. After an incubation period of 16–18 da, a slight cold, sore throat, and fever appear. Suboccipital, postauricular, and cervical lymph nodes are enlarged. A fine pink rash begins on the head and spreads to the rest of the body, usually fading away after 2 da. From the respiratory tract, the rubella virus spreads through the lymphatic system. In the case of a damaged fetus, it is thought that this virus is noncytocidal: the infected cells continue to divide but are abnormal.

Immunity to rubella is lifelong, and vaccination of young children is suggested in order to reduce the incidence of rubella infection. In recent years, the greater percentage of cases has occurred in nonimmunized or improperly immunized older teenagers and young adults. Rubella vaccine is a live attenuated vaccine; a single dose leads to a minor rubella infection with minimal symptoms. Vaccination is not suggested once pregnancy has been determined.

Laboratory diagnosis of rubella is made by the isolation of the virus from a patient's nose or throat (the virus produces a cytopathic effect in green monkey kidney ([Vero]), baby hamster ([BHK-21]), and rabbit kidney ([RK-13] cells) or serologically by demonstrating a rise in antibody titer in the hemagglutination inhibition assay in two specimens 5–10 da apart is diagnostic. IgM immunoglobulin rather than IgG to rubella is indicative of a recent infection. For congenital rubella syndrome, rubella IgM in cord blood is diagnostic. For more serologic information, see the accompanying table.

Also called *German measles* and, in French and Spanish, *rubeola.* See also *congenital r. syndrome* under *rubella* and *togavirus.*

congenital r. syndrome, infection of the fetus with rubella virus from an infected mother, who lacks protective immunity. Viral infection of the fetal cells slows their growth rate; the earlier the infection in fetal life, the greater the damage to the fetus. Infection of the fetus in its first month causes abnormalities in 80 per cent of cases.

The infant with congenital rubella syndrome may have one or more defects of the heart, great vessels, eyes, and brain. About 20 per cent of those infected die at birth; those who do not may shed virus to all contacts for as long as 18 mo after birth.

rubella antibody tests assays for antibody to rubella virus. The most common tests include passive hemagglutination (PHA), hemagglutination inhibition (HI), and complement fixation (CF). Sensitive techniques such as radioimmunoassay, enzyme-linked immunosorbent assay, single radial hemolysis, and fluorometry are being developed but are not yet in widespread clinical use. For the PHA and HI tests, sheep erythrocytes are coated with soluble rubella antigen. In the PHA test, dilutions of the test serum are assayed for their ability to agglutinate the antigen-coated erythrocytes. In the HI assay, dilutions of the test serum are incubated with the hemagglutinating antigen and pigeon erythrocytes are added. The HI titer is the highest dilution of serum that inhibits the antigen from agglutinating the erythrocytes. For both of these assays, a fourfold rise in titer is significant.

The presence of antibody in serum indicates im-

RUBELLA. RECOMMENDED TESTS FOR RUBELLA SEROLOGIC DIAGNOSIS IN SPECIFIC SITUATIONS

CLINICAL SITUATION	PRIMARY METHOD	BACK-UP METHOD
Acute rubella illness (paired sera)	HAI	CF, HAI-IgM*
Acute rubella illness (convalescent-phase serum only)	HAI-IgM*	
Immune status (single serum specimen)	HAI, PHA	
Exposure/no illness (single serum specimen within 7 days) (follow-up serum specimen if negative)	HAI	CF
Exposure/no illness (serum, 7-21 days after exposure plus convalescent-phase > 1 month after exposure)	HAI	CF, HAI-IgM*
Congenital rubella		
Birth–3 months old (single serum specimen)	HAI-IgM*	HAI†
3–6 months old (infant and maternal serum specimen)	HAI	HAI-IgM*
6–12 months old (single serum specimen)	HAI	
Over 12 months old‡ (single serum specimen)	HAI	

NOTE: HAI—hemagglutination inhibition, CF—complement fixation, IgM—immunoglobulin, and PHA—passive hemagglutination.

* Other comparable rubella IgM antibody may be used.
† Follow-up testing required.
‡ Antibody present may be result of acquired natural infection or rubella vaccination.
From Lennette, E. H., and Schmidt, N. J.: Diagnostic Procedures for Viral, Rickettsial and Chlamydial Infections. 5th ed. Washington DC, American Public Health Association, 1970, p. 758.

munity to rubella. Individuals without detectable antibody are usually susceptible to rubella infection, although some adults may be immune in the absence of detectable HI antibody. These individuals often have neutralizing antibody.

Assessment of immunity to rubella infection by the evaluation of antibody titers is important in women of childbearing age because the disease, if contracted during pregnancy, is of potential risk to the fetus; females who are not immune and capable of childbearing should be vaccinated after it has been ascertained they are not pregnant.

rubella virus a single-stranded RNA virus, 50–70 nm in diameter, that is the causative agent of rubella. See also *rubella.*

rubeola (roo-be′o-lah, roo″be-o′lah) [L. *ruber* red] a synonym for *measles* in English and for *rubella* in French and Spanish.

rubidium (Rb) (roo-bid′e-um) [L. *rubidus* red, from a red spectral line] a soft, silvery-white metallic element; atomic number 37; atomic mass 85.4678; Group I of the periodic table (the alkali metals); oxidation state +1.

Metallic rubidium reacts with air and vigorously with water; it is a fire and explosion hazard, as well as a caustic irritant to tissues. Ionic rubidium is a nonessential trace element; it can substitute for potassium as an enzyme activator and in many physiologic processes. Rubidium toxicity has not been observed in humans.

rubidomycin (rou-bid′o-mi″sin) see *daunorubicin.*

Rubin test (roo′bin) [Isidor Clinton *Rubin,* New York physician, 1883–1958] see *tubal insufflation.*

rubivirus (roo′bĭ-vi″rus) a group of togaviruses containing only the rubella virus.

rubredoxin an iron-sulfide protein of *Clostridium.* See also *iron-sulfide protein.*

rubriblast (roo′brĭ-blast) see pronormoblast under *normoblast.*

rudimentary bone a bone that has developed only partially.

ruga (roo′gah), pl. *rugae* [L.] a ridge, wrinkle, or fold, as of mucous membrane.

rugae of stomach, longitudinal folds of mucous membrane observed in the empty contracted stomach; they are most obvious in the greater curvature and near the pyloric antrum.

rugae of urinary bladder folds of mucous membrane seen in the contracted urinary bladder, except in the area of the trigone.

Rumpel-Leede test (room′pel-la′dĕ) [Theodor *Rumpel,* German physician, 1862–1923; Stockbridge Carl *Leede,* German physician, born 1882] see *tourniquet test.*

runt disease see *wasting disease.*

Runyon's classification a classification of mycobacteria based on the pigmentation and growth condition of the organisms. See also *mycobacterium.*

Russell body (rus′el) [William *Russell,* physician in Edinburgh, 1852–1940] a spherical inclusion body of plasma cells. These structures are variable in size and may stain a blue-violet or pink in color, yet often appear as colorless vacuoles owing to the fixation and staining procedures. If present in large numbers, the plasma cell becomes a Mott cell. Russell bodies result from the accumulation of mucopolysaccharides and globins in the sacs of the rough endoplasmic reticulum (RER) and the Golgi apparatus. See also *Mott cell.*

Russell viper venom (rus′el) [Patrick *Russell,* Aleppo physician, 1727–1805] the active ingredient in a one-stage prothrombin time test called the Stypven time. Russell viper venom is used to distinguish between Factor VII and Factor X deficiency, serving as a thromboplastin. The Stypven time is prolonged in deficiencies of Factors II, V, and X, but is normal in Factor VII deficiencies, as Russell viper venom bypasses this factor. The Stypven time test is no longer used in most coagulation laboratories, having been replaced by specific factor assays that use commercially available deficient plasma.

ruthenium (Ru) (roo-the′ne-um) [L. *Ruthenia* Russia] a hard, lustrous, silvery-white metallic element of the platinum group; atomic number 44; atomic mass 101.07; a 4d transition element; oxidation states +1 through +8 (+2, +3, +4 are common). It is used in corrosion-resistant alloys.

ruthenium red an ammoniated ruthenium oxychloride, $Ru_2(OH)_2Cl_4 \cdot 7NH_3 \cdot 3H_2O$, used for staining complex glyco- or mucoproteins, such as the sialic acid coating of the outside of the plasma membrane, by light or electron microscopy.

rutherford (ruth′er-ford) [Ernest *Rutherford,* British physicist, 1871–1937] a unit of radioactivity equal to 1 million disintegrations per second. One curie equals 3700 rutherfords.

Rutherford scattering elastic scattering of a particle (e.g., an alpha or beta particle) by an atomic nucleus.

rutin (roo′tin) a bioflavonoid (coumarin derivative) extracted from buckwheat. It was formerly used to decrease capillary fragility (the so-called vitamin P activity).

RV abbrev. See *residual volume.*

RV time abbrev. for Russell viper time. See under *Stypven time.*

R wave a positive deflection that occurs during the QRS complex of the electrocardiogram. The first positive deflection is termed the R wave; the second positive deflection R prime (R′). The term R wave is part of a terminology representative of the order and polarity of the deflections making up the QRS complex, and by itself does not denote a specific physiologic event.

S

S symbol for *entropy,* mean dose per unit cumulated activity (see under *dose estimate*), *serine,* a standard normal deviate, the chemical element *sulfur,* sum of an arithmetic series.

***S*-** [L. *sinister* left] a stereodescriptor used to indicate the configuration at an asymmetric carbon atom, e.g., (*S*)-2-amino-3-hydroxypropanoic acid (L-serine). See also *isomerism.*

***S*$_f$** abbrev. See *Svedberg flotation unit.*

s symbol for atomic orbital with angular momentum quantum number 0, distance, sample standard deviation, (chromosomal) *satellite, second.*

$\bar{s}$ abbrev. for *sine* (without).

Σ the Greek capital letter *sigma;* used in mathematics to indicate summation of a series: $\Sigma_i \overset{n}{=} 1\ x_i$ means $x_1 + x_2 + x_3 + \ldots + x_n - 1 + x_n$; i is the summation index and 1 and n are the lower and upper summation limits.

σ the Greek lower case letter *sigma;* symbol for: (1) population standard deviation, (2) surface tension, (3) wavenumber, (4) a type of molecular orbital or bond.

Sabethes a genus of mosquitoes, of which the species *S. chloropterus* is involved in the transmission of jungle yellow fever in South and Central America, the West Indies, and Africa.

Sabin vaccine (sa'bin) [Albert Bruce *Sabin,* American virologist, born 1906] an oral vaccine for poliomyelitis, which contains live attenuated strains of three antigenically different types of poliomyelitis virus. The virus multiples in the gastrointestinal tract, stimulating both systemic and local antibody production.

Sabin-Feldman dye test a dye test for the detection of *Toxoplasma gondii* antibody. In the procedure, the organism is mixed with serum and stained with methylene blue. With normal serum the organism takes up the stain and appears blue, but if the antibody is present, the organism does not stain. This test is used by the World Health Organization to titer standard reference sera, but its routine use in most laboratories is not feasible in view of the requirement for live organisms.

Sabouraud's dextrose agar (sab'oo-rōz) [Raymond Jacques Adrien *Sabouraud,* French dermatologist, 1864–1938] see *Sabouraud's dextrose a.* under *agar.*

sac (sak) [L. *saccus;* Gr. *sakkos*] a pouch; a baglike organ or structure. For more information, see the specific sac.

sacchar/o (sak'ah-ro) [L. *saccharum;* Gr. *sakcharon* sugar] a word element used in combining form to denote relationship to sugar, e.g., saccharolytic.

saccharase (sak'ah-rās) see *β-fructofuranosidase.*

saccharic acid (sak-ah'rik) D-glucaric acid; 2,3,4,5-tetrahydroxyhexanedioic acid. It exists as white needles derived from oxidation of cane sugar, glucose, or starch by nitric acid.

saccharin (sak'ah-rin) [USP], a nonnutritive sweetener used as a sugar substitute in such substances as drugs and diet foods. Animal tests have shown it to be a weak carcinogen, and products containing saccharin are now required to have warning labels.

saccharoid (sak'ah-roid) [L. *saccharum;* Gr. *sakcharon* sugar] a nonglucose-reducing substance that, if present in analytical specimens, may interfere with those procedures for determining glucose that are based on the reducing action of glucose in alkaline solution. Glutathione and ergothioneine in erythrocytes, and urate, creatinine, and oxo acids in plasma are examples of saccharoids that are detected by the above-mentioned nonspecific methods for glucose, and thus increase the apparent glucose value unless they are removed prior to analysis.

Saccharomyces (sak"ah-ro-mi'sēz) [*saccharo-* + Gr. *mykēs* fungus] a genus of yeast fungi belonging to the family Saccharomycetaceae. These yeasts are oval and unicellular and can have a haploid or diploid nucleus, depending on the stage of the life cycle. *Saccharomyces* divides by budding and is characterized by forming one to four ascospores per ascus that are global to ellipsoidal in form. Some species are used in baking breads and in brewing beer because of the cell's capability of alcoholic fermentation. Rarely, *Saccharomyces* has been found to cause pulmonary and gastrointestinal diseases among brewery workers. For more information on species of *Saccharomyces,* see the species under the current nomenclature, e.g., *Candida albicans, Cryptococcus neoformans,* and *Pityrosporon ovale.*

S. cerevisiae, a species with oval or spherical cells, known as brewers' or bakers' yeast. It causes alcoholic fermentation and is a very rare cause of lung disease, vulvovaginitis, and thrush; it has also been reported in the urine of diabetics.

saccharomycosis any fungal infection caused by an organism belonging to the genus *Saccharomyces.*

L-saccharopine (sak'ah-ro-pēn") an intermediate in the metabolism of lysine, named after its role as an intermediate of lysine synthesis in *Saccharomyces.*

saccharopine dehydrogenase (sak'ah-ro-pēn" de-hi'dro-jen-ās) an enzyme of the oxidoreductase class (EC 1.5.1.7) that catalyzes the reaction L-saccharopine + NAD^+ + H_2O ⇄ L-lysine + 2-oxoglutarate + NADH. A genetic deficiency in the enzyme leads to hyperlysinemia, a disease characterized by increased blood lysine with overflow into the urine. Also called *lysine ketoglutarate reductase* and *lysine-2-oxoglutaryl reductase.*

saccharopinuria a disorder of lysine metabolism, presumably transmitted as an autosomal recessive trait, that is characterized by mental and physical retardation and spastic diplegia. It is speculated that this disorder may be due to a relative or absolute deficiency of saccharopine cleavage enzyme saccharopine dehydrogenase, or to aminoadipic semialdehyde glutamate reductase. Increases of lysine, histidine, saccharopine, and citrulline in blood and urine are seen. This disorder can be detected in utero. Also called *hyperlysinemia.* See also *aminoacidopathy.*

Saccomanno's fixative a solution of polypropylene glycol 1540 carbowax in 50 percent ethanol, used in cytology for the fixation of fluid specimens. The polypropylene glycol infiltrates the cell spaces, thus preserving them and preventing collapse during air drying.

saccule (sak′ūl) [L. *sacculus*] 1. a little bag or sac.
2. a spherical, endolymph-filled chamber that lies anterior and medial to the utricle in the membranous labyrinth of the vestibule. In addition to its role as part of the vestibular apparatus, it may sense low-frequency vibrational (auditory) stimuli. Also called sacculus.

sacr/o (sa′kro) [L. *sacrum* sacred] a word element used in combining form to denote the sacrum, e.g., sacralgia.

sacral (sa′kral) [L. *sacralis*] pertaining to or situated near the sacrum.

sacralization (sa″kral-i-za′shun) a congenital malformation that results in the fusion of the fifth lumbar vertebra, or parts of it, to the first segment of the sacrum.

sacral plexus (sa′kral plek′sus) [L. *sacralis*] a plexus arising from the last two lumbar nerves (the lumbosacral trunk) and the first four sacral nerves. It innervates the pelvic structures, buttocks, and lower limbs.

sacral region the region of the back that overlies the sacrum.

sacroiliac joint (sa″kro-il′e-ak) the articulation between the sacrum and ilium. The joint is synovial in type but allows little movement.

sacrum (sa′krum) [L. "sacred"] the triangle-shaped bone at the base of the spine above the coccyx, formed by five fused vertebrae wedged between the two hip bones.

safety can a container for flammable or combustible liquids that is especially designed to resist spillage, breakage, or rupture from exposure to fire; it has a spring-closing lid and spout cover, and is designed to relieve internal pressure safely when subjected to fire exposure. Many safety cans are equipped with flash arrestors in the pouring spouts so that a flame cannot flash back into the container during a pouring operation. Safety cans used in the United States usually bear the label of Underwriters Laboratories or the Factory Mutual System.

safety glasses see under *eye and face protection.*

safety program a program recommended for laboratories by the NFPA (National Fire Protection Association, regulation 56C-1980) that should include the following points of safety information: a clear definition of safety responsibilities; the orientation of new employees; the periodic education of laboratory personnel in recognizing hazards, emergency procedures, and use of protective equipment; the surveillance of the hazards of chemicals, compressed gases, electrical equipment, and other laboratory activities; and a review of unsafe conditions observed or reported.

safety responsibility a responsibility for safety instruction and for ensuring that safe procedures and equipment are provided and used by those taught or supervised; this responsibility is assumed concurrently by everyone who teaches others or supervises, orients, or directs their activities.

safety shower a deluge shower located adjacent to any work area where users of chemicals may be splashed with and need to flush from the body chemicals that are irritating, corrosive, or toxic. The shower should have an assured supply of water, a quick-opening valve that will stay open until manually closed, and a pull-chain or cord that can be reached by persons of any height, including those in wheelchairs. A drain is also desirable to remove the water conveniently, as flushing for at least 15 min is recommended in cases of chemical splash. The water can be cold, which will cool the burns and moderate any skin reaction.

safflower oil an oily liquid (triglycerides) extracted from the seeds of the safflower, *Carthamus tinctorius,* used as a dietary supplement in the management of hypercholesterolemia and as a vehicle for medicines, paints, and varnishes. It is an important food oil, and has a relatively high content of linoleic acid in its constituent fatty acids.

safranin O a basic aniline dye that produces a red color; C.I. 50240. It is used as a nuclear stain and as a counterstain for gram-negative organisms in the Gram stain.

sagittal (saj′ĭ-tal) [L. *sagittalis,* from *sagitta* arrow] shaped like or resembling an arrow; straight.

sagittal plane a vertical plane passing through the body from front to back, parallel to the median sagittal (midsagittal) plane.

sagittal sinus, superior a venous channel between the two layers of the dura in the attached convex margin of the falx cerebri. Blood within it runs posteriorly to the internal occipital protuberance, where it deviates, usually to the right, to continue as the transverse sinus of that side.

sagittal suture the suture between the two parietal bones of the skull, so named because of the triangular anterior fontanelle at its front end and the diamond-shaped posterior fontanelle at its posterior end.

SAH abbrev. See *S-adenosyl-L-homocysteine.*

Saint Anthony's fire 1. ergotism. See under *ergot.*
2. an infection of the skin and subcutaneous tissues.

Saint Vitus' dance see *Sydenham's c.* under *chorea.*

Saksenaea a genus of fungi that belongs to the order Mucorales. The sporangium is flask-shaped and has a necklike extension.

salaam attacks see *infantile spasms.*

salicylamide (sal″ĭ-sil′ah-mīd) an analgesic drug related to aspirin, used in pain relievers.

salicylate (sah-lis′ĭ-lāt, sal″ĭ-sil′āt) a salt or ester of salicylic acid. The salicylates used as drugs include acetylsalicylic acid (aspirin), choline salicylate, methyl salicylate, magnesium salicylate, sodium salicylate, and choline magnesium trisalicylate. All have analgesic, antipyretic, and antiinflammatory activity and are used for relief of mild pain. See also *acetylsalicylic acid.*

salicylate assays a colorimetric determination based on the violet- or red-brown–colored complex formed by the interaction of ferric ions and phenols. Ketone bodies and phenothiazines also form colored products, but interference can be eliminated. The ferric nitrate–mercuric chloride reagent (Trinder's) is added to a serum or urine sample. The sample is centrifuged, and the salicylate concentration is determined from the absorbance at 540 nm. A urine blank is set up by adding H_3PO_4 to the specimen followed by Trinder's reagent. This method is accurate to within 5 percent. A reagent strip for the detection of salicylates, using the same reaction, is available for urine screening tests.

Therapeutic serum levels of salicylate are usually below 20 mg/dl; toxic symptoms appear at 30 mg/dl; lethal levels are usually greater than 60 mg/dl.

See also *acetylsalicylic acid.*

salicylic acid (sal″ĭ-sil′ik) 2-hydroxybenzoic acid, used as a keratolytic agent to induce peeling of the skin or skin lesions; M.W. 138.12.

salicylsalicylic acid (sal′i-sil-sal″i-sil″ik) see *salsalate.*

saline (sa′lēn) [L. *salinus, sal* salt] salty; of the nature of a salt; containing a salt or salts.

saline agglutinin an antibody that agglutinates cells in a saline solution containing no additional proteinaceous substances.

saline solution an aqueous solution of a salt, particularly of sodium chloride.

physiologic s. s., see *isotonic s. c. solution* under *sodium chloride.*

saline technique see under *antibody detection.*

saliva (sah-li′vah) [L.] the clear, alkaline, somewhat viscid secretion from the parotid, submaxillary, sublingual, and smaller mucous glands of the mouth, of which about 0.8–1.2 l is secreted each day. It moistens and softens the food, keeps the mouth moist, and contains amylase (ptyalin), a digestive enzyme that converts starch into maltose. The saliva also contains mucin, proteins, leukocytes, and epithelial debris. Secretors of the Lewis and ABH blood group substances are identified by testing the saliva for the presence or absence of the Lewis and H substances. Saliva has been analyzed in clinical practice to determine the sodium/potassium ratio, which is altered in aldosteronism; it has also been used to ascertain the presumed free concentrations of various therapeutic drugs, which are similar in saliva and serum. Analysis of saliva for sodium and chloride has been advocated as a test for the diagnosis of cystic fibrosis.

salivary gland (sal′ĭ-ver-e) [L. *salivarius*] one of three paired masses of glandular tissue—the parotid, sublingual, and submandibular glands—and many small discrete lobules in the cheeks, palate, and tongue. These glands, which form the enzyme salivary amylase, produce a mixture of serous and mucous secretions that pass by ducts to the oral cavity, where they help to lubricate and digest food during mastication.

salivary gland functional study a procedure in nuclear medicine for imaging the salivary glands; it uses a scintillation scanner. After films showing the pertechnetate concentration have been made, lemon juice or sodium perchlorate is given to the patient to enhance pertechnetate excretion. This procedure is also used to follow the course of Sjögren's syndrome and other diseases that cause inflammation of the salivary glands and are characterized by loss of concentrating and excreting ability.

salivary gland scan a procedure in nuclear medicine for imaging the salivary glands; it uses a rectilinear scanner. Sodium pertechnetate Tc 99m is administered intravenously; like other large anions, the pertechnetate is actively trapped by the salivary gland intralobular ductules.

On lateral views obtained from each side using a medium-energy, fine-focus collimator, the normal parotid and submandibular glands are clearly delineated. Most tumors appear as cold lesions (scanning defects). Benign masses usually have distinct edges; malignant lesions have more irregular edges. Some tumors, such as papillary cystadenoma lymphomatosum (Warthin's tumor) and pleomorphic adenoma (mixed tumor), may also appear as hot lesions.

Potassium perchlorate is given to block pertechnetate uptake by the thyroid and gastrointestinal tract. Atropine may be given to reduce salivation and increase pertechnetate concentration.

salivary gland tumors neoplasms of the salivary gland; their incidence in the United States is roughly 2 per 100,000 persons, with a slight female predominance. The tumors are uncommon in young children, and the malignant forms are usually seen in older adults. Etiologic factors are not understood, but there is no evidence that antecedent inflammation predisposes to the development of cancer.

Most tumors occur within the parotid glands, 10 percent involve the submandibular glands, and another 10 percent arise in minor salivary glands, particularly those of the palate, lip, and cheek. Sublingual tumors are uncommon. Connective tissue neoplasms and lymphoma/leukemia may occur within the major glands, particularly the parotid.

Epithelial salivary tumors may be benign (adenoma) or malignant (carcinoma). The adenomas can be monomorphic, as in the basal cell adenoma; much more frequently, however, they more commonly are seen in the form of a mixed tumor, also called a pleomorphic adenoma.

Mixed Tumor. The designation of mixed tumor emphasizes its dual composition of epithelial and mesenchymal tissues. Most mixed tumors are less than 5 cm in size when excised; typically, they are firm, lobulated lesions with apparent encapsulation, and a broad range of histologic patterns, as reflected in the synonym for mixed tumor, i.e., pleomorphic adenoma. Epithelial and myoepithelial cells in a variety of patterns lie within a connective tissue framework that ranges from mucinous through fibrous to cartilaginous. Most mixed tumors grow slowly and behave as benign lesions, but recurrence is common if the tumor is not adequately excised. A small number of mixed tumors are malignant and infiltrate aggressively and may metastasize.

Mucoepidermoid Carcinoma. Up to 5 percent of salivary gland neoplasms are composed of irregular nests and strands of cells that display a transition from epidermoid features to mucin-rich cytoplasm. The relative proportions of the two components vary, and ultrastructurally, frequent transitional forms can be seen. Some mucoepidermoid tumors behave in a benign fashion and do not recur; others are locally aggressive and may metastasize.

Adenoid Cystic Carcinoma. This tumor represents about 6 percent of salivary tumors. It is composed of solid nests or cords of small epithelial cells enclosing round or oval cavities to form a cribriform pattern. The epithelial cells are sharply demarcated from the intervening strands of stromal connective tissue. Invasion along perineural spaces is typical and may extend far beyond the apparent margins of the tumor. Adenoid cystic carcinoma arises with greater frequency in minor salivary glands. Recurrences are common and eradication is usually difficult. Most adenoid cystic salivary gland tumors ultimately metastasize.

ACINIC CELL TUMOR. Acinic cell tumors make up 1 percent of all salivary tumors; 90 percent occur in the parotid. Most are less than 5 cm in diameter when excised, and may be cystic. The tumor cells form diffuse sheets, broad trabeculae, or small, acinus-like groupings. Ultrastructurally, the cells contain large, dense granules within their cytoplasm and resemble normal serous cells. Although some acinic cell tumors do not recur following removal, they are nevertheless regarded as potentially malignant neoplasms. The histologic appearance does not indicate the subsequent behavior. At least 10 percent recur, some many years after surgery, and metastases are occasionally reported.

CARCINOMA. Some malignant epithelial tumors of the salivary tissues cannot be categorized histologically and are termed carcinomas without further classification.

Salk vaccine (sahlk) [Jonas Edward *Salk,* American physician and virologist, born 1914] a vaccine for poliomyelitis that consists of formalin-killed poliomyelitis virus; it is administered in three subcutaneous doses.

Salmonella (sal″mo-nel′ah) [Daniel *Salmon,* American pathologist, 1850–1914] a genus of bacteria of the family Enterobacteriaceae, consisting of gram-negative facultatively anaerobic, nonspore-forming rods. Most strains are aerogenic, motile with peritrichous flagella, and able to use citrate as a sole carbon source. They ferment glucose but not sucrose or lactose (with some exceptions), and usually produce H_2S on triple sugar iron agar.

The *Salmonella* genus is exceedingly complex; for this reason and because of their great medical importance, the salmonellae have been subjected to continuous and intensive study for the past 40 yr. During this period there have been series of changes in taxonomy and nomenclature as new knowledge was gained. The early, predominantly biochemical basis for classification gradually gave way to primary dependence on antigenic analysis or serotyping.

Salmonellae contain two kinds of antigens that are used in serotyping: cellular or somatic (O) antigen, and flagellar (H) antigen in motile organisms. H antigen in *Salmonella* is biphasic, meaning that in any culture some of the cells possess flagella with one or more antigens (phase 1), whereas other cells contain a different set of antigens (phase 2). As there are many phase 1 and 2 H antigens, as well as O antigens, many combinations (serotypes) are possible; about 1500 serotypes are currently recognized.

Nevertheless, clinically useful serotyping is an entirely practical procedure for the average clinical microbiology laboratory. It became so with the development of good, commercially prepared antisera. Simple agglutination tests with pooled (polyvalent) antisera for groups A, B, C_1, C_2, D, and E can detect 95 percent of the serotypes that cause salmonellosis in the United States. The laboratory reports any isolate agglutinated by one of these sera as "Salmonella Group ——," provided the corresponding biochemical reactions are *Salmonella*-like. All presumptive *Salmonella* isolates should be forwarded to a *Salmonella* reference laboratory for verification and precise serotyping.

Bergey's Manual of Determinative Bacteriology (Williams & Wilkins Co.) recognizes four subgenera of *Salmonella* and 11 species; it also lists 1500 serotypes or quasi-species. However, many clinical microbiologists follow the 1972 Edwards and Ewing classification of the U.S. Public Health Service Centers for Disease Control, which lists only three species: *S. typhi, S. cholerae-suis,* and *S. enteritidis.* The last-named contains all the 1500 serotypes except the first two named above. *S. typhi* and *S. cholerae-suis* can be definitely and conveniently identified when freshly isolated by the use of commercial monospecific antisera.

The genus contains pathogenic species causing enteric fevers (typhoid and paratyphoid), septicemias, and gastroenteritis. The most frequent clinical manifestation is food poisoning. *Salmonella* species are widely distributed among, and frequently produce disease in, lower animals.

See also *Enterobacteriaceae.*

S. arizonae, formerly a species of the genus *Salmonella,* now generally classified as a separate genus; see *Arizona.*

S. cholerae-suis, a group C species, the most frequent cause of prolonged *Salmonella* septicemia. It does not ferment arabinose and trehalose and does not produce H_2S.

S. enteritidis, a group D species, one of the three species most frequently isolated from human specimens. It contains more than 1500 different serotypes, which also are often known by their individual names. These organisms ferment trehalose and arabinose, produce H_2S on triple sugar iron agar, and can utilize citrate as a sole carbon source. Various serotypes are the causative agents of typhoid and paratyphoid fevers, septicemia, and acute gastroenteritis.

S. enteritidis* serotype *agona, a frequently isolated group B serotype. Also called *S. agona.*

S. enteritidis* serotype *heidelberg, a frequently isolated group B serotype. Also called *S. heidelberg.*

S. enteritidis* serotype *hirschfeldii, a group C serotype that causes paratyphoid fever. Also called *S. paratyphi C* and *S. hirschfeldii.*

S. enteritidis* serotype *infantis, a frequently isolated group C serotype. Also called *S. infantis.*

S. enteritidis* serotype *montevideo, a frequently isolated group C serotype. Also called *S. montevideo.*

S. enteritidis* serotype *newport, a frequently isolated group C serotype. Also called *S. newport.*

S. enteritidis* serotype *paratyphi A, a group A serotype that causes paratyphoid fever. The organisms do not ferment xylose, produce little H_2S on TSI (triple sugar iron) agar, and cannot use citrate as a sole carbon source. They are pathogenic only for humans. Also called *S. paratyphi A.*

S. enteritidis* serotype *schottmülleri, a group B serotype that is one of the most common causes of paratyphoid fever in the United States. Also called *S. paratyphi B* and *S. schottmülleri.*

S. enteritidis* serotype *typhimurium, a group B serotype. In the United States, it is the most frequently isolated serotype of *Salmonella* and the most frequent cause of food poisoning. Blood cultures are generally negative, but the organism can be cultured from stool specimens. It also causes paratyphoid fever. Also called *S. typhimurium.*

S. typhi, a group D species, the cause of typhoid fever. The organism cannot utilize citrate as a sole carbon source and does not produce gas from glucose fermentation. Transmitted by food or water contaminated by human excreta, *S. typhi* is pathogenic in humans, causing typhoid fever; it is not pathogenic in animals.

salmonellosis (sal″mo-nel-lo′sis) an infection with a species of the genus *Salmonella,* usually caused by the ingestion of contaminated food or water. It results in enteric fever (typhoid or paratyphoid), septicemia, or acute gastroenteritis (food poisoning).

salping/o (sal-ping′go) [Gr. *salpinx* tube] a word element used in combining form to denote a tube, specifically the fallopian, or auditory tubes, e.g., salpingotomy.

salpingitis (sal″pin-ji′tis) [*salpingo-* + *-itis* inflammation] an acute or chronic inflammation of the fallopian tubes secondary to infection, which occurs predominantly in young, sexually active females. Symptoms include severe, nonradiating lower abdominal pain, fever, adnexal tenderness, and leukorrhea. Usually there is a history of recent intercourse, childbirth, abortion, or insertion of an IUD. Most often, salpingitis is due to sexually transmitted *Neisseria gonorrhoeae;* however, *Chlamydia trachomatis,* T mycoplasma, and other organisms are now being implicated with increasing frequency.

Cervical and urethral swabs should be taken for Gram-stain examination and culture on Thayer-Martin medium to detect *N. gonorrhoeae* or any other pathogen. The usual laboratory findings include a white count >20,000/μl and an increased erythrocyte sedimentation rate (ESR). Radiographic examination may show tubal occlusion.

Chronic salpingitis can lead to tubal obstruction, tubal abscess, hydrosalpinx, and infertility.

See also *sexually transmitted diseases.*

salpinx (sal′pinks) [Gr.] a tube, generally a uterine tube. Also called *fallopian tube.*

-salpinx (sal′pinks) [Gr. *salpinx* tube] a suffix word element to denote the fallopian tubes, e.g., hematosalpinx.

Salpix trademark for a radiopaque contrast medium used in hysterosalpingography. It is a mixture of povidone, a suspending agent; acetrizoate sodium, a contrast agent; EDTA, a chelating agent; and potassium phosphate. See also *acetrizoate.*

salsalate (sal′sah-lāt) an ester of salicylic acid hydrolyzed after absorption to produce free salicylate, used as an analgesic antiinflammatory agent.

salt (sawlt) [L. *sal;* Gr. *hals*] 1. an ionic chemical compound formed by replacing the hydrogen of an acid by a metal ion or its equivalent (e.g., an ammonium ion).

2. see *sodium chloride.*

saltation (sal-ta′shun) [L. *saltatio* from *saltare* to jump] 1. leaping or dancing, as in chorea. The term is often used to refer to conduction along myelinated nerve fibers, as the impulse jumps from node to node.

2. in genetics, an abrupt variation in species; a mutation.

Saltatoria a suborder of grasshoppers and crickets. Several species may be occasional intermediate hosts of helminths that are parasitic in humans.

saltatory conduction (sal′tah-to″re) [L. *saltare* to jump] the rapid and efficient manner by which a wave of depolarization travels from one node to the next along a myelinated nerve fiber. The myelin sheath insulates the fiber at the internodes. Thus, resting and action potentials are generated only at low-threshold areas of plasma membrane at the nodes. Saltatory conduction permits myelinated axons to conduct at velocities 50 times faster than unmyelinated fibers.

salt bridge a tube containing a concentrated potassium chloride or sodium chloride solution, which is used to connect the two half cells of an electrolytic cell.

salting-in the addition of small amounts of ionic solutes, such as Na^+, Cl^-, NH_4^+, or SO_4^{2-}, to a protein suspension, which effects solubilization of the protein by decreasing the protein-protein interaction. The solute ions bind to the charged side-chains of the protein molecules, breaking protein-protein bonds. Water molecules follow the ions and, by forming new water-protein bonds, stabilize the separated protein units.

salting-out the separation of mixtures of proteins in solution (e.g., serum, plasma) into fractions by stepwise precipitation, using increasing concentrations of one or more neutral salts. The added salt ions hydrate at the expense of protein-bound water. This exposes the hydrophobic sections of the protein molecules, making them less soluble and amenable to protein-protein aggregation and precipitation. See also *protein.*

salt-losing syndrome vomiting, dehydration, hypotension, and sudden death due to very large sodium losses from the body. It may be seen in cases of abnormal losses of sodium into the urine (as in congenital adrenal hyperplasia, adrenocortical insufficiency, or one of the forms of salt-losing nephritis), or in large extrarenal sodium losses, usually from the gastrointestinal tract or in the abnormal sweat characteristic of cystic fibrosis.

Salzman method a test that measures platelet adhesion (retention). A platelet count is performed on a whole blood sample before and after it is passed through a glass-bead column. Although it is the method of choice, many variables (including length of filter, quality and quantity of beads, and flow rate) decrease its value as a routine laboratory procedure. Results are expressed as the percentage of platelets retained by the glass-bead column. The reference value is 56.3 ± 13.1 percent. Also called *glass-bead retention method* and *platelet retention test.* See also *platelet adhesiveness test.*

SAM abbrev. See *S-adenosyl-L-methionine.*

samarium (Sm) (sah-mar′e-um) [from the mineral *samarskite*] a hard, silvery metallic element; atomic number 62; atomic weight 150.4; a 4f transition element (lanthanide rare earth); oxidation states +2, +3. See also *rare earth elements.*

sample (sam′p'l) [L. *exemplum* example] a representative subset of a population or portion of a material object obtained in order to estimate the characteristics of the whole. See also *random sample.*

sample interaction in a flow system, the effect of the preceding samples in the moving stream on a sample reading, caused by the incomplete separation of the samples.

sampler 1. an electronic circuit that produces a pulsed output representing the value of a continuous input at a discrete series of points in time.

2. a device used to obtain small samples of material for chemical analysis.

3. a mechanical device for sequentially aspirating aliquots of liquid samples and delivering them to an automated chemical analyzer.

sample steady state in an AutoAnalyzer, the period of time (after the wash-in of a sample into the flow-through cuvet) during which the transmittance has a small rate of change. This time period varies with the interaction in the system and with the sample aspiration time; i.e., in analyses with high interaction, a longer sample aspiration may be required to reach a steady state. Also called plateau.

sandalwood oil (san′dal-wood) see *santal oil.*

sandfly (sand′fli) any of various two-winged flies, especially those of the genus *Phlebotomus.* See also *Phlebotomus.*

sandfly fever see *phlebotomus fever.*

Sandhoff's disease (sand′hofs) a disorder of sphingolipid metabolism, transmitted as an autosomal recessive trait; it is due to a relative or absolute deficiency of both hexosaminidase A and B, and results in the accumulation of globoside and ganglioside G_{M2}. Clinically, the disease is a variant of Tay-Sachs disease, with identical signs, symptoms, and pathology, but it differs biochemically and genetically. Tay-Sachs disease is a deficiency of hexosaminidase A only, and is seen primarily in Ashkenazi Jews, whereas Sandhoff's disease has no ethnic restriction. See also *sphingolipidoses* and *Tay-Sachs disease.*

Sanfilippo's syndrome a rare genetic disorder, transmitted as an autosomal recessive trait; it is characterized by abnormal mucopolysaccharide metabolism, leading to progressive and severe mental deficiencies with relatively minor somatic abnormalities, including dwarfism and hepatosplenomegaly. Increased urinary excretion of heparan sulfate is seen. At least two phenotypically identical types of this syndrome exist: type A is characterized by a deficiency of the enzyme heparan *N*-sulfatase, and type B by a deficiency of the enzyme *N*-acetyl-α-D-glucosaminidase.

Diagnosis of Sanfilippo's syndrome prenatally and postnatally depends on the demonstration of enzyme deficiency and increased intracellular mucopolysaccharides in cultured cells.

Also called mucopolysaccharidosis III (MPS III). See also *mucopolysaccharidoses.*

sanguivorous myiasis (sang-gwiv′o-rus) [L. *sanguis* blood + *vorare* to eat] a type of myiasis in which the mosquitos attach superficially during bloodsucking.

sanitization (san″ĭ-ti-za′shun) a cleaning or sterilizing process used to lower bacterial count, especially of utensils used for eating and drinking. It may include, but not necessarily, the use of an antimicrobial chemical. Cf. *sterilization.*

San Joaquin Valley fever see *coccidioidomycosis.*

SA node see *sinoatrial n.* under *node.*

santal oil (san′tal) [L. *santalum oleum*] a pale yellow, somewhat viscid oily liquid with the characteristic odor and taste of sandalwood. It is distilled with steam from the dried heartwood of *Santalum album* and is used as a clearing agent for histologic specimens. The main constituents are the sesquiterpene alcohols, α- and β-santalol.

santonin (san-to′nin) a drug extracted from flowers of *Artemisia cina;* formerly used to treat ascariasis.

Santorini's cartilage (sahn″to-re′nēz) [Giovanni Domenico *Santorini,* Italian anatomist, 1681–1737] small conical nodules of cartilage at the apex of the arytenoid cartilages. Also called corniculate cartilage.

saphenous (sah-fe′nus) pertaining to or associated with the saphenous veins.

saphenous nerve a branch of the femoral nerve. It descends through the adductor canal and provides sensory innervation for the skin of the medial side of the leg and foot.

saphenous opening an aperture in the deep fascia through which the long saphenous vein passes, below the inguinal ligament. The opening is covered by the cribriform fascia.

saphenous veins a system of superficial veins in the lower extremity. Its main components are the long saphenous vein, which begins on the medial side of the foot and ends in the femoral vein below the inguinal ligament, and the short saphenous vein, which begins behind the lateral malleolus and runs up the back of the leg to end in the popliteal vein.

saponifiable fraction (sah-pon″ĭ-fi′ah-b′l) [L. *sapo* soap + *facere* to make] the portion of total lipid that, after treatment with hot alkali, is soluble in water and insoluble in ether. Cf. *nonsaponifiable fraction.*

saponification (sah-pon″ĭ-fĭ-ka′shun) [L. *sapo* soap + *facere* to make] the chemical reaction of a fat (triglyceride) with an alkali, yielding glycerol and salts of fatty acids (soaps). The reaction is irreversible and goes to completion. More generally, the term refers to any hydrolysis of a fatty acid ester followed by neutralization to produce a soap.

saponin (sap′o-nin) [from *Saponaria* the soapwart] any of a group of varied triterpene or steroid glycosides occurring in many plants. Saponins are characterized by their ability to form a durable foam when shaken with water and by their ability to lyse red blood cells at very great dilutions. Many are toxic to fish but not to humans, except for the lysing of red blood cells on venous injection.

steroid s., a saponin having a steroid aglycone residue.

triterpenoid s., a saponin having a 1,2,7-trimethylnaphthalene aglycone residue.

Sappinea (sah-pin′e-ah) a genus of free-living coprozoic amebae, of which the species *S. diploidea* has been identified in human feces.

sapr/o (sap′ro) [Gr. *sapros* rotten] a word element used in combining form to denote rotten, putrid, or decaying, e.g., saprozoite.

saprobe (sa′prōb) [*sapro-* + Gr. *-bios* life] an organism that lacks the ability of photosynthesis, and lives on dead or decaying organic matter; a saprophyte.

sapronosis (sap″ro-no′sis) an imprecise term to describe a disease caused by organisms of the environment, in distinction to one that occurs in both humans and lower animals (e.g., tuberculosis) and is acquired by a recognized route of transmission. Urban listeriosis of humans is an example: the causative organism, *Listeria monocytogenes,* is frequently present on plants and in soil in areas where infections occur, and animal contact is unlikely.

saprophyte (sap′ro-fīt) [*sapro-* + Gr. *phyton* plant] an organism, such as a bacterium, that lives upon dead or decaying organic matter.

saramycetin an investigational polypeptide antifungal agent. It is effective against *Histoplasma* *capsulatum, Blastomyces dermatitidis,* and species of *Aspergillus.*

sarc/o (sar′ko) [Gr. *sarx, sarkos* flesh] a word element used in combining form to denote flesh (connective tissue), e.g., sarcoma.

Sarcina (sar-si′nah) [L. "bundles"] a genus of cocci that characteristically adhere in square tetrads and cubical packets after division in two or three perpendicular planes. They are gram-positive and strict anaerobes, and are found in soil, on grains, and occasionally in clinical specimens.

sarcina (sar′sĭ-nah), pl. *sarcinae* [L. "bundles"] 1. any coccal bacterium that remains adhered in square tetrads or cubical packets; this formation results from the failure of daughter cells to separate following division in two or three perpendicular planes.

2. an organism of the genus *Sarcina.*

sarcocyst (sar′ko-sist) [*sarco-* + Gr. *kystis* bladder] 1. any member of the genus *Sarcocystis.*

2. a cylindric cyst containing a large number of crescentic trophozoites (Rainey's corpuscles), found in the muscles of individuals infected with *Sarcocystis.*

sarcocystin (sar″ko-sis′tin) a toxic by-product secreted by species of the genus *Sarcocystis* (a sporozoan), which affects the central nervous system, heart, adrenals, and intestinal wall.

Sarcocystis (sar″ko-sis′tis) [*sarco-* + Gr. *kystis* bladder] a genus of sporozoa. The species *S. lindemanni* occasionally infects humans, and represents a "dead-end" stage of an *Isospora* species. Infection is acquired by the ingestion of undercooked, infected meat and is generally asymptomatic, but it may give rise to eosinophilia and intermittent focal myositis, with fever, malaise, and bronchospasms.

It has also been found that *Isospora hominis* (now known as *Sarcocystis hominis* and *S. suihominis*), shed as sporulated sporocysts, represents the sexual stage of two species of *Sarcocystis* (of cattle and of swine), of which humans are the final hosts.

Sarcodina (sar″ko-di′nah) [Gr. *sarkōdēs* fleshlike] a subphylum of Protozoa that includes free-living and parasitic amebae. These protozoa lack a thick cell membrane; their locomotion is achieved by means of pseudopodia. This subphylum includes the class Rhizopoda.

sarcoidosis (sar″koi-do′sis) a chronic, progressive, generalized, granulomatous reticulosis of unknown etiology, involving almost any organ or tissue, but particularly lungs, lymph nodes, and skin. It is characterized histologically by the presence in affected organs of noncaseating epithelioid cell granulomas. Laboratory findings may include hypo- or hypercalcemia and hypergammaglobulinemia; there is usually diminished or absent reactivity to tuberculin, and in most cases a positive Kveim reaction. Formerly called benign lymphogranulomatosis, *Besnier-Boeck disease, Boeck's disease,* and sarcoid of Boeck. See also *granuloma* and *Kveim test.*

sarcolemma (sar″ko-lem′ah) [*sarco-* + Gr. *lemma* husk] the cell membrane of a muscle fiber.

sarcoma (sar-ko′mah), pl. *sarcomas* or *sarcomata* [*sarco-* + *-oma*] a malignant soft tissue tumor; a malignant tumor of cells of mesodermal origin. Sarcomas are usually designated by prefixing the tissue type (e.g., rhabdomyosarcoma, fibrosarcoma, liposarcoma, leiomyosarcoma), but some are named descriptively because their histogenesis is uncertain (e.g., epithelioid sarcoma, alveolar soft part sarcoma). The etiology of most sarcomas is unknown, but a fibrosarcoma occasionally occurs in a previously irradiated area, and a lymphangiosarcoma may develop in a lymphedematous arm following radical mastectomy.

It is sometimes difficult to decide from the histologic pattern whether a particular soft tissue tumor is benign or a low-grade sarcoma. Some locally aggressive tumors (certain of the fibromatoses) cause considerable damage to adjacent structures by local infiltration and may be difficult to eradicate surgically, but as they do not metastasize they are not considered to be sarcomas. Atypical fibrous histiocytoma (xanthoma) of the skin and dermatofibrosarcoma protuberans are examples of soft tissue tumors that are generally benign in their behavior, but occasionally metastasize.

A tumor may be suspected to be of soft tissue origin on the basis of the clinical findings (e.g., a rapidly growing mass in the soft tissues of the thigh), but confirmation and classification require biopsy and histologic examination. Needle biopsies are not generally suitable for this purpose; their application to soft tissue neoplasms should be limited to providing tissue for electron microscopy or confirming a suspected recurrence of a previously diagnosed tumor. An open biopsy of a large lesion or total excision of a small or superficial tumor is recommended so that the pathologist may have sufficient tissue for examination.

Classification of a soft tissue tumor is based on the appearance and histologic arrangement of the component cells. Special staining procedures are of limited value, although they can be useful on occasion, e.g., for examining the connective tissue pattern with a reticulin stain or for demonstrating the presence of cytoplasmic glycogen. Histochemistry is more applicable when the differential diagnosis includes poorly differentiated carcinoma or melanoma.

At least one sarcoma in three cannot be classified by light microscopy because of lack of specific histologic features. Ultrastructural examination can reveal the cell type in some tumors that cannot be diagnosed by light microscopy. Some sarcomas are composed of poorly differentiated mesenchymal cells with no specific organization into definable histologic patterns. In such tumors, the value of electron microscopy is then limited to excluding other possible diagnoses that might be considered after light microscopy.

Sarcomas spread by local infiltration and by distant metastases through blood vessels and, in some instances, the lymphatics. The extent to which the pathologist can predict the behavior of a sarcoma from its histologic features is relatively limited. Grading based on the standard criteria of cell pleomorphism and mitotic activity can be very misleading. Assessment should take into consideration the cell type, age of patient, and tumor size and location. For example, a rhabdomyosarcoma may spread to regional lymph nodes, whereas a fibrosarcoma in an infant only rarely metastasizes. As a general rule, the larger the sarcoma, the more likelihood there is of distant spread. Superficial atypical tumors of fat cells generally behave in a benign fashion, in contrast to many deeply located liposarcomas.

See also *soft tissue tumor* for classification of neoplasms.

Sarcomastigophora a subphylum of Protozoa that includes the class Zoomastigophorea.

sarcomere (sar′ko-mēr) [*sarco-* + Gr. *meros* part] the part of a myofibril between two Z lines. See also *skeletal m.* under *muscle.*

Sarcophaga (sar-kof′ah-gah) [*sarco-* + Gr. *phagein* to eat] a genus of flies (the fleshflies) of the family Sarcophagidae. The adults feed on either filth or flowers. Larvae of the species *S. haemorrhoidalis,* found on fruit or meat, cause intestinal myiasis in humans when ingested.

Sarcophagidae (sar″ko-faj′ĭ-de) a family of flies of the order Diptera, including the genera *Sarcophaga* and *Wohlfahrtia.*

sarcoplasm (sar′ko-plazm) [*sarco-* + Gr. *plasma* anything formed or molded] the cytoplasm of a striated muscle fiber.

sarcoplasmic reticulum (sar″ko-plaz′mik) a system of connected tubes within a muscle fiber. Around each sarcomere (in mammalian cells, at the junction of the A and I bands) runs a T tubule, on each side of which there is a terminal cisterna formed from the endoplasmic reticulum. The terminal cisternae and T tubule constitute a triad. Terminal cisternae are connected by tubules, which run longitudinally over the A bands and form an irregular network over the H band. See also *muscle.*

Sarcoptes (sar-kop′tēz) [*sarco-* + Gr. *koptein* to cut] a genus of mites (the itch mites). The species *S. scabiei* causes scabies in humans, and is often transmitted through sexual contact. The female measures 330–450 μ long by 250–350 μ wide; the male, 200–240 μ by 150–200 μ.

Laboratory diagnosis requires microscopic identification of the mites from lesions. See also *scabies* and the illustration under *mite.*

sarcoptic mange (sar-kop′tic mānj) see *scabies.*

Sarcoptidae a family of mites of the class Arachnida that includes the genus *Sarcoptes.*

sarcoptidosis (sar-kop″tĭ-do′sis) an infestation with mites of the genus *Sarcoptes.*

Sarcoptoidea a superfamily of mites of the order Acari that includes the genus *Sarcoptes.*

sarcosine (sar′ko-sēn) an amino acid, *N*-methylglycine, that occurs as an intermediate between glycine and dimethyl glycine in the one-carbon cycle.

sarcosine dehydrogenase (sar′ko-sēn de-hi′dro-jen-ās) an enzyme of the oxidoreductase class (EC 1.5.99.1) that catalyzes the reaction sarcosine + acceptor + $H_2O \rightleftharpoons$ glycine + HCHO + reduced acceptor, which is an important reaction in the metabolism of methyl groups. A genetic defect resulting in sarcosinemia, transmitted as an autosomal recessive trait, appears to be caused by a deficiency of sarcosine dehydrogenase.

sarcosinemia (sar″ko-sēn-e′me-ah) see *hypersarcosinemia.*

Sarcosporidia (sar″ko-spo-rid′e-ah) an order of sporozoa that includes the genus *Sarcocystis,* which occasionally parasitizes humans.

satellite (sat′ĕ-līt) [L. *satelles* companion] 1. (abbrev. s), the portion of an acrocentric chromosome distal to the secondary constriction.

2. a structure that has a subsidiary relationship to a larger structure, such as an accompanying vein of an artery or a small lesion near a larger one.

satellite cell 1. one of the flattened, epithelium-like supporting cells that surround the neurons in some peripheral ganglia (dorsal root ganglia and the sensory ganglia of some cranial nerves). Satellite cells are similar to Schwann cells. Also called *amphicyte* and *capsule cell.*

2. a small cell with scanty cytoplasm that lies between the basal lamina and sarcolemma of a skeletal muscle fiber. The muscle fiber nuclei do not divide, but during muscle growth or hypertrophy, satellite cells undergo mitosis and are incorporated into the fibers; they are thus facultative myoblasts.

satellite colony a microbial colony that requires a growth factor secreted by a second microorganism and thus grows only in the vicinity of the other organism.

satellite DNA highly repeated short DNA nucleotide sequences, originally named because of results obtained with cesium chloride buoyant density centrifugation. Generally, when DNA is purified, it is broken into moderately sized pieces that accumulate in a thin layer during centrifugation, forming a band corresponding to its density. The portion of DNA that forms bands distinct from the main band is satellite DNA. Human DNA, however, forms density bands that are usually too close to the main band to be detected by cesium chloride centrifugation. See also *repeated DNA sequences.*

saturated (sach′ĕ-rāt″ed) 1. having all the chemical affinities satisfied. The term saturated hydrocarbon refers to the absence of double or triple bonds (unsaturation) in a hydrocarbon, e.g., hexane.

2. unable to dissolve any more of a given substance, as in a saturated solution.

saturated fatty acid a fatty acid of the general formula $C_nH_{2n+1}COOH$, and having all chemical affinities in the alkyl chain satisfied either by single bonds to carbon or by bonds to hydrogen.

saturation (sach′ĕ-ra′shun) [L. *saturāre* to satiate] 1. the act of saturating or the condition of being saturated.

2. the condition of a system in which a further change of some parameter has no effect.

3. the condition of a solution in which no more solute can dissolve at a given temperature and pressure.

4. the condition of an atom (especially carbon) that has an equal number of valence bonds and bonded atoms. Unsaturated linkages involve multiple bonds between two atoms.

5. the substrate concentration at which all enyzme-active sites are occupied and, consequently, at which the reaction velocity is maximal; it also refers to the complete occupation of sites of a binding protein, a hormone, or a drug receptor.

6. the condition of maximal magnetization of a magnetic material. See under *ferromagnetic.*

7. the intensity of a color; mixing a color with white decreases its saturation.

saturation current the maximal electric current for a device operating under certain specified conditions. In an x-ray tube, the term refers to the space-charge–limited current at which all the electrons emitted by the filament are collected at the anode; an increase in kilovoltage increases the hardness of the x-ray beam but does not increase the milliamperage.

In an ion-collection radiation detector, the term refers to the current produced when the voltage is sufficient to collect all the ion pairs formed by radiation. All the positive ions move to the cathode, and all the electrons move to the anode; a small voltage increase produces no increase in current. A large voltage increase, however, causes gas amplification, the production of secondary ion pairs.

S. aureus see *S. aureus* under *Staphylococcus.*

Sb [L. *stibium*] symbol for the chemical element *antimony.*

SBE abbrev. for *subacute bacterial endocarditis;* see *subacute infective e.* under *endocarditis.*

SBN_2 abbrev. See *single-breath nitrogen test.*

σ bond see *sigma b.* under *bond.*

Sc symbol for the chemical element *scandium.*

scabies (ska'bēz) [L., from *scabere* scratch] a skin disease caused by the itch mite (*Sarcoptes scabiei*), which burrows into the skin and causes extreme itching and eczema. These mites are common in crowded environments with poor sanitary conditions. Infection is spread through contact among people; scabies is frequently a sexually transmitted disease. Untreated cases usually resolve spontaneously within a few months. Also called *gale, Norwegian itch, sarcoptic mange,* and *7-year itch.*

scala (ska'lah), pl. *scalae* [L. "staircase"] a stairlike structure; especially applied to the three spiral passages of the cochlea.

s. media, an endolymph-filled lumen, part of the membranous labyrinth, which, as it ascends the spiral turns of the bony canal of the cochlea, separates the upper scala vestibuli from the lower scala tympani. Also called *cochlear duct.*

s. tympani, [NA], one of the perilymph-filled divisions of the bony canal of the cochlea, which terminates near the round window of the tympanic cavity. At the apex of the cochlea it communicates with the scala media through a small opening.

s. vestibuli, [NA], the lowermost of the two divisions of the cochlear canal, which are separated from the scala tympani by the spiral lamina and scala media. It arises from the vestibule of the osseous labyrinth.

scalar product a type of multiplication of vectors indicated $c = \mathbf{A} \cdot \mathbf{B}$. In terms of the components $c = a_1 b_1 + a_2 b_2 + \ldots + a_n b_n$. For three-dimensional vectors, $c = |\mathbf{A}| \cdot |\mathbf{B}| \cdot \cos\theta$, where $|\mathbf{A}|$ and $|\mathbf{B}|$ are the magnitudes of **A** and **B** and θ is the angle between them. Also called *dot product.* See also *vector product.*

scalded skin syndrome (SSS) a group of dermatologic manifestations that are due to coagulase-positive staphylococci, primarily in bacteriophage group II. There are three clinical forms: Ritter's disease, bullous impetigo, and scarlet skin syndrome. All are characterized by the production of staphylococci exotoxin, which leads to exfoliation through the intraepidermal cleavage of the desmosomes.

The generalized exfoliative form, known as Ritter's disease, is characterized by diffuse erythema, extremely painful skin, the formation of large flaccid bullae, and red streaking of antecubital, neck, inguinal, and axillary skin folds. Within several days of onset, these conditions are accompanied by shedding of the upper epidermis in large sheets, especially when lightly stroked (Nikolsky's sign). This condition occurs most frequently in neonates but may also be seen in adults; it usually abates within several weeks, and heals without scarring. Also called toxic epidermal necrolysis, Lyell's disease, and pemphigus neonatorum.

In the second form of the syndrome, bullous impetigo, large, flaccid, fluid-filled bullae are sharply demarcated, with exfoliation occurring only at the rim of the lesion. This localized form commonly appears in the diaper area and on the trunk.

The third form, scarlet skin syndrome, is the scarlatiniform rash pattern. It is a mild variant that clinically resembles scarlet fever and is not associated with exfoliation or bullae formation.

Diagnosis is based on clinical appearance and positive skin cultures. Blood cultures for staphylococci are rarely positive. Antibiotic therapy is often instituted for 7–10 da.

scale (skāl) 1. [Fr. *escala* husk], a thin, compacted, platelike structure, as of cornified epithelial cells, either on the surface of the body or shed from the skin.

2. [L. *scala* ladder, *scalae* stairs], a measuring device or measuring scheme. In physics, the term refers to a correspondence between numbers and a physical quantity, for example, a temperature scale. In measurement theory, it refers to one of four possible ways to impose a measurement structure on a sample space: (1) A nominal scale (the weakest) is a qualitative classification of the sample space into separate categories so that each possible result belongs to only one category. A dichotomous scale is a nominal scale with two categories. Nominal data are also called *categorical data.* (2) An ordinal scale is an ordered nominal scale. The sample points are numbers, but only their order (relative size) is significant. A classification of disease symptoms as being mild [1], moderate [2], or severe [3] would be an ordinal scale. Ordinal data are also called *ranked data.* (3) An interval scale is an ordinal scale with a distance measure. The sample points are numerical but the zero point of the scale is arbitrary (as in the Celsius and Fahrenheit temperature scales). Interval data also called *metric data.* (4) A ratio scale is an interval scale with a meaningful zero point (such as mass or length), so that products involving the data points (like volume or density) make sense. *Ratio data* are also called *metric data.*

For more information, see the specific scale.

scaler (skāl'er) see *counter.*

scaler-timer an electronic device containing a counter circuit and a frequency standard (a tuned oscillator) that can count the number of input pulses received in a preset time interval (scaler mode); it can also measure the time between input pulses (timer mode) by counting the oscillator output.

scalloped (skol'op'd, skal'op'd) wavy, having curved projections; used in describing the margin of a part. Also called *undulating.*

scalp (skalp) that part of the skin and muscles of the head, exclusive of the face and ears, that is normally covered with hair.

scan (skan) 1. to move a beam of light, an electron beam, or a detector over an object to produce or sense an image, as in a scanning electron microscope, a rectilinear scanner, a CT scanner, or an oscilloscope.

2. the image produced by a scan, colloquially ap-

plied also to other images, such as scintillation photographs.

scandium (Sc) (skan′de-um) [L. *Scandia* Scandinavia] a silvery-white metallic element; atomic number 21; atomic weight 44.9559; a 3d transition element; oxidation state +3.

scan information density the count density of a rectilinear scanner.

scanner (skan′er) 1. an instrument that produces an image by scanning, such as an optical scanner or rectilinear scanner.
2. see *multiplexer.*

scanning (skan′ning) the motion of the beam or detector in making a scan.

scanning electron microscope (SEM) see under *electron microscope.*

scanning sequence the order in which the points of an object are scanned, e.g., the back-and-forth pattern of a rectilinear scanner.

scanography (skan-og′rah-fe) the radiographic measurement of the length of internal organs, particularly the long bones, using parallel beams at all points along the length of the organ so that size distortion is eliminated.

slit s., a method of scanography in which the x-ray beam is collimated with a narrow slit (about 1/16 in.). This fan-shaped beam is scanned along the length of the organ, while the milliamperage or scan speed is adjusted to vary the exposure. There is no distortion in direction of the scan; the divergence of the beam perpendicular to the scan produces distortion of the width.

spot s., a method of scanography of long bones, in which a narrowly coned beam is used. Exposures are made only of the joints, using parallel beams.

scaphocephaly (skaf″o-sef′ah-le) [Gr. *skaphē* skull + *kephalē* head] a long, narrow skull, resulting from early closure of the sagittal suture. See also *craniostenosis.*

scapul/o (skap′u-lo) [L. *scapula* shoulder] a word element used in combining form to denote the scapula, e.g., scapulodynia.

scapula (skap′u-lah), pl. *scapulae* [L.] a triangular, thin, flat bone that lies in the upper part of the back opposite the second to seventh ribs. It has a body and three processes, the spine, acromion, and coracoid process. Its lateral angle is truncated and thickened, and the surface is hollowed to form the glenoid cavity that articulates with the head of the humerus.

scapular (skap′u-lar) of or pertaining to the scapula.

scapular line a vertical line on either side of the surface of the back that passes through the inferior angle of the scapula.

scapular region the region of the back that overlies the scapula.

scar (skahr) [Gr. *eschara* the scar or eschar on a wound caused by a burning] cicatrix; a mark that remains after the healing of a wound. See also *repair.*

scarabiasis see *canthariasis.*

scarlet fever (skar′let) an infection with group A β-hemolytic streptococci that is characterized by pharyngitis and tonsillitis concurrent with an erythematous skin rash. The streptococci produce an erythrogenic toxin responsible for the rash. The clinical manifestations include a red papillar tongue, a toxic erythematous rash progressing from the trunk to the extremities and face, and a flushed red face with a pale area around the mouth. Petechiae may be present. After 6–9 da of illness, the erythema disappears and the skin begins desquamation. The severity of scarlet fever varies greatly.

Microbiologic diagnosis is based on culture of throat swab material on sheep blood agar anaerobically at 37°C for 24 hr, with a filter disk containing bacitracin. This allows for the presumptive identification of group A β-hemolytic streptococci. Serologically, antistreptococcal antibodies do not appear until 10–20 da after onset; thus, the detection of these antibodies is especially useful in determining a previous illness caused by streptococci. A fluorescent-antibody technique is available for the identification of isolated streptococci from the throat. The treatment of choice is penicillin.

See also *erythrogenic toxin* and *streptococcus.*

scarlet skin syndrome see under *scalded skin syndrome.*

Scatchard equation an equation that describes protein-ligand binding, e.g., of the steroid receptor or antibody-antigen reactions. In the latter case, the formula is $r/c = K(n - r)$, where K is the intrinsic association constant (equilibrium constant) measuring the affinity of one Ab binding site for a univalent ligand, c is the concentration of free ligand molecules, n is the number of binding sites per Ab molecule (the Ab valence), and r is the average number of ligand molecules bound to an Ab molecule.

Scatchard plot a plot of the ratio of bound to free ligand (B/F), the y coordinate, versus the concentration of bound ligand (B), the x coordinate, used for ligand-binding assays, e.g., radioimmunoassay or radioligand receptor assay. When nonspecific binding is removed, the Scatchard equation applies and the plot is linear with a slope equal to $-K_d$, the negative of the dissociation constant and an x-intercept equal to B_{max}, the concentration of available binding sites.

scatter (skat′er) the diffusion of deviation of x-rays produced by passage through a medium.

scatter diagram see *scatterplot.*

scattered radiation in radiology, the secondary x-rays generated in the patient and surrounding objects by the scattering of the primary x-rays.

scattergram (skat′er-gram) see *scatterplot.*

scattering (skat′er-ing) a change in the direction in which a particle is moving, caused by a collision with a particle or atomic nucleus. See also *Compton scattering, interaction of radiation with matter,* and *Rutherford scattering.*

elastic s., a scattering process in which no kinetic energy is absorbed by the ionization or excitation of one of the colliding particles or by the emission of secondary particles. Kinetic energy is usually transferred from the scattered particles to the target particle, but the total kinetic energy of the two is unchanged.

inelastic s., a scattering process that is not elastic. Some of the particle kinetic energy is absorbed.

scatterplot (skat′er-plot) a plot of a random sample of observations of a two-dimensional random variable, each point on the plot indicating the X and Y values of one observation. Examination of the scatterplot may suggest a linear or curvilinear relationship (a regression curve) among the variables; clustering of the observations may suggest that several different subpopulations are represented in the sample. Also called *scatter diagram* and *scattergram.*

Scaurus a genus of beetles of which the species *S. striatus* is an obligatory intermediate host of the rat tapeworm *Hymenolepis diminuta.*

scavenger (skav′en-jer) in chemistry, a substance added to a material to remove or inactivate trace impurities, or added to a reaction to absorb undesired species or inhibit their activity. Water and oxygen molecules, heavy metal ions, and free radicals are common targets of scavengers.

SCBA abbrev. See *breathing apparatus.*

SCD abbrev. See *subacute combined degeneration of the s. c.* under *spinal cord.*

Scedosporium a genus of fungi. *S. apiospermum* is the anamorph (asexual stage) of *Petriellidium boydii* (*Allescheria boydii*). Also called (incorrectly) *Monosporium.*

Schales and Schales method for chloride see *chloride methods.*

Schatzki's ring a thin mucosal fold, located 3–5 cm above the gastroesophageal junction, that may narrow the lumen of the esophagus and cause intermittent dysphagia. Barium x-ray examinations of the esophagus usually reveal the ring's presence. Also called lower esophageal ring.

Scheie's syndrome (shāz) a genetic disorder, transmitted as an autosomal recessive trait, that appears to be a clinical and allelic variant of Hurler's syndrome. There is abnormal metabolism of mucopolysaccharides, with excretion of large amounts of dermatan sulfate and heparan sulfate in the urine. There is a relative or absolute deficiency of α-L-iduronidase, which leads to stiff joints, corneal clouding, and aortic regurgitation. Life span and intelligence are nearly normal. Prenatal diagnosis, using cultured amniotic fluid cells, may soon be available. Also called mucopolysaccharidosis I S (MPS-I S). See also *mucopolysaccharidoses.*

Scheloribates a genus of mites of which the species *S. laevigatus* is a host of the tapeworm *Bertiella studeri.*

schematic (ske-mat′ik) [Gr. *schēma* form, shape] 1. pertaining to a scheme or diagram.

2. a diagram of an electric circuit showing the components as standard symbols and the wiring as lines connecting the components. Some of the more common circuit component symbols are shown in the accompanying illustration.

Schick test (shik) [Béla *Schick,* Hungarian pediatrician in the United States, born 1877] a test for measuring immunity to diphtheria. It involves the intracutaneous injection of diphtheria toxin: 0.1 ml of 1/50 of the minimal lethal dose. After 24–48 hr, the area of skin injected is observed for erythema and edema. A positive response indicates a lack of immunity to diphtheria; a negative response indicates the presence of antitoxin. One-thirteenth of a unit of antitoxin per cubic centimeter of blood is sufficient to neutralize the injected toxin and is also sufficient to protect most individuals from diphtheria.

Schiff base (shif) [Hugo (Ugo) *Schiff,* German chemist in Florence, 1834–1915] a class of compounds, aldimines, derived by chemical reaction (condensation) of aldehydes or ketones with primary amines; the general formula is $RR'C = NR''$. Such compounds may be formed by amino acids during metabolism; some substrates probably form these compounds with an enzyme amino group during an enzymatic reaction. For example, transamination that involves the cofactors pyridoxal and pyridoxamine is believed to proceed through a Schiff-base mechanism.

Schiff reagent [Hugo (Ugo) *Schiff*] a histochemical reagent used to demonstrate aldehydes. Free aldehydes do not occur naturally in tissues; the Schiff reagent is used following procedures that have produced free aldehydes in certain tissue components. The most common of these are oxidation in periodic acid and hydrolysis in weak hydrochloric acid (see below).

The Schiff reagent is produced from a triphenylmethane dye, such as basic fuchsin or pararosaniline, by reduction with sulfurous acid (H_2SO_3). First, a triphenylmethylsulfonic acid (ϕ_3CSO_3H) is produced (ϕ being an aminoaryl) group, e.g., *p*-aminophenyl is pararosaniline). This compound is colorless because the double bonds are not all conjugated (alternated with single bonds) as they are in the quinoid resonance structure of the original dye. Another one or two sulfite groups are subsequently added to the arylamino groups (ϕNH_2) to produce arylaminosulfinic acid groups ($\phi NHSO_2H$); this decolorized fuchsin (leukofuchsin) is the Schiff reagent.

Aldehydes (RCHO) produce an addition product (ϕNH—SO_2—CHOH—R) with the aminosulfinic acid groups, which is believed to undergo molecular rearrangement to the aminoalkylsulfonic acid (ϕNH—CHR—SO_3H) form. The product is unstable and spontaneously loses the sulfonic acid group, which restores the quinoic structure and color (the original magenta or a slightly bluer reddish-purple) to the dye.

Similar leuko compounds can be made with other dyes that have at least one primary arylamino (ϕ NH_3) group, which is necessary to form the aldehyde-reactive arylaminosulfinic acid group. Thus, Schiff reagents can be made from thiozine dyes (such as methylene blue or thionine), oxazine dyes (such as celestine blue or cresyl violet), and acridine fluorochrome dyes (such as auramine O or acriflavin).

The most commonly used oxidative Schiff method is the periodic acid–Schiff (PAS) technique. Periodic acid oxidizes the 1,2-diol(—CHOH—CHOH—) group found in glucose and other hexoses, breaking the carbon-carbon bond to produce a dialdehyde; it also produces aldehydes by oxidation of the 1-hydroxy-2-amino group (found in glucosamine and other hexosamines and in the phospholipid sphingomyelin) and of the double bonds of unsaturated fatty acids. It releases aldehyde by the hydrolysis of plasmalogens (phosphatidyl compounds); however, these phospholipids are removed by normal paraffin processing.

These chemical groups are responsible for the PAS-reactivity of polysaccharides, proteoglycans, glycoproteins, and complex lipids. PAS-positive polysaccharides include glycogen, found in animal tissues (particularly liver and muscle) and in cellulose; starch; and chitosan, found in the cell walls of bacteria and fungi. Epithelia and connective tissues

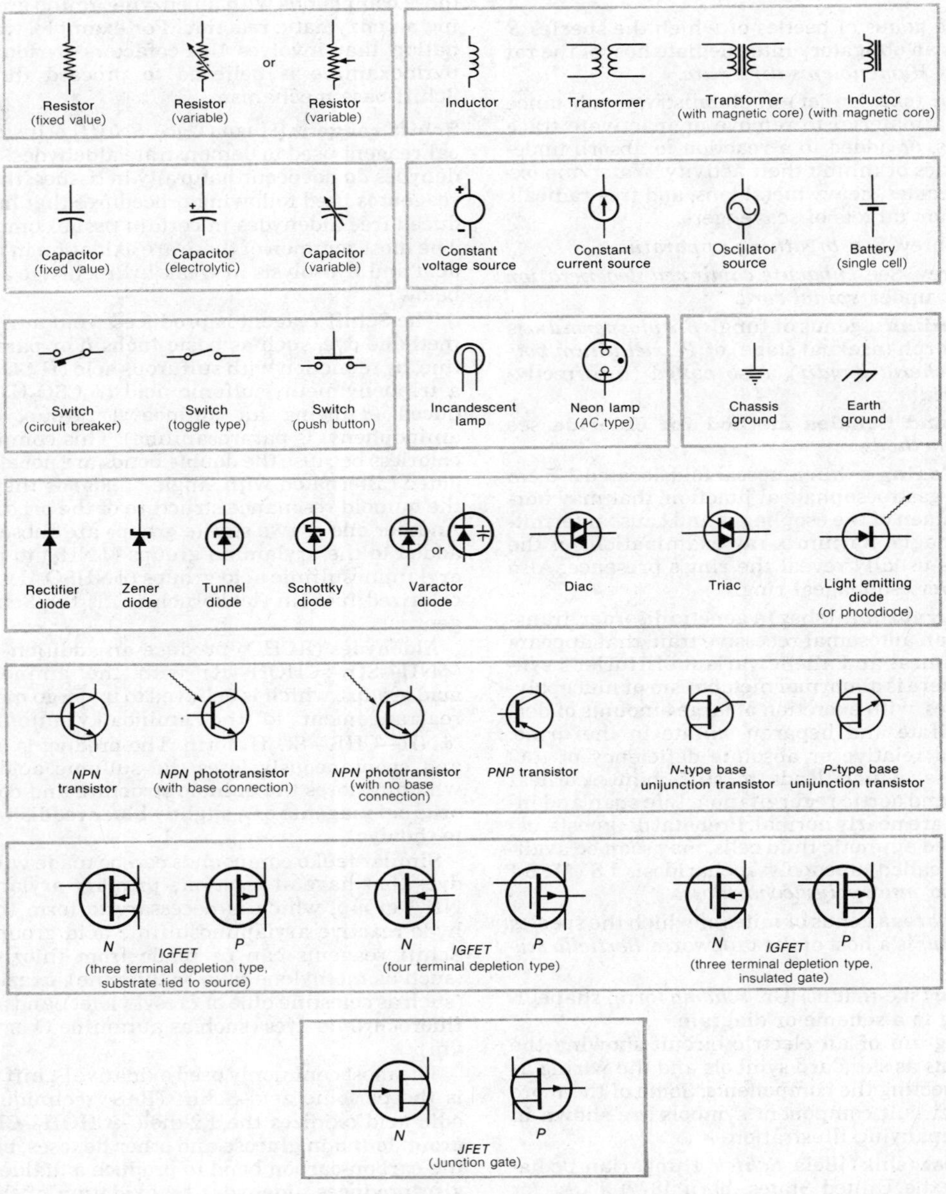

Schematic. **Common circuit component symbols. (Compiled from Diefenderfer, A. J.: Principles of Electronic Instruments. 2nd ed. Philadelphia, W. B. Saunders Co., 1979.)**

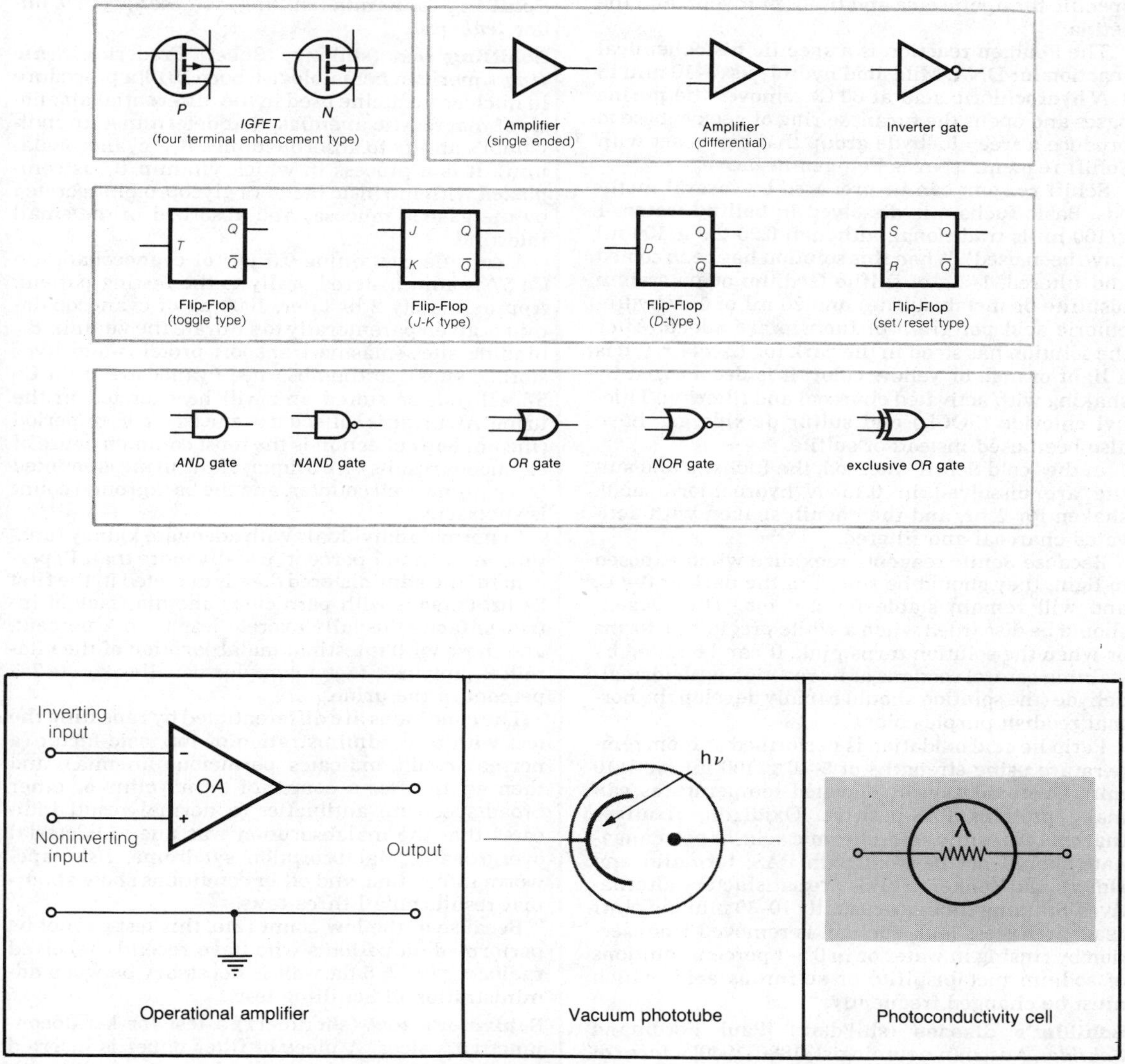

Schematic. (continued)

are especially reactive owing to PAS-positive proteoglycans and glycosaminoglycans (mucopolysaccharides) found in mucins, basement membrane, cell coats, and reticulum. Some glycoproteins, particularly hyaluronic acid and chondroitin sulfate (acid mucopolysaccharides), are PAS-negative. Glycoprotein hormones, such as follicle-stimulating hormone (FSH), luteinizing hormone (LH), thyroid-stimulating hormone (TSH), and thyroglobulin, produce the PAS-reactivity of thyroid colloid and the β cells (basophils) of the adenohypophysis. Noncarbohydrate PAS-positive substances contain glycolipids (such as gangliosides in the gray matter of the nervous system and cerebrosides in the white matter) or unsaturated lipids (such as lipofuscin pigments).

Because so many substances are PAS-reactive, blockade or enzymatic digestion techniques are used to obtain more definitive results. Acetylation esterifies the hydroxyl groups of 1,2-diols and 1-hydroxy-2-amino groups, thus blocking PAS reactivity that occurs owing to the carbohydrates. This distinguishes polysaccharides, proteoglycans, and glycoproteins from lipids. Glycogen is positively identified by enzymatic digestion with α-amylase (which is specific for glycogen), and diastase or ptyalin (which also digest starch).

Other oxidizing reagents have been used in place of periodic acid. These include chromic acid (the Bauer reaction), potassium permanganate (the Casella reaction), lead tetraacetate, sodium bismuthate, and hydrogen peroxide. Because all of these can overoxidize the aldehydes produced from carbohydrates to form unreactive carboxylic acid groups, they are rarely used. Performic acid and peracetic acid oxidize only the double bonds of un-

saturated lipids. Thus, the performic acid–Schiff (PFAS) reaction or peracetic acid–Schiff reaction is specific for lipofuscins and lipids of myelin and the retina.

The Feulgen reaction is a specific histochemical reaction for DNA. Mild acid hydrolysis (5–10 min in 1 *N* hydrochloric acid at 60°C) removes the purine bases and opens the furanose ring of deoxyribose to produce a free aldehyde group that can react with Schiff reagent. RNA is Feulgen-negative.

Schiff reagent can be prepared by several methods. Basic fuchsin is dissolved in boiling water (1 g/100 ml is traditional, although 0.25–2.0 g/100 ml have been used). When this solution has been cooled and filtered, 1–2 g of sulfite (sodium or potassium bisulfite or metabisulfite) and 20 ml of 1 *N* hydrochloric acid per gram of fuchsin are added. After the solution has stood in the dark for 12–24 hr, it has a light orange or yellow color; it is decolorized by shaking with activated charcoal and filtering. Thionyl chloride ($SOCl_2$) and sulfur dioxide gas have also been used instead of sulfite.

In the "cold Schiff" method, the fuchsin, and sulfite are dissolved in 0.15 *N* hydrochloric acid, shaken for 2 hr, and then again shaken with activated charcoal and filtered.

Because Schiff reagents reoxidize when exposed to light, they should be stored in the dark at 0–4°C, and will remain stable for 2–6 mo. The reagent should be discarded when a white precipitate forms or when the solution turns pink. It can be tested by staining control sections or by reaction with formaldehyde (the solution should rapidly develop the normal reddish-purple color).

Periodic acid oxidation is performed at room temperature using strengths of 5–10 g/100 ml for 5–10 min. Overoxidation or elevated temperatures can make proteins PAS-positive. Oxidizing fixatives that contain osmic adic, chromic acid, or permanganate should not be used with PAS; formalin and Helly's and Zenker's fluids are satisfactory alternatives. Staining times are usually 10–30 min in Schiff reagent. Excess leukofuchsin is removed from section by rinsing in water or in 0.5–1 percent solutions of sodium metabisulfite or sulfurous acid, which must be changed frequently.

Schilder's disease (shil′derz) [Paul Ferdinand *Schilder,* Austrian neurologist, 1886–1940] a form of diffuse sclerosis of the cerebral hemisphere that is characterized by the massive destruction of myelin. This results in bilateral spasticity, pseudobulbar palsy, visual field defects, cortical blindness, optic atrophy, and dementia. White matter cavitation and glial scarring are common. Of unknown cause, this disease primarily affects children and adolescents; most patients die within 1–2 yr, although some survive much longer. Schilder's disease may be a form of multiple sclerosis in some instances. Cases of adrenoleukodystrophy were originally included as examples of Schilder's disease but are now classified separately. Also called encephalitis periaxialis diffusa and Heubner-Schilder syndrome.

Schiller's test (shil′erz) [Walter *Schiller,* Austrian pathologist in the United States, 1887–1960] a solution of iodine used to detect lesions of cervical or vaginal epithelium. The solution is painted on the epithelial surface of interest. Normal areas, which tend to be rich in glycogen, take on a mahogany color. In contrast, glycogen-poor epithelium, such as dysplastic epithelium and carcinoma in situ, appears pale or unstained.

Schilling leukemia (shil′ing) see *monocytic l.* under *leukemia.*

Schilling test (shil′ing) [Robert Frederick *Schilling,* American hematologist, born 1919] a procedure in nuclear medicine used in the differential diagnosis of macrocytic anemias, that determines an individual's ability to absorb vitamin B_{12} (cyanocobalamin). It is a process in which vitamin B_{12} is complexed with intrinsic factor (a glycoprotein secreted by the gastric mucosa) and absorbed in the small intestine.

A capsule containing 0.5 μCi of cyanocobalamin Co 57 is administered orally to the fasting patient. Approximately 2 hr later, 1000 μg of cyanocobalamin is given parenterally to saturate the vitamin B_{12} binding sites (plasma transport proteins and liver storage sites), so the absorbed cyanocobalamin Co 57 will not be stored and will be excreted in the urine. All urine is collected over a 24- or 48-hr period (incomplete collection is the most common cause of erroneous results). An aliquot of the urine is counted in a gamma-well counter, and the background count is subtracted.

In normal individuals with adequate kidney function, more than 7 percent (usually more than 10 percent) of the administered dose is excreted in the first 24 hr. Persons with pernicious anemia (lack of intrinsic factor) usually excrete less than 2 percent, and those with intestinal malabsorption of the vitamin B_{12} intrinsic factor complex usually excrete 3–5 percent in the urine.

The conditions are differentiated by repeating the test with oral administration of intrinsic factor (a normal result indicates pernicious anemia), and then again after a course of tetracycline or other broad-spectrum antibiotics (a normal result indicates that the malabsorption was due to bacterial overgrowth). Malabsorption syndrome, fish tapeworm infestation, and other conditions show abnormal results on all three tests.

Because of the low count rate, this test cannot be performed on patients who have recently received radioactivity. A 5-da wait is necessary between administration of Schilling tests.

Schirmer's test (sher′merz) a test for keratoconjunctivitis sicca. A piece of filter paper is inserted into the conjunctival sac over the lower eyelid with the end of the paper hanging down on the outside. Deficient tear formation is indicated if the projecting paper remains dry after 15 min.

schist/o (skis′to) [Gr. *schistos* split] a word element used in combining form to denote split or cleft, e.g., schistoglossia.

schistocyte see *schizocyte.*

Schistosoma (skis″to-so′mah) [*schisto-* + Gr. *sōma* body] a genus of trematodes, commonly known as blood flukes. The three major species that are parasitic in humans are *S. haematobium, S. mansoni,* and *S. japonicum.* A fourth species, *S. intercalatum,* causes an intestinal form of the disease in persons living in certain areas of Central Africa.

S. haematobium, a species that inhabits the vesical and pelvic plexuses of the venous circulation and the veins of the lower colon and rectum in humans. This parasite is commonly found in Africa and the Middle East. The adult worms are diecious;

the males measure 10–15 mm long, the females about 20 mm. Also called *Bilharzia haematobia* and formerly called *Distoma haematobium*.

Infection results from contact with infested waters containing fork-tailed cercariae discharged by infected snails. In North Africa and the Middle East, the chief intermediate hosts are the freshwater snails of the genus *Bulinus*. In South Africa, the subgenus *Physopsis* is the common host.

The cercariae penetrate the skin and enter the blood stream. The young worms mature in the portal vein, where their metabolites cause an acute inflammatory reaction; they then migrate into the vesical and pelvic plexuses. The eggs of the mature female are discharged into the venules, causing trauma, hemorrhage, and fibrosis, and eventually calcification of the bladder wall. The incidence of bladder cancer is high in persons living in areas where this infection is endemic.

Laboratory diagnosis requires microscopic identification of the eggs (112–170 μm long by 40–70 μm wide with a terminal spine or knob on the shell) in the urine, feces, seminal fluid, or cervical smears.

S. intercalatum, a species that causes intestinal schistosomiasis. It is parasitic in humans and is found in West Central Africa. The male adult worms measure 11.5–14.5 mm long; the female worms, 13–24 mm.

Infection is caused by penetration of the skin by the cercariae, which are found in waters contaminated with infected snails of the genus *Bulinus*. The eggs, measuring 140 by 36.7 μm, are deposited in the mesenteric venules and break through to the lumen of the intestines.

Laboratory diagnosis requires identification of the terminal-spined eggs in the feces or in mucosal snips from the rectum. The eggshells are positive for Ziehl-Neelsen staining in histologic sections.

S. japonicum, a species that causes Oriental schistosomiasis, which is found in the Far East, including Japan, China, Taiwan, the Phillipines, Thailand, Laos, Cambodia, and Malaysia. The male adult worms measure 12–20 mm long; the females, about 26 mm. Also called *Oriental blood fluke* and *Sinobilharzia japonica*.

Human infection results from bathing or wading in waters containing cercariae that are discharged from infected snails of the genus *Oncomelania*.

The eggs, measuring 70–90 by 50–70 μm, are broad and oval and have an enclosed miracidium. These are deposited in the venules of the small and large intestines, and break into the lumen. The eggs may also be carried to the liver by the portal blood, causing abscesses and scars. The common clinical features of chronic infection are portal hypertension and ascites.

Laboratory diagnosis requires identification of the eggs in the feces or in a rectal biopsy speciman. Complement-fixation and intradermal tests are valuable when eggs cannot be found.

S. mansoni, a species that causes an endemic disease characterized by abdominal and dysenteric symptoms and splenomegaly. This parasite is distributed throughout Africa, the West Indies, and South America. The adult worms resemble *S. haematobium* but are smaller (the males measure 6.4–12 mm long; the females, 7.2–17 mm). Also called *Schistosomum americanum*.

Human infection is acquired by penetration of the skin by eggs while bathing or wading in water (contaminated from the feces of infected persons) that contains the eggs. The freshwater snails of the genus *Biomphalaria* are intermediate hosts.

Following the penetration of the skin, the eggs are deposited in the capillaries and venules of the large intestine or are carried to the liver by the blood stream. The intestinal wall becomes thickened, and polyps protrude into the lumen. Cirrhosis and portal obstruction develop, causing splenomegaly and ascites. Occasionally, the worms migrate to the spinal cord, where they deposit their eggs, producing lesions and resulting in paralysis.

Laboratory diagnosis requires identification of the eggs in the feces; they are lateral-spined with a yellowish-brown, transparent shell measuring 114–175 μ long by 45–68 μ wide. The method of choice for egg detection is the acid-sodium sulfate-Triton-ether concentration method. The modified Kato thick-smear technique is also used. If the eggs cannot be found and *S. mansoni* infection is suspected, the complement-fixation, intradermal, or circumoval tests may be diagnostic.

Schistosomatidae a family of trematodes (blood flukes), including the species *Schistosoma haematobium, S. intercalatum, S. japonicum,* and *S. mansoni*.

Schistosomatoidea a superfamily of trematodes including the family Schistosomatidae.

schistosome (skis′to-sōm) any member of the genus *Schistosoma*.

schistosomiasis (skis″to-so-mi′ah-sis) the condition of being infected with flukes of the genus *Schistosoma*. Also called bilharziasis. For more information, see the individual species under *Schistosoma*.

schistosomicidal (skis″to-so″mĭ-si′dal) destructive to schistosomes.

schistosomicide (skis″to-so′mĭ-sīd) any chemical or agent that destroys schistosomes.

schiz/o (skiz′o) [Gr. *schizein* to divide] a word element used in combining form to denote division, e.g., schizogony.

schizocyte (skiz′o-sīt) [*schizo-* + *-cyte*] an erythrocyte whose abnormal morphology is the result of the deformation of red cells and the adhesion of apposing parts of the red cell membrane. This occurs when erythrocytes are trapped in a meshwork of fibrin strands as in microangiopathic anemia, on valve prostheses, and in the uremic-hemolytic syndrome, disseminated intravascular coagulation, vasculitis, renal graft rejection, severe burns, and possibly other conditions. The irreversibly adherent portions of the red cell membrane are removed, presumably in the spleen. Also called *helmet cell*.

schizogony (skĭ-zog′o-ne) [*schizo-* + Gr. *gonē* seed] the asexual life cycle of Sporozoa, especially of the genus *Plasmodium* (the malarial parasite). Cf. *sporogony*.

schizomycetes (skiz″o-mi-se′tēz) [*schizo-* + Gr. *mykēs* fungus] 1. a group of bacteria that cause mycetoma. An actinomycetoma may be caused by *Nocardia, Actinomyces, Actinomadura,* or *Streptomyces*. Botryomycosis, a purulent granulomatous infection in some mammals, may be due to *Staphylococcus, Streptococcus, Escherichia, Pseudomonas, Proteus,* or *Actinobacillus*.

2. a term, formerly used in some classification systems, which comprises the bacteria (fission fungi).

schizont (skiz′ont) [*schizo-* + Gr. *ōn, ontos* being] a stage in the development of the malarial parasite (*Plasmodium*) following the trophozoite. When the trophozoite's vacuole is filled in, its ameboid motility is reduced; with its nucleus divided by mitosis, it becomes a mature schizont. The mature schizont goes through erythrocytic schizogony, dividing into erythrocytic merozoites.

Schizophora a series of flies of the suborder Cyclorrhapha of the order Diptera, including the families Drosophilidae, Chloropidae, Oscinidae, Calliphoridae, Glossinidae, Sarcophagidae, and Cuterebridae.

Schlemm's canal (shlemz) [Friedrich S. *Schlemm,* German anatomist, 1795–1858] a circular channel coursing circumferentially at the junction of the sclera and cornea, which functions to eliminate aqueous humor from the eye. Obstruction of this canal system results in increased intraocular pressure and eventually in glaucoma.

Schmidt-Lanterman cleft (shmit′ lahn″ter-mahn′) [Henry D. *Schmidt,* American anatomist, 1823–1888; A.J. *Lanterman,* American anatomist, 19th century] see under *myelin sheath.*

Schmitt trigger a type of bistable multivibrator used as a voltage discriminator or pulse shaper. The output is switched on when the input rises above the upper trigger level; it is switched off when the input falls below the lower trigger level. Thus, any input waveform is turned into a train of rectangular pulses.

Schmorl reaction see *ferric ferricyanide reduction test.*

Schüffner dots (shif′ner) [Wilhelm August Paul *Schüffner,* German pathologist, 1867–1949] numerous small, uniform, pink granules. Usually found in erythrocytes infected with *Plasmodium vivax* and *P. ovale,* they are absent when the organisms are *P. malariae* and *P. falciparum.* They appear orange-pink or pink when stained with Romanowsky's stain. The dots may not be evident in improperly stained slides and in cells infected with ring forms. Also called punctuation, Schüffner granules, or stippling.

Schüller position 1. a radiographic position used to obtain a submentovertical (basal, axial) projection of the skull. The patient is supine with the torso elevated and the chin extended. The central ray is perpendicular to the (nearly horizontal) infraorbitomeatal line and passes through the pituitary fossa (about 2 cm anterior to the external auditory meatuses).

2. a position used to obtain the verticosubmental projection (the central ray passes exactly opposite to the direction given above). The patient is supine with the chin extended.

3. a position used to obtain a semiaxial lateral projection of the mastoid process and petrous regions of the temporal bone. See under *Henschen position.*

Schultz-Dale test (shoolts dāl) [Werner *Schultz,* German internist, 1878–1947; Sir Henry Hallett *Dale,* British physiologist and pharmacologist, born 1875] an in vitro biologic test for immediate hypersensitivity. Tissue from the uterus or ileum of a guinea pig is passively sensitized with appropriate antiserum. When specific antigen is added to the tissue, the antigen-antibody complexes cause the release of histamine and other similar substances into smooth muscle cells, resulting in contractions.

Schwann cell (shvon) [Theodor *Schwann,* German anatomist and physiologist, 1810–1882; professor of anatomy at Louvain, and the founder of cell theory] a cell that during development wraps around a nerve cell axon to produce a sheath of cytoplasm, and in myelinated nerve axons, of myelin.

schwannoma (shwah-no′mah) a benign tumor of Schwann cells. It may arise intracranially, most often in the cerebellopontine angle from the eighth cranial nerve, or at any location in the peripheral nervous system including the roots of the spinal nerves. Histologically, the predominant appearances are parallel arrays of cells that are typically elongated with tapering cytoplasm (called Antoni type-A tissue) within which the nuclei are frequently arranged in a palisading pattern (Verocay bodies), or a loose-textured fabric of slender fusiform cells (Antoni type-B pattern). The tumor cells have long cytoplasmic extensions that often branch elaborately, contain longitudinally aligned microfilaments and varying numbers of microtubules, and are invested by a basal lamina.

Symptoms indicating the presence of a schwannoma vary with the size and location of the tumor. If the eighth cranial nerve is involved, there may be hearing loss; headache; disturbances of balance and gait; facial weakness, numbness, or pain; and tinnitus. Schwannomas may be unilateral or bilateral.

Also called neurilemmoma, neurinoma, and neurolemmoma, but schwannoma is the logical term. See also *neurofibroma.*

sciatic (si-at′ik) [L. *sciaticus*] pertaining to or located near the ischium; the term is used especially to refer to the sciatic nerve.

sciatica (si-at′ĭ-kah) [L. *sciaticus*] a syndrome characterized by pain that radiates along the distribution of the sciatic nerve (the posterior aspect of the thigh, postero- and anterolateral aspects of the leg, and into the foot). Paresthesias and weakness may also occur. This condition is due to a variety of pathologic processes that affect the fifth lumbar and first sacral nerve roots (which make up the sciatic nerve). Such processes include herniation of a lumbosacral disk, chronic arthritis, spondylosis, spinal neoplasms, and spinal fractures. The precise cause of sciatica may be difficult to localize, but radiography, computerized tomographic scanning, myelography, and electromyography may be useful.

sciatic nerve the thickest nerve in the body. It arises from the sacral plexus and leaves the pelvis through the greater sciatic foramen to run down the back of the thigh. Above the knee joint, it divides into its terminal branches, the tibial (medial popliteal) and common peroneal (lateral popliteal) nerves.

science (si′ens) [L. *scientia* knowledge] 1. the branch of knowledge that produces theoretical explanations of natural phenomena based on experiments and observations.

2. an area of such knowledge that is restricted to explaining a limited class of phenomena or to a particular type of theoretical models.

scientific (si-en-tif′-ik) pertaining to science.

scientific notation the expression of numbers in the form $a \times 10^n$, where a is a number greater than or equal to 1 and less than 10 and n is an integer exponent. To convert from scientific notation to regular numbers, the decimal point in the factor (a) is moved n places to the right (or if n is negative, $|n|$ places to the left).

scientist (si′en-tist) a person who is trained in the experimental techniques and theoretical principles of a science and who works to expand the scope of scientific knowledge.

scint/i (sin′ti) [L. *scintilla* spark] a word element used in combining form to denote a spark, e.g., scintillation, scintiscan.

scintigram (sin′tĭ-gram) a general term for an image produced by a rectilinear scanner or scintillation camera.

scintigraphy (sin-tig′rah-fe) a general term for a nuclear medicine imaging procedure.

scintillation (sin″tĭ-la′shun) [L. *scintillatio*] 1. a spark or a flash of light.

2. the perception of seeing sparks.

3. the flash of light produced by a phosphor or fluor when struck by a particle of ionizing radiation.

scintillation camera an imaging system used in nuclear medicine; see Figure 1 for a block diagram of the camera. Gamma rays, emitted by a radiopharmaceutical localized in certain tissues of the patient, are detected by their absorption in a large, thallium-activated sodium iodide crystal (about 12 mm thick and up to 420 mm in diameter). A collimator permits the gamma rays emitted from a particular point to reach only a small region of the crystal. Thus, the scintillations produced in the crystal when gamma rays are absorbed form an image of the distribution of the radiopharmaceutical in the patient. The image is the same size if the collimator holes are parallel, enlarged if the collimator holes converge toward a point in the patient, or reduced if the collimator holes diverge.

The light emitted in each scintillation is detected by a hexagonal array of photomultiplier tubes placed behind the crystal. There is one tube at the center of the crystal back, surrounded by close-packed hexagons of 6, 12, 18 tubes, etc. Most cameras have 37 tubes, as shown in Figure 2; some have 19 or 61. Each scintillation produces a large output pulse from the nearest photomultiplier tube and smaller pulses from surrounding tubes.

The outputs of the photomultipliers are preamplified if they are above the level of random circuit noise and are summed by five resistor networks. The Z output is the sum of all the photomultiplier outputs, being roughly proportional to the energy of the absorbed gamma ray. Because of statistical variations in the amount of light emitted by the crystal, in the fraction of this light that falls on each photomultiplier, and in the photomultiplier gain, monoenergetic gamma rays produce Z outputs varying

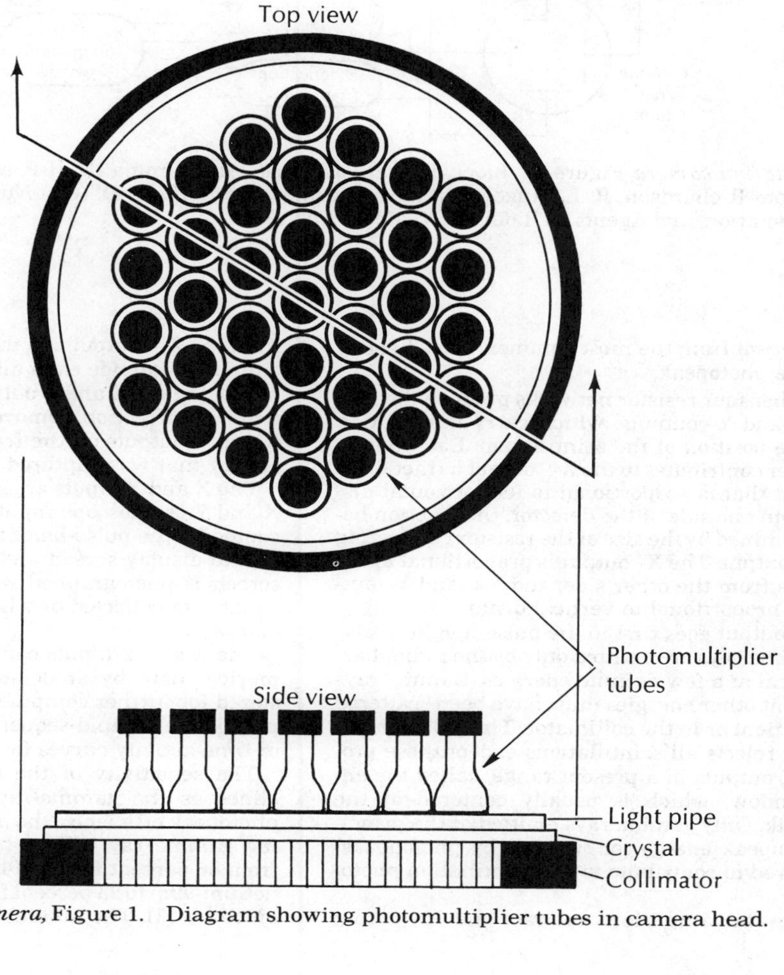

Scintillation camera, Figure 1. Diagram showing photomultiplier tubes in camera head.

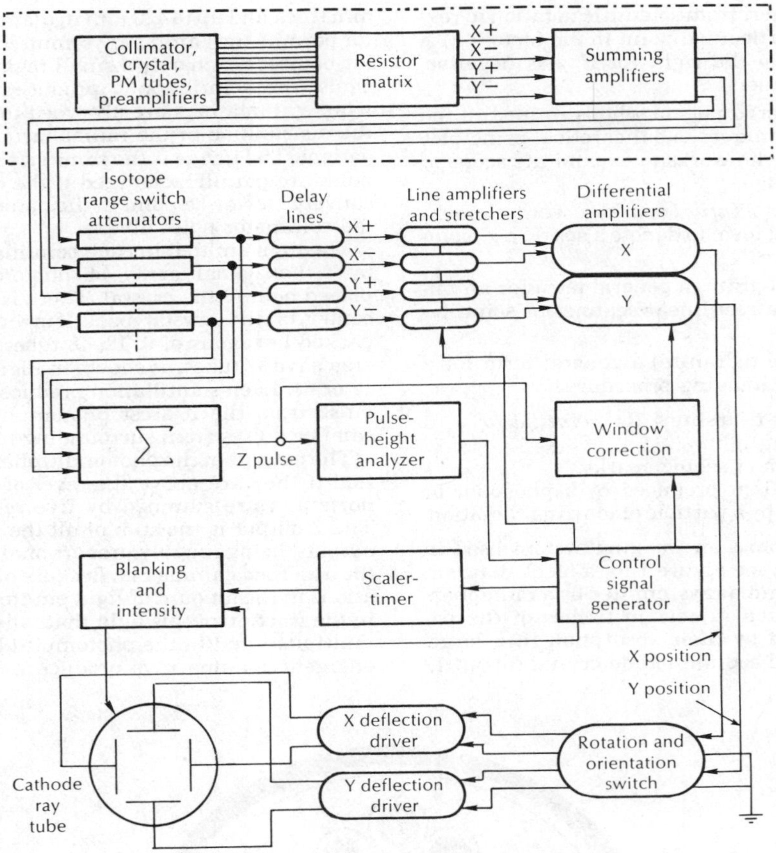

Scintillation camera, Figure 2. Block diagram of Searle Pho/Gamma III, H-P, and IV scintillation cameras. (From Richardson, R. L.: Anger scintillation camera. In Rollo, F. D. (ed.) Nuclear Medicine Physics, Instrumentation, and Agents. St. Louis, C.V. Mosby Co., 1977.)

10–15 percent from the most common pulse height, called the photopeak.

The other four resistor networks produce the X+, X–, Y+, and Y– outputs, which carry information about the position of the scintillation. Each photomultiplier contributes to the X+ output a fraction of its output that is proportional to its horizontal distance from one side of the detector, the fraction being determined by the size of the resistor connecting it to the output. The X– output is proportional to the distances from the other side, and Y+ and Y– outputs are proportional to vertical distances.

The Z output goes first to the pulse-height analyzer. Gamma rays are emitted only by the radiopharmaceutical at a few definite energies. Gamma rays detected at other energies must have been scattered in the patient or in the collimator. The pulse-height analyzer rejects all scintillations except those producing Z outputs in a present range, called the energy window, which is usually centered at the photopeak. Only gamma rays emitted at the principal photopeak energy (or two nearby photopeaks) are allowed to contribute to the scintillation photograph.

Differential amplifiers subtract the X– output from the X+ output and the Y– output from the Y+ output, and divide each difference by the Z output, producing the X and Y outputs. This process, called window correction, removes the dependence of the X and Y outputs on the fraction of the gamma-ray energy that was captured by the photomultipliers.

The X and Y inputs are generally used directly as X and Y oscilloscope inputs. Every scintillation accepted by the pulse-height analyzer produces a dot on the display screen and is counted. The display screen is photographed while a preset number of counts are collected or while a preset time interval elapses.

The X and Y inputs can also be converted to numerical data by analog-to-digital converters and stored for further computer processing, such as the production of rapid-sequence images or the plotting of time-activity curves for a region of interest.

The sensitivity of the scintillation camera declines as the gamma-ray energy increases. The photopeak efficiency, the probability that an incoming gamma ray will be totally absorbed, declines from 86 percent for the 140-keV photopeak of technetium-99m to 23 percent for the 364-keV photopeak of iodine-131. The inherent spatial resolution of the scintillation camera increases with the gamma-ray energy, because there is more light produced in each scintillation, and thus less statistical fluctuation in the responses of the photomultiplier tubes to scintillations. The inherent spatial resolution is maximal at energies above 300 keV and becomes unsatisfactory below 70 keV. At the 140-keV photopeak of technetium-99m, where the trade-off between resolution and sensitivity is optimal, most cameras have an inherent resolution of 5–8 mm (the full-width half-maximal value of the line-spread function).

The collimator's spatial resolution, which varies with the patient-detector distance and the type of collimator, has a range of 8–13 mm. Because these two factors combine like standard deviations, the overall resolution of the camera system is 9–15 mm (13–18 mm when scattering in the patient is also considered). When a focused collimator is used, the best resolution is obtained if the imaged organ is in the focal plane of the collimator. With the parallel-hole collimator, the best resolution is obtained when the collimator makes skin contact with the patient, because collimator resolution deteriorates with distance from the collimator face.

The scintillation camera can produce whole-body images with an accessory that consists of a moving table on which the patient is positioned and a circuit that moves the image across the oscilloscope screen in synchrony with the table movement. Although any particular point in the patient moves past the detector, a gamma ray emitted there is always recorded at the same point on the photograph. Because the camera's field of view is usually not as wide as the patient's body, two or three side-by-side passes are required.

Also called *gamma camera.* See also *collimator, computer data analysis,* and *quality control.*

scintillation counter a radiation counter used to measure gamma radiation in nonimaging nuclear medicine procedures, such as the venous thrombosis scan or the renogram.

The detector (or probe) is a thallium-activated sodium iodide [(NaI(Tl)] crystal attached to the face of a photomultiplier tube (PMT). Gamma rays absorbed in the crystal produce scintillations and the light produces an electronic pulse in the PMT. The pulse height is approximately proportional to the energy of the gamma-ray photon. The PMT output is amplified and goes to a pulse-height analyzer (PHA), a circuit that passes only those pulses corresponding to photons with energies within a present range (the energy window). A counter circuit records the PHA output. The energy window is usually set so that only gamma rays with the principal photopeak energy for the radionuclide of interest are counted.

scintillation crystal a solid-state scintillator used in the radiation detectors of scintillation counters, scintillation cameras, and rectilinear scanners. The most widely used scintillator for counting gamma rays is a sodium iodide crystal containing as a trace impurity about 1 percent thallium, which is referred to as a thallium-activated sodium iodide [(NaI(Tl)] crystal. Other scintillators, such as anthracene or plastic fluors, are used for beta-particle counting.

Low-energy gamma rays interact with the NaI(Tl) crystal primarily by photoelectric absorption; medium-energy gamma rays may undergo several Compton scattering interactions before escaping from the crystal or being absorbed in a photoelectric interaction. Both interactions produce high-energy electrons that travel a short distance, losing their energy by ionization, excitation, and collision processes. The deexcitation of the thallium atoms produces 3-eV visible light photons (410-nm peak wavelength). The size of the light flash is approximately proportional to the gamma-ray energy; 20–30 photons are produced per kiloelectron volt of energy absorbed by the crystal.

One face of the crystal is coupled to a photomultiplier tube (PMT) through an optical window having a high index of refraction to minimize reflection. The other faces are coated with aluminum oxide powder, which reflects light back into the crystal. Only about 30 percent of the light photons reach the PMT photocathode, and only about 15 percent of these produce photoelectrons that reach the first dynode. A 140-keV photon totally absorbed in the crystal produces only about 185 photoelectrons. The Poissonian statistical fluctuation in the number of photoelectrons reaching the first dynode is about 7 percent.

Because some gamma rays are not completely absorbed and some of the absorbed energy is lost as heat or x-rays, the overall variation is higher. The energy resolution of the large 0.5-in. thick crystals used in scintillation cameras is about 14 percent FWHM at 140 keV. The fraction of incident gamma rays that are totally absorbed (the photopeak efficiency) is about 86 percent at 140 keV and falls off at higher energies (to 23 percent at 364 keV).

Cf. *solid-state radiation detector.*

scintillator (sin'til-a-tor) material that emits flashes when struck by particles of ionizing radiation.

scintiscan (sin'tĭ-skan) an image produced by a rectilinear scanner.

scirrh/o (skir'o) [Gr. *skirrhos* hard] a word element used in combining form to denote hard, e.g., scirrhous.

scirrhous (skir'us) [L. *scirrhosus*] hard or indurated.

scirrhous carcinoma a carcinoma, with a particularly hard consistency, that reflects the prominent dense fibrous stroma supporting the tumor cells. The term is particularly applied to infiltrating intraductal carcinomas of the breast with these features.

SCJ abbrev. See *squamocolumnar junction.*

scler/o (skle'ro) [Gr. *sklēros* hard] a word element used in combining form to indicate hard, often used especially to denote the sclera of the eyes, e.g., scleritis.

sclera (skle'rah) [L.; Gr. *skleros* hard] [NA], the compact, fibrous, white outer tunic of the eyeball. It covers the posterior four-fifths of the eye, and is continuous with the cornea anteriorly and the sheath of the optic nerve posteriorly.

scleral spur (skle'ral sper) a short inward projection of scleral tissue in the anterior eye from which the ciliary muscle arises.

sclerema (skle-re'mah) a complication developing in severely ill, very young infants, characterized by hard, cold, yellow thickenings of subcutaneous fat. Infants suffering from diarrhea, severe infections, or marked prematurity are at risk. The changes are due to biochemical alteration of the highly cellular subcutaneous fetal fat. Also called *Underwood's disease.*

scleroderma (skle″ro-der′mah) [*sclero-* + Gr. *derma* skin] a connective tissue disease in which fibrosis occurs within multiple organs and in blood vessels; it most often involves the arms and hands, and Raynaud's phenomenon is present. Systemic involvement (systemic sclerosis) can produce a broad range of clinical manifestations, the most serious of which is the occasional occurrence of severe hypertension. In localized scleroderma, including morphea, linear scleroderma, and acrosclerosis, only the skin is involved. This form is more common in middle life and primarily affects females. The histology is dominated by the formation of excess collagen. The involved skin appears thick and tight with a diminution or loss of normal folds; the constricting effect of the encasing dermal collagen may in time produce secondary bone resorption and joint immobilization. These changes are particularly evident in the hands, where the radiographic appearance can be characteristic and even diagnostic.

The clinical course is variable. Chronic progression with occasional partial remissions may occur, but patients with systemic (e.g., pulmonary, cardiac, renal) involvement are likely to show more rapid progression that may continue to a fatal outcome. There is no specific treatment, but careful care of the hands is important to preserve their function and minimize the risk of infection and ulceration.

For the systemic manifestations, see *progressive systemic s.* under *sclerosis.*

scleromyxedema (skle″ro-mik″sĕ-de′mah) a variant of lichen myxedematosus that is characterized by a generalized eruption of the nodules and a diffuse thickening of the skin.

sclerosing (skle-rōs′ing) causing or undergoing sclerosis.

sclerosing adenosis (skle-rōs′ing ad″ĕ-no′sis) see *a. of breast* under *adenosis.*

sclerosis (skle-ro′sis) [Gr. *sklērōsis* hardness] a general term used to describe hardening or induration, especially when applied to hardening that is due to inflammation or the proliferation of connective tissue rich in collagen.

amyotrophic lateral s. (ALS), a degenerative disease characterized by muscle weakness, fasciculations, and wasting due to the progressive destruction of anterior horn cells, as well as spasticity and hyperreflexia due to lesions in the corticospinal tracts. Sensory perception and cerebral function are not affected. This disease usually affects adults over age 40 and tends to cause death within 2–5 yr, usually from respiratory complications.

bone s., in osteoarthritis, the thickening of the subchondral bone resulting from degeneration of the articular cartilage. The radiographic density of the bone is much greater than normal. Also called *eburnation.*

disseminated s., see *multiple s.*

multiple s. (MS), a slowly progressive disease of the central nervous system of unknown cause, usually beginning in early adult life, that is characterized by disseminated, patchy demyelination of the brain and spinal cord. It results in a variety of neurologic symptoms and signs that may relapse and remit over long periods. The nature of the clinical deficit depends on the location of the demyelinated regions.

A variety of etiologic agents have been implicated in MS, including slow viruses, but the precise cause remains unclear. An environmental agent may be involved in the pathogenesis, as the incidence of this disease is more common in individuals who have spent their early years in temperate rather than tropical climates, and migration after the age of 15 yr does not alter the risk. A genetic predisposition may exist, and the incidence of MS increases in those who possess certain HLA antigens (e.g., A3, A7, and B18).

The onset of illness can be precipitated by a variety of factors, including infection and trauma. In fully established cases, there are signs of CNS involvement at multiple sites. Slurred speech, nystagmus, ataxia, pyramidal weakness, optic neuritis, diplopia, and incontinence may all occur. Individual attacks may abate but generally leave some neurologic deficit. As further attacks take place, the degree of permanent disability increases. In fully established cases, the neurologic deficit cannot be explained on a single anatomic basis. The average duration of the disease may exceed a 20-yr period; the eventual course is downhill, but the time-course and the degree of ultimate disability are unpredictable.

Absent waveforms, reduced amplitude and/or prolonged peaks, and interpeak latencies in auditory, somatosensory, and visual evoked potentials often occur in the absence of clinical signs, and may provide evidence for a multiplicity of lesions when clinical signs are not evident. Thus, changes in evoked potentials, along with exclusion of other treatable diseases by appropriate tests, represent a means of early diagnosis as well as a possible means of assessing the results of treatment. No specific treatment for MS is available. Death is usually due to some intercurrent disease.

Also called *disseminated s.*

progressive systemic s. (PSS), a chronic disease of the connective tissue, characterized by diffuse fibrosis, inflammatory and degenerative changes of the skin and viscera, and vascular abnormalities. It usually occurs in persons aged 20–60 yr; females are affected two to three times more often than males. The disease may occur in a benign form that is compatible with a long life or in a rapidly progressive form in which visceral function is compromised and death occurs in a few years. The etiology is unknown, but associated serologic abnormalities have linked PSS to the rheumatic diseases.

The presenting abnormalities usually include Raynaud's phenomenon, gradual thickening and tightening of the skin of the fingers, and swelling of the distal extremities. Intestinal complaints or polyarthralgia may also be present. As the disease progresses, the skin becomes taut and shiny, and telangiectasias, subcutaneous calcifications, and flexion contractures of the fingers (sclerodactyly) appear. Dysphagia, peptic esophagitis, and sacculations of the colon may occur. Fibrosis of the lungs leads to restrictive and obstructive ventilatory disease; fibrosis in the myocardium can lead to cardiac arrhythmias and conduction disturbances. The abrupt onset of malignant hypertension is followed by the development of rapidly progressive and irreversible renal disease, a major cause of death.

Hematologic studies may show anemia. Urinalysis is normal, except in the presence of renal disease when there is proteinuria, microscopic hematuria, and increased numbers of casts. Mild hypergammaglobulinemia (IgG) is a frequent finding, as is the presence of antinuclear antibodies. Between 25 and 33 percent of those affected have positive tests for syphilis; positive LE cell reactions also occur. Pulmonary function tests may show increased residual volume and decreased maximal breathing capacity. X-ray examinations show esophageal hypomotility and diverticuli. Treatment has been attempted with dimethylsulfoxide (DMSO) and D-penicillamine; however, the inefficacy has not been proved. The prognosis is variable and depends on the degree of visceral involvement.

Also called *scleroderma.*

tuberous s., a genetic disease, transmitted as a dominant trait, that may be characterized by mental retardation, convulsive seizures, and adenoma sebaceum of the skin. Despite their name, the lesions of the skin are not true adenomas, but rather fibromas, appearing as pink nodules, especially over the cheeks, nasolabial folds, and chin. Other cutaneous manifestations include areas of hypopigmentation or subepidermal fibrosis, and subungual fibromas. Rhabdomyoma of the heart is an occasional accompaniment. Other malformations may be found in the kidneys, liver, and pancreas. Neurologically, there are local or generalized seizures and mental retardation. Obstructive hydrocephalus sometimes occurs and relates to abnormal gliomatous deposits. Neoplastic transformations of abnormal glial cells may be noted.

Radiographs of the skull may reveal calcified nodules. The cerebrospinal fluid is often normal, but the electroencephalogram is usually abnormal, showing single or multiple spikes, spike and slow-wave complexes, or slow-wave foci. CT scans may show deformity of the ventricular system and tumor deposits.

Also called *Bourneville's disease* and epiloia.

-sclerosis (skle-ro'sis) [Gr. *sklērōsis* hardness] a suffix word element to denote hardening, e.g., arteriosclerosis.

sclerotium (skle-ro'she-um) a hard, blackish mass of hyphae formed by certain fungi.

SCM abbrev. See *Society of Computer Medicine.*

scolecoid (sko'le-koid) [Gr. *skōlekoeidēs* vermiform] 1. resembling a worm; vermiform.
2. resembling a scolex; hydatid.

scolex (sko'leks), pl. *scoleces* [Gr. *skōlēx* worm] the attachment organ of a tapeworm from which the proglottids develop. The organ anchors the worm to the intestinal wall of its host.

scoli/o (sko'le-o) [Gr. *skolios* twisted] a word element used in combining form to denote crooked or bent, e.g., scoliosis.

scoliosis (sko"le-o'sis) [Gr. *skoliōsis* curvation] a lateral curvature of the spine. Most cases have no known cause; some may be associated with neuromuscular disease, pulmonary disease, and major thoracic surgery. There is a primary lateral curvature with a compensatory secondary curve in the opposite direction (as in the upper and lower halves of the letter S).

Diagnosis is based on physical examination with radiographic profiles. Compromise of pulmonary function rarely occurs. Treatment may consist of orthopedic appliances or surgical procedures.

Cf. *kyphosis* and *lordosis.*

S colony abbrev. See *smooth c.* under *colony.*

Scolopendra (sko"lo-pen'drah) [Gr. *skolops* anything pointed] a genus of centipedes. The venom of the species *S. cingulata, S. morsitans,* and *S. subspinipes* may cause a painful burning sensation in humans.

scop/o (sko'po) a word element used in combining form to denote examination (usually visual), e.g., scopometer, scopophilia.

-scope (skōp) [Gr. *skopein* to view, examine] a suffix word element to denote an instrument for visual examination, e.g., endoscope.

scopolamine (sko-pol'ah-mēn) an alkaloid, similar to atropine, that is extracted from plants of the family Solanaceae. It is used as an anticholinergic and antispasmodic and as a preanesthetic to reduce secretions. Also called *hyoscine.*

s. hydrobromide, [USP], a salt of scopolamine used as scopolamine.

Scopulariopsis (skop"u-la"re-op'sis) a genus of fungi belonging to the family Moniliaceae, order Moniliales, and characterized by penicillate conidial structures. The colonies appear wrinkled and powdery, and range in color from white to light beige to gray and brown. Microscopically, thick-walled conidia with truncate bases are produced on annellophores. The species *S. brevicaulis* sometimes causes onychomycosis.

scopulariopsosis (skop"u-la"re-op-so'sis) any fungal infection caused by the genus *Scopulariopsis.*

-scopy (skop'e) [Gr. *skopein* to examine] a suffix word element to denote examining, e.g., endoscopy, microscopy.

score (skōr) a rating, usually expressed numerically, that is based on specific achievement or the degree to which certain qualities are manifest.

Scorpio a genus of scorpions found in North Africa. These scorpions have neurotoxic venom and are extremely dangerous.

Scorpiones an order of scorpions, including the genera *Buthus, Centrurus,* and *Vejovis.*

scot/o (sko'to) [Gr. *skotos* darkness] a word element used in combining form to denote darkness, e.g., scotoma.

Scotch tape method a method for the recovery of eggs or female worms from the perianal region in humans. It is used primarily for obtaining eggs of the species *Enterobius vermicularis* (pinworm). The speciman should be taken in the morning before bathing or a bowel movement.

The sample is obtained by using a strip of Scotch tape, adhesive side out, which is held on a wooden tongue depressor or looped on a microscope slide. After a swabbing of the perianal region is taken, the tape is placed adhesive side down on a slide. A drop of toluene or xylol placed on the slide before the tape is placed may help in clearing. The slide is then examined microscopically for eggs.

Also called *cellophane tape method.*

scotochromogen (sko"to-kro'mo-jen) [*scoto-* + Gr. *chroma* color + *gennan* to produce] a microorganism that produces pigmented colonies that develop color in dark or light.

scotoma (sko-to'mah), pl. *scotomata* [Gr. *skotōma*] a localized region of impaired vision within the visual fields of one or both eyes. Scotomata may be due to lesions affecting the eye or optic pathway or any point along its course. Many diverse conditions result in scotomata, including CNS neoplasms, inflammation, and infections, and nutritional deficiencies. Diagnosis requires examination of the eyes and visual fields.

scotopic (sko-top′ik) pertaining to vision at a low level of illumination, i.e., in the dark. See also *scotopic vision.*

scotopic vision vision under night conditions, which depends on rod receptor functioning; colors are not well differentiated.

Scott's tap water substitute an alkaline solution, composed of sodium or potassium bicarbonate and magnesium sulfate dissolved in distilled water, that is used in blueing sections after staining with hematoxylin if the available tap water is acidic. Thymol crystals may be added as a preservative.

SCR abbrev. See *silicon-controlled rectifier.*

scratch-pad memory a computer memory, with short access time and small size, used by the central processing unit for the storage of temporary results.

scratch test a test for hypersensitivity in which a minute amount of the substance in question is inserted in small scratches made in the skin. A positive reaction is swelling and reddening at the site within 30 min. Scratch tests are used in allergy testing. See also *skin test* and *wheal and erythema skin test.*

screen (skrēn) 1. a thin sheet of material used as a protection or shield against light, x-rays, etc.

2. in radiology, a thin sheet of material coated with phosphors that emit visible light when excited by x-rays. See also *fluoroscopic screen* and *intensifying screen.*

3. an agent applied to the skin to protect against the sun's rays (a solar screen or sun screen) or other effects.

4. to routinely test an individual or segment of the population for a specific disease.

screen burn an area of damaged phosphor on an oscilloscope screen produced when a bright image is left on the screen for too long a time.

screen lag see *afterglow.*

screen speed in radiology, the amount of amplification of x-ray energy by an intensifying screen. It is usually a number that gives the necessary exposure time relative to other screens: the lower the number, the faster the screen. Screen speed is sometimes given as slow (or detail), medium, or fast speed.

scrofuloderma (skrof″u-lo-der′mah) [*scrofula* + Gr. *derma* skin] suppurating abscesses and fistulous passages opening on the skin; they are secondary to tuberculosis of the lymph nodes, especially those of the neck (scrofula).

scrotum (skro′tum) [L. "bag"] the fibromuscular pouch that contains the testes, epididymides, and distal portion of the spermatic cords.

SCS abbrev. See *silicon-controlled switch.*

scurvy (skur′ve) [L. *scorbutus*] a connective tissue disorder, due to a deficiency of vitamin C, that is characterized by the failure to form collagen, impaired formation of the osteroid matrix of bones, and a hemorrhagic diathesis. It most often affects older individuals and children between 6 mo and 2 yr who are lacking in supplementary vitamin C. X-ray examination of the long bones shows transverse thickening and increased density at the ends, followed by an area appearing as a small fracture medially. Evidence of subperiosteal hemorrhage is common. Capillary resistance is reduced, and serum and white cell ascorbic acid levels are lowered. Treatment involves the administration of ascorbic acids.

Scutigera a genus of centipedes, several species of which have been accidental parasites of the human digestive tract.

SD abbrev. See *standard deviation.*

SD antigen abbrev. See *serologically defined antigen.*

SDH abbrev. for sorbitol dehydrogenase. See *iditol dehydrogenase.*

SDS abbrev. See *sodium dodecyl sulfate.*

SDS–gel electrophoresis a technique in which charged complexes of protein with sodium dodecyl sulfate (SDS) are subjected to zone electrophoresis in a gel of uniform porosity, the rate of migration increasing as the molecular weight decreases. The relationship between the molecular weight of the protein and its mobility is linear, and can be used to estimate the protein's molecular weight. SDS denatures the protein and dissociates it into its subunits to form long, rodlike SDS-polypeptide complexes. For a similar technique, see also *SDS–gel filtration chromatography.*

SDS–gel filtration chromatography a technique in which charged complexes of a protein with sodium dodecyl sulfate (SDS) are chromatographed through a gel of uniform porosity used to estimate the molecular weight of the protein. Solutions of SDS serve as eluting solvent. This technique is similar to SDS–gel electrophoresis.

S. dysenteriae see *S. dysenteriae* under *Shigella.*

Se symbol for the chemical element *selenium.*

sealed envelope technique a method for assigning subjects admitted to a randomized clinical trial to the treatment and control groups. Serially numbered envelopes are used, which are opened serially as patients are entered into the trial. Each envelope contains a card designating the treatment assignment for the patient; the assignment sequence is arranged in random order, often in a permuted block design.

search (serch) in computer programming, the examination of the records of a random or ordered file until a record having a particular key identifier is found.

seatworm (sēt′werm) see *E. vermicularis* under *Enterobius.*

seb/o (seb′o) a word element used in combining form to denote sebum, e.g., seborrhea.

sebaceous (sĕ-ba′shus) [L. *sebaceus*] pertaining to or secreting sebum, as in sebaceous cysts.

sebaceous cyst a benign retention cyst of a sebaceous gland containing the fatty secretion of the gland. These cysts may occur anywhere on the body except the palms of the hands and soles of the feet; they are most common on the scalp, back, and scrotum. A sebaceous cyst may be a source of irritation or infection and may rupture if not excised. Also called *wen.*

sebaceous glands holocrine glands of the skin that secrete an oily substance, sebum. They are found in the dermis in most areas of the body other than the palms or soles. Secretion is under hormonal (particularly androgenic) control.

seborrhea (seb″o-re′ah) [*sebo-* + Gr. *rhoia* flow] excessive discharge from the sebaceous glands, forming greasy scales or cheesy plugs on the body. It is generally accompanied by itching or burning.

sebum (se′bum) [L.] the secretion of the sebaceous glands; a thick, semifluid substance composed of a mixture of lipids.

sec abbrev. See *second.*

sec- (sek) see under *secondary.*

secobarbital (se″ko-bar′bĭ-tal) [USP], a short-acting barbiturate used as a sedative. See also *barbiturate.* Trademark, *Seconal.*

s. sodium, [USP], the salt; given by injection or capsule.

second (sek′und) [L. *pars minuta secunda* the second small part (of an hour or degree of arc)] 1. (abbrev. s, sec), the International System (SI) unit of defined time, with the use of the cesium atomic clock, as 9 192 631 770 periods of the microwave radiation emitted in a transition between two hyperfine levels of the ground state of cesium-133. Note that the abbreviation sec corresponds to those for minute (min), hour (hr), and day (da); the official SI symbol for second is s (e.g., μs, m/s^2).

2. (symbol ″), one-sixtieth of a minute of arc.

3. (abbrev. 2nd), the ordinal number next in succession after first.

secondary (sek′un-der″e) [L. *secondarius; secundus* second] in organic chemistry, a term used in several contexts. A secondary carbon has two carbon atoms attached to it, as in R—CH$_2$—R′. A secondary substituent is one in which the point of attachment to the parent compound is a secondary carbon; it may be named with the prefix "sec-," as in sec-butyl (systematically named as 1-methylpropyl). A secondary amine is one having a nitrogen atom with two carbon atoms and one hydrogen atom attached. A secondary alcohol is one in which the OH is attached to a secondary carbon. See also *secondary structure.*

secondary active transport see under *active transport.*

secondary coil the output coil of a transformer.

secondary constriction a narrow region of uncoiled chromatin in the short arm of an acrocentric autosome (human chromosomes 13, 14, 15, 21, and 22) that separates the main part of the chromosome from the satellite. It is believed to contain the highly repetitive DNA sequence of the nucleolar organizer site.

secondary culture see *secondary c.* under *culture.*

secondary granule see *specific granule.*

secondary lysosome a digestive vacuole formed by fusion of primary lysosomes within a membrane-bound sac of material to be digested. See also *autophagic vacuole, heterophagic vacuole,* and *lysosome.*

Secondary Reference Materials see under *reference materials.*

secondary sex character see under *character.*

secondary structure the folding of part of a long-chain macromolecule (biopolymer) into an ordered structure such as an α-helix or β-pleated sheet; it is the result of hydrogen bonding between adjacent segments of the chain. The distinction between secondary and tertiary structure is somewhat arbitrary (see *tertiary structure*). Although the term usually is applied to proteins, it can be applied to other polymers, e.g., the cloverleaf structure of transfer RNA.

secondary x-rays x-rays produced in an object by the absorption of the primary x-ray beam. They may be produced by elastic scattering of the primary x-rays or by characteristic fluorescence of atoms from which inner shell electrons have been ejected by the primary x-rays. The secondary rays emerge from the object in all directions and produce a background fog on radiographs, which can be reduced by use of a grid.

second-order reaction see under *kinetics.*

second-set phenomenon the accelerated and intensified rejection by the recipient of a second graft of tissue from the same donor as a consequence of the primary immune response, i.e., antibody production and cell-mediated immunity, induced by the first graft.

secretin (se-kre′tin) a basic polypeptide secreted by S cells of the duodenal mucosa and the upper jejunum. It consists of a single chain of 27 amino acids (similar in structure to glucagon). The entire fragment is essential for biologic activity via a cAMP-mediated mechanism.

Secretin release is stimulated by intestinal acidification mostly due to gastric HCl, but fatty acids and amino acids can also elicit the secretory response. Secretin stimulates the pancreas to release a watery, alkaline, pancreatic juice high in salt (particularly bicarbonate) and low in enzyme content. It is also a potent inhibitor of gastric acid secretion and a weak stimulant for bile and intestinal secretion. The amount of secretin released is directly proportional to the amount of acid introduced into the intestines. Secretin release is maximal when the pH is less than 3.5 and does not occur when the pancreatic juice increases the pH of duodenal content to greater than 4.5; it is also inhibited by somatostatin from the hypothalamus.

Secretin stimulates pepsinogen secretion by the stomach, and stimulates bicarbonate and water secretion in the intra- and extrahepatic biliary ducts and by Brunner's glands. Its actions include the inhibition of smooth muscle contraction in the small and large intestines, stomach, and esophageal sphincter.

secretin test a direct measure of pancreatic function that determines the rate of bicarbonate output and the secretion rate of pancreatic juice in response to stimulation with secretin. The test is of value to demonstrate pancreatic dysfunction (e.g., in fibrocystic disease) and to aid in the differentiation of steatorrhea of pancreatic origin from that due to sprue or celiac disease. Over an 80-min period, normal individuals will secrete more than 80–100 ml of pancreatic juice, which in the first 30 min contains more than 15 mmol of HCO_3^-.

secretion (se-kre′shun) [L. *secretio,* from *secernere* to secrete] 1. the process of elaborating a specific product as a result of the activity of a gland.

2. any substance produced by the process of secretion.

secretor (se-kre′tor) an individual possessing the secretor phenotype.

secretor factor a hereditary trait, transmitted as an autosomal dominant trait, that involves the ability to secrete A, B, or H red cell antigens (ABO blood group antigens) in the saliva and other body fluids.

secretor gene (*Se*) a dominant allele that confers the ability to secrete the A,B. or H red cell antigens in the saliva. The recessive allele (*se*) has no known function. The secretor gene is linked to the Lutheran blood group locus and the myotonic dystrophy locus.

secretor phenotype an individual who secretes the A, B, or H red cell anitgens in the saliva. This phenotype corresponds to the *Se*/ *Se* or *Se*/ *se* genotype.

secretory (se-kre'to-re) pertaining to secretion.

secretory component a polypeptide carbohydrate complex synthesized by epithelial cells near mucous membranes; M.W. 70,000. It binds to the IgA immunoglobulin during formation of secretory IgA. Also called secretory piece and T piece. See also *immunoglobulin*.

secretory granule a small saccule pinched off from the Golgi membrane of an endocrine or exocrine gland cell, which contains a protein or hormone. The saccule fuses with the plasma membrane of the cell, and the contents are released from the cell.

The granules may accumulate in the cytoplasm, where they are a distinctive ultrastructural diagnostic feature. The caliber of the granules varies to some degree with the cell type. The largest (600 nm or greater in diameter) are seen in exocrine gland cells, whereas the smallest (150 nm or less) occur in small cell carcinomas, such as those of the lung, and in neuroblastomas and neuroendocrine carcinomas, where they are comparable with adrenergic synaptic vesicles. An intermediate size group is seen in the polypeptide-forming endocrine cells, which are often collectively designated APUD (an acronym from *a*mine, *p*recursor *u*ptake, and *d*ecarboxylation) cells. The granules in a particular cell type generally fall within a relatively narrow range of diameters, but in pathologic conditions such as hyperplasia or neoplasia the granules may vary more than normal or be smaller than usual. Granules in an actively secreting cell are smaller and fewer than those in a resting cell of the same type.

Most secretory granules are spherical, and in ultrastructural diagnosis they must be distinguished from primary lysosomes. A tumor should not be assumed to possess secretory granules unless they are present in many cells, are relatively numerous in at least some cells, and fall within a narrow range of diameters. The granules are ovoid, with eccentrically positioned cores in cells of a pheochromocytoma; the dense core may be crystalline in pancreatic islet β-cell neoplasms.

See also *gland*.

secretory IgA a class of immunoglobulin found in some of the body's secretions (e.g., saliva, nasal secretions, sweat, breast milk, colostrum). Each secretory IgA molecule consists of two four-chain basic immunoglobulin units, a secretory component, and a J chain. Secretory IgA is responsible for local immunity in mucosa and body secretions. The reference range for secretory IgA in saliva and tears is $\approx$5–10 mg/dl; in colostrum, $\approx$450. See also *immunoglobulin*.

secti/o (sek'she-o) a word element used in combining form to denote cutting, e.g., section.

section (sek'shun) [L. *sectio*] 1. an act of cutting.

2. a cut surface.

3. in anatomy, a segment or subdivision of an organ.

4. in histology, a thin slice of tissue prepared for microscopic examination.

section cutting 1. the cutting of routine paraffin blocks on a rotary microtome. Serial sections (usually 4–6 μm thick) are cut. The pressure of the knife edge joins the sections end-to-end in a ribbon. This is moved to a warm water bath (flotation bath) to smooth out wrinkles. The sections to be mounted are separated from the ribbon and picked up with a glass slide. Usually, the flotation bath contains gelatin, which makes the sections adhere more securely to the slide.

2. the cutting of plastic, ultrathin sections (about 70 nm) for electron microscopy or 1-μ plastic sections for light microscopy, using an ultramicrotome. See also *electron microscope*.

section freeze substitution technique a histologic method for preparing frozen, dried cryostat sections using quick freezing in liquid nitrogen and fixation in cold acetone. This technique is particularly good for the demonstration of water-diffusible enzymes.

sedation (se-da'shun) [L. *sedatio*] the production of a sedative effect; the act or process of calming of an individual.

sedation threshold in electroencephalography, a procedure sometimes used to define the relationship between intravenously administered amylobarbitone sodium and the integrated amount of beta activity (15–30 Hz) as recorded on the electroencephalogram. Although there are marked differences in the various psychiatric disorders, the individual variation is such that the technique has little, if any, diagnostic significance.

sedative (sed'ah-tiv) [L. *sedativus* calming] 1. calming; reducing excitement.

2. a drug that produces sedation; a central nervous system depressant used to produce sedation. This type of drug is also called a hypnotic or sedative-hypnotic. Cf. *hypnotic*.

sediment (sed'ĭ-ment) [L. *sedimentum*] a solid material that has settled out of a suspension or solution.

sedimentation (sed"ĭ-men-ta'shun) the act of causing the deposit of sediment, especially in a centrifuge.

sedimentation coefficient the speed at which a particle settles out of a solution (sedimentation velocity) divided by the applied accelerating field (in a centrifuge, the relative centrifugal force). The commonly used unit is the svedberg (S), which is equal to 10^{-13} sec.

The sedimentation coefficient depends on the density and shape of the particle. For spherical molecules, a sedimentation coefficient of 2S corresponds to a mass of about 10,000 daltons; 4S to 50,000 daltons; 8S to 160,000 daltons; and 16S to 400,000 daltons. For long, thin molecules the corresponding molecular masses are several times larger.

Sedimentation coefficients are not additive; for example, in ribosomal synthesis a 41S rRNA particle is cleaved to yield 23S and 26S particles. The sedimentation velocity is determined by observing the fall of the particles from top to bottom of an ultracentrifuge cell, using ultraviolet light absorption to visualize the particles.

Also called sedimentation constant.

sedimentation equilibrium a technique for determining the molecular weight of macromolecules, especially proteins, using the analytical ultracentrifuge. On centrifugation, the equilibrium distribution of particles is a characteristic for each protein and depends, among other things, on the molecular weight of the protein. The molecular weight may be calculated mathematically from sedimentation equilibrium data.

sedimentation rate (SR) the rate at which a sediment settles out of solution, as during centrifugation. See also *erythrocyte sedimentation rate.*

sedimentation techniques cytologic methods for isolating cells from small fluid specimens with a sparse cell population, e.g., cerebrospinal fluid. In one method, in which the fluid is absorbed by filter paper, the specimen is placed in a glass tube, which rests on a piece of hard filter paper on a glass slide. There is a hole in the paper under the tube opening. Weights placed on the paper slow the fluid absorption. If the rate is very slow, cells settle on the slide and are not drawn under the tube wall into the filter paper. The slide is stained and examined when all the fluid is absorbed.

sedimentation velocity-diffusion a technique for determining the molecular weight of a protein using the analytical ultracentrifuge. On monitoring the rate of sedimentation in a centrifugal field by one of several methods, the molecular weight is calculated by a mathematical equation that utilizes both sedimentation and diffusion constants.

sedoheptulose-7-phosphate the 7-phosphate derivative of a 2-ketoheptulose, a 7-carbon sugar; an important intermediate of the pentose shunt of glucose metabolism.

segmented cell a mature (polymorphonuclear) neutrophil.

Segmentina (seg″men-ti′nah) a genus of mollusks that may serve as hosts for the fluke *Fasciolopsis buski* in China, North Vietnam, and Taiwan.

Segmentininae a subfamily of mollusks of the family Planorbidae, including the genera *Segmentina* and *Hippeutis.*

segregation (seg″re-ga′shun) in genetics, the separation of allelic genes during meiosis when the homologous chromosomes on which the genes are located are passed to separate gametes.

Seitz filter see *Seitz f.* under *filter.*

seizure (se′zhur) 1. a sudden attack of a disease.

2. an epileptic fit, i.e., a sudden transient disturbance of cerebral function due to an abnormal neuronal discharge in the brain. The clinical features of seizures can range from loss of consciousness and jerking movements in all extremities, as in a tonic-clonic (grand mal) attack, to subtle changes in actions or behavior that may make diagnosis very difficult, as in an absence (petit mal) attack.

Seizures have numerous causes. In many cases (e.g., idiopathic epilepsy), the cause is unknown, although it is sometimes believed to be related to an earlier unrecognized injury to the central nervous system. Other causes include metabolic abnormalities such as hypoglycemia, hyponatremia, or hypocalcemia. Seizures may also occur in drug or alcohol withdrawal states, with infectious diseases involving the CNS, and with focal cerebral lesions (such as neoplasms, abscesses, hemorrhage, infarction, or scarring.

There are several types of seizures, which vary in their symptoms, severity, and response to treatment. Generalized seizures are the most common, involve both cerebral hemispheres, and are exemplified by tonic-clonic and absence attacks. In tonic-clonic convulsions, the individual often gives a brief cry as consciousness is lost, becomes rigid (tonic phase), and then exhibits clonic rhythmic movements of the extremities. Urinary or fecal incontinence may occur. Following the seizure, the individual recovers consciousness and may go into a period of sleep, has further convulsions without recovering consciousness (status epilepticus), or recovers consciousness and then has additional (serial seizures). In absence attacks there is a brief loss of external awareness accompanied by minimal motor signs for about 5–10 sec with no change in body tone. This type of attack is most frequently seen in children.

In contrast to generalized seizures, focal seizures initially show localized symptoms, although these may become generalized secondarily. In focal motor seizures, the tonic or clonic movements begin in one extremity and may spread to the rest of the body. In sensory seizure, a person experiences sensory symptoms in an extremity or has special sensory symptoms (e.g., visual). A complex type of focal seizure is the so-called psychomotor attack, which is frequently preceded by an aura that often consists of visual, auditory, or olfactory hallucinations. During the seizure there is generally an impairment of consciousness with loss of full awareness of external events, and there may be ideational disturbances.

In the diagnosis of seizures, a good clinical history is most important. In addition to a detailed description of the events during the attack, the age and the medical background of the patient are significant. Initial laboratory studies should include a complete blood count and determinations of serum glucose, calcium, sodium, and potassium concentrations for evidence of underlying metabolic abnormalities. An electroencephalogram (EEG) is extremely useful, as it often shows characteristic abnormalities. Skull radiographs, CT brain scans, and examination of the cerebrospinal fluid are used to document structural brain lesions, infectious diseases, and unusual CNS diseases.

febrile s., a convulsion occurring in a child younger than 5 yr during the course of a high fever. A few children with febrile seizures later develop epilepsy, but most do not. During the week after the seizure the electroencephalogram may be slowed, but epileptiform activity is found only occasionally. Paroxysmal activity subsequently develops in some individuals but is of little predictive value. Risk factors for development of epilepsy following febrile seizures include a family history of febrile seizures; preexisting neurologic abnormality; and an initial seizure lasting more than 15 min, recurring within 24 hr, or having focal features.

jacksonian motor s., see *jacksonian e.* under *epilepsy.*

Selas filter see under *bacterial f.* under *filter.*

Seldinger technique percutaneous arterial catheter technique, which involves the passage of a plastic catheter over a thin wire placed in the lumen of a vessel after needle puncture. The method is also used in radiology for the replacement of one catheter by another.

selection (sĕ-lek′shun) 1. a process that acts to change the gene frequencies of a population; see also *evolution*.

2. see *ascertainment*.

s. against dominant mutations, the selection against a harmful dominant genotype. Most deleterious dominant mutations have fitness values between 0 and 1. Therefore, individuals that carry dominant mutations reproduce less, and their offspring have reduced fitness. The mutation can be lost through selection at a rate proportional to the loss of fitness of heterozygotes. This occurs in genetic diseases, such as achondroplasia and Huntington's chorea.

s. against heterozygotes, the selection against the heterozygote genotype by loss of the alleles; the homozygotes are more fit. The relative frequencies of the alleles are decreased to a level lower than the frequency of the rarest allele. The Rh blood group system demonstrates such selection: for example, some Dd infants would die or be physically damaged if Rh hemolytic disease of the newborn were not treated.

s. against homozygotes, the selection against the homozygote genotype; the heterozygote is more fit than either homozygote in its given environment. A classic example of selection against homozygotes is sickle cell anemia. In tropical areas, sickle cell heterozygotes have more resistance to malaria than either homozygote.

s. against recessive mutations, the selection against a harmful recessive genotype. Complete selection against the homozygous recessives, to reduce the frequency from 0.10 to 0.05, takes 10 generations. Frequencies of recessive mutations, e.g., in genetic diseases such as cystic fibrosis and Tay-Sachs disease, decline only very slowly under selection.

coefficient of s., the measure of the loss of fitness (f); $s = 1 - f$.

directional s., the selection toward one extreme phenotype, not at the mean of the population. The concept of directional selection is basic to darwinian evolution mechanisms.

natural s., the process by which evolution takes place. Most species produce offspring in numbers greater than are necessary to maintain a constant population. Mutation and recombination produce a large degree of variation in the characteristics of members of a species. Those individuals that by chance are well adapted to their environmental niche are, on the average, more able to survive and to produce offspring than those less well adapted. Thus, genes that cooperate well with the rest of the genome to produce fit individuals become more prevalent in each succeeding generation.

Darwin defined fitness as "success in leaving progeny," but the term can also be explained in terms of differences in the physical, chemical, or biologic efficiency of individuals in coping with their environment.

Darwin's phrase "the struggle for existence" is often thought to mean direct competition between conspecific individuals for food, mates, and territory, and the struggle to escape predators and disease. However, the indirect competition of better adaptation to an environmental niche is, in many cases, more important—as with the tapeworm, which became well adapted to its niche in being reduced to little more than intestines and gonads.

selection pressure acting to produce changes in gene frequencies. See also *natural s.* under *selection*.

selectivity (sĕ-lek-tiv′ĭ-te) the ability of an analytic instrument independently to measure separate components of the sample. In gas chromatography, the term refers to the distance between peaks.

selectivity ratio see under *glass electrode*.

selenium (Se) (sĕ-le′ne-um) [Gr. *selēnē* moon] a nonmetallic, semiconducting element having several allotropic forms; atomic number 34; atomic weight 78.96; Group VI of the periodic table; oxidation states +4, +6, −2. It is chemically similar to sulfur. The electric resistance of selenium varies under the influence of light. Livestock feeding on plants grown in seleniferous soils can suffer cirrhosis of the liver, anemia, sterility, and emaciation as a result of chronic selenium toxicity. Selenium is an essential mineral (a constituent of the enzyme glutathione peroxidase); human deficiencies, however, are unknown.

Hydrogen selenide (H_2Se) (a gas with a disagreeable odor resembling garlic), selenium dioxide, and some other selenium compounds used in industry are highly toxic.

See also *selenium cell*.

selenium-75 (Se 75, ^{75}Se) a reactor-produced radionuclide that decays by electron capture to arsenic-75 with a half-life of 120 da. The principal energies of gamma rays emitted by ^{75}Se are 121, 136, 265, and 280 keV; the last two are generally used for imaging. Because of its long half-life, the radiation dose of ^{75}Se is relatively high.

selenium assays atomic absorption spectrophotometry that utilizes a urine specimen. The selenium, as well as copper and zinc, is complexed with sodium diethyldithiocarbamate. Copper and zinc complexes are first extracted into methyl isobutyl ketone under alkaline conditions; the selenium complex is then extracted under acid conditions, aspirated into an acetylene flame, and read at 196.1 nm. Normal concentrations in a 24-hr specimen are less than 150 μg/l.

selenocyte see *crescent cell*.

selenoid body see *selenocyte*.

selenomethionine Se 75 (sel″en-o-mĕ-thi′o-nēn) an analog of the amino acid methione, with selenium-75 replacing the sulfur atom, used in scanning of the pancreas and the parathyroid glands.

self-absorption in flame photometry, absorption of emitted radiation by other atoms of the same element, which causes low readings. Self-absorption is reduced by diluting the specimen.

self-contained breathing apparatus (SCBA) an emergency device for providing respiratory protection to persons who enter toxic atmospheres in which the concentration of toxic material is unknown but likely to be dangerous. Such an apparatus is needed by those who clean up spills of toxic solvents with hazardous or unknown concentrations, or who enter laboratories after fires or spills for search and rescue purposes. The device has a supply of breathing air, usually compressed in a gas cylinder, as well as a harness, regulator, and facepiece.

According to safety standards, two SCBA devices

plus spare cylinders should be purchased, and users should be medically qualified and provided with initial and periodic training and practice under simulated emergency conditions. Cooperation with local emergency services is also desirable.

self-dose in dose estimation, the radiation dose received by a target organ from a radioactive source localized in the same organ. See also *dose estimate.*

selfing (self′ing) continuous cross-fertilization between different proglottids of the same tapeworm.

selfwise (self′wīz) developing in a previously determined manner despite transplantation to a new and strange location; said of embryonic cells or tissue.

Seliwanoff reagent [Feodor Fedorovich *Seliwanoff,* Russian chemist, born 1859] a solution used as a color reagent for fructose, which contains resorcinol in diluted HCl.

sella turcica (sel′ah tur′si-ka), pl. *sellae turcicae* [L. "Turkish saddle"] [NA], a transverse, saddle-shaped depression containing the hypophysis. It is situated in the midline on the superior surface of the body of the sphenoid bone.

SEM abbrev. See *scanning e. m.* under *electron microscope.*

semantics (se-man′tiks) [Gr. *sēmantikos* significant, from *sēma* a sign] the meaning of the statements in any computer language. Cf. *syntax.*

semeiography (se″mi-og′rah-fe) [Gr. *sēmeion* sign + *graphein* to write] a description of the signs and symptoms of a disease.

semen (se′men) [L. "seed"] 1. any seed or seedlike fruit.

2. the thick, whitish secretions of the reproductive organs of the male. Semen is composed of spermatozoa and an array of mucoproteins, proteolytic enzymes, prostaglandins, acids, bases, and sugars that are produced in the prostate and seminal vesicles. Also called *seminal fluid.*

semen examination analysis of semen, usually part of a comprehensive investigation of both partners when the cause of suspected infertility is being sought. The gross examination includes notation of its physical characteristics, coagulation and liquefaction, and volume. Freshly ejaculated semen is an opaque, white, viscid coagulum, which spontaneously liquefies within 10–20 min to form a translucent, viscous fluid with a pH of 7.7. The average volume is 3.5 ml (normal range, 1.5–5.0).

Microscopic examination of sperm determines the count, motility, and morphology. Sperm count is determined with a hemocytometer, the reference interval being 60–150 $\times 10^9$/l. Sperm motility is determined by examining at least 200 spermatozoa, focusing throughout the full depth of a high-power microscope field; normally, at least 60 percent are motile. Sperm morphology is evaluated by performing a differential count on a Papanicolaou-stained smear; at least 200 spermatozoa are examined, the reference value being at least 70 percent normal, mature spermatozoa.

semi- (sem′e) [L. *semis* half] a prefix word element to denote half, e.g., semiconscious.

semiaxial (sem″e-ak′se-al) pertaining to a radiographic projection in which the central ray is neither perpendicular nor parallel to the long axis of the part; the angulation is usually specified.

semicarbazide hydrochloride a crystalline solid, $H_2NCONHNH_2 \cdot HCl$, used as a reagent for aldehydes and ketones, with which it forms semicarbazones; $RCHO + H_2NNHCONH_2 \rightarrow RCH{=}NNHCONH_2$, where RCHO is any carbonyl compound.

semicircular canal a part of the osseous labyrinth of the inner ear, one of the three bony, tubular extensions that arise from the recesses of the vestibule to form two-thirds of a circle and return to the vestibule. Each perilymph-filled canal is oriented at right angles to the two others, and is named superior, lateral, or posterior according to its relative position.

semicircular duct one of a series of endolymph-filled tubes, part of the membranous labyrinth of the ear, that loosely occupies corresponding spaces in the semicircular canals. The expanded ends of these tubes contain regions of specialized neuroepithelial cells (cristae) which, as part of the vestibular apparatus, are stimulated by the angular acceleration of the head.

semiconductor (sem″e-kon-duk′tor) 1. a crystalline solid that has thermal and electric conductivities between those of metals and insulators. At room temperature only a few thermally excited electrons are free to move like the electrons in metals; the rest are tightly bound to an atom. The conductivity increases with increasing temperature.

2. any one of the group of chemical elements that form semiconducting crystals at room temperature, e.g., silicon or arsenic.

extrinsic s., a semiconductor that is an almost pure crystal, a doped crystal usually of a tetravalent element (such as silicon), containing a very small amount of an impurity element (0.01–0.1 percent).

A pentavalent (or donor impurity) atom has an extra electron that does not bond to one of the four surrounding silicon atoms; this electron is free to carry electric current and increases the conductivity of the material.

A trivalent (or acceptor impurity) atom has an adjacent silicon atom to which it cannot bond. It can acquire a bonding electron from a neighboring atom passing on the deficit, a process called hole conduction.

intrinsic s., a pure substance that is a semiconductor, e.g., silicon or gallium arsenide.

***n*-type s.,** an extrinsic semiconductor that has been doped with a donor impurity. Electrons are the current carriers.

***p*-type s.,** an extrinsic semiconductor that has been doped with an acceptor impurity. Holes are the current carriers.

semiconductor device an electronic circuit component made from a semiconductor; usually a silicon or germanium crystal having regions of *n*-type and *p*-type doping. See also *diode, integrated circuit,* and *transistor.*

semidominance the production in heterozygotes of a phenotype intermediate between that produced in either homozygote, used especially for phenotypes not detected biochemically. Also called *incomplete dominance.* Cf. *codominance.*

semierect see *semirecumbent.*

semiinterquartile range (sem″e-in″ter-kwor′tīl) a measure of dispersion or variation of a probability distribution or a sample of observations; the difference between the third and first quartiles.

semilunar (sem″e-lu′nar) [L. *semilunaris,* from *semi-* + *luna* moon] resembling a crescent or half-moon, e.g., semilunar cartilage.

semilunar cartilage one of the pair of crescent-shaped fibrocartilages in the knee joint that rest on the articular surface of the tibia and are attached to the margins of the tibial condyles by coronary ligaments.

seminal (sem′ĭ-nal) [L. *seminalis*] 1. pertaining to seed or semen.
2. original, constituting a source.

seminal fluid see *semen.*

seminal vesicle (sem′ĭ-nal ves′ĭ-k′l) [L. *seminalis;* L. *vesicula,* dim. of *vesica* bladder] one of the paired sacculated pouches attached to the posterior part of the urinary bladder. The duct of each joins the ipsilateral vas deferens to form the ejaculatory duct. The slightly alkaline secretion produced here is rich in fructose and provides the bulk of the seminal fluid.

seminiferous (se″mĭ-nif′er-us) [*semen* + L. *ferre* to bear] producing or conveying semen.

seminiferous epithelium (se″mĭ-nif′er-us ep″ĭ-the′le-um), pl. *epithelia,* the stratified epithelium that lines the seminiferous tubules in the testes. Internal to the basement membrane, there are two populations of cells: supporting Sertoli cells and germ cells.

seminiferous tubule a delicate, contorted canal within a lobule of the testes. Spermatozoa develop from germ cells within its lumen. See also *testis.*

seminoma (se″mĭ-no′mah) [*semen* + *-oma*] a germ cell tumor that generally arises in the testes, but also occurs in extragonadal locations such as the retroperitoneum and mediastinum. It usually affects males over age 30 yr. Seminomas frequently are pure neoplasms, but they may be admixed with embryonal cell carcinoma or choriocarcinoma, or may form part of a teratoma. The tumor cells are spherical and of moderate size, with plentiful cytoplasm that contains sparse organelles but much glycogen. The cells form diffuse sheets devoid of any architectural patterns. Extension of a seminoma to the spermatic cord may be followed by retroperitoneal lymph node involvement and more distant metastases. Histologically and histogenetically, the seminoma is the counterpart of the dysgerminoma in the female.

semipermeable (sem″e-per′me-ah-b′l) permitting the passage of certain sizes or kinds of molecules and preventing the passage of others.

semipermeable membrane a membrane through which solvent molecules and some solute particles can freely pass, but which stops or hinders the passage of other solute particles. A strictly semipermeable membrane passes only the solvent, whereas a partially semipermeable membrane also allows some small molecules and ions to pass, yet stops passage of all macromolecules. See also *osmosis.*

semipronation (sem″e-pro-na′shun) the pronation of the hand or foot through an angle of approximately 45°.

semiprone (sem″e-prōn′) lying chest down with the head and hips rotated toward one side and the knees slightly flexed. Also called Sims's position.

semiquantitative (sem″e-kwon′tĭ-ta′tiv) pertaining to a numerical measurement having limited precision. Cf. *qualitative* and *quantitative.*

semiquantitative analysis see *semiquantitative a.* under *analysis.*

semiquinone (sem″e-kwin-ōn′) a free radical derived by careful oxidation of hydroquinones or by controlled reduction of quinones or quinone imines in basic solution.

semirecumbent (sem″e-re-kum′bent) approximately halfway between erect and recumbent, referring to a position in which the long axis of the part being radiographed makes a 45° angle with the horizon. Also called *semierect.*

semisupination (sem″e-su″pi-na′shun) the supination of the hand or foot through an angle of approximately 45°.

semustine (sĕ-mus′-tēn) a cancer chemotherapeutic drug. For more information, see *Appendix A.*

senna (sen′ah) [USP], dried leaves of *Cassia senna,* an irritant cathartic used in laxatives. See also *sennoside.*

sennoside (sen′o-sīd) either of two anthraquinone glucosides, sennoside A and B, extracted from senna. Sennoside is an irritant cathartic more powerful than casanthranol. The anthraquinones are absorbed in the small intestine and excreted in the large intestine, where they increase peristalsis by irritation of the mucosa.

sense (sens) [L. *sensus,* from *sentire* to think] a faculty by which the conditions or properties of things are perceived. There are five major senses: vision, hearing, smell, taste, and touch.

sense organ an organ that receives stimuli in different forms of energy, including light, vibration, chemicals, and pressure, and translates them to nerve impulses that are perceived as sensations. Such structures may be neuroepithelial, epithelial, or neuronal.

sense strand the strand of double-stranded DNA that codes for a gene product. The antisense strand is complementary to it.

sensibility (sen″si-bil′ĭ-te) [L. *sensibilitas*] susceptibility of feeling; ability to feel or perceive.

sensitivity (sen″sĭ-tiv′ĭ-te) 1. a state of acute or abnormal responsiveness to stimuli.
2. in clinical chemistry and toxicology, the smallest concentration of a substance that can be reliably detected by a particular assay method.
3. in nuclear medicine, the number of counts per second recorded by an imaging system per unit of activity in the field of view.
4. for a measuring device, the response to a signal input in scale divisions per unit of input.
5. referring to a voltmeter, the reciprocal of the current drawn by the meter in producing a full-scale deflection expressed in ohms per volt (Ω/V). It is used in calculating the input resistance; e.g., a multimeter with a sensitivity of 2500 Ω/V has an input resistance of 25 kΩ on the 10-V range.
6. the ability of a clinical test to identify correctly those persons having a disease; the conditional probability that a person with the disease will have a positive test result. Cf. *specificity.*

sensitization (sen″sĭ-tĭ-za′shun) 1. the initial exposure of an individual to a specific antigen, resulting in an immune response; subsequent exposure then induces a much stronger immune response. It is said that such exposure results in a hypersensitivity reaction.

2. the coating of cells with antibody as a preparatory step in eliciting an immune reaction.

3. the preparation of a tissue or organ by one hormone so that it will respond functionally to the action of another.

4. the modification of cell surfaces, as by treatment with trypsin, to make them more sensitive to participation in an immune reaction.

active s., the sensitization that results from the injection of a dose of antigen into an animal.

passive s., the sensitization that results when the blood serum of a sensitized animal is injected into a normal animal.

sensor (sen′sor) a device that measures a physical quantity, such as temperature, pressure, light, or sound level, and converts it to an electric signal that can be observed on a readout, recorded, or processed by a computer.

sensory (sen′so-re) [L. *sensorius*] pertaining to sensation.

sensory epithelium the epithelium of a sensory end organ, e.g., olfactory epithelium.

sensory ganglion (sen′so-re gang′gle-on), pl. *ganglia* [L. *sensorius;* Gr. "knot"] a group of sensory nerve cell bodies located outside the central nervous system, which function to receive and transmit sensory impulses.

sensory receptor the specialized peripheral termination of a sensory axon that is concerned with the transduction of various energy forms into neural impulses.

sentinel node an enlarged supraclavicular node containing metabolic carcinoma that is often the first sign of an abdominal carcinoma. Also called *signal node* and *Virchow's node.*

SEP abbrev. for somatosensory evoked potential. See *somatosensory e. p.* under *evoked potential.*

separatory funnel a funnel, with a stopper at the top of the cone and a stopcock at the bottom, used for solvent extractions. Two immiscible solvents are shaken together, which separate on standing; the dissolved solutes are partitioned according to their solubilities in each solvent. The lower layer is then drained out (separated from the upper lobe) by opening the stopcock.

Sephadex (sef′ah-deks) trademark. See *dextran.*

seps/o (sep′so) [Gr. *sēpsis* decay] a word element used in combining form to denote infection, e.g., sepsis, septicemia.

Sepsidae a family of flies that may cause intestinal myiasis in humans.

sepsis (sep′sis) [Gr. *sēpsis* decay] see *septicemia.*

septal (sep′tal) pertaining to a septum, especially the septa of the heart.

septal defect an abnormal opening in the septum of the heart that forms a direct passage between the right and left chambers. See also *atrial septal defect* and *ventricular septal defect.*

septate (sep′tāt) divided by a septum.

septic (sep′tik) [L. *septicus;* Gr. *sēptikos*] characterized by septicemia.

septicemia (sep″tĭ-se′me-ah) [*septic* + Gr. *haima* blood] a systemic infectious condition caused by pathogenic microorganisms (bacteria, fungi, parasites, viruses) or their by-products (endotoxins, exotoxins, or enzymes) in the blood. Clinical symptoms include chills, fever, malaise, hyperventilation, and prostration. Often the septic individual has an occult infection in the body, evidence that the microorganisms have multiplied despite any immune response; eventually, these microorganisms become disseminated and appear in the blood stream. Septicemia, which should not be confused with bacteremia, is a serious condition that, if unsuccessfully treated, can lead to renal failure, vascular collapse, disseminated intravascular coagulation, and death. In septicemia, organisms may be transported to various tissues where they may seed new sites of infection, resulting in such conditions as arteritis, meningitis, and pyelonephritis.

In the blood, endotoxin, a lipopolysaccharide from the outer membrane of gram-negative bacteria, causes fever, chills, hypotension, and septic shock; minute (nanogram) quantities can produce these effects. Owing to their large molecular weight ($>10^6$), endotoxins are not cleared by the glomeruli of the kidneys and must be removed by the reticuloendothelial system (macrophages). The various enzymes and toxins produced by gram-positive bacteria (streptococci and staphylococci) can result in a similar clinical picture.

Viruses, fungi, parasites, and bacteria often enter the blood stream after trauma or a mild infection, causing a transient bacteremia. This situation is usually cleared up promptly by the host's immune system. Only under conditions of a more severe infectious process or an impaired immune system does the bacteremia persist and septicemia develop.

Because of the serious outcome of unsuccessful treatment, precise identification, of the etiologic agent and its antibiotic susceptibilities are most important. Several (as many as six) blood cultures should be collected aseptically as soon as possible after the onset of chills. Leukocytosis usually accompanies a bacterial infection. In general, polymorphonuclear leukocytes are associated with bacteria and monocytes, and macrophages, with viruses. The blood cultures should be incubated at 37°C, both aerobically and anaerobically, for at least 7 da. For patients with subacute bacterial endocarditis, blood cultures should be kept for 14 da.

The premature and indiscriminate use of antimicrobial therapy before necessary laboratory test samples are collected may delay the initiation of specific antimicrobial treatment. Sometimes blood cultures are negative, although the patient shows clincial signs of septicemia. This may be due to growth-inhibitory factors in the blood, the inability of a microorganism to escape from a local infection, or a drug fever that mimics septicemia.

See also *bacteremia, disseminated intravascular coagulation, endotoxinemia, fungemia, parasitemia, septic shock, toxemia,* and *viremia.*

Septra trademark for a combination of *sulfamethoxazole* and *trimethoprim.*

septum (sep′tum), pl. *septa* [L.] 1. [NA], in anatomy, a general term for a dividing wall or partition.

2. in mycology, the wall that sometimes divides fungal hyphae, resulting in multicellular hyphae.

3. in nuclear medicine, the lead wall between holes of a multihole collimator for a scintillation camera.

4. in instrumentation analysis, the rubber covering of the injection port of a gas chromatograph.

5. in bacteriology, the wall formed during cell division that divides the parent cell into two daughter cells. Also called *cross wall.*

alveolar s., the partition that separates adjacent pulmonary alveoli. It is formed by the alveolar lining cells (pneumocytes) of each alveolus, their basal laminae, and a slender sheet of intervening collagen with a few fibroblasts, some macrophages, and a network of capillaries. The partition is perforated by pores of Kohn.

atrioventricular s., the combined interatrial and interventricular septa that together separate the right and left sides of the heart.

deviated s., the alteration of the normal structure of the nasal septum by developmental irregularities or trauma. Obstruction, infections (especially sinusitis), and bleeding are common complications.

interatrial s., the partition between the right and left atria of the heart.

intermuscular s., a sheet of deep fascia intervening between groups of limb muscles.

interventricular s., the partition between the right and left ventricles of the heart.

s. lucidum, a vertical median partition between the lateral ventricles of the brain. Consisting of a portion of laminae separated by a slender cavity, the septum lucidum separates their anterior horns and central portions. Also called *s. pellucidum.*

nasal s., the thin sheet of cartilage covered by mucosa that separates the right and left sides of the nasal cavity.

s. pellucidum, see *s. lucidum.*

s. primum, in the embryonic heart, a partition that develops to partially separate the right and left atria. See also *s. secundum.*

rectovesical s., a sheet of fascia that extends from the peritoneum, forming the floor of the rectovesical pouch, to the perineal body. It separates the lower part of the rectum from the seminal vesicles and vasa deferentia and from the prostate, and fuses with the fascia covering the prostate.

scrotal s., a partition that separates the two halves of the scrotal sac.

s. secundum, in the embryonic heart, a partition that develops following the appearance of the septum primum. It is an incomplete partition, with a free inferior margin, that lies alongside the septum primum and eventually fuses with it. Imperfect fusion results in the creation of an interatrial septal defect.

s. spurium, in the embryonic heart, a fold formed at the sinoatrial orifice by fusion of the right and left venous valves; ultimately it becomes incorporated into the interatrial septum.

tracheoesophageal s., in the embryo, the respiratory diverticulum (lung bud) develops from the anterior wall of the foregut and grows downward in the mesoderm; the partition separating the two is the trachoeseophageal septum. Normally they retain patency only at the entrance to the larynx, but occassionally the distal esophagus communicates with the trachea just above its bifurcation, forming a trachoesophageal fistula. See also *esophageal a.* under *atresia* and *tracheoesophageal f.* under *fistula.*

s. transversum, in the embryo, a thickened sheet of mesoderm and muscle that separates the foregut from the body wall contributes to the formation of the pericardium and diaphragm.

urorectal s., in the embryo, a partition that forms to divide the cloaca into an anterior portion, the primitive urogenital sinus, and a posterior part, the anorectal canal.

sequela (se-kwel′lah), pl. *sequelae*[L.] a morbid condition that follows or occurs as a consequence of another condition or event, e.g., nephritis following streptococcal pharyngitis.

sequence (se′kwens) a connected series of items or events.

sequential pertaining to a sequence.

sequential access pertaining (1) to a computer storage device, such as magnetic tape, from which data are recalled in the order that they were stored or (2) to file residence on such a device from which records must be recalled in sequence. Cf. *direct access.*

sequential analysis a statistical technique in which the sample size is not fixed in advance. As each observation is collected, a decision is made either to collect more data or to stop data collection and decide whether to reject the null hypothesis. In an open design, the experiment can continue indefinitely, whereas in a restricted design, the maximum possible size is known at the start.

sequestered antigen an antigenic determinant that is physically hidden so that it cannot combine with antibody or elicit an immune response to make specific antibody.

Ser abbrev. See *serine.*

Serentil trademark. See *mesoridazine besylate.*

Sereny test a test to determine the ability of a bacterium to invade tissue. The organism is inoculated into the eye of a guina pig; invasiveness is determined by the organism's ability to produce conjunctivitis. The test is used particularly for determining the invasiveness of strains of *Escherichia coli* and *Listeria monocytogenes.*

serial (se′re-al) arranged in or forming a series.

serial data transmission the transmission of data over a single transmission line as a train of pulses. See *asynchronous data transmission* and *synchronous data transmission.*

serial films a series of radiographs of the same aspect of the same structure (either a rapid sequence or one taken over a period of days or weeks).

serial operation in digital logic circuitry, the processing of one item (e.g., bit, word, line, channel) at a time.

serial printer see *typewriter terminal.*

Sericopelma a genus of spiders found in tropical America. The species *S. communis* is a large black spider that has a painful but not dangerous bite, the effects of which are local, not general.

series (sēr′ez) [L. "row"] 1. a group of objects that are related in a sequential order either by temporal succession or by a regularly varying one-dimensional characteristic.

2. in mathematics, the sum of an ordered set of numbers. The sum of an infinite series is the limit of the sequence of partial sums.

series circuit an electric circuit in which the components are connected in series, i.e., in which the current flows through each component in turn. The current is the same in all components, and the sum of the voltage drops across the components is the applied voltage. Resistors connected in series are equivalent to one resistor having the sum of their resistances; inductances add in the same way. Capacitors connected in series combine differently, however. The reciprocal of the equivalent capacitance is the sum of the reciprocals of the individual capacitances ($1/C_{eq} = 1/C_1 + 1/C_2 + \ldots$). Cf. *parallel circuit.*

serine (Ser or S) (ser′ēn) [L. *sericus* silken] 2-amino-3-hydroxypropanoic acid, $HOCH_2CH(NH_2)COOH$, a naturally occurring, nonessential amino acid; M.W. 105.09. It may be synthesized from glucose and is interconvertible with glycine. Serine is a substrate in the formation of cystathionine. Present in many proteins, it provides a side-chain hydroxyl group, which permits modification of the protein by phosphorylation or glycosylation. Serine can provide carbons for the one-carbon pool. It is used as a dietary supplement and feed additive, in biologic studies and tests, and in culture media. See also under *amino acids.*

seroconversion (se″ro-kon-ver′shun) the development of detectable antibodies in the serum as a result of infection, vaccine administration, or previous exposure to an antigen.

serodiagnosis (se″ro-di″ag-no′sis) a diagnosis determined from the analysis of various reactions in blood serum. One common type utilizes the detection of antigens or antibodies in serum for the diagnosis of infectious disease and other immunologic diseases.

serologic (se″ro-loj′ik) pertaining to serology.

serologically defined (SD) antigen an antigen present on the membranes of most mammalian cells, as the genes of the major histocompatibility complex control the expression of this antigen. This antigen can be identified with appropriate antibody. In contrast, LD antigens are detected by cellular typing reactions.

serologic test for syphilis (STS) any of a number of tests for syphilis performed on serum, including the VDRL, RPR (rapid plasma reagin), and fluorescent treponemal antibody–absorbed (FTA–ABS) tests.

serology (se-rol′o-je) [*serum* + *-logy*] the study of antigen-antibody reactions, using a variety of immunologic methods. Originally, the term denoted the study of antibodies to infectious agents, but it is currently used in a broader context to include most antibody-mediated reactions.

seroma (sēr-o′mah) a collection of serosanguineous fluid in the body, which produces a tumorlike mass.

α_1-seromucoid (se″ro-mu′koid) see *orosomucoid.*

seronegative (se″ro-neg′ah-tiv) showing negative results on serologic examination, commonly used to refer to negative reactions to the VDRL test and similar tests for syphilis.

serophilic (se″ro-fil′ik) a term used to describe a bacterium whose growth is enhanced in the presence of serum.

seropositive (se″ro-poz′ĭ-tiv) showing positive results on serologic examination.

serotonin (ser″o-to′nin) 3-(2-aminoethyl)-5-hydroxyindole, a powerful vasoconstrictor and a metabolite of L-tryptophane; M.W. 176.21. Formed primarily in the enterochromaffin cells of the gastrointestinal mucosa, serotonin can also be found in serum and many tissues of the body, including platelets, pineal gland, lungs, and central nervous system. It is stored and transported by platelets and is released on platelet aggregation.

In addition to its vasoconstrictor function, serotonin aids in blood coagulation, possesses neurotransmitter activity, and stimulates prolactin and growth hormone release. It is a stimulant for smooth muscle contraction and may be involved in the peristaltic reflex.

Serotonin is converted to melatonin in the pineal gland, is oxidized in the lungs to 5-hydroxyindoleacetic acid (5-HIAA, its primary end-stage metabolite), and is excreted as such. Owing to its instability in sampling and its occurrence in small quantities (0.05–0.3 μg/l of blood), changes in serotonin output are usually evaluated by assaying changes in urine 5-HIAA output.

Blood serotonin levels are elevated (0.5–2.7 μg/l) in persons with metastatic carcinoid tumors (argentaffinomas); smaller increases are seen in those with nontropical sprue and as a result of release from tissues by the drug reserpine. Serotonin levels are depressed in conditions of renal insufficiency, Down's syndrome, and (occasionally) phenylketonuria.

Also called *5-hydroxytryptamine (5-HT).* See also *5-hydroxyindoleacetic acid.*

serotonin assays the quantitation of serotonin, used for the confirmation of a carcinoid tumor, is generally done by measuring the urinary excretion of 5-hydroxyindole acetic acid (5-HIAA), the major metabolite of serotonin. See also *5-hydroxyindole acetic acid assay.*

serotype (se′ro-tīp) the type of a microorganism or bacterium as determined by the kinds of antigens present in the cell. Serotyping is performed by reactions with specific antiserum and is frequently used for the identification of species within a bacterial genus, e.g., *Salmonella.*

serous (se′rus) [L. *serosus*] 1. pertaining to serum; thin and watery, like serum.
2. producing or containing serum.

serous cell a roughly cuboidal cell associated with an acinar lumen, found in the salivary glands. Serous cells secrete a watery, albuminous fluid that is rich in proteins and contains enzymes.

serous fluid the normal fluid in a serous cavity, such as the pleural, pericardial, and peritoneal cavities. See also *pericardial fluid, peritoneal fluid,* and *pleural fluid.*

serous gland an aggregation of cells that produce a watery, albuminous secretion that often contains enzymes. See also *serous cell.*

serpent infection see *dracunculiasis.*

serpent worm see *D. medinensis* under *Dracunculus.*

serrate (ser′āt) [L. *serratus,* from *serra* saw] having a jagged, saw-toothed edge or margin. Also called serrated.

Serratia (sĕ-ra′she-ah) [named for Serafino *Serrati,* an Italian physicist of the 18th century] a genus of bacteria in the family Enterobacteriaceae, which consists of gram-negative, facultatively anaerobic motile rods. The organisms are DNAase-positive, and some strains produce pink-to-red pigments. Most strains do not ferment lactose or do so slowly. Serotyping and bacteriocin typing are used also for species identification. The organisms are opportunistic pathogens and cause infections of the endocardium, blood, wounds, and urinary and respiratory tracts. The infections frequently are due to contaminated equipment or personnel and usually occur in otherwise debilitated individuals. Three species are recognized, *S. marcescens* being by far the most commonly encountered in clinical specimens. See also *Enterobacteriaceae.*

S. liquefaciens, a species that ferments sorbitol, arabinose, and raffinose, and is positive for ornithine decarboxylase.

S. marcescens, the type species; by classic description it produces a bright red pigment, but most clinical isolates are nonpigmented. Sorbitol is fermented but not arabinose, raffinose, or rhamnose; it is positive for ornithine decarboxylase.

Because of its hardy nature and comparative resistance to the commonly used antibiotics, *S. marcescens* has become an important cause of nosocomial infections in the last decade. Outbreaks of epidemic proportions, involving nurseries and inhalation therapy equipment, continue to occur.

Antibiotic susceptibility patterns are unpredictable, so that each organism isolated should be tested. Some strains produce drug-resistant plasmids.

S. rubidaea, a species that ferments arabinose and raffinose but not sorbitol or rhamnose, and is negative for ornithine decarboxylase.

Sertoli cell (ser-to'lē) [Enrico *Sertoli,* Italian histologist, 1842–1910] a tall columnar cell in the seminiferous tubules of the testes, which extends from the basal lamina to the lumen. Adjacent Sertoli cells are united by tight junctions to form the blood-testis barrier that seals off the more apical cells from the base of the tubule. The cells are also joined by gap junctions through which ions and small molecules can pass from one cell to another.

Sertoli cells support and nourish the developing spermatozoa, and the precursors of the mature spermatozoan nestle within indentations of the Sertoli cells. Degenerating cells are phagocytosed by the Sertoli cells. The synthesis of androgens, primarily testosterone, is another function of Sertoli cells. See also *testis.*

Sertoli–Leydig cell tumors ovarian or testicular neoplasms composed of Sertoli and Leydig cells in variable proportions. Occasionally, a pure Sertoli cell tumor occurs. Most Sertoli–Leydig cell tumors occur in young females in one ovary, and the prognosis following surgical removal is good. The tumors display a broad range of histologic appearances from a well-differentiated tubular neoplasm to a sarcoma-like spindle cell tumor. Functional effects consist of progressive defeminization, followed by masculinizing symptoms. The ovarian tumors are also called arrhenoblastomas or androblastomas, but only the latter term is used as a synonym for testicular tumors. See also *ovarian tumors* and *testicular tumors.*

serum (se'rum), pl. *sera, serums* [L. "whey"] the clear, yellowish fluid that separates from blood when it is allowed to clot. Formed from blood plasma from which the fibrin has been precipitated, it closely resembles plasma except for the absence of some coagulation factors. Cf. *plasma.*

serum glutamate oxaloacetate transaminase (SGOT) see *aspartate aminotransferase.*

serum glutamate pyruvate transaminase (SGPT) see *alanine aminotransferase.*

serum hepatitis see under *hepatitis.*

serum protein electrophoresis (SPE) see *protein electrophoresis.*

serum prothrombin conversion accelerator (SPCA) deficiency see under *Factor VII.*

serum prothrombin conversion accelerator (SPCA) factor see *Factor VII.*

serum prothrombin time see *prothrombin consumption test.*

serum sickness a type of immune complex disease that results from the injection of foreign serum. The foreign serum elicits an immune response that forms antigen-antibody complexes deposited intravascularly. These immune complexes lead to inflammation including complement fixation, release of vasoactive amines, increased vascular permeability, infiltration of polymorphonuclear leukocytes, and deposition of fibrin. Clinically, by 3 da–3 wk after injection of foreign serum, an individual will develop fever, malaise, skin rash, lymphadenopathy, and splenomegaly. These symptoms may last up to 2 wk.

servomechanism (ser'vo-mek"ah-nizm) an automatic control system in which feedback is used to control the movement of a servomotor.

servomotor (ser'vo-mo"tor) [L. *servus* slave + *motor*] an electric or hydraulic motor in which the position of the output shaft is controlled by the electric input. Also called servo.

seryl (sēr'il, ser'il) the acyl radical derived from or relating to serine.

sesame oil [USP], the refined fixed oil obtained from the seed of one or more cultivated varieties of *Sesamum indicum;* used as a solvent for drugs. It has also been used internally as a laxative and externally as a skin softener.

sesamoid bone (ses'ah-moid) [L. *sesamoides;* Gr. *sēsamon* sesame + *eidos* to form] an ovoid nodular bone, often small, that is embedded in a tendon or joint capsule. These bones are mainly found in the hands or feet.

sesquiterpene (ses"kwe-ter'pēn) an isoprenoid compound with 15 carbon atoms in three isoprene units.

sessile (ses'il) [L. *sessilis*] attached by a base; not pedunculated or stalked. Cf. *pedunculated.*

set (set) 1. to align bones or bone fragments, as in reducing a fracture.

2. to set a binary logic circuit to the 1 state. Cf. *reset.*

3. the input line of a flip-flop to which a set signal is applied.

4. in mathematics, a collection of distinct objects called elements of the set. A set is denoted by a list of its elements in curly brackets, e.g., $\{1,2,3\}$, or by the form {typical element of the set | defining relation}, e.g., $\{y \mid 1<y<3\}$. The set with no elements is called the empty set, $\emptyset = \{\ \}$.

Membership in a set is denoted $a \in \{a, b\}$, read a is an element of $\{a, b\}$. Inclusion in a set is denoted $\{a\} \subseteq \{a, b\}$, read $\{a\}$ is a subset of $\{a, b\}$. If two sets A and B are subsets of each other, they have the same elements, $A = B$. If $A \subseteq B$ but $A \neq B$, then $A \subsetneq B$, read A is a proper subset of B.

There are three operations on sets: the intersection of two sets $A \cap B$ (the set of elements that are members of both A and B), the union of two sets $A \cup B$ (the set of elements that are members of either A or B or both), and the complement of a set $\bar{A}$ (the set of elements in a specified universe of discourse that are not elements of A).

See also *Venn diagram.*

set point the desired value at which the output (controlled variable) of a control system is maintained. Any deviation from the set point (error signal) is applied as negative feedback to return the output to the set point. See also *control system.*

seven-segment display a digital readout in which the digits are formed from seven straight lines forming a figure eight when all segments are on. This is the usual type of light-emitting diode (LED) or liquid crystal readout seen in pocket calculators and digital instruments.

7-year itch see *scabies.*

Sever's disease (se'verz) [James Warren *Sever,* Boston orthopedic surgeon, born 1878] see under *osteochondritis juvenilis.*

sex [L. *sexus*] a characteristic of an individual based on the type of gametes it produces. The female sex produces macrogametes, or ova; the male sex produces microgametes, or sperm.

sex cords cords of proliferating epithelial cells, separated by layers of mesenchyme, that form the cortex of the primitive gonad.

sex cord–stromal tumor see *ovarian tumors* and *testicular tumors.*

sex determination the process by which genetic make-up and/or environmental influences dictate the phenotypic sex of an individual.

In mammals, the chromosomal genes are of primary importance in determining gonadal sex. Typically, females have two X chromosomes and are the homogametic sex, as they produce only one kind of gamete. Males usually have one X and one Y chromosome; they are the heterogametic sex, producing both X and Y gametes. The Y chromosome is much smaller than the X chromosome and, except for the gene(s) for maleness, appears to be composed primarily of highly repeated DNA sequences of little informational consequence.

Sexual differentiation of undifferentiated gonads into testes and ovaries occurs late in the development of mammals. In the male, the Y chromosome promotes testicular development and carries a gene that codes for or regulates the synthesis of the membrane-bound H-Y antigen that is believed to promote testicular differentiation. This antigen is a histocompatibility antigen bound to the plasma membranes of all male gonadal cells. An individual can develop as a male even without the Y chromosome, as evidenced by the sex-reversed (Sxr) mutation, and H-Y antigen is found in such individuals. Chromosomal XX females carrying the Sxr mutation are phenotypically male, possibly because of the presence of the H-Y antigen.

The fetal testis promotes development of the male secondary sex structures and inhibits development of the female structures. At least two types of hormones from the fetal testes are needed for normal male development: testosterone (a steroid with androgenic activity) and the müllerian-inhibiting hormone, which promotes degeneration of the müllerian duct.

In mammalian females, sexual differentiation prior to birth does not require a specific stimulus. It proceeds normally in embryos that are genetically XX or XY (without the H-Y antigen or other male determinants), in embryos whose gonads spontaneously fail to develop, and in embryos whose gonads are removed at the sexually undifferentiated stage. In normal males, gonadal activity relies on the normal pituitary release of gonadotropins in a continuous pattern. Females, however, require cyclic stimulation of gonadotropin output.

A wide variety of sex chromosome patterns exist among animals whose sex determination is primarily genetic or chromosomal. Certain mammals have two different X chromosomes (X_1, X_2) — males have one copy of both (X_1, X_2, Y), and females have two copies (X_1, X_1, X_2, X_2). There are also species with one X and two Y chromosomes (X, Y_1, Y_2) in males and two X chromosomes in females (XX). Either of these situations results in an unequal number of chromosomes.

An altered number of sex chromosomes frequently produces anomalies of sexual differentiation in humans. Individuals with one X and no Y (XO) chromosomes, a situation caused by the nondisjunction of the XX chromosomes, develop into female fetuses with specific defects (Turner's syndrome): webbing of the neck and other dysmorphic features, sexually juvenile development without secondary sex characteristics, but no impaired intelligence. They lack sex chromatin (the Barr body) in their somatic cells.

Individuals with karyotype XXX are also female and have two Barr bodies. They are generally fertile with relatively normal sex differentiation. If there are more than three X chromosomes, the individual is usually severely retarded.

Nondisjunction of the XY chromosomes leads to Klinefelter's syndrome (XXY); those affected are sterile phenotypic males, some being mentally retarded. Testes are present but small, and there is some degree of testicular degeneration in early adulthood. The phenotypic characteristics of this syndrome appear in individuals with more than two X chromosomes in combination with one Y chromosome.

Individuals with XYY karyotype are males who are taller than average but otherwise relatively normal. Surveys of newborn infants suggest that about 0.1 percent of all male fetuses are XYY.

Hermaphroditism results in ambiguity of genital structures due to incomplete müllerian duct inhibition and/or incomplete androgenic masculinization. Individuals referred to as pseudohermaphrodites have definite male or female gonads in addition to other ambiguous reproductive organs.

See also *congenital a. h.* under *adrenal hyperplasia* and *testicular feminization syndrome.*

sexivalent (sek-siv'ah-lent) [L. *sex* six + *valere* to have power] in chemistry, having a valence of 6. Also called *hexivalent.*

sexually transmitted diseases (STD) those infectious diseases acquired through sexual contact. Initially, there were five classic venereal diseases: gonorrhea (caused by *Neisseria gonorrhoeae*), syphilis (*Treponema pallidum*), chancroid (*Hemophilus ducreyi*), lymphogranuloma venereum (*Chlamydia trachomatis*), and granuloma inguinale (*Calymmatobacterium granulomatis*). Gradually, as contraceptives became more common and human sexual behavior changed, the reported frequency and variety of venereal diseases increased. Advances in the field led to the discovery of additional etiologic agents associated with sexually transmitted diseases; a list of these agents and the diseases they produce is shown in the accompanying table. At present, venereal diseases may be divided into three common clinical syndromes: male urethritis, female lower genitourinary tract infection, and vaginitis.

Many of these diseases manifest themselves in the form of skin lesions, which may be ulcerative or nonulcerative. When nonulcerative genital lesions are observed, a sexually transmitted disease should be suspected, such as infection with *Candida,* certain bacteria, or scabies. Ulcerative lesions suggest herpes simplex type 2 infection, chancroid, syphilis, lymphogranuloma venereum, or granuloma inguinale.

MALE URETHRITIS. This disease is either gonococcal or nongonococcal. About half the nongonococcal urethritis infections are due to *Chlamydia trachomatis;* the remainder are due to *Ureaplasma urealyticum* or herpes simplex virus. Usually there is a urethral discharge from which diagnosis can be made. A Gram-stained smear of the discharge can be diagnostic for gonorrhea, if gram-negative diplococci are demonstrated within neutrophils.

FEMALE LOWER GENITOURINARY TRACT INFECTION. Symptoms include burning on urination, dyspareunia, vulvar irritation, and occasionally a vaginal discharge (infection of this region is often localized as cystitis, urethritis, vaginitis, or cervicitis). There are some important differences in etiology. Vulvitis is often due to *Candida albicans* or herpes simplex virus; cervicitis to *N. gonorrhoeae* or *C. trachomatis,* or to herpes simplex virus if vaginitis is absent. *C. trachomatis* cervicitis is demonstrated by

SEXUALLY TRANSMITTED DISEASES. SEXUALLY TRANSMITTED AGENTS AND DISEASES THEY CAUSE

ETIOLOGICAL AGENT	DISEASE OR SYNDROME
BACTERIAL	
Neisseria gonorrhoeae	Urethritis, cervicitis, proctitis, pharyngitis, conjunctivitis, endometritis, pelvic inflammatory disease, perihepatitis Bartholinitis, amniotic infection syndrome, disseminated gonococcal infection
Treponema pallidum	Syphilis
Haemophilus ducreyi	Chancroid
Gardnerella (Hemophilus) vaginalis	? Nonspecific vaginitis
Calymmatobacterium granulomatis	Granuloma inguinale
Clostridium difficile	? Nonspecific urethritis
Ureaplasma urealyticum	? Nonspecific urethritis
Corynebacterium genitalium	? Nonspecific urethritis
Chlamydia trachomatis	Nongonococcal urethritis, epididymitis, cervicitis, salpingitis, inclusion conjunctivitis, infant pneumonia, trachoma, lymphogranuloma venereum
Group B beta-hemolytic streptococci	Neonatal sepsis, neonatal meningitis
Shigella species and other Enterobacteriaceae	Shigellosis, etc., in homosexual men
VIRAL	
Herpesvirus hominis	Primary and recurrent genital herpes, aseptic meningitis, neonatal herpes, ? cervical carcinoma
Cytomegalovirus	Heterophile-negative infectious mononucleosis, congenital birth defects, ? cervicitis
Genital wart virus	Condyloma acuminatum, ? laryngeal papilloma
Molluscum contagiosum virus	Genital molluscum contagiosum
Hepatitis B virus	Classic hepatitis, fulminant hepatitis, chronic active hepatitis, submassive hepatic necrosis, persistent (unresolved) hepatitis, polyarteritis nodosa, chronic membranous glomerulonephritis
PROTOZOAN	
Trichomonas vaginalis	Trichomonal vaginitis
Giardia lamblia	Giardiasis in homosexual men
Entamoeba histolytica	Amebiasis in homosexual men
FUNGAL	
Candida albicans	Vulvovaginitis, penile candidiasis
ARTHROPODS	
Phthirus pubis	Pubic lice infestation
Sarcoptes scabiei	Scabies

Note: Evidence for sexual transmission of some of these agents is circumstantial or is limited to homosexual males.

Modified from Lennette, E. H., et al.: Manual of Clinical Microbiology. 3rd ed. Washington, DC, American Society for Microbiology, 1980, p. 345.

isolation of the organism in tissue culture. Nongonococcal cervicitis without an ulcerative lesion is also assumed to be due to *C. trachomatis.*

VAGINITIS. There are three clinical types of sexually transmitted vaginitis: those caused by *Trichomonas* and *Candida,* and nonspecific vaginitis. (1) Vaginitis due to *T. vaginalis* is often asymptomatic but may cause a malodorous discharge that is yellow-green owing to the high concentration of polymorphonuclear leukocytes. Diagnosis is made by demonstration of motile trichomonads in vaginal secretions, and treatment involves administration of nitroimidazoles. (2) *C. albicans* vaginitis causes an itching, odorless white discharge. The diagnosis is made by microscopic observation of yeast cells and by culturing *C. albicans.* (3) Nonspecific vaginitis may be attributed to *Hemophilus vaginalis.* This is verified by microscopic and cultural procedures.

For more information, see the specific disease.

Sézary syndrome a leukemic dissemination of T lymphocytes associated with cutaneous infiltrates of similar cells identical to the skin lesions of mycosis fungoides. The circulating cells are referred to as Sézary cells; like those in the skin, they have markedly irregular (cerebriform) nuclei. See also *Sézary cell.*

SFEMG abbrev. See *single-fiber e.* under *electromyography.*

SG abbrev. See *specific gravity.*

SGAW abbrev. See *specific a. c.* under *airway conductance.*

SGOT abbrev. for serum glutamate oxaloacetate transminase. See under *aspartate aminotransferase.*

SGPT abbrev. for serum glutamate pyruvate transaminase. See *alanine aminotransferase.*

shadow (shad′o) the image of an object produced by its blocking of a beam of light or radiation, as the image of a radiopaque structure in a radiograph.

shadow-casting (shad″o kast′ing) the application of a thin coating of gold or other heavy metal for the purpose of increasing the contrast of certain electron-microscopy specimens. Applied at a low angle, these vaporized atoms of metal impart a three-dimensional quality to the specimen.

sharp and slow-wave complex in electroencephalograpy, a sequence consisting of a sharp wave (i.e., a wave with a pointed peak and 70–200 msec in duration) associated with a slow wave (i.e., a wave longer than 125 msec in duration). The diagnostic value of this complex depends on the clinical context in which it is found. See also *sharp w.* under *wave.*

Sharpey's fibers (shar′pēz) [William *Sharpey,* English anatomist and physiologist, 1802–1880] bundles of collagen that penetrate the surface of a bone or tooth to anchor a tendon or ligament. Also called perforating fibers of Sharpey.

sharpness (sharp′nes) in radiography, the definition or clarity of detail and the lack of blurring of the radiographic image. See also *definition.*

S Hb (Hb S) abbrev. See *sulfhemoglobin.*

sheath (shēth) [L. *vagina;* Gr. *thēkē*] a tubular structure surrounding one organ or part.

rectus s., a sheath, formed by the aponeuroses of the oblique and transverse muscles of the abdomen, that envelops the rectus abdominis muscle.

tendon s., a double-walled cylinder of fibrous connective tissue lined by specialized surface cells through which tendons pass. The concentric layers are continuous at their ends, and the sheath contains a thin film of synovial fluid.

Sheehan's syndrome see *postpartum pituitary n.* under *necrosis.*

sheep cell agglutination test see *Rose-Waaler test.*

shell (shel) 1. a hard covering or encasement, such as a turtle shell or an eggshell.

2. a grouping of atomic electron states by the electron energy. The shells are labeled by letters: K shell (containing at most two electrons), L (8 electrons), M (18), N (32), O (50), etc.

shield (shēld) a device used to protect personnel from radiation.

gonadal s., a piece of lead foil placed over the gonads during diagnostic x-ray examinations of the pelvic region. It should be at least 1 mm thick. The radiation from the primary beam is blocked from reaching the gonads, but there is some exposure from secondary x-rays.

syringe s., a shield made of high-density material, such as depleted uranium or tungsten, used to shield syringes containing radiopharmaceuticals.

tabletop s., a shield made of lead with a leaded glass insert, used to protect personnel during radiopharmaceutical dose preparation and calibration.

shielding (shēl′ding) the protection of personnel from ionizing radiation by surrounding the source with a layer of absorbing material. High-density materials such as lead, leaded glass, tungsten, and depleted uranium are most commonly used.

The effectiveness of the shielding material is stated in terms of the half-value layer (HVL), which is the thickness of material that will absorb half the x-rays or gamma rays emitted by the source. The HVL varies with the energy of the radiation.

shift (shift) a change or deviation.

chloride s., the simultaneous exchange of chloride and bicarbonate ions between plasma and red blood cells. Chloride diffuses from the cell as bicarbonate enters in order to maintain the balance of ions on both sides of the red cell membrane, thus maintaining the electric potential across the red cell membrane. This mechanism permits a greater concentration of bicarbonate ions to be carried in the plasma.

s. to the left, a deviation in the normal distribution of granulocytes in a blood smear, in which there is a relative increases in the number of bands and other less mature neutrophils. It is usually an indication of infection and is accompanied by neutrophilic leukocytosis. See also Arneth count.

s. to the right, an alteration in the normal distribution of blood neutrophils, in which immature forms such as bands are absent and only mature segmental neutrophils are present. This change can be seen in pernicious anemia. See also Arneth count.

shift register a digital electronic circuit used to store binary data. The data can be entered or removed in parallel (when bits are set or read out simultaneously) or in the serial mode (when each bit is shifted to the next bit position on every clock pulse, and the last bit is output). Shift left means toward the most significant bit; shift right is toward the least significant bit.

Shiga's bacillus (she′gahz) [Kiyoshi *Shiga,* Japanese physician, 1870–1957] see *S. dysenteriae* type 1 under *Shigella.*

Shigella (shĭ-gel′ah) [Kiyoshi *Shiga*] a genus of gram-negative bacilli in the family Enterobacteriaceae composed of four species: *S. boydii, S. dysenteriae, S. flexneri,* and *S. sonnei.* The major differential biochemical characteristics are a lack of motility, an inability to utilize citrate as a sole carbon source, and the fermentation of carbohydrates with acid but not gas production. The normal habitat is the intestinal tract of humans and higher monkeys; all four species cause dysentery. See also *Enterobacteriaceae.*

S. boydii, a species that causes dysentery; it has 15 serologic types. The organisms ferment mannitol but not lactose, and are variable for ornithine decarboxylase.

S. dysenteriae, a highly pathogenic species that causes a particularly severe dysentery; it has 10 serologic types. *S. dysenteriae* type 1 produces a potent neurotoxin and is the etiologic agent of an epidemic dysentery that can be fatal in children. The organisms do not ferment lactose or mannitol and are negative for ornithine decarboxylase. See also *exotoxins.*

S. flexneri, a species that sometimes causes a severe dysentery; it has six serologic types. The organisms ferment mannitol but not lactose, and are negative for ornithine decarboxylase.

S. sonnei, the least pathogenic *Shigella* species, which causes a milder dysentery. The organisms ferment mannitol and are positive for ornithine decarboxylase; most strains ferment lactose slowly.

shigellosis (shĭ″gel-lo′sis) infection by *Shigella* bacteria. The organisms invade the intestinal epithelial cells and cause a dysentery that ranges from mild to potentially fatal. Shigellosis has played a major role in military history. Available documents indicate that dystentery and its sister disease, typhus, had more to do with the outcome of land-based campaigns before the twentieth century than did the strategy of generals. In modern times the disease is most prevalent in institutions where overcrowding and poor sanitation prevail.

All four species can produce bacillary dysentery. Although some strains produce a toxin, the capacity to invade intestinal cells seems to be the decisive factor for pathogenicity. The lesions are limited to the terminal ileum and colon; they develop into ulcerations of the mucosa, but seldom penetrate deeper than the submucosa. An enterotoxin is responsible for much of the local tissue damage. In addition, *S. dysenteriae* type 1 produces a neurotoxin giving these infections another clinical dimension. The bacilli must be cultured promptly from stool specimens for laboratory diagnosis. Ampicillin is considered the drug of choice.

Also called *bacillary dysentery.*

shingles (shing′g′lz) [L. *cingulus,* belt] a viral disease caused by herpes zoster. It is a reactivation of a varicella zoster virus that has remained dormant in a spinal ganglion since a previous attack of chickenpox. The vesicular eruptions on the skin follow nerve root distribution. Activation of the latent herpes zoster virus is most commonly seen in patients with secondary depressed cell–mediated immunity, such as in Hodgkin's disease, in other malignancy, or in the debilitated elderly.

shistocyte (shis′to-sit) see *schizocyte.*

shock (shok) a serious condition that occurs when blood pressure falls to extremely low levels because of bleeding, heart failure, or other disorders, in which case an adequate supply of blood (and therefore, oxygen and nutrients) cannot reach the body's tissues, resulting in damage to vital organs. The brain, heart, lungs, kidneys, and liver are particularly sensitive to injury and may be permanently damaged if shock is not treated quickly and appropriately; death may follow.

The different types of shock are classified according to the event that triggered the drop in blood pressure. Certain signs and symptoms, however, are characteristic of all types, for example, low blood pressure, rapid and weak pulse, pale complexion, sweating, and confusion. Treatment consists of immediate efforts to restore blood pressure to normal and to correct the condition that initially caused the shock. A complete blood count, urinalysis (especially specific gravity), blood urea nitrogen (BUN), and serum glucose determinations are helpful in the initial assessment and management of patients in shock. Serum electrolytes are monitored as an aid in fluid replacement therapy. A major complication of shock is the development of acidosis secondary to tissue hypoxia. Therefore, oxygen is given to persons in shock, and arterial blood gases are followed closely.

Normal blood pressure is dependent on three conditions: adequate blood volume, a functioning heart, and an intact functioning vascular system. Failure of any one of these factors results in the fall in blood pressure that leads to a specific type of shock.

NANETTE SMITH, M.D.

cardiogenic s., the state that occurs when blood pressure falls because the heart cannot maintain an adequate (cardiac) output. Cardiac output is the product of stroke volume and heart rate, and a serious fall in either can result in cardiogenic shock. A reduced stroke volume can result from impaired myocardiac contractility, as occurs with myocardial ischemia and/or infarction secondary to coronary vascular insufficiency, from primary myocardial muscle diseases (cardiomyopathies), or from marked changes in rhythm (severe bradycardia or tachycardia).

hypovolemic s., the drop in blood pressure that results from a loss of circulating blood volume, as in blood loss following trauma, or fluid loss from the gut, kidneys, or severely burned skin. Initial therapy involves replacement of circulating volume with an isotonic solution, such as normal saline, or with whole blood. A central venous pressure catheter (CVP line) may be used for monitoring volume status. The MAST suit is frequently used by emergency medical personnel to increase blood pressure during prehospital treatment.

neurogenic s., the condition that exists when blood pressure falls because peripheral blood vessels have lost their normal sympathetic tone. Arteriolar resistance falls, arterial and venous blood pooling begins, and blood pressure can be maintained only by increasing cardiac output or by increasing circulatory blood volume with blood or fluid infusions. When these compensatory adjustments fail, hypotension and, ultimately, shock ensue. The usual cause is injury to the spinal cord, although neurogenic shock may be transiently seen during anesthesia.

osmotic s., see *osmotic shock.*

septic s., a type of shock that results from septicemia, and is usually caused by endotoxin, produced by a gram-negative bacteremia, in the circulating blood. The fact that shock occurs with gram-positive bacteremia indicates that a substance or substances other than endotoxin may cause similar symptoms. Endotoxin can cause cell injury by at least four mechanisms: direct cell membrane damage, release of lysosomal enzymes from white blood cells, activation of the complement system, and tissue anoxia. These mechanisms affect the small blood vessels, resulting in immobilization of blood, inadequate tissue perfusion, and anoxia. Endotoxin promotes the activation of bradykinin, a vasodilator, which leads to the pooling of blood in peripheral tissue and a decrease in the circulating blood volume and cardiac output.

Clinically, symptoms of septic shock include chills, fever, nausea, tachycardia, cold and clammy skin, a weak pulse, and hypotension. An inadequate blood supply to the kidneys, lungs, or heart can lead to respiratory failure, coma, or heart failure. Complications of septic shock may include disseminated intravascular coagulation, a deficiency of several clotting factors, which causes the formation of fibrin-platelet aggregates.

Laboratory diagnostic studies usually reveal an elevated hematocrit falling to less than normal when blood volume deficit is corrected, leukocytosis, a decreased platelet count, and abnormal coagulation values. Respiratory alkalosis with a low P_{CO_2} and high arterial pH may be present. Microbiologic studies of the blood may not reveal bacteremia, as a consequence either of antimicrobial therapy or of the transient or erratic presence of the microorganisms in the blood. Endotoxin can be measured by the Limulus lysate assay (see Limulus test under *pyrogen*).

See also *endotoxin* and *septicemia.*

toxic s., see *toxic shock syndrome.*

shock artifact see under *artifact.*

shock lung a lung that has been damaged by the hemodynamic consequences of advanced hemorrhagic shock. The primary effect of shock on the lung is damage to the capillary endothelium. Microaggregates of leukocytes and platelets congest the capillaries, release hydrolytic enzymes that destroy endothelial cells. The result is an increased capillary permeability leading to pulmonary interstitial edema. Inadequate surfactant production (possibly due to the low pulmonary blood flow) perpetuates the edema. Pulmonary venoconstriction stimulated by tissue hypoxia may also add to the capillary congestion. The overall pathologic changes in shock lung thus may include the following: pulmonary edema, hyaline membrane formation, atelectasis, bronchial pneumonia, alveolar hemorrhage, pronounced dilation of the capillaries, and extensive vascular congestion.

Shope papilloma see *rabbit papilloma.*

short bone a bone whose main dimensions are approximately equal, e.g., one of the bones of the carpus or tarsus.

short circuit see *short c.* under *circuit.*

shoulder joint (shōl′der) the ball-and-socket synovial joint formed by the head of the humerus and the glenoid cavity of the scapula.

shunt (shunt) 1. to turn to one side, divert, or bypass.

2. a precision resistor connected across the terminals of an ammeter to increase the current indicated by a full-scale deflection.

3. pertaining to an electronic component connected in parallel with some specified component or with the input or output.

4. the hexose monophosphate shunt; see *pentose phosphate pathway.*

5. a passage or anastomosis between two blood vessels. Such structures may be formed physiologically (e.g., to bypass a thrombosis), through abnormal development, or by surgery.

anatomic s., a vascular communication between the systemic and pulmonary circulations that diverts blood from alternate channels. Anatomic shunts can occur pathologically when normal fetal circulatory communications fail to close postnatally; as the result of abnormal development; or following trauma.

Left-to-right shunts divert blood from the systemic to the pulmonary circulation. Examples are atrial, ventricular, and aortopulmonary septal defects, and patent ductus arteriosus. Venous-to-arterial or right-to-left shunts divert venous blood (which has not equilibrated with alveolar gas) into the arterial circulation. In the healthy individual, a small percentage of cardiac output flows through right-to-left shunts that normally operate to transfer blood from the thebesian veins into the left heart, and from the bronchial veins into the postcapillary pulmonary circulation.

arteriovenous (A-V) s., 1. connections between small arteries and veins that bypass the capillary beds. Under sympathetic stimulation, communicating vessel constricts and blood is channeled through the capillaries. Such connections are present in the skin of the nose, lips, and external ears; erectile tissue; mucous membranes; and other locations.

2. A U-shaped plastic tube inserted between an artery and a vein, thus bypassing the capillary network. This procedure is commonly performed to allow repeated access to the arterial system for the purpose of hemodialysis.

physiologic s., the flow of blood through the pulmonary capillaries that accompanies completely unventilated alveoli. Oxygenation of this blood does not occur; as a result, the P_{O_2} of the arterial blood is lowered below that of the pulmonary capillary blood that has equilibrated with alveolar gas. The condition may be the consequence of normal regional differences in pulmonary compliance and airway resistance during the respiratory cycle, or it may occur as the result of lung disease.

total s., the lack of contact between mixed venous blood and alveolar gas that is due to absolute (venous-to-arterial) shunt and to an additional component representing the excess perfusion of hypoventilated alveoli with a low ventilation-perfusion ratio (often called venous admixture), which produces a shuntlike effect.

The relative quantities of blood contributing to the total shunt from venous admixture and venous-to-arterial shunts can be distinguished by a 100 percent O_2 test. After approximately 20 min of breathing 100 percent O_2, any venous admixture is corrected and any residual arterial hypoxemia (or abnormally widened $P(A\text{-}a)O_2$) can be attributed to the presence of venous-to-arterial shunt.

The total shunt, or wasted pulmonary blood flow can be calculated as: $\dot{Q}_{va}/\dot{Q}_t = Ca_{O_2} - Ci_{O_2}/Cv_{O_2} - Ci_{O_2}$, where $\dot{Q}_{va}/\dot{Q}_t$ is the ratio between the venous admixture and total blood flow, Ca_{O_2} and Cv_{O_2} are the oxygen content of the arterial and mixed venous blood, and Ci_{O_2} is the ideal O_2 content of arterial blood (if Pa_{O_2} were to equal PA_{O_2}). It normally amounts to less than 5 percent of the cardiac output in healthy individuals.

See also *ventilation-perfusion ratio.*

venous-to-arterial s., a pathway that permits unoxygenated mixed venous blood to flow from the right to the left side of the heart, bypassing the pulmonary capillaries and thus the alveolar air. Blood shunted in this manner will not be oxygenated, and contributes continuously to the venous admixture of blood that has been arterialized by passage through normal lung.

In the healthy individual, about 2 percent of cardiac output flows through right-to-left shunt pathways (the bronchial and thebesian vessels). For this reason, systemic arterial blood normally has a lower Po_2 than the blood just equilibrated with alveolar gas.

Abnormal right-to-left shunts occur through interseptal defects (congenital heart disease), through channels such as pulmonary arteriovenous fistulas, or between the bronchial and pulmonary arteries in bronchiectasis. The degree of arterial hypoxemia that results depends on the magnitude of the shunt.

Also called *absolute* or *right-to-left s.* See also *total s.* under *shunt.*

Shwartzman's phenomenon (shwartz'manz) [Gregory *Shwartzman,* Russian bacteriologist in the U.S., 1896–1965] a combination of skin necrosis and generalized kidney, heart, and liver disease that is the result of a second dose of bacterial endotoxin. No immunologic mechanisms have been shown to explain this phenomenon. See also *lipopolysaccharide.*

SI abbrev. for *Système International* d'Unités. See *International System.*

Si symbol for the chemical element *silicon.*

sial/o (si'ah-lo) [Gr. *sialon* saliva] a word element used in combining form to denote saliva, e.g., sialogenous.

sialaden/o (si"al-ad'e-no) a word element used in combining form to denote the salivary glands, e.g., sialadenitis.

sialic acid (si-al'ik) [Gr. *sialikos*] a class of important carbohydrate derivatives that contain nine carbon atoms (ketononoses) and are acylated derivatives of neuraminic acid, a condensation product of L-pyruvic acid and mannosamine. Sialic acids are distributed in bacteria and animal tissues as constituents of lipids, polysaccharides, glycoproteins, and mucoproteins. The sialic acids of most mammals may be either *N*-acetyl or *N*-glycolyl (—CO—CH_2-OH) derivatives; diacetyl derivatives have also been isolated.

sialidase (si-al'ĭ-dās) see *neuraminidase.*

sialidase digestion a histochemical technique for the removal of sialomucins by the hydrolysis of sialic acid. A test slide is treated with sialidase, an extract of *Vibrio cholerae* cultures, and then stained for mucosubstances. Slides negative for mucosubstances when compared with a control slide indicate the presence of sialomucins.

sialography (si"ah-log'rah-fe) [*sialo-* + Gr. *graphein* to write] the radiologic examination of the salivary ducts and alveoli following the injection of a water-soluble iodinated contrast medium (e.g., diatrizoate) into a salivary duct. It is used to demonstrate inflammatory lesions, neoplasms, fistulas, calculi, diverticula, or strictures. Anteroposterior, lateral, or lateral-oblique films are taken after the filling of the duct. A delayed film taken 5–10 min later verifies the emptying of the duct.

sialomucin (si"ah-lo-mu'sin) mucin in which the polysaccharide contains sialic acids and hexoseamines. See also *mucin.*

sib (sib) [A.S. "kin"] a brother and/or sister. Sibs are individuals sharing the same parents. Also called *sibling.*

Sibine a genus of caterpillars of which the species *S. stimulea,* the saddle-back caterpillar, is commonly found in the United States. These creatures possess spinelike poisonous hairs.

Sibley-Lehninger (SL) unit an empirical unit for expressing aldolase activity, defined as the quantity of enzyme in 1.0 ml of specimen that will split 1.0 μl (1/22.4 μmol) of D-fructose-1,6-diphosphate into D-glyceraldehyde-3-phosphate and dihydroxyacetone in 60 min, under the conditions of the test. The relation to International Units is given by 1.0 SL unit = 0.74 mU/ml.

sibling (sib'ling) [A.S. *sib* kin + *-ling* diminutive ending] see *sib.*

sibling species a species that is morphologically almost indistinguishable from another.

sibship (sib'ship) a group of siblings.

Sicariidae a family of spiders, including the genus *Loxosceles,* that causes necrotic arachnidism.

siccus (sik'us) [L.] dry.

sickle cell anemia see under *hemoglobinopathy.*

sickle cell beta-thalassemia see under *thalassemia.*

sickle cell diseases see under *hemoglobinopathy.*

sickle cell hemoglobin C disease see under *hemoglobinopathy.*

sickle cell hemoglobin D_{Punjab} disease see under *hemoglobinopathy.*

sickle cell trait see under *hemoglobinopathy.*

sickled cell an erythrocyte that has undergone shape deformation resulting from the deoxygenation and semisolid gelation of hemoglobin S, forming spiculated bipolar, holly-leaf, and irregularly spiculated shapes. Upon reoxygenation, the erythrocyte reassumes its normal biconcave disk shape. Also called *drepanocyte.* See also *irreversibly sickled cell.*

sickling tests (sik'ling) 1. sickle cell preparation. This method is used to demonstrate the presence of hemoglobin S (Hb S) in erythrocytes by depriving the red cell of oxygen. This can be done by sealing a coverslip over a drop of fresh blood and observing the rapidity with which the cells sickle; the time will vary with the amount of Hb S present. The reaction can be expedited by mixing a reducing substance, such as sodium metabisulfite ($Na_2S_2O_5$) with whole blood.

2. solubility test for sickle cell screening. Whole

blood is placed in a high concentration of phosphate buffer. When the sickle hemoglobin is released from the red cells by the addition of saponin, it becomes insoluble and forms crystals, producing a cloudy solution. The test is not entirely specific for Hb S, as hemoglobins C_{Harlem}, $C_{Zinguinchor}$, and S_{Travis} also give positive results. Hemoglobins A, C, D, F, G, I, J, and O_{Arab} give negative results. No information is available on other hemoglobins. Consequently, whenever possible, hemoglobin electrophoresis should be used for screening.

sickness any condition or episode marked by pronounced deviation from the normal heathy state; illness. See also *disease.*

sick sinus syndrome dysfunction of the sinoatrial node that can manifest itself as syncope or chest pain with accompanying bradycardia or tachycardia. Hypertension or arteriosclerotic heart disease is often the underlying cause. Electrocardiographic monitoring, stress testing, and the monitoring of cardiac response to drug administration can be useful in diagnosis.

side-effect (sīd′ef-fekt″) a consequence other than the ones for which an agent or measure is used. It particularly refers to the direct effect a drug produces that has no therapeutic value for the condition it is being administered to treat (e.g., drowsy and dry mouth conditions caused by antihistamines). Serious or deleterious side-effects are usually called adverse reactions.

sider/o (sid′er-o) [Gr. *sidēros* iron] a word element used in combining form to denote iron, e.g., siderosis, hemosiderosis.

sideramine (sid′er-ah-mēn″) a derivative of hydroxamic acid ($R—CONH_2OH$) that binds ferric iron. Sideramines secreted by certain bacterial cells function in the active transport of iron into the bacterial cell. See also *mycobactin* and *siderophore.*

sideroachrestic anemia see *sideroblastic a.* under *anemia.*

sideroblast (sid′er-o-blast″) a normoblast that contains nonhemoglobin iron (ferritin) and is stainable with Prussian blue. All normal normoblasts and reticulocytes contain ferritin either dispersed or in siderosomes when examined with the electron microscope, but only 30–70 percent have aggregates that stain with Prussian blue.

Pathologic sideroblasts may contain excessive amounts of siderosomes or may contain ferritin in mitochondria which, if sufficiently massive, become stainable with Prussian blue. Because mitochondria tend to arrange themselves concentrically around the nucleus, sideroblasts containing large amounts of ferritin are characterized by a ring of Prussian blue–positive material around the nucleus and are called "ringed sideroblasts."

sideroblastic anemia see *sideroblastic a.* under *anemia.*

siderochrome (sid′er-o-krōm″) see *siderophore.*

siderocyte (sid′er-o-sīt″) an erythrocyte with particles of nonhemoglobin iron (ferritin) either in siderosomes or within mitochondria. These cells are not generally visible after staining with Giemsa or Wright stain, but only after an iron stain. Nucleated red cells always contain dispersed ferritin and siderosomes, but normal red cells do not. Ferritin is never identifiable microscopically in mitochondria in the normal erythroblast or reticulocyte. Consequently, siderosomes in mature red cells or mitochondrial iron in nucleated red cells are pathologic. They are found in refractory, sideroblastic, and dyserythropoietic anemias, particularly after splenectomy, and also in thalassemia.

Occasionally, small basophilic granules are seen after staining with Giemsa-type dyes that stain the protein matrix holding the iron particle. These granules, called Pappenheimer bodies, represent secondary lysosomes that give a positive reaction for iron.

See also *ringed sideroblast.*

siderocytic granule an aggregate of iron-containing ferritin molecules normally found in polychromatophilic normoblasts. It appears blue after staining with Perls' Prussian blue stain. These granules are occasionally found in reticulocytes and are not seen in normal mature erythrocytes. Pathologic siderocytic granules are composed of hemosiderin- or iron-filled mitochondria, and are seen in disturbances of hemoglobin synthesis such as thalassemia or refractory anemia. Also called *siderosome.*

sideroderma (sid″er-o-der′mah) bronzed coloration of the skin resulting from disordered iron metabolism, as in advanced hemochromatosis.

siderofibrosis (sid″er-o-fi-bro′sis) the fibrosis that is associated with abnormal tissue deposits of iron.

sideromycin (sid″er-o-mi′sin) an antibiotic synthesized by certain actinomycetes. Sideromycins are nonchelating analogs of sideramines that interfere with the uptake of sideramine-iron complexes by bacterial cells.

sideropenia (sid″er-o-pe′ne-ah) [*sidero-* + Gr. *penia* poverty] a deficiency of iron in the body or blood.

sideropenic dysphagia see *Plummer-Vinson syndrome.*

siderophilin (sid′er-of″ĭ-lin) see *transferrin.*

siderophore (sid′er-o-fōr″) a compound that binds iron. These compounds are produced by certain bacteria (e.g., species of mycobacteria and enterobacteria) and secreted into the medium. The ferric iron chelate compound formed is actively transported into the bacteria, where it is hydrolyzed and the iron utilized for intracellular processes. Also called *siderochrome.* See also *sideramine.*

siderosis (sid″er-o′sis) [*sider-* + *-osis* condition] 1. an increase in the storage of iron in the body. See also *hemosiderosis.*

2. a chronic, fibrotic pneumoconiosis due to prolonged exposure to iron oxides or metallic iron. Inhalation of the former leads to fibrosis and red discoloration of the lungs, whereas inhalation of the latter leads to red discoloration and symptoms referable to silicosis. See also *pneumoconiosis* and *silicosis.*

3. in the liver, the presence of stainable iron in the absence of fibrosis and cirrhosis. Cf. *hemochromatosis.*

siderosome an aggregate of ferritin surrounded by a limiting membrane, normally seen in developing erythroblasts but absent in mature erythrocytes. All but the smallest siderosomes can be seen by light microscopy using Perl's stain. These bodies are usually arranged around the nucleus in a concentric manner and are responsible for the appearance of "ringed sideroblasts." Siderosomes are associated with lead poisoning, sideroblastic anemias, and dyserythropoietic anemias. In pathologic states, mitochondria may fill with micelles of amorphous iron.

siderotic (sid″er-ot′ik) pertaining to or characterized by siderosis.

siderotic granule the particulate iron normally found in the normoblast. It stains blue with Perls' Prussian blue stain. These granules are occasionally found in reticulocytes and are absent in normal mature erythrocytes.

Electron microscopy shows the granules to consist of ferruginous micelles, ferritin surrounded by a membrane (siderosome). Iron is normally transported to the mitochondria, where hemoglobin synthesis occurs. The particulate iron becomes visible in mitochondria only under pathologic conditions.

See also *Pappenheimer body, ringed s.* under *sideroblast, sideroblast,* and *siderosome.*

siderotic nodules see *Gamna-Gandy bodies.*

SIDS abbrev. See *sudden infant death syndrome.*

sievert (Sv) (se′vert) the proposed new International System (SI) unit of radiation dose equivalent to 1 J/kg. One sievert equals 100 rem.

Siggaard-Andersen alignment nomogram a nomogram that allows calculation of: (1) the base excess if two of the following parameters are known: tCO_2 (or HCO_3^-), pH, or Pco_2 together with the hemoglobin; and (2) any of the following parameters if two of these are known: tCO_2 (or HCO_3^-), pH, or Pco_2. The nomogram is based on the *Henderson-Hasselbalch equation.* See also the accompanying illustration.

sigma (Σ, σ) (sig′mah) the eighteenth letter of the *Greek alphabet.*

sigma rhythm see *s. spindle* under *sleep.*

sigmoid/o (sig-moi′do) a word element used in combining form to denote the sigmoid colon, e.g., sigmoidoscope.

sigmoid (sig′moid) [Gr. *sigma* the letter *s* + *eidos* resemblance] 1. S-shaped.

2. the sigmoid colon.

sigmoidoscope (sig-moi′do-skōp) [*sigmoido-* + Gr. *skopein* to examine] an endoscope (usually 25 cm long) that consists of a light source, a magnifying eyepiece, and attachments for aspiration, biopsy, electrodesiccation, and swabbing of the mucosa. Newer fiberoptic designs are now being used to modify existing rigid sigmoidoscopes.

sigmoidoscopy (sig″moi-dos′ko-pe) a diagnostic procedure performed to examine the distal sigmoid colon and proximal rectum by means of a rigid tubular instrument called a sigmoidoscope. This procedure is useful for examination of the gastrointestinal tract for a distance of some 25 cm from the anus. Occasionally, it may not be possible to employ this technique because of difficulties in passing the instrument from the proximal rectum to the distal sigmoid colon.

The diagnostic value of this technique has become increasingly evident; it can demonstrate 90 percent of all neoplasms of the rectum and rectosigmoid area. Rectal biopsy is painless. In addition, more than half of all neoplasms of the large intestine lie within the 25-cm range of this procedure, in areas where barium x-ray demonstration of tumors is particularly difficult.

This procedure is also useful in the diagnosis of ulcerative colitis, dysentery, and amebic colitis. The longer, flexible sigmoidoscopes (60 cm) can be used for examination of the colon beyond the range of the rigid sigmoidoscope.

Also called *proctosigmoidoscopy.*

sigmoid sinus (sig′moid si′nus) a direct continuation of the transverse sinus beginning at the tentorium and leaving the cranial cavity through the jugular foramen as the internal jugular vein.

signal (sig′nel) 1. a physical process, such as a light, sound, or electrical wave, that carries information.

2. the information carried over a communications channel.

signal averaging a process for removing noise from a periodic signal. The waveforms for a large number of periods are electronically averaged. The signal, the same in each period, is unchanged, but the noise tends to cancel out. The effective noise level is divided by the square root of the number of periods over which the signal is averaged. In most clinical laboratory applications, the signal is at a constant level or is slowly changing so that high-frequency random noise is easily removed by simple algorithms.

signal level the measured signal at some point in a communications system, usually given in decibels referred to an arbitrary reference level.

signal node see *sentinel node.*

signal-to-noise ratio (SNR, S/N) the ratio of the amplitude of a signal to the amplitude of the superimposed random noise.

signature (sig′nah-chūr) [L. *signatura,* from *signare* to write] see under *prescription.*

signed magnitude a representation of numbers used in computers in the form of a sign and an absolute value. For binary numbers in n-bit words, the low-order n–1 bits represent the absolute value, and the high-order bit represents the sign. Cf. *two's complement.*

signed rank test a nonparametric statistical test used to analyze matched pair data. The differences $\{d_i\}$ between the responses of matched pairs of treatment and control subjects are assumed to have a continuous symmetric distribution with median Δ. The test statistic is the Wilcoxson signed rank statistic T^+, constructed as follows: the differences are ranked in order of increasing absolute value, and T^+ is the sum of the ranks of the positive differences.

Under the null hypothesis ($\Delta = 0$), T^+ has a symmetric distribution with mean $\mu = n(n + 1)/4$ and variance $\sigma^2 = n(n + 1)(2n + 1)/24$, where n is the sample size. The exact sampling distribution of T^+ under the null hypothesis is tabulated for small sample sizes. For large samples, the normal approximation is used: the upper tail probabilities are approximated by the area under the normal curve to the right of $(T^+ - \frac{1}{2} - \mu)/\sigma$. The null hypothesis is rejected, and the alternative $\Delta > 0$ is accepted if T^+ exceeds the upper α percentile point of the null distribution. The alternative $\Delta \neq 0$ is accepted if T^+or $n(n + 1)/2 - T^+$ exceeds the upper $\alpha/2$ percentile point.

When the distribution of the differences is discrete, ties can occur. Differences equal to zero are discarded from the sample and the sample size is reduced accordingly; average ranks are used for tied nonzero differences.

The signed rank test is a nonparametric competitor of the student t test for matched pairs which is

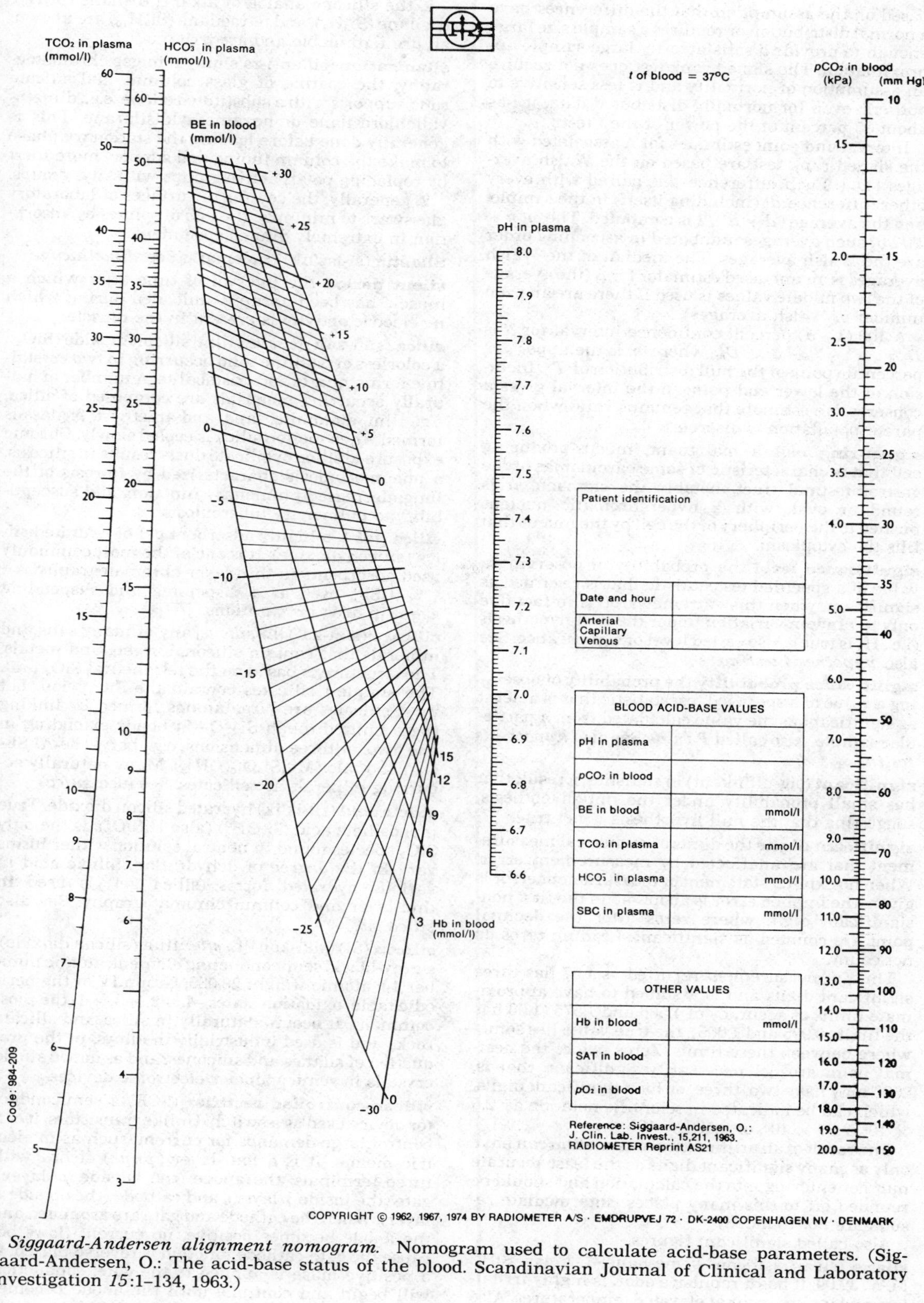

Siggaard-Andersen alignment nomogram. Nomogram used to calculate acid-base parameters. (Siggaard-Andersen, O.: The acid-base status of the blood. Scandinavian Journal of Clinical and Laboratory Investigation *15*:1–134, 1963.)

based on the assumption that the differences have a normal distribution or requires a sample size large enough to provide a satisfactorily large sample approximation. The signed rank test does not require an assumption of normality and is less sensitive to outliers; even for normally distributed data, it has about 95 percent of the power of the t test.

Interval and point estimates for Δ associated with the signed rank test are based on the Walsh averages $\{D_k\}$. Each difference d is paired with every other difference d' (including itself) in the sample, and the average $(d + d')/2$ is computed. The $n(n + 1)/2$ of such averages numbered in ascending order are the Walsh averages. The median of the Walsh averages is an unbiased estimator for Δ (the average of the two middle values is used if there are an even number of Walsh averages).

A 100 $(1 - \alpha)$ percent confidence interval for Δ is $D_{n(n+1)+1-m} - \Delta < D_m$, where m is the upper $\alpha/2$ percentile point of the null distribution of T^+. Inclusion of the lower end point in the interval gives a conservative estimate that remains valid when the parent population is discrete.

signet-ring cell a malignant, mucus-producing cell that is characteristic of some carcinomas of the gastrointestinal tract, notably the stomach. It is round or oval, with a hyperchromatic nucleus pushed to the periphery of the cell by the mucus that fills the cytoplasm.

significance level the probability of observing a value of a specified test statistic that is regarded as significant, when this extreme value is in fact due only to random variation under the null hypothesis (i.e., H_0 is true). Also called level of significance. See also *hypothesis testing.*

significance probability the probability of observing a value of a specified test statistic that is at least as significant as the value calculated from a particular sample. Also called *P value.* See also *hypothesis testing.*

significant (sig-nif'ĭ-kant) in statistics, a result that has small probability under the null hypothesis, suggesting that the null hypothesis is not true.

significant digits the digits of numerical measurement that are unaffected by measurement error. When no explicit statement of measurement error is given, the implied error is about ±5 in the first nonsignificant digit, where zeros after the decimal point are counted as significant. Leading zeros do not count.

Thus, a measurement reported as 1.57 has three significant digits and is assumed to have approximate limits of accuracy of 1.565 and 1.575 (1.00 has the limits 0.995 and 1.005); the true value lies somewhere between these limits. Zeros before the decimal point are not necessarily significant; that is, 2500 may have two, three, or four significant digits, which can be indicated in scientific notation as: 2.5×10^3, 2.50×10^3, or 2.500×10^3.

The result of an arithmetical calculation can have only as many significant digits as the least accurate number entering into the calculation and should be rounded off to this many places (intermediate results are not rounded).

Also called significant figures.

silane (sil'ān) [silicon + methane] 1. a gas, SiH_4; M.W. 32.09. It has a repulsive odor, is highly irritating, and ignites in air at elevated temperatures. Also called monosilane.

2. the silicone analog of alkane; disilane (Si_2H_6), trisilane (Si_3H_8), and tetrasilane (Si_4H_{10}) are known; all are flammable and are irritants.

silanization (sil"an-ĭ-za'shun) 1. in gas chromatography, the coating of glass columns and silicate solid supports with a substituted silane, e.g., dimethyldichlorosilane or hexamethyldisilazane. This is generally done before loading the stationary phase to make the column tubing and support more inert by replacing polar, active groups with silyl groups.

2. generally, the coating of surfaces of laboratory glassware to minimize the loss of solutes by adsorption in extremely diluted specimens.

Silastic (sĭ-las'tik) trademark. See *dimethicone.*

silent period the interval of time after which a muscle has been abruptly unloaded during which no electric activity is present in the muscle.

silica (sil'ĭ-kah) [L. *silex* flint] silicon dioxide (SiO_2); a colorless crystalline solid occurring in two crystalline forms, quartz and cristobalite. A number of naturally occurring materials are composed of silica, e.g., flint, diatomite, sand, and amethyst. A glass is formed when molten silica is cooled slowly. Chronic exposure to silica or silicate dusts results in silicosis, a pneumoconiosis characterized by fibrosis of the lung, decreased pulmonary function, and susceptibility to pulmonary tuberculosis.

silica gel 1. a highly adsorbent gel of hydrated silica (silicon dioxide). It is one of the most commonly used adsorbents in thin-layer chromatography.

2. [USP], used as a dispersing and suspending agent in drug preparations.

silicate (sil'ĭ-kāt) [L. *silicus*] any of many salts and minerals that contain silicon, oxygen, and metals. The structure is based on the tetrahedral SiO_4 unit. The simplest silicates contain the SiO_4^{4-} ion, but most silicates are large anions formed by linking these units through Si—O—Si bonds extending in one, two, or three dimensions, e.g., beryl ($Be_3Al_2Si_6O_{18}$) and talc ($Mg_3Si_4O_{10}(OH)_2$). Many naturally occurring minerals are silicates. See also *silica.*

silicic acid (sil-ik'ik) hydrated silicon dioxide. True monosilicic acid, $Si(OH_4)$ (also H_4SiO_4), is the only SiO_2 species found in neutral solution. Other forms vary in the degree of dehydration. Silicic acid in various hydrated forms (silica gel) is used in thin-layer and column chromatography. See also *silica gel.*

silicon (Si) (sil'ĭ-kon) [L. *silex* flint (silicon dioxide)] a gray-black, semiconducting element; atomic number 14; atomic weight 28.086; Group IV of the periodic table; oxidation states –4, +2, +3, +4 (the most common). It occurs naturally in silica and silicate rocks and is used industrially in alloys, in the production of silanes and silicones, and as doped single crystals in semiconductor electronic devices.

silicon-controlled rectifier (SCR) a semiconductor device used as a switch. Unlike transistors, it can control large demands for current, such as in electric motors. It is a four-layer (*pnpn*) device with three terminals: the anode (the outside *p* layer), gate (the inside *p* layer), and cathode (the outside *n* layer). When the cathode and gate are grounded and the anode becomes positive, no current flows because the gate-cathode junction is reverse-biased. If a positive pulse is applied to the gate, conduction will begin and continue until the anode becomes negative. Then, no current will flow until the anode is again positive and another gate pulse applied. Because it is necessary to reverse-bias the anode to switch off the current, the SCR is usually employed to control alternating current devices.

silicon-controlled switch (SCS) a semiconductor device used as a switch. Like the silicon-controlled rectifier (SCR), it is a four-layer (*pnpn*) device, but each is attached to a terminal. In order these are the anode, anode gate, cathode gate (which corresponds to the SCR gate), and cathode. An SCS operates exactly like an SCR, except that it can be switched off without reversing the anode polarity: by applying a positive pulse to the anode gate, it cuts off conduction by reverse-biasing the anode-anode gate junction.

silicon dioxide a colorless crystalline or amorphous solid, SiO_2; M.W. 60.09. See also *silica.*

colloidal s. d., [NF], used as a tablet diluent and suspending agent.

silicone (sil′ĭ-kōn) any of a large group of stable, inert polymers. Simple silicones have the repeating structural unit $—R_2Si—O—$, where R is a hydrocarbon group (such as methyl, ethyl, or phenyl). Cross-linked silicones have oxygen bridges between silicon atoms in different chains.

Silicones are water-repellent, good lubricants, and stable at high temperatures. They are commonly used as greases or sealants; as the stationary phase in gas chromatography; and to coat glassware used for blood collection (to reduce platelet loss). Elastomeric silicone (silicon rubber) is biologically inert and is used in surgical prostheses.

See also *dimethicone* and *simethicone.*

silicosis (sil″i-ko′sis) [L. *silex* flint + *-osis*] a chronic, fibrotic pneumoconiosis due to prolonged exposure (2–20 yr) to free silica (i.e., quartz or silicon dioxide) dust. It is an occupational hazard in the hard rock mining, sandblasting, iron molding, and ceramic industries. Chronic inhalation of the silica particles (greater than 5 μ in diameter) leads to discrete nodular pulmonary fibrosis, conglomerate fibrosis, and respiratory impairment. Radiographs of the chest usually reveal bilateral, symmetric interstitial fibrosis, hilar adenopathy, and "eggshell" calcifications of hilar lymph nodes. The disease may remain asymptomatic for years after lesions become radiographically visible. Tuberculosis and recurrent respiratory infections are common complications. Emphysema is often associated with silicosis and leads to increased radiolucency of the lungs, especially at the bases. There is no effective therapy. See also *pneumoconiosis.*

silo-filler's disease pulmonary inflammation, often with acute pulmonary edema, due to inhalation of the irritant gases (especially oxides of nitrogen) that collect in recently filled silos.

silver (Ag) (sil′ver) [A.S. *siolfor* ultimately from Akkadian *sarpu;* L. *argentum*] a lustrous, ductile, white metallic element; atomic number 47; atomic weight 107.868; a 4d transition element; oxidation state +1, and, rarely, +2, +3.

Silver has the highest thermal and electric conductivity of all metals. It is used in jewelry and tableware, as a catalyst, and in photography. During the photographic developing process, silver halide salts become activated when exposed to light or x-rays and are easily reduced to metallic silver.

Ingestion or inhalation of silver or its salts can cause argyria (argyrosis), the deposition of insoluble silver sulfide in the elastic fibers of the dermis, which causes a patchy blue-black pigmentation of the skin and sometimes the cornea and conjunctiva of the eye. It also deposits in other organs, particularly the lungs.

Silver salts are used medicinally as antiseptics and as bacteriostatic agents. The silver(I) ion binds to active groups in microbial enzymes, thus inactivating them.

mild s. protein, a silver proteinate complex, less irritating then soluble salts, that is used as an antiseptic for skin and mucous membranes. It can produce argyria (see under *silver*). Trademark, Argyrol.

s. nitrate, [USP], a soluble silver salt used as a topical antiseptic; in stronger solutions it is used as a caustic. Routinely, 1 percent solution is administered to the eyes of all newborns for the prevention of ophthalmia neonatorum (gonococcal conjunctivitis).

silver sulfadiazine (sul″fah-di′ah-zēn) a broad-spectrum antimicrobial agent applied topically to burns and wounds to prevent infection. Trademark, Silvadene.

silvex (sil′veks) one of the chlorophenoxy herbicides, 2-(2,4,5-trichlorophenoxy)propionic acid (2,4,5-TCPPA), used as a defoliant. See also *chlorophenoxy herbicides.*

silylation (sil″il-a′shun) in gas chromatography, the derivatization of a compound by replacement of a reactive hydrogen (as in acids, amines, or alcohols) with a trimethylsilyl group (TMS, $—Si(CH_3)_3$). The derivative is usually more volatile, less polar, and more stable at a high temperature than the parent compound, and will chromatograph more quickly and with less tailing.

Silylation is accomplished by reaction with a silylation reagent, such as bis-trimethylsilyltrifluoroacetamide (BSTFA) or bis-trimethylsilylacetamide (BSA), in an unreactive, dry solvent such as acetonitrile, dimethylsulfoxide, tetrahydrofuran, or pyridine.

simethicone (si-meth′ĭ-kōn) [USP], a mixture of dimethyl polysiloxanes and silica gel used as an antiflatulent. It releases gas by altering surface tension.

simian crease (sĭm′ē-an) a single transverse crease on the palm, instead of the usual multiple diagonal and transverse creases. It is found in 1 percent of normal whites, in a larger percentage of normal Orientals, in 70 percent of those affected with Down's syndrome, and in an intermediate percentage of children with other congenital malformations.

Simmonds' disease (sim′ondz) [Morris *Simmonds,* Hamburg physician, 1855–1925] panhypopituitarism that leads to a true pituitary cachexia. It follows the destruction of the pituitary following surgery, infection, trauma, or neoplastic invasion. See also *panhypopituitarism.*

simple epithelium an epithelium composed of a single layer of cells.

simple protein (sim′p′l pro′te-in) [L. *simplex;* Gr. *prōtos* first] a group of proteins in an older classification system; those that yield only α-amino acids on complete hydrolysis. This class includes albumins, globulins, glutelins, alcohol-soluble proteins, albuminoids (scleroproteins), histones, and protamines.

Simulated Matrix Reference Materials see under *reference materials.*

simulation (sim″u-la′shun) [L. *simulatio*] 1. the mimicking of one disease by another.

2. the modeling of the behavior of physical process by means of a computer program or another physical process with analogous behavior.

simulator (sim′u-la″tor) a piece of diagnostic x-ray equipment that exactly reproduces the movements and capabilities of a radiation therapy treatment machine, with the single exception that it does not produce a treatment beam. In place of the treatment beam it carries a diagnostic x-ray tube and fluoroscopy unit, which allows the radiation treatment planned to be visualized. The patient can then be transferred to a treatment unit where the treatment can be carried out in exactly the prescribed manner. Such equipment allows careful planning without the use of the treatment machine.

Simuliidae (si″mu-le′ĭ-de) a family of flies, including the genus *Simulium,* that is known to transmit *Onchocerca volvulus.* These flies are small, with a humped back and short, stubbed antennae. This family contains approximately 1200 species of worldwide distribution, known variously as black flies, buffalo gnats or turkey gnats.

sin abbrev. See *sine.*

sincalide (sin′kah-lid) the C-terminal octapeptide residue of the intestinal hormone cholecystokinin-pancreozymin (CCK-PZ). It can be synthesized and some evidence suggests that it may exist as a natural hormone. Sincalide stimulates contraction of the gallbladder within 5–15 min after intravenous injection and is a powerful stimulator of pancreatic enzyme secretion. It is used in combination with secretin, in a test of pancreatic function, as a diagnostic in cholecystography, or in the collection of bile samples by duodenal intubation. The common side-effects, abdominal pain and an urge to defecate, are normal hormonal actions. Trademark, *Kinevac.* See also *cholagogue.*

sine (sīn) [L. *sinus* fold, a mistranslation of Ar. *jayb* chord and also fold] a trigonometric function, $\sin \theta = \chi / s$, where θ is the angle formed by two radii of a circle, s is the length of the arc, and χ is the length of the chord between the radii. See also *sine w.* under *wave.*

Sinequan (sin′ĕ-kwan) trademark. See *doxepin.*

singers' nodules see *laryngeal nodules.*

single-blind pertaining to an experiment in which the subjects do not know whether they are in the treatment group or the control group. See also *clinical trials.*

single-breath nitrogen test (SBN_2) a procedure used to detect the uneven distribution of ventilation that is based on measurement of the change in the percentage of nitrogen (N_2) in maximal expiration following a single deep inspiration of 100 percent oxygen (O_2). The change in the N_2 content of the expired air is monitored with a rapid N_2 analyzer; simultaneous measurements of respiratory flow (pneumotachographic) and volume (spirometric) are made. The N_2 percentage, which should be unchanged if the inspired O_2 is distributed evenly to each of the alveoli, is by convention measured between 750 and 1250 ml of the expired air.

The change in nitrogen percentage varies from 0–1.5 percent in healthy, young subjects to often greater than 10 percent in those with obstructive lung disease or with markedly uneven distribution of ventilation to functioning respiratory units.

single diffusion test see *Oudin test.*

single-phase (sing′g'l fāz) pertaining to ordinary alternating current as opposed to *three-phase current.*

sink (singk) a device or region in which some physical quantity, such as energy or heat, is removed from a system. See also *heat sink.* Cf. *source.*

sinoatrial (si″no-a′tre-al) pertaining to the sinus venosus and the atrium of the heart.

sinoatrial block the absence of atrioventricular depolarization resulting from the blockage of a normally formed sinus node impulse. Sinoatrial block may be caused by diseases of the atrium, by hyperkalemia, or by certain antiarrhythmic drugs; it may also follow myocardial infarction.

sinoatrial node see *sinoatrial n.* under *node.*

Sinografin trademark for a radiopaque contrast medium used in hysterosalpingography. It is a mixture of diatrizoate meglumine and iodipamide meglumine.

sinus/o (si′nŭ-so) a word element used in combining form to denote sinus or cavity, e.g., sinusoid.

sinus (si′nus), pl. *sinus* or *sinuses* [L. "a hollow"] 1. [NA], a general term for such spaces as the dilated channels for venous blood in the cranial cavity, or the air cavities in the skull bones. For more information, see the specific sinus.

2. an abnormal channel or tract.

sinus arrest the intermittent absence of sinus node depolarization, resulting in a long pause between cardiac contractions, and notable on physical examination or electrocardiography.

sinus arrhythmia (si′nus ah-rith′me-ah) variability of the heart rhythm due to lack of regularity in the firing of the sinoatrial node. The most common form is a regular variation in heart rate that is synchronized to the phases of the respiratory cycle; it is a phenomenon that frequently occurs in the normal human heart. The heart rate may increase and decrease by a much as 30 percent with each cycle of inspiration and expiration. Sinus arrhythmia is usually the result of several cardiopulmonary reflexes that effect a cyclic change through the autonomic nerves to the heart. It may also result from disease of the AV node.

sinus bradycardia a heart rate of fewer than 60 beats/min, with electric impulses originating from the sinoatrial node (the normal pacemaker of the heart). Sinus bradycardia may be associated with hypothyroidism, hypothermia, myocardial infarction, and certain drugs. Bradycardia may be a sign of sinoatrial node disease, or even an ominous sign of increasing intracranial pressure from an intracranial tumor or other disease processes. Often, however, it is a normal change in rate found in deep sleep, and during waking in well-conditioned athletes.

sinusitis (si″nŭ-si′tis) an acute or chronic inflammation of one or all of the sinus cavities. Acute sinusitis commonly follows an upper respiratory tract infection, nasal allergy, or dental infection. Pain and swelling occur at the involved sinuses, with nasal congestion and purulent discharge. Fever, chills, and malaise may accompany the infection. Staphylococci and streptococci are frequently involved. Chronic sinusitis resembles the acute form and may result from recurrent acute attacks. In both forms, there may be an elevated white blood cell count, and the etiologic agent may be cultured from nasal secretions. Radiographs of the skull reveal cloudy opacification of the involved sinuses.

sinus node see *sinoatrial n.* under *node.*

sinusoid (si′nŭ-soid) [*sinus* + Gr. *eidos* form] 1. resembling a sinus.

2. thin-walled, irregular vascular spaces that conform in shape to the interstices among the epithelial elements of the perfused organ. Some are lined by reticuloendothelial cells.

sinus venosus (si′nus ven-o′sus) in the embryo, the caudal segment of the primitive heart tube that develops into the portion of the atrium receiving the venae cavae.

Siphonaptera (si″fo-nap′ter-ah) [Gr. *siphon* tube + *apteros* wingless] an order of fleas. They are small, wingless ectoparasites of mammals and birds, with a range of 1.5–4.0 mm in length and are laterally compressed and highly chitinized. More than 1900 species and subspecies have been described. The order consists of six or more families, of which two, the Pulicidae and Tungidae, are of medical importance. Fleas are known transmitters of *Rickettsia typhi* (which causes murine typhus), reservoirs of *Yersinia pestis* (the causal agent for bubonic plague), and intermediate hosts of several tapeworms. Some fleas have extremely annnoying bites that may result in dermatitis.

Siphunculina (si-fun″ku-li′nah) a genus of flies, the eye gnats, of the family Chloropidae. The species *S. funicola,* the eye fly, is commonly found in India and is thought to transmit the causative agent of conjunctivitis.

Sipple's syndrome see *MEN II* under *MEN.*

Sirius red 4B a red water- and alcohol-soluble dye, often used in amyloid stains; C.I. 28160.

SIRS abbrev. See *soluble immune response suppressor.*

Sisyrosea a genus of urticating caterpillars of the family Limacodidae. The species *S. textula,* commonly found in the eastern United States, possesses spine-type poisonous hairs.

sitosterols (si″to-ster′olz) [NF], a preparation of plant sterols used in the treatment of hyperlipoproteinemia. It produces small decreases in serum cholesterol and triglyceride levels by interfering with cholesterol absorption. Trademark, Cytellin.

situs (si′tus), pl. *situs* [L.] site or position.

s. inversus, the transposition of the viscera of the thorax and abdomen, as in a mirror image; the transposition may be complete or partial.

six-Hertz spike and slow waves in electroencephalography, a complex appearing as bilaterally synchronous bursts of spike and slow-wave activity at 5–7 Hz. The amplitude of this complex is variable, and the activity is generally confined to, or most conspicuous over, either the anterior or posterior region of the head. The diagnostic significance of this complex is controversial. Also called *phantom spike and wave.*

6/60 see *SMA 6/60.*

size-exclusion chromatography see under *chromatography.*

Sjögren's syndrome (sho′grenz) [Henrik Samuel Conrad *Sjögren,* Swedish ophthalmologist, born 1899] a chronic inflammatory disease characterized by the lack of lacrimal and salivary secretions, and usually associated with a systemic connective tissue disease. The ducts of the involved secretory glands narrow, followed by an infiltrate of lymphocytes (both T- and B-), plasma cells, and macrophages. The duct-lining cells proliferate and are involved in the replacement and destruction of acinar cells.

The mechanism causing the cellular infiltrate is unclear; however, antibody-dependent cellular cytotoxicity activity is probably involved. This immune reaction may be due to viral antigens or abnormal autoantigens.

skatole (skat′ōl) [Gr. *skōr, skatos* dung] β-methylindole, a strong-smelling crystalline amine occurring in human feces. It is produced by the bacterial decomposition of digested protein in the intestine, and is derived from tryptophan by several different pathways involving indole and indoleacetic acid as intermediates.

skatoxyl (skah-tok′sil) β-hydroxymethylindole, an oxidation product of skatole, formed by the bacterial action on indoleacetic acid. It is found in the urine of individuals having certain diseases of the large intestine.

skeletal (skel′e-tal) pertaining to the skeleton.

skeletal muscle see *skeletal m.* under *muscle.*

skeleton (skel′ĕ-ton) [Gr. "a dried body, mummy"] the hard framework of the animal body, especially the bony framework of higher vertebrate animals. The term is also used to refer collectively to the bones of the body; see also the accompanying illustration.

skew (sku) deviating from a straight line; in statistics, deviation from symmetry for a frequency distribution.

skewed distribution a probability distribution that is not symmetric. Cf. *probability distribution* and *symmetric distribution.*

skewness (sku′nes) the characteristic of asymmetry of a probability distribution, or any measure of the degree of asymmetry of a distribution.

skiagraph (ski′ah-graf) see *radiograph.*

skiametry (ski-am′ĕ-tre) see *retinoscopy.*

skin the tissue that forms the external covering of the body. It consists of an outer epithelial layer, the epidermis, supported by an underlying connective tissue layer, the dermis. The skin helps the body control its internal environment by aiding in regulation of temperature and fluid balance. The dermis lies on the subcutaneous fat, which varies in thickness in different parts of the body.

The epidermis is composed of stratified squamous epithelium, which undergoes continuous and relatively rapid turnover of epidermal cells. Much of the mitotic activity takes place within the single layer of basal cells that rest on the basal lamina at the epidermal-dermal junction. The more superficial squamous cells, constituting the stratum spinosum, become progressively flattened as they approach the surface, and accumulate granules of keratohyalin within their cytoplasm (stratum granulosum). The surface layer (stratum corneum) is composed of a compact mass of flattened cells that have lost their nuclei and organelles. This surface layer of keratin serves to protect the skin from friction.

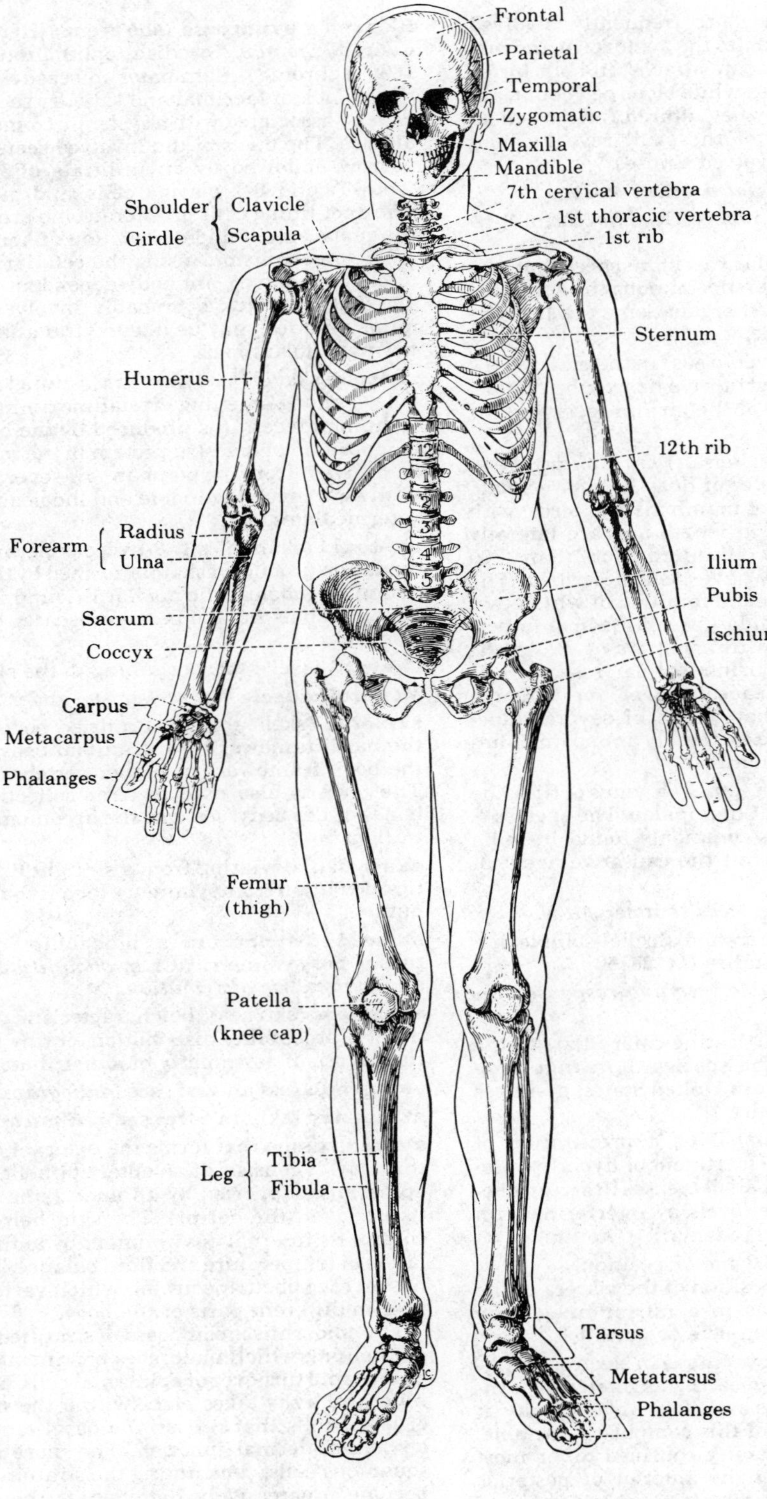

Skeleton. Anterior view of the human skeleton. (From Dorland's Illustrated Medical Dictionary. 26th ed. Philadelphia, W. B. Saunders Co., 1981.)

Within the stratum spinosum, the squamous cells are united by numerous desmosomes with associated bundles of prekeratin or tonofilaments. These cells also form membrane-limited granules, which are extruded toward the surface of the epidermis to aid in cell cohesion.

The epidermis does not contain capillaries, receiving nutriment by diffusion from the dermis. Ducts of the dermal sweat glands and hair shafts pierce the epidermis to reach the surface. In addition to keratin-forming cells, the epidermis contains pigment-producing melanocytes and Langerhans cells. The epidermis varies in thickness in different parts of the body: it is thinnest on a surface exposed to little abrasion, such as the eyelid, and is thickest on surfaces exposed to wear and tear, such as the sole of the foot, which is heavily keratinized. The dermis consists of interwoven collagen elastic fibers and fibroblasts. In the more superficial or papillary dermis, the collagen fibers are not as dense as in the thicker reticular dermis. The papillary dermis fills the ridges formed by the undulating undersurface of the epidermis, producing the dermal papillae. There is not always a sharp demarcation between the deep aspect of the dermis and the subcutaneous areolar tissue.

Vessels and nerves enter the dermis through the subcutaneous tissue and ramify in its deeper levels, sending branches upward toward the dermal-epidermal junction. Some sensory nerves terminate as fine ramifications, whereas others have specialized receptors at their tips, e.g., pacinian and Meissner corpuscles and Merkel cells.

The skin hairs emerge from follicles within the dermis or upper subcutaneous tissue. The material of the hair is formed by concentric layers of cells within the matrix of the follicle. Each hair has an outer cuticle, cortex, and central medulla. Bundles of smooth muscle cells constitute the arrector pili muscles, which can elevate the hairs. Sebaceous glands surround the hair follicles and express their secretion through a short duct into the canal of the follicle.

The eccrine sweat glands have a coiled secretory portion within the dermis leading into a simple tubular duct that pierces the epidermis. Apocrine glands in the human are confined to the axilla, urogenital area, nipple, eyelid (Moll's glands), and external auditory canal (ceruminous glands).

skin-film distance (sfd, SFD) in radiology, the distance between the skin of the subject and the x-ray film or cassette. See also *object-film distance.*

skin reactive factor (SRF) a complex of lymphokines that may be responsible for the evolution of a skin reaction similar to delayed hypersensitivity reactions. SRF may be a combination of migration inhibitory factor (MIF) and monocyte and neutrophil chemotactic factors, as well as factors that increase vascular permeability.

skin test a procedure that uses delayed hypersensitivity to detect an antigen for investigating an infectious disease or to detect an individual's immunocompetence. Skin tests are commonly used to detect tuberculosis or various fungal diseases or to observe an allergy to specific antigens.

Freshly prepared antigen is injected intradermally, and erythema and induration are measured at intervals of 24 and 48 hr. Induration of 5 mm or greater is considered a positive skin test. If the patient is expected to be anergic, dinitrochlorobenzene (DNCB) is applied 7–10 da prior to skin testing. This results in increased sensitivity to challenge doses of new antigen. If the patient reacts excessively to a skin test, an injection of corticosteroids will moderate the reaction.

skin tumors tumors of epidermal cells, which are the most common neoplasms affecting the human body. Exposure to sunlight is a known etiologic factor. Squamous cell and basal cell carcinomas are predominantly seen on noncovered areas of the body. Tumors of pigmented cells of the skin include various forms of nevi and malignant melanoma. A broad range of histologic features is seen among adnexal neoplasms, reflecting the developmental potential of the cells of origin. Primary lymphoma/leukemia may involve the dermis, and in this location exhibit distinctive clinical and histologic features, e.g., mycosis fungoides. Similarly, most soft tissue neoplasms seen elsewhere in the body can occur in the skin; a few, notably dermatofibrosarcoma protuberans and Kaposi's sarcoma, have characteristic clinical appearances and histologic features. For more information, see the specific tumor.

Skiodan (ski'o-dan) trademark. See *methiodal sodium.*

skull (skul) the skeleton of the head and face. It is made up of 22 bones, 21 of which (excluding the mandible) are firmly united in the mature individual to form a single unit. They enclose the cranial cavity, which houses the brain and its supporting membranes. Smaller cavities formed by the skull bones are the nasal cavity, orbits, air sinuses, and cavities of the middle and internal ears. The flat skull bones are made up of two plates of bone enclosing a narrow cavity (the diplöe). Some of the bones of the skull are paired and others are unpaired. The paired bones are the parietal, temporal, nasal, lacrimal, inferior nasal conchae, maxillary, zygomatic, and palatine. The unpaired bones are the frontal, ethmoid, sphenoid, occipital, vomer, and mandible. The terms skull and cranium denote the bones of the head excluding the mandible, although cranium was formerly used to indicate the part of the head covered with hair. The term calvaria refers to the top part of the skull.

The cranial features are logically described by viewing the exterior of the skull from above (norma verticalis), from the front (norma frontalis), from the back (norma occipitalis), from the side (norma lateralis), and from below (norma basalis). To view the upper surface of the base of the skull, the cranial cavity must be opened by removing its roof. When this is done, the floor of the cranial cavity is seen to be arranged in three broad depressions or fossae: the anterior, middle, and posterior cranial fossae.

slant (slant) a sloping surface of agar in a test tube used for bacterial cultures. See also *slant c.* under *culture.*

SLE abbrev. See *systemic l. erythematosus* under *lupus.*

sleep (slēp) a behavioral state marked by a reversible decrease in motor activity and sensitivity to external stimuli; changes in autonomic function; and characteristic electroencephalographic patterns.

There are two sleep states in humans, slow-wave sleep (SWS) and rapid eye movement (REM) or desynchronized sleep (DS). SWS is characterized by high-voltage slow activity in the electroencephalogram (EEG) and decreased (as compared with wakefulness) but regular respiration, heart rate, and blood pressure. REM sleep is characterized by low-voltage electric activity of variable frequency in the EEG. Because this activity resembles that recorded on the EEG during wakefulness, this stage is often referred to as paradoxical sleep (PS). Heart rate, blood pressure, and respiration are accelerated and irregular, muscle tone is reduced, and small muscle twitches may occur. Penile erection and REM also occur episodically. Humans awakened during this stage of sleep frequently recall dreaming.

In mammals, the alternation between sleep and wakefulness is an endogenous circadian rhythm independent of ambient temperature, but one that can be entrained to a 24-hr light-dark cycle. Although the sleep-wakefulness cycle depends on an intact hypothalamus, it does not require the presence of the pituitary, pineal, thyroid, gonadal, or adrenal glands.

In the human infant, a greater proportion of sleep consists of REM sleep than in later life. During the first year of life, the periods of wakefulness during the day gradually lengthen, and age appears to be the single most important determinant of the sleep pattern of an individual. With age, the total amount of daily sleep and of daily REM sleep declines.

Clinical observations have shown that partial removal of the cerebral hemispheres does not disrupt the sleep-wakefulness cycle, whereas lesions of the diencephalon may produce alterations in the cycle.

From experimental studies conducted on laboratory animals, it can be shown that sleep is an active process mediated by two parallel central nervous system pathways. One system located in the medial tegmentum projects to the hypothalamus and thalamus, and then to the frontal and temporal cortex. The primary neurotransmitter of this system is 5-hydroxtryptamine (5-HT). Activation of this system leads to hypersomnia with increases in both SWS and DS.

The parallel system is found in the lateral tegmentum, and includes the locus ceruleus and substantia nigra. These areas contain large amounts of the neurotransmitter norepinephrine; destruction of these areas results in a suppression of DS. The phasic muscle and eye movements of DS are mediated by the vestibular nuclei.

The mechanism regulating the suppression or activation of these two systems in the intact animal has not been determined. There appears to be a biologic need for sleep, for sleep-deprived laboratory animals die within a few days and sleep-deprived humans exhibit disturbed behavior, but the physiologic role of sleep is still unknown.

See also *hypersomnia* and *insomnia.*

s. apnea, see *hypersomnia–sleep apnea syndrome.*

s. deprivation, the systematic deprivation of a human or laboratory animal of all sleep or of one of the phases of sleep (SWS or REM). In the normal individual, when undisturbed sleep is again permitted, there is an increase or rebound in the phase of sleep that has been interrupted. If the person has been deprived of all sleep for 24 hr before sleep is again permitted, there is first an increase in SWS, and a rebound in REM sleep is delayed until the second or third night of undisturbed sleep.

A subject deprived of sleep may experience irritability, impaired concentration in attention and memory, poor muscle coordination, and visual or tactile hallucinations. Such symptoms usually disappear once sleep is again allowed.

Sleep deprivation is used as an activation technique in electroencephalography to provoke abnormalities in the electric activity of the brain. The technique is harmless and may be helpful in the evaluation of those suspected of having epilepsy.

drug-induced s., an activation technique used in human electroencephalography. Drugs commonly used to induce sleep include barbiturates (e.g., pentobarbital), and nonbarbiturates (e.g., glutethimide and chlorpromazine). Barbiturates, in particular, produce an EEG characterized by symmetric beta activity (18–24 Hz) that predominates in the frontocentral regions of the head. Except during the intravenous administration of baribturates and during drug-induced necrosis, other activity resembles that of spontaneous sleep. Consistent asymmetry of induced activity may be of clinical significance in suggesting the possibility of lateralized pathologic change. In addition, the procedure may activate epileptiform activity and is sometimes helpful in the evaluation of patients with suspected epilepsy.

s. spindle, in electroencephalography, a burst of 11- to 15-Hz activity that occurs symmetrically over the anterior and central regions of the head during light sleep (Stage 2) in normal adults and children. Tha amplitude is variable (usually less than 50 μV) but of higher voltage when recorded from the central areas than elsewhere. In some forms of insomnia, sleep spindles may occur abnormally during REM sleep. Also called *sigma rhythm.*

s. stages, in human electroencephalography, those characteristic changes in the electric activity of the brain that occur progressively and repeatedly during sleep.

There are five stages. During Stage 1 (*drowsiness*), the EEG shows attenuation of the alpha rhythm and a background of theta and beta activity.

During Stage 2 (*light sleep*), the EEG shows spontaneous sleep spindles on a low-voltage background activity of 3- to 6-Hz frequency, and K complexes or vertex sharp waves occur spontaneously and in response to sensory stimuli.

During Stage 3 (*intermediate sleep*), the EEG shows high-voltage delta and theta waves, with superimposed K complexes and sleep spindles.

During Stage 4 (*deep sleep*), the EEG shows more profuse and continuous high-voltage delta waves, and the individual cannot be easily aroused by external stimuli.

During the fifth stage (*REM*), the EEG show low-voltage fast activity resembling that of wakefulness, and in addition there are rapid eye movements. The muscle tone is generally low, although periodic muscle jerks may occur, and the respiratory and heart rates are irregular. Persons awakened during this sleep often report dreaming. Also called *desynchronized sleep, paradoxical sleep,* and *rapid eye movement* (*REM*) *sleep.*

To determine the contribution of the various stages of sleep to total sleep time, the EEG record can be divided into time blocks or epochs that usually last between 10 sec and 2 min. The epoch is then characterized by the predominating sleep stage.

In humans, sleep progresses from Stage 1 through Stage 4, then reversing through Stages 3 and 2 to Stage REM. Stage REM alternates with non-REM sleep every 90–100 min. In a normal young adult, an average 450-min sleep period consists of 5–10 percent Stage 1, 50 percent Stage 2, 15 percent Stage 3, 10 percent Stage 4, and 20 percent Stage REM. Stages 3 and 4 usually occur predominantly during the first third of the sleep period, with Stage REM increasing in duration as sleep time progresses.

In mammals such as the cat, monkey, and rat, sleep stages can also be identified, but high-voltage, slow-wave activity is usually termed *slow-wave sleep* (*SWS*) or *synchronous sleep.*

sleeping disease see *narcolepsy.*

sleeping sickness see *African t.* under *trypanosomiasis.*

sleep terror disorder see *p. nocturnus* under *pavor.*

sleepwalking see *somnambulism.*

slide (slid) a rectangular glass plate on which tissue sections are mounted for microscopic examination.

slope (slōp) 1. an inclined plane.

2. the tangent of the angle made by a given line and the horizontal plane. If the line is represented by the equation $y = mx + b$, m is the slope. The slope of a curved line at a given point is the slope of the tangent line at that point.

slot exhaust a specially designed exhaust system for sweeping contaminants to an exhaust inlet at the back of a laboratory bench or other work surface. A slot exhaust is suitable for materials of moderate toxicity if the total system of exhaust and supply of air is designed so that the slot exhaust is effective. See also *local exhaust* under *ventilation.*

slow activity in electroencephalography, any pattern of electric activity that has a frequency less than 8 Hz.

slow-fused transient see *posterior slow w.* under *wave.*

"slow" hemoglobins those hemoglobins that are less mobile than normal adult Hb A on electrophoresis (at pH 8.6 in barbital buffer), such as Hb S and Hb D.

slow neutron a neutron having a kinetic energy of less than 100 eV. Slow and thermal neutrons undergo neutron capture reactions.

slow-reacting substance of anaphylaxis (SRS-A) a vasoactive amine induced by type-1 anaphylactic reactions. SRS-A is an acidic lipid that increases vascular permeability, contracts smooth muscle; M.W. 400–500. It does not exist in a preformed state, but rather is formed as a result of antigen-antibody interactions with mast cells. It is the chief mediator of prolonged bronchospasms of asthma with a half-life of hours and is not inhibited by antihistamines. After SRS-A is released from basophilic granules, its biologic activity may be inhibited by diethylcarbamazine. The smooth muscle contractions caused by SRS-A can be inhibited with epinephrine. Eosinophilic granules contain arylsulfatase, which divides SRS-A into two inactive fragments. See also *anaphylaxis.*

slow viruses viruses that, after a long incubation period, cause a slowly progressive and usually lethal disease. The four viruses in this group (those causing scrapie, transmissible mink encephalopathy, kuru, and Creutzfeldt-Jakob disease) that cause subacute spongiform encephalopathies have not been well characterized, but have similar characteristics. These agents are not typical virions, as they are highly resistant to inactivation by the usual chemical and physical sterilizing agents such as formaldehyde, β-propiolactone, protease, nuclease (RNases and DNases), ultraviolet irradiation, and heat at 80°C.

Electron-microscopic examination of infected cerebral tissues and virus concentrated in cesium chloride or sucrose gradient has not revealed the presence of viral particles, nor have infectious nucleic acid or viral antigens been detected. It has been suggested that the agent may be a membrane-associated "viroid" rather than an orthodox virus. Nevertheless, these agents are filterable and can cause similar disease in chimpanzees and other primates by transmission. One of the most unusual characteristics of slow viruses has been their inability to induce host immune response, so that the host has no mechanism to control the multiplication and pathologic effects of these agents.

See also *Creutzfeldt-Jakob disease* and *kuru.*

slow-wave sleep (SWS) see under *sleep* and *s. stages.*

Sly disease see *β-D-glucuronidose deficiency.*

Sm symbol for the chemical element *samarium.*

SMA 6/60 [acronym from *S*equential *M*ultiple *A*nalyzer] trademark for an automated chemistry system that performs six different tests on serum in 60 min and reports results in a fixed sequence; the tests include determination of creatinine or glucose, urea nitrogen, chloride, carbon dioxide, sodium, and potassium concentrations. See also *clinical chemistry automation.*

SMA 12/60 trademark for an automated chemistry system that performs 12 different tests on serum and reports results in a fixed sequence; the tests include measurement of calcium, inorganic phosphorus, glucose, urea nitrogen, uric acid, cholesterol, total protein, albumin, total bilirubin, alkaline phosphatase, lactate dehydrogenase, and aspartate aminotransferase levels. See also *clinical chemistry automation.*

SMAF abbrev. See *specific macrophage-arming factor.*

small airways disease a term used to denote a form of chronic obstructive bronchitis in which most of the affected airways (bronchi and bronchioles) are of a diameter smaller than 2 mm. See also *chronic obstructive bronchitis.*

small cell carcinoma a descriptive and nonspecific term for a carcinoma composed of small round cells lacking architectural organization; it may be used as a synonym for bronchogenic small cell (oat cell) undifferentiated carcinoma.

small cell tumor a nonspecific designation for a heterogeneous group of neoplasms, histogenetically unrelated, that have in common the histologic appearance of sheets of small round or ovoid cells, generally with little or no architectural organization. The differential diagnosis may include rhabdomyosarcoma, neuroblastoma, lymphoma-leukemia, Ewing's tumor, and small cell carcinoma. The age of the patient and location of the tumor may be of some assistance in determining its histogenetic type. Electron microscopy and immunoperoxidase staining may be useful for this purpose. Also called small round cell neoplasm.

small intestine the more proximal of the two sections of the intestine, comprising the duodenum, jejunum, and ileum, and extending from the pylorus to the ileocecal valve. Also called small bowel. See also *duodenum, ileum,* and *jejunum.*

small intestine tumors neoplasms of the small intestine; they constitute fewer than 5 percent of all neoplasms arising in the gastrointestinal tract. Adenomas are relatively uncommon and may be symptomless. Malignant small intestinal neoplasms are most common in the ileum and least frequent in the jejunum, where they most commonly occur close to the ligament of Treitz. Symptoms from the malignant tumors consist predominantly of pain, bleeding, and obstruction. Diagnosis is suggested by radiologic findings. At the time of surgery, most patients have metastases. Fewer than 25 percent of those affected survive beyond 5 yr.

Most endocrine tumors arising in the small bowel involve the distal ileum, and form submucosal nodules that are multiple in one-third of the patients. The larger tumors are prone to metastasize, and all endocrine small intestinal tumors should be viewed as potentially malignant. Most are labeled as carcinoids from their histologic and ultrastructural features, but immunocytochemical studies are necessary to establish which hormonal polypeptides are being formed by the tumor cells.

The most common mesenchymal tumor in the small bowel is of smooth muscle origin; more than half are malignant. They are most common in the ileum and light microscopy may show epithelioid transformation. Electron-microscopically, smooth muscle features may not be evident in the tumor cells. The histologic appearance of smooth muscle tumors does not give a good indication of how they are likely to behave. Five-year survival rates of 50 percent have been reported for leiomyosarcomas of the small intestine.

smallpox (smawl′poks) an acute, highly contagious, febrile viral disease characterized by vesicular and pustular cutaneous eruptions. It is due to a poxvirus, one of a group of large DNA-containing viruses with a common antigen, for which a vaccine has been developed. A global effort by the World Health Organization (WHO) to promote vaccination against smallpox has successfully eliminated smallpox. As there are no longer any animal vectors, the only source of the virus now is in medical laboratories.

Also called *variola.*

S. marcescens see *S. marcescens* under *Serratia.*

smart terminal see *intelligent terminal.*

smear (smēr) a specimen for microscopic study prepared by spreading the material thinly across a glass slide with a swab, a loop, or the edge of another slide.

peripheral blood s., a thin film of blood (usually venous) for microscopic study, prepared by spreading the blood across a glass slide. A variety of staining procedures may be employed.

s. preparation and staining for blood parasites, the procedure for preparing blood films for examination.

PREPARATION. It is essential first to clean the microscopic slides and coverslips, which should be washed in alcohol and dried with a clean towel. New slides must be used for permanent stain preparation.

EXAMINATION OF FRESH BLOOD. Although not a routine procedure, microscopic examination of fresh blood may be useful in the detection of trypanosomes and microfilariae. Trypanosomes with rapid undulating and twisting motion may be detected under a high-dry objective with reduced illumination. Low power is used for microfilariae that possess a whiplike movement.

Because these parasites are very small, it is essential to avoid covering thin films with several layers of red blood cells. A small drop of blood is placed on a slide and covered with a coverslip to prevent clotting. Normal saline may be used as a diluent if the preparation is too thick.

PERMANENT PREPARATIONS. Permanent slides may be prepared from thin or thick films for specific identification of malarial parasites, trypanosomes, and microfilariae. Peripheral blood (e.g., fingerstick) is preferred in making permanent slides, which should be prepared quickly to prevent clotting. Heparin or other anticoagulants must be added when using venous blood. It should be noted that preparations from venous blood are usually distorted.

A thin film is prepared as for the blood smear, its chief advantage being that the structure of the parasite is preserved with minimal distortion. As malarial parasites are intracellular parasites, a single cell layer is extremely important so that they can be detected and their morphologic characteristics distinguished.

Thick films are prepared by placing three small drops of blood on one end of a slide. The corner of another slide is used to mix the drops, with continuous stirring for 30 sec to prevent formation of fibrin strands, and allowed to dry.

The films are then laked to remove the hemoglobin. This can be accomplished by immersing the slide in a buffer solution prior to staining. The two most common stains used for permanent slides are Wright and Giemsa. If Giemsa stain is used, the laking and fixation steps are eliminated. The advantage of thick films is that more parasites are likely to be present in a field, although this method produces more distortions of the parasite than with thin films. Permanent stains are examined under high-dry objective and oil immersion.

smear background materials such as cellular debris, blood, mucus, or inflammatory cells that are present on a slide, in addition to the specimen, for microscopic study. Smear background may interfere with viewing of the specimen. See also *smear.*

smegma (smeg′mah) [Gr. *smēgma* soap] a sebaceous material secreted by small glands on the glans and neck of the penis (preputial glands).

Smith-Strang disease (smith strang) see *m. malabsorption syndrome,* under *methionine.*

smoldering leukemia see *acute myelogenous l.* under *leukemia.*

smooth endoplasmic reticulum see under *endoplasmic reticulum.*

smoothing (smoo′thing) the statistical analysis of measurements taken through time (e.g., in the electroencephalogram or electrocardiogram) or space (e.g., CT scans) for the purpose of averaging out sharp fluctuations and thus, in some cases, reducing random noise and enhancing signal detection. In effect, smoothing filters out high-frequency components of the signal. Some of the statistical procedures useful for smoothing include exponential smoothing, moving averages, periodogram or autocorrelation, and power spectrum analysis.

smooth muscle see *smooth m.* under *muscle* and *nonstriated muscle.*

smooth-rough (S-R) variation a type of mutation or a response to environmental factors seen in bacteria. It is most often evidenced by a change in the surface of colonies from smooth (S, glossy) to rough (R, dull). The change correlates with pathogenicity, S strains being generally more virulent and R strains less so. The cells in S colonies have polysaccharide capsules and are more antigenically complete; R cells contain little or no capsule. The term may also refer to other structures such as flagella and somatic antigens, as well as susceptibility to bacteriophage. Many such variations are reversible and tend to result in mixed types on repeated subculture.

SMR abbrev. for standard mortality ratio or standard morbidity ratio. See *adjusted r.* under *rate.*

S/N abbrev. See *signal-to-noise ratio.*

Sn [L. *stannum*] symbol for the chemical element *tin.*

sn- see under *stereospecific numbering.*

snail (snāl) a mollusk of the class Gastropoda. Several freshwater snails in tropical regions are intermediate hosts of parasitic trematodes (flukes). See also *Gastropoda.*

snake (snāk) a limbless reptile of the suborder Ophidia, containing many poisonous species. Important venomous snakes found in the United States include rattlesnakes (species of *Crotalus* and *Sistrurus*), the copperhead (*Agkistrodon contortrix*), and the water moccasin (*Agkistrodon piscivorus*), all of which belong to the family Crotalidae (the pit vipers), and the coral snake (*Micrurus fulvius*), which belongs to the Elapidae.

snakebite (snāk′bīt) injury caused by venom injected during the bite of a poisonous snake. The pit viper venoms are both hemotoxic and necrotoxic. The victim experiences immediate severe pain, swelling, and edema at the site of the bite. There is also a profound fall in blood pressure and a weak, rapid pulse. If the victim survives for several hours, there is development of hemolytic anemia, hemoglobinuria, and extensive tissue necrosis. Coral snake venom is primarily neurotoxic. After such bites, the victim experiences little immediate pain, but within 20 min there is disorientation, difficulty in swallowing, and skeletal paralysis, followed by respiratory paralysis. Treatment for snakebite consists of removal of injected venom, symptomatic supportive therapy, and administration of specific antivenin (see under *antivenin*).

snapback DNA see *palindrome.*

snare (snār) a wire loop for removing polyps and other pedunculated growths by cutting (snaring) them off at the stalk, which connects the polyp to the underlying mucosa.

Snellen chart (snel′en) [Hermann *Snellen,* ophthalmologist in Utrecht, 1834–1908] a chart printed with block letters of gradually decreasing sizes, which is used in testing visual acuity.

Snell's law (snelz) [Willebrod Van Roijen *Snell,* Dutch astronomer and mathematician, 1591–1626] see under *refraction.*

SNM abbrev. See *Society of Nuclear Medicine.*

SNOBOL (sno′bawl) [acronym from *S*tring-*O*riented *S*ymbolic *L*anguage] a high-level list processing computer language for symbol manipulation.

SNR abbrev. See *signal-to-noise ratio.*

snuffles (snuf′elz) the catarrhal discharge from the nasal mucous membrane that occurs in newborns with congenital syphilis.

SO_2 abbrev. for fractional saturation of hemoglobin with oxygen; see *blood gas analysis.*

soap (sop) [L. *sapo*] the salt of a long-chain fatty acid. Commonly, the term describes water-soluble salts in which the cation of the salt is sodium or potassium; sodium salts are referred to as "hard" soaps, potassium salts as "soft" soaps. They are prepared by the alkaline hydrolysis of fats, which are esters of fatty acids. Such soaps are emulsifying agents and are used as cleansers. Soap is also employed in liniments and enemas and has mild purgative, antacid, and antiseptic properties.

The term also refers to water-insoluble salts of fatty acids in which heavier metals (such as aluminum and zinc) are the cation. They are used in greases, gel thickeners, etc.

SOB abbrev. for shortness of breath.

Society of Computer Medicine (SCM) a professional organization for practitioners of computer medicine.

Society of Nuclear Medicine (SNM) a professional organization of nuclear medicine physicians.

sodium (Na) (so′de-um) [Fr. *soda* sodium carbonate (Na_2CO_3); modern L. *natrium,* from Gr. *natrūm,* from *nitron* sodium carbonate] a soft, silvery white metallic element; atomic number 11; atomic weight 22.98977; Group I of the periodic table (the alkali metals); oxidation state +1. It oxidizes spontaneously in air, turning dull gray, and reacts spontaneously with water, releasing hydrogen. Sodium metal is an extremely caustic tissue irritant and a fire hazard. Sodium is present naturally in minerals in ionic form and occurs dissolved in sea water (about 3 g/dl).

Sodium is the major cation of the extracellular fluid. The reference range for sodium in human serum is 135–148 mmol/l (138–150 mmol/l for cerebrospinal fluid); in contrast, the extracellular concentration of all other cations combined is normally only about 12 mEq/l. Sweat contains about 30–80 mmol/l; saliva 6–40. The stool normally contains almost no sodium except in diarrhea. Sodium ingested in excess of these losses is excreted by the kidneys. Urine normally contains 30–280 mmol/da, depending on the diet.

Sodium plays an important role in kidney function. The glomerular filtrate (protein-free plasma) passes into the proximal convoluted tubule, where sodium (Na^+) is actively transported out of the tubular lumen by the epithelial cells. Chloride (Cl^-) follows to maintain electric neutrality, and water follows so that the luminal fluid remains isoosmotic. The concentration of Na^+ and Cl^-, both in the loop of Henle and in the interstitial fluid and blood, increases going from the top (renal cortex) to the bottom (renal pelvis) of the medulla. The descending loop of Henle is impervious to Na^+ and Cl^-; therefore, water flows out of the luminal fluid by osmosis and the concentration of the luminal fluid increases from about 300 mOsm/l at the top to about 1000 mOsm/l at the bottom. The ascending limb is impermeable to water, and Na^+ and Cl^- diffuse out of the lumen in the thin portion of the limb and are pumped out by active transport of Cl^- in the thick portion. This is the source of the medullary concentration gradient.

Entering the distal tubules, the urine is dilute (about 100 mOsm/l). As it passes down the collecting tubules, water can flow out by osmosis because of the medullary concentration gradient, which can increase the urine osmolality back up to 1000 mOsm/l. The amount of water leaving the tubular urine (and thus its osmolality) is controlled by antidiuretic hormone. Also in the collecting tubules, Na^+ is actively transported out of the urine coupled with potassium (K^+) transported into the urine; this process is controlled by the hormone aldosterone.

See also *action potential, active transport, aldosterone,* and *potassium.*

sodium and potassium assays 1. emission flame photometry. Serum (plasma) specimens must be free from hemolysis, because erythrocytes have some 20–25 times the serum potassium concentraton. Lithium (or cesium) ions are added to the specimens as an internal standard. Solutions containing alkali ions, after dilution with internal standard, are aspirated into the flame; each atom present in the flame (Na^+, K^+, Li^+, Cs^+) emits light of one or more distinctive wavelengths (generally 589, 768, 671, 852 nm, respectively). These light emissions are measured directly or indirectly. Because emission energy varies with flame temperature and other properties, the emission ratios (e.g., Na^+/Li^+, K^+/Cs^+) are used, as they vary minimally with flame fluctuations. Lithium (cesium) atoms also serve as radiation buffers; the transfer of energy from sodium to potassium atoms (mutual excitation) causes the potassium emission to vary with sodium concentration, but a high Li^+ concentration prevents this. The Na^+ and K^+ concentrations are determined by comparing the emission ratios with those of appropriate standards.

2. electrochemical measurement with ion-specific electrodes. This is the newest technique, used in several proprietary automated systems. The sodium ion concentration (activity) is determined, using an Na^+ glass electrode, which selectively responds to Na^+. The potassium ion concentration (activity) is determined using a type of liquid ion-exchange membrane electrode, in which the antibiotic valinomycin is used as a neutral carrier for K^+ ion. Both these electrodes have selectivity ratios relative to each other as low as 10^{-3}; hence, interference effects are very small and the measured electrode potential is essentially proportional to the logarithm of the ion activity being measured.

3. atomic absorption flame spectrophotometry. The comments for emission flame photometry apply, except that the amount of light absorbed (as opposed to emitted) is measured. The increased sensitivity of this technique is not needed; emission flame photometry is more convenient and provides the precision required for clinical laboratory analysis.

4. precipitation and isolation as complex salts. Na^+ can be precipitated as the sodium zinc uranyl acetate or as the pyroantimonate, and potassium as the cobaltinitrite, followed by gravimetric, volumetric, or colorimetric quantitation. These methods are now considered obsolete.

sodium chloride a colorless or white crystalline solid, NaCl, common table salt used medicinally and as a laboratory reagent; M.W. 58.44.

isotonic s. c. solution, [USP], a 0.9 percent aqueous solution of sodium chloride, $\approx$0.155 mol/l, used to restore blood volume and as a vehicle for intravenous medications. Also (incorrectly) referred to as physiologic saline solution and normal saline solution.

sodium chromate Cr 51 a radiopharmaceutical used to label red blood cells for the determination of red cell volume and survival time.

sodium dodecyl sulfate (SDS) (so′de-um do″des′il sul′fāt) [L. *natrium;* Gr. *dodeka* twelve; L. *sulphas*] a surfactant used industrially and in laboratories. As it denatures proteins and dissociates them into subunits, it is predominantly utilized in the preparation of SDS gels for the electrophoretic or gel-filtration chromatographic study of proteins.

sodium fluoroacetate a white powder, sodium fluoroethanoate, used as rat poison; M.W. 100.02. It is highly toxic; ingestion of 2–5 mg/kg of body weight may be fatal. Also called 1080. See also *fluoroacetate assay.*

sodium fluorosilicate a white granular powder, Na_2SiF_6, that is highly toxic when ingested or inhaled; M.W. 188.05. It is used as a disinfectant, preservative, and rat and insect poison. Also called *sodium hexafluorosilicate* and *sodium silicofluoride.*

sodium hexafluorosilicate see *sodium fluorosilicate.*

sodium iodide (NaI) a white crystalline powder with a salty taste, used in the diet as a source of iodine and in radiology as a radiopaque contrast medium for cystography; M.W. 149.92. In this procedure, a 5–20 percent solution is used to opacify the bladder; mucosal irritation is avoided by irrigation of the bladder and washing out the iodide after the cystograms are made.

sodium iodide crystal a thallium-activated sodium iodide [NaI(Tl)] crystal, the scintillator used in many gamma-ray detectors. See under *scintillation crystal.*

sodium iodide I 123 [USP], a radiopharmaceutical used for thyroid imaging.

sodium iodide I 125 a radiopharmaceutical used rarely for thyroid imaging and uptake tests. Its principal uses are for the in vitro labeling of compounds for radioimmunoassay procedures and, in vivo, as a label for human serum albumin.

sodium iodide I 131 a radiopharmaceutical used for thyroid imaging and uptake tests, and also for the treatment of some cases of hyperthyroidism or carcinoma of the thyroid. See also *iodine-131 therapy.*

sodium nitroprusside (so′de-um ni″tro-prus′īd) [USP], sodium nitrosylpentacyanoferrate (III), sodium nitroferricyanide, $Na_2Fe(CN)_5NO \cdot 2H_2O$, a ruby-red crystalline salt; M.W. 261.91. It is used in clinical chemistry for the detection of cysteine in urine or renal calculi. Pharmacologically, it is an immediate-acting hypotensive agent administered by infusion for the reduction of blood pressure in hypertensive crises and for the production of controlled hypotension during surgery. The duration of action is short (1–10 min) owing to enzymatic conversion to thiocyanate in the liver.

Toxicity resulting from the extended use of nitroprusside at high dosage can be indirectly monitored by determining the serum thiocyanate or cyanide concentration.

sodium pertechnetate Tc-99m [USP], a radiopharmaceutical; see under *technetium-99m.*

sodium phosphate P 32 a radiopharmaceutical used for the localization of eye tumors and also for the treatment of polycythemia vera, chronic myelogenous leukemia, and chronic lymphocytic leukemia. It is administered intravenously and is distributed like nonradioactive inorganic phosphate. After several days, the concentration in the bone marrow, liver, and spleen is about 10 times that in other tissues. The bones receive 10–15 rad/mCi of administered ^{32}P. The primary use is for maintenance of the venous hematocrit in polycythemia vera as an alternative to repeated venesection.

sodium silicofluoride see *sodium fluorosilicate.*

soft chancre see *chancroid.*

soft tissue tumor a neoplasm of cells of the soft tissues of the body. In the broad sense these tumors are of mesodermal origin, but lymphopoietic and hematopoietic tumors are not included, and tumors with bone or cartilage differentiation are grouped with the soft tissue tumors only when they occur in extraskeletal locations.

Soft tissue tumors may be benign or malignant. Benign tumors are named by combining the name of the tissue of origin with the suffix -oma, e.g., fibroma. Certain tumors (e.g., dermatofibrosarcoma protuberans) usually behave in a benign fashion but infrequently give rise to metastases. Some lesions, notably the aggressive fibromatoses, do not metastasize but nevertheless cause considerable morbidity through local infiltration. Histologically it sometimes is not possible to decide whether a particular tumor is benign or a low-grade sarcoma. Nonneoplastic soft tissue proliferation, notably nodular fasciitis and proliferative myositis, may be mistaken for sarcomas histologically, but correlation of the clinical features and histologic features of such lesions should aid in their identification.

Biopsy is usually necessary to establish the diagnosis of a soft tissue tumor. The gross appearance of the specimen may be suggestive of the diagnosis, but confirmation requires histologic examination. In some cases, notably some of the sarcomas, subclassification (determination of cell type) is not possible because of lack of specific histologic features. Special staining procedures are usually of limited value, but electron microscopy may be helpful.

The behavior of a soft tissue tumor depends on several factors, including location, age of patient, histologic type, and whether it is benign or malignant. Benign soft tissue tumors are generally encapsulated or well circumscribed, typically slow-growing, and frequently asymptomatic. However, a strategically located benign tumor can produce serious complications by pressure or encroachment on adjacent structures, e.g., intestinal intussusception or obstruction of respiratory or biliary passages.

Most of the defined entities, benign and malignant, among soft tissue tumors are listed in the accompanying table. Any classification must be regarded as tentative, as the histogenesis of some of these neoplasms is not known.

SOFT TISSUE TUMOR. CLASSIFICATION OF SOFT TISSUE TUMORS

CATEGORY/TUMOR
Tumors of fibroblasts
Fibromatosis
Fibroma
Fibrous histiocytoma (xanthoma)
Dermatofibrosarcoma protuberans
Fibrosarcoma
Malignant fibrous histiocytoma
Tumors of fat cells
Lipoma
Angiolipoma
Hibernoma
Liposarcoma
Tumors of smooth muscle cells
Leiomyoma
Glomus tumor
Myoepithelial cell tumor
Leiomyosarcoma
Tumors of skeletal muscle cells
Rhabdomyoma
Rhabdomyosarcoma
Tumors of synovium
Synovial sarcoma, biphasic and monophasic
Tumors of vasoformative cells
Hemangioma
Lymphangioma
Angiosarcoma
Kaposi's sarcoma
Hemangiopericytoma
Tumors of Schwann cells
Schwannoma
Neurofibroma
Schwann cell sarcoma
Extraskeletal tumors with osteoblastic or chondroblastic differentiation
Chordoma
Chondroma
Chondrosarcoma
Osteosarcoma
Tumors of uncertain histogenesis
Malignant giant cell tumor
Epithelioid sarcoma
Granular cell tumor
Alveolar soft part sarcoma
Clear cell sarcoma
Soft tissue tumor resembling Ewing's tumor of bone
Carcinosarcoma and mixed mesodermal tumors

Courtesy of Bruce Mackay, M.D., Ph.D.

software in a computer, the programs, particularly the operating system, assembler, compilers, and library subprograms, which are usually supplied by the vendor and are treated by the user as part of the machine. Cf. *firmware* and *hardware.*

sol (sol) a colloidal state in which a solid (dispersed phase) is suspended throughout a liquid (continuous phase). Sols can be classified as lyophilic colloids (e.g., a solution of a protein, like gelatin, or a carbohydrate, like starch, in water); association colloids (e.g., a solution of soap in water); or lyophobic colloids (e.g., an alumina sol in water). Hot gelatin is a sol, cold gelatin a gel. See also *colloid* and *gel.*

solanine (so'lah-nēn) a steroidal glycoalkaloid derived from several *Solanum* species, and composed of solanidine coupled to three sugars. The aglycone is very toxic.

solanocyte (so-lah'no-sīt) see *flame cell.*

Solanum (so-la'num) [L. "nightshade"] a genus of solanaceous plants, including the potato, tomato, and eggplant, and several nightshades. Many species have poisonous fruit or foliage.

solenoid (so'le-noid) [L. *solanum* potato + Gr. *eidos* form] 1. a coil of insulated wire used to produce a magnetic field.

2. a coil surrounding a movable iron core that is pulled in when the coil is energized. It can be used to perform some mechanical work, such as opening a valve.

Solenopsis (so″lĕ-nop'sis) a genus of stinging ants, including the fire ants, that attack humans; they cause extremely painful, burning stings and occasionally produce a severe local inflammatory reaction.

The species *S. saevissima richteri,* the black imported fire ant, and *S. invicta,* the red imported fire ant, are commonly found in the United States.

solid (sol'id) [L. *solidus*] 1. not fluid or gaseous; not hollow.

2. a state of matter in which the constituent atoms or molecules are bound in a regular periodic array (a crystal lattice). The molecules do not move except in virbration about their rest positions.

3. any material such as an amorphous solid (glass) in which fluid flow of the molecules is so slow as to be imperceptible.

solid angle the geometric figure formed by the rays (half lines) projecting from one point (the vertex) through each point of the boundary of a surface. The measure of a solid angle in steradians (sr) is given by the area of the region inside the solid angle on the unit sphere centered at the vertex. Any surface that totally encloses the vertex subtends a solid angle of 4πsr. A radiant source emits equal intensities into equal solid angles.

solid-phase radioimmunoassay an RIA procedure in which the antibody is either adsorbed or covalently bound to an inert matrix, thereby facilitating the separation of bound and free radioactively labeled antigen. Inert matrices that have been used include polypropylene tubes, glass beads, Sephadex particles, and various polymers. See also *radioimmunoassay.*

solid state 1. pertaining to the physics of matter in the solid (crystalline) state.

2. pertaining to electronic devices or components such as transistors or semiconductor diodes, the properties of which are explained by solid-state physics.

solid-state radiation detector a solid-state electronic device that is in essence a reverse-biased junction diode used for detecting charged particles or gamma rays.

An ionizing particle entering the depletion region interacts with the semiconductor material (silicon or germanium), producing electron-hole pairs that carry a current pulse proportional to the energy lost by the particle in the depletion region. Because of the low atomic number of silicon, it is not suitable for gamma detectors. Germanium detectors have enough sensitivity to detect gamma rays, but they must be operated at liquid nitrogen temperature (–196°C).

Solid-state detectors have much better detector response and energy resolution than do conventional detectors. The response time is about 1 ns, as opposed to about 1 μs for thallium-activated sodium iodide [NaI(Tl)] crystal detectors used in scintillation counters, scintillation cameras, and rectilinear scanners, and 1 ms for ion-collection detectors (proportional counters, Geiger counters). The full-width half-maximum (FWHM) energy resolution is about 5 percent, as opposed to 14 percent for NaI(Tl) crystal detectors. Because of the small size of these devices, less than 20 cm^2 in area with a depletion region less than 1 cm thick, they have a low sensitivity and at present only limited application.

There are three types of solid-state detectors: surface barrier, lithium-drifted, and cadmium telluride detectors. In the surface barrier detector, there is a thin layer of *p*-type silicon or germanium at the detector face with a thicker *n*-type layer below. The lithium-drifted detector is similar, but lithium ions are diffused into the depletion layer, so that the charge of the acceptor impurity atoms is compensated and the depth of the depletion layer can be increased without producing Zener breakdown. The cadmium telluride detector is operated at room temperature; because of the high atomic numbers of cadmium and tellurium it has high sensitivity. A 2-mm thick CdTe detector absorbs 85 percent of 100-keV gamma rays entering the detector.

Cf. *scintillation crystal.*

solubility (sol″u-bil'ĭ-te) the ability of one substance to dissolve in another; the concentration of a saturated solution. Also called (when referring to liquid-liquid solutions) *miscibility.* See also the accompanying table.

solubility coefficient see *Bunsen coefficient.*

solubility product (K_{sp}) the equilibrium constant for the equilibrium between the excess solid phase of a partially soluble ionic solid and a saturated solution of its ions. It is the product of the concentration of each ion raised to the power equal to the subscript of that ion in the chemical formula of the salt, e.g., for $Mg(OH)_2$, $K_{sp} = [Mg^{2+}][OH^-]^2$.

solubilize (sol'u-bĭ-līz) to make soluble a material normally not soluble, e.g., by addition of a detergent, emulsifier, or sulfhydryl agent.

solubilizer a substance that stabilizes a solution of a substance that is by itself insoluble.

soluble (sol'u-b'l) [L. *solubilis*] susceptible of being dissolved (in a given solvent). Cf. *insoluble.*

soluble immune response suppressor (SIRS) a glycoprotein found in concanavalin A–stimulated mouse spleen cells; M.W. 35,000–67,000. It nonspecifically suppresses the antigen response to such antigens as sheep red blood cells and dinitrophenol-ficoll. SIRS does not affect the mixed lymphocyte reaction or the DNA synthesis induced by T-cell mitogens or allogenic cells; it does suppress DNA synthesis induced by the B-cell mitogen lipopolysaccharide. Its apparent target cell is the macrophage. This factor does not have an antigen-binding site.

SOLUBILITY. SOLUBILITY EXPRESSED IN THE USUAL USP FORMAT

USP DESCRIPTIVE SOLUBILITY TERM	SYMBOL	PARTS OF SOLVENT/ ONE PART SOLUTE	MG OF SOLUTE/ 100 ML OF SOLVENT	G OF SOLUTE/ 100 ML OF SOLVENT
Very	vs	<1	over 100,000	100
Freely	fs	1–10	100,000–10,000	100–10
Soluble	s	10–30	10,000–3,333	10–3.3
Sparingly	ss	30–100	3,333–1,000	3.3–1.0
Slightly	sls	100–1,000	1,000–100	1.0–0.1
Very slightly	vsl	1,000–10,000	100–10	0.1–0.01
Insoluble	in	>10,000		
Miscible	mis			

Modified from United States Pharmacopeia XIX. Rockville, MD, United States Pharmacopeial Convention, 1975, p. xiv.

solute (so'lūt) a substance dissolved in a solvent. A solution consists of a solute and a solvent. Cf. *solvent.*

solution (so-lu'shun) [L. *solutio*] 1. in chemistry, a homogeneous mixture (in a single phase) of two or more substances, in which the molecules, atoms, or ions of each substance are distributed randomly and uniformly throughout the volume of the solution. Usually one (or more) component(s) of the solution is/are termed the solute, and another (or several), present in greater amount, the solvent. In general, solution occurs when solvent-solute interactions are sufficiently greater than solvent-solvent and solute-solute forces and because the dispersion of solute in solvent represents an increase in entropy.

The solute may be a gas, solid, or liquid, as may be the solvent. Gases are infinitely miscible with other gases. Liquids of similar molecular structure, and consequently affected by similar intermolecular forces, are infinitely miscible, but dissimilar liquids most commonly are not. This is expressed in the aphorism "like dissolves like." Solids that may be infinitely miscible have identical crystal structures and are composed of similar molecular radii, or they contain atoms with identical ionic radii, so that they combine into the crystal lattice without distortion.

Solutions of a solid, liquid, or gas (the solute) in a liquid (the solvent) that are in equilibrium with excess pure solute at a given temperature and pressure are called saturated solutions. Supersaturated solutions (formed by cooling of a saturated solution) are more concentrated than saturated solutions. They are unstable as their temperature is below the point at which crystallization should occur. The excess solute precipitates rapidly when a small seed crystal is added. Unsaturated solutions are those that have less solute than a saturated solution.

In all but a few cases, the solubility of a solid in a liquid increases with temperature; the solubility of a gas in a liquid increases with pressure but decreases with increasing temperature. Within groups of similar compounds, the solubility of solids increases with decreasing melting point, and the solubility of gases increases with increasing boiling point.

For more information, see the specific solution.

2. the process of forming a chemical solution.

3. the state of a solute (being in solution).

4. the answer to a problem; in mathematics, the values that satisfy an equation.

5. the process of solving a problem.

ideal s., a solution in which solvent-solute, solvent-solvent, and solute-solute forces are all the same. When the solute is dissolved in an ideal solution, there is no heat produced by mixing nor any change in volume. An ideal solution exactly obeys Raoult's law and Henry's law. Such conditions are seldom completely realized for real solutions.

nonideal s., a solution whose properties deviate from those predicted theoretically for so-called "ideal solutions," in which no molecule interacts in any way with any other molecule and in which properties such as osmotic pressure and conductivity are proportional to the concentration of solutes. In nonideal solutions, such properties are proportional to the activity (the effective concentration) of the solute, which can be less or greater than the concentration. Activity coefficients (activity divided by concentration), however, approach unity with increasing dilution of solute, and solutions approach "ideality." In moderately concentrated solutions (between 0.1 and 1.0 mol/l), activity coefficients of electrolyte solutions are less than 0.8, reflecting considerable deviation from the ideal state (ion hydration, ion association, ion complexes). At very high concentrations, activity coefficients may be greater than unity.

solvate (sol'vāt) 1. a solid compound that includes in its crystal structure at least one molecule of the solvent from which it crystallized.

2. to undergo solvation.

solvation (sol-va'shun) the stabilizing interaction of a solvent with a solute or of a solvent with functional groups at the surface of an insoluble material.

solve (solv) [L. *solvere* to loosen] to find the answer to a problem; to produce a solution of a mathematical equation.

solvent (sol'vent) [L. *solvens*] a liquid that dissolves or is capable of dissolving; the component of a solution that is present in greater amount. Cf. *solute.*

solvent extraction see under *extraction.*

solvolysis (sol-vol'i-sis) a reaction involving substances in solution, in which the solvent reacts with the dissolved substance (solute), breaking one or more bonds in the solute (e.g., alcoholysis).

soma (so'mah) [Gr. *sōma* body] 1. the body as distinguished from the mind.

2. the body tissue as distinguished from the germ cells.

3. the cell body of a neuron.

somasthenia (sōm″as-the′ne-ah) [*soma* + *a* neg. + Gr. *sthenos* strength + *-ia*] body weakness that is the result of poor appetite and lack of sleep.

somat/o (so′mah-to) [Gr. *sōma, sōmatos* body] a word element used in combining form to denote the body, e.g., somatic.

somatesthesia (so″mat-es-the′ze-ah) see *somesthesia.*

somatic (so-mat′ik) [Gr. *sōmatikos*] pertaining to the body or main part of a cell.

somatic cell the diploid cells of an organism, which include all the cells except the gametes (germ cells).

somatomedin C (so″mah-to-me′din) an insulinlike basic peptide growth factor controlled by the secretion of growth hormone; M.W. 7500. Increased concentrations are observed in acromegaly; decreases may be seen in hypopituitarism, hypothyroidism, chronic illness, and nutritional deficiency. Somatomedins possess insulinlike activity and compete with insulin for insulin-binding sites. They have also been shown to stimulate certain cells derived from extraskeletal tissues, e.g., myoblasts, fetal liver cells, and ovarian tumor cells. Also called *sulfation factor.*

somatomedins a family of peptides with similar biologic activities; M.W. 6000–9000. They are stimulated by growth hormone, and in turn stimulate cartilage growth by inducing the synthesis of collagen and other proteins. The reference ranges for somatomedin C in serum are: for adults, 0.4–2.0 U/ml; and for children: birth–5 yr, 0.2–1.8; 5–8 yr, 0.4–2.0; and 8–18 yr, 0.8–6.0. See also *somatomedin C.*

somatosensory pertaining to the senses of the body.

somatosensory evoked potential (SEP) see *somatosensory e. p.* under *evoked potential.*

somatostatin (so″mah-to-stat′in) see *growth hormone–release-inhibiting hormone.*

somatotopic (so″mah-to-top′ik) related to particular areas of the body; referring to the phenomenon in which different points on the body are spatially represented in their motor and sensory connections with the central nervous system. For example, a specific area of the motor cortex controls movement of a specific part of the body.

somatotropin (so″mah-to-tro′pin) [*somatō* + Gr. *tropos* a turning] a substance that has a stimulating effect on body nutrition and growth. The term commonly refers to *growth hormone.*

somesthesia (so″mes-the′ze-ah) [Gr. *sōma* body + *aisthesis* perception + *-ia*] the sensation of temperature (coolness and warmth), touch-pressure, pain, and/or joint position elicited by stimulation of receptors other than those involved with vision, hearing, taste, or smell. Somesthesia results from the differential stimulation of one or several of the following sensory receptors: Meissner's corpuscle (touch), Krause's end bulb (cold), Ruffini's end organs (warmth), pacinian corpuscle (deep pressure), bare nerve endings (pain), and Merkel's disks (touch).

Generally, afferent somatic sensory information is relayed from the receptor to the thalamus, which in turn projects to the postcentral gyrus of the cerebral cortex (sensory cortex). However, there are two major subdivisions in the prethalamic afferent system that are associated with somesthesia—the lemniscal and anterolateral systems. The lemniscal system, in which there is rapid transmission and precise representation of body form, is composed of large, myelinated fibers (4–6 μm) that project from the somatic receptors to the dorsal column nuclei and other sensory nuclei of the brain stem. These nuclei project via the medial lemnisci to the ventrobasilar nuclei of the thalamus, and then to the sensory cortex. This system subserves discriminative mechanoreception.

The anterolateral system originates in the dorsal horn of the spinal cord, where small myelinated (A-delta) and unmyelinated (C) fibers from mechanical, pain, and temperature receptors initiate segmental reflexes. In the spinal cord, fibers from the dorsal horn ascend within the contralateral anterolateral column. Within the brain stem, two paths are followed: one via the thalamic nuclei to specific sensory cortex; and the other, less localized, via nonspecific thalamic nuclei to less clear cortical destinations.

Also called *somatesthesia.*

somite (so′mīt) in the developing embryo, one pair of the blocklike masses formed by the subdivision of the thickened mesoderm alongside the neural tube. Somites are added progressively from the head toward the tail as the embryo develops, forming the vertebral column and segment musculature.

somn/o (som′no) [L. *somnus* sleep] a word element used in combining form to denote sleep, e.g., somnolence.

somnambulism (som-nam′bu-lizm) [L. *somnambulismus; somn-* + *ambulare* to walk] a disorder of sleep characterized by motor activity in which the individual arises from bed and walks about the room or performs a familiar task. The eyes are open, and the sight of unfamiliar objects may awaken the person. There may be vocalization but no vocal response to a question or command. The following morning, the individual usually has no recollection of the episode. This disorder occurs more frequently in children than in adults and is usually associated with sleep Stages 3 and 4.

somnolence (som′no-lens) [L. *somnolentia*] sleepiness.

Somogyi unit (of amylase activity) defined as the quantity of catalytic activity able to liberate from a starch substrate reducing substances equivalent to 1.0 mg of glucose in a 30-min reaction period at 40°C.

son/o (so-no′) a word element used in combining form to denote sound, e.g., ultrasonic.

sonication (son″ĭ-ka′shun) the exposure to audible sound waves (of a frequency less than 15,000 cps). Cf. *ultrasonication.*

sonogram (son′o-gram) an image produced by diagnostic ultrasonography. Also called *echogram* and *ultrasonogram.*

sonographer (so-nog′rah-fer) an individual who performs diagnostic ultrasound procedures under the supervision of a physician, who directs the examination and interprets the sonograms.

sonolucent (son″o-loo′sent) in ultrasonography, referring to areas of a sonogram that are transparent to ultrasound (producing no echoes). Also called *echolucent.*

Sopor (so′por) trademark. See *methaqualone.*

sorbefacient (sōr″bĕ-fa′shent) [L. *sorbere* to suck + *facere* to make] 1. promoting absorption.

2. an agent that promotes absorption; in particular, an agent that aids the absorption of medication.

sorbent (sor′bent) a general term used to refer nonspecifically to either an adsorbent or an absorbent.

sorbitol (sor′bĭ-tol) a crystalline hexahydric alcohol, first found in the ripe berries of the mountain ash tree *Sorbus aucuparia;* it also occurs in small quantities in other fruits such as berries, cherries, plums, and pears. Sorbitol is formed as an intermediate in the conversion of glucose to fructose in human semen; it is also associated with lens deposits and cataracts in persons with diabetes mellitus. Sorbitol is used as a flavoring agent, an osmotic diuretic, and a sugar substitute for diabetics. Also called *glucitol.*

sorbitol dehydrogenase (SDH) see *iditol dehydrogenase.*

sorption (sorp′shun) [L. *sorbere* to suck in] a general term covering the surface processes of adsorption, absorption, and ion exchange.

SOS repair system see under *DNA repair.*

sound (sownd) [L. *sonus*] 1. a physical phenomenon consisting of pressure waves in a fluid, or of vibrational waves in an elastic, medium. The sound wave travels at a velocity, the speed of sound, determined by the physical properties of the medium. Sound waves with frequencies above the human range of hearing (20 kHz) are termed ultrasonic; those with frequencies below the human range of hearing are termed subsonic or infrasonic.

2. the sensation produced in the ear and nervous system by sound waves.

3. a slender instrument introduced into body passages or cavities, especially for the dilation of strictures or detection of foreign bodies.

4. a noise, normal or abnormal, emanating from within the body.

source (sōrs) 1. an object that emits energy or matter, such as a radioactive source.

2. an electric device or circuit from which a signal or power is drawn, such as a signal generator or a power line.

3. one of the terminals of a field effect transistor.

source language the language in which the programmer codes a computer program.

source program a computer program in a user language, which requires translation by an assembler, compiler, or interpreter.

source statement a single statement of a computer language, often one line of code.

Southern blot technique a method used in gene cloning to separate and identify specific DNA fragments. After separation by agarose gel electrophoresis, a nitrocellulose film is placed on the gel surfaces and dry blotting material on the nitrocellulose. Liquid is thus transported from a reservoir beneath the gel through the gel and nitrocellulose filter. The film adsorbs DNA fragments, which are then visualized using a complementary DNA or RNA radioactive probe.

sp. abbrev. See *species.*

space (spās) 1. the three-dimensional continuum in which the objects of the physical universe are located.

2. a bounded area or volume.

3. a cavity in the body. For more information, see the specific space.

4. the character in a digital computer's alphanumeric character set that denotes a blank space.

space charge the electric charge contained in a given volume.

spacer a nucleotide sequence between genes, usually arranged in tandem fashion. Spacers can be either transcribed or nontranscribed. Transcribed spacer regions, as in the 18S/28S rRNA genes, are then degraded. Nontranscribed spacers have been observed in genes for 5S, 18S, and 28S rRNA, tRNA, and histones. Spacers are theorized to be one of the molecular mechanisms that control gene expression; they are removed during RNA processing.

sparganosis (spar″gah-no′sis) a disease caused by the migration of the larvae, or spargana, of the genus *Spirometra,* which are accidental parasites of humans. This disease commonly occurs in Japan, China, and Indonesia.

Human infection is caused by ingestion of copepods or amphibians contaminated with the larvae. These larvae invade the subcutaneous tissues primarily and mature there, causing inflammation, swelling, and fibrosis. Marked eosinophilia is usually present.

Laboratory diagnosis is difficult. Most cases are identified after surgical removal of the tapeworms. In Japan, an indirect fluorescent antibody test has been used successfully as a diagnostic aid.

Sparganum (spar-ga′num) [Gr. *sparganon* swaddling clothes] a genus of tapeworms related to *Diphyllobothrium.* Spargana occur in copepods and a variety of amphibious animals including frogs; they may be infective to humans if ingested. Most sparganosis in humans is probably caused by larvae of *Spirometra mansonoides,* which are collectively known as *Sparganum mansoni.*

spark a flash of light accompanied by a crackling sound made by the discharge of electricity.

sparteine (spar′te-in) [L. *spartium* broom] an alkaloid extracted from legumes of the genera *Cytisus* (broom) and *Lupinus* (lupin bean); it has been used to induce labor.

spasm/o (spaz′mo) [L. *spasmus;* Gr. *spasmos*] a word element used in combining form to denote the sudden contraction of muscles and twitching, e.g., spasmogen.

spasm (spazm) [L. *spasmus;* Gr. *spasmos*] 1. a sudden, violent, involuntary contraction of a muscle or group of muscles, attended by pain and interference with function, producing involuntary movement and distortion.

2. a sudden but transitory constriction of a passage, canal, or orifice.

spastic colitis see *irritable bowel syndrome.*

spatial (spa′shal) pertaining to space.

spatial distortion an imperfection in the performance of an imaging system in which parallel straight lines curve or diverge in the image. A scintillation camera is checked for spatial distortion by imaging a bar phantom or an orthogonal hole phantom. There is commonly edge packing or barreling of the image at the edge of the field of view, but the central 90 percent of the field should be free of distortion.

spatial frequency the frequency of repetition of a periodic image (e.g., a pattern of stripes) measured in cycles per unit length. In digital image processing, the image is decomposed by Fourier analysis into sinusoidally varying components. Large objects and fuzzy edges produce components with low spatial frequency; small objects, sharp edges, and background noise produce components with high spatial frequency. Removal of high-frequency components reduces noise (but not distortion) but also causes some loss of definition (image sharpness).

The spatial resolution of an imaging system can be described in terms of the modulation transfer function, which gives the image contrast as a function of object spatial frequency. The representation of an image in terms of its spatial frequencies is also used in reconstruction tomography algorithms that utilize Fourier transform techniques.

spatial resolution the ability of an imaging device to separate the images of nearby points. For a scintillation camera or rectilinear scanner, a commonly used measure of spatial resolution is the full width of the line-spread function at half-maximum height (FWHM). Spatial resolution is routinely checked for quality control purposes by imaging a bar phantom.

The intrinsic (or inherent) resolution is limited by the detector (or the scan spacing in a scanner); it is measured with the collimator removed. The total (or overall, or detector) resolution is the square root of the sum of the squares of the intrinsic resolution and the collimator resolution. The resolution is affected by the design of the collimator and the distance of the object from the focal plane (for focusing collimators).

In computed tomography, the spatial resolution is measured in the same way (FWHM). It depends on the width of the pixels and on the number of photons passing through each voxel of the subject.

SPCA abbrev. for serum prothrombin conversion accelerator factor. See *Factor VII.*

SPE abbrev. for serum protein electrophoresis. See under *protein electrophoresis.*

Spearman's rank correlation coefficient see *rank correlation coefficient.*

speciation (spe″se-a′shun) the evolutionary process by which new species arise. It is generally assumed that most, if not all, new species arise by allopatric speciation, geographic isolation of a small population from the rest of the species for a time during which random mutations and natural selection produce isolating mechanisms—such as differences in anatomy, physiology, behavior, or ecologic strategy—that prevent reproduction between the two groups.

It is possible that species may also arise by sympatric speciation: isolating mechanisms develop between two groups that have overlapping geographical ranges but that inhabit different ecologic zones.

See also *evolution.*

species (sp., spp.) (spe′shēz, spe′sēz) [L.] a taxonomic category surbordinate to a genus composed of individuals with common characteristics that distinguish them from other groups of the same taxonomic level. The scientific binomial nomenclature of an organism gives both the genus (capitalized) and species (lower case), because the species name is not unique, e.g., *Buteo borealis,* a hawk, and *Quercus borealis,* an oak.

specific (spĕ-sif′ik) [L. *specificus*] 1. pertaining to a species.

2. produced by a single kind of microorganism.

3. restricted in application, effect, etc., to a particular structure, function, etc.

4. a remedy especially indicated for any particular disease.

5. in immunology, pertaining to the special affinity of antigen for the corresponding antibody.

specific dynamic action the extra heat produced by the organism, over and above the basal heat production, as a result of food ingestion. Of the energy of food ingested, it represents about 30 percent for proteins, 6 percent for carbohydrates, and 4 percent for lipids.

specific granule the characteristic granule of the later stages of neutrophilic granulocytes beginning with myelocytes (which are present in addition to azurophilic or primary granules produced in myeloblasts and promyelocytes). They stain beige with Romanowsky-type stains (e.g., Wright-Giemsa); the individual granules usually are not discernible with the light microscope because of their small size. The specific granules contain acid ribonuclease, cathepsin and, in some species, alkaline phosphatase. (In humans, alkaline phosphatase is found in the lighter membrane fraction.) Although they are also called neutrophilic granules the term specific or secondary granules is preferred, because neutrophils also contain azurophilic granules. Also called *secondary granule.* See also *granules of developing neutrophils.*

specific gravity (SG, sp. gr.) the ratio of the density of a substance to the density of a standard substance (usually water) at a specified temperature. The measurement of the specific gravity of urine is a standard component in routine urinalysis. It is a screening test that provides information about the concentrating and diluting ability of the renal tubules.

The reference range for a 24-hr urine specimen is 1.015–1.025, but values in a random specimen may have a range of 1.002–1.030, depending on the fluid intake. A value higher than 1.025 after fluid restriction indicates a normal ability to concentrate urine.

The specific gravity and osmolality are related measurements; both reflect the concentration of dissolved substances, although not always proportionally. The measurement of osmolality is more precise and informative, but that of specific gravity is simpler and faster to perform.

A urinometer is a hydrometer specifically calibrated for the measurement of the specific gravity of urine. The observed reading is corrected by adding 0.001 for each 3°C that the temperature exceeds the calibration temperature, by subtracting 0.001 for each 3°C below the calibration temperature, and by subtracting 0.003 for each 1 g/dl of protein and 0.004 for each 1 g/dl of glucose in the urine.

The specific gravity and refractive index correlate well with urine that has a low protein content. Refractometers are available that give readings in specific gravity values, although they actually measure the refractive index.

specificity (spec″ĭ-fis′ĭ-te) the ability of a clinical test to identify correctly those persons not having a disease; the conditional probability that a person without disease will have a negative test result. Cf. *sensitivity.*

specific macrophage-arming factor (SMAF) a product of stimulated T cells that have interacted with specific tumor antigen; it activates macrophages to kill that specific tumor. The arming is cytophilic. It can be absorbed either by macrophages or by the specific tumor that induced it. SMAF may be a unique cytophilic receptor that is shed into the culture supernatant by the activated lymphocyte.

specific rotation see *optical activity.*

specimen (spes'ĭ-men) 1. a sample or part taken to show or determine the character of the whole.

2. a preparation of a tissue, organ, or organism for the study of its structure.

3. see *clinical bacteriologic specimens.*

spectinomycin (spek"tĭ-no-mi'sin) an aminocyclitol antibiotic that has some chemical, pharmacologic, and antibacterial properties similar to those of the aminoglycosides. Protein synthesis is inhibited, but the antibiotic is bacteriostatic only.

Although spectinomycin has a broad spectrum of activity against gram-negative bacilli, its clinical use is restricted in other organisms. Spectinomycin is used for treatment of uncomplicated gonococcal urethritis, cervicitis, and proctitis in individuals with penicillin allergy or in patients who fail to respond to penicillin treatment, particularly when their condition is due to beta-lactamase–producing *Neisseria gonorrhoeae.*

See also *aminoglycosides* and *antibacterial agents.*

spectral (spek'tral) pertaining to a spectrum; performed by means of a spectrum.

spectral interference in flame photometry, emission by two different elements at wavelengths too close to be separated by the monochromator.

spectral resolution the average wavelength of two absorption peaks that can just be distinguished by a spectrophotometer divided by the difference in the wavelengths of the two peaks.

spectral response the variation of the response of a photosensitive detector with the wavelength of the light.

spectrin (spek'trin) a protein found at the inner surface of the erythrocyte membrane, a structural protein that also serves as a part of a contractile apparatus. See also *erythrocyte membrane.*

spectrofluorometer (spek"tro-floo"or-om'ĕ-ter) see under *fluorometry.*

spectrometer (spek-trom'ĕ-ter) a spectroscope that measures the wavelengths emitted from a given source or their intensity. See also *spectroscope.*

spectrometry (spek-trom'ĕ-tre) [L. *spectrum* image + *metrum* measure] the determination of the spectral lines emitted from a source.

spectrophotometer (spek"tro-fo-tom'ĕ-ter) [*spectrum* + *photometer*] an optical instrument that measures the light energy transmitted through a solution (or a gas) at any given wavelength throughout the continuous band of wavelengths. The term is generally applied only to ultraviolet/visible (UV/visible) light instruments operating in the electromagnetic wavelength range of 200–800 nm, although the term does cover those instruments operating in the infrared range (wavelength, 0.75–25 μm; wavenumber, 13,000–400 cycles/cm). For precision instruments, the energy bandpass is narrow, 0.1–10 nm, although some instruments use a 20-nm bandpass. The principal components of a spectrophotometer are a stable light source, monochromator (grating or prism), cuvet, adjustable slit, energy detector, and recording or printing device.

To obtain measurements in the UV/visible range, an ordinary tungsten lamp may be used as the light source, whereas for measurements in the UV region, mercury, hydrogen, or deuterium lamps are available. Spectrophotometers are differentiated from photometers, which contain no monochromators, but instead use color absorption or interference filters for a partial separation of wavelength bands.

In high-precision instruments, diffraction gratings are used most commonly as monochromators, because they are less expensive. Furthermore, prisms large enough for very fine resolution are difficult to obtain. The light source or the grating (prisms) are moved relative to each other so that the collated beam of light energy of narrow bandwidth passes first through the slit and then through the cuvet to the detector.

The cuvet is the specimen holder; its volume may vary from 0.10 to 7.0 ml or more, and its cross-sectional shape may vary from a square or rectangle to a circle (round test tube form). Effective light paths may vary from 1 mm to 0.5, 1.0, 2.0 cm or more. The most commonly used form has a square cross section, plane-parallel sides, with a light path of 10 mm. Glass cuvets are used for work in the long UV/visible region, 330 to about 900 nm. Glass absorbs all light below 320 nm. Quartz or silica cuvets are used in the UV range (190–400 nm) and can be used in the visible region. Special cuvets (made of NaCl or KBr) are used in the far infrared region because glass and quartz have limited transparency in this region.

The most common types of detectors used in routine instruments are the barrier–layer cell type, whereas photomultiplier tubes (PMTs) are encountered in high-precision instruments. The PMTs are far more sensitive to weak energy input and have a faster response than do barrier-cell detectors.

In a single-beam instrument, only one light beam from source to detector is used. The meter measuring the current from the detector is adjusted to read zero (0) percent *T* (transmittance) with no light reaching the detector, and 100 percent *T* with a cuvet containing the reagent blank inserted in the light path. When measurements are made, the latter cuvet is replaced with one containing the treated specimen, and the change in meter reading is noted. In a double-beam instrument, the light beam is split into two equal beams by a chopper or half-silvered mirror, with one beam passing through the reagent blank to its detector and the other through the specimen to its detector. The meter measures the difference in the current produced by the two beams, automatically compensating for variations in light source or detector response.

A recording UV/visible spectrophotometer is a double-beam instrument that automatically scans the entire spectrum and produces a graph relating percentage *T* (or *A* for absorbance) as a function of wavelength.

Important performance parameters for spectrophotometers include the wavelength range over which measurements can be made; bandpass (the width of wavelengths transmitted by the monochromator); wavelength accuracy and repeatability; sensitivity (the maximal detectable absorbance); photometric accuracy (linearity of response of the detector and readout); and percentage stray light (the amount of scattered or reflected light reaching the detector that does not pass through the cuvet or that is not of the proper wavelength).

spectrophotometric assays analytic methods using spectrophotometry for the quantitation of chemical species (analytes). The visible wavelength range is used most frequently, but many analytes are measured in the ultraviolet range and some even in the infrared range. Spectrophotometric assays are the basis of many procedures used in the clinical laboratory and in biochemical analysis in general. If the analyte itself is pigmented, it can be measured directly, although at times simple or involved procedures may be required to isolate it from the specimen matrix (e.g., carotene). If not pigmented, the analyte is caused to undergo reaction to form some colored product, the concentration of which is proportional to the analyte. The intensity of colored material present is a measure of the quantity of analyte. Usually, the color intensity is measured at the wavelength of maximal absorbance of the chromogen; in the presence of interfering materials, or if the procedure is too sensitive at that wavelength, some other appropriate wavelength may be used.

The parameter measured by the spectrophotometer is the transmittance (T), i.e., the ratio of the intensity of light that has been transmitted through the specimen cuvet to the intensity of the light transmitted through the reagent blank (reference) cuvet. Because T varies exponentially with concentration, another quantity, the absorbance (A), defined as: $\log_{10}(1/T) = 2 - \log_{10}$ (percent T) is used. Beer's law states that $A = k \times b \times C$, where k is a proportionality constant, b is light path, and C is concentration of analyte. When $b = 1$ cm, and $C = 1$ g/l, $k = a$, the specific absorptivity. When $C = 1$ mol/l, $k = \epsilon$, the molar absorptivity.

Beer's law is followed precisely only if monochromatic light is used and if there is no interaction between solute (analyte) molecules and solvent molecules, and between solute molecules. The noninteraction conditions are realized or approximated only in solutions of low concentration. With routine laboratory spectrophotometers, Beer's law is followed only to a limited extent because of such chemical interactions and because of the nonmonochromatic nature of light obtained. The range of concentration of analyte for which Beer's law holds, i.e., the linear portion of the calibration curve, must be determined for each analytic procedure using a series of standards. The absorbances of analytes and standards are read against that of a reagent blank (reference) containing all chemical constituents present in the test cuvet, except the analyte.

For solutions obeying Beer's law, the concentration of analyte is given by the equation $C_U = C_S \times A_U/A_S$, where C_U and C_S stand for the concentration of solute in the unknown and standard cuvets, and A_U and A_S stand for the corresponding absorbances. For solutions that do not obey Beer's law, the concentration is determined from a calibration curve obtained by plotting the absorbances of a series of standards against their concentrations, usually chosen to cover the range of concentration of clinical interest.

Absorbance curves of chemical species are highly specific for a compound or for a genus of compounds. Thus, absorbance spectra can be used to identify unknown chemicals but only if present in a fairly pure state. Inasmuch as most clinical specimens are highly complex mixtures, identification procedures are seldom practical. However, some drugs that can be isolated from mixtures by simple procedures, such as barbiturates and glutethimide (Doriden), can often be identified. The absorbance spectra of barbiturates in the ultraviolet region change in a characteristic way as one goes from the di-ionized to the mono- and nonionized forms.

JOHN F. KACHMAR, Ph.D.

spectrophotometric assays (toxicology) the identification and quantitation of toxic compounds by their light absorption.

In assays for the drugs that do not absorb strongly, or if other substances interfere, an absorbing reaction product is formed. It may be an oxidation product (e.g., benzophenone formed from phenytoin or methadone), or it may be a complex with a specific color reagent. In some assays, the same or a similar reaction may also occur with other substances present. For this reason, spectrophotometric assays generally are not considered a means of absolutely characterizing specific substances.

Some drugs, however, can be positively identified by the different absorbance spectra seen under varying conditions. For example, barbiturates are identified by the different absorbances of the free acid, the singly ionized form, and the doubly ionized form, whereas glutethimide is identified by the disappearance of its absorption peak as it is hydrolyzed.

spectrophotometry (spek″tro-fo-tom′ĕ-tre) 1. a technique used to study and establish the absorption spectra of chemical entities.

2. the measurement of absorbances of solutions, liquids, or solids at specific wavelengths as part of an analytic procedure.

infrared s., the characterization or identification of the infrared absorption spectra of chemical compounds, used primarily to determine the molecular structure of pure samples of unknown compounds. Absorption in this region (wavenumbers of approximately 4000–400 cm^{-1}) is due to vibrational modes of the molecule, involving either bond-bending or bond-stretching motions. Specific absorption bands characterize different functional groups. The infrared spectrum of a compound can be used to determine whether specific functional groups are present or absent, and also to identify compounds by comparing their spectra with those in a library of pure compounds. In a more limited sense, infrared spectrophotometry refers to the measurement of the intensity of absorption at a given wavenumber to quantitate a given compound.

ultraviolet/visible s., the measurement of the ultraviolet/visible absorption spectra of chemical compounds. This procedure is used both for the identification of chemical compounds by their characteristic absorption bands and for the determination of the concentrations of compounds by their absorbance at a particular wavelength, usually an absorption maximum (by Beer's law the absorbance is proportional to the concentration).

Absorption in this region (approximately 200–800 nm) is due to electronic transitions. In organic compounds, the strong absorption bands are due to transitions of π electrons in double and triple bonds and n (nonbonding) electrons in the unshared electron pairs of hetero atoms (nitrogen, oxygen, sulfur, and the halogens) to higher antibonding π^* orbitals.

These bands will be in the UV spectrum unless the excited state is stabilized by resonance; this occurs where two double bonds are separated by one single bond (—C═C—C═C—) or where a hetero atom is bonded to a double-bonded carbon (as in an arylamine). Thus, alkanes have no UV/visible absorption; unsaturated compounds and compounds containing hetero atoms absorb in the UV spectrum; and compounds containing large, conjugated π-electron systems, e.g., eight or more conjugated double bonds, absorb in the visible spectrum. In inorganic compounds, additional strong bands are due to transitions of *d*-shell and *f*-shell electrons; these are responsible for the colors of compounds of the transition metals and the rare earths.

spectrum (spek′trum), pl. *spectra* [L. "apparition"] 1. the pattern produced by passing a beam of white light through a prism. The degree of refraction depends on the wavelength; thus, the colors are spread out in a band. From the longest visible wavelength (770 nm) to the shortest (390 nm), these are, in order: red, orange, yellow, green, blue, and violet.

2. any graph of the intensity of detected radiation against one of the related quantities: wavelength, frequency, or energy; the absorption spectrum of a chemical compound; the emission spectrum of an element; or the gamma-ray spectrum of a radionuclide.

3. a range of frequencies, wavelengths, or energies, e.g., the ultraviolet spectrum, 4–400 nm.

For more information, see the specific spectrum.

spectrum analyzer an electronic instrument that produces a plot of the amplitude of the sinusoidal components of a complex waveform as a function of frequency. The output is produced on a cathode-ray tube (CRT) or chart recorder. Cf. *wave analyzer.*

speculum (spek′u-lum), pl. *specula* [L. "mirror"] an instrument for opening or distending a body orifice or cavity to permit visual inspection, e.g., a nasal or vaginal speculum.

Spelotrema a genus of trematodes (flukes) of the family Microphallidae. The species *S. brevicaeca* has been found in lesions of the heart and brain in humans in the Philippines. The adults measure 0.5–0.7 mm long by 0.3–0.4 mm wide. The eggs (measuring 15–16 μ long by 9.4–10 μ wide) are small, yellowish, and operculated.

spermat/o (sper′mah-to) [Gr. *sperma, spermatos* seed] a word element used in combining form to denote spermatozoa, e.g., spermatogenic, spermatocele.

spermatic (sper-mat′ik) [L. *spermaticus;* Gr. *spermatikos*] pertaining to the semen; seminal.

spermatic cord the structure that suspends the testis in the scrotum; it extends from the inguinal ring and is composed of the vas deferens, testicular artery, veins, nerves, and lymph vessels enclosed within a sheath of connective tissue and fibers of cremasteric muscle.

spermatid (sper′mah-tid) the precursor cell of a spermatozoon. At this stage in spermiogenesis, the acrosome is formed, the nucleus condenses, and the flagellum develops. See also *gametogenesis.*

spermatocele (sper′mah-to-sēl″) [*spermato-* + Gr. *kēlē* tumor] a cystic swelling produced by an accumulation of semen within an efferent duct in the head of the epididymus.

spermatocyte (sper′mah-to-sīt″) [*spermato-* + *-cyte*] the stage in the maturation of the spermatozoon at which meiotic nuclear division takes place, resulting in the formation of spermatids. See also *gametogenesis* and *spermatogenesis.*

spermatogenesis (sper″mah-to-jen′ĕ-sis) [*spermato-* + Gr. *genesis* production] the process by which spermatogonia divide and differentiate, ultimately to produce the spermatozoon or sperm. See also under *gametogenesis.*

spermatogonium (sper″mah-to-go′ne-um), pl. *spermatogonia* [*spermato-* + Gr. *gonē* generation] the undifferentiated stem cell of the male, situated along the basement membrane of the seminiferous tubules. These large, rounded cells are the progenitors of the spermatozoa.

spermatozoon (sper″mah-to-zo′on), pl. *spermatozoa* [*spermato-* + Gr. *zōon* animal] the male gamete or sperm; a highly specialized motile cell composed of an expanded head connected by a neck to the tail portion, which is a complex flagellum subdivided into middle, principal, and end pieces. A sperm is approximately 60 μm long. The head consists of a dense nucleus covered over its anterior two-thirds by a thin, enzyme-containing acrosomal cap. The neck is a narrow constriction that joins the head to the tail. An axoneme of 9 + 2 microtubules, surrounded by a ring of nine outer dense fibers and a helical sheath of flattened mitochondria, extends along most of the tail.

end piece of s., the distal portion of the tail of the spermatozoon. It consists only of an axoneme and flagellar membrane.

middle piece of s., the second part of the tail of a spermatozoon. It is characterized by an axoneme of 9 + 2 microtubules, surrounded by nine outer dense fibers and a sheath of circumferentially oriented mitochondria arranged in a tight helix.

neck of s., the proximal region of the spermatozoon tail. Immediately below the connecting piece, which attaches the flagellum to the head, is a dense capitulum. Below the capitulum is a transversely oriented proximal centriole. The microtubules of the centriole are embedded in nine segmented columns, which are continuous with the nine outer dense fibers that course along the flagellum through its middle piece.

outer dense fibers of s., electron-dense columns of fibers that run longitudinally along the tail of a spermatozoon, forming a ring outside the axoneme.

principal piece of s., the major region of the tail of a spermatozoon. It is an axoneme of 9 + 2 microtubules and asymmetrically arranged outer dense fibers.

spermidine (sper′mĭ-din) $NH_3^+(CH_2)_4NH_2^+(CH_2)_3$-$NH_3^+$, a polyamine present in cells. See also *polyamine.*

spermine (sper′min) $NH_2(CH_2)_3NH_2^+(CH_2)_4NH_2^+(CH_2)_3NH_3^+$, a polyamine present in cells. See also *polyamine.*

spermiogenesis (sper″me-o-jen′ĕ-sis) the sequence of events that results in the differentiation of immature spermatids into spermatozoa.

sp. gr. abbrev. See *specific gravity.*

sphaceloderma (sfas″ĕ-lo-der′mah) [L. *sphacelus,* from Gr. *sphakelos* gangrene + Gr. *derma* skin] gangrene of the skin.

S phase the phase of DNA synthesis as measured by

nuclear incorporation of tritiated thymidine. See also *cell cycle.*

sphen/o (sfe'no) [Gr. *sphēn* wedge] a word element used in combining form to denote wedge-shaped or the sphenoid bone, e.g., sphenoiditis.

sphenoid bone (sfe'noid) [*spheno-* + Gr. *eidos* form] the bone that forms the central part of the floor of the cranial cavity. It lies between the frontal and occipital bones, and articulates laterally with the temporal bones. The sphenoid has a body and three pairs of processes, the greater and lesser wings and the pterygoid processes. The body contains the sphenoid air sinus, and houses the sella turcica. Each lesser wing projects laterally, and together with the greater wing encloses the superior orbital fissure. The greater wing contains the foramina rotundum, ovale, and spinosum. Each pterygoid process projects downward and consists of a lateral and a medial plate that are fused anteriorly, enclosing the pterygoid fossa between them.

spher/o (sfe'ro) [Gr. *sphaira* a ball or globe] a word element used in combining form to denote globe-shaped or round, e.g., spherocytosis.

sphere (sfēr) [Gr. *sphaira*] 1. a ball, globe, or orb. 2. in mathematics, the surface consisting of all points equidistant from a fixed point (the center).

spherical (sfēr'ĭ-kal) [Gr. *sphairikos*] having the shape of a sphere; pertaining to a sphere. A spherical object has the same outline, a circle, in all views. See also the illustration accompanying *contour.*

spherical aberration the distortion of an image produced by a lens or mirror with spherical surfaces because rays at different distances from the center are focused at different points.

spherocyte (sfe"ro-sīt) [*sphero-* + Gr. *kytos* cell] a small diameter erythrocyte recognizable in smears by the absence of the usual central pallor and, as a rule, the presence of an increased MCHC (36 or higher). Spherocytes have a markedly increased fragility to hypotonic solutions, as demonstrated by the osmotic fragility test. Under electron-microscopic examination the cells are seen to have markedly increased thickness, but with preservation of a small dimple, indicative of their still minimally discoid rather than truly spherocytic shape.

Microspheres, true spherocytes, arise as result of intravascular red cell fragmentation by fibrin strands on the altered wall of the vessels. Small fragments have a tendency to fuse and form true spheres.

Spherocytes are characteristically found in patients with hereditary spherocytosis, but are also observed in those with familial or congenital hemolytic anemia and acquired hemolytic anemia.

Also called *prelytic sphere.*

spherocytic (sfe"ro-sit'ik) characterized by the presence of spherocytes.

spheroid (sfēr'oid) [*sphero-* + Gr. *eidos* form] a globular body, or one resembling a sphere.

spheroidal (sfe-roi'dal) having the form or shape of a sphere.

spheroplast (sfer'o-plast) a membrane-bound spherical form that results from only partial removal of cell wall constituents after enzymatic treatment of a bacterial, yeast, or fungus cell in a hypertonic medium. Cf. *protoplast.*

spherule (sfer'ūl) 1. a small sphere. 2. a thick-walled, spherical, multinucleated cell that is characteristic of the fungus *Coccidioides immitis.* The spherule develops from a barrel-shaped arthrospore to a mature spherule that produces endospores through progressive cleavage. Eventually, the spherule wall breaks, releasing uninucleate endospores into the environments. Spherules are useful in the histologic diagnosis of coccidioidomycosis.

spherulin an antigen, prepared from *Coccidioides immitis,* that is used in delayed hypersensitivity skin testing for coccidioidomycosis.

sphincter (sfingk'ter) [L.; Gr. *sphinktēr* that which binds tight] a ringlike band of circular muscle fibers that contricts a passage or closes a natural orifice.

anal s., a thickened band of muscles surrounding the anal canal. It is divided into two parts, an internal sphincter that surrounds the upper three-quarters of the anal canal and an external sphincter that surrounds the entire length of the anal canal.

s. of Oddi, the thickened, circular muscle surrounding the lower end of the common bile duct, the ampulla, and the terminal region of the pancreatic duct. Also called sphincter of the hepatopancreatic ampulla.

pupillary s., a flat, circular band of smooth muscle in the iris. It surrounds the pupil and functions in constricting it.

pyloric s., a thickening of the circular muscle of the stomach that surrounds the opening into the duodenum. See also *pylorus.*

sphing/o (sfing'go) [Gr. *sphingein* to bind fast] a word element used in combining form to denote relationship to sphingosine or a sphingolipid, e.g., sphingomyelin.

sphinganine see *dihydrosphingosine.*

sphingenine see *sphingosine.*

sphingolipid (sfing"go-lip'id) [*sphingo-* + *lipid*] a lipid molecule that contains a structural residue of sphingosine, dihydrosphingosine, or a closely similar molecule.

sphingolipidoses (sfing"go-lip"ĭ-do'sēz) a group of inherited lipid storage diseases caused by the accumulation within the nervous system of a specific substrate owing to the absence or deficiency of a lysosomal hydrolytic enzyme needed to catalyze the step-by-step degradation of sphingolipids.

The concept of inborn errors of catabolism caused by a mutation of a lysosomal enzyme was first formulated by Hers in 1965. Lysosomes are cytoplasmic organelles surrounded by a lipoprotein membrane. They contain acid hydrolases that have intracellular disgestive activities. Normal functioning of lysosomal enzymes has a vital physiologic role in the catabolism of endogenous as well as exogenous material; thus, they are essential to the orderly renewal of cell constituents and the removal of large macromolecules.

The critical catabolic role of the acid hydrolases was first realized in two neuronal storage disorders, Gaucher's disease and Niemann-Pick disease. The demonstration of the specific enzymatic lesion was made possible by the identification and chemical characterization of the sphinogolipids, a group of lipids that contain a moiety called ceramide. Ceramide contains a complex long-chain amino alcohol, sphingosine, bound at carbon-2 by an amide bond to a long-chain fatty acid. The type of group covalently bonded to carbon-1 of the sphingosine portion of the ceramide determines the class of sphingolipid. The use of the substrates labeled with radioactive elements in a particular portion of the molecule provided the technique needed for the precise identification of enzyme activity.

The clinical signs of this group of diseases are caused by the progressive and excessive accumulation of cerebral lipids within the body of nerve or glial cells, accompanied by varying degrees of demyelination and storage in other organs. Abnormalities of lipid metabolism are clinically characterized in infants by decreased mental development, frequently associated with splenomegaly, and hepatomegaly. Diagnosis of the disease process in these patients may be extremely difficult; prenatal diagnosis is available for many of the sphingolipidoses. Although the type of sphingolipidosis can be identified on the basis of clinical findings, laboratory tests are needed to determine the exact enzymatic defect. Tissue biopsy and enzymatic assay using labeled substrates were used initially but are difficult and expensive. Artificial substrates are now used with a much more accessible enzyme source, such as washed leukocytes, serum samples, or cultured skin fibroblasts.

Among the sphingolipidoses, the basic biochemical defect in each disorder has been identified. The accompanying table lists the nine principal disorders and identifies for each the site of the metabolic block, as well as the enzyme defect and the major sphingolipid that is stored. Ethnic and geographic considerations have an important role in the delineation of the variants of each disorder.

One of the major breakthroughs in the understanding of the sphingolipidoses was the identification of a deficiency of hexosaminidase A as the basic genetic defect causing Tay-Sachs disease (formerly known as infantile amaurotic idiocy). The reduced or absent activity of hexosaminidase A was demonstrated in leukocytes and serum of affected children. Significantly, a partial deficiency was shown to exist in serum and white blood cells of obligate heterozygotes for the Tay-Sachs disease gene, and the enzymatic defect was clearly definable in cultured skin fibroblasts and amniotic fluid cells. These accomplishments led to the first successful public heterozygote screening program. See also *genetic screening.*

For more information, see the specific sphingolipid storage disease.

MURIEL GLUCKSON, M.S.

sphingolipid storage disease see *sphingolipidoses.*

sphingolipodystrophy (sfing″go-lip″o-dis′tro-fe) any of a group of disorders of sphingolipid metabolism; see *sphingolipidoses.*

sphingomyelin (sfing″go-mi′ĕ-lin) a general designation for a group of phospholipids or sphingolipids (phosphocholine derivatives of ceramide) that differ from one another in the nature of the fatty acyl group joined to the amino group of sphingosine. On hydrolysis, they yield phosphoric acid, choline, sphingosine or a sphingosine-like base, and a fatty acid that may have 16–24 carbons. Sphingomyelin occurs primarily in nervous tissue and generally in membranes.

sphingomyelinase (sfing″go-mi′e-li-nās) see *sphingomyelin phosphodiesterase.*

sphingomyelin phosphodiesterase (sfing″go-mi′ĕ-lin fos″fo-di-es′ter-ās) an enzyme of the hydrolase class, sphingomyelin cholinephosphohydrolase (EC 3.1.4.12) that catalyzes the reaction: sphingomyelin + $H_2O \rightleftarrows$ *N*-acylsphingosine + choline phosphate. A genetic disorder, which is known as Niemann-Pick disease and is due to the absence (deficiency) of the enzyme, leads to sphingolipidosis, the accumulation of sphingomyelin in the tissues. Also called *sphingomyelinase.* See also *sphingolipidoses.*

sphingosine (sfing′go-sin) D(+)-*erythro*-1, 3-dihydroxy-2-amino-4-*trans*-octadecane; a long-chain, C_{18} mono-unsaturated, aliphatic amino alcohol present in a variety of sphingolipids. Sphingosine present as a CoA derivative is synthesized in animal tissues (e.g., brain) from palmitoyl CoA and L-serine. Also called *sphingenine.*

sphygm/o (sfig′mo) [Gr. *sphygmos* pulse] a word element used in combining form to denote pulse, e.g., sphygmoscopy, sphygmomanometer.

sphygmic (sfig′mik) [Gr. *sphygmikos*] pertaining to the pulse.

spicule (spik′ūl) [L. *spiculum*] a sharp, needlelike body, especially a small fragment of spongy bone.

spider (spi′der) 1. an arthropod of the class Arachnida.

2. a spiderlike nevus; a telangiectasis that is composed of small vessels radiating from a central arteriole, the whole resembling spider legs. It usually occurs in children and pregnant females, and also in persons with liver disease, most often on the upper arms and chest. Also called spider nervus.

Spiegler-Fendt sarcoid see *pseudolymphoma of Spiegler-Fendt.*

Spielmeyer-Vogt syndrome [Walter *Spielmeyer,* 1879-1935; Heinrich *Vogt,* born 1875] see *juvenile amaurotic familial i.* under *idiocy.*

spike (spīk) 1. any sharp upward deflection in a curve or tracing.

2. in electrophysiology, the electric activity that can be recorded from a single nerve fiber or muscle cell with the passage of an impulse (i.e., an action potential).

3. in electroencephalography, a transient wave 20–70 msec in duration, characterized by a pointed peak when recorded at a paper speed of 30 mm/sec. The diagnostic value of the viewing of spikes in the electroencephalogram depends on their appearance and the clinical context in which they are found.

See also *action potential* and *epilepsy.*

s. and dome complex, see *s. and slow-wave complex.*

s. and slow-wave complex, in electroencephalography, a sequence consisting of a spike followed by a slow wave. Also called *s. and dome complex.*

s. and slow-wave rhythm, repetitive spike and slow-wave complexes. See also *three-Hertz spike and slow waves.*

spill control procedures developed for responding appropriately to spills of fluids that cause slipping hazards or exposures to microorganisms, flammable vapors, or vapors that may be irritating, corrosive, or toxic. Among such action plans should be steps for the evacuation of personnel and for the clean-up of the spill by personnel trained and equipped with spill control material and self-contained breathing apparatus. As spill residues are

SPHINGOLIPIDOSES

Condition	Enzyme Defect	Major Lipid Accumulation	Mode of Inheritance*
Angiokeratoma, diffuse (Fabry's disease)	Ceramide trihexosidase (α-galactosidase)	Cer-β-Glc-β-Gal-α-Gal ceramide trihexoside	X-linked
Gm_1 gangliosidosis (generalized gangliosidosis)	β-D-Galactosidase (Gm_1-ganglioside-β-galactosidase)	Cer-β-Glc-β-Gal-β-GalNAc-β-Gal ganglioside Gm_1	AR
Gm_2 gangliosidosis I (Tay-Sachs disease)	Hexosaminidase A (β-*N*-acetyl-D-galactosaminidase)	Cer-β-Glc-β-Gal-β-GalNAc ganglioside Gm_2	AR
Gm_2 gangliosidosis II (Sandhoff's disease)	Hexosaminidase A and B (β-*N*-acetyl-D-galactosaminidase)	Cer-β-Glc-β-Gal-α-Gal-β-GalNAc globoside (also ganglioside Gm_2)	AR
Galactosyl ceramide lipidosis (Krabbe's disease)	Galactosylceramidase (galactocerebroside β-galactosidase)	Cer-β-Gal galactocerebroside	AR
Glucosyl ceramide lipidosis (Gaucher's disease)	Glucosylceramidase (glucocerebroside β-glucosidase)	Cer-β-Glc glucocerebroside	AR
Lipogranulomatosis (Farber's disease)	Acylsphingosine deacylase (ceramidase)	Cer ceramide	AR
Metachromatic leukodystrophy	Arylsulfatase A (sulfatidase)	Cer-β-Gal-SO_4 ceramide-galactose-3-sulfate (sulfatide)	AR
Sphingomyelin lipidosis (Niemann-Pick disease)	Sphingomyelin phosphodiesterase (sphingomyelinase)	Cer-pCh sphingomyelin	AR

* AR = autosomal recessive.

likely to be considered hazardous wastes, spill control plans should include disposal.

spill control kit a package of spill control supplies with the capacity to control the volume of material that may be spilled in the laboratory. Personnel should have training in how to apply and pick up the spilled material effectively and safely, including use of self-contained breathing apparatus.

spill residue residues of spills, which are considered to be hazardous waste if the material spilled is regarded as hazardous waste.

spin/o (spi'no) a word element used in combining form to denote the spine, e.g., spinifugal.

spina bifida (spi'nah bif'ĭ-dah) a developmental anomaly characterized by the defective closure of the bony encasement of the spinal cord, through which the cord and the meninges may or may not protrude.

s. b. cystica, a congenital malformation of the spinal column characterized by defective closure of the vertebral arches with a cystic swelling through the opening, involving the meninges (meningocele), spinal cord (myelocele), or both (meningomyelocele). Severe cases may result in complete rachischisis in which the lumbar arches are absent, the cord is aplastic, and the neural elements have no covering. Spina bifida and anencephaly are considered to be a single entity; see *neural tube defects.* Also called rachischisis posterior, spina bifida aperta, and spina bifida manifesta.

s. b. occulta, a congenital malformation of the spinal column, usually in the lumbar or sacral region, characterized by a defective closure of the vertebral arches without protrusion of the spinal cord or meninges. It is usually asymptomatic. About 10 percent of radiographs of the lumbosacral vertebra show this malformation.

spinal (spi'nal) [L. *spinalis*] pertaining to a spine or the vertebral column, and to the spinal cord and the nerves that emerge from it.

spinal cord the portion of the central nervous system that lies within the upper two-thirds of the vertebral canal and connects with the medulla at the foramen magnum. It is approximately 45 cm long and ends at the level of the upper border of the second lumbar vertebra. A slender band of connective tissue, the filum terminale, extends from the lower end of the cord to the coccyx. The cord is wider than it is thick, and expands in the cervical and lumbar regions because of the outflows to the upper and lower extremities. The right and left sides of the cord are almost completely separated by an anterior median fissure and a posterior median sulcus and septum. A slender central canal lies at its center.

In cross section, the gray matter of the cord is roughly H-shaped and is surrounded by the nerve fibers of the white matter. The anterior limbs of the H constitute the anterior gray columns, and the posterior limbs are the posterior gray columns. Small lateral gray columns are present at the thoracic level. The cells in the anterior gray columns give rise to motor axons that leave the cord in the spinal nerves through the anterior (ventral) nerve roots. Sensory fibers enter the cord through the posterior (dorsal) roots. The lower spinal nerves must descend within the vertebral canal to reach the vertebral foramen through which they exit.

The white matter of the cord consists of tracts of nerve fibers, which include afferent fibers from the dorsal root ganglia, motor fibers from the cells in the ventral and lateral gray columns, tracts of long ascending or descending fibers connecting with the brain stem, and fibers that unite segments of the cord for reflex pathways. Blood vessels within the cord are branches of longitudinal systems of arteries and veins.

Also called spinal medulla.

subacute combined degeneration (SCD) of the s. c., degeneration of the spinal cord that is associated with pernicious anemia (vitamin B_{12} deficiency). Characterized by the destruction of myelin and the proliferation of glial cells, primarily in the posterior and lateral columns of the spinal cord, SCD manifests itself with ataxia, abnormal deep tendon reflexes, loss of vibration sense, paresthesias, weakness, and spasticity, usually in a symmetric distribution and often involving only the lower extremities. Changes in personality ranging from emotional instability to psychosis may also occur, as may visual impairment and occasionally a mild peripheral neuropathy. The neurologic manifestations of vitamin B_{12} deficiency, although responsive to B_{12} therapy, are often not entirely reversed, especially when diagnosis has been delayed.

spinal cord tumors neoplasms of neuroglial, ependymal, and meningeal cells of the spinal cord. The tumors are histologically similar to those arising within the brain. The cord is also vulnerable by virtue of its location to a broad range of primary and metastatic neoplasms involving the vertebral and paravertebral tissues.

Astrocytomas of the spinal cord are most common in the cervical and thoracic regions, where they may form elongated fusiform swellings. Only occasionally do oligodendrogliomas involve the cord. More than half the gliomas affecting the cord are ependymal tumors. Meningiomas in the spinal canal are most common in the thoracic region and are usually firmly adherent to the dura. Schwann cell neoplasms of the spinal nerve roots are seen most frequently in the lumbar region.

spinal fluid see *cerebrospinal fluid.*

spinal nerve a nerve composed of nerve fibers arising from the spinal cord. There are 31 pairs (8 cervical, 12 thoracic, 5 lumbar, 5 sacral, 1 coccygeal). Each spinal nerve is formed by the union of a ventral and dorsal spinal nerve root. A spinal nerve emerges from the vertebral canal through an intervertebral foramen and divides into dorsal and ventral rami.

spinal puncture see *lumbar puncture.*

spinal somatosensory evoked potential see *spinal somatosensory evoked p.* under *potential.*

spinal tap see *lumbar puncture.*

spindle (spin'd'l) 1. in anatomy and histology, any fusiform structure; one resembling a cylinder with tapered ends.

2. an organelle existing only during the division of eukaryotic cells. It consists of two types of microtubules that run between the centrioles and between the centrioles and chromosomes: continuous microtubules that grow out from each centriole toward the other one, passing around the chromosomes and enmeshing them in a bundle of microtubules and appearing to push the centrioles apart and toward the poles of the cell; and chromosomal microtubules that appear to grow out from the chromosomes, one set growing out from each chromatid with each set

going to a different centriole. During anaphase, the chromatids separate and are drawn to the poles by the spindle fibers. The mechanism of this motion probably involves the two types of microtubules being pulled past one another. Also called achromatic spindle and mitotic spindle.

3. in electroencephalography, any group of rhythmic waves that gradually increase and then decrease in amplitude. Cf. *s. spindle* under *sleep.*

barbiturate s., a spindle recorded in patients or laboratory animals anesthetized with barbiturates. Barbiturate spindles may have their origin in alternating excitatory and inhibitory postsynaptic potentials of cells of nonspecific thalamic nuclei.

bipolar s., a normal mitotic spindle.

multipolar s., a mitotic spindle with more than two poles, which is formed in rare mutant cells having multiple centrioles.

muscle s., see *muscle spindle.*

spindle attachment see *centromere.*

spindle cell a narrow, elongated fusiform cell with its cytoplasm terminating in thin points at either end. The length-to-width ratio may be as great as 50:1. Spindle-shaped cells may be epithelial or nonepithelial, and either benign or malignant.

In cytology, spindle cells of squamous origin with benign nuclei occur in inflammatory conditions, whereas spindle cells with less marked nuclear abnormality than occurs in squamous carcinoma may be found in dysplasia and carcinoma in situ.

See also *fiber cell* and *spindly squamoid cell.*

spindle cell lipoma a lipoma composed of predominantly fusiform cells.

spindle cell nevus see *spindle n.* under *nevus.*

spindle nevus see *spindle n.* under *nevus.*

spindling (spind′ling) 1. in radiology, appearing to have a weakened thin section, as the radiographic architecture of a bone. See also the illustration accompanying *contour.*

2. in pathology, the tendency for cells to become elongated and tapered. Spindling may occur in certain neoplasms, making it difficult or impossible to determine whether the cells in question are epithelial or mesenchymal.

spindly squamoid cell a narrow, elongated, needle-shaped cell, usually 10–40 μm long, that is characteristic of invasive epidermoid carcinoma of the cervix. The nucleus is large, elongated, and hyperchromatic.

Because benign spindly squamous cells are occasionally observed in cervical smears, nuclear abnormalities must be present for the cell to be classified as cancerous. The presence of malignant spindly squamoid cells may be the only factor permitting correct cytologic classification of an anaplastic carcinoma as epidermoid in origin.

spine (spīn) 1. a thornlike process or projection.

2. the spinal column.

anterior inferior iliac s., a blunt, bony process that projects forward from the anterior border of the ilium above the acetabulum.

anterior superior iliac s., a blunt, bony projection on the anterior border of the ilium that forms the anterior end of the iliac crest.

ischial s., a heavy process of bone that projects down and medially from the posterior surface of the ischium. It serves as a point of attachment for the sacrospinous ligament and the coccygeus and levator ani muscles.

posterior inferior iliac s., a wide, bony projection from the posterior border of the ilium that indicates the limit of the posterior border above the greater sciatic notch.

posterior superior iliac s., a broad, bony projection on the posterior border of the ilium that forms the posterior limit of the iliac crest.

spine apparatus an aggregate of vesicular or saclike structures found together with bands of electron-dense material in many dendritic spines. Its function is unknown.

spinocerebellar (spi″no-ser″e-bel′ar) pertaining to the spinal cord and cerebellum.

spinocerebellar degeneration a group of hereditary diseases, transmitted as either dominant or recessive traits, that are characterized by degeneration of the spinal cord and cerebellum, often involving also the brain stem, peripheral nerves, and other parts of the neuraxis. These diseases may occur fully expressed or as formes frustes. Most commonly, ataxia, dysmetria, tremor, rigidity, and sensory and motor impairment are seen. There is no general agreement as to which disorders may be regarded as spinocerebellar degenerative diseases, but among those often included are Friedreich's ataxia, olivopontocerebellar degeneration, Marie's ataxia, and Strümpell-Lorrain disease.

spir/o (spi′ro) [Gr. *speira* coil; L. *spirare* to breathe] 1. a word element used in combining form to denote spiral form, e.g., spirochete, or a relation to breathing, e.g., spirometer.

2. a prefix word element in organic chemistry to denote a compound having two rings that share a single atom, e.g., spiro[2.3]hexane.

spiral lamina (spi′ral lam′ĭ-nah) a bony plate that spirals around and projects from the modiolus, incompletely dividing the cochlear canal into two parts, the lower scala tympani and the upper scala media.

spiral organ see *organ of Corti.*

Spirillaceae (spi″ril-la′se-e) a family of spiral and curved bacteria containing two genera, *Spirillum* and *Campylobacter.*

Spirillum (spi-ril′um) [L. *spirillum* a small spiral] a genus of bacteria of the family Spirillaceae, consisting of spiral rods that are short, rigid, and gram-negative and that have bipolar flagella. The organisms are motile, microaerophilic, or aerobic, and are found in fresh and salt water that contains organic matter.

S. minor, the species that causes the sodoku form of rat-bite fever in humans. The organism cannot be cultivated on artificial media. Laboratory diagnosis is made by direct microscopic demonstration of *S. minor* in wet mounts of exudates from skin eruptions or of blood; blood films may also be stained with Giemsa or Wright stain. Animal inoculation is used in cases when the organism cannot be demonstrated directly.

spirochete (spi′ro-kēt) [*spiro-* + Gr. *chaete* hair] a flexuous, helically coiled, motile bacterium of the Spirochaetaceae family. Of the five genera within the family, three contain species that are pathogenic for humans: *Treponema, Borrelia,* and *Leptospira.* Individual cells can be as long as 300 μm and so slender as to escape detection by ordinary light microscopy. They are, however, readily detectable by darkfield microscopy.

STRUCTURE. All spirochetes possess a cell membrane, a thin cell wall layer of peptidoglycan responsible for the helical form, and an outer membrane. The cytoplasm contains ribosomes, nonmembrane-bound nuclear material, mesosomes, and inclusions. In some spirochetes, cytoplasmic tubules of unknown function are present. Axial fibrils, chemically and structurally resembling flagella, are located between the outer membrane and the peptidoglycan layer. These are attached subterminally near each end of the cell, and extend toward or beyond the opposite pole of the cell. There are three different types of motility—a rapid rotation about the long axis, flexion of part or all of the cell, and a serpentine movement—that are sufficiently consistent among species to be of some presumptive diagnostic value.

GROWTH REQUIREMENTS. Nutritional requirements of spirochetes are generally complex. *Leptospira, Borrelia,* and *Treponema* require long-chain saturated and unsaturated fatty acids for growth. *Leptospira* species are aerobic and can be cultivated in vitro in a medium containing 10 percent rabbit serum. *B. recurrentis* and some other *Borrelia* species can be cultivated in Kelly's medium, a complex mixture of components including rabbit serum.

Many nonpathogenic *Treponema* species have been cultivated in vitro, including the Reiter strain, an extract of which is employed as a sorbent in the fluorescent treponemal antibody absorption (FTA-ABS) test for syphilis. However, the treponemes pathogenic for humans have not yet been cultivated, either in artificial media or tissue culture, although they can be propagated in rabbit testicles.

TREPONEMES. Nonpathogenic treponemes inhabit the human oral cavity, as well as the gastrointestinal and genitourinary tracts. The treponemes pathogenic for humans are similar both immunologically and structurally, appearing as tightly wound, tapered spirals that have three axial filaments at each end.

The important human treponemal diseases are syphilis, which is transmitted sexually, and yaws and pinta, the nonvenereal infections found in the tropics. All three are chronic diseases that exhibit characteristic clinical stages.

Syphilis, caused by *T. pallidum,* is found worldwide. Although usually acquired venereally, it may also be transmitted by direct contact with infectious lesions or infectious material and transplacentally from mother to fetus. Primary syphilis is characterized by the chancre, a nonpainful, self-limited lesion that appears at the site of contact. The secondary stage of syphilis, appearing several weeks later, involves the skin and mucous membranes, producing a rash. A tertiary or late stage occurring after a latent period that may last for years affects a small number of infected individuals. The destructive lesions of tertiary syphilis can affect any organ of the body, but the aorta and central nervous system are particularly susceptible.

Because treponemes usually cannot be observed in stained smears owing to their thinness, darkfield examination of lesions is used to diagnose primary and secondary stages of syphilis. Serous exudates of chancres, saline aspirates of lymph nodes, or skin lesions of secondary syphilis must be examined immediately. Darkfield microscopy reveals tightly wound spirochetes with characteristic bending and flexing motility. Lesions suspected of being caused by syphilis (especially oral lesions) may contain nonpathogenic treponemes that may be difficult to distinguish from pathogenic organisms.

Serologic tests include nonspecific nontreponemal reaginic tests used for screening and specific treponemal antibody tests used to confirm a positive screening test. Most useful of the currently available tests are: (1) nontreponemal (reaginic) tests, including the venereal disease research laboratory (VDRL) test, rapid plasma reagin (RPR) card test, and automated reagin test (ART); and (2) specific treponemal antibody tests, including the treponemal immobilization (TPI) test, fluorescent treponemal antibody absorption (FTA-ABS) test, and *T. pallidum* hemagglutination (TPHA) test.

The antigen used in the reaginic tests is cardiolipin-cholesterol-lecithin. Cardiolipin is a phospholipid obtained from beef livers or hearts. The VDRL test is the standard reaginic antibody test in which serum or spinal fluid is tested for the ability to flocculate a fine suspension of the antigen. The rapid methods (RPR, ART) are used by many serology laboratories for routine screening.

Biologic false-positive reactions with nontreponemal tests may occur in many infectious diseases and in a variety of other conditions such as autoimmune diseases, pregnancy, drug addiction, and old age.

Specific treponemal antibody tests are used to confirm the results of nontreponemal antibody tests. The most specific in the TPI test, but it requires viable rabbit-virulent treponemes and is therefore performed in only a few specialized laboratories. The FTA-ABS test is an indirect fluorescent antibody test, utilizing the Nichols strain of *T. pallidum* as antigen and a suspension of nonpathogenic Reiter treponemes to remove cross-reacting antibody from serum. A hemogglutination test is also available for specific antibody testing.

All serologic tests are positive in secondary syphilis. Adequate treatment of syphilis does not affect the results of specific antibody tests, but the titers of reaginic tests do decrease following successful treatment, and thus are used to monitor response to therapy. The VDRL test is performed as a definitive test on spinal fluid when a diagnosis of neurosyphilis is being considered, because serum antibody does not penetrate the normal blood-brain barrier. Serial VDRL titers are used for the diagnosis of congenital syphilis.

Nonvenereal treponemal diseases are endemic in tropical areas. They occur in syphilis-like stages, but unlike syphilis do not affect the internal organs. They primarily infect children.

Yaws is a disease involving the skin and bones. It is caused by *T. pertenue,* which is transmitted when traumatized skin comes into contact with infectious lesion exudates. *T. carateum* causes pinta, a disfiguring skin disease infecting individuals in remote rural areas of tropical South and Central America. The mode of transmission is the same.

Diagnosis of the nonvenereal treponemal diseases is based on the clinical manifestations, a history of residence in an endemic area, and darkfield examination of lesions. Because of immunologic similarities among the organisms, both nontreponemal and treponemal antibodies are produced.

BORRELIA. The genus *Borrelia* consists of arthropod-borne spirochetes, which appear as loosely wound spirals with 12–15 axial filaments at each end. *Borrelia* species cause relapsing fever, a disease characterized by recurrent episodes of fever and spirochetemia separated by febrile periods in which spirochetes are not present in the blood. There are two types of relapsing fever: louse-borne or epidemic, and tick-borne or endemic. Epidemic relapsing fever, caused by *B. recurrentis,* is transmitted from person to person by the body louse (*Pediculus humanus*); there is no animal reservoir. The disease is endemic in parts of Africa and South America, and can become epidemic in the conditions of overcrowding and poor personal hygiene associated with wars and large-scale national disasters.

Endemic relapsing fever is caused by any one of many *Borrelia* species. Ticks of the genus *Ornithodoros* transmit spirochetes to humans from various animal reservoirs, especially rodents and other small animals. United States outbreaks occur most often in the West or Southwest, areas in which the species *O. hermsii* and *O. turicata* are endemic.

Definitive diagnosis involves the demonstration of loosely wound spirochetes in the peripheral blood of febrile patients. Both thick and thin smears may be stained by Giemsa or Wright stains.

The relapses and recurrent nature of relapsing fever are a striking clinical feature, the immunologic mechanism of which is unique among bacteria, both in frequency and degree. Each recurrence is caused by outgrowth of a mutant strain that is quite different antigenically from those causing the preceding attacks. Remission results despite elaboration of new antibodies because the high mutation rate among *Borrelia* gives rise to a new antigenic variant that is beyond the current range of specificity.

LEPTOSPIRA. *Leptospira* are tightly wound spirals with their ends bent into hooks and one axial filament at each end. *L. biflexa* is a saphrophytic leptospira found primarily in fresh water and rarely in sea water. *L. interrogans,* the pathogenic species, is actually a designation for a large heterogeneous complex of related spirochetes that are presently being arranged into genetic groups and serologic aggregates called serovars. Leptospirosis is primarily a zonosis. Rodents and a variety of wild and domestic animals serve as infected hosts as well as reservoirs. The organisms have a predilection for the lumen of nephritic tubules, where they are shed into the urine. Humans become infected following occupational exposure by indirect contact with water or soil containing contaminated urine, or by direct contact with infected animals. The organism enters the body through skin abrasions, mucosal surfaces of the nasopharynx and esophagus, or the eyes. After an initial stage of spirochetemia, the organism may be found in kidney tubules. Clinical manifestations range from a mild, catarrh-like illness to aseptic meningitis, and to a severe form with jaundice, hemorrhaging, and kidney involvement (Weil's disease).

Definitive diagnosis rests either on isolation of the organism, or on demonstration of a fourfold or greater rise in antibody titer in the presence of clinical findings suggestive of leptospirosis. The organism can be observed in infectious specimens by darkfield microscopy. Diagnosis cannot be made solely on results obtained by darkfield microscopy because of the difficulty in distinguishing the finely wound spirals from artifacts seen in clinical specimens. Leptospira grow aerobically in appropriate artificial media. Microscopic and macroscopic agglutination tests are used for antibody detection. Serologic mutants can be identified by agglutination tests performed in reference laboratories.

spirogram (spi'ro-gram) [*spiro-* + Gr. *gramma* a writing] the record obtained from spirometry, a tracing or graph of the volume or velocity of expired air.

spirometer (spi-rom'ĕ-ter) [*spiro-* + L. *metrum* measure] 1. an instrument for measuring the air taken into and exhaled from the lungs.

2. an instrument for delivering a quantity of radioactive gas to the lungs for a pulmonary perfusion scan. The gas can be rebreathed until equilibrium is reached, and collected for disposal.

Spirometra (spi″ro-met'rah) a genus of tapeworms naturally parasitic in a variety of carnivores. Human infection is caused by ingestion of the infected *Cyclops* or the infected flesh of a second intermediate host (fish, snakes, or amphibians). The eggs (measuring 57–66 μ long by 33–37 μ wide) are ellipsoidal and possess a rounded, conical operculum. Several species may infect humans, causing sparganosis.

spirometric (spi″ro-met'rik) pertaining to spirometry or the spirometer.

spirometry (spi-rom'ĕ-tre) the use of the spirometer to measure (and record) changes in the gas volume in the lungs with time, and thus the extent of abnormality in ventilatory capacity and mechanical factors in breathing. The parameters of pulmonary function that are obtained by spirometry can be compared with predicted values that are adjusted for the patient's age, height, and sex (pulmonary function prediction nomograms).

In addition to measurements of respiratory frequency and tidal volume, three basic maneuvers are generally performed during a spirometric examination: vital capacity (VC), forced vital capacity (FVC), and maximal voluntary ventilation (MVV). These procedures are carried out before and 15–30 min after administration of a bronchodilator.

In the VC maneuver, following a maximal inspiration, the patient exhales as forcefully as possible into the spirometer mouthpiece. This results in exhalation of about 80 percent of the air in the lungs (the VC). Even though a reduced VC suggests the presence of an abnormality in ventilatory function, the VC maneuver alone cannot be used to establish the precise underlying pathologic mechanism.

A FVC maneuver is performed in a manner similar to the VC, but in addition the patient is instructed to exhale as quickly as possible from the maximal inspiration. The FVC is the total volume of air delivered into the mouthpiece. The spirogram obtained from this maneuver is a curve that relates the changes in the forced expired volume to the time required for expiration; the slope of the curve at any volume or volume interval represents the expiratory flow at that point.

It is possible to determine various timed expiratory volumes by analyzing the forced expiratory spirogram, such as the total volumes exhaled at 0.5, 1, 2, and 3 sec of the forced expiration (the FEV-0.5, FEV-1, FEV-2, and FEV-3, respectively). The points at which 25, 50, and 75 percent of the FVC have been exhaled (and 75, 50, and 25 percent remain in the lungs, respectively) are also identified on the spirogram. The forced expiratory flows during intervals of the expiration (for example, during the first 25 percent, the FEF_{25}; or during the midportion, the FEF_{25-75}) can then be calculated as the slope of the curve between various combinations of these points. Finally, when the volume is between 200 and 1200 ml of expired air (the maximal expiratory flow rate, 200–1200), the slope of the curve can also be calculated from the forced expiratory spirogram. All parameters obtained from the forced expiratory spirogram are useful indicators of the extent of limitation to expiratory flow, whether caused by a loss of elastic recoil forces, by intrinsic airway obstruction, or by chest wall or diaphragmatic weakness. See also the illustration accompanying *lung volume.*

To obtain a measure of the MVV, the patient is instructed to breath as forcefully and rapidly as possible into and out of the spirometer mouthpiece for a period of 12–15 sec. The calculation volume breathed per minute, the MVV, reflects intrinsic properties of the respiratory system (the strength and stamina of the respiratory muscles and the resistance to airflow), as well as nonpulmonary variables such as the extent of patient cooperation. Thus, like the VC, it is useful only when considered in combination with other parameters of pulmonary function.

In addition to the values measured or calculated during the three basic maneuvers, there are five diagnostic signs that may be identified on a spirogram: (1) the air-trapping sign (when the FVC decreases in magnitude during serial measurements, an indication of obstructive airway disease); (2) the emotional stress pattern (a pattern of respiration consisting of hyperventilation interspersed with deep, irregular, sighing inspirations, exacerbated by emotional stress); (3) the airway collapse pattern (a notching and sudden reduction in flow in the initial expired segments of the MVV or FVC curve); (4) the penmanship sign (the rapid, shallow, extremely regular respirations seen when the VC is diminished by conditions such as diffuse pulmonary fibrosis); and (5) an elevation of the end-expiratory level (seen during the initial breaths of the MVV measurement, an indication of increased airway resistance).

spironolactone (spi-ro″no-lak′tōn) [USP], a mild diuretic, a steroid similar to aldosterone. It acts as an aldosterone receptor antagonist, which reduces the reabsorption of sodium and water in the distal tubules of the kidney. Unlike other diuretics (except triamterene), it does not cause potassium depletion. It is used to treat edema, particularly that due to cirrhosis of the liver, and to treat hypertension. Trademark, *Aldactone.*

Spirurata a suborder of nematodes, including the family Spiruridae.

Spirurida an order of nematodes, including the suborder Spirurata.

Spiruridae a family of nematodes, including the superfamilies Spiruroidea and Filarioidea.

Spiruroidea (spi″roo-roi′de-ah) a superfamily of nematodes, including the genera *Gnathostoma, Physaloptera, Thelazia,* and *Cheilospirura.*

Spitz nevus see *spindle n.* under *nevus.*

splanchnic (splank′nik) [Gr. *splanchnikos;* L. *splanchnicus*] see *visceral.*

splanchnic nerves the nerve trunks of the autonomic nervous system that arise from various levels of the sympathetic trunk or from the anterior rami of the spinal nerves to provide autonomic innervation to the viscera.

greater s. n., a nerve of preganglionic and visceral afferent fibers that arises from the fifth to the ninth thoracic ganglia of the sympathetic trunk. Branches of this nerve invest the thoracic aorta while the main trunk pierces the diaphragm to end in the celiac ganglion. A few fibers pass the celiac ganglion to end in the aorticorenal ganglion and the adrenal gland.

lesser s. n., a small sympathetic nerve formed of fibers from the ninth through eleventh thoracic ganglia. It penetrates the diaphragm and terminates in the aorticorenal ganglion.

lowest s. n., a small sympathetic nerve that arises from the lowest thoracic ganglion of the sympathetic trunk and ends in the renal plexus.

lumber s. n.'s, sympathetic nerves that arise from one or more of the four lumbar ganglia and end in the celiac, intermesenteric, and superior hypogastric plexuses.

pelvic s. n.'s, the parasympathetic nerves to the viscera that arise from the anterior rami of the second, third, and fourth sacral spinal nerves. Their action influences the rectum, bladder wall, colon, and erectile tissue of the penis and clitoris.

spleen (splēn) [Gr. *splēn;* L. *splen*] a highly vascular hematopoietic organ derived from the dorsal mesogastrium and located within the left upper quadrant of the peritoneal cavity; it weighs 100–200 g in adults. Although the spleen has long been considered mysterious, the microcirculation and function have recently been elucidated.

The splenic parenchyma consists of two distinct components, the red and white pulps. The splenic red pulp is the main phagocytic or "reticuloendothelial" constituent of the body. It is a complex, blood-filled, loose meshwork composed of an intricate series of anastomosing endothelium-lined vascular channels (sinuses), which are separated by solid thin partitions, the Billroth or pulp cords. The red pulp cords are rich in macrophages, as well as a variety of other cells, including supporting reticulum cells, fibroblasts, plasma cells, leukocytes, platelets, and erythrocytes; these cells are irregularly separated in the pulp cords by extracellular reticulin and basement membrane–like material. Recent studies on the precise microcirculation within the red pulp have demonstrated that the splenic arterioles, after supplying the white pulp, either terminate in the interface between the red and white pulps (marginal zone) or enter the red pulp to discharge within the cords. Formed blood elements can pass into adjacent sinuses from the cords via a series of fenestrations in the basement membranes separating the pulp cords from sinus endothelial cells. The fenestrations provide an effective filtration system. Normal erythrocytes pass readily through the apertures of the basement membranes; senescent or pathologic red cells, however, are unable to traverse this passage and are subject to phagocytosis by macrophages within the cords. The phagocytosis of the formed blood elements is referred to as the culling function of the spleen. The spleen also has the unique capacity to remove abnormal inclusions from red cells such as Howell-Jolly bodies (nuclear remnants) with subsequent release of the intact erythrocytes into the circulation, a phenomenon termed the pitting function. Splenic cordal macrophages also may phagocytose other particulate matter such as antigens and opsonized bacteria. In addition to its phagocytic function, the red pulp provides a reservoir function (with storage of up to one-third of the total platelets), serves as a source of extramedullary hematopoiesis both in utero and in certain disease conditions, and synthesizes two opsonizing agents–tuftsin and properdin.

The white pulp of the spleen is a modified lymphoid organ and consists of a series of small lymphoid aggregates, often referred to as malpighian bodies, surrounding splenic arterial vessels and set within the red pulp. The white pulp contains both thymic-processed (T) and bone marrow–derived (B) lymphocytes, in addition to plasma cells, macrophages, and supporting reticulum cells. The T lymphocytes are mainly found in the periarteriolar lymphoid sheaths, whereas the B lymphocytes are located predominantly adjacent to the sheaths as eccentric lymphoid nodules. Similar to lymph nodes, the B-cell nodules may form secondary reactive germinal centers. The white pulp also functions similarly to lymph nodes in producing specialized antibodies for immunologic defense. The area adjacent to the white pulp, which separates it from the red pulp, is the ill-defined marginal zone that is important for antigen trapping and antigen-antibody interaction.

Despite the important functions described above, adults may live quite normally without a spleen, e.g., following surgical removal (splenectomy) as a result of trauma. Curiously, splenic function may return after traumatic removal; this is due to the overgrowth of hertertopic splenic fragments of damaged spleen implanted on the peritoneal surfaces during the traumatic episode. This phenomenon is referred to as splenosis or the born-again spleen. In children, however, splenectomy may be hazardous, owing to an increased risk of septicemic infection by encapsulated bacteria, such as pneumococci. This risk of infection also is found among individuals whose spleens have ceased to function (functional asplenia or hyposplenism). Hyposplenism may occur, for example, following radiation therapy to the spleen or in patients with sickle cell anemia.

More common than hyposplenism is increased splenic phagocytic function or hypersplenism, a hematologic term that refers to the premature destruction of blood cells by the spleen. Primary features of hypersplenism consist of (1) blood cytopenia, (2) corresponding hyperplasia of bone marrow precursors, (3) splenic enlargement (splenomegaly), and (4) relief of the cytopenia by splenectomy. The pathogeneses of hypersplenism are varied. Causes include the production of an antibody by the spleen against a specific blood element such as platelets in idiopathic thrombocytopenic purpura; the excess trapping of blood elements within the pulp cords because of an inherent cellular defect, as found in red cells in hereditary spherocytosis; an increase in splenic cordal macrophages, commonly occurring in association with increased pressure in the portal vein due to cirrhosis of the liver; and the various malignancies affecting the white or red pulps, including lymphomas and leukemias. Splenomegaly also may be found in a variety of other conditions, not necessarily associated with hypersplenism, such as infections (malaria, infectious mononucleosis), the various lipid histiocytoses, and the rare primary splenic vascular tumors (hemangiomas, angiosarcomas). The major histologic categories of diseases found in North America involving the splenic white and red pulps and associated with splenomegaly and/or hypersplenism are listed in the accompanying table.

SPLEEN. MAJOR HISTOLOGIC CATEGORIES OF SPLENIC DISEASES ASSOCIATED WITH SPLENOMEGALY

CATEGORY
White Pulp
Reactive hyperplasia
Malignant lymphomas
Chronic lymphocytic leukemia and related lymphoproliferative disorders
Red Pulp
Congestion
Infections
Histiocytic proliferations
Leukemias and lymphoproliferative disorders
Nonhematopoietic tumors

Courtesy of Jerome S. Burke, M.D.

Also called *lien.* See also *splenic tumors.*
JEROME S. BURKE, M.D.

spleen scan either of two procedures in nuclear medicine for imaging the spleen. The more commonly performed procedure uses the imaging agent technetium Tc 99m sulfur colloid, which is taken up (by phagocytosis) from the blood by macrophages in the spleen, liver, and bone marrow. The other procedure uses heat-damaged autologous red blood cells labeled with either ^{51}chromium or ^{99m}technetium, agents sequestered only by the spleen. Posterior, left lateral, and anterior views of the upper left quadrant of the abdomen are made with a scintillation camera or a rectilinear scanner (the whole abdomen is imaged in searching for accessory splenic tissue).

These procedures are used for the evaluation of focal lesions of spleen (infarction, hematoma, cyst, abscess, metastatic malignancy), palpaple upper quadrant masses, spleen size (splenomegaly), and spleen function—either the permanent (autosplenectomy) or correctable (functional asplenia) loss of function seen in sickle cell anemia. They are also used to locate the spleen in determining radiation therapy treatment portals. The red cell scan is used to locate accessory splenic tissue that has become enlarged after splenectomy.

The colloid scan is begun 10 min after injection of the agent; the red cell scan 1–24 hr after injection. The heat-damaged red cells are prepared by drawing 10–15 ml of blood from the patient and adding acid-citrate-dextrose (ACD) and sodium chromate Cr 51 (the chromate binds to hemoglobin). This is then incubated at 50°C for 20 min, and ascorbic acid is added to reduce the unbound chromium to the trivalent state, which cannot enter red cells. After cooling to 37°C, the red cells are injected intravenously.

splen/o (sple'no) [Gr. *splēn* spleen] a word element used in combining form to denote the spleen, e.g., splenomegaly.

splenic (splen'ik) [Gr. *splēnikos*, L. *splenicus*] pertaining to the spleen; lienal.

splenic anemia of infants see *kala-azar.*

splenic artery one of the three terminal branches of the celiac artery. It runs along the upper border of the pancreas to the spleen.

splenic cords the masses of red pulp, rich in macrophages, that surround the venous sinusoids of the spleen. Also called *cords of Billroth.*

splenic corpuscle an aggregation of lymphatic tissue, primarily T lymphocytes, that ensheaths the arteries of the spleen to form the white pulp.

splenic tumors neoplasms of the spleen, rarely encountered apart from lymphomas and leukemias in which the spleen is frequently involved as part of a multicentric process. The most common tumors are angiosarcomas and benign hemangiomas or lymphangiomas. Patients with angiosarcomas have a poor prognosis, most dying in less than 1 yr, from metastases to the liver or lungs. In some patients, spontaneous rupture of the spleen occurs, leading to hemoperitoneum. Other benign and malignant splenic tumors are exceedingly rare; occasional fibrosarcomas and malignant fibrous histiocytomas have been recorded.

splenic vein the vein that drains the spleen. It runs to the right, behind the body of the pancreas and below the splenic artery, and meets the superior mesenteric vein behind the neck of the pancreas to form the portal vein.

splenohepatomegaly (sple"no-hep"ah-to-meg'ah-le) [*spleno-* + Gr. *hēpar* liver + *megas* large] the enlargement of the spleen and liver.

splenomegaly (sple"no-meg'ah-le) [*spleno-* + Gr. *megas* large] a condition characterized by an enlarged spleen. The etiology is greatly varied because of the circulation of the spleen and its hemopoietic and immunologic functions. Splenomegaly is most commonly secondary to cirrhosis of the liver and portal hypertension, but several vascular deformities may contribute, including portal vein thrombosis and stenosis and aneurysm of the splenic artery. Other causes include reactive hyperplasmia due to infection or inflammation (mononucleosis and tuberculosis), metabolic-infiltrative disorders (Gaucher's disease and Niemann-Pick disease), lymphoproliferative diseases (leukemias and lymphomas), connective tissue diseases (systemic lupus erythematosus and rheumatoid arthritis), and hemolytic anemias. A common clinical manifestation is hypersplenism.

Diagnosis is based on abdominal palpation, clinical signs, and laboratory tests on the blood components. Radionuclide scans using technetium and angiography are helpful in determining spleen size.

See also *Felty's syndrome* and *hypersplenism.*

splenoportography see *splenoportal v.* under *venography.*

splenosis (sple-no'sis) see under *spleen.*

splicing (spli'sing) 1. the introduction of donor DNA sequences into a vector for cloning. See also *gene splicing.* 2. the excision of introns from messenger RNA precursors during posttranscriptional processing.

split gene a gene that contains intervening sequences (introns) of DNA between coding sequences (exons). The introns are removed and the exons spliced together before translation begins. See also *RNA processing.*

spondyl/o (spon'di-lo) [Gr. *spondylos* vertebra] a word element used in combining form to denote the vertebrae, e.g., spondylolisthesis.

spondylitis (spon"dĭ-li'tis) a general term used to describe an inflammation of the vertebrae. It may occur as a result of infection or trauma, or may be of unknown cause (e.g., ankylosing spondylitis).

ankylosing s., chronic, progressive inflammation of the vertebral and sacroiliac joints. It may also involve the hip and shoulder joints. Young males between the ages of 15 and 40 yr are most commonly affected. Early signs include low back pain, tenderness in the joints, and muscle spasms. Later symptoms include stiffening of the joints and ligaments, marked distortion of posture, and decreased chest expansion, at times to the point of interfering with breathing. The vertebrae finally fuse, connected by bony bridges called syndesmophytes.

In a large majority of cases, mild anemia and an increased erythrocyte sedimentation rate are noted; hypergammaglobulinemia and antinuclear antibodies are not present. There are certain clinical similarities between ankylosing spondylitis and diseases such as osteoarthritis of the spine and rheumatoid arthritis. Diagnosis is based on the presence of the clinical and radiologic signs of each disease.

There is apparently a strong genetic component underlying the development of ankylosing spondylitis. More than four-fifths of those with the disease have the HLA-B27 antigen. An immunologic mechanism may be involved, but has not been identified at this time. Antiinflammatory agents and physical therapy are the present treatment of choice.

Also called rheumatic spondylitis and *von Bechterew's disease.*

tuberculous s., see *Pott's disease.*

spondylolisthesis (spon"dĭ-lo-lis'the-sis) [*spondyl-* + Gr. *olisthanein* to slip] the forward displacement of one vertebra (body, pedicle, and superior articular facet) over another. It most frequently occurs as a slippage of L5 over the sacrum, or L4 over L5. There is limitation of movement and pain in the lower back, which radiates to the thighs. The nerve roots may be affected. Diagnosis may be aided by plain x-ray, electromyography, or myelography. Severe cases may lead to shortening of the trunk and protrusion of the abdomen.

spondylosis (spon"dĭ-lo'sis) a general term used to describe degenerative changes in the vertebral bodies of the spine.

cervical s., degeneration of the cervical vertebrae, leading to compression of the cervical portion of the spinal cord and/or of the cervical nerve roots.

Cervical radiculopathy, compression of one or more nerve roots, is usually associated with radicular pain, weakness, and numbness. Neurologic examination and electromyography may document segmental dysfunction in the appropriate distribution. Oblique x-rays of the cervical spine may demonstrate narrowing of cervical intervertebral foramina.

Cervical spondylotic myelopathy, compression of

the cervical spinal cord, is usually painless and produces abnormal strength and sensation of the lower extremities, often with associated bladder dysfunction. Hyperreflexia and spasticity may be present in the legs, and a narrowed anteroposterior diameter of the cervical spinal canal (less than 12 mm) is usually seen on plain radiographs. Diagnosis is established by cervical myelography.

lumbar s., degeneration of the lumbar vertebrae, leading to compression of the lumbar segment of the spinal cord, the lumbar nerve roots, or the cauda equina. The most common symptom is back pain after prolonged standing or effort. Muscle weakness, sensory abnormalities, and bladder dysfunction may also be seen. Diagnosis, based on radiographic demonstration of stenosis of the lumbar spinal canal or narrowed neural foramina, usually requires CT scanning and/or myelography.

spongioblast (spun′je-o-blast″) [L., Gr. *spongia* sponge + Gr. *blastos* germ] see *glioblast.*

spongy bone the spongy interior portion of mature bone. It consists of intercommunicating spaces containing bone marrow in between a three-dimensional lattice of branching bony spicules or trabeculae. Also called *cancellous bone* and trabecular bone. Cf. *compact bone.*

spontaneous (spon-ta′ne-us) [L. *spontaneous,* voluntary] 1. having no apparent cause.

2. occurring without external influence owing to the inherent properties of an object.

spontaneous activity the electric activity recorded in the absence of any external stimulus from a fully relaxed muscle or a nerve after the activity generated by electrode insertion has ceased. The action potentials thus recorded can be normal or of pathologic origin. For specific types of spontaneous activity, see also *end-plate noise, f. potential* under *fasciculation, f. potential* under *fibrillation, myotonic discharge,* and *positive sharp wave.*

SPOOL (acronym from *s*imultaneous *p*eripheral *o*peration *o*n-*l*ine) a method of handling input-output (I/O) in a data processing system in which the I/O from slow-speed devices (card readers, printers, remote terminals) is temporarily stored in a disk file or buffer. User programs do not have to wait for the I/O devices, and the operating system can work the devices efficiently.

spor/o- (spo′ro) [Gr. *sporos* seed] a word element used in combining form to denote relationship to a spore, e.g., sporocyst.

sporangiophore (spo-ran′je-o-fōr) a hypha that bears a sporangium.

sporangiospore (spo-ran′je-o-spōr) a spore that is contained and borne within a sporangium.

sporangium (spo-ran′je-um), pl. *sporangia*[*spor-* + Gr. *angeron* vessel] a cell within which spores or sporelike bodies are borne. Generally, it is an asexual structure of certain fungi.

spore (spōr) [L. *spora;* Gr. *sporos* seed] a reproductive element produced by certain fungi, algae, and bacteria. It is inactive, resistant to environmental factors, and unusually dehydrated.

bacterial s., a spore formed most readily under conditons of nutritional deprivation by certain species of bacteria, such as *Bacillus, Clostridium,* and *Sarcina.* The bacterial spore is not reproductive but is rather a dehydrated concentration of cell constituents admirably suited for surviving long exposure to adverse conditions. Spores are highly resistant to heat, drying, freezing, toxic chemicals, and radiation, but can be destroyed by autoclaving. They may survive for months or years in a dry environment.

Bacterial spores are formed within normal bacterial cells. Sporulation is generally initiated by a limitation in the supply of nutrients. The material is converted to an axial filament, and one chromosome migrates to the end of the cell, causing asymmetric cell division with the ingrowth of the cytoplasmic membranes to form a spore septum. This septum finally surrounds the chromosome and adjacent cytoplasm in a double membrane to form a forespore at one end of the cell, which is visible as an area of increased refractility.

A large amount of material is formed between the layers of the cytoplasmic membrane, producing a thick envleope. the spore cell wall consists of a thin inner membrane and a thick layer, the cortex, which contains many layers of peptidoglycan. Surrounding this cell wall is the coat, composed of an impervious, keratin-like protein with many S-S linkages; it is responsible for the spore's chemical resistance. In some cases, a delicate lipoprotein membrane surrounds the coat. When mature, the endospore is freed by autolysis of the mother cell wall (the sporangium). The spore then enters a stage of dormancy until conditions are favorable for the resumption of normal vegetative growth, when it is capable of initiating a new generation of the organism. The freed spore contains all the material necessary for resuming growth: DNA, small amounts of ribosomes, tRNAs, accessory factors and enzymes for protein synthesis, storage materials of proteins, ribonucleosides, and 3-phosphoglycerate, a high-energy phosphate source.

The process of converting a spore into a single vegetative cell is known as generation and involves three stages: activation, generation proper, and outgrowth. Activation may occur spontaneously upon aging when the spore is placed in a favorable medium, or it may requre a traumatic agent such as heat, low pH, or a sulfhydryl compound. Damage to the impervious cell coat appears to be essential for activation. This stage is followed by generation proper (initiation), which requires the presence of water and specific generating agents, such as various metabolites or inorganic ions. These penetrate the damaged cell coat, the cortex barrier of peptidoglycans breaks down, and the cell rapidly takes up water, potassium, and magnesium. The storage materials are hydrolyzed to provide amino acids and energy. In a favorable medium, generation is followed immediately by the outgrowth stage and a gradual resumption of the normal vegetative reproductive growth of the organism.

Also called endospore. See also *bacterium* and *spore form.*

fungal s., the reproductive element of fungi. There are two classes: sexual spores, which are produced by the fusion of two nuclei, and asexual spores, which develop by the differentiation of spore-bearing hyphae. In certain fungi (Zygomycetes), asexual spores are formed within a sporangium. In higher molds, asexual spores are not contained within a sporangium but rather are borne on the tips of hyphae or produced by segmentation of hyphae. Asexual spores produced by budding hyphae are called conidia.

Aleuriospores resemble conidia, although they

are borne directly from hyphae and not on conidiophores. The dermatophytes (*Trichophyton, Microsporum,* and *Epidermophyton*) produce aleuriospores. Arthrospores are produced by fragmentation of preformed mycelium, resulting in a chain of spores. *Coccidioides* is an example of a genus with arthrospores. Chlamydospores are large, thick-walled spores formed within or at the ends of the hyphae. They are irregular in form and size and may be produced by certain dermatophytes.

spore form the dehydrated resting form produced by some bacteria. It develops from an endospore that is contained within the cell. Gradually, the cytoplasm disappears, leaving a refractile, thick-walled spore. Also called mature spore or naked spore. See also *bacterial s.* under *spore* and *bacterium.*

spore strips spores of *Bacillus stearothermophilus* impregnated onto paper strips and used to monitor the sterilization effectiveness of autoclaves. *B. subtilis niger* may be used to monitor gas sterilizers or dry-heat sterilizers. Spores are also available in ampules.

sporoblast (spo′ro-blast) [*sporo-* + Gr. *blastos* germ] one of the bodies developed from nuclear division within the oocyst of the malarial parasite (*Plasmodium*) in the mosquito. Other genera with similar stages are *Eimeria, Isospora,* and *Toxoplasma.*

sporocyst (spo′ro-sist) [*sporo-* + Gr. *kystis* sac, bladder] 1. a stage formed from a sporoblast as a sporozoan. Within the oocyst, the sporoblast secretes a cystic membrane around itself and becomes a sporocyst.

2. a saclike organism that develops from a miracidium in the body of a snail host; it contains germ cells that give rise to other sporocysts in the life cycle of certain trematodes.

sporogony (spo-rog′o-ne) [*sporo-* + Gr. *goneia* generation] the sexual cycle of sporozoa (multiplication takes place following the fertilization of female cells by the male), which occurs in the life cycle of the malarial parasite (*Plasmodium*) in the body and stomach of the mosquito. Cf. *schizogony.*

Sporothrix (spo′ro-thriks) a genus of fungi that are hyphomycetes and the cause of sporotrichosis. This dimorphic fungus forms cigar-shaped yeast cells and blastospores at 37°C; at 25°C, its hyphae are thin, septate, and branching. The conidiophores expand at the apex to form denticulate vesicles. Isolates of *S. schenckii* are rarely encountered in the clinical laboratory unless they are associated with sporotrichosis. See also *sporotrichosis.*

sporotrichosis (spo″ro-tri-ko′sis) a chronic, subcutaneous, lymphatic (rarely respiratory) mycosis caused by the fungus *Sporothrix schenkii,* and taking three forms: lymphatic, disseminated, and respiratory. The lymphatic form of sporotrichosis is the most common one observed clinically. The disease has been called "alcoholic–rose gardener's" disease. This infection is associated with injuries caused by thorns or splinters. Handlers of peat moss are susceptible to this disease, especially when working in rose gardens. The fungus also grows saprophytically on mine timbers, as well as on other pieces of wood; the greatest outbreak occurred in the gold mines of South Africa, where more than 2800 native miners became infected following skin injuries acquired in the mines.

Clinical Diagnosis. The lymphatic form of sporotrichosis has characteristic pustules, papules, or nodules at the site of invasion, which can develop into multiple painless granulomas and break down to ulcers and cold abcesses. The disseminated form is a generalized disease involving bones, joints, lungs, and the central nervous system. The respiratory form is a result of the inhalation of fungal spores, and presents as a chronic granulomatous mycosis.

Laboratory Diagnosis. The causative agent, *S. schenkii,* may be identified by growth as a dimorphic fungus. At 37°C the organism exists as a cigar-shaped yeast, whereas at 25°C it is mold; *Sporothrix* is resistant to cyclohexamide. Microscopically, the mold phase has characteristic thin, septate, and branching hyphae bearing at their tips clusters of conidia in flowerlike arrangements.

A fluorescent antibody staining technique is available for the identification of *S. schenkii.* Two of the most sensitive identification tests are the yeast cell and the latex particle agglutination tests. The yeast cell agglutination test utilizes lyophilized whole yeast cells in a buffer suspension and several dilutions of patient serum with agglutinations checked after 1 hr. There is also a skin test available that uses a derivative of *S. schenkii* called sporotrichin, which produces a tuberculin-type reaction.

Sporozoa (spo″ro-zo′ah) [*sporo-* + Gr. *zōon* animal] a subphylum of protozoa characterized by the lack of organelles for locomotion in the adult stage, and a complex life cycle with alternating asexual (schizogony) and sexual (sporogony) multiplication. It includes the classes Telosporea, Toxoplasmea, and Haplosporea.

sporozoite (spo″ro-zo′īt) [*sporo-* + Gr. *zōon* animal] a sickle-shaped or wormlike spore in the oocyst following nuclear and cytoplasmic division of the sporocyst. In malaria, the sporozoites are liberated from the oocyst and accumulate in the salivary glands of the mosquito. These are transferred to humans when the mosquito bites.

spot-film device a device incorporated in the frame of a fluoroscopic screen that rapidly moves a cassette and grid over the patient, automatically switches the tube voltage and current from the fluoroscopic exposure values to the preset radiographic values, and makes the exposure. A phototimer usually controls the exposure time.

spot-film radiography the instantaneous production of radiographs during fluoroscopy.

spot test any simple qualitative procedure in which a specific test reagent is added directly to the test sample (e.g., an aliquot of blood, urine, gastric content, emesis fluid, or food residue) without a lengthy extraction procedure. These tests are often performed using a spot plate, a white tile plate with several wells into which a few milliliters of specimen and a few drops of the reagent are placed. A positive test result is shown by a color change.

spp abbrev. See *species.*

spreading factor see *hyaluronidase.*

spread plate (spred plāt) a culture of bacteria made by spreading a measured volume of inoculum evenly over the surface of an agar plate. Its uses are to determine bacterial count, to obtain an even lawn of growth, and (more often) to obtain well-isolated colonies for identification and pure culture study.

sprinkler system see under *fire extinguishing system.*

sprue (sproo) a disease of the small intestine characterized by impaired absorption.

celiac s., a chronic familial intestinal disorder in which ingestion of gluten (found in wheat and rye proteins) causes the development of a malabsorption syndrome. The disorder usually develops during the first year of life; symptoms may reappear intermittently throughout life.

Jejunal biopsy shows a lack of villi, increased numbers of lymphocytes in the lamina propria and abnormal epithelial cells, and elongated crypts. Other laboratory findings are identical to those found in the malabsorption syndrome. Treatment involves administration of a gluten-free diet.

Also called *gluten-sensitive enteropathy* and *nontropical sprue.* See also *malabsorption syndrome.*

nontropical s., see *celiac s.*

tropical s., a disorder of unknown etiology, possibly infectious, characterized by malabsorption and, in the advanced stages, the development of megaloblastic anemia due to a deficiency of vitamin B_{12} and folic acid. Diarrhea, anorexia, and weight loss occur. Jejeunal biopsy may show changes in villous height, damage to epithelial cells, elongated crypts, and large numbers of lymphocytes in the lamina propria. Radiologic examination of the small intestine shows intestinal dilation. See also *malabsorption syndrome.*

Spumavirinae a subfamily of Retroviridae that consists of syncytial and foamy viruses of humans, monkeys, cattle, and cats. See also *Retroviridae.*

spur cell (sper) see *acanthocyte.*

spurious (spu're-us) [L. *spurius*] simulated; not genuine; false.

spurious parasite a free-living parasite or one that parasitizes hosts other than humans. Such organisms can be recovered in the living or dead state from human stools.

sputum (spu'tum) [L.] a serous or mucoid fluid mixture of secretions and particulates ejected from the lungs, bronchi, and trachea by coughing. The tracheobronchial secretions are a variable mixture of mucin, protein, and electrolytes. The particulates are primarily composed of pus and exfoliated cells. Sputum specimens also contain nasal and salivary gland secretions and bacteria from the mouth. Sputum is 95 percent water. The solids primarily contain carbohydrate, protein, and lipids.

sputum examination the combined physical, chemical, microscopic, and microbiologic evaluation of a sample of sputum. The specimen is collected by coughing up sputum from deep in the bronchial tree. Production of sputum may be induced with aerosols containing 10 percent sodium chloride or acetylcysteine combined with a bronchodilator.

The volume, consistency, color, and odor are noted on physical examination. Cheesy masses, bronchial casts, lung stones, solid plugs, foreign bodies, bronchial epithelial cells, blood cells, alveolar macrophages, eosinophils, pus cells, parasites, and mycetomas may be observed microscopically.

Chemical assays performed on sputum include those for neuraminic acid to monitor the viscosity of sputum, and for alpha$_1$-antitrypsin. Increased IgG and IgA in sputum has been reported in association with bronchogenic carcinoma. CEA and a high-molecular-mass ACTH have also been associated with the tumor.

A variety of bacteria and fungi can be identified microscopically in gram-stained smears and agar plate streak cultures (see *Gram stain*).

In the presence of bronchogenic carcinoma and other carcinomas involving the lungs, malignant epithelial cells can frequently be identified in sputum samples. The sensitivity of the tests is increased by examining a minimum of three to five early morning specimens.

squalene (skwal'ēn) an unsaturated terpene hydrocarbon $[(CH_3)_2C{:}CH(CH_2)_2C(CH_3){:}CH(CH_2)_2(C(CH_3){:}CH\cdot CH_2]_2$, from the liver oil of sharks and some other fishes. It is an intermediate in cholesterol biosynthesis in animals.

squam/o (skwa'mo) a word element used in combining form to denote scale, e.g., squamatization.

squama (skwa'mah), pl. *squamae* [L.] a scale or scalelike substance.

squamocolumnar junction (SCJ) (skwa"mo-kolum'nar) the area of transition from squamous to columnar epithelium, as occurs in the cervix and other organs when columnar epithelium meets squamous epithelium. The cervical SCJ may be located at the external os, on the portio, or within the endocervical canal. This last location is more common in postmenopausal females. It is often the site of the origin of carcinoma of the uterine cervix. See also *transformation zone.*

squamous (skwa'mus) [L. *squamosus* scaly] scaly or platelike.

squamous cell a flat, scalelike epithelial cell, e.g., the endothelial cell. In stratified squamous epithelium, only the surface cells are flattened, although the underlying spherical cells also are collectively designated as squamous cells. See also *skin.*

squamous cell carcinoma a malignant neoplasm that arises from stratified squamous epithelium on the skin or from mucosal surfaces. On the skin, it is much more common in sun-exposed areas, and it may be preceded by actinic keratosis. The verrucous form of squamous carcinoma grows slowly, and rarely gives rise to metastases.

The initial metastases from a squamous carcinoma are typically to regional lymph nodes, but larger tumors may be found to have distant spread. The primary site of a metastatic squamous carcinoma cannot be determined from its histologic appearance.

Also called *epidermoid carcinoma.*

intraepidermal, s. c. c., a neoplastic disorder of the epidermis in which the atypical cells are confined by an intact basal lamina. It is usually a solitary lesion and can involve the skin in any location; lesions with similar histologic features also occur on mucosal surfaces. It appears as a slowly enlarging area of erythema with sharply defined margins, usually with overlying crusting. Histologically, varying degrees of acanthosis, loss of polarity, and cytologic atypia may be seen. Also called *Bowen's disease* (on the body epidermis), erythroplasia of Queyrat (on certain mucosal surfaces), and squamous carcinoma in situ.

squamous cell index a quantitation of squamous cell maturation or other morphologic characteristics of morphology in vaginal smears with some relationship to hormonal status. The Maturation Index (see below) is generally considered the most useful of the indices. A single examination is unreliable. If all requirements are not followed, the method is subject to considerable error.

crowded cell i., a value that represents the relationship of mature squamous cells, lying in clusters of four or more cells, to all mature squamous cells.

eosinophilic i. (EI), a value that expresses the percentage relationship of mature squamous cells with eosinophilic cytoplasm (Papanicolaou stain) among all mature squamous cells counted. The peak EI (50–75 percent) coincides with the peak karyopyknotic index (KI) at the time of ovulation. Shorr's stain is often preferred to the Papanicolaou stain for this evaluation.

folded-cell i., a value that represents the percentage of mature folded (i.e., not flat) squamous cells among all mature squamous cells.

karyopyknotic i. (KI), a value that expresses the percentage relationship of superficial squamous cells with pyknotic nuclei among all mature squamous cells. Some 200–400 cells in three or four fields are evaluated. The peak of the KI (50–85 percent) coincides with the time of ovulation.

maturation i. (MI), a value that expresses the maturation of the squamous epithelium as percentages of parabasal, intermediate, and superficial cells among cells counted, expressed in that order. For example, the MI at the time of ovulation may be 0:35:65, indicating that most of the cells (65 percent) are superficial type.

squamous epithelium an epithelium composed of squamous cells. The name is given because of the scalelike appearance of flattened squamous cells in a simple squamous epithelium where the cells are a single layer thick. In stratified squamous epithelium, the flattened cells are seen only toward the surface.

squamous pearl a concentric arrangement of superficial keratinized squamous cells. Such structures may be seen in both benign and malignant squamous epithelium. A round anuclear mass of keratin, which stains orange in the Papanicolaou stain, may be observed in the center of a squamous pearl of either benign or malignant squamous epithelial origin.

square (skwār) 1. a polygon with four equal sides and four equal angles.

2. the product of a number multiplied by itself.

square root the divisor of a quantity that will yield that quantity when multiplied by itself.

squeak phenomenon in electroencephalography, the increase in mean frequency (by up to about 2 Hz) of the alpha rhythm that may occur immediately after closure of the eyes.

squill (skwil) [L. *scilla;* Gr. *skilla*] the fleshy inner scales of the white variety of *Urginea maritima* (*Scilla maritima*), a plant in the lily family. Containing several cardiac glycosides (including glucoscillaren A, scillaren A, and proscillaridin A), squill was formerly used as a diuretic, emetic, expectorant, and cardiotonic.

red s., the bulbs of the red variety of *Urginea maritima,* which contain, in addition to cardiac glycosides, a powerful central-acting emetic. Ingestion of large doses produces vomiting, blurred vision, cardiac arrhythmias, and convulsions. It is used as a selective rat poison: because it does not produce vomiting in rats, it is much more toxic to rats than to humans.

squint (skwint) see *strabismus.*

SR abbrev. See *sedimentation rate, sensitivity response.*

Sr symbol for the chemical element *strontium.*

sr abbrev. see *steradian.*

SRAW abbrev. See *specific a. r.* under *airway resistance.*

SRF abbrev. See *skin reactive factor.*

SRM abbrev. See *standard r. m.* under *reference materials.*

SRS-A abbrev. See *slow-reacting substance of anaphylaxis.*

S-R variation see *smooth-rough variation.*

SSEP abbrev. See *somatosensory e. p.* under *evoked potential.*

SSPE abbrev. See *subacute sclerosing p.* under *panencephalitis.*

SSS abbrev. See *scalded skin syndrome.*

St abbrev. See *stoke.*

stabile (sta'bil) [L. *stabilis* stable] 1. not moving, resistant to chemical change.

2. in reference to a nuclide or elementary particle, not undergoing decay.

stability (stah-bil'ĭ-te) 1. resistance to change; the maintenance of a steady state in the presence of perturbing forces.

2. the maintenance of steady operating characteristics of an electronic component or device during changes in temperature and load and as it ages.

stable (sta'b'l) not moving, fixed, firm; resistant to change.

stable factor see *Factor VII.*

stable factor deficiency see under *Factor VII.*

stable fly see *Stomoxys.*

stachybotryotoxicosis a type of mycotoxicosis caused by the toxin-producing fungus *Stachybotrys alterans.* Stachybotryotoxicosis is associated with people who frequently come into contact with hay.

stachyose (stak'e-ōs) an indigestible tetrasaccharide, α-Gal-(1 → 6)-α-Gal-(1 → 6)-α-Glc-(1 → 2)-β-Fru, which is similar in structure and occurrence to raffinose.

stack (stak) 1. an area of computer memory used for temporary data storage.

2. a data structure that provides last in, first out (LIFO) access to the data. Only the last data item placed in the stack is available. As each item is removed, the item below it becomes available. Because stacks are very useful to compilers, some computers have hardware-implemented stack memories. Cf. *queue.*

stage (stāj) 1. a period or distinct phase in the course of a disease, the life history of an organism, or any biologic process.

2. the platform of a microscope on which a slide is placed for viewing of the specimen.

3. referring to the anatomic extent of a malignant neoplasm; see *tumor staging.*

staggered (stag'erd) pertaining to the most stable conformation of ethane (or one of its derivatives) in which the hydrogen atoms (or substituent groups) have the maximal separation. See also *conformation.*

staging (sta′jing) see *tumor staging.*

Stagnicola a genus of mollusks that serve as hosts of dermatitis-producing schistosome cercariae.

stain (stān) 1. any dye, reagent, or other material used in producing coloration; the term particularly refers to a biologic stain, a substance used in coloring tissues or microorganisms for microscopic study. For more information, see the specific stains.

2. a superficial discoloration or an artificially colored spot in the skin.

staining (stān′ing) in histology, the artificial coloration of tissues, microorganisms, or other cells, generally to facilitate their examination under the microscope. See also *dye.*

bacterial s., the process of treating bacterial cells with solutions that contain one or more specific dyes. A thin layer of cells on a glass slide is treated with heat or chemicals (e.g., ethanol, formalin, or methanol) for fixation to the slide. The smear is then treated with a specific dye or with sequential dyes, and the excess dye is removed by washing.

In negative staining, the background rather than the bacterial cell is stained to demonstrate a particular feature, e.g., bacterial capsules. Silver salts are used to stain specific features (e.g., flagella) and organisms (e.g., *Legionella*). Certain chemicals may be used to bind dyes to specific structures (mordant), e.g., certain tannates.

See also specific stains (e.g., *Gram stain*) and specific bacterial species.

bipolar s., in bacteriology, uneven staining of rod-shaped cells in which only the ends are colored.

histologic s., the process of selectively coloring certain tissue elements by soaking cut tissue sections in solutions containing one or more dyes. Before staining, the embedding medium is removed: paraffin by dissolving it in xylene (deparaffinization), or Carbowax by dissolving it in water.

In progressive staining, the sections are removed from the dye when the desired intensity of color is attained. In regressive staining, sections are overstained; the excess dye is then selectively removed, usually under microscopic control (a process called differentiation). This involves dipping the sections in alcohol, acid alcohol, or mordant solution. When two different stains are used, the second is called a counterstain. After staining, the sections are dehydrated, cleared, and mounted.

For more information, see specific stains (e.g., *hematoxylin*) and tissue components; for automated methods, see *tissue processing.*

staircase phenomenon the gradual increase in the force of muscle contraction that occurs with repetitive low-frequency stimulation. Also called *treppe.*

stalk (stawk) a pedicle; an elongated, more or less slender anatomic structure resembling the stalk of a plant. See also *polyp.*

-stalsis (stal′sis) a suffix word element to denote constriction, e.g., peristalsis.

standard (stan′dard) something established as a norm with which similar things are compared, e.g., a standard solution in quantitative analytical work, a standard of purity for reagents, or a standard of performance.

standard curve see *calibration curve.*

standard deviation (σ) in statistics, a measure of dispersion in a distribution of values; the square root of the average squared deviation from the mean (variance). It is the most common measure of the dispersion (spread) of statistical data. In computing the standard deviation of a sample set of n observations, the sum of the squared deviations is usually divided by $n-1$ rather than n, to obtain an unbiased average, followed by extraction of the square root. See also *variance.*

standard electrode potential the voltage produced in an electrochemical cell composed of a specified electrode and a hydrogen electrode at the standard state. All solids and liquids are pure; solute concentrations are 1 M; gases have a partial pressure of 1 atm; and the temperature is 298K (25°C). Also called *standard reduction potential.* See also *Nernst equation.*

standard enthalpy of formation the enthalpy of reaction for the formation of a specified allotropic form of a substance from elements in their standard state. Also called heat of formation.

standard free energy ($G°$) the free energy for a chemical reaction when all reactants are in their standard states (temperature of 25°C; pressure of 1 atm for gases; concentration of 1 mol/l for substances in solution). The free energy (G) for a chemical reaction not at standard conditions can be related to the standard free energy by the equation: $G = G° + RT \ln Q$, where R is the gas constant, T is absolute temperature, and Q is the reaction quotient for the reaction.

standardization (stan″dard-ĭ-za′shun) 1. the process of determining or adjusting the concentration of a secondary standard solution.

2. the preparation of a standard curve for an analytic method relating concentration to some measurable parameter or calculating an equivalent numerical factor.

standardize (stan′dard-īz) to compare with or conform to a standard; to establish standards.

standardized deviate (Z or z) a value obtained by normalizing a datum point (X) by subtracting the mean (μ) of the parent population and dividing by the standard deviation (σ): $Z = (X - \mu)/\sigma$. If the data (raw scores) are a random sample from a normal distribution, the standardized deviates are a random sample from a standard normal distribution. Also called *standard score* and *Z score.*

standard reduction potential see *standard electrode potential.*

standard score see *standardized deviate.*

standard solution a solution containing a known concentration of a specified constituent, which is used in standardizing an analytic method. It may be prepared by dissolving a weighed amount of a pure, dry substance in a known volume of solvent or by comparing a solution of unknown concentration with a primary standard. See also *primary standard* and *reference materials.*

standard state the most stable state (solid, liquid, or vapor) of a substance at a pressure of 1 atmosphere and at a specified temperature, usually 298 K (about 77°F).

standard temperature and pressure (STP) a temperature of 0°C (273.16 K) and a pressure of 1 atm. At STP, 1 mole of an ideal gas occupies a volume of 22.41383 l.

stannic (stan′ik) pertaining to the tin(IV) cation, Sn^{4+}.

stannous (stan′us) pertaining to the tin(II) cation, Sn^{2+}.

stapes (sta′pēz) [L. "stirrup"] [NA], the most medial of the three auditory ossicles. Its base fits against the fenestra vestibuli.

Staph abbrev. See *Staphylococcus.*

staphyl/o (staf′ĭ-lo) [Gr. *staphylē* a bunch of grapes] a word element used in combining form to denote resemblance to clusters of grapes, e.g., staphylococcus.

staphylococcal (staf″ĭ-lo-kok′al) pertaining to or caused by staphylococci.

staphylococcal clumping test see under *fibrin(fibrinogen) degradation products methods.*

staphylococcin (staf″ĭ-lo-kok′sin) a bacteriocin produced under plasmid control by certain strains of *Staphylococcus aureus.* It is a heat-stable protein that inhibits the growth of many gram-positive organisms.

Staphylococcus (Staph) (staf″ĭ-lo-kok′us) [*staphylo-* + Gr. *kokkus* berry] a genus in the family Micrococcaceae. Members of this genus are gram-positive cocci that exhibit a tendency to grow in bunches as well as in pairs or tetrads. Staphylococci are nonmotile, nonspore-forming, catalase-positive, facultative anaerobes. Although they are common inhabitants of the skin and mucous membranes, they may cause serious opportunistic infections. Staphylococci are generally hardy organisms, surviving drying and temperature changes and able to grow on simple nutrient media. They are more resistant than most bacteria to disinfectants. *S. aureus* can grow in the presence of high salt concentrations (7–10 percent). Tests used to differentiate *Staphylococcus* species from *Micrococcus* species include acid production from glucose anaerobically, sensitivity to lysostaphin, and acid production from glycerol in the presence of erythromycin. All three are positive for staphylococci.

STAPHYLOCOCCUS AUREUS. This species is the most important member of the genus because of its ability to cause serious suppurative infections; it is present in the anterior nares, skin, and mucous membranes of about 30 percent of human adults who act as carriers. Carriage of the organism may be transient or permanent. Staphylococcal disease is spread by direct or airborne contact. Conditions predisposing individuals to *S. aureus* infection include: impaired host defense (impaired humoral or cellular immunity), damaged skin, viral infections of the lungs, age (neonates and the elderly), metabolic disturbances (such as diabetes), steroid or radiation therapy, and antibiotic therapy (especially with agents to which the staphylococci are resistant).

The most frequently encountered staphylococcal lesion is a cutaneous abscess or boil. Staphylococci may cause systemic disease by spreading from a local site via the blood stream or the lymphatic system. *S. aureus* may be isolated from 17–40 percent of all surgical wound infections. The presence of foreign bodies such as sutures, prosthetic devices, or drainage tubes predisposes patients to infections at these sites. *S. aureus* is also an important cause of septicemia in drug addicts. About 70 percent of osteomyelitis cases and 55 percent of acute arthritis cases are caused by this organism.

Several diseases are caused by exotoxins elaborated by certain strains of *S. aureus.* Scalded skin syndrome, caused by toxin-producing strains of *S. aureus,* primarily affects neonates and infants. The organism is also a major cause of food poisoning, which results from the ingestion of preformed, heat-stable enterotoxin. Foods involved generally are high-protein foods contaminated by enterotoxin-producing organisms shed from food handlers. Improper storage of contaminated food results in elaboration of enterotoxin, ingestion of which causes short-incubation, self-limiting gastroenteritis. Toxic shock syndrome, characterized by fever, rash, and hypotension, is observed primarily in young females; the syndrome has been associated with the use of tampons during menstruation. Although, in a high percentage of those with this syndrome, *S. aureus* can be isolated from the vagina, the systemic effects are presumably caused by a toxin that has not yet been characterized.

Bacteriophage typing may be used for epidemiologic studies of *S. aureus* infections. The predominant phage types currently observed are the group III and 94/96 complexes. Cultures implicated in an outbreak of staphylococci disease may be forwarded to the Department of Health of the particular state or to the Centers for Disease Control in Atlanta, Georgia.

S. aureus produces several extracellular enzymes and toxins that contribute to its pathogenicity. Extracellular coagulase, associated with virulence, clots the plasma, possibly contributing to the ability of the organism to protect itself from phagocytic cells. Other extracellular staphylococcal enzymes include staphylokinase (which causes dissolution of clots), nucleases, lipases, and hyaluronidase (which causes hydrolysis of connective tissue). Such enzymes may contribute to the spread of the organism through tissue.

S. aureus may produce one or more chemically and serologically distinct hemolysins, designated α, β, γ, and δ, which also damage cells other than red blood cells. The most potent hemolysin is alpha (α) toxin which, upon injection into laboratory animals, causes dermal necrosis (when injected locally) or death (when injected systemically). Its mode of action is unknown.

Exfoliation toxin is an epidermolytic toxin that causes several "scalded skin" syndromes, including exfoliative dermatitis in newborns and infants, impetigo, and a form of scarlatinal rash. The toxin is produced by certain strains of *S. aureus* that belong to phage group II. Specific antibody from early exposure may account for the uncommon occurrence of these syndromes in adults.

About 50 percent of *S. aureus* isolates produce a heat-stable enterotoxin, ingestion of which causes food poisoning. There are five serologically distinct enterotoxins, designated by the letters A–E. Enterotoxins cause both local and central nervous system effects; enterotoxin B has been associated with staphylococcal pseudomembranous colitis.

S. aureus produces beta lactamases, enzymes that destroy the penicillin group of antibiotics, resulting in resistance. Only about 20 percent of *S. aureus* isolates are sensitive to penicillin. Rarely, the organism may be resistant to the beta-lactamase–resistant penicillin group of antibiotics, such as methicillin, nafcillin, or oxacillin. Such resistance can be detected by incubation of in vitro susceptibility tests at 35°C.

OTHER STAPHYLOCOCCAL SPECIES. Species other than *S. aureus* may be referred to collectively as

Staphylococcus. TESTS FOR IDENTIFICATION OF *Staphylococcus* SPECIES

TEST	*S. aureus*	*S. epidermidis*	*S. saprophyticus*
Coagulase	+	−	−
Hemolysis[1]	+	−, ±	−
Novobiocin resistance[2]	−	−	+
Phosphatase[3]	+	+	−, ±
Acid from:[4]			
D-Trehalose	+	−	+
D-Mannitol	+	−	+, −
Xylitol	−	−	+, ±, −

[1] Beta hemolysis on sheep or bovine blood agar.
[2] Using a 5-μg susceptibility disk.
[3] Hydrolysis of 0.005 M of phenolphthalein monophosphate in citrate buffer, pH 5.8.
[4] Aerobic production of acid in carbohydrate-containing purple broth or agar base.

coagulase-negative staphylococci. The clinical importance of *S. epidermidis* and *S. saprophyticus* have been well documented. Other species isolated from human infections include *S. hominis, S. hemolyticus,* and *S. simulans.* The staphylococcal species other than *S. aureus* are an important cause of infection in the presence of foreign bodies such as prosthetic devices and shunts. Therefore, growth of coagulase-negative staphylococci in blood cultures should not always be interpreted as contamination. *Staphylococcus* species may cause septicemia, endocarditis, or osteomyelitis in heroin addicts. *S. saprophyticus* has been implicated in urinary tract infections in children and young females. *S. epidermidis* is a part of the normal flora of skin and the most frequent cause of minor (stitch) abscesses.

SPECIES IDENTIFICATION. On nonselective media such as blood, nutrient, or trypticase soy agars, staphylococci grow abundantly in 18–24 hr at 34°–37°C. At 24 hr, the colonies are generally 1–3 mm in diameter and are circular, smooth, and convex. *S. aureus* and *S. saprophyticus* may exhibit a golden pigment on primary isolation; infrequently, *S. epidermidis* colonies are pigmented.

The coagulase test is of primary importance for the differentiation of *S. aureus* from other *Staphylococcus* species. Two types of tests are available, both using citrated rabbit plasma: EDTA (ethylenediaminetetraacetate), a rapid slide test that detects cell-bound coagulase or "clumping factor," and a tube test that detects free as well as bound coagulase. The latter is used to confirm a negative slide test.

A novobiocin disk test can differentiate the resistant *S. saprophyticus,* frequently isolated from urine, from other species of *Staphylococcus.*

A battery of tests may be used to identify accurately the *Staphylococcus* species of clinical importance: coagulase; hemolysis; novobiocin resistance; phosphatase; acid (aerobically) from trehalose, mannitol, maltose, sucrose, xylose or arabinose, and xylitol; and anaerobic growth in thioglycolate. The accompanying table lists results obtained for *S. aureus, S. epidermidis,* and *S. saprophyticus.*

S. albus, see *S. epidermidis.*

S. aureus, the type species that often occurs harmlessly on the skin and mucous membranes, yet is also an important and potentially severe pathogen. Cultures are coagulase-positive, and on blood agar typically show beta hemolysis and a characteristic golden-yellow pigment. Various strains can be identified by bacteriophage typing. A few strains are encapsulated but most are not. Identification of *S. aureus* in the laboratory is based primarily on the ability to clot plasma. See also the accompanying table.

Several types of hemolytic toxins are produced, the most potent being alpha toxin. Among the virulence-related enzymes produced by most strains are several lipases and hyaluronidase.

When penicillin was first used clinically, most strains of *S. aureus* were susceptible, but currently up to 90 percent of isolates in the same institution may be resistant to the antibiotic. This resistance is due to the staphylococcal production of penicillinase, a plasmoid-coded enzyme, beta lactamase. Penicillin-resistant strains are usually susceptible to methicillin or oxacillin.

See also *coagulase.*

S. epidermidis, a species that is coagulase-negative, producing colonies that are usually white in color and that produce hemolysis. The organisms are phosphatase-positive and susceptible to novobiocin. *S. epidermidis* is frequently found on normal skin but is potentially pathogenic, causing systemic disease such as postoperative endocarditis and infections associated with cerebrospinal fluid shunts.

S. saprophyticus, a species that is coagulase-negative and ferments glucose weakly. It is phosphatase-negative and resistant to novobiocin. The species is generally regarded as a harmless commensal, but recent observations have suggested that it may be pathogenic, causing urinary tract infections.

***Staphylococcus aureus* neutral proteinase** an enzyme of the hydrolase class (EC 3.4.24.4) that catalyzes the conversion of plasminogen to plasmin. It is an extracellular enzyme produced by certain strains of *Staphylococcus.* It acts on the plasma of certain animal species, but not on human plasma. Also called *staphylokinase.*

staphylokinase (staf″ĭ-lo-ki′nās) see *Staphylococcus aureus neutral proteinase.*

staphyloma (staf″ĭ-lo′mah) [Gr. *staphylōma* a defect in the eye inside the cornea] protrusion of the sclera or cornea, usually lined with uveal tissue, due to inflammation.

starch (starch) [L. *amylum*] the storage carbohydrate of plants. It consists of two discrete kinds of glucan chains: amylose and amylopectin. Amylose

Staphylococcus aureus. SOME DISTINGUISHING CHARACTERISTICS OF CLINICALLY IMPORTANT MEMBERS OF THE GENUS *Staphylococcus*

CHARACTERISTIC	*S. aureus*	*S. saprophyticus*	*S. epidermidis*
Coagulase production	+	−	−
Pigment	gold	−	variable
Nitrate reduction	+	−	variable
Mannitol, acid aerobic	+	+	−
Trehalose, acid aerobic	+	+	−
Phosphatase	+	−	+
DNAse	+	−	−
Novobiocin			
5-μg disk[a]	S	R	S

[a] S (sensitive) is indicated by a zone of inhibition greater than 5 mm. R (resistant) is indicated by a zone of inhibition less than 5 mm.

From Treagan, L., and Pulliam, L. Medical Microbiology Laboratory Procedures. Philadelphia, W. B. Saunders Co., 1982, p. 6.

is a chain of α-(1→4)-linked glucose units that form a large, linear homopolymer. Amylopectin is also a homopolymer of glucose but, in addition to α-(1→4)-linkages, it has branches formed by α-(1→6)-links. Amylopectin is similar to glycogen in structure but is less highly branched (24–30 residues per branch). It is a major fuel in the diet of humans, and is used as a dusting powder and tablet disintegrant in pharmaceuticals. Amylose chains are polydisperse; their molecular weights vary from 4,000 to 100,000, whereas the molecular weight of amylopectin complexes ranges from 50,000 to many million. Amylose stains blue with iodine; amylopectin stains red.

Starling's hypothesis, law (star′lingz) [Ernest Henry *Starling,* English physiologist, 1866–1927] stated as: at all points along the length of the capillary, the hydrostatic pressure on the surface is opposed by the osmotic pressure exerted by the plasma proteins. It is the classic concept explaining the mechanism and dynamics of the exchange of fluid between the plasma in the capillary and the interstitial fluid surrounding it.

Starling's law of the heart [Ernest Henry *Starling*] stated as: the principle that describes the intrinsic ability of the heart to adjust itself to varying loads of incoming venous blood (the venous return). It is based on the fact that in cardiac muscle, as in all striated muscle, the force of contraction varies directly with the fiber length just prior to contraction, until an optimal length is exceeded.

For muscle fibers in the walls of the heart, the fiber length prior to contraction (systole) increases as the diastolic volume increases during venous filling. The force of, or external work done by, contraction is related to the resulting stroke volume. Starling's law thus holds that the volume of blood ejected into the aorta with each systole (the stroke volume) is directly proportional to the end-diastolic volume. The right heart, which supplies the pulmonary circulation, also obeys this law.

Also called *Frank-Starling mechanism.*

start codon the codon (AUG, or rarely, GUG) that always begins the transcription of a polypeptide. A special transfer RNA (tRNA) recognizes this codon and starts the chain with the amino acid methionine (met) or rarely, valine, in the cytosol of eukaryotes or with *N*-formyl methionine (F-met) in prokaryotes, mitochondria, and chloroplasts. A different tRNA reads AUG as met in the middle of a chain.

starvation (star-va′shun) the long, continued deprival of the body of food. Remarkable adaptations in the metabolism of fuels occur during starvation. With the fairly rapid depletion of the carbohydrate reserves of glycogen, the body increasingly utilizes fatty acids for fuel, notably those present in muscles and liver cells. In the liver, the oxidation of fatty acids produces ketone bodies, which are exported to the muscles for fuel and, as starvation is prolonged, are exported in increasing quantities to the brain.

The fatty acid oxidation in the liver also produces energy in the form of ATP needed to drive gluconeogenesis at that site. Gluconeogenesis utilizes the carbon skeletons of the amino acids mobilized from muscle protein and transported to the liver to make glucose, which is the preferred energy source for the brain and is required for vital metabolic reactions.

With fatty acid oxidation and gluconeogenesis proceeding, fatty acid synthesis and lipogenesis are essentially halted and adipose triglycerides are depleted. Because of the increased use of amino acids from protein for gluconeogenesis, the body goes into negative nitrogen balance. The rapid production of ketone bodies results in some ketosis, with excretion of ketone bodies in urine.

When these major changes in the utilization of fuels occur, there are adaptations in the activity of groups of enzymes: pancreatic enzymes decrease; enzymes of fatty acid synthesis and glucose utilization (liver) decrease; and enzymes of fatty acid utilization and gluconeogenesis increase.

stasis (sta′sis) [Gr. "a standing still"] 1. a stoppage or diminution of the flow of blood or other body fluid in any part.

2. a state of equilibrium among opposing forces.

-stasis a suffix word element used in combining form to denote control or stop, e.g., hemostasis.

Stasisia a genus of flies. In West Africa, the species *S. rodhaini* has been found to cause human myiasis.

stat abbrev. for L. *statim,* immediately; frequently used to identify an emergency laboratory request.

state (stāt) [L. *status*] a condition; a situation, or stage of a process; status.

statement (stāt′ment) a single step in a high-level language computer program, the smallest unit that is syntactically independent of the rest of the program, such as a sentence in a natural language. A program consists of a sequence of statements.

static (stat′ik) [L. *staticus*, causing to stand] at rest; unchanging; in equilibrium; not in motion.

-static (stat′ik) a suffix word element used in combining form to denote stopping or controlling, e.g., hemostatic.

stationary (sta′shun-er″e) [L. *stationarius*] not subject to variations or to change of place.

stationary phase see *stationary p.* under *phase.*

statistic (stah-tis′tik) 1. a sample datum.

2. a function computed from the sample data, such as the sample mean.

statistical (stah-tis′tĭ-kal) pertaining to (1) the area of study of statistical theory and/or statistical technique, or (2) the numerical nature of a set of facts or data.

statistical symbols mathematical signs and abbreviations used in the representation of numerical data. Some of the more common are listed in the accompanying table.

statistics (stah-tis′tiks) [Ger. *Statistik*, the political science of facts and figures, from L. *status* state] 1. a collection of numerical data.

2. the mathematical science dealing with the collection, analysis, and interpretation of data. Statistical methods are used to determine what can be inferred about the characteristics of an aggregate of individuals (the population) from the characteristics of a part of the population (a sample). See also

STATISTICAL SYMBOLS

SYMBOL	MEANING
ANOVA	Analysis of variance
α	Probability of Type I error; significance level
β	Probability of Type II error
$1-\beta$	Power of a statistical test
$_nC_k$; $\binom{n}{k}$	Binomial coefficient; the number of combinations of *n* things taken *k* at a time
χ^2	Chi-squared statistic
E	Expected frequency in a cell of a contingency table
$E(X)$	Expected value of the random variable X
F	F statistic (variance ratio)
f	Frequency
H_0	Null hypothesis
H_1	Alternative hypothesis
μ	Population mean
N	Population size
n	Sample size
O	Observed frequency in a contingency table
p	Probability of success in independent trials
P	Probability
$P(A)$	Probability that event A occurs
$P(A\|B)$	Conditional probability that A occurs given that B has occurred
r	Sample correlation coefficient, usually the Pearson product-moment correlation
r^2	Coefficient of determination
r_S	Spearman rank correlation coefficient
ρ	Population correlation coefficient
s	Sample standard deviation
s^2	Sample variance
SE	Standard error of estimate
σ	Population standard deviation
σ^2	Population variance
$\Sigma_{i=1}^{n} x_i$	$x_1 + x_2 + \ldots + x_n$
t	Student's t statistic
U	Mann-Whitney rank sum statistic
W	Wilcoxson rank sum statistic
$\overline{X}$	Sample mean
z	Standard score
$\sqrt{x}$	Square root of x
$n!$	n factorial
$\|x\|$	Absolute value of x
$=$	Equal
$\neq$	Not equal
$\approx$	Approximately equal
$>$	Greater than
$<$	Less than
$\geq$	Greater than or equal to
$\leq$	Less than or equal to
∞	Infinity

confidence interval estimate, hypothesis testing, and *probability.*

stat test a laboratory test to be performed without any delay. Stat tests are frequently classified as those whose test results will immediately determine or influence a therapeutic decision.

status (sta'tus) [L.] a state or condition.

status asthmaticus see under *asthma.*

status epilepticus 1. in clinical neurology, the continuation of a seizure for an enduring length of time, or the occurrence of repeated seizures so frequently that recovery between attacks does not occur.

2. in electroencephalography, the occurrence of continuous seizure activity as recorded on the electroencephalogram during a specified time interval.

See also *epilepsy.*

STD abbrev. See *sexually transmitted diseases.*

steady state the condition in which certain properties of a system do not change with time.

steady-state condition a point in time of an enzymatic reaction in progress when the enzyme-substrate complex concentration [ES] is constant: i.e., the rate of change of [ES] is zero; the quantity of ES formed is equal to the quantity decomposed to E + P (products).

steapsin (ste-ap'sin) see *lipase.*

stearate (ste'ah-rāt) octadecanoate; any salt, ester, or ionic form of stearic acid. See also *stearic acid.*

stearic acid octadecanoic acid, a saturated fatty acid, $CH_3(CH_2)_{16}COOH$, widely distributed in plant and animal fats. As a pharmaceutical preparation of solid organic acids obtained from fats, stearic acid consists chiefly of stearic and palmitic acids, and is used as a constituent of glycerin suppositories.

stearin (ste'ah-rin) see *tristearin.*

steat/o (ste'ah-to) [Gr. *stear, steatos* fat] a word element used in combining form to denote fat, e.g., steatorrhea.

steatomatosis (ste"ah-to"mah-to'sis) the presence of numerous sebaceous cysts on the body.

steatosis (ste"ah-to'sis) see *fatty liver.*

Stefan-Boltzmann law see under *blackbody radiation.*

Stegobium a genus of beetles. The species *S. paniceum* is an obligatory intermediate host of *Hymenolepis diminuta.*

Stegomyia (steg"o-mi'yah) [Gr. *stegos* roof + *myia* fly] a subgenus of mosquitoes. The species *S. argenteus, S. calopus,* and *S. fasciatus* are now classified with *Aedes aegypti.*

Steinert's disease see *myotonic dystrophy.*

Stein-Leventhal syndrome (stīn lev'en-thal) [Irving F. *Stein,* Sr., American gynecologist, born 1887; Michael Leo *Leventhal,* American obstetrician and gynecologist, born 1901] a group of related syndromes characterized by bilateral polycystic ovaries, secondary amenorrhea, infertility, and often hirsutism and obesity; it is usually found in females with a history of menstrual irregularity. Although the etiology is unknown the endocrine disturbance associated with this condition is due to a continuous secretion of follicle-stimulating hormone (FSH) and luteinizing hormone (LH) by the hypothalamo-hypophyseal axis, in contrast to the normal sequential release of these hormones. Palpation of enlarged ovaries, culdoscopy, and laparoscopy are useful in establishing the diagnosis. Laboratory findings may include increased levels of plasma testosterone and urinary 17-ketosteroids.

Stelazine (stel-ah-zēn) trademark. See *trifluoperazine.*

Stellantchasmus a genus of flukes. In Hawaii and

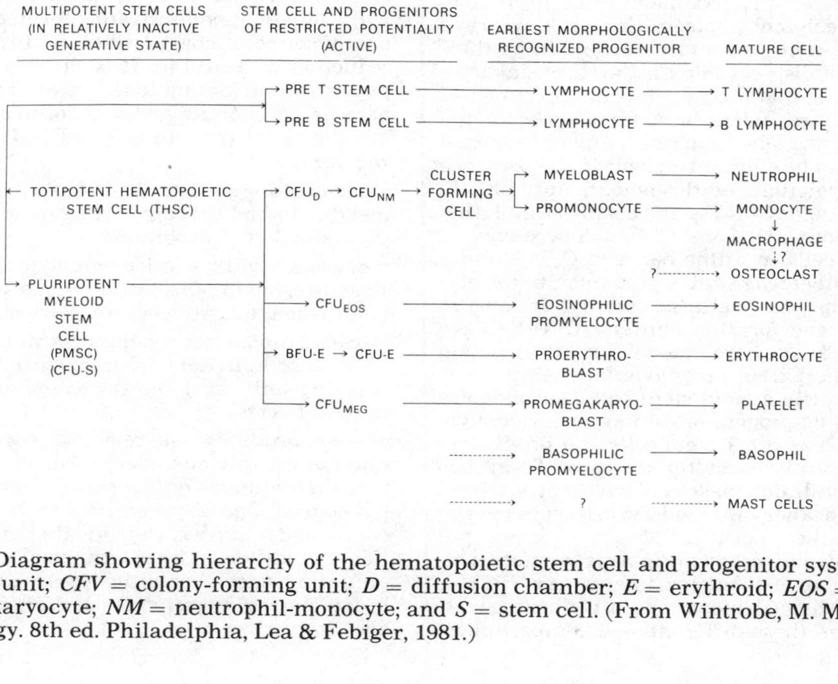

Stem cell. Diagram showing hierarchy of the hematopoietic stem cell and progenitor systems; *BFU* = burst-forming unit; *CFV* = colony-forming unit; *D* = diffusion chamber; *E* = erythroid; *EOS* = eosinophil; *MEG* = megakaryocyte; *NM* = neutrophil-monocyte; and *S* = stem cell. (From Wintrobe, M. M., et al.: Clinical Hematology. 8th ed. Philadelphia, Lea & Febiger, 1981.)

Japan, the species *S. falcatus* is known to cause human infection.

stellate (stel′āt) [L. *stellatus*] shaped like a star; arranged in a rosette or rosettes.

stem cell 1. any precursor cell.

2. a hematopoietic stem cell; any blood cell progenitor characterized by the capacity for both self-replication (production of progeny identical in appearance and potential that maintain the stem cell pool) and differentiation (production of more specialized progeny, such as stem cells of more restricted potential or precursors of mature cells). Stem cells give rise to the various morphologically recognizable precursors of the different blood cell lines, such as the proerythroblast and myeloblast, which cannot self-replicate and must differentiate into more mature daughter cells.

Current models of the hematopoietic stem cell compartment designate the cell that is totipotent for all blood cells as the totipotent hematopoietic stem cell (THSC) or pluripotent stem cell. Progeny of the THSC have more restricted potential and differentiation into at least two cell lines, one giving rise to the lymphoid system and the other to the myeloid system (through the pluripotent myeloid stem cell, MMSC).

No assay has yet been developed for the THSC, although its existence is demonstrated by induced chromosome defects in mice: when marrow is transplanted from irradiated mice into isogeneic recipients, the same chromosome defect is sometimes found in both myeloid and lymphoid cells. The existence of common antigens on B lymphocytes and the CFU_{NM} stem cell also provides evidence for the existence of the THSC in humans.

The various classes of demonstrated stem cells are characterized by specific assay systems, as they all are morphologically alike and resemble a lymphocyte that is small to medium in size. The pluripotent myeloid stem cell (PMSC) is usually referred to as CFU-S, for colony-forming unit–spleen. This refers to the assay in which marrow cells injected into isogeneic lethally irradiated mice form colonies on the recipient's spleen. Each colony arises from a single stem cell and may contain erythrocytes, neutrophils, eosinophils, and megakaryocytes, indicating that the CFU-S is the precursor of all four cell lines. There is now no assay for the CFU-S in humans. The stem cells of more restricted potentiality can be cultured on agar in the presence of specific poietins, erythropoietin for BFU-E, thrombopoietin for CFU_{MEG}, and colony-stimulating factor (CSF) for CFU_{NM} and CFU_{EOS}. There may be several stem cells in a line between CFU-S and a morphologically recognizable precursor. In the erythroid line, one forming large colonies or "bursts" (BFU-E) and one forming clusters (CFU-E) have been identified. They are presumably intermediate stages having a parent-progeny relationship.

A pluripotent lymphoid stem cell also undoubtedly exists, as do progenitors of more restricted potentiality, such as pre-T stem cells and pre-B stem cells, which can also be cultured on agar. Stem cells for the basophil and mast cell have not yet been identified, and other intermediate cell types may be discovered in the other cell lines.

Normally, hematopoiesis is in a steady state. Differentiated stem cell compartments (e.g., BFU-E and CFU_{NM}) replenish blood cells lost by senescence. It is only when these differentiated compartments are damaged or when there is an increased demand for mature blood cells that the multipotential stem cells, such as CFU-S, begin to proliferate and differentiate, thus increasing the numbers of differentiated stem cells.

See also the accompanying illustration.

stemline (stem-līn) a population of cells in a tumor having a stemline number (S) that is more prevalent than the adjacent chromosome counts S + 1 and S – 1. In a histogram of distribution of chromosome numbers, the modal counts are stemline numbers. The common adult solid tumors have aneuploid stemline numbers. Many have two distant stemlines; frequently one arises by doubling—the stemline numbers are S and 2S.

Stenoglossa a suborder of snails of the class Gastropoda that possesses poisonous glands.

stenosis (stĕ-no′sis) [Gr. *stenōsis*] a tightening or stricture of a duct or canal,, e.g., pyloric stenosis, obstruction of the pyloric opening. For more information, see the specific type of stenosis.

Stenvers position a radiographic position used to obtain an anterior profile view of the petrous portion of the temporal bone. The head is tilted 45° toward the face, with the infraorbitomeatal line parallel to the transverse axis of the film and a localization point 2.5 cm anterior to the dependent external auditory meatus centered to the midpoint of the film. The central ray has a 12° cranial angulation. This projection demonstrates the mastoid cells, mastoid antrum, tympanic cavity, labyrinth, internal auditory meatus, and petrous apex.

step function a mathematical function that is discontinuous at a discrete set of points and constant on the intervals between.

Stephenson-Gibbs reference see *sternospinal reference e.* under *electrode.*

steradian (sr) (ste-ra′de-an) [Gr. *stereos* solid + *radian*] the unit of measurement of solid angle, defined as $1/4\pi$ of a full sphere.

stercobilin (ster″ko-bi′lin) [L. *stercus* dung + *bilin*] a bile pigment derivative formed by air oxidation of stercobilinogen, which in turn is derived by reduction of bilirubin. It is the brown-orange-red pigment contributing to the color of feces and perhaps urine. Urobilin and stercobilin appear similar, but the latter is more reduced (4H). See also *bile pigment.*

stercobilinogen (ster″ko-bi-lin′o-jen) a bilirubin metabolite and precursor of stercobilin, formed by the reduction of urobilinogen.

stereo- a prefix word element to denote a solid structure, having three dimensions, or being firmly established, e.g., stereogram, stereology.

stereocampimeter (ster″e-o-kam-pim′ĕ-ter) [*stereo-* + L. *campus* field + *metrum*] an instrument for studying unilateral central scotomata and central retinal defects.

stereochemistry (ste″re-o-kem′is-tre) a subdiscipline of organic chemistry devoted to the study of the three-dimensional spatial configurations of molecules. One aspect deals with stereoisomers, compounds that have identical chemical constitution but differ in the arrangement of atoms or groups in space. Stereoisomers are divided into two broad classes: enantiomers and diastereomers. See also *isomerism.*

stereocilia (ste″re-o-sil′e-ah, pl. of *stereocilium*) an established misnomer for the elongated microvilli that occur on the lining of the epididymis and on the hair cells of the cochlea.

stereocinefluorography (ste″re-o-sin″ĕ-floo″or-og′rah-fe) recording by motion picture camera of images observed by steroscopic fluoroscopy, affording three-dimensional visualization.

stereognosis (ster″e-og-no′sis) [*stereo-* + Gr. *gnōsis* knowledge] the perception and understanding of the form and nature of objects through the sense of touch.

stereoisomer (ster″e-o-i′so-mer) one of a group of compounds related by stereoisomerism. See also *isomerism.*

stereoisomerism (ster″e-o-i-som′er-izm) [*stereo-* + *isomerism*] the relationship between different chemical compounds that have their atoms bonded together in the same sequence. Their molecules differ only in the spatial positions of their atoms. See also *isomerism.*

stereology (ste″re-ol′o-je) the study of the three-dimensional architecture of objects customarily seen in only two dimensions.

stereoscope (ster′e-o-skōp″) [*stereo-* + Gr. *skopein* to examine] an instrument for producing a three-dimensional image of an object. Photographs are taken of the object from two different angles, with each eye viewing only one photograph. See also *stereoscopic radiography.*

stereoscopic radiography (ste″re-o-skop′ik) a procedure for obtaining a three-dimensional x-ray view of an object. One film is exposed and, while the body part remains immobilized, the tube is shifted and another film is exposed at the same position. The films are then viewed with a stereoscope. The optimal tube shift distance is equal to the interpupillary distance of the viewer multiplied by the ratio of the target-film distance to the viewing distance. Also called stereoradiography and stereoscopy.

stereospecific numbering (ste″re-o-spĕ-sif′ik) a system used in designating the enantiomers of asymmetric glyceryl lipids. In the Fischer projection of the chiral center, carbon number 2 (the number 2 carbon atom) is given the L configuration by convention (OH to the left). The carbon above the chiral center is numbered 1 and the one at the bottom is numbered 3. When this convention is used, the prefix *sn-* is attached to the name, as in *sn*-1-acylglycerol and *sn*-3-acylglycerol. In the accompanying illustration, compound A is *sn*-1-acylglycerol or L-1-acylglycerol or D-3-acylglycerol, and its enantiomer compound B is *sn*-3-acylglycerol or L-3-acylglycerol or D-1-acylglycerol.

stereotactic (ste″re-o-tak′tik) 1. pertaining to or characterized by precise positioning in space. 2. exhibiting stereotaxis.

stereotactic instrument an apparatus consisting of a calibrated framework to fix the head in one position and to carry one or more electrode holders, so that electrodes can be placed accurately in a particular anatomic location in the brain using three-dimensional coordinates. In animals, the head is fixed by placing bars in the external ear canals, on the infraorbital bone ridges and against the upper teeth. The framework is calibrated in rectangular or polar coordinates. Using the ear bar location as a zero reference, brain structures can be located by their distance in front of or behind, and above or below, ear bar zero and the distance from brain midline. In human stereotactic surgery, electrode placement in reference to the brain ventricles can be determined by radiography. Also called *Horsley-Clarke apparatus.*

stereotactic surgery the placement of a discrete lesion in a precisely localized region of the brain by the use of an apparatus that permits localization of the target using three-dimensional coordinates.

stereotaxis (ste″re-o-tak′sis) movement (taxis) in response to contact with a solid or rigid surface.

steric (ste′rik) pertaining to the arrangement of atoms in space; pertaining to stereochemistry.

steric hindrance nonbonded repulsions between atoms or groups of atoms in a molecule or transition state. For example, steric hindrance is greater in *cis*-2-butene than in *trans*-2-butene because of the closeness of the two methyl groups in the former. The *cis-* isomer is less stable as a consequence. In a bimolecular substitution reaction, greater steric hindrance in the transition state (compared with some reference compound) results in a slower reaction rate.

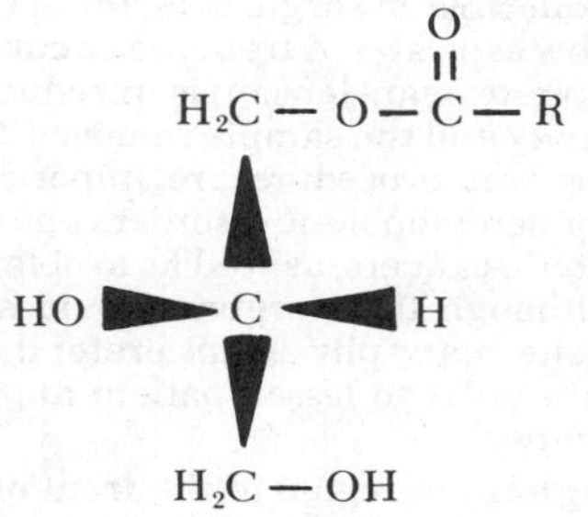

A

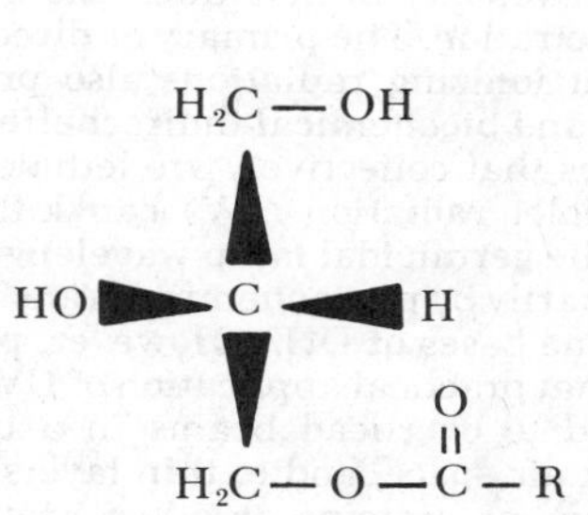

B

Stereospecific numbering. Formulas representing enantiomers: *A*, sn-1-acylglycerol; and *B*, sn-3-acylglycerol. (From Tietz, N. W.: Fundamentals of Clinical Chemistry. 2nd ed. Philadelphia, W. B. Saunders Co., 1976.)

sterigma (ste-rig′mah), pl. *sterigmata* [Gr. *stērigma* support] a structure, found at the end of a hyphal branch, which supports a sporangium, a conidium, or a basidiospore. Examples of fungi with sterigmata include *Aspergillus* and *Penicillium.* Cf. *annellophore* and *phialide.*

sterile (ster′il) [L. *sterilis*] 1. not fertile; unable to produce offspring.

2. aseptic; free from living microorganisms.

sterility (stĕ-ril′ĭ-te) [L. *sterilitas*] 1. the inability to produce offspring: the inability either to conceive or to induce conception. See also *infertility.*

2. the state of being aseptic, or free from microorganisms.

sterilization (ster″ĭ-li-za′shun) 1. any procedure by which an individual is made incapable of reproduction, e.g., castration, vasectomy, salpingectomy, and so forth.

2. in the microbiologic sense, a process that destroys all living microoganisms. Some foods, many biologicals, and a great variety of small medical and personal hygiene articles are presterilized by the manufacturer to eliminate microbial contamination. In hospitals, sterilization of reusable instruments and associated materials is mandatory for aseptic surgery. Most medical and surgical supplies are sterilized with a physical agent, heat, or radiation; chemical sterilization is employed as a substitute when physical methods cannot or should not be used. Liquids containing heat-labile substances are sterilized by filtration.

Autoclaving is the usual and fastest method of heat sterilization. The process consists of admitting supersaturated steam under pressure into a chamber until the temperature reaches 121°C, and then leaving it for 30 min. In the 1960s, high-vacuum–steam sterilizers were introduced, which have the distinct advantage of a shorter cycle: 3 min at 135°C. Smaller autoclaves are available for use in clinics and medical offices. When operated according to the manufacturer's directions and with adequate quality control, autoclaving guarantees sterility, i.e., the destruction of all life. Materials that cannot be autoclaved (e.g., oils) may be sterilized with dry air. The hot air oven cycles are 160°C for 2 hr or 170°C for 1 hr.

A large variety of commercial medical and personal hygiene products are presterilized by ionizing radiation. The principal agent is β-radiation in the form of electrons (cathode rays) accelerated to a very high velocity in machines, thereby acquiring deep penetration. The primary or direct effect is on DNA, but ionizing radiations also produce many physical and biochemical indirect effects in microorganisms that collectively are lethal.

Ultraviolet radiation (UV) can kill microoganisms in the germicidal lamp wavelength of 220–300 nm, primarily by photochemical transformations of pyrimidine bases of DNA. However, penetration is so poor that practical application of UV sterilization is limited to overhead beams in a confined and high-risk air space, and to thin layers of liquids.

Solutions of proteins or other heat-denaturable substances may be sterilized by filtration. Bacteria-free filtrates are obtained with filters that have a maximal pore size not exceeding 1 nm (which does allow passage of virus particles). Early types of bacterial filters were made of asbestos or diatomaceous earth; subsequently, unglazed porcelain and sintered glass were developed. However, these have been replaced by disposable nitrocelluose membrane filters available in carefully graded porosities, and are now employed widely in the pharmaceutical industry and in hospitals and research laboratories.

A few chemical compounds are sufficiently sporicidal in concentrations that do not badly damage materials, and are thus useful as chemical sterilants. These agents, however, of which ethylene oxide (EO) gas is the most important, require exposure times of 6 hr or longer and are comparatively expensive to use. Despite these inconveniences, many manufactured medical items are presterilized this way. EO is also used in hospitals to sterilize endoscopes and other reusable instruments that have a high infection-risk potential. The procedure involves a chamber that is first partially evacuated and then filled wth moist air to a relative humidity of about 30 percent and with EO gas to a concentration of at least 450 mg/l. A common cycle is 8 hr at 130°–140°C.

Three other chemical sterilants are recommended by Center for Disease Control guidelines (1981): aqueous 2 percent glutaraldehyde, 8 percent formaldehyde–70 percent alcohol, and aqueous 6 percent stabilized hydrogen peroxide. The specified exposure times are 10, 18, and 6 hr, respectively. Articles exposed to these toxic chemicals should be well aerated or carefully rinsed before they contact tissues.

Cf. *antisepsis* and *disinfection.*

sterilize (ster′ĭ-līz) 1. to render aseptic; to free from microorganisms.

2. to render incapable of reproduction.

sterilizer (ster′i-līz″er) an apparatus, such as an autoclave, that uses heat for the destruction of all forms of microorganisms, e.g., to achieve sterility. Sterility can also be achieved with a gas sterilizer, provided adequate concentration and time are employed. Currently, the most commonly used gas sterilant is ethylene oxide.

stern/o (ster′no) [Gr. *sternon* breast] a word element used in combining form to denote the sternum, e.g., sternodynia.

sternal (ster′nal) [L. *sternalis*] pertaining to the sternum.

sternal notch the jugular notch of the sternum; the point at the top of the breast bone between the clavicular notches. Also called suprasternal notch.

sternal puncture a surgical technique to obtain bone marrow aspirates. A trephine or cutting needle (such as a Westerman-Jensen) is introduced into the marrow cavity and the sample removed. Specimens obtained by this procedure are important for the diagnosis of hematopoietic disorders and of primary and metastatic cancers, as well as to obtain cells for culture. Although the sternum provides an easily accessible site, many physicians prefer the posterior iliac crest in order to lessen patient apprehension. See also *biopsy.*

sternal region the region of the front of the chest that overlies the sternum.

Sternberg-Reed cell (stern′berg rēd) [Carl *Sternberg;* Dorothy *Reed,* American pathologist] see *Reed-Sternberg cell.*

sternoxiphoid plane (ster″no-zif′oid) the horizontal plane that intersects the trunk at the level of the xiphisternal joint and the fifth costal cartilages.

STEROID. SUFFIXES AND PREFIXES FOR STEROIDS

SUFFIX OR PREFIX	MEANING
Suffix	
-ane	Saturated hydrocarbon
-ene	Unsaturated hydrocarbon
-ol	Hydroxyl group, as in alcohol or phenol
-one	Ketone group
Prefix	
hydroxy- (oxy-)	Hydroxyl group
keto- (oxo-)	Ketone group
deoxy-	Loss of an oxygen atom
dehydro-	Loss of two hydrogen atoms
dihydro-	Gain of two hydrogen atoms
cis-	Refers to spatial arrangement of two groups on the same side of the molecule
trans-	Refers to spatial arrangement of two groups on opposite sides of the molecule
α-	Refers to group which is *trans* to the methyl at C-10
β-	Refers to group which is *cis* to the methyl at C-10
epi-	Isomeric in configuration to a reference compound; specifically α at location C-3
iso-	Similar to epi-, but not restricted to C-3
allo-	Differing from reference compound in having 5α instead of 5β configuration; rings A and B in *trans* instead of *cis* relation to each other
etio-	Refers to final degradation product of a more complex molecule which still retains the essential chemical character of the original molecule
nor-	Refers to compound similar chemically to reference substance, but having one less carbon atom in side-chain
Δ	Indicates position of unsaturated linkage

From Cantarow, A., and Schepartz, B.: Biochemistry. 4th ed. Philadelphia, W. B. Saunders Co., 1967, p. 683.

sternum (ster′num) [L.; Gr. *sternon* breast] [NA], a dagger-shaped bone, 6–8 in. long, that lies in the anterior wall of the thorax in the median plane. The clavicles articulate with its upper end, and cartilages of the upper seven pairs of ribs attach to its lateral borders. It has three main parts: a manubrium, a body consisting of four fused segments, and a xiphoid process made up of cartilage with a core of bone.

steroid (ste′roid) the name for a group of compounds that contain a hydrogenated cyclopentanophenanthrene ring system. There are three six-sided rings (A, B, and C) that constitute the phenanthrene nucleus and an additional cyclopentane ring (D). They are derived from cholesterol.

Some of the common steroids are adrenocortical hormones, sex hormones, bile acids, sterols, and cardiac aglycones. Almost all steroids have an oxygen function (ketone or alcohol) at position C-3, and generally the methyl groups C-19 and C-18 are substituted at C-10 and C-13, respectively. Chains of various lengths are added at C-17 in the synthesis of sterols, bile acids, and some of the adrenocortical steroids.

In addition to being hormones and important intermediates in steroid biosynthesis, steroids are also used pharmacologically as antiinflammatory agents, immunosuppressive agents, and antiarrhythmic agents. Vitamin D metabolites are also derived from the steroid nucleus.

See also *adrenocortical hormones, androgen, bile acids, cardiac glycoside, estrogen,* and *sterol,* and the accompanying illustration and table.

steroid-21-hydroxylase see *steroid-21-monooxygenase.*

steroid-21-monooxygenase (ste′roid mon″o-ok′sĭ-jen-ās) an enzyme of the oxidoreductase class (steroid, hydrogen-donor:oxygen oxidoreductase [21-hydroxylating], EC 1.14.99.10) that catalyzes the reaction steroid + hydrogen donor (H_2) + O_2 ⇄ a 21-hydroxysteroid + hydrogen donor + H_2O. The enzyme system also involves cytochrome P_{450} and flavoprotein. A genetic deficiency in this enzyme is the most common cause of adrenogenital syndrome, marked by lack of cortisol and increased urinary 17-ketogenic steroids, especially pregnanetriol. Also called *steroid-21-hydroxylase.*

steroid-receptor complex a complex formed by a highly specific binding between a particular steroid and a high-affinity protein receptor. This complex occurs in the cytoplasm of a target cell; the activated cytoplasmic receptor complex is then transferred to the nucleus, where it stimulates gene transcription. Specific molecules of mRNA are formed, resulting in the production of proteins characteristic of that cell.

sterol (ste′rol) [Gr. *stereos* solid + L. *oleum* oil] a steroid with long (8–10 carbons) aliphatic side-chains at position 17 and at least one alcoholic hydroxyl group, usually at position 3. It has a lipidlike solubility. Examples are cholesterol and ergosterol.

sterol carrier proteins see under *carrier protein.*

steth/o (steth′o) [Gr. *stēthos* chest] a word element used in combining form to denote the chest, e.g., stethoscope.

Stevens-Johnson syndrome (ste′venz jon′son) [Albert Mason *Stevens,* American pediatrician, 1884–1945; Frank Chambliss *Johnson,* American pediatrician, 1894–1934] a severe form of erythema multi-

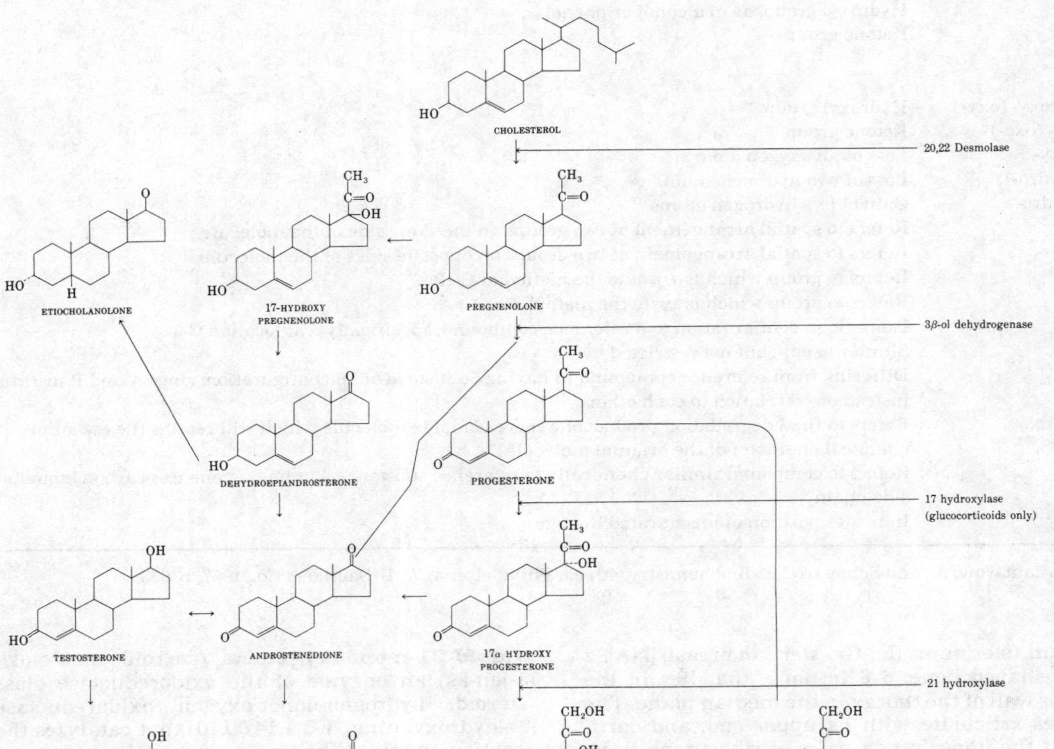

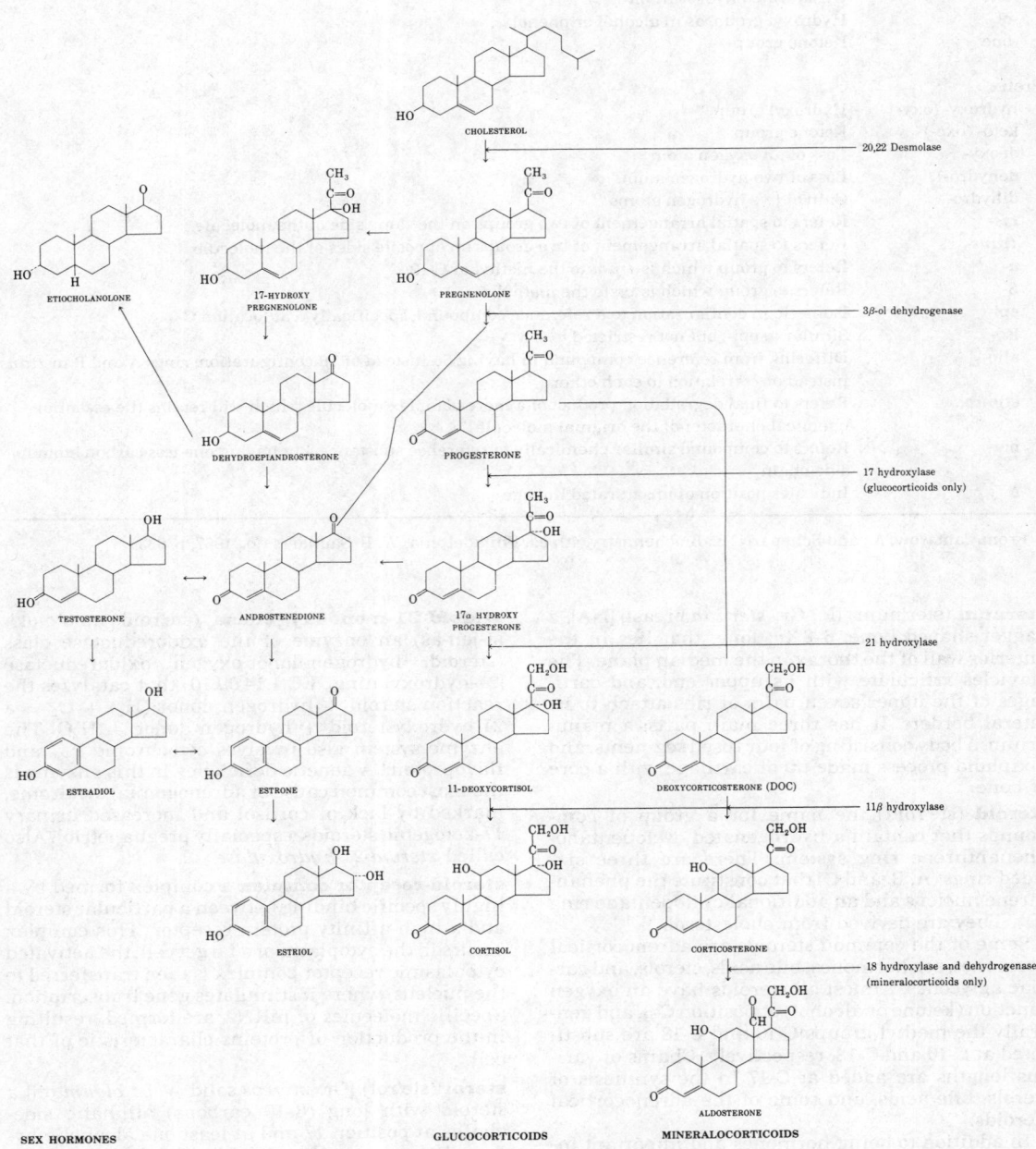

Steroid. Simplified pathways of adrenocortical hormone synthesis. (From Henry, J. B.: Clinical Diagnosis and Management. 16th ed. Philadelphia, W. B. Saunders Co., 1979.)

forme characterized by vesiculobullous and urticarial lesions of the mucosal membranes and skin of the hands and feet. Inflammatory lesions with hemorrhagic crusts are seen, and the "target" lesion —with a clear center and concentric erythematous ring—is often considered pathognomonic. There often are systemic signs, including toxicity, arthralgia, fever, malaise, and nausea. Onset is usually rapid, and the disease may last several weeks. Fatal cases have been recorded. This syndrome is thought to occur as an adverse reaction to a variety of drugs, including sulfonamides, thiazide diuretics, phenytoin, tetracycline, barbiturates, salicylates, and certain penicillins.

Stewart-Treves syndrome an angiosarcoma arising in a lymphedematous upper extremity. It may appear in an arm rendered chronically lymphedematous by an axillary lymph node dissection performed as part of a radical mastectomy.

-sthenia (sthe′ne-ah) [Gr. *sthenos* strength] a suffix word element to denote strength, e.g., asthenia.

STI abbrev. See *systolic time interval.*

stibine (stĭb′ēn) antimony hydride, a colorless, highly toxic gas, SbH_3; M.W. 124.78. The symptoms of poisoning are similar to those for *arsine.*

stiff-man syndrome a condition of unknown etiology marked by progressive stiffness and spasms of axial and limb muscles in the absence of signs of cerebral and spinal cord disease, but with continuous electromyographic activity.

stilbestrol (stil-bes′trol) see *diethylstilbestrol.*

stimulator (stim″u-la′tor) 1. any agent that excites functional activity.

2. in electroencephalography and electromyography, an instrument used to generate and apply pulses of current (stimulus) to identify or evoke a response from a nerve, muscle, or discrete area of the central nervous system, or to diagnose a neuromuscular disorder. The stimulator allows for control of the specific duration, intensity, and frequency of the applied stimulus. The stimulator output is generally insulated from the common ground connection through use of an isolation unit, and is synchronized with the beam of an oscilloscope.

stimulus (stim′u-lus), pl. *stimuli* [L. "goad"] 1. any internal or external agent, state, or act that can elicit or influence the activity of a cell, receptor, tissue, or organism.

2. in neurophysiologic studies, an electric stimulus of known intensity, duration, and frequency applied to a muscle, nerve, or other excitable tissue to evoke a measurable response.

adequate s., 1. the specific energy form to which a sensory receptor is most sensitive (i.e., exhibits the lowest threshold).

2. a stimulus sufficient to trigger a particular reflex action or response.

maximal s., a stimulus of just sufficient strength to excite all the axons in a nerve or all the fibers in a muscle, each of which may have varying thresholds. Any further increase in the stimulus strength produces no additional increase in the strength of the muscle contraction or in the amplitude of the evoked action potential.

submaximal s., a stimulus with an intensity between that of the threshold and of maximal stimuli.

subthreshold s., a stimulus of less than threshold strength.

supramaximal s., a stimulus of an intensity exceeding that of the stimulus necessary for complete activation of the given nerve or muscle.

threshold s., a stimulus of just sufficient intensity to elicit response. In neurophysiologic studies, an electric stimulus of threshold magnitude that evokes a nerve or muscle action potential.

stimulus artifact see under *artifact.*

stipple cell (sti′p′l) an erythrocyte containing granules that take a basic or bluish stain with Wright stain. The granules are RNA, mitochondria, or iron, and are seen in lead poisoning, thalassemia, and other disorders.

stippling (stip′pling) a spotted or granulated condition or appearance. See also *basophilic stippling.*

stochastic (sto-kas′tik) [Gr. *stochastikos* conjectural] pertaining to a random process, used particularly to refer to a time series of random variables. See *random.*

stock culture see *stock c.* under *culture.*

stoichiometry (stoi″ke-om′ĕ-tre) [Gr. *stoicheion* element + *metron* measure] originally, the study of the combining proportions of the chemical elements; now, the derivation from the chemical formula or equation of the numerical relationships in terms of mass, volume, or amount of substance (moles) of the elements in a compound or of the products and reactants in a reaction.

stoke (St) (stōk) [Sir George Gabriel *Stokes,* British mathematician and physicist, 1819–1903] the centimeter-gram-second (CGS) unit of kinematic viscosity, 1 poise · ml/g.

Stokes' law (stōks) an approximate formula, accurate at low velocities, for the viscous drag on a spherical object: $F = 6\,\pi v \eta \rho$, where F is the force, v is the velocity, η is the viscosity, and ρ is the radius of the sphere.

Stokes shift the phenomenon by which luminescent or fluorescent substances emit light at longer wavelengths than the exciting wavelength at which the light is absorbed. See also *fluorescence.*

Stoll's dilution egg count technique a technique used for estimating the worm burden of an individual infected with hookworm, *Ascaris,* or *Trichuris.* Sodium hydroxide, feces, and glass beads are mixed and allowed to stand for several hours. After mixing thoroughly, a sample is drawn and counted on a slide under a microscope.

stoma (sto′mah), pl. *stomas, stomata* [Gr. "mouth"] 1. any minute pore, orifice, or opening on a free surface.

2. a created permanent or semipermanent opening in the abdominal wall, e.g., colostomy, ureterostomy.

stomach (stum′ak) [L. *stomachus;* Gr. *stomachos*] the expanded segment of the alimentary canal in the upper part of the abdominal cavity that receives food from the esophagus through the cardiac sphincter, retains it while the food is exposed to mechanical churning from muscular contractions of the gastric wall and to the digestive actions of the gastric juice, and then passes the food on through the pyloric sphincter into the duodenum.

In the embryo, the stomach develops from a simple tube that expands, the posterior wall growing more rapidly so that the greater curvature of the stomach is longer than the lesser curvature. In addition, there is a partial rotation in which the posterior wall moves to the left, while the distal end of the stomach swings to the right of the midline. The stomach thus has anterior and posterior walls and is slung across the upper abdomen, suspended from the liver by the lesser omentum. The greater omentum hangs from the greater curvature. The stomach is derived from the foregut, and therefore receives its blood supply from branches of the celiac artery through two arterial arches that run along the curvatures. Innervation of the smooth muscle and blood vessels in the wall of the stomach is through the vagus nerves. Because of the embryologic rotation of the stomach, the left vagus passes from the left side of the esophagus onto its anterior wall, whereas the right vagus supplies the posterior wall.

The wall of the stomach is organized in the same basic way as the rest of the alimentary canal, with certain unique modifications. Its wall is thicker than that of the intestine because of the presence of three rather than two layers of muscle, and the entire surface is covered by peritoneum. The submucosa supports the mucosa, which comprises the thin muscularis mucosae, the loose connective tissue of the lamina propria, and the epithelium. The lining of the stomach forms a series of longitudinal folds, the rugae, that disappear when the organ is distended. The surface of the mucosa is studded by myriads of tiny depressions (foveolae) into each of which several tubular glands open.

The gastric epithelium is simple columnar in type. The surface cells produce a neutral mucoprotein that bathes the interior of the stomach and protects the mucosa from the acidic gastric juice. Cells in the necks of the gastric glands form mucus. Within the glands, in addition to mucus-forming cells, there are chief cells that produce pepsinogen, and parietal cells that elaborate hydrochloric acid at a concentration of 0.17 mmol/l. The parietal cells also secrete intrinsic factor, a glycoprotein that combines with vitamin B_{12} to form an active complex necessary for the normal maturation of red blood cells. There are scattered endocrine cells in the epithelium that form gastrin, serotonin, and other hormones.

Up to 1500 ml of gastric juice is formed in a 24-hr period under the stimulus of gastrin, which is produced in the distal stomach and proximal duodenum. Vagal stimulation promotes the release of gastrin. Enterogastrone from the upper small bowel mucosa inhibits gastric secretion.

Food leaves the stomach when the pyloric sphincter relaxes. The rate at which the stomach empties is controlled by a number of factors, including the volume, consistency, and acidity of its contents.

See also *chief cell, enterogastrone, gastrin, intrinsic factor, parietal cell, pepsin, serotonin,* and *vitamin* B_{12}.

stomach tumors gastric tumors, of which approximately 90 percent are carcinomas, 3 percent are lymphomas, and 2 percent are sarcomas (the majority of which are leiomyosarcomas). Benign neoplasms represent approximately 5 percent of the total.

A high incidence of adenocarcinoma of the stomach is found in individuals in some countries such as Japan and Iceland; this is probably related to dietary factors. Older adults, particularly males, are most frequently affected by carcinoma of the stomach. Conditions producing mucosal atrophy have been related to the development of gastric adenocarcinoma. Fifty percent of the tumors arise in the pyloric region and another 25 percent on the lesser curvature. The tumor is most frequently ulcerated, but malignant change rarely occurs in a benign chronic ulcer. Histologically, adenocarcinomas of the stomach show evidence of mucin production to varying degrees. Particularly in the linitis plastica type, there are many individual cells with a signet ring configuration.

Typically, adenocarcinomas of the stomach are aggressive, and metastasis to regional lymph nodes is found at the time of diagnosis in more than 80 percent of patients. The frequency of nodal metastases can be related to the size of the primary tumor. Metastases occur in fewer than half the tumors that are under 4 cm in size. The prognosis is best for those patients who have had an early diagnosis and surgical resection. For patients with metastases, the 5-yr survival rate is below 15 percent.

Most soft tissue neoplasms arising in the stomach are of smooth muscle origin, but tumors of fibroblasts and Schwann cells also occur. Small leiomyomas are common and not unusual. Larger leiomyomas of the stomach frequently tend to contain bizarre areas. The designation of leiomyoblastoma has been suggested for such tumors that appear atypical in their histology, often with areas of epithelioid change, but the term does not provide an adequate indication of their behavior, as some behave in a malignant manner. Leiomyosarcomas of the stomach make up about 1 percent of all gastric neoplasms.

stomat/o (sto′mah-to) [Gr. *stoma, stomatos* mouth] a word element used in combining form to denote mouth, e.g., stomatology, stomatitis.

stomatitis (sto-mah-ti′tis), pl. *stomatitides* [*stomato-* + *-itis*] a nonspecific inflammation of the mouth, which can be caused by a number of agents including bacteria (e.g., streptococci), viruses (e.g., herpes simplex), spirochetes (e.g., syphilis), mechanical trauma (e.g., ill-fitting dentures), avitaminosis (e.g., scurvy or vitamin B_{12} deficiency), and systemic lupus erythematosus.

Culture of a smear obtained directly from the lesion may be useful in diagnosis of an infectious process; darkfield microscopic examination is indicated to rule out syphilis. Blood counts and other laboratory studies may be useful in the detection of systemic disorders.

See also *aphthous stomatitis.*

stomatocyte (sto′mah-to-sīt) a cup-shaped erythrocyte produced by antibodies or hydrocytosis; in smears it appears as a red cell with a central zone of pallor that is slitlike rather than the usual circular shape. Stomatocytes are seen in hereditary spherocytosis, hereditary stomatocytosis, alcoholism, cirrhosis, obstructive liver disease, erythrocyte sodium pump defect, and Rh null cells. They also occur as an artifact due to transformation of the normal discocytes induced by drugs and a decrease in the pH.

Stomoxys (sto-mok′sis) a genus of bloodsucking flies of the family Muscidae. The species *S. calcitrans* is of cosmopolitan distribution; it frequently attacks humans and causes a sharp, stabbing pain. These flies breed in decaying hay, straw, grass, marine grass, rotting grain, or stable manure. Also called *biting house fly, dog fly,* or *stable fly.*

stone (stōn) see *calculus.*

stool the fecal discharge from the bowels. See also *feces.*

stool culture the bacteriologic analysis of a specimen of fecal material for diagnosing infectious diseases of the gastrointestinal tract. Often, GI tract disorders present as abdominal pain, diarrhea, and/or neurologic complications. Stools have an extremely high number of bacteria that are normal flora, more than 99.9 percent of which are anaerobic. Generally, the normal flora of stools includes *Bifidobacterium, Eubacterium,* and *Bacteroides* species, anaerobic cocci, *Clostridium* species, streptococci including enterococci, and many members of the Enterobacteriaceae (e.g., *Escherichia coli*).

Bacteriologic examination of stools for pathogens requires separation of the normal flora from the pathogens. Some common pathogens that can be recovered from stools in infected individuals include *Salmonella, Shigella, Campylobacter,* certain *Clostridium* species, enteropathogenic and enterotoxic *Escherichia coli, Vibrio* species, *Yersinia enterocolitica,* certain pathogenic staphylococci, and *Mycobacterium tuberculosis.* Stool specimens should be collected in sterile plastic containers and transported to the microbiology laboratory as soon as possible to avoid destruction of the bacteria (often through dehydration). If it is not practical to obtain a stool specimen for culture, a rectal swab is a less desirable alternative.

Stool specimens are plated on special selective media, as well as on differential media. Selective media are used to inhibit normal flora, especially many gram-positive bacteria; differential media distinguish lactose-fermenting from nonlactose-fermenting gram-negative bacilli. Most enteric pathogens do not ferment lactose. Because stool specimens contain a large variety and a huge number of normal flora bacteria, as well as possible pathogens, no single medium is sufficiently differential and selective. Although Enterobacteriaceae generally grow well aerobically at 37°C, some enteric pathogens such as *Yersinia* and *Campylobacter* grow better in a different atmosphere or at another temperature.

See also *Gram stain* and *normal flora.*

stopcock (stop′kok) a small valve for stopping or regulating the flow of a fluid through a pipe, such as the device that regulates the outflow from a buret or a separatory funnel.

stop codon see *termination codon.*

storage (stor′ij) 1. the part of a computer that stores data and programs. Also called *memory.*

2. the movement of information into storage. Also called *store.*

external s., any medium except the main memory of a computer used to store data in a machine-readable form. This usually refers to magnetic tape, disk, or drum, but may also refer to punched cards used as a back-up storage medium.

internal s., the main memory of a computer.

storage allocation the assignment of an area of computer memory to a particular variable name or other data label.

dynamic s. a., allocation of storage space when a main program or subroutine is entered or by execution of statements in the program.

static s. a., allocation of storage space that is not altered during program execution.

storage cabinet see *flammable liquid storage cabinet.*

storage capacity the amount of information, measured in bits, bytes, or words, that can be contained in a computer memory or other storage device.

storage limits see *flammable liquid storage limits.*

storage location the part of a computer memory referred to by a particular address. It contains one byte or one word of information.

storage room see *flammable liquid storage room.*

store (stōr) 1. to place data in a computer memory or other storage device such as a disk, drum, or magnetic tape.

2. an instruction that causes the transfer of data from a register to memory.

storiform (stor′ĭ-form) [from L. *storia*] spread out; a matting of plaited straw or rushes. The term is frequently applied in histopathology to describe the whorled or pinwheel arrangement of tumor cells in certain soft tissue neoplasms, e.g., benign and malignant forms of fibrous histiocytoma.

stork bite see *vascular n.* under *nevus.*

Stovall-Black method a staining method for cytoplasmic inclusion bodies, especially Negri bodies, in brain tissue. The sections are stained in alcoholic ethyl eosin, counterstained with methylene blue, and differentiated with dilute acetic acid. The Negri bodies appear red, cytoplasm pink, and nuclei pale blue.

STP abbrev. See *2,5-dimethoxy-methylamphetamine* or *standard temperature and pressure.*

STPD conditions of a gas a volume of gas that is at standard temperature (0°C) and pressure (760 torr) and that contains no water vapor (dry).

strabismus (strah-biz′mus) [Gr. *strabismos* a squinting] a muscle imbalance that results in the improper alignment and deviation of one eye from the other. Nonparalytic (concomitant) strabismus is due to unequal ocular muscle tone and is primarily an ophthalmologic condition. Paralytic (noncomitant) strabismus is due to paralysis of one or more of the ocular muscles and thus is primarily a neurologic condition. There is limited eye movement and double vision (diplopia). If the condition is congenital, diplopia is almost always absent, owing to early suppression of vision in the affected eye. All forms of strabismus, when diagnosed by physical examination, require complete neurologic and ophthalmologic evaluation. Also called *squint.*

Strachan's syndrome a disorder of the peripheral and optic nerves, dominated by sensory symptoms and signs. It is considered to be due to a nutritional deficiency, although the deficient factor has not yet been determined. The associated amblyopia is accompanied by ataxia and tingling and loss of sensation in the extremities as the most common manifestations. Mucocutaneous lesions (orogenital syndrome) also are frequently observed. This syndrome primarily affects individuals in underdeveloped populations, but may be seen in alcoholics and in individuals with chronic liver disease and nontropical sprue in developed countries.

strain (strān) 1. to filter out solids from a solution.

2. an overstretching or overexertion of some part of the musculature.

3. a pure culture of organisms within a species, characterized by one or more particular phenotypic

or genotypic property, such as serologic type or biochemical reaction, that is retained in a relatively stable manner during repeated subculture.

4. in physics, the deformation produced in an object by an applied force. See also *stress.*

stratification (strat″ĭ-fĭ-ka′shun) [L. *stratum* layer + *facere* to make] an arrangement of structures in layers.

stratified (strat′ĭ-fīd) more than one layer. Cf. *pseudostratified.*

stratified epithelium an epithelium consisting of more than a single layer of cells. Stratified squamous epithelium is found in the epidermis and in mucosal surfaces that are subjected to friction, such as the oral cavity, esophagus, and vagina. See also *epithelium.*

stratigraphy (strah-tig′rah-fe) [L. *stratum* layer + Gr. *graphein* to write] a type of body-section radiography. See also under *tomography.*

Stratiomyidae a family of flies, the larvae of which may cause intestinal myiasis in humans.

stratum (stra′tum), pl. *strata* [L.] [NA], a general term for a sheetlike mass of substance of nearly uniform thickness, particularly when the layer is one of several associated layers.

s. basale, the deepest layer of cells in the epidermis, usually called the basal layer.

s. corneum, the horny layer of the epidermis; the outermost cornified layer of the skin, consisting predominantly of keratin. Also called the cornified or horny layer.

s. granulosum, 1. a relatively thick layer of squamous cells, containing pre-keratin, between the stratum spinosum and the stratum corneum of the epidermis.

2. the layer of follicular cells that surrounds the follicular cavity of an ovarian follicle and lines the theca folliculi. After ovulation, these cells develop into the corpus luteum.

s. lucidum, a clear, translucent layer of the skin immediately above the granular layer, seen best on the palm or sole. It is rich in protein-bound phospholipids, which resist water penetration.

s. spinosum, a layer, several cells thick, between the stratum basale and the stratum granulosum in the epidermis. The cells are connected by numerous desmosomes.

strawberry cervix the clinical appearance of the uterine cervix during infection with *Trichomonas vaginalis,* marked by distention of the superficial blood vessels and focal hemorrhages. "Double hairpin" capillaries are evident colposcopically.

strawberry foot rot see *dermatophilosis.*

strawberry nevus see *vascular n.* under *nevus.*

straw itch see under *predaceous mites.*

stray light in a spectrophotometer, any light from outside the instrument, or from scattering within the instrument, that falls on the detector and causes errors in the measured absorbance.

streak (strēk) in bacteriology, the act of inoculating a culture to produce separated colonies. Also called streaking. See also *streak c.* under *culture.*

Strengeria a genus of crabs that serve as intermediate hosts for the fluke *Paragonimus caliensis* in Central and South America.

strength-duration curve (S-D curve) a graph that relates the intensity of an electrical stimulus (Y axis) to its duration (X axis) when the current is applied to the motor point of a muscle and elicits a minimal contraction. As the duration of the stimulus is shortened, a greater current strength must be used to stimulate the muscle effectively. A point is reached at which the duration is so brief that a response does not occur no matter what stimulus intensity is used. Likewise, with stimuli of sufficiently weak intensity, no contraction is produced no matter how long the stimulating current is allowed to flow.

By convention, the minimal stimulus strength of infinitely long duration necessary to produce a muscle contraction is called the rheobase. The chronaxie is the current duration necessary to elicit a minimal contraction at twice the rheobase intensity.

When the strength-duration curve is determined for a completely or partially denervated muscle, the curve has a different shape from that for normally innervated muscle; it may be shifted partly or entirely to the right along the X axis and will exhibit a great increase in the chronaxie.

Strep abbrev. See *Streptococcus.*

strept/o (strep′to) [Gr. *streptos* twisted] a word element used in combining form to denote twisted, e.g., streptobacteria, streptothrix.

Streptobacillus (strep″to-bah-sil′us) [*strepto-* + Gr. *bacillus* small rod] a genus of bacteria composed of gram-negative, facultatively anaerobic, rod-shaped organisms, and consisting of a single species, *S. moniliformis.* The organisms occur frequently in chains and long, looped filaments. Cells are pleomorphic with L-phase variant formation. The organism grows on the surface of blood cultures in the form of "fluff balls." Reactions to catalase and oxidase are negative, and positive to phosphatase. The organism is a normal inhabitant of rodents, and a cause of rat-bite and Haverhill fevers in humans.

Streptococcaceae (strep″to-kok-ka′se-e) a family of bacteria containing facultatively anaerobic gram-positive cocci that occur in pairs, chains, or tetrads. It includes five genera: *Aerococcus, Gemella, Leuconostoc, Pediococcus,* and *Streptococcus.*

Streptococcus (strep″to-kok′us) [*strepto-* + Gr. *kokkos* berry] a genus in the family Streptococcaceae. Members of the genus are gram-positive cocci with a tendency to grow in pairs or chains. Streptococci are cytochrome-, oxidase-, and catalase-negative organisms that are nonmotile, nonspore-forming, and facultative anaerobes; some species are microaerophilic. Streptococci are homofermentative; for example, lactic acid is the end product of fermentation under both aerobic and anaerobic conditions.

CLASSIFICATION. Streptococci may be classified in several ways, including: (1) patterns of hemolysis on blood agar, (2) antigenic composition, and (3) physiologic and biochemical characteristics.

Hemolysis is useful for preliminary identifications. The terms alpha, beta, and gamma were introduced in 1818 as descriptors of the types of hemolytic reactions observed when streptococci grow on or in blood agar. With alpha hemolysis, the colonies are surrounded by a zone of incomplete clearing in which some residual intact erythrocytes can be seen. Outside this zone there may be an additional zone of complete hemolysis, which is called alpha-prime hemolysis. Also characteristic of alpha hemolysis is an area of greenish discoloration of the medium around the colony. Streptococci that exhibit this type of hemolysis on blood agar are known as alpha-hemolytic or viridans streptococci; *S. salivarius* is an example. The colonies of beta-hemolytic streptococci produce clear, colorless zones of complete (beta) hemolysis; there is no greening. *S. pyogenes* is the prototype species. The term gamma hemolysis is confusing, for it refers to the absence of a hemolytic reaction on blood agar. Nonhemolytic streptococci are sometimes called gamma streptococci. Nonhemolytic strains of *S. faecalis* are frequently isolated from clinical specimens.

Beta-hemolytic streptococci have been classified according to differences in their cell wall carbohydrate antigens; these are known as group-specific, or simply group, antigens. They are designated by letters A–O (Table 1).

Physiologic and biochemical characteristics are used as an accessory means of classification because hemolysis and antigenic composition are neither sufficient nor entirely satisfactory. The pneumococcus or *S. pneumoniae,* for example, is alpha hemolytic, but this is not a primary feature in its identification, which is based on its capsule (unrelated to beta-hemolytic group antigens) and solubility in bile. Similarly, group D streptococci cannot be identified by hemolysis alone, nor is group identification adequate.

CLINICAL SIGNIFICANCE. Streptococci constitute a large part of the normal flora of the oral cavity, and some varieties are regularly present in the intestinal tract. Certain species, however, are highly virulent for humans, notably *S. pyogenes* and *S. pneumoniae,* causing acute, severe infections. A number of other species, although less virulent, are nevertheless of great clinical importance.

S. pneumoniae, formerly *Diplococcus pneumoniae,* is a major respiratory tract pathogen. It is the most common cause of community-acquired pneumonia and is frequently responsible for meningitis, acute otitis media in children, and peritonitis in both children and adults.

Between 40 and 70 percent of all healthy adults carry one or more pneumococcal types in their throats, but growth of the pneumococcus in the throat is limited by the action of alpha-hemolytic streptococci. The lower respiratory tract also contains effective defense mechanisms. Certain individuals are particularly susceptible to pneumococcal disease, notably neonates, the elderly, individuals with splenectomies or sickle cell disease, infants and children with hereditary immunodeficiencies, and patients with hematologic malignancies.

More than 80 serologic types of pneumococci have been identified by differences in their capsular polysaccharides (Quellung reaction). The polysaccharide capsule plays an important role in the virulence of the organism by allowing it to evade phagocytic cells. Antibodies formed to the capsular polysaccharide are type-specific and protective—the basis for the pneumococcal vaccine now available.

Group A streptococcus (*S. pyogenes*) is one of the most important bacterial pathogens of humans. It causes not only a wide range of suppurative diseases, but also some serious nonsuppurative sequelae. The suppurative diseases include pharyngitis ("strep throat"), scarlet fever, peritonsillar cellulitis and abscesses, otitis media, sinusitis, cervical lymphadenitis, meningitis, brain abscess, pneumonia, endocarditis, osteomyelitis, puerperal sepsis, impetigo, and erysipelas. The most serious nonsuppurative sequelae, especially of group A streptococcal pharyngitis, are acute rheumatic fever and acute glomerulonephritis. They appear to be immunologically mediated, involving the deposition of immune complexes. Owing to the risk of sequelae, early diagnosis and treatment of streptococcal disease is important.

Group A streptococci are divided into about 55 serotypes on the basis of the antigenic differences in M-protein molecules localized at the cell surface and associated with the fimbriae. M protein is the major virulence antigen of group A streptococci,

Streptococcus, TABLE 1. SOME DISTINGUISHING CHARACTERISTICS OF CLINICALLY IMPORTANT MEMBERS OF THE GENUS *Streptococcus*

LANCEFIELD GROUP	HEMOLYSIS (SHEEP BLOOD)	BACITRACIN SENSITIVITY	HIPPURATE HYDROLYSIS	CAMP FACTOR	BILE ESCULIN HYDROLYSIS	6.5% NaCl TOLERANCE
A (*Strep. pyogenes*)	β^a	+	–	–[b]	–	–
B (*Strep. agalactiae*)	β	–[c]	+	+	–	–
D (Enterococcus)	α, β, γ	–	variable	–	+	+
D (Non-enterococcus)	α, γ	–	–	–	+	–
C, G, F, H, K and other viridans streptococci	α, β, γ	–[c]	–	–	variable	variable

[a] Rare strains of *S. pyogenes* may not be β-hemolytic.
[b] Group A positive under anaerobic conditions.
[c] Occasional strain positive.

From Treagan, L., and Pulliam, L.: Medical Microbiology Laboratory Procedures. Philadelphia, W. B. Saunders Co., 1982, p. 13.

and contributes to the resistance of the organism to phagocytosis by polymorphonuclear leukocytes. Antibodies formed to M protein provide type-specific immunity. The hyaluronic acid capsule is another antiphagocytic factor, and lipoteichoic acid appears to be responsible for the adherence of *S. pyogenes* to epithelial cells.

These streptococci elaborate extracellular toxins and harmful enzymes. A few strains of *S. pyogenes* produce erythrogenic toxin, which is responsible for the rash of scarlet fever; most strains produce streptolysin S and streptolysin O, both of which damage the membranes of red blood cells and leukocytes. Streptolysin S, which is oxygen-stable, is not immunogenic. Streptolysin O is inactivated by atmospheric oxygen. Patients recovering from streptococcal disease usually have antibodies to streptolysin O in their serum.

Four serologically and electrophoretically distinct deoxyribonucleases are produced, designated A, B, C, and D. Detection of antibody to deoxyribonuclease B has been used for the diagnosis of streptococcal infection, particularly in individuals with pyoderma, a disease in which the antistreptolysin O response is unreliable. Certain group A types produce hyaluronidase, an enzyme thought by some to play a role in the spread of the organism through connective tissue; many recovering from streptococcal pharyngitis or pyoderma have antibodies to this enzyme. Oher extracellular products include diphosphopyridine nucleotidase and streptokinase.

Group B streptococcus *S. agalactiae* is found primarily in the genital and intestinal tracts of apparently healthy infants and adults. Most, but not all, isolates are beta hemolytic, the exceptions being nonhemolytic. Although group B infections can occur at all ages, a large majority of isolates are from infants younger than 3 mo. In this age group, *S. agalactiae* meningitis and septicemia are frequent complications. The colonization rate among infants is sometimes high in hospital nurseries, and outbreaks of clinical infections do occur. The most likely source of the group B streptococci that colonize infants is the mother's vagina, as two-thirds of vaginal cultures taken at term are positive. Group B streptococci are also isolated from individuals with urinary tract infections, wound infections, and otitis media.

Group C streptococci occur in the human pharynx, vagina, and skin, and are sometimes recovered from blood cultures. The pathogenicity of group C streptococci for humans is not known. *S. equisimilis* is the only group C species found frequently in human specimens.

Group D streptococci may exhibit beta or alpha hemolysis, or hemolysis may be absent. These streptococci are divided for diagnostic purposes into two groups, enterococci and nonenterococci, on the basis of the enterococci's ability to grow in broth containing 6.5 percent NaCl (Table 2). The enterococci includes *S. faecalis, S. faecium, S. durans,* and *S. avium;* nonenterococcal species include *S. bovis* and *S. equinus.* Differentiation of group D streptococci into enterococci and nonenterococci is important to the clinician because of the high resistance of enterococci to penicillin. Group D streptococci cause approximately 10–20 percent of human subacute bacterial endocarditis.

Group F streptococci (*S. anginosus*) are microaerophilic organisms found in the pharynx, vagina, and intestinal tracts of healthy individuals; they have also been isolated from the wounds, abscesses, and blood of infected persons.

Group G streptococci (sometimes called *S. canis*) colonize the pharynx, and have been isolated from wound infections and from the blood of septic patients. The role of these organisms in causing pharyngitis is not known. Beta-hemolytic streptococci belonging to groups other than those discussed above rarely cause human infection.

Viridans streptococci (alpha-hemolytic streptococci) represents a group of several species without well-defined group antigens (Table 3). They are identified on the basis of biochemical reactions. Viridans streptococci differ from the pneumococci by their resistance to bile solubility, and from enterococci by their inability to grow in 6.5 percent NaCl broth.

Viridans streptococci make up a large part of the normal flora of the upper respiratory tract and may have a protective role in the pharynx. Nevertheless, they cause or participate in a number of important diseases. Two species, *S. mutans* and *S. sanguis,* are involved in—and may be the primary cause of—dental caries, and members of the viridans group are responsible for 50–70 percent of bacterial endocarditis. Viridans streptococci frequently escape from their natural habitat: they can often be recovered from the blood during the first 30 min after a tooth extraction and after the simple act of chewing paraffin. Thus, when interpreting blood cultures containing alpha-hemolytic streptococci, care must

Streptococcus, TABLE 2. DIFFERENTIAL CHARACTERISTICS OF LANCEFIELD GROUP D *Streptococcus*

	ENTEROCOCCUS			NON-ENTEROCOCCUS	
CHARACTERISTIC	*S. faecalis*	*S. faecium*	*S. durans*	*S. bovis*	*S. equinus*
Hemolysis	α, β, γ	α, γ	α, β, γ	α, γ	α, γ
6.5% NaCl	G	G	G	NG	NG
Bile esculin	G	G	G	G	G
Litmus milk	A/C	A/C	A/C	A/C	–
Starch	–	–	–	+	–
Glycerol	+	–	–	–	–
Sorbitol	+	–(+)	–	–	NR

G = growth; NG = no growth; A/C = acid/clot; NR = no reaction.
Modified from Treagan, L., and Pulliam, L.: Medical Microbiology Laboratory Procedures. Philadelphia, W. B. Saunders Co., 1982, p. 14.

be taken to distinguish transient bacteremia from the persistent bacteremia of endocarditis.

Nonhemolytic streptococcus is a descriptive term with little meaning, but it has clinical significance, as some enterococcal colonies are nonhemolytic in blood agar. These and other streptococci are not to be confused with the obligately anaerobic cocci in the family Peptococcaceae.

IDENTIFICATION. Direct microscopic examination of clinical specimens is of little value in the identification of streptococci, an exception being the Quellung test performed on body fluids that contain pneumococci.

Streptococci are fastidious with respect to nutritional requirements. Complex media should be used, such as trypticase soy, heart infusion, or Todd-Hewitt, and supplemented with blood. For the isolation of *S. pyogenes* from throat specimens, a medium containing 5 percent sheep blood is recommended. Pour plates or streaked and stabbed plates are used to detect beta hemolysis. Selective media are available for isolating enterococci and group A or B streptococci from specimens containing mixed flora.

The presumptive identification of streptococci includes observation of the colony morphology and hemolysis, as well as several simple tests. After a 24-hr incubation period, colonies of beta-hemolytic streptococci are typically translucent and smooth with an entire edge. Group A streptococcal colonies may be somewhat smaller than group B colonies and may be surrounded by a larger zone of beta hemolysis. Some strains of group B are nonhemolytic. Group D streptococci may exhibit beta or alpha hemolysis, or hemolysis may be absent. Colonies of group F streptococci are generally minute, although some strains of groups A and G are also very small. Colonies of viridans streptococci vary in size and may be surrounded by a zone of alpha hemolysis or no hemolysis. As the culture ages, the centers of the pneumococcal colonies become depressed as a result of autolysis.

Further identification depends on several procedures. Susceptibility to bacitracin may be used for the presumptive identification of group A streptococci. Using a pure culture, an inhibitory zone of any size around a 0.04-unit disk (not the more concentrated susceptibility disk) is considered positive. False-positive results may be obtained with some strains of groups B, C, or G. The CAMP test is useful for presumptive identification of beta-hemolytic or nonhemolytic group B streptococci. Group B streptococci produce a substance, called CAMP factor, which results in an increase in the zone of hemolysis produced by a *Staphylococcus* culture producing beta-lysin.

Serologic grouping of beta-hemolytic streptococci and nonhemolytic groups B and D utilizes the group-specific cell wall carbohydrate antigen. Antigen extracted by a variety of methods is tested against antisera to groups A–D, F, and G. The presence and identity of these antigens can be detected by a precipitation or agglutination procedure. Latex agglutination and coagglutination slide test reagents are commercially available. Groups A and B streptococci can also be identified by direct immunofluorescence using specific antisera conjugated with fluorescein isothiocyanate. See also *anti-DNase B (ADN-B) assay* and *antihyaluronidase (AH) assays.*

Pneumococcal colonies may be identified by the Quellung test using pooled and monovalent sera. They may be presumptively differentiated from viridans streptococci either by the bile solubility test, in which pneumococcal colonies lyse in the presence of sodium deoxycholate, or by optochin susceptibility, in which pneumococcal colonies are inhibited by a disk containing optochin. When 6-mm optochin disks are used, the zone of inhibition must be at least 14 mm in diameter to be considered positive. Equivocal results should be confirmed with a bile solubility test.

Group D streptococci may be presumptively identified by the bile-esculin test, in which group D streptococci hydrolyze esculin in the presence of 4 percent bile in a special culture medium. Enterococci should be differentiated from the group D nonenterococci because of their pencillin resis-

Streptococcus, TABLE 3. DIFFERENTIAL CHARACTERISTICS OF "VIRIDANS," OR MICROAEROPHILIC, STREPTOCOCCI

CHARACTERISTIC	*S. mutans*	*S. intermedius MG-anginosus*	*S. constellatus*	*S. mitis*	*S. salivarius*	*S. morbillorum*	*S. sanguis I*	*S. sanguis II*
Hemolysis	α,β,γ	α,β,γ	α,β,γ	α/γ	γ	γ	α,γ	α,γ
Inulin	+	−	−	−	+	−	+	−
Lactose	+	+	−	+	+	−	+	+
Mannitol	+	−	−	−	−	−	−	−
Raffinose	+	−/+	−	−	+	−	−/+	+
Esculin hyd.	+	+	+	−	+	−	+	−
Litmus milk	A/C	A/C	A/no clot	A/C	A/C	−	A/C	A/C
5% sucrose agar	adherent	nonadh.	nonadh.	nonadh.	nonadh. gummy colony	nonadh.	adherent	adherent

A/C = acid/clot.

From Treagan, L., and Pulliam, L.: Medical Microbiology Laboratory Procedures. Philadelphia, W. B. Saunders Co., 1982, p. 16.

tance; enterococci grow in broth in the presence of 6.5 percent NaCl. Group D streptococci and viridans streptococci may be identified to the species level by biochemical tests.

streptodornase (strep″to-dor′nās) an enzyme produced by hemolytic streptococci that catalyzes the depolymerization of deoxyribonucleic acid (DNA). Formerly called streptococcal deoxyribonuclease. See also *deoxyribonuclease I.*

streptokinase (strep″to-ki′nās) [*strepto-* + *kinase*] a proteolytic enzyme of the hydrolase class (EC 3.4) that catalyzes the conversion of plasminogen to plasmin. It is produced extracellularly by group A streptococci and may be related to the invasiveness of the organism. See also under *thrombolytic agents.*

streptokinase-streptodornase a mixture of proteolytic enzymes elaborated by hemolytic streptococci; used as a proteolytic and fibrinolytic agent. The term streptodornase is applied to the mixture of enzymes, whereas streptokinase refers specifically to the enzyme that converts ("activates") plasminogen to plasmin. Trademark, Veridase.

streptolysin (strep-tol′ĭ-sin) [*strepto*coccus + hemo*lysin*] an exotoxin produced by most strains of group A streptococci that lyses red blood cells, and is thus responsible for the hemolytic activity of the organism. Two forms have been identified, streptolysin S and O. See also *exotoxins.*

s. O, an oxygen-labile and antigenic form. In such diseases as rheumatic carditis, it is believed that streptolysin O combines with antistreptolysin O (antibody); some myocardial substrates also combine with antistreptolysin O, resulting in immune complexes deposited in the heart. See also *antistreptolysin O tests.*

s. S, an oxygen-stable and nonantigenic form. It cannot be detected serologically with antibodies. In normal serum, there is a lipoprotein that inhibits the lytic activity of streptolysin S. However, decreased amounts of this lipoprotein are found in individuals with rheumatic fever and rheumatoid arthritis.

Streptomyces (strep″to-mi′sēz) [*strepto-* + Gr. *mykēs* fungus] a genus of funguslike bacteria within the Actinomycetes. Most of the more than 450 recognized species have been isolated from soil. It appears that some of them may produce a chronic, actinomycotic-type infection that usually occurs in the upper respiratory tract. *Streptomyces* is a bacterium with many fungal characteristics, such as nonfragmented aerial mycelia with chains of spores produced within the hyphal element. It is strictly aerobic and nonacid-fast. Mature spore-bearing hyphae form spirals. Cell walls contain L-diaminopimelic acid and glycine and do not contain major amounts of arabinose (cell wall type 1 of Lechevalier). *Streptomyces* is the source of more than 500 antimicrobial compounds, including at least 90 percent of the therapeutically useful antibiotics. This genus consists of scavengers capable of breaking down a myriad of large organic molecules into simple compounds that restore fertility to the soil.

Streptomycetaceae (strep″to-mi″se-ta′se-e) a family of bacteria of the order Actinomycetales. It consists of four genera: *Streptomyces, Streptoverticillium, Sporichthya,* and *Microellobosporia.*

streptomycin (strep″to-mi′sin) a bactericidal antibiotic derived from *Streptomyces griseus* and belonging to the aminoglycoside group. Streptomycin is effective against gram-negative bacilli and against *Mycobacterium tuberculosis* and *M. bovis* in vitro. It may be used in the treatment of tuberculosis, especially with isoniazid-resistant strains. Streptomycin is highly effective in the treatment of tularemia, plague, and brucellosis. See also *aminoglycosides* and *antibacterial agents.*

streptomycosis (strep″to-mi-ko′sis) any infection caused by an organism of the genus *Streptomyces.*

Streptothrix (strep′to-thriks) 1. a genus of sheathed bacteria.

2. a former name for the genus *Dermatophilus;* the species *S. bovis* is now called *D. congolensis.*

streptotrichosis (strep″to-tri-ko′sis) see *dermatophilosis.*

streptozocin (strep″to-zo′sin) a cancer chemotherapeutic drug; trademark, Zanosar. For more information, see *Appendix A.*

streptozyme test see under *antistreptolysin O tests.*

stress (stres) 1. in biology, a stimulus having sufficient magnitude to produce the breakdown of normal homeostatic regulatory mechanisms.

2. in physics, a force producing a deformation in an object. Cf. *strain.*

stress reticulocyte see *stress r.* under *reticulocyte.*

stress testing a clinical procedure that introduces physiologic stress through exercise to increase cardiac output and myocardial oxygen consumption, thus determining the available coronary arterial reserve. Utilizing such a technique, the clinician can stress an individual in a safe environment. Exercise stress testing is indicated to evaluate chest discomfort, a therapy course for coronary artery disease, and the effectiveness of drug therapy, as well as to follow the course of rehabilitation after myocardial infarction and surgical procedures.

Among the tests often performed during and following exercise stress are the electrocardiogram, isotope scintigraphy, and oxygen consumption. Exercising may be accomplished by having the patient use a treadmill, bicycle, or two-step staircase. The time course of such exercise is variable and may be matched to the individual being tested. Open-ended tests include exercise to a fixed heart rate, to a rate proportional to estimated maximal heart rate, or to a point at which the patient is unable to continue.

Controversy surrounds stress testing, except in specific circumstances, because of a significant number of false-positive and false-negative results. Nonetheless, exercise stress testing remains a valuable technique for evaluating physiologic response to increased performance demands; as such, it is a very useful tool for evaluating high-risk individuals and as a clinical follow-up after coronary disease and subsequent treatment.

stria (stri′ah), pl. *striae* [L. "a furrow, groove"] 1. a streak or line.

2. a narrow, bandlike structure.

3. [NA], a general term for visible bundles of nerve fibers in the brain.

striated (stri′āt-ed) [L. *striatus*] marked by striae; possessing a transversely banded structure, as in a skeletal muscle fiber.

striated border see *brush border.*

striated muscle a muscle whose fibers have transverse striations by light microscopy, because of the band arrangement of myofilaments. Cardiac and skeletal muscles are striated. See also *muscle*.

striation (stri-a'shun) 1. the quality of being marked by stripes or striae.
2. a streak or scratch.
basal s.'s., marked infoldings of basal cell membrane seen in certain actively transporting cells, such as those of the proximal convoluted tubule cells of the kidney and ducts of certain glands.

stridor (stri'dor) [L.] a harsh, high-pitched respiratory sound heard during inspiration in upper airway obstruction, especially in infancy.
laryngeal s., stridor due to laryngeal obstruction. A congenital form, marked by stridor and dyspnea, is due to an infolding of a congenitally flabby epiglottis and aryepiglottic folds during inspiration; it is usually outgrown by age 2 yr.

Strigeata a suborder of flatworms of the class Trematoda.

string (string) in computer programming, a data type that consists of a sequence of zero or more items of the same type, such as a bit string or a character string.

stringent response the mechanism resulting from a deficiency of an amino acid to such a level that transfer RNA (tRNA) for that amino acid is not kept fully charged. Under these conditions the concentration of guanosine-5'-diphosphate-3'-diphosphate (ppGpp) increases. Metabolic changes mediated by ppGpp include the termination of ribosomal and tRNA synthesis and the accelerated production of amino acids.

strip-chart recorder see *chart recorder*.

stripped nucleus a nucleus of a cell, the cytoplasm of which has disintegrated. It is commonly observed in cytologic preparations of uterine endocervical cells. Columnar cells from other anatomic sites exhibit similar cytoplasmic fragility.

strobe light a bright light that flashes periodically and appears to stop the motion of an object rotating at the same frequency as the light pulses; used in the laboratory for calibrating the speed of a centrifuge.

strobila (stro-bi'lah), pl. *strobilae* [L.; Gr. *strobilos* anything twisted up] the entire chain of proglottids that make up the body of an adult tapeworm.

stroke (strōk) a lay term for the sudden and dramatic loss of neurologic function due to the destruction of cerebral tissue by the effects of cerebrovascular disease; for more information see *cerebrovascular accident*.

stroke volume the amount of blood ejected from a ventricle of the heart as it empties during systole (contraction), equal to 70–80 ml in the normal male at rest in the supine position. The various factors that bring about changes in ventricular end-diastolic volume (the preload), aortic pressure (the afterload), and the contractility of the heart will alter the stroke volume.

stroke work the amount of energy converted to work by each ventricle to raise the pressure of the blood from a low venous pressure to a high arterial pressure during each beat of the heart. For the left ventricle, it is equivalent to the stroke volume × (left ventricular mean ejection pressure – left atrial pressure). Because the right ventricle pumps against a smaller systolic pressure, it must perform less stroke work than the left side.

stroma (stro'mah), pl. *stromata* [Gr. *strōma* anything laid out for lying or sitting on] 1. the supporting tissue or matrix of an organ, as distinguished from its functional element, or parenchyma.
2. the supporting connective tissue of a tumor.
3. the portion of the erythrocyte remaining after hemolysis.

stromal sarcoma (stro'mal) a malignant tumor that arises from the supporting connective tissue cells of an organ such as the uterus or breast.

Strongylata a suborder of nematodes of the order Rhabditida, including the superfamilies Strongyloidea, Trichostrongyloidea, and Metastrongyloidea.

Strongylidae (stron-jil'ĭ-de) a family of nematodes of the order Rhabditida, including the genera *Ternidens* and *Oesophagostomum*.

Strongyloidea (stron'jĭ-loi'de-ah) a superfamily of nematodes of the suborder Strongylata, order Rhabditida, including the genera *Ancylostoma, Necator, Ternidens,* and *Oesophagostomum*.

Strongyloididae a family of nematodes of the order Rhabditida, including the genus *Strongyloides*.

strontium (Sr) (stron'she-um) [*Strontian* a village in Scotland] a silvery white metal; atomic number 38; atomic weight 87.62; Group II of the periodic table (the alkaline earths); oxidation state +2. Strontium rapidly oxidizes and turns yellow in air; it also reacts with water, releasing hydrogen.

strontium-90 (^{90}Sr, Sr 90) a beta-emitting isotope of strontium with a half-life of 38 yr. It occurs in nuclear reactor waste and in nuclear weapons fallout. When ingested or inhaled, strontium-90 is deposited in bone, in which it can cause a malignant neoplasm.

structural (struk'tūr-al) pertaining to or affecting structure.

structural gene a gene containing coded information for the synthesis of specific proteins. See also *gene* and *regulatory gene*.

structural protein one of a group of protein molecules that meet structural requirements in tissues. These proteins often have a high ratio of length to diameter and are constructed to form fibers by associating side-by-side. Both the dermis and the epidermis illustrate supporting structures formed by fibers embedded in an amorphous matrix. The physical properties of biologic combinations of fibers and matrix vary with the materials in the two phases. The fibers may range from flexible shafts to rigid rods, and the matrix may be a hard casting or a resilient bed. Materials in fibers and matrix include proteins and polysaccharides.

Examples of structural proteins include keratin, collagen, and elastin. Disturbances in the formation of structural protein can result in one of a number of distinct disease entities.

structure (struk'chur) [L. *struere* to build] the configuration, composition, or arrangement of the components of a complex entity.

β-structure see *pleated sheet*.

struma (stroo'mah) [L.] an enlargement of the thyroid gland; see *goiter*.
s. lymphomatosa, see *chronic t.* under *thyroiditis*.

struma ovarii a teratoma of the ovary that contains thyroid tissue.

Strümpell-Lorrain disease see *spinocerebellar degeneration.*

strychnine (strik'nīn) [Gr. *strychnos* nightshade] an extremely toxic alkaloid extracted from seeds of the tropical genus *Strychnos.* It was once used medicinally as a stimulant and tonic and is now employed commercially as a rodent poison. The primary mode of action is blockade of postsynaptic inhibitors in nervous tissue.

Strychnine poisoning produces tonic convulsions that last about 1 min and soon cause death by respiratory paralysis. Artificial respiration and oxygen administration are used to prevent respiratory failure and short-acting barbiturates, and muscle relaxants are used to stop the convulsions.

strychnine assays 1. color reaction. Strychnine is extracted from alkalinized samples into chloroform. The solvent is evaporated, and Mandelin's reagent is added to the residue. If strychnine is present, the color changes from blue to violet to red-orange.

2. ultraviolet spectrophotometry. A chloroform extract (as above) is reextracted into acid. The absorbance at 286 nm is proportional to the strychnine concentration.

STS abbrev. See *serologic test for syphilis.*

S-T segment the portion of the electrocardiogram (ECG) between the end of the S wave and the beginning of the T wave. S-T segment changes take place during a variety of cardiac disorders: S-T segment elevation is a common EKG finding subsequent to acute myocardial infarction, left ventricular aneurysm, or Prinzmetal's (variant) angina. Depression of the segment may occur with myocardial ischemia.

Stuart factor see *Factor X.*

Stuart-Prower factor see *Factor X.*

student's t test see *t test.*

stupor (stu'por) [L.] a state of unresponsiveness from which temporary arousal is possible only by vigorous and repeated stimulation. Most stuporous patients have organic neurologic disease, but psychologic factors occasionally are implicated in some, with the "stupor" relating to hysteria, depressive illness, or schizophrenia. See also *consciousness disorder.*

Sturge-Weber syndrome (sterg web'er) [William Allen *Sturge,* British physician, 1850–1919; Frederick Parkes *Weber,* British physician, 1863–1962] a rare congenital disorder thought to result from the faulty development of select mesodermal and ectodermal elements. It is characterized by an extensive vascular nevus in the cutaneous area served by the trigeminal nerve, associated with an ipsilateral meningeal angioma. Cerebral involvement may lead to seizures, motor or sensory deficits, visual field defects, and mental retardation; blindness may occur as a result of glaucoma.

Calcium bands develop in the cortex subadjacent to the meninges, presenting a characteristic "railroad track" radiographic picture. Radiopacities of the skull are also observed. The electroencephalogram sometimes shows decreased background activity on the affected side, but this cannot be directly correlated to the degree of cerebral calcification. Focal slow activity may also be present unilaterally.

Also called *encephalotrigeminal syndrome.*

sty (sti), pl. *styes* a staphylococcal abscess (hordeolum) of a sebaceous gland that occurs on an eyelid. An internal hordeolum affects the meibomian gland, whereas an external hordeolum is an abscess of the gland of Moll or Zeis. Also called *hordeolum.*

styloid (sti'loid) [Gr. *stylos* pillar + *eidos* form] resembling a pillar; long and pointed.

styloid process a long, slender projection that juts down and slightly forward from the inferior surface of the temporal bone.

S. typhi see *S. typhi* under *Salmonella.*

styptic (stip'tik) [Gr. *styptikos*] 1. astringent; arresting hemorrhage.

2. an astringent and hemostatic agent.

Stypven time (stip'ven) see under *Russell viper venom.*

styramate (sti'rah-māt) a drug chemically related to meprobamate, formerly used as a central skeletal muscle relaxant.

styrene (sti'rēn) a liquid hydrocarbon with penetrating odor, vinyl benzene, $C_6H_5 \cdot CH{:}CH_2$. Its main use is in the manufacture of polystyrene, a familiar plastic.

sub- (sub) [L. *sub* under] a prefix word element to denote under or below, e.g., subclavian.

subacute (sub"ah-kūt') somewhat acute; between acute and chronic.

subacute bacterial endocarditis (SBE) see *subacute infective e.* under *endocarditis.*

subaortic stenosis a cardiac malformation that produces obstruction to left ventricular outflow at a site below the aortic valve. Also called subvalvular stenosis.

discrete s. s., subaortic stenosis due to a membranous or fibrous lesion in the outflow tract below the aortic valve, creating a pressure gradient across the obstructive site. The symptoms may include dyspnea, angina, or syncope; dilation of the ascending aorta or mild aortic regurgitation also are commonly observed.

Left ventricular angiocardiography can be used to identify the specific site of obstruction. Echocardiography and the recording of intracardiac pressures are techniques frequently used to differentiate between this condition and valvular or hypertrophic subvalvular aortic stenosis. Surgical excision of the obstructive lesion may bring about a complete cure or an improvement in the hemodynamic state of the afflicted individual.

idiopathic hypertrophic s. s. (IHSS), a cardiomyopathy associated with a pronounced thickening of the septum and/or free wall of the left ventricle. It is of uncertain etiology, although believed to be transmitted as an autosomal dominant trait. A systolic anterior motion (SAM) of the anterior leaflet of the mitral valve may be present; this motion may create obstruction to left ventricular ejection (by opposing the leaflet to the hypertrophied septum) that commonly is associated with the condition.

The symptoms include dyspnea, angina, and syncope; overt congestive heart failure, dizziness, and palpitation are less commonly observed. Clinical manifestations of IHSS include an abnormal electrocardiogram, a midsystolic murmur best heard between the apex and left sternal border, a loud fourth heart sound, an exaggerated a wave in the apexcardiogram and in the jugular venous pulse, and a "spike-and-dome" complex in the carotid pressure tracing.

Echocardiographic techniques may reveal a small ventricular cavity, an abnormal septal-to-free wall ratio (greater than 1.3), a narrowing of the left ventricular outflow tract, or a partial midsystolic closure or pronounced fluttering of the aortic valve. Cardiac catheterization may reveal a pressure gradient within the left ventricle. Bizarrely shaped, hypertrophied, and disarrayed myocardial cells may be present on pathologic examination.

subarachnoid space a narrow space between the arachnoid mater and pia mater that contains the cerebrospinal fluid.

subbasal projection (sub-ba′sal) an axial radiographic projection of the base of the skull (verticosubmental or submentovertical) that is not a full basal view. Various angulations are used to obtain projections of the jugular or carotid foramina or of parts of the ear that are not obscured by other structures. Cf. *basal projection.*

subclavian (sub-kla′ve-an) situated under the clavicle.

subclavian artery the main artery to the upper limb. The right artery arises from the brachiocephalic trunk, and the left arises directly from the arch of the aorta. At the outer border of the first rib, the subclavian becomes the axillary artery.

subclavian steal syndrome brain stem ischemia that results from the diversion of blood flow from the basilar artery to the subclavian artery in the presence of occlusive disease of the proximal portion of the subclavian artery. If neurologic symptoms develop, they do so following exercise of the arm on the affected side. Diagnosis may be suggested by the absence of pulses in the upper extremity on the affected side.

subclavian vein the continuation of the axillary vein in the thorax. It extends from the outer border of the first rib to the medial border of the scalenus anterior, where it joins with the internal jugular to form the brachiocephalic vein.

subcostal (sub-kos′tal) situated beneath the ribs.

subcostal line the line on the surface of the abdomen in the subcostal plane. Also called *infracostal line.*

subcostal margin the lower border of the rib cage.

subcostal plane the horizontal plane that intersects the trunk at the level of the lower margin of the tenth costal cartilages.

subculture (sub′kul-tūr) 1. a culture of bacteria derived from another culture.

2. the act of preparing a fresh culture from an existing one.

subcutaneous (sub″ku-ta′ne-us) beneath the skin.

subcutis (sub-ku′tis) [*sub-* + L. *cutis* skin] a layer of fat beneath the dermis, the subcutaneous tissue.

subdural space a potential space between the arachnoid mater and dura mater that contains a thin film of fluid.

subharmonic (sub″har-mon′ik) in acoustics, pertaining to a waveform having a frequency that is an integral submultiple of a reference frequency (fundamental).

subjacent (sub-ja′sent) [*sub-* + L. *jacere* to lie] lying just beneath or underneath.

sublimation (sub″lĭ-ma′shun) [L. *sublimatio*] the transformation of a substance directly from the solid state to the gaseous state without passing through the liquid state. Above the critical temperature, solids sublime as the pressure is reduced; below it they become liquids, then vapors.

Sublimaze (sub′lĭ-māz) trademark. See *fentanyl citrate.*

sublingual (sub-ling′gwal) located beneath the tongue.

submaxill/o (sub-mak′sil-o) a word element used in combining form to denote the mandible, e.g., submaxillary.

submaxillary (sub-mak′sĭ-ler″e) situated beneath the maxilla.

submaxillary glycoprotein a glycoprotein of the saliva that is particularly rich in carbohydrate. That from sheep contains more than 800 disaccharide units—one for every six amino acid residues, on the average—amounting to about 40 percent of its mass. Most of the carbohydrate residues are *N*-acetylneuraminate and *N*-acetylglycosamine, attached to either serine or threonine of the protein.

submaxillary region the region of the front of the neck on either side of the submental region and below the mandible.

submental (sub-men′tal) [*sub-* + L. *mentum* chin] below the chin.

submental region the region of the front of the neck beneath the chin.

submentovertical (sub-men″to-ver′tĭ-kal) pertaining to a basal or subbasal radiographic projection in which the central ray passes from the base to the vertex. Cf. *verticosubmental.*

submetacentric (sub″met-ah-sen′trik) pertaining to a mitotic chromosome having the centromere closer to one end than the other, so that one arm is appreciably longer than the other. Cf. *metacentric, subtelocentric,* and *telocentric.*

submucosa (sub″mu-ko′sah) a layer of areolar tissue beneath a mucous membrane.

submucosal (sub″mu-ko′sal) pertaining to the submucosa, or situated beneath the mucous membrane.

subroutine (sub′roo-tēn) a computer program, or program segment, that is executed at the command of a user program to perform a specific task. When finished, a subroutine returns control to the program that invoked it at the point of invocation. Data may be exchanged between the calling program and subroutines. Local subroutines are contained in the user program; global or system subroutines are part of the operating system and available to all programs. See also *variable passing.*

subscript (sub′skript) 1. a distinguishing letter, number, or formula written below and to the right of a symbol. In mathematics, a subscript serves to indicate a particular element of a set, such as a component of a vector, a term in a sequence, or a particular value of a variable. In a chemical formula, subscripts indicate the number of atoms of each element in a molecule or substituent group; e.g., Na_2CO_3 containing two atoms of sodium, one of carbon, and three of oxygen. Cf. *superscript.*

2. see under *subscripted variable.*

subscripted variable in high-level computer languages, a variable name associated with a set of values. A particular value is specified by a "subscript," which is usually written in parentheses after the variable name: e.g., B(10) refers to the tenth value associated with the variable B. Many languages allow multiple subscripts: imagine a rectangular array of values; then, B(R,C) might refer to the value in the R-th row and C-th column.

subscription (sub-skrip′shun) [*sub-* + L. *scribere* to write] see under *prescription.*

subspecies (sub′spe-sēz) see *race.*

substance (sub′stans) [L. *substantia*] 1. in anatomy, the material constituting an organ or body.

2. in chemistry, an element or compound. Also called pure substance.

3. in physics, matter, especially a complex mixture of pure chemical substances.

substantia nigra (sub-stan′she-ah ni′grah), pl. *substantiae* [L.] [NA], a layer of darkly pigmented gray matter that separates the tegmentum from the crus cerebri. These melanin-containing, multipolar neurons are connected with the cerebral cortex, spinal cord, hypothalamus, and basal ganglia.

substituent (sub-stich′u-ent) in the systematic nomenclature of organic chemistry, an atom or group of atoms in a chemical compound considered as having replaced a hydrogen atom in the parent compound (an unbranched aliphatic hydrocarbon or an unsubstituted aromatic ring). The position of the substituent is indicated by a locant (usually a number) preceding the prefix for the substituent. For example, in 1-chloro-2-methylbutane, butane is the parent compound and chlorine and the methyl group are substituents.

substitution (sub″stĭ-tu′shun) [L. *substitutio,* from *sub* under + *statuere* to place] the act of putting one thing in place of another, especially the chemical replacement of an atom or group in a substrate by another atom or group.

substitution reaction a chemical reaction in which one substituent (atom or group of atoms) in a compound is replaced by another substituent. In organic chemistry, a reaction in which a substituent on a carbon atom is replaced, e.g., $CH_4 + Br_2 \rightarrow CH_3Br + HBr$. See also *addition reaction* and *elimination reaction.*

substrate (sub′strāt) [*sub-* + L. *stratum* layer] 1. a substance on which an enzyme acts or, more specifically, the chemical entity whose transformation to a product or products is catalyzed by an enzyme. Frequently, an enzymatic reaction requires two substances, and the designation of one of the reactants as the major substrate is an arbitrary choice.

2. the supporting surface on which a printed circuit or integrated circuit is fabricated.

3. in biology, the surface on which or the liquid in which an organism grows.

substrate level phosphorylation the creation of a high-energy phosphate linkage in a metabolite, rather than by electron flow on the mitochondrial membrane. An example is the formation of 1,3-bisphospho-D-glycerate from D-glyceraldehyde-3-phosphate and inorganic phosphate by the enzyme glyceraldehyde phosphate dehydrogenase. The high-energy phosphate of the bisphosphoglycerate can be transferred by a kinase enzyme to ADP to form ATP.

subsynchronous (sub″sin′kro-nus) operating at a frequency that is a submultiple of the source frequency, e.g., a subsynchronous motor.

subtelocentric (sub-tel″o-sen′trik) pertaining to a mitotic chromosome having the centromere near one end, so that one arm is much longer than the other. Also called *acrocentric.* Cf. *acrocentric, metacentric, submetacentric,* and *telocentric.*

subtraction methods in radiology, procedures by which obscuring shadows are canceled out of a radiograph. A radiograph (called the zero film, base film, or control film) is made of the obscuring structures. Without any movement by the patient, the contrast medium is then injected, opacifying the structure to be demonstrated (e.g., in angiography, the blood vessels), and a series of radiographs is made.

A positive transparency (called the reversal film, positive mask, or diapositive) is made from the base film; this changes the radiopaque obscuring structures, such as bones, from white in the base film to black in the reversal film. The reversal film is then registered (precisely superimposed) over a selected film of the series, and a print (the subtraction film) is made. Because of the imprecision of the developing process, densities in reversal film will not be exactly the opposite of the control film. To achieve perfect cancellation, the base film and reversal film are registered and a print showing the difference in densities is made. The diapositive of this print (called the secondary mask or correction mask) is registered over the base film and the film of the opacified structure. Prints made by this technique (called second-order subtraction) have nearly perfect cancellation of obscuring structures.

See also *digital radiography.*

succinic acid (suk′sĭ-nik) 1,4-butanedioic acid, $COOH(CH_2)_2COOH$, occurring in amber, lichens, and fossils, and in certain hydatid cysts. Succinic acid was formerly used both in the treatment of diabetic ketosis and, combined with salicylates, in the treatment of rheumatic fever and arthritis. It is an intermediate of the tricarboxylic acid cycle. In human plasma it has a concentration of 0.1–0.6 mg/dl (8–50 μmol/l). Both succinic acid and its salts are used as buffers in the pH range of 3.2–6.6 ($pK'_{a_1} = 4.2$; $pK'_{a_2} = 5.6$).

succinylcholine chloride (suk″sĭ-nil-ko′lēn) [USP], a depolarizing neuromuscular blocking drug used to induce skeletal muscle relaxation during surgery and also during electroconvulsive therapy. It is rapidly hydrolyzed to choline and succinic acid by the plasma enzyme pseudocholinesterase. Individuals having low levels of this enzyme due to severe liver disease, to insecticide poisoning by cholinesterase inhibitors, or to a recessive hereditary trait should be given minimal doses. Adverse reactions, primarily respiratory depression, are caused by excessive action of the drug; its effect usually disappears in 5–10 min, unless repeated doses are administered. See also *cholinesterase assays* and *pseudocholinesterase deficiency.*

succinylcoenzyme A (suk″sĭ-nil-ko′en-zīm) the succinate thioester of coenzyme A, $COOH(CH_2)_2$-COSCoA. It is notably an intermediate in the tricarboxylic acid cycle but also occurs elsewhere, as in the metabolism of fatty acid and valine and in the synthesis of protoporphyrin, methionine, and lysine.

sucking louse see *Anoplura* and *Pediculus.*

Sucquet-Hoyer canal (sik-a′ oy-ār) a regulatory anastomosis between small peripheral arteries and veins, especially in the hands and feet, but also found is some viscera. See also *glomus.*

sucrase (su′krās) an enzyme of the hydrolase class (sucrose α-D-glucohydrolase, EC 3.2.1.48, one of the disaccharidases) that catalyzes the hydrolysis of α-D-glucoside linkages in sucrose, maltose, and isomaltose. A congenital deficiency of the enzyme results in sucrose intolerance and/or inadequate utilization of disaccharides. See also *disaccharide deficiency, sucrose,* and *sucrose α-D-glucohydrolase.*

sucrose (su′krōs) [L. *sucrosum*] a nonreducing disaccharide composed of glucose and fructose units. It is an α-D-glucopyranosyl-β-D-fructofuranoside. Unlike most disaccharides, sucrose is abundant in the plant world. Sucrose is readily hydrolyzed to glucose and fructose by acid or by the enzyme invertase.

Sucrose is soluble in water and is often used as a food-sweetening agent and in pharmaceutical products. It is involved in the development of dental caries with the formation of a microbial plaque. *Streptococcus mutans* will utilize sucrose to synthesize a dextranlike extracellular capsule that helps the organism to adhere to teeth, an important factor in the development of dental plaque.

Sucrose, among other sugars, is used in bacteriology in the identification of individual organisms in fermentation tests.

See also *sugar.*

sucrose α-D-glucohydrolase (su′krōs gloo″ko-hi′dro-lās) an enzyme of the hydrolase class (EC 3.2.1.48) that catalyzes the hydrolysis of sucrose and maltose by an α-D-glucosidase–type action. The enzyme is isolated from the intestinal mucosa as a complex and also displays activity toward isomaltose. See also *sucrase.*

sucrose hemolysis test a screening test for paroxysmal nocturnal hemoglobinuria (PNH). In the procedure, red cells from a patient are placed in a fresh serum and isotonic sucrose solution, which promotes the binding of complement components to the red cells; hemolysis is virtually diagnostic for PNH. This is because in PNH some red cells have abnormal sensitivity to complement-mediated lysis.

sucrose intolerance a rare inborn error of metabolism characterized by various degrees of gastrointestinal distress on the ingestion of sucrose. It is caused by a deficiency of the enzyme β-D-fructofuranosidase in the intestinal mucosa. See also *disaccharidase deficiency.*

suction (suk′shun) [L. *sugere* to suck] the aspiration of material into a tube drawn by a partial vacuum in the tube.

Suctoria (suk-to′re-ah) a class of protozoa of the subphylum Ciliophora. These protozoa have cilia only during the larval stage. Most are free-living and are occasionally parasitic in mammals.

Sudafed (soo′dah-fed) trademark. See *pseudoephedrine hydrochloride.*

sudamen (soo-da′men), pl. *sudamina* [L.] a small, whitish vesicle caused by retention of sweat in the layers of the epidermis.

Sudan (su-dan′) any of a large group of fat-soluble disazo dyes, used as histologic stains for neutral fats. See also *fat stains.*

S. I, an orange disazo dye; C.I. 12055.

S. II, an orange-yellow monoazo dye; C.I. 12140.

S. III, an orange-red dye, phenylazophenylazo-β-naphthol; C.I. 26100.

S. IV, a red dye, *o*-tolylazo-*o*-tolylazo-β-naphthol; C.I. 26105. Also called *scarlet red.*

S. black B, a black, fat-soluble disazo dye; C.I. 26150. The dye also contains two secondary amine groups and can act as a basic dye for staining connective tissue. It is less suitable for the staining of neutral fats than other stains such as oil red O, but it is superior to other fat stains for the demonstration of phospholipids and cerebrosides. Provided that proper fixation is obtained, these compounds can be demonstrated with Sudan black in paraffin sections.

sudanophil (soo-dan′o-fil) a tissue component that stains readily with Sudan.

sudanophilia affinity for Sudan or other oil-soluble dyes. Sudanophilia generally indicates the presence of lipids.

sudanophilic (soo-dan″o-fil′ik) staining readily with Sudan dyes.

sudden infant death syndrome (SIDS) the unexpected sudden death of an infant who was previously well, and whose death cannot be explained following an adequate autopsy. The incidence is between 1 and 3 deaths per 1000 live births. Infants are usually between 2 and 4 mo of age, and some have been premature births. Males are affected more frequently than females, and the occurrence is more common in the lower social strata and under conditions of poor maternal care.

Death often occurs during the night, but when an observer has been present, the child is said to simply stop breathing and become limp. The mechanism is not understood, but sudden interruption of the central mechanism for control of respiratory or cardiac function has been postulated. Another possibility is occlusion of the respiratory passages as, for example, by laryngeal spasm. Such deaths are more common in cold weather, and respiratory or other infections have been implicated, including botulinum toxin in a small number of cases. There are no specific pathologic findings, but thickening of the walls of small arteries in the lungs has been reported.

Also called cot death and crib death.

Sudeck's disease (soo′deks) [Paul Hermann Martin *Sudeck,* Hamburg surgeon, 1866–1938] a form of regional osteoporosis that is due to reflex sympathetic dystrophy and vasomotor changes, and most commonly occurs in the hands, wrists, and feet. There may be pain, tenderness, and swelling of underlying tissues. Sudeck's disease occurs following fractures or other trauma; it is often episodic and recurrent and may terminate in permanent skeletal injury. In severe cases, regional sympathectomy may be required. X-rays reveal punched-out areas of bony rarefaction. Also called Sudeck-Leriche syndrome.

sufficient condition in logic, a proposition that is sufficient for another to hold. That A is a sufficient condition for B means if A is true, then B is true; however, if A is false, B may be either true or false. Equivalent statements are "A implies B" and "B if A." Cf. *necessary condition.*

sugar (shoog′ar) [L. *saccharum;* Gr. *sakcharon*] 1. a general term meaning any carbohydrate, although the term is usually reserved for the simpler carbohydrates, the mono- and disaccharides, which are sweet and crystalline. See also *carbohydrate.*

2. common table sugar; see also *sucrose.*

invert s., a mixture of glucose (dextrose) and fructose (levulose), in a ratio of approximately 1:1 that is obtained by the hydrolysis of sucrose. Honey is mostly invert sugar. The name arises from the fact that, whereas the original sucrose has a positive sign of rotation, the hydrolysis product mixture has a net negative sign; the sign of rotation has been inverted.

sugar acid a compound formed by the oxidation of a monosaccharide to a carboxylic acid or a dicarboxylic acid. The most important members of this class are the acids derived from oxidation of an aldose at the carbon-1 aldehyde carbon (an aldonic acid), at the terminal hydroxymethyl group (a uronic acid), or at both carbons (an aldaric acid). Examples are gluconic acid, glucuronic acid, and saccharic (glucaric) acid.

sulcus (sul'kus), pl. *sulci* [L.] 1. [NA], a general term for a groove, trench, or furrow, especially one on the surface of the brain, between the gyri.

2. a linear depression or valley in the occlusal surface of a tooth.

sulfabenzamide (sul″fah-benz'ah-mīd) one of the sulfonamide group of antibacterial drugs, *N*-sulfanilylbenzamide. See also *sulfonamide*.

sulfacetamide (sul″fah-se'tah-mīd) one of the sulfonamide group of antibacterial drugs, *N*-sulfanilylacetamide. See also *sulfonamide*.

s. sodium, [USP], a salt used in ophthalmic ointments and solutions to treat ocular infections.

sulfadiazine (sul″fah-di'ah-zēn) [USP], one of the sulfonamide group of antibacterial drugs, 2-sulfanilamidopyrimidine, used in the treatment of urinary tract infections. See also *antibacterial agents* and *sulfonamide*.

sulfa drug (sul'fah) see *sulfonamide*.

sulfaguanidine (sul″fah-gwan'ĭ-dēn) one of the sulfonamide group of antibacterial drugs. See also *antibacterial agents* and *sulfonamide*.

sulfamerazine (sul″fah-mer'ah-zēn) [USP], one of the sulfonamide group of antibacterial drugs. See also *antibacterial agents* and *sulfonamide*.

sulfameter (sul'fah-me″ter) a long-acting member of the sulfonamide group of antibacterial drugs, 5-methoxysulfadiazine, used in the treatment of urinary tract infections. Trademark, Sulla. See also *sulfonamide*.

sulfamethazine (sul″fah-meth'a-zēn) [USP], one of the sulfonamide group of antibacterial drugs. See also *antibacterial agents* and *sulfonamide*.

sulfamethizole (sul″fah-meth'ĭ-zōl) [USP], one of the sulfonamide group of antibacterial drugs, 2-sulfanilamido-5-methyl-1,3,4-thiadiazole, used in the treatment of urinary tract infections. Trademark, *Thiosulfil*. See also *antibacterial agents* and *sulfonamide*.

sulfamethoxazole (sul″fah-meth-oks'ah-zōl) [USP], one of the sulfonamide group of antibacterial compounds, 3-sulfanilamido-5-methylisoxazole, used alone and in combination with trimethoprim (to block two steps in the synthesis of folinic acid) in the treatment of urinary tract infections, otitis media, and acute bronchial infections. Trademarks, Gantanol and, in combinations with trimethoprim, *Bactrim* and *Septra*. See also *antibacterial agents* and *sulfonamide*.

sulfanilamide (sul″fah-nil'ah-mīd) a white crystalline solid, *p*-aminobenzenesulfonamide; M.W. 172.21. The first sulfa drug, it has now been replaced by more effective and less toxic derivatives. See also *antibacterial agents* and *sulfonamide*.

sulfanilic acid (sul″fah-nil'ik) a white crystalline solid, *p*-aminobenzenesulfonic acid, $H_2NC_6H_4SO_3H$; M.W. 173.84. It is utilized in organic synthesis and as an analytic reagent; for example, Ehrlich's diazo reagent, used for the detection and quantitation of bilirubin, and Pauly's reagent, used to detect histidine, other imidazoles, tyrosine, and other phenolic compounds in thin-media chromatography.

sulfapyridine (sul″fah-pir'ĭ-dēn) [USP], one of the sulfonamide group of antibacterial drugs. See also *antibacterial agents* and *sulfonamide*.

sulfatase (sul'fah-tās) one of a sub-subclass of enzymes (sulfuric ester hydrolases, EC 3.1.6) of the hydrolase class that catalyzes the hydrolysis of a sulfuric acid ester into sulfuric acid and an alcohol. See also *arylsulfatase*.

sulfate (sul'fāt) [L. *sulphas*] pertaining to the SO_4^{2-} ion or to a compound containing this ion.

sulfathiazole (sul″fah-thi'ah-zōl) one of the sulfonamide group of antibacterial drugs, 2-sulfanilamidothiazole. See also *sulfonamide*.

sulfatidase see *arylsulfatase*.

sulfatide (sul'fah-tīd) a glycosphingolipid with a sulfate ester at one of the sugar hydroxyls, usually the hydroxyl group at carbon 3. Phrenosin sulfate is an example, containing D-galactose-3-sulfate, and the 2-hydroxy fatty acid, cerebronic acid. See also *cerebroside sulfatide*.

sulfatide lipidosis see *metachromatic l.* under *leukodystrophy*.

sulfatide sulfatase see *arylsulfatase*.

sulfation (sul-fa'shun) 1. the oxidation of a sulfide to a sulfate.

2. the addition of a sulfate group to a chemical compound; the conversion of a chemical compound to a sulfate.

3. a process by which substituents in tissues containing alcohol groups are converted to sulfuric acid monoesters. This process renders neutral compounds acidic and increases their basophilia.

sulfation factor see *somatomedin C*.

sulfhemoglobin (sulf″he-mo-glo'bin) a greenish substance that arises in vitro from the interaction of hemoglobin with hydrogen sulfide in the presence of an oxidizing agent. Not normally found in blood, it can be caused by the same drugs that cause the formation of methemoglobin (e.g., phenacetin, sulfonamides, and acetanilid), but it can also arise without drug exposure. Why some individuals form methemoglobin and others form sulfhemoglobin is not known. Sulfhemoglobin cannot carry oxygen nor can it be reconverted to hemoglobin. The characteristic spectral absorbance peak is at 620 nm; it cannot be converted to cyanmethemoglobin on the addition of cyanide. Also called *sulfmethemoglobin*.

sulfhemoglobinemia (sulf″he-mo-glo″bin-e'me-ah) the presence of sulfhemoglobin in the blood, which results in cyanosis. See also *sulfhemoglobin*. Cf. *methemoglobinemia*.

sulfhydryl group (sulf-hi'dril) the univalent radical, —SH.

sulfide (sul'fīd) 1. a compound containing sulfur in the –2 oxidation state, such as hydrogen sulfide (H_2S).

2. an organic sulfide, R—S—R'; also called *thio-*

ether. In IUPAC nomenclature, sulfides are named like ethers, such as methyl sulfide, $(CH_3)_2S$, and ethyl methyl sulfide, $C_2H_5SCH_3$. *Chemical Abstracts* does not use the term sulfide; these compounds are called thiobismethane and (methylthio)ethane.

sulfinic acid (sul-fin′ik) an organic acid that contains the functional group $—SO_2H$. Cf. *sulfonic acid.*

sulfinpyrazone (sul″fin-pi′rah-zōn) [USP], a uricosuric drug, used to treat the hyperuricemia of chronic and intermittent gouty arthritis, although not during acute attacks. It is a pyrazolone derivative related to phenylbutazone. Major side-effects are gastrointestinal intolerance and hypersensitivity; blood dyscrasias including thrombocytopenia may also occur. Trademark, Anturane.

sulfinyl (sul′fĭ-nil) the functional group —SO—. See also *sulfoxide* and *sulfinic acid.*

sulfisoxazole (sul″fĭ-sok′sah-zōl) [USP], one of the sulfonamide group of antibacterial drugs, 5-sulfanilamido-3,4-dimethylisoxazole, used in the treatment of urinary tract infections. Trademark, *Gantrisin.* See also *antibacterial agents* and *sulfonamide.*

s. acetyl, a tasteless derivative digested to sulfisoxazole.

s. diolamine, a salt used in ophthalmic solutions and ointments to treat ocular infections; it is also used in injectable preparations.

sulfite (sul′fīt) [L. *sulfis*] pertaining to the SO_3^{2-} ion or to a compound containing this ion.

sulfite oxidase an enzyme of the oxidoreductase class (EC 1.8.3.1) that catalyzes the reaction sulfite $+ O_2 + H_20 \rightleftarrows$ sulfate $+ H_2O_2$. The enzyme contains molybdenum and a hemoprotein, and is important in brain metabolism.

sulfite oxidase deficiency a disorder of cysteine metabolism, transmitted as an autosomal recessive trait, that is due to a relative or absolute deficiency of the enzyme sulfite oxidase. Those affected have increased levels of *S*-sulfo-L-cysteine sulfite, and thiosulfite in the urine. The most common clinical manifestations include mental retardation, central nervous system dysfunction with a decerebrate posture, and dislocation of lenses. See also *aminoacidopathy.*

sulfmethemoglobin (sulf″met-he″mo-glo′bin) see *sulfhemoglobin.*

sulfo- (sul′fo) a prefix word element to denote the $—SO_3H$ group when it must be treated as a substituent in a polyfunctional compound, e.g., sulfoacetic acid, HO_3SCH_2COOH.

sulfobromophthalein sodium (sul″fo-bro″mo-thal′e-in) [USP], phenol-tetrabromphthalein-disodium sulfonate; M.W. 838.05. It is an indicator-type material used to evaluate the capacity of the liver to conjugate and excrete foreign materials present in the blood, and is available in ampoules containing 3.0 or 7.5 ml of a solution with 50 mg of indicator per 1.0 ml. Trademark, *Bromsulphalein.* Also called bromosulfophthalein. See also *dye excretion tests.*

***S*-sulfoglutathione** (sul″fo-gloo″tah-thi′ōn) an analog of glutathione, which occurs in the lens of the eye. In the analog, cysteine is replaced by *S*-sulfocysteine.

L-sulfoiduronate sulfatase see *iduronic sulfatase.*

sulfolipid (sul″fo-lip′id) a lipid of the cerebroside type that contains one or more sulfate groups.

sulfomucin (sul″fo-mu′sin) mucin that contains sulfated glycosaminoglycans in the polysaccharide component. See also *mucin.*

sulfonamide (sul-fon′ah-mid) 1. an organic compound that contains the functional group $—SO_2NH_2$.

2. Any of a large class of antibacterial drugs, derivatives of sulfonanilamide (*p*-aminobenzenesulfonamide, $H_2NC_6H_4SO_2NH_2$), which is similar to *p*-aminobenzoic acid (PABA), a substance required by bacteria for folic acid synthesis. Most have a pyrimidine or thiazole ring or an acyl group bound to the sulfonamide nitrogen. The sulfonamides are bacteriostatic only and inhibit the incorporation of PABA into dihydropteroic acid, PABA being a precursor of folic acid and a coenyzme involved in DNA synthesis. The ultimate result of decreased folic acid synthesis is a decrease in bacterial nucleotide concentration.

Many chemical modifications of the sulfonamides have been made, but fewer than 20 are useful clinically, having been replaced largely by more effective and less toxic antibacterial agents. Among the more important sulfonamides are sulfadiazine, sulfamethoxazole, and the poorly absorbed phthalylsulfathiazole and sulfaguanidine.

ANTIMICROBIAL ACTIVITY. Organisms synthesizing folic acid are susceptible to sulfonamides, whereas those requiring preformed folic acid are resistant. In vitro, sulfonamides exhibit inhibitory activity against a variety of gram-positive and gram-negative species. The in vitro antimicrobial susceptibility to sulfonamides is influenced by inoculum size and test medium composition. High concentrations of PABA and thymidine in test media inhibit sulfonamide activity.

RESISTANCE. Resistance to sulfonamides is due either to microbial overproduction of PABA or to a structural change in the target enzyme that lowers affinity for sulfonamides. Decreased permeability to sulfonamides can result in bacterial resistance.

CLINICAL USE. Sulfonamides have several uses, including: (1) the treatment of acute urinary tract infections due to susceptible bacteria; (2) the treatment of infections due to *Nocardia asteroides;* (3) the prophylaxis of patients against recurrent rheumatic fever associated with group A streptococci; (4) the prophylaxis of close contacts of patients with meningitis due to *Neisseria meningitidis;* and (5) the treatment of toxoplasmosis, dermatitis herpetiformis, lymphogranuloma venereum, chancroid, trachoma-inclusion conjunctivitis, and nongonococcal urethritis. Sulfonamides are often used in conjunction with trimethoprim.

The most common adverse reactions are headache, apathy, nausea, vomiting, crystalluria, photosensitization, and skin rashes. Serious toxic reactions include hypersensitivity reactions, lowering of blood cell count, and oliguria or hematuria due to the deposition of insoluble crystals of the drug in the renal tubules.

Sulfonamides are excreted in the urine; one fraction is unchanged, another is acetylated by the liver. The acetylated form has no bacteriostatic activity and is less soluble than the unchanged drug.

Also called *sulfa drug.* See also *antibacterial agents.*

sulfonamide assays 1. a color test. Urine is streaked on newspaper and covered with hydrochloric acid. An intense yellow or orange color indicates the presence of a sulfonamide, aminosalicylic acid, or another primary aryl amine. As little as 2 μg of drug can be detected.

2. ultraviolet spectrophotometry. Protein is removed from urine or blood samples by precipitation with trichloroacetic acid and filtration. Sodium nitrite, ammonium sulfamate, and then *N*-(1-naphthyl)-ethlenediamine dihydrochloride are added to the filtrate, and the reaction proceeds in the dark for 15 min, forming a diazo derivative. The absorbance at 550 nm is proportional to the free sulfonamide concentration in the sample. The total (free plus acetylated) sulfonamide may be determined by subjecting the filtrate to acid hydrolysis before preparation of the diazo derivative. Other primary aryl amines interfere.

sulfonation (sul″fo-na′shun) the introduction of a sulfo group (—SO_3H) into a chemical compound, which produces a sulfonic acid.

sulfone (sul′fōn) an organic compound that contains the sulfonyl functional group —SO_2—. The nomenclature is analogous to that for sulfoxides.

sulfones (sul′fōns) a group of synthetic antibacterial agents containing the sulfonyl group (R—SO_2—R). They are effective against many gram-negative and gram-positive bacteria by the same mechanism as that of the sulfonamides, but they have limited clinical usage because of their toxicity. The most important of the sulfones is dapsone, which is used in the treatment of leprosy. See also *antibacterial agents.*

sulfonethylmethane (sul″fōn-eth″il-meth-ān) a drug, 2,2-bis(ethyl sulfonyl) butane, which has been used as a hypnotic.

sulfonic acid (sul-fon′ik) an organic compound containing the functional group —$SO_2(OH)$, linking carbon to sulfur, such as ethanesulfonic acid, CH_3-CH_2—SO_2OH. Sulfonic acid derivatives include sulfonyl chlorides (R—SO_2—Cl), sulfonate esters (R—SO_2—OR′), and sulfonamides (R—SO_2—NH_2). Cf. *sulfinic acid.*

sulfonmethane (sul″fōn-meth′ān) a drug, 2,2-bis-(ethyl sulfonyl) propane, which has been used as a hypnotic.

sulfonyl (sul′fo-nil) the functional group —SO_2—. See also *sulfone* and *sulfonic acid.*

sulfonylurea (sul″fo-nil-u-re′ah) one of a group of oral hypoglycemic drugs that contain the functional group —$SO_2NHCONH$—, e.g., acetohexamide, chlorpropamide, tolazamide, or tolbutamide.

Sulfonylureas are used to lower the blood sugar in selected cases of patients with mild adult-onset diabetes mellitus who are not prone to ketosis and who do not require large doses of insulin. One mode of action is stimulation of insulin secretion by the beta cells of the pancreas; there is also a reduction in the glucose output of the liver.

Adverse reactions include gastrointestinal intolerance, severe hypoglycemia, hypersensitivity, low blood count, and alcohol intolerance (similar to that produced by disulfiram).

sulfonylurea assays gas chromatography using a flame ionization detector and a nonpolar silicone stationary phase is the preferred technique. Sulfonylureas are extracted from plasma or urine samples into toluene at pH 5.2. Reaction with trimethylanilinium hydroxide (TMAH) produces a dimethylsulfonamide derivative. The concentration of the drug in the sample is proportional to the ratio of the peak areas in the chromatogram of the sulfonylurea derivative and the internal standard (aprobarbital). Tolazamide and tolbutamide produce the same derivative and are not separately identified.

sulfoprotein (sul″fo-pro′te-in) [L. *sulphos*] a protein that has been modified by the conversion of a hydroxyl group to a sulfate ester or of an amino group to a sulfate amide. Gastrin II contains such a tyrosyl side-chain with sulfate. See also *phosphoprotein.*

sulfoxide (sul-fok′sīd) an organic compound that contains the functional group —SO—, such as dimethyl sulfoxide, $(CH_3)_2SO$. *Chemical Abstracts* names sulfoxides as sulfinyl derivatives, e.g., sulfinylbismethane, $(CH_3)_2SO$, or methylsulfinylethane, $CH_3SOC_2H_5$.

sulfur (S) (sul′fur) [L.] a yellow, solid, nonmetallic element; atomic number 16; atomic weight 32.06; Group VI of the periodic table; oxidation states –2, +4, +6. It occurs in many allotropic forms including rhombic and monoclinic crystals, and an amorphous polymeric plastic.

In biologic systems, sulfur occurs in thiol (R—SH), disulfide (R—S—S—R), thioether (R—S—R), and thioester (R—C—O—SR) groups (e.g., in the two amino acids cysteine and methionine, and in coenzyme A); in organic sulfates R—SO_4^- (e.g., in sulfated proteoglycans); and as inorganic sulfite (SO_3^{2-}) and sulfate (SO_4^{2-}) produced by the metabolism of these compounds.

Sulfur is used medicinally, often in preparations with benzoyl peroxide or salicylic acid, as a topical antiseptic for the treatment of scabies, seborrheic dermatitis, or acne vulgaris.

s. dioxide, a colorless gas, SO_2, with a pungent, suffocating odor; M.W. 64.07. Its solution in water produces sulfurous acid, H_2SO_3. It is a common air pollutant produced by the smelting of ores and the burning of sulfur-containing coal or oil. SO_2 is a strong reducing agent but may also act as a mild oxidant. It is used as a bleach, antioxidant, disinfectant, and food additive. Sulfur dioxide is highly irritating to the eyes and mucous membranes. Chronic exposure causes bronchitis and nasopharyngitis, pulmonary edema, airway obstruction, and reduced resistance to respiratory tract infection.

precipitated s., [USP], microcystalline sulfur, used in ointments as a scabicide.

sublimed s., [USP], powdered sulfur, used as a scabicide.

s. trioxide, a solid with three isotropic forms, SO_3, the anhydride of sulfuric acid; M.W. 80.06. Sulfur trioxide is used in the manufacture of sulfuric acid and organic sulfonic acids. It is highly toxic, a strong oxidizing agent, and a tissue irritant.

sulfur granules the small yellow granules found in the pus of an abscess or in the sputum of individuals with actinomycosis. The granules consist of small clusters of colonies of actinomycetes, are often associated with other organisms, and range in size from barely visible to several millimeters in diameter. Detection of the presence of the granules in the pus or an abscess is an indication of infection by an actinomycete. Formed by nonpathogenic actinomycetes, sulfur granules are also seen frequently as an incidental finding in the crypts of tonsils removed because of hyperplasia or chronic inflammation.

sulfuric acid (sul-fu′rik) a clear, colorless, nearly odorless, dense, oily liquid, H_2SO_4; M.W. 98.08. It is extremely corrosive and can cause severe burns on contact; inhalation of the vapor can produce lung damage. Concentrated solutions of sulfuric acid are strong acids; they are very effective dehydrating agents, as well as moderately strong oxidizing agents, especially when hot. Note that sulfuric acid should always be diluted by slowly adding the acid to water (or other diluent): the high heat of hydration can cause explosive spattering of hot water and acid, so that water should never be added to acid.

sulfurous acid (sul-fu′rus) a weak acid, H_2SO_3, once assumed to be formed when SO_2 is dissolved in water. However, it is now known that only very small amounts of H_2SO_3 are present; most of the SO_2 does not combine with water. Salts of H_2SO_3 containing the bisulfite, HSO_3^-, and sulfite, SO_3^{2-}, ions are stable.

sulindac (sul-in′dak) a nonsteroidal, antiinflammatory drug, which is used in the treatment of osteoarthritis, rheumatoid arthritis, acute gouty arthritis, ankylosing spondylitis, acute subacromial bursitis, and supraspinatus tendinitis. An indene derivative, it is similar to indomethacin but with a longer serum half-life. Sulindac inhibits platelet function, although less so than does aspirin. Common adverse reactions include gastrointestinal intolerance (pain, nausea, diarrhea, constipation), rash, and dizziness. Trademark, *Clinoril.*

Sulkowitch test (sul′ko-wich) [Hirsh Wolf *Sulkowitch,* American physician, born 1906] see under *calcium assays.*

sunburn (sun′bern) see *photodermatitis.*

sunstroke (sun′strōk) insolation, or thermic fever; a condition produced by exposure to the sun, and marked by convulsions, coma, and a high skin temperature. Also called *coup de soleil.* Cf. *heat stroke:* see *systemic h.* under *hyperthermia.*

super- (soo′per) [L. *super* above] a prefix word element to denote above or excess, e.g., supersaturated.

supercooled (soo″per-ko͞old) pertaining to a liquid that has been cooled to a temperature below its freezing point without freezing. A very pure liquid can be supercooled well below the freezing point (for example, water can be cooled to –40°C). On the addition of a seed crystal or other crystallization nuclei such as dust particles, the supercooled liquid rapidly freezes solid.

superdominance (soo″per-dom′ĭ-nans) see *overdominance.*

superfemale (soo″per-fe′māl) a sex chromosome abnormality, XXX karyotype, observed in females. Those affected have two Barr bodies and are usually fertile, although they have a tendency toward small breasts and juvenile sexual maturation. The occurrence of more than three X chromosomes generally leads to mental retardation. See also *sex determination.*

superficial (soo″per-fish′al) [L. *superficialis*] at or near the surface.

superheated (soo″per-he′ted) pertaining to a liquid that has been heated to a temperature above its boiling point without boiling. Care must be exercised to ensure that there are no sharp edges in the container, dust particles, or other centers where bubbles can form. Such a situation produces a metastable state, which will "bump," or bubble rapidly, once the boiling begins.

superinfection (soo″per-in-fek′shun) an infection occurring during or immediately after a course of chemotherapy that is caused by an organism resistant to antimicrobial agents. Superinfection is common when antimicrobial agents are administered in large doses, when several agents are used together, or when broad-spectrum agents are used. These secondary infections are characterized by the appearance of new symptoms and the culture of resistant organisms from new sites of inflammation.

The microbial agents involved in superinfections are often normal flora and include staphylococci, gram-negative enteric bacilli, anaerobes, and fungi. This process may be enhanced when indigenous normal flora (especially gram-negative enteric bacteria) possess R-transfer factors that mediate antimicrobial resistance.

Cf. *reinfection.*

superior (soo-pe′re-or) [L. "upper"] situated above or directed upward.

supernatant (soo″per-na′tant) [*super-* + L. *natare* to swim] 1. situated over or on top of something.

2. a liquid floating on top of another liquid or a solid sediment or precipitate.

supernumerary (soo″per-nu′mer-ăr″e) [L. *supernumerarius*] in excess of the regular number.

supernumerary breast see *polymastia.*

supernumerary nipple a congenital malformation that results in accessory nipples from the persistence of fragments of the mammary line; the nipples usually develop along the mammary line in the axillary or inner thigh regions. This condition occurs in about 1 percent of females and less frequently in males. See also *polymastia.*

superoinferior (soo″per-o-in-fe′re-or) pertaining to a radiographic projection in which the central ray passes through the part from top to bottom (not necessarily in a vertical direction).

superoxide (soo″per-oks′īd) [*super-* + L. *oxidum*] an anion formed by the reduction of a molecule of oxygen by one electron: $O_2 + e^- \rightarrow O_2^-$. This anion is produced by a number of agents and enzymes in body tissues. To prevent undue buildup of O_2^-, a threat to living systems, this ion is removed by the action of dismutases.

superoxide dismutase an enzyme of the oxidoreductase class (superoxide: superoxide oxidoreductase, EC 1.15.1.1) that catalyzes the reaction $O_2^- + O_2^- + 2H^+ \rightarrow H_2O_2 + O_2$; M.W. 32,500. The enzyme is present in all living organisms, being absent only in obligate anaerobic bacteria. The superoxide anion, O_2^-, is deleterious to living systems and may be the mutagenic agent formed by ionizing radiation. The above reaction ensures its removal. The enzyme contains two Cu^{2+} and two Zn^{2+} per molecule. It is identical with proteins previously isolated and named hemocuprein, erythrocuprein, cerebrocuprein, and hepatocuprein.

supersaturated (soo″per-sach′ĕ-rāt″ed) pertaining to a solution in a metastable, nonequilibrium state that has a higher concentration of solute than it can hold at true equilibrium conditions.

superscript (soo′per-skript) a distinguishing letter, number, or formula written above and usually to the right of a symbol. In mathematics, a superscript generally indicates a power or the order of a derivative. In a chemical formula, a superscript to the right indicates the ionic charge, e.g., SO_4^{2-}, and a superscript to the left shows the mass number of an isotope, e.g., ^{14}C. Cf. *subscript.*

superscription (soo″per-skrip′shun) [L. *superscriptio*] see under *prescription.*

supersonic (soo″per-son′ik) 1. faster than the speed of sound.

2. see *ultrasonic.*

Superstitionia a genus of scorpions found in Mexico and southwestern United States whose bite produces a local reaction in humans.

supervoltage (soo″per-vol′tij) see *megavoltage.*

supination (soo″pĭ-na′shun) [L. *supinatio*] 1. the act of assuming the supine position, or the state of being supine.

2. the act of turning the forearm so that the palm faces upward (superiorly).

3. the movement of the foot so that the medial margin and the longitudinal arch are raised.

Cf. *pronation.*

supine (soo′pin) [L. *supinus*] lying on the back, face up.

support (sup-port′) 1. an appliance that helps maintain a part in position.

2. in chromatography, an inert solid on which a liquid stationary phase is absorbed.

suppression (sŭ-presh′un) [L. *suppressio*] in genetics, the restoration of a lost function by a second mutation, either in a gene other than that involved in the primary mutation (intergenic suppression) or at a different site within the same gene (intragenic suppression).

suppression-burst activity a description of an electroencephalogram characterized by alternating periods of high-amplitude, low-frequency activity (theta and/or delta waves), sometimes mixed with faster activity, and periods of quiescence with relatively low-voltage activity or apparent electric inactivity. The periods of apparent inactivity can last as long as 15 min or so.

This pattern of cerebral electric activity is commonly observed during deep anesthesia or intoxication with central nervous system depressant drugs, and after anoxia, cardiac arrest, and some head injuries.

Also called *burst-suppression.*

suppressor gene a mutant gene that reverses the effect of a type of mutation occurring in other genes, e.g., a suppressor tRNA gene.

suppressor T lymphocyte see *suppressor T l.* under *lymphocyte.*

suppuration (sup″u-ra′shun) [L. *sub* under + *puris* pus] the formation or discharge of pus.

suppurative (sup′u-ra″tiv) producing pus, or associated with suppuration.

suppurative inflammation inflammation characterized by the formation of pus. When the pus is sequestered in a localized collection, it is termed an abscess. A suppurative inflammation is often seen in response to infection with pyogenic bacteria, especially the *Staphylococcus.* Also called purulent inflammation. See also *abscess* and *inflammation.*

supra- (soo′prah) [L. "above"] a prefix word element to denote above or over, e.g., supratentorial.

supraclavicular (soo″prah-klah-vik′u-lar) situated above the clavicle.

supraclavicular region the region of the front of the neck above a clavicle.

supraorbital (soo″prah-or′bi-tal) situated above the orbit.

supraorbital projection a radiographic projection used in cerebral angiography in which the supraorbital ridges are superimposed on the petrous ridges. In both posterior and posterior oblique (20°) views, the central ray is parallel to and 2 cm above a plane that passes through the supraorbital ridges and through points 2 cm above the external auditory meatuses.

supraorbital region the region of the head above the eyebrow.

suprapubic (soo″prah-pu′bik) situated or performed above the pubic arch.

suprapubic needle aspiration a general technique performed to obtain a urine specimen directly from the bladder, which is uncontaminated by urethral bacteria. Used primarily to determine whether bacteria are present in the bladder, this method is especially useful in infants. To obtain the specimen, a needle is inserted through aseptic suprapubic skin into the distended bladder, and the urine obtained is subjected to quantitative culture. See also *catheterization, clean-catch midstream urine specimen, quantitative culture,* and *urinary tract infection.*

suprarenal glands (soo″prah-re′nal) [*supra-* + L. *ren* kidney] see *adrenal glands.*

suprascapular (soo″prah-skap′u-lar) situated on or above the upper part of the scapula.

suprascapular region the area on either side of the back above the scapular region.

suprasternal (soo″prah-ster′nal) situated above the sternum.

suprasternal plane the horizontal plane that intersects the trunk at the level of the sternal notch.

supravital (soo″prah-vi′tal) denoting a staining method in which dye is added to unfixed cells removed from a living organism.

supravital staining the staining of a living tissue sample by incubation at 37°C in a stain that does not kill the cells. The term is used loosely to include vital staining, in which the tissue is perfused with the dye before removal. Both procedures have been used with methylene blue for staining nerve endings, and also with Janus green B, diethylsafranin, and other dyes for staining mitochondria and for demonstrating phagocytosis in macrophages.

sural (su′ral) pertaining to the calf of the leg; used especially to refer to the sural nerve.

sural nerve a branch of the tibial nerve. It receives a communication from the common peroneal nerve, then runs down the lateral side of the Achilles tendon, behind the lateral malleolus. It innervates the skin of the lateral side of the leg and foot.

suramin (soo′rah-min) an aromatic polysulfonate, which is used to treat early cases of *Trypanosoma rhodesiense* and *T. gambiense;* the drug has no effect after the development of the sleeping sickness state. Proteinuria is known to develop with use of suramin, and treatment should be discontinued if this appears. Administered intravenously, the drug is toxic; it should not be given to patients with renal disease. A few individuals may experience nausea, vomiting, loss of consciousness, and seizures; other side-effects include fever, hepatitis, rash, pruritus, edema, blepharitis, conjunctivitis, photophobia, tearing, and painful palms and soles. Suramin is also used in treating onchocerciasis.

surface (sur′fis) the outer part or the external aspect of an object.

surface-active agent see *surfactant.*

surface-barrier detector a type of charged particle radiation detector. See under *solid-state radiation detector.*

surface tension the force tending to minimize the surface area of a liquid, which makes small droplets spherical. This occurs because of the greater attraction of liquid molecules at the surface by molecules in the interior than by gas molecules above the surface. Specifically, it refers to the force of contraction acting across a line of unit length on the surface measured in newtons per meter (N/m). Liquids with stronger intermolecular forces have a higher surface tension and flow less readily.

surfactant (sur-fak′tant) compounds with soaplike detergent action. The molecules contain both a hydrophilic and a hydrophobic portion, and reduce the surface tension. By forming micelles and layers in which the hydrophilic portion of the molecule is in contact with water, they solubilize hydrophobic molecules or structures.

Synthetic detergents can be anionic, non-ionic, or cationic; cationic detergents such as quaternary ammonium compounds are employed as antiseptics and disinfectants. Also called *surface-active agent.* See also *disinfection.*

pulmonary s., a complex lipoprotein, containing a high percentage of the phospholipid dipalmitoyl lecithin, that is mostly secreted by type II alveolar cells. Pulmonary surfactant is distributed in a monomolecular film at the alveolar lining fluid–alveolar air interface, and acts to reduce the interfacial tension in the alveoli as they decrease in size. This counteracts the inherent instabiliy of the alveoli and minimizes the effect of surface tension in causing the collapse of smaller air spaces into larger ones.

A disturbance in the balance between the removal (by alveolar macrophages) and renewal of surfactant in the alveolar surface film occurs in pathologic conditions such as hyaline membrane disease, alveolar proteinosis, and shock lung.

surgeon (sur′jun) [L. *chirurgio;* Fr. *chirurgien*] 1. a physician who specializes in surgery.

2. the senior medical officer of a military unit.

surgical (sur′je-kal) pertaining to surgery.

surgical pathology see *surgical p.* under *pathology.*

suroplantar (sur″o-plan′tar) [L. *sura* calf + *planta* sole] pertaining to a radiographic projection, in which the central ray passes from the calf to the sole of the foot. Also called *dorsoplantar.*

surveillance (sur-vāl′ans) in immunologic theory, the constant monitoring of the body tissues by the immune system for abnormal cells.

survey (sur′va) 1. to make a detailed and comprehensive examination.

2. in statistics, an observational study of a population of subjects or objects in which there is no treatment or manipulation of the subjects. The goal of the survey is to determine or estimate certain characteristics of the population, such as a mean or a correlation, by sampling or taking a census of the population.

survey meter a portable radiation detector, usually an ionization chamber detector, used to monitor personnel and facilities to detect hazardous ionizing radiation.

survey program see *proficiency survey.*

survival the act of surviving.

survival curve in a survivorship study, a graph of the probability of survival versus time; for example, if X is the relapse-free survival time, the survival curve is a plot of $Pr(X > t)$. When there are censored observations, conditional probability of a relapse in each time period is the ratio of the subjects relapsing during the interval to the subjects still under observation at the beginning of the interval (i.e., those that have not yet relapsed and have not left the trial without relapse). The conditional probability of no relapse during the interval is one minus the probability of relapse. The survival probability from time zero to the end of a specified interval is given by the product of the conditional probability of no relapse for all intervals up to and including the specified interval. This is called the actuarial method for computing the survival curve.

susceptibility (sus-sep″tĭ-bil′ĭ-te) the state of being readily affected or acted upon. In immunology, the condition may be acquired, familial, individual, inherited, racial, specific, etc., the same as is immunity.

susceptibility testing see *antibacterial agent susceptibility testing.*

suspension (sus-pen′shun) [L. *suspensio*] in chemistry, a mixture of solid or liquid particles (the dispersed phase) in a liquid or gas (the continuous phase) in which the particles are aggregates of molecules small enough not to settle out. Cf. *colloid* and *solution.*

suture (su′chur) [L. *sutura* a seam] 1. a type of fibrous joint in which the opposed surfaces are closely united, such as in the skull.

2. the material used in closing a surgical or accidental wound with stitches.

3. a stitch or series of stitches made to secure apposition of the edges of a surgical or accidental wound.

4. the act or process of uniting a wound by stitches.

SV40 [from *s*imian *v*acuolating virus *40*] a small papovavirus that causes tumors in laboratory animals; it is noteworthy because its ability to cause tumors is dependent on the production of a specific protein tumor, the T- antigen, which is synthesized during the early phase of the viral replicative cycle. Its smaller circular DNA genome has provided a useful model for biologic studies.

Svedberg (S) (sfed′berg) [Theodor *Svedberg,* Swedish chemist, 1884–1971, inventor of the ultracentrifuge; winner of the Nobel Prize for chemistry in 1926 for his work on disperse systems] a unit equal to 10^{-13} sec, used for expressing sedimentation coefficients. Also called *Svedberg unit.*

Svedberg flotation unit (S_f) a unit equal in magnitude but opposite in sign to the svedberg; i.e., it measures the rate at which a substance rises (flotation rate) rather than that at which it sinks (sedimentation rate). Also called negative sedimentation Svedberg unit.

Svedberg unit see *svedberg.*

swab (swob) a small amount of cotton, calcium alginate, or polyester wrapped around the end of a thin wooden stick or wire. Swabs are used for obtaining specimens for microbiologic examination or for inoculating a culture plate.

nasopharyngeal s., a specimen obtained by swabbing the pharyngonasal cavity.

throat s., a specimen obtained by swabbing the pharyngolaryngeal cavity. See also *throat culture.*

Swan-Ganz catheter (swan gantz) a soft, flow-directed catheter with balloon tip, used in hemodynamic monitoring. It is introduced into the vascular system via a peripheral vein, and then into the vena cava, right atrium, and right ventricle until it reaches a branch of the pulmonary artery.

The most useful version is a triple-lumen type. One lumen is used to inflate the balloon; the others open into the pulmonary artery and right atrium when the catheter is properly positioned. Pressure measurements can be made in the right atrium, right ventricle, and pulmonary artery, as well as pulmonary capillary wedge pressures when the balloon is inflated. Blood withdrawn through the lumen at the tip is used to determine mixed venous oxygen content. A thermistor at the tip is used to determine cardiac output by the thermal dilution method.

swarm (sworm) a thin, spreading growth of microorganisms that forms on the surface of moist agar. Swarms are especially seen in cultures of *Proteus.*

S wave any negative deflection that follows an R wave (a positive deflection) of the QRS complex of the electrocardiogram. The term S wave is part of a terminology representative of the order and polarity of the deflections making up the QRS complex, and by itself does not denote a specific physiologic event.

sweat (swet) perspiration. Secreted by the two sweat glands, this liquid has a salty taste and a pH with a range of 4.5–7.5. The sweat produced by the eccrine sweat glands is clear, has a faint characteristic odor, and contains water, sodium chloride, and traces of albumin, urea, and other compounds. Its composition varies with many factors, such as fluid intake, external temperature and humidity, and hormonal activity. The sweat produced by the larger, deeper apocrine sweat glands of the axillae additionally contains organic material which, on bacterial decomposition, produces an offensive odor.

Through evaporation, the secretion of sweat is one of the major mechanisms for cooling the body. Unreplaced loss of large volumes of perspiration may result in hypertonic contraction of voluntary muscle. In cystic fibrosis, a congenital defect involving most or all of the glandular epithelial structures of the body, sweat and tears characteristically have a higher than normal concentration of NaCl. This analytic difference is striking enough to be diagnostic.

Cf. *perspiration.*

sweat glands glands that secrete sweat; situated in the subcutaneous layer of the skin, each communicates with the body surface via a duct. There are two types, eccrine and apocrine. Eccrine sweat glands, the most important cutaneous glands, are unbranched, coiled tubular glands that are distributed over most of the body. They play a major role in thermoregulation by providing the fluid for evaporative cooling. Apocrine sweat glands are branched, specialized glands that empty their secretions into the upper portions of hair follicles through ducts. The apocrine glands are primarily restricted to the axillae, anogenital region, mammary areolae, ear canals, and eyelids. They are under adrenergic control.

sweat test a diagnostic test for cystic fibrosis that is based on determination of the concentrations of sodium and chloride in sweat. Sweat, which is induced by the iontophoresis of pilocarpine, is collected on gauze or filter paper and assayed using ion-specific electrodes for chloride and sodium, flame photometry for sodium, and mercurometric or amperometric titration for chloride.

In children, sweat chloride concentrations greater than 60 mmol/l and sodium concentrations greater than 80 mmol/l are indicative of cystic fibrosis.

Sweet method a radiographic method of localizing foreign bodies in the eye. It uses an apparatus that immobilizes the patient's head with the median sagittal plane held parallel to the film tunnel; a localizer device holds a small metal ball exactly 10 mm from the center of the cornea and a cone exactly 15 mm lateral to the ball.

Two exposures are made while the patient gazes directly forward, with the central ray passing vertically through the ball and cone in the first film and with a 10°–25° cranial angulation in the second. The position of the foreign body in a side view of the eye is taken directly from the first film, and the perpendicular elevation above or below the center of the cornea is transferred to a front view. A point is plotted in the front view above or below the ball at the apparent distance taken from the second film and a similar point above or below the cone. The intersection of the line through these points (representing the x-ray through the foreign body) and the horizontal line at the true elevation locates the foreign body in the front view. The position in the horizontal section is found using the front-to-back position from the side views and the side-to-side position from the front view.

See also *foreign body localization.* Cf. *Pfeiffer-Comberg method.*

swelling (swel'ing) 1. a transient abnormal enlargement or increase in volume of a body part or area that is not caused by proliferation of cells. See also *edema.*

2. an eminence or elevation.

Swift's disease (swifts) [H. *Swift,* Australian physician] see *acrodynia.*

switch (swich) an electronic or mechanical device that opens or closes a current path.

SWS abbrev. for slow-wave sleep. See under *sleep* and *s. stages.*

sycosis (si-ko'sis) [Gr. *sykōsis,* from *sykon* fig] a papulopustular inflammation of the hair follicles, usually of the beard, e.g., sycosis barbae (tinea barbae).

Sydenham's chorea (sid'en-hams) [Thomas *Sydenham,* English physician, 1624–1689] see *Sydenham's c.* under *chorea.*

Sylvest's disease (sil-vests') [Ejnar *Sylvest,* Norwegian physician, 1880–1931] see *epidemic p.* under *pleurodynia.*

sym- (sim) 1. a prefix word element to denote together or with, e.g., symbiosis.

2. a prefix word element in organic chemistry to denote one of several constitutional isomers that are symmetric, e.g., *sym*-dichloroethane (1,2-dichloroethane, CH_2ClCH_2Cl), *sym*-dichloroacetone (1,3-dichloro-2-propanone, $CH_2ClCOCH_2Cl$), or *sym*-di-

chlorodifluoroethane (1,2-dichloro-1,2-difluoroethane, CHClFCHClF). Cf. *asym-*.

symbiont (sim′bi-ont, sim′be-ont) [*sym-* + Gr. *bioun* to live] an organism that lives in the state of symbiosis.

symbiosis (sim″bi-o′sis) [Gr. *symbiōsis*] the living together of two individuals or populations of different species. If the association is beneficial to both organisms, the relationship is referred to as mutualism. If the parasite derives benefit without effect on the other, it is commensalism. When the relationship is beneficial to the parasite and detrimental to the other, it is parasitism.

symbol (sim′bul) [Gr. *symbolon,* from *symballein* to interpret] 1. a mark or character representing some quality or relation.

2. in chemistry, a letter or combination of letters representing an atom or a group of atoms.

symmetric (si-met′rik) pertaining to or exhibiting symmetry.

symmetric distribution a probability distribution of a random variable X for which $X - \mu$ and $\mu - X$ have the same distribution, where μ is the central point of the distribution (μ is a median; the mean, if it exists, is also μ). Cf. *probability distribution* and *skewed distribution.*

symmetry (sim′ĕ-tre) [Gr. *symmetria; syn-* same + *metron* measure] 1. a property of an object, such as a molecule or a crystal, which consists of its having identical structures on opposite sides of a reflection plane or at multiples of a given angle of rotation about an axis. See also *symmetry operation.*

2. in neurophysiology, the equal distribution of potentials of opposite polarity about the isopotential axis.

3. in electroencephalography, the distribution of waveforms of approximately equal amplitude, frequency, and shape over homologous areas on both sides of the head.

bilateral s., the approximate identity of structures on the left and right sides of an object (such as the human body). The median plane is a symmetry plane.

radial s., the regular arrangement of parts around a rotation axis, such as the approximate fivefold rotational symmetry of a starfish.

symmetry element see under *symmetry operation.*

symmetry group see under *symmetry operation.*

symmetry operation a rotation, reflection, translation, or combination thereof that leaves the form of an object, such as a molecule or crystal, unchanged. The set of all the symmetry elements of an object in its symmetry group.

Every molecule belongs to one of 32 point groups (symmetry groups composed of rotations and reflections). The point groups are composed of two types of symmetry element: the *n*-fold proper rotation axis (symbol C_n), in which rotation by 360°/ n about the axis is a symmetry operation, and the *n*-fold improper rotation axis (S_n), in which rotation by 360°/ n followed by a reflection through a plane perpendicular to the axis is a symmetry operation. Three special cases of these types are the identity operation (E), C_1, a 360° rotation; the reflection (σ), S_1, a mirror plane; and inversion (i), S_2, reflection in three mutually perpendicular planes.

Every crystal lattice belongs to one of 230 space groups. These contain two types of symmetry elements in addition to those of point groups. They are translations by multiples of lattice vectors (which move unit cells onto unit cells) and *n*-fold screw axes (rotations by 180°, 120°, or 60°, followed by a translation along the rotation axis by a fraction of a lattice vector).

symmetry plane a reflection plane that divides an object into two mirror-image halves, which are reflections of each other in the symmetry plane.

sympathectomy (sim″pah-thek′to me) [*sympathetic* + Gr. *ektomē* excision] the ablation or interruption of some portion of the sympathetic nervous pathway, a procedure to promote improved circulation. It is also effective treatment for causalgia in those patients who improve with sympathetic blockade by a local anesthetic.

sympathetic nervous system a division of the autonomic nervous system. Its peripheral efferent component originates between the first thoracic and the second or third lumbar segments of the spinal cord. Myelinated preganglionic (B) fibers branch from the spinal nerves at these levels and pass via white rami communicantes to join a chain of ganglia (paravertebral sympathetic chains) on either side of the spinal cord. The fibers synapse in these ganglia or pass through to synapse with postganglionic neurons in collateral ganglia in the abdominal or thoracic cavity or with cells in the adrenal medulla.

The neurotransmitter of the preganglionic fiber is acetylcholine. The postganglionic fibers are unmyelinated, and innervate cardiac muscle, smooth muscle, or glandular tissue; their neurotransmitter is either acetylcholine or norepinephrine. The adrenal medulla does not have a postganglionic fiber, and its cells release epinephrine and norepinephrine directly into the systemic circulation. These anatomic characteristics result in rather widespread physiologic effects when the sympathetic system is stimulated. Such stimulation generally produces responses that facilitate increased muscle activity. Specifically, stimulation of particular sympathetic fibers effects the following: dilation of the pupils; contraction of the pilomotor muscles; vasoconstriction of the blood vessels of the skin and viscera; vasodilation of the blood vessels of skeletal muscles, cardiac muscle, and skin of the face; activation of adenyl cyclase, which is necessary to promote the breakdown of glycogen to glucose in the liver; and contraction of the splenic capsule, which results in the expulsion of erythrocytes into the systemic circulation. It also increases sweat secretion, inhibits peristalsis and secretion of some digestive enzymes, increases the blood level of free fatty acids, increases the release of renin from the kidney juxtaglomerular cells, increases the heart rate (tachycardia) and force of contraction (positive chronotropic and ionotropic effects), and promotes ejaculation of semen in the male.

See also *autonomic nervous system* and its accompanying illustration.

sympathomimetic (sim′pah-tho-mi-met′ik) [*sympathetic* + Gr. *mimētikos* imitative] a compound or drug that, when administered, produces physiologic and pharmacologic responses resembling those produced by stimulation of the sympathetic nervous system. These responses can be described generally as excitation of smooth muscle of the blood vessels of the skin, mucous membranes, and certain glands (e.g., salivary and sweat glands); inhibition of the smooth muscle of the gut, bronchial tree, and blood vessels of skeletal muscle; an increase in the force of contraction and rate of the heart; an increase in glycogenolysis and lipolysis; central nervous system stimulation of respiration; an increase in wakefulness; and a reduction of appetite. The duration and intensity of these responses vary among different sympathomimetic drugs, reflecting their chemical structure, the number of possible sites of drug action, and the responses of other homeostatic or compensatory reflex mechanisms.

Sympathomimetics directly stimulate α- and/or β-adrenergic receptors in effector tissue, or they indirectly stimulate these receptors by affecting intact intraneural norepinephrine stores. Most sympathomimetics are derivatives of β-phenylethylamine, a benzene ring with ethylamine side-chain.

Clinically, sympathomimetics are administered to increase systemic arterial blood pressure during certain hypotensive states; to produce mucosal decongestion when applied locally; to reduce bleeding of superficial wounds by topical application; to relax bronchial smooth muscle in asthmatic individuals with bronchospasm; and to relax the uterus during dysmenorrhea and premature labor. They have also been prescribed to increase wakefulness and to suppress appetite in the treatment of obesity. Epinephrine, norepinephrine, isoproterenol, phenylephrine, methoxamine, amphetamine, tyramine, and metamphetamine are examples of some commonly used sympathomimetics.

See also *adrenergic receptor* and *catecholamine*.

symphysis (sim′fĭ-sis), pl. *symphyses* [Gr. "a growing together, natural union"] a site or line of union; a type of cartilaginous joint in which the apposed bony surfaces are firmly united by a fibrocartilage plate.

s. menti, the line of fusion between the two halves of the mandible, usually completed during fetal development.

s. pubis, the thick, fibrocartilaginous joint that joins the medial surfaces of the pubic bones.

sympodia (sim-po′de-ah) [*syn-* + Gr. *pous* foot + *-ia*] a rare congenital malformation that results in abnormal fusion of the lower extremities. Also called sirenomelia. Cf. *syndactyly.*

symport (sim′port) a transport protein that simultaneously moves two substances in the same direction. See also *active transport.* Cf. *antiport* and *uniport.*

symptom (simp′tum) [L. *symptoma;* Gr. *symptōma* anything that has befallen one] any subjective evidence of disease or of a patient's condition, i.e., such evidence as perceived by the patient; a change in a patient's condition indicative of some bodily or mental state.

symptomatic (simp″to-mat′ik) [Gr. *symptomatikos*] 1. pertaining to or of the nature of a symptom.

2. indicative (of a particular disease or disorder).

3. exhibiting the symptoms of a particular disease but having a different cause.

4. directed at the allaying of symptoms, as symptomatic treatment.

syn- (sin) [Gr. *syn* with, together] 1. a prefix word element to denote union or association.

2. a prefix word element in organic chemistry to denote the relationship of the three substituents attached to a carbon-nitrogen double bond (as in oximes). For example, for oximes derived from aldehydes, the hydroxyl group and hydrogen are on the same side of the double bond in the *syn* isomer. The other configuration is denoted by the prefix *anti-*. See also *isomerism.*

synapse (sin′aps) [Gr. *synapsis* a conjunction, connection] the functional contact of a neuron with another neuron, an effector (muscle or gland) or a sensory receptor, for the purpose of transmitting information.

Most synapses are chemically mediated by a neurotransmitter, such as acetylcholine, norepinephrine, γ-aminobutyric acid, or dopamine, which is released from the axon terminal of the presynaptic element into the synaptic cleft. Neurotransmitters are stored in membrane-bound vesicles in the presynaptic terminal; when released in response to an action potential, they diffuse across the cleft to affect the postsynaptic membrane.

Synapses can be either excitatory or inhibitory. Electric synapses called gap junctions also occur. Characterized by a very narrow cleft and no transmitter vesicles, gap junctions are areas of low electric resistance that permit electric potentials to flow from one neuron to another.

synapsis (sĭ-nap′sis) [Gr. "conjunction"] the pairing of homologous chromosomes during the zygotene stage of the first meiotic prophase. The chromosomes make contact at one or several points, then join in zipper fashion so that the homologous points on each chromosome are adjacent. The resulting structure is called a bivalent or tetrad. A special cell organelle, the synaptonemal complex, mediates this pairing. Also called *pairing.*

synaptic cleft (sĭ-nap′tik) a space, usually 20–30 nm wide, between the membranes of pre- and postsynaptic cells. Neurotransmitter diffuses rapidly across this space to affect the postsynaptic cell.

synaptic transmission the communication of a neural impulse from one neuron to another neuron, a muscle fiber, or a gland across a synapse.

synaptic transmitter see *neurotransmitter.*

synaptic vesicles small membranous sacs in the terminal bouton, which contain neurotransmitter substance. They are found clustered against the presynaptic membrane.

synaptonemal complex (sĭ-nap″to-ne′mal) the structure that forms between homologous chromosome pairs and is seen during the zygotene and pachytene stages of meiotic prophase. The homologous chromosomes (each composed of two sister chromatids) are separated by a space of 150–200 nm, and are aligned (synapsed) so that homologous points (chromomeres) are adjacent to each other.

The complex is a flat ribbon with a low-density medial element at the center and lateral elements 20–80 nm wide on the sides; it is composed primarily of basic proteins. At the edges it is joined to the axes of the homologous chromosomes by fine fibrils that contain DNA.

synaptosome (sin-ap′to-sōm) a laboratory preparation of particulate neuron synapse substance, made by homogenizing brain or spinal cord tissue. The membranes of the nerve cell terminals snapped off in the procedure reseal to form artifactual organelles, which are osmotically active, maintain internal K^+ and Na^+ levels, and show a normal potential difference across the membrane.

synarthrosis (sin″ar-thro′sis), pl. *synarthroses* [*syn-* + Gr. *arthrōsis* joint] see *fibrous j.* under *joint.*

synchronized (sin′kro-nīzd) occurring at the same time.

synchronized culture see *synchronized c.* under *culture.*

synchronous (sin′kro-nus) [*syn-* + Gr. *chronos* time] occurring at the same time; operating in step or in phase.

synchronous data transmission a method of coordinating the data transmission between a computer and peripheral device. A regularly spaced clock signal is transmitted along with the data, and the receiving device is operated in step with the clock signal. Cf. *asynchronous data transmission.*

synchronous sleep see *s. stages* under *sleep.*

syncopal (sin′ko-pal) pertaining to or characterized by syncope.

syncope (sing′ko-pe) [Gr. *synkopē*] 1. a temporary suspension of consciousness due to cerebral ischemia.

2. fainting. Syncope may occur for a variety of reasons. It may relate to a temporary reduction of blood flow to the brain, which in turn may relate to a decrease in peripheral resistance, hypovolemia, reduced cardiac output, or mechanical reduction in venous return to the heart. Alternately, it may relate to an abnormality in the state of the blood (e.g., anemia, hypoxia, hypoglycemia) or to emotional factors.

cardiac s., a syncopal episode brought about by a cardiac disorder that produces a sudden reduction in cardiac output and thus an inadequate cerebral blood flow. The most common of these cardiac disorders include massive myocardial infarction, aortic valvular or subvalvular stenosis, pulmonary stenosis, pulmonary hypertension, cardiac tamponade, bradyarrhythmias (e.g., complete atrioventricular block), or tachyarrhythmias (e.g., ventricular tachycardia).

carotid sinus s., syncope due to hypersensitivity of the carotid sinus reflex (carotid sinus syndrome).

exertional s., a form of cardiac syncope brought on by physical exertion in individuals with cardiac disorders such as severe coronary artery disease, valvular lesions (idiopathic hypertrophic subaortic stenosis or aortic stenosis), or congenital heart disease (tetralogy of Fallot). The onset of the syncopal episodes may be caused by normal exercise vasodilation combined with relatively fixed cardiac output that fails to rise normally during exercise. Other episodes are associated with transient arrhythmias, perhaps due to an inadequate blood flow through the coronary arteries.

micturition s., a temporary loss of consciousness, during or immediately after micturition, that is most common in males who have abruptly arisen from bed in the middle of the night. This form of syncopal attack may represent a form of postural syncope (associated with a sudden shift from a recumbent to a standing position); alcohol consumption and the warmth of the bed may exacerbate the orthostatic hypotension. A peripheral vasodilation brought about by vasomotor reflexes arising from the bladder may also contribute to the onset of these attacks.

syncytiotrophoblast (sin-sit″e-o-trof′o-blast) in the developing embryo, the outer layer of the trophoblast, composed of multinucleated cells without distinct cell boundaries. Also called *syncytium.* Cf. *cytotrophoblast.*

syncytium (sin-sish′e-um) a multinucleate mass of protoplasm produced by the fusion of uninucleate cells.

syndactyly (sin-dak′tĭ-le) [*syn-* + Gr. *daktylos* finger] the most common congenital deformity of the hand, involving the fusion of the bone or flesh of two or more digits, causing a webbed appearance. The middle and third digits are most commonly involved. The anomaly may also occur in the foot.

syndesm/o (sin-des′mo) [Gr. *syndesmos* band or ligament] a word element used in combining form to denote a ligament, e.g., syndesmophyte.

syndrome (sin′drōm) [Gr. *syndromē* concurrence] a set of symptoms or findings that occur together; the sum of signs of any morbid state. For more information, see the particular syndrome. Cf. *disease.*

synechia (sĭ-nek′e-ah), pl. *synechiae* [Gr.] adhesion, as of the iris to the cornea or the lens.

syneresis (sĭ-ner′ĕ-sis) [Gr. *synairesis* a drawing together] a drawing together of the particles of the dispersed phase of a gel, with separation of some of the disperse medium and shrinkage of the gel, such as occurs in the clotting of blood. See also *clot retraction.*

synergism (sin′er-jizm) the phenomenon of two causes having a combined effect greater than the sum of their individual effects, as in the use of a combination of antibacterial agents in the treatment of infection.

synergist (sin′er-jist) 1. an adjuvant, a medicine that enhances the effect of another medicine.

2. one of a group of muscles or organs that act in concert. Cf. *antagonist.*

synergistic (sin″er-jis′tik) pertaining to or exhibiting synergy.

synergy (sin′er-je) [L. *synergia;* Gr. *syn-* + *ergon* work] the cooperative interaction of two or more causes, agents, or drugs.

Syngamidae (sin-gam′ĭ-de) a family of nematodes of the order Rhabditida, including the genus *Syngamus.*

syngamy (sin′gah-me) [*syn-* + Gr. *gamos* marriage] the union of the male and female pronuclei after fertilization, producing the diploid zygote nucleus.

syngeneic (sin″jĕ-ne′ik) denoting individuals or tissues that have identical genotypes, i.e., identical twins or animals of the same inbred strain. Also called *isogeneic.*

syngeneic graft see *isogeneic g.* under *graft.*

syngraft (sin′graft) see *isogeneic g.* under *graft.*

synkaryon (sin-kar′e-on) [*syn-* + Gr. *karyon* nucleus] the zygote nucleus produced by the fusion of the male and female pronuclei.

synophthalmia (sin″of-thal′me-ah) [*syn-* + Gr. *ophthalmos* eye + *-ia*] see **cyclopia.**

Synosternus a genus of fleas of the family Pulicidae. The species *S. pallidus* attacks humans in Dakar and West Africa.

synovi/o (sĭ-no′ve-o) a word element used in combining form to denote membrane lining and joint fluid, e.g., synovitis, synovioma.

synovia (si-no've-ah) [L.; Gr. *syn-* + *oon* egg] the transparent, viscid fluid secreted by the synovial membrane and found in joint cavities, bursae, and tendon sheaths.

synovial (si-no've-al) [L. *synovialis*] pertaining to a synovial joint or to its lining membrane.

synovial bursa a closed sac of synovial membrane situated between closely apposed surfaces that allows smooth movement between these surfaces. The location may be subcutaneous, subtendinous, subfascial, or submuscular.

synovial fluid a fluid found in the joint cavities, bursae, and tendon sheaths that is transparent, alkaline, viscid, and straw-colored. Its electrolyte composition is that of a transudate from plasma. Synovial fluid contains proteoglycans formed by cells of the synovium; the pH is 7.3–7.4, the specific gravity 1.010, and the protein concentration is about 1 percent with an albumin/globulin ratio of approximately 4.0. No fibrinogen is present. Electrolytes and readily diffusible substances of synovial fluid exchange with plasma, whereas larger particles can leave the intraarticular space only via lymphatics. Synovial fluid is an extension of interstitial fluid and is not a product of secretion. Synovial fluid is often examined under polarized light for crystals, which are present in conditions such as gout and pseudogout.

Also called synovia.

synovial fluid examination a procedure performed after the removal of synovial fluid from a joint capsule for diagnostic and prognostic information; the knee is the most common site for withdrawal of the fluid. Normally, joint fluid is clear, transparent, and sterile. It should contain less than 200 white blood cells/ml (predominantly mononuclear leukocytes), and have a glucose content nearly equal to that of blood.

A variety of disease processes can change the synovial fluid profile. Noninflammatory joint diseases, such as osteochondritis, osteochondromatosis, and degenerative joint disease, may increase the amount of synovial fluid, which often has a yellow tinge. White blood cell counts also increase, up to 3000 cells/μl. The crystals associated with crystal-induced arthritis—e.g., apatite, monosodium urate (MSU), calcium pyrophosphate dihydrate (CPPD, the cause of pseudogout), talcum crystals, and crystals of corticosteroid drugs injected into the joint—can be identified under polarized light microscopy.

Inflammatory joint diseases such as rheumatoid arthritis, gout, ankylosing spondylitis, rheumatic fever, and scleroderma produce increased amounts of synovial fluid, which may be yellow and opaque. The white blood cell count increases up to 100,000 cells/μl, more than half of them being polymorphonuclear leukocytes. The glucose concentration may be decreased by 25–50 mg/dl below the plasma level, and the protein concentration elevated above normal. In the investigation of rheumatoid arthritis and systemic lupus erythematosus, immunologic tests for rheumatoid factor, antinuclear antibodies, and complement may be helpful in making a diagnosis. Rheumatoid arthritis cells can be identified using phase contrast microscopy.

Septic joint disease, such as that due to bacterial infection, yields increased amounts of fluid, which is usually opaque and yellow-green. The white blood cell count frequently exceeds 10,000 cells/μl, of which 75 percent are polymorphonuclear leukocytes. Glucose concentrations are below 25 mg/dl. Specimens are cultured for bacteria and the sediment is examined with Gram-stained or acid-fast stained smears; cultures are often positive for the infectious agent.

synovial joint a type of articulation between two bones in which the ends of the bones are united by a short, wide tube of strong, fibrous connective tissue. The tube surrounds a space between the two bones that is filled by synovial fluid, which is secreted by the membrane that lines the connective tissue tube (synovial membrane). The synovial membrane does not cover the articular cartilages.

synovial membrane the layer of loose connective tissue and surface cells that lines the nonarticular parts of synovial joints. This membrane is also responsible for the formation of synovial fluid.

synovial sarcoma a malignant soft tissue tumor, so named because of supposed derivation from or differentiation toward the synovium. Frequently the tumor arises some distance from the nearest synovial joint. Its histogenesis is therefore open to question; nevertheless, there is some similarity between the epithelial component of the typical biphasic synovial sarcoma and normal synovium. The epithelial cells form branching tubes, sheets, or glandlike aggregates, and the lining cells are usually columnar, although they can be flattened in some of the larger clefts. The stromal component of the biphasic tumors is composed of spindle cells with less cytoplasm and fewer organelles than fibroblasts; these cells are closely packed in most areas, but interspersed collagen and foci of calcification are common.

In some synovial sarcomas, only the stromal component, the so-called monophasic variant, is present. Most synovial sarcomas occur in the limbs of young and middle-aged adults but they occasionally are found in the trunk or neck tissues. Synovial sarcoma may grow slowly, but local recurrence is frequent; those that are aggressive frequently metastasize, typically to the lungs.

synovial villi slender, fingerlike projections along the inner surface of the synovial membrane.

synovitis (sin"o-vi'tis) [*synovia* + *-itis* inflammation] a general term used to describe inflammation of a synovial membrane. It may produce pain, especially on movement, and various degrees of swelling. Synovitis may be due to systemic disease (rheumatoid arthritis, gout) or bacterial infection. Diagnosis of the specific cause of synovitis may require examination of the synovial fluid. See also *synovial fluid examination.*

pigmented villonodular s., a benign, subacute, inflammatory disorder of the joints that occurs most frequently in young males. It most commonly affects the knees: there is pain, swelling, and motion limitation. The synovium may become covered with large villi, which fuse to become pedunculated nodules. The synovial fluid is brown, and synovial cells and interstitial spaces contain hemosiderin, cholesterol crystals, and multinucleate giant cells. X-rays reveal synovial thickening, narrowing of joint spaces, bone erosion, and subchondral cysts. A similar process can affect the sheath of tendons; when present in this location, it is called giant cell tumor of tendon sheath. The cause is unknown. Also called villonodular synovitis.

syntax (sin′taks) the formal rules that specify the forms of valid statements in any computer language (the grammar of computer language). Cf. *semantics.*

syntax error an incorrect formatting of a computer language statement.

syntenic being located on the same chromosome. The syntenic relationships, without linkage distances, of the structural genes for many human enzymes have been determined using somatic cell genetics.

synteny (sin′tĕ-ne) the relationship of genes that are on the same chromosome, regardless of whether the linkage is large enough to measure. Cf. *linkage.*

synthase (sin′thās) any enzyme of the lyase class (EC 4) that catalyzes the synthesis of a compound by the joining together of two molecules without the necessary cleavage of a high-energy phosphate bond, e.g., cystathionine synthase. See also *lyase.*

synthesis (sin′thĕ-sis) [Gr. "a combination"] 1. the union of disparate elements to form a coherent whole. Cf. *analysis.*

2. in chemistry, the process or the sequence of chemical reactions, purifications, and procedures required to produce a compound or other chemical material from one or more raw materials.

synthetase (sin′thĕ-tās) the common name for an enzyme of the ligase class (EC 6). These enzymes catalyze the synthesis of a compound by the joining together of two molecules coupled with hydrolysis of the terminal pyrophosphate bond in adenosine triphosphate (ATP) or a similar triphosphate, e.g., glutathione synthetase and carbamoyl-phosphate synthetase. See also *ligase.*

synthetic (sin-thet′ik) [L. *syntheticus;* Gr. *synthetikos*] 1. pertaining to, of the nature of, or participating in, synthesis.

2. produced by synthesis; artificial.

synthetic lethal a lethal genetic chromosome produced by the crossing over of homologous chromosomes, e.g., when one of the chromosomes has an inversion and cross-over occurs in the inversion, producing a duplication deficiency.

syntrophism (sin′trōf-izm) [*syn-* + Gr. *trophē* nourishment] the stimulation of the growth of a microorganism resulting from the provision of a growth factor or nutrient from another microorganism growing nearby, e.g., the growth of *Hemophilus influenzae* as satellite colonies of *Staphylococcus.*

syntropic (sin-trop′ik) [*syn-* + Gr. *trepein* to turn] 1. turning or pointing in the same direction, as the ribs or the vertebral spines.

2. denoting the correlation of several factors, as the relation of one disease to the development or incidence of another disease.

Syphacia (si-fa′se-ah) a genus of nematodes that is parasitic in rodents and occasionally in humans. The species *S. muris* and *S. obvelata* have been identified in human feces. Infection is thought to be accidental.

syphilis (sif′ĭ-lis) [*Syphilus,* the name of a shepherd infected with the disease in the poem of Fracastorius (1530), in which the term first appears. Derived perhaps from Gr. *syn* together + *philein* to love or from Gr. *siphlos* crippled, maimed] a contagious venereal disease, with forms ranging from subacute to chronic, that is caused by the spirochetal bacterium *Treponema pallidum.* Syphilis is acquired primarily through sexual contact with an infected individual or in utero (congenital syphilis); it is also possible to acquire the disease through blood transfusions from infected individuals.

There is complex immunologic reaction to *Treponema pallidum,* resulting in a long-term host-parasite relationship. Untreated syphilis waxes and wanes through three stages—primary, secondary, and tertiary—also known as early, infectious, and late syphilis, respectively.

In the late fifteenth century an epidemic of syphilis occurred in Europe, and the crew of Christopher Columbus was blamed for importing the disease to Europe from the West Indies. It was not until the sixteenth century that syphilis was determined to be transmitted by means of sexual contact. Initial treatment of syphilis involved heavy metals (mercury), which were minimally effective. In 1910, Ehrlich developed a new chemotherapeutic agent, arsphenamine ("magic bullet"), which was mixed with bismuth salts and administered over a 2-yr period. Finally, in the 1940s, penicillin became available and proved to be effective against the causative organism, *T. pallidum.*

CLINICAL DISEASE. *Treponema pallidum* can penetrate small abrasions in the epithelium or normal mucosal membranes. In the primary stage, a lesion, called a chancre, usually appears at the portal of entry after an incubation period of 10–90 da (with an average of 21 da). Initially, this lesion is a painless papule, surrounded by an inflammatory cuff, which breaks and forms an ulcer. The lesion may persist for 2–6 wk and heal spontaneously. This sequence represents the primary or early stage of syphilis and is infectious. In the secondary stage, the individual may develop a low-grade fever, headache, malaise, lymphadenopathy, and reappearance of syphilitic lesions after a latent period of several weeks. After 2–6 wk, the secondary infectious lesions heal and the symptoms disappear spontaneously. Any time thereafter, the tertiary stage, late syphilis, may develop, taking one of three forms: a benign tertiary lesion, which involves skin, bones, and viscera; cardiovascular syphilis; or neurosyphilis.

The benign tertiary lesions arise 3–10 yr after the initial infection, with the appearance of a chronic granulomatous reaction. These lesions may be localized in various organs or tissues, forming a soft, gummy tumor (gumma), which increases slowly in size, and is finally replaced after healing by a scar. Cardiovascular syphilis results from *T. pallidum,* growing in blood vessels 10–25 yr after the initial infection. The inflammatory response of this infection results in endarteritis of the vasa vasorum, which leaves scars in the wall of the aorta. Neurosyphilis may be asymptomatic or may produce headaches, dizziness, lassitude, stiffness of the neck, and cranial nerve palsies. Parenchymatous neurosyphilis may progress to convulsions and epileptic attacks.

LABORATORY DIAGNOSIS. The primary lesion may be examined for the presence of spirochetes by means of darkfield microscopy. The lesion surface should first be cleaned with a saline solution and gauze, before serous fluid from the lesion is applied to a glass slide. The chancre of syphilis must be differentiated from lesions of herpes (multiple, vesicular, painful), chancroid (painful, multiple, exudative), lymphogranuloma venereum (small, papular), and granuloma inguinale (redder, more granular).

Serologic studies for the diagnosis of syphilis may be divided into nontreponemal (cardiolipin) and treponemal tests. The nontreponemal tests include the VDRL (Venereal Disease Research Laboratory) and rapid plasma reagin (RPR) tests. The VDRL test utilizes a buffered saline suspension of cardiolipin-lecithin-cholesterol antigen and the individual's serum. Flocculation is observed microscopically. This test is simple, inexpensive, and rapid; it is often used for screening large numbers of people and is capable of detecting 75 percent of all primary syphilis cases. The disadvantage of this test is its low specificity; i.e., it can produce false-positive results. Treponemal antibody tests include the FTA-ABS (fluorescent treponemal antibody absorption) and TPHA (treponemal passive hemagglutination) tests. The former measures antibodies that react with killed *T. pallidum* after absorption with the patient's serum. It is useful for investigating false-positive results; because of its high sensitivity, it also aids in diagnosing late syphilis. The latter test or its modification, microhemagglutination–*Treponema pallidum* (MHA-TP), is simple, rapid, and reproducible. This hemagglutination assay is highly specific although it does not work well in the diagnosis of early syphilis; for the serology of untreated cases of syphilis, see the accompanying illustration.

See also *spirochete.*

syring/o (sĭ-ring′go) [Gr. *syrinx* pipe, tube, fistula] a word element used in combining form to denote tube, e.g., syringomyelia.

syringe (sĭ-rinj′, sir′inj) [L. *syrinxe*] an instrument for injecting liquids into or withdrawing them from any vessel or cavity.

syringocystadenoma (sĭ-ring″go-sis″tad-ē-no′mah) a benign neoplasm originating from cells of either apocrine or eccrine glands in the skin. It is seen most frequently on the head and scalp and appears as a hyperkeratotic plaque or nodule. The lesion is characterized by papillary epidermal hyperplasia, which forms papillae that invaginate into the dermis. A dense plasma cell infiltrate is common, and basal cell carcinoma may be associated with this benign neoplasm. Also called syringocystadenoma papilliferum.

syringoma (sir″ing-go′mah) [*syring-* + Gr. *oma* tumor] a multiple, benign dermal neoplasm that is thought to arise from the intraepidermal portion of eccrine glands. Syringomas appear after puberty, localizing on the face and abdomen. Keratin-filled cysts, ductal structures, and a fibrous stroma are found.

syringomyelia (sĭ-ring″go-mi-e′le-ah) a condition in which cavitation occurs in several segments of the spinal cord. It may be developmental in origin or arise secondary to trauma, infection, or tumor. Syringomyelia differs in degree from hydromyelia, which is merely dilation of the central canal. When the cavities involve the medulla, the term syringobulbia is used.

syringomyelocele (si-ring″go-mi′ĕ-lo-sēl″) [*syringo-* + Gr. *myelos* marrow + *kēlē* tumor] hernial protrusion of the spinal cord through the bony defect in spina bifida; the mass containing a cavity connected with the central canal of the spinal cord. Also called hydromyelocele and myelocystocele.

Syrphidae (sir′phĭ-de) a family of flies, the hover flies, of the order Diptera, which may cause intestinal myiasis in humans.

system (sis′tem) [Gr. *systerna* a complex or organized whole] 1. a group of interconnected, interdependent, or interacting objects regarded as a collective entity performing a common function, e.g., the circulatory system, the nervous system, or a computer system.

2. an organized collection of ideas, rules, theories, or methods, e.g., the International System of measuring units.

3. in physics, a region of space and the matter and energy it contains. A closed system is one that is isolated from its surroundings; no matter or energy crosses its boundary. An open system is one that is not closed.

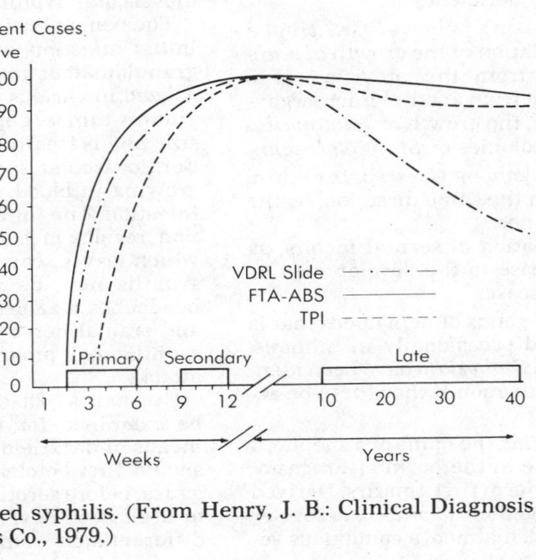

Syphilis. Serology of untreated syphilis. (From Henry, J. B.: Clinical Diagnosis and Management. 16th ed. Philadelphia, W. B. Saunders Co., 1979.)

systematic (sis″te-mat′ik) [Gr. *systematikos*] pertaining to or according to a system.

systematic error an error in a measurement process that remains constant in a series of measurements under identical conditions. Systematic errors introduce a constant bias that cannot be detected by statistical methods. Cf. *random error.*

systematization (sis-tem″ah-ti-za′shun) arrangement according to a system.

systemic (sys-tem′ik) affecting the body as a whole; distributed throughout the body.

systemic lupus erythematosus (SLE) see *systemic l. erythematosus* under *lupus.*

systole (sis′to-le) [Gr. *systolē* a drawing together, contraction] the contraction or period of contraction of the heart chambers, particularly that of the ventricles. Ventricular systole follows that of the atria, and is commonly divided into periods of isometric (isovolumic) contraction and ejection. The duration of systole, an average of about 0.3 sec, can be measured clinically as the brief time interval between the first heart sound (closure of the A-V valves) and the second heart sound (closure of the aortic and pulmonic valves). Cf. *diastole.*

systolic (sis-tol′ik) pertaining to or produced by systole; occurring along with ventricular systole.

systolic murmur see under *murmur.*

systolic pressure see under *arterial pressure.*

systolic time interval (STI) the duration of electromechanical events that occur during ventricular contraction. The measurement of these intervals, commonly made through combined use of the phonocardiogram, carotid pressure tracing, and electrocardiogram (EKG), is useful as a noninvasive technique for the quantitative evaluation of left ventricular performance.

Three intervals are measured. The duration of ejection, the left ventricular ejection time (LVET), is measured from the beginning of the rise in carotid pressure to the dicrotic notch. The duration of total electromechanical systole ($Q–S_2$) is the interval between the beginning of the QRS complex of the EKG and that of the high-frequency vibrations produced by closure of the aortic valve (A_2 of the phonocardiogram). The preejection period (PEP) is the interval between the onset of the QRS complex and that of ejection, encompassing both the electrical and mechanical events leading to the left ventricular ejection. It is calculated indirectly as the difference between the $Q–S_2$ and the LVET. The values for these intervals are adjusted to compensate for differences in heart rate.

Although the $Q–S_2$ is fairly constant, the duration of the PEP and the LVET can vary markedly (and in opposing directions) with different cardiac disorders and hemodynamic factors, and with the use of pharmacologic agents that exert inotropic effects. Thus, the ratio PEP/LVET is the most useful relationship between the systolic time intervals for assessment of the degree of compromise in left ventricular performance caused by a particular cardiac disease.

T

T symbol for *absolute temperature, period* (time), *tera-, tesla, threonine, thymidine, torque, transmittance.*

2,4,5-T one of the chlorophenoxy herbicides (2,4,5-trichlorophenoxy) acetic acid; M.W. 255.49. See also *chlorophenoxy herbicides* and *dioxin.*

T_C the generation time of a cell cycle; $T_C = tG + tS + tG_2 + tM$. See also *cell cycle.*

T_D the time required to double the number of cells in a given population. $T_D = T_C$ when every cell in the population is cycling and all daughter cells survive. See also *cell cycle.*

$T\frac{1}{2}$, $t\frac{1}{2}$ symbol for *half-life.*

T_3 abbrev. See *triiodothyronine.*

T_4 abbrev. See *thyroxine.*

t symbol for student's t variable (see under *t-test*), *time, translocation.*

τ the Greek lower case letter *tau;* symbol for relaxation time.

Ta symbol for the chemical element *tantalum.*

tabanid (tab′ah-nid) any fly of the family Tabanidae, which includes the genera *Tabanus* and *Chrysops.*

Tabanidae (tah-ba′nĭ-de) a family of flies (the horseflies, gadflies, deerflies, and mango flies) of worldwide distribution, which includes the genera *Tabanus* and *Chrysops.*

Tabanus (tah-ba′nus) [L. "gadfly"] a genus of blood-sucking flies of worldwide distribution. They are large flies with heavy bodies and mouth parts that inflict a painful wound. Several species are known to transmit trypanosomes. Also called *gadfly* or *horsefly.*

tabes (ta′bēz) [L. *tabes* "wasting away," "decay," "melting"] a general term used to describe the progressive wasting or atrophy of a body part, usually the limbs. Causes include neurologic damage by neoplasms, infection, or systemic disorders such as syphilis.

tabes dorsalis (ta′bēz dor-sa′lis) [L. "wasting away, decay, melting"; "of the back,"from *dorsum* back] a complication of late tertiary syphilis characterized by chronic, progressive degeneration of the posterior columns, dorsal roots, and dorsal root ganglia. Clinical signs include impaired position and vibration sense, optic atrophy, hypotonia, hyporeflexia, disturbances of bladder function, trophic joint degeneration (Charcot's joints), painful visceral crises, and recurrent shooting pain in the leg muscles.

Early in the course of the disease, serologic tests for syphilis are strongly positive, and the cerebrospinal fluid may reveal increased numbers of white cells (3–200/μl) and protein levels; these may return to normal after antisyphilitic treatment.

See also *syphilis.*

table (ta′b′l) [L. *tabula*] 1. in anatomy, a flat layer or surface.

2. a display of data, usually printed in a rectangular array.

3. a collection of data in a computer program in which each item is located by its position rather than by content.

tablet (tab′let) [O.F. *tablete,* diminutive of *table* table] a solid dosage form of a drug for oral administration. Cf. *pill.*

tache (tahsh) [Fr.] a spot or blemish.

tachometer (tah-kom′ĕ-ter) [Gr. *tachos* speed + *metron* measure] a device that measures the angular speed (usually in revolutions per minute) of a rotating shaft.

tachy- (tak′e) [Gr. *tachys* swift] a prefix word element to denote fast, e.g., tachycardia.

tachyarrhythmia (tak″e-ah-rith′me-ah) [*tachy-* + *a-* neg. + Gr. *rhythmos* rhythm] an arrhythmia with a heart rate in adults of more than 100 beats/min. The term encompasses both supraventricular and ventricular tachycardias; the former includes sinus tachycardia, atrial flutter and fibrillation with rapid ventricular response, and atrial tachycardia.

tachycardia (tak″e-kar′de-ah) [*tachy-* + Gr. *kardia* heart] a term referring to a heart rate more rapid than 100 beats/min in adults. Most often the mechanism is sinus rhythm (governed by the sinoatrial node), and the rapid rate is secondary to factors such as emotions, exercise, anemia, drug effects, and fever. Other mechanisms include atrial tachycardias, atrial fibrillation and flutter, and ventricular tachycardia. Differentiation among the varying types of tachycardia is based on the ECG tracings.

atrial t., a rapid, regular, abnormal rhythm of the heartbeat conforming to normal sinus origin, with a rate between 160 and 190 beats/min.

junctional t., see *nodal t.*

nodal t., a rapid heart rate (in excess of 100 beats/min) resulting from impulses that originate in or near the atrioventricular node. It is less common than atrial or ventricular tachycardia, and is usually of minor hemodynamic significance because of the relatively slow rate (usually less than 130 beats/min). Also called *junctional t.*

ventricular t., three or more premature ventricular contractions in a series and with a rate above 100 beats/min. Ventricular tachycardia can be paroxysmal or sustained. Reentry is thought to be the cause. See also *reentry.*

tachyphylaxis (tak″e-fi-lak′sis) [*tachy-* + Gr. *phylaxis* protection] 1. the rapid acquisition of tolerance to a drug or toxin.

2. see *drug sensitization.*

tachypnea (tak″ip-ne′ah) [*tachy-* + Gr. *pnoia* breath] a rapid pattern of respiration that is usually but not always shallow. The tachypnea that can accompany pulmonary congestion and edema is thought to be a reflex response to stimulation of the pulmonary J receptors. Also called *polypnea.*

tactile (tak′til) [L. *tactilis*] pertaining to the touch.

tadpole cell (tad′pōl) an elongated, club-shaped epithelial cell with one broad and one narrow end, somewhat resembling the shape of a tadpole. It is a characteristic pleomorphic cell type associated with invasive keratinizing squamous carcinoma.

Taenia (te′ne-ah) [L. "a flat band," "bandage,"

"tape"] a genus of large tapeworms of the family Taeniidae.

T. africana, a species of "unarmed" tapeworms. The strobila measures 1.3 m long, and the proglottids are broader than they are long. This species has been reported only occasionally to infect humans.

T. canina, see *D. caninum* under *Dipylidium.*

T. confusa, a species of "unarmed" tapeworms occasionally found in the United States (the Mississippi Valley) and East Africa. The adult worms measure 5–8 m in length. The eggs are not distinctive and measure 33 by 42 μ. It is thought that this species is a variant of *T. saginata.* Also called *T. bremneri.*

T. diminuta, see *H. diminuta* under *Hymenolepis.*

T. lata, see *D. latum* under *Diphyllobothrium.*

T. murina, see *H. nana* under *Hymenolepis.*

T. nana, see *H. nana* under *Hymenolepis.*

T. saginata, a large tapeworm, the beef tapeworm, of cosmopolitan distribution. The adult worms measure 10–15 m in length (under favorable conditions, they may attain lengths of 25 m). They are characterized by a scolex lacking a rostellum and hooks (which distinguishes them from *T. solium*). The eggs are spherical to ovoid, measure 31–43 μm in diameter, and are indistinguishable from those of *T. solium.*

Human infection is caused by eating infected raw or improperly cooked beef. Following ingestion, the parasite attaches itself to the wall of the small intestines and requires a maturation period of 10–12 wk.

Laboratory diagnosis requires identification of eggs in the stool (indicating that the individual is infected with a species of *Taenia*). Diagnosis of *T. saginata* infection requires identification of mature proglottids. The proglottids are pressed between two glass slides and examined under a dissecting microscope in order to enumerate the number of main lateral uterine branches. *T. saginata* has 15–20 uterine branches on each side (averaging 18), whereas *T. solium* has 7–13 on each side (averaging 9). Also called *beef tapeworm, T. inermis, T. mediocanellata,* and *Taeniarhynchus mediocanellata.*

T. solium, the pork tapeworm of cosmopolitan distribution. The adult worms measure 2–7 m in length. Their scolex bears a prominent terminal rostellum with two circular rows of hooklets. The eggs are spherical in shape, measure 31–43 μm in diameter, and are indistinguishable from those of *T. saginata.*

Human infection may be caused by the ingestion of infected pork containing larvae, or by the ingestion of eggs from exogenous sources or from one's own stools. The larva becomes attached to the wall of the small intestine and develops into a mature worm in 5–12 wk, whereas some of the eggs penetrate the mucosa, enter the circulation, and give rise to cysticercosis.

Laboratory diagnosis first requires identification of eggs of the genus *Taenia.* Whether the infection is caused by *T. solium* or *T. saginata* is determined by microscopic examination of the mature proglottids in the stools. The proglottids are pressed between two slides and the number of main lateral uterine branches are counted. *T. solium* has 7–13 uterine branches on each side (averaging 9), whereas *T. saginata* has 15–20 on each side (averaging 18).

Also called *pork tapeworm, T. armata umana, T. cucurbitina, T. pellucida,* and *T. vulgaris.*

Taeniarhynchus (te″ne-ah-ring′kus) the former genus name for beef tapeworms, which includes the species *T. mediocanellata.* See also *T. saginata* under *Taenia.*

taeniasis (te-ni′ah-sis) [*Taenia* + *-iasis*] infection with tapeworms of the genus *Taenia.*

Taeniasis caused by *T. solium,* the pork tapeworm, has a cosmopolitan distribution. Human infection is acquired by the ingestion of raw or undercooked pork contaminated with the eggs of *T. solium.* The infection produces gastric and abdominal pain, an increased appetite, hunger pains, weakness, and weight loss. An infection with *T. solium* is potentially dangerous because of the possibilities of developing cysticercosis.

Taeniasis caused by *T. saginata,* the beef tapeworm, has worldwide distribution. Human infection is acquired in the same manner as that of *T. solium.* Most infections are asymptomatic, but some individuals experience abdominal pains, malaise, weight loss, and increased appetite.

Laboratory diagnosis requires detection of characteristic *Taenia* eggs in the stools. Specific species identification is obtained by finding gravid proglottids: the number of main lateral uterine branches on the proglottids counted under a dissecting microscope can differentiate the species (*T. saginata* possesses 15–20 on each side; *T. solium,* 7–13).

See also *T. saginata* and *T. solium* under *Taenia.*

Taeniidae (te-ni′ĭ-de) a family of tapeworms parasitic in humans, including the genera *Taenia, Multiceps,* and *Echinococcus.*

Taenzer-Unna stain (ten′zer ōō′nah) [Paul R. *Taenzer,* 1859–1919, German dermatologist; Paul Gerson *Unna,* 1850–1929, German dermatologist] a stain for elastic fibers. See under *acid orcein.*

tag (tag) 1. a small appendage, flap, or polyp.

2. a term in common usage for label, i.e., an immunofluorescent label or a radiolabel.

Tagamet (tag′ah-met) trademark. See *cimetidine.*

tail (tāl) [L. *cauda;* Gr. *oura*] 1. any slender appendage. Also called *cauda.*

2. the appendage that extends from the posterior trunk of many animals.

tailing (ta′ling) in gas chromatography, the phenomenon caused by chemical interaction of the component with active sites on the solid support and exhibited as a peak that has a sharp rise and gradual fall.

tail poikilocyte see *teardrop cell.*

Takayasu's arteritis (tok″ah-yah′sōōz) an inflammatory disease of unknown origin that principally involves the thoracic aorta and proximal segments of its major branches, with round cell infiltration and fibrosis in the media and adventitia. Females aged 10–50 yr are most commonly affected. The manifestations vary, depending on the degree of arterial obstruction, and include hypertension, lack of pulse in the arms or necks, intermittent claudication, visual disturbances, and syncope.

Laboratory findings include an elevated erythrocyte sedimentation rate (ESR), moderate leukocytosis, transient eosinophilia, and thrombocytosis. Hypergammaglobulinemia (IgA, IgG, and IgM), positive test for rheumatoid factor, LE cells, and antinuclear antibodies have also been found. In the early stages of the disease, the administration of corticosteroids has produced remission; in the chronic stages, however, bypass grafts of the involved vessels are necessary.

talc (talk) [USP], a native, hydrous magnesium silicate, sometimes containing a small proportion of aluminum silicate, used as a dusting powder. Also called purified talc.

talipes (tal′ĭ-pēz) [N.L. "clubfoot," from *talus* ankle + *pes* foot] a congenital abnormality of the foot characterized by a distortion of shape or position. The most frequent form is equinovarus, in which the foot is plantar flexed, inverted, and adducted. Early care may normalize the position. Other forms include talipes calcaneovalgus (dorsiflexed), talipes valgus (everted), and talipes cavus (high longitudinal arch). Also called *clubfoot.*

talus (ta′lus), pl. *tali* [L. "ankle"] the ankle bone. It rests on the upper surface of the calcaneus, and is clasped by and articulates with the inner surfaces of the lateral and medial malleoli and the lower surface of the tibia.

tamoxifen citrate (tah-mok′sĭ-fen) a cancer chemotherapeutic drug; trademark, Nolvadex. For more information, see *Appendix A.*

tamponade (tam″pon-ād′) [Fr. *tamponner* to stop up] 1. the surgical use of a tampon.

2. the pathologic compression of a part.

cardiac t., see *cardiac tamponade.*

Tamulus (tam′u-lus) a genus of scorpions found in India. Their neurotoxic venom makes them extremely dangerous.

tan (tan) abbrev. See *tangent.*

tangent (tan′jent) [L. *linea tangens* touching line] 1. a straight line that touches but does not intersect a smooth curve; the tangent at a given point is the line that passes through that point but no neighboring point on the curve.

2. (abbrev. tan), a trigonometric function, the sine of an angle divided by the cosine: $\tan(\theta) = \sin(\theta)/\cos(\theta)$.

tangential projection (tan-jen′shal) a radiographic projection in which the central ray passes along a tangent to the surface of an organ or part, e.g., carpal tunnel or carpal bridge, scapular spine, mastoid process, or parotid gland.

Tangier disease (tan-jēr′) [from *Tangier* Island, in Chesapeake Bay, where the disease was first discovered] a rare genetic disorder, transmitted as an autosomal recessive trait, that is characterized by a relative or absolute deficiency of alpha lipoproteins (also known as high-density lipoproteins, HDLs) in the serum. Onset occurs in childhood with the excessive storage of cholesterol esters in reticuloendothelial cells, leading to hepatosplenomegaly, lymphadenopathy, and a characteristic yellow-orange tonsillar enlargement. In addition, there may be corneal opacities and a recurrent polyneuropathy with severe, progressive, cutaneous anesthesia to pain and temperature over the face, scalp, and proximal limbs.

Laboratory testing reveals that total plasma cholesterol and beta lipoproteins are decreased, while prebeta lipoproteins, chylomicrons, and triglycerides may be increased. HDL deficiencies are demonstrable by electrophoretic or ultracentrifugal techniques. Heterozygotes have HDL concentrations that are lower than normal. There is no known treatment.

Also called familial alpha-lipoprotein deficiency.

tanned red cell hemagglutination inhibition test see under *fibrin (fibrinogen) degradation products methods.*

tannic acid (tan′ik) a lustrous powder, yellow to light-brown in color, that is found in tree bark (particularly oak), fruits, leaves, and tea. It is used medicinally as an astringent, commercially in tanning hides, and as a dye mordant.

tantalum (Ta) (tan′tah-lum) [*Tantalus* a figure in Greek mythology condemned in Hades to stand up to his neck in water without being able to drink it] a hard, ductile, gray metallic element; atomic number 73; atomic weight 180.9479; a 5d transition element; oxidation states +1, +2, +3, +4, +5 (the most common).

Tantalum is not attacked by acids, is completely corrosion-resistant at normal temperatures, and is used surgically for intracranial plates to repair cranial defects, for wire sutures, and in the production of prosthetic appliances. Inhalation of tantalum dusts may produce benign pulmonary lesions; no other toxic effects are known.

T antigen (tumor antigen) a large protein found in the nucleus of tumor cells transformed with DNA viruses; M.W. 90,000–100,000. It was first demonstrated by complement-fixation tests with sera from hamsters with SV40-induced tumors. Its nuclear location can be demonstrated by immunofluorescence tests. The term T antigen should not be confused with the term tumor-specific antigen.

tape (tāp) see *magnetic tape* and *paper tape.*

tape drive a computer peripheral device used to read and write data on magnetic tape.

tape mark a special end-of-file character used with magnetic tape. It is a uniquely readable character on a tape, typically indicating the beginning and ending of a file.

tape transport the mechanism that moves the magnetic tape past the tape heads of a tape recorder or tape drive.

tapeworm (tāp′werm) a parasitic intestinal cestode worm, which has a flattened, bandlike form. Those tapeworms primarily responsible for human infection include the genera *Diphyllobothrium, Dipylidium, Echinococcus, Hymenolepis,* and *Taenia.* See also *cestode.*

TARA abbrev. See *tumor-associated rejection antigen.*

Taractan (tar-ak′tan) trademark. See *chlorprothixene.*

tare (tār) [Fr.] 1. the weight of the vessel in which a substance is weighed.

2. to weigh a vessel in which a substance is weighed to allow for its weight.

target (tar′get) an object or material subjected to bombardment by radiation, such as the area of the anode of an x-ray tube where x-rays are produced by electron bombardment, or the material irradiated by particles from an accelerator or nuclear reactor in order to produce radioisotopes.

target cell 1. in hematology, a hypochromic erythrocyte with increased surface-volume ratio. Scanning electron microscopy shows the cell to be a thin-walled cup, shaped like a bell. In stained smears the top of the bell collapses, producing the appearance of a central accumulation of hemoglobin with a narrow, pale circle between the central "target" or "bull's-eye," and the peripheral rim of hemoglobin. Another appearance in smears is that of a sombrero. Target cells commonly occur in thalassemia, iron deficiency, lecithin-cholesterol-acyl transferase (LCAT) deficiency, the postsplenectomy state, hemoglobin SC disease, and other conditions. Also called *codocyte.*

2. in immunology, an altered or foreign cell such as a tumor cell or virus-infected cell, or any antigenically different cell from another individual that is subject to immune assault. It particularly refers to interaction with a cytotoxic T lymphocyte.

target organ the organ or tissue affected by a particular hormone.

tar oil the volatile oil from pine tar rectified by steam distillation. It is used in veterinary medicine: internally as a stimulant expectorant and externally as an antipruritic, antiseptic, and stimulant for skin diseases.

tarsal (tahr′sal) [L. *tarsalis*] pertaining to the tarsus.

tarsal tunnel syndrome a peripheral entrapment neuropathy that occurs when the posterior tibial nerve is compressed in the tarsal tunnel as a result of trauma to the ankle, the presence of a ganglion or varix on the vasculature passing through the tunnel, tendon sheath cysts, or hypertrophy of the abductor hallucis muscle. The most prominent clinical manifestations, a burning pain and paresthesia in the foot, are most severe at night.

tarsus (tahr′sus) [N.L.; Gr. *tarsos* a frame or flat basket of wickerwork; any broad, flat surface] the seven bones that make up the skeleton of the posterior half of the foot. The talus and calcaneus lie posterior to the medial, intermediate, and lateral cuneiforms, cuboid, and navicular. Together with the metatarsus, the bones of the tarsus create intersecting longitudinal and transverse arches that diffuse the weight of the body.

tartaric acid (tar″tar′ik) 2,3-dihydroxybutanedioic acid, HOOC—$(CHOH)_2$—COOH; M.W. 150.09. With two like chiral centers, it exists in three isomeric forms: D-tartaric acid (levorotatory, (–), or unnatural tartaric acid); L-tartaric acid (dextrorotatory, (+), or natural tartaric acid); and meso-tartaric acid (internally compensated tartaric acid, which is optically inactive). DL-Tartaric acid (racemic or paratartaric acid), an equimolar mixture of D- and L-tartaric acids, is also optically inactive. In its natural form, L-(+)-tartaric acid is found in grape juice, in the lees of winemaking, and in various plant fluids. Only small quantities of the D-(–) and DL-form are found in nature. Tartaric acid is used in baking and tanning; in the preparation of soft drinks, confectionary products, ceramics, and lacquers (diethyl, dibutyl derivatives); and as a chemical agent.

tart cell a cell formed by the ingestion by a neutrophil of an entire lymphocyte. Tart cells can be confused with lupus erythematosus (LE) cells, but the events that lead to their formation are different and tart cells have no significance. In a tart cell, the entire cell is first ingested, and the nucleus is homogenized only later, if at all, by the influence of enzymes released into the digestion vacuole, whereas an LE cell is formed by ingestion of one or more rounded off, already homogenized fragments of a nucleus. Cf. *lupus erythematosus cell.*

tartrate (tar′trāt) [L. *tartras*] any salt or ester of tartaric acid.

tartrazine (tar′trah-zēn) a yellow acid dye, 3-carboxy-5-hydroxy-1-*p*-sulfophenyl-4-*p*-sulfophenylazopyrazole trisodium salt; C.I. 19140. It is used in histology as a plasma stain, and also is commonly employed as a dye for foods and drugs. Also called *FD & C Yellow No. 5.*

task (task) in a multiprogramming system, a group of programs, data sets, and control messages that constitute one complete unit of work for the operating system.

taste (tāst) [Old French *taster* to taste] the peculiar sensation caused by contact of a soluble substance with the tongue and its contained receptors or taste buds. There are four basic tastes: sweet, salt, sour, and bitter.

taste bud a minute, barrel-shaped chemosensory structure composed of modified epithelial elements. Found throughout the buccal cavity and associated pharynx, these structures are most numerous around the circumvallate papillae on the tongue. Each bud is a group of outer supporting cells surrounding inner sensory cells.

tau (Τ, τ) (tou, taw) the nineteenth letter of the *Greek alphabet.*

taurine (taw′rēn) a crystallizable acid, 2-aminoethanesulfonic acid, $NH_2(CH_2)_2SO_2OH$, present in bile in the form of peptide bond conjugates with bile acids. Taurine is present in the brain (75 mg/100 g) and in small quantities in the lungs, muscles, and serum. It is derived from cysteine via oxidation to cysteine sulfinic acid, followed by decarboxylation and another oxidation.

taurochenodeoxycholate (taw″ro-ke″no-de-ok″se-ko′lat) any salt, ester, or dissociated form of taurochenodeoxycholic acid. See also *taurochenodeoxycholic acid.*

taurochenodeoxycholic acid (taw″ro-ke″no-de-ok″se-ko′lic) *N*-chenodeoxycholoyl taurine, the amide conjugate of chenodeoxycholic acid with taurine (2-aminoethanesulfonic acid). It is formed in the liver and appears in the bile.

taurocholate (taw″ro-ko′lāt) any salt, ester, or dissociated form of taurocholic acid. See also *taurocholic acid.*

taurocholic acid (taw″ro-ko′lic) *N*-choloyl-taurine, the amide conjugate of cholic acid with taurine (2-aminoethanesulfonic acid). It is the chief ingredient of the bile of carnivorous animals.

taurodeoxycholic acid (taw″ro-de-ok″se-ko′lik) a bile acid conjugate in which the carboxyl group of deoxycholic acid and the amino group of taurine are joined by an amide linkage. It is formed in the liver from deoxycholic acid produced in the gut by bacterial dehydroxylation of cholic acid and returned via the enterohepatic circulation.

taurolithocholic acid (taw″ro-lith″o-ko′lic) a bile acid conjugate in which the carboxyl group of lithocholic acid and the amino group of taurine are joined by an amide linkage. It is formed in the liver from lithocholic acid produced in the gut by bacterial dehydroxylation of chenodeoxycholic acid and returned via the enterohepatic circulation.

Taussig-Bing syndrome (taw′sig bing) [Helen Brooke *Taussig,* American pediatrician, born 1898; Richard J. *Bing,* American surgeon, born 1909] a rare congenital condition in which both the aorta and pulmonary artery arise from the right ventricle. A subpulmonic ventricular septal defect is invariably present. The main symptom is cyanosis, the degree of which also depends on the presence or absence of pulmonary stenosis. Diagnosis is based on clinical signs and angiocardiographic analysis. Also called *incomplete transposition of great arteries.*

tautomer (tau'to-mer) any of several compounds related by tautomerism.

tautomerism (tau-tom'er-izm) [Gr. *tauto-* from *to auto* the same + *meros* part] the dynamic equilibrium that exists between two isomers that can be readily interconverted. See also *isomerism.*

keto-enol t., proton tautomerism in which the keto tautomer contains a carbonyl group (—CO—CHR—) and the enol tautomer has a hydroxyl group and a double bond (—COH═CR—). The keto form is more stable unless the enol form is stabilized by conjugation of the enol double bond or by intramolecular hydrogen bonding.

proton t., a type of tautomerism involving the transfer of an acidic proton from one atom (usually nitrogen or oxygen) to another atom. Examples of proton tautomerism are keto-enol, nitro–*aci*-nitro, imine-enamine, and nitroso-oxime tautomerism.

ring-chain t., a type of tautomerism in which the two forms are an open chain and a ring. Many sugars exhibit this type. The open-chain form is a hydroxyketone or hydroxyaldehyde, and the five- or six-membered ring (furanose or pyranose) is a hemiacetal or hemiketal.

valence t., a type of tautomerism occurring especially in ring compounds in which no part of the molecule is detached from the rest in the reaction that converts one tautomer to the other.

tax/o (tak'so) [Gr. *taxis* arrangement] a word element used in combining form to denote order or coordination, e.g., ataxia.

taxis (tak'sis) [Gr. "a drawing up in rank and file"] an orientation movement of a motile organism in response to an external stimulus. The movement may be positive (toward) or negative (away from) the stimulus.

-taxis a suffix word element to denote a stimulus, e.g., chemotaxis, phototaxis.

taxon (tak'son), pl. *taxa* [*taxis* + *-on*] a particular group or taxonomic category into which related organisms are classified on the basis of mutual characteristics, e.g., family, tribe, genus. See also *taxonomy.*

taxonomy (tak-son'o-me) [*taxo-* + Gr. *nomos* law] the science of biologic classification; the orderly classification of organisms in a hierarchy of categories (taxa) on the basis of mutual characteristics with the application of suitable and correct names. Schemes of taxonomy fulfill two purposes. A purely descriptive taxonomy groups organisms of like characteristics and describes the criteria of groupings. Such a system is used in the description of microorganisms (bacteria, fungi, viruses), so that application of successive criteria leads to the correct identification of an unknown specimen. Taxonomy in higher organisms (plants, animals) is also phylogenetic, in which the classification aims at reflecting evolutionary development. Categories used in taxonomy include, in descending order: kingdom, phylum or division, class, order, family, tribe, genus, species. In bacteriology, a species may be subdivided into several *strains.* See also *classification.*

Tay-Sachs disease (ta saks') [Warren *Tay,* English physician, 1843–1927; Bernard *Sachs,* New York neurologist, 1858–1944] a rare metabolic disease, transmitted as an autosomal recessive trait, that occurs primarily among Jewish individuals of northeastern European descent (Ashkenazi), in whom the carrier rate in heterozygotes is 1 in 30. It is characterized by a lack of the enzyme hexosaminidase A. The enzyme deficiency leads to the accumulation of a sphingolipid (ganglioside G_{M2}) in nerve cells. The accumulation destroys the nerve cells and causes the proliferation of glial cells and the degeneration of myelin. Onset of the disease occurs within the first 4 or 5 mo of life and leads to psychomotor disabilities, hypotonia, seizures, dementia, blindness (with cherry-red retinal spots), paralysis and death by age 3–4 yr. There is no known cure.

Diagnosis is based on blood analysis for hexosaminidase A activity; a deficiency of the enzyme can also be detected in cultured cells. Abnormal electroencephalographic recordings accompany the development of neurologic abnormalities, and are characterized by high-voltage delta activity or triphasic waveforms occurring on irregular background activity of 1.5–6 Hz. Abnormalities in visual evoked potentials may also be recorded in response to flash stimuli.

Mass screening programs have helped identify heterozygous carriers of the genetic trait; antenatal diagnostic tests by amniocentesis at about 18 wk of gestation should be performed if both parents are known heterozygotes.

Also called *G_{M2} gangliosidosis.* See also *Sandhoff's disease* and *sphingolipidoses.*

TB abbrev. See *tuberculosis.*

Tb symbol for the chemical element *terbium.*

T banding (telomere or terminal banding) a chromosome banding technique that preferentially stains telomeres. For a description of frequently used banding techniques, see *chromosome banding.*

TBG abbrev. See *thyroxine-binding globulin*

TBG cap abbrev. for T_4-binding capacity of TBG. See under *thyroxine-binding globulin assays.*

TBH abbrev. See *total body h.* under *hematocrit.*

TBI abbrev. for total-body irradiation.

TBII abbrev. for TSH-binding inhibitory immunoglobulin; see under *thyroid-stimulating immunoglobulins.*

T bili abbrev. for total bilirubin; see under *bilirubin assays.*

TBPA abbrev. See *thyroxine-binding prealbumin.*

TC abbrev. for to contain. See under *pipet.*

T_4(C) abbrev. for serum thyroxine (T_4) measured by the column chromatographic technique. See under *thyroxine assays.*

Tc symbol for the chemical element *technetium.*

TCA abbrev. See *tricarboxylic acid cycle, trichloroacetic acid.*

TCBS agar [acronym from *t*hiosulfate-*c*itrate-*b*ile *s*alts] an agar medium containing thiosulfate-citrate-bile salts, used as a selective medium in the primary isolation of pathogenic vibrios, especially *Vibrio cholerae.*

TCDD abbrev. for tetrachlorodibenzodioxin. See *dioxin.*

TC detector abbrev. for thermal conductivity detector. See under *gas chromatography.*

T cell see *T l.* under *lymphocyte.*

T-cell replacing factor (TRF) a glycoprotein produced by T cells, presumably helper cells; M.W. 30,000. TRF gives a differential signal to intermediary B cells, which turn into IgM- or IgG-producing plasma cells.

TCP abbrev. See *tricresyl phosphate.*

tcRNA abbrev. See *translation control RNA.*

TD abbrev. for to deliver. See under *pipet.*

T_4(D) abbrev. for serum thyroxine (T_4) measured by displacement analysis, a type of competitive binding assay. See under *thyroxine assays.*

TDA abbrev. for TSH-displacing antibody; see under *thyroid-stimulating immunoglobulins.*

TDE an insecticide; 1,1-dichloro-2,2-bis(*p*-chlorophenyl)ethane, formerly tetrachlorodiphenylethane; similar to DDT. See also *chlorinated hydrocarbon pesticides.*

TDI abbrev. See *toluene 2,4-diisocyanate.*

***t* distribution** the exact sampling distribution of the random variable $T_n = Z/S$, where Z and S are independent random variables, Z has the standard normal distribution, and nS^2 has the chi-squared distribution with n degree of freedom.

If $\overline{X}$ and s are the sample mean and standard deviation of a random sample of size n from a normal distribution with mean μ and standard deviation σ, $(\overline{X} - \mu)/(\sigma/\sqrt{n})$ has the standard normal distribution and $(n-1)s^2/\sigma^2$ has the chi-squared distribution with $n-1$ degrees of freedom. Thus, $T_{n-1} = (X - \mu)/(s/\sqrt{n})$ has the t distribution with $n-1$ degrees of freedom. The upper α percentile point is written $t_{\alpha,\, n-1}$; $P(T_{n-1} > t_{\alpha,\, n-1}) = \alpha$.

The points $X \pm t_{\alpha/2,\, n-1} \cdot s/\sqrt{n}$ are the upper and lower confidence limits for a $100(1-\alpha)$ confidence interval for μ. In hypothesis tests, the null hypothesis that μ is the true population mean is rejected at the α significance level if $T_{n-1} > t_{\alpha,\, n-1}$ for a one-tailed test against the alternative hypothesis that the true mean is different from μ. It is rejected if $|T_{n-1}| > t_{\alpha/2,\, n-1}$ for a two-tailed test against the alternative hypothesis that the true mean is different from μ.

For data that consist of the same measurement performed on n matched pairs of treated subjects and controls, the n differences between each subject and its control are normally distributed if both measurements are normally distributed. The same tests and confidence intervals are calculated using the mean and standard deviation of the differences.

For two independent random samples from normal distributions with different means but the same standard deviation, $[(X_1 - X_2) - (\mu_1 - \mu_2)]/\sigma\sqrt{1/n_1 + 1/n_2}$ has the standard normal distribution and $[(n_1 - 1)s_1^2/\sigma^2] + [(n_2 - 1)s_2^2/\sigma^2]$ has the chi-squared distribution with $n_1 + n_2 - 2$ degrees of freedom; thus,

$$T_{n_1 + n_2 - 2} = \frac{(X_1 - X_2) - (\mu_1 - \mu_2)}{\sqrt{\dfrac{\frac{1}{n_1} + \frac{1}{n_2}}{n_1 + n_2 + 2}\left[(n_1 - 1)s_1^2 + (n_2 - 2)s_2^2\right]}}$$

has the t distribution with $n_1 + n_2 - 2$ degrees of freedom and can be used to construct confidence intervals or hypothesis tests for the difference of the means.

TDT abbrev. for terminal deoxynucleotidyl transferase. See *DNA nucleotidylexotransferase.*

Te symbol for the chemical element *tellurium.*

tear (tēr) [A.S. *tēar* L. *lacrima;* Gr. *dakrya*] 1. a watery secretion of the lacrimal glands, which serves to moisten the conjunctiva; the secretion is slightly alkaline and contains protein (0.6–0.8 g/dl), which lowers the surface tension, permitting wetting of the epithelial surfaces. This film improves the optical properties of the eye; microscopic irregularities in the corneal epithelium are abolished, producing a smooth optical surface. The film also protects the eye from damage by small foreign bodies such as dust or airborne bacteria. Lysozyme, which is present in tears, hydrolyzes the muramic acid–containing mucopeptide in the polysaccharide of the cell walls of many airborne cocci. Also called *lacrimal fluid.*

2. a small, naturally formed, droplike mass of a gum or resin.

tear (tār) a laceration.

teardrop cell an erythrocyte found in myelofibrosis and other myelproliferative disorders and infrequently in thalassemia. It is distorted or fragmented, small, and often hypochromic; the cell takes its name from its resemblance to a teardrop.

technetium (Tc) (tek-ne'she-um) [N.L., from Gr. *technētos* artificial] a synthetic, radioactive metallic element; atomic number 43; most stable isotope ^{97}Tc (half-life, 2.6 million years); a 4d transition element; oxidation states +1 through +7 (+4, +7 are most common). ^{99}Tc produced by the decay of ^{99m}Tc (used in nuclear medicine) has a half-life of 212,000 yr.

technetium-99m (^{99m}Tc, Tc 99m) the most widely used radionuclide in nuclear medicine. It decays by isomeric transition with a half-life of 6.03 hr, emitting 140.5-keV gamma rays. This photon energy provides good detector sensitivity and resolution for both scintillation cameras and rectilinear scanners. No other radiation is produced.

^{99m}Tc is generator-produced when a reactor-produced nuclide, molybdenum-99, undergoes positron beta decay with a 67-hr half-life, producing ^{99m}Tc. The two nuclides are separated by column chromatography; sterile isotonic sodium chloride is used for elution. The ^{99}Mo remains bound to the alumina column packing, while the ^{99m}Tc is eluted as pertechnetate (TeO_4^-). The eluate (sodium pertechnetate Tc 99m, USP) is used as an imaging agent for thyroid, salivary gland, blood pool, and brain scans, and also in the preparation of other ^{99m}Tc radiopharmaceuticals.

The physiologic distribution of pertechnetate is similar to that of iodide. It is loosely bound by plasma proteins, taken up but not organified by the thyroid, and also taken up by the choroid plexus, salivary glands, and gastric mucosa. Administration of the perchlorate ion (ClO_4^-) blocks uptake in these organs by competitive inhibition. Pertechnetate is excreted by both the gastrointestinal tract and the kidneys.

technetium Tc-99m aggregated albumin [USP], a radiopharmaceutical used for pulmonary perfusion imaging. Also called ^{99m}Tc macroaggregated albumin and Tc-99m-MAA. See also *aggregated a.* under *albumin.*

technetium Tc-99m albumin microspheres a radiopharmaceutical used for pulmonary perfusion imaging. See also *a. microspheres* under *albumin.*

technetium Tc-99m dihydrothiotic acid a lipid-soluble agent used for imaging the biliary system and the gallbladder. It localizes in the parenchymal cells of the liver and is excreted in the bile.

technetium Tc-99m dimercaptosuccinic acid (Tc-99m-DMSA) a kidney-imaging agent. It has greater kidney concentration than Tc-99m-glucoheptonate, but is somewhat less stable.

technetium Tc-99m diphosphonate any of several bone-imaging agents in which ^{99m}Tc is complexed with a diphosphonate using the stannous ion as the complexing and reducing agent.

Diphosphonates are rapidly cleared from the blood, and are primarily taken up by bone or excreted; they are not broken down by enzymes, although some elution of the label occurs. The approved diphosphonates are ^{99m}Tc medronate methylene diphosphonate, also called MDP) and ^{99m}Tc etidronate (ethane-1-hydroxy-1,1-diphosphonate, also called EHPD and HEDSPA); both are prepared using sterile reagent kits.

technetium Tc-99m etidronate sodium see under *technetium Tc-99m diphosphonate.*

technetium Tc-99m glucoheptonate a complex of technetium with glucoheptonic acid (glucose-monocarboxylic acid), used for kidney imaging. Its distribution in the body is similar to ^{99m}Tc iron-ascorbate and it is more stable. Also called Tc-99m glucoheptonate.

technetium Tc-99m iron ascorbate complex a kidney-imaging agent prepared by reducing pertechnetate with ascorbic acid in the presence of ferric iron. It is filtered and bound by the renal tubules. The sterile reagent kit preparation, technetium Tc-99m iron ascorbate pentetic acid complex (Tc-99m-iron-ascorbate-DTPA), has the same distribution in the body.

technetium Tc-99m medronate sodium see under *technetium Tc-99m diphosphonate.*

technetium Tc-99m pentetic acid (Tc-99m-DTPA, Tc-99m-Sn-DTPA) a chelate, prepared with a sterile reagent kit, used in measuring the glomerular filtration rate. It is also one of the agents used for brain scans. Pertechnetate is reduced by stannous chloride and chelated by pentetate (DPTA). This agent is rapidly cleared from the blood by the kidneys.

technetium Tc-99m pertechnetate see under *technetium-99m.*

technetium Tc-99m polyphosphate a bone-imaging agent similar to Tc-99m pyrophosphate. The polyphosphate is a linear chain containing 46–50 phosphate monomers.

technetium Tc-99m pyrophosphate a bone-imaging agent which is a stable technetium-tin-pyrophosphate complex, and is prepared using a sterile reagent kit. The agent is primarily taken up by bone or is excreted. The blood clearance is slower than with diphosphonates, and the pyrophosphate is broken down by phosphatase enzymes. ^{99m}Tc pyrophosphate is the preferred agent for imaging acute myocardial infarctions.

technetium Tc-99m red blood cells an imaging agent used for blood pool imaging. It is prepared by adding a reducing agent containing the stannous ion to the patient's packed red cells and then adding pertechnetate, which is reduced and bound intracellularly. When the cell membrane is damaged by heat or by large amounts of the stannous ion, the denatured cells are sequestered by the spleen and are used for spleen imaging.

technetium Tc-99m serum albumin (Tc-99m-HSA) a radiopharmaceutical preparation of ^{99m}Tc, complexed with human serum albumin, that is used for blood pool imaging, particularly of the cardiovascular pools. The technetium ion is reduced either chemically or electrolytically and is strongly bound to the albumin. Some unbound technetium is localized in the kidneys and bladder.

technetium Tc-99m sulfur colloid [USP], a radiopharmaceutical prepared by reducing thiosulfate to sulfur in an acidic solution with heat. It is the agent of choice for obtaining images of the liver, spleen, and bone marrow. With use of a sterile reagent kit, colloidal particles 0.1–2 μm in size form and trap pertechnetate ions. As with other colloids, ^{99m}Tc sulfur colloid is taken up by reticuloendothelial cells.

technic (tek′nik, tek-nēk′) [Gr. *technikos* technical, systematic] 1. the theory and principles of an applied science.

2. see *technique.*

technical (tek′nĭ-kal) pertaining to technique.

technician (tek-nish′un) a person skilled in preforming the technical or procedural aspects of a health care profession. Generally, the minimal preparation for this role is an associate (2-yr) degree. The technician carries out the routine work of the profession under the supervision of a physician, therapist, technologist, or other health care professional.

technique (tek-nēk′) [Fr., from Gr. *technikos* systematic] a systematic, detailed procedure for performing some activity, such as a test or assay in clinical chemistry or the processing of tissue sections in histology, also described as a procedure or method. Also spelled technic.

technologic life (tek″no-loj′ik) the period of time until a technologically superior piece of equipment becomes available and makes an existing piece of equipment obsolete.

technologist (tek-nol′o-jist) a person skilled in the theory and practice of a technical profession. In several allied health fields, technologist is the highest professional rank. Generally, the minimal preparation for this role is a baccalaureate (4-yr) degree. In additon to routine work, the technologist is involved in problem-solving and implementing new procedures. See also *medical technologist.*

technology (tek-nol′o-je) [Gr. *technē* art + *logos* reason, discourse] 1. an applied science e.g., medical laboratory technology.

2. a specific technical method or engineering design. The term usually refers to the instrumentation or equipment involved in a procedure rather than the basic method. Cf. *method.*

3. the instruments and devices used in the application of science and engineering.

tectorial (tek-to′re-al) [L. *tectorius,* from *tectum* roof] of the nature of a roof or covering.

tectorial membrane in the ear, a membrane formed of delicate fibers distributed throughout a gelatinous mass and resting on the spiral organ of Corti. Hair cell stereocilia are firmly attached to the membrane, which is wider and thicker apically in the cochlea than at its basal end.

tectum (tek′tum) [L. "roof"] a rooflike structure, especially the posterior part of the midbrain.

TED abbrev. See *threshold erythema d.* under *dose.*

Teflon (tef′lon) trademark for polytetrafluoroethylene (TFE), fluorocarbon polymers available in the form of molding, extrusion powders, aqueous dispersions, film, finishes, and multifilament yarn or fiber. The name also applies to fluorinated ethylene-propylene polymer (FEP) resins available in the same forms. Teflon is inert and not affected by heat. It is used in the manufacture of stopcocks, stoppers, and the tips of forceps and tongs for laboratory use. Other uses of Teflon include surgical implantation, valve packing, machine bearings, filters, electric insulation, high-temperature industrial plastics, cooking utensils, and plumbing sealants.

tegafur (teg′ah-fur) a cancer chemotherapeutic drug; trademark, Ftorafur. For more information, see *Appendix A.*

tegmen (teg′men), pl. *tegmina* [L. "cover"] a general term to designate a covering structure or roof.

tegmentum (teg-men′tum), pl. *tegmenta* [L.] 1. a covering.

2. [NA], the dorsal part of the cerebral peduncles situated above the substantia nigra. Continuous posteriorly with the pontine tegmentum, it includes fibers of the reticular formation, the medial longitudinal fasciculus, and nuclei of cranial nerves III (oculomotor), IV (trochlear), and V (mesencephalic nucleus of the trigeminal).

tegmen tympani (teg′men tim′pah-ne) [NA], a thin layer of compact bone that forms part of the petrous portion of the temporal bone and separates the tympanic cavity from the cranial cavity.

teichoic acid (ti′ko-ik) a macromolecule on the surfaces of all gram-positive organisms. These are polymers of glycerol or ribitol in phosphodiester linkage. Alanine and some monosaccharides may be in ester or glycoside linkage, respectively, to glycerol molecules in the polymer. There is evidence that teichoic acids are in phosphodiester linkage with the carbon-6 of *N*-acetylmuramic acid in peptidoglycans of many bacteria.

tel/o (tel′o) [Gr. *telos* end] a word element used in combining form to denote an end, e.g., telocentric.

tela (te′lah), pl. *telae* [L. "something woven," "web"] [NA], a general term for a thin membrane resembling a web.

t. choroidea of fourth ventricle, a double layer or fold of pia mater situated between the cerebellum and roof of the fourth ventricle. The vascular fringes of the tela choroidea form the choroid plexus.

t. choroidea of lateral ventricles, an extension of the tela choroidea of the third ventricle laterally into the lateral ventricles of the brain. Vascular folds invade the ventricular ependyma to form the choroid plexuses in this area.

t. choroidea of third ventricle, a fold of pia mater that combines with ventricular ependyma to form the roof of the third ventricle. This roof is invaginated by the vascular fringes of the tela choroidea to produce the choroid plexus.

telangiectasia (tel-an″je-ek-ta′ze-ah) [*tel-* + Gr. *angeion* vessel + *ektasis* dilation] the dilation of superficial blood vessels (arterioles, capillaries, and venules) that creates small, focal, red lesions, usually in the skin and mucous membranes. Enlargement of vessel caliber is seen, and may represent congenital anomalies or acquired deformation of existing blood vessels.

Telangiectasia may be associated with erythema in systemic lupus erythematosus, dermatomyositis, and psoriasis. It may be scattered and discrete in scleroderma, consist of sharply outlined red macules or papules in Rendu-Weber-Osler disease, generalized in mastocytosis, or occur in fine lines following solar damage to the skin. A special form of telangiectasia, the spider nevus, may be seen, often in association with liver disease. Telangiectasia is a prominent clinical finding and diagnostic feature of ataxia telangiectasia (Louis-Bar syndrome).

hereditary hemorrhagic t., a familial condition, transmitted as an autosomal dominant trait, that is characterized by multiple, dilated, thin-walled veins with aneurysms (telangiectases) in the skin and mucous membranes. These lesions appear as small areas, red to purple in color, that blanch on pressure and tend to bleed with minimal trauma. They can be present at birth on an infant's face, mouth, nose, or hands; they may be responsible for profuse blood loss, often through the nose and gastrointestinal tract, and especially in persons over 30 yr of age. Pulmonary arteriovenous fistulas and secondary iron deficiency anemia may also occur.

Laboratory findings are used to rule out other causes of bleeding and diagnosis is made on clinical grounds. There is no known cure. Long-term iron therapy is recommended and multiple blood transfusions may be required.

Also called heredofamilial angiomatosis, Osler's syndrome, and *Rendu-Weber-Osler disease.*

telangiectasis (tel-an″je-ek′tah-sis), pl. *telangiectases* the spot formed, most commonly on the skin, by a dilated capillary or other small vessel. See also *telangiectasia.*

Teldrin (tel′drin) trademark. See *chlorpheniramine maleate.*

tele/o (tel′e-o) 1. [Gr. *telos* end], a word element used in combining form to denote end, final cause, e.g., telecanthus.

2. [Gr. *tēle* far, off, at a distance], a word element used in combining form to denote at a distance or far away, e.g., telecurietherapy.

telecardiography (tel″ĕ-kar″de-og′rah-fe) [*tele-* + Gr. *kardia* heart + *graphein* to write] the recording of an electrocardiogram by transmission of impulses to a site at a distance from the patient.

telemetry (tĕ-lem′ĕ-tre) [*tele-* + Gr. *metron* measure] the making of measurements at a distance, the data being transmitted via a radio link or telephone line from measurement apparatus at a remote location, as in the transmission of the electrocardiogram of a patient en route to a hospital to the physician in the emergency room.

teleomorph (tel′e-o-morf″) [*teleo-* + Gr. *morphē* form] a reproductive organ that is specialized morphologically or karyologically for generating meiospores or their homologues, whether by normal sexual or parthenogenetic means. The teleomorphic name should be the name for the whole fungus (holomorph). Cf. *anamorph.*

teleonomy (tel″e-on′o-me) [*teleo-* + Gr. *nomos* law] the doctrine that the genetic characteristics of an organism exist because of evolutionary adaptation to the environment.

Telepaque (tel′ĕ-pāk) trademark. See *iopanoic acid.*

teleroentgenography (tel″e-rent″gen-og′rah-fe) [*tele-* + *roentgenography*] the use in radiography of a long focal-film distance (6 ft or more) to produce nearly parallel x-rays, and thus minimal unsharpness and geometric image distortion.

teletherapy (tel″ĕ-ther′ah-pe) [*tele-* + Gr. *therapeia* treatment] radiation therapy using an external radiation source, an x-ray or gamma-ray machine or a particle accelerator. See also *radiation therapy.*

tellurate (tel′u-rāt) a salt of telluric acid.

tellurite (tel′u-rīt) any salt of tellurous acid.

tellurite medium a bacterial culture medium that contains potassium tellurite (K_2TeO_3), used for the culture of *Corynebacterium.*

tellurium (Te) (tĕ-lu′re-um) [L. *tellus* the planet earth] a silvery-white, lustrous, semiconducting element; atomic number 52; atomic weight 127.60; Group VI of the periodic table; oxidation states −2, +2, +4, +6. It is used industrially in alloys, batteries, and catalysts. Tellurium is similar to selenium in toxicity. Poisoning causes decreased sweating, scaling and itching skin, nausea, vomiting, and central nervous system depression; the breath and urine have a garlic odor, caused by excretion of dimethyl telluride.

tellurium assays a variation of the Reinsch test. Heavy metals are deposited from acidified specimens onto metallic copper. Tellurium, selenium, and sulfur can be dissolved in potassium cyanide solution. In the presence of copper and after the addition of cadmium acetate reagent and ethanol, tellurium forms a black precipitate. Selenium and sulfur form orange or yellow precipitates under these conditions. This is a qualitative test only.

telocentric (tel″o-sen′trik) [*telo-* + Gr. *kentrikos* pertaining to the center] pertaining to a mitotic chromosome having the centromere at one end so that the chromosome has only a long arm and no short arm. Such chromosomes may be formed by chromosome breakage at the centromere. Cf. *metacentric, submetacentric,* and *subtelocentric.*

telodendron (tel″o-den′dron) [*telo-* + Gr. *dendron* tree] one of the fine endings in the terminal arborization of a neuron.

telomere (tel′o-mēr) [*telo-* + Gr. *meros* part] the chromeric tips of chromosome arms.

telophase (tel-o-fāz) [*telo-* + Gr. *phasis* appearance] the last stage of cell division during which the two daughter nuclei are formed and cleavage into two cells occurs. See also *meiosis* and *mitosis.*

TEM abbrev. See *transmission e. m.* under *electron microscope.*

temperate phage (tem′per-at fāj) [L. *temperatus,* p. p. of *temperare* to be moderate; Gr. *phagein* to eat] a bacteriophage capable of lysogenization, i.e., of being inserted into the cellular DNA of the host bacterium as a prophage, and of replicating indefinitely within the bacterial chromosome without producing virions.

temperature (tem′per-ah-chūr) [L. *temperatura* due measure, proportion] a measure of hotness or coldness; a property of a system in thermodynamic equilibrium, which is a linear function of the internal energy of the system.

For an ideal gas at constant pressure, the temperature varies linearly with the volume. This makes possible the construction of a thermometer in which the volume of the gas (or a liquid with a relatively constant coefficient of thermal expansion, such as mercury) indicates the temperature. Traditionally, temperature is measured not in units but on a scale divided into degrees. Absolute temperature (T) is measured on a scale that has a zero point corresponding to absolute zero.

Customary temperature (t) is measured on a scale having some other zero point. The absolute temperature scales are Kelvin and Rankine. The conversion formulas are: $T(°K) = t(°C) - 273.15$ and $T(°R) = t(°F) - 459.68$. The customary temperature scales are Celsius (formerly called centigrade scale) and Fahrenheit. The formulas for conversion are: $t(°F) = 32 + (9/5)t(°C)$ and $t(°C) = (5/9)(t(°F) - 32)$. (See also the accompanying table.)

For absolute temperature, the terms degree and scale have been abandoned, and temperature is measured in terms of a unit, the kelvin (K), like other quantities. Measurement in kelvins is numerically the same as using the Kelvin scale, 273 K, not 273°K.

Clinically, body temperature is usually measured with an oral thermometer, and has a reference range of 96.4°–99.1°F (35.8°–37.3°C). Rectal temperature is measured occasionally in adults and often in young children—it is usually higher by approximately 1°F (0.5°C) than an oral temperature; axillary temperatures are 1°F (0.5°C) lower. The body temperature varies among individuals, and also with the time of day in the same individual (diurnal variation).

See also *fever* and *hypothermia.*

maximal growth t., in bacteriology, the temperature above which growth does not occur.

minimal growth t., in bacteriology, the temperature below which growth does not occur.

normal body t., the average body temperature, 37°C (98.6°F) measured orally; see also *temperature.*

optimal growth t., the temperature that promotes the most rapid growth of a given species of microorganism, or the temperature at which an enzyme operates at maximal velocity.

room t., the ordinary temperature of a room, 18°–24°C (64.4°–75.2°F).

temperature coefficient the change in a physical quantity per degree of temperature change. In pH measurement, the term is used to indicate the change in output of the pH electrode per measured pH unit per degree of temperature: 0.198 mV/pHu·°C.

temperature programming see under *gas chromatography.*

template (tem′plat) a nucleic acid sequence used to synthesize the complementary nucleic acid sequence. in DNA replication, each strand serves as a template for a new daughter strand; in transcription, one strand serves as a template for a messenger RNA.

temple (tem′p′l) [L. *tempula,* dim. of *tempora,* pl. of *tempus*] the region on each side of the head above the zygomatic arch.

temporal (tem′po-ral) [L. *temporalis*] 1. pertaining

TEMPERATURE. TABLE OF EQUIVALENTS OF CELSIUS (CENTIGRADE) AND FAHRENHEIT TEMPERATURE SCALES

CELSIUS (°)	FAHR. (°)	CELSIUS (°)	FAHR. (°)	CELSIUS (°)	FAHR. (°)
–40	–40.0	9	48.2	57	134.6
–39	–38.2	10	50.0	58	136.4
–38	–36.4	11	51.8	59	138.2
–37	–34.6	12	53.6	60	140.0
–36	–32.8	13	55.4	61	141.8
–35	–31.0	14	57.2	62	143.6
–34	–29.2	15	59.0	63	145.4
–33	–27.4	16	60.8	64	147.2
–32	–25.6	17	62.6	65	149.0
–31	–23.8	18	64.4	66	150.8
–30	–22.0	19	66.2	67	152.6
–29	–20.2	20	68.0	68	154.4
–28	–18.4	21	69.8	69	156.2
–27	–16.6	22	71.6	70	158.0
–26	–14.8	23	73.4	71	159.8
–25	–13.0	24	75.2	72	161.6
–24	–11.2	25	77.0	73	163.4
–23	–9.4	26	78.8	74	165.2
–22	–7.6	27	80.6	75	167.0
–21	–5.8	28	82.4	76	168.8
–20	–4.0	29	84.2	77	170.6
–19	–2.2	30	86.0	78	172.4
–18	–0.4	31	87.8	79	174.2
–17	+1.4	32	89.6	80	176.0
–16	3.2	33	91.4	81	177.8
–15	5.0	34	93.2	82	179.6
–14	6.8	35	95.0	83	181.4
–13	8.6	36	96.8	84	183.2
–12	10.4	37	98.6	85	185.0
–11	12.2	38	100.4	86	186.8
–10	14.0	39	102.2	87	188.6
–9	15.8	40	104.0	88	190.4
–8	17.6	41	105.8	89	192.2
–7	19.4	42	107.6	90	194.0
–6	21.2	43	109.4	91	195.8
–5	23.0	44	111.2	92	197.6
–4	24.8	45	113.0	93	199.4
–3	26.6	46	114.8	94	201.2
–2	28.4	47	116.6	95	203.0
–1	30.2	48	118.4	96	204.8
0	32.0	49	120.2	97	206.6
+1	33.8	50	122.0	98	208.4
2	35.6	51	123.8	99	210.2
3	37.4	52	125.6	100	212.0
4	39.2	53	127.4	101	213.8
5	41.0	54	129.2	102	215.6
6	42.8	55	131.0	103	217.4
7	44.6	56	132.8	104	219.2
8	46.4				

From Dorland's Illustrated Medical Dictionary. 26th ed. Philadelphia, W. B. Saunders Co., 1981, p. 1173.

to the lateral region of the head, above the zygomatic arch.

2. pertaining to time; temporary.

temporal artery, deep two temporal arteries, the anterior and posterior, which are branches of the second part of the maxillary artery. They ascend between the temporal muscle and the underlying bone.

temporal artery, middle a branch of the superficial temporal artery. It ascends over the posterior root of the zygoma and pierces the temporal muscle.

temporal artery, superficial a terminal branch of the external carotid artery. It arises behind the neck of the mandible, gives off the middle temporal artery, and ascends behind the zygomatic arch to divide into branches that run to the frontal and parietal eminences.

temporal bone one of the paired bones located in the lower half of the side of the skull and the lateral part of its base. Each temporal bone has an expanded squamous part that projects upward as part of the lateral wall of the cranial cavity, a petrous part that encloses the internal ear, a mastoid process that projects downward behind the ear, and a tympanic part that forms part of the wall of the external auditory meatus. The temporal bone has two processes: the zygomatic process, which projects forward from the base of the squamous part and forms the posterior part of the zygomatic arch, and the slender styloid process, which projects downward and forward.

temporal dispersion the lengthening of the duration of an evoked potential. It occurs when a nerve segment contains fibers with differing degrees of pathologically slowed conduction velocities.

temporal lobe the lower lateral of the four lobes of the cerebral hemisphere. It lies below the posterior ramus of the lateral sulcus, lateral to the collateral sulcus, and merges posteriorly with the occipital lobe.

temporal lobe epilepsy a form of epilepsy characterized by partial seizures arising in the temporal lobe of the brain. See *partial e.* and *psychomotor e.* under *epilepsy.*

ten/o, tend/o, tendin/o (ten'o, ten'do, ten'dĭ-no) [Gr. *tenōn*; L. *tendo* tendon] a word element used in combining form to denote the tendon, e.g., tendinoplasty.

tenaculum (te-nak'u-lum) [L.] 1. a hooklike instrument for seizing and holding tissues.

2. any fibrous band for maintaining structures in place.

tendinitis (ten″dĭ-ni'tis) [*tendin-* + *-itis* inflammation] acute or chronic inflammation of a tendon and its muscle attachment, characterized clinically by inflammation, pain, and limited joint mobility. It frequently occurs in the infrapatellar tendon, the Achilles tendon, and the supraspinatus and infraspinatus tendons. Calcification of the affected tendon also is often observed, leading to a characteristic radiographic appearance of diffuse opacities deposited linearly along the length of the tendon. See also *tenosynovitis.*

tendo (ten'do), pl. *tendines* [L.] see *tendon.*

tendo calcaneus (ten'do kal-ka'ne-us) see *Achilles t.* under *tendon.*

tendon (ten'dun) [L. *tendo,* from *tendere* to stretch] a strong cord or band of dense, fibrous connective tissue that attaches a muscle to bone.

Achilles t., the powerful tendon extending from midcalf to heel that joins the soleus and gastrocnemius muscles to the posterior surface of the calcaneus. Also called calcaneal tendon, tendo Achillis, and *tendo calcaneus.*

central t. of diaphragm, a thin, trilobar aponeurosis located near the center of the dome of the diaphragm.

conjoined t., the medial portion of the fused aponeuroses of the transverse and internal oblique abdominal muscles, which attaches to the crest and pecten of the pubis. Also called inguinal falx.

hamstring t.'s, the posterior femoral muscles—semitendinosus, semimembranosus, and biceps femoris. Their tendons form the lateral and medial borders of the popliteal fossa.

patellar t., a tendon that joins the common tendon of the quadriceps femoris to insert this muscle group on the tuberosity of the tibia. It contains the patella, a sesamoid bone.

Tenebrio (tĕ-ne′bre-o) [L. *tenebrae* darkness] a genus of arthropods, of which larvae of the species *T. molitor* serve as obligatory intermediate hosts of the rat tapeworm *Hymenolepis diminuta* and the dwarf tapeworm *H. nana.*

tenia (te′ne-ah), pl. *teniae* [L. "a flat band," "bandage," "tape"] 1. [NA], a flat band or strip of soft tissue. Also called taenia.

2. see *Taenia.*

teniae coli, [NA], three longitudinal bands of smooth muscle arranged along the surface of the large intestine up to the rectum. Because these bands are shorter than the intestine, they cause puckering (haustra of colon).

t. of fourth ventricle, a narrow white ridge that serves as the line of attachment of the tela choroidea of the fourth ventricle to the caudal region of the ependyma in the floor of the fourth ventricle.

tennis elbow see *epicondylitis.*

tennis racket cell see *teardrop cell.*

ten/o (ten′o) [Gr. *tenōn, tenontos* tendon] a word element used in combining form to denote relationship to a tendon, e.g., tenodynia.

tenosynovitis (ten″o-sin″o-vi′tis) [*teno-* + *synovia* + *-itis* inflammation] inflammation of a tendon sheath. Causes include trauma, tendon stress, bacterial disease (gonorrhea, tuberculosis), rheumatic disease, and gout. Common sites are the shoulder capsule, hip capsule, hamstring muscles, and Achilles tendon. The tendon sheaths become inflamed and painful, and accumulate fluid. Joint mobility is usually reduced. Friction rubs may be felt or heard (with a stethoscope) on movement. Calcium deposits may occur in the tendon and its sheath, leading to opacities on radiographs of the affected area. See also *tendinitis.*

tension (ten′shun) [L. *tensio;* Gr. *tonos*] 1. the act of stretching.

2. the condition of being stretched.

3. a force that tends to stretch or lengthen an object. Cf. *compression.*

4. the partial pressure of a gas in a mixture of gases or when dissolved in a liquid.

tension cyst of breast a cyst, derived from a mammary lobule, that is lined by metaplastic apocrine-type epithelial cells and contains fluid under pressure as a result of obstruction to its outflow tract. See also *cystic disease of breast.*

tentorium (ten-to′re-um), pl. *tentoria* [L. "tent"] an anatomic part resembling a tent or covering.

tentorium cerebelli (ten-to′re-um ser″ĕ-bel′i) [NA], a crescent-shaped layer of dura mater that covers the cerebellum and supports the occipital lobes. The anterior border is free, whereas the posterior and lateral borders are attached to the skull.

10-20 system see *International 10-20 System.*

TEPP a highly toxic organophosphate insecticide, tetraethyl pyrophosphate. See also *organophosphate compounds.*

tera- (T) (ter′ah) [L. *ter* three times] a prefix attached to International System (SI) units of measurement to make a unit that is equal to 1 trillion of the basic units (10^{12} units).

terahertz (THz) (ter′ah-herts) a unit of frequency equal to 1 trillion hertz (10^{12} Hz).

terat/o (ter′ah-to) [Gr. *teras,* gen. *teratos* monster] a word element used in combining form to denote structural malformation, e.g., teratogenesis.

teratogen (ter′ah-to-jen) [*terato-* + Gr. *gennan* to produce] an agent or factor, e.g., thalidomide or rubella virus, that causes the production of congenital defects. Cf. *mutagen.*

teratogenesis (ter″ah-to-jen′ĕ-sis) [*terato-* + Gr. *genesis* production] the production of malformations in the developing embryo.

teratogenic (ter″ah-to-jen′ik) pertaining to teratogenesis.

teratology (ter″ah-tol′o-je) the division of embryology and pathology that deals with abnormal development and congenital malformations.

teratoma (ter″ah-to′mah), pl. *teratomas, teratomata* [Gr. *terata* monsters + *-oma* a swelling] a neoplasm, which may be benign or malignant, that is derived from multipotential cells capable of forming tissues of a variety of types often representing all three germ layers. The most common locations are the testis and ovary, but extragonadal teratomas occasionally occur. See also *ovarian tumors* and *testicular tumors.*

terbium (Tb) (ter′be-um) [from *Ytterby,* the Swedish town where the element was discovered] a silvery-gray metallic element; atomic number 65; atomic weight 158.9254; a 4f transition element (lanthanide rare earth); oxidation states +3, +4. See also *rare earth elements.*

terbutaline sulfate (ter-bu′tah-lēn) [USP], a sympathomimetic amine used as a bronchodilator in the treatment of bronchial asthma and of bronchospasm associated with bronchitis or emphysema. It is a beta-adrenergic receptor blocking agent with a preferential effect on the β_2-receptors in bronchial smooth muscle but also on the β_1-receptors in the heart. Adverse reactions include nervousness, tremor, palpitations, drowsiness, and gastrointestinal intolerance. Trademark, *Brethine.*

term (term) [L. *terminus,* from Gr. *terma*] 1. a word or combination of words commonly used to designate a specific entity.

2. a limit or boundary.

3. a definite period or specified time of duration, such as the culmination of pregnancy at the end of 9 mo.

terminal (ter′mĭ-nal) [L. *terminalis,* from *terminus* boundary] 1. forming or pertaining to an end or extremity; placed at an end, as in the amino-terminal end of a peptide chain.

2. a post, lug, or screw to which electric connections are made.

3. a computer input-output device such as a teletype or video terminal.

amino t. (N. t.), the end of a peptide having a free amino group. The final amino acid on this end has its carboxyl group involved in a peptide bond, but not its α-amino group.

carboxyl t. (C. t.), the end of a peptide having a free carboxyl group. The final amino acid on this end has its α-amino group involved in a peptide bond, but not its carboxyl group.

terminal addition enzyme see *DNA nucleotidylexotransferase.*

terminal airway unit the portion of the airways distal to the terminal bronchioles. It consists of two to three orders of respiratory bronchioles, each of which gives rise to several alveolar ducts, which in turn subdivide into a number of alveolar sacs. Each sac is divided into approximately 20 alveoli by interalveolar septae.

terminal bar a band in the apical cytoplasm of a columnar epithelial cell of the intestine, which is formed by a bundle of actin filaments that insert on the zonula adherens and extend up into the microvilli.

terminal cisterna see under *sarcoplasmic reticulum.*

terminal deletion see under *deletion.*

terminal deoxynucleotidyl transferase (TDT, TdT) see *DNA nucleotidylexotransferase.*

terminal deoxyribonucleotidyl transferase see *DNA nucleotidylexotransferase.*

terminalization (ter″mĭ-nal″ĭ-za′shun) the process occurring during the diakinesis stage of meiotic prophase in which the chiasmata move to the ends of the chromosomes. See also *meiosis.*

terminal latency see *distal l.* under *latency.*

termination (ter″mĭ-na′shun) [L. *terminatio,* from *terminare* to set boundries, limit] 1. a distal end; a cessation.

2. the release of the completed peptide chain from the ribosome and from the final tRNA in the translation process. Termination requires the presence of termination codons, specific release factors (only one in eukaryotes), and hydrolysis of guanosine triphosphate (GTP) in both eukaryotes and prokaryotes. See also *translation.*

3. the completion of RNA synthesis. The exact DNA sequence that signals termination is unknown but appears to include a sequence of T's (thymidines); in prokaryotes, a specific protein factor, rho (ρ), is needed with the RNA polymerase. See also *transcription.*

termination codon a codon that stops the translation of mRNA into a polypeptide—UAA, UAG, or UGA. These codons do not code for any amino acid. Also called *stop codon.*

termination factor any of several specific proteins involved in the ending of protein synthesis on a ribosome once the termination codon on the messenger RNA is reached.

Termination factors, along with the peptidases of 50S ribosome, are responsible for the hydrolysis of the completed polypeptide chain from its ester linkage with transfer RNA (tRNA). After the release of the free polypeptide and the emptied tRNA from the ribosome, the latter is then free to dissociate from messenger RNA by combination of the light subunit with initiation factors, so that it is ready to begin the entire sequence once more.

termination sequence a nucleotide sequence, generally found at the end of a transcription unit of DNA, where the stability of the DNA double helix suddenly decreases—a short GC-rich sequence followed by an AT-rich sequence.

ternary acid an acid that contains three elements, e.g., H_2SO_4.

Ternidens (ter-ni′denz) a genus of strongylid nematodes, one species of which, *T. deminutus,* is occasionally parasitic for humans in East and South Africa. The adult male of *T. deminutus* measures 9.5 mm by 0.56 mm; the female, 12–16 mm by 0.65–0.73 mm. The eggs are ovoid and transparent; they resemble human hookworm eggs, but are much larger (51–84 μ).

T. deminutus inhabits the large intestine and may produce cystic nodules. Because these worms are blood suckers, heavy infections usually produce anemia.

terpene (ter′pēn) [from *terpentin,* an old form of *turpentine*] 1. any hydrocarbon of the formula $C_{10}H_{16}$, derived chiefly from essential oils, resins, and other vegetable aromatic products. Such hydrocarbons may be acyclic, bicyclic, or monocyclic.

2. more generally, a compound with a carbon skeleton, which is formally divisible into 5-carbon atom isoprene units. The broad class of terpenes may be subdivided into C_{10} compounds (terpenes or monoterpenes), C_{15} compounds (sesquiterpenes), C_{20} compounds (diterpenes), C_{30} compounds (triterpenes), etc. Other terpene compounds, such as natural rubber, are high polymers of isoprene units. Although originally the term referred only to hydrocarbons, it now may refer to compounds with other functional groups, such as hydroxyl and carbonyl groups.

terpin hydrate (ter′pin) a terpin used in cough syrups, which reduces bronchial inflammation and secretions, and acts as an irritant and astringent.

tert- (tert) see under *tertiary.*

tertiary (ter′she-ar-e) [L. *tertiarius* containing a third part, from *tertius* third] 1. third in order.

2. in organic chemistry, a term used in several contexts: a tertiary carbon has three carbon atoms attached to it, as in CHR_3; a tertiary substituent is one in which the point of attachment to the parent compound is a tertiary carbon, and it may have the prefix *tert-,* as in *tert*-butyl (systematically named as the 1,1-dimethylethyl substituent); a tertiary amine is one having a nitrogen with three bonds to carbon and no hydrogens attached, as in R_3N; and a tertiary alcohol is one in which the OH is attached to a tertiary carbon. See also *tertiary structure.*

tertiary structure the complete form assumed by a long-chain macromolecule (biopolymer); the combination of the various secondary structures and nonordered segments. It is the result of interactions between various parts of the chain, which may be due to hydrogen bonds, van der Waals forces, hydrophobic bonds, or disulfide bonds. The distinction between secondary and tertiary structure is somewhat arbitrary. Secondary structure results from interactions between parts of the chain that are close to each other; tertiary structure, between parts that are far apart. Although the term is usually applied to proteins, it can be applied to other polymers, e.g., transfer RNA.

tesla (T) (tes′la) [Nikola *Tesla,* Croatian-born American electrical engineer, 1856–1943] the International System (SI) unit of magnetic flux density defined as 1 weber per square meter (1 Wb/m²). Cf. *gauss.*

test/o (tes'to) a word element used in combining form to denote the testis, e.g., testicular.

test (test) [Old French "crucible," from L. *testum* earthenware pot] 1. an examination or procedure for determining the presence or absence of a disease. For more information, see under the particular test.

2. a qualitative, quantitative, semiquantitative, or semiqualitative procedure for detecting the presence or measuring the quantity of a chemical constituent. Cf. *assay.* For information, see under the particular test.

3. in statistics, a rule that determines the acceptance or rejection of a hypothesis based on the value of some statistic.

4. the operation of a piece of equipment in order to determine whether it is functioning properly.

5. in invertebrate zoology, a hard shell, such as the exoskeleton of an insect or an oyster shell. Also called testa.

Tes-Tape (tes'tāp) see under *glucose assays.*

testcross the mating of a heterozygote of unknown genotype to an individual homozygous for the recessive genes in question. Cf. *backcross.*

testicular (tes-tik'u-lar) pertaining to a testis.

testicular artery one of the paired slender arteries that convey blood to the testes. These arteries arise anteriorly from the abdominal aorta below the origin of the renal arteries, and run obliquely down the posterior abdominal wall, each to its corresponding inguinal canal, which they traverse to reach the scrotum.

testicular feminization syndrome (TFM) a form of pseudohermaphroditism in humans and animals that results from an X-linked mutation. It renders normal androgen-sensitive target tissue totally unresponsive because of a lack of functional androgen receptors.

Such afflicted XY karotypic individuals develop testes and secrete normal concentrations of androgens, but because their tissues do not respond to androgens, they are phenotypically female externally. Except for a blind vagina, no female ducts are present, owing to the normal secretion of müllerian-inhibiting hormone. At puberty, enough estrogen is produced by the testes to support female secondary sex characteristic differentiation (because of the absence of testicular androgenic effects). Breast development and body contours are normal, and except for lack of menstruation, sterility, and sparse or missing pubic and axillary hair, these genetic males function psychologically and sexually as females. Occasionally, corrective surgery is needed to lengthen the shallow vagina.

See also *pseudohermaphroditism* and *sex determination.*

testicular tumors neoplasms of the testis. Histologically identical tumors occasionally arise in extragonadal locations. Most testicular tumors are malignant neoplasms of germ cell origin, some containing more than a single histologic component. Cells of the stroma of the testis can also give rise to tumors (gonadal stromal tumors).

The incidence of testicular tumors in North America is just over 2 per 100,000; these tumors are responsible for fewer than 1 percent of the male cancer death rate, although the percentage rises to above 10 percent for those in their second through fourth decades. Little is known concerning the etiology. Tumors are more common in ectopic testes, and genetic factors are believed to be involved in some instances. A testicular tumor may possess hormonal activity; e.g., human chorionic gonadotropin (hCG) may be demonstrable in a germ cell tumor, and a Leydig cell tumor can elaborate corticosteroids or progesterone. Approximately 40 percent of primary testicular tumors contain more than a single histologic pattern, and each component should be specified in the pathologic diagnosis, as the elements present influence the management and clinical course. Some 35 percent of patients have metastases at the time of diagnosis. The TNM system may be used for clinical staging, but the ABC system is sometimes employed (in stage A, the tumor is confined to the testis; in stage B, metastases are present only below the diaphragm; and in stage C, metastases exist above the level of the diaphragm.

A seminoma is the most common primary germ cell tumor of the testis. Those affected are usually older than 30 yr (this tumor is hardly ever seen in children). Seminomas are often histologically pure; occasionally a pure seminoma displays more than one component in metastases. Cells of a seminoma are moderately large and typically uniform, and form diffuse sheets. The cell borders are smooth, the nuclei are central, the organelles are sparse, and the cytoplasm contains plentiful glycogen. Occasional giant cells of syncytiotrophoblastic type may be present, and the stroma can display a lymphoid or a granulomatous response. Cells of the anaplastic variant of seminoma are larger with irregular cytologic features; in some reports, this form has been found to be more aggressive and prone to give rise to metastases. Spermatocytic seminomas make up fewer than 10 percent of the total, and those affected are usually older than 40 yr. The tumor is often large and soft, and the cells include secondary spermatocytes and large mononuclear cells.

Pure seminoma offers a more favorable prognosis than other primary germ cell tumors of the testis: with appropriate therapy, the 5-yr survival rate should exceed 95 percent. Spermatocytic seminoma has a particularly good prognosis, whereas the presence of syncytiotrophoblastic elements and a high mitotic index are unfavorable prognostic indicators.

Embryonal carcinoma is a type of germ cell tumor with variable histopathology, which makes up roughly 20 percent of testicular tumors. The cells may form tubules, glands, papillary fronds, or solid sheets, and often display considerable anaplasia. The adult type of embryonal carcinoma is seen more commonly in the second and third decades, and is an aggressive tumor. The infantile form is the most common testicular tumor found in children; this tumor is also called endodermal sinus tumor, juvenile embryonal carcinoma, and yolk sac tumor. Ultrastructurally, the cells contrast with those of seminoma in their variability in size and shape, irregular nuclear profiles, number of organelles, tight junctions, and microvilli. Alpha$_1$-fetoprotein can be demonstrated in the cells of approximately 70 percent of embryonal carcinomas using the immunoperoxidase procedure. Embryonal carcinoma usually metastasizes in pure form. The 5-yr survival rates are less than 65 percent.

Polyembryoma represents an extremely rare

form of primary testicular tumor. It is composed of embryoid bodies less than 1 mm in diameter, within a myxoid matrix. These embryoid bodies vary considerably in composition but essentially resemble an embryo of one to two weeks gestation; they may form a component of an embryonal carcinoma or teratoma.

Choriocarcinoma is a neoplasm composed of trophoblastic elements. Like its gestational counterpart, a testicular choriocarcinoma can contain both cyto- and syncytiotrophoblastic elements. It may form a component of seminoma, embryonal carcinoma, or malignant teratoma, and is only rarely seen in pure form as a primary testicular tumor. Choriocarcinomas are aggressive, spreading to the lungs and other organs via the blood stream, and less frequently via lymphatics. When a choriocarcinoma forms one component of a mixed germ cell tumor, all histologic elements should be specified in the diagnosis. This tumor is not radiosensitive, and most patients die within a year after diagnosis.

A teratoma, which makes up fewer than 10 percent of primary testicular tumors, is a neoplasm that contains histologic elements from more than one germ layer. The components may be mature or immature (primitive). Immature components may be derived from any of the three germ layers, and they can form recognizable tissues or organoid structures. Testicular teratomas in young children are often mature. Metastasis is primarily through lymphatics to the periaortic and iliac lymph nodes; less frequently involved are the liver or lungs. Teratomas can occur at any age, but most of those affected are under 30 yr. One patient in four with malignant teratoma has metastases when first seen. The 5-yr survival rate is approximately 70 percent, but an admixture of embryonal carcinoma or choriocarcinoma lowers this figure.

Gonadal stromal tumors are neoplasms that arise from the specialized stromal elements of the testis. Usually a single cell type is present, but mixtures occur; the rare gonadoblastoma contains both germ cell and stromal portions.

A Leydig (interstitial) cell tumor is one that arises from the cells of the same name. There is considerable variability in the histologic pattern, which ranges from sheets of uniform cells to the formation of nests and cords. At least 90 percent of Leydig cell tumors are benign. These tumors may form corticosteroids or progesterone and can produce functional effects, e.g., precocious puberty, gynecomastia. At least 5 percent are bilateral.

Other gonadal stromal tumors are rare. They may be derived from primitive specialized stromal cells or mesenchymal cells and can consist of Sertoli cells, granulosa cells, theca-like cells, or mixtures thereof. Leydig cells may also be present.

testicular vein the vein that drains the pampiniform plexus of the spermatic cord. It runs across the wall of the pelvis and up the posterior wall of the abdomen with the testicular artery. The left vein ends in the left renal vein; the right vein enters the inferior vena cava.

testis (tes′tis), pl. *testes* [L.] [NA], the male gonad, one of a pair of ovoid structures, 4 cm long in the adult. The testis develops in the embryo on the posterior wall of the coelomic cavity, and migrates down through the inguinal canal to its permanent location within the scrotum. During its descent, it carries with it vessels, nerves, fibers of the cremaster muscle, the vas deferens, and an invagination of peritoneum; these structures form the spermatic cord. The covering of peritoneum lines the wall of the cavity of the scrotum, and its visceral layer (the tunica vaginalis) clothes the epididymis, testis, and the lower portion of the cord. The epididymis lies along the posterior border of the testis lateral to the lower end of the cord and vas deferens, and is continuous with these structures. A small body on the upper end of the testis, the appendix testis, is a remnant of the mesonephric duct and corresponds to the infundibulum of the uterine tube.

The capsule of the testis, the tunica albuginea, is a dense coat of fibrous connective tissue. Slender partitions of connective tissue extend into the interior of the testis to subdivide it into many compartments, each occupied by a seminiferous tubule. The tubules are highly convoluted; if straightened, each would be about 50 cm long. There are several hundred tubules in each testis, lined by the layers of cells that form the spermatozoa. The sequence of maturation of spermatozoa takes more than 2 mo and occurs in several stages, during which meiotic as well as mitotic divisions occur. The stem cells, or spermatogonia, are attached to the basal lamina. Development proceeds through spermatocytes and spermatids to the mature spermatozoa. The seminiferous tubules empty into tubules of the rete testis.

The germ cells of the testis are supported by tall Sertoli cells that rest on the basal lamina of the seminiferous tubule, and unite with neighboring Sertoli cells through specialized intercellular junctions to form a barrier that limits the transport of material from vessels in the connective tissue surrounding the tubule and its lumen. This is the anatomic basis for the so-called blood-testis barrier. Maturing germ cells indent the cytoplasm of adjacent Sertoli cells and probably derive nutrients from them. Sertoli cells are involved in the production of estrogen and the synthesis of androgen-binding protein, which are secreted into the testicular tubular lumens, and pass into the epididymis and possibly into the blood stream. Testosterone is also produced by the Leydig or interstitial cells arranged in small groups in the connective tissue between the seminiferous tubules. Through its gonadotropic hormones, the anterior lobe of the pituitary gland participates in controlling the synthesis of androgen and the maturation of the germ cells.

See also *gametogenesis, germ cell, Leydig cells, Sertoli cell testicular tumors,* and *testosterone.*

test meal a meal containing material given for the specific purpose of aiding diagnostic examination of the stomach, as by radiography or by subsequent chemical analysis of stomach contents.

testolactone (tes″to-lak′tōn) a cancer chemotherapeutic drug; trademark, Teslac. For more information, see *Appendix A.*

testosterone (tes-tos′tĕ-rōn) [*test*es + *ster*ol + *-one*] 17β-hydroxyandrost-4-en-3-one, the principal male sex hormone; M.W. 288.41. Testosterone is a C_{19} androgen synthesized from cholesterol by the interstitial or Leydig cells of the testes. It promotes the growth and function of the epididymis, vas deferens, prostate gland, seminal vesicles, and penis.

In males almost all the circulating testosterone is from the testes, with a small amount from the adrenals; in females the hormone is secreted by the ovaries and adrenals. The production of testosterone in males is controlled by pituitary luteinizing hormone via hypothalamic luteinizing-releasing hormone in conjunction with free serum testosterone through a negative feedback mechanism, whereas in females this regulatory mechanism does not exist. Approximately 98 percent of circulating testosterone is bound to a testosterone-estradiol–binding globulin (TeBG, or sex hormone–binding globulin, SHBG) and albumin, the remainder existing as the biologically active free testosterone. In some target tissues, testosterone is metabolized to dehydrotestosterone (DHT), a more potent hormone than testosterone. The action of both testosterone and DHT is mediated by a specific high-affinity cytosol receptor.

Testosterone is metabolized in the liver to its glucuronide and sulfate and also is converted to androsterone and etiocholanolone. These compounds are measured as urinary 17-ketosteroids and thereby reflect testicular function. Direct determinations of serum testosterone are a better indicator of testicular function than either 17-ketosteroids or urinary testosterone determinations.

Increased testosterone concentrations are observed in females with Stein-Leventhal syndrome (polycystic ovarian disease), ovarian tumors, adrenal tumors, and adrenal hyperplasia. Decreased testosterone concentrations in males are seen in hypogonadism, orchidectomy, Klinefelter's syndrome, hypopituitarism, and estrogen therapy; increased concentrations in males can be caused by testicular tumors.

Reference values for testosterone in serum and plasma are: for prepubertal males, less than 100 ng/dl; for prepubertal females, less than 40; for adult males, 300–1000; and for adult females, 20–80.

See also *dihydrotestosterone* and *luteinizing hormone.*

free t., testosterone that is not bound to a plasma protein. It is this form that is biologically active and can diffuse through the membranes of its target cells, where it is bound to a specific high-affinity cytosol receptor.

testosterone propionate a cancer chemotherapeutic drug; trademark Oreton. For more information, see *Appendix A.*

test statistic a function of the sample data that determines the result of a statistical hypothesis test. See also under *hypothesis testing.*

test tube a cylindric glass tube with a closed rounded bottom and an open top, used in chemistry and biology laboratories.

tetanic contraction the sustained contraction of a muscle without intervals of relaxation. A decrease in calcium ions, which are important in altering the membrane potential, can increase the membrane permeability to sodium ions, resulting in spontaneous impulses and muscular spasm. In addition to hypocalcemia, tetanic contractions can be caused by alkalosis, potassium deficiency, and hypomagnesemia.

tetanolysin (tet″ah-nol′ĭ-sin) [Gr. *tetanos,* from *teinein* to stretch + *lysin*] a hemolytic exotoxin produced by *Clostridium tetani,* the causative organism of tetanus. It is not known to contribute to the pathogenicity of the organism.

tetanospasmin (tet″ah-no-spas′min) [*tetanus* + L. *spasmus* spasm + *-in*] a highly potent neurotoxin elaborated by germinating spores of *Clostridium tetani;* M.W. 160,000. Structurally, this toxin is a polypeptide with two subunits, α and β. Although there are several different antigenic types of *C. tetani,* there is only one immunotype of tetanospasmin. It is this toxin that is responsible for the clinical manifestations of tetanus; thus, immunity to the disease is achieved only with antibody to this neurotoxin.

After the toxin is produced in an anaerobic local infected wound, it migrates to the central nervous system. Although it is unclear whether tetanospasmin travels along axons in the peripheral nerves in retrograde fashion or via the blood stream, it is certain that once the toxin reaches the spinal cord, it travels within the cord. When tetanospasmin reaches the CNS, the β-chain subunit of the toxin binds to a ganglioside (consisting of sialic acid, stearic acid, sphingosine, glucose, galactose, and *N*-acetylgalactosamine) on a synaptosome membrane. Tetanus toxoid prevents tetanospasmin activity by inhibiting the binding of toxin to gangliosides.

Once bound, however, tetanospasmin causes a spasmogenic effect by preventing the release of an inhibitory transmitter, glycine, which controls the normal postsynaptic inhibition of spinal motor neurons. Without the glycine, excitatory impulses continue unchecked, resulting in muscular spasms.

See also *exotoxins.*

tetanus (tet′ah-nus) [Gr. *tetanos,* from *teinein* to stretch] an acute and often fatal bacterial disease caused by *Clostridium tetani. C. tetani* is a strict anaerobe that can form an endospore; it is found in soil and animal feces. The bacterial spores most commonly enter the body through puncture wounds, although burns, cutaneous ulcers, wounds, and injection sites of narcotic addicts are also portals of entry. If the locally infected tissue becomes anaerobic and necrotic, the spores germinate and *C. tetani* multiplies. This bacterium produces two toxins, tetanospasmin and tetanolysin. Tetanospasmin is a potent neurotoxin that causes generalized muscular spasms.

The incubation period of tetanus ranges from a few days to several weeks. If a wound is clean, remains aerobic, and contains no necrotic tissue, it may heal with *C. tetani* spores remaining locally. As a result, later nonpuncture trauma to the area can result in tetanus. The shorter the incubation period and time from onset of symptoms to muscle spasms, the more severe the disease and the higher the mortality rate.

There are two forms of tetanus, generalized and local. Generalized tetanus is the more common and involves severe, painful spasms and rigidity of the voluntary muscles. Lockjaw and involvement of the pharyngeal muscles cause difficulty in swallowing, and death usually results from respiratory failure. If one does recover from tetanus, there are no sequelae, regardless of the severity of the disease.

Local tetanus is less common and involves localized twitching and muscle spasms. Although the condition may persist for months, it eventually subsides.

The diagnosis of tetanus may be made clinically and bacteriologically. Cultures of the infected site should be incubated anaerobically for isolation of *C. tetani.*

As antitoxin blocks the binding of tetanospasmin to gangliosides of the central nervous system, toxin that is already bound cannot be neutralized. Tetanus toxoid is combined with the diphtheria and pertussis prophylactic (DPT) immunization usually given to children during the first year of life. A booster injection of toxoid given 1 yr after initial immunization results in protective antibody levels for 10–20 yr. When there is a suspicion of tetanus, severely injured individuals should receive either a booster of toxoid (if previously immunized) or the tetanus immune globulin (if not previously immunized).

See also *tetanospasmin.*

tetany (tet′ah-ne) a special form of cramp, particularly affecting the flexor muscles of the hands and fingers; it is found in association with laryngospasm and hypocalcemia. Tetany can be differentiated from other cramp patterns produced electromyographically by the characteristic rhythmic grouping of the discharge potentials. See also *hypocalcemia.*

tetra- (T) (tet′rah) [Gr., from *tettares* four] a prefix attached to International System (SI) units to make a unit that is equal to 1 trillion of the basic units (10^{12} unit).

tetracaine (tet′rah-kān) [USP], a local anesthetic used topically; it is about 10 times as potent as procaine.

t. hydrochloride, [USP], a soluble salt used for both topical and spinal anesthesia. Trademark, Pontocaine.

tetrachlorethane (tet″rah-klōr-eth′ān) a heavy, colorless, nonflammable liquid with a sweet, chloroform-like odor, $CHCl_2CHCl_2$; M.W. 167.86. It is used as an industrial solvent. Symptoms of tetrachlorethane poisoning resemble those of carbon tetrachloride except that it is much more damaging to the liver; it is considered to be the most toxic of the common chlorinated hydrocarbons.

tetrachloroethylene (tet″rah-klo″ro-eth′ĭ-lēn) [USP], a colorless, nonflammable liquid with an ethereal odor, tetrachloroethene, $CCl_2{=}CCl_2$; M.W. 165.85. Tetrachloroethylene is used as a dry-cleaning solvent and a degreasing agent. The vapors, which are readily absorbed in the lungs, are narcotic at high concentrations and are also irritating to the eyes, skin, and upper respiratory tract. Also called *perchloroethylene* and tetrachloroethene.

***n*-tetracosanoic acid** (tet″rah-kos-ah-no′ik) see *lignoceric acid.*

tetracyclines (tet″rah-si′klēns) a group of antibiotics whose basic structure consists of a hydronaphthacene nucleus containing four fused ring structures. Tetracyclines are bacteriostatic. Protein synthesis is inhibited through affinity for the 30S ribosomal subunit of bacteria, with resultant blocking of the binding of aminoacyl–transfer RNA to the acceptor site on the messenger RNA–ribosome complex. Resistance can be mediated by loss of permeability to tetracyclines or by alterations in the target site on the ribosome. Resistance among enteric organisms can be mediated by transferable plasmids.

Tetracyclines are broad-spectrum antibiotics. In vitro, they are effective against gram-positive and gram-negative aerobic and anaerobic bacteria, spirochetes, mycoplasmas, rickettsiae, chlamydiae, and some protozoa. The antimicrobial spectra of all tetracyclines—chlortetracycline, oxytetracycline, tetracycline, demeclocycline, methocycline, doxycycline, minocycline — are similar; however, there are some differences in the degree of activity and pharmacokinetics. For the disk diffusion test, the tetracycline disk is used to evaluate susceptibility for all tetracycline analogs.

See also *antibacterial agents.*

tetrad (tet′rad) [Gr. *tetra* four] 1. a group of four similar or related entities.

2. in genetics, the structure composed of four homologous chromatids joined at their centromeres, which is produced in the pachytene stage of meiosis by the separation of the sister chromatids of a bivalent.

3. a square of cells produced by the division of certain cocci in two planes.

tetrahydrobiopterin (tet″rah-hi″dro-bi-op′ter-in) a pterin cofactor for the phenylalanine hydroxylase reaction in which tyrosine and dihydrobiopterin (a quinoid compound) are formed. Cf. *tetrahydrofolic acid.*

tetrahydrocannabinol (THC) (tet″rah-hi″dro-kah-nab′ĭ-nol) the active principle of marijuana. Two isomers occur, Δ^8-THC and Δ^9-THC; both are psychoactive, but Δ^9-THC is the major component. Both are rapidly metabolized to the 11-hydroxy THC form which is more potent than either parent compound. Some metabolites of THC remain in the body for as long as 8 da. See also *C. sativa* under *Cannabis.*

tetrahydro-compound S (THS) see *tetrahydro-11-deoxycortisol.*

tetrahydrocortisol (tet″rah-hi″dro-kor′tĭ-sol) one of the major metabolites of cortisol produced in the liver by the reduction of cortisol, yielding a $3\alpha,5\alpha$- and a $3\alpha,5\beta$-tetrahydrocortisol. These substances are further reduced to allocortol and cortol, respectively. Also called *urocortisol.* See also *cortisol.*

tetrahydro-11-deoxycortisol (tet″rah-hi′dro de-ok″se-kor′tĭ-sol) a major metabolite of 11-deoxycortisol (compound S). It is produced by a reduction of compound S in the liver and subsequently excreted as glucuronide conjugates in the urine. Virilizing adrenal hyperplasia leading to hypertension results in an increased THS owing to an 11β-hydroxylase defect. Decreases are observed in Addison's disease or in a hypofunctioning pituitary. Measurement of THS in the urine following administration of metyrapone is useful in assessing pituitary reserve. Reference values in urine are less than 1 mg/da. Also called *tetrahydro-compound S (THS).* See also *adrenal hyperplasia, 11-deoxycortisol,* and *metyrapone test.*

tetrahydrofolate dehydrogenase (tet″rah-hi″-dro-fo′lāt) an enzyme of the oxidoreductase class (5,6,7,8-tetrahydrofolate:NADP$^+$ oxidoreductase, EC 1.5.1.3) that catalyzes the reaction 5,6,7,8-tetrahydrofolate + NADP$^+$ $\rightleftarrows$ 7,8-dihydrofolate + NADPH. The reaction is essential in the synthesis of nucleotides; it is inhibited by the antineoplastic drug methotrexate (a derivative of folate). Also called *dihydrofolate reductase* and *folate reductase.*

tetrahydrofolic acid (tet″rah-hi″dro-fo′lik) a reduced pteridine, tetrahydropteroylglutamate, which is a pteridine linked to *p*-aminobenzoic acid linked to glutamic acid. This cofactor has the specific function of carrying one-carbon units and does not participate in mixed-function oxidase reactions. See also *folic acid.* Cf. *tetrahydrobiopterin.*

tetrahydrofuran (THF) (tet″rah-hi″dro-fu′ran) a colorless liquid, $CH_2CH_2CH_2CH_2O$, with an ethereal odor, used as a solvent for natural and synthetic resins and as a chemical intermediate and monomer.

tetrahydropteroylglutamate methyltransferase (tet″rah-hi″dro-ter″o-il-gloo′tah-māt meth″il-trans′fer-ās) an enzyme of the transferase class (EC 2.1.1.13) that catalyzes the reaction 5-methyltetrahydropteroyl-L-glutamate + L-homocysteine ⇄ tetrahydropteroylglutamate + L-methionine. It is a step in the biosynthesis of methionine and requires methylcobalamin as a coenzyme. A defect in synthesis of the coenzyme, transmitted as an autosomal recessive trait, results in homocystinuria (type III). Also called methionine synthase.

tetralogy (tě-tral′o-je) [Gr. *tetralogia* a group of four plays presented together at a dramatic festival, from *tetra-* + *logos* discourse] a combination of four elements or factors, such as four concurrent symptoms or defects.

tetralogy of Fallot a combination of congenital cardiac defects consisting of pulmonary stenosis, interventricular septal defect, dextroposition of the aorta so that it overrides the interventricular septum and receives both venous and arterial blood, and right ventricular hypertrophy.

tetramastigote (tet″rah-mas′tĭ-gōt) [*tetra-* + Gr. *mastix* lash] any organism possessing four flagella.

tetramer (tet′rah-mer) [*tetra-* + Gr. *meros* part] 1. an oligomer composed of four monomers, e.g., hemoglobin and lactate dehydrogenase isoenzymes.
2. a viral capsomere composed of four polypeptide units; see under *capsid.*

Tetramitidae (tet″rah-mi′tĭ-de) a family of flagellate protozoa that includes the genus *Enteromonas.*

tetraplegia (tet″rah-ple′je-ah) [*tetra-* + Gr. *plēgē* stroke] see *quadriplegia.*

tetraploid (4n) (tet′rah-ploid) [Gr. *tetraploos* fourfold, from *tetra-* + *ploos* fold, + *eidos* form] 1. referring to an increase in the chromosome number (and, by extension, to the nuclear DNA content) twice that of the value in postmitotic diploid cells. Cf. *polyploid.*
2. an individual or cell that has four homologous sets of chromosomes. ($4n$).

tetraploidy (tet″rah-ploi′de) having four times the normal haploid chromosome number ($4n$).

tetrasomic (tet″rah-so′mik) characterized by or pertaining to tetrasomy.

tetrasomy (tet′rah-so″me) [*tetra-* + Gr. *soma* body] the presence of two homologous chromosomes in excess of the normal diploid set, making a total of four homologous chromosomes.

Tetratrichomonas (tet″rah-trik-om′o-nas) a genus of flagellate protozoa. See *T. tenax* under *Trichomonas.*
T. buccalis, see *T. tenax* under *Trichomonas.*
T. hominis, see *T. tenax* under *Trichomonas.*

tetravalent (tet″rah-va′lent) see *quadrivalent.*

tetrazolium salts colorless, water-soluble substances used in histochemical techniques to demonstrate localized enzymatic reactions. Following reduction with a hydrogen donor, as in dehydrogenation, these salts yield a highly colored pigment.

tetrodotoxin (tet″ro-do-tok′sin) a pure, crystalline, highly lethal neurotoxic substance in the livers of numerous species of puffer fish. Within minutes, ingestion results in malaise, dizziness, and tingling about the mouth, which may be followed by ataxia, convulsions, respiratory paralysis, and death.

tetrose (tet′rōs) a monosaccharide that contains four carbon atoms in a molecule; e.g., erythrose, threose, and erythrulose.

TFE see *Teflon.*

TFM abbrev. See *testicular feminization syndrome.*

tG$_1$ the time required to complete the G_1 phase of the cell cycle. See also *cell cycle.*

tG$_2$ the time required to complete the G_2 phase of the cell cycle. See also *cell cycle.*

TGT abbrev. See *thromboplastin generation test.*

Th symbol for the chemical element *thorium.*

Θ the Greek capital letter *theta.*

θ the Greek lower case *theta;* used in mathematics as an angular coordinate variable.

thalam/o (thal′ah-mo) [Gr. *thalamos* inner chamber] a word element used in combining form to denote the thalamus, e.g., thalamocoele.

thalamus (thal′ah-mus), pl. *thalami* [L.; Gr. *thalamos* inner chamber] the paired masses of gray matter on each side of the third ventricle in the diencephalon. The thalamus consists of seven nuclei and numerous fiber tracts that collectively serve as a major relay center for information projecting between the cerebral cortex and the lower areas of the central nervous system. See also *brain.*

thalass/o (thah-las′o) [Gr. *thalassa* sea] a word element used in combining form to denote the sea, e.g., thalassemia.

thalassemia (thal″ah-se′me-ah) [Gr. *thalassa* sea (because it was observed originally in persons of Mediterranean stock) + *haima* blood + *-ia*] a group of hereditary hemoglobinopathies characterized by a quantitative decrease in the production or total absence of a normal globin chain. Normal hemoglobin contains two alpha and two non-alpha ($\alpha_2\beta_2$ or $\alpha_2\gamma_2$) chains. The clinically significant disorders are those in which the synthesis of the alpha- and beta-globin chains is affected; they are designated alpha thalassemia and beta thalassemia. As with other hemoglobinopathies, the disorder occurs in both the homozygous and the heterozygous states and has many variants.

Historically, the first of these syndromes was called Mediterranean anemia because of the geographic origin of those affected by the disease. The distribution is actually worldwide, with pockets of high incidence of a particular type seen in certain populations. Examples include beta thalassemia in Chinese and Mediterranean peoples, and alpha thalassemia in Southeast Asians (Thais).

The severity of the anemia varies according to the degree of alpha- or beta-chain depression; when present, the anemia is microcytic (mean corpuscular volume 60–70) and hypochromic. The pathophysiology of these disorders is due to an imbalance in globin chain synthesis. The excess globin chain found in alpha thalassemia (excess beta chain) or in beta thalassemia (excess alpha chain) will precipitate, either with heme still attached or as a free globin. These precipitates, Heinz bodies, can render the red cell more vulnerable to fragmentation and lysis, and shorten the red cell survival.

BETA THALASSEMIA. A heterogeneous group of disorders, beta thalassemia is attributed to deficient or absent beta-chain synthesis. Molecularly, the structural beta genes are present, but either mRNA production is inefficient or the mRNA is degraded rapidly, resulting in quantitatively abnormal beta-chain synthesis. Beta thalassemia is classified according to the degree of beta-chain suppression, the pattern of inheritance (heterozygous trait or homozygous disease), and the resulting clinical severity. The degree of beta-chain suppression results in β° thalassemia, denoting a complete absence of beta-chain production from the affected gene, and β^{+} thalassemia, denoting a decrease in beta-chain production from the affected gene. The types of beta thalassemia include thalassemia major, thalassemia minor (thalassemia trait), thalassemia intermedia, delta-beta thalassemia, gamma thalassemia, and hemoglobin Lepore syndrome.

The homozygous state (thalassemia major, homozygous beta thalassemia, Cooley's anemia, Mediterranean anemia) is characterized by the absence (β°) or marked decrease (β^{+}) in beta-chain production, an excess of alpha chains, and continued high production of gamma chains (elevated Hb F). Hemoglobin electrophoresis reveals 20–100 percent Hb F, 3.6–7.0 percent Hb A_2, and 0–80 percent Hb A. The peripheral blood smear exhibits hypochromia, microcytosis, extreme poikilocytosis, target cells, ovalocytes, Cabot rings, Howell-Jolly bodies, nuclear fragments, siderocytes, anisochromia, anisocytosis, and normoblastosis. The homozygous state is almost always associated with severe anemia, ineffective erythropoiesis, and massive hypertrophy of the bone marrow, liver, and spleen. Organ damage associated with anemia, bony abnormalities, and fractures are present, as is mongoloid facies. This form is manifested during the first few months of life and becomes progressively more severe, requiring repeated transfusions for survival. In the past, the disease was usually fatal in childhood as a result of cardiac complications associated with iron overload from repeated transfusions, but chelation therapy to rid the body of excess iron now prolongs the life of many patients.

A variant of homozygous beta thalassemia is thalassemia intermedia, a less severe impairment in beta-globin synthesis, with fewer alpha-chain inclusions. Patients with thalassemia intermedia maintain a hemoglobin concentration of 6–10 g/dl without transfusion, except during periods of severe stress, such as infections or surgery. The condition ranges from a very mild disease despite moderately severe anemia to a more severe disease state. The peripheral blood demonstrates a picture similar to that of homozygous beta thalassemia. Hemoglobin electrophoresis shows 20–100 perent Hb F, up to 7 percent Hb A_2, and 0–80 percent Hb A, depending on the genotype of the patient. Iron overload is still a complication in these cases because of the markedly accelerated, although ineffective, erythropoiesis, with an increase in plasma iron turnover and increased gastrointestinal iron absorption.

Beta-thalassemia trait occurs in individuals heterozygous for a mutation responsible for beta-globin synthesis. It is a microcytic, mildly hypochromic anemia, with targeting and elliptocytosis. Bone marrow erythroid hyperplasia is mild to moderate. Characteristically, patients with beta-thalassemia trait have elevated Hb A_2 or Hb F, or both.

Beta-thalassemia trait has been classified according to the level of Hb A_2 and Hb F, and includes (1) High Hb A_2–beta thalassemia, the most common syndrome, which demonstrates Hb A_2 levels of 3.5–8.0 percent and Hb F levels of $<$1–5 percent. Homozygosity leads to thalassemia major and, in rare instances, to thalassemia intermedia. (2) High Hb A_2–high Hb F thalassemia, which demonstrates Hb A_2 levels elevated to 4 percent and Hb F levels of 5–20 percent. Homozygosity for the syndrome leads to thalassemia intermedia syndrome. (3) Heterozygosity for delta-beta thalassemia, which demonsrates low Hb A_2 levels and increased Hb F levels of 5–20 percent. Homozygosity results in a mild thalassemia intermedia syndrome with complete absence of Hb A and Hb A_2, but the presence of Hb F.

Delta-beta thalassemia (δ-β thalassemia), a variant of beta thalassemia, is caused by the deletion of most or all of the beta and delta structural genes. In the homozygous state, only Hb F is present but is variably distributed, with many cells having very little Hb F; Hb A and Hb A_2 are absent. The heterozygous state is clinically milder than that of beta-thalassemia minor, with elevated Hb F levels (5–20 percent) and normal or slightly reduced Hb A_2 levels. The red cells are hypochromic and microcytic. Delta-beta–thalassemia trait can coexist with Hb C and Hb S trait.

Gamma-thalassemia trait has been reported in a newborn with severe hypochromic microcytic red cells. This disorder is due to either deletion or malfunction of a gamma gene and is self-limited, as the normal increased production of beta-globin chains by age 3 mo maintains the normal hemoglobin concentrations. Homozygous gamma thalassemia would probably be incompatible with life.

Hemoglobin Lepore (Hb Lepore) syndrome is another variant of beta thalassemia. This form has normal alpha-chain subunits, with a nonalpha chain composed of a cross-over between the normal C-terminal structure hemoglobin a beta chain at one end and the N-terminal structure of a delta chain at the other end of the molecule. At least three different Lepore hemoglobins have been described, which vary in the point at which the cross-over occurs between the delta- and beta-chain structural genes. Hemoglobin Lepore is produced at a markedly reduced rate. The homozygous state is clinically similar to severe thalassemia major (or thalassemia intermedia); the Hb F level is 75 percent, the Hb Lepore level is 10–20 percent, and, since these individuals fail to synthesize either delta- or beta-globin chains, there is no hemoglobin A or A_2. The heterozygous state is clinically indistinguishable from thalassemia minor: the Hb Lepore level is 6–15 percent, the Hb A_2 level is decreased, and the Hb F level is slightly increased. Hb Lepore has the same electrophoretic mobility as Hb S. It can be associated with other hemoglobin variants.

Alpha Thalassemia. This form of thalassemia includes a group of disorders whose most common molecular defect is alpha-globin gene deletion. Although there are two alleles of a single gene that control beta-chain production, there are two genes and four alleles responsible for alpha-chain regulation. As one, two, three, or four alleles may be missing, various alpha-thalassemia syndromes can be inherited. The two genotypes of alpha thalassemia are characterized either by the deletion (–) of a single **alpha-globin locus** ($-\alpha$) on a single chromosome or by the deletion of both alpha-globin loci (– –) on a single chromosome. There is a less common non-deletion type $(\alpha\alpha)^{th}$ that may result in alpha thalassemia. Additionally, a chain termination mutation (e.g., Hb Constant Spring, $\alpha\alpha^{CS}$) may result in the decreased production of the alpha-globin chain, producing alpha-thalassemia syndrome. The four clinical syndromes of alpha thalassemia classified according to their genotypes are: (1) the silent carrier state (silent alpha thalassemia or alpha thalassemia–2), $-\alpha/\alpha\alpha$, $\alpha\alpha^{CS}/\alpha\alpha$, which is asymptomatic and difficult to diagnose outside the newborn period; (2) heterozygous alpha thalassemia (alpha-thalassemia trait), $--/\alpha\alpha$, $\alpha\alpha^{CS}/\alpha\alpha^{CS}$, $\alpha\alpha^{th}/\alpha\alpha$, or $-\alpha/-\alpha$, which is microcytic and hypochromic with mild anemia; (3) hemoglobin H disease, $--/-\alpha$, $--/\alpha\alpha^{CS}$, or $--/\alpha\alpha^{th}$, which causes mild to moderately severe hemolytic anemia but is compatible with life—hemoglobin H (β_4) is demonstrated by hemoglobin found on electrophoresis; and (4) homozygous alpha thalassemia $(--/--)$. Because no alpha-globin chains are produced in homozygous alpha thalassemia, gamma chains form tetramers (γ_4) called Bart's hemoglobin (Hb Bart's). No Hb A is produced. The γ_4 chains are unable to transport oxygen, causing fetal death at or around birth from hydrops fetalis. Electrophoresis of cord blood samples shows 1–3 percent Hb Bart's in silent carriers and 3–6 percent Hb Bart's in alpha-thalassemia trait. However, this γ_4 hemoglobin cannot be detected after the first few weeks of life. Restrictive endonuclease gene-mapping techniques can identify each gene deletion variant of alpha thalassemia and have been used for prenatal diagnosis on fibroblasts obtained by amniocentesis.

Alpha-thalassemia trait is characterized by marked microcytosis and hypochromia of the red cell associated with mild anemia and erythrocytosis; Hb A_2 and Hb F levels are normal or low. The diagnosis of alpha-thalassemia trait can be made if red cell abnormalities are present, iron deficiency is absent, and beta-thalassemia trait has been ruled out.

Hemoglobin H disease is characterized by hypochromia, microcytosis, red cell fragmentation, and a fast migrating hemoglobin component on electrophoresis. The hemoglobin component Hb H is composed of four beta chains and makes up 5–30 percent of the total hemoglobin. Hemoglobin Bart's is present at birth and makes up approximately 20 percent; by the age of 3 mo Hb Bart's (γ_4) disappears and is replaced by Hb H (β_4). In splenectomized individuals, incubation of blood with brilliant cresyl blue causes the formation of many small inclusion bodies in the red cells owing to the susceptibility of Hb H to oxidation. The erythrocytes containing Hb H are also sensitive to oxidative stress, with enhanced destruction occurring when oxidant drugs such as sulfonamides are administered. Hemoglobin H disease is primarily a hemolytic anemia because with age the red cells lose their capacity to withstand oxidant stress, the Hb H is precipitated, and the cell is prematurely destroyed. Acquired hemoglobin H disease has been reported in individuals with erythroleukemia.

Hemoglobin Constant Spring has one or two slowly migrating components associated with Hb H, accounting for 3–5 percent of the total hemoglobin. Structurally, the hemoglobin contains a normal beta chain but an elongated alpha chain—additional amino acids attached to the C-terminal end of the alpha chain. Phenotypically, heterozygotes for Hb Constant Spring and silent carrier $(\alpha\alpha^{CS}/-\alpha)$ are similar to individuals with alpha-thalassemia trait $(-\alpha,-\alpha$ or $--,\alpha\alpha)$, one parent with silent carrier $(-\alpha,\alpha\alpha)$ and the other parent apparently hematologically normal except for the presence of 1 percent Hb Constant Spring $(\alpha\alpha^{CS},\alpha\alpha)$ on electrophoresis. Because the degree of imbalance in production rates of alpha and beta globin determines clinical severity, coinheritance of alpha- and beta-globin thalassemia defects results in milder clinical and laboratory manifestations than does inheritance of either one alone.

HEMOGLOBIN VARIANTS ASSOCIATED WITH THALASSEMIA: Thalassemia interacts with globin structural variants. The most important beta-thalassemia globin interactions are with the genes for β^S, β^C, and β^E globins. Clinically, these disorders resemble the disease patterns found in individuals homozygous for the structural mutation. The most important alpha-thalassemia globin interaction is with the gene for hemoglobin Q.

Sickle cell beta (S/β) thalassemia is the second most common genetic variant of sickle cell disease. In this disease, the beta-thalassemia gene is inherited from one parent and the hemoglobin S gene from the other.

The β°-type of S/β thalassemia closely resembles sickle cell anemia both clinically and electrophoretically, with the mean corpuscular hemoglobin concentration and mean corpuscular volume lower than those values found in sickle cell anemia, whereas Hb A_2 levels are higher. Hemoglobin electrophoresis reveals primarily Hb S with no Hb A. A familial study is usually required for the diagnosis of S/β° thalassemia.

The β^+ type of S/β thalassemia is easier to detect, with 15–30 percent of normal adult hemoglobin and the rest Hb S. The clinical and hematologic abnormalities may be very mild. On routine electrophoresis, Hb S will be higher than Hb A, which is the exact opposite of the sickle cell trait picture. Patients with homozygous sickle cell anemia/alpha thalassemia are less symptomatic than those with homozygous sickle cell anemia. It is difficult to recognize alpha-thalassemia trait in the presence of sickle cell anemia; however, in the absence of iron deficiency, studies of sickle cell patients with low mean corpuscular volume and mild clinical courses should exclude beta-thalassemia trait, and gene-mapping techniques should be performed. Family studies may be helpful in this regard. It is possible to detect individuals possessing both sickle cell trait and alpha-thalassemia trait owing to the unusually low level of Hb S (36 percent, with the remainder Hb A).

Hemoglobin E–beta thalassemia is a disorder found in individuals in Southeast Asia, with a clinical and hematologic picture similar to that of mild-to-severe thalassemia major. On electrophoresis, Hb E values have a range of 15–95 percent; Hb F has a range of 5–85 percent, with nearly a complete absence of Hb A. Hemoglobin E–beta thalassemia can be confused with homozygous Hb E; however, in individuals with Hb E, the hematologic parameters are close to normal.

Hemoglobin C–beta thalassemia is a hematologic disorder with little clinical evidence of disease. The mean corpuscular hemoglobin and mean corpuscular volume are reduced, with hypochromic target cells, fragmented red cells, and microspherocytes seen on peripheral blood smears. With Hb electrophoresis, Hb C values have a range of 65–95 percent, the Hb F is variable, and the Hb A is about 20 percent. Hb A_2 levels cannot be determined when Hb C is present because the two hemoglobins cannot be separated satisfactorily by electrophoresis.

Hemoglobin Q–alpha thalassemia is a hemoglobin disorder with moderate hemolytic anemia. The red cells are microcytic and hypochromic, and contain Hb H (β_4), Hb Bart's (γ_4), Hb Q ($\alpha_2{}^Q\beta_2$), and Hb Q_2($\alpha_2{}^Q\delta_2$). One parent has alpha-thalassemia trait; the other, Hb Q.

Alpha- and beta-thalassemia mutation interactions have been described. Individuals doubly heterozygous for alpha-thalassemia trait and typical beta-thalassemia trait usually exhibit symptoms similar to those of thalassemia trait.

See also *hemoglobinopathy.*

thalidomide (thah-lid'o-mīd) a sedative and hypnotic compound whose use during early pregnancy was frequently followed by the birth of infants showing serious developmental deformities, notably malformation of a limb or limbs.

thallium (Tl) (thal'e-um) [L. *thallus* green shoot, from Gr. *thallos,* from a green spectral line] a bluish-white, soft, leadlike metallic element; atomic number 81; atomic weight 204.37; Group III of the periodic table; oxidation states +1, +3.

Thallium is employed in alloys; its salts are used as reagents, catalysts, and rat poison. Human symptoms of acute poisoning from thallium salts include gastrointestinal irritation, joint pain, hair loss, paralysis, and mental confusion. The lethal dose of thallium sulfate is 8–12 mg/kg. Chronic subacute poisoning causes lesions of the liver, kidneys, lungs, and nervous system; this form also can be fatal.

When poisoning is suspected, brown granules of thallium iodide can be detected in iodine–potassium iodide–stained tissue sections of nervous tissue. Also, the medulla of the hair root is grossly enlarged.

t. sulfate, a highly toxic, water-soluble thallium salt used as a rat poison.

thallium-201 a cyclotron-produced radionuclide that decays by electron capture to ^{201}Hg, emitting gamma rays at 69, 80, 135, and 168 keV. The thallium(I) ion, like potassium(I), is taken up into muscle and other cells by active transport, and it is, therefore, useful for myocardial scanning procedures. See *myocardial scan.*

thallium assays 1. colorimetric screening method. Organic matter from a specimen of urine, tissue, or stomach contents is removed by acid digestion and the thallium oxidized by bromine to thallium(III), which forms a blue, benzene-extractable complex with the dye methyl violet. Detergents, mercury, iodine, and vanadium can cause false-positive results.

2. atomic absorption spectrophotometry. Specimens are digested, oxidized, and aspirated into an acetylene-air flame of the spectrophotometer. The specimen thallium concentration is proportional to the absorbance at 277 nm.

thallium scan see *myocardial scan.*

thallospore (thal'o-spōr) [*thallus* + Gr. *sporos* seed] any type of asexual spore that is produced on a fungal thallus by septation of a hypha, i.e., an arthrospore, blastospore, or chlamydospore.

thallous chloride Tl 201 a radiopharmaceutical used in myocardial imaging. See also *thallium-201.*

thallus (thal'us) [L. "green shoot", from Gr. *thallos*] in mycology, a mycelial mat of the vegetative body; a loose network of hyphae.

THAM see *tris(hydroxymethyl)aminomethane.*

Thaumetopoea (thaw"mĕ-to-pe'ah) a genus of caterpillars of the family Thaumetopoeidae, of which the species *T. processionea, T. pinivora,* and *T. pityocampa* are found in Europe and Africa. They possess poisonous hairs, which on contact with human skin cause cutaneous wheals and severe itching.

Thaumetopoeidae (thaw"mĕ-to-pe'ĭ-de) a family of urticating caterpillars that possess poisonous hairs. They are commonly found in Europe and Africa.

Thayer-Martin agar see *Thayer-Martin a.* under *agar.*

THC abbrev. See *tetrahydrocannabinol.*

thebaine (the-ba'ēn) [L. *Thebae,* the Egyptian city of Thebes, where opium was once produced, from Gr. *Thebai*] a poisonous alkaloid derived from raw opium. It has properties similar to those of strychnine. Also called dimethyl morphine or paramorphine.

thec/o (the'ko) [L. *theca*] a word element used in combining form to denote a sheath, e.g., thecoma.

theca (the'kah), pl. *thecae* [L.; Gr. *thēkē*] an enclosing case or sheath.

theca cell a cell of the corpus luteum that originates from the theca interna of the ovarian follicle.

theca cell tumor see under *ovarian tumors.*

theca folliculi an envelope, formed from the stromal cells of the ovarian cortex, surrounding an ovarian follicle.

thecoma (the-ko'mah) [*thec-* + Gr. *-ōma* tumor] an ovarian tumor composed of theca cells. Varying degrees of admixture of theca and granulosa cells are present in the spectrum of granulosa-theca cell tumors. See also *ovarian tumors.*

thel/o (the'lo) [Gr. *thēlē* nipple] a word element used in combining form to denote the nipple, e.g., theleplasty, thelorrhagia.

thelarche (the-lar'ke) [*thel-* + Gr. *archē* beginning] a condition characterized by premature development of the female breast, unaccompanied by the development of other sexual characteristics. Cf. *precocious p.* under *puberty* and *pubarche.*

Thelazia (the-la'ze-ah) a genus of nematode worms that are parasites of the conjunctiva of dogs, rabbits, and humans. The species *T. callipaeda* is found in India, China, Korea, and Russia. These threadlike, creamy white worms measure 4.5–13 mm long by 0.25–0.75 mm wide (males) and 6.2–17 mm long by 0.3–0.85 mm wide (females). The eggs range in size from 54–60 by 34–37 μ and are hyaline, thin-shelled and ovoid. Laboratory diagnosis requires microscopic identification of the worms from the conjunctival sac.

thelaziasis (the"la-zi'ah-sis) infection of the eye with the nematode worms of the genus *Thelazia.* They inhabit the conjunctival sac, causing lacrimation, paralysis of lower eyelid muscles, excruciating pain, and severe nervous symptoms. When the worms migrate across the corneal conjunctiva, they cause corneal irritation, scars, and fibrous opacity of the region.

thenyldiamine hydrochloride (then″il-di′ah-mēn) an antihistamine formerly used in bronchial decongestant sprays.

theobroma oil (the″o-bro′mah) [Gr. *theos* god + *broma* food] [USP], the fat obtained from the roasted seed of *Theobroma cacao,* used as a base in suppositories. Also called *cacao oil* or *cocoa butter.*

theobromine (the″o-bro′mēn) an alkaloid, 3,7-dimethylxanthine, related to caffeine and theophylline, that occurs in chocolate, cola, and tea. It has been used as a diuretic, vasodilator, and smooth muscle relaxant. Derivatives such as theobromine calcium salicylate, theobromine sodium salicylate, and theobromine calcium gluconate are used to increase solubility.

theophylline (the-of′ĭ-lēn) [N.L. *thea* tea + *phyllon* leaf] [USP], an alkaloid, 1,3-dimethylxanthine, that occurs in tea. It inhibits the enzyme phosphodiesterase, which breaks down cyclic AMP, and theophylline monoethanolamine and theophylline sodium glycinate are used as bronchodilators in the treatment of bronchial asthma, chronic bronchitis, and emphysema. Side-effects include central nervous system stimulation, diuresis, and increased blood pressure and cardiac output. Typical therapeutic serum concentrations are 10–20 μg/ml; higher levels may cause gastrointestinal irritation, irritability, headache, convulsions, tachycardia, and palpitations.

Theophylline increases the toxicity of digitalis derivatives and of sympathomimetic amines, e.g., ephedrine. Macrolide antibiotics (e.g., erythromycin) increase the serum concentrations.

See also *aminophylline, dyphylline,* and *oxtriphylline.*

theophylline assays 1. ultraviolet spectrophotometry. The sample is extracted with chloroform, and this is followed by reextraction into a buffer of pH 9.0. The absorbance at 280 nm is compared with that of a reference solution. Other xanthines (from coffee, tea, or chocolate), furosemide, sulfathiazole, phenylbutazone, and probenecid interfere.

2. gas chromatography. The method involves use of a flame ionization detector and a silicone column packing having intermediate polarity. A methylene chloride extract is evaporated to dryness, redissolved in toluene, and extracted into ammonium hydroxide solution. An *n*-butyl derivative of theophylline is prepared. The peak heights of this derivative and the internal standard, alphenal, are compared. The sensitivity limit is about 1 μg/ml.

3. high-pressure liquid chromatography. Plasma is deproteinized by addition of acetonitrile. The supernatant is injected onto a reversed-phase column, and theophylline and an internal standard (β-hydroxyethyltheophylline) are detected at 254 nm.

theorem (the′o-rem) [Gr. *theōrēma* a principle arrived at by speculation, from *theōrein* to see, consider] a mathematical statement that is proved to be a logical consequence of explicitly stated assumptions.

theoretical (the″o-ret′ĭ-kal) [Gr. *theōrētikos* contemplative] 1. determined by a particular theory. Cf. *empirical.*

2. not yet having any practical application.

theoretical plate in gas chromatography, a measure of column efficiency, the degree of separation produced by a perfect distillation. The number of theoretical plates (N) is given by the formula: $N = 16\,(t/w)^2$, where t is the corrected retention time of a peak (the time the component is delayed owing to interaction with the stationary phase) and w is the peak width at the baseline (the base of the triangle formed by drawing tangents to the sides of the peak). The height equivalent to a theoretical plate (HETP) is the column length divided by N.

theory (the′o-re) [Gr. *theōria* contemplation as opposed to practice, from *theōrein* to see, contemplate] 1. an explanation of the behavior of a class of phenomena by rules or laws that predict the phenomena as effects of a number of other phenomena (causes).

2. abstract knowledge, doctrine, or principles, as opposed to practice.

therapeutic (ther″ah-pu′tik) [Gr. *therapeutikos* inclined to serve] pertaining to or effective in the treatment of disease.

therapeutic ratio a measure of the relative safety and effectiveness of a drug. Originally the term referred to the maximal tolerated dose divided by the minimal curative dose; now it refers to the median lethal dose (LD_{50}) divided by the median effective dose (ED_{50}). This meaning is less informative but statistically more reliable, and is widely used.

therapist (ther′ah-pist) an individual skilled in the corrective treatment of disease or other types of disorders. In several allied health fields, therapist is the highest professional rank. Generally, the minimal preparation for this role is a baccalaureate degree; in the mental health field, therapists often possess master's and Ph.D. degrees. The therapist generally has both a theoretical and a practical knowledge of the profession, and can plan and implement a program of therapy appropriate for each patient.

therapy (ther′ah-pe) [Gr. *therapeia* service done to the sick] a suffix word element to denote treatment, e.g., hydrotherapy, chemotherapy.

therm/o (ther′mo) [Gr. *thermē* heat] a word element used in combining form to denote relationship to heat, e.g., thermodynamics, thermohyperesthesia.

thermal (ther′mal) [Gr. *thermē* heat] pertaining to heat.

thermal conductivity (TC) detector see under *gas chromatography.*

thermal death point the lowest temperature at which a broth culture of microorganisms can be heat-killed in a 10-min exposure time.

thermal death time the time required at a given temperature for the heat-killing of a broth culture of microorganisms.

thermal neutron a neutron having a kinetic energy of about 0.025 eV, the average kinetic or vibrational energy of a molecule at room temperature. Slow and thermal neutrons undergo neutron capture reactions.

thermionic (therm″i-on′ik) pertaining to charged particles emitted by a substance at an elevated temperature.

thermionic emission the liberation of electrons from the surface of a hot electric conductor, as occurs at the cathode or filament of a vacuum tube.

thermistor (ther-mis′tor) [*therm-* + res*istor*] an electric resistor, used as a thermometer, that has a large increase in conductivity with increasing temperature. It is usually a semiconductor device employed for measuring small temperature changes, as in an osmometer.

Thermoactinomyces (ther″mo-ak″tĭ-no-mi′sēz) [*thermo-* + *actinomyces*] a genus of microorganisms of the family Micromonosporaceae, order Actinomycetales. One of the actinomycetes, the genus consists of thermophilic (45°–60°C) organisms bearing single spores on the aerial and substrate mycelium.

T. vulgaris, a species of the genus that has been isolated from soils, manure, and hay. It is one of the causative organisms of farmer's lung. Formerly called *Micromonospora vulgaris.*

thermocouple (ther′mo-kup″l) a device that serves as a temperature-to-voltage transducer. It consists of two wires of different metals or metal alloys joined at the ends. When the two junctions are held at different temperatures, a current will flow in the circuit. If a high-resistance precision voltmeter is inserted in the circuit, the measured (open-circuit) voltage is approximately proportional to the temperature difference between the junctions. By holding one junction at a known reference temperature (e.g., the ice point), the temperature of the other junction can be accurately determined from the voltage with the use of calibration tables.

thermodilution (ther″mo-dĭ-lu′shun) see under *cardiac output measurements.*

thermoduric (ther″mo-du′rik) [*thermo-* + L. *durus* enduring] capable of withstanding high temperature, especially used to describe bacteria that are resistant to temperatures lethal to most microorganisms.

thermodynamics (ther″mo-di-nam′iks) [*thermo-* + Gr. *dynamis* power] the science that deals with the relations between heat, work, and the properties of matter.

thermograph (ther′mo-graf) 1. an instrument for recording variations in temperature (heat).

2. the apparatus or device employed in thermography.

thermography (ther-mog′rah-fe) [*thermo-* + Gr. *graphein* to write] an imaging technology in which heat radiation is used to make a thermogram, an image that indicates the temperatures of each point of the body surface.

Any object at body temperature emits heat radiation (black-body radiation) in the infrared region of the spectrum. A thermographic image is made by an infrared television camera and displayed on a cathode-ray tube (CRT) with different shades of gray (or different colors), indicating the temperature. The full-scale range of temperatures displayed is usually about 5°C.

Thermography has been used as a screening procedure for breast cancer, although there is a high false-negative rate, because only superficial tumors produce enough elevation of the skin temperature to be detected; it also produces a high false-positive rate because other lesions, e.g., abscesses, mastitis, and fibrocystic disease of the breast, may have a higher temperature than that of normal tissue. It is also used to evaluate peripheral vascular disease; areas with adequate blood supply are differentiated from those with poor blood supply on the basis of relative surface temperature of the respective areas.

thermolabile (ther″mo-la′bil) [*thermo-* + L. *labilis* liable to fall] easily altered or destroyed by heat.

thermoluminescence (ther″mo-lu-mĭ-nes′ens) [*thermo-* + L. *lumen* light] the production of light by a substance when its temperature is increased.

thermoluminescent detector see *thermoluminescent d.* under *dosimeter.*

thermometer (ther-mom′ĕ-ter) [*thermo-* + Gr. *metron* measure] a device for measuring temperature, such as the familiar mercury and alcohol thermometers in which the liquid expands with increasing temperature and rises in the capillary tube. See also *thermocouple.*

clinical t., a thermometer used to measure human body temperature.

oral t., a clinical thermometer that is placed under the tongue. It characteristically has an elongated bulb.

rectal t., a clinical thermometer that is inserted into the rectum. It characteristically has a pear-shaped bulb.

thermometry (ther-mom′ĕ-tre) the measurement of temperature.

thermophile (ther′mo-fīl) [*thermo-* + Gr. *philos* loving] a microorganism, usually a bacterium, with an optimal growth temperature within the range of 50°–70°C and the ability to survive temperatures as high as 90°C. A well-known example is *Bacillus stearothermophilus,* whose highly resistant spores are used to monitor sterilization procedures. Cf. *mesophile* and *psychrophile.*

thermoresistant (ther″mo-re-zis′tant) not greatly affected by heat.

thermotaxis (ther″mo-tak′sis) [*thermo-* + Gr. *taxis* arrangement] 1. the movement of an organism toward or away from an increase in temperature. Also called *thermotropism.*

2. the regulation of heat production or dissipation.

thermotropism (ther″mo-tro′pizm) [*thermo-* + Gr. *tropē* turn] see *thermotaxis.*

thesaurismosis (the-saw″riz-mo′sis) [Gr. *thēsauros* treasure] a metabolic disorder in which some substance (such as fats, proteins, or carbohydrates) accumulates in certain cells in abnormal amounts.

thesaurocyte (the-sawr′o-sīt) see *Mott cell.*

theta (Θ, θ) (tha′tah) the eighth letter of the *Greek alphabet.*

theta antigen see *Thy-1 antigen.*

theta band in electroencephalography, electric activity having a frequency of from 4 to just under 8 Hz.

theta rhythm in electroencephalography, electric activity of the brain having a frequency of 4–7 Hz. In humans, theta activity is especially prominent in the electroencephalogram of infants and children, and decreases with maturation. Some theta activity may be seen in young adults, especially during hyperventilation, but otherwise is not common in healthy adults except during drowsiness or sleep.

Focal or lateralized theta activity suggests the presence of a localized cerebral disorder, whereas diffuse theta activity may accompany a variety of generalized neurologic disorders or indicate a change in the state of arousal.

THF abbrev. See *tetrahydrofuran.*

thia- (thi′ah) [Gr. *theion* sulfur] a prefix word element in organic chemistry to denote the replacement of a methylene group (—CH_2—) by a sulfur atom (—S—), e.g., thiabenzene.

thial (thi′al) see *thioaldehyde.*

thiamine (thi′ah-mēn) the generic term for compounds having vitamin B_1 activity, all salts of the 3-[(4-amino-2-methyl-5-pyrimidinyl)-methyl]-5-(2-hydroxyethyl)-4-methylthiazolium ion. A deficiency of the thiamine affects mainly the neuromuscular system. Clinical symptoms are peripheral neuritis and extreme muscular weakness, as well as anxiety and mental confusion. The heart may become enlarged and the pericardium edematous. Congestive heart failure may develop because of weakening of the heart muscle itself. Deficiency may result in beriberi. A water-soluble vitamin, thiamine is found in almost all food sources, particularly in liver, heart and kidney foods, and in whole cereal grains.

t. hydrochloride, [USP], the hydrochloride of thiamine, 3-[(4-amino-2-methyl-5-pyrimidinyl)-methyl]5-(2-hydroxyethyl)-4-methylthiazolium chloride monohydrochloride; M.W. 337.28. This substance occurs as white crystals or a crystalline powder. It is used as a vitamin supplement in the prophylaxis and treatment of thiamine deficiency.

t. mononitrate, [USP], 3-(4-amino-2-methylpyrimidyl-5-methyl)-4-methyl-5-hydroxyethylthiazolium nitrate; M.W. 327.36. This compound is prepared by exchanging the chloride ions from thiamine hydrochloride with the nitrate ion. It is chemically more stable than the hydrochloride analog and is used as a supplement in the prophylaxis and treatment of thiamine deficiency.

phosphorylated t., the active form of thiamine, which serves as the cofactor in reactions involving oxidative decarboxylation of certain important intermediates in carbohydrate metabolism, such as pyruvate or α-ketoglutarate. Thiamine pyrophosphate also acts as a coenzyme of transketolase in the pentose phosphate pathway.

thiamine assays 1. fluorometric thiochrome method. Thiamine is oxidized to thiochrome by alkaline potassium ferricyanide. The thiochrome formed, which is extracted into isobutanol, exhibits an intense blue fluorescence and is measured fluorometrically. The presence of a variety of interfering substances necessitates purification of the specimen by ion-exchange chromatography. The amount of thiamine in the specimen is calculated in reference to a known standard.

2. microbiologic assay. The growth of *Lactobacillus viridescens* is thiamine-dependent. Cultures of this inoculum are grown in the presence of increasing amounts of pure thiamine, which is used as a standard, and in the unknown specimen. The culture is harvested and the absorbance determined at 620 nm. A standard curve is prepared by plotting the thiamine concentration against the absorbance, from which the amount of thiamine in the specimen is derived.

thiamine deficiency see under *Wernicke-Korsakoff syndrome.*

thiamphenicol (thi″am-fen′ĭ-kōl) an antibiotic chemically related to chloramphenicol. The two antibiotics are similar in their uses and in the adverse reactions they produce.

thiamphenicol assays gas chromatography using an electron-capture detector and a moderately polar silicone stationary phase. The drug is extracted from blood samples into ethyl acetate and silylated using bis-trimethyl-silylacetamide (BSA). The thiamphenicol concentration in the sample is proportional to the peak height ratio in the chromatogram of the silylated derivatives of thiamphenicol and the internal standard (chloramphenicol).

thiamylal sodium (thi-am′ĭ-lal) [USP], an ultrashort-acting thio-substituted barbiturate, used as an injected general anesthetic. See also *barbiturate.*

Thiara (thi-ar′ah) a genus of freshwater snails of worldwide distribution. The species *T. granifera, T. toucheana,* and *T. tuberculata* serve as hosts for several trematode parasites, including *Paragonimus, Metagonimus,* and *Haplorchis.*

Thiaridae (thi-ar′ĭ-de) a family of snails that includes the genus *Thiara.*

thiazide diuretics (thi′ah-zīd) a group of benzothiadiazine sulfonamide derivatives. They function primarily by inhibiting H_2O and Cl^- reabsorption in the cortical thick-walled portion of the ascending limb of the loop of Henle; they are also weak carbonic anhydrase inhibitors.

Thiazide diuretics are used to treat hypertension and edema due to congestive heart failure or kidney disease. The primary adverse effect is potassium depletion as a result of increased secretion in the distal renal tubules; the serum levels of other electrolytes, uric acid, and glucose can also be disturbed. This group includes bendroflumethiazide, benzthiazide, chlorothiazide, cyclothiazide, hydrochlorothiazide, hydroflumethiazide, methylclothiazide, polythiazide, and trichlormethiazide. Chlorthalidone and quinethazone are related sulfonamides that have similar effects.

thiazinamium chloride (thi″ah-zin′ah-me-um) a phenothiazine compound with antihistaminic and anticholinergic properties.

thiazol yellow G (thi′ah-zōl) see *titan yellow.*

thiethylperazine maleate (thi-eth″il-per′ah-zēn) [USP], a phenothiazine used in the treatment of nausea, vertigo, and vomiting. It is contraindicated in pregnancy, for severely depressed patients, and for children younger than 12 yr. Adverse reactions include drowsiness, hypotension, and potentiation of the sedative effects of alcohol and other central nervous system depressants. Trademark, Torecan.

thigh (thi) [Anglo-Saxon *thioh*] the portion of the lower extremity situated between the hip and the knee.

thigh bone see *femur.*

thimerosal (thi-mer′o-sal) [USP], a mercurial topical antiseptic, also used as a preservative in drug preparations. Trademark, *Merthiolate.*

thin-layer chromatography a method of chromatography in which the stationary phase is a thin layer of an adsorbent (e.g., silica gel, alumina, kieselguhr, polyacrylamide gel, starch gel, or microcellulose) coated on a glass plate or sheet of plastic, and the mobile phase is a solvent or a solvent mixture. Often, some fluorescing material is added to the adsorbent to assist the visualization of components of the sample after completion of the chromatographic separation.

The sample, dissolved in a solvent, is applied to the plate in a small spot (or fine streak) and dried. The plate is then placed on edge in a covered developing tank, with the lower edge dipping into the (developing) solvent, the level of which should be slightly below the point of application. Before the plate is inserted into the tank, the tank atmosphere is equilibrated with vapor phase of the solvent. As the solvent rises by capillary action through the pores in the adsorbent, the sample separates into its components as a result of differences in solubility in the solvent components and differences in the affinity for the adsorbent. When the solvent approaches the upper edge of the plate, the plate is removed and dried. In two-dimensional chromatography, the plate is dried, rotated 90°, and rechromatographed with a different solvent. After drying, the components are visualized by staining or examination under ultraviolet light.

The ratio of the distance that a sample has moved from the point of application to the distance that the solvent has moved from the point of application is called the R_f value. For a specific adsorbent and developing solvent, the R_f value is a characteristic of a substance and may be compared with those established for known standards.

Thin-layer chromatography is used in the clinical laboratory to separate and identify urinary sugars, barbiturates, and amino acids, and in screening studies for drugs and poisons. For sugars, a pyridine-butanol or pyridine-ethyl acetate mixture is used as the solvent, and the spots (sample components) are visualized by spraying the plate with dinitrosalicylic acid. For drugs, various mixtures of chloroform, methanol, ethyl acetate, isopropyl ether, and ammonia are used as solvents, and the spots are visualized by examination under ultraviolet light or by spraying with iodoplatinate, ninhydrin, mercuric sulfate, or furfural. Thin-layer chromatography is also used to identify components of lipids, e.g., the lecithin/sphingomyelin ratio.

thio- (thi′o) [Gr. *theion* sulfur] 1. a prefix word element to denote the presence of sulfur.

2. a prefix word element in bacteriology to denote a sulfur-metabolizing bacterium, e.g., *Thiobacillus.*

3. a word element in chemistry to denote compounds containing sulfur in several senses: as a prefix in some classes of compounds (e.g., thiols, thioketones, thioethers) and in a few specific compounds (e.g., thioacetic acid, thioacetone) to indicate the replacement of an oxygen atom by a sulfur atom; as a prefix in naming thioethers of symmetric structure (e.g., 3,3′-thiodipropanoic acid for $HO_2CCH_2CH_2SCH_2CH_2CO_2H$); as a part of several suffixes used when certain sulfur-containing groups are the principal functional group, e.g., methanethiol (CH_3SH), ethanthial (CH_3CHS); and as a part of several prefixes used when certain sulfur-containing functional groups are named as substituents, e.g., methylthiopropane ($CH_3SCH_2CH_2CH_3$), 2-thioxopropanoic acid (CH_3CSCO_2H).

thio acid (thi′o) in inorganic chemistry, an acid derived from an oxo acid by replacing one or more oxygen atoms with sulfur atoms, such as thiophosphoric (monothiophosphoric) acid (H_3PO_3S) and dithiophosphoric acid ($H_3PO_2S_2$); in organic chemistry, there is some ambiguity in the term because it does not specify which of the two oxygens in a carboxylic acid is replaced. When the oxygen in the OH is replaced, the acid can be named in several ways, as in CH_3COSH: thioloacetic acid, thioacetic acid, or thiolacetic acid. If the oxygen in the carbonyl group is replaced by sulfur, CH_3CSOH, it is called thionoacetic acid.

thioaldehyde (thi″o-al′dĕ-hīd) an organic compound with the generic formula R—CHS, i.e., an aldehyde in which the carbonyl oxygen is replaced by a sulfur atom. Also called *thial.*

thiobarbiturate (thi″o-bar-bit′u-rāt) a group of ultrashort-acting barbiturates (thiopental, thiamylal) in which S replaces O at the 2 position of the pyrimidine ring. See also *barbiturate.*

thiocarbonyl group (thi″o-kar′bon-il) a carbonyl group with oxygen replaced by sulfur. The rare compounds containing this group are named *thioketones* (*thiones*) or *thioaldehydes* (*thials*).

thiochrome (thi″o-krōm) [*thio-* + Gr. *chrōma* color] a compound having blue fluorescence and obtained from thiamine by the action of mild oxidants. This procedure serves as the basis for the measurement of thiamine concentration in biologic materials.

thioctic acid (thi-ok′tik) 1,2-dithiolane-3-pentanoic acid; M.W. 206.32. Thioctic acid participates as a coenzyme in the oxidative decarboxylation of pyruvate to acetate. No symptoms of thioctic acid deficiency in humans are known. Also called *lipoic acid.*

thiocyanate (thi″o-si′ah-nāt) pertaining to the SCN^- ion or to a compound containing this ion.

thioester (thi″o-es′ter) an ester of a carboxylic acid and a thiol, R_1—CO—S—R_2. See also *functional group.*

thioethanolamine (thi″o-eth″ah-nol′ah-mēn) see *β-mercaptoethylamine.*

thioether (thi″o-e′ther) the generic name for an organic sulfide, R—S—R′. See also *sulfide.*

thioflavine T a blue-white, basic thiazole fluorochrome dye; C.I. 49005. It is used for the fluorescent staining of amyloid.

thioglycolate (thi″o-gli′ko-lāt) a salt or ester of thioglycolic acid. Various salts are used in permanent wave solutions for treating hair and in depilatories. Sodium thioglycolate is used in some culture media for growing anaerobic bacteria; it removes free oxygen and inactivates mercurial antiseptics by chelating the mercury.

thioglycolic acid (thi″o-gli-kol′ik) a colorless liquid with a strong unpleasant odor, $HSCH_2COOH$; M.W. 92.12. It is very corrosive, causing burns and blisters on skin contact. Thioglycolic acid is used as a sulfhydryl reagent and as a reducing agent in the assays for iron, molybdenum, silver, and tin. Also called *mercaptoacetic acid.*

thioguanine (thi″o-gwah′nēn) a cancer chemotherapeutic drug. For more information, see *Appendix A.*

thioketone (thi″o-ke′tōn) an organic compound with the generic formula R—CS—R′, i.e., a ketone in which the carbonyl oxygen is replaced by a sulfur atom. Also called *thione.*

thiol (thi′ol) a compound containing the —SH functional group (not attached to a carbonyl or other functional group). Thiols are named systematically as alcohols with the suffix -thiol, which replaces -ol. The analog of ethanol (C_2H_5OH) is ethanethiol (C_2H_5SH).

thiolaminopropionic acid (thi″ol-ah-me″no-pro″pe-on′ik) see *cysteine.*

thiolysis (thi-ol′ĭ-sis) [*thio-* + Gr. *lysis*] the splitting of a bond in a molecule by a thiol aided by enzymatic catalysis. An example is the cleavage of 3-ketohexadecanoyl coenzyme A by HSCoA and the enzyme acyl CoA thiolase to yield myristoyl CoA and acetyl CoA.

thione (thi′ōn) see *thioketone.*

thionin (thi′o-nin) a metachromatic thiazin dye; C.I. 52000. It is used in histology to stain mucin and connective tissue. Its orthochromatic color is violet and its metachromatic color is red.

thiopental sodium (thi″o-pen′tal) [USP], an ultra-short-acting thio-substituted barbiturate, used as an injected general anesthetic or to control convulsions. See also barbiturate. Trademark, *Pentothal.*

thiopropazate hydrochloride (thi″o-pro′pah-zāt) [USP], a piperazine-type phenothiazine major tranquilizer. See also *phenothiazine tranquilizers.*

thioproperazine mesylate (thi″o-pro-per′ah-zēn) a phenothiazine compound that has been used as an antiemetic and antianxiety agent.

thioredoxin (thi″o-re-dok′sin) a small protein factor found in *Escherichia coli.* It contains two adjacent cysteine groups and functions in the reduction of ribonucleotides to deoxyribonucleotides.

thioridazine (thi″o-rid′ah-zēn) [USP], a piperidine-type phenothiazine major tranquilizer used in the management of psychotic and other psychiatric disorders. The free base is administered orally in suspensions. See also *phenothiazine tranquilizers.* Trademark, *Mellaril.*

t. hydrochloride, [USP], the salt of thioridazine, administered orally.

thioridazine assays 1. urine ferric chloride screening test; see *phenothiazine tranquilizer assays.*

2. spectrophotofluorometry. Thioridazine is extracted from an alkalinized blood or urine sample into heptane and reextracted into acid. It is oxidized by hydrogen peroxide to produce the sulfoxide, which fluoresces at 430 nm when excited at 352 nm. The difference in relative fluorescence between the specimen and a reference sample is proportional to the thioridazine concentration.

thiosulfate (thi″o-sul′fāt) pertaining to the $S_2O_3^{2-}$ ion or to a compound containing this ion.

thiotepa (thi″o-te′pah) [USP], a nitrogen mustard cytotoxic alkylating agent used as a cancer chemotherapeutic drug. For more information, see *Appendix A.*

thiothixene (thi″o-thik′sēn) [USP], one of the thioxanthene major tranquilizers used in the treatment of psychotic disorders. It is similar to the piperazine-type phenothiazines. The free base is administered orally. See also *phenothiazine tranquilizers.* Trademark, *Navane.*

t. hydrochloride, the salt of thiothixene, used for oral and intramuscular administration.

thioxanthene tranquilizers (thi″o-zan′thēn) a group of major tranquilizers. See under the related *phenothiazine tranquilizers.*

third-degree heart block see *third-degree A-V b.* under *atrioventricular (A-V) block.*

thixotropic (thik″so-trop′ik) pertaining to or characterized by thixotropy.

thixotropy (thik-sot′ro-pe) [Gr. *thixis* a touch + *tropos* a turning] a property of certain gels, such as synovial fluid, which liquefy or become less viscous when shaken or subjected to shearing stress, and solidify again when left standing. The mucin clot test for synovial fluid depends on thixotropic properties.

Thomsen's disease (tom′senz) [Asmus Julius Thomas *Thomsen,* Danish physican, 1815–1896] see *m. congenita* under *myotonia.*

Thoms method see under *pelvimetry.*

thonzylamine hydrochloride (thon-zil′ah-měn) an antihistamine used in cold preparations.

thorac/o (tho′rah-ko) [Gr. *thōrax,* genitive *thōrakos* chest] a word element used in combining form to denote the chest, e.g., thoracoplasty.

thoracentesis (tho″rah-sen-te′sis) [*thoraco-* + Gr. *kentēsis* a pricking] the aspiration of fluid from the thoracic cavity. It may be performed to obtain fluid for diagnostic studies (e.g., in infections and neoplasms), to drain pleural effusions, or to reexpand a collapsed lung. The site of entry of the needle or trocar into the thoracic cavity is determined by physical or radiographic findings, but is most frequently at the seventh interspace in the posterior axillary line. See also *pleural fluid examination.*

Also called pleurocentesis and thoracocentesis.

thoracic (tho-ras′ik) [L. *thoracicus;* Gr. *thōrakikos,* from *thōrax*] pertaining to the chest.

thoracic outlet syndrome a variety of disorders characterized by compression of the neurovascular bundle as it courses between the clavicle and the first rib. The compression is usually caused by a fibrous band attached to the transverse process of the seventh cervical vertebra. When the brachial plexus is involved, there is numbness over the ulnar aspect of the hand and forearm with thenar weakness and wasting, although pain is often absent or moderate in severity. Adson's maneuver may be positive in up to 70 percent of normal individuals and must be interpreted with caution. Electromyography and x-rays may be useful in diagnosis; arteriograms are only minimally helpful.

thoracostomy (tho″rah-kos′to-me) [*thoraco-* + Gr. *stoma* mouth] a surgical incision to create an opening in the chest wall.

thoracotomy (tho″rah-kot′o-me) [*thoraco-* + Gr. *tomē* a cutting] a general term used to describe surgical incision of the chest wall. See also *thoracostomy.*

thorax (tho′raks), pl. *thoraces* [Gr. thōrax] [NA], a framework of bones and cartilages (thoracic vertebrae, ribs, costal cartilages, sternum) that encloses the thoracic cavity. Its upper, open end, or inlet, is kidney-shaped. The shape of the thorax alters with respiration. Also called *chest.*

-thorax (tho′raks) [Gr. *thōrax*] a suffix word element to denote the pleural cavity, e.g., pneumothorax.

Thorazine (thor′ah-zēn) trademark. See *chlorpromazine.*

thorium (Th) (thor′e-um, tho′re-um) [*Thor* a Norse god] a soft, silvery, metallic radioactive element; atomic number 90; atomic weight 232.0381; a 5f transition element (actinide series); oxidation state +4.

Thorium occurs naturally; ^{232}Th has a half-life of 14.1 billion yr. It is used as fuel for nuclear reactors (^{232}Th is converted in the reactor to fissionable ^{233}U by neutron capture). Thorium and its decay products are carcinogenic radioactive poisons when ingested or inhaled.

Thr abbrev. See *threonine.*

three-Hertz spike and slow waves in electroencephalography, a type of paroxysmal activity that consists of a regular sequence of spike and slow waves repeated at intervals of 3–3.5 Hz. The amplitude of the complex may vary but is often maximal over the frontal areas. The complex appears bilaterally and is then symmetric and synchronous over the two sides of the head. Similar activity that does not conform to the above criteria is called atypical repetitive spike and slow waves. Also called *spike and slow-wave rhythm.*

three-phase current a three-wire source of alternating current. The voltage across each of the three pairs of wires is the same, but the waveforms are 120° out of phase. Because the peaks are evenly spaced over a full cycle, full-wave rectification produces a pulsed direct current output with six overlapping pulses in each cycle, as opposed to the two pulses produced from a single-phase input. At the same peak voltage, the three-phase system produces 60 percent more power and has much less ripple voltage.

three-point cross see under *genetic mapping.*

threo- (thre′o) a prefix word element in chemistry to denote a stereoisomer that has a structure similar to threose, as in *threo*-2-deoxypentose. The term is used to specify the configuration of compounds with two chiral carbons that have only two similar groups on each carbon. If the similar groups are on the same side in the Fischer projection formula, the molecule is labeled *threo.* Cf. *erythro-.*

threonin (Thr or T) (thre′o-nēn) 2-amino-3-hydroxy butanoic acid, $CH_3CH(OH)CH(NH_2)COOH$, a naturally occurring essential amino acid; M.W. 119.12. In proteins, its hydroxyl group serves to bind phosphate groups or oligosaccharide chains in glycoproteins. See also under *amino acids.*

threonyl (thre′o-nil) the acyl radical derived from or relating to threonine.

threose (thre′ōs) an aldotetrose sugar, isomeric with erythrose.

threshold (thresh′old) 1. a certain critical value at which a stimulus just evokes a response or reaches the limit of perception.

2. in neurophysiology, the critical level of depolarization (reduction in membrane potential difference) beyond which a propagated action potential is triggered. Threshold is reached at a transmembrane potential of about –30 to –55 mV in an excitable cell.

3. the minimal level of a physical quantity needed to produce some effect; the minimal input that produces an output.

4. see *renal threshold.*

threshold limit values (TLV) the recommended guidelines for limiting inhalation exposures to chemicals in the workplace. These values are reviewed and revised annually by the American Conference of Governmental Industrial Hygienists (ACGIH), which defines threshold limits as "airborne concentrations of substances [which] represent conditions under which it is believed that nearly all workers may be repeatedly exposed day after day without adverse effect. Because of wide variation in individual susceptibility, however, a small percentage of workers may experience discomfort from some substances at concentrations at or below the threshold limit; a smaller percentage may be affected more seriously by aggravation of a preexisting condition or by development of an occupational illness." These limits include three categories: ceiling limits, which should not be exceeded even for an instant; tentative short-term exposure limits, which should not be exceeded for more than 15 min at a time and not more than four times a day; and time-weighted average concentrations, which are for a normal 8-hr workday or 40-hr workweek.

It should be noted that although TLV are published for many chemicals commonly used in laboratories, many of the limits are not based on toxicity; the ACGIH specifically states in the preface of its annual listing that the values "are not intended for use, or for modification for use, as a relative index of hazard or toxicity. . . ."

thrill (thril) a palpable vibration accompanying loud cardiac murmurs, which can be described as the feel of a cat's purr, that is transmitted through the chest wall. Thrills are felt over the aortic, pulmonic, apical, or ventricular areas of the precordium, depending on the etiology of the murmur. They are most frequently present in aortic stenosis, mitral stenosis, ventricular septal defects, and pulmonic stenosis.

-thrix (thriks) [Gr.] a suffix word element to denote the hair, e.g., *Erysipelothrix.*

throat (thrōt) 1. the area that includes the larynx and pharynx.

2. the fauces.

3. the anterior part of the neck.

throat culture a microbiologic examination of a pharyngeal specimen, which is useful in the diagnosis of upper respiratory tract infections as well as in identifying infectious disease carriers. The throat has a normal bacterial flora that includes α-hemolytic streptococci, certain *Neisseria* species, coagulase-negative staphylococci, *Hemophilus* species, pneumococci, and diphtheroid bacilli. A throat culture is considered normal when there is a good mixture of these bacteria present in addition to other less commonly identified nonpathogenic bacteria. When one or more pathogenic species predominate and the normal flora is modified, it is an indication that a bacterial infection is present.

The most dangerous pathogen of the throat is β-hemolytic group A streptococcus, the causative agent of "strep" throat. Infection with β-hemolytic group A streptococcus carries the risk of subsequently developing rheumatic heart disease. Other pathogens commonly isolated from throat cultures in patients with infections of the pharynx include *Bordetella pertussis, Candida albicans, Corynebacterium diphtheriae, Fusobacterium nucleatum, Neisseria meningitidis,* and *N. gonorrhoeae.*

A throat culture is best obtained with a swab: the patient's tongue is depressed and the posterior pharynx (back of the throat) and areas of inflammation are touched by the swab. The swab should then be transported to the microbiology laboratory in an appropriate transport medium.

See also *Gram stain.*

thromb/o (throm′bo) [Gr. *thrombos* clot] a word element used in combining form to denote a clot, e.g., thrombophlebitis.

thrombasthenia (throm″bas-the′ne-ah) [*thromb-* + Gr. *astheneia* weakness] a rare but severe congenital bleeding disorder, transmitted as an autosomal recessive trait, in which the platelets function abnormally, although they are usually normal in number. Characteristics of the disorder include weak or absent platelet aggregation with adenosine diphosphate (ADP), collagen, epinephrine, thrombin, ristocetin and arachidonic acid; absent or incomplete clot retraction; prolonged bleeding time; abnormal platelet retention; and normal clotting factors. Genetic heterogeneity seems apparent. Also called Glanzmann-Naegeli's disease and *Glanzmann's thrombasthenia.*

thrombin (throm′bin) an enzyme of the hydrolase class (EC 3.4.21.5) formed from prothrombin by its proenzyme, the hydrolytic action of activated Factor X. It catalyzes the hydrolysis of Arg-Gly bonds in fibrinogen with the release of active fibrin.

In the course of this reaction, two peptides (fibrinopeptides A, FPA, and fibrinopeptide B, FPB) are cleaved from fibrinogen, leaving fibrin monomers that polymerize, forming the insoluble fibrin strands that form the elements of the clot. Activated by the thrombin, Factor XIII then stabilizes the clot in the presence of Ca^{++} by the formation of covalent bonds. Besides converting fibrinogen to fibrin and activating Factor XIII, thrombin stimulates platelet aggregation and secretion, increases the coagulant activity of Factors IV and V, and participates in a positive feedback system that greatly accelerates the rate of clotting.

Thrombin is rapidly generated through the extrinsic system but in low concentration. The intrinsic generation of thrombin is slow but can result in very high concentrations of the substance.

thrombin clotting time (TCT) a test that quantitates the antithrombin activity of heparin. It measures the capacity of heparin to inactivate a standardized quantity of thrombin with the results calculated from a heparin reference curve. Fibrin (fibrinogen) degradation products and low fibrinogen levels will also prolong the TCT. The reference range for a patient not receiving heparin is 8–10 sec.

thrombin time test a measure of the end stage of coagulation, the conversion of fibrinogen to fibrin. In this procedure, buffered human thrombin is added to plasma and the clotting time is measured; normal time is 16–18 sec. The results may be prolonged in the presence of heparin, fibrin degradation products, or any substance that inhibits the conversion of fibrinogen to fibrin.

thromboangiitis (throm″bo-an″je-i′tis) [*thrombo-* + Gr. *angeion* vessel + *-itis*] inflammation of a blood vessel with thrombosis.

thromboangiitis obliterans (throm″bo-an″je-i′tis ob-lit′ĕ-rans) [*thrombo-* + Gr. *angeion* vessel + *-itis;* L. *obliterare* to blot out] a disease of uncertain etiology that usually occurs in young males who smoke; it is characterized by segmental, thrombosing inflammatory changes in small- and medium-sized blood vessels. Onset may be sudden or gradual, with involvement of both arms and legs. The symptoms are primarily due to ischemia. The affected extremities are pale and cold and may demonstrate absent pulses, intermittent claudication, ulceration, and gangrene. Cessation of smoking is imperative.

thrombocyte (throm′bo-sīt) [*thrombo-* + Gr. *kytos* hollow vessel] see *platelet.*

thrombocythemia (throm″bo-sĭ-the′me-ah) [*thrombocyte* + Gr. *haima* blood + *-ia*] an increase in the number of circulating blood platelets. Cf. *thrombocytosis.*

essential t., a myeloproliferative disorder characterized by the proliferation of megakaryocytes and an increase in platelets in the bone marrow. The peripheral blood demonstrates thrombocytosis, neutrophilic leukocytosis, and a mild erythrocytosis. The elevation in platelet count is at least three times normal, and may reach into the millions per cubic millimeter.

Clinically, spontaneous, excessive, recurrent bleeding is frequent but purpura is not. Splenic enlargement is a common characteristic. The disease must be distinguished from thrombocytosis attributed to other causes.

Treatment is achieved by whole-body irradiation using ^{32}P or by chemotherapy. Essential thrombocytopenia is potentially lethal, and complications arising from hemorrhagic episodes are always a danger. Transformation to more acute disease, including granulocytic leukemia, is not uncommon.

Also called hemorrhagic thrombocythemia and idiopathic thrombocythemia. Cf. *acute megakaryoblastic l.* under *leukemia.*

thrombocytic series (throm″bo-sit′ik) the morphologically recognizable precursors of platelets: megakaryoblast, promegakaryocyte, and megakaryocyte. See under *thrombocytopoiesis.*

thrombocytin (throm″bo-si′tin) see *serotonin.*

thrombocytopenia (throm″bo-si″to-pe′ne-ah) [*thrombocyte* + Gr. *penia* poverty] a decrease in the number of blood platelets.

thrombocytopoiesis (throm″bo-si″to-poi-e′sis) [*thrombocyte* + Gr. *poiēsis* a making] the process of platelet formation. Platelets (thrombocytes) are formed by the fragmentation of megakaryocytes, which are multinucleate giant cells found in the bone marrow. These platelets develop from committed stem cells called colony-forming units, CFU_{MEG} (see also *stem cells*). CFU_{MEG} differentiates into the earliest morphologically recognizable precursor, the megakaryoblast, which is 20–30 μm in diameter with basophilic cytoplasm and an irregular, lobulated nucleus. The megakaryoblast matures into the promegakaryocyte (basophilic megakaryocyte), which has a spherical nucleus and contains azurophilic granules that develop first near the nucleus. The promegakaryocyte develops into the mature (acidophilic or granular) megakaryocyte, in which the cytoplasm is no longer basophilic and the azurophilic granules are distributed throughout the cytoplasm. Megakaryocytes are polyploid with chromosome numbers of 8N–64N; the degree of ploidy, however, does not correspond to the number of lobes. Megakaryocytes extend long pseudopodia into the venous sinuses of the bone marrow. Fragmentation of the pseudopodia produces the platelets, each megakaryocyte being responsible for the formation of 2000–4000 platelets.

thrombocytosis (throm″bo-si-to′sis) an elevation of the platelet count above normal levels. Thrombocytosis often occurs in a benign, secondary form as a temporary and self-limited event in infections, anemia, iron deficiency, or malignant lymphoma; after hemorrhage or surgery (particularly splenectomy); or as a response to exercise. It is usually asymptomatic and abnormal bleeding is rarely observed. Platelet function tests and platelet morphology are generally normal; diagnosis depends on demonstration of the underlying disorder. Treatment is frequently unnecessary, owing to the absence of symptoms.

The primary neoplastic form of this condition, essential thrombocythemia, is considered one of the myeloproliferative disorders. It can be differentiated from secondary thrombocytosis by the associated blood abnormalities.

Cf. *thrombocythemia.*

thromboembolism (throm″bo-em′bo-lizm) the dislodgment and movement of a thrombus that was formed in the heart, arteries, or veins. Such emboli often lodge in smaller arteries or arterioles, producing infarction of the tissue supplied by the occluded vessels.

thromboendarterectomy (throm″bo-end″ar-ter-ek′to-me) [*thrombo-* + Gr. *endō* within + *artēria* artery + *ektomē* a cutting out] the surgical removal of an obstructing thrombus from an artery.

thromboendarteritis (throm″bo-end-ar″ter-i′tis) inflammation of the intima of an artery, with thrombus formation.

thromboendocarditis (throm″bo-en″do-kar-di′tis) [*thrombo-* + Gr. *endō* within + *kardia* heart + *-itis*] formation of a thrombus on the endocardium, usually on a heart valve that has bacterial or nonbacterial vegetations.

thrombolysis (throm-bol′i-sis) [*thrombo-* + *lysis* dissolution] the phenomenon by which preformed thrombi are lysed by a complex series of events, the most important of which involves the local action of plasmin confined within the substance of the thrombus.

thrombolytic (throm″bo-lit′ik) dissolving or splitting up a thrombus.

thrombolytic agents substances that activate the plasminogen circulating in the plasma and adsorbed to the thrombus, which induce fibrinolysis. In the treatment of thrombosis, these agents have been directed toward the plasminogen adsorbed to the thrombus. Activation in the plasma results in the destruction of fibrinogen, Factor V, and Factor VIII, and may cause a severe hermorrhagic diathesis.

ANCROD. Ancrod is a thrombolytic agent extracted from the venom of the Malayan pit viper, *Agkistrodon rhodostoma.* It has thrombin-like proteolytic enzymatic action that converts fibrinogen into an abnormal soluble fibrin polymer, which is then lysed by endogenous fibrinolytic enzymes. Ancrod has been used in therapeutic defibrination.

STREPTOKINASE. Streptokinase is a thrombolytic agent produced by certain β-hemolytic streptococci. It activates the fibrinolytic system by converting inactive plasminogen to plasmin. It is highly antigenic, and predominantly activates circulating plasminogen.

UROKINASE. an enzyme of the hydrolase class (EC 3.4.21.31) that catalyzes the cleavage of peptide bonds containing arginine and valine in plasminogen, thus converting it to plasmin. Urokinase has been isolated from urine and from renal tubular cells, and is part of the complex plasminogen activator system. Also called plasminogen activator.

thrombophlebitis (throm″bo-fle-bi′tis) [*thrombo-* + Gr. *phleps* vein + *-itis*] thrombosis within a vein, frequently accompanied by an inflammatory response. Venous thrombosis usually occurs in the lower extremities or pelvis. The most common precipitating factor is stasis with pooling of blood in these locations, as occurs in individuals who are immobilized or at bed rest. Changes in the coagulability of blood may also be a factor, although definite laboratory evidence of this is lacking in most cases. Certain persons are at particular risk for thrombophlebitis, including those who have had recent surgery or a myocardial infarction, those with cancer or inflammatory bowel disease, and females taking supplemental estrogens. Less commonly, thrombophlebitis is due to chemical irritation and/or infection induced by an indwelling catheter or intravenous solution. In hospitalized patients, the prevalence of venous thrombi is in the range of 4–75 percent, depending on the clinical setting. It is highest in patients with hip fractures and recent myocardial infarctions. About half of all patients dying in the hospital are found at autopsy to have premortem clots in the legs or pelvis.

The presence of venous thrombosis is frequently asymptomatic. When symptomatic, the most common presentation of thrombophlebitis is leg swelling, sometimes accompanied by pain and redness. Swelling is most easily detected by comparison of the circumferences of both legs at several levels. When a superficial vein is involved, an inflamed, tender vein is usually present over the thigh or calf. When a deep vein is affected, the symptoms may be more subtle: 20–30 percent have a tender, swollen leg. The degree of swelling depends on the level of thrombosis. Many have tenderness on dorsiflexion of the foot (Homan's sign), and occasionally a tender, cordlike vein is palpable. Thrombophlebitis must be differentiated from cellulitis, lymphatic obstruction, trauma, and ruptured popliteal cyst.

Confirmation of diagnosis frequently requires performance of a diagnostic procedure. The simplest is Doppler examination, which is relatively sensitive for detecting obstruction of the deep veins of the calf or thigh. Radionuclide venography is more sensitive than Doppler examination for detecting disease in the thigh and pelvis, but is less accurate in detecting deep venous thrombosis (DVT) of the calf. Impedance plethysmography also has a high degree of accuracy. The most sensitive noninvasive test employs ^{125}I-labeled fibrinogen, but is prone to false-positive results and is still considered a research tool. The definitive diagnostic tool for DVT is contrast venography, but its use is limited by expense, patient discomfort, and a significant risk of thrombophlebitis that may be induced by the procedure.

The most worrisome complication of DVT is pulmonary thromboembolism, which occurs when part of the thrombus breaks off and lodges in the lung. This problem may be life-threatening when the embolus is very large and occludes a major pulmonary artery. Pulmonary embolism is most frequently associated with pelvic and thigh thrombophlebitis, and rarely results from isolated disease in the calf.

The second major complication is the postphlebitic syndrome, a consequence of pelvic or thigh thrombosis. This is caused by damage to venous valves that renders them incompetent, and by the failure of the thrombus to recanalize along with inadequate collateral circulation. Those affected with this syndrome are plagued by chronic pain and swelling of the affected extremity.

Recurrent thrombosis is also a problem, requiring a conscientious effort by the patient to avoid circumstances that predispose to stasis, such as prolonged sitting.

In most instances, the thrombophlebitis resolves without sequelae, and patients are able to resume normal activity without impairment.

For high-risk patients in the hospital, prophylaxis against DVT is often indicated. This usually consists of the subcutaneous administration of low doses of heparin. In addition, postoperative patients need to be ambulated early.

Also called *phlebitis.* See also *thrombosis.*

STEPHAN D. FIHN, M.D., M.P.H.

thromboplastin (throm″bo-plas′tin) a substance having procoagulant properties or activity.

thromboplastin generation test (TGT) a test for measuring the efficiency with which prothrombinase (plasma thromboplastin) is formed from a mixture of normal serum (containing Factors XII, XI, X, IX, and VII), adsorbed plasma (containing Factors XII, XI, VIII, and V and fibrinogen), and platelets or a platelet substitute. Its intensity can be measured by adding the mixture to normal plasma at various times after incubation together with calcium. Normal adsorbed plasma and normal serum are substituted, distinguishing a deficiency of Factor VIII (present only in plasma) from Factor IX (present only in serum), as well as Factor XI (present in both), provided the one-stage prothrombin time is not prolonged.

The test is cumbersome, however, when compared with the factor assay test, which uses commercially available plasma deficient in specific coagulation factors. Although the TGT has also been used to identify functional platelet deficiencies, it has been largely replaced for that purpose by aggregation and adhesiveness tests and tests for platelet factor, β-thromboglobulin, and others.

thrombopoietin (throm″bo-poi′e-tin) [*thrombo-* + Gr. *poiētēs* maker + *-in*] one or more poorly characterized substances, found in the plasma of platelet-deficient animals, that induce thrombopoiesis when administered to animal recipients. The assumption is that the thrombopoietin acts on the committed stem cell CFU_{MEG}.

thrombosis (throm-bo′sis) [Gr. *thrombōsis*] the formation, development, or presence of a solid mass (thrombus) in a blood vessel or in the heart. It is composed of fibrin, platelets, and (in most instances) erythrocytes. The major causes of thrombosis include injury to the endothelium of the blood vessel and exposure of the subendothelial wall to the blood, with subsequent platelet adhesion to the exposed basement membrane, underlying collagen or microfibrils, and platelet aggregation; alteration in normal blood flow, including stasis, which is produced by prolonged inactivity; and alterations in blood coagulability, which arise from the increased activities or concentration of various procoagulants, from the presence of activated coagulation factors in the blood, and from the quantitative increase or qualitative alteration in platelet activity.

The body possesses some natural defenses against thrombosis: e.g., inhibitors of the coagulation factors and the clearing of activated coagulation factors by the reticuloendothelial system, as well as the antithrombins and the fibrinolytic system.

thrombosthenin (throm″bo-sthe′nin) [*thrombo-* + Gr. *sthenos* strength + *-in*] a contractile protein similar to actomyosin of muscle but present in the platelet membrane. It is active in clot retraction.

thromboxane A_2 (TXA_2) (throm-bok′sān) an unstable prostaglandin that deviates from the basic prostaglandin structure by possessing an unusual oxane-oxetane ring instead of the cyclopentane ring; M.W. 353.48. TXA_2 is a powerful vasoconstrictor as well as a potent platelet-aggregating agent.

TXA_2 is formed mainly in platelets from prostaglandin endoperoxides, and rapidly (half-life, 30 sec) decomposes to its stable, inactive metabolite, TXB_2. TXA_2 is also formed by pulmonary fibroblasts, the spleen, and the brain. Because it has not yet been isolated, determination of TXA_2 is based on the appearance of the stable metabolite, TXB_2.

thromboxane B_2 (TXB_2) a hemiacetal derivative of 8-(1-hydroxy-3-oxopropyl)-9,12-dihydroxy-5,10-heptadecadienoic acid, a metabolite of thromboxane A_2 with no apparent biologic activity.

thrombus (throm′bus), pl. thrombi [Gr. *thrombos* clot] an aggregation of blood elements, particularly platelets and fibrin with entrapment of cellular elements in the heart, arteries, or veins. Thrombi may enlarge and occlude the vessel at the point of formation, may dislodge and travel to occlude a smaller vessel, or may undergo organization or resolution. When an artery or arteriole becomes blocked by a thrombus, ischemic necrosis or infarction of the tissue supplied by that vessel may occur if there is inadequate collateral circulation. Also called *clot.* See also *infarction.* Cf. *embolism.*

thrush (thrush) [Danish *tröske* rotten wood] an infection of the mucous membranes of the mouth caused by *Candida albicans;* oral candidiasis. See also *candidiasis.*

THS abbrev. for tetrahydro-compound S. See *tetrahydro-11-deoxycortisol.*

thulium (Tm) (thu′le-um) [*Thule,* in ancient times, the legendary northernmost point of the world] a lustrous, silvery-white metallic element; atomic number 69; atomic weight 168.9342; a 4f transition element (lanthanide or rare earth); oxidation state +3. See also *rare earth elements.*

thumb (thum) [L. *pollex, pollux*] the first and most lateral digit of the hand. It contains only two phalanges and is apposable to the other digits of the hand. Also called *pollex.*

thumbprinting (thum′prin-ting) having surface indentations resembling thumbprints, as the radiographic appearance of the barium-filled colon in ischemic colitis. See also the illustration under *contour.*

Thy-1 antigen a surface alloantigen found on thymocytes and peripheral T lymphocytes. In mice it is also present on brain tissue. Also called *theta antigen.*

thym/o (thi′mo) [N.L. *thymus,* from Gr. *thymos*] a word element used in combining form to denote the thymus gland, e.g., thymolysis.

thyme oil (tīm) [L. *thymum;* Gr. *thymon*] the volatile oil distilled from the flavoring plant *Thymus vulgaris,* used as a flavoring agent for drugs. It has also been used as a rubefacient, expectorant, counterirritant, antiseptic, and carminative.

thymic (thi′mik) [L. *thymicus*] pertaining to the thymus.

thymic factor a low molecular weight peptide believed to be secreted by thymic epithelial cells. In mice, thymic factor increases the Thy-1 antigen and concanavalin A responsiveness of bone marrow cells and increases cAMP levels in cells; it also increases T-cell immunity in thymectomized animals. Its effects in humans have not been defined.

thymic humoral factor a polypeptide, isolated from mouse and calf thymus. In animals it is capable of enhancing a variety of T-cell functions, as well as cooperation between T and B cells in antibody production. Its effects in humans have not been defined.

thymic replacing factor a substance that restores the immune responsiveness of cultures deprived of T cells to T-cell mitogens or T-dependent antigens; M.W. 45,000–60,000.

thymic tumors neoplasms of the thymus. Such tumors include thymoma, malignant lymphoma, germ cell tumors, carcinoid tumor, and metastatic carcinoma. See also *thymoma.*

thymidine (T) (thi′mĭ-dēn) thymine-2-deoxyriboside, a nucleoside, $C_{10}H_{14}N_2O_5$, isolable from deoxyribonucleotide.

t. diphosphate (dTDP), a nucleotide involved in metabolic reactions; formed hydrolytically from dTTP.

t. monophosphate, see *thymidine-5′-phosphate.*

t. triphosphate (dTTP), an energy-rich compound analagous to adenosine triphosphate (ATP).

thymidine-5′-phosphate (dTMP) (thi′mĭ-dēn fos′fāt) a mononucleotide formed from thymine, 2-deoxyribose, and phosphoric acid. Also called *thymidine monophosphate* and *thymidylic acid.* See also under *nucleotide.*

thymidylic acid (thī″mĭ-dil′ic) see *thymidine-5′-phosphate.*

thymidylyl (thi″mĭ-dĭl′il) a name for thymidylic acid (thymidine-5′-phosphate) when it is being named as a substituent of some parent group or as an ester, e.g., thymidylyl sulfate, thymidylyltransferase, or the thymidylyl group. It is attached to the other moiety at the 5′ position.

thymin (thi′min) see *thymopoietin.*

thymine (thī′mēn) a crystalline base, 5-methyluracil, $C_5H_6N_2O_2$, found in animal and plant tissues as a pyrimidine base constituent of DNA, which pairs with adenine. It is not used in mRNA. The transcribed base for adenine in mRNA is uracil. Thymine is present in some thymidylyl compounds in tissues: ribothymidylic acid and the deoxyribose compounds dTMP, dTDP, and dTTP. It may also be found as a free base in body fluids.

t. ribonucleoside, a nucleoside that contains thymine and ribose residues.

thymine-2-deoxyriboside (thi′min de-ok″se-ri′bo-sīd) see *thymidine.*

thymine ribonucleoside-5′-phosphate (TMP) (thi′mēn ri′bo-nu″kle-o-sīd fos′fāt) a mononucleotide formed from thymine, ribose, and phosphoric acid. Also called *ribothymidylic acid.* See also under *nucleotide.*

thymocytotoxic autoantibody (throm″bo-si-to-tok′sik) an antibody, found in New Zealand mice, that is cytotoxic for T lymphocytes in the presence of complement. The antibody is of the IgM class and is reactive in the cold. A similar antilymphocytic antibody is found in some humans with systemic lupus erythematosus.

thymol (thi′mol) [occurs in the herb *thyme*] a white, aromatic, crystalline solid, 5-methyl-2-isopropyl-1-phenol, which has been used as an antiseptic and as a preservative (antibacterial agent) for reagents and biologic specimens such as urine.

thymol blue a pH indicator, thymolsulfonphthalein, with an acid pH range of 1.2 (red)–2.8 (yellow) and an alkaline pH range of 8.0 (yellow)–9.6 (blue).

thymolphthalein (thi″mol-thal′ēn) a pH indicator with a pH range of 9.3 (colorless)–10.5 (blue). As monophosphate, it is used as a substrate for acid phosphatase activity measurements.

thymol turbidity test an obsolete test of hepatic function based on the formation of a precipitate with the addition of the reagent to serum in the presence of increased concentrations of serum gamma globulin, especially when accompanied by decreased albumin. Positive tests are also obtained with sera containing increased amounts of lipoproteins and lipids. The degree of turbidity is increased in individuals with hepatocellular disease but is usually normal in those with obstructive jaundice. It is a nonspecific test and has been replaced by more sensitive and specific tests of hepatocellular function.

thymoma (thi-mo′mah) [*thym-* + *-oma*] a neoplasm of thymic epithelial cells; the most common tumor arising in the upper anterior mediastinum. It occurs occasionally in the neck, and exceptionally in the posterior mediastinum. Typically, thymomas are located in the midline. The majority are encapsulated and under 10 cm. A lymphocytic component is usually present and may dominate the histologic picture, but epithelial cells must be present for the diagnosis; pure epithelial thymomas, however, constitute less than 5 percent of all thymomas. Most patients are older adults; children are rarely affected. A minority of those with thymomas have the clinical manifestations of myasthenia gravis.

The histologic appearance of a thymoma depends on the relative proportions of epithelial cells and lymphocytes, and the shape of epithelial cells. The epithelial cells are usually round to ovoid, but they are occasionally spindled. Typically, groups of epithelial cells and small lymphocytes are intermingled. The differential diagnosis often includes lymphoma (demonstration by electron microscopy of the cell junctions between the epithelial cells serves to distinguish the two), metastatic carcinoma, mediastinal germ cell tumors, and the carcinoid tumor. Hassall's corpuscles are seen in fewer than 15 percent of thymomas, and lymphoid follicles in less than 10 percent. In large tumors, cystic areas or foci of necrosis may be found.

The behavior of the tumor cannot be predicted from its histologic appearance, but incidence of invasion at the time of surgery indicates a malignant neoplasm. Fewer than 20 percent of thymomas are invasive and distant metastases are rarely seen. Most thymomas grow slowly and behave as benign tumors.

thymopoietin (thi″mo-poi′ĕ-tin) [*thymo-* + Gr. *poiētēs* maker + *-in*] a substance, presumably produced by thymic epithelial cells, whose function is not clearly defined. It was first isolated from animals with thymitis and myasthenia. Thymopoietin can result in impaired neuromuscular transmission. It has been shown to induce mouse bone marrow cells to acquire Thy-1 antigen and responsiveness to concanavalin A in vitro, but the in vivo effects on human cells are not defined. Formerly called *thymin.*

thymosin (thi′mo-sin) a protein hormone produced by the thymus; M.W. 12,000. It promotes the growth of thymus-dependent peripheral lymphoid tissues and enhances the maturation of prothymocytes to mature T cells. It can restore T-cell immunity in thymectomized animals and has been used to enhance T-cell immunity in immunodeficient patients.

thymus (thi′mus) [N.L., from Gr. *thymos* soul, mind] [NA], a bilobed gland located in the upper part of the anterior mediastinum. It weighs about 40 g at the time of puberty but progressively diminishes in size through adult life. The base of the gland rests on the pericardium, and the upper poles of its lobes are in apposition to the trachea and thyroid. The lobes develop from the third branchial pouch, and migrate down through the neck to meet and partially fuse in the upper mediastinum. Small groups of thymic cells are often left along the track of migration and may be encountered during surgical procedures on the thyroid or parathyroid glands.

The thymus has a continuous, branching medulla whose fingerlike projections are capped by a cortex composed largely of closely packed lymphocytes. The predominant cell in the medulla is the thymic epithelial cell, which is larger than the lymphocyte and has cytoplasmic projections that unite with the processes of adjacent cells through prominent desmosomes. Tonofilaments attached to the desmosomes form bundles within the cells and are particularly abundant in the epithelial cells that form the concentric layers of Hassall's corpuscles. Keratin is also present in the corpuscles. Lymphoid follicles are not normally found in the thymus.

One of the two major populations of lymphocytes (T lymphocytes) depends on the thymus for the induction of immunologic competence. These lymphocytes are formed in the bone marrow but migrate to the thymus; there they proliferate and in some manner are influenced by a humoral factor formed by the epithelial cells (thymosin) to become T lymphocytes capable of participating in cell-mediated immune responses.

See also *thymic tumors.*

thymus-dependent antigen an antigen that must interact with a T lymphocyte before B lymphocytes can mount an antibody response to it. It is generally a complex antigen such as a cell, serum protein, or hapten-carrier complex; In the case of the last-named it is believed that helper T cells interact with the carrier, and B cells recognize the hapten.

thymus-independent antigen an antigen that elicits an antibody response by interacting directly with B cells and not requiring the help of T cells. It is usually a less complex antigen with many repeating determinants, such as a polysaccharide. Many, but not all, thymus-independent antigens are B-cell mitogens.

thymus-leukemia antigen an antigen expressed on the surface of the thymocytes of mice that carry the TL-positive gene, or on malignant, neoplastic T cells of TL-negative mice. It is lost as the thymocyte matures. Also called *TL antigen.*

thyr/o (thi′ro) [Gr. *thyreoeidēs* thyroid] a word element used in combining form to denote the thyroid gland, e.g., thyrotoxic.

thyristor (thi-ris′tor) [from *thyr*atron tube + trans*istor*] any of several solid-state electronic components used as high-current switches. See *silicon-controlled rectifier, silicon-controlled switch,* and *triac.*

thyrocalcitonin (thi″ro-kal″sĭ-to′nin) see *calcitonin.*

thyrocervical trunk (thi″ro-ser′vĭk′l) a short, wide artery that arises from the front of the first part of the subclavian artery and almost immediately divides into three branches: the inferior thyroid, suprascapular, and superficial cervical arteries.

thyroglobulin (thi-rō-glob′u-lin) 1. a thyroid glycoprotein that contains 120 tyrosine residues; M.W. 660,000. It serves as an acceptor to the organified iodide in the biosynthesis of mono- and diiodotyrosine, as well as triiodothyronine (T_3) and thyroxine (T_4).

2. [USP], a purified extract from the hog, *Sus scrofa domesticus,* containing thyroid hormones. It is used for replacement therapy in hypothyroidism.

thyroglossal (thi″ro-glos′al) pertaining to the thyroid gland and tongue.

thyroglossal duct see *thyroglossal d.* under *duct.*

thyroid (thi′roid) [Gr. *thyreoeidēs; thyreos* shield + *eidos* form] 1. resembling a shield; scutiform.

2. see *thyroid gland.*

3. [USP], an extract of the thyroid glands of domesticated food animals, which has been cleaned, dried, and assayed for iodine content, to be used for replacement therapy in hypothyroidism.

thyroidal clearance (thi-roi′d′l) the rate (expressed in milliliters per minute) at which plasma is cleared of iodide by the thyroid gland, equivalent to the rate of increase of ^{131}I activity in the thyroid divided by the concentration of ^{131}I activity in the plasma. Increased uptake may indicate hyperthyroidism. This rate is seldom measured clinically but is estimated by the thyroid uptake at fixed times, especially the 24-hr uptake. See *thyroid uptake tests.*

thyroid artery, superior a branch of the external carotid artery that supplies the thyroid gland and adjacent muscles.

thyroid crisis a severe acute form of hyperthyroidism characterized by delirium, extreme tachycardia, fever, vomiting, nausea, diarrhea, and dehydration. It may be precipitated by infection, surgery, emotional stress, or childbirth. Therapy must be implemented rapidly to avoid a fatal outcome. Also called *thyroid storm.*

thyroid gland the gland located in the lower anterior neck within the pretracheal fascia. It weighs approximately 25 g in the adult. The right and left lobes are connected at their lower poles through an isthmus that lies in front of the second and third tracheal rings. In the embryo the gland develops with the tongue, and the cells migrate down through the anterior neck past the hyoid bone to the permanent location of the gland. A rest of thyroid cells may occasionally persist in the tongue (lingual thyroid) or along the course of the thyroglossal duct.

The epithelial cells of the thyroid form follicles that contain colloid; the size of the follicles and follicular cells reflects the degree of functional activity. In the hyperfunctioning gland, small follicles are lined by columnar cells. A rich capillary network permeates the stroma of the gland.

The follicular cells are activated by pituitary thyrotropin (TSH). The thyroglobulin synthesized by the follicular cells is bound to iodine, which is actively transported across the basal cell membrane. In response to TSH stimulation, the cells develop long microvilli that project into the colloid to facilitate the endocytosis of iodinated thyroglobulin. Lysosomes fuse with the colloid droplets, and their enzymes release the thyroid hormones (T_3 and T_4), which leave the follicular cell and enter adjacent capillaries in the stroma. Both triiodothyronine (T_3) and tetraiodothyronine (thyroxine, T_4) appear to have similar functions in elevating cell metabolism. Nerve terminals have been demonstrated on thyroid follicular cells, and it is possible that sympathetic stimulation may promote release of the thyroid hormones.

The peptide hormone calcitonin is formed by the parafollicular or C cells that are scattered throughout the gland, lying within the follicular basal lamina. They contain dense core granules and are the cell of origin of medullary carcinoma. There is a reciprocal relationship between the secretion of calcitonin and parathyroid hormone, regulated by the serum calcium level.

The gland receives its arterial supply through the inferior thyroid branch of the thyrocervical trunk and the superior thyroid branch of the external carotid artery.

thyroiditis (thi″roi-di′tis) a general term used to describe an inflammation of the thyroid. On the basis of clinical and histologic features, specific types have been identified, which include acute, subacute, chronic, and invasive fibrous thyroiditis. Rarely, the inflammation may represent a component of a systemic disease such as sarcoidosis, tuberculosis, deep mycosis, syphilis, or amyloidosis.

acute t., a relatively rare form of thyroiditis. It usually represents thyroid involvement in individuals with bacterial infections of the pharynx or upper respiratory tract. The predominant inflammatory cell is the polymorphonuclear leukocyte. The inflammation may be localized or diffuse, and the disease may subside or progress to abscess formation. Bacteria most frequently responsible for acute thyroiditis include *Staphylococcus aureus,* hemolytic streptococci (usually group A), and pneumococci.

Typical laboratory findings include a granulocytosis and elevated sedimentation rate. Tests of thyroid function are usually within normal limits unless significant necrosis of the thyroid parenchyma occurs.

chronic t., the most common form of thyroiditis. It occurs at any age, although usually between ages 35 and 55 yr; it is 5–10 times more frequent in females then in males and is thought to be of autoimmune origin. The initial symptom is usually painless enlargement of the thyroid, which may develop over a period of many months or years. If the thyroid becomes sufficiently large, it may produce symptoms of compression including dysphagia, choking, and dyspnea.

Grossly, the thyroid is typically enlarged. Involvement is generally diffuse, although the enlargement may be nodular; in some cases the lesion may occur as a solitary nodule. Histologically, this disease is characterized by an intense infiltration of the thyroid stroma and follicles by lymphocytes and plasma cells, and by degeneration and regeneration of the thyroid parenchyma. In areas of parenchymal degeneration, the follicles become reduced in size, the colloid is diminished, and chronic inflammatory cells may be seen in follicular lumens and infiltrating the epithelium. If there is regeneration, the follicles are lined by large active cells or are replaced by masses of proliferating epithelial cells, many of which are in mitosis. Characteristically, numerous oxyphil cells (Hürthle or Askanazy cells) are seen throughout the thyroid. These cells represent metaplasia of the follicular epithelium to large polygonal cells with a strongly eosinophilic granular cytoplasm and large nuclei. In addition to the inflammatory component of lymphocytes (which may be aggregated to form lymphoid follicles and plasma cells), fibrosis is usually present, although it varies in degree from case to case.

The clinical course is not predictable; the process may regress, remain stationary, or progress. If sufficient fibrous replacement of thyroid parenchyma occurs, the patient may become hypothyroid. Laboratory studies usually reveal the presence of circulating antibodies to thyroid antigens (microsomal antigens and thyroglobulin). Tests of thyroid function including T_3 and T_4 levels, T_3-resin uptake, and ^{131}I uptake are usually in the range of low to normal; in such cases, the most sensitive test for hypothyroidism is measurement of TSH levels.

Also called *autoimmune thyroiditis, Hashimoto's thyroiditis, lymphoadenoid goiter, lymphocytic thyroiditis,* and *struma lymphomatosa.*

invasive fibrous t., a rare, destructive, and fibrosclerotic lesion of the thyroid. It usually occurs in individuals between ages 35 and 55 yr, and is four times more frequent in females than in males. The etiology is unknown, but the condition is thought to be related to similar forms of fibrosclerosis seen in the retroperitoneum, mediastinum, and orbit. The first symptom is usually thyroid enlargement, which may be asymmetric. Frequently there is local pain or referred pain to the ear and neck. Later symptoms result from pressure on adjacent structures. The disease may be self-limited, but more often the fibrosis progresses, resulting in extension to adjacent structures in the neck and producing complications of compression. The fibrosis may destroy the thyroid to the extent that hypothyroidism develops.

Grossly, the thyroid is woody hard. Histologically, involved areas of thyroid parenchyma are replaced by dense collagenous tissue. The fibrosis frequently extends through the capsule with adhesions to adjacent structures. Scattered inflammatory cells are seen but giant cells are absent. Tests of thyroid function are usually within normal limits unless the thyroid replacement has progressed to the point of producing hypothyroidism.

Also called fibrosclerosis, *fibrous thyroiditis,* ligneous thyroiditis, and *Riedel's thyroiditis.*

subacute t., a form somewhat more common than acute thyroiditis. It is usually seen in adults and is three to four times more frequent in females than in males. Because this form is usually preceded by a prodromal viral respiratory infection, measles, or mumps, it is assumed to be of viral origin. The onset is typically characterized by thyroid tenderness, fever, and dysphagia. The thyroid is usually enlarged, tender, and indurated.

Histologically, the lesions are characterized by local or diffuse destruction of follicular epithelium and inflammation, which is predominantly acute. Older lesions are characterized by epithelial regeneration, fibrosis, chronic inflammation, and the presence of multinucleated foreign body–type giant cells. As a result of fibrosis, the thyroid may become adherent to adjacent structures, particularly muscles.

The acute inflammation of the thyroid during the early stages of this disease produces a markedly elevated sedimentation rate, and parenchymal damage results in the release of stored thyroid hormone into the circulation, which may render the patient temporarily hyperthyroid. During this stage, the ^{131}T uptake is usually depressed while T_3 and T_4 levels are elevated and the T_3-resin uptake is increased. During the recovery phase, ^{131}I uptake may be increased to levels above normal, T_3 and T_4 levels and T_3-resin uptake fall into the hypothyroid range, and thyroid-stimulating hormone (TSH) becomes elevated. The disease usually lasts 2–8 wk. Approximately 10 percent of patients experience some degree of permanent hypothyroidism.

Also called acute nonsuppurative thyroiditis, *de Quervain's thyroiditis, giant cell thyroiditis,* and *granulomatous thyroiditis.*

thyroid microsomal antibodies autoantibodies (predominantly IgG) to a membrane lipoprotein, probably in the smooth endoplasmic reticulum of follicular epithelial cells. They are seen in about 85 percent of patients with Hashimoto's thyroiditis, in about 40 percent of patients with Graves' disease, in less than 15 percent of patients with other thyroid disorders, and in less than 5 percent of normal individuals. Thyroid microsomal antibodies are demonstrated in serum using complement-fixation, immunofluorescence, or hemagglutination tests; they can be demonstrated in tissue by immunofluorescence or immunoperoxidase methods. Also called *antimicrosomal antibodies.*

thyroid scan the gamma-ray imaging of the thyroid gland. The preferred radionuclides are ^{123}I as iodide and ^{99m}TC as pertechnetate; both are suitable for use with the scintillation camera or rectilinear scanner. The pertechnetate ion is only trapped, not organified, by the thyroid, so a somewhat different picture results. Because it is more readily available than ^{123}I, ^{131}I is still used frequently. Scanning is used to evaluate the position, size, and functioning of the thyroid gland, as well as the functioning of nodules or a goiter, and to follow the progress of therapy. See also *fluorescent scan.*

thyroid-stimulating hormone (hTSH, TSH) a glycoprotein hormone synthesized and released by the anterior pituitary gland; M.W. about 30,000. The target organ is the thyroid, which is stimulated to synthesize and release thyroxine (T_4) and triiodothyronine (T_3). The hormone is composed of two subunits, α and β, with all the specificity of action deriving from the β-subunit. Secretion of TSH by the pituitary is determined partially by the level of circulating thyroid hormone and partially by hypothalamic thyrotropin-releasing hormone (TRH). The negative feedback control of thyrotropin secretion exercised by circulating thyroid hormone is exerted primarily at the pituitary level.

TSH stimulates iodine uptake, tyrosine iodination, increased synthesis of thyroglobulin (Tg), iodotyrosine and iodothyronine formation, thyroxine and triiodotyrosine release from the thyroid gland, and increases metabolic activity. As with other hormones, it is assumed that it binds to specific receptors on the thyroid gland to activate adenylate cyclase; the cyclic AMP formed may activate synthesis of the enzymes involved in T_4 synthesis, either directly or through its effect on protein synthesis at the nuclear level. Elevations of TSH give rise to hyperthyroidism.

TSH is used clinically to differentiate between primary hypothyroidism (myxedema) and secondary hypothyroidism (pituitary insufficiency). Reference ranges for TSH in plasma are, for adults, 0–3 ng/ml or 2–8 μIU/ml.

Also called thyrotropic hormone and *thyrotropin.*

thyroid-stimulating hormone assay radioimmunoassay for TSH in serum. This measurement is most useful in distinguishing primary hypothyroidism (in which serum concentrations of TSH are increased) from secondary or tertiary hypothyroidism, characterized by a low TSH concentration.

Current TSH assays are not sufficiently sensitive to distinguish reliably between normal and subnormal basal levels of TSH. Definitive diagnosis can be established by demonstrating a subnormal response to exogenous TRH in the case of intrinsic pituitary disease, and a normal, but retarded, response in the case of hypothalamic disease.

thyroid-stimulating immunoglobulins (TSI) IgG immunoglobulins found in the blood of 85–90 percent of patients with active Graves' disease. TSI can be measured by its ability to stimulate adenylate cyclase activity in human thyroid tissue. Radioreceptor assays have also shown that TSI is capable of blocking the binding of TSH to specific binding sites on human thyroid cell membranes. In this case, alternate (and preferable) names include TSH-displacing antibody (TDA) and TSH-binding inhibitory immunoglobulin (TBII). Unfortunately, results from these two tests do not correlate well with one another, leading to the theory that the thyroid-related IgG immunoglobulins in autoimmune thyroid disease are a heterogeneous group of antibodies directed at varying sites within the thyroid cell membrane.

thyroid storm see *thyroid crisis.*

thyroid tumors neoplasms of the thyroid. Most solitary nodules of the thyroid are adenomas. Clinically they often cannot be distinguished from colloid nodules of nodular goiter. Histologically, adenomas are encapsulated and have a uniform histologic appearance that is often similar to that of a normal gland but may be microfollicular. The cells may undergo oncocytic transformation (Hürthle cell adenoma).

Fewer than 0.5 percent of deaths from cancer are due to thyroid carcinoma; however, the incidence of this disease is higher than this figure would indicate, as many cases are clinically silent and detected only incidentally at autopsy.

Two-thirds of malignant thyroid neoplasms are derived from the follicular epithelium. They typically exhibit a papillary, follicular, or mixed papillary and follicular architecture. Areas of Hürthle cell change may be present. Pure follicular tumors make up approximately 20 percent of the total. Aggressive anaplastic carcinomas make up 10 percent, and carcinomas of the parafollicular cells constitute less than 10 percent of malignant thyroid neoplasms. The differentiated papillary and follicular carcinomas may be relatively indolent in their behavior. At least half of those affected have regional node metastases at the time of diagnosis, but even with metastases the survival may be relatively long. In contrast, anaplastic tumors, which are made up of spindle and bizarre cells, are characterized by highly aggressive behavior with rapid growth, local recurrence, and early metastases, and result in a poor prognosis.

Medullary or C-cell tumors of the thyroid are derived from the parafollicular calcitonin-forming cells. They differ in their histologic appearance from the follicular epithelial carcinomas and are usually formed of nests and sheets of round cells; in some instances, distinction between the two tumors is difficult by light microscopy. A C-cell carcinoma may have amyloid in its stroma, which is uncommon in the follicular cell tumors. Ultrastructurally, the cells of a C-cell carcinoma contain cytoplasmic granules indicating their endocrine nature: these must be distinguished from the lysosomes that are customarily present within the cells of follicular carcinoma. C-cell carcinoma of the thyroid may coexist with pheochromocytoma and parathyroid hyperplasia or adenoma in the MEN syndrome, type II (Sipple's syndrome), or mucosal neuromas may replace the parathyroid lesion (MEN III, or IIb). C-cell carcinomas tend to pursue a relentless course, invading local tissues and metastasizing to regional nodes and to distant sites via the blood stream. The 5-yr survival rate is about 50 percent.

An increase in the incidence of thyroid cancer in the last two decades is believed to be related to the former therapeutic practice of radiotherapy to the neck in children.

In the investigation of a thyroid nodule, the uptake of a radioisotope (such as radioiodine) is determined. Areas of the thyroid failing to take up radioiodine (cold nodules) particularly require further investigation, as the likelihood of a cold nodule representing a thyroid cancer is significantly greater than that of a "hot" or "warm" nodule.

See also *thyroid scan.*

thyroid uptake tests the determination of the amount of an administered dose of iodine taken up by the thyroid gland. In the radioactive iodine (RAI) uptake test, ^{131}I is administered as iodide. The uptake is measured 24 hr later by counting the radioactivity of the thyroid with a scintillation probe. Corrections are made for the decay rate of ^{131}I and for the background radioactivity of the patient. This test indicates the ability of the thyroid to trap and organify the iodide.

Several variations of this test use the same procedure. The uptake can be measured after suppression of the thyroid by administration of triiodothyronine (T_3), which is the T_3 suppression test; a lack of suppression indicates hyperthyroidism. The uptake can be measured after the administration of thyroid-stimulating hormone (TSH) or thyrotropin-releasing hormone (TRH); these are the TSH and TRH stimulation tests. Patients with secondary hypothyroidism show an increased RAI uptake after stimulation; this test has been replaced by radioimmunoassay for TSH. Stimulation by TSH but not by TRH distinguishes secondary from tertiary hypothyroidism. Administration of perchlorate 1–2 hr after the ^{131}I blocks further uptake and flushes iodide from the thyroids of patients who have defective organification of iodide; this is the perchlorate discharge test. The 20-min ^{99m}Tc-pertechnetate uptake measures only the trapping function of the thyroid.

thyrotoxic (thi″ro-tok′sik) marked by toxic activity of the thyroid (hyperthyroidism).

thyrotoxic heart disease heart disease associated with hyperthyroidism, often marked by atrial fibrillation, cardiac enlargement, and congestive heart failure. Also called thyrocardiac disease.

thyrotoxicosis (thi″ro-tok″sĭ-ko′sis) see *hyperthyroidism.*

thyrotropin (thi-rot′ro-pin) [*thyro-* + Gr. *tropē* a turning + -in] the generic drug name for thyroid-stimulating hormone (TSH), which is used as a diagnostic aid.

thyrotropin-releasing hormone (TRH) a tripeptide. It consists of pyroglutamic acid, histidine, and an amide derivative of proline. Both the *N*-terminal pyroglutamyl (cyclized glutamic acid) and the carboxy terminus proline amide residues are essential for full biologic activity. TRH is synthesized in several hypothalamic nuclei and is transported to the pituitary via the hypophyseal portal system. TRH stimulates the release of thyrotropin (TSH) from the anterior pituitary. The stimulation is calcium-dependent and does not require protein synthesis. It is used clinically to evaluate the TSH-releasing capacity of the pituitary and also to distinguish between hypothalamic and pituitary lesions. TRH is known to stimulate the secretion of prolactin and also the release of GH in persons with acromegaly. Also called *TSH-releasing factor* and *TSH-releasing hormone.* Generic drug name, *protirelin.*

thyrotropin-releasing hormone stimulation test the determination of the amount of thyroid-stimulating hormone (TSH) released by the pituitary gland in response to the administration of a dose of thyrotropin-releasing hormone (TRH). TSH is determined by radioimmunoassay or by its effect on the thyroid uptake of radioiodine.

thyroxine (T_4) (thi-rok′sēn) 3,5,3′,5′-L-tetraiodothyronine, a hormone produced and released by the thyroid gland; M.W. 776.93. The biosynthesis involves three main steps: the active uptake of iodide into the thyroid; the oxidation of iodide by iodide-peroxidase and the iodination of the tyrosyl residue with thyroglobulin, yielding the intermediate products monoiodotyrosine (MIT) and diiodotyrosine (DIT); and the coupling of these iodotyrosines to form the biologically active iodothyronines T_4 and triiodothyronine (T_3).

Iodine peroxidase is a key enzyme of T_4 synthesis that catalyzes the oxidation, iodination, and coupling reactions. The principal hormone synthesized in the thyroid gland is T_4, and it is therefore the primary secretory product. The normal thyroid gland contains about 200 $\mu g/g$ and 15 $\mu g/g$ of T_4 and T_3, respectively. Most of the T_3 in the plasma is derived from T_4, a conversion occurring in peripheral tissues. On metabolic demand, the thyroglobulin is resorbed by the thyroid cell and subjected to proteolysis by lysosomal enzymes. The liberated T_4 and T_3 are secreted into the blood stream where they are bound to carrier proteins, namely, thyroxine-binding globulins (TBG), thyroxine-binding prealbumin (TBPA), and albumin. TBG, a protein synthesized in the liver, has the highest affinity for T_4 and T_3 but a low capacity among the binding proteins, whereas TBPA has a lower affinity but a very high capacity. Of the two hormones, T_4 has higher affinity for both TBG and TBPA than T_3, which accounts for its higher serum levels and longer half-life. About 99.96 percent of T_4 and 99.6 percent of T_3 are protein-bound. It should be noted that only the free hormones, which are present in minute amounts and in equilibrium with protein-bound hormone, are biologically active. Iodine is extracted and reutilized from any unused MIT and DIT released after proteolysis of thyroglobulin.

All steps in the biosynthesis and release of T_3 and T_4 are stimulated by thyrotropin (TSH). TSH is released by the adenohypophysis, a process stimulated by thyrotropin-releasing hormone (TRH). The action of TSH on the thyroid cell is initiated by its binding to specific receptor sites on the cell membrane and activation of adenylate kinase, leading to the synthesis of cyclic AMP. Circulating T_4 and T_3 regulate the synthesis and secretion of TSH by the pituitary and the hypothalamic release of TRH by a negative feedback process.

T_3, principally derived from T_4 by monodeiodination at the 5′-position of the thyronine ring in the peripheral tissues, is about four times more active than T_4. T_4 is also converted to a relatively inactive metabolite by a monodeiodination process at the 5-position of the ring; this product is known as reverse T_3. The precise mechanisms of regulation of synthesis of these two products of T_4, one active and another relatively inactive, are not yet understood.

Thyroid hormones have a variety of effects on the body. They stimulate calorigenesis due to increased ATP consumption, facilitate protein synthesis by binding to specific receptors on the chromatin of target cells, thereby increasing mRNA synthesis and translation of the mRNA ribosomes, increase carbohydrate and lipid turnover, increase calcium mobilization from the bones, and stimulate the metabolism of vitamins. T_4 has a latent period of 2–3 da before it manifests its activity. This, together with the diversity of the effects caused by the hormone, suggests that these actions are secondary to a more fundamental mechanism, as yet unknown. It has been suggested, however, that increased mitochondrial oxidation might be the cause of an increase in the overall metabolism in the various tissues.

Reference ranges for plasma/serum T_4 by protein-binding assay [T_4(D) or T_4(RIA)] are: for adults, 5–12 μg/dl; and for newborns, 10–21. Reference ranges for the other T_4 parameters in adults are: for T_4(C), 2.8–6.4 μg of T_4-I/dl; for PBI, 4.0–8.0 μg/dl; for BEI, 3.2–6.4 μg I/dl; for FT_4, 0.8–2.5 ng/dl; and for FT_4 index, values arbitrary, depending on procedures used.

N. V. BHAGAVAN, PH.D.

free t. (**FT_4**), the portion of T_4 not bound to plasma proteins (less than 0.05 percent of total T_4). As FT_4 is the metabolically active fraction, its concentration is more indicative of the clinical state of the thyroid than is total T_4. See under *thyroxine assays.*

thyroxine assays 1. competitive protein-binding assay, which measures total serum T_4. The serum T_4 competes in a reaction mixture with radioactive T_4 for binding sites on added thyroxine-binding globulin (TBG) (T_4(D)) or on an antibody specific for T_4 (T_4(RIA)). By measuring the radioactivity bound to the TBG or T_4 antibody and comparing it with standards, the total concentration of T_4 can be calculated. These two tests are sensitive and independent of the presence of other iodine compounds, and have largely replaced the other less accurate quantitative assays, such as protein-bound iodine (PBI) and butanol-extractable iodine (BEI).

2. serum thyroxine by column chromatography, T_4(C). T_4 and T_3 are separated by anion exchange chromatography and the iodine content of the final column eluates is analyzed by chemical methods.

3. protein-bound iodine (PBI). The amount of iodine bound to precipitated plasma proteins (most of which is contained in T_4) is measured by chemical means after protein digestion. Any iodine that is bound to protein, regardless of whether organic or inorganic, will be detected. If a butanol extraction is added to remove some forms of iodine contamination, the iodine measured is called butanol-extractable iodine (BEI).

4. free thyroxine, FT_4, that percentage of serum T_4 not bound to plasma proteins. It is determined by adding labeled T_4 to the sample, measuring the radioactivity in the dialysate after equilibrium dialysis, and dividing by the amount of radioactivity in the sample before dialysis. The absolute concentration of FT_4 can be calculated by multiplying the percent FT_4 by total T_4 concentration as determined by T_4(RIA).

5. free thyroxine index, FT_4 index, is an empirical, arbitrary index of FT_4 activity calculated from values for total T_4 and the T_3 resin uptake test. See *triiodothyronine resin uptake test.*

thyroxine-binding albumin a minor thyroid hormone (T_3 and T_4) carrier protein of blood plasma. This protein carries a small amount of T_3 and T_4 compared with thyroxine-binding globulin (TBG) and thyroxine-binding prealbumin (TBPA).

thyroxine-binding globulin (TBG) an α-globulin–type protein, a glycoprotein, which is a carrier for T_4 and T_3 in plasma; M.W. 50,000. TBG has one high-affinity binding site, which binds T_4 better than T_3. TBG is responsible for transporting most of the T_4 in plasma and is by far the major determinant of the total T_4 in plasma. Reference ranges are: for TBG, 12–30 μg/ml; for resin T_3 uptake, T_3 (RU), 26–35 percent; and for TBG capacity, 12–20 μg of T_4 per deciliter.

thyroxine-binding globulin (TBG) assays 1. radioimmunoassay, which directly measures the serum concentration of TBG.

2. the triiodothyronine (T_3) uptake test, which indirectly measures free TBG-binding sites; see *triiodothyronine uptake test.*

3. electrophoretic protein separation. Radioactive T_4 is added to the specimen to allow for binding with the carrier proteins. After electrophoretic separation of the proteins, the protein-bound T_4 label is measured radiometrically and is assumed to be a measure of the available TBG binding sites.

Maximal binding capacity for T_4 (TBG cap) is quantitated by comparing specimens to which varying amounts of labeled and unlabeled T_4 have been added.

thyroxine-binding prealbumin (TBPA) a plasma carrier protein that transports T_4 but does not bind T_3; M.W. approximately 50,000. TBPA has one binding site with lower affinity than TBG, but higher capacity of binding T_4 owing to its higher plasma levels (25 mg/dl), which can bind up to 200 μg of T_4. TBPA exists in part as a complex with retinol (vitamin A)–binding protein.

THz abbrev. See *terahertz.*

Ti symbol for the chemical element *titanium.*

TIA abbrev. See *transient ischemic attack.*

TIBC abbrev. for total iron-binding capacity. See under *iron-binding capacity tests.*

tibi/o (tib′e-o) a word element used in combining form to denote the tibia, e.g., tibiofemoral.

tibia (tib′e-ah) [L.] [NA], the shin bone; the medial and larger of the two bones of the leg. The upper end is expanded and has two articular facets for the femur. A roughened elevation in front of the upper end is the tubercle, which provides attachment for the patellar tendon. The anterior border of the tibial shaft is sharp and readily palpable. A curving, roughened line on the posterior surface is the soleal line. The lower end of the tibia articulates with the talus and has a pointed projection, the medial malleolus.

tibial (tib′e-al) [L. *tibialis*] pertaining to the tibia.

tibial artery, anterior a terminal branch of the popliteal artery. It arises at the lower border of the popliteus muscle, passes forward between the two heads of tibialis posterior, descends on the front of the interosseous membrane, and becomes the dorsalis pedis artery on the dorsal surface of the foot.

tibial artery, posterior one of the two terminal branches of the popliteal artery. It begins at the lower border of the popliteus muscle, runs down the back of the leg, and passes behind the medial malleolus to divide into medial and lateral plantar arteries.

tibial nerve a terminal branch of the sciatic nerve. It arises above the knee joint, and descends through the popliteal fossa and leg and behind the medial malleolus to form the plantar nerves.

tic (tik) [Fr.] a spasmodic, involuntary twitch that is recurrent and can easily be imitated. Tics tend to occur particularly about the face, can be voluntarily suppressed for short periods, and are worsened by stress. They are especially common in children, but their origin and nature are unclear. A syndrome of chronic multiple tics, or Tourette's disease, develops in childhood but is a chronic lifelong disorder with multiple somatic and phonic tics that may seriously interfere with an individual's social and professional life.

-tic (tik) a suffix word element to denote pertaining to, e.g., plastic.

ticarcillin (ti″kar-sil′in) a semisynthetic penicillin with a spectrum similar to that of carbenicillin. In vitro, it is more active than carbenicillin against *Pseudomonas aeruginosa.* A pharmacologic advantage of ticarcillin over carbenicillin is the deliverance of a lower sodium load. See also *antibacterial agents* and *penicillins.*

tic douloureux (tēk doo″loo-roo′) see *trigeminal n.* under *neuralgia.*

tick (tik) a blood-sucking ascarid parasite of the order Acarina, superfamily Ixodoidea, which lacks body segmentation, antennae, and wings. Ticks are divided into two families: The Argasidae, the soft ticks, and the Ixodidae, the hard ticks.

The former includes the genera *Argas, Ornithodoros, Antricola,* and *Otobius.* Several species of *Ornithodoros* are known to harbor the spirochete *Borrelia,* which causes human relapsing fever. The genera *Argas* and *Ornithodoros* are known transmitters of various viruses.

The family Ixodidae includes medically important genera such as *Ixodes, Haemaphysalis, Amblyomma, Dermacentor, Hyalomma,* and *Rhipicephalus.* Species of *Ixodes* are transmitters of viruses that cause Russian spring-summer encephalitis and tick-borne encephalitis. Other species are irritating pests in the tropics.

In the genus *Haemaphysalis,* several species are transmitter viruses that cause Kyasanur Forest encephalitis, Russian spring-summer encephalitis, and tick-borne encephalitis. These ticks are best known as vectors of the *Rickettsia* species that causes spotted fever group typhus diseases in Africa, Asia, and the Americas. Species of the genus *Amblyomma* also transmit rickettsiae of the spotted fever group in Africa and the Americas.

Dermacentor species are vectors of spotted fever group rickettsiae, Colorado tick fever virus, and the Russian spring-summer encephalitis virus complex. In the genus *Hyalomma,* Q fever (*Coxiella burnetii*) has been isolated from several species.

Species of the genus *Rhipicephalus* have been found to be infected with several viruses, including Crimeon-Congo hemorrhagic fever, and Thogoto and Kyasanur Forest disease. These ticks are also transmitters of spotted fever group rickettsiae.

Approximately 20 species in the genera *Argas, Ornithodoros, Ixodes, Haemaphysalis, Dermacentor, Amblyomma,* and *Rhipicephalus* are known to cause tick paralysis. The paralysis usually begins 1–2 da after the tick attaches. Ataxia and areflexia are common. In most cases, the patient improves once the tick is removed. It is thought that the paralysis is due to a toxin released when the tick bites.

See also the accompanying illustration.

tick fever pertaining to fevers caused by tick-transmitted pathogens, e.g., Rocky Mountain spotted fever, Q fever, relapsing fever, and Colorado tick fever. See also *Rickettsiaceae.*

tid abbrev. for *ter in die* (three times daily).

tidal volume (V_T) the volume of gas inhaled or exhaled with each respiratory cycle, normally equal to 400–500 ml in the young adult.

tidal wave a small systolic peak between the percussion wave and dicrotic notch of the central arterial pulse, attributed to a reflection of the pressure wave from the peripheral vessels. It can be recorded but is rarely palpable under normal conditions.

Tietze's syndrome (tēt′sez) [Alexander *Tietze,* Breslau surgeon, 1864–1927] a painful enlargement, swelling, and tenderness of the upper costal cartilages of unknown cause. This condition usually affects a single costochondral junction, or multiple junctions unilaterally. Onset may be gradual or acute and may be associated with trauma. Those affected may interpret the pain as angina.

tiglium oil (tig′le-um) [L.] see *croton oil.*

time (*t*) (tīm) [Gr. *chronos;* L. *tempus*] the dimension of space-time (the physical universe) that is measured with a clock. A point in time is called an epoch; a point in space-time, an event. The International System (SI) unit of time is the second (s).

mean generation t., the time required for a doubling of bacterial mass in a liquid culture.

thermal death t., see *thermal death time.*

time of flight the time interval between the emission of a particle and its detection.

timer (ti′mer) 1. an electronic or mechanical clock used to turn a device on or off automatically at a preset time.

2. an electronic circuit that generates timing pulses, used to synchronize the operation of other circuits.

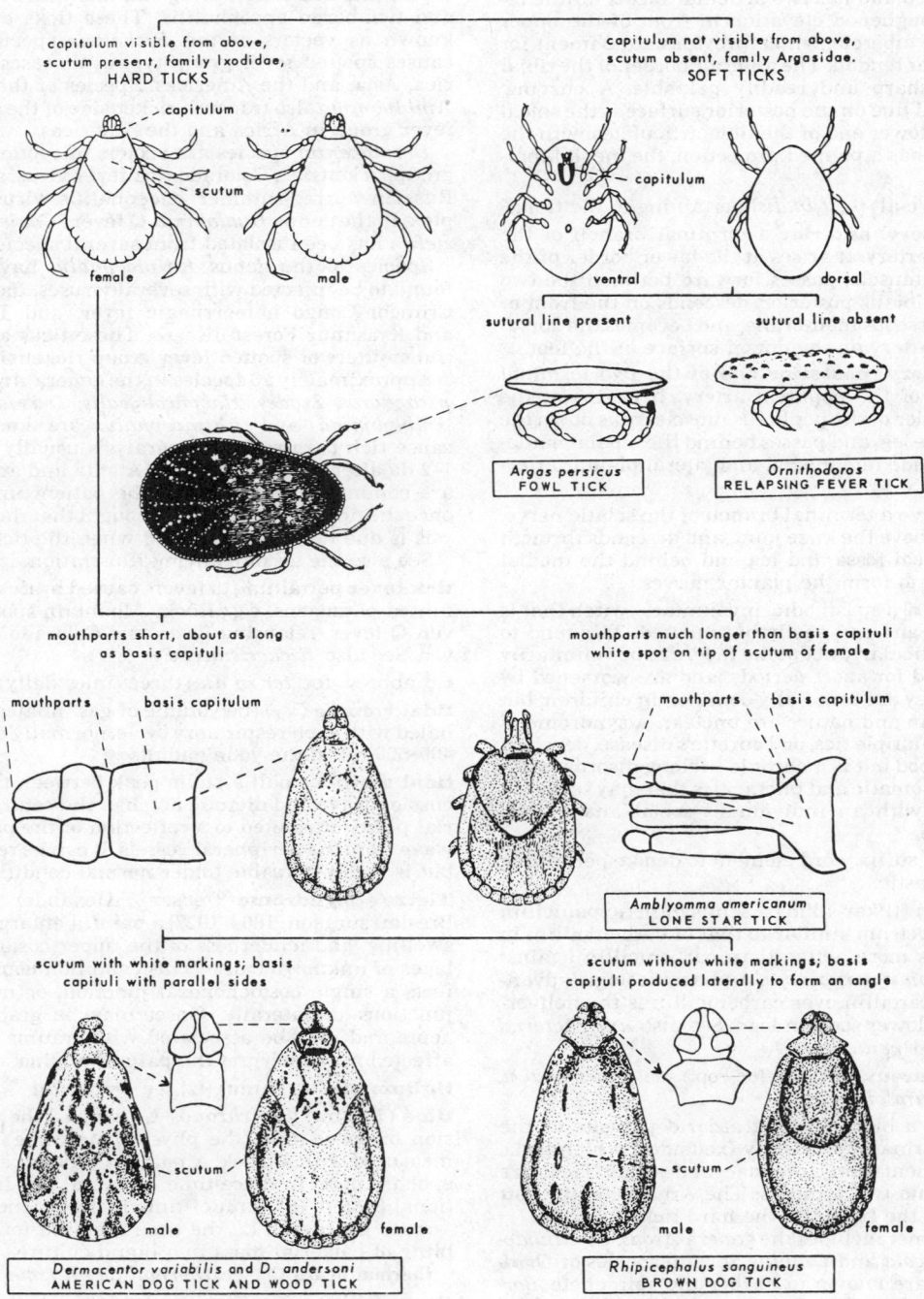

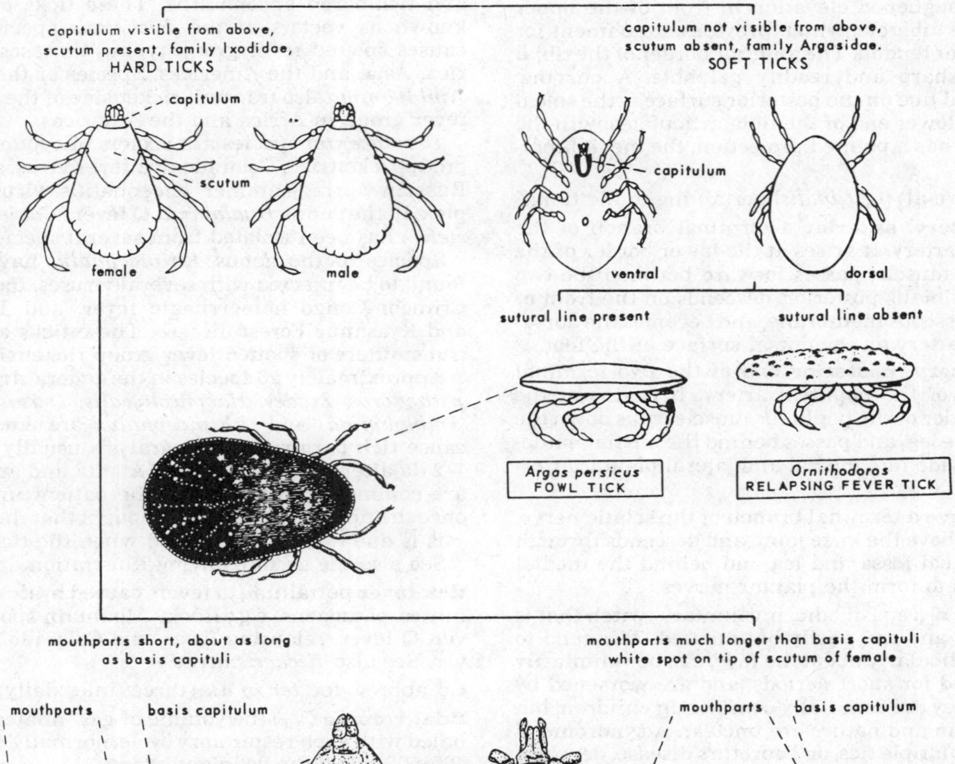

Tick. Pictorial key to some common ticks. (Courtesy of Centers for Disease Control, Public Health Service, U.S. Department of Health and Human Services, Atlanta, Georgia.)

time-sharing the simultaneous use of an interactive computer system from several terminals.

timolol maleate (ti′mo-lōl) a beta-adrenergic receptor-blocking drug. It is used in eye drops for the reduction of intraocular pressure in patients with glaucoma, or those with significant ocular hypertension who are at risk of developing glaucoma. Trademark, Timoptic.

Timoptic (ti-mop′tik) trademark. See *timolol maleate.*

TIN abbrev. See *tubulointerstitial nephropathy.*

tin (Sn) (tin) [A.S. *tin;* L. *stannum*] a silvery white, ductile metallic element; atomic number 50; atomic weight 118.69; Group IV of the periodic table; oxidation states +4, +2, –4.

Tin is used industrially in alloys and in tin-plated steel. Organic tin compounds are toxic; many can cause severe central nervous system injury. Chronic inhalation of tin dusts causes stannosis, a benign pneumoconiosis.

Tinactin (tin-ak′tin) trademark. See *tolnaftate.*

Tinca (ting′kah) [L.] a genus of fish. The species *T. tinca* (tench) serves as host for the fluke *Opisthorchis felineus* and is the main source of human infection by this fluke.

tinctorial (tink-tor′e-al) pertaining to dyeing or staining.

tincture (tink′tūr) [L. *tingere* to wet] in pharmacology, an alcoholic solution of a drug.

Tindal (tin′dal) trademark. See *acetophenazine maleate.*

Tinea (tin′e-ah) [L. "moth"] a genus of moths. The species *T. granella* and *T. pellionella* are intermediate hosts of the rat tapeworm *Hymenolepis diminuta.*

tinea (tin′e-ah) [L. "grub, larva, worm"] a term used to describe various cutaneous fungal infections usually caused by the dermatophytic fungus *Epidermophyton, Microsporum,* or *Trichophyton.* The specific type of tinea infection is described by a modifying term.

t. unguium, a disease of the nails of the fingers and toes caused by a dermatophyte, i.e., *Epidermophyton floccosum,* or *Trichophyton* or *Microsporum* species. *Candida albicans* and saprophytic fungi such as *Scopulariopsis brevicaulis* and *Hendersonula toruloidea* can also cause a similar disease (onychomycosis) in which the nails become opaque, white, thickened, friable, and brittle. See also *onychomycosis.*

tinea barbae (tin′e-ah bar′be) a dermatophytic fungal infection of the bearded areas of the face and neck. The lesions of tinea barbae are either superficial or deep. This fungal infection is usually the result of close contact with infected animals. Both zoophilic and anthropophilic dermatophytes can cause tinea barbae; anthropophilic organisms, however, produce a more severe infection. The organisms most commonly involved in tinea barbae include *Trichophyton mentagrophytes, T. verrucosum, T. rubrum,* and *Microsporum canis.* The cutaneous lesion resembles that of tinea corporis, with central scaling and a vesiculopustular border. These pustular lesions contain fungal arthrospores, and the hair shafts also contain fungal elements.

Diagnosis is made by the combination of a history of close contact with animals, the presence of inflamed pustular cutaneous lesions, the identification of fungal elements in scrapings of the lesion on a KOH slide, and, if *M. canis* is involved, the presence of fluorescence. If the infection is not severe, spontaneous resolution will occur. More severe infections can last from 3 wk to several months.

Also called *barber's itch* and *tinea sycosis.*

tinea capitis (tin′e-ah kap′ĭ-tis) a dermatophyte infection of the scalp caused by species of *Microsporum* and *Trichophyton.* The fungus causes erythematous, scaly lesions that lead to inflammation and ulceration. Tinea capitis is divided into two classes, ectothrix and endothrix. An ectothrix infection is characterized by fungal mycelia and spores on the outside of the hair shaft, whereas endothrix describes the fragmentation of fungal hyphae inside the hair shaft. Examination of affected areas with a Wood's lamp distinguishes these two classes.

Pathologically, tinea capitis assumes three forms: (1) Gray-patch ringworm, the result of ectothrix tinea capitis with *Microsporum* species. The most common species involved are *M. audouinii, M. canis,* and *M. gypseum.* During infection, the hair breaks off and the *Microsporum* spreads concentrically on the scalp. In gray-patch ringworm there is usually little inflammation, and spontaneous cures are common. (2) Black-dot ringworm, an endothrix infection with *Trichophyton* species. The most common species involved are *T. tonsurans* and *T. violaceum.* The lesions are relatively small, and the few hairs that are infected break off, leaving a short, spore-filled hair shaft that is black in color. Endothrix *Trichophyton* tinea capitis causes a more severe inflammation than *Microsporum* tinea capitis, with kerion formation and substantial scarring. These infections tend to continue through adult life rather than ceasing at puberty. (3) Ectothrix *Trichophyton* infections. The most common species involved are *T. mentagrophytes, T. verrucosum,* and *T. megnini.* These infections result in considerable inflammation, but are less common than other forms of tinea capitis. This variety of tinea capitis is usually transmitted indirectly from animals and can be found in persons from rural areas who have frequent contact with animals.

tinea circinata (tin′e-ah ser″sĭ-na′tah) see *tinea corporis.*

tinea corporis (tin′e-ah kor′por-is) a dermatophytic fungal infection of glabrous (hair-free) skin involving the stratum corneum of the epidermis. The fungi produce toxins and allergens that can result in erythema and deep granulomata. Tinea corporis is a common disease of humans that occurs throughout the world, including the Arctic. Although any species of *Trichophyton* or *Microsporum* can cause tinea corporis, *T. rubrum* and *T. mentagrophytes* are most commonly involved.

Infection may be initiated directly by contact with an infected person or animal, or indirectly via contaminated clothing and furniture. The infected lesions spread centrifugally; with time, the centers of the lesions heal, resulting in rings of infections. In these rings, there may be two types of lesions. One, most often caused by *T. rubrum* and *Epidermophyton floccosum,* is dry, scaly, and annular with red, elevated areas of inflammation. The other lesion is characterized by irregular, crusted vesicles that may become pustular. There are a few reports of atypical deep forms of tinea corporis. How an organism normally producing only superficial skin damage can invade deep tissues has not been explained.

Diagnosis is established by direct microscopic examination of the scales and lesions. The presence of septate hyphae and arthrospores is indicative of tinea corporis. The lesions should also be cultured for fungal growth.

Also called *ringworm* (of the body), *tinea circinata*, and *tinea glabrosa*.

tinea cruris (tin′e-ah kroo′ris) a dermatophytic fungal infection of the groin and perianal region. The resultant lesions characteristically are sharply demarcated with a raised red margin and thin, dry epidermal scaling. The most common causative organisms of tinea cruris are *Epidermophyton floccosum* and *Trichophyton rubrum*. This infection begins as a small area of inflammation, spreading at different rates. Factors predisposing to tinea usually include living conditions, humidity, and irritation of skin folds.

Diagnosis is based on the observation of characteristic eczema marginatum with a raised border and the demonstration of fungal elements in the lesions.

Also called *jock itch* and *ringworm* (of the groin).

tinea favosa (tin′e-ah fa-vo′sah) see *favus*.

tinea glabrosa (tin′e-ah gla-bro′sah) see *tinea corporis*.

tinea pedis (tin′e-ah pe′dis) a dermatophyte infection of the feet. Tinea pedis is the most common fungal disease of humans, affecting people of all ages worldwide. The organisms most often involved are *Trichophyton mentagrophytes, T. rubrum*, and *Epidermophyton floccosum*. Clinical manifestations vary from the chronic intertriginous form with peeling and maceration to the acute ulcerative form with eczematoid vesiculopustular lesions.

Diagnosis is made by clinical observation, direct microscopic examination of scrapings of the lesion, and confirmation by culture on selective media. In more severe cases, there is often a secondary bacterial infection.

Also called *athlete's foot* and *ringworm of the foot*.

tinea sycosis (tin′e-ah si-ko′sis) see *tinea barbae*.

tinea versicolor (tin′e-ah ver′sĭ-kul″or) a type of superficial mycosis; a chronic, mild, noninflammatory infection of the stratum corneum caused by the opportunistically pathogenic fungus *Malassezia furfur* (*Pityrosporum orbiculare*). A common and world-wide disease occurring in both males and females, tinea versicolor is a cosmetic problem with no serious pathologic consequences; living tissue is not affected. The resultant lesions are discrete, discolored areas of skin of variable size and color. Their color depends on the pigmentation of the normal skin and may range from whitish to fawn to brown. The scalp, chest, upper limbs, and back are most often infected.

M. furfur may be part of the normal flora of the skin. It is a lipophilic yeast, requiring specific fatty acids for growth. The pathogenesis of this infection is not understood, although it may relate to a decrease in the epithelial cellular turnover rate. Exposure to sunlight appears to be an inciting factor.

Diagnosis of tinea versicolor is made by direct examination of skin scrapings (in potassium hydroxide preparation—see the accompanying illustration). *M. furfur* is characterized by round or oval budding yeast cells and hyphal elements. A Wood's lamp examination reveals a reddish- to orange-colored fluorescence of the infected area.

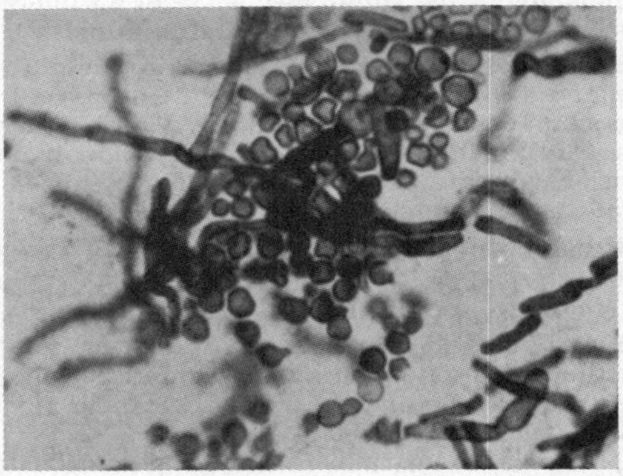

Tinea versicolor. Skin scraping; Periodic acid–Schiff stain, ×1200. (From Lennette, E. H., et al. Manual of Clinical Microbiology. 3rd ed. Washington DC, American Society for Microbiology, 1980.)

Also called *liver spots* and *pityriasis versicolor*.

Tinel's sign (tin-elz′) [Jules *Tinel*, French neurologist, 1879–1952] a radiating, tingling sensation in the cutaneous distribution of an injured nerve when the nerve trunk is lightly percussed. It indicates regeneration of sensory nerve fibers.

tine test (tīn) a tuberculin skin test, employing a multiple-puncture, disposable device. It is especially useful in the mass screening of children, although it is less accurate than the Mantoux test. Any doubtful reaction to the test should be rechecked by a Mantoux test before a follow-up chest x-ray is recommended. Tine tests are read 48–72 hr after injection.

tinnitus (tĭ-ni′tus) [L. "a ringing"] a subjective phenomenon reported as a noise in the ears such as a ringing, buzzing, roaring, or hissing sound. A frequent symptom in adults, it is invariably due to disease of the middle ear or eustachian tube.

tissue (tish′u) [Fr. *tissu*] an aggregation of similarly specialized cells united in the performance of a particular function. For more information, see the specific tissue.

tissue culture the growth of differentiated cellular tissue in a chemically defined basal medium containing all the major ions, sugars, amino acids, etc., needed for cellular survival. The medium is supplemented and fortified with undefined additives such as serum and embryo extract or pituitary extract. Tissue cultures differ from cell cultures in the level of organization maintained in the explanted cultures; see also *cell culture*.

Early techniques in tissue culturing were imprecise: tissue fragments were placed on plasma clots and covered with a medium consisting of a mixture of saline, serum, and embryo extract; satisfactory growth can now be maintained on glass, using the proper culture medium. Trypsin may be used to release cells from the glass for subculturing.

tissue factor see *Factor III*.

tissue processing the preparation of histologic specimens for microscopic examination. Routine processing consists of several stages, each a process in itself. Fixation is the first step and involves chemically treating the specimen to harden the tissue by denaturing the proteins. Fixation is followed by dehydration, during which water is removed by moving the specimens through graded alcohols up to 100 percent. In the clearing procedure that follows, the alcohol is replaced with a wax solvent. In the infiltration process, the specimen is immersed in melted paraffin, followed by casting, blocking, or embedding, which encloses it in a solid block of wax. The specimen is then ready for the sectioning procedure, in which thin sections (usually 4–5 μm) are cut from the wax block with a microtome. The final steps in the process are the staining and mounting of sections on slides.

For more information, see the specific process.

automatic t. p., the procedure in which tissue specimens are moved by an automated machine through the solutions used in the first four stages of tissue processing. The specimens are carried in wire baskets from one solution to another on a preset schedule.

A typical schedule for routine paraffin tissue processing is: 10 percent buffered neutral formalin, 4 hr; 70 percent ethanol, 1 hr; 80 percent ethanol, 1 hr; 95 percent ethanol, 1 hr; 100 percent ethanol—three changes, 1 hr each; xylene, toluene, or chloroform—three changes, 1 hr each; and melted paraffin or Paraplast—two changes, 2 hr each.

tissue slice a very thin slice of fresh tissue used for in vitro metabolic studies.

tissue thromboplastin see *Factor III.*

titanium (Ti) (ti-ta′ne-um) [N.L., from Gr. *Titan* + N.L. *-ium*] a metallic element occurring as a silvery solid or dark-gray powder; atomic number 22; atomic weight 47.90; a 3d transition element; oxidation states −1, +2, +3, +4 (the most stable).

Titanium is used to make incandescent lamp filaments and strong, lightweight, corrosion-resistant alloys for surgical appliances.

titan yellow (ti′tan) a yellow organic dye that forms a colored lake with magnesium in body fluids and tissues; C.I. 19540. Tests using this principle are rarely made today. Also called *thiazol yellow G.*

titer (ti′ter) [Fr. *titre* standard] 1. the quantity of a substance required to produce a reaction with a given volume of another substance.

2. agglutination titer, the greatest dilution of serum that produces agglutination of microorganisms or particulate antigens.

titrant (ti′trant) a standard solution of known concentration used in a titration.

titration (ti-tra′shun) [Fr. *titre* standard] in quantitative chemical analysis, the determination of the unknown concentration of a substance in solution from the volume of a standard solution of another substance that will completely react with it. The point at which chemically equivalent amounts of the two substances have been mixed (the end point or equivalence point) is frequently indicated by a color change, either the disappearance of a colored reactant or a change in the color of an added indicator dye. More precise titrations use electric endpoint indications, such as the conductivity of the solution as determined by amperometry or conductometry or the pH of the solution as determined by a pH meter.

titration technique in hematology, a semiquantitative method to determine the strength of a particular red cell antibody in serum. The known antibody is serially diluted and reacted with known red cells. The greatest dilution that still produces a detectable reaction with the red cell reflects the strength of the antibody, which is expressed as the reciprocal of this dilution.

titrimetric (ti″trĭ-met′rik) [*titer* + Gr. *metron* measure] pertaining to analysis by titration.

Tityus (tit′e-us) a genus of scorpions. The species *T. bahiensis* and *T. serrulatus* possess neurotoxic venom and are extremely dangerous.

Tl symbol for the chemical element *thallium.*

TL antigen see *thymus-leukemia antigen.*

TLC abbrev. for *thin-layer chromatography* and *total lung capacity.*

TLD abbrev. See *thermoluminescent d.* under *dosimeter* and *tumor lethal d.* under *dose.*

TLV abbrev. See *threshold limit values.*

Tm symbol for the chemical element *thulium.*

tM the time required to complete the M phase of the cell cycle. See also *cell cycle.*

TMA abbrev. See *trimethoxyamphetamine.*

TMP abbrev. See *thymine ribonucleoside-5′-phosphate.*

Tn element see *transposon.*

TNF abbrev. See *tumor necrosis factor.*

TNM abbrev. for tumor, nodes, and metastases. See under *tumor staging.*

TNT abbrev. See *2,4,6-trinitrotoluene.*

toad toxins (tōd tok′sinz) glycoside poisons secreted by the skin glands of all toads, although only the river toad (*Bufo alvarius*) and the marine toad (*B. marinus*) are highly poisonous. The toxins are similar in action to the cardiac glycosides; some also produce hemolysis. Young children may be poisoned by putting their fingers in their mouths after handling toads; symptoms of poisoning are profuse salivation, cardiac arrhythmias and hypertension, pulmonary edema, and convulsions.

Tobie, von Brand, and Mehlman's diphasic medium a medium consisting of a solid phase and a liquid overlay for the cultivation of *Trypanosoma cruzi* and *T. rangeli,* and of *Leishmania tropica, L. brasiliensis,* and *L. donovani.* The solid phase is composed of beef and peptone agar with inactivated rabbit's blood. The liquid overlay consists of sodium chloride, potassium chloride, calcium chloride, monobasic potassium phosphate, and dextrose diluted in distilled water.

tobramycin (to″brah-mi′sin) [USP], a bactericidal aminoglycoside antibiotic derived from a species of *Streptomyces.* The antibacterial spectrum is similar to that of gentamicin; however, it is more active against *Pseudomonas aeruginosa* and less active against *Serratia marcescens.* Tobramycin is used clinically for the treatment of serious infections caused by susceptible gram-negative bacilli. Synergism can often be observed with penicillin. Nephrotoxicity and ototoxicity are adverse reactions. See also *aminoglycosides* and *antibacterial agents.*

toc/o (to′ko) a word element used in combining form to denote childbirth or labor, e.g., tocomania.

-tocia (to′se-ah) [Gr. *tokos* childbirth] a suffix word element to denote labor or birth, e.g., dystocia.

-tocin (to′sin) a suffix word element to denote labor or delivery, e.g., oxytocin.

α-tocopherol (to-kof′er-ol) [*toco-* + Gr. *pherein* to carry] see *vitamin E.*

TOCP abbrev. See *tri-o-cresyl phosphate.*

toe (to) any of the five digits of the foot.

Tofranil (to-fra′nil) trademark. See *imipramine.*

togavirus (to″gah-vi′rus) any of a group of single-stranded RNA viruses that includes the genera *Alphavirus, Flavivirus, Rubivirus,* and *Pestivirus.* The togaviruses multiply in the cytoplasm of their hosts (primarily arthropods) and are released from the cell by budding. The togavirus group is the smallest in size of the enveloped animal viruses and is responsible for rubella, hemorrhagic fevers with a biphasic temperature curve, and mosquito-borne diseases.

Alphaviruses and flaviviruses are best identified by viral neutralization techniques, whereas *Rubivirus* identification depends on the specific clinical situation.

toggle (tog′l) 1. in reference to digital logic circuitry, the change from one state to another.

2. see *flip-flop.*

toggle switch a two-position snap switch used to make or break an electric circuit.

tolazamide (tol-az′ah-mīd) [USP], one of the sulfonylureas, used as an oral hypoglycemic agent in the control of mild, maturity-onset diabetes mellitus. Trademark, *Tolinase.* See also *sulfonylurea.*

tolazoline hydrochloride (tol-az′o-lēn) [NF], an alpha-adrenergic blocking drug that also stimulates gastric secretion, used in peripheral vascular disorders. Adverse reactions include cardiac arrhythmia, anginal pain, hypertension, and aggravation of peptic ulcer.

tolbutamide (tol″bu′tah-mīd) [USP], a phenylsulfonylurea derivative used as an oral hypoglycemic agent in the control of mild, maturity-onset diabetes mellitus. Also used by intravenous injection as a test for the detection of insulinoma. Trademark, *Orinase.* See also *sulfonylurea.*

Tolectin (tol′ek-tin) trademark. See *tolmetin sodium.*

tolerance (tol′er-ans) [L. *tolerantia*] 1. the ability to endure without ill effect or to be less responsive to a stimulus, e.g., a drug, poison, or noxious stimulus.

2. in pharmacology, a state in which a higher dose of a drug is required to produce a specific effect. With many drugs, tolerance is associated with physical dependence (occurrence of withdrawal symptoms when the drug is withheld).

3. in clinical chemistry, the ability to normally metabolize or otherwise dispose of a standard dose of a substance, e.g., glucose tolerance.

4. in immunology, the specific immunologic nonreactivity to a particular antigen that, under other conditions, can elicit a humoral or cell-mediated immune response. Tolerance may be induced by exposing an individual to the antigen in fetal or early postnatal life, or by administering very high or very low doses of certain antigens to an adult. The most obvious importance of tolerance lies in its prevention of individuals from mounting an immune response to their own tissues (self-tolerance). When self-tolerance breaks down, autoimmunity results.

Under appropriate conditions, almost any antigen can act as a tolerogen, a substance capable of inducing tolerance. Many factors influence whether an antigen will act as a tolerogen or an immunogen, a substance that induces an immune response. One important factor is the dose of the antigen. Every antigen has an optimal immunogenic range; larger amounts of the antigen induce high-zone tolerance. With T-dependent antigens (those requiring the interaction of T cells with B cells for a response) but not with T-independent antigens (those capable of stimulating B cells directly), low amounts can induce low-zone tolerance. Another factor influencing tolerance induction is the physical state of the antigen. Aggregated molecules tend to be immunogenic, whereas soluble molecules tend to be tolerogenic. Complex antigens such as whole bacteria or viruses are poor tolerogens; simpler antigens such as proteins are better tolerogens. The route of administration of the antigen also is important. Injecting an antigen into a tissue tends to elicit immunity, whereas intravenous injection often induces tolerance. The genetics and immunocompetence of the individual also determine whether an antigen will induce tolerance. The ability to become tolerant to a particular antigen varies among species. For example, rabbits are more easily made tolerant to serum proteins than are guinea pigs. Strain variation exists within a particular species; for example, C57B1/6 mice can be rendered tolerant to human gamma globulin, whereas Balb/c mice cannot. The immunocompetence of the individual is also important. Immature individuals with poorly developed immune systems or those who are immunosuppressed are more easily made tolerant.

The mechanisms of tolerance induction are not clearly understood. With T-independent antigens, tolerance results from the unresponsiveness of B cells rather than T cells. With T-dependent antigens, tolerance is the result of the unresponsiveness of either B or T cells. For some unknown reason, T cells are made tolerant more easily than are B cells. T-cell tolerance is established sooner, lasts longer, and can be induced with lower amounts of antigen than can B-cell tolerance.

Two major theories have been advanced to explain how tolerance occurs: (1) clonal deletion, in which particular clones of B or T cells are eliminated; and (2) suppression, in which the necessary clones are present but their activity is blocked by the action of suppressor T cells or soluble suppressive factors.

The hypothesized mechanism for clonal deletion is most easily understood in tolerance induction of the fetus or newborn. B cells have specific immunoglobulins on their surface that act as receptors for the antigen. Once the antigen binds to this immunoglobulin, the membrane surface of the B cell undergoes modulation, a process that involves the aggregation of the antigen-antibody complex on the surface of the cell (capping) and the subsequent internalization of the complex. Adult lymphocytes have the capacity to regenerate the surface immunoglobulin once this process has occurred so that the cell can once again interact with the antigen. Immature lymphocytes lack this capacity, however, so that when immature B cells come into contact with an antigen, they lose their receptors and are incapable of further interaction with that antigen. This inactivation of B cells at a critical stage of their differentiation is known as clonal deletion, or clonal abortion. Although clonal deletion also occurs with adult B lymphocytes, the mechanism is not well understood. T-cell unresponsiveness may be the result of clonal deletion of a set of helper T cells, but the nature of the T-cell antigen receptor is unknown and the mechanism is unclear.

The second major mechanism of tolerance induction is the presence of excess suppressor T cells. This was first discovered when it was shown that tolerance to sheep red blood cells in mice could be transferred from a tolerant mouse to a normal one by transferring T cells. Why an antigen preferentially stimulates T-suppressor rather than T-helper cells is not clear; complex interactions between macrophages and T cells seems to be involved.

Tolerance is not an irreversible phenomenon. It can be broken or terminated in a number of ways. Persistence of the antigen is necessary for the maintenance of tolerance. New B and T cells are constantly developing from stem cells to replace the tolerant cells. The duration of high-dose tolerance depends on the rate of breakdown of the antigen in tissues. For example, many polysaccharides are not broken down in mammalian tissues, and a single high dose of this type of antigen results in life-long tolerance. Conversely, proteins usually are broken down, and thus tolerance to this type of antigen is of relatively short duration. Tolerance can also be abrogated by exposing the individual to a closely related, cross-reacting antigen. The mechanism for this phenomenon appears to be that helper T cells that are specific for the antigenic determinants unique to the second cross-reacting antigen will react with B cells specific for the unique as well as the common determinants of the tolerogen and the cross-reacting antigen.

This last concept is particularly important as a mechanism of autoimmunity—mounting an immunologic response to a person's own tissues. In those with rheumatic fever, for example, antigens on the group A streptococci cross react with antigens on heart tissue; thus, individuals' tolerance to their heart tissue is broken and they mount an immune response to it. Any process such as infection by bacteria or viruses or inflammation that damages tissues (which results in exposure of new antigenic determinants) or changes the tissue (which creates new antigenic determinants) can produce the breakdown of tolerance and autoimmunity.

Methods for inducing tolerance artificially may one day be useful in tissue transplantation. The recipient could be made tolerant to the transplantation antigens present on the donated organ. The recipient would then not mount an immune response to the organ and it would not be rejected. This type of treatment is far from the stage of development required for clinical use, however. At this point, tolerance is a phenomenon that may aid in understanding the complex interactions and mechanisms of the immune system, rather than having a direct clinical application.

See also *autoimmunity* and *immunocompetence*.

drug t., the decreased responsiveness of an individual to a drug so that higher-than-normal doses are required to produce a response. Many drugs such as opiates, barbiturates, and alcohol induce a tolerance with chronic use. Cf. *addiction* and *dependence*.

tolerance interval in statistics, a type of interval estimate that has a specified probability of covering a specified fraction of the parent population. The end points of the interval are statistics calculated from the sample data called the upper and lower tolerance limits (U and L). If $F(X)$ is the distribution function of the parent distribution, $F(U) - F(L)$ is the fraction of the parent population covered by the interval (L, U). If U and L are defined so that $P[F(U) - F(L) \geq \beta] = \gamma$, then U and L are called 100 β percent tolerance limits at probability level γ.

tolerogen (tol′er-o-jen) an antigen that induces specific immunologic unresponsiveness (tolerance) to subsequent challenging doses of the antigen.

***o*-tolidine** (tol′ĭ-dēn) a white or reddish crystalline solid, 4,4′-diamino-3,3′-dimethylbiphenyl; M.W. 212.28. It is used in the manufacture of dyes and as a reagent for the detection of hemoglobin in urine or feces.

Tolinase (tōl′in-ās) trademark. See *tolazamide*.

tolmetin sodium (tol′met-in) an antiinflammatory, antipyretic, and analgesic nonsteroidal drug used for symptomatic relief in rheumatoid arthritis. The drug inhibits prostaglandin synthetase and reduces the level of prostaglandin in the blood, which may be responsible for its antiinflammatory action. The most common side-effects are gastrointestinal intolerance (nausea, indigestion, heartburn), headache, dizziness, skin rashes, and tinnitus. Trademark, *Tolectin*.

tolnaftate (tol-naf′tāt) [USP], an antifungal agent used effectively for treating most cutaneous infections caused by dermatophytes, but not for tinea capitis or tinea unguium. Insoluble in water, tolnaftate is a synthetic chemical agent that should be applied only topically. Trademark, *Tinactin*.

toluene (tol′u-ēn) the hydrocarbon, $C_6H_5{\cdot}CH_3$, methylbenzene; a colorless liquid obtainable from coal tar. It is used as starting material in chemical synthesis and as a solvent. Also called *toluol*. See also *benzene assays*.

toluene 2,4-diisocyanate (TDI) (tol′u-ēn di″i-so-si′an-āt) a white or pale yellow liquid with a sharp, pungent odor, used in the manufacture of polyurethanes; M.W. 174.15. TDI is highly irritating to the eyes and upper respiratory tract, and causes bronchial asthma; it also is a potent skin sensitizer and produces allergic eczema.

toluic acid (to-lu′ik) one of three isomeric compounds, $CH_3{\cdot}C_6H_4{\cdot}COOH$ (ortho, meta, and para; 2-methylbenzoic acid, 3-methylbenzoic acid, and 4-methylbenzoic acid).

toluidine (tol-u′ĭ-dēn) methylbenzenamine, used in the manufacture of dyes and other chemicals; M.W. 107.15. There are three isomers: *o*-toluidine (a yellow liquid), *m*-toluidine (a colorless liquid), and *p*-toluidine (a white solid). All are toxic by inhalation, ingestion, and skin absorption and produce hematuria as a result of hemorrhagic cystitis and methemoglobinemia.

toluidine blue a metachromatic thiazin dye; C.I. 52040. Its orthochromatic color is blue and its metachromatic color is purple-red.

toluol (tol′u-ol) see *toluene*.

tolyl- (tol′il) a prefix word element in organic chemistry to denote a methylphenyl substituent group ($CH_3C_6H_4$—). *o*-Tolyl denotes 2-methylphenyl; *m*-tolyl denotes 3-methylphenyl; and *p*-tolyl denotes 4-methylphenyl.

tom/o (to′mo) [Gr. *tomē* a cutting] a word element

used in combining form to denote a cutting, e.g., tomography.

tome (tōm) [Gr. *tomē* a cutting] a suffix word element to denote an instrument to cut, e.g., dermatome.

Tomes' fibers (tōmz) [Sir John *Tomes,* English dentist, 1815–1895] apical processes of the odontoblast that extend into the dentinal tubule.

tomogram (to'mo-gram) [*tomo-* + Gr. *gramma* mark, drawing] the image produced by any method of tomography, particularly a wide-angle, body-section radiograph. See also *zonogram.*

tomography (to-mog'rah-fe) [*tomo-* + Gr. *graphein* to write] any method of producing an image of a body section. In one method, reconstruction tomography, a computer program produces the image from views of the section (slice) looked at on edge. More precisely, the image is reconstructed from readings of the average density along many rays crossing the slice. These readings can be obtained by using narrow beams or fans of x-rays (see *computed tomography*). A pair of gamma rays is emitted in opposite directions from a positron decay. A ring of detectors can be used in counting the number of decays that occur along the ray connecting each detector pair, which indicates the radioisotope density along the ray (see *positron emission tomography*).

Other tomographic methods produce images in which features lying in the body section (called the focal plane, layer, cut, or zone) are in sharp focus, but features above or below the section are out of focus and blurred. In nuclear medicine, this effect is produced by using a focusing collimator on a rectilinear scanner (see *multiplane tomographic scanner* and *rectilinear scanner*). In conventional radiology, the effect is produced by moving the x-ray tube and film holder (or film and object) during the exposure. The preferred generic names for this method are *body section radiography* and *tomography.* Specific technical methods have been called *laminagraphy, planigraphy,* and *stratigraphy.*

The usual method of body-section radiography uses a linear motion of the x-ray tube and film tray. Both are attached to a metal rod that pivots around a fixed fulcrum, which is adjusted up or down to set the height of the focal plane. The angle through which the rod swings during the exposure is called the exposure angle. The rod moves the tube and film in opposite directions; thus, features on the axis of rotation (the pivot) remain between the focal spot of the tube and a single point of the film. Other features in the focal plane are slightly blurred, and features above and below the focal plane are more blurred. The amount of blurring increases with the distance from the focal plane and with the exposure angle.

Because tomography overlays images of objects viewed from different angles, the outlines (structural contours) of objects are lost, and the contrast is lower than in a conventional radiograph. Wide-angle tomography uses an exposure angle greater than 10° (usually 20°–60°). The layer of tissue in sharp focus is only 1–5 mm thick, and is used to separate thin, high-contrast objects from nearby obscuring structures; only very thin objects show sharp margins. Narrow-angle tomography (zonography) uses an exposure angle less than 10° (usually 2°–10°). The thicker focal plane cut (called a zone) is 10–25 mm thick, and is used to preserve some structural contours and detail of extended objects, particularly low-contrast soft tissues.

Because out-of-focus objects are smeared out along the direction of the tube motion (along the length of the table), long, thin objects aligned in this direction produce streaks called parasite lines. For example, in a chest tomogram the spine produces a long streak, whereas the ribs are totally erased. This problem can be avoided with special equipment (e.g., a Multiplanigraph), which uses a pattern of tube movement (e.g., circular, elliptic, spiral, or figure-of-eight) that provides blurring in both directions. These units are more expensive than linear tomographs, however; they also have longer exposure times and lower contrast, and still produce some phantom images, particularly in circular zonography.

See also the accompanying illustration.

axial transverse t., a method of producing body-section radiographs of a transverse plane through the body. The x-ray beam projects through the patient at the level of the transverse plane, and is inclined at an angle of 10°–45° to the horizontal transverse plane and x-ray film. The tomographic blurring is produced by the synchronous rotation on a vertical axis of both the patient and the film, or by the simultaneous revolution of both the x-ray tube and the film around the patient's body axis. Axial transverse tomograms have relatively poor contrast and detail. Also called *transversal t.*

computed t., see *computed tomography.*

panoramic t., a radiographic technique for producing a distortion-free lateral view of the teeth, maxilla, mandible, and temporomandibular joints. The x-ray beam is collimated by a narrow vertical slit. It passes through a thin vertical section of the jaw and through another slit, which removes secondary radiation, to the film. The patient and film (or tube and film) rotate so that the jaw and film move synchronously through the beam. Also called *panography, pan-oral radiography, pantotomography,* and *rotational t.*

plesiosectional t., see under *simultaneous multifilm t.*

rotational t., see *panoramic t.*

simultaneous multifilm t., a type of body-section radiography in which tomograms of several adjacent tissue cuts are made with one exposure by use of multiscreen cassettes.

The book cassette contains three to seven films sandwiched between intensifying screens. The films are separated 5–10 mm by plastic sponges. Absorption and scattering in the upper layers of the book necessitate an increase in screen speed in the lower layers. This maintains the same radiographic density, but the radiographic quality decreases owing to increased fogging. The tissue sections have the same separation as the films in the cassette, and the top layer is at the fulcrum height.

A plesiocassette has four films and no spacers, so that the sections are only 1 mm apart; it is used primarily in (plesiosectional) tomography of the ear.

transversal t., see *axial transverse t.*

tomolaryngography (to"mo-lar"ing-gog'rah-fe) [*tomo-* + Gr. *larynx* larynx + *graphein* to write] a tomographic examination of the larynx and pharynx. See also *laryngography.*

-tomy (to'me) [Gr. *tomē* a cutting] a suffix word ele-

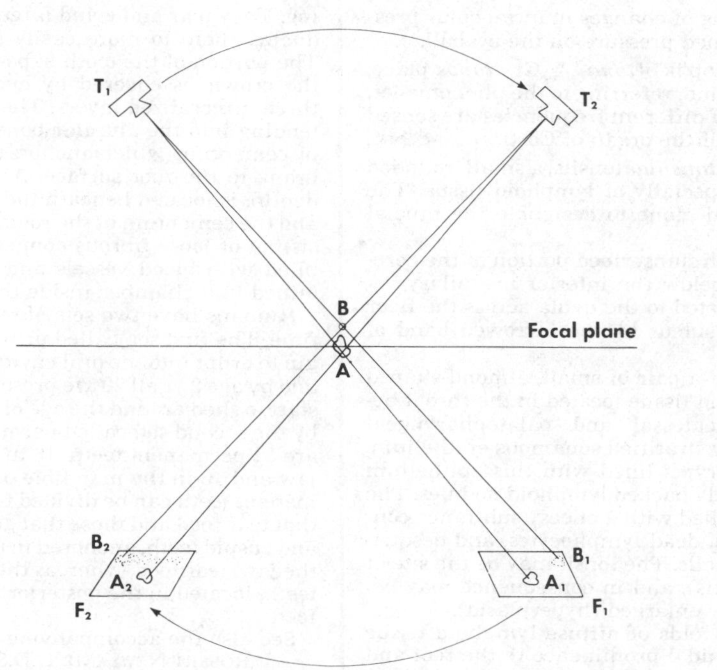

Tomography. Tomographic principle. (From Books, J.: Tomography. *In* Ballinger, P. W. Merrill's Atlas of Radiographic Positions and Radiologic Procedures. 5th ed. St. Louis, C. V. Mosby Co., 1982.)

ment to denote cutting, an incision, or to cut into, e.g., laparotomy.

ton/o (ton′o) [Gr. *tonos* tension] a word element used in combining form to denote relationship to tone or tension, e.g., tonometry.

tone (tōn) [Gr. *tonos;* L. *tonus*] 1. the normal degree of vigor and tension. In muscle, the resistance to a passive elongation or stretch.

2. a healthy state of a part; tonus.

3. a particular quality of sound or of voice.

4. to make permanent, or to change, the color of a silver stain by chemical treatment, usually with a heavy metal.

toner (to′ner) a blue powder used to produce an electrostatic image. See also under *xeroradiography.*

tongue (tung) [L. *lingua,* Gr. *glōssa*] the movable muscular organ in the mouth and pharynx that is associated with taste, chewing and swallowing, and speech. Also called *lingua.*

tongue-tie (tung′ti″) see *ankyloglossia.*

tongue worms see *Pentastomida.*

tonic-clonic attack (ton′ik clon′ik) [Gr. *tonos* tension; *klonos* confused motion] a form of seizure characterized by a sudden loss of consciousness, the patient exhibiting tonic and then clonic muscle movements of the trunk and limbs. These events may be accompanied by sphincter relaxation and other autonomic disorders. After motor manifestations have ceased, the patient may remain comatose for a short time (30 min or so), following which there may be drowsiness, mental confusion, and headache.

The interictal electroencephalogram (EEG) may include bursts of generalized, bilaterally synchronous spike or slow-wave and spike activity. During the tonic phase of the seizure itself, low-voltage fast activity is first seen in the EEG; this gradually becomes slower and more conspicuous until generalized, high-amplitude synchronous spikes of 8–12 Hz are present. During the clonic phase, these spikes become intermixed with slow waves of 1.5–3 Hz. After the attack, there is usually a transient attenuation of the background and then irregular polymorphic slow activity, often for several hours, before the EEG returns to the interictal pattern.

The usual prophylactic treatment of tonic-clonic attacks includes the administration of phenobarbital, phenytoin (Dilantin), carbamazepine, or other drugs.

Formerly called *grand mal attack.* See also *epilepsy.*

tonicity (to-nis′ĭ-te) 1. the state of tissue tone or tension.

2. the osmolality of a solution as compared with that of blood plasma, e.g., hypotonic, isotonic, or hypertonic.

tonofibril (ton′o-fi″bril) [tono- + N.L. *fibrilla* dim. of *fibra* fiber] a small fiber seen with the light microscope in some epithelial cells. Together, tonofibrils make up the cell web. With the electron microscope, tonofibrils can be seen to be bundles of tonofilaments, which attach to desmosomes. See also *cell junction.*

tonofilament (ton″o-fil′ah-ment) [*tono-* + L. *filamentum* thread] intermediate filaments (about 10 nm in diameter) that provide structural support in cells. Some insert on desmosomes. Cf. *microfilament.*

tonography (to-nog′rah-fe) [*tono-* + Gr. *graphein* to

write] the recording of changes in intraocular pressure due to sustained pressure on the eyeball.

tonotopic (ton″o-top′ik) [*tono-* + Gr. *topos* place, area] related to sound; referring to the phenomenon in which sounds of different frequencies are sensed by specific areas of the organ of Corti.

tonsil (ton′sil) [L. *tonsillae* tonsils] a small, rounded mass of tissue, especially of lymphoid tissue. The term is often used alone to designate the faucial tonsil.

cerebellar t., a circumscribed portion of the cerebellum that lies below the inferior medullary velum, and is connected to the uvula across the floor of the vallecular sulcus by the furrowed band of cerebellar cortex.

faucial t., one of a pair of small, almond-shaped masses of lymphoid tissue located in the throat between the palatoglossal and palatopharyngeal arches, covered by stratified squamous epithelium. Each tonsil has crypts lined with this epithelium and contains closely packed lymphoid nodules. The crypts are often filled with a cheesy substance consisting of bacteria, dead lymphocytes, and desquamated epithelial cells. The tonsil may be the site of infection (tonsillitis), and in consequence may become considerably enlarged (hyperplasia).

pharyngeal t.'s, folds of diffuse lymphoid tissue that form a pyramidal prominence in the roof and posterior wall of the nasopharynx near the midline. They are prominent in young children and they often atrophy in adults.

tonsill/o (ton′sĭ-lo) a word element used in combining form to denote the tonsils, e.g., tonsillitis.

tonsillitis (ton″sĭ-li′tis) [*tonsill* + *-itis*] an inflammation of the tonsils. The term most often refers to inflammation of the faucial tonsils but may also include the pharyngeal and lingual tonsils. For descriptive purposes, tonsillitis is often divided into exudative and nonexudative forms. The clinical manifestations include sore throat, fever, mucopurulent nasal discharge, headache, malaise, and erythema.

Viruses are the most common etiologic agent. The adenovirus is isolated in 25 percent of those with tonsillitis. Other viruses causing tonsillitis include herpes simplex, coxsackie virus A, and echovirus. The most important bacterium causing tonsillitis is group A β-hemolytic streptococcus. Other responsible bacteria include *Corynebacterium diphtheriae, Neisseria gonorrhoeae, N. meningitidis, Hemophilus influenzae* type B, and group B, C, or G β-hemolytic streptococci. The tonsils may be infected with *Mycoplasma pneumoniae* during mycoplasmal upper respiratory tract disease.

Infections of the tonsils can be spread through the air, by contaminated food or liquid, or by direct person-to-person contact. Once the microorganisms have entered the oropharynx, the tonsils are relatively ineffective in controlling potential pathogens in the upper respiratory tract.

Diagnosis is made by observation of the clinical signs and symptoms, and by a microbiologic throat culture. Antistreptococcal serologic analysis of serum is also a useful diagnostic tool.

tooth (to͞oth), pl. *teeth* [Anglo-Saxon tōth] one of the highly specialized mineralized organs attached to the alveolar processes of the jaw bones by a band of dense fibrous connective tissue, the periodontal membrane. Teeth function in mastication or chewing. They tear and grind large particles of food, reducing them to more easily digestible fragments. The portion of the tooth exposed to the oral cavity, the crown, is covered by enamel, the hardest of three mineralized layers. The part of the tooth extending into the alveolar bone, the root, is covered by cementum, which anchors the periodontal membrane to the root surface. A third calcified layer, dentin, is located beneath the enamel of the crown and the cementum of the root. The dental pulp, consisting of loose fibrous connective tissue well supplied with blood vessels and nerve fibers, is contained in a chamber inside the dentin.

Humans have two sets of teeth during their lifetime. The first set, called primary or deciduous, begin to erupt into the oral cavity at about 6 mo of age and by age 2 yr all 20 are present. The primary teeth start to shed around the age of 6 yr and are replaced by the second set, called permanent or adult. There are 32 permanent teeth, 16 in the maxilla or upper jaw and 16 in the mandible or lower jaw. The permanent teeth can be divided functionally into those that tear food and those that grind food. The incisor and cuspid teeth, anchored in the anterior portion of the jaw, tear food, whereas the premolar and molar teeth, located in the posterior part of the jaw, grind food.

See also the accompanying illustration.

J. Robert Newland, D.D.S.

top/o (top′o) [Gr. *topos* place] a word element used in combining form to denote a place, position, or location, e.g., topography.

tophus (to′fus), pl. *tophi* [L. "porous stone"] a deposit of urates in relatively avascular structures that are rich in acid mucopolysaccharides, such as joint capsules, bursae, tendons, skin, and the soft tissues of the external ear. Histologically, the tophus is characterized by "sheaves-of-wheat"–urate crystal deposits surrounded by epithelioid cells and multinucleated giant cells. See also *gout.* Cf. *pseudogout* (chondrocalcinosis).

topographic (top″o-graf′ik) describing or pertaining to special regions; of or related to topography.

topography (to-pog′rah-fe) [*topo-* + Gr. *graphein* to write] 1. the description of an anatomic region or a specific part.
2. in electroencephalography, the distribution of amplitudes of electric activity recorded from the scalp, cerebral cortex, or deep brain structures.

torocyte (tor′o-sīt) a red cell artifact. The central area of pallor is sharply set off against the narrow peripheral rim of hemoglobin rather than shading into it gradually. Torocytes are produced when traces of water are mixed with the fixative solution or when the blood smear is dried too slowly; they must not be confused with leptocytes, in which the area of central pallor is increased, but the transition between it and the peripheral hemoglobin is still gradual. Cf. *leptocyte.*

torpor (tor′por) [L.] sluggishness.

torque (T) (tork) [L. *torquere* to twist] the moment of a force about an axis of rotation, the cause of a torsion or angular acceleration. It is defined as the product of the length of the lever arm (the perpendicular from the point of application of the force to the axis) and the component of the force perpendicular to the lever arm. The International System (SI) unit of torque is the newton-meter (N·m).

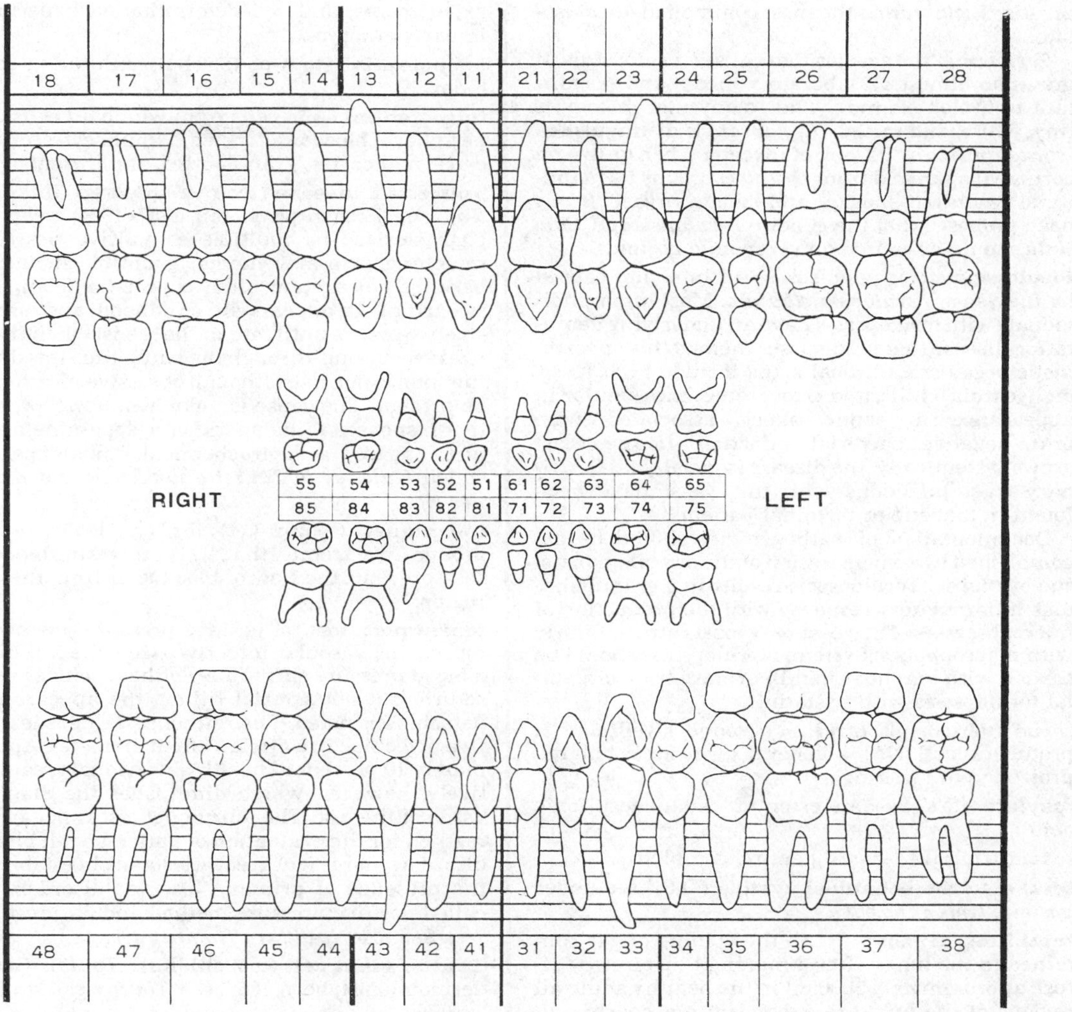

Tooth. Diagram of permanent and deciduous teeth according to the internationally used numbering system. The deciduous teeth are shown in the center. (Courtesy of University of Texas at Houston Dental Branch, J. Robert Newland, D.D.S.)

torr (tor) [after Evangelista *Torricelli,* Italian mathematician, 1608–1647] a unit of pressure, 133.3224 pascal (Pa), equal to 1/760 atomosphere (atm) and to the millimeter of mercury (mmHg) to within 1 part per million (ppm).

torsion (tor′shun) [L. torsio, from *torquere* to twist] a twisting; the deformation produced when the two ends of an object are rotated in opposite directions, or one end rotates while the other remains fixed. Torsion may occur in certain organs (for example, testis, ovary, gallbladder, or a loop of small intestine) and, if uncorrected, may produce necrosis secondary to obstruction of blood flow at the site of torsion.

torso (tor′so) the trunk without the head or extremities.

torticollis (tor″ti-kol′is) [L. *tortus* twisted + *collum* neck] wryneck, a contracted state of the cervical muscles, producing torsion of the neck. The deformity may be congenital, but in most cases the pathogenesis is unknown.

Torula (tor′u-lah) [L. "*roll*"] a genus of dematiacious fungi. A number of medically important fungi have been erroneously classified in this genus; e.g., *Torula* is the former name for *Cryptococcus,* and *T. capsulatus* and *T. histolytica* are now *Cryptococcus neoformans. Torula* is seldom isolated in the clinical laboratory.

Torulopsis (tor″u-lop′sis) [L. *torulus* tuft + Gr. *opsis* appearance] a genus of fungi that is synonymous with *Candida.* This fungus belongs to the family Cryptococcaceae, order Moniliales, and is morphologically similar to *Cryptococcus* without a capsule. In the healthy individual, *Torulopsis* is nonpathogenic; in the debilitated host, however, it can cause pneumonia, septicemia, meningitis, and pyelonephritis. *T. glabrata* is the most common medical isolate.

T. glabrata, the species that causes torulopsosis. It grows on almost all laboratory media and is resistant to cyclohexamide. The colony morphology is tiny, white, and raised. *T. glabrata* is distinguished from *Candida* by its lack of mycelia when grown on cornmeal agar, and from *Cryptococcus* by its inability to assimilate inositol and lack of urease. It has been proposed that the genera *Torulopsis* and *Candida* should be united on taxonomic grounds.

torulopsosis (tor″u-lop-so′sis) an infection caused by the yeast *Torulopsis glabrata.* Most often, individuals with torulopsosis have an underlying debilitating disease that predisposes them to this opportunistic organism. Clinical signs include high fever, tachycardia, chills, and rigors sometimes similar in appearance to septic shock associated with gram-negative bacterial infection. If the yeast grows systemically, the disease is usually fatal. Urinary tract infections with this yeast have been found in diabetic or terminal patients.

Documentation of pathogenicity should be accomplished by demonstration of the organism in tissue by biopsy. Torulopsosis results in a granulomatous inflammatory response with the production of microabscesses. The yeast may exist intracellularly with macrophages. Systemic torulopsosis should be treated with amphotericin B; urinary tract or genital torulopsosis with nystatin.

torus (to′rus), pl. *tori* [L. "a round swelling," "a protuberance"] [NA], a general term for a bulging projection or swelling.

tosylate (to′sĭ-lāt) an ester of *p*-toluenesulfonic acid.

total (to′tal) [L. *totus* all] entire, complete.

total electromechanical systole (Q-S_2) see under *systolic time interval.*

total lung capacity (TLC) the volume of gas contained in the lungs after a maximal inspiratory effort, approximately 5800 ml in the healthy adult; all regions of the lung are expanded to a nearly uniform degree at full inspiration (TLC). It is equal to the sum of the inspiratory and functional residual capacities, or to the sum of the vital capacity and residual volume.

total peripheral resistance the impediment to blood flow provided by the entire systemic vasculature, normally equal to approximately 1 peripheral resistance unit (PRU). The total peripheral resistance, along with the cardiac output, is one of the primary determinants of the magnitude of the arterial blood pressure. See also *resistance.*

total ventilation the amount of air exchanged through the nose and mouth with each breath (tidal volume) or during each minute (minute ventilation). Cf. *alveolar ventilation.*

totipotency (to″tĭ-po′ten-se) [L. *totus* all + *potentia* power] the ability of a single cell to form a complete fertile organism: the cell thus retains all genetic information necessary to differentiate into a mature adult. Differentiated cells from various organisms have been shown to possess this property, e.g., carrot phloem cells, amphibian nuclei, mammalian blastomeres, *Drosophila* blastoderm, and tobacco pith cells. Totipotency is imperative for successful embryo fusion experiments, nuclear transplantation experiments, and cell determination experiments in early embryos.

totipotential (to″tĭ-po-ten′shal) exhibiting totipotency.

totipotential cells cells from which all cells of the peripheral blood are formed (lymphocytes, erythrocytes, monocytes, granulocytes, and thrombocytes).

Tourette's disease (too-retz′) [George Gilles de la *Tourette,* French physician, 1857–1904] a condition characterized by multiple convulsive tics (facial twitching, arm movements); grunting, shouting, or barking noises; and often coprolalia (compulsive swearing). It appears in childhood and progressively worsens until late in the teens, when it stabilizes, recurring throughout adult life. Intellectual function is normal, although obsessive ideation may be present. The cause is unknown; however, objective responses to haloperidol, a dopamine antagonist, suggest a neurochemical imbalance. Also called *Gilles de la Tourette syndrome* and *maladie des tics.*

tourniquet (toor′nĭ-ket) [Fr.] a device applied around an extremity that, by compressing blood vessels, prevents the flow of blood to or from the distal region.

tourniquet test a positive-pressure method for measuring vascular integrity. After the inflation of a blood pressure cuff to a level that occludes venous return, but not arterial filling, the appearance of petechiae is noted. The reference value is less than five petechiae in a circle 3 cm in diameter. Approximately 10 percent of healthy individuals react positively, however, which diminishes the diagnostic value of the test. The tourniquet test is not a useful method for the evaluation of patients with bleeding disorders, nor is it of great assistance in establishing the presence of primary vascular disorders. Also called positive pressure method and *Rumpel-Leede test.* See also *capillary fragility test.*

Touton giant cell (toot′on) [Karl *Touton,* German dermatologist, born 1858] see *Touton g. c.* under *giant cell.*

tower skull see *acrocephaly.*

Towne projection a projection used in radiography of the cranium and in pneumoencephalography. The patient is in the brow-up position and the central ray is angled 25°–35° caudad. Also called half-axial anteroposterior projection.

reverse T. p., the projection opposite to the Towne projection. The patient is in the brow-down position and the central ray is inclined 25°–35° cranially.

tox/o (tok′so) [Gr. *toxikon;* L. *toxinum* poison] a word element used in combining form to denote a toxin or poison, e.g., toxanemia.

toxaphene (toks′ah-fēn) an insecticide, a mixture of polychlorinated camphenes. See also *chlorinated hydrocarbon pesticides.*

toxemia (tok-se′me-ah) [*tox-* + Gr. *haima* blood + *ia*] the presence in the blood of toxic substances. These can be microbial products, ingested or injected chemicals, or by-products of metabolic processes.

t. of pregnancy, see *preeclampsia.*

toxic (tok′sik) pertaining to, due to, or of the nature of a poison; poisonous.

toxic/o (tok′sĭ-ko) [Gr. *toxikon* poison] a word element used in combining form to denote poison, e.g., toxicology.

toxicant (toks'ĭ-kant) [L. *toxicans* poison] 1. poisonous; toxic.

2. a poisonous agent.

toxic chemical handling recommended procedures for handling toxic chemicals, which emphasize preventing the exposure of laboratory personnel by any route of entry, with particular attention to facilities and procedures for ventilation and for washing of the hands and other potentially exposed skin surfaces. Facilities are also needed so that food and beverages can be stored and ingested away from possible toxic exposures.

toxic granulation see *toxic granule.*

toxic granule a dark purple–staining granule in polymorphonuclear leukocytes, containing peroxidase and acid hydrolases, that is found in inflammatory disorders (often together with cytoplasmic vacuoles and occasionally Dohle bodies).

toxicity (tok-sis-ĭ-te) the capacity of a toxic substance (toxicant) to cause tissue damage, disease, or death. The degree of toxicity depends on the dosage and route of exposure of the agent (whether by ingestion, inhalation, or absorption through contact with the skin). It may also depend on the physical state and the chemical properties (such as solubility) of the agent (e.g., ionic mercury is more dangerous than the metal, and certain metals are dangerous only as dusts or fumes). Acute toxicity refers to the effects of a single intense exposure, whereas chronic toxicity refers to the cumulative effect of repeated exposure to small amounts over a long time.

One index of toxicity is lethality, usually expressed as LD_{50}, the dose that kills 50 percent of a population under specified conditions of exposure. Although LD_{50} is determined for a given species from animal experiments, it can also be estimated for humans from data obtained from accidental human poisonings.

The toxicity of many chemicals has been summarized in *Registry of Toxic Effects of Chemicals,* a report published by the National Institute for Occucational Safety and Health. The safety standards and exposure limits that apply to some toxic agents may provide another indication of toxicity; these include some of the threshold-limit values (TLV) for occupational exposure to a selected list of chemicals, which are published annually by the American Conference of Governmental Industrial Hygienists.

See also *threshold limit values.*

toxicologic (tok″sĭ-ko-loj'ik) pertaining to toxicology.

toxicologist (tok″sĭ-kol'o-jist) one who specializes in toxicology.

toxicology (tok″sĭ-kol'o-je) the science of poisons; the study of their effects, mechanism of action, metabolism, and mode of excretion. It also includes the study of analytical methods for the detection and quantitation of poisons and antidotes and the treatment of poisoning, as well as determination of the limits of safe use of hazardous materials.

analytical t., a branch of chemistry that deals with the determination of drugs and poisons in various matrices.

clinical t., the branch of medical science that deals with the diagnosis and treatment of poisoning; in particular, with methods of identification and quantitation of the toxic agent, with specific antidotes or antagonists, and with methods of preventing further absorption or of increasing excretion of the toxic agent. Drug abuse screening and therapeutic drug monitoring may be included in the practice of clinical toxicology.

environmental t., the branch of toxicology concerned with the detection and quantitation of pollutants in the environment and the investigation of their toxic effects on living organisms.

forensic t., the branch of toxicology concerned with the application of toxicologic principles to the purposes of the law, particularly with respect to medico-legal investigations of deaths in cases of suspected poisoning.

industrial t., a branch of toxicology concerned with the hazards of industrial chemicals, particularly in regard to the occupational diseases they can cause and the safety standards for their use.

toxicosis (tok″sĭ-ko'sis) [*toxic-* + *-osis*] a condition due to poisoning; the term was formerly used to refer to a condition of dehydration, fever, and threatening collapse due to infectious diarrhea in infancy or early childhood.

toxic shock syndrome a rare but serious condition thought to be caused by toxins produced by the bacterium *Staphylococcus aureus,* and associated with specific environmental situations such as the use of highly absorbent tampons and suture materials. Clinically, toxic shock syndrome involves fever, profound multisystem dysfunction, acute erythroderma, and shock. Because the exact etiology of the disease is still unclear, there is no laboratory test or animal model available for diagnosis.

toxic waste chemicals disposed of directly as waste or as spill residue and defined as toxic waste by the Environmental Protection Agency (EPA) in the regulations of the Resource Conservation and Recovery Act; examples include acetone, ethyl ether, methanol, toluene, trichloroethylene, and xylene.

toxigenic (tok″sĭ-jen'ik) capable of producing or elaborating a toxin.

toxigenicity (tok″sĭ-jĕ-nis'ĭ-te) disease-producing ability based on the production of a soluble toxin, which accounts for at least part of the virulence of a parasite. A measurement of toxigenicity is thus similar to a measurement of virulence if the toxin produced is pathogenic.

toxin (tok'sin) [L. *toxicum* poison, from Gr. *toxikos* of or for the bow] a poison; the term is frequently used to refer specifically to a substance produced by a plant, animal, fungus, or bacterium that is highly toxic. Such substances are differentiated from chemical poisons by their high molecular weight, by their antigenicity, and by the ability of some varieties to be converted to nontoxic but still antigenic toxoids. See also *endotoxin* and *exotoxins.*

Toxocara (tok″so-ka'rah) a genus of nematode worms of the superfamily Ascaridoidea. The species *T. canis* (a parasite in the intestines of dogs) and *T. cati* (a parasite of cats) cause visceral larva migrans in humans. See also *larva migrans.*

T. canis, a species parasitic in the intestines of dogs. The male worms are 4–6 cm long; the females, 6.5–10 cm long. The eggs (measuring $85 \times 75\ \mu$) are dark brown or dark gray and are unembryonated when passed. Human infection is caused by the ingestion of the eggs from close association with contaminated dogs, or from contact with the eggs in the soil or feces. As humans are not a natural host, the infections rarely reach maturity.

T. cati, a species commonly found in cats. The male worms are 4–6 cm long; the females, 4–12 cm long. *T. cati* eggs are thin-shelled and measure 65–70 μ. Also called *Belascaris cati, B. mystax,* and *T. mystax.*

T. mystax, see *T. cati.*

toxocariasis (tok″so-kār-i′ah-sis) an infection with nematode worms of the genus *Toxocara.* See also *larva migrans.*

toxoid (tok′soid) [*toxo-* + Gr. *eidos* form] a bacterial exotoxin that has lost its toxicity without losing its antigenicity. This phenomenon was discovered to occur spontaneously with toxic filtrates left at room temperature. The transformation of toxin molecules into toxoid can be accelerated by the addition of many different chemicals, but formaldehyde is the substance used almost universally for the commercial production of toxoids for immunization. Toxoids are most valuable for active immunization against bacterial species whose exotoxins are largely responsible for the pathologic changes produced by the infection. The outstanding examples are *Corynebacterium diphtheriae* and *Clostridium tetani.*

Methods have been developed for the purification and concentration of toxoids. They are available in unprecipitated or fluid form and in precipitated or adsorbed form. Alum, aluminum hydroxide, and aluminum phosphate are useful precipitating agents. As they are relatively insoluble, precipitated toxoids are absorbed slowly following injection; the longer persistence in tissue is generally thought to produce higher levels of immunity than fluid toxoids.

The *U.S. Pharmacopeia* contains essential data concerning the various toxoid preparations available commercially.

Toxoplasma (toks″o-plaz-mah) [*toxo-* + Gr. *plasma* anything formed or molded] a genus of sporozoa. The species *T. gondii* causes toxoplasmosis and is an intracellular parasite of humans and animals of worldwide distribution. The cat is the definitive host, with the sexual cycle taking place in this host's intestinal epithelial cells. *Toxoplasma* are small organisms, measuring 2–3 μm wide by 4–6 μm long. They are usually grouped in pseudocysts (ranging from 10–50 μm). Humans serve as intermediate hosts, human infection being caused by ingestion of improperly cooked or raw meat containing toxoplasma cysts, or accidental ingestion of oocysts from cat feces.

Laboratory diagnosis is usually based on histologic or serologic procedures. Hematoxylin-eosin, Romanowsky, or Giemsa stains may be used to demonstrate cysts in biopsy specimens. For isolation, minced tissue or body fluids may be inoculated intraperitoneally into mice. Serologic procedures include the Sabin-Feldman dye, complement-fixation, indirect fluorescent antibody, and indirect hemagglutination tests. An enzyme-linked immunosorbent assay (ELISA) has also been developed for serologic diagnosis of toxoplasmosis.

Toxoplasmea a class of sporozoa, of which the genus *Toxoplasma* is a member.

toxoplasmosis (tok″so-plaz-mo′sis) a disease caused by *Toxoplasma gondii,* which varies in severity from a benign infection to a severe systemic disease leading to encephalitis and death. The parasites spread via the blood stream to various organs and tissues, where they invade the cells, multiply, and disrupt them. Cysts are usually formed in the muscles and brain.

Congenital toxoplasmosis occurs through transplacental transmission following an acute maternal infection. It may be fatal or cause hydrocephalus, retinochoroiditis, and encephalomyelitis, usually resulting in blindness and mental retardation. The acquired form may give rise to (1) an acute lymphadenopathy; (2) a severe illness characterized by myocarditis, pneumonitis, hepatitis, or meningoencephalitis; or (3) an ocular disease, depending on the immune status of the host.

TP abbrev. for total protein; see under *protein assays.*

TPI abbrev. for *Treponema pallidum* immobilization.

TPR abbrev. for temperature, pulse, and respiration.

TPS abbrev. See *trypsin.*

trabecula (trah-bek′u-lah), pl. *trabeculae* [L. dim of *trabs* a beam] [NA], a supporting or anchoring sheet of connective tissue.

trabeculae of bone, bony spicules in cancellous bone that form a meshwork of intercommunicating spaces filled with bone marrow.

trabeculae carneae, the rounded or irregular muscular ridges, bands, or columns of myocardium on the interior walls of the ventricles of the heart.

trabecular (trah-bek′u-lar) pertaining to a trabecula.

trabecular carcinoma an uncommon skin neoplasm formed of anatomosing cords of cells containing dense-core granules. Its relation to the Merkel cell tumor is unclear but it may be a variant with the same histogenesis. See also *Merkel cell tumor.*

trace (trās) 1. a line recording the passage of an object.

2. the line drawn by the electron beam on the face of a cathode-ray tube (CRT).

3. the graphic output of a recording device such as an electrocardiograph.

4. a very small or barely perceptible amount.

5. to follow the execution of a computer program by displaying some intermediate results to pin down the location of a bug.

6. the output of a trace routine.

7. in mathematics, the sum of the diagonal elements of a matrix.

tracé alternant the discontinuous pattern of electric activity recorded from the brain of full-term infants during quiet sleep. The pattern consists of 3- to 5-sec bursts of delta activity (1–3 Hz) intermixed with theta and beta activity. These bursts appear on a relatively quiescent background of mixed frequency.

tracé discontinu the discontinuous pattern of electric activity recorded from the brain of normal preterm infants during quiet sleep. The pattern consists of bursts of activity at 1–3 Hz (delta activity) and/or brushes (8- to 20-Hz rhythmic activity superimposed on slow waves) on a low-amplitude, quiescent background.

trace element a chemical element present in small quantities in a substance. Trace elements found in the human body can be divided into essential mineral nutrients, and nonessential trace elements that perform no known function but are ingested in food, water, and air. The latter category includes aluminum, antimony, arsenic, bismuth, boron, cadmium, germanium, gold, lead, mercury, silver, and titanium. Several of these, especially the heavy metals, are toxic. See also *mineral nutrients.*

tracer (trās'er) 1. a foreign substance added to a given substance so that its distribution in the body or passage through the body can be followed. The most common type of tracer is a compound labeled with a radioactive isotope. Other types include compounds labeled with stable isotopes of low natural abundance and (for fluids) chemical dyes.

2. a dissecting instrument used for isolating blood vessels and nerves.

trace routine a computer program, usually part of the software supplied by the manufacturer, that traces computer programs written in a particular language by printing out the results of every assignment statement, test, or branch and loop, or of all three types of operation.

trache/o (tra'ke-o) a word element used in combining form to denote the trachea, e.g., tracheotomy.

trachea (tra'ke-ah) [L.; Gr. *tracheia artēria*] the air passage that begins at the lower border of the cricoid cartilage and ends by bifurcating at the level of the sternal angle. About 10 cm long and less than 2 cm wide, it lies in the median plane, with the bifurcation slightly to the right of the midline. Its patency is maintained by a series of horseshoe-shaped cartilages. At the bifurcation the trachea divides to form the right and left main bronchi. The ridge between the two bronchi is the carina. The mucosa of the trachea is lined by pseudostratified ciliated columnar (respiratory) epithelium, and mucous glands in the submucosal connective tissue pass their secretion through slender ducts to the surface.

tracheostomy (tra"ke-os'to-me) [*tracheo-* + Gr. *stomoun* to furnish with an opening or mouth] a surgical creation of an opening in the trachea through the neck. It may be indicated to relieve a supratracheal obstruction in the respiratory pathway, to clear tracheobronchial secretions, for the administration of anesthesia, or to place the larynx at rest.

tracheotomy (tra"ke-ot'o-me) [*tracheo-* + Gr. *tomē* a cutting] a general term used to describe the surgical incision of the trachea. It may be performed to remove a foreign body or lesion, obtain a biopsy, relieve an acute airway obstruction, or carry out an exploratory procedure. See also *tracheostomy.*

trachoma (trah-ko'mah), pl. trachomata [Gr. *trachōma* roughness] an eye disease characterized by a chronic keratoconjunctivitis, preceded by acute inflammatory changes in the conjunctiva and cornea, which progresses to scarring and blindness over a period of years. It is the single greatest cause of blindness in the world today. In endemic areas, the initial chlamydial infection occurs early in childhood and is often mixed with a bacterial conjunctivitis. It has been estimated that more than 400 million people are infected by this agent and that as a consequence some 20 million people are blind. The disease occurs primarily in Asia, Africa, and the Mediterranean area. It is associated with poor sanitation and hygiene practices. See also *Chlamydia.*

tracing (trās'ing) a graphic record produced by copying another, or scribed by an instrument capable of making a visual record of movements.

tract (trakt) [L. *tractus*] 1. a region, principally one of some length; specifically, a collection or bundle of nerve fibers having the same origin, function, and termination.

2. a number of organs, arranged in series, subserving a common function.

traction (trak'shun) [L. *tractio*] the act of drawing or exerting a pulling force, as along the long axis of a structure. In orthopedics, traction is applied to an extremity with a fractured bone or dislocation to help reestablish and maintain normal position; in obstetrics, it is used to assist in delivery of the fetus.

tragi (tra'ji) [L., pl. of *tragus*] [NA], the hair growing on the pinna of the external ear, especially on the cartilaginous projection anterior to the meatus (tragus).

tragus (tra'gus), pl. *tragi* [L.; Gr. *tragos* goat] [NA], the small, curved, cartilaginous projection anterior to and partially covering the external auditory meatus.

trait (trāt) any genetically determined character. See also *character.*

tranquilizer (tran"kwĭ-līz'er) [L. *tranquillus* quiet, calm + *-ize* verb ending meaning to make + *-er* agent] a drug that acts to reduce anxiety, tension, or agitation without producing sedation or hypnosis. Also called *ataractic* and ataraxic.

major t., see *antipsychotic drug.*

minor t., see *antianxiety drug.*

trans- (trans, tranz) [L. "through"] 1. a prefix word element to denote through, across, or beyond, e.g., transection.

2. (*trans-*), a prefix word element in organic chemistry to designate the relative geometric positions of two substituent groups on different carbon atoms in a molecule. *Trans*-substituents on a double bond lie on opposite sides of a plane that contains the doubly-bound atoms and that is perpendicular to the plane of the molecule. In a compound containing a saturated ring, *trans*-substituents lie on opposite sides of a plane containing the atoms of the ring. Nonplanar rings (e.g., substituted cyclohexanes) are usually expressed in a planar conformation for the application of this definition. See also *isomerism.* Cf. *cis-*.

transaldolase (trans-al'do-lās) an enzyme of the transferase class (EC 2.2.1.2) that catalyzes the reaction sedoheptulose-7-phosphate + D-glyceraldehyde 3-phosphate ⇄ D-erythrose-4-phosphate + D-fructose-6-phosphate. Also called *aldotransferase* and *dihydroxyacetone-transferase.*

transaminase (trans-am'ĭ-nās) see *aminotransferase.*

transamination (trans"am-ĭ-na'shun) the enzymatically catalyzed transfer of an amino group from one carbon skeleton (amino acid) to another carbon skeleton (oxo acid) and vice versa. The enzymes involved are the aminotransferases, formerly called transaminases. See also *alanine aminotransferase* and *aspartate aminotransferase.*

trans configuration (trans con-fig"u-ra'-tion) the location of two alleles on different homologous chromosomes. Cf. *cis configuration.*

transcortin (trans-kor'tin) an α-globulin of serum; M.W. 52,000. It has a single cortisol binding site per molecule; the binding of cortisol with the protein ensures a ready source of available circulating hormone and protects it from inactivation. Transcortin also binds progesterone, deoxycorticosterone, corticosterone, and some but not all synthetic corticosteroid analogs (e.g., prednisolone). Transcortin is produced in the liver; its concentration is reduced in liver disease and nephrosis, and is elevated by thyroid hormone and estrogen. Also called *corticosteroid-binding globulin.*

transcript (tran′skript) [L. *transcriptum,* past participle of *transcribere* to copy] a sequence of RNA ready for posttranscriptional processing and/or translation.

transcription (tran-skrip′shun) the synthesis of RNA molecules from a DNA template. Genetic information contained in the DNA cannot act directly as a template for protein synthesis but must first be transcribed into messenger RNA (mRNA). In addition to mRNA, which makes up 5–10 percent of the total RNA, other RNAs are required for the very complex process of translating a four-base code into a sequence of 20 amino acids: ribosomal RNA (rRNA) and transfer RNA (tRNA), which account for 75–80 percent and 10–20 percent, respectively, of the rest of the cell's RNA. RNA is synthesized by the enzyme RNA polymerase. Generally, the rate of expression of a particular gene is controlled by the frequency with which RNA polymerase begins the transcription of that gene.

The transcripts synthesized by RNA often are not the final products utilized by the cell. To become functionally competent, the primary transcripts must be modified by a series of chemical alterations known as processing. There are three main types of modification in the processing of RNA: (1) the cleavage of large precursor RNAs into smaller RNAs; (2) the terminal addition of nucleotides to eukaryotic mRNAs with the addition of a poly A segment to the 3′ end and the "cap" nucleotides to the 5′ end; and (3) nucleotide modifications, such as methylation of the bases, common in tRNA and rRNA.

In Prokaryotes. Only one strand of DNA serves as a template. The RNA polymerase enzyme catalyzes the formation of RNA from the four ribonucleotide triphosphates (A, U, G, C) according to the Watson-Crick base-pairing rules. A complete molecule of RNA polymerase (holoenzyme) is formed from several polypeptides: two α-chains, 40,000 daltons; one β-chain, 155,000; one β'-chain, 165,000; one σ-chain, 95,000. The sigma (σ) factor is bound loosely to the rest of the enzyme and the $\beta\beta'\alpha_2$ is called the core polymerase. The factor is required for recognition of the correct initiation signals on DNA.

The start signals on DNA are called promoters. Promoters have AT-rich regions centered some 10 bases before the first base transcribed into mRNA. The binding of the sigma subunit of RNA polymerase to a promoter region leads to the local unwinding of the DNA helix; after the initiation of transcription, the sigma dissociates from the rest of the enzyme, which continues the process. The sigma can be used in the transcription of other RNA molecules. The binding of RNA polymerase to its promoter is a crucial step in the regulation of gene expression, as repressors can bind to specific sequences of DNA (operators) that overlap the promoter, turning off the expression of a given set of genes by preventing the binding of RNA polymerase.

Actual RNA synthesis starts with elongation. During elongation, RNA polymerase copies the DNA sequence of one strand proceeding in the $5' \rightarrow 3'$ direction (the same direction used in DNA replication and protein synthesis). The first nucleotide incorporated is always A or G.

Termination of transcription occurs when the RNA polymerase arrives at a stop signal on the DNA. A termination factor of rho (ρ) factor causes the release of the transcribed RNA molecules. Rho factor is a protein tetramer of 200,000 daltons. Isolated and purified rho has an ATPase activity that seems to be required for proper termination. The termination signal recognized by RNA polymerase on DNA is a GC-rich region followed by a series of AT residues.

The net result is the production of an RNA polynucleotide strand whose base sequence is complementary to that of the DNA from which it was transcribed. In prokaryotes, transcription is coupled to protein synthesis: as soon as mRNA transcription by RNA polymerase begins, the ribosomes become attached to the mRNA to initiate protein synthesis.

In Eukaryotes. Transcription in eukaryotes is more complex and is carried out by three RNA polymerases (I, II, III), each having between 6 and 10 protein subunits. The enzyme structure consists of two large and several small subunits, which are different for each enzyme type except for two small polypeptides of 19,000 and 29,000 daltons that are common to all three RNA polymerases. RNA polymerase I is located in the nucleolus, whereas polymerases II and III are localized in the nucleoplasm of the nucleus.

In addition to nuclear DNA, eukaryotic cells also contain DNA in the mitochondria and chloroplasts, which is transcribed by a different enzyme. Mitochondrial RNA polymerase is a simple enzyme formed by a single peptide.

In fully transcribing genes, RNA polymerases may be very close together, with one RNA chain completed every 10 sec. The nascent RNA becomes associated with proteins as it is being transcribed, producing ribonucleoprotein rather than free RNA. The processing of the initial transcripts into smaller RNAs can also begin before the RNA chains are completed.

In eukaryotes the nuclear envelope introduces a barrier between transcription and protein synthesis. The mRNA must be transported into the cytoplasm before it is translated.

See also *protein synthesis, RNA,* and *RNA polymerase.* Cf. *translation.*

inhibitors of t., substances that affect RNA production. The antibiotic actinomycin D inhibits RNA synthesis by intercalating between the DNA bases, especially in GC-rich regions, preventing RNA polymerase from functioning at these sites. Its action not only prevents the transcription of mRNA but also prevents the synthesis of rRNA and tRNA.

The antibiotic rifampin works by binding to bacterial RNA polymerase and inhibiting the initiation of transcription. Eukaryotic mitochondrial RNA polymerase is also sensitive to this drug, but because eukaryotic nuclear enzyme is not, the antibiotic can be used for medical treatment.

The mushroom toxin α-amanitin inhibits transcription in eukaryotes by inhibition of RNA polymerase II. Higher concentrations also inhibit RNA polymerase III, which inhibits rRNA synthesis.

transcription unit a sequence of genes transcribed at one time, e.g., the genes for the 18S and 28S rRNA arranged in tandem fashion along the DNA molecule. In this case, each transcription unit contains spacer regions interspersed between the 18S and 28S rRNA genes. These regions are transcribed into RNA that is later degraded.

transducer (trans-dūs′er) [L. *transducere* to lead across] any device that converts information or energy from one form to another, particularly a device that converts a physical effect, such as sound, light, temperature, or pressure, into an electric signal (or the reverse).

electroacoustic t., a transducer that converts electric signals to sound waves or vice versa. In diagnostic ultrasonography, the transducer uses a piezoelectric crystal, such as barium titanate or lead zirconate, to produce the ultrasound and to receive the echoes.

The transducer is held so that the acoustic lens, which focuses the sound produced by the crystal, is in contact with the body surface. The crystal emits short pulses of ultrasound and receives echoes during the interval between pulses.

See also the accompanying illustration.

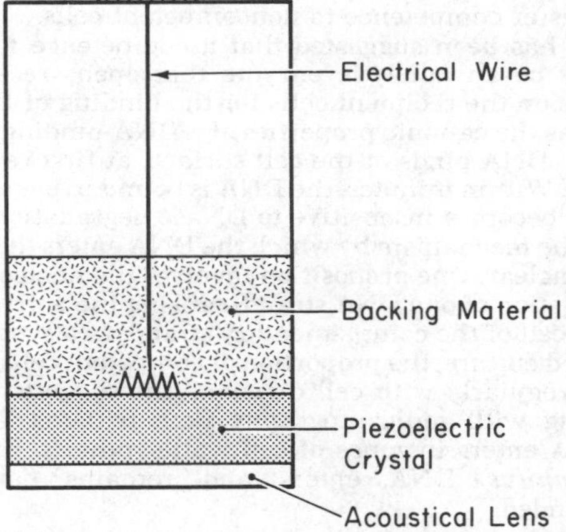

Electroacoustic transducer. Diagram of the probe housing the transducer crystal. (From Griffiths, H. J., and Sarno, R. C.: Contemporary Radiology. Philadelphia, W. B. Saunders Co., 1979.)

transduction (trans-duk′shun) [L. *transducere* to lead across] the transfer of bacterial genetic material from one cell (donor) to another (recipient), a process mediated by defective bacteriophage particles. A wide variety of bacterial viruses transduce bacterial DNA; transduction has been reported in a wide range of bacteria including *Escherichia, Salmonella, Shigella, Pseudomonas, Proteus, Bacillus, Klebsiella,* and *Staphylococcus.* The process of transduction can be used to map the bacterial chromosome, and two types are distinguished—generalized and specialized (restricted). See also *bacterial g.* under *genetics.*

generalized t., the transfer of any donor gene or plasmid contained within the donor. It is usually carried out with a high-titer phage lysate obtained either by lytic infection of the donor population or by induction of lysogenic cells. The lysate is used to infect the recipient cells.

During phage development in the donor cells, donor chromosomes are fragmented. As the phage matures, donor DNA fragments are packaged into the phage coat usually in place of phage DNA. When the donor cells lyse, the lysate is mixed with the recipient population, and the phage transfers the donor genes to the recipient cells. There must be a low multiplicity of infection (MOI < 1) so that cell lysis is prevented; it is unlikely that a phage will enter a cell already infected with a donor fragment. Although almost any gene may be transduced, only closely linked markers can be cotransduced by the same phage particle because the piece of bacterial DNA must fit inside the phage head and thus be similar in size to the phage DNA (i.e., approximately 1–2 percent of the bacterial DNA).

Although some transduced bacterial DNA segments become stably incorporated into the recipient cell chromosomes, many transduced fragments do not integrate into the host genome. Such abortive transductants are incapable of autonomous replication. Because they can be transcribed the genes may be expressed, but the markers are segregated to one daughter cell at each cell division, becoming diluted during cell growth.

specialized t., the transfer of genes from only a small region of the host chromosome adjacent to the prophage site. This type of transduction only occurs following induction of a lysogenic bacteriophage. The transduced genes are incorporated into the phage genome by abnormal excision of the prophage.

In a lysate from a normal lysogenic culture, only a very small proportion of the defective virions are transducing; thus, the lysate causes low-frequency transduction (LFT). The transducing virions differ from one another in the precise DNA replacements because they arise by independent recombination events.

Defective transducing particles can replicate in a mixed infection with a wild-type phage as a helper to complement the defective virions' missing functions. Both defective and normal phage genomes can integrate with the recipient chromosome to form a double lysogen. The cells then yield a high-frequency transduction (HFT) lysate, in which about half the particles are normal phage and half defective phage. In contrast to LFT lysates, HFT lysates contain a high proportion of identical transducing particles (with the exception of mutants).

transfection (trans-fek′shun) the uptake of intact double-stranded DNA extracted from a bacteriophage or plasmid by competent bacterial or mammalian cells. Infection with a helper phage or brief exposure to $CaCl_2$ can cause a transient change in cell permeability to allow entry of DNA in several genera of bacteria, including *Escherichia, Pseudomonas,* and *Proteus.* The DNA is usually precipitated with $CaPO_4$ for transfection of mammalian cells. This process is essentially the same as transformation, except for the route of entry of the DNA. See also *transformation.*

transfer (trans′fer) [*trans-* + L. *ferre* to carry] 1. the movement of information or a material substance from one place to another.

2. in a computer program, an instruction in an assembly language program (usually called a

branch or jump) or a statement in a high-level language program (often called a transfer of control) that causes some statement or instruction other than the next in sequence to be executed.

transferase (trans'fer-ās) any of a class of enzymes (EC 2) consisting of those that catalyze reactions not involving oxidation and reduction, in which a group containing C, N, P, or S is transferred from one substrate to another. Clinically important enzymes of the group include alanine aminotransferase (ALT), aspartate aminotransferase (AST), γ-glutamyltransferase (GGT), and ornithine carbamoyltransferase (OCT). This class includes enzymes variously known as transaminases, transketolases, transaldolases, transmethylases, transacetylases, glycosyltransferases, and phosphotransferases.

transfer factor a substance isolated from disrupted blood leukocytes that transfers delayed antigenic hypersensitivity from one individual to another. Transfer factor (M.W. <4000) is dialyzable and is inactivated by heat (56°C for 30 min) but not by trypsin, DNase, or RNase. Its exact chemical nature is unknown. Recipients become reactive to the antigen 1–7 da after receiving the extract; sensitivity can persist for years.

Clinical trials indicate that transfer factor may be effective therapeutically in patients with cell-mediated immune deficiencies. This is especially evident in some children with chronic mucocutaneous candidiasis: after receiving transfer factor from *Candida*-sensitive donors, *Candida* infections and skin lesions in some patients subside, and the recipients become skin test–positive. Nonspecific effects are sometimes observed, i.e., the recipients react to antigens to which the donor did not respond.

transfer factor of lungs for CO a more precise term for the diffusing capacity of the lungs for CO. In the presence of lung disease that produces a sizeable $\dot{V}/\dot{Q}$ imbalance, CO uptake is reduced, even in instances in which diffusion of CO is unimpaired. The uptake of CO in these instances is not an accurate test or measure of diffusion across the alveolar membrane, but is instead an overall index of the efficiency of gas exchange (i.e., a transfer factor for CO). See also *d. c. of the l. for carbon monoxide* under *diffusing capacity of the lungs.*

transfer function the relation between the input of a system and the output. See also *black box.*

transferrin (trans-fer'rin) [*trans-* + L. *ferrum* iron + *-in*] a single-chain serum β-globulin, a glycoprotein; M.W. 76,500. It contains 5.3 percent carbohydrate, which functions in the transport of iron from the intestinal tract to the sites of hemoglobin synthesis. Transferrin can bind two Fe^{3+} ions per molecule; up to 1.43 g of Fe can be bound per gram of transferrin. The usual serum concentration of transferrin is about 2–4 g/l, but only about one-third is saturated with iron. A number of genetic variants are recognized, as is a disease characterized by a congenital absence of transferrin. Also called iron-binding protein and siderophilin.

transferrin assays performed either by direct methods, such as nephelometry, radial immunodiffusion, or electroimmunodiffusion; or by indirect methods, such as total iron-binding capacity using colorimetric or radiometric procedures. The average concentration in plasma (serum) is about 290 mg/dl (about 30 μmol/l).

transferrin saturation the percentage or fraction of the total iron-binding protein of serum that is saturated with iron. See also under *iron-binding capacity.*

transfer RNA see under *ribonucleic acid.*

transformation (trans"for-ma'shun) [*trans-* + L. *formatio* a shaping] 1. a change of form or structure, a conversion from one form to another.

2. in oncology, the change undergone by a normal cell in becoming malignant.

3. in mathematics, a function that maps one set onto another set.

4. in genetics, a mode of bacterial genetic exchange in which a DNA fragment of one bacterial cell (donor) is transferred to another (recipient). Following uptake by the recipient cell, the incoming DNA undergoes recombination with the recipient chromosome. Many genera (including *Streptococcus, Staphylococcus, Hemophilus, Neisseria, Bacillus, Moraxella,* and *Acinetobacter*) have been shown to be capable of transformation.

Demonstrated first in *Streptococcus pneumoniae,* transformation is observed with double-stranded DNA fragments M.W. 10^5–10^7.

Cells that can take up DNA are said to be competent. The establishment of competence in a recipient cell appears to involve certain proteins called competence factors, which differ among genera. A competence factor of *S. pneumoniae* can activate noncompetent cells to become competent; a competence factor of *Bacillus subtilis* appears unable to transfer competence to noncompetent cells.

It has been suggested that a competence factor may be an autolytic enzyme that opens receptor sites on the recipient cells for the binding of DNA; it has the cationic properties of a DNA-binding protein. DNA binds at the cell surface, at first reversibly. Within minutes, the DNA is bound irreversibly and becomes insensitive to DNase degradation.

The mechanism by which the DNA enters the cell is unclear. One proposition involves the nucleolytic digestion of one DNA strand, causing the entry into the cell of the complementary strand. In a synchronized culture, the proportion of competent cells varies regularly with cell division; this suggests that, along with radioautography with tritiated DNA, DNA enters in zones of cell wall synthesis. In *Hemophilus,* DNA enters and remains double-stranded.

Recombination within the recipient cells occurs only if there are regions of homology between donor and recipient DNA; therefore, most transformations are intraspecific. A single-stranded fragment of recipient DNA is excised and replaced by transforming DNA, resulting in hybrid regions of DNA. Replication does not appear to be a prerequisite to recombination. Transformant cells can be detected by plating on media selective for certain donor markers.

Artificial transformation can be accomplished through modification of the cell envelope, first performed with spheroplasts, with calcium chloride to increase DNA permeability. Transformation in enteric bacteria has been achieved with this method.

See also *bacterial g.* under *genetics* and *transfection.*

transformation zone a term used by colposcopists to describe the area of squamous metaplasia and reserve cell hyperplasia between the ectocervical squamous mucosa and the endocervical columnar mucosa. It may be located entirely on the portio so that the entire squamocolumnar junction (SCJ) is visualized colposcopically, or it may also involve the endocervix, precluding satisfactory examination of the SCJ. See also *squamocolumnar junction.*

transformer (trans-for′mer) [*trans-* + L. *formere* to shape] an electric component used to change the voltage of alternating current. It essentially consists of two electromagnets coupled by mutual induction. Alternating current passes through the primary coil wound around an iron core, and produces an alternating magnetic field in the core. The magnetic field then produces alternating current in the secondary coil, also wound around the core.

The magnetic flux is proportional to the product of the voltage and the number of windings of coil, so that the ratio of the voltages in the two coils is the inverse of the ratio of the number of turns in the coils. Because the power is transferred through the transformer with only slight losses, the current ratio is proportional to the winding ratio. For example, if the voltage is stepped up by a factor of 10, the current is cut to 1/10.

step-down t., a transformer used to decrease the input voltage.

step-up t., a transformer used to increase the input voltage.

transfusion (trans-fu′zhun) [L. *transfusio,* from *trans-* + *fundere* to pour] the infusion of blood or blood components directly into the circulation of a recipient. Indications include replacement of red blood cells or restoration of blood volume; increasing the number of circulating platelets in individuals with thrombocytopenia; correction of deficiencies in coagulation factors; and increasing granulocyte counts in individuals with leukopenia. Components such as granulocytes and platelets must be prepared fresh, as they have a very short shelf-life. Certain coagulation factors can be given as fresh frozen plasma. Packed red cells can be preserved for several weeks as can whole blood.

autologous t., see under *autologous transfusion.*

coagulation factor t., the infusion of the coagulation factor or factors in plasma, plasma fractions, or concentrates necessary to correct deficiencies in those factors in order to achieve adequate hemostasis. Examples of factor replacement include the transfusion of fresh frozen plasma to correct Factor V deficiencies; the infusion of prothrombin complex to halt hemorrhage from Factor II, VIII, IX, and X deficiencies; and the transfusion of Factor VIII in the form of cryoprecipitate to arrest bleeding in individuals with hemophilia and von Willebrand's disease.

exchange t., a procedure performed as a treatment for hemolytic disease of the newborn. Fetal blood is withdrawn and replaced with blood not reacting with the maternal antibody present in the serum of newborns. To maximize the effect of the transfusion, donor blood should be free of hemoglobin S, less than 5 da old, and crossmatched with the mother's serum. Exchange transfusions have also been used successfully in treating renal failure, hepatic coma, thrombotic thrombocytopenic purpura, myasthenia gravis, and other disorders.

intrauterine t., the introduction of red blood cells in utero into the abdominal cavity of a fetus suffering from a severe case of hemolytic disease of the newborn. The volume of cells transfused should be adjusted to fetal size; the cells should be type O and compatible with the mother's serum. Once initiated, transfusions are usually repeated every 2 wk until delivery.

leukocyte t., the introduction of granulocytes directly into the circulation of a recipient. This procedure is indicated for patients on cytotoxic therapy for malignant neoplasms or for those with severe neutropenia who have infections that do not respond to antibiotics. Typing and matching for HLA characteristics may improve the efficacy of the transfusion and help to prevent the development of leukocyte antibodies, but it is seldom practicable.

massive t., the transfusion of a large amount of blood, approaching or even exceeding the patient's normal blood volume. This may result from surgical and medical emergencies and surgical procedures involving extracorporeal circulation. Problems associated with massive transfusion of banked blood include depletion of platelets and coagulation factors, thrombocytopenia, and a diminished ability of the cells to deliver oxygen because of low 2,3-DPG.

platelet t., the transfusion of platelet concentrates to prevent or stop the bleeding associated with thrombocytopenia and qualitative platelet disorders. Platelet concentrates are harvested from unrefrigerated fresh whole blood; preferably, the donor plasma should be ABO-compatible with the recipient's red cells.

transfusion reaction any adverse effect that occurs after the transfusion of blood or blood components. Reactions can occur in many forms and range from acute hemolytic reaction, which is the most severe (and life-threatening), to the relatively benign allergic reaction.

acute hemolytic t. r., a reaction to transfused blood that results in hemolysis of the donor red blood cells. Symptom onset occurs soon after or during the transfusion. Usually commencing with chills and fever, the symptoms may also include chest pain, nausea, hemoglobinuria, shock, flushing, and generalized bleeding. The life-threatening effects usually include shock, acute renal failure, and disseminated intravascular coagulation.

The reaction is initiated by the formation of an antigen-antibody complex. This complex activates Hageman factor (Factor XIIa), which induces the production of bradykinin. Bradykinin affects the vascular system, lowering the blood pressure by increasing capillary permeability and dilating the arterioles. The resulting hypotension stimulates the sympathetic nervous system to constrict the renal, splanchnic, pulmonary, and cutaneous vascular beds. Antigen-antibody complexes also activate the complement system, which induces mast cells to release histamine and 5-hydroxytryptamine (serotonin).

Coagulation may be initiated through the Hageman factor or it may be induced by circulating red cell stroma. This results in disseminated intravascular coagulation with consumption of many of the coagulation factors, the formation of microemboli, and, in some cases, uncontrolled bleeding. An acute hemolytic transfusion reaction is usually the result of ABO incompatibility, failure to recognize which most commonly results from a clerical error that leads to the transfusion of the wrong blood type. Extravascular destruction of red cells occurs more slowly and is more often observed in Rh incompatibility.

There are two tests that can be rapidly performed to confirm or rule out a suspected hemolytic reaction. After all labels and records have been carefully checked to ensure that the patient received the correct blood type, a sample of the patient's posttransfusion serum or plasma should be compared with a pretransfusion sample to detect obvious hemolysis. Simultaneously, a direct antiglobulin test should be performed on the posttransfusion sample and examined closely for agglutinated red cells.

If such a reaction has occurred, treatment of hypotension and maintenance of renal circulation are of paramount importance. If disseminated intravascular coagulation DIC occurs, heparin therapy may be indicated to induce intravascular clotting.

allergic t. r., a nonhemolytic reaction associated with transfusion and characterized by localized erythema, urticaria, and itching. It is suspected that this reaction is caused by allergy to some soluble product in the donor plasma; treatment consists of antihistamine administration.

anaphylactic t. r., an immediate reaction to the transfusion of very small quantities of blood or plasma. No fever ensues, but there is coughing, respiratory distress, nausea, diarrhea, vascular instability, shock, and unconsciousness. This reaction most commonly occurs in IgA-deficient patients having circulating anti-IgA antibodies.

Immediate treatment calls for stopping the transfusion and treating the hypotension with fluids and epinephrine. After diagnosis of IgA deficiency by immunoelectrophoresis, further transfusions must be performed only with IgA-deficient donor blood, deglycerolized blood, or autologous blood.

bacterial t. r., a rare, highly dangerous reaction caused by bacterial contamination of the donor blood, usually the result of endotoxins produced by cold-growing, gram-negative bacteria. It is characterized by fever, shock, hemoglobinuria, renal failure, and disseminated intravascular coagulation (DIC).

delayed hemolytic t. r., a reaction to transfused blood that results in hemolysis of the donor red blood cells and occurs from 1 da to several weeks after transfusion. There are two types of delayed reaction. The first is the result of primary alloimmunization to the transfused red cells. Usually occurring several weeks or more after transfusion, it may be diagnosed by an unexpected fall in hemoglobin, a positive direct antiglobulin test, or the appearance of a red cell alloantibody. The second and more severe type results from an anamnestic response to transfused red cell antigens. It usually occurs within 5 da of the transfusion and involves the destruction of large numbers of transfused cells. Clinical manifestations include fever, a fall in hemoglobin, and mild jaundice; rarely, there is renal involvement, which should be monitored. Treatment is seldom necessary.

febrile nonhemolytic t. r., a reaction associated with transfusion characterized by a rise in temperature ($>1°C$) without any evidence of hemolysis or red cell sensitization. The reaction appears to result from cytotoxic or agglutinating antibodies in the patient's plasma against lymphocytes, granulocytes, or platelets in the transfused blood.

Most commonly occurring in those who have had repeated transfusions or in multiparous females, the reaction is not dangerous and usually responds to antipyretics. The use of leukocyte-poor blood usually prevents a recurrence.

hemolytic t. r., the hemolysis of transfused red blood cells, a potentially life-threatening transfusion reaction that may lead to hemoglobinemia, hemoglobinuria, hypotension, disseminated intravascular coagulation (DIC), acute renal failure, and death. The hemolysis may occur immediately and intravascularly (due to complement fixation of the cells) or be delayed and extravascular (due to phagocytosis of antibody-sensitized red blood cells). In all cases of immediate hemolytic reaction, postreaction anticoagulated blood should be examined for hemolysis and a direct antiglobulin test performed. If the result is positive, a complete evaluation of the compatibility testing should be initiated.

transglutaminase (tranz″gloo-tam′in-ās) see *glutaminyl-peptide γ-glutamyltransferase.*

transient (tran′shent) [L. *transiens,* present participle of *transire* to go across] in electroencephalography, an isolated wave or complex that can be distinguished from background activity.

transient derepression the process of plasmid transfer regulation that initially enhances the spread of the plasmids but ultimately results in low frequency of transfer.

The initial recipient of the transfer lacks any repressor, and the transfer operon of the incoming plasmid is active, resulting in transient high-frequency transfer (Hft). Eventually, however, the recipient accumulates repressor, and low-frequency transfer results. See *p. transfer* under *plasmid* and *transfer o.* under *operon.*

transient hypogammaglobulinemia an immunologic deficiency of gamma globulins, which may extend beyond 18 mo of age. A physiologic temporary form occurs in normal infants at about 3 mo of age. Transient hypogammaglobulinemia is rare and probably results from an exaggerated tendency to physiologic hypogammaglobulinemia.

transient ischemic attack (TIA) a focal neurologic disturbance of sudden onset and brief duration (less than 24 hr); it is due to cerebral ischemia and resolves without permanent residual damage. The usual cause is occlusion of intracranial vessels either by emboli (from the heart or proximally situated atherosclerotic plaques) or thrombosis, or by reduced cerebral blood flow due to a fall in cardiac output. Attacks occur most commonly in the elderly and may precede a cerebrovascular accident (stroke).

Affected individuals may experience several to hundreds of attacks per year. Consciousness remains throughout the episodes, and symptoms depend on the region of the brain affected: for example, ischemia in the territory of the internal carotid artery may lead to unilateral (ipsilateral) blindness and contralateral hemiparesis, whereas vertebral-basilar artery insufficiency may result in confusion, vertigo, dysarthria, weakness, and other symptoms. Hypertension, diabetes, heart disease, atherosclerotic vascular disease, anemia, and polycythemia are predisposing factors.

Diagnosis rests on the patient's history and the findings on clinical examination. Angiography and ultrasound may help determine the degree of patency and amount of blood flow in the cerebral arteries. Treatment may involve anticoagulant or aspirin therapy, or surgery for localized and accessible atherosclerotic vascular disease.

transistor (tran-sis′tor) a three-terminal semiconductor device used as an amplifier or switch. Although it can be a discrete component, it is now more frequently manufactured as part of a single integrated circuit (IC) formed on a small silicon crystal chip, along with diodes, resistors, other transistors, and sometimes capacitors.

field effect t. (FET), a type of transistor that has a much higher input resistance than the junction transistor. Two of the terminals (called the source and drain) are connected by a narrow channel. The width of the channel (and thus its resistance) is controlled by the voltage applied to an adjacent region (called the gate) from which it is electrically insulated. Thus, the current from the source to the drain is controlled by the gate bias voltage. The FET basically functions as a voltage amplifier. It has higher input resistance and lower output resistance than a common emitter junction transistor amplifier, but has less voltage gain. Because of its high input impedance, it is used as the input stage for some high-quality operational amplifiers.

insulated gate field effect t. (IGFET), see *metal oxide semiconductor field effect t.*

junction t., the original and most common type of transistor, with two configurations: *npn* and *pnp.* The *npn* transistor consists of a very thin (1–10 μm) layer of lightly doped *p*-type semiconductor (called the base). This is sandwiched between two regions of *n*-type semiconductor, one heavily doped (the emitter) and one lightly doped (the collector).

The base-emitter junction operates like a diode; when it is forward-biased, the base current is proportional to the bias voltage. The collector-base junction is always reverse-biased; when the majority current carriers of the emitter (electrons) cross the base-emitter junction, only a few can combine with majority carriers in the base (holes) to become part of the base current; most, attracted by the high voltage applied to the collector, drift across the thin base region without combining, and become the collector current. The ratio of the collector current to the base current (called the current gain) is practically independent of the current and is a characteristic of the particular transistor (usually between 20 and 100).

A transistor thus functions basically as a current amplifier; a small change in the emitter current controls a large change in the collector current. The *pnp* transistor is identical to the *npn* transistor, except that the dopants (*n*-type and *p*-type), majority current carriers (holes and electrons), and bias voltage polarities are interchanged.

There are three transistor amplifier configurations—common emitter, common collector (also called emitter follower), and common base—named according to the terminal common to both the input and the output (the base is always one of the input leads and the collector one of the output leads). All three configurations provide power amplification, but only the common emitter provides both voltage and current amplification. It has moderate input and output resistance, and is used for typical amplifier stages and in digital logic circuits. The common collector has a voltage gain of less than one, high input resistance, and low output resistance. It is used as an input or output amplifier stage in order to match the impedance of the source or load. The common base has a current gain less than one, low input resistance, and high output resistance. It is used infrequently.

Also called bipolar junction t.

junction field effect t. (JFET), a type of field effect transistor in which the drain, source, and channel are a connected region of one type of doping (*n* or *p*) and the gate (two electrically connected regions on either side of the channel) is of the other type. The junction between the gate and the channel is always reverse-biased. As in a diode, an increase in the bias voltage widens the depletion layer. In the JFET, the depletion zones surrounding the gate regions constrict the channel and increase its resistance as they expand. The two doping configurations are called *n*-channel and *p*-channel JFETs. Also called junction-gate field effect t.

metal oxide semiconductor field effect t. (MOSFET), a type of field effect transistor in which the source and drain are two regions of one type of doping (*n* or *p*) diffused into a large substrate of the opposite-type material. The connecting channel may be doped like the drain and source but less heavily (a depletion mode MOSFET), or may be unchanged substrate (an enhancement mode MOSFET). The channel is covered with an oxidized layer of the semiconductor material, then a nitride layer, and then the metal gate. This insulating layer produces an input impedance of 10^9–$10^{14}\Omega$.

An *n*-channel MOSFET (of either mode) has *n*-type source and drain and *p*-type substrate. In a depletion mode MOSFET, a negative charge on the gate repels electrons (majority carriers in the source drain and channel) and decreases the current in the channel; a positive charge increases the current. In an enhancement mode MOSFET, a positive charge on the gate attracts electrons from the rest of the substrate into the channel (where they are in this case minority carriers) and increases the current in the channel; a negative charge stops conduction. A *p*-channel MOSFET is identical to an *n*-channel MOSFET except that the dopants and charges on the gate are reversed in polarity and that holes are the current carriers.

These transistors are widely used in computer memory circuits (MOS memory).

Also called insulated gate field effect t.

unijunction t. (UJT), a three-terminal semiconductor device used primarily in relaxation oscillators. Two terminals (base 1 and base 2) are connected by uniformly doped *n*-type material near the middle of which is implanted a probe of *p*-type material (the third terminal, called the emitter). A voltage is applied between the bases, and the emitter voltage is controlled by a charging capacitor. When the emitter-base 1 bias reaches a fraction η (the intrinsic standoff ratio, a parameter of the particular UJT) of the base-base voltage, the *pn*-junction becomes forward-biased and the emitter draws current, discharging the capacitor. The UJT exhibits negative-resistance behavior; the emitter current increases as the voltage decreases until the cutoff point is reached and conduction stops. The waveform at the emitter is a sawtooth.

transistor-transistor logic (TTL) the most widely used type of logic circuitry. TTL gates are integrated circuits (ICs) containing several junction transistors, which are operated either at saturation "full on" or in the off condition. The switching speed is therefore slower than that of emitter-coupled logic (ECL), which uses nonsaturating operation. TTL, however, is less complex and less expensive. See also *complementary metal oxide semiconductor logic.*

transition (tran-zish′un) [L. *transitio* a going across] 1. in molecular genetics, a point mutation that replaces a purine base with a purine base or a pyrimidine base with a pyrimidine base. Cf. *transversion.*

2. in quantum mechanics, a change from one energy state to another.

transitional cell papilloma an uncommon benign lesion of the bladder in which fronds of lamina propria are covered by histologically normal transitional epithelium.

transitional cell tumors neoplasms of urothelial cells arising in areas of the urinary tract lined by transitional epithelium (renal pelvis, ureter, bladder). A transitional cell type of cloacogenic carcinoma also occurs.

TRANSITIONAL CELL PAPILLOMA. This neoplasm is a benign papillary lesion of a urothelial surface in which the transitional epithelium covering the fronds is not more than six layers thick and shows normal maturation from base to surface. In some instances the lesion is reported to precede development of carcinoma. (Such neoplasms are only occasionally seen by the surgical pathologist, and some are fulgurated by cystoscopy.)

TRANSITIONAL CELL CARCINOMA IN SITU. This lesion involves the presence of focal or diffuse malignant cells within the confines of the urothelium; papillary lesions are usually excluded. The involved surface may appear normal by cystoscopy, or it can mimic acute or chronic cystitis because of inflammatory changes in the subjacent lamina propria. In histologic sections, the number of cell layers varies from normal to two or three times this number, the surface is irregular, and the epithelial cells display cytologic features of malignancy. The basal lamina is, by definition, intact. Attempts have been made to grade these in situ tumors, and it has been claimed that the grading has clinical relevance. Transitional cell carcinoma in situ may be the only finding on biopsy, but its presence should raise the possibility of the presence of occult invasive carcinoma.

TRANSITIONAL CELL CARCINOMA. This is a malignant neoplasm of urothelial cells, constituting more than 90 percent of tumors arising from surfaces clothed by transitional epithelium. The tumor may contain areas of squamous or adenocarcinomatous change. Most transitional cell carcinomas have a papillary configuration, but some are sessile lesions. Roughly 30 percent are invasive when diagnosed, and depth of infiltration, involvement of muscularis, and presence of lymphatic or vascular invasion are prognostic factors. The histologic grade is also significant: a three-grade scale based on the degree of cellular anaplasia and mitotic activity is commonly used. A four-grade system is also employed, but offers little advantage, as tumors that are grades 3 and 4 behave similarly. In one study with an 8-yr follow-up period, patients with grade 1 tumors had zero mortality, but the statistics rose to 50 percent mortality for those with grade 2 tumors and 90 percent for those with grade 3 and 4 carcinoma. Grade 1 tumors are rarely invasive when first detected, whereas 80 percent of grade 3 tumors show invasion. Chromosome and blood group antigen studies have been reported to have prognostic significance.

transitional epithelium a stratified epithelium composed of round cells that do not become flattened toward the surface, as do cells in a stratified squamous epithelium. Transitional epithelium is adapted to stretching and is found in the urinary passages (renal pelvis, ureter, bladder) and in a small band at the anorectal junction.

transition state in a one-step reaction, the state at the top of the potential energy profile leading from reactants to products. Multistep reactions can be treated as a series of one-step reactions with a transition state for each step. Also called activated complex.

transketolase (trans-ke′to-lās) an enzyme of the transferase class (EC 2.2.1.1) that catalyzes the reaction sedoheptulose-7-phosphate + D-glyceraldehyde-3-phosphate = D-ribose-5-phosphate + D-xylulose-5-phosphate. This enzyme is important in the metabolism of pentose phosphates and catalyzes the transfer of two-carbon units from one sugar to another, converting two pentose phosphates into a triose phosphate and a heptose phosphate. Also called *ketotransferase.*

transketolase assays determination of the transketolase enzyme activity in whole blood, used as an indirect measure of thiamine deficiency. In each of several methods that have been developed, a hemolyzed, buffered blood specimen is incubated with ribose-5-phosphate. In the Brin procedure, aliquots are removed at three intervals, and the ribose-5-phosphate is measured colorimetrically at 580 nm using the orcinol reagent. Sedoheptulose, a product of the reaction, also gives a color with some absorbance at 580 nm and maximal absorbance at 670 nm. The enzyme activity can be calculated using both readings and solving simultaneous equations.

In the Horecker procedure, the rate of formation of a product, glyceraldehyde-3-phosphate, is measured at 340 nm via conversion to dihydroxyacetone-phosphate and reduction to glycero-3-phosphate.

In other methods, the rate of formation of fructose (anthrone reaction) or sedoheptulose (reaction with cysteine and sulfuric acid) is measured. The enzyme requires thiamine pyrophosphate (TPP) for maximal activity. The reaction is carried out with and without added TPP. Any increase in activity over 25 percent (some authors claim >10 percent) with added TPP indicates vitamin B_1 deficiency in the red cells and in the patient.

translation (trans-la′shun) [*trans-* + L. *latus* carried] 1. a change of position.

2. the process of transforming a message or text encoded in one language or code into an equivalent message in another language or code. In computer science, this refers to the translation of a program from one computer language to another, as occurs in assembly or compilation.

3. protein synthesis; the formation of a peptide chain from individual amino acids, which involves four major steps: activation, initiation, elongation, and termination.

ACTIVATION. The first step in protein synthesis is the activation of the 20 different amino acids and their attachment to tRNA, which contains anticodons capable of complementary base-pairing with the codons of mRNA. More than 20 different aminoacyl-tRNA synthetases recognize the 20 amino acids (some amino acids have more than one tRNA), activate them with ATP to form AMP–amino acid complexes, and attach the activated amino acids to tRNA molecules that contain anticodons. Amino acid attachment occurs at the 3′ end of the tRNA to the base sequence, CCA-3′OH, by an ester linkage forming an aminoacyl-tRNA.

INITIATION. For protein synthesis to occur, an initiation complex of mRNA, large and small ribosomal subunits, and the initiator tRNA (fMet-tRNA in prokaryotes or Met-tRNA in eukaryotes) carrying the first amino acid must be made. The first amino acid in a prokaryotic peptide is *N*-formylmethionine; in eukaryotes the first amino acid is methionine.

In prokaryotes, three initiation factors (IF-1, IF-2, and IF-3) function catalytically to form the initiation complex at the expense of the hydrolysis of GTP. The initiation stage involves the formation of a complex consisting of 30S and 50S ribosomal subunits, mRNA, and the initiator tRNA with bound *N*-formylmethionine (fMet-$tRNA^{Met}$). The final product is the 70S initiation complex.

In the eukaryote, numerous factors are needed for assembly of the initiation complex. One molecule each of Met-tRNA, guanosine triphosphate (GTP), and eIF-2 (eukaryotic initiation factor 2) form a complex, which attaches to the 40S ribosomal subunit and eIF-3. Messenger RNA is then attached to the 40S complex by several additional initiation factors (eIF-4a, eIF-4d, eIF-1), and ATP is hydrolyzed by eIF-4. Formation of the completed 80S initiation complex is achieved by linking the 60 ribosomal subunit to the 40S complex, requiring hydrolysis of the GTP by 3IF-5. All initiation factors are displaced when the 80S complex is formed. Recent data suggest that the 7-methylguanosine caps of the 5′ end of mRNA play an important role in proper attachment of the mRNA to the initiation complex. Removal of the caps greatly reduces initiation.

ELONGATION. Growth of the peptide chain is referred to as elongation. In prokaryotes, each 70S ribosome has two sites for aminoacyl-tRNA attachment, called the A and P sites. At the beginning of elongation, the fMet-$tRNA^{Met}$ is at the P site, where it attaches during the initiation process. The initial attachment of all other amino acids occurs at the A site and is mediated by elongation factor (EF-Tu) and the hydrolysis of GTP.

The actual elongation begins with attachment at the A site of the second aminoacyl-tRNA. The anticodon of the tRNA is brought into proximity to the second codon of the mRNA. Peptide bond formation between the two amino acids is catalyzed by a peptide transferase. The new dipeptide remains attached at its carboxyl end to the tRNA that brought the second amino acid to the ribosome. This tRNA is then translocated to the P site, displacing the tRNA that had carried the *N*-formylmethionine. The translocation requires EF-G and the hydrolysis of GTP.

The tRNA carrying the next amino acid coded for the mRNA enters the A site, and the carboxyl end of the dipeptide is bonded to the free amino end of the amino acid. The tRNA moves to the P site, freeing the A site for the next aminoacyl-tRNA. This process continues until the chain reaches full length. The hydrolysis of the two GTP, EF-Tu, EF-G, and peptidyl transferase, plus EF-Ts, are required for each amino acid added to the chain.

In eukaryotes, EG-1 is needed to bind the aminoacyl-tRNA to the A site, and EF-2 is involved in the translocation of the tRNA to the P site. The hydrolysis of two GTP is still necessary. In eukaryotes, the actual assembly of the protein is similar to the assembly in prokaryotes.

TERMINATION. Termination of the chain occurs when a termination codon (UAA, UAG, or UGA) enters the A site. The completed peptide chain is released from the ribosome and the final tRNA to which it was attached by the presence of specific release factors (in prokaryotes) and the hydrolysis of GTP. Only one release factor (RF) has been identified in eukaryotes.

Nonsense mutations can convert an amino acid codon into a termination codon, resulting in an incomplete protein. Such mutations can also convert termination codons into amino acid–specifying codons, resulting in the formation of an abnormally long protein whose growth continues until the next termination codon is reached.

Also called *protein synthesis.* See also *inhibitors of t.* Cf. *transcription.*

inhibitors of t., substances that affect protein synthesis. The drug cycloheximide, which is active only in eukaryotic systems, binds to the 60S ribosomal subunit and blocks the process of chain elongation. It also inhibits peptide chain initiation.

The agent puromycin, active in both prokaryotic and eukaryotic systems, has a structure similar to the 3′ end of the aminoacyl-tRNA and binds to the A site of the large ribosomal subunit. The puromycin does not attach to the P site; no more amino acids are added. This results in the premature termination of the peptide chain. Vinca alkaloids and L-asparaginase interfere with the supply of amino acids.

Many antibiotics used for bacterial infections bind bacterial ribosomes: chloramphenicol, which blocks peptidyl transferase; streptomycin, which affects the initiation complex and prevents normal triplet recognition; and tetracycline, which blocks binding of aminoacyl-tRNAs.

Diphtheria toxin inhibits elongation in eukaryotes by catalyzing the transfer of part of NAD to EF-2, rendering it nonfunctional.

translation control RNA (tcRNA) a hypothesized special class of cytoplasmic RNA molecules believed to function in the control of message translation. Two types have been reported: the first is found in a particular initiation factor fraction and is claimed to inhibit translation of heterologous messages; the second type appears to affect the availability of messages for translation.

translator (trans′la-tor) in computer hardware, a computer circuit that translates information coded in one form into another code. The term is also used in computer software for a program that translates a high-level computer language into an intermediate-level computer language.

translocation (t) (trans″lo-ka′shun) [*trans-* + L. *locare* to place] in genetics, a chromosomal aberration caused by the transfer of a segment of one chromosome to a nonhomologous chromosome. The most common type is the reciprocal translocation in which the chromosomes exchange segments; this may be further classified as equal or unequal, referring to the length of the exchanged segments. Nonreciprocal translocations are less common. See also *reciprocal t.* and *robertsonian t.*

translocation factor a specific protein involved in

the movement of a ribosome along the messenger RNA during protein synthesis and coding. The enzymatic hydrolysis of guanosine triphosphate with the resultant dissociation of the translocation factor causes the conformational shift by which the ribosome moves.

translucent (trans-lu′sent) [trans- + L. *lucens* shining] permitting the passage of light but scattering it. Only diffuse light, not images, is transmitted. Cf. *opaque* and *transparent.*

transmandibular projection (trans″man-dib′u-lar) a radiographic projection of the jugular foramen through the ramus of the mandible. The central ray is angled 15°–20° medially and 25° cranially.

transmethylase (trans-meth′ĭ-lās) see *methyltransferase.*

transmethylation (trans″meth-ĭ-la′shun) the transfer of a methyl group (CH_3—) from one compound to another. Commonly, the methyl group donor is *S*-adenosylmethionine and the transfer reaction is enzyme-catalyzed.

transmissible (trans-mis′ĭ-b′l) 1. capable of being transmitted from one individual or one species to another.

2. in bacteriology, referring to a bacterial strain that is capable of causing a demonstrable infection in a given animal host.

transmission (trans-mish′un) [*trans-* + L. *missio* a sending] 1. the transfer, as of a disease, from one person to another.

2. the passing on of hereditary qualities from parent to offspring.

transmission electron microscope see under *electron microscope.*

transmission scan a procedure in nuclear medicine used primarily to delineate the silhouette of the body or an organ to provide anatomic markers for another procedure, such as heart blood pool scan, liver scan, or radionuclide cisternography. The method involves 140-keV gamma rays from a ^{99m}technetium flood source being passed through the patient and imaged by a scintillation camera (the detector is 1–2 m from the source). The images are similar to radiographs, but the resolution is much lower, and only objects adjacent to air are outlined. Unlike radiographs there is no magnification or distortion. When this procedure is used in conjunction with another, the two scans can be superimposed if the patient is not moved.

transmittance (T) (trans-mit′tans) [L. *transmittere* to send through] the ratio of the radiant energy transmitted through a medium to the total radiant energy incident on the medium.

peak t., the transmittance of a filter or other monochromator at the nominal wavelength (the wavelength with the maximum transmittance).

transmural (trans-mu′ral) [*trans-* + L. *muralis,* from *murus* wall] through the wall of an organ; extending through or affecting the entire thickness of the wall of an organ or cavity.

transmural pressure the force exerted against the inner (luminal) surface of the wall of a blood vessel, a duct, or any of the hollow viscera when measured relative to the ambient pressure at the outer surface; the difference in pressure across the wall.

transmutation (trans″mu-ta′shun) [*trans-* + L. *mutatio* change] a nuclear reaction in which one chemical element is changed into another; this occurs when matter is irradiated with heavy particles that are captured by nuclei.

transonic (tran-son′ik) in ultrasonography, pertaining to material that does not attentuate sound waves.

transoral projection (trans-or′al) [*trans-* + L. *os, oris* mouth] pertaining to a radiograph in which the parts of interest are projected through the open mouth. See also *open-mouth position.*

transorbital (trans-or′bĭ-tal) through the bony socket of the eye.

transorbital projection a radiographic projection used in cerebral angiography in which the central ray passes through the center of the orbit at a cranial inclination of 20°. Both posterior and posterior oblique (30°) views are employed.

transparent (trans-păr′ent) [trans- + L. *parere* to appear] permitting the passage of light with some absorption or reflection but little scattering, so that images are clearly transmitted. Cf. *opaque, radiolucent,* and *translucent.*

transphosphorylase (trans″fos-for′ĭ-lās) see *phosphotransferase.*

transplant (trans-plant′, trans′plant) 1. to transfer tissue from one part to another.

2. an organ or tissue taken from the body for grafting into another area of the same body or into another individual.

transplantation (trans″plan-ta′shun) [*trans-* + L. *plantare* to plant] the process in which diseased or damaged tissue and organs in an individual are replaced by healthy grafts taken from other parts of the same person's body or from other members of the same or different species.

Transplants are categorized as being autografts, isografts, allografts, and xenografts. Autografts represent a condition in which the transplant donor is also the transplant recipient, e.g., skin grafting in burn patients. Isografts or syngeneic grafts refer to a situation in which the donor and recipient are of identical genetic background, as is the case in tissue transplanted between identical twins or members of the same inbred animal strain. Isografts are very successful because they are genetically histocompatible and elicit no rejection response. Allografts are transplants exchanged between members of the same species but of different genetic make-up. This situation is nearly always encountered in the transplantation of tissues such as kidneys, heart, liver, and bone marrow; it provides the most formidable problem in transplantation, as genetic differences in tissue compatibility rapidly lead to the immunologic destruction of such grafts. Xenografts, the fourth type, are sometimes referred to as heterografts, and involve tissue transplants between individuals of different species, such as animal to human. These grafts always incite very strong rejection reactions and are used only as a short-term treatment procedure until suitable allografts can be found.

Immunocompetent individuals respond to the transplantation of foreign tissue by recognizing structures known as histocompatibility antigens. Histocompatibility antigens are glycoproteins and are present at various densities on nearly every cell of the body. Recognizing histocompatibility antigens on foreign grafts, recipient lymphocytes respond by producing antibodies and cytotoxic killer cells directed against the histocompatability antigens that are capable of attacking and destroying the foreign tissue. The strongest rejection responses are directed against antigens coded for by an area of the genome referred to as the major histocompatibility complex (MHC). The MHC in outbred populations is extremely polymorphic, and the chances of any two related individuals being identically histocompatible are astronomically low.

Critical for successful graft survival is provision of the potential organ recipient with the most closely matched donor allograph. To accomplish this task, a clinical laboratory test known as tissue typing is performed on all potential organ graft recipients and prospective donors. The test involves extracting lymphocytes from the peripheral blood of both recipient and donor in the case of living related kidney donors, or from the spleen or lymph nodes in the case of cadaver donors for kidneys and other organs. Lymphocytes are used because they are readily obtainable and possess the same histocompatibility antigens present on most body cells. The lymphocytes are incubated with a series of antibodies directed against known histocompatibility antigens followed by incubation with rabbit complement. Reaction of antibody with complement results in the lysis of the cell and its subsequent permeability to staining with various vital dyes such as trypan blue or eosin. Reactions are then read microscopically, and stained cells are matched with antibody specificities and the tissue type of the individual determined.

Computerized national and international registries are available for cadaver donor organs to be matched with the most suitable recipients. When an acceptable match is found, the kidney and a lymphocyte cell suspension are shipped to the particular center that has the best recipient, and a crossmatch is performed using donor cells and recipient lymphocytes. When a negative cytotoxic reaction indicates that the recipient possesses no antibodies to the donor kidney, the transplant is performed.

Sources of typing antibodies include previously transplanted patients who have rejected their kidneys and are thus sensitized to the previous graft antigens, multiparous females who have made antibodies to the paternal complement of antigens present in their fetuses, patients who have received multiple transfusions, and volunteers who have been injected with lymphocytes of known antigenic specificity. Typing sera is readily available to define antigenic specificities coded for at the A, B, and C alleles of the human MHC. A fourth locus, termed the D or MLR (mixed leukocyte reaction) locus, was classically defined by mixing two lymphocyte cell populations together in tissue culture. Incompatibility at the D locus resulted in the proliferation of lymphocytes measured by incorporating a radioactive label. Because this test requires up to 1 wk to perform, it is not practical for predicting cadaver donor compatibility. However, this test can be used for living related donors, usually family members of the recipient. Considerable evidence indicates that matching at the D locus is very important for graft success, and thus a great deal of current transplantation research is directed toward developing serologic methods for defining these specificities.

In addition to the major difficulty of finding compatible grafts, the technical problems must be considered, such as procurement, preparation, and long- or short-term storage of organs harvested from cadaver donors. Generally, organs are transplanted within 72 hr of procurement. Various methods have been devised to perfuse harvested organs to ensure that they are viable and well oxygenated.

Even with the best matching facilities, complete compatibility between donor and recipient is rarely achieved, both because of the extreme polymorphism of the major histocompatibility system and the lack of proper reagents to define completely all possible antigenic specificities coded for by genes within that complex. Because of these difficulties, the 1-yr graft survival rate for cadaver organs at most transplant centers ranges between 40 and 50 percent. Living related allografts, however, are extremely successful, and 1-yr survival rates of up to 90 percent are not uncommon.

In addition to proper matching for MHC antigens, the success of allografts depends on the continued use of immunosuppressive drug treatment. This is necessary because matching is rarely complete and because of the presence of numerous minor histocompatibility antigens that may result in a slow, chronic rejection of the grafted tissue. Most of these drugs work by inhibiting the development of immune effector cells. Such agents include alkylating agents (e.g., cytoxan), folic acid antagonists (e.g., aminopterin), and purine and pyrimidine analogs (e.g., azathioprine), as well as steroids and antilymphocyte serum.

Patients undergoing continued immunosuppression are in danger of developing a number of viral and fungal infections, as well as an increased susceptibility to certain reticuloendothelial malignancies.

See also *alloantigen, allograft, histocompatibility,* and *major histocompatibility complex.*

GARY FAGAN, B.S.

transplantation antigen an alloantigen on the surface of a nucleated cell that is responsible for the cell being recognized as foreign by a genetically different individual. It is important in the survival of tissue or organ grafts between allogeneic individuals. Transplantation antigens are analogous to major and minor histocompatibility antigens. Also called *histocompatibility antigen.* See also *histocompatibility, major histocompatibility complex, minor histocompatibility complex,* and *transplantation.*

transport (trans′port) [L. *transportare* to carry across] the movement of materials in biologic systems, particularly between organs, into and out of cells, and across epithelial layers. See also *active transport* and *passive transport.*

transport disease a group of diseases that result from inherited deficiencies of the proteins responsible for transporting substrate across cell membranes, chiefly involving the epithelial cells of the kidneys and intestine. Examples include certain of the aminoacidurias, familial vitamin D–resistant rickets, renal glycosuria, glucose-galactose malabsorption, and Fanconi's syndrome.

transport medium in bacteriology, a medium used for the transport of specimens from patient collection to the clinical laboratory. See also under *clinical bacteriologic specimens.*

transposable element a sequence of DNA capable of movement from one locus in the genome to another. These elements contain terminal direct or inverted repeat sequences (80–1700 bp), which are probably involved in the insertion mechanism. They can transfer genes from chromosomes to plasmids and thus, for example, enable resistance to antibiotics to be transferred between species of bacteria. See also *bacterial g.* under *genetics, insertion sequence,* and *transposon.*

transposition (trans″po-zish′un) [trans- + L. *positio* placement] 1. a change of position.

2. the exchange of position of two atoms within a molecule.

3. the operative procedure that involves moving a tissue flap from one position to another, severing the connection only after it is united at its new location.

4. the location of a viscus on the opposite side from normal.

5. the reversal of the position of the aorta and pulmonary trunk. Also called transposition of the great vessels.

6. the movement of a DNA sequence from one locus in the genome to another locus.

complete t. of great arteries, a congenital anomaly in which the aorta originates from the right ventricle and the pulmonary artery from the left—an arrangement incompatible with life. However, almost all affected infants have additional blood shunts to maintain circulation; these include ventricular septal defects, a patent ductus arteriosus, and a patent foramen ovale. Major signs include right ventricular hypertrophy, increased pulmonary blood flow, and cyanosis.

Diagnosis is made using clinical signs, electrocardiography, echocardiography, x-rays, and, most definitively, angiocardiography. Treatment is surgical, to redirect blood flow. The condition is fatal for a majority of such infants in the first year of life.

incomplete t. of great arteries, see *Taussig-Bing syndrome.*

transposon (tranz-po′zon) a type of transposable element, incapable of autonomous existence, that is responsible, for instance, for the transfer of bacterial genes for drug resistance. These DNA sequences transpose genetic material back and forth between cell chromosomes and smaller replicons such as plasmids. Also called *Tn element.* See also *bacterial g.* under *genetics, insertion sequence,* and *transposable element.*

transpulmonary pressure (P_L) the pressure difference across the lungs, equal to the difference between alveolar pressure and the pressure surrounding the alveoli (intrapleural pressure) at a given lung volume. The individual components of transpulmonary pressure are the pressures necessary to overcome the frictional resistance and elasticity of the lung-chest wall system. It is normally lower at the apex than at the base of the lung.

transpyloric plane (trans-pi-lor′ik) a horizontal plane passing midway between the upper border of the sternum and the upper border of the pubic symphysis, or roughly between the xiphisternal junction and the umbilicus. It separates the epigastric zone of the abdomen from the umbilical zone and passes through the pylorus, neck of the pancreas, hili of the kidneys, and lower border of the first lumbar vertebra. See also *Addison's planes.*

transsexualism (trans-sek′shu-ah-lizm) a disturbance of gender identity in which the person has an overwhelming desire to be of the opposite sex, often seeking hormonal and surgical treatment to achieve this goal.

transtubercular plane (trans″tu-ber′ku-lar) a transverse (horizontal) plane that passes midway between the transpyloric plane and the upper margin of the pubic symphysis (the center of the front of the pelvis). It divides the hypogastric zone of the abdomen from the umbilical zone and lies at about the level of the fifth lumbar vertebra. Alternatively, it has been defined as the transverse plane passing through the tubercles of the iliac crest. Also called *intertubercular plane.* See also *Addison's planes.*

transudate (trans′u-dāt) [*trans-* + L. *sudare* to sweat] an effusion of fluid into a serous cavity, produced by mechanical factors (osmotic or hydrostatic pressure), which influences the formation or resorption of fluid, e.g., decreased serum albumin levels, increased venous pressure, or both. The recommended laboratory criteria for distinguishing transudates from exudates vary with the type of serous cavity. For more information, see *pericardial fluid, peritoneal fluid,* and *pleural fluid.* Cf. *exudate.*

transudation (trans″u-da′shun) the process of forming a transudate. See also *transudate.*

transverse (trans-vers′) [L. *transversus*] placed crosswise, at right angles to the long axis.

transverse plane a horizontal plane through the body or a plane perpendicular to the axis of a structure.

transversion (trans-ver′zhun) in molecular genetics, a point mutation that replaces a purine base with a pyrimidine base or vice versa. Cf. *transition.*

tranylcypromine sulfate (tran″il-si′pro-mēn) [NF], an antidepressant; see under *monoamine oxidase inhibitors.*

trauma (traw′mah), pl. *traumas* or *traumata* [L., from Gr.] a wound or injury, especially damage produced by external force.

Treacher Collins syndrome [Treacher *Collins,* English ophthalmologist, 1862–1932] a congenital malformation, transmitted as an autosomal dominant trait, that involves abnormalities of the first branchial arch. Characteristics of the syndrome include malar hypoplasia with antimongoloid obliquity of the palpebral fissures; defects of the lower eyelid, including coloboma; hypoplasia of the mandible; and ear deformities. The abnormality may be caused by insufficient migration of the neural crest cells of the first arch. Treatment involves regional reconstructive surgery. Also called *mandibulofacial dysostosis.* See also *first arch syndrome.*

trehalose (tre-ha′lōs) a nonreducing disaccharide, α-D-glucopyranosyl-α-D-glucopyranoside, that serves as the storage and transport fuel in insects. Trehalose also occurs esterified with mycolic acids as the cord factor of *Mycobacterium tuberculosis.*

trematode (trem′ah-tōd) [Gr. *trēmatōdēs* having holes, from *trēma* hole + *eidos* form] an individual of the class Trematoda. This class includes all the flukes that are parasitic in humans. Medically important trematodes include the genera *Schistosoma, Echinostoma, Fasciolopsis, Clonorchis, Fasciola, Opisthorchis,* and *Paragonimus.*

tremor (trem′or, tre′mor) [L., from *tremere* to shake] an involuntary, regular oscillation of a body part due to rhythmic contractions of opposing muscle groups. The distal parts of the limbs and head are the body parts most commonly affected. Tremor is classified according to rate, rhythm, and distribution. Rapid fine tremor occurs at 8–10 oscillations/sec, whereas coarse slow tremor occurs at 3–5 oscillations/sec. Tremor may be further classified as intentional (arising during or increased by voluntary movement), rest (present during rest and decreasing during movement), and static (occurring while the position of a body part fixed without support is maintained).

Diverse etiologies may produce tremor. Physiologic tremor may appear in normal persons as the result of hunger, exercise, chills, or excitement, or it may be present in an inherited pattern or in old age without associated disorder (benign essential and senile tremors). Diseases affecting the cerebellum and its connections (e.g., Friedreich's ataxia, mercury intoxication) usually produce intention tremor or action tremor. Diseases that affect the basal ganglia and their connections usually produce a coarse slow tremor, which is most noticeable at rest (e.g., parkinsonism).

trench fever (trench' fe'ver) a self-limiting febrile disease due to infection with *Rickettsia* (*Rochalimaea*) *quintana* and transmitted to humans by the body louse. It was formerly quite common in military populations and wartime civilians, and is currently endemic in Central America. Following an incubation period of 2–4 wk, fever, headache, weakness, and leg and back pains occur. A transient maculopapular rash and hepatosplenomegaly may be noted. Multiple relapses are to be expected.

R. quintana is the only rickettsia that can be cultured on artificial media without living cells (blood agar and 10 percent fresh blood). Diagnosis is aided by complement-fixation, hemagglutination, and immunofluorescent tests; the Weil-Felix reaction is negative. Xenodiagnosis is a useful diagnostic aid. The patient generally recovers without treatment.

Also called His-Werner disease, quintan fever, shin bone fever, and Wolhynia fever. See also *Rickettsiaceae.*

trench foot see *immersion syndrome.*

trench mouth see *fusospirochetosis.*

Trendelenburg position (tren-del'en-burg) [Friedrich *Trendelenburg,* German surgeon, 1844–1924] any recumbent position (usually supine or prone) in which the table is tilted so that the head is lower than the pelvis. The angle of tilt is usually specified; the full Trendelenburg position is at a 45° angle.

Treponema (trep"o-ne'mah) [Gr. *trepein* to turn + *nēma* thread] a genus of bacteria belonging to the order of Spirochaetales, family Spirochaetaceae. These bacteria are characterized as gram-negative, microaerophilic, spirochete-shaped microorganisms that exhibit motility with a flexing, bending, snapping motion, and divide by transverse fission. The outer surfaces of *Treponema* have polar flagella or axial filaments that wind around the microorganism.

Nonpathogenic species of *Treponema* may be found in the oral, intestinal, and genital mucosa. There are three pathogenic species of *Treponema: T. pallidum,* which causes syphilis; *T. pertenue,* which causes yaws; and *T. carateum,* which causes pinta. All species are susceptible to penicillin and are immunologically cross-related, so that infection with one (e.g., *T. pertenue*) produces protective antibodies to another (in this instance, *T. pallidum*).

Because *Treponema* species cannot be grown in culture, diagnosis must be made by clinical observations, darkfield microscopy, and serologic methods. *Treponema* infections are chronic, with an early stage lasting 2 yr followed by later stages; asymptomatic periods are common.

See also *spirochetes.*

T. carateum, the species that is the etiologic agent of pinta. See also *pinta.*

T. pallidum, the species that is the etiologic agent of both venereal and nonvenereal syphilis in humans. See also *syphilis.*

T. pertenue, the species that is the etiologic agent of yaws in humans. See also *yaws.*

***Treponema pallidum* immobilization (TPI) test** a specific immunologic test for the identification of *Treponema pallidum,* the causative agent of syphilis. The procedure involves incubating a live, motile, and virulent strain (Nichol strain) of syphilitic spirochetes with the patient's serum and complement. If the serum contains specific antisyphilitic antibody, it will combine with the spirochetes. The organisms become immobilized and die. This loss of motility is observed under the darkfield microscope: a positive reaction means no motility is seen. A negative reaction means motility of the organisms is observed; other *Treponema* spirochetal diseases (e.g., yaws) may give positive reactions. The primary disadvantages of this test are that it is expensive, it is difficult to perform accurately, live spirochetes must be used, and an animal colony is necessary. Because of these drawbacks, the TPI test is not suitable for routine use by most laboratories.

treponematosis (trep"o-ne-mah-to'sis) any infection with the genus *Treponema.*

trepopnea (trep"op-ne'ah) [Gr. *trepein* to turn + *pnoia* breath] a condition in which respiration is more comfortable with the individual turned in a definite recumbent position.

treppe (trep'ĕ) [Ger. "staircase"] see *staircase phenomenon.*

-tresia (tre'ze-ah) [Gr. *trēsis* perforation] a suffix word element to denote an opening, e.g., atresia.

TRF abbrev. See *T-cell replacing factor.*

TRH abbrev. See *thyrotropin-releasing hormone.*

TRH stimulation test see *thyrotropin-releasing hormone stimulation test.*

tri- (tri) [L. or Gr. *tri-*] a prefix word element to denote three, e.g., trigone.

T_3(RIA) see under *triiodothyronine assays.*

T_4(RIA) abbrev. for serum thyroxine (T_4) measured by radioimmunoassay. See under *thyroxine assays.*

triac (tri'ak) a three-terminal semiconductor device that is equivalent to two silicon-controlled rectifiers connected in parallel in reversed directions with the gates wired together. When a positive pulse is applied to the gate, it conducts in either direction until the applied voltage drops to zero.

triacetin (tri-as'ĕ-tin) triacetylglycerol, used as a solvent and topical antifungal agent.

triacetyloleandomycin (tri"as-ĕ-til-o"le-an-do-mi'sin) one of the macrolide group of antibiotics. See also *antibacterial agents* and *macrolides.*

triacylglycerol (tri-as"il-glis'er-ol) the systematic name for triglyceride.

triacylglycerol lipase an enzyme of the esterase class (triacylglycerol acylhydrolase, EC 3.1.1.3) that catalyzes the reaction triacylglycerol + $H_2O \rightleftarrows$ diacylglycerol + a fatty acid anion. The reaction is important in the metabolism of dietary fats. Serum lipase determination is used in the clinical diagnosis of pancreatic disorders. See also *lipase.*

triage (tre-ahzh') [Fr. "sorting"] a procedure that involves the sorting out and classification of injured or acutely or severely ill patients, undertaken at a hospital emergency room or a military advanced station hospital or during other disaster situations in order to determine priority of need and the proper place of treatment.

triamcinolone (tri″am-sin'o-lōn) [USP], a synthetic antiinflammatory corticosteroid (9α-fluoro-16α-hydroxyprednisolone), a potent glucocorticoid with no mineralocorticoid activity. See also *corticosteroid.*

triamterene (tri-am'ter-ēn) [USP], a diuretic that reduces the reabsorption of sodium and water in the distal tubules of the kidney and does not cause potassium depletion. It is used to treat hypertension and edema resulting from congestive heart failure. Trademark, *Dyrenium.*

triangle (tri'ang-g'l) [*tri-* + L. *angulus* angle] 1. a three-cornered area, figure, or object.

2. in mathematics, a three-sided polygon, a figure with three straight sides.

triangular (tri-ang'gu-lar) [L. *triangularis*] having the shape of a triangle, or having three angles or corners. See also the illustration accompanying *contour.*

Triatoma (tri-at'o-mah) a genus of bloodsucking bugs. Several species are known vectors of *Trypanosoma cruzi* (which causes Chagas' disease) in Mexico, Central and South America, and the United States. Also called *assassin bug, cone-nosed bug, kissing bug,* and *Mexican bedbug.*

Triatomidae (tri″ah-to'mĭ-de) a family of bugs that includes the genus *Triatoma* (a known vector of *Trypanosoma curzi*).

tribasic acid an acid that contains three replaceable hydrogen atoms, e.g., H_3PO_4.

tribe (trīb) [L. *tribus*] a taxonomic group of organisms within a family; it may be further subdivided into genera. See also *taxonomy.*

tricarboxylic acid (tri″car-bok-sil'ik) an acid with three carboxyl groups, most commonly citric acid.

tricarboxylic acid (TCA) cycle a part of the aerobic oxidation of fuels that require the participation of two other metabolically interrelated processes, namely, electron transport and oxidative phosphorylation. All these processes occur in mitochondria. The TCA cycle consists of the cyclic metabolic mechanism by which the complete oxidation of the acetyl moiety (two-carbon fraction) of acetyl coenzyme A (CoA) is effected. The acetyl CoA is derived from the major fuels (e.g., amino acids, carbohydrates, and fats). The oxidation of the acetyl groups to CO_2 and H_2O accounts for roughly two-thirds of the total oxygen consumption and ATP production in most animals.

The cycle begins with the condensation of acetyl CoA with oxaloacetate to produce citrate and CoASH. The citrate undergoes a series of discrete oxidative steps, producing CO_2, the generation of reducing equivalents (electrons) as NADH + H^+ and $FADH_2$, and the regeneration of oxaloacetate. The transfer of the electrons via the mitochondrial electron transport chain to molecular O_2 results in the formation of high-energy phosphate bonds as ATP and the production of H_2O. The sum of all the reactions of the cycle itself adds up to the formal stoichiometry: acetyl CoA + 3 NAD^+ + FAD + GDP + P_i + 2 $H_2O \rightarrow$ 2 CO_2 + 3 NADH + 2 H^+ + $FADH_2$ + GTP + CoA.

In addition to its catabolic role, the TCA cycle is utilized for anabolic purposes (e.g., α-ketoglutarate, a TCA cycle intermediate, is a direct precursor of the amino acid L-glutamate).

Also called *citric acid cycle* and *Krebs' cycle.*

Tricercomonas (tri″ser-kom'o-nas) a genus of protozoa now called *Enteromonas;* the species *T. intestinalis* is now called *E. hominis.*

trich/o (trik'o) [Gr. *thrix, trichos* hair] a word element used in combining form to denote the hair, e.g., trichobezoar.

Trichinella (trik″ĭ-nel'ah) [Gr. *trichinos* of hair] a genus of nematode parasites of the superfamily Trichuroidea.

T. spiralis, a tissue-inhabiting nematode that causes trichinosis. *T. spiralis* is a white roundworm; the adult male measures 1.4–1.6 mm long by 40–60 μm wide; the female, 3–4 mm long by 60–90 μm wide.

Infection is caused by ingestion of uncooked or undercooked pork or pork products contaminated with encysted larvae. These larvae are liberated upon digestion of the cyst in the digestive tract, and penetrate the upper intestine, where the parasites mature and mate. The females penetrate the mucosa and liberate larvae, which are carried via the blood stream to muscles or various tissues that they then penetrate.

Also called *pork worm.* See also *trichinosis.*

trichinosis (trik″ĭ-no'sis) a disease caused by the presence of *Trichinella spiralis,* the trichina worm. Trichinosis is distributed worldwide wherever pork or pork products are eaten. Occasionally, an outbreak appears to be associated with the eating of walrus or bear meat. Human infection is acquired by ingestion of undercooked pork contaminated with larvae encysted in the muscles. Once in the small intestine, the larvae excyst, penetrate the duodenal epithelium, and mature. The adult female becomes fertilized and invades the intestinal mucosa to produce new larvae. If large numbers of larvae are produced, they enter the blood stream and invade various other tissues and body cavities. Only those reaching skeletal muscle develop and become encysted.

Trichinosis causes localized inflammation and necrosis in muscle. In severe cases the myocardium may be damaged, resulting in cellular infiltration and necrosis. The disease may be fatal owing to toxemia, secondary pneumonia, and myocardial failure.

Clinical characteristics are generally divided into several stages. Following ingestion of viable larvae, individuals commonly experience fever, gastrointestinal symptoms, muscle swelling, and eosinophilia. Once muscle penetration begins, there is also edema, an irregular fever, and myositis. It is during this stage that the eosinophil count usually is markedly increased. Serum transaminases are elevated in the invasive stage. The last stage is characterized by neurotoxic symptoms and occasionally myocarditis.

Diagnosis is dependent on a history of consumption of raw pork or pork products, and on immunodiagnostic tests and demonstration of the parasite in muscle biopsy (or spinal fluid when there is heavy infection). Some of the immunodiagnostic tests available include intradermal, complement-fixation, bentonite flocculation, indirect hemagglutination, latex, indirect fluorescent antibody, and precipitin tests.

See also *T. spiralis* under *Trichinella.*

trichlorfon (tri-klōr′fon) a moderately toxic organophosphate insecticide, *O,O*-dimethyl 2,2,2-trichloro-1-hydroxyethylphosphonate. See also *organophosphate compounds.*

trichlormethiazide (tri-klōr″mĕ-thi′ah-zīd) [USP], see under *thiazide diuretics.*

trichloroacetic acid (TCA) (tri-klo″ro-ah-se′tik) a hygroscopic, crystalline substance, CCl_3COOH; M.W. 163.38. TCA is a strong acid with a pungent odor, used in analytic procedures to precipitate proteins. It is a strong irritant, highly toxic when ingested or inhaled, corrosive, capable of causing severe skin burns.

1,1,1-trichloroethane (tri″klo-ro-eth′ān) a colorless, nonflammable liquid, CH_3CCl_3, widely used as a solvent and degreasing agent; M.W. 133.42. It is less toxic than most other chlorinated hydrocarbons, but it is irritating to the eyes and mucous membranes and causes narcosis at high concentrations. Also called *methyl chloroform.*

1,1,2-trichloroethane an isomer of 1,1,1-trichloroethane, with similar properties. It is used less widely, however, because it is more toxic, especially to the liver and kidneys. Also called *vinyl trichloride.*

trichloroethanol (tri″klo-ro-eth′ah-nol) a viscous, flammable liquid with an ethereal odor, CCl_3CH_2OH; M.W. 149.42. It is a metabolite of chloral hydrate, which has been used as a hypnotic and sedative.

trichloroethylene (tri″klo-ro-eth′ĭ-lēn) a nonflammable, colorless liquid, $CHCl{=}CCl_2$, formerly used as an inhalation anesthetic. It is widely employed as a solvent and degreasing agent. Also called *acetylene trichloride.*

(2,4,5-trichlorophenoxy)acetic acid (tri-klo″ro-phen-ok″se-ah-se′tik) see *2,4,5-T.*

Trichobilharzia (trik″o-bil-har′ze-ah) a genus of flukes that are parasitic in birds and whose cercariae cause schistosome dermatitis.

trichocephaliasis (trik″o-sef″ah-li′ah-sis) see *trichuriasis.*

trichochrome (trik′o-krōm) [*tricho-* + Gr. *chrōma* color] a brilliant red, melanin-type polymer. Trichochromes have a relatively lower molecular weight than do the eumelanins and pheomelanins, and also contain sulfur. They are probably of less importance than pheomelanins in the pigmentation of red hair. See also *melanin.*

trichoepithelioma (trik″o-ep″ĭ-the-le-o′mah) a nodular benign skin lesion usually affecting the face and commonly seen in adolescents. It is typically multiple, but occasionally solitary. The tumor shows differentiation toward cells of the hair follicle. Histologically, horn cysts of varying size are present in the dermis, together with islands of cells similar to those seen in basal cell carcinoma. Also called *epithelioma adenoides cysticum.*

Trichomonas (trik″o-mo′nus) [*tricho-* + Gr. *monas* unit] a genus of flagellate protozoa. The trophozoites are pear-shaped, possessing four free anterior flagella and a fifth one that parallels the body along the outer surface of the undulating membrane. Three species occur in humans: *T. hominis, T. tenax,* and *T. vaginalis.*

T. hominis, a nonpathogenic species commonly found in the human intestines. The trophozoites measure 7–15 μ long and move rapidly in a nondirectional motion. Filth and flies transmit these organisms. Humans may ingest the trophic forms in contaminated food or drink.

Identification is made from fecal films by observing the characteristic wavelike movements of the undulating membrane and an axostyle protruding through the posterior portion of the body.

Also called *T. confusa* and *Tritrichomonas hominis.*

T. tenax, a nonpathogenic commensal of the human mouth, which lives in the tartar of the teeth, in cavities, or in necrotic mucosal cells. It is a small organism, measuring 6–10 μ long. Also called *T. buccalis, T. elongata, T. hominis,* and *Tetratrichomonas buccalis.*

T. vaginalis, a species found in the vagina and prostate gland of humans. The organism is found only as a trophozoite, measuring 12–26 μ long. *T. vaginalis* is transmitted (as a trophozoite) during sexual intercourse. In females, infections cause a profuse vaginal discharge, associated with burning, itching, or chafing. In males, the infection is usually asymptomatic.

Laboratory diagnosis requires identification of the trichomonads in wet film preparations from a vaginal swab or from urethral discharge (in males). The organism is a characteristic motile, pear-shaped flagellate. *T. vaginalis* may also be seen during urinary sediment examination.

See also *vaginitis.*

trichomoniasis (trik″o-mo-ni′ah-sis) an infection with flagellate protozoa of the genus *Trichomonas.* See also *vaginitis.*

trichomycosis (trik″o-mi-ko′sis) [*tricho-* + Gr. *mykēs* fungus] any disease of the hair due to infection by a fungus.

t. axillaris, a disease characterized by small, soft nodules of different colors (red, yellow, or black), on the affected hair shafts in the axillary and pubic areas. The causative organism has long been mistaken for a fungus; it is now believed to be *Nocardia*-like bacteria.

Trichophyton (tri-kof′ĭ-ton) [*tricho-* + Gr. *phyton* plant] a genus of fungi belonging to the family Moniliaceae, order Moniliales. Its perfect stage is *Arthroderma.* Trichophyton is considered to be a dermatophyte in that it infects the hair, skin, and nails. When the hair is infected with *Trichophyton,* arthrospores may be found within (endothrix) or outside (ectothrix) the hair shaft; when the skin or nails are infected, branching, segmented mycelial elements may be seen, which are similar to *Microsporum* and *Epidermophyton.* See also the accompanying table.

T. concentricum, a fungus that causes tinea imbricata, a disease characterized by a series of concentrically located rings of a papular and scaly nature involving the stratum corneum of hairless (glabrous) skin. *T. concentricum* is geographically distributed in Asia, the Pacific, and South America.

TRICHOPHYTON. DIFFERENTIAL CHARACTERISTICS OF SOME *Trichophyton* SPECIES

ORGANISM	COLONY MORPHOLOGY	MICROSCOPIC MORPHOLOGY	PHYSIOLOGIC CHARACTERISTICS
Trichophyton mentagrophytes	Flat, cream or yellowish powdery colony; concentric rings may be present	Small, spherical grape-like microconidia; coiled spirals; cigar-shaped macroconidia may be present	Hydrolysis of urea in 48 hours
T. rubrum	Fluffy, white colony with deep red pigment on the undersurface	Long strands of hyphae with lateral, tear-shaped microconidia; arthroconidia; pencil-shaped macroconidia	
T. tonsurans	Flat, powdery, tan, brown or red colony; undersurface of the colony may be yellow to tan	Abundant microconidia, club- or balloon-shaped. Many arthroconidia; spiral coils may be present. Blunt, thick-walled macroconidia may be present	Requires thiamine

Modified from Treagan, L., and Pulliam, L.: Medical Microbiology Laboratory Procedures. Philadelphia, W. B. Saunders Co., 1982, p. 127.

The colony morphology is deeply folded and convoluted; it is white at first, turning brown or red with time, and has a fuzzy growth. Microscopically, convoluted hyphae without spores and branching mycelia are seen.

T. gourvilii, a dermatophytic fungus that causes an inflammatory scarring and ringworm of the scalp with an endothrix invasion of the hair and hair follicles. *T. gourvilii* is endemic in West Africa. The colony morphology is heaped and waxy, and pink to red in color. It is similar microscopically to other *Trichophyton* species, but does not require histidine and thiamine for growth.

T. mentagrophytes, a medium-size–spored ectothrix species that causes infections of the hair, skin, and nails. The zoophilic variety, *T. mentagrophytes mentagoaphytes,* invades the hair follicles, causing an extremely inflammatory infection; it has a granular appearance in culture. The anthropophilic variety, *T. mentagrophytes interdigitale,* causes tinea pedis, a chronic infection of the foot; it is more downy in culture and produces fewer conidia.

T. rubrum, a dermatophytic fungus that can cause tinea corporis, tinea cruris, tinea manus, tinea pedis, and tinea unguium. *T. rubrum* is the most common dermatophyte occurring in humans, and results in a psoriasis-like lesion of smooth skin. The colony morphology appears downy-white on the surface, usually lacking spores; the reverse side of the colony is red. Microscopically, teardrop-shaped microaleuriospores are seen clustered in a "pine tree" arrangement.

T. simii, a dermatophytic fungus that causes ringworm in monkeys and chickens. Infection in humans is uncommon and results in an ecto/endothrix type of hair invasion; it is commonly isolated from soil. The perfect state of *Trichophyton simii* is *Arthroderma simii.* The colony morphology appears flat and granular, and creamy to white on the surface, while the undersurface of the colony is often red. Microscopically, fusiform macroaleuriospores are seen with 4–10 septa.

T. verrucosum, a dermatophytic fungus that can cause tinea barbae and tinea corporis in humans and tinea in cattle. *T. verrucosum* causes an ectothrix infection of hair and hair follicles. The colony morphology is knoblike, heaped, and gray-white or yellow in color. Microscopically, distorted hyphae are noted with antlerlike branching. No spores are seen.

T. violaceum, a dermatophytic fungus that causes black dot endothrix infection on both the scalp and smooth skin. *T. violaceum* is an anthropophilic fungus endemic in South America, Mexico, Europe, Asia, Africa, and occasionally the United States. The colony morphology appears faviform, waxy, and deep violet in color; the underside of the colony is purple. Microscopically, the hyphae are distorted, and aleuriospores are often lacking. The hyphae contain cytoplasmic granules.

Trichoprosopon (trik″o-prŏ-so′pon) [*tricho* + Gr. *prosōpon* face] a genus of mosquitoes. The species *T. frontosum* is believed to be involved in the transmission of yellow fever among humans in Europe and North Africa.

Trichosporon (trik-kos′po-ron) [*tricho-* + Gr. *sporos* seed] a genus of fungi that belongs to the family Cryptococcaceae, order Moniliales; it is characterized by hyphae, pseudohyphae, blastoconidia, and arthroconidia, and rapid growth at 37°C. Its perfect stage is being associated with Basidiomycetes. It can cause white piedra (superficial nodules on distal hair shafts) or mucous membrane infections. Medically, the most important species is *T. beigelii,* which is the etiologic agent of white piedra.

trichostrongyliasis (trik″o-stron″jĭ-li′ah-sis) an infection caused by intestinal nematodes of the genus

5′-monodeiodination of T_4 in the peripheral tissues. T_4 and T_3, both calorigenically active hormones, differ significantly in several properties, namely, volume of distribution, fractional turnover rate, affinity for binding proteins, and biologic potency. T_3 is about four times more biologically active than T_4.

The peripheral (extrathyroidal) synthesis of T_3 from T_4 is decreased in a number of chronic and acute situations, e.g., acute starvation, chronic caloric deprivation, hepatic cirrhosis, anorexia nervosa, renal failure, and stress related to surgery. However, in these conditions the patients remain in a euthyroid state, which presumably is due to the intrinsic biologic activity of T_4.

T_3 is frequently decreased in hospitalized euthyroid patients. It is not normally measured to determine hypothyroidism, but rather to confirm hyperthyroidism in cases in which the level of T_4 is marginally elevated. Additionally, T_3 is elevated in a condition known as T_3 thyrotoxicosis, in which T_4 is normal and the patient is clinically hyperthyroid.

The reference range for T_3 in serum is, for adults, 120–195 ng/dl.

See also *thyroxine.* Generic drug name, *liothyronine sodium.*

free T_3, the T_3 that is not bound to plasma proteins. See under *triiodothyronine assays.*

triiodothyronine assays radioimmunoassay for T_3 in serum T_3 (RIA). Free T_3 (FT_3) and the FT_3 index are determined by the same method as that for FT_4 and the FT_4 index; see under *thyroxine assays* and *triiodothyronine uptake test.*

triiodothyronine resin uptake (T_3U) test a laboratory method for the relative quantitation of available thyroid hormone–binding sites on thyroxine-binding globulin (TBG). The name of this test is a misnomer because actual T_3 (triiodothyronine) is not measured and is used only as a reagent in the procedure. An excess of radioactive exogenous T_3 is added to the sample and followed by the addition of a resin that also binds T_3. A portion of the radioactive T_3 binds to the binding sites on TBG not already occupied by endogenous thyroxine, whereas the remainder, not bound to the TBG, binds to the resin. The amount of radioactivity bound to the resin (i.e., T_3 resin uptake) is inversely proportional to the number of unoccupied binding sites on TBG in the sample.

Results of this test are interpreted in conjunction with a T_4 determination. By means of a mathematical manipulation (i.e., $T_3U \times T_4$), an estimate can be made of the biologically active (free) T_4, termed free thyroxine index. Individuals with normal TBG concentrations have decreased T_3U values in hypothyroidism and increased T_3U values in hyperthyroidism. However, certain conditions that alter the level of TBG can result in abnormal T_3U values for euthyroid individuals.

Increased TBG, and thus decreased T_3U values, may have genetic causes or may be due to pregnancy or to the use of oral contraceptives or other estrogen-containing preparations. Decreased TBG, and thus increased T_3U values, may result from severe renal or hepatic disease, and certain medications (anticoagulants, salicylates, phenylbutazone, phenytoin, and androgens), or may have genetic causes. In the above cases, thyroid status can be estimated by the free thyroxine index or direct determinations of free T_4.

The reference range for T_3U is 25–35 percent or 0.85–1.14 (ratio of measured percent uptake/mean percent uptake of reference range). The test is now being replaced by the direct immunochemical determination of TBG.

Also called T_3 uptake and abbreviated T_3RU, RT_3U, and T_3U. See also *thyroxine* and *triiodothyronine.*

triiodothyronine suppression test see under *thyroid uptake tests.*

Trilafon (tri′lah-fon) trademark. See *perphenazine.*

trimeprazine tartrate (tri-mep′rah-zēn) [USP], a phenothiazine drug used for symptomatic relief of itching. It may cause drowsiness, and it increases the sedation caused by alcohol and other central nervous system depressants. Trademark, Temaril.

trimer (tri′mer) [*tri-* + Gr. *meros* part] 1. an oligomer composed of three monomers.

2. a viral capsomere composed of three polypeptide units; see under *capsid.*

trimethadione (tri″meth-ah-di′ōn) [USP], an anticonvulsant drug related to paramethadione, used for the control of absence (petit mal) seizures that are not controlled by other drugs. Trademark, Tridione. See also *oxazolidinedione compounds.*

trimethaphan camsylate (tri-meth′ah-fan) a ganglionic blocking drug used to produce controlled hypotension during surgery and for emergency treatment of hypertensive emergencies.

trimethobenzamide hydrochloride (tri″meth-o-ben′zah-mīd) [USP], a drug used to control nausea and vomiting by depressing the chemoreceptor trigger zone (CTZ) of the medulla oblongata. It may cause drowsiness. In view of the possibility that centrally acting antiemetics may unfavorably alter the course of Reye's syndrome, they should not be used for uncomplicated vomiting in children. Trademark, Tigan.

trimethoprim (tri-meth′o-prim) [USP], an antibacterial agent, 2,4,-diamino-5-(3′,4′,5′-trimethoxybenzyl) pyrimidine, generally used in combination with a sulfonamide. Trimethoprim inhibits bacterial dihydrofolate reductase, the next enzymatic step in folic acid synthesis following the one inhibited by sulfonamides. When trimethoprim and a sulfonamide are used in combination, the sequential blockade of the folic acid synthetic pathway results in synergistic activity against a broad spectrum of microorganisms. The optimal ratio for in vitro synergy of trimethoprim-sulfamethoxazole is 1:20.

In vitro, trimethoprim is active against most gram-positive cocci and most gram-negative bacilli except *Pseudomonas aeruginosa* and *Bacteroides* species. Thymidine in test media will inhibit the in vitro activity of trimethoprim. Resistance may result from the emergence of thymine dependence or from modification of the target enzyme.

Trimethoprim is used for the treatment of acute urinary tract infections due to susceptible organisms. For recurrent or chronic urinary tract infections due to susceptible organisms, trimethoprim-sulfamethoxazole (1:5) is effective. The combination is also useful in bacterial prostatitis, otitis media, and *Shigella* and *Pneumocystis carinii* infections.

See also *antibacterial agents.*

trimethoxyamphetamine (TMA) (tri″mĕ-thok″-

se-am-fet'ah-mēn) a potent hallucinogen occurring in nutmeg oil. It produces effects similar to those of LSD.

trimipramine maleate (tri-mip'rah-mēn) one of the tricyclic antidepressants, used in treatment of depression. Trademark, Surmontil.

2,4,6-trinitrotoluene (TNT) (tri"ni-tro-tol'u-ēn) a yellow crystalline solid, $CH_3C_6H_2(NO_2)_3$, a "safe" high explosive that detonates only from a high-velocity shock; M.W. 227.13. TNT is toxic when ingested, inhaled, or absorbed through the skin, and produces headache and weakness; in severe poisoning, it produces massive necrosis of the liver and aplastic anemia.

tri-*o*-cresyl phosphate (TOCP) (tri"o-kres'il) a highly toxic isomer of tricresyl phosphate. Ingestion produces nausea, vomiting, and diarrhea. It also is a delayed neurotoxin, producing axonal degeneration followed by demyelination; severe poisoning causes peripheral neuropathy that leads to paralysis. Also called tri-*o*-tolyl phosphate.

triol (tri'ol) an alcohol having three hydroxyl groups, i.e., a trihydric alcohol such as glycerol, $CH_2OHCHOHCH_2OH$.

-triol (tre-ol) a suffix word element to denote the presence of three alcoholic groups in a molecule, e.g., pregnanetriol.

trioleandomycin (tri-o"le-an"do-mi'sin) see under *macrolides.*

triolein I 131 (tri'o-lēn) a radioiodine-labeled fat. See *fat absorption test.*

triose (tri'ōs) a monosaccharide having three carbon atoms in a molecule, e.g., glyceraldehyde and dihydroxyacetone.

triosephosphate an intermediate formed from the glycolytic metabolism of glucose, specifically, glyceraldehyde-3-phosphate and dihydroxyacetone phosphate. It is formed by the action of fructose bisphosphate aldolase on fructose-1,6-bisphosphate.

triosephosphate dehydrogenase see *glyceraldehyde-phosphate dehydrogenase.*

triosephosphate isomerase (TPI) an enzyme of the isomerase class (D-glyceraldehyde-3-phosphate ketol-isomerase, EC 5.3.1.1) that catalyzes the reaction D-glyceraldehyde-3-phosphate ⇄ dihydroxyacetone phosphate. The reaction is a step in the metabolism of pyruvate formed from glucose in the Embden-Meyerhof pathway.

triosephosphate isomerase (TPI) assays determination of the TPI activity in erythrocytes. In the assay, the TPI reaction is coupled to the α-glycerophosphate dehydrogenase reaction, which causes conversion of the dihydroxyacetonephosphate to α-glycerophosphate with concomitant oxidation of NADH to NAD^+. The decrease of NADH can be measured either spectrophotometrically at 340 nm or by a loss of fluorescence.

triosephosphate isomerase deficiency a rare genetic disorder, transmitted as an autosomal recessive trait, that is charcterized by hemolytic anemia, neuromuscular dysfunction, and recurrent infection. Affected individuals have only 6 percent of the normal red cell triosephosphate isomerase activity and 20 percent of the normal white cell TPI activity.

2,6,8-trioxypurine (tri"ok-se-pu'rin) see *uric acid.*

tripelennamine (tri"pĕ-len'ah-mēn) an antihistamine used to treat vasomotor rhinitis, allergic rhinitis, and other allergic reactions. The most common side-effects are drowsiness; dizziness; dryness of the mouth, nose, and throat; and thickening of bronchial secretions. Trademark, PBZ.

t. citrate, [USP], a salt used in elixirs. It is more palatable than tripelennamine hydrochloride.

t. hydrochloride, [USP], a salt used in tablets, capsules, and ointments.

triphenylmethane dyes (tri-fen"il-meth'ān) an important group of dyes used in biologic stains. These dyes include pararosaniline and many of its derivatives, such as new fuchsin (trimethylpararosaniline) and crystal violet (*N*-hexamethylpararosaniline). See also *fuchsin* and *Schiff reagent.*

triple-blind pertaining to an experiment in which all subjects, persons administering treatment, and evaluators of response to treatment are unaware which subjects are receiving the treatment and which are receiving the placebo. See also *clinical trials.*

triple bond an unsaturated bond of three covalent linkages between two adjacent atoms, as in acetylenic compounds (—C≡C—), nitriles (—C≡N), and diazonium salts (—N^+≡N:).

triple point the temperature and pressure (i.e., the point of the thermodynamic phase diagram) at which the solid, liquid, and vapor phases of a substance are in equilibrium. The triple point of water (273.16 K and 4.6 mmHg) is used to define the kelvin, the unit of absolute temperature. Cf. *ice point.*

triplet (trip'let) 1. one of three individuals produced at the same birth.

2. a set of three objects of one kind.

3. three consecutive bases along a nucleic acid chain. Also called *codon.*

triploid (trip'loid) [Gr. *triploos* threefold + *eidos* form] 1. pertaining to triploidy.

2. an individual or cell that has three homologous sets of chromosomes. See also *polyploid.*

triploidy (trip'loi-de) the state of having three times the normal haploid chromosome number (3n).

triprolidine hydrochloride (tri-pro'lĭ-dēn) an antihistamine used in the treatment of vasomotor rhinitis, allergic rhinitis, and other allergic reactions. Common side-effects include drowsiness; dizziness; dryness of the mouth, nose, and throat; and thickening of bronchial secretions. Trademarks, *Actidil* and, combined with pseudoephedrine hydrochloride, *Actifed.*

TRIS see *tris(hydroxymethyl)aminomethane.*

tris (hydroxymethyl) aminomethane (TRIS, THAM) a white crystalline solid, 2-amino-2-hydroxymethyl--1,3-propanediol, $H_2NC(CH_2OH)_3$; M.W. 121.14, a weak base used in chemistry as a buffer. TRIS has a high temperature coefficient (pK at room temperature, approximately 8.1; at body temperature, 7.8). It is also used in chemistry as a primary acid-base standard, in physiologic chemistry as a buffer, and in medicine as an intravenously administered agent for the correction of systemic acidosis. Generic drug name, *tromethamine.*

trisomic (tri-so'mik) 1. pertaining to or characterized by trisomy.

2. an individual or cell exhibiting trisomy.

trisomy (tri'so"me) [*tri-* + Gr. *sōma* body] the presence of one additional chromosome in excess of the normal diploid number. The most common genetic disorders due to trisomy are Down's syndrome (trisomy 21, occurring in 1 in 600–1000 births), trisomy 18 (1 in 5000), and trisomy 13 (1 in 6000); trisomy 8 and trisomy 22 also occur.

These disorders generally involve mental retardation, shortened life span, and anatomic malformations. They can also be caused by partial trisomy due to an unbalanced translocation or duplication. They arise in less severe form in mosaics having two cell lines, one trisomic and one normal.

double t., the presence of two nonhomologous chromosomes in addition to the normal diploid set.

partial t., the presence of part of a chromosome, arising from translocation or duplication, in excess of the normal two homologous chromosomes. The excess part is usually attached to a nonhomologous chromosome.

primary t., trisomy. Three homologous chromosomes are present.

secondary t., partial trisomy in which an isochromosome is present in addition to a normal set.

translocation t., partial trisomy resulting from a translocation.

trisomy D syndrome see *trisomy 13 syndrome.*

trisomy E syndrome see *trisomy 18 syndrome.*

trisomy 13 syndrome the condition of multiple congenital malformations in infants that results from the presence of an extra chromosome 13. The most common characteristics include low-set ears, bilateral cleft lip and palate, microcephaly with sloping forehead, multiple eye anomalies (colobomas, microphthalmia, anophthalmia, or hypertelorism), hemangiomas, mental retardation, deafness, convulsions, hernias, and ventricular septal defects. Also reported are rotation of the thumbs, flexion deformities of the hands and feet, polydactyly, syndactyly, dextrorotation of the heart, rotation of the bowel, absence of the gallbladder, the presence of an accessory spleen, and infantile arteriosclerosis.

Trisomy 13 syndrome results from nondisjunction of chromosome 13, producing 47 chromosomes instead of the normal 46. About .30 per 1000 newborn infants are affected.

Treatment is symptomatic and surgical when feasible, but abnormalities are such that death usually occurs before age 1 yr.

Also called Patau's syndrome and *trisomy D syndrome.*

trisomy 18 syndrome the condition of multiple congenital malformations in infants that results from the presence of an extra chromosome 18. The most common characteristics include failure to thrive, mental retardation, low-set malformed ears, micrognathia, flexion deformities of the fingers, low arch dermal ridge patterning on the fingertips, hypertonicity, and eye abnormalities. Also reported are "rocker-bottom" feet, congenital heart defects, umbilical and/or inguinal hernia, short sternum, small pelvis, hypertrichosis of forehead, corneal opacities, and urinary tract anomalies.

Trisomy 18 syndrome results from nondisjunction during oogenesis, which is caused by increased maternal age or translocation of part of chromosome 18. About 0.23–2.0 per 1000 newborn infants are affected, with a male-to-female ratio of 1 to 3.

There is no treatment; the life span is short and very few of those affected reach early childhood.

Also called *Edwards-Patau syndrome, trisomy E syndrome,* and trisomy 17-18 syndrome.

trisomy 21 syndrome see *Down's syndrome.*

tristate logic (trī'stāt loj'ik) a type of logic circuitry in which the logic elements (gates) have three possible outputs: the usual binary outputs one and zero, plus an additional "high Z" state activated when a control signal is not present at the enable input. When many tristate gates are connected to a common data bus, only those in the enabled condition draw current from the bus; the other gates are in effect disconnected so that the signal on the bus is not degraded.

tristearin (tri-ste'ah-rin) [*tri-* + Gr. *stear* hard fat + *-in*] a white crystalline fat, glyceryl tristearate, that is found in the harder fats such as tallow. Also called *stearin.*

tritanomaly (tri"tah-nom'ah-le) [Gr. *tritos* third + *anōmalia* irregularity] defective color vision of the trichromatic type in which blue vision is anomalous (weak).

tritanopia (tri"tah-no'pe-ah) [Gr. *tritos* third + *an-* neg. + *ōpē* sight + *-ia*] defective color vision of the dichromatic type in which blue cones are lacking and the color blue cannot be perceived.

triterpene (tri"ter'pēn) a subclass of terpene compounds having 30 carbon atoms in six isoprene units, an isoprenoid compound.

tritium (^{3}H,T) (trit'e-um, trish'e-um) [Gr. *tritos* third] hydrogen 3, a radionuclide with a half-life of 12.26 yr, which decays by beta emission. It has been used as a label in radioimmunoassay and for experimental biologic research. Tritium occurs in the environment, and is also produced by cosmic rays, nuclear explosions, and nuclear reactors. Cf. *deuterium* and *protium.*

Triton-X 100 (tri'ton) trademark for a neutral surfactant compound; one member of the Triton-X series; iso-octyl phenoxy polyethoxy ethanol. It is a non-ionic liquid used as a surfactant, detergent, wetting agent, and emulsifier.

trivalent (tri-va'lent) [*tri-* + L. *valens* powerful] 1. in chemistry, having a valence of 3.

2. in genetics, the object formed by synapsis of three partially homologous chromosomes during meiosis. See also *robertsonian translocation.*

tRNA abbrev. for transfer ribonucleic acid. See under *ribonucleic acid.*

tRNA suppressor a mutation in a tRNA gene producing a tRNA with a base substitution in the anticodon. Thus, it matches a different codon (usually a terminator codon) and inserts its amino acid instead of terminating the chain.

trochanter (tro-kan'ter) [L.; Gr. *trochantēr*] one of the two processes below the neck of the femur: the greater trochanter provides a point of insertion for the muscles of the gluteal region; the lesser trochanter is the site of insertion for the psoas major.

trochlea (trok'le-ah), pl. *trochleae* [L.; Gr. *trochileia* pulley] a general term for a pulley-shaped part or structure.

t. of humerus, the medial part of the distal end of the humerus that fits into the trochlear notch of the ulna.

t. of orbit, a fibrocartilaginous ring attached to the bony wall of the orbit near its anteromedial corner. The slender tendon of the superior oblique muscle passes through it. A synovial sheath covers the tendon, lining the pulley and a fibrous sheath that extends over the tendon from the lateral margin of the trochlea.

trochlear (trok′le-ar) 1. pertaining to a trochlea. 2. pertaining to the fourth cranial nerve.

trochlear nerve cranial nerve IV; a motor nerve whose fibers arise in the midbrain, run forward in the lateral wall of the cavernous sinus, and enter the orbit to supply the superior oblique muscle. See also *cranial nerves.*

Troglotrema (trog″lo-tre′mah) [Gr. *trōglē* hole + *trēma* hole] a genus of flukes.

T. salmincola, a small, pyriform worm (0.8–1.1 mm by 0.3–0.5 mm), which is a digenetic trematode and is parasitic in the kidneys of fish (especially trout and salmon). It serves as a vector of *Neorickettsia helmintheca,* a rickettsia causing salmon poisoning. Human infection with *N. helmintheca* is acquired by eating raw fish contaminated with the rickettsia. The disease is frequently fatal. Also called *Nanophyetus salmincola.*

Troglotrematidae (trog″lo-tre-mat′ĭ-de) a family of trematodes including the species *Troglotrema salmincola* and *Paragonimus westermani.*

Trojan Horse inhibitor see under *affinity labeling.*

Trombicula (trom-bik′u-lah) a genus of ascarine mites of the family Trombiculidae. Medically, these mites are important, as all species cause an irritating dermatitis in humans, and a few species are known vectors of *Rickettsia tsutsugamushi,* the etiologic agent of scrub typhus. The mites act as reservoirs as transovarial transmission of the *Rickettsia* occurs.

The adult mite is approximately 1 mm long; most species are reddish in color or have red, orange, or black spots. They have a cosmopolitan distribution, but also are commonly found in tropical and subtropical regions.

Also called *chigger, harvest mite, kedani mite, red bug, red mite,* and *trombiculid mite.* See also *chigger.*

T. akamushi, the kedani mite, commonly found in Japan, whose larvae transmit *Rickettsia tsutsugamushi,* the causative agent of scrub typhus.

T. alfreddugèsi, see *E. alfreddugèsi* under *Eutrombicula.*

T. autumnalis, a mite, found in Europe, that causes dermatitis and whose larvae are common pests to humans in the fall months during harvest season.

T. deliensis, a species whose larvae transmit *Rickettsia tsutsugamushi,* the causative agent of scrub typhus; it is found from Pakistan and India through Indonesia to New Guinea and Austrailia, and is more characteristically associated with forests.

T. irritans. see *E. alfreddugèsi* under *Eutrombicula.*

T. pallida, a carrier of *Rickettsia tsutsugamushi,* the causative agent of scrub typhus.

T. scutellaris, a carrier of *Rickettsia tsutsugamushi,* the causative agent of scrub typhus.

trombiculiasis (trom-bik″u-li′ah-sis) an infestation with mites of the genus *Trombicula.*

trombiculid (trom-bik′u-lid) a mite of the genus *Trombicula.*

Trombiculidae (trom″bik-u′li-de) a family of mites, of which the genus *Trombicula* is a member.

trombiculid mite see *Trombicula.*

Trombidoidea (trom′bĭ-doi′de-ah) a superfamily of mites, including the genus *Trombicula.*

tromethamine (tro-meth′ah-mēn) [NF], generic drug name. See *tris(hydroxymethyl)aminomethane.*

troph/o (trof′o) [Gr. *trophē* nutrition] a word element used in combining form to denote food or nourishment, e.g., dystrophia.

trophic (trof′ik) [Gr. *trophikos*] pertaining to nutrition.

trophic nucleus see *macronucleus.*

trophoblast (trof′o-blast) [*tropho-* + Gr. *blastos* germ] in the developing embryo, the extraembryonic ectodermal capsule covering the blastocyst. It is responsible for establishing the attachment between ovum and uterus, and for the development of the chorion, amnion, and placenta.

trophonucleus (trof″o-nu′kle-us) see *macronucleus.*

trophotaxis (trof″o-tak′sis) [*tropho-* + Gr. *taxis* a drawing up in rank and file] the orientation movement of motile organisms in response to the stimulus of nutritive materials.

trophozoite (trof″o-zo′īt) [*tropho-* + Gr. *zōon* animal] the active or motile feeding stage of a protozoan organism, as contrasted with the resting or nonmotile encysted stage. In the malarial parasite, it is the stage of schizogony between the merozoites and the mature schizont. In red cells, a trophozoite is uninucleate, ring-shaped, more or less ameboid, and vacuolated. As it grows, its nucleus divides by mitosis and its vacuole is filled; with its ameboid motility curbed, it becomes a mature schizont.

The trophozoites of *Toxoplasma gondii,* also known as tachyzoites, are crescentic in shape. They are quickly multiplying forms responsible for the initial spread of infection and tissue destruction.

trophy (tro′fe) a suffix word element to denote nourishment and development, e.g., atrophy and hypertrophy.

-tropia (tro′pe-ah) [Gr. *tropē* a turning] a suffix word element to denote turn, e.g., heliotropia.

-tropic [L. *tropicus* of a turn, from Gr. *tropikos* of the solstice] a suffix word element to denote a turn or change, e.g., enterotropic.

Tropicorbis (trop″ĭkor′bis) a genus of snails, of which the species *T. centimetralis* and *T. havanesis,* found in Brazil and Louisiana, respectively, are hosts for the blood fluke *Schistosoma mansoni.*

-tropin (tro′pin) a suffix word element denoting to nourish, develop, or stimulate, e.g., gonadotropin.

tropism (tro′pizm) [Gr. *tropē* a turn, turning] the tendency of an organism to respond to an external stimulus by growth or movement. Such response may be positive (toward the stimulus) or negative (away from the stimulus). See also *chemotropism* and *phototropism.*

tropocollagen (tro″po-kol′ah-jen) [Gr. *tropē* a turning + *collagen*] a triple-stranded helical polypeptide chain rich in glycine and some 5-hydroxylysine and 4-hydroxyproline. Tropocollagen is rod-shaped and one of the longest proteins; it has a length of 300 nm and a diameter of 1.5 nm. The three chains are in a cablelike structure; tropocollagen chains associate in a specific manner and then become cross-linked to stabilize large fibers of collagens. Collagen fibers have a quarter-staggered arrangement of tropocollagen molecules.

tropoelastin (tro″po-e-las′tin) the globular submits of elastin, which are irregularly arranged in three-dimensional sheets; M.W. 67,000.

tropomyosin (tro″po-mi′o-sin) a regulatory muscle protein that prevents myosin heads from attaching to myosin. It is bound to troponin and is deflected when troponin binds with Ca^{++}.

troponin (tro′po-nin) a muscle protein bound to tropomyosin that inhibits muscular contraction unless removed by binding with Ca^{++}.

Trousseau's sign (troo-sōz′) [Armand *Trousseau,* French physician, 1801–1867] 1. thrombophlebitis migrans in association with visceral cancer. See also *t. migrans* under *thrombophlebitis.*

2. a sign occurring in association with tetany, whereby carpopedal spasm may be elicited by compression of the upper arm with a tourniquet or blood pressure cuff for approximately 3 min. It may also arise in association with an alkalotic state and in a small percentage of individuals in the normal population.

Trp abbrev. See also *tryptophan.*

true oxygen the amount of oxygen, expressed as a percentage change, that is removed from inhaled air and becomes available for tissue consumption. It may be calculated in the following manner: true $O_2 = F_{I_{O_2}} \times (F_{E_{N_2}}/F_{I_{N_2}}) - F_{E_{O_2}}$. Under standard conditions, this percentage change, multiplied by minute ventilation, is the calculated oxygen consumption per minute. It would appear that the percentage change could be easily obtained by subtracting the mixed expired oxygen from the inhaled value (usually room air). However, this subtraction is accurate only when the respiratory quotient (RQ) is equal to 1. When it is less than 1, the amount of CO_2 eliminated in exhaled air is less, milliliter for milliliter, than the amount of oxygen absorbed. Thus, the size of each exhaled breath is smaller than the preceding inhaled breath, and the percentage of oxygen in the mixed expired air has been altered by this volume difference, independent of the amount of oxygen consumed caused by a respiratory quotient less than unity.

True oxygen is a percentage figure calculated to correct for this volume change effect. The correction is based on the fact that the amount of nitrogen in inspired and expired air remains constant although the percentage of nitrogen does not, with the percentage change being proportional to the volume change.

truncate (trung′kāt) [L. *truncare* to cut off from *truncus* torso] 1. to amputate or cut off squarely.

2. in biology, having a blunt, squared-off end.

3. in mathematics, to reduce the precision of a numerical value by truncation. See also *rounding* and *truncation.*

truncation (trung-ka′shun) 1. in numerical analysis and computer programming, the process of dropping low-order digits of a numerical value. This results in a number with specified precision (number of significant digits), as opposed to a rounded-off number, in which the number with the specified precision closest to the original value is chosen (e.g., $\pi = 3.141592\ldots$ rounded to five digits is 3.1416 but truncated to five places is 3.1415.

In both the worst case and the average, truncation produces twice the error that rounding does, but the arithmetic operations of most computers truncate results to achieve greater speed. Rounding is used mostly for output of floating-point variables.

2. in statistics, ignoring or disregarding all measurements or observations beyond a prespecified cutoff point.

truncus (trung′kus), pl. *trunci* [L. "trunk"] [NA], a general term for the main part of the body, to which the head and limbs are attached.

t. arteriosus, an arterial trunk connected to the fetal heart that gives rise to the aortic arches; it develops into the aorta and pulmonary trunk.

trunk (trungk) [L. *truncus*] 1. the main part of the body, to which head and limbs are attached.

2. a major, undivided, and usually short portion of a nerve, blood or lymphatic vessel, or other duct.

See also *truncus.*

pulmonary t., the large vessel that conveys unoxygenated blood to the lungs from the right ventricle; it divides beneath the aortic arch into the right and left pulmonary arteries.

truth table the analog of a multiplication table for a logical operation, which gives the result for each possible pair of operands.

trypan blue (tri′pan) an acid disazo dye; C.I. 23850. It has been used as a supravital stain and as an amyloid stain. This anionic dye also has an important application in immunology, e.g., the study of cytotoxicity in lymphocytes. Trypan blue may be used to count dead cells, as it penetrates and stains those cells whose cell membranes are damaged; the intact cells remain unstained. Also called blue 3B and direct blue 3B.

trypanocidal (tri-pan″o-si′dal) see *trypanosomicidal.*

Trypanosoma (trip″ah-no-so′mah) [Gr. *trypanon* borer + *sōma* body] a genus of flagellate protozoan parasites of the family Trypanosomatidae. These parasites inhabit the blood and tissues of human hosts. In their life cycle these species may have amastigote, promastigote, epimastigote, and trypomastigote stages, and live in vertebrate and invertebrate hosts.

The adult parasite has a characteristic elongated body with a whiplike posterior flagellum, which is attached to the cell by a delicate undulating membrane that runs the length of the body. This adult stage usually occurs only in the vertebrate host. Several species are pathogenic for humans.

T. ariarii, see *T. rangeli.*

T. brucei, a species of the genus *Trypanosoma.* It consists of three subspecies: *T. brucei brucei,* which, although it apparently does not infect humans, does produce a relatively mild disease in African game animals and a severe infection in many domestic animals (e.g., trypanosomiasis [nagana] in cattle); *T. brucei gambiense,* which causes Gambian or West African sleeping sickness; and *T. brucei rhodesiense,* which causes Rhodesian or East African sleeping sickness. Some authorities prefer to grant specific status to *T. gambiense* and *T. rhodesiense.*

T. castellani, see *T. gambiense.*

T. cruzi, a pleomorphic trypanosome that causes trypanosomiasis or Chagas' disease in individuals in the Western hemisphere. The parasite has two phases in its life cycle: one in humans or reservoir hosts and one in the transmitting insects. In the mammalian host, *T. cruzi* has two morphologic forms, a trypomastigote form present in the blood and an amastigote form with transformation stages present in the reticuloendothelial and other tissue cells.

In its trypomastigote form, *T. cruzi* is spindle-shaped, is approximately 20 μm in length, and may be long and slender or short and broad. In its amastigote form, when it loses its flagellum and undulating membrane, it is round or ovoidal in shape, with a range of 1.5–4.0 μ in diameter. In the transmitting insects, the parasite is commonly in the epimastigote and metacyclic trypomastigote forms.

T. cruzi is transmitted from human to human by reduviid bugs of the genera *Panstrongylus, Triatoma,* and *Rhodnius.* When the insect bites, it defecates, and the contaminated fecal material is rubbed into the puncture wound. The insect becomes infected from biting an infective host.

Laboratory diagnosis requires identification of the parasite in blood or tissues by animal inoculation, cultivation, xenodiagnosis, or serologic procedures. In peripheral blood smears stained with Giemsa stain, the trypomastigote has a centrally located nucleus in the body and a large kinetoplast, and assumes a characteristic C- or U-shape. Only in early infections can *T. cruzi* be detected in the blood. A skeletal muscle biopsy may show leishmanial forms in muscle cells. These have a large red nucleus and a dark purple kinetoplast when stained.

Animals may be inoculated with 5–10 ml of the patient's blood and the animal's blood checked periodically for 2 mo to demonstrate infection.

T. cruzi is easily cultivated on NNN medium or in blood broth. The individual's blood is inoculated on the medium or in broth. Most forms found in culture are morphologically similar to those in the transmitting insects. The forms are usually infective to animals used experimentally.

Examination of aspirations from lymph nodes, bone marrow, or splenic punctures may yield positive results.

Xenodiagnosis is a technique used in chronic infections. Laboratory-bred reduviid bugs feed on suspected infected individuals. When infection is present, the transformed epimastigotes multiply in the bug's intestines, and examination of its intestinal contents demonstrates metacyclic forms.

Complement-fixation tests, such as the Machado-Guerreiro test or Kelser's test, use a *T. cruzi* antigen, and positive results are obtained in 95 percent of infections.

Also called *Schizotrypanum cruzi* and *T. triatomae.* See also *American t.* under *trypanosomiasis.*

T. gambiense, a polymorphic trypanosome that causes African trypanosomiasis, or West African sleeping sickness, in individuals in tropical areas of Africa. The life cycle of this parasite has two phases, one in the vertebrate host (which includes humans) and another in the invertebrate host (in trypomastigote and epimastigote forms). In the blood of the vertebrate host, *T. gambiense* occurs in three forms: a long, slender trypomastigote form possessing a flagellum; a short, broad form without a flagellum; and an intermediate form. Trypomastigotes may also be found in the lymph and tissues of the central nervous system. They have a range of 8–30 μm in length.

Human infection is acquired through the bites of infected tsetse flies of the genus *Glossina.* The insect transmits the parasite through its salivary glands as it bites its victims.

Laboratory diagnosis requires identification of the parasite in the blood or aspirates or by animal inoculation. Blood smears stained with Giemsa or Wright stains show slender flagellates with a granular cytoplasm; they stain pale blue with dark blue granules. Trypomastigotes may be identified microscopically in stained smears of aspirates from lymph nodes and liver biopsy material. Cerebrospinal fluid can be examined as stained smears or wet preparations. Animals can be inoculated with emulsified tissue and their blood checked daily for the presence of infection.

Also called *Castellanella gambiense, T. castellani, T. hominis, T. nigeriense,* and *T. ugandense.* See also *African t.* under *trypanosomiasis.*

T. hominis, see *T. gambiense.*

T. nigeriense, see *T. gambiense.*

T. rangeli, a nonpathogenic hemoflagellate that occurs in Venezuela, Colombia, and Guatemala, being transmitted by the reduviid bug *Rhodnius prolixus.* Because this species causes an asymptomatic infection in humans and is often found in association with *T. cruzi,* it is important clinically to differentiate the two species in blood, in the reduviid bug's intestine, and in culture.

T. rangeli organisms in the peripheral blood are approximately 30 μm long, with an anterior nucleus and a small kinetoplast. In the transmitting insect, the flagellates are found in the hemolymph; following reproduction they invade the salivary glands and produce metacyclic trypomastigotes.

Also called *T. ariarii.*

T. rhodesiense, a species of hemoflagellates that causes African trypanosomiasis, or East African sleeping sickness, in individuals in southeastern regions of Africa. Infection is transmitted from human to human by flies of the genus *Glossina. T. rhodesiense* has a range of 14–33 μm in length, is long and slender, and possesses a single flagellum.

In the mammalian host, *T. rhodesiense* inhabits the blood, lymph nodes, and cerebrospinal fluid and tissues in the trypomastigote stage. In the transmitting flies, the parasite multiplies in the intestines and is transmitted through the salivary duct and glands of the fly when it bites its victim.

Laboratory diagnosis requires identification of the trypomastigotes in the blood, in fluid aspirates (lymph nodes, cerebrospinal fluid), and by animal inoculation. Blood smears stained by Giemsa or Wright stain show characteristic trypomastigotes in positive cases during the febrile stage of the disease.

Also called *Castellanella castellani.*

T. triatomae, see *T. cruzi.*

T. ugandense, see *T. gambiense.*

Trypanosomatidae (trip″ah-no-so-mat′ĭ-de) a family of flagellate protozoa that inhabits the blood and tissues of the human host. It consists of six genera, including two of medical importance, *Leishmania* and *Trypanosoma.*

trypanosome (trĭ-pan′o-sōm) any member of the genus *Trypanosoma.*

trypanosomiasis (trip″ah-no-so-mi′ah-sis) an infection with the blood and tissue flagellates of the genus *Trypanosoma.* Trypanosomal infections in humans include the Gambian and Rhodesian forms of African trypanosomiasis and American trypanosomiasis (Chagas' disease).

African t., a disease with both acute and chronic forms, caused by the hemoflagellates of the genus *Trypanosoma*. It is transmitted from human to human by the tsetse flies of the genus *Glossina* and is common in tsetse fly–infested areas of Africa.

Two subspecies of *Trypanosoma brucci* are known to cause African trypanosomiasis. *T. b. gambiense* (the causative agent of Gambian trypanosomiasis or West African sleeping sickness) is transmitted by flies of the groups *Glossina palpalis* and *G. tachinoides* and causes the chronic form of the disease. *T. b. rhodesiense* (the etiologic agent of Rhodesian trypanosomiasis or East African sleeping sickness) is a parasite of wild animals, humans being an accidental host, and is transmitted by flies of the species *Glossina morsitans*, causing the acute form of the disease. The distribution of both Gambian and Rhodesian trypanosomiasis is dependent on its reservoir and vector. For example, Gambian trypanosomiasis is confined to the forest belt in mid- or western Africa because it has no animal reservoir and its vector is an inhabitant of that area.

The acute form of the disease (caused by *T. b. rhodesiense*) is characterized by fever, lymphadenitis, rash, transitory edemas, and myocarditis. The nervous system symptoms that occur in the chronic form are lacking or less evident. Most acute infections result in death within a year. The chronic form of the disease (caused by *T. b. gambiense*) runs a milder, chronic course and results in death after a duration of several years as a result of central nervous system involvement.

In human infections, the infective metacyclic trypanosomes are introduced into the host while the flies feed. The parasites lodge in the tissue of the bite wound, causing a local inflammatory reaction that lasts approximately 1–2 wk. In the first stage of the disease, the parasites enter the blood stream and localize in the lymph nodes, causing proliferation of lymphoid tissue and enlargement of the cervical lymph nodes (Winterbottom's sign in Gambian trypanosomiasis). The tissue cells are not invaded per se, but the parasite has injurious effects on the tissues and organs.

In the second stage of the disease, CNS involvement may occur early (Rhodesian type) with no evident symptoms of sleeping sickness, or it may develop several months or years later (Gambian type). The Gambian type is characterized by tremors (of the tongue and fingers), headaches, hysteria, delusions, and other signs of meningoencephalitis and meningomyelitis. Sleepiness develops and is so pronounced that the affected individual may fall asleep while eating, standing, or sitting. One of the immunologic disorders includes marked elevation of the immunoglobins, especially IgM, which often exceeds IgG by a factor of 3:1; yet both cellular and humoral immunity are depressed in individuals with this form of trypanosomiasis. Histologic examination often reveals lymphoid tissue disorganization and the presence of characteristic mononuclear cells with eccentric nuclei known as morular (mulberry) cells of Mott.

Diagnosis is made by identification of the trypanosomes in blood or spinal fluid early in the disease. Various serologic tests are also used, such as the ELISA test.

Also called *African sleeping sickness, Gambian t., Rhodesian t.,* and *sleeping sickness.* See also *T. gambiense* and *T. rhodesiense.*

American t., an acute, subacute, or chronic disease caused by infection with blood and tissue flagellates of the species *Trypanosoma cruzi*, a pleomorphic trypanosome. The disease is characterized by the presence of trypomastigotes in the blood and amastigotes (leishmania) in the tissues. The disease is prevalent in individuals in rural areas and is distributed throughout the Western hemisphere except for Canada, Surinam, and Guyana.

T. cruzi is transmitted from human to human by the reduviid bug of the genera *Panstrongylus, Triatoma,* and *Rhodnius.* When the bug bites, the feces, which contain metacyclic trypomastigotes, contaminate the puncture site and the parasites multiply rapidly, causing a severe inflammatory reaction. The parasites invade the body's fat cells (resulting in lipogranulomas), blood, reticuloendothelial cells, and cardiac and skeletal muscle.

Within the cell the parasites proliferate by binary fusion, filling the cytoplasm with amastigotes and producing leishmanial pseudocysts. When these burst, the amastigote invades a new host cell. Several amastigotes may develop into trypomastigotes (becoming enlongated and producing a flagellum), which may enter the blood stream; this stage is accompanied by fever. Because the trypomastigotes do not multiply, the pathogenicity of the disease stems from the ability of the amastigotes to proliferate. When the parasite is intracellular, the inflammatory response is minimal. Only when the pseudocyst ruptures or the amastigote dies (liberating toxic products) is an inflammatory response induced.

The clinical manifestations of the disease vary. In the acute form (prevalent in children) the disease is characterized by high fever; a swollen face (with edema of the eyelids, Romaña's sign); swelling of the lacrimal glands; enlarged lymph nodes, liver, and spleen; and meningoencephalic irritation. Death may occur in 2–4 wk from myocardial insufficiency or extensive CNS damage; if it does not, the disease may resolve completely within a few weeks or pass into the subacute or chronic stages.

The subacute form may last for several months or years and is characterized by a mild fever, severe asthenia, and generalized lymphadenopathy.

Most chronic cases are found in young adults or children who survive the acute stages. Chronic stage symptoms are usually myocardial-related, with meningoencephalitic, myxedematous, pseudomyxedematous, or suprarenal types, depending on the localization of the intracellular parasite. Megaesophagus and megacolon are common complications.

Also called *Brazilian t.,* and *Chagas' disease.* See also *T. cruzi* under *Trypanosoma.*

Brazilian t., see *American t.*
Gambian t., see *African t.*
Rhodesian t., see *African t.*

trypanosomicide (trip″ah-no-so′mĭ-sīd) [*trypanosome* + L. *caedere* to kill] any substance that is destructive to or kills trypanosomes.

tryparsamide (trip-ar′sah-mīd) an aromatic, synthetic arsenical, monosodium *N*-phenyl-glycineamide-*p*-arsonate, used intravenously to treat African trypanosomiasis (sleeping sickness). Treatment must be long-term to be effective. Trypanosomes become resistant to the drug in approximately 80 percent of individuals treated. As it also has a tendency to cause optic atrophy, it has been gradually replaced by melarsoprol.

Trypetidae (trĭ-pe'tĭ-de) a family of flies that may cause intestinal myiasis in humans.

trypsin (trip'sin) [Gr. *tryein* to rub + pe*psin*] a proteolytic enzyme of the hydrolase class (EC 3.4.21.4) that catalyzes the hydrolysis of peptides (and other compounds) at bonds involving the carboxyl group of arginine or lysine, forming smaller peptide (or other) units. It is synthesized by the pancreas in the inactive trypsinogen form and secreted into the duodenum, where it is converted to the active trypsin by enterokinase or by preformed trypsin. It has an important function in protein digestion. Determination of trypsin activity has limited clinical importance as a measure of pancreatic function in fibrocystic disease.

trypsin assays 1. the x-ray film test, a semiquantitative determination of trypsin activity in infant stool specimens. Serial doubling dilutions of a stool or duodenal fluid specimen in pH 8 buffer are spotted on unexposed x-ray film and incubated for 30 min at 37°C. The trypsin activity is indicated by the highest dilution that can digest the gelatin on the film, leaving a cleared area.

2. quantitative enzyme assay. Trypsin can be distinguished from other peptidases in specimens by its ability to hydrolyze not only peptide bonds involving arginine and lysine, but also ester and amide linkages. Various synthetic substrates have been used, with the reaction products being determined photometrically or by titration.

trypsin inhibitor a class of small proteins that can bind to the active trypsin molecule, inhibiting its proteolytic activity. One form of the inhibitor (Inhibitor I) is present in pancreatic fluid. The inhibitors found in plasma (alpha$_1$-antitrypsin) are synthesized in the liver. All show a broad-spectrum inhibitory activity against proteolytic enzymes, namely, trypsin, chymotrypsin, elastin, and neutral proteases. Alpha$_1$-antitrypsin deficiency has been associated with two disorders: emphysema and a form of hepatitis, sometimes progressing to cirrhosis, in infants and children and, occasionally, in adults.

trypsinogen (trip-sin'o-jen) [*trypsin* + Gr. *gennan* to produce] the inactive precursor of trypsin. It is synthesized by the pancreas and secreted into the duodenum, where it is converted to trypsin by enterokinase or preformed trypsin. See also *trypsin.*

tryptamine (trip'tah"mēn) a minor product of the metabolism of tryptophan formed by the action of aromatic amino acid decarboxylase activity in the liver. It is present in small quantities in normal urine, and its excretion is increased in pellagrins.

tryptophan (Trp or W) (trip'to-fan) [*trypsin* + Gr. *phanes* appearing] 2-amino-3-indolylpropanoic acid, $(C_8H_6N)CH_2CH(NH_2)COOH$, a naturally occurring essential amino acid; M.W. 204.22. Existing in proteins, it is a precursor of serotonin and nicotinate. The presence of tryptophan in the diet may compensate for deficiencies of niacin, and thus mitigate pellagra. It is present in many diet proteins but is low in some food such as corn or maize. See also under *amino acids.*

t. malabsorption syndrome, see *blue diaper syndrome.*

tryptophanemia (trip"to-fah-ne'me-ah) an increase in the concentration of tryptophan in the blood, which is due to disorders that affect the normal metabolism of tryptophan. See also *aminoacidopathies* and *tryptophanuria.*

tryptophanuria (trip"to-fan-u're-ah) a disorder of tryptophan metabolism, transmitted as an X-linked trait, that is due to a relative or absolute deficiency of the enzyme tryptophan pyrrolase. This results in dwarfism, decreased pigmentation of the optic fundus leading to photosensitivity, and ataxia. Levels of tryptophan are slightly increased in blood and greatly increased in urine. See also *aminoacidopathies* and *tryptophanemia.*

tryptophyl (trip'to-fil) the acyl radical derived from or relating to tryptophan.

TS abbrev. for total solids (in urine), which are measured by specific gravity with a urine meter or by refractometry.

tS the time required to complete the S phase of the cell cycle. See also *cell cycle.*

tsetse fly (tset'se) a fly common in Africa that belongs to the genus *Glossina* and is known to transmit *Trypanosoma gambiense* and *T. rhodesiense,* the etiologic agents of African trypanosomiasis.

TSH abbrev. See *thyroid-stimulating hormone.*

TSH-binding inhibitory immunoglobulin (TBII) see under *thyroid-stimulating immunoglobulins.*

TSH-displacing antibody (TDA) see under *thyroid-stimulating immunoglobulins.*

TSH-releasing hormone see *thyrotropin-releasing hormone* (*TRH*).

TSH stimulation test see under *thyroid uptake tests.*

TSI abbrev. See *thyroid-stimulating immunoglobulins.*

TSI agar abbrev. See *triple sugar iron a.* under *agar.*

T-strain mycoplasma see *T-strain m.* under *mycoplasma.*

tsutsugamushi fever (disease) (soot"soo-gah-moosh'e) [Japanese "dangerous bug"] see *scrub t.* under *typhus.*

TTD abbrev. See *tissue tolerance d.* under *dose.*

t test any hypothesis test based on the t distribution. See also *t distribution.*

TTL abbrev. See *transistor-transistor logic.*

T tube a T-shaped rubber tube used for postoperative drainage and cholangiography.

T tubule [the T stands for transverse relative to the long axis of a myofibril] see under *sarcoplasmic reticulum.*

tuaminoheptane sulfate (too-am"ĭ-no-hep'tān) [USP], a sympathomimetic amine used as a nasal decongestant. Trademark, Tuamine.

tubal (too'bal) pertaining to, like, or occurring in a tube.

tubal insufflation an office diagnostic procedure employed in the diagnostic evaluation of infertility to determine whether the fallopian tubes are patent. It is most successfully performed during the preovulatory period. Carbon dioxide is used to inflate the tubes; shoulder pain and abdominal auscultation of gas passing through the tubes are positive proof of patency. Also called *Rubin test.*

tube (tūb) [L. *tubus*] an elongated, hollow, cylindric organ or instrument. For more information, see the specific tube.

tube current in radiology, the current drawn from the high-voltage supply by the x-ray tube. See also *milliamperage.*

tube dilution test see under *antibacterial agent susceptibility testing.*

tubeless gastric analysis test an obsolete procedure for the indirect detection of hydrochloric acid in the stomach. Gastric stimulation is produced by giving the patient caffeine, followed by a compound of blue dye and a cation exchange resin. Excess HCl in the stomach causes the resin complex to release the dye, which is then excreted in the urine and causes a measurable blue color. The test is subject to many sources of error, and so is of limited value.

tube-rating chart a graph that indicates the maximal exposure values that may be used without damage to the x-ray tube. For a series of kilovoltages (separated by 10 kV), the chart gives the maximal permissible milliamperage as a function of the exposure time. There is a different chart for each combination of tube type, focal spot size, and kind of rectification.

tubercle (too′ber-k'l) [L. *tubercula,* diminutive of *tuber* swelling] 1. a nodule, especially a solid elevation of the skin, which is larger than a papule.

2. a small, rounded nodule produced by the tubercle bacillus (*Mycobacterium tuberculosis*) in an affected tissue. It is made up of epithelioid cells and multinucleated giant cells and may contain foci of caseation necrosis. See also *granulomatous i.* under *inflammation* and *M. tuberculosis* under *Mycobacterium.*

3. a nodule or small eminence, especially one on a bone, for attachment of a tendon.

tuberculin (too-ber′ku-lin) a sterile liquid that contains the growth products of, or specific substances extracted from, the tubercle bacillus (*Mycobacterium tuberculosis*). It is used as a skin test antigen to test for delayed hypersensitivity to tubercle bacilli. See also *Mantoux test.*

tuberculin test see *Mantoux test.*

tuberculoma (too-ber″ku-lo′mah) a tumorlike mass formed by the confluence of caseated tubercles.

tuberculosis (TB) (too-ber″ku-lo′sis) a chronic infectious disease caused by the acid-fast bacterium *Mycobacterium tuberculosis.* It also is rarely caused by *M. bovis, M. avium, M. kansasii,* or *M. intracellulare.* The disease is transmitted through the air when droplet nuclei are excreted from an infected individual; it also may rarely be obtained through direct cutaneous inoculation. Generally, the droplet nuclei (less than 5 μm in diameter) reach the lower respiratory tract, where the microorganism grows to form a colony, producing little immunologic response and no symptoms. The bacteria enter the blood stream and spread to the lymphatic system.

CLINICAL DISEASE. Initially, pulmonary tuberculosis is asymptomatic. After lesions appear in the lungs, symptoms due to an inflammatory response become apparent. There is a cough caused by irritations and secretions in the lungs. The sputum increases in volume, and may be green and purulent or yellowish and mucoid; it also may contain blood. Chest pain and difficulty in breathing develop with advanced tuberculosis. Symptoms may be intermittent over long periods of time because the infection can be rendered inactive by the host's immune response.

PATHOGENESIS. Tuberculosis is a prototype of infectious diseases in which cellular immunity is responsible for a large part of the pathogenesis. An initial infection with *M. tuberculosis* can progress for 3–6 wk before lymphocytes bring the infection under control. The lymphocytes are activated by mycobacterial antigens to produce lymphokines that, in turn, are chemotactic and stimulatory to macrophages. These activated macrophages differentiate into epithelioid cells and then to fibroblasts, halting multiplication of the bacteria. The activity of the lymphocytes is also responsible for local tissue hypersensitivity, resulting in necrosis. This immune response is bacteriostatic, not bactericidal. Therefore, *M. tuberculosis* may be inactive for years, later becoming reactivated. Less than 10 percent of diagnosed cases of tuberculosis represent new infections. The course of the disease depends on the lymphocyte-bacteria balance: an increase in lymphocytes and decrease in bacteria results in inactivity; the reverse results in the development of exudative lesions that progress to caseous necrosis. *M. tuberculosis* is a slow-growing bacterium (doubling every day or two) that requires oxygen and carbon dioxide (5–10 percent) for steady growth.

LABORATORY DIAGNOSIS. Sputum or gastric washings are stained for acid-fast mycobacteria. Direct staining without concentration may yield false-negative results. For best results, an early morning sputum should be tested; this allows for the accumulation of exudate overnight, resulting in an increased concentration of mycobacteria. The sputum should be liquefied with 0.1 N sodium hydroxide at 37°C and then centrifuged for concentration. The organism can be cultured on egg yolk–enriched agar or oleic acid–albumin agar and incubated at 37°C for 6 wk. If there is growth, the microorganism should be tested for the production of catalase and niacin and for susceptibility to isoniazid. *M tuberculosis* is positive for catalase and niacin, and susceptible to isoniazid. Isoniazid-resistant mutants of *M. tuberculosis* do not produce catalase. *M. bovis* is catalase-positive and niacin-negative.

There is also a tuberculin skin test for detecting delayed hypersensitivity with a purified protein derivative (see *Mantoux test*). It involves the intradermal injection of antigen and the observation of an inflammatory response within 48–72 hr. The tuberculin skin test is subject to false-positive results, owing to the lack of specificity and the possibility of cross-reactivity of the antigen.

See also *Mycobacterium* and *mycobacterium.*

central nervous system t., a form of tuberculosis that develops when *M. tuberculosis* progresses from the subependym to the subarachnoid space. It is often a complication of miliary tuberculosis. This form of tuberculosis is most common among children (age 1–5 yr); symptoms include headache, drowsiness, or coma.

endobronchial t., a progressive complication of pulmonary tuberculosis in which the bronchial mucosa becomes infected with *Mycobacterium tuberculosis* as a result of dissemination from cavitary tuberculosis of the lung.

extrapulmonary t., a type of tuberculosis that results from lymphohematogenous spread. The lungs are usually the primary site of extrapulmonary infection.

gastrointestinal t., a form of tuberculosis that can result from pulmonary tuberculosis or the ingestion of contaminated milk. Signs of GI tuberculosis include ulceration of the tongue and mouth, and infection and inflammation of the esophagus, stomach, small intestine, and colon. At any of these sites, the infected lesions can perforate and produce abscesses and fistulas.

laryngeal t., a complication of progressive pulmonary tuberculosis in which the *M. tuberculosis* infection spreads to the larynx. Symptoms and signs include hoarseness, pain, and difficulty in breathing; there may also be a hematogenous spread to the lungs. Individuals with laryngeal tuberculosis have an extremely poor prognosis, but the effectiveness of modern antibiotics has made this form of the disease uncommon.

miliary t., a type of tuberculosis in which the metastatic foci from the initial pulmonary lesions spread to locations near blood vessel lumens, where hypersensitivity and necrosis cause morbidity. A high temperature and meningeal complications often result.

pericardial t., a form of tuberculosis that results from the passage of *M. tuberculosis* from mediastinal nodes to the pericardium. It is often associated with pleural tuberculosis and is quite serious. Owing to the location of infection, diagnosis is sometimes difficult. Also called *tuberculous pericarditis.*

pleural t., a type of tuberculosis that occurs when subpleural foci of *M. tuberculosis,* which form during the early asymptomatic stages of the disease, break down and enter the pleural space. The resultant cellular immune response then causes a serofibrinous pleurisy with effusion.

pulmonary t., the most common form of tuberculosis, in which the primary infection is located in the lungs. Childhood pulmonary tuberculosis causes hilar lymphadenopathy and pleural involvement, as well as hypersensitivity reactions. Adult pulmonary tuberculosis begins in the apices of the lungs, spreading to the lower portions. Eventually, there is caseous necrosis, liquefaction, and cavity formation.

tuberculostearic acid (too-ber″ku-lo″ste′ah-rik) 10-methylstearic acid, a part of the lipids of the tubercle bacillus and of tuberculosis lesions.

tuberosity (too″bĕ-ros′ĭ-te) an elevation or protuberance.

ischial t., a large, rough, bony elevation along the inferior part of the posterior margin of the ischium. It is a site of attachment of several muscles.

pubic t., a rounded projection on the lateral extremity of the pubic crest situated at the superior border of the superior ramus of the pubic bone. It provides a point of attachment for the inguinal ligament. Also called pubic tubercle.

tibial t., a narrow, elongated, raised triangular area along the anterior crest of the proximal tibia. It is a point of attachment for the patellar ligament.

tuberous (too′ber-us) [L. *tuberosus,* from *tuber* swelling] knobby.

tuberous sclerosis see *tuberous s.* under *sclerosis.*

tube voltage in radiology, the high voltage applied across the x-ray tube, measured in *kilovolts.*

Tubifera (too-bĭ′fĕ-rah) [L. *tubus* tube + *-fer* bearer] a genus of flies, of which the species *T. tenax* (the drone fly) has been incriminated in the accidental production of intestinal myiasis in humans.

tubocurarine (too″bo-ku-rah′rēn) a toxic alkaloid isolated from trees of the genus *Chondodendron* native to South America; it is the active principle of curare.

t. chloride, [USP], a nondepolarizing neuromuscular blocking drug used to produce relaxation of the skeletal muscles during surgery and also during electroconvulsive therapy. Adverse reactions, primarily respiratory depression, are due to excessive muscle relaxation. A cholinesterase inhibitor such as neostigmine or edrophonium is administered to antagonize the effects or to assist recovery. See also *metocurine iodide.*

tubovillous adenoma an adenoma with a histologic pattern intermediate between that of tubular adenoma and villous adenoma. Also called papillary adenoma and villoglandular adenoma. See also *colon tumors* and *polyp.*

tubular (too′bu-lar) [L. *tubularis*] shaped like a tube; pertaining to a tubule.

tubular adenoma see *adenomatous p.* under *polyp.*

tubular interstitial nephritis see *tubulointerstitial nephropathy.*

tubule (too′būl) [L. *tubulus*] a small tube.

tubulin (too′bu-lin) [L. *tubulus*] a protein that is the major constituent of microtubules; M.W. 54,000. Tubulin exists as α- and β-tubulin, which must unite as dimers to form microtubules. Tubulin resembles actin in that it will bind with nucleotides and will combine with an ATPase, but it is a much larger molecule.

tubulointerstitial nephropathy (TIN) (tu″bu-lo-in″ter-stĭ′shul neph-rop′ah-the) a general term used to describe disease entities that primarily affect the renal tubules and interstitium. It is caused by a large number of unrelated diseases with different etiologies, such as infections, chemicals, immunologic reactions, physical damage, and congenital lesions, as listed in the accompanying table. These diseases range in frequency from the rare and exotic to the common bacterial pyelonephritis. In some cases of tubulointerstitial disease, a specific etiologic diagnosis can be made, but in many instances no cause can be identified even after a thorough clinical study has been made, cultures taken, and a renal biopsy performed. Most tubulointerstitial diseases are associated with an inflammatory infiltrate. TIN can be divided into acute and chronic types based mainly on the clinical course and, to a lesser extent, on the histologic pattern.

Acute TIN (acute tubulointerstitial nephritis) is characterized clinically by the abrupt onset of renal failure. The most important causes of acute TIN are acute pyelonephritis and drug-induced hypersensitivity; less frequently, it is caused by septicemia and myeloma. Histologically, there is interstitial edema, and a variable number of lymphocytes, plasma cells, and neutrophils are present in the interstitium. Eosinophils may be present in some cases, and can be numerous in the interstitial nephropathies caused by hypersensitivity to drugs and chemicals. In acute TIN, the tubules may be infiltrated with inflammatory cells and may be necrotic. When this pattern of tubular necrosis occurs, morphologic distinction from acute tubular necrosis (vasoactive nephropathy) is impossible.

TUBULOINTERSTITIAL NEUROPATHY. SOME CAUSES OF TUBULOINTERSTITIAL NEUROPATHY

CAUSE	TYPE OF NEPHROPATHY
Bacterial infections	Acute pyelonephritis Chronic and granulomatous pyelonephritis Reflux and obstruction
Drug reactions	Acute interstitial nephropathy Penicillin and its analogs Sulfonamides Cephalothin Tetracyclines Thiazides Chronic interstitial nephropathy Analgesics Lithium
Immune complex depositions	Primary tubulointerstitial immunologic injury Secondary to glomerulopathy
Metabolic factors	Urates and oxalates Hypercalcemia
Miscellaneous factors	Heavy metals Hereditary and congenital Radiation Idiopathic

Courtesy of Richard L. Kempson, M.D.

A wide variety of conditions can cause chronic TIN (chronic tubulointerstitial nephritis), the most important and frequent of which is chronic pyelonephritis. Vesicoureteral reflux, metabolic disturbances such as oxalate and urate nephropathies, and analgesic nephropathies are also prominent causes. Individuals with chronic TIN generally have a more prolonged course than those with acute TIN, and progress more slowly into renal failure. Histologically, there is less edema, and increased fibrous tissue separates the tubules. The tubules often demonstrate varying degrees of atrophy rather than necrosis, and tubular casts may be abundant. The inflammatory infiltrate is predominantly composed of lymphocytes and plasma cells; neutrophils and eosinophils generally are not present or are inconspicuous. Focally, the inflammatory infiltrate may be dense and associated with extensive renal parenchymal destruction. In far-advanced chronic TIN, the glomeruli demonstrate periglomerular fibrosis or obsolescence.

The functional abnormalities in TIN vary from mild and subtle tubular dysfunction to hematuria, proteinuria, oliguria with renal failure, and a clinical picture very similar to that of the primary glomerulopathies. Functional impairment may be localized in the proximal tubules, the distal tubules, the medulla, or combinations of these. In general, the more severe and diffuse the inflammatory changes, particularly in chronic TIN, the more severe the functional impairment. In far-advanced cases, there is striking impairment of glomerular function with reduction in the glomerular filtration rate (GFR) and proteinuria.

The prognosis in TIN appears to depend on the severity of the inflammatory response. When edema is prominent and extensive fibrosis is absent, complete recovery is the rule if treatment is promptly instituted and the offending agent removed. When extensive scarring and glomerular destruction have occurred, residual impairment of renal function can be expected even after successful removal of the cause of the nephropathy.

Also called tubular interstitial disease and *tubular interstitial nephritis.*

RICHARD L. KEMPSON, M.D.

tuftsin (tuft′sin) the peptide responsible for the biologic activity of leukokinin. Its amino acid sequence is threonine-lysine-proline-arginine. Tuftsin is believed to be produced in the spleen, which may be one of the reasons why persons who have had a splenectomy are more susceptible to certain infections. See also *leukokinin.*

tuftsin deficiency a rare condition characterized by the lack of tuftsin, a phagocytosis-stimulating tetrapeptide. The disorder may be familial, or it may occur in splenectomized persons. Those affected are subject to severe local and systemic infections. There is no known treatment for tuftsin deficiency, although gamma-globulin therapy seems to be beneficial.

tularemia (too″lah-re′me-ah) [*Tulare* a district in California, where the disease was first described] an infectious zoonotic disease of rodents, resembling plague, which is acquired by the bites of deerflies and ticks, and more often by handling contaminated animals or their products. Rabbits, muskrats, and squirrels are the most frequent sources. The etiologic agent is *Francisella tularensis,* a small, pleomorphic, nonmotile, gram-negative bacillus with only one serologic type. There are two varieties of this organism: a virulent strain found only in North America, designated Jellson type A, and an avirulent strain, Jellson type B. The cottontail rabbit commonly carries *F. tularensis* in the blood and liver. The infectious agent enters the host through skin wounds, inhalation, or ingestion. As a result, there are several different forms of tularemia: ulceroglandular, oculoglandular, typhoidal, and pneumonic.

Once in the body, *F. tularensis* reaches the blood via the lymphatics. This bacterium may grow and multiply intracellularly after phagocytosis, which eventually leads to granulomatous lesions. The macrophage is the predominant phagocyte. Progressive tularemia can lead to caseous necrosis and abscess formation in infected tissues. There is an incubation period of 2–10 da, after which headache, fever, regional lymph node enlargement, myalgia, and prostration develop. Pneumonia sometimes occurs.

Diagnosis is based on bacteriologic and serologic tests. Laboratory personnel should be cautious in handling specimens from individuals suspected of having tularemia because of the highly infectious nature of *F. tularensis.* The microorganism grows on blood glucose–cysteine agar. Multiple blood specimens should be collected and transported in a medium without anticoagulants. Ulcers, if present, should also be cultured. The cultures are incubated in a CO_2 atmosphere at 37°C for 18 hr. For the serologic identification of tularemia, an agglutination test can identify serum antigens after 1 wk of infection. A titer of 1:40 or greater or a rise of antibody titer with time is diagnostic. There is also a skin test utilizing delayed hypersensitivity; 48 hr after purified *F. tularensis* antigen is injected intradermally, an erythematous reaction is indicative of tularemia. The skin test will be positive after 1 wk of infection and will remain positive for years.

oculoglandular t., a form of tularemia that involves eye contamination and results in pain, photophobia, itching, lacrimation, and a mucopurulent discharge. Granulomatous lesions may form on the cornea. Regional lymph nodes are enlarged; if this disease progresses, corneal perforation and optic atrophy may occur.

pneumonic t., a form of tularemia in which lung infection results from bacteremia or from inhalation of the etiologic agent. Clinical manifestations include a nonproductive cough, headache, fever, malaise, and substernal pain. The sputum can be bloody and mucoid. Physical findings may be minimal, even with extensive involvement of the lung fields.

typhoidal (enteric) t., an unusual form of tularemia in which large numbers of *F. tularensis* are swallowed, producing abdominal pain, high fever, and symptoms similar to those of typhoid fever.

ulceroglandular t., the most frequent form of human tularemia. Infection begins as an erythematous papule at the site of entry, generally the skin. As the local lesion develops into a pustule and then an ulcer, there is enlargement of regional lymph nodes, which often suppurate, accompanied by systemic manifestations. Pneumonia may be a complication.

tumor (too′mor) [L. from *tumere* to swell] 1. a swelling. Tumor was one of Galen's four cardinal signs of inflammation.

2. see *neoplasm* and the specific tumor.

tumor antigen see *T antigen.*

tumor-associated rejection antigen (TARA) a highly polymorphic tumor-associated antigen present in cells transformed by chemical carcinogens to which an immune response can be mounted, resulting in rejection of the tumor. The same carcinogen can induce expression of different TARAs on individual tumors in the same animal.

tumor cell kinetics see *chemotherapy* and *neoplastic growth.*

tumor grading a method of predicting the biologic behavior of malignant neoplasms (i.e., likelihood of recurrence, metastases, or both) and, by extension, of prognosticating patient outcome from the assessment of certain cytologic and histologic features of the neoplasm. Typically, the results of such an evaluation are expressed on a scale of three or four grades, grade 1 representing tumors with the best differentiation, and the highest grade representing tumors with the poorest differentiation. In general, the poorer the degree of differentiation (the higher the number), the more aggressive the tumor and the worse the prognosis.

Current tumor grading systems incorporate many concepts of earlier systems, relying heavily on cytologic features such as the frequency of mitosis, degree of nuclear hyperchromasia and pleomorphism, and ratio of nuclear to cytoplasmic diameter to determine tumor grade. Recently, increasing attention has been paid to tumor architecture, as well as to other morphologic features in tumor grading. For example, in adenocarcinoma of the breast, architectural features (e.g., degree of structural disarray, presence or absence of papillary structures, extent of necrosis, percentage of glandular elements present, presence or absence of vascular invasion, nature of the advancing border of the tumor) as well as features of host response (e.g., accumulation of lymphocytes and plasma cells and stromal proliferation) have been taken into consideration. No single system of histologic grading is applicable to all malignant neoplasms. For some neoplasms, tumor morphology and tumor behavior are poorly correlated and tumor grading is of little or no value. For other tumors, histologic grading is useful to varying degrees, depending on the tissue of origin and the histologic subtype of the tumor in question.

A major obstacle to making greater use of tumor grading is the need for better definition of the criteria necessary to achieve reproducible results from one observer to another. Despite the limitations of the technique, histologic grading has proved valuable for certain tumor types, and it may be of particular clinical use for those tumors in which it has prognostic value when surgical staging is not available.

Also called *histologic grading.* Cf. *tumor staging.*

tumorlet (too′mor-let) a term for a small nodule of the lung produced by proliferation of serotonin-forming argentaffin (Kulchitsky) cells. Tumorlets are often multiple and may occur in association with pulmonary fibrosis. Histologically, their oval or elongated cells are similar to those of a carcinoid tumor.

tumor markers metabolically and biologically active products released by tumors (tumor-derived markers) or produced by the cells of uninvolved organs or tissues in response to the presence, physical or chemical, of a tumor in the body (tumor-associated markers).

Tumor-derived and tumor-associated markers can be detected in the blood, the urine, and other body fluids. Tumor-derived markers can also be detected in or on the tumor cells of origin with appropriate immunohistochemical techniques (see *immunoperoxidase technique*).

In general, tumor markers may be categorized as: (1) hormones and their subunits, (2) oncofetal antigens and other so-called "antigens," (3) enzymes and isoenzymes, and (4) other macromolecules. Some examples of tumor-derived markers and the characteristic tumors that produce them are shown in the accompanying table.

TUMOR MARKERS

PRODUCT	TYPICAL CARCINOMAS
Hormones and their subunits	
ACTH and related MSH, LPH	Bronchus
ADH	Bronchus
Hypothalamic releasing factors	Bronchus
Calcitonin	Bronchus, breast
HCG and subunits	Bronchus, teratoma
PTH	Bronchus
Prostaglandins	Breast, colon
Oncofetal products and other 'antigens'	
CEA and related materials	Gastrointestinal
AFP	Hepatoma, teratoma
FSA	Gastric
Ferritin (α_2-HFP)	Many
BOFA	Many
Cancer basic protein	All
Pregnancy associated proteins	Breast, teratoma
Placental type enzymes	Many
Enzymes	
Prolyl hydroxylase	Hepatoma, breast
Sialyl transferase	Many
Phosphatases	Prostate, hepatoma
Other macromolecules	
Milk protein	Breast
Polyamines	Many
Nucleosides	Many
Paraproteins	Myeloma

From Woolf, N., and Anthony, P. P.: Recent Advances in Histopathology. 10th ed. Edinburgh, Churchill Livingstone, 1979, p. 24.

The application of tumor markers to oncology includes their use in deriving a functional classification of neoplasms; as an aid in the diagnosis, staging, and monitoring of malignant neoplasms; and in explaining certain systemic effects of cancer.

tumor necrosis factor (TNF) a factor that causes a hemorrhagic necrosis of tumors in vivo, and cytotoxic effects on transformed and tumor cells in vitro, while not affecting normal cells; M.W. 62,000. TNF probably is produced by mononuclear cells and is not species-specific.

tumor promoter see *tumor p.* under *promoter.*

tumor registry see under *registry.*

tumor-specific antigen an antigen that is expressed by tumor cells transformed by chemical carcinogens; it is not expressed by normal cells. In laboratory animals, it has been shown that immunity to transplanted tumors can be induced in syngeneic recipients by pretreating the recipient with tumor cells.

tumor staging a technique for describing the anatomic extent of a malignant neoplasm in a common language that can be understood anywhere in the world. The practice of dividing cancer cases into groups according to so-called stages arose from the finding that survival rates were better for patients in whom the maligant neoplasm was localized than for those in whom the tumor had extended beyond the site or organ of origin. From these observations, staging systems have been developed with the objectives of providing a basis for: (1) assisting the clinician in planning treatment; (2) providing an estimate of the prognosis; (3) establishing criteria to be used in evaluating the prognosis; (4) facilitating the exchange of information between treatment centers; and (5) contributing to the continuing research on human cancer.

Most staging systems are based both on assessment of anatomic spread and on pathologic findings. The majority have as a basic limitation the fact that they do not include the degree of histologic differentiation of the cancer. The notable exception to this is the method for staging non-Hodgkin's malignant lymphomas, in which morphologic classification is weighted as heavily as the extent of the disease in arriving at the tumor stage.

Although many staging systems have been proposed, some unique to specific organs or neoplasms, the method that has received the most widespread acceptance is the TNM system. In this system, T defines the primary tumor (numerals are added to indicate either the size or degree of penetration into surrounding tissues); N describes the number of regional lymph nodes in proximity to the primary tumor that are found microscopically to contain metastatic tumor; and M indicates whether distant metastases have been detected. By thus grouping the characteristics of a tumor into its TNM classes, stages of diseases have been defined, which allow for universal communication and data accrual. Tables 1 and 2 are representative examples illustrating how cancer of the stomach is staged. Analysis of this example indicates that adequate staging requires careful inspection and surgical removal of suspected malignant tumor, and biopsy sampling of regional lymph nodes. Examination must include a complete pathologic review of all submitted specimens. Finally, appropriate modern diagnostic studies must be undertaken as clinically indicated to search for distant metastases.

Hodgkin's disease and the non-Hodgkin's malignant lymphomas are examples of neoplasms in which histopathologic classification is the major basis for international data accumulation and study. These classifications, as well as their implications for prognosis, have been altered many times, yet undergo continued revision as newer laboratory techniques for studying these lymphomas become available. The most current Working Formulation of Non-Hodgkin's Lymphomas for Clinical Usage incorporates the prognostic significance of each entity (see the table under *lymphoma*). The extent of disease in both Hodgkin's disease and non-Hodgkin's malignant lymphoma shares a similar staging system, as shown in Table 3. Meticulous staging of these diseases by a broad array of diag-

TUMOR STAGING, TABLE 1. TNM CLASSIFICATION FOR CANCER OF THE STOMACH

Stage	Involvement
Primary Tumor (T)	
TX	Degree of penetration of stomach wall not determined
T0	No evidence of primary tumor
T1	Tumor limited to mucosa and submucosa regardless of its extension or location
T2	Tumor involvement of mucosa, submucosa (including muscularis propria), and extension to or into serosa, but without penetration through serosa
T3	Tumor penetration through serosa without invasion of contiguous structures
T4	Tumor penetration through serosa and invasion of contiguous structures
Nodal Involvement (N)	
NX	Metastases to intraabdominal lymph nodes not determined (e.g., laparotomy not performed)
N0	No metastases to regional lymph nodes
N1	Involvement of perigastric lymph nodes within 3 cm of primary tumor along lesser or greater curvature
N2	Involvement of regional lymph nodes more than 3 cm from primary tumor, which are removed or removable at operation, including those located along left gastric, splenic, celiac, and common hepatic arteries
N3	Involvement of other intraabdominal lymph nodes that are not removable at operation, such as paraaortic, hepatoduodenal, retropancreatic, and mesenteric nodes
Distant Metastases (M)	
MX	Not assessed
M0	No (known) distant metastasis
M1	Distant metastasis present

Courtesy of Richard J. Cohen, M.D.

nostic tests is mandatory for the successful application of specific treatment programs.

RICHARD J. COHEN, M.D.

Tunga (tung'gah) a genus of fleas, of which the species *T. penetrans*, distributed throughout the tropical regions of America and Africa, causes dermatitis in humans. Also called burrowing flea, chigoe, *jigger*, nigua, and sand flea.

tungiasis (tung-gi'ah-sis) an infection with fleas of the species *Tunga penetrans*. Human infestation is acquired from contact with earth or sand contaminated by infested pigs or dogs. These animals drop flea eggs to the ground, where the insect develops through the larvae, pupae and unfed adult stages of its life cycle. A gravid female flea then burrows into the skin of a host (usually beneath the nails of the toes and fingers) and engorges itself, becoming distended by blood and developing eggs. The sites develop into festering sores with intense itching and inflammation. Usually they become secondarily in-

TUMOR STAGING, TABLE 2. STAGE GROUPING

Stage	Clinical-Diagnostic Staging	Postsurgical Treatment Pathologic Staging
I	cT1 N0 M0	pT1 N0 M0
II	cT2 N0 M0 cT3 N0 M0	pT2 N0 M0 pT3 N0 M0
III	cTX–3 N1–3 M0	pT1–3 N1 M0 pT1–3 N2 M0 pT1–3 N3 M0 (resected for cure)
IV	cT4 NX–3 M0 (probably not resectable) cTX–4 NX–3 M1	pT1–3 N3 M0 pT4 N0–3 M0 (not resectable) pT1–4 or pTX or N0–3 or NX M1

Courtesy of Richard J. Cohen, M.D.

TUMOR STAGING, TABLE 3. ANN ARBOR STAGING CLASSIFICATION OF LYMPHOMA AND HODGKIN'S DISEASE

STAGE	INVOLVEMENT
I	Single lymph node region (I) or localized involvement of single extranodal organ/site (I_E)
II	More than one lymph node region on same side of diaphragm (II) or one or more lymph node regions and localized involvement of an extralymphatic organ/site (II_E) on same side of diaphragm
III	Lymph node regions on both sides of diaphragm (III), which may be accompanied by splenic involvement (III_S), by localized involvement of an extralymphatic organ/site (III_E), or by both (III_{SE})
IV	Diffuse or disseminated involvement of one or more extralymphatic organs/sites with or without lymph node involvement

Courtesy of Richard J. Cohen, M.D.

fected, leading to ulceration, abscesses, tetanus, or gas gangrene.

Infestation is treated by surgically removing the flea aseptically with a needle, or bathing the area in Lysol, puncturing the wound, and repeating the Lysol bath to kill the eggs and sterilize the wound.

Tungidae (tun′gĭ-de) a family of fleas including the genera *Echidnophaga* and *Tunga.*

tungsten (W) (tung′sten) [Swed. "heavy stone"; Ger. *wolfram*] a hard, gray metallic element; atomic number 74; atomic weight 183.85; a 5d transition element; oxidation states −2, +1 through +6.

Tungsten has the highest melting point of all metals (3410°C) and is used to make filaments for incandescent lights and electron tubes, anodes in x-ray tubes, tungsten steel (a high-strength alloy), and tungsten carbide, WC, an extremely strong material used for cutting tools and abrasives. Individuals involved in the production of tungsten carbide are at risk for developing hard-metal pneumoconiosis caused by cobalt in ore dusts.

tungstic acid (tung′stik as′id) a yellow crystalline compound, H_2WO_4, used in analytic procedures as a protein precipitant. It is insoluble in water or acid but is slowly soluble in alkali. In the Folin-Wu type of protein-free filtrate, the proteins are precipitated by tungstic acid formed in situ after mixing a solution of Na_2WO_4 and H_2SO_4.

tunica (too′nĭ-kah), pl. *tunicae* [L.] [NA], a general term for a covering or coat; the thin membrane or other structure that covers or lines a body part or organ.

t. adventitia, the fibrous connective tissue outer layer of an artery or vein.

t. albuginea of the spleen, the dense fibroelastic covering of the spleen.

t. albuginea of the testis, [NA], a dense, bluish-white fibrous coat that invests the testis beneath the visceral layer of the tunica vaginalis.

t. intima, see *intima.*

t. media, the muscular middle layer of a blood vessel. It is composed of muscle cells, elastic fibers, and the external elastic lamina.

t. vaginalis testis, [NA], the serous membrane that covers the front and sides of the testis and epididymis; the distal extremity of the processus vaginalis.

Turbatrix (tur-ba′triks) a genus of rhabditoid nematodes, of which the species *T. aceti* has been recovered from the urine or vaginal exudate of females who accidentally introduced the worm into the vagina when using vinegar as a vaginal douche. This worm exhibits some potentialities of becoming a parasite but cannot establish itself permanently in the vagina. Also called vinegar eel.

turbidimeter (tur″bĭ-dim′ĕ-ter) a colorimeter used for measuring turbidity.

turbidimetric (tur″bid-ĭ-met′rik) performed with a turbidimeter.

turbidimetric immunoassays see *nonradioisotopic i.* under *immunoassays.*

turbidimetry (tur″bĭ-dim′ĕ-tre) the measurement of turbidity. It is generally performed using an instrument (a spectrophotometer or colorimeter) that measures the ratio of the intensity of the light transmitted through a dispersion to the intensity of the incident light. The measurement is affected by light absorbed by solvent and particles, as well as light scattered by the particles in the suspension.

turbidity (tur″bid′ĭ-te) [L. *turbidus* muddy] the cloudiness of a solution caused by suspended particles that scatter light. The amount of light scattered is related in a complex way to the concentration of the particles and to their sizes and shapes. Turbidity measurements can be very sensitive methods of analysis but, because they are highly dependent on experimental conditions, reproducibility is often poor. See also *nephelometry* and *turbidimetry.*

Turcot's syndrome (tur-koz′) [J. *Turcot*] a rare association of adenomas of the colon and tumors of the central nervous system, thought to be transmitted as an autosomal recessive trait. See also *multiple p.* under *polyposis.*

Türk's irritation leukocyte see *Türk's irritation l.* under *leukocyte.*

turnaround time (turn′ah-round′ tīm′) 1. in laboratory medicine, the length of time between submission of a specimen for analysis and the availability of the results to the clinician.

2. in computer processing, the length of time between the submission of a job for processing and the return of the results.

Turnbull blue (turn′bul) a dark blue dye, ferrous ferricyanide, $Fe_3(Fe(CN)_6)_2$, formed in a reaction to demonstrate ferrous iron in tissue; M.W. 591.45. See under *iron-positive pigment demonstration.*

Turner's syndrome (tur′nerz) [Henry Hubert *Turner,* American endocrinologist, born 1892] an abnormality of the sex chromosome, resulting from nondisjunction of an X chromosome; the sexual karyotype is XO. Individuals are phenotypic females and lack sex chromatin. Typical features of Turner's syndrome include short stature, sparse pubic hair, sexual infantilism, webbing of the neck, cubitus valgus, and broad chest with widely spaced nipples. Early embryonic development of the ovaries is normal, but degeneration leads to a whitish streak of ovarian tissue in connective tissue prior to birth.

About 15 percent of all those affected with Turner's syndrome are mosaics, XO/XX, XO/XXX, and XO/XY being the most common.

Also called *gonadal dysgenesis.* See also *sex determination.*

turnkey system (turn′ke sis′tem) a computer installation for which the vendor supplies all the necessary software. It is ready to perform its intended function as delivered; no user programming is necessary.

turnover (turn′o-ver) 1. the replacement of atoms or molecules in a structure or tissue by identical atoms and molecules, thus maintaining a dynamic steady state.

2. the maximal number of substrate molecules that can be consumed per minute by an enzyme under optimal conditions. Also called *turnover number.*

turnover number see *turnover.*

turpentine oil (tur′pen-tīn) [L. *terebinthinus,* of the turpentine tree, from *terebinthus* turpentine tree] the volatile oil distilled from an oleoresin obtained from *Pinus palustris* and other species of *Pinus;* used as a counterirritant and rubefacient. When ingested or otherwise absorbed, it produces abdominal pain and depression of the central nervous system; if aspirated, it may produce pulmonary edema and pneumonitis. Turpentine oil may impart to urine a smell resembling that of violets.

rectified t. o., turpentine oil that has been rectified by the addition of sodium hydroxide, used as an inhalation expectorant.

T wave the deflection in the electrocardiogram that is the result of recovery (repolarization) of the ventricles. An inversion in the polarity of the T wave is commonly seen with diseases affecting the ventricles.

Tween (twēn) trademark. See *polysorbate.*

12/60 see *SMA 12/60.*

twin (twin) one of two offspring produced in the same pregnancy.

conjoined t.'s, monozygotic twins produced by an incomplete split of the original embryo, occurring relatively late in development. This takes place with a frequency of 1 in 120,000 births or 1 in 400 monozygotic twin births. Conjoined twins can be separated if they have no vital organs or parts in common.

dizygotic t.'s, twins developed from two separate ova fertilized at the same time. Genetically, they are no more closely related to each other than to other full siblings. Also called *fraternal t.'s.*

fraternal t.'s, see *dizygotic t.'s.*

heterokaryotic t.'s, monozygotic twins with different karyotypes. Such twins are rare and are thought to originate in zygotic nondisjunction preceded, followed, or accompanied by twinning.

identical t.'s, see *monozygotic t.'s.*

monozygotic t.'s, genetically identical twins developed from a single fertilized ovum. Also called *identical t.'s.*

Twining position (twīn′ing) a radiographic position used to obtain a lateral projection in which the cervicothoracic vertebrae are not obscured by the shoulders. The patient is erect, and the film is parallel to the median sagittal plane and centered to the adjacent axilla. The shoulder nearer the film is rotated forward and elevated by placing the hand on top of the head; the farther shoulder is depressed and rotated back. The central ray is horizontal or, if the shoulder cannot be depressed, directed toward the feet at an angle of up to 15°.

twitch (twich) a single, brief contraction of a skeletal muscle that is elicited by a synchronous volley of impulses arriving in the motor neurons that supply it.

two-dimensional chromatography see *paper chromatography.*

two's complement (tooz′ com′plĕ-ment) a representation of binary numbers used in computers in which negative numbers are obtained by subtracting their absolute value from zero. If the word size is n, then the numbers from 1 to $2^{n-1} - 1$ represent themselves, and the numbers from 2^{n-1} to 2^n represent negative numbers. The representation $2^n - x$ corresponds to the number $-x$. The most significant bit indicates the sign of the number: if this bit is "1," the number is negative; otherwise, it is positive. Cf. *signed magnitude.*

two-sided alternative (too′sīd″ed awl-ter′nah-tiv) an alternative hypothesis that a population parameter differs from the value specified by the null hypothesis. A two-tailed hypothesis test is used based on a test statistic estimating the parameter. See also *hypothesis testing* and *two-tailed test.* Cf. *one-sided alternative.*

two-tailed test (too′tāld″ test′) a statistical hypothesis test in which the critical region consists of all values of the test statistic below a specified lower critical value and of all values above an upper critical value. Usually, both tails are assigned the same probability $\alpha/2$, where α is the significance level, especially when the test statistic has a symmetric distribution. See also *hypothesis testing.* Cf. *one-tailed test.*

Tylenol (ti′lĕ-nol) trademark. See *acetaminophen.*

tympan/o (tim′pah-no) a word element used in combining form to denote the eardrum or middle ear, e.g., tympanosclerosis.

tympanic (tim-pan′ik) [L. *tympanicus*] of or pertaining to the tympanic cavity.

tympanic cavity an irregular, air-filled space within the temporal bone that contains the auditory ossicles. It is enclosed laterally by the tympanic membrane and medially by the wall of the inner ear, and communicates posteriorly with the mastoid air cells and anteriorly with the pharyngotympanic tube. This latter connection provides a route for the spread of upper respiratory tract infections to the middle ear. Also called *middle ear* and *tympanum.*

tympanic membrane the membrane between the external acoustic meatus and the tympanic cavity of the ear. It is a fibrous sheet covered externally by ectodermal epithelium and internally by entoderm, with a plexus of blood vessels lying between the two.

The tympanic membrane is connected to the inner ear by the auditory ossicles. See also *ear.*

tympanography (tim″pah-nog′rah-fe) see *eustachianography.*

tympanosclerosis (tim″pah-no-sklĕ-ro′sis) [*tympano-* + Gr. *sklĕrōsis* hardening] a condition characterized by the presence of masses of hard, dense connective tissue around the auditory ossicles in the middle ear.

tympanum (tim′pah-num) [L., from Gr. *tympanon* drum] see *tympanic cavity.*

Tymphonotonus (tim″fo-not′ŏ-nus) see *Cerithidia.*

type (tīp) [L. *typus,* from Gr. *typos* mark] the general or prevailing character, as of an individual, a species, or a particular case of disease.

type culture a standard strain of bacteria or other microorganisms maintained in pure culture at various laboratories in many countries. The most extensive collection in the United States is kept by the American Type Culture Collection (ATCC) in Bethesda, Maryland. See also *American Type Culture Collection.*

Type I error in statistical hypothesis testing, rejection of the null hypothesis when it is in fact true. See also *hypothesis testing.*

Type II error in statistical hypothesis testing, acceptance of the null hypothesis when it is in fact false. See also *hypothesis testing.*

type species in bacteriology, the species that characterizes a genus. When reclassification occurs, the type species always retains the generic name, except when two genera are combined. Type species are designated by the *International Journal of Systematic Bacteriology.*

type strain a strain of bacteria or other microorganisms that is maintained in culture as the standard type species of the genus. See also *American Type Culture Collection.*

typewriter terminal (tīp′rī″ter ter′mĭ-nal) a slow-speed printer (20–60 lines/min) that prints text a character at a time. A new line is generated by line feed and carriage return. Special code characters received by the terminal from the computer. Cf. *line printer.*

typhoid fever (ti′foid) [Gr. *typhōdes* like smoke; delirious] a generalized febrile illness caused by the gram-negative bacterium *Salmonella typhi.* Typhoid fever is a systemic disease; the portal of entry is the gastrointestinal tract. *S. typhi* is transmitted by contaminated food and water through flies, fingers, and fomites. As the organism grows only within humans, occurrence of the disease indicates the presence of a carrier.

Once ingested, *S. typhi* microorganisms invade the intestinal mucosa and spread via the lymphatics to the blood stream. Large numbers of bacteria ($> 10^7$) are usually necessary for production of the disease because many are killed in gastric acid. After bacteremia is established, the bacteria multiply within macrophages and monocytic cells and subsequently spread to various organs.

The duration of typhoid fever is variable, usually 4 wk; the length of the incubation period (7–14 da) depends on the size of the inoculating dose. Clinical manifestations during the first week include fever, headache, abdominal pains, an enlarged spleen, and a rose spot rash. This may be followed by a period of mental deterioration, including delirium and even coma. During the third week of illness, all previous symptoms progress and diarrhea and intestinal hemorrhage may begin. During the fourth week of illness, the previous symptoms subside, with the patient experiencing fatigue and weight loss.

Certain individuals may become carriers of typhoid fever after acute infection has subsided. Most often this happens when *S. typhi* organisms persist in the gallbladder and are shed periodically. A carrier who is a food handler is especially dangerous.

To establish diagnosis, *S. typhi* should be cultured from the individual. The best specimen source depends on the stage of the disease. Initially, *S. typhi* is found only in the blood. As the disease progresses, it is rarely found in the blood but may be isolated from the stool. During the third week of illness, the organisms are often found in the urine. Suspected carriers should have cultures of bile, stool, and urine specimens.

See also *Salmonella.*

typhous (ti′fus) pertaining to typhus.

typhus (ti′fus) [Gr. *typhos* stupor arising from fever] a general term used to describe a group of infectious diseases caused by rickettsial organisms. Typhus causes a high fever, skin rash, and mental debilitation. On the basis of the epidemiology, etiologic agent, and clinical manifestations, typhus may be separated into three forms: epidemic louse-borne, recrudescent (Brill-Zinsser), and endemic murine. See also *Rickettsiaceae* and the specific form of typhus.

endemic murine t., an acute febrile illness transmitted from a rodent to a human through a rat flea (*Xenopsylla cheopsis*) vector. The etiologic agent of murine typhus is *Rickettsia mooseri* (*R. typhus*), which contains an antigen in common with *Proteus* OX19 strains. This disease is a zoonosis with symptoms similar to, but milder than, epidemic louse-borne typhus. The incubation period for murine typhus is 6–14 da. Often there is a history of association with locations where rats or mice are numerous. The prognosis and prevention are similar to those for epidemic typhus. See also *Rickettsiaceae.*

epidemic louse-borne t., an ancient disease, the etiologic agent of which is *Rickettsia prowazekii,* a small pleomorphic bacterium that is an obligate intracellular parasite. First described in 1546, the disease has changed the course of history through epidemics in military personnel during World War I and, to a lesser extent, World War II. The rickettsiae are transmitted by the human body louse, *Pediculus humanus,* although not by louse bite. They grow in the gut of the louse (up to 10^8 bacteria per louse) and are excreted in the feces. The contaminated feces enters the human body through minor skin lesions. *R. prowazekii* will kill the louse within 2 wk. Epidemic typhus is most likely to occur under conditions predisposing to lousiness.

CLINICAL DISEASE. The clinical manifestations of epidemic typhus begin after an incubation period of 8–12 da. The prodromal phase of the disease involves malaise, headache, and myalgia followed by an acute onset of fever, back and leg pain, and chills. The fever remains constant: 39°–41°C. Eventually the headache becomes intensely severe, and the individual's mental state is altered. Cough, nausea, and weakness may also be present. A macular rash appears on the first febrile day, beginning on the trunk and spreading to the extremities. If untreated, the disease progresses to stupor, delirium, and cranial nerve impairment. Death usually occurs between da 9 and da 18 of the illness. Secondary bacterial infections and "superinfections" are common complications.

LABORATORY DIAGNOSIS. Laboratory tests are similar to those for all rickettsial infections. Serologic identification is the safest approach, owing to the infectious hazards of isolating the organism. However, antibodies are not formed until the individual has been infected for about 1 wk. The Weil-Felix test is an agglutination test using OX strains of *Proteus* species containing an antigen shared with rickettsiae and the patient's serum. It is a simple, inexpensive, and standard test for suspected rickettsial disease, although a minor drawback is its nonspecificity. Antibodies from primary louse-borne typhus agglutinate the OX19 strain of *Proteus.* Another assay for rickettsiae is the complement-fixation test, in which rickettsial antigens are used to screen patient sera for antibodies. The indirect fluorescent-antibody technique is an alternate and useful serologic procedure.

The prevention and control of typhus depends on elimination of the louse. Nonimmune persons are quite susceptible to typhus; should a typhus-infected individual require hospitalization, it is essential to decontaminate the clothing, blankets, and skin to remove all louse feces. Proper hygienic procedures, together with the application of insecticides to the skin, help to reduce the incidence of typhus. If untreated, the death rate of typhus has a range of 10–60 percent.

See also *Rickettsiaceae.*

recrudescent t., a reactivation of epidemic louse-borne typhus, which can occur months or years after the initial infection. The etiologic agent, *Rickettsia prowazekii,* persists in the body tissue in an inactive state (for as long as 70 yr), with humans as the reservoir.

Unlike epidemic louse-borne typhus, recrudescent typhus produces a lower fever of shorter duration. In a primary (epidemic louse-borne) typhus infection, the immediate antibody response involves IgM immunoglobulins; however, the secondary long-term antibody response involves IgG immunoglobulins. Therefore, serologic diagnosis is accomplished with the identification of IgG antibodies. See also the information on laboratory diagnosis under *epidemic louse-borne t.*

Also called *Brill's disease* and *Brill-Zinsser disease.* See also *Rickettsiaceae.*

scrub t., a typhuslike disease caused by *Rickettsia tsutsugamushi* (*R. orientalis*), which is transmitted by the bite of larval trombiculid mites (chiggers). Scrub typhus is most often seen in Asia and the southern Pacific. A small, painless papule forms at the site of the chigger bite, becoming enlarged with an area of central necrosis. Regional lymphadenopathy is characteristic of scrub typhus. Other clinical symptoms include headache, fever, anorexia, weakness, malaise, and splenomegaly. As scrub typhus progresses, meningoencephalitis and focal myocarditis appear. All abnormalities reverse in nonfatal cases.

The diagnosis of scrub typhus depends on physical examination, on rickettsial serology (see under *epidemic louse-borne t.*) and sometimes on isolation within white mice.

Also called *tsutsugamushi fever.* See also *Rickettsiaceae.*

typhus antibody tests assays for antibody to rickettsia that cause typhus. The most common tests include the indirect immunofluorescence, indirect hemagglutination, and Weil-Felix tests, which are performed in the same manner as for Rocky Mountain spotted fever. See also *Rocky Mountain spotted fever antibody tests* and information on laboratory diagnosis under *epidemic louse-borne t.*

typing (tīp′ing) in bacteriology, the characterization of bacteria to distinguish between closely related strains of a species. Methods used include antigen-antibody reactions to immune sera (serotyping), demonstration of susceptibility to various bacteriophages (phage typing), and susceptibility to certain colicins (colicin typing).

Tyr abbrev. See *tyrosine.*

tyramine (ti′rah-mēn) the decarboxylation product of tyrosine, which occurs in ripe cheese, ergot, and decayed animal tissue. Tyramine stimulates the release of the neurotransmitter noradrenalin in the nervous system.

Tyroglyphidae (ti″ro-glif′ĭ-de) [Gr. *tyros* cheese + *glyphein* to cut + -idae sons of] a family of mites that includes the genus *Tyrophagus.*

tyropanoate (ti″ro-pah-no′āt) a radiopaque contrast medium used in oral cholecystography. It is a water-soluble triiodobenzene derivative. Trademark for t. sodium, *Bilopaque.*

Tyrophagus (ti-rof′ah-gus) [Gr. *tyros* cheese + *phagein* to eat] a genus of mites of cosmopolitan distribution found in cereals, grains, and various other stored products. In copra handlers, the species *T. castellanii* causes a condition known as copra itch. *T. longior* may contaminate cheese and thus may be ingested, but it does not produce a true intestinal infection.

tyrosine (Tyr or Y) (ti′ro-sin) [Gr. tyros cheese] 2-amino-3-(4-hydroxyphenyl)propanoic acid, $HOC_6H_4CH_2CH(NH_2)COOH$, a naturally occurring, nonessential amino acid; M.W. 181.19. It is found in most proteins and is synthesized metabolically from phenylalanine. Tyrosine is essential in the diets of persons with phenylketonuria because of its deficient synthesis. It is a precursor of thyroxine, triiodothyronine, epinephrine, norepinephrine, and melanin. See also under *amino acids.*

tyrosine assays 1. fluorometric method for the detection or quantitation of tyrosine in serum or tyrosine and some of its metabolites in urine. A trichloroacetic acid extract of serum or urine is treated with 1-nitroso-2-naphthol, sodium nitrite, and nitric acid; tyrosine and its metabolite *p*-hydroxyphenylpyruvic acid form a yellow pigment, which can be extracted into ethylene dichloride and quantitated spectrofluorometrically with excitation at 460 nm and measurement at 570 nm.

2. the Millon reaction, a qualitative test for tyrosine and other phenols. Urine mixed or underlayered with Millon's reagent (mercury dissolved in nitric or sulfuric acid) gives an orange-red color in the presence of tyrosine by its derivative *p*-hydroxyphenylpyruvic acid and other phenols. Proteins also give a positive test.

3. thin-layer chromatography of amino acids. This detects an excess of tyrosine in serum and urine or *p*-hydroxyphenylpyruvic acid in urine.

4. high-pressure liquid chromatography (HPLC) and ion-exchange chromatography.

tyrosinemia (ti″ro-sĭ-ne′me-ah) 1. a hereditary disorder of tyrosine metabolism, transmitted as an autosomal recessive trait, that is marked by an excess of tyrosine in the blood and by tyrosyluria (*p*-hydroxyphenyllactic acid and *p*-hydroxyphenylpyruvic acid predominate). The specific enzyme defect is still open to question, but may be a relative or absolute deficiency of *p*-hydroxyphenylpyruvate dioxygenase. Tyrosinemia is characterized by severe nodular cirrhosis of the liver and renal tubular defects. See also *aminoacidopathies.*

2. transient or neonatal tyrosinemia, which is a benign condition of elevated blood tyrosine levels that occurs in about 10 percent of newborns, especially low-birth-weight infants.

3. see *hypertyrosinemia, Oregon type.*

tyrosinuria (ti″ro-sĭ-nu′re-ah) [*tyrosine* + Gr. *ouron* urine + *-ia*] the presence of excessive tyrosine in the urine, caused by various disorders that affect the normal metabolism of tyrosine. See also *aminoacidopathies* and *tyrosinemia.*

tyrosyl (ti′ro-sil) the acyl radical derived from or relating to tyrosine.

tyrosyluria (ti″ro-sil-u′re-ah) the increased excretion of *p*-hydroxyphenyl compounds derived from tyrosine, as occurs in tyrosinemia.

Tzanck's test (tsankz) [Arnault *Tzanck,* Russian-born dermatologist living in Paris, 1886–1954] the cytologic examination of scrapings from the base of vesicular or bullous herpetic lesions, a useful procedure in the diagnosis of herpes simplex, herpes genitalis, herpes zoster, varicella, or pemphigus. The scrapings are fixed on a slide with absolute or methyl alcohol for 10 min and stained with Giemsa stain. The finding of multinucleated giant cells or typical eosinophilic intranuclear inclusions is diagnostic of herpesvirus infection.

U

U symbol for International Unit of enzyme activity, the chemical element *uranium, uridine.*

u symbol for unified atomic mass unit.

U/A abbrev. See *uric acid, urinalysis.*

UBG abbrev. See *urobilinogen.*

ubiquinol (u-bik′wĭ-nol) a form of the mitochondrial electron transport cofactor ubiquinone (CoQ) that has accepted two protons and two electrons. During electron transport, it converts ubiquinone to dihydroubiquinone (ubiquinol or QH_2). See also *ubiquinone.*

ubiquinone (u-bik′wĭnōn) one of a group of related quinone compounds with a variable number of isoprenoid groups in the side-chain. These molecules, which occur in the lipid fraction of mitochondria along with mitochondrial cytochromes, also serve as an intermediate in electron transport. Vitamin E, vitamin K, and plastoquinone found in chloroplasts have structures similar to ubiquinone. Also called *coenzyme Q* (Co Q).

ubisemiquinone (u″bi-sem″e-kwi′nōn) a form of the mitochondrial electron transport cofactor ubiquinone (CoQ) that has accepted one proton and one electron, which converts ubiquinone to a free radical (QH·) during electron transport. See also *ubiquinone.*

UDP abbrev. See *uridine diphosphate.*

UDP-*N*-acetyl-D-galactosamine (as′e-til gah-lak-tōs′ah-mēn″) uridine diphosphate-*N*-acetyl-D-galactosamine, an *N*-acetyl-galactosamine donor molecule for the synthesis of polysaccharides. It is interconvertible with UDP-*N*-acetyl-D-glucosamine.

UDP-*N*-acetyl-D-glucosamine (as′e-til gloo-kōs′-ah-mēn″) uridine diphosphate-*N*-acetyl-D-glucosamine, an *N*-acetyl-glucosamine donor molecule for the synthesis of polysaccharides. It is interconvertible with UDP-*N*-acetyl-D-galactosamine.

UDP-bilirubin glucuronosyltransferase see *UDP–glucuronate:bilirubin–glucuronosyltransferase.*

UDP-galactose (gah-lak′tos) uridine diphosphate galactose, an important nucleotide sugar that is involved in galactose metabolism in humans, and also the biologic interconversion of galactose and glucose.

UDP-glucose (gloo′kōs) uridine diphosphate glucose, an important nucleotide sugar that is used in the synthesis of glycogen, UDP-glucuronate, UDP-xylose, and UDP-L-iduronate. It is also used in the biologic interconversion of glucose and galactose.

UDP-glucose-hexose-1-phosphate uridylyltransferase an enzyme of the transferase class (UDP-glucose:α-D-galactose-1-phosphate uridylyltransferase, EC 2.7.7.12) that catalyzes the reaction UDP-glucose + α-D-galactose-1-phosphate ⇄ α-D-glucose-1-phosphate + UDP-galactose. A genetic deficiency of this enzyme causes galactosemia. Also called *uridyl transferase.* See also under *galactosemia.*

UDP-glucose-hexose-1-phosphate uridylyltransferase assays 1. quantitative enzyme assays. The physiologic substrates galactose-1-phosphate and uridine diphosphoglucose (UDPG) are added to a hemolyzed whole blood specimen and incubated at pH 8.1 and 37°C. The transferase reaction produces glucose-1-phosphate and UDP-galactose (UDP-Gal).

In one method, the UDPG consumed is determined using the coupled reaction catalyzed by the NAD-dependent enzyme UDP-glucose dehydrogenase. In another method, the UDP-Gal produced is determined using the coupled reaction catalyzed by the NAD-dependent enzyme UDP-glucose-4-epimerase, which converts UDP-Gal to UDPG. The progress of the reaction in both methods is determined from the NADH absorbance at 340 nm. In a third method, radioactive 1-^{14}C-galactose-1-phosphate is used as the substrate for the transferase reaction. The ^{14}C-UDP-galactose produced is determined by adsorbing it on charcoal, eluting with ethanol-ammonia solution, and measuring the radioactivity.

2. a screening test for galactosemia. A reaction mixture containing a hemolyzed blood specimen, galactose-1-phosphate, UDPG, NADP, and pH 8.0 buffer is spotted on filter paper and incubated. Glucose-1-phosphate produced by the transferase reaction is converted to glucose-6-phosphate, which enters the pentose phosphate pathway and reduces NADP to NADPH, which is detected by its fluorescence under ultraviolet light.

UDP-glucuronate (gloo-ku′ro-nāt) uridine diphosphate glucuronate, an important nucleotide sugar donor molecule and biosynthetic intermediate. A donor molecule in mucopolysaccharide and glucuronide conjugate biosynthesis, it is also an intermediate in the formation of UDP-xylose, UDP-L-iduronate, and ascorbic acid in some animal species.

UDP-glucuronate:bilirubin-glucuronosyltransferase an enzyme of the transferase class (EC 2.4.1.76) that catalyzes the reaction UDP-glucuronate + bilirubin ⇄ UDP + bilirubin-glucuronoside. The conjugation is a two-step reaction that occurs in the liver and converts bilirubin to the more soluble bilirubin-glucuronoside, which is then secreted into the bile.

The enzyme may be insufficiently developed in premature infants, resulting in jaundice and possibly brain damage. A genetic deficiency of the enzyme results in a severe form of congenital familial nonhemolytic jaundice (Crigler-Najjar syndrome, transmitted as an autosomal recessive trait), or a mild form (Crigler-Najjar syndrome type II, transmitted as an autosomal dominant trait).

Also called *glucuronyl transferase, UDP-bilirubin glucuronosyltransferase,* and *UDP-glucuronyl transferase.* See also *Crigler-Najjar syndrome.*

UDP-glucuronic acid (gloo-ku′ro-nik) uridine diphosphate glucuronic acid, formed from UDP-glucose by a two-step NAD^+-mediated oxidation. It can be converted to UDP-xylose and UDP-galacturonic acid; hydrolysis results in free D-glucuronate, which can be metabolized to L-xylulose or to L-ascorbic acid. It is the source of "active" glucuronide, which is used in the liver to form glucuronic acid conjugates, such as bilirubin diglucuronide and steroid glucuronides, that can be found in urine.

UDP-glucuronyl transferase see *UDP-glucuronate:bilirubin-glucuronosyltransferase.*

UDP-L-iduronate (ĭ-du′ro-nāt) uridine diphosphate-L-iduronate, a hexose sugar donor molecule. It is used in forming the polysaccharide portion of some proteoglycans.

UDP-iduronic acid (ĭ-du′ro-nik) uridine diphosphate iduronic acid synthesized from UDP-glucuronic acid. It is an iduronic acid donor molecule used for the formation of some proteoglycans.

UDP-xylose (zi′lōs) uridine diphosphate xylose, a pentose sugar donor molecule. It is used in forming the polysaccharide portion of proteoglycans.

UFA abbrev. for unesterified fatty acids. See *nonesterified f. a.* under *fatty acids.*

UIBC abbrev. for unsaturated iron-binding capacity. See under *iron-binding capacity tests.*

UIP abbrev. for usual interstitial pneumonitis. See *pulmonary f.* under *fibrosis.*

ulatrophy (u-lat′ro-fe) [Gr. *oulon* gum + *atrophy*] a retraction or shrinkage of the gums secondary to trauma, diminished blood supply, malposition of the teeth, or deposition of plaque.

ulcer (ul′ser) [L. *ulcus;* Gr. *helkosis*] a local defect or excavation on the surface of a tissue or organ caused by the sloughing of necrotic inflamed tissue.

acute u., an ulcer of short duration. Histologically, it shows destruction of tissue and associated acute and chronic inflammation, but minimal fibrosis. When superficial, it may be termed an acute erosion.

amebic u., an ulcer resulting from tissue invasion by amebae (usually *Entamoeba histolytica*). It may occur on the skin, but is most common in the terminal ileum and colon. In the intestine it is typically a small, flask-shaped defect in the mucosa that overlies a more extensive area of submucosal necrosis. See also *amebiasis.*

aphthous u., a shallow defect of the oral mucosa with a regular, flat, reddened periphery. Although stress, certain diseases, and some foods seem to be associated with this type of ulcer, the cause is not known. The lesions are often multiple and painful, but they usually heal spontaneously within two to three weeks. Also called *aphtha* and *canker sore.*

Barrett's u., a peptic ulcer found in the lower esophagus at a site of heterotopic (abnormally located) gastric epithelium. Occurring singly or multiply, such ulcers often produce stricture formation and may be a result of reflux esophagitis.

Buruli u., a large, persistent, progressively destructive cutaneous ulcer, usually found on the extremities, that is caused by infection with *Mycobacterium ulcerans.* It is so named because it occurs in individuals in the Buruli district of northern Africa; it is also found in Australia but rarely in other locations.

chancroidal u., see *chancroid.*

chronic u., an ulcer that has been present for some time. The surrounding tissues show chronic inflammation and fibrosis, and healing is accompanied by variable degrees of scarring.

corneal u., a superficial defect of the cornea that may result from trauma, including irritation by a foreign body, or from bacterial or viral (especially herpes simplex) infection.

Curling's u., an ulceration of the gastric mucosa that occurs following severe burns, sepsis, trauma, or major surgery. The lesions are often small, multiple, circular ulcers that can occur anywhere in the stomach. They are not associated with hyperacidity, and may be due to elevated corticosteroid levels.

Cushing's u., an ulceration of the mucosa of the stomach, or, less frequently, the duodenum or esophagus, that can accompany acute brain damage or follow a neurosurgical procedure.

decubitus u., an area of ulceration commonly occurring on the buttocks of bedridden patients as a result of pressure-induced ischemia complicating erosion of the skin. Also called bed sore.

dendritic u., a descriptive term for a corneal ulcer produced by herpes simplex virus infection.

diabetic u., an ulcer of the lower extremities, particularly the foot, that occurs in diabetic individuals. It is usually preceded by formation of a blister or callus, or by a wound of the skin. Development of the ulcer is promoted by the presence of diabetic neuropathy, which decreases the patient's awareness of pain and may cause an abnormal distribution of weight bearing on the foot, and by a diminished blood supply to the limbs as a result of vascular disease. Secondary infection can occur and may lead to gangrene.

duodenal u., an ulcer that occurs in the duodenum, usually on the anterior or posterior wall of the first part of the duodenum. Duodenal ulcers are more common in males than in females and have a peak occurrence around age 35 yr. In most instances, the ulcer can be related to gastric hyperacidity. Endoscopy and radiography are used to demonstrate the ulcer crater or to show a deformed duodenal cap. See also *peptic u.*

gastric u., an ulcer that occurs in the stomach, commonly a peptic ulcer associated with gastric hyperacidity, usually on or near the lesser curvature, particularly on the posterior wall within 5 cm of the pyloric sphincter. Gastric ulcers are more common in males than in females and have a peak occurrence around age 50 yr. Other causes include aspirin intake, steroid therapy, smoking, and alcohol abuse. Some gastric adenocarcinomas may appear as ulcers. Radiography and endoscopy are used to visualize the ulcer, and a gastroscopic biopsy may be performed, particularly if malignancy is suspected. See also *peptic u.*

Hines' u., an ulcer commonly located on the lateral aspect of the leg or ankle, that is seen occasionally in hypertensive patients. It develops from a hemorrhagic bleb that loses its surface, creating an ulcer with reddish-purple margins. More common in females, this ulcer can be exceedingly painful.

Hunner's u., an ulceration of the bladder mucosa that occurs as one of the morphologic alterations in interstitial (Hunner's) cystitis. It may excavate deeply into the bladder wall.

malignant u., an ulcerated malignant neoplasm that involves the skin or a mucosal surface. It tends to be larger than a benign ulcer and has an irregular elevated margin. Biopsy of the margin of the ulcer can be performed to confirm its neoplastic nature.

marginal u., ulceration of the mucosa of the jejunum adjacent to the anastomosis of a gastroenterostomy. Gastroscopy or endoscopy may reveal the ulcer.

neuropathic u., a cutaneous ulcer of the foot that occurs in individuals with sensory denervation as a result of a peripheral neuropathy. See also *diabetic u.,*

peptic u., an ulcer that occurs in the mucosa of the gastrointestinal tract in the portion bathed by gastric secretion. It is most frequently found in the first part of the duodenum, less frequently in the stomach, and rarely in a Barrett's esophagus or Meckel's diverticulum. Intractable peptic ulceration is associated with excessive gastrin secretion in Zollinger-Ellison syndrome.

Most peptic ulcers are small and have a punched out appearance with sharply defined margins, which contrasts with the elevated, rolled, or undermined edges of a malignant ulcer. A superficial area of peptic ulceration that does not extend through the muscularis mucosa is termed an acute erosion.

Duodenal ulcer is more commonly found in most countries than gastric ulcer, but in some countries, e.g., Japan, gastric ulcers are more common than duodenal ulcers. A number of factors predisposing to peptic ulceration have been identified, including autosomal dominant transmission of elevated pepsinogen levels and possession of blood group O. Psychologic factors may be implicated in the genesis of peptic ulceration, and certainly influence the clinical course.

Diagnosis is based on history, demonstration of gastric hyperacidity, and radiographic and endoscopic studies including biopsy. The development of adenocarcinoma within a peptic ulcer is probably rare, but ulcerated carcinomas are common and must be considered as a diagnostic possibility in all gastric ulcers.

Complications of peptic ulcer include hemorrhage, perforation, and obstruction. Bleeding may be manifested as hematemesis or melena. Perforation, when it occurs, is usually into the main peritoneal cavity or lesser sac; posterior duodenal ulcers can erode into the pancreas. Gastric obstruction may result from scarring and superimposed spasm produced by a prepyloric or duodenal ulcer.

perforating u., a deeply invasive ulcer of an anatomic structure, involving its entire thickness and creating an opening on both surfaces. It can occur, for example, in the foot of an individual with peripheral neuropathy and sensory denervation, and in the stomach of a person with untreated or unresponsive peptic ulcer.

phagedenic u., an acute cutaneous ulcer that results from infection with *Borrelia vincentii* or *Bacteroides.* It develops from a small blister, usually below the knee and often at the site of a small wound or insect bite. The blister ruptures, creating a circular ulcer with a raised edge. It can extend around the leg and aggressively erode underlying tissue, in some cases extending to bone. Despite its depth, the ulcer usually heals spontaneously within several months. Also called tropical phagedenic ulcer.

serpiginous u., a descriptive term for an ulcer with wandering margins.

Siberian u., one of many synonyms for the skin lesion of anthrax.

stasis u., a cutaneous ulcer caused by impaired venous return. It is usually found on the inner or anterior aspect of the leg above the ankle.

stercoral u., an ulcer in the rectum or lower colon that develops as a consequence of fecal impaction. Associated inflammation is usually mild, and healing occurs rapidly following correction of the impaction.

stress u., an acute peptic ulcer, commonly an extension of acute erosive gastritis, associated with stress, steroid therapy, and smoking.

trophic u., an ulcer that occurs as a result of inadequate nutrition of the involved tissue, e.g., a stasis ulcer.

varicose u., a cutaneous ulcer on the lower leg that occurs as a sequela of varicose veins.

ulcerate (ul′sĕ-rāt) [L. *ulceratus*, past participle of *ulcerare*] to form an ulcer or ulcers.

ulceration (ul″sĕ-ra′shun) [L. *ulceratio*] 1. the process of forming an ulcer.
2. an ulcer.

ulcerative (ul′ser-a″tiv) a term used to describe those disorders that produce ulcers.

ulcerative colitis see *ulcerative c.* under *colitis.*

ulcerogenic (ul″ser-o-jen′ik) [*ulcer* + Gr. *gennan* to produce] causing ulceration; leading to the production of ulcers.

ulcerogenic tumor a tumor of pancreatic islet cells that produces large amounts of gastrin, which in turn stimulates the secretion of gastric acid. Occasionally these tumors arise in the duodenum. Those affected develop ulcers of the duodenum, or infrequently the stomach, and show the symptoms of peptic ulcer disease. There may also be severe diarrhea.

Laboratory diagnosis relies primarily on detection of increased levels of fasting serum gastrin, usually over 500 pg/ml. The response of the serum gastrin level to infusions of calcium or of the hormone secretin is also helpful in making a diagnosis.

Also called *gastrinoma.* See also *Zollinger-Ellison syndrome.*

ulceromembranous (ul″ser-o-mem′brah-nus) a term used to describe a process or disorder that forms an ulcer with a pseudomembrane (of fibrin and cell debris). Such a lesion may be seen in the throats of those afflicted with diphtheria.

ulcerous (ul′ser-us) [L. *ulcerosus*] 1. like an ulcer.
2. having ulcers.

-ule (ūl) [L. *-ulus, -ula, -ulum,* diminutive suffixes] a suffix word element to denote little or small, e.g., minuscule.

Ullmann's line (ul′manz) [Emerich *Ullmann,* Hungarian surgeon, 1861–1937] an imaginary line drawn from the anterior edge of the first sacral vertebra to the superior surface of the sacrum. If the line is extended superiorly and passes through the body of the fifth lumbar vertebra, this indicates that the vertebral body has slipped forward over the sacrum.

uln/o (ul′no) a word element used in combining form to denote the ulna, e.g., ulnoradial.

ulna (ul′nah), pl. *ulnae* [L. "the arm"] [NA], the more medial of the two bones of the forearm. Its upper end has two projections that give it a clawlike appearance, and they enclose the trochlear notch that clasps the trochlea of the humerus in the elbow joint. The head of the radius rotates within a sling that is attached to the margins of the radial notch of the ulna. The lower end of the ulna is smaller and includes the head, separated by an articular disk from carpal bones, and the short styloid process.

ulnar (ul′nar) [L. *ulnaris*] related to the ulna, e.g., ulnar deformity (deformity of the ulna) or ulnar deviation (deviation of structures toward the ulnar side of the forearm).

ulnar artery one of the two terminal branches of the brachial artery. It begins just below the elbow joint, runs down the medial side of the forearm, and then crosses the palm as the superficial palmar arch.

ulnar nerve a nerve that arises from the medial cord of the brachial plexus. It runs down the medial side of the arm and forearm, passing behind the medial epicondyle. Above the wrist it gives off a dorsal branch, then continues over the flexor retinaculum into the palm, where its terminal branches supply the medial one and one-half digits.

ultimobranchial bodies (ul″tĭ-mo-brang′ke-al) paired parapharyngeal structures in avian and other species, composed of calcitonin-forming cells (C cells). In mammals, these C cells migrate from the fifth branchial pouch to the thyroid gland, where they become dispersed throughout its substance. See also *thyroid.*

ultra- (ul′trah) [L. *ultra*] a prefix word element to denote beyond or excess, e.g., ultrasound.

ultrabrachycephalic (ul″trah-brak″e-sĕ-fal′ik) [*ultra-* + Gr. *brachys* short + *kephalē* head] a term used to describe a head with an extremely high ratio of width to length, i.e., that has a cephalic index [(width/length) × 100] of more than 90.

ultracentrifuge (ul″trah-sen′trĭ-fūj) a very high speed centrifuge capable of rotating at speeds of 30,000–100,000 rpm and generating a relative centrifugal force (RCF) of 50,000–500,000 *g.*

analytic u., a precision ultracentrifuge used for the quantitative separation and analysis of samples. It is used in research laboratories to determine plasma lipoprotein fractions.

ultradolichocephalic (ul″trah-dol″ĭ-ko-sĕ-fal′ik) [*ultra-* + Gr. *dolichos* long + *kephalē* head] a term used to describe a head that is extremely long, i.e., that has a cephalic index [(width/length) × 100] of less than 80.

ultrafilter (ul″trah-fil′ter) a material or apparatus used to separate true solutes from colloidal material or to separate colloidal material of different sizes. In the clinical laboratory, ultrafilters are used to separate solutes from proteins in body fluids (e.g., serum, urine, cerebrospinal fluid). Most often, the material used in the separation consists of membranes of various types or special molecular sieve columns.

ultrafiltrate (ul″trah-fil′trāt) the liquid that has passed through an ultrafilter.

ultrafiltration (ul″trah-fil-tra′shun) filtration through filters with pores small enough to permit separation of macromolecular (colloidal) solutes from small molecular solutes. By selection of a specific pore size, some control over the size of molecules in the ultrafiltrate is possible. Ultrafiltration occurs naturally, as in the filtration of plasma at the capillary membrane, and the glomerular filtration in the kidney. In the laboratory, it is used especially to separate and concentrate proteins in urine and cerebrospinal fluid and to separate free ions or metabolites from those that are protein-bound. The filtration process may be accelerated by use of pressure or centrifugal force.

ultramicroanalysis (ul″trah-mi″kro-ah-nal′ĭ-sis) chemical analysis using samples less than 10 μl in size or 10 μg in mass.

ultramicrotome (ul″trah-mi′kro-tōm) an instrument used to cut ultrathin sections of plastic-embedded tissues for electron microscopy. The basic principle of operation is similar to that of microtomes used in light-microscopic histotechnology, but a number of modifications are incorporated, including a binocular stereomicroscope to allow viewing of the sectioning process, illumination of the knife edge, and a precision advance mechanism, which may be thermal or mechanical. The excursion of the tissue block past the knife edge and through its return stroke generally has a two-speed control to allow slow sectioning and a more rapid return cycle.

ultrasonic (ul″trah-son′ik) [*ultra-* + L. *sonus* sound] pertaining to sound waves having frequencies above the range of human hearing, i.e., above about 20 kHz. Also (improperly) called *supersonic.*

ultrasonication (ul″trah-son″ĭ-ka′shun) the exposure to ultrasonic sound waves (of a frequency greater than 15,000 cps). The process denatures proteins and is used to disintegrate cells for experimental purposes. Cf. *sonication.*

ultrasonogram (ul″trah-son′o-gram) see *sonogram.*

ultrasonography (ul″trah-son-og′rah-fe) a radiologic technique that uses high-frequency sound to produce images of sections of the body. No x-rays are involved, and no adverse reactions or side-effects have been reported.

The technique is an offshoot of the development of SONAR and was first adapted for medical diagnostic work in the late 1950s. It employs a transducer that produces very short pulses of very-high-frequency sound that are transmitted into the body. Echoes from interfaces within the body are detected and displayed on a television screen so that the normal and abnormal internal structures of the body can be viewed. The picture is similar to that which would be obtained if one were actually to slice the body like a loaf of bread and look at one of the slices. These "slices" can be produced in any plane desired—transversely, longitudinally, or obliquely. A complete scan is made up of a series of slices parallel to each other, and then repeated in several planes. The three-dimensional form of the internal organs can be determined from this series of two-dimensional slices.

Whereas standard radiographs are particularly useful for demonstrating the difference between air, organ, and bone densities, ultrasound is unfortunately useless when there is any intervening air or bone. However, it is particularly good at demonstrating the solid organs of the body and is exceptionally good at detecting accumulations of fluid. It is useful for differentiating solid lesions, such as tumors, from fluid-filled structures, such as cysts. It can be used to determine the cause of jaundice and to detect gallbladder disease and gallstones. In pregnant females, ultrasound can be used to determine the number of fetuses, the age and sex of the fetus, and the position of the placenta; fetal abnormalities also may detected. It has been found particularly useful for evaluating the structures within the heart (as the blood is clearly differentiated from the myocardium and valves) and at assessing the size of the heart chambers and the functioning of the valves.

In superficial organs such as the eyes, thyroid, breast, and scrotum, ultrasound can easily detect masses and differentiate solid tumors from cystic structures. The technique is useful in detecting hemorrhage and enlarged ventricles of the brain of newborns. Along with other imaging techniques, ultrasound can locate the position of a tumor within the body as an aid to directing the surgeon in obtaining a biopsy.

The major advantages of ultrasound are that it is completely noninvasive, is not uncomfortable, and has no known harmful effects. Ultrasound has added significantly to the imaging armamentarium as an aid in the diagnosis of structural abnormalities within the body.

Also called *echography.*

PETER L. COOPERBERG, M.D.

A-mode (amplitude modulation) u., a type of ultrasound scanning in which echoes are represented on an oscilloscope trace, the distance between echogenic interfaces being represented by the distance between blips, and the strength of the echo being represented by the height of the blip. This mode is used in echoencephalography. See also the accompanying illustration.

B-mode (brightness modulation) u., a type of ultrasound scanning in which echoes are represented on the oscilloscope screen as bright spots, the distance between the spots representing the distance between echogenic interfaces. A scan is built up from many scan lines. The transducer is moved by hand so that the ultrasound beam sweeps over the section of the body to be scanned. Potentiometers in a mechanical arm holding the transducer indicate its position and angle of orientation. The composite of all the scan lines produces an image of a section of the body called a (compound) B scan.

Early scanners used a bistable display mode; strong echoes were spots of a uniform brightness against a blank background. Newer models use gray-scale display; the strength of the echo is represented by the optical brightness of the spot on the screen.

Doppler u., a type of ultrasonography that uses the Doppler effect to detect the movement of blood flow or tissue interfaces. The Doppler shift (the difference between the frequencies of the transmitted and reflected waves) is an audible frequency. Thus, the velocities of motions inside the body are converted to sounds, and the structures in the ultrasound can be identified by their characteristic movements. It is used to examine the blood flow in peripheral vessels, to detect the fetal heartbeat, and to localize the placenta. The depth of the movement can also be measured by devices using Doppler ultrasound.

M-mode (motion mode) u., a type of simple B-mode ultrasound used in echocardiography. The distance between echogenic objects, e.g., the heart valves and walls of the heart chambers, is represented by the distance between the spots along the x-axis. The y-axis is the time axis; the dots sweep along in the y-direction at a constant rate, moving back and forth in the x-direction and producing a trace of the motion of each echogenic object.

real time u., a type of B-mode scan in which an array of many detectors is used so that each scan can be built up very rapidly, producing a motion picture usually at a rate of 30 frames/sec.

ultrasound (u/s) (ul'trah-sownd) 1. sound waves

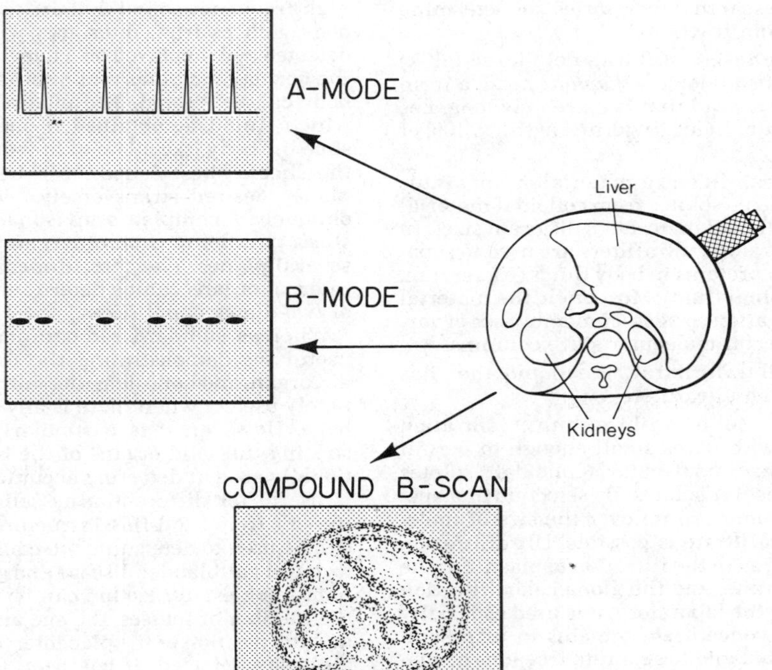

Ultrasonography. Illustration of A-mode, B-mode, and compound B-scan images of the abdomen. (From Griffiths, H. J., and Sarno, R. C.: Contemporary Radiology. Philadelphia, W. B. Saunders Co., 1979.)

having a frequency above the limit of human hearing, 20 kHz.

2. see *ultrasonography.*

ultrastructure (ul″trah-struk′chur) 1. the arrangement of the smallest elements making up a tissue.

2. cell structure beyond the resolving power of the light microscope, i.e., structure visible only with an electron microscope. Also called *fine structure.*

ultraviolet (UV) (ul″trah-vi′o-let) pertaining to ultraviolet radiation, i.e., electromagnetic radiation in the range of 4–400 nm. This range is beyond the violet spectrum of visible light.

ultraviolet light electromagnetic radiation, with wavelengths between 4 and 400 nm, that is absorbed by atoms and molecules in electronic transitions.

ultraviolet radiation (UVR) electromagnetic radiation having wavelengths of 4–400 nm, shorter than visible light and longer than x-rays. Ultraviolet radiation in the region of 260 nm is strongly absorbed by purine and pyrimidine bases in nucleic acids, causing the formation of thymine dimers and distortion of the DNA duplex. This inhibits replication and transcription, resulting in genetic mutations, and inactivation and destruction of bacteria, phages, and viruses.

Ultraviolet radiation is sometimes used in special laboratory cabinets to reduce contamination and protect workers, and to "sterilize" the air in operating rooms, hospital rooms, and public areas.

umbilical (um-bil′ĭ-kal) [L. *umbilicalis*] associated with or related to the umbilicus.

umbilical artery one of the paired arteries that passes through the umbilical cord of the fetus to invest the placenta. These arteries are continuous with the internal iliac arteries, which ascend on the anterior wall of the abdomen to enter the umbilicus. After birth, the pelvic portion of the arteries persists as the internal iliac artery and a portion of the superior vesical artery, while the remainder becomes the fibrous medial umbilical ligament.

umbilical cord the flexible cord that connects the developing fetus with the placenta. The cord contains the umbilical arteries and vein, surrounded by a mucoid connective tissue (Wharton's jelly).

umbilical region 1. the central region of the abdomen surrounding the umbilicus.

2. the region of the abdomen below the transpyloric plane, above the transtubercular plane, and between the lateral sagittal planes; used in radiographic positioning. See illustration under *abdominal regions.*

umbilical vein one of a pair of veins that carry blood from the placenta to the fetus. In later fetal life, the right vein disappears. The left vein enters the abdomen at the umbilicus and travels in the falciform ligament to join the left branch of the portal vein. In adults, the umbilical vein remains as a fibrous cord, the ligamentum teres.

umbilical zone the part of the abdomen between the transpyloric and transtubercular planes. It consists of the umbilical (mesogastric) and left and right lumbar (lateral) regions. Also called *mesogastric zone.*

umbilicate (um-bil′ĭ-kāt) [L. *umbilicatus*] a term used to describe a lesion or structure that has a depression or dimple resembling the umbilicus, e.g., the lesions of molluscum contagiosum.

umbilicus (um-bil′ĭ-kus, um″bĭ-li′kus) [L.] [NA], the navel; the healed site of attachment of the umbilical cord in the fetus.

umbra (um′bra) a region in full shadow. Cf. *penumbra.*

umbrella cell a superficial cell of the transitional epithelium of the urinary bladder, so named because it straddles several underlying cells.

UMP abbrev. See *uridine-5′-phosphate.*

unattended laboratory operation as defined by NFPA (National Fire Protection Association) standards for laboratories for the purposes of specifying needed safety precautions, "a laboratory procedure or operation at which there is no person present who is *knowledgeable* regarding the operation and emergency shutdown procedures." This includes absence even for short periods without coverage by a knowledgeable person.

unblanking pulse a square wave voltage pulse applied to a cathode ray tube (CRT) to turn on the electron beam.

uncertainty principle a conclusion drawn from quantum mechanics stating that it is impossible to determine precisely the values of complementary pairs of physical variables, such as position and linear momentum, angle and angular momentum, or time and energy. The product of the measurement errors for complementary variables must be at least of the order of magnitude of Planck's constant.

An electronic orbital in an atom is a state of definite energy. The point in time when an atom is in such a state cannot be determined; any measurement attempt would cause a transition to some other state. Neither the position nor the momentum of an orbital electron is precisely defined; quantum theory gives only the probabilities of observing particular values of the electron's position or momentum.

Also called Heisenberg uncertainty principle.

Uncinaria (un″sĭ-na′re-ah) [L. *uncus* hook] a former name for a genus of nematode worms.

U. americana, see *N. americanus* under *Necator.*

U. duodenalis, see *A. duodenale* under *Ancylostoma.*

uncinariasis (un″sin-ah-ri′ah-sis) an infection with hookworms. See also *hookworm.*

unconditional jump in a digital computer, a machine-language instruction that specifies the address of the next instruction and thus alters the normal execution of instructions in sequence. Also called branch. Cf. *conditional jump.*

unconscious (un-kon′shus) 1. a term that describes those states in which a person, incapable of responding to sensory stimulation, is unaware of his or her surroundings; the term applies both to sleep and to coma. There is no exact division between unconsciousness and consciousness, as there are states of altered consciousness that form a continuum between the two extremes.

2. in psychiatry, the drives, repressed memories, and knowledge of which an individual is normally unaware but which are still powerful behavioral influences.

uncus (ung′kus) [L. "hook"] [NA], the medially curved anterior end of the parahippocampal gyrus that covers the amygdala.

undecaprenol a 55-carbon polyprenol found in the liver and functioning also in bacteria as undecaprenol phosphate, a sugar carrier molecule, participating in the synthesis of bacterial cell-wall oligosaccharides.

u. phosphate, undecaprenol that is esterified by its terminal hydroxyl group to phosphoric acid.

underflow (un'der-flo) in a computer, an error condition raised by the execution of a floating-point arithmetic operation, which produces a result too small to be represented in floating-point format (the exponent would be too large a negative number). The computer is usually programmed to ignore underflows by taking the result to be zero. Cf. *overflow.*

Underwood's disease (un'der-woodz) [Michael *Underwood,* London obstetrician and pediatrician, 1737–1820] see *sclerema.*

undifferentiated characterized by the absence or lack of differentiation; anaplastic. See also *tumor grading.*

undifferentiation (un-dif-er-en"she-a'shun) see *anaplasia.*

undulant fever (un'du-lant) [L. *undula,* dim. of *unda* wave] see *brucellosis.*

undulating (un'du-la"ting) wavy, rippling; used in describing the margin of a part. Also called *scalloped.*

undulating membrane a protoplasmic membrane found in some protozoa, which runs along the body and ends at the flagellum.

ungu/o (ung'gwo) a word element used in combining form to denote the nail, e.g., ungulate.

uni- (u'nĭ) [L. *unus* one] a prefix word element to denote one, e.g., unicellular or unilateral.

unicameral bone cyst (u"ni-kam'er-al) [*uni-* + L. *camera* chamber] a simple, solitary bone cyst, of unknown etiology, that commonly occurs in the long bones and usually first appears during childhood or adolescence. Also called simple bone cyst and solitary cyst.

unicellular (u"nĭ-sel'u-lar) [*uni-* + L. *cellula* cell] pertaining to a single-celled organism, e.g., a bacterium or protist.

unidirectional (u"nĭ-di-rek'shun-al) flowing or radiating in only one direction, such as direct current.

uniflagellate (u"nĭ-flaj'ĕ-lāt) possessing one flagellum.

unigravida (u"nĭ-grav'ĭ-dah) [*uni-* + L. *gravida* pregnant] see *primigravida.*

unilocular (u"nĭ-lok'u-lar) [*uni-* + L. *loculus*] having a single loculus or compartment.

unilocular cyst a type of hydatid cyst (forming single or multiple, expanding cysts) common in infections with tapeworms of the species *Echinococcus granulosus.* These cysts are characterized by an external laminated cuticula and an interior germinative membrane, and are distended with hydatid fluid. If the germinative membrane epithelium is fertile, it will produce daughter cysts that bud off. The free daughter cysts in the hydatid fluid may produce granddaughter cysts. See also *hydatid.*

unilocular echinococcosis see under *hydatid.*

unimodal (u"nĭ-mo'dal) having a single mode.

union (ūn'yun) [L. *unio*] in medicine, the healing of bone, tissue, or the edges of a wound. See also *healing.*

delayed primary u., healing by third intention, which occurs when a wound is left open to allow formation of granulation tissue and then is closed with sutures or tape.

faulty u., malunion, which refers to a fracture of bone that does not realign correctly in healing.

primary u., healing by first intention, which describes the healing of a wound whose edges have been brought together and in which no infection or other complication occurs.

secondary u., healing by secondary intention, which occurs when the wound is left open and closes by filling of the defect with granulation tissue.

uniovular (u"ne-ov'u-lar) [*uni-* + L. *ovum* egg] a term that refers to twins arising from one ovum or egg (monozygotic twins).

unipara (u-nip'ah-rah) [*uni-* + L. *parere* to bring forth] see *primipara.*

unipolar (u"nĭ-po'lar) [*uni-* + L. *polus* pole] 1. having but one pole, polarity, or process.

2. in anatomy, pertaining to a neuron having only one process.

3. in electronics, pertaining to an amplifier, power supply, or waveform in which the voltage is always positive or always negative.

uniport (u"nĭ-port') a transport protein that mediates the transport of one substance, as opposed to the coupled transport of two substances. See also *active transport.* Cf. *antiport* and *symport.*

unit (u'nit) [L. *unus* one] 1. a single entity, particularly one regarded as a functional constituent of a larger object.

2. a module or assembly that performs a definite function and is part of a larger system.

3. in measurement, a precisely defined quantity of some physical property used as a standard in terms of which other quantities can be specified, e.g., the meter, second, volt. See also *International System* and the specific unit.

unit cell a parallelepiped that is the repeating unit of a crystal lattice.

United States Adopted Name (USAN) a nonproprietary designation for a drug established since June 1961 by negotiation between the manufacturer and the USAN council, which is sponsored jointly by the American Medical Association, the American Pharmaceutical Association, and the United States Pharmacopeial Convention, or by its predecessor, the AMA-USP Nomenclature Committee. In the United States, the USAN is the official generic name of a drug.

United States Pharmacopeia (USP) a legally recognized compendium of monographs on drugs giving methods of preparation and standards, tests, and assays for strength, quality, and purity. This volume, containing monographs on both USP and NF drug preparations, is published by the United States Pharmacopeial Convention, Inc., which in 1974 acquired the National Formulary (NF). Since 1980 the two compendia have been published in a single volume that is revised every 5 yr.

unit membrane the three-layered image seen in cross sections of cellular membranes when viewed with the transmission electron microscope. There are two electron-dense layers each 2 nm thick separated by a 3.5-nm light layer. This image is not strictly related to the structure of the membrane but represents deposit of the electron-dense stain on the membrane surface. See also *cell membrane.*

asymmetric u. m., a specialized cell membrane of the superficial cells of the transitional epithelium that lines the urinary bladder. It is approximately 12 nm thick and is composed of two components of uneven thickness, the thicker facing the lumen. The asymmetric unit membrane is also found in elongated vesicles within the superficial cytoplasm, which are believed to provide a reserve of membrane for incorporation into the plasma membrane as the cell adapts to changes in configuration of the bladder.

univalent (u″nĭ-va′lent) [*uni-* + L. *valere* to be strong] 1. in genetics, the single unpaired chromosome lacking a homologous chromosome to synapse with during the zygotene stage of meiotic prophase. 2. see *monovalent.*

univitelline (u″nĭ-vi-tel′in) pertaining to or derived from a single ovum.

unmedullated (un-med′u-lāt″ed) a term used to describe nerve fibers that have no outer myelin sheath. Also called *unmyelinated.*

unmyelinated (un-mi′ĕ-lĭnāt″ed) not having a myelin sheath. Also called *nonmyelinated;* see under *nerve.*

unpack (un-pak′) in computer programming, to convert data to a form that requires more storage. See also *pack.*

unresolved hepatitis see under *hepatitis.*

unsaturated (un-sach′-e-ra-ted) 1. not saturated. 2. a chemical compound in which two or more atoms are united by double or triple bonds, which are bonds having two or three pairs of shared electrons. In the molecular orbital terminology, these bonds are formed when two carbons having electrons in *p* orbitals combine to form π bonds in which the *p* orbitals overlap. Such compounds may still add atoms or groups to the unsaturated bonding atoms up to the limit of bonding power (saturation). The term most commonly refers to carbon-carbon bonds, as in unsaturated fatty acids. Cf. *monounsaturated* and *polyunsaturated.* 3. a solution in which more solute can be dissolved at a specified temperature and pressure. Cf. *saturated.*

Unschuld's sign (oon′shooldz) [Paul *Unschuld,* German internist, born 1835] muscular cramping in the calves as a result of diabetes.

unsharpness (un-sharp′ness) any indistinctness, blurring, or lack of detail in a radiograph due to motion of the part during the exposure or to magnification of the image. Unsharpness is minimized by reducing object motion, focal spot size, and the object-film distance as much as possible.

A formula that gives the quantity of unsharpness (the distance over which points of the object are smeared in the image) is $U = (dF + Dm)/(D - d)$, where U is unsharpness, d is the object-film distance, D is the focal-film distance, F is the optical focal spot diameter, and m is the distance a part moves during the exposure. U is increased by about 0.15 mm when a screen is used. The term $dF/(D - d)$ by itself is called the geometric unsharpness; it is the width of the penumbra.

unstable hemoglobin an abnormal hemoglobin with decreased stability, which precipitates, forms Heinz bodies, and eventually leads to hemolysis of the erythrocytes. The anemia that results was originally designated Heinz body anemia but is now referred to as unstable hemoglobin hemolytic anemia. Heinz body formation may be absent in the presence of the spleen and may become marked after splenectomy.

The abnormality of the hemoglobin in Heinz body anemia had remained undetected until relatively recently because of the neutral amino acid substitution, usually in the beta chain, which caused no change in electrophoretic mobility. Since 1966, however, more than 70 unstable hemoglobins have been identified. Mild degrees of instability may be clinically silent; see also *hemoglobinopathy.*

unstable hemoglobin disease see under *hemoglobinopathy.*

unwinding protein a protein with a high affinity for single-stranded DNA, which is found in bacteria. It is needed during the unwinding of small, circular chromosomes to hold the strands apart physically for replication. Eukaryotic cells contain similar unwinding proteins.

update (up′dāt) in automatic data processing, to search a file for a particular record and modify the record to reflect a specified transaction affecting that record.

upsilon (Υ, υ) (up′sĭ-lon) the twentieth letter of the *Greek alphabet.*

uptake (up′tāk) the absorption of a substance by a cell or tissue as the result of passive or energy-dependent processes. The measurement of the uptake of a substance may be an indicator of the activity or metabolic rate of the tissue. Rapidly growing tissues, or organs with a high output of their end product, may show an increased uptake of needed precursors or nutrients.

uptime the part of the scheduled operating time during which a piece of equipment is in use or available for use. Cf. *downtime.*

ur/o (u′ro) [Gr. *ouron* urine] a word element used in combining form to denote urine or the urinary tract, e.g., urokinase, urolith.

urachus (u′rah-kus) [Gr. *ourachos*] in the fetus, the elongated tube that leads from the bladder to the umbilicus, serving as a means of excretion. After birth it remains as a cord, known as the middle umbilical ligament. Rarely, part of it remains patent as a urachal cyst.

uracil (u′rah-sil) a crystalline base, 2,4-dioxypyrimidine, $C_4H_4N_2O_2$, found in animal and plant tissues as a pyrimidine base constituent of ribonucleic acids (RNA). Its complementary base on the template DNA is adenine. Uracil is present in the uridylyl compounds: UMP, dUMP, UDP, UTP, and others. It may be found as a free base in body fluids.

uracrasia (u″rah-kra′se-ah) [*ur-* + Gr. *akrasia* bad mixture] a disorder of urine composition.

uragogue (u′rah-gog) [*ur-* + Gr. *agōgos* leading] a substance that increases the formation or flow of urine; a diuretic.

uranium (U) (u-ra′ne-um) [from the planet *Uranus*] a ductile, malleable, dense, silvery-white, metallic radioactive element; atomic number 92; atomic weight 238.029; a 5f transition element (actinide series); oxidation states +3 through +6 (the most common).

The naturally occurring isotopes of uranium are ^{238}U (half-life, 4.51 billion yr, 99.3 percent abundance), ^{235}U (half-life, 0.713 billion yr, 0.7 percent abundance), and ^{234}U (half-life, 248,000 yr, 0.006 percent abundance). In addition, 10 artificial isotopes are known. ^{235}U is fissionable and is used as nuclear reactor fuel and in the manufacture of atomic bombs; ^{238}U can be converted in a reactor to fissionable ^{239}Pu.

Uranium is a highly toxic radiation hazard; exposure to uranium dust and decay products (especially radon) is associated with an increased incidence of lung cancer and other tumors. Soluble compounds are highly nephrotoxic; uranium ions damage the proximal convoluted tubules of the kidney by chemically disrupting the cell membranes.

uranyl (u′rah-nil) pertaining to the UO_2^{2+} ion, the most common form in which uranium is found (e.g., $UO_2(NO_3)_2$ and $Na_2(UO_2)(SO_4)_2$). Most uranyl salts are characteristically soluble in organic solvents. Such salts are nephrotoxic agents, and the U.S. Public Health Service standards for drinking water limit radioactivity to 5 pCi/l.

urate (ūr′āt) [L. *uras*] a salt of uric acid.

urate crystals crystals of urate salts. The most common forms are monosodium urate (MSU) crystals, which occur in normal acid urine; large numbers may indicate urate nephropathy. MSU crystals are often present in the joints of individuals with gouty arthritis.

uratemia (u″rah-te′me-ah) [*urate* + Gr. *haima* blood + *-ia*] the presence of urates in the blood. The average level varies with age, increasing after puberty at different rates for males and females. Serum urate levels may also be affected by renal function and variations in the rate of production (due to biochemical abnormalities or changes in rates of cell turnover). Normally, reference ranges for urates in serum are: for males, 2.1–7.8 mg/100 ml; and for females, 2.0–6.4.

uratohistechia (u″rah-to-his-tek′e-ah) [*urate* + Gr. *histos* tissue + *echein* to hold + *-ia*] the presence of an abnormally high amount of urate, urea, or uric acid in the tissues.

uratoma (u″rah-to′mah) a tophus (inorganic mass), a concretion composed of urates. Such masses may be found in the subcutaneous tissues, bones, cartilage, or joints, and may accompany high serum concentrations of uric acid.

Urbach-Oppenheim disease (ur′bak op′en-hīm) [Erich *Urbach,* Philadelphia dermatologist, 1893–1946; Maurice *Oppenheim,* Chicago dermatologist, 1876–1949] see *n. lipoidica diabeticorum* under *necrobiosis.*

urea (u-re′ah) 1. the diamide of carbonic acid or amide of carbamic acid, $NH_2{\cdot}CO{\cdot}NH_2$, a white, tasteless, crystallizable substance found in the urine, blood, lymph, and all body fluids. It is the chief nitrogenous constituent of urine, nonprotein nitrogenous compound in plasma, and nitrogenous end product of the metabolism of proteins. Urea is formed in the liver from nitrogens of ammonia and aspartate and from $HCO_3^-(CO_2)$. Most of the nitrogen is derived from amino acids, some from pyrimidines, and only a small part from purines. Formation of urea prevents accumulation of potentially toxic NH_3. Efficient synthesis of urea and its excretion is important in the maintenance of the nitrogen balance or equilibrium of the body. See also *carbamide, urea cycle,* and *urea nitrogen.*

2. [USP], a preparation containing 99–100 percent urea, occasionally used as a diuretic. It is also used to lower intracranial pressure in cerebral edema.

urea clearance an infrequently used measure of total renal function (both glomerular filtration and tubular absorption). The tubular reabsorption of urea varies with the urine flow rate. At flow rates over 2 ml/min, the maximal clearance (C_m) is used. Corrected for body surface area, it is given by the formula: $C_m = U/P \times V \times 1.73/A$, where U and P are the urine and plasma urea concentrations, V is the urine flow rate in milliliters per minute, A is the body surface area in square meters, and 1.73 is the body surface area of the average adult. At flow rates of 1–2 ml/min, the standard clearance C_s is used; it is given by the formula for C_m with $\sqrt{V}$ substituted for V. Reference ranges are: for C_s, 41–68 ml/min; and for C_m, 64–99. Also called *blood urea clearance.*

urea cycle a cyclic series of enzyme reactions in which ornithine is utilized and regenerated during the synthesis of urea. It is the major cyclic pathway in which ammonia, a toxic product, is detoxified in humans. The urea cycle involves five enzymes. Part of the pathway is also used for the synthesis of arginine. The complete pathway occurs in the liver. Also called *Krebs-Henseleit cycle.* See also *urea synthesis.*

urea nitrogen the nitrogen content in urea, two atoms per molecule, constituting 46.64 percent of urea mass; in clinical chemistry, it is the nitrogen of urea, particularly in serum, plasma, blood, and other body fluids. The reference range for plasma (serum) for young adults is 2.5–6.5 mmol/l in terms of urea or 5.0–13.0 mmol/l in terms of urea nitrogen. These values, in terms of mass concentration, are 15–39 mg of urea or 7–18 mg of urea-N/dl of serum. The serum or plasma urea nitrogen still is often, but incorrectly, referred to as BUN (from blood urea nitrogen). Serum (plasma) urea nitrogen is approximately 12 percent higher than the blood urea nitrogen concentration because of the greater protein content of red blood cells. Increases in blood or serum urea nitrogen are referred to as azotemia and may have prerenal, renal, or postrenal causes.

urea nitrogen assays 1. direct method. Diacetyl (CH_3—CO—CO—CH_3) condenses with urea in a strongly acid solution to form a predominantly yellow diazine, which is quantitated photometrically at 540 nm. Because diacetyl is unstable, most methods use diacetyl monoxime, which is hydrolyzed to diacetyl and hydroxylamine by heat and oxidants. Various reagents are used to remove the hydroxylamine and intensify the color of the condensation product.

2. indirect methods. The enzyme urease hydrolyzes urea at neutral pH, producing ammonium carbonate. The liberated ammonia is quantitated by one of a variety of manual or automated methods. In manual methods, the ammonia is detected by the indophenol reaction of Berthelot (ammonia reacts with phenol and sodium hypochlorite in the presence of nitroprusside to form blue indophenol, which is measured photometrically at 630 nm), or by nesslerization. Both techniques can be automated and both are essentially specific, as no other appreciable sources of ammonia are present in serum. See also *Nessler reaction.*

3. enzymatic method. Ammonia released by urease reacts with glutarate in the presence of gluta-

mate dehydrogenase and NAD to form glutamate and NADH, which is measured at 340 nm.

4. ion-selective electrode method. The ammonia formed in the urease reaction can be measured potentiometrically using an ammonia electrode. In some cases, electrodes contain a built-in immobilized urease, thus eliminating the need for separate incubation with urease.

Ureaplasma (u-re′ah-plaz″ma) a genus of bacteria-like microorganisms of the family Mycoplasmataceae, one of the Mollicutes. It is closely related to the *Mycoplasma* but hydrolyzes urea. The organism is a common inhabitant of the genitourinary tract but has also been isolated from the blood in systemic infections. The genus contains a single species, *U. urealyticum,* which can cause a sexually transmitted disease classified as nongonococcal urethritis. See also *mycoplasma* and *sexually transmitted diseases.*

ureapoiesis (u-re″ah-poi-e′sis) [*urea* + Gr. *poiein* to make] the formation of urea, which usually occurs by the hydrolysis of arginine in the liver by the enzyme arginase.

urease (u′re-ās) an enzyme of the hydrolase class (EC 3.5.1.5) that catalyzes the reaction urea + $H_2O \rightleftarrows CO_2 + 2\ NH_3$. It is produced by certain microorganisms, especially *Bacillus pasteurii,* and by some of the intestinal bacteria. Urease was the first enzyme prepared in the crystalline state. It is utilized in analytic methods to measure urea.

urease test a test for the production of urease by bacterial cultures. A peptone agar medium containing urea concentrate and phenol red is prepared in slants. After inoculation of the surface and incubation, urease-positive cultures produce an alkaline reaction (red color) in the medium. *Proteus* cultures show an early urease-positive reaction; other genera may have a delayed response.

urea synthesis (u′re′ah sin′thĕ-sis) the formation of urea from ammonia, CO_2, and the nitrogen of aspartic acid by a series of five enzymatic reactions and the cyclic utilization and regeneration of ornithine. This reaction sequence is also the source of arginine for metabolic needs.

Synthesis of carbamoyl phosphate and citrulline occurs in the mitochondrial matrix of the liver. Four ATP molecules are consumed in the reaction. The first ATP molecule is used to convert HCO_3^- to enzyme-bound carboxy-phosphate, which reacts with NH_4^+ to form enzyme-bound carbamate. This, with the energy of the second ATP molecule, forms carbamoyl phosphate. The third ATP molecule is required for argininosuccinate synthesis, and the fourth to recover the high-energy P lost in the hydrolysis of pyrophosphate.

The five enzyme disorders of urea synthesis of clinical interest are carbamoyl phosphate synthetase deficiency, ornithine transcarbamylase deficiency, citrullinemia, argininosuccinic aciduria, and argininemia. All are characterized by hyperammonemia, with toxic effects that include episodes of vomiting, lethargy, and coma after ingestion of protein.

For more information, see the accompanying illustration.

uremia (u-re′me-ah) [*ur-* + Gr. *haima* blood + *-ia*] symptoms of anorexia, nausea, vomiting, acidosis, water and electrolyte imbalance, anemia, and neuropsychiatric changes; stupor and coma ensue at urea nitrogen concentrations near 200 mg/dl. See also *renal failure.*

uremic (u-re′mik) related to or caused by uremia.

ureotelic (u″re-o-tel′ik) [*urea* + Gr. *telikos* belonging to the completion, or end] having urea as the chief excretory product of nitrogen metabolism.

ureter/o (u-re′ter-o) [Gr. *ourētēr* the duct that conveys urine from the kidney to the bladder] a word element used in combining form to denote the ureter, e.g., ureterostenosis.

ureter (u-re′ter) [Gr. *ourētēr*] [NA], the fibromuscular tube lined by transitional epithelium and 25–30 cm long, that extends from the funnel-shaped renal pelvis to the base of the bladder.

ureterectasia (u-re″ter-ek-ta′se-ah) the dilation of a ureter, often the result of obstruction distally in the urinary tract by a stone or tumor. It is usually accompanied by hydronephrosis. Also called hydroureter.

ureteritis (u″re-ter-i′tis) inflammation of a ureter.

ureterocele (u-re′ter-o-sēl″) a dilated ureter that protrudes into the bladder, often with the resulting obstruction of the urinary tract on that side of the body. Such obstruction may lead to damage or failure of the kidney on that side. Ureteroceles are most common in young females with a congenital duplication of the ureter on the side of the lesion. A simple ureterocele is a ureteral dilation protruding into the trigone of the bladder, and is usually associated with a normally placed but stenotic ureteral orifice.

ureterolith (u-re′ter-o-lith″) [*uretero-* + Gr. *lithos* stone] a calculus or stone formed or lying within a ureter. See also *kidney stone.*

ureterolysis (u-re″ter-ol′ĭ-sis) [*uretero-* + Gr. *lysis* dissolution] 1. the tearing of a ureter.

2. the paralysis of a ureter.

3. the surgical freeing of a ureter from adhesions to surrounding structures.

ureteropathy (u-re″ter-op′ah-the) [*uretero-* + Gr. *pathos* disease] a general term for diseases of the ureter.

ureteropyelitis (u-re″ter-o-pi-ĕ-li′tis) [*uretero-* + Gr. *pyelos* pelvis + *-itis*] an inflammation of the renal pelvis and its ureter, most often due to infection. Also called ureteropyelonephritis.

ureterostenosis (u-re″ter-o-stĕ-no′sis) [*uretero-* + Gr. *stenōsis* narrowing] a narrowing or stricture of the ureter, which may be congenital or due to ureteral inflammation or tumor, or to retroperitoneal fibrosis or tumor.

urethan (u′rĕ-thān) a white crystalline substance, ethyl carbamate, $NH_2COOC_2H_5$; M.W. 89.09.

urethr/o (u-re′thro) [Gr. *ourēthra* the tube by which urine is discharged from the bladder] a word element used in combining form to denote the urethra, e.g., urethropexy.

urethra (u-re′thrah) [Gr. *ourēthra*] the mucous membrane–lined canal that conveys urine from the bladder to the urinary meatus.

female u., a canal, 4 cm long, that exits the bladder and traverses the anterior vaginal wall to emerge at the vulva, immediately in front of the vagina.

male u., a canal, 18–20 cm long, that connects the bladder with the urinary meatus. It is divided into three regions: prostatic, membranous, and pendulous.

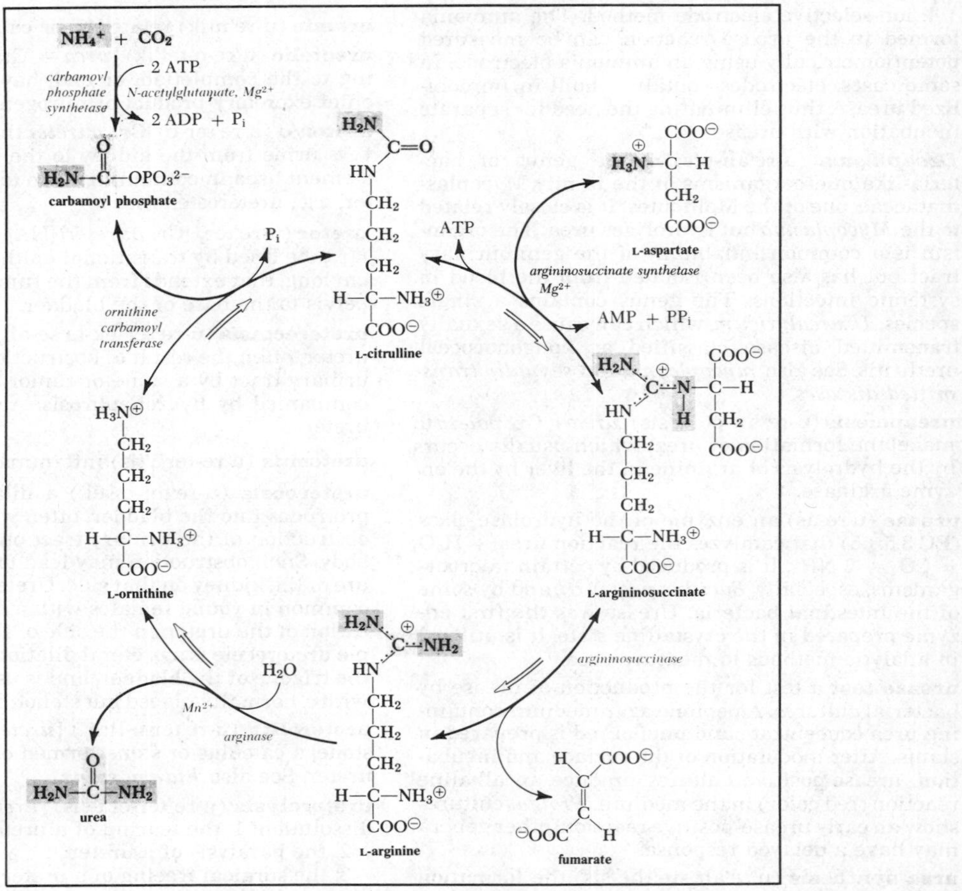

Urea synthesis. The synthesis of urea by the Krebs-Henseleit cycle. (From McGilvery, R. W.: Biochemistry: A Functional Approach. Philadelphia, W. B. Saunders Co., 1979.)

urethral obstruction (u-re′thral) a partial or complete obstruction to the flow of urine from the bladder, more common in males than in females. Complete obstruction leads to acute urinary retention; chronic partial obstruction manifests itself by burning on urination, hesitation, terminal dribbling, and a weak, slow urinary stream. In males, the condition may be produced by benign prostatic hyperplasia, chronic prostatitis, prostatic cancer, or urethral meatal stenosis.

urethritis (u″rĕ-thri′tis) an inflammation of the urethra due to chemical, bacterial, viral, or other infectious agents. In females it is often caused by an ascending infection of the urethra; in males it may be associated with an infection or inflammation of the prostate. Urethritis may also be caused by *Neisseria gonorrhoeae,* which is transmitted through sexual contact with an infected partner. Nongonococcal infectious urethritis is often caused by bacteria of the genus *Chlamydia.*

Laboratory diagnosis is aided by a culture and smear of urethral discharge or by a culture of urine. The first urine voided often shows evidence of inflammation and infection (e.g., white blood cells), whereas later specimens taken at the same voiding show little or no abnormality in the absence of infection higher in the urinary tract.

urethrocele (u-re′thro-sēl) [*urethro-* + Gr. *kēlē* tumor] a bulging of the female urethra that prolapses through the external urinary meatus.

urethrocystography (u-re″thro-sis-tog′rah-fe) [*urethro-* + Gr. *kystis* bladder + *graphein* to write] the radiologic examination of both the urethra and bladder, using a radiologic contrast agent. This procedure may be accomplished as part of urography or, in males primarily, by introduction of a radiopaque agent through a urethral catheter into the urethra and bladder (retrograde urethrocystography). See also *cystography* and *urography.*

urethrography (u″rĕ-throg′rah-fe) the radiologic examination of the urethra after injection of a radiopaque contrast medium. See also *cystourethrography.*

urethrostenosis (u-re″thro-stĕ-no′sis) [*urethro-* + Gr. *stenōsis* stricture] a narrowing of the urethra, which may result from congenital stricture, inflammation and scarring, or traumatic injury.

uretic (u-ret′ik) [L. *ureticus;* Gr. *ourētikos*] related to urine or having the properties of a diuretic.

urhidrosis (ur″hid-ro′sis) [*ur-* + Gr. *hidrōs* sweat]

the excretion in sweat of substances normally found in the urine, including urea or urates. This may be seen in severe renal failure, when the blood levels of urates rise to high concentrations.

URI abbrev. for upper respiratory infection.

-uria (u're-ah) [Gr. *ouron* urine + *-ia* state] a suffix word element to denote urination or urine, e.g., pyuria.

uric acid (U/A) (u'rik) [Gr. *ourikos*] a crystallizable acid, 2,6,8-trioxypurine, $C_5H_4N_4O_3$, present in the urine of humans and animals. It is the main end product of purine metabolism in humans and some animals. Nearly insoluble in water, alcohol, and ether, it is soluble in solutions of alkaline salts. Uric acid forms a large portion of certain renal calculi, and its accumulation in the blood and in joints leads to gout. Also called *lithic acid.*

uric acid assays 1. photometry. Uric acid in protein-free serum filtrates or in urine can be oxidized to allantoin by phosphotungstic acid, and the tungsten blue formed is measured photometrically.

2. enzymatic methods. Uric acid, which has a characteristic absorption at 293 nm, is oxidized by uricase to allantoin, which has no absorption at this wavelength. Thus, measurement of absorption before and after oxidation of the specimen with uricase provides a measure of uric acid. Alternatively, hydrogen peroxide, a product of the enzymatic reaction, can be measured in a second coupled reaction involving catalase and the formation of a chromophore, or the oxygen consumed in the uricase reaction can be measured with an O_2 electrode. Both the nonspecific chemical methods and the enzymatic assays have been adapted to automated analysis.

3. the microscopic demonstration of sodium urate crystals in fluid aspirated by syringe from an affected joint, which provides important diagnostic information for the diagnosis of gout.

uric acid crystals crystals of uric acid that may be found in normal acid urine, as they are insoluble at normal urine pH. Large numbers occur in association with uricacidemia and with some forms of cancer chemotherapy. See also *urate crystals.*

uricacidemia (u″rik-as″ĭ-de'me-ah) [*uric acid* + Gr. *haima* blood + *-ia*] see *uricemia.*

uricemia (u″rĭ-se'me-ah) the presence of an elevated concentration of uric acid in the blood. Reference ranges for uric acid in serum differ with the method employed; phosphotungstate methods usually give values for males of 4.5–8.2 mg/dl, and for females, 3.0–6.5, whereas methods employing uricase give values of 3.5–7.2 and 2.6–6.0, respectively. Higher concentrations may be related to unusually large dietary intake of precursors of uric acid, or may be due to defects in uric acid metabolism (e.g., gout), impaired renal function, or neoplastic disorders (leukemia). Also called *hyperuricemia* and *uricacidemia.*

uricosuria (u″ri-ko-su're-ah) the presence of an elevated concentration of uric acid in the urine. Normal excretion values are 0.2–0.7 g/24 hr; higher concentrations may lead to the formation of uric acid stones, a frequent complication of metabolic or neoplastic disorders that produce high systemic levels of urates.

uricosuric (u″rĭ-ko-su'rik) an agent or drug, such as probenecid or sulfinpyrazone, that increases the urinary excretion of uric acid.

uridine (U) (u'rĭ-dēn) a nucleoside, uracil riboside, a crystalline compound obtainable from nucleic acid (RNA) hydrolyzates. It can be degraded to CO_2, ammonia, and amino acid compounds in the body.

uridine diphosphate (UDP) (u'rĭ-dēn dī-fos'fāt) a compound that has both a precursor and a product relationship with uridine triphosphate (UTP). Many carbohydrate derivatives of UDP are involved in carbohydrate metabolism and sugar transfer reactions.

uridine monophosphate (u'ri-dēn mon'o-fos'fāt) see *uridine-5′-phosphate.*

uridine-5′-phosphate (UMP) (u'rĭ-dēn fos'fāt) a mononucleotide formed from uracil, ribose, and phosphoric acid. Also called *uridine monophosphate* and *uridylic acid.* See also under *nucleotide.*

uridine triphosphate (UTP) (u'rĭ-dēn trī-fos'fāt) an energy-rich compound, analogous to adenosine triphosphate (ATP). It is a biosynthetic intermediate of cytidine triphosphate. UTP forms important sugar donor molecules for biosynthetic and metabolic purposes.

uridylic acid (u'rĭ-dil'ik) see *uridine-5′-phosphate.*

uridyl transferase (u'ri-dil trans'fer-ās) see UDP-glucose-hexose-1-phosphate uridyltransferase.

uridylyl (u'rĭ-dĭ-lil) a term for uridylic acid when it is being named as a substituent on some parent group or as an ester.

urin/o (u-rĭ-no) [L. *urina*] a word element used in combining form to denote relationship to urine, e.g., urinalysis, urinometer.

urinalysis (U/A) (ur″ĭ-nal'ĭ-sis) the performance of clinical laboratory tests on urine specimens. Routine urinalysis typically consists of observing any unusual color or odor, determining specific gravity, performing chemical screening tests, screening for bacteriuria, and examining the sediment microscopically.

The usual chemical tests are qualitative or semiquantitative tests for pH, protein or albumin, glucose or reducing substances, ketone bodies, occult blood, bilirubin, urobilinogen, and nitrite. These tests are performed using reagent tablets or multiple or separate reagent strips. The pH can be determined to an accuracy of about half a unit by means of an acid-base indicator dye, or it may be measured to within 0.1 with a pH electrode. The protein test is based on the "protein error" of acid-base indicators such as bromphenol blue; it becomes positive at a concentration of 10–20 mg/dl of albumin. The glucose test uses the glucose oxidase-peroxidase method and becomes positive at a glucose concentration of 40–100 mg/dl, depending on which reagent strip is used. The ketone bodies test is based on the nitroprusside method and detects 5–10 mg/dl of acetoacetic acid. The *o*-tolidine test for occult blood is sensitive to 0.05–0.3 mg/dl of hemoglobin or myoglobin. Tests for bilirubin, urobilinogen, and nitrite all use azo dye methods. These tests normally respond to concentrations of approximately 0.2–0.5 mg/dl of bilirubin, 0.1 Ehrlich units/dl of urobilinogen, and 0.05–0.075 mg/dl of nitrite. The nitrite test is a screening test for bacteriuria. Reducing substances are detected using the copper reduction test for sugars (Benedict's), a screening test for inborn errors of metabolism in infants.

More specific procedures routinely performed include microscopic examination of an uncentrifuged urine specimen and of a Gram-stained smear. A quantitative culture using the calibrated loop streak-plate method may be performed if bacteria are detected.

The centrifuged urine sediment is examined for formed elements—cells, casts, and crystals. The sediment is examined on a microscopic slide, either stained or unstained, and the number of cells of each type counted in a high-power microscope field. Types of cells usually encountered include erythrocytes, leukocytes, and renal tubular epithelial, transitional epithelial, or squamous epithelial cells and other cells of the genitourinary tract. Casts and crystals are counted in a low-power microscope field. Hyaline (only in large numbers), red blood cell, tubular epithelial cell, granular, fatty, and waxy casts signify renal disease. Crystals found may include urate, oxalate, cystine, tyrosine, and crystals of certain drugs.

Positive results in some routine tests require confirmation and/or identification by a more specific procedure. The presence of proteins is confirmed by a quantitative method and further identified by electrophoresis or immunochemical tests; sugars are further identified by chromatography. Cystine crystals are confirmed by a chemical test. In addition to these routine procedures, many special tests may also be performed when indicated, such as tests for aminoacidurias when inborn errors of metabolism are suspected.

Urinalysis is most commonly performed on a random specimen, although for some specific tests other specimens are better suited. The first morning specimen is the most concentrated and is therefore better than others for the detection of protein or the examination of formed elements. This specimen is also preferred because the long incubation in the bladder is helpful in detecting bacteriuria. The specimen for bacteriologic examination, in order to be free of contamination from the external genitalia, should be collected by the clean-catch method or, if necessary, via suprapubic aspiration or transurethral catheterization. A postprandial specimen is better for the detection of glucose in screening for diabetes, and an afternoon specimen (taken between 2 and 4 pm) is better for urobilinogen testing. For quantitative assays, 24-hr specimens are used to eliminate the effects of diurnal variation in excretion of constituents of interest.

See also *clean-catch collection method, crystals in urine sediment, urinary cast,* and the specific tests and assays.

urinary (u′ri-ner″e) pertaining to the urine; containing or secreting urine.

urinary bladder see *urinary b.* under *bladder.*

urinary cast an aggregate composed of material deposited in renal tubules. When a cast is washed out in the urine, its shape is that of the lumen in which it was deposited. The matrix of a cast is protein, primarily Tamm-Horsfall mucoprotein, but it can also be plasma protein, especially when proteinuria is present. Casts are classified according to the materials trapped in their matrices.

bacterial u. c., a urinary cast made up of bacteria or containing a large number of bacteria.

broad u. c., a urinary cast formed in the collecting tubules. Although usually of the waxy or epithelial variety, broad casts of almost any composition may be seen. They usually suggest severe renal disease, and in large numbers imply a grave prognosis. For this reason they have been termed renal failure casts.

crystal u. c., a urinary cast that contains crystals such as urate or oxalate.

epithelial cell u. c., a urinary cast that contains tubular epithelial cells. These casts usually indicate acute tubular necrosis.

fatty u. c., a urinary cast composed of fat droplets. These occur along with free oval fat bodies in nephrotic syndrome. They have been associated with a variety of nephropathies.

granular u. c., a urinary cast that contains granules of material from plasma proteins or degenerated cells. These casts may be associated with several forms of renal diseases, such as pyelonephritis, viral disease, and chronic lead poisoning.

hyaline u. c., a transparent urinary cast composed of glycoprotein and possibly globulins. These casts are associated with aciduria and proteinuria. In small numbers they are not clinically meaningful, but in large numbers they usually indicate renal parenchymal disease.

red blood cell u. c., a urinary cast that contains red blood cells. These casts usually indicate glomerular disease or renal infarction. If the cells have degenerated, the cast is called a blood cast or a hemoglobin cast.

waxy u. c., a smooth, yellow urinary cast thought to result from the further degeneration of a granular cast. It is associated with decreased urine flow or oliguria, as seen in chronic renal failure or in allograft rejection.

white blood cell u. c., a urinary cast that contains white blood cells. These casts usually indicate tubulointerstitial disease, most commonly pyelonephritis.

urinary sediment substances that separate from freshly voided urine upon standing or after light centrifugation. Normally, such sediment includes: (1) a flocculent material consisting of a small amount of nucleoprotein or mucoprotein, together with some epithelial cells of the lining of the genitourinary tract and (rarely) leukocytes, erythrocytes, and some hyaline casts; (2) in alkaline urine, a mixture of calcium phosphate and ammonium magnesium phosphate (triple phosphate), and (occasionally) urates and calcium oxalate, which redissolve on acidification; and (3) in acidic urine, urates and/or uric acid and (rarely) cystine.

In disease states, inspection of urinary sediments can be of significant diagnostic aid, e.g., in disclosing the presence of large numbers of leukocytes, erythrocytes, and abnormal casts. Crystals may also appear in urine in cases of drug treatment.

urinary tract infection (UTI) infection of the urinary tract, a common infection in humans. Females are generally affected 10 times more often than males; in infants, however, boys are infected more often than girls. In infants, the route of infection is usually through the blood stream or the lymphatics; in adults, it is usually ascending. Predisposing factors include physiologic or anatomic obstruction to the flow of urine; in females, intercourse has been related to acute infection (honeymoon cystitis). Gram-negative organisms are the primary pathogens in bacterial UTI, *Escherichia coli* being the most common. *Klebsiella, Proteus, Enterobacter,* and *Pseudomonas* are also encountered.

To determine the extent of infection, urine must be quantitatively cultured. It is usually collected by

(1) the clean-catch collection (the most common method); (2) suprapubic needle aspiration, which allows the collection of urine without urethral contaminants; or (3) catheterization, which identifies an active significant infection with 95 percent accuracy when quantitative culture reveals more than 100,000 bacteria of a single species per milliliter of urine. The urine should be cultured and examined within 1 hr of collection if fresh, or within 18 hr if refrigerated. Microscopic examination showing greater than 10 bacteria per high power field suggests significant infection (>100,000 cells/ml of urine). A Gram stain should be routinely performed.

Acute lower UTI is characterized by pain or burning on urination and lower abdominal pain; acute upper UTI produces costovertebral angle tenderness, nausea, headache, and malaise. Laboratory studies are needed to demonstrate bacteriuria and pyuria. Upper UTI also is often accompanied by proteinuria and leukocytosis with a shift to the left.

Chronic, recurrent UTI is characterized by chronic significant bacteriuria. Urologic examination, including voiding cystourethrograms, cystoscopy, excretory urograms, and retrograde pyelography, help to identify underlying and contributory abnormalities of the urinary tract. Laboratory studies may indicate decreased renal function. Antibiotic susceptibility tests should be performed on cultured organisms.

urinate (u′rĭ-nāt) to void or discharge urine. Also called *micturate.*

urination (u″rĭ-na′shun) the process of discharging or voiding urine from the urinary bladder. As the bladder fills and the tension in its wall reaches a critical value, a nervous reflex is initiated. Unless it can be voluntarily overridden, this reflex causes muscular contractions that empty the bladder and allow passage of urine out through the urethra. Also called *micturition.*

urine (u′rin) [L. *urina*; Gr. *ouron*] a fluid, containing water and metabolic products, that is secreted by the kidneys, stored in the bladder, and discharged by way of the urethra. In healthy individuals, urine has an amber color, a slight acid reaction and a distinctive odor. The largest component of urine by weight is water and the second largest is urea, followed by sodium chloride, phosphate, sulfate, and uric acid; other normal components include potassium, calcium, magnesium, and various organic compounds.

urine culture the bacteriologic analysis of urine as an aid in the diagnosis and treatment of urinary tract infections (UTIs) and certain renal parenchymal infections such as active pyelonephritis. The increasing use of indwelling urinary catheters in hospitalized patients is associated with a corresponding rise in the number of UTIs. Because bladder urine is normally sterile, specimens from catheterized patients should be sterile. If the urine is collected without special preparation (clean catch, suprapubic aspiration, or catheterization), it will not be sterile, and several different nonpathogenic bacteria may be isolated. Voided urine is considered to contain pathogens when the colony count is greater than 10^5/ml. Bacteria present in smaller numbers are probably picked up from the surrounding tissue while the patient is voiding.

The urine is an excellent medium for the growth of urinary tract pathogens. Thus, when a urine specimen is collected in a sterile container, its processing (including transportation and plating) should be completed as soon as possible (within 1 hr if fresh or 18 hr if refrigerated); otherwise, the growth of bacteria leads to an incorrect estimate of the numbers of bacteria present.

Examples of nonpathogenic bacteria often associated with voided urine in low numbers are coagulase-negative staphylococci, diptheroids, coliform bacteria, and lactobacilli. Common pathogens of the urinary tract include *Escherichia coli, Streptococcus faecalis* (enterococci), *Proteus* species, *Klebsiella* species, *Enterobacter, Serratia, Pseudomonas,* and *Staphylococcus aureus.*

See also *Gram stain.*

urine specimen collection see *clean-catch collection method.*

urinometer (u″rĭ-nom′ĕ-ter) [*urino-* + Gr. *metron* measure] a hydrometer used to measure the specific gravity of urine.

urinophilous (u″rĭ-nof′ĭ-lus) [*urino-* + Gr. *philein* to love] having an affinity for urine, e.g., a microorganism that grows well in urine.

urobenzoic acid (u″ro-ben-zo′ik) see *hippuric acid.*

urobilin (u″ro-bi′lin) [*uro-* + L. *bilis* bile] an amorphous, orange-red to red-brown pigment found in the feces and sometimes in urine that has been left standing exposed to air. It is an oxidized form of the colorless urobilinogen that is initially derived from reduction of bilirubin in the intestinal tract.

urobilin assays the zinc fluorescence test for collectively determining *d*-urobilin, *i*-urobilin, and *l*-stercobilin in urine. Urobilinogen is first converted to urobilin by oxidation with iodine. A zinc-urobilin complex showing green fluorescence is formed by adding alcoholic zinc acetate solution to the urine. A number of other substances give fluorescence of differing colors. This test is more sensitive and specific than Ehrlich's *p*-dimethylaminobenzaldehyde reaction for urobilinogen, which measures urobilin after reduction to urobilinogen, e.g., with ferrous sulfate and NaOH.

urobilinogen (UBG) (u″ro-bi-lin′o-jen) [*urobilin* + Gr. *gennan* to produce] one of several colorless reduction products of bilirubin formed by the action of intestinal microorganisms. *d*-Urobilinogen, *i*-urobilinogen (mesobilirubinogen), and *l*-urobilinogen (stercobilinogen) vary in their degree of saturation, having, 6, 8, and 12 more hydrogen atoms than bilirubin. They can be oxidized by air to yellowish-brown *d*-urobilin, *i*-urobilin, or *l*-stercobilin.

Increases in urinary and fecal urobilinogen levels occur in hemolytic jaundice and early hepatitis. Decreases occur in obstructive jaundice, posthepatic biliary obstruction, and most other liver diseases. Timed 24-hr or early afternoon 2-hr urine specimens are used for quantitative assays. Reference ranges are: for urine, 0.5–2.5 mg/da or 0.5–4.0 Ehrlich Units (EU)/da or 0.1–1.0 EU/2 hr; for stool, 50–275 mg/da.

urobilinogen assays 1. the Watson-Schwartz test for urobilinogen and porphobilinogen in urine. Ehrlich's reagent (*p*-dimethylaminobenzaldehyde in hydrochloric acid) is added to the specimen, followed immediately by saturated sodium acetate solution. Urobilinogen, porphobilinogen, and other Ehrlich chromogens form a product that is pink to red. The urobilinogen color can be extracted into chloroform, whereas the porphobilinogen color remains in the aqueous phase.

2. reagent strip tests, which use either Ehrlich's reaction or an azo coupling reaction with 4-methoxybenzene-diazonium-tetrafluoroborate.

3. quantitative assay for urobilinogen in urine or feces. Urobilins are reduced to urobilinogens with alkaline ferrous sulfate, and extracted into petroleum ether. Ehrlich's reagent and sodium acetate are added and the absorbance measured at 562 nm. The concentration is determined by comparison with a stercobilin standard or with a phenolsulfonphthalein or Pontacyl dye standard.

urobilinogenuria (u″ro-bi-lin″o-je-nu′re-ah) the excretion of elevated concentrations of urobilinogens in the urine. The normal rate of excretion of urobilinogens varies between 0.1 and 1.0 Ehrlich units/100 ml. These levels may increase with the increased destruction of red blood cells, as in hemolytic anemia.

urocanic acid (u″ro-kan′ik) an intermediate product of histidine metabolism formed by the removal of one molecule of NH_3 from the side-chain by the enzyme histidine ammonia-lyase. The genetic deficiency of this enzyme gives rise to histidinemia.

urocele (u′ro-sēl) [*uro-* + Gr. *kēlē* hernia] a scrotal distention caused by the escape of urine into the scrotum, often found in association with traumatic tears of the urethra; the urine may flow into the pelvis and also up into the abdominal wall.

urochrome (u′ro-krōm) [*uro-* + Gr. *chrōma* color] a yellow pigment found in urine that gives it its usual amber color.

urocortisol see *tetrahydrocortisol.*

uroerythrin (u″ro-er′ĭ-thrin) [*uro-* + Gr. *erythros* red] a dark-red coloring matter that imparts the red color to some urine urate sediments. Uroerythrin is believed to be a product of melanin metabolism. Also called purpurin.

urogram (u′ro-gram) the radiologic visualization of the urinary tract following intravenous injection of a radiopaque contrast agent. Also called excretory urogram.

urography (u-rog′rah-fe) radiography of the urinary tract after introduction of an opaque contrast medium. Pyelography, although it refers only to the pelvis of the kidney, is a term commonly used as an equivalent to urography; both include examination of the calyces and pelvis of the kidney, ureters, bladder, and, when indicated, a voiding study of the urethra. Cystography applies only to radiographic examination of the bladder and urethra. See also *nephrotomography* and *pneumocystography.*

ascending u., urography in which the contrast medium is introduced into the pelvis and calyces of the kidney by urinary catheter with the aid of a ureterocystoscope. Also called ascending, cystoscopic, and retrograde pyelography, and retrograde urography.

descending u., urography in which the contrast medium is introduced intravenously, either by injection or by infusion, and filtered by the kidney into the urinary tract. Also called descending, excretory, and intravenous pyelography, and excretory and intravenous urography.

percutaneous antegrade u., the radiologic examination of the urinary tract after percutaneous injection of a water-soluble iodinated contrast medium directly into the renal calyces and pelvis. This method is generally used in examining individuals with hydronephrosis. Also called percutaneous antegrade pyelography.

urokinase (u″ro-ki′nās) an enzyme of the hydrolase class (EC 3.4.21.31) that catalyzes the cleavage of peptide bonds between arginine and valine in plasminogen, thus converting it to plasmin. Urokinase has been isolated from urine and from renal tubular cells, and is part of the complex plasminogen activator system. Also called plasminogen activator. See also *thrombolytic agents.*

urolith (u′ro-lith) [*uro-* + Gr. *lithos* stone] a urinary stone. See also *kidney stone.*

urolithiasis (u″ro-lĭ-thi′ah-sis) the presence of calculi or stones in the urinary tract or urine. This condition is associated with disorders of metabolism and/or urinary tract anatomy, as well as urinary tract infection. The calculi of urolithiasis are usually formed of calcium salts, although cystine, xanthine, and uric acid stones are also found. The condition may result in decreased renal function, infection, or urinary obstruction.

urologic (u″ro-loj′ik) related to urology.

urologist (u-rol′o-jist) a physician specializing in urology.

urology (u-rol′o-je) [*uro-* + *-logy*] the branch of medicine dealing with the diagnosis and treatment, both medical and surgical, of diseases and disorders of the genitourinary system.

uromucoid (u″ro-mu′koid) an insoluble mucoprotein found in urine; it is not as yet well characterized. It occurs as polymers (M.W. 7×10^6 and 28×10^6) and as a monomer of smaller size. Uromucoid may be a normal excretion product of the cells that line the renal tubules. One form or variant is identified as the Tamm-Horsfall protein. Its concentration in urine is increased in inflammation of the urinary tract and in renal lithiasis and decreased when tubular defects are present.

uromucoid assays 1. acetic acid sedimentation test. Acetic acid is added drop by drop to diluted urine until precipitation stops. The same amount of acetic acid plus five to seven additional drops is added to another aliquot. Normally, both tubes produce the same amount of precipitate. If excess mucoprotein is present, the second tube shows a decreased amount of precipitate.

2. immunoassay using specific antisera for uromucoid. After uromucoid is dissociated into monomeric forms using sodium dodecyl sulfate, it is determined by radial immunodiffusion or electroimmunodiffusion.

uron/o (u-ron′o) [Gr. *ouron* urine] a word element used in combining form to denote urine or the urinary tract, e.g., uronophile.

uronephrosis (u″ro-nĕ-fro′sis) see *hydronephrosis.*

uronic acid (u-ro′nik) any of certain aldehyde acids derived from simple sugars by oxidation of the alcohol end of the chain. See also *glucuronic acid.*

uronophile (u-ron′o-fīl) [*urono-* + Gr. *philein* to love] in microbiology, an organism that can grow in a medium containing urine.

uropepsin (u″ro-pep′sin) gastric pepsin that has entered the blood stream and been excreted in the urine, predominantly in the form of the proenzyme uropepsinogen. See also under *pepsin A.*

uropepsinogen (u″ro-pep-sin′o-jen) pepsinogen that occurs in the urine.

uropepsinogen assays see *pepsinogen assays.*

uroporphyrin (u″ro-por′fĭ-rin) one of a group of compounds produced from uroporphyrinogen by oxidation. The pyrrole groups, linked by methyne bridges, each have an acetate (A) and propionate (P) side-chain present in the order APAPAPAP in uroporphyrin I, but are reversed at one of the pyrrole rings in uroporphyrin type III (APAPAPPA). In hepatic porphyria, urinary concentrations of uroporphyrin, which are normally very low (up to 25 μg/da), may be increased.

uroporphyrin assays see under *porphyrin assays.*

uroporphyrinogen (u″ro-por″fĭ-rin′o-jen) one of a group of porphyrins formed enzymatically by the condensation of four porphobilinogen molecules. Uroporphyrinogens can be air oxidized to uroporphyrins or precursors thereof, and converted to coproporphyrinogens by loss of four CO_2 molecules. Excessive amounts of uroporphyrinogen I are formed in individuals with hereditary erythropoietic porphyria, and increased amounts are excreted in some forms of hepatic porphyria. See also *uroporphyrin.*

uroporphyrinogen III cosynthase a protein cofactor required for the reaction porphobilinogen ⇄ uroporphyrinogen III + 4 NH_3 catalyzed by uroporphyrinogen I synthase (EC 4.3.1.8). Uroporphyrinogen III cosynthase permits the isomerization of an intermediate formed by the action of uroporphyrinogen I synthase on porphobilinogen. An extremely rare genetic deficiency of this factor, transmitted as an autosomal recessive trait, causes congenital erythropoietic porphyria (Günther's disease).

uroporphyrinogen decarboxylase an enzyme of the lyase class (EC 4.1.1.37) that catalyzes the reaction uroporphyrinogen III ⇄ coproporphyrinogen + 4 CO_2. A deficiency of this enzyme causes porphyria cutanea tarda, which is transmitted as an autosomal dominant trait and is associated with increased amounts of urinary uroporphyrin.

uroporphyrinogen I synthase an enzyme of the lyase class (EC 4.3.1.8) that catalyzes the reaction 4-porphobilinogen ⇄ uroporphyrinogen I + 4 NH_3. A deficiency of this enzyme leads to acute intermittent porphyria, which is transmitted as an autosomal dominant trait and is the most common type of inherited porphyria. Also called *porphobilinogen deaminase.*

uroschesis (u-ros′kĕ-sis) [*uro-* + Gr. *schesis* holding] urine retention. It may be due to simple obstruction of the lower urinary tract, anticholinergic medications, or diseases and conditions affecting the nerve supply to the bladder such as spinal cord injury, diabetic neuropathy, or other peripheral neuropathies.

urorosein (u″ro-ro′ze-in) a rose-colored pigment found in the urine of individuals with typhoid fever, nephritis, pulmonary tuberculosis, and other diseases. Its excretion is related to the ingestion of indole compounds. Also called urorrhodin.

urticaria (ur″tĭ-ka′re-ah) [L. *urtica* stinging nettle + *-ia*] a disorder affecting the upper layer of the dermis and characterized by the eruption of well-circumscribed wheals with erythematous, raised borders and blanched centers. The lesions are pruritic and may occur anywhere on the body. Individual lesions spontaneously remit over a period of 48 hr, but in some forms they may be chronic. Urticaria can result from many different stimuli and may have immunologic or nonimmunologic causes. Most commonly it is due to a type I hypersensitivity response, which is mediated by IgE and a variety of substances (principally histamine) that are released from basophils and mast cells and are capable of producing urticarial lesions. Other causes of this disorder include drugs, insect bites, bee stings, and physical factors (heat, cold, sunlight, and pressure). Allergies to penicillin, molds, animal products, foods (such as shellfish and strawberries), vaccines, and chemicals (including cosmetics) may evoke episodes of urticaria.

Histologically, there is secondary histamine release, to massive edema of the dermis and separation of collagen bundles. Lymphocyte, eosinophil, and neutrophil infiltrates are seen in the dermis, and blood levels of eosinophils may be elevated. Diagnosis can be confirmed by testing with suspected causative agents to determine whether one or more cause a wheal-and-flare reaction in affected patients. The lesions of urticaria must be differentiated from contact sensitivity and atopic dermatitis. Also called *hives.*

u. pigmentosa, mastocytosis manifested as persistent pink-to-brown macules or soft plaques of various size, the irritation of which results in localized pruritus and urtication (Darier's sign).

Juvenile urticaria pigmentosa is present at birth or occurs within the first few weeks of life. It may take the form of a single tumor or nodule (solitary mastocytoma), often on the back of the hand, or it may appear as a disseminated eruption of yellowish-brown to yellowish-red macules, plaques, or bullae.

Persons affected may experience pruritus, flushing, headaches, diarrhea, and peptic ulcers. Factors that precipitate attacks may be mechanical (hot baths or exercise) or pharmacologic (codeine or aspirin), all of which lead to mast cell degranulation. The condition usually disappears before puberty.

urticate (ur′ti-kāt) marked by the presence of wheals.

urticating caterpillar any caterpillar of the order Lepidoptera that possesses poisonous hairs that cause urticating dermatitis in humans.

u/s abbrev. See *ultrasound.*

USAN (u′san) acronym. See *United States Adopted Name.*

useful life the period of time during which it is intended that a piece of equipment be used, i.e., the period over which an asset will be depreciated for purposes of financial accounting.

USP abbrev. See *United States Pharmacopeia.*

ustilaginism (us″tĭ-laj′ĭ-nizm) a syndrome of edema, redness or cyanosis, and painful burning or itching sensations affecting the extremities. It is produced by eating maize contaminated with the fungus *Ustilago maydis.*

uta (oo′tah) naso-oral leishmaniasis. See *mucocutaneous l.* under *leishmaniasis.*

uter/o (u′ter-o) a word element used in combining form to denote the uterus, e.g., uterosalpingography.

uterine (u′ter-in) [L. *uterinus*] pertaining to the uterus.

uterine artery a branch of the anterior trunk of the internal iliac artery. It runs medially on the levator ani toward the cervix, ascends the side of the uterus in the broad ligament, and courses laterally toward the ovary, where it unites with the ovarian artery.

uterine bleeding any bleeding, including normal menstrual bleeding, that originates from the uterus, usually from the endometrium.

dysfunctional u. b., any abnormal uterine bleeding that has no identifiable cause such as a neoplasm, abortion, or inflammation. It occurs most commonly during menarche and menopause. Alterations in the normal hormonal cycle due to exogenous or excess endogenous estrogen cause the abnormal bleeding, which is usually anovulatory. Excess endogenous estrogen may be associated with conditions such as Stein-Leventhal syndrome and estrogen-producing neoplasms. Laboratory studies are not diagnostic.

premenopausal abnormal u. b., any uterine bleeding that occurs between menstrual cycles, or any menstrual flow that is abnormally prolonged or profuse in premenopausal females. The abnormal bleeding may be due to any of several disorders, including endometrial and cervical polyps, endometrial cancer, salpingitis, early abortion, and thyroid problems.

uterine tube see *fallopian tube.*

uterine tumors neoplasms of the uterus; generally classified according to site of origin, e.g., the cervix, endometrium, and myometrium.

CERVIX. Neoplastic changes in the cervix include those with differentiation toward squamous cells, such as cervical intraepithelial neoplasia (CIN I-III), invasive squamous carcinoma, adenocarcinoma, and mixed adenosquamous carcinoma. The concept of cervical intraepithelial neoplasia embraces those epithelial lesions conventionally considered to represent precursors of invasive squamous cell carcinoma. It is defined as a spectrum of intraepithelial histologic and cytologic alterations that have been defined traditionally as beginning with mild dysplasia (CIN I), progressing through moderate dysplasia (CIN II), to severe dysplasia and carcinoma in situ (CIN III).

Invasive squamous carcinoma represents more than 90 percent of invasive carcinomas of the cervix; it is the third most common invasive malignant lesion of the genital organs following carcinoma of the endometrium and ovary. The incidence rate of invasive squamous carcinoma of the cervix has dropped dramatically in recent years due to cytologic screening, but inasmuch as approximately half of adult females have never had a cervical smear for cytologic evaluation, the frequency is still relatively high. Approximately one-third of patients present with Grade I tumors, one-third with Grade II, one-third with Grade III, and a small percentage with Grade IV. Squamous cell carcinoma of the cervix spreads by direct local invasion to the adjacent tissues, and by the lymphatics to the regional lymph nodes. The 5-yr survival rates are approximately 85–90 percent for those with Grade I tumors, 70–75 percent for Grade II, 30–35 percent for Grade III, and 10 percent for Grade IV.

A special subcategory of Grade I squamous carcinoma of the cervix is microinvasive carcinoma. Some authors reserve this term for tumors with invasion less than 1 mm into the cervical stroma, others for tumors with invasion of fewer than 3 mm, and still others for those with invasion of fewer than 5 mm. Precision in the use of the term microinvasive carcinoma, preferably with quantitation of the depth of invasion, is important. Tumors with invasion of less than 1 mm have little, if any, propensity for local or distant metastasis, whereas tumors with invasion of 1–3 mm have been reported as being associated with a mortality of 4–7 percent.

Adenocarcinoma of the cervix represents approximately 5–8 percent of all invasive carcinomas of the cervix. The majority of such tumors are well differentiated, forming caricatures of normal endocervical glands, and are capable of mucus production. Transitions to in situ adenocarcinoma of the endocervix occurs in approximately 40 percent of cases. Spread is similar to the pattern of invasive squamous carcinoma of the cervix; however, it is generally held that local extension and lymph node metastases occur earlier. The overall 5-yr survival rate for adenocarcinoma of the cervix is somewhat lower than that for squamous carcinoma of the cervix.

ENDOMETRIUM. Benign neoplasms of the endometrium are relatively rare. They are represented by papillary adenofibromas characterized by cystic spaces lined by a single layer of epithelial cells into which project papillary structures covered by a similar type of epithelium. Malignant neoplasms of the endometrium are primarily adenocarcinomas of the endometrium. Adenocarcinomas of the endometrium tend to mimic the pattern of normal endometrial glands (endometrioid adenocarcinoma). Other histologic patterns of endometrial adenocarcinoma include clear cell and mucinous, papillary, mixed adenosquamous, squamous cell, and undifferentiated. Distinction between well-differentiated adenocarcinoma and hyperplasia with atypia is often difficult, as there is a continuous histopathologic spectrum from adenomatous hyperplasia with mild atypia, through severe adenomatous hyperplasia, to well-differentiated adenocarcinoma. Adenocarcinomas of the endometrium require histologic grading as well as pathologic staging, as the prognosis depends to a great extent on the degree of differentiation and extent of invasion. However, certain endometrial carcinomas, e.g., clear cell, squamous, and undifferentiated, are particularly aggressive and carry an unfavorable prognosis.

A role of exogenously administered estrogen in the development of endometrial adenocarcinoma has been postulated but not yet proven. It is well documented, however, that adenocarcinomas of the endometrium are frequently associated with or are preceded by endometrial hyperplasia and are associated with hyperestrogenic states including Stein-Leventhal syndrome and functioning ovarian tumors.

MYOMETRIUM. Leiomyomas—benign neoplastic proliferations of smooth muscle—are present in at least 20 percent of females and are frequently multiple. Those with unusually increased cellularity are frequently designated as cellular leiomyomas, whereas those composed of bizarre epithelioid cells are referred to as epithelioid leiomyomas. Distinction of atypical and cellular leiomyomas from leiomyosarcoma is based on the frequency of mitotic figures. Malignant tumors of the uterus (uterine sarcomas) include leiomyosarcoma, malignant mixed müllerian tumor, müllerian adenosarcoma, and endometrial stromal sarcoma. Leiomyosarcoma is the most common malignant neoplasm involving the myometrium.

Diagnosis is based on the degree of cellularity, cytologic atypia, and frequency of mitotic figures. Malignant mixed müllerian tumor recapitulates the embryologic derivation of the uterus from the müllerian ducts, which are composed of glandular epithelium supported by mesenchyme. These neoplasms contain malignant epithelial elements (adenocarcinoma, squamous carcinoma, or undifferentiated carcinoma) admixed with malignant homologous elements (leiomyosarcoma or stromal sarcoma) or with malignant heterologous elements (osteosarcoma, chondrosarcoma, or rhabdomyosarcoma). Approximately 12–15 percent of patients with mixed malignant müllerian tumors have had prior pelvic irradiation. The overall survival is approximately 30 percent at 5 yr. Also called *carcinosarcoma* and malignant mixed mesodermal tumor.

Müllerian adenosarcoma is a uterine malignancy characterized by benign epithelium admixed with a sarcomatous stroma that is a much less aggressive tumor than malignant mixed müllerian tumor. Most patients reported to date have survived for a relatively long period.

Stromal sarcoma is a term that encompasses low-grade (endolymphatic stromal myosis) and high-grade stromal sarcoma. Both are composed of neoplastic proliferations of endometrial stromal cells. Endolymphatic stromal myosis is characterized histologically by proliferation of stromal elements in vascular spaces throughout the myometrium. When this tumor is confined to the uterus with few or no mitotic figures, it rarely metastasizes or recurs. However, when it is found beyond the uterus at the time of surgery and is associated with an increased number of mitotic figures, recurrence rates are high and metastases do occur. High-grade stromal sarcoma is a frankly infiltrating malignant neoplasm with greater than 10 mitotic figures per 10 high-power fields; it is associated with infiltrating margins, extension beyond the uterus, and metastasis. The overall 5-yr survival rate is approximately 30–40 percent.

uterosalpingography (u″ter-o-sal″ping-gog′rah-fe) see *hysterosalpingography.*

uterus (u′ter-us), pl. *uteri* [L.; Gr. *hystera*] a hollow, thick-walled, epithelium-lined muscular organ situated in the pelvis of the female that houses the developing conceptus during its 9-mo gestation. The uterus consists of a cervix, the lower uterine segment or isthmus, and a body (corpus). The cervix is divided into three areas: exocervix (which is in continuity with the vaginal wall), transformation zone, and endocervical canal. The isthmus connects the cervix to the uterine body. The uterine body makes up the major part of the adult uterus; it is a roughly triangular structure that is flattened in the anteroposterior direction. Its base extends laterally to form the uterine cornua (which merge with the fallopian tubes), and its apex merges with the isthmus. The uterine cavity is a flattened, slitlike space in continuity with the lumina of the intrauterine intramural portion of the fallopian tubes superiorly and the endocervical canal inferiorly. The latter opening is termed the internal cervical os; the vaginal opening is the external cervical os.

The uterine wall is composed of a thin mucosa that lines the uterine cavity, a bulky muscularis, and a thin serosa. The serosa is a continuation of the peritoneum covering the broad ligament and fallopian tubes, and is absent over those portions of the uterus that attach to the pelvic floor and side wall. The term used to denote the layers of the uterine wall depends on the portion of the uterus being considered.

The surface of the exocervix is covered by a stratified squamous epithelium, which is rich in glycogen and differs from skin by the absence of a keratohyaline granular layer. The endocervix is lined by columnar, nonstratified, mucin-secreting epithelium. The transformation zone bridges the endocervical and exocervical mucosa, and typically contains a mixture of a columnar and squamous epithelium. The boundaries of this zone change during reproductive life by the process of squamous metaplasia, the effect of which is to replace columnar epithelium with squamous epithelium. The most significant pathologic processes involving the cervix arise in this zone (e.g., dysplasia, invasive squamous carcinoma). The bulk of the cervix is made up of cervical stroma, a mixture of smooth muscle and collagen.

The mucosal lining of the uterine body (endometrium) is composed of glands set within a specialized spindled stroma. During the reproductive years, the endometrium undergoes cyclic morphologic changes in response to changing blood levels of ovarian steroids. Over the course of approximately 1 mo, the endometrium is sloughed and then reconstituted. During the proliferative phase, which lasts approximately 14 da, glands and stroma develop synchronously under the stimulus of estrogen secreted by the developing ovarian follicles. The secretory phase (lasting 14 da) begins after ovulation and is directed by the progesterone and estrogen elaborated by the ovarian corpus luteum. This phase is marked by endometrial glandular secretion and stromal predecidual change. Should implantation occur, the stromal changes are accentuated to form decidua. In the absence of implantation, a coordinated series of hemodynamic changes results in the sloughing of the fully developed secretory endometrium (menstruation). After several days of bleeding, the cycle is continued by the initiation of a new proliferative phase.

The wall of the uterine body (myometrium) is composed of spindled smooth muscle cells. During pregnancy there is a dramatic increase in the myometrial bulk, which is due to both hyperplasia and hypertrophy of the smooth muscle cells.

The uterus houses the conceptus during gestation. Full secretory development of the endometrium is essential for normal implantation, and the dramatic increase in uterine wall thickness is essential for the coordinated contractions that expel the newborn at term. The uterine vasculature greatly expands during gestation to accommodate the increased blood flow to the placental circulation. The cervix elaborates large quantities of mucin to form the mucous plug; this is reflected morphologically in the marked hyperplasia of the endocervical lining mucosa that occurs during pregnancy. Before and after the reproductive years, the uterus is in a quiescent state; in the postmenopausal years (in the absence of disease), it is normally atrophic.

See also *menstruation* and *uterine tumors.*

MICHAEL R. HENDRICKSON, M.D.

UTI abbrev. See *urinary tract infection.*

UTP abbrev. See *uridine triphosphate.*

utricle (u′trĭ-k′l) [L. *utriculus*] 1. any small sac.

2. the oblong, endolymph-filled sac, part of the membranous labyrinth, which communicates with the three semicircular ducts and their ampullae in the posterosuperior region of the vestibule. As an organ of the vestibular apparatus, it contains a neuroepithelium that senses the position of the head relative to the direction of gravitational and linear acceleratory forces. Also called utriculus.

utriculitis (u-trik″u-li′tis) 1. an inflammation of the utricle of the prostate.

2. an inflammation of the utricle of the inner ear.

UV abbrev. See *ultraviolet.*

μV abbrev. See *microvolt.*

uve/o (u′ve-o) a word element used in combining form to denote the vascular layer of the eye, e.g., uveitis.

uvea (u′ve-ah) the middle pigmented layer and vascular coat of the eyeball. It includes the iris, ciliary body, and choroid, which function in control of light entering the eye, accommodation, and nutrition of ocular tissues, respectively.

uveitis (u″ve-i′tis) [*uvea* + *-itis*] an inflammation of the uvea. Uveitis may involve one or both eyes and may be limited to the anterior uvea (iris and ciliary body) or the posterior uvea (choroid), or may involve the entire choroid with extension to the retina or sclera. It may be associated with trauma, with noninfectious inflammatory diseases, or with invasion by infective organisms. Organisms commonly involved include herpes simplex virus, herpes zoster virus, *Histoplasma capsulatum, Toxoplasma gondii, Mycobacterium tuberculosis,* and *Treponema pallidum.*

Diagnosis is aided by slit-lamp examination, the presence of visible precipitates of keratin often associated with the disease, and the characteristic dilated vessels surrounding the perimeter of the cornea.

uveomeningitis (u′ve-o-men″in-ji′tis) a disease characterized by uveitis, meningitis, hearing disturbances, depigmentation of hair and skin, and loss of eyelashes; it may be precipitated by a viral infection that triggers a self-destructive immunologic response in an immunogenetically predisposed individual. Cerebrospinal fluid examination findings are consistent with an aseptic meningitis. In Harada's disease, the uveitis is posterior and retinal separation is more common, but skin and hair changes are rare. See also *Harada's syndrome* and *Vogt-Koyanagi disease.*

uveoparotid fever (u″ve-o-pah-rot′id) an inflammation of the uvea and the parotid salivary glands associated with fever; it is a manifestation of sarcoidosis, a granulomatous inflammatory disease of unknown origin. Uveal involvement leads to chronic iridocyclitis and to impairment of vision. The swelling and inflammation in the parotid glands may affect nerves passing through these glands, producing facial muscle paralysis and other nerve palsies. Also called uveoparotitis.

UVR see *ultraviolet radiation.*

uvula (u′vu-lah), pl. *uvulae* [L. "little grape"] a pendent, fleshy mass; the term is generally used alone to designate the palatine uvula.

u. of bladder, a rounded elevation at the neck of the bladder in adult males, caused by the median lobe of the prostate.

palatine u., the small, fleshy projection that hangs from the soft palate above the roof of the tongue.

uvulitis (u″vu-li′tis) [*uvula* + *-itis*] inflammation of the uvula.

U wave an undulating deflection, usually of low amplitude, that immediately follows the T wave on an electrocardiogram (ECG). It is an inconstant finding in the normal ECG, but commonly becomes more prominent in a variety of conditions, such as hypokalemia or spontaneous intracranial or subarachnoid hemorrhage.

V

V symbol for *valine,* the chemical element *vanadium, vector, volt, voltage, volume.*

v symbol for specific volume, *velocity* (also V).

$\dot{V}_A$ abbrev. See *alveolar ventilation.*

V_C abbrev. See *pulmonary capillary blood volume.*

V_E abbrev. See *respiratory minute volume.*

V_T abbrev. See *tidal volume.*

V_{O_2} abbrev. See *oxygen consumption, oxygen uptake.*

VA abbrev. See *volt-ampere.*

vaccenic acid (vak′sēn-ik) an unsaturated fatty acid, *trans*-11-octadecenoic acid $CH_3(CH_2)_5CH{:}CH(CH_2)_9COOH$, isomeric with oleic acid; it is found in butterfat.

vaccinate (vak′sĭ-nāt) to inoculate with vaccine for the purpose of producing immunity.

vaccination (vak″si-na′shun) [L. *vacca* cow] the administration of an immunogen (vaccine) or antibody to an immunogen for the purpose of establishing resistance to an infectious disease in the recipient. Vaccination is one of the most powerful tools used in the prevention of disease.

There are two forms of immunization—active and passive. Only active immunization generates immunity by means of inoculation with vaccine. The vaccine can take the form of a killed organism or some fraction of it, an avirulent attenuated living mutant, or an inactivated toxin associated with that organism. The immune system generates the same response to the antigen on the surface of a pathogen whether the pathogen is in a living virulent state, or is an attenuated mutant or a killed organism. Although immunity from natural infection with the virulent strain is usually most effective, a high level of immunity can be achieved with a living attenuated mutant. A modest degree of immunity is usually accomplished with killed vaccine. The immunity conferred by active vaccination often approaches 100 percent and may give lifelong protection, whereas protection by passive immunization is less successful and is short-lived. Vaccines are also less expensive to prepare than the sera used in passive immunization.

Passive immunization is used when the organism has not been grown in the laboratory and a vaccine is unavailable. Either whole immune serum or the gamma-globulin fraction of immune serum from an individual who has had the disease is administered, thus passively transferring preformed antibody that will persist only a few weeks or months. Two forms of gamma-globulin preparation are available. Human immune serum globulin (ISG) for general use is an alcohol fractionation of pooled human sera that removes most serum proteins as well as any viruses present. It is available for intramuscular injection only, because high-molecular-weight aggregates are present, which produce systemic reactions in about 2 out of every 1000 injections. Special human immune serum globulin with known antibody content is also available for specific illnesses.

ADENOVIRUS. Types 7, 4, and 3 are frequently the cause of epidemics of acute respiratory and ocular diseases. Type 4 is primarily responsible for acute respiratory disease in military recruits and is rarely seen in civilians.

To prevent outbreaks among infants and young children in closed populations, a vaccine containing types 1 through 7 may be useful. Vaccine for military personnel should contain types 3, 4, 7, and 21.

Adenoviruses types 3 and 7 are oncogenic for animals and, although there are no data to suggest that they are also oncogenic for humans, it may be unwise to use adenovirus vaccine to prevent mild, self-limiting illnesses.

CHOLERA. After recovery from cholera, an individual has a high level of resistance to the homologous organism but not to heterologous organisms; therefore, a suspension of killed vibrios, including multivalent antigenic types, is used for vaccination. Immunity induced by the killed vaccine persists for only a few months and must be followed by booster injections every 6 mo during times of possible exposure. International travelers may be required to have vaccinations against cholera, as well as smallpox and yellow fever.

INFLUENZA. Vaccination with appropriate variant strains can reduce the incidence of influenza by up to 70 percent. Vaccines are produced by propagating viruses in chick embryos, partially purifying them, and then inactivating the viruses with formalin. They are effective as long as the virus used contains hemagglutinin and neuraminidase glycoproteins that are immunologically related to the prevalent strain. The currently employed vaccines are a mixture of several influenza A and B strains. As influenza is under global surveillance, the new major antigenic variants can be identified as they emerge.

A single subcutaneous injection of at least 300 chick cell agglutinating (CCA) units usually confers immunity in 2–4 wk. Several factors, however, have limited the usefulness of influenza vaccination. Pyrogenic reactions and symptoms similar to those of mild influenza are common in young children and infants. In addition, a subcutaneous injection of the vaccine only induces low levels of secretory IgA in the respiratory tract, which may be insufficient for complete resistance. Immunity is often lost 6 mo after vaccination.

MEASLES. A highly contagious disease, measles may be associated with encephalitis, permanent neurologic sequelae, or death. A highly effective, live, attenuated Edmonston B strain vaccine is available. It can be administered either alone or in combination with vaccines for rubella and mumps. It is recommended that children be immunized at age 15 mo. However, if there is a risk of exposure to measles, they may be immunized at age 6 mo, and again at 15 mo.

MENINGOCOCCUS. Currently, a polysaccharide vaccine is available for meningococcus types A and C; there is no vaccine for type B, however, which is presently responsible for most disease. Polysaccharide vaccines are type-specific and thus offer very little protection against other strains. Because of its limited efficacy, isolated incidences of the disease, and successful antibiotic prophylaxis, routine vaccination is not recommended. The vaccine should be considered during epidemics involving types A and C and for travelers.

TYPHOID FEVER. Typhoid fever remains a major health problem in developing countries. Although the disease usually confers lifelong immunity, the nature of the immunity is not well understood. Acetone-inactivated dried vaccine is more effective than heat- or alcohol-killed vaccine. In the United States typhoid vaccine is not recommended for general use, nor for use in controlling outbreaks from a common source or from natural disaster such as a flood. The vaccine should be administered to individuals who are in intimate exposure to a documented typhoid carrier, or given to persons traveling to high-risk areas of exposure to typhoid.

Primary immunizations in individuals 10 yr or older should be administered subcutaneously in two doses (0.5 ml each) 3 wk apart, or in three doses at weekly intervals; children aged 6 mo to 10 yr should be given 0.25 ml of vaccine. Reimmunization every 3 yr is recommended if there is continued risk of exposure. The vaccine is given intradermally (0.1 ml) in the flexor surface of the forearm, or subcutaneously (0.5 ml for those older than 10 yr and 0.25 ml for those younger than 10 yr). Reactions to the vaccine include local pain, malaise, headache, and fever. A new live, attenuated oral vaccine is currently being evaluated in clinical trials.

CYTOMEGALOVIRUS (CMV). Two live attenuated virus vaccines are currently being studied. The vaccines have induced specific cell-mediated immunity in seronegative recipients, but have not been able to prevent CMV infection. The capacity of CMV to transform cells has created concern that a vaccine may be oncogenic.

HEPATITIS. An adjuvant-supplemented hepatitis B vaccine is newly available commercially. Prepared from formalin-inactivated HbsAg collected from the serum of injected individuals, this vaccine is recommended for high-risk populations of homosexuals and individuals undergoing hemodialysis; research on other indications is under way. Two doses are given intramuscularly 1 mo apart, and a booster is given 6 mo later. Hepatitis A infection may be prevented by passive immunization with standard ISG, which should be administered as soon as possible after close exposure to an infected person. The benefit of passive immunization against hepatitis B is not clear. Hepatitis B immune globulin (HBIG) is sufficient to lessen the effects of the diesase; however, it permits infection, thereby establishing active immunity.

SMALLPOX. Successful immunization against smallpox requires the use of a live vaccinia virus vaccine, which is a stable hybrid of smallpox and cowpox. The vaccine is administered by breaking the epidermis under a drop of vaccine or by jet injection. A vesicle should appear 4 da later; if not, vaccine should be readministered. Protection develops in 7–10 da, which is rapid enough if contacts of smallpox cases are vaccinated shortly after exposure. Protection lasts for 3–7 yr. With the apparent global eradication of smallpox, the risk of serious or fatal complications of vaccination (1 in 100,000 and 1 in 10 million vaccinated individuals, respectively) outweigh the advantages of general vaccination.

VARICELLA-ZOSTER. Varicella (chickenpox) is usually a mild, self-limiting disease in young children. In adults, the disease is more severe—mortality may be as high as 20 percent. Herpes zoster is recurrent, has a low incidence, and is predominantly confined to persons aged 20 yr and older. An attenuated virus vaccine has been developed but not yet fully tested. Chickenpox can be prevented or modified with administration of high-titer IgG to contacts within 72 hr of exposure. Prophylaxis is useful for susceptible adults and children with impaired immunity.

ROCKY MOUNTAIN SPOTTED FEVER. Since 1970, a formalin-inactivated vaccine, prepared from *Rickettsia rickettsii* grown in chick embryo fibroblasts and purified by sucrose density gradient, has been studied. The vaccine has been highly immunogenic and protective in guinea pigs and rhesus monkeys; results of preliminary human trials have been encouraging.

TYPHUS. A formalin-inactivated vaccine prepared from *Rickettsia prowazekii* grown in embryonated eggs is available. The vaccine is protective against louse-borne typhus only and not mouse, murine, or scrub typhus. Typhus vaccine is recommended for individuals who visit or live in areas with typhus, and for laboratory personnel who work with *R. prowazekii*.

Q FEVER. There is no effective vaccine against Q fever.

MUMPS. Generally a benign illness, mumps may result in meningoencephalitis or meningitis in 0.5–10 percent of all affected individuals. A highly effective attenuated live vaccine is available using the Jeryl-Lynn strain. Some argue that mumps is severe enough to warrant a vaccine.

DIPHTHERIA. The diphtheria toxin can be treated with formaldehyde to convert it to the toxoid, which is devoid of toxicity. The toxoid is given in two doses 1 mo apart for the primary immunization. Booster injections are given approximately yearly during childhood.

WHOOPING COUGH. Immunization against whooping cough (pertussis) usually begins at age 2–4 mo, along with that against diphtheria and tetanus. There is a high incidence of severe reaction to the pertussis vaccine, ranging from fever, periods of screaming in infants, and convulsions, to frank encephalopathy and thrombocytopenic purpura. Children who experience severe reactions should not receive further immunizations. Protection is not long-lasting.

TETANUS. Tetanus toxoid is given during the first year of life. Three injections of fluid or alum-precipitated toxoid are given in the initial immunization. A single booster injection should be administered to children a year later and again when they enter elementary school. Also, after sustaining a potentially dangerous wound, a booster of toxoid should be given to a previously immunized person. However, prophylactic human tetanus immune globulin (250 U) is given to a previously unimmunized individual. The combined diphtheria-pertussis-tetanus (DPT) vaccine is usually administered during the first year of life.

PLAGUE. Short-term immunity is achieved by immunization with killed or attenuated vaccines, or with fractions of the bacilli. It is recommended that persons entering endemic areas or working in laboratories with *Yersinia pestis* receive formalin-treated vaccine.

PNEUMOCOCCUS. A 14-valent polysaccharide vaccine is made from purified capsular material of pneumococci extracted separately from 14 American types. Each dose contains 50 mg of each type. The vaccine is not recommended for healthy individuals. It may benefit children older than age 2 yr with sickle cell disease or other splenic dysfunction, and individuals with diabetes mellitus, chronic cardiorespiratory disease, hepatic dysfunction, or renal disease. Field trials have shown an 80 percent reduction in the incidence of infection in immunized individuals; the duration of protection is unknown.

POLIOMYELITIS. An inactivated virus vaccine (Salk vaccine) and a live attenuated virus vaccine (Sabin vaccine) are available. The inactivated vaccine has high potency and moderate purity. It is safe and remarkably effective when properly used. However, it has several disadvantages, such as the requirement for booster injections and the failure to eliminate intestinal infection and fecal excretions. The live attenuated vaccine is the vaccine of choice in the United States. The vaccine produces an infection of the gastrointestinal canal and excretion of virus in high titer for 4–5 wk. It results in synthesis and excretion of IgA antibody into the GI tract, thus producing alimentary tract resistance and decreasing spread within the population. The disadvantages of this vaccine are reversion to increased virulence of the virus and dissemination of the virus to unvaccinated contacts. The vaccine is given orally, preferably during the period from age 3 mo to age 18 mo, and a booster is advised when children enter elementary school.

RABIES. The vaccine currently used in the United States is produced from rabies virus propagated in a human diploid cell line of WI-38 fibroblasts. This vaccine carries virtually no risk of inducing allergic encephalomyelitis, unlike earlier vaccines. Two doses 1 wk apart, followed by a third dose 2–3 wk later, are recommended in preexposure situations. Advanced texts on microbiology or infectious disease should be consulted for specific details and indications for postexposure vaccination. The older duck embryo vaccine is inferior to human diploid vaccine and should not be used.

RUBELLA. Rubella vaccine is given not to protect the recipient, but rather to protect an unborn fetus. Two strategies are used: (1) immunization of teenagers who may be prospective mothers; or (2) immunization of children aged 1–12 yr who are major viral transmitters—this procedure protects pregnant females. Immunization is recommended for all females of childbearing age. Following immunization, effective birth control must be rigidly practiced for 2–3 mo. The vaccines are produced from live attenuated viruses administered in a single injection and are immunogenic in at least 95 percent of the recipients.

TUBERCULOSIS. The BCG (bacille Calmette-Guérin) vaccine is derived from an attenuated strain of *Mycobacterium bovis.* The rationale of its use is to prevent tuberculosis by conferring cell-mediated immunity against an attenuated strain of mycobacteria immunologically similar to *Mycobacterium tuberculosis.* The live vaccine can induce an increase in resistance to tuberculosis, but not complete protection. There is evidence that the BCG vaccine prevents the establishment of a latent infection when recipients are subsequently challenged with live tubercle bacilli, thus preventing not only primary tuberculosis but also reactivation. Vaccination has a major disadvantage in that inducing tuberculin hypersensitivity destroys the usefulness of the tuberculin test. The prevalence of tuberculosis in the United States is too low to justify widespread vaccination. The identification and prophylactic treatment of individuals whose tuberculin skin tests have converted to positive has proved to be safe and effective.

In the United States, it is recommended that BCG be considered only for infants who are skin test–negative to tuberculin but who will have repeated exposure to individuals with sputum-positive pulmonary tuberculosis, and for individuals in areas where skin-test conversion exceeds 1 percent per yr and the usual surveillance and treatment have failed. BCG is given only to individuals who are skin test–negative: 5 tuberculin units of purified protein derivation (PPD). Infants younger than 28 da should receive one-half the recommended adult dose. Both intradermal and percutaneous vaccines are licensed in the United States. If the skin test 2–3 mo after immunization is negative and the indications for BCG remain, a second dose should be given. BCG should not be administered to individuals with impaired immunity, and it should also be avoided during pregnancy unless there is an excessive and unavoidable exposure to infectious tuberculosis. BCG immunization is also used as a means of stimulating cell-mediated immunity as one form of immunotherapy for patients with certain forms of cancer.

TULAREMIA. An attenuated live vaccine is available and indicated for individuals such as laboratory personnel who are likely to be exposed to *Francisella tularensis.* The vaccine causes a local reaction at the intradermal injection site; however, it provides protection against respiratory, not cutaneous, challenge.

For more information on childhood immunization, see the accompanying tables.

vaccine (vak'sēn) [L. *vaccinus*] a suspension of attenuated or killed microorganisms (bacteria, viruses, or rickettsiae), administered for the prevention, amelioration, or treatment of infectious diseases.

vaccinia (vak-sin'e-ah) [L., from *vacca* cow] a viral disease of the skin caused by a poxvirus that had been passed in cow and induced to generate protective immunity against smallpox. Despite the common belief that vaccinia virus is cowpox or a closely related derivative, its true identity remains a mystery. Jenner believed that his strain was horsepox ("grease"), which had been passed in cows before transfer to humans. Laboratory markers show that current vaccinia strains differ from cowpox, as well as other known members of the poxvirus group. Some investigators suggest that it is a recombinant of cowpox and smallpox.

Subcutaneous introduction of the vaccinia virus into nonimmune individuals results in a papule that becomes vesicular and pustular and resolves with formation of crust. Complications that result from vaccination include rashes, skin lesions, secondary bacterial infections, and encephalomyelitis. Vaccination against smallpox was once so common and successful that now it is indicated only for laboratory personnel who have contact with smallpox virus and for those traveling to countries where vaccination is required for entry. It should never be administered to persons with impaired immunity or to those receiving chemo- or radiotherapy (which can lead to immunosuppression). It also is not recom-

VACCINATION, TABLE 1. RECOMMENDED SCHEDULE FOR THE ACTIVE IMMUNIZATION OF NORMAL INFANTS AND CHILDREN

RECOMMENDED AGE	VACCINE(S)	COMMENTS
2 mo	DTP,[1] OPV[2]	Can be initiated earlier in areas of high endemicity
4 mo	DTP, OPV	2-mo interval desired for OPV to avoid interference
6 mo	DTP (OPV)	OPV optional for areas where polio might be imported (e.g., some areas of southwest United States)
12 mo	Tuberculin Test[3]	May be given simultaneously with MMR at 15 mo
15 mo	Measles, Mumps, Rubella (MMR)[4]	MMR preferred
18 mo	DTP, OPV	Consider as part of primary series—DTP essential
4–6 yr[5]	DTP, OPV	
14–16 yr	Td[6]	Repeat every 10 yr for lifetime

[1] DTP—Diphtheria and tetanus toxoids with pertussis vaccine.
[2] OPV—Oral, attenuated poliovirus vaccine contains poliovirus types 1, 2, and 3.
[3] Tuberculin test—Mantoux (intradermal PPD) preferred. Frequency of tests depends on local epidemiology. The Committee on Infectious Diseases of the American Academy of Pediatrics recommends annual or biennial testing unless local circumstances dictate less frequent or no testing.
[4] MMR—Live measles, mumps, and rubella viruses in a combined vaccine.
[5] Up to the seventh birthday.
[6] Td—Adult tetanus toxoid (full dose) and diphtheria toxoid (reduced dose) in combination.

For all products used, consult manufacturer's brochure for instructions for storage, handling, and administration. Biologics prepared by different manufacturers may vary, and those of the same manufacturer may change from time to time. The package insert should be followed for a specific product.

From Report of the Committee on Infectious Diseases. 19th ed. Evanston, IL, American Academy of Pediatrics, 1981, p. 7. Copyright American Academy of Pediatrics, 1982.

mended for individuals who have eczema or other severe skin disorders or for pregnant females.

vacuolation (vak″u-o-la′shun) the process of forming vacuoles; the condition of being vacuolated. Also called *vacuolization.*

vacuole (vak′u-ōl) [L. *vacuus* empty + *-ole* diminutive ending] any small space or cavity formed in the protoplasm of a cell. For more information, see the specific vacuole.

vacuolization (vak″u-o-li-za′shun) see *vacuolation.*

vacuum (vak′u-um, vak′ūm), pl. *vacuums, vacua* [L., neuter of *vacuus* empty] 1. in physics, empty space containing no matter or energy.

2. an enclosure from which enough gas has been evacuated to enable some process to be performed.

high v., a vacuum having a gas pressure range of approximately 10^{-3}–10^{-6} torr.

ultrahigh v., a vacuum having a gas pressure of approximately 10^{-10} torr.

vacuum breaker a device interposed in a water line to prevent the backsiphonage of contaminated water into a water supply line through a hose or other outlet that may be submerged in contaminated water. Vacuum breakers or other backflow preventers are usually required on every potable water outlet to which a hose may be connected.

vacuum gauge an instrument that indicates the absolute gas pressure in an evacuated enclosure.

vacuum tube a type of active electronic component, now largely replaced by semiconductor devices, in which a stream of electrons flows between two electrodes, the cathode and the anode (plate), the flow being controlled by the voltage on one or more electrodes (called grids) through which the electron stream passes. A diode has only two electrodes (the plate and cathode) and functions as a rectifier. The triode has one grid, which controls the plate current so that the tube functions as an amplifier. Tetrodes and pentodes have additional grids that improve the operating characteristics of the tube by increasing the plate resistance and permitting higher amplification factors to be obtained.

vacuum tube voltmeter (VTVM) a voltmeter in which the measured voltage is amplified so that very little current is drawn from the circuit being tested. Most vacuum tube voltmeters measure DC and AC voltage and resistance. See also *electronic voltmeter.*

vagabond's disease (vag′ah-bondz) a skin condition of persons who continuously harbor lice: the skin becomes hardened and deeply pigmented as the result of chronic irritation by dirt, sweat, lice, and vermin. See also *pediculosis.*

vagin/o (vaj′ĭ-no) a word element used in combining form to denote the vagina, e.g., vaginoplasty.

vagina (vah-ji′nah), pl. *vaginae* [L. "sheath"] 1. a general anatomic term for a sheath or sheathlike structure.

2. [NA], the fibromuscular tube that extends from the vulva to the uterine cervix, which is lined with stratified squamous epithelium. The vagina functions as the female organ of copulation, the exit site for the menses, and the birth canal.

vaginal tumors neoplasms of the vagina. Primary carcinoma of the vagina is uncommon. Most are squamous cell carcinomas, but an occasional adenocarcinoma arises in foci of vaginal adenosis or in mesonephric remnants (clear cell carcinoma). A polypoid lesion of the vagina in a young child may be a botryoid rhabdomyosarcoma, but the diagnosis must be confirmed histologically, as some benign polyps have a pseudosarcomatous appearance.

Because of its location, the vagina can be secondarily involved by extension of a cervical squamous carcinoma, lymphatic spread of endometrial or ovarian carcinoma, or extension from a rectal adenocarcinoma.

vaginismus (vaj″ĭ-niz′mus) an uncontrolled conditioned spasm of the muscles surrounding the vagina in response to attempted penetration. A form of sexual dysfunction, vaginismus is thought to be a result of a past real or imagined, painful, or frightening sexual experience, and may occur even in the presence of full sexual responsiveness.

VACCINATION, TABLE 2. RECOMMENDED IMMUNIZATION SCHEDULES FOR INFANTS AND CHILDREN NOT INITIALLY IMMUNIZED AT THE USUAL RECOMMENDED TIMES IN EARLY INFANCY

TIMING	RECOMMENDED SCHEDULES				COMMENTS
	Preferred Schedule	*Alternatives*			
		#1	*#2*	*#3*	
First visit	DTP #1, OPV #1, Tuberculin test (PPD)	MMR, PPD	DTP #1, OPV #1, PPD	DTP #1, OPV #1, MMR, PPD	MMR should be given no younger than 15 mo old
1 mo after first visit	MMR	DTP #1, OPV #1,	MMR, DTP #2	DTP #2	
2 mo after first visit	DTP #2, OPV #2	—	DPT #3, OPV #2	DTP #3, OPV #2	—
3 mo after first visit	(DTP #3)	DTP #2, OPV #2	—	—	In preferred schedule, DTP #3 can be given if OPV #3 is not to be given until 10–16 mo
4 mo after first visit	DTP #3 (OPV #3)	—	(OPV #3)	(OPV #3)	OPV #3 optional for areas for likely importation of polio (e.g., some southwestern states)
5 mo after first visit	—	DTP #3 (OPV #3)	—	—	
10–16 mo after last dose	DTP #4, OPV #3 or OPV #4	DTP #4, OPV #3 or OPV #4	DTP #4, OPV #3 or OPV #4	DTP #4, OPV #3 or OPV #4	—
Preschool	DTP #5, OPV #4 or OPV #5	DTP #5, OPV #4 or OPV #5	DTP #5, OPV #4 or OPV #5	DTP #5, OPV #4 or OPV #5	Preschool dose not necessary if DTP #4 or #5 given after fourth birthday
14–16 yr old	Td	Td	Td	Td	Repeat every 10 yr.

Alternative #1 can be used in those more than 15 months old if measles is occurring in the community.
Alternative #2 allows for more rapid DTP immunization.
Alternative #3 should be reserved for those whose access to medical care is compromised by poor compliance.
DTP = Diphtheria and tetanus toxoids with pertussis vaccine.
OPV = Oral, attenuated poliovirus vaccine contains types 1, 2, and 3.
Tuberculin test = Mantoux (intradermal PPD) preferred. Frequency of tests depends on local epidemiology. The Committee on Infectious Diseases of the American Academy of Pediatrics recommends annual or biennial testing unless local circumstances dictate less frequent or no testing.
MMR = Live measles, mumps, and rubella viruses in a combined vaccine.
Td = Adult tetanus toxoid (full dose) and diphtheria toxoid (reduced dose) in combination.
For all products used, consult manufacturer's brochure for instructions for storage, handling, and administration. Biologics prepared by different manufacturers may vary, and those of the same manufacturer may change from time to time. The package insert should be followed for a specific product.
From Report of the Committee on Infectious Diseases. 19th ed. Evanston, IL, American Academy of Pediatrics, 1981, pp. 18–19. Copyright American Academy of Pediatrics, 1982.

vaginitis (vaj″ĭ-ni′tis) [*vagin-* + *-itis*] an inflammation of the vagina (with or without a purulent discharge) that is characterized by irritation of the vulva, pain with urination or with sexual intercourse, and itching or burning sensations. Vaginitis is most often due to infection; common causative organisms include *Trichomonas vaginalis, Candida albicans, Neisseria gonorrhoeae,* herpesvirus, and *Chlamydia trachomatis.*

Laboratory diagnosis of infectious vaginitis rests on demonstration of the organism(s) involved. Motility of *T. vaginalis* is often revealed in wet mounts of vaginal secretions. *H. vaginalis* infection is suggested by the presence of epithelial cells covered with gram-negative rods ("clue" cells), *C. albicans* infection by demonstration of KOH on a wet mount, or gonorrhea by demonstration of intracellular gram-negative diplococci in neutrophils. Culture on Sabouraud's or other media may also be used to identify *C. albicans.* Vaginitis may be promoted by systemic disease, especially diabetes mellitus, and by hormonal insufficiency due to decreased endogenous production of estrogen.

See also *sexually transmitted diseases.*

vaginomycosis (vaj″ĭ-no-mi-ko′sis) [*vagin-* + Gr. *mykēs* fungus] any fungal infection of the vagina. The most common agent is *Candida albicans,* although *Torulopsis glabrata,* and rarely other fungi, may also be found. Vaginomycoses may be an indication of systemic disease (e.g., diabetes mellitus), or may be associated with pregnancy or the use of systemic antibiotics.

vagolysis (va-gol′ĭ-sis) [*vagus* + Gr. *lysis* dissolution] see *vagotomy.*

vagotomy (va-got′o-me) [*vagus* + Gr. *tomē* a cutting] the surgical division of the vagus nerve or any of its branches, or the pharmacologic blocking of vagal impulse traffic. Vagotomy can be used in an effort to control peptic ulcer disease. Surgical division of the vagus diminishes or ends the vagal stimulation of gastric acid secretion, important in the pathogenesis of this condition.

Selective cooling of one or both vagi in steps to 0°C (vagal cold block) can be used to perform a functional vagotomy to study the activity of individual components of this mixed nerve (different fibers are blocked at different temperatures). The laboratory test for the evaluation of the completeness of vagotomy is the *insulin hypoglycemia test* (Hollander test).

Also called *vagolysis.*

vagotonia (va″go-to′ne-ah) [*vagus* + Gr. *tonos* tension + *-ia*] a condition of excess activity or irritability of the vagus nerve, resulting in autonomic imbalance, hyperperistalsis, and vasomotor instability.

vagus nerve (va′gus) [L. "wandering"] cranial nerve X; a mixed motor and sensory nerve with an extensive distribution: motor to the muscles of the heart, trachea, and bronchi, and much of the alimentary tract; secretory to the liver, pancreas, and kidney; and sensory to the dura, external auditory meatus, and respiratory and alimentary organs. It also conveys taste fibers from the epiglottis. The vagus nerve emerges from the skull through the jugular foramen in company with the cranial root of the accessory nerve (XI), descends through the neck behind the carotid arteries, enters the thorax, descends along the side of the trachea to the back of the main bronchus, then continues along the esophagus to the abdominal viscera. See also *cranial nerves.*

Vahlkampfia (vahl-kamp′fe-ah) a genus of free-living amebae that are coprozoic (living in fecal material) and common contaminants of passed feces or of water used in making fecal films. They possess no flagellate state in their development. The trophozoites are characterized by one or more contractile vacuoles and, in the encysted state, by a thick cyst wall. The species *V. lobospinosa* and *V. punctata* have been identified from human feces and fecal films.

Val abbrev. See *valine.*

valence (va′lens) [L. *valentia* strength] 1. the combining power of a particular element, i.e., the number of bonds it makes to other atoms; used in this sense, the number is always positive. An element may have one or more different valences. The term valence has now been replaced by the more precise concept of oxidation number and molecular orbitals, but it may still be used to indicate the charge of both monoatomic and polyatomic ions or the number of covalent bonds formed by an atom in a molecule. 2. in immunology, the number of antigen-binding sites possessed by an antibody molecule, for example, IgG, IgA, IgD, and IgE each have two sites, and IgM has 10.

valence electrons the electrons in the outer shell (occasionally in the two outer shells) of an atom. The outer shell electrons are easiest to remove and are often involved in bonding. Specifically, an atom's electrons can be considered in two categories: those that have the same configuration as the noble gas element with the nearest lower atomic number, and the remaining ones. The latter group are the outer shell or valence electrons.

valeric acid (vah-le′rĭk) an organic acid with an unpleasant odor; $CH_3(CH_2)_3COOH$, *n*-valeric acid, pentanoic acid.

valine (Val, V) (va′lēn) 2-amino-3-methylbutanoic acid, $(CH_3)_2CHCH(NH_2)COOH$, a naturally occurring essential amino acid; M.W. 117.15. It is a constituent of proteins, and in some bacteria can be used for the synthesis of branched-chain fatty acids. Its source is from dietary proteins. See also under *amino acids.*

valine aminotransferase (va′lēn ah″me″no-trans′-fer-ās) one of several enzymes of varied specificity. Branched-chain amino acid, 2-oxoglutarate aminotransferase (EC 2.6.1.42), transfers the amino group between oxoglutarate and any of the three branched-chain amino acids. L-Valine:3-methyl-2-oxovalerate aminotransferase (EC 2.6.1.32) is more specific, transferring NH_2 between valine and isoleucine. A genetic deficiency leads to valinemia, a disease characterized by elevated levels of valine in blood. Also called *valine transaminase.*

valinemia (val″ĭ-ne′me-ah) see *hypervalinemia.*

valine transaminase (va′lēn trans-am′i-nās) see *valine aminotransferase.*

valinuria (val″ĭ-nu′re-ah) the excretion of excessive amounts of valine in the urine, as in hypervalinemia.

Valium (val′e-um) trademark. See *diazepam.*

valley fever see *coccidioidomycosis.*

valproic acid (val-pro′ik) an anticonvulsant, 2-propylpentanoic acid, used particularly for the treatment of absence attacks or myoclonic seizures, and sometimes for generalized tonic-clonic attacks or partial seizures.

Fatal liver failure has occurred in rare instances during valproic acid therapy, so liver function tests should be performed at frequent intervals during therapy. As valproic acid may increase the serum phenobarbital concentration and thereby lead to central nervous system depression, patients should be closely monitored during concomitant phenobarbital (or primidone) therapy; the serum phenytoin concentration is also affected by the drug. Valproic acid and clonazepam used in conjunction can produce absence status.

The most common side-effects of valproic acid are gastrointestinal intolerance, sedation, transient hair loss, and weight gain. Gas chromatography or EMIT assays are used for monitoring valproic acid serum concentration. The therapeutic reference range is 50–100 $\mu g/ml$.

Valsalva maneuver (val-sal′vah) [Antonio Maria *Valsalva,* Italian anatomist, 1666–1723] a voluntary maximal contraction of the abdominal and thoracic muscles (a forced expiratory effect) against a closed glottis (or nose and mouth). The Valsalva maneuver is used in tests of cardiovascular function, particularly in dynamic auscultation; for example, the systolic murmur of idiopathic subaortic stenosis is intensified during a Valsalva maneuver.

The contractile effort involved in this procedure elevates intraabdominal and intrathoracic pressures to as high as 200 mmHg. In the initial phase, this maneuver causes an increase in systemic arterial blood pressure. In the subsequent phase, as venous return (and cardiac output) are reduced by the high intrathoracic pressure, mean arterial blood pressure decreases; it then overshoots when the maneuver is stopped (swing to influx into the heart of the blood previously pooled in the venous bed) before returning to normal.

A similar maneuver is performed during certain kinds of muscular effort and during attempts to move the bowels.

modified V. m., an effort at exhalation against the closed mouth and nose (as if attempting to open the eustachian tubes to clear the ears).

value (val'u) a numerical quantity; the number produced by a measurement.

valv/o (val'vo) a word element used in combining form to denote a valve, e.g., valvulotomy, valvotomy.

valve (valv) a membranous fold in a canal or passage that prevents reflux of the contents passing through it.

anal v.'s, crescent-shaped folds of mucous membrane that join the lower ends of the anal columns.

aortic v., the outflow valve of the left ventricle. It consists of three semilunar cusps that prevent reflux of blood from the aorta into the left ventricle during diastole. See also *bicuspid aortic valve* and *heart.*

bicuspid v., see *mitral v.*

v. of coronary sinus, a thin, semicircular fold of endocardium that covers the lower part of the opening of the coronary sinus into the right atrium. It serves to prevent the reflux of blood into the sinus during atrial contraction.

ileocecal v., a valve with a pair of semilunar flaps of colonic mucosa that project into the lumen of the bowel at the ileocecal junction. Circular muscle from the terminal ileum extends into these flaps. Also called ileocolic valve.

v. of inferior vena cava, a semilunar flap of endocardium at the junction of the inferior vena cava and the right atrium. A rudimentary structure in the adult, it is important in the fetus in directing blood through the foramen ovale into the left atrium.

mitral v., the valve between the left atrium and left ventricle. Originally thought to possess two leaflets, it actually consists of a continuous apron of tissue surrounding the orifice, which prevents the regurgitation of blood into the atrium during ventricular contraction. Also called *bicuspid v.* See also *heart.*

pulmonary v., the valve between the right ventricle and the pulmonary trunk. Composed of three semilunar leaflets, it prevents the backflow of blood into the ventricle after contraction. See also *heart.*

spiral v., elevated folds of mucous membrane arranged in a spiral manner along the lumen of the cytic duct. Also called *Heister's valve.*

tricuspid v., the valve between the right atrium and the right ventricle. Composed of three cusps (anterior, posterior, and septal), it prevents the backflow of blood during ventricular contraction. See also *heart.*

venous v., a fold of the intima, strengthened with connective tissue, which prevents the backflow of blood in the veins. When distended, these semilunar flaps take on a pouchlike appearance.

valvotomy (val-vot'o-me) [*valvo-* + Gr. *tomē* a cutting] the surgical dilation or division of a stenotic, narrowed heart valve with a finger, knife, or other instrument. It may be performed under direct vision during open heart surgery, or without visualization of the valve (closed valvotomy). Valvotomies may be performed on any of the four cardiac valves. Also called *valvulotomy.*

valvulitis (val"vu-li'tis) [L. *valvula,* dim. of *valva* valve + *-itis*] an inflammation of a valve or valves, particularly those of the heart, due to infection (bacterial endocarditis) or an immunologic reaction by the body against valve tissues (rheumatic valvulitis). Such inflammation may lead to scarring, deformity, calcification, and dysfunction of the valve. See also *rheumatic heart disease.*

valvulotomy (val"vu-lot'o-me) see *valvotomy.*

valyl (val'il, va'lil) the acyl radical derived from or relating to valine.

vanadium (V) (vah-na'de-um) [*Vanadis* a name of Freya, Norse goddess of love] a silvery-white, ductile metallic element; atomic number 23; atomic weight 50.9414; a 3d transition element; oxidation states +2, +3, +4, +5 (the most stable). Vanadium is used industrially in the manufacture of steel alloys and vanadium compounds. Inhalation of the dusts of vanadium compounds, particularly vanadium pentoxide, causes bronchitis; other toxic effects include irritation of the skin, eyes, and gastrointestinal tract.

van Bogaert's disease see *cerebrotendinous xanthomatosis.*

van Buren's disease (van bu'renz) [William Holme *van Buren,* American surgeon, 1819–1883] see *Peyronie's disease.*

vancomycin (van'ko-mi"sin) an antibiotic, a complex glycopolypeptide obtained from *Streptomyces* species. This bactericidal antibiotic inhibits biosynthesis of cell wall peptidoglycan by binding to the acyl-D-alanyl-D-alanine terminus of peptidoglycan precursor molecules. The peptidoglycan chain extension is inhibited. Vancomycin is active against gram-positive bacteria including *Staphylococcus* species, even those that produce β-lactamase, and spirochetes in vitro.

Vancomycin has been used to treat antibiotic-associated pseudomembranous colitis due to *Clostridium difficile* and severe staphylococcal infections, especially those caused by methicillin and cephalothin-resistant organisms. It may be used to treat endocarditis caused by enterococci when patients are allergic to penicillin.

See also *antibacterial agents.*

van der Waals equation (van der wawlz) [Johannes D. *van der Waals,* Dutch chemist] an equation that gives a good approximation to the behavior of a nonideal gas: $(P + an^2/V^2)(V - nb) = nRT$, where P is pressure, V is volume, T is absolute temperature, R is the gas constant (8.314 J/mol · K), n is the number of moles of gas present, and a and b are the van der Waals constants, which are different for different gases. The constant b accounts for the finite volume of the gas molecules, and a accounts for the strength of intermolecular attractions. If *a* and *b* are zero, the van der Waals equation reduces to the ideal gas law.

van der Waals forces [Johannes D. *van der Waals*] weak, short-range intermolecular forces or forces between nonbonded atoms within a single molecule, which are commonly divided into three types: dipole-dipole forces (the electrostatic attraction between molecules with permanent dipole moments), dipole-induced dipole (forces between molecules with permanent dipoles and those without them), and London forces (the much weaker electrostatic attractions between nonpermanent, induced dipoles in molecules). Sometimes, although not usually, hydrogen bonds are included in this category. Van der Waals forces play an important role in the deviation of gases from ideal behavior, liquefaction, and the stability of non-ionic crystals.

van Gieson's stain (van ge'sonz) [Ira *van Gieson,* New York neuropathologist, 1865–1913] a combination of acid fuchsin, which stains collagen bright red, and of picric acid, which stains other tissue components yellow; used as a counterstain with iron hematoxylin and with elastic stains. Also called van Gieson's picrofuchsin.

vanillic acid (vah-nil'ik) [*vanillin,* the fragrant constituent of vanilla] 4-hydroxy-3-methoxy benzoic acid, $C_6H_3(OCH_3)(OH)(COOH)$, obtained by the oxidation of vanillin. It is a minor catabolite of the catecholamines norepinephrine and epinephrine, formed via methylation and then oxidation to 4-hydroxy-3-methoxy mandelic aldehyde, followed by reduction to the glycol and subsequent oxidation of the latter to vanillic acid. Vanillic acid appears in urine, primarily in conjugated form, as the sulfate.

vanillylmandelic acid (VMA) (vah-nil″il-mandel'ik) 4-hydroxy-3-methoxymandelic acid; M.W. 198.17. VMA is an end product, via *o*-methylation and oxidative deamination, in the metabolism of both epinephrine and norepinephrine. It is excreted in urine in the free form and is frequently increased in pheochromocytomas, neuroblastomas, and ganglioneuromas. The reference range for VMA is 1.8–7.1 mg/da or 1.5–7.0 μg/mg of creatinine. Also called vanylmandelic acid. See also *catecholamine, epinephrine, norepinephrine,* and *pheochromocytoma.*

V antigen an antigen expressed by viruses and virus-infected cells.

vapor (va'por), pl. *vapores, vapors* [L. "steam"] 1. a gas. The term is technically used to refer to the gas phase of substances that are normally liquid or solid at room temperature; more generally, it refers to visible particles of moisture suspended in the air as fog, mist, or steam. The terms gas and vapor are sometimes used interchangeably.

2. an aerosol, any dispersion of a substance in air or another gas.

3. in medicine, a vaporized substance administered by inhalation.

vaporization (va″por-ĭ-za'shun) the conversion of molecules from the solid or liquid phase of a system into the gas phase.

vaporize (va'por-iz) to convert into vapor or be transformed into vapor.

vapor-phase chromatography (VPC) see *gas chromatography.*

vapor pressure the pressure exerted by the vapor of a substance in equilibrium with some other phase (or phases) of the substance at a particular temperature. Both solids and liquids have vapor pressures.

vapor pressure depression osmometer see under *osmometer.*

$\dot{V}_A/\dot{Q}_C$ ratio abbrev. see *ventilation-perfusion ratio.*

var abbrev. for variant or variety; the term is also used in microbiology to differentiate a distinctive strain of a bacterial species.

variable (var'e-ah-b'l) [L. *variabilis,* from *variare* to change] 1. changing from time to time.

2. in mathematics, a symbol that represents an arbitrary element of a set (e.g., x or y in the equation $y = x + 2$).

3. in high-level computer language, a memory location that is referred to by a symbolic variable name and is assigned to contain a particular type of data (e.g., real number, integer, logical variable, character string). The value of the variable can be changed by assignment statements (the statement $x = x + 1$ increases the value of the variable x by one) or by input statements (the statement "get (x)" reads in a new value of x from the input file).

variable region the aminoterminal region of the heavy or light chain of the immunoglobulin molecule; it has heterogeneous amino acid sequences and determines the antigen-binding specificity of the molecule. See also *immunoglobulin.*

variance (văr'e-ans) in statistics, the average squared deviation from the mean. The expectation of $(X - \mu)^2$ is variance (symbol σ^2) of the probability distribution of X, defined for a discrete distribution by $\sigma^2 = \Sigma_x (x - \mu)^2 p_x$ and for a continuous distribution by $\sigma^2 = \int (x - \mu)^2 f(x) dx$; σ^2 is often referred to as the population variance. The sample variance (symbol s^2) is usually defined by $s^2 = \Sigma_k (X_k - \overline{X})^2 / (n - 1)$, where $\overline{X}$ is the sample mean, n is the sample size, and the X_k is the sample observation. (For some purposes, s^2 is defined as $\Sigma_k (X_k - \overline{X})^2 / n$.) The sample variance is a statistic with a probability distribution having a mean of σ^2, the population variance; i.e., s^2 is an unbiased estimate of σ^2. The square root of the variance is called the (population or sample) standard deviation.

variant (var.) (văr'e-ant) [L. *varians,* from *variare* to change] 1. something that differs in some characteristic from others in its class, such as a variant of a disease or a bacterial species. See also *microbial v.* under *variation.*

2. exhibiting such variation.

variation (va″re-a'shun) in genetics, differences not due to age or sex that exist between members of the same species. This includes both genetic variation (phenotypic differences due to genetic factors) and environmental variation (phenotypic differences due to the particular environment of an individual).

meristic v., a variation in a discrete character (one that can be counted).

microbial v., the range of characteristics within a species used in identification and differentiation. Many of these alterations, generally reversible, are not inherited. Studies on microbial variation broadened the concepts of genetic mechanisms when it became evident that variability need not be due to random selection of spontaneous genetic mutants, but may be induced by changes in the environment.

varic/o (var'ĭ-co) [L. *varix* dilated vein] a word element used in combining form to denote a dilated vein, e.g., varicocele.

varicella (var″ĭ-sel′ah) [N.L., dim. of M.L. *variola* smallpox] see *chickenpox*.

varicella-zoster antibody tests assays for antibodies against varicella-zoster viruses. The most commonly used is the complement-fixation test, but it is relatively insensitive. Indirect immunofluorescence for antibody against membrane antigen is a specific sensitive test. Dilutions of the test serum are incubated with varicella-zoster–infected human embryonic lung cells. Fluorescein-labeled antihuman globulin is then added and the cells observed for a characteristic ring of fluorescence around them. Antibody can be detected in normal individuals 2 da after the onset of a rash, or at 2 wk in immunosuppressed patients. This test is used to determine patients at risk for infection or to screen donors for zoster immune globulin.

varicella-zoster virus human herpesvirus 3, the etiologic agent of varicella (chickenpox) and herpes zoster (shingles). See also under *herpesvirus*.

varicelliform (var″ĭ-sel′ĭ-form) a term referring to rashes having an appearance like that of varicella (chickenpox). Classically described as "a dewdrop on a rose petal," the rash of varicella has a raised red base with a central vesicle or pustule.

varicocele (var′ĭ-ko-sēl″) [*varico-* + Gr. *kēlē* tumor] a condition characterized by dilation of the veins of the spermatic cord owing to a diminished blood flow from the spermatic vein into the renal vein. Most commonly observed on the left side, a varicocele may be caused by pressure from abdominal organs on the spermatic vein or by poor valvular function; it may also be the initial sign of a neoplasm of the kidney. Clinical manifestations include infertility due to retrograde flow that increases the temperature in the scrotum. Diagnosis is made on physical examination; treatment is surgical correction.

varicose (var′ĭ-kōs) [L. *varicosus*] a term used to describe a dilated winding vessel. See also *varix*.

varicosity (var″ĭ-kos′ĭ-te) 1. a varix.
2. the state of having varicose vessels.

variety (vah-ri′ĕ-te) [L. *varietas*, from *varius* diverse] a taxonomic subcategory of a species, particularly used for selectively bred plants (cultivars). Cf. *race* and *subspecies*.

variola (vah-ri′o-lah) [L.] see *smallpox*.

varix (vār′iks), pl. *varices* [L.] an enlarged and tortuous vein, artery, or lymphatic vessel.

esophageal v.'s, varicosities of the submucosal veins of the esophagus, which occur in individuals with portal hypertension. These enlarged veins anastomose with the portal veins, thus providing collateral communication between the portal vein and the superior and inferior venae cavae (systemic veins).

vas/o (vas′o) [L. *vas* vessel] a word element used in combining form to denote a vessel or duct, e.g., vasectomy.

vas (vas), pl. *vasa* [L.] [NA], a general term for a vessel; a canal that conveys fluid.

v. deferens, see *d. deferens* under *ductus*.

vasa recta, long, U-shaped vessels arising from the efferent arterioles of juxtamedullary nephrons. They supply the renal medulla and contribute to the capillary plexuses associated with the loop of Henle.

vasa vasorum, [NA], small arteries or veins that nourish the walls of the large blood vessels. These conduits may be branches of the main vessel or of neighboring vessels; they seldom penetrate deeply into the tunica media.

vascular (vas′ku-lar) pertaining to blood vessels or indicative of a copious blood supply.

vascular resistance the hydraulic resistance (R) to fluid flow in a vessel; see under *resistance*.

vasculature (vas′ku-lah-tūr) the vascular system of the body or any part of it.

vasculitis (vas″ku-li′tis) [L. *vasculum* vessel + *-itis*] an acute or chronic inflammation of blood vessels that is thought to be caused primarily by immunologic reactions, especially immune complex disposition. It is characterized by endothelial edema, proliferation, and hemorrhage, leading to ischemia of the supplied tissues. The varying clinical features may be due to differences in antigens or antibodies involved.

Vasculitis may involve long portions of a vessel or affect it segmentally, or it may be confined to vessels of a certain size or solely to arteries (arteritis). The symptoms and signs are referable to ischemia of the organs involved, and include headaches, abdominal pain, angina, muscle weakness and pain, and pain in the fingers or toes. Complete loss of blood supply leads to tissue necrosis, resulting in stroke, myocardial infarction, intestinal infarction, or gangrene of the fingers or toes.

Laboratory findings vary with each type of vasculitis, but the erythrocyte sedimentation rate is almost always markedly elevated above the normal maximum of 20 mm/hr.

Vasculitis is the primary pathologic alteration in many so-called autoimmune diseases, especially systemic lupus erythematosus, Wegener's granulomatosis, polyarteritis nodosa, and chronic hepatitis.

hypersensitivity v., a necrotizing inflammation of the small vessels (arterioles, capillaries, and venules), thought to be caused by an immunologic response to an antigen with possible deposition of antigen-antibody complexes in the vessels. Small vessel vasculitis causes systemic manifestations involving all organ systems. Headache, malaise, abdominal pain and bleeding, fever, hemorrhagic skin lesions, and renal abnormalities may occur, especially in younger individuals; in addition, there may be pulmonary and cardiac involvement, and nervous system damage may manifest itself by confusion, delirium, and coma. The vasculitis may be preceded by a respiratory infection or ingestion of drugs, or may be associated with systemic lupus erythematosus (SLE), rheumatoid arthritis, or infection with hepatitis B.

Laboratory diagnosis is aided by findings of elevated erythrocyte sedimentation rates, anemia, moderate leukocytosis, and possibly reduced complement levels. When associated with other disease (e.g., SLE), findings consistent with that disease are sought.

vasectomy (vah-sek′to-me) [*vas* + Gr. *ektomē* excision] the removal of all or part of the vas deferens, usually to prevent the passage of sperm. When performed bilaterally, vasectomy results in sterility.

vasoactive (vas″o-ak′tiv) exerting an effect on the caliber of blood vessels.

vasoconstriction (vas″o-kon-strik′shun) constriction of a vessel, especially constriction of an arteriole, which leads to decreased blood flow. The sympathetic vasoconstrictor system, controlled by the vasomotor center in the pons and medulla, innervates all the vascular beds of the body and is important in maintaining vasomotor tone and in adjusting peripheral resistance in the alarm reaction. Vasoconstriction is mediated by norepinephrine released at sympathetic nerve terminals or by epinephrine or norepinephrine released by the adrenal medulla.

vasoconstrictive (vas″o-kon-strik′tiv) pertaining to, characterized by, or producing vasoconstriction.

vasoconstrictor (vas″o-kon-strik′tor) 1. an agent that causes vasoconstriction, e.g., angiotensin; vasopressin; and epinephrine, norepinephrine, and α-adrenergic agonists.

2. a motor nerve that causes vasoconstriction.

vasodilation (vas″o-di-la′shun) dilation of a vessel, especially dilation of arterioles, which leads to increased blood flow to a part. Most blood vessels do not have vasodilating efferent neurons, and dilation is achieved through reduction in sympathetic vasoconstrictor tone. Nerve-mediated vasodilation is, however, reported to occur in arteries within skeletal muscle receiving a cholinergic sympathetic innervation, in some exocrine glands when secretory efferent stimuli induce the release of bradykinin, and in the skin when afferent neurons produce axon reflexes through their collaterals to vessels.

vasodilator (vas″o-di-la′tor) 1. an agent that causes vasodilation, e.g., bradykinin, serotonin, histamine, prostaglandins, organic nitrites used for treatment of angina, α-adrenergic blockers such as prazosin, and β-adrenergic agonists such as isoxsuprine and nylidrin.

2. a motor nerve that causes vasodilation.

vasomotor (vas-o-mo′tor) [*vaso-* + L. *motor* mover] 1. affecting the caliber of a vessel, especially of a blood vessel.

2. any element or agent that affects the caliber of a blood vessel.

vasopressin (vas″o-pres′in) see *antidiuretic hormone.*

vasopressor (vas″o-pres′or) [*vaso-* + *pressus* from L. *premere* to press + *-or*] that which increases the blood pressure.

VBP abbrev. for vinblastine, bleomycin, and Platinol, a major established cancer chemotherapy drug regimen. For more information, see the specific drug (listed under its generic name) and *Appendix A.*

VC abbrev. See *vital capacity.*

V-Cillin trademark. See *p. V* under *penicillins.*

VD abbrev. for venereal disease. See *sexually transmitted diseases.*

V deflection the deflection in the His bundle electrogram that is the result of depolarization of the upper ventricular septum.

VDRL test [acronym from *V*enereal *D*isease *R*esearch *L*aboratory] a slide microagglutination test used as an aid in the diagnosis of syphilis. The principle of this test is based on the Wassermann reaction. It is susceptible to false-positive results because cardiolipin, the antigen used in this test, is present in various mammalian tissues and in some microorganisms. The value of the VDRL test lies in its high sensitivity, not its specificity (which is low).

vector (vek′tor) [L. "one who carries," from *vehere* to carry] 1. a carrier involved in the spread of an infectious disease from one host to another, such as a fly, mosquito, tick, or louse. A distinction may be drawn between an intermediate host, such as the *Anopheles* mosquito in malaria, in which the pathogen passes through one or more developmental states in its life cycle, and a vector, in which the pathogen does not develop. The same distinction exists between a biologic vector, in which the pathogen develops, and a mechanical vector, a passive carrier not essential to the pathogen's life cycle.

2. a physical quantity having both magnitude and direction, such as velocity, force, or electric field intensity. Vectors are indicated by boldface type ($\boldsymbol{V}$) or by an arrow ($V\rightarrow$). Multiplication of a vector by a scalar (a real number) gives a vector having the same direction but a magnitude multiplied by the scalar. The addition of vectors gives a vector that sometimes is called the resultant. Two vectors and their sum form three sides of a triangle. Vectors can be represented mathematically by a set of numbers called components: $V = (v_1, v_2, \ldots, v_n)$; then, scalar multiplication is performed by multiplying each component by the scalar: $X = aY$, if $x_i = ay_i$. Vector addition is performed by addition of components: $X = Y + Z$, if $x_i = y_i + z_i$.

3. a one-dimensional array. See also *array.*

4. a DNA sequence capable of autonomous replication in a bacterial cell (a plasmid or temperate phage) used in gene cloning to replicate a DNA segment. The DNA segment to be reproduced is spliced into the vector.

vectorcardiogram (vek″tor-kar′de-o-gram″) a graphic representation, usually a photograph of the loop inscribed on an oscilloscope, that represents the instantaneous vectors generated within the heart. See also *vectorcardiography.*

vectorcardiograph (vek″tor-kar′de-o-graf″) an instrument used to record the moment-to-moment changes in the direction and magnitude of electric currents generated by the heart. See also *vectorcardiography.*

vectorcardiography (vek″tor-kar″de-og′rah-fe) the recording of the sequence of instantaneous changes in electrical activity in a complete cardiac cycle. Appearing as a loop display, this technique measures the direction and magnitude, i.e., the vector, of the action potentials as they travel through the heart muscle.

The heart functions as a single fixed location dipole within the chest. This cardiac dipole acts as an instantaneous current generator with its associated vectors that may be measured. These potentials, which are recorded from the body surface, are plotted anterior-posterior (sagittally), head-to-foot (vertically) and left-to-right (transversely) across the heart. One lead is connected to the horizontal grids of a cathode ray oscilloscope, with the other lead connected to its vertical grids. The resulting loop represents the path of the action potentials as the course of these potentials through the heart is displayed on the oscilloscope.

A commonly employed electrode placement scheme utilizes seven electrodes placed on the surface of the body. One of these electrodes or a combination can then be connected as a lead to the oscilloscope. The first five electrodes are placed at the fifth intercostal space. Electrodes A and I are placed at the left and right midaxillary line, respectively, with E at the midsternal line, M at the midvertebral line, and C at 45° between the midsternal and left midaxillary line. The other two electrodes go to the neck (H) and the left foot (F). Combinations of electrodes that can be connected to the oscilloscope to demonstrate the components of the heart's electric activity are: the sagittal leads, consisting of IEC and AM; the vertical leads, consisting of MF and H; and the transverse leads, consisting of ACE and I.

The large recorded loop presents a dynamic representation of ventricular activation and is referred to as the QRS loop. The electric axis of the heart is graphically portrayed on the oscilloscope; with the use of the three lead configurations it is possible to determine regions of abnormal activity and the type of abnormality. An abnormal position of the heart, hypertrophy, bundle branch blocks, ischemia, and infarction result in changes in the vectorcardiogram. Coupled with electrocardiography, vectorcardiography is a useful tool in diagnosing abnormal and pathologic conditions of the heart.

vector product a type of multiplication of three-dimensional vectors, indicated $\boldsymbol{C} = \boldsymbol{A} \times \boldsymbol{B}$. The component equations are $c_1 = a_2b_3 - a_3b_2$, $c_2 = a_3b_1 - a_1b_3$, and $c_3 = a_1b_2 - a_2b_1$. The magnitude of $\boldsymbol{C}$, $|\boldsymbol{C}|$, is equal to $|\boldsymbol{A}| \cdot |\boldsymbol{B}| \cdot \sin\theta$, where θ is the angle between $\boldsymbol{A}$ and $\boldsymbol{B}$. The vector product is anticommutative: $\boldsymbol{A} \times \boldsymbol{B} = -\boldsymbol{B} \times \boldsymbol{A}$. Also called *cross product.* See also *scalar product.*

vegan (vej'an) a strict vegetarian who eats only plant products, avoiding eggs and dairy products as well as meat and fish. See also *vegetarian.*

vegetation (vej″e-ta'shun) [L. vegetatio] any plant-like fungoid neoplasm or growth; a luxurious, funguslike growth of pathologic tissue, particularly one occurring on the valve cusps of the heart.

bacterial v., a small, irregular excrescence found on the cardiac valves or endocardium in association with endocarditis; these growths are caused by fibrin and platelet deposits around the bacteria. See also *endocarditis.*

vegetative (vej'e-ta″tiv) 1. concerned with growth and nutrition.

2. functioning involuntarily or unconsciously.

3. in bacteriology, referring to the growing form of the cell. Cf. *spore form.*

vegetative multiplication division of the entire cell, as with the binary fission of bacteria.

vehicle (ve'ĭ-k'l) [L. *vehiculum,* from *vehere* to carry] 1. an excipient, a relatively inert substance added to a drug in order to obtain a suitable consistency or form. It may be a liquid or a solid, such as a powder.

2. any medium through which an impulse is propagated.

Veillonella (va″yon-el'ah) [A. *Veillon,* French bacteriologist, 1864–1931] a genus of bacteria of the family Veillonaceae, the only one of clinical significance. The small, gram-negative, anaerobic cocci occur in pairs or short chains. Nitrate is reduced by this organism but other biochemical test reactions are negative. *Veillonella* is found in the mouth and intestinal tract; it is not considered pathogenic. The type species is *V. parvula.*

Veillonaceae (va-yo-na'se-e) a family of gram-negative anaerobic cocci that includes the genera *Veillonella, Acidaminococcus,* and *Megasphaera,* of which only *Veillonella* has clinical importance.

vein (vān) [L. vena] a vessel that conveys blood from various organs or parts to or toward the heart, or from the wall of the heart. All veins except the pulmonary veins carry blood that has given up most of its oxygen. Many veins have valves that prevent the backward flow of the blood away from the heart; see also *valve.* For more information, see the specific vein and the accompanying illustrations.

velocity (V or v) (vě-los'ĭ-te) [L. *velocitas,* from *velox* swift] the time rate of change of position with which an object moves through space. In International System (SI) units, velocity is measured in meters per second (m/sec).

velum (ve'lum), pl. *vela* [L.] [NA], a general term for a veil or veil-like structure.

ven/o (ve'no) [L. *vena* vein] a word element used in combining form to denote a vein, e.g., venography.

Vena (ve'nah) a genus of nematode worms. For a description of the species *V. medinensis,* see *D. medinensis* under *Dracunculus.*

vena cava, inferior (ve'nah ca'vah) [N.L. "hollow vein"] the vein formed in front of the fifth lumbar vertebra by the junction of the two common iliac veins. It ascends in front of the vertebral column to the front of the aorta, passes behind the liver and through the central tendon of the diaphragm, and enters the right atrium. A single valve cusp positioned at its orifice is functional in the fetus.

vena cava, superior the vein that drains blood from the upper half of the body. It is about 7 cm long and is formed by the union of the brachiocephalic veins. It begins behind the first right costal cartilage and ends in the right atrium opposite the third right costal cartilage.

venacavography (ve″nah-ka-vog'rah-fe) the radiologic examination of the inferior vena cava after introduction of a contrast medium.

venae cordis minimae (ve'nā cor'dis min'ĭ-mā) [L.] small veins in the wall of the heart that open independently into the chambers, principally the right atrium.

venereal (ve-ne're-al) [L. *venereus,* having to do with *Venus* the goddess of love] a term describing any condition or disease caused or spread by sexual contact.

venereal disease a term once used to describe five infectious diseases (syphilis, gonorrhea, chancroid, lymphogranuloma venereum, and granuloma inguinale) that have been known for many decades to be transmitted from one individual to another through sexual activity. However, advances in microbiology in the 1960s and 1970s revealed that an increasing number of diseases are transmitted by sexual contact; this group of diseases is now more accurately referred to by the term sexually transmitted diseases. See also *sexually transmitted diseases.*

venesection (ven″ĕ-sek'shun) [L. *vena* vein + *sectio* cutting] see *phlebotomy.*

venipuncture (ven″ĭ-pungk'tūr) the puncture of a vein for therapeutic purposes or for collection of blood specimens.

Venn diagram (ven) [John *Venn,* English logician, 1834–1923] a diagram showing the logical relationship among several sets, which are represented by

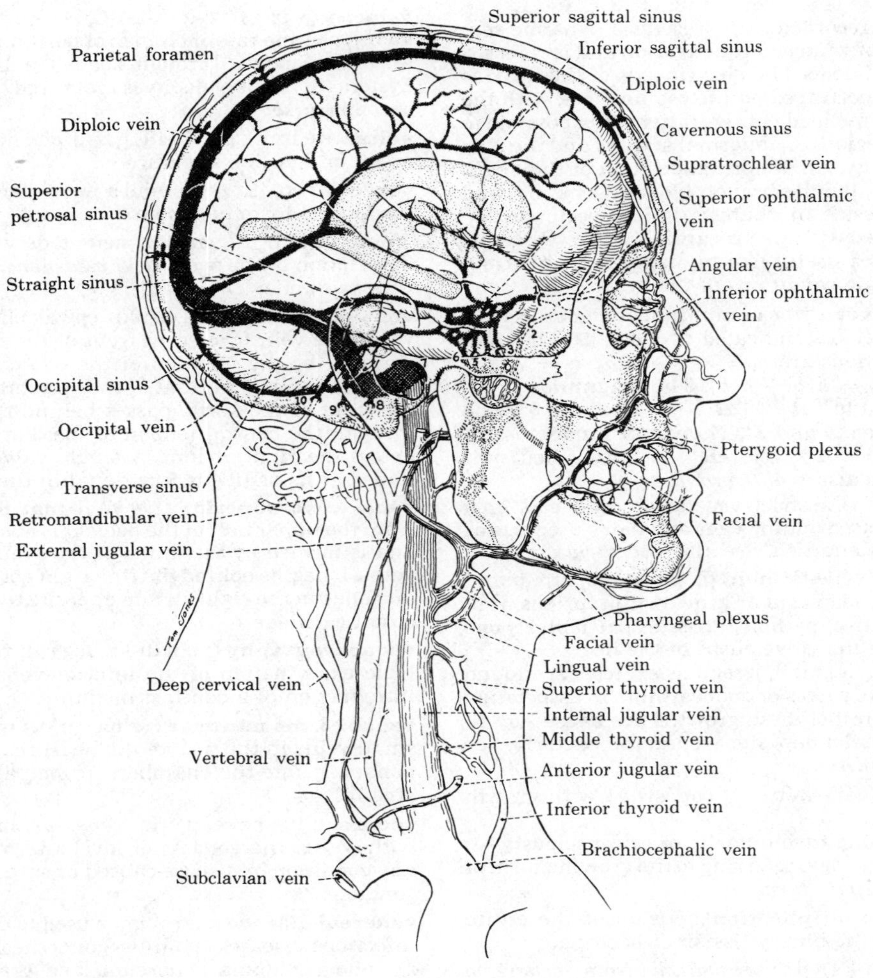

Vein, Figure 1. **Veins of the head and neck. (From Dorland's Illustrated Medical Dictionary. 26th ed. Philadelphia, W. B. Saunders Co., 1981.)**

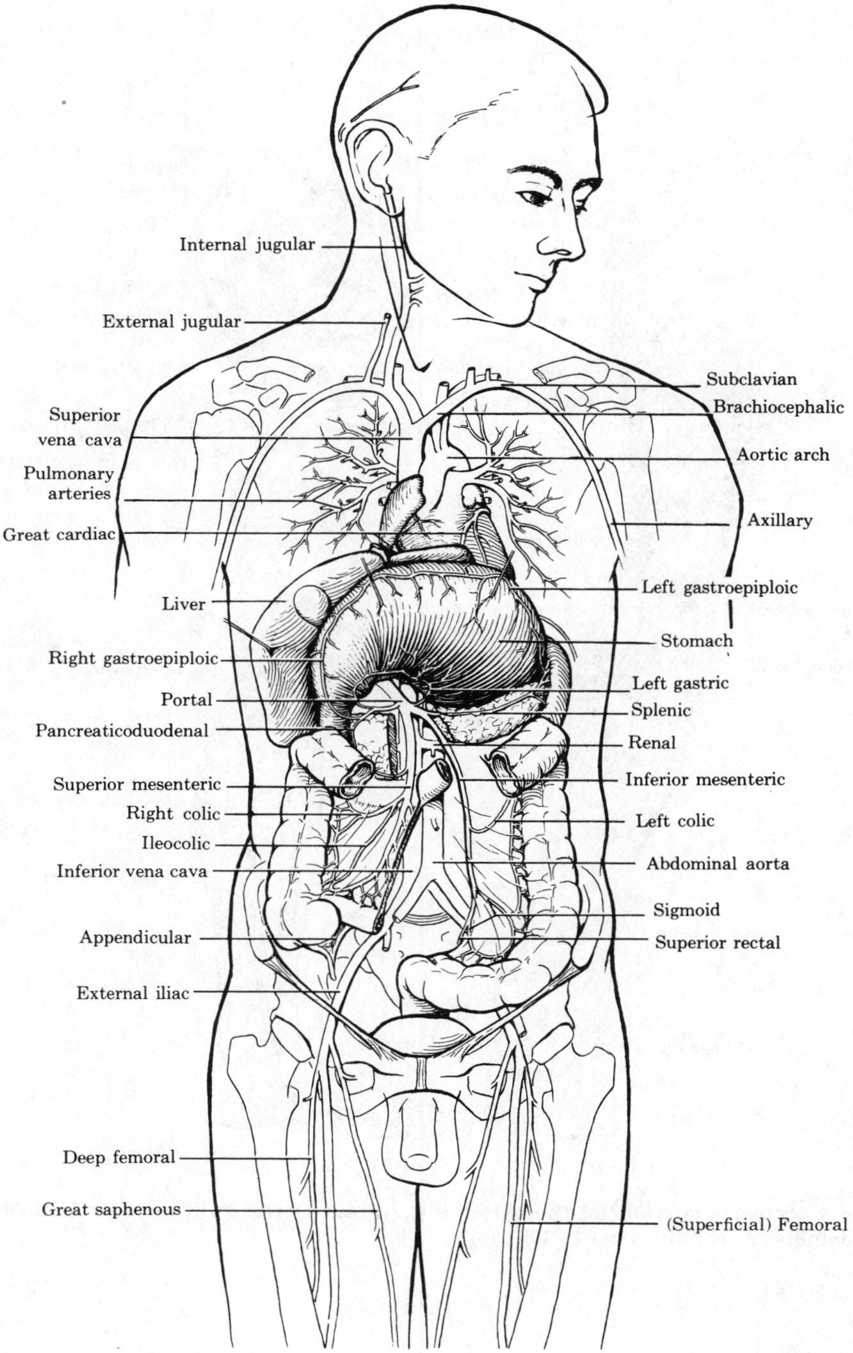

Vein, Figure 2. Principal veins of the body. (From Dorland's Illustrated Medical Dictionary. 26th ed. Philadelphia, W. B. Saunders Co., 1981.)

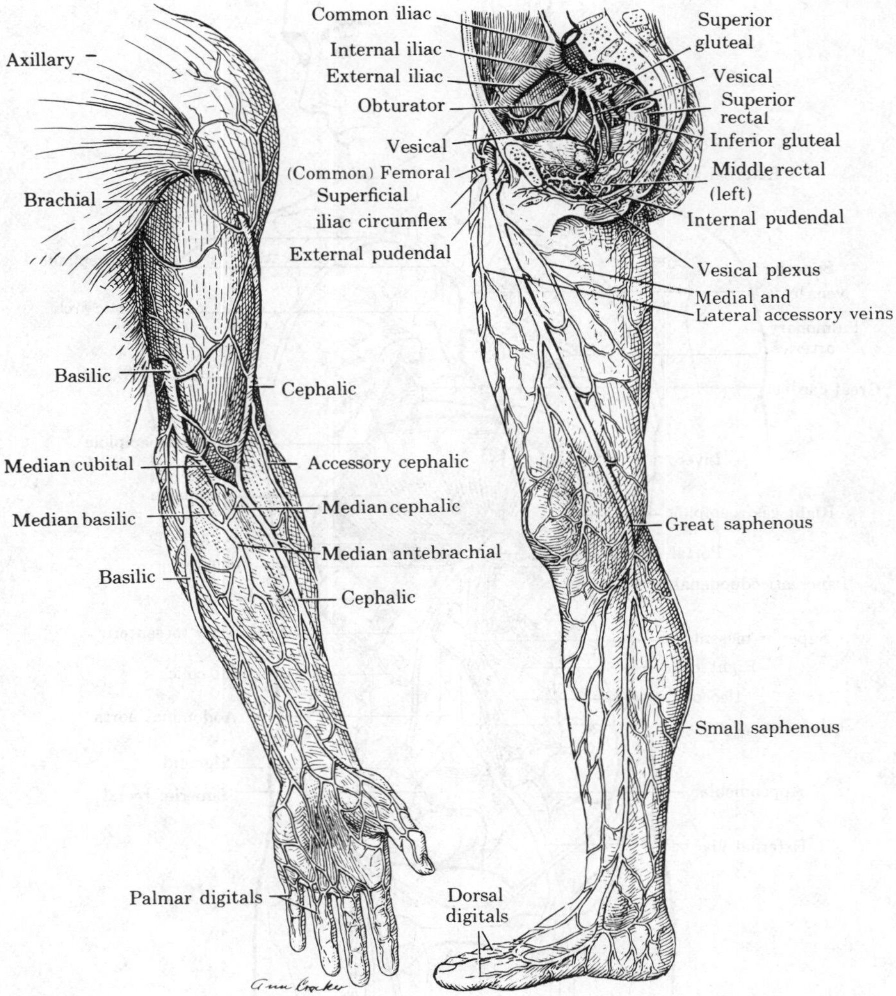

Vein, Figure 3. Superficial veins of the extremities. (From Dorland's Illustrated Medical Dictionary. 26th ed. Philadelphia, W. B. Saunders Co., 1981.)

the areas within closed curves, usually circles. For example, if there are two circles representing the sets *A* and *B*, then the intersection $A \cap B$ is the area of overlap, if any (if there is no overlap $A \cap B$ is the empty set), and the union $A \cap B$ is the area contained within both circles. The complement of *A*, denoted *A*, is the area outside the circle containing *A*.

venogram (ve′no-gram) [*veno-* + Gr. *gramma* drawing] a radiograph of an opacified vein, in particular a cerebral angiogram demonstrating the venous circulation. Also called *phlebogram.*

venography (ve-nog′rah-fe) [*veno-* + Gr. *graphein* to write or draw] 1. a radiologic examination of the veins after the introduction of a radiopaque contrast medium.

2. scintiphotography of the deep veins of the thighs and pelvis for the detection of thrombophlebitis. Technetium Tc-99m macroaggregated albumin or Tc-99m albumin microspheres solution is injected into the dorsal veins of the feet and is directed into the deep veins by tourniquets above the ankles. An anterior scintigram is made as the circulation carries the isotope through the field of view. The procedure is repeated to obtain overlapping views covering the thighs and pelvis. See also *venous thrombosis scanning.*

peripheral v., venography of the extremities, commonly used to examine the deep veins of the legs for thrombophlebitis or occlusions.

portal v., radiologic examination of the hepatic circulation after injection of a contrast medium directly into the portal vein during surgery.

splenoportal v., radiologic examination of the splenic and portal circulation after percutaneous injection of a water-soluble radiopaque contrast medium directly into the pulp of the spleen. It is used to demonstrate esophageal varices or abnormalities of the intrahepatic vessels. Also called *splenoportography.*

venom (ven′om) [L. *venenum* poison] poison, especially a toxic substance normally secreted by a snake, insect, or other animal. Most venoms are complex mixtures containing several toxic substances, which are usually enzymes that attack cellular structures or are polypeptides that inhibit enzymes in the victim.

venostasis (ve″no-sta′sis) [*veno-* + Gr. *stasis* stopping] the blockage or slowing of blood flow through a vein due to obstruction or to incompetent valves superior to the area of stasis.

venous (ve′nus) [L. *venosus*] of or pertaining to the veins.

venous admixture the dilution of oxygenated arterial blood with unoxygenated mixed venous blood. This effect occurs when blood bypasses the pulmonary capillaries and thus the ventilated alveoli (venous-to-arterial shunt), or when it passes through lung regions with a low ventilation/perfusion ratio. See also *total s.* and *venous-to-arterial s.* under *shunt* and *ventilation-perfusion ratio.*

venous pressure the pressure within the venous portion of the vascular tree. Venous pressures vary widely, from negative values to as high as 90 mmHg, depending on variables including the pumping activity of the heart, other factors influencing central venous pressure, the position of the vein with respect to gravity and to anatomic structures that would act to compress it, and the degree of skeletal muscle activity.

For example, as a result of hydrostatic pressure, the venous pressure tends to increase or decrease by a factor of 0.77 mmHg for every centimeter of distance below or above the right atrium, respectively. Pressure thus tends to be maximum in the veins of the lower leg of the standing adult, an effect that is opposed by the pumping action of any skeletal muscle activity. The negative pressure of the thorax is transmitted to the great veins within, the most negative pressures being reached during inspiration.

central v. p., the pressure in the great veins at their point of entrance into the right atrium, an average of 0–6 mmHg. It is influenced by changes in blood flow returning from the peripheral veins, by the contraction of the right atrium, and by the pumping action of the right ventricle. It fluctuates during different portions of the cardiac and respiratory cycles.

venous return the volume of blood that enters the right atrium from the systemic circulation each minute. In the effectively pumping heart, it is equal to the cardiac output (CO) when evaluated over a prolonged time interval, and is one of the primary factors that determines the magnitude of the CO.

venous sinuses of dura mater the venous channels between the two layers of the dura mater that drain the blood from the brain and the bones of the cranium.

venous thrombosis scanning a procedure in nuclear medicine for the detection of deep-vein thrombosis of the legs and pelvis. Iodinated I-125 fibrinogen is injected intravenously and circulates in the blood until it is incorporated into a clot or active inflammation. At a series of points along the deep vein of the leg, the radioactivity is measured as a percentage of the precordial count rate, using a portable thin-window scintillation counter. An increase of a reading by 20 percent over previous scans indicates a thrombus. Scanning can be repeated for up to 14 da or as long as the precordial rate exceeds 100 counts/sec. Lugol's iodine or potassium perchlorate is administered orally before the procedure in order to block thyroid uptake of free iodide released from the fibrinogen.

ventilation (ven″tĭ-la′shun) [L. *ventilatio*, from *ventilare* to fan] 1. the replacement of gas in a space.

2. the movement of gases into and out of the lungs.

3. (symbol V), the air exchanged between the lungs and the atmosphere, measured in liters per minute (l/min). See also *alveolar ventilation, maximal voluntary ventilation,* and *total ventilation.*

4. the process of supplying a room with fresh air. The ventilation of laboratories is an important factor in laboratory safety, needed to control temperatures; to provide clean, fresh air within acceptable limits of humidity; and to remove and disperse released contaminants. The choice of air quality supplied to the laboratory should be based on the conditions necessary for the satisfactory operation of equipment and performance of personnel; air intake location and velocity and direction of delivery of the air to the laboratory are significant factors.

Laboratories in which specimens and chemicals are handled usually need to have special ventilation to capture and remove contaminants that may otherwise adversely affect personnel, equipment, and facilities. Special ventilation mechanisms may include local exhaust ventilation, enclosures such as glove boxes and biological safety cabinets, and laboratory hoods. The only air captured from contaminant ventilation that can safely be recirculated is the exhaust from HEPA filters, which are certifiably effective in capturing particulate contamination. Air captured from local exhaust systems and laboratory hoods cannot safely be recirculated: tests have shown that absorption filters such as activated carbon retain captured solvent vapors in limited quantity and only for limited times.

NFPA (National Fire Protection Association) regulations 56C-1980 and 45-1981 may be consulted for additional requirements and for information on ventilation.

local exhaust v., a method of capturing contaminants close to their point of release and exhausting them from the workplace. Local exhaust ventilation may include flexible exhaust ducts that allow the inlet to be positioned close to the source of contaminant release, slotted exhaust inlets at the back of laboratory work surfaces, or special enclosures or equipment that release aerosols, vapors, or other contaminants. Local exhaust ventilation is a more effective means of controlling contaminants than general (dilution) ventilation, and may be more efficient than laboratory hoods for many contaminants that are not particularly toxic or irritating.

ventilation-perfusion ratio ($\dot{V}_A/\dot{Q}_C$) the ratio between gas distribution (alveolar ventilation) and blood distribution (pulmonary capillary perfusion) in the lungs. The $\dot{V}_A/\dot{Q}_C$ ratio is used as an indication of the degree of uniformity between the air and blood flow within lung units, and thus the extent of alveolocapillary gas exchange and the resulting arterialization of the pulmonary capillary blood.

Ideally, the $\dot{V}_A/\dot{Q}_C$ ratio is uniform throughout, with each alveolus receiving a share of the pulmonary blood flow that is exactly matched to its ventilation; the P_{CO_2} and PO_2 of the blood leaving all alveoli is equal and optimal. In reality, however, the $\dot{V}_A/\dot{Q}_C$ ratio is nonuniform throughout even the healthy lung. In a healthy individual in the standing position, various physical factors (particularly the effect of gravity on intravascular pressures) result in $\dot{V}_A/\dot{Q}_C$ ratios that vary from 0.5–1.0 at the base or dependent portion of the lung to 2–3 at the apex. However, the mean ratio for the lungs as a whole in normal persons under basal conditions is close to 0.8, reflecting a resting average alveolar ventilation of 4 l/min and an average capillary blood flow of 5 l/min. Many lung units have a ratio close to this value.

Various cardiopulmonary disease conditions lead to nonuniformities in alveolar ventilation and/or perfusion. The resulting mismatching of gas and blood is an important cause of the chronic arterial hypoxemia and hypercapnia (CO_2 retention) that is often secondary to these conditions.

When lung units receiving a normal blood flow are underventilated (relative hyperperfusion, or low $\dot{V}_A/\dot{Q}_C$ ratio), the blood leaving these units has a relatively unchanged composition, similar to that of mixed venous blood. When it joins the mixed arterial blood in the left heart, it lowers its O_2 content even if compensation is attempted by increasing ventilation to the surrounding healthy units. Because hemoglobin is nearly fully saturated during normal ventilation, no amount of hyperventilation can correct this condition of low arterial saturation. However, because these low $\dot{V}_A/\dot{Q}_C$ regions are hyperperfused relative to their ventilation, the pulmonary capillary blood flowing through them removes more oxygen from the alveolar gas, which results in a regional hypoxemia. The hypoxemia, in turn, leads to a regional vasoconstriction, diverting the blood flow to other more adequately ventilated regions.

Capillary blood leaving regions with a low $\dot{V}_A/\dot{Q}_C$ ratio has a high P_{CO_2}. Hyperventilation of normal lung units, a reflex response integrated by the respiratory centers in response to the initial hypercapnia, brings about a compensatory decrease in P_{CO_2} to normal levels. Chronic hypercapnia occurs only when the regions of low $\dot{V}_A/\dot{Q}_C$ ratio are extensive, and blood leaving the remaining alveoli contributes so little to the CO_2 content of the arterial blood that compensation is ineffective.

Low $\dot{V}_A/\dot{Q}_C$ ratios may result from any of the various disease states that lead to an uneven airway resistance (asthma, emphysema, bronchitis, bronchiolitis, pulmonary edema, tumors), uneven lung compliance (emphysema, pneumothorax, pulmonary congestion, pulmonary edema, or pleural effusion or thickening), or factors contributing to an increase in the distance of the alveolocapillary diffusion pathway.

The ventilation to relatively underperfused regions (with a high $\dot{V}_A/\dot{Q}_C$ ratio) is essentially wasted, as it contributes little to the arterialization of the mixed venous blood. (This wasted ventilation, or alveolar dead space, together with the anatomic dead space, defines the physiologic dead space.) If these regions are not extensive, they result in relatively little change in arterial CO_2 or O_2 tensions. When enough high $\dot{V}_A/\dot{Q}_C$ units are present, however, hypoxemia and hypercapnia result unless Pa_{CO_2} and Pa_{O_2} are maintained by a compensatory increase in respiratory minute volume.

Alveolar P_{CO_2} is low in regions with a high $\dot{V}_A/\dot{Q}_C$ ratio. This condition induces a regional bronchoconstriction that directs ventilation away from underperfused areas, tending to equalize the $\dot{V}_A/\dot{Q}_C$ ratio throughout the lungs.

Conditions that lead to underperfusion of the lungs and thus to regionally high $\dot{V}_A/\dot{Q}_C$ ratios include embolization of the pulmonary circulation, occlusion, compression, kinking or localized congestion of the pulmonary vessels, the closure of pulmonary vessels subsequent to severe hypotension and shock, the destruction of vessels due to emphysema or fibrosis, tension cysts, or anatomic venous-to-arterial shunts.

Various methods are available for measuring the presence of inequalities in the ventilation-perfusion ratio. Physiologic dead space can be calculated from the Bohr equation. $\dot{V}_A/\dot{Q}_C$ inequality can be detected from a single-breath CO_2 test, in which the CO_2 content of the expired alveolar gas from a single expiration is continually monitored by a CO_2 analyzer. A variation in the $\dot{V}_A/\dot{Q}_C$ ratio is indicated by a much higher CO_2 content in the last portion of the expired gas relative to the first. A difference between the P_{N_2} in the alveolar gas and arterial blood also indicates a mismatching; gas chromatography can be used to measure Pa_{N_2}.

Techniques such as bronchospirometry and radioisotopes such as ^{133}Xe are used to locate the specific regions in which unevenness in the $\dot{V}_A/\dot{Q}_C$ ratio occurs. Bronchospirometry is used to measure the O_2 uptake and ventilation of each lung. A decrease in O_2 uptake and a normal ventilation to one lung indicates an abnormal perfusion. In the second method, radioactive xenon is inhaled or injected intravenously; its rate of appearance in various regions of the lung is detected by external counters (placed on selected locations on the chest surface) or by Anger scintillation camera. The regional rates of blood flow and ventilation are related to the concentration or rate of appearance and disappearance of the xenon.

ventilator (ven′tĭ-la′tor) an automatic cycling machine used to assist in or control alveolar ventilation by delivering an appropriate volume of gas to the respiratory airways. Air supplied by the ventilator can be delivered to the patient's airways by means of mouthpiece, mask, tracheostomy, or endotracheal tubes, or via a spirometer. Almost any pattern of ventilation can be provided by a mechanical ventilator when the machine's settings for cycling frequency and amplitude, inspiratory and expiratory flow rates, and peak inspiratory pressures are properly adjusted. These parameters can also be adjusted to override a patient's spontaneous (and inadequate) pattern of breathing.

Ventilators are designed so that the inspiratory phase of the respiratory cycle is initiated by the machine (in the apneic patient) and/or by the patient's own effort when operated in the assist mode. They are classified according to the manner in which the inspiratory phase is terminated. Volume-cycled ventilators end the inspiration when a predetermined tidal volume has been delivered. Because they deliver this volume regardless of the level of peak inspiratory pressure achieved, these ventilators are particularly useful in the condition of decreased lung and chest wall compliance, such as occurs in those with adult respiratory distress syndrome (ARDS), flail chest, or extreme obesity. Pressure-cycled ventilators end inspiration and initiate expiration when a preset airway pressure is achieved, regardless of the actual volume of gas that has been delivered. A disadvantage of this type of ventilator is that the tidal volume delivered may not be constant or otherwise adequate in patients with stiff lungs (increased pulmonary compliance) who need greater airway pressures to inflate the lungs adequately. Time-cycled ventilators terminate when a predetermined inspiratory flow has been supplied for a prescheduled length of time.

Also called *respirator.*

ventr/o (ven′tro) [L. *venter* belly or abdomen] a word element used in combining form to denote the stomach or front side of the body, e.g., ventrofixation.

ventral (ven′tral) [L. *ventralis*] 1. pertaining to the abdomen or to the belly of a muscle.

2. denoting a position or direction toward the front of the body. Also called *anterior.* Cf. *dorsal.*

ventral pontine syndrome a condition caused by a pathologic process, usually infarct or hemorrhage, that destroys the basis pontis or ventral pontine regions of the brain bilaterally. Bilateral midbrain lesions may produce a similar disorder. Individuals are rendered tetraplegic and mute, but higher mental function is preserved. They are usually able to communicate by voluntary movements of the eyes or eyelids. The electroencephalogram of these patients when awake and nonrapid eye movement sleep is usually unremarkable. Also called *deefferented states.*

ventricle (ven′trĭ-k'l) [L. *ventriculus,* dim. of *venter* belly] a small cavity or chamber, such as one of the chambers of the heart or one of the cavities in the brain. See also under *brain* and *heart.*

v. of larynx, see *ventricle of l.* under *larynx.*

ventricul/o (ven-trik′u-lo) a word element used in combining form to denote a ventricle, e.g., ventriculogram.

ventricular (ven-trik′u-lar) pertaining to a ventricle.

ventricular escape the occurrence of one or more escape beats initiated in the ventricle. See also *escape beats.*

ventricular fibrillation see *ventricular f.* under *fibrillation.*

ventricular premature beat (VPB) see *premature ventricular contraction.*

ventricular premature contraction (VPC) see *premature ventricular contraction.*

ventricular premature depolarization (VPD) see *premature ventricular contraction.*

ventricular septal defect a congenital anomaly characterized by an abnormal opening in the ventricular septum, between the left and right ventricles. The membranous portion of the ventricle is the most common location of such defects. Small defects are asymptomatic, but larger openings create a left-to-right shunt that eventually leads to left and right ventricular hypertrophy. Clinical manifestations, which increase with age, may include holosystolic murmur, split second heart sound, pulmonary hypertension, dyspnea, heart block, and bacterial endocarditis; cardiac failure may result. If the pulmonary hypertension is great enough, a right-to-left shunt results, causing cyanosis.

Diagnosis is made on the basis of clinical signs, electrocardiography, echocardiography, angiocardiography, and x-ray. Surgical correction of the defect may be recommended but must be done before severe pulmonary hypertension develops. See also *Roger's disease.*

ventriculography (ven-trik″u-log′rah-fe) [*ventriculō* + Gr. *graphein* to write] the radiologic examination of the ventricles of the brain or of a ventricle of the heart. Ventriculography of the brain usually utilizes air as the contrast medium; see *cerebral p.* under *pneumoradiography.*

cardiac v., examination of the left or right ventricle of the heart after introduction of a contrast medium directly into the ventricle. Also called left ventriculography or right ventriculography. See also *angiocardiography.*

contrast v., examination of the ventricles of the brain after introduction of a contrast medium (usually iophendylate) into the ventricles, either by direct injection through a burr hole in the cranium or via lumbar puncture.

Venturi mask (ven-tu′ri) [G. B. *Venturi,* Italian physicist, 1746–1822] a face mask used in inhalation therapy to deliver inspired oxygen at a constant, known concentration (24, 28, 35, or 40 percent O_2). This device operates on the Venturi principle, entraining a fixed amount of air to combine with the O_2 supplied to the mask. When oxygen flows into the mask at a specified rate, the air entrainment is constant and predictable, and the O_2 concentration to the patient is constant and specific.

venule (ven'ūl) [L. *venula*, dim. of *vena* vein] a small vessel that drains blood from a capillary plexus and joins other venules to form a vein.

postcapillary v., any of the small vessels that collects blood from the capillary plexuses to which they are immediately adjacent. These structures are important sites of fluid exchange and leukocyte migration. In lymph nodes, they are a major pathway whereby T lymphocytes enter the paracortical zone of the node.

VEP abbrev. for visual evoked potential. See *visual e. p.* under *evoked potential*.

verapamil (ver-ap'ah-mil) a calcium channel blocking agent, administered intravenously, for the treatment of cardiac arrhythmias, particularly supraventricular tachycardias. The excitation wave is propagated in the heart by the movement of sodium ions in the fast channel, which is blocked by lidocaine, procainamide, and other drugs; and by calcium ions in the slow channel, which is blocked by verapamil.

The primary effect of the drug is to slow the rate of SA node discharge and the conduction velocity through the A-V node. Adverse reactions include hypotension, bradycardia, A-V block, and ventricular fibrillation.

Trademarks, Isoptin and Calan.

verbascose (ver-bas'cōs) an oligosaccharide present in the edible seeds of some leguminous plants such as beans, peas, and soybeans, which has (1,6)-linked galactose residues that cannot be hydrolyzed for absorption from the intestine. It may be regarded as three galactose residues linked by a (1,6)-bond to the glucose residue of sucrose. The indigestibility of the carbohydrate results in flatus following ingestion.

Verhoeff's stain (ver'hefz) [Fredrick Herman *Verhoeff*, American ophthalmologist, 1874–1968] a permanent iodine-iron hematoxylin stain for elastic fibers. Paraffin sections fixed in formalin or Zenker's fluid are stained in Verhoeff's solution for 15–45 min and then differentiated in 2 percent aqueous ferric chloride. Elastic fibers are stained black; the nuclei, gray-black. Eosin or van Gieson's picrofuchsin may be used as a counterstain.

Verhoeff's solution consists of hematoxylin dissolved in hot absolute alcohol, which is then added to a solution of aqueous ferric chloride and Lugol's solution.

vermicular (ver-mik'u-lar) [L. *vermicularis*, from *vermis* worm] wormlike in shape or appearance.

vermifuge (ver'mĭ-fūj) [*vermis* + *fugare* to put to flight] an agent that expels worms or intestinal parasites; an anthelmintic.

vermis (ver'mis) [L.] a worm or wormlike structure; often used alone to designate the vermis cerebelli, the median part of the cerebellum.

Verner-Morrison syndrome a disorder characterized by chronic watery diarrhea, hypokalemia, and hypochlorhydria or achlorhydria, often accompanied by hyperglycemia, hypercalcemia, hypotension, and episodic flushing. Individuals with this syndrome most commonly have solitary nonbeta-pancreatic islet cell tumors, more than 50 percent of which are malignant. Diffuse hyperplasia of the pancreatic islet cells, or extrapancreatic tumors, have also been observed. Classically, the syndrome has been attributed to the overproduction of vasoactive intestinal polypeptide (VIP). A few cases, however, have been associated with normal or minimal elevation of VIP levels in blood but very high levels of circulating pancreatic polypeptide (PP). Such reports strongly indicate that, in some cases at least, Verner-Morrison syndrome can be manifested by PP excess. It is probable that other polypeptide hormones also are involved in the pathogenesis of the syndrome. Also called pancreatic cholera, WDAH syndrome, and WDHH syndrome.

Vernet's syndrome (ver-nāz') [Maurice *Vernet*, French neurologist, born 1887] a syndrome characterized by disruption of function of the ninth, tenth, and eleventh cranial nerves. It is most frequently due to neoplasms and aneurysms in the region of the jugular foramen. Persons affected experience hoarseness of the voice, difficulty in swallowing, palatal and pharyngeal weakness, impaired pharyngeal sensation, and weakness of the sternocleidomastoid and trapezius muscles.

vernier (ver'ne-ā) [Pierre *Vernier*, French physicist, 1580–1637] an auxiliary scale on a measuring device that is used to read off fractions of a scale division on the main scale. In the accompanying illustration, the vernier indicates a reading of 3.6. The zero on the vernier is six-tenths of the way between the 3 and the 4 on the main scale; this is indicated by the 6 being the scale division on the vernier that is lined up with a main scale division.

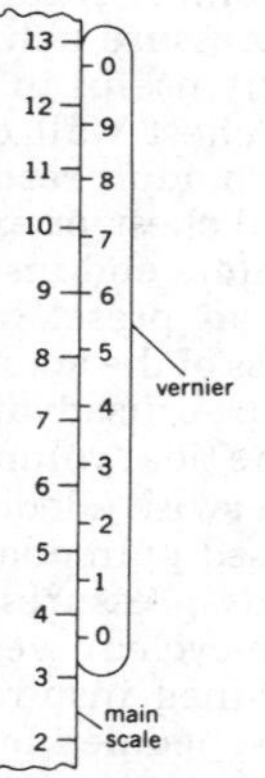

Vernier. Direct vernier scale (reading, 3.6). (Modified from McGraw-Hill Dictionary of Scientific and Technical Terms. New York, McGraw-Hill Book Co., 1976.)

vernier dial a type of dial used for precision adjustment in which the control knob turns several revolutions to produce a full-scale dial movement.

vernix (ver'niks) [L.] varnish.

vernix caseosa [L. "cheesy varnish"] a cheesy or caseous covering of fetal epidermis, composed of superficial cornified cells, sebaceous secretions, and the remains of the periderm. Its function is to protect the underlying epidermis from the amniotic fluid; it is shed shortly after birth.

Verocay body (ver'o-ka) [José *Verocay*, Prague pathologist, 1876–1927] a histologic pattern characterized by palisading nuclei; seen in schwannomas and infrequently in certain other soft tissue tumors.

verruca (vě-roo′kah), pl. *verrucae* [L.] 1. a lobulated elevation of the epidermis, which may occur anywhere on the skin, or on the mucous membranes. The lesions are believed to be caused by an intranuclear papillomavirus and tend to recur after removal. Clinically, the symptoms associated with a verruca depend on the location. Most are not painful, with the notable exception of those on the sole of the foot (plantar warts, verruca plantaris). Itching is not common except with anal or genital warts; however, their appearance is upsetting enough to encourage "picking" or scratching, which then spreads the virus to other areas.

Treatment usually involves removal by surgical or chemical (e.g., liquid nitrogen) means.

Also called common wart, verruca vulgaris, and *wart*.

2. a term loosely applied to any wartlike lesion of the skin.

v. peruana, see *bartonellosis.*

v. plana, a flat, skin-colored elevation of the skin, common on the face, neck, chest, backs of the hands, elbows, and shins. It is thought to be caused by the same papillomavirus that causes verruca vulgaris, the common wart. Also called flat wart and verruca plana juvenilis.

v. plantaris, see *plantar wart.*

v. seborrheica, see *seborrheic k.* under *keratosis.*

verrucous (ver′oo-kus) having a wartlike appearance.

verrucous hyperplasia epithelial hyperplasia that is characterized by acanthosis, papillomatosis, and accentuation of the granular layer, which resembles a verruca.

vertebr/o (ver′tě-bro) [L. *vertebra,* from *vertere* to turn] a word element used in combining form to denote the vertebrae, e.g., vertebrochondral.

vertebra (ver′tě-brah), pl. *vertebrae* [L.] one of the bones in the chain that forms the vertebral column. A typical vertebra has an expanded anterior portion or body, and a posterior arch that encircles the vertebral foramen through which the spinal cord passes. Foramina between adjacent vertebral arches transmit the spinal nerves and vessels. Each vertebral arch has a narrow anterior part, the pedicle, and a broader posterior portion, the lamina. Paired transverse processes and a single spine project from the vertebral arch, and pairs of facets articulate with those of the vertebrae above and below.

vertebral (ver′te-bral) [N.L. *vertebralis*] of or pertaining to the vertebral column or its component vertebrae or disks.

vertebral artery a branch of the subclavian artery that ascends through the foramina in the transverse processes of the sixth through first cervical vertebrae, passes through the foramen magnum into the skull, and, with the vertebral artery from the opposite side, forms the basilar artery at the lower border of the pons.

vertebral column the columnar chain of vertebrae that extends from the foramen magnum to the tip of the coccyx. It consists of 33 bones in five regions (7 cervical, 12 thoracic, 5 lumbar, 5 [fused] sacral, and 4 [fused] coccygeal vertebrae). Flexible joints with fibrocartilaginous disks separate the adjacent nonfused vertebrae. The vertebral column is about 70 cm long in the adult male. It possesses two primary curves (thoracic and pelvic) that are concave ventrally, and two secondary or compensatory (cervical and lumbar) curves. Also called *spine.* See also *vertebra.*

Vertebrata (ver″tě-bra′tah) a subphylum of the Chordata comprising all animals that have a vertebral column (the vertebrates): mammals, birds, reptiles, amphibians, and fishes.

vertex (ver′teks), pl. *vertices* [L.] 1. the highest point or summit, particularly the vertex of the cranium, the highest point of the skull.

2. the point of intersection of the sides of an angle, two sides of a polygon, or three or more edges of a polyhedron.

vertex sharp transient (V wave) in electroencephalography, a sharp potential that occurs spontaneously during nonrapid eye movement (non-REM) sleep or in response to sensory stimuli of any modality during sleep or wakefulness. Its amplitude is usually $\leq 250\ \mu V$ and the potential is recorded maximally from the vertex of the skull, where it is negative relative to other areas. When induced by sensory stimuli, V waves have a latency of 65 ± 25 msec. They can usually be recognized in infants after the fifth month of life. Also called *biparietal hump* and *vertex sharp wave.*

vertex sharp wave see *vertex sharp transient.*

vertical (ver′tĭ-kal) [M. L. *verticalis,* from *vertex*] 1. straight up and down, perpendicular to the horizon. Cf. *horizontal.*

2. pertaining to a vertex.

vertical ray pertaining to a radiographic projection in which the central ray passes through the part in the vertical direction (perpendicular to the table).

verticosubmental (ver″tĭ-ko-sub-men′tal) pertaining to a basal or subbasal radiographic projection in which the central ray passes from the vertex to the base. Cf. *submentovertical.*

vertigo (ver′tĭ-go, ver-ti′go) [L., from *vertere* to turn] a sensation of rotation, either of the surroundings or of the affected person, often experienced in combination with nausea and vomiting, pallor, and perspiration. Occasionally there is a feeling of being drawn off balance, with the surroundings tilting or otherwise changing in perspective.

Vertigo may be associated with many disorders, including lesions of the inner ear, the eighth cranial nerve, or the brain stem and overindulgence in alcoholic beverages. Benign and unexplained vertigo may also occur.

verumontanum (ve″ru-mon-ta′num) [L. "mountain ridge"] a thickened elevated area of the urethral mucosa within the prostatic urethra. It is the entrance site of the ejaculatory duct.

very high frequency (VHF) pertaining to radio waves in the wavelength range of 1–10 m (frequency range, 30–300 MHz).

very-large-scale integration (VSLI) integrated circuit technology in which more than 10^4 logic circuits are placed on a single chip, as in the new 16- and 32-bit microprocessors and the 16- to 64 K-byte memories.

very-low-density lipoprotein see *very-low-density l.* under *lipoprotein.*

vesic/o (ves′ĭ-ko) [L. *vesica* bladder] a prefix word

element to denote a bladder, particularly the urinary bladder, e.g., vesicocele.

vesical (ves′ĭ-kal) pertaining to a bladder, particularly the urinary bladder.

vesical artery, inferior a branch of the anterior trunk of the internal iliac artery, often arising in common with the middle rectal artery. Fine branches of the inferior vesical artery ramify to supply the fundus of the bladder, prostate, seminal vesicles, and distal ureter. It may contribute the artery to the ductus deferens.

vesical artery, superior a branch of the anterior trunk of the internal iliac artery, providing numerous branches to the upper part of the bladder and ureter. It may contribute the artery to the ductus deferens.

vesical blood fluke see *S. haematobium* under *Schistosoma.*

vesicle (ves′ĭ-k′l) [L. *vesicula,* dim. of *vesica* bladder] 1. a small bladder or sac that contains liquid or gas; also called vesicula.

2. a small blister, which is a separation of the epidermis raised by the exudation of pus or serous fluid. Diseases that produce a rash with vesicles include coxsackie, herpes simplex, and varicella infections, and congenital syphilis. Cf. *bleb* and *bulla.*

3. any membrane-bound cytoplasmic sac, such as a saccule of the Golgi apparatus or a pericytotic vesicle. For more information, see the specific vesicle.

vesicul/o (vĕ-sik′u-lo) a word element used in combining form to denote the seminal vesicles, e.g., vesiculogram.

vesicular (vĕ-sik′u-lar) 1. composed of or relating to small, saclike bodies.

2. pertaining to or made up of vesicles on the skin.

vesicular nucleus a nucleus that has a distinct chromatinic membrane and is pale staining centrally. The structure can also be described as uniformly, finely granular.

vesicular pharyngitis see *herpangina.*

vesiculin (vĕ-sik′u-lin) a highly acidic protein present in the numerous coated vesicles in synaptosomes; M.W. 10,000. Each vesicle contains 2000–4000 molecules of acetylcholine and one-fifth as many molecules of adenosine triphosphate.

vesiculography (vĕ-sik″u-log′rah-fe) [*vesiculo-* + Gr. *graphein* to write or draw] radiologic examination of the seminal vesicles to investigate conditions such as cysts, tumors, orchitis, or obstruction. A water-soluble iodinated contrast medium is injected into the deferent ducts or, by catheterization, into the ejaculatory ducts. See also *epididymovesiculography.*

Vesprin (ves′prin) trademark. See *triflupromazine.*

vessel (ves′el) any channel for carrying a fluid, such as the blood or lymph. See also *vas.*

vestibular (ves-tib′u-lar) pertaining to a vestibule.

vestibular apparatus the sensory organ of the inner ear concerned with the maintenance of equilibrium. It sends information to the central nervous system concerning the position of the head with respect to gravity and its state of linear or angular acceleration. The vestibular apparatus is composed of specialized neuroepithelia of the walls of the utricle, saccule, and semicircular ducts; of the corresponding spaces of the osseous labyrinth in which these structures reside; and of the endolymph and perilymph contained in and surrounding them.

vestibular membrane see *Reissner's membrane.*

vestibule (ves′tĭ-būl) [L. *vestibulum*] a space or cavity at the entrance to a canal, such as the entrance to the nose, mouth, inner ear, or female genital tract.

v. of ear, an irregularly oval cavity, the most expanded portion of the tortuous canals of the osseous labyrinth. Located medial to the tympanic cavity, its lateral wall is penetrated by the round window.

v. of larynx, the part of the laryngeal cavity between the inlet and the vestibular folds.

v. of mouth, a narrow space within the oral cavity bounded by the lips and cheeks on one side and the gums and teeth on the other.

v. of vagina, the space between the labia minora within which the vaginal and urethral orifices are situated.

vestibulocochlear nerve (ves-tib″u-lo-kok′le-ar) cranial nerve VIII; consisting of two nerves, the cochlear and vestibular, both sensory and united into a single trunk. The cochlear nerve is the nerve of hearing; its fibers arise in the spiral organ of the internal ear. The vestibular nerve is the nerve of equilibration, and its fibers arise in the utricle, saccule, and semicircular canals of the internal ear. The united nerve traverses the internal auditory meatus and enters the pons. See also *cranial nerves.*

vestigial (ves-tij′e-al) [L. *vestigium* footprint] rudimentary; pertaining to a relic or a vestige, a remnant, a rudimentary or imperfectly developed organ that is not functional but was functional in the embryo or fetus or in some ancestral evolutionary form.

V factor an accessory substance required for the growth of certain species of *Hemophilus,* replaceable by NAD or NADP and present in red blood cells. Chocolate agar rather than blood agar is the medium of choice to supply V factor. See also *Hemophilus.*

VHF abbrev. See *very high frequency.*

viability (vi″ah-bil′ĭ-te) [Fr. *vie* life, from L. *vita*] in genetics, the relative number of individuals of one phenotype able to live in a specified environment as compared with those of another standard phenotype.

viable (vi′ah-b′l) alive, capable of living; especially said of a fetus that has reached a stage of development when it can live outside the uterus, or of microorganisms that have the ability to grow and multiply.

vial (vi′al) [Gr. *phialē*] a small bottle.

Vi antigen a bacterial antigen, the presence of which is used in the serologic classification of certain enteric bacteria, especially *Salmonella.* It is a polysaccharide that forms a partial layer on the cell surface, and was originally thought to be related to virulence in *S. typhi.* Vi cells can be agglutinated only by anti-H or anti-Vi antibodies. Destruction of Vi and H antigens by boiling allows agglutination by O antibodies.

vibration (vi-bra′shun) [L. *vibratio,* from *vibrare* to shake] 1. a rapid movement to and fro; tremor or quivering.

2. an oscillation; any periodic motion.

Vibrio (vib′re-o) [L. *vibro* move rapidly, vibrate] a genus of bacteria of the family Vibrionaceae that consists of gram-negative, facultatively anaerobic, straight or curved rods. The organisms are motile with a single polar flagellum. Oxidase and catalase reactions are positive; glucose is fermented with the production of acid but not gas. The genus contains the highly pathogenic nonhalophilic species *V. cholerae,* the cause of cholera. Five of the marine halophilic species described so far have been recovered from clinical specimens; they are sometimes associated with diarrheal illnesses, and occasionally with septicemia and wound infection.

V. alginolyticus, a halophilic species found in seawater and seafoods that is sometimes associated with diarrheal outbreaks, wound infections, and septicemias, but is not considered a major pathogen. The organism produces yellow colonies on thiosulfate-citrate-bile salts (TCBS) agar, may require as much as 7 percent NaCl for growth, and is oxidase- and sucrose-positive and lactose-negative.

V. cholerae, the causative agent of cholera. The organisms produce yellow colonies on TCBS agar and grow without NaCl. In stool specimens and primary cultures, the cells are characteristically curved, which is the reason this species was originally termed *V. comma.* It grows rapidly in media that are so alkaline (pH 9.0–9.6) as to inhibit most other bacteria. Reactions to lactose, sucrose, and oxidase are positive. The highly pathogenic epidemic strain secretes the potent cholera enterotoxin choleragen, and agglutinates with polyvalent 01 antiserum. Rapid identification may be made by a slide agglutination test.

This strain consists of two biotypes, the classic type, which produces severe cholera, and the El Tor vibrio, which usually produces a milder disease. At least 72 serotypes have been identified that are not agglutinated by 01 antiserum; non-01 strains exhibit a wide range of virulence, but in general cause mild, cholera-like diarrheal disease. Non-01 *V. cholerae* serotypes are unrelated to the halophilic vibrios.

See also *cholera, choleragen,* and *El Tor vibrio.*

V. fetus, see *C. fetus* under *Campylobacter.*

***V.* group F (EF-6),** a halophilic species isolated from individuals with diarrheal illness but not identified as a causative agent of human illness. The organism produces yellow colonies on TCBS agar, does not react with 01 antiserum, and requires 3–7 percent NaCl for growth. It is oxidase-negative, sucrose-positive, and lactose-variable.

V. metschnikovii, a halophilic species, found in rivers and sewage, that is not known to be pathogenic for humans. It produces yellow colonies on TCBS agar, does not react with 01 antiserum, and requires 3–7 percent NaCl for growth. It is oxidase-negative and sucrose-positive. Reactions to lactose are variable.

V. parahaemolyticus, a halophilic species, a major cause of the gastroenteritis in individuals in Japan and other countries that is due to eating raw or improperly cooked fish. The organism produces blue-green colonies on TCBS agar, requires 2–7 percent NaCl for growth, and is oxidase-positive and lactose- and sucrose-negative. Most strains produce β-hemolysis on special blood agar plates (Kanagawa phenomenon). Serotyping by O and K antigens is available.

V. vulnificus, a halophilic species found in seawater and seafoods. This organism has caused fatal septicemia in individuals with liver disease, and also wound infections following contact with infected water or seafood. The species produces blue-green colonies on TCBS agar, does not react with 01 antiserum, and requires 6 percent NaCl for growth. It is oxidase- and lactose-positive and sucrose-negative.

Vibrionaceae (vib″re-o-na′se-e) a family of facultatively anerobic, motile, straight or curved rods. It consists of five genera: *Vibrio, Acromonas, Plesiomonas, Photobacterium,* and *Lucibacterium.*

vic- a prefix word element to denote an organic compound having usually identical substituent groups on adjacent carbon atoms of a ring or chain.

vicinal (*vic-*) (vis′ĭ-nal) [L. *vicinus* neighboring] pertaining to organic compounds having substituent groups bonded to adjacent carbon atoms of a ring or chain. Cf. *geminal.*

Vidal's disease (ve-dahlz′) [Jean Baptiste Emile *Vidal,* Parisian dermatologist, 1825–1893] see *l. simplex chronicus* under *lichen.*

vidarabine (vi-dăr′ah-bēn) [USP], adenine arabinoside (ara-A), an antiviral agent that is an analog of purine nucleoside. Ara-A is effective against herpesvirus, poxvirus, and possibly hepatitis B virus groups. See also *antiviral agent.*

view (vu) in radiology, a radiograph. View refers to the orientation of the radiograph with the radiologist looking at the film as though looking at the patient. It has the opposite alignment to projection, which refers to the direction of the passage of the central ray through the patient; e.g., a posteroanterior (or posterior) view is produced by an anteroposterior projection.

view box (vu′ boks″) 1. in blood banking, a lighted box equipped with a translucent, heated horizontal surface, which is utilized for Rh slide agglutination. The surface of the box should be maintained at 40°–50°C to provide the proper temperature for reaction between red blood cells and antisera.

2. in radiology, a lighted box or panel of boxes used for viewing and interpreting radiographs.

Villaret syndrome (ve-lar-ā′) [Maurice *Villaret,* French neurologist, 1877–1946] a syndrome characterized by the disruption of function of the ninth through twelfth cranial nerves and the sympathetic pathway. It is most frequently due to lesions of the retroparotid space, including neoplasms of the parotid gland, carotid body, and regional lymph nodes. Those affected experience ipsilateral weakness or paralysis of the palatal, pharyngeal, laryngeal, sternocleidomastoid, trapezius, and lingual muscles, as well as signs and symptoms of Horner's syndrome. See also *Horner's syndrome.*

villous adenoma see *villous p.* under *polyp.*

villus (vil′lus), pl. *villi* [L. "tuft of hair"] [NA], a general term for a small, vascularized protrusion or projection from the free surface of a membrane. For more information, see the specific villus.

vinblastine sulfate (vin-blas′tēn) [USP], a cancer chemotherapeutic drug; trademark, Velban. For more information, see *Appendix A.*

Vincent's stomatitis (Vin′sents) [Henri Vincent, physician in Paris, 1862–1950] see *necrotizing ulcerative g.* under *gingivostomatitis.*

vincristine sulfate (vin-kris′tēn) [USP], a cancer chemotherapeutic drug; trademark, Oncovin. For more information, see *Appendix A.*

vindesine (vin′dĕ-sēn) a cancer chemotherapeutic drug; trademark, Eldesine. For more information, see *Appendix A.*

vinegar acid (vin′e-gar) [Fr. *vinaigre* sour wine] see *acetic acid.*

vinyl- (vi′nil) [L. *vinum* wine + *-yl*] a prefix word element in organic chemistry to denote the ethenyl group ($CH_2{=}CH{-}$), e.g., vinyl chloride, 17α-vinyl-19-nortestosterone.

vinyl chloride (vi′nil klo′rīd) a highly flammable, colorless gas with an ethereal odor, chloroethylene, $CH_2{=}CHCl$, used in the production of polyvinyl chloride plastic; M.W. 62.50. It is probably carcinogenic; an increased incidence of angiosarcoma of the liver has been associated with exposure to vinyl chloride.

vinyl polymers (vi′nil pol′ĭ-merz) the most common addition polymers. Various vinyl monomers are used to produce many high polymers, e.g., Plexiglas, polystyrene, polyethylene, and many ion exchange resins.

vinyl trichloride (vi′nil tri-klo′rid) see *1,1,2-trichloroethane.*

violet (vi′o-let) [L. *viola*] a spectral color that corresponds to the perceived hue of monochromatic light having a wavelength between 390 and 455 nm (i.e., between near-ultraviolet and blue).

viomycin (vi″o-mi′sin) an antibiotic produced by *Streptomyces puniceus.* It is an aminoglycoside and a strong base, effective against acid-fast organisms and used mainly in the treatment of tuberculosis. Viomycin may cause damage to the kidneys and to the cranial nerve. See also *antibacterial agents.*

viosterol (vi-os′ter-ol) see *ergocalciferol.*

VIP abbrev. See *vasoactive intestinal p.* under *polypeptide.*

vir/o (vi′ro) a word element used in combining form to denote virus, e.g., virology.

viral (vi′ral) pertaining to or caused by a virus.

viral inclusion an intracellular mass of new material formed as the viral multiplication cycle proceeds. These substances generally represent viral synthesis that consists either of virions or of unassembled viral components. As shown in the accompanying illustration, inclusions can be in the nucleus (e.g., adenovirus), cytoplasm (e.g., rabies virus—Negri bodies), or both (e.g., measles). Certain bodies may disrupt the structure and function of the cells and contribute to their death. Other inclusion bodies do not contain detectable virions or their components but are residues left by earlier viral multiplication, e.g., the eosinophilic, intranuclear inclusion bodies that eventually appear in cells infected by herpes simplex virus. Inclusions may have some diagnostic value but are not unique for viral infections, because certain chemicals and bacteria, especially *Chlamydia,* also produce inclusion bodies.

Virchow's node (vēr′kōz) [Rudolph Ludwig Karl *Virchow,* German pathologist, 1821–1902] see *sentinel node.*

Virchow-Robin space (vēr′ko ro-ba′) [Rudolf Ludwig Karl *Virchow;* Charles Philippe *Robin,* French anatomist, 1821–1885] a prolongation of the subarachnoid space around a vessel as it enters the brain.

viridans streptococcus (vir′ĭ-dans strep″to-kok′us) see *S. viridans group* under *Streptococcus.*

virilism (vir′ĭ-lizm) [L. *virilis* masculine, from *vir* man] masculinity; the development of masculine

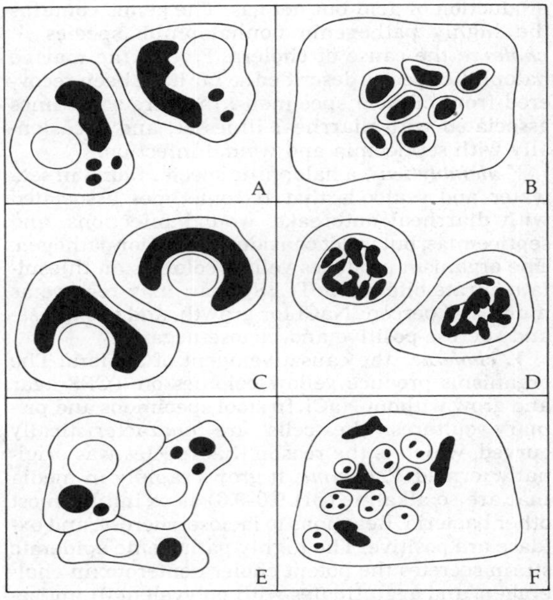

Viral inclusion. Inclusion bodies in virus-infected cells. *A,* Vaccinia virus: intracytoplasmic acidophilic inclusion (Guarnieri body). *B,* Herpes simplex virus: intranuclear acidophilic inclusion (Cowdry type A); cell fusion produces syncytium. *C,* Reovirus: perinuclear intracytoplasmic acidophilic inclusion. *D,* Adenovirus: intranuclear basophilic inclusion. *E,* Rabies virus: intracytoplasmic acidophilic inclusions (Negri bodies). *F,* Measles virus: intranuclear and intracytoplasmic acidophilic inclusions; cell fusion produces syncytium. (From Fenner, F. J., and White, D. O.: Medical Virology. 2nd ed. New York, Academic Press, 1976.)

traits in the female. See also *adrenogenital syndrome.*

virilization (vir″ĭ-li-za′shun) the abnormal development of secondary male sex characteristics in the female, along with the suppression of many female sex characteristics. This disorder may lead to changes such as hair proliferation (hirsutism), amenorrhea, hoarse voice, acne, clitoral enlargement, breast size regression, and changes in body mass distribution. The etiology may be broadly divided into two categories: adrenal virilization, leading to consistently elevated 17-ketosteroid levels; and virilization from other causes, including ovarian disorders (Stein-Leventhal syndrome, theca luteinization, and arrhenoblastoma), hypothalamic-pituitary disorders, choriocarcinoma, adrenocortical hyperplasia and neoplasms, and thymic neoplasms.

Adrenal exploration and hysterosalpinography, pelvic pneumography, and laparoscopy may be required for diagnosis. Elevated 17-ketosteroid concentrations suppressible by dexamethasone suggest either an adrenocortical or an ovarian stromal neoplasm; elevated luteinizing hormone (LH) concentrations are consistent in Stein-Leventhal syndrome. Testosterone determinations should also be performed.

See also *adrenogenital syndrome* and *congenital a. h.* under *adrenal hyperplasia.*

adrenal v., a group of syndromes, congenital or acquired, that lead to an excessive synthesis and release of adrenal androgens. Symptoms are related to the age of onset of the disorder. In the prenatal period and in childhood, excess elaboration of adrenal androgens may be due to adrenogenital syndrome with congenital adrenal hyperplasia. In the adult female, the classic signs of virilization are typically present and are caused by adrenal hyperplasia or an adrenocortical neoplasm. Adrenal hyperplasia leads to a dexamethasone-suppressible increase in 17-ketosteroids, usually due to a metabolic defect. Adrenal neoplasms, including adenomas and adenocarcinomas, cause an increase in 17-ketosteroids that is not suppressible by dexamethasone.

Although 17-ketosteroid and pregnanetriol concentrations are normally assayed in the diagnosis of this disorder, plasma 11-deoxycortisol (compound S) and 17-hydroxyprogesterone determinations are becoming more available and more frequently used. Adrenal tomography, intravenous urograms, adrenal angiograms, retroperitoneal pneumograms, and computerized tomography also are used to confirm the diagnosis.

See also *adrenogenital syndrome* and *congenital a. h.* under *adrenal hyperplasia.*

virion (vi're-on) a complete extracellular virus particle that consists of an enclosed nucleic acid core of DNA or RNA, a surrounding capsid, and sometimes an envelope. A virion may or may not be infectious.

virology (vi-rol'o-je) the science and study of viruses and viral infections. These intracellular parasites have been the source of much information in the field of molecular biology, particularly in studies of DNA and RNA. Viral infections can have many effects on the host, ranging from asymptomatic infection to acute disease, or to induction of tumor.

virulence (vir'u-lens) [L. *virulentia,* from *virus* poison] the degree of pathogenicity of a microorganism as indicated by the severity of the infection of the host and/or its ability to invade the host tissue. Virulence is sometimes expressed quantitatively as LD_{50} (median lethal dose) and ED_{50} (median effective dose).

virulent (vir'u-lent) [L. *virulentus*] pertaining to virulence; exceedingly pathogenic or noxious.

virus (vi'rus) a parasitic microorganism that consists of a core of a single type of nucleic acid (either deoxyribonucleic acid or ribonucleic acid) and a protein envelope. In general, viruses lack enzymes to reproduce and utilize the enzymes of cells they infect for reproduction; i.e., viruses cannot multiply on artificial culture media. Viruses are not sensitive to conventional antibiotics and are affected only by specific antiviral compounds. For more information, see the specific virus, *antiviral agents,* and the accompanying tables.

viscer/o (vis'er-o) [L. *viscus,* pl. *viscera*] a word element used in combining form to denote the internal organs, e.g., visceromegaly, visceroptosis.

visceral (vis'er-al) [L. *visceralis,* from *viscus*] pertaining to the viscera. Also called *splanchnic.*

visceral membrane that portion of a serous membrane (pleura, peritoneum, pericardium) that invests the surface of a viscus, in contradistinction to the parietal portion of the membrane.

viscid (vĭ-sid) [L. *viscidus*] glutinous, sticky, or adhesive.

viscosimeter (vis″ko-sim′ĕ-ter) a device used to measure the viscosity of a fluid, such as blood or serum. In a capillary viscosimeter (such as an Ostwald viscosimeter), the viscosity is determined from the time taken for a quantity of the fluid to drain through a capillary tube as compared with the time taken by a standard fluid. In a rotational viscosimeter, the viscosity is determined from the frictional drag on a rotating cylinder immersed in the fluid.

viscosity (vis-kos'ĭ-te) a physical property of fluids; the internal resistance to laminar (streamline) flow. A liquid with low viscosity, such as water, flows freely, whereas a fluid with high viscosity, such as molasses, does not.

absolute v. (η), the frictional resistance in a fluid generated by two parallel planes flowing at different velocities. It is defined as the frictional force per unit area of the planes multiplied by the separation of the planes and then divided by their relative velocity. The centimeter-gram-second (CGS) unit of viscosity is the poise (1 $dyn \cdot sec/cm^2$). Also called *dynamic v.*

dynamic v., see *absolute v.*

kinematic v. (ν), the absolute viscosity divided by the density of the fluid. The CGS unit of kinematic viscosity is the stoke (1 $cm^2/sec.$)

viscous (vis'kus) [L. *viscosus*] having a high viscosity; viscid or sticky.

viscus (vis'kus), pl. *viscera* [L.] an organ situated in a body cavity, particularly the major organs of the circulatory, digestive, endocrine, respiratory, and urogenital systems located in the abdominal and thoracic cavities.

visible (viz'ĭ-b'l) [L. *visibilis,* from *visus* past participle of *videre* to see] capable of being seen; perceptible by the sight.

visible light light having wavelengths 390–770 nm, the range in which the human eye is sensitive.

vision (vizh'un) [L. *visio,* from *videre* to see] the faculty of seeing; sight.

Vistaril (vis'tah-ril) trademark. See *hydroxyzine.*

visual (vizh'u-al) [L. *visualis,* from *videre* to see] pertaining to vision or sight.

visual evoked potential see *visual e. p.* under *evoked potential.*

vit/a, vit/o (vi'tah, vi'to) [L. *vita* life] a word element used in combining form to denote life, e.g., vitality, vitochemical.

vital capacity (VC) (vi'tal) [L. *vitalis,* from *vita* life] the maximal volume of air that can be forcefully expelled from the lungs, with no limit to the duration of expiration, following a maximal inspiratory effort. It is equal to the sum of the inspiratory capacity and the expiratory reserve volume, and amounts to approximately 3100–4600 ml in the normal young adult. The strength of the respiratory muscles, the body position of the individual during vital capacity measurement, and conditions causing a change in pulmonary compliance are major factors that affect the size of the vital capacity.

vital dye a dye that penetrates living cells and col-

VIRUS, TABLE 1. LABORATORY DIAGNOSIS OF VIRAL DISEASE

Virus	Specimen	Host	Recognition
Papovaviridae			
PML	PM (brain), urine	CC	CPE
Warts	Biopsy	Nil	Nucl incl, EM (virions)
Adenoviridae, types 1–31	Throat, feces, conjunctiva	CC hu	Slow CPE, nucl incl (B)
Herpesviridae			
Herpes simplex	Vesicle, throat, cornea, brain	CC hu	Rapid focal CPE, nucl incl (A), fluor
Varicella	Vesicle, throat, PM (lung)	CC hu fibro	Slow focal CPE, syncytia, nucl incl, fluor
Cytomegalovirus	Throat, leukocytes, urine, PM	CC hu fibro	Slow focal CPE, giant cells, nucl cyt incl
Infectious mononucleosis (EBV)	Serum	Nil	Heterophil agglutinins
	Lymphocytes	Cocultivation	Fluor
Poxviridae			
Smallpox, Vaccinia	Vesicle fluid	Nil	EM (virus), CF, gel diff
		Egg CAM	Pocks
		CC primate	Focal CPE, fluor
	Vesicle scrapings	Nil	Cyt incl (A), fluor
Picornaviridae			
Poliovirus, types 1–3	Feces, throat, PM (CNS)	CC primate	Rapid CPE
Coxsackie A, types 1–24	Feces, throat, vesicle, CSF	Newborn mouse	Generalized myositis
		CC monk kid, hu fibro	CPE (some types)
Coxsackie B, types 1–6	Feces, throat, CSF, PM (heart)	CC primate kid	Rapid CPE
		Newborn mouse	Myositis, encephalitis
Echovirus, types 1–33 and Enterovirus 68–71	Feces, throat, CSF	CC primate kid, hu fibro	CPE (often incomplete)
Rhinovirus, > 100 types	Nose	CC hu kid or fibro or HeLa	Slow CPE (often incomplete)
Togaviridae and Bunyaviridae, > 200 types	Blood, PM (brain)	Newborn mouse	Encephalitis
		CC Vero, BHK21	CPE, hemadsorption
	Serum	Nil	Serology (HI, neut)

Reoviridae, types 1–3	Feces, throat	CC primate kid	Slow CPE, cyt incl (A)
		Newborn mouse	Steatorrhea, hepatitis, encephalitis
Rotavirus	Feces	Nil	EM (virus)
Orthomyxoviridae			
Influenza A, B	Throat, PM (lung)	CC primate kid	Hemadsorption
		Egg amnion	Hemagglutination
Paramyxoviridae			
Measles	Throat, urine	CC primate kid	Syncytia, cyt nucl incl (A), fluor
	Leukocytes	Nil	Fluor
Mumps	Throat, saliva, CSF, urine	CC primate kid	Hemadsorption, syncytia, cyt incl, fluor
Parainfluenza, types 1–4	Throat	CC primate kid	Hemadsorption, cyt incl (A), fluor
Respiratory syncytial (RS)	Throat, PM (lung)	CC HEp2, hu fibro	Syncytia, cyt incl (A), fluor
Coronaviridae	Throat, nose	CC hu fibro	Incomplete CPE
Arenaviridae	Blood, CSF, PM (organs)	Newborn mouse	Encephalitis
Rhabdoviridae			
Rabies	PM (brain)	Nil	Fluor
Unclassified			
Rubella	Serum	Nil	HI
	Throat, urine, PM (organs)	RK13, Vero, SRIC	Slow focal CPE, fluor
Hepatitis A	Feces	Nil	Immuno-EM (virus)
Hepatitis B	Serum	Nil	RIA, reverse passive HA, CIEP
Norwalk agent	Feces	Nil	Immuno-EM (virus)

Note: Tests for antibody in the patient's serum have been omitted, except where the available techniques of viral isolation are unreliable. Abbreviations: A, acidophilic; B, basophilic; cyt, cytoplasmic; CC, cell culture; CAM, chorioallantoic membrane; CF, complement fixation; CIEP, counterimmunoelectrophoresis; CPE, cytopathic effect; CSF, cerebrospinal fluid; egg, embryonated hen's egg; EM, electron microscopy; fibro, fibroblastic; fluor, immunofluorescence; gel diff, gel diffusion; HI, hemagglutination inhibition; hu, human; immuno-EM, immunoelectron microscopy; incl, inclusion body; kid, kidney; monk, monkey; nucl, nuclear; neut, neutralization; PM, post-mortem; and RIA, radioimmunoassay.
From Fenner, F., and White, D.: Medical Virology. 2nd ed. New York, Academic Press, 1976, pp. 282–283.

VIRUS, TABLE 2. MEMBERS OF VIRUS FAMILIES, WITH EMPHASIS ON VIRUSES THAT INFECT HUMANS

FAMILY	GENUS	COMMON SPECIES	NO. OF MEMBERS
Picornaviridae	*Enterovirus*	Polioviruses	3
		Coxsackieviruses	23
		Echoviruses	31
		Enteroviruses 68–71	4
		Viruses of other vertebrates	34
		Viruses of invertebrates	3
		Possible member: hepatitis A virus	1
	Cardiovirus	Encephalomyocarditis (EMC) virus and Mengo virus; mouse encephalomyelitis (ME)	2
	Rhinovirus	Virus types 1A–114	>115
		Viruses of cattle	2
	Aphthovirus (foot-and-mouth disease virus)	Aphthoviruses of cattle and other cloven-hoofed animals	7
Caliciviridae	*Calicivirus*	Vesicular exanthema of swine virus (VESV)	13
		Viruses of cats, sea lions	Many
		Possible member: human calicivirus	
Reoviridae	*Reovirus*	Types 1–3	3
		Viruses of birds	5
	Orbivirus	Seventeen subgroups, including Colorado tick fever and Kemerovo viruses as well as African horse sickness virus and bluetongue virus of sheep	>80
	Rotavirus	Human rotavirus	4
		Rotaviruses of many mammals, including SA-11 virus of monkeys and Nebraska calf diarrhea virus	Many
Togaviridae	*Alphavirus* (arbovirus group A)	Sindbis virus and many other mosquito-borne viruses, including the viruses of eastern equine, Venezuelan, and western equine encephalitis, and Semliki Forest virus	22
	Flavivirus (arbovirus group B)	Yellow fever virus, and other mosquito-borne viruses, including the viruses of dengue, Japanese, Murray Valley, and St. Louis encephalitis, and West Nile fever	25
		Tick-borne viruses, including the viruses of Kyasanur Forest disease, Omsk hemorrhagic fever, European and Far Eastern tick-borne encephalitis; louping ill of sheep	11
		Viruses whose vectors are unknown	17
	Rubivirus	Rubella virus	1
	Pestivirus	Viruses of cattle and pigs	>3
Orthomyxoviridae	*Influenzavirus*	Influenza virus type A	Many
		Influenza virus type B	Several
		Influenza virus type C	1
Paramyxoviridae	*Paramyxovirus*	Parainfluenza virus	4
		Mumps virus	1
		Viruses of avian Newcastle disease and other diseases of birds and mammals	>6
	Morbillivirus	Measles virus	1
		Viruses of rinderpest (cattle) and distemper (dogs)	2

VIRUS, TABLE 2. (*Continued*)

FAMILY	GENUS	COMMON SPECIES	NO. OF MEMBERS
	Pneumovirus	Respiratory syncytial (RS) virus	1
		Respiratory disease viruses of cattle and mice	?
Rhabdoviridae	*Vesiculovirus*	Vesicular stomatitis virus of horses, cattle, swine, with some human infections also	Several
		Other viruses of various vertebrate species	Several
	Lyssavirus	Rabies virus	1
		Other viruses of various vertebrate species	Several
Retroviridae			
Oncovirinae (RNA tumor virus group)[a]	Type C oncovirus group	Sarcoma and leukemia viruses of mice, cats, cattle, birds, snakes, and primates	Many
	Type B oncovirus group	Mammary tumor virus of mice (and humans?)	
Spumavirinae		Syncytial and foamy viruses of humans, monkeys, cattle, cats	
Lentivirinae		Visna virus of sheep	
Arenaviridae	*Arenavirus*	Lymphocytic choriomeningitis virus	1
		Lassa fever virus	1
		Tacaribe complex viruses, including Junin and Machupo viruses of South American hemorrhagic fevers	8
Coronaviridae	*Coronavirus*	Human coronavirus	1
		Viruses of mouse hepatitis, avian infectious bronchitis (IBV), pig gastroenteritis, pig hemagglutinating encephalitis, and others	>4
Bunyaviridae	*Bunyavirus*	Bunyamwera virus	
		California encephalitis viruses	>11
		Twelve other groups of antigenically related viruses plus ungrouped agents	>102
	(Ungrouped genus or genera)	Eleven other serological groupings plus ungrouped agents; included are viruses of the Uukuniemi group and well-known human pathogens such as the Crimean hemorrhagic fever-Congo group, phlebotomus fever group, Rift Valley fever virus—as well as Nairobi sheep disease virus and other agents	>95
Parvoviridae	*Parvovirus*	Viruses of rodents, pigs, cattle	Many
		Possible members:	
		Norwalk gastroenteritis virus	2
		Aleutian mink disease virus	1
	Adeno-associated virus group	AAV (adeno-satellite virus)	4
		Viruses of cattle, dogs, birds	>4
Papovaviridae	*Papovavirus* A	Wart virus	Several
		Papilloma viruses of numerous animal species	Several
	Papovavirus B	BK and JC viruses	2
		Polyoma virus (mice)	1
		Simian virus 40 (monkey)	1
		Viruses of other species	3
Adenoviridae	*Mastadenovirus*	Virus types 1–34	34
		Viruses of numerous mammal species	45
	Aviadenovirus	Viruses of birds	13

VIRUS, TABLE 2. (*Continued*)

FAMILY	GENUS	COMMON SPECIES	NO. OF MEMBERS
Herpesviridae			
Alphaherpesvirinae[a]		Herpes simplex virus	2
		Varicella-zoster virus	1
		Viruses of monkeys, cattle, pigs, horses, cats	>7
Betaherpesvirinae		Cytomegalovirus	1
		Viruses of mice, pigs, and other species	>4
Gammaherpésvirinae		Epstein-Barr virus	1
		Viruses of monkeys, birds, rabbits	>5
Iridoviridae		African swine fever virus	Many
Poxviridae			
Chordopoxvirinae[a]	*Orthopoxvirus*	Smallpox virus (variola)	1
		Vaccinia virus	1
		Cowpox, monkeypox, and viruses of other species	6
	Parapoxvirus	Virus of milker's node	1
		Orf virus and other viruses of ungulates	?
	Avipoxvirus	Fowlpox virus and other bird viruses	8
	Capripoxvirus	Viruses of sheep pox, goat pox, and lumpy skin disease	3
	Leporipoxvirus	Myxoma virus of hares	
		Fibroma virus of rabbits and squirrels	2
	Suipoxvirus	Swinepox virus	1
Entomopoxvirinae		Poxviruses of insects	>24

[a] Where subfamilies have been established, their names are included in this column, e.g., Oncovirinae.
From Lennette, E. H., et al. Manual of Clinical Microbiology. 3rd ed. Washington, DC, American Society for Microbiology, 1980, pp. 775–777.

ors certain structures without serious injury to the cells.

vital red an acid disazo dye; C.I. 23570. It is used as a supravital stain to demonstrate phagocytic and pinocytic activity in living tissues. It is also used in amyloid staining.

vital signs a term for the measurements of blood pressure, pulse, respiratory rate, and body temperature, parameters commonly recorded on patients during an initial physical examination, either on an outpatient basis or as part of the hospital admission process. The measurement of vital signs is often repeated periodically during a hospital stay, as these signs are important in evaluating physiologic changes during the hospital stay. See also *blood pressure, fever, pulse,* and *respiration.*

vital staining the staining of living cells by a dye that does not kill them. See also *supravital staining.*

vitamin (vi'tah-min) [*vit-* + *amine*] a general term for a number of unrelated organic substances that occur in many foods in small amounts and that are necessary for the normal metabolic functioning of the body. They may be water-soluble or fat-soluble. For more information, see the designated vitamin below or the specific compound.

vitamin A all-*trans*-retinol, a light yellow isoprenoid pigment, $C_{20}H_{30}O$; M.W. 286.44. It is a fat-soluble vitamin found free and esterified to fatty acids in the tissues (liver, fat depots, lung, kidney) of many vertebrates, especially fish. It is synthesized in the intestinal wall and liver from carotenes (pro-vitamin A) found in most plants. β-Carotene yields two molecules of retinol per molecule, α- and γ-carotene only one. The vitamin exists and functions also as the aldehyde retinal, and as the carboxylic acid retinoic acid.

Vitamin A is essential for the integrity of epithelial cells. It plays a vital role in the visual cycle; the visual pigment rhodopsin consists of the protein opsin, linked to *cis*-retinal, which undergoes reversible reduction to *trans*-retinol. Vitamin A deficiency leads to night blindness and, if protracted, to keratomalacia and xerophthalmia (dryness, greasiness of the cornea). Vitamin A is essential for normal membrane function and proper growth. Normal values for plasma vitamin A levels are 35–70 μg/dl. Excessive quantities of the vitamin produce hyperkeratosis and can be toxic.

vitamin A_1 retinol; the form of vitamin A found in mammals; see also *retinol.*

vitamin A_1 aldehyde retinal or vitamin A_1 aldehyde. It occurs in two forms: retinene$_1$, the aldehyde of retinol, and retinene$_2$, the aldehyde of dehydroretinol. Formerly called *retinene.* See also under *vitamin A.*

vitamin A_2 an analog of vitamin A_1 in which there is an additional double bond in the ring; the form of vitamin A found in freshwater fish. Also called dehydroretinol and retinol$_2$.

vitamin A and carotene assays spectrophotometry. Vitamin A and β-carotene are extracted from a serum specimen into petroleum ether. The β-carotene concentration is proportional to the absorbance at 450 nm. If vitamin A is also to be determined, the above petroleum ether extract is evaporated, and the residue is dissolved in chloroform and reacted with trifluoroacetic acid (or antimony trichloride). As both vitamin A and β-carotene form a blue color that absorbs at 620 nm, a correction for β-carotene must be made. The correction factor F is the ratio of the absorbance of β-carotene at 450 nm to the absorption of the color product at 620 nm as determined with a carotene standard solution. The vitamin A concentration is proportional to $A_{620} - F \times A_{450}$.

vitamin A clearance test a method for determining the presence of malabsorption. An individual in the fasting state is given 7500 IU of vitamin A palmitate per kilogram of body weight, and vitamin A determinations are carried out before, and at intervals of 4, 5, and 6 hr after administration of the vitamin. Individuals with malabsorption have only a slight increase in serum levels of vitamin A, whereas those with normal absorption show a peak increase up to 80 μmol/l.

vitamin B_1 see *thiamine.*

vitamin B_2 see *riboflavin.*

vitamin B_3 see *niacin.*

vitamin B_6 a group of water-soluble vitamins, including pyridoxine, pyridoxal, and pyridoxamine, found in most foods, especially meats, liver, vegetables, whole-grain cereals, and egg yolk. The vitamin B_6 group functions as coenzymes, and participate in the metabolism of amino acids (during their decarboxylation, transamination, deamination, or the modification of their side-chains), the degradation of tryptophan, and the breakdown of glycogen to glucose-1-phosphate. Daily requirements are: for adults, 1.6–20 mg/da; for pregnant females, 2.5; and for infants, 0.3. Deficiencies in vitamin B_6 are observed in a variety of conditions including chronic alcoholism, malnutrition, malabsorption, pregnancy, and gestational diabetes. Reference values for vitamin B_6 are 4–18 ng/ml. See also *pyridoxal, pyridoxamine,* and *pyridoxine.*

vitamin B_6 assay enzymatic assay using radiolabeled substrate. Deproteinized EDTA plasma and aqueous vitamin B_6 standards are incubated with tyrosine apodecarboxylase. The resulting activated enzyme catalyzes the decarboxylation of an L-tyrosine-1-^{14}C substrate. The $^{14}CO_2$ that is formed is then released from solution by the addition of HCl and is trapped on a KOH-soaked paper wick; the wick is subsequently added to scintillation fluid and counted in a suitable beta counter. This method is considered the most reliable indicator of vitamin B_6 status.

Other methods for the measurement of vitamin B_6 include: direct assessment in urine or blood utilizing microbiologic assays with specific strains of microorganisms (e.g., *Saccharomyces carlsbergensis*); fluorometric assays after condensation of vitamin B_6 with a fluorophore such as methyl anthranilate; indirect assessment by the measurement of urinary tryptophan metabolites, particularly xanthurenic acid, following an oral load of L-tryptophan (vitamin B_6 is an important coenzyme in several of the reactions forming tryptophan metabolites); and indirect assessment by measuring the activation of erythrocyte aspartate or alanine aminotransferase activity after addition of vitamin B_6.

vitamin B_7 see *biotin.*

vitamin B_{12} cyanocobalamin, a hematopoietic vitamin; M.W. 1355.42. It is a red-colored material and consists of two main parts: a porphyrin-like corrin ring system and a 2,3-dimethylbenzene imidazole nucleotide A. Cobalt ion is chelated to the corrin ring, to the nucleotide via the imidazole, and to a cyanide ion. B_{12} is produced by microorganisms and occurs in some seafood and in egg yolk. It is found in the body in the liver, kidneys, and heart. The term B_{12} is used as a generic name for a family of cobalamin vitamins, all analogous to cyanocobalamin, in which ligands other than cyanide are chelated to the cobalt. These include hydroxocobalamin (vitamin B_{12a}), aquocobalamin (vitamin B_{12b}), nitrocobalamin, and methylcobalamin. B_{12} is absorbed in the intestine (ileum) after binding with a specific glycoprotein, called the intrinsic factor.

B_{12} deficiency, which arises from the absence of effective intrinsic factor (secreted by the gastric mucosa), is known as pernicious anemia. Other B_{12} deficiencies lead to megaloblastic (macrocytic) anemias, which result from the improper maturation of erythrocytes. The more complex deoxyadenosyl- and methyl-derivatives of B_{12} (cobalamides, with no CN^-) serve as true coenzymes in methylation and methyl transfer reactions; a deficiency of B_{12} is associated with methylmalonic aciduria. Vitamin B_{12} is also implicated in the maintenance of the myelin of the nervous system (see *subacute combined degeneration* of the *s. c.* under *spinal cord*). True B_{12} levels in serum are assayed using RIA techniques.

Reference ranges for vitamin B_{12} are: for newborns, 160–900 pg/ml; and for adults; 140–700.

See also *cyanocobalamin.*

vitamin B_{12} absorption test see *Schilling test.*

vitamin B_{12} assays 1. radioassay using intrinsic factor as the binding protein. This is the most accurate and preferred method and is based on the principles of competitive protein binding. The sample is added to ^{57}Co-labeled vitamin B_{12} and after inactivation of endogenous binding proteins, intrinsic factor (IF) is added to the mixture as binder. After an incubation period, the bound and free fractions of vitamin B_{12} are separated, and either fraction is counted in a gamma-scintillation counter. Levels of vitamin B_{12} in the samples are determined by interpolation from a suitable calibration curve constructed with results obtained from calibration standards included in the assay.

If the IF is not highly purified, it may contain R proteins, which will bind B_{12} as well as related metabolically inactive compounds (B_{12} analogs) that may be present in the sample, thereby causing artificially elevated B_{12} results. To measure only metabolically active B_{12} ("true B_{12}") in CPB assays, the IF must be highly purified, or cobinamide (B_{12} analog) must be added to the IF to saturate all binding sites on the R-proteins. Cobinamide is not bound by IF since IF is highly specific for true B_{12}.

2. microbiologic assay utilizing *Euglena gracilis* or *Lactobacillus leichmannii.* This method is not frequently used because it may give falsely low values in the presence of antibiotics or tranquilizers, and also because it is time consuming.

3. deoxyuridine suppression test. This test is performed on bone marrow cells aspirated from the patient. Vitamin B_{12} deficiency is shown if there is reduction in the suppression of radioactive iododeoxyuridine incorporation into DNA by deoxyuridine; the reduction can be corrected by vitamin B_{12} but not by folic acid.

4. the Schilling test. This is a measure of the absorption of vitamin B_{12} by administering radioactive B_{12} and measuring the urinary excretion. Malabsorption of vitamin B_{12} occurs when less than 9 percent of the radioactivity is found in the first 24-hr urine collection. See also *Schilling test.*

vitamin B_c the former name for *folic acid.*

vitamin B_x see *p-aminobenzoic acid.*

vitamin B complex a group of water-soluble vitamins including thiamine (B_1), riboflavin (B_2), niacin (B_3), pyridoxine (B_6), cyanocobalamin (B_{12}), pantothenic acid, folic acid, and biotin.

vitamin C see *ascorbic acid.*

vitamin D a generic name for structurally related, fat-soluble sterols that have the biologic activity of ergocalciferol (vitamin D_2) or cholecalciferol (vitamin D_3). These sterols are converted in the body first to 25-hydroxyvitamin D, the major circulating form of vitamin D, and then by the kidneys to 1,25-dihydroxyvitamin D, the most active hormone. The latter acts on target tissues such as intestine and bone to maintain the plasma calcium and phosphate concentration. Vitamin D deficiency causes rickets in children and osteomalacia and osteoporosis in adults and may lead to hypocalcemic tetany. Also called *calciferol.*

vitamin D assays 1. assays for 25-hydroxyvitamin D (25-OH-D). Fat-soluble D vitamins are extracted from serum or plasma and then added to gel filtration columns (e.g., Sephadex LH-20) to separate 25-OH-D from other metabolites and lipophilic contaminants. The eluent containing 25-OH-D is then assayed using a competitive protein-binding assay, using a specific protein binder from rat kidney or serum. Alternatively, the purified eluent containing both 25-OH-D_3 (25-hydroxycholecalciferol) and 25-OH-D_2 (25-hydroxyergocholecalciferol) may be resolved and quantitated using high-pressure liquid chromatography (HPLC) and UV detection at 254 nm.

2. assays for 1,25-dihydroxycholecalciferol (1,25-OH-D_3). Isolation of 1,25-OH-D_3 from serum or plasma requires multiple solvent extractions and purification by HPLC. The resulting eluent can then be assayed by a receptor assay that uses chick intestinal cytosol as the specific protein binder.

vitamin E α-tocopherol, a fat-soluble vitamin, 2,5,7,8-tetramethyl-2-(4′,8′,12′-tri-methyltridecyl)-6-chromanol; M.W. 430.69. Vitamin E behaves as a strong antioxidant and prevents lipid peroxidation, particularly that of polyunsaturated fatty acids. It is necessary in the diet of many species for normal reproduction, development of muscle, and resistance of erythrocytes to hemolysis.

Vitamin E is acquired from such dietary sources as eggs, muscle, liver, fish, chicken, oatmeal, corn, soya, cotton, wheat, and rice seed oils, and products containing these oils. Other members of the tocopherol family (β, γ, δ, ϵ) containing fewer methyl groups on the benzene portion of the chroman structure also possess vitamin E activity, but less so than α-tocopherol. Reference ranges for vitamin E in blood are 361–412 μg/dl.

vitamin E assays fluorometric methods in which, following a protein precipitation, vitamin E is extracted into hexane and quantitated by determining its fluorescence relative to pure standards.

vitamin H the former name for vitamin B_7; see *biotin.*

vitamin K a group of fat-soluble vitamins, all derivatives of 2-methyl-1,4-naphthoquinone, including vitamins K_1, K_2, and K_3, that promote clotting of the blood. All forms have methyl groups at position 2, but K_1 and K_2 have different isoprene polymer side-chains at position 3. K vitamins play a key role in the posttranslational transformation of Factors II (prothrombin), VII, IX, and X from precursors to their biologically active forms in hepatocytes. They mediate the γ-carboxylation of glutamic acid residues that are clustered near the amino-terminal end of these factors. The modified residues serve as binding sites for calcium ions, which are necessary for their activity. K vitamins are acquired naturally from dietary sources, such as plants (K_1) and fish and meat (K_2), and are also synthesized by intestinal bacteria (K_2). A deficiency in vitamin K leads to hemorrhagic disorders. These vitamins, especially K_3, are used clinically in the treatment of prothrombin deficiency in obstructive jaundice and other liver diseases, and in the treatment of hemorrhagic states associated with intestinal diseases and the hypoprothrombinemia of the newborn. For more information, see the individual forms of vitamin K.

vitamin K_1 a naturally occurring, fat-soluble vitamin, 2-methyl-3-phytyl-1,4-naphthoquinone, obtained from plants; M.W. 450.68. Vitamin K_1 promotes the clotting of blood and is also essential to the phosphorylation processes involved in photosynthesis in green plants. Vitamin K_1 is used as a prothrombinogenic agent, and in veterinary medicine as an antidote for warfarin poisoning. Also called *phylloquinone.*

vitamin K_1 oxide 2-methyl-3-phytyl-1,4-naphthoquinone-2,3-oxide, one of the active forms of vitamin K_1; M.W. 466.68.

vitamin K_2 menaquinone, 2-methyl-3-all-*trans*-polyprenyl-1,4-naphthoquinone; one of the class of K vitamins obtained from fish meal and possessing polyisoprenyl side-chains that have a range of 30–60 carbons in length; thus, vitamin $K_2(30)$ is 2-methyl-3-hexaprenyl-1,4-naphthoquinone.

vitamin K_3 [NF], menadione, 2-methyl-1,4-naphthoquinone; a bright yellow, crystalline powder used as a substitute for vitamin K. It is almost as effective, on a molar basis, as vitamin K_1.

vitamin K assays a colorimetric assay in which an ethanolic solution of vitamin K is mixed with solutions of sodium diethyldithiocarbamate and sodium ethylate. Vitamin K_1 gives a deep cobalt blue color, with absorbance at 575 nm.

vitellin (vi-tel′in) [L. *vitellus* yolk] a phosphoprotein found in the yolk of eggs.

vitelline (vi-tel′in) [L. *vitellus* yolk] resembling or pertaining to the yolk of an egg or ovum.

vitelline duct see *omphalomesenteric d.* under *duct.*

vitellointestinal duct (vi-tel″o-in-tes′tĭ-nal) see *omphalomesenteric d.* under *duct.*

vitiligo (vit″ĭ-li′go) [L.] a loss of pigmentation usually occurring as small white spots that gradually enlarge. These lesions are generally limited to certain areas of the body, e.g., a dermatome, or the extensor surfaces, bony prominences, eyes, and mouth. Occasionally the loss of pigmentation extends to involve much of the body. Sometimes there is some repigmentation. Melanocytes are absent or markedly reduced in the affected areas.

The disorder has no known cause, although it may be associated with several endocrine disorders, candidiasis, pernicious anemia, and alopecia areata. In 30 percent of cases a genetic or familial pattern of transmission has been noted.

vitre/o (vit′re-o) [L. *vitrium* glass] a word element used in combining form to denote glassy, e.g., vitreodentin.

vitreous (vit′re-us) [L. *vitreus* glassy] 1. glasslike or hyaline.

2. the transparent substance that fills the eyeball between the lens and the retina. Also called vitreous body.

Vivactil (vi-vak′til) trademark. See *protriptyline.*

vivax malaria (vi′vaks mah-lār′e-ah) see *P. vivax* under *Plasmodium.*

Viviparidae (vi″vĭ-pār′ĭ-de) [L. *vivus* alive + *parere* to bear + Gr. *-idae* sons of] a family of freshwater snails, including the genus *Viviparus.*

Viviparus (vi-vip′ah-rus) a genus of freshwater snails. In Java, the species *V. javanicus* is found as a secondary intermediate host of the fluke *Echinostoma ilocanum.*

VLDL abbrev. for very-low-density lipoprotein. See *very-low-density l.* under *lipoprotein.*

VLSI abbrev. see *very-large-scale integration.*

VMA abbrev. See *vanillylmandelic acid.*

vocal (vo′kal) [L. *vocalis,* from *vox* voice] pertaining to the voice.

vocal cord one of the paired folds of mucous membrane within the larynx. The false vocal cords are found superiorly to the true vocal cords and separate the laryngeal vestibule from the ventricle, whereas the true vocal cords form the inferior boundary of the laryngeal ventricle and are concerned with phonation.

vocal fold a true vocal cord.

Voges-Proskauer test (vo′jes pros′kow-er) [Otto *Voges,* German physician, born 1867; Bernard *Proskauer,* German hygienist, 1851–1915] a widely used procedure for the differentiation of Enterobacteriaceae species. It tests for the production of acetylmethylcarbinol, which is oxidized to diacetyl. This reacts with creatine in the culture medium to form a pink compound. Also called the V-P test; one of the *IMVIC tests.*

Vogt-Koyanagi disease [Alfred *Vogt,* Swiss ophthalmologist, 1879–1943; Yosizo *Koyanagi,* Japanese ophthalmologist, born 1880] a form of uveomeningitis that is associated with vitiligo, poliosis, alopecia, and deafness, usually in young Oriental adults. See also *uveomeningitis.*

vol abbrev. See *volume.*

volatile (vol′ah-til) [L. *volatilis,* from *volare* to fly] having an appreciable vapor pressure at room temperature, i.e., appreciable volumes of liquid enter the gaseous state, evaporating or subliming readily.

volatile oil an oil that evaporates readily. Volatile oils occur in aromatic plants, to which they give odor and other characteristics. Most volatile oils consist of a mixture of two or more terpenes or a mixture of an eleopten with a stearopten. Many have been used as abortifacients, but their high toxicity, particularly to the liver and kidney, preclude their use with safety. Also called distilled oil, essential oil, and ethereal oil.

volatile organic substances assay see *head space analysis.*

volatility (vol″ah-til′ĭ-te) the property of being volatile, i.e., evaporating rapidly.

volatilization (vol″ah-til-ĭ-za′shun) conversion into a vapor.

vole bacillus (vōl bah-sil′lus) see *M. microti* under *Mycobacterium.*

Volkmann's canals (fōlk′mahnz) [Alfred Wilhelm *Volkmann,* German physiologist, 1800–1877] transverse channels in bone that connect the haversian canals.

Volkmann's paralysis (folk′mahnz) [Richard von *Volkmann,* German surgeon, 1830–1889] see *Volkmann's p.* under *paralysis.*

volt (V) (vōlt) [Alessandro *Volta,* Italian physiologist and physicist, 1745–1827] the International System (SI) unit of electric potential equal to 1 joule per coulomb (1 J/C).

voltage (V) (vōl′tij) the energy required to move a unit charge between two points of an electric circuit; measured in volts. Also called *electric potential difference* and *electromotive force.*

voltage divider two resistors connected in series across a voltage source. The output voltage is taken across one of the resistors. It is the same fraction of the input voltage as the output resistor is of the sum of the two resistances. A potentiometer (variable resistor) can be used to make an adjustable voltage divider.

voltage drop the voltage produced across an electrical component. See also *IR drop.*

voltage-regulating transformer a saturated-core transformer that produces an output constant to within about 5 percent when the input voltage is varied by up to 20 percent.

voltage regulator a device that maintains the output voltage of a generator or regulated power supply despite changes in the input voltage or load.

electronic v. r., the circuit in a regulated power supply that maintains a preset output voltage despite changes in the load or line voltage. It operates by comparing a fraction of the output voltage with a reference voltage (usually produced by a Zener diode). Any difference is amplified and used to control a variable load (e.g., a power transistor) placed in series (a series regulator) or in parallel (a shunt regulator) with the load across the output terminals. The variable load is adjusted until the error difference is corrected.

IC v. r., a complete electronic voltage regulator on an integrated circuit chip.

voltage-regulator tube a glow-discharge tube, a gas-filled electron tube in which the voltage drop is nearly independent of the current over a wide range of current values.

voltage-to-frequency converter an electronic circuit that produces an output that is a train of equal-width rectangular pulses at a frequency proportional to the input voltage level. The input voltage is integrated, and the integrator output is compared with a reference voltage. When the reference voltage is exceeded, a comparator circuit resets the integrator to zero and triggers a monostable multivibrator, which produces an output pulse.

volt-ampere (VA) (vōlt′ am′pēr) a unit of apparent power in alternating current circuits equal in magnitude to 1 watt.

voltmeter (vōlt′me-ter) an instrument for measuring the electric potential difference (voltage) between two points. See also *digital voltmeter, electronic voltmeter, vacuum tube voltmeter,* and *volt-ohm-milliammeter.*

volt-ohm-milliammeter (VOM) (vo′lt′ ōm′ mil″e-am′me-ter) a portable, electric test instrument for measuring voltage, resistance, and current. It is composed of a D'Arsonval meter, series and shunt resistances that can be switched into the circuit to provide different measuring ranges, and a battery to provide the current for resistance measurement. Also called *multimeter.*

volume (vol′ūm) [L. *volumen* scroll] 1. (abbrev. V.), the capacity or size of an object or region of space. The coherent International System (SI) unit of volume is the cubic meter (m^3). The liter (l), a noncoherent derived unit of a more convenient size, 10^{-3} m^3, has also been adopted as an SI unit. For more information, see the specific volume.

2. in data processing, a unit of external storage that is all on-line at one time, e.g., a magnetic tape or a disk pack.

volume conduction the spread of current through the electrolytic conducting medium of the body fluid, especially in inactive fluid-filled tissues.

volumetric (vol″u-met′rik) 1. pertaining to or accompanied by measurement in volumes.

2. used for measuring volumes as in volumetric glassware, e.g., burets, pipets, and graduated cylinders.

voluntary (vol′un-tār″e) [L. *voluntas* will] accomplished with willed effort; the term is generally used in reference to consciously controlled muscle contraction.

voluntary activity the electric and mechanical activity that can be recorded during a muscle contraction initiated and controlled through conscious effort. The degree of effort used and the resulting strength of contraction should be specified in relative or absolute terms as an accompaniment to the electromyographic record.

voluntary muscle any part of the skeletal musculature that is under direct voluntary control.

volutin (vo-lu′tin) a bacterial polymer of orthophosphate. Occurring as cytoplasmic granular inclusions (metachromatic granules), volutin serves as an intracellular phosphate reserve and has a marked affinity for basic dyes such as methylene blue. These granules are present in abundance in diphtheria bacilli, especially when grown in nutrient-deficient media.

volvulus (vol′vu-lus) [L. *volvere* to twist round] a rotation of a length of bowel about an axis that passes through the mesentery. This rotation first produces bowel obstruction, accompanied by continuous pain of varying intensity, abdominal enlargement, and vomiting. As rotation continues, the blood supply to the involved bowel is cut off, and death of that segment occurs, with contamination of the peritoneal cavity and a high mortality rate.

Two major groups are affected: infants, who acquire volvulus through a failure of the gut (in development) to rotate to its usual position; and older adults, who, because of congenital anomalies, poor patterns of elimination, or high-residue diets, may develop volvulus of the cecum or large intestine.

Diagnosis is made by the history of symptoms attributable to intestinal obstruction, physical examination, and x-ray findings, which vary with the segment of bowel involved.

VOM abbrev. See *volt-ohm-milliammeter.*

vomer (vo′mer) [L. "plowshare"] an unpaired bone of the skull, roughly trapezoidal in shape, that forms the posterior part of the nasal septum.

vomit (vom′it) [L. *vomitare*] 1. the material brought up from the gut and out through the mouth. Such material may be from the stomach, as caused by food poisoning or toxins, etc., or from lower in the gastrointestinal tract when there is obstruction of the bowel distal to the stomach.

2. to bring up material from the gut; the process is caused by stimulation of vomiting centers in the central nervous system.

vomiting (vom′it-ing) a common general symptom in which food and other contents of the gastrointestinal tract are expelled through the mouth. Vomiting may be simply the result of food or alcohol abuse, food poisoning, or other gastrointestinal disturbances associated with nausea, or it may be severe and prolonged, reflecting a serious systemic disorder such as uremia. The vomiting center is located in the medulla; it may be centrally stimulated by increased intracranial pressure, toxins, and central emetics such as morphine. Peripheral, afferent stimulation of the vomiting center may reflect GI disturbance or disorders in other organs. Also called *emesis.*

vomitus (vom′ĭ-tus) [L.] the material vomited or brought up from the stomach.

von Bechterew's disease (bek-ter′yevs) [Vladimir Mikhailovich *von Bechterew,* Russian neurologist, 1857–1927] see *ankylosing s.* under *spondylitis.*

von Gierke's disease (gēr′kez) [Edgar Otto Konrad von *Gierke,* German pathologist, 1877–1945] a hereditary disease of glycogen metabolism, transmitted as an autosomal recessive trait, that is due to a relative or absolute deficiency of the specific enzyme glucose-6-phosphatase. This disease is characterized by an excess storage of glycogen within the liver and kidneys (hepatorenal form). It usually becomes manifest during the first year of life, with convulsions related to hypoglycemia, hyperlipemia, and lipid deposits. The kidneys and liver are enlarged, with glycogen and fat deposits. Infants with this disease fail to thrive and have retarded growth and large abdomens; many die from intercurrent infections. Also called glycogen storage disease I. See also *glycogenoses.*

von Hippel's disease (hip′elz) [Eugen *von Hippel,* German ophthalmologist, 1867–1939] retinal capillary angiomas associated with von Hippel–Lindau disease. See also *von Hippel–Lindau disease.*

von Hippel–Lindau disease (hip′el lin′dow) [Eugen *von Hippel;* Arvid *Lindau,* Swedish pathologist, born 1892] a genetic disease, transmitted as an autosomal dominant trait, that is characterized by vascular malformations, primarily retinal capillary angiomas (von Hippel's disease), and cerebellar hemangioblastomas (Lindau's disease). The retinal neoplasms lead to a slowly progressive loss of vision. The cerebral neoplasms are often multiple and cystic, and lead to dizziness, ataxia, and increased intercranial pressure. Polycythemia is commonly found. A variety of other neoplasms are seen in this syndrome, including renal adenocarcinomas and cystic angiomas of the kidneys, pancreas, and liver. Pheochromocytomas have been reported in association with this disease. Also called *Lindau–von Hippel.*

von Kossa's method (kos′az) [Julius *von Kossa,* Hungarian pharmacologist, born 1865] see under *calcium deposit demonstration.*

von Meyenburg's complex (mi′en-burgz) a microhamartoma of the liver, which is of no clinical significance. The lesion is typically small, round, and well circumscribed, and is usually located adjacent to portal tracts. It is composed of irregular, dilated bile ducts set in a mature connective tissue stroma. In affected individuals, several complexes may be found in the same biopsy. There is a frequent association with congenital cystic disease of the liver and polycystic disease of the kidneys. Also called bile duct hamartoma, cholangial adenoma, congenital hyperplasia of the interlobular ducts, and multiple microhamartomatosis.

von Recklinghausen's disease (rek′ling-how″-zenz) [Friedrich Daniel *von Recklinghausen,* German pathologist, 1833–1910] see *neurofibromatosis.*

Von Recklinghausen's disease of bone [Friedrich Daniel *von Recklinghausen*] see *osteitis fibrosa cystica.*

von Willebrand antigen (vil′ĕ-brand) [Erik Adolf *von Willebrand,* Finnish physician, 1870–1949] an antigen precipitated by a rabbit antibody to Factor VIII; it is absent in von Willebrand's disease, but is present both in normal plasma and in the plasma of hemophiliacs. Also called Factor VIII_{AGN} or Factor VIII–related antigen.

von Willebrand's disease [E. A. *von Willebrand*] a bleeding disorder, transmitted as an autosomal dominant trait, that is characterized by a prolonged bleeding time, impaired platelet adhesiveness, impaired ristocetin aggregation, and a concordant decrease in the levels of antihemophiliac Factor VIII, von Willebrand factor (VIII_{VWF}), and Factor VIII antigen (VIII_{AGN}). Many variants have been described, leading to several expressions of the disorder and wide fluctuation in laboratory results. The bleeding tends to be mucosal and cutaneous, and in severe cases may be excessive.

von Willebrand factor [E. A. *von Willebrand*] the property of Factor VIII that is necessary for normal platelet function. It is distinct from the coagulant and antigenic properties of the antihemophiliac factor molecule and is probably required for a normal bleeding time. Also called Factor VIII_{VWF}, Factor VIII-vwf, *ristocetin cofactor,* VWF factor, and VIII-rist. See also *Factor VIII.*

vortex (vor′teks), pl. *vortices* [L. "whirl"] 1. a whorled arrangement, design, or pattern, as of muscle fibers, or of the ridges or hairs on the skin.

2. [NA], a general term for a structure having a whorled arrangement, design, or pattern.

VPB abbrev. for *v*entricular *p*remature *b*eat; see *premature ventricular contraction.*

VPC abbrev. for vapor-phase chromatography (see *gas chromatography*), *v*entricular *p*remature *c*ontraction (see *premature ventricular contraction*).

VPD abbrev. for *v*entricular *p*remature *d*epolarization; see *premature ventricular contraction.*

VP test see *Voges-Proskauer test.*

Vr abbrev. See *relaxation volume.*

VTVM abbrev. See *vacuum tube voltmeter.*

vulv/o (vul′vo) [L. *vulva* covering, womb] a word element used in combining form to denote the vulva, e.g., vulvovaginitis, vulvectomy.

vulva (vul′vah) [L. "covering, womb"] the external genitalia of the female. Also called *pudendum femininum* and *pudendum muliebre.*

vulvar tumors (vul′var) neoplasms of the vulva. Abnormalities of the stratified squamous epithelium of the vulva range from mild dysplasia to invasive carcinoma. Carcinoma in situ may be multifocal, or may be present at the edge of an infiltrating tumor; it must be distinguished from a condyloma, which is a papilloma of viral etiology. The prognosis for invasive squamous carcinoma of the vulva depends on the size and depth of the primary lesion and on the presence or absence of lymph node metastases. Five-year survival rates in excess of 70 percent have been reported, but the rate drops below 50 percent when there is nodal involvement.

Paget's disease of the vulva is histologically similar to that of the nipple, although an underlying carcinoma may not be found. Primary melanoma of the vulva is histologically similar to malignant melanoma seen on cutaneous surfaces, but it has a relatively poor prognosis.

Hidradenoma papilliferum is an adenoma of apocrine sweat glands that can be mistaken histologically for an adenocarcinoma.

vulvitis (vul-vi′tis) [*vulv-* + *-itis* inflammation] an inflammation of the vulva. It may be due to a mechanical irritation by certain fabrics, chemical irritation, an allergic reaction to underclothes or medications, or the extension of infection from a vaginitis. Local moisture and heat may combine to produce a pruritic vulvitis, especially in obese women. Vulvitis may also be associated with atrophy or dystrophy of the vulvar skin, as in lichen sclerosis, or with neoplastic disorders. See also *vaginitis.*

vulvovaginitis (vul″vo-vaj″ĭ-ni′tis) an inflammation of the vulva and vagina that is characterized by pruritus, pain on intercourse, and vaginal discharge; it may occur in females of any age. In children, the condition is usually due to a foreign body lodged in the vagina; in adults, it is usually due to infection. Possible pathogens include *Neisseria gonorrhoeae, Candida albicans, Hemophilis vaginalis, Trichomonas vaginalis,* and herpes simplex virus type 2. Cultures of any discharge should be made to isolate the etiologic agent, which should then be treated appropriately.

v/v abbrev. for volume of solute per volume of solution; e.g., a 70 percent (v/v) solution contains 70 volumes of one solvent or liquid per 100 volumes of total solution. This form is no longer recommended and should be replaced by liter of solute per liter of total solution.

V wave abbrev. See *vertex sharp transient.*

v wave see under *jugular venous pulse.*

W

W symbol for *tryptophan,* the chemical element *tungsten* (wolfram), *watt, work.*

Waardenburg's syndrome (var'den-bergz) [Petrus Johannes *Waardenburg,* Dutch ophthalmologist, born 1872] a form of albinism, transmitted as an autosomal dominant trait, that is characterized by deafness, a broad nasal bridge, irregular coloration of the irises, white eyelashes, and white forelock. Those affected may show only one or two of the characteristics.

wakefulness (wāk'ful-nes) a behavioral state marked by high sensitivity to external stimuli and characteristic low-voltage, high-frequency electric activity in the brain.

Waldenström's macroglobulinemia (vahl'den-stremz mac″ro-glob″u-lĭ-ne'me-ah) [Johan Henning *Waldenström,* orthopedic surgeon in Stockholm, born 1877] a rare, slowly progressive malignant neoplastic disorder of B lymphocytes, with plasmacytic morphology, in which the lymphocytes secrete IgM components. It is observed particularly in males older than 50 yr. It is associated with the proliferation of plasmacytic B lymphocytes that form IgM paraprotein. Clinical features include adenopathy, hepatomegaly, splenomegaly, hemorrhagic phenomena, anemia, neurologic sequelae, and lymphocytosis and plasmacytosis of the bone marrow.

Patients frequently present with symptoms and signs resulting from serum hyperviscosity; a relative serum viscosity of >3.0 units is associated with moderate symptoms and >7.0 with severe symptoms. Factors contributing to the hyperviscosity include the serum concentration of IgM, rouleaux formation, cryoprecipitation, antibody against serum proteins, and vascular factors. The IgM usually is in the pentameric 19S form, although many with the disorder have monomeric 7S IgM due to a biosynthetic abnormality of the malignant clone. Ten percent of those affected have Bence Jones proteinuria.

Waldeyer's ring (vahl'di-erz) [Heinrich Wilhelm Gottfried von *Waldeyer,* anatomist in Berlin, 1836–1921] a circular band of lymphoid tissue, consisting of the palatine, tubal, lingual, and pharyngeal tonsils, that surrounds the back of the oropharynx.

Wallenberg's syndrome (vahl'en-bergz) [Adolf *Wallenberg,* German physician, 1862–1949] a neurologic syndrome caused by occlusion of one vertebral or posterior inferior cerebellar artery. On the side of the blocked vessel, there is numbness of the face and limbs, unsteadiness and incoordination of the limbs, Horner's syndrome, and a paralyzed vocal cord. On the contralateral side, appreciation of pain and temperature is impaired over the limbs and trunk.

wallerian degeneration (wol-le're-an) [Augustus Volney *Waller,* English physician, 1816–1870] the sequence of degenerative changes that occurs in the distal portion of a sectioned peripheral nerve. A few hours or days after severance from its cell body, an axon undergoes a progressive disintegration and resorption that begins with the degeneration of the neurilemmal cells and axis cylinder, and is followed by a dissolution into globules of the myelin sheath. After several days, macrophages appear to ingest the myelin globules and other fragments of the disintegrating fibers until all remnants of the axis cylinder and myelin sheath are removed and only cords of neurilemmal cells remain. The process of regeneration may begin simultaneously with this degeneration.

Conduction velocity is slowed throughout either the entire length or distal portion of a nerve undergoing wallerian degeneration. Following degeneration, distal stimulation of a motor nerve evokes a muscle action potential that is decreased in both amplitude and area, until conduction fails completely and no response can be obtained (7–10 da).

Also called *axonal degeneration* and *axonal reaction.*

Walsh average (wawlsh) see under *signed rank test.*

Walthard rests [Max *Walthard,* Swiss gynecologist, 1867–1933] serosal epithelial nodules located in the subserosa of the fallopian tubes—usually 1 to 2 mm in diameter, commonly found incidentally during routine pathologic examination. They are of no clinical significance but are of interest because of their uncertain histogenesis and a resemblance to Brenner tumors of the ovary. Their origin is generally attributed to epithelial metaplasia of mesothelial cell–lined inclusion cysts of the fallopian tube derived from the fallopian tube serosa. Because Brenner tumors are found in the ovary but not the fallopian tubes and because glycogen is present in cells of the Brenner tumor but not cells forming Walthard rests, it is argued that there is no histogenetic relationship despite the cytologic similarity between cells of these two entities. See also *Brenner tumor.*

warble fly (wor'b'l) see *Dermatobia.*

warbles (war'b'lz) a common name for flies of the genus *Hypoderma,* whose larvae parasitize domestic and wild animals, and occasionally humans.

warfarin (war'fah-rin) [named for *Wisconsin Alumni Research Foundation*] one of the coumarin group of anticoagulant drugs used to treat venous thrombosis, pulmonary embolism, atrial fibrillation with embolization, and transient cerebral ischemic attacks.

Warfarin inhibits the synthesis of the prothrombin complex of coagulation factors (Factors II, VII, IX, and X). The active factors are formed in the liver by carboxylation of precursor proteins accompanied by oxidation of vitamin K; warfarin blocks the reduction of oxidized vitamin K back to the active form. The anticoagulant effect is thus delayed until the prothrombin complex factors and vitamin K are cleared from the blood. The dosage is then adjusted until the desired prothrombin time is achieved.

The most common adverse reaction is hemorrhage due to excessive depletion of prothrombin. The anticoagulant effect is increased by the presence of drugs (e.g., phenylbutazone, clofibrate) that displace warfarin bound to plasma proteins, and is decreased by barbiturates, which induce an increase in warfarin metabolism.

Warfarin is also one of the most widely used and safest of rodent poisons. Because of the delay in the effect, the single lethal dose is about 100 times the lethal continuous daily dose.

w. potassium, [USP], the potassium salt of warfarin. Trademark, Athrombin-K.

w. sodium, [USP], the sodium salt of warfarin. Trademarks, *Coumadin* and Panwarfin.

warfarin assays 1. fluorimetry. Warfarin is extracted from plasma samples into acetone. Warfarin and some of its metabolites fluoresce at 400 nm when excited at 340 nm. The concentration of the drug in the sample is proportional to the difference between the fluorescence of the extract before and after it is quenched with acid.

2. high-pressure liquid chromatography (HPLC). Warfarin and an internal standard, *p*-chlorowarfarin, are extracted from acidified plasma into ether. The concentrated extract is analyzed by reverse-phase liquid chromatography, with detection at 308 nm.

warm antibody any blood group antibody that reacts optimally at 37°C.

wart (wort) [L. *verruca*] see *verruca.*

Warthin's tumor (war′thinz) [Alfred Scott *Warthin,* American pathologist, 1866–1931] see *c. lymphomatosum* under *cystadenoma.*

Warthin-Finkeldey cells (war′thin fing′kel-da) [Alfred Scott *Warthin;* W. *Finkeldey,* 20th century German pathologist] multinucleated giant cells of lymphoreticular origin, seen in various organs, e.g., the lung and appendix, during the prodromal phase of measles.

washed red blood cells red blood cells washed with physiological saline solution (as many as six times) to remove leukocytes and/or blood plasma proteins. Washed cells are indicated for patients with severe febrile transfusion reactions and for those with anti-IgA. The cells are also produced by the deglycerolization of frozen red blood cells.

wash time in an AutoAnalyzer, the length of time during which plain water is introduced into the moving stream between samples. A sample-to-wash ratio of 2:1 is commonly used.

wasserhelle cell (vos′er-hel″ĕ) [Ger. "water-clear cell"] a subtype of the parathyroid gland chief cell. Its clear appearance is due to an abundance of intracytoplasmic glycogen, which is removed on routine histologic processing. This cell type is distinct from the water-clear cells seen in wasserhelle (water-clear cell) hyperplasia of the parathyroid gland. Also called *water-clear cell.*

wasserhelle hyperplasia see *wasserhelle h.* under *hyperplasia.*

Wassermann antigen (vos′er-man) [August Paul von *Wassermann,* bacteriologist in Berlin, 1866–1925] see *cardiolipin.*

Wassermann reaction [August Paul von *Wassermann*] a complement-fixation test used for the diagnosis of syphilis. Individuals with active syphilis produce antibodies that react with cardiolipin from mitochondrial membranes of beef heart. See also *VDRL test.*

waste (wāst) 1. gradual loss, decay, or diminution of bulk; worn out or used up.

2. useless and effete material, unfit for further use within the organism; material excreted from the body as urine or feces.

3. to become weak or enfeebled.

4. by-products of technologic processing.

waste product 1. a chemical compound produced by metabolic processes in excess of metabolic requirements, or an end product of metabolism. Both are normally excreted.

2. the nonusable product of manufacturing or industrial and engineering processes.

wasting disease a condition that occurs in certain strains of neonatally thymectomized mice and is characterized by runting, marked lymphadenopathy, impaired cellular immunity, and, ultimately, death. The human counterpart occurs with graft-versus-host reactions following transplantation or, rarely, at birth as a result of the passage of maternal cells into an immunoincompetent fetus. The term is also used in a general sense to refer to a chronic disease process associated with cachexia. Also called *runt disease.*

water (wah′ter) a colorless, odorless, tasteless liquid with the composition hydrogen dioxide, H_2O; M.W. 18.016. The H—O—H bond angles are each 105°. The water molecule is highly polar in electronic configuration and has a large dipole moment (1.86 D). Hydrogen bonding gives rise to strong intermolecular forces in water and ice; each molecule is bonded to a maximum of four other molecules.

Water freezes at 0°C and boils at 100°C at 760 mmHg. The common solid form (ice) has a density of 0.915 g/ml, and the liquid has its maximal density of 1.0000 at 3.98°C.

Water dissolves all ionic compounds to some extent. A water molecule interposes itself between anion and cation and aligns itself so that its dipole moment cancels some of the interionic forces. Water forms coordination complexes with many cations to form cation hydrates (e.g., $K^+(H_2O)_4$). Water dissolves most polar covalent compounds with which it can form hydrogen bonds (such as carboxylic acids, alcohols, sugars, polypeptides). Nonpolar organic compounds are generally insoluble.

Pure water is only very slightly dissociated into its component ions. The dissociation constant, $K_w = [H^+][OH^-]$ is 1.008×10^{-14} ($pK_w = 13.96$) at 25°C.

All life is based on water as solvent and reaction medium; water makes up some 70 percent of body mass.

water bath 1. in film processing, a tray filled with water in which the film is briefly immersed after it is removed from the developer.

2. in the clinical laboratory, a tray or tank filled with water maintained within a narrow range of a specific temperature by thermostatic controls. The advantages of a warming or cooling water bath over an incubator or refrigerator are that the contents of tubes or flasks placed in a water bath quickly reach the temperature of the fluid in which they are immersed, and are readily available for observation and manipulation.

3. in histotechnology, a device used for flotation of paraffin-embedded tissue sections on hot water to eliminate wrinkles and distortion of the specimen prior to the transfer of the section onto a glass microscope slide.

water-clear cell see *wasserhelle cell.*

water-clear-cell hyperplasia see *wasserhelle h.* under *hyperplasia.*

water gas a mixture of carbon monoxide and hydrogen prepared by passing a mixture of steam and air through hot, incandescent coke. Water gas is used as an industrial raw material and formerly as a fuel for domestic heating.

Waterhouse-Friderichsen syndrome (waw'ter-hous frid"er-ik'sen) [Rupert *Waterhouse,* British physician, 1873–1958; Carl *Friderichsen,* Danish physician, born 1886] a severe hemorrhage in both adrenal glands that is usually associated with septicemia, most often with meningococcemia. Overwhelming infection with *Hemophilus influenzae,* staphylococci, or pneumococci also may occasionally be responsible. Acute adrenal insufficiency leads to collapse, vomiting, and low blood pressure. See also *primary h.* under *hypoadrenocorticism.*

Waters position (waw'terz) a position used in radiography of the facial bones or maxillary sinuses. The patient's chin rests on the film, which makes a 37° angle with the orbitomeatal line and is perpendicular to the midsagittal plane; the central ray projects vertically through the acanthion (a parietoacanthal projection). At this angle the maxillary sinuses are not overshadowed by the petrous portions of the temporal bone.

Watsonius (wot-so"ne-us) [Malcolm *Watson,* British physician, 1873–1955] a genus of trematodes, of which the species *W. watsoni* occasionally infects humans. The adult worms are pear-shaped and reddish-yellow, and have a translucent, glistening appearance; they measure 8–10 mm long by 4–5 mm wide. The eggs are ovoidal in shape and operculate, measuring 122–130 μ long by 75–80 μ wide. Infection, which is acquired by ingesting contaminated vegetation, causes a severe toxic diarrhea in humans.

watt (W) (wot) [James *Watt,* Scottish engineer and inventor, 1736–1819] the International System (SI) unit of power equal to 1 joule per second (1 J/s) or 1 volt-ampere (1 V·A).

wave (wāv) 1. any physical disturbance that propagates through space with a definite velocity, such as a light wave or a sound wave. A wave propagating in one dimension has the form $f(x - vt)$, where x is distance, t is time, v is wave velocity, and f is any arbitrary function.

2. a graphic representation of a change in the potential difference between a pair of electrodes in an electrophysiologic recording. The wave may have a characteristic configuration, duration, or frequency of repetition.

alpha w., in electroencephalography, a wave having a frequency of 8–13 Hz.

delta w., in electroencephalography, a wave with a duration of more than 0.25 sec.

diphasic w., a wave composed of two phases on alternate sides of the baseline. Also called biphasic wave.

fast w., in electroencephalography, any wave with a duration of less than 0.08 sec (i.e., under 1/13 sec).

monophasic w., a wave consisting of a single phase on one side of the baseline.

periodic w., a wave having a waveform that is a periodic function of the time: $f(x) = f(x + vT)$, where T is the period of the oscillation, x is distance, and v is wave velocity.

polyphasic w., a wave composed of two or more phases alternating about the baseline. In electromyography, the term is generally restricted to waves or action potentials that have five or more phases.

positive rolandic sharp w., a sharp wave recorded from the scalp over the rolandic area and characterized by a high-amplitude positive wave (25–200 μV) that may be preceded by a low-voltage negative wave. This electroencephalographic pattern is well described in infants with intraventricular hemorrhage. See also *sharp w.*

posterior slow w., in electroencephalography, electric activity in the delta and theta ranges that can be recorded from posterior (occipital) regions of the skull. It is common in children of all ages, especially during drowsiness. Two forms of posterior slow wave—parietal theta (4–6 Hz) and occipital delta (2–4 Hz)—occur with particular frequency in children affected with centrencephalic seizures and absence attacks (petit mal attacks). Occipital slow waves intermixed with ongoing alpha activity are called slow-fused transients, and may be mistakenly regarded as epileptiform by the inexperienced electroencephalographer.

sawtooth w., an electric waveform in which the voltage has a linear rise and instantaneous fall, or a linear fall and instantaneous rise.

sharp w., in electroencephalography, a wave of variable amplitude, which is 70–200 msec in duration and has a pointed peak when recorded at a paper speed of 3 cm/sec. See also *positive rolandic sharp w.* Cf. *spike.*

sine w., a wave having a sinusoidal waveform described by the function $A \sin(kx - \omega t + \delta)$, where A is wave amplitude, x is position, t is time, k is wave number, ω is angular frequency, and δ is phase angle. Single-frequency light and sound waves and alternating current electricity are examples.

slow w., in electroencephalography, a wave of greater than 1/8 sec in duration, i.e., having a frequency below the alpha range.

square w., an electric waveform in which the voltage periodically jumps between two values.

theta w., in electroencephalography, a wave that has a duration in the range of 1/4 to just over 1/8 sec.

triangular w., an electric waveform in which the voltage rises and falls linearly at the same rate between two values.

triphasic w., a wave composed of three phases alternating about the baseline.

wave amplitude the maximal displacement from equilibrium produced by a wave.

wave analyzer see *spectrum analyzer.*

waveform (wāv'form) the shape of a wave, the graph of the deviation of the wave at a given point as a function of the time.

waveguide (wāv'gīd) a metallic tube that conducts microwave radiation, which is contained by the conducting walls.

wavelength (λ) (wāv'length) the distance that a periodic wave propagates in one period or the distance between wave crests. Wavelength equals velocity times period or velocity divided by frequency: $\lambda = vT$ or $\lambda = v/f$.

wavelength accuracy the average deviation of the wavelength reading of a spectrometer from the true wavelength of light passing through the sample.

wavelength repeatability a measure of the variation in the true wavelength of light passing through the sample when a spectrophotometer is repeatedly set at a specific wavelength reading.

wave number 1. (abbrev. σ), the reciprocal of the wavelength: $\sigma = 1/\lambda$.

2. (abbrev. k), the quotient of 2π and the wavelength: $k = 2\pi / \lambda$. Also called circular wave number.

wave velocity the velocity at which a wave propagates. Also called phase velocity. See under *wave.*

wax (waks) [L. *cera*] a term originally applied only to beeswax, but now referring to any low-melting substance with a waxy feel. Natural waxes include animal waxes (e.g., beeswax), vegetable waxes (e.g., carnauba wax), and mineral waxes (e.g., paraffin wax). Synthetic waxes include polymers (e.g., Carbowax) and chloronaphthalenes. The natural animal and vegetable waxes are esters of fatty acids with long-chain alcohols, usually monohydric (e.g., cetyl alcohol). Other waxes are cholesterol esters, vitamin A esters, and vitamin D esters. The wax of pharmacy is principally yellow-wax (beeswax), the material of which the honeycomb is made. It consists chiefly of cerotic acid and myricin and is used in making such substances as ointments and cerates. When yellow wax is bleached, it becomes white (white wax). Also called *cera.*

wax D a glycolipid, containing mycolic acid and a glycopeptide, that is found in the basal cell wall of *Mycobacterium tuberculosis.* It can be used instead of whole mycobacteria in Freund's adjuvant.

Wayson stain a method used to demonstrate polar staining. A smear is treated with a mixture of basic fuchsin and methylene blue with phenol, washed with water, and dried. It is used especially to demonstrate *Yersinia pestis* in specimens from tissues and lymph nodes.

Wb abbrev. See *weber.*

WBC abbrev. for *w*hite *b*lood *c*ell. See *leukocyte.*

WDHA syndrome [acronym from *w*atery, *d*iarrhea, *h*ypokalemia, and *a*chlorhydria] see *Verner-Morrison syndrome.*

web (web) a tissue or membrane that connects or bridges two structures or surfaces.

cell w., the network of tonofibrils that provides internal support for cells.

terminal w., the part of the cell web that lies just below the free surface of absorbing or secreting epithelial cells and is attached to the terminal bar. It is composed of actin filaments that insert on the zonula adherens. See also *cell j.* under *junction.*

weber (Wb) (web′er) [Wilhelm Edward *Weber,* German physicist, 1804–1891] the International System (SI) unit of magnetic flux defined as the magnetic flux that, in linking a circuit of one turn, produces in it an electric potential difference of 1 volt while it is uniformly reduced to zero in 1 second. In other words, a rate of change of 1 weber per second in the flux through an *n* turn coil produces an output of *n* volts. Dimensionally, a weber equals a volt-second (V·s). Cf. *maxwell.*

Weber's test (va′berz) [Friedrich Eugen *Weber,* German otologist, 1832–1891] a simple hearing test designed to differentiate conductive hearing loss from sensorineural hearing loss. A tuning fork (preferably at 512 cps) is set in vibration, and the stem is placed on the midline of the skull on or a central incisor. The patient is asked in which ear the sound is loudest. In normal individuals, the sound is equally loud in both ears. In unilateral conduction deafness, however, the sound is louder in the affected ear (for reasons not entirely understood); in unilateral sensorineural hearing loss, the stimulus is louder in the unaffected ear, as the fork stimulates both inner ears equally. Thus, the person perceives the sound more clearly in the ear having the more sensitive, unaffected end organ and eighth cranial nerve. Cf. *Rinne's test.*

Weber-Christian disease (web′er kris′chan) [Frederick Parkes *Weber,* British physician, 1863–1962; Henry Asbury *Christian,* U.S. physician, 1876–1951] a disorder characterized by widespread inflammation of subcutaneous fat with the formation of multiple, tender red nodules. The cause is not known, but some patients may have evidence of visceral disease, and this is rarely fatal. If only the skin is involved, the prognosis is good, and a series of exacerbations and remissions may lead to permanent remission.

Laboratory diagnosis is aided by the findings of elevated plasma amylase and lipase levels.

Also called nodular panniculitis. See also *panniculitis.*

WEE abbrev. See *western equine e.* under *encephalitis.*

Wegener's granulomatosis [F. *Wegener,* German pathologist, 20th century] a disease characterized by the triad of necrosis of the upper respiratory tract and lungs, necrotizing angiitis of veins and arteries, and focal glomerulitis. It occurs primarily in males, with an average age at onset of 40 yr. The etiology is unknown, but may relate to an immune mechanism.

Laboratory tests are not specific for this disorder, although the sedimentation rate is often used to monitor its course and severity. If left untreated, the disease runs a rapidly fatal course; however, the use of immunosuppressive agents (e.g., cyclophosphamide) has dramatically improved the survival rate.

See also *lethal midline g.* under *granuloma.*

Weibel-Palade body rod-shaped granules considered to be ultrastructural markers for endothelial cells. These bodies are 0.1 μm thick by 3 μm long and consist of several tubules, each approximately 15 nm thick, embedded in a dense matrix.

weighing (wa′ing) the process of determining an unknown mass by comparison with calibrated weights.

weight (wāt) the force with which an object is attracted by the earth's gravity, measured in units of force, such as newtons or pounds. Weight is distinguished from mass, the quantity of matter in an object, measured in units of mass, such as kilograms, atomic mass units (daltons), or slugs.

weight-bearing coalition view a radiographic projection of the heel in which the patient stands on the film with the knees slightly flexed, and the central ray is inclined anteriorly at a 45° angle. This view demonstrates tarsal coalition, the fusion of two or more tarsal bones (usually a talocalcaneal bridge or calceonavicular bar), which is a congenital anomaly associated with rigid flatfoot.

weight-bearing view a radiographic view of a body part that shows the response to the stresses of a natural posture. Lateral (horizontal ray) and dorsoplantar (15° posterior and 25° anterior central ray angulations) weight-bearing views of the foot are useful in studying flatfoot or cave foot. An anteroposterior weight-bearing projection of the knee demonstrates narrowing of the joint space, or varus or valgus deformity, occurring in some arthritic knees.

weighted average a statistic of the form $\Sigma_{i=1}^{N} a_i X_i$, where $X_i, X_2, \ldots, X_N$ are the data points, and $a_1, a_2, \ldots, a_N$ are a set of weights arbitrarily specified subject to the conditions $0 < a_i < 1, i = 1, 2, \ldots,$ N, and $\Sigma_{i=1}^{N} a_i = 1$.

weights (wāts) 1. a set of objects of known mass used in weighing unknown masses with an analytic balance or in calibrating another set of weights.

2. in statistics, a set of constants between zero and one, which sum to one, used to specify the contribution that each datum point makes to a statistic, as in a weighted average. Weighting is also used in linear regression.

Weil's disease (vīlz) [Adolf *Weil,* physician in Wiesbaden, 1848–1916] a form of severe leptospirosis in which there is jaundice, swelling of the liver, fever, and (occasionally) nephritis and meningitis. See also *leptospirosis* and *spirochete.*

Weil-Felix test (vīl fa′liks) [Edmund *Weil,* German physician in Prague, 1880–1922; Arthur *Felix,* Prague bacteriologist, 1887–1956] the agglutination of certain (OX) strains of *Proteus vulgaris* by cross-reacting antibodies in the serum of individuals with rickettsial disease. The three types of OX antigens (OX-2, OX-19, OX-K) have different relationships to antigens in the various rickettsiae; consequently, the reaction can be used diagnostically. See also *Rocky Mountain spotted fever antibody tests.*

Weinman's medium (wīn-mans) a medium, consisting of sodium chloride, citrated human plasma, and human hemoglobin, that is used for the cultivation of *Trypanosoma gambiense.*

wen (wen) see *sebaceous cyst.*

Wenckebach block (ven′kĕ-bahk) [Karel Frederik *Wenckebach,* Dutch internist in Vienna, 1864–1940] a progressive atrioventricular (A-V) conduction delay and block, most commonly in the A-V node, that is characterized by a Wenckebach periodicity of A-V conduction and successive R-R intervals. The P-R interval gradually lengthens during each of several beats (A-V conduction progressively slows), until A-V conduction is completely blocked, causing a long R-R interval. (A junctional escape beat may end this pause in the cycle.) The next P wave is followed by a QRS complex, and the P-R interval of this first beat is the shortest one of the Wenckebach cycle. The magnitude of the increment in the P-R interval gradually lessens with each beat, however, causing a progressive shortening of the R-R interval until the complete block again occurs.

A Wenckebach-type block is frequently associated with infarctions of the inferior wall of the left ventricle, or digitalis intoxication. Atropine treatment often restores a normal 1:1 A-V conduction ratio. Also called Mobitz type I second-degree atrioventricular block.

Werdnig-Hoffman paralysis (verd′nig hof′man) [Guido *Werdnig,* Austrian neurologist; Ernst *Hoffman,* German neurologist, born 1868] a syndrome of progressive muscular weakness and atrophy, usually transmitted as an autosomal recessive trait, that involves limb, bulbar, and respiratory muscles. The muscular atrophy results from a degeneration of motor neurons in the spinal cord, the cause of which is unknown.

The disease is usually found in infants, although onset may occur somewhat later in life. Often the disease ends in death, especially in the types with an early onset, usually from repeated respiratory infection.

Wermer syndrome (wer′mer) [Paul *Wermer,* U.S. physician, 20th century] see *MEN I* under *MEN.*

Wernicke's syndrome (ver′nĭ-kez) [Karl *Wernicke,* German neurologist, 1848–1905] see *Wernicke-Korsakoff syndrome.*

Wernicke-Korsakoff syndrome (ver′nĭ-kē kor-sak′of) [Karl *Wernicke;* Sergei Sergeevich *Korsakoff,* Russian neurologist, 1854–1900] a disease that occurs primarily in malnourished chronic alcoholics and is characterized by encephalopathy (Wernicke's syndrome) and psychosis (Korsakoff's syndrome). The deficient nutritional factor is thiamine (vitamin B_1).

Wernicke's encephalopathy consists of ocular disturbances, an ataxia primarily of stance and gait, mental confusion, and, occasionally, polyneuropathy. The ocular disturbance consists of bilateral weakness or paralysis of the lateral rectus muscles, horizontal and vertical nystagmus, and impairment of conjugate gaze. Pathologically, nerve cell loss, hemorrhage, and glial and endothelial reactions are symmetrically located in the mamillary bodies and terminal fornices; in parts of the thalamus and hypothalamus; in the floor of the fourth ventricle; and in the periaqueductal gray matter and superior vermis.

Korsakoff's psychosis very frequently is found in individuals with Wernicke's encephalopathy. It is characterized by an impairment of memory, inability to retain new information, and other abnormalities of cognitive function. Confabulation may also be a conspicuous feature.

The onset of this syndrome is sudden. During the acute phase, mortality may exceed 15 percent. The patient responds dramatically to the administration of thiamine and the ocular signs improve within several days while the ataxia resolves more slowly (ultimately disappearing in about half the patients). However, Korsakoff's psychosis may persist in as many as two of every three individuals.

Also called cerebral beriberi.

Wesenberg-Hamazaki body a small oval or needlelike body that is yellow or brown when stained with hematoxylin-eosin and is usually periodic acid–Schiff positive. Such bodies are found principally in the sinuses of lymph nodes, either lying free or in the cytoplasm of histiocytes. They are thought to represent lysosomes that contain hemolipofuscin. Originally it was claimed that they were diagnostic for sarcoidosis, but it is now recognized that they have no etiologic or diagnostic significance. Also called *yellow body* and yellow-brown body.

Westergren sedimentation rate method (west′-er-gren) [Alf *Westergren,* Swedish physician] a test that measures the speed at which erythrocytes settle (erythrocyte sedimentation rate, ESR). One volume of a sodium citrate solution is added to four volumes of anticoagulated whole blood and placed in a Westergren sedimentation tube. The tube (30 cm long and 2.5 mm in internal diameter, calibrated in millimeters from 0 to 200) is open at both ends. It is placed vertically in a rack and the erythrocyte level read at the end of 1 hr. Modified methods have been described. Reference values are: for males, 0–10 mm/hr; and for females, 0–20. See also *erythrocyte sedimentation rate.* Cf. *Wintrobe sedimentation rate method* and *zeta sedimentation method.*

West Nile fever a mosquito-borne illness due to group B arbovirus, found in Asia and Africa; it is endemic in Egypt. Those affected experience fever, malaise, headaches, myalgia, maculopapular rash, and lymphadenopathy. Leukopenia, and cerebrospinal fluid involvement, with increased cells and protein, may occur. Diagnosis is based on viral culture and isolation, or on demonstration of a rising specific antibody titer. Recovery is the rule, but symptoms may persist for several weeks. Treatment is limited to symptomatic therapy.

wet mount a histologic preparation in which a specimen (a fluid or suspended in a fluid) is placed on a slide and covered by a coverslip rather than being dehydrated and embedded in a permanent mounting medium.

wetting agent a substance (surfactant) that lowers the surface tension of water, used to promote wetting of solutes and particles by water.

WGA abbrev. See *wheat germ agglutinin.*

Wharton's jelly (hwar'tunz) [Thomas *Wharton,* English physician and anatomist, 1614–1673] the myxoid connective tissue of the umbilical cord. It is soft and jellylike, and contains mesenchymal cells and sparse collagen fibers.

wheal (hwēl, wēl) a round, red elevated lesion due to localized edema in the upper dermis, seen in urticaria, a skin manifestation of allergic reaction often caused by drugs or food.

wheal-and-erythema skin tests tests for an immediate hypersensitivity (allergic) response to a particular antigen, which involve cutaneous or intracutaneous injections of the test allergen and observation for any reddening (erythema) and swelling (wheal) of the skin at the site of injection.

The cutaneous test is performed by pricking or scratching the skin (usually on the back) and applying the antigen. The antigen is wiped off after 20 min and the reaction recorded.

The intracutaneous test is more sensitive, but it may cause a dangerous systemic reaction in highly sensitive individuals and should be performed only on the extremities. A small amount of sterile antigen (0.01 ml or less) is injected intracutaneously and the reaction read in 20 min. Concentration of the allergen is critical, as a high dose of some allergens may cause a reaction in nonallergic individuals, giving a false-positive reaction.

wheat germ agglutinin (WGA) a lectin originating from wheat germ that will cause the clumping (agglutination) of malignant cells, but not benign cells. Possible mechanisms include increased lectin receptors or clustering of receptor sites on malignant cells.

wheat germ oil oil derived from the germ of wheat kernels and rich in vitamin E.

Wheatstone bridge (hwēt'stōn) [Sir Charles *Wheatstone,* English physicist, 1802–1875] an electric circuit used for highly accurate measurements of resistance. One side of the bridge consists of two known resistances in series; the other side has a variable resistor in series with the unknown resistance. The two sides are connected in parallel across a voltage source, and a galvanometer is connected between the junctions of the resistors on the two sides. When the potentiometer is adjusted so that the ratio of the resistance of the potentiometer and the unknown is the same as that of the two resistors on the other side, the bridge is in balance and no current flows through the galvanometer.

whiplash (hwip'lash) a hyperextension of the neck that may occur as the result of an automobile accident or fall. It is a common mechanism of injury to the spinal cord.

Whipple's disease (hwip'elz) [George Hoyt *Whipple,* U.S. pathologist, born 1878; cowinner with George R. Minot and William P. Murphy of the Nobel Prize in medicine and physiology, 1934] a rare disorder of insidious onset, occurring primarily in males aged 30–60 yr, characterized by steatorrhea, malabsorption, anemia, increased skin pigmentation, and a migratory arthritis. The etiology is uncertain; however, jejunal biopsy shows a lamina propria infiltrated with PAS-positive macrophages that contain bacteria, and the usual villous architecture of the small intestine is lost. Laboratory tests reveal findings of the malabsorption syndrome.

Whipple's operation [Allen O. *Whipple,* United States surgeon, 1881–1963] the surgical removal of the distal stomach, gallbladder with the common bile duct, duodenum, and much of the pancreas. The procedure is performed in some cases for bile duct or pancreatic cancer.

Whipple's triad a triad of clinical manifestations seen with some insulin-producing islet cell tumors and other causes of hypoglycemia. It consists of symptomatic hypoglycemia, associated low fasting blood glucose, and prompt alleviation of symptoms on administration of glucose. See also *pancreatic tumors.*

whipworm (hwip'werm) see *Trichuris.*

whipworm infection see *trichuriasis.*

white blood cell (WBC) see *leukocyte.*

white blood cell count the number of white blood cells in a representative blood sample; see *blood cell count.*

whitehead see *milium.*

white lead see *input terminal 2.*

white line see *l. alba* under *linea.*

white matter the white tissue of the central nervous system. The pinkish-white opalescence that characterizes the white matter is imparted by the myelinated nerve fibers that constitute this conducting portion of the brain and spinal cord.

white muscle pale muscle that is rich in sarcoplasmic reticulum and phosphorylases, but deficient in mitochondria and oxidative enzymes. These muscles have a well-developed anaerobic metabolism, and react quickly for short bursts of activity. See also *muscle.* Cf. *red muscle.*

white pulp the lymphoid tissue of the spleen, organized into sheaths around the arterioles and their branches.

white ramus see under *ramus communicans.*

whitlow (hwit'lo) [M.E. *whitflawe,* from *whit* white + *flawe* flaw] a purulent infection in the tightly closed fascial layers of the fingertip, usually the result of trauma (as by a prick with a thorn). The expanding infection presses on surrounding blood vessels and may cut off blood supply in this area, resulting in osteomyelitis and tissue necrosis. Tenderness, pain, and edema accompany the infection.

Incision of the fingertip over the whitlow usually prevents necrosis and enables the infection to drain. Also called *felon.*

WHO abbrev. See *World Health Organization.*

whole-arm fusion see *robertsonian translocation.*

whole blood anticoagulated donor blood. It contains the cellular and plasma components of the donor, as well as anticoagulant and preservative solution. It is indicated in patients with both a symptomatic deficit in oxygen-carrying capacity and hypovolemic shock. Whole blood less than 5 da old, with hematocrit adjusted by removing plasma, is suitable for neonatal exchange transfusion. Platelet function in whole blood rapidly declines with storage.

whole blood clotting time a measure of the activity of the intrinsic system of blood coagulation. Venous blood is collected and allowed to rest in test tubes. The clotting time is measured from the time blood first appears in the syringe during blood withdrawal until the tube can be inverted without spilling. Reference values vary with technique (4–8 min); prolongation of the clotting time occurs with marked coagulation factor deficiencies or in the presence of circulating anticoagulants, such as heparin. It can be used to monitor heparin therapy, although the activated partial thromboplastin time is the preferred method. Size of clot, clot retraction, and clot lysis can also be studied by continued observation. Also called *Lee-White clotting test.*

whooping cough (hōōp′ing kawf′) an acute, highly infectious respiratory disease of humans, which occurs primarily in infants younger than age 2 yr. It is characterized by a 2-wk catarrhal stage (malaise, anorexia, cough) and a later paroxysmal cough, ending in a high-pitched "whoop" on inspiration (from which the disease's common name arose).

Infection is the result of inhaling droplets contaminated with *Bordetella pertussis* and the closely related *B. parapertussis.* It is a superficial infection limited to the ciliated bronchial epithelium, although subepithelial inflammation and necrosis occur from action of the liberated toxins. The characteristic lymphocytosis of 15,000–20,000/μl is attributed to a lymphocyte promoting factor (LPF), which also has a number of other effects.

Bacteriologic diagnosis is made by culturing nasopharyngeal swabs on a Bordet-Gengou agar plate. The once-popular "cough-plate" procedure has been replaced by the flexible wire swab technique. A rapid, definitive bacteriologic diagnosis can sometimes be made by the direct staining of nasopharyngeal smears with fluorescein-labeled antibody.

Active immunization with pertussis vaccine (as part of the DPT vaccine) is recommended for all infants.

Also called *pertussis.*

wicket rhythm see *mu rhythm.*

Widal test (ve′dahl) [Georges *Widal,* French physician, 1862–1929] a bacterial agglutination test to detect serum antibodies to *Salmonella* antigens. When it was first introduced, the term applied specifically to the organism of typhoid fever, but with time, *Salmonella* antigens other than those of *S. typhi* were added; thus, the term is seldom used today. See also *febrile agglutination test.*

Wilcoxon rank sum statistic (wil′koks-on) [Frank *Wilcoxon,* Irish-born U.S. chemist, b. 1892] see under *rank sum test.*

Wilcoxon signed rank statistic [Frank *Wilcoxon*] see under *signed rank test.*

wild type in genetics, a phenotype normal for the species; in some cases it is an arbitrarily designated, frequently occurring type.

wild-type gene the normal allele (often symbolized as +).

Wilms' tumor (vilmz) [Marx *Wilms,* German surgeon, 1867–1918] see *nephroblastoma.*

Wilson central terminal (wil′sun) a reference electrode system used in electrocardiography that is formed by connecting each limb lead to a common negative pole through a 50,000-Ω resistance. This effectively provides a relatively unchanging (and approximately zero) reference voltage for comparison with that recorded from the exploring (positive) electrode, positioned on one of the extremities, on the chest, or elsewhere on or in the body.

In Goldberger's modification of the central terminal, which is used in the augmented limb lead system, the connection to the central terminal of the limb on which the exploring electrode is positioned is eliminated; this results in approximately 50 percent increased amplitude of the recorded electrocardiographic deflections.

Wilson's disease (wil′sunz) [Samuel Alexander Kinnier *Wilson,* English neurologist, 1878–1936] a rare hereditary disorder, transmitted as an autosomal recessive trait, that results in the excessive accumulation of copper, primarily in the liver and brain. This condition is associated with a low serum concentration of total copper and of ceruloplasmin, increased 24-hr urinary copper excretion, and a concentration of copper greater than 250 μg/g of dry weight in a liver biopsy. Owing to excess copper in tissue, the functions of the brain, liver, and kidneys are affected. In childhood, those affected commonly present with jaundice, hepatosplenomegaly, and cirrhosis. In older children and young adults, tremor, chorea, dystonia, athetosis, ataxia, dysarthria, dysphagia, and behavioral abnormalities are common, and Kayser-Fleischer rings may be found in the eyes owing to the deposition of copper in the deepest layer of the cornea.

Treatment is with penicillamine, a copper-chelating agent. A low copper diet is advised, and potassium sulfide prescribed to reduce copper absorption from the gastrointestinal tract. Other family members should be screened for the disorder.

Also called *hepatolenticular degeneration.*

Wilson-Mikity syndrome [Miriam Geisendorfer *Wilson,* U.S. pediatrician, born 1922; Victor G. *Mikity,* U.S. radiologist, born 1919] a condition of respiratory distress, of unknown cause, that occurs primarily in premature infants of less than 32 wks' gestation and weighing less than 1500 g. It is characterized by an insidious onset of dyspnea, tachypnea, and cyanosis in the first month of life. Occasionally, the condition may be seen in full-term infants who have had a history of oxygen toxicity or prolonged respirator exposure. Affected infants may develop cough, rales, and wheezes. Lung collapse or right-sided heart failure may occur.

Diagnosis is accomplished by x-rays, which reveal bilateral infiltrates that are coarse, reticular, and streaky, and that may progress to the appearance of homogeneous opacity. Lung immaturity with overinflation and a translucent bubbly appearance may also be seen with progression of the condition. Treatment consists of supportive care and supplementary oxygen. Although those affected may have recurrent pulmonary infections during childhood, pulmonary function usually becomes entirely normal with maturity.

Also called bronchopulmonary dysplasia, bubbly lung syndrome, and interstitial pulmonary fibrosis of prematurity.

window (win′do) [Old Norse *vindauga* wind-eye] in a gamma-ray detector (such as a scintillation camera, rectilinear scanner, or scintillation counter), an interval of photon energies that selects the gamma rays contributing to the image or count. A circuit called the pulse height analyzer rejects the pulses produced by photons with energies outside the window. The window is set by adjusting the upper and lower discriminator levels of the pulse height analyzer. These are not adjusted independently; the instrument controls adjust the window centerline energy and window width.

Wintrobe hematocrit tube (win′trōb) a thick-walled glass tube used in the macro method of hematocrit determination. It has a uniform internal bore and flattened bottom and is calibrated in millimeters from 0 to 105. See also *hematocrit.*

Wintrobe sedimentation rate method a test that measures the speed at which erythrocytes settle (erythrocyte sedimentation rate, ESR). Anticoagulated whole blood is placed in a Wintrobe hematocrit tube (EDTA is now the accepted anticoagulant). The tube is placed in a rack in a vertical position, and the erythrocyte level read at the end of 1 hr. The volume of packed leukocytes and platelets (VPRC) and icterus index can also be read from this tube. Reference ranges are: for males, 0–10 mm/hr; and for females, 0–20. See also *erythrocyte sedimentation rate.* Cf. *Westergren sedimentation rate method* and *zeta sedimentation ratio method.*

Wirsung's duct (vēr′soongz) [Johann Georg *Wirsung,* German physician, 1600–1643] the main pancreatic duct.

Wiskott-Aldrich syndrome (wis′kot awl′drich) [Alfred *Wiskott,* German pediatrician, born 1898; Robert A. *Aldrich,* U.S. pediatrician, born 1917] a genetic disorder, transmitted as an X-linked trait, characterized by thrombocytopenia, hemorrhagic tendencies, eczema, and immunodeficiency. Thrombocytopenia is present at birth and results in a bleeding tendency that becomes less severe with age. Hypercatabolism of immunoglobulins occurs early. Recurrent infections, usually with polysaccharide-containing organisms (e.g., pneumococcus, meningococcus, and *Hemophilus influenzae*), begin after 6 mo of age and result in pneumonia, meningitis, and otitis media. As affected individuals age, they become susceptible to recurrent viral infections, especially herpes and warts. Eczema appears in affected children by approximately age 1 yr. In older persons who survive the infectious illnesses, the incidence of lymphoreticular malignancies, especially of the central nervous system, is high.

Measurement of serum immunoglobulins reveals low levels of IgM, normal or elevated levels of IgA and IgG, and very high levels of IgE. Antibody responses to polysaccharide antigens are poor, whereas responses to protein antigens are normal. Cellular immune responses are often abnormal and decrease with age. Cutaneous anergy is common. Platelet counts are frequently in the range of 5000–100,000 cells/μl. The platelets are small in contrast to those in other disorders involving thrombocytopenia (in such diseases, the platelets are larger than normal). Anemia is often present. Treatment involves controlling infections with antibiotics and platelet transfusions in severe thrombocytopenia. Splenectomy is contraindicated because it makes the patient even more immunosuppressed. Bone marrow transplants have been employed successfully.

witch hazel (wich ha′zel) [A.S. *wych* elm + *hazel*]

1. a shrub, *Hamamelis virginiana.*

2. an alcoholic extract of the bark and leaves of this shrub, which is applied topically as an astringent. Also called *hamamelis water.*

withdrawal (with-draw′al) 1. the abstinence from a drug or drugs and the associated symptoms and signs that signify physical dependence. Withdrawal is often characterized by symptoms of altered central nervous system function. Function of the autonomic nervous system also is often affected, resulting in gastrointestinal disorders and other visceral complaints.

The severity and type of withdrawal symptoms depend on the substance abused, amount used, and duration of use. Withdrawal from stimulants, for example, may produce lethargy or somnolence, whereas withdrawal from alcohol, a CNS depressant, may produce irritability or convulsions. Death may occur in up to 15 percent of those withdrawing from alcohol who also experience delirium tremens; withdrawal from other drugs often is not as severe.

2. the retreat from reality or from social contact that is associated with psychiatric disorders. Withdrawal may be found, for example, in neglected children and in suicidal, depressed, or psychotic individuals. See also *addiction* and *habituation.*

wobble hypothesis an explanation of how a specific transfer RNA (tRNA) molecule can translate different codons in a messenger RNA template: there is some looseness in the alignment that allows the third base of the anticodon to pair with a base other than its normal complementary base. Other than the normal complementary pairs of guanine (G) with cytosine (C) and adenine (A) with uracil (U), G pairs with U, U pairs with G, and I (inosine) pairs with A, U, or C, where the first base of these pairs is the third base of the anticodon. One exception to these pairing rules is $tRNA^{GlyIII}$ with anticodon CCA, which recognizes the codon GGC.

Wohlfahrtia (vōl-fahr′te-ah) a genus of flies (the fleshflies) of the family Sarcophagidae.

W. magnifica, a large fleshfly found in the Mediterranean region, in the Near East, and throughout the USSR. The adult flies deposit their larvae in skin lesions, nasal sinuses, sores of the tongue and eyes, and the vagina. These larvae are large and produce serious disfigurement unless removed immediately. Also called Old World fleshfly.

W. vigil, a North American species; the adults deposit their larvae in skin lesions, which produces swelling. The fly is attracted by foul odors from secretions of the eyes and nose; soiled diapers may also be implicated, as the flies are particularly attracted to young children. Permanent disfiguration is prevented by surgical removal of the larvae. Also called Nearctic fleshfly.

wolffian body (woolf'e-an) [Kaspar Friedrich *Wolff*, German anatomist and embryologist, 1733–1794] see *mesonephros.*

wolffian duct (woolf'e-an) [Kaspar Friedrich *Wolff*] see *mesonephric d.* under *duct.*

Wolff-Parkinson-White (WPW) syndrome [Louis *Wolff*, U.S. cardiologist, born 1898; Sir John *Parkinson*, British physician, born 1885; Paul Dudley *White*, American cardiologist, 1886–1973] a disorder of conduction of the electrical impulses of the heart, in which normally formed sinoatrial impulses are conducted to the ventricles both by way of the atrioventricular (A-V) node and by an abnormal conductive pathway (the bundle of Kent). Conduction is more rapid through the abnormal pathway, and as a result ventricular activation begins earlier than usual; this produces a short PR interval followed by a characteristic delta wave (an initial slow upstroke of the R wave or downstroke of the S wave of the QRS complex). Most ventricular depolarization occurs as a result of normal conduction through the A-V node, bundle of His, bundle branches, and myocardial tissue, so the remainder of the QRS complex is normal.

A common complication of the syndrome is the development of supraventricular tachycardia secondary to reentry involving the dual conduction pathways. With rapid atrial rates, as in atrial flutter and fibrillation, dangerously rapid ventricular rates may result in decreased cardial output severe enough to be life threatening.

WPW syndrome is often diagnosed on a routine electrocardiogram, and suspected when an individual has symptoms and signs of paroxysmal tachycardia. Electrophysiologic studies can help define the anatomic variants. Although most patients have no symptoms or only minor arrhythmias, a rare patient requires surgical division of the accessory pathway.

Wolman's disease (wol'man) [Moshe *Wolman*, Israeli pathologist, born 1914] a primary familial xanthomatosis, which appears in the first weeks of life. It is due to abnormal lipid metabolism following a severe enzymatic deficiency of acid lipase. As a result, large amounts of neutral lipids, cholesterol esters, and glycerides accumulate in the body tissues. Symptoms include spleen and liver enlargement, adrenal calcification, steatorrhea, vomiting, growth disturbances, and the presence of lipid-containing histiocytes (foam cells) in the bone marrow and other tissue. No specific therapy exists and death usually occurs within 6 mo. There is also a juvenile form (see *cholesterol ester storage disease*). Both carrier detection and prenatal diagnosis are thought to be possible.

Wood's lamp (woodz) [Robert W. *Wood*, American physicist, 1868–1953] a light source that emits long-wave ultraviolet light of about 365 nm, used to detect the fluorescence of colonies of dermatophytes and some bacteria (*Pseudomonas, Bacteroides*) in infections of the hair and scalp. Also called Wood's filter and Wood's light.

word (werd) 1. a measure of data-storage capacity. 2. a unit of data in a computer. In many small computers, a word consists of 16 binary bits; it may be divided into two bytes of eight bits each. In most computers, data are handled as complete bytes or words: a given location in memory will store one word or one byte.

When measuring memory size, "K" is an abbreviation for 1024 (2^{10}); thus, a 32K-word memory contains 32,768 words.

word length the number of bits in a computer word.

word processing a term applied to typing or editing a document using a word-processing typewriter or computer that stores the text on magnetic cards or tape so that the text can be edited without retyping.

word salad an incomprehensible mix of phrases and words, a manifestation of the abnormal thought processes found in those suffering from severe schizophrenia.

work (W) (werk) a transfer of energy produced by the movement of a force against a resistance. It is the line integral, taken along the path of the movement, of the tangential component of the force. For a constant force, the work is force times distance ($W = F \cdot s$); for a constant torque, the work is torque times the angle of rotation ($W = L \cdot \theta$); for a constant pressure, the work is pressure times the change in volume ($W = p \, \Delta \, V$). The International System (SI) unit of work is the joule (J).

working distance (werk'ing dis'tans) in microscopy, the distance when the instrument is correctly focused between the objective lens of a microscope and the object.

work of breathing the energy expended by the respiratory muscles in expanding the lungs and thoracic cage during each breathing cycle. The work of inspiration is needed to overcome the elastic recoil of the lung-chest wall system (65 percent) and the frictional resistance to airflow in the respiratory passageways and viscous resistance of the lung tissues (35 percent). Expiration is normally passive, resulting from release of the energy stored in the system during inspiration.

The work of breathing is equal to the cumulative product of the pressure (P) or force per unit area developed by the respiratory muscles and the volume (V) of air moved during each instant of the respiratory cycle. It is calculated from pressure-volume curves as $\int$ PdV.

The energy expended during breathing varies from the normal value of 0.5 kg/m/min found during resting respiration when a change in alveolar ventilation occurs. The elastic component of work increases with increasing tidal volumes, whereas the resistive component increases with increases in the respiratory rate. Thus, slow deep breathing helps to overcome the increased airway resistance that is present in conditions such as asthma, and shallow breathing reduces the additional elastic work caused by stiffening of the lungs in conditions such as pulmonary interstitial fibrosis.

work-up (werk'up) the procedures done to arrive at a diagnosis, including the taking of a clinical history, doing a physical examination, and obtaining laboratory tests and radiographs.

World Health Organization (WHO) an agency of the United Nations with headquarters in Geneva. It was established in 1948, its purpose stated as "the attainment by all peoples of the highest possible level of health." The organizational structure of WHO in Geneva is a world health assembly of 155 member states that meets once a year, an executive committee that meets twice a year, and a permanent secretariat headed by a director-general.

The operation of WHO programs is largely in the hands of six regional offices covering the Americas, the eastern Mediterranean, Europe, Southeast Asia, and the western Pacific. Associated with each regional office are technical and advisory committees.

Smallpox has been stamped out completely by a program initiated and carried out by WHO. Notable progress has also been made in checking other infectious diseases, among them poliomyelitis, leprosy, cholera, malaria, and tuberculosis. At present, a major effort of WHO is the control of the whole spectrum of diarrheal diseases.

wound (wōōnd) [L. *vulnus*] an injury involving separation or disorganization of the anatomic structures normally present. This term is usually applied to injuries of the skin, which can involve the underlying tissues. See also *healing* and *union.*

woven bone bony tissue found in the embryo, in young children, and in various pathologic conditions in adults, in which the bone fails to show the oriented arrangement of collagen fibers characteristic of lamellated bone. Also called primitive bone.

Wright peak flow meter (rīt) [Barbara Evelyn *Wright,* U.S. biochemist, born 1926] an instrument used to record the rate of airflow during the early moments of a maximal forced expiration. See also *peak expiratory flow rate.*

Wright stain (rīt) [James Homer *Wright,* Boston pathologist, 1871–1928] a polychromatic Romanowsky-type stain, one of the most commonly used stains for blood cells. It contains a solution of eosin and a complex mixture of several metachromatic thiazin dyes (methylene blue, azure B, and their derivatives) in methyl alcohol. When stained, red cells appear pink; nuclei of white cells, blue to purple; cytoplasmic granules of granulocytes, red-orange (in eosinophils), tan (in neutrophils), or dark blue to purple (in basophils); cytoplasm of lymphocytes, light blue, and that of monocytes, a faint bluish tinge.

wrist (rist) the region of the joint between the hand and forearm. It is formed by a series of articulations between the distal ends of the radius and ulna, the carpal bones, and the proximal surface of the metacarpals.

wrist joint the biaxial synovial joint formed by the radius and an articular disc with the scaphoid, lunate, and triquetral bones. Also called *radiocarpal joint.*

write (rīt) 1. to transfer data from computer memory to an output device, or the operation or statement of a program that accomplishes this transfer.

2. to transfer data from a register to the memory of a computer. This operation is usually called a *store.*

Wuchereria (voo″ker-er′e-ah) [Otto *Wucherer,* German physician in Brazil, 1820–1873] a genus of filarial nematodes (roundworms) indigenous throughout the warm regions of the world.

W. bancrofti, a tissue-inhabiting nematode that causes lymphangitis, hydrocele, and elephantiasis. The adult worms are minute, creamy white, and threadlike with rounded, blunt ends. The males measure approximtely 40 mm long by 0.1 mm wide; the females, 65–100 mm by 0.24–0.3 mm.

Also called *Filaria bancrofti, F. nocturna, F. sanguinis hominis,* and *W. pacifica.*

W. malayi, see *B. malayi* under *Brugia.*

W. pacifica, see *W. bancrofti.*

wuchereriasis (voo-ker″e-ri′ah-sis) infection with nematodes of the genus *Wuchereria.*

w/v abbrev. for weight of solute per volume of solution; e.g., a 70 percent (w/v) solution contains 70 g of solute per 100 ml of solution. This form is no longer recommended and should be replaced by mass of solute per liter of solution, or moles of solute per liter of solution. The latter conforms to the SI system. See also *mass concentration.*

w/w abbrev. for weight of solute per weight of total solution; e.g., a 70 percent (w/w) solution contains 70 masses of solute per 100 masses of solution. This form is no longer recommended and should be replaced by mass of solute per kilogram of total solution or by mole fraction, which is moles of solute per total moles of solute plus solvent. The latter conforms to the SI system.

Wyeomyia (we″o-mi′yah) a genus of culicine mosquitoes. The species *W. arthrostigma* is believed to be involved in the transmission of yellow fever.

X

X symbol for reactance.

$\bar{X}$, $\bar{x}$ symbol for the sample mean. See also *mean.*

Ξ the Greek capital letter *xi.*

ξ the Greek lower case letter *xi.*

xanth/o (zan′tho) [Gr. *xanthos* yellow] a word element used in combining form to denote yellow, e.g., xanthoma, xanthochromia.

xanthelasma (zan″thel-az′mah) [*xanth-* + Gr. *elasma* plate] a type of xanthoma; a deposit of lipids in the skin of the eyelids. Xanthelasmas, which usually are soft, yellow, elevated plaques, are the most common form of xanthoma. See also *xanthoma.*

xanthine (zan′thēn) [Gr. *xanthos* yellow: named from the yellow color of its nitrate] 1. a white, amorphous compound, 2,6,-dioxopurine, $C_5H_4N_4O_2$. Obtained from most of the body tissues and fluids, and certain plants, it is formed by the oxidation of hypoxanthine and is itself oxidized to uric acid; xanthine oxidase catalyzes both reactions. A hereditary deficiency of the enzyme xanthine oxidase causes the condition of xanthinuria, which is also seen in individuals being treated for gout with allopurinol, a xanthine oxidase inhibitor widely used in clinical medicine to prevent the conversion of xanthine to uric acid. Xanthine renal calculi are seen but are rare. Xanthine is a stimulant to muscular tissue, especially that of the heart.

2. a general term for any of the drugs caffeine, theobromine, and theophylline, which are dimethyl- or trimethylxanthines.

xanthinuria (zan″thin-u′re-ah) [*xanthine* + Gr. *ouron* urine] a rare hereditary disorder of purine metabolism, transmitted as an autosomal recessive trait, that is caused by a deficiency of the enzyme xanthine oxidase. This results in an excess of xanthine in the urine, which may lead to the formation of xanthine calculi in the urinary tract and a reduction of uric acid concentration in serum and urine. Also called *xanthuria.*

xanthochromia (zan″tho-kro′me-ah) [*xantho-* + Gr. *chrōma* color *-ia*] any yellow discoloration, as of skin. Its presence in the cerebrospinal fluid is often an indication of a previous intracranial hemorrhage.

xanthochromic (zan″tho-kro′mik) having a yellow color; applied almost exclusively to cerebrospinal fluid. Also called xanthochromatic.

xanthogranuloma (zan″tho-gran″u-lo′mah) a term that has been used for a lesion characterized by the presence of proliferating fibroblasts together with histiocytic cells with foamy cytoplasm, some of them multinucleated. Retroperitoneal or mediastinal lesions with this appearance may in fact be true fibrous histiocytomas, and as the connotation of the term is imprecise, it has little practical value.

juvenile x., a reactive lesion of the skin, usually characterized by the presence of one or more nodules that are soft, elevated, small, and yellow. Rarely, the iris is also involved. In the early stages there is a uniform infiltrate of foamy histiocytes or macrophages; in later stages the histiocytic infiltrate is accompanied by multinucleated Touton giant cells, lymphocytes, and eosinophils. The lesion may be present at birth, but usually arises in early infancy and then regresses spontaneously after several months. It is important to differentiate this condition from histiocytosis X. Formerly called *nevoxanthoendothelioma.*

xanthoma (zan-tho′mah) [*xanth-* + Gr. *-oma* tumor] an orange or yellow deposit of lipids, usually in the skin or tendons, that is associated with abnormally high concentrations of serum lipids. When found in the skin, the deposits are often flattened and surrounded by a reddened base; those in the tendons are tuberous (rounded). Disorders producing abnormal concentrations of serum lipids include lipoprotein lipase deficiency, dysbetalipoproteinemia, hypercholesterolemia, and hypertriglyceridemia, all of which are familial disorders. Many other disorders may secondarily produce high serum lipid concentrations. See also *xanthelasma.*

xanthoma cell see *foam cell.*

xanthomatosis (zan″tho-mah-to′sis) the occurrence of multiple yellowish plaques, most often on the eyelids, neck, and trunk, which are histologically similar to xanthomas. Xanthomatosis is often associated with lymphomas, multiple myeloma, and other malignancies. See also *cerebrotendinous xanthomatosis, systemic h.* under *histiocytosis* (*Hand-Schüller-Christian disease*), and *Wolman's disease.*

xanthomatous (zan-tho′mah-tus) like a xanthoma or related to xanthomas. See *xanthoma.*

xanthopterin (zan-thop′ter-in) [*xantho-* + Gr. *pteron* wing] a yellow pteridine pigment, 2-amino-4,6-pteridinediol, $C_6H_5N_5O_2$, from the integument of wasps and hornets and from butterfly wings. Xanthopterin has some hematopoietic stimulating activity in anemic animals. It is an inhibitor of xanthine oxidase. See also *pterin.*

xanthosine (zan′tho-sēn) a nucleoside, xanthine-9-ribofuranoside, that on hydrolysis yields xanthine and ribose. It is formed catabolically from xanthylic acid, an intermediate in the formation of guanylic acid from adenylic acid.

xanthosine monophosphate (XMP) see *xanthosine-5′-phosphate.*

xanthosine-5′-phosphate a mononucleotide composed of xanthine, ribose, and phosphoric acid. It is an intermediate in the formation of guanylic acid from adenylic acid. Also called *xanthosine monophosphate* and *xanthylic acid.*

xanthurenic acid (zan″thu-ren′ik) a metabolite of tryptophan, $C_9H_5N(OH)_2COOH$, present in normal urine and found in increased amounts in pyridoxine (vitamin B_6) deficiency. Kynurenine is a precursor.

xanthurenic aciduria (zan″thu-ren′ik as″id-u′re-ah) a rare hereditary disorder, transmitted as an autosomal recessive trait, that is due to the diminished activity or absence of kynureninase (L-kynurenine hydrolase, EC 3.7.1.3). In the normal pathway for the metabolism of tryptophan in the liver, kynurenine and 3-hydroxykynurenine are formed and are hydrolyzed by the enzyme kynureninase to alanine and anthranilic acid or 3-hydroxyanthranilic acid. In the absence of this enzyme, the hydroxykynurenine accumulates and is converted in the extrahepatic tissues (kidney) to xanthurenic acid, which accumulates and is excreted in the urine along with the kynurenines. The enzyme requires pyridoxal phosphate as cofactor; if a person's dietary intake of pyridoxine is deficient, the activity of the enzyme is depressed, resulting also in the formation and excretion of xanthurenic acid. Pregnancy, with its high demand for pyridoxine, may also be accompanied by temporary xanthurenic aciduria.

xanthuria (zan-thu're-ah) [*xanth-* + Gr. *ouron* urine + *-ia*] see *xanthinuria.*

xanthylic acid (zan'thil-ik) see *xanthosine-5'-phosphate.*

x-axis the horizontal axis of a rectangular (Cartesian) coordinate system, i.e., the line $y = 0$.

X chromosome (eks' kro'mo-sōm) one of the sex chromosomes of the XX/XY sex chromosome pattern. Generally, the mammalian female sexual karyotype is XX and the male is XY, but variations exist.

In the somatic cells of the XX female, one of the X chromosomes is inactivated. It is believed the inactivation ensures that both males and females have the same ratio of functional X chromosomal genes to autosomal genes. Both X chromosomes are needed in the human female, as the absence of one results in congenital abnormalities (Turner's syndrome).

The Lyon hypothesis suggests that one of the X chromosomes is inactivated randomly in each cell during early development. The inactive X chromosome can be either paternal or maternal in different cells of the same individual, but all clonal descendants of the cell have the same inactive X. X chromosome inactivation is permanent in at least somatic cells.

There appears to be a small region of the human X that is not inactivated in either homologue, which is suggested by the X-linked Xg blood group system. Heterozygotes and homozygotes for the blood antigen Xg^a have the same phenotype. Also, individuals with more or less than two X chromosomes exhibit abnormalities that would not be expected if all but one X chromosome were totally inactivated.

The nuclei of female cells contain dark-staining regions of chromatin (Barr body); the number of Barr bodies is one less than the number of X chromosomes. Normal female cells contain one, and normal male cells have none.

The two X chromosomes of female mammals do not replicate at the same time in the cell cycle. The X chromosome that forms the Barr body replicates later in the S period than does the other.

See also *sex determination* and *XX/XY sex chromosome pattern.*

Xe the symbol for the chemical element *xenon.*

xen/o (zen'o) [Gr. *xenos* a guest-friend; any stranger or foreigner] a word element used in combining form to denote foreign material, e.g., xenoparasite.

xenobiotic (zen"o-bi-ot'ik) [*xeno-* + Gr. *biōtikos* pertaining to life] a chemical not normally present in biologic systems, such as certain environmental pollutants.

xenodiagnosis (zen"o-di-ag-no'sis) [*xeno-* + *diagnosis*] a special method of animal inoculation that employs laboratory-bred bugs and animals in the diagnosis of certain parasitic infections when it has not been possible to demonstrate the organism in blood films. This method was originally used in the diagnosis of *Trypanosoma cruzi* infections (Chagas' disease) and has been used for *Trichinella spiralis* infections.

In the original method, bugs are fed patients' blood, or are offered aliquots of patients' blood through a moistened membrane (e.g., cat gut). Approximately 10–30 da after the blood meal, the feces or intestinal contents of the bugs are examined for the presence of any of the organisms. For the diagnosis of trichinosis, muscle tissue from patients may be fed to laboratory rats to detect larvae.

xenogeneic (zen"o-jĕ-ne'ik) [*xeno-* + Gr. *gennan* to produce] pertaining to the genotypes of two individuals from different species. Also called *heterologous.*

xenogeneic graft see *heterologous g.* under *graft.*

xenograft (zen'o-graft) see *heterologous g.* under *graft.*

xenology (ze-nol'o-je) the study of the relationships of parasites to their hosts.

xenon (Xe) (ze'non) [Gr. *xenos* stranger] a colorless, odorless, unreactive gaseous element; atomic number 54; atomic weight 131.30; group O of the periodic table; oxidation numbers +2, +4, +6, +8. It is used in electric discharge lamps and in lasers. Many xenon compounds are strong oxidizing agents (e.g., XeF_2, XeO_3, and XeO_4, the last two of which are explosively unstable). XeF_2 and XeF_4 are fluorinating agents.

xenon-127 (Xe 127, ^{127}Xe) an accelerator-produced radionuclide, which decays by electron capture with a half-life of 36.4 da; it also emits gamma rays. The principal gamma photon (203 keV) permits better resolution in scintillation photographs than when Xe-133 is used (81 keV); however, this nuclide is not generally available.

xenon-133 (Xe 133, ^{133}Xe) a reactor-produced radionuclide, which decays by beta decay with a half-life of 5.27 da; it also emits gamma rays at 81 keV (used for imaging) and 31 keV. This is the most commonly used radioactive gas, particularly for pulmonary ventilation scans and for blood flow studies.

xenoparasite (zen"o-par'ah-sīt) an organism not ordinarily parasitic in the host, but which may become so in a host that is compromised.

Xenopsylla (zen"op-sil'ah) [*xeno-* + Gr. *psylla* flea] a genus of fleas, of which several species are known transmitters of disease-producing microorganisms and parasites.

X. astia, a rat flea, commonly found in Ceylon and India, that has been incriminated in the transmission of plague.

X. brasiliensis, a rat flea, with distribution in Africa, Brazil, and India, that has been implicated in the transmission of plague.

X. cheopis, the Oriental rat flea that transmits

plague and murine typhus. *X. cheopsis* is a host of the rat tapeworm, *Hymenolepis diminuta,* and the dwarf tapeworm, *H. nana.* See also the illustration under *flea.*

xer/o (ze'ro) [Gr. *xēros* dry] a word element used in combining form to denote dry, e.g., xerophthalmia.

xeroderma (ze"ro-der'mah) [*xero-* + Gr. *derma* skin] a generalized dryness and roughness of the skin, often accompanied by changes in coloration. This disorder is the result of hyperkeratinization of the skin, i.e., the buildup of the superficial layer of dead cells.

x. pigmentosum, a hereditary condition, transmitted as an autosomal recessive trait, that is characterized by a markedly increased disposition to the development of malignancies of the skin, specifically of skin exposed to sunlight. The biochemical defect is the lack of an enzyme involved in releasing thymine dimers (formed by ultraviolet (UV) radiation) from DNA. Affected individuals are therefore deficient in the ability to repair DNA that has been damaged by UV radiation. Multiple subgroups are known.

xerography (ze-rog'rah-fe) [*xero-* + Gr. *graphein* to write] the making of photographs or photocopies by means of a dry electrostatic process. See also under *xeroradiography.*

xerophthalmia (ze"rof-thal'me-ah) [*xero-* + Gr. *ophthalmos* eye + *-ia*] an abnormal condition characterized by the formation of a dry, greasy cornea, which often becomes thickened and denuded. Small foamy spots may develop on the bulbar conjunctiva. If untreated, there may be progression to keratomalacia, characterized by corneal ulceration, necrosis, secondary infection, and eventual loss of vision. Night blindness is an early prodromal finding. This disorder is caused by a deficiency of vitamin A and may be reversible by proper therapeutic intake of the vitamin. It is a common cause of blindness in some underdeveloped countries. See also *h. A* under *hypovitaminosis.*

xeroradiography (ze"ro-ra"de-og'rah-fe) a radiologic technique in which the x-ray image is recorded by xerography rather than by conventional photographic techniques. A xeroradiograph records a wider latitude (range of radiographic density) than does conventional x-ray film; it also shows more detail and more contrast owing to edge enhancement effect.

This technique is primarily used in mammography and other soft-tissue radiography, and in orthopedic radiology. Xeromammographs more clearly show vessels, subcutaneous tissues, tumors, and calcifications. Xeroradiographs of bone and muscle more clearly show the periosteum and trabeculae of bone, and differentiate between the soft-tissue planes. Because at present it requires 1.5–2 times the normal radiation dose, xeroradiography is not used for routine radiographic procedures.

In the procedure, the x-ray image is recorded in a layer of amorphous selenium vacuum that has been deposited on an aluminum plate. An electrostatic charge of 600–800 V is applied uniformly over the selenium layer. When the plate is exposed to x-rays, the photoconduction electrons produced discharge the selenium layer. The discharge in any small area is proportional to the x-ray exposure to the area; this makes a latent electrostatic image. The image is made visible by applying a fine, blue, electrically charged powder (the toner), which clings to the charged areas of the plate by electrostatic attraction.

At any sharp line of demarcation between high-density and low-density areas of the image, toner is attracted across the line to the high-density side. This effect, called edge enhancement, exaggerates the contrast of contours relative to the contrast of the latent image. A permanent image is produced by applying photographic paper to the plate, transferring the toner to the paper, applying a charge to the paper, and melting the powder into the surface of the paper.

xerostomia (ze"ro-sto'me-ah) [*xero-* + Gr. *stoma* mouth + *-ia*] a dryness of the mouth due to the decreased production of saliva, especially that associated with xerophthalmia in Sjögren's syndrome. In this syndrome the salivary glands become infiltrated with lymphocytes, with the gradual destruction and hyalinization of these glands. Manifestations include difficulty in swallowing, fissures of the mouth, and decreased taste sensation. See also *Sjögren's syndrome* and *xerophthalmia.*

X factor (eks'fak'tor) an accessory substance required for the aerobic growth of certain species of *Hemophilus,* replaceable by hemin or other iron porphyrin compounds and present in red blood cells. It is heat-stable and not destroyed by autoclaving. See also *Hemophilus.*

xi (Ξ, ξ) (zi, ksi, kse) the fourteenth letter of the *Greek alphabet.*

X-inactivation (eks"in-ak"tĭ-va'shun) the mechanism by which only one of the two X chromosomes in the cells of female mammals remains active; the other chromosome is condensed (forming the Barr body) and cannot be used as a template for protein synthesis. The single X of males appears to be inactivated during spermatogenesis. See also *Lyon hypothesis.*

xiphisternal joint (zif"ĭ-ster'nal) the fibrocartilaginous joint between the body and xiphoid process of the sternum.

xiphisternum (zif"ĭ-ster'num) [Gr. *xiphos* sword + *sternon* sternum] see *xiphoid process.*

xiphoid process (zif'oid) [*xipho-* + Gr. *eidos* form] [NA], the pointed process of cartilage supported by a core of bone, at the lower end of the sternum.

X karyotype see *XO karyotype.*

XLD agar abbrev. See *xylose-lysine-deoxycholate a.* under *agar.*

XMP abbrev. for xanthosine monophosphate. See *xanthosine-5'-phosphate.*

XO karyotype an abnormal karyotype of the female in the XX/XY sex chromosome pattern. One X chromosome is missing, resulting in the phenotypic characteristics of Turner's syndrome in humans. It is also the normal karyotype of male hemiptera and certain nematodes. See also *sex determination, Turner's syndrome,* and *X chromosome.*

XOR abbrev. See *exclusive OR.*

x-ray (eks-rā) [translation of Ger. *X Strahlen,* so named by their discoverer, Dr. Roentgen, because their nature was unknown] the ionizing radiation composed of high-energy (about 1 keV–1 MeV) photons produced when high-energy electrons collide with atoms. Diagnostic x-rays are usually in the range of 30–150 keV. Therapeutic x-rays range from the Grenz rays (5–10 keV) used in superficial therapy to the very-high-energy x-rays (1 MeV and above) used in supervoltage therapy.

The electrons striking the tungsten target of an x-ray tube have an energy equal to the product of their charge and the tube voltage (e.g., 100 keV if the kilovoltage is 100 kVp). X-ray photons are produced with all energies up to the electron energy by two processes.

Bremsstrahlung is a continuous spectrum of x-rays, which has one peak (at about 25 keV for 50-keV electrons).

Characteristic x-rays are produced when a K-shell electron is ejected by a colliding electron (which requires an electron energy of at least 70 keV for tungsten). Electrons drop down primarily from the L and M shells, producing 59- and 67.5-keV x-rays. (Characteristic x-rays produced by ejection of electrons from higher shells are soft and are filtered out of the beam.)

The x-rays emitted from the target are filtered by passing them through aluminum. Because x-ray absorption is inversely proportional to the cube of the energy, the softer x-rays are absorbed more strongly. This reduces the radiation dose to the skin produced by soft x-rays, but has little effect on the radiograph, which records the differential absorption of the harder x-rays.

x-ray crystallography the determination of crystal structure by means of x-ray diffraction. A monoenergetic x-ray beam is reflected by a crystal only at certain Bragg angles, forming a pattern of spots on a photographic film, which characterizes the lattice structure of the crystal. The positions of the spots are determined by the orientations of regularly spaced planes of atoms in the crystal; the intensities of the spots are determined by the density of electrons around the atoms in the planes. See also *Bragg reflection.*

x-ray machine a device for producing x-rays. It has three primary components: x-ray tube, high-voltage generator, and control console, each usually in a separate housing. A variety of x-ray devices are used for routine and special radiographic examinations and for fluoroscopy. In addition, there are mobile x-ray units for bedside examinations, and special high-energy (megavoltage) machines used in radiation therapy.

The tube is mounted inside a protective housing that acts as an electric insulator and radiation shield. The x-ray beam exits the housing through an adjustable-aperture collimator that limits the beam to the desired size. The x-ray tube is a vacuum tube with two electrodes, the cathode (or filament) and the anode, which are enclosed in an evacuated glass envelope. The filament is a small coil of tungsten wire, which is heated by alternating current to incandescence so that it emits a cloud of electrons. One end of the filament is grounded and a high positive voltage (30–40 kVp) is applied to the anode. Electrons accelerated to high speed by this voltage strike the anode, producing x-rays.

The energy of the x-rays depends on the electron kinetic energy, which in turn depends on the anode voltage (also called tube voltage or kilovoltage). The quantity of x-rays depends on the number of electrons striking the anode (the tube current or milliamperage). Because the tube is operated at saturation with all the electrons thermionically emitted from the cathode traveling to the anode, the tube current is controlled by the filament current.

About 99 percent of the beam energy is dissipated as heat. Cooling the anode is a problem solved differently by the two types of tubes, the stationary and rotating anode tubes. The stationary anode, a large copper bar, passes through the glass envelope and conducts heat out of the tube to the oil in which the tube is immersed. The rotating anode, a tungsten disk, rotates at 3000–10,000 rpm, becoming white-hot and thus losing heat by radiation. In both types of tubes, the area struck by the electron beam (the target) is beveled at an angle of 15°–20°. In the stationary anode, the target is a tungsten plate fused to the copper bar.

In some low-kilovoltage tubes used for mammography, molybdenum targets are employed. The electron beam is focused by a focusing cup around the filament, which has a negative charge and repels electrons. The beam strikes a rectangular area of the target, termed the actual focal spot. The x-ray beam leaves the target at a low angle; its cross-sectional area at the target, termed the effective focal spot, is approximately square.

Many tubes have dual filaments, permitting selection of two different focal spot sizes (often 2.0 mm and 0.3 mm); some tubes have focal spot sizes as small as 0.12 mm. The size of the focal spot is a compromise between image sharpness (definition) and the ability of the tube to dissipate the heat. Rotating anode tubes have the smallest focal spots.

The high voltage applied to the tube is rectified alternating current (pulsating direct current). In single-phase equipment, the voltage drops to zero twice a cycle. The intensity of the x-ray beam is below half of maximum two-thirds of the time. In three-phase, six-pulse equipment, the voltage only drops to 87 percent of the peak; in three-phase, 12-pulse equipment it only drops to 92 percent of peak. The intensity of the x-ray beam remains near the maximum, and much shorter exposure times can be used.

The high-voltage generator contains the high-voltage step-up transformer, the filament transformer, and the silicon diode full-wave rectifier. These components are immersed in oil for electric insulation.

The operating console contains switches that select the kilovoltage, milliamperage, and exposure time, and may contain meters to monitor the kilovoltage and milliamperage and phototiming circuitry. The controls select the kilovoltage and milliamperage by tapping different voltages from an autotransformer, which are sent to the primaries of the transformers in the high-voltage generator. The control console also contains line compensation circuitry, which adjusts for variations in line voltage by varying the number of coils of the autotransformer across which the line voltage is applied.

See also the accompanying illustration.

x-ray therapy see *radiation therapy.*

XX karyotype the normal sex karyotype of the female organism in the XX/XY sex chromosome pattern. See also *sex determination* and *X chromosome.*

XXX karyotype an abnormal karyotype of the female in the XX/XY sex chromosome pattern. An extra chromosome and Barr body are present, which may result in a mildly altered phenotype. Also called *superfemale.* See also *sex determination.*

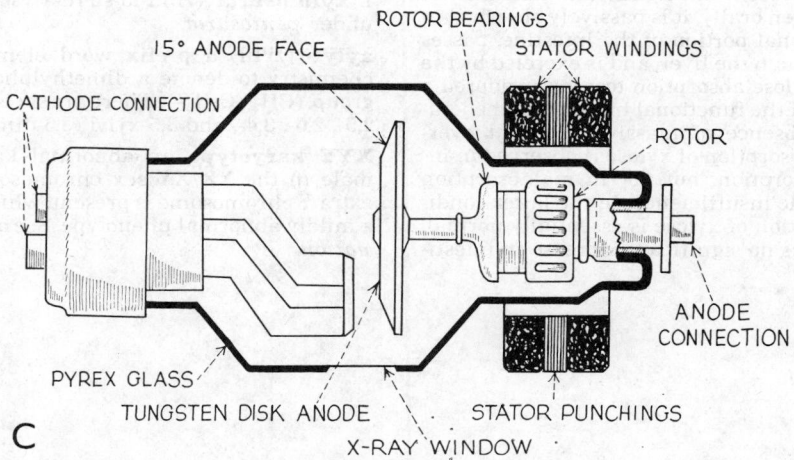

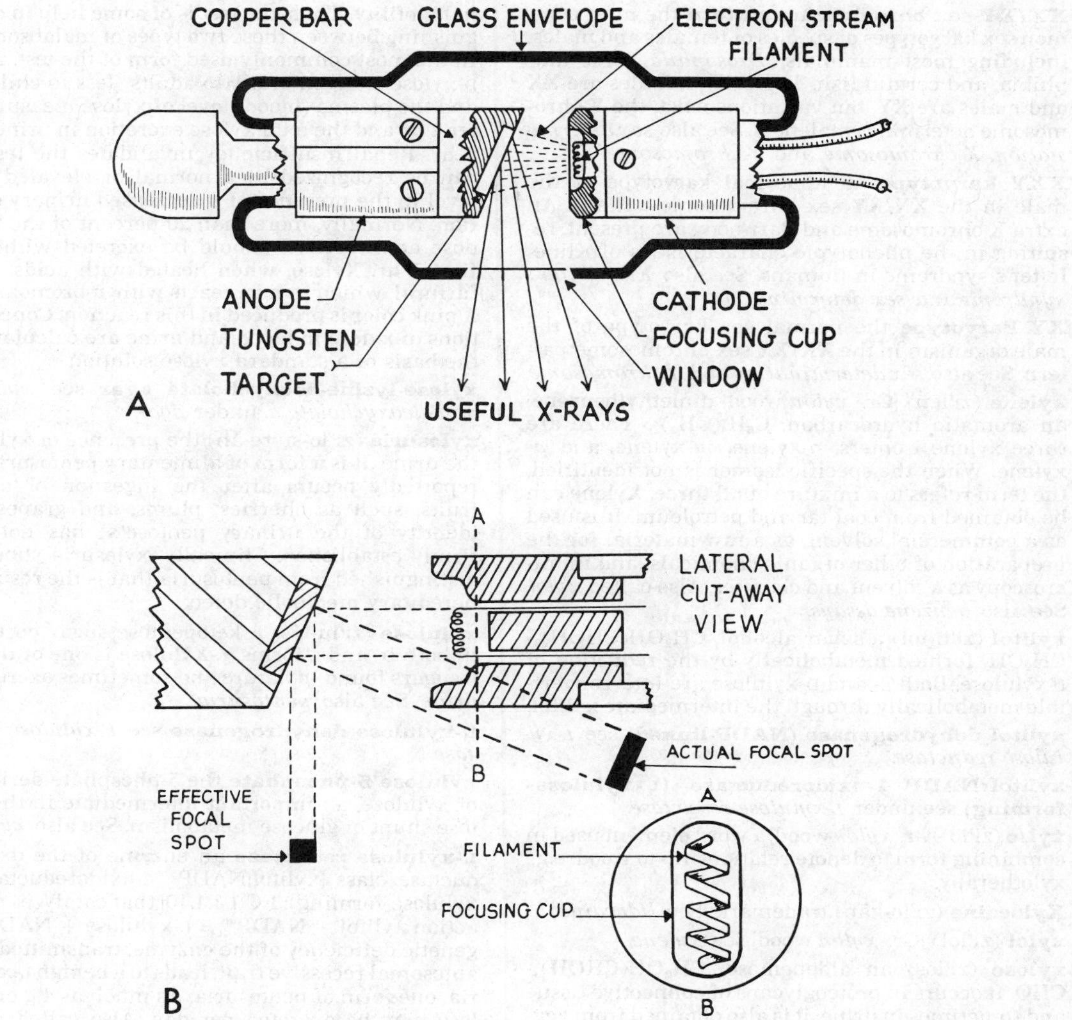

X-ray machine. Diagrams of common components: *A*, standard stationary anode x-ray tube; *B*, focusing cup and filament; and *C*, rotating anode x-ray tube. (From Meschan, I.: Radiographic Positioning and Related Anatomy. 2nd ed. Philadelphia, W. B. Saunders Co., 1978.)

XX/XY sex chromosome pattern the most common sex karyotypes of species of females and males, including most mammals, *Drosophila,* some amphibia, and certain fish. Typically, females are XX and males are XY, but variations exist; the Y chromosome determines maleness. See also *sex determination, X chromosome,* and *Y chromosome.*

XXY karyotype an abnormal karyotype of the male in the XX/XY sex chromosome pattern. An extra X chromosome and Barr body are present, resulting in the phenotypic characteristics of Klinefelter's syndrome in humans. See also *Klinefelter's syndrome* and *sex determination.*

XY karyotype the normal sex karyotype of the male organism in the XX/XY sex chromosome pattern. See also *sex determination* and *Y chromosome.*

xylene (zi'lēn) [Gr. *xylon* wood] dimethylbenzene; an aromatic hydrocarbon, $C_6H_4(CH_3)_2$. There are three xylene isomers, *o*-xylene, *m*-xylene, and *p*-xylene. When the specific isomer is not identified, the term refers to a mixture of all three. Xylene can be obtained from coal tar and petroleum. It is used as a commercial solvent, as a raw material for the preparation of other organic chemicals, and in microscopy as a solvent and clarifier. Also called *xylol.* See also *benzene assays.*

xylitol (zi'lĭ-tol) a sugar alcohol, $CH_2OH(CHOH)_3$-CH_2OH, formed metabolically by the reduction of L-xylulose. Both L- and D-xylulose are interconvertible metabolically through the intermediate xylitol.

xylitol dehydrogenase (NADP-linked) see *L-xylulose reductase.*

xylitol:NADP$^+$4-oxidoreductase (L-xylulose-forming) see under *L-xylulose reductase.*

xyl/o (zi'lo) [Gr. *xylon* wood] a word element used in combining form to denote relationship to wood, e.g., xylotherapy.

Xylocaine (zi'lo-kān) trademark. See *lidocaine.*

xylol (zi'lol) [Gr. *xylon* wood] see *xylene.*

xylose (zi'lōs) an aldopentose, $CH_2OH(CHOH)_3$-CHO. It occurs in proteoglycans of connective tissue and sometimes in urine; it is also obtained from vegetable gums, beechwood, and jute.

xylose absorption test D-xylose is an aldopentose not normally present in significant amounts in blood. When given orally, it is passively absorbed in the duodenojejunal portion of the intestine, passes unchanged through the liver, and is excreted by the kidneys. The xylose absorption test is considered a reliable index of the functional integrity of the jejunum (in the absence of massive bacterial overgrowth). Low absorption of xylose is observed in intestinal malabsorption, but not in malabsorption due to pancreatic insufficiency. In the latter condition, the absorption of xylose is essentially normal, provided there is no significant increase in intestinal motility. Thus, the test is of some help in distinguishing between these two types of malabsorption. In the most commonly used form of the test, 25 g of D-xylose is given orally to adults (less to children), and the plasma (blood) level of xylose measured after 2 hr and the total xylose excretion in urine after 5 hr. Renal insufficiency invalidates the test and can be recognized by a normal or elevated blood level in the presence of a decreased urinary excretion. Normally, more than 20 percent of the xylose dose administered should be excreted within the first 5 hr. Xylose, when heated with acids, forms furfural, which in turn reacts with *p*-bromoaniline. A pink color is produced in this reaction. Concentrations of xylose in blood and urine are calculated on the basis of a standard xylose solution.

xylose-lysine-deoxycholate agar see *xylose-lysine-deoxycholate a.* under *agar.*

xylosuria (zi"lo-su're-ah) the presence of xylose in the urine. It is a form of alimentary pentosuria that reportedly occurs after the ingestion of certain fruits, such as cherries, plums, and grapes. The identity of the urinary pentose(s) has not been firmly established. Clinically, xylosuria should be distinguished from pentosuria that is the result of a hereditary metabolic defect.

xylulose (zi'lu-lōs) a ketopentose sugar occurring in both D- and L-forms. L-Xylulose is one of the few L-sugars found in nature and sometimes excreted in urine. See also *pentosuria.*

L-xylulose dehydrogenase see *L-xylulose reductase.*

xylulose 5-phosphate the 5-phosphate derivative of xylulose, an important intermediate in the pentose shunt of glucose metabolism. See also *xylulose.*

L-xylulose reductase an enzyme of the oxidoreductase class [xylitol:NADP$^+$ 4-oxidoreductase (L-xylulose-forming); EC 1.1.1.10] that catalyzes the reaction xylitol + NADP$^+$ $\rightleftarrows$ L-xylulose + NADPH. A genetic deficiency of the enzyme, transmitted as an autosomal recessive trait, leads to a benign L-xylosuria, one form of pentosuria. As much as 4 g of xylulose may be excreted per day. Also called *xylitol dehydrogenase* and *L-xylulose dehydrogenase* (L-XDH). See also *pentosuria.*

L-xylulosuria (zi"lu-lo-su're-a) see *idiopathic p.* under *pentosuria.*

xylyl- (zi'lil) a prefix word element in organic chemistry to denote a dimethylphenyl substituent group, $(CH_3)_2C_6H_3$—. There are six isomers: 2,3-, 2,4-, 2,5-, 2,6-, 3,4-, and 3,5-xylyl (3,5-dimethylphenyl).

XYY karyotype an abnormal karyotype of the male in the XX/XY sex chromosome pattern. An extra Y chromosome is present, which may result in a mildly abnormal phenotype. See also *sex determination.*

Y

Y symbol for one of the coordinate axes in a plane, *tyrosine,* the chemical element *yttrium.*

-y a suffix word element to denote a condition or process, e.g., polydactyly.

Υ the Greek capital letter *upsilon.*

υ the Greek lower case letter *upsilon.*

yaws (yawz) an endemic infectious disease, limited primarily to tropical regions, that is caused by the spirochete *Treponema pertenue.* The organism is spread by body contact. When it enters a break in the skin, it produces granulomatous lesions of the skin, bones, and mucous membranes. The initial lesion appears after 3–4 wk as a painless papule, which ulcerates and produces a regional lymphadenopathy. About 6–12 wk later, there is a generalized eruption of soft granulomas, which heal slowly and may relapse. Keratotic lesions often appear on the feet and lead to painful ulcerations. Chronic yaws is characterized by skin destruction, bone changes (contraction), and disfigurement. The gummatous lesions of late yaws and syphilis are clinically similar. Yaws usually is not fatal and rarely involves the central nervous system, the cardiovascular system, or other viscera.

Diagnosis is based on the clinical symptoms and positive VDRL and FTA-ABS test results, although the latter are indistinguishable from those in other treponemal infections. Microscopically, early lesions may be darkfield-positive for spirochetes, which are indistinguishable from *T. pallidum.* Penicillin therapy may resolve the infection with residual scar formation within the cutaneous lesions.

Also called bouba, frambesia, parangi, patek, and pian. See also *spirochete.*

forest y., see *American l.* under *leishmaniasis.*

y-axis the vertical axis of a rectangular (Cartesian) coordinate system, i.e., the line $x = 0$.

Yb symbol for the chemical element *ytterbium.*

Y chromosome one of the sex chromosomes of the XX/XY sex chromosome pattern. Generally, the mammalian female sexual karyotype is XX and the male is XY, but variations exist. The Y chromosome specifies maleness. Studies have suggested the presence of an H-Y antigen structural or regulator gene on the Y chromosome. It is this antigen that may be responsible for testicular development; in its absence, XY individuals are phenotypic females. See also *H-Y antigen, sex determination,* and *XX/XY sex chromosome pattern.*

yeast (yēst) a unicellular fungus, 3–5 μm in diameter and oval or spherical in shape. As with all fungi, yeasts are eukaryotic and thus contain several chromosomes, mitochondria, and an endoplasmic reticulum complex. The cell wall of yeasts contains glucan (β-1,6-linked D-glucose residues with β-1,3 branches) and mannan (α-1,6-linked D-mannose with α-1,2 and α-1,3 branches). Many yeast cell walls also contain chitin (*N*-acetylglucosamine residues linked by β-1,4 glycosidic bonds).

Although most yeasts reproduce by budding, a few have been shown to reproduce by fission. When single yeast cells adhere to each other, they form chains known as pseudohyphae. Certain yeasts (*Cryptococcus,* for example) have an exteral capsular polysacchsaride.

Most yeasts are saprophytic and can be useful in the preparation of food and beverages (*Saccharomyces cerevisiae*). A few, however, are pathogenic to humans. These medically important yeasts, which consist of seven genera, belong to the class Deuteromycetes (Fungi Imperfecti), order Moniliales, family Cryptococcaceae: *Cryptococcus, Torulopsis, Pityrosporum, Rhodotorula, Candida, Trichosporon,* and *Geotrichum.* However, sexual stages have been found in some species that subsequently have been assigned to perfect genera.

See also the accompanying table.

bakers' y., *Saccharomyces cerevisiae,* a yeast used in brewing beer, making alcoholic liquors, and baking bread. Also called brewers' yeast. See also *Saccharomyces cerevisiae.*

dried y., the dry cells of any suitable strain of *Saccharomyces cerevisiae,* usually a by-product of the brewing industry. It is used as a natural source of protein and B-complex vitamins.

imperfect y., a yeast whose perfect (sexual) stage is unknown.

perfect y., a yeast whose perfect (sexual) stage is known.

yellow (yel'o) [Anglo Saxon *geolu*] a spectral color that corresponds to the perceived hue of monochromatic light having a wavelength between 577 and 597 nm (i.e., between green and orange).

yellow body see *Wesenberg-Hamazaki body.*

yellow fever a viral hemorrhagic fever characterized by fever, jaundice, hemorrhage, albuminuria, severe headache, myalgia, and chills. The etiologic agent is a group B arbovirus. There are two epidemiologic transmissions of yellow fever: an urban form that is passed from one viremic indivdual to a nonimmune host by a mosquito (*Aedes aegypti*) vector, and a sylvatic (jungle) form that involves a zoonosis in which a mosquito carries the infection from a primate animal to a nonimmune human host. Clinically, the disease is most often a mild, nonspecific febrile illness, but it can occur as a severe syndrome with a 3-da viremic period followed by a remission period.

Laboratory diagnosis is based on the findings of a prolonged blood clotting time with depressed clotting Factors II, V, VII, VIII, IX, X, and XI; increased serum bilirubin; increased serum glutamic oxaloacetic transaminase (SGOT) and serum glutamic pyruvic transaminase (SGPT) levels; the presence of albumin and bile in urine; and the serologic demonstration of antibodies to group B arbovirus.

Fifty percent of patients with the uncommon, severe form of the disease die; treatment is nonspecific and symptomatic, owing to a lack of antiviral chemotherapy.

See also *arbovirus.*

Yersinia (yer-sin'e-ah) [Alexandre John Emile *Yersin,* French bacteriologist, 1863–1943] a genus of gram-negative, facultatively anaerobic, rod- or ovoid-shaped bacteria of the family Enterobacteria-

YEAST. CULTURAL AND BIOCHEMICAL CHARACTERISTICS OF YEASTS FREQUENTLY ISOLATED FROM CLINICAL SPECIMENS[a]

							Assimilation												Fermentation								
	Growth at 37°C	Pellicle in Broth	Pseudo/True Hyphae	Chlamydospores	Germ Tubes	Capsule, India Ink	*Glucose*	*Maltose*	*Sucrose*	*Lactose*	*Galactose*	*Melibiose*	*Cellobiose*	*Inositol*	*Xylose*	*Raffinose*	*Trehalose*	*Dulcitol*	*Glucose*	*Maltose*	*Sucrose*	*Lactose*	*Galactose*	*Trehalose*	Urease	KNO_3 Utilization	Phenol Oxidase
Candida albicans	+	−	+	+	+	−	+	+	+	−	+	−	−	−	+	−	+	−	F	F	−	−	F	F	−	−	−
C. famata (Torulopsis candida)	+	−	−	−	−	−	+	+	+	+	+	+	+	−	+	+	+	+	W	−	W	−	−	W	−	−	−
C. glabrata (T. glabrata)	+	−	−	−	−	−	+	−	−	−	−	−	−	−	−	−	+	−	F	−	−	−	−	F	−	−	−
C. guilliermondii	+	−	+	−	−	−	+	+	+	−	+	+	+	−	+	+	+	+	F	−	F	−	F*	F	−	−	−
C. krusei	+	+	+	−	−	−	+	−	−	−	−	−	−	−	−	−	−	−	F	−	−	−	−	−	+*	−	−
C. parapsilosis	+	−	+	−	−	−	+	+	+	−	+	−	−	−	+	−	+	−	F*	−	−	−	F*	−*	−	−	−
C. pintolopesii	+[b]	−	−	−	−	−	+	−	−	−	−	−	−	−	−	−	−	−	F	−	−	−	−	−	−	−	−
C. pseudotropicalis	+	−	+	−	−	−	+	−	+	+	+	−	+	−	+*	+	−	−	F	−	F	F	F	−	−	−	−
C. rugosa	+	−	+	−	−	−	+	−	−	−	+	−	−	−	+	−	−	−	−	−	−	−	−	−	−	−	−
C. stellatoidea	+	−	+	+	+	−	+	+	−	−	+	−	−	−	+	−	+*	−	F	F	−	−	−	−	−	−	−
C. tropicalis	+	+	+	−[c]	−	−	+	+	+	−	+	−	+*	−	+	−	+	−	F	F	F	−	F	F	−	−	−
Cryptococcus neoformans	+	−	R	−	−	+	+	+	+	−	+	−	+	+	+	+*	+	+	−	−	−	−	−	−	+	−	+
C. albidus var. *albidus*	−*	−	R	−	−	+	+	+	+	+	+*	−*	+	+	+	+	+	+*	−	−	−	−	−	−	+	+	−
C. albidus var. *diffluens*	+*	−	−	−	−	+	+	+	+	−	−*	+*	+	+	+	+	+	+*	−	−	−	−	−	−	+	+	−
C. gastricus	−	−	−	−	−	+	+	+	+*	−	+	−	+	+	+	−	+	−	−	−	−	−	−	−	+	−	−
C. laurentii	+*	−	−	−	−	+	+	+	+	+	+	+*	+	+	+	+*	+	+	−	−	−	−	−	−	+	−	−
C. luteolus	−	−	−	−	−	−	+	+	+	−	+	+	+	+	+	+	+	+	−	−	−	−	−	−	+	−	−
C. terreus	−*	−	−	−	−	+	+	+*	−	+*	+*	−	+	+	+	−	+	−*	−	−	−	−	−	−	+	+	−
C. uniguttulatus	−	−	−	−	−	+	+	+	+	−	−*	−	−*	+	+	+*	−*	−	−	−	−	−	−	−	+	−	−
Rhodotorula glutinis	+	−	−	−	−	−*	+	+	+	−	+*	−	+	−	+	+	+	−	−	−	−	−	−	−	+	+	−
R. rubra	+	−	−	−	−	−*	+	+	+	−	+	−	+*	−	+	+	+	−	−	−	−	−	−	−	+	−	−
Saccharomyces cerevisiae	+	−	−*	−	−	−	+	+	+	−	+	−	−	−	−	+	+*	−	F	F	F	−	F	F*	−	−	−
Trichosporon beigelii	+*	+	+	−	−	−	+	+	+	+	+*	+*	+*	+*	+	+*	+*	+*	−	−	−	−	−	−	+*	−	−
T. pullulans	+*	+	+	−	−	−	+	+	+	+*	+	+*	+	+	+*	+*	+	−	−	−	−	−	−	−	+	+	−
Geotrichum candidum	−*	+	+	−	−	−	+	−	−	−	+	−	−	−	+	−	−	−	−	−	−	−	−	−	−	−	−

a Asterisks indicate strain variation; R, rare. Under Assimilation, plus signs indicate growth greater than that of the negative control. Under Fermentation, F indicates that the sugar is fermented (i.e., gas is produced); W, weak fermentation.

b *C. pintolopesii* is a thermophilic yeast capable of growth at 40°–42°C.

c Occasional strains of *C. tropicalis* produce teardrop-shaped chlamydospores.

Modified from Lennette, E. H., et al.: Manual of Clinical Microbiology. 3rd ed. Washington, DC, American Society for Microbiology, 1981, p. 563: based on the data of Ahearn, D. G., and Schlitzer, R. L. (eds.): Yeast infections, in Balows, A. (ed): Diagnostic Procedures in Bacterial, Mycotic, and Parasitic Infections, 6th ed., Washington, DC, American Public Health Association, 1980; and Lodder, J. (ed.): The Yeasts: A Taxonomic Study, 2nd ed., Amsterdam, North-Holland Publishing Co., 1970.

ceae. The organisms are nonmotile at 37°C, produce β-galactosidase, ferment glucose with no production of gas, and are oxidase-, Voges-Proskauer–, and lysine decarboxylase–negative. Hydrogen sulfide (H_2S) is not produced on triple sugar iron agar. The genus contains the organism responsible for bubonic plague; other species cause gastroenteritis and mesenteric lymphadenitis. Species identification depends on biochemical reactions. Antigenic analysis may be performed with specific antisera. See also *Enterobacteriaceae.*

Y. enterocolitica, a species that causes acute gastroenteritis and mesenteric lymphadenitis, especially in young children. The organism is ubiquitous and has been isolated from mammals, birds, and frogs, and from material contaminated by feces. Transmission occurs via infected food and water and from person-to-person contact. Cells from cultures grown below 30°C are motile with peritrichous flagella, are not encapsulated, and are ornithine decarboxylase–positive at 25°C. Unlike *Y. pestis* and *Y. pseudotuberculosis,* this species acidifies both the slant and butt of triple sugar iron agar.

Y. pestis, the bacillus that causes bubonic or pneumonic plague. The organism is transmitted by fleas from rats to humans. It may be cultured from tissues or infected lymph nodes. The cells are nonmotile, are sometimes encapsulated, and stain in a characteristic bipolar "safety-pin" fashion. Colonies are small, brown, and nonhemolytic. Positive identification is most rapid with fluorescent antibody staining. Unlike other *Yersinia* species, *Y. pestis* is urease-negative.

Y. pseudotuberculosis, a species commonly present in the intestinal tracts of birds and domestic and wild animals. Humans are infected by consuming food contaminated with animal excreta or by direct contact. Mesenteric lymphadenitis without gastroenteritis is the most frequent clinical manifestation.

yield (yēld) the amount of substance produced by a chemical synthesis. The theoretical yield is the amount that would have been produced if every reaction step went to completion, if no side-reactions occurred, and if none of the product were lost in handling and purification, i.e., the amount predicted by stoichiometric considerations. The actual yield is usually expressed as a percentage of the theoretical yield.

***y*-intercept** the point at which the graph of a linear equation crosses the *y*-axis. If the equation is $y = mx + b$, b is the *y*-intercept.

-yl (il) [Gr. *hylē* matter or substance] a suffix word element in organic chemistry to indicate a substituent group, e.g., methyl (CH_3—) as in 2-methylpropane, or a free radical or ion, e.g., methyl radical ($CH_3\cdot$), methyl cation (CH_3^+), methyl anion (CH_3^-).

-yne (īn) a suffix word element in organic chemistry to denote the presence of a carbon-carbon triple bond in the parent chain, e.g., propyne ($CH_3C{\equiv}CH$). A multiplying prefix denotes the number of triple bonds, e.g., 1,3-butadiyne ($CH{\equiv}C{-}C{\equiv}CH$). Cf. *-ane* and *-ene.*

yohimbine (yo-him′bēn) an alkaloid that occurs in *Rauwolfia serpentina.* It is an α-adrenergic blocker and was formerly used as a local anesthetic and mydriatic.

Yokogawa's fluke (yo″ko-gah′waz) [Sadamu *Yokagawa,* Japanese microbiologist, 20th century] see *M. yokogawai* under *Metagonimus.*

yolk sac (yōk) [L. *vitellus*] in the embryo, a sac of extraembryonic entoderm that is continuous with the embryonic midgut at the umbilical opening. The connection between the two narrows, forming the vitelline duct, which may partially persist as a Meckel's diverticulum attached to the terminal ileum. The yolk sac has a nutritive function in lower animals, but in mammals is mainly vestigial after the early stages of development. Primitive blood cells and vessels develop in its wall (see *blood island*). A primary yolk sac of cells derived from the cytotrophoblast (Heuser's membrane) precedes the formation of the secondary yolk sac described above. See also *embryo.*

yolk sac tumor see *endodermal sinus tumor.*

ytterbium (Yb) (ĭ-ter′be-um) [from *Ytterby,* the Swedish town where the element was discovered] a silvery ductile metallic element; atomic number 70; atomic weight 173.04; a 4f transition element (lanthanide or rare earth element): oxidation states 0, +2, +3. See also *rare earth elements.*

ytterbium-169 (Yb 169, ^{169}Yb) a cyclotron-produced radionuclide with a half-life of 31.8 da. It decays by electron capture, emitting gamma rays; the 177-keV and 198-keV energies are used for imaging.

ytterbium Yb 169 pentetate sodium a radiopharmaceutical used in radionuclide cisternography. Also called ytterbium-169-DTPA and pentetate calcium trisodium Yb 169.

yttrium (Y) (ĭ′tre-um) [from *Ytterby,* the Swedish town where the element was discovered] a dark-gray metallic element; atomic number 39; atomic weight 88.9059; a 4d transition element; oxidation state +3. It is chemically similar to the lanthanide elements and occurs with them in nature.

Z

Z symbol for *atomic number, impedance, ionic charge number.*

Z- [Ger. *zusammen* together] a stereodescriptor used to indicate the configuration at a double bond, e.g., (*Z*)-2-butene(*cis*-2-butene); see also *isomerism.*

z symbol for an algebraic unknown or space coordinate; a standard normal deviate; the z-axis, perpendicular to the plane of the x- and y-axis.

ζ the Greek lower case letter *zeta.*

Zahn's infarct (zahnz) [Friedrich Wilhelm *Zahn*, Swiss pathologist, 1845–1904] one of the multiple congested areas seen on the cut surface of the liver in individuals with portal vein thrombosis. The hepatocytes show varying degrees of degenerative change, but the lesions are not true infarcts.

Zahn's lines [Friedrich Wilhelm *Zahn*] the visible, alternating layers of coagulated blood and platelets enmeshed in fibrin that are found in arterial thrombi.

Zarontin (zah-ron'tin) trademark. See *ethosuximide.*

z-axis the axis of a three-dimensional rectangular (Cartesian) coordinate system, i.e., the line $x = 0$, $y = 0$.

Zebrina (ze-bri'nah) a genus of land snails. The species *Z. detrita* may serve as an intermediate host of the lancet fluke, *Dicrocoelium dendriticum.*

Zeeman effect (tse'man) [Pieter *Zeeman*, Dutch physicist, 1865–1943] a splitting of spectral lines for electronic transitions by an applied magnetic field, caused by the interaction between the field and the electron magnetic moment.

Zellballen alveolar aggregates of uniform cells of a paraglioma, each surrounded and separated by a richly vascular fibrous stroma.

Zener breakdown (ze'ner) [Clarence Melvin *Zener*, U.S. physicist, born 1905] the process by which a semiconductor diode conducts at sufficiently high reverse bias owing to an avalanche of current carriers. Also called Zener effect. See also *Zener d.* under *diode.*

Zenker's diverticulum (zeng'kerz) [Friedrich Albert von *Zenker*, German pathologist, 1825–1898] see *pharyngoesophageal d.* under *diverticulum.*

Zenker's fluid (zeng'kerz) [Konrad *Zenker*, German histologist, died 1884] a mercuric chloride–dichromate fixative; see under *fixative.*

zeolite (ze'o-līt) [N.L. *zeolites*, from Gr. *zein* to boil + *-lite*, from Gr. *lithos* stone] a hydrated aluminum silicate used as an ion-exchange resin to remove calcium and magnesium from hard water.

zero (zēr'o) [Ital. "naught"] 1. a number that when added to another number gives that number itself.
2. a digit (0) indicating the number zero.
3. in digital logic circuitry, the low-level voltage used to indicate the logical value "false."
4. to calibrate or adjust a measuring device so that it reads out zero when there is no input.

zero-order reaction see under *kinetics.*

zeta (Z, ζ) (za'tah) the sixth letter of the *Greek alphabet.*

zeta potential the electric potential across the interface between a solid and a liquid; more precisely, the potential across the layer of ions that surround charged colloidal particles in the liquid.

zeta sedimentation ratio (ZSR) method a test that measures the degree of red cell sedimentation under low centrifugal force. In a special centrifuge called the Zetafuge, capillary tubes filled with anticoagulated blood are kept in a fixed vertical position so that red cells migrate across the diameter of the tube for a 45-sec initial cycle. At the end of the cycle, the position of the tubes is changed by 180° so that the red cells then sediment toward the opposite wall of the capillary. The same reversal of the tubes occurs at each of the first three cycles; the Zetafuge stops after the fourth 45-sec cycle.

The degree of sedimentation that has taken place is read in the same manner as a hematocrit in a suitable reader called zetacrit. The ZSR is the percent zetacrit divided by percent hematocrit. Reference ranges for both males and females are 41–54 percent. In contrast to the Westergren and Wintrobe techniques, the ZSR is unaffected by the degree of anemia.

Cf. *Westergren sedimentation rate method* and *Wintrobe sedimentation rate method.*

Ziehl-Neelsen stain (zēl nēl-sen) [Franz *Ziehl*, German bacteriologist, 1857–1926; Friederich Karl Adolf *Neelsen*, 1854–1894] a stain used to demonstrate acid-fast organisms, especially species of *Mycobacterium.* A heat-fixed smear is flooded with carbolfuchsin, heated to steaming for 3–5 min, and cooled. The slide is washed, decolorized with acid alcohol, washed again, and then counterstained with methylene blue; acid-fast organisms appear red against a blue background. A modified method is also used for staining *Actinomyces* in tissues and for *Brucella.* See also *acid-fast* staining methods and *mycobacterium.*

ZIG abbrev. See *zoster immune globulin.*

Zimmermann reaction (zim'er-mahn) [Wilhelm *Zimmermann*, German physiologic chemist and physician, born 1910] the most common colorimetric reaction used for the determination of 17-ketosteroids. The reaction is based on the treatment of 17-ketosteroids with *m*-dinitrobenzene in alcoholic alkali to produce a reddish-purple color, with maximal absorption at 520 nm.

zinc (Zn) (zingk) [Ger. *Zink*] a blue-white, lustrous metallic element; atomic number 30; atomic weight 65.37; a 3d transition element; oxidation state +2. Zinc is used in alloys and plating (galvanized steel). It is an essential trace mineral and a component of enzymes such as DNA polymerase, RNA polymerase, carbonic anhydrase, carboxypeptidase, alcohol dehydrogenase, and aldolase.

The recommended daily allowance of 0.3 mg/kg (15 mg for adults, 20 mg for pregnant females, and 25 mg for lactating females) is obtained from a normal diet. Zinc deficiency retards growth and sexual development; it also produces anemia and enlargement of the liver and spleen. Deficiency in humans is generally seen only in individuals with diets rich in cereals (phytates) that bind zinc.

Inhalation of the fumes of zinc salts can cause metal fume fever and irritation of the skin as well as of the respiratory and gastrointestinal tracts. Oral poisoning (uncommon), caused by drinking from galvanized cans, also produces fever and GI distress.

Reference ranges for zinc are: in serum, 50–150 μg/dl; in blood, 400–1200 μg/dl; and in urine, 150–1250 μg/24 hr.

zinc assays atomic absorption spectrophotometry. Serum or urine specimens are aspirated directly into the burner of the spectrophotometer; the zinc concentration is obtained from a standard curve, the absorbance being proportional to the concentration. Ion-free water and plastic labware are used to minimize external zinc contamination.

zinc oxide [USP], a white powder, ZnO, used medicinally in ointment form as a topical protectant and astringent, and industrially as a white pigment.

zinc phosphide a highly toxic rat poison, Zn_3P_2, which evolves phosphine by reaction with acids, as in the stomach. See also *phosphine* and *phosphorus assays.*

zinc-sulfate flotation method a concentration method to demonstrate the presence of the cysts and eggs of parasites in fecal specimens. This method is especially useful for detecting cysts of amebae and flagellates; *Strongyloides* larvae can also be recovered.

In the procedure, a small sample of feces is mixed with water and strained through gauze. This fecal suspension is mixed with water and centrifuged. The supernate is discarded, and the pellet is mixed with more water and recentrifuged. After the supernate is decanted, the remaining sediment is resuspended with zinc-sulfate, specific gravity 1.18, and centrifuged. In the last centrifugation, any cysts or eggs present that float to the top of the suspension can be removed with a wire loop and placed on a slide with iodine solution for microscopic examination.

zinc-sulfate turbidity test an obsolete diagnostic test of liver function. It is nonspecific and its result is predominantly affected by changes in the concentration of serum gamma-globulin.

zirconium (Zr) (zir-ko′ne-um) [Ger. *Zircon* ($ZrSiO_4$), Fr. *jargon,* It. *giargone,* Arabic *zarqūn,* Persian *zargūn* gold-colored] a metallic element that occurs as a lustrous, grayish-white solid or a bluish-black powder; atomic number 40; atomic weight 91.22; a 4d transition element; oxidation states +1, +2, +3, +4 (the most stable and most common). Zirconium has low toxicity. It is used as a catalyst and in alloys.

Z line [Ger. *Zwischenscheibe* intermediate disk] the disk that separates sarcomeres. See also *skeletal m.* under *muscle.*

Zn symbol for the chemical element *zinc.*

zo/o (zo′o) [Gr. *zōon* animal] a word element used in combining form to denote animal life, e.g., zoology.

Zollinger-Ellison syndrome (zol′lin-jer el′lĭ-son) [Robert Milton *Zollinger,* U.S. physician, born 1903; Edwin H. *Ellison,* U.S. physician, born 1918] a disorder characterized by extensive gastrointestinal ulceration, elevated levels of serum gastrin and gastric acid, and the formation of gastrinomas, usually of the pancreas. Other endocrine disorders such as hyperparathyroidism are often present. Males are affected slightly more often than females; the age of onset is usually between 20 and 50 yr. The gastrinomas produce gastrin, a hormone that stimulates the growth and activity of the parietal cells. Acid produced by the parietal cells results in ulceration of the GI tract in common and uncommon sites. Associated findings may include diarrhea, GI bleeding, and perforation of an ulcer into adjacent structures.

Diagnosis is established by radioimmunoassay determination of serum gastrin levels (as >300 pg/ml, but usually 3500–350,000). Gastric hypersecretion (>15 mEq/hr) is evident by gastric analysis (acid secretion >20 mmol/hr; BAO/PAO >60 percent), and the intravenous administration of secretin or calcium will cause a very high increase in serum gastrin.

Cf. *peptic u.* under *ulcer.*

zona (zo′nah), pl. *zonae* [L. "a girdle"] [NA], a general term for an area with a specific boundary or characteristic; a zone: an encircling region or area.

z. fasciculata, the thick middle layer of the adrenal cortex. See also *adrenal.*

z. glomerulosa, the thin outer layer of the adrenal cortex whose cells form aldosterone. See also *adrenal.*

z. pellucida, a layer of gel-like neutral protein-polysaccharide, 50–80 μm in diameter, that becomes visible around oocytes. It is secreted by either the ovum or the surrounding follicular cells.

z. reticularis, the inner layer of the adrenal cortex. See *adrenal.*

zonogram (zo′no-gram) a narrow-angle, body-section radiograph. Cf. *tomogram.*

zonography (zo-nog′rah-fe) a method of body-section radiography in which a narrow exposure angle (2°–10°) is used, producing a focal zone 10–25 mm thick. See also *tomography.*

stereoscopic z., the making of a pair of zonograms that view the patient from two different angles, viewed with a stereoscope. The tomography is shifted or the patient is rotated about 5° between exposures.

zonula (zōn′u-lah), pl. *zonulae* [L., dim. of *zona*] a small zone, or zonule.

zonula adherens, pl. *zonulae adherentes* a cell junction, one of the components of the junctional complex that unites cells of simple columnar epithelium at their luminal margins. It lies between the tight junction and desmosome, and is formed at the site where the microfilaments of the terminal web insert to the inner aspects of the lateral cell membranes. A gap of approximately 20 nm separates the cells.

zonula occludens, pl. *zonulae occludentes* a type of cell junction in which the apposed cell membranes come into contact through a series of tiny ridges, hence the synonym tight junction. A zonula occludens forms the outermost component of the junctional complex that unites adjacent simple columnar epithelial cells such as in the small intestine: it forms a bandlike seal that prevents extracellular material from passing into the intercellular space. Also called *macula occludens* and tight junction.

zooanthroponoses (zo″o-an″thro-po-no′sēs) [*zoo-* + Gr. *anthrōpos* human being + *nosos* disease] diseases primarily of human origin, although they may be acquired by other vertebrates.

Potential Host Distribution of Selected Zoonoses

	DOMESTIC ANIMALS									WILD ANIMALS									
															MAMMALS				
	Horses	Cattle	Sheep	Goats	Swine	Dogs	Cats	Lab rodents	Poultry	Invertebrates	Fish	Amphibians	Reptiles	Birds	Rodents	Primates	Carnivores	Ungulates	Other
VIRUS DISEASES																			
Arbovirus encephalitis	X	X	X	X	X				X	X			X	X	X			X	X
Cat-scratch disease (virus suspected)							X										X		
Lymphocytic choriomeningitis						X		X							X				
Newcastle									X					X					
Rabies	X	X	X	X	X	X	X	X							X	X	X	X	X
Vesicular stomatitis	X	X			X					X									
Yellow Fever										X					X	X			X
RICKETTSIAL DISEASES																			
Q fever		X	X	X										X	X				
Rocky Mountain spotted fever			X	X				X		X					X				
SPIROCHETAL DISEASES																			
Leptospirosis	X	X	X	X	X	X	X	X							X	X	X	X	X
Rat-bite fever						X		X							X		X		
BACTERIAL DISEASE																			
Anthrax	X	X	X	X	X	X	X	X	X					X	X		X	X	X
Brucellosis	X	X	X	X	X	X	X	X	X						X		X	X	X
Erysipelas					X			X	X		X			X	X				
Hemorrhagic septicemia	X	X	X	X	X	X	X	X	X										
Listeriosis	X	X	X	X	X	X			X					X	X		X		
Melioidosis	X	X	X	X	X	X	X	X							X				
Plague			X	X		X	X	X						X	X		X		X
Pseudotuberculosis			X	X	X	X		X	X										
Psittacosis									X					X					
Salmonellosis	X	X	X	X	X	X	X	X	X	X	X	X	X	X	X	X	X	X	X
Scarlet fever		X				X													
Septic sore throat		X																	
Staphylococcosis		X																	
Tetanus	X												X					X	
Tuberculosis	X	X	X	X	X	X	X	X	X		X			X		X	X	X	X
Tularemia		X	X	X	X	X	X							X	X		X	X	X
Vibriosis		X	X	X															
FUNGUS DISEASES																			
Actinomycosis	X	X	X	X	X	X	X								X		X	X	X
Aspergillosis	X	X	X	X	X		X	X						X					
Coccidioidomycosis	X	X	X	X	X	X									X	X	X	X	
Cryptococcosis	X	X	X	X	X	X	X		X					X		X	X	X	
Epizootic lymphangitis	X																		
Histoplasmosis	X	X	X	X	X	X	X	X	X					X	X		X		X
Nocardiosis	X	X	X	X	X	X	X								X				X
North American blastomycosis	X					X													
Rhinosporidiosis	X	X																	
Ringworm	X	X	X	X	X	X	X	X	X						X	X	X	X	X
Sporotrichosis	X	X				X		X											
Streptothricosis	X	X	X	X		X												X	
PROTOZOAN																			
Amebiasis																X			
Balantidiasis					X											X			
Leishmaniasis						X									X		X		
Plasmodium (malaria)																X			
Sarcocystis	X	X	X	X				X							X				X
Toxoplasmosis		X				X	X	X						X	X		X		X
Trypanosomiasis	X	X	X	X	X	X	X	X		X								X	X

Reference: Fowler, M.E.: Curr. Probl. Pediatr., *4*:3, 1974.

Zoonoses. **Potential host distribution of selected zoonoses. (Reproduced with permission from Fowler, M. E.: Diseases of children acquired from nondomestic animals. *In* Gluck, L., et al. (eds.): Current Problems in Pediatrics. Copyright © 1974 by Year Book Medical Publishers, Inc., Chicago.)**

Zoomastigophorea (zo″o-mas″tĭ-go-for′e-ah) [*zoo-* + Gr. *mastix* whip + *phoros* bearing] a class of flagellate protozoa, including all flagellates that parasitize higher animals. Members of this class lack chromatophores, and usually have a single nucleus and a neuromotor apparatus. Reproduction is asexual, by longitudinal binary fission.

Two major groups are medically important: (1) those organisms that inhabit the digestive tract and genitalia, being transmitted from person to person without a biologic vector, e.g., *Giardia, Trichomonas, Chilomastix, Retortamonas,* and *Enteromonas;* (2) parasites of the blood stream and tissues that require a bloodsucking invertebrate as a biologic vector, e.g., *Leishmania* and *Trypanosoma.*

zoonosis (zo″o-no′sis), pl. *zoonoses* [*zoo-* + Gr. *nosos* disease] any infection or infectious disease of animals transmissible to humans under natural conditions. For a list of the more common examples, see the accompanying table.

zoophilic (zo″o-fil′ik) [*zoo-* + Gr. *philos* loving] preferring animals to humans as a host.

zooprophylaxis (zo″o-pro″fĭ-lak′sis) [*zoo-* + Gr. *prophylax* guard] a means of protecting humans from mosquito-borne diseases by diverting the mosquitoes from humans to animals (e.g., cattle). Although this method is rarely practiced deliberately, it is nonetheless effective.

zoster (zos′ter) [Gr. *zōstē* girdle] a girdle, encircling structure, or pattern.

zoster immune globulin (ZIG) the antibody passively administered to immunoincompetent individuals who have been exposed to varicella or herpes zoster. The immune globulin is prepared from the sera of patients convalescing from a herpes zoster infection. It should be given to immunocompromised children under 15 yr who have been exposed for longer than 1 hr to a person with a known case of varicella zoster, or to neonates whose mothers develop varicella within 4 da before or 48 hr after delivery. The immune globulin modifies the course of the disease but may not affect the development of immunity.

Plasma from convalescents, which is collected 1–5 wk after onset of herpes zoster infection, is available at some blood banks; it is effective at intravenous doses of 7–10 ml/kg of body weight. If the immune globulin or convalescent plasma is not available, normal immune serum globulin at intramuscular doses of 0.6–1.2 ml/kg may modify the illness. Rarely, allergic-type reactions develop to the immune globulin, especially in individuals deficient in immunoglobulins. Immune globulin prepared for intramuscular usage must never be administered intravenously, as the globulins are usually aggregated and may cause anaphylactic reactions.

Zr symbol for the chemical element *zirconium.*

Z score see *standardized deviate.*

ZSR abbrev. See *zeta sedimentation ratio method.*

Zuckerkandl's organs (tsook′er-kan″d′lz) [Emil *Zuckerkandl,* German anatomist, 1849–1910] extraadrenal aggregates of norepinephrine-secreting chromaffin tissue situated along each side of the abdominal aorta in association with the sympathetic ganglia. Found primarily in young children, they subserve the adrenal medulla as an additional source of catecholamines.

zwischenferment (tsvish″en-fer′ment) [Ger.] see *glucose-6-phosphate dehydrogenase.*

zwitterion (tsvit′er-i″on) see under *ion.*

zyg/o (zi′go) [Gr. *zygon* yoke] a word element used in combining form to denote yoked, joined, or junction, e.g., zygosity.

zygoma (zi-go′mah) [Gr. *zygōma* bolt or bar] referring to the zygomatic arch, process, or bone.

zygomatic (zi″go-mat′ik) pertaining to the zygoma.

zygomatic bone one of the paired skull bones that lie below and lateral to the orbit and form the prominence of the cheek. A temporal process projects backward to articulate with the zygomatic process of the temporal bone and form the zygomatic arch.

Zygomycetes (zi″go-mi-se′tēz) [*zygo-* + Gr. *mykēs* fungus] a class of fungi that includes the orders Mucorales and Entomophthorales. Common genera that belong to this fungal class include *Absidia, Basidiobolus, Conidiobolus, Cunninghamella, Mucor, Rhizomucor, Rhizopus,* and *Saksenaea.*

zygomycosis (zi″go-mi-ko′sis) [*zygo-* + Gr. *mykēs* fungus + *-osis*] any fungal infection in which the etiologic agent is a zygomycete; the infection is usually either opportunistic or limited to the subcutaneous tissue. See also *mucormycosis.*

zygonema (zi″go-ne′mah) see *zygotene.*

zygote (zi′gōt) [Gr. *zygōtos* yoked together] the diploid cell that results from the union of haploid male and female gametes; the fertilized ovum. The term also refers to the organism that develops from this cell.

zygotene (zi′go-tēn) [Gr. *zygōtos* yolked together] the second stage of prophase in meiosis I during which homologous chromosomes synapse to form bivalents. Also called *zygonema.* See also *meiosis.*

zym/o (zi′mo) [Gr. *zymē* leaven] a word element used in combining form to denote an enzyme, catalyst, or fermentation, e.g., zymogen.

zymogen (zi′mo-jen) [*zymo-* + Gr. *gennan* to produce] an inactive precursor that is converted to an active agent by the action of acid, alkali, or an enzyme. Also called *proenzyme.*

zymogenic (zi″mo-jen′ik) causing or pertaining to fermentation; enzyme-producing.

zymogenic cell see *chief cell.*

Appendix A

TABLE 1. COMMERCIALLY AVAILABLE CANCER CHEMOTHERAPY DRUGS

DRUG	FORMULATION	MAJOR INDICATIONS	ACUTE TOXICITY	DELAYED TOXICITY
ALKYLATING AGENTS				
Busulfan (Myleran)	Oral	Chronic granulocytic leukemia; polycythemia vera	Nausea and vomiting; rare diarrhea	*Bone marrow depression;* pulmonary fibrosis; hyperpigmentation; cutaneous reactions; alopecia; gynecomastia; amenorrhea; menopausal symptoms; sterility; azoospermia; leukemia; chromosome aberrations; cataracts; hyperuricemia
Chlorambucil (Leukeran)	Oral	Chronic lymphocytic leukemia; Hodgkin's disease; non-Hodgkin's lymphoma; ovarian carcinoma		*Bone marrow depression;* pulmonary fibrosis; leukemia
Cyclophosphamide (Cytoxan)	Oral, intravenous	Acute lymphocytic leukemia; chronic lymphocytic leukemia; breast carcinoma; bronchogenic carcinoma; Ewing's sarcoma; Hodgkin's disease; multiple myeloma; neuroblastoma; non-Hodgkin's lymphoma; ovarian carcinoma; rhabdomyosarcoma; sarcomas (general); uterine cervix carcinoma	*Nausea and vomiting;* anaphylaxis	*Bone marrow depression; alopecia;* hemorrhagic pulmonary cystitis; sterility (may be temporary); pulmonary fibrosis hyperpigmentation; secondary malignancies; nonspecific dermatitis
Mechlorethamine (nitrogen mustard; HN_2; Mustargen)	Intravenous	Bronchogenic carcinoma; Hodgkin's disease; non-Hodgkin's lymphoma	*Nausea and vomiting;* local reaction and phlebitis	*Bone marrow depression;* alopecia diarrhea; oral ulcers
Melphalan (1-phenylalanine mustard; Alkeran)	Oral	Breast carcinoma; malignant melanoma; multiple myeloma; ovarian carcinoma; testicular seminoma	Mild nausea; hypersensitivity reactions	*Bone marrow depression;* (especially platelets); possible pulmonary fibrosis; interstitial pneumonitis; leukemia
Thiotepa (triethylenethiophosphoramide; Thiotepa)	Intravenous	Bladder cancer (intravesically); breast carcinoma; Hodgkin's disease; ovarian cancer	*Nausea and vomiting;* local pain	*Bone marrow depression;* alopecia (one case)
ANTIMETABOLITES				
Cytarabine HCl (cytosine arabinoside; Cytosar-U)	Intravenous	Acute granulocytic leukemia; acute lymphocytic leukemia	*Nausea and vomiting;* diarrhea; anaphylaxis	*Bone marrow depression;* megaloblastosis; oral ulceration; hepatic damage

TABLE 1. COMMERCIALLY AVAILABLE CANCER CHEMOTHERAPY DRUGS (*Continued*)

DRUG	FORMULATION	MAJOR INDICATIONS	ACUTE TOXICITY	DELAYED TOXICITY
Floxuridine (FUDR)	Intraarterial	Liver metastases from gastrointestinal malignancies	*Nausea and vomiting;* diarrhea	*Oral and gastrointestinal ulcerations; bone marrow depression;* neurologic defects, usually cerebellar; pigmentation; alopecia; dermatitis
Fluorouracil (5-FU; Fluorouracil; Adrucil)	Intravenous	Bladder carcinoma; breast carcinoma; colorectal carcinoma; gastric adenocarcinoma; hepatoma; ovarian carcinoma; pancreatic adenocarcinoma; uterine cervix carcinoma; basal cell and squamous cell skin carcinoma (topically)	*Nausea and vomiting;* diarrhea	*Oral and gastrointestinal ulcers; bone marrow depression;* increased lacrimation; neurologic defects, usually cerebellar; pigmentation; alopecia; dermatitis
Mercaptopurine (6-MP; Purinethol)	Oral	Acute granulocytic leukemia; acute lymphocytic leukemia; chronic granulocytic leukemia	*Nausea and vomiting;* diarrhea	*Bone marrow depression; cholestasis and rarely hepatic necrosis; oral and intestinal ulcers;* chromosoma; aberrations; anorexia; hyperuricemia
Methotrexate (MTX; Methotrexate; Mexate)	Oral, intravenous	Acute lymphocytic leukemia; breast carcinoma; bronchogenic carcinoma; choriocarcinoma; medulloblastoma; mycosis fungoides; osteogenic sarcoma; rhabdomyosarcoma; squamous cell carcinoma of head and neck; testicular carcinoma; uterine cervix carcinoma	*Nausea and vomiting;* diarrhea; fever; anaphylaxis	*Oral and gastrointestinal ulceration* (perforation may occur); *bone marrow depression;* hepatic toxicity including cirrhosis and acute hepatic necrosis; renal toxicity; pulmonary infiltrates; osteoporosis; chills, fever; alopecia; depigmentation; cutaneous reactions; infertility; menstrual dysfunction; aphasia; paresis; convulsions
Thioguanine (6-TG; Thioguanine)	Oral	Acute granulocytic leukemia; acute lymphocytic leukemia	Occasional *nausea and vomiting*	*Bone marrow depression;* possible hepatic damage; stomatitis
NATURAL PRODUCTS				
Asparaginase (Elspar); source: enzyme	Intravenous	Acute lymphocytic leukemia	*Nausea and vomiting; fever,* chills; headache; *hypersensitivity,* possible anaphylaxis; abdominal pain; hyperglycemia leading to coma	CNS depression or hyperexcitability; acute hemorrhagic pancreatitis; coagulation defects; renal damage; hepatic damage

TABLE 1. (*Continued*)

DRUG	FORMULATION	MAJOR INDICATIONS	ACUTE TOXICITY	DELAYED TOXICITY
Bleomycin (Blenoxane); source: antibiotic	Intravenous	Hodgkin's disease; non-Hodgkin's lymphoma; penile carcinoma; squamous cell carcinoma of head and neck; testicular carcinoma; uterine cervix carcinoma	*Nausea and vomiting; fever;* anaphylaxis and other allergic reactions	*Pneumonitis and pulmonary fibrosis; cutaneous reactions;* stomatitis; alopecia; hyperpigmentation; Raynaud's phenomenon
Dactinomycin (actinomycin D; Cosmegen); source: antibiotic	Intravenous	Choriocarcinoma; Ewing's sarcoma; osteogenic sarcoma; rhabdomyosarcoma; sarcomas (general); testicular carcinoma; Wilms' tumor	*Nausea and vomiting;* diarrhea; local reaction and phlebitis	*Stomatitis; oral ulceration; bone marrow depression;* alopecia folliculitis
Daunorubicin (Daunomycin; Cerubidine); source: antibiotic	Intravenous	Acute granulocytic leukemia; acute lymphocytic leukemia	*Nausea and vomiting;* red urine (not hematuria); severe local tissue damage and necrosis on extravasation; transient ECG changes	*Bone marrow depression; cardiotoxicity; alopecia;* stomatitis; cutaneous toxicity; hyperuricemia; anorexia; diarrhea; fever and chills
Doxorubicin (Adriamycin); source: antibiotic	Intravenous	Acute granulocytic leukemia; acute lymphocytic leukemia; bladder carcinoma; breast carcinoma; bronchogenic carcinoma; endometrial carcinoma; Ewing's sarcoma; hepatoma; Hodgkin's disease; neuroblastoma; non-Hodgkin's lymphoma; osteogenic sarcoma; prostate carcinoma; rhabdomyosarcoma; sarcomas (general); squamous cell carcinoma of the head and neck; testicular carcinoma; thyroid carcinoma; Wilms' tumor	*Nausea and vomiting;* red urine (not hematuria); severe local tissue damage and necrosis on extravasation; diarrhea; transient ECG changes; ventricular arrhythmia; hypertensive encephalopathy; angioneurotic edema	*Bone marrow depression; cardiotoxicity* (may be irreversible); alopecia; stomatitis; cutaneous toxicity; hyperuricemia; anorexia; diarrhea; fever, chills; urticaria; anaphylaxis; conjunctivitis; lacrimation
Mithramycin (Mithracin); source: antibiotic	Intravenous	Testicular carcinoma	*Nausea and vomiting;* diarrhea; fever	*Hemorrhagic diathesis; bone marrow depression* (thrombocytopenia); hepatic damage; hypocalcemia and hypokalemia; stomatitis; cutaneous reactions
Mitomycin (Mutamycin) source: antibiotic	Intravenous	Breast carcinoma; colorectal carcinoma; gastric carcinoma; lung carcinoma; pancreatic carcinoma	*Nausea and vomiting;* local reaction if extravasation; fever	*Bone marrow depression* (cumulative); stomatitis; renal toxicity; alopecia; pulmonary fibrosis; hepatotoxicity at high doses

TABLE 1. COMMERCIALLY AVAILABLE CANCER CHEMOTHERAPY DRUGS (*Continued*)

Drug	Formulation	Major Indications	Acute Toxicity	Delayed Toxicity
Vinblastine sulfate (Velban); source: plant	Intravenous	Breast carcinoma; choriocarcinoma; Hodgkin's disease; non-Hodgkin's lymphoma; testicular carcinoma	*Nausea and vomiting;* local reaction and phlebitis if extravasation	*Bone marrow* depression; alopecia; stomatitis; loss of deep tendon reflexes; jaw pain; paralytic ileus
Vincristine sulfate (Oncovin); source; plant	Intravenous	Acute lymphocytic leukemia; breast carcinoma; Ewing's sarcoma; Hodgkin's disease; neuroblastoma; non-Hodgkin's lymphoma; rhabdomyosarcoma; sarcomas (general); Wilms' tumor	Local reaction if extravasation	*Peripheral neuropathy* (loss of deep tendon reflexes, numbness, tingling and muscle weakness); neuritic pain; *alopecia;* mild bone marrow depression; constipation leading to paralytic ileus
MISCELLANEOUS DRUGS				
Carmustine (BCNU; BiCNU)	Intravenous	Brain tumors; colorectal carcinoma; gastric carcinoma; hepatoma; Hodgkin's disease; multiple myeloma; non-Hodgkin's lymphoma	*Nausea and vomiting;* local phlebitis	*Delayed leukopenia and thrombocytopenia* (may be prolonged); pulmonary fibrosis (may be irreversible); delayed renal damage; gynecomastia
Cisplatin (Cis-Diammine-dichloroplatinum; Cis-DDP; Platino)	Intravenous	Bladder carcinoma; osteogenic sarcoma; ovarian cancer; squamous cell carcinoma of the head and neck; testicular carcinoma; uterine cervix carcinoma	*Nausea and vomiting;* anaphylactic-like reactions; fever	*Renal damage;* bone marrow depression; ototoxicity; hemolysis; hypomagnesemia; hyperuricemia; peripheral neuropathy; hypocalcemia; hypokalemia
Dacarbazine (DTIC; DIC)	Intravenous	Hodgkin's disease; malignant melanoma; sarcomas (general)	*Nausea and vomiting;* anaphylaxis; pain on administration	*Bone marrow depression;* influenza-like syndrome; alopecia; renal impairment; hepatic necrosis; facial flushing, paresthesia; rash; photosensitivity
Hydroxyurea (Hydrea)	Oral	Chronic granulocytic leukemia	*Nausea and vomiting;* allergic reactions to tartrazine dye	*Bone marrow depression;* hyperkeratosis and hyperpigmentation; stomatitis; dysuria, alopecia, neurologic disturbances rare
Lomustine (CCNU; CeeNU)	Oral	Brain tumors; bronchogenic carcinoma; colorectal carcinoma; Hodgkin's disease	*Nausea and vomiting*	*Delayed (4–6 wk) leukopenia and thrombocytopenia* (may be prolonged); stomatitis; alopecia; transient elevation of transaminase activity; neurologic reactions

TABLE 1. (*Continued*)

DRUG	FORMULATION	MAJOR INDICATIONS	ACUTE TOXICITY	DELAYED TOXICITY
Mitotane (*o,p'*-DDD; Lysodren)	Oral	Adrenocortical carcinoma	*Nausea and vomiting;* diarrhea	*CSN depression;* dermatitis; visual disturbances; adrenal insufficiency; brain damage with long-term high dosage; hematuria, hemorrhagic cystitis, albuminuria; hypertension; orthostatic hypotension
Procarbazine HCl (Matulane)	Oral	Brain tumors; Hodgkin's disease; non-Hodgkin's lymphoma	*Nausea and vomiting;* CNS depression	*Bone marrow depression;* stomatitis; dermatitis; peripheral neuropathy; pneumonitis
HORMONES				
Corticosteroids				
Prednisone or prednisolone	Oral	Acute lymphocytic leukemia; chronic lymphocytic leukemia; breast carcinoma; multiple myeloma; Hodgkin's disease; non-Hodgkin's lymphoma		Mental aberrations; gastric ulcers; glucose intolerance; osteoporosis; hypertension; cataract formation
Dexamethasone (Decadron)	Oral, intramuscular, intravenous	Brain tumors (cerebral edema reduced)		
Estrogens				
Diethylstilbestrol (DES)	Oral	Breast carcinoma; prostate carcinoma	*Nausea and vomiting;* cramps	*Fluid retention;* hypercalcemia; feminization; uterine bleeding; if given during pregnancy, may cause vaginal carcinoma in offspring; increased frequency of vascular accidents
Ethinyl estradiol (Estinyl; others)	Oral	Breast carcinoma; prostate carcinoma		*Fluid retention;* hypercalcemia; feminization; uterine bleeding; increased incidence of vascular accidents
Androgens				
Dromostanolone propionate (Drolban)	Intramuscular	Breast carcinoma		*Fluid retention; masculinization;* hypercalcemia
Fluoxymesterone (Halotestin)	Oral	Breast carcinoma		*Fluid retention; masculinization;* cholestatic jaundice; hypercalcemia; painful hypertrophy of clitoris; hirsutism
Testolactone (Teslac)	Intramuscular	Breast carcinoma	Local pain, inflammation at injection site	Hypercalcemia; rare alopecia

TABLE 1. COMMERCIALLY AVAILABLE CANCER CHEMOTHERAPY DRUGS (*Continued*)

Drug	Formulation	Major Indications	Acute Toxicity	Delayed Toxicity
Testosterone propionate (Oreton; others)	Intramuscular	Breast carcinoma		*Fluid retention; masculinization;* hypercalcemia
Progestins				
Hydroxyprogesterone caproate (Delalutin)	Intramuscular	Endometrial carcinoma	Local abscess, pain	Hypercalcemia; cholestatic jaundice
Medroxyprogesterone acetate (Provera; others)	Oral	Breast carcinoma; endometrial carcinoma; renal cell carcinoma	Orally: nausea (rare) IM: local pain, abscess at injection site	Fluid retention; hypercalcemia
Megestrol acetate (Megace)	Intramuscular	Endometrial carcinoma	Allergic reactions to tartrazine dye	Fluid retention; thromboembolism
Antiestrogen				
Tamoxifen citrate (Nolvadex)	Oral	Breast carcinoma	*Nausea and vomiting;* hot flashes; transient increased bone or tumor pain	*Vaginal bleeding and discharge;* rash; hypercalcemia; retinopathy; corneal changes; decreased visual acuity; peripheral edema; depression; dizziness; headache

Courtesy of Stephen K. Carter, M.D.

TABLE 2. SOME INVESTIGATIONAL DRUGS

DRUG	FORMULATION	POTENTIAL INDICATIONS	ACUTE TOXICITY	DELAYED TOXICITY
Aminoglutethimide	Intravenous	Breast carcinoma	Skin rash; lethargy	Hypothyroidism (rare); bone marrow depression; fever, chills; gastrointestinal toxicity
Amsacrine (AMSA; 4′-(9-acridinylamino)methanesulfon-*m*-anisidide)	Intravenous	Acute granulocytic leukemia	*Nausea and vomiting;* diarrhea; pain or phlebitis on infusion	*Bone marrow depression;* hepatic injury; convulsions; stomatitis, ventricular fibrillation; alopecia
5-Azacytidine	Intravenous	Acute granulocytic leukemia	*Nausea and vomiting;* diarrhea; fever	*Leukopenia* (may be prolonged); thrombocytopenia; hepatic damage; rash; muscle pain and weakness
Estramustine (Estracyt; Emcyt)	Oral	Prostatic carcinoma	*Nausea and vomiting*	Mild gynecomastia
Etoposide (VP16-213)	Oral, intravenous	Acute granulocytic leukemia; small cell bronchogenic carcinoma; testicular carcinoma	*Nausea and vomiting;* diarrhea; fever	*Bone marrow depression;* alopecia; peripheral neuropathy
Hexamethylmelamine (HMM)	Oral	Bronchogenic carcinoma; ovarian carcinoma	*Nausea and vomiting*	*Bone marrow depression;* CNS depression; peripheral neuritis; visual hallucinations
Ifosfamide (Cyfos)	Intravenous	Same as cyclophosphamide (see Table 1)	*Nausea and vomiting*	*Bone marrow depression; hemorrhagic cystitis;* alopecia; sterility (may be temporary)
Prednimustine	Intravenous	Breast carcinoma; chronic lymphocytic leukemia; non-Hodgkin's lymphoma	Nausea and vomiting	Myelosuppression
Razoxane	Oral	Blast crisis of chronic myelogenous leukemia; colorectal carcinoma	Nausea and vomiting	Bone marrow depression
Semustine (methyl-CCNU)	Oral	Brain tumors; colorectal carcinoma; gastric carcinoma; Hodgkin's disease; malignant melanoma	Nausea and vomiting	Delayed leukopenia and thrombocytopenia (may be prolonged); pulmonary fibrosis; leukemia; renal failure
Streptozocin (streptozotocin; Zanosar)	Intravenous	Hodgkin's disease; islet cell carcinoma; malignant carcinoid	Nausea and vomiting; local pain; chills	Renal damage; hyperglycemia
Tegafur (Ftorafur)	Oral, intravenous	Same as fluorouracil (see Table 1)	Nausea and vomiting; CNS symptoms including dizziness and lethargy	Stomatitis; bone marrow depression; pigmentation; alopecia; dermatitis
Vindesine (Eldesine)	Intravenous	Acute lymphocytic leukemia; breast carcinoma; malignant melanoma	Local reaction if extravasation; fever; nausea and vomiting; diarrhea	Bone marrow depression; alopecia; peripheral neuropathy; rash

Courtesy of Stephen K. Carter, M.D.

TABLE 1. COLLECTION OF SPECIMENS FOR BACTERIOLOGICAL CULTURE[a]

Specimen	Preparation	No., Type Volume	Container	Technique	Helpful Clinical Information	Comments[b]
Anaerobic cultures						
Actinomycosis	Use gauze dressing for sulfur granules.	Aspirated pus	Anaerobic transport medium (TN) or syringe	Aspirate with syringe from sinus tract or from swollen abscess areas. Granules may be recovered from secretion in dressing and examined microscopically.	History of "lumpy jaw" chronic infection	Fistulating chronic infections often in the neck, jaw, and upper chest area. Sometimes also abdominal lesions.
Body fluids, secretions, pus	Decontaminate skin.	1 ml if possible	Syringe or gassed-out tubes	Aspirate without air, leave needle on, and cover with plastic sleeve or rubber stopper.	Foul-smelling discharge, abdominal surgery, septic abortion	Do not refrigerate; immediately transport to lab; indicator in TN should remain colorless.
Respiratory tract	Transtracheal aspirate, pleural or empyema fluid only	1 ml if possible	Anaerobic container or syringe	Collected by physician	Foul-smelling sputum, history of aspiration	
Tissue	Surgery	1 cm^3 if possible	Anaerobic container	Put in gassed-out tube. Hold upright.	As above, gas gangrene	Do not add fluid. Larger specimens (>1 cm^3) tolerate short exposure to air.
Autopsy material						
Blood		10 ml of right heart blood	Sterile tube or Vacutainer with anticoagulant	From right heart either through skin and chest wall or (through unopened heart) from right ventricle after removal of sternum	Clinical diagnosis; postmortem interval; autopsy impression; previous positive cultures; suspected infection	Autopsy cultures are often contaminated with bacteria from the water faucet and with enteric bacteria.
Tissue	Best collected before body is handled too much or opened. Decontaminate skin or sear surface of heart or other organ before inserting needle or cutting out tissue block.	6-cm^3 cube (if possible) with one serosal or other surface; this large size is preferred because aseptic collection is difficult.	Sterile container	In the laboratory, aseptically cut a 1-cm^3 cube from suspicious area including some normal tissue.		A block of spleen tissue may be submitted in lieu of a blood culture. N.B. Coccidiomycosis and TB are discovered often at autopsy only.
Blood						
Peripheral	Skin decontamination with 0.5% tincture of iodine followed by 70% alcohol.	10 ml (adults and older child); 1–2 ml (infants); 3 samples per 24 h or 4 to 6 in 48 h for FUO	Culture bottle for direct inoculation or Vacutainer with SPS	Sterile venipuncture; specimens should not be drawn through catheter or cannulas.	Clinical diagnosis; anti-biotic and chemotherapy; immune status	Incubate immediately; do not refrigerate. (1)

Bone marrow	Same as above	1 ml or more	Same as above	Sterile percutaneous aspiration	Same as above	Direct smears should be made. Recommended by many authorities for diagnosis of systemic histoplasmosis and for other fungus infections. Also, for diagnosis of miliary TB.
Body fluids (other than blood, urine, CSF)						
Bile	Surgery	Several ml (First ml from post-op drain site often contains contaminants.)	Sterile container	Aspiration with syringe during surgery, from post-op drainage site, or via nasogastric tube from duodenum	Possible *Salmonella* or *Clostridia* infection	Sample may contain gall stones, which should be examined. Duodenal aspirates are sometimes submitted for special tests (overgrowth of coliforms).
Hematomas	Skin decontamination	Several ml	Sterile tube or Vacutainer	Sterile aspiration with syringe	Suspected abscess	May clot; when in doubt use anticoagulant (SPS)
Joint fluid	Same	Several ml	Same	Same	History of trauma, previous surgery, or infection (GC)	Often proteinaceous, may clot. Do not add acetic acid or other fluid which may precipitate protein; this makes cell evaluation impossible. Distilled sterile water is acceptable.
Pericardial fluid	Same as above	Several ml	Sterile jar or tube	Same as above	History of TB or previous surgery	
Peritoneal fluid	Same	Several ml or more	Sterile tube or jar	Sterile aspiration, may be quite proteinaceous or clot	History of TB, surgery, or cancer	Same as for joint fluids; consider also GC; specimen may be peritoneal dialysis fluid. (5)
Pleural fluid	Same	Several ml or more	Sterile tube or jar	Sterile aspiration with syringe		
Breast milk	Skin decontamination of nipple	Several ml; first few may be contaminated	Sterile tube or jar	Pump or manual expression	Suspected abscess	Often submitted for presence of *Staphylococcus aureus* and/or hemolytic streptococci

Table 1. (*Continued*)

Specimen	Preparation	No., Type Volume	Container	Technique	Helpful Clinical Information	Comments(b)
Catheter tips						
Foley catheter		Not recommended				Foley catheters or tips should not be cultured except unused, as sterility check.
Vascular cannulae, central venous pressure lines, umbilical or intravenous catheters	Skin decontamination	2- to 3-inch (ca. 5- to 7.5-cm) catheter: 1 segment of 2 inches (ca. 5 cm); 8- to 24-inch (ca. 20- to 60-cm) catheter: 2 segments of 2 inches (ca. 5 cm), 1 from skin interface and 1 from within vessel	Sterile jar or tube	Sever aseptically just inside skin interface	History of infection	Occasionally are removed because of sepsis or fever that is kept going because of a colonized catheter tip. Yeasts are the most common isolates from hyperalimentation lines.
Central nervous system						
Brain biopsy	Surgery	See tissue	As for anaerobic cultures	As for anaerobic cultures	Suspected abscess or cryptococcosis	Needs coordination with pathology and virus laboratories (Herpes)
CSF	Skin decontamination	Several ml if possible	Sterile, clean, screw-capped tube	Sterile lumbar puncture; ventricular or suboccipital tap	Tentative clinical diagnosis and/or suspicion	Since cultures yield more from a larger volume, an alternate method is to pool all tubes collected (after cell count). The supernatant goes to chemistry and serology.
Meningomyelocele fluid	Same	Often only one specimen will be submitted.	Same	Sterile aspiration through the skin	Suspected infection	Fluid is more frequently contaminated or infected than regular spinal fluid.
Shunt fluid	Skin and catheter decontamination	Often only one tube	Same	Sterile aspiration through shunt	Suspected infected	Often contaminated or infected with skin flora
Ear						
Internal	Cleanse external canal with mild antiseptic.	Most often swabs; if volume allows, submit fluid	Sterile clean tube; TN for swabs	Collect specimen through sterile funnel from ear drum or beyond.	History of acute or chronic otitis media	If eardrum is not perforated, specimen should be collected by otolaryngologist or other physician.
External	Cleanse external canal with mild detergent.	Swab, scraping, or fluid aspiration	Sterile tube, TN for swabs	Obtain specimen from active margin, preferably including fresh secretion from deeper areas.	Clinical suspicion	Surface swabbing might miss streptococcal cellulitis or erysipelas.

Eye						
Internal	Surgery	Volume of specimen usually suboptimal	Sterile tube	Surgical technique; label carefully whether left or right eye	History of trauma or post-op infection	Since specimen is usually small and obtained under great difficulty, speed in transport and care in handling are very important.
External	Cleanse skin around eye with mild antiseptic. Gently remove make-up and ointment with sterile cotton and saline.	For most cases moistened swabs are used. For diagnosis of viral or chlamydial infections and for cytology, conjunctival and/or corneal scrapings are necessary. Make 2 slides per lesion.	Moist sterile swabs in sterile tubes with a small amount of nutrient broth; alcohol-cleaned glass slides for scrapings; sterile tube for scrapings to be cultured (AFB, fungi)	Swabbing: Pass moistened swab 2 times over lower conjunctiva. Avoid eyelid border and lashes. (Culture these separately in a similar fashion if indicated.) Scrapings: use local anesthetic and platinum spatula. Rub spatula with scrapings gently over small area on slide. If too dry use very small amount of water.	History and suspected problem: e.g., bacterial, fungal, AFB, inclusion bodies (viral or chlamydial), GC only, allergic (vernal)	Handle carefully; transport to laboratory immediately. Often only a few microorganisms present. Scraping should be done by ophthalmologist. Consult with physician about any unclarity of terms or the handling of the specimen (OD=right eye, OS=left eye). Giemsa and Gram stains are frequently requested.
Genital tract—female						
Amniotic fluid		Uncontaminated fluid	Sterile tube	Aspirate with syringe.	Premature rupture of membranes >24 h	Treat as any other normally sterile body fluid; may contain *Neisseria gonorrhoeae*
Cervix (endocervix)	Wipe cervix clean of vaginal secretion and mucus. Use speculum and no lubricant.	Uncontaminated endocervical secretions; take two swabs.	Sterile container with TN; for *N. gonorrhoeae,* immediate planting or Transgrow is preferred.	Under direct vision, gently compress cervix with blades of speculum and use a rotating motion with swab. Obtain exudate from endocervical glands.	Venereal disease, postpartum infection	Viability of *N. gonorrhoeae* held in Amies or modified Stuart transport medium decreases substantially after several hours.
Cul de sac (culdocentesis)	Surgical procedure	Fluid, secretions	See anaerobic culture	Aspiration through posterior vaginal vault.	Venereal disease, pelvic inflammatory disease	Pelvic inflammatory disease
Endometrium	As for cervix	Curettings or aspiration	Sterile container, anaerobic conditions	If swabs are to be used, insertion through a sterile tube sheath will help avoid contamination with vaginal flora.	Postpartum fever, venereal disease	Likelihood of external contamination is high for cultures obtained through the vagina.
Intrauterine device	Surgical	Entire device plus secretion, pus	Sterile container	Surgical removal; consider anaerobic culture.	History of bleeding	Unusual organisms may be isolated, e.g., *Actinomyces, Torulopsis,* and other yeasts.

TABLE 1. (*Continued*)

SPECIMEN	PREPARATION	NO., TYPE VOLUME	CONTAINER	TECHNIQUE	HELPFUL CLINICAL INFORMATION	COMMENTS(b)
Lymph nodes (inguinal)	Skin decontamination	Biopsy or needle aspirate	Sterile container	Aspiration of lymph nodes with syringe and needle or excision	History of venereal disease	Needs arrangements with special lab for lymphogranuloma venereum cultures. See Tissue.
Products of conception (fetal tissue, placenta, membranes, lochia)	Surgical	Tissue or aspirates	Sterile container	Sample suspicious areas of tissue; if contaminated, use autopsy tissue sampling technique.		Occasionally this type of specimen is expelled into toilet and is grossly contaminated.
Urethra	Wipe clean with sterile gauze or swab	Swab with urethral secretion or free discharge	Transgrow or sterile container with TN (if held less than 2 h)	Collect 1 h or more after urinating; if discharge cannot be obtained by "milking" the urethra, use swabs to collect material from about 2 cm inside urethra.	History of discharge	Discharge may be stimulated by gently stripping and massaging the urethra against pubic symphysis through the vagina. (3)
Tubes, ovaries	Surgery	Tissue, aspirates or swabs	Sterile container; see anaerobic cultures	Surgical	Salpingo-oophoritis	Consider venereal, fungal, anaerobic, and AFB infection.
Vagina	Use speculum without lubricant	Aspirate or swab, Gram stains and wet mounts	Swab with TN, Transgrow	Simple aspiration or swabbing; swab mucosa high in vaginal canal.	History of discharge	Ulcerations should be checked out for syphilis, soft chancre, or genital herpes. Yeast common. For GC, cervical specimen is preferred. Wet mount is for yeast and *Trichomonas*. "Clue cells" and role of *Corynebacterium vaginale* in vaginitis are controversial
Vaginal cuff		Aspirate of abscess	See anaerobic culture		Postsurgery	
Vulva (including labia, Bartholin glands)	Do not use alcohol for mucous membranes. Skin prep for regular skin sites.	Swab or aspirate (Bartholin gland abscess)	Swab with TN. See anaerobic culture for aspirate.	Collect with swab or aspirate abscesses with syringe and needle.	Discharge	Same as above.
Lesion (dark field, for *Treponema pallidum*)	1- to 2-h soaking with sterile saline on gauze	Several slide preparations, or aspirate fluid into capillary tube.	Slide and cover slip or capillary tube	Abrade lesion with sterile dry sponge, gently remove blood, collect serous exudate. (i) Touch cover slip to fluid and place on slide, or (ii) collect into sterile capillary tube.		Transport to lab immediately. Motility is seen only on warm material. Seal cover slip or capillary tube with lanolin or petrolatum.

Genital tract-male						
Lymph nodes			Same as for female genital tract			
Penile lesion	Do not use alcohol for mucous membranes. Skin prep for regular skin sites.				Duration of lesion, pain, discomfort	Special culture/ microscopic techniques are required for chancroid and granuloma inguinale.
Culture		Swab	Swab with TN if pus			
Dark field (for *T. pallidum*)			Same as for female genital tract			
Prostatic fluid		Secretion for smear and culture	Sterile tube or swab with TN	Digital massage through rectum	History of chronic UTI	Not recommended for GC cultures, but helpful in some chronic UTI
Urethra	Same as for female		Secretion, slide, and/or swab	Same as for females; thin urethrogenital alginate swabs are preferred	History and duration of painful discharge	In males the diagnosis of gonorrhea can often be made by microscopic examination of a Gram-stained smear. (3)
Pus/abscess			See Anaerobic culture and Skin (Deep suppurative lesion)			May be labeled "incision and drainage" ("I&D")
Intestinal						
Duodenal contents	Through tube	Several ml	Sterile tube	Aspiration	Travel, food	Examine for bacterial overgrowth, *Salmonella typhi*, and parasites.
Feces		1 g; 3 consecutive specimens	Clean, waxed cardboard container with tight cover	If collected in sterile bedpan, must not be contaminated with urine or residual soap or disinfectants	Travel, food, suspected etiology	Transport to laboratory immediately. If delayed, use buffered-glycerol transport medium.
Rectal swab		3 consecutive specimens	Swab with TN	Swabs of lesions of rectal wall during proctoscopy or sigmoidoscopy preferred	As above	Not useful for detection of carriers
Gastric aspirate, neonate		Enough for smear and culture	Sterile container	Collected by physician	History of ruptured membranes	May visualize and isolate causative agent of septicemia before blood cultures become positive.

TABLE 1. (*Continued*)

Specimen	Preparation	No., Type Volume	Container	Technique	Helpful Clinical Information	Comments(b)
Respiratory tract						
Throat/pharynx		Swab	Swab with TN	Swab areas of exudation, membrane formation, or inflammation. Rub tonsillar crypts vigorously.	Agent suspected (e.g., group A streptococci, *N. gonorrhoeae*)	Do not touch oral mucosa or tongue with swab.
Epiglottis		Swab				Do not swab throat in cases of acute epiglottitis unless prepared for tracheostomy.
Nasal sinuses			See Anaerobic cultures: Body fluids			
Nasopharynx		Swab	Thin wire or flexible pernasal swab with TN	Swab is passed through nose gently and into nasopharynx. Stay near septum and floor of nose. Rotate and remove.	Agent suspected (e.g., *Bordetella pertussis*)	Transport to laboratory immediately.
Nose			Swab with TN	Insert swab about 1 inch (ca. 2.5 cm) into nose, gently rotate against nasal mucosa, and remove.		Used mainly for staphylococcal carriers
Oral cavity						
Mucosal surface of gums or teeth	Rinse mouth	Scraping, swab	Swab, tongue depresser, or slide in sterile container	Scrape, swab	Duration, agent suspected	Culture for yeast. Smear for yeast or organisms of Vincent's angina.
Dental abscess, root abscess	Rinse mouth, prep with dry sterile gauze	Exudate	See anaerobic culture	Aspirate with needle and syringe		Predominant pathogens are anaerobes including *Actinomyces* and various streptococci.
Bronchoscopy		Brushings, transbronchial biopsies, bronchial secretions	Sterile container	Aspirated through inner chamber of bronchoscope	Agent(s) suspected	See (5).
Lung aspirate/biopsy	Skin decontamination	See anaerobic culture	See anaerobic culture	Performed by physician; needle inserted through chest wall, transbronchoscopic needle biopsy, or thoracotomy	Underlying disease	Invasive procedure; process immediately. (5)
Expectorated sputum	May require ultrasonic nebulization, hydration, physiotherapy, or postural drainage	Sputum, not saliva	Sterile container	Patient must cough deeply. Best under direct supervision of physician or respiratory therapist	Pneumonia	May be refrigerated overnight. (5)
Tracheal aspirate		Sputum	Sterile container		Pneumonia	Cellular composition may be misleading due to inflammatory reaction caused by endotracheal tube. May be refrigerated. (5)

Transtracheal aspirate (infralaryngeal aspirate)	Skin is cleansed and anesthetized		Sterile container. See anaerobic culture	Performed by physician. A 14 gauge needle is inserted through skin of the neck and the cricothyroid membrane into the trachea. A small sterile catheter is passed through the needle, and exudate aspirated.	Pneumonia, aspiration, TB	Process immediately. (5)
Skin						
Superficial wound	Clean wound surface with 70% alcohol	Pus, biopsy	Aspirate or swab with transport medium	Swab or aspirate deep areas rather than lesion surface.	Animal bite or trauma, duration, travel	
Extensive burns or decubiti	Clean wound surface with 70% alcohol	For quantitative culture, 3- to 4-mm dermal punch	Sterile container	Punch biopsy		Consider quantitative culture .
Deep suppurative lesion						
Closed abscess	Clean and treat with antiseptic	Pus, ≥1 ml if possible	Syringe or anaerobic container	Aspirate directly into syringe	Duration, location	See Anaerobic Cultures.
Fistula, sinus tract	Clean surface	Pus, ≥1 ml if possible	Syringe or swab with TN	Swab or aspirate deeply	Duration, location	See Actinomycosis.
Rash	Clean surface with 70% alcohol	Pus, fluid	Syringe	Aspirate directly into syringe; if no fluid, instill small amount of sterile saline and aspirate saline.		
Umbilicus	No cleaning	Swab	Swab with TN	Swab	Culture for *S. aureus*	Used to determine *S. aureus* colonization
Tissue						
Surgical or biopsy	Surgery	5- to 10-mm^3 cube or aspirate	Sterile container with TN	Collected by physician		See also Anaerobic Culture. Do not discard leftover tissue. Freeze in sterile broth until culture and pathology are completed.

TABLE 1. (*Continued*)

Specimen	Preparation	No., Type Volume	Container	Technique	Helpful Clinical Information	Comments [b]
Urine						
Clean-voided	Instruct carefully; early morning specimen is best.	Urine, 1 ml; 2 consecutive specimens may be necessary in females.	Sterile wide-mouthed container	Clean genital area well. Void 20- to 25-ml, then collect specimen without stopping the stream.		Do not culture 24-h pooled urine. Must be planted within 2 h of collection unless refrigerated. (2)
Catheter or ileal loop collection	Disinfect tubing with alcohol	Urine, 1 ml	Sterile container	Aspirate through tubing with a syringe.		Same as above
Bladder urine (suprapubic or cystoscopic)		Urine, 1 ml	Sterile container	Collected by physician by needle aspiration or cystoscopy		Same as above

[a] Abbreviations: TN, transport medium; TB, tuberculosis; FUO, fever of unknown origin; SPS, sodium polyethanol sulfonate; post-op, postoperation; GC, *Neisseria gonorrhoeae;* and UTI, urinary tract infection.

[b] Numbers in parentheses indicate reference to previous Cumitech papers: Cumitech 1, Blood Cultures (October 1974); Cumitech 2, Laboratory Diagnosis of Urinary Tract Infections (April 1975); Cumitech 4, Laboratory Diagnosis of Gonorrhea (October 1976); Cumitech 5, Practical Anaerobic Bacteriology (April 1977); and Cumitech 7, Laboratory Diagnosis of Lower Respiratory Tract Infections (September 1978). Cumitech series (Cumulative Techniques and Procedures in Clinical Microbiology). Washington, DC, American Society for Microbiology.

Modified from Isenberg, H. D., et al.: Cumitech 9, Collection and Processing of Bacteriological Specimens. Washington, DC, American Society for Microbiology, 1979, pp. 7–14.

TABLE 2. BACTERIA FOR WHICH SPECIAL PROCEDURES ARE REQUIRED FOR ISOLATION OR DETECTION IN CLINICAL SPECIMENS

ORGANISM	DISEASE	SPECIMENS	ISOLATION MEDIA	COMMENTS
GRAM-POSITIVE BACTERIA				
Clostridium difficile	Pseudomembranous colitis	Feces	Cycloserine-cefoxitin-fructose agar	Test isolate and stool supernatant for toxin
Corynebacterium diphtheriae	Diphtheria	Nasopharyngeal swab; throat swab; skin scrapings; rarely, swabs of conjunctivae, middle ear, vagina	Loeffler or Pai slant; cystine-tellurite agar	Isolate must be tested for diphtheria toxin production
Gardnerella vaginale	Nonspecific vaginitis	Vaginal discharge	Vaginalis (V) agar	Wet mount shows "clue" cells; "fishy" odor with addition of 10% KOH to discharge
GRAM-NEGATIVE BACTERIA				
Bordetella pertussis	Whooping cough	Nasopharyngeal swabs or aspirates; bronchial washings, transtracheal aspirates	Bordet-Gengou medium with and without methicillin	Direct fluorescent antibody technique
Calymmatobacterium granulomatis	Granuloma inguinale	Scrapings or biopsy of ulcer	Yolk sac inoculation; egg yolk slants	Smears stained with Wright or Giemsa for Donovan bodies
Campylobacter fetus fetus subsp. jejuni	Gastroenteritis	Feces	Skirrow medium	
Francisella tularensis	Tularemia	Biopsy or aspirate of lesion or draining lymph node; conjunctival scrapings; sputum and gastric aspirates	Glucose-cysteine agar with thiamine or cystine heart agar; Thayer-Martin or supplemented chocolate agar	
Hemophilus ducreyi	Chancroid	Lesion exudate; aspirates of inguinal lymph nodes	Chocolate agar supplemented with IsoVitaleX with and without vancomycin	Smears stained with Giemsa, or Wright stains for "schools of fish"
Legionella	Legionellosis	Lung biopsies; pleural fluid; transtracheal aspirates; bronchial washings	Buffered charcoal–yeast extract agar	Direct fluorescent antibody technique
Spirillum minor	Rat-bite fever	Lesion or lymph node exudates; blood	Mouse or guinea pig inoculation	Smears stained with Giemsa or Wright stain; darkfield microscopy
Streptobacillus moniliformis	Rat-bite fever	Blood, joint fluid; wound exudate	Heart infusion broth with horse serum and yeast extract	Gram and Giemsa or Wayson stained smears
Vibrio species	Cholera or gastroenteritis; septicemia and wound infections	Feces, vomitus Wounds, blood	Blood agar; thiosulfate-citrate bile salts agar; tellurite taurocholate gelatin agar	Test *V. cholerae* for toxin
SPIROCHETES				
Borrelia species	Relapsing fever	Blood	Kelly medium	Wright or Giemsa stain blood smears (thick and thin films); darkfield microscopy
Leptospira interrogans	Leptospirosis	Blood and spinal fluid (first week); urine (thereafter)	Media containing serum (e.g., Fletcher) or albumin and fatty acids	Darkfield microscopy; serology
Treponema species	Syphilis, endemic syphilis, yaws, pinta	Serous exudate from lesions	Noncultivatable in vitro	Darkfield microscopy; syphilis serology
MYCOPLASMA				
M. pneumoniae	Respiratory infections	Sputum, throat	Diphasic broth; E-agar	Complement fixation
M. hominis *Ureaplasma urealyticum*	Urogenital infections	Urine; genital	E-agar	

TABLE 2. (*Continued*)

ORGANISM	DISEASE	SPECIMENS	ISOLATION MEDIA	COMMENTS
CELL WALL–DEFECTIVE BACTERIA	Suggested role in relapsing or unresolving infections	Tissues and body	Hypertonic medium (20% sucrose)	
CHLAMYDIAE				
C. psittaci	Psittacosis, ornithosis	Sputum, blood, tissue	Tissue culture (McCoy cells); yolk sac of embryonated eggs	Giemsa-stained smears for inclusions; complement fixation
C. trachomatis	Lymphogranuloma venereum	Aspirates or biopsies of inguinal lymph nodes; pus	Same as above	Direct examination not recommended; complement fixation
	Ocular and genital infections; infant pneumonia	Conjunctival scrapings; urethral and cervical specimens; tracheal aspirates; nasopharyngeal swabs	Same as above	Giemsa-stained smears or immunofluorescence for inclusions (especially useful for infant conjunctivitis)
RICKETTSIAE	Arthropod-borne rickettsial diseases	Blood, tissues; arthropods	Yolk sacs of embryonated eggs; guinea pig inoculation	Giménez-stained smears; rickettsial serology (complement fixation, agglutination)

Appendix C

REFERENCE RANGES AND LABORATORY VALUES OF CLINICAL IMPORTANCE*

Norbert W. Tietz, Ph.D.

INTRODUCTION

Reference ranges are valuable guidelines for the clinician, but they should not be regarded as absolute indicators of health and disease. There are several reasons for using reference ranges with caution, some of which are listed in Ch. 547. Most importantly, values for "healthy" individuals often overlap significantly with values for persons afflicted with disease. In addition, laboratory values may vary significantly due to methodologic differences and mode of standardization. This is especially true for immunologic tests, which utilize antibodies that may have different characteristics. As a result, laboratory values in individual institutions may differ from those listed in this chapter.

For those laboratory tests in which clearly established differences among the ages and sexes exist, all values are listed. Values without any age specification should be considered as those for the adult individual in the fasting state.

All laboratory values are given in conventional units, as well as in international units. In general, the international units given conform to the SI system (Système International d'Unités). However, in some cases the recommendations of the International Union of Pure and Applied Chemistry (IUPAC) and the Commission on World Standards of the World Association of Societies of Pathology (COWS of WASP) are used where these have found wider acceptance in clinical laboratories and offer advantages over the units recommended in the SI system.

Throughout this chapter, we have used the prefixes for units as approved by the CGPM (Conférence Générale des Poids et Mésures), 1964, and the International Congress of Clinical Chemistry, 1966. The pertinent prefixes denoting the decimal factors are listed below.

Prefixes Denoting Decimal Factors

Prefix	*Symbol*	*Factor*
mega	M	10^{6}
kilo	k	10^{3}
hecto	h	10^{2}
deka	da	10^{1}
deci	d	10^{-1}
centi	c	10^{-2}
milli	m	10^{-3}
micro	μ	10^{-6}
nano	n	10^{-9}
pico	p	10^{-12}
femto	f	10^{-15}

For convenience and to preserve space, we have used standard abbreviations commonly used in laboratory medicine. Less common abbreviations and some nonstandard abbreviations are given below.

Abbreviations

AU	Arbitrary Units
BMD	Boehringer Mannheim Diagnostics, Inc.
G-D	General Diagnostics
GPIMH	Guinea Pig Intestinal Mucosal Homogenate
ICSH	International Committee for Standardization in Hematology
IFA	Immunofluorescent Assay
IRP-2-hMG	2nd International Reference Preparation of Human Menopausal Gonadotropin
IU	International Unit (of hormone activity)
NEFA	Nonesterified Fatty Acids (Free Fatty Acids)
Occup.	Occupational
P-5-P	Pyridoxal-5′-Phosphate
RIA	Radioimmunoassay
RID	Radialimmunodiffusion
RT	Room Temperature
U	International Unit (of enzyme activity)
WHO	World Health Organization

ACKNOWLEDGMENT. We thankfully acknowledge the assistance of Nancy M. Logan, B.A., and Karen D. Reeves in the preparation of this material.

REFERENCES

Beutler E: Hemolytic Anemia in Disorders of Red Cell Metabolism. New York, Plenum Publishing Company, 1978.
Brown SS, Mitchell FL, Young DS (eds.): Chemical Diagnosis of Disease. Amsterdam, Elsevier/North-Holland Biomedical Press, 1979.
Conn HF, Conn RB (eds.): Current Diagnosis. 6th ed. Philadelphia, W. B. Saunders Company, 1980.
Gilman AG, Goodman L, Gilman A (eds.): The Pharmacological Basis of Therapeutics. 6th ed. New York, Macmillan, 1980.
Henry JB (ed.): Todd-Sanford-Davidsohn Clinical Diagnosis and Management by Laboratory Methods. 16th ed. Philadelphia, W. B. Saunders Company, 1979.
Mabry CC, Tietz NW: Tables of normal laboratory values. *In* Nelson WE, Vaughan VC, McKay RJ, Behrman RE (eds.): Nelson Textbook of Pediatrics. 11th ed. Philadelphia, W. B. Saunders Company, 1979.
Miale JB: Laboratory Medicine: Hematology. 5th ed. St. Louis, C. V. Mosby Company, 1977.
Tietz NW (ed.): Fundamentals of Clinical Chemistry. 2nd ed. Philadelphia, W. B. Saunders Company, 1976.
Tietz NW, Blackburn RH (eds.): Reference Ranges and General Information. Clinical Laboratories, A. B. Chandler Medical Center, University of Kentucky, Lexington, Kentucky, July, 1981.
Williams WJ, Beutler E, Erslev AJ, Rundles RW: Hematology. 2nd ed. New York, McGraw-Hill Book Company, 1977.

*** From Wyngaarden, J. B., and Smith, L. H., Jr.: Cecil Textbook of Medicine. 16th ed. Philadelphia, W. B. Saunders Co., 1982, pp. 2320–2354.**

HEMATOLOGY, COAGULATION, AND RED CELL ENZYMES*

Test	Specimen	Reference Range	Reference Range (International Units)
Acidified Serum Test (Ham's Test)	Whole blood (without anticoagulant)	<5% lysis	Lysed fraction <0.05
Activated Coagulation Time (ACT)	Whole blood (no anticoagulant; drawn into tubes containing celite)	107±13 s (1 SD)	107±13 s (1 SD)
Activated Partial Thromboplastin Time (APTT)	Whole blood (Na citrate); remove plasma immediately	25–35 s (differs with method)	25–35 s
Microtechnique (Miale)	Capillary blood (siliconized micropipets; Na citrate)	Infants: <90 s Reaches adult levels by 2–6 mo.	<90 s
Alkaline Phosphatase, Leukocyte, see *Neutrophil Alkaline Phosphatase*			
Anti-DNA antibodies			
Indir. fluorescence	Serum	Neg in 1:10 dilution	Neg. in 1:10 dilution
Farr	Serum	<20% of DNA bound	Fraction DNA bound: <0.20
Ginsberg/Keiser	Plasma (EDTA, oxalate, or heparin)	≤1 μg DNA bound/mL plasma	≤1000 μg DNA bound/L plasma
Anti-thrombin III (AT-III)			
Radialimmunodiffusion (RID)	Plasma (citrate)	21–30 mg/dL	210–300 mg/L
	Serum	17–25 mg/dL	170–250 mg/L
Amidolytic (chromogenic)	Plasma	85–115% of standard	85–115 AU
	Serum	55–80% of standard	55–80 AU
Bleeding Time (BT)	Blood from skin puncture		
Ivy		Normal: 2–7 min	2–7 min
		Borderline: 7–11 min	7–11 min
Simplate (G-D)		2.75–8 min	2.75–8 min
Blood Volume	Whole blood (heparin)	M: 52–83 mL/kg	M: 0.052–0.083 L/kg
		F: 50–75 mL/kg	F: 0.050–0.075 L/kg
Bone Marrow, Differential Count	Bone marrow aspirate		
		% (mean)	*Number fraction (mean)*
Myeloblasts		0.3–5.0 (2.0)	0.003–0.05 (0.02)
Promyelocytes		1.0–8.0 (5.0)	0.01–0.08 (0.05)
Myelocytes: Neutrophilic		5.0–19.0 (12.0)	0.05–0.19 (0.12)
Eosinophilic		0.5–3.0 (1.5)	0.005–0.03 (0.015)
Basophilic		0.0–0.5 (0.3)	0.00–0.005 (0.003)
Metamyelocytes		13.0–32.0 (22.0)	0.13–0.32 (0.22)
Polymorphonuclear neutrophils		7.0–30.0 (20.0)	0.07–0.30 (0.20)
Polymorphonuclear eosinophils		0.5–4.0 (2.0)	0.005–0.04 (0.02)
Polymorphonuclear basophils		0.0–0.7 (0.2)	0.00–0.007 (0.002)
Lymphocytes		3.0–17.0 (10.0)	0.03–0.17 (0.10)
Plasma cells		0.0–2.0 (0.4)	0.00–0.02 (0.004)
Monocytes		0.5–5.0 (2.0)	0.005–0.05 (0.02)
Reticulum cells		0.1–2.0 (0.2)	0.001–0.02 (0.002)
Megakaryocytes		0.03–3.0 (0.1)	0.0003–0.03 (0.001)
Pronormoblasts		1.0–8.0 (4.0)	0.01–0.08 (0.04)
Normoblasts		7.0–32.0 (18.0)	0.07–0.32 (0.18)
Clot Lysis, 37°C	Whole clotted blood	48–72 h	48–72 h
Clot Retraction			
Screen	Whole blood (no anticoagulant)	Retraction begins at 1 h, maximum at 24 h	Retraction begins at 1 h, maximum at 24 h
Semi-quantitative	Whole blood (no anticoagulant); two-syringe technique	At 2 h:	At 2 h:
		% serum extruded	*fraction serum extruded*
		0: none	0: none
		1+: 5–10	1+: 0.05–0.10
		2+: 10–20	2+: 0.10–0.20
		3+: 20–35	3+: 0.20–0.35
		Normal	
		4+: >35	4+: >0.35
		Firm clot; retraction from three sides	Firm clot; retraction from three sides
Quantitative (plasma recalcification)	Platelet-rich plasma (EDTA) collected in plastic tube	56±14 mg (weight of clot)	56±14 mg (weight of clot)

(*Continued*)

*The material in this appendix was partially extracted from *Clinical Guide to Laboratory Tests,* NW Tietz, ed., PR Finley, asst. ed.; Philadelphia, W.B. Saunders Company, 1982 (in press). The main contributors are RV Blanke and RA Blouin: Drugs and Toxicology; C Hougie: Coagulation; HP Lehmann: International Units; J Leonard: Endocrinology; W Mertz and RV Blanke: Trace Metals; DA Nelson: Hematology; SE Ritzmann: Proteins; and HE Sauberlich: Vitamins. A portion of the values was generated in the clinical laboratories of the University of Kentucky Medical Center. Other sources are listed under references at the end of this chapter.

HEMATOLOGY, COAGULATION, AND RED CELL ENZYMES (*Continued*)

Test	Specimen	Reference Range	Reference Range (International Units)
Clotting Time			
Lee-White, 37°C	Whole blood (no anticoagulant)	Glass tubes: 5–8 min (5–15 min at RT) Silicon tubes: about 30 min prolonged	Glass tubes: 5–8 min (5–15 min at RT) Silicon tubes: about 30 min prolonged
Clotting Time, Plasma	Plasma (citrate)	Platelet-rich plasma: 100–150 s	Platelet-rich plasma: 100–150 s
Coagulation Factor Assays	Plasma (citrate)		
Factor II		0.5–1.5 U/mL or 60–150% of normal Cord: 25–85%	0.5–1.5 kU/L or 60–150 AU 25–85 AU
Factor II antigen		75–125% of normal	75–125 AU
Factor V		0.5–2.0 U/mL or 60–150% of normal	0.5–2.0 kU/L or 60–150 AU
Factor VII	Perform test immediately after collection	65–135% of normal Cord: 25–85%	65–135 AU 25–85 AU
Factor VIII		60–145% of normal	60–145 AU
Factor VIII antigen		50–200% of normal	50–200 AU
Factor IX		60–140% of normal Cord: 15–42%	60–140 AU 15–42 AU
Factor X		60–130% of normal	60–130 AU
Factor XI		65–135% of normal Cord: ~30%	65–135 AU ~30 AU
Factor XII		65–150% of normal Cord: 11–83%	65–150 AU 11–83 AU
Factor XIII (Fibrin Stabilizing Factor, FSF)	Whole blood (citrate or oxalate)	Minimal hemostatic level: 0.02–0.05 U/mL or 1–2% of normal	20–50 U/L or 1–2 AU
Differential Count, see *Bone Marrow, Leukocyte Differential,* and *Synovial Fluid Differential Count,* respectively			
2,3 Diphosphoglycerate (2,3 DPG)	Whole blood (ACD, EDTA, or heparin)	12.27±1.87 μmol/g Hb (1 SD); lower in newborns	0.79±0.12 mol/mol Hb (1 SD)
Eosinophil Count	Whole blood (EDTA or heparin); capillary blood	50–350 cells/mm³ (μL)	50–350 × 10^6 cells/L
Erythrocyte Count (RBC Count)	Whole blood (EDTA)	*millions of cells/mm³ (μL)*	× 10^{12} *cells/L*
		Birth: 5.0–6.3	5.0–6.3
		3–14 y: 3.7–5.2	3.7–5.2
		Adult M: 4.3–5.9	4.3–5.9
		F: 3.5–5.5	3.5–5.5
Erythrocyte Sedimentation Rate (ESR)		*mm/h*	*mm/h*
Westergren, modified	Whole blood (EDTA)	Child: 0–10	0–10
		Adult: M, <50 y: 0–15	0–15
		>50 y: 0–20	0–20
		F, <50 y: 0–20	0–20
		>50 y: 0–30	0–30
Wintrobe		Child: 0–13	0–13
		Adult: M, 0–9	0–9
		F, 0–20	0–20
ZETA		41–54%	41–54 AU
Erythropoietin			
Hemagglutination	Serum	25–125 mIU/mL	25–125 IU/L
RIA	Serum	<5–20 mIU/mL	<5–20 IU/L
Euglobulin Clot Lysis	Whole blood (citrate)	Lysis in 2–4 h	Lysis in 2–4 h
Ferritin, see *Chemistry section*			
Ferrohemoglobin Solubility Test	Whole blood (EDTA)	*Hb* — *% Solubility in phosphate buffer*	*Solubility in phosphate buffer (unit: mass fraction)*
		AA, AD >90	>0.90
		AC, CC >90	>0.90
		AS, CS 40–50	0.4–0.5
		SS 6–23	0.06–0.23
Fibrin Degradation Products			
Agglutination (Thrombo-Wellco test)	Whole blood; special tube containing thrombin and proteolytic inhibitor	<10 μg/mL	<10 mg/L
	Urine; 2 mL in special tube (see above)	<0.25 μg/mL	<0.25 mg/L
Staphylococcal clumping	Whole blood, collected with thrombin and ε-aminocaproic acid	<10 μg/mL	<10 mg/L

(*Continued*)

HEMATOLOGY, COAGULATION, AND RED CELL ENZYMES (*Continued*)

Test	Specimen	Reference Range	Reference Range (International Units)
Fibrin Lysis Time	Plasma	>60 min	>60 min
Fibrinogen	Whole blood (Na citrate)	200–400 mg/dL	2.00–4.00 g/L
Glucose-6-phosphate Dehydrogenase (G-6-PD) in Erythrocytes *WHO and ICSH methods*	Whole blood (ACD, EDTA, or heparin)	12.1±2.09 U/g Hb (1 SD)	0.78±0.13 MU/mol Hb (1 SD)
Glutathione, Reduced (GSH)	Whole blood (ACD, EDTA, or heparin)	6.57±1.04 μmol/g Hb; values are higher in newborns	0.42±0.07 mol/mol Hb
Glutathione Reductase in Erythrocytes	Whole blood (ACD, EDTA, or heparin)	Reaction without added flavin adenine dinucleotide, FAD: 7.18±1.09 U/g Hb (1 SD) Reaction using FAD: 10.4±1.5 U/g Hb (1 SD)	Reaction without added flavin adenine dinucleotide, FAD: 0.46±0.07 MU/mol Hb (1 SD) Reaction using FAD: 0.67±0.10 MU/mol Hb (1 SD)
Ham's Test, see *Acidified Serum Test*			
Haptoglobin (Hp)	Serum; avoid hemolysis		
RID		40–180 mg Hb bound/dL of serum or: 30–175 mg/dL	6.20–27.90 μmol Hb bound/L of serum or: 300–1750 mg/L
Nephelometry		25–175 mg/dL	250–1750 mg/L
Hematocrit (HCT, Hct) *Calculated from MCV and RBC (electronic displacement or laser)*	Whole blood (EDTA)	*% of packed red cells (V red cells/V whole blood × 100)* 1–3 d (cap): 45–67 2 mo: 28–42 6–12 y: 35–45 12–18 y, M: 37–49 F: 36–46 18–49 y, M: 41–53 F: 36–46	*Volume fraction (V red cells/V whole blood)* 0.45–0.67 0.28–0.42 0.35–0.45 0.37–0.49 0.36–0.46 0.41–0.53 0.36–0.46
Hemoglobin (Hb)	Whole blood (EDTA)	*g/dL* 1–3 d (cap:) 14.5–22.5 2 mo: 9.0–14.0 6–12 y: 11.5–15.5 12–18 y, M: 13.0–16.0 F: 12.0–16.0 18–49 y, M: 13.5–17.5 F: 12.0–16.0	*mmol/L* 2.25–3.49 1.40–2.17 1.78–2.40 2.02–2.48 1.86–2.48 2.09–2.71 1.86–2.48
	Plasma (heparin, ACD, or EDTA)	1–4 mg/dL	0.16–0.62 μmol/L
Hemoglobin A	Whole blood (EDTA, citrate, or heparin)	>95%	*Mass fraction* >0.95
Hemoglobin A_2 (HbA_2)	Whole blood (EDTA, oxalate)	Adult: 1.5–3.5% (2 SD) Lower in infants <1 y	*Mass fraction* 0.015–0.035 (2 SD)
Hemoglobin (Hb) Electrophoresis	Whole blood (EDTA, citrate, or heparin)	HbA >95% HbA_2 1.5–3.5% HbF <2%	*Mass fraction* HbA >0.95 HbA_2 0.015–0.035 HbF <0.02
Hemoglobin F *Alkali denaturation (White)*	Whole blood (EDTA)	*% HbF* 1 day: 77.0±7.3 6 mo: 4.7±2.2 Adult: <2.0	*Mass fraction HbF* 0.77±0.073 0.047±0.022 <0.020
Hemoglobin H (HbH) *Isopropanol precipitation*	Whole blood (ACD, EDTA, or heparin)	No precipitation at 40 min	No precipitation at 40 min
Leukocyte Count (WBC Count)	Whole blood (EDTA)	*× 1000 cells/mm³ (μL)* Birth: 9.0–30.0 24 h: 9.4–34.0 1 mo: 5.0–19.5 1–3 y: 6.0–17.5 4–7 y: 5.5–15.5 8–13 y: 4.5–13.5 Adult: 4.5–11.0	*Cells × 10⁹/L* 9.0–30.0 9.4–34.0 5.0–19.5 6.0–17.5 5.5–15.5 4.5–13.5 4.5–11.0
	CSF	0–5 mononuclear cells/μL	0–5 × 10^6 cells/L

(*Continued*)

HEMATOLOGY, COAGULATION, AND RED CELL ENZYMES (*Continued*)

Test	Specimen	Reference Range		Reference Range (International Units)	
Leukocyte Differential Count	Whole blood (EDTA)	*%*	*Cells/mm³ (μL)*	*Number fraction*	*Cells × 10⁶ /L*
Myelocytes		0	0	0	0
Neutrophils—'bands'		3–5	150–400	0.03–0.05	150–400
Neutrophils—'segs'		54–62	3000–5800	0.54–0.62	3000–5800
Lymphocytes		25–33	1500–3000	0.25–0.33	1500–3000
Monocytes		3–7	285–500	0.03–0.07	285–500
Eosinophils		1–3	50–250	0.01–0.03	50–250
Basophils		0–0.75	15–50	0–0.0075	15–20
Leukocyte Differential Count	CSF	*%*		*Number fraction*	
Lymphocytes		62±34		0.62±0.34	
Monocytes (includes pia-arachnoid mesothelial cells)		36±20		0.36±0.20	
Neutrophils		2±5		0.02±0.05	
Histocytes		Rare		Rare	
Ependymal cells		Rare		Rare	
Eosinophils		Rare		Rare	
Lysozyme (Muramidase)	Serum, plasma (EDTA)	*μg/mL* M: 11±2.75 (1 SD) F: 9.6±1.3 (1 SD)		*mg/L* 11.0±2.75 (1 SD) 9.6±1.3 (1 SD)	
	Urine	<2.0 μg/mL		<2.0 mg/L	
Mean Corpuscular Hemoglobin (MCH)	Whole blood (EDTA)		*pg/cell*	*fmol/cell*	
		Child, birth:	28–42	0.43–0.65	
		1 mo:	30–42	0.47–0.65	
		3 mo:	27–39	0.42–0.61	
		6 mo:	25–35	0.39–0.54	
		9 mo:	23–34	0.36–0.53	
		1–7 y:	22–32	0.34–0.50	
		8–14 y:	23–34	0.36–0.53	
		Adults:	25.4–34.6	0.39–0.54	
Mean Corpuscular Hemoglobin Concentration (MCHC)	Whole blood (EDTA)	*%Hb/cell or gHb/dL RBC* Adults and children: 31–36		*mmol Hb/L RBC* 4.81–5.58	
Mean Corpuscular Volume (MCV)	Whole blood (EDTA)		*μm³*	*fL*	
		1–3 d (cap):	95–121	95–121	
		0.5–2 y:	70–86	70–86	
		6–12 y:	77–95	77–95	
		12–18 y, M:	78–98	78–98	
		F:	78–102	78–102	
		18–49 y, M:	80–100	80–100	
		F:	80–100	80–100	
Methemalbumin	Whole blood (heparin)	Negative		Negative	
Methemoglobin (MetHb)	Whole blood (EDTA, heparin, or ACD)	0.06–0.24 g/dL or 0.78±0.37% of total Hb		9.3–37.2 μmol/L 0.0078±0.0037 (mass fraction)	
NADH Methemoglobin Reductase (NADH Diaphorase) *Hegesh method*	Whole blood (ACD, EDTA, or heparin)	3.40±0.5 U/g Hb (1 SD); lower in newborns		0.22±0.03 MU/mol Hb (1 SD)	
Neutrophil Alkaline Phosphatase (Leukocyte Alkaline Phosphatase)	Finger-stick blood	Score: 13–130			
Osmotic Fragility Test (RBC Fragility) *pH 7.4, 20°C*	Whole blood (heparin)	*% NaCl (g/dL)*	*% Hemolysis*	*NaCl (g/L)*	*Hemolyzed fraction*
		0.30	97–100	3.0	0.97–1.00
		0.35	90–99	3.5	0.90–0.99
		0.40	50–95	4.0	0.50–0.95
		0.45	5–45	4.5	0.05–0.45
		0.50	0–6	5.0	0.00–0.06
		0.55	0	5.5	0.00
Sterile incubation at 37°C		*% NaCl (g/dL)*	*% Hemolysis*	*NaCl (g/L)*	*Hemolyzed fraction*
		0.20	95–100	2.0	0.95–1.00
		0.30	85–100	3.0	0.85–1.00
		0.35	75–100	3.5	0.75–1.00
		0.40	65–100	4.0	0.65–1.00
		0.45	55–95	4.5	0.55–0.95
		0.50	40–85	5.0	0.40–0.85
		0.55	15–70	5.5	0.15–0.70
		0.60	0–40	6.0	0.00–0.40
		0.65	0–10	6.5	0.00–0.10
		0.70	0–5	7.0	0.00–0.05
		0.85	0	8.5	0.00

(*Continued*)

HEMATOLOGY, COAGULATION, AND RED CELL ENZYMES (*Continued*)

Test	Specimen	Reference Range	Reference Range (International Units)
Partial Thromboplastin Time (PTT)	Whole blood (Na citrate)		
Nonactivated		60–85 s (Platelin)	60–85 s
Activated		25–35 s (differs with method)	25–35 s
Phosphofructokinase (PFK) in Erythrocytes (ICSH method)	Whole blood (ACD, EDTA, or heparin)	9.05±1.89 U/g Hb (1 SD) 317±66 U/10^{12} RBC 3.17±0.7 U/mL RBC Lower in newborns	0.58±0.12 MU/mol Hb (1 SD) 0.32±0.07 nU/RBC 3.17±0.7 kU/L RBC
Plasma Volume	Plasma (heparin)	M: 25–43 mL/kg F: 28–45 mL/kg	M: 0.025–0.043 L/kg F: 0.028–0.045 L/kg
Platelet Count (Thrombocyte Count)	Whole blood (EDTA)	*× 10^3/mm³ (μL)* Newborn: 84–478 (After 1 wk, same as adult) Adult: 150–400	*× 10^9/L* 84–478 150–400
Prothrombin Consumption (PCT, Serum Prothrombin Time)	Whole blood (no anticoagulant)	>30 s or >80% consumed in 1 h	>30 s >0.80 (fraction consumed)
Prothrombin Time			
One-stage (Quick)	Whole blood (Na citrate)	In general: 11–15 s (varies with type of thromboplastin) Newborn: prolonged by 2–3 s	11–15 s prolonged by 2–3 s
Two-stage modified (Ware and Seegers)	Whole blood (Na citrate)	18–22 s	18–22 s
RBC Count, see *Erythrocyte Count*			
RBC Fragility, see *Osmotic Fragility*			
Red Cell Volume	Whole blood (heparin)	M: 20–36 mL/kg F: 19–31 mL/kg	M: 0.020–0.036 L/kg F: 0.019–0.031 L/kg
Reticulocyte Count	Whole blood (EDTA, heparin, or oxalate)	Adults: 0.5–1.5% of erythrocytes or 25,000–75,000/mm³ (μL)	0.005–0.015 (number fraction) 25,000–75,000 × 10^6/L
Sulfhemoglobin	Whole blood (EDTA, heparin, or ACD)	≤1.0% of total Hb	≤0.010 of total Hb (mass fraction)
Synovial Fluid Differential Count	Synovial fluid	%	*Number fraction*
Polymorphonuclear cells		0–25	0–0.25
Monocytes		0–71	0–0.71
Lymphocytes		0–78	0–0.78
Clasmatocytes		0–26	0–0.26
Unclassified		0–21	0–0.21
Synovial cells		0–12	0–0.12
Thrombin Time	Whole blood (Na citrate)	Control time ± 2 s when control is 9–13 s	Control time ± 2 s when control is 9–13 s
Thromboplastin Time, activated, see *Activated Partial Thromboplastin Time (APTT)*			
Tourniquet Test (Capillary Fragility)		<5–10 petechiae on forearm (halfway between systolic and diastolic pressure) 0–8 petechiae in 6 cm circle (50 torr for 15 min) 10–20 petechiae in 5 cm circle (80 mm Hg)	<5–10 petechiae on forearm (halfway between systolic and diastolic pressure) 0–8 petechiae in 6 cm circle (50 torr for 15 min) 10–20 petechiae in 5 cm circle (80 mm Hg)

CLINICAL CHEMISTRY, TOXICOLOGY, SEROLOGY

Test	Specimen	Reference Range	Reference Range (International Units)
Acetaldehyde	Whole blood	<0.2 mg/L Toxic: 1–2 mg/L	<4.5 μmol/L 23–45 μmol/L
Acetoacetate			
Semiquantitative	Serum or plasma (fluoride/oxalate) Urine	Negative (<3 mg/dL) Negative	Negative (<0.3 mmol/L) Negative
Acetone			
Semiquantitative *Quantitative*	Serum or plasma (oxalate)	Negative (<3 mg/dL) 0.3–2.0 mg/dL	Negative (<0.5 mmol/L) 0.05–0.34 mmol/L
Semiquantitative	Urine	Negative	Negative
Adrenocorticotropic Hormone (ACTH)	Plasma (EDTA)	Adult, 0800 h: 25–100 pg/mL 1800 h: <50 pg/mL	 25–100 ng/L <50 ng/L
Adrenocorticotropic Hormone Stimulation Test (Prolonged Infusion)	Urine, 24 h	17-KGS: 2- to 4-fold rise 17-KS: 2-fold rise 17-OHCS: 2- to 5-fold rise	17-KGS: 2- to 4-fold rise 17-KS: 2-fold rise 17-OHCS: 2- to 5-fold rise
Dose: 500 μg Cortrosyn/d × 3	Serum	Cortisol: 25–50 μg/dL	Cortisol: 0.7–1.4 μmol/L
Adrenocorticotropic Hormone Stimulation Test (Rapid Test)	Serum, fasting, 30 and 60 min after stimulation	Cortisol Baseline: >5.0 μg/dL After cortrosyn: 2× baseline	 Baseline: >0.14 μmol/L After cortrosyn: 2× baseline
Alanine	Urine, 24 h	10 d–2 wks: 4–10 mg/d 3–12 y: 9–39 mg/d Adult: 8–48 mg/d	0.04–0.1 mmol/d 0.1–0.44 mmol/d 0.09–0.54 mmol/d
Alanine Aminotransferase (ALT, GPT)	Serum	Newborn/Infant: 5–28 U/L Adult: 8–20 U/L >60 y: 6–24 U/L	5–28 U/L 8–20 U/L 6–24 U/L
Albumin	Serum	Adult: 3.5–5.0 g/dL >60 y: 3.4–4.8 g/dL Avg. ~ 0.3 g/dL higher in ambulatory individuals	35–50 g/L 34–48 g/L Avg. ~ 3 g/L higher in ambulatory individuals
	CSF Urine	10–30 mg/dL <80 mg/d	100–300 mg/L <80 mg/d
Aldolase	Serum	1.0–7.5 U/L (30°C) 0.3–3.0 U/L at bed rest 1.5–12.0 U/L (37°C)	1.0–7.5 U/L (30°C) 0.3–3.0 U/L at bed rest 1.5–12.0 U/L (37°C)
Aldosterone	Plasma (heparin, EDTA) or serum	*ng/dL* 3–11 y: 5–70 11–15 y: <5–50 Adult, *average sodium diet* supine: 3–10 ng/dL upright, F: 5–30 ng/dL M: 6–22 ng/dL 2–3× higher during pregnancy; adrenal vein: 200–800 ng/dL *Low sodium diet:* increases 2 to 5-fold; Florinef suppression: <4 ng/dL ACTH or angiotensin stimulation, 1 h: 2 to 5-fold	*nmol/L* 0.14–1.9 <0.14–1.4 0.08–0.3 nmol/L 0.14–0.8 nmol/L 0.17–0.61 nmol/L 5.5–22 nmol/L <0.1 nmol/L
	Urine, 24 h	*Total Urinary Na (mmol/d)* — *Plasma renin activity (ng AI/mL/h)* — *Urinary aldosterone (μg/d)* <20 — 5–24 — >35–80 50 — 2–7 — 13–33 100 — 1–5 — 5–24 150 — 0.5–4 — 3–19 200 — — 1–16 250 — — 1–13 (assuming normal serum Na, K, and extracellular vol)	*Urinary aldosterone (nmol/d)* >97–220 36–91 14–66 8–53 3–44 3–36
α-Amino Acid Nitrogen (AAN)	Plasma (EDTA) Urine, 24 h	3.2–5.5 mg/dL 50–200 mg/d	2.28–3.93 mmol/L 3.57–14.3 mmol/d
δ-Aminolevulinate Dehydratase	Erythrocytes (heparin)	139–211 U/mL erythrocytes	139–211 kU/L
δ-Aminolevulinic Acid (δ-ALA)	Serum Urine	15–23 μg/dL; lower in children 1.3–7.0 mg/d	1.1–1.8 μmol/L 9.9–53.4 μmol/d

(*Continued*)

CLINICAL CHEMISTRY, TOXICOLOGY, SEROLOGY (*Continued*)

Test	Specimen	Reference Range	Reference Range (International Units)
Ammonium Chloride Loading Test	Hourly urine between 1000 and 1600 h	pH should fall to ≤5.2 between 2 and 8 h after the dose	H^+ concentration should increase to >6 µmol/L between 2 and 8 h after the dose
Ammonia Nitrogen *Resin or Enzymatic*	Serum or plasma (Na-heparin)	*µg N/dL* Newborn: 90–150 >1 mo: 29–70 Adult: 15–45	*µmol NH_3/L* 53–88 17–41 8.8–26
	Urine, 24 h	500–1200 mg/d	29–70 mmol/d
Amylase *(Beckman; BMD)*	Serum	Adult: 25–125 U/L >70 y: 20–160 U/L	25–125 U/L 20–160 U/L
	Urine, timed specimen	1–17 U/h	1–17 U/h
Androstenedione	Serum	*ng/dL (mean ±1 SE)* *M* / *F* Cord: 85±27 / 93±28 1–3 mo: 34±11 / 19±4 Adult: 107±25 / 151±38	*nmol/L (mean ±1 SE)* *M* / *F* 2.9±0.94 / 3.2±1.0 1.2±0.4 / 0.66±0.14 3.74±0.87 / 5.27±1.33
Angiotensin I	Peripheral venous plasma (K-EDTA)	11–88 pg/mL	11–88 ng/L
Angiotensin II	Plasma (K-EDTA)	Arterial blood: 2.4±1.2 ng/dL Venous blood: 50–75% of arterial blood concentration	24±12 ng/L Fraction of arterial blood conc.: 0.50–0.75
Anion Gap [Na − (Cl + CO_2)]	Plasma (heparin)	7–16 mmol/L	7–16 mmol/L
α_1-Antichymotrypsin (α_1AC)	Serum	Newborn: ~1 mg/dL Adult: 30–60 mg/dL	~10 mg/L 300–600 mg/L
Anti-Deoxyribonuclease B Titer (Anti-DNAse Titer)	Serum	≤170 units	≤170 units
Antidiuretic Hormone (hADH, Vasopressin)	Plasma (EDTA)	*Plasma (mOsmol/kg)* / *Plasma ADH (pg/mL)* 270–280: <1.5 280–285: <2.5 285–290: 1–5 290–295: 2–7 295–300: 4–12	*Plasma ADH (ng/L)* <1.5 <2.5 1–5 2–7 4–12
Antidiuretic Hormone–Water Deprivation Stimulation Test (Miller Test)	Serum (0600 h) and hourly urine for osmolality; when urine osmolality plateaus after fluid restriction, measure serum osmolality and ADH	Max. urine osmolality before vasopressin admin. > serum osmolality; at end of test, serum osmolality: <300 mOsmol/kg, urine osmolality: >500 mOsmol/kg, ADH levels: see table under hADH; 1 h after vasopressin admin. <5% increase in urine osmolality over previous specimen	
Anti-Hyaluronidase Titer (AH Titer)	Serum	≤128 units	≤128 units
Anti-Streptolysin-O Titer (ASO Titer)	Serum	≤166 Todd Units; 170–330 Todd Units in school-aged children	
α_1-Antitrypsin	Serum	Newborn: 145–270 mg/dL Adult: 105–200 mg/dL	32.2–60.0 µmol/L 23.3–44.4 µmol/L
Arsenic	Whole blood (heparin)	*µg/dL* 0.2–6.2 Chronic poisoning: 10–50 Acute poisoning: 60–93	*µmol/L* 0.03–0.82 1.33–6.65 7.98–12.37
	Urine, 24 h	5–50 µg/d	0.067–0.665 µmol/d
Ascorbic Acid, see *Vitamin C*			
Aspartate Aminotransferase (AST, SGOT, 30°C)	Serum	Newborn/Infant: 5–40 U/L Adult: 8–20 U/L >60 y: 10–25 U/L With P-5-P: 12–29 U/L	5–40 U/L 8–20 U/L 10–25 U/L 12–29 U/L
Base Excess	Whole blood (heparin)	*mmol/L* Newborn: (−10)–(−2) Infant: (−7)–(−1) Child: (−4)–(+2) Adult: (−3)–(+3)	*mmol/L* (−10)–(−2) (−7)–(−1) (−4)–(+2) (−3)–(+3)

(*Continued*)

CLINICAL CHEMISTRY, TOXICOLOGY, SEROLOGY (*Continued*)

Test	Specimen	Reference Range	Reference Range (International Units)
Bicarbonate	Serum	Art.: 21–28 mmol/L Ven.: 22–29 mmol/L	Art.: 21–28 mmol/L Ven.: 22–29 mmol/L
Bile Acids, Total	Serum, fasting Serum, 2 h postprandial Feces	0.3–2.3 μg/mL 1.8–3.2 μg/mL 120–225 mg/d	0.3–2.3 mg/L 1.8–3.2 mg/L 120–225 mg/d
Bilirubin *Total*	Serum	*Premature* / *Full Term* *mg/dL* / *mg/dL* Cord: <2.0 / <2.0 0–1 d: <8.0 / <6.0 3–5 d: <16.0 / <12.0 Thereafter: <2.0 / 0.2–1.0	*Premature* / *Full Term* *μmol/L* <34 / <34 <137 / <103 <274 / <205 <34 / 3.4–17.1
	Urine	Negative	Negative
Conjugated (direct)	Serum	0–0.2 mg/dL	0–3.4 μmol/L
Bromosulfophthalein (BSP) Test (5 mg/kg)	Serum	<6% retention at 45 min	Fraction dye retained: <0.06
Brucellosis, Agglutinins	Serum	≤1:8	≤1:8
C-Peptide	Serum	Adult: ≤4.0 ng/mL >60 y, M: 1.5–5.0 ng/mL F: 1.4–5.5 ng/mL	≤4.0 μg/L 1.5–5.0 μg/L 1.4–5.5 μg/L
C-Reactive Protein	Serum	Cord blood: 10–350 ng/mL Adult: 68–8200 ng/mL	10–350 μg/L 68–8200 μg/L
Calcitonin (hCT)	Serum or plasma (heparin or EDTA)	*pg/mL* *Newborn, term,* cord: 30–240 48 h: 91–580 7 d: 77–293 Adult, M: <100 F: 4 times lower (increases in pregnancy) Concentrations decrease with age	*ng/L* 30–240 91–580 77–293 <100
Calcitonin-Calcium Infusion Stimulation Test *Dose: 15 mg Ca (as gluconate)/kg, IV infusion/4 h*	Serum or plasma (heparin or EDTA); fasting, 3 and 4 h for hCT	Peak hCT level: M: <265 pg/mL F: <120 pg/mL	M: <265 ng/L F: <120 ng/L
Calcium, Ionized (iCa)	Serum, plasma or whole blood (heparin)	*mg/dL* Cord: 5.5±0.3 Newborn, 3–24 h: 4.3–5.1 24–48 h: 4.0–4.7 Adults: 4.48–4.92 or 2.24–2.46 mEq/L	*mmol/L* 1.37±0.07 1.07–1.27 1.00–1.17 1.12–1.23
Calcium, Total	Serum	*mg/dL* Child: 8.8–10.8 Adult: 8.4–10.2 M, >60 y: 8.4–10.0	*mmol/L* 2.2–2.70 2.1–2.55 2.1–2.50
	Urine, 24 h	*Ca in diet* *mg/d* Free Ca: 5–40 Low to average: 50–150 Average (20 mmol/d): 100–300	*mmol/d* 0.13–1.0 1.25–3.8 2.5–7.5
	CSF	2.1–2.7 mEq/L or 4.2–5.4 mg/dL	1.05–1.35 mmol/L 1.05–1.35 mmol/L
	Feces	Avg.: 0.64 g/d	16 mmol/d
Carbon Dioxide, Partial Pressure (Pco_2)	Whole blood (heparin)	*mm/Hg* Newborn: 27–40 Infant: 27–41 Adult, M: 35–48 F: 32–45	*kPa* 3.6–5.3 3.6–5.5 4.7–6.4 4.3–6.0
Carbon Dioxide, Total (Tco_2)	Serum or plasma (heparin)	*mmol/L* Cord: 14–22 Newborn: 17–24 Infant: 20–28 Child: 20–28 Adult: 23–30 >60 y: 23–31	*mmol/L* 14–22 17–24 20–28 20–28 23–30 23–31
Carbon Monoxide	Whole blood (EDTA)	Nonsmokers: <2% CO Hb Smokers: <10% CO Hb Lethal: >50% CO Hb	CO Hb fraction: <0.02 <0.10 >0.5

(*Continued*)

CLINICAL CHEMISTRY, TOXICOLOGY, SEROLOGY (*Continued*)

Test	Specimen	Reference Range	Reference Range (International Units)
Carboxyhemoglobin, see *Carbon Monoxide*			
Carcinoembryonic Antigen (CEA)	Plasma (EDTA)	1.34±0.16 ng/mL	1.34±0.16 μg/L
β-Carotene	Serum	Infant: 20–70 μg/dL Child: 40–130 μg/dL Adult: 60–200 μg/dL	0.37–1.30 μmol/L 0.74–2.42 μmol/L 1.12–3.72 μmol/L
Carotene Absorption Test	Serum	Increase by ≥35 μg/dL	Increase by ≥0.65 μmol/L
Catecholamines, Fractionated	Urine, 24 h	Norepinephrine *μg/d* 1–4 y: 0–29 4–10 y: 8–65 10–15 y: 15–80 Adult: 0–100 Epinephrine *μg/d* 1–4 y: 0–6.0 4–10 y: 0–10.0 10–15 y: 0.5–20 Adult: 0–15 Dopamine *μg/d* 1–4 y: 40–260 4 y–adult: 65–400	*nmol/d* 0–170 47–380 89–470 0–590 *nmol/d* 0–33 0–55 2.7–110 0–82 *nmol/d* 260–1700 425–2610
Catecholamines, Free	Plasma (EDTA-sodium metabisulfite)	*pg/mL* Epinephrine, random: <88 Norepinephrine, random: 104–548 Dopamine, random: <136	*pmol/L* <480 615–3240 <888
Catecholamines, Total	Urine, 24 h	<110 μg/d	<650 nmol/d
Cerebrospinal Fluid Pressure	CSF	70–180 mm water	70–188 mm water
Cerebrospinal Fluid Volume	CSF	Child: 60–100 mL Adult: 100–160 mL	0.006–0.10 L 0.1–0.16 L
Ceruloplasmin	Serum	*mg/dL* Newborn: 1–30 6 mo–1 y: 15–50 1–12 y: 30–65 Thereafter: 14–40	*μmol/L* 0.06–1.99 0.99–3.31 1.99–4.30 0.93–2.65
Chenodeoxycholic Acid, Total	Serum, fasting	0.31±0.32 μg/mL	0.79±0.81 μmol/L
Chenodeoxycholylglycine, Conjugated	Serum, fasting	0.2±0.03 μmol/L	0.2±0.03 μmol/L
Chloride	Serum or plasma (heparin) CSF Urine, 24 h Sweat	98–106 mmol/L 118–132 mmol/L *mmol/d* Infant: 2–10 Child: 15–40 Thereafter: 110–250 (vary greatly with Cl intake) *mmol/L* Normal (homozygote): 0–35 Marginal: 30–70 Cystic fibrosis: 60–200	98–106 mmol/L 118–132 mmol/L *mmol/d* 2–10 15–40 110–250 *mmol/L* 0–35 30–70 60–200
Cholesterol, Total	Serum or plasma (EDTA)	*mg/dL* Cord: 45–100 Newborn: 45–150 Infant: 70–175 Child: 120–200 Adolescent: 120–210 Adult: 140–310 Recommended (desirable) range for adults: 140–250	*mmol/L* 1.17–2.59 1.17–3.89 1.81–4.53 3.11–5.18 3.11–5.44 3.63–8.03 3.63–6.48
Cholic Acid, Total	Serum, fasting	0.20±0.17 μg/mL	0.49±0.42 μmol/L
Cholinesterase II (Pseudocholinesterase) *RID* *DuPont ACA*	 Serum	 0.5–1.5 mg/dL 7–19 U/mL Dibucaine: 84±3% inhibition Fluoride: 49±5% inhibition	 5–15 mg/L 7–19 kU/L Fraction of activity inhibited: 0.84±0.03 0.49±0.05

(*Continued*)

CLINICAL CHEMISTRY, TOXICOLOGY, SEROLOGY (*Continued*)

Test	Specimen	Reference Range	Reference Range (International Units)
Chorionic Gonadotropin, β-Subunit (β-hCG)	Serum or plasma (EDTA)	M: nondetectable	
		F, postconception: *mIU/mL*	*IU/L*
		7–10 d: >5.0	>5.0
		30 d: >100	>100
		40 d: >2000	>2000
		10 wks: 50,000–100,000	50,000–100,000
		14 wks: 10,000–20,000	10,000–20,000
		Trophoblastic disease: >100,000	>100,000
Citrulline	Serum	*µmol/L*	*µmol/L*
		Newborn, 1 d: 9–29	9–29
		2–6 mo: 31–50	31–50
		6–18 y: 19–52	19–52
		Adult: 12–55	12–55
	Urine, 24 h	Adult: 0.4–8 mg/d or 2±1 mg/g creatinine	2.3–46 µmol/d or 1.3±0.64 mmol/mol creatinine
Complement			
Total hemolytic complement activity	Plasma (EDTA)	75–160 U/mL or 40–85 CH_{50} Units/mL	75–160 kU/mL
Total complement decay rate (functional)	Plasma (EDTA)	~10–20%	
		Deficiency: >50%	
Classic pathway components:		*mg/dL*	*µmol/L*
C1q	Serum	5.7–8.1	0.14–0.20
C1r	Serum	2.5–3.8	0.15–0.22
C1s (C1 esterase)	Serum	2.5–3.8	0.28–0.42
C2	Serum	2.0–3.0	0.17–0.25
C3 (β-1-C globulin)	Serum	80–170	4.4–9.4
C4 (β-1-E globulin)	Serum	15–45	0.73–2.18
C5 (β-1-F globulin)	Serum	5.5–8.0	0.31–0.45
C6	Serum	5.4–7.2	0.60–0.80
C7	Serum	4.9–7.0	0.45–0.64
C8	Serum	4.3–6.3	0.26–0.39
C9	Serum	4.7–6.9	0.59–0.86
Alternative pathway components:			
C4 binding protein	Serum	18.0–32.0	180–320 mg/L
Factor B (C3 proactivator)	Serum	20.0–42.0	2.16–4.54 µmol/L
Properdin	Serum	2.8±0.4	0.13±0.02 µmol/L
Regulatory proteins			
β1H globulin (C3b inactivator accelerator)	Serum	37.0–69.0	370–690 mg/L
C1 inhibitor (Esterase inhibitor)	Plasma (EDTA)	13–29	1.2–2.8 mg/L
C1 inhibitor by complement decay rate (functional)	Plasma (EDTA)	~10–20%	
		Deficiency: >50%	
C3b inactivator (KAF)	Serum	2.9–4.0 mg/dL	29–40 mg/L
S protein	Serum	41.8–60.0 mg/dL	418–600 mg/L
Copper	Serum	*µg/dL*	*µmol/L*
		Birth–6 mo: 20–70	3.14–10.99
		6 y: 90–190	14.13–29.83
		Adult, M: 70–140	10.99–21.98
		F: 80–155	12.56–24.34
		Pregnancy at term: 118–302	18.53–47.41
	Erythrocytes (heparin)	90–150 µg/dL	14.13–23.55 µmol/L
	Urine, 24 h	15–30 µg/d	0.24–0.47 µmol/d
Coproporphyrin	Urine, 24 h	34–234 µg/d	51–351 nmol/d
	Feces, 24 h	<30 µg/g dry wt	<45 nmol/g dry wt
		400–1200 µg/d	600–1800 nmol/d
Corticobinding Globulin (CBG), see *Transcortin*			
Corticosterone	Serum or plasma (heparin, EDTA, or oxalate)	0.13–2.3 µg/dL	3.75–66 nmol/L
Cortisol	Serum or plasma (heparin)	0800 h: 5–23 µg/dL	138–635 nmol/L
		1600 h: 3–15 µg/dL	82–413 nmol/L
		2000 h: ≤50% of 0800 h	Fraction of 0800 h: ≤0.50
Cortisol, Free	Urine, 24 h	Child: 2–27 µg/d	5.5–74 nmol/d
		Adolescent: 5–55 µg/d	14–152 nmol/d
		Adult: 10–100 µg/d	27–276 nmol/d
Creatine	Serum or plasma	M: 0.17–0.70 mg/dL	M: 13–54 µmol/L
		F: 0.35–0.93 mg/dL	F: 27–71 µmol/L
	Urine	M: 0–40 mg/d	M: 0–307 µmol/d
		F: 0–80 mg/d	F: 0–615 µmol/d

(*Continued*)

CLINICAL CHEMISTRY, TOXICOLOGY, SEROLOGY (*Continued*)

Test	Specimen	Reference Range	Reference Range (International Units)
Creatine Kinase (CK, 30°C)			
Total	Serum	*U/L*	*U/L*
		Newborn: 10–200	10–200
		Adult, M: 12–70	12–70
		F: 10–55	10–55
		Ambulatory,	
		M: 25–90	25–90
		F: 10–70	10–70
		Higher after exercise	
Isoenzymes	Serum	Fraction 2 (MB) <5% of total	Fraction of total: <0.05
Creatinine			
Jaffe, kinetic or enzymatic	Serum or plasma	*mg/dL*	*µmol/L*
		Cord: 0.6–1.2	53–106
		Child: 0.3–0.7	27–62
		Adult, M: 0.6–1.2	53–106
		F: 0.5–1.1	44–97
Jaffe, manual	Serum or plasma	0.8–1.5 mg/dL	70–133 µmol/L
	Urine, 24 h	*mg/kg/d*	*µmol/kg/d*
		Child: 8–22	71–195
		Adult: 14–26	124–230
		or: *mg/d*	*mmol/d*
		M: 800–2000	7–18
		F: 600–1800	5.3–16
Creatinine Clearance (Endogenous)	Serum or plasma and urine	<40 y, M: 97–137 mL/min	
		F: 88–128 mL/min	
		Decreases ~6.5 mL/min/decade	
Cyanide	Serum	Nonsmokers: 0.004 mg/L	0.15 µmol/L
		Smokers: 0.006 mg/L	0.22 µmol/L
		Nitroprusside therapy:	
		0.01–0.06 mg/L	0.37–2.21 µmol/L
		Toxic: >0.1 mg/L	>3.7 µmol/L
	Whole blood (oxalate)	Nonsmokers: 0.016 mg/L	0.59 µmol/L
		Smokers: 0.041 mg/L	1.52 µmol/L
		Nitroprusside therapy:	
		0.05–0.5 mg/L	1.9–19 µmol/L
		Toxic: >1 mg/L	>37 µmol/L
Cyclic AMP	Plasma (EDTA)	M: 17–33 nmol/L	M: 17–33 nmol/L
		F: 11–27 nmol/L	F: 11–27 nmol/L
	Urine, 24 h	1000–11,500 nmol/d	1000–11,500 nmol/d
		<6000 nmoles cAMP/g creatinine	<6000 nmoles cAMP/g creatinine
Cystine or Cysteine			
Qualitative	Urine, random	Negative	Negative
Quantitative	Urine, 24 h	10–100 mg/d	83–830 µmol/d
Dehydroepiandrosterone (DHEA)	Serum	*ng/mL*	*nmol/L*
		Cord: 5.6–20.0	19.4–69.3
		Child: 1.0–3.0	3.5–10.4
		Adult, M: 1.7–4.2	5.9–14.6
		F: 2.0–5.2	6.9–18.0
		Pregnancy: 0.5–12.5	1.7–43.3
	Urine, 24 h	*mg/d*	*µmol/d*
		Child, 0–1 y: <0.1	<0.35
		10–15 y: <0.4	<1.4
		Adult, M: 0–2.3	0–8.0
		F: 0–1.2	0–4.2
Dehydroepiandrosterone Sulfate ($DHEA-SO_4$)	Serum or plasma (heparin or EDTA)	*µg/mL*	*µmol/L*
		Newborn: <300	<780
		1–4 d: <20	<52
		Child: 0.60–2.54	1.6–6.6
		Adult, M: 1.99–3.34	5.2–8.7
		F, premenopausal: 0.82–3.38	2.1–8.8
		Postmenopausal: 0.11–0.61	0.3–1.6
		Pregnancy, term: 0.23–1.17	0.6–3.0
Deoxycholic Acid, Total	Serum, fasting	0.22±0.13 µg/mL	0.56±0.33 µmol/L
11-Deoxycortisol (Compound S)	Plasma (heparin, EDTA, or oxalate)	*µg/dL*	*nmol/L*
		<1 without metyrapone	<30
		>7 after metyrapone	>200
11-Deoxycorticosterone (DOC)	Serum or plasma (heparin, EDTA, or oxalate)	Ad lib diet, 0800 h: 4.3–12.3 ng/dL	0.13–0.37 nmol/L

(*Continued*)

CLINICAL CHEMISTRY, TOXICOLOGY, SEROLOGY (*Continued*)

Test	Specimen	Reference Range	Reference Range (International Units)
Dexamethasone Suppression Test (Standard)	Serum, 0800 h Control, day 2, day 3	Cortisol: suppression on day 3 to <50% of baseline or to <5 μg/dL	Cortisol: suppression on day 3; fraction of baseline: <0.50 or <138 nmol/L
Low dose, adult: 0.5 mg q 6 h × 8	Urine, 24 h Day 1, 2, and 3	17-KGS: Suppression on day 2 to <7.5 mg/d 17-OHCS: Suppression on day 2 to <4.5 mg/d	17-KGS: Suppression on day 2 to <26 μmol/d 17-OHCS: Suppression on day 2 to <12.4 μmol/d
High dose, adult: 2.0 mg q 6 h × 8		Cortisol, 17-KGS, 17-OHCS: suppression on day 3 to <50% of baseline	Cortisol, 17-KGS, 17-OHCS: suppression on day 3; fraction of baseline: <0.50
Dexamethasone Single Dose Overnight Suppression Test *Dose: 1 mg orally at 2300 or 2400 h*	Serum for cortisol, 0800 h following morning	Suppression to 5–10 μg/dL or to <50% of baseline	Suppression to 138–276 nmol/L or fraction of baseline: <0.50
Dihydrotestosterone (DHT)	Serum	*ng/dL* *M* *F*	*nmol/L* *M* *F*
		Pubertal stage I: <10 <10	<0.34 <0.34
		II: <20 <15	<0.7 <0.5
		III: <35 <25	<1.2 <0.86
		IV–V: <75 <25	<2.6 <0.86
		Adult: 60–300 10–40	2–10.3 0.34–1.4
Erythropoietin			
RIA	Serum	<5–20 mU/mL	<5–20 U/L
Hemagglutination		25–125 mU/mL	25–125 U/L
Bioassay		5–18 mU/mL	5–18 U/L
Estradiol	Serum or plasma (heparin or EDTA)	*pg/mL*	*pmol/L*
		Adult, M: 8–36	29–132
		F,	
		Follicular: 10–90	37–330
		Midcycle: 100–500	370–1835
		Luteal: 50–240	184–880
		Postmenopausal: 10–30	37–110
	Urine, 24 h	*μg/d*	*nmol/d*
		Adult, M: 0–6	0–22
		F,	
		Follicular: 0–3	0–11
		Ovulatory peak: 4–14	15–51
		Luteal: 4–10	15–37
		Postmenopausal: 0–4	0–15
Estriol (E_3), Free	Serum	*Weeks of gestation* *μg/L*	*nmol/L*
		25: 3.5–10.0	12–34.7
		28: 4.0–12.5	14–43.3
		30: 4.5–14.0	16–48.5
		32: 5.0–16.0	17–55.5
		34: 5.5–18.5	19–64.1
		36: 7.0–25.0	24–86.7
		37: 8.0–28.0	28–97.1
		38: 9.0–32.0	31–111
		39: 10.0–34.0	35–118
		40–41: 10.5–25.0	36–86.7
Estriol (E_3), Total	Serum	*ng/mL*	*nmol/L*
		Pregnancy (wks),	
		24–28: 30–170	104–590
		28–32: 40–220	140–760
		32–36: 60–280	208–970
		36–40: 80–350	280–1210
		Adult, M and nonpregnant F: <2	<7
	Urine, 24 h	*mg/d*	*μmol/d*
		Pregnancy (wks),	
		30: 6–18	21–62
		35: 9–28	31–97
		40: 13–42	45–146
		Decrease of >40% of previous value suggests fetus at risk	Fraction of previous value of <0.60 suggests fetus at risk

(*Continued*)

CLINICAL CHEMISTRY, TOXICOLOGY, SEROLOGY (*Continued*)

Test	Specimen	Reference Range	Reference Range (International Units)
Estrogens, Total	Serum	*pg/mL*	*ng/L*
		M: 40–115	40–115
		F, cycle-days	
		1–10 d: 61–394	61–394
		11–20 d: 122–437	122–437
		21–30 d: 156–350	156–350
		Prepubertal and postmenopausal: ≤40	≤40
	Urine, 24 h	*μg/d*	*μg/d*
		M: 5–25	5–25
		F, Preovulation: 4–25	4–25
		Ovulation: 28–100	28–100
		Luteal peak: 22–80	22–80
		Pregnancy: <45000	<45000
		Postmenopause: <10	<10
Estrogen Receptor Assay (ERA)	0.5–1 g tissue	*fmol/mg protein*	*nmol/kg protein*
		Negative: <3.0	<3.0
		Borderline positive: 3–10	3–10
		Positive >10.0	>10.0
Estrone (E_1)	Serum	*pg/mL*	*pmol/L*
		M, Pubertal stage I: 11	41
		II: 16	59
		III: 21	78
		Adult: 30–170	111–630
		F, Pubertal stage I: 0–29	0–107
		II: 10–35	37–130
		III: 15–45	55–166
		IV: 20–80	74–296
		Follicular: 20–150	74–555
	Urine, 24 h	*μg/d*	*nmol/d*
		Adult, M: 3–8	11–30
		F, Ovulatory peak: 11–31	41–115
		Luteal: 10–23	37–85
		Postmenopausal: 1–7	3.7–26
Fat, Fecal	Feces, 72 h	*g/d*	*g/d*
		Infant, breast-fed: <1	<1
		0–6 y: <2	<2
		Adult: <7	<7
		Adult (fat-free diet): <4	<4
Fatty Acid Profile	Serum or plasma (heparin)	*% of Total Nonesterified Fatty Acids*	*Fraction of Total Nonesterified Fatty Acids*
		Oleic: 26–45	0.26–0.45
		Palmitic: 23–25	0.23–0.25
		Stearic: 10–14	0.10–0.14
		Linoleic: 8–16	0.08–0.16
Fatty Acids, Nonesterified (Free)	Serum or plasma (heparin)	*mg/dL*	*mmol/L*
		Adults: 8–25	0.30–0.90
		Children and obese adults: Up to 31	<1.10
Fatty Acids, Total	Serum	190–420 mg/dL	7–15 mmol/L
Ferritin	Serum	*ng/mL*	*μg/L*
		Newborn: 25–200	25–200
		1 mo: 200–600	200–600
		2–5 mo: 50–200	50–200
		6 mo-15 y: 7–140	7–140
		Adult, M: 15–200	15–200
		F: 12–150	12–150
α_1-Fetoprotein	Serum	Adult: <40 ng/mL	<40 μg/L
		Mean: 2.6±1.6 (1 SD) ng/mL	2.6±1.6 (1 SD) μg/L
		Fetal: peak of 200–400 mg/dL in first trimester	Peak of 2–4 g/L in first trimester
		1 y: <30 ng/mL	<30 μg/L
	Amniotic fluid	*weeks* — *mg/dL median* — *±2 log SD*	*mg/L median* — *±2 log SD*
		11–12 — 24 — 10–50	240 — 100–500
		13–14 — 23 — 13–41	230 — 130–410
		15–16 — 18 — 9–35	180 — 90–350
		17–18 — 15 — 6–33	150 — 60–330
		19–20 — 10 — 5–25	100 — 50–250
		21–25 — 7 — 4–14	70 — 40–140
		26–30 — 6 — 3–10	60 — 30–100
		31–35 — 2 — 0.5–7	20 — 5–70
		36–40 — 1 — 0.2–3	10 — 2–30

(*Continued*)

CLINICAL CHEMISTRY, TOXICOLOGY, SEROLOGY (*Continued*)

Test	Specimen	Reference Range	Reference Range (International Units)
Fibrinogen, see *Hematology section*			
FIGLU *Dose: 5 g histidine q 4 h × 3*	Urine, 24 h, after initial dose of histidine	<35 mg/d	<200 μmol/d
Fluoride	Plasma (heparin) Urine	0.01–0.2 μg/mL 0.2–1.1 μg/mL Occup. exposure: 4–5 μg/mL	0.5–10 μmol/L 10–58 μmol/L Occup. exposure: 200–260 μmol/L
Folate	Serum Erythrocyte (EDTA)	1.8–9 ng/mL >60 y: 1.8–12 ng/mL 150–450 ng/mL cells >60 y: 95–500 ng/mL cells	4.1–20.4 nmol/L 4.1–27.2 nmol/L 340–1020 nmol/L cells 215–1132 nmol/L cells
Folate Absorption Test	Urine, 24 h	45±7% of dose	Fraction of dose: 0.45±0.07
Follicle Stimulating Hormone (hFSH)	Serum or plasma (heparin) Urine, 24 h	*mIU/mL* Adult, M: 4–25 F, Premenopause: 4–30 Midcycle peak: 10–90 Pregnancy: low to undetectable Postmenopause: 40–250 *IU/d (IRP-2-hMG)* Birth-1 y, F: <0.5–1.4 1–8 y, M: <0.5–4.5 F: <0.5–4.0 9–10 y, M: 1–5 F: 1–4 11–12 y, M: 1.5–5 F: 1–8 13–14 y, M: 2–12 F: 1–10 Adult, M: 4–18 F: 3–12 Higher in males >60 y	*IU/L* 4–25 4–30 10–90 Low to undetectable 40–250 *IU/d (IRP-2-hMG)* <0.5–1.4 <0.5–4.5 <0.5–4.0 1–5 1–4 1.5–5 1–8 2–12 1–10 4–18 3–12 Higher in males >60 y
Free Thyroxine Index (FT_4I) *with normalized T_3RU*	Serum	*FT_4 Index* 1.2–5.0 1–3 d: 9.3–26.6 1–4 wk: 7.6–20.8 1–4 mo: 7.4–17.9 4–12 mo: 6.1–14.5 1–6 y: 5.7–13.3 6–10 y: 5.5–10.0 >10 y: 5.5–10.0 Borderline low: 4.8 Borderline high: 14.0	
Free Triiodothyronine, see *Triiodothyronine, Free*			
Fructose	Serum Urine	1–6 mg/dL <60 mg/d	55.5–333.0 μmol/L <333 μmol/d
Fructose Loading Test	Serum Urine	Peak: 15–25 mg/dL 1–2% of administered dose	Peak: 0.83–1.39 mmol/L Fraction of administered dose: 0.01–0.02
Galactose	Serum Urine	Newborn: 0–20 mg/dL Thereafter: <5 mg/dL Newborn: ≤60 mg/dL Thereafter: <14 mg/d	0–1.11 mmol/L <0.28 mmol/L ≤3.33 mmol/L <0.08 mmol/d
Gastric Acid	Gastric contents	Fasting: 0–5 mmol/L Post stimul.: 10–60 mmol/L	0–5 mmol/L 10–60 mmol/L
Gastric Content	Gastric contents	Volume: 20–100 mL pH: 1.5–3.5	0.02–0.1 L H^+ concentration: 32–316 μmol/L
Gastric Secretion Rate	Total gastric contents, six 15 min spec.	BAO: 0–5 mmol/h PAO: 1–20 mmol/h (post Pentagastrin) BAO/PAO: 0.20	0–5 mmol/h 1–20 mmol/h (post Pentagastrin) 0.20
Gastrin	Serum	<60 y: <100 pg/mL >60 y: upper 15%: 100–800 pg/mL	<100 ng/L Upper 0.15 fraction of population: 100–800 ng/L

(*Continued*)

CLINICAL CHEMISTRY, TOXICOLOGY, SEROLOGY (*Continued*)

Test	Specimen	Reference Range	Reference Range (International Units)
Gastrin-Calcium Infusion Stimulation Test	Serum	Gastrin: Slight or no increase Z.E. syndrome: >450 pg/mL	Gastrin: Slight or no increase Z.E. syndrome: >450 ng/L
Gastrin-Secretin Stimulation Test *IV dose: 5 U secretin/kg*	Serum, fasting, at 15 min intervals for 1 h	No response or slight suppression Z. E. syndrome: Increase >110 pg/mL if base level 80–500 pg/mL	No response or slight suppression Z. E. syndrome: Increase >110 ng/L if base level 80–500 ng/L
Glomerular Selectivity Test (IgG/Albumin Clearance)	Urine	<0.16 indicates high selectivity	<0.16 indicates high selectivity
Glucagon	Plasma (heparin or EDTA)	*pg/mL* 30–210 Big glucagon: 113±79 Proglucagon: 11±16 Glucagon: 31±29 Small glucagon: 26±18	*ng/L* 30–210 113±79 11±16 31±29 26±18
Glucose	Serum	*mg/dL* Cord: 45–96 Premature: 20–60 Neonate: 30–60 Newborn, 1 d: 40–60 >1 d: 50–80 Child: 60–100 Adult: 70–105 >60 y: 80–115	*mmol/L* 2.5–5.3 1.1–3.3 1.7–3.3 2.2–3.3 2.8–4.4 3.3–5.5 3.9–5.8 4.4–6.4
	Whole blood (heparin)	Adult: 65–95	3.6–5.3
	CSF	Adult: 40–70	2.2–3.9
Quant., enzymatic	Urine	<0.5 g/d	<2.8 mmol/d
Qual.	Urine	Negative	Negative
Glucose, 2 h Postprandial	Serum	<120 mg/dL Diabetes: see *Glucose Tolerance Test, Oral*	<6.7 mmol/L
Glucose Tolerance Test (GTT) with Cortisone *Dose: 50 mg, 8.5 and 2 h before test*	Plasma (fluoride oxalate), fasting, 1, 1½, 2 h after glucose ingestion	*Glucose* *mg/dL* Fasting: 70–105 1 h: <200 1½ h: <200 2 h: <140	*mmol/L* 3.9–5.8 <11 <11 <7.8
Glucose Tolerance Test (GTT) *Oral*	Serum	*mg/dL* Adults, *Normal* *Diabetic* Fasting: 70–105 >115 60 min: 120–170 >200 90 min: 100–140 >200 120 min: 70–120 >140	*mmol/L* *Normal* *Diabetic* 3.9–5.8 >6.4 6.7–9.4 >11 5.6–7.8 >11 3.9–6.7 >7.8
I.V.	Serum	5 min: ~250 mg/dL 90 min: below fasting concentration or K = >1.5%	5 min: ~13.9 mmol/L
Glutamine	CSF	6–16 mg/dL	0.41–1.10 mmol/L
γ-Glutamyltransferase (GGT), 37°C	Serum	M: 9–50 U/L F: 8–40 U/L	M: 9–50 U/L F: 8–40 U/L
Glycerol, Free	Plasma	*mg/dL* 3–10 y: 0.56–2.14 11–80 y: 0.29–1.72	*mmol/L* 0.061–0.232 0.032–0.187
Glycine	Urine, 24 h	*mg/d* 10 d–2 wks: 15–59 3–12 y: 12–107 Adult: 59–294 or: 60±24 mg/g creatinine	*mmol/d* 0.20–0.79 0.16–1.43 0.79–3.92 or: 90±36 mmol/mol creatinine
Glycolic Acid	Urine, 24 h	Adult: 15–60 mg/d	0.20–0.79 mmol/d
Gold	Serum	<10 μg/dL Therap. range: 38–500 μg/dL	<0.51 μmol/L Therap. range: 1.93–25.40 μmol/L
	Urine, 24 h	<1 μg/d	<5 nmol/d
Gonadotropins, see *Pregnancy Tests* and *Chorionic Gonadotropin, β-Subunit*			

(*Continued*)

CLINICAL CHEMISTRY, TOXICOLOGY, SEROLOGY (*Continued*)

Test	Specimen	Reference Range	Reference Range (International Units)
Growth Hormone (hGH, Somatotropin)	Serum or plasma (EDTA, heparin)	*ng/mL* Cord: 10–50 Newborn: 15–40 Child: <1–20 Adult, M: <2 F: <10 >60 y, M: 0.4–10 F: 1–14	*μg/L* 10–50 15–40 <1–20 <2 <10 0.4–10 1–14
Growth Hormone-Arginine Stimulation Test	Serum, fasting, 30 min intervals for 2 h	Fasting: <5 ng/mL; rise to >7 ng/mL during test (peak range 8–35 ng/mL) at 30–60 min	Fasting: <5 μg/L; rise to >7 μg/L during test (peak range 8–35 μg/L) at 30–60 min
Growth Hormone-Glucagon Stimulation Test	Serum, fasting, then hourly for 3–4 h	>7 ng/mL after stimulation or >5 ng/mL rise above baseline	>7 μg/L after stimulation or >5 μg/L rise above baseline
Growth Hormone-L-Dopa Stimulation Test *Dose, adult: 500 mg L-dopa, orally; child: 10 mg/kg*	Serum, fasting, 30, 60, 90, 120, and 180 min after L-dopa	Peak: >7 ng/mL or >5 ng/mL rise above baseline	>7 μg/L or >5 μg/L rise above baseline
Haptoglobin, see *Hematology section*			
HDL-Cholesterol (HDLC)	Serum or plasma (EDTA)	*mg/dL* (*M* / *F*) Mean: 45 / 55 Range, cord blood: 5–50 / 5–50 <19 y: 30–65 / 30–70 20–29 y: 30–70 / 30–75 40+ y: 30–70 / 30–85 Values for blacks ~10 mg/dL higher *HDLC, % of total cholesterol:* (*M* / *F*) *CHD Risk* Dangerous: <7 / <12 High: 7–15 / 12–18 Average: 15–25 / 18–27 Below average: 25–37 / 27–40 Protection probable: >37 / >40	*mmol/L* (*M* / *F*) 1.17 / 1.42 0.13–1.30 / 0.13–1.30 0.78–1.68 / 0.78–1.81 0.78–1.81 / 0.78–1.94 0.78–1.81 / 0.78–2.20 *Fraction HDLC of CHOL* (*M* / *F*) <0.07 / <0.12 0.07–0.15 / 0.12–0.18 0.15–0.25 / 0.18–0.27 0.25–0.37 / 0.27–0.40 >0.37 / >0.40
Hemoglobin	Serum or plasma (EDTA) Urine, fresh random	<3 mg/dL with butterfly set-up and 18 g needle Negative	<0.47 μmol/L with butterfly set-up and 18 g needle Negative
Hemoglobin A_{1c} *Electrophoresis* *Column*	Whole blood (heparin, EDTA, or oxalate)	 5.6–7.5% of total Hb 6–9% of total Hb	 Fraction of Hb: 0.056–0.075 0.06–0.09
Homocystine	Urine, random	Negative	Negative
Homovanillic Acid (HVA)	Urine, 24 h	Child: 3–16 μg/mg creatinine Adult: <15 mg/d	1.9–10 mmol/mol creatinine <82 μmol/d
β-Hydroxybutyric Acid	Serum or plasma	Undetectable	Undetectable
17-Hydroxycorticosteroids (17-OHCS)	Urine, 24 h	*mg/d* 0–1 y: 0.5–1.0 Child: 1.0–5.6 Adult, M: 3.0–10.0 F: 2.0–8.0 or: 3–7 mg/g creatinine	*μmol/d* 1.4–2.8 2.8–15.5 8.2–27.6 5.5–22 or: 0.9–2.5 mmol/mol creatinine (conv. factor based on hydrocortisone, M.W. 362)
5-Hydroxyindole Acetic Acid (5-HIAA) *Qual.* *Quant.*	 Fresh random urine Urine, 24 h	 Negative 2–8 mg/d	 Negative 10.5–42 μmol/d
17-Hydroxyprogesterone (17-OHP)	Serum	*ng/mL* M, Pub. stage I: 0.1–0.3 Adult: 0.2–1.8 F, Pub. stage I: 0.2–0.5 Follicular: 0.2–0.8 Luteal: 0.8–3.0 Postmenopausal: 0.04–0.5	*nmol/L* 0.3–0.9 0.6–5.4 0.6–1.5 0.6–2.4 2.4–9.0 0.12–1.5

(*Continued*)

CLINICAL CHEMISTRY, TOXICOLOGY, SEROLOGY (*Continued*)

Test	Specimen	Reference Range	Reference Range (International Units)
Hydroxyproline	Serum	*µmol/L* Premature, 1 d: 40±40 6–18 y, M: 0–50 F: 0–44 Adult, M: 0–42 F: 0–34	*µmol/L* 40±40 0–50 0–44 0–42 0–34
	Urine, 24 h	*mg/d* 1–5 y: 20–65 6–10 y: 35–99 11–14 y: 63–180 18–21 y: 20–55 >21 y: 15–43 Free hydroxyproline 2–5% of total	*µmol/d* 150–496 270–750 480–1370 150–420 114–330 Free hydroxyproline fraction of total: 0.02–0.05
Immunoglobulin A (IgA)	Serum	*mg/dL* Cord: 0–5 Newborn: 0–2.2 ½–6 mo: 3–82 6 mo–2 y: 14–108 2–6 y: 23–190 6–12 y: 29–270 12–16 y: 81–232 Adults: 60–380	*mg/L* 0–50 0–22 30–820 140–1080 230–1900 290–2700 810–2320 600–3800
	CSF	0–0.6 mg/dL	0–6 mg/L
Immunoglobulin D (IgD)	Serum	Newborn: None detected Adult: 0–8 mg/dL	None detected 0–0.44 µmol/L
Immunoglobulin E (IgE)	Serum	Adult, M: 0–230 IU/mL F: 0–170 IU/mL	0–230 kIU/L 0–170 kIU/L
Immunoglobulin G (IgG)	Serum	*mg/dL* Cord: 760–1700 Newborn: 700–1480 ½–6 mo: 300–1000 6 mo–2 y: 500–1200 2–6 y: 500–1300 6–12 y: 700–1650 12–16 y: 700–1550 Adults: 600–1600 (higher in blacks)	*g/L* 7.6–17 7–14.8 3–10 5–12 5–13 7–16.5 7–15.5 6–16
	CSF	0.5–5 mg/dL	5–50 mg/L
Immunoglobulin G/Albumin Ratio	CSF and serum	0.3–0.7	0.3–0.7
Immunoglobulin G Synthesis Rate	CSF and serum	(−)9.9 to (+)3.3 mg/d	(−)9.9 to (+)3.3 mg/d
Immunoglobulin M (IgM)	Serum	*mg/dL* Cord: 4–24 Newborn: 5–30 ½–6 mo: 15–109 6 mo–2 y: 43–239 2–6 y: 50–199 6–12 y: 50–260 12–16 y: 45–240 Adults: 40–345 Results vary with std. preparation	*mg/L* 40–240 50–300 150–1090 430–2390 500–1990 500–2600 450–2400 400–3450
	CSF	0–1.3 mg/dL	0–13 mg/L
Insulin (12 h Fasting)	Serum	Newborn: 3–20 µU/mL Adult: 7–24 µU/mL >60 y: 6–35 µU/mL	3–20 mU/L 7–24 mU/L 6–35 mU/L
Insulin Antibodies	Serum	Undetectable	Undetectable
Insulin and Glucose Suppression Test	Serum, every 6–12 h	>50 mg glucose/dL during a 72 h period of fasting with values slightly lower in females Insulin: <4 µU/mL or undetectable Normal fasting insulin-glucose ratio: <0.3	>2.8 mmol glucose/L during a 72 h period of fasting with values slightly lower in females Insulin: <4 mU/L or undetectable Normal fasting insulin-glucose ratio: <5.4

(*Continued*)

CLINICAL CHEMISTRY, TOXICOLOGY, SEROLOGY (*Continued*)

Test	Specimen	Reference Range	Reference Range (International Units)
Insulin with Oral Glucose Tolerance Test	Serum	*Min* *Insulin, μU/mL*	*mU/L*
		0: 7–24	7–24
		30: 25–231	25–231
		60: 18–276	18–276
		120: 16–166	16–166
		180: 4–38	4–38
Insulin Tolerance Test	Serum	Glucose: Decrease ~50% of the fasting level by 30 min and return to normal fasting limits by 90–120 min	Fractional decrease in glucose ~0.50 of the fasting level by 30 min and return to normal fasting limits by 90–120 min
		hGH: Increase of >5 ng/mL within 60 min of hypoglycemia	hGH: Increase of >5 μg/L within 60 min of hypoglycemia
		Cortisol: Increase of >6 μg/dL with peak of >20 μg/dL	Cortisol: Increase of >165 nmol/L with peak of >552 nmol/L
Intrinsic Factor, see *Vitamin B_{12} Intrinsic Factor*			
Inulin Clearance Test	Serum and urine	*Mean (±2 SD) mL/min*	
		M *F*	
		20–29 y: 132 (90–174) 119 (84–156)	
		30–39 y: 128 (88–168) 116 (82–150)	
		40–49 y: 120 (78–162) 114 (82–146)	
		50–59 y: 110 (68–152) 104 (66–142)	
		60–69 y: 97 (57–137) 94 (58–130)	
		70–79 y: 82 (42–122) 83 (45–121)	
		80–89 y: 67 (39–105)	
Iron	Serum	*μg/dL*	*μmol/L*
		Newborn: 100–250	17.90–44.75
		Infant: 40–100	7.16–17.90
		Child: 50–120	8.95–21.48
		Adult, M: 50–160	8.95–28.64
		F: 40–150	7.16–26.85
Iron-Binding Capacity, Total (TIBC)	Serum	*μg/dL*	*μmol/L*
		Infant: 100–400	17.90–71.60
		Thereafter: 250–400	44.75–71.60
Iron Saturation	Serum	20–55%	Fraction saturation 0.20–0.55
Isocitrate Dehydrogenase (ICD), 30°C	Serum	1.2–7.0 U/L	1.2–7.0 U/L
Isoleucine	Serum	*μmol/L*	*μmol/L*
		Premature, 1 d: 40±20	40±20
		Newborn, 1 d: 27–53	27–53
		1–3 mo: 59±14	59±14
		Adult: 37–98	37–98
	Urine, 24 h	*mg/d*	*μmol/d*
		10 d–2 wks: trace–0.4	trace–3
		3–12 y: 2–7	15–53
		Adult: 2–24	15–180
		or: 3±1 mg/g creatinine	
17-Ketogenic Steroids (17-KGS)	Urine, 24 h	*mg/d*	*μmol/d*
		0–1 y: <1.0	<3.5 (conv. factor based on DHEA, M.W. 288)
		1–10 y: <5	<17
		11–14 y: <12	<42
		Adult, M: 5–23	17–80
		F: 3–15	10–52
		>70 y, M: 3–15	10–52
		F: 3–13	10–45
Ketone bodies			
Qualitative	Serum	Negative	Negative
	Urine, random	Negative	Negative
Quantitative	Serum	0.5–3.0 mg/dL	5–30 mg/L

(*Continued*)

CLINICAL CHEMISTRY, TOXICOLOGY, SEROLOGY (*Continued*)

Test	Specimen	Reference Range			Reference Range (International Units)	
17-Ketosteroids (17 KS), Total	Urine, 24 h		*mg/d*		*μmol/d*	
Zimmerman reaction		14 d–2 y:	<1		<3.5	(conv. factor based on DHEA, M.W. 288)
		2–6 y:	<2		<7	
		6–10 y:	1–4		3.5–14	
		10–12 y:	1–6		3.5–21	
		12–14 y:	3–10		10–35	
		14–16 y:	5–12		17–42	
		Adult, M, 18–30:	9–22		31–76	
		M, >30:	8–20		28–70	
		F:	6–15		21–52	
		Decreases with age			Decreases with age	
Chromatography	Urine, 24 h	Adult, M:	5.0–12.0		Adult, M: 17–42	
		F:	3.0–10.0		F: 10–35	
17-Ketosteroid (KS) Fractionation	Urine, 24 h		*mg/d*		*μmol/d*	
Androsterone		0–1 y:	<0.1		<0.3	
		1–5 y:	<0.3		<1	
		6–9 y:	0.1–1.0		0.3–3.4	
		10–15 y, M:	0.2–2.0		0.7–6.9	
		10–15 y, F:	0.5–3.0		1.7–10.3	
		Adult, M:	2.2–5.0		7.6–17.2	
		F:	0.5–2.4		1.7–8.3	
Dehydroepiandrosterone		0–5 y:	<0.1		<0.35	
		6–9 y:	<0.2		<0.7	
		10–15 y, M and F:	<0.4		<1.4	
		Adult, M:	<2.3		<8.0	
		F:	<1.5		<5.2	
Etiocholanolone		0–1 y:	<0.1		<0.35	
		1–2 y:	<0.4		<1.4	
		3–5 y:	<0.7		<2.4	
		6–9 y:	0.3–1.0		1–3.4	
		10–15 y, M:	0.1–1.6		0.3–5.5	
		10–15 y, F:	0.7–3.1		2.4–10.7	
		Adult, M:	1.9–4.7		6.5–16.2	
		F:	1.1–3.5		3.8–12.0	
11-β-Hydroxyandrosterone		0–2 y:	<0.3		<1	
		3–5 y:	<0.4		<1.3	
		6–9 y:	0.4–1.0		1.3–3.3	
		10–15 y, M:	0.1–1.1		0.3–3.6	
		10–15 y, F:	0.2–1.0		0.7–3.3	
		Adult, M:	0.5–1.3		1.6–4.2	
		F:	0.2–0.6		0.7–2.0	
11-β-Hydroxyetiocholanolone		0–2 y:	<0.1		<0.3	
		3–5 y:	<0.4		<1.3	
		6–9 y:	0.1–0.5		0.3–1.6	
		10–15 y, M:	<0.3		<1	
		10–15 y, F:	0.1–0.5		0.3–1.6	
		Adult, M:	0.3–0.7		1–2.3	
		F:	0.2–0.6		0.7–2.0	
11-Ketoandrosterone		≤15 y:	<0.1		<0.3	
		Adult, M:	0.2–1.0		0.7–3.3	
		F:	0.2–0.8		0.7–2.6	
11-Ketoetiocholanolone		0–2 y:	<0.1		<0.3	
		3–5 y:	<0.4		<1.3	
		6–9 y:	0.1–0.7		0.3–2.3	
		10–15 y, M:	0.2–0.6		0.7–2.0	
		10–15 y, F:	0.1–0.6		0.3–2.0	
		Adult, M:	0.2–1.0		0.7–3.3	
		F:	0.2–0.8		0.7–2.6	
17-Ketosteroid (17 KS) Fractions	Urine, 24 h					
Beta-Alpha ratio		<0.2			<0.2	
Alpha-Beta ratio		>5			>5	
LDL-Cholesterol (LDLC)	Serum or plasma (EDTA)		*mg/dL*		*mmol/L*	
			M	*F*	*M*	*F*
		Cord blood:	10–50	10–50	0.26–1.30	0.26–1.30
		0–19 y:	60–140	60–150	1.55–3.63	1.55–3.89
		20–29 y:	60–175	60–160	1.55–4.53	1.55–4.14
		30–39 y:	80–190	70–170	2.07–4.92	1.81–4.40
		40–49 y:	90–205	80–190	2.33–5.31	2.07–4.92
		50–59 y:	90–205	90–220	2.33–5.31	2.33–5.70
		60–69 y:	90–215	100–235	2.33–5.57	2.59–6.09
		70+ y:	90–190	95–215	2.33–4.92	2.46–5.57
		Recommended (desirable) range for adults: 65–175 mg/dL			1.68–4.53	

(*Continued*)

CLINICAL CHEMISTRY, TOXICOLOGY, SEROLOGY (*Continued*)

Test	Specimen	Reference Range	Reference Range (International Units)
Lactate	Whole blood (heparin)	*mmol/L*	*mmol/L*
		Venous: 0.5–2.2	0.5–2.2
		Arterial: 0.5–1.6	0.5–1.6
		Inpatients,	
		Venous: 0.9–1.7	0.9–1.7
		Arterial: <1.25	<1.25
Lactate Dehydrogenase (LDH), 30°C	Serum	*U/L*	*U/L*
Total (L→P)		Newborn: 290–500	290–500
		Neonate: 300–1500	300–1500
		Infant: 100–250	100–250
		Child: 60–170	60–170
		Adult: 45–90	45–90
		>60 y: 55–102	55–102
Total (P→L)		85–190	85–190
	CSF	~10% of serum value	~0.10 fraction of serum value
			Fraction of total:
Isoenzymes	Serum	Fraction 1: 15–29%	0.15–0.29
		Fraction 2: 28–45%	0.28–0.45
		Fraction 3: 16–27%	0.16–0.27
		Fraction 4: 5–15%	0.05–0.15
		Fraction 5: 3–12%	0.03–0.12
Lactate/Pyruvate Ratio	Whole blood (heparin)	10/1	10/1
Lactose	Serum	<0.5 mg/dL	<14.6 μmol/L
	Urine	12–40 mg/dL	350–1168 μmol/L
Lead	Whole blood (heparin)	Child: <30 μg/dL	<1.45 μmol/L
		Adult: <40 μg/dL	<1.93 μmol/L
		Toxic: ≥100 μg/dL	≥4.83
	Urine, 24 h	<80 μg/L	<0.39 μmol/L
Leucine	Serum	*μmol/L*	*μmol/L*
		Premature, 1 d: 70±25	70±25
		Newborn, 1 d: 47–109	47–109
		1–3 mo: 104±30	104±30
		Adult: 75–175	75–175
	Urine, 24 h	*mg/d*	*μmol/d*
		10 d–2 wks: 0.9–2.0	6.9–15
		3–12 y: 3–11	23–84
		Adult: 3–70	23–530
		or: 4±2 mg/g creatinine	or: 3.4±1.7 mmol/mol creatinine
Lipase	Serum		
Tietz method		0.1–1.0 U/mL	28–280 U/L
BMD		<180 U/L	<180 U/L
Lipoprotein Electrophoresis	Serum	Distinct beta band; negligible chylomicron and pre-beta bands	
Long-Acting Thyroid Stimulating Hormone (LATS)	Serum	Undetectable	Undetectable
Luteinizing Hormone (hLH)	Serum or plasma (heparin)	*mIU/mL*	*IU/L*
		M, 10–13 y: 4–12	4–12
		12–14 y: 6–12	6–12
		12–17 y: 6–16	6–16
		15–18 y: 7–19	7–19
		Adult: 6–23	6–23
		F, 8–12 y: 2.0–11.5	2.0–11.5
		9–14 y: 2.0–14.0	2.0–14.0
		12–18 y: 3.0–29.0	3.0–29.0
		F, Follicular phase: 5–30	5–30
		Midcycle: 75–150	75–150
		Luteal: 3–40	3–40
		Postmenopausal: 30–200	30–200
	Urine	*IU/d*	*IU/d*
		11–13 y: 0.48–11.28	0.48–11.28
		13–15 y: 2.6–27.6	2.6–27.6
		15–17 y: 4.6–24.0	4.6–24.0
		Adult, M: 13–60	13–60
		F, Follicular phase: 7.2–23.5	7.2–23.5
Lysozyme	Serum or plasma (EDTA)	5–15 μg/mL	5–15 mg/L
Magnesium	Serum	1.3–2.1 mEq/L	0.65–1.05 mmol/L
	Urine, 24 h	6.0–10.0 mEq/d	3.00–5.00 mmol/d

(*Continued*)

CLINICAL CHEMISTRY, TOXICOLOGY, SEROLOGY (*Continued*)

Test	Specimen	Reference Range	Reference Range (International Units)
Mercury	Whole blood (EDTA)	<5.0 µg/dL	<0.25 µmol/L
	Urine, 24 h	<20 µg/L	<0.1 µmol/L
		Toxic: >150 µg/L	>0.75 µmol/L
Metanephrine, Total	Urine, 24 h	*µg/mg creatinine*	*mmol/mol creatinine*
		<1 y: 0.001–4.60	0.0006–2.64
		1-2 y: 0.27–5.38	0.15–3.08
		2-5 y: 0.35–2.99	0.20–1.71
		5-10 y: 0.43–2.70	0.25–1.55
		10-15 y: 0.001–1.87	0.0006–1.07
		15-18 y: 0.001–0.67	0.0006–0.38
		Adult: 0.05–1.20	0.03–0.69
Methanol	Whole blood (fluoride/oxalate)	<0.15 mg/dL	<160 µmol/L
		Toxic con.: >20 mg/dL	>6.24 mmol/L
	Urine	Occup. exposure: <5.0 mg/dL	<1.6 mmol/L
	Breath	Occup. exposure: <0.08 mg/L	<2.5 µmol/L
Methionine	Serum	*µmol/L*	*µmol/L*
		Premature, 1 d: 35±5	35±5
		Newborn, 1 d: 9-41	9-41
		1-3 mo: 21±9	21±9
		Adult: 6-40	6-40
	Urine, 24 h	*mg/d*	*µmol/d*
		10 d-2 wks: 0.8–2.0	5.4-13
		3-12 y: 3–14	20-94
		Adult: trace-9	trace-60
		or: 4.5±2.5 mg/g creatinine	or: 3.4±1.9 mmol/mol creatinine
Metyrapone (Metopyrone) Stimulation Test	Serum	11-Deoxycortisol: >7.0 µg/dL	11-Deoxycortisol: >200 nmol/L
	Serum	Cortisol: <8 µg/dL	Cortisol: <220 nmol/L
Dose, adult: 750 mg q 4 h × 6	Urine, 24 h	17-KGS: 2.5–3-fold rise, but at least 10 mg/d	17-KGS: 2.5–3-fold rise, but at least 35 µmol/d
Dose, child: 300 mg/m²	Urine, 24 h	17-KS: >2× base level	17-KS: >2× base level
	Urine, 24 h	17-OHCS: 3–5× base level	17-OHCS: 3–5× base level
Single Dose Metyrapone Test—Dose: 30 mg/kg orally with milk or snack at midnight	Serum for 11-deoxycortisol determination at 0800 h following morning	>7 µg/dL	>200 nmol/L
Microsomal Antibodies, Thyroid, see *Thyroid Microsomal Antibodies*			
Myelin Basic Protein	CSF	<4 ng/mL	<4 µg/L
Myoglobin	Serum	6–85 ng/mL	6–85 pg/L
	Urine, random	Negative	Negative
Nitrogen, Total	Feces	Infants: 0.11–0.52 g N/d	7.9-37 mmol N/d
		Adults: Up to 2 g N/d	Up to 140 mmol N/d
Normetanephrine, Total	Plasma (EDTA—sodium metabisulfite)	Normotensive: 1.2 ng/mL ± 0.1 (SEM)	6.5 nmol/L ± 0.55
Occult Blood	Feces, random	Negative (<2 mL blood/d in ~100–200 g stool)	Negative
	Urine, random	Negative	Negative
Oleic Acid-^{131}I Absorption Test	Plasma	1.7% of administered dose/L after 4–6 h	Fraction of administered dose: 0.017
Dose: 50 µCi in milk	Feces, 72 h	Less than 5% of administered dose in 72 h specimen	Fraction of administered dose: <0.05
Orosomucoid	Serum	55–140 mg/dL	12.5–31.8 µg/L
Osmolality	Serum	Child, adult: 275–295 mOsmol/kg	
	Urine, random	50–1400 mOsmol/kg, depending on fluid intake	
		After 12 h fluid restriction: >850 mOsmol/kg	
	Urine, 24 h	≃300–900 mOsmol/kg	

(*Continued*)

CLINICAL CHEMISTRY, TOXICOLOGY, SEROLOGY (*Continued*)

Test	Specimen	Reference Range	Reference Range (International Units)
Osmolality Ratio, Urine/Serum	Urine and serum	1.0–3.0 >3 after 12 h fluid restriction	1.0–3.0 >3 after 12 h fluid restriction
Oxalate	Serum	1–2.4 μg/mL Ethylene glycol poisoning: >20 μg/mL	11–27 μmol/L Ethylene glycol poisoning: >200 μmol/L
	Urine	8–40 μg/mL Ethylene glycol poisoning: >150 μg/mL	90–445 μmol/L Ethylene glycol poisoning: >1670 μmol/L
Oxygen, Partial Pressure (Po_2)	Whole blood (heparin), arterial	83–108 mmHg (decreases with age)	11–14.4 kPa
Oxygen Saturation	Whole blood (heparin), arterial	95–99%	Fraction saturated: 0.95–0.99
Oxytocin	Plasma (EDTA)	<3.2 μU/mL	<3.2 mU/L
Po_2, see *Oxygen, Partial Pressure*			
Parathyroid Hormone (hPTH)	Serum	Vary with laboratory, e.g., Mayo Clinic, Bioscience: N-terminal 230–630 pg/mL C-terminal 410–1760 pg/mL Nichols Institute: C-terminal 40–100 μLEq/mL	 230–630 ng/L 410–1760 ng/L
pH	Whole blood (heparin), arterial	7.35–7.45 Must be corrected for body temperature	H^+ concentration: 36–44 nmol/L
	Urine, random	Newborn/neonate: 5–7 Thereafter: 4.5–8 (average ≃6)	0.1–10 μmol/L 0.01–32 μmol/L (average ≃1.0 μmol/L)
Pentoses	Urine, 24 h	Total pentoses: 2–5 mg/kg/d or 225 mg/d L-Xylulose: <60 mg/d D-Ribose: <15 mg/d D-Ribulose: traces	 13.3–33.3 μmol/kg/d 1.50 mmol/d <400 μmol/d <100 μmol/d
	Serum	L-Xylulose: <2 mg/dL	<133.2 μmol/L
Pepsinogen (PG I)	Serum	*ng/mL* Cord: 26±2 1–10 y: 95±10 11–14 y: 107±11 19–38 y: 133±9 Women at delivery: 127±11	*μg/L* 26±2 95±10 107±11 133±9 127±11
Phenols	Urine	*mg/L* Phenol: 5–8 *p*-Cresol: 20–200 Toxic, Phenol: >10 *o*-Cresol: >2 *m*-Cresol: >2 *p*-Cresol: >200	*μmol/L* 50–85 185–1850 >110 >18 >18 >1850
Phenylalanine	Serum	*mg/dL* Premature: 2.0–7.5 Newborn: 1.2–3.4 Adult: 0.8–1.8	*mmol/L* 0.12–0.45 0.07–0.21 0.05–0.11
	Urine, 24 h	*mg/d* 10 d–2 wks: 1–2 3–12 y: 4–18 Adult: trace–17 or: 6±2 mg/g creatinine	*μmol/d* 6–12 24–110 trace–103 or: 4.1±1.4 mmol/mol creatinine
Phenylpyruvic Acid, Qualitative	Urine, fresh random	Negative by $FeCl_3$ test	Negative by $FeCl_3$ test
Phosphatase, Acid *Prostatic (RIA)* *Roy, Brower, and Hayden, 37°C*	 Serum	 <3.0 ng/mL 0.11–0.60 U/L	 <3.0 μg/L 0.11–0.60 U/L
Phosphatase, Alkaline *(p-nitrophenyl phosphate, carbonate buffer: 30°C)* *Bowers and McComb (30°C)*	Serum	Infant: 50–165 U/L Child: 20–150 U/L Adult: 20–70 U/L 25–90 U/L	50–165 U/L 20–150 U/L 20–70 U/L 25–90 U/L

(*Continued*)

CLINICAL CHEMISTRY, TOXICOLOGY, SEROLOGY (*Continued*)

Test	Specimen	Reference Range	Reference Range (International Units)
Phospholipids, Total	Serum or plasma (EDTA)	*mg/dL*	*g/L*
		Newborn: 75–170	0.75–1.70
		Infant: 100–275	1.00–2.75
		Child: 180–295	1.80–2.95
		Adult: 125–275	1.25–2.75
		Adult, >65 y: 196–366	1.96–3.66
Phosphorus, Inorganic	Serum	*mg/dL*	*mmol/L*
		Cord: 3.7–8.1	1.2–2.6
		Child: 4.5–6.5	1.45–2.1
		Thereafter: 3.0–4.5	0.97–1.45
		>60 y, M: 2.3–3.7	0.74–1.2
		F: 2.8–4.1	0.90–1.3
	Urine, 24 h	Adults on diet containing 0.9–1.5 g P and 10 mg Ca/kg: <1.0 g/d	Adults on diet containing 29–48 mmol P and 0.25 mmol Ca/kg: <32 mmol/d
		On nonrestricted diet: 0.4–1.3 g/d	On nonrestricted diet: 13–42 mmol/d
Placental Lactogen (hPL)	Serum	*μg/mL*	*mg/L*
		Nonpregnant F: <0.5	<0.5
		Wks of pregnancy,	
		22: 1.0–3.8	1.0–3.8
		26: 1.5–4.5	1.5–4.5
		30: 2.8–5.8	2.8–5.8
		34: 3.4–6.9	3.4–6.9
		38: 3.6–8.2	3.6–8.2
		42: 3.0–8.0	3.0–8.0
Porphobilinogen (PBG)			
Quantitative	Urine, 24 h	0–2.0 mg/d	0–8.8 μmol/d
Qualitative	Urine, fresh random	Negative	Negative
Post-Heparin Lipolytic Activity	Plasma (heparin)	0.24–0.57 μmol NEFA/min/mL	240–570 U/L
Potassium	Serum	*mmol/L*	*mmol/L*
		Newborn: 3.7–5.0	3.7–5.0
		Infant: 4.1–5.3	4.1–5.3
		Child: 3.4–4.7	3.4–4.7
		Thereafter: 3.5–5.1	3.5–5.1
	Plasma (heparin)	3.5–4.5 mmol/L	3.5–4.5 mmol/L
	Urine, 24 h	2.5–125 mmol/d; varies with diet	2.5–125 mmol/d; varies with diet
Pregnancy Tests			
Chorionic Gonadotropin (hCG) Tube Test (Semi-quantitative)	Serum or urine	Negative	Negative
		Positive by 4th–8th d after expected menstrual period	Positive by 4th–8th d after expected menstrual period
		Peak values up to 120,000 mIU/mL	Peak values up to 120,000 IU/L
Chorionic Gonadotropin (β-hCG), see *Chorionic Gonadotropin, β-Subunit*			
Radio Receptor Assay (RRA)	Serum	Negative; pregnancy can be detected 6–8 d after conception	Negative; pregnancy can be detected 6–8 d after conception
Pregnanediol	Urine, 24 h	*mg/d*	*μmol/d*
		<2 y: <0.1	<0.3
		6–9 y: <0.5	<1.5
		M, 10–15 y: 0.1–0.7	0.3–2.2
		Adult: 0.6–1.5	1.9–4.7
		F, 10–15 y: 0.1–1.2	0.3–3.7
		Adult,	
		Follicular: <1.0	<3.1
		Luteal: 2–7	6.2–22
		Postmenopausal: 0.2–1.0	0.6–3.1
		Weeks of pregnancy,	
		16: 5–21	16–65
		20: 6–26	19–81
		24: 12–32	37–100
		28: 19–51	59–160
		32: 22–66	69–206
		36: 13–77	41–240
		40: 23–63	72–197
Pregnanetriol	Urine, 24 h	*mg/d*	*μmol/d*
		2 wk–2 y: 0.02–0.2	0.06–0.6
		2–5 y: <0.5	<1.5
		5–15 y: <1.5	<4.5
		>15 y: <2.0	<5.9

(*Continued*)

CLINICAL CHEMISTRY, TOXICOLOGY, SEROLOGY (*Continued*)

Test	Specimen	Reference Range	Reference Range (International Units)
Pregnenolone	Serum	Adult: 0.3–2 ng/mL	0.9–6.3 nmol/L
Progesterone	Serum	*ng/mL*	*nmol/L*
		M, Pub. stage I: 0.11–0.26	0.35–0.83
		Adult: 0.12–0.3	0.38–1
		F, Pub. stage I: 0–0.3	0–1
		II: 0–0.46	0–1.5
		III: 0–0.6	0–2
		IV: 0.05–13.0	0.16–41
		Follicular: 0.02–0.9	0.06–2.9
		Luteal: 6.0–30.0	19–95
Progesterone Receptor Assay (PRA)	Tumor tissue	*fmol/mg protein*	*nmol/kg protein*
		Normal, or benign and nonresponsive tumor: ≤5	≤5
		Positive: >10	>10
Proinsulin	Serum	<30% of total immunoreactive insulin-like material, or <0.2 ng/mL	Fraction of immunoreactive insulin-like material: 0.30, or <0.2 μg/L
Prolactin (hPRL)	Serum	*ng/mL*	*μg/L*
		Adults, M: up to 20	up to 20
		F, Follicular phase: up to 23	up to 23
		Luteal phase: 5–40	5–40
		Pregnancy,	
		1st trimester: <80	<80
		2nd trimester: <160	<160
		3rd trimester: <400	<400
		Newborn: >10-fold adult levels	
Prolactin-Insulin Stimulation Test	Serum	Peak values: 1.4–19.0 × baseline within 35–75 min after stimulation	Peak values: 1.4–19.0 × baseline within 35–75 min after stimulation
Properdin	Serum	*mg/dL (± 1 SD)*	*nmol/L*
		Cord: 1.50±0.1	68.2±4.5
		1 mo: 1.4±0.4	63.6±18.2
		6 mo: 1.9±0.3	86.4±13.6
		Adult: 2.8±0.4	127.3±18.2
Protein			
Total	Serum	*g/dL*	*g/L*
		Premature: 4.3–7.6	43.0–76.0
		Newborn: 4.6–7.4	46.0–74.0
		Child: 6.2–8.0	62.0–80.0
		Ambulatory: 6.4–8.3	64.0–83.0
		Recumbent: 6.0–7.8	60.0–78.0
		>60 y: slightly lower (≃0.2)	∼2
		∼0.5 g higher in ambulatory patients	∼5 g higher in ambulatory patients
Electrophoresis		*g/dL*	*g/L*
		Albumin,	
		Adult: 3.5–5.0	35–50
		>60 y: 3.7–4.7	37–47
		α_1-Globulin,	
		Adult: 0.2–0.3	2–3
		>60 y: 0.2–0.5	2–5
		α_2-Globulin,	
		Adult: 0.4–0.8	4–8
		>60 y: 0.5–1.1	5–11
		β-Globulin,	
		Adult: 0.5–0.9	5–9
		>60 y: 0.5–1.2	5–12
		γ-Globulin,	
		Adult: 0.7–1.2	7–12
		>60 y: 0.6–1.6	6–16
Total	Urine, 24 h	1–14 mg/dL	10–140 mg/L
		50–80 mg/d (at rest)	50–80 mg/d
		<250 mg/d after intense exercise	<250 mg/d after intense exercise
Electrophoresis		*Average % of Total Protein*	*Fraction of Total*
		Alb. 37.9	0.379
		α_1 27.3	0.273
		α_2 19.5	0.195
		β 8.8	0.088
		γ 3.3	0.033

(*Continued*)

CLINICAL CHEMISTRY, TOXICOLOGY, SEROLOGY (*Continued*)

Test	Specimen	Reference Range	Reference Range (International Units)
Protein (*Continued*)			
Total	CSF		
Column			
Turbidimetry		Lumbar: 8–32 mg/dL	80–320 mg/L
		Lumbar,	
		Adult: 15–45 mg/dL	150–450 mg/L
		Newborn: 20–120 mg/dL	200–1200 mg/L
Electrophoresis		*% of Total*	*Fraction of Total*
		Prealbumin: 2–7	0.02–0.07
		Albumin: 56–76	0.56–0.76
		α_1-Globulin: 2–7	0.02–0.07
		α_2-Globulin: 4–12	0.04–0.12
		β-Globulin: 8–18	0.08–0.18
		γ-Globulin: 3–12	0.03–0.12
Electrophoresis	Synovial fluid	Albumin: 63	0.63
		α_1-Globulin: 7	0.07
		α_2-Globulin: 7	0.07
		β-Globulin: 9	0.09
		γ-Globulin: 14	0.14
		Fibrinogen: 0	0
Prostaglandins	Plasma (heparin)		
E		25–200 pg/mL	71–564 pmol/L
F		25–150 pg/mL	71–423 pmol/L
Protoporphyrin	Whole blood (heparin or EDTA)	<50 μg/dL RBC	<0.89 μmol/L RBC
	Feces, 24 h	≤60 μg/g dry wt or <1500 μg/d	<2.67 μmol/d
Pseudocholinesterase (PCHE), see *Cholinesterase II*			
Pyruvic Acid	Whole blood (heparin)	0.3–0.9 mg/dL	0.034–0.102 mmol/L
Renal Plasma Flow (RPF)	Plasma and urine	M: 560–830 mL/min	
		F: 490–700 mL/min	
		or: 390 mL/min/m² body surface	
		>40 y: decreases ~75 mL/decade	
Renin	Plasma (EDTA)	*Normal sodium diet:*	
		ng/mL/h	*μg/L/h*
		Supine: 1.6±1.5	1.6±1.5
		Standing: (4 h): 4.5±2.9	4.5±2.9
		Low sodium:	
		Supine: 3.2±1.1	3.2±1.1
		Standing: (4 h): 9.9±4.3	9.9±4.3
Reverse Triiodothyronine (rT_3)	Serum	*ng/dL*	*nmol/L*
		1–5 y: 15–71	0.23–1.1
		5–10 y: 17–79	0.26–1.2
		10–15 y: 19–88	0.29–1.36
		Adults: 30–80	0.46–1.23
Riboflavin (Vitamin B_2)	Urine, random, fasting	*μg/g creatinine*	*μmol/mol creatinine*
		Adult: 80–269	24–81
		Pregnancy: 90–120	27–36
Schilling Test (Intrinsic Factor Test) *Dose: 0.5–1 μCi ⁵⁸Co-Vitamin B₁₂*	Urine, 24 h	>7.5% of dose	Fraction of dose: 0.075
Secretin	Serum or plasma (heparin or EDTA)	37±8 pg/mL	37±8 ng/L
Sediment	Urine, fresh random		
Casts		Hyaline: occasional (0–1) casts/hpf	Hyaline: occasional (0–1) casts/hpf
		RBC: not seen	RBC: not seen
		WBC: not seen	WBC: not seen
		Tubular epithelial: not seen	Tubular epithelial: not seen
		Transitional and squamous epithelial: not seen	Transitional and squamous epithelial: not seen
Cells		RBC: 0–2/hpf	RBC: 0–2/hpf
		WBC,	WBC,
		Males: 0–3/hpf	Males: 0–3/hpf
		Females and children: 0–5/hpf	Females and children: 0–5/hpf
		Epithelial: few; more frequent in newborn	Epithelial: few; more frequent in newborn
		Bacteria,	Bacteria,
		Unspun: no organisms/oil immersion field	Unspun: no organisms/oil immersion field
		Spun: <20 organisms/hpf	Spun: <20 organisms/hpf

(*Continued*)

CLINICAL CHEMISTRY, TOXICOLOGY, SEROLOGY (*Continued*)

Test	Specimen	Reference Range		Reference Range (International Units)	
Selenium	Whole blood (heparin)	10–34 μg/dL Serum approx. 20% lower		1.27–4.32 μmol/L	
	Urine, 24 h	10–100 μg/L		0.13–1.27 μmol/L	
Semen Analysis (Sperm Count)	Ejaculate	Volume: 2–4 mL Sperm count: >20 million/mL Motility: >60% Morphology: >60% normal forms		Volume: 0.002–0.004 L Sperm count: >20 × 10^9/L Motility: Fraction of total: >0.60 Morphology: Fraction of total: >0.60 normal forms	
Serotonin	Whole blood (EDTA)	39–361 ng/mL		0.22–2.05 μmol/L	
	Platelets	~314 ng/10^9 platelets			
Sodium	Serum or plasma (heparin)		*mmol/L*	*mmol/L*	
		Newborn:	134–144	134–144	
		Infant:	139–146	139–146	
		Child:	138–145	138–145	
		Thereafter:	136–146	136–146	
	Urine, 24 h	40–220 mmol/L (diet dependent)		40–220	
	Sweat	10–40 mmol/L		10–40 mmol/L	
Somatomedin C	Plasma (EDTA)	0.4–2.0 U/mL		400–2000 U/L	
Specific Gravity	Urine, random	Adult: 1.002–1.030 After 12 h fluid restriction: >1.025		Adult: 1.002–1.030 After 12 h fluid restriction: >1.025	
	Urine, 24 h	1.015–1.025			
Sucrose	Serum or plasma	Mean: 0.06 mg/dL		1.75 μmol/L	
	Urine	Mean: 2.2 mg/dL		64.26 μmol/L	
Testosterone, Free	Serum	*ng/dL(mean ± 1SE)*	*% of total*	*pmol/L(mean ± 1SD)*	*Fraction of total*
		Cord,			
		M: 1.0±0.4	2.9±0.6	34.6±14	0.029±0.006
		F: 0.89±0.29	3.0±0.5	31±10	0.03±0.005
		1–15 d,			
		M: 0.8±0.8	1.3±0.2	28±28	0.013±0.002
		F: 0.14±0.06	1.2±0.2	4.9±2	0.012±0.002
		Prepubertal,			
		M: 0.04±0.01	0.7±0.2	1.4±0.35	0.007±0.002
		F: 0.04±0.01	0.7±0.1	1.4±0.35	0.007±0.001
		Adult,			
		M: 7.9±2.3	1.4±0.3	274±80	0.014±0.003
		F: 0.31±0.07	0.9±0.2	11±2	0.009±0.002
Testosterone, Total	Serum		*ng/dL*	*nmol/L*	
		Prepubertal,			
		M:	6.6±2.5	0.23±0.09	
		F:	6.6±2.5	0.23±0.09	
		Adult, M:	572±135	19.8±4.7	
		F:	37±10	1.3±0.3	
	Urine, 24 h	*Pubertal stage*	*μg/kg body weight*	*nmol/kg body weight*	
		I, M:	0.25	0.87	
		F:	0.16	0.55	
		II, M:	0.34	1.18	
		F:	0.16	0.55	
		III, M:	0.37	1.28	
		F:	0.16	0.55	
			μg/d	*nmol/d*	
		20–50 y, M:	50–135	173–470	
		F:	2–12	7–42	
		>50 y, M:	40–60	139–210	
		F:	2–8	7–28	
Tetrahydrocortisol (THF)	Urine, 24 h	Adult: 0.5–1.5 mg/d		Adult: 1.4–4.1 μmol/d	
Tetrahydrodeoxycortisol	Urine, 24 h	<1000 μg/d		<2.9 μmol/d	
Thyroglobulin (Tg)	Serum	Up to 50 ng/mL		Up to 50 μg/L	
Thyroid Antibodies	Serum	Adults: ≤1:10 dilution Children: ≤1:4		Adults: ≤1:10 dilution Children: ≤1:4	
Thyroid Microsomal Antibodies	Serum	Nondetectable (Hemagglutination) or <1:10 (IFA)		Nondetectable (Hemagglutination) or <1:10 (IFA)	

(*Continued*)

CLINICAL CHEMISTRY, TOXICOLOGY, SEROLOGY (*Continued*)

Test	Specimen	Reference Range	Reference Range (International Units)
Thyroid-Stimulating Hormone (hTSH)	Serum or plasma	*μU/mL* Cord: 3–12 Child: 4.5±3.6 Adult: 2–10 >60 y, M: 2–7.3 F: 2–16.8	*mU/L* 3–12 4.5±3.6 2–10 2–7.3 2–16.8
Thyroid-Stimulating Hormone—Response to TRH	Serum	30 min after stimulation: Child: 11–35 μU/mL Adult, M: 15–30 μU/mL F: 20–40 μU/mL	30 min after stimulation: Child: 11–35 mU/L Adult, M: 15–30 mU/L F: 20–40 mU/L
Thyroid Uptake of Radioactive Iodine	Activity over thyroid gland	2 h: <6% 6 h: 3–20% 24 h: 8–30%	Fractional uptake: 2 h: <0.06 6 h: 0.03–0.20 24 h: 0.08–0.30
Thyroid Uptake of $^{99m}TcO_4^-$	Activity over thyroid gland	After 24 h: 0.4–3.0%	Fractional uptake: 0.004–0.03
Thyrotropin-Releasing Hormone	Plasma	5–60 pg/mL	14–165 pmol/L
Thyrotropin-Releasing Hormone Stimulation Test *Dose, adult: 500 μg TRH, I.V.*	Serum	TSH within 30 min, <40 y: >6 μU/mL rise >40 y, M: >2 μU/mL rise hPRL: 3–5-fold rise above baseline (diminishes with age)	TSH within 30 min, <40 y: >6 mU/L rise >40 y, M: >2 mU/L rise hPRL: 3–5-fold rise above baseline (diminishes with age)
Thyroxine (T_4), Total	Serum	*μg/dL* Cord: 8–13 Newborn: 10–21 Neonate: 9–18 Infant: 7–15 1–5 y: 7.3–15 5–10 y: 6.4–13.3 Thereafter: 5–12 Pregnant, last 5 mo: 6.1–17.6 >60 y, M: 5.0–10.0 F: 5.5–10.5	*nmol/L* 103–167 130–270 116–230 90–193 94–193 82–170 64–155 79–227 64–129 71–135
Thyroxine-Binding Globulin (TBG)	Serum	15.0–34.0 μg/mL	15.0–34.0 mg/L
Thyroxine Ratio, Effective (ETR)		0.86–1.13	0.86–1.13
Thyroxine, Free (FT_4)	Serum	0.8–2.4 ng/dL	10–31 pmol/L
Thyroxine, Free, Index, see *Free Thyroxine Index*			
Thyroxine/TBG Ratio	Serum	0.2–0.5 T_4(μg/dL)/TBG(μg/mL)	2.7–6.4 T_4(nmol/L)/TBG(mg/L)
Transcortin	Serum	*mg/dL* M: 1.5–2.0 F, Follicular: 1.7–2.0 Luteal: 1.6–2.1 Postmenopausal: 1.7–2.5 Pregnancy, 21–28 wks: 4.7–5.4 33–40 wks: 5.5–7.0	*mg/L* 15–20 17–20 16–21 17–25 47–54 55–70
Transferrin	Serum	Adults: 200–400 mg/dL >60 y: 210–350 mg/dL	2.0–4.0 g/L 2.1–3.5 g/L
Transketolase	Whole blood (heparin)	9–12 μmol/h/mL whole blood 2.1–2.4 μmol/h/10^9 red cells	50–200 U/L whole blood 0.035–0.040 U/10^9 red cells
Triglycerides (TG)	Serum, after ≥12 h fast	*mg/dL* M / F Cord blood: 10–98 / 10–98 0–5 y: 30–86 / 32–99 6–11 y: 31–108 / 35–114 12–15 y: 36–138 / 41–138 16–19 y: 40–163 / 40–128 20–29 y: 44–185 / 40–128 30–39 y: 49–284 / 38–160 40–49 y: 56–298 / 44–186 50–59 y: 62–288 / 55–247 Values decrease slightly above age 60 Levels for blacks: 10–20 mg/dL lower *Recommended* (desirable) levels for adults: Male: 40–160 mg/dL Female: 35–135 mg/dL	*g/L* M / F 0.10–0.98 / 0.10–0.98 0.30–0.86 / 0.32–0.99 0.31–1.08 / 0.35–1.14 0.36–1.38 / 0.41–1.38 0.40–1.63 / 0.40–1.28 0.44–1.85 / 0.40–1.28 0.49–2.84 / 0.38–1.60 0.56–2.98 / 0.44–1.86 0.62–2.88 / 0.55–2.47 Values decrease slightly above age 60 Levels for blacks: 0.10–0.20 g/L lower *Recommended* (desirable) levels for adults: Male: 0.40–1.60 g/L Female: 0.35–1.35 g/L

(*Continued*)

CLINICAL CHEMISTRY, TOXICOLOGY, SEROLOGY (*Continued*)

Test	Specimen	Reference Range	Reference Range (International Units)
Triiodothyronine (T_3-RIA)	Serum	*ng/dL* Cord: 30–70 Newborn: 90–170 1–5 y: 100–260 5–10 y: 90–240 10–15 y: 80–210 Thereafter: 115–190 >60 y, M: 105–175 F: 108–205	*nmol/L* 0.5–1.1 1.4–2.6 1.5–4.0 1.4–3.7 1.2–3.2 1.8–2.9 1.6–2.7 1.7–3.1
Triiodothyronine, Free	Serum	*mean pg/dL* Cord: 130±10 (SE) 1–3 d: 410±20 6 wk: 400±20 Adults (20–50 y): 230–660 pg/dL	*mean pmol/L* 2.0±0.15 (SE) 6.3±0.3 6.1±0.3 3.5–10 pmol/L
Triiodothyronine, Free, Index	Serum	1–5 y: 165 5–10 y: 150 10–15 y: 130	
Triiodothyronine Resin Uptake Test (T_3RU)	Serum	Newborn: 27–32% Adult: 26–35% >60 y: 23–32%	Fractional uptake: Newborn: 0.27–0.32 Adult: 0.26–0.35 >60 y: 0.23–0.32
Triolein-^{131}I Absorption Test	Plasma	1.7% of administered dose/L after 4–6 h	Fraction of administered dose: 0.017/L
Dose: 50 μCi in milk	Feces, 72 h	<5% of administered dose in 72 h specimen	Fraction of administered dose: 0.05/72
Tubular Reabsorption of Phosphate (TRP)	Urine, 4 h (8–12 AM), and serum	82–95%	Fraction reabsorbed: 0.82–0.95
Tyrosine	Serum	*mg/dL* Premature: 7.0–24.0 Newborn: 1.6–3.7 Adult: 0.8–1.3	*mmol/L* 0.39–1.32 0.088–0.20 0.044–0.07
Urea Nitrogen	Serum or plasma	*mg/dL* Cord: 21–40 Premature (1 wk): 3–25 Newborn: 4–18 Infant/child: 5–18 Adult: 7–18 >60 y: 8–21	*mmol urea/L* 7.5–14.3 1.1–9 1.4–6.4 1.8–6.4 2.5–6.4 2.9–7.5
	Urine	12–20 g/d	430–710 mmol urea/L
Urea Nitrogen/Creatinine Ratio	Serum	12/1 to 20/1	12/1 to 20/1
Uric Acid *Phosphotungstate*	Serum	*mg/dL* Adult, M: 4.5–8.2 F: 3.0–6.5 >60 y, M: 4.2–8.0 F: 3.2–7.3	*μmol/L* 268–488 178–387 250–476 190–434
Uricase		M: 3.5–7.2 F: 2.6–6.0 Child: 2.0–5.5	208–428 155–357 119–327
	Urine, 24 h	*mg/d* Free purine diet, M: <420 F: slightly lower Low purine diet, M: <480 F: <400 High purine diet, <1000	*mmol/d* <2.5 <2.86 <2.38 <5.9
Urinary Sediment, see *Sediment*			
Urine Volume	Urine, 24 h	M: 800–1800 mL/d F: 600–1600 mL/d (Varies with intake and other factors)	M: 0.800–1.800 L/d F: 0.600–1.600 L/d
Urobilinogen	Urine, 2 h Urine, 24 h Feces	0.1–1.0 EU/2 h 0.5–4.0 EU/d 75–275 EU/100 g 75–400 EU/d 40–280 mg/d	0.1–1.0 EU/2 h 0.5–4.0 EU/d 75–275 EU/100 g 75–400 EU/d 40–280 mg/d

(*Continued*)

CLINICAL CHEMISTRY, TOXICOLOGY, SEROLOGY (*Continued*)

Test	Specimen	Reference Range	Reference Range (International Units)
Uroporphyrin	Urine, 24 h	<50 μg/d	<60 nmol/d
	Feces, 24 h specimen	10–40 μg/d	12–48 nmol/d
	Erythrocyte (heparin or EDTA)	Negative	Negative
Valine	Serum	*μmol/L*	*μmol/L*
		Premature, 1 d: 130±50	130±50
		Newborn, 1 d: 80–246	80–246
		1–3 mo: 194±49	194±49
		Adult: 141–317	141–317
	Urine, 24 h	*mg/d*	*μmol/d*
		10 d–2 wks: 1–3	8.5–26
		3–12 y: 2–6	17–51
		Adult: 2–12	17–102
		or: 4±1 mg/g creatinine	or: 4±1 mmol/mol creatinine
Vanillylmandelic Acid (Vanilmandelic Acid)	Urine, 24 h	*mg/d*	*μmol/d*
		Newborn: <1.0	<5.0
		Infant: <2.0	<10.1
		Child: 1–3	5–15
		Adolescent: 1–5	5–25
		Thereafter: 2–7	10–35
		or 1.5–7 μg/mg creatinine	or 0.86–4 mmol/mol creatinine
Vasoactive Intestinal Polypeptide (VIP)	Plasma (heparin)	20–53 pg/mL	20–53 ng/L
Viscosity	Serum	1.10–1.22 Centipoise	1.10–1.22 mPa·s
Vitamin A	Serum	30–65 μg/dL	1.05–2.27 μmol/L
Vitamin A Tolerance Test *Dose: 5000 U vit. A in oil/kg orally*	Serum	3 and/or 6 h: 200–600 μg vit. A/dL	7–21 μmol/L
Vitamin B_2, see *Riboflavin*			
Vitamin B_6	Plasma (EDTA)	3.6–18 ng/mL	14.6–72.8 nmol/L
Vitamin B_{12}	Serum	140–700 pg/mL	103–517 pmol/L
		>60 y: 110–800 pg/mL	81–590 pmol/L
Vitamin B_{12} Intrinsic Factor	Gastric juice	50–400% enhancement of ^{57}Co-B_{12} uptake by GPIMH	Fractional increase in ^{57}Co-B_{12} uptake by GPIMH: 0.50–4.00
Vitamin C	Plasma (oxalate, heparin, or EDTA)	0.6–2.0 mg/dL	34–113 μmol/L
	Buffy coat (heparin)	20–53 μg/10^8 WBC	114–301 nmol/10^8 WBC
Vitamin C Saturation Test	Urine, 24 h	60–80% of test dose excreted	Fraction test dose excreted: 0.60–0.80
Vitamin D_3, 25-hydroxy	Plasma (heparin)	Summer: 15–80 ng/mL	37–200 nmol/L
		Winter: 14–42 ng/mL	35–105 nmol/L
Vitamin D_3, 1,25-dihydroxy	Serum	25–45 pg/mL	60–108 nmol/L
Vitamin E	Serum	5.0–20 μg/mL	11.6–46.4 μmol/L
Xylose Absorption Test	Whole blood (Na-fluoride)	*mg/dL*	*mmol/L*
		Child, 1 h: >30	>2.00
		Adult, 2 h: >25	>1.67
	Urine, 5 h	Child: 16–33% of ingested dose	Fraction ingested dose: 0.16–0.33
		Adult, *g/5 h*	*mmol/5 h*
		5 g dose: >1.2	>8.00
		25 g dose: >4.0	>26.64
		>65 y: >3.5	>23.31

DRUGS—THERAPEUTIC AND TOXIC

NOTE: The values for the therapeutic and toxic concentration of drugs are according to present knowledge. Additional experience with these drugs may lead to revised values. Where no therapeutic or toxic level is given, it was felt by the author that there are presently no reliable data available.

Test	Specimen	Reference Range	Reference Range (International Units)
Acetaminophen	Serum, plasma (heparin, EDTA)	Therap. conc.: 10–30 μg/mL Toxic conc.: >200 μg/mL	66–200 μmol/L >1300 μmol/L
Amikacin	Serum, plasma (EDTA)	*μg/mL* Therap. conc., peak: 25–35 trough (less severe infection): 1–4 (life-threatening infection): 4–8 Toxic conc., peak: >35–40 trough: >10–15	*μmol/L* 43–60 1.7–6.8 6.8–13.7 >60–68 >17–26
ε-Aminocaproic Acid	Serum, plasma (heparin, EDTA); collect at trough conc.	Therap. conc.: >130 μg/mL	>990 μmol/L
Amitriptyline	Serum, plasma (heparin, EDTA); collect at trough conc.	Therap. conc.: 120–250 ng/mL Toxic conc.: >500 ng/mL	430–900 nmol/L >1800 nmol/L
Amobarbital, quant.	Serum	Therap. conc.: 1–5 μg/mL Toxic conc.: 10–30 μg/mL	4.4–22.1 μmol/L 44.2–132.6 μmol/L
Amphetamine	Serum, plasma (heparin, EDTA)	Therap. conc.: 20–30 ng/mL Toxic conc.: >200 ng/mL	150–220 nmol/L >1500 nmol/L
Bromide	Serum	*mg/dL* Child: <1.0 Adult: 0.8–1.5 Therap. conc.: 7.5–10.0 Toxic conc.: >50	*μmol/L* <12.5 10–19 94–125 >625
Caffeine	Serum, plasma (heparin, EDTA)	Therap. conc.: 3–15 μg/mL Toxic conc.: >50 μg/mL	15–77 μmol/L >260 μmol/L
Carbamazepine	Serum, plasma (heparin, EDTA); collect at trough conc.	Therap. conc.: 8–12 μg/mL Toxic conc.: >15 μg/mL	34–51 μmol/L >63 μmol/L
Carbenicillin	Serum, plasma (heparin, EDTA)	Therap. conc.: dependent on minimum inhibitory conc. of specific organism Toxic conc.: >250 μg/mL (neurotoxicity)	 >660 μmol/L
Chloral Hydrate	Serum	As Trichloroethanol: Therap. conc.: 2–12 μg/mL Toxic conc.: >20 μg/mL	 13–80 μmol/L >134 μmol/L
Chloramphenicol	Serum, plasma (heparin, EDTA); collect at trough conc.; separate immed.	Therap. conc.: 10–25 μg/mL Toxic conc.: >25 μg/mL	31–77 μmol/L >77 μmol/L
Chlordiazepoxide	Serum, plasma (heparin, EDTA); collect at trough conc.	Therap. conc.: 700–1000 ng/mL Toxic conc.: >5000 ng/mL	2.34–3.34 μmol/L >16.7 μmol/L
Chlorpromazine	Serum, plasma (heparin, EDTA); collect at trough conc.	Therap. conc.: 50–300 ng/mL Toxic conc.: >750 ng/mL	157–940 nmol/L >2350 nmol/L
Cimetidine	Serum, plasma (heparin, EDTA); collect at trough conc.	Therap. conc.: >1.0 μg/mL	>4.0 μmol/L
Clonazepam	Serum, plasma (heparin, EDTA); collect at trough conc.	Therap. conc.: 15–60 ng/mL Toxic conc.: >80 ng/mL	48–190 nmol/L >250 nmol/L
Clonidine	Serum, plasma (heparin, EDTA)	Therap. conc.: 1.0–2.0 ng/mL	4.3–8.7 nmol/L
Clorazepate	Serum, plasma (heparin, EDTA)	Therap. conc.: 0.12–1.0 μg/mL (as desmethyl-diazepam)	0.44–3.7 μmol/L
Cocaine	Serum, plasma (heparin, EDTA); store on ice; assay within 1 h	Therap. conc.: 100–500 ng/mL Toxic conc.: >1000 ng/mL	330–1650 μmol/L >3300 μmol/L
Desipramine	Serum, plasma (heparin, EDTA); collect at steady-state trough conc. at least 12 h after dose	Therap. conc.: 75–160 ng/mL Toxic conc.: >1000 ng/mL	280–600 nmol/L >3750 nmol/L
Desmethylmethsuximide	Serum	Therap. conc.: 10–40 μg/mL	53–210 μmol/L

(*Continued*)

DRUGS—THERAPEUTIC AND TOXIC (*Continued*)

Test	Specimen	Reference Range	Reference Range (International Units)
Diazepam	Serum, plasma (heparin, EDTA); collect at trough conc.	Therap. conc.: 100–1000 ng/mL Toxic conc.: >5000 ng/mL	350–3500 nmol/L >17,500 nmol/L
Digitoxin	Serum, plasma (heparin, EDTA); collect at least 6 h after dose	Therap. conc.: 20–35 ng/mL Toxic conc.: >45 ng/mL	26–46 nmol/L >59 nmol/L
Digoxin	Serum, plasma (heparin, EDTA); collect at least 12 h after dose	*ng/mL* Therap. conc., CHF: 0.8–1.5 Arrhythmias: 1.5–2.0 Toxic conc., adult: >2.5 child: >3.0	*nmol/L* 1–1.9 1.9–2.6 >3.2 >3.8
Diphenylhydantoin, see *Phenytoin*			
Disopyramide	Serum, plasma (heparin, EDTA); collect at trough conc.	Arrhythmias, Atrial: 2.8–3.2 μg/mL Ventricular: 3.3–7.5 μg/mL	 8.2–9.4 μmol/L 9.7–22 μmol/L
Doxepin	Serum, plasma (heparin, EDTA); collect at trough conc. at least 12 h after dose	Therap. conc.: 30–150 ng/mL Toxic conc.: >500 ng/mL	107–540 nmol/L >1800 nmol/L
Ethanol	Whole blood (oxalate), serum	Toxic conc.: 50–100 mg/dL Depression of CNS: >100 mg/dL	11–22 mmol/L >22 mmol/L
Ethchlorvynol	Serum, plasma (heparin, EDTA); collect during postdistribution phase	Therap. conc.: 2–8 μg/mL Toxic conc.: >20 μg/mL	14–55 μmol/L >140 μmol/L
Ethosuximide	Serum, plasma (heparin, EDTA); collect at trough conc.	Therap. conc.: 40–100 μg/mL Toxic conc.: >150 μg/mL	280–700 μmol/L >1060 μmol/L
Fenoprofen	Plasma (EDTA)	Therap. conc.: 20–65 μg/mL	80–270 μmol/L
Furosemide	Serum	Therap. conc.: 1–2 μg/mL, 30 min after last dose	3–6 μmol/L
Gentamicin	Serum, plasma (EDTA)	*μg/mL* Therap. conc., peak (less severe infections): 5–8 (severe infections): 8–10 trough (less severe infections): <1 (moderate infections): <2 (severe infections): <2–4 Toxic conc., peak: >10–12 trough: >2–4	*μmol/L* 10.7–17 17–21 <2 <4.3 <4.3–8.5 >21–26 >4.3–8.5
Glutethimide	Serum	Therap. conc.: 2–6 μg/mL Toxic conc.: 5–120 μg/mL	9–28 μmol/L 23–550 μmol/L
Imipramine	Serum, plasma (heparin, EDTA); collect at trough conc. at least 12 h after dose	Therap. conc.: 125–250 ng/mL Toxic conc.: >500 ng/mL	450–900 nmol/L >1800 nmol/L
Isoniazid	Serum, plasma (heparin, EDTA)	Therap. conc.: 1–7 μg/mL Toxic conc.: 20–710 μg/mL	7.3–50 μmol/L 145–5200 μmol/L
Kanamycin	Serum, plasma (EDTA)	*μg/mL* Therap. conc., peak: 25–35 trough, (less severe infection): 1–4 (life threatening infection): 4–8 Toxic conc., peak: >35–40 trough: >10–15	*μmol/L* 52–72 2.1–8.2 8.2–16.5 >72–82 >21–31
Lidocaine	Serum, plasma (heparin, EDTA); at least 45 min following bolus dose	*μg/mL* Therap. conc.: 1.5–6.0 Toxic conc., CNS, cardiovascular depression: 6–8 Seizures, obtundation, decreased cardiac output: >8	*μmol/L* 6.4–25 25–34 >34
Lithium	Serum, plasma (heparin, EDTA); at least 12 h after last dose	Therap. conc.: 0.6–1.2 mmol/L Toxic conc.: >2 mmol/L	0.6–1.2 mmol/L >2 mmol/L

(*Continued*)